British Pharmacopoeia 1998

Volume II

Published on the recommendation of the Medicines Commission pursuant to the Medicines Act 1968 and notified in draft to the European Commision in accordance with Directive 83/189/EEC (as amended)

Effective date: 1 December 1998

London: The Stationery Office

DEPARTMENT OF HEALTH
SCOTTISH OFFICE
WELSH OFFICE
DEPARTMENT OF HEALTH AND SOCIAL SERVICES FOR NORTHERN IRELAND

Published by The Stationery Office under licence from the Controller of Her Majesty's Stationery Office for the Department of Health on behalf of the Health Ministers

ISBN 0 11 322100 2

British Pharmacopoeia Commission

Office:

Market Towers
1 Nine Elms Lane
London SW8 5NQ

Telephone: +44 (0)171 273 0561
Facsimile: +44 (0)171 273 0566

Laboratory:

Government Buildings
Block 2, Honeypot Lane
Stanmore
Middlesex HA7 1AY

Telephone: +44 (0)171 972 3609
Facsimile: +44 (0)181 951 3069

Printed in the United Kingdom by The Stationery Office Limited under the authority and superintendence of the Controller of Her Majesty's Stationery Office and the Queen's Printer of Acts of Parliament

J27073 C115 3/98

Contents

PAGE

Contents of Volume I

NOTICES	vi
PREFACE	vii
BRITISH PHARMACOPOEIA COMMISSION	ix
INTRODUCTION	xv
GENERAL NOTICES	1
MONOGRAPHS	
Medicinal and Pharmaceutical Substances	29

Contents of Volume II

NOTICE	xl
GENERAL NOTICES	1391
MONOGRAPHS	
Formulated Preparations: General Monographs	1419
Formulated Preparations: Specific Monographs	1463
Blood Products	1999
Immunological Products	2027
Radiopharmaceutical Preparations	2101
Surgical Materials	2253
INFRARED REFERENCE SPECTRA	S1
APPENDICES	A1
CONTENTS OF THE APPENDICES	A3
SUPPLEMENTARY CHAPTERS	A315
INDEX	A347

Notices

Monographs of the European Pharmacopoeia are distinguished by a chaplet of stars against the title. The term European Pharmacopoeia, used without qualification, means the third edition of the European Pharmacopoeia comprising, unless otherwise stated, the main volume, published in 1996 as amended by any subsequent supplements and revisions.

Patents

In this Pharmacopoeia certain drugs and preparations have been included notwithstanding the existence of actual or potential patent rights. In so far as such substances are protected by Letters Patent their inclusion in this Pharmacopoeia neither conveys, nor implies, licence to manufacture.

General Notices

Contents of the General Notices

Part I
Italic introduction
European Pharmacopoeia

Part II
Italic introduction
Official Standards
Expression of Standards
Temperature
Weights and Measures
Atomic Weights
Constant Weight
Expression of Concentrations
Water Bath
Reagents
Indicators
Caution Statements
Titles
Chemical Formulae
Definition
Production
Manufacture of Formulated Preparations
Freshly and Recently Prepared
Methods of Sterilisation
Water
Excipients
Colouring Agents
Antimicrobial Preservatives
Characteristics
Solubility
Identification
Assays and Tests
Biological Assays and Tests
Storage
Labelling
Action and Use
Crude Drugs

Part III
Italic introduction
General Notices of the European Pharmacopoeia

1.1 General Statements
Conventional terms

1.2 Other Provisions Applying to General Chapters and Monographs
Quantities
Apparatus and procedures
Water-bath
Drying and ignition to constant mass
Reagents
Solvents
Expression of content
Temperature

1.3 General Chapters
Containers

1.4 Monographs
Titles
Relative atomic and molecular masses
Definition
Limits of content
Vegetable drugs
Production
Characters
Solubility
Identification
Tests and assays
Scope
Calculation
Limits
Indication of permitted limits of impurities
Vegetable drugs
Equivalents
Storage
Labelling
Warnings
Impurities
Critical physical properties
Reference substances, reference preparations and reference spectra
Chemical reference substances
Biological reference preparations
Reference spectra

1.5 Abbreviations and Symbols

1.6 Units of the International System (SI) Used in the Pharmacopoeia and Equivalence With Other Units

General Notices

Part I

The British Pharmacopoeia comprises the entire text within this publication. The word 'official' is used in the Pharmacopoeia to signify 'of the Pharmacopoeia'. It applies to any title, substance, preparation, method or statement included in the general notices, monographs and appendices of the Pharmacopoeia. The abbreviation for British Pharmacopoeia is BP.

European Pharmacopoeia

Monographs of the European Pharmacopoeia are reproduced in this edition of the British Pharmacopoeia by incorporation of the text published under the direction of the Council of Europe (Partial Agreement) in accordance with the Convention on the Elaboration of a European Pharmacopoeia (Treaty Series No. 32 (1974) CMND 5763) as amended by the Protocol to the Convention (Treaty Series No MISC16 (1990) CMND 1133). They are included for the convenience of users of the British Pharmacopoeia. In cases of doubt or dispute reference should be made to the Council of Europe text.

Monographs of the European Pharmacopoeia are distinguished by a chaplet of stars against the title and by an italicised statement preceding the Definition. The beginnning and end of text from the European Pharmacopoeia are denoted by means of horizontal lines with the symbol '*Ph Eur*' ranged left and right, respectively.

Inclusion of a triangle within the chaplet of stars denotes monographs that have been adopted by the European Pharmacopoeia Commission following their preparation according to a procedure of harmonisation agreed between the bodies responsible for the European Pharmacopoeia and those of Japan and the United States of America.

The general provisions of the European Pharmacopoeia relating to different types of dosage form are included in the appropriate general monograph in that section of the British Pharmacopoeia entitled Monographs: Formulated Preparations. These general provisions apply to all dosage forms of the type defined, whether an individual monograph is included in the British Pharmacopoeia or not.

Texts of the European Pharmacopoeia are governed by the General Notices of the European Pharmacopoeia. These are reproduced as Part III of these notices.

Part II

The following general notices apply to the statements made in the monographs of the British Pharmacopoeia other than those reproduced from the European Pharmacopoeia and to the statements made in the Appendices of the British Pharmacopoeia other than when a method, test or other matter described in an appendix is invoked in a monograph reproduced from the European Pharmacopoeia.

Official Standards The requirements stated in the monographs of the Pharmacopoeia apply to articles that are intended for medicinal use but not necessarily to articles that may be sold under the same name for other purposes. An article intended for medicinal use that is described by means of an official title must comply with the requirements of the relevant monograph. A formulated preparation must comply throughout its assigned shelf-life (period of validity). The subject of any other monograph must comply throughout its period of use.

A monograph is to be construed in accordance with any general monograph or notice or any appendix, note or other explanatory material that is contained in this edition and that is applicable to that monograph. All statements contained in the monographs, except where a specific general notice indicates otherwise and with the exceptions given below, constitute standards for the official articles. An article is not of Pharmacopoeial quality unless it complies with all of the requirements stated. This does not imply that a manufacturer is obliged to perform all the tests in a monograph in order to assess compliance with the Pharmacopoeia before release of a product. The manufacturer may assure himself that a product is of Pharmacopoeial quality by other means, for example, from data derived from validation studies of the manufacturing process, from in-process controls or from a combination of the two. Parametric release in appropriate circumstances is thus not precluded by the need to comply with the Pharmacopoeia. The general notice on Assays and Tests indicates that analytical methods other than those described in the Pharmacopoeia may be employed for routine purposes.

Requirements in monographs have been framed to provide appropriate limitation of potential impurities rather than to provide against all possible impurities. Material found to contain an impurity not detectable by means of the prescribed tests is not of Pharmacopoeial quality if the nature or amount of the impurity found is incompatible with good pharmaceutical practice.

The status of any statement given under the side-headings Definition, Production, Characteristics, Storage, Labelling or Action and use is defined within the general notice relating to the relevant side-heading. In addition to any exceptions indicated by one of the general notices referred to above, the following parts of a monograph do not constitute standards: (a) a graphic or molecular formula given at the beginning of a monograph; (b) a molecular weight; (c) a Chemical Abstracts Service Registry Number; (d) any information given at the end of a monograph concerning impurities known to be limited by that monograph; (e) information in any annex to a monograph. Any statement containing the word 'should' constitutes non-mandatory advice or recommendation.

The expression 'unless otherwise justified and authorised' means that the requirement in question has to be met, unless a competent authority authorises a modification or exemption where justified in a particular case. The term 'competent authority' means the national, supranational or international body or organisation vested with the authority for making decisions concerning the issue in question. It may, for example, be a licensing authority or an official control laboratory. For a formulated preparation that is the subject of monograph in the British Pharmacopoeia any justified and authorised modification to, or exemption from, the requirements of the relevant general monograph of the European Pharmacopoeia is stated in the individual monograph. For example, the general monograph for Tablets requires that Uncoated Tablets, except for chewable tablets, disintegrate within 15 minutes; for Calcium Lactate Tablets a time of 30 minutes is permitted.

Many of the general monographs for formulated preparations include statements and requirements additional to those of the European Pharmacopoeia that are applicable to the individual monographs of the British Pharmacopoeia. Such statements and requirements apply to all monographs for that dosage form included in the Pharmacopoeia unless otherwise indicated in the individual monograph.

Where a monograph on a biological substance or preparation refers to a strain, a test, a method, a substance, *etc.*, using the qualifications 'suitable' or 'appropriate' without further definition in the text, the choice of such strain, test, method, substance, *etc.*, is made in accordance with any international agreements or national regulations affecting the subject concerned.

Expression of Standards Where the standard for the content of a substance described in a monograph is expressed in terms of the chemical formula for that substance an upper limit exceeding 100% may be stated. Such an upper limit applies to the result of the assay calculated in terms of the equivalent content of the specified chemical formula. For example, the statement 'contains not less than 99.0% and not more than 101.0% of '$C_{20}H_{24}N_2O_2$,HCl' implies that the result of the assay is not less than 99.0% and not more than 101.0%, calculated in terms of the equivalent content of $C_{20}H_{24}N_2O_2$,HCl.

Where the result of an assay or test is required to be calculated with reference to the dried, anhydrous or ignited substance, the substance free from a specified solvent or to the peptide content, the determination of loss on drying, water content, loss on ignition, content of the specified solvent or peptide content is carried out by the method prescribed in the relevant test in the monograph.

Temperature The Celsius thermometric scale is used in expressing temperatures.

Weights and Measures The metric system of weights and measures is employed; SI Units have generally been adopted. Metric measures are required to have been graduated at 20° and all measurements involved in the analytical operations of the Pharmacopoeia are intended, unless otherwise stated, to be made at that temperature. Graduated glass apparatus used in analytical operations should comply with Class A requirements of the appropriate specification issued by the British Standards Institution.

Atomic Weights The atomic weights adopted are the values given in the Table of Relative Atomic Weights 1989 published by the International Union of Pure and Applied Chemistry. The values are based on the carbon-12 scale (Appendix XXII).

Constant Weight The term 'constant weight', used in relation to the process of drying or the process of ignition, means that two consecutive weighings do not differ by more than 0.5 milligram, the second weighing being made after an additional period of drying or ignition under the specified conditions appropriate to the nature and quantity of the residue (1 hour is usually suitable).

Expression of Concentrations The term 'per cent' or more usually the symbol '%' is used with one of four different meanings in the expression of concentrations according to circumstances. In order that the meaning to be attached to the expression in each instance is clear, the following notation is used.

Per cent w/w (% w/w) (percentage weight in weight) expresses the number of grams of solute in 100 g of product.

Per cent w/v (% w/v) (percentage weight in volume) expresses the number of grams of solute in 100 ml of product.

Per cent v/v (% v/v) (percentage volume in volume) expresses the number of millilitres of solute in 100 ml of product.

Per cent v/w (% v/w) (percentage volume in weight) expresses the number of millilitres of solute in 100 g of product.

Usually the strength of solutions of solids in liquids is expressed as percentage weight in volume, of liquids in liquids as percentage volume in volume and of gases in liquids as percentage weight in weight.

When the concentration of a solution is expressed as parts per million (ppm), it means weight in weight, unless otherwise specified.

When the concentration of a solution is expressed as parts of dissolved substance in parts of the solution, it means parts by weight (g) of a solid in parts by volume (ml) of the final solution; or parts by volume (ml) of a liquid in parts by volume (ml) of the final solution; or parts by weight (g) of a gas in parts by weight (g) of the final solution.

When the concentration of a solution is expressed in molarity designated by the symbol M preceded by a number, it denotes the number of moles of the stated solute contained in sufficient Purified Water (unless otherwise stated) to produce 1 litre of solution.

Water Bath The term 'water bath' means a bath of boiling water, unless water at some other temperature is indicated in the text. An alternative form of heating may be employed providing that the required temperature is approximately maintained but not exceeded.

Reagents The reagents required for the assays and tests of the Pharmacopoeia are defined in appendices. The descriptions set out in the appendices do not imply that the materials are suitable for use in medicine.

Indicators Indicators, the colours of which change over approximately the same range of pH, may be substituted for one another but in the event of doubt or dispute as to the equivalence of indicators for a particular purpose, the indicator specified in the text is alone authoritative.

The quantity of an indicator solution appropriate for use in acid—base titrations described in assays or tests is 0.1 ml unless otherwise stated in the text.

Any solvent required in an assay or test in which an indicator is specified is previously neutralised to the indicator, unless a blank test is prescribed.

Caution Statements A number of materials described in the monographs and some of the reagents specified for use in the assays and tests of the Pharmacopoeia may be injurious to health unless adequate precautions are taken. The principles of good laboratory practice and the provisions of any appropriate regulations such as those issued in the United Kingdom in accordance with the Health and Safety at Work *etc.* Act (1974) should be observed at all times in carrying out the assays and tests of the Pharmacopoeia.

Attention is drawn to particular hazards in certain monographs by means of an italicised statement; the absence of such a statement should not however be taken to mean that no hazard exists.

Titles Subsidiary titles, where included, have the same significance as the main titles. An abbreviated title constructed in accordance with the directions given in Appendix XXI A has the same significance as the main title.

Titles that are derived by the suitable inversion of words of a main or subsidiary title, with the addition of a preposition if appropriate, are also official titles. Thus, the following are all official titles: Aspirin Tablets, Tablets of Aspirin; Ginger Tincture, Tincture of Ginger; Atropine Injection, Injection of Atropine.

A title of a formulated preparation that includes the full nonproprietary name of the active ingredient or ingredients, where this is not included in the title of the monograph, is also an official title. For example, the title Amitriptyline Embonate Oral Suspension has the same significance as Amitriptyline Oral Suspension and the title Brompheniramine Maleate Tablets has the same significance as Brompheniramine Tablets.

Where the English title at the head of a monograph in the European Pharmacopoeia is different from that at the head of the text incorporated into the British Pharmacopoeia, the European Pharmacopoeia title is given in an italicised statement at the head of the incorporated text. The titles and subsidiary titles (if any) of such incorporated texts have been declared Approved Synonyms in accordance with section 65(8) of the Medicines Act 1968 and are thus official titles. A cumulative list of such Approved Synonyms is provided in Appendix XXI B.

Where the names of Pharmacopoeial substances, preparations and other materials occur in the text they are printed with capital initial letters and this indicates that materials of Pharmacopoeial quality must be used. Words in the text that name a reagent or other material, a physical characteristic or a process that is described or defined in an appendix are printed in italic type, for example, *methanol*, *absorbance*, *gas chromatography*, and these imply compliance with the requirements specified in the appropriate appendix.

Chemical Formulae When the chemical composition of an official substance is known or generally accepted, the graphic and molecular formulae, the molecular weight and the Chemical Abstracts Service Registry Number are normally given at the beginning of the monograph for information. This information refers to the chemically pure substance and is not to be regarded as an indication of the purity of the official material. Elsewhere, in statements of standards of purity and strength and in descriptions of processes of assay, it is evident from the context that the formulae denote the chemically pure substances.

Where the absolute stereochemical configuration is specified, the International Union of Pure and Applied Chemistry (IUPAC) *R*/*S* and *E*/*Z* systems of designation have been used. If the substance is an enantiomer of unknown absolute stereochemistry the sign of the optical rotation, as determined in the solvent and under the conditions specified in the monograph, has been attached to the systematic name. An indication of sign of rotation has also been given where this is incorporated in a trivial name that appears on an IUPAC preferred list.

All amino acids, except glycine, have the L-configuration unless otherwise indicated. The three-letter and one-letter symbols used for amino acids in peptide and protein sequences are those recommended by the Joint Commission on Biochemical Nomenclature of the International Union of Pure and Applied Chemistry and the International Union of Biochemistry.

In the graphic formulae the following abbreviations are used:

Me	$-CH_3$	Bu^s	$-CH(CH_3)CH_2CH_3$
Et	$-CH_2CH_3$	Bu^n	$-CH_2CH_2CH_2CH_3$
Pr^i	$-CH(CH_3)_2$	Bu^t	$-C(CH_3)_3$
Pr^n	$-CH_2CH_2CH_3$	Ph	$-C_6H_5$
Bu^i	$-CH_2CH(CH_3)_2$	Ac	$-COCH_3$

Definition Statements given under the side-heading Definition constitute an official definition of the substance, preparation or other article that is the subject of the monograph. They constitute instructions or requirements and are mandatory in nature.

Certain medicinal or pharmaceutical substances and other articles are defined by reference to a particular method of manufacture. A statement that a substance or article *is* prepared or obtained by a certain method constitutes part of the official definition and implies that other methods are not permitted. A statement that a substance *may be* prepared or obtained by a certain method, however, indicates that this is one possible method and does not imply that other methods are proscribed.

Additional statements concerning the definition of formulated preparations are given in the general notice on Manufacture of Formulated Preparations.

Production Statements given under the side-heading Production draw attention to particular aspects of the manufacturing process but are not necessarily comprehensive. They constitute mandatory instructions to manufacturers. They may relate, for example, to source materials, to the manufacturing process itself and its validation and control, to in-process testing or to testing that is to be carried out by the manufacturer on the final product (bulk material or dosage form) either on selected batches or on each batch prior to release. These statements cannot necessarily be verified on a sample of the final product by an independent analyst. The competent authority may establish that the instructions have been followed, for example, by examination of data received from the manufacturer, by inspection or by testing appropriate samples.

The absence of a section on Production does not imply that attention to features such as those referred to above is not required. A substance, preparation or article described in a monograph of the Pharmacopoeia is to be manufactured in accordance with the principles of good manufacturing practice and in accordance with relevant international agreements and supranational and national regulations governing medicinal products.

Where in the section under the side-heading Production a monograph on a vaccine defines the characteristics of the vaccine strain to be used, any test methods given for confirming these characteristics are provided as examples of suitable methods. The use of these methods is not mandatory.

Additional statements concerning the production of formulated preparations are given in the general notice on Manufacture of Formulated Preparations.

Manufacture of Formulated Preparations Attention is drawn to the need to observe adequate hygienic precautions in the preparation and dispensing of pharmaceutical formulations. The principles of good pharmaceutical manufacturing practice should be observed.

The Definition in certain monographs for pharmaceutical preparations is given in terms of the principal ingredients only. Any ingredient, other than those included in the Definition, must comply with the general notice on Excipients and the product must conform with the Pharmacopoeial requirements.

The Definition in other monographs for pharmaceutical preparations is presented as a full formula. No deviation from the stated formula is permitted except those allowed by the general notices on Colouring Agents and Antimicrobial Preservatives. Where additionally directions are given under the side-heading Extemporaneous Preparation these are intended for the extemporaneous preparation of relatively small quantities for short-term supply and use. When so prepared, no deviation from the stated directions is permitted. If, however, such a pharmaceutical preparation is manufactured on a larger scale with the intention that it may be stored, deviations from the stated directions are permitted provided that the final product meets the following criteria:

(1) compliance with all of the requirements stated in the monograph;

(2) retention of the essential characteristics of the preparation made strictly in accordance with the directions of the Pharmacopoeia.

Monographs for yet other pharmaceutical preparations include both a Definition in terms of the principal ingredients and, under the side-heading Extemporaneous Preparation, a full formula together with, in some cases, directions for their preparation. Such full formulae and directions are intended for the extemporaneous preparation of relatively small quantities for short-term supply and use. When so prepared, no deviation from the stated formula and directions is permitted. If, however, such a pharmaceutical preparation is manufactured on a larger scale with the intention that it may be stored, deviations from the formula and directions stated under the side-heading Extemporaneous Preparation are permitted provided that any ingredient, other than those included in the Definition, complies with the general notice on Excipients and that the final product meets the following criteria:

(1) accordance with the Definition stated in the monograph;

(2) compliance with all of the requirements stated in the monograph;

(3) retention of the essential characteristics of the preparation made strictly in accordance with the formula and directions of the Pharmacopoeia.

In the manufacture of any official preparation on a large scale with the intention that it should be stored, in addition to following any instruction under the side-heading Production, it is necessary to ascertain that the product is satisfactory with respect to its physical and chemical stability and its state of preservation over the claimed shelf-life. This applies irrespective of whether the formula of the Pharmacopoeia and any instructions given under the side-heading Extemporaneous Preparation are followed precisely or modified. Provided that the preparation has been shown to be stable in other respects, deterioration due to microbial contamination may be inhibited by the incorporation of a suitable antimicrobial preservative. In such circumstances the label states appropriate storage conditions, the date after which the product should not be used and the identity and concentration of the antimicrobial preservative.

Freshly and Recently Prepared The direction, given under the side-heading Extemporaneous Preparation, that a preparation must be freshly prepared indicates that it must be made not more than 24 hours before it is issued for use. The direction that a preparation should be recently prepared indicates that deterioration is likely if the preparation is stored for longer than about 4 weeks at 15° to 25°.

Methods of Sterilisation The methods of sterilisation used in preparing the sterile materials described in the Pharmacopoeia are given in Appendix XVIII. For aqueous preparations, steam sterilisation (heating in an autoclave) is the method of choice wherever it is known to be suitable. Any method of sterilisation must be validated with respect to both the assurance of sterility and the integrity of the product and to ensure that the final product complies with the requirements of the monograph.

Water The term Water used without qualification in formulae for formulated preparations means either potable water freshly drawn direct from the public supply and suitable for drinking or freshly boiled and cooled Purified Water. The latter should be used if the public supply is from a local storage tank or if the potable water is unsuitable for a particular preparation.

Excipients Where an excipient for which there is a Pharmacopoeial monograph is used in preparing an official preparation it shall comply with that monograph. Any substance added in preparing an official preparation shall be innocuous, shall have no adverse influence on the therapeutic efficacy of the active ingredients and shall not interfere with the assays and tests of the Pharmacopoeia. Particular care should be taken to ensure that such substances are free from harmful organisms.

Colouring Agents If in a monograph for a formulated preparation defined by means of a full formula a specific colouring agent or agents is prescribed, suitable alternatives approved in the country concerned may be substituted.

Antimicrobial Preservatives When the term 'suitable antimicrobial preservative' is used it is implied that the preparation concerned will be effectively preserved according to the appropriate criteria applied and interpreted as described in the test for *efficacy of antimicrobial preservation* (Appendix XVI C). In certain monographs for formulated preparations defined by means of a full formula, a specific antimicrobial agent or agents may be prescribed; suitable alternatives may be substituted provided that their identity and concentration are stated on the label.

Characteristics Statements given under the side-heading Characteristics are not to be interpreted in a strict sense and are not to be regarded as official requirements. Statements on taste are provided only in cases where this property is a guide to the acceptability of the material (for example, a material used primarily for flavouring). The status of statements on solubility is given in the general notice on Solubility.

Solubility Statements on solubility given under the side-heading Characteristics are intended as information on the approximate solubility at a temperature between 15° and 25°, unless otherwise stated, and are not to be considered as official requirements.

Statements given under side-headings such as Solubility in ethanol express exact requirements and constitute part of the standards for the substances under which they occur.

The following table indicates the meanings of the terms used in statements of approximate solubilities.

Descriptive term	Approximate volume of solvent in millilitres per gram of solute
very soluble	less than 1
freely soluble	from 1 to 10
soluble	from 10 to 30
sparingly soluble	from 30 to 100
slightly soluble	from 100 to 1000
very slightly soluble	from 1000 to 10,000
practically insoluble	more than 10,000

The term 'partly soluble' is used to describe a mixture of which only some of the components dissolve.

Identification The tests described or referred to under the side-heading Identification are not necessarily sufficient to establish absolute proof of identity. They provide a means of verifying that the identity of the material being examined is in accordance with the label on the container.

Unless otherwise prescribed, identification tests are carried out at a temperature between 15° and 25°.

When tests for infrared absorption are applied to material extracted from formulated preparations, strict concordance with the specified reference spectrum may not always be possible, but nevertheless a close resemblance between the spectrum of the extracted material and the specified reference spectrum should be achieved.

Assays and Tests The assays and tests described are the official methods upon which the standards of the Pharmacopoeia depend. The analyst is not precluded from employing alternative methods, including methods of microanalysis, in any assay or test if it is known that the method used will give a result of equivalent accuracy. Local reference materials may be used for routine analysis, provided that these are calibrated against the official reference materials. In the event of doubt or dispute, the methods of analysis, the reference materials and the reference spectra of the Pharmacopoeia are alone authoritative.

Where the solvent used for a solution is not named, the solvent is Purified Water.

Unless otherwise prescribed, the assays and tests are carried out at a temperature between 15° and 25°.

A temperature in a test for Loss on drying, where no temperature range is given, implies a range of ± 2° about the stated value.

Visual comparative tests, unless otherwise prescribed, are carried out using identical tubes of colourless, transparent, neutral glass with a flat base and an internal diameter of 16 mm. Equal volumes of the liquids to be compared are examined down the vertical axis of the tubes against a white background or, if necessary, against a black background. The examination is carried out in diffuse light.

Where a direction is given that an analytical operation is to be carried out 'in subdued light', precautions should be taken to avoid exposure to direct sunlight or other strong light. Where a direction is given that an analytical operation is to be carried out 'protected from light', precautions should be taken to exclude actinic light by the use of low-actinic glassware, working in a dark room or similar procedures.

For preparations other than those of fixed strength, the quantity to be taken for an assay or test is usually expressed in terms of the active ingredient. This means that the quantity of the active ingredient expected to be present and the quantity of the preparation to be taken are calculated from the strength stated on the label.

In assays the approximate quantity to be taken for examination is indicated but the quantity actually used must not deviate by more than 10% from that stated. The quantity taken is accurately weighed or measured and the result of the assay is calculated from this exact quantity. Reagents are measured and the procedures are carried out with an accuracy commensurate with the degree of precision implied by the standard stated for the assay.

In tests the stated quantity to be taken for examination must be used unless any divergence can be taken into account in conducting the test and calculating the result. The quantity taken is accurately weighed or measured with the degree of precision implied by the standard or, where the standard is not stated numerically (for example, in tests for Clarity and colour of solution), with the degree of precision implied by the number of significant figures stated. Reagents are measured and the procedures are carried out with an accuracy commensurate with this degree of precision.

The limits stated in monographs are based on data obtained in normal analytical practice; they take account of normal analytical errors, of acceptable variations in manufacture and of deterioration to an extent considered acceptable. No further tolerances are to be applied to the limits prescribed to determine whether the article being examined complies with the requirements of the monograph.

In determining compliance with a numerical limit, the calculated result of a test or assay is first rounded to the number of significant figures stated, unless otherwise prescribed. The last figure is increased by one when the part rejected is equal to or exceeds one half-unit, whereas it is not modified when the part rejected is less than a half-unit.

In certain tests, the concentration of impurity is given in parentheses either as a percentage or in parts per million by weight (ppm). In chromatographic tests such concentrations are stated as a percentage irrespective of the limit. In other tests they are usually stated in ppm unless the limit exceeds 500 ppm. In those chromatographic tests in which a secondary spot or peak in a chromatogram obtained with a solution of the substance being examined is described as corresponding to a named impurity and is compared with a spot or peak in a chromatogram obtained with a reference solution of the same impurity, the percentage given in parentheses indicates the limit for that impurity. In those chromatographic tests in which a spot or peak in a chromatogram obtained with a solution of the substance being examined is described in terms other than as corresponding to a named impurity (commonly, for example, as any (other) *secondary spot* or *peak*) but is compared with a spot or peak in a chromatogram obtained with a reference solution of a named impurity, the percentage given in parentheses indicates an impurity limit expressed in terms of a nominal concentration of the named impurity. In chromatographic tests in which a comparison is made between spots or peaks in chromatograms obtained with solutions of different concentrations of the substance being examined, the percentage given in parentheses indicates an impurity limit expressed in terms of a nominal concentration of the medicinal substance itself. In some monographs, in particular those for certain formulated preparations, the impurity limit is expressed in terms of a nominal concentration of the active moiety rather than of the medicinal substance itself. Where necessary for clarification the terms in which the limit is expressed are stated within the monograph.

In all cases where an impurity limit is given in parentheses, the figures given are approximations for information only; conformity with the requirements is determined on the basis of compliance or otherwise with the stated test.

The use of a proprietary designation to identify a material used in an assay or test does not imply that another equally suitable material may not be used.

Biological Assays and Tests

Methods of assay described as Suggested methods are not obligatory, but when another method is used its precision must be not less than that required for the Suggested method.

For those antibiotics for which the monograph specifies a microbiological assay the potency requirement is expressed in the monograph in International Units (IU) per milligram. The material is not of pharmacopoeial quality if the upper fiducial limit of error is less than the stated potency. For such antibiotics the required precision of the assay is stated in the monograph in terms of the fiducial limits of error about the estimated potency.

For other substances and preparations for which the monograph specifies a biological assay, unless otherwise stated, the precision of the assay is such that the fiducial limits of error, expressed as a percentage of the estimated potency, are within a range not wider than that obtained by multiplying by a factor of ten the square roots of the limits given in the monograph for the fiducial limits of error about the stated potency.

In all cases fiducial limits of error are based on a probability of 95% ($P = 0.95$).

Where the biological assay is being used to ascertain the purity of the material, the stated potency means the potency stated on the label in terms of International Units (IU) or other Units per gram, per milligram or per millilitre. When no such statement appears on the label, the stated potency means the fixed or minimum potency required in the monograph. This interpretation of stated potency applies in all cases except where the monograph specifically directs otherwise.

Where the biological assay is being used to determine the total activity in the container, the stated potency means the total number of International Units (IU) or other Units stated on the label or, if no such statement appears, the total activity calculated in accordance with the instructions in the monograph.

Wherever possible the primary standard used in an assay or test is the respective International Standard or Reference Preparation established by the World Health Organization for international use and the biological activity is expressed in International Units (IU).

In other cases, where Units are referred to in an assay or test, the Unit for a particular substance or preparation is, for the United Kingdom, the specific biological activity contained in such an amount of the respective primary standard as the appropriate international or national organisation indicates. The necessary information is provided with the primary standard.

Unless otherwise directed, animals used in an assay or a test are healthy animals, drawn from a uniform stock, that have not previously been treated with any material that will interfere with the assay or test. Unless otherwise stated, guinea-pigs weigh not less than 250 g or, when used in systemic toxicity tests, not less than 350 g. When used in skin tests they are white or light coloured. Unless otherwise stated, mice weigh not less than 17 g and not more than 22 g.

Certain of the biological assays and tests of the Pharmacopoeia are such that in the United Kingdom they may be carried out only in accordance with the Animals (Scientific Procedures) Act 1986. Instructions included in such assays and tests in the Pharmacopoeia, with respect to the handling of animals, are therefore confined to those concerned with the accuracy and reproducibility of the assay or test.

Storage Statements under the side-heading Storage constitute non-mandatory advice. The substances and preparations described in the Pharmacopoeia are to be stored under conditions that prevent contamination and, as far as possible, deterioration. Precautions that should be taken in relation to the effects of the atmosphere, moisture, heat and light are indicated, where appropriate, in the monographs. Further precautions may be necessary when some materials are stored in tropical climates or under other severe conditions. The expression 'protected from moisture' means that the product is to be stored in an airtight container. Care is to be taken when the container is opened in a damp atmosphere. A low moisture content may be maintained, if necessary, by the use of a desiccant in the container provided that direct contact with the product is avoided. The expression 'protected from light' means that the product is to be stored either in a container made of a material that absorbs actinic light sufficiently to protect the contents from change induced by such light or in a container enclosed in an outer cover that provides such protection or stored in a place from which all such light is excluded. The expression 'tamper-evident container' means a closed container fitted with a device that reveals irreversibly whether the container has been opened.

Labelling The labelling requirements of the Pharmacopoeia are not comprehensive and laws governing the statements to be declared on labels of official articles should also be met. In the United Kingdom the provisions of regulations issued in accordance with the Medicines Act 1968, together with those of regulations for the labelling of hazardous materials, should be met.

Only those statements in monographs given under the side-heading Labelling that are necessary to demonstrate compliance or otherwise with the monograph are mandatory. Any other statements are included as recommendations.

Such matters as the exact form of wording to be used and whether a particular item of information should appear on the primary label and additionally, or alternatively, on the package or exceptionally in a leaflet are, in general, outside the scope of the Pharmacopoeia. When the term 'label' is used in Labelling statements of the Pharmacopoeia, decisions as to where the particular statement should appear should therefore be made in accordance with relevant legislation.

The label of every official article states (i) the name at the head of the monograph and (ii) a reference consisting of either figures or letters, or a combination of figures and letters, by which the history of the article may be traced.

The label of every official formulated preparation other than those of fixed strength also states the content of the active ingredient or ingredients expressed in the terms required by the monograph. Where the content of active ingredient is required to be expressed in terms other than the weight of the official medicinal substance used in making the formulation, this is specifically stated under the side-heading Labelling. Thus, where no specific requirement is included under the side-heading Labelling, it is implied that the content of active ingredient is expressed in terms of the weight of the official medicinal substance used in making the formulation. For example, for Ampicillin Injection, which contains Ampicillin Sodium but for which the content is expressed in terms of the equivalent amount of ampicillin, a specific requirement to this effect is included under the side-heading Labelling. For Amitriptyline Tablets which contain Amitriptyline Hydrochloride and for which the result of the assay is expressed in terms of amitriptyline hydrochloride no specific statement is included under the side-heading Labelling; these Tablets are thus labelled with the nominal weight of Amitriptyline Hydrochloride.

These requirements do not necessarily apply to the labelling of articles supplied in compliance with a prescription.

Action and Use The statements given under this side-heading in monographs are intended only as information on the principal pharmacological actions or the uses of the materials in medicine or pharmacy. It should not be assumed that the substance has no other action or use. The statements are not intended to be binding on prescribers or to limit their discretion.

Crude Drugs The macroscopical characteristics of a crude drug includes those features that can be seen by the unaided eye or by the use of a hand lens.

Vegetable drugs are required to be free from insects and other animal matter, and from animal excreta. Not more than traces of foreign organic matter may be present in powdered vegetable drugs. Microbial contamination should be minimal.

In determining the content of active principle, Acid-insoluble ash, Ash, Extractive soluble in ethanol, Loss on drying, Sulphated ash, Water, Water-soluble ash and Water-soluble extractive of vegetable drugs, the calculations are made with reference to the drug that has not been specially dried unless otherwise prescribed in the monograph.

In the assays for alkaloids in crude drugs and their preparations, definite quantities of solvents are specified. The quantities are given as being suitable for typical cases; they may, however, be varied where necessary to overcome the difficulties that may be encountered in special instances, provided that the effect of the prescribed directions is ensured.

When it is found necessary to dry a crude drug before it can be reduced to powder for the purpose of assay, a correction is made for the loss on drying and the alkaloidal content is calculated with reference to the undried drug.

Part III

Monographs and other texts of the European Pharmacopoeia that are incorporated in this edition of the British Pharmacopoeia are governed by the general notices of the European Pharmacopoeia; these are reproduced below.

GENERAL NOTICES OF THE EUROPEAN PHARMACOPOEIA

Text in [ ] does not form part of the General Notices of the European Pharmacopoeia but has been added for the convenience of the user of the British Pharmacopoeia.

1.1. GENERAL STATEMENTS

The General Notices apply to all monographs and other texts of the European Pharmacopoeia.

In the texts of the European Pharmacopoeia, the word 'Pharmacopoeia' without qualification means the European Pharmacopoeia. The official abbreviation Ph. Eur. may be used to indicate the European Pharmacopoeia.

The use of the title or the subtitle of a monograph implies that the article complies with the requirements of the relevant monograph. Such references to monographs in the texts of the Pharmacopoeia are shown using the monograph title and serial number in *italics*.

A pharmaceutical preparation must comply throughout its period of validity. The subject of any other monograph must comply throughout its period of use. The period of validity that is assigned to any given article and the time from which that period is to be calculated are decided by the competent authority in the light of experimental results of stability studies.

Unless otherwise indicated in the General Notices or in the monographs, statements in monographs constitute mandatory requirements. General chapters [Appendices] become mandatory when referred to in a monograph, unless such reference is made in a way that indicates that it is not the intention to make the text referred to mandatory but rather to cite it for information or guidance.

The active ingredients (medicinal substances), excipients (auxiliary substances), pharmaceutical preparations and other articles described in the monographs are intended for human and veterinary use (unless explicitly restricted to one of these uses). An article is not of Pharmacopoeia quality unless it complies with all the requirements stated in the monograph. This does not imply that performance of all the tests in a monograph is necessarily a prerequisite for a manufacturer in assessing compliance with the Pharmacopoeia before release of a product. The manufacturer may obtain assurance that a product is of Pharmacopoeia quality from data derived, for example, from validation studies of the manufacturing process and from in-process controls. Parametric release in circumstances deemed appropriate by the competent authority is thus not precluded by the need to comply with the Pharmacopoeia.

The tests and assays described are the official methods upon which the standards of the Pharmacopoeia are based. With the agreement of the competent authority, alternative methods of analysis may be used for control purposes, provided that the methods used enable an unequivocal decision to be made as to whether compliance with the standards of the monographs would be achieved if the official methods were used. In the event of doubt or dispute, the methods of analysis of the Pharmacopoeia are alone authoritative.

Certain materials that are the subject of a pharmacopoeial monograph may exist in different grades suitable for different purposes. Unless otherwise indicated in the monograph, the requirements apply to all grades of the material. In some monographs, particularly those on excipients, a list of critical properties that are important for the use of the substance may be appended to the monograph for information and guidance. Test methods for determination of one or more of these critical properties may be given, also for information and guidance.

The general monographs on dosage forms apply to all preparations of the type defined. The requirements are not necessarily comprehensive for a given specific preparation and requirements additional to those prescribed in the general monograph may be imposed by the competent authority.

Conventional terms The term 'competent authority'means the national, supranational or international body or organisation vested with the authority for making decisions concerning the issue in question. It may, for example, be a national pharmacopoeia authority, a licensing authority or an official control laboratory.

The expression 'unless otherwise justified and authorised' means that the requirements have to be met, unless the competent authority authorises a modification or an exemption where justified in a particular case.

Statements containing the word 'should' are informative or advisory.

In certain monographs or other texts, the terms 'suitable' and 'appropriate' are used to describe a reagent, micro-organism, test method etc.; if criteria for suitability are not described in the monograph, suitability is demonstrated to the satisfaction of the competent authority.

1.2. OTHER PROVISIONS APPLYING TO GENERAL CHAPTERS [APPENDICES] AND MONOGRAPHS

Quantities In tests with numerical limits and assays, the quantity stated to be taken for examination is approximate. The amount actually used, which may deviate by not more than 10 per cent from that stated, is accurately weighed or measured and the result is calculated from this exact quantity. In tests where the limit is not numerical, but usually depends upon comparison with the behaviour of a reference in the same conditions, the stated quantity is taken for examination. Reagents are used in the prescribed amounts.

Quantities are weighed or measured with an accuracy commensurate with the indicated degree of precision. For weighings, the precision corresponds to plus or minus 5 units after the last figure stated (for example, 0.25 g is to be interpreted as 0.245 g to 0.255 g). For the measurement of volumes, if the figure after the decimal point is a zero or ends in a zero (for example, 10.0 ml or 0.50 ml), the volume is measured using a pipette, a volumetric flask or a burette, as appropriate; otherwise, a graduated measuring cylinder or a graduated pipette may be used. Volumes stated in microlitres are measured using a micropipette or microsyringe. It is recognised, however, that in certain cases the precision with which quantities are stated does not correspond to the number of significant figures stated in a specified numerical limit. The weighings and measurements are then carried out with a sufficiently improved accuracy.

Apparatus and procedures Volumetric glassware complies with Class A requirements of the appropriate International Standard issued by the International Organisation for Standardisation.

Unless otherwise prescribed, analytical procedures are carried out at a temperature between 15°C and 25°C.

Unless otherwise prescribed, comparative tests are carried out using identical tubes of colourless, transparent, neutral glass with a flat base and an internal diameter of 16 mm. Equal volumes of the liquids to be compared are examined down the vertical axis of the tubes against a white background, or if necessary against a black background. The examination is carried out in diffuse light.

Any solvent required in a test or assay in which an indicator is to be used is previously neutralised to the indicator, unless a blank test is prescribed.

Water-bath The term 'water-bath' means a bath of boiling water unless water at another temperature is indicated. Other methods of heating may be substituted provided the temperature is near to but not higher than 100°C or the indicated temperature.

Drying and ignition to constant mass The terms 'dried to constant mass' and 'ignited to constant mass' mean that two consecutive weighings do not differ by more than 0.5 mg, the second weighing following an additional period of drying or of ignition respectively appropriate to the nature and quantity of the residue.

Where drying is prescribed using one of the expressions 'in a desiccator' or '*in vacuo*', it is carried out using the conditions described under *2.2.32. Loss on drying* [Appendix IX D].

Reagents The proper conduct of the analytical procedures described in the Pharmacopoeia and the reliability of the results depend, in part, upon the quality of the reagents used. The reagents are described in general chapter 4 [Appendix I]. It is assumed that reagents of analytical grade are used; for some reagents, tests to determine suitability are included in the specifications.

Solvents Where the name of the solvent is not stated, the term 'solution' implies a solution in water. Where the use of water is specified or implied in the analytical procedures described in the Pharmacopoeia or for the preparation of reagents, water complying with the requirements of the monograph on *Purified water (8)* is used. The term 'distilled water' indicates purified water prepared by distillation.

The term 'ethanol' without qualification means absolute alcohol. The term 'alcohol' without qualification means alcohol containing about 96 per cent *V/V* of ethanol (C_2H_6O). Other dilutions of ethanol are indicated by the term 'alcohol' followed by a statement of the percentage by volume of ethanol (C_2H_6O) required.

Expression of content In defining content, the expression 'per cent' is used according to circumstances with one of two meanings:

- per cent *m/m* (percentage, mass in mass) expresses the number of grams of substance in 100 grams of final product.
- per cent *V/V* (percentage, volume in volume) expresses the number of millilitres of substance in 100 millilitres of final product.

The expression 'parts per million (ppm)' refers to mass in mass, unless otherwise specified.

Temperature Where an analytical procedure describes temperature without a figure, the general terms used have the following meaning:

In a deep-freeze		below	−15°C
In a refrigerator	2°C	to	8°C
Cold or cool	8°C	to	15°C
Room temperature	15°C	to	25°C

1.3. GENERAL CHAPTERS [incorporated in the Appendices of the British Pharmacopoeia]

Containers Materials used for containers are described in general chapter 3 [Appendix XX]. General names used for materials, particularly plastics materials, each cover a range of products varying not only in the properties of the principal constituent but also in the additives used. The test methods and limits for materials depend on the formulation and are therefore applicable only for materials whose formulation is covered by the preamble to the specification. The use of materials with different formulations and the test methods and limits applied to them are subject to agreement by the competent authority.

The specifications for containers in general chapter 3 [Appendix XIX], have been developed for general application to containers of the stated category but in view of the wide variety of containers available and possible new developments, the publication of a specification does not exclude the use, in justified circumstances, of containers that comply with other specifications, subject to agreement by the competent authority.

Reference may be made within the monographs of the Pharmacopoeia to the definitions and specifications for containers provided in this section. The general monographs for pharmaceutical dosage forms may, under the heading Definition/Production, require the use of certain types of container; certain other monographs may, under the heading Storage, indicate the type of container that is recommended for use.

1.4. MONOGRAPHS

Titles Monograph titles are in English and French in the respective versions [published by the Council of Europe] and there is a Latin subtitle which may be used in place of the English or French title as may any synonyms declared equivalent by the competent authority [see Approved Synonyms, Appendix XXI B].

Relative atomic and molecular masses The relative atomic mass (A_r) or the relative molecular mass (M_r) is shown, as and where appropriate, at the beginning of each monograph. The relative atomic and molecular masses and the molecular and graphic formulae do not constitute analytical standards for the substances described.

Definition Statements under the heading Definition constitute an official definition of the substance, preparation or other article that is the subject of the monograph.

Limits of content Where limits of content are prescribed, they are those determined by the method described under Assay.

Vegetable drugs In monographs on vegetable drugs, the definition indicates whether the subject of the monograph is, for example, the whole drug or the drug in powdered form. Where a monograph applies to the drug in several states, for example both to the whole drug and the drug in powdered form, the definition states this.

Production Statements under the heading Production draw attention to particular aspects of the manufacturing process but are not necessarily comprehensive. They constitute instructions to manufacturers. They may relate, for example, to source materials, to the manufacturing process itself and its validation and control, to in-process testing or to testing that is to be carried out by the manufacturer on the final article either on selected batches or on each batch prior to release. These statements cannot necessarily be verified on a sample of the final article by an independent analyst. The competent authority may establish that the instructions have been followed, for example, by examination of data received from the manufacturer, by inspection of manufacture or by testing appropriate samples.

The absence of a section on Production does not imply that attention to features such as those referred to above is not required. A product described in a monograph of the Pharmacopoeia is manufactured in accordance with the principles of good manufacturing practice and in accordance with relevant international agreements and supranational and national regulations governing products for human or veterinary use.

Where in the section under the heading Production a monograph on a vaccine defines the characteristics of the vaccine strain to be used, any test methods given for confirming these characteristics are provided for information as examples of suitable methods.

Characters The statements under the heading Characters are not to be interpreted in a strict sense and are not requirements.

Solubility. In statements of solubility in the section headed Characters, the terms used have the following significance referred to a temperature between 15 °C and 25 °C.

Descriptive term	Approximate volume of solvent in millilitres per gram of solute			
Very soluble	less than	1		
Freely soluble	from	1	to	10
Soluble	from	10	to	30
Sparingly soluble	from	30	to	100
Slightly soluble	from	100	to	1000
Very slightly soluble	from	1000	to	10,000
Practically insoluble	more than			10,000

The term 'partly soluble' is used to describe a mixture where only some of the components dissolve. The term 'miscible' is used to describe a liquid that is miscible in all proportions with the stated solvent.

Identification The tests given in the identification section are not designed to give a full confirmation of the chemical structure or composition of the product; they are intended to give confirmation, with an acceptable degree of assurance, that the article conforms to the description on the label.

Certain monographs have subdivisions entitled 'First identification' and 'Second identification'. The test or tests that constitute the 'Second identification' may be used instead of the test or tests of the 'First identification' provided it can be demonstrated that the substance or preparation is fully traceable to a batch certified to comply with all the requirements of the monograph.

Tests and assays **Scope** The requirements are not framed to take account of all possible impurities. It is not to be presumed, for example, that an impurity that is not detectable by means of the prescribed tests is tolerated if common sense and good pharmaceutical practice require that it be absent. See also below under Impurities.

Calculation Where the result of a test or assay is required to be calculated with reference to the dried or anhydrous substance or on some other specified basis, the determination of loss on drying, water content or other property is carried out by the method prescribed in the relevant test in the monograph.

Limits The limits prescribed are based on data obtained in normal analytical practice; they take account of normal analytical errors, of acceptable variations in manufacture and compounding and of deterioration to an extent considered acceptable. No further tolerances are to be applied to the limits prescribed to determine whether the article being examined complies with the requirements of the monograph.

In determining compliance with a numerical limit, the calculated result of a test or assay is first rounded to the number of significant figures stated, unless otherwise prescribed. The last figure is increased by one when the part rejected is equal to or exceeds one half-unit, whereas it is not modified when the part rejected is less than a half-unit.

Indication of permitted limit of impurities The approximate content of impurity tolerated, or the sum of impurities, may be indicated in parentheses for information only. If the use of a reference substance for the named impurity is not prescribed, this content may be expressed as a nominal concentration of the substance used to prepare the reference solution specified in the monograph, unless otherwise described. Acceptance or rejection is determined on the basis of compliance or non-compliance with the stated test.

Vegetable drugs For vegetable drugs, the sulphated ash, total ash, water-soluble matter, alcohol-soluble matter, water content, content of essential oil and content of active principle are calculated with reference to the drug that has not been specially dried, unless otherwise prescribed in the monograph.

Equivalents Where an equivalent is given, for the purposes of the Pharmacopoeia only the figures shown are to be used in applying the requirements of the monograph.

Storage The information and recommendations given under the heading Storage do not constitute a pharmacopoeial requirement but the competent authority may specify particular storage conditions that must be met.

The articles described in the Pharmacopoeia are stored in such a way as to prevent contamination and, as far as possible, deterioration. Where special conditions of storage are recommended, including the type of container (see General Notice on Containers above) and limits of temperature, they are stated in the monograph.

The following expressions are used in monographs under Storage with the meaning shown.

Protected from moisture means that the product is stored in an airtight container. Care is to be taken when the container is opened in a damp atmosphere. A low moisture content may be maintained, if necessary, by the use of a desiccant in the container provided that direct contact with the product is avoided.

Protected from light means that the product is stored either in a container made of a material that absorbs actinic light sufficiently to protect the contents from change induced by such light or in a container enclosed in an outer cover that provides such protection or stored in a place from which all such light is excluded.

Labelling In general, labelling is subject to supranational and national regulation and to international agreements. The statements under the heading Labelling therefore are not comprehensive and, moreover, for the purposes of the Pharmacopoeia only those statements that are necessary to demonstrate compliance or non-compliance with the monograph are mandatory. Any other labelling statements are included as recommendations. When the term 'label' is used in the Pharmacopoeia, the labelling statements may appear on the container, the package or a leaflet accompanying the package, as decided by the competent authority.

Warnings Materials described in monographs and reagents specified for use in the Pharmacopoeia may be injurious to health unless adequate precautions are taken. The principles of good quality control laboratory practice and the provisions of any appropriate regulations are to be observed at all times. Attention is drawn to particular hazards in certain monographs by means of a warning statement; absence of such a statement is not to be taken to mean that no hazard exists.

Impurities A list of all known and potential impurities that have been shown to be controlled by the tests in a monograph may be given for information. The list may be divided into two sublists entitled 'Qualified impurities'and 'Other detectable impurities'. Qualified impurities are those previously accepted by the competent authority as being qualified; impurities deemed qualified by other means (for example, impurities which occur as natural metabolites) may also be included. Other detectable impurities are those potential impurities that have not been detected in any samples of the substance during elaboration of the monograph or that occur in amounts below 0.1 per cent, but that have been shown to be limited by the tests.

Critical physical properties A list of critical physical properties that are not the subject of official requirements but which are nevertheless important for the use of a substance may be appended to a monograph, for information and guidance (see also above 1.1. General statement).

Reference substances, reference preparations and reference spectra Certain monographs require the use of a reference substance, a reference preparation or a reference spectrum. These are chosen with regard to their intended use as prescribed in the monographs of the Pharmacopoeia and are not necessarily suitable in other circumstances. The European Pharmacopoeia Commission does not accept responsibility for any errors arising from use other than as prescribed.

The reference substances, the reference preparations and the reference spectra are established by the European Pharmacopoeia Commission and may be obtained from the Technical Secretariat. They are the official reference materials to be used in cases of arbitration. A list of reference substances, reference preparations and reference spectra may be obtained from the Technical Secretariat.

Local reference materials may be used for routine analysis, provided they are calibrated against the materials established by the European Pharmacopoeia Commission.

Any information necessary for proper use of the reference substance or reference preparation is given on the label or in the accompanying leaflet or brochure. Where no drying conditions are stated in the leaflet or on the label, the substance is to be used as received. No certificate of analysis or other data not relevant to the prescribed use of the product are provided. No expiry date is indicated: the products are guaranteed to be suitable for use when despatched and can normally be used for not less than 6 months after receipt if the containers are stored unopened as described in the accompanying leaflet; beyond this period, it is necessary to seek advice from the Technical Secretariat. The stability of the contents of opened containers cannot be guaranteed.

Chemical Reference Substances The abbreviation CRS indicates a Chemical Reference Substance established by the European Pharmacopoeia Commission. Some Chemical Reference Substances are used for the microbiological assay of antibiotics and their activity is stated, in International Units, on the label or on the accompanying leaflet and defined in the same manner as for Biological Reference Preparations.

Biological Reference Preparations The majority of the primary biological reference preparations referred to in the European Pharmacopoeia are the appropriate International Standards and Reference Preparations established by the World Health Organisation. Because these reference materials are usually available only in limited quantities, the Commission has established Biological Reference Preparations (indicated by the abbreviation BRP) where appropriate. Where applicable, the potency of the Biological Reference Preparations is expressed in International Units. For some Biological Reference Preparations, where an international standard or reference preparation does not exist, the potency is expressed in European Pharmacopoeia Units.

Reference spectra The reference spectrum is accompanied by information concerning the conditions used for sample preparation and recording the spectrum.

1.5 ABBREVIATIONS AND SYMBOLS

A	Absorbance
$A^{1\ \mathrm{per\ cent}}$	Specific absorbance
A_l	Relative atomic mass
$[\alpha]_D^{20}$	Specific optical rotation
bp	Boiling point
BRP	Biological Reference Preparation
CRS	Chemical Reference Substance
d_{20}^{20}	Relative density
I.U.	International Unit
l	Wavelength
M	Molarity
M_r	Relative molecular mass
mp	Melting point
n_D^{20}	Refractive index
Ph. Eur. U.	European Pharmacopoeia Unit
ppm	Parts per million
R	Substance or solution defined under "Reagents"
R_f	Used in chromatography to indicate the ratio of the distance travelled by a substance to the distance travelled by the solvent front
R_{st}	Used in chromatography to indicate the ratio of the distance travelled by a substance to the distance travelled by a reference substance
RV	Substance used as a primary standard in volumetric analysis

ABBREVIATIONS USED IN THE MONOGRAPHS ON IMMUNOGLOBINS, IMMUNOSERA AND VACCINES

LD_{50}	The statistically determined quantity of a substance that, when administered by the specific route, may be expected to cause the death of 50 per cent of the test animals within a given period.
MLD	Minimum lethal dose
L+/10 dose	The smallest quantity of a toxin that, in the condition of the test, when mixed with 0.1 I.U. of antitoxin and administered by the specific route, causes the death of the test animals within a given period.
L+ dose	The smallest quantity of a toxin that, in the condition of the test, when mixed with 1 I.U. of antitoxin and administered by the specific route, causes the death of the test animals within a given period.
Lr/100 dose	The smallest quantity of a toxin that, in the condition of the test, when mixed with 0.01 I.U. of antitoxin and injected intracutaneously causes a characteristic reaction at the site of injection within a given period.
Lp/10 dose	The smallest quantity of a toxin that, in the condition of the test, when mixed with 0.1 I.U. of antitoxin and administered by the specific route, causes paralysis in the test animals within a given period.
Lo/10 dose	The largest quantity of a toxin that, in the condition of the test, when mixed with 0.1 I.U. of antitoxin and administered by the specific route, does not cause symptoms of toxicity in the test animals within a given period.

Lf dose	The quantity of toxin or toxoid that flocculates in the shortest time with 1 I.U. of antitoxin.
$CCID_{50}$	The statistically determined quantity of virus that may be expected to infect 50 per cent of the cell cultures to which it is added.
EID_{50}	The statistically determined quantity of virus that may be expected to infect 50 per cent of fertilised eggs into which it is inoculated.
ID_{50}	The statistically determined quantity of virus that may be expected to infect 50 per cent of the animals into which it is inoculated.
PD_{50}	The statistically determined dose of a vaccine that, in the conditions of the tests, may be expected to protect 50 per cent of the animals against a challenge dose of the micro-organisms or toxins against which it is active.
ED_{50}	The statistically determined dose of a vaccine that, in the conditions of the tests, may be expected to induce specific antibodies in 50 per cent of the animals for the relevant vaccine antigens.
PFU	Pock-forming units or plaque-forming units.
SPF	Specified-pathogen-free.

COLLECTIONS OF MICRO-ORGANISMS

ATTC	American Type Culture Collection 12301 Parklawn Drive Rockville, MD 20852, USA
C.I.P.	Collection de l'Institut Pasteur (strains of bacteria)
I.P.	Institut Pasteur (strains of other micro-organisms) Service de la Collection Nationale de Culture de Micro-organismes (C.N.C.M.) 25, rue du Docteur-Roux F-75015 Paris, France
NCIMB	National Collection of Industrial and Marine Bacteria Ltd 23 St Machar Drive Aberdeen AB2 1RY, Great Britain
NCPF	National Collection of Pathogenic Fungi London School of Hygiene & Tropical Medicine Keppel Street London WC1E 7HT, Great Britain
NCTC	National Collection of Type Cultures Central Public Health Laboratory Colindale Avenue London NW9 5HT, Great Britain
NCYC	National Collection of Yeast Cultures AFRC Food Reserach Institute Colney Lane Norwich NR4 7UA, Great Britain
S.S.I.	Statens Serum Institut 80 Amager Boulevard, Copenhagen, Denmark

[See also Appendix XXIV]

1.6. UNITS OF THE INTERNATIONAL SYSTEM (SI) USED IN THE PHARMACOPOEIA AND EQUIVALENCE WITH OTHER UNITS

International System of Units (SI)

The International System of Units comprises three classes of units, namely base units, derived units and supplementary units.[1] The base units and their definitions are set out in Table 1.6-1.

The derived units may be formed by combining the base units according to the algebraic relationships linking the corresponding quantities. Some of these derived units have special names and symbols. The SI units used in the European Pharmacopoeia are shown in Table 1.6-2.

Some important and widely used units outside the International System are shown in Table 1.6-3.

The prefixes shown in Table 1.6-4 are used to form the names and symbols of the decimal multiples and submultiples of SI units.

[1]The definitions of the units used in the International System are given in the booklet *Le Système International d'Unités (SI)* published by the Bureau International des Poids et Mesures, Pavillon de Breteuil, F-92310 *Sevres*, France

TABLE 1.6.-1. — *SI Base Units*

Quantity		Unit		Definition
Name	Symbol	Name	Symbol	
Length	*l*	metre	m	The metre is the length of the path travelled by light in a vacuum during a time interval of 1/299,792,458 of a second.
Mass	*m*	kilogram	kg	The kilogram is equal to the mass of the international prototype of the kilogram.
Time	*t*	second	s	The second is the duration of 9,192,631,770 periods of the radiation corresponding to the transition between the two hyperfine levels of the ground state of the caesium-133 atom.
Electric current	*I*	ampere	A	The ampere is that constant current which, maintained in two straight parallel conductors of infinite length, of negligible circular cross-section and placed 1 metre apart in vacuum would produce between these conductors a force equal to 2×10^{-7} newton per metre of length.
Thermodynamic temperature	*T*	kelvin	K	The kelvin is the fraction 1/273.16 of the thermodynamic temperature of the triple point of water.
Amount of substance	*n*	mole	mol	The mole is the amount of substance of a system containing as many elementary entities as there are atoms in 0.012 kilogram of carbon-12*
Luminous intensity	I_v	candela	cd	The candela is the luminous intensity in a given direction of a source emitting monochromatic radiation with a frequency of 540×10^{12} hertz and whose energy intensity in that direction is 1/683 watt per steradian.

*When the mole is used, the elementary entities must be specified and may be atoms, molecules, ions, electrons, other particles or specified groups of such particles.

TABLE 1.6.-2. — *SI Units used in the European Pharmacopeia and Equivalence with Other Units*

Quantity		Unit				Conversion of other units into SI units
Name	Symbol	Name	Symbol	Expression in SI base units	Expression in other SI units	
Wave number	ν	one per metre	1/m	m^{-1}		
Wavelength	λ	micrometre	µm	10^{-6} m		
		nanometre	nm	10^{-9}m		
Area	*A, S*	square metre	m^2	m^2		
Volume	*V*	cubic metre	m^3	m^3		1 ml = 1 cm^2 = 10^{-6} m^3
Frequency	ν	hertz	Hz	s^{-1}		
Density	*ρ*	kilogram per cubic metre	kg/m^3	kg·m^{-3}		1g/ml = 1g/ m^3 = 10^3 kg·m^{-3}
Velocity	ν	metre per second	m/s	m· s^{-1}		
Force	*F*	newton	N	m·kg· s^{-2}		1 dyne = 1g·cm· s^{-2} = 10^{-5} N 1kp = 9.806 65 N
Pressure	ρ	pascal	Pa	m^{-1}·kg· s^{-2}	N·m^{-2}	1 dyne/cm^2 = 10^{-1} Pa = 10^{-1} N·m^{-2} 1 atm = 101 325 Pa = 101.325 kPa 1 bar = 105 Pa = 0.1 MPa 1 mm Hg = 133.322 387 Pa 1 Torr = 133.322 368 Pa 1 psi = 6.894 757 kPa
Dynamic viscosity	η	pascal second	Pa·s	m^{-1}·kg· s^{-1}	N·s·m^{-2}	1 P = 10^{-1} Pa·s = 10^{-1} N·s·m^{-2} 1 cP = 1 mPa·s
Kinematic viscocity	ν	square metre per second	$m^{\cdot 1}$ /s	m^2· s^{-1}	Pa·s·m^3·kg $^{-1}$ N·s·m·kg $^{-1}$	1 St = 1 cm^2·s $^{-1}$ = 10^{-4} m^2· s^{-1}
Energy	*W*	joule	J	m^2·kg· s^{-2}	N·m	1 erg = 1 cm^2·g·s^{-2} = 1 dyne·cm = 10^{-1} J 1 cal = 4.1868 J
Power Radiant flux	*P*	watt	W	m^2·kg· s^{-3}	N·m·s^{-1} J·s^{-1}	1 erg/s = 1 dyne·cm·s^{-1} = 10^{-7} W = 10^{-7} N·m·s^{-1} = 10^{-7} J·s^{-1}
Absorbed dose (of radiant energy)	*D*	gray	Gy	m^2·s^{-2}	J·kg^{-1}	1 rad = 10^{-2} Gy
Wave number	ν	one per metre	1/m	m^{-1}		
Electrical potential electromotive force	*U*	volt	V	m^2·kg·s^{-3}·A^{-1}	W·A^{-1}	
Electrical resistance	*R*	ohm	Ω	m^2·kg·s^{-3}·A^{-2}	V·A^{-1}	
Quantity of electricity	*Q*	coulomb	C	A·s		
Activity of a radionuclide	*A*	becquerel	Bq	s^{-1}		1Ci = 37 × 10^9 Bq = 37 × 10^9 s^{-1}
Concentration (of amount of substance)						
Molar concentration	*c*	mole per cubic metre	mol/m^3	mol·m^{-3}		1 mol/1 = 1M = 1 mol/dm^3 = 10^3 mol·m^{-3}
Mass concentration	*ρ*	kilogram per cubic metre	kg/m^3	kg·m^{-3}		1 g/l = 1 g/dm^3 = 1kg·m^{-3}

TABLE 1.6.-3. — *Units used with the International System*

Quantity	Unit Time	Symbol	Value in SI units
Time	minute	min	1 min = 60 s
	hour	h	1 h = 60 mins = 3600 s
	day	d	1 d = 24 h = 86 4000 s
Plane angle	degree	°	1° = (π/180) rad
Volume	litre	l	1 l = 1 dm^3 = 10^{-3} m^3
Mass	tonne	t	1 t = 10^3 kg
Rotational frequency	revolution per minute	r/min	1 r/min = (1/60) s^{-3}

TABLE 1.6.-4. — *Decimal Multiples and Sub-multiples of Units*

Factor	Prefix	Symbol	Factor	Prefix	Symbol
10^{18}	exa	E	10^{-1}	deci	d
10^{15}	peta	P	10^{-2}	centi	c
10^{12}	tera	T	10^{-3}	milli	m
10^{9}	giga	G	10^{-6}	micro	µ
10^{6}	mega	M	10^{-9}	nano	n
10^{3}	kilo	k	10^{-12}	pico	p
10^{2}	hecto	h	10^{-15}	femto	f
10^{1}	deca	da	10^{-18}	atto	a

NOTES

1. In the Pharmacopoeia the Celsius temperature is used (symbol *t*). This is defined by the equation

$$t = T - T_o$$

where T_o = 273.15 K by definition. The Celsius or centigrade temperature is expressed in degree Celsius (symbol °C). The unit "degree Celsius" is equal to the unit "kelvin".

2. The practical expressions of concentrations used in the Pharmacopoeia are defined in the General Notices.
3. The radian is the plane angle between two radii of a circle which cut off on the circumference an arc equal in length to the radius.
4. In the Pharmacopoeia conditions of centrifugation are defined by reference to the acceleration due to gravity (*g*): $g = 9.806\ 65\ mvs^{-2}$
5. Certain quantities without dimensions are used in the Pharmacopoeia: relative density *(2.2.5)*, absorbance *(2.2.25)*, specific absorbance *(2.2.25)* and refractive index *(2.2.6)* as well as quantities expressed in other units such as the specific optical rotation *(2.2.7)*.
6. The microkatal is defined as the enzymic activity which, under defined conditions, produces the transformation (e.g. hydrolysis) of 1 micromole of the substrate per second.

Monographs

Formulated Preparations: General Monographs

CAPSULES

Capsules comply with the requirements of the 3rd edition of the European Pharmacopoeia [0016]. These requirements are reproduced after the heading 'Definition' below.

Ph Eur

The requirements of this monograph do not necessarily apply to preparations that are presented as capsules intended for use other than by oral administration. Requirements for such preparations may be found, where appropriate, in other general monographs, for example Rectal preparations (1145) and Vaginal preparations (1164).

DEFINITION

Capsules are solid preparations with hard or soft shells of various shapes and capacities, usually containing a single dose of active ingredient. They are intended for oral administration.

The capsule shells are made of gelatin or other substance, the consistency of which may be adjusted by the addition of substances such as glycerol or sorbitol. Excipients such as surface-active agents, opaque fillers, antimicrobial preservatives, sweeteners, colouring matter authorised by the competent authority and flavouring substances may be added. The capsules may bear surface markings.

The contents of capsules may be solid, liquid or of a paste-like consistency. They consist of one or more active ingredients with or without excipients such as solvents, diluents, lubricants and disintegrating agents. The contents do not cause deterioration of the shell. The shell, however, is attacked by the digestive fluids and the contents are released.

Where applicable, containers for capsules comply with the requirements *of Materials Used for the Manufacture of Containers* (*3.1* and subsections) and *Containers* (*3.2* and subsections).

Several categories of capsules may be distinguished:

- hard capsules,
- soft capsules,
- gastro-resistant capsules,
- modified-release capsules.

PRODUCTION

In the manufacture, packaging, storage and distribution of capsules, suitable means are taken to ensure their microbial quality; recommendations on this aspect are provided in the text on *Microbial Quality of Pharmaceutical Preparations (5.1.4)*.

TESTS

Uniformity of content (*2.9.6*). Unless otherwise prescribed or justified and authorised, capsules with a content of active ingredient less than 2 mg or less than 2 per cent of the total mass comply with test B for uniformity of content of single-dose preparations. If the preparation has more than one active ingredient, the requirement applies only to those ingredients which correspond to the above conditions. The test is not required for multivitamin and trace-element preparations.

Uniformity of mass (*2.9.5*). Capsules comply with the test for uniformity of mass of single-dose preparations. If the test for uniformity of content is prescribed for all the active ingredients, the test for uniformity of mass is not required.

Dissolution A suitable test may be carried out to demonstrate the appropriate release of the active ingredient(s), for example one of the tests described in *Dissolution Test for Solid Dosage Forms* (*2.9.3*).

Where a dissolution test is prescribed, a disintegration test may not be required.

STORAGE

Store in a well-closed container, at a temperature not exceeding 30°C.

LABELLING

The label states the name of any added antimicrobial preservative.

Hard Capsules

DEFINITION

Hard capsules have shells consisting of two prefabricated cylindrical sections one end of which is rounded and closed, the other being open.

PRODUCTION

The active ingredient(s) usually in solid form (powder or granules) are filled into one of the sections which is then closed by slipping the other section over it. The security of the closure may be strengthened by suitable means.

TESTS

Disintegration Hard capsules comply with the test for disintegration of tablets and capsules (*2.9.1*). Use *water R* as the liquid. When justified and authorised, *0.1M hydrochloric acid* or *artificial gastric juice R* may be used as the liquid medium. If the capsules float on the surface of the water, a disc may be added. Operate the apparatus for 30 min, unless otherwise justified and authorised and examine the state of the capsules. The capsules comply with the test if all six have disintegrated.

Soft Capsules

DEFINITION

Soft capsules have thicker shells than those of hard capsules. The shells consist of one part and are of various shapes.

PRODUCTION

Soft capsules are usually formed, filled and sealed in one operation but for extemporaneous use, the shell may be prefabricated. The shell material may contain an active ingredient.

Liquids may be enclosed directly; solids are usually dissolved or dispersed in a suitable vehicle to give a solution or dispersion of a somewhat paste-like consistency.

There may be partial migration of the constituents from the capsule contents into the shell and vice versa because of the nature of the materials and the surfaces in contact.

TESTS

Disintegration Soft capsules comply with the test for disintegration of tablets and capsules (*2.9.1*). Use *water R* as the liquid. When justified and authorised, *0.1M hydrochloric acid* or *artificial gastric juice R* may be used as the liquid medium. Add a disc to each tube. Liquid medicinal substances dispensed in soft capsules may attack the disc;

in such circumstances and where authorised, the disc may be omitted. Operate the apparatus for 30 min, unless otherwise justified and authorised and examine the state of the capsules. If the capsules fail to comply because of adherence to the discs, repeat the test on a further six capsules omitting the discs. The capsules comply with the test if all six have disintegrated.

Gastro-Resistant Capsules

DEFINITION

Gastro-resistant capsules are modified release capsules that are intended to resist the gastric fluid and to release their active ingredient or ingredients in the intestinal fluid. They are prepared by providing hard or soft capsules with a gastro-resistant shell (enteric capsules) or by filling capsules with granules or with particles covered with a gastro-resistant coating.

PRODUCTION

For capsules filled with granules or filled with particles covered with a gastro-resistant coating, a suitable test is carried out to demonstrate the appropriate release of the active ingredient(s).

TESTS

Disintegration For capsules with a gastro-resistant shell carry out the test for disintegration (*2.9.1*) with the following modifications. Use *0.1M hydrochloric acid* as the liquid and operate the apparatus for 2 h, or other such time as may be authorised, without the discs. Examine the state of the capsules. The time of resistance to the acid medium varies according to the formulation of the capsules to be examined. It is typically 2 h to 3 h but even with authorised deviations it must not be less than 1 h. No capsule shows signs of disintegration or rupture permitting the escape of the contents. Replace the acid by *phosphate buffer solution pH 6.8 R*. When justified and authorised, a buffer solution of pH 6.8 with added pancreas powder (for example, 0.35 g of *pancreas powder R* per 100 ml of buffer solution) may be used. Add a disc to each tube. Operate the apparatus for 60 min and examine the state of the capsules. If the capsules fail to comply because of adherence to the discs, repeat the test on a further six capsules omitting the discs. The capsules comply with the test if all six have disintegrated.

Modified-Release Capsules

DEFINITION

Modified-release capsules are hard or soft capsules in which the contents or the shell or both contain special excipients or are prepared by a special process designed to modify the rate or the place at which the active ingredient(s) are released.

PRODUCTION

A suitable test is carried out to demonstrate the appropriate release of the active ingredient(s).

Ph Eur

Capsules of the British Pharmacopoeia

In addition to the above requirements of the European Pharmacopoeia, the following statements apply to those capsules that are the subject of an individual monograph in the British Pharmacopoeia.

When presented as granules the contents of the requisite number of capsules should be mixed and powdered before performing the Assay and tests described in the monograph.

Content of active ingredient in capsules The range for the content of active ingredient stated in the monograph is based on the requirement that 20 capsules, or such other number as may be indicated in the monograph, are used in the Assay. In the circumstances where 20 capsules cannot be obtained, a smaller number, which must not be less than 5, may be used, but to allow for sampling errors the tolerances are widened in accordance with Table I.

The requirements of Table I apply when the stated limits are 90 to 110%. For limits other than 90 to 110%, proportionately smaller or larger allowances should be made.

Disintegration For those Hard Capsules or Soft Capsules for which a requirement for Dissolution is included in the individual monograph, the requirement for Disintegration does not apply.

Uniformity of content Details of the analytical method to be employed for determining the content of active ingredient may be included in certain monographs. Unless otherwise stated in the monograph the limits are as given in the test for *uniformity of content*, Appendix XII H.

Any capsules that when examined individually show a gross deviation from the prescribed or stated content are not official.

Labelling The label states (1) the quantity of the active ingredient contained in each Capsule; (2) the date after which the Capsules are not intended to be used; (3) the conditions under which the Capsules should be stored.

The following capsules are the subject of an individual monograph in the British Pharmacopoeia.

Amantadine Capsules
Amoxicillin Capsules
Ampicillin Capsules
Azapropazone Capsules
Bromocriptine Capsules
Calcitriol Capsules

Table I

Weight of active ingredient in each capsule	Subtract from the lower limit for samples of			Add to the upper limit for samples of		
	15	10	5	15	10	5
0.12 g or less	0.2	0.7	1.6	0.3	0.8	1.8
More than 0.12 and less than 0.3 g	0.2	0.5	1.2	0.3	0.6	1.5
0.3 g or more	0.1	0.2	0.8	0.2	0.4	1.0

Cefalexin Capsules
Cefradine Capsules
Chloramphenicol Capsules
Chlordiazepoxide Capsules
Clindamycin Capsules
Clobazam Capsules
Clofazimine Capsules
Clofibrate Capsules
Clomethiazole Capsules
Clomipramine Capsules
Cloxacillin Capsules
Co-danthrusate Capsules
Co-fluampicil Capsules
Demeclocycline Capsules
Dextropropoxyphene Capsules
Diazepam Capsules
Disopyramide Capsules
Disopyramide Phosphate Capsules
Dosulepin Capsules/Dothiepin Capsules
Doxepin Capsules
Doxycycline Capsules
Erythromycin Estolate Capsules
Estramustine Phosphate Capsules
Ethosuximide Capsules
Etodolac Capsules
Fenbufen Capsules
Flucloxacillin Capsules
Flurazepam Capsules
Gemfibrozil Capsules
Halibut-liver Oil Capsules
Haloperidol Capsules
Hydroxycarbamide Capsules
Indometacin Capsules
Ketoprofen Capsules
Levodopa Capsules
Lincomycin Capsules
Lomustine Capsules
Lymecycline Capsules
Mefenamic Acid Capsules
Metyrapone Capsules
Mexiletine Capsules
Naftidrofuryl Capsules
Nifedipine Capsules
Nitrazepam Capsules
Nortriptyline Capsules
Oxytetracycline Capsules
Pentazocine Capsules
Phenoxybenzamine Capsules
Phenytoin Capsules
Piroxicam Capsules
Rifampicin Capsules
Tetracycline Capsules
Triamterene Capsules

MEDICATED CHEWING GUMS

Medicated Chewing Gums comply with the requirements of the 3rd edition of the European Pharmacopoeia [1239]. These requirements are reproduced after the heading 'Definition' below.

Ph Eur

DEFINITION

Medicated chewing gums are solid, single-dose preparations with a base consisting mainly of gum that are intended to be chewed but not swallowed.

They contain one or more active ingredients which are released by chewing. After dissolution or dispersion of the active ingredient(s) in saliva, chewing gums are intended to be used for:

— local treatment of mouth diseases,
— systemic delivery after absorption through the buccal mucosa or from the gastrointestinal tract.

PRODUCTION

Medicated chewing gums are made with a tasteless masticatory gum base that consists of natural or synthetic elastomers. They may contain other excipients such as fillers, softeners, sweetening agents, flavouring substances, stabilisers and plasticisers and authorised colouring matter.

Medicated chewing gums are manufactured by compression or by softening or melting the gum bases and adding successively the other substances. In the latter case, chewing gums are then further processed to obtain the desired gum presentation. The medicated chewing gums may be coated, for example, if necessary to protect from humidity and light.

Unless otherwise justified and authorised, a suitable test is carried out to demonstrate the appropriate release of the active ingredient(s).

In the manufacture, packaging, storage and distribution of medicated chewing gums, suitable means must be taken to ensure their microbial quality; recommendations related to this aspect are provided in the general chapter on *Microbiological quality of pharmaceutical preparations* (*5.1.4*).

TESTS

Uniformity of content (*2.9.6*). Unless otherwise prescribed or justified and authorised, medicated chewing gums with a content of active ingredient less than 2 mg or less than 2 per cent of the total mass comply with test A for uniformity of content of single-dose preparations. If the preparation contains more than one active ingredient, the requirement applies only to those ingredients which correspond to the above conditions.

Uniformity of mass (*2.9.5*). Uncoated medicated chewing gums and, unless otherwise justified and authorised, coated medicated chewing gums comply with the test for uniformity of mass of single-dose preparations. If the test for uniformity of content is prescribed for all the active ingredients, the test for uniformity of mass is not required.

STORAGE

Store uncoated medicated chewing gums protected from humidity and light.

Ph Eur

LIQUIDS FOR CUTANEOUS APPLICATION

Liquids for Cutaneous Application comply with the requirements of the 3rd edition of the European Pharmacopoeia [0927]. These requirements are reproduced after the heading 'Definition' below.

Ph Eur

DEFINITION

Liquids for cutaneous application are liquid preparations of varying viscosity intended to be applied to the skin (including the scalp) or nails in order to obtain a local effect. They are solutions, emulsions or suspensions which may contain one or more active ingredients in a suitable vehicle. They may contain suitable antimicrobial preservatives, antioxidants and other excipients such as stabilisers, emulsifiers and thickeners.

Emulsions may show evidence of phase separation but are easily reformed on shaking. Suspensions may show a sediment which is readily dispersed on shaking to give a suspension which is sufficiently stable to enable a homogeneous preparation to be delivered.

Where applicable, containers for liquids for cutaneous application comply with the requirements for *Materials Used for the Manufacture of Containers* (*3.1* and subsections) and *Containers* (*3.2* and subsections).

When liquids for cutaneous application are dispensed in pressurised containers, the containers comply with the requirements of the monograph on *Pressurised Pharmaceutical Preparations* (*523*).

Preparations specifically intended for use on severely injured skin are sterile.

Several categories of liquids for cutaneous application may be distinguished:
— shampoos,
— cutaneous foams.

Certain designations such as 'lotions' or 'liniments' are sometimes used.

PRODUCTION

During the development of a liquid for cutaneous application, the formulation for which contains an antimicrobial preservative, the effectiveness of the chosen preservative shall be demonstrated to the satisfaction of the competent authority. A suitable method of test together with criteria for judging the preservative properties of the formulation are provided in the text on *Efficacy of Antimicrobial Preservation* (*5.1.3*).

In the manufacture, packaging, storage and distribution of liquids for cutaneous application, suitable means are taken to ensure their microbial quality; recommendations on this aspect are provided in the text on *Microbial Quality of Pharmaceutical Preparations* (*5.1.4*).

Sterile liquids for cutaneous application are prepared using materials and methods designed to ensure sterility and to avoid the introduction of contaminant and the growth of micro-organisms; recommendations on this aspect are provided in the text on *Methods of preparation of sterile products* (*5.1.1*).

In the manufacture of liquids for cutaneous application containing dispersed particles measures are taken to ensure a suitable and controlled particle size with regard to the intended use.

TESTS

Sterility (*2.6.1*). Where the label indicates that the preparation is sterile, it complies with the test for sterility.

STORAGE

Store in a well-closed container. If the preparation is sterile, store in a sterile, airtight, tamper-proof container.

LABELLING

The label states:
— the name of any added antimicrobial preservative,
— where applicable, that the preparation is sterile.

Shampoos

DEFINITION

Shampoos are liquid or, occasionally semi-liquid preparations intended for application to the scalp and subsequent washing away with water. Upon rubbing with water they usually form a foam.

They are emulsions, suspensions or solutions. Shampoos normally contain surface active agents.

Cutaneous Foams

DEFINITION

Cutaneous foams comply with the requirements of the monograph on *Medicated foams (1105)*.

Ph Eur

Liquids for Cutaneous Application of the British Pharmacopoeia

In addition to the above requirements of the European Pharmacopoeia, the following statements apply to any application, collodion, liniment, lotion or paint that is the subject of an individual monograph in the British Pharmacopoeia and to the solutions listed below.

APPLICATIONS

Labelling The label states (1) that the Application is intended for external use only; (2) the date after which the Application is not intended to be used; (3) the conditions under which the Application should be stored; (4) the directions for using the Application; (5) any special precautions associated with the use of the Application.

COLLODIONS

Definition Collodions are Liquids for Cutaneous Application, usually containing Pyroxylin in a mixture of Ether and Ethanol. When they are allowed to dry, a flexible film is formed at the site of application.

Storage Collodions should be stored at temperatures not exceeding 25° and remote from fire.

Labelling The label states (1) that the Collodion is intended for external use only; (2) the date after which the Collodion is not intended to be used; (3) the conditions under which the Collodion should be stored; (4) the directions for using the Collodion; (5) any special precautions associated with the use of the Collodion.

LINIMENTS

Definition Liniments are Liquids for Cutaneous Application that are intended to be applied to the unbroken skin with friction.

Storage Certain plastic containers, such as those made from polystyrene, are unsuitable for Liniments.

Labelling The label states (1) the names and concentrations of the active ingredients; (2) that the Liniment is intended for external use only; (3) if appropriate, that the contents of the container should be shaken before use; (4) the date after which the Liniment is not intended to be used; (5) the conditions under which the Liniment should be stored; (6) the directions for using the Liniment; (7) any special precautions associated with the use of the Liniment.

LOTIONS

Definition Lotions are Liquids for Cutaneous Application that are intended to be applied to the unbroken skin without friction.

Labelling The label states (1) the names and concentrations of the active ingredients; (2) that the Lotion is intended for external use only; (3) that the Lotion should be shaken before use; (4) the date after which the Lotion is not intended to be used; (5) the conditions under which the Lotion should be stored; (6) the directions for using the Lotion; (7) any special precautions associated with the use of the Lotion.

PAINTS

Definition Paints are solutions or dispersions of one or more active ingredients. They are intended for application to the skin or, in some cases, mucous membranes.

Storage Paints should be kept in airtight containers.

Labelling The label states (1) the names and concentrations of the active ingredients; (2) the date after which the Paint is not intended to be used; (3) the conditions under which the Paint should be stored; (4) the directions for using the Paint; (5) any special precautions associated with the use of the Paint.

The following liquids for cutaneous application are the subject of an individual monograph in the British Pharmacopoeia.

Applications
Benzyl Benzoate Application
Betamethasone Valerate Scalp Application
Selenium Sulphide Scalp Application

Collodions
Flexible Collodion
Salicylic Acid Collodion

Liniments
Methyl Salicylate Liniment
White Liniment

Lotions
Benzoyl Peroxide Lotion
Betamethasone Valerate Lotion
Calamine Lotion
Carbaryl Lotion
Crotamiton Lotion
Zinc Sulphate Lotion

Paints
Podophyllin Paint, Compound

Solutions
Note: Certain formulated preparations other than the ones listed below are the subject of an individual monograph in the British Pharmacopoeia with the title Solution. As confirmed by the absence of a cross reference to the general monograph for Liquids for Cutaneous Application, such solutions are outside the scope of this general monograph.

Adrenaline Solution/Epinephrine Solution
Cetrimide Solution
Chlorinated Lime and Boric Acid Solution
Chloroxylenol Solution
Iodine Solution, Alcoholic
Lidocaine Solution, Sterile
Povidone—Iodine Solution
Sodium Chloride Solution
Sodium Hypochlorite Solution, Dilute
Tretinoin Solution

EAR PREPARATIONS

Ear Preparations comply with the requirements of the 3rd edition of the European Pharmacopoeia [0652]. These requirements are reproduced after the heading 'Definition' below.

Ph Eur

DEFINITION

Ear preparations are liquid, semi-solid or solid preparations intended for instillation, for spraying, for insufflation, for application to the auditory meatus or as an ear wash.

Ear preparations usually contain one or more active ingredients in a suitable vehicle. They may contain excipients, for example, to adjust tonicity or viscosity, to adjust or stabilise the pH, to increase the solubility of the active ingredients, to stabilise the preparation or to provide adequate antimicrobial properties. The excipients do not adversely affect the intended medicinal action of the preparation or, at the concentrations used, cause toxicity or undue local irritation.

Preparations for application to the injured ear, particularly where the ear-drum is perforated, or prior to surgery are sterile, free from antimicrobial preservatives and supplied in single-dose containers.

Unless otherwise justified and authorised, aqueous ear preparations supplied in multidose containers contain a suitable antimicrobial preservative at a suitable concentration, except where the preparation itself has adequate antimicrobial properties.

Where applicable, containers for ear preparations comply with the requirements of *Materials Used for the Manufacture of Containers* (*3.1* and subsections) and *Containers* (*3.2* and subsections).

Several categories of ear preparations may be distinguished:
— ear-drops and sprays,
— semi-solid ear preparations,
— ear powders,
— ear washes,
— ear tampons.

PRODUCTION

During the development of an ear preparation, the formulation for which contains an antimicrobial preservative, the effectiveness of the chosen preservative shall be demonstrated to the satisfaction of the competent authority. A suitable test method together with criteria for judging the preservative properties of the formulation are provided in the text on *Efficacy of Antimicrobial Preservation* (*5.1.3*).

In the manufacture, packaging, storage and distribution of ear preparations, suitable means are taken to ensure their microbial quality; recommendations on this aspect are provided in the text on *Microbial Quality of Pharmaceutical Preparations* (*5.1.4*).

Sterile ear preparations are prepared using materials and methods designed to ensure sterility and to avoid the introduction of contaminants and the growth of micro-organisms; recommendations on this aspect are provided in the text on *Methods of Preparation of Sterile Products* (*5.1.1*).

In the manufacture of ear preparations containing dispersed particles measures are taken to ensure a suitable and controlled particle size with regard to the intended use.

TESTS

Sterility (*2.6.1*). Where the label indicates that the ear preparation is sterile, it complies with the test for sterility.

STORAGE

Store in a well-closed container. If the preparation is sterile, store in a sterile, airtight, tamper-proof container.

LABELLING

The label states:
— the name of any added antimicrobial preservative,
— where applicable, that the preparation is sterile.

Ear-Drops and Sprays

DEFINITION

Ear-drops and sprays are solutions, emulsions or suspensions of one or more active ingredients in liquids suitable for application to the auditory meatus without exerting harmful pressure on the ear-drum (for example, water, glycols or fatty oils). They may also be placed in the auditory meatus by means of a tampon impregnated with the liquid.

Emulsions may show evidence of phase separation but are easily reformed on shaking. Suspensions may show a sediment which is readily dispersed on shaking to give a suspension which remains sufficiently stable to enable the correct dose to be delivered.

Ear-drops and sprays are usually supplied in multi-dose containers fitted with an appropriate applicator. When sprays are supplied in pressurised containers, these comply with the requirements of the monograph on *Pressurised pharmaceutical preparations (523)*.

Semi-Solid Ear Preparations

DEFINITION

Semi-solid ear preparations are intended for application to the external auditory meatus, if necessary by means of a tampon impregnated with the preparation.

Semi-solid ear preparations comply with the requirements of the monograph on *Topical semi-solid preparations (132)*.

They are supplied in containers fitted with a suitable applicator.

Ear Powders

DEFINITION

Ear powders comply with the requirements of the monograph on *Topical powders (1166)*.

They are supplied in containers fitted with a suitable device for application or insufflation.

Ear Washes

DEFINITION

Ear-washes are preparations intended to cleanse the external auditory meatus. They are usually aqueous solutions with a pH within physiological limits.

Ear Tampons, Medicated

DEFINITION

Ear tampons are intended to be inserted into the external auditory meatus. They comply with the requirements of the monograph on *Medicated tampons (1155)*.

Ph Eur

Ear Preparations of the British Pharmacopoeia

In addition to the above requirements of the European Pharmacopoeia, the following statements apply to those ear drops that are the subject of an individual monograph in the British Pharmacopoeia.

EAR DROPS

Storage Ear Drops are supplied in containers of glass or suitable plastic that are fitted with an integral dropper or with a screw cap of suitable materials incorporating a dropper and rubber or plastic teat. Alternatively, such a cap assembly is supplied separately.

Labelling The label states (1) the names and concentrations of the active ingredients; (2) that the Ear Drops are intended for external use only; (3) the date after which the Ear Drops are not intended to be used; (4) the conditions under which the Ear Drops should be stored.

The following ear drops are the subject of an individual monograph in the British Pharmacopoeia.

Almond Oil Ear Drops
Aluminium Acetate Ear Drops
Chloramphenicol Ear Drops
Choline Salicylate Ear Drops
Hydrocortisone Acetate and Neomycin Ear Drops
Olive Oil Ear Drops
Sodium Bicarbonate Ear Drops

EXTRACTS

Extracts comply with the requirements of the 3rd edition of the European Pharmacopoeia [0765]. These requirements are reproduced after the heading 'Definition' below.

Ph Eur

DEFINITION

Extracts are concentrated preparations of liquid, solid or intermediate consistency, usually obtained from dried vegetable or animal matter. For some preparations, the matter to be extracted may undergo a preliminary treatment, for example, inactivation of enzymes, grinding or defatting.

Extracts are prepared by maceration, percolation or other suitable, validated methods using ethanol or another suitable solvent. After extraction, unwanted matter is removed, if necessary.

PRODUCTION

Production by percolation If necessary, reduce the matter to be extracted to pieces of suitable size. Mix thoroughly with a portion of the prescribed extraction solvent and allow to stand for an appropriate time. Transfer to a percolator and allow the percolate to flow slowly making sure that the matter to be extracted is always covered with the remaining extraction solvent. The residue may be pressed out and the expressed fluid combined with the percolate.

Production by maceration Unless otherwise prescribed, reduce the matter to be extracted to pieces of suitable size, mix thoroughly with the prescribed extraction solvent and allow to stand in a closed container for an appropriate time. The residue is separated from the extraction solvent, and if necessary, pressed out. In the latter case, the two liquids obtained are combined.

Concentration to the intended consistency is carried out using suitable methods, generally under reduced pressure and at a temperature at which deterioration of the constituents is at a minimum. The residual solvents in the extract do not exceed the prescribed limits.

Standardised extracts are adjusted to the defined content of constituents using suitable inert materials or using another extract of the vegetable or animal matter used for the preparation.

Liquid Extracts

DEFINITION

Liquid extracts are fluid preparations of which, in general, one part by mass or volume is equivalent to one part by mass of the original dried drug. These preparations are adjusted, if necessary, so that they satisfy the requirements for content of solvent, for constituents or for dry residue.

Liquid extracts may be prepared by the methods described above using only ethanol of suitable concentration or water or by dissolving a soft or dry extract in one of these solvents and, if necessary, filtering; whatever their method of preparation, the extracts obtained have a comparable composition. A slight sediment may form on standing and that is acceptable as long as the composition is not changed significantly.

Liquid extracts may contain suitable antimicrobial preservatives.

TESTS

Relative density *(2.2.5)*. Where applicable, the liquid extract complies with the limits prescribed in the monograph.

Ethanol content *(2.9.10)*. For alcoholic liquid extracts, carry out the determination of ethanol content. The ethanol content complies with that prescribed.

Methanol and 2-propanol *(2.9.11)*. For alcoholic liquid extracts, not more than 0.05 per cent *V/V* of methanol and not more than 0.05 per cent *V/V* of 2-propanol, unless otherwise prescribed.

Dry residue Where applicable, the liquid extract complies with the limits prescribed in the monograph. In a flat-bottomed dish about 50 mm in diameter and about 30 mm in height, introduce rapidly 2.00 g or 2.0 ml of the extract to be examined. Evaporate to dryness on a water-bath and dry in an oven at 100°C to 105°C for 3 h. Allow to cool in a desiccator over *diphosphorus pentoxide R* and weigh. Calculate the result as a mass percentage or in grams per litre.

STORAGE

Store in a well-closed container, protected from light.

LABELLING

The label states:
— the vegetable or animal matter used,
— where applicable, that fresh vegetable or animal matter was used,
— the name and the ethanol content in per cent *V/V* of the solvent used for the preparation,
— where applicable, the ethanol content in per cent *V/V* in the final extract,
— the content of active principle and/or the ratio of starting material to final liquid extract,
— the name and concentration of any added antimicrobial preservative.

Soft Extracts

DEFINITION

Soft extracts are preparations of an intermediate consistency, between liquid and dry extracts. They are obtained by partial evaporation of the solvent used for preparation. Only ethanol of suitable concentration or water is used. Soft extracts generally have a dry residue of not less than 70 per cent by mass. They may contain suitable antimicrobial preservatives.

TESTS

Dry residue Where applicable, the soft extract complies with the limits prescribed in the monograph. In a flat-bottomed dish about 50 mm in diameter and about 30 mm in height, weigh rapidly 2.00 g of the extract to be examined. Heat to dryness on a water-bath and dry in an oven at 100°C to 105°C for 3 h. Allow to cool in a desiccator over *diphosphorus pentoxide R* and weigh. Calculate the result as a mass percentage.

STORAGE

Store in a well-closed container, protected from light.

LABELLING

The label states:
— the vegetable or animal matter used,
— where applicable, that fresh vegetable or animal matter was used,
— the name and the ethanol content in per cent *V/V* of the

solvent used for the preparation,
— the content of active principle and/or the ratio of starting material to final soft extract,
— the name and concentration of any added antimicrobial preservative.

Dry Extracts

DEFINITION

Dry extracts are solid preparations obtained by evaporation of the solvent used for their production. Dry extracts generally have a dry residue of not less than 95 per cent by mass. Suitable inert materials may be added.

Standardised dry extracts are adjusted to the defined content of constituents, using suitable inert materials or a dry extract of the vegetable or animal matter used for the preparation.

Where applicable, the monograph on a dry extract prescribes a limit test for the solvent used for extraction.

TESTS

Loss on drying (*2.2.32*). Where applicable, the dry extract complies with the limits prescribed in the monograph. In a flat-bottomed dish about 50 mm in diameter and about 30 mm in height, weigh rapidly 0.50 g of the extract to be examined, finely powdered. Dry in an oven at 100°C to 105°C for 3 h. Allow to cool in a desiccator over *diphosphorus pentoxide R* and weigh. Calculate the result as a mass percentage.

STORAGE

Store in an airtight container, protected from light.

LABELLING

The label states:
— the name and amount of any inert material used,
— the vegetable or animal matter used,
— where applicable, that fresh vegetable or animal matter was used,
— the name and the ethanol content in per cent *V*/*V* of the solvent used for the preparation,
— the content of active principle and/or the ratio of starting material to final dry extract.

Ph Eur

Extracts of the British Pharmacopoeia

The following extracts are the subject of an individual monograph in the British Pharmacopoeia. Those distinguished by the symbol '☆' in the list below are monographs of the European Pharmacopoeia.

Aloes Dry Extract, Standardised ☆
Belladonna Dry Extract
Cascara Dry Extract
Frangula Bark Dry Extract, Standardised ☆
Hyoscyamus Dry Extract
Ipecacuanha Liquid Extract
Liquorice Liquid Extract
Quillaia Liquid Extract
Senna Leaf Dry Extract, Standardised ☆
Senna Liquid Extract
Squill Liquid Extract

EYE PREPARATIONS

Eye Preparations comply with the requirements of the 3rd edition of the European Pharmacopoeia [1163]. These requirements are reproduced after the heading 'Definition' below.

Ph Eur

DEFINITION

Eye preparations are sterile, liquid, semi-solid or solid preparations intended for administration upon the eyeball and/or to the conjunctiva or to be inserted in the conjunctival sac.

Where applicable, containers for eye preparations comply with the requirements of *Materials Used for the Manufacture of Containers* (*3.1* and subsections) and *Containers* (*3.2* and subsections).

Several categories of eye preparations may be distinguished:
— eye drops,
— eye lotions,
— semi-solid eye preparations,
— ophthalmic inserts.

PRODUCTION

During the development of an eye preparation, the formulation for which contains an antimicrobial preservative, the effectiveness of the chosen preservative shall be demonstrated to the satisfaction of the competent authority. A suitable method of test together with criteria for judging the preservative properties of the formulation are provided in the text on *Efficacy of Antimicrobial Preservation (5.1.3)*.

Eye preparations are prepared using materials and methods designed to ensure sterility and to avoid the introduction of contaminants and the growth of micro-organisms; recommendations on this aspect are provided in the text on *Methods of Preparation of Sterile Products* (*5.1.1*).

In the manufacture of eye preparations containing dispersed particles measures are taken to ensure a suitable and controlled particle size with regard to the intended use.

TESTS

Sterility (*2.6.1*). Eye preparations comply with the test for sterility. Applicators supplied separately also comply with the test for sterility. Remove the applicator with aseptic precautions from its package and transfer it to a tube of culture medium so that it is completely immersed. Incubate and interpret the results as described in the test for sterility.

STORAGE

Unless otherwise prescribed, store in a sterile, airtight, tamper-proof container.

LABELLING

The label states the name of any added antimicrobial preservative.

Eye-drops

DEFINITION

Eye-drops are sterile, aqueous or oily solutions or suspensions of one or more active ingredients intended for instillation into the eye. When the stability of the final preparation requires it, the medicinal substances may be supplied in a dry, sterile form to be dissolved or suspended in an appropriate sterile liquid immediately before use.

Eye-drops may contain excipients, for example, to adjust the tonicity or the viscosity of the preparation, to adjust or stabilise the pH, to increase the solubility of the active ingredient, or to stabilise the preparation. These substances do not adversely affect the intended medicinal action or, at the concentrations used, cause undue local irritation.

Aqueous preparations supplied in multidose containers contain a suitable antimicrobial preservative in appropriate concentration except when the preparation itself has adequate antimicrobial properties. The antimicrobial preservative chosen are compatible with the other ingredients of the preparation and remain effective throughout the period of time during which eye-drops are in use.

If eye-drops are prescribed without antimicrobial preservatives they are supplied wherever possible in single-dose containers. Eye-drops intended for use in surgical procedures do not contain antimicrobial preservatives and are supplied in single-dose containers.

Eye-drops that are solutions, examined under suitable conditions of visibility, are practically clear and practically free from particles.

Eye-drops that are suspensions may show a sediment that is readily dispersed on shaking to give a suspension which remains sufficiently stable to enable the correct dose to be delivered.

Multidose preparations are supplied in containers that allow successive drops of the preparation to be administered. The containers contain at most 10 ml of the preparation, unless otherwise justified and authorised.

TESTS

Particle size Eye-drops in the form of a suspension comply with the following test: introduce a suitable quantity of the suspension into a counting cell or with a micropipette onto a slide, as appropriate, and scan under a microscope an area corresponding to 10 µg of the solid phase. For practical reasons, it is recommended that the whole sample is first scanned at low magnification (e.g. ×50) and particles greater than 25 µm are identified. These larger particles can then be measured at a large magnification (e.g. ×200 to ×500). Not more than twenty particles have a maximum dimension greater than 25 µm, and not more than two of these particles have a maximum dimension greater than 50 µm. None of the particles has a maximum dimension greater than 90 µm.

LABELLING

The label states that for multidose containers, the period after opening the container after which the contents must not be used. This period does not exceed 4 weeks, unless otherwise justified and authorised.

Eye Lotions

DEFINITION

Eye lotions are sterile aqueous solutions intended for use in washing or bathing the eye or for impregnating eye dressings.

Eye lotions may contain excipients, for example to adjust the tonicity or the viscosity of the preparation or to adjust or stabilise the pH. These substances do not adversely affect the intended action or, at the concentrations used, cause undue local irritation.

Eye lotions supplied in multidose containers contain a suitable antimicrobial preservative in appropriate concentration except when the preparation itself has adequate antimicrobial properties. The antimicrobial preservative chosen is compatible with the other ingredients of the preparation and remains effective throughout the period of time during which the eye lotions are in use.

If eye lotions are prescribed without an antimicrobial preservative, they are supplied in single-dose containers. Eye lotions intended for use in surgical procedures or in first-aid treatment do not contain an antimicrobial preservative and are supplied in containers intended for use on one occasion only.

Eye lotions examined under suitable conditions of visibility, are practically clear and practically free from particles.

The containers for multidose preparations do not contain more than 200 ml of eye lotion, unless otherwise justified and authorised.

LABELLING

The label states:

— for single-dose preparations, that the contents are to be used on one occasion only,
— for multidose preparations, the period after opening the container after which the contents must not be used. This period does not exceed 4 weeks, unless otherwise justified and authorised.

Semi-Solid Eye Preparations

DEFINITION

Semi-solid eye preparations are sterile ointments, creams or gels intended for application to the conjunctiva. They contain one or more active ingredients dissolved or dispersed in a suitable basis. They have a homogeneous appearance.

Semi-solid eye preparations comply with the requirements of the monograph on *Topical semi-solid preparations (132)*. The basis is non-irritant to the conjunctiva.

Semi-solid eye preparations are packed in small, sterilised collapsible tubes fitted or provided with a cannula and having a content of not more than 5 g of the preparation. The tubes must be well-closed to prevent microbial contamination. Semi-solid eye preparations may also be packed in suitably designed single-dose containers.

TESTS

Particle size Semi-solid eye preparations containing dispersed solid particles comply with the following test: spread gently a quantity of the preparation corresponding to at least 10 µg of solid active ingredient as a thin layer. Scan under a microscope the whole area of the sample. For practical reasons, it is recommended that the whole sample is first scanned at a small magnification (e.g. ×50) and particles greater than 25 µm are identified. These larger particles can then be measured at a larger magnification (e.g. ×200 to ×500). For each 10 µg of solid active ingredient, not more than twenty particles have a maximum dimension greater than 25 µm, and not more than two of these particles have a maximum dimension greater than 50 µm. None of the particles has a maximum dimension greater than 90 µm.

Ophthalmic Inserts

DEFINITION

Ophthalmic inserts are sterile, solid or semi-solid preparations of suitable size and shape, designed to be inserted in the conjunctival sac, to produce an ocular effect. They generally consist of a reservoir of active ingredient embedded in a matrix or bounded by a rate-controlling membrane. The active ingredient, which is more or less soluble in physiological fluids, is released over a determined period of time.

Ophthalmic inserts are individually distributed into sterile containers.

PRODUCTION

In the manufacture of ophthalmic inserts means must be taken to ensure a suitable dissolution behaviour.

TESTS

Uniformity of content (*2.9.6*). Ophthalmic inserts comply, where applicable, with test A for uniformity of content.

LABELLING

The label states:
— where applicable, the total quantity of active ingredient per insert,
— where applicable, the dose released per unit time.

Ph Eur

Eye Preparations of the British Pharmacopoeia

In addition to the above requirements of the European Pharmacopoeia, the following statements apply to any eye drops, eye lotion or eye ointment that is the subject of an individual monograph in the British Pharmacopoeia.

EYE DROPS

Definition Definition of particular Eye Drops as a solution or suspension in Purified Water does not preclude the inclusion of suitable additional substances where necessary for the purposes referred to above under the requirements of the European Pharmacopoeia. However if buffering agents are used in preparations intended for use in surgical procedures great care should be taken to ensure that the nature and concentration of the chosen agent are suitable.

Where the active ingredient is susceptible to oxidative degradation appropriate precautions such as the addition of a suitable antioxidant should be taken. If an antioxidant is added care should be taken to ensure compatibility between the antioxidant and the antimicrobial preservative.

Production Methods of sterilisation that may be used in the manufacture of Eye Drops are described in Appendix XVIII.

Storage Eye Drops are supplied in tamper-evident containers. The compatibility of plastic or rubber components should be confirmed before use.

Containers for multidose Eye Drops are fitted with an integral dropper or with a sterile screw cap of suitable materials incorporating a dropper and rubber or plastic teat. Alternatively such a cap assembly is supplied, sterilised, separately.

Labelling The label states (1) the names and percentages of the active ingredients; (2) the date after which the Eye Drops are not intended to be used; (3) the conditions under which the Eye Drops should be stored.

For multidose containers the label states that care should be taken to avoid contamination of the contents during use.

Single-dose containers that because of their size bear only an indication of the active ingredient and the strength of the preparation do so by use of an approved code, Appendix XIX D, together with an expression of the percentage present. When a code is used on the container, the code is also stated on the package.

EYE OINTMENTS

Definition Eye Ointments of the British Pharmacopoeia that are intended to be used solely or primarily as a suitable eye-ointment basis contain no active ingredient.

Production Methods of sterilisation that may be used in the manufacture of Eye Ointments are described in Appendix XVIII.

In preparing Eye Ointments in tropical or subtropical countries where the prevailing high temperatures otherwise make the basis too soft for convenient use, the proportions of Yellow Soft Paraffin and Liquid Paraffin specified in the individual monograph may be varied, or Hard Paraffin may be added but the proportions of active ingredients must not be changed.

Storage Single-dose containers for Eye Ointments, or the nozzles of tubes, are of such a shape as to facilitate administration without contamination. The former type of container is individually wrapped. Tubes are tamper-evident.

Unless otherwise indicated Eye Ointments should be stored at a temperature not exceeding 25°.

Labelling The label states (1) the names and percentages of the active ingredients; (2) the date after which the Eye Ointment is not intended to be used; (3) the conditions under which the Eye Ointment should be stored.

The following eye preparations are the subject of an individual monograph in the British Pharmacopoeia.

Eye Drops

Adrenaline Eye Drops/Epinephrine Eye Drops
Atropine Eye Drops
Betamethasone Eye Drops
Carteolol Eye Drops
Chloramphenicol Eye Drops
Cyclopentolate Eye Drops
Fluorescein Eye Drops
Fluorometholone Eye Drops
Flurbiprofen Eye Drops
Gentamicin Eye Drops
Homatropine Eye Drops
Hydrocortisone Acetate and Neomycin Eye Drops
Hyoscine Eye Drops
Hypromellose Eye Drops
Idoxuridine Eye Drops
Levobunolol Eye Drops
Neomycin Eye Drops
Phenylephrine Eye Drops
Pilocarpine Hydrochloride Eye Drops
Pilocarpine Nitrate Eye Drops
Prednisolone Sodium Phosphate Eye Drops

Proxymetacaine Eye Drops
Sodium Chloride Eye Drops
Sodium Citrate Eye Drops
Sulfacetamide Eye Drops
Tetracaine Eye Drops/Amethocaine Eye Drops
Timolol Eye Drops
Tropicamide Eye Drops
Zinc Sulphate Eye Drops

Eye Lotions

Sodium Bicarbonate Eye Lotion
Sodium Chloride Eye Lotion

Eye Ointments

Aciclovir Eye Ointment
Atropine Eye Ointment
Chloramphenicol Eye Ointment
Chlortetracycline Eye Ointment
Hydrocortisone Acetate and Neomycin Eye Ointment
Neomycin Eye Ointment
Oxyphenbutazone Eye Ointment
Polymyxin and Bacitracin Eye Ointment
Simple Eye Ointment
Sulfacetamide Eye Ointment

MEDICATED FOAMS

Medicated Foams comply with the requirements of the 3rd edition of the European Pharmacopoeia [1105]. These requirements are reproduced after the heading 'Definition' below.

Additional requirements for medicated foams may be found, where appropriate, in other general monographs, for example on Rectal preparations (1145), Vaginal preparations (1164) and Liquids for cutaneous application (927).

Ph Eur

DEFINITION

Medicated foams are preparations consisting of large volumes of gas dispersed in a liquid generally containing one or more active ingredients, a surfactant ensuring their formation and various other excipients. Medicated foams are usually intended for application to the skin or mucous membranes.

Medicated foams are usually formed at the time of administration from a liquid preparation in a pressurised container. The container is equipped with a device consisting of a valve and a push button suitable for the delivery of the foam.

Medicated foams intended for use on severely injured skin and on large open wounds are sterile.

Medicated foams supplied in pressurised containers comply with the requirements in the monograph for *Pressurised pharmaceutical preparations (523)*.

PRODUCTION

Sterile medicated foams are prepared using materials and methods designed to ensure sterility and to avoid the introduction of contaminants and the growth of micro-organisms; recommendations on this aspect are provided in the text on *Methods of preparation of sterile products (5.1.1)*.

TESTS

Relative foam density Maintain the container at about 25°C for at least 24 h. Taking care not to warm the container, fit a rigid tube 70 mm to 100 mm long and about 1 mm in internal diameter onto the push button. Shake the container to homogenise the liquid phase of the contents and dispense 5 ml to 10 ml of foam to waste. Tare a flat-bottomed dish of about 60 ml volume and about 35 mm high. Place the end of the rigid tube attached to the push button in the corner of the dish, press the push button and fill the dish uniformly, using a circular motion. After the foam has completely expanded, level off by removing the excess foam with a slide. Weigh. Determine the mass of the same volume of *water R* by filling the same dish with *water R*.

The relative foam density is equivalent to the ratio:

$$\frac{m}{e}$$

m = mass of test sample of foam in grams,

e = mass of same volume of *water R* in grams.

Carry out three measurements. None of the individual values deviate by more than 20 per cent from the mean value.

Duration of expansion The apparatus (Fig. 1105-1) consists of a 50 ml burette, 15 mm in internal diameter, with 0.1 ml graduations and fitted with a 4 mm single bore stopcock. The graduation corresponding to 30 ml is at least 210 mm from the axis of the stopcock. The lower part of the burette is connected by means of a plastic tube not longer than 50 mm and 4 mm in internal diameter to the foam-generating container equipped with a push button fitted to this connection. Maintain the container at about 25°C for at least 24 h. Shake the container, taken care not to warm it, to homogenise the liquid phase of the contents and dispense 5 ml to 10 ml of the foam to waste.

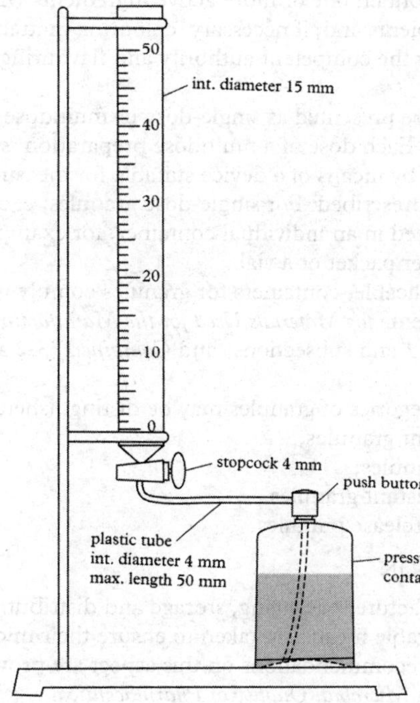

Fig. 1

Connect the push button to the outlet of the burette. Press the button and introduce about 30 ml of foam in a single delivery. Close the stopcock and at the same time start the chronometer and read the volume of foam in the burette. Every 10 s read the growing volume until the maximum volume is reached.

Carry out three measurements. None of the times needed to obtain the maximum volume is more than 5 min.

Sterility (*2.6.1*). When the label indicates that the preparation is sterile, it complies with the test for sterility.

LABELLING

The label states, where applicable, that the preparation is sterile.

Ph Eur

GRANULES

Granules comply with the requirements of the 3rd edition of the European Pharmacopoeia [0499]. These requirements are reproduced after the heading 'Definition' below.

Ph Eur

Requirements for granules to be used for the preparation of oral solutions or suspensions are given in the monograph on Liquids for Oral Use (672).

DEFINITION

Granules are preparations consisting of solid, dry aggregates of powder particles sufficiently resistant to withstand handling. They are intended for oral administration. Some are swallowed as such, some are chewed and some are dissolved or dispersed in water or another suitable liquid before being administered.

Granules contain one or more active ingredients with or without excipients and, if necessary, colouring matter authorised by the competent authority and flavouring substances.

Granules are presented as single-dose or multidose preparations. Each dose of a multidose preparation is administered by means of a device suitable for measuring the quantity prescribed. For single-dose granules, each dose is enclosed in an individual container, for example a sachet, a paper packet or a vial.

Where applicable, containers for granules comply with the requirements *for Materials Used for the Manufacture of Containers* (*3.1* and subsections) and *Containers* (*3.2* and subsections).

Several categories of granules may be distinguished:

— effervescent granules,
— coated granules,
— gastro-resistant granules,
— modified-release granules.

PRODUCTION

In the manufacture, packaging, storage and distribution of granules, suitable means are taken to ensure their microbial quality; recommendations on this aspect are provided in the text on *Microbial Quality of Pharmaceutical Preparations* (*5.1.4*).

TESTS

Uniformity of content (*2.9.6*). Unless otherwise prescribed or justified and authorised, single-dose granules with a content of active ingredient less than 2 mg or less than 2 per cent of the total mass comply with test B for uniformity of content of single-dose preparations. If the preparation has more than one active ingredient, the requirement applies only to those ingredients which correspond to the above conditions. The test is not required for multivitamin and trace-element preparations.

Uniformity of mass (*2.9.5*). Single-dose granules except for coated granules comply with the test for uniformity of mass of single-dose preparations. If the test for uniformity of content is prescribed for all the active ingredients, the test for uniformity of mass is not required.

STORAGE

Store in a well-closed container or, if the preparation contains volatile ingredients or the contents have to be protected, store in an airtight container.

Effervescent Granules

DEFINITION

Effervescent granules are uncoated granules generally containing acid substances and carbonates or hydrogen carbonates which react rapidly in the presence of water to release carbon dioxide. They are intended to be dissolved or dispersed in water before administration.

TESTS

Disintegration Place one dose of the effervescent granules in a beaker containing 200 ml of *water R* at 15°C to 25°C; numerous bubbles of gas are evolved. When the evolution of gas around the individual grains ceases, the granules have disintegrated, being either dissolved or dispersed in the water. Repeat the operation on five other doses. The preparation complies with the test if each of the six doses used disintegrates within 5 min.

STORAGE

Store in an airtight container.

Coated Granules

DEFINITION

Coated granules are usually multidose preparations and consist of granules coated with one or more layers of mixtures of various excipients.

PRODUCTION

The substances used as coatings are usually applied as a solution or suspension in conditions in which evaporation of the vehicle occurs.

TESTS

Dissolution A suitable test may be carried out to demonstrate the appropriate release of the active ingredient(s), for example one of the tests described in *Dissolution Test for Solid Dosage Forms* (*2.9.3*).

Gastro-Resistant Granules

DEFINITION

Gastro-resistant granules are modified-release granules that are intended to resist the gastric fluid and to release the active ingredient(s) in the intestinal fluid. These properties are achieved by covering the granules with a gastro-resistant material (enteric coated granules) or by other suitable means.

PRODUCTION

A suitable test is carried out to demonstrate the appropriate release of the active ingredient(s) or ingredients.

Modified-Release Granules

DEFINITION

Modified-release granules are coated or uncoated granules prepared using special excipients or special procedures which, separately or together, are designed to modify the rate or the place at which the active ingredient or ingredients are released.

PRODUCTION

A suitable test is carried out to demonstrate the appropriate release of the active ingredient(s).

Ph Eur

Granules of the British Pharmacopoeia

In addition to the above requirements of the European Pharmacopoeia, the following statements apply to those granules that are the subject of an individual monograph in the British Pharmacopoeia.

Labelling For single-dose containers the label states the name and amount of active ingredient per container and for multidose containers the label states the name and amount of active ingredient in a suitable quantity by weight.

The label also states (1) the date after which the Granules are not intended to be used; (2) the conditions under which the Granules should be stored; (3) the instructions for using the Granules.

The following granules are the subject of an individual monograph in the British Pharmacopoeia.

Colestipol Granules
Methylcellulose Granules
Pancreatin Granules
Senna Granules, Standardised
Sterculia Granules

INFUSIONS

Definition Infusions are dilute solutions containing the readily-soluble constituents of crude drugs. They are usually prepared by diluting one volume of a concentrated Infusion to ten volumes with Water.

For dispensing purposes, Infusions should be used within 12 hours of their preparation.

Storage Infusions should be kept in well-closed containers.

Labelling The label states (1) the time after which the Infusion is not intended to be used; (2) the conditions under which the Infusion should be stored.

The following infusions are the subject of an individual monograph in the British Pharmacopoeia.

Gentian Infusion, Compound
Orange Peel Infusion

PREPARATIONS FOR INHALATION

Preparations for Inhalation comply with the requirements of the 3rd edition of the European Pharmacopoeia [0671]. These requirements are reproduced after the heading 'Definition' below.

Ph Eur

DEFINITION

Preparations for inhalation are liquid or solid preparations intended for administration as vapour, aerosols or powders to the lower respiratory tract in order to obtain a local or systemic effect. They contain one or more active ingredients dissolved or dispersed in a suitable vehicle.

Preparations for inhalation may, dependent on the type of preparation, contain propellants, co-solvents, antimicrobial preservatives and solubilising and stabilising agents. The excipients do not adversely affect the functions of the mucosa of the respiratory tract or its cilia.

Preparations for inhalation are supplied in multidose or single-dose containers. When supplied in pressurised containers, they comply with the requirements of the monograph on *Pressurised pharmaceutical preparations (523)*.

Preparations intended to be administered as aerosols (dispersions of solid or liquid particles in a gas) are administered by one of the following devices depending on the type of preparation:
— nebuliser,
— pressurised metered-dose inhaler,
— dry-powder inhaler.

Several categories of preparations for inhalation may be distinguished:
— liquid preparations for inhalation,
— liquids for nebulisation,
— pressurised metered-dose preparations for inhalation,
— powders for inhalation.

PRODUCTION

During the development of a preparation for inhalation, the formulation for which contains an antimicrobial preservative, the effectiveness of the chosen preservative shall be demonstrated to the satisfaction of the competent authority. A suitable method of test together with criteria for judging the preservative properties of the formulation are provided in the text on *Efficacy of antimicrobial preservation (5.1.3)*.

The size of aerosol particles to be inhaled is controlled so a significant fraction is deposited in the lower respiratory tract. The fine-particle fraction of preparations for inhalation is determined by suitable method for aerodynamic assessment of fine particles (*2.9.18*).

Pressurised metered-dose inhalers are tested for leakage and for extraneous particulate contamination.

TESTS

Uniformity of dose The test is intended to control the dose delivered by the device, i.e. the dose received by the patient. However, for pressurised metered-dose inhalers, the uniformity of dose metered from the valve is substituted, and for capsules and other pre-dispensed dose forms intended for inhalation, the variation in dose in these units may be substituted. In all cases, a dosage unit is the number of units or actuations of the device given on the label required to provide the recommended dose.

For preparations for inhalation containing more than one active ingredient, carry out the test for uniformity of dose for each active ingredient.

LABELLING

The label states:

— where applicable, the number of actuations of the device to provide the recommended dose,

— where applicable, the name of any added antimicrobial preservative.

Liquid Preparations for Inhalation

DEFINITION

Three categories of liquid preparations for inhalation may be distinguished:

— preparations intended to be converted into vapour,

— liquids for nebulisation,

— pressurised metered-dose preparations for inhalation.

Liquid preparations for inhalation are solutions or dispersions.

Dispersions are readily dispersible on shaking and they remain sufficiently stable to enable the correct dose to be delivered. Suitable co-solvents or solubilisers may be used.

Preparations intended to be converted into vapour are solutions, dispersions or solid preparations. They are usually added to hot water and the vapour generated is inhaled.

Liquids for Nebulisation

DEFINITION

Liquids for inhalation intended to be converted into aerosols by nebulisers at a specified rate are aqueous solutions, suspensions or emulsions.

Liquids for nebulisation in concentrated form are diluted to the prescribed volume with the prescribed liquid before use.

Suitable co-solvents or solubilisers may be used to increase the solubility of the active ingredients.

The pH of the liquid, if aqueous, is not lower than 3 and not higher than 8.5.

Suspensions and emulsions are readily dispersible on shaking and they remain sufficiently stable to enable the correct dose to be delivered.

Aqueous preparations for inhalation supplied in multidose containers may contain a suitable antimicrobial preservative at a suitable concentration except where the preparation itself has adequate antimicrobial properties.

Nebulisers are devices that convert liquids into aerosols by high-pressure gases, ultrasonic vibration or other methods. They allow the dose to be inhaled at an appropriate rate and particle size which ensure deposition of the preparation in the lower respiratory tract.

PRODUCTION

The aerodynamic assessment of fine particles of liquids for nebulisation converted into aerosols by nebulisers may be carried out using the impingement apparatus and procedure *(2.9.18)*.

Pressurised Metered-Dose Preparations for Inhalation

DEFINITION

Pressurised metered-dose preparations for inhalation are solutions, suspensions or emulsions supplied in special containers equipped with a metering valve and which are held under pressure with suitable propellants or suitable mixtures of liquefied propellants, which can act also as solvents. Suitable co-solvents or solubilisers may be added.

TESTS

Uniformity of dose Containers usually operate in an inverted position. For containers that operate in an upright position, an equivalent test is applied using methods that ensure the complete collection of the dose emitted from the valve.

A. ***Uniformity of delivered dose*** Use this test if the label claim is based on the delivered dose.

Use an apparatus capable of quantitatively retaining the dose leaving the actuator of the inhaler.

The following apparatus and procedure may be used:

Mount a 500 ml separating funnel in a horizontal position and plug the stopcock end with a wad of absorbent cotton moistened with a suitable solvent. By means of a suitable pump, adjust the air flow through the funnel to 30 litres per minute. Close the stopcock and spray the inside of the funnel with the solvent.

Shake the inhaler for 5 s and discharge once to waste. Wait for not less than 5 s, shake for 5 s and discharge again to waste. Repeat this procedure for a further three actuations. Open the stopcock and, after 2 s, fire the inverted inhaler into the funnel, depressing the valve for 1 s. Shake the inhaler for 5 s and repeat the procedure until the number of actuations that constitute a dosage unit have been sampled. Close the stopcock and collect the contents of the funnel by successive rinses. Determine the content of active ingredient in the combined rinses.

Repeat the procedure for a further nine containers.

Unless otherwise justified and authorised, the preparation complies with the test if nine out of ten results lie between 75 per cent and 125 per cent of the average value and all lie between 65 per cent and 135 per cent. If two or three values lie outside the range of 75 per cent to 125 per cent, repeat the test for twenty more containers. Not more than three of the thirty values lie outside the range 75 per cent to 125 per cent and no value lies outside the range 65 per cent to 135 per cent.

B. ***Uniformity of metered dose*** Use this test if the label claim is based on the metered dose (that is, the dose delivered by the device when the actuator is not attached).

The following apparatus and procedure may be used:

Take one container. Remove the pressurised container from the actuator and remove all labels and markings, which may be present on the container, with a suitable solvent. Dry the container, replace in its actuator and shake for 5 s. Discharge once to waste, wait for not less than 5 s, shake for 5 s and discharge again to waste. Repeat for three further actuations. Remove the pressurised container from its actuator, clean the valve stem (internally and externally) and the valve ferrule by washing with a suitable solvent. Dry the complete valve assembly.

Place a suitable holder made of inert material in a small vessel suitable for shaking. (A holder with three legs and a central indentation with a hole tapered in a downward direction is suitable). Add a volume of suitable solvent such that discharge takes place at least 25 mm below the surface.

Shake the pressurised container for about 5 s and place it inverted in the vessel. Maintaining the pressurised container in the vertical plane, discharge the inhaler through the hole in the centre of the holder. Repeat the procedure for the number of actuations which constitute a dosage unit. Remove the pressurised container, wash the inside of the valve stem and all external surfaces with solvent and determine the amount of active ingredient in the combined solvent and washings.

Repeat the procedure for a further nine containers.

Unless otherwise justified and authorised, the preparation complies with the test if nine out of ten results lie between 75 per cent and 125 per cent of the average value and all lie between 65 per cent and 135 per cent. If two or three values lie outside the range of 75 per cent to 125 per cent, repeat the test for twenty more containers. Not more than three of the thirty values lie outside the range 75 per cent to 125 per cent and no value lies outside the range 65 per cent to 135 per cent.

Aerodynamic assessment of fine particles *(2.9.18)*. Carry out the test using a suitable impingement device.

Number of deliveries per container Take one container and discharge the contents to waste, actuating the valve at intervals of not less than 5 s. The total number of deliveries so discharged from the pressurised container is not less than the number stated on the label.

Powders for Inhalation

DEFINITION

Powders for inhalation are presented as single-dose powders, multidose powders or as powders derived from a solid compact. To facilitate their use, active ingredients may be combined with a suitable carrier. They are generally administered by dry-powder inhalers. For single-dose powders, the inhaler is loaded with powders predispensed

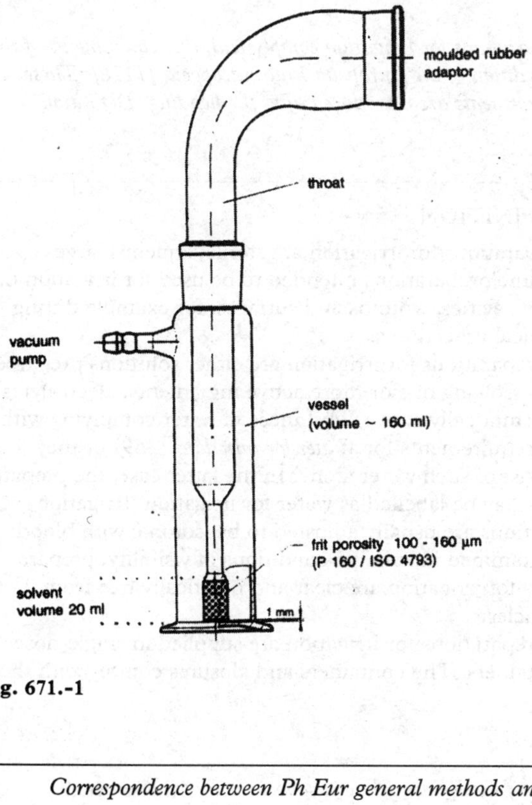

Fig. 671.-1

in capsules or other suitable pharmaceutical form. For multidose powders, the dose is created by a metering unit within the inhaler, or by the use of an assembly of pre-dispensed powders.

TESTS

Uniformity of dose

A. ***Uniformity of delivered dose*** Use this test for single-dose powders with a label claim based on the delivered dose and for multidose powders.

Use an apparatus capable of quantitatively retaining the content of active ingredient of the dose leaving the powder inhaler.

A suitable apparatus is shown in 671.-1; the following procedure may be used.

Prepare the inhaler for use and fire to waste by using a suitable pump. Repeat this procedure for a further four doses. Prepare the inhaler for use and connect it to the apparatus using an adaptor which ensures a good seal. Switch on the pump and draw 3 litres of air through the inhaler at a suitable flow rate, for example 60 litres per minute. Repeat the procedure until the number of deliveries which constitute a dosage unit have been sampled. Dismantle the apparatus, wash all internal surfaces and determine the amount of active ingredient in the washings.

Repeat the procedure for a further nine inhalers.

The preparation complies with the test if not more than one of the ten values deviates from the average value by more than 35 per cent and no value deviates by more than 50 per cent. If two or three values deviate by more than 35 per cent and none deviate by more than 50 per cent, test a further twenty inhalers. The preparation complies with the test if not more than three of the thirty values deviate by more than 35 per cent and no value deviates by more than 50 per cent.

B. ***Uniformity of pre-dispensed dose*** If the label claim is based on a pre-dispensed dose in the form of capsules, blisters, etc., the preparation complies with test B for *Uniformity of Content of Single-Dose Preparations (2.9.6)*.

Aerodynamic assessment of fine particles *(2.9.18)*. Carry out the test using a suitable impingement device.

Number of deliveries per container for multidose containers Discharge doses from the device at an appropriate flow rate. Record the deliveries discharged. The total number of doses delivered is not less than the number stated on the label.

Ph Eur

Preparations for Inhalation of the British Pharmacopoeia

In addition to the above requirements of the European Pharmacopoeia, the following statements apply to any inhalation, powder for inhalation, pressurised inhalation or solution for nebulisation that is the subject of an individual monograph in the British Pharmacopoeia.

INHALATIONS

Definition Inhalations are solutions or dispersions of one or more active ingredients which may contain an inert, suspended, diffusing agent. They are intended to release volatile constituents for inhalation either when placed on a pad or when added to hot, but not boiling, water.

Labelling The label on the container states (1) the names and concentrations of the active ingredients; (2) that the Inhalation is not to be taken by mouth; (3) the date after which the Inhalation is not intended to be used; (4) the conditions under which the Inhalation should be stored.

POWDERS FOR INHALATION

Labelling The label on the container states (1) the date after which the Powder for Inhalation is not intended to be used; (2) the conditions under which the Powder for Inhalation should be stored.

Where the Powder for Inhalation is supplied in a capsule, the label also states (3) the quantity of the active ingredient contained in each capsule; (4) that the capsules are intended for use in an inhaler and are not to be swallowed.

PRESSURISED INHALATIONS

Definition Pressurised Inhalations are Pressurised Metered-dose Preparations for Inhalation. They are intended to be inhaled in controlled amounts.

Production The formulation of the inhalation and the components of the delivery device (that is the pressurised container with its integral metering valve and the actuator) should be designed and, where appropriate, the particle size of the active ingredient should be controlled so that, when the pressurised inhalation is used in accordance with the manufacturer's recommendations, an adequate proportion of the active ingredient is made available for inhalation. A proportion of the active ingredient is deposited on the inner surface of the actuator; the amount available for inhalation is therefore less than the amount released by actuation of the valve.

Pressurised Inhalations should be manufactured in conditions designed to minimise microbial and particulate contamination.

Content of active ingredient delivered by actuation of the valve Prepare the container, prime the metering valve and use the vessel and holder described in test B for Uniformity of dose under Pressurised Metered-dose Preparations for Inhalation. Use the volume of the solvent specified in the monograph.

Shake the pressurised container for about 30 seconds and place it inverted in the vessel. Discharge 10 deliveries below the surface of the solvent actuating the valve at intervals of not less than 5 seconds, maintaining the pressurised container in the vertical plane and discharging the pressurised inhalation through the hole in the centre of the base plate. (It may be necessary because of the nature of the formulation to shake the pressurised container between each actuation of the valve; where this is the case shaking should be carried out without removing the pressurised container from its inverted position in the vessel.) Remove the pressurised container, wash it with the specified solvent and dilute the combined solution and washings to the volume specified in the monograph. Determine the amount of active ingredient by the method described under the Assay and calculate the amount delivered from each actuation of the valve. The result lies within the range for the content of active ingredient stated in the monograph.

Storage Pressurised Inhalations are supplied in suitable containers fitted with an appropriate metering valve that forms an integral part of the container. Metal containers comply with the relevant requirements of British Standard 3914: Part 1:1974 (Non-returnable metal containers up to 1400 cm^3 and 85 mm diameter). The containers are usually supplied with an appropriate actuator.

Labelling The label states (1) the name of the active ingredient or ingredients; (2) the amount of active ingredient or ingredients delivered by each actuation of the valve and the number of deliveries available from the container; (3) the instructions for using the Pressurised Inhalation; (4) the date after which the Pressurised Inhalation is not intended to be used; (5) the conditions under which the Pressurised Inhalation should be stored; (6) any special precautions associated with the use of the Pressurised Inhalation.

SOLUTIONS FOR NEBULISATION

Labelling The label states (1) the date after which the solution for nebulisation is not intended to be used; (2) the conditions under which the solution for nebulisation should be stored.

The following preparations for inhalation are the subject of an individual monograph in the British Pharmacopoeia.

Inhalations
Benzoin Inhalation
Menthol and Benzoin Inhalation

Powders for Inhalation
Sodium Cromoglicate Powder for Inhalation

Pressurised Inhalations
Beclometasone Pressurised Inhalation
Ipratropium Pressurised Inhalation
Salbutamol Pressurised Inhalation

Solutions for Nebulisation
Tribavirin Solution for Nebulisation

PREPARATIONS FOR IRRIGATION

Preparations for Irrigation comply with the requirements of the 3rd edition of the European Pharmacopoeia [1116]. These requirements are reproduced after the heading 'Definition' below.

Ph Eur

DEFINITION

Preparations for irrigation are sterile, aqueous large volume preparations intended to be used for irrigation of body cavities, wounds and surfaces, for example during surgical procedures.

Preparations for irrigation are either solutions prepared by dissolving one or more active ingredients, electrolytes or osmotically active substances in water complying with the requirements for *Water for injections (169)* or they consist of such water alone. In the latter case, the preparation may be labelled as water for irrigation. Irrigation solutions are usually adjusted to be isotonic with blood.

Examined in suitable conditions of visibility, preparations for irrigation are clear and practically free from particles.

Preparations for irrigation are supplied in single-dose containers. The containers and closures comply with the requirements for containers for preparations for parenteral use (*3.2.1 and 3.2.2*) but the administration port of the container is incompatible with intravenous administration equipment and does not allow the preparation for irrigation to be administered with such equipment.

PRODUCTION

Preparations for irrigation are prepared using materials and methods designed to ensure sterility and to avoid the introduction of contaminants and the growth of micro-organisms; recommendations on this aspect are provided in the text on *Methods of Preparation of Sterile Products* (*5.1.1*).

TESTS

Sterility (*2.6.1*). Preparations for irrigation comply with the test for sterility.

Bacterial endotoxins (*2.6.14*). Not more than 0.5 I.U. of endotoxin per millilitre.

Pyrogens (*2.6.8*). Preparations for which a validated test for bacterial endotoxins cannot be carried out comply with the test for pyrogens. Inject per kilogram of the rabbits mass, 10 ml of the preparation, unless otherwise justified and authorised.

LABELLING

The label states:

— that the preparation is not to be used for injection,

— that the preparation is to be used for one occasion only and that any unused portion of preparation is to be discarded.

Ph Eur

Preparations for Irrigation of the British Pharmacopoeia

In addition to the above requirements of the European Pharmacopoeia, the following statements apply to those irrigation solutions that are the subject of an individual monograph in the British Pharmacopoeia.

IRRIGATION SOLUTIONS

Labelling The label states (1) the names and concentrations of the active ingredients; (2) the date after which the Irrigation Solution is not intended to be used; (3) the conditions under which the irrigation solution should be stored.

The following irrigation solutions are the subject of an individual monograph in the British Pharmacopoeia.

Chlorhexidine Irrigation Solution
Glucose Irrigation Solution
Glycine Irrigation Solution
Sodium Citrate Irrigation Solution
Water for Irrigation

MOUTHWASHES

Definition Mouthwashes are aqueous solutions containing one or more active ingredients. They are intended for use in contact with the mucous membranes of the oral cavity, usually after dilution with warm water. They may contain excipients such as suitable antimicrobial preservatives.

Storage Mouthwashes should be kept in well-closed containers.

Labelling The label states (1) directions for the dilution of the Mouthwash for use, if appropriate; (2) that large quantities of the Mouthwash should not be swallowed; (3) the date after which the Mouthwash is not intended to be used; (4) the conditions under which the Mouthwash should be stored.

The following mouthwashes are the subject of an individual monograph in the British Pharmacopoeia.

Benzydamine Mouthwash
Hydrogen Peroxide Mouthwash
Sodium Chloride Mouthwash, Compound

NASAL PREPARATIONS

Nasal Preparations comply with the requirements of the 3rd edition of the European Pharmacopoeia [0676]. These requirements are reproduced after the heading 'Definition' below.

Ph Eur

DEFINITION

Nasal preparations are liquid, semi-solid or solid preparations intended for administration to the nasal cavities to obtain a systemic or local effect. They contain one or more active ingredients. Nasal preparations are as far as possible non-irritating and do not adversely affect the functions of the nasal mucosa and its cilia. Aqueous nasal preparations are usually isotonic.

Nasal preparations are supplied in multidose or single-dose containers, provided, if necessary, with a suitable administration device which may be designed to avoid the introduction of contaminants.

Unless otherwise justified and authorised, aqueous nasal preparations supplied in multidose containers contain a suitable antimicrobial preservative in appropriate concentration, except where the preparation itself has adequate antimicrobial properties.

Where applicable, the containers comply with the requirements of *Materials Used for the Manufacture of Containers* (*3.1* and subsections) and *Containers* (*3.2* and subsections).

Several categories of nasal preparations may be distinguished:

— nasal drops and liquid nasal sprays,

— nasal powders,

— semi-solid nasal preparations,

— nasal washes,

— nasal sticks.

PRODUCTION

During the development of a nasal preparation, the formulation for which contains an antimicrobial preservative, the effectiveness of the chosen preservative shall be demonstrated to the satisfaction of the competent authority. A suitable test method together with criteria for judging the preservative properties of the formulation are provided in the text on *Efficacy of Antimicrobial Preservation*

(*5.1.3*).

In the manufacture, packaging, storage and distribution of nasal preparations, suitable means are taken to ensure their microbial quality; recommendations on this aspect are provided in the text on *Microbial Quality of Pharmaceutical Preparations* (*5.1.4*).

Sterile nasal preparations are prepared using materials and methods designed to ensure sterility and to avoid the introduction of contaminants and the growth of micro-organisms; recommendations on this aspect are provided in the text on *Methods of Preparation of Sterile Products* (*5.1.1*).

In the manufacture of nasal preparations containing dispersed particles measures are taken to ensure a suitable and controlled particle size with regard to the intended use.

TESTS

Sterility (*2.6.1*). Where the label states that the preparation is sterile, it complies with the test for sterility.

STORAGE

Store in a well-closed container. If the preparation is sterile, store in a sterile, airtight, tamper-proof container.

LABELLING

The label states:
— the name of any added antimicrobial preservative,
— where applicable, that the preparation is sterile.

Nasal Drops and Liquid Nasal Sprays

DEFINITION

Nasal drops and liquid nasal sprays are solutions, emulsions or suspensions intended for instillation or spraying into the nasal cavities.

Emulsions may show evidence of phase separation but are easily reformed on shaking. Suspensions may show a sediment which is readily dispersed on shaking to give a suspension which remains sufficiently stable to enable the correct dose to be delivered.

Nasal drops are usually supplied in multidose containers provided with a suitable applicator.

Liquid nasal sprays are supplied in containers with atomising devices or in pressurised containers fitted with a suitable adaptor and with or without a metering dose valve, which comply with the requirements of the monograph on *Pressurised pharmaceutical preparations* (*523*).

The size of droplets of the spray is such as to localise their deposition in the nasal cavity.

TESTS

Unless otherwise prescribed or justified and authorised, nasal drops supplied in single dose containers and single doses of metered nasal sprays intended for systemic action, comply with the following tests.

Uniformity of mass. Nasal drops that are solutions comply with the following test: Weigh individually the contents of ten containers emptied as completely as possible, and determine the average mass. Not more than two of the individual masses deviate by more than 10 per cent from the average mass and none deviates by more than 20 per cent.

Metered dose nasal sprays that are solutions comply with the following test: Discharge once to waste. Wait for not less than 5 seconds and discharge again to waste. Repeat this procedure for a further three actuations. Weigh the mass of the container, discharge once to waste and weigh the remaining mass of the container. Calculate the difference between the two masses. Repeat the procedure for a further nine containers. They comply with the test if not more than two of the individual values deviate by more than 25 per cent from the average value and none deviates by more than 35 per cent.

Uniformity of content. Nasal drops that are suspensions or emulsions comply with the following test: Empty each container as completely as possible and carry out the test on the individual content. They comply with test B of uniformity of content (*2.9.6*).

Uniformity of delivered dose. Metered dose nasal sprays that are suspensions or emulsions comply with the following test: Use an apparatus capable of quantitatively retaining the dose leaving the actuator of the atomising device.

Shake a container for 5 seconds and discharge once to waste. Wait for not less than 5 seconds, shake for 5 seconds and discharge again to waste. Repeat this procedure for a further three actuations. After 2 seconds, fire one dose of the metered dose nasal spray into the collecting vessel by actuating the atomising device. Collect the contents of the collecting vessel by successive rinses. Determine the content of active ingredient in the combined rinses.

Repeat the procedure for a further nine containers.

Unless otherwise justified and authorised, the preparation complies with the test if not more than one of the individual contents is outside the limits of 75 per cent to 125 per cent and none is outside the limits of 65 per cent and 135 per cent of the average content.

If two or three individual contents are outside the limits of 75 per cent to 125 per cent but within the limits of 65 per cent to 135 per cent, repeat the test for twenty more containers. The preparation complies with the test if not more than three individual contents of the thirty individual contents are outside the limits of 75 per cent to 125 per cent and none is outside the limits of 65 per cent to 135 per cent of the average content.

Nasal Powders

DEFINITION

Nasal powders are powders intended for insufflation into the nasal cavities by means of a suitable device.

They comply with the requirements of the monograph on *Topical powders (1166)*.

The size of the particles is such as to localise their deposition in the nasal cavity and verified by adequate methods of particle-size determination.

Semi-Solid Nasal Preparations

DEFINITION

Semi-solid nasal preparations comply with the requirements of the monograph on *Topical semi-solid preparations* (*132*).

The containers are adapted to deliver the product to the site of application.

Nasal Washes

DEFINITION

Nasal washes are generally aqueous isotonic solutions intended to cleanse the nasal cavities.

Nasal washes intended for application to injured parts or prior to a surgical operation are sterile.

Nasal Sticks

DEFINITION

Nasal sticks comply with the monograph on *Sticks (1154)*.

Ph Eur

Nasal Preparations of the British Pharmacopoeia

In addition to the above requirements of the European Pharmacopoeia, the following statements apply to any intranasal solution, intranasal suspension, nasal drops or nasal spray that is the subject of an individual monograph in the British Pharmacopoeia.

INTRANASAL SOLUTIONS AND INTRANASAL SUSPENSIONS

Definition Intranasal Solutions and Intranasal Suspensions are intended for administration to the nostrils for local or systemic effects. When supplied in a container fitted with a spray mechanism, they may be entitled Nasal Spray.

Labelling The label states (1) the name and quantity of the active ingredient; (2) the name and quantity of any added substance; (3) that the preparation is for intranasal administration; (4) the date after which the preparation is not intended to be used; (5) the conditions under which the preparation should be stored.

NASAL DROPS

Labelling The label states (1) the name and quantity of the active ingredient; (2) the instructions for using the Nasal Drops; (3) the date after which the Nasal Drops are not intended to be used; (4) the conditions under which the Nasal Drops should be stored.

The following nasal preparations are the subject of an individual monograph in the British Pharmacopoeia.

Intranasal Solutions

Desmopressin Intranasal Solution

Nasal Drops

Ephedrine Nasal Drops

Xylometazoline Nasal Drops

Nasal Sprays

Beclometasone Nasal Spray

ORAL LIQUIDS

Oral Liquids comply with the requirements of the 3rd edition of the European Pharmacopoeia for Liquids for oral use [0672]. These requirements are reproduced after the heading 'Definition' below.

Ph Eur

DEFINITION

Liquids for oral use are usually solutions, emulsions or suspensions containing one or more active ingredients in a suitable vehicle; some liquids for oral administration may consist of liquid active ingredients as such.

They are intended to be swallowed either undiluted or after dilution. These preparations may also be prepared before use from concentrated liquid preparations, or from powders, granules or tablets for the preparation of oral solutions or suspensions using a suitable vehicle.

Liquids for oral use may contain suitable antimicrobial preservatives, antioxidants and other excipients such as dispersing, suspending, thickening, emulsifying, buffering, wetting, solubilising, stabilising, flavouring and sweetening agents and colouring matter authorised by the competent authority.

Emulsions may show evidence of phase separation but are easily reformed on shaking. Suspensions may show a sediment which is readily dispersed on shaking to give a suspension which remains sufficiently stable to enable the correct dose to be delivered.

Liquids for oral use are supplied in multidose or single-dose containers. They are administered either in volumes such as 5 ml or multiples thereof or in small volumes (drops). Each dose of a multidose preparation is administered by means of a device suitable for measuring the prescribed volume.

Where applicable, containers for liquids for oral use comply with the requirements of *Materials Used for the Manufacture of Containers* (*3.1* and subsections) and *Containers* (*3.2* and subsections).

PRODUCTION

During the development of a liquid for oral use, the formulation for which contains an antimicrobial preservative, the effectiveness of the chosen preservative shall be demonstrated to the satisfaction of the competent authority. A suitable method of test together with criteria for judging the preservative properties of the formulation are provided in the text on *Efficacy of Antimicrobial Preservation (5.1.3)*.

In the manufacture, packaging, storage and distribution of liquids for oral use, suitable means are taken to ensure their microbial quality; recommendations on this aspect are provided in the text on *Microbial Quality of Pharmaceutical Preparations (5.1.4)*.

In the manufacture of liquids for oral use containing dispersed particles measures are taken to ensure a suitable and controlled particle size with regard to the intended use.

TESTS

Uniformity of content Unless otherwise prescribed or justified and authorised, single-dose liquids that are suspensions comply with the following test. After shaking, empty each container as completely as possible and carry out the test on the individual contents. They comply with test B for *Uniformity of Content of Single-dose Preparations (2.9.6)*.

Uniformity of mass Single-dose liquids that are solutions or emulsions comply with the following test: weigh individually the contents of twenty containers, emptied as completely as possible, and determine the average mass. Not more than two of the individual masses deviate by more than 10 per cent from the average mass and none deviates by more than 20 per cent.

Dose and uniformity of dose of oral drops Into a suitable, graduated cylinder, introduce by means of the dropping device the number of drops usually prescribed for one dose or introduce by means of the measuring device, the usually prescribed quantity. The dropping speed does not exceed two drops per second. Weigh the liquid, repeat the addition, weigh again and carry on repeating the addition and weighing until a total of ten masses are obtained. No single mass deviates by more than 10 per cent from the average mass. The total of ten masses does not differ by more than 15 per cent from the nominal mass of ten doses. If necessary, measure the total volume of ten doses. The volume does not differ by more than 15 per cent from the nominal volume of ten doses.

STORAGE

Store in a well-closed container.

LABELLING

The label states:
- the name of any added antimicrobial preservative,
- the label for oral drops includes a statement of the number of drops per millilitre of preparation or per gram of preparation if the dose is measured in drops.

Powders and Granules for Oral Solutions and Suspensions

DEFINITION

Powders and granules for the preparation of solutions or suspensions for oral use generally conform to the definitions in the monographs on *Oral Powders (1165)* and *Granules (499)* respectively. They may contain excipients in particular to facilitate dispersion or dissolution and to prevent caking.

After dissolution or suspension, they comply with the requirements for oral solutions or oral suspensions, as appropriate.

TESTS

Uniformity of content (*2.9.6*). Unless otherwise prescribed or justified and authorised, single-dose powders and single-dose granules with a content of active ingredient less than 2 mg or less than 2 per cent of the total mass comply with the test B for *Uniformity of Content of Single-dose Preparations* (*2.9.6*). If the preparation has more than one active ingredient, the requirement applies only to those ingredients that correspond to the above conditions. The test is not required for multivitamin and trace-element preparations.

Uniformity of mass (*2.9.5*). Single-dose powders and single-dose granules comply with the test for uniformity of mass of single-dose preparations. If the test for uniformity of content is prescribed for all the active ingredients, the test for uniformity of mass is not required.

STORAGE

Store in a well-closed container.

LABELLING

The label states:
- the method of preparation of the solution or suspension,
- the conditions and the duration of storage after constitution.

Ph Eur

Oral Liquids of the British Pharmacopoeia

In addition to the above requirements of the European Pharmacopoeia, the following statements apply to any elixir, linctus, mixture, oral drops, oral emulsion, oral solution or oral suspension, that is the subject of an individual monograph in the British Pharmacopoeia.

Syrups, defined by the separate monograph of that title, are not Oral Liquids since they are not intended to be administered as such but are used as vehicle ingredients for their flavouring and sweetening properties.

Definition The vehicle for any particular Oral Liquid should be chosen having regard to the nature of the active ingredient or ingredients and to provide organoleptic characteristics appropriate to the intended use of the preparation.

Oral Liquids other than Oral Emulsions may be supplied as liquids or prepared just before issue for use by dissolving or dispersing granules or powder in the liquid stated on the label.

Storage Oral Liquids should be kept in well-closed containers.

Labelling The label states (1) the date after which the Oral Liquid is not intended to be used; (2) the conditions under which the Oral Liquid should be stored; (3) for Oral Emulsions, Oral Suspensions and, where appropriate, for Mixtures, that the bottle should be shaken before use.

If the Oral Liquid is supplied as granules or powder to be constituted just before issue for use the label states (1) that the contents of the container are granules or powder for the preparation of an Oral Liquid; (2) the strength as the amount of the active ingredient in a suitable dose-volume of the constituted preparation; (3) the directions for preparing the Oral Liquid including the nature and quantity of liquid to be used.

ELIXIRS

Definition Elixirs are clear, flavoured Oral Liquids containing one or more active ingredients dissolved in a vehicle that usually contains a high proportion of Sucrose or a suitable polyhydric alcohol or alcohols and may also contain Ethanol (96 per cent) or a Dilute Ethanol.

LINCTUSES

Definition Linctuses are viscous Oral Liquids that may contain one or more active ingredients in solution. The vehicle usually contains a high proportion of Sucrose, other sugars or a suitable polyhydric alcohol or alcohols. Linctuses are intended for use in the treatment or relief of cough, and are sipped and swallowed slowly without the addition of water.

MIXTURES

Definition Mixtures are Oral Liquids containing one or more active ingredients dissolved, suspended or dispersed in a suitable vehicle. Suspended solids may separate slowly on standing but are easily redispersed on shaking.

ORAL DROPS

Definition Oral Drops are Oral Liquids that are intended to be administered in small volumes with the aid of a suitable measuring device.

ORAL EMULSIONS

Definition Oral Emulsions are Oral Liquids containing one or more active ingredients. They are stabilised oil-in-water dispersions, either or both phases of which may contain dissolved solids. Solids may also be suspended in Oral Emulsions.

When issued for use, Oral Emulsions should be supplied in wide-mouthed bottles.

Extemporaneous preparation In Oral Emulsions prepared according to the formula and directions given for Extemporaneous preparation, the quantity of emulsifying agent specified in individual monographs may be reduced to yield a preparation of suitable consistency provided that by so doing the stability of the preparation is not adversely affected.

ORAL SOLUTIONS

Definition Oral Solutions are Oral Liquids containing one or more active ingredients dissolved in a suitable vehicle.

ORAL SUSPENSIONS

Definition Oral Suspensions are Oral Liquids containing one or more active ingredients suspended in a suitable vehicle. Suspended solids may slowly separate on standing but are easily redispersed.

The following oral liquids are the subject of an individual monograph in the British Pharmacopoeia.

Elixirs
Chloral Elixir, Paediatric
Ephedrine Elixir
Phenobarbital Elixir
Piperazine Citrate Elixir

Linctuses
Codeine Linctus
Codeine Linctus, Paediatric
Methadone Linctus
Pholcodine Linctus
Pholcodine Linctus, Strong
Simple Linctus
Simple Linctus, Paediatric
Squill Linctus, Opiate
Squill Linctus, Paediatric Opiate
Tolu Linctus, Paediatric Compound

Mixtures
Ammonia and Ipecacuanha Mixture
Ammonium Chloride Mixture
Chloral Mixture
Gentian Mixture, Acid
Gentian Mixture, Alkaline
Ipecacuanha Emetic Mixture, Paediatric
Kaolin and Morphine Mixture
Kaolin Mixture
Magnesium Carbonate Mixture, Aromatic
Magnesium Hydroxide Mixture
Magnesium Sulphate Mixture
Magnesium Trisilicate Mixture
Potassium Citrate Mixture

Oral Emulsions
Liquid Paraffin Oral Emulsion
Liquid Paraffin and Magnesium Hydroxide Oral Emulsion

Oral Solutions
Alimemazine Oral Solution, Paediatric/Trimeprazine Oral Solution, Paediatric
Alimemazine Oral Solution, Strong Paediatric/ Trimeprazine Oral Solution, Strong Paediatric
Amantadine Oral Solution
Atenolol Oral Solution
Baclofen Oral Solution
Bumetanide Oral Solution
Calciferol Oral Solution
Chlorphenamine Oral Solution/Chlorpheniramine Oral Solution
Chlorpromazine Oral Solution
Cimetidine Oral Solution
Clemastine Oral Solution
Clomethiazole Oral Solution
Cloxacillin Oral Solution
Co-amilozide Oral Solution
Codeine Phosphate Oral Solution
Diazepam Oral Solution
Dicycloverine Oral Solution/Dicyclomine Oral Solution
Digoxin Oral Solution, Paediatric
Dihydrocodeine Oral Solution
Diphenhydramine Oral Solution
Etamivan Oral Solution
Ethosuximide Oral Solution
Ferrous Sulphate Oral Solution, Paediatric
Flucloxacillin Oral Solution
Haloperidol Oral Solution
Haloperidol Oral Solution, Strong
Iodine Oral Solution, Aqueous
Metoclopramide Oral Solution
Neomycin Oral Solution
Orciprenaline Oral Solution
Paracetamol Oral Solution, Paediatric
Phenoxymethylpenicillin Oral Solution
Prochlorperazine Oral Solution
Promethazine Oral Solution
Ranitidine Oral Solution
Sodium Valproate Oral Solution
Temazepam Oral Solution
Thioridazine Oral Solution
Triclofos Oral Solution

Oral Suspensions
Aciclovir Oral Suspension
Aluminium Hydroxide Oral Suspension
Amitriptyline Oral Suspension
Amoxicillin Oral Suspension
Ampicillin Oral Suspension
Barium Sulphate Oral Suspension
Benorilate Oral Suspension
Cefalexin Oral Suspension
Cimetidine Oral Suspension
Co-fluampicil Oral Suspension
Co-magaldrox Oral Suspension
Co-trimoxazole Oral Suspension
Co-trimoxazole Oral Suspension, Paediatric
Erythromycin Ethyl Succinate Oral Suspension
Ferrous Fumarate Oral Suspension
Flucloxacillin Oral Suspension

Fusidic Acid Oral Suspension
Ibuprofen Oral Suspension
Magaldrate Oral Suspension
Nabumetone Oral Suspension
Nalidixic Acid Oral Suspension
Naproxen Oral Suspension
Nitrazepam Oral Suspension
Nitrofurantoin Oral Suspension
Nystatin Oral Suspension
Paracetamol Oral Suspension
Phenytoin Oral Suspension
Primidone Oral Suspension
Rifampicin Oral Suspension
Sulfadimidine Oral Suspension, Paediatric
Thioridazine Oral Suspension

ORAL POWDERS

Oral Powders comply with the requirements of the 3rd edition of the European Pharmacopoeia [1165]. These requirements are reproduced after the heading 'Definition' below.

Ph Eur

Requirements for powders to be used for the preparation of oral solutions or suspensions are given in the monograph for Liquids for oral use (672).

DEFINITION

Oral powders are preparations consisting of solid, loose, dry particles of varying degrees of fineness. They contain one or more active ingredients, with or without excipients and, if necessary, colouring matters authorised by the competent authority and flavouring substances. They are generally administered in or with water or another suitable liquid. They may also be swallowed directly. They are presented as single-dose or multidose powders.

Where applicable, containers for oral powders comply with the requirements *of Materials used for the Manufacture of Containers* (*3.1* and subsections) and *Containers* (*3.2* and subsections). Multidose oral powders require the provision of a measuring device capable of delivering the quantity prescribed. Each dose of a single-dose powder is enclosed in an individual container, for example a sachet, a paper packet or a vial.

PRODUCTION

In the manufacture, packaging, storage and distribution of oral powders, suitable means are taken to ensure their microbial quality; recommendations on this aspect are provided in the text on *Microbial Quality of Pharmaceutical Preparations* (*5.1.4*).

TESTS

Fineness If prescribed, the fineness of a powder is determined by the sieve test (*2.9.12*) or another appropriate method.

Uniformity of content (*2.9.6*). Unless otherwise prescribed or justified and authorised, single-dose oral powders with a content of active ingredient less than 2 mg or less than 2 per cent of the total mass comply with test B for *Uniformity of Content of Single-dose Preparations*. If the preparation has more than one active ingredient, the requirement applies only to those ingredients which correspond to the above conditions. The test is not required for multivitamin and trace-element preparations.

Uniformity of mass (*2.9.5*). Single-dose oral powders comply with the test for uniformity of mass of single-dose preparations. If the test for uniformity of content is prescribed for all the active ingredients, the test for uniformity of mass is not required.

STORAGE

Store in a well-closed container or, if the preparation contains volatile ingredients, store in an airtight container.

Effervescent Powders

Effervescent powders are presented as single-dose or multidose powders and generally contain acid substances and carbonates or hydrogen carbonates which react rapidly in the presence of water to release carbon dioxide. They are intended to be dissolved or dispersed in water before administration.

STORAGE

Store in an airtight container.

Ph Eur

Oral Powders of the British Pharmacopoeia

In addition to the above requirements of the European Pharmacopoeia, the following statements apply to those oral powders that are the subject of an individual monograph in the British Pharmacopoeia.

Labelling For single dose containers the label states the name and quantity of active ingredient per container. For multidose containers the label states the name and quantity of active ingredient in a suitable amount by weight.

The label also states (1) the name and proportions of any antimicrobial preservative; (2) the directions for use of the Oral Powder; (3) the date after which the Oral Powder is not intended to be used; (4) the conditions under which the Oral Powder should be stored.

The following oral powders are the subject of an individual monograph in the British Pharmacopoeia.

Compound Magnesium Trisilicate Oral Powder
Oral Rehydration Salts
Sodium Picosulfate Oral Powder
Vigabatrin Oral Powder

PARENTERAL PREPARATIONS

Parenteral Preparations comply with the requirements of the 3rd edition of the European Pharmacopoeia [0520]. These requirements are reproduced after the heading 'Definition' below.

Ph Eur

The requirements of this monograph do not necessarily apply to products derived from human blood, from immunological preparations, radiopharmaceutical preparations or to prostheses to be implanted.

DEFINITION

Parenteral preparations are sterile preparations intended for administration by injection, infusion or implantation into the human or animal body.

Parenteral preparations may require the use of excipients, for example to make the preparation isotonic with blood, to adjust the pH, to increase solubility, to prevent deterioration of the active ingredients or to provide adequate antimicrobial properties but not to adversely affect the intended medicinal action of the preparation or, at the concentrations used, to cause toxicity or undue local irritation.

Containers for parenteral preparations are made as far as possible from materials that are sufficiently transparent to permit the visual inspection of the contents, except for implants and in other justified and authorised cases.

Where applicable, the containers for parenteral preparations comply with the requirements for *Materials Used for the Manufacture of Containers* (*3.1* and subsections) and *Containers* (*3.2* and subsections). Parenteral preparations are supplied in glass containers (*3.2.1*) or in other containers such as plastic containers (*3.2.2, 3.2.7 and 3.2.9*) and prefilled syringes complying with the requirements of the competent authority. The tightness of the container is ensured by suitable means. Closures ensure a good seal, prevent the access of micro-organisms and other contaminants and usually permit the withdrawal of a part or the whole of the contents without removal of the closure. The plastic materials or elastomers (*3.2.9*) of which the closure is composed are sufficiently firm and elastic to allow the passage of a needle with the least possible shedding of particles. Closures for multidose containers are sufficiently elastic to ensure that the puncture is resealed when the needle is withdrawn.

Several categories of parenteral preparations may be distinguished:

— injections,
— intravenous infusions,
— concentrates for injections or intravenous infusions,
— powders for injections or intravenous infusions,
— implants.

PRODUCTION

During the development of a parenteral preparation, the formulation for which contains an antimicrobial preservative, the effectiveness of the chosen preservative shall be demonstrated to the satisfaction of the competent authority. A suitable method of test together with criteria for judging the preservative properties of the formulation are provided under *Efficacy of Antimicrobial Preservation* (*5.1.3*).

Parenteral preparations are prepared using materials and methods designed to ensure sterility and to avoid the introduction of contaminants and the growth of micro-organisms; recommendations on this aspect are provided in the text on *Methods of Preparation of Sterile Products* (*5.1.1*).

Water used in the manufacture of parenteral preparations complies with the requirements of water for injections in bulk stated in the monograph on *Water for injections (169)*.

TESTS

Bacterial endotoxins (*2.6.14*). The test for bacterial endotoxins may replace the test for pyrogens in the following circumstances:

— for a preparation that is the subject of a monograph in the Pharmacopoeia, the test may be prescribed in the monograph,
— in any other cases, the test conditions and the requirements are to be authorised by the competent authority,
— where a test for bacterial endotoxins is prescribed or authorised, a test for pyrogens is not required unless justified by special circumstances.

Sterility (*2.6.1*). Parenteral preparations comply with the test for sterility.

STORAGE

Store in a sterile, airtight, tamper-proof container.

LABELLING

The label states the name and concentration of any added antimicrobial preservative.

Injections

DEFINITION

Injections are sterile solutions, emulsions or suspensions. They are prepared by dissolving, emulsifying or suspending the active ingredient and any added substances in *Water for injections (169)*, in a suitable, sterile non-aqueous liquid or in a mixture of these vehicles.

Solutions for injection, examined under suitable conditions of visibility, are clear and practically free from particles.

Emulsions for injection do not show any evidence of phase separation. Suspensions for injection may show a sediment which is readily dispersed on shaking to give a suspension which remains sufficiently stable to enable the correct dose to be withdrawn.

Single-dose preparations. The volume of the injection in a single-dose container is sufficient to permit the withdrawal and administration of the nominal dose using a normal technique.

Multidose preparations. Multidose aqueous injections contain a suitable antimicrobial preservative at an appropriate concentration except when the preparation itself has adequate antimicrobial properties. When it is necessary to present a preparation for parenteral use in a multidose container, the precautions to be taken for its administration and more particularly for its storage between successive withdrawals are given.

Antimicrobial preservatives. Aqueous preparations which are prepared using aseptic precautions and which cannot be terminally sterilised may contain a suitable antimicrobial preservative in an appropriate concentration.

No antimicrobial preservative is added when:

— the volume to be injected in a single dose exceeds 15 ml, unless otherwise justified,
— the preparation is intended for administration by routes where, for medical reasons, an antimicrobial preservative is not acceptable, such as intracisternally or by any route giving access to the cerebrospinal fluid, or intra-or retro-ocularly.

Such preparations are presented in single-dose containers.

PRODUCTION

In the manufacture of injections containing dispersed particles measures are taken to ensure a suitable and controlled particles size with regard to the intended use.

TESTS

Uniformity of content (*2.9.6*). Unless otherwise prescribed or justified and authorised, single-dose suspensions for injection with a content of active ingredient less than 2 mg or less than 2 per cent of the total mass comply with test A for uniformity of content of single-dose preparations. If the preparation has more than one active ingredient, the requirement applies only to those ingredients that correspond to the above conditions. The test is not required for multivitamin and trace-element preparations.

Pyrogens (*2.6.8*). When the volume to be injected in a single dose is 15 ml or more, and no test for bacterial endotoxins is prescribed or authorised, the preparation complies with the test for pyrogens, unless otherwise justified and authorised. When the volume to be injected in a single dose is less than 15 ml, the label states that the preparation is pyrogen-free and no test for bacterial endotoxins is prescribed or authorised, the preparation complies with the test for pyrogens.

Intravenous Infusions

DEFINITION

Intravenous infusions are sterile, aqueous solutions or emulsions with water as the continuous phase; they are free from pyrogens and are usually made isotonic with blood. They are principally intended for administration in large volume. Intravenous infusions do not contain any added antimicrobial preservative.

Solutions for intravenous infusion, examined under suitable conditions of visibility, are clear and practically free from particles.

Emulsions for intravenous infusion do not show any evidence of phase separation.

PRODUCTION

In the manufacture of intravenous infusions containing dispersed particles measures are taken to ensure a suitable and controlled particle size with regard to the intended use.

The volume of the intravenous infusion in the container is sufficient to permit the withdrawal and administration of the nominal dose using a normal technique (*2.9.17*).

TESTS

Pyrogens (*2.6.8*). When no test for bacterial endotoxins is prescribed or authorised, they comply with the test for pyrogens, unless otherwise justified and authorised. Inject 10 ml per kilogram of body mass into each rabbit, unless otherwise justified and authorised.

Concentrates for Injections or Intravenous Infusions

DEFINITION

Concentrates for injections or intravenous infusions are sterile solutions intended for injection or infusion after dilution. They are diluted to a prescribed volume with a prescribed liquid before administration. After dilution, they comply with the requirements for injections or for intravenous infusions.

TESTS

Pyrogens (*2.6.8*). When no test for bacterial endotoxins is prescribed or authorised, they comply with the test for pyrogens prescribed for injections or for parenteral infusions, as appropriate, after dilution to a suitable volume.

Powders for Injections or Intravenous Infusions

DEFINITION

Powders for injections or intravenous infusions are solid, sterile substances distributed in their final containers and which, when shaken with the prescribed volume of a prescribed sterile liquid, rapidly form either clear and practically particle-free solutions or uniform suspensions. After dissolution or suspension, they comply with the requirements for injections or for intravenous infusions.

Freeze-dried products for parenteral use are considered as powders for injections or intravenous infusions.

TESTS

Uniformity of content (*2.9.6*). Unless otherwise prescribed or justified and authorised, powders for injections or intravenous infusions with a content of active ingredient less than 2 mg or less than 2 per cent of the total mass or with a unit mass equal to or less than 40 mg comply with test A for uniformity of content of single-dose preparations. If the preparation has more than one active ingredient, the requirement applies only to those ingredients that correspond to the above conditions. The test is not required for multivitamin and trace-element preparations.

Uniformity of mass (*2.9.5*). Powders for injections or intravenous infusions comply with the test for uniformity of mass of single-dose preparations. If the test for uniformity of content is prescribed for all the active ingredients, the test for uniformity of mass is not required.

Pyrogens (*2.6.8*). When no test for bacterial endotoxins is prescribed or authorised, they comply with the test for pyrogens prescribed for injections or for intravenous infusions, as appropriate, after dissolution or suspension in a suitable volume of liquid.

Implants

DEFINITION

Implants are sterile, solid preparations of a size and shape suitable for parenteral implantation and release the active ingredients over an extended period of time. They are provided individually in sterile containers.

Ph Eur

Parenteral Preparations of the British Pharmacopoeia

In addition to the above requirements of the European Pharmacopoeia, the following statements apply to any injection, intravenous infusion or implant that is the subject of an individual monograph in the British Pharmacopoeia.

Definition Definition of a particular Parenteral Preparation as a solution, emulsion or suspension in Water for Injections does not preclude the inclusion of suitable excipients where necessary for the purposes referred to in the requirements of the European Pharmacopoeia above. In particular, aqueous Parenteral Preparations for administration by the subcutaneous, intradermal, intramuscular, or, in the case of larger volumes, intravenous route, should if possible be made isotonic with blood by the addition of Sodium Chloride or other suitable substances. However if buffering agents are used in preparations intended for intra-ocular or intracardiac injection, or in preparations that may gain access to the cerebrospinal fluid, great care should be taken to ensure that the nature and concentration of the chosen agent are suitable for the intended route of administration.

Where the active ingredient is susceptible to oxidative degradation appropriate precautions, such as the addition of a suitable antioxidant or storage under oxygen-free nitrogen or other suitable inert gas, should be taken.

Production Methods of sterilisation that may be used in the manufacture of Parenteral Preparations are described in Appendix XVIII.

Where a direction is given to use Water for Injections in the manufacture of a Parenteral Preparation, Water for Injections in bulk is used. Where the use of Water for Injections free from dissolved air or Water for Injections free from dissolved carbon dioxide is specified, water freshly prepared by the process described under Water for Injections is boiled for at least 10 minutes with as little exposure to air as possible, cooled with precautions to exclude air and carbon dioxide, and sterilised by *heating in an autoclave*.

Particulate contamination Where stated in individual monographs, solutions to be injected that are supplied in containers with a nominal content of 100 ml or more comply with the test for *sub-visible particles*, Appendix XIII A.

Storage Closures used for containers of oily parenteral preparations should be made of oil-resistant materials.

Labelling Where appropriate the label states the strength of the parenteral preparation in terms of the amount of active ingredient in a suitable dose-volume.

The label also states (1) the name of any added substance; (2) the date after which the Parenteral Preparation is not intended to be used; (3) the conditions under which the Parenteral Preparation should be stored.

The label of a single-dose parenteral preparation states that any portion of the contents remaining should be discarded.

INTRAVENOUS INFUSIONS

Labelling The label states the nominal volume of the contents.

POWDERS FOR INJECTIONS

Uniformity of weight When required for the Assay of a powder for injection, determine the weight of the contents of 10 containers as described in the test for *uniformity of weight*, Appendix XII G.

Labelling The label states (1) that, when dissolved or suspended, the contents of the sealed container are intended for parenteral use; (2) the amount of active ingredient contained in the sealed container; (3) the directions for the preparation of the Injection or Intravenous Infusion.

If a container of the liquid for constituting the parenteral preparation is supplied with the powder for injections, the label of this container states the composition of this liquid.

CONCENTRATED SOLUTIONS FOR INJECTIONS

Labelling The label states (1) the name of the concentrated solution; (2) that the solution must be diluted before use; (3) the directions for the preparation of the Injection or Intravenous Infusion.

The following parenteral preparations are the subject of an individual monograph in the British Pharmacopoeia. Those distinguished by the symbol in '☆' in the list below are monographs of the European Pharmacopoeia.

Implants

Testosterone Implants

Injections

Acetylcysteine Injection
Adrenaline Injection/Epinephrine Injection
Adrenaline Injection 1 in 10,000, Dilute/Epinephrine Injection 1 in 10,000, Dilute
Aminophylline Injection
Amoxicillin Injection
Ampicillin Injection
Aprotinin Injection
Ascorbic Acid Injection
Atenolol Injection
Atropine Injection
Azlocillin Injection
Benzatropine Injection
Benzylpenicillin Injection
Betamethasone Injection
Bretylium Injection
Bumetanide Injection
Bupivacaine Injection
Bupivacaine and Adrenaline Injection/Bupivacaine and Epinephrine Injection
Calciferol Injection
Calcitonin (Pork) Injection
Calcitonin (Salmon) Injection/Salcatonin Injection
Calcium Gluconate Injection
Capreomycin Injection
Carbenicillin Injection
Cefazolin Injection
Cefotaxime Injection
Cefoxitin Injection
Ceftriaxone Injection
Cefuroxime Injection
Chloramphenicol Sodium Succinate Injection
Chlormethine Injection/Mustine Injection
Chloroquine Sulphate Injection
Chlorphenamine Injection/Chlorpheniramine Injection
Chlorpromazine Injection
Chorionic Gonadotrophin Injection
Cimetidine Injection
Cisplatin Injection
Clindamycin Injection
Clonazepam Injection
Clonidine Injection
Cloxacillin Injection
Colistimethate Injection
Cyanocobalamin Injection
Cyclizine Injection
Cyclophosphamide Injection
Cytarabine Injection
Dacarbazine Injection
Desferrioxamine Injection
Desmopressin Injection
Dextromoramide Injection
Diamorphine Injection
Diazepam Injection
Diazoxide Injection
Digoxin Injection
Digoxin Injection, Paediatric
Dihydrocodeine Injection

Dimercaprol Injection
Dinoprost Injection
Doxapram Injection
Doxorubicin Injection
Droperidol Injection
Edrophonium Injection
Ergometrine Injection
Ergometrine and Oxytocin Injection
Ergotamine Injection
Erythromycin Ethyl Succinate Injection
Estradiol Injection
Etamiphylline Injection
Ethanolamine Oleate Injection
Flucloxacillin Injection
Fluorescein Injection
Fluorouracil Injection
Flupenthixol Injection
Fluphenazine Decanoate Injection
Furosemide Injection/Frusemide Injection
Gallamine Injection
Gentamicin Injection
Glucagon Injection
Gonadorelin Injection
Haloperidol Injection
Heparin Injection
Hyaluronidase Injection
Hydralazine Injection
Hydrocortisone Acetate Injection
Hydrocortisone Sodium Phosphate Injection
Hydrocortisone Sodium Succinate Injection
Hydroxocobalamin Injection
Hydroxyprogesterone Injection
Hyoscine Butylbromide Injection
Hyoscine Injection
Insulin Preparations ☆
Biphasic Insulin Injection ☆
Biphasic Isophane Insulin Injection ☆
Insulin Injection ☆
Insulin Zinc Suspension ☆
Insulin Zinc Suspension (Amorphous) ☆
Insulin Zinc Suspension (Crystalline) ☆
Isophane Insulin Injection ☆
Inulin Injection
Iodised Oil Fluid Injection
Iophendylate Injection
Iron Dextran Injection
Iron Sorbitol Injection
Isoniazid Injection
Isoprenaline Injection
Kanamycin Injection
Ketamine Injection
Labetalol Injection
Lidocaine Injection
Lidocaine and Adrenaline Injection/Lidocaine and Epinephrine Injection
Lorazepam Injection
Lypressin Injection ☆
Magnesium Sulphate Injection
Meglumine Amidotrizoate Injection
Meglumine Iodipamide Injection
Meglumine Iotalamate Injection
Melphalan Injection
Menadiol Phosphate Injection
Menotrophin Injection
Meptazinol Injection
Metaraminol Injection
Methadone Injection
Methohexital Injection
Methotrexate Injection
Methoxamine Injection
Methyldopate Injection
Methylprednisolone Acetate Injection
Metoclopramide Injection
Metoprolol Injection
Mexiletine Injection
Midazolam Injection
Morphine Sulphate Injection
Morphine and Atropine Injection
Naloxone Injection
Naloxone Injection, Neonatal
Nandrolone Decanoate Injection
Nandrolone Phenylpropionate Injection
Neostigmine Injection
Nikethamide Injection
Noradrenaline Injection/Norepinephrine Injection
Oxytocin Injection
Pancuronium Injection
Papaveretum Injection
Paraldehyde Injection
Pentagastrin Injection
Pentamidine Injection
Pentazocine Injection
Pethidine Injection
Phenobarbital Injection
Phenol Injection, Oily
Phenol and Glycerol Injection
Phentolamine Injection
Phenylephrine Injection
Phenytoin Injection
Phytomenadione Injection
Potassium Chloride Concentrate, Sterile
Prilocaine Injection
Procainamide Injection
Procaine Benzylpenicillin Injection/Procaine Penicillin Injection
Procaine Benzylpenicillin Injection, Fortified/Procaine Penicillin Injection, Fortified
Prochlorperazine Injection
Procyclidine Injection
Progesterone Injection
Promazine Injection
Promethazine Injection
Propranolol Injection
Propyliodone Injection
Propyliodone Oily Injection
Protamine Sulphate Injection
Pyridostigmine Injection
Ranitidine Injection
Ritodrine Injection
Salbutamol Injection
Sodium Aurothiomalate Injection
Sodium Amidotrizoate Injection
Sodium Etacrynate Injection
Sodium Iodide Injection
Sodium Iotalamate Injection
Sodium Stibogluconate Injection
Sodium Tetradecyl Sulphate Injection
Sodium Thiosulphate Injection
Somatropin Injection [incorporating Somatropin For Injection ☆]

Sotalol Injection
Spectinomycin Injection
Streptokinase Injection
Streptomycin Injection
Sulfadiazine Injection
Sulfadimidine Injection
Suxamethonium Chloride Injection
Testosterone Propionate Injection
Tetracosactide Injection
Tetracosactide Zinc Injection
Thiamine Injection
Thiopental Injection
Thiotepa Injection
Tobramycin Injection
Tranexamic Acid Injection
Triamcinolone Acetonide Injection
Urofollitropin Injection
Vancomycin Injection
Verapamil Injection
Vinblastine Injection
Vincristine Injection
Vitamins B and C Injection
Zuclopenthixol Acetate Injection
Zuclopenthixol Decanoate Injection

Intravenous Infusions

Aciclovir Intravenous Infusion
Amiodarone Intravenous Infusion
Calcium Chloride Intravenous Infusion
Ciprofloxacin Intravenous Infusion
Clomethiazole Intravenous Infusion
Co-trimoxazole Intravenous Infusion
Dextran 40 Intravenous Infusion
Dextran 70 Intravenous Infusion
Dextran 110 Intravenous Infusion
Disodium Pamidronate Intravenous Infusion
Dopamine Intravenous Infusion
Erythromycin Lactobionate Intravenous Infusion
Foscarnet Intravenous Infusion
Fructose Intravenous Infusion
Glucose Intravenous Infusion
Mannitol Intravenous Infusion
Metronidazole Intravenous Infusion
Potassium Chloride and Glucose Intravenous Infusion
Potassium Chloride and Sodium Chloride Intravenous Infusion
Potassium Chloride, Sodium Chloride and Glucose Intravenous Infusion
Sodium Bicarbonate Intravenous Infusion
Sodium Calcium Edetate Intravenous Infusion
Sodium Chloride and Glucose Intravenous Infusion
Sodium Chloride Intravenous Infusion
Sodium Lactate Intravenous Infusion
Sodium Lactate Intravenous Infusion, Compound
Sodium Nitroprusside Intravenous Infusion
Sorbitol Intravenous Infusion
Tetracycline Intravenous Infusion
Trisodium Edetate Intravenous Infusion

PRESSURISED PHARMACEUTICAL PREPARATIONS

Pressurised Pharmaceutical Preparations comply with the requirements of the 3rd edition of the European Pharmacopoeia [0523]. These requirements are reproduced after the heading 'Definition' below.

Additional requirements for preparations presented in pressurised containers may be found, where appropriate, in other general monographs, for example; Preparations for inhalation (671), Liquids for cutaneous application (927), Topical powders (1166), Nasal preparations (676) and Ear preparations (652).

Ph Eur

DEFINITION

Pressurised pharmaceutical preparations are presented in special containers under pressure of a gas and contain one or more active ingredients. The preparations are released from the container, upon actuation of an appropriate valve, in the form of an aerosol (dispersion of solid or liquid particles in a gas, the size of the particles being adapted to the intended use) or of a liquid or semisolid jet such as a foam. The pressure for the release is generated by suitable propellants. The preparations consist of a solution, an emulsion or a suspension and are intended for local application to the skin or to mucous membranes of various body orifices, or for inhalation. Suitable excipients may also be used, for example solvents, solubilisers, emulsifying agents, suspending agents and lubricants for the valve to prevent clogging.

Propellants. The propellants are either gases liquefied under pressure or compressed gases or low-boiling liquids. Liquefied gases are, for example, fluorinated hydrocarbons and low-molecular-mass hydrocarbons (such as propane and butane). Compressed gases are, for example, carbon dioxide, nitrogen and nitrous oxide.

Mixtures of these propellants may be used to obtain optimal solution properties and desirable pressure, delivery and spray characteristics.

Containers. The containers are tight and resistant to the internal pressure and may be made of metal, glass, plastic or combinations of these materials. They are compatible with their contents. Glass containers are protected with a plastic coating.

Spraying device. The valve keeps the container tightly closed when not in use and regulates the delivery of the contents during use. The spray characteristics are influenced by the type of spraying device, in particular by the dimensions, number and location of orifices. Some valves provide a continuous release, others ("metering dose valves") deliver a defined quantity of product upon each valve actuation.

The various valve materials in contact with the contents are compatible with them.

Requirements for pressurised pharmaceutical preparations Pressurised preparations are provided with a delivery device appropriate for the intended application.

Special requirements may be necessary for the selection of propellants, for particle size and the single-dose delivered by the metering valves.

LABELLING

The label states:
— the method of use,
— any precautions to be taken,
— for a container with a metering dose valve, the amount of active ingredient in a unit-spray.

Ph Eur

RECTAL PREPARATIONS

Rectal preparations comply with the requirements of the 3rd edition of the European Pharmacopoeia [1145]. These requirements are reproduced after the heading 'Definition' below.

Ph Eur

DEFINITION

Rectal preparations are intended for rectal use in order to obtain a systemic or local effect, or they may be intended for diagnostic purposes.

Where applicable, containers for rectal preparations comply with the requirements for *Materials Used for the Manufacture of Containers* (*3.1* and subsections) and *Containers* (*3.2* and subsections).

Several categories of rectal preparations may be distinguished:
— suppositories,
— rectal capsules,
— rectal solutions and suspensions,
— powders and tablets for rectal solutions and suspensions,
— semi-solid rectal preparations,
— rectal foams,
— rectal tampons.

PRODUCTION

During the development of a rectal preparation, the formulation for which contains an antimicrobial preservative, the effectiveness of the chosen preservative shall be demonstrated to the satisfaction of the competent authority. A suitable method of test together with criteria for judging the preservative properties of the formulation are provided in the text on *Efficacy of Antimicrobial Preservation* (*5.1.3*).

In the manufacture, packaging, storage and distribution of rectal preparations, suitable means are taken to ensure their microbial quality; recommendations on this aspect are provided in the text on *Microbial Quality of Pharmaceutical Preparations* (*5.1.4*).

In the manufacture of semi-solid and liquid rectal prparations containing dispersed particles measures are taken to ensure a suitable and controlled particle size with regard to the intended use.

TESTS

Uniformity of content (*2.9.6*). Unless otherwise prescribed or justified and authorised, solid single-dose preparations with a content of active ingredient less than 2 mg or less than 2 per cent of the total mass comply with test A (tablets) or test B (suppositories, rectal capsules) for uniformity of content of single-dose preparations. If the preparation contains more than one active ingredient, this requirement applies only to those ingredients that correspond to the above conditions.

Uniformity of mass (*2.9.5*). Solid, single-dose preparations comply with the test for uniformity of mass. If the test for uniformity of content is prescribed for all active ingredients, the test for uniformity of mass is not required.

Dissolution A suitable test may be required to demonstrate the appropriate release of the active ingredient(s) from solid, single-dose preparations, for example the dissolution test for suppositories and soft capsules (*2.9.3*).

Where a dissolution test is prescribed, a disintegration test may not be required.

LABELLING

The label states the name of any added antimicrobial preservative.

Suppositories

DEFINITION

Suppositories are solid, single-dose preparations. The shape, volume and consistence of suppositories are suitable for rectal administration.

They contain one or more active ingredients dispersed or dissolved in a simple or compound excipient which may be soluble or dispersible in water or may melt at body temperature. Excipients such as diluents, adsorbents, surface-active agents, lubricants, antimicrobial preservatives and colouring matter, authorised by the competent authority, may be added if necessary.

PRODUCTION

Suppositories are prepared by compression or moulding. If necessary, the active ingredient(s) are previously ground and sieved through a suitable sieve. When prepared by moulding, the medicated mass, sufficiently liquefied by heating, is poured into suitable moulds. The suppository solidifies on cooling. Various excipients are available for this process, such as hard fat, macrogols, cocoa butter, and various gelatinous mixtures consisting, for example, of gelatin, water and glycerol.

A suitable test is carried out to demonstrate the appropriate release of the active ingredient(s) from suppositories intended for modified release or for prolonged local action.

TESTS

Disintegration Unless intended for modified release or for prolonged local action, they comply with the test for disintegration of suppositories and pessaries (*2.9.2*). For suppositories with a fatty base, examine after 30 min and for suppositories with a water-soluble base after 60 min, unless otherwise justified and authorised.

STORAGE

Store in a well-closed container.

Rectal Capsules

DEFINITION

Rectal capsules (shell suppositories) are solid, single-dose preparations generally similar to soft capsules as defined in the monograph on *Capsules* (*16*) except that they may have lubricating coatings. They are of elongated shape, are smooth and have a uniform external appearance.

PRODUCTION

A suitable test is carried out to demonstrate the appropriate release of the active ingredient(s) from rectal capsules intended for modified release or for prolonged local action.

TESTS

Disintegration Unless intended for modified release or for prolonged local action, they comply with the test for disintegration of suppositories and pessaries (*2.9.2*). Examine the state of the capsules after 30 min, unless otherwise justified and authorise.

Rectal Solutions and Suspensions

DEFINITION

Rectal solutions and suspensions (enemas) are liquid preparations intended for rectal use in order to obtain a systemic or local effect, or they may be intended for diagnostic purposes.

They are single-dose preparations containing one or more active ingredients dissolved or dispersed in water, glycerol or macrogols. Suspensions may show sediment which is readily dispersible on shaking to give a suspension which remains sufficiently stable to enable the correct dose to be delivered.

Rectal solutions and suspensions may contain excipients, for example to adjust the viscosity of the preparation, to adjust or stabilise pH, to increase the solubility of the active ingredient(s) or to stabilise the preparation. These substances do not adversely affect the intended medical action or, at the concentrations used, cause undue local irritation.

Rectal solutions and suspensions are supplied in containers containing a volume in the range of 2.5 ml to 2000 ml. The container is adapted to deliver the preparation to the rectum or it is accompanied by a suitable applicator.

TESTS

Uniformity of content (*2.9.6*). Unless otherwise prescribed or justified and authorised, rectal suspensios comply wit the following test: Empty each container as completely as possible and arry out the test on the individual contents. They comply with test B

Uniformity of mass Rectal solutions comply with the following test: Weigh individually the contents of twenty containers emptied as completely as possible, and determine the average mass. For containers weighing not more than 100 g, not more than two of the individual masses deviate by more than 10 per cent from the average mass and none deviates by more than 20 per cent. For containers weighing more than 100 g, not more than two of the individual masses deviate by more than 5 per cent from the average mass and none deviates by more than 10 per cent.

Powders and Tablets for Rectal Solutions and Suspensions

DEFINITION

Powders and tablets intended for the preparation of rectal solutions or suspensions are single-dose preparations which are dissolved or dispersed in water at the time of administration. They may contain excipients to facilitate dissolution or dispersion or to prevent aggregation of the particles.

After dissolution or suspension, they comply with the requirements for rectal solutions or rectal suspensions, as appropriate.

TESTS

Disintegration Tablets for rectal solutions or suspensions disintegrate within 3 min when tested according to the test for disintegration of tablets and capsules (*2.9.1*) but using *water R* at 15°C to 25°C.

LABELLING

The label states:

— the method of preparation of the rectal solution or suspension,

— the conditions and duration of storage of the solution or suspension after constitution.

Semi-Solid Rectal Preparations

DEFINITION

Semi-solid rectal preparations are ointments, creams or gels.

They are often supplied as single-dose preparations in containers provided with a suitable applicator.

Semi-solid rectal preparations comply with the requirements in the monograph on *Topical semi-solid preparations (132)*.

Rectal Foams

DEFINITION

Rectal foams are comply with the requirements in the monograph on *Medicated foams (1105)*.

Rectal Tampons

DEFINITION

Rectal tampons are solid, single-dose preparations intended to be inserted into the lower part of the rectum for a limited time.

They comply with the requirements in the monograph on *Medicated tampons (1155)*.

Ph Eur

Rectal Preparations of the British Pharmacopoeia

In addition to the above requirements of the European Pharmacopoeia, the following statements apply to any enema, rectal solution or suppositories that is the subject of an individual monograph in the British Pharmacopoeia.

ENEMAS

Labelling The label states (1) the names and concentrations of the active ingredients; (2) that the preparation should not be swallowed; (3) the date after which the Enema is not intended to be used; (4) the conditions under which the Enema should be stored; (5) the directions for using the Enema.

RECTAL SOLUTIONS

Labelling The label states (1) the names and concentrations of the active ingredients; (2) that the preparation should not be swallowed; (3) the date after which the

Rectal Solution is not intended to be used; (4) the conditions under which the Rectal Solution should be stored; (5) the directions for using the Rectal Solution.

SUPPOSITORIES

Labelling The label states (1) the names and concentrations of the active ingredients; (2) that the preparation should not be swallowed; (3) the date after which the Suppositories are not intended to be used; (4) the conditions under which the Suppositories should be stored.

The following rectal preparations are the subject of an individual monograph in the British Pharmacopoeia.

Enemas
Arachis Oil Enema
Phosphates Enema
Prednisolone Enema

Rectal Solutions
Diazepam Rectal Solution

Suppositories
Bisacodyl Suppositories
Chlorpromazine Suppositories
Etamiphylline Suppositories
Glycerol Suppositories
Indometacin Suppositories
Metronidazole Suppositories
Morphine Suppositories
Naproxen Suppositories
Pentazocine Suppositories

SPIRITS

Definition Spirits are solutions of one or more substances in Ethanol (96 per cent) or a Dilute Ethanol. They may contain a proportion of Water.

Storage Spirits should be kept in well-closed containers of glass or other suitable materials and stored at temperatures not exceeding 25°.

Labelling The label states (1) the date after which the Spirit is not intended to be used; (2) the conditions under which the Spirit should be stored.

The following spirits are the subject of an individual monograph in the British Pharmacopoeia.

Ammonia Spirit, Aromatic
Benzaldehyde Spirit
Chloroform Spirit
Lemon Spirit
Orange Spirit, Compound
Peppermint Spirit
Soap Spirit
Surgical Spirit

STICKS

Sticks comply with the requirements of the 3rd edition of the European Pharmacopoeia [1154]. These requirements are reproduced after the heading 'Definition' below.

Ph Eur

Additional requirements for sticks may be found, where appropriate, in other general monographs, for example in the monograph on Nasal preparations (676).

DEFINITION

Sticks are solid preparations intended for local application. They are rod-shaped or conical preparations consisting of one or more active ingredients alone or which are dissolved or dispersed in a simple or compound excipient which may dissolve or melt at body temperature.

Urethral sticks and sticks for insertion into wounds are sterile.

PRODUCTION

In the manufacture, packaging, storage and distribution of sticks, suitable means are taken to ensure their microbial quality; recommendations on this aspect are provided in the text on *Microbial Quality of Pharmaceutical Preparations (5.1.4)*.

Urethral sticks and other sterile sticks are prepared using materials and methods designed to ensure sterility; recommendations on this aspect are provided in the text on *Methods of Preparation of Sterile Products (5.1.1)*.

In the manufacture of sticks means are taken to ensure that the preparation complies with a test for mass uniformity or, where appropriate, a test for uniformity of content.

TESTS

Sterility (*2.6.1*). Urethral sticks and sticks for insertion into wounds comply with the test for sterility.

LABELLING

The label states:
— the quantity of active ingredient(s) per stick,
— for urethral sticks and sticks to be inserted into wounds that they are sterile.

Ph Eur

SYRUPS

Definition Syrups are concentrated aqueous solutions of Sucrose, other sugars or sweetening agents, to which small quantities of suitable polyhydric alcohols may be added to retard crystallisation or to increase the solubility of the other ingredients. Syrups usually contain aromatic or other flavouring materials. They do not usually contain active ingredients. They should be recently prepared unless they contain suitable antimicrobial preservatives.

Storage Syrups should be kept in well-closed containers and stored at temperatures not exceeding 30°.

Labelling The label states (1) the date after which the Syrup is not intended to be used; (2) the conditions under which the Syrup should be stored.

The following syrups are the subject of an individual monograph in the British Pharmacopoeia.

Black Currant Syrup
Invert Syrup
Lemon Syrup
Orange Syrup
Syrup
Tolu Syrup

TABLETS

Tablets comply with the requirements of the 3rd edition of the European Pharmacopoeia [0478]. These requirements are reproduced after the heading 'Definition' below.

Ph Eur

The requirements of this monograph do not necessarily apply to preparations that are presented as tablets intended for use other than by oral administration. Requirements for such preparations may be found, where appropriate, in other general monographs, for example; Rectal preparations (1145) and Vaginal preparations (1164).

DEFINITION

Tablets are solid preparations each containing a single dose of one or more active ingredients and obtained by compressing uniform volumes of particles. They are intended for oral administration. Some are swallowed whole, some after being chewed, some are dissolved or dispersed in water before being administered and some are retained in the mouth where the active ingredient is liberated.

The particles consist of one or more active ingredients with or without excipients such as diluents, binders, disintegrating agents, glidants, lubricants, substances capable of modifying the behaviour of the preparations in the digestive tract, colouring matter authorised by the competent authority and flavouring substances.

Tablets are usually right, circular solid cylinders, the end surfaces of which are flat or convex and the edges of which may be bevelled. They may have lines or break-marks and may bear a symbol or other markings. Tablets may be coated.

Where applicable, containers for tablets comply with the requirements for *Materials used for the manufacture of containers* (*3.1* and subsections) and *Containers* (*3.2* and subsections).

Several categories of tablets for oral use may be distinguished:
— uncoated tablets,
— coated tablets,
— effervescent tablets,
— soluble tablets,
— dispersible tablets,
— gastro-resistant tablets,
— modified-release tablets,
— tablets for use in the mouth.

PRODUCTION

Tablets are prepared by compressing uniform volumes of particles or particle aggregates produced by granulation methods. In the manufacture of tablet cores, means are taken to ensure that they possess a suitable mechanical strength to resist handling without crumbling or breaking. This may be demonstrated by examining the *Friability of uncoated tablets* (*2.9.7*) and the *Resistance to crushing* (*2.9.8*). Chewable tablets are prepared to ensure that they are easily crushed by chewing.

In the manufacture, packaging, storage and distribution of tablets, suitable means are taken to ensure their microbial quality; recommendations on this aspect are provided in the text on *Microbiological quality of pharmaceutical preparations* (*5.1.4*).

TESTS

Uniformity of content (*2.9.6*). Unless otherwise prescribed or justified and authorised, tablets with a content of active ingredient less than 2 mg or less than 2 per cent of the total mass comply with test A for uniformity of content of single-dose preparations. If the preparation has more than one active ingredient, the requirement applies only to those ingredients which correspond to the above conditions. The test is not required for multivitamin and trace-element preparations.

Uniformity of mass (*2.9.5*). Uncoated tablets and, unless otherwise justified and authorised, film-coated tablets comply with the test for uniformity of mass of single-dose preparations. If the test for uniformity of content is prescribed for all the active ingredients, the test for uniformity of mass is not required.

Dissolution. A suitable test may be carried out to demonstrate the appropriate release of the active ingredient(s), for example one of the tests described in *Dissolution test for solid dosage forms* (*2.9.3*).

Where a dissolution test is prescribed, a disintegration test may not be required.

STORAGE

Store in well-closed container, protected from crushing and mechanical shock.

Uncoated Tablets

DEFINITION

Uncoated tablets include single-layer tablets resulting from a single compression of particles and multi-layer tablets consisting of concentric or parallel layers obtained by successive compression of particles of different composition. The excipients used are not specifically intended to modify the release of the active ingredient in the digestive fluids.

Uncoated tablets conform to the general definition of tablets. A broken section, when examined under a lens, shows either a relatively uniform texture (single-layer tablets) or a stratified texture (multi-layer tablets) but no signs of coating.

TESTS

Disintegration. Uncoated tablets comply with the test for disintegration of tablets and capsules (*2.9.1*). Use *water R* as the liquid. Add a disc to each tube. Operate the apparatus for 15 min, unless otherwise justified and authorised, and examine the state of the tablets. If the tablets fail to comply because of adherence to the discs, repeat the test on a further six tablets omitting the discs. The tablets comply with the test if all six have disintegrated.

Chewable tablets are not required to comply with the test.

Coated Tablets

DEFINITION

Coated tablets are tablets covered with one or more layers of mixtures of various substances such as natural or synthetic resins, gums, gelatin, inactive and insoluble fillers, sugars, plasticisers, polyols, waxes, colouring matter authorised by the competent authority and sometimes flavouring substances and active ingredients. The substances used as coatings are usually applied as a solution or suspension in conditions in which evaporation of the vehicle occurs. When the coating is a very thin polymeric coating, the tablets are known as film-coated tablets.

Coated tablets have a smooth surface which is often coloured and may be polished; a broken section, when examined under a lens, shows a core surrounded by one or more continuous layers with a different texture.

TESTS

Disintegration. Coated tablets other than film-coated tablets comply with the test for disintegration of tablets and capsules (*2.9.1*). Use *water R* as the liquid. Add a disc to each tube. Operate the apparatus for 60 min, unless otherwise justified and authorised, and examine the state of the tablets. If any of the tablets has not disintegrated, repeat the test on a further six tablets, replacing *water R* in the beaker with *0.1M hydrochloric acid.* The tablets comply with the test if all six have disintegrated in the acid medium.

Film-coated tablets comply with the disintegration test prescribed for uncoated tablets except that the apparatus is operated for 30 min, unless otherwise justified and authorised.

If coated tablets or film-coated tablets fail to comply because of adherence to the discs, repeat the test on a further six tablets omitting the discs. The tablets comply with the test if all six have disintegrated.

Chewable coated tablets are not required to comply with the test.

Effervescent Tablets

DEFINITION

Effervescent tablets are uncoated tablets generally containing acid substances and carbonates or hydrogen carbonates which react rapidly in the presence of water to release carbon dioxide. They are intended to be dissolved or dispersed in water before administration.

TESTS

Disintegration. Place a tablet in a beaker containing 200 ml of *water R* at 15°C to 25°C; numerous bubbles of gas are evolved. When the evolution of gas around the tablet or its fragments ceases the tablet has disintegrated, being either dissolved or dispersed in the water so that no agglomerates of particles remain. Repeat the operation on five other tablets. The tablets comply with the test if each of the six tablets used disintegrates in the manner prescribed within 5 min, unless otherwise justified and authorised.

Soluble Tablets

DEFINITION

Soluble tablets are uncoated or film-coated tablets. They are intended to be dissolved in water before administration. The solution produced may be slightly opalescent due to the added substances used in the manufacture of the tablets.

TESTS

Disintegration. Soluble tablets disintegrate within 3 min when examined by the test for disintegration of tablets and capsules (*2.9.1*), using *water R* at 15°C to 25°C.

Dispersible Tablets

DEFINITION

Dispersible tablets are uncoated or film-coated tablets intended to be dispersed in water before administration giving a homogeneous dispersion.

TESTS

Disintegration. Dispersible tablets disintegrate within 3 min when examined by the test for disintegration of tablets and capsules (*2.9.1*), using *water R* at 15°C to 25°C.

Fineness of dispersion. Place two tablets in 100 ml of *water R* and stir until completely dispersed. A smooth dispersion is produced, which passes through a sieve screen with a nominal mesh aperture of 710 µm.

Gastro-Resistant Tablets

DEFINITION

Gastro-resistant tablets are modified release tablets that are intended to resist the gastric fluid and to release their active ingredient(s) in the intestinal fluid. They are prepared by covering tablets with a gastro-resistant coating (enteric-coated tablets) or from granules or particles already covered with a gastro-resistant coating.

Tablets covered with a gastro-resistant coating conform to the definition of coated tablets.

PRODUCTION

For tablets prepared from granules or particles already covered with a gastro-resistant coating, a suitable test is carried out to demonstrate the appropriate release of the active ingredient(s).

TESTS

Disintegration. For tablets covered with a gastro-resistant coating carry out the test for disintegration (*2.9.1*) with the following modifications. Use 0.1M *hydrochloric acid* as the liquid. Operate the apparatus for 2 h, or other such time as may be authorised, without the discs and examine the state of the tablets. The time of resistance to the acid medium varies according to the formulation of the tablets to be examined. It is typically 2 h to 3 h but even with authorised deviations is not less than 1 h. No tablet shows signs of either disintegration (apart from fragments of coating) or cracks that would allow the escape of the contents. Replace the acid by *phosphate buffer solution pH 6.8 R* and add a disc each tube. Operate the apparatus for 60 min and examine the state of the tablets. If the tablets fail to comply because of adherence to the discs, repeat the test on a further six tablets omitting the discs. The tablets comply with the test if all six have disintegrated.

Modified-Release Tablets

DEFINITION

Modified-release tablets are coated or uncoated tablets containing special excipients or prepared by special procedures which, separately or together, are designed to modify the rate or the place at which the active ingredient(s) are released.

PRODUCTION

A suitable test is carried out to demonstrate the appropriate release of the active ingredient(s).

Tables for Use in the Mouth

DEFINITION

Tablets for use in the mouth are usually uncoated tablets.

They are formulated to effect a slow release and local action of the active ingredient(s) or the release and absorption of the active ingredient or ingredients at a defined part of the mouth.

Ph Eur

Tablets of the British Pharmacopoeia

In addition to the above requirements of the European Pharmacopoeia, the following statements apply to those tablets that are the subject of an individual monograph in the British Pharmacopoeia.

Definition Unless otherwise stated in the individual monograph, tablets of the British Pharmacopoeia are solid, right circular cylinders the end surfaces of which are flat or convex and the edges of which may be bevelled.

Tablets of the British Pharmacopoeia may contain flavouring only when indicated in the individual monograph.

Tablets that are the subject of individual monographs in the British Pharmacopoeia may be uncoated, compression-coated, film-coated or sugar-coated unless otherwise indicated in the monograph. Tablets for which the monograph states 'They are coated' are compression-coated or film-coated or sugar-coated. Tablets may be made gastro-resistant by enteric-coating or by other means only where this is specifically indicated in the monograph. When presented as coated formulations it may be necessary to remove the coating before performing the Assay and tests described in the monograph.

In preparing Tablets for which Chocolate Basis is specified, the active ingredient may be incorporated with a mixture of 15 parts of non-alkalinised cocoa powder of commerce, 15 parts of Sucrose and 70 parts of Lactose.

Content of active ingredient of tablets The range for the content of active ingredient stated in the monograph is based on the requirement that 20 tablets, or such other number as may be indicated in the monograph, are used in the Assay. In circumstances where 20 tablets cannot be obtained, a smaller number, which must not be less than five, may be used, but to allow for sampling errors the tolerances are widened in accordance with Table I.

The requirements of Table I apply when the stated limits are 90 to 110%. For limits other than 90 to 110%, proportionately smaller or larger allowances should be made.

Disintegration For those Uncoated or Coated Tablets for which a requirement for Dissolution is included in the individual monograph, the requirement for Disintegration does not apply.

Uniformity of content Details of the analytical method to be employed for determining the content of active ingredient may be included in certain monographs. Unless otherwise stated in the monograph the limits are as given in the test for *Uniformity of content*, AppendixXII H.

Any tablets that when examined individually show a gross deviation from the prescribed or stated content are not official.

Labelling The label states (1) the quantity of the active ingredient contained in each tablet; (2) 'enteric-coated' for tablets coated in this manner; (3) the date after which the Tablets are not intended to be used; (4) the conditions under which the Tablets should be stored.

The following tablets are the subject of an individual monograph in the British Pharmacopoeia.

Acenocoumarol Tablets
Acetazolamide Tablets
Aciclovir Tablets
Alimemazine Tablets/Trimeprazine Tablets
Allopurinol Tablets
Aloxiprin Tablets
Aluminium Hydroxide Tablets
Amiloride Tablets
Aminophylline Tablets
Amiodarone Tablets
Amitriptyline Tablets
Ascorbic Acid Tablets
Aspirin and Caffeine Tablets
Aspirin Tablets
Aspirin Tablets, Dispersible
Aspirin Tablets, Effervescent Soluble
Atenolol Tablets
Atropine Tablets
Azapropazone Tablets
Azathioprine Tablets
Baclofen Tablets
Bendroflumethiazide Tablets/Bendrofluazide Tablets
Benorilate Tablets
Benzatropine Tablets
Betamethasone Sodium Phosphate Tablets
Betamethasone Tablets
Bisacodyl Tablets
Bromocriptine Tablets
Brompheniramine Tablets
Bumetanide Tablets
Bumetanide and Slow Potassium Tablets
Busulfan Tablets
Calciferol Tablets
Calcium Gluconate Tablets

TABLE I

Weight of active ingredient in each tablet	Subtract from the lower limit for samples of			Add to the upper limit for samples of		
	15	10	5	15	10	5
0.12 g or less	0.2	0.7	1.6	0.3	0.8	1.8
More than 0.12 and less than 0.3 g	0.2	0.5	1.2	0.3	0.6	1.5
0.3 g or more	0.1	0.2	0.8	0.2	0.4	1.0

Calcium Gluconate Tablets, Effervescent
Calcium Lactate Tablets
Captopril Tablets
Carbamazepine Tablets
Carbimazole Tablets
Cascara Tablets
Cefuroxime Axetil Tablets
Cefalexin Tablets
Chlorambucil Tablets
Chlordiazepoxide Hydrochloride Tablets
Chloroquine Phosphate Tablets
Chloroquine Sulphate Tablets
Chlorothiazide Tablets
Chlorphenamine Tablets/Chlorpheniramine Tablets
Chlorpromazine Tablets
Chlorpropamide Tablets
Chlortalidone Tablets
Choline Theophyllinate Tablets
Cimetidine Tablets
Ciprofloxacin Tablets
Clemastine Tablets
Clomifene Tablets
Clonidine Tablets
Co-amilofruse Tablets
Co-amilozide Tablets
Co-amoxiclav Tablets
Co-careldopa Tablets
Co-codamol Tablets
Co-codaprin Tablets
Co-codaprin Tablets, Dispersible
Co-dergocrine Tablets
Co-dydramol Tablets
Co-magaldrox Tablets
Co-proxamol Tablets
Co-tenidone Tablets
Co-triamterzide Tablets
Co-trimoxazole Tablets
Co-trimoxazole Tablets, Dipersible
Co-trimoxazole Tablets, Paediatric
Codeine Phosphate Tablets
Colchicine Tablets
Colistin Tablets
Cortisone Tablets
Cyanocobalamin Tablets
Cyclizine Tablets
Cyclopenthiazide Tablets
Cyclophosphamide Tablets
Cyproheptadine Tablets
Dapsone Tablets
Debrisoquine Tablets
Desipramine Tablets
Dexamethasone Tablets
Dexamfetamine Tablets
Dextromoramide Tablets
Diazepam Tablets
Diazoxide Tablets
Dichlorophen Tablets
Diclofenac Tablets
Diclofenac Tablets, Slow
Dicycloverine Tablets/Dicyclomine Tablets
Diethylstilbestrol Tablets
Diflunisal Tablets
Digitoxin Tablets
Digoxin Tablets
Dihydrocodeine Tablets
Diloxanide Tablets
Dimenhydrinate Tablets
Dipipanone and Cyclizine Tablets
Dipyridamole Tablets
Disulfiram Tablets
Docusate Tablets
Dosulepin Tablets/Dothiepin Tablets
Droperidol Tablets
Dydrogesterone Tablets
Ephedrine Hydrochloride Tablets
Ergometrine Tablets
Erythromycin Ethyl Succinate Tablets
Erythromycin Stearate Tablets
Erythromycin Tablets
Estropipate Tablets
Etacrynic Acid Tablets
Ethambutol Tablets
Ethinylestradiol Tablets
Ethylestrenol Tablets
Etodolac Tablets
Fenbufen Tablets
Fenoprofen Tablets
Ferrous Fumarate and Folic Acid Tablets
Ferrous Fumarate Tablets
Ferrous Gluconate Tablets
Ferrous Sulphate Tablets
Flavoxate Tablets
Flucytosine Tablets
Fludrocortisone Tablets
Fluphenazine Tablets
Flurbiprofen Tablets
Fluvoxamine Tablets
Folic Acid Tablets
Furosemide Tablets/Frusemide Tablets
Gemfibrozil Tablets
Glibenclamide Tablets
Gliclazide Tablets
Glipizide Tablets
Gliquidone Tablets
Glyceryl Trinitrate Tablets
Griseofulvin Tablets
Guanethidine Tablets
Haloperidol Tablets
Hydralazine Tablets
Hydrochlorothiazide Tablets
Hydroflumethiazide Tablets
Hydrotalcite Tablets
Hydroxychloroquine Tablets
Hyoscine Butylbromide Tablets
Hyoscine Tablets
Ibuprofen Tablets
Imipramine Tablets
Indoramin Tablets
Inositol Nicotinate Tablets
Iopanoic Acid Tablets
Isoniazid Tablets
Isosorbide Dinitrate Tablets
Labetalol Tablets
Levodopa Tablets
Levonorgestrel and Ethinylestradiol Tablets
Levothyroxine Tablets
Liothyronine Tablets
Lithium Carbonate Tablets
Lithium Carbonate Tablets, Slow
Loprazolam Tablets
Lorazepam Tablets
Lormetazepam Tablets
Magnesium Trisilicate Tablets, Compound
Mebeverine Tablets

Megestrol Tablets
Melphalan Tablets
Menadiol Phosphate Tablets
Meptazinol Tablets
Mepyramine Tablets
Mercaptopurine Tablets
Metformin Tablets
Methadone Tablets
Methotrexate Tablets
Methylcellulose Tablets
Methyldopa Tablets
Methylprednisolone Tablets
Methysergide Tablets
Metoclopramide Tablets
Metoprolol Tartrate Tablets
Metronidazole Tablets
Mianserin Tablets
Minocycline Tablets
Mitobronitol Tablets
Morphine Tablets
Moxisylyte Tablets/Thymoxamine Tablets
Nabumetone Tablets
Nalidixic Acid Tablets
Naproxen Tablets
Neomycin Tablets
Neostigmine Tablets
Niclosamide Tablets
Nicotinamide Tablets
Nicotinic Acid Tablets
Nicotinyl Alcohol Tablets
Nitrazepam Tablets
Nitrofurantoin Tablets
Norethisterone Tablets
Nortriptyline Tablets
Nystatin Tablets
Orciprenaline Tablets
Orphenadrine Hydrochloride Tablets
Oxazepam Tablets
Oxprenolol Tablets
Oxymetholone Tablets
Oxytetracycline Tablets
Pancreatin Tablets
Paracetamol Tablets
Paracetamol Tablets, Dispersible
Paracetamol Tablets, Soluble
Penicillamine Tablets
Pentaerythritol Tetranitrate Tablets
Pentazocine Tablets
Pentobarbital Tablets
Perphenazine Tablets
Pethidine Tablets
Phenelzine Tablets
Phenindamine Tablets
Phenindione Tablets
Phenobarbital Sodium Tablets
Phenobarbital Tablets
Phenoxymethylpenicillin Tablets
Phenytoin Tablets
Phytomenadione Tablets
Pindolol Tablets
Piperazine Phosphate Tablets
Pizotifen Tablets
Poldine Tablets
Polythiazide Tablets
Potassium Chloride Tablets, Effervescent
Potassium Chloride Tablets, Slow
Potassium Iodate Tablets
Prazosin Tablets
Prednisolone Tablets
Prednisolone Tablets, Enteric-coated
Prednisone Tablets
Primidone Tablets
Probenecid Tablets
Procainamide Tablets
Prochlorperazine Tablets
Procyclidine Tablets
Proguanil Tablets
Promazine Tablets
Promethazine Hydrochloride Tablets
Promethazine Teoclate Tablets
Propantheline Tablets
Propranolol Tablets
Propylthiouracil Tablets
Protriptyline Tablets
Pseudoephedrine Tablets
Pyrazinamide Tablets
Pyridostigmine Tablets
Pyridoxine Tablets
Pyrimethamine Tablets
Quinidine Sulphate Tablets
Quinine Bisulphate Tablets
Quinine Sulphate Tablets
Ranitidine Tablets
Ritodrine Tablets
Salbutamol Tablets
Senna Tablets
Sodium Bicarbonate Tablets, Compound
Sodium Chloride Tablets
Sodium Citrate Tablets
Sodium Valproate Tablets
Sodium Valproate Tablets, Enteric-coated
Sotalol Tablets
Spironolactone Tablets
Stanozolol Tablets
Sulindac Tablets
Sulfadimidine Tablets
Sulfinpyrazone Tablets
Tamoxifen Tablets
Terbutaline Tablets
Tetracycline Tablets
Thiamine Tablets
Thioridazine Tablets
Tiabendazole Tablets
Timolol Tablets
Tioguanine Tablets
Tocopheryl Succinate Tablets, Alpha
Tolazamide Tablets
Tolbutamide Tablets
Tranexamic Acid Tablets
Tranylcypromine Tablets
Triamcinolone Tablets
Trifluoperazine Tablets
Trihexyphenidyl Tablets/Benzhexol Tablets
Trimethoprim Tablets
Trimipramine Tablets
Triprolidine Tablets
Verapamil Tablets
Vigabatrin Tablets
Warfarin Tablets
Zuclopenthixol Tablets

Lozenges

Amphotericin Lozenges

MEDICATED TAMPONS

Medicated tampons comply with the requirements of the 3rd edition of the European Pharmacopoeia [1155]. These requirements are reproduced after the heading 'Definition' below.

Ph Eur

Additional requirements for medicated tampons may be found, where appropriate, in other general monographs, for example; Rectal preparations (1145), Vaginal preparations (1164), and Ear preparations (652).

DEFINITION

Medicated tampons are solid, single-dose preparations intended to be inserted into the body cavities for a limited period of time. They consist of a suitable material such as cellulose, collagen or silicone impregnated with one or more active ingredients.

PRODUCTION

In the manufacture, packaging, storage and distribution of medicated tampons, suitable means are taken to ensure their microbial quality; recommendations on this aspect are provided in the text on *Microbial Quality of Pharmaceutical Preparations (5.1.4)*.

LABELLING

The label states the quantity of active ingredient(s) per tampon.

Ph Eur

TINCTURES

Tinctures comply with the requirements of the 3rd edition of the European Pharmacopoeia [0792]. These requirements are reproduced after the heading 'Definition' below.

Ph Eur

DEFINITION

Tinctures are liquid preparations usually obtained from dried vegetable or animal matter. For some preparations, the matter to be extracted may undergo a preliminary treatment, for example, inactivation of enzymes, grinding or defatting.

Tinctures are prepared by maceration, percolation or other suitable, validated methods, using alcohol of suitable concentration. Tinctures may also be obtained by dissolving or diluting extracts in alcohol of suitable concentration.

Tinctures are usually obtained using either 1 part of drug and 10 parts of extraction solvent or 1 part of drug and 5 parts of extraction solvent. Tinctures are usually clear. A slight sediment may form on standing and that is acceptable as long as the composition is not changed significantly.

PRODUCTION

Production by percolation If necessary, reduce the matter to be extracted to pieces of suitable size. Mix thoroughly with a portion of the prescribed extraction solvent and allow to stand for an appropriate time. Transfer to a percolator and allow the percolate to flow slowly making sure that the matter to be extracted is always covered with the remaining extraction solvent. The residue may be pressed out and the expressed fluid combined with the percolate.

Production by maceration Unless otherwise prescribed, reduce the matter to be extracted to pieces of suitable size, mix thoroughly with the prescribed extraction solvent and allow to stand in a closed container for an appropriate time. The residue is separated from the extraction solvent and, if necessary, pressed out. In the latter case, the two liquids obtained are combined.

Production from extracts The tincture is prepared by dissolving or diluting an extract, using alcohol of appropriate concentration. The content of alcohol and constituents or, where applicable, the content of alcohol and of dry residue correspond to that of tinctures obtained by maceration or percolation.

Adjustment of the constituents Adjustment of the content of constituents may be carried out, if necessary, either by adding the extraction solvent of suitable concentration or by adding another tincture of the vegetable or animal matter used for the preparation.

TESTS

Relative density *(2.2.5)*. Where applicable, the tincture complies with the limits prescribed in the monograph.

Ethanol content *(2.9.10)*. The ethanol content complies with that prescribed.

Methanol and 2-propanol *(2.9.11)*. Not more than 0.05 per cent *V/V* methanol and not more than 0.05 per cent *V/V* of 2-propanol, unless otherwise prescribed.

Dry residue Where applicable, the tincture complies with the limits prescribed in the monograph. In a flat-bottomed dish about 50 mm in diameter and about 30 mm in height, introduce rapidly 2.00 g or 2.0 ml of the tincture. Evaporate to dryness on a water-bath and dry in an oven at 100°C to 105°C for 3 h. Allow to cool in a desiccator over *diphosphorus pentoxide R* and weigh. Calculate the result as a mass percentage or in grams per litre.

STORAGE

Store in a well-closed container, protected from light.

LABELLING

The label states:

- the vegetable or animal matter used,
- where applicable, that fresh vegetable or animal matter was used,
- the concentration of alcohol used for the preparation,
- the concentration of alcohol in the final tincture,
- the content of active principle and/or the ratio of starting material to extraction fluid or of starting material to final tincture.

Ph Eur

Tinctures of the British Pharmacopoeia

In addition to the above requirements of the European Pharmacopoeia, the following statements apply to those tinctures that are the subject of an individual monograph in the British Pharmacopoeia.

Definition Certain preparations of the British Pharmacopoeia entitled Tinctures do not conform strictly to the definition of the European Pharmacopoeia and consequently application of some of the above requirements is inappropriate. Any necessary exceptions are stated in the relevant individual monographs.

The following tinctures are the subject of an individual monograph in the British Pharmacopoeia.

Belladonna Tincture
Benzoin Tincture, Compound
Cardamom Tincture, Aromatic
Cardamom Tincture, Compound
Chloroform and Morphine Tincture
Ginger Tincture, Strong
Ginger Tincture, Weak
Ipecacuanha Tincture
Opium Tincture
Opium Tincture, Camphorated
Opium Tincture, Concentrated Camphorated
Orange Tincture
Quillaia Tincture
Rhubarb Tincture, Compound

TOPICAL POWDERS

Topical Powders comply with the requirements of the 3rd edition of the European Pharmacopoeia [1166]. These requirements are reproduced after the heading 'Definition' below.

Ph Eur

DEFINITION

Topical powders are preparations consisting of solid, loose, dry particles of varying degrees of fineness. They contain one or more active ingredients, with or without excipients and, if necessary, colouring matters authorised by the competent authority.

Topical powders are presented as single-dose powders or multidose powders. They are free from grittiness. Powders specifically intended for use on large open wounds or on severely injured skin are sterile.

Multidose topical powders may be dispensed in sifter-top containers, containers equipped with a mechanical spraying device or in pressurised containers.

Powders dispensed in pressurised containers comply with the requirements of *Pressurised pharmaceutical preparations (523)*.

Where applicable, containers for powders comply with the requirements of *Materials used for the manufacture of containers* (*3.1* and subsections) and *Containers* (*3.2* and subsections).

PRODUCTION

In the manufacture, packaging, storage and distribution of topical powders, suitable means are taken to ensure their microbial quality; recommendations on this aspect are provided in the text on *Microbial quality of pharmaceutical preparations* (*5.1.4*).

Sterile topical powders are prepared using materials and methods designed to ensure sterility and to avoid the introduction of contaminants and the growth of micro-organisms; recommendations on this aspect are provided in the text on *Methods of preparation of sterile products* (*5.1.1*).

TESTS

Fineness If prescribed, the fineness of a powder is determined by the sieve test (*2.9.12*) or another appropriate method.

Uniformity of content (*2.9.6*). Unless otherwise prescribed or justified and authorised, single-dose topical powders with a content of active ingredient less than 2 mg or less than 2 per cent of the total mass comply with test B for Uniformity of Content of single-dose Preparations. If the preparation has more than one active ingredient, the requirement applies only to those ingredients which correspond to the above conditions. The test is not required for multivitamin and trace-element preparations.

Uniformity of mass (*2.9.5*). Single-dose topical powders comply with the test for uniformity of mass of single-dose preparations. If the test for uniformity of content is prescribed for all the active ingredients, the test for uniformity of mass is not required.

Sterility (*2.6.1*). Where the label indicates that the preparation is sterile, it complies with the test for sterility.

STORAGE

Store in a well-closed container.

LABELLING

The label states:
— that the preparation is for external use,
— where applicable, that the preparation is sterile.

Ph Eur

Topical Powders of the British Pharmacopoeia

In addition to the above requirements of the European Pharmacopoeia, the following statements apply to those dusting powders that are the subject of an individual monograph in the British Pharmacopoeia.

DUSTING POWDERS

Definition Dusting Powders are finely divided powders that are intended to be applied to the skin for therapeutic, prophylactic or lubricant purposes.

Storage Dusting Powders should be stored in a dry place.

Labelling The label states (1) the date after which the Dusting Powder is not intended to be used; (4) the conditions under which the Dusting Powder should be stored.

The following dusting powders are the subject of an individual monograph in the British Pharmacopoeia.

Hexachlorophene Dusting Powder
Talc Dusting Powder

TOPICAL SEMI-SOLID PREPARATIONS

Topical Semi-solid Preparations comply with the requirements of the 3rd edition of the European Pharmacopoeia [0132]. These requirements are reproduced after the heading 'Definition' below.

Ph Eur

The requirements of this monograph apply to all topical semi-solid preparations. Where appropriate, additional requirements specific to semi-solid preparations intended to be applied to particular surfaces or mucous membranes may be found in other general monographs, for example Ear preparations (652), Eye preparations (1163), Nasal preparations (676), Rectal preparations (1145) and Vaginal preparations (1164).

DEFINITION

Topical semi-solid preparations are intended to be applied to the skin or to certain mucous surfaces for local action or percutaneous penetration of active ingredients, or for their emollient or protective action. They are of homogeneous appearance.

Topical semi-solid preparations consist of a simple or compound basis in which, usually, one or more active ingredients are dissolved or dispersed. According to its composition, the basis may influence the action of the preparation and the release of the active ingredient(s).

The bases may consist of natural or synthetic substances and may be single-phase or multiphase systems. According to the nature of the basis, the preparation may have hydrophilic or hydrophobic (lipophilic) properties; it may contain suitable additives such as antimicrobial preservatives, antioxidants, stabilisers, emulsifiers and thickeners.

Topical semi-solid preparations intended for use on large open wounds or on severely injured skin are sterile.

Where applicable, containers for topical semi-solid preparations comply with the requirements for *Materials Used for the Manufacture of Containers* (*3.1* and subsections) and *Containers* (*3.2* and subsections).

Several categories of topical semi-solid preparations may be distinguished:
— ointments,
— creams,
— gels,
— pastes.

PRODUCTION

During the development of a topical semi-solid preparation, the formulation for which contains an antimicrobial preservative, the effectiveness of the chosen preservative shall be demonstrated to the satisfaction of the competent authority. A suitable method of test together with criteria for judging the preservative properties of the formulation are provided in the text on *Efficacy of Antimicrobial Preservation* (*5.1.3*).

In the manufacture, packaging, storage and distribution of topical semi-solid preparations, suitable means are taken to ensure their microbial quality; recommendations on this aspect are provided in the text on *Microbial Quality of Pharmaceutical Preparations* (*5.1.4*).

Sterile topical semi-solid preparations are prepared using materials and methods designed to ensure sterility and to avoid the introduction of contaminants and the growth of microorganisms; recommendations on this aspect are provided in the text on *Methods of Preparation of Sterile Products (5.1.1)*.

In the manufacture of topical semi-solid preparations containing dispersed particles measures are taken to ensure a suitable and controlled particle size with regard to the intended use.

TESTS

Sterility (*2.6.1*). Where the label indicates that the preparation is sterile, it complies with the test for sterility.

STORAGE

Store in a well-closed container or, if the preparation contains water or other volatile ingredients, store in an airtight container. The containers are preferably collapsible metal tubes from which the preparation may be readily extruded. If the preparation is sterile, store in a sterile, airtight, tamper-proof container.

LABELLING

The label states:
— the name of any added antimicrobial preservative,
— where applicable, that the preparation is sterile.

Ointments

DEFINITION

An ointment consists of a single-phase basis in which solids or liquids may be dispersed.

Hydrophobic Ointments

Hydrophobic (lipophilic) ointments can absorb only small amounts of water. Typical substances used for their formulation are hard, soft and liquid paraffins, vegetable oils, animal fats, synthetic glycerides, waxes and liquid polyalkylsiloxanes.

Water-Emulsifying Ointments

Water-emulsifying ointments can absorb larger amounts of water. Their bases are those of hydrophobic ointments, incorporating water-in-oil emulsifying agents such as wool fat, wool alcohols, sorbitan esters, monoglycerides and fatty alcohols.

Hydrophilic Ointments

Hydrophilic ointments are preparations having bases that are miscible with water. The bases usually consist of mixtures of liquid and solid macrogols (polyethylene glycols). They may contain appropriate amounts of water.

Creams

DEFINITION

Creams are multiphase preparations consisting of a lipophilic phase and an aqueous phase.

Hydrophobic Creams

Hydrophobic creams have as the continuous phase the lipophilic phase. They contain water-in-oil emulsifying agents such as wool fat, sorbitan esters and monoglycerides.

Hydrophilic Creams

Hydrophilic creams have as the continuous phase the aqueous phase. They contain oil-in-water emulsifying agents such as sodium or triethanolamine soaps, sulphated fatty alcohols and polysorbates, combined, if necessary, with water-in-oil emulsifying agents.

Gels

DEFINITION

Gels consist of liquids gelled by means of suitable gelling agents.

Hydrophobic Gels

Hydrophobic gels (oleogels) are preparations whose bases usually consist of liquid paraffin with polyethylene or fatty oils gelled with colloidal silica or aluminium or zinc soaps.

Hydrophilic Gels

Hydrophilic gels (hydrogels) are preparations whose bases usually consist of water, glycerol or propylene glycol gelled with suitable gelling agents such as tragacanth, starch, cellulose derivatives, carboxyvinyl polymers and magnesium-aluminium silicates.

Pastes

DEFINITION

Pastes are semi-solid preparations containing large proportions of solids finely dispersed in the basis.

Ph Eur

Topical Semi-solid Preparations of the British Pharmacopoeia

In addition to the above requirements of the European Pharmacopoeia, the following statements apply to any cream, gel, ointment or paste that is the subject of an individual monograph in the British Pharmacopoeia. Eye ointments are described in the monograph on Eye Preparations.

CREAMS

Definition Creams are formulated to provide preparations that are essentially miscible with the skin secretion. They are intended to be applied to the skin or certain mucous membranes for protective, therapeutic or prophylactic purposes especially where an occlusive effect is not necessary.

Creams should not normally be diluted. However, should dilution be necessary care should be taken, in particular, to prevent microbial contamination. The appropriate diluent should be used and heating should be avoided during mixing. Excessive dilution may affect the stability of some creams. If diluted, creams should normally be used within two weeks of their preparation.

Storage Creams should be stored at temperatures not exceeding 25° unless otherwise authorised. They should not be allowed to freeze.

Labelling The label states (1) the date after which the Cream is not intended to be used; (2) the conditions under which the Cream should be stored.

GELS

Storage Gels should be stored at temperatures not exceeding 25° unless otherwise prescribed. They should not be allowed to freeze.

Labelling The label states (1) the date after which the Gel is not intended to be used; (2) the conditions under which the Gel should be stored.

OINTMENTS

Definition Ointments are formulated to provide preparations that are immiscible, miscible or emulsifiable with the skin secretion. Hydrophobic ointments and water-emulsifying ointments are intended to be applied to the skin or certain mucous membranes for emollient, protective, therapeutic or prophylactic purposes where a degree of occlusion is desired. Hydrophilic ointments are miscible with the skin secretion and are less emollient as a consequence.

In tropical and subtropical countries varying quantities of Arachis Oil, White Beeswax, Wool Fat, Hard Paraffin, White Soft Paraffin, Yellow Soft Paraffin or Liquid Paraffin may be used in the preparation of the Ointments of the Pharmacopoeia when prevailing high temperatures otherwise make them too soft for convenient use, but the specified proportions of the active ingredients must be maintained.

Ointments should not normally be diluted. However, should dilution be necessary care should be taken in the selection of diluents to avoid risk of incompatibility or instability.

Storage Ointments should be stored at a temperature not exceeding 25° unless otherwise authorised.

Labelling The label states (1) the date after which the Ointment is not intended to be used; (2) the conditions under which the Ointment should be stored.

PASTES

Definition Pastes are usually intended to be applied to small, localised areas of the skin.

Storage Pastes should be stored at a temperature not exceeding 25° unless otherwise authorised.

Labelling The label states (1) the date after which the Paste is not intended to be used; (2) the conditions under which the Paste should be stored.

The following topical semi-solid preparations are the subject of an individual monograph in the British Pharmacopoeia.

Creams

Aciclovir Cream
Aqueous Cream
Beclometasone Cream
Benzoyl Peroxide Cream
Benzydamine Cream
Betamethasone Valerate Cream
Betamethasone and Clioquinol Cream
Buffered Cream
Calamine Cream, Aqueous
Cetrimide Cream
Clioquinol Cream
Clobetasol Cream
Clobetasone Cream
Clotrimazole Cream
Crotamiton Cream
Diethylamine Salicylate Cream
Diflucortolone Cream
Diflucortolone Oily Cream
Dithranol Cream
Econazole Cream
Fluocinolone Cream
Fluocinonide Cream
Fluocortolone Cream

Fluorouracil Cream
Fluticasone Cream
Gentamicin Cream
Hydrocortisone Cream
Hydrocortisone Acetate Cream
Hydrocortisone and Clioquinol Cream
Hydrocortisone and Neomycin Cream
Ibuprofen Cream
Mexenone Cream
Miconazole Cream
Potassium Hydroxyquinoline Sulphate and Benzoyl Peroxide Cream
Triamcinolone Cream
Urea Cream
Zinc Cream
Zinc and Ichthammol Cream

Gels

Benzoyl Peroxide Gel
Choline Salicylate Dental Gel
Ibuprofen Gel
Lidocaine Gel
Lidocaine and Chlorhexidine Gel
Metronidazole Gel
Piroxicam Gel
Tretinoin Gel

Ointments

Beclometasone Ointment
Benzoic Acid Ointment, Compound
Betamethasone Valerate Ointment
Betamethasone and Clioquinol Ointment
Calamine Ointment
Calamine and Coal Tar Ointment
Cetomacrogol Emulsifying Ointment
Cetrimide Emulsifying Ointment
Chlortetracycline Ointment
Clobetasol Ointment
Clobetasone Ointment
Diflucortolone Ointment
Dithranol Ointment
Emulsifying Ointment
Fluocinolone Ointment
Fluocinonide Ointment
Fluocortolone Ointment
Fluticasone Ointment
Gentamicin Ointment
Hydrocortisone Ointment
Hydrocortisone Acetate Ointment
Hydrocortisone and Clioquinol Ointment
Hydrous Ointment
Macrogol Ointment
Methyl Salicylate Ointment
Nystatin Ointment
Paraffin Ointment
Salicylic Acid Ointment
Simple Ointment
Sodium Fusidate Ointment
Tar and Salicylic Acid Ointment, Coal
Tar and Zinc Ointment, Coal
Triamcinolone Ointment
Wool Alcohols Ointment
Zinc Ointment
Zinc and Castor Oil Ointment

Pastes

Aluminium Paste, Compound
Dithranol Paste
Magnesium Sulphate Paste
Tar Paste, Coal
Triamcinolone Dental Paste
Zinc Paste, Compound
Zinc and Coal Tar Paste
Zinc and Salicylic Acid Paste

TRANSDERMAL PATCHES

Transdermal Patches comply with the requirements of the 3rd edition of the European Pharmacopoeia [1011]. These requirements are reproduced after the heading 'Definition' below.

Ph Eur

DEFINITION

Transdermal patches are flexible pharmaceutical preparations of varying sizes, containing one or more active ingredients. They are intended to be applied to the unbroken skin in order to deliver the active ingredient(s) to the systemic circulation after passing through the skin barrier.

Transdermal patches normally consist of an outer covering which supports a preparation which contains the active ingredient(s). The transdermal patches are covered on the site of the release surface of the preparation by a protective liner, which is removed before applying the patch to the skin.

The outer covering is a backing sheet impermeable to the active ingredient(s) and normally impermeable to water, designed to support and protect the preparation. The outer covering may have the same dimensions as the preparation or it may be larger. In the latter case the overlapping border of the outer covering is covered by pressure-sensitive adhesive substances which assure the adhesion of the patch to the skin.

The preparation contains the active ingredient(s) together with excipients such as stabilisers, solubilisers or substances intended to modify the release rate or to enhance transdermal absorption. It may be a single layer or multi-layer solid or semi-solid matrix, and in this case it is the composition and structure of the matrix which determines the diffusion pattern of the active ingredient(s) to the skin. The matrix may contain pressure-sensitive adhesives which assure the adhesion of the preparation to the skin. The preparation may exist as a semi-solid reservoir one side of which is a membrane which controls the release and the diffusion of the active ingredient(s) from the preparation. The pressure-sensitive adhesive substances may, in this case, be applied to some or all parts of the membrane, or only around the border of the membrane of the outer covering.

When applied to the dried, clean and unbroken skin, the transdermal patch adheres firmly to the skin by gentle pressure of the hand or the fingers and can be peeled off without causing appreciable injury to the skin or detachment of the preparation from the outer covering. The patch must not be irritant or sensitising to the skin, even after repeated applications.

The protective liner generally consists of a sheet of plastic or metal material. When removed, the protective liner does not detach the preparation (matrix or reservoir) or the adhesive from the patch.

Transdermal patches are normally individually enclosed in sealed sachets.

PRODUCTION

In the manufacture, packaging, storage and distribution of transdermal patches suitable means are taken to ensure their microbial quality; recommendations on this aspect are provided in the text on *Microbial Quality of Pharmaceutical Preparations* (*5.1.4*).

TESTS

Uniformity of content (*2.9.6*). Unless otherwise prescribed or justified and authorised, transdermal patches comply with test C for uniformity of content of single-dose preparations.

Dissolution. A suitable test may be required to demonstrate the appropriate release of the active ingredient(s), for example one of the tests described in *Dissolution Test for Transdermal Patches* (*2.9.4*). The disc assembly method, the cell method or the rotating cylinder method may be used, as suitable, according to the composition, dimensions and shape of the patch. A membrane may be used. It can be of various materials, such as inert porous cellulose or silicones, and must not affect the release kinetics of the active ingredient(s) from the patch. Furthermore, it must be free of substances that may interfere with its performance (for example grease). The membrane may be suitably treated before the tests, for example, by maintaining it in the medium to be used in the test for 24 h. Apply the membrane above the releasing surface of the patch, avoiding the formation of air bubbles.

The test conditions and the requirements are to be authorised by the competent authority.

STORAGE

Store at room temperature, unless otherwise indicated.

LABELLING

The label states, where applicable, the total quantity of active ingredient(s) per patch, the dose released per unit time and the area of the releasing surface.

Ph Eur

VAGINAL PREPARATIONS

Vaginal preparations comply with the requirements of the 3rd edition of the European Pharmacopoeia [1164]. These requirements are reproduced after the heading 'Definition' below.

Ph Eur

DEFINITION

Vaginal preparations are liquid, semi-solid or solid preparations intended for administration to the vagina usually in order to obtain a local effect. They contain one or more active ingredients in a suitable basis.

Where appropriate, containers for vaginal preparations comply with the requirements for *Materials used for the Manufacture of Containers* (*3.1* and subsections) and *Containers* (*3.2* and subsections).

Several categories of vaginal preparations may be distinguished:

— moulded pessaries,
— vaginal tablets,
— vaginal capsules,
— vaginal foams,
— vaginal tampons.

PRODUCTION

In the manufacturing, packaging, storage and distribution of vaginal preparations, suitable means are taken to ensure their microbial quality; recommendations on this aspect are provided in the text on *Microbial Quality of Pharmaceutical Preparations* (*5.1.4*).

TESTS

Uniformity of content (*2.9.6*). Unless otherwise prescribed or justified and authorised, solid single-dose preparations with a content of active ingredient less than 2 mg or less than 2 per cent of the total mass comply with test A (vaginal tablets) or test B (moulded pessaries, vaginal capsules) for uniformity of content of single-dose preparations. If the preparation has more than one active ingredient, the requirement applies only to those ingredients which correspond to the above conditions.

Uniformity of mass (*2.9.5*). Solid single-dose preparations comply with the test for uniformity of mass of single-dose preparations. If the test for uniformity of content is prescribed for all the active ingredients, the test for uniformity of mass is not required.

Dissolution A suitable test may be carried out to demonstrate the appropriate release of the active ingredient(s) from solid single-dose preparations, for example one of the tests described in *Dissolution Test for Solid Dosage Forms* (*2.9.3*).

Where a dissolution test is prescribed, a disintegration test may not be required.

Moulded Pessaries

DEFINITION

Moulded pessaries are solid, single-dose preparations. They have various shapes, usually ovoid, with a volume and consistence suitable for insertion into the vagina. Apart from their shape they conform to the definition of moulded suppositories in the monograph on *Rectal preparations (1145)*.

Moulded pessaries are prepared using the method and excipients described for moulded suppositories in the monograph on *Rectal preparations (1145)*. The active ingredient(s) are dispersed or dissolved in a simple or compound basis, which may be soluble, insoluble but melting at body temperature or dispersible in water.

Vaginal preparations which conform to the definition of moulded pessaries may be prepared by compression. They comply with the requirements for moulded pessaries.

PRODUCTION

A suitable test is carried out to demonstrate the appropriate release of the active ingredient(s) from pessaries intended for modified release or prolonged local action.

TESTS

Disintegration Unless intended for modified release or for prolonged local action, they comply with the test for *Disintegration of Suppositories and Pessaries (2.9.2)*. Examine the state of the pessaries after 60 min, unless otherwise justified and authorised.

STORAGE

Store in a well-closed container.

Vaginal Tablets

DEFINITION

Vaginal tablets (compressed pessaries) are solid, single-dose preparations. They generally conform to the definitions of uncoated or film-coated tablets given in the monograph on *Tablets (478)*.

PRODUCTION

A suitable test is carried out to demonstrate the appropriate release of the active ingredient(s) from vaginal tablets intended for modified release or prolonged local action.

TESTS

Disintegration Unless intended for modified release or prolonged local action, they comply with the test for *Disintegration of suppositories and pessaries* (special method for vaginal tablets, *2.9.2*). Examine the state of the tablets after 30 min, unless otherwise justified and authorised.

Vaginal Capsules

DEFINITION

Vaginal capsules (shell pessaries) are solid, single dose preparations. They are generally similar to soft capsules, differing only in their shape and size. Vaginal capsules have various shapes, usually ovoid. They are smooth and have a uniform external appearance.

PRODUCTION

A suitable test is carried out to demonstrate the appropriate release of the active ingredient(s) from vaginal capsules intended for modified release or prolonged local action.

TESTS

Disintegration Unless intended for modified release or prolonged local action, they comply with the test for *Disintegration of Suppositories and Pessaries (2.9.2)*. Examine the state of the capsules after 30 min, unless otherwise justified and authorised.

Vaginal Foams

DEFINITION

Vaginal foams comply with the requirements in the monograph on *Medicated foams (1105)*.

Vaginal Tampons

DEFINITION

Vaginal tampons are solid, single-dose preparations intended to be inserted in the vagina for a limited time.

They comply with the requirements in the monograph on *Medicated tampons (1155)*.

Ph Eur

Vaginal Preparations of the British Pharmacopoeia

In addition to the above requirements of the European Pharmacopoeia, the following statements apply to those pessaries that are the subject of an individual monograph in the British Pharmacopoeia.

PESSARIES

Labelling The label states (1) the names and concentrations of the active ingredients; (2) that the preparation should not be swallowed; (3) the date after which the Pessaries are not intended to be used; (4) the conditions under which the Pessaries should be stored.

The following pessaries are the subject of an individual monograph in the British Pharmacopoeia.

Clotrimazole Pessaries
Diethylstilbestrol Pessaries
Econazole Pessaries
Lactic Acid Pessaries
Nystatin Pessaries

AROMATIC WATERS

Definition Aromatic Waters are saturated solutions of volatile oils or other aromatic substances in water, usually employed for their flavouring rather than their medicinal properties. Aromatic Waters prepared as described below contain a small amount of Ethanol.

Production Aromatic Waters are normally prepared by diluting a concentrated, ethanolic solution of the aromatic substance with Water.

Labelling The label states (1) the date after which the Aromatic Water is not intended to be used; (2) the conditions under which the Aromatic Water should be stored.

The following aromatic waters are the subject of an individual monograph in the British Pharmacopoeia.

Anise Water, Concentrated
Camphor Water, Concentrated
Chloroform Water
Chloroform Water, Double-strength
Cinnamon Water, Concentrated

Monographs

Formulated Preparations: Specific Monographs

FORMULATED PREPARATIONS: SPECIFIC MONOGRAPHS

Acenocoumarol Tablets

Definition Acenocoumarol Tablets contain Acenocoumarol.

The tablets comply with the requirements stated under Tablets and with the following requirements.

Content of acenocoumarol, $C_{19}H_{15}NO_6$ 92.5 to 107.5% of the prescribed or stated amount.

Identification

A. Heat a quantity of the powdered tablets containing 50 mg of Acenocoumarol with 30 ml of *acetone* under a reflux condenser for 5 minutes, filter and wash the residue with two 10-ml quantities of *acetone*. Evaporate the combined filtrate and washings to 5 ml, add *water* drop-wise until the solution becomes turbid, heat on a water bath until the solution is clear and allow to stand. Filter, wash the crystals with a mixture of equal volumes of *acetone* and *water* and dry at 100° at a pressure of 2 kPa for 30 minutes. The *infrared absorption spectrum* of the residue, Appendix II A, is concordant with the *reference spectrum* of acenocoumarol.

B. The *light absorption*, Appendix II B, of the final solution obtained in the Assay exhibits maxima at 283 nm and 306 nm.

C. Heat 25 mg of the residue obtained in test A with 2.5 ml of *glacial acetic acid*, 0.5 ml of *hydrochloric acid* and 0.2 g of *zinc powder* on a water bath for 5 minutes, cool and filter. To the filtrate add 0.05 ml of *sodium nitrite solution* and add the mixture to 10 ml of a 1% w/v solution of *2-naphthol* containing 3 ml of 5M *sodium hydroxide*. A bright red precipitate is produced.

Related substances Carry out the method for *thin-layer chromatography*, Appendix III A, using *silica gel GF_{254}* as the coating substance and a mixture of 20 volumes of *glacial acetic acid*, 50 volumes of *chloroform* and 50 volumes of *cyclohexane* as the mobile phase. Apply separately to the plate 20 µl of each of the following solutions. For solution (1) shake a quantity of the powdered tablets containing 20 mg of Acenocoumarol with 5 ml of *acetone*, centrifuge and use the supernatant liquid. For solution (2) dilute 1 volume of solution (1) to 200 volumes with *acetone*. After removal of the plate, allow it to dry in air and immediately examine under *ultraviolet light (254 nm)*. Any *secondary spot* in the chromatogram obtained with solution (1) is not more intense than the spot in the chromatogram obtained with solution (2) (0.5%).

Uniformity of content Tablets containing 4 mg or less of Acenocoumarol comply with the requirements stated under Tablets using the following method of analysis. Finely crush one tablet, add 30 ml of *methanol*, stir the mixture for 30 minutes and filter through sintered glass, washing the residue with three 15-ml quantities of *methanol*. To the combined filtrate and washings add 10 ml of 1M *hydrochloric acid* and sufficient *methanol* to produce 100 ml. If necessary dilute further with a solvent prepared by diluting 1 volume of 1M *hydrochloric acid* to 10 volumes with *methanol* to produce a solution containing about 0.001% w/v of Acenocoumarol. Measure the *absorbance* of the resulting solution at the maximum at 306 nm, Appendix II B. Calculate the content of $C_{19}H_{15}NO_6$ taking 521 as the value of A(1%, 1 cm) at the maximum at 306 nm.

Assay Weigh and powder 20 tablets. To a quantity of the powder containing 1 mg of Acenocoumarol add 30 ml of *methanol*, stir the mixture for 30 minutes and filter through sintered glass, washing the residue with three 15-ml quantities of *methanol*. To the combined filtrate and washings add 10 ml of 1M *hydrochloric acid* and sufficient *methanol* to produce 100 ml and measure the *absorbance* of the resulting solution at the maximum at 306 nm, Appendix II B. Calculate the content of $C_{19}H_{15}NO_6$ taking 521 as the value of A(1%, 1 cm) at the maximum at 306 nm.

When nicoumalone tablets are prescribed or demanded, Acenocoumarol Tablets shall be dispensed or supplied.

Acetazolamide Tablets

Definition Acetazolamide Tablets contain Acetazolamide.

The tablets comply with the requirements stated under Tablets and with the following requirements.

Content of acetazolamide, $C_4H_6N_4O_3S_2$ 95.0 to 105.0% of the prescribed or stated amount.

Identification

A. Shake a quantity of the powdered tablets containing 0.5 g of Acetazolamide with 2 ml of 1M *sodium hydroxide* and filter. Neutralise the filtrate with *glacial acetic acid*, filter and dry the resulting precipitate at 105°. The *infrared absorption spectrum* of the residue, Appendix II A, is concordant with the *reference spectrum* of acetazolamide.

B. Triturate a quantity of the powdered tablets containing 0.5 g of Acetazolamide with a mixture of 5 ml of *water* and 1 ml of 1M *sodium hydroxide*, transfer to a test tube, add 0.2 g of *zinc powder* and 0.5 ml of *hydrochloric acid* and immediately place a piece of *lead acetate paper* over the mouth of the tube. The paper exhibits a brownish black colour.

C. To a quantity of the powdered tablets containing 25 mg of Acetazolamide add 5 ml of *water*, 0.15 ml of 1M *sodium hydroxide* and 0.1 ml of *weak copper sulphate solution*. A greenish blue colour or precipitate is produced.

Related substances Carry out the method for *thin-layer chromatography*, Appendix III A, using *silica gel GF_{254}* as the coating substance and a freshly prepared mixture of 50 volumes of *propan-2-ol*, 30 volumes of *ethyl acetate* and 20 volumes of 13.5M *ammonia* as the mobile phase. Use the tank without lining the walls and allow to saturate for 1 hour before development. Apply separately to the plate 20 µl of each of the following solutions. For solution (1) shake a quantity of the powdered tablets containing 50 mg of Acetazolamide for 20 minutes with 10 ml of a mixture of equal volumes of *ethanol (96%)* and *ethyl acetate* and filter. For solution (2) dilute 1 volume of solution (1) to 100 volumes with the same solvent mixture. After removal of the plate, allow it to dry in air and examine under *ultraviolet light (254 nm)*. Any *secondary spot* in the chromatogram obtained with solution (1) is not more intense than the spot in the chromatogram obtained with solution (2) (1%).

Assay Weigh and powder 20 tablets. To a quantity of the powder containing 0.4 g of Acetazolamide add 90 ml of *dimethylformamide* and carry out Method II for *non-aqueous titration*, Appendix VIII A, using 0.1M *tetrabutylammonium hydroxide VS* as titrant and determining the end point potentiometrically. Each ml of 0.1M *tetrabutylammonium hydroxide VS* is equivalent to 22.22 mg of $C_4H_6N_4O_3S_2$.

Acetylcysteine Injection

Definition Acetylcysteine Injection is a sterile solution in Water for Injections of acetylcysteine sodium, prepared by the interaction of Acetylcysteine with Sodium Hydroxide.

The injection complies with the requirements stated under Parenteral Preparations and with the following requirements.

Content of acetylcysteine, $C_5H_9NO_3S$ 95.0 to 105.0% of the prescribed or stated amount.

Identification To a volume containing the equivalent of 0.8 g of Acetylcysteine add 3M *hydrochloric acid* until the pH of the solution is 2. Add, while stirring continuously, two 200-mg portions of finely powdered *sodium chloride* followed, if necessary, by further 25-mg portions of *sodium chloride* until a precipitate begins to appear. Allow to stand for 15 minutes, filter and dry the residue at 70° at a pressure not exceeding 0.7 kPa for 2 hours. The *infrared absorption spectrum* of the residue, Appendix II A, is concordant with the *reference spectrum* of acetylcysteine. Examine as discs prepared using *potassium bromide*.

Acidity or alkalinity pH, 6.5 to 7.5, Appendix V L.

Specific optical rotation +21° to +27°, Appendix V F. Use a solution prepared by diluting a volume containing the equivalent of 1.25 g of Acetylcysteine with a mixture of 1 ml of a 0.1% w/v solution of *disodium edetate* and 7.5 ml of 1M *sodium hydroxide* and add sufficient *mixed phosphate buffer pH 7.0* to produce 25 ml.

Related substances Carry out the method for *liquid chromatography*, Appendix III D, using the following solutions. With the exception of solution (3), the solutions should be prepared immediately before use. For solution (1) dilute the injection with the mobile phase to produce a solution containing the equivalent of 0.2% w/v of Acetylcysteine. Solution (2) is a 0.2% w/v solution of N-*acetyl-L-cysteine* in the mobile phase. Prepare solution (3) in the same manner as solution (2) but store at room temperature for at least 2 hours before use. For solution (4) dissolve 20 mg of *L-cysteine* and 20 mg of *L-cystine* in 10 ml of 1M *hydrochloric acid*, add 40 mg of N-*acetyl-L-cysteine* and immediately dilute to 100 ml with the mobile phase. Dilute 10 ml of the resulting solution to 200 ml with the mobile phase.

The chromatographic procedure may be carried out using (a) a stainless steel column (25 cm × 5 mm) packed with *stationary phase C* (5 μm) (Lichrosorb RP18 is suitable), (b) as the mobile phase with a flow rate of 1 ml per minute a mixture of 10 volumes of *methanol* and 90 volumes of a 0.5% w/v solution of *ammonium sulphate* containing 0.02M *sodium pentanesulphonate*, the solution being adjusted to pH 2 using 2M *hydrochloric acid*, and (c) a detection wavelength of 205 nm.

Inject 20 μl of solution (4). The chromatogram obtained shows three peaks with retention times of about 3.6 minutes (cystine), about 4 minutes (cysteine) and about 6 minutes (acetylcysteine). Adjust the sensitivity so that the height of the peak due to cysteine is about 20% of full-scale deflection. The test is not valid unless, in the chromatogram obtained with solution (4), the height of the trough separating the peaks due to cysteine and cystine is less than one quarter of the height of the peak due to cysteine. Inject 20 μl of solutions (2) and (3) and allow the chromatography to continue for three times the retention time of acetylcysteine. In the chromatogram obtained with solution (3) a peak due to acetylcysteine disulphide appears which has a retention time of about 13 minutes. The area of this peak is greater than the area of any corresponding peak in the chromatogram obtained with solution (2).

In the chromatogram obtained with solution (1) the area of any peak corresponding to acetylcysteine disulphide is not greater than the area of the peak due to acetylcysteine in the chromatogram obtained with solution (4) (1%), the area of any peak due to cysteine or cystine is not greater than the corresponding peak in the chromatogram obtained with solution (4) (0.5%) and the sum of the areas of any other *secondary peaks* is not greater than the area of the peak due to acetylcysteine in the chromatogram obtained with solution (4) (1%).

Pyrogens Complies with the *test for pyrogens*, Appendix XIV D. Use per kg of the rabbit's weight a volume containing the equivalent of 0.3 g of Acetylcysteine.

Assay Add 20 ml of *glacial acetic acid* to a volume containing the equivalent of 0.4 g of Acetylcysteine and titrate with 0.05M *iodine VS* until a permanent pale yellow colour is obtained. Each ml of 0.05M *iodine VS* is equivalent to 16.23 mg of $C_5H_9NO_3S$.

Storage Acetylcysteine Injection should be protected from light.

Labelling The strength is stated in terms of an equivalent percentage w/v of Acetylcysteine.

Aciclovir Cream

Definition Aciclovir Cream contains Aciclovir in a suitable basis.

The cream complies with the requirements stated under Topical Semi-solid Preparations and with the following requirements.

Content of aciclovir, $C_8H_{11}N_5O_3$ 95.0 to 105.0% of the prescribed or stated amount.

Identification

A. The *light absorption*, Appendix II B, in the range 230 to 350 nm of the solution prepared in the Assay exhibits a maximum at 255 nm and a broad shoulder at about 274 nm.

B. In the test for Guanine, the principal spot in the chromatogram obtained with solution (2) is similar in position and intensity to that in the chromatogram obtained with solution (3).

Guanine Carry out the method for *thin-layer chromatography*, Appendix III A, using *cellulose F_{254}* as the coating substance (Merck cellulose F plates are suitable). Apply separately to the plate 10 µl of each of the following solutions. For solution (1) transfer a quantity of the well-mixed cream containing 30 mg of Aciclovir into a 10-ml graduated, stoppered centrifuge tube, add 3 ml of 0.1M *sodium hydroxide* and shake to disperse the cream. Add 5 ml of a mixture of 1 volume of *chloroform* and 2 volumes of *propan-1-ol*, shake well, centrifuge and dilute the upper aqueous layer to 5 ml with 0.1M *sodium hydroxide*, mix, centrifuge and use the upper aqueous layer. For solution (2) dilute 1 volume of solution (1) to 10 volumes with 0.1M *sodium hydroxide*. For solution (3) dissolve 6.0 mg of *aciclovir BPCRS* in 10 ml of 0.1M *sodium hydroxide*. For solution (4) dissolve 6.0 mg of *guanine* in 100 ml of 0.1M *sodium hydroxide*. Use *ethyl acetate* for the first mobile phase but allow the solvent front to ascend to the top of the plate. After removal of the plate, dry it in a current of air and repeat the development in the same direction using a mixture of 10 volumes of *propan-1-ol*, 30 volumes of 13.5M *ammonia* and 60 volumes of a 5% w/v solution of *ammonium sulphate* as the mobile phase and allowing the solvent front to ascend 8 cm above the line of application. After removal of the plate, allow it to dry in air and examine under *ultraviolet light (254 nm)*. Any *secondary spot* corresponding to guanine in the chromatogram obtained with solution (1) is not more intense than the spot in the chromatogram obtained with solution (4) (1.0%). Disregard any spot that appears just below the solvent front.

Assay Shake a quantity of the well-mixed cream containing about 7.5 mg of Aciclovir with 50 ml of 0.5M *sulphuric acid*. Shake well with 50 ml of *ethyl acetate*, allow to separate and collect the clear lower aqueous layer. Wash the organic layer with 20 ml of 0.5M *sulphuric acid* and dilute the combined washings and the aqueous layer to 100 ml with 0.5M *sulphuric acid*. Mix well and filter (Whatman GF/F is suitable). Discard the first few ml of filtrate and to 10 ml of the filtrate add sufficient *water* to produce 50 ml. Measure the *absorbance* of the resulting solution at the maximum at 255 nm, Appendix II B. Calculate the content of $C_8H_{11}N_5O_3$ taking 562 as the value of A(1%, 1 cm) at the maximum at 255 nm.

Storage Aciclovir Cream should be stored at a temperature not exceeding 25°.

Aciclovir Eye Ointment

Definition Aciclovir Eye Ointment is a sterile preparation containing Aciclovir in a suitable basis.

The eye ointment complies with the requirements stated under Eye Ointments and with the following requirements.

Content of aciclovir, $C_8H_{11}N_5O_3$ 95.0 to 105.0% of the prescribed or stated amount.

Identification

A. The *light absorption*, Appendix II B, in the range 230 to 350 nm of the solution prepared in the Assay exhibits a maximum at 255 nm and a broad shoulder at about 274 nm.

B. In the test for Guanine, the principal spot in the chromatogram obtained with solution (2) is similar in position and intensity to that in the chromatogram obtained with solution (3).

Guanine Complies with the test described under Aciclovir Intravenous Infusion but preparing solution (1) in the following manner. Disperse a quantity of the eye ointment containing 30 mg of Aciclovir in 100 ml of *hexane*, extract with 5 ml of 0.1M *sodium hydroxide*, allow to separate and retain the lower aqueous layer.

Assay Disperse a quantity of the eye ointment containing 10 mg of Aciclovir in 60 ml of *hexane*. Extract with three 30-ml quantities of 0.1M of *sodium hydroxide*, add sufficient 0.1M *sodium hydroxide* to produce 100 ml and filter. To 15 ml of this solution add 5 ml of 2M *hydrochloric acid* and sufficient *water* to produce 100 ml. Measure the *absorbance* of the resulting solution at the maximum at 255 nm, Appendix II B. Calculate the content of $C_8H_{11}N_5O_3$ taking 560 as the value of A(1%, 1 cm) at the maximum at 255 nm.

Aciclovir Intravenous Infusion

Definition Aciclovir Intravenous Infusion is a sterile solution of aciclovir sodium in Water for Injections. It is prepared by dissolving Aciclovir Sodium for Intravenous Infusion in the requisite amount of Water for Injections before use.

The intravenous infusion complies with the requirements stated under Parenteral Preparations and with the following requirements.

Bacterial endotoxins Carry out the test for *bacterial endotoxins*, Appendix XIV C. The endotoxin limit concentration of the intravenous infusion, diluted, if necessary, with *water BET* to give a solution containing the equivalent of 25 mg of Aciclovir per ml is 4.37 IU per ml. Carry out the test using the maximum valid dilution of the above defined solution calculated from the declared sensitivity of the lysate used in the test.

Storage Aciclovir Intravenous Infusion should be used within the period recommended by the manufacturer when prepared and stored strictly in accordance with the manufacturer's instructions.

Labelling The strength is stated as the equivalent amount of Aciclovir in a suitable dose-volume.

ACICLOVIR SODIUM FOR INTRAVENOUS INFUSION

Definition Aciclovir Sodium for Intravenous Infusion is a sterile material prepared from Aciclovir with the aid of a suitable alkali. It may contain excipients. It is supplied in a sealed container.

The contents of the sealed container comply with the requirements for Powders for Injections stated under Parenteral Preparations and with the following requirements.

Content of aciclovir, $C_8H_{11}N_5O_3$ 95.0 to 105.0% of the prescribed or stated amount.

Identification

A. The *light absorption*, Appendix II B, in the range 230 to 350 nm of the solution prepared in the Assay exhibits a maximum at 255 nm and a broad shoulder at about 274 nm.

B. In the test for Guanine, the principal spot in the chromatogram obtained with solution (2) is similar in position and intensity to that in the chromatogram obtained with solution (3).

C. Yield reaction A characteristic of *sodium salts*, Appendix VI.

Alkalinity Dissolve the contents of a sealed container in sufficient *water for injections* to produce a solution containing the equivalent of 2.5% w/v of Aciclovir (solution A). The pH of solution A is 10.7 to 11.7, Appendix V L.

Clarity and colour of solution Solution A is not more opalescent than *reference suspension II*, Appendix IV A, and not more intensely coloured than *reference solution* Y_6, Appendix IV B, Method II.

Guanine Carry out the method for *thin-layer chromatography*, Appendix III A, using *cellulose* F_{254} as the coating substance (Merck cellulose F plates are suitable) and a mixture of 10 volumes of *propan-1-ol*, 30 volumes of 13.5M *ammonia* and 60 volumes of a 5% w/v solution of *ammonium sulphate* as the mobile phase but allowing the solvent front to ascend 12 cm above the line of application. Apply separately to the plate 10 µl of each of the following solutions. For solution (1) dissolve the contents of a sealed container in sufficient 0.1M *sodium hydroxide* to produce a solution containing the equivalent of 0.5% w/v of Aciclovir. For solution (2) dilute 1 volume of solution (1) to 10 volumes with 0.1M *sodium hydroxide*. For solution (3) dissolve 5 mg of *aciclovir BPCRS* in 10 ml of 0.1M *sodium hydroxide*. For solution (4) dissolve 5 mg of *guanine* in 100 ml of 0.1M *sodium hydroxide*. After removal of the plate, allow it to dry in air and examine under *ultraviolet light (254 nm)*. Any *secondary spot* corresponding to guanine in the chromatogram obtained with solution (1) is not more intense than the spot in the chromatogram obtained with solution (4) (1%). Disregard any spot that appears just below the solvent front.

Related substances Carry out the method for *thin-layer chromatography*, Appendix III A, using *silica gel* GF_{254} as the coating substance and a mixture of 2 volumes of 13.5M *ammonia*, 20 volumes of *methanol* and 80 volumes of *dichloromethane* as the mobile phase but allowing the solvent front to ascend 10 cm above the line of application. Apply separately to the plate 2 µl of each of the following freshly prepared solutions. For solution (1) dissolve the contents of a sealed container in sufficient *dimethyl sulphoxide* to produce a solution containing the equivalent of 2.5% w/v of Aciclovir. For solution (2) dilute 1 volume of solution (1) to 200 volumes with *dimethyl sulphoxide*. After removal of the plate, allow it to dry in air and examine under *ultraviolet light (254 nm)*. In the chromatogram obtained with solution (1) any *secondary spot* with an Rf value greater than that of the principal spot is not more intense than the spot in the chromatogram obtained with solution (2) (0.5%).

Assay Determine the weight of the contents of 10 containers as described in the test for Uniformity of weight under Parenteral Preparations, Powders for Injections.

Dissolve the total contents of 10 containers in sufficient 0.1M *hydrochloric acid* to produce 500 ml. Dilute 3 ml of the resulting solution to 100 ml with 0.1M *hydrochloric acid* and dilute 5 ml of the resulting solution with the same solvent to produce a solution containing the equivalent of 0.0015% w/v of Aciclovir. Measure the *absorbance* at the maximum at 255 nm, Appendix II B. Calculate the content of $C_8H_{11}N_5O_3$ taking 560 as the value of A(1%, 1 cm) at the maximum at 255 nm.

Storage The sealed container should be stored at a temperature not exceeding 25°.

Labelling The label of the sealed container states the quantity of aciclovir sodium in terms of the equivalent amount of Aciclovir.

Aciclovir Oral Suspension

Definition Aciclovir Oral Suspension is a suspension of Aciclovir in a suitable flavoured vehicle.

The oral suspension complies with the requirements stated under Oral Liquids and with the following requirements.

Content of aciclovir, $C_8H_{11}N_5O_3$ 95.0 to 105.0% of the prescribed or stated amount.

Identification

A. The *light absorption*, Appendix II B, in the range 230 to 250 nm of the solution prepared in the Assay before the final dilution exhibits a maximum at 255 nm and a broad shoulder at about 274 nm.

B. In the test for Guanine, the principal spot in the chromatogram obtained with solution (2) is similar in position and intensity to that in the chromatogram obtained with solution (3). If the Rf values of the principal spots in the chromatograms obtained with solutions (2) and (3) are different, the oral suspension complies if the chromatogram obtained with solution (5) shows a single, compact spot.

Acidity pH, 4.5 to 7.0, Appendix V L.

Guanine Carry out the test described under Aciclovir Intravenous Infusion but applying 5 µl of each of the following solutions. For solution (1) add 20 ml of 0.1M *sodium hydroxide* to a quantity of the oral suspension containing 0.6 g of Aciclovir, shake to disperse and add sufficient *absolute ethanol* to produce 100 ml. Mix well and allow any suspended material to settle before application to the plate. For solution (2) dilute 1 volume of solution (1) to 10 volumes with a mixture of 35 volumes of 0.1M *sodium hydroxide* and 65 volumes of *absolute ethanol*. For solution (3) dissolve 6 mg of *aciclovir BPCRS* in 10 ml of a mixture of 35 volumes of 0.1M *sodium hydroxide* and 65 volumes of *absolute ethanol*. For solution (4) dissolve 6 mg of *guanine* in 100 ml of a mixture of 35 volumes of 0.1M *sodium hydroxide* and 65 volumes of *absolute ethanol* (1%). Solution (5) contains equal volumes of solutions (2) and (3).

Assay To a weighed quantity containing 0.4 g of Aciclovir add 400 ml of *water* and 25 ml of 1M *sulphuric acid*, shake well, disperse with the aid of ultrasound for 10 minutes and add sufficient *water* to produce 500 ml. Filter the resulting solution, discard the first few ml of filtrate and dilute 5 ml of the filtrate to 200 ml with 0.05M *sulphuric acid*. Add 10 ml of the resulting solution to 5 ml of a 0.01% w/v solution of *cetrimide* in 0.05M *sulphuric acid*, add sufficient 0.05M *sulphuric acid* to produce 100 ml and measure the *fluorescence* Appendix II E, using an excitation wavelength of 308 nm and an emission wavelength of 415 nm. Set the instrument to zero using a 0.0005% w/v solution of *cetrimide* in 0.05M *sulphuric acid*. Calculate the content of $C_8H_{11}N_5O_3$ in the oral suspension from the *fluorescence* obtained by carrying out the operation at the same time using a mixture prepared by adding 10 ml of a

0.002% w/v solution of *aciclovir BPCRS* in 0.05M *sulphuric acid* and beginning at the words 'to 5 ml of a 0.01% w/v solution of *cetrimide* ...'. Determine the *weight per ml* of the oral suspension, Appendix V G, and calculate the content of $C_8H_{11}N_5O_3$, weight in volume, using the declared content of $C_8H_{11}N_5O_3$ in *aciclovir BPCRS*.

Storage Aciclovir Oral Suspension should be stored at a temperature not exceeding 25°.

Aciclovir Tablets

Definition Aciclovir Tablets contain Aciclovir.

With the exception of the requirements for shape, the tablets comply with the requirements stated under Tablets and with the following requirements.

Content of aciclovir, $C_8H_{11}N_5O_3$ 95.0 to 105.0% of the prescribed or stated amount.

Identification

A. The *light absorption*, Appendix II B, in the range 230 to 350 nm of the solution prepared in the Assay exhibits a maximum at 255 nm and a broad shoulder at about 274 nm.

B. In the test for Guanine, the principal spot in the chromatogram obtained with solution (2) is similar in position and intensity to that in the chromatogram obtained with solution (3).

Guanine Comply with the test described under Aciclovir Intravenous Infusion but preparing solution (1) in the following manner. Shake a quantity of the powdered tablets containing 0.25 g of Aciclovir with 25 ml of 0.1M *sodium hydroxide* for 10 minutes. Add a sufficient quantity of 0.1M *sodium hydroxide* to produce 50 ml, allow to stand and allow any undissolved material to settle before application to the plate.

Related substances Carry out the method for *thin-layer chromatography*, Appendix III A, using *silica gel GF_{254}* as the coating substance and a mixture of 2 volumes of 13.5M *ammonia*, 20 volumes of *methanol* and 80 volumes of *dichloromethane* as the mobile phase but allowing the solvent front to ascend 10 cm above the line of application. Apply separately to the plate 2 µl of each of the following freshly prepared solutions. For solution (1) shake a quantity of the powdered tablets containing 0.25 g of Aciclovir with 10 ml of *dimethyl sulphoxide* for 15 minutes and filter. For solution (2) dilute 0.7 volumes of solution (1) to 100 volumes with *dimethyl sulphoxide*. After removal of the plate, allow it to dry in air and examine under *ultraviolet light (254 nm)*. In the chromatogram obtained with solution (1) any *secondary spot* with an Rf value greater than that of the principal spot is not more intense than the spot in the chromatogram obtained with solution (2) (0.7%).

Assay Weigh and finely powder 20 tablets. To a quantity of the powdered tablets containing 0.1 g of Aciclovir add 60 ml of 0.1M *sodium hydroxide* and disperse with the aid of ultrasound for 15 minutes. Add a sufficient quantity of 0.1M *sodium hydroxide* to produce 100 ml, mix well and filter. To 15 ml of the filtrate add 50 ml of *water* and 5.8 ml of 2M *hydrochloric acid* and sufficient *water* to produce 100 ml. To 5 ml of the solution add sufficient 0.1M *hydrochloric acid* to produce 50 ml and mix well. Measure the *absorbance* of the resulting solution at the maximum at 255 nm, Appendix II B, using 0.1M *hydrochloric acid* in the reference cell. Calculate the content of $C_8H_{11}N_5O_3$ taking 560 as the value of A(1%, 1 cm) at the maximum at 255 nm.

Storage Aciclovir Tablets should be stored at a temperature not exceeding 25°.

Adrenaline Eye Drops
Epinephrine Eye Drops

Neutral Adrenaline Eye Drops
Neutral Epinephrine Eye Drops

For the purposes of product labelling in the United Kingdom, the pair of names given above shall be used together (see Introduction, Changes in title).

Definition Adrenaline Eye Drops are a sterile solution of Adrenaline in Purified Water.

The eye drops comply with the requirements stated under Eye Preparations and with the following requirements.

Content of adrenaline, $C_9H_{13}NO_3$ 95.0 to 110.0% of the prescribed or stated amount.

Identification

A. In the Assay, the retention time of the principal peak in the chromatogram obtained with solution (2) is the same as that of the principal peak in the chromatogram obtained with solution (1).

B. To 1 ml of a dilution of the eye drops containing 0.1% w/v of Adrenaline adjusted, if necessary, to a neutral or slightly acidic pH add, dropwise, a 0.25% w/v solution of *iron(III) chloride hexahydrate* until a green colour is produced. On the gradual addition of *sodium hydrogen carbonate solution*, the solution changes first to blue and then to red.

C. To 1 ml of a dilution of the eye drops containing 0.1% w/v of Adrenaline add 2 ml of a 10% w/v solution of *disodium hydrogen orthophosphate* and sufficient *iodinated potassium iodide solution* to produce a brown colour. Remove excess iodine by adding 0.2M *sodium thiosulphate* dropwise. A red colour is produced.

Acidity or alkalinity pH, 5.5 to 7.6, Appendix V L.

Noradrenaline Complies with the test described under Adrenaline but using as solution (2) the eye drops diluted with the mobile phase to contain 0.1% w/v of Adrenaline.

Assay Carry out the method for *liquid chromatography*, Appendix III D, using the following solutions. Solution (1) contains 0.2% w/v of *adrenaline acid tartrate BPCRS* in the mobile phase. For solution (2) dilute the eye drops with sufficient mobile phase to produce a solution containing 0.1% w/v of Adrenaline. Solution (3) contains 0.2% w/v of *adrenaline acid tartrate BPCRS* and 0.2% w/v of *noradrenaline acid tartrate* in the mobile phase.

The chromatographic procedure may be carried out using (a) a stainless steel column (10 cm × 4.6 mm) packed with *stationary phase C* (5 µm) (Nucleosil C18 is suitable), (b) as the mobile phase with a flow rate of 2 ml per minute, a solution prepared by adding 4.0 g of *tetramethylammonium hydrogen sulphate*, 1.1 g of *sodium heptanesulphonate* and 2 ml of 0.1M *disodium edetate* to a mixture of 950 ml of *water* and 50 ml of *methanol*, the pH of the mixture being adjusted to 3.5 with 1M *sodium hydroxide* and (c) a detection wavelength of 205 nm.

The test is not valid unless the *resolution factor* between the two principal peaks in the chromatogram obtained with solution (3) is at least 2.0.

Calculate the content of $C_9H_{13}NO_3$ in the eye drops using the declared content of $C_9H_{13}NO_3$ in *adrenaline acid tartrate BPCRS*.

Storage Adrenaline Eye Drops should be protected from light.

Labelling The label states 'Adrenaline Eye Drops' and 'Epinephrine Eye Drops'.

Adrenaline Injection
Epinephrine Injection

Adrenaline Tartrate Injection
Epinephrine Tartrate Injection

For the purposes of product labelling in the United Kingdom, the pair of names given above shall be used together (see Introduction, Changes in title).

Definition Adrenaline Injection is a sterile, isotonic solution containing 0.18% w/v of Adrenaline Acid Tartrate in Water for Injections.

The injection complies with the requirements stated under Parenteral Preparations and with the following requirements.

Content of adrenaline, $C_9H_{13}NO_3$ 0.09 to 0.11% w/v.

Characteristics A colourless solution.

Identification

A. In the Assay, the principal peak in the chromatogram obtained with solution (2) has the same retention time as that in the chromatogram obtained with solution (1).

B. To 1 ml add a 0.25% w/v solution of *iron(III) chloride hexahydrate* dropwise until a green colour is produced. On the gradual addition of *sodium hydrogen carbonate solution*, the solution changes first to blue and then to red.

C. To 10 ml add 2 ml of a 10% w/v solution of *disodium hydrogen orthophosphate* and sufficient *iodinated potassium iodide solution* to produce a brown colour and remove excess iodine by adding 0.1M *sodium thiosulphate* dropwise. A red colour is produced.

Acidity pH, 2.8 to 3.6, Appendix V L.

Noradrenaline Carry out the method for *liquid chromatography*, Appendix III D, using the following solutions. Solution (1) contains 0.0018% w/v of *noradrenaline acid tartrate* in the mobile phase. For solution (2) use the injection. Solution (3) contains 0.0018% w/v of *adrenaline acid tartrate BPCRS* and 0.0018% w/v of *noradrenaline acid tartrate* in the mobile phase.

The chromatographic procedure may be carried out using (a) a stainless steel column (10 cm × 4.6 mm) packed with *stationary phase C* (5 μm) (Nucleosil C18 is suitable), (b) as the mobile phase with a flow rate of 2 ml per minute a solution containing 4.0 g of *tetramethylammonium hydrogen sulphate*, 1.1 g of *sodium heptanesulphonate* and 2 ml of 0.1M *disodium edetate* in a mixture of 950 ml of *water* and 50 ml of *methanol* and adjusting the pH to 3.5 with 1M *sodium hydroxide* and (c) a detection wavelength of 205 nm.

The test is not valid unless the *resolution factor* between the two principal peaks in the chromatogram obtained with solution (3) is at least 2.0.

In the chromatogram obtained with solution (2) the area of any peak corresponding to noradrenaline is not greater than the area of the principal peak in the chromatogram obtained with solution (1).

Assay Carry out the method for *liquid chromatography*, Appendix III D, using the following solutions. Solution (1) contains 0.02% w/v of *adrenaline acid tartrate BPCRS* in the mobile phase. For solution (2) dilute 1 volume of the injection to 10 volumes with the mobile phase. Solution (3) contains 0.02% w/v of *adrenaline acid tartrate BPCRS* and 0.02% w/v of *noradrenaline acid tartrate* in the mobile phase.

The chromatographic procedure may be carried out using (a) a stainless steel column (10 cm × 4.6 mm) packed with *stationary phase C* (5 μm) (Nucleosil C18 is suitable), (b) as the mobile phase with a flow rate of 2 ml per minute a solution prepared by adding 4.0 g of *tetramethylammonium hydrogen sulphate*, 1.1 g of *sodium heptanesulphonate* and 2 ml of 0.1M *disodium edetate* to a mixture of 950 ml of *water* and 50 ml of *methanol* and adjusting the pH of the mixture to 3.5 with 1M *sodium hydroxide* and (c) a detection wavelength of 205 nm.

The test is not valid unless the *resolution factor* between the two principal peaks in the chromatogram obtained with solution (3) is at least 2.0.

Calculate the content of $C_9H_{13}NO_3$ in the injection using the declared content of $C_9H_{13}NO_3$ in *adrenaline acid tartrate BPCRS*.

Storage Adrenaline Injection should be protected from light.

Labelling The label states (1) 'Adrenaline Injection' and 'Epinephrine Injection'.

The quantity of active ingredient is stated in terms of the equivalent amount of adrenaline (epinephrine).

Adrenaline Injection contains the equivalent of adrenaline (epinephrine), 1 in 1000 (1 mg in 1 ml).

Dilute Adrenaline Injection 1 in 10,000
Dilute Epinephrine Injection 1 in 10,000

For the purposes of product labelling in the United Kingdom, the pair of names given above shall be used together (see Introduction, Changes in title).

Definition Dilute Adrenaline Injection 1 in 10,000 is a sterile, isotonic solution containing either 0.018% w/v of Adrenaline Acid Tartrate or 0.01% w/v of adrenaline hydrochloride, prepared by the interaction of Adrenaline and Hydrochloric Acid, in Water for Injections.

The injection complies with the requirements stated under Parenteral Preparations and with the following requirements.

Content of adrenaline, $C_9H_{13}NO_3$ 0.009 to 0.011% w/v.

Characteristics A colourless or almost colourless solution.

Identification A. In the Assay, the chromatogram obtained with solution (1) shows a peak with the same retention time as the principal peak in the chromatogram obtained with solution (2).

B. To 10 ml add 2 ml of a 10% w/v solution of *disodium hydrogen orthophosphate* and sufficient *iodinated potassium iodide solution* to produce a brown colour and remove excess iodine by adding 0.1M *sodium thiosulphate* dropwise. A red or pink colour is produced.

Acidity pH, 2.2 to 5.0, Appendix V L.

Noradrenaline Carry out the method for *liquid chromatography*, Appendix III D, using the following solutions. Solution (1) contains 0.00018% w/v of *noradrenaline acid tartrate* in the mobile phase. For solution (2) use the injection. Solution (3) contains 0.00018% w/v of *adrenaline acid tartrate BPCRS* and 0.00018% w/v of *noradrenaline acid tartrate* in the mobile phase.

The chromatographic procedure may be carried out using (a) a stainless steel column (10 cm × 4.6 mm) packed with *stationary phase C* (5 µm) (Nucleosil C18 is suitable), (b) as the mobile phase with a flow rate of 2 ml per minute a solution containing 4.0 g of *tetramethylammonium hydrogen sulphate*, 1.1 g of *sodium heptanesulphonate* and 2 ml of 0.1M *disodium edetate* in a mixture of 950 ml of *water* and 50 ml of *methanol* and adjusting the pH to 3.5 with 1M *sodium hydroxide* and (c) a detection wavelength of 205 nm.

The test is not valid unless, in the chromatogram obtained with solution (3), the *resolution factor* between the two principal peaks is at least 2.0.

In the chromatogram obtained with solution (2) the area of any peak corresponding to noradrenaline is not greater than the area of the principal peak in the chromatogram obtained with solution (1) (1%, calculated with respect to the content of adrenaline).

Assay Carry out the method for *liquid chromatography*, Appendix III D, using the following solutions. Solution (1) contains 0.02% w/v of *adrenaline acid tartrate BPCRS* in the mobile phase. Solution (2) is the injection. Solution (3) contains 0.02% w/v of *adrenaline acid tartrate BPCRS* and 0.02% w/v of *noradrenaline acid tartrate* in the mobile phase.

The chromatographic procedure may be carried out using (a) a stainless steel column (10 cm × 4.6 mm) packed with *stationary phase C* (5 µm) (Nucleosil C18 is suitable), (b) as the mobile phase with a flow rate of 2 ml per minute a solution prepared by adding 4.0 g of *tetramethylammonium hydrogen sulphate*, 1.1 g of *sodium heptanesulphonate* and 2 ml of 0.1M *disodium edetate* to a mixture of 950 ml of *water* and 50 ml of *methanol* and adjusting the pH of the mixture to 3.5 with 1M *sodium hydroxide* and (c) a detection wavelength of 205 nm.

The test is not valid unless, in the chromatogram obtained with solution (3), the *resolution factor* between the two principal peaks is at least 2.0.

Calculate the content of $C_9H_{13}NO_3$ in the injection using the declared content of $C_9H_{13}NO_3$ in *adrenaline acid tartrate BPCRS*.

Storage Dilute Adrenaline Injection 1 in 10,000 should be protected from light.

Labelling The label states 'Dilute Adrenaline Injection (1 in 10,000)' and 'Dilute Epinephrine Injection 1 in 10,000'.

The quantity of active ingredient is stated in terms of the equivalent amount of adrenaline (epinephrine).

Dilute Adrenaline Injection contains the equivalent of adrenaline (epinephrine), 1 in 10,000 (100 µg in 1 ml).

Adrenaline Solution
Epinephrine Solution

Adrenaline Tartrate Solution
Epinephrine Tartrate Solution

For the purposes of product labelling in the United Kingdom, the pair of names given above shall be used together (see Introduction, Changes in title).

Definition Adrenaline Solution is an isotonic *cutaneous solution* containing 0.18% w/v of Adrenaline Acid Tartrate with a suitable combination of an antioxidant and an antimicrobial preservative in Purified Water.

The solution complies with the requirements stated under Liquids for Cutaneous Application and with the following requirements.

Content of adrenaline, $C_9H_{13}NO_3$ 0.09 to 0.11% w/v.

Characteristics A clear, colourless solution.

Identification

A. In the Assay, the principal peak in the chromatogram obtained with solution (2) has the same retention time as that in the chromatogram obtained with solution (1).

B. To 1 ml add a 0.25% w/v solution of *iron(III) chloride hexahydrate* dropwise until a green colour is produced. On the gradual addition of *sodium hydrogen carbonate solution*, the solution changes first to blue and then to red.

C. To 10 ml add 2 ml of a 10% w/v solution of *disodium hydrogen orthophosphate* and sufficient *iodinated potassium iodide solution* to produce a brown colour and remove excess iodine by adding 0.1M *sodium thiosulphate* dropwise. A red colour is produced.

Acidity pH, 2.7 to 3.6, Appendix V L.

Noradrenaline Complies with the test described under Adrenaline but using the preparation being examined as solution (2).

Assay Carry out the method for *liquid chromatography*, Appendix III D, using the following solutions. Solution (1) contains 0.02% w/v of *adrenaline acid tartrate BPCRS* in the mobile phase. For solution (2) dilute 1 volume of the preparation being examined to 10 volumes with the mobile phase. Solution (3) contains 0.02% w/v of *adrenaline acid tartrate BPCRS* and 0.02% w/v of *noradrenaline acid tartrate* in the mobile phase.

The chromatographic procedure may be carried out using (a) a stainless steel column (10 cm × 4.6 mm) packed with *stationary phase C* (5 µm) (Nucleosil C18 is suitable), (b) as the mobile phase with a flow rate of 2 ml per minute a solution prepared by adding 4.0 g of *tetramethylammonium hydrogen sulphate*, 1.1 g of *sodium heptanesulphonate* and 2 ml of 0.1M *disodium edetate* to a mixture of 950 ml of *water* and 50 ml of *methanol* and adjusting the pH of the mixture to 3.5 with 1M *sodium hydroxide* and (c) a detection wavelength of 205 nm.

The test is not valid unless the *resolution factor* between the two principal peaks in the chromatogram obtained with solution (3) is at least 2.0.

Calculate the content of $C_9H_{13}NO_3$ in the preparation being examined using the declared content of $C_9H_{13}NO_3$ in *adrenaline acid tartrate BPCRS*.

Storage Adrenaline Solution should be kept in a well-filled, well-closed, glass container suitable for parenteral preparations, Appendix XIX B, and should be protected from light.

Labelling The label states (1) 'Adrenaline Solution' and 'Epinephrine Solution'; (2) the date after which the solution is not intended to be used; (3) the conditions under which it should be stored.

The quantity of active ingredient is stated in terms of the equivalent amount of adrenaline (epinephrine).

The label indicates the pharmaceutical form as 'cutaneous solution'.

Adrenaline Solution contains the equivalent of adrenaline (epinpehrine), 1 in 1000 (1 mg in 1 ml).

When a solution of adrenaline hydrochloride is prescribed or demanded, a solution complying with the requirements of this monograph may be dispensed or supplied.

Paediatric Alimemazine Oral Solution
Paediatric Trimeprazine Oral Solution

For the purposes of product labelling in the United Kingdom, the pair of names given above shall be used together (see Introduction, Changes in title).

Definition Paediatric Alimemazine Oral Solution is a solution containing 0.15% w/v of Alimemazine Tartrate in a suitable flavoured vehicle.

The oral solution complies with the requirements stated under Oral Liquids and with the following requirements.

Content of alimemazine tartrate, $C_{36}H_{44}N_4S_2$, $C_4H_6O_6$ 0.135 to 0.165% w/v.

Identification Dilute 50 ml with 175 ml of *water* and add 7 ml of 1M *sodium hydroxide*. Extract with 100 ml of *ether*, wash the ether layer with 15 ml of *water* and dry over *anhydrous sodium sulphate* (solution A).

A. Evaporate 30 ml of solution A to dryness and dissolve the residue in 100 ml of a mixture of 1 volume of 5M *ammonia* and 99 volumes of *methanol*. Dilute 4 ml of the resulting solution to 100 ml with the same solvent mixture. The *light absorption* of the resulting solution, Appendix II B, in the range 230 to 350 nm exhibits a maximum at 255 nm and a less well-defined maximum at 301 nm.

B. Evaporate 30 ml of solution A to dryness and dissolve the residue in 0.2 ml of *chloroform*. The *infrared absorption spectrum* of the resulting solution, Appendix II A, is concordant with the *reference spectrum* of alimemazine.

C. Evaporate 30 ml of solution A to dryness and add 0.05 ml of a mixture of 0.1 ml of *formaldehyde solution* and 1 ml of *sulphuric acid* to the residue. A purple colour is produced.

Related substances Complies with the test for *related substances in phenothiazines*, Appendix III A, using *mobile phase A* and the following freshly prepared solutions. For solution (1) dilute 15 ml with an equal volume of *water*, add 2 ml of 1M *sodium hydroxide* and extract with two 15-ml quantities of *chloroform*. Dry the chloroform extracts with *anhydrous sodium sulphate*, filter and evaporate the filtrate to dryness. Dissolve the residue as completely as possible in 1 ml of a mixture of 95 volumes of *methanol* and 5 volumes of *diethylamine*. For solution (2) dilute 1 volume of solution (1) to 50 volumes with the same solvent mixture.

Assay Carry out the following procedure protected from light. To a weighed quantity containing 15 mg of Alimemazine Tartrate add 25 ml of *water* and 5 ml of a 5% w/v solution of *sodium hydroxide*. Extract the mixture with two 50-ml quantities of *chloroform*, shaking vigorously for 1 minute each time, evaporate the combined extracts to dryness at about 30° at a pressure of 2 kPa and dissolve the residue in sufficient 0.1M *hydrochloric acid* to produce 50 ml (solution B). Dilute 10 ml of solution B to 50 ml with *water* (solution C). To a further 10 ml of solution B add 5 ml of *peroxyacetic acid solution*, allow to stand for 10 minutes and add sufficient *water* to produce 50 ml (solution D). Measure the *absorbance* of solution D at the maximum at 340 nm, Appendix II B, using solution C in the reference cell and measure the *absorbance* of solution C at the same wavelength using *water* in the reference cell. Repeat the procedure using a 0.03% w/v solution of *alimemazine tartrate BPCRS* in 0.1M *hydrochloric acid* in place of solution B and beginning at the words 'Dilute 10 ml of ...'. Determine the *weight per ml* of the oral solution, Appendix V G, and calculate the content of $C_{36}H_{44}N_4S_2,C_4H_6O_6$, weight in volume, using the declared content of $C_{36}H_{44}N_4S_2,C_4H_6O_6$ in *alimemazine tartrate BPCRS*. The result is not valid if the absorbance of solution C is more than 0.10.

Storage Paediatric Alimemazine Oral Solution should be protected from light.

Labelling The label states 'Paediatric Alimemazine Oral Solution' and 'Paediatric Trimeprazine Oral Solution'.

Paediatric Alimemazine Oral Solution contains in 5 ml 7.5 mg of Alimemazine Tartrate (Trimeprazine Tartrate).

Strong Paediatric Alimemazine Oral Solution
Strong Paediatric Trimeprazine Oral Solution

For the purposes of product labelling in the United Kingdom, the pair of names given above shall be used together (see Introduction, Changes in title).

Definition Strong Paediatric Alimemazine Oral Solution is a solution containing 0.6% w/v of Alimemazine Tartrate in a suitable flavoured vehicle.

The oral solution complies with the requirements stated under Oral Liquids and with the following requirements.

Content of alimemazine tartrate, $C_{36}H_{44}N_4S_2$, $C_4H_6O_6$ 0.54 to 0.66% w/v.

Identification Complies with the tests stated under Paediatric Alimemazine Oral Solution but using 15 ml of the oral solution to prepare solution A.

Related substances Complies with the test for *related substances in phenothiazines*, Appendix III A, using *mobile phase A* and the following freshly prepared solutions. For solution (1) dilute 5 ml with 15 ml of *water*, add 2 ml of 1M *sodium hydroxide* and extract with two 15-ml quantities of *chloroform*. Dry the chloroform extracts with *anhydrous sodium sulphate*, filter and evaporate the filtrate to dryness. Dissolve the residue as completely as possible in 1 ml of a mixture of 95 volumes of *methanol* and 5 volumes of *diethylamine*. For solution (2) dilute 1 volume of solution (1) to 50 volumes with the same solvent mixture.

Assay Carry out the Assay described under Paediatric Alimemazine Oral Solution but using as solution B a solution prepared in the following manner. To a weighed quantity containing 30 mg of Alimemazine Tartrate add 25 ml of *water* and 5 ml of a 5% w/v solution of *sodium hydroxide*. Extract the mixture with two 50-ml quantities of *chloroform*, shaking vigorously for 1 minute each time, evaporate the combined extracts to dryness at about 30° at a pressure of 2 kPa and dissolve the residue in sufficient 0.1M *hydrochloric acid* to produce 100 ml.

Storage Strong Paediatric Alimemazine Oral Solution should be protected from light.

Labelling The label states 'Strong Paediatric Alimemazine Oral Solution' and 'Strong Paediatric Trimeprazine Oral Solution'.

Strong Paediatric Alimemazine Oral Solution contains in 5 ml 30 mg of Alimemazine Tartrate (Trimeprazine Tartrate).

Alimemazine Tablets
Trimeprazine Tablets

For the purposes of product labelling in the United Kingdom, the pair of names given above shall be used together (see Introduction, Changes in title).

Definition Alimemazine Tablets contain Alimemazine Tartrate.

The tablets comply with the requirements stated under Tablets and with the following requirements.

Content of alimemazine tartrate, $C_{36}H_{44}N_4S_2$, $C_4H_6O_6$ 92.5 to 107.5% of the prescribed or stated amount.

Identification

A. To a quantity of the powdered tablets containing 40 mg of Alimemazine Tartrate add 10 ml of *water* and 2 ml of 1M *sodium hydroxide*, shake and extract with 15 ml of *ether*. Wash the ether layer with 5 ml of *water*, dry with *anhydrous sodium sulphate* and evaporate the ether to dryness. Dissolve the residue in 0.4 ml of *chloroform*. The *infrared absorption spectrum* of the resulting solution, Appendix II A, is concordant with the *reference spectrum* of alimemazine.

B. To a quantity of the powdered tablets containing 1 mg of Alimemazine Tartrate add 1 ml of a mixture of equal volumes of *formaldehyde solution* and *sulphuric acid*. A purple colour is produced.

Related substances Comply with the test for *related substances in phenothiazines*, Appendix III A, using *mobile phase A* and applying separately to the plate 20 µl of each of the following freshly prepared solutions. For solution (1) extract a quantity of the powdered tablets containing 0.1 g of Alimemazine Tartrate with 10 ml of a mixture of 95 volumes of *methanol* and 5 volumes of *diethylamine* and filter. For solution (2) dilute 1 volume of solution (1) to 200 volumes with the same solvent mixture.

Assay Carry out the following procedure protected from light. Add 150 ml of 0.1M *hydrochloric acid* to 10 tablets, shake for 10 minutes, mix with the aid of ultrasound for 1 minute, dilute with 0.1M *hydrochloric acid* to produce a solution containing 0.050% w/v of Alimemazine Tartrate and filter (solution A). Dilute 10 ml of solution A to 100 ml with *water* (solution B). To a further 10 ml of solution A add 2 ml of *peroxyacetic acid solution*, mix, allow to stand for 5 minutes and add sufficient *water* to produce 100 ml (solution C). Measure the *absorbance* of solution C at the maximum at 342 nm, Appendix II B, using solution B in the reference cell and measure the *absorbance* of solution B at the same wavelength using *water* in the reference cell. Repeat the procedure using a 0.05% w/v solution of *alimemazine tartrate BPCRS* in 0.1M *hydrochloric acid* in place of solution A, beginning at the words 'Dilute 10 ml of solution A ...' and calculate the content of $C_{36}H_{44}N_4S_2,C_4H_6O$ using the declared content of $C_{36}H_{44}N_4S_2,C_4H_6O$ in *alimemazine tartrate BPCRS*. The test is not valid if the absorbance of solution B is more than 0.10.

Labelling The label states 'Alimemazine Tablets' and 'Trimeprazine Tablets'.

Allopurinol Tablets

Definition Allopurinol Tablets contain Allopurinol.

The tablets comply with the requirements stated under Tablets and with the following requirements.

Content of allopurinol, $C_5H_4N_4O$ 92.5 to 107.5% of the prescribed or stated amount.

Identification

A. The *light absorption*, Appendix II B, in the range 230 to 350 nm of the solution obtained in the Assay exhibits a maximum only at 250 nm.

B. Shake a quantity of the powdered tablets containing 0.1 g of Allopurinol with 5 ml of 1.25M *sodium hydroxide* and add 3 ml of *lithium and sodium molybdotungstophosphate solution* and 5 ml of a 20% w/v solution of *sodium carbonate*. A greyish blue colour is produced.

Related substances Carry out the method for *thin-layer chromatography*, Appendix III A, using *silica gel GF_{254}* as the coating substance and a mixture of 60 volumes of *butan-2-one*, 20 volumes of 13.5M *ammonia* and 20 volumes of *2-methoxyethanol* as the mobile phase. Apply separately to the plate 10 µl of each of the following solutions. For solution (1) shake a quantity of the powdered tablets containing 0.25 g of Allopurinol with 10 ml of a 10% v/v solution of *diethylamine* and filter. Solution (2) contains 0.0050% w/v of *5-aminopyrazole-4-carboxamide hydrogen sulphate EPCRS* in 13.5M *ammonia*. After removal of the plate, allow it to dry in a current of air and examine under *ultraviolet light (254 nm)*. Any *secondary spot* in the chromatogram obtained with solution (1) is not more intense than the spot in the chromatogram obtained with solution (2).

Assay Weigh and powder 20 tablets. Shake a quantity of the powder containing 0.1 g of Allopurinol with 20 ml of 0.05M *sodium hydroxide* for 20 minutes, add 80 ml of 0.1M *hydrochloric acid*, shake for 10 minutes, add sufficient 0.1M *hydrochloric acid* to produce 250 ml, filter and dilute 10 ml of the filtrate to 250 ml with 0.1M *hydrochloric acid*. Measure the *absorbance* of the resulting solution at the maximum at 250 nm, Appendix II B, using 0.1M *hydrochloric acid* in the reference cell. Calculate the content of $C_5H_4N_4O$ taking 563 as the value of A(1%, 1 cm) at the maximum at 250 nm.

Almond Oil Ear Drops

Definition Almond Oil Ear Drops are Almond Oil in a suitable container.

The ear drops comply with the requirements stated under Ear Preparations and with the following requirements.

Identification Carry out the test for the *identification of fixed oils by thin-layer chromatography*, Appendix X N. The chromatogram obtained from the oil being examined shows spots corresponding to those in the *typical chromatogram* for almond oil.

Acid value Not more than 2.0, Appendix X B. Use 5 g dissolved in 50 ml of the prescribed mixture of solvents.

Peroxide value Not more than 10, Appendix X F.

Relative density 0.911 to 0.920, Appendix V G.

Unsaponifiable matter Not more than 0.7% w/w, Appendix X H, Method II. Use 5 g.

Apricot-kernel oil and peach-kernel oil Shake 2 ml for 5 minutes with a mixture of 1 ml of *fuming nitric acid* and 1 ml of *water* and allow to separate. No pink or brown colour develops in either layer.

Foreign fixed oils Carry out the test for *foreign oils by gas chromatography*, Appendix X N. The fatty-acid fraction of the oil has the following composition.
Saturated fatty acids of chain length less than C_{16} Not more than 0.1%.
Palmitic acid 4.0 to 9.0%.
Palmitoleic acid (equivalent chain length on polyethylene glycol adipate, 16.3) Not more than 0.6%.
Margaric acid Not more than 0.2%.
Stearic acid Not more than 3.0%.
Oleic acid (equivalent chain length on polyethylene glycol adipate, 18.3) 62.0 to 86.0%.
Linoleic acid (equivalent chain length on polyethylene glycol adipate, 18.9) 20.0 to 30.0%.
Linolenic acid (equivalent chain length on polyethylene glycol adipate, 19.7) Not more than 0.4%.
Arachidic acid Not more than 0.1%.
Gadoleic acid (equivalent chain length on polyethylene glycol adipate, 20.3) Not more than 0.1%.
Behenic acid Not more than 0.1%.
Erucic acid (equivalent chain length on polyethylene glycol adipate, 22.3) Not more than 0.1%.

Sterols Carry out the test for *sterols in fatty oils*, Appendix X N. The sterol fraction of the oil has the following composition.
Cholesterol Not more than 0.7%.
Campesterol Not more than 4.0%.
Stigmasterol Not more than 3.0%.
β-Sitosterol 73.0% to 87.0%.
Δ5-Avenasterol At least 10.0%.
Δ7-Avenasterol Not more than 3.0%.
Δ7-Stigmastenol Not more than 3.0 per cent.
Fucosterol Not more than 2.0 per cent.
Brassicasterol Not more than 0.3%.

Sesame oil Shake 10 ml with 5 ml of a mixture of 0.5 volume of a 0.35% v/v solution of *furfuraldehyde* in *acetic anhydride* and 4.5 volumes of *acetic anhydride* for 1 minute, filter through a filter paper impregnated with *acetic anhydride* and add 0.2 ml of *sulphuric acid*. No bluish green colour develops.

Storage Almond Oil Ear Drops should be kept in a well-filled, well-closed container and protected from light.

Standardised Aloes Dry Extract

Standardised Aloes Dry Extract complies with the requirements of the 3rd edition of the European Pharmacopoeia [0259]. These requirements are reproduced after the heading 'Definition' below.

Ph Eur

DEFINITION

Standardised aloes dry extract is prepared from Barbados aloes or Cape aloes, or a mixture of the two, by treatment with boiling water. It is adjusted, if necessary, to contain not less than 19.0 per cent and not more than 21.0 per cent of hydroxyanthracene derivatives, expressed as barbaloin ($C_{21}H_{22}O_9$; M_r 418.4) and calculated with reference to the dried extract.

CHARACTERS

A brown or yellowish-brown powder, sparingly soluble in boiling water.

IDENTIFICATION

A. Examine by thin-layer chromatography (*2.2.27*), using *silica gel G R* as the coating substance.

Test solution. To 0.25 g of the preparation to be examined add 20 ml of *methanol R* and heat to boiling in a water-bath. Shake for a few minutes and decant the solution. Store at about 4°C and use within 24 h.

Reference solution. Dissolve 25 mg of *barbaloin R* in *methanol R* and dilute to 10 ml with the same solvent.

Apply separately to the plate as bands 20 mm by not more than 3 mm 10 µl of each solution. Develop over a path of 10 cm using a mixture of 13 volumes of *water R*, 17 volumes of *methanol R* and 100 volumes of *ethyl acetate R*. Allow the plate to dry in air, spray with a 100 g/l solution of *potassium hydroxide R* in *methanol R* and examine in ultraviolet light at 365 nm. The chromatogram obtained with the test solution shows in the central part a zone of yellow fluorescence (barbaloin) similar in position to the zone corresponding to barbaloin in the chromatogram obtained with the reference solution and in the lower part there is a zone of light blue fluorescence (aloesine). In the lower part of the chromatogram obtained with the test solution two zones of yellow fluorescence (aloinosides A and B) (Cape aloes) and one zone of violet fluorescence just below the zone corresponding to barbaloin (Barbados aloes) may be present.

B. Shake 1 g of the preparation to be examined with 100 ml of boiling *water R*. Cool, add 1 g of *talc R* and filter. To 10 ml of the filtrate add 0.25 g of *disodium tetraborate R* and heat to dissolve. Pour 2 ml of the solution into 20 ml of *water R*. A yellowish-green fluorescence appears which is particularly marked in ultraviolet light at 365 nm.

TESTS

Loss on drying Not more than 4.0 per cent *m*/*m*, determined as prescribed in the monograph on *Extracts (765)* (Dry extracts).

Total ash (*2.4.16*). Not more than 2.0 per cent.

ASSAY

Carry out the assay protected from bright light.

Introduce 0.400 g into a 250 ml conical flask. Moisten with 2 ml of *methanol R*, add 5 ml of *water R* warmed to about 60°C, mix, add a further 75 ml of *water R* at about 60°C and shake for 30 min. Cool, filter into a volumetric flask, rinse the conical flask and filter with 20 ml of *water R*, add the rinsings to the volumetric flask and dilute to 1000.0 ml with *water R*. Transfer 10.0 ml of this solution to a 100 ml round-bottomed flask containing 1 ml of a 600 g/l solution of *ferric chloride R* and 6 ml of *hydrochloric acid R*. Heat in a water-bath under a reflux condenser for 4 h, with the water level above that of the liquid in the flask. Allow to cool, transfer the solution to a separating funnel, rinse the flask successively with 4 ml of *water R*, 4 ml of *1M sodium hydroxide* and 4 ml of *water R*, and add the rinsings to the separating funnel. Shake the contents of the separating funnel with three quantities, each of 20 ml, of *ether R*. Wash the combined ether layers with two quantities, each of 10 ml, of *water R*. Discard the washings and dilute the organic phase to 100.0 ml with *ether R*. Evaporate 20.0 ml carefully to dryness on a water-bath and dissolve the residue in 10.0 ml of a 5 g/l solution of *magnesium acetate R* in *methanol R*. Measure the absorbance (*2.2.25*) at 512 nm using *methanol R* as the compensation liquid.

Calculate the percentage content of hydroxyanthracene derivatives, as barbaloin, from the expression:

$$\frac{A \times 19.6}{m}$$

i.e. taking the specific absorbance of barbaloin to be 255.

A = absorbance at 512 nm,

m = mass of the substance to be examined in grams.

STORAGE

See the monograph on *Extracts (765)* (Dry extracts).

LABELLING

See the monograph on *Extracts (765)* (Dry extracts).

Ph Eur

Aloxiprin Tablets

Definition Aloxiprin Tablets contain Aloxiprin.

With the exception of the requirements for shape, the tablets comply with the requirements stated under Tablets and with the following requirements.

Content of total salicylates 92.5 to 107.5% of the stated amount, calculated as *O*-acetylsalicylic acid, $C_9H_8O_4$.

Identification To 0.5 g of the powdered tablets add 5 ml of *hydrochloric acid*, boil, cool and filter. Wash the residue with 20 ml of *water* and combine the filtrate and washings. The resulting solution yields the reactions characteristic of *aluminium* and, after neutralisation with 1M *sodium hydroxide*, yields reaction A characteristic of *salicylates*, Appendix VI.

Disintegration Maximum time, 5 minutes, Appendix XII A.

Free salicylates To a quantity of the powdered tablets containing the equivalent of 0.6 g of total salicylates add 50 ml of dry *ether* and shake for 30 minutes. Filter rapidly through fluted filter paper and wash the paper with several portions of dry *ether*. To the combined filtrate and washings add 10 ml of 1M *sodium hydroxide*, swirl to mix and evaporate the ether on a water bath. Cool, adjust the pH to between 2.40 and 2.50 with 1M *hydrochloric acid* and dilute to 100 ml with *water*. To 20 ml of the resulting solution add 4 ml of *iron(III) chloride solution* and dilute to 50 ml with *acetate buffer pH 2.45*. Allow to stand for 30 minutes, filter, if necessary, through a pair of fluted filter papers and measure the *absorbance* of the solution at the maximum at 530 nm, Appendix II B, using in the reference cell a solution prepared by diluting 4 ml of *iron(III) chloride solution* to 50 ml with *acetate buffer pH 2.45*. The absorbance is not more than that obtained using 5 ml of a 0.036% w/v solution of *salicylic acid* diluted to 20 ml with *water* in place of the solution being examined and beginning at the words 'add 4 ml of *iron(III) chloride solution* ...' (1.5%, calculated with reference to the content of total salicylates).

Combined salicylate Not more than 15.0%, calculated as salicylic acid, $C_7H_6O_3$, with reference to the content of total salicylates when determined by the following method. To a quantity of the finely powdered tablets containing the equivalent of 0.15 g of total salicylates add 40 ml of a 0.5% w/v solution of *sodium fluoride* in 0.1M *hydrochloric acid* and shake for 5 minutes. Allow the mixture to stand for 10 minutes, shaking at frequent intervals, extract with six 20-ml quantities of *chloroform*, filter the combined extracts through *anhydrous sodium sulphate*, wash with 30 ml of *chloroform* and dilute to 200 ml with *chloroform*. Dilute 20 ml of the solution to 100 ml with *chloroform* and measure the *absorbance* of the resulting solution at the maximum at 308 nm, Appendix II B. Calculate the content of $C_7H_6O_3$ taking 293 as the value of A(1%, 1 cm) at the maximum at 308 nm.

Assay Weigh and finely powder 20 tablets. To a quantity of the powder containing the equivalent of 0.3 g of total salicylates add 50 ml of 1M *sodium hydroxide* and boil gently for 15 minutes with occasional swirling. Cool, adjust the pH of the mixture to between 2.40 and 2.50 with 1M *hydrochloric acid* and dilute to 500 ml with *water*. Filter a portion of the suspension; to 5 ml of the filtrate add 35 ml of *acetate buffer pH 2.45* and 4 ml of *iron(III) chloride solution* and dilute to 50 ml with *water*. Allow to stand for 30 minutes and measure the *absorbance* of the resulting solution at the maximum at 530 nm, Appendix II B, using in the reference cell a solution prepared by diluting 4 ml of *iron(III) chloride solution* to 50 ml with *acetate buffer pH 2.45*. Calculate the content of total salicylates as *O*-acetylsalicylic acid, $C_9H_8O_4$, from the *absorbance* obtained by repeating the procedure using 4 ml of a 0.05% w/v solution of *salicylic acid* in place of the solution being examined and beginning at the words 'add 35 ml of *acetate buffer pH 2.45* ...'. Each g of salicylic acid is equivalent to 1.305 g of $C_9H_8O_4$.

Labelling The quantity of active ingredient is stated both as the amount of Aloxiprin and in terms of the equivalent amount of total salicylates calculated as *O*-acetylsalicylic acid, $C_9H_8O_4$.

Compound Aluminium Paste

Baltimore Paste

Definition Compound Aluminium Paste contains 20% w/w of Aluminium Powder and 40% w/w of Zinc Oxide in a suitable hydrophobic liquid basis.

Extemporaneous preparation The following formula and directions apply.

Aluminium Powder	200 g
Zinc Oxide	400 g
Liquid Paraffin	400 g

Mix the Aluminium Powder and the Zinc Oxide with the Liquid Paraffin until smooth.

The paste complies with the requirements stated under Topical Semi-solid Preparations and with the following requirements.

Content of aluminium, Al 15.8 to 20.0% w/w.

Content of zinc oxide, ZnO 37.0 to 42.0% w/w.

Identification

A. To 5 ml of solution A prepared in the Assay for aluminium add 2 ml of *ammonia buffer pH 10.9*, centrifuge and reserve the supernatant liquid. Dissolve the residue in the minimum quantity of 2M *hydrochloric acid* and add 0.25 ml of *ammonium acetate solution* and 0.25 ml of a 0.1% w/v solution of *mordant blue 3*. An intense purple colour is produced.

B. Add 2 ml of *sodium sulphide solution* to the supernatant liquid reserved in test A, centrifuge, dissolve the sediment in the minimum volume of 1M *sulphuric acid* and add 0.05 ml of a 0.1% w/v solution of *copper(II) sulphate* and 2 ml of *ammonium mercurithiocyanate reagent*. A violet precipitate is produced.

Assay

For aluminium Disperse 1 g in a mixture of 20 ml of *hydrochloric acid* and 20 ml of *water* with the aid of gentle heat, filter, wash the filter with *water*, cool the combined filtrate and washings and dilute to 100 ml with *water* (solution A). Neutralise 10 ml of solution A to *congo red paper* with 5M *sodium hydroxide*, add 50 ml of 0.05M *disodium edetate VS*, heat on a water bath for 30 minutes, cool, add 3 g of *hexamine* and titrate the excess of disodium edetate with 0.05M *lead nitrate VS*, using *xylenol orange solution* as indicator, to a purplish red colour. Add 1 g of *sodium fluoride* to the resulting solution, heat on a water bath for 15 minutes, cool and continue the titration to a purplish red colour. The volume of 0.05M *lead nitrate VS* used in the second titration represents the amount of disodium edetate liberated from the complex. Each ml of 0.05M *disodium edetate VS* is equivalent to 1.349 mg of Al.

For zinc oxide The difference between the volume of 0.05M *disodium edetate VS* added in the Assay for aluminium and the total volume of 0.05M *lead nitrate VS* used represents the amount of zinc present. Each ml of 0.05M *disodium edetate VS* is equivalent to 4.068 mg of ZnO.

Aluminium Acetate Ear Drops

Definition

Aluminium Sulphate	225 g
Calcium Carbonate	100 g
Tartaric Acid	45 g
Acetic Acid (33 per cent)	250 ml
Purified Water	750 ml

Extemporaneous preparation The following directions apply.

Dissolve the Aluminium Sulphate in 600 ml of the Purified Water, add the Acetic Acid and then the Calcium Carbonate mixed with the remainder of the Purified Water and allow to stand for not less than 24 hours in a cool place, stirring occasionally. Filter, add the Tartaric Acid to the filtrate and mix.

The ear drops comply with the requirements stated under Ear Preparations and with the following requirements.

Content of aluminium, Al 1.7 to 1.9% w/v.

Characteristics A clear liquid.

Weight per ml 1.06 to 1.08 g, Appendix V G.

Assay Dilute 10 ml to 100 ml with *water*. To 10 ml of the resulting solution add 40 ml of 0.05M *disodium edetate VS*, 90 ml of *water* and 0.15 ml of *methyl red solution*. Neutralise by the dropwise addition of 1M *sodium hydroxide* and warm on a water bath for 30 minutes. Cool, add 1 ml of 2M *nitric acid* and 5 g of *hexamine* and titrate with 0.05M *lead nitrate VS* using 0.5 ml of *xylenol orange solution* as indicator. Each ml of 0.05M *disodium edetate VS* is equivalent to 1.349 mg of Al.

Storage Aluminium Acetate Ear Drops should be kept in a well-filled container and stored at a temperature not exceeding 25°.

When aluminium acetate solution or Burow's Solution is prescibed or demanded a solution complyimg with the requirements of this monograph shall be dispensed or supplied.

Aluminium Chloride Solution

Definition Aluminium Chloride Solution is a *cutaneous solution*. It contains Aluminium Chloride Hexahydrate in a suitable ethanolic vehicle.

Production In making Aluminium Chloride Solution, Industrial Methylated Spirits may be used provided that the law and the statutory regulations governing the use of Industrial Methylated Spirits are observed.

The solution complies with the requirements stated under Liquids for Cutaneous Application and with the following requirements.

Content of aluminium chloride hexahydrate, $AlCl_3$, $6H_2O$ 95.0 to 105.0% of the prescribed or stated amount.

Identification Dilute the solution with *water* to produce a solution containing 2% w/v of Aluminium Chloride Hexahydrate. The solution yields reaction A characteristic of *aluminium salts* and reaction A characteristic of *chlorides*, Appendix VI.

Iron Dilute the solution being examined with *water* to produce a solution containing 10.0% w/v of Aluminium Chloride Hexahydrate. 10 ml of this solution complies with the *limit test for iron*, Appendix VII (10 ppm, determined with respect to the content of aluminium chloride hexahydrate).

Ethanol Not less than 70.0% v/v, Appendix VIII F.

Assay To a weighed quantity containing about 0.4 g of Aluminium Chloride Hexahydrate add 25 ml of *water* and carry out the *complexometric titration of aluminium*, Appendix VIII D. Each ml of 0.1M *disodium edetate VS* is equivalent to 24.14 mg of $AlCl_3,6H_2O$.

If the declared content is in terms of weight in volume, determine the *weight per ml* of the solution, Appendix V G, and hence calculate the content of $AlCl_3,6H_2O$, weight in volume.

Storage Aluminium Chloride Solution should be stored at a temperature not exceeding 25°. The container should be kept upright.

Labelling The label states (1) the date after which the solution is not intended to be used; (2) the conditions under which it should be stored; (3) that the solution is flammable.

The label states indicates the pharmaceutical form as 'cutaneous solution'.

Aluminium Hydroxide Oral Suspension

Definition Aluminium Hydroxide Oral Suspension is an aqueous suspension of hydrated aluminium oxide together with varying quantities of basic aluminium carbonate. It contains the equivalent of 4% w/w of aluminium oxide and has a peppermint flavour.

The oral suspension complies with the requirements stated under Oral Liquids and with the following requirements.

Content of aluminium oxide, Al_2O_3 The equivalent of 3.5 to 4.4% w/w.

Characteristics A white suspension from which small amounts of clear liquid may separate on standing. It may exhibit thixotropic properties.

Identification A solution in 2M *hydrochloric acid* yields the reactions characteristic of *aluminium salts*, Appendix VI.

Alkalinity pH, when diluted with an equal volume of *carbon dioxide-free water*, not more than 7.5, Appendix V L.

Neutralising capacity Disperse 5 g in 100 ml of *water*, heat to 37°, add 100 ml of 0.1M *hydrochloric acid VS* previously heated to 37° and stir continuously, maintaining the temperature at 37°. The pH of the solution, at 37°, after 10, 15 and 20 minutes, is not less than 1.8, 2.3 and 3.0 respectively and at no time during this period is it more than 4.0. Add 10 ml of 0.5M *hydrochloric acid VS* previously heated to 37°, stir continuously for 1 hour maintaining the temperature at 37° and titrate the solution with 0.1M *sodium hydroxide VS* to pH 3.5. Not more than 50 ml of 0.1M *sodium hydroxide VS* is required.

Ammonium salts To 25 g in an ammonia-distillation apparatus add 25 ml of 5M *sodium hydroxide* and 250 ml of *water*, distil about 100 ml, collecting the distillate in 25 ml of 0.1M *hydrochloric acid VS*, and titrate the excess of acid with 0.1M *sodium hydroxide VS* using *methyl red solution* as indicator. Not less than 20.0 ml of 0.1M *sodium hydroxide VS* is required.

Arsenic Dissolve 2.0 g in 18 ml of *brominated hydrochloric acid* and 32 ml of *water*. 25 ml of the resulting solution complies with the *limit test for arsenic*, Appendix VII (1 ppm).

Heavy metals Dissolve 2.0 g in 20 ml of 1M *hydrochloric acid* and 10 ml of *water*, add 0.5 ml of *nitric acid* and boil for about 30 seconds. Cool, add 2 g of *ammonium chloride* and 2 g of *ammonium thiocyanate* and extract with two 10-ml quantities of a mixture of equal volumes of *amyl alcohol* and *ether*. To the aqueous layer add 2 g of *citric acid* and dilute to 40 ml with *water*. 12 ml of the resulting solution complies with *limit test A for heavy metals*, Appendix VII. Use *lead standard solution (1 ppm Pb)* to prepare the standard (20 ppm).

Chloride Dissolve 0.30 g in 2 ml of 2M *nitric acid*, boil, cool, dilute to 250 ml with *water* and filter. 15 ml of the filtrate complies with the *limit test for chlorides*, Appendix VII (0.3%).

Sulphate Dissolve 0.50 g in 5 ml of 2M *hydrochloric acid*, boil, cool, dilute to 200 ml with *water* and filter. 12.5 ml of the filtrate, diluted to 15 ml with 2M *hydrochloric acid*, complies with the *limit test for sulphates*, Appendix VII (0.5%).

Microbial contamination Carry out a quantitative evaluation for Enterobacteriaceae and certain other Gram-negative bacteria, Appendix XVI B1. 0.01 ml of the preparation gives a negative result, Table I (most probable number of bacteria per gram fewer than 10^2).

Assay Dissolve 5 g in 3 ml of *hydrochloric acid* by warming on a water bath, cool to below 20° and dilute to 100 ml with *water*. To 20 ml of this solution add 40 ml of 0.05M *disodium edetate VS*, 80 ml of *water* and 0.15 ml of *methyl red solution* and neutralise by the dropwise addition of 1M *sodium hydroxide*. Heat on a water bath for 30 minutes, add 3 g of *hexamine* and titrate with 0.05M *lead nitrate VS* using 0.5 ml of *xylenol orange solution* as indicator. Each ml of 0.05M *disodium edetate VS* is equivalent to 2.549 mg of Al_2O_3.

Storage Aluminium Hydroxide Oral Suspension should be kept at a temperature not exceeding 30°. It should not be allowed to freeze.

Aluminium Hydroxide Tablets

Definition Aluminium Hydroxide Tablets contain, in each, 500 mg of Dried Aluminium Hydroxide in a suitable basis with a peppermint flavour.

The tablets comply with the requirements stated under Tablets and with the following requirements.

Content of aluminium oxide, Al_2O_3 Not less than the equivalent of 0.225 g.

Identification The powdered tablets yield the reactions characteristic of *aluminium salts*, Appendix VI, and have the odour and taste of peppermint.

Disintegration The requirement for Disintegration does not apply to Aluminium Hydroxide Tablets.

Neutralising capacity Pass a sufficient quantity of the powder prepared for use in the Assay through a sieve with a nominal mesh aperture of 150 µm. Mix a quantity of the powder containing 0.5 g of dried aluminium hydroxide with a small quantity of *water* to give a smooth paste and slowly add further quantities of *water* to a total volume of 100 ml. Warm to 37°, add 100 ml of 0.1M *hydrochloric acid VS* previously heated to 37° and stir continuously, maintaining the temperature at 37°. The pH of the solution at 37° after 10, 15 and 20 minutes is not less than 1.6, 1.8 and 2.2 respectively and at no time during this period is it more than 4.0. Add 10 ml of 0.5M *hydrochloric acid VS* previously heated to 37°, stir continuously for 1 hour maintaining the temperature at 37° and titrate the solution with 0.1M *sodium hydroxide VS* to pH 3.5. Subtract the volume of 0.1M *sodium hydroxide VS* from 150 to obtain the number of ml of 0.1M *hydrochloric acid VS* required for the neutralisation. Calculate the number of ml of 0.1M *hydrochloric acid VS* required for the total weight of the tablets taken for the Assay and divide by the number of tablets. The result is not less than 115.

Assay Weigh and powder 20 tablets, avoiding frictional heating. Dissolve a quantity of the powder containing 0.4 g of Dried Aluminium Hydroxide as completely as possible in a mixture of 3 ml of *hydrochloric acid* and 3 ml of *water* by warming on a water bath, cool to below 20° and dilute to 100 ml with *water*. To 20 ml of this solution add 40 ml of 0.05M *disodium edetate VS*, 80 ml of *water* and 0.15 ml of *methyl red solution* and neutralise by the dropwise addition of 1M *sodium hydroxide VS*. Heat on a water bath for 30 minutes, add 3 g of *hexamine* and titrate with 0.05M *lead nitrate VS* using 0.5 ml of *xylenol orange solution* as indicator. Each ml of 0.05M *disodium edetate VS* is equivalent to 2.549 mg of Al_2O_3.

Storage Aluminium Hydroxide Tablets should be stored at a temperature not exceeding 25°.

Labelling The label states that the tablets should be chewed before swallowing.

Amantadine Capsules

Definition Amantadine Capsules contain Amantadine Hydrochloride.

The capsules comply with the requirements stated under Capsules and with the following requirements.

Content of amantadine hydrochloride, $C_{10}H_{17}N,HCl$ 95.0 to 105.0% of the prescribed or stated amount.

Identification

A. Shake a quantity of the contents of the capsules containing 200 mg of Amantadine Hydrochloride in 10 ml of 0.1M *hydrochloric acid* on a water bath and filter. Add 1 ml of 5M *sodium hydroxide* to the filtrate, extract with 5 ml of *dichloromethane*, filter the dichloromethane layer through *anhydrous sodium sulphate*, wash the sodium sulphate with 2 ml of *dichloromethane* and evaporate the solution to dryness. The *infrared absorption spectrum* of the residue, Appendix II A, is concordant with the *reference spectrum* of amantadine.

B. The contents of the capsules yield the reactions characteristic of *chlorides*, Appendix VI.

Related substances Carry out the method for *gas chromatography*, Appendix III B, using 1 µl or other suitable volume of the following solution. Dissolve a quantity of the contents of the capsules containing 0.1 g of Amantadine Hydrochloride in 2 ml of *water*, add 2 ml of a 20% w/v solution of *sodium hydroxide* and 2 ml of *chloroform* and shake for 10 minutes. Separate the chloroform layer, dry over *anhydrous sodium sulphate* and filter.

The chromatographic procedure may be carried out using a glass column (1.8 m × 2 mm) containing a packing material prepared in the following manner. Mix 19.5 g of *silanised diatomaceous support* (Chromosorb G/AW/DMCS is suitable) with 60 ml of a 0.33% w/v solution of *potassium hydroxide* in *methanol* and evaporate the solvent under reduced pressure while slowly rotating the mixture. Dissolve 0.4 g of *low-vapour pressure hydrocarbons (type L)* (Apiezon L is suitable) in 60 ml of *toluene* (dissolution requires up to 5 hours), add this solution to the prepared silanised diatomaceous support and evaporate the solvent under reduced pressure while slowly rotating the mixture. Program the temperature of the column to increase from 100° to 200° at a constant rate of 6° per minute with the inlet port at 220° and the detector at 300°. Use a flow rate of 30 ml per minute for the carrier gas. Record the chromatogram for at least 2.5 times the retention time of the principal peak.

The area of any *secondary peak* is not greater than 0.3% and the sum of the areas of any secondary peaks is not greater than 1% by *normalisation*.

Assay Dissolve a quantity of the mixed contents of 20 capsules containing 0.5 g of Amantadine Hydrochloride as completely as possible in 10 ml of *water* by heating on a water bath while shaking and cool. Add 10 ml of 5M *sodium hydroxide* and 50 ml of *hexane*, shake gently for 15 minutes and centrifuge. To 10 ml of the supernatant liquid add 30 ml of *anhydrous acetic acid* and carry out Method I for *non-aqueous titration*, Appendix VIII A, determining the end point potentiometrically. Each ml of 0.1M *perchloric acid VS* is equivalent to 18.77 mg of $C_{10}H_{17}N,HCl$.

Storage Amantadine Capsules should be kept in an airtight container and protected from light.

Amantadine Oral Solution

Definition Amantadine Oral Solution is a solution of Amantadine Hydrochloride in a suitable flavoured vehicle.

The oral solution complies with the requirements stated under Oral Liquids and with the following requirements.

Content of amantadine hydrochloride, $C_{10}H_{17}N$, HCl 95.0 to 105.0% of the prescribed or stated amount.

Identification

A. Acidify a volume of the oral solution containing 0.1 g of Amantadine Hydrochloride with 1M *hydrochloric acid* and extract with three 15-ml quantities of *ether*. Discard the ether layer, add 2M *sodium hydroxide* to the aqueous layer until it is just alkaline, extract with two 10-ml quantities of *dichloromethane*, filter the dichloromethane layer through *anhydrous sodium sulphate*, evaporate the filtrate to dryness under reduced pressure and dry the residue at room temperature over *phosphorus pentoxide* at a pressure of 2 kPa for 1 hour. The *infrared absorption spectrum* of the dried residue, Appendix II A, is concordant with the *reference spectrum* of amantadine.

B. In the Assay, the retention time of the principal peak in the chromatogram obtained with solution (1) corresponds to that of the principal peak in the chromatogram obtained with solution (2).

Related substances Carry out the method described under Assay using 1 µl of the following solution. Mix, with swirling, a volume of the oral solution containing 0.1 g of Amantadine Hydrochloride with 4 ml of a 20% w/v solution of *sodium hydroxide*, add 10 ml of *toluene*, shake the mixture for 10 minutes, allow the layers to separate and use the upper layer.

The area of any *secondary peak* is not greater than 0.3% and the sum of the areas of any *secondary peaks* is not greater than 1% by *normalisation*.

Assay Prepare a 0.6% w/v solution of *naphthalene* (internal standard) in *toluene* (solution A). Carry out the method for *gas chromatography*, Appendix III B, using 1 µl of each of the following solutions. For solution (1) mix, with swirling, a weighed quantity of the oral solution containing 0.1 g of Amantadine Hydrochloride with 4 ml of a 20% w/v solution of *sodium hydroxide* and add 10 ml of solution A. Shake the mixture for 10 minutes, allow the layers to separate and use the upper layer. Prepare solution (2) in the same manner but using 0.1 g of *amantadine hydrochloride BPCRS* in 10 ml of *water* in place of the preparation being examined.

The chromatographic procedure may be carried out using a glass column (1.5 m × 4 mm) packed with *silanised diatomaceous support* (Chromosorb WHP is suitable) and coated with 10% polyethylene glycol compound (Carbowax 20 M is suitable) previously treated with a 5% w/v solution of *potassium hydroxide* in *methanol*. Maintain at 150° with the inlet port at 180° and the detector at 250° and use a flow rate of 40 ml per minute for the carrier gas.

Calculate the content of $C_{10}H_{17}N$,HCl using the ratios of the area of the peak corresponding to Amantadine Hydrochloride to the area of the peak due to the internal standard in the chromatograms obtained with solutions (1) and (2) and using the declared content of $C_{10}H_{17}N$, HCl in *amantadine hydrochloride BPCRS*.

Amiloride Tablets

Definition Amiloride Tablets contain Amiloride Hydrochloride.

With the exception of the requirements for shape, the tablets comply with the requirements stated under Tablets and with the following requirements.

Content of anhydrous amiloride hydrochloride, $C_6H_8ClN_7O$,HCl 90.0 to 110.0% of the prescribed or stated amount.

Identification

A. Extract a quantity of the powdered tablets containing the equivalent of 0.5 mg of anhydrous amiloride hydrochloride with 100 ml of 0.1M *hydrochloric acid* and filter. The *light absorption* of the filtrate, Appendix II B, in the range 230 to 380 nm exhibits two maxima, at 285 nm and at 361 nm.

B. Carry out the method described under Related substances applying separately to the plate 1 µl of each of the following solutions. For solution (1) shake a quantity of the powdered tablets containing the equivalent of 10 mg of anhydrous amiloride hydrochloride with 10 ml of *methanol* and centrifuge. Solution (2) contains 0.1% w/v of *amiloride hydrochloride BPCRS* in *methanol*. The principal spot in the chromatogram obtained with solution (1) corresponds to that in the chromatogram obtained with solution (2).

Related substances Carry out the method for *liquid chromatography*, Appendix III D, using the following four solutions. For solution (1) shake a quantity of the powdered tablets containing the equivalent of 17.5 mg of anhydrous amiloride hydrochloride with 10 ml of a mixture of 1 volume of *acetonitrile* and 3 volumes of *water*, disperse with the aid of ultrasound for 5 minutes and centrifuge. For solution (2) dilute 1 volume of solution (1) to 100 volumes with a mixture of 1 volume of *acetonitrile* and 3 volumes of *water*. For solution (3) dilute 1 volume of solution (2) to 10 volumes with a mixture of 1 volume of *acetonitrile* and 3 volumes of *water*. Solution (4) contains 0.0010% w/v of *methyl 3,5-diamino-6-chloropyrazine-2-carboxylate EPCRS* in a mixture of 1 volume of *acetonitrile* and 3 volumes of *water*.

The chromatographic procedure may be carried out using (a) a stainless steel column (25 cm × 4.6 mm) packed with *stationary phase C* (5 µm) (Nucleosil C18 is suitable), (b) as the mobile phase with a flow rate of 1 ml per minute, a mixture of 5 volumes of *tetramethylammonium hydroxide solution*, 250 volumes of *acetonitrile* and 745 volumes of *water*, the pH of the mixture being adjusted to 7.0 using a mixture of 1 volume of *orthophosphoric acid* and 9 volumes of *water*, and (c) a detection wavelength of 254 nm.

Inject 20 µl of solution (4) and adjust the concentration of acetonitrile so that the retention time of methyl 3,5-diamino-6-chloropyrazine-2-carboxylate is 5 to 6 minutes (an increase in the concentration of acetonitrile reduces the retention time). Inject 20 µl of solution (2) and adjust the concentrations of tetramethylammonium hydroxide and orthophosphoric acid so that the retention time of amiloride is 9 to 12 minutes keeping the pH at 7.0 (an increase in the concentrations reduces the retention time).

Inject 20 µl of solution (3). The test is not valid unless the *signal-to-noise ratio* of the peak due to amiloride in the chromatogram obtained is at least 5.0.

Inject 20 µl of each of solutions (1) and (4) and record the chromatograms for 5 times the retention time of amiloride. In the chromatogram obtained with solution (1) the sum of the areas of any *secondary peaks* is not greater than the area of the peak due to methyl 3,5-diamino-6-chloropyrazine-2-carboxylate in the chromatogram obtained with solution (4) (0.6%). Disregard any peak with an area less than 10% of the area of the peak due to methyl 3,5-diamino-6-chloropyrazine-2-carboxylate in the chromatogram obtained with solution (4) (0.06%).

Assay Weigh and powder 20 tablets. To a quantity of the powder containing the equivalent of 10 mg of anhydrous amiloride hydrochloride add 10 ml of *methanol* and shake for 10 minutes. Add 60 ml of 0.1M *sodium hydroxide*, shake for 30 minutes and dilute to 100 ml with 0.1M *sodium hydroxide*. Immediately transfer 4 ml of the resulting solution to a stoppered centrifuge tube and add 10 ml of 0.1M *sodium hydroxide* and 20 ml of *tributyl orthophosphate* that has been washed with *water* before use. Shake vigorously for 2 minutes and centrifuge for 5 minutes. Remove the upper layer and repeat the extraction with a further 20 ml of the water-washed tributyl orthophosphate. To the combined extracts add 2 ml of *methanol* and sufficient of the water-washed tributyl orthophosphate to produce 50 ml and centrifuge to remove traces of water. Measure the *absorbance* of the resulting solution at the maximum at 363 nm, Appendix II B, using in the reference cell a mixture of 48 volumes of the water-washed tributyl orthophosphate and 2 volumes of *methanol*. Calculate the content of $C_6H_8ClN_7O,HCl$ taking 692 as the value of (1%, 1 cm) at the maximum at 363 nm.

Labelling The quantity of active ingredient is stated in terms of the equivalent amount of anhydrous amiloride hydrochloride.

Aminophylline Injection

Definition Aminophylline Injection is a solution of Aminophylline or Aminophylline Hydrate in Water for Injections free from carbon dioxide.

The injection complies with the requirements stated under Parenteral Preparations and with the following requirements.

Content of ethylenediamine, $C_2H_8N_2$ Not more than 0.295 g for each g of anhydrous theophylline, $C_7H_8N_4O_2$, determined in the Assay for theophylline.

Content of theophylline, $C_7H_8N_4O_2$ 73.25 to 88.25% of the prescribed or stated amount of aminophylline.

Identification

A. To a volume containing 0.1 g of aminophylline add 0.5 ml of 2M *hydrochloric acid* with constant stirring, allow to stand for a few minutes and filter. Wash the residue with small quantities of cold *water*, recrystallise from hot *water* and dry at 105°. The *infrared absorption spectrum* of the residue, Appendix II A, is concordant with the *reference spectrum* of theophylline.

B. To a volume containing 0.1 g of aminophylline add 2 ml of a 1% w/v solution of *copper(II) sulphate* and shake. A purplish blue colour is produced.

C. Evaporate a volume containing 60 mg of aminophylline to dryness in a porcelain dish. To the residue add 1 ml of *hydrochloric acid* and 0.1 g of *potassium chlorate* and evaporate to dryness. A reddish residue is produced, which becomes purple on exposure to the vapour of 5M *ammonia*.

Alkalinity pH, 8.8 to 10.0, Appendix V L.

Assay

For theophylline To a volume containing 0.1 g of aminophylline add sufficient 0.01M *sodium hydroxide* to produce 250 ml, dilute 5 ml to 250 ml with 0.01M *sodium hydroxide* and measure the *absorbance* of the resulting solution at the maximum at 275 nm, Appendix II B. Calculate the content of $C_7H_8N_4O_2$ taking 650 as the value of A(1%, 1 cm) at the maximum at 275 nm.

For ethylenediamine To a volume containing 0.5 g of aminophylline add, if necessary, sufficient *water* to produce 20 ml and titrate with 0.05M *sulphuric acid VS*, using *bromocresol green solution* as indicator, until the colour changes from blue to green. Each ml of 0.05M *sulphuric acid VS* is equivalent to 3.005 mg of $C_2H_8N_2$. Calculate the weight of $C_2H_8N_2$ present for each g of $C_7H_8N_4O_2$ found.

Labelling When the injection is prepared from Aminophylline Hydrate, Theophylline or Theophylline Hydrate the strength is stated as the equivalent amount of aminophylline in a suitable dose-volume.

Aminophylline Tablets

Definition Aminophylline Tablets contain Aminophylline.

The tablets comply with the requirements stated under Tablets and with the following requirements.

Content of theophylline, $C_7H_8N_4O_2$ 80.6 to 90.8% of the prescribed or stated amount of Aminophylline.

Content of ethylenediamine, $C_2H_8N_2$ Not less than 10.9% of the prescribed or stated amount of Aminophylline.

Identification

A. Shake a quantity of the powdered tablets containing 0.5 g of Aminophylline with 20 ml of *water*, filter, add to the filtrate with constant stirring 1 ml of 2M *hydrochloric acid*, allow to stand for a few minutes and again filter. Reserve the filtrate for test C. Wash the residue with small quantities of cold *water*, recrystallise from hot *water* and dry at 105°. The *melting point* of the residue is about 271°, Appendix V A.

B. The *infrared absorption spectrum* of the residue obtained in test A, Appendix II A, is concordant with the *reference spectrum* of theophylline.

C. To the filtrate reserved in test A add 0.2 ml of *benzoyl chloride*, make alkaline with 5M *sodium hydroxide* and shake vigorously. Filter, wash the residue with cold *water* and recrystallise from a mixture of 1 volume of *water* and 3 volumes of *ethanol (96%)*. The *melting point* of the crystals, after drying at 100°, is about 250°, Appendix V A.

D. Shake a quantity of the powdered tablets containing 0.25 g of Aminophylline with 5 ml of *water* and filter. To 2 ml of the filtrate add 2 ml of a 1% w/v solution of *copper(II) sulphate* and shake. A purplish blue colour is produced.

Dissolution *For theophylline* Comply with the *dissolution test for tablets and capsules*, Appendix XII D, using Apparatus II. Use as the medium 900 ml of *phosphate buffer pH 7.0* and rotate the paddle at 50 revolutions per minute. Withdraw a sample of 10 ml of the medium and filter. Carry out the method for *liquid chromatography*, Appendix III D, using the following solutions. Solution (1) is a 0.001% w/v solution of *theophylline EPCRS* in *phosphate buffer pH 7.0*. Use the filtered dissolution medium as solution (2), diluted with *phosphate buffer pH 7.0*, if necessary.

The chromatographic procedure may be carried out using (a) a stainless steel column (10 cm × 4.6 mm) packed with particles of silica the surface of which has been modified with chemically-bonded phenyl groups (5 µm) (Apex Phenyl is suitable), (b) a mixture of 45 volumes of *methanol* and 55 volumes of *water* as the mobile phase with a flow rate of 2 ml per minute and (c) a detection wavelength of 273 nm.

Calculate the total content of theophylline, $C_7H_8N_4O_2$, in the medium taking 100% as the content of $C_7H_8N_4O_2$ in *theophylline EPCRS*.

Assay

For theophylline Weigh and powder 20 tablets. Shake a quantity of the powder containing 80 mg of Aminophylline with a mixture of 20 ml of 0.1M *sodium hydroxide* and 60 ml of *water* for 10 minutes, add sufficient *water* to produce 200 ml, mix and filter. Dilute 5 ml of the filtrate to 250 ml with 0.01M *sodium hydroxide* and measure the *absorbance* of the resulting solution at the maximum at 275 nm, Appendix II B. Calculate the content of $C_7H_8N_4O_2$ taking 650 as the value of A(1%, 1 cm) at the maximum at 275 nm.

For ethylenediamine Weigh and powder 20 tablets. Shake a quantity of the powder containing 0.3 g of Aminophylline with 20 ml of *water*, heat to 50° for 30 minutes and titrate with 0.05M *sulphuric acid VS*, using *bromocresol green solution* as indicator, until the colour changes from blue to green. Each ml of 0.05M *sulphuric acid VS* is equivalent to 3.005 mg of $C_2H_8N_2$.

Storage Aminophylline Tablets should be kept in an airtight container and protected from light.

Amiodarone Intravenous Infusion

Definition Amiodarone Intravenous Infusion is a sterile solution of Amiodarone Hydrochloride in Water for Injections. It is prepared immediately before use by diluting Sterile Amiodarone Concentrate with Glucose Intravenous Infusion in accordance with the manufacturer's instructions.

The intravenous infusion complies with the requirements stated under Parenteral Preparations and with the following requirement.

Particulate contamination When the volume of the constituted intravenous infusion is 100 ml or more, it complies with the test for *sub-visible particles*, Appendix XIII A.

STERILE AMIODARONE CONCENTRATE

Definition Sterile Amiodarone Concentrate is a sterile solution of Amiodarone Hydrochloride in Water for Injections.

The concentrate complies with the requirements for Concentrated Solutions for Injections stated under Parenteral Preparations and with the following requirements.

Content of amiodarone hydrochloride, $C_{25}H_{29}I_2NO_3$, HCl 95.0 to 105.0% of the prescribed or stated amount.

Identification

A. Extract a volume of the concentrate containing 0.3 g of Amiodarone Hydrochloride with three 25-ml volumes of *dichloromethane*. Dry the combined extracts over *anhydrous sodium sulphate*, filter and evaporate to dryness. To the residue add 2 ml of 1M *sodium hydroxide* and extract with 25 ml of *ether*. Dry the extract over *anhydrous sodium sulphate*, filter and evaporate to dryness. Dry the residue obtained under reduced pressure over *phosphorus pentoxide* and dissolve in 2.5 ml of *dichloromethane*. The *infrared absorption spectrum* of the resulting solution, Appendix II A, is concordant with the *reference spectrum* of amiodarone.

B. In the Assay, the principal peak in the chromatogram obtained with solution (1) has the same retention time as the peak in the chromatogram obtained with solution (2).

Colour of solution Not more intense than *reference solution GY_5*, Appendix IV B, Method II.

Iodides Prepare solutions (1) and (2) simultaneously. Dilute a volume of the concentrate with *water* to produce a solution containing 3.0% w/v of Amiodarone Hydrochloride (solution A).

Solution (1) To 15 ml of solution A add 1 ml of 0.1M *hydrochloric acid* and 1 ml of 0.05M *potassium iodate*. Dilute to 20 ml with *water*. Allow to stand protected from light for 4 hours.

Solution (2) To 15 ml of solution A add 1 ml of 0.1M *hydrochloric acid*, 1 ml of a 0.00882% w/v solution of *potassium iodide* and 1 ml of 0.05M *potassium iodate*. Dilute to 20 ml with *water*. Allow to stand protected from light for 4 hours.

Measure the *absorbances* of the solutions at 420 nm, Appendix II B, using in the reference cell a mixture of 15 ml of solution A and 1 ml of 0.1M *hydrochloric acid* diluted to 20 ml with *water*. The *absorbance* of solution (1) is not greater than half the *absorbance* of solution (2) (150 ppm).

Related substances Carry out the method for *thin-layer chromatography*, Appendix III A, using *silica gel GF_{254}* as the coating substance and a mixture of 5 volumes of *anhydrous formic acid*, 10 volumes of *methanol* and 85 volumes of *dichloromethane* as the mobile phase. Pre-wash the plate with the mobile phase and allow to dry in air before use. Apply separately to the plate 10 µl of each of the following solutions. For solution (1) dilute a volume of the concentrate containing 50 mg of Amiodarone Hydrochloride to 20 ml with *methanol*. For solution (2) dilute 1 volume of solution (1) to 200 volumes with *methanol*. Solution (3) contains 0.00125% w/v of *2-butyl-3-(4-hydroxy-3,5-di-iodobenzoyl)benzofuran BPCRS* in *methanol*. Solution (4) contains 0.1% w/v of *benzyl alcohol* in *methanol*. After removal of the plate, allow it to dry in air and examine under *ultraviolet light (254 nm)*. In the chromatogram obtained with solution (1) any spot corresponding to 2-butyl-3-(4-hydroxy-3,5-di-iodobenzoyl)-benzofuran is not more intense than the spot in the chromatogram obtained with solution (3) (0.5%) and any other *secondary spot*, other than any spot corresponding to benzyl alcohol, is not more intense than the spot in the chromatogram obtained with solution (2) (0.5%).

Assay Carry out the method for *liquid chromatography*, Appendix III D, using the following solutions. For solution (1) dilute a volume of the concentrate containing 50 mg of Amiodarone Hydrochloride to 50 ml with the mobile phase and dilute 10 ml of this solution to 100 ml with the mobile phase. Solution (2) contains 0.01% w/v of *amiodarone hydrochloride BPCRS* in the mobile phase. Solution (3) contains 0.01% w/v of *amiodarone hydrochloride BPCRS* and 0.01% w/v of *benzyl alcohol* in the mobile phase.

The chromatographic procedure may be carried out using (a) a stainless steel column (7.5 cm × 3.9 mm) packed with silica particles the surface of which have been modified by chemically-bonded nitrile groups (4 µm) (Nova-Pak CN HP is suitable), (b) as the mobile phase with a flow rate of 1.0 ml per minute a mixture of 45 volumes of 0.01M *sodium perchlorate* and 55 volumes of *acetonitrile*, the pH of the mixture being adjusted to 3.0 with 2M *orthophosphoric acid* and (c) a detection wavelength of 244 nm.

Calculate the content of $C_{25}H_{29}I_2NO_3,HCl$ using the declared content of $C_{25}H_{29}I_2NO_3,HCl$ in *amiodarone hydrochloride BPCRS.*

Storage Sterile Amiodarone Concentrate should be protected from light.

Labelling The label states (1) 'Sterile Amiodarone Concentrate'; (2) that the solution must be diluted with Glucose Intravenous Infusion.

Amiodarone Tablets

Definition Amiodarone Tablets contain Amiodarone Hydrochloride.

The tablets comply with the requirements stated under Tablets and with the following requirements.

Content of amiodarone hydrochloride, $C_{25}H_{29}I_2NO_3$, HCl 95.0 to 105.0% of the prescribed or stated amount.

Identification

A. Shake a quantity of the powdered tablets containing 0.3 g of Amiodarone Hydrochloride with 25 ml of *dichloromethane*, filter and evaporate the filtrate to dryness. To the residue add 2 ml of 1M *sodium hydroxide* and extract with 25 ml of *ether*. Dry the extract over *anhydrous sodium sulphate*, filter and evaporate to dryness. Dry the residue obtained under reduced pressure over *phosphorus pentoxide* and dissolve in 2.5 ml of *dichloromethane*. The *infrared absorption spectrum* of the resulting solution, Appendix II A, is concordant with the *reference spectrum* of amiodarone.

B. In the Assay, the principal peak in the chromatogram obtained with solution (2) has the same retention time as the peak in the chromatogram obtained with solution (1).

Related substances Carry out the method for *thin-layer chromatography*, Appendix III A, using *silica gel GF_{254}* as the coating substance and a mixture of 5 volumes of *anhydrous formic acid,* 10 volumes of *methanol* and 85 volumes of *dichloromethane* as the mobile phase. Pre-wash the plate with the mobile phase and allow to dry in air before use. Apply separately to the plate 10 µl of each of the following solutions. For solution (1) shake a quantity of the powdered tablets containing 50 mg of Amiodarone Hydrochloride with 20 ml of *methanol* and filter. For solution (2) dilute 1 volume of solution (1) to 200 volumes with *methanol.* Solution (3) contains 0.00125% w/v of *2-butyl-3-(4-hydroxy-3,5-di-iodobenzoyl)benzofuran BPCRS* in *methanol*. After removal of the plate, allow it to dry in air and examine under *ultraviolet light (254 nm)*. In the chromatogram obtained with solution (1) any spot corresponding to 2-butyl-3-(4-hydroxy-3,5-di-iodobenzoyl)benzofuran is not more intense than the spot in the chromatogram obtained with solution (3) (0.5%) and any other *secondary spot* is not more intense than the spot in the chromatogram obtained with solution (2) (0.5%).

Assay Weigh and finely powder 20 tablets. Carry out the method for *liquid chromatography*, Appendix III D, using the following solutions. For solution (1) dissolve 0.1 g of *amiodarone hydrochloride BPCRS* in 70 ml of *methanol*, cool and dilute to 100 ml with the same solvent. Mix and dilute 10 ml of the resulting solution to 100 ml with the mobile phase. For solution (2) disperse a quantity of the finely powdered tablets containing 0.1 g of Amiodarone Hydrochloride in 70 ml of *methanol* with the aid of ultrasound for 15 minutes, cool and dilute to 100 ml with the same solvent. Mix, filter and dilute 10 ml of the filtrate to 100 ml with the mobile phase.

The chromatographic procedure may be carried out using (a) a stainless steel column (7.5 cm × 3.9 mm) packed with silica particles the surface of which have been modified by chemically-bonded nitrile groups (4 µm) (Nova-Pak CN HP is suitable), (b) as the mobile phase with a flow rate of 1.0 ml per minute a mixture of 45 volumes of 0.01M *sodium perchlorate* and 55 volumes of *acetonitrile*, the pH of the mixture being adjusted to 3.0 with 2M *orthophosphoric acid* and (c) a detection wavelength of 244 nm.

Calculate the content of $C_{25}H_{29}I_2NO_3,HCl$ using the declared content of $C_{25}H_{29}I_2NO_3,HCl$ in *amiodarone hydrochloride BPCRS.*

Storage Amiodarone Tablets should be protected from light.

Amitriptyline Oral Suspension

Definition Amitriptyline Oral Suspension is a suspension of Amitriptyline Embonate in a suitable flavoured vehicle.

The oral suspension complies with the requirements stated under Oral Liquids and with the following requirements.

Content of amitriptyline, $C_{20}H_{23}N$ 90.0 to 110.0% of the prescribed or stated amount.

Identification

A. Evaporate to dryness 5 ml of the dichloromethane extract obtained in the Assay, dissolve the residue in 1 ml of *methanol* and add 1 ml of a 2.5% w/v solution of *sodium hydrogen carbonate*, 1 ml of a 2% w/v solution of *sodium periodate* and 1 ml of a 0.3% w/v solution of *potassium permanganate*. Allow to stand for 15 minutes, acidify the solution with 1M *sulphuric acid* and extract with 10 ml of *2,2,4-trimethylpentane*. The *light absorption* of the resulting solution, Appendix II B, in the range 230 to 350 nm exhibits a maximum only at 265 nm.

B. Shake a quantity containing the equivalent of 50 mg of amitriptyline with 20 ml of *chloroform*, allow to separate, add 10 ml of 2M *sodium hydroxide* to the chloroform layer, shake and allow to separate. When examined under ultraviolet light, the aqueous layer exhibits a green fluorescence.

Acidity or alkalinity pH, 5.0 to 7.0, Appendix V L.

Related substances Carry out the method for *thin-layer chromatography*, Appendix III A, protected from light, using *silica gel G* as the coating substance and a mixture of 3 volumes of *diethylamine*, 15 volumes of *ethyl acetate* and 85 volumes of *cyclohexane* as the mobile phase but allowing the solvent front to ascend 14 cm above the line of application in an unlined tank. Apply separately to the plate 10 µl of each of the following solutions. For solution (1) extract a quantity containing the equivalent of 20 mg of amitriptyline with 5 ml of *chloroform* and use the chloroform layer. Solution (2) contains 0.0010% w/v of *dibenzosuberone EPCRS* in *chloroform*. Solution (3) contains 0.004% w/v of *cyclobenzaprine hydrochloride EPCRS* in *chloroform*. After removal of the plate, allow it to dry in air, spray with a freshly prepared mixture of 4 volumes of *formaldehyde* and 96 volumes of *sulphuric acid*, heat at 100° to 105° for 10 minutes and examine under *ultraviolet light (365 nm)*. Any spot corresponding to dibenzosuberone in the chromatogram obtained with solution (1) is not more intense than the spot in the chromatogram obtained with solution (2) (0.25%). Examine the plate under *ultraviolet light (254 nm)*. Any other *secondary spot* in the chromatogram obtained with solution (1) is not more intense than the spot in the chromatogram obtained with solution (3) (1%).

Assay To a weighed quantity containing the equivalent of 4 mg of amitriptyline add 20 ml of *water*, mix well, extract with four 20-ml quantities and one 15-ml quantity of *dichloromethane* and dilute the combined extracts to 100 ml with *dichloromethane*. To 20 ml of the solution add 10 ml of 1M *sodium hydroxide*, shake, allow to separate, filter the dichloromethane layer through absorbent cotton, discarding the first portion of the filtrate, and evaporate 10 ml of the clear filtrate to dryness on a water bath in a current of nitrogen. Dissolve the residue in sufficient 0.1M *hydrochloric acid* to produce 50 ml and measure the *absorbance* of the resulting solution at the maximum at 239 nm, Appendix II B, using 0.1M *hydrochloric acid* in the reference cell. Calculate the content of $C_{20}H_{23}N$ taking 510 as the value of A(1%, 1 cm) at the maximum at 239 nm. Determine the *weight per ml* of the oral suspension, Appendix V G, and calculate the content of $C_{20}H_{23}N$, weight in volume.

Labelling The quantity of active ingredient is stated in terms of the equivalent amount of amitriptyline.

Amitriptyline Tablets

Definition Amitriptyline Tablets contain Amitriptyline Hydrochloride. They are coated.

The tablets comply with the requirements stated under Tablets and with the following requirements.

Content of amitriptyline hydrochloride, $C_{20}H_{23}N$, HCl 90.0 to 110.0% of the prescribed or stated amount.

Identification

A. Shake a quantity of the powdered tablets containing 5 mg of Amitriptyline Hydrochloride with 20 ml of *methanol* and filter. To 1 ml of the filtrate add 1 ml of a 2.5% w/v solution of *sodium hydrogen carbonate*, 1 ml of a 2% w/v solution of *sodium periodate* and 1 ml of a 0.3% w/v solution of *potassium permanganate*, allow to stand for 15 minutes, acidify with 1M *sulphuric acid* and extract with 10 ml of *2,2,4-trimethylpentane*. The *light absorption* of the resulting solution, Appendix II B, in the range 230 to 350 nm exhibits a maximum only at 265 nm.

B. Triturate a quantity of the powdered tablets containing 0.1 g of Amitriptyline Hydrochloride with 10 ml of *chloroform*, filter and evaporate the filtrate to a low volume. Add *ether* until a turbidity is produced and allow to stand. Dissolve 50 mg of the precipitate in 3 ml of *water* and add 0.05 ml of a 2.5% w/v solution of *quinhydrone* in *methanol*. No red colour is produced within 15 minutes (distinction from nortriptyline).

C. The precipitate obtained in test B yields reaction A characteristic of *chlorides*, Appendix VI.

Related substances Carry out the method for *thin-layer chromatography*, Appendix III A, protected from light, using *silica gel G* as the coating substance and a mixture of 3 volumes of *diethylamine*, 15 volumes of *ethyl acetate* and 85 volumes of *cyclohexane* as the mobile phase but allowing the solvent front to ascend 14 cm above the line of application in an unlined tank. Apply separately to the plate 10 µl of each of the following solutions. For solution (1) extract a quantity of the powdered tablets containing 20 mg of Amitriptyline Hydrochloride with 5 ml of a mixture of 1 volume of 2M *hydrochloric acid* and 9 volumes of *ethanol (96%*, centrifuge and use the supernatant liquid. Solution (2) contains 0.0010% w/v of *dibenzosuberone EPCRS* in *chloroform*. Solution (3) contains 0.0040% w/v of *cyclobenzaprine hydrochloride EPCRS*. After removal of the plate, allow it to dry in air, spray with a freshly prepared mixture of 4 volumes of *formaldehyde* and 96 volumes of *sulphuric acid*, heat at 100° to 105° for 10 minutes and examine under *ultraviolet light (365 nm)*. Any spot corresponding to dibenzosuberone in the chromatogram obtained with solution (1) is not more intense than the spot in the chromatogram obtained with solution (2) (0.25%). Examine the plate under *ultraviolet light (254 nm)*. Any other *secondary spot* in the chromatogram obtained with solution (1) is not more intense than the spot in the chromatogram obtained with solution (3) (1%).

Assay Carry out the method for *liquid chromatography*, Appendix III D, using the following solutions. For solution (1) dissolve 50 mg of *amitriptyline hydrochloride BPCRS* in 10 ml of *methanol* and dilute to 200 ml with *methanol (50%)*. For film-coated tablets, prepare solution (2) in the following manner. Add 50 ml of 0.1M *hydrochloric acid* to 20 tablets, shake vigorously until the tablets are completely disintegrated, add 100 ml of *methanol* and shake for 30 minutes. Dilute the suspension to 200 ml with *methanol*, centrifuge and dilute a volume of the supernatant liquid containing 25 mg of Amitriptyline Hydrochloride to 100 ml with *methanol (50%)*. For sugar-coated tablets prepare solution (2) in the following manner. Weigh and powder 20 tablets. Shake a quantity of the powder containing 50 mg of Amitriptyline Hydrochloride with 50 ml of 0.1M *hydrochloric acid* for 30 minutes, add 100 ml of *methanol* and shake for 30 minutes. Dilute the suspension to 200 ml with *water*, centrifuge and use the supernatant liquid.

The chromatographic procedure may be carried out using (a) a stainless steel column (20 cm × 4.6 mm) packed with *stationary phase C* (10 µm) (Nucleosil C18 is

suitable), (b) as the mobile phase with a flow rate of 2 ml per minute 0.03M *sodium hexanesulphonate* in a mixture of equal volumes of *water* and *acetonitrile*, adjusted to pH 4.5 by the addition of *glacial acetic acid*, and (c) a detection wavelength of 239 nm.

Calculate the content of $C_{20}H_{23}N,HCl$ using the declared content of $C_{20}H_{23}N,HCl$ in *amitriptyline hydrochloride BPCRS*.

Ammonia and Ipecacuanha Mixture

Ammonia and Ipecacuanha Oral Solution

Definition Ammonia and Ipecacuanha Mixture is an *oral solution* containing 2% w/v of Ammonium Bicarbonate and 3% v/v of Ipecacuanha Tincture in a suitable vehicle containing Liquorice Liquid Extract with a flavour of anise and camphor.

Extemporaneous preparation It is recently prepared according to the following formula.

Ammonium Bicarbonate	20 g
Ipecacuanha Tincture	30 ml
Concentrated Anise Water	5 ml
Concentrated Camphor Water	10 ml
Liquorice Liquid Extract	50 ml
Double-strength Chloroform Water	500 ml
Water	sufficient to produce 1000 ml

The mixture complies with the requirements stated under Oral Liquids and with the following requirements.

Content of ammonium bicarbonate, NH_4HCO_3 1.90 to 2.12% w/v.

Identification Carry out the method for *thin-layer chromatography*, Appendix III A, using *silica gel G* as the coating substance and a mixture of 90 volumes of *chloroform* and 10 volumes of *diethylamine* as the mobile phase. Apply separately to the plate 10 µl of each of the following solutions. For solution (1) add 10 ml of 1M *sulphuric acid* to 10 ml of the mixture, mix, extract with two 10-ml quantities of *chloroform* and discard the chloroform extracts. Add sufficient 5M *ammonia* to make the aqueous solution alkaline to *litmus paper*, extract with four 10-ml quantities of *chloroform*, filter, evaporate the combined filtrates to dryness and dissolve the residue in 0.5 ml of *ethanol (96%)*. Solution (2) contains 0.1% w/v of *cephaeline hydrochloride EPCRS* in *ethanol (96%)*. Solution (3) contains 0.1% w/v of *emetine hydrochloride EPCRS* in *ethanol (96%)*. After removal of the plate, heat it at 105° for 30 minutes, allow to cool and spray with *dilute potassium iodobismuthate solution*. The principal spots in the chromatogram obtained with solution (1) correspond in colour and position to the spots in the chromatograms obtained with solutions (2) and (3).

Assay Transfer 10 ml to an ammonia-distillation apparatus, dilute to 200 ml with *water* and add 1 g of *heavy magnesium oxide* suspended in 10 ml of *water*. Distil into 50 ml of 0.05M *sulphuric acid VS*, boil to remove carbon dioxide, cool and titrate the excess sulphuric acid with 0.1M *sodium hydroxide VS* using *methyl red solution* as indicator. Repeat the operation without the mixture being examined. The difference between the titrations represents the amount of acid required. Each ml of 0.05M *sulphuric acid VS* is equivalent to 7.906 mg of NH_4HCO_3.

Labelling The label indicates the pharmaceutical form as 'oral solution'.

Aromatic Ammonia Solution

Sal Volatile Solution

Definition

Ammonium Bicarbonate	25 g
Nutmeg Oil	0.3 ml
Lemon Oil	0.5 ml
Ethanol (90 per cent)	37.5 ml
Strong Ammonia Solution	67.5 ml
Purified Water, freshly boiled and cooled	sufficient to produce 1000 ml

Extemporaneous preparation The following directions apply.

Dissolve the Ammonium Bicarbonate in 800 ml of the Purified Water. Separately dissolve the Lemon Oil and the Nutmeg Oil in the Ethanol (90 per cent). Add the ethanolic solution to the aqueous solution and add the Strong Ammonia Solution and sufficient Purified Water to produce 1000 ml. Add 25 g of previously sterilised Purified Talc, shake, allow to stand for a few hours, shaking occasionally, and filter.

Content of free ammonia, NH_3 1.12 to 1.25% w/v.

Content of ammonium carbonate, $(NH_4)_2CO_3$ 2.76 to 3.24% w/v.

Ethanol content 2.6 to 3.5% v/v, Appendix VIII F.

Weight per ml 0.980 to 1.005 g, Appendix V G.

Assay

For free ammonia To 20 ml add 50 ml of 1M *hydrochloric acid VS*, boil, cool and titrate the excess of acid with 1M *sodium hydroxide VS* using *methyl red solution* as indicator. Each ml of 1M *hydrochloric acid VS*, after subtraction of the volume of 1M *sodium hydroxide VS* required in the Assay for ammonium carbonate, is equivalent to 17.03 mg of NH_3.

For ammonium carbonate To 20 ml add 25 ml of 1M *sodium hydroxide VS* and 40 ml of *barium chloride solution*, heat on a water bath for 15 minutes, cool, add 10 ml of *formaldehyde solution* previously neutralised to *thymol blue solution* and titrate the excess of alkali with 1M *hydrochloric acid VS*, using *thymol blue solution* as indicator, to the grey colour indicative of pH 8.8. Each ml of 1M *sodium hydroxide VS* is equivalent to 48.04 mg of $(NH_4)_2CO_3$.

Storage Aromatic Ammonia Solution should be kept in a well-closed container and stored at a temperature not exceeding 25°.

Labelling The label states (1) the date after which the solution is not intended to be used; (2) the conditions under which it should be stored.

Dilute Ammonia Solution

Definition Dilute Ammonia Solution contains 10% w/w of ammonia. It is prepared by diluting Strong Ammonia Solution with freshly boiled and cooled Purified Water.

Content of ammonia, NH_3 9.5 to 10.5% w/w.

Relative density 0.958 to 0.962, Appendix V G.

Assay Weigh 6 g into 50 ml of 1M *hydrochloric acid VS* and titrate the excess of acid with 1M *sodium hydroxide VS* using *methyl red solution* as indicator. Each ml of 1M *hydrochloric acid VS* is equivalent to 17.03 mg of NH_3.

Storage Dilute Ammonia Solution should be kept in a well-closed container.

Labelling The label states (1) the date after which the solution is not intended to be used; (2) the conditions under which it should be stored.

When ammonia solution is prescribed or demanded, Dilute Ammonia Solution shall be dispensed or supplied.

Aromatic Ammonia Spirit

Sal Volatile Spirit

Definition

Nutmeg Oil	3 ml
Lemon Oil	5 ml
Ethanol (90 per cent)	750 ml
Ammonium Bicarbonate	25 g
Strong Ammonia Solution	67.5 ml
Purified Water	sufficient to produce 1000 ml

Extemporaneous preparation The following directions apply.

Distil a mixture of the Lemon Oil, the Nutmeg Oil, the Ethanol (90 per cent) and 375 ml of Purified Water. Reserve the first 875 ml of distillate. Distil a further 55 ml and add the Ammonium Bicarbonate and the Strong Ammonia Solution to the distillate. Heat on a water bath to 60° in a sealed bottle of not less than 120-ml capacity, shaking occasionally, until solution is complete, cool, filter through absorbent cotton, mix the filtrate with the reserved distillate, add sufficient Purified Water to produce 1000 ml and mix.

The spirit complies with the requirements stated under Spirits and with the following requirements.

Content of free ammonia, NH_3 1.12 to 1.30% w/v.

Content of ammonium carbonate, $(NH_4)_2CO_3$ 2.76 to 3.24% w/v.

Ethanol content 64 to 70% v/v, Appendix VIII F.

Weight per ml 0.880 to 0.893 g, Appendix V G.

Assay

For free ammonia To 20 ml add 50 ml of 1M *hydrochloric acid VS*, boil, cool and titrate the excess of acid with 1M *sodium hydroxide VS* using *methyl red solution* as indicator. Each ml of 1M *hydrochloric acid VS*, after subtraction of the volume of 1M *sodium hydroxide VS* required in the Assay for ammonium carbonate, is equivalent to 17.03 mg of NH_3.

For ammonium carbonate To 20 ml add 25 ml of 1M *sodium hydroxide VS* and 40 ml of *barium chloride solution*, heat on a water bath for 15 minutes, cool, add 10 ml of *formaldehyde solution* previously neutralised to *thymol blue solution* and titrate the excess of alkali with 1M *hydrochloric acid VS*, using *thymol blue solution* as indicator, to the grey colour indicative of pH 8.8. Each ml of 1M *sodium hydroxide VS* is equivalent to 48.04 mg of $(NH_4)_2CO_3$.

Strong Ammonium Acetate Solution

Definition

Ammonium Bicarbonate	470 g
Glacial Acetic Acid	453 g
Strong Ammonia Solution	a sufficient quantity
Purified Water, freshly boiled and cooled	sufficient to produce 1000 ml

Extemporaneous preparation The following directions apply.

Dissolve the Ammonium Bicarbonate by adding gradually to the Glacial Acetic Acid diluted with 350 ml of Purified Water. Add Strong Ammonia Solution until 0.05 ml of the resulting solution diluted with 0.5 ml of *water* gives a full blue colour with 0.05 ml of *bromothymol blue solution R3* and a full yellow colour with 0.05 ml of *thymol blue solution*; about 100 ml of Strong Ammonia Solution is required. Add sufficient Purified Water to produce 1000 ml.

Content of ammonium acetate, $C_2H_7NO_2$ 55.0 to 60.0% w/v.

Acidity or alkalinity pH of a 10% v/v solution, 7.0 to 8.0, Appendix V L.

Weight per ml 1.085 to 1.095 g, Appendix V G.

Assay To 5 ml add 50 ml of *water* and 12 ml of *formaldehyde solution* previously neutralised to *phenolphthalein solution R1* and titrate with 1M *sodium hydroxide VS* using *phenolphthalein solution R1* as indicator. Each ml of 1M *sodium hydroxide VS* is equivalent to 77.08 mg of $C_2H_7NO_2$.

Storage Strong Ammonium Acetate Solution should be kept in lead-free glass containers.

Labelling The label states (1) the date after which the solution is not intended to be used; (2) the conditions under which it should be stored.

When ammonium acetate solution or dilute ammonium acetate solution is prescribed or demanded, Strong Ammonium Acetate Solution diluted to eight times its volume with freshly boiled and cooled Purified Water, shall be dispensed or supplied.

Ammonium Chloride Mixture

Ammonium Chloride Oral Solution

Definition Ammonium Chloride Mixture is an *oral solution* containing 10% w/v of Ammonium Chloride in a suitable vehicle containing Aromatic Ammonia Solution and Liquorice Liquid Extract.

Extemporaneous preparation It is recently prepared according to the following formula.

Ammonium Chloride	100 g
Aromatic Ammonia Solution	50 ml
Liquorice Liquid Extract	100 ml
Water	sufficient to produce 1000 ml

The mixture complies with the requirements stated under Oral Liquids and with the following requirements.

Content of ammonium chloride, NH_4Cl 9.50 to 10.66% w/v.

Assay To 1 ml add 20 ml of *water* and titrate with 0.1M *silver nitrate VS* determining the end point potentiometrically. Each ml of 0.1M *silver nitrate VS* is equivalent to 5.349 mg of NH_4Cl.

Labelling The label indicates the pharmaceutical form as 'oral solution'.

Amoxicillin Capsules

Definition Amoxicillin Capsules contain Amoxicillin Trihydrate.

The capsules comply with the requirements stated under Capsules and with the following requirements.

Content of amoxicillin, $C_{16}H_{19}N_3O_5S$ 92.5 to 110.0% of the prescribed or stated amount.

Identification Shake a quantity of the contents of the capsules containing the equivalent of 0.5 g of amoxicillin with 5 ml of *water* for 5 minutes, filter, wash the residue first with *absolute ethanol* and then with *ether* and dry at a pressure not exceeding 0.7 kPa for 1 hour. The residue complies with the following tests.

A. The *infrared absorption spectrum*, Appendix II A, is concordant with the *reference spectrum* of amoxicillin trihydrate.

B. Carry out the method for *thin-layer chromatography*, Appendix III A, using a silica gel precoated plate (Merck silica gel 60 plates are suitable). Impregnate the plate by spraying it with a 0.1% w/v solution of *disodium edetate* in a 5% w/v solution of *sodium dihydrogen orthophosphate*, allow the plate to dry in air and heat at 105° for 1 hour. Use as the mobile phase a mixture of 50 volumes of *butyl acetate*, 30 volumes of *glacial acetic acid*, 10 volumes of a 0.1% w/v solution of *disodium edetate* in a 5% w/v solution of *sodium dihydrogen orthophosphate* and 5 volumes of *butan-1-ol*. Apply separately to the plate 1 µl of each of two solutions in *phosphate buffer pH 7.0* containing (1) 0.20% w/v of the residue and (2) 0.20% w/v of *amoxicillin trihydrate BPCRS*. After removal of the plate, allow it to dry in air, heat at 105° for 10 to 15 minutes and spray with a mixture of 100 volumes of *starch mucilage*, 6 volumes of *glacial acetic acid* and 2 volumes of a 1% w/v solution of *iodine* in a 4% w/v solution of *potassium iodide*. The principal spot in the chromatogram obtained with solution (1) corresponds to that in the chromatogram obtained with solution (2).

Assay To a quantity of the mixed contents of 20 capsules containing the equivalent of 0.15 g of amoxicillin add sufficient *water* to produce 500 ml, shake for 30 minutes and filter. Transfer 10 ml of the filtrate to a 100-ml graduated flask, add 10 ml of *boric buffer pH 9.0* followed by 1 ml of *acetic anhydride—dioxan solution*, allow to stand for 5 minutes and add sufficient *water* to produce 100 ml. Place two 2-ml quantities of this solution in separate stoppered tubes. To one tube add 10 ml of *imidazole—mercury reagent*, mix, stopper the tube and immerse in a water bath at 60° for exactly 25 minutes, swirling occasionally. Remove from the water bath and cool rapidly to 20° (solution A). To the second tube add 10 ml of *water* and mix (solution B). Without delay measure the *absorbances* of solutions A and B at the maximum at 325 nm, Appendix II B, using in the reference cell a mixture of 2 ml of *water* and 10 ml of *imidazole—mercury reagent* for solution A and *water* for solution B. Calculate the content of $C_{16}H_{19}N_3O_5S$ from the difference between the absorbances of solutions A and B, from the difference obtained by repeating the operation using 0.17 g of *amoxicillin trihydrate BPCRS* in place of the substance being examined and from the declared content of $C_{16}H_{19}N_3O_5S$ in *amoxicillin trihydrate BPCRS*.

Labelling The quantity of active ingredient is stated in terms of the equivalent amount of amoxicillin.

When amoxycillin capsules are prescribed or demanded Amoxicillin Capsules shall be dispensed or supplied.

Amoxicillin Injection

Definition Amoxicillin Injection is a sterile solution of Amoxicillin Sodium in Water for Injections. It is prepared by dissolving Amoxicillin Sodium for Injection in the requisite amount of Water for Injections immediately before use.

The injection complies with the requirements stated under Parenteral Preparations.

Storage Amoxicillin Injection should be used immediately after preparation.

AMOXICILLIN SODIUM FOR INJECTION

Definition Amoxicillin Sodium for Injection is a sterile material consisting of Amoxicillin Sodium with or without excipients. It is supplied in a sealed container.

The contents of the sealed container comply with the requirements for Powders for Injections stated under Parenteral Preparations and with the following requirements.

Content of amoxicillin $C_{16}H_{19}N_3O_5S$ 90.0 to 105.0% of the prescribed or stated amount.

Identification

A. The *infrared absorption spectrum*, Appendix II A, is concordant with the *reference spectrum* of amoxicillin sodium.

B. Carry out the method for *thin-layer chromatography*, Appendix III A, using *silanised silica gel H* as the coating substance and a mixture of 10 volumes of *acetone* and 90 volumes of a 15.4% w/v solution of *ammonium acetate* adjusted to pH 5.0 with *glacial acetic acid* as the mobile phase. Apply separately to the plate 1 µl of each of three solutions in a 4.2% w/v solution of *sodium hydrogen carbonate* containing (1) sufficient of the contents of the sealed container to give a solution containing the equivalent of 0.25% w/v of amoxicillin, (2) 0.25% w/v of *amoxicillin trihydrate BPCRS* and (3) 0.25% w/v of *amoxicillin trihydrate BPCRS* and 0.25% w/v of *ampicillin trihydrate BPCRS*. After removal of the plate, allow it to dry in air, expose it to iodine vapour until spots appear and examine in daylight. The principal spot in the chromatogram obtained with solution (1) is similar in position, colour and size to that in the chromatogram obtained with solution (2). The test is not valid unless the chromatogram obtained with solution (3) shows two clearly separated spots.

C. Yield the reactions characteristic of *sodium salts*, Appendix VI.

Alkalinity pH of a 10% w/v solution, 8.0 to 10.0, Appendix V L.

***N,N*-Dimethylaniline** Not more than 20 ppm with respect to the content of Amoxicillin Sodium when determined by the following method. Prepare a 0.005% w/v solution of *naphthalene* (internal standard) in *cyclohexane* (solution A). Mix 50 mg of N,N-*dimethylaniline* with 2 ml of *hydrochloric acid* and 20 ml of *water*, shake to dissolve, add sufficient *water* to produce 50 ml and dilute 5 ml of the resulting solution to 250 ml with *water* (solution B). Carry out the method for *gas chromatography*, Appendix III B, injecting 1 µl of each of the following solutions. For solution (1) add 5 ml of 1M *sodium hydroxide* and 1 ml of solution A to 1 ml of solution B, shake vigorously for 1 minute, centrifuge if necessary and use the clear, upper layer. For solution (2) dissolve a quantity of the contents of the sealed container containing the equivalent of 0.95 g of amoxicillin in 5 ml of 1M *sodium hydroxide*, add 1 ml of *cyclohexane*, shake vigorously for 1 minute, centrifuge if necessary and use the clear, upper layer. Prepare solution (3) in the same manner as solution (2) but adding 1 ml of solution A in place of the cyclohexane.

The chromatographic procedure may be carried out using a glass column (2 m × 2 mm) packed with *acid-washed, silanised diatomaceous support* (Gas Chrom Q is suitable) coated with 3% w/w of phenyl methyl silicone fluid (50% phenyl) (OV-17 is suitable) and maintained at 120° with the inlet port and the detector at 150° and using 30 ml per minute as the flow rate of the carrier gas.

Degradation products Not more than 9.0% with respect to the content of Amoxicillin Sodium when determined by the following method. To a quantity of the contents of the sealed container containing the equivalent of 0.24 g of amoxicillin add 25 ml of *boric buffer pH 9.0* and 0.5 ml of *acetic anhydride*, stir for 3 minutes, add 10 ml of *acetate buffer pH 4.6* and titrate immediately with 0.02M *mercury(II) nitrate VS*. Determine the end point potentiometrically using a platinum or mercury indicator electrode and a mercury—mercury(I) sulphate reference electrode. Disregard any preliminary inflection on the titration curve. Each ml of 0.02M *mercury(II) nitrate VS* is equivalent to 7.748 mg of degradation products, calculated as $C_{16}H_{18}N_3NaO_5S$.

Water Not more than 4.0% w/w, Appendix IX C. Use 0.3 g.

Pyrogens Comply with the *test for pyrogens*, Appendix XIV D. Use per kg of the rabbit's weight 1 ml of a solution in *water for injections* containing 20 mg per ml.

Assay Determine the weight of the contents of 10 containers as described in the test for Uniformity of weight under Parenteral Preparations, Powders for Injections.

Dissolve 0.17 g of the mixed contents of the 10 containers in sufficient *water* to produce 500 ml. Transfer 10 ml of the resulting solution to a 100-ml graduated flask, add 10 ml of *boric buffer pH 9.0* followed by 1 ml of *acetic anhydride—dioxan solution*, allow to stand for 5 minutes and add sufficient *water* to produce 100 ml. Place two 2-ml quantities of the solution in separate stoppered tubes. To one tube add 10 ml of *imidazole—mercury reagent*, stopper the tube and place in a water bath at 60° for exactly 25 minutes, swirling occasionally. Remove the tube from the water bath and cool rapidly to 20° (solution A). To the second tube add 10 ml of *water* and mix (solution B). Without delay measure the *absorbances* of solutions A and B at the maximum at 325 nm, Appendix II B, using in the reference cell a mixture of 2 ml of *water* and 10 ml of *imidazole—mercury reagent* for solution A and *water* for solution B. Calculate the content of $C_{16}H_{19}N_3O_5S$ in a container of average content weight from the difference between the absorbances of solutions A and B, from the difference obtained by repeating the operation using 0.17 g of *amoxicillin trihydrate BPCRS* in place of the preparation being examined and from the declared content of $C_{16}H_{19}N_3O_4S$ in *amoxicillin trihydrate BPCRS*.

Storage The sealed container should be stored at a temperature not exceeding 25°.

Labelling The label of the sealed container states the quantity of Amoxicillin Sodium contained in it in terms of the equivalent amount of amoxicillin.

When amoxycillin injection or amoxycillin sodium for injection is prescribed or demanded Amoxicillin Injection or Amoxicillin Sodium for Injection shall be dispensed or supplied.

Amoxicillin Oral Suspension

Definition Amoxicillin Oral Suspension is a suspension of Amoxicillin Trihydrate in a suitable flavoured vehicle. It is prepared by dispersing the dry ingredients in the specified volume of Water just before issue for use.

The dry ingredients comply with the requirements for Powders and Granules for the Preparation of Oral Liquids stated under Oral Liquids.

Storage The dry ingredients should be stored at a temperature not exceeding 25°.

For the following tests prepare the Oral Suspension as directed on the label. The suspension, examined immediately after preparation unless otherwise indicated, complies with the requirements stated under Oral Liquids and with the following requirements.

Content of amoxicillin, $C_{16}H_{19}N_3O_5S$ When freshly constituted not more than 120.0% of the prescribed or stated amount. When stored at the temperature and for the period stated on the label during which the Oral Suspension may be expected to be satisfactory for use, not less than 80.0% of the prescribed or stated amount.

Identification Complies with test B for Identification described under Amoxicillin Capsules using the following solutions. For solution (1) dilute a volume of the oral suspension containing the equivalent of 0.125 g of amoxycillin to 100 ml with *phosphate buffer pH 7.0*. Solution (2) contains 0.14% w/v of *amoxicillin trihydrate BPCRS* in *phosphate buffer pH 7.0*.

Acidity or alkalinity pH, 4.0 to 7.0, Appendix V L.

Assay To a weighed quantity of the oral suspension containing the equivalent of 0.15 g of amoxicillin, add sufficient *water* to produce 500 ml, shake for 30 minutes, filter and complete the Assay described under Amoxicillin Capsules, beginning at the words 'Transfer 10 ml of the filtrate ...'. Determine the *weight per ml* of the oral suspension, Appendix V G, and calculate the content of $C_{16}H_{19}N_3O_5S$, weight in volume.

Repeat the procedure using a portion of the oral suspension that has been stored at the temperature and for the period stated on the label during which it may be expected to be satisfactory for use.

Storage The Oral Suspension should be kept at the temperature and used within the period stated on the label.

Labelling The quantity of active ingredient is stated in terms of the equivalent amount of amoxicillin.

When amoxycillin oral suspension is prescribed or demanded, Amoxicillin Oral Suspension shall be dispensed or supplied.

Amphotericin Lozenges

Definition Amphotericin Lozenges contain Amphotericin. They are prepared by compression.

The lozenges comply with the requirements stated under Tablets and with the following requirements.

Identification

A. To a quantity of the powdered lozenges containing the equivalent of 12.5 mg of amphotericin B add 2.5 ml of *dimethyl sulphoxide* and shake for 5 minutes. Add 15 ml of *methanol*, shake for a further 10 minutes, add sufficient *methanol* to produce 25 ml and filter. Dilute 1 ml of the filtrate to 100 ml with *methanol*. The *light absorption* of the resulting solution, Appendix II B, in the range 300 to 450 nm exhibits three maxima, at 362, 381 and 405 nm. The ratio of the *absorbance* at the maximum at 362 nm to that at the maximum at 381 nm is 0.5 to 0.6. The ratio of the *absorbance* at 381 nm to that at the maximum at 405 nm is about 0.9.

B. Shake a quantity of the powdered lozenges containing the equivalent of 5 mg of amphotericin B with 1 ml of *dimethyl sulphoxide* and add 5 ml of *orthophosphoric acid* to form a lower layer. A blue ring is produced immediately at the junction of the liquids. Mix; an intense blue colour is produced. Add 15 ml of *water* and mix; a pale straw colour is produced.

Content of tetraenes Not more than 13.3% w/w of the prescribed or stated amount of amphotericin B when determined by the method described under Amphotericin but preparing solution (1) in the following manner. To a quantity of the powdered lozenges containing the equivalent of 37.5 mg of amphotericin B add 5 ml of *dimethyl sulphoxide* and 25 ml of *methanol*, shake for 10 minutes, add sufficient *methanol* to produce 50 ml, mix thoroughly and filter. Dilute 4 ml of the filtrate to 50 ml with *methanol*.

Disintegration The requirement for disintegration does not apply to Amphotericin Lozenges.

Assay Weigh and powder 20 lozenges. Triturate a quantity of the powder containing the equivalent of 10 mg of amphotericin B with 10 ml of *water*, add sufficient *dimethyl sulphoxide* to produce 100 ml, shake for 20 minutes and filter. Carry out the *biological assay of antibiotics*, Appendix XIV A. The precision of the assay is such that the fiducial limits of error are not less than 95% and not more than 105% of the estimated potency.

Calculate the content of amphotericin B in the lozenges taking each 1000 IU found to be equivalent to 1 mg of amphotericin B. The upper fiducial limit of error is not less than 90.0% and the lower fiducial limit of error is not more than 120.0% of the prescribed or stated content.

Storage Amphotericin Lozenges should be protected from light.

Labelling The quantity of active ingredient is stated in terms of the equivalent amount of amphotericin B.

Ampicillin Capsules

Definition Ampicillin Capsules contain Ampicillin or Ampicillin Trihydrate.

The capsules comply with the requirements stated under Capsules and with the following requirements.

Content of ampicillin, $C_{16}H_{19}N_3O_4S$ 92.5 to 107.5% of the prescribed or stated amount.

Identification The contents of the capsules comply with the following tests.

A. Comply with the test for Identification described under Ampicillin Oral Suspension using the following solutions. For solution (1) shake a quantity containing 0.125 g of ampicillin with sufficient *phosphate buffer pH 7.0* to produce 100 ml and filter. Solution (2) contains 0.14% w/v of *ampicillin trihydrate BPCRS* in *phosphate buffer pH 7.0*.

B. Suspend 10 mg in 1 ml of *water* and add 2 ml of a mixture of 2 ml of *cupri-tartaric solution R1* and 6 ml of *water*. A magenta-violet colour is produced immediately.

Assay To a quantity of the mixed contents of 20 capsules containing 0.15 g of ampicillin add sufficient *water* to produce 500 ml, shake for 30 minutes and filter. Transfer 10 ml of the filtrate to a 100-ml graduated flask, add 10 ml of *boric buffer pH 9.0* followed by 1 ml of *acetic anhydride—dioxan solution*, allow to stand for 5 minutes and add sufficient *water* to produce 100 ml. Place two 2-ml aliquots of this solution in separate stoppered tubes. To one tube add 10 ml of *imidazole—mercury reagent*, mix, stopper the tube and immerse in a water bath at 60° for exactly 25 minutes, swirling occasionally. Remove from the water bath and cool rapidly to 20° (solution A). To the second tube add 10 ml of *water* and mix (solution B). Without delay measure the *absorbances* of solutions A and B at the maximum at 325 nm, Appendix II B, using in the reference cell a mixture of 2 ml of *water* and 10 ml of *imidazole—mercury reagent* for solution A and *water* for solution B. Calculate the content of $C_{16}H_{19}N_3O_4S$ from the difference between the absorbances of solutions A and B, from the difference obtained by repeating the operation using 0.17 g of *ampicillin trihydrate BPCRS* in place of the substance being examined and from the declared content of $C_{16}H_{19}N_3O_4S$ in *ampicillin trihydrate BPCRS*.

Labelling When the active ingredient is Ampicillin Trihydrate, the quantity is stated in terms of the equivalent amount of ampicillin.

Ampicillin Injection

Definition Ampicillin Injection is a sterile solution of Ampicillin Sodium in Water for Injections. It is prepared by dissolving Ampicillin Sodium for Injection in the requisite amount of Water for Injections immediately before use.

The injection complies with the requirements stated under Parenteral Preparations.

Storage Ampicillin Injection should be used immediately after preparation.

AMPICILLIN SODIUM FOR INJECTION

Definition Ampicillin Sodium for Injection is a sterile material consisting of Ampicillin Sodium, with or without excipients. It is supplied in a sealed container.

The contents of the sealed container comply with the requirements for Powders for Injections stated under Parenteral Preparations and with the following requirements.

Content of ampicillin, $C_{16}H_{19}N_3O_4S$ 95.0 to 105.0% of the prescribed or stated amount.

Identification

A. The *infrared absorption spectrum*, Appendix II A, is concordant with the *reference spectrum* of ampicillin sodium. If the spectra are not concordant carry out the following procedure. Dissolve 0.25 g of the contents in 5 ml of *water*, add 0.5 ml of 2M *acetic acid*, mix and allow to stand for 10 minutes in ice. Filter through a sintered-glass filter (BS porosity No. 3), wash the residue with 2 to 3 ml of a mixture of 9 volumes of *acetone* and 1 volume of *water*, dry at 60° for 30 minutes and prepare a new spectrum of the residue. The spectrum of the residue is concordant with the *reference spectrum* of ampicillin trihydrate.

B. Carry out the method for *thin-layer chromatography*, Appendix III A, using *silanised silica gel H* as the coating substance and a mixture of 10 volumes of *acetone* and 90 volumes of a 15.4% w/v solution of *ammonium acetate* adjusted to pH 5.0 with *glacial acetic acid* as the mobile phase. Apply separately to the plate 1 µl of each of three solutions in a 4.2% w/v solution of *sodium hydrogen carbonate* containing (1) sufficient of the contents of the sealed container to give a solution containing the equivalent of 0.25% w/v of ampicillin, (2) 0.25% w/v of *ampicillin trihydrate BPCRS* and (3) 0.25% w/v of *ampicillin trihydrate BPCRS* and 0.25% w/v of *amoxicillin trihydrate BPCRS*. After removal of the plate, allow it to dry in air, expose it to iodine vapour until spots appear and examine in daylight. The principal spot in the chromatogram obtained with solution (1) is similar in position, colour and size to that in the chromatogram obtained with solution (2). The test is not valid unless the chromatogram obtained with solution (3) shows two clearly separated spots.

C. Yield the reaction characteristic of *sodium salts*, Appendix VI.

Alkalinity pH of a 10% w/v solution, 8.0 to 10.0, Appendix V L, measured within 10 minutes of preparing the solution.

***N,N*-Dimethylaniline** Not more than 20 ppm with respect to the content of Ampicillin Sodium when determined by the following method. Prepare a 0.005% w/v solution of *naphthalene* (internal standard) in *cyclohexane* (solution A). Carry out the method for *gas chromatography*, Appendix III B, injecting 1 µl of each of the following solutions. For solution (1) dissolve a quantity of the contents of the sealed container containing the equivalent of 0.95 g of ampicillin in 5 ml of 1M *sodium hydroxide*, add 1 ml of solution A, shake vigorously for 1 minute, centrifuge if necessary and use the clear, upper layer. For solution (2) dissolve 50 mg of N,N-*dimethylaniline* in a mixture of 2 ml of *hydrochloric acid* and 20 ml of *water* with shaking, add sufficient *water* to produce 50 ml and dilute 5 ml of the resulting solution to 250 ml with *water*. To 1 ml of this solution add 5 ml of 1M *sodium hydroxide* and 1 ml of solution A, shake vigorously for 1 minute, centrifuge if necessary and use the upper layer.

The chromatographic procedure may be carried out using a glass column (2 m × 2 mm) packed with *acid-washed, silanised diatomaceous support* (Gas Chrom Q is suitable) coated with 3% w/w of phenyl methyl silicone fluid (50% phenyl) (OV-17 is suitable) and maintained at 120° with the inlet port and the detector at 150° and using 30 ml per minute as the flow rate of the carrier gas. Inject 1 µl of each solution.

Iodine-absorbing substances Dissolve 0.25 g in sufficient *water* to produce 100 ml. To 10 ml add 0.5 ml of 1M *hydrochloric acid* and 10 ml of 0.01M *iodine VS* and titrate with 0.02M *sodium thiosulphate VS* using *starch mucilage*, added towards the end of the titration, as indicator. Repeat the titration without the substance being examined. The difference between the titrations represents the amount of iodine-absorbing substances present. Each ml of 0.02M *sodium thiosulphate VS* is equivalent to 0.7392 mg of iodine-absorbing substances. Calculate the percentage of iodine-absorbing substances in the substance being examined. The sum of the percentage of iodine-absorbing substances and that of ampicillin sodium, both calculated with reference to the anhydrous substance, is not less than 97.5%. Each mg of $C_{16}H_{19}N_3O_4S$, as determined in the Assay, is equivalent to 1.063 mg of ampicillin sodium, $C_{16}H_{18}N_3NaO_4S$.

Water Not more than 2.0% w/w, Appendix IX C. Use 0.3 g.

Bacterial endotoxins Carry out the *test for bacterial endotoxins*, Appendix XIV C. Dissolve the contents of the sealed container in *water BET* to give a solution containing 10 mg per ml (solution A). The endotoxin limit concentration of solution A is 1.5 IU per ml. Carry out the test using the maximum valid dilution of solution A calculated from the declared sensitivity of the lysate used in the test.

Assay Determine the weight of the contents of 10 containers as described in the test for Uniformity of weight under Parenteral Preparations, Powders for Injections.

Dissolve 0.17 g of the mixed contents of the 10 containers in sufficient *water* to produce 500 ml. Transfer 10 ml of the resulting solution to a 100-ml graduated flask, add 10 ml of *boric buffer pH 9.0* followed by 1 ml of *acetic anhydride—dioxan solution*, allow to stand for 5 minutes and add sufficient *water* to produce 100 ml. Place two 2-ml quantities of this solution in separate stoppered tubes. To one tube add 10 ml of *imidazole—mercury reagent*, mix, stopper the tube and place in a water bath at 60° for exactly 25 minutes, swirling occasionally. Remove the tube from the water bath and cool rapidly to 20° (solution A). To the second tube add 10 ml of *water* and mix (solution B). Without delay measure the *absorbances* of solutions A and B, Appendix II B, at the maximum at 325 nm using in the reference cell a mixture of 2 ml of *water* and 10 ml of *imidazole—mercury reagent* for solution A and *water* for solution B. Calculate the percentage content of $C_{16}H_{19}N_3O_4S$ and the content of $C_{16}H_{19}N_3O_4S$ in a container of average content weight from the difference between the absorbances of solutions

A and B, from the difference obtained by repeating the operation using 0.17 g of *ampicillin trihydrate BPCRS* in place of the substance being examined and from the declared content of $C_{16}H_{19}N_3O_4S$ in *ampicillin trihydrate BPCRS*.

Storage The sealed container should be stored at a temperature not exceeding 25°.

Labelling The label of the sealed container states the quantity of Ampicillin Sodium contained in it in terms of the equivalent amount of ampicillin.

Ampicillin Oral Suspension

Definition Ampicillin Oral Suspension is a suspension of Ampicillin or Ampicillin Trihydrate in a suitable flavoured vehicle. It is prepared by dispersing the dry ingredients in the specified volume of Water just before issue for use.

The dry ingredients comply with the requirements for Powders and Granules for the Preparation of Oral Liquids stated under Oral Liquids.

Storage The dry ingredients should be stored at a temperature not exceeding 25°.

For the following tests prepare the Oral Suspension as directed on the label. The suspension, examined immediately after preparation unless otherwise indicated, complies with the requirements stated under Oral Liquids and with the following requirements.

Content of ampicillin, $C_{16}H_{19}N_3O_4S$ When freshly constituted not more than 120.0% of the prescribed or stated amount. When stored at the temperature and for the period stated on the label during which the Oral Suspension may be expected to be satisfactory for use, not less than 80.0% of the prescribed or stated amount.

Identification Carry out the method for *thin-layer chromatography*, Appendix III A, using a silica gel pre-coated plate (Merck silica gel 60 plates are suitable). Impregnate the plate by spraying it with a 0.1% w/v solution of *disodium edetate* in a 5% w/v solution of *sodium dihydrogen orthophosphate*, allow the plate to dry in air and heat at 105° for 1 hour. Use as the mobile phase a mixture of 50 volumes of *butyl acetate*, 30 volumes of *glacial acetic acid*, 10 volumes of a 0.1% w/v solution of *disodium edetate* in a 5% w/v solution of *sodium dihydrogen orthophosphate* and 5 volumes of *butan-1-ol*. Apply separately to the plate 1 µl of each of the following solutions. For solution (1) dilute a quantity of the oral suspension containing 0.125 g of ampicillin to 100 ml with *phosphate buffer pH 7.0*. Solution (2) contains 0.14% w/v of *ampicillin trihydrate BPCRS* in *phosphate buffer pH 7.0*. After removal of the plate, allow it to dry in air, heat at 105° for 10 to 15 minutes and spray with a mixture of 100 volumes of *starch mucilage*, 6 volumes of *glacial acetic acid* and 2 volumes of a 1% w/v solution of *iodine* in a 4% w/v solution of *potassium iodide*. The principal spot in the chromatogram obtained with solution (1) corresponds to that in the chromatogram obtained with solution (2).

Acidity or alkalinity pH, 4.0 to 7.0, Appendix V L.

Assay To a quantity of the oral suspension containing 0.15 g of ampicillin add sufficient *water* to produce 500 ml, shake for 30 minutes, filter and complete the Assay described under Ampicillin Capsules, beginning at the words 'Transfer 10 ml of the filtrate ...'. Determine the *weight per ml* of the oral suspension, Appendix V G, and calculate the content of $C_{16}H_{19}N_3O_4S$, weight in volume.

Repeat the procedure using a portion of the oral suspension that has been stored at the temperature and for the period stated on the label during which it may be expected to be satisfactory for use.

Storage The Oral Suspension should be stored at the temperature and used within the period stated on the label.

Labelling When the active ingredient is Ampicillin Trihydrate, the quantity is stated in terms of the equivalent amount of ampicillin.

Concentrated Anise Water

Definition

Anise Oil	20 ml
Ethanol (90 per cent)	700 ml
Water	sufficient to produce 1000 ml

Extemporaneous preparation The following directions apply.

Dissolve the Anise Oil in the Ethanol (90 per cent) and add gradually, with vigorous shaking after each addition, sufficient Water to produce 1000 ml. Add 50 g of previously sterilised Purified Talc, or other suitable filtering aid, allow to stand for a few hours, shaking occasionally, and filter.

The water complies with the requirements stated under Aromatic Waters and with the following requirements.

Ethanol content 60 to 64% v/v, Appendix VIII F.

Weight per ml 0.898 to 0.908 g, Appendix V G.

Aprotinin Injection

Definition Aprotinin Injection is a sterile solution of Aprotinin or a sterile dilution of Aprotinin Concentrated Solution in Water for Injections.

The injection complies with the requirements stated under Parenteral Preparations and with the following requirements.

Content of aprotinin 90.0 to 110.0% of the stated number of IU.

Characteristics A colourless solution.

Identification

A. Carry out the method for *thin-layer chromatography*, Appendix III A, using *silica gel G* as the coating substance and a 10% w/v solution of *sodium acetate* in a mixture of 50 volumes of *glacial acetic acid* and 40 volumes of *water* as the mobile phase but allowing the solvent front to ascend 12 cm above the line of application. Apply separately to the plate 10 µl of each of the following solutions. For solution (1) use the undiluted injection. For solution (2) dilute *aprotinin solution EPBRP* with sufficient *water* to give a solution containing the same number of IU per ml as solution (1). After removal of the plate, allow it to dry in air and spray with a solution containing 0.1 g of *ninhydrin* in a mixture of 70 ml of *absolute ethanol*, 21 ml of *glacial acetic acid* and 6 ml of a 1% w/v solution of *copper(II) chloride*. Dry the plate at 60°. The principal spot in the chromatogram obtained with solution (1) corresponds in position, colour and size to that in the chromatogram obtained with solution (2).

B. Dilute a volume of the injection containing 15 IU to 50 ml with *phosphate buffer pH 7.2*. Mix 1 ml of the resulting solution with 1 ml of a solution containing 0.01% w/v of *trypsin EPCRS* in 0.002M *hydrochloric acid* and allow to stand for 10 minutes. Add 1 ml of a 0.2% w/v solution of *casein* in *phosphate buffer pH 7.2* and incubate at 35° for 30 minutes. Cool in ice and add 0.5 ml of a mixture of 50 volumes of *absolute ethanol*, 49 volumes of *water* and 1 volume of *glacial acetic acid*. Shake and allow to stand at room temperature for 15 minutes; the solution becomes cloudy. Repeat the operation using *phosphate buffer pH 7.2* in place of the diluted injection; the solution remains clear.

Acidity or alkalinity pH, 5.0 to 7.0, Appendix V L.

Proteins of higher molecular weight Carry out the method for *size-exclusion chromatography*, Appendix III C, equilibrating the column with 3M *acetic acid*. Freeze dry a volume of the injection containing 300 IU at –30° at a pressure of 2.7 Pa; the procedure, including a period of drying at 15° to 25°, should take 6 to 12 hours. Dissolve the residue thus obtained in 1 ml of 3M *acetic acid* and apply to the top of the column.

The chromatographic procedure may be carried out using (a) a column (80 to 100 cm × 25 mm) packed with a cross-linked dextran suitable for fractionation of proteins in the range of molecular weights from 1,500 to 30,000 (Sephadex G-50-SF is suitable), (b) 3M *acetic acid* as the mobile phase and (c) a detection wavelength of 277 nm.

Collect the eluate in 2-ml fractions. No peak is eluted in advance of the principal peak.

Histamine Not more than 0.2 µg of histamine per 3 IU when determined by the *test for histamine*, Appendix XIV G.

Pyrogens Complies with the test for *pyrogens*, Appendix XIV D. Use per kg of the rabbit's weight a volume containing 15 IU.

Assay Carry out the Assay described under Aprotinin.

Storage Aprotinin Injection should be protected from light and stored at a temperature not exceeding 25°.

Labelling The label states the number of IU (Units) per ml.

Aqueous Cream

Definition

Emulsifying Ointment	300 g
Phenoxyethanol	10 g
Purified Water, freshly boiled and cooled,	sufficient to produce 1000 g

The suitability of the Cream for use as a diluent should be confirmed before use.

Extemporaneous preparation Aqueous Cream may be prepared in the following manner.

Dissolve the Phenoxyethanol in sufficient Purified Water at about 60° to produce a total weight of about 700 g. Melt the Emulsifying Ointment, add the phenoxyethanol solution when both are at about 60° and mix. Stir gently until cool, add sufficient of the Purified Water to produce 1000 g and mix.

The cream complies with the requirements stated under Topical Semi-solid Preparations.

Arachis Oil Enema

Definition Arachis Oil Enema is Arachis Oil in a suitable container.

The enema complies with the requirements stated under Rectal Preparations and with the following requirements.

Identification Carry out the test for *identification of fixed oils by thin-layer chromatography*, Appendix X N. The chromatogram obtained from the oil being examined shows spots corresponding to those in the *typical chromatogram* for arachis oil.

Acid value Not more than 0.6, Appendix X B.

Alkaline impurities Complies with the test for *alkaline impurities*, Appendix X N.

Peroxide value Not more than 5.0, Appendix X F.

Relative density 0.912 to 0.918, Appendix V G.

Unsaponifiable matter Not more than 1.0% w/w, Appendix X H, Method II. Use 5 g.

Foreign fixed oils Carry out the test for *foreign oils by gas chromatography*, Appendix X N. The fatty-acid fraction of the oil has the following composition.

Saturated fatty acids of chain length less than C_{16} Not more than 0.4%.
Palmitic acid 7.0 to 16.0%.
Stearic acid 1.3 to 6.5%.
Oleic acid 35.0 to 72.0%.
Linoleic acid (equivalent chain length on polyethylene glycol adipate 18.9) 13.0 to 43.0%.
Linolenic acid (equivalent chain length on polyethylene glycol adipate 19.7) Not more than 0.6%.
Arachidic acid 1.0 to 3.0%.
Gadoleic acid (equivalent chain length on polyethylene glycol adipate 20.3) 0.5 to 2.1%.
Behenic acid 1.0 to 5.0%.
Erucic acid (equivalent chain length on polyethylene glycol adipate 22.3) Not more than 0.5%.
Lignoceric acid 0.5 to 3.0%.
The ratio of linoleic acid to behenic acid is not more than 15.

Semi-drying oils To 1.0 g of the oil being examined add 5 ml of a mixture of 3 volumes of 2M *ethanolic potassium hydroxide* and 1 volume of *ethanol (96%)*, boil under a reflux condenser for 5 minutes, add 1.5 ml of 5M *acetic acid* and 50 ml of *ethanol (70%)* and heat until the solution is clear. Allow to cool or cool very slowly with a thermometer in the liquid. The temperature at which the liquid begins to become cloudy is not lower than 36°.

Sesame oil Shake 10 ml with 5 ml of a mixture of 0.5 volume of a 0.35% v/v solution of *furfuraldehyde* in *acetic anhydride* and 4.5 volumes of *acetic anhydride* for 1 minute, filter the solution through a filter paper impregnated with *acetic anhydride* and add 0.2 ml of *sulphuric acid*. No bluish green colour develops.

Ascorbic Acid Injection

Definition Ascorbic Acid Injection is a sterile solution of Ascorbic Acid in Water for Injections containing Sodium Bicarbonate.

The injection complies with the requirements stated under Parenteral Preparations and with the following requirements.

Content of ascorbic acid, $C_6H_8O_6$ 95.0 to 105.0% of the prescribed or stated amount.

Characteristics A colourless liquid.

Identification

A. Carry out the method for *thin-layer chromatography*, Appendix III A, using a silica gel F_{254} precoated plate (Merck silica gel 60 F_{254} plates are suitable) and a mixture of 120 volumes of *ethanol (96%)* and 20 volumes of *water* as the mobile phase. Apply separately to the plate 2 µl of each of the following solutions. For solution (1) dilute the injection, if necessary, with *water* to contain 0.5% w/v of Ascorbic Acid. Solution (2) contains 0.5% w/v of *ascorbic acid EPCRS* in *water*. After removal of the plate, allow it to dry in air and examine under *ultraviolet light (254 nm)*. The principal spot in the chromatogram obtained with solution (1) corresponds to that in the chromatogram obtained with solution (2).

B. To a volume containing 50 mg of Ascorbic Acid add 0.2 ml of 2M *nitric acid* and 0.2 ml of 0.1M *silver nitrate*. A grey precipitate is produced.

Acidity pH, 5.0 to 6.5, Appendix V L.

Oxalic acid Dilute a volume containing 0.25 g to 5 ml with *water*, neutralise to *litmus paper* with 2M *sodium hydroxide*, add 1 ml of 2M *acetic acid* and 0.5 ml of *calcium chloride solution* and allow to stand for 1 hour. Any opalescence produced is not more intense than that in a solution prepared at the same time and in the following manner. Dissolve 70 mg of *oxalic acid* in 500 ml of *water* and to 5 ml of the resulting solution add 1 ml of 2M *acetic acid* and 0.5 ml of *calcium chloride solution* (0.3%).

Assay To a volume containing 0.2 g add 5 ml of 2M *sulphuric acid* and titrate with 0.05M *iodine VS* using *starch mucilage* as indicator. Each ml of 0.05M *iodine VS* is equivalent to 8.806 mg of $C_6H_8O_6$.

Storage Ascorbic Acid Injection should be protected from light and stored at a temperature of 2° to 8°.

When vitamin C injection is prescribed or demanded, Ascorbic Acid Injection shall be dispensed or supplied.

Ascorbic Acid Tablets

Definition Ascorbic Acid Tablets contain Ascorbic Acid.

The tablets comply with the requirements stated under Tablets and with the following requirements.

Content of ascorbic acid, $C_6H_8O_6$ 95.0 to 107.5% of the prescribed or stated amount.

Identification

A. Carry out the method for *thin-layer chromatography*, Appendix III A, using a silica gel F_{254} precoated plate (Merck silica gel 60 F_{254} plates are suitable) and a mixture of 120 volumes of *ethanol (96%)* and 20 volumes of *water* as the mobile phase. Apply separately to the plate 2 µl of each of the following solutions. For solution (1) shake a quantity of the powdered tablets containing 50 mg of Ascorbic Acid with 10 ml of *water* for 15 minutes and filter. Solution (2) contains 0.5% w/v of *ascorbic acid EPCRS* in *water*. After removal of the plate, allow it to dry in air and examine under *ultraviolet light (254 nm)*. The principal spot in the chromatogram obtained with solution (1) corresponds to that in the chromatogram obtained with solution (2).

B. Shake a quantity of the powdered tablets with *water* and filter. The filtrate is acidic to *litmus solution*, decolorises *2,6-dichlorophenolindophenol solution* and reduces *silver nitrate solution* immediately at room temperature producing a black precipitate.

Disintegration The requirement for Disintegration does not apply to Ascorbic Acid Tablets containing 500 mg or more of Ascorbic Acid.

Assay Weigh and powder 20 tablets. Dissolve a quantity of the powder containing 0.15 g of Ascorbic Acid as completely as possible in a mixture of 30 ml of *water* and 20 ml of 1M *sulphuric acid* and titrate with 0.1M *ammonium cerium(IV) sulphate VS* using *ferroin solution* as indicator. Each ml of 0.1M *ammonium cerium(IV) sulphate VS* is equivalent to 8.806 mg of $C_6H_8O_6$.

Storage Ascorbic Acid Tablets should be kept free from contact with metal and protected from light and moisture.

Labelling For tablets containing 500 mg or more of Ascorbic Acid the label states that the tablets should be chewed before swallowing.

When vitamin C tablets are prescribed or demanded, Ascorbic Acid Tablets shall be dispensed or supplied.

Aspirin Tablets

Acetylsalicylic Acid Tablets

Definition Aspirin Tablets contain Aspirin.

The tablets comply with the requirements stated under Tablets and with the following requirements.

Content of aspirin, $C_9H_8O_4$ 95.0 to 105.0% of the prescribed or stated amount.

Identification Boil 0.5 g of the powdered tablets for 2 to 3 minutes with 10 ml of 5M *sodium hydroxide*, cool and add an excess of 1M *sulphuric acid*; a crystalline precipitate is produced and the odour of acetic acid is detectable. To a solution of the precipitate in *water* add *iron(III) chloride solution R1*; a deep violet colour is produced.

Salicylic acid Shake a quantity of the powdered tablets containing 0.20 g of Aspirin with 4 ml of *ethanol (96%)* and dilute to 100 ml with *water* at a temperature not exceeding 10°. Filter immediately, transfer 50 ml of the filtrate to a *Nessler cylinder*, add 1 ml of freshly prepared *ammonium iron(III) sulphate solution R1*, mix and allow to stand for 1 minute. Any violet colour produced is not more intense than that obtained by adding 1 ml of freshly prepared *ammonium iron(III) sulphate solution R1* to a mixture of 3 ml of a freshly prepared 0.010% w/v solution of *salicylic acid*, 2 ml of *ethanol (96%)* and sufficient *water* to produce 50 ml contained in a second *Nessler cylinder* (0.3%).

Dissolution Comply with the *dissolution test for tablets and capsules*, Appendix XII D, using Apparatus II. Use as the medium 500 ml of a pH 4.5 buffer prepared by mixing 29.9 g of *sodium acetate* and 16.6 ml of *glacial acetic acid* with sufficient *water* to produce 10 litres and rotate the paddle at 50 revolutions per minute. Withdraw a sample of 20 ml of the medium and filter. Immediately measure the *absorbance* of the filtrate, Appendix II B, diluted with the dissolution medium if necessary, at 265 nm using dissolution medium in the reference cell. Measure the *absorbance* of a suitable solution of *aspirin BPCRS* in the dissolution medium and calculate the total content of aspirin, $C_9H_8O_4$, in the medium using the declared content of $C_9H_8O_4$ in *aspirin BPCRS*.

Assay Weigh and powder 20 tablets. To a quantity of the powder containing 0.5 g of Aspirin add 30 ml of 0.5M *sodium hydroxide VS*, boil gently for 10 minutes and titrate the excess of alkali with 0.5M *hydrochloric acid VS* using *phenol red solution* as indicator. Repeat the operation without the substance being examined. The difference between the titrations represents the amount of sodium hydroxide required. Each ml of 0.5M *sodium hydroxide VS* is equivalent to 45.04 mg of $C_9H_8O_4$.

Labelling The label states that the tablets contain Aspirin, unless this word appears in the name of the tablets. This requirement does not apply in countries where exclusive proprietary rights in the name Aspirin are claimed.

Dispersible Aspirin Tablets

Definition Dispersible Aspirin Tablets contain Aspirin in a suitable dispersible basis.

The tablets comply with the requirements stated under Tablets and with the following requirements.

Content of aspirin, $C_9H_8O_4$ 95.0 to 105.0% of the prescribed or stated amount.

Identification Disperse a quantity of the powdered tablets containing 50 mg of Aspirin in 10 ml of warm *water*, boil and add 0.5 ml of *iron(III) chloride solution R1*. A violet-red colour is produced.

Salicylic acid To a quantity of the powdered tablets containing 0.50 g of Aspirin add 50 ml of *chloroform*, 2 ml of 2.5M *sulphuric acid* and shake vigorously for 2 minutes. Filter the chloroform extract through a dry filter paper containing 1 g of *anhydrous sodium sulphate* and evaporate 5 ml of the filtrate to dryness at room temperature using a rotary evaporator. Dissolve the residue in 2 ml of *ethanol (96%)*, transfer to a *Nessler cylinder* with a further 1 ml of *ethanol (96%)*, dilute to 50 ml with *water* at a temperature not exceeding 10°, add 1 ml of freshly prepared *ammonium iron(III) sulphate solution R1*, mix and allow to stand for 1 minute. Any violet colour produced is not more intense than that obtained by adding 1 ml of freshly prepared *ammonium iron(III) sulphate solution R1* to a mixture of 3 ml of a freshly prepared 0.010% w/v solution of *salicylic acid*, 3 ml of *ethanol (96%)* and sufficient *water* to produce 50 ml contained in a second *Nessler cylinder* (0.6%).

Assay Weigh and powder 20 tablets. Dissolve a quantity of the powder containing 0.3 g of Aspirin in 10 ml of 1M *sulphuric acid* and boil under a reflux condenser for 1 hour. Cool, transfer to a separating funnel, rinsing the flask and condenser with small quantities of *water* and extract the liberated salicylic acid with four 20-ml quantities of *ether*. Wash the combined ether extracts with two 5-ml quantities of *water*, evaporate the ether in a current of air at a temperature not exceeding 30°, dissolve the residue in 20 ml of 0.5M *sodium hydroxide VS* and dilute to 200 ml with *water*. Transfer 50 ml to a stoppered flask, add 50 ml of 0.05M *bromine VS* and 5 ml of *hydrochloric acid*, protect the solution from light, shake repeatedly during 15 minutes and allow to stand for 15 minutes. Add 20 ml of *dilute potassium iodide solution*, shake thoroughly and titrate with 0.1M *sodium thiosulphate VS*, using *starch mucilage*, added towards the end point, as indicator. Each ml of 0.05M *bromine VS* is equivalent to 3.003 mg of $C_9H_8O_4$.

Storage Dispersible Aspirin Tablets should be kept in a well-closed container and stored at a temperature not exceeding 25°.

Labelling The label states (1) that the tablets contain Aspirin, unless this word appears in the name of the tablets (this requirement does not apply in countries where exclusive proprietary rights in the name Aspirin are claimed); (2) that the tablets should be dispersed in water immediately before use.

When Dispersible Aspirin Tablets are prescribed or demanded, no strength being stated, tablets containing 300 mg shall be dispensed or supplied.

When soluble aspirin tablets are prescribed, Dispersible Aspirin Tablets shall be dispensed.

Effervescent Soluble Aspirin Tablets

Effervescent Aspirin Tablets

Definition Effervescent Soluble Aspirin Tablets contain Aspirin in a suitable soluble, effervescent basis.

The tablets comply with the requirements stated under Tablets and with the following requirements.

Content of aspirin, $C_9H_8O_4$ 95.0 to 105.0% of the prescribed or stated amount.

Identification

A. Dissolve with vigorous effervescence on the addition of warm *water* to produce a clear solution.

B. Dissolve a quantity of the powdered tablets containing 50 mg of Aspirin in 10 ml of warm *water*, boil and add 0.5 ml of *iron(III) chloride solution R1*. A violet-red colour is produced.

Disintegration Comply with the requirement for Effervescent Tablets stated under Tablets.

Salicylic acid Comply with the test described under Dispersible Aspirin Tablets but using a quantity of the powdered tablets containing 0.10 g of Aspirin (3.0%).

Assay Carry out the Assay described under Dispersible Aspirin Tablets.

Storage Effervescent Soluble Aspirin Tablets should be kept in a well-closed container and stored at a temperature not exceeding 25°.

Labelling The label states (1) that the tablets contain Aspirin, unless this word appears in the name of the tablets (this requirement does not apply in countries where exclusive proprietary rights in the name Aspirin are claimed); (2) that the tablets should be dissolved in water immediately before use.

When Effervescent Soluble Aspirin Tablets are prescribed or demanded, no strength being stated, tablets containing 300 mg shall be dispensed or supplied.

When soluble aspirin tablets are prescribed, Dispersible Aspirin Tablets shall be dispensed.

Aspirin and Caffeine Tablets

Definition Aspirin and Caffeine Tablets contain, in each, 350 mg of Aspirin and 30 mg of Caffeine.

The tablets comply with the requirements stated under Tablets and with the following requirements.

Content of aspirin, $C_9H_8O_4$ 330 to 370 mg .

Content of caffeine, $C_8H_{10}N_4O_2$ 27.5 to 32.5 mg .

Identification

A. Boil 1 g of the powdered tablets with 10 ml of 1M *sodium hydroxide*, cool and filter. Acidify the filtrate with 1M *sulphuric acid*; a white precipitate is produced. To a solution of the precipitate add *iron(III) chloride solution R1*; a deep violet colour is produced.

B. Shake 0.5 g of the powdered tablets with 10 ml of *water* for 5 minutes, filter and add 10 ml of 1M *sodium hydroxide*. Extract with three 30-ml quantities of *chloroform*, washing each extract with the same 10 ml of *water*. Filter the combined extracts through absorbent cotton and evaporate the filtrate to dryness. Reserve a quantity of the residue for test C. Dissolve 10 mg of the residue in 1 ml of *hydrochloric acid*, add 0.1 g of *potassium chlorate* and evaporate to dryness in a porcelain dish. A reddish residue remains which becomes purple on exposure to ammonia vapour.

C. The *light absorption*, Appendix II B, in the range 240 to 350 nm of a 0.001% w/v solution of the residue reserved in test B exhibits a maximum at 273 nm.

Salicylic acid To a quantity of the powdered tablets containing 0.50 g of Aspirin add 50 ml of *chloroform* and 10 ml of *water*, shake well and allow to separate. Filter the chloroform layer through a dry filter paper and evaporate 10 ml of the filtrate to dryness at room temperature using a rotary evaporator. To the residue add 4 ml of *ethanol (96%)*, stir well, dilute to 100 ml with *water* at a temperature not exceeding 10°, filter immediately, rapidly transfer 50 ml to a *Nessler cylinder*, add 1 ml of freshly prepared *ammonium iron(III) sulphate solution R1*, mix and allow to stand for 1 minute. Any violet colour produced is not more intense than that obtained by adding 1 ml of freshly prepared *ammonium iron(III) sulphate solution R1* to a mixture of 3 ml of a freshly prepared 0.010% w/v solution of *salicylic acid*, 2 ml of *ethanol (96%)* and sufficient *water* to produce 50 ml contained in a second *Nessler cylinder* (0.6%).

Dissolution Comply with the *dissolution test for tablets and capsules* with respect to the content of Aspirin, Appendix XII D, using Apparatus II. Use as the medium 500 ml of a pH 4.5 buffer prepared by mixing 29.9 g of *sodium acetate* and 16.6 ml of *glacial acetic acid* with sufficient *water* to produce 10 litres and rotate the paddle at 50 revolutions per minute. Withdraw a sample of 20 ml of the medium and filter. Immediately measure the *absorbance* of the filtrate, Appendix II B, diluted with the dissolution medium if necessary, at 265 nm using dissolution medium in the reference cell. Measure the *absorbance* of a suitable solution of *aspirin BPCRS* in the dissolution medium and calculate the total content of aspirin, $C_9H_8O_4$, in the medium using the declared content of $C_9H_8O_4$ in *aspirin BPCRS*.

Assay Weigh and powder 20 tablets.

For aspirin To a quantity of the powder containing 0.7 g of Aspirin add 20 ml of *water* and 2 g of *sodium citrate* and boil under a reflux condenser for 30 minutes. Cool, wash the condenser with 30 ml of warm *water* and titrate with 0.5M *sodium hydroxide VS* using *phenolphthalein solution R1* as indicator. Each ml of 0.5M *sodium hydroxide VS* is equivalent to 45.04 mg of $C_9H_8O_4$.

For caffeine To a quantity of the powder containing 30 mg of Caffeine add 200 ml of *water* and shake for 30 minutes. Add sufficient *water* to produce 250 ml and filter. To 10 ml of the filtrate add 10 ml of 1M *sodium hydroxide* and extract immediately with five 30-ml quantities of *chloroform*, washing each extract with the same 10 ml of *water*. Filter the combined chloroform extracts, if necessary, through absorbent cotton previously moistened with *chloroform*. Evaporate the solution to dryness and dissolve the residue as completely as possible in *water*, warming gently if necessary. Cool, add sufficient *water* to produce 100 ml, mix and filter if necessary. Measure the *absorbance* of the resulting solution at the maximum at 273 nm, Appendix II B. Calculate the content of $C_8H_{10}N_4O_2$ taking 504 as the value of A(1%, 1 cm) at the maximum at 273 nm.

Labelling The label states that the tablets contain Aspirin, unless this word appears in the name of the tablets. This requirement does not apply in countries where exclusive proprietary rights in the name Aspirin are claimed.

Atenolol Injection

Definition Atenolol Injection is a sterile solution of Atenolol in Water for Injections containing Citric Acid Monohydrate and Sodium Chloride.

The injection complies with the requirements stated under Parenteral Preparations and with the following requirements.

Content of atenolol, $C_{14}H_{22}N_2O_3$ 90.0 to 110.0% of the prescribed or stated amount.

Identification To a volume of the injection containing 5 mg of Atenolol add sufficient 1M *sodium hydroxide* to make it alkaline (about 0.5 ml) and extract with three 10-ml quantities of a mixture of 1 volume of *propan-2-ol* and 3 volumes of *chloroform*. Filter the combined extracts through *anhydrous sodium sulphate* and evaporate to dryness in a current of nitrogen. The *infrared absorption spectrum* of the residue, Appendix II A, is concordant with the *reference spectrum* of atenolol.

Acidity pH, 5.5 to 6.5, Appendix V L.

Related substances Carry out the method for *liquid chromatography*, Appendix III D, using the following solutions. For solution (1) use the injection being examined. For solution (2) dilute 1 volume of solution (1) to 200 volumes with the mobile phase. For solution (3) dissolve 10 mg of *atenolol impurity standard BPCRS* in 0.1 ml of *dimethyl sulphoxide*, with the aid of gentle heat, and dilute to 20 ml with the mobile phase.

The chromatographic procedure may be carried out using (a) a stainless steel column (15 cm × 4.6 mm) packed with *stationary phase C* (5 μm) (Spherisorb ODS 2 is suitable), (b) as the mobile phase with a flow rate of 1.0 ml per minute a mixture of 20 volumes of *tetrahydrofuran*, 180 volumes of *methanol* and 800 volumes of 0.025M *potassium dihydrogen orthophosphate* containing 1.0 g of *sodium octanesulphonate* and 0.4 g of *tetrabutylammonium hydrogen sulphate* per litre and adjusted to pH 3.0 with *orthophosphoric acid* and (c) a detection wavelength of 226 nm.

The test is not valid unless the chromatogram obtained with solution (3) resembles the reference chromatogram provided with *atenolol impurity standard BPCRS* in that the peak due to bis ether precedes, and is separated from, that due to tertiary amine, which is normally a doublet. If necessary, adjust the concentration of sodium octanesulphonate in the mobile phase; increasing the concentration increases the retention time of the tertiary amine.

In the chromatogram obtained with solution (1) the area of any peak corresponding to blocker acid is not greater than the area of the peak in the chromatogram obtained with solution (2) (0.5%) and the area of any peak corresponding to either tertiary amine or bis ether is not greater than half of the area of the peak in the chromatogram obtained with solution (2) (0.25%).

Assay Dilute a volume of the injection containing 10 mg of Atenolol to 100 ml with *methanol* and measure the *absorbance* at the maximum at about 275 nm, Appendix II B. Calculate the content of $C_{14}H_{22}N_2O_3$ taking 53.7 as the value of A(1%, 1 cm) at the maximum at 275 nm.

Storage Atenolol Injection should be protected from light.

Atenolol Oral Solution

Definition Atenolol Oral Solution is a solution of Atenolol in a suitable aqueous vehicle.

The oral solution complies with the requirements stated under Oral Liquids and with the following requirements.

Content of atenolol, $C_{14}H_{22}N_2O_3$ 94.0 to 106.0% of the prescribed or stated amount.

Identification

A. Carry out the method for *thin-layer chromatography*, Appendix III A, using *silica gel GF_{254}* as the coating substance and a mixture of 1 volume of 18M *ammonia* and 99 volumes of *methanol* as the mobile phase. Apply separately to the plate 10 μl of each of the following solutions. For solution (1), make a volume of the oral solution containing 50 mg of Atenolol alkaline with 1M *sodium hydroxide* (about 0.5 ml), extract with three 10-ml quantities of a mixture of 1 volume of *propan-2-ol* and 3 volumes of *chloroform*, filter the combined extracts through *anhydrous sodium sulphate*, evaporate to dryness under reduced pressure with gentle heat and dissolve the residue in 0.5 ml of *methanol*. Solution (2) contains 1.0% w/v of *atenolol BPCRS* in *methanol*. After removal of the plate, allow it to dry in air and examine under *ultraviolet light (254 nm)*. The principal spot in the chromatogram obtained with solution (1) corresponds in position, size and intensity to that in the chromatogram obtained with solution (2). Disregard any spots due to excipients at Rf values of 0.69 and 0.80.

B. In the Assay, the principal peak in the chromatogram obtained with solution (1) has the same retention time as that in the chromatogram obtained with solution (2).

Acidity pH, 5.5 to 6.5, Appendix V L.

Related substances Carry out the method for *liquid chromatography*, Appendix III D, using the following solutions. For solution (1) dilute the oral solution with the mobile phase to produce a solution containing 0.2% w/v of Atenolol. For solution (2) dilute 1 volume of solution (1) to 200 volumes with the mobile phase. For solution (3) dissolve 10 mg of *atenolol impurity standard BPCRS* in 0.1 ml of *dimethyl sulphoxide*, with the aid of gentle heat, and dilute to 20 ml with the mobile phase.

The chromatographic procedure described under Atenolol Injection may be used.

The test is not valid unless the chromatogram obtained with solution (3) resembles that of the reference chromatogram provided with *atenolol impurity standard BPCRS* in that the peak due to bis ether precedes, and is separated from, that due to tertiary amine, which is normally a doublet. If necessary adjust the concentration of sodium octanesulphonate in the mobile phase; increasing the concentration increases the retention time of the tertiary amine.

In the chromatogram obtained with solution (1) the area of any peak corresponding to blocker acid is not greater than the area of the peak in the chromatogram obtained with solution (2) (0.5%) and the area of any peak corresponding to either tertiary amine or bis ether is not greater than half of the area of the peak in the chromatogram obtained with solution (2) (0.25%). Allow the chromatography to proceed for twice the retention time of the blocker acid.

Assay Carry out the method for *liquid chromatography*, Appendix III D, using the following solutions. For solution (1) dilute the oral solution with the mobile phase to produce a solution containing 0.025% w/v of Atenolol. Solution (2) contains 0.025% w/v of *atenolol BPCRS* in the mobile phase.

The chromatographic procedure may be carried out using (a) a stainless steel column (20 cm × 4.6 mm) packed with *stationary phase C* (5 μm) (Hypersil ODS is suitable), (b) as the mobile phase with a flow rate of 1.5 ml per minute a mixture of 1 volume of *sulphuric acid (10%)*, 25 volumes of *acetonitrile* and 74 volumes of *water* containing 0.93 g per litre of *sodium octyl sulphate* adjusted to pH 3 with 2M *sodium hydroxide* and (c) a detection wavelength of 275 nm. For solution (1) allow the chromatography to proceed for at least 30 minutes.

Calculate the content of $C_{14}H_{22}N_2O_3$ in the oral solution using the declared content of $C_{14}H_{22}N_2O_3$ in *atenolol BPCRS*.

Atenolol Tablets

Definition Atenolol Tablets contain Atenolol.

The tablets comply with the requirements stated under Tablets and with the following requirements.

Content of atenolol, $C_{14}H_{22}N_2O_3$ 92.5 to 107.5% of the prescribed or stated amount.

Identification

A. Heat a quantity of the powdered tablets containing 0.1 g of Atenolol with 15 ml of *methanol* to 50°, shake for 5 minutes, filter (Whatman No. 42 paper is suitable) and evaporate the filtrate to dryness on a water bath. Warm the residue with 10 ml of 0.1M *hydrochloric acid,* shake and filter. Add to the filtrate sufficient 1M *sodium hydroxide* to make it alkaline, extract with 10 ml of *chloroform,* dry by shaking with *anhydrous sodium sulphate,* filter, evaporate the filtrate to dryness on a water bath and dry the residue at 105° for 1 hour. The *infrared absorption spectrum* of the residue, Appendix II A, is concordant with the *reference spectrum* of atenolol.

B. The *light absorption,* Appendix II B, in the range 230 to 350 nm of the solution obtained in the Assay exhibits maxima at 275 nm and 282 nm.

Related substances Carry out the method for *liquid chromatography,* Appendix III D, using the following solutions. For solution (1) shake a quantity of the powdered tablets containing 25 mg of Atenolol with 25 ml of the mobile phase, mix with the aid of ultrasound for 20 minutes, filter (Whatman GF/C filter paper is suitable) and use the filtrate. For solution (2) dilute 1 volume of solution (1) to 200 volumes with the mobile phase. For solution (3) dissolve 10 mg of *atenolol impurity standard BPCRS* in 0.1 ml of *dimethyl sulphoxide,* with the aid of gentle heat, add 10 ml of the mobile phase and mix.

The chromatographic procedure may be carried out using (a) a stainless steel column (15 cm × 4.6 mm) packed with *stationary phase C* (5 µm) (Spherisorb ODS 2 is suitable), (b) as the mobile phase with a flow rate of 1 ml per minute a mixture prepared as described below and (c) a detection wavelength of 226 nm. For the mobile phase dissolve 0.8 g of *sodium octanesulphonate* and 0.4 g of *tetrabutylammonium hydrogen sulphate* in 1 litre of a mixture of 20 volumes of *tetrahydrofuran,* 180 volumes of *methanol* and 800 volumes of a 0.34% w/v solution of *potassium dihydrogen orthophosphate;* adjust the pH to 3.0 with *orthophosphoric acid.* Inject 20 µl of each solution.

The test is not valid unless the chromatogram obtained with solution (3) resembles the reference chromatogram provided with *atenolol impurity standard BPCRS* in that the peak due to bis ether precedes, and is separated from, that due to tertiary amine, which is normally a doublet. If necessary, adjust the concentration of sodium octanesulphonate in the mobile phase; increasing the concentration increases the retention time of the tertiary amine.

In the chromatogram obtained with solution (1) the area of any peak corresponding to blocker acid is not greater than the area of the peak in the chromatogram obtained with solution (2) (0.5%) and the area of any peak corresponding to either tertiary amine or bis ether is not greater than half of the area of the peak in the chromatogram obtained with solution (2) (0.25%).

Assay Powder 20 tablets. Transfer the powder to a 500-ml flask using 300 ml of *methanol,* heat the resulting suspension to 60° and shake for 15 minutes. Cool, dilute to 500 ml with *methanol,* filter through a fine glass microfibre filter paper (Whatman GF/C is suitable) and dilute a suitable volume of the filtrate with sufficient *methanol* to produce a solution containing 0.01% w/v of Atenolol. Measure the *absorbance* of the resulting solution at the maximum at 275 nm, Appendix II B. Calculate the content of $C_{14}H_{22}N_2O_3$ taking 53.7 as the value of A(1%, 1 cm) at the maximum at 275 nm.

Atropine Eye Drops

Definition Atropine Eye Drops are a sterile solution of Atropine Sulphate in Purified Water.

The eye drops comply with the requirements stated under Eye Preparations and with the following requirements.

Content of atropine sulphate, $(C_{17}H_{23}NO_3)_2,H_2SO_4,H_2O$ 90.0 to 110.0% of the prescribed or stated amount.

Identification

A. Comply with test A for Identification described under Atropine Injection, using for the preparation of solution (1) a volume of the eye drops containing 5 mg of Atropine Sulphate.

B. In the Assay, the chromatogram obtained with solution (1) exhibits a peak with the same retention time as the peak due to atropine sulphate in the chromatogram obtained with solution (2).

Assay Carry out the method for *liquid chromatography,* Appendix III D, using the following solutions.

For eye drops containing less than 0.1% w/v of Atropine Sulphate For solution (1) use the eye drops being examined. Solution (2) contains 0.05% w/v of *atropine sulphate BPCRS* and 0.05% w/v of *homatropine hydrobromide BPCRS* in the mobile phase. Inject 100 µl.

For eye drops containing 0.1% w/v of Atropine Sulphate or more For solution (1) dilute the eye drops to contain 0.1% w/v of Atropine Sulphate with *water.* Solution (2) contains 0.1% w/v of *atropine sulphate BPCRS* and 0.1% w/v of *homatropine hydrobromide BPCRS* in the mobile phase. Inject 20 µl.

The chromatographic procedure may be carried out using (a) a stainless steel column (10 cm × 4.6 mm) packed with *stationary phase C* (5 µm) (Nucleosil C18 is suitable), (b) as the mobile phase with a flow rate of 2 ml per minute a solution containing 0.01M *sodium acetate* and 0.005M *dioctyl sodium sulphosuccinate* in *methanol (60%)* adjusted to pH 5.5 with *glacial acetic acid* and (c) a detection wavelength of 257 nm.

The test is not valid unless, in the chromatogram obtained with solution (2), the *resolution factor* between the peaks due to atropine sulphate and homatropine hydrobromide is at least 2.5.

Calculate the content of $(C_{17}H_{23}NO_3)_2,H_2SO_4,H_2O$ in the eye drops using the declared content of $(C_{17}H_{23}NO_3)_2,H_2SO_4,H_2O$ in *atropine sulphate BPCRS.*

Atropine Eye Ointment

Definition Atropine Eye Ointment is a sterile preparation containing Atropine Sulphate in a suitable basis.

The eye ointment complies with the requirements stated under Eye Preparations and with the following requirements.

Content of atropine sulphate, $(C_{17}H_{23}NO_3)_2,H_2SO_4,H_2O$ 92.5 to 105.0% of the prescribed or stated amount.

Identification

A. Complies with test A for Identification described under Atropine Injection but preparing solution (1) in the following manner. Dissolve a quantity of the ointment containing 10 mg of Atropine Sulphate as completely as possible in 10 ml of *petroleum spirit (boiling range, 40° to 60°)* and extract with two 10-ml quantities of 0.05M *sulphuric acid*, washing each acid solution with the same 5 ml of *petroleum spirit (boiling range, 40° to 60°)*. Mix the acid solutions, make alkaline with 5M *ammonia* and extract with two 15-ml quantities of *chloroform*. Evaporate the chloroform and dissolve the residue in 2 ml of *ethanol (96%)*.

B. In the Assay, the chromatogram obtained with solution (1) exhibits a peak with the same retention time as the peak due to atropine sulphate in the chromatogram obtained with solution (2).

Assay Carry out the method for *liquid chromatography*, Appendix III D, using the following solutions. For solution (1) dissolve a quantity of the eye ointment containing 10 mg of Atropine Sulphate in 10 ml of *ether* and extract with two 10-ml quantities of 0.01M *hydrochloric acid*. Use the combined extracts. Solution (2) contains 0.05% w/v of *atropine sulphate BPCRS* and 0.05% w/v of *homatropine hydrobromide BPCRS* in the mobile phase. Inject 100 µl.

The chromatographic procedure may be carried out using (a) a stainless steel column (10 cm × 4.6 mm) packed with *stationary phase C* (5 µm) (Nucleosil C18 is suitable), (b) as the mobile phase with a flow rate of 2 ml per minute a solution containing 0.01M *sodium acetate* and 0.005M *dioctyl sodium sulphosuccinate* in *methanol (60%)* adjusted to pH 5.5 with *glacial acetic acid* and (c) a detection wavelength of 257 nm.

The test is not valid unless, in the chromatogram obtained with solution (2), the *resolution factor* between the peaks due to atropine sulphate and homatropine hydrobromide is at least 2.5.

Calculate the content of $(C_{17}H_{23}NO_3)_2,H_2SO_4,H_2O$ in the eye ointment using the declared content of $(C_{17}H_{23}NO_3)_2,H_2SO_4,H_2O$ in *atropine sulphate BPCRS*.

Atropine Injection

Definition Atropine Injection is a sterile solution of Atropine Sulphate in Water for Injections.

The injection complies with the requirements stated under Parenteral Preparations and with the following requirements.

Content of atropine sulphate, $(C_{17}H_{23}NO_3)_2,H_2SO_4,H_2O$ 90.0 to 110.0% of the prescribed or stated amount.

Identification

A. Carry out the method for *thin-layer chromatography*, Appendix III A, using *silica gel G* as the coating substance and a mixture of 50 volumes of *chloroform*, 40 volumes of *acetone* and 10 volumes of *diethylamine* as the mobile phase. Apply separately to the plate 5 µl of each of the following solutions. For solution (1) evaporate a volume of the injection containing 5 mg of Atropine Sulphate to dryness on a water bath, triturate the residue with 1 ml of *ethanol (96%)*, allow to stand and use the supernatant liquid. Solution (2) contains 0.5% w/v of *atropine sulphate BPCRS* in *ethanol (96%)*. After removal of the plate, heat it at 105° for 20 minutes, allow to cool and spray with *potassium iodobismuthate solution R1*. The spot in the chromatogram obtained with solution (1) corresponds to that in the chromatogram obtained with solution (2).

B. In the Assay, the chromatogram obtained with solution (1) exhibits a peak with the same retention time as the peak due to atropine sulphate in the chromatogram obtained with solution (2).

Acidity pH, 2.8 to 4.5, Appendix V L.

Assay Carry out the method for *liquid chromatography*, Appendix III D, using the following solutions.

For injections containing less than 0.1% w/v of Atropine Sulphate For solution (1) use the injection being examined. Solution (2) contains 0.05% w/v of *atropine sulphate BPCRS* and 0.05% w/v of *homatropine hydrobromide BPCRS* in the mobile phase. Inject 100 µl.

For injections containing 0.1% w/v or more of Atropine Sulphate For solution (1) dilute the injection, if necessary, to contain 0.1% w/v of Atropine Sulphate with *water*. Solution (2) contains 0.1% w/v of *atropine sulphate BPCRS* and 0.1% w/v of *homatropine hydrobromide BPCRS* in the mobile phase. Inject 20 µl.

The chromatographic procedure may be carried out using (a) a stainless steel column (10 cm × 4.6 mm) packed with *stationary phase C* (5 µm) (Nucleosil C18 is suitable), (b) as the mobile phase with a flow rate of 2 ml per minute a solution containing 0.01M *sodium acetate* and 0.005M *dioctyl sodium sulphosuccinate* in *methanol (60%)* adjusted to pH 5.5 with *glacial acetic acid* and (c) a detection wavelength of 257 nm.

The test is not valid unless, in the chromatogram obtained with solution (2), the *resolution factor* between the peaks due to atropine sulphate and homatropine hydrobromide is at least 2.5.

Calculate the content of $(C_{17}H_{23}NO_3)_2,H_2SO_4,H_2O$ in the injection using the declared content of $(C_{17}H_{23}NO_3)_2,H_2SO_4,H_2O$ in *atropine sulphate BPCRS*.

Atropine Tablets

Definition Atropine Tablets contain Atropine Sulphate.

The tablets comply with the requirements stated under Tablets and with the following requirements.

Content of atropine sulphate, $(C_{17}H_{23}NO_3)_2,H_2SO_4,H_2O$ 90.0 to 110.0% of the prescribed or stated amount.

Identification

A. Comply with test A for Identification described under Atropine Injection using as solution (1) the supernatant liquid obtained by shaking a quantity of the powdered tablets containing 10 mg of Atropine Sulphate with 2 ml of *ethanol (96%)* and centrifuging.

B. In the test for Uniformity of content, the chromatogram obtained with solution (1) exhibits a peak with the same retention time as the peak due to atropine sulphate in the chromatogram obtained with solution (2).

Uniformity of content Tablets containing 600 µg of Atropine Sulphate comply with the requirements stated under Tablets using the following method of analysis. Carry out the method for *liquid chromatography*, Appendix III D, using the following solutions. For solution (1) shake 1 tablet with 2 ml of the mobile phase with the aid of ultrasound until fully disintegrated and filter. Solution (2) contains 0.03% w/v of *atropine sulphate BPCRS* and 0.03% w/v of *homatropine hydrobromide BPCRS* in the mobile phase.

The chromatographic procedure may be carried out using (a) a stainless steel column (10 cm × 4.6 mm) packed with *stationary phase C* (5 µm) (Nucleosil C18 is suitable), (b) as the mobile phase with a flow rate of 2 ml per minute a solution containing 0.01M *sodium acetate* and 0.005M *dioctyl sodium sulphosuccinate* in *methanol (60%)* adjusted to pH 5.5 with *glacial acetic acid* and (c) a detection wavelength of 257 nm.

The test is not valid unless, in the chromatogram obtained with solution (2), the *resolution factor* between the peaks due to atropine sulphate and homatropine hydrobromide is at least 2.5.

Calculate the content of $(C_{17}H_{23}NO_3)_2,H_2SO_4,H_2O$ in each tablet using the declared content of $(C_{17}H_{23}NO_3)_2,H_2SO_4,H_2O$ in *atropine sulphate BPCRS*.

Assay Use the average of the 10 individual results determined in the test for Uniformity of content.

Azapropazone Capsules

Definition Azapropazone Capsules contain Azapropazone.

The capsules comply with the requirements stated under Capsules and with the following requirements.

Content of azapropazone, $C_{16}H_{20}N_4O_2,2H_2O$ 95.0 to 105.0% of the prescribed or stated amount.

Identification

A. The *infrared absorption spectrum* of the contents of the capsules, Appendix II A, is concordant with the *reference spectrum* of azapropazone.

B. In the Assay, the principal peak in the chromatogram obtained with solution (1) has the same retention time as that in the chromatogram obtained with solution (2).

Related substances The contents of the capsules comply with the test described under Azapropazone.

Assay Carry out the following operations in subdued light using low-actinic glassware without delay. Carry out the method for *liquid chromatography*, Appendix III D, using the following solutions. For solution (1) shake a quantity of the mixed contents of 20 capsules containing 20 mg of Azapropazone with 40 ml of a mixture of 1 volume of *phosphate buffer pH 4.0* and 3 volumes of *methanol* (solvent A) and add sufficient solvent A to produce 100 ml. Solution (2) contains 0.02% w/v of *azapropazone BPCRS* in solvent A.

The chromatographic procedure may be carried out using (a) a stainless steel column (30 cm × 3.9 mm) packed with *stationary phase C* (10 µm) (µBondapak C18 is suitable), (b) a mixture of 1 volume of *glacial acetic acid*, 36 volumes of *methanol* and 63 volumes of a 0.068% w/v solution of *sodium butanesulphonate* in *water* as the mobile phase at a flow rate of 2.5 ml per minute and (c) a detection wavelength of 254 nm.

Calculate the content of $C_{16}H_{20}N_4O_2,2H_2O$ using the declared content of $C_{16}H_{20}N_4O_2,2H_2O$ in *azapropazone BPCRS*.

Storage Azapropazone Capsules should be protected from light.

Azapropazone Tablets

Definition Azapropazone Tablets contain Azapropazone.

With the exception of the requirements for shape, the tablets comply with the requirements stated under Tablets and with the following requirements.

Content of azapropazone, $C_{16}H_{20}N_4O_2,2H_2O$ 95.0 to 105.0% of the prescribed or stated content.

Identification

A. Shake a quantity of the powdered tablets containing 0.1 g of Azapropazone with 10 ml of *methanol*, filter (Whatman GF/C paper is suitable), evaporate the filtrate and dry the residue at 60° for 1 hour. The *infrared absorption spectrum* of the residue, Appendix II A, is concordant with the *reference spectrum* of anhydrous azapropazone.

B. The *light absorption*, Appendix II B, in the range 210 to 350 nm of solution (1) obtained in the Assay is concordant with that of solution (2).

Related substances Carry out the method for *liquid chromatography*, Appendix III D, using the following solutions in a mixture of 1 volume of *phosphate buffer pH 4.0* and 3 volumes of *methanol* (solvent A). For solution (1) shake a quantity of the powdered tablets containing 0.1 g of Azapropazone with 70 ml of solvent A, dilute to 100 ml and filter. Solution (2) contains 0.00025% w/v of *azapropazone impurity A BPCRS*. Solution (3) contains 0.00075% w/v of *azapropazone impurity C BPCRS*. For solution (4) dilute 10 ml of solution (1) to 100 ml and dilute 1 ml of the resulting solution to 100 ml. Solution (5) contains 0.1% w/v of *azapropazone impurity standard BPCRS*. For solution (6) dilute 1 volume of solution (4) to 2 volumes.

The chromatographic procedure may be carried out using (a) a stainless steel column (30 cm × 3.9 mm) packed with *stationary phase C* (10 µm) (µBondapak C18 is suitable), (b) a mixture of 1 volume of *glacial acetic acid*, 36 volumes of *methanol* and 63 volumes of a 0.068% w/v solution of *sodium butanesulphonate* in *water* as the mobile phase with a flow rate of 2.5 ml per minute and (c) a detection wavelength of 254 nm.

Inject solution (5) and continue the chromatography for 5 times the retention time of the principal peak. The test is not valid unless the chromatogram obtained with solution (5) closely resembles the reference chromatogram. If necessary adjust the proportion of methanol in the mobile phase to give the required retention times.

In the chromatogram obtained with solution (1) the area of any peaks corresponding to azapropazone impurities A and C are not greater than the areas of the corresponding peaks in the chromatograms obtained with solutions (2) and (3) (0.25% and 0.75% respectively). The area of any other *secondary peak* other than any peak corresponding to azapropazone impurity B is not greater than the area of the peak in the chromatogram obtained with solution (4) (0.1%). Calculate the content of impurities A and C using the respective reference solutions and the content of any unnamed impurities using solution (4). The total content of impurities is not greater than 1%. Disregard any peak with an area less than the area of the peak in the chromatogram obtained with solution (6) (0.05%).

Assay Carry out the following operations in subdued light using low-actinic glassware without delay. Weigh and powder 20 tablets. To a quantity of the powdered tablets containing 0.6 g of Azapropazone add 20 ml of *water,* shake for 30 minutes, add 60 ml of *methanol,* shake for 10 minutes and dilute to 100 ml with *water.* Centrifuge a portion of the solution at 3000 revolutions per minute for 10 minutes and filter the supernatant liquid through a 0.45-μm membrane filter. Dilute 5 ml of the filtrate to 500 ml with *water* and further dilute 15 ml of the resulting solution to 200 ml with *water.* Measure the *absorbance* of the resulting solution at the maximum at 253 nm, Appendix II B. Calculate the content of $C_{16}H_{20}N_4O_2,2H_2O$, taking 1033 as the value of A(1%, 1 cm) at the maximum at 253 nm.

Storage Azapropazone Tablets should be protected from light.

Azathioprine Tablets

Definition Azathioprine Tablets contain Azathioprine.

The tablets comply with the requirements stated under Tablets and with the following requirements.

Content of azathioprine, $C_9H_7N_7O_2S$ 92.5 to 107.5% of the prescribed or stated amount.

Identification

A. Carry out the method described under the test for 5-Chloro-1-methyl-4-nitroimidazole and 6-mercaptopurine applying separately to the plate 5 μl of each of the following solutions. For solution (1) shake a quantity of the powdered tablets containing 0.2 g of Azathioprine with 50 ml of 6M *ammonia,* filter through a glass microfibre paper (Whatman GF/C is suitable) and use the filtrate. Solution (2) contains 0.4% w/v of *azathioprine EPCRS* in 6M *ammonia.* The principal spot in the chromatogram obtained with solution (1) corresponds to that in the chromatogram obtained with solution (2).

B. Heat a quantity of the powdered tablets containing 20 mg of Azathioprine with 100 ml of *water* and filter. To 5 ml of the filtrate add 1 ml of *hydrochloric acid* and 10 mg of *zinc powder* and allow to stand for 5 minutes; a yellow colour is produced. Filter, cool in ice, add 0.1 ml of a 10% w/v solution of *sodium nitrite* and 0.1 g of *sulphamic acid* and shake until the bubbles disappear. Add 1 ml of *2-naphthol solution*; a pale pink precipitate is produced.

5-Chloro-1-methyl-4-nitroimidazole and 6-mercaptopurine Carry out the method for *thin-layer chromatography,* Appendix III A, using *cellulose F_{254}* as the coating substance and *butan-1-ol* saturated with 6M *ammonia* as the mobile phase. Apply separately to the plate 5 μl of each of the following solutions prepared immediately before use. For solution (1) shake a quantity of the powdered tablets containing 0.20 g of Azathioprine with 10 ml of 6M *ammonia* and filter through a glass microfibre filter paper (Whatman GF/C is suitable). Solution (2) contains 2.0% w/v of *azathioprine EPCRS* and 0.020% w/v of *6-mercaptopurine* in 6M *ammonia.* Solution (3) contains 0.020% w/v of *6-mercaptopurine* in 6M *ammonia.* Solution (4) contains 0.020% w/v of *chloromethylnitroimidazole EPCRS* in 6M *ammonia.* After removal of the plate, dry it at 50° and examine under *ultraviolet light (254 nm).* Any spot in the chromatogram obtained with solution (1) corresponding to 6-mercaptopurine in the chromatogram obtained with solution (2) is not more intense than the spot in the chromatogram obtained with solution (3). Any spot corresponding to 5-chloro-1-methyl-4-nitroimidazole in the chromatogram obtained with solution (1) is not more intense than the spot in the chromatogram obtained with solution (4).

Assay Weigh and powder 20 tablets. Shake a quantity of the powder containing 0.15 g of Azathioprine with 20 ml of *dimethyl sulphoxide* for 15 minutes and dilute to 500 ml with 0.1M *hydrochloric acid.* Avoid heating or the use of ultrasound. Filter, dilute 25 ml of the filtrate to 1000 ml with 0.1M *hydrochloric acid* and measure the *absorbance* of the resulting solution at the maximum at 280 nm, Appendix II B. Calculate the content of $C_9H_7N_7O_2S$ taking 628 as the value of A(1%, 1 cm) at the maximum at 280 nm.

Storage Azathioprine Tablets should be protected from light.

Azlocillin Injection

Definition Azlocillin Injection is a sterile solution of Azlocillin Sodium in Water for Injections. It is prepared by dissolving Azlocillin Sodium for Injection in the requisite amount of Water for Injections immediately before use.

The injection complies with the requirements stated under Parenteral Preparations.

Storage Azlocillin Injection should be used immediately after preparation but, in any case, within the period recommended by the manufacturer when prepared and stored strictly in accordance with the manufacturer's instructions.

AZLOCILLIN SODIUM FOR INJECTION

Definition Azlocillin Sodium for Injection is a sterile material consisting of Azlocillin Sodium with or without excipients. It is supplied in a sealed container.

The contents of the sealed container comply with the requirements for Powders for Injections stated under Parenteral Preparations and with the following requirements.

Content of azlocillin, $C_{20}H_{23}N_5O_6S$ 90.0 to 105.0% of the prescribed or stated amount.

Identification

A. The *infrared absorption spectrum,* Appendix II A, is concordant with the *reference spectrum* of azlocillin sodium.

B. In the Assay, the principal peak in the chromatogram obtained with solution (1) has the same retention time as the principal peak in the chromatogram obtained with solution (2).

C. Yield reaction A characteristic of *sodium salts,* Appendix VI.

Acidity or alkalinity pH of a 10% w/v solution, 6.0 to 8.0, Appendix V L.

Clarity and colour of solution A 10.0% w/v solution is *clear,* Appendix IV A, and not more intensely coloured than *reference solution BY_4,* Appendix IV B, Method I.

Related substances Carry out the method for *liquid chromatography,* Appendix III D, using the following solutions. For solutions (1) and (2) dissolve a sufficient quantity of the contents of the sealed container in *water* to produce solutions containing the equivalent of (1) 0.050% w/v and (2) 0.0010% w/v of azlocillin respectively.

The chromatographic procedure may be carried out using (a) a stainless steel column (12.5 cm × 4.6 mm) packed with *stationary phase C* (5 μm) (Hypersil ODS is suitable), (b) as the mobile phase with a flow rate of 1.6 ml per minute a mixture of 145 volumes of *acetonitrile* and 855 volumes of a solution containing 0.58 g of *dipotassium hydrogen orthophosphate* and 4.09 g of *potassium dihydrogen orthophosphate* in 1000 ml of *water* and (c) a detection wavelength of 210 nm. Carry out the procedure at 40°.

Adjust the system so that the height of the principal peak in the chromatogram obtained with solution (2) is at least 20% of the full scale of the recorder. When recorded under the prescribed conditions the retention time of azlocillin is about 5 minutes. If necessary adjust the composition of the mobile phase.

The test is not valid unless the *column efficiency* determined on the peak due to azlocillin in the chromatogram obtained with solution (2) is at least 24,000 *theoretical plates* per metre and the *symmetry factor* of the principal peak is 0.9 to 2.0.

In the chromatogram obtained with solution (1): the sum of the areas of any peaks due to the 5*R* and 5*S* epimers of azlocillin penicilloate (retention times relative to azlocillin, 0.22 and 0.27) is not greater than 1.5 times the area of the principal peak in the chromatogram obtained with solution (2) (3%); the area of any peak due to ampicillin (retention time relative to azlocillin, 0.29) is not greater than 1.25 times the area of the principal peak in the chromatogram obtained with solution (2) (2.5%) and the area of any peak due to the epimers of azlocillin penilloate, which may appear as a doublet, (retention time relative to azlocillin, 0.73) is not greater than the area of the principal peak in the chromatogram obtained with solution (2) (2%).

Water Not more than 2.5% w/w, Appendix IX C. Use 0.25 g.

Bacterial endotoxins Carry out the *test for bacterial endotoxins*, Appendix XIV C. Prepare a solution in *water BET* containing the equivalent of 10 mg of azlocillin per ml (solution A). The endotoxin limit concentration of solution A is 0.7 IU of endotoxin per ml. Carry out the test using the maximum valid dilution of solution A calculated from the declared sensitivity of the lysate used in the test.

Assay Determine the weight of the contents of 10 containers as described in the test for Uniformity of weight under Parenteral Preparations, Powders for Injections.

Carry out the method for *liquid chromatography*, Appendix III D, using the following solutions. For solution (1) dissolve a quantity of the mixed contents of the 10 containers in sufficient *water* to produce a solution containing the equivalent of 0.05% w/v of azlocillin. Solution (2) contains 0.05% w/v of *azlocillin sodium BPCRS* in *water*.

The chromatographic procedure may be carried out using the conditions described under Related substances.

Calculate the content of $C_{20}H_{23}N_5O_6S$ in a container of average content weight from the declared content of $C_{20}H_{23}N_5O_6S$ in *azlocillin sodium BPCRS*.

Storage The sealed container should be stored at a temperature not exceeding 25°.

Labelling The label of the sealed container states the quantity of Azlocillin Sodium contained in it in terms of the equivalent amount of azlocillin.

Baclofen Oral Solution

Definition Baclofen Oral Solution is a solution of Baclofen in a suitable aqueous vehicle.

The oral solution complies with the requirements stated under Oral Liquids and with the following requirements.

Content of baclofen, $C_{10}H_{12}ClNO_2$ 95.0 to 105.0% of the prescribed or stated amount.

Identification

A. Carry out the method for *thin-layer chromatography*, Appendix III A, using *silica gel G* as the coating substance and a mixture of 20 volumes of *glacial acetic acid*, 20 volumes of *water* and 80 volumes of *butan-1-ol* as the mobile phase but allowing the solvent front to ascend 10 cm above the line of application. Apply separately to the plate 5 μl of each of the following solutions. For solution (1) dilute a volume of the oral solution containing 5 mg of Baclofen to 100 ml with a mixture of 35 volumes of *acetonitrile* and 65 volumes of *water*. Solution (2) contains 0.005% w/v of *baclofen BPCRS* in the same solvent mixture. After removal of the plate, allow the solvent to evaporate. Place an evaporating dish containing a mixture of 4 ml of *water*, 1 ml of 7M *hydrochloric acid* and 0.5 g of *potassium permanganate* in a chromatography tank, close the tank and allow to stand for 2 minutes. Place the plate in the tank, close the tank and leave the plate in contact with the vapour for 1 minute. After removal of the plate, place it in a current of cold air until an area of coating below the line of application shows only a faint blue colour on the addition of 0.05 ml of *potassium iodide and starch solution*. Spray the plate with *potassium iodide and starch solution* and examine in daylight. The chromatogram obtained with solution (1) exhibits a spot that corresponds to the spot in the chromatogram obtained with solution (2).

B. In the Assay, the chromatogram obtained with solution (1) shows a peak with the same retention time as the principal peak in the chromatogram obtained with solution (2).

Lactam Carry out the method for *liquid chromatography*, Appendix III D, using the following solutions. For solution (1) use solution (1) prepared for the Assay. Solution (2) contains 0.0002% w/v of *baclofen lactam BPCRS* in the mobile phase. Solution (3) contains 0.01% w/v of *baclofen BPCRS*, 0.0003% w/v of *propyl 4-hydroxybenzoate*, 0.0003% w/v of *methyl 4-hydroxybenzoate* and 0.0002% w/v of *baclofen lactam BPCRS* in the mobile phase.

The chromatographic procedure described under Assay may be used.

The test is not valid unless the chromatogram obtained with solution (3) shows four clearly separated peaks.

In the chromatogram obtained with solution (1) the area of any peak corresponding to baclofen lactam is not greater than the area of the peak in the chromatogram obtained with solution (2) (2%).

Assay Carry out the method for *liquid chromatography*, Appendix III D, using the following solutions. For solution (1) dilute a weighed quantity of the oral solution containing 5 mg of Baclofen to 50 ml with the mobile phase. Solution (2) contains 0.01% w/v of *baclofen BPCRS* in the mobile phase. Solution (3) contains 0.01% w/v of *baclofen BPCRS*, 0.0003% w/v of *propyl 4-hydroxybenzoate* and 0.0002% w/v of *baclofen lactam BPCRS* in the mobile phase.

The chromatographic procedure may be carried out using (a) a stainless steel column (25 cm × 4.6 mm) packed with *stationary phase C* (10 µm) (Nucleosil C18 is suitable), (b) as the mobile phase with a flow rate of 1.5 ml per minute a solution prepared by dissolving 5 g of *sodium dodecyl sulphate* in a mixture of 5 ml of *orthophosphoric acid* and 650 ml of *water* and diluting to 1000 ml with *acetonitrile* and (c) a detection wavelength of 218 nm.

The test is not valid unless the chromatogram obtained with solution (3) shows three clearly separated peaks.

Determine the *weight per ml* of the oral solution, Appendix V G, and calculate the content of $C_{10}H_{12}ClNO_2$, weight in volume, using the declared content of $C_{10}H_{12}ClNO_2$ in *baclofen BPCRS*.

Storage Baclofen Oral Solution should be stored below 25° and protected from light. It should not be refrigerated.

Baclofen Tablets

Definition Baclofen Tablets contain Baclofen.

The tablets comply with the requirements stated under Tablets and with the following requirements.

Content of baclofen, $C_{10}H_{12}ClNO_2$ 90.0 to 110.0% of the prescribed or stated amount.

Identification

A. Carry out the method for *thin-layer chromatography*, Appendix III A, using *silica gel G* as the coating substance and a mixture of 80 volumes of *butan-1-ol*, 20 volumes of *glacial acetic acid* and 20 volumes of *water* as the mobile phase. Apply separately to the plate 5 µl of each of the following solutions. For solution (1) shake a quantity of the powdered tablets containing 20 mg of Baclofen with 20 ml of a mixture of 4 volumes of *absolute ethanol* and 1 volume of *glacial acetic acid* for 30 minutes and filter. Solution (2) contains 0.1% w/v of *baclofen BPCRS* in a mixture of 4 volumes of *absolute ethanol* and 1 volume of *glacial acetic acid*. After removal of the plate, allow it to dry in air, spray with *ninhydrin solution* and heat at 100° for 10 minutes. The principal spot in the chromatogram obtained with solution (1) corresponds to that in the chromatogram obtained with solution (2).

B. In the Assay, the chromatogram obtained with solution (1) shows a peak with the same retention time as the principal peak in the chromatogram obtained with solution (2).

Lactam Carry out the method for *liquid chromatography*, Appendix III D, using the following solutions. For solution (1) mix with the aid of ultrasound a quantity of the powdered tablets containing 0.10 g of Baclofen with 20 ml of the mobile phase for 30 minutes, shaking occasionally to disperse the sample, and filter through a glass-fibre filter (Whatman GF/C is suitable). For solution (2) dilute 1 volume of solution (1) to 50 volumes with the mobile phase. For solution (3) heat 20 mg of *baclofen BPCRS* at 170° for 75 minutes, allow to cool, shake with 20 ml of the mobile phase for 10 minutes and filter if necessary.

The chromatographic procedure may be carried out using (a) a stainless steel column (25 cm × 4.6 mm) packed with *stationary phase C* (10 µm) (Spherisorb ODS 1 is suitable), (b) as the mobile phase with a flow rate of 2 ml per minute a mixture of 5 volumes of *glacial acetic acid*, 440 volumes of *methanol* and 560 volumes of *water*, the mixture containing 1.822 g per litre of *sodium hexanesulphonate* and (c) a detection wavelength of 266 nm.

In the chromatogram obtained with solution (1) the area of any peak corresponding to the principal peak in the chromatogram obtained with solution (3) (lactam) is not greater than the area of the peak in the chromatogram obtained with solution (2) (2%).

Dissolution Comply with the *dissolution test for tablets and capsules*, Appendix XII D, using Apparatus II. Use as the medium 900 ml of 0.1M *hydrochloric acid* and rotate the paddle at 50 revolutions per minute. Withdraw a sample of 20 ml of the medium and filter through a membrane filter with a nominal pore size not greater than 0.45 µm, discarding the first 10 ml of filtrate. Carry out the method for *liquid chromatography*, Appendix III D, using the following solutions. Solution (1) contains 0.001% w/v of *baclofen BPCRS* in the mobile phase. Solution (2) is the filtrate from the dissolution vessel.

The chromatographic conditions described under Assay may be used.

Calculate the total content of baclofen, $C_{10}H_{12}ClNO_2$, in the medium from the declared content of $C_{10}H_{12}ClNO_2$ in *baclofen BPCRS*.

Assay Carry out the method for *liquid chromatography*, Appendix III D, using the following solutions. For solution (1) add a quantity of whole tablets containing 0.1 g of Baclofen to 25 ml of a mixture of 100 volumes of *water* and 1 volume of *glacial acetic acid* and disperse with the aid of ultrasound. Dilute to 50 ml with *methanol*, filter and use the filtrate. Solution (2) contains 0.2% w/v of *baclofen BPCRS* in a mixture of 100 volumes of *methanol*, 100 volumes of *water* and 1 volume of *glacial acetic acid*.

The chromatographic procedure may be carried out using (a) a stainless steel column (20 cm × 4.6 mm) packed with *stationary phase C* (10 µm) (Nucleosil C18 is suitable), (b) 0.01M *sodium hexanesulphonate* in a mixture of 100 volumes of *methanol*, 100 volumes of *water* and 1 volume of *glacial acetic acid* as the mobile phase with a flow rate of 2 ml per minute and (c) a detection wavelength of 265 nm.

Calculate the content of $C_{10}H_{12}ClNO_2$ using the declared content of $C_{10}H_{12}ClNO_2$ in *baclofen BPCRS*.

Barium Sulphate Oral Suspension

Definition Barium Sulphate Oral Suspension is a suspension of Barium Sulphate for Suspension in a suitable aqueous vehicle.

The oral suspension complies with the requirements stated under Oral Liquids and with the following requirements.

Content of barium sulphate, $BaSO_4$ Not less than 75.0% w/v.

Characteristics A smooth, white or creamy white suspension.

Identification Evaporate 1 ml to dryness and ignite to

constant weight. The residue complies with the following tests.

A. To 0.2 g add 5 ml of a 50% w/v solution of *sodium carbonate* and boil for 5 minutes, add 10 ml of *water* and filter. Reserve the residue for test B. Acidify the filtrate with 2M *hydrochloric acid*. The resulting solution yields the reactions characteristic of *sulphates*, Appendix VI.

B. Wash the residue reserved in test A with *water*, add 5 ml of 2M *hydrochloric acid*, mix well and filter. Add 0.3 ml of 1M *sulphuric acid* to the filtrate. A white precipitate is produced which is insoluble in 2M *hydrochloric acid*.

Acidity or alkalinity pH, 4.5 to 7.0, Appendix V L.

Soluble barium compounds To 10.0 g add 10 ml of 2M *hydrochloric acid* and 90 ml of *water*. Boil for 10 minutes, cool and filter. Wash the residue with *water* and dilute the combined filtrate and washings to 100 ml with *water*. Carefully evaporate 50 ml of the resulting solution to avoid charring, add 0.1 ml of 2M *hydrochloric acid* and 10 ml of hot *water* to the residue and filter. To the clear filtrate add 0.5 ml of 1M *sulphuric acid* and allow to stand for 30 minutes. The solution is *clear*, Appendix IV A.

Assay Evaporate 0.9 g in a platinum dish to dryness on a water bath and carry out the Assay described under Barium Sulphate for Suspension, beginning at the words 'add 5 g of *sodium carbonate* ...'. Determine the *weight per ml* of the oral suspension, Appendix V G, and calculate the percentage of $BaSO_4$, weight in volume.

Beclometasone Cream

Definition Beclometasone Cream contains Beclometasone Dipropionate in a suitable basis.

The cream complies with the requirements stated under Topical Semi-solid Preparations and with the following requirements.

Content of beclometasone dipropionate, $C_{28}H_{37}ClO_7$ 90.0 to 110.0% of the prescribed or stated amount.

Identification

A. Carry out the method for *thin-layer chromatography*, Appendix III A, using *silica gel G* as the coating substance and a mixture of 100 volumes of *chloroform*, 10 volumes of *acetone* and 5 volumes of *absolute ethanol* as the mobile phase. Apply separately to the plate 10 µl of each of the following solutions. For solution (1) disperse a quantity of the preparation being examined containing 0.5 mg of Beclometasone Dipropionate in 20 ml of *methanol (80%)* by heating on a water bath until the methanol begins to boil. Shake vigorously, cool in ice for 30 minutes and centrifuge. Mix 10 ml of the supernatant liquid with 3 ml of *water* and 5 ml of *chloroform*, shake vigorously, allow the layers to separate, evaporate the chloroform layer to dryness in a current of nitrogen with gentle heating and dissolve the residue in 1 ml of *chloroform*. Solution (2) contains 0.025% w/v of *beclometasone dipropionate BPCRS* in *chloroform*. Solution (3) is a mixture of equal volumes of solutions (1) and (2). After removal of the plate, allow it to dry in air until the odour of solvent is no longer detectable, heat at 105° for 5 minutes and, while hot, spray with *alkaline tetrazolium blue solution*. The principal spot in the chromatogram obtained with solution (1) corresponds to that in the chromatogram obtained with solution (2). The principal spot in the chromatogram obtained with solution (3) appears as a single compact spot.

B. In the Assay, the chromatogram obtained with solution (2) shows a peak with the same retention time as the peak due to beclometasone dipropionate in the chromatogram obtained with solution (1).

Assay Carry out the method for *liquid chromatography*, Appendix III D, using the following solutions.

For creams containing 0.025% w/w of Beclometasone Dipropionate prepare solution (1) by mixing 10 ml of *methanol (80%)* containing 0.01% w/v of *beclometasone dipropionate BPCRS* and 0.0005% w/v of *beclometasone 17-propionate BPCRS* with 2 ml of a 0.05% w/v solution of *testosterone propionate* (internal standard) in *methanol (80%)* and diluting to 50 ml with the same solvent. For solution (2) disperse a quantity of the preparation being examined containing 1 mg of Beclometasone Dipropionate in 20 ml of hot *methanol (90%)*, add 25 ml of *2,2,4-trimethylpentane*, cool, shake the mixture and filter the lower layer through a small plug of absorbent cotton previously washed with *methanol (80%)*. Repeat the extraction of the trimethylpentane solution with two further 10-ml quantities of *methanol (80%)*, filtering the extracts through the absorbent cotton. Combine the extracts and add sufficient *methanol (80%)* to produce 50 ml. If the resulting solution is more than slightly cloudy, filter. Prepare solution (3) in the same manner as solution (2) but add 2 ml of a 0.05% w/v solution of the internal standard in *methanol (80%)* before diluting to 50 ml.

For creams containing 0.5% w/w of Beclometasone Dipropionate prepare solution (1) by mixing 25 ml of *methanol (80%)* containing 0.04% w/v of *beclometasone dipropionate BPCRS* and 0.002% w/v of *beclometasone 17-propionate BPCRS* with 20 ml of a 0.05% w/v solution of *testosterone propionate* (internal standard) in *methanol (80%)* and dilute to 200 ml with the same solvent. For solution (2) add 100 ml of *methanol (80%)* to a quantity of the preparation being examined containing 10 mg of Beclometasone Dipropionate and heat on a water bath, with swirling, until the preparation has dispersed. Cool, dilute to 200 ml with *methanol (80%)* and filter. Prepare solution (3) in the same manner as solution (2) but add 20 ml of a 0.05% w/v solution of the internal standard in *methanol (80%)* before diluting to 200 ml.

The chromatographic procedure may be carried out using (a) a stainless steel column (10 cm × 5 mm) packed with *stationary phase C* (5 µm) (Spherisorb ODS 1 is suitable) and maintained at 60°, (b) as the mobile phase with a flow rate of 2 ml per minute a mixture of *methanol* and *water* such that the *resolution factor* between the peaks due to beclometasone 17-propionate (retention time about 1.5 minutes) and beclometasone dipropionate (retention time about 2 minutes) is more than 2.0 (a mixture of 70 volumes of *methanol* and 30 volumes of *water* is usually suitable) and (c) a detection wavelength of 238 nm.

Calculate the content of $C_{28}H_{37}ClO_7$ in the preparation being examined using the declared content of $C_{28}H_{37}ClO_7$ in *beclometasone dipropionate BPCRS*.

Storage Beclometasone Cream should be protected from light.

When beclomethasone cream is prescribed or demanded, Beclometasone Cream shall be dispensed or supplied.

Beclometasone Nasal Spray

Definition Beclometasone Nasal Spray is a suspension of Beclometasone Dipropionate in a suitable liquid in a suitable pressurised container fitted with a suitable nasal delivery system.

The intranasal solution complies with the requirements stated under Nasal Preparations and with the following requirements.

Content of beclometasone dipropionate, $C_{28}H_{37}ClO_7$ 80.0 to 120.0% of the amount stated to be delivered by actuation of the valve.

Identification Complies with the test described under Beclometasone Pressurised Inhalation.

Related substances Complies with the test described under Beclometasone Pressurised Inhalation when determined on the residue collected from a sufficient number of discharges.

Assay Carry out the Assay described under Beclometasone Pressurised Inhalation.

Labelling The label states the amount of active ingredient delivered by each actuation of the valve and the number of deliveries available from the container.

When beclomethasone nasal spray is prescribed or demanded, Beclometasone Nasal Spray shall be dispensed or supplied.

Beclometasone Ointment

Definition Beclometasone Ointment contains Beclometasone Dipropionate in a suitable basis.

The ointment complies with the requirements stated under Topical Semi-solid Preparations and with the following requirements.

Content of beclometasone dipropionate, $C_{28}H_{37}ClO_7$ 90.0 to 110.0% of the prescribed or stated amount.

Identification

A. Complies with test A for Identification described under Beclometasone Cream using the following as solutions (1) and (2). For solution (1) dissolve a quantity of the ointment containing 0.5 mg of Beclometasone Dipropionate in 2 ml of *chloroform* by heating on a water bath, add 10 ml of *methanol* and heat on the water bath until the mixture begins to boil. Shake vigorously, cool in ice for 30 minutes and filter. Evaporate the filtrate to dryness in a current of nitrogen with gentle heating and dissolve the residue in 1 ml of *chloroform*. Solution (2) contains 0.05% w/v of *beclometasone dipropionate BPCRS* in *chloroform*.

B. In the Assay the chromatogram obtained with solution (2) shows a peak with the same retention time as the peak due to beclometasone dipropionate in the chromatogram obtained with solution (1).

Assay Carry out the Assay described under Beclometasone Cream, preparing the solutions in the following manner. For solution (1) mix 10 ml of *methanol (80%)* containing 0.01% w/v of *beclometasone dipropionate BPCRS* and 0.0005% w/v of *beclometasone 17-propionate BPCRS* with 2 ml of a 0.05% w/v solution of *testosterone propionate* (internal standard) in *methanol (80%)* and dilute to 50 ml with the same solvent. For solution (2) disperse a quantity of the ointment containing 1 mg of Beclometasone Dipropionate in 25 ml of hot *2,2,4-trimethylpentane*, cool and extract the mixture with successive quantities of 20, 10 and 10 ml of *methanol (80%)*, filtering each extract in turn through a small plug of absorbent cotton previously washed with *methanol (80%)*. Combine the filtrates and dilute to 50 ml with *methanol (80%)*. Prepare solution (3) in the same manner as solution (2) but add 2 ml of a 0.05% w/v solution of the internal standard in *methanol (80%)* before diluting to 50 ml.

Storage Beclometasone Ointment should be protected from light.

When beclomethasone ointment is prescribed or demanded, Beclometasone Ointment shall be dispensed or supplied.

Beclometasone Pressurised Inhalation

Definition Beclometasone Pressurised Inhalation is a suspension of Beclometasone Dipropionate in a suitable liquid in a suitable pressurised container.

The pressurised inhalation complies with the requirements stated under Preparations for Inhalation and with the following requirements.

Content of beclometasone dipropionate, $C_{28}H_{37}ClO_7$ 80.0 to 120.0% of the amount stated to be delivered by actuation of the valve.

Identification

A. The *infrared absorption spectrum*, Appendix II A, is concordant with the appropriate *reference spectrum* of beclometasone dipropionate. Examine the substance as a dispersion in *potassium bromide* prepared in the following manner. Discharge the container a sufficient number of times, under conditions of very low relative humidity (less than 5%), into a mortar to obtain 2 mg of Beclometasone Dipropionate. Heat at 110° for 2 hours at a pressure of 2 kPa, cool, grind the residue thoroughly with 0.1 g of *potassium bromide*, add a further 0.2 g of *potassium bromide* and mix thoroughly.

B. In the Assay, the principal peak in the chromatogram obtained with solution (2) corresponds to the peak due to beclometasone dipropionate in the chromatogram obtained with solution (1).

Related substances Carry out the method for *thin-layer chromatography*, Appendix III A, using *silica gel G* as the coating substance and a mixture of 3 volumes of *methanol* and 97 volumes of *1,2-dichloroethane* as the mobile phase. Apply separately to the plate the whole of solution (1) and 10 µl of each of solutions (2), (3) and (4). For solution (1) discharge the container into a small, dry flask a sufficient number of times to obtain 0.5 mg of Beclometasone Dipropionate and dissolve the residue in 2 ml of *acetone*. Evaporate the solution to a volume such that the whole solution can be applied to the plate. Solution (2) contains 0.1% w/v of *beclometasone dipropionate BPCRS* in *acetone*. For solution (3) dilute 1 volume of solution (2) to 2 volumes with *acetone*. For solution (4) dilute 1 volume of solution (2) to 4 volumes with *acetone*.

After removal of the plate, allow it to dry in air, spray with *alkaline tetrazolium blue solution* and heat at 50° for 5 minutes. Cool and spray again with *alkaline tetrazolium blue solution*. Any *secondary spot* in the chromatogram obtained with solution (1) is not more intense than the spot in the chromatogram obtained with solution (2) (2%), not more than one such spot is more intense than the spot in the chromatogram obtained with solution (3) (1%) and any other *secondary spot* is not more intense than the spot in the chromatogram obtained with solution (4) (0.5%). Disregard any spot with an Rf value of more than 0.85.

Deposition of the emitted dose Carry out the test for *aerodynamic assessment of fine particles*, Appendix XII F, using apparatus A with 7 ml of *methanol* in the upper impingement chamber and 30 ml of *methanol* in the lower impingement chamber but determining the content of active ingredient as described below. Use *methanol* to wash the coupling tube, E, and transfer the combined solution and washings in the lower impingement chamber to a flask containing sufficient *testosterone propionate EPCRS* (internal standard) in *methanol* that, on dilution to volume with appropriate amounts of *water* and *methanol*, the final solution contains 0.00015% w/v each of testosterone propionate and beclometasone dipropionate in the methanol—water mixture in the proportions 70:30 by volume (solution A).

Carry out the method for *liquid chromatography*, Appendix III D, using the following solutions. Solution (1) contains 0.00015% w/v each of *testosterone propionate EPCRS* and *beclometasone dipropionate BPCRS* in the mobile phase. For solution (2) use the diluted solution from the lower impingement chamber.

The chromatographic procedure may be carried out using the conditions described under the Assay.

Calculate the amount of beclometasone dipropionate, $C_{28}H_{37}ClO_7$, delivered to the lower impingement chamber per actuation of the valve using the declared content of $C_{28}H_{37}ClO_7$ in *beclometasone dipropionate BPCRS*. For pressurised inhalations containing 50 µg and 100 µg of Beclometasone Dipropionate, not less than 35% of the average amount of beclometasone delivered per actuation of the valve, calculated as the average of the three results determined in the Assay, is deposited in the lower impingement chamber. For pressurised inhalations containing 200 µg and 250 µg of Beclometasone Dipropionate, not less than 25% of the average amount of beclometasone dipropionate delivered per actuation of the valve, calculated as the average of the three results determined in the Assay, is deposited in the lower impingement chamber.

Assay Determine the content of active ingredient delivered by the first 10 successive combined actuations of the valve after priming. Carry out the procedure for Content of active ingredient delivered by actuation of the valve described under Pressurised Inhalations, beginning at the words 'Remove the pressurised container from the actuator ...' and ending at the words '... to the volume specified in the monograph', using 35 ml of *methanol* in the vessel. Transfer the combined solution and washings obtained from the set of 10 combined actuations to a flask containing sufficient *testosterone propionate EPCRS* (internal standard) in *methanol* that, on dilution to volume with appropriate amounts of *water* and *methanol*, the final solution contains 0.00015% w/v each of testosterone propionate and beclometasone dipropionate in the methanol—water mixture in the proportions 70:30 by volume (solution A). Determine the content of active ingredient in the 10 combined actuations using the following method of analysis.

Carry out the method for *liquid chromatography*, Appendix III D, using the following solutions. Solution (1) contains 0.00015% w/v each of *testosterone propionate EPCRS* and *beclometasone dipropionate BPCRS* in the mobile phase. For solution (2) use solution A.

The chromatographic procedure may be carried out using (a) a stainless steel column (10 cm × 4.6 mm) packed with *stationary phase C* (5 µm) (Spherisorb ODS 1 is suitable) and maintained at 50°, (b) as the mobile phase with a flow rate of 2 ml per minute a mixture of 70 volumes of *methanol* and 30 volumes of *water*, adjusted if necessary so that the *resolution factor* between the peaks due to beclometasone dipropionate and testosterone propionate is not less than 2.0 and (c) a detection wavelength of 239 nm.

The test is not valid unless the *resolution factor* between the two principal peaks in the chromatogram obtained with solution (1) is at least 2.0.

Calculate the average content of $C_{28}H_{37}ClO_7$ delivered by a single actuation of the valve using the declared content of $C_{28}H_{37}ClO_7$ in *beclometasone dipropionate BPCRS*.

Determine the content of active ingredient a second and third time by repeating the procedure on the middle 10 and on the last 10 successive combined actuations of the valve, as estimated from the number of deliveries available from the container as stated on the label. For each of the three determinations the average content of $C_{28}H_{37}ClO_7$ delivered by a single actuation of the valve is within the limits stated under Content of beclometasone dipropionate.

When beclomethasone pressurised inhalation is prescribed or demanded, Beclometasone Pressurised Inhalation shall be dispensed or supplied.

Belladonna Dry Extract

Definition Belladonna Dry Extract is prepared by extracting Belladonna Herb with Ethanol (70 per cent) and removing the solvent. It contains not less than 0.95% and not more than 1.05% w/w of alkaloids, calculated as hyoscyamine.

In making Belladonna Dry Extract, Ethanol (70 per cent) may be replaced by Industrial Methylated Spirit[1] diluted so as to be of equivalent ethanolic strength.

Extemporaneous preparation The following formula and directions apply.

Belladonna Herb, in *moderately coarse powder*	1000 g
Belladonna Herb, in *fine powder*, dried at 80°	a sufficient quantity
Ethanol (70 per cent)	a sufficient quantity

Percolate the Belladonna Herb in *moderately coarse powder* with Ethanol (70 per cent) until 4000 ml of percolate has been obtained.

Determine the proportion of total solids in the percolate by evaporating 20 ml, drying the residue at 80° and weighing. Determine also the proportion of alkaloids in the percolate by the Assay described under Belladonna Tincture, using 50 ml, and the proportion of alkaloids present in the Belladonna Herb in *fine powder*. From the results of the three determinations, calculate the amount of Belladonna Herb in *fine powder* that must be added to the percolate to produce a dry extract containing 1.0% of alkaloids.

Add to the percolate a slightly smaller amount of Belladonna Herb in *fine powder* than calculation has shown to be necessary, remove the ethanol, evaporate to dryness under reduced pressure at a temperature not exceeding 60° and dry in a current of air at 80°. Powder the residue, add the final necessary amount of Belladonna Herb in *fine powder* and triturate in a dry, slightly warmed mortar until thoroughly mixed. Pass the powdered Extract through a sieve with a nominal mesh aperture of 710 µm and mix.

The extract complies with the requirements stated under Extracts and with the following requirements.

Loss on drying Not more than 5.0%.

Assay Weigh 3 g and wash into a separating funnel with 12 ml of a mixture of equal volumes of *ethanol (96%)* and *water*, allow to stand for 30 minutes, shaking frequently, add 2 ml of 5M *ammonia* and 25 ml of *chloroform* and complete the Assay described under Belladonna Tincture, beginning at the words 'Shake well, allow to separate ...'.

Storage Belladonna Dry Extract should be kept in a small, wide-mouthed, airtight container.

[1]The law and the statutory regulations governing the use of Industrial Methylated Spirit must be observed.

Belladonna Tincture

Definition

Belladonna Herb, in *moderately coarse powder*	100 g
Ethanol (70 per cent)	a sufficient quantity

Extemporaneous preparation The following directions apply.

Prepare about 900 ml of a tincture by *percolation*, Appendix XI F. Determine the proportion of alkaloids in this tincture by the Assay and add, if necessary, sufficient Ethanol (70 per cent) to produce a Tincture containing 0.03% w/v of alkaloids, calculated as hyoscyamine.

The tincture complies with the requirements stated under Tinctures and with the following requirements.

Content of alkaloids 0.028 to 0.032% w/v, calculated as hyoscyamine.

Identification Carry out the method for *thin-layer chromatography*, Appendix III A, using *silica gel G* as the coating substance and a mixture of 3 volumes of 13.5M *ammonia*, 7 volumes of *water* and 90 volumes of *acetone* as the mobile phase but allowing the solvent front to ascend 10 cm above the line of application. Apply separately to the plate 20 µl of solution (1) and 10 µl of solution (2). For solution (1) dilute 1 volume of the tincture being examined to 10 volumes with *water* and mix 10 ml of this solution with 10 ml of 1M *sulphuric acid*, shake with two 10-ml quantities of *chloroform*, discarding the chloroform extracts. Add 5M *ammonia* until the aqueous solution is distinctly alkaline to *litmus paper*. Shake with four 10-ml quantities of *chloroform*, evaporate the combined chloroform extracts to dryness and dissolve the residue in 0.5 ml of *ethanol (96%)*. Solution (2) contains 0.1% w/v of *hyoscyamine sulphate* in *ethanol (96%)*.

After removal of the plate, dry it at 100° to 105° for 15 minutes, allow to cool and spray with 10 ml of *potassium iodobismuthate solution R2* until the spots become visible as orange or brown on a yellow background. The spot in the chromatogram obtained with solution (1) corresponds in position to that in the chromatogram obtained with solution (2). Spray the plate with a freshly prepared 10% w/v solution of *sodium nitrite* until transparent and examine after 15 minutes. Any orange spot in the lower third of the chromatogram changes from orange to brown but not to greyish blue (atropine); any secondary bands are no longer visible.

Ethanol content 64 to 69% v/v, Appendix VIII F, Method III.

Relative density; Dry residue The requirements for Relative density and Dry residue do not apply to Belladonna Tincture.

Assay Evaporate 100 ml on a water bath to about 10 ml and transfer to a separating funnel with the aid of 25 ml of *chloroform* and a mixture of 10 ml of *water* and 3 ml of 5M *ammonia*. Shake well, allow to separate and filter the chloroform layer into a second separating funnel through a plug of absorbent cotton previously moistened with *chloroform*. Continue the extraction with further 25-ml quantities of *chloroform* until *complete extraction* of the alkaloids is effected, Appendix XI G, filtering each chloroform solution through the same plug of absorbent cotton. Extract the combined chloroform solutions with successive quantities of a mixture of 3 volumes of 0.1M *sulphuric acid* and 1 volume of *ethanol (96%)* until *complete extraction* of the alkaloids is effected, filtering each extract through absorbent cotton previously moistened with *water*. Wash the mixed acid solutions with successive quantities of 10, 5 and 5 ml of *chloroform*, extracting each chloroform solution with the same 20 ml of 0.05M *sulphuric acid*, and discard the chloroform. Combine the acid solutions, neutralise with 5M *ammonia*, add 5 ml in excess and shake with successive 25-ml quantities of *chloroform* until *complete extraction* of the alkaloids is effected. Wash each chloroform solution with the same 10 ml of *water* and filter into a flask through absorbent cotton previously moistened with *chloroform*. Distil most of the chloroform from the combined extracts and transfer the remainder of the solution to a shallow, open dish. Evaporate the remainder of the chloroform without the aid of a current of air, heat the residue in an oven at 100° for 15 minutes, dissolve in a little *chloroform*, evaporate to dryness without the aid of a current of air and again heat in an oven at 100° for 15 minutes. Dissolve the residue in 2 ml of *chloroform*, add 5 ml of 0.025M *sulphuric acid VS*, warm to remove the chloroform, cool and titrate the excess of acid with 0.05M *sodium hydroxide VS* using *methyl red solution* as indicator. Each ml of 0.025M *sulphuric acid VS* is equivalent to 14.47 mg of alkaloids, calculated as hyoscyamine.

Bendroflumethiazide Tablets
Bendrofluazide Tablets

For the purposes of product labelling in the United Kingdom, the pair of names given above shall be used together (see Introduction, Changes in title).

Definition Bendroflumethiazide Tablets contain Bendroflumethiazide.

The tablets comply with the requirements stated under Tablets and with the following requirements.

Content of bendroflumethiazide, $C_{15}H_{14}F_3N_3O_4S_2$ 92.5 to 107.5% of the prescribed or stated amount.

Identification Carry out the method for *thin-layer chromatography*, Appendix III A, using *silica gel GF_{254}* as the coating substance and *ethyl acetate* as the mobile phase. Apply separately to the plate 5 µl of each of the following solutions. For solution (1) shake a quantity of the powdered tablets containing 10 mg of Bendroflumethiazide with 10 ml of *acetone* for 10 minutes and filter. Solution (2) contains 0.1% w/v of *bendroflumethiazide EPCRS* in *acetone*. After removal of the plate, allow it to dry in air, examine under *ultraviolet light (254 nm)* and then reveal the spots by *Method I*. By each method of visualisation the principal spot in the chromatogram obtained with solution (1) corresponds in colour and intensity to that in the chromatogram obtained with solution (2).

Related substances Carry out the method for *thin-layer chromatography*, Appendix III A, using *silica gel G* as the coating substance and *ethyl acetate* as the mobile phase. Apply separately to the plate 10 µl of each of the following solutions. For solution (1) shake a quantity of the powdered tablets containing 25 mg of Bendroflumethiazide with 25 ml of *acetone* for 10 minutes, filter, evaporate the filtrate to dryness and dissolve the residue in 2.5 ml of *acetone*. For solution (2) dilute 1 volume of solution (1) to 100 volumes with *acetone*. After removal of the plate, allow it to dry in air and reveal the spots by *Method I*. Any *secondary spot* in the chromatogram obtained with solution (1) is not more intense than the spot in the chromatogram obtained with solution (2).

Assay Weigh and powder 20 tablets. Mix a quantity of the powder containing 15 mg of Bendroflumethiazide with 50 ml of 0.1M *sodium hydroxide* with the aid of ultrasound for 10 minutes and dilute to 100 ml with 0.1M *sodium hydroxide*. Mix, filter, dilute 10 ml of the filtrate to 100 ml with *water* and measure the *absorbance* of the resulting solution at the maximum at 275 nm, Appendix II B. Calculate the content of $C_{15}H_{14}F_3N_3O_4S_2$ taking 410 as the value of A(1%, 1 cm) at the maximum at 275 nm.

Labelling The label states 'Bendroflumethiazide Tablets' and 'Bendrofluazide Tablets'.

Benorilate Oral Suspension

Definition Benorilate Oral Suspension is a suspension of Benorilate in a suitable flavoured vehicle.

The oral suspension complies with the requirements stated under Oral Liquids and with the following requirements.

Content of benorilate, $C_{17}H_{15}NO_5$ 95.0 to 105.0% of the prescribed or stated amount.

Identification To a quantity of the oral suspension containing 0.5 g of Benorilate add 10 ml of *water*, mix and extract with 50 ml of *dichloromethane*. Wash the extract with 10 ml of *water*, shake with *anhydrous sodium sulphate*, filter and evaporate the filtrate to dryness. The residue complies with the following tests.

A. The *infrared absorption spectrum*, Appendix II A, is concordant with the *reference spectrum* of benorilate.

B. To 10 mg add 10 ml of 6M *hydrochloric acid* and boil until completely dissolved. To 5 ml of the resulting solution add 0.1 ml of *strong 1-naphthol solution*, mix and add sufficient 1M *sodium hydroxide* to make the solution just alkaline. A blue colour is produced which can be extracted into *butan-1-ol*.

C. *Melting point*, about 179°, Appendix V A.

Acidity pH, 4.5 to 5.5, Appendix V L.

Related substances Carry out the method for *thin-layer chromatography*, Appendix III A, using a silica gel HF_{254} precoated plate (Analtech plates are suitable) and a mixture of 80 volumes of *dichloromethane*, 15 volumes of *ether* and 5 volumes of *glacial acetic acid* as the mobile phase. Apply separately to the plate 40 µl of solution (1) and 10 µl of each of solutions (2), (3), (4) and (5). For solution (1) add 20 ml of *methanol* to a quantity of the oral suspension containing 0.40 g of Benorilate, mix well, add 20 ml of *chloroform*, shake and filter. For solutions (2), (3) and (4) dilute 1 volume of solution (1) with *methanol* to 12.5 volumes, 25 volumes and 125 volumes respectively. Solution (5) contains 0.0080% w/v of *paracetamol* in *methanol*. After removal of the plate, allow it to dry in air and develop in a second mobile phase consisting of a mixture of 45 volumes of *ether*, 45 volumes of *2,2,4-trimethylpentane* and 10 volumes of *formic acid*. After removal of the plate, allow it to dry in air and examine under *ultraviolet light (254 nm)*. Any spot corresponding to paracetamol in the chromatogram obtained with solution (1) is not more intense than the spot in the chromatogram obtained with solution (5). Any *secondary spot* in the chromatogram obtained with solution (1) with an Rf value slightly higher than that of the principal spot is not more intense than the principal spot in the chromatogram obtained with solution (3). Any other *secondary spot* in the chromatogram obtained with solution (1) is not more intense than the spot in the chromatogram obtained with solution (2) and not more than one such spot is more intense than the spot in the chromatogram obtained with solution (4). Disregard any spot with an Rf value higher than 1.5 relative to benorilate in the chromatograms obtained with solutions (1), (2), (3) and (4).

Salicylic acid Carry out the method for *liquid chromatography*, Appendix III D, using the following solutions. For solution (1) dilute the oral suspension with *methanol (80%)* to produce a solution containing 0.40% w/v of Benorilate. Solution (2) contains 0.00040% w/v of *salicylic acid* in *methanol (80%)*. Solution (3) contains 0.0010% w/v of *salicylic acid* and 0.020% w/v of *sorbic acid* in *methanol (80%)*.

The chromatographic procedure may be carried out using (a) a stainless steel column (15 cm × 4.6 mm) packed with particles of silica 5 µm in diameter the surface of which has been modified with chemically bonded hexyl groups (Spherisorb hexyl is suitable), (b) as the mobile phase with a flow rate of 2 ml per minute a mixture of 5 volumes of a 9.0% w/v solution of *disodium hydrogen orthophosphate* adjusted to pH 6.5 with *orthophosphoric acid*, 30 volumes of *acetonitrile* and 65 volumes of *water*, the mixture adjusted to pH 2.2 with *orthophosphoric acid*, and (c) a detection wavelength of 305 nm.

The test is not valid unless the *resolution factor* between the peaks due to salicylic acid and sorbic acid in the chromatogram obtained with solution (3) is at least 2.

In the chromatogram obtained with solution (1) the area of any peak corresponding to salicylic acid is not greater than the area of the peak in the chromatogram obtained with solution (2) (0.1%).

Assay To a quantity of the oral suspension containing 0.25 g of Benorilate, add 10 ml of *water*, mix, extract with two 40-ml quantities of *dichloromethane* filtering each extract successively through a plug of absorbent cotton saturated with *dichloromethane* and wash the plug with 10 ml of *dichloromethane*. Combine the extracts and washings and dilute to 100 ml with *dichloromethane*. Dilute 5 ml to 50 ml with *absolute ethanol* and dilute 2 ml of the resulting solution to 50 ml with *absolute ethanol*. Measure the *absorbance* of the final solution at the maximum at 240 nm, Appendix II B. Calculate the content of $C_{17}H_{15}NO_5$ taking 740 as the value of A(1%, 1 cm) at the maximum at 240 nm. Determine the *weight per ml* of the oral suspension, Appendix V G, and calculate the percentage of $C_{17}H_{15}NO_5$, weight in volume.

When benorylate oral suspension is prescribed or demanded, Benorilate Oral Suspension shall be dispensed or supplied.

Benorilate Tablets

Definition Benorilate Tablets contain Benorilate.

With the exception of the requirements for shape, the tablets comply with the requirements stated under Tablets and with the following requirements.

Content of benorilate, $C_{17}H_{15}NO_5$ 95.0 to 105.0% of the prescribed or stated amount.

Identification Shake a quantity of the powdered tablets containing 1 g of Benorilate with 30 ml of a mixture of 9 volumes of *chloroform* and 1 volume of *methanol* for 10 minutes, filter and evaporate the filtrate to dryness. The residue complies with the following tests.

A. The *infrared absorption spectrum*, Appendix II A, is concordant with the *reference spectrum* of benorilate.

B. To 10 mg add 10 ml of 6M *hydrochloric acid* and boil until completely dissolved. To 5 ml of the resulting solution add 0.1 ml of *strong 1-naphthol solution*, mix and add sufficient 1M *sodium hydroxide* to make the solution just alkaline. A blue colour is produced which can be extracted into *butan-1-ol*.

C. *Melting point*, about 179°, Appendix V A.

4-Aminophenol Shake a quantity of the powdered tablets containing 2.5 g of Benorilate with 100 ml of *water* for 15 minutes and filter. If the filtrate is opalescent, warm on a water bath until it becomes clear and allow to cool. Carry out the test described under Benorilate beginning at the words 'To 20 ml of the filtrate ...'.

Salicylic acid Shake a quantity of the powdered tablets containing 0.5 g of Benorilate with 20 ml of *water* for 15 minutes and filter. If the filtrate is opalescent, warm on a water bath until it becomes clear and allow to cool. Carry out the test described under Benorilate beginning at the words 'Transfer 10 ml of the filtrate ...'.

Related substances Comply with the test for Related substances described under Benorilate, preparing solutions (1), (2) and (3) using the residue obtained in the tests for Identification.

Assay Weigh and powder 20 tablets. Shake a quantity of the powder containing 0.1 g of Benorilate with 100 ml of *absolute ethanol* for 30 minutes and filter. Dilute 5 ml of the filtrate to 250 ml with *absolute ethanol* and measure the *absorbance* of the resulting solution at the maximum at 240 nm, Appendix II B. Calculate the content of $C_{17}H_{15}NO_5$ taking 740 as the value of A(1%, 1 cm) at the maximum at 240 nm.

Storage Benorilate Tablets should be kept in a well-closed container.

When benorylate tablets are prescribed or demanded, Benorilate Tablets shall be dispensed or supplied.

Benzaldehyde Spirit

Definition

Benzaldehyde	10 ml
Ethanol (90 per cent)	800 ml
Purified Water	sufficient to produce 1000 ml

Extemporaneous preparation The following directions apply.

Dissolve the Benzaldehyde in the Ethanol (90 per cent) and add sufficient Purified Water to produce 1000 ml.

The spirit complies with the requirements stated under Spirits and with the following requirements.

Content of benzaldehyde, C_7H_6O 0.85 to 1.05% v/v.

Ethanol content 69 to 72% v/v, Appendix VIII F.

Weight per ml 0.870 to 0.885 g, Appendix V G.

Assay Carry out the method for the *determination of aldehydes*, Appendix X K, but using 10 ml and titrating with 0.1M *ethanolic potassium hydroxide VS*. Each ml of 0.1M *ethanolic potassium hydroxide VS* is equivalent to 10.61 mg of C_7H_6O. Calculate the percentage content of C_7H_6O, volume in volume, taking 1.046 mg as its weight per ml.

Storage Benzaldehyde Spirit should be kept in a well-filled container and protected from light.

Benzatropine Injection

Definition Benzatropine Injection is a sterile solution of Benzatropine Mesilate in Water for Injections.

The injection complies with the requirements stated under Parenteral Preparations and with the following requirements.

Content of benzatropine mesilate, $C_{21}H_{25}NO, CH_4O_3S$ 90.0 to 110.0% of the prescribed or stated amount.

Identification

A. Dilute a suitable volume with sufficient 2M *hydrochloric acid* to produce a solution containing 0.1% w/v of Benzatropine Mesilate. The *light absorption* of the resulting solution, Appendix II B, exhibits maxima at 253 nm and 258 nm and inflections at 249, 264 and 268 nm.

B. To a volume containing 10 mg of Benzatropine Mesilate add 5 ml of *picric acid solution R1*, mix and allow to stand for 1 hour. The *melting point* of the precipitate, after drying at 105°, is about 185°, Appendix V A.

Acidity or alkalinity pH, 5.0 to 8.0, Appendix V L.

Tropine Carry out the method for *thin-layer chromatography*, Appendix III A, using *silica gel G* as the coating substance and a mixture of 75 volumes of *ethanol (96%)* and 15 volumes of 13.5M *ammonia* as the mobile phase. Apply separately to the plate 20 µl of each of the following solutions. For solution (1) evaporate to dryness using a rotary evaporator a volume containing 10 mg of Benzatropine Mesilate, extract the residue with two 2-ml quantities of *acetone* and evaporate the combined extracts to dryness. Dissolve the residue in 0.5 ml of *acetone*. Solution (2) contains 0.010% w/v of *tropine* in *acetone*. After removal of the plate, allow it to dry in air and spray with *sodium iodobismuthate solution* and then with a 0.4% w/v solution of *sulphuric acid*. Any spot corresponding to tropine in the chromatogram obtained with solution (1) is not more intense than the spot in the chromatogram obtained with solution (2).

Assay To a volume containing 25 mg of Benzatropine Mesilate add 10 ml of 5M *sodium hydroxide*, 10 ml of *water* and an excess of *sodium chloride*. Extract with four 25-ml quantities of *ether*, combine the ether extracts and extract with four 10-ml quantities of 2M *hydrochloric acid*, remove any residual ether from the combined extracts in a current of air, dilute to 50 ml with 2M *hydrochloric acid* and measure the *absorbance* of the resulting solution at the maximum at 258 nm, Appendix II B. Calculate the content of $C_{21}H_{25}NO,CH_4O_3S$ from the *absorbance* obtained by repeating the operation using 25 mg of *benzatropine mesilate BPCRS* beginning at the words 'add 10 ml of 5M *sodium hydroxide* ...' and from the declared content of $C_{21}H_{25}NO,CH_4O_3S$ in *benzatropine mesilate BPCRS*.

When benztropine injection is prescribed or demanded, Benzatropine Injection shall be dispensed or supplied.

Benzatropine Tablets

Definition Benzatropine Tablets contain Benzatropine Mesilate.

The tablets comply with the requirements stated under Tablets and with the following requirements.

Content of benzatropine mesilate, $C_{21}H_{25}NO,CH_4O_3S$ 90.0 to 110.0% of the prescribed or stated amount.

Identification

A. Shake a suitable quantity of the powdered tablets with 2M *hydrochloric acid* and filter. Dilute the filtrate with sufficient 2M *hydrochloric acid* to produce a solution containing 0.1% w/v of Benzatropine Mesilate. The *light absorption* of the resulting solution, Appendix II B, in the range 230 to 350 nm exhibits two maxima, at 253 nm and 258 nm.

B. Extract a quantity of the powdered tablets containing 10 mg of Benzatropine Mesilate with 10 ml of *ethanol (96%)* and filter. Evaporate the filtrate to about 2 ml, pour into 5 ml of hot *picric acid solution R1* and allow to cool. The *melting point* of the precipitate, after drying at 105°, is about 185°, Appendix V A.

Tropine Carry out the method for *thin-layer chromatography*, Appendix III A, using *silica gel G* as the coating substance and a mixture of 75 volumes of *ethanol (96%)* and 15 volumes of 13.5M *ammonia* as the mobile phase. Apply separately to the plate 20 µl of each of the following solutions. For solution (1) shake a quantity of the powdered tablets containing 20 mg of Benzatropine Mesilate with 4 ml of *acetone* for 5 minutes, centrifuge, evaporate 2 ml of the supernatant liquid to dryness and dissolve the residue in 0.5 ml of *acetone*. Solution (2) contains 0.010% w/v of *tropine* in *acetone*. After removal of the plate, allow it to dry in air and spray with *sodium iodobismuthate solution* and then with a 0.4% w/v solution of *sulphuric acid*. Any spot corresponding to tropine in the chromatogram obtained with solution (1) is not more intense than the spot in the chromatogram obtained with solution (2).

Uniformity of content Tablets containing 2 mg or less of Benzatropine Mesilate comply with the requirement stated under Tablets using the following method of analysis. Carry out the method for *liquid chromatography*, Appendix III D, using the following solutions. Solution (1) contains 0.02% w/v of *benzatropine mesilate BPCRS* in the mobile phase. For solution (2) shake one tablet with 8 ml of the mobile phase for 5 minutes, add sufficient of the mobile phase to produce 10 ml, centrifuge for 5 minutes and use the supernatant liquid.

The chromatographic procedure may be carried out using (a) a stainless steel column (25 cm × 4.6 mm) packed with *stationary phase B* (10 µm) (Lichrosorb RP8 or Spherisorb C8 is suitable), (b) a mixture of 65 volumes of *acetonitrile* and 35 volumes of *octylamine phosphate buffer pH 3.0* as the mobile phase with a flow rate of 1.3 ml per minute and (c) a detection wavelength of 259 nm.

Calculate the content of $C_{21}H_{25}NO,CH_4O_3S$ in each tablet using the declared content of $C_{21}H_{25}NO,CH_4O_3S$ in *benzatropine mesilate BPCRS*.

Assay Weigh and powder 30 tablets. To a quantity of the powder containing 50 mg of Benzatropine Mesilate add 50 ml of *water* and shake for 15 minutes. Add 10 ml of a 50% w/v solution of *sodium hydroxide* and an excess of *sodium chloride* and extract with successive quantities of 50, 25, 25 and 25 ml of *ether*. Extract the combined ether layers with successive quantities of 25, 25, 25 and 15 ml of 2M *hydrochloric acid*, dilute the combined extracts to 100 ml with 2M *hydrochloric acid*, mix and filter if necessary. Measure the *absorbance* of the resulting solution at the maximum at 258 nm, Appendix II B. Calculate the content of $C_{21}H_{25}NO,CH_4O_3S$ from the *absorbance* obtained by repeating the operation using 50 mg of *benzatropine mesilate BPCRS* in place of the powdered tablets and from the declared content of $C_{21}H_{25}NO,CH_4O_3S$ in *benzatropine mesilate BPCRS*.

When benztropine tablets are prescribed or demanded, Benzatropine Tablets shall be dispensed or supplied.

Compound Benzoic Acid Ointment

Whitfield's Ointment

Definition Compound Benzoic Acid Ointment contains 6.0% w/w of Benzoic Acid and 3.0% w/w of Salicylic Acid in a suitable emulsifying basis.

Extemporaneous preparation The following formula and directions apply.

Benzoic Acid, in *fine powder*	60 g
Salicylic Acid, in *fine powder*	30 g
Emulsifying Ointment	910 g

Triturate the Benzoic Acid and the Salicylic Acid with a portion of the Emulsifying Ointment until smooth and gradually incorporate the remainder of the Emulsifying Ointment.

The ointment complies with the requirements stated under Topical Semi-solid Preparations and with the following requirements.

Content of benzoic acid, $C_7H_6O_2$ 5.7 to 6.3% w/w.

Content of salicylic acid, $C_7H_6O_3$ 2.7 to 3.3% w/w.

Identification Carry out the method for *thin-layer chromatography*, Appendix III A, using a silica gel F_{254} precoated plate (Merck silica gel 60 F_{254} plates are suitable) and a mixture of 80 volumes of *toluene* and 20 volumes of *glacial acetic acid* as the mobile phase. Apply separately to the plate 2 µl of each of the following solutions. For solution (1) warm 1 g of the ointment with 10 ml of *chloroform*, cool and filter. Solution (2) contains 0.6% w/v of *benzoic acid* and 0.3% w/v of *salicylic acid* in *chloroform*. After removal of the plate, allow the solvent to evaporate in a current of air and examine under *ultraviolet light (254 nm)*. The chromatogram obtained with solution (1) shows spots corresponding in colour and position to those in the chromatogram obtained with solution (2). Examine under *ultraviolet light (365 nm)*. The chromatogram obtained with solution (1) shows a blue fluorescent spot corresponding in colour and position to that in the chromatogram obtained with solution (2). Spray the plate with *iron(III) chloride solution R1*. The chromatogram obtained with solution (1) shows a purple spot corresponding in position to the blue fluorescent spot observed under ultraviolet light (365 nm) and corresponding in colour and position to the spot in the chromatogram obtained with solution (2).

Assay

For benzoic acid To 2 g add 150 ml of *water*, warm until melted and titrate with 0.1M *sodium hydroxide VS* using *phenolphthalein solution R1* as indicator. Reserve the solution for the Assay for salicylic acid. After the subtraction of 1 ml for each 13.81 mg of $C_7H_6O_3$ found in the Assay for salicylic acid, each ml of 0.1M *sodium hydroxide VS* is equivalent to 12.21 mg of $C_7H_6O_2$.

For salicylic acid Cool the titrated solution obtained in the Assay for benzoic acid, dilute to 250 ml with *water* and filter. To 5 ml of the filtrate add sufficient *iron(III) nitrate solution* to produce 50 ml. Filter, if necessary, to remove haze and measure the *absorbance* of the resulting solution at the maximum at 530 nm, Appendix II B, using *iron(III) nitrate solution* in the reference cell. Calculate the content of $C_7H_6O_3$ from the absorbance obtained by repeating the operation using 5 ml of a 0.024% w/v solution of *salicylic acid* and beginning at the words 'add sufficient *iron(III) nitrate solution* ...'.

Benzoic Acid Solution

Definition

Benzoic Acid	50 g
Propylene Glycol	750 ml
Purified Water, freshly boiled and cooled	sufficient to produce 1000 ml

Extemporaneous preparation The following directions apply.

Dissolve the Benzoic Acid in the Propylene Glycol and add sufficient Purified Water, in small quantities and with constant stirring, to produce 1000 ml.

Content of benzoic acid, $C_7H_6O_2$ 4.75 to 5.25% w/v.

Identification

A. To 5 ml add 30 ml of 1M *sulphuric acid* and extract the precipitated acid with three 25-ml quantities of *petroleum spirit (boiling range, 40° to 60°)*. Wash the combined extracts with three 25-ml quantities of *water*, filter through absorbent cotton and evaporate to dryness. The *infrared absorption spectrum* of the residue, Appendix II A, is concordant with the *reference spectrum* of benzoic acid.

B. *Melting point* of the residue obtained in test A, about 121°, Appendix V A.

Weight per ml 1.045 to 1.055 g, Appendix V G.

Assay To 10 ml add 20 ml of *ethanol (96%)* previously neutralised to *phenolphthalein solution R1* and titrate with 0.1M *sodium hydroxide VS* using *phenolphthalein solution R1* as indicator. Each ml of 0.1M *sodium hydroxide VS* is equivalent to 12.21 mg of $C_7H_6O_2$.

Labelling The label states (1) the date after which the solution is not intended to be used; (2) the conditions under which it should be stored.

Benzoin Inhalation

Definition

Benzoin Inhalation is an *inhalation vapour, solution*.

Sumatra Benzoin, crushed	100 g
Prepared storax, of commerce	50 g
Ethanol (96 per cent)	sufficient to produce 1000 ml

In making Benzoin Inhalation, Ethanol (96 per cent) may be replaced by Industrial Methylated Spirit[1].

Extemporaneous preparation The following directions apply.

Macerate the crushed Sumatra Benzoin and the prepared storax with 750 ml of Ethanol (96 per cent) for 24 hours. Filter and pass sufficient Ethanol (96 per cent) through the filter to produce 1000 ml.

The inhalation complies with the requirements stated under Preparations for Inhalation and with the following requirements.

Content of total balsamic acids Not less than 3.0% w/v, calculated as cinnamic acid, $C_9H_8O_2$.

Total solids 9.0 to 12.0% w/v when determined by drying at 105° for 4 hours, Appendix XI A. Use 2 ml.

Assay Carry out the Assay described under Sumatra Benzoin using 10 ml of the inhalation. Each ml of 0.1M *sodium hydroxide VS* is equivalent to 14.82 mg of total balsamic acids, calculated as cinnamic acid, $C_9H_8O_2$.

Labelling The label indicates the pharmaceutical form as 'inhalation vapour'.

[1]The statutory regulations governing the use of Industrial Methylated Spirit must be observed.

Compound Benzoin Tincture

Friars' Balsam

Definition

Barbados Aloes or Cape Aloes	20 g
Prepared storax, of commerce	100 g
Sumatra Benzoin, crushed	100 g
Ethanol (90 per cent)	sufficient to produce 1000 ml

Extemporaneous preparation The following directions apply.

Macerate the Barbados Aloes or Cape Aloes, the prepared storax and the Sumatra Benzoin with 800 ml of Ethanol (90 per cent) in a closed vessel for not less than 2 days, shaking occasionally, filter and pass sufficient Ethanol (90 per cent) through the filter to produce 1000 ml.

The tincture complies with the requirements stated under Tinctures and with the following requirements.

Content of total balsamic acids Not less than 4.5% w/v, calculated as cinnamic acid, $C_9H_8O_2$.

Ethanol content 70 to 76% v/v, Appendix VIII F, Method III.

Dry residue 15 to 19% w/v.

Relative density 0.880 to 0.910, Appendix V G.

Assay Carry out the Assay described under Sumatra Benzoin using 10 ml of the tincture. Each ml of 0.1M *sodium hydroxide VS* is equivalent to 14.82 mg of total balsamic acids, calculated as cinnamic acid, $C_9H_8O_2$.

Benzoyl Peroxide Cream

Definition Benzoyl Peroxide Cream contains Hydrous Benzoyl Peroxide in a suitable basis.

The cream complies with the requirements stated under Topical Semi-solid Preparations and with the following requirements.

Content of anhydrous benzoyl peroxide, $C_{14}H_{10}O_4$ 90.0 to 110.0% of the prescribed or stated amount.

Identification Carry out the method for *thin-layer chromatography*, Appendix III A, using *silica gel GF_{254}* as the coating substance and a mixture of 50 volumes of *toluene*, 2 volumes of *dichloromethane* and 1 volume of *glacial acetic acid* as the mobile phase. Apply separately to the plate 5 µl of each of the following solutions. For solution (1) shake a quantity of the preparation being examined containing the equivalent of 50 mg of anhydrous benzoyl peroxide with 10 ml of *chloroform* and filter. Solution (2) contains 0.5% w/v of *benzoyl peroxide* in *chloroform*. After removal of the plate, allow it to dry in air and examine under *ultraviolet light (254 nm)*. The principal spot in the chromatogram obtained with solution (1) corresponds to that in the chromatogram obtained with solution (2).

Related substances Carry out the method for *liquid chromatography*, Appendix III D, using the following solutions. For solution (1) dilute 2 volumes of solution (2) to 100 volumes with the mobile phase. For solution (2) disperse a quantity of the preparation being examined containing the equivalent of 0.10 g of anhydrous benzoyl peroxide in 25 ml of *acetonitrile*, add sufficient *water* to produce 50 ml, mix and filter. Solution (3) contains 0.020% w/v of *benzoic acid* in the mobile phase. Solution (4) contains 0.0020% w/v of *ethyl benzoate* in the mobile phase. Solution (5) contains 0.0020% w/v of *benzaldehyde* in the mobile phase.

The chromatographic procedure may be carried out using (a) a stainless steel column (20 cm × 4.6 mm) packed with *stationary phase C* (10 µm) (Spherisorb ODS 1 is suitable), (b) a mixture of 500 volumes of *acetonitrile*, 500 volumes of *water* and 1 volume of *glacial acetic acid* as the mobile phase with a flow rate of 1 ml per minute and (c) a detection wavelength of 235 nm.

In the chromatogram obtained with solution (2) the areas of any peaks corresponding to benzoic acid, ethyl benzoate and benzaldehyde are not greater than the areas of the principal peaks in the chromatograms obtained with solutions (3), (4) and (5) respectively. The area of any other *secondary peak* is not greater than half of the area of the principal peak in the chromatogram obtained with solution (1).

Assay Mix a quantity of the preparation being examined containing the equivalent of 0.25 g of anhydrous benzoyl peroxide with 50 ml of *acetone* and add sufficient *acetone* to produce 100 ml. To 10 ml add 25 ml of a 20% w/v solution of *potassium iodide*, mix, stopper the flask and allow to stand for 15 minutes protected from light. Add 25 ml of *acetone* and titrate with 0.01M *sodium thiosulphate VS* using *starch mucilage*, added towards the end of the titration, as indicator. Repeat the operation without the substance being examined. The difference between the titrations represents the amount of sodium thiosulphate required. Each ml of 0.01M *sodium thiosulphate VS* is equivalent to 1.211 mg of $C_{14}H_{10}O_4$.

Labelling The quantity of active ingredient is stated in terms of the equivalent amount of anhydrous benzoyl peroxide.

Benzoyl Peroxide Gel

Definition Benzoyl Peroxide Gel is a solution of Hydrous Benzoyl Peroxide in a suitable water-soluble basis.

The gel complies with the requirements stated under Topical Semi-solid Preparations and with the following requirements.

Content of anhydrous benzoyl peroxide, $C_{14}H_{10}O_4$ 90.0 to 110.0% of the prescribed or stated amount.

Identification; Related substances Complies with the tests described under Benzoyl Peroxide Cream.

Assay Carry out the Assay described under Benzoyl Peroxide Cream.

Labelling The quantity of active ingredient is stated in terms of the equivalent amount of anhydrous benzoyl peroxide.

Benzoyl Peroxide Lotion

Definition Benzoyl Peroxide Lotion is a *cutaneous suspension.* It contains Hydrous Benzoyl Peroxide in a suitable non-greasy vehicle.

The lotion complies with the requirements stated under Liquids for Cutaneous Application and with the following requirements.

Content of anhydrous benzoyl peroxide, $C_{14}H_{10}O_4$ 90.0 to 110.0% of the prescribed or stated amount.

Identification; Related substances Complies with the tests described under Benzoyl Peroxide Cream.

Assay Carry out the Assay described under Benzoyl Peroxide Cream.

Labelling The quantity of active ingredient is stated in terms of the equivalent amount of anhydrous benzoyl peroxide.

The label indicates the pharmaceutical form as 'cutaneous suspension'.

Benzydamine Cream

Definition Benzydamine Cream contains Benzydamine Hydrochloride in a suitable basis.

The cream complies with the requirements stated under Topical Semi-solid Preparations and with the following requirements.

Content of benzydamine hydrochloride, $C_{19}H_{23}N_3O,HCl$ 92.5 to 107.5% of the prescribed or stated amount.

Identification

A. Heat a quantity of the cream containing 25 mg of Benzydamine Hydrochloride with 50 ml of *absolute ethanol* until the cream is completely dissolved and place in an ice-bath until a white precipitate forms. Allow to warm to 20°, dilute to 100 ml with *absolute ethanol* and filter. Dilute 10 ml of the filtrate to 100 ml with *absolute ethanol.* The *light absorption* of the resulting solution, Appendix II B, in the range 230 to 350 nm exhibits a maximum at 308 nm.

B. In the test for 1-Benzyl-1*H*-indazol-3-ol, the principal spot in the chromatogram obtained with solution (1) corresponds to that in the chromatogram obtained with solution (2).

1-Benzyl-1*H*-indazol-3-ol Carry out the method for *thin-layer chromatography,* Appendix III A, using *silica gel* GF_{254} as the coating substance and a mixture of 30 volumes of *triethylamine* and 80 volumes of *toluene* as the mobile phase. Apply separately to the plate 40 µl of each of the following solutions. For solution (1) extract a quantity of the cream containing 60 mg of Benzydamine Hydrochloride with 25 ml of hot *methanol,* cool the solution in ice and filter; repeat the extraction twice, filtering each extract and evaporate the combined extracts to dryness using a rotary evaporator; dissolve the residue in 5 ml of *methanol.* Solution (2) contains 1.2% w/v of *benzydamine hydrochloride BPCRS* in *methanol.* Solution (3) contains 0.0024% w/v of *1-benzyl-1*H*-indazol-3-ol BPCRS* in *methanol.* After removal of the plate, allow it to dry in air and examine under *ultraviolet light (254 nm* and *365 nm).* By each method of visualisation, any *secondary spot* in the chromatogram obtained with solution (1) is not more intense than the spot in the chromatogram obtained with solution (3) (0.2%).

Assay To a quantity of the cream containing 25 mg of Benzydamine Hydrochloride add 50 ml of *ethanol (96%),* heat until the cream is completely dissolved and cool in an ice-bath until a white precipitate forms. Allow to warm to 20°, dilute to 100 ml with *ethanol (96%)* and filter. Dilute 10 ml of the filtrate to 100 ml with *ethanol (96%)* and measure the *absorbance* of the resulting solution at the maximum at about 308 nm, Appendix II B, using *ethanol (96%)* in the reference cell. Calculate the content of $C_{19}H_{23}N_3O,HCl$ from the *absorbance* obtained with a solution containing 0.0025% w/v of *benzydamine hydrochloride BPCRS* in *ethanol (96%)* and using the declared content of $C_{19}H_{23}N_3O,HCl$ in *benzydamine hydrochloride BPCRS.*

Benzydamine Mouthwash

Definition Benzydamine Mouthwash is a solution of Benzydamine Hydrochloride in a suitable flavoured and coloured vehicle.

The mouthwash complies with the requirements stated under Mouthwashes and with the following requirements.

Content of benzydamine hydrochloride, $C_{19}H_{23}N_3O,HCl$ 92.5 to 107.5% of the prescribed or stated amount.

Identification

A. Carry out the method for *thin-layer chromatography,* Appendix III A, using a silica gel F_{254} precoated plate (Merck silica gel 60 F_{254} plates are suitable) and a mixture of 30 volumes of *triethylamine* and 80 volumes of *toluene* as the mobile phase. Apply separately to the plate 50 µl of each of the following solutions. For solution (1) dilute the mouthwash, if necessary, with *absolute ethanol* to contain 0.15% w/v of Benzydamine Hydrochloride. Solution (2) contains 0.15% w/v of *benzydamine hydrochloride BPCRS* in *absolute ethanol.* After removal of the plate, allow it to dry in air and examine under *ultraviolet light (254 nm).* The principal spot in the chromatogram obtained with solution (1) corresponds to that in the chromatogram obtained with solution (2).

B. In the Assay, the chromatogram obtained with solution (2) shows a peak with the same retention time as the principal peak in the chromatogram obtained with solution (1).

pH 5.0 to 7.0, Appendix V L.

1-Benzyl-1*H*-indazol-3-ol Carry out the method for *thin-layer chromatography,* Appendix III A, using *silica gel* GF_{254} as the coating substance and a mixture of 10 volumes of *glacial acetic acid,* 20 volumes of *chloroform* and 70 volumes of *cyclohexane* as the mobile phase. Apply separately to the plate 20 µl of each of the following solutions. For solution (1) extract a quantity of the mouthwash containing 15 mg of Benzydamine Hydrochloride with seven 90-ml quantities of *chloroform.* Filter each extract through phase separating paper, evaporate the combined extracts to dryness and dissolve the residue in 10 ml of *methanol.* Solution (2) contains 0.0015% w/v of *1-benzyl-1*H*-indazol-3-ol BPCRS* in *methanol.* After removal of the plate, allow it to dry in air and examine under *ultraviolet light (365 nm).* Any *secondary spot* in the chromatogram obtained with solution (1) is not more intense than the spot in the chromatogram obtained with solution (2) (1%).

Assay Carry out the method for *gas chromatography*, Appendix III B, using the following solutions. Prepare a 0.075% w/v solution of *1-benzyl-3-(3-diethylamino-propoxy)-1*H*-indazole BPCRS* (internal standard) in *water* (solution A). For solution (1) add 10 ml of solution A, 5 ml of *water*, 5 ml of 1M *sodium hydroxide* and 20 ml of *chloroform* to 5 ml of a solution containing 0.15% w/v of *benzydamine hydrochloride BPCRS* in *water*, shake for 5 minutes, centrifuge and use the chloroform layer. Prepare solution (2) in the same manner as solution (1) but using a volume of the mouthwash containing 7.5 mg of Benzydamine Hydrochloride, diluted, if necessary, to 5 ml with *water* in place of the 5 ml of solution containing 0.15% w/v of *benzydamine hydrochloride BPCRS* in *water*.

The chromatographic procedure may be carried out using a glass column (2 m × 2 mm) packed with *acid-washed, diatomaceous support* (80 to 100 mesh) coated with 3% w/w of phenyl methyl silicone fluid (50% phenyl) (OV-17 is suitable) and maintained at 260° with a flame ionisation detector.

Calculate the content of $C_{19}H_{23}N_3O,HCl$ using the declared content of $C_{19}H_{23}N_3O,HCl$ in *benzydamine hydrochloride BPCRS*.

Labelling The label states, where appropriate, that the preparation is also suitable for use as a gargle.

Benzydamine Oromucosal Spray

Definition Benzydamine Oromucosal Spray is a solution of Benzydamine Hydrochloride in a suitable flavoured vehicle in a suitable metered-dose container.

The oromucosal spray complies with the following requirements and, where appropriate, with the requirements stated under Pressurised Pharmaceutical Preparations.

Content of benzydamine hydrochloride, $C_{19}H_{23}N_3O,HCl$ 92.5 to 107.5% of the prescribed or stated amount.

Identification A. Carry out the method for *thin-layer chromatography*, Appendix III A, using a silica gel F_{254} precoated plate (Merck silica gel 60 F_{254} plates are suitable) and a mixture of 30 volumes of *triethylamine* and 80 volumes of *toluene* as the mobile phase. Apply separately to the plate 50 µl of each of the following solutions. For solution (1) dilute the oromucosal spray, if necessary, with *absolute ethanol* to contain 0.15% w/v of Benzydamine Hydrochloride. Solution (2) contains 0.15% w/v of *benzydamine hydrochloride BPCRS* in *absolute ethanol*. After removal of the plate, allow it to dry in air and examine under *ultraviolet light (254 nm)*. The principal spot in the chromatogram obtained with solution (1) corresponds to that in the chromatogram obtained with solution (2).

B. In the Assay, the chromatogram obtained with solution (2) shows a peak with the same retention time as the principal peak in the chromatogram obtained with solution (1).

pH 5.0 to 7.0, Appendix V L.

Uniformity of weight Weigh one unit. Fire one shot and reweigh the unit. Repeat four times, then repeat the entire process with 3 more units (20 shots). Determine the average weight delivered per shot. Not more than two of the individual weights deviate from the average weight by more than 10% and none deviates by more than 20%.

1-Benzyl-1*H*-indazol-3-ol Carry out the method for *thin-layer chromatography*, Appendix III A, using *silica gel GF_{254}* as the coating substance and a mixture of 10 volumes of *glacial acetic acid*, 20 volumes of *chloroform* and 70 volumes of *cyclohexane* as the mobile phase. Apply separately to the plate 20 µl of each of the following solutions. For solution (1) extract a quantity of the oromucosal spray containing 15 mg of Benzydamine Hydrochloride with seven 90-ml quantities of *chloroform*. Filter each extract through phase separating paper, evaporate the combined extracts to dryness and dissolve the residue in 10 ml of *methanol*. Solution (2) contains 0.0015% w/v of *1-benzyl-1*H*-indazol-3-ol BPCRS* in *methanol*. After removal of the plate, allow it to dry in air and examine under *ultraviolet light (365 nm)*. Any *secondary spot* in the chromatogram obtained with solution (1) is not more intense than the spot in the chromatogram obtained with solution (2) (1%).

Assay Carry out the method for *gas chromatography*, Appendix III B, using the following solutions. Prepare a 0.075% w/v solution of *1-benzyl-3-(3-diethylamino-propoxy)-1*H*-indazole BPCRS* (internal standard) in *water* (solution A). For solution (1) add 10 ml of solution A, 5 ml of *water*, 5 ml of 1M *sodium hydroxide* and 20 ml of *chloroform* to 5 ml of a solution containing 0.15% w/v of *benzydamine hydrochloride BPCRS* in *water*, shake for 5 minutes, centrifuge and use the chloroform layer. Prepare solution (2) in the same manner as solution (1) but using a quantity of the oromucosal spray containing 7.5 mg of Benzydamine Hydrochloride, diluted, if necessary, to 5 ml with *water* in place of the 5 ml of solution containing 0.15% w/v of *benzydamine hydrochloride BPCRS* in *water*.

The chromatographic procedure may be carried out using a glass column (2 m × 2 mm) packed with *acid-washed, diatomaceous support* (80 to 100 mesh) coated with 3% w/w of phenyl methyl silicone fluid (50% phenyl) (OV-17 is suitable) and maintained at 260°, with a flame ionisation detector.

Calculate the content of $C_{19}H_{23}N_3O,HCl$ from the chromatograms obtained using the declared content of $C_{19}H_{23}N_3O,HCl$ in *benzydamine hydrochloride BPCRS*.

Labelling The label states (1) the date after which the oromucosal spray is not intended to be used; (2) the conditions under which it should be stored.

Benzyl Benzoate Application

Definition Benzyl Benzoate Application is a *cutaneous emulsion*. It contains 25% w/v of Benzyl Benzoate in a suitable oil-in-water emulsified basis.

Extemporaneous preparation The following formula and directions apply.

Benzyl Benzoate	250 g
Emulsifying Wax	20 g
Purified Water, freshly boiled and cooled	sufficient to produce 1000 ml

Melt the Emulsifying Wax, add the Benzyl Benzoate and mix. Pour the mixture into sufficient warm Purified Water to produce 1000 ml and stir thoroughly until cold.

The application complies with the requirements stated under Liquids for Cutaneous Application and with the following requirements.

Content of benzyl benzoate, $C_{14}H_{12}O_2$ 23.1 to 26.9% w/v.

Assay Carry out the method for *liquid chromatography*, Appendix III D, using the following solutions. Solution (1) contains 0.0050% w/v of *benzyl benzoate BPCRS* in the mobile phase. For solution (2) dissolve 1 g of the application in sufficient of the mobile phase to produce 100 ml and dilute 1 volume of the resulting solution to 50 volumes with the mobile phase.

The chromatographic procedure may be carried out using (a) a stainless steel column (20 cm × 4.6 mm) packed with *stationary phase C* (10 µm) (Nucleosil C18 is suitable), (b) a mixture of 70 volumes of *acetonitrile* and 30 volumes of *water* as the mobile phase with a flow rate of 1.5 ml per minute and (c) a detection wavelength of 230 nm.

Determine the *weight per ml* of the application, Appendix V G, and calculate the content of $C_{14}H_{12}O_2$, weight in volume, using the declared content of $C_{14}H_{12}O_2$ in *benzyl benzoate BPCRS*.

Labelling The label states that the contents of the container should be shaken before use.

The label indicates the pharmaceutical form as 'cutaneous emulsion'.

Benzylpenicillin Injection

Definition Benzylpenicillin Injection is a sterile solution of Benzylpenicillin Potassium or Benzylpenicillin Sodium in Water for Injections. It is prepared by dissolving Benzylpenicillin for Injection in the requisite amount of Water for Injections.

The injection complies with the requirements stated under Parenteral Preparations.

Storage Benzylpenicillin Injection should be used immediately after preparation but, in any case, within the period recommended by the manufacturer when prepared and stored strictly in accordance with the manufacturer's instructions.

BENZYLPENICILLIN FOR INJECTION

Definition Benzylpenicillin for Injection is a sterile material consisting of Benzylpenicillin Potassium or Benzylpenicillin Sodium with or without excipients. It is supplied in a sterile container.

The contents of the sealed container comply with the requirements for Powders for Injections stated under Parenteral Preparations and with the following requirements.

Content of penicillins, calculated as $C_{16}H_{18}N_2O_4S$ 95.0 to 105.0% of the content of benzylpenicillin stated on the label.

Identification

A. The *infrared absorption spectrum*, Appendix II A, is concordant with the spectrum of *benzylpenicillin potassium EPCRS* or *benzylpenicillin sodium EPCRS* as appropriate.

B. Carry out the method for *thin-layer chromatography*, Appendix III A, using *silanised silica gel H* as the coating substance and a mixture of 30 volumes of *acetone* and 70 volumes of a 15.4% w/v solution of *ammonium acetate* adjusted to pH 5.0 with *glacial acetic acid* as the mobile phase. Apply separately to the plate 1 µl of each of three solutions in *water* containing (1) sufficient of the contents of the sealed container to give a solution containing 0.5% w/v of Benzylpenicillin Sodium or Benzylpenicillin Potassium, (2) 0.5% w/v of *benzylpenicillin sodium EPCRS* or 0.5% w/v of *benzylpenicillin potassium EPCRS*, as appropriate, and (3) 0.5% w/v of *benzylpenicillin sodium EPCRS* or 0.5% w/v of *benzylpenicillin potassium EPCRS*, as appropriate, and 0.5% w/v of *phenoxymethylpenicillin potassium EPCRS*. After removal of the plate, allow it to dry in air, expose to iodine vapour until spots appear and examine in daylight. The principal spot in the chromatogram obtained with solution (1) is similar in position, colour and size to that in the chromatogram obtained with solution (2). The test is not valid unless the chromatogram obtained with solution (3) shows two clearly separated spots.

C. Yield reaction A characteristic of *potassium salts* or reaction A characteristic of *sodium salts*, Appendix VI, as appropriate.

Acidity or alkalinity pH of a 10% w/v solution, 5.5 to 7.5, Appendix V L.

Loss on drying When dried to constant weight at 105°, lose not more than 1.0% of their weight. Use 1 g.

Pyrogens Comply with the *test for pyrogens*, Appendix XIV D. Use per kg of the rabbit's weight 1 ml of a solution in *water for injections* containing the equivalent of 1.5 mg of benzylpenicillin per ml.

Assay Determine the weight of the contents of 10 containers as described in the test for Uniformity of weight under Parenteral Preparations, Powders for Injections.

Dissolve a quantity of the mixed contents of the 10 containers containing the equivalent of 0.1 g of benzylpenicillin in sufficient *water* to produce 500 ml and dilute 25 ml to 100 ml with *water*. Place two 2-ml quantities of the resulting solution in separate stoppered tubes. To one tube add 10 ml of *imidazole—mercury reagent*, mix, stopper the tube and place in a water bath at 60° for exactly 25 minutes, swirling occasionally. Remove from the water bath and cool rapidly to 20° (solution A). To the second tube add 10 ml of *water* and mix (solution B). Without delay measure the *absorbances* of solutions A and B at the maximum at 325 nm, Appendix II B, using in the reference cell a mixture of 2 ml of *water* and 10 ml of *imidazole—mercury reagent* for solution A and *water* for solution B. Calculate the content of penicillins as $C_{16}H_{18}N_2O_4S$ in a container of average content weight from the difference between the absorbances of solutions A and B, from the difference obtained by repeating the procedure using 0.15 g of *benzylpenicillin sodium EPCRS* in place of the contents of the sealed containers and from the declared content of $C_{16}H_{18}N_2O_4S$ in *benzylpenicillin sodium EPCRS*.

Storage The sealed container should be stored at a temperature not exceeding 30°.

Labelling The label of the sealed container states (1) whether the contents are Benzylpenicillin Potassium or Benzylpenicillin Sodium; (2) the quantity of Benzylpenicillin Potassium or Benzylpenicillin Sodium contained in it in terms of the equivalent amount of benzylpenicillin..

Betamethasone Valerate Scalp Application

Definition Betamethasone Valerate Scalp Application is a *cutaneous solution*. It contains Betamethasone Valerate in a suitable liquid basis.

The application complies with the requirements stated under Liquids for Cutaneous Application and with the following requirements.

Content of betamethasone, $C_{22}H_{29}FO_5$ 90.0 to 115.0% of the prescribed or stated amount.

Identification

A. Complies with test A for Identification described under Betamethasone Valerate Lotion, preparing solution (1) by diluting a suitable volume of the application with *absolute ethanol* to give a solution containing the equivalent of 0.04% w/v of betamethasone.

B. In the Assay, the chromatogram obtained with solution (2) shows a peak with the same retention time as the peak due to betamethasone valerate in the chromatogram obtained with solution (1).

Assay Carry out the Assay described under Betamethasone Valerate Lotion, preparing solutions (2) and (3) in the following manner. For solution (2) dilute a quantity of the application containing the equivalent of 3 mg of betamethasone to 25 ml with *ethanol (65%)*. For solution (3) add 5 ml of a 0.11% w/v solution of the internal standard to a quantity of the application containing the equivalent of 3 mg of betamethasone and dilute to 25 ml with *ethanol (65%)*.

Storage Betamethasone Valerate Scalp Application should be protected from light.

Labelling The quantity of active ingredient is stated in terms of the equivalent amount of betamethasone.

The label indicates the pharmaceutical form as 'cutaneous solution'.

Betamethasone Valerate Cream

Definition Betamethasone Valerate Cream contains Betamethasone Valerate in a suitable basis.

The cream complies with the requirements stated under Topical Semi-solid Preparations and with the following requirements.

Content of betamethasone, $C_{22}H_{29}FO_5$ 90.0 to 110.0% of the prescribed or stated amount.

Identification

A. Complies with test A for Identification described under Betamethasone Valerate Lotion using the following solutions. For solution (1) disperse a quantity of the cream containing the equivalent of 0.5 mg of betamethasone in 20 ml of *methanol (80%)* by heating on a water bath until the methanol begins to boil. Shake vigorously, cool in ice for 30 minutes and centrifuge. Mix 10 ml of the supernatant liquid with 3 ml of *water* and 5 ml of *chloroform*, shake vigorously, allow the layers to separate and evaporate the chloroform layer to dryness in a current of nitrogen with gentle heating. Dissolve the residue in 1 ml of *chloroform*. Solution (2) contains 0.03% w/v of *betamethasone valerate BPCRS* in *chloroform*.

B. In the Assay, the chromatogram obtained with solution (2) shows a peak with the same retention time as the peak due to betamethasone valerate in the chromatogram obtained with solution (1).

Assay Carry out the method for *liquid chromatography*, Appendix III D, using the following solutions. For solution (1) mix 10 ml of a solution containing 0.024% w/v of *betamethasone valerate BPCRS* and 0.0012% w/v of *betamethasone 21-valerate BPCRS* in *ethanol (80%)* with 5 ml of a 0.072% w/v solution of *beclomethasone dipropionate BPCRS* (internal standard) in *ethanol (80%)* and dilute to 50 ml with the same solvent. For solution (2) shake a quantity of the cream containing the equivalent of 2 mg of betamethasone with 100 ml of hot *hexane* for 2 minutes, cool, extract the mixture with 20 ml of *ethanol (96%)* and filter the lower, ethanolic layer through absorbent cotton previously washed with *ethanol (75%)*. Repeat the extraction of the hexane mixture with two 10-ml quantities of *ethanol (75%)*, filtering each extract in turn through the absorbent cotton and dilute the combined filtrates to 50 ml with *ethanol (75%)*. Prepare solution (3) in the same manner as solution (2) but add 5 ml of a 0.072% w/v solution of the internal standard in *ethanol (80%)* before diluting to 50 ml.

The chromatographic procedure may be carried out using (a) a stainless steel column (10 cm × 5 mm) packed with *stationary phase C* (5 μm) (Spherisorb ODS 1 is suitable) and maintained at 60°, (b) as the mobile phase with a flow rate of 2 ml per minute a mixture of *absolute ethanol* and *water* adjusted so that the *resolution factor* between the peaks due to betamethasone valerate (retention time about 5 minutes) and betamethasone 21-valerate (retention time about 7 minutes) is more than 1.0 (a mixture of 42 volumes of *absolute ethanol* and 58 volumes of *water* is usually suitable) and (c) a detection wavelength of 238 nm.

Calculate the content of $C_{22}H_{29}FO_5$ in the cream using the declared content of $C_{22}H_{29}FO_5$ in *betamethasone valerate BPCRS* and using peak areas.

Storage Betamethasone Valerate Cream should be protected from light.

Labelling The quantity of active ingredient is stated in terms of the equivalent amount of betamethasone.

Betamethasone and Clioquinol Cream

Definition Betamethasone and Clioquinol Cream contains Betamethasone Valerate and Clioquinol, the latter in *very fine powder*, in a suitable basis.

The cream complies with the requirements stated under Topical Semi-solid Preparations and with the following requirements.

Content of betamethasone, $C_{22}H_{29}FO_5$ 90.0 to 110.0% of the prescribed or stated amount.

Content of clioquinol, C_9H_5ClINO 90.0 to 110.0% of the prescribed or stated amount.

Identification

A. Carry out the method for *thin-layer chromatography*, Appendix III A, using *silica gel G* as the coating substance and a mixture of 5 volumes of *absolute ethanol*, 10 volumes of *acetone* and 100 volumes of *chloroform* as the mobile phase. Apply separately to the plate 10 μl of each of the following solutions. For solution (1) disperse a quantity of the preparation being examined containing the equivalent of 0.5 mg of betamethasone in 20 ml of *methanol (80%)* by heating on a water bath until the methanol begins to boil. Shake vigorously, cool in ice and centrifuge. Transfer 10 ml of the supernatant liquid to a separating funnel, add 3 ml of *water* and 5 ml of *chloroform*, shake vigorously, allow the layers to separate and evaporate the chloroform layer to dryness in a current of *nitrogen* with gentle heating. Dissolve the residue in 1 ml of *chloroform*. Solution (2) contains 0.03% w/v of *betamethasone valerate BPCRS* in *chloroform*. After removal of the plate, allow it to dry in air, heat at 105° for 5 minutes and spray while hot with *alkaline tetrazolium blue solution*. The principal spot in the chromatogram obtained with solution (1) corresponds to that in the chromatogram obtained with solution (2).

B. In the Assay for betamethasone the chromatogram obtained with solution (2) shows a peak with the same retention time as the peak due to betamethasone valerate in the chromatogram obtained with solution (1).

C. In the Assay for clioquinol the chromatogram obtained with solution (2) shows a peak with the same retention time as the peak due to clioquinol in the chromatogram obtained with solution (1).

Assay

For betamethasone Carry out the method for *liquid chromatography*, Appendix III D, using the following solutions. For solution (1) mix 10 ml of a solution containing 0.024% w/v of *betamethasone valerate BPCRS* and 0.0012% w/v of *betamethasone 21-valerate BPCRS* in *ethanol (80%)* with 5 ml of a 0.072% w/v solution of *beclomethasone dipropionate BPCRS* (internal standard) in *ethanol (80%)* and dilute to 50 ml with the same solvent. For solution (2) shake a quantity of the cream containing the equivalent of 2 mg of betamethasone with 100 ml of hot *hexane* for 2 minutes, cool, extract the mixture with 20 ml of *ethanol (96%)* and filter the lower, ethanolic layer through absorbent cotton previously washed with *ethanol (75%)*. Repeat the extraction of the hexane mixture with two 10-ml quantities of *ethanol (75%)*, filtering each extract in turn through the absorbent cotton and dilute the combined filtrates to 50 ml with *ethanol (75%)*. Prepare solution (3) in the same manner as solution (2) but add 5 ml of a 0.072% w/v solution of the internal standard in *ethanol (80%)* before diluting to 50 ml.

The chromatographic procedure may be carried out using (a) a stainless steel column (10 cm × 5 mm) packed with *stationary phase C* (5 µm) (Spherisorb ODS 1 is suitable) and maintained at 60°, (b) as the mobile phase with a flow rate of 2 ml per minute a mixture of *absolute ethanol* and *water* adjusted so that the *resolution factor* between the peaks due to betamethasone valerate (retention time about 5 minutes) and betamethasone 21-valerate (retention time about 7 minutes) is more than 1.0 (a mixture of 42 volumes of *absolute ethanol* and 58 volumes of *water* is usually suitable) and (c) a detection wavelength of 238 nm.

Calculate the content of $C_{22}H_{29}FO_5$ in the cream using the declared content of $C_{22}H_{29}FO_5$ in *betamethasone valerate BPCRS* and using peak areas.

For clioquinol Carry out the method for *liquid chromatography*, Appendix III D, using the following solutions. For solution (1) mix 5 ml of a solution containing 0.024% w/v of *clioquinol BPCRS* in an 80% v/v solution of *2-methoxyethanol* and 1 ml of a solution containing 1% w/v of *nickel(II) chloride hexahydrate* in *water* and dilute to 50 ml with the mobile phase. For solution (2) add 80 ml of a hot 80% v/v solution of *2-methoxyethanol* to a quantity of the cream containing 30 mg of Clioquinol and heat on a water bath for 5 minutes, swirling vigorously. Cool to room temperature, dilute to 100 ml with the same solvent, mix and filter. To 5 ml of the filtrate add 1 ml of a solution containing 1% w/v of *nickel(II) chloride hexahydrate* and dilute to 50 ml with the mobile phase.

The chromatographic procedure may be carried out using (a) a column (25 cm × 4.6 mm) packed with particles of silica the surface of which has been modified with chemically bonded phenyl groups (5 µm) (Spherisorb Phenyl is suitable), (b) a solution containing 0.024% w/v of *nickel(II) chloride hexahydrate* in a mixture of 2 volumes of *methanol*, 3 volumes of *acetonitrile* and 5 volumes of *water* as the mobile phase with a flow rate of 1.5 ml per minute and (c) a detection wavelength of 273 nm.

Calculate the content of C_9H_5ClINO in the cream using the declared content of C_9H_5ClINO in *clioquinol BPCRS*.

Storage Betamethasone and Clioquinol Cream should be protected from light.

Labelling The quantity of active ingredient with respect to Betamethasone Valerate is stated in terms of the equivalent amount of betamethasone.

Betamethasone Eye Drops

Definition Betamethasone Eye Drops are a sterile solution of Betamethasone Sodium Phosphate in Purified Water.

The eye drops comply with the requirements stated under Eye Preparations and with the following requirements.

Content of betamethasone sodium phosphate, $C_{22}H_{28}FNa_2O_8P$ 90.0 to 110.0% of the prescribed or stated amount.

Identification

A. Carry out the method for *thin-layer chromatography*, Appendix III A, using *silica gel GF_{254}* as the coating substance and a mixture of 60 volumes of *butan-1-ol*, 20 volumes of *acetic anhydride* and 20 volumes of *water*, prepared immediately before use, as the mobile phase. Apply separately to the plate 10 µl of each of the following solutions. For solution (1) use the eye drops, diluted if necessary with *water* to contain 0.1% w/v of Betamethasone Sodium Phosphate. Solution (2) contains 0.1% w/v of *betamethasone sodium phosphate BPCRS* in *water*. Solution (3) is a mixture of equal volumes of solutions (1) and (2). Solution (4) is a mixture of equal volumes of solution (2) and a 0.1% w/v solution of *prednisolone sodium phosphate BPCRS* in *water*. After removal of the plate, allow it to dry in air, heat at 110° for 10 minutes and examine under *ultraviolet light (254 nm)*. The chromatograms obtained with solutions (1), (2) and (3) show single principal spots with similar Rf values. The chromatogram obtained with solution (4) shows two principal spots with almost identical Rf values.

B. In the Assay, the chromatogram obtained with solution (2) shows a peak with the same retention time as the peak due to betamethasone sodium phosphate in the chromatogram obtained with solution (1).

C. To a volume containing 0.2 mg of Betamethasone Sodium Phosphate, add slowly 1 ml of *sulphuric acid* and allow to stand for 2 minutes. A brownish yellow colour but no red colour or yellowish green fluorescence is produced.

Acidity or alkalinity pH, 7.0 to 8.5, Appendix V L.

Related substances Carry out the method for *liquid chromatography*, Appendix III D, protected from light, using the following three solutions in the mobile phase. For solution (1) dilute 1 volume of solution (2) to 50 volumes with *water*. For solution (2) dilute the eye drops if necessary to give a solution containing 0.10% w/v of Betamethasone Sodium Phosphate. Solution (3) contains 0.0060% w/v each of *betamethasone sodium phosphate BPCRS* and *betamethasone*.

The chromatographic procedure may be carried out using (a) a stainless steel column (20 cm × 4.6 mm) packed with *stationary phase C* (10 µm) (Spherisorb ODS 1 is suitable) and maintained at 60°, (b) a mixture of 60 volumes of *citro-phosphate buffer pH 5.0* and 40 volumes of *methanol* as the mobile phase with a flow rate of 2 ml per minute and (c) a detection wavelength of 241 nm.

Inject 20 µl of solution (3). The test is not valid unless the *resolution factor* between the peaks due to betamethasone sodium phosphate and betamethasone is at least 3.5.

Inject separately 20 µl of each of solutions (1) and (2) and record the chromatogram for three times the retention time of the principal peak. In the chromatogram obtained with solution (2) the area of any peak corresponding to betamethasone is not greater than 1.3 times the area of the principal peak in the chromatogram obtained with solution (1), the area of any other *secondary peak* is not greater than 1.5 times the area of the principal peak in the chromatogram obtained with solution (1) and the sum of the areas of all the *secondary peaks* is not greater than 2.5 times the area of the principal peak in the chromatogram obtained with solution (1). Disregard any peak the area of which is less than 0.05 times the area of the principal peak in the chromatogram obtained with solution (1).

Assay Carry out the method for *liquid chromatography*, Appendix III D, using the following solutions. Solution (1) is a mixture of 5 ml of a 0.1% w/v solution of *betamethasone sodium phosphate BPCRS* in *water* (solution A) and 10 ml of a 0.06% w/v solution of *hydrocortisone* (internal standard) in *methanol* and sufficient *water* to produce 25 ml. For solution (2) mix a quantity of the eye drops containing 5 mg of Betamethasone Sodium Phosphate with 10 ml of *methanol* and dilute to 25 ml with *water*. Prepare solution (3) in the same manner as solution (2) but using 10 ml of the internal standard solution in place of the methanol.

The chromatographic procedure may be carried out using (a) a stainless steel column (20 cm × 5 mm) packed with *stationary phase C* (10 µm) (Spherisorb ODS 1 is suitable) and maintained at 60°, (b) a mixture of 55 volumes of *citro-phosphate buffer pH 5.0* and 45 volumes of *methanol* as the mobile phase with a flow rate of 2 ml per minute and (c) a detection wavelength of 241 nm.

Calculate the content of $C_{22}H_{28}FNa_2O_8P$ in solution A by measuring the *absorbance*, Appendix II B, of an aliquot diluted with *water* to contain 0.002% w/v of Betamethasone Sodium Phosphate at the maximum at 241 nm and taking 297 as the value of A(1%, 1 cm) at the maximum at 241 nm. Calculate the content of $C_{22}H_{28}FNa_2O_8P$ in the eye drops using peak areas.

Storage Betamethasone Eye Drops should be protected from light and stored at a temperature not exceeding 25°.

Betamethasone Injection

Definition Betamethasone Injection is a sterile solution of Betamethasone Sodium Phosphate in Water for Injections.

The injection complies with the requirements stated under Parenteral Preparations and with the following requirements.

Content of betamethasone, $C_{22}H_{29}FO_5$ 92.5 to 107.5% of the prescribed or stated amount.

Identification

A. To a volume containing the equivalent of 4 mg of betamethasone add 1 ml of *water* and sufficient *absolute ethanol* to produce 40 ml. Place 2 ml of the solution in a stoppered tube, add 10 ml of *phenylhydrazine—sulphuric acid solution*, mix, warm in a water bath at 60° for 20 minutes and cool immediately. The *absorbance* of the resulting solution at the maximum at 450 nm is not more than 0.1, Appendix II B.

B. Carry out the method for *thin-layer chromatography*, Appendix III A, using *silica gel GF_{254}* as the coating substance and a mixture of 60 volumes of *butan-1-ol*, 20 volumes of *acetic anhydride* and 20 volumes of *water*, prepared immediately before use, as the mobile phase. Apply separately to the plate 5 µl of each of the following solutions. For solution (1) use the injection, if necessary diluted with *water* to contain the equivalent of 2 mg of betamethasone per ml. Solution (2) contains 0.25% w/v solution of *betamethasone sodium phosphate BPCRS* in *water*. Solution (3) is a mixture of equal volumes of solutions (1) and (2). Solution (4) is a mixture of equal volumes of solution (1) and a 0.25% w/v solution of *prednisolone sodium phosphate BPCRS* in *water*. After removal of the plate, allow it to dry in air, heat at 110° for 10 minutes and examine under *ultraviolet light (254 nm)*. The chromatograms obtained with solutions (1), (2) and (3) show single spots with similar Rf values. The chromatogram obtained with solution (4) shows two principal spots with almost identical Rf values. *Secondary spots* due to excipients may also be observed in the chromatograms obtained with solutions (1), (3) and (4).

C. Evaporate a volume containing the equivalent of 2 mg of betamethasone to dryness on a water bath, dissolve the residue in 2 ml of *sulphuric acid* and allow to stand for 2 minutes. No red colour is produced.

Alkalinity pH, 8.0 to 9.0, Appendix V L.

Colour The injection, diluted if necessary with *water* to contain the equivalent of 2 mg of betamethasone per ml, is not more intensely coloured than *reference solution BY_4*, Appendix IV B, Method I.

Related substances Complies with test described under Betamethasone Eye Drops using the following three solutions. For solution (1) dilute 1 volume of solution (2) to 50 volumes with the mobile phase. For solution (2) dilute the injection with the mobile phase to give a solution containing the equivalent of 0.10% w/v of betamethasone. Solution (3) contains 0.0060% w/v each of *betamethasone sodium phosphate BPCRS* and *betamethasone*.

Assay Dilute a volume containing the equivalent of 20 mg of betamethasone with sufficient *water* to produce 200 ml. To 25 ml add 2.5 g of *sodium chloride*, dissolve, add 1 ml of *hydrochloric acid* and shake with three 25-ml quantities of *chloroform*. Wash each chloroform layer with 1 ml of 0.1M *hydrochloric acid*, add the washings to the aqueous solution and discard the chloroform solutions. Extract the aqueous solution with two 10-ml quantities of *tributyl orthophosphate* and dilute the combined extracts to 25 ml with *methanol*. To 2 ml add 10 ml of *isoniazid solution*, heat in a stoppered tube at 50° for 3 hours, protecting the solution from light, cool and measure the *absorbance* of the resulting solution at the maximum at 405 nm, Appendix II B, using in the reference cell a solution prepared in the same manner but omitting the preparation. Repeat the operation using 25 ml of a solution of *betamethasone sodium phosphate BPCRS* containing the equivalent of 0.01% w/v of betamethasone and beginning at the words 'add 2.5 g ...'. Calculate the content of $C_{22}H_{29}FO_5$ in the preparation from the absorbances obtained and the exact strength of the solution of the betamethasone sodium phosphate BPCRS, determined by diluting 1 volume of the preparation to 5 volumes with *water*, measuring the *absorbance* of the resulting solution at the maximum at 241 nm and calculating the content of $C_{22}H_{29}FO_5$ taking 391 as the value of A(1%, 1 cm) at the maximum at 241 nm.

Storage Betamethasone Injection should be stored at a temperature not exceeding 30° and protected from light.

Labelling The quantity of active ingredient is stated in terms of the equivalent amount of betamethasone in a suitable dose-volume.

Betamethasone Valerate Lotion

Definition Betamethasone Valerate Lotion is a *cutaneous solution*. It contains Betamethasone Valerate in a suitable vehicle.

The lotion complies with the requirements stated under Liquids for Cutaneous Application and with the following requirements.

Content of betamethasone, $C_{22}H_{29}FO_5$ 90.0 to 110.0% of the prescribed or stated amount.

Identification

A. Carry out the method for *thin-layer chromatography*, Appendix III A, using *silica gel G* as the coating substance and a mixture of 100 volumes of *chloroform*, 10 volumes of *acetone* and 5 volumes of *absolute ethanol* as the mobile phase. Apply separately to the plate 10 µl of each of the following solutions. For solution (1) disperse a quantity of the preparation being examined containing the equivalent of 1 mg of betamethasone with 5 ml of *methanol (80%)* by heating on a water bath until the methanol begins to boil. Shake vigorously, cool in ice and filter. Transfer the filtrate to a separating funnel and add 0.5 ml of *water* and 1 ml of *chloroform*. Shake vigorously, allow the layers to separate and use the chloroform layer. Solution (2) contains 0.05% w/v of *betamethasone valerate BPCRS* in *chloroform*. Solution (3) is a mixture of equal volumes of solutions (1) and (2). After removal of the plate, allow it to dry in air until the odour of solvent is no longer detectable, heat at 105° for 5 minutes and spray while hot with *alkaline tetrazolium blue solution*. The principal spot in the chromatogram obtained with solution (1) corresponds to that in the chromatogram obtained with solution (2). The spot in the chromatogram obtained with solution (3) appears as a single compact spot.

B. In the Assay, the chromatogram obtained with solution (2) shows a peak with the same retention time as the peak due to betamethasone valerate in the chromatogram obtained with solution (1).

Assay Carry out the method for *liquid chromatography*, Appendix III D, using the following solutions. For solution (1) mix 20 ml of a solution containing 0.018% w/v of *betamethasone valerate BPCRS* and 0.0010% w/v of *betamethasone 21-valerate BPCRS* in *ethanol (65%)* with 5 ml of a 0.11% w/v solution of *beclomethasone dipropionate BPCRS* (internal standard) in *ethanol (65%)*. For solution (2) disperse a quantity of the preparation being examined containing the equivalent of 3 mg of betamethasone in a mixture of 10 ml of *ethanol (65%)* and 50 ml of *hexane*, shake for 2 minutes and filter the lower, ethanolic layer through absorbent cotton previously washed with *ethanol (65%)*. Repeat the extraction of the hexane mixture with two 5-ml quantities of *ethanol (65%)*, filtering the ethanol extracts through the absorbent cotton, add 5 ml of *ethanol (65%)* to the combined filtrates and mix. Prepare solution (3) in the same manner as solution (2) but adding 5 ml of a 0.11% w/v solution of the internal standard in *ethanol (65%)* in place of the 5 ml of ethanol (65%).

The chromatographic procedure may be carried out using (a) a stainless steel column (10 cm × 5 mm) packed with *stationary phase C* (5 µm) (Spherisorb ODS 1 is suitable) and maintained at 60°, (b) as the mobile phase with a flow rate of 2 ml per minute a mixture of *absolute ethanol* and *water* adjusted so that baseline separation is obtained between betamethasone valerate (retention time about 5 minutes) and betamethasone 21-valerate (retention time about 7 minutes) and between betamethasone 21-valerate and beclomethasone dipropionate (retention time about 8 minutes) (a mixture of 42 volumes of *absolute ethanol* and 58 volumes of *water* is usually suitable) and (c) a detection wavelength of 238 nm.

Calculate the content of $C_{22}H_{29}FO_5$ in the preparation being examined using the declared content of $C_{22}H_{29}FO_5$ in *betamethasone valerate BPCRS*.

Storage Betamethasone Valerate Lotion should be protected from light.

Labelling The quantity of active ingredient is stated in terms of the equivalent amount of betamethasone.

The label states that pharmaceutical form as 'cutaneous solution'.

Betamethasone Valerate Ointment

Definition Betamethasone Valerate Ointment contains Betamethasone Valerate in a suitable basis.

The ointment complies with the requirements stated under Topical Semi-solid Preparations and with the following requirements.

Content of betamethasone, $C_{22}H_{29}FO_5$ 90.0 to 110.0% of the prescribed or stated amount.

Identification

A. Complies with test A for Identification described under

Betamethasone Valerate Lotion preparing solution (1) in the following manner. Disperse a quantity of the ointment containing the equivalent of 1 mg of betamethasone in 10 ml of *methanol* by heating on a water bath until the methanol begins to boil, shake vigorously, cool in ice for 30 minutes and filter. Evaporate the filtrate to dryness in a current of nitrogen with gentle heating and dissolve the residue in 0.5 ml of *chloroform*. Solution (2) contains 0.24% w/v of *betamethasone valerate BPCRS* in *chloroform*.

B. In the Assay, the chromatogram obtained with solution (2) shows a peak with the same retention time as the peak due to betamethasone valerate in the chromatogram obtained with solution (1).

Assay Carry out the method for *liquid chromatography*, Appendix III D, using the following solutions. For solution (1) mix 10 ml of a solution containing 0.024% w/v of *betamethasone valerate BPCRS* and 0.0012% w/v of *betamethasone 21-valerate BPCRS* in *ethanol (65%)* with 5 ml of a 0.072% w/v solution of *beclomethasone dipropionate BPCRS* (internal standard) in *ethanol (65%)* and dilute to 50 ml with *ethanol (65%)*. For solution (2) disperse a quantity of the ointment containing the equivalent of 2 mg of betamethasone in 100 ml of hot *hexane*, cool, extract with 20 ml of *ethanol (65%)* and filter the lower, ethanolic layer through absorbent cotton previously washed with *ethanol (65%)*; repeat the extraction of the hexane mixture with two 10-ml quantities of *ethanol (65%)*, filtering each extract in turn through the absorbent cotton and dilute the combined filtrates to 50 ml with *ethanol (65%)*. Prepare solution (3) in the same manner as solution (2) but add 5 ml of the 0.072% w/v solution of the internal standard in *ethanol (65%)* before diluting to 50 ml.

The chromatographic procedure may be carried out using (a) a stainless steel column (10 cm × 5 mm) packed with *stationary phase C* (5 µm) (Spherisorb ODS 1 is suitable) and maintained at 60°, (b) as the mobile phase with a flow rate of 2 ml per minute a mixture of *absolute ethanol* and *water* adjusted so that the *resolution factor* between the peaks due to betamethasone valerate (retention time about 5 minutes) and betamethasone 21valerate (retention time about 7 minutes) is more than 1.0 (a mixture of 42 volumes of *absolute ethanol* and 58 volumes of *water* is usually suitable) and (c) a detection wavelength of 238 nm.

Calculate the content of $C_{22}H_{29}FO_5$ in the ointment using the declared content of $C_{22}H_{29}FO_5$ in *betamethasone valerate BPCRS*.

Storage Betamethasone Valerate Ointment should be protected from light.

Labelling The quantity of active ingredient is stated in terms of the equivalent amount of betamethasone.

Betamethasone and Clioquinol Ointment

Definition Betamethasone and Clioquinol Ointment contains Betamethasone Valerate and Clioquinol, the latter in *very fine powder*, in a suitable basis.

The ointment complies with the requirements stated under Topical Semi-solid Preparations and with the following requirements.

Content of betamethasone, $C_{22}H_{29}FO_5$ 90.0 to 110.0% of the prescribed or stated amount.

Content of clioquinol, C_9H_5ClINO 90.0 to 110.0% of the prescribed or stated amount.

Identification

A. Complies with test A for Identification described under Betamethasone and Clioquinol Cream but preparing the solutions in the following manner. For solution (1) disperse a quantity of the ointment containing the equivalent of 1 mg of betamethasone with 10 ml of *methanol* by heating on a water bath until the methanol begins to boil. Shake vigorously, cool in ice and filter. Evaporate the filtrate to dryness in a current of nitrogen and dissolve the residue in 0.5 ml of *chloroform*. Solution (2) contains 0.24% w/v of *betamethasone valerate BPCRS* in *chloroform*.

B. In the Assay for betamethasone the chromatogram obtained with solution (2) shows a peak with the same retention time as the peak due to betamethasone valerate in the chromatogram obtained with solution (1).

C. In the Assay for clioquinol the chromatogram obtained with solution (2) shows a peak with the same retention time as the peak due to clioquinol in the chromatogram obtained with solution (1).

Assay

For betamethasone Carry out the method for *liquid chromatography*, Appendix III D, using the following solutions. For solution (1) mix 10 ml of a solution containing 0.024% w/v of *betamethasone valerate BPCRS* and 0.0012% w/v of *betamethasone 21-valerate BPCRS* in *ethanol (65%)* with 5 ml of a 0.072% w/v solution of *beclomethasone dipropionate BPCRS* (internal standard) in *ethanol (65%)* and dilute to 50 ml with *ethanol (65%)*. For solution (2) disperse a quantity of the ointment containing the equivalent of 2 mg of betamethasone in 100 ml of hot *hexane*, cool, extract with 20 ml of *ethanol (65%)* and filter the lower, ethanolic layer through absorbent cotton previously washed with *ethanol (65%)*; repeat the extraction of the hexane mixture with two 10-ml quantities of *ethanol (65%)*, filtering each extract in turn through the absorbent cotton and dilute the combined filtrates to 50 ml with *ethanol (65%)*. Prepare solution (3) in the same manner as solution (2) but add 5 ml of the 0.072% w/v solution of the internal standard in *ethanol (65%)* before diluting to 50 ml.

The chromatographic procedure may be carried out using (a) a stainless steel column (10 cm × 5 mm) packed with *stationary phase C* (5 µm) (Spherisorb ODS 1 is suitable) and maintained at 60°, (b) as the mobile phase with a flow rate of 2 ml per minute a mixture of *absolute ethanol* and *water* adjusted so that the *resolution factor* between the peaks due to betamethasone valerate (retention time about 5 minutes) and betamethasone 21-valerate (retention time about 7 minutes) is more than 1.0 (a mixture of 42 volumes of *absolute ethanol* and 58 volumes of *water* is usually suitable) and (c) a detection wavelength of 238 nm.

Calculate the content of $C_{22}H_{29}FO_5$ in the ointment using the declared content of $C_{22}H_{29}FO_5$ in *betamethasone valerate BPCRS*.

For clioquinol Carry out the Assay described under Betamethasone and Clioquinol Cream.

Storage Betamethasone and Clioquinol Ointment should be protected from light.

Labelling The quantity of active ingredient with respect to Betamethasone Valerate is stated in terms of the equivalent amount of betamethasone.

Betamethasone Tablets

Definition Betamethasone Tablets contain Betamethasone.

The tablets comply with the requirements stated under Tablets and with the following requirements.

Content of betamethasone, $C_{22}H_{29}FO_5$ 90.0 to 110.0% of the prescribed or stated amount.

Identification

A. Shake a quantity of the powdered tablets containing 25 mg of Betamethasone with 150 ml of *dichloromethane* for 30 minutes, filter, wash the filtrate with 20 ml of *water*, dry over *anhydrous sodium sulphate*, evaporate the solution to dryness and dry the residue at 105° for 2 hours. The *infrared absorption spectrum* of the residue, Appendix II A, is concordant with the *reference spectrum* of betamethasone.
B. The residue obtained in test A complies with the test for the *identification of steroids*, Appendix III A, using *impregnating solvent I* and *mobile phase A*. At a fourth point apply to the plate 2 µl of a mixture of equal volumes of solution (1) and a 0.25% w/v solution of *dexamethasone EPCRS* in a mixture of 9 volumes of *chloroform* and 1 volume of *methanol*. The chromatogram obtained with this solution shows two principal spots with almost identical Rf values.

C. In the Assay, the chromatogram obtained with solution (2) shows a peak with the same retention time as the peak due to betamethasone in the chromatogram obtained with solution (1).

Uniformity of content Tablets containing less than 2 mg of Betamethasone comply with the requirements stated under Tablets using the following method of analysis. Carry out the method for *liquid chromatography*, Appendix III D, protected from light using the following solutions. Solution (1) contains 0.0025% w/v of *betamethasone BPCRS* and 0.002% w/v of *hydrocortisone* (internal standard) in *methanol (50%)*. For solution (2) finely crush one tablet, add 20 ml of a 0.002% w/v solution of *hydrocortisone* in *methanol (50%)*, shake for 10 minutes and filter through a glass-fibre filter paper (Whatman GF/C is suitable).

The chromatographic procedure may be carried out using (a) a stainless steel column (20 cm × 5 mm) packed with *stationary phase C* (10 µm) (Spherisorb ODS 1 is suitable), (b) a mixture of 53 volumes of *water* and 47 volumes of *methanol* as the mobile phase with a flow rate of 1.4 ml per minute and (c) a detection wavelength of 238 nm.

Calculate the content of $C_{22}H_{29}FO_5$ in each tablet taking 100.0% as the content of $C_{22}H_{29}FO_5$ in *betamethasone BPCRS*.

Assay Carry out the method for *liquid chromatography*, Appendix III D, protected from light using the following solutions. Solution (1) contains 0.0125% w/v of *betamethasone BPCRS* and 0.010% w/v of *hydrocortisone* (internal standard) in *methanol (50%)*. For solution (2) weigh and powder 20 tablets; to a quantity of the powder containing 2.5 mg of Betamethasone add 20 ml of *methanol (50%)*, shake for 10 minutes and filter through a glass-fibre filter paper (Whatman GF/C is suitable). Prepare solution (3) in the same manner as solution (2) but use 20 ml of a 0.01% w/v solution of *hydrocortisone* in *methanol (50%)* in place of the 20 ml of methanol (50%).

The chromatographic conditions described under Uniformity of content may be used.

Calculate the content of $C_{22}H_{29}FO_5$ in the tablets from the declared content of $C_{22}H_{29}FO_5$ in *betamethasone BPCRS*.

Storage Betamethasone Tablets should be protected from light.

Betamethasone Sodium Phosphate Tablets

Definition Betamethasone Sodium Phosphate Tablets contain Betamethasone Sodium Phosphate.

The tablets comply with the requirements stated under Tablets and with the following requirements.

Content of betamethasone, $C_{22}H_{29}FO_5$ 90.0 to 110.0% of the prescribed or stated amount.

Identification

A. Carry out the method for *thin-layer chromatography*, Appendix III A, using *silica gel G* as the coating substance and a mixture of 60 volumes of *butan-1-ol*, 20 volumes of *acetic anhydride* and 20 volumes of *water* prepared immediately before use as the mobile phase. Apply separately to the plate 5 µl of each of the following solutions. For solution (1) dissolve a quantity of the powdered tablets containing the equivalent of 2 mg of betamethasone in 25 ml of *water*, add 2.5 g of *sodium chloride* and 1 ml of *hydrochloric acid*, extract with 25 ml of *chloroform* and discard the chloroform layer. Extract with 25 ml of *tributyl orthophosphate* and discard the aqueous layer. Prepare solution (2) in the same manner as solution (1) but using 2.5 mg of *betamethasone sodium phosphate BPCRS* in place of the powdered tablets. Solution (3) is a mixture of equal volumes of solutions (1) and (2). Solution (4) is a mixture of equal volumes of solution (1) and a solution prepared in the same manner as solution (1) but using 2.5 mg of *prednisolone sodium phosphate BPCRS* in place of the powdered tablets. After removal of the plate, allow it to dry in air, heat at 110° for 10 minutes, spray the hot plate with *ethanolic sulphuric acid (20%)* and again heat at 110° for 10 minutes. The chromatograms obtained with solutions (1), (2) and (3) show single spots with similar Rf values. The chromatogram obtained with solution (4) shows two principal spots with almost identical Rf values.

B. Mix a quantity of the powdered tablets containing the equivalent of 0.4 mg of betamethasone with 1 ml of *sulphuric acid* and allow to stand for 5 minutes. A pale yellow colour is produced (distinction from prednisolone sodium phosphate tablets).

Disintegration Maximum time, 5 minutes, Appendix XII A.

Uniformity of content Tablets containing less than the equivalent of 2 mg of betamethasone comply with the requirements stated under Tablets using the following method of analysis. Carry out the method for *liquid chromatography*, Appendix III D, using the following solutions protected from light. Solution (1) is a mixture of equal volumes of a solution containing 0.0065% w/v of *betamethasone sodium phosphate BPCRS* in *water* and a solution containing 0.006% w/v of *hydrocortisone* in *methanol* (internal standard solution). For solution (2) dissolve one tablet as completely as possible in 5 ml of *water* and add 5 ml of *methanol*. For solution (3) dissolve one tablet as completely as possible in 5 ml of *water* and add 5 ml of the internal standard solution.

The chromatographic procedure may be carried out using (a) a stainless steel column (20 cm × 4.6 mm) packed with *stationary phase C* (10 µm) (Spherisorb ODS 1 is suitable) and maintained at 60°, (b) a mixture of 55 volumes of *citro-phosphate buffer pH 5.0* and 45 volumes of *methanol* as the mobile phase with a flow rate of 2 ml per minute and (c) a detection wavelength of 241 nm.

Calculate the content of $C_{22}H_{29}FO_5$ in each tablet.

Assay Weigh and powder 20 tablets. Dissolve a quantity of the powder containing the equivalent of 5 mg of betamethasone in sufficient *water* to produce 50 ml and carry out the Assay described under Betamethasone Injection beginning at the words 'To 25 ml add 2.5 g of *sodium chloride* ...'.

Storage Betamethasone Sodium Phosphate Tablets should be protected from light.

Labelling The quantity of active ingredient is stated in terms of the equivalent amount of betamethasone.

Bisacodyl Suppositories

Definition Bisacodyl Suppositories contain Bisacodyl in a suitable suppository basis.

The suppositories comply with the requirements stated under Rectal Preparations and with the following requirements.

Content of bisacodyl, $C_{22}H_{19}NO_4$ 90.0 to 110.0% of the prescribed or stated amount.

Identification

A. Carry out the method described under Related substances applying to the plate 2 µl of each solution and using as solution (2) a 1% w/v solution of *bisacodyl EPCRS* in *acetone*. The principal spot in the chromatogram obtained with solution (1) corresponds to that in the chromatogram obtained with solution (2).

B. Dissolve a quantity of the suppositories containing 0.15 g of Bisacodyl as completely as possible in 150 ml of *petroleum spirit (boiling range, 40° to 60°)*, filter, wash the residue with *petroleum spirit (boiling range, 40° to 60°)* until free from fatty material and dry at about 100°. Wash with a very small quantity of warm *chloroform* and dissolve the residue in 10 ml of a 0.5% v/v solution of *sulphuric acid*. To 2 ml of the solution add 0.05 ml of *potassium tetraiodomercurate solution*. A white precipitate is produced.

C. To 2 ml of the solution obtained in test B add *sulphuric acid*. A reddish violet colour is produced.

D. Boil 2 ml of the solution obtained in test B with a little *nitric acid*; a yellow colour is produced. Cool and add 5M *sodium hydroxide*; the colour becomes yellowish brown.

Related substances Carry out the method for *thin-layer chromatography*, Appendix III A, using *silica gel GF_{254}* as the coating substance and a mixture of equal volumes of *butan-2-one* and *xylene* as the mobile phase. Apply separately to the plate 10 µl of each of the following solutions. For solution (1) shake a quantity of the suppositories containing 20 mg of Bisacodyl with 20 ml of *petroleum spirit (boiling range, 40° to 60°)*, filter, wash the residue with *petroleum spirit (boiling range, 40° to 60°)* until free from fat and dissolve in 2 ml of *acetone*. For solution (2) dilute 3 volumes of solution (1) to 100 volumes with *acetone*. After removal of the plate, allow it to dry in air and examine under *ultraviolet light (254 nm)*. Any *secondary spot* in the chromatogram obtained with solution (1) is not more intense than the spot in the chromatogram obtained with solution (2).

Assay To a quantity of the suppositories containing 0.1 g of Bisacodyl add 80 ml of *anhydrous acetic acid* previously neutralised with 0.02M *perchloric acid VS* to *1-naphtholbenzein solution*, warm gently until solution is complete and immediately carry out Method I for *non-aqueous titration*, Appendix VIII A, using 0.02M *perchloric acid VS* and determining the end point potentiometrically. Each ml of 0.02M *perchloric acid VS* is equivalent to 7.228 mg of $C_{22}H_{19}NO_4$. Calculate the average content of bisacodyl, $C_{22}H_{19}NO_4$, in the suppositories.

Bisacodyl Tablets

Definition Bisacodyl Tablets contain Bisacodyl. They are made gastro-resistant by enteric-coating or by other means.

The tablets comply with the requirements stated under Tablets and with the following requirements.

Content of bisacodyl, $C_{22}H_{19}NO_4$ 95.0 to 105.0% of the prescribed or stated amount.

Identification

A. Carry out the method described under Related substances applying to the plate 2 µl of each solution and using as solution (2) a 1% w/v solution of *bisacodyl EPCRS*. The principal spot in the chromatogram obtained with solution (1) corresponds to that in the chromatogram obtained with solution (2).

B. Extract a quantity of the powdered tablets containing 50 mg of Bisacodyl with *chloroform*, filter, evaporate the filtrate to dryness and dissolve the residue in 10 ml of a 0.5% v/v solution of *sulphuric acid*. To 2 ml of the solution add 0.05 ml of *potassium tetraiodomercurate solution*. A white precipitate is produced.

C. To 2 ml of the solution obtained in test B add *sulphuric acid*. A reddish violet colour is produced.

D. Boil 2 ml of the solution obtained in test B with a little *nitric acid*; a yellow colour is produced. Cool and add 5M *sodium hydroxide*; the colour becomes yellowish brown.

Disintegration Tablets made gastro-resistant by enteric-coating comply with the *disintegration test for enteric-coated tablets*, Appendix XII B, using a 1.5% w/v solution of *sodium hydrogen carbonate* in place of the mixed phosphate buffer pH 6.8.

Related substances Carry out the method for *thin-layer chromatography*, Appendix III A, using *silica gel GF_{254}* as the coating substance and a mixture of equal volumes of *butan-2-one* and *xylene* as the mobile phase. Apply separately to the plate 10 µl of each of the following solutions. For solution (1) shake a quantity of the powdered tablets containing 20 mg of Bisacodyl with 2 ml of *acetone* for 10 minutes, centrifuge and use the supernatant liquid. For solution (2) dilute 3 volumes of solution (1) to 100 volumes with *acetone*. After removal of the plate, allow it to dry in air and examine under *ultraviolet light (254 nm)*. Any *secondary spot* in the chromatogram obtained with solution (1), other than any spot (due to tablet excipient) with an Rf value of 1.3 relative to the principal spot, is not more intense than the spot in the chromatogram obtained with solution (2).

Assay Weigh and powder 20 tablets. Shake a quantity of the powder containing 40 mg of Bisacodyl with 70 ml of *chloroform* for 30 minutes, dilute to 100 ml with *chloroform*, mix, filter and dilute 10 ml of the filtrate to 100 ml with *chloroform*. Measure the *absorbance* of the resulting solution at the maximum at 264 nm, Appendix II B. Calculate the content of $C_{22}H_{19}NO_4$ taking 148 as the value of A(1%, 1 cm) at the maximum at 264 nm.

Black Currant Syrup

Definition Black Currant Syrup is prepared either from the clarified juice of Black Currant or from concentrated black currant juice of commerce. It contains a suitable antioxidant. Permitted food grade colours may be added.

Production It is prepared by dissolving 700 g of Sucrose either in 560 ml of clarified juice, previously diluted with Water to a weight per ml of 1.045 g, or in 560 ml of a solution of the same weight per ml prepared from the concentrated juice of commerce and Water, and adding to this solution sufficient Benzoic Acid to give a final concentration of not more than 800 ppm, or sufficient Sodium Metabisulphite or other suitable sulphite to give a final concentration of not more than 350 ppm of sulphur dioxide.

The syrup complies with the requirements stated under Syrups and with the following requirements.

Content of ascorbic acid[1], $C_6H_8O_6$ Not less than 0.055% w/w.

Sulphur dioxide Not more than 350 ppm, Appendix IX B.

Weight per ml 1.27 to 1.30 g, Appendix V G.

Assay Mix 5 g with 25 ml of a freshly prepared 20% w/v solution of *metaphosphoric acid*, add 20 ml of *acetone* and dilute to 100 ml with *water*. To four 3-ml quantities of this solution add 0.4, 0.5, 0.6 and 0.7 ml, respectively, of *double-strength standard 2,6-dichlorophenolindophenol solution*, mix well by agitation with a fine stream of carbon dioxide, add 3 ml of *chloroform*, agitate for a further 15 seconds, examine the solutions against a white background and select the two that are on either side of the end point (that is, one colourless and one pink). Prepare a further six solutions as directed above, but adding to the first an amount of dye solution equal to that added to the selected colourless solution, successively increasing this volume by 0.02-ml increments in the second to the fifth solutions and adding to the sixth solution a volume equal to that added to the selected pink solution. Select the solution exhibiting the faintest pink colour. Each ml of *double-strength standard 2,6-dichlorophenolindophenol solution* added to this solution is equivalent to 0.200 mg of $C_6H_8O_6$.

Storage Black Currant Syrup should be kept in a well-filled, well-closed container, protected from light and stored at a temperature not exceeding 25°.

Black Currant Syrup contains, in 10 ml, about 7.5 mg of ascorbic acid.

---

[1]The requirement for Content of ascorbic acid does not apply when Black Currant Syrup is used as a flavouring agent for pharmaceutical purposes.

Bretylium Injection

Definition Bretylium Injection is a sterile solution of Bretylium Tosilate in Water for Injections.

The injection complies with the requirements stated under Parenteral Preparations and with the following requirements.

Content of bretylium tosilate, $C_{18}H_{24}BrNO_3S$ 95.0 to 105.0% of the prescribed or stated amount.

Characteristics A clear, colourless solution.

Identification

A. Dry a quantity of the injection containing 50 mg of Bretylium Tosilate over *phosphorus pentoxide* at a pressure not exceeding 0.7 kPa for 16 hours. The *infrared absorption spectrum* of the residue, Appendix II A, is concordant with the *reference spectrum* of bretylium tosilate. If the spectra are not concordant, dissolve a sufficient quantity of the residue in the minimum volume of *acetone* by heating on a water bath at 50°, evaporate to dryness at room temperature under a current of nitrogen and prepare a new spectrum of the residue.

B. Carry out the method for *thin-layer chromatography*, Appendix III A, using *silica gel GF_{254}* as the coating substance and a mixture of 15 volumes of *glacial acetic acid*, 30 volumes of *water* and 75 volumes of *butan-1-ol* as the mobile phase. Apply separately to the plate 10 µl of each of the following solutions. For solution (1) dilute the injection with *water*, if necessary, to contain 5.0% w/v of Bretylium Tosilate. Solution (2) contains 5.0% w/v of *bretylium tosilate BPCRS* in *water*. After removal of the plate, dry it in a current of air and examine under *ultraviolet light (254 nm)*. In the chromatogram obtained with solution (1) the two principal spots correspond to those in the chromatogram obtained with solution (2).

Acidity or alkalinity pH, 5.0 to 7.0, Appendix V L.

Related substances Carry out the method for *liquid chromatography*, Appendix III D, using the following solutions. For solution (1) dilute the injection with sufficient of the mobile phase to produce a solution containing 0.2% w/v of Bretylium Tosilate. For solution (2) dilute 1 volume of solution (1) to 100 volumes with the mobile phase. Solution (3) contains 0.05% w/v of *bretylium tosilate BPCRS* and 0.05% w/v of *2-bromobenzyldimethylamine hydrochloride BPCRS* in the mobile phase.

The chromatographic procedure may be carried out

using (a) a stainless steel column (25 cm × 4.6 mm) packed with particles of silica the surface of which has been modified by chemically-bonded phenyl groups (5 µm) (Spherisorb Phenyl is suitable), (b) as the mobile phase with a flow rate of 2 ml per minute a mixture of 0.5 volume of *triethylamine*, 2 volumes of *glacial acetic acid*, 19 volumes of *acetonitrile* and 81 volumes of 0.01M *sodium octanesulphonate* and (c) a detection wavelength of 265 nm.

The test is not valid unless, in the chromatogram obtained with solution (3), the *resolution factor* between the two principal peaks is at least 6.

In the chromatogram obtained with solution (1) the area of any *secondary peak* is not greater than half the area of the peak in the chromatogram obtained with solution (2) (0.5%) and the sum of the areas of any such peaks is not greater than the area of the peak in the chromatogram obtained with solution (2) (1%). Disregard any peak due to tosilate (retention time, about 2 minutes) and any peak with an area less than 0.05 times the area of the peak in the chromatogram obtained with solution (2) (0.05%).

Assay Carry out the method for *liquid chromatography*, Appendix III D, using the following solutions. For solution (1) dilute the injection with sufficient of the mobile phase to produce a solution containing 0.05% w/v of Bretylium Tosilate. Solution (2) contains 0.05% w/v of *bretylium tosilate BPCRS* in the mobile phase. Solution (3) contains 0.05% w/v of *bretylium tosilate BPCRS* and 0.05% w/v of *2-bromobenzyldimethylamine hydrochloride BPCRS* in the mobile phase.

The chromatographic conditions described under Related substances may be used.

The test is not valid unless the *resolution factor* between the two principal peaks in the chromatogram obtained with solution (3) is at least 6.

Calculate the content of $C_{18}H_{24}BrNO_3S$ in the injection from the area of the peaks corresponding to bretylium and using the declared content of $C_{18}H_{24}BrNO_3S$ in *bretylium tosilate BPCRS*.

Storage Bretylium Injection should be protected from light and stored at a temperature not exceeding 25°.

IMPURITIES

The impurities limited by the requirements of this monograph include those listed in the monograph for Bretylium Tosilate.

Bromocriptine Capsules

Definition Bromocriptine Capsules contain Bromocriptine Mesilate.

The capsules comply with the requirements stated under Capsules and with the following requirements.

Content of bromocriptine, $C_{32}H_{40}BrN_5O_5$ 90.0 to 110.0% of the prescribed or stated amount.

Identification

A. Shake a quantity of the contents of the capsules containing the equivalent of 10 mg of bromocriptine with 50 ml of *methanol* for 30 minutes, centrifuge and dilute 5 ml of the supernatant liquid to 20 ml with *methanol*. The *light absorption* of the resulting solution, Appendix II B, in the range 230 to 380 nm exhibits a maximum at 305 nm and a minimum at 270 nm.

B. In the test for Related substances, the principal band in the chromatogram obtained with solution (2) corresponds to that in the chromatogram obtained with solution (6).

C. In the Assay, the retention time of the principal peak in the chromatogram obtained with solution (1) is the same as that of the principal peak in the chromatogram obtained with solution (2).

Related substances Carry out the method for *thin-layer chromatography*, Appendix III A, using *silica gel G* as the coating substance and as the mobile phase a mixture of 0.1 volume of 13.5M *ammonia*, 1.5 volumes of *water*, 3 volumes of *propan-2-ol*, 88 volumes of *dichloromethane* and 100 volumes of *ether*. Apply separately to the plate as 10-mm bands 50 µl of each of the following six solutions prepared immediately before use. For solution (1) shake a quantity of the contents of the capsules containing the equivalent of 20 mg of bromocriptine with 10 ml of *methanol* for 20 minutes and centrifuge. For solution (2) dilute 1 volume of solution (1) to 10 volumes with *methanol*. For solution (3) dilute 3 volumes of solution (1) to 100 volumes with *methanol*. For solution (4) dilute 1 volume of solution (1) to 100 volumes with *methanol*. For solution (5) dilute 1 volume of solution (1) to 200 volumes with *methanol*. Solution (6) contains 0.023% w/v of *bromocriptine mesilate BPCRS* in *methanol*. Apply solution (1) as the last solution and develop the chromatograms immediately in an unsaturated tank. After removal of the plate, dry it in a current of cold air for 2 minutes, spray with *ammonium molybdate solution R3* and heat at 100° until bands appear (about 10 minutes). In the chromatogram obtained with solution (1) any *secondary band* is not more intense than the band in the chromatogram obtained with solution (3) (3%). Not more than one such band is more intense than the band in the chromatogram obtained with solution (4) (1%) and not more than a further two such bands are more intense than the band in the chromatogram obtained with solution (5) (0.5%). Disregard any band within 20 mm of the line of application.

Assay Prepare the solutions in subdued light. Carry out the method for *liquid chromatography*, Appendix III D, using the following solutions. Solution (1) contains 0.011% w/v of *bromocriptine mesilate BPCRS* in *methanol (50%)*. For solution (2) mix a quantity of the mixed contents of 20 capsules containing the equivalent of 10 mg of bromocriptine with 70 ml of *methanol (50%)* with the aid of ultrasound for 5 minutes, filter and dilute to 100 ml with the same solvent. For solution (3) heat a 0.011% w/v solution of *bromocriptine mesilate BPCRS* in a mixture of 1 volume of 1M *acetic acid* and 9 volumes of *methanol* at 60° for 90 minutes and cool to room temperature.

The chromatographic procedure may be carried out using (a) a stainless steel column (10 cm × 4 mm) packed with *stationary phase C* (5 µm) (Spherisorb ODS 1 is suitable), (b) a mixture of 55 volumes of *acetonitrile* and 45 volumes of a 0.08% w/v solution of *ammonium carbonate* as the mobile phase with a flow rate of 1 ml per minute and (c) a detection wavelength of 300 nm.

The assay is not valid unless the *resolution factor* between the two peaks obtained with solution (3) is not less than 3.0.

Calculate the content of $C_{32}H_{40}BrN_5O_5$ using the declared content of $C_{32}H_{40}BrN_5O_5$ in *bromocriptine mesilate BPCRS*.

Storage Bromocriptine Capsules should be kept in an airtight container and protected from light.

Labelling The quantity of active ingredient is stated in terms of the equivalent amount of bromocriptine.

Bromocriptine Tablets

Definition Bromocriptine Tablets contain Bromocriptine Mesilate.

The tablets comply with the requirements stated under Tablets and with the following requirements.

Content of bromocriptine, $C_{32}H_{40}BrN_5O_5$ 90.0 to 110.0% of the prescribed or stated amount.

Identification

A. Shake a quantity of the powdered tablets containing the equivalent of 10 mg of bromocriptine with 50 ml of *methanol* for 30 minutes, centrifuge and dilute 5 ml of the supernatant liquid to 20 ml with *methanol*. The *light absorption* of the resulting solution, Appendix II B, in the range 230 to 380 nm exhibits a maximum at 305 nm and a minimum at 270 nm.

B. In the test for Related substances, the principal band in the chromatogram obtained with solution (2) corresponds to that in the chromatogram obtained with solution (6).

C. In the Assay, the retention time of the principal peak in the chromatogram obtained with solution (1) is similar to that of the principal peak in the chromatogram obtained with solution (2).

Related substances Carry out the method described under Bromocriptine Capsules applying separately to the plate, as 10-mm bands, 20 µl of each of the following solutions. For solution (1) shake a quantity of the powdered tablets containing the equivalent of 10 mg of bromocriptine with 25 ml of a mixture of equal volumes of *chloroform* and *methanol* for 30 minutes, filter through a sintered-glass filter (BS porosity No. 4) and wash the residue with two 5-ml quantities of the solvent mixture. Evaporate the filtrate and washings to dryness at 25° at a pressure of 2 kPa, dissolve the residue in 2 ml of the solvent mixture and centrifuge. For solution (2) dilute 1 volume of solution (1) to 10 volumes, for solution (3) dilute 3 volumes of solution (2) to 10 volumes, for solution (4) dilute 1 volume of solution (2) to 10 volumes and for solution (5) dilute 1 volume of solution (2) to 20 volumes, each with a mixture of equal volumes of *chloroform* and *methanol* as the diluent. Solution (6) contains 0.055% w/v of *bromocriptine mesilate BPCRS* in the same solvent mixture. In the chromatogram obtained with solution (1) any *secondary band* is not more intense than the band in the chromatogram obtained with solution (3) (3%). Not more than one such band is more intense than the band in the chromatogram obtained with solution (4) (1%) and not more than a further two such bands are more intense than the band in the chromatogram obtained with solution (5) (0.5%). Disregard any band within 20 mm of the line of application.

Uniformity of content Tablets containing less than the equivalent of 2 mg of bromocriptine comply with the requirements stated under Tablets using the following method of analysis. Mix one tablet with 50 ml of *ethanol (50%)* with the aid of ultrasound until disintegrated, shake for 30 minutes and centrifuge. Measure the *absorbance* of the supernatant liquid at the maximum at 305 nm, Appendix II B. Calculate the content of $C_{32}H_{40}BrN_5O_5$ taking 144 as the value of A(1%, 1 cm) at the maximum at 305 nm.

Assay Weigh and powder 20 tablets. Carry out the Assay described under Bromocriptine Capsules but preparing solution (2) in the following manner. Mix a quantity of the powdered tablets containing the equivalent of 10 mg of bromocriptine with 70 ml of *methanol (50%)* with the aid of ultrasound for 5 minutes, shake for 30 minutes, filter and dilute to 100 ml with the same solvent mixture.

Storage Bromocriptine Tablets should be kept in an airtight container and protected from light.

Labelling The quantity of active ingredient is stated in terms of the equivalent amount of bromocriptine.

Brompheniramine Tablets

Definition Brompheniramine Tablets contain Brompheniramine Maleate.

The tablets comply with the requirements stated under Tablets and with the following requirements.

Content of brompheniramine maleate, $C_{16}H_{19}BrN_2$, $C_4H_4O_4$ 95.0 to 105.0% of the prescribed or stated amount.

Identification In the test for Related substances the retention time of the principal peak in the chromatogram obtained with solution (2) is similar to that of the principal peak in the chromatogram obtained with solution (3).

Related substances Carry out the method for *gas chromatography*, Appendix III B, using the following solutions. For solution (1) shake a quantity of the powdered tablets containing 20 mg of Brompheniramine Maleate with 5 ml of *water* for 5 minutes, make the resulting suspension alkaline by adding 13.5M *ammonia* dropwise, add 2.5 ml of *toluene*, shake for a further 5 minutes, centrifuge and use the upper, toluene layer. For solution (2) dilute 1 volume of solution (1) to 50 volumes with *dichloromethane*. Solution (3) is a 0.016% w/v solution of *brompheniramine maleate EPCRS* in *dichloromethane*. Solution (4) contains 0.5% w/v *brompheniramine maleate EPCRS* and 0.25% w/v *chlorphenamine maleate EPCRS* in *dichloromethane*.

The chromatographic procedure may be carried out using a glass column (2.3 m × 2 mm) packed with *acid- and base-washed, silanised diatomaceous support* (135 µm to 175 µm) (Chromosorb W AW-DMCS is suitable) impregnated with 3% w/w of *polymethylphenylsiloxane (50% phenyl)* (OV 17 is suitable) and maintaining the temperature of the column at 205° and that of the injection port and the detector at 250°.

Inject 1 µl of each solution. The test is not valid unless in the chromatogram obtained with solution (4) the *resolution factor* between the peaks corresponding to brompheniramine and chlorpheniramine is at least 1.5. After injecting solution (1), continue the chromatography for at least 2.5 times the retention time of the principal peak. In the chromatogram obtained with solution (1) the sum of the areas of any *secondary peaks* is not greater than 1% of the area of the principal peak and no *secondary peak* has an area greater than 0.4% of the area of the principal peak. Disregard any peak with an area less than 0.1% of that of the principal peak in the chromatogram obtained with solution (1).

Assay Weigh and powder 20 tablets. Shake a quantity of the powder containing 4 mg of Brompheniramine Maleate with 50 ml of *water* for 10 minutes, adjust the pH to 11.0 with 0.1M *sodium hydroxide* and cool to room temperature. Extract the mixture with two 75-ml quantities of *petroleum spirit (boiling range, 40° to 60°)*. Extract the combined extracts with three 50-ml quantities of 1M *hydrochloric acid*, combine the acidic extracts and add sufficient 1M *hydrochloric acid* to produce 200 ml. Measure the *absorbance* of the resulting solution at the maximum at 265 nm, Appendix II B. Calculate the content of $C_{16}H_{19}BrN_2,C_4H_4O_4$ taking 199 as the value of A(1%, 1 cm) at the maximum at 265 nm.

Storage Brompheniramine Tablets should be protected from light.

Buffered Cream

Definition

Emulsifying Ointment	300 g
Disodium Hydrogen Phosphate Dodecahydrate	25 g
Citric Acid Monohydrate	5 g
Chlorocresol	1 g
Purified Water, freshly boiled and cooled, sufficient to produce	1000 g

If another antimicrobial preservative replaces Chlorocresol in this formulation, the suitability of the Cream as a diluent should be confirmed before use.

Extemporaneous preparation Melt the Emulsifying Ointment with the aid of gentle heat. In a vessel that can be closed, heat about 650 g of Purified Water to about 60°; add the Chlorocresol and, when it melts, vigorously shake the closed vessel to effect dissolution. Dissolve the Disodium Hydrogen Phosphate Dodecahydrate and the Citric Acid Monohydrate in the chlorocresol solution. Add the aqueous phase to the melted ointment when both are at about 60°. Stir gently until cool, add sufficient Purified Water to produce 1000 g and mix.

The cream complies with the requirements stated under Topical Semi-solid Preparations and with the following requirements.

Acidity pH, 5.7 to 6.3, determined directly on the cream, Appendix V L.

Storage If Buffered Cream is kept in aluminium tubes, their inner surfaces should be coated with a suitable lacquer.

Bumetanide Injection

Definition Bumetanide Injection is a sterile solution of Bumetanide in Water for Injections.

The injection complies with the requirements stated under Parenteral Preparations and with the following requirements.

Content of bumetanide, $C_{17}H_{20}N_2O_5S$ 95.0 to 105.0% of the prescribed or stated amount.

Identification

A. Shake a quantity of the injection containing 10 mg of Bumetanide with 20 ml of *ether*, filter the ether layer through *anhydrous sodium sulphate* and evaporate to dryness using a rotary evaporator. The *infrared absorption spectrum* of the residue, Appendix II A, is concordant with the *reference spectrum* of bumetanide.

B. In the Assay, the retention time of the principal peak in the chromatogram obtained with solution (1) is similar to that of the principal peak in the chromatogram obtained with solution (2).

Acidity or alkalinity pH, 6.0 to 7.8, Appendix V L.

Related substances Carry out the method for *thin-layer chromatography*, Appendix III A, using a silica gel F_{254} precoated plate (Merck silica gel 60 F_{254} plates are suitable) and a mixture of 2.5 volumes of *methanol*, 10 volumes of *glacial acetic acid*, 10 volumes of *cyclohexane* and 80 volumes of *chloroform* as the mobile phase. Apply separately to the plate 25 µl of each of the following solutions. For solution (1) adjust the pH of a quantity of the injection containing 5 mg of Bumetanide to 12 using 0.1M *sodium hydroxide* and extract with two 20-ml quantities of *ether*. Discard the ether, adjust the pH to 4 using 1M *acetic acid*, extract with two further 20-ml quantities of *ether*, dry the ether by filtering through *anhydrous sodium sulphate*, wash the filter with 5 ml of *ether* and evaporate the combined filtrate and washings to dryness using a rotary evaporator. Dissolve the residue in 5 ml of *methanol* and centrifuge. Evaporate the supernatant liquid to dryness using a rotary evaporator and dissolve the residue in 0.5 ml of *methanol*. For solution (2) dilute 1 volume of solution (1) to 10 volumes with *methanol* and further dilute 1 volume of this solution to 30 volumes with *methanol*. For solution (3) dilute 1 volume of solution (2) to 3 volumes with *methanol*. Solution (4) contains 0.005% w/v of *3-amino-4-phenoxy-5-sulphamoylbenzoic acid BPCRS* in *methanol*. After removal of the plate, allow it to dry in air and examine under *ultraviolet light (365 nm)*. Any *secondary spot* in the chromatogram obtained with solution (1) corresponding to 3-amino-4-phenoxy-5-sulphamoylbenzoic acid is not more intense than the spot in the chromatogram obtained with solution (4) (0.5%), any other *secondary spot* is not more intense than the spot in the chromatogram obtained with solution (2) (0.3%) and not more than two other such spots are more intense than the spot in the chromatogram obtained with solution (3) (0.1%).

Assay Carry out the method for *liquid chromatography*, Appendix III D, using the following solutions. For solution (1) dilute a quantity of the injection containing 2.5 mg of Bumetanide to 20 ml using a mixture of 2 volumes of *glacial acetic acid*, 5 volumes of *tetrahydrofuran* and 45 volumes of *methanol*. For solution (2) dilute 10 ml of a 0.025% w/v solution of *bumetanide BPCRS* in a mixture of 2 volumes of *glacial acetic acid*, 5 volumes of *tetrahydrofuran* and 45 volumes of *methanol* to 20 ml with *water*. Inject 20 µl of each solution. Solution (3) contains 0.0125% w/v of *3-amino-4-phenoxy-5-sulphamoylbenzoic acid BPCRS* in solution (2).

The chromatographic procedure may be carried out using (a) a stainless steel column (30 cm × 4 mm) packed with *stationary phase C* (10 µm) (µBondapak ODS is suitable), (b) a mixture of 2 volumes of *glacial acetic acid*, 5 volumes of *tetrahydrofuran*, 45 volumes of *water* and 50 volumes of *methanol* as the mobile phase with a flow rate of 1 ml per minute and (c) a detection wavelength of 254 nm.

The Assay is not valid unless, in the chromatogram obtained with solution (3), the *resolution factor* between the two principal peaks is at least 15.

Calculate the content of $C_{17}H_{20}N_2O_5S$ using the declared content of $C_{17}H_{20}N_2O_5S$ in *bumetanide BPCRS*.

Bumetanide Oral Solution

Definition Bumetanide Oral Solution is a solution of Bumetanide in a suitable flavoured vehicle.

The oral solution complies with the requirements stated under Oral Liquids and with the following requirements.

Content of bumetanide, $C_{17}H_{20}N_2O_5S$ 95.0 to 105.0% of the prescribed or stated amount.

Identification

A. In the test for Related substances, the principal spot in the chromatogram obtained with solution (2) corresponds to that in the chromatogram obtained with solution (5).

B. In the Assay, the retention time of the principal peak in the chromatogram obtained with solution (1) is similar to that of the peak in the chromatogram obtained with solution (2).

Related substances Carry out the method for *thin-layer chromatography*, Appendix III A, using a silica gel F_{254} precoated plate (Merck silica gel 60 F_{254} plates are suitable) and a mixture of 2.5 volumes of *methanol*, 10 volumes of *glacial acetic acid*, 10 volumes of *cyclohexane* and 80 volumes of *chloroform* as the mobile phase. Apply separately to the plate 25 µl of each of the following solutions. For solution (1) mix a quantity of the oral solution containing 2 mg of Bumetanide with 10 ml of *water* and 0.6 ml of 1M *hydrochloric acid*, add 5 ml of *ethyl acetate*, shake for 15 minutes, centrifuge and decant the ethyl acetate. Add a further 5 ml of *ethyl acetate* to the residue, shake for 15 minutes, centrifuge and decant the ethyl acetate. Evaporate the combined ethyl acetate extracts to dryness using a rotary evaporator and dissolve the residue in 0.5 ml of *methanol*. For solution (2) dilute 1 volume of solution (1) to 10 volumes with *methanol*. For solution (3) dilute 1 volume of solution (2) to 10 volumes with *methanol* and further dilute 1 volume of this solution to 3 volumes with *methanol*. For solution (4) dilute 1 volume of solution (2) to 100 volumes with *methanol*. Solution (5) contains 0.040% w/v of *bumetanide BPCRS* in *methanol*. Solution (6) contains 0.002% w/v of *3-amino-4-phenoxy-5-sulphamoylbenzoic acid BPCRS* in *methanol*. After removal of the plate, allow it to dry in air and examine under *ultraviolet light (365 nm)*. Any *secondary spot* in the chromatogram obtained with solution (1) corresponding to 3-amino-4-phenoxy-5-sulphamoylbenzoic acid is not more intense than the spot in the chromatogram obtained with solution (6) (0.5%), any other *secondary spot* is not more intense than the spot in the chromatogram obtained with solution (3) (0.3%) and not more than two other such spots are more intense than the spot in the chromatogram obtained with solution (4) (0.1%).

Assay Carry out the method for *liquid chromatography*, Appendix III D, using the following solutions. For solution (1) mix a quantity of the oral solution containing 2.5 mg of Bumetanide with 12.5 ml of *water* and 0.8 ml of 1M *hydrochloric acid*, add 10 ml of *ethyl acetate*, shake for 15 minutes, centrifuge and decant the ethyl acetate. Repeat the extraction procedure twice using a further two 10-ml quantitites of *ethyl acetate* and beginning at the words 'add 10 ml of ... '. Evaporate the combined ethyl acetate extracts to dryness using a rotary evaporator, dissolve the residue in 10 ml of a mixture of 2 volumes of *glacial acetic acid*, 5 volumes of *tetrahydrofuran* and 45 volumes of *methanol* and dilute to 20 ml with *water*. For solution (2) dilute 5 ml of a 0.025% w/v solution of *bumetanide BPCRS* in a mixture of 2 volumes of *glacial acetic acid*, 5 volumes of *tetrahydrofuran* and 45 volumes of *methanol* and dilute to 10 ml with *water*. Inject 20 µl of each solution. Solution (3) contains 0.0125% w/v of *3-amino-4-phenoxy-5-sulphamoylbenzoic acid BPCRS* in solution (2).

The chromatographic procedure may be carried out using (a) a stainless steel column (30 cm × 4 mm) packed with *stationary phase C* (10 µm) (µBondapak ODS is suitable), (b) a mixture of 2 volumes of *glacial acetic acid*, 5 volumes of *tetrahydrofuran*, 45 volumes of *water* and 50 volumes of *methanol* as the mobile phase with a flow rate of 1 ml per minute and (c) a detection wavelength of 254 nm.

The Assay is not valid unless, in the chromatogram obtained with solution (3), the *resolution factor* between the two principal peaks is at least 15.

Determine the *weight per ml* of the oral solution, Appendix V G, and calculate the content of $C_{17}H_{20}N_2O_5S$, weight in volume, using the declared content of $C_{17}H_{20}N_2O_5S$ in *bumetanide BPCRS*.

Bumetanide Tablets

Definition Bumetanide Tablets contain Bumetanide.

The tablets comply with the requirements stated under Tablets and with the following requirements.

Content of bumetanide, $C_{17}H_{20}N_2O_5S$ 95.0 to 105.0% of the prescribed or stated amount.

Identification

A. Shake a quantity of the powdered tablets containing 50 mg of Bumetanide with 25 ml of *ether*, filter through *anhydrous sodium sulphate* and evaporate the filtrate to dryness using a rotary evaporator. The *infrared absorption spectrum* of the residue, Appendix II A, is concordant with the *reference spectrum* of bumetanide.

B. In the Assay, the retention time of the principal peak in the chromatogram obtained with solution (1) is similar to that of the peak in the chromatogram obtained with solution (2).

Related substances Carry out the method for *thin-layer chromatography*, Appendix III A, using a silica gel F_{254} precoated plate (Merck silica gel 60 F_{254} plates are suitable) and a mixture of 2.5 volumes of *methanol*, 10 volumes of *glacial acetic acid*, 10 volumes of *cyclohexane* and 80 volumes of *chloroform* as the mobile phase. Apply separately to the plate 10 µl of each of the following solutions. For solution (1) shake mechanically a quantity of the powdered tablets containing 12.5 mg of Bumetanide with 25 ml of *acetone* for 10 minutes, centrifuge for 10 minutes, evaporate the supernatant liquid to dryness using a rotary evaporator and dissolve the residue in 0.5 ml of *methanol*. For solution (2) dilute 1 volume of solution (1) to 100 volumes with *methanol* and further dilute 3 volumes of this solution to 10 volumes with *methanol*. For solution (3) dilute 1 volume of solution (1) to 10 volumes with *methanol* and further dilute 1 volume of this solution to 100 volumes with *methanol*. After removal of the plate, allow it to dry in air and examine under *ultraviolet light (254 nm)*. Any *secondary spot* in the chromatogram obtained with solution (1) is not more intense than the spot in the chromatogram obtained with solution (2) (0.3%) and not more than three such spots are more intense than the spot in the chromatogram obtained with solution (3) (0.1%).

Uniformity of content Tablets containing less than 2 mg of Bumetanide comply with the requirements stated under Tablets using the following method of analysis. Carry out the method for *liquid chromatography*, Appendix III D, using the following solutions. For solution (1) dissolve one tablet in 10 ml of a mixture of 2 volumes of *glacial acetic acid*, 5 volumes of *tetrahydrofuran* and 45 volumes of *methanol*, shake with the aid of ultrasound for 5 minutes, dilute to 20 ml with *water*, filter and use the filtrate. For solution (2) dilute 10 ml of a 0.010% w/v solution of *bumetanide BPCRS* in a mixture of 2 volumes of *glacial acetic acid*, 5 volumes of *tetrahydrofuran* and 45 volumes of *methanol* to 20 ml with *water*.

The chromatographic procedure described under Assay may be used.

Calculate the content of $C_{17}H_{20}N_2O_5S$ in each tablet using the declared content of $C_{17}H_{20}N_2O_5S$ in *bumetanide BPCRS*.

Assay Carry out the method for *liquid chromatography*, Appendix III D, using the following solutions. For solution (1) dissolve a quantity of the powdered tablets containing 2.5 mg of Bumetanide in 10 ml of a mixture of 2 volumes of *glacial acetic acid*, 5 volumes of *tetrahydrofuran* and 45 volumes of *methanol*, shake with the aid of ultrasound for 5 minutes, dilute to 20 ml with *water*, filter and use the filtrate. For solution (2) dilute 10 ml of a 0.025% w/v solution of *bumetanide BPCRS* in a mixture of 2 volumes of *glacial acetic acid*, 5 volumes of *tetrahydrofuran* and 45 volumes of *methanol* to 20 ml with *water*. Inject 20 µl of each solution. Solution (3) contains 0.0125% w/v of *3-amino-4-phenoxy-5-sulphamoylbenzoic acid BPCRS* in solution (2).

The chromatographic procedure may be carried out using (a) a stainless steel column (30 cm × 4 mm) packed with *stationary phase C* (10 µm) (µBondapak ODS is suitable), (b) a mixture of 2 volumes of *glacial acetic acid*, 5 volumes of *tetrahydrofuran*, 45 volumes of *water* and 50 volumes of *methanol* as the mobile phase with a flow rate of 1 ml per minute and (c) a detection wavelength of 254 nm.

The Assay is not valid unless, in the chromatogram obtained with solution (3), the *resolution factor* between the two principal peaks is at least 15.

Calculate the content of $C_{17}H_{20}N_2O_5S$ using the declared content of $C_{17}H_{20}N_2O_5S$ in *bumetanide BPCRS*.

Bumetanide and Slow Potassium Tablets

Definition Bumetanide and Slow Potassium Tablets contain Bumetanide and Potassium Chloride. They are formulated so that the Potassium Chloride is released over a period of several hours.

With the exception of the requirements for shape, the tablets comply with the requirements stated under Tablets and with the following requirements.

Content of bumetanide, $C_{17}H_{20}N_2O_5S$ 92.5 to 107.5% of the prescribed or stated amount.

Content of potassium chloride, KCl 95.0 to 105.0% of the prescribed or stated amount.

Identification

A. In the test for Related substances the spot in the chromatogram obtained with solution (1) is similar in position, size and intensity to the spot in the chromatogram obtained with solution (2).

B. Examine the filtrate obtained in the test for Uniformity of content by *fluorescence spectrophotometry*, Appendix II E, using an excitation wavelength of 350 nm. The solution emits light at 445 nm.

C. Dissolve a quantity of the powdered tablets containing 0.1 g of Potassium Chloride as completely as possible in 2 ml of *water* and filter. The filtrate yields reaction A characteristic of *potassium salts*, Appendix VI.

D. Dissolve a quantity of the powdered tablets containing 0.02 g of Potassium Chloride as completely as possible in 2 ml of *water* and filter. The filtrate yields reaction A characteristic of *chlorides*, Appendix VI.

Dissolution

For bumetanide Comply with the *dissolution test for tablets and capsules*, Appendix XII D, using Apparatus II. Use as the medium 900 ml of *water* and rotate the paddle at 100 revolutions per minute. Withdraw a sample of 10 ml of the medium, filter and measure the *fluorescence*, Appendix II E, using an excitation wavelength of 350 nm and an emission wavelength of 445 nm and *water* in the reference cell. Measure the *fluorescence* of a 0.04% w/v solution of *bumetanide BPCRS* in *ethanol (96%)* diluted to a suitable concentration with *water* under the same conditions and calculate the total content of $C_{17}H_{20}N_2O_5S$ in the medium from the fluorescences obtained and from the declared content of $C_{17}H_{20}N_2O_5S$ in *bumetanide BPCRS*.

For potassium chloride Carry out the *dissolution test for tablets and capsules*, Appendix XII D, using Apparatus II. Use as the medium 900 ml of *water* and rotate the paddle at 100 revolutions per minute. Withdraw a sample of 10 ml of the medium after 1, 2 and 6 hours and treat each sample in the following manner. Add to the sample 25 ml of *water*, 5 ml of a 25% v/v solution of *acetic acid* and 0.1 ml of a saturated solution of *potassium sulphate*. Titrate with 0.01M *silver nitrate VS* determining the end point potentiometrically. Each ml of 0.01M *silver nitrate VS* is equivalent to 0.7455 mg of KCl. The amount of potassium chloride released after 1 hour is not more than 50%, after 2 hours is not less than 25% and not more than 75% and after 6 hours is not less than 75%, calculated with reference to the declared content of Potassium Chloride.

Related substances Carry out the method for *thin-layer chromatography*, Appendix III A, using a high-performance silica gel F_{254} plate (Merck 5629 plates are suitable) and a mixture of 2.5 volumes of *methanol*, 10 volumes of *glacial acetic acid*, 10 volumes of *cyclohexane* and 80 volumes of *chloroform* as the mobile phase but allowing the solvent front to ascend 8 cm above the line of application. Apply separately to the plate 10 µl of each of solutions (1) and (2) and 5 µl of solution (3). For solution (1) add 10 ml of a 0.1% w/v solution of *citric acid* to a number of whole tablets containing, in total, 1 mg of Bumetanide, shake for 10 minutes, remove and discard the cores, extract the solution with two 20-ml quantities of *ether*, evaporate the combined extracts to dryness under reduced pressure and dissolve the residue in 0.5 ml of *ethyl acetate*. For solution (2) add 2 ml of a 0.20% w/v solution of *bumetanide BPCRS* in *ethyl acetate* to 10 ml of a 0.1% w/v solution of *citric acid*, shake for 15 minutes, centrifuge and use the ethyl acetate layer. For solution (3) mix 1 ml of a 0.20% w/v solution of *3-amino-4-phenoxy-5-sulphamoylbenzoic acid BPCRS* in *ethyl acetate* and 1 ml of a 0.20% w/v solution of *bumetanide BPCRS* in *ethyl acetate*, add sufficient *ethyl acetate* to produce 100 ml, add 2 ml of this solution to 10 ml of a 0.1% w/v solution of *citric acid*, shake for 15 minutes and use the ethyl acetate layer. After removal of the plate, allow it to dry in air and examine under *ultraviolet light (365 nm)*. Any *secondary spot* in the chromatogram obtained with solution (1) corresponding to 3-amino-4-phenoxy-5-sulphamoylbenzoic acid is not more intense than the corresponding spot in the chromatogram obtained with solution (3) (0.5%) and any other *secondary spot* is not more intense than the spot due to bumetanide in the chromatogram obtained with solution (3) (0.5%).

Uniformity of content Tablets containing less than 2 mg of Bumetanide comply with the requirements stated below. Carry out the method for *liquid chromatography*, Appendix III D, using the following solutions. For solution (1) shake one tablet in 0.5 ml of *methanol* for 3 minutes, add 9 ml of the mobile phase and shake for 30 minutes. Filter to remove the tablet core, add sufficient of the mobile phase to produce 10 ml, centrifuge for 15 minutes and use the supernatant liquid. If the supernatant liquid is cloudy, filter through a 0.45-µm membrane filter (Millipore Millex is suitable), discarding the first 2 ml of filtrate. For solution (2) dilute 5 ml of a 0.1% w/v solution of *bumetanide BPCRS* in *methanol* to 100 ml with the mobile phase.

The chromatographic procedure described under Assay may be used.

Calculate the content of $C_{17}H_{20}N_2O_5S$ in each tablet using the declared content of $C_{17}H_{20}N_2O_5S$ in *bumetanide BPCRS*. The tablets comply with the test if not more than one of the individual values is outside the range 85% to 115% of the average value and none is outside the limits 75% to 125% of the average value. If two or three individual values are outside the limits 85% to 115% of the average value and none is outside the limits 75% to 125%, repeat the determination on a further 20 tablets taken at random. The tablets comply with the test if in the total number of tablets tested not more than three individual values are outside the limits 85% to 115% and none is outside the limits 75% to 125% of the average value.

Assay

For bumetanide Carry out the method for *liquid chromatography*, Appendix III D, using the following solutions. For solution (1) shake a number of whole tablets containing 5 mg of Bumetanide in 5 ml of *methanol* for 3 minutes, add 90 ml of the mobile phase and shake for 30 minutes. Filter to remove the tablet cores, add sufficient of the mobile phase to produce 100 ml, centrifuge for 15 minutes and use the supernatant liquid. If the supernatant liquid is cloudy, filter through a 0.45-µm membrane filter (Millipore Millex is suitable), discarding the first 2 ml of filtrate. For solution (2) dilute 5 ml of a 0.1% w/v solution of *bumetanide BPCRS* in *methanol* to 100 ml with the mobile phase. Solution (3) contains 0.005% w/v of *3-amino-4-phenoxy-5-sulphamoylbenzoic acid BPCRS* in solution (2).

The chromatographic procedure may be carried out using (a) a stainless steel column (12.5 cm × 4 mm) packed with *stationary phase C* (5 µm) (Lichrospher 100 RP-18 is suitable), (b) a mixture of 2 volumes of *glacial acetic acid*, 5 volumes of *tetrahydrofuran*, 45 volumes of *water* and 50 volumes of *methanol* as the mobile phase with a flow rate of 1 ml per minute and (c) a detection wavelength of 254 nm. Inject separately 20 µl of each solution.

The Assay is not valid unless, in the chromatogram obtained with solution (3), the *resolution factor* between the two principal peaks is at least 15.

Calculate the content of $C_{17}H_{20}N_2O_5S$ in the tablets using the declared content of $C_{17}H_{20}N_2O_5S$ in *bumetanide BPCRS*.

Labelling The label states that the tablets should be swallowed whole and not chewed.

Bupivacaine Injection

Definition Bupivacaine Injection is a sterile solution of Bupivacaine Hydrochloride in Water for Injections.

The injection complies with the requirements stated under Parenteral Preparations and with the following requirements.

Content of anhydrous bupivacaine hydrochloride, $C_{18}H_{28}N_2O,HCl$ 92.5 to 107.5% of the prescribed or stated amount.

Characteristics A colourless or almost colourless solution.

Identification

A. To a volume of the injection containing the equivalent of 25 mg of anhydrous bupivacaine hydrochloride add 2 ml of 13.5M *ammonia*, shake and filter. Wash the precipitate with *water* and dry at 60° at a pressure of 2 kPa for 16 hours. The *infrared absorption spectrum* of the dried residue, Appendix II A, is concordant with the *reference spectrum* of bupivacaine.

B. To a volume of the injection containing the equivalent of 50 mg of anhydrous bupivacaine hydrochloride add 2 ml of a 10% w/v solution of *disodium hydrogen orthophosphate* and sufficient *iodinated potassium iodide solution* to produce a distinct brown colour. Remove the excess iodine by adding 0.1M *sodium thiosulphate*. No pink colour is produced.

Acidity pH, 4.0 to 6.5, Appendix V L.

2,6-Dimethylaniline To a volume of the injection containing the equivalent of 25 mg of anhydrous bupivacaine hydrochloride add sufficient *water*, if necessary, to produce 10 ml, add 2M *sodium hydroxide* until the solution is just alkaline and extract with three 5-ml quantities of *chloroform*. Dry the combined chloroform extracts over *anhydrous sodium sulphate*, filter, wash with a further 5 ml of *chloroform* and evaporate the filtrate to dryness using a rotary evaporator. Dissolve the residue in 2 ml of *methanol*, add 1 ml of a 1% w/v solution of *4-dimethylaminobenzaldehyde* in *methanol* and 2 ml of *glacial acetic acid* and allow to stand at room temperature for 10 minutes. The yellow colour produced is not more intense than the colour produced by repeating the operation using 10 ml of a solution in *water* containing 1 µg of *2,6-dimethylaniline* per ml in place of the injection (400 ppm).

Related bases Carry out the method for *thin-layer chromatography*, Appendix III A, using *silica gel G* as the coating substance and a mixture of 0.1 volume of 13.5M *ammonia* and 100 volumes of *methanol* as the mobile phase but allowing the solvent front to ascend 10 cm above the line of application. Apply separately to the plate 10 µl of each of the following solutions. For solution (1) evaporate a volume of the injection containing the equivalent of 0.1 g of anhydrous bupivacaine hydrochloride using a rotary evaporator, add sufficient *methanol* to the residue to produce 2 ml, mix, centrifuge and use the supernatant liquid. For solution (2) dilute 1 volume of solution (1) to 100 volumes with *methanol*. After removal of the plate, allow it to dry in air and spray with *dilute potassium iodobismuthate solution*. Any *secondary spot* in the chromatogram obtained with solution (1) is not more intense than the spot in the chromatogram obtained with solution (2) (1%).

Assay Carry out the method for *liquid chromatography*, Appendix III D, using the following solutions. For solution (1) dilute a quantity of the injection with sufficient of the mobile phase to produce a solution containing 0.0025% w/v of anhydrous bupivacaine hydrochloride. Solution (2) contains 0.0025% w/v of *bupivacaine hydrochloride BPCRS* in the mobile phase. For solution (3) prepare a 0.1% w/v solution of *2,6-dimethylaniline* in *acetonitrile*, dilute 10 volumes to 20 volumes with the mobile phase and then dilute 1 volume of the resulting solution to 100 volumes with solution (2).

The chromatographic procedure may be carried out using (a) a stainless steel column (30 cm × 3.9 mm) packed with *stationary phase C* (10 µm) (µBondapak C18 is suitable), (b) a mixture of 40 volumes of *phosphate buffer pH 8.0* and 60 volumes of *acetonitrile* as the mobile phase with a flow rate of 1 ml per minute and (c) a detection wavelength of 240 nm. Inject 20 µl of each solution.

The test is not valid unless in the chromatogram obtained with solution (3) the *resolution factor* between the two principal peaks is at least 8.

Calculate the content of $C_{18}H_{28}N_2O,HCl$ in the injection using the declared content of $C_{18}H_{28}N_2O,HCl$ in *bupivacaine hydrochloride BPCRS*.

Labelling The strength is stated in terms of the equivalent amount of anhydrous bupivacaine hydrochloride in a suitable dose-volume.

Bupivacaine and Adrenaline Injection
Bupivacaine and Epinephrine Injection

For the purposes of product labelling in the United Kingdom, the pair of names given above shall be used together (see Introduction, Changes in title).

Definition Bupivacaine and Adrenaline Injection is a sterile solution of Bupivacaine Hydrochloride and Adrenaline Acid Tartrate in Water for Injections.

The injection complies with the requirements stated under Parenteral Preparations and with the following requirements.

Content of anhydrous bupivacaine hydrochloride, $C_{18}H_{28}N_2O,HCl$ 92.5 to 107.5% of the prescribed or stated amount.

Content of adrenaline, $C_9H_{13}NO_3$ 80.0 to 120.0% of the prescribed or stated amount.

Characteristics A colourless or almost colourless solution.

Identification

A. Carry out the method for *thin-layer chromatography*, Appendix III A, using a silica gel pre-coated plate (Merck silica gel G60 plates are suitable) and a mixture of 5 volumes of *methanol* and 95 volumes of *dichloromethane* as the mobile phase. Apply separately to the plate 5 µl of each of the following solutions. For solution (1) dilute a quantity of the injection, if necessary, with *water* to produce a solution containing 0.2% w/v of Bupivacaine Hydrochloride. Solution (2) contains 0.2% w/v of *bupivacaine hydrochloride BPCRS* in *water*. Solution (3) contains 0.2% w/v of *bupivacaine hydrochloride BPCRS* and 0.2% w/v of *lidocaine hydrochloride BPCRS* in *water*. After removal of the plate, dry it in a current of cold air, heat at 110° for 1 hour, place the hot plate in a tank of chlorine gas prepared by the addition of *hydrochloric acid* to a 5% w/v solution of *potassium permanganate* contained in a beaker placed in the tank and allow to stand for 2 minutes. Dry the plate in a current of cold air until an area of the plate below the line of application gives at most a very faint blue colour with a 0.5% w/v solution of *potassium iodide* in *starch mucilage*; avoid prolonged exposure to cold air. Spray the plate with a 0.5% w/v solution of *potassium iodide* in *starch mucilage*. The principal spot in the chromatogram obtained with solution (1) corresponds to that in the chromatogram obtained with solution (2). The test is not valid unless the chromatogram obtained with solution (3) shows two clearly separated principal spots.

B. In the Assay for adrenaline, the chromatogram obtained with solution (2) shows a peak with the same retention time as the principal peak in the chromatogram obtained with solution (1).

Acidity pH, 3.0 to 5.5, Appendix V L.

2,6-Dimethylaniline; Related bases Complies with the requirements stated under Bupivacaine Injection.

Assay

For anhydrous bupivacaine hydrochloride Carry out the Assay described under Bupivacaine Injection.

For adrenaline Dissolve 8.0 g of *tetramethylammonium hydrogen sulphate*, 2.2 g of *sodium heptanesulphonate* and 2 ml of 0.1M *disodium edetate* in a mixture of 900 ml of *water* and 100 ml of *methanol*, adjust the pH to 3.5 with 1M *sodium hydroxide* and filter through glass microfibre paper under reduced pressure (solution A). Carry out the method for *liquid chromatography*, Appendix III D, using the following solutions. For solution (1) dilute 5 ml of a 0.001% w/v solution of *adrenaline acid tartrate BPCRS* to 10 ml with solution A. For solution (2) dilute the injection, if necessary, to produce a solution containing the equivalent of 0.0005% w/v of adrenaline and dilute 5 ml of the resulting solution to 10 ml with solution A. For solution (3) mix 5 ml of solution (1) with 5 ml of a 0.001% w/v solution of *noradrenaline acid tartrate* in the mobile phase.

The chromatographic procedure may be carried out using (a) a stainless steel column (10 cm × 4.6 mm) packed with *stationary phase C* (5 μm) (Nucleosil C18 is suitable), (b) as the mobile phase with a flow rate of 2 ml per minute a solution prepared by adding 4.0 g of *tetramethylammonium hydrogen sulphate*, 1.1 g of *sodium heptanesulphonate* and 2 ml of 0.1M *disodium edetate* to a mixture of 950 ml of *water* and 50 ml of *methanol* and adjusting the pH of the mixture to 3.5 with 1M *sodium hydroxide* and (c) a detection wavelength of 205 nm.

The test is not valid unless the *resolution factor* between the two principal peaks in the chromatogram obtained with solution (3) is at least 2.0.

Calculate the content of $C_9H_{13}NO_3$ in the injection using the declared content of $C_9H_{13}NO_3$ in *adrenaline acid tartrate BPCRS*.

Storage Bupivacaine and Adrenaline Injection should be protected from light.

Labelling The label states 'Bupivacaine and Adrenaline Injection' and 'Bupivacaine and Epinephrine Injection'.

The quantities of the active ingredients are stated in terms of the equivalent amounts of anhydrous bupivacaine hydrochloride and adrenaline (epinephrine).

Busulfan Tablets

Definition Busulfan Tablets contain Busulfan. They are coated.

The tablets comply with the requirements stated under Tablets and with the following requirements.

Content of busulfan, $C_6H_{14}O_6S_2$ 90.0 to 115.0% of the prescribed or stated amount.

Identification

A. Shake a quantity of the powdered tablets containing 10 mg of Busulfan with 10 ml of hot *acetone*, filter and evaporate the filtrate to dryness. Dry the residue at 60° at a pressure not exceeding 0.7 kPa for 1 hour. The *infrared absorption spectrum* of the residue, Appendix II A, is concordant with the *reference spectrum* of busulfan.

B. In the Assay the retention time of the principal peak in the chromatogram obtained with solution (3) is similar to that of the principal peak in the chromatogram obtained with solution (1).

Disintegration Maximum time, 15 minutes, Appendix XII A.

Uniformity or content Tablets containing less than 2 mg of Busulfan comply with the requirements stated under Tablets using the following method of analysis. Carry out the method for *gas chromatography*, Appendix III B, using the following solutions. Prepare a 0.0001% w/v solution of *1,5-di-iodopentane* (internal standard) in *acetone* (solution A). For solution (1) add 5 ml of a 30% w/v solution of *sodium iodide* in *acetone* to 5 ml of a 0.0001% w/v solution of *busulfan BPCRS* in *acetone*, stopper the flask lightly and heat in a water bath at 50° for 90 minutes. Cool, add 10 ml of solution A, mix, add 10 ml of *water* and 20 ml of *hexane*, shake vigorously for 1 minute and allow to separate. Use the hexane layer. Prepare solution (2) in the same manner as solution (3) but using 10 ml of *acetone* in place of solution A. For solution (3) add 1 ml of *water* to one tablet in a 50-ml graduated flask and mix with the aid of ultrasound until completely dispersed. Add 30 ml of *acetone*, shake for 15 minutes and dilute to 50 ml with *acetone*. Centrifuge and dilute a quantity of the supernatant liquid with *acetone* to produce a solution containing 0.0001% w/v of Busulfan. To 5 ml of the resulting solution add 5 ml of a 30% w/v solution of *sodium iodide* in *acetone*, stopper the flask lightly and heat in a water bath at 50° for 90 minutes. Cool, add 10 ml of solution A, mix, add 10 ml of *water* and 20 ml of *hexane*, shake vigorously for 1 minute and allow to separate. Use the hexane layer.

The chromatographic procedure may be carried out using a glass column (1.5 m × 4 mm) packed with *acid-washed, diatomaceous support* (80 to 100 mesh) coated with 3% w/w of phenyl methyl silicone fluid (50% phenyl) (OV-17 is suitable) and maintained at 140° with an electron capture detector.

Calculate the content of $C_6H_{14}O_6S_2$ using the declared content of $C_6H_{14}O_6S_2$ in *busulfan BPCRS*.

Assay Weigh and powder 20 tablets. Carry out the method of analysis described under Uniformity of content but prepare solution (3) in the following manner. Add 5 ml of *water* to a quantity of powdered tablets containing 2.5 mg of Busulfan and mix with the aid of ultrasound until completely dispersed. Add 150 ml of *acetone*, shake for 15 minutes and dilute to 250 ml with *acetone*. Centrifuge and dilute 10 ml of the supernatant liquid to 100 ml with *acetone*. To 5 ml of the resulting solution add 5 ml of a 30% w/v solution of *sodium iodide* in *acetone*, stopper the flask lightly and heat in a water bath at 50° for 90 minutes. Cool, add 10 ml of solution A, mix, add 10 ml of *water* and 20 ml of *hexane*, shake vigorously for 1 minute and allow to separate. Use the hexane layer.

Calculate the content of $C_6H_{14}O_6S_2$ using the declared content of $C_6H_{14}O_6S_2$ in *busulfan BPCRS*.

When busulphan tablets are prescribed or demanded, Busulfan Tablets shall be dispensed or supplied.

Aqueous Calamine Cream

Definition Aqueous Calamine Cream contains 4% w/w of Calamine and 3% w/w of Zinc Oxide in a suitable oil-in-water emulsified basis.

Extemporaneous preparation The following formula and directions apply.

Calamine	40 g
Zinc Oxide	30 g
Liquid Paraffin	200 g
Self-emulsifying Glyceryl Monostearate	50 g
Cetomacrogol Emulsifying Wax	50 g
Phenoxyethanol	5 g
Purified Water, freshly boiled and cooled,	sufficient to produce 1000 g

Melt the Cetomacrogol Emulsifying Wax with the Self-emulsifying Glyceryl Monostearate, add the Liquid Paraffin and heat to about 60°. Dissolve the Phenoxyethanol in about 620 g of Purified Water at about 60°, add the oily phase to the phenoxyethanol solution and mix. Stir until cool, add sufficient Purified Water to produce 930 g and mix. Triturate the Calamine and the Zinc Oxide and incorporate in the cream.

The cream complies with the requirements stated under Topical Semi-solid Preparations and with the following requirements.

Content of zinc, Zn 4.3 to 5.2% w/w.

Identification The residue obtained in the Assay is yellow when hot and white when cool.

Assay Gently heat 4 g, taking precautions to avoid loss caused by spitting, until the basis is completely volatilised or charred, increase the temperature until the carbon is removed and ignite the residue to constant weight. Each g of residue is equivalent to 0.8034 g of Zn.

Calamine Lotion

Definition

Calamine Lotion is a *cutaneous suspension.*

Calamine	150 g
Zinc Oxide	50 g
Bentonite	30 g
Sodium Citrate	5 g
Liquefied Phenol	5 ml
Glycerol	50 ml
Purified Water, freshly boiled and cooled	sufficient to produce 1000 ml

Extemporaneous preparation The following directions apply.

Triturate the Calamine, the Zinc Oxide and the Bentonite with a solution of the Sodium Citrate in about 700 ml of the Purified Water and add the Liquefied Phenol, the Glycerol and sufficient Purified Water to produce 1000 ml.

The lotion complies with the requirements stated under Liquids for Cutaneous Application and with the following requirements.

Identification

A. To 2 ml add 2 ml of *periodic acid reagent*, shake, centrifuge and add 0.5 ml of the supernatant liquid to 2 ml of *ammoniacal silver nitrate solution* in a test tube. A silver mirror is produced on the side of the tube.

B. Mix 2 ml with 50 ml of *water*, centrifuge and decant the supernatant liquid. Suspend the residue in 20 ml of *water*, add 1 ml of *hydrochloric acid*, mix and filter. 5 ml of the filtrate, after neutralisation by dropwise addition of 2M *sodium hydroxide*, yields the reaction characteristic of *zinc salts*, Appendix VI.

Residue on ignition 14.5 to 18.0% w/w when determined by the following method. Evaporate 5 g to dryness and ignite until, after further ignition, two successive weighings do not differ by more than 0.2% of the weight of the residue.

Labelling The label indicates the pharmaceutical form as 'cutaneous suspension'.

Calamine Ointment

Definition Calamine Ointment contains 15% w/w of Calamine in a suitable hydrophobic basis.

Extemporaneous preparation The following formula and directions apply.

Calamine, finely sifted	150 g
White Soft Paraffin	850 g

Triturate the Calamine with part of the White Soft Paraffin until smooth and gradually incorporate the remainder of the White Soft Paraffin.

The ointment complies with the requirements stated under Topical Semi-solid Preparations and with the following requirements.

Content of zinc, Zn 7.8 to 9.4% w/w.

Identification The residue obtained in the Assay is yellow when hot and white when cool.

Assay Gently heat 1 g until the basis is completely volatilised or charred, increase the heat until all the carbon is removed and ignite the residue until, after further ignition, two successive weighings do not differ by more than 0.2% of the weight of the residue. Each g of residue is equivalent to 0.8034 g of Zn.

Calamine and Coal Tar Ointment

Compound Calamine Ointment

Definition Calamine and Coal Tar Ointment contains 12.5% w/w each of Calamine and Zinc Oxide and 2.5% w/w of Strong Coal Tar Solution in a suitable water-emulsifying basis.

Extemporaneous preparation The following formula and directions apply.

Calamine, finely sifted	125 g
Zinc Oxide, finely sifted	125 g
Strong Coal Tar Solution	25 g
Hydrous Wool Fat	250 g
White Soft Paraffin	475 g

Melt together the Hydrous Wool Fat and the White Soft Paraffin. Triturate the Calamine and Zinc Oxide in the melted basis and stir gently, when cooled, to about 40°.

Gradually incorporate the Strong Coal Tar Solution and stiruntil cold.

The ointment complies with the requirements stated under Topical Semi-solid Preparations and with the following requirements.

Content of zinc compounds, calculated as ZnO 19.8 to 22.8% w/w.

Identification The residue obtained in the Assay is yellow when hot and white when cool.

Assay Gently heat 1 g until the basis is completely volatilised or charred. Increase the heat until the carbon is removed and ignite the residue of ZnO until, after further ignition, two successive weighings do not differ by more than0.2% of the weight of the residue. Each g of residue is equivalent to 0.8034 g of Zn.

Storage Calamine and Coal Tar Ointment should be kept in a container that minimises evaporation losses.

Calciferol Injection

Definition Calciferol Injection is a sterile solution containing 0.75% w/v of Colecalciferol or Ergocalciferol in Ethyl Oleate.

The title Colecalciferol Injection may be used for an injection containing Colecalciferol and the title Ergocalciferol Injection may be used for an injection containing Ergocalciferol.

The injection complies with the requirements stated under Parenteral Preparations and with the following requirements.

Content of colecalciferol or ergocalciferol 0.67 to 0.83% w/v.

Characteristics A pale yellow, oily liquid.

Identification To 1 ml of a 0.2% v/v solution of the injection in *ethanol-free chloroform* add 9 ml of *antimony trichloride solution*. The *light absorption* of the resulting solution, Appendix II B, exhibits a maximum at 500 nm.

Assay Carry out the following procedure in subdued light. Dilute 0.1 g of the injection to 50 ml with dry *1,2-dichloroethane* that has been purified by passing it through a column of *silica gel*. To 1 ml of this solution add rapidly 9 ml of *antimony trichloride in 1,2-dichloroethane solution* and measure the *absorbance* of the solution at 500 and 550 nm, Appendix II B, 90 to 120 seconds after adding the reagent. Repeat the operation using 1 ml of a 0.002% w/v solution of *cholecalciferol EPCRS* or *ergocalciferol EPCRS* in the dry, purified 1,2-dichloroethane, beginning at the words 'add rapidly 9 ml of ... '. Calculate the result of the assay from the difference between the absorbances at 500 and 550 nm using the declared content of $C_{27}H_{44}O$ in *cholecalciferol EPCRS* or of $C_{28}H_{44}O$ in *ergocalciferol EPCRS,* as appropriate. Calculate the percentage w/v of colecalciferol or ergocalciferol taking 0.87 g as the value of the weight per ml of the injection.

Storage Calciferol Injection should be protected from light and stored at a temperature not exceeding 25°.

Labelling The label on the container states that the preparation is for intramuscular use only.

When Calciferol Injection is prescribed or demanded, an injection described as Colecalciferol Injection or as Ergocalciferol Injection may be dispensed or supplied.

Calciferol Oral Solution

Calciferol Oral Drops

Definition Calciferol Oral Solution is a 0.0075% w/v solution of Colecalciferol or Ergocalciferol in a suitable vegetable oil.

The title Colecalciferol Oral Solution may be used for an oral solution containing Colecalciferol and the title Ergocalciferol Oral Solution may be used for an oral solution containing Ergocalciferol.

Production Calciferol Oral Solution may be prepared by warming to 40° a 1% w/v suspension of Colecalciferol or Ergocalciferol in a suitable vegetable oil, such as Arachis Oil, Carbon Dioxide being bubbled through it to facilitate solution, and adding a sufficient quantity of the oil to produce a solution containing 0.0075% w/v of Colecalciferol or Ergocalciferol.

The oral solution complies with the requirements stated under Oral Liquids and with the following requirements.

Content of colecalciferol or ergocalciferol 0.00635 to 0.00900% w/v.

Characteristics A pale yellow, oily liquid; odour, slight but not rancid.

Identification To 1 ml of a 20% v/v solution in *ethanol-free chloroform* add 9 ml of *antimony trichloride solution*. The *light absorption* of the resulting solution, Appendix II B, exhibits a maximum at 500 nm.

Assay Carry out the following procedure in subdued light. To about 1.5 g, accurately weighed, add 0.1 g of *hydroquinone* and 25 ml of 0.5M *ethanolic potassium hydroxide*, boil under a reflux condenser for 20 minutes, cool and add 50 ml of *water*. Extract with three 30-ml quantities of *ether*, wash the combined ether extracts with 20 ml of *water*, then with 20 ml of 0.5M *potassium hydroxide* and finally with successive 20-ml quantities of *water* until the washings are no longer alkaline to *phenolphthalein solution R1*. Filter the ether solution through absorbent cotton, wash with two 10-ml quantities of *ether* and evaporate the combined extracts and washings to dryness under *oxygen-free nitrogen* by immersion in a water bath at 50°. Dissolve the residue in about 10 ml of *hexane*, transfer to a column (20 cm × 1 cm) packed with *deactivated aluminium oxide* and elute continuously with a 15 to 20% v/v solution of *ether* in *hexane*, using a flow rate of 1 to 2 ml per minute and collecting the fraction that contains the calciferol (this fraction may be identified conveniently by testing aliquots of successive 10-ml fractions with *antimony trichloride solution*). Evaporate the solvent under *oxygen-free nitrogen* at a temperature not exceeding 50° and dissolve the residue in 5 ml of *ethanol-free chloroform*. Using duplicate 1-ml portions of this solution add rapidly 9 ml of *antimony trichloride solution* and measure the *absorbance* of each solution at 500 and 550 nm, 90 to 120 seconds after adding the reagent, Appendix II B. Repeat the operation using duplicate 1-ml portions of a solution containing a known amount of *cholecalciferol EPCRS* or *ergocalciferol EPCRS* in *ethanol-free chloroform* and beginning at the words 'add rapidly 9 ml of *antimony trichloride solution ...*'. Calculate the results of the assay from the difference between the absorbances at 500 and 550 nm using the declared content of $C_{27}H_{44}O$ in *cholecalciferol EPCRS* or of $C_{28}H_{44}O$ in *ergocalciferol EPCRS,* as appropriate. Determine the *weight per ml* of the oral solution, Appendix V G, and calculate the percentage of colecalciferol or ergocalciferol, weight in volume.

Storage Calciferol Oral Solution should be kept in a well-filled, well-closed container, protected from light and stored at a temperature not exceeding 25°.

Labelling The label states the number of IU (Units) of antirachitic activity (vitamin D) in 1 ml.

Each microgram of colecalciferol or ergocalciferol is equivalent to 40 IU of antirachitic activity (vitamin D).

When Calciferol Oral Solution or Calciferol Oral Drops is prescribed or demanded, a preparation described as Colecalciferol Oral Solution, as Ergocalciferol Oral Solution, as Colecalciferol Oral Drops or as Ergocalciferol Oral Drops may be dispensed or supplied.

Calciferol Tablets

Definition Calciferol Tablets contain Colecalciferol or Ergocalciferol.

The title Colecalciferol Tablets may be used for tablets containing Colecalciferol and the title Ergocalciferol Tablets may be used for tablets containing Ergocalciferol.

The tablets comply with the requirements stated under Tablets and with the following requirements.

Content of colecalciferol or ergocalciferol 90.0 to 125.0% of the prescribed or stated amount.

Identification

A. In the test for Uniformity of content, the retention time of the principal peak in the chromatogram obtained with solution (2) is a similar to that of the principal peak in the chromatogram obtained with solution (1).

B. Extract a tablet, in powder, with 5 ml of *ethanol-free chloroform*, filter and to 1 ml of the filtrate add 9 ml of *antimony trichloride solution*. A brownish red colour is produced.

Uniformity of content Tablets containing less than 2 mg of Colecalciferol or Ergocalciferol comply with the requirements stated under Tablets using the following method of analysis. Carry out the method for *liquid chromatography*, Appendix III D, using the following solutions. Solution (1) contains 0.001% w/v of *cholecalciferol EPCRS* or *ergocalciferol EPCRS*, as appropriate, in *hexane*. For tablets containing more than 0.25 mg prepare solution (2) in the following manner. Add 4 ml of *water* to one tablet in an amber flask and disperse with the aid of ultrasound. Add 12 ml of *dimethyl sulphoxide*, mix, extract with 100 ml of *hexane* by shaking for 30 minutes, centrifuge the hexane layer and use the clear supernatant liquid. For tablets containing 0.25 mg or less carry out the same procedure but using 2 ml of *water*, 6 ml of *dimethyl sulphoxide* and 25 ml of *hexane*. For solution (3) dissolve 0.5 g of *cholecalciferol for performance test EPCRS* in 2 ml of *toluene* and dilute to 10 ml with the mobile phase; heat under a reflux condenser in a water bath at 90° for 45 minutes and cool.

The chromatographic procedure may be carried out using (a) a stainless steel column (20 cm × 4.6 mm) packed with *stationary phase A* (5 µm) (Partisil is suitable), (b) a mixture of 992 volumes of *hexane* and 8 volumes of *pentan-1-ol* as the mobile phase with a flow rate of 2 ml per minute and (c) a detection wavelength of 254 nm.

Inject a suitable volume of solution (3) and record the chromatogram using a sensitivity such that the height of the peak due to colecalciferol is more than 50% of full-scale deflection. When the chromatogram is recorded under the prescribed conditions, approximate retention times relative to colecalciferol are 0.4 for precolecalciferol and 0.5 for *trans*-colecalciferol. The *resolution factor* for precolecalciferol and *trans*-colecalciferol should be not less than 1.0; if necessary, adjust the proportions of the constituents and the flow rate of the mobile phase to obtain this resolution.

Inject a suitable volume of solution (1) and record the chromatogram using a sensitivity such that the the height of the peak due to colecalciferol or ergocalciferol, as appropriate, is more than 50% of full-scale deflection. Repeat the operation using solution (2) and injecting the same volume.

Calculate the content of colecalciferol, $C_{27}H_{44}O$, or ergocalciferol, $C_{28}H_{44}O$, using the declared content of $C_{27}H_{44}O$ in *cholecalciferol EPCRS* or of $C_{28}H_{44}O$ in *ergocalciferol EPCRS*, as appropriate, and using peak heights.

Assay Carry out the following procedure in subdued light. Weigh and powder 25 tablets, or more if necessary. To a quantity of the powder containing 6 mg of Colecalciferol or Ergocalciferol add 50 ml of *ethanol (96%)*, 14 ml of *glycerol* and 20 ml of a 50% w/v solution of *potassium hydroxide*. Boil under a reflux condenser for 30 minutes, swirling occasionally, add 110 ml of *water* and allow to stand for 10 minutes with occasional stirring. Cool and add sufficient *ethanol (96%)* to produce 250 ml. Shake 5 ml with 25 ml of *petroleum spirit (boiling range, 40° to 60°)* for 3 minutes and evaporate duplicate 5-ml portions of the extract to dryness in a current of *oxygen-free nitrogen*. Dissolve each residue in 1 ml of *ethanol-free chloroform*, add rapidly 9 ml of *antimony trichloride solution* and measure the *absorbance* of each solution at 500 nm and at 550 nm, 90 to 120 seconds after adding the reagent, Appendix II B. Repeat the operations using duplicate 1-ml portions of a solution containing a known amount of *cholecalciferol EPCRS* or *ergocalciferol EPCRS*, as appropriate, in *ethanol-free chloroform* and beginning at the words 'add rapidly 9 ml of *antimony trichloride solution* ...'. Subtract the absorbance at 550 nm from that at 500 nm and calculate the content of colecalciferol or ergocalciferol in mg from the average value so obtained and from the amount of colecalciferol or ergocalciferol in the reference solution using the declared content of $C_{27}H_{44}O$ in *cholecalciferol EPCRS* or of $C_{28}H_{44}O$ in *ergocalciferol EPCRS*, as appropriate.

Storage Calciferol Tablets should be stored at a temperature not exceeding 25°.

When calciferol tablets qualified by a descriptor relating to strength are prescribed or demanded, the intention of the prescriber or purchaser with respect to the strength expressed in micrograms or milligrams per tablet should be ascertained.

Each microgram of Colecalciferol or Ergocalciferol is equivalent to 40 IU of antirachitic activity (vitamin D).

When Calciferol Tablets are prescribed or demanded, tablets described as Colecalciferol Tablets or as Ergocalciferol Tablets may be dispensed or supplied.

Calcitonin (Pork) Injection

Definition Calcitonin (Pork) Injection is a sterile solution of Calcitonin (Pork) in a suitable liquid. It is prepared by dissolving Calcitonin (Pork) for Injection in the liquid stated on the label.

The injection complies with the requirements stated under Parenteral Preparations.

Storage Calcitonin (Pork) Injection should be used immediately after preparation but, in any case, within the period recommended by the manufacturer when prepared and stored strictly in accordance with the manufacturer's instructions.

CALCITONIN (PORK) FOR INJECTION

Definition Calcitonin (Pork) for Injection is a sterile material consisting of Calcitonin (Pork) with or without excipients. It is supplied in a sealed container.

The contents of the sealed container comply with the requirements for Powders for Injections stated under Parenteral Preparations and with the following requirements.

Characteristics A white, or almost white, friable solid.

Identification Comply with the test described under Calcitonin (Pork), using a freshly prepared solution prepared by dissolving the contents of the sealed container in sufficient mobile phase B to give a solution containing 30 IU per ml.

Acidity Dissolve the contents of the sealed container in the specified volume of the liquid stated on the label (solution A). The pH is 3.5 to 5.5, Appendix V L.

Clarity of solution Solution A is *clear*, Appendix IV A.

Bacterial endotoxins Carry out the *test for bacterial endotoxins*, Appendix XIV C. Dissolve the contents of the sealed container in *water BET* to give a solution containing 40 IU of Calcitonin per ml (solution B). The endotoxin limit concentration of solution B is 43.75 IU of endotoxin per ml. In order to eliminate interference, carry out the test using a lysate with a declared sensitivity not less sensitive than 0.0625 IU of endotoxin per ml, and using the maximum valid dilution of solution B calculated from the declared sensitivity of the lysate used in the test.

Assay Carry out the *biological assay of calcitonin (pork)* described under Calcitonin (Pork). The estimated potency is not less than 80% and not more than 125% of the stated potency. The fiducial limits of error are not less than 64% and not more than 156% of the stated potency.

Storage The sealed container should be protected from light and stored at a temperature not exceeding 25°. Under these conditions the contents may be expected to retain their potency for not less than 3 years.

Labelling The label of the sealed container states (1) the total number of IU (Units) in the sealed container; (2) that the preparation is for subcutaneous or intramuscular use only.

Calcitonin (Salmon) Injection
Salcatonin Injection

For purposes of product labelling in the United Kingdom, the pair of names given above shall be used together (see Introduction, Changes in title).

Definition Calcitonin (Salmon) Injection is a sterile solution of Calcitonin (Salmon) in Water for Injections.

The injection complies with the requirements stated under Parenteral Preparations and with the following requirements.

Content of calcitonin (salmon), $C_{145}H_{240}N_{44}O_{48}S_2$ 90.0 to 115.0% of the prescribed or stated amount of the peptide.

Characteristics A colourless solution.

Identification In the Assay, the retention time of the principal peak in the chromatogram obtained with solution (1) is similar to that of the principal peak in the chromatogram obtained with solution (2).

Acidity pH, 3.9 to 4.5, Appendix V L.

Calcitonin C Carry out the method for *liquid chromatography*, Appendix III D, injecting 0.2 ml of the following solutions. For solution (1) dilute the injection, if necessary, with a 0.1M solution of *sodium dihydrogen orthophosphate* adjusted to pH 4.0 with *orthophosphoric acid* to give a final concentration of 10 µg of calcitonin (salmon) per ml. Solution (2) contains 10 µg of *calcitonin (salmon) BPCRS* per ml in the sodium dihydrogen orthophosphate solution. For solution (3) heat the injection at 75° for 15 hours and, if necessary, dilute as described for solution (1).

The chromatographic procedure may be carried out using (a) a stainless steel column (25 cm × 4.6 mm) packed with *stationary phase C* (5 µm) (Vydac C18, 300 Å wide pore column for proteins and peptides is suitable) maintained at 40°, (b) as the mobile phase with a flow rate of 1 ml per minute a mixture of 100 volumes of a 0.363% w/v solution of *tetramethylammonium hydroxide pentahydrate* and 150 volumes of *acetonitrile* adjusted to pH 2.5 with *orthophosphoric acid* (mobile phase A) and a mixture of 450 volumes of a 0.402% w/v solution of *tetramethylammonium hydroxide pentahydrate* and 50 volumes of *acetonitrile* adjusted to pH 2.5 with *orthophosphoric acid* (mobile phase B) and (c) a detection wavelength of 220 nm.

Equilibrate the column with a mixture of 35 volumes of mobile phase A and 65 volumes of mobile phase B. Operate by gradient elution increasing continuously and linearly the proportion of mobile phase A to 57% over a period of 21 minutes.

In the chromatogram obtained with solution (3) the peak due to calcitonin C is the largest peak to elute after the injection buffer salts and before the principal peak with a relative retention to that of calcitonin (salmon) of between 0.5 and 0.6.

The test is not valid unless the *resolution factor* between the peaks due to calcitonin C and calcitonin (salmon) in the chromatogram obtained with solution (3) is at least 3.0.

In the chromatogram obtained with solution (1) the area of any peak corresponding to calcitonin C is not greater than 7% by *normalisation.*

Assay Carry out the method described under the test for Calcitonin C.

Calculate the content of calcitonin (salmon) from the areas of the peak due to calcitonin (salmon) and that of any peak due to calcitonin C, using the declared content of $C_{145}H_{240}N_{44}O_{48}S_2$ in *calcitonin (salmon) BPCRS*.

Storage Calcitonin (Salmon) Injection should be protected from light and stored at a temperature of 2° to 8°. Under these conditions it may be expected to retain its potency for not less than 2 years.

Labelling The label states (1) 'Calcitonin (Salmon) Injection' and 'Salcatonin Injection'; (2) the strength as the number of IU (Units) per ml. The label also states the equivalent number of micrograms of the peptide per ml.

Calcitriol Capsules

Definition Calcitriol Capsules contain a solution of Calcitriol in a suitable fixed oil.

The capsules comply with the requirements stated under Capsules and with the following requirements.

Content of calcitriol, $C_{27}H_{44}O_3$ 90.0 to 110.0% of the prescribed or stated amount.

Identification In the Assay, the chromatogram obtained with solution (1) shows a peak with the same retention time as the peak due to calcitriol in the chromatogram obtained with solution (2).

Assay Carry out the method for *liquid chromatography*, Appendix III D, in subdued light using the following solutions. For capsules containing 0.25 µg or less, use the mixed contents of 10 capsules as solution (1). For capsules containing more than 0.25 µg, prepare solution (1) by diluting a quantity of the mixed contents of 10 capsules containing 1.5 µg of Calcitriol to 1 ml with the mobile phase. Solution (2) contains 0.00015% w/v of *calcitriol EPCRS* in the mobile phase.

The chromatographic procedure may be carried out using (a) a stainless steel column (25 cm × 4.6 mm) packed with *stationary phase A* (5 µm) (Lichrosorb Si60 is suitable), (b) a mixture of 1 volume of *propan-1-ol*, 2 volumes of *methanol*, 40 volumes of *hexane* and 60 volumes of *ethyl acetate* as the mobile phase with a flow rate of 1.2 ml per minute and (c) a detection wavelength of 265 nm. If necessary, adjust the composition of the mobile phase so that the principal peak in the chromatogram obtained with solution (1) is clearly separated from the tail of the peak due to the excipient.

Calculate the content of calcitriol, $C_{27}H_{44}O_3$, using the declared content of $C_{27}H_{44}O_3$ in *calcitriol EPCRS*.

Calcium Chloride Intravenous Infusion

Calcium Chloride Injection

Definition Calcium Chloride Intravenous Infusion is a sterile solution of Calcium Chloride in Water for Injections.

The infusion complies with the requirements stated under Parenteral preparations and with the following requirements.

Content of calcium chloride The equivalent of 95.0 to 105.0% of the prescribed or stated amount of calcium chloride dihydrate, $CaCl_2,2H_2O$.

Identification

A. 1 ml yields reaction C characteristic of *calcium salts*, Appendix VI.

B. Dilute 1 volume of the intravenous infusion to 50 ml with *water*. The resulting solution yields reaction A characteristic of *chlorides*, Appendix VI.

Acidity or alkalinity pH 5.0 to 8.0, Appendix V L.

Colour of solution The intravenous infusion is not more intensely coloured than *reference solution BY_6*, Appendix IV B, Method II.

Assay Carry out the *complexometric titration of calcium*, Appendix VIII D. Use a volume of the intravenous infusion containing about 0.3 g of Calcium Chloride.

Labelling The label states (1) the percentage w/v of Calcium Chloride; (2) the concentration of calcium ion as millimoles in a suitable volume; (3) the concentration of chloride ion as millimoles in a suitable volume; (4) that the infusion should be used in accordance with the manufacturer's instructions; (5) that solutions containing visible solid particles must not be used.

Calcium Gluconate Injection

Definition Calcium Gluconate Injection is a sterile solution of Calcium Gluconate for Injection in Water for Injections. Not more than 5.0% of the Calcium Gluconate may be replaced with calcium D-saccharate, or other suitable calcium salt, as a stabilising agent.

The injection complies with the requirements stated under Parenteral Preparations and with the following requirements.

Content of calcium, Ca 8.5 to 9.4% of the content of Calcium Gluconate stated on the label.

Identification

A. To 1 ml add 0.05 ml of *iron(III) chloride solution R1*. An intense yellow colour is produced.B. Warm a volume containing the equivalent of 0.5 g of Calcium Gluconate, add 0.65 ml of *glacial acetic acid* and 1 ml of *phenylhydrazine*. Heat on a water bath for 30 minutes, allow to cool and induce crystallisation. Filter, dissolve the residue in 10 ml of hot *water*, add a few mg of *activated charcoal*, shake, filter, allow the filtrate to cool and induce crystallisation. A white, crystalline precipitate is produced. The *melting point* of the crystals, after drying, is about 200°, with decomposition, Appendix V A.

C. Yields the reactions characteristic of *calcium salts*, Appendix VI.

Pyrogens Complies with the *test for pyrogens*, Appendix XIV D. Use per kg of the rabbit's weight a volume containing the equivalent of 0.2 g of Calcium Gluconate.

Assay To a volume containing the equivalent of 0.5 g of Calcium Gluconate add 300 ml of *water* and carry out the *complexometric titration of calcium*, Appendix VIII D, beginning at the words 'add 6 ml of ...'.

Labelling The label states (1) the percentage w/v of Calcium Gluconate equivalent to the total amount of calcium present; (2) that solutions containing visible solid particles must not be used; (3) the name and the percentage of any added stabilising agent.

Calcium Gluconate Tablets

Definition Calcium Gluconate Tablets contain Calcium Gluconate. Tablets that are intended to be chewed before swallowing are prepared using Chocolate Basis or other suitable basis with a chocolate flavour.

The tablets comply with the requirements stated under Tablets and with the following requirements.

Content of calcium gluconate, $C_{12}H_{22}CaO_{14},H_2O$ 95.0 to 105.0% of the prescribed or stated amount.

Identification

A. Extract five tablets, finely powdered, with two 25-ml quantities of *petroleum spirit (boiling range, 40° to 60°)*, discard the extracts and repeat the extraction with three 10-ml quantities of *water*, again discarding the extracts. Dissolve the residue as completely as possible in 30 ml of hot *water*, filter and to 0.5 ml of the filtrate add 0.05 ml of *iron(III) chloride solution R1*. An intense yellow colour is produced.

B. To a volume of the filtrate obtained in test A containing 0.5 g of Calcium Gluconate add 0.65 ml of *glacial acetic acid* and 1 ml of *phenylhydrazine*, heat on a water bath for 30 minutes, cool and induce crystallisation. Filter, dissolve the residue in 10 ml of hot *water*, add a few mg of *activated charcoal*, shake, filter, allow the filtrate to cool and induce crystallisation. A white, crystalline precipitate is produced. The *melting point* of the crystals, after drying, is about 201°, with decomposition, Appendix V A.

C. The powdered tablets yield the reactions characteristic of *calcium salts*, Appendix VI.

Disintegration The requirement for Disintegration does not apply to Calcium Gluconate Tablets intended to be chewed. Tablets intended to be swallowed whole comply with the test for disintegration of uncoated tablets.

Dissolution Comply with the *dissolution test for tablets and capsules*, Appendix XII D, using Apparatus II. Use as the medium 900 ml of *water* and rotate the paddle at 50 revolutions per minute. Withdraw a sample of 20 ml of the medium and filter. Carry out the method for *atomic absorption spectrophotometry*, Appendix II D, measuring at 422.7 nm using a calcium hollow-cathode lamp as the radiation source, an air—acetylene flame and the following solutions.

Test solution Use the filtered dissolution medium diluted, if necessary, with *water* to give a concentration suitable for the instrument used.

Standard solutions Use *calcium standard solution (100 ppm Ca)* suitably diluted with *water*.

Determine the total content of calcium in the dissolution medium and calculate the content of calcium gluconate taking each mg of calcium to be equivalent to 11.21 mg of $C_{12}H_{22}CaO_{14},H_2O$.

Assay Weigh and powder 20 tablets. Ignite a quantity of the powder containing 0.5 g of Calcium Gluconate, cool and dissolve the residue with gentle heat in 5 ml of 2M *hydrochloric acid*. Filter, wash the residue on the filter with *water* and dilute the combined filtrate and washings to 50 ml with *water*. Neutralise with 5M *ammonia*, using *methyl orange solution* as indicator, add 5 ml of 8M *sodium hydroxide* and titrate with 0.05M *disodium edetate VS* using *calconcarboxylic acid triturate* as indicator. Each ml of 0.05M *disodium edetate VS* is equivalent to 22.42 mg of $C_{12}H_{22}CaO_{14},H_2O$.

Labelling The label states, where appropriate, that the tablets should be chewed before swallowing.

When Calcium Gluconate Tablets are prescribed or demanded, no strength being stated, tablets containing 600 mg shall be dispensed or supplied.

Effervescent Calcium Gluconate Tablets

Definition Effervescent Calcium Gluconate Tablets contain Calcium Gluconate in a suitable effervescent basis.

The tablets comply with the requirements stated under Tablets and with the following requirements.

Content of calcium gluconate, $C_{12}H_{22}CaO_{14},H_2O$ 95.0 to 105.0% of the prescribed or stated amount.

Identification

A. Dissolve a quantity of the powdered tablets containing 1 g of Calcium Gluconate in 20 ml of hot *water*, cool and filter. To 0.5 ml of the filtrate add 0.05 ml of *iron(III) chloride solution R1*. An intense yellow colour is produced.

B. To 5 ml of the filtrate obtained in test A add 0.65 ml of *glacial acetic acid* and 1 ml of *phenylhydrazine*, heat on a water bath for 30 minutes, allow to cool and induce crystallisation. Filter, dissolve the residue in 10 ml of hot *water*, add a suitable quantity of *activated charcoal*, shake, filter, allow the filtrate to cool and induce crystallisation. A white, crystalline precipitate is produced. The *melting point* of the crystals, after drying, is about 201°, with decomposition, Appendix V A.

C. The powdered tablets yield reaction B characteristic of *calcium salts*, Appendix VI.

D. The tablets effervesce on the addition of *water*.

Assay Weigh and powder 20 tablets. Ignite a quantity of the powder containing 0.5 g of Calcium Gluconate, cool and dissolve the residue with gentle heat in 5 ml of 2M *hydrochloric acid*. Filter, wash the residue on the filter with *water* and dilute the combined filtrate and washings to 50 ml with *water*. Neutralise with 5M *ammonia*, using *methyl orange solution* as indicator, add 5 ml of 8M *sodium hydroxide* and titrate with 0.05M *disodium edetate VS* using *calconcarboxylic acid triturate* as indicator. Each ml of 0.05M *disodium edetate VS* is equivalent to 22.42 mg of $C_{12}H_{22}CaO_{14},H_2O$.

Storage Effervescent Calcium Gluconate Tablets should be kept in a well-closed container and stored at a temperature not exceeding 25°.

Labelling The label states that the tablets should be dissolved in water immediately before use.

Calcium Hydroxide Solution

Lime Water

Definition

Calcium Hydroxide	10 g
Purified Water, freshly boiled and cooled	sufficient to produce 1000 ml

Extemporaneous preparation The following directions apply.

Shake together thoroughly and repeatedly; allow to stand until clear. Siphon off the clear solution as required.

Content of calcium hydroxide, $Ca(OH)_2$ Not less than 0.15% w/v.

Characteristics A colourless liquid. It absorbs carbon dioxide from the air, a film of calcium carbonate being formed on the surface of the liquid. It becomes turbid when boiled and clear again on cooling.

Identification Yields the reactions characteristic of *calcium salts*, Appendix VI.

Assay Titrate 25 ml with 0.1M *hydrochloric acid VS* using *phenolphthalein solution R1* as indicator. Each ml of 0.1M *hydrochloric acid VS* is equivalent to 3.705 mg of $Ca(OH)_2$.

Storage Calcium Hydroxide Solution should be kept in a well-filled and well-closed container.

Labelling The label states (1) the date after which the solution is not intended to be used; (2) the conditions under which it should be stored.

Calcium Lactate Tablets

Definition Calcium Lactate Tablets contain Calcium Lactate Pentahydrate or Calcium Lactate Trihydrate.

The tablets comply with the requirements stated under Tablets and with the following requirements.

Content of calcium lactate, calculated as $C_6H_{10}CaO_6,5H_2O$ 95.0 to 105.0% of the prescribed or stated amount.

Identification

A. Triturate a quantity of the powdered tablets containing 0.3 g of Calcium Lactate Pentahydrate or its equivalent with 5 ml of *methanol* and filter. To 0.2 ml of the filtrate add 2 ml of *sulphuric acid*, heat at 85° for 2 minutes, cool and add 4 mg of *4-hydroxybiphenyl*. A violet-red colour is produced.

B. The powdered tablets, when moistened with *hydrochloric acid* and introduced on a platinum wire into a flame, impart a brick red colour to the flame.

Disintegration Maximum time, 30 minutes, Appendix XII A.

Assay Weigh and powder 20 tablets. Dissolve a quantity of the powder containing 0.3 g of Calcium Lactate Pentahydrate or its equivalent as completely as possible in 50 ml of *water* and titrate with 0.05M *disodium edetate VS* to within a few millilitres of the expected end point. Add 8 ml of 5M *sodium hydroxide* and 0.1 g of *solochrome dark blue mixture* and continue the titration until the colour changes from pink to full blue. Each ml of 0.05M *disodium edetate VS* is equivalent to 15.41 mg of $C_6H_{10}CaO_6$, $5H_2O$.

Labelling When the active ingredient is Calcium Lactate Trihydrate the quantity is stated in terms of the equivalent amount of Calcium Lactate Pentahydrate.

Concentrated Camphor Water

Definition

Racemic Camphor	40 g
Ethanol (90 per cent)	600 ml
Water	sufficient to produce 1000 ml

Extemporaneous preparation The following directions apply.

Dissolve the Racemic Camphor in the Ethanol (90 per cent) and add, gradually, with vigorous shaking after each addition, sufficient Water to produce 1000 ml.

The water complies with the requirements stated under Aromatic Waters and with the following requirement.

Ethanol content 51 to 55% v/v, Appendix VIII F.

Capreomycin Injection

Definition Capreomycin Injection is a sterile solution of Capreomycin Sulphate in Water for Injections. It is prepared by dissolving Capreomycin Sulphate for Injection in the requisite amount of Water for Injections immediately before use.

The injection complies with the requirements stated under Parenteral Preparations.

Storage Capreomycin Injection should be used immediately after preparation but, in any case, within the period recommended by the manufacturer when prepared and stored strictly in accordance with the manufacturer's instructions.

CAPREOMYCIN SULPHATE FOR INJECTION

Definition Capreomycin Sulphate for Injection is a sterile material consisting of Capreomycin Sulphate, with or without excipients. It is supplied in a sealed container.

The contents of the sealed container comply with the requirements for Powders for Injections stated under Parenteral Preparations and with the following requirements.

Identification

A. The *light absorption*, Appendix II B, in the range 230 to 350 nm of a 0.004% w/v solution in 0.1M *hydrochloric acid* exhibits a maximum only at 268 nm. The *absorbance* at 268 nm is about 1.2.

B. The *light absorption*, Appendix II B, in the range 230 to 350 nm of a 0.004% w/v solution in 0.1M *sodium hydroxide* exhibits a maximum only at 287 nm. The *absorbance* at 287 nm is about 0.8.

C. Comply with test C for Identification described under Capreomycin Sulphate.

Acidity or alkalinity pH of a 3% w/v solution, 4.5 to 7.5, Appendix V L.

Capreomycin I Comply with the test described under Capreomycin Sulphate. For solution (1) dissolve a quantity of the contents of the container in *water* to produce a solution containing 0.025% w/v of Capreomycin Sulphate.

Loss on drying When dried at 100° at a pressure not exceeding 0.7 kPa for 4 hours, lose not more than 10.0% of their weight. Use 1 g.

Pyrogens Comply with the *test for pyrogens*, Appendix XIV D. Use per kg of the rabbit's weight 1 ml of a solution in *water for injections* containing 7000 IU per ml.

Assay Determine the weight of the contents of each of 10 containers as described in the test for Uniformity of weight under Parenteral Preparations, Powders for Injections.

Mix the contents of the 10 containers and carry out the *biological assay of antibiotics*, Appendix XIV A. The precision of the assay is such that the fiducial limits of error are not less than 95% and not more than 105% of the estimated potency. For a container of average content weight, the upper fiducial limit of error is not less than 95.0% and the lower fiducial limit of error is not more than 115.0% of the prescribed or stated number of IU.

Storage The sealed container should be stored at a temperature not exceeding 15°.

Labelling The label states (1) the total number of IU (Units) contained in it; (2) the number of IU (Units) per mg.

Captopril Tablets

Definition Captopril Tablets contain Captopril.

With the exception of the requirements for shape, the tablets comply with the requirements stated under Tablets and with the following requirements.

Content of captopril, $C_9H_{15}NO_3S$ 95.0 to 105.0% of the prescribed or stated amount.

Identification

A. Dissolve a quantity of the powdered tablets containing 0.1 g of Captopril in 25 ml of *methanol* with the aid of ultrasound and filter. Mix 1 ml of the filtrate with 0.5 g of *potassium bromide*, dry at room temperature at 2 kPa, grind to a uniform mixture and prepare a disc. The *infrared absorption spectrum*, Appendix II A, is concordant with the *reference spectrum* of captopril.

B. In the Assay, the principal peak in the chromatogram obtained with solution (1) has the same retention time as the peak due to captopril in the chromatogram obtained with solution (2).

Captopril disulphide Carry out the method for *liquid chromatography*, Appendix III D, using the following solutions. For solution (1) transfer a quantity of the powdered tablets containing 25 mg of Captopril to a centrifuge tube, add 25 ml of *methanol*, centrifuge for 15 minutes and use the supernatant liquid. Solution (2) contains 0.0020% w/v of *captopril disulphide BPCRS* in *methanol*. For solution (3) dilute 1 volume of solution (1) to 100 volumes with solution (2).

The chromatographic procedure may be carried out using (a) a stainless steel column (25 cm × 4.6 mm) packed with *stationary phase C* (5 µm) (Nucleosil C18 is suitable), (b) a mixture of 0.5 volume of *orthophosphoric acid*, 450 volumes of *water* and 550 volumes of *methanol* as the mobile phase with a flow rate of 1 ml per minute and (c) a detection wavelength of 220 nm.

The test is not valid unless the *resolution factor* between the peaks due to captopril and captopril disulphide in the chromatogram obtained with solution (3) is at least 2.0.

In the chromatogram obtained with solution (1) the area of any peak corresponding to captopril disulphide is not greater than the area of the peak in the chromatogram obtained with solution (2) (2%).

Assay Weigh and powder 20 tablets. Carry out the method for *liquid chromatography*, Appendix III D, using the following solutions. For solution (1) transfer a quantity of the powdered tablets containing 25 mg of Captopril to a centrifuge tube, add 25 ml of the mobile phase, mix with the aid of ultrasound for 15 minutes and centrifuge. Dilute 1 volume of the supernatant liquid to 10 volumes with the mobile phase. Solution (2) contains 0.01% w/v of *captopril BPCRS* and 0.0005% w/v of *captopril disulphide BPCRS* in the mobile phase.

The chromatographic procedure may be carried out using (a) a stainless steel column (25 cm × 4.6 mm) packed with *stationary phase C* (10 µm) (Nucleosil C18 is suitable), (b) a mixture of 0.5 volume of *orthophosphoric acid*, 450 volumes of *water* and 550 volumes of *methanol* as the mobile phase with a flow rate of 1 ml per minute and (c) a detection wavelength of 220 nm.

The test is not valid unless, in the chromatogram obtained with solution (2), the *resolution factor* between the peaks due to captopril and captopril disulphide is at least 2.0.

Calculate the content of $C_9H_{15}NO_3S$ using the declared content of $C_9H_{15}NO_3S$ in *captopril BPCRS*.

Carbamazepine Tablets

Definition Carbamazepine Tablets contain Carbamazepine.

The tablets comply with the requirements stated under Tablets and with the following requirements.

Content of carbamazepine, $C_{15}H_{12}N_2O$ 95.0 to 105.0% of the prescribed or stated amount.

Identification

A. Boil a quantity of the powdered tablets containing 0.2 g of Carbamazepine with 15 ml of *acetone*, filter the hot solution, wash the filter with two 5-ml quantities of hot *acetone*, evaporate the combined filtrates to 5 ml and cool in ice. The *melting point* of the crystals, after washing with *acetone* and drying at 70° at a pressure of 2 kPa for 30 minutes, is about 191°, Appendix V A.

B. The powdered tablets exhibit an intense blue fluorescence under ultraviolet light (365 nm).

C. Heat 0.1 g of the crystals obtained in test A with 2 ml of *nitric acid* in a water bath for 3 minutes. An orange-red colour is produced.

Related substances

A. Carry out the method for *thin-layer chromatography*, Appendix III A, using *silica gel G* as the coating substance and a mixture of 14 volumes of *methanol* and 90 volumes of *toluene* as the mobile phase, but allowing the solvent front to ascend 8 cm above the line of application using a tank appropriate to the dimensions of the plate. Apply separately to a plate (100 mm × 100 mm) 2 µl of each of the following solutions. For solution (1) shake a quantity of powdered tablets containing 0.25 g of Carbamazepine with three 10-ml quantities of *chloroform*, filtering each extract successively; evaporate the combined extracts to a small volume and dilute to 5 ml with *chloroform*. For solution (2) dilute 1 volume of solution (1) to 100 volumes with *chloroform* and dilute 1 volume of the resulting solution to 100 volumes with *chloroform*. Solution (3) contains 0.0050% w/v of *iminodibenzyl* in a mixture of equal volumes of *chloroform* and *ethanol (96%)*. After removal of the plate, allow it to dry in air for 15 minutes and spray with a 0.5% w/v solution of *potassium dichromate* in 1M *sulphuric acid*. Any spot corresponding to iminodibenzyl in the chromatogram obtained with solution (1) is not more intense than the spot in the chromatogram obtained with solution (3) (0.1%). Heat the plate at 140° for 15 to 20 minutes and examine under *ultraviolet light (254 nm)*. Any *secondary spot* in the chromatogram obtained with solution (1) with an Rf value less than that of the principal spot is not more intense than the spot in the chromatogram obtained with solution (2) (0.01%).

B. Carry out the method for *liquid chromatography*, Appendix III D, using the following solutions. Prepare a mixture of 1 volume of *ethanol (96%)* and 9 volumes of *methanol* (solvent A). For solution (1) add 25 ml of a mixture of 1 volume of solvent A to a quantity of the powdered tablets containing 0.15 g of Carbamazepine, disperse with the aid of ultrasound for 5 minutes, dilute to 50 ml with *water* and filter. For solution (2) add 5 ml of solvent A to 1 ml of solution (2) and dilute to 10 ml with *water*. For solution (3) add 25 ml of solvent A to 1 ml of solution (2) and dilute to 50 ml with *water*. For solution (4) dissolve 6 mg of *10,11-dihydrocarbamazepine* in 5 ml of solvent A and dilute to 10 ml with *water*. For solution (5) mix 1 ml of each of solutions (3) and (4), add 10 ml of solvent A and dilute to 25 ml with *water*.

The chromatographic procedure may be carried out using (a) a stainless steel column (25 cm × 4 mm) packed under pressure with a suspension in *methanol* of silica gel chemically bonded to alcoholic hydroxyl groups (Lichrosorb DIOL is suitable), (b) a mixture of 5 volumes of *acetonitrile*, 5 volumes of *methanol* and 90 volumes of a 0.05% v/v solution of *anhydrous acetic acid* as the mobile phase with a flow rate of 1.0 ml per minute and (c) a detection wavelength of 230 nm.

Inject 10 µl of solution (5). The test is not valid unless the *resolution factor* between the peaks due to carbamazepine and 10,11-dihydrocarbamazepine is greater than 1.5. If necessary reduce the amounts of both acetonitrile and methanol in the mobile phase or increase their proportions to 7.5 volumes and adjust the proportion of acetic acid solution accordingly.

Inject separately 10 µl of each of solutions (1) and (3) and adjust the sensitivity so that the height of the principal peak in the chromatogram obtained with solution (3) is at least 30% of full-scale deflection. Record the chromatograms for 3 times the retention time of carbamazepine (about 18 minutes). In the chromatogram obtained with solution (1) the area of any *secondary peak* is not greater than the area of the principal peak in the chromatogram obtained with solution (3) (0.2%) and the sum of the areas of any such peaks is not greater than 2.5 times the area of the principal peak in the chromatogram obtained with solution (3) (0.5%). Disregard any peak the area of which is less than 25% of the area of the principal peak in the chromatogram obtained with solution (3) (0.05%).

Assay Weigh and powder 20 tablets. Boil a quantity of the powder containing 60 mg of Carbamazepine with 25 ml of *ethanol (96%)* for a few minutes, stir the hot mixture in a closed flask for 10 minutes and filter through sintered glass, washing the flask and filter with *ethanol (96%)* and adding sufficient *ethanol (96%)* to the cooled filtrate to produce 100 ml. Dilute 5 ml to 250 ml with *ethanol (96%)* and measure the *absorbance* of the resulting solution at the maximum at 285 nm, Appendix II B. Calculate the content of $C_{15}H_{12}N_2O$ taking 490 as the value of A(1%, 1 cm) at the maximum at 285 nm.

Carbaryl Lotion

Definition Carbaryl Lotion is a *cutaneous solution*. It contains Carbaryl in a suitable vehicle.

The lotion complies with the requirements stated under Liquids for Cutaneous Application and with the following requirements.

Content of carbaryl, $C_{12}H_{11}NO_2$ 90.0 to 110.0% of the prescribed or stated amount.

Identification

A. Carry out the method for *thin-layer chromatography*, Appendix III A, using *silica gel GF_{254}* as the coating substance and a mixture of 0.5 volume of *water*, 10 volumes of *methanol* and 90 volumes of *chloroform* as the mobile phase. Apply separately to the plate 5 µl of each of the following solutions. For solution (1) disperse a quantity of the preparation being examined containing 4 mg of Carbaryl in a solution containing 10 ml of a saturated solution of *sodium chloride* and 50 ml of *ether*, shake, allow the layers to separate, wash the ether layer with two 10-ml quantities of *water*, filter through *anhydrous sodium sulphate* and evaporate the filtrate to dryness using a rotary evaporator. Dissolve the residue in 1 ml of *absolute ethanol*. Solution (2) contains 0.4% w/v of *carbaryl BPCRS* in *absolute ethanol*. After removal of the plate, allow it to dry in air and examine under *ultraviolet light (254 nm)*. The principal spot in the chromatogram obtained with solution (1) corresponds to that in the chromatogram obtained with solution (2).

B. In the Assay, the chromatogram obtained with solution (1) shows a peak with the same retention time as that of the principal peak in the chromatogram obtained with solution (2).

1-Naphthol Carry out the method for *liquid chromatography*, Appendix III D, using the following solutions. For solution (1) dilute a quantity of the preparation being examined with sufficient *acetonitrile* to produce a solution containing 0.1% w/v of Carbaryl. Solution (2) contains 0.003% w/v of *1-naphthol* in the mobile phase. Solution (3) contains 0.005% w/v of *carbaryl BPCRS* and 0.005% w/v of *1-naphthol* in the mobile phase.

The chromatographic conditions described under Assay may be used.

The test is not valid unless in the chromatogram obtained with solution (3) the *resolution factor* between the two principal peaks is at least 2.0.

In the chromatogram obtained with solution (1) the area of any peak corresponding to 1-naphthol is not greater than the area of the principal peak in the chromatogram obtained with solution (2) (3%).

Assay Carry out the method for *liquid chromatography*, Appendix III D, using the following solutions. For solution (1) dilute a quantity of the preparation being examined with sufficient *methanol* to produce a solution containing 0.005% w/v of Carbaryl. Solution (2) contains 0.005% w/v of *carbaryl BPCRS* in *methanol*. Solution (3) contains 0.005% w/v of *carbaryl BPCRS* and 0.005% w/v of *1-naphthol* in the mobile phase.

The chromatographic procedure may be carried out using (a) a stainless steel column (10 cm × 4.6 mm) packed with *stationary phase C* (5 µm) (Spherisorb ODS 2 is suitable), (b) a mixture of 1 volume of *glacial acetic acid*, 25 volumes of *acetonitrile* and 75 volumes of *water* as the mobile phase with a flow rate of 2.5 ml per minute and (c) a detection wavelength of 280 nm.

Inject 20 µl of each solution. The test is not valid unless in the chromatogram obtained with solution (3) the *resolution factor* between the two principal peaks is at least 2.0.

Calculate the content of $C_{12}H_{11}NO_2$ using the declared content of $C_{12}H_{11}NO_2$ in *carbaryl BPCRS*.

Storage Carbaryl Lotion should be protected from light and stored at a temperature not exceeding 25°.

Labelling The label indicates the pharmaceutical form as 'cutaneous solution'.

Carbenicillin Injection

Definition Carbenicillin Injection is a sterile solution of Carbenicillin Sodium in Water for Injections. It is prepared by dissolving Carbenicillin Sodium for Injection in the requisite amount of Water for Injections.

The injection complies with the requirements stated under Parenteral Preparations.

Storage Carbenicillin Injection should be used immediately after preparation but, in any case, within the period recommended by the manufacturer when prepared and stored strictly in accordance with the manufacturer's instructions.

CARBENICILLIN SODIUM FOR INJECTION

Definition Carbenicillin Sodium for Injection is a sterile material consisting of Carbenicillin Sodium with or without excipients. It is supplied in a sealed container.

The contents of the sealed container comply with the requirements for Powders for Injections stated under Parenteral Preparations and with the following requirements.

Content of carbenicillin, $C_{17}H_{18}N_2O_6S$ 95.0 to 105.0% of the prescribed or stated amount.

Identification

A. The *infrared absorption spectrum*, Appendix II A, is concordant with the *reference spectrum* of carbenicillin sodium.

B. Yield the reactions characteristic of *sodium salts*, Appendix VI.

Acidity or alkalinity pH of a 5% w/v solution, 5.5 to 7.5, Appendix V L.

Total carbenicillin sodium, benzylpenicillin sodium, iodine-absorbing substances and water 96.0 to 102.0% when determined by adding together the percentages of carbenicillin sodium (corrected for benzylpenicillin sodium), benzylpenicillin sodium, iodine-absorbing substances (all calculated with reference to the undried material) and water found by the methods described below.

Benzylpenicillin sodium Not more than 5.0%, determined by *liquid chromatography*, Appendix III D, using the following solutions. For solution (1) dissolve a quantity of the mixed contents of the 10 containers used in the Assay in sufficient *water* to produce a solution containing 0.4% w/v of carbenicillin sodium (calculated by multiplying the declared content of carbenicillin by 1.116). Solution (2) contains 0.02% w/v of *benzylpenicillin sodium EPCRS* in *water*. Solution (3) contains 0.01% w/v of *carbenicillin sodium EPCRS* and 0.01% w/v of *benzylpenicillin sodium EPCRS* in *water*.

The chromatographic procedure may be carried out using (a) a column (25 cm × 4.6 mm) packed with *stationary phase C* (5 µm) (Hypersil ODS is suitable), (b) as the mobile phase with a flow rate of 1.5 ml per minute a mixture of 60 volumes of a 0.41% w/v solution of *anhydrous sodium acetate*, adjusted to pH 7.0 with 2M *acetic acid* and 40 volumes of *methanol*, (c) a detection wavelength of 230 nm and (d) a 10-µl loop injector.

Inject solution (3). Adjust the sensitivity to obtain peaks with a height of at least half the full-scale deflection on the recorder. The test is not valid unless the *resolution factor* between the peaks corresponding to benzylpenicillin and carbenicillin is at least 5. If necessary, adjust the methanol content of the mobile phase.

Inject separately solutions (1) and (2). Calculate the percentage content of benzylpenicillin sodium from the areas of the peaks for benzylpenicillin sodium in the chromatograms obtained with solutions (1) and (2) and from the declared content of $C_{16}H_{17}N_2NaO_4S$ in *benzylpenicillin sodium EPCRS*.

Iodine-absorbing substances Not more than 8.0%, calculated with reference to the anhydrous substance, when determined by the following method. Dissolve 0.125 g of the mixed contents of the 10 containers used in the Assay in sufficient *mixed phosphate buffer pH 7.0* to produce 25 ml. To 10 ml add 10 ml of *mixed phosphate buffer pH 4.0* and 10 ml of 0.01M *iodine VS* and titrate immediately with 0.01M *sodium thiosulphate VS* using *starch mucilage*, added towards the end of the titration, as indicator. Repeat the operation without the substance being examined. The difference between the titrations represents the amount of iodine-absorbing substances present. Each ml of 0.01M *sodium thiosulphate VS* is equivalent to 0.489 mg of iodine-absorbing substances.

Water Not more than 5.5% w/w, Appendix IX C. Use 0.3 g of the mixed contents of the 10 containers used in the Assay.

Bacterial endotoxins Carry out the *test for bacterial endotoxins*, Appendix XIV C. Dissolve the contents of the sealed container in *water BET* to give a solution containing 10 mg per ml (solution A). The endotoxin limit concentration of solution A is 0.5 IU of endotoxin per ml. Carry out the test using the maximum valid dilution of solution A calculated from the declared sensitivity of the lysate used in the test.

Assay Determine the weight of the contents of 10 containers as described in the test for Uniformity of weight under Parenteral Preparations, Powders for Injections.

Dissolve 0.25 g (w_1) of the mixed contents of the 10 containers in sufficient *water* to produce 500 ml and dilute 10 ml to 100 ml with *water*. Place two 2-ml quantities of the resulting solution in separate stoppered tubes. To one tube add 10 ml of *imidazole—mercury reagent*, mix, stopper the tube and immerse in a water bath at 60° for exactly 25 minutes, swirling occasionally. Remove from the water bath and cool rapidly to 20° (solution B). To the second tube add 10 ml of *water* and mix (solution C). Without delay measure the *absorbances* of solutions B and C at the maximum at 325 nm, Appendix II B, using in the reference cell a mixture of 2 ml of *water* and 10 ml of *imidazole—mercury reagent* for solution B and *water* for solution C. Calculate the difference (S_1) between the absorbances of solutions B and C.

Repeat the procedure using 0.21 g (w_2) of *benzylpenicillin sodium EPCRS* in place of the substance being examined. Calculate the difference (S_2) between the *absorbances* of solutions B and solution C.

Calculate the percentage of total penicillins from the expression $1.185 S_1 w_2 F / S_2 w_1$, where F is the declared content of $C_{16}H_{17}N_2NaO_4S$ in *benzylpenicillin sodium EPCRS*. Subtract the percentage of benzylpenicillin sodium, determined by the test described above, multiplied by 1.185. The difference is the content of carbenicillin sodium, $C_{17}H_{16}N_2Na_2O_6S$.

Calculate the content of carbenicillin, $C_{17}H_{18}N_2O_6S$, in a container of average content weight. Each mg of $C_{17}H_{16}N_2Na_2O_6S$ is equivalent to 0.896 mg of $C_{17}H_{18}N_2O_6S$.

Storage The sealed container should be stored at a temperature of 2° to 8°.

Labelling The label of the sealed container states the quantity of Carbenicillin Sodium contained in it in terms of the equivalent amount of carbenicillin.

Carbimazole Tablets

Definition Carbimazole Tablets contain Carbimazole.

The tablets comply with the requirements stated under Tablets and with the following requirements.

Content of carbimazole, $C_7H_{10}N_2O_2S$ 90.0 to 110.0% of the prescribed or stated amount.

Identification

A. Extract a quantity of the powdered tablets containing 50 mg of Carbimazole with two 5-ml quantities of *chloroform*. Combine the chloroform extracts, filter and evaporate the filtrate to dryness. The *infrared absorption spectrum*, Appendix II A, of the residue after drying at 60° at a pressure not exceeding 0.7 kPa for 30 minutes is concordant with the *reference spectrum* of carbimazole.

B. To a small quantity of the powdered tablets add 0.05 ml of *dilute potassium iodobismuthate solution*. A scarlet colour is produced.

Methimazole and other related substances Carry out the method for *thin-layer chromatography*, Appendix III A, using *silica gel GF_{254}* as the coating substance and a mixture of 20 volumes of *acetone* and 80 volumes of *dichloromethane* as the mobile phase. Apply separately to the plate 20 µl of each of the following solutions. For solution (1) shake a quantity of the powdered tablets containing 50 mg of Carbimazole with 10 ml of *dichloromethane* for 5 minutes and filter. For solution (2) dilute 1 volume of solution (1) to 200 volumes with *dichloromethane*. Solution (3) contains 0.0050% w/v of *methimazole* in *dichloromethane*. After removal of the plate, allow it to dry in air for 30 minutes and examine under *ultraviolet light (254 nm)*. Any spot corresponding to methimazole in the chromatogram obtained with solution (1) is not more intense than the spot in the chromatogram obtained with solution (3) (1%) and any other *secondary spot* is not more intense than the principal spot in the chromatogram obtained with solution (2) (0.5%).

Assay Weigh and powder 20 tablets. To a quantity of the powder containing 80 mg of Carbimazole, add 400 ml of *water* warmed to a temperature not exceeding 35°, shake for 5 minutes, add 200 ml of *water*, shake again and add sufficient *water* to produce 1000 ml. Filter, dilute 50 ml of the filtrate to 500 ml with *water* and measure the *absorbance* of the resulting solution at the maximum at 291 nm, Appendix II B. Calculate the content of $C_7H_{10}N_2O_2S$ taking 557 as the value of A(1%, 1 cm) at the maximum at 291 nm.

Aromatic Cardamom Tincture

Definition

Cardamom Oil	3 ml
Caraway Oil	10 ml
Cinnamon Oil	10 ml
Clove Oil	10 ml
Strong Ginger Tincture	60 ml
Ethanol (90 per cent)	sufficient to produce 1000 ml

The tincture complies with the requirements stated under Tinctures and with the following requirements.

Ethanol content 84 to 87% v/v, Appendix VIII F, Method III.

Relative density 0.825 to 0.845, Appendix V G.

Compound Cardamom Tincture

Definition

Cardamom Oil	0.450 ml
Caraway Oil	0.400 ml
Cinnamon Oil	0.225 ml
Cochineal, in *moderately coarse powder*	7 g
Glycerol	50 ml
Ethanol (60 per cent)	sufficient to produce 1000 ml

Extemporaneous preparation The following directions apply.

Moisten the Cochineal with a sufficient quantity of Ethanol (60 per cent) and prepare 900 ml of tincture by *percolation*, Appendix XI F. Add the Cardamom Oil, the Caraway Oil, the Cinnamon Oil and the Glycerol and sufficient Ethanol (60 per cent) to produce 1000 ml ; mix. Filter, if necessary.

The tincture complies with the requirements stated under Tinctures and with the following requirements.

Ethanol content 52 to 57% v/v, Appendix VIII F, Method III.

Glycerol 4.5 to 5.5% v/v when determined by the following method. Dilute 20 ml to 100 ml with *water*. To 20 ml of this solution add 100 ml of *water* and 1 g of *activated charcoal* and boil under a reflux condenser for 15 minutes. Filter and wash the filter and charcoal with sufficient *water* to produce 150 ml. Add 0.25 ml of *bromocresol purple solution* and neutralise with 0.1M *sodium hydroxide* or 0.05M *sulphuric acid* to the blue colour of the indicator. Add 1.4 g of *sodium periodate* and allow to stand for 15 minutes. Add 3 ml of *propane-1,2-diol,* shake and allow to stand for 5 minutes. Add 0.25 ml of *bromocresol purple solution* and titrate with 0.1M *sodium hydroxide VS* to the same blue colour. Each ml of 0.1M *sodium hydroxide VS* is equivalent to 9.210 mg of glycerol. Calculate the percentage v/v of glycerol, taking its weight per ml to be 1.260 g.

Relative density 0.925 to 0.937, Appendix V G.

Carteolol Eye Drops

Definition Carteolol Eye Drops are a sterile solution of Carteolol Hydrochloride in Purified Water.

The eye drops comply with the requirements stated under Eye Preparations and with the following requirements.

Content of carteolol hydrochloride, $C_{16}H_{24}N_2O_3$,HCl
95.0 to 105.0% of the prescribed or stated amount.

Identification

A. Carry out the method for *thin-layer chromatography,* Appendix III A, using *silica gel GF_{254}* as the coating substance and a mixture of 1 volume of 13.5M *ammonia,* 20 volumes of *methanol* and 50 volumes of *chloroform* as the mobile phase but allowing the solvent front to ascend 12 cm above the line of application. Apply separately to the plate 2 µl of each of the following solutions. For solution (1) dilute the eye drops with *water,* if necessary, to contain 0.5% w/v of Carteolol Hydrochloride. Solution (2) contains 0.5% w/v of *carteolol hydrochloride BPCRS* in *water.* After removal of the plate, allow it to dry in air and examine under *ultraviolet light (254 nm).* The principal spot in the chromatogram obtained with solution (1) corresponds to that in the chromatogram obtained with solution (2).

B. In the Assay, the principal peak in the chromatogram obtained with solution (1) has the same retention time as that of the principal peak in the chromatogram obtained with solution (2).

Acidity pH, 6.2 to 7.2, Appendix V L.

Related substances Carry out the method for *liquid chromatography,* Appendix III D, using the following solutions. For solution (1) dilute the eye drops with the mobile phase to contain 0.20% w/v of Carteolol Hydrochloride. For solution (2) dilute 1 volume of solution (1) to 100 volumes with the mobile phase. For solution (3) dilute 1 volume of solution (1) to 100 volumes with the mobile phase and dilute 1 volume of this solution to 10 volumes with the mobile phase.

The chromatographic procedure may be carried out using (a) a stainless steel column (25 cm × 4.6 mm) packed with *stationary phase C* (5 µm) (YMC-PACK ODS-A is suitable), (b) as the mobile phase a mixture of 1 volume of *methanol,* 20 volumes of *acetonitrile* and 79 volumes of a 0.282% w/v solution of *sodium hexanesulphonate* at a flow rate such that the retention time of carteolol hydrochloride is about 14 minutes (1 ml per minute may be suitable) and (c) a detection wavelength of 252 nm.

The test is not valid unless the *column efficiency,* determined on the principal peak in the chromatogram obtained with solution (2), is at least 6000 *theoretical plates* per metre.

In the chromatogram obtained with solution (1), the area of any *secondary peak* is not greater than twice the area of the peak in the chromatogram obtained with solution (3) (0.2%), the area of not more than one such peak is greater than the area of the principal peak in the chromatogram obtained with solution (3) (0.1%) and the sum of the areas of all such peaks is not greater than 0.6 times the area of the principal peak in the chromatogram obtained with solution (2) (0.6%).

Assay Carry out the method for *liquid chromatography,* Appendix III D, using the following solutions in *water.* For solution (1) dilute the eye drops to contain 0.002% w/v of Carteolol Hydrochloride. Solution (2) contains 0.002% w/v of *carteolol hydrochloride BPCRS.*

The chromatographic procedure may be carried out using (a) a stainless steel column (12.5 cm × 4 mm) packed with *stationary phase B* (5 µm) (Lichrosphere C8 is suitable), (b) as the mobile phase at a flow rate of 1 ml per minute a solution containing 1.0 g of *potassium dihydrogen orthophosphate* in a mixture of 80 ml of *acetonitrile* and 400 ml of *water* and (c) a detection wavelength of 252 nm.

The test is not valid unless the *column efficiency,* determined on the principal peak in the chromatogram obtained with solution (2), is at least 6000 *theoretical plates* per metre.

Calculate the content of $C_{16}H_{24}N_2O_3$,HCl in the eye drops from the chromatograms obtained and from the declared content of $C_{16}H_{24}N_2O_3$,HCl in *carteolol hydrochloride BPCRS.*

Cascara Dry Extract

Definition Cascara Dry Extract is prepared by extracting Cascara with Purified Water and removing the solvent. It contains not less than 13.5% of hydroxyanthracene derivatives, of which not less than 40% consists of cascarosides, both calculated as cascaroside A with reference to the dried substance.

The extract complies with the requirements stated under Extracts and with the following requirements.

Frangula Carry out the method for *thin-layer chromatography,* Appendix III A, using *silica gel G* as the coating substance and a mixture of 100 volumes of *ethyl acetate,* 17 volumes of *methanol* and 13 volumes of *water* as the mobile phase. Apply separately to the plate 10 µl of each of two solutions prepared in the following manner. For solution (1) boil a quantity containing the equivalent of 32 mg of total hydroxyanthracene derivatives with 5 ml of *ethanol (70%),* cool and centrifuge. Decant the supernatant liquid and use within 30 minutes. For solution (2) dissolve 20 mg of *barbaloin* in 10 ml of *ethanol (70%).* After removal of the plate, dry it in a current of air until the odour of solvent is no longer detectable, spray immediately with a 0.1% w/v solution of N,N-*dimethyl*-p-*nitrosoaniline* in *pyridine,* then spray with a 5% w/v solution of *potassium hydroxide* in *ethanol (50%)* and heat at 105°

for 15 minutes. In the chromatogram obtained with solution (1) no spot is observed with an Rf value of 1.7 to 1.8 relative to the principal spot in the chromatogram obtained with solution (2).

Loss on drying Not more than 7.0%.

Assay Carry out the following procedure protected from light. To 0.5 g add 80 ml of *ethanol (70%)*, shake, allow to stand overnight, add sufficient *ethanol (70%)* to produce 100 ml, shake and filter. Transfer 10 ml of the filtrate to a separating funnel, add 0.1 ml of 1M *hydrochloric acid* and shake with two 20-ml quantities of *carbon tetrachloride*. Wash the combined carbon tetrachloride layers with 5 ml of *water* and add the washings to the aqueous solution. Extract the aqueous solution with four 30-ml quantities of water-saturated ethyl acetate, freshly prepared by shaking 150 ml of *ethyl acetate* with 15 ml of *water* for 3 minutes and allowing to separate. Use the combined ethyl acetate extracts for the determination of hydroxyanthracene glycosides other than cascarosides and the aqueous solution for the determination of cascarosides.

For hydroxyanthracene glycosides other than cascarosides Remove the solvent from the combined ethyl acetate extracts and evaporate just to dryness. Dissolve the residue in 0.5 ml of *methanol*, transfer to a flask with the aid of warm *water*, cool and add sufficient *water* to produce 50 ml. Add 20 ml to a mixture of 2 g of *iron(III) chloride hexahydrate* and 12 ml of *hydrochloric acid* and heat under a reflux condenser in a water bath for 4 hours, maintaining the level of the water above that of the liquid in the flask. Allow to cool, transfer to a separating funnel, wash the flask successively with 4 ml of 1M *sodium hydroxide* and 4 ml of *water* and add the washings to the separating funnel. Extract with three 30-ml quantities of *carbon tetrachloride*, wash the combined carbon tetrachloride layers with two 10-ml quantities of *water*, discard the washings and add sufficient *carbon tetrachloride* to produce 100 ml. Evaporate 20 ml to dryness on a water bath, dissolve the residue in 10 ml of a 0.5% w/v solution of *magnesium acetate* in *methanol* and measure the *absorbance* of the resulting solution at 440 nm and at 515 nm, Appendix II B, using *methanol* in the reference cell.

Calculate the content of hydroxyanthracene glycosides, as cascaroside A, from the absorbance at 515 nm taking 169 as the value of A(1%, 1 cm). The result of the assay is not valid unless the ratio of the absorbance at 515 nm to that at 440 nm is at least 2.6.

For cascarosides To the aqueous solution reserved from the preliminary extraction add sufficient *water* to produce 50 ml and carry out the Assay for hydroxyanthracene glycosides other than cascarosides, beginning at the words 'Add 20 ml ...'. Calculate the content of cascarosides, as cascaroside A, from the *absorbance* at 515 nm, Appendix II B, taking 169 as the value of A(1%, 1 cm). The result of the assay is not valid unless the ratio of the absorbance at 515 nm to that at 440 nm is at least 2.7.

Storage Cascara Dry Extract should be kept in a well-closed container.

Labelling The label states the percentage of total hydroxyanthracene derivatives.

Cascara Tablets

Definition Cascara Tablets contain Cascara Dry Extract. They are coated.

The tablets comply with the requirements stated under Tablets and with the following requirements.

Content of total hydroxyanthracene derivatives 17.0 to 23.0 mg , of which not less than 40% consists of cascarosides, both calculated as cascaroside A.

Disintegration Comply with the requirements stated under Tablets but for sugar-coated tablets the maximum time is 120 minutes.

Frangula Comply with the requirements stated under Cascara Dry Extract, but preparing solution (1) with a quantity of the powdered tablets containing 32 mg of total hydroxyanthracene derivatives.

Assay Weigh and powder 20 tablets. Carry out the Assay described under Cascara Dry Extract using a quantity of the powder containing 75 mg of total hydroxyanthracene derivatives.

Cefalexin Capsules

Definition Cefalexin Capsules contain Cefalexin.

The capsules comply with the requirements stated under Capsules and with the following requirements.

Content of anhydrous cefalexin, $C_{16}H_{17}N_3O_4S$ 92.5 to 110.0% of the prescribed or stated amount.

Identification

Shake a quantity of the contents of the capsules containing the equivalent of 0.5 g of anhydrous cefalexin with 1 ml of *water* and 1.4 ml of 1M *hydrochloric acid*, filter and wash the filter with 1 ml of *water*. Add slowly to the filtrate a saturated solution of *sodium acetate* until precipitation occurs. Add 5 ml of *methanol*, filter and wash the precipitate with two 1-ml quantities of *methanol*. The residue, after drying at a pressure not exceeding 0.7 kPa, complies with the following tests.

A. The *infrared absorption spectrum*, Appendix II A, is concordant with the *reference spectrum* of cefalexin.

B. Carry out the method for *thin-layer chromatography*, Appendix III A, using *silanised silica gel HF_{254}* as the coating substance and a mixture of 15 volumes of *acetone* and 85 volumes of a 15.4% w/v solution of *ammonium acetate*, previously adjusted to pH 6.2 with 5M *acetic acid* as the mobile phase. Apply separately to the plate 1 µl of each of the following solutions. For solution (1) shake a quantity of the contents of the capsules containing the equivalent of 0.2 g of anhydrous cefalexin with 25 ml of a mixture of equal volumes of *methanol* and 0.067M *mixed phosphate buffer pH 7.0*, dilute to 50 ml with the same solvent mixture, filter and use the filtrate. Solution (2) contains 0.4% w/v of *cefalexin EPCRS* in a mixture of equal volumes of *methanol* and 0.067M *mixed phosphate buffer pH 7.0*. Solution (3) contains 0.4% w/v of *cefalexin EPCRS* and 0.4% w/v of *cefradine EPCRS* in a mixture of equal volumes of *methanol* and 0.067M *mixed phosphate buffer pH 7.0*. After removal of the plate, allow it to dry and examine under *ultraviolet light (254 nm)*. The principal spot in the chromatogram obtained with solution (1) is similar in position and size to that in the chromatogram obtained with solution (2). The test is not valid unless the chromatogram obtained with solution (3) shows two clearly separated spots.

C. Mix 20 mg with 0.25 ml of a 1% v/v solution of *glacial acetic acid* and add 0.1 ml of a 1% w/v solution of *copper(II) sulphate* and 0.1 ml of 2M *sodium hydroxide*. An olive-green colour is produced.

Disintegration Maximum time, 15 minutes, using a 0.6% v/v solution of *hydrochloric acid* in place of *water*, Appendix XII A.

Related substances Carry out the method for *thin-layer chromatography*, Appendix III A, using *silica gel G* as the coating substance and a mixture of 3 volumes of *acetone*, 80 volumes of a 7.2% w/v solution of *disodium hydrogen orthophosphate* and 120 volumes of a 2.1% w/v solution of *citric acid* as the mobile phase. Impregnate the plate by development with a 5% v/v solution of *n-tetradecane* in *hexane*. Allow the solvent to evaporate and carry out the chromatography in the same direction as the impregnation. Apply separately to the plate 5 µl of each of the following solutions. For solution (1) shake a quantity of the contents of the capsules containing the equivalent of 0.25 g of anhydrous cefalexin with 10 ml of 2M *hydrochloric acid*, filter and use the filtrate. For solution (2) dilute 1 volume of solution (1) to 100 volumes with 2M *hydrochloric acid*. Solution (3) contains 0.025% w/v of *7-aminodesacetoxycephalosporanic acid EPCRS* in 2M *hydrochloric acid*. Solution (4) contains 0.025% w/v of *DL-phenylglycine* in 2M *hydrochloric acid*. Solution (5) contains 2.5% w/v of *cefalexin EPCRS* and 0.025% w/v of each of *7-aminodesacetoxycephalosporanic acid EPCRS* and *DL-phenylglycine* in 2M *hydrochloric acid*. After removal of the plate, dry it at 90° for 3 minutes, spray the hot plate with a 0.1% w/v solution of *ninhydrin* in the mobile phase, heat the plate at 90° for 15 minutes and allow to cool. In the chromatogram obtained with solution (1) any spot corresponding to 7-aminodesacetoxycephalosporanic acid is not more intense than the spot in the chromatogram obtained with solution (3) (1%), any spot corresponding to DL-phenylglycine is not more intense than the spot in the chromatogram obtained with solution (4) (1%) and any other *secondary spot* is not more intense than the spot in the chromatogram obtained with solution (2) (1%). The test is not valid unless the chromatogram obtained with solution (5) shows three clearly separated spots.

Assay Carry out the method for *liquid chromatography*, Appendix III D, using the following solutions. For solution (1) shake a quantity of the powdered, mixed contents of 20 capsules containing the equivalent of 0.25 g of anhydrous cefalexin with 100 ml of *water* for 30 minutes, add sufficient *water* to produce 250 ml and filter. Dilute 25 ml of the filtrate to 50 ml with *water*. Solution (2) contains 0.05% w/v of *cefalexin EPCRS* in *water*. Solution (3) contains 0.01% w/v each of *cefalexin EPCRS* and *cefradine EPCRS* in *water*.

The chromatographic procedure may be carried out using (a) a column (25 cm × 4.6 mm) packed with *stationary phase C* (5 µm) (Nucleosil C18 is suitable), (b) a mixture of 2 volumes of *methanol*, 5 volumes of *acetonitrile*, 10 volumes of a 1.36% w/v solution of *potassium dihydrogen orthophosphate* and 83 volumes of *water* as the mobile phase with a flow rate of 1.5 ml per minute and (c) a detection wavelength of 254 nm. Adjust the sensitivity so that the height of the peaks in the chromatogram obtained with solution (3) is at least half the full-scale deflection on the chart recorder.

The assay is not valid unless the *resolution factor* between the peaks corresponding to cephalexin and cephradine in the chromatogram obtained with solution (3) is at least 4; if necessary adjust the acetonitrile content of the mobile phase. Make six injections of solution (2); the assay is not valid if the relative standard deviation for the peak area of cephalexin is greater than 1.0%.

Inject solutions (1) and (2) alternately and calculate the percentage content of $C_{16}H_{17}N_3O_4S$ from the declared content of $C_{16}H_{17}N_3O_4S$ in *cefalexin EPCRS*.

Storage Cefalexin Capsules should be stored at a temperature not exceeding 30°.

Labelling The quantity of active ingredient is stated in terms of the equivalent amount of anhydrous cefalexin.

When cephalexin capsules are prescribed or demanded, Cefalexin Capsules shall be dispensed or supplied.

Cefalexin Oral Suspension

Definition Cefalexin Oral Suspension is a suspension of Cefalexin in a suitable flavoured vehicle. It is prepared by dispersing the dry ingredients in the specified volume of Water just before issue for use.

The dry ingredients comply with the requirements for Powders and Granules for the Preparation of Oral Liquids stated under Oral Liquids.

Storage The dry ingredients should be kept in a well-closed container, protected from light and stored at a temperature not exceeding 30°.

For the following tests prepare the Oral Suspension as directed on the label. The suspension, examined immediately after preparation unless otherwise indicated, complies with the requirements stated under Oral Liquids and with the following requirements.

Content of anhydrous cefalexin, $C_{16}H_{17}N_3O_4S$ When freshly constituted, not more than 120.0% of the prescribed or stated amount. When stored at the temperature and for the period stated on the label during which the Oral Suspension may be expected to be satisfactory for use, not less than 80.0% of the prescribed or stated amount.

Identification

A. Complies with test B described under Cefalexin Capsules but preparing solution (1) in the following manner. Shake a quantity of the oral suspension containing the equivalent of 0.2 g of anhydrous cefalexin with 70 ml of *methanol*, filter, evaporate to dryness using a rotary evaporator and dissolve the residue in sufficient 0.5M *hydrochloric acid* to produce 50 ml.

B. Shake a quantity of the oral suspension containing the equivalent of 0.1 g of anhydrous cefalexin with 70 ml of *methanol*, filter and evaporate the filtrate to dryness using a rotary evaporator. Dissolve the residue in the minimum volume of a 1% v/v solution of *glacial acetic acid*, decolorise if necessary by the addition of sufficient *activated charcoal*, shake and filter. To 0.25 ml of the resulting solution add 0.1 ml of a 1% w/v solution of *copper(II) sulphate* and 0.05 ml of 2M *sodium hydroxide*. An olive-green colour is produced.

Assay Carry out the Assay described under Cefalexin Capsules but using as solution (1) a solution prepared in the following manner. Shake a weighed quantity of the oral suspension containing the equivalent of 0.25 g of anhydrous cefalexin with 100 ml of *water* for 30 minutes, add sufficient *water* to produce 250 ml, filter and dilute 25 ml of the filtrate to 50 ml with *water*.

Determine the *weight per ml* of the oral suspension, Appendix V G, and calculate the content of $C_{16}H_{17}N_3O_4S$, weight in volume.

Storage The Oral Suspension should be stored at the temperature and used within the period stated on the label.

Labelling The quantity of active ingredient is stated in terms of the equivalent amount of anhydrous cefalexin.

When cephalexin oral suspension is prescribed or demanded, Cefalexin Oral Suspension shall be dispensed or supplied.

Cefalexin Tablets

Definition Cefalexin Tablets contain Cefalexin.

With the exception of the requirements for shape, the tablets comply with the requirements stated under Tablets and with the following requirements.

Content of anhydrous cefalexin, $C_{16}H_{17}N_3O_4S$ 92.5 to 110.0% of the prescribed or stated amount.

Identification

Remove any coating. Shake a quantity of the powdered tablet cores containing the equivalent of 0.5 g of anhydrous cefalexin with 1 ml of *water* and 1.4 ml of 1M *hydrochloric acid*, add 0.1 g of *activated charcoal*, shake, filter and wash the filter with 1 ml of *water*. Add slowly to the filtrate a saturated solution of *sodium acetate* until precipitation occurs. Add 5 ml of *methanol*, filter and wash the precipitate with two 1-ml quantities of *methanol*. The residue, after drying at a pressure not exceeding 0.7 kPa, complies with the following tests.

A. The *infrared absorption spectrum*, Appendix II A, is concordant with the *reference spectrum* of cefalexin.

B. Complies with test B described under Cefalexin Capsules but preparing solution (1) in the following manner. Shake 0.2 g with 25 ml of a mixture of equal volumes of *methanol* and 0.067M *mixed phosphate buffer pH 7.0*, dilute to 50 ml with the same solvent mixture, filter and use the filtrate.

C. Mix 20 mg with 0.25 ml of a 1% v/v solution of *glacial acetic acid* and add 0.1 ml of a 1% w/v solution of *copper(II) sulphate* and 0.1 ml of 2M *sodium hydroxide*. An olive-green colour is produced.

Disintegration Maximum time, 30 minutes, Appendix XII A.

Related substances Comply with the test described under Cefalexin Capsules but using the following solutions. For solution (1) shake a quantity of the powdered tablets containing the equivalent of 0.25 g of anhydrous cefalexin with 10 ml of 2M *hydrochloric acid*, filter and use the filtrate. For solution (2) dilute 1 volume of solution (1) to 100 volumes with 2M *hydrochloric acid*. Solution (3) contains 0.025% w/v of *7-aminodesacetoxycephalosporanic acid EPCRS* in 2M *hydrochloric acid*. Solution (4) contains 0.025% w/v of *DL-phenylglycine* in 2M *hydrochloric acid*. Solution (5) contains 2.5% w/v of *cefalexin EPCRS* and 0.025% w/v of each of *7-aminodesacetoxycephalosporanic acid EPCRS* and *DL-phenylglycine* in 2M *hydrochloric acid*.

Assay Weigh and powder 20 tablets. Carry out the Assay described under Cefalexin Capsules but using as solution (1) a solution prepared in the following manner. Shake a quantity of the powdered tablets containing the equivalent of 0.25 g of anhydrous cefalexin with 100 ml of *water* for 30 minutes, add sufficient *water* to produce 250 ml, filter and dilute 25 ml of the filtrate to 50 ml with *water*.

Storage Cefalexin Tablets should be stored at a temperature not exceeding 30°.

Labelling The quantity of active ingredient is stated in terms of the equivalent amount of anhydrous cefalexin.

When cephalexin tablets are prescribed or demanded, Cefalexin Tablets shall be dispensed or supplied.

Cefazolin Injection

Definition Cefazolin Injection is a sterile solution of Cefazolin Sodium in Water for Injections. It is prepared by dissolving Cefazolin Sodium for Injection in the requisite amount of Water for Injections.

The injection complies with the requirements stated under Parenteral Preparations.

Storage Cefazolin Injection should be used immediately after preparation but, in any case, within the period recommended by the manufacturer when prepared and stored strictly in accordance with the manufacturer's instructions.

CEFAZOLIN SODIUM FOR INJECTION

Definition Cefazolin Sodium for Injection is a sterile material consisting of Cefazolin Sodium with or without excipients. It is supplied in a sealed container.

The contents of the sealed container comply with the requirements for Powders for Injections stated under Parenteral Preparations and with the following requirements.

Content of cefazolin, $C_{14}H_{14}N_8O_4S_3$ 90.0 to 105.0% of the prescribed or stated amount.

Identification

A. Carry out the method for *thin-layer chromatography*, Appendix III A, using *silanised silica gel HF_{254}* as the coating substance and as the mobile phase a mixture of 15 volumes of *acetonitrile* and 85 volumes of a 15% w/v solution of *ammonium acetate*, previously adjusted to pH 6.2 with 5M *acetic acid*. Apply separately to the plate 1 µl of each of the following solutions. For solution (1) dissolve a quantity of the contents of a sealed container in sufficient of a mixture of equal volumes of *methanol* and *0.067M mixed phosphate buffer pH 7.0* to produce a solution containing the equivalent of 0.4% w/v of cefazolin. Solution (2) contains 0.4% w/v of *cefazolin sodium EPCRS* in a mixture of equal volumes of *methanol* and *0.067M mixed phosphate buffer pH 7.0*. Solution (3) contains 0.4% w/v each of *cefazolin sodium EPCRS* and *cefoxitin sodium EPCRS* in a mixture of equal volumes of *methanol* and *0.067M mixed phosphate buffer pH 7.0*. After removal of the plate, allow it to dry in a current of warm air and examine under *ultraviolet light (254 nm)*. The principal spot in the chromatogram obtained with solution (1) corresponds to that in the chromatogram obtained with solution (2). The test is not valid unless the chromatogram obtained with solution (3) shows two clearly separated principal spots.

B. Yield reaction A characteristic of *sodium salts*, Appendix VI.

Acidity pH of a solution containing the equivalent of 10.0% w/v of cefazolin, 4.0 to 6.0, Appendix V L.

Clarity of solution A solution containing the equivalent of 10.0% w/v of cefazolin in *carbon dioxide-free water* is *clear*, Appendix IV A. The *absorbance* of the solution measured at 430 nm is not greater than 0.15, Appendix II B.

Related substances Carry out the method for *thin-layer chromatography*, Appendix III A, using *silica gel GF_{254}* as the coating substance and a mixture of 10 volumes of *glacial acetic acid*, 10 volumes of *water*, 20 volumes of *acetone* and 50 volumes of *ethyl acetate* as the mobile phase. Apply separately to the plate 5 µl of each of the following solutions under a stream of nitrogen. For solution (1) dissolve a quantity of the contents of a sealed container in sufficient *water* to produce a solution containing the equivalent of 5.0% w/v of cefazolin. For solution (2) dilute 1 volume of solution (1) to 100 volumes with *water*. After removal of the plate, allow it to dry in air and examine under *ultraviolet light (254 nm)*. Expose the plate to iodine vapour in an airtight tank until the spots appear and examine again. For each examination any *secondary spot* in the chromatogram obtained with solution (1) is not more intense than the spot in the chromatogram obtained with solution (2) (1%).

Water Not more than 6.0% w/w, Appendix IX C, Method I. Use 0.3 g.

Bacterial endotoxins Carry out the *test for bacterial endotoxins*, Appendix XIV C. Dissolve the contents of the sealed container in *water BET* to give a solution containing the equivalent of 10 mg of cefazolin per ml (solution A). The endotoxin limit concentration of solution A is 1.5 IU per ml. Carry out the test using the maximum valid dilution of solution A calculated from the declared sensitivity of the lysate used in the test.

Assay Determine the weight of the contents of 10 containers as described in the test for Uniformity of weight under Parenteral Preparations, Powders for Injections.

Carry out the method for *liquid chromatography*, Appendix III D, using the following solutions in *water*. For solution (1) dissolve a quantity of the mixed contents of the 10 containers to produce a solution containing the equivalent of 0.1% w/v of cefazolin. Solution (2) contains 0.1% w/v of *cefazolin sodium EPCRS*. Solution (3) contains 0.005% w/v of *cefuroxime sodium EPCRS* and 0.01% w/v of *cefazolin sodium EPCRS*.

The chromatographic procedure may be carried out using (a) a stainless steel column (25 cm × 4.6 mm) packed with *stationary phase C* (5 µm to 10 µm) (Spherisorb ODS 1 is suitable), (b) as the mobile phase with a flow rate of 1 ml per minute a mixture of 10 volumes of *acetonitrile* and 90 volumes of a solution containing 0.277% w/v of *disodium hydrogen orthophosphate* and 0.186% w/v of *citric acid* and (c) a detection wavelength of 270 nm. Inject 20 µl of each solution.

Inject solution (3). Adjust the sensitivity of the detector so that the heights of the peaks are at least 50% of the full scale of the recorder. The test is not valid unless the *resolution factor* between the peaks corresponding to cefazolin and cefuroxime is at least 2.0. If necessary, adjust the concentration of acetonitrile in the mobile phase. Inject alternately solution (1) and solution (2).

Calculate the content of $C_{14}H_{14}N_8O_4S_3$ in a container of average content weight from the declared content of $C_{14}H_{13}N_8NaO_4S_3$ in *cefazolin sodium EPCRS*. Each mg of $C_{14}H_{13}N_8NaO_4S_3$ is equivalent to 0.9539 mg of $C_{14}H_{14}N_8O_4S_3$.

Storage The sealed container should be protected from light and stored at a temperature not exceeding 30°.

Labelling The label on the sealed container states the quantity of Cefazolin Sodium contained in it in terms of the equivalent amount of cefazolin.

When cephazolin injection or cephazolin sodium for injection are prescribed or demanded, Cefazolin Injection or Cefazolin Sodium for Injection shall be dispensed or supplied.

Cefotaxime Injection

Definition Cefotaxime Injection is a sterile solution of Cefotaxime Sodium in Water for Injections. It is prepared by dissolving Cefotaxime Sodium for Injection in the requisite amount of Water for Injections immediately before use.

The injection complies with the requirements stated under Parenteral Preparations.

Storage Cefotaxime Injection should be used immediately after preparation but, in any case, within the period recommended by the manufacturer when prepared and stored strictly in accordance with the manufacturer's instructions.

CEFOTAXIME SODIUM FOR INJECTION

Definition Cefotaxime Sodium for Injection is a sterile material consisting of Cefotaxime Sodium with or without excipients. It is supplied in a sealed container.

The contents of the sealed container comply with the requirements for Powders for Injections stated under Parenteral Preparations and with the following requirements.

Content of cefotaxime, $C_{16}H_{17}N_5O_7S_2$ 90.0 to 110.0% of the prescribed or stated amount.

Identification

A. The *infrared absorption spectrum*, Appendix II A, is concordant with the *reference spectrum* of cefotaxime sodium.

B. Carry out the method for *thin-layer chromatography*, Appendix III A, using *silanised silica gel HF_{254}* as the coating substance and as the mobile phase a mixture of 15 volumes of *acetone* and 85 volumes of a 15.4% w/v solution of *ammonium acetate*, previously adjusted to pH 6.2 with *glacial acetic acid*. Apply separately to the plate 1 µl of each of the following solutions. For solution (1) dissolve a quantity of the contents of the sealed container in sufficient of a mixture of equal volumes of *methanol* and *0.067M mixed phosphate buffer pH 7.0* to produce a solution containing the equivalent of 0.4% w/v of cefotaxime.

Solution (2) contains 0.4% w/v of *cefotaxime sodium EPCRS* in a mixture of equal volumes of *methanol* and *0.067M mixed phosphate buffer pH 7.0*. Solution (3) contains 0.4% w/v each of *cefotaxime sodium EPCRS* and *cefoxitin sodium EPCRS* in a mixture of equal volumes of *methanol* and *0.067M mixed phosphate buffer pH 7.0*. After removal of the plate, allow it to dry in air and examine under *ultraviolet light (254 nm)*. The principal spot in the chromatogram obtained with solution (1) corresponds to that in the chromatogram obtained with solution (2). The test is not valid unless the chromatogram obtained with solution (3) shows two clearly separated principal spots.

C. Yields reaction characteristic of *sodium salts*, Appendix VI.

Acidity pH of a 10.0% w/v solution, 4.5 to 6.5, Appendix V L.

Clarity of solution A 10.0% w/v solution in *carbon dioxide-free water* is *clear*, Appendix IV A. The *absorbance* of the solution at 430 nm is not greater than 0.60, Appendix II B.

Related substances Carry out the method for *liquid chromatography*, Appendix III D, using the following freshly prepared solutions. For solution (1) dissolve a quantity of the contents of the sealed container in sufficient of the mobile phase to produce a solution containing the equivalent of 0.1% w/v of cefotaxime. Solution (2) contains 0.001% w/v of *cefotaxime sodium EPCRS* in the mobile phase.

The chromatographic conditions described under Assay may be used.

Inject 10 µl of each solution. Allow the chromatography to proceed for at least 8 times the retention time (about 6 minutes) of cefotaxime. In the chromatogram obtained with solution (1) the area of any *secondary peak* is not greater than the area of the principal peak in the chromatogram obtained with solution (2) (1%) and the sum of the areas of all the *secondary peaks* is not greater than 4 times the area of the principal peak in the chromatogram obtained with solution (2) (4%).

Loss on drying When dried in an oven at 100° to 105°, lose not more than 3.0% of their weight. Use 1 g.

Bacterial endotoxins Carry out the *test for bacterial endotoxins*, Appendix XIV C. Dissolve the contents of the sealed container in *water BET* to give a solution containing the equivalent of 10 mg of cefotaxime per ml (solution A). The endotoxin limit concentration is 0.5 IU per ml. Carry out the test using the maximum valid dilution of solution A calculated from the declared sensitivity of the lysate used in the test.

Assay Determine the weight of the contents of 10 containers as described in the test for Uniformity of weight under Parenteral Preparations, Powders for Injections.

Carry out the method for *liquid chromatography*, Appendix III D, using the following freshly prepared solutions. For solution (1) dissolve a quantity of the mixed contents of the 10 containers in sufficient of the mobile phase to produce a solution containing 0.01% w/v of cefotaxime. Solution (2) contains 0.01% w/v of *cefotaxime sodium EPCRS* in the mobile phase. For solution (3) add 1 ml of 2M *hydrochloric acid* to 4 ml of solution (1), heat the solution at 40° for 2 hours, add 5 ml of *phosphate buffer pH 6.6* and 1 ml of 2M *sodium hydroxide* and mix.

The chromatographic procedure may be carried out using (a) a stainless steel column (25 cm × 4.6 mm) packed with *stationary phase C* (5 µm) (Hypersil 5µ ODS is suitable), (b) as the mobile phase with a flow rate of 1 ml per minute a mixture prepared in the following manner: dissolve 3.5 g of *potassium dihydrogen orthophosphate* and 11.6 g of *disodium hydrogen orthophosphate* in 1000 ml of *water* at pH 7.0 and add 375 ml of *methanol*, and (c) a detection wavelength of 235 nm. Inject 10 µl of each solution.

Inject solution (2) and solution (3). Adjust the sensitivity of the detector so that the heights of the peaks in the chromatogram obtained with solution (3) are at least 50% of the full scale of the recorder. The test is not valid unless cefotaxime is eluted as the second of the principal peaks and the *resolution factor* between the two principal peaks is at least 3.5. The test is not valid unless the *symmetry factor* of the principal peak in the chromatogram obtained with solution (2) is less than 2.0. When the chromatograms are recorded under the prescribed conditions the retention time of the principal peak is about 6 minutes. If necessary use another stationary phase or adjust the concentration of *methanol* in the mobile phase.

Calculate the content of $C_{16}H_{17}N_5O_7S_2$ in a container of average content weight from the declared content of $C_{16}H_{16}N_5NaO_7S_2$ in *cefotaxime sodium EPCRS*. Each mg of $C_{16}H_{16}N_5NaO_7S_2$ is equivalent to 0.9539 mg of $C_{16}H_{17}N_5O_7S_2$.

Storage The sealed container should be protected from light and stored at a temperature not exceeding 25°.

Labelling The label on the sealed container states the quantity of Cefotaxime Sodium contained in it in terms of the equivalent amount of cefotaxime.

Cefoxitin Injection

Definition Cefoxitin Injection is a sterile solution of Cefoxitin Sodium in Water for Injections. It is prepared by dissolving Cefoxitin Sodium for Injection in the requisite amount of Water for Injections.

The injection complies with the requirements stated under Parenteral Preparations.

Storage Cefoxitin Injection should be used immediately after preparation but, in any case, within the period recommended by the manufacturer when prepared and stored strictly in accordance with the manufacturer's instructions.

CEFOXITIN SODIUM FOR INJECTION

Definition Cefoxitin Sodium for Injection is a sterile material consisting of Cefoxitin Sodium with or without excipients. It is supplied in a sealed container.

The contents of the sealed container comply with the requirements for Powders for Injections stated under Parenteral Preparations and with the following requirements.

Content of cefoxitin, $C_{16}H_{17}N_3O_7S_2$ 95.0 to 105.0% of the prescribed or stated amount.

Identification

A. The *infrared absorption spectrum*, Appendix II A, is concordant with the *reference spectrum* of cefoxitin sodium.

B. Carry out the method for *thin-layer chromatography*, Appendix III A, using *silanised silica gel HF_{254}* as the coating substance and as the mobile phase a mixture of 10 volumes of *tetrahydrofuran* and 90 volumes of a 15.4% w/v solution of *ammonium acetate* previously adjusted to pH 6.2 with 5M *acetic acid*. Apply separately to the plate 1 µl of each of the following solutions. For solution (1) dissolve a quantity of the contents of a sealed container in sufficient of a mixture of equal volumes of *methanol* and *0.067M mixed phosphate buffer pH 7.0* to produce a solution containing the equivalent of 0.4% w/v of cefoxitin. Solution (2) contains 0.4% w/v of *cefoxitin sodium EPCRS* in a mixture of equal volumes of *methanol* and *0.067M mixed phosphate buffer pH 7.0*. Solution (3) contains 0.4% w/v of each of *cefoxitin sodium EPCRS* and *cefazolin sodium EPCRS* in a mixture of equal volumes of *methanol* and *0.067M mixed phosphate buffer pH 7.0*. After removal of the plate, allow it to dry in a current of warm air and examine under *ultraviolet light (254 nm)*. The principal spot in the chromatogram obtained with solution (1) corresponds to that in the chromatogram obtained with solution (2). The test is not valid unless the chromatogram obtained with solution (3) shows two clearly separated principal spots.

C. Yield reaction A characteristic of *sodium salts*, Appendix VI.

Acidity or alkalinity pH of a solution containing the equivalent of 1.0% w/v of cefoxitin, 4.2 to 7.0, Appendix V L.

Clarity of solution A solution containing the equivalent of 10.0% w/v of cefoxitin in *carbon dioxide-free water* is *clear*, Appendix IV A, and not more intensely coloured than intensity 5 of the range of reference solutions of the most appropriate colour, Appendix IV B, Method II.

Related substances Carry out the method for *thin-layer chromatography*, Appendix III A, using *silica gel GF_{254}* as the coating substance and as the mobile phase a mixture of 10 volumes of *glacial acetic acid*, 10 volumes of *water*, 20 volumes of *acetone* and 50 volumes of *ethyl acetate*. Apply separately to the plate 5 µl of each of the following solutions. For solution (1) dissolve a quantity of the contents of a sealed container in sufficient *water* to produce a solution containing the equivalent of 2.5% w/v of cefoxitin. For solution (2) dilute 0.5 volume of solution (1) to 100 volumes with *water*. After removal of the plate, allow it to dry in air and examine under *ultraviolet light (254 nm)*. Any *secondary spot* in the chromatogram obtained with solution (1) is not more intense than the spot in the chromatogram obtained with solution (2) (0.5%).

Water Not more than 1.0% w/w, Appendix IX C, Method I. Use 0.5 g.

Bacterial endotoxins Carry out the *test for bacterial endotoxins*, Appendix XIV C. Dissolve the contents of the sealed container in *water BET* to give a solution containing the equivalent of 10 mg of cefoxitin per ml (solution A). The endotoxin limit concentration of solution A is 1.3 IU per ml. Carry out the test using the maximum valid dilution of solution A calculated from the declared sensitivity of the lysate used in the test.

Assay Determine the weight of the contents of 10 containers as described in the test for Uniformity of weight under Parenteral Preparations, Powders for Injections.

Carry out the method for *liquid chromatography*, Appendix III D, using the following solutions in *water*. For solution (1) dissolve a quantity of the mixed contents of the 10 containers to produce a solution containing the equivalent of 0.1% w/v of cefoxitin. Solution (2) contains 0.1% w/v of *cefoxitin sodium EPCRS*. Solution (3) contains 0.08% w/v of *2-(2-thienyl)acetic acid*. For solution (4) mix 1 volume of solution (2) and 5 volumes of solution (3).

The chromatographic procedure may be carried out using (a) a stainless steel column (25 cm × 4.6 mm) packed with *stationary phase C* (5 µm to 10 µm) (Hypersil ODS is suitable), (b) as the mobile phase with a flow rate of 1 ml per minute a mixture of 1 volume of 5M *acetic acid*, 19 volumes of *acetonitrile* and 81 volumes of *water* and (c) a detection wavelength of 254 nm. Inject 20 µl of each solution.

Inject solution (4). Adjust the sensitivity of the detector so that the heights of the peaks in the chromatogram obtained are at least 50% of the full scale of the recorder. The test is not valid unless the *resolution factor* between the two principal peaks is at least 3.5. If necessary, adjust the concentration of acetonitrile in the mobile phase. Inject alternately solution (1) and solution (2).

Calculate the content of $C_{16}H_{17}N_3O_7S_2$ in a container of average content weight from the declared content of $C_{16}H_{16}N_3NaO_7S_2$ in *cefoxitin sodium EPCRS*. Each mg of $C_{16}H_{16}N_3NaO_7S_2$ is equivalent to 0.9510 mg of $C_{16}H_{17}N_3O_7S_2$.

Storage The sealed container should be protected from light and stored at a temperature not exceeding 30°.

Labelling The label on the sealed container states the quantity of Cefoxitin Sodium contained in it in terms of the equivalent amount of cefoxitin.

Cefradine Capsules

Definition Cefradine Capsules contain Cefradine.

The capsules comply with the requirements stated under Capsules and with the following requirements.

Content of cephalosporins, calculated as the sum of cefradine, ($C_{16}H_{19}N_3O_4S$) and cefalexin ($C_{16}H_{17}N_3O_4S$) 90.0 to 105.0% of the prescribed or stated amount of Cefradine.

Identification

A. The *infrared absorption spectrum* of the contents of the capsules, Appendix II A, is concordant with the *reference spectrum* of cefradine. If the spectra are not concordant, dissolve a quantity of the contents containing 30 mg of Cefradine in 10 ml of *methanol*, evaporate to dryness at 40° at a pressure of 2 kPa and prepare a new spectrum.

B. Carry out the method for *thin-layer chromatography*, Appendix III A, using a silica gel G precoated plate (Analtech plates are suitable) and the mobile phase and method of visualisation described under Related substances. Impregnate the plate as described under Related substances and apply separately 5 µl of each of the following solutions. For solution (1) shake a quantity of the contents of the capsules containing 0.1 g of Cefradine with 25 ml of 0.01M *ammonia* for 45 minutes and dilute 1 ml of the resulting solution to 10 ml with 0.01M *ammonia*. Solution (2) contains 0.040% w/v of *cefradine EPCRS* in 0.01M *ammonia*. The principal spot in the chromatogram obtained with solution (1) corresponds to that in the chromatogram obtained with solution (2).

Dissolution Comply with the *dissolution test for tablets and capsules*, Appendix XII D, using as the medium 900 ml of

0.12M *hydrochloric acid* and rotating the basket at 100 revolutions per minute. Withdraw a sample of 10 ml of the medium and filter. Measure the *absorbance* of the filtered solution, diluted if necessary with 0.12M *hydrochloric acid,* at the maximum at 255 nm, Appendix II B, using 0.12M *hydrochloric acid* in the reference cell. Calculate the total content of cefradine, $C_{16}H_{19}N_3O_4S$, in the medium from the *absorbance* obtained from a 0.0025% w/v solution of *cefradine EPCRS* and using as the declared content the sum of the contents of $C_{16}H_{19}N_3O_4S$ and cephalexin, $C_{16}H_{17}N_3O_4S$, in *cefradine EPCRS.*

Related substances Carry out the method for *thin-layer chromatography,* Appendix III A, using a silica gel G precoated plate (Analtech plates are suitable) and using a mixture of 3 volume of *acetone,* 80 volumes of 0.2M *anhydrous disodium hydrogen orthophosphate* and 120 volumes of 0.1M *citric acid* as the mobile phase. Impregnate the plate by placing it in a tank containing a shallow layer of a 5% w/v solution of n-*tetradecane* in n-*hexane,* allowing the impregnating solvent to ascend to the top, removing the plate from the tank and allowing the solvent to evaporate; use with the flow of the mobile phase in the same direction as the impregnation was carried out. Apply separately to the plate, as bands about 3 cm wide, 40 µl of each of the following freshly prepared solutions. For solution (1) shake a quantity of the contents of the capsules containing 0.1 g of Cefradine with 25 ml of 0.01M *ammonia* for 45 minutes. For solution (2) dilute 1 ml of solution (1) to 100 ml with 0.01M *ammonia.* Solution (3) contains 0.0040% w/v of *cyclohexa-1,4-dienylglycine EPCRS* and 0.0040% w/v of *7-aminodesacetoxycephalosporanic acid EPCRS* in 0.01M *ammonia.* Solution (4) contains 0.040% w/v of *cefalexin EPCRS* in 0.01M *ammonia.*

After removal of the plate, heat at 90° for 2 to 3 minutes and spray the hot plate with a 0.1% w/v solution of *ninhydrin* in the mobile phase. Heat at 90° for 15 minutes in a circulating air oven with the plates parallel to the airflow, cool for 15 minutes protected from light and examine in daylight. In the chromatogram obtained with solution (1) any bands corresponding to cyclohexa-1,4-dienylglycine and 7-aminodesacetoxycephalosporanic acid are not more intense than the corresponding bands in the chromatogram obtained with solution (3) (1%) and any other *secondary band* is not more intense than the band in the chromatogram obtained with solution (2) (1%). Disregard any band that corresponds to the band in the chromatogram obtained with solution (4).

Cefalexin Not more than 10.0%, calculated as the percentage of $C_{16}H_{17}N_3O_4S$ in the sum of $C_{16}H_{19}N_3O_4S$ and $C_{16}H_{17}N_3O_4S$ determined in the Assay.

Loss on drying The contents of the capsules, when dried at 60° at a pressure not exceeding 0.7 kPa for 3 hours, lose not more than 7.0% of their weight. Use 1 g.

Assay Carry out the method for *liquid chromatography,* Appendix III D, injecting 20 µl of each of the following solutions in the mobile phase. For solution (1) dissolve a quantity of the powdered mixed contents of 20 capsules to produce a solution containing 0.05% w/v of Cefradine. Solution (2) contains 0.05% w/v of *cefradine EPCRS.* Solution (3) contains 0.005% w/v each of *cefradine EPCRS* and *cefalexin EPCRS.*

The chromatographic procedure may be carried out using (a) a stainless steel column (25 cm × 4.6 mm) packed with *stationary phase C* (5 µm or 10 µm) (Hypersil ODS is suitable), (b) as mobile phase with a flow rate of 1 ml per minute, a mixture of 1 volume of 5M *acetic acid,* 17 volumes of a 3.62% w/v solution of *sodium acetate,* 200 volumes of *methanol* and 782 volumes of *water* and (c) a detection wavelength of 254 nm.

Inject solution (3). Adjust the sensitivity to obtain peaks with a height of at least 50% of the full-scale deflection on the recorder. The test is not valid unless the *resolution factor* between the peaks corresponding to cefalexin and cefradine is at least 5.0. If necessary, adjust the methanol content in the mobile phase. Inject separately solutions (1) and (2).

Calculate the content of cephalosporins by determining the sum of the contents of $C_{16}H_{19}N_3O_4S$ and $C_{16}H_{17}N_3O_4S$, using the declared contents of $C_{16}H_{19}N_3O_4S$ in *cefradine EPCRS* and $C_{16}H_{17}N_3O_4S$ in *cefalexin EPCRS* respectively.

When cephradine capsules are prescribed or demanded, Cefradine Capsules shall be dispensed or supplied.

Ceftriaxone Injection

Definition Ceftriaxone Injection is a sterile solution of ceftriaxone sodium in Water for Injections. It is prepared by dissolving Ceftriaxone Sodium for Injection in the requisite amount of Water for Injections.

The injection complies with the requirements stated under Parenteral Preparations.

Storage Ceftriaxone Injection should be used immediately after preparation but, in any case, within the period recommended by the manufacturer when prepared and stored strictly in accordance with the manufacturer's instructions.

CEFTRIAXONE SODIUM FOR INJECTION

Definition Ceftriaxone Sodium for Injection is a sterile material prepared from Ceftriaxone Sodium with or without excipients. It is supplied in a sealed container.

The contents of the sealed container comply with the requirements for Powders for Injections stated under Parenteral Preparations and with the following requirements.

Content of ceftriaxone, $C_{18}H_{18}N_8O_7S_3$ 92.0 to 108.0% of the prescribed or stated amount.

Identification

A. The *infrared absorption spectrum,* Appendix II A, is concordant with the *reference spectrum* of ceftriaxone sodium.

B. In the Assay, the principal peak in the chromatogram obtained with solution (1) has the same retention time as that of the principal peak in the chromatogram obtained with solution (2).

C. Yield reaction A characteristic of *sodium salts,* Appendix VI.

Acidity or alkalinity pH of a solution containing the equivalent of 12.0% w/v of ceftriaxone, 6.0 to 8.0, Appendix V L.

Clarity of solution A solution containing the equivalent of 1.20% w/v of ceftriaxone in *carbon dioxide-free water* is *clear,* Appendix IV A, and not more intensely coloured than *reference solution* Y_5 or BY_5, Appendix IV B.

Related substances Carry out the method for *liquid chromatography*, Appendix III D, using solutions (1) and (4) as described under Assay.

The chromatographic conditions described under Assay may be used.

Inject 20 µl of each solution. Allow the chromatography to proceed for at least twice the retention time of the principal peak. In the chromatogram obtained with solution (1) the area of any *secondary peak* is not greater than the area of the principal peak in the chromatogram obtained with solution (4) (1%) and the sum of the areas of all the *secondary peaks* is not greater than 5 times the area of the principal peak in the chromatogram obtained with solution (4) (5%). Disregard any peak with an area less than 0.1 times the area of the principal peak in the chromatogram obtained with solution (4) (0.1%).

Water Not more than 11.0% w/w, Appendix IX C, Method I. Use 0.1 g.

Bacterial endotoxins Carry out the *test for bacterial endotoxins*, Appendix XIV C. Dissolve the contents of the sealed container in *water BET* to give a solution containing the equivalent of 10 mg of ceftriaxone per ml (solution A). The endotoxin limit concentration of solution A is 2.0 IU per ml. Carry out the test using the maximum valid dilution of solution A calculated from the declared sensitivity of the lysate used in the test.

Assay Determine the weight of the contents of 10 containers as described in the test for Uniformity of weight under Parenteral Preparations, Powders for Injections.

Carry out the method for *liquid chromatography*, Appendix III D, using the following solutions in the mobile phase. For solution (1) dissolve a quantity of the mixed contents of the 10 containers to produce a solution containing the equivalent of 0.030% w/v of ceftriaxone. Solution (2) contains 0.030% w/v of *ceftriaxone sodium EPCRS*. Solution (3) contains 0.0050% w/v each of *ceftriaxone sodium EPCRS* and *ceftriaxone sodium E-isomer EPCRS*. For solution (4) dilute 1 volume of solution (1) to 100 volumes.

The chromatographic procedure may be carried out using (a) a stainless steel column (25 cm × 4.6 mm) packed with *stationary phase C* (5 µm) (Lichrosphere RP-18 is suitable), (b) as the mobile phase with a flow rate of 1.5 ml per minute, a mixture prepared in the following manner: dissolve 2 g of *tetradecylammonium bromide* and 2 g of *tetraheptylammonium bromide* in a mixture of 440 ml of *water*, 55 ml of *0.067M mixed phosphate buffer pH 7.0*, 5 ml of a citrate buffer solution pH 5.0 prepared by dissolving 20.17 g of *citric acid* in 800 ml of *water*, adjusting to pH 5.0 with 10M *sodium hydroxide* and diluting to 1000 ml with *water*, and 500 ml of *acetonitrile*, and (c) a detection wavelength of 254 nm. Inject 20 µl of each solution.

Inject solution (3). Adjust the sensitivity of the detector so that the heights of the peaks are at least 50% of the full scale of the recorder. The test is not valid unless the *resolution factor* between the two principal peaks is at least 3.0. Inject alternately solution (1) and solution (2).

Calculate the content of $C_{18}H_{18}N_8O_7S_3$ in a container of average content weight from the declared content of $C_{18}H_{16}N_8Na_2O_7S_3,3\frac{1}{2}H_2O$ in *ceftriaxone sodium EPCRS*. Each mg of $C_{18}H_{16}N_8Na_2O_7S_3,3\frac{1}{2}H_2O$ is equivalent to 0.8383 mg of $C_{18}H_{18}N_8O_7S_3$.

Storage The sealed container should be stored at a temperature not exceeding 30°.

Labelling The label on the sealed container states the quantity of Ceftriaxone Sodium contained in it in terms of the equivalent amount of ceftriaxone.

Cefuroxime Injection

Definition Cefuroxime Injection is a sterile solution or suspension of Cefuroxime Sodium in Water for Injections. It is prepared by dissolving or suspending Cefuroxime Sodium for Injection in the requisite amount of Water for Injections immediately before use.

The injection complies with the requirements stated under Parenteral Preparations.

Storage Cefuroxime Injection should be used immediately after preparation but, in any case, within the period recommended by the manufacturer when prepared and stored strictly in accordance with the manufacturer's instructions.

CEFUROXIME SODIUM FOR INJECTION

Definition Cefuroxime Sodium for Injection is a sterile material consisting of Cefuroxime Sodium with or without excipients. It is supplied in a sealed container.

The contents of the sealed container comply with the requirements for Powders for Injections stated under Parenteral Preparations and with the following requirements.

Content of cefuroxime, $C_{16}H_{16}N_4O_8S$ 90.0 to 105.0% of the prescribed or stated amount.

Identification

A. The *infrared absorption spectrum*, Appendix II A, is concordant with the *reference spectrum* of cefuroxime sodium.

B. Carry out the method for *thin-layer chromatography*, Appendix III A, using *silanised silica gel HF_{254}* as the coating substance and as the mobile phase a mixture of 10 volumes of *tetrahydrofuran* and 90 volumes of a 15.0% w/v solution of *ammonium acetate*, previously adjusted to pH 6.2 with *glacial acetic acid*. Apply separately to the plate 1 µl of each of the following solutions. For solution (1) dissolve a quantity of the contents of a sealed container in sufficient of a mixture of equal volumes of *methanol* and *0.067M mixed phosphate buffer pH 7.0* to produce a solution containing the equivalent of 0.4% w/v of cefuroxime. Solution (2) contains 0.4% w/v of *cefuroxime sodium EPCRS* in a mixture of equal volumes of *methanol* and *0.067M mixed phosphate buffer pH 7.0*. Solution (3) contains 0.4% w/v each of *cefuroxime sodium EPCRS* and *cefoxitin sodium EPCRS* in a mixture of equal volumes of *methanol* and *0.067M mixed phosphate buffer pH 7.0*. After removal of the plate, allow it to dry in a current of warm air and examine under *ultraviolet light (254 nm)*. The principal spot in the chromatogram obtained with solution (1) corresponds to that in the chromatogram obtained with solution (2). The test is not valid unless the chromatogram obtained with solution (3) shows two clearly separated principal spots.

C. Yield reaction A characteristic of *sodium salts*, Appendix VI.

Acidity pH of a 10.0% w/v solution, 5.5 to 8.5, Appendix V L.

Clarity of solution A 10.0% w/v solution in *carbon dioxide-free water* is not more opalescent than *reference suspension II*, Appendix IV A.

Related substances Carry out the method for *liquid chromatography*, Appendix III D, using solutions (1), (3) and (4) described under Assay.

The chromatographic conditions described under Assay may be used.

Inject 20 µl of each solution. Allow the chromatography to proceed for at least 3 times the retention time of the principal peak. In the chromatogram obtained with solution (1) the area of any peak corresponding to descarbamoyl-cefuroxime (located by comparison with the chromatogram obtained with solution (3)) is not greater than the area of the principal peak in the chromatogram obtained with solution (4) (1%), the area of any other *secondary peak* is not greater than the area of the principal peak in the chromatogram obtained with solution (4) (1%) and the sum of the areas of all the *secondary peaks* is not greater than 3 times the area of the principal peak in the chromatogram obtained with solution (4) (3%). Disregard any peak with an area less than 0.1 times the area of the principal peak in the chromatogram obtained with solution (4) (0.1%).

Water Not more than 3.5% w/w, Appendix IX C. Use 0.4 g.

Bacterial endotoxins Carry out the *test for bacterial endotoxins*, Appendix XIV C. Dissolve the contents of the sealed container in *water BET* to give a solution containing the equivalent of 10 mg of cefuroxime per ml (solution A). The endotoxin limit concentration is 1.0 IU per ml. Carry out the test using the maximum valid dilution of solution A calculated from the declared sensitivity of the lysate used in the test.

Assay Determine the weight of the contents of 10 containers as described in the test for Uniformity of weight under Parenteral Preparations, Powders for Injections.

Carry out the method for *liquid chromatography*, Appendix III D, using the following solutions in *water*. For solution (1) dissolve a quantity of the mixed contents of the 10 containers to produce a solution containing the equivalent of 0.1% w/v of cefuroxime. Solution (2) contains 0.1% w/v of *cefuroxime sodium EPCRS*. For solution (3) heat 20 ml of solution (2) in a water bath at 60° for 10 minutes, cool and inject immediately. For solution (4) dilute 1 volume of solution (1) to 100 volumes.

The chromatographic procedure may be carried out using (a) a stainless steel column (12.5 cm × 4.6 mm) packed with particles of silica the surface of which has been modified with chemically-bonded hexylsilyl groups (5 µm) (Spherisorb S5 C6 is suitable), (b) as the mobile phase with a flow rate of 1.5 ml per minute a mixture of 1 volume of *acetonitrile* and 99 volumes of *acetate buffer pH 3.4* and (c) a detection wavelength of 273 nm. Inject 20 µl of each solution.

Inject solution (3). The chromatogram obtained shows peaks corresponding to cefuroxime and descarbamoyl-cefuroxime. The assay is not valid unless the *resolution factor* between the two principal peaks is at least 2.0. If necessary adjust the concentration of *acetonitrile* in the mobile phase.

Inject solution (4). Adjust the sensitivity of the detector so that the height of the principal peak is not less than 25% of the full scale of the recorder. The assay is not valid unless the *symmetry factor* of the cefuroxime peak is 1.5 or less.

Calculate the content of $C_{16}H_{16}N_4O_8S$ in a container of average content weight from the declared content of $C_{16}H_{15}N_4NaO_8S$ in *cefuroxime sodium EPCRS*. Each mg of $C_{16}H_{15}N_4NaO_8S$ is equivalent to 0.9508 mg of $C_{16}H_{16}N_4O_8S$.

Storage The sealed container should be protected from light and stored at a temperature not exceeding 25°.

Labelling The label on the sealed container states the quantity of Cefuroxime Sodium contained in it in terms of the equivalent amount of cefuroxime.

Cefuroxime Axetil Tablets

Definition Cefuroxime Axetil Tablets contain Cefuroxime Axetil. They are coated.

With the exception of the requirement for shape, the tablets comply with the requirements stated under Tablets and with the following requirements.

Content of cefuroxime, $C_{16}H_{16}N_4O_8S$ 92.5 to 105.0% of the prescribed or stated amount.

Identification

A. Extract a quantity of the powdered tablets containing the equivalent of 0.1 g of cefuroxime with 5 ml of *dichloromethane*, filter and evaporate the filtrate to dryness. The *infrared absorption spectrum* of the residue, Appendix II A, is concordant with the *reference spectrum* of cefuroxime axetil.

B. In the Assay, the retention times of the principal peaks in the chromatogram obtained with solution (1) correspond to those of the peaks due to diastereoisomers A and B of cefuroxime axetil in the chromatogram obtained with solution (4).

Related substances Carry out the method for *liquid chromatography*, Appendix III D, using the procedure described under Assay. In the chromatogram obtained with solution (1) the sum of the areas of the pair of peaks corresponding to the pair of principal impurity peaks in the chromatogram obtained with solution (3) is not greater than 1.5% by *normalisation,* the area of any peak corresponding to the peak of the principal impurity in the chromatogram obtained with solution (2) is not greater than 2.0% by *normalisation* and the area of any other *secondary peak* is not greater than 1.0%, by *normalisation.*

Dissolution Comply with the *dissolution test for tablets and capsules*, Appendix XII D, using Apparatus II. Use as the medium 900 ml of 0.1M *hydrochloric acid* and rotate the paddle at 50 revolutions per minute. Withdraw a sample of 10 ml of the medium and filter. Measure the *absorbance* of the filtered sample, diluted if necessary with 0.1M *hydrochloric acid*, at the maximum at 278 nm, Appendix II B, using 0.1M *hydrochloric acid* in the reference cell, and compare with that of a standard solution in 0.1M *hydrochloric acid* having a known concentration of *cefuroxime axetil BPCRS* equivalent to about 10 to 20 µg of $C_{16}H_{16}N_4O_8S$ per ml. Calculate the total content of cefuroxime axetil, $C_{16}H_{16}N_4O_8S$, in the medium.

Assay Carry out the Assay described under Cefuroxime Axetil but using a flow rate of 1.2 ml per minute and the following solutions in place of solutions (1) and (4). For solution (1) disperse 10 tablets in 0.2M *ammonium dihydrogen orthophosphate,* previously adjusted to pH 2.4 with *orthophosphoric acid,* using 10 ml per g of the stated content of cefuroxime. Immediately add sufficient *methanol* to produce a solution containing the equivalent of 0.5% w/v of cefuroxime and shake vigorously. Filter (Whatman GF/C is suitable) and dilute a quantity of the filtrate with sufficient of the mobile phase to produce a solution containing the equivalent of 0.025% w/v of cefuroxime. Solution (4) contains 0.03% w/v of *cefuroxime axetil BPCRS* in the mobile phase. Each mg of $C_{20}H_{22}N_4O_{10}S$ is equivalent to 0.8313 mg of $C_{16}H_{16}N_4O_8S$.

Labelling The quantity of active ingredient is stated in terms of the equivalent amount of cefuroxime.

Cetomacrogol Emulsifying Ointment

Definition

White Soft Paraffin	500 g
Cetomacrogol Emulsifying Wax	300 g
Liquid Paraffin	200 g

Extemporaneous preparation The following directions apply.

Melt together and stir until cold.

The ointment complies with the requirements stated under Topical Semi-solid Preparations.

Cetomacrogol Emulsifying Wax

Non-ionic Emulsifying Wax

Definition

Cetostearyl Alcohol	800 g
Cetomacrogol 1000	200 g

Extemporaneous preparation The following directions apply.

Melt together and stir until cold.

Characteristics A white or almost white, waxy solid or flakes melting when heated to a clear almost colourless liquid; odour faint and characteristic of cetostearyl alcohol.

Practically insoluble in *water*, producing an emulsion; moderately soluble in *ethanol (96%)*; partly soluble in *ether*.

Identification

A. Incinerate at a temperature not exceeding 450° until free from carbon and cool. The residue is negligible (distinction from Emulsifying Wax).

B. Complies with the test for Sulphated ash.

Acid value Not more than 0.5, Appendix X B.

Refractive index At 60°, 1.435 to 1.439, Appendix V E.

Solidifying point 45° to 53°, Appendix V B, using the following modifications. Place in the inner test tube sufficient of the melted substance to fill the tube to a depth of about 50 mm. Stir the substance gently and steadily, without scraping the wall of the tube, while the tube and its contents are allowed to cool. The temperature at which the level of the mercury in the thermometer remains stationary for a short time is regarded as the solidifying point.

Alkalinity Dissolve 10 g in 10 ml of *water* and 10 ml of *ethanol (96%)*. Not more than 0.5 ml of 0.1M *hydrochloric acid VS* is required for neutralisation using *phenolphthalein solution R1* as indicator.

Hydroxyl value 175 to 192, Appendix X D. Use 3.5 g.

Saponification value Not more than 2.0, Appendix X G. Use 20 g.

Sulphated ash Not more than 0.1%, Appendix IX A.

Cetrimide Cream

Definition Cetrimide Cream contains the stated percentage w/w of Cetrimide in a suitable basis.

Extemporaneous preparation The following formula and directions apply.

Cetrimide	5 g, or a sufficient quantity
Cetostearyl Alcohol	50 g
Liquid Paraffin	500 g
Purified Water, freshly boiled and cooled	sufficient to produce 1000 g

Melt the Cetostearyl Alcohol and heat with the Liquid Paraffin to about 60°. Dissolve the Cetrimide in sufficient Purified Water to produce about 450 g. Add the aqueous solution to the oily phase when both are at about 60° and mix. Stir gently until cool, add sufficient of the Purified Water to produce 1000 g and mix.

The cream complies with the requirements stated under Topical Semi-solid Preparations and with the following requirements.

Content of cetrimide, $C_{17}H_{38}BrN$ 88.0 to 106.0% of the prescribed or stated amount.

Identification

Mix 1 g with 50 ml of *water*. The diluted cream complies with the following tests.

A. To 10 ml add 2 ml of *potassium hexacyanoferrate(III) solution*. A yellow precipitate is produced.

B. Shake 3 ml of *water* with 1 ml of 1M *sulphuric acid,* 2 ml of *chloroform* and 0.5 ml of *methyl orange solution*. Add 2 ml of the diluted cream, shake and allow to separate. A yellow colour develops in the chloroform layer.

Assay To a quantity containing 5 mg of Cetrimide add 10 ml of hot *water* and shake gently until dispersed. Add 5 ml of 1M *sulphuric acid*, 20 ml of *chloroform* and 0.25 ml of *dimethyl yellow solution* and titrate with 0.001M *dioctyl sodium sulphosuccinate VS*. Each ml of 0.001M *dioctyl sodium sulphosuccinate VS* is equivalent to 0.3364 mg of $C_{17}H_{38}BrN$.

Labelling The strength is stated as the percentage w/w of Cetrimide.

When Cetrimide Cream is prescribed or demanded, no strength being stated, a cream containing 5% w/v shall be dispensed or supplied.

Cetrimide Emulsifying Ointment

Definition

White Soft Paraffin	500 g
Cetostearyl Alcohol	270 g
Liquid Paraffin	200 g
Cetrimide	30 g

Extemporaneous preparation The following directions apply.

Melt together the White Soft Paraffin, Cetostearyl Alcohol and Liquid Paraffin, add the Cetrimide and stir until cold.

The ointment complies with the requirements stated under Topical Semi-solid Preparations and with the following requirements.

Content of cetrimide, $C_{17}H_{38}BrN$ 2.5 to 3.3% w/w.

Assay To 0.3 g in a stoppered cylinder, add 10 ml of hot *water* and shake until the solid is dispersed. Add 5 ml of 1M *sulphuric acid*, 20 ml of *chloroform* and 1 ml of *dimethyl yellow—oracet blue B solution* and titrate with 0.001M *sodium dodecyl sulphate VS*. Each ml of 0.001M *sodium dodecyl sulphate VS* is equivalent to 0.3364 mg of $C_{17}H_{38}BrN$.

Cetrimide Solution

Definition Cetrimide Solution is a 1% w/v *cutaneous solution* of cetrimide prepared by appropriately diluting Strong Cetrimide Solution with Purified Water. Cetrimide Solution is freshly prepared.

The solution complies with the requirements stated under Liquids for Cutaneous Application and with the following requirements.

Content of cetrimide, $C_{17}H_{38}BrN$ 0.90 to 1.10% w/v.

Identification

A. To 10 ml add 2 ml of a 5% w/v solution of *potassium hexacyanoferrate(III)*. A yellow precipitate is produced.

B. Shake together 5 ml of *water*, 1 ml of 1M *sulphuric acid*, 2 ml of *chloroform* and 0.05 ml of *methyl orange solution*; the chloroform layer is colourless. Add 2 ml of the solution being examined and shake; a yellow colour is produced slowly in the chloroform layer.

C. Yields reaction A characteristic of *bromides*, Appendix VI.

Assay To 100 ml of the solution add 25 ml of *chloroform*, 10 ml of 0.1M *sodium hydroxide* and 10 ml of a freshly prepared 8.0% w/v solution of *potassium iodide*. Shake well, allow to separate and discard the chloroform layer. Wash the aqueous layer with three 10-ml quantities of *chloroform* and discard the washings. Add 40 ml of *hydrochloric acid*, cool and titrate with 0.05M *potassium iodate VS* until the deep brown colour is almost discharged. Add 2 ml of *chloroform* and continue the titration, with shaking, until the chloroform layer no longer changes colour. Carry out a blank titration on a mixture of 10 ml of the freshly prepared 8.0% w/v potassium iodide solution, 20 ml of *water* and 40 ml of *hydrochloric acid*. The difference between the titrations represents the amount of potassium iodate required. Each ml of 0.05M *potassium iodate VS* is equivalent to 0.03364 g of $C_{17}H_{38}BrN$.

Labelling The label states that the solution should not be used later than 1 week after the container is first opened.

The label indicates the pharmaceutical form as 'cutaneous solution'.

STERILE CETRIMIDE SOLUTION

Definition Sterile Cetrimide Solution is Cetrimide Solution that has been sterilised by *heating in an autoclave*.

Content of cetrimide; Identification Complies with the requirements stated under Cetrimide Solution.

Assay Carry out the Assay described under Cetrimide Solution.

Sterility Complies with the *test for sterility*, Appendix XVI A.

Labelling The label states (1) 'Sterile Cetrimide Solution'; (2) that the solution is not intended for injection; (3) that the contents should not be used later than 1 week after the container is first opened; (4) the date after which the solution is not intended to be used; (5) the conditions under which it should be stored.

The label indicates the pharmaceutical form as 'cutaneous solution'.

Paediatric Chloral Elixir

Paediatric Chloral Oral Solution

Definition Paediatric Chloral Elixir is an *oral solution* containing 4% w/v of Chloral Hydrate in a suitable vehicle with a blackcurrant flavour.

Extemporaneous preparation It is recently prepared according to the following formula and directions.

Chloral Hydrate	40 g
Water	20 ml
Black Currant Syrup	200 ml
Syrup	sufficient to produce 1000 ml

Dissolve the Chloral Hydrate in the Water, add the Black Currant Syrup and sufficient Syrup to produce 1000 ml and mix.

The elixir complies with the requirements stated under Oral Liquids and with the following requirements.

Content of chloral hydrate, $C_2H_3Cl_3O_2$ 3.80 to 4.20% w/v.

Identification To 5 ml add 2 ml of 5M *sodium hydroxide* and mix. A liquid with the odour of chloroform separates.

Assay To 3 g add 2.5 g of *zinc powder*, 15 ml of *glacial acetic acid* and 30 ml of *water*, boil under a reflux condenser for 30 minutes, cool, filter through absorbent cotton, wash the residue with *water* and combine the filtrate and washings. Add 20 ml of 2M *nitric acid* and 30 ml of 0.1M *silver nitrate VS*, shake vigorously, filter, wash the residue with *water* and titrate the excess of silver nitrate with 0.1M *ammonium thiocyanate VS* using *ammonium iron(III) sulphate solution R2* as indicator. Each ml of 0.1M *silver nitrate VS* is equivalent to 5.513 mg of $C_2H_3Cl_3O_2$. Determine the *weight per ml* of the elixir, Appendix V G, and calculate the content of $C_2H_3Cl_3O_2$, weight in volume.

Labelling The label indicates the pharmaceutical form as 'oral solution'.

Chloral Mixture

Chloral Oral Solution; Chloral Hydrate Mixture

Definition Chloral Mixture is an *oral solution* containing 10% w/v of Chloral Hydrate in a suitable vehicle. It is intended to be diluted with water before use.

Extemporaneous preparation It is recently prepared according to the following formula.

Chloral Hydrate	100 g
Syrup	200 ml
Water	sufficient to produce 1000 ml

The mixture complies with the requirements stated under Oral Liquids and with the following requirements.

Content of chloral hydrate, $C_2H_3Cl_3O_2$ 9.40 to 10.55% w/v.

Identification To 5 ml add 2 ml of 10M *sodium hydroxide* and mix. Chloroform separates as a liquid, recognisable by its odour.

Assay To 1 g add 2.5 g of *zinc powder*, 15 ml of *glacial acetic acid* and 30 ml of *water*, boil under a reflux condenser for 30 minutes, cool, filter through absorbent cotton and wash the residue with *water*. Combine the filtrate and washings, add 20 ml of 2M *nitric acid* and 30 ml of 0.1M *silver nitrate VS*, shake vigorously, filter, wash the residue with *water* and titrate the excess of silver nitrate in the combined filtrate and washings with 0.1M *ammonium thiocyanate VS* using *ammonium iron(III) sulphate solution R2* as indicator. Each ml of 0.1M *silver nitrate VS* is equivalent to 5.513 mg of $C_2H_3Cl_3O_2$. Determine the *weight per ml* of the mixture, Appendix V G, and calculate the content of $C_2H_3Cl_3O_2$, weight in volume.

Labelling The label states that the mixture should be well diluted with water before use.

The label indicates the pharmaceutical form as 'oral solution'.

Chlorambucil Tablets

Definition Chlorambucil Tablets contain Chlorambucil. They are coated.

The tablets comply with the requirements stated under Tablets and with the following requirements.

Content of chlorambucil, $C_{14}H_{19}Cl_2NO_2$ 90.0 to 110.0% of the prescribed or stated amount.

Identification Shake a quantity of the powdered tablets containing 10 mg of Chlorambucil with 10 ml of 2M *hydrochloric acid*, allow to stand for 30 minutes, shaking occasionally, and filter. To 5 ml of the filtrate add 0.5 ml of *potassium tetraiodomercurate solution*; a precipitate is produced. To the remainder of the filtrate add 0.15 ml of *dilute potassium permanganate solution*; the colour of the permanganate is discharged.

Uniformity of content Tablets containing 2 mg or less of Chlorambucil comply with the requirements stated under Tablets using the following method of analysis. Carry out the method for *liquid chromatography*, Appendix III D, using the following solutions. Solution (1) contains 0.0020% w/v of *chlorambucil BPCRS* in a mixture of 9 volumes of *acetonitrile* and 1 volume of 0.1M *hydrochloric acid*. For solution (2) dissolve one tablet as completely as possible in 10 ml of 0.1M *hydrochloric acid*, add 40 ml of *acetonitrile* and mix for 5 minutes with the aid of ultrasound. Add sufficient *acetonitrile* to produce a solution containing 0.002% w/v of Chlorambucil, filter through a glass microfibre filter paper (Whatman GF/C is suitable), discarding the first 20 ml of filtrate, and use the filtrate.

The chromatographic procedure may be carried out using (a) a stainless steel column (30 cm × 4 mm) packed with *stationary phase C* (10 µm) (µBondapak C18 and Spherisorb ODS 1 are suitable), (b) a mixture of 60 volumes of *acetonitrile* and 40 volumes of 0.02M *potassium dihydrogen orthophosphate* as the mobile phase with a flowrate of 2 ml per minute and (c) a detection wavelength of 254 nm.

Calculate the content of $C_{14}H_{19}Cl_2NO_2$ in the tablet using the declared content of $C_{14}H_{19}Cl_2NO_2$ in *chlorambucil BPCRS*.

Assay Carry out the method for *liquid chromatography*, Appendix III D, using the following solutions. Solution (1) contains 0.0020% w/v of *chlorambucil BPCRS* in a mixture of 9 volumes of *acetonitrile* and 1 volume of 0.1M *hydrochloric acid*. For solution (2) dissolve as completely as possible a quantity of the powdered tablets containing 10 mg of Chlorambucil in a mixture of 25 ml of 0.1M *hydrochloric acid* and 100 ml of *acetonitrile* by mixing for 10 minutes with the aid of ultrasound. Dilute to 250 ml with *acetonitrile*, filter through a glass microfibre filter paper (Whatman GF/C is suitable), discarding the first 20 ml of filtrate, and dilute 50 ml to 100 ml with a mixture of 9 volumes of *acetonitrile* and 1 volume of 0.1M *hydrochloric acid*.

The chromatographic procedure described under Uniformity of content may be used.

Calculate the content of $C_{14}H_{19}Cl_2NO_2$ using the declared content of $C_{14}H_{19}Cl_2NO_2$ in *chlorambucil BPCRS*.

Chloramphenicol Capsules

Definition Chloramphenicol Capsules contain Chloramphenicol.

The capsules comply with the requirements stated under Capsules and with the following requirements.

Content of chloramphenicol, $C_{11}H_{12}Cl_2N_2O_5$ 95.0 to 105.0% of the prescribed or stated amount.

Identification

Suspend a quantity of the contents of the capsules containing 0.1 g of Chloramphenicol in 60 ml of *water* and extract with two 20-ml quantities of *petroleum spirit (boiling range, 120° to 160°)*. Wash the combined extracts with two 15-ml quantities of *water*, add the washings to the aqueous layer, extract with four 50-ml quantities of *ether* and evaporate the combined ether extracts. The residue complies with the following tests.

A. Carry out the method for *thin-layer chromatography*, Appendix III A, using *silica gel GF_{254}* as the coating substance and a mixture of 90 volumes of *chloroform*, 10 volumes of *methanol* and 1 volume of *water* as the mobile phase. Apply separately to the plate 1 µl of each of two solutions in *ethanol (96%)* containing (1) 1% w/v of the residue and (2) 1% w/v of *chloramphenicol EPCRS*. After removal of the plate, allow it to dry in air and examine under *ultraviolet light (254 nm)*. The principal spot in the chromatogram obtained with solution (1) corresponds to that in the chromatogram obtained with solution (2).

B. Dissolve 10 mg in 2 ml of *ethanol (50%)*, add 4.5 ml of 1M *sulphuric acid* and 50 mg of *zinc powder* and allow to stand for 10 minutes. Decant the supernatant liquid or filter if necessary. Cool the resulting solution in ice and add 0.5 ml of *sodium nitrite solution* and, after 2 minutes, 1 g of *urea* followed by 1 ml of *2-naphthol solution* and 2 ml of 10M *sodium hydroxide*; a red colour is produced. Repeat the test omitting the zinc powder; no red colour is produced.

Dissolution Comply with the *dissolution test for tablets and capsules*, Appendix XII D, using as the medium 900 ml of 0.1M *hydrochloric acid* and rotating the basket at 100 revolutions per minute. Withdraw a sample of 10 ml of the medium. Measure the *absorbance* of the filtered sample, suitably diluted if necessary, at the maximum at 278 nm, Appendix II B. Calculate the total content of chloramphenicol, $C_{11}H_{12}Cl_2N_2O_5$, in the medium taking 297 as the value of A(1%, 1 cm) at the maximum at 278 nm.

2-Amino-1-(4-nitrophenyl)propane-1,3-diol Carry out the method for *liquid chromatography*, Appendix III D, using the following solutions. Solution (1) contains 0.0002% w/v of *2-amino-1-(4-nitrophenyl)propane-1,3-diol BPCRS* in the mobile phase. For solution (2) shake a quantity of the contents of the capsules containing 40 mg of Chloramphenicol with 100 ml of the mobile phase for 10 minutes, add sufficient mobile phase to produce 200 ml, mix and filter.

The chromatographic procedure may be carried out using (a) a stainless steel column (10 cm × 4.6 mm), packed with *stationary phase C* (5 µm) (Nucleosil C18 is suitable), (b) a mixture of 85 volumes of a 0.21% w/v solution of *sodium pentanesulphonate*, 15 volumes of *acetonitrile* and 1 volume of *glacial acetic acid* as the mobile phase with a flow rate of 2 ml per minute and (c) a detection wavelength of 272 nm.

In the chromatogram obtained with solution (2) the area of any peak corresponding to 2-amino-1-(4-nitrophenyl)-propane-1,3-diol is not greater than the area of the peak in the chromatogram obtained with solution (1).

Assay Dissolve a quantity of the mixed contents of 20 capsules containing 0.2 g of Chloramphenicol in 800 ml of *water*, warming if necessary to effect solution, and add sufficient *water* to produce 1000 ml. Dilute 10 ml to 100 ml with *water* and measure the *absorbance* of the resulting solution at the maximum at 278 nm, Appendix II B. Calculate the content of $C_{11}H_{12}Cl_2N_2O_5$ taking 297 as the value of A(1%, 1 cm) at the maximum at 278 nm.

Chloramphenicol Ear Drops

Definition Chloramphenicol Ear Drops are a solution of Chloramphenicol in a suitable vehicle.

The ear drops comply with the requirements stated under Ear Preparations and with the following requirements.

Content of chloramphenicol, $C_{11}H_{12}Cl_2N_2O_5$ 90.0 to 110.0% of the prescribed or stated amount.

Identification

A. Carry out the method for *thin-layer chromatography*, Appendix III A, using *silica gel GF_{254}* as the coating substance and a mixture of 90 volumes of *chloroform*, 10 volumes of *methanol* and 1 volume of *water* as the mobile phase. Apply separately to the plate 1 µl of each of the following solutions. For solution (1) dilute a volume of the ear drops containing 0.1 g of Chloramphenicol to 10 ml with *ethanol (96%)*. Solution (2) contains 1% w/v of *chloramphenicol EPCRS* in *ethanol (96%)*. After removal of the plate, allow it to dry in air and examine under *ultraviolet light (254 nm)*. The principal spot in the chromatogram obtained with solution (1) corresponds to that in the chromatogram obtained with solution (2).

B. Dilute a volume of the ear drops containing 50 mg of Chloramphenicol to 10 ml with *ethanol (50%)*. To 2 ml add 4.5 ml of 1M *sulphuric acid* and 50 mg of *zinc powder* and allow to stand for 10 minutes. Decant the supernatant liquid or filter if necessary. Cool the resulting solution in ice and add 0.5 ml of *sodium nitrite solution* and, after 2 minutes, 1 g of *urea* followed by 1 ml of *2-naphthol solution* and 2 ml of 10M *sodium hydroxide*; a red colour is produced. Repeat the test omitting the zinc powder; no red colour is produced.

2-Amino-1-(4-nitrophenyl)propane-1,3-diol Comply with the test described under Chloramphenicol Eye Drops using the following solutions. For solution (1) dilute the ear drops with the mobile phase to contain 0.050% w/v of Chloramphenicol. Solution (2) contains 0.0025% w/v of *2-amino-1-(4-nitrophenyl)propane-1,3-diol BPCRS* in the mobile phase.

Assay Dilute a quantity containing 25 mg of Chloramphenicol to 250 ml with *water*. Dilute 10 ml to 100 ml with *water* and measure the *absorbance* of the resulting solution at the maximum at 278 nm, Appendix II B. Calculate the content of $C_{11}H_{12}Cl_2N_2O_5$ taking 297 as the value of A(1%, 1 cm) at the maximum at 278 nm.

Storage Chloramphenicol Ear Drops should be protected from light.

Chloramphenicol Eye Drops

Definition Chloramphenicol Eye Drops are a sterile solution of Chloramphenicol in Purified Water.

The eye drops comply with the requirements stated under Eye Preparations and with the following requirements.

Content of chloramphenicol, $C_{11}H_{12}Cl_2N_2O_5$ 90.0 to 110.0% of the prescribed or stated amount.

Identification

To a volume containing 50 mg of Chloramphenicol add 15 ml of *water* and extract with four 25-ml quantities of *ether*. Combine the extracts and evaporate to dryness. The dried residue complies with the following tests.

A. Carry out the method for *thin-layer chromatography*, Appendix III A, using *silica gel GF_{254}* as the coating substance and a mixture of 90 volumes of *chloroform*, 10 volumes of *methanol* and 1 volume of *water* as the mobile phase. Apply separately to the plate 1 µl of each of two solutions in *ethanol (96%)* containing (1) 1% w/v of the residue and (2) 1% w/v of *chloramphenicol EPCRS*. After removal of the plate, allow it to dry in air and examine under *ultraviolet light (254 nm)*. The principal spot in the chromatogram obtained with solution (1) corresponds to that in the chromatogram obtained with solution (2).

B. Dissolve 10 mg in 2 ml of *ethanol (50%)*, add 4.5 ml of 1M *sulphuric acid* and 50 mg of *zinc powder* and allow to stand for 10 minutes. Decant the supernatant liquid or filter if necessary. Cool the resulting solution in ice and add 0.5 ml of *sodium nitrite solution* and, after 2 minutes, 1 g of *urea* followed by 1 ml of *2-naphthol solution* and 2 ml of 10M *sodium hydroxide*; a red colour is produced. Repeat the test omitting the zinc powder; no red colour is produced.

Acidity or alkalinity pH, 7.0 to 7.5, Appendix V L.

2-Amino-1-(4-nitrophenyl)propane-1,3-diol Carry out the method for *liquid chromatography*, Appendix III D, using the following solutions. For solution (1) dilute the eye drops with the mobile phase to contain 0.050% w/v of Chloramphenicol. Solution (2) contains 0.0040% w/v of *2-amino-1-(4-nitrophenyl)propane-1,3-diol BPCRS* in the mobile phase.

The chromatographic procedure may be carried out using (a) a stainless steel column (10 cm × 4.6 mm), packed with *stationary phase C* (5 µm) (Nucleosil C18 is suitable), (b) a mixture of 85 volumes of a 0.21% w/v solution of *sodium pentanesulphonate*, 15 volumes of *acetonitrile* and 1 volume of *glacial acetic acid* as the mobile phase with a flow rate of 2 ml per minute and (c) a detection wavelength of 272 nm.

In the chromatogram obtained with solution (1) the area of any peak corresponding to 2-amino-1-(4-nitrophenyl)propane-1,3-diol is not greater than the area of the peak in the chromatogram obtained with solution (2).

Assay Dilute a volume containing 25 mg of Chloramphenicol to 250 ml with *water*. Dilute 10 ml to 100 ml with *water* and measure the *absorbance* of the resulting solution at the maximum at 278 nm, Appendix II B. Calculate the content of $C_{11}H_{12}Cl_2N_2O_5$ taking 297 as the value of A(1%, 1 cm) at the maximum at 278 nm.

Storage Chloramphenicol Eye Drops should be protected from light.

Chloramphenicol Eye Ointment

Definition Chloramphenicol Eye Ointment is a sterile preparation containing Chloramphenicol in a suitable basis.

The eye ointment complies with the requirements stated under Eye Preparations and with the following requirements.

Content of chloramphenicol, $C_{11}H_{12}Cl_2N_2O_5$ 95.0 to 105.0% of the prescribed or stated amount.

Identification

Mix a quantity containing 30 mg of Chloramphenicol with 10 ml of *petroleum spirit (boiling range, 40° to 60°)*, centrifuge and discard the supernatant liquid. Repeat this procedure using three 10-ml quantities of the same solvent. The dried residue complies with the following tests.

A. Carry out the method for *thin-layer chromatography*, Appendix III A, using *silica gel GF_{254}* as the coating substance and a mixture of 90 volumes of *chloroform*, 10 volumes of *methanol* and 1 volume of *water* as the mobile phase. Apply separately to the plate 1 µl of each of two solutions in *ethanol (96%)* containing (1) 1% w/v of the residue and (2) 1% w/v of *chloramphenicol EPCRS*. After removal of the plate, allow it to dry in air and examine under *ultraviolet light (254 nm)*. The principal spot in the chromatogram obtained with solution (1) corresponds to that in the chromatogram obtained with solution (2).

B. Dissolve 10 mg of the residue in 2 ml of *ethanol (50%)*, add 4.5 ml of 1M *sulphuric acid* and 50 mg of *zinc powder* and allow to stand for 10 minutes. Decant the supernatant liquid or filter if necessary. Cool the resulting solution in ice and add 0.5 ml of *sodium nitrite solution* and, after 2 minutes, 1 g of *urea* followed by 1 ml of *2-naphthol solution* and 2 ml of 10M *sodium hydroxide*; a red colour is produced. Repeat the test omitting the zinc powder; no red colour is produced.

2-Amino-1-(4-nitrophenyl)propane-1,3-diol Complies with the test described under Chloramphenicol Eye Drops using the following solutions. For solution (1) add 25 ml of a 0.21% w/v solution of *sodium pentanesulphonate* to a quantity of the eye ointment containing 10 mg of Chloramphenicol and heat in a water bath until melted. Stir thoroughly with a glass rod, cool until the ointment base solidifies and filter through absorbent cotton. Repeat the extraction with a further 20 ml the sodium pentanesulphonate solution and dilute to 50 ml with the same solution. Solution (2) contains 0.00020% w/v of *2-amino-1-(4-nitrophenyl)propane-1,3-diol BPCRS* in the mobile phase.

Assay Suspend a quantity containing 10 mg of Chloramphenicol in 50 ml of *petroleum spirit (boiling range, 40° to 60°)* and extract with successive quantities of 50, 50, 50 and 30 ml of warm *water*. Combine the extracts, dilute to 200 ml with *water*, mix well and filter, discarding the first 20 ml of the filtrate. Dilute 10 ml of the filtrate to 50 ml with *water* and measure the *absorbance* of the resulting solution at the maximum at 278 nm, Appendix II B. Calculate the content of $C_{11}H_{12}Cl_2N_2O_5$ taking 297 as the value of A(1%, 1 cm) at the maximum at 278 nm.

Chloramphenicol Sodium Succinate Injection

Definition Chloramphenicol Sodium Succinate Injection is a sterile solution of Chloramphenicol Sodium Succinate in Water for Injections. It is prepared by dissolving Chloramphenicol Sodium Succinate for Injection in the requisite amount of Water for Injections.

The injection complies with the requirements stated under Parenteral Preparations.

Storage Chloramphenicol Sodium Succinate Injection should be used immediately after preparation but, in any case, within the period recommended by the manufacturer when prepared and stored strictly in accordance with the manufacturer's instructions.

CHLORAMPHENICOL SODIUM SUCCINATE FOR INJECTION

Definition Chloramphenicol Sodium Succinate for Injection is a sterile material consisting of Chloramphenicol Sodium Succinate with or without excipients. It is supplied in a sealed container.

The contents of the sealed container comply with the requirements for Powders for Injections stated under Parenteral

Preparations and with the following requirements.

Content of chloramphenicol sodium succinate, calculated as $C_{11}H_{12}Cl_2N_2O_5$ 95.0 to 105.0% of the prescribed or stated amount.

Characteristics A white or yellowish white solid; hygroscopic.

Identification

A. Carry out the method for *thin-layer chromatography*, Appendix III A, using *silica gel GF_{254}* as the coating substance and a mixture of 1 volume of 2M *acetic acid*, 14 volumes of *methanol* and 85 volumes of *chloroform* as the mobile phase. Apply separately to the plate 2 µl of each of three solutions in *acetone* containing (1) 1% w/v of the contents of the container, (2) 1% w/v of *chloramphenicol sodium succinate EPCRS* and (3) 1% w/v of *chloramphenicol EPCRS*. After removal of the plate, allow it to dry in air and examine under *ultraviolet light (254 nm)*. The two principal spots in the chromatogram obtained with solution (1) are similar in position and size to those in the chromatogram obtained with solution (2) and their positions are different from that of the principal spot in the chromatogram obtained with solution (3).

B. Dissolve 10 mg in 1 ml of *ethanol (50%)*, add 3 ml of a 1% w/v solution of *calcium chloride* and 50 mg of *zinc powder* and heat on a water bath for 10 minutes. Filter the hot solution, allow to cool, add 0.1 ml of *benzoyl chloride* and shake for 1 minute. Add 0.5 ml of *iron(III) chloride solution R1* and 2 ml of *chloroform* and shake. The aqueous layer is light violet-red to purple.

C. Yields reaction A characteristic of *sodium salts*, Appendix VI.

Acidity or alkalinity pH of a 25% w/v solution, 6.0 to 7.0, Appendix V L.

Chloramphenicol and chloramphenicol disodium disuccinate Carry out the method for *liquid chromatography*, Appendix III D, using four solutions in the mobile phase containing (1) 0.00050% w/v of *chloramphenicol disodium disuccinate EPCRS*, (2) 0.00050% w/v of *chloramphenicol EPCRS*, (3) sufficient of the contents of the sealed container to give a solution containing the equivalent of 0.025% w/v of chloramphenicol and (4) 0.00050% w/v each of *chloramphenicol disodium disuccinate EPCRS* and *chloramphenicol EPCRS* and sufficient of the contents of the sealed container to give a solution containing the equivalent of 0.025% w/v of chloramphenicol.

The chromatographic procedure may be carried out using (a) a column (25 cm × 4.6 mm) packed with *stationary phase C* (5 µm) (Lichrosorb RP-18, Hypersil ODS and Polygosil C18 5 mm are suitable), (b) a mixture of 5 volumes of a 2% w/v solution of *orthophosphoric acid*, 40 volumes of *methanol* and 55 volumes of *water* as the mobile phase with a flow rate of 1 ml per minute and (c) a detection wavelength of 275 nm.

Inject 20 µl of each solution. The test is not valid unless the two peaks in the chromatogram obtained with solution (4) corresponding to those in the chromatograms obtained with solutions (1) and (2) are clearly separated from the peaks corresponding to the two principal peaks in the chromatogram obtained with solution (3). If necessary, adjust the methanol content of the mobile phase.

In the chromatogram obtained with solution (3) the areas of any peaks corresponding to chloramphenicol and chloramphenicol disodium disuccinate are not greater than those of the principal peaks in the chromatograms obtained with solutions (2) and (1) respectively (2% of each).

Water Not more than 5.0% w/w, Appendix IX C. Use 0.5 g.

Pyrogens Comply with the *test for pyrogens*, Appendix XIV D. Use per kg of the rabbit's weight 2 ml of a solution in *water for injections* containing the equivalent of 0.25% w/v of chloramphenicol.

Assay Determine the weight of the contents of 10 containers as described in the test for Uniformity of weight under Parenteral Preparations, Powders for Injections.

Dissolve 0.2 g of the mixed contents of the 10 containers in *water* and add sufficient *water* to produce 500 ml. Dilute 5 ml of this solution to 100 ml with *water* and measure the *absorbance* of the resulting solution at the maximum at 276 nm, Appendix II B. Calculate the content of chloramphenicol sodium succinate expressed as chloramphenicol, $C_{11}H_{12}Cl_2N_2O_5$, in a container of average content weight taking 297 as the value of A(1%, 1 cm) at the maximum at 276 nm.

Storage The sealed container should be protected from light.

Labelling The label of the sealed container states the quantity of Chloramphenicol Sodium Succinate contained in it in terms of the equivalent amount of chloramphenicol.

Chlordiazepoxide Capsules

Definition Chlordiazepoxide Capsules contain Chlordiazepoxide Hydrochloride.

The capsules comply with the requirements stated under Capsules and with the following requirements.

Content of chlordiazepoxide hydrochloride, $C_{16}H_{14}ClN_3O,HCl$ 92.5 to 107.5% of the prescribed or stated amount.

Identification

A. Dilute 1 volume of the final solution obtained in the Assay to 2 volumes with 0.1M *hydrochloric acid*. The *light absorption*, Appendix II B, in the range 230 to 350 nm exhibits two maxima, at 246 nm and 308 nm.

B. Shake a quantity of the contents of the capsules containing 25 mg of Chlordiazepoxide Hydrochloride with 2.5 ml of *water*, add 0.5 ml of 6M *ammonia*, mix, allow to stand for 5 minutes and filter. The filtrate, after making acidic with 2M *nitric acid*, yields reaction A characteristic of *chlorides*, Appendix VI.

Related substances Carry out in subdued light the method for *thin-layer chromatography*, Appendix III A, using *silica gel GF_{254}* as the coating substance and a mixture of 85 volumes of *chloroform*, 14 volumes of *methanol* and 1 volume of 13.5M *ammonia* as the mobile phase. Prepare the following solutions immediately before use in *acetone* containing 2% v/v of 13.5M *ammonia* and 8% v/v of *water*. For solution (1) shake a quantity of the contents of the capsules containing 0.10 g of Chlordiazepoxide Hydrochloride with 10 ml of the solvent mixture, allow to settle and use the clear supernatant liquid. For solution (2) dilute 3 volumes of solution (1) to 100 volumes with the same solvent mixture. Solution (3) contains 0.0010% w/v of *2-amino-5-chlorobenzophenone*. Apply separately to the plate 2-µl and 20-µl quantities of solution (1), 2 µl of solution (2) and 20 µl of solution (3). After removal of the plate, allow it to dry in air and examine under *ultraviolet light (254 nm)*. Any *secondary spot* in the chromatogram obtained with 2 µl of solution (1) is not more intense than the spot in the chromatogram obtained with solution (2). Spray the plate with a freshly prepared 1% w/v solution of *sodium nitrite* in 1M *hydrochloric acid*, dry it in a current of cold air and spray with a 0.4% w/v solution of N-*(1-naphthyl)ethylenediamine dihydrochloride* in *ethanol (96%)*. Any violet spot corresponding to 2-amino-5-chlorobenzophenone in the chromatogram obtained with 20 µl of solution (1) is not more intense than the spot in the chromatogram obtained with solution (3).

Dissolution Carry out the *dissolution test for tablets and capsules*, Appendix XII D, using as the medium 900 ml of 0.1M *hydrochloric acid* and rotating the basket at 100 revolutions per minute. Measure the *absorbance* of a layer of suitable thickness of the filtered sample, suitably diluted, if necessary, with 0.1M *hydrochloric acid* at the maximum at 308 nm, Appendix II B. Calculate the total content of chlordiazepoxide hydrochloride, $C_{16}H_{14}ClN_3O,HCl$, in the medium taking 292 as the value of A(1%, 1 cm) at the maximum at 308 nm.

Assay Carry out the following procedure protected from light. Shake a quantity of the mixed contents of 20 capsules containing 20 mg of Chlordiazepoxide Hydrochloride with 150 ml of 0.1M *hydrochloric acid* for 20 minutes. Add sufficient 0.1M *hydrochloric acid* to produce 200 ml and filter. Dilute 10 ml of the filtrate to 50 ml with 0.1M *hydrochloric acid* and measure the *absorbance* of the resulting solution at the maximum at 308 nm, Appendix II B. Calculate the content of $C_{16}H_{14}ClN_3O,HCl$ taking 292 as the value of A(1%, 1 cm) at the maximum at 308 nm.

Storage Chlordiazepoxide Capsules should be protected from light.

Chlordiazepoxide Hydrochloride Tablets

Definition Chlordiazepoxide Hydrochloride Tablets contain Chlordiazepoxide Hydrochloride.

The tablets comply with the requirements stated under Tablets and with the following requirements.

Content of chlordiazepoxide, $C_{16}H_{14}ClN_3O$ 90.0 to 110.0% of the prescribed or stated amount.

Identification

A. Dilute 1 volume of the final solution obtained in the Assay to 2 volumes with 0.1M *hydrochloric acid*. The *light absorption*, Appendix II B, in the range 230 to 350 nm exhibits two maxima, at 246 nm and 308 nm.

B. To a quantity of the powdered tablets containing the equivalent of 0.2 g of chlordiazepoxide add 4 ml of hot 2M *hydrochloric acid*, heat at 100° for 10 minutes, cool and filter. 2 ml of the filtrate yields the reaction characteristic of *primary aromatic amines*, Appendix VI, producing a reddish precipitate.

C. Shake a quantity of the powdered tablets containing the equivalent of 25 mg of chlordiazepoxide with 2.5 ml of *water*, add 0.5 ml of 6M *ammonia*, mix, allow to stand for 5 minutes and filter. The filtrate, after making acidic with 2M *nitric acid*, yields reaction A characteristic of *chlorides*, Appendix VI.

Related substances Carry out in subdued light the method for *thin-layer chromatography*, Appendix III A, using *silica gel GF_{254}* as the coating substance and a mixture of 85 volumes of *chloroform*, 14 volumes of *methanol* and 1 volume of 13.5M *ammonia* as the mobile phase. Prepare the following solutions immediately before use in *acetone* containing 2% v/v of 13.5M *ammonia* and 8% v/v of *water*. For solution (1) shake a quantity of the powdered tablets containing the equivalent of 0.10 g of chlordiazepoxide with 10 ml of the solvent mixture, allow to settle and use the supernatant liquid. For solution (2) dilute 5 volumes of solution (1) to 100 volumes with the same solvent mixture. For solution (3) dilute 1 volume of solution (1) to 100 volumes with the same solvent. Solution (4) contains 0.0010% w/v of *2-amino-5-chlorobenzophenone*. Apply separately to the plate 2-µl and 20-µl quantities of solution (1), 2 µl of each of solutions (2) and (3) and 20 µl of solution (4). After removal of the plate, allow it to dry in air and examine under *ultraviolet light (254 nm)*. Any *secondary spot* in the chromatogram obtained with 2 µl of solution (1) is not more intense than the spot in the chromatogram obtained with solution (2) and not more than one such spot is more intense than the spot in the chromatogram obtained with solution (3). Spray the plate with a freshly prepared 1% w/v solution of *sodium nitrite* in 1M *hydrochloric acid*, dry it in a current of cold air and spray with a 0.4% w/v solution of N-*(1-naphthyl)ethylenediamine dihydrochloride* in *ethanol (96%)*. Any violet spot corresponding to 2-amino-5-chlorobenzophenone in the chromatogram obtained with 20 µl of solution (1) is not more intense than the spot in the chromatogram obtained with solution (4).

Assay Shake 10 whole tablets with 150 ml of 0.1M *hydrochloric acid* for 20 minutes, add sufficient 0.1M *hydrochloric acid* to produce 250 ml and filter. Dilute 10 ml of the filtrate with sufficient 0.1M *hydrochloric acid* to produce a solution containing the equivalent of 0.0020% w/v of chlordiazepoxide and measure the *absorbance* of the resulting solution at the maximum at 308 nm, Appendix II B. Calculate the content of $C_{16}H_{14}ClN_3O$ taking 327 as the value of A(1%, 1 cm) at the maximum at 308 nm.

Storage Chlordiazepoxide Hydrochloride Tablets should be stored at a temperature not exceeding 25°.

Labelling The quantity of active ingredient is stated in terms of the equivalent amount of chlordiazepoxide.

Chlorhexidine Irrigation Solution

Definition Chlorhexidine Irrigation Solution is either a sterile aqueous solution of Chlorhexidine Acetate or a sterile aqueous dilution of Chlorhexidine Gluconate Solution.

Production Chlorhexidine Irrigation Solution intended to be used for the irrigation of body cavities, for the flushing of wounds or operation cavities or for the irrigation of the urogenital system is prepared using Water for Irrigation.

The solution complies with the requirements stated under Preparations for Irrigation and with the following requirements.

Content of chlorhexidine acetate, $C_{22}H_{30}Cl_2N_{10}$, $2C_2H_4O_2$ or chlorhexidine gluconate, $C_{22}H_{30}Cl_2N_{10}$, $2C_6H_{12}O_7$ 95.0 to 105.0% of the prescribed or stated amount.

Identification *Chlorhexidine Irrigation Solution prepared using Chlorhexidine Acetate complies with tests A, B and C. Chlorhexidine Irrigation Solution prepared using Chlorhexidine Gluconate Solution complies with tests A and B only.*

A. In the Assay, the retention time of the principal peak in the chromatogram obtained with solution (2) is the same as that of the peak due to chlorhexidine in the chromatogram obtained with solution (1).

B. To 10 ml of the irrigation solution add 5 ml of a warm 1% w/v solution of *cetrimide*, 1 ml of 5M *sodium hydroxide* and 1 ml of *bromine water*. A deep red colour is produced.

C. Evaporate or dilute a volume of the irrigation solution containing the equivalent of about 5 mg of chlorhexidine to about 5 ml. The resulting solution yields reaction B characteristic of *acetates*, Appendix VI.

Acidity pH, 5.0 to 6.5, Appendix V L.

Related substances Carry out the method for *liquid chromatography*, Appendix III D, using the following solutions. For solution (1) dilute 3 volumes of the irrigation solution to 100 volumes with the mobile phase. For solution (2) use the irrigation solution. Solution (3) contains 0.10% w/v of *chlorhexidine for performance test EPCRS* in the mobile phase.

The chromatographic procedure may be carried out using (a) a stainless steel column (20 cm × 4 mm) packed with *stationary phase C* (10 μm) (Nucleosil C18 is suitable), (b) as the mobile phase with a flow rate of 1 ml per minute, a solution containing 2.0 g of *sodium octanesulphonate* in a mixture of 730 ml of *methanol* and 270 ml of *water* and sufficient *glacial acetic acid* (120 ml may be suitable) to produce with solution (3) a chromatogram resembling that reproduced in the monograph for Chlorhexidine Acetate, measuring the volumes of the solvents separately to avoid errors from changes in volume on mixing, and (c) a detection wavelength of 254 nm.

Pass the mobile phase through the column for at least 1 hour before starting the analysis.

The principal peak (peak A in the reference chromatogram) in the chromatogram obtained with solution (3), recorded at a chart speed of 5 mm per minute for 30 minutes, should have a retention time of between 5.5 and 8 minutes and there should be a peak (peak D) with a retention time of between 20 and 25 minutes. The height of peak B should be at least 75% of full-scale deflection on the chart paper and peaks B and C should be at least partly resolved. If this pattern is not obtained, adjust the concentration of *glacial acetic acid* in the mobile phase; increasing the concentration decreases the retention times and decreasing the concentration increases the retention times. If peaks B and C are not resolved when satisfactory retention times have been obtained for the principal peak and peak D the column should be equilibrated for a further 12 hours and if the required resolution is still not obtained, inject ten 20-μl quantities of solution (3) in quick succession. If after this treatment a chromatogram resembling that in the monograph for Chlorhexidine Acetate cannot be obtained the column is not suitable.

In the chromatogram obtained with solution (2) the sum of the areas of any *secondary peaks* is not greater than the area of the principal peak in the chromatogram obtained with solution (1).

Assay Carry out the method for *liquid chromatography*, Appendix III D, using the following solutions. Solution (1) contains 0.008% w/v of *chlorhexidine acetate BPCRS* in the mobile phase. For solution (2) dilute a quantity of the solution being examined containing 4 mg of Chlorhexidine Acetate or 5 mg of chlorhexidine gluconate with sufficient of the mobile phase to produce 50 ml.

The chromatographic procedure described under Related substances may be used.

Calculate the content of $C_{22}H_{30}Cl_2N_{10},2C_2H_4O_2$ or $C_{22}H_{30}Cl_2N_{10},2C_6H_{12}O_7$ from the declared content of $C_{22}H_{30}Cl_2N_{10}$ in *chlorhexidine acetate BPCRS*. Each mg of chlorhexidine, $C_{22}H_{30}Cl_2N_{10}$, is equivalent to 1.238 mg of $C_{22}H_{30}Cl_2N_{10},2C_2H_4O_2$ or 1.775 mg of $C_{22}H_{30}Cl_2N_{10},2C_6H_{12}O_7$.

Storage Chlorhexidine Irrigation Solution should be protected from light.

Labelling The label on the container states whether the preparation contains Chlorhexidine Acetate or chlorhexidine gluconate.

Chlormethine Injection
Mustine Injection

For the purposes of product labelling in the United Kingdom, the pair of names given above shall be used together (see Introduction, Changes in title).

Definition Chlormethine Injection is a sterile solution of Chlormethine Hydrochloride in Water for Injections or Sodium Chloride Intravenous Infusion. It is prepared by dissolving Chlormethine Hydrochloride for Injection in the requisite amount of Water for Injections or Sodium Chloride Intravenous Infusion immediately before use.

The injection complies with the requirements stated under Parenteral Preparations.

Storage Chlormethine Injection deteriorates rapidly on storage and should be used immediately after preparation.

Labelling The label states 'Chlormethine Injection' and 'Mustine Injection'.

CHLORMETHINE HYDROCHLORIDE FOR INJECTION
MUSTINE HYDROCHLORIDE FOR INJECTION

For the purposes of product labelling in the United Kingdom, the pair of names given above shall be used together (see Introduction, Changes in title).

Definition Chlormethine Hydrochloride for Injection is a sterile material consisting of Chlormethine Hydrochloride with or without excipients. It is supplied in a sealed container.

The contents of the sealed container comply with the requirements for Powders for Injections stated under Parenteral Preparations and with the following requirements.

Content of chlormethine hydrochloride, $C_5H_{11}Cl_2N$, HCl 90.0 to 110.0% of the prescribed or stated amount.

Identification Dissolve the contents of a sealed container in 1 ml of *water* and add 0.02 ml of *potassium tetra-iodomercurate solution*. A cream precipitate is produced.

Uniformity of content The content of chlormethine hydrochloride, $C_5H_{11}Cl_2N,HCl$, in each of 10 individual containers as determined in the Assay is not less than 80.0% and not more than 120.0% of the average amount.

Assay Dissolve the contents of a sealed container in 2 ml of *ethanol (96%)* previously neutralised to *phenolphthalein solution R1*, add 0.1 ml of *phenolphthalein solution R1* and titrate with 0.01M *sodium hydroxide VS* (carbonate-free). Each ml of 0.01M *sodium hydroxide VS* is equivalent to 1.925 mg of $C_5H_{11}Cl_2N,HCl$. Calculate the content of $C_5H_{11}Cl_2N,HCl$ in the sealed container. Repeat the procedure with a further nine sealed containers. Calculate the average content of $C_5H_{11}Cl_2N,HCl$ per container from the 10 individual results thus obtained.

Labelling The label of the sealed container states (1) 'Chlormethine Hydrochloride for Injection' and 'Mustine Hydrochloride for Injection'; (2) the amount of the active ingredient contained in it; (2) that the contents are strongly vesicant.

Chloroform Spirit

Definition

Chloroform	50 ml
Ethanol (90 per cent)	sufficient to produce 1000 ml

The spirit complies with the requirements stated under Spirits and with the following requirements.

Ethanol content 83 to 87% v/v, Appendix VIII F.

Weight per ml 0.856 to 0.862 g, Appendix V G.

Chloroform and Morphine Tincture

Chlorodyne

Definition

Chloroform	125 ml
Morphine Hydrochloride	2.29 g
Peppermint Oil	1 ml
Ether	30 ml
Purified Water	50 ml
Ethanol (90 per cent)	125 ml
Liquorice Liquid Extract	125 ml
Treacle, of commerce	125 ml
Syrup	sufficient to produce 1000 ml

Extemporaneous preparation The following directions apply.

Dissolve the Peppermint Oil in the Ethanol (90 per cent), add the Purified Water, dissolve the Morphine Hydrochloride in the mixture and add the Chloroform and the Ether. Separately, mix the Liquorice Liquid Extract and the treacle with 400 ml of Syrup. Mix the two solutions, add sufficient Syrup to produce 1000 ml and mix.

The tincture complies with the requirements stated under Tinctures and with the following requirements.

Content of anhydrous morphine, $C_{17}H_{19}NO_3$ 0.157 to 0.191% w/v.

Chloroform content 11.25 to 13.75% v/v when determined by the following method. Carry out the method for *gas chromatography*, Appendix III B, using the following solutions. Solution (1) contains 5% v/v of *chloroform* and 5% v/v of *propan-1-ol* (internal standard) in a mixture of 2 volumes of *methanol* and 1 volume of *water*. For solution (2) dilute 40 ml of the tincture to 100 ml with a mixture of 2 volumes of *methanol* and 1 volume of *water*. For solution (3) dilute 40 ml of the tincture and 5 ml of *propan-1-ol* to 100 ml with *methanol*.

The chromatographic procedure may be carried out using a glass column (1.5 m × 4 mm) packed with porous polymer beads (80 to 100 mesh) (Chromosorb 101 is suitable) and maintained at 120°.

Calculate the content of $CHCl_3$ from the areas of the peaks due to chloroform and propan-1-ol in the chromatograms obtained with solutions (1) and (3).

Ethanol content 12 to 15% v/v when determined by the method described under Chloroform content but using for solution (1) a solution containing 5% v/v of *absolute ethanol* and 5% v/v of *propan-1-ol* (internal standard) in a mixture of 2 volumes of *methanol* and 1 volume of *water*.

Calculate the content of C_2H_6O from the areas of the peaks due to ethanol and propan-1-ol in the chromatograms obtained with solutions (1) and (3).

Relative density 1.22 to 1.26, Appendix V G.

Assay To 13 g add 1 ml of 5M *ammonia* and 4 ml of *water*, extract with 30 ml of a mixture of equal volumes of *ethanol (96%)* and *chloroform* and then with two 22.5-ml quantities of a mixture of 2 volumes of *chloroform* and 1 volume of *ethanol (96%)*. Wash each extract with the same 20 ml of a mixture of equal volumes of *ethanol (96%)* and *water* and evaporate the combined extracts to dryness. Dissolve the residue in 100 ml of 1M *hydrochloric acid*, dilute to 500 ml with *water* and filter. Dilute 10 ml of the filtrate with 10 ml of *water*, add 8 ml of a freshly prepared 1% w/v solution of *sodium nitrite*, allow to stand in the dark for 15 minutes, add 12 ml of 5M *ammonia* and dilute to 50 ml with *water*. Measure the *absorbance* of a 4-cm layer of the resulting solution at the maximum at 442 nm, Appendix II B, using in the reference cell a solution prepared in the same manner and at the same time but using 8 ml of *water* in place of the solution of sodium nitrite. Calculate the content of $C_{17}H_{19}NO_3$ from a calibration curve prepared from quantities of 2, 4, 6 and 8 ml of a 0.008% w/v solution of *anhydrous morphine* in 0.1M *hydrochloric acid*, each diluted to 20 ml with 0.1M *hydrochloric acid* and using the method described above beginning at the words 'add 8 ml...'. Using the *weight per ml* of the tincture, calculate the content of $C_{17}H_{19}NO_3$, weight in volume.

Storage Chloroform and Morphine Tincture should be kept in an airtight container.

Labelling The label states that the tincture must be shaken well before use.

Chloroform Water

Definition

Chloroform	2.5 ml
Purified Water, freshly boiled and cooled	sufficient to produce 1000 ml

Extemporaneous preparation The following directions apply.

Dissolve the Chloroform in the Purified Water by shaking.

The water complies with the requirements stated under Aromatic Waters.

Double-strength Chloroform Water

Definition

Chloroform	5 ml
Purified Water, freshly boiled and cooled	sufficient to produce 1000 ml

Extemporaneous preparation The following directions apply.

Dissolve the Chloroform in the Purified Water by shaking.

The water complies with the requirements stated under Aromatic Waters.

Chloroquine Phosphate Tablets

Definition Chloroquine Phosphate Tablets contain Chloroquine Phosphate. They are coated.

The tablets comply with the requirements stated under Tablets and with the following requirements.

Content of chloroquine phosphate, $C_{18}H_{26}ClN_3$, $2H_3PO_4$ 92.5 to 107.5% of the prescribed or stated amount.

Identification

A. Dissolve a quantity of the powdered tablets containing 0.1 g of Chloroquine Phosphate in a mixture of 10 ml of *water* and 2 ml of 2M *sodium hydroxide* and extract with two 20-ml quantities of *chloroform*. Wash the chloroform extracts with *water*, dry with *anhydrous sodium sulphate*, evaporate to dryness and dissolve the residue in 2 ml of *chloroform IR*. The *infrared absorption spectrum* of the resulting solution, Appendix II A, is concordant with the *reference spectrum* of chloroquine.

B. Extract a quantity of the powdered tablets containing 25 mg of Chloroquine Phosphate with 20 ml of *water*, filter and add 8 ml of *picric acid solution R1* to the filtrate. The *melting point* of the precipitate, after washing successively with *water*, *ethanol (96%)* and *ether*, is about 207°, Appendix V A.

C. Extract a quantity of the powdered tablets containing 0.5 g of Chloroquine Phosphate with 25 ml of *water* and filter. To the filtrate add 2.5 ml of 5M *sodium hydroxide* and extract with three 10-ml quantities of *ether*. The aqueous layer, after neutralisation with 2M *nitric acid*, yields the reactions characteristic of *phosphates*, Appendix VI.

Dissolution Comply with the *dissolution test for tablets and capsules*, Appendix XII D, using as the medium 900 ml of 0.1M *hydrochloric acid* and rotating the basket at 100 revolutions per minute. Withdraw a sample of 10 ml of the medium. Measure the *absorbance* of a layer of suitable thickness of the filtered sample, suitably diluted if necessary, at the maximum at 344 nm, Appendix II B. Calculate the total content of chloroquine phosphate, $C_{18}H_{26}ClN_3,2H_3PO_4$, in the medium taking 371 as the value of A(1%, 1 cm) at the maximum at 344 nm.

Related substances Carry out the method for *thin-layer chromatography*, Appendix III A, using *silica gel GF_{254}* as the coating substance and a mixture of 50 volumes of *chloroform*, 40 volumes of *cyclohexane* and 10 volumes of *diethylamine* as the mobile phase. Apply separately to the plate 2 µl of each of the following solutions. For solution (1) shake a quantity of the powdered tablets containing 1 g of Chloroquine Phosphate with 20 ml of *water* for 30 minutes, centrifuge and use the supernatant liquid; if necessary filter through a glass fibre paper. For solution (2) dilute 1 ml of solution (1) to 100 ml with *water*. For solution (3) dilute 25 ml of solution (2) to 50 ml with *water*. After removal of the plate, allow it to dry in air and examine under *ultraviolet light (254 nm)*. Any *secondary spot* in the chromatogram obtained with solution (1) is not more intense than the spot in the chromatogram obtained with solution (2) and not more than one such spot is more intense than the spot in the chromatogram obtained with solution (3).

Assay Weigh and powder 20 tablets. Dissolve a quantity of the powder containing 0.5 g of Chloroquine Phosphate in 20 ml of 1M *sodium hydroxide* and extract with four 25-ml quantities of *chloroform*. Combine the chloroform extracts and evaporate to a volume of about 10 ml. Add 40 ml of *anhydrous acetic acid* and carry out Method I for *non-aqueous titration*, Appendix VIII A, determining the end point potentiometrically. Each ml of 0.1M *perchloric acid VS* is equivalent to 25.79 mg of $C_{18}H_{26}ClN_3$, $2H_3PO_4$.

250 mg of Chloroquine Phosphate is approximately equivalent to 155 mg of chloroquine.

Chloroquine Sulphate Injection

Definition Chloroquine Sulphate Injection is a sterile solution of Chloroquine Sulphate in Water for Injections.

The injection complies with the requirements stated under Parenteral Preparations and with the following requirements.

Content of chloroquine, $C_{18}H_{26}ClN_3$ 95.0 to 105.0% of the prescribed or stated amount.

Identification

A. To a volume containing the equivalent of 60 mg of chloroquine add 2 ml of 2M *sodium hydroxide* and extract with two 20-ml quantities of *chloroform*. Wash the chloroform extracts with *water*, dry with *anhydrous sodium sulphate*, evaporate to dryness and dissolve the residue in 2 ml of *chloroform*. The *infrared absorption spectrum* of the resulting solution, Appendix II A, is concordant with the *reference spectrum* of chloroquine.

B. Dilute a volume containing the equivalent of 15 mg of chloroquine to 20 ml with *water* and add 8 ml of *picric acid solution R1*. The *melting point* of the precipitate, after washing successively with *water*, *ethanol (96%)* and *ether*, is about 207°, Appendix V A.

C. Yields the reactions characteristic of *sulphates*, Appendix VI.

Acidity pH, 4.0 to 5.5, Appendix V L.

Related substances Carry out the method for *thin-layer chromatography*, Appendix III A, using *silica gel* GF_{254} as the coating substance and a mixture of 10 volumes of *diethylamine*, 40 volumes of *cyclohexane* and 50 volumes of *chloroform* as the mobile phase but allowing the solvent front to ascend 12 cm above the line of application. Apply separately to the plate 2 µl of each of the following three solutions. For solution (1) use the injection being examined. For solution (2) dilute 1 volume of solution (1) to 100 volumes with *water*. For solution (3) dilute 1 volume of solution (2) to 2 volumes with *water*. After removal of the plate, allow it to dry in air and examine under *ultraviolet light (254 nm)*. Any *secondary spot* in the chromatogram obtained with solution (1) is not more intense than the spot in the chromatogram obtained with solution (2) (1%) and not more than one such spot is more intense than the spot in the chromatogram obtained with solution (3) (0.5%).

Assay To a volume containing the equivalent of 0.4 g of chloroquine add 20 ml of 1M *sodium hydroxide* and extract with four 25-ml quantities of *chloroform*. Combine the chloroform extracts and evaporate to a volume of about 10 ml. Add 40 ml of *anhydrous acetic acid* and carry out Method I for *non-aqueous titration*, Appendix VIII A, determining the end point potentiometrically. Each ml of 0.1M *perchloric acid VS* is equivalent to 15.99 mg of $C_{18}H_{26}ClN_3$.

Labelling The strength is stated as the equivalent amount of chloroquine in a suitable dose-volume.

40 mg of chloroquine is approximately equivalent to 55 mg of Chloroquine Sulphate.

Chloroquine Sulphate Tablets

Definition Chloroquine Sulphate Tablets contain Chloroquine Sulphate. They are coated.

The tablets comply with the requirements stated under Tablets and with the following requirements.

Content of chloroquine sulphate, $C_{18}H_{26}ClN_3$, H_2SO_4,H_2O 92.5 to 107.5% of the prescribed or stated amount.

Identification

A. Dissolve a quantity of the powdered tablets containing 0.1 g of Chloroquine Sulphate in a mixture of 10 ml of *water* and 2 ml of 2M *sodium hydroxide* and extract with two 20-ml quantities of *chloroform*. Wash the chloroform extracts with *water*, dry with *anhydrous sodium sulphate*, evaporate to dryness and dissolve the residue in 2 ml of *chloroform IR*. The *infrared absorption spectrum* of the resulting solution, Appendix II A, is concordant with the *reference spectrum* of chloroquine.

B. Shake a quantity of the powdered tablets containing 0.1 g of Chloroquine Sulphate with 10 ml of *water* and 1 ml of 2M *hydrochloric acid* and filter. To the filtrate add 1 ml of *barium chloride solution*. A white precipitate is produced.

Dissolution Comply with the *dissolution test for tablets and capsules*, Appendix XII D, using as the medium 900 ml of 0.1M *hydrochloric acid* and rotating the basket at 100 revolutions per minute. Withdraw a sample of 10 ml of the medium. Measure the *absorbance* of a layer of suitable thickness of the filtered sample, suitably diluted if necessary, at the maximum at 344 nm, Appendix II B. Calculate the total content of chloroquine sulphate, $C_{18}H_{26}ClN_3$,H_2O_4,H_2O, in the medium taking 450 as the value of A(1%, 1 cm) at the maximum at 344 nm.

Related substances Carry out the method for *thin-layer chromatography*, Appendix III A, using *silica gel* GF_{254} as the coating substance and a mixture of 50 volumes of *chloroform*, 40 volumes of *cyclohexane* and 10 volumes of *diethylamine* as the mobile phase. Apply separately to the plate 2 µl of each of the following solutions. For solution (1) shake a quantity of the powdered tablets containing 2.0 g of Chloroquine Sulphate with 50 ml of *water* for 30 minutes, centrifuge and use the supernatant liquid; if necessary filter through a glass fibre paper. For solution (2) dilute 1 ml of solution (1) to 100 ml with *water*. For solution (3) dilute 25 ml of solution (2) to 50 ml with *water*. After removal of the plate, allow it to dry in air and examine under *ultraviolet light (254 nm)*. Any *secondary spot* in the chromatogram obtained with solution (1) is not more intense than the spot in the chromatogram obtained with solution (2) and not more than one such spot is more intense than the spot in the chromatogram obtained with solution (3).

Assay Weigh and powder 20 tablets. Dissolve a quantity of the powder containing 0.5 g of Chloroquine Sulphate in 20 ml of 1M *sodium hydroxide* and extract with four 25-ml quantities of *chloroform*. Combine the chloroform extracts and evaporate to a volume of about 10 ml. Add 40 ml of *anhydrous acetic acid* and carry out Method I for *non-aqueous titration*, Appendix VIII A, determining the end point potentiometrically. Each ml of 0.1M *perchloric acid VS* is equivalent to 20.90 mg of $C_{18}H_{26}ClN_3$,H_2SO_4.

200 mg of Chloroquine Sulphate is approximately equivalent to 146 mg of chloroquine.

Chlorothiazide Tablets

Definition Chlorothiazide Tablets contain Chlorothiazide.

The tablets comply with the requirements stated under Tablets and with the following requirements.

Content of chlorothiazide, $C_7H_6ClN_3O_4S_2$ 95.0 to 105.0% of the prescribed or stated amount.

Identification Carry out the method for *thin-layer chromatography*, Appendix III A, using *silica gel* GF_{254} as the coating substance and *ethyl acetate* as the mobile phase. Apply separately to the plate 5 µl of each of the following solutions. For solution (1) triturate a quantity of the powdered tablets containing 10 mg of Chlorothiazide with 10 ml of *acetone* and filter. Solution (2) contains 0.1% w/v of *chlorothiazide EPCRS* in *acetone*. After removal of the plate, allow it to dry in air, examine under *ultraviolet light (254 nm)* and then reveal the spots by

Method I. By each method of visualisation the principal spot in the chromatogram obtained with solution (1) corresponds in colour and intensity to that in the chromatogram obtained with solution (2).

Related substances Carry out the method for *thin-layer chromatography*, Appendix III A, using *silica gel G* as the coating substance and a mixture of 85 volumes of *ethyl acetate* and 15 volumes of *propan-2-ol* as the mobile phase. Apply separately to the plate 5 µl of each of the following solutions. For solution (1) shake vigorously a quantity of the powdered tablets containing 50 mg of Chlorothiazide with 50 ml of *acetone*, filter, evaporate the filtrate to dryness and dissolve the residue in 10 ml of *acetone*. For solution (2) dilute 1 volume of solution (1) to 100 volumes with *acetone*. After removal of the plate, dry it in a current of air and reveal the spots by *Method I*. Any *secondary spot* in the chromatogram obtained with solution (1) is not more intense than the spot in the chromatogram obtained with solution (2).

Assay Weigh and powder 20 tablets. Shake a quantity of the powder containing 0.2 g of Chlorothiazide with 50 ml of 0.1M *sodium hydroxide* for 10 minutes and dilute to 100 ml with 0.1M *sodium hydroxide*. Mix, filter and dilute 10 ml of the filtrate to 100 ml with *water*. Dilute 10 ml of this solution to 100 ml with *water* and measure the *absorbance* of the resulting solution at the maximum at 292 nm, Appendix II B. Calculate the content of $C_7H_6ClN_3O_4S_2$ taking 435 as the value of A(1%, 1 cm) at the maximum at 292 nm.

Chloroxylenol Solution

Definition Chloroxylenol Solution is a *cutaneous solution*.

Chloroxylenol	50.0 g
Potassium Hydroxide	13.6 g
Oleic Acid	7.5 ml
Castor Oil	63.0 g
Terpineol	100 ml
Ethanol (96 per cent)	200 ml
Purified Water, freshly boiled and cooled	sufficient to produce 1000 ml

In making Chloroxylenol Solution, the Ethanol (96 per cent) may be replaced by Industrial Methylated Spirit[1].

Extemporaneous preparation The following directions apply.

Dissolve the Potassium Hydroxide in 15 ml of Purified Water, add a solution of the Castor Oil in 63 ml of Ethanol (96 per cent), mix, allow to stand for 1 hour or until a small portion of the mixture remains clear when diluted with 19 times its volume of Purified Water and then add the Oleic Acid. Mix the Terpineol with a solution of the Chloroxylenol in the remainder of the Ethanol (96 per cent), pour into the soap solution and add sufficient Purified Water to produce 1000 ml.

The solution complies with the requirements stated under Liquids for Cutaneous Application and with the following requirements.

Content of chloroxylenol, C_8H_9ClO 4.75 to 5.25% w/v.

Ethanol content 16 to 21% v/v, Appendix VIII F.

Assay Dissolve 0.4 g of *4-chloro-o-cresol* (internal standard) in sufficient *chloroform* to produce 50 ml (solution A). Carry out the method for *gas chromatography*, Appendix III B, using solutions prepared in the following manner. For solution (1) dissolve 0.10 g of *chloroxylenol BPCRS* in 10 ml of solution A and dilute to 20 ml with *chloroform*. For solution (2) place 4 ml of the solution being examined in a separating funnel, add 20 ml of *chloroform*, mix, add 4 ml of 2M *hydrochloric acid* and shake. Extract with two further 10-ml quantities of *chloroform*. Combine the chloroform extracts, dry by shaking with *anhydrous sodium sulphate* and filter. Prepare solution (3) in the same manner as solution (2) but adding 20 ml of solution A in place of the 20 ml of chloroform.

The chromatographic procedure may be carried out using a glass column (1.5 m × 4 mm) packed with *acid-washed, silanised diatomaceous support* (80 to 100 mesh) coated with 3% w/w of polyethylene glycol (Carbowax 20M is suitable) and maintained at 160°.

Calculate the content of C_8H_9ClO using the declared content of C_8H_9ClO in *chloroxylenol BPCRS*.

Storage Chloroxylenol Solution should be kept in a well-closed container.

Labelling The label states (1) the date after which the solution is not intended to be used; (2) the conditions under which it should be stored.

The label indicates the pharmaceutical form as 'cutaneous solution'.

[1]The law and statutory regulations governing the use of Industrial Methylated Spirit must be observed.

Chlorphenamine Injection
Chlorpheniramine Injection

For the purposes of product labelling in the United Kingdom, the pair of names given above shall be used together (see Introduction, Changes in title).

Definition Chlorphenamine Injection is a sterile solution of Chlorphenamine Maleate in Water for Injections free from dissolved air.

The injection complies with the requirements stated under Parenteral Preparations and with the following requirements.

Content of chlorphenamine maleate, $C_{16}H_{19}ClN_2,C_4H_4O_4$ 90.0 to 110.0% of the prescribed or stated amount.

Characteristics A colourless solution.

Identification Carry out the method for *thin-layer chromatography*, Appendix III A, using *silica gel GF_{254}* as the coating substance and a mixture of 20 volumes of 1M *acetic acid*, 30 volumes of *methanol* and 50 volumes of *ethyl acetate* as the mobile phase. Heat the plate at 105° for 30 minutes before use. Apply separately to the plate 2 µl of each of the following solutions. For solution (1) evaporate an appropriate volume to dryness in a current of nitrogen using the minimum amount of heat, dissolve the residue as completely as possible in sufficient *chloroform* to produce a solution containing 0.5% w/v of Chlorphenamine Maleate and centrifuge. Solution (2) contains 0.5% w/v of *chlorphenamine maleate BPCRS* in *chloroform*. After removal of the plate, allow it to dry in air and examine under *ultraviolet light (254 nm)*. The two principal spots in the chromatogram obtained with solution (1) correspond to those in the chromatogram obtained with solution (2). Spray the plate with *dilute potassium iodobismuthate solution*. The principal spot in the chromatogram obtained with solution (1) corresponds to that in the chromatogram obtained with solution (2).

Acidity pH, 4.0 to 5.2, Appendix V L.

Related substances Carry out the method for *thin-layer chromatography*, Appendix III A, using *silica gel GF_{254}* as the coating substance and a mixture of 10 volumes of *diethylamine*, 40 volumes of *chloroform* and 50 volumes of *cyclohexane* as the mobile phase but allowing the solvent front to ascend 12 cm above the line of application. Apply separately to the plate 10 µl of each of the following solutions. For solution (1) evaporate a suitable volume of the injection to dryness in a current of nitrogen using the minimum amount of heat, dissolve the residue as completely as possible in sufficient *chloroform* to produce a solution containing 5% w/v of Chlorphenamine Maleate and centrifuge. For solution (2) dilute 1 volume of solution (1) to 500 volumes with *chloroform*. After removal of the plate, allow it to dry in air and examine under *ultraviolet light (254 nm)*. Any *secondary spot* in the chromatogram obtained with solution (1) is not more intense than the spot in the chromatogram obtained with solution (2) (0.2%). Disregard any spot remaining on the line of application.

Assay Dilute a volume containing 10 mg of Chlorphenamine Maleate to 500 ml with 0.25M *sulphuric acid* and measure the *absorbance* of the resulting solution at the maximum at 265 nm, Appendix II B. Calculate the content of $C_{16}H_{19}ClN_2,C_4H_4O_4$ taking 212 as the value of A(1%, 1 cm) at the maximum at 265 nm.

Storage Chlorphenamine Injection should be protected from light.

Labelling The label states 'Chlorphenamine Injection' and 'Chlorpheniramine Injection'.

Chlorphenamine Oral Solution
Chlorpheniramine Oral Solution

For the purposes of product labelling in the United Kingdom, the pair of names given above shall be used together (see Introduction, Changes in title).

Definition Chlorphenamine Oral Solution is a solution of Chlorphenamine Maleate in a suitable flavoured vehicle.

The oral solution complies with the requirements stated under Oral Liquids and with the following requirements.

Content of chlorphenamine maleate, $C_{16}H_{19}ClN_2$, $C_4H_4O_4$ 90.0 to 110.0% of the prescribed or stated amount.

Identification In the test for Related substances, the principal spot in the chromatogram obtained with solution (3) corresponds to the spot in the chromatogram obtained with solution (4).

Related substances Carry out the method for *thin-layer chromatography*, Appendix III A, using *silica gel G* as the coating substance and a mixture of 50 volumes of *ethyl acetate*, 30 volumes of *methanol* and 20 volumes of 1M *acetic acid* as the mobile phase. Apply separately to the plate 10 µl of each of the following solutions. For solution (1) dilute a volume of the oral solution containing 10 mg of Chlorphenamine Maleate with an equal volume of *water*, add 20 ml of a 10% w/v solution of *sodium hydroxide* and extract with four 15-ml quantities of *chloroform*. Add 1 g of *anhydrous sodium sulphate* to the combined extracts, filter, evaporate at a temperature not exceeding 40° at a pressure of 2kPa and dissolve the residue in 1 ml of *chloroform*. For solution (2) dilute 1 volume of solution (1) to 500 volumes with *chloroform*. For solution (3) dilute 1 volume of solution (1) to 10 volumes with *chloroform*. Solution (4) contains 0.1% w/v of *chlorphenamine maleate BPCRS* in *chloroform*. After removal of the plate, allow it to dry in air and spray with *dilute potassium iodobismuthate solution*. Any *secondary spot* in the chromatogram obtained with solution (1) is not more intense than the spot in the chromatogram obtained with solution (2).

Assay Carry out the method for *gas chromatography*, Appendix III B, using the following solutions. Solution (1) contains 0.15% w/v of *chlorphenamine maleate BPCRS* and 0.15% w/v of N-*phenylcarbazole* (internal standard) in *chloroform*. Prepare solution (2) in the same manner as solution (3), but omitting the internal standard. For solution (3) add 10 ml of a 10% w/v solution of *sodium hydroxide* in *methanol* and 5 ml of a 0.060% w/v solution of N-*phenylcarbazole* in *chloroform* to a quantity of the oral solution containing 3 mg of Chlorphenamine Maleate, extract with four 25-ml quantities of *chloroform* and wash each extract with the same 10 ml of *water*. Combine the chloroform extracts, shake with *anhydrous sodium sulphate*, filter, evaporate at a temperature not exceeding 40° at a pressure of 2kPa and dissolve the residue in 2 ml of *chloroform*.

The chromatographic procedure may be carried out using a glass column (1.5 m × 4 mm) packed with *acid-washed, silanised diatomaceous support* (100 to 120 mesh) (Gas Chrom Q or Diatomite CQ is suitable) coated with 3% w/w of dimethyl silicone fluid (OV-101 is suitable) and maintained at 220° with the inlet port at 250°.

Calculate the content of $C_{16}H_{19}ClN_2,C_4H_4O_4$ using the declared content of $C_{16}H_{19}ClN_2,C_4H_4O_4$ in *chlorphenamine maleate BPCRS*.

Storage Chlorphenamine Oral Solution should be protected from light and stored at a temperature not exceeding 25°.

Labelling The label states 'Chlorphenamine Oral Solution' and 'Chlorpheniramine Oral Solution'.

Chlorphenamine Tablets
Chlorpheniramine Tablets

For the purposes of product labelling in the United Kingdom, the pair of names given above shall be used together (see Introduction, Changes in title).

Definition Chlorphenamine Tablets contain Chlorphenamine Maleate.

The tablets comply with the requirements stated under Tablets and with the following requirements.

Content of chlorphenamine maleate,

$C_{16}H_{19}ClN_2,C_4H_4O_4$ 92.5 to 107.5% of the prescribed or stated amount.

Identification Comply with the test described under Chlorphenamine Injection using as solution (1) a solution prepared in the following manner. Extract a quantity of the powdered tablets containing 5 mg of Chlorphenamine Maleate with *chloroform*, filter, evaporate to dryness and dissolve the residue in 1 ml of *chloroform*.

Related substances Carry out the method for *thin-layer chromatography*, Appendix III A, using *silica gel GF_{254}* as the coating substance and a mixture of 10 volumes of *diethylamine*, 40 volumes of *chloroform* and 50 volumes of *cyclohexane* as the mobile phase but allowing the solvent front to ascend 12 cm above the line of application. Apply separately to the plate 10 µl of each of the following solutions. For solution (1) extract a quantity of the powdered tablets containing 50 mg of Chlorphenamine Maleate with *chloroform*, filter, evaporate the filtrate to dryness and dissolve the residue in 1 ml of *chloroform*. For solution (2) dilute 1 volume of solution (1) to 500 volumes with *chloroform*. After removal of the plate, allow it to dry in air and examine under *ultraviolet light (254 nm)*. Any *secondary spot* in the chromatogram obtained with solution (1) is not more intense than the spot in the chromatogram obtained with solution (2) (0.2%). Disregard any spot remaining on the line of application.

Assay Weigh and powder 20 tablets. Shake a quantity of the powder containing 3 mg of Chlorphenamine Maleate with 20 ml of 0.05M *sulphuric acid* for 5 minutes, add 20 ml of *ether*, shake carefully and filter the acid layer into a second separating funnel. Extract the ether layer with two 10-ml quantities of 0.05M *sulphuric acid*, filter each acid layer into the second separating funnel and wash the filter with 0.05M *sulphuric acid*. Make the combined acid extracts and washings just alkaline to *litmus paper* with 1M *sodium hydroxide*, add 2 ml in excess and extract with two 50-ml quantities of *ether*. Wash each ether extract with the same 20 ml of *water* and extract with successive quantities of 20, 20 and 5 ml of 0.25M *sulphuric acid*. Dilute the combined acid extracts to 50 ml with 0.25M *sulphuric acid*, dilute 10 ml to 25 ml with 0.25M *sulphuric acid* and measure the *absorbance* of the resulting solution at the maximum at 265 nm, Appendix II B. Calculate the content of $C_{16}H_{19}ClN_2,C_4H_4O_4$ taking 212 as the value of A(1%, 1 cm) at the maximum at 265 nm.

Labelling The label states 'Chlorphenamine Tablets' and 'Chlorpheniramine Tablets'.

Chlorpromazine Injection

Definition Chlorpromazine Injection is a sterile solution of Chlorpromazine Hydrochloride in Water for Injections free from dissolved air.

The injection complies with the requirements stated under Parenteral Preparations and with the following requirements.

Content of chlorpromazine hydrochloride, $C_{17}H_{19}ClN_2S,HCl$ 95.0 to 105.0% of the prescribed or stated amount.

Characteristics A colourless or almost colourless solution.

Identification

A. To a volume containing 0.1 g of Chlorpromazine Hydrochloride add 20 ml of *water* and 2 ml of 10M *sodium hydroxide*. Shake and extract with 25 ml of *ether*. Wash the ether layer with two 5-ml quantities of *water*, dry with *anhydrous sodium sulphate*, evaporate the ether and dissolve the residue in 1 ml of *chloroform*. The *infrared absorption spectrum* of the resulting solution, Appendix II A, is concordant with the *reference spectrum* of chlorpromazine.

B. Complies with the test for *identification of phenothiazines*, Appendix III A. For solution (1) dilute the injection with *water* to give a solution containing 0.2% w/v of Chlorpromazine Hydrochloride.

Acidity pH, 5.0 to 6.5, Appendix V L.

Related substances Carry out the test for *related substances in phenothiazines*, Appendix III A, using *mobile phase A* and applying separately to the plate 20 µl of each of the following freshly prepared solutions. For solution (1) dilute a volume of the injection, if necessary, with sufficient of a mixture of 95 volumes of *methanol* and 5 volumes of *diethylamine* to produce a solution containing 0.5% w/v of Chlorpromazine Hydrochloride. For solution (2) dilute 1 volume of solution (1) to 20 volumes with the same solvent. For solution (3) dilute 1 volume of solution (1) to 200 volumes with the same solvent. Any *secondary spot* in the chromatogram obtained with solution (1) is not more intense than the spot in the chromatogram obtained with solution (2) and not more than one such spot is more intense than the spot in the chromatogram obtained with solution (3).

Assay Carry out the following procedure protected from light. Dilute a suitable volume with sufficient 0.1M *hydrochloric acid* to produce a solution containing 0.0005% w/v of Chlorpromazine Hydrochloride and measure the *absorbance* at the maximum at 254 nm, Appendix II B. Calculate the content of $C_{17}H_{19}ClN_2S,HCl$ taking 915 as the value of A(1%, 1 cm) at the maximum at 254 nm.

Storage Chlorpromazine Injection should be protected from light.

Chlorpromazine Oral Solution

Chlorpromazine Elixir

Definition Chlorpromazine Oral Solution is a solution of Chlorpromazine Hydrochloride in a suitable flavoured vehicle.

The oral solution complies with the requirements stated under Oral Liquids and with the following requirements.

Content of chlorpromazine hydrochloride, $C_{17}H_{19}ClN_2S,HCl$ 90.0 to 110.0% of the prescribed or stated amount.

Identification Carry out the method for *identification of phenothiazines*, Appendix III A. For solution (1) dilute a suitable volume of the oral solution with *water* to give a solution containing 0.2% w/v of Chlorpromazine Hydrochloride.

Related substances Carry out the method for *thin-layer chromatography*, Appendix III A, protected from light under an atmosphere of nitrogen using *silica gel GF_{254}* as the coating substance and a mixture of 10 volumes of *acetone*, 10 volumes of *diethylamine* and 80 volumes of *cyclohexane* as the mobile phase but allowing the solvent front to ascend 12 cm above the line of application. Apply separately to the plate 10 µl of each of the following freshly prepared solutions. For solution (1) add 40 ml of *water* and 5 ml of a 20% w/v solution of *sodium hydroxide* to a quantity of the oral solution containing 20 mg of Chlorpromazine Hydrochloride in a separating funnel and swirl to mix. Extract with two 25-ml quantities of *chloroform*, combine the chloroform extracts and filter through *anhydrous sodium sulphate*. Wash the sodium sulphate with a further 25 ml of *chloroform* and evaporate the combined filtrate and washings to dryness at about 30° in a gentle current of *nitrogen*. Dissolve the residue in 2 ml of a mixture of 95 volumes of *methanol* and 5 volumes of *diethylamine*. For solution (2) dilute 1 volume of solution (1) to 200 volumes with the same solvent. Solution (3) is a 0.030% w/v solution of *chlorpromazine sulphoxide BPCRS* in the same solvent. After removal of the plate, allow it to dry in air, spray with a 20% w/w solution of *perchloric acid* and heat at 100° for 5 minutes. In the chromatogram obtained with solution (1) any spot corresponding to chlorpromazine sulphoxide is not more intense than the spot in the chromatogram obtained with solution (3) and any other *secondary spot* is not more intense than the spot in the chromatogram obtained with solution (2). Disregard any spot remaining on the line of application.

Assay Carry out the following procedure protected from light. Dilute a quantity containing 0.1 g of Chlorpromazine Hydrochloride to 500 ml with 2M *hydrochloric acid*. To 10 ml of this solution add 20 ml of *water*, make distinctly alkaline to *litmus paper* with 13.5M *ammonia* and extract with six 25-ml quantities of *ether*. Extract the combined ether solutions with four 25-ml quantities of a mixture containing 1 volume of *hydrochloric acid* and 99 volumes of *water*, discard the ether, remove any dissolved ether from the combined extracts with a current of air and dilute to 250 ml with a mixture containing 1 volume of *hydrochloric acid* and 99 volumes of *water*. Measure the *absorbance* of the resulting solution at the maximum at 254 nm, Appendix II B. Calculate the content of $C_{17}H_{19}ClN_2S,HCl$ taking 914 as the value of A(1%, 1 cm) at the maximum at 254 nm.

Storage Chlorpromazine Oral Solution should be protected from light.

Chlorpromazine Suppositories

Definition Chlorpromazine Suppositories contain Chlorpromazine in a suitable suppository basis.

The suppositories comply with the requirements stated under Rectal Preparations and with the following requirements.

Content of chlorpromazine, $C_{17}H_{19}ClN_2S$ 95.0 to 105.0% of the prescribed or stated amount.

Identification Comply with the test for *identification of phenothiazines*, Appendix III A. For solution (1) dissolve a quantity of the suppositories containing 0.1 g of Chlorpromazine in 50 ml of *chloroform*. Use *chlorpromazine hydrochloride EPCRS* to prepare solution (2).

Related substances Comply with the test for *related substances in phenothiazines*, Appendix III A, using *mobile phase A* and the following freshly prepared solutions. For solution (1) dissolve a quantity of the suppositories containing 0.2 g of Chlorpromazine in sufficient *chloroform* to produce 20 ml. For solution (2) dilute 1 volume of solution (1) to 200 volumes with *chloroform*.

Assay Weigh five suppositories. Dissolve a quantity containing 0.5 g of Chlorpromazine in sufficient *chloroform* to produce 100 ml and dilute 20 ml to 100 ml with *ethanol (96%)*. Dilute 10 ml of this solution to 100 ml with *ethanol (96%)* and further dilute 5 ml of this solution to 100 ml with the same solvent. Measure the *absorbance* of the resulting solution at the maximum at 258 nm, Appendix II B, using *ethanol (96%)* in the reference cell. Calculate the content of $C_{17}H_{19}ClN_2S$ taking 1150 as the value of A(1%, 1 cm) at the maximum at 258 nm.

Storage Chlorpromazine Suppositories should be protected from light.

Chlorpromazine Tablets

Definition Chlorpromazine Tablets contain Chlorpromazine Hydrochloride. They are coated.

The tablets comply with the requirements stated under Tablets and with the following requirements.

Content of chlorpromazine hydrochloride, $C_{17}H_{19}ClN_2S,HCl$ 92.5 to 107.5% of the prescribed or stated amount.

Identification

A. To a quantity of the powdered tablets containing 40 mg of Chlorpromazine Hydrochloride add 10 ml of *water* and 2 ml of 10M *sodium hydroxide*. Shake and extract with 15 ml of *ether*. Wash the ether layer with two 5-ml quantities of *water*, dry with *anhydrous sodium sulphate* and evaporate the ether. Dissolve the residue in 0.4 ml of *chloroform*. The *infrared absorption spectrum* of the resulting solution, Appendix II A, is concordant with the *reference spectrum* of chlorpromazine.

B. Comply with the test for *identification of phenothiazines*, Appendix III A. For solution (1) shake a quantity of the powdered tablets with sufficient *chloroform* to produce a solution containing 0.20% w/v of Chlorpromazine Hydrochloride, centrifuge and use the supernatant liquid.

Related substances Comply with the test for *related substances in phenothiazines*, Appendix III A, using *mobile phase A* and the following freshly prepared solutions. For solution (1) extract a quantity of the powdered tablets containing 0.1 g of Chlorpromazine Hydrochloride with 10 ml of a mixture of 95 volumes of *methanol* and 5 volumes of *diethylamine* and filter. For solution (2) dilute 1 volume of solution (1) to 200 volumes with the same solvent mixture.

Dissolution Comply with the *dissolution test for tablets and capsules*, Appendix XII D, using Apparatus II, protected from light. Use as the medium 900 ml of 0.1M *hydrochloric acid* and rotate the paddle at 50 revolutions per minute. Withdraw a sample of 10 ml of the medium, filter and dilute a suitable volume of the filtrate with 0.1M *hydrochloric acid* to produce a solution containing 0.0005% w/v of Chlorpromazine Hydrochloride. Measure the *absorbance* of this solution, Appendix II B, at 254 nm using 0.1M *hydrochloric acid* in the reference cell. Calculate the total content of $C_{17}H_{19}ClN_2S,HCl$ in the medium taking 914 as the value of A(1%, 1 cm) at the maximum at 254 nm.

Assay Carry out the following procedure protected from light. Powder 10 tablets without loss, triturate the powder with 10 ml of *absolute ethanol,* add about 300 ml of 0.1M *hydrochloric acid* and shake for 15 minutes. Add sufficient 0.1M *hydrochloric acid* to produce 500 ml , filter, dilute a volume of the filtrate containing 5 mg of Chlorpromazine Hydrochloride to 100 ml with 0.1M *hydrochloric acid* and further dilute 10 ml to 100 ml with the same solvent. Measure the *absorbance* of the resulting solution at the maximum at 254 nm, Appendix II B. Calculate the content of $C_{17}H_{19}ClN_2S,HCl$ taking 915 as the value of A(1%, 1 cm) at the maximum at 254 nm.

Chlorpropamide Tablets

Definition Chlorpropamide Tablets contain Chlorpropamide.

The tablets comply with the requirements stated under Tablets and with the following requirements.

Content of chlorpropamide, $C_{10}H_{13}ClN_2O_3S$ 92.5 to 107.5% of the prescribed or stated amount.

Identification Extract a quantity of the powdered tablets containing 1 g of Chlorpropamide with five 4-ml quantities of *acetone,* filter and evaporate the filtrate carefully to dryness on a water bath. The *infrared absorption spectrum* of the residue, Appendix II A, is concordant with the *reference spectrum* of chlorpropamide.

Dissolution Comply with the *dissolution test for tablets and capsules,* Appendix XII D, using as the medium 900 ml of a 0.68% w/v solution of *potassium dihydrogen orthophosphate* adjusted to pH 6.8 by the addition of 1M *sodium hydroxide* and rotating the basket at 100 revolutions per minute. Withdraw a 10-ml sample of the medium and measure the *absorbance* of the filtered sample, suitably diluted if necessary, at the maximum at 230 nm, Appendix II B. Calculate the total content of chlorpropamide, $C_{10}H_{13}ClN_2O_3S$, in the medium taking 469 as the value of A(1%, 1 cm) at the maximum at 230 nm.

Related substances Carry out the method for *thin-layer chromatography,* Appendix III A, using *silica gel 60* as the coating substance and a mixture of 11.5 volumes of 13.5M *ammonia,* 30 volumes of *cyclohexane,* 50 volumes of *methanol* and 100 volumes of *dichloromethane* as the mobile phase. Apply separately to the plate 5 µl of each of the following solutions. For solution (1) shake a quantity of the powdered tablets containing 0.5 g of Chlorpropamide with 10 ml of *acetone* for 10 minutes and filter (Whatman GF/C filter paper is suitable). Solution (2) contains 0.015% w/v of *4-chlorobenzenesulphonamide* in *acetone.* Solution (3) contains 0.015% w/v of *1,3-dipropylurea* in *acetone.* For solution (4) dilute 0.3 volume of solution (1) to 100 volumes with *acetone.* For solution (5) dilute 1 volume of solution (4) to 3 volumes with *acetone.* After removal of the plate, dry it in a current of cold air and heat at 110° for 10 minutes. Place the hot plate in a tank of chlorine gas prepared by the addition of *hydrochloric acid* to a 5% w/v solution of *potassium permanganate* contained in a beaker placed in the tank and allow to stand for 2 minutes. Dry it in a current of cold air until the excess of chlorine is removed and an area of the plate below the line of application gives at most a very faint blue colour with a 0.5% w/v solution of *potassium iodide* in *starch mucilage;* avoid prolonged exposure to cold air. Spray the plate with a 0.5% w/v solution of *potassium iodide* in *starch mucilage.* In the chromatogram obtained with solution (1) any spot corresponding to 4-chlorobenzenesulphonamide is not more intense than the spot in the chromatogram obtained with solution (2) (0.3%), any spot corresponding to 1,3-dipropylurea is not more intense than the spot in the chromatogram obtained with solution (3) (0.3%), any other *secondary spot* is not more intense than the spot in the chromatogram obtained with solution (4) (0.3%) and not more than two such spots are more intense than the spot in the chromatogram obtained with solution (5) (0.1%).

Assay Weigh and powder 20 tablets. Shake a quantity of the powder containing 0.25 g of Chlorpropamide with 40 ml of *methanol* for 20 minutes, add sufficient *methanol* to produce 50 ml, mix, filter and dilute 5 ml of the filtrate to 100 ml with 0.1M *hydrochloric acid.* Dilute 10 ml of this solution to 250 ml with 0.1M *hydrochloric acid* and measure the *absorbance* of the resulting solution at the maximum at 232 nm, Appendix II B. Calculate the content of $C_{10}H_{13}ClN_2O_3S$ taking 598 as the value of A(1 cm, 1%) at the maximum at 232 nm.

Chlortalidone Tablets

Definition Chlortalidone Tablets contain Chlortalidone.

The tablets comply with the requirements stated under Tablets and with the following requirements.

Content of chlortalidone, $C_{14}H_{11}ClN_2O_4S$ 92.5 to 107.5% of the prescribed or stated amount.

Identification Heat a quantity of the powdered tablets containing 0.2 g of Chlortalidone with 20 ml of *acetone* on a water bath for 10 minutes, cool and filter. Add 40 ml of *water* to the filtrate and heat on a water bath for 20 minutes using a gentle current of air to remove the acetone. Cool the solution to room temperature, allow to stand, filter and dry the crystals at 105° for 4 hours. The *infrared spectrum* of the crystals, Appendix II A, is concordant with the *reference spectrum* of chlortalidone.

Related substances Carry out the method for *thin-layer chromatography,* Appendix III A, using *silica gel GF_{254}* as the coating substance and a mixture of 10 volumes of *toluene,* 10 volumes of *xylene,* 20 volumes of 18M *ammonia,* 30 volumes of *1,4-dioxan* and 30 volumes of *propan-2-ol* as the mobile phase. Apply separately to the plate 5 µl of each of the following solutions. For solution (1) add a quantity of the powdered tablets containing 0.1 g of Chlortalidone to 5 ml of *ethanol (96%),* mix with the aid of ultrasound for 15 minutes, centrifuge and use the supernatant liquid. For solution (2) dilute 1 volume of solution (1) to 200 volumes with *ethanol (96%).* Solution (3) contains 0.020% w/v of *2-(4-chloro-3-sulphamoylbenzoyl)benzoic acid EPCRS* in *ethanol (96%).* After removal of the plate, allow it to dry in air and examine under *ultraviolet light (254 nm).* Any spot corresponding to 2-(4-chloro-3-sulphamoylbenzoyl)benzoic acid in the chromatogram obtained with solution (1) is not more intense than the spot in the chromatogram obtained with solution (3) (1%) and any other *secondary spot* is not more intense than the spot in the chromatogram obtained with solution (2) (0.5%).

Assay Weigh and powder 20 tablets. Boil a quantity of the powder containing 0.1 g of Chlortalidone under a reflux condenser with 30 ml of *methanol* for 5 minutes, shake vigorously for 15 minutes, cool and filter. Wash the residue and filter with *methanol* and dilute the combined filtrate and washings to 100 ml with *methanol.* To 5 ml add 2 ml of 1M *hydrochloric acid* and sufficient *methanol* to produce 50 ml and measure the *absorbance* of the resulting solution at the maximum at 275 nm, Appendix II B. Calculate the content of $C_{14}H_{11}ClN_2O_4S$ taking 57.4 as the value of A(1%, 1 cm) at the maximum at 275 nm.

When chlorthalidone tablets are prescribed or demanded, Chlortalidone Tablets shall be dispensed or supplied.

Chlortetracycline Eye Ointment

Definition Chlortetracycline Eye Ointment is a sterile preparation containing Chlortetracycline Hydrochloride in a suitable basis.

The eye ointment complies with the requirements stated under Eye Preparations and with the following requirements.

Content of chlortetracycline hydrochloride, $C_{22}H_{23}ClN_2O_8$,HCl 90.0 to 110.0% of the prescribed or stated amount.

Identification

A. Disperse a quantity of the eye ointment containing 10 mg of Chlortetracycline Hydrochloride in 10 ml of *dichloromethane,* extract with two 10-ml quantities of 0.01M *hydrochloric acid,* filter and dilute the filtrate to 100 ml with 0.01M *hydrochloric acid.* Dilute 20 ml of the resulting solution to 100 ml with 0.01M *hydrochloric acid.* The *light absorption* of the resulting solution, Appendix II B, in the range 220 to 420 nm exhibits two maxima, at 266 nm and 368 nm.

B. Carry out the method for *thin-layer chromatography,* Appendix III A, using *silica gel H* as the coating substance and a mixture of 6 volumes of *water,* 35 volumes of *methanol* and 59 volumes of *dichloromethane* as the mobile phase. Adjust the pH of a 10% w/v solution of *disodium edetate* to 8.0 with 10M *sodium hydroxide* and spray the solution evenly onto the plate (about 10 ml for a plate 100 mm × 200 mm). Allow the plate to dry in a horizontal position for at least 1 hour. At the time of use, dry the plate in an oven at 110° for 1 hour. Apply separately to the plate 1 µl of each of the following solutions. For solution (1) disperse a quantity of the eye ointment containing 25 mg of Chlortetracycline Hydrochloride in 25 ml of *dichloromethane,* extract with two quantities of 0.01M *hydrochloric acid,* filter the aqueous layer and dilute to 50 ml with *water.* Solution (2) contains 0.05% w/v of *chlortetracycline hydrochloride EPCRS* in *water.* Solution (3) contains 0.05% w/v of each of *chlortetracycline hydrochloride EPCRS, tetracycline hydrochloride EPCRS* and *metacycline hydrochloride EPCRS* in *water.* Allow the plate to dry in a stream of air and examine under *ultraviolet light (365 nm)*. The principal spot in the chromatogram obtained with solution (1) corresponds to that in the chromatogram obtained with solution (2). The test is not valid unless the chromatogram obtained with solution (3) shows three clearly separated spots.

C. To a quantity of the eye ointment containing 0.5 mg of Chlortetracycline Hydrochloride add 2 ml of *sulphuric acid;* a deep blue colour is produced, which becomes bluish green. Add 1 ml of *water;* a brown colour is produced.

Tetracycline hydrochloride and 4-epichlortetracycline hydrochloride Not more than 8.0% and 6.0% respectively, determined as described under Assay. Inject separately solutions (1) and (4).

Assay Carry out the method for *liquid chromatography,* Appendix III D, using the following solutions. For solution (1) disperse a quantity of the eye ointment containing 25 mg of Chlortetracycline Hydrochloride in 20 ml of *chloroform* and 50 ml of 0.01M *hydrochloric acid* and shake for 15 minutes, dilute to 100 ml with 0.01M *hydrochloric acid,* mix thoroughly, allow to separate and filter the aqueous layer. For solution (2) dissolve 25 mg of *chlortetracycline hydrochloride EPCRS* in 20 ml of *chloroform* and 50 ml of 0.01M *hydrochloric acid* and treat in the same manner as solution (1) beginning at the words 'and shake for 15 minutes...'. Solution (3) contains 0.025% w/v of each of *chlortetracycline hydrochloride EPCRS* and *4-epichlortetracycline hydrochloride EPCRS* in 0.01M *hydrochloric acid.* Solution (4) contains 0.002% w/v of *tetracycline hydrochloride EPCRS* and 0.0015% w/v of *4-epichlortetracycline hydrochloride EPCRS* in 0.01M *hydrochloric acid.*

The chromatographic procedure may be carried out using (a) a stainless steel column (25 cm × 4.6 mm) packed with *stationary phase C* (10 µm) (Nucleosil C18 is suitable) and maintained at 40°, (b) as the mobile phase with a flow rate of 2 ml per minute a mixture of 80 volumes of 0.1M *oxalic acid* the pH of which has been adjusted to 2.2 with *triethylamine* and 20 volumes of *dimethylformamide* and (c) a detection wavelength of 355 nm.

The assay is not valid unless the *resolution factor* between the two principal peaks in the chromatogram obtained with solution (3) is at least 1.5.

Calculate the content of $C_{22}H_{23}ClN_2O_8$,HCl in the eye ointment using the declared content of $C_{22}H_{23}ClN_2O_8$, HCl in *chlortetracycline hydrochloride EPCRS.*

Storage Chlortetracycline Eye Ointment should be protected from light and stored at a temperature not exceeding 25°.

Chlortetracycline Ointment

Definition Chlortetracycline Ointment contains Chlortetracycline Hydrochloride in a suitable basis.

The ointment complies with the requirements stated under Topical Semi-solid Preparations and with the following requirements.

Content of chlortetracycline hydrochloride, $C_{22}H_{23}ClN_2O_8$,HCl 90.0 to 110.0% of the prescribed or stated amount.

Identification

A. Disperse a quantity of the ointment containing 10 mg of Chlortetracycline Hydrochloride in 10 ml of *dichloromethane,* extract with two 10-ml quantities of 0.01M *hydrochloric acid,* combine the aqueous extracts, filter and extract the filtrate with two 10-ml quantities of *ether.* Discard the ether extracts and dilute the aqueous layer to

100 ml with 0.01M *hydrochloric acid.* Dilute 20 ml of the resulting solution to 100 ml with 0.01M *hydrochloric acid.* The *light absorption* of the resulting solution, Appendix II B, in the range 220 to 420 nm exhibits two maxima, at 266 nm and 368 nm.

B. Complies with test B for Identification described under Chlortetracycline Eye Ointment but using the following solutions. For solution (1) disperse a quantity of the ointment containing 25 mg of Chlortetracycline Hydrochloride in 25 ml of *dichloromethane,* extract with two quantities of 0.01M *hydrochloric acid,* filter the aqueous layer and dilute to 50 ml with *water.* Solution (2) contains 0.05% w/v of *chlortetracycline hydrochloride EPCRS* in *water.* Solution (3) contains 0.05% w/v each of *chlortetracycline hydrochloride EPCRS, tetracycline hydrochloride EPCRS* and *metacycline hydrochloride EPCRS* in *water.*

C. To a quantity of the ointment containing 0.5 mg of Chlortetracycline Hydrochloride add 2 ml of *sulphuric acid*; a deep blue colour is produced, which becomes bluish green. Add 1 ml of *water*; a brown colour is produced.

Tetracycline hydrochloride and 4-epichlortetracycline hydrochloride Not more than 8.0% and 6.0% respectively, determined as described under Assay. Inject separately solutions (1) and (4).

Assay Carry out the Assay described under Chlortetracycline Eye Ointment but using the following solutions. For solution (1) disperse a quantity of the ointment containing 25 mg of Chlortetracycline Hydrochloride in 20 ml of *chloroform* and 50 ml of 0.01M *hydrochloric acid* and shake for 15 minutes, dilute to 100 ml with 0.01M *hydrochloric acid,* mix thoroughly, allow to separate and filter the aqueous layer. For solution (2) dissolve 25 mg of *chlortetracycline hydrochloride EPCRS* in 20 ml of *chloroform* and 50 ml of 0.01M *hydrochloric acid* and treat in the same manner as solution (1) beginning at the words 'and shake for 15 minutes...'. Solution (3) contains 0.025% w/v each of *chlortetracycline hydrochloride EPCRS* and *4-epichlortetracycline hydrochloride EPCRS* in 0.01M *hydrochloric acid.* Solution (4) contains 0.002% w/v of *tetracycline hydrochloride EPCRS* and 0.0015% w/v of *4-epichlortetracycline hydrochloride EPCRS* in 0.01M *hydrochloric acid.*

The assay is not valid unless the *resolution factor* between the two principal peaks in the chromatogram obtained with solution (3) is at least 1.5.

Calculate the content of $C_{22}H_{23}ClN_2O_8$,HCl in the ointment using the declared content of $C_{22}H_{23}ClN_2O_8$, HCl in *chlortetracycline hydrochloride EPCRS.*

Storage Chlortetracycline Ointment should be protected from light and stored at a temperature not exceeding 25°.

Choline Salicylate Ear Drops

Definition Choline Salicylate Ear Drops are a solution of choline salicylate in Propylene Glycol. They are prepared by diluting Choline Salicylate Solution.

The ear drops comply with the requirements stated under Ear Preparations and with the following requirements.

Content of choline salicylate, $C_{12}H_{19}NO_4$ 95.0 to 105.0% of the prescribed or stated amount.

Identification

A. Heat 2 ml with *sodium hydroxide* until fumes are evolved. The odour of trimethylamine is produced.

B. Dilute a quantity containing 2 g of choline salicylate to 20 ml with *water.* The resulting solution yields the reactions characteristic of *salicylates,* Appendix VI.

Assay To a quantity containing 0.4 g of choline salicylate add 50 ml of *1,4-dioxan* and 5 ml of *acetic anhydride* and carry out Method I for *non-aqueous titration,* Appendix VIII A, using 0.25 ml of *methyl orange—xylene cyanol FF solution* as indicator. Each ml of 0.1M *perchloric acid VS* is equivalent to 24.13 mg of $C_{12}H_{19}NO_4$.

Labelling The strength is stated as the percentage w/v of choline salicylate.

Choline Salicylate Dental Gel

Definition Choline Salicylate Dental Gel is a solution of choline salicylate in a suitable water-miscible basis. It is prepared from Choline Salicylate Solution.

The dental gel complies with the requirements stated under Topical Semi-solid Preparations and with the following requirements.

Content of choline salicylate, $C_{12}H_{19}NO_4$ 90.0 to 110.0% of the prescribed or stated amount.

Identification

A. Mix a quantity containing 0.1 g of choline salicylate with 9 ml of *water* (solution A). To 1 ml of solution A add 1 ml of *ammonium reineckate solution,* filter and wash the precipitate produced. The precipitate is pink.

B. 1 ml of solution A yields reaction A characteristic of *salicylates,* Appendix VI.

C. Mix a quantity containing 0.2 g of choline salicylate with 15 ml of *water,* heat on a water bath for 15 minutes and filter. The filtrate yields reaction B characteristic of *salicylates,* Appendix VI.

Assay To a quantity containing 0.5 g of choline salicylate in a conical flask add 25 ml of *1,4-dioxan* and 5 ml of *acetic anhydride.* Shake well until the gel has completely dispersed and wash the inside wall of the flask with 25 ml of *1,4-dioxan.* Carry out Method I for *non-aqueous titration,* Appendix VIII A, using 0.25 ml of *methyl orange—xylene cyanol FF solution* as indicator. Each ml of 0.1M *perchloric acid VS* is equivalent to 24.13 mg of $C_{12}H_{19}NO_4$.

Labelling The quantity of active ingredient is stated as the amount of choline salicylate.

Choline Theophyllinate Tablets

Definition Choline Theophyllinate Tablets contain Choline Theophyllinate. They are coated.

The tablets comply with the requirements stated under Tablets and with the following requirements.

Content of choline theophyllinate, $C_{12}H_{21}N_5O_3$ 95.0 to 105.0% of the prescribed or stated amount.

Identification

A. Shake a quantity of the powdered tablets containing 0.1 g of Choline Theophyllinate with 20 ml of *absolute ethanol* for 10 minutes, filter and evaporate the filtrate to dryness. The *infrared absorption spectrum* of the residue, Appendix II A, is concordant with the *reference spectrum* of choline theophyllinate.

B. The *light absorption* of the final solution obtained in the Assay, Appendix II B, exhibits a maximum at 275 nm.

Related substances Carry out the method for *thin-layer chromatography*, Appendix III A, using *silica gel HF_{254}* as the coating substance and a mixture of 95 volumes of *chloroform* and 5 volumes of *ethanol (96%)* as the mobile phase. Apply separately to the plate 5 µl of each of the following solutions. For solution (1) shake a quantity of the powdered tablets containing 0.1 g of Choline Theophyllinate with 10 ml of *ethanol (96%)* for 10 minutes and filter. For solution (2) dilute 1 volume of solution (1) to 100 volumes with *ethanol (96%)*. After removal of the plate, allow it to dry in air and examine under *ultraviolet light (254 nm)*. Any *secondary spot* in the chromatogram obtained with solution (1) is not more intense than the spot in the chromatogram obtained with solution (2).

Assay Weigh and powder 20 tablets. To a quantity of the powder containing 0.1 g of Choline Theophyllinate add 500 ml of *water* shake vigorously for 2 minutes, dilute to 1000 ml with *water*, mix and filter. To 10 ml of the filtrate add 10 ml of 0.1M *sodium hydroxide* and dilute to 100 ml with *water*. Measure the *absorbance* of the resulting solution at the maximum at 275 nm, Appendix II B. Calculate the content of $C_{12}H_{21}N_5O_3$ taking 415 as the value of A(1%, 1 cm) at the maximum at 275 nm.

Storage Choline Theophyllinate Tablets should be protected from light and stored at a temperature not exceeding 25°.

Chorionic Gonadotrophin Injection

Definition Chorionic Gonadotrophin Injection is a sterile solution of Chorionic Gonadotrophin in Water for Injections. It is prepared by dissolving Chorionic Gonadotrophin for Injection in the requisite amount of Water for Injections immediately before use.

The injection complies with the requirements stated under Parenteral Preparations.

Storage Chorionic Gonadotrophin Injection should be used immediately after preparation.

CHORIONIC GONADOTROPHIN FOR INJECTION

Definition Chorionic Gonadotrophin for Injection is a sterile material consisting of Chorionic Gonadotrophin with or without excipients. It is supplied in a sealed container.

The contents of the sealed container comply with the requirements for Powders for Injections stated under Parenteral Preparations and with the following requirements.

Characteristics A white or almost white, amorphous powder.

Identification Cause an increase in the weight of the seminal vesicles or the prostate glands of immature male rats when administered as directed under the Assay.

Acidity or alkalinity pH of a 1% w/v solution, 6.0 to 8.0, Appendix V L.

Clarity and colour of solution A 1.0% w/v solution is *clear*, Appendix IV A, and *colourless*, Appendix IV B, Method I.

Pyrogens Comply with the *test for pyrogens*, Appendix XIV D. Use per kg of the rabbit's weight 1 ml of a solution in *sodium chloride injection* containing 300 IU per ml.

Assay Carry out the Assay described under Chorionic Gonadotrophin. The estimated potency is not less than 80% and not more than 125% of the stated potency. The fiducial limits of error are not less than 64% and not more than 156% of the stated potency.

Storage The sealed container should be protected from light and stored at a temperature not exceeding 20°. Under these conditions, the contents may be expected to retain their potency for not less than 3 years.

Labelling The label of the sealed container states the number of IU (Units) contained in it.

Cimetidine Injection

Definition Cimetidine Injection is a sterile solution in Water for Injections of cimetidine hydrochloride, prepared by the interaction of Cimetidine and Hydrochloric Acid.

The injection complies with the requirements stated under Parenteral Preparations and with the following requirements.

Content of cimetidine, $C_{10}H_{16}N_6S$ 95.0 to 105.0% of the prescribed or stated amount.

Identification

A. The *light absorption*, Appendix II B, in the range 210 to 310 nm of solution A used in the Assay exhibits a maximum at about 218 nm.

B. In the test for Related substances, the principal spot in the chromatogram obtained with solution (2) corresponds to that in the chromatogram obtained with solution (8).

Acidity or alkalinity pH, 4.5 to 6.0, Appendix V L.

Related substances Carry out the method for *thin-layer chromatography*, Appendix III A, using *silica gel GF_{254}* as the coating substance and using the following solutions. For solution (1) dilute a quantity of the injection with sufficient *methanol* to give a solution containing the equivalent of 5.0% w/v of Cimetidine. For solution (2) dilute 1 volume of solution (1) to 10 volumes with *methanol*. For solution (3) dilute 1 volume of solution (1) to 100 volumes with *methanol* and dilute 20 volumes of the resulting solution to 100 volumes with *methanol*. For solution (4) dilute 5 volumes of solution (3) to 10 volumes with *methanol*. For solution (5) dilute 5 volumes of solution (4) to 10 volumes with *methanol*. For solution (6) dissolve 2.24 mg of *2-carbamoyl-1-methyl-3-[2-(5-methylimidazol-4-yl-methylthio)ethyl]guanidine dihydrochloride BPCRS* ('amide' impurity) in 5 ml of a 1.65% w/v solution of *sodium chloride* in *methanol (50%)*. For solution (7) dissolve 6.6 mg of *1-methyl-3-[2-(5-methylimidazol-4-yl-methylthio)ethyl]-guanidine dihydrochloride BPCRS* ('guanidine' impurity) in 5 ml of a 1.65% w/v solution of *sodium chloride in methanol (50%)*. For solution (8) dissolve 5.0 mg of *cimetidine BPCRS* in 1 ml of *methanol*. Carry out the following tests.

A. Apply separately to the plate 4 µl of each solution. Allow the plate to stand for 15 minutes in the tank saturated with vapour from the mobile phase which consists of a mixture of 15 volumes of 13.5M *ammonia*, 20 volumes of *methanol* and 65 volumes of *ethyl acetate*. After development and removal of the plate, dry it in a current of cold air, expose to iodine vapour until maximum contrast of the spots has been obtained and examine under *ultraviolet light (254 nm)*.

B. Apply separately to the plate 4 µl of each solution. Develop using a mixture of 8 volumes of 13.5M *ammonia*, 8 volumes of *methanol* and 84 volumes of *ethyl acetate*. After removal of the plate, dry it in a current of cold air, expose to iodine vapour until maximum contrast of the spots has been obtained and examine under *ultraviolet light (254 nm)*.

The following limits apply to both methods. Any spot in the chromatogram obtained with solution (1) corresponding to the 'amide' impurity is not more intense than the principal spot in the chromatogram obtained with solution (6) (0.7%, calculated as the 'amide' base and with reference to cimetidine) and any spot corresponding to the 'guanidine' impurity is not more intense than the principal spot in the chromatogram obtained with solution (7) (2%, calculated as the 'guanidine' base and with reference to cimetidine). Any other *secondary spot* is not more intense than the principal spot in the chromatogram obtained with solution (3) (0.2%) and not more than two such spots are more intense than the principal spot in the chromatogram obtained with solution (4) (0.1% each). The tests are not valid unless the chromatograms obtained with solution (5) show clearly visible spots.

Assay Dilute a volume containing the equivalent of 0.5 g of Cimetidine with sufficient 0.05M *sulphuric acid* to produce a solution containing 0.001% w/v (solution A). Prepare a 0.001% w/v solution of *cimetidine BPCRS* in 0.05M *sulphuric acid* (solution B). Measure the *absorbance* of solutions A and B at the maximum at 218 nm and at 260 nm, Appendix II B. Calculate the content of $C_{10}H_{16}N_6S$ using the difference between the absorbances of solutions A and B at the two wavelengths and the declared content of $C_{10}H_{16}N_6S$ in *cimetidine BPCRS*.

Labelling The strength is stated in terms of the equivalent amount of Cimetidine in a suitable dose-volume.

Cimetidine Oral Solution

Definition Cimetidine Oral Solution is a solution containing Cimetidine in a suitable flavoured vehicle.

The oral solution complies with the requirements stated under Oral Liquids and with the following requirements.

Content of cimetidine, $C_{10}H_{16}N_6S$ 90.0 to 105.0% of the prescribed or stated amount.

Identification

A. Carry out the method for *thin-layer chromatography*, Appendix III A, using *silica gel GF_{254}* as the coating substance and a mixture of 15 volumes of 13.5M *ammonia*, 20 volumes of *methanol* and 65 volumes of *ethyl acetate* as the mobile phase. Apply separately to the plate 5 µl of each of the following solutions. For solution (1) dilute a volume of the preparation with *methanol* to contain 0.04% w/v of Cimetidine. Solution (2) contains 0.04% w/v of *cimetidine BPCRS* in *methanol*. After removal of the plate, allow it to dry and expose it to iodine vapour until maximum contrast between the spots is obtained. The principal spot in the chromatogram obtained with solution (1) corresponds to that in the chromatogram obtained with solution (2).

B. In the Assay, the principal peak in the chromatogram obtained with solution (1) has the same retention time as the principal peak in the chromatogram obtained with solution (2).

Acidity pH, 5.0 to 6.5, Appendix V L.

Related substances Carry out the method for *liquid chromatography*, Appendix III D, using the following solutions. For solution (1) dilute a volume of the preparation with the mobile phase to contain 0.050% w/v of Cimetidine. Solutions (2) to (6) are solutions in the mobile phase containing (2) 0.0020% w/v of *1-methyl-3-(2-(5-methylimidazol-4-yl-methylthio)ethyl)guanidine dihydrochloride BPCRS* ('guanidine' impurity), (3) 0.0019% w/v of *2-carbamoyl-1-methyl-3-(2-(5-methylimidazol-4-yl-methylthio)ethyl)guanidine dihydrochloride BPCRS* ('amide' impurity), (4) 0.0015% w/v of *2-cyano-1-methyl-3-(2-(5-methylimidazol-4-yl-methylsulphinyl)ethyl)-guanidine BPCRS* ('sulphoxide' impurity) and (5) 0.00025% w/v each of 'guanidine', 'amide' and 'sulphoxide' reference substances and 0.0002% w/v of *saccharin*. For solution (6) dilute 1 volume of solution (1) to 200 ml with the mobile phase.

The chromatographic procedure may be carried out using (a) a stainless steel column (30 cm × 4.6 mm) packed with particles of silica (10 µm) the surface of which has been modified with chemically bonded phenyl groups (µBondapak phenyl is suitable) and maintained at 40°, (b) as the mobile phase with a flow rate of 1 ml per minute a mixture of 4 volumes of *acetonitrile* and 96 volumes of a 0.25% v/v solution of *orthophosphoric acid*, the pH of the mixture being adjusted to 3.0 using 10M *potassium hydroxide* and (c) a detection wavelength of 228 nm. For solution (1) allow the chromatography to proceed for 3 times the retention time of the peak due to cimetidine.

The test is not valid unless the chromatogram obtained with solution (5) shows four clearly separated peaks.

The areas of any peaks in the chromatogram obtained with solution (1) corresponding to 'guanidine' and 'amide' are not greater than the areas of the principal peaks in the chromatograms obtained with solutions (2) and (3) respectively (3% each, calculated as the bases and with reference to cimetidine). The areas of any other *secondary peaks* in the chromatogram obtained with solution (1), except that of any peak corresponding to saccharin, are not greater than the area of the principal peak in the chromatogram obtained with solution (6) (0.5%). Calculate the content of the individual named impurities using the respective reference solutions and the content of unnamed impurities using solution (6). The total content of impurities is not greater than 4.0%.

Assay Carry out the method for *liquid chromatography*, Appendix III D, using the following solutions. For solution (1) dilute a weighed quantity of the preparation containing 0.2 g of Cimetidine with sufficient of the mobile phase to produce 200 ml. Dilute 5 ml of this solution to 100 ml with the mobile phase. Solution (2) contains 0.005% w/v of *cimetidine BPCRS* in the mobile phase. Solution (3) contains 0.004% w/v of *saccharin* in solution (2).

The chromatographic procedure described under Related substances may be used.

The test is not valid unless the chromatogram obtained with solution (3) shows two clearly separated principal peaks.

Determine the *weight per ml* of the preparation, Appendix V G, and calculate the content of $C_{10}H_{16}N_6S$ using the declared content of $C_{10}H_{16}N_6S$ in *cimetidine BPCRS*.

Storage Cimetidine Oral Solution should be protected from light and stored at a temperature not exceeding 25°.

Cimetidine Oral Suspension

Definition Cimetidine Oral Suspension is a suspension containing Cimetidine in a suitable flavoured vehicle.

The oral suspension complies with the requirements stated under Oral Liquids and with the following requirements.

Content of cimetidine, $C_{10}H_{16}N_6S$ 90.0 to 105.0% of the prescribed or stated amount.

Identification Complies with the tests described under Cimetidine Oral Solution. For test A prepare solution (1) in the following manner. Shake a volume of the oral suspension containing 40 mg of Cimetidine with 50 ml of *methanol*, dilute to 100 ml with *methanol*, mix and filter.

Alkalinity pH, 7.0 to 8.5, Appendix V L.

Related substances Carry out the method for *liquid chromatography*, Appendix III D, using the conditions and solutions (2) to (6) described under Cimetidine Oral Solution. For solution (1) use the filtrate obtained in the assay.

The area of any peak in the chromatogram obtained with solution (1) corresponding to the 'sulphoxide' impurity is not greater than the area of the principal peak in the chromatogram obtained with solution (4) (3%). The areas of any other *secondary peaks* in the chromatogram obtained with solution (1), except that of the peak due to saccharin, are not greater than the area of the principal peak in the chromatogram obtained with solution (6) (0.5%). Calculate the content of the individual named impurities using the respective reference solutions and the content of unnamed impurities using solution (6). The total content of impurities is not greater than 4.0%.

Assay Carry out the Assay described under Cimetidine Oral Solution preparing solution (1) in the following manner. To a weighed quantity of the oral suspension containing 0.1 g of Cimetidine add 100 ml of the mobile phase and shake for 10 minutes. Dilute to 200 ml with the mobile phase, mix and filter through a Whatman GF/F filter paper. Dilute 5 ml of the filtrate to 50 ml with the mobile phase.

Storage Cimetidine Oral Suspension should be protected from light and stored at a temperature not exceeding 25°.

Cimetidine Tablets

Definition Cimetidine Tablets contain Cimetidine.

With the exception of the requirements for shape, the tablets comply with the requirements stated under Tablets and with the following requirements.

Content of cimetidine, $C_{10}H_{16}N_6S$ 95.0 to 105.0% of the prescribed or stated amount.

Identification

A. Shake a quantity of the powdered tablets containing 0.10 g of Cimetidine with 10 ml of *methanol* for 10 minutes, filter (Whatman GF/A is suitable) and evaporate to dryness on a rotary evaporator using gentle heat. Dissolve the residue in 5 ml of *chloroform* and evaporate to dryness with the aid of a current of air. Dry the residue at 60° at a pressure not exceeding 0.7kPa. The *infrared absorption spectrum* of the residue, Appendix II A, is concordant with the *reference spectrum* of cimetidine.

B. In the test for Related substances, the principal spot in the chromatogram obtained with solution (2) corresponds to that in the chromatogram obtained with solution (6).

Related substances Carry out the method for *thin-layer chromatography*, Appendix III A, using *silica gel GF_{254}* as the coating substance and using the following solutions. For solution (1) add 20 ml of *methanol* to a quantity of the powdered tablets containing 1 g of Cimetidine, mix with the aid of ultrasound for 2 minutes, shake for 3 minutes and filter using a suitable 0.2-μm filter. For solution (2) dilute 1 volume of solution (1) to 10 volumes with *methanol*. For solution (3) dilute 1 volume of solution (2) to 20 volumes with *methanol*. For solution (4) dilute 1 volume of solution (1) to 100 volumes with *methanol* and dilute 20 volumes of this solution to 100 volumes with *methanol*. For solution (5) dilute 5 volumes of solution (4) to 10 volumes with *methanol*. Solution (6) contains 0.50% w/v of *cimetidine BPCRS* in *methanol*. Carry out the following tests.

A. Apply separately to the plate 4 μl of each solution. Allow the plate to stand for 15 minutes in the tank saturated with vapour from the mobile phase which consists of a mixture of 15 volumes of 13.5M *ammonia*, 20 volumes of *methanol* and 65 volumes of *ethyl acetate*. After development and removal of the plate, dry it in a current of cold air, expose to iodine vapour until maximum contrast of the spots has been obtained and examine under *ultraviolet light (254 nm)*.

B. Apply separately to the plate 4 μl of each solution. Develop using a mixture of 8 volumes of 13.5M *ammonia*, 8 volumes of *methanol* and 84 volumes of *ethyl acetate*. After removal of the plate, dry it in a current of cold air, expose to iodine vapour until maximum contrast of the spots has been obtained and examine under *ultraviolet light (254 nm)*.

The following limits apply to both methods. Any *secondary spot* in the chromatogram obtained with solution (1) is not more intense than the principal spot in the chromatogram obtained with solution (3) (0.5%) and not more than two such spots are more intense than the principal spot in the chromatogram obtained with solution (4) (0.2% of each). The tests are not valid unless the chromatograms obtained with solution (5) show clearly visible spots.

Assay Weigh and finely powder 20 tablets. Shake a quantity of the powdered tablets containing 0.1 g of Cimetidine with 300 ml of 0.05M *sulphuric acid* for 20 minutes, add sufficient 0.05M *sulphuric acid* to produce 500 ml and filter (Whatman GF/C is suitable). Dilute 5 ml of the filtrate to 100 ml with 0.05M *sulphuric acid* (solution A). Prepare a 0.001% w/v solution of *cimetidine BPCRS* in 0.05M *sulphuric acid* (solution B). Measure the *absorbance* of solutions A and B at the maximum at 218 nm and at 260 nm, Appendix II B. Calculate the content of $C_{10}H_{16}N_6S$ using the difference between the absorbances of solutions A and B at the two wavelengths and the declared content of $C_{10}H_{16}N_6S$ in *cimetidine BPCRS*.

Concentrated Cinnamon Water

Definition

Cinnamon Oil	20 ml
Ethanol (90 per cent)	600 ml
Water	sufficient to produce 1000 ml

Extemporaneous preparation The following directions apply.

Dissolve the Cinnamon Oil in the Ethanol (90 per cent) and add gradually, with vigorous shaking after each addition, sufficient Water to produce 1000 ml. Add 50 g of previously sterilised Purified Talc, or other suitable filtering aid, allow to stand for a few hours, shaking occasionally, and filter.

The water complies with the requirements stated under Aromatic Waters and with the following requirements.

Ethanol content 52 to 56% v/v, Appendix VIII F.

Weight per ml 0.914 to 0.922 g, Appendix V G.

Ciprofloxacin Intravenous Infusion

Definition Ciprofloxacin Intravenous Infusion is a sterile solution in Sodium Chloride Intravenous Infusion of ciprofloxacin lactate prepared by the interaction of Ciprofloxacin and Lactic Acid.

The intravenous infusion complies with the requirements stated under Parenteral Preparations and with the following requirements.

Content of ciprofloxacin, $C_{17}H_{18}FN_3O_3$ 95.0 to 105.0% of the prescribed or stated amount.

Identification A. Carry out the method for *thin-layer chromatography*, Appendix III A, using a silica gel F_{254} high-performance precoated plate (Merck silica gel 60 F_{254} HPTLC plates are suitable) and a mixture of 10 volumes of *acetonitrile*, 20 volumes of 13.5M *ammonia*, 40 volumes of *dichloromethane* and 40 volumes of *methanol* as the mobile phase. Apply separately to the plate, as bands, 10 µl of each of the following solutions. For solution (1) dilute a quantity of the intravenous infusion with sufficient *water* to produce a solution containing the equivalent of 0.05% w/v of Ciprofloxacin. Solution (2) contains 0.058% w/v of *ciprofloxacin hydrochloride EPCRS* in *water*. For solution (3) mix 1 volume of solution (1) and 1 volume of solution (2). After removal of the plate, allow it to dry in air for 15 minutes and examine under *ultraviolet light (254 nm* and *365 nm)*. The principal band in the chromatogram obtained with solution (1) corresponds to that in the chromatogram obtained with solution (2). The principal band in the chromatogram obtained with solution (3) appears as a single, compact band.

B. In the Assay, the retention time of the principal peak in the chromatogram obtained with solution (1) is the same as that of the principal peak in the chromatogram obtained with solution (2).

Acidity pH, 3.9 to 4.5, Appendix V L.

Colour of solution The intravenous infusion is not more intensely coloured than *reference solution GY_6*, Appendix IV B, Method II.

Related substances Carry out the method for *liquid chromatography*, Appendix III D, using solutions (1) and (4) described under Assay.

The chromatographic conditions described under Assay may be used.

In the chromatogram obtained with solution (1) the area of any peak corresponding to 7-[(2-aminoethyl)amino]-1-cyclopropyl-6-fluoro-1,4-dihydro-4-oxoquinoline-3-carboxylic acid (ciprofloxacin impurity C) is not greater than the area of the peak due to ciprofloxacin impurity C in the chromatogram obtained with solution (4) (0.5%), the area of any other *secondary peak* is not greater than 0.4 times the area of the peak due to ciprofloxacin impurity C in the chromatogram obtained with solution (4) (0.2%) and the total area of any such peaks is not greater than the area of the peak due to ciprofloxacin impurity C in the chromatogram obtained with solution (4) (0.5%). Disregard any peak with an area less than 0.1 times the area of the peak due to ciprofloxacin impurity C in the chromatogram obtained with solution (4) (0.05%).

Bacterial endotoxins The endotoxin limit concentration is 0.5 IU per ml, Appendix XIV C.

Particulate contamination When supplied in a container with a nominal content of 100 ml or more, complies with the *test for sub-visible particles*, Appendix XIII A.

Assay Carry out the method for *liquid chromatography*, Appendix III D, using the following solutions. For solution (1) dilute a quantity of the intravenous infusion with sufficient of the mobile phase to produce a solution containing the equivalent of 0.05% w/v of Ciprofloxacin. Solution (2) contains 0.058% w/v of *ciprofloxacin hydrochloride EPCRS* in the mobile phase. Solution (3) contains 0.025% w/v of *ciprofloxacin impurity C EPCRS* (ethylenediamine compound) in solution (2). For solution (4) dilute 1 volume of solution (3) to 100 volumes with the mobile phase.

The chromatographic procedure may be carried out using (a) a stainless steel column (12.5 cm × 4 mm) packed with *stationary phase C* (5 µm) (Nucleosil C18 is suitable), (b) as the mobile phase with a flow rate of 1.5 ml per minute a mixture of 13 volumes of *acetonitrile* and 87 volumes of a 0.245% w/v solution of *orthophosphoric acid* the pH of which has been adjusted to 3.0 with *triethylamine* and (c) a detection wavelength of 278 nm. Maintain the temperature of the column at 40°.

The Assay is not valid unless, in the chromatogram obtained with solution (3), the *resolution factor* between the peaks due to ciprofloxacin and ciprofloxacin impurity C is at least 1.5.

Calculate the content of $C_{17}H_{18}FN_3O_3$ in the intravenous infusion using the declared content of $C_{17}H_{19}ClFN_3O_3$ in *ciprofloxacin hydrochloride EPCRS*. Each mg of $C_{17}H_{19}ClFN_3O_3$ is equivalent to 0.9010 mg of $C_{17}H_{18}FN_3O_3$.

Storage Ciprofloxacin Intravenous Infusion should be protected from light. It should not be refrigerated.

Labelling The quantity of active ingredient is stated in terms of the equivalent amount of Ciprofloxacin.

Ciprofloxacin Tablets

Definition Ciprofloxacin Tablets contain Ciprofloxacin Hydrochloride.

With the exception of the requirements for shape, the tablets comply with the requirements stated under Tablets and with the following requirements.

Content of ciprofloxacin, $C_{17}H_{18}FN_3O_3$ 95.0 to 105.0% of the prescribed or stated amount.

Identification A. Carry out the method for *thin-layer chromatography*, Appendix III A, using a silica gel F_{254} high-performance precoated plate (Merck silica gel 60 F_{254} HPTLC plates are suitable) and a mixture of 10 volumes of *acetonitrile*, 20 volumes of 13.5M *ammonia*, 40 volumes of *dichloromethane* and 40 volumes of *methanol* as the mobile phase. Apply separately to the plate, as bands, 10 µl of each of the following solutions. For solution (1) use solution (1) described under Assay. Solution (2) contains 0.058% w/v of *ciprofloxacin hydrochloride EPCRS* in *water*. For solution (3) mix 1 volume of solution (1) and 1 volume of solution (2). After removal of the plate, allow it to dry in air for 15 minutes and examine under *ultraviolet light (254 nm* and *365 nm)*. The principal band in the chromatogram obtained with solution (1) corresponds to that in the chromatogram obtained with solution (2). The principal band in the chromatogram obtained with solution (3) appears as a single, compact band.

B. In the Assay, the retention time of the principal peak in the chromatogram obtained with solution (1) is the same as that of the principal peak in the chromatogram obtained with solution (2).

Dissolution Carry out the *dissolution test for tablets and capsules*, Appendix XII D, using Apparatus II. Use as the medium 900 ml of *water* and rotate the paddle at 50 revolutions per minute. After 30 minutes withdraw a sample of 10 ml of the medium and filter, discarding the first few ml of filtrate. Dilute the filtered solution, if necessary, with *water* to give a solution expected to contain the equivalent of about 0.011% w/v of ciprofloxacin. Measure the *absorbance* of the solution at the maximum at 276 nm, Appendix II B, using *water* in the reference cell. Calculate the total content of ciprofloxacin, $C_{17}H_{18}FN_3O_3$, in the medium from the *absorbance* obtained from a 0.013% w/v solution of *ciprofloxacin hydrochloride EPCRS* in *water* and using the declared content of $C_{17}H_{18}FN_3O_3$ in *ciprofloxacin hydrochloride EPCRS*. Each mg of $C_{17}H_{19}ClFN_3O_3$ is equivalent to 0.9010 mg of $C_{17}H_{18}FN_3O_3$. The amount of ciprofloxacin released is not less than 80% of the prescribed or stated amount.

Related substances Carry out the method for *liquid chromatography*, Appendix III D, using solutions (1) and (4) described under Assay.

The chromatographic conditions described under Assay may be used.

In the chromatogram obtained with solution (1) the area of any peak corresponding to 7-[(2-aminoethyl)amino]-1-cyclopropyl-6-fluoro-1,4-dihydro-4-oxoquinoline-3-carboxylic acid (ciprofloxacin impurity C) is not greater than the area of the peak due to ciprofloxacin impurity C in the chromatogram obtained with solution (4) (0.5%), the area of any other *secondary peak* is not greater than 0.4 times the area of the peak due to ciprofloxacin impurity C in the chromatogram obtained with solution (4) (0.2%) and the total area of any such peaks is not greater than the area of the peak due to ciprofloxacin impurity C in the chromatogram obtained with solution (4) (0.5%). Disregard any peak with an area less than 0.1 times the area of the peak due to ciprofloxacin impurity C in the chromatogram obtained with solution (4) (0.05%).

Assay Carry out the method for *liquid chromatography*, Appendix III D, using the following solutions. Weigh and powder 20 tablets. For solution (1) add a quantity of the powdered tablets containing the equivalent of 2 g of ciprofloxacin to 750 ml of *water*, mix with the aid of ultrasound for 20 minutes, add sufficient *water* to produce 1000 ml and mix. Centrifuge a portion of the resulting suspension and dilute the clear supernatant liquid with sufficient *water* to produce a solution containing the equivalent of 0.05% w/v of ciprofloxacin. Solution (2) contains 0.058% w/v of *ciprofloxacin hydrochloride EPCRS* in the mobile phase. Solution (3) contains 0.025% w/v of *ciprofloxacin impurity C EPCRS* (ethylenediamine compound) in solution (2). For solution (4) dilute 1 volume of solution (3) to 100 volumes with the mobile phase.

The chromatographic procedure may be carried out using (a) a stainless steel column (25 cm × 4.6 mm) packed with *stationary phase C* (7 µm) (Nucleosil C18 is suitable), (b) as the mobile phase at a flow rate of 1.5 ml per minute a mixture of 13 volumes of *acetonitrile* and 87 volumes of a 0.245% w/v solution of *orthophosphoric acid* the pH of which has been adjusted to 3.0 with *triethylamine* and (c) a detection wavelength of 278 nm. Maintain the temperature of the column at 40°.

The Assay is not valid unless in the chromatogram obtained with solution (3) the *resolution factor* between the peaks due to ciprofloxacin and ciprofloxacin impurity C is at least 3.

Calculate the content of $C_{17}H_{18}FN_3O_3$ in the tablets using the declared content of $C_{17}H_{19}ClFN_3O_3$ in *ciprofloxacin hydrochloride EPCRS*. Each mg of $C_{17}H_{19}ClFN_3O_3$ is equivalent to 0.9010 mg of $C_{17}H_{18}FN_3O_3$.

Labelling The quantity of active ingredient is stated in terms of the equivalent amount of ciprofloxacin.

Cisplatin Injection

Definition Cisplatin Injection is a sterile solution of Cisplatin in Water for Injections. It is prepared by dissolving Cisplatin for Injection in the requisite amount of Water for Injections immediately before use.

The injection complies with the requirements stated under Parenteral Preparations.

Characteristics A bright yellow solution.

Storage Cisplatin Injection should be used immediately after preparation but, in any case, within the period recommended by the manufacturer when prepared and stored strictly in accordance with the manufacturer's instructions.

CISPLATIN FOR INJECTION

Definition Cisplatin for Injection is a sterile material consisting of Cisplatin with Mannitol and Sodium Chloride. It is supplied in a sealed container.

The contents of the sealed container comply with the requirements for Powders for Injections stated under Parenteral Preparations and with the following requirements.

Content of cisplatin, $Cl_2H_6N_2Pt$ 95.0 to 105.0% of the prescribed or stated amount.

Identification

A. The *light absorption*, Appendix II B, in the range 230 to 350 nm of a solution containing 0.1% w/v of Cisplatin in 0.1M *hydrochloric acid* exhibits a maximum only at 300 nm.

B. Apply 0.05 ml of a saturated solution of *thallium(I) nitrate* to a filter paper (Whatman grade 1 is suitable). Add three 0.05-ml volumes of a solution of the constituted injection containing 0.1% w/v of Cisplatin followed by a further 0.05 ml of the thallium nitrate solution. Dry the paper between the applications. Wash the filter paper with 2M *ammonia* and dry. Add 0.05 ml of *tin(II) chloride solution R2*. A yellowish orange spot is produced.

C. In the test for Related substances the principal spot in the chromatogram obtained with solution (2) corresponds to that in the chromatogram obtained with solution (4).

Acidity pH of a solution containing 0.1% w/v of Cisplatin, 3.5 to 6.5, Appendix V L.

Related substances Carry out the method for *thin-layer chromatography*, Appendix III A, using *microcrystalline cellulose* as the coating substance, activating the plate by heating at 150° for 1 hour and using a mixture of 90 volumes of *dimethylformamide* and 10 volumes of *acetone* as the mobile phase. Apply separately to the plate 20 µl of each of the following solutions. For solution (1) shake the contents of one vial with *dimethylformamide* to produce a solution containing 0.5% w/v of Cisplatin, mix with the aid of ultrasound for 10 minutes and filter. For solution (2) dilute 1 volume of solution (1) to 10 volumes with *dimethylformamide*. For solution (3) dilute 1 volume of solution (1) to 50 volumes with *dimethylformamide*. Solution (4) contains 0.05% w/v of *cisplatin EPCRS* in *dimethylformamide*. After removal of the plate, allow it to dry in air and spray with a 5% w/v solution of *tin(II) chloride* in 1M *hydrochloric acid*. After 1 hour, the chromatogram obtained with solution (1) shows no *secondary spot* with an Rf value lower than that of the principal spot and any *secondary spot* with an Rf value higher than that of the principal spot is not more intense than the spot in the chromatogram obtained with solution (3) (2%).

Assay Carry out the method for *liquid chromatography*, Appendix III D, using the following solutions. Solution (1) contains 0.1% w/v of *cisplatin EPCRS* in a 0.9% w/v solution of *sodium chloride*. For solution (2) dissolve the contents of a sealed container in sufficient *water* to produce a solution containing 0.1% w/v of Cisplatin. Solution (3) contains 0.05% w/v of *cisplatin EPCRS* and 0.005% w/v of *transplatin BPCRS* in a 0.9% w/v solution of *sodium chloride*; shake for 30 minutes to effect dissolution.

The chromatographic procedure may be carried out using (a) a stainless steel column (25 cm × 4.6 mm) packed with particles of silica the surface of which has been modified by chemically bonded amine groups (Lichrosorb NH_2 is suitable), (b) 10 volumes of *water* and 90 volumes of *acetonitrile* as the mobile phase with a flow rate of 1.5 ml per minute and (c) a detection wavelength of 220 nm. Inject 5 µl of each solution. Peaks with long retention times may appear in any of the chromatograms.

The test is not valid unless the *resolution factor* between the peaks due to cisplatin and transplatin in the chromatogram obtained with solution (3) is at least 10.

Calculate the content of $Cl_2H_6N_2Pt$ in the sealed container using the declared content of $Cl_2H_6N_2Pt$ in *cisplatin EPCRS*. Repeat the procedure with a further nine sealed containers. Calculate the average content of $Cl_2H_6N_2Pt$ per container from the 10 individual results thus obtained.

Storage The sealed container should be protected from light and stored at a temperature of 15° to 25°. It should not be refrigerated.

Clemastine Oral Solution

Definition Clemastine Oral Solution contains Clemastine Fumarate in a suitable vehicle.

The oral solution complies with the requirements stated under Oral Liquids and with the following requirements.

Content of clemastine, $C_{21}H_{26}ClNO$ 90.0 to 105.0% of the prescribed or stated amount.

Identification

A. In the test for Related substances, the principal spot in the chromatogram obtained with solution (2) corresponds to that in the chromatogram obtained with solution (3).

B. In the Assay, the retention time of the principal peak in the chromatogram obtained with solution (1) is the same as that of the principal peak in the chromatogram obtained with solution (2).

4-Chloro-1,1-diphenylethanol Carry out the method for *liquid chromatography*, Appendix III D, using the following solutions. For solution (1) dilute a quantity of the oral solution containing the equivalent of 0.5 mg of clemastine to 25 ml with a mixture of 25 volumes of *acetonitrile* and 75 volumes of a 1% w/v solution of *ammonium dihydrogen orthophosphate*. Solution (2) contains 0.00008% w/v of *4-chloro-1,1-diphenylethanol BPCRS* in a mixture of 25 volumes of *acetonitrile* and 75 volumes of a 1% w/v solution of *ammonium dihydrogen orthophosphate*. Solution (3) contains 0.000335% w/v of *clemastine fumarate BPCRS* and 0.00008% w/v of *4-chloro-1,1-diphenyl-*

ethanol BPCRS in a mixture of 25 volumes of *acetonitrile* and 75 volumes of a 1% w/v solution of *ammonium dihydrogen orthophosphate*.

The chromatographic procedure described under Assay may be used. Inject 100 µl of each solution.

The test is not valid unless the *resolution factor* between the peaks due to clemastine fumarate and 4-chloro-1,1-diphenylethanol in the chromatogram obtained with solution (3) is at least 2.2.

In the chromatogram obtained with solution (1) the area of any peak corresponding to 4-chloro-1,1-diphenylethanol is not greater than the area of the peak in the chromatogram obtained with solution (2) (3%, calculated with reference to clemastine fumarate).

Related substances Carry out the method for *thin-layer chromatography*, Appendix III A, using a silica gel 60 F_{254} precoated plate (Merck plates are suitable) and a mixture of 1 volume of 13.5M *ammonia*, 20 volumes of *methanol* and 80 volumes of *stabiliser-free tetrahydrofuran* as the mobile phase. Apply separately to the plate 10 µl of each of the following solutions. For solution (1) add 20 ml of *water*, 20 ml of a saturated solution of *sodium chloride* and 2 ml of 13.5M *ammonia* to a quantity of the oral solution containing the equivalent of 8 mg of clemastine, extract with four 40-ml quantities of *dichloromethane*, washing each extract with the same 40-ml of *water*, filter the dichloromethane extracts and evaporate to dryness at a temperature of 30° to 40° under reduced pressure. Dissolve the residue in 50 ml of *methanol*, evaporate to dryness under the same conditions and dissolve the residue in 4 ml of *methanol*. For solution (2) dilute 1 volume of solution (1) to 10 volumes with *methanol*. Solution (3) contains 0.027% w/v of *clemastine fumarate BPCRS* in *methanol*. Solution (4) contains 0.00135% w/v of *clemastine fumarate BPCRS* in *methanol*. Solution (5) contains 0.0135% w/v of each of *clemastine fumarate BPCRS* and *diphenhydramine hydrochloride EPCRS* in *methanol*. Solution (6) contains 0.0054% w/v of *2-(2-hydroxyethyl)-1-methylpyrrolidine BPCRS* in *methanol*. After removal of the plate, dry it in a current of cold air for 5 minutes, spray with a freshly prepared mixture of 1 volume of *potassium iodobismuthate solution* and 10 volumes of 2M *acetic acid* and then with *hydrogen peroxide solution (10 vol)*. Cover the plate immediately with a glass plate of the same size and examine the chromatograms after 2 minutes. In the chromatogram obtained with solution (1) any spot corresponding to 2-(2-hydroxyethyl)-1-methylpyrrolidine is not more intense than the spot in the chromatogram obtained with solution (6) (2%, with reference to clemastine fumarate) and any orange-brown *secondary spot* is not more intense than the spot in the chromatogram obtained with solution (4) (0.5%, with reference to clemastine fumarate). Disregard any spot remaining on the line of application and any spot with an Rf value greater than that of the principal spot. The test is not valid unless the chromatogram obtained with solution (5) shows two clearly separated spots.

Assay Carry out the method for *liquid chromatography*, Appendix III D, using the following solutions. For solution (1) dilute a quantity of the oral solution containing the equivalent of 0.5 mg of clemastine to 20 ml with a mixture of 25 volumes of *acetonitrile* and 75 volumes of a 1% w/v solution of *ammonium dihydrogen orthophosphate*. Solution (2) contains 0.00335% w/v of *clemastine fumarate BPCRS* in a mixture of 25 volumes of *acetonitrile* and 75 volumes of a 1% w/v solution of *ammonium dihydrogen orthophosphate*.

The chromatographic procedure may be carried out using (a) a stainless steel column (10 cm × 4.6 mm) packed with *stationary phase C* (5 µm) (Nucleosil C18 is suitable), (b) a mixture of 0.1 volume of *orthophosphoric acid*, 45 volumes of *acetonitrile* and 55 volumes of a 1% w/v solution of *ammonium dihydrogen orthophosphate* as the mobile phase with a flow rate of 1 ml per minute and (c) a detection wavelength of 220 nm. Inject 10 µl of each solution.

Determine the *weight per ml* of the oral solution, Appendix V G, and calculate the content of $C_{21}H_{26}ClNO$, weight in volume, using the declared content of $C_{21}H_{26}ClNO$ in *clemastine fumarate BPCRS*.

Storage Clemastine Oral Solution should be stored at a temperature not exceeding 25°.

Labelling The quantity of the active ingredient is stated in terms of the equivalent amount of clemastine.

Clemastine Tablets

Definition Clemastine Tablets contain Clemastine Fumarate.

The tablets comply with the requirements stated under Tablets and with the following requirements.

Content of clemastine, $C_{21}H_{26}ClNO$ 93.0 to 105.0% of the prescribed or stated amount.

Identification

A. In the test for Related substances, the principal spot in the chromatogram obtained with solution (2) corresponds to that in the chromatogram obtained with solution (3).

B. In the test for 4-Chloro-1,1-diphenylethanol, the retention time of the principal peak in the chromatogram obtained with solution (1) is the same as that of the peak in the chromatogram obtained with solution (3).

4-Chloro-1,1-diphenylethanol Carry out the method for *liquid chromatography*, Appendix III D, using the following solutions. For solution (1) add to a quantity of the powdered tablets containing the equivalent of 10 mg of clemastine 200 ml of a mixture of 25 volumes of *acetonitrile* and 75 volumes of a 1% w/v solution of *ammonium dihydrogen orthophosphate*, shake vigorously for 45 minutes, centrifuge at a speed of at least 400 revolutions per minute for 10 minutes and use the supernatant liquid. Solution (2) contains 0.0000335% w/v of *4-chloro-1,1-diphenylethanol BPCRS* in a mixture of 25 volumes of *acetonitrile* and 75 volumes of a 1% w/v solution of *ammonium dihydrogen orthophosphate*. Solution (3) contains 0.0067% w/v of *clemastine fumarate BPCRS* in a mixture of 25 volumes of *acetonitrile* and 75 volumes of a 1% w/v solution of *ammonium dihydrogen orthophosphate*. Solution (4) contains 0.000335% w/v of *clemastine fumarate BPCRS* and 0.000064% w/v of *4-chloro-1,1-diphenylethanol BPCRS* in a mixture of 25 volumes of *acetonitrile* and 75 volumes of a 1% w/v solution of *ammonium dihydrogen orthophosphate*.

The chromatographic procedure described under Assay may be used. Inject 100 µl of each solution.

The test is not valid unless the *resolution factor* between the peaks due to clemastine fumarate and 4-chloro-1,1-

diphenylethanol in the chromatogram obtained with solution (4) is at least 2.2.

In the chromatogram obtained with solution (1) the area of any peak corresponding to 4-chloro-1,1-diphenylethanol is not greater than the area of the peak in the chromatogram obtained with solution (2) (0.5%, calculated with reference to clemastine fumarate).

Related substances Carry out the method for *thin-layer chromatography*, Appendix III A, using a silica gel 60 F_{254} precoated plate (Merck plates are suitable) and a mixture of 1 volume of 13.5M *ammonia*, 20 volumes of *methanol* and 80 volumes of *stabiliser-free tetrahydrofuran* as the mobile phase. Apply separately to the plate 20 µl of each of the following solutions. For solution (1) shake a quantity of the powdered tablets containing the equivalent of 8 mg of clemastine with 4 ml of *methanol* for 15 minutes, centrifuge at 4000 revolutions per minute for 10 minutes and use the supernatant liquid. For solution (2) dilute 1 volume of solution (1) to 10 volumes with *methanol*. Solution (3) contains 0.027% w/v of *clemastine fumarate BPCRS* in *methanol*. Solution (4) contains 0.00135% w/v of *clemastine fumarate BPCRS* in *methanol*. Solution (5) contains 0.0135% w/v of each of *clemastine fumarate BPCRS* and *diphenhydramine hydrochloride EPCRS* in *methanol*. Solution (6) contains 0.00135% w/v of *2-(2-hydroxyethyl)-1-methylpyrrolidine BPCRS* in *methanol*. After removal of the plate, dry it in a current of cold air for 5 minutes, spray with a freshly prepared mixture of 1 volume of *potassium iodobismuthate solution* and 10 volumes of 2M *acetic acid* and then with *hydrogen peroxide solution (10 vol)*. Cover the plate immediately with a glass plate of the same size and examine the chromatograms after 2 minutes. In the chromatogram obtained with solution (1) any spot corresponding to 2-(2-hydroxyethyl)-1-methylpyrrolidine is not more intense than the spot in the chromatogram obtained with solution (6) (0.5%, with reference to clemastine fumarate) and any orange-brown *secondary spot* is not more intense than the spot in the chromatogram obtained with solution (4) (0.5%, with reference to clemastine fumarate). Disregard any spot remaining on the line of application and any spot with an Rf value greater than that of the principal spot. The test is not valid unless the chromatogram obtained with solution (5) shows two clearly separated spots.

Uniformity of content Tablets containing the equivalent of less than 2 mg of clemastine comply with the requirements stated under Tablets using the following method of analysis. Carry out the method for *liquid chromatography*, Appendix III D, using the following solutions. For solution (1) vigorously shake one tablet with 40 ml of a mixture of 25 volumes of *acetonitrile* and 75 volumes of a 1% w/v solution of *ammonium dihydrogen orthophosphate* for 45 minutes and centrifuge until a clear supernatant liquid is obtained. Solution (2) contains 0.00335% w/v of *clemastine fumarate BPCRS* in a mixture of 25 volumes of *acetonitrile* and 75 volumes of a 1% w/v solution of *ammonium dihydrogen orthophosphate*.

The chromatographic procedure may be carried out using (a) a stainless steel column (10 cm × 4.6 mm) packed with *stationary phase C* (5 µm) (Nucleosil C18 is suitable), (b) a mixture of 0.1 volume of *orthophosphoric acid*, 50 volumes of *acetonitrile* and 50 volumes of a 1% w/v solution of *ammonium dihydrogen orthophosphate* as the mobile phase with a flow rate of 1 ml per minute and (c) a detection wavelength of 220 nm. Inject 10 µl of each solution.

Calculate the content of $C_{21}H_{26}ClNO$ in each tablet using the declared content of $C_{21}H_{26}ClNO$ in *clemastine fumarate BPCRS*.

Assay

For tablets containing the equivalent of 2 mg or more of clemastine Weigh and powder 20 tablets. Carry out the method for *liquid chromatography*, Appendix III D, using the following solutions. For solution (1) add to a quantity of the powdered tablets containing the equivalent of 10 mg of clemastine 200 ml of a mixture of 25 volumes of *acetonitrile* and 75 volumes of a 1% w/v solution of *ammonium dihydrogen orthophosphate*, shake vigorously for 45 minutes, centrifuge at a speed of at least 400 revolutions per minute for 10 minutes and use the supernatant liquid. Solution (2) contains 0.0067% w/v of *clemastine fumarate BPCRS* in a mixture of 25 volumes of *acetonitrile* and 75 volumes of a 1% w/v solution of *ammonium dihydrogen orthophosphate*.

The chromatographic procedure may be carried out using (a) a stainless steel column (10 cm × 4.6 mm) packed with *stationary phase C* (5 µm) (Nucleosil C18 is suitable), (b) a mixture of 0.1 volume of *orthophosphoric acid*, 45 volumes of *acetonitrile* and 55 volumes of a 1% w/v solution of *ammonium dihydrogen orthophosphate* as the mobile phase with a flow rate of 1 ml per minute and (c) a detection wavelength of 220 nm. Inject 10 µl of each solution.

Calculate the content of $C_{21}H_{26}ClNO$ in the tablets using the declared content of $C_{21}H_{26}ClNO$ in *clemastine fumarate BPCRS*.

For tablets containing the equivalent of less than 2 mg of clemastine Use the average of the individual results obtained in the test for Uniformity of content.

Labelling The quantity of the active ingredient is stated in terms of the equivalent amount of clemastine.

Clindamycin Capsules

Definition Clindamycin Capsules contain Clindamycin Hydrochloride.

The capsules comply with the requirements stated under Capsules and with the following requirements.

Content of clindamycin, $C_{18}H_{33}ClN_2O_5S$ 90.0 to 110.0% of the prescribed or stated amount.

Identification

A. Shake a quantity of the contents of the capsules containing the equivalent of 30 mg of clindamycin with 15 ml of *chloroform*, filter and evaporate the filtrate to dryness. The *infrared absorption spectrum* of the residue, Appendix II A, is concordant with the *reference spectrum* of clindamycin hydrochloride.

B. In the Assay, the retention time of the principal peak derived from clindamycin hydrochloride in the chromatogram obtained with solution (3) is the same as the retention time of the principal peak derived from *clindamycin hydrochloride BPCRS* in the chromatogram obtained with solution (1).

Water The contents of the capsules contain not more than 7.0% w/w of water, Appendix IX C. Use 1 g.

Assay Carry out the method for *gas chromatography*, Appendix III B, using the following solutions. For solution (1) add 1 ml of *trifluoroacetic anhydride* to 50 mg of *clindamycin hydrochloride BPCRS,* swirl to dissolve and allow to stand at room temperature for 30 minutes. Add 20 ml of a 0.15% w/v solution of *hexacosane* (internal standard) in *1,2-dichloroethane* and mix. For solution (2) add 1 ml of *trifluoroacetic anhydride* to a quantity of the mixed contents of 20 capsules containing the equivalent of 45 mg of clindamycin, swirl to dissolve and allow to stand at room temperature for 30 minutes. Add 20 ml of *1,2-dichloroethane* and mix. Prepare solution (3) in the same manner as solution (2) but using 20 ml of a 0.15% w/v solution of the internal standard in *1,2-dichloroethane* in place of the 20 ml of 1,2-dichloroethane.

The chromatographic procedure may be carried out using a glass column (1.5 m × 4 mm) packed with *acid-washed, silanised diatomaceous support* (80 to 100 mesh) coated with 1% w/w of phenyl methyl silicone fluid (50% phenyl) (OV-17 is suitable) and maintained at 170°.

Calculate the content of $C_{18}H_{33}ClN_2O_5S$ using the declared content of $C_{18}H_{33}ClN_2O_5S$ in *clindamycin hydrochloride BPCRS*.

Labelling The quantity of active ingredient is stated in terms of the equivalent amount of clindamycin.

Clindamycin Injection

Definition Clindamycin Injection is a sterile solution of Clindamycin Phosphate in Water for Injections.

The injection complies with the requirements stated under Parenteral Preparations and with the following requirements.

Content of clindamycin $C_{18}H_{33}ClN_2O_5S$ 90.0 to 105.0% of the prescribed or stated amount.

Characteristics An almost colourless solution.

Identification

A. Carry out the method for *thin-layer chromatography*, Appendix III A, using *silica gel GF_{254}* as the coating substance and a mixture of 1.5 volumes of 18M *ammonia*, 30 volumes of *toluene* and 70 volumes of *methanol* as the mobile phase. Apply separately to the plate 10 µl of each of two solutions in *methanol* containing (1) a volume of the injection containing the equivalent of 50 mg clindamycin diluted to 10 ml and (2) 0.5% w/v of *clindamycin phosphate BPCRS*. After removal of the plate, allow it to dry in air and spray with *dilute potassium iodobismuthate solution*. The principal spot in the chromatogram obtained with solution (1) corresponds to that in the chromatogram obtained with solution (2).

B. In the Assay, the chromatogram obtained with solution (1) shows a peak with the same retention time as the peak due to clindamycin phosphate in the chromatogram obtained with solution (2).

Acidity or alkalinity pH, 5.5 to 7.0, Appendix V L.

Related substances Carry out the method for *liquid chromatography*, Appendix III D, using the following solutions. For solution (1) dilute a volume of the injection with the mobile phase to contain the equivalent of 0.3% w/v of clindamycin. Solution (2) contains 0.012% w/v of *lincomycin hydrochloride EPCRS*, 0.024% w/v of *clindamycin phosphate BPCRS* and 0.0015% v/v of *benzyl alcohol* in the mobile phase.

The chromatographic conditions described under Assay may be used. The order of the peaks in the chromatogram obtained with solution (2) is lincomycin hydrochloride, clindamycin phosphate and benzyl alcohol.

The test is not valid unless the *resolution factor* between the peaks due to lincomycin hydrochloride and clindamycin phosphate is at least 7.

In the chromatogram obtained with solution (1) the sum of the areas of any *secondary peaks* is not greater than 8.0% by *normalisation*. Disregard any peak due to benzyl alcohol.

Bacterial endotoxins Carry out the *test for bacterial endotoxins*, Appendix XIV C. Dilute the injection in *water BET* to give a solution containing the equivalent of 10 mg of clindamycin per ml (solution A). The endotoxin limit concentration of solution A is 6 Units of endotoxin per ml. Carry out the test using the maximum valid dilution of solution A calculated from the declared sensitivity of the lysate used in the test.

Assay Carry out the method for *liquid chromatography*, Appendix III D, using the following solutions. For solution (1) dilute a volume of the injection with the mobile phase to contain the equivalent of 0.015% w/v of clindamycin. Solution (2) contains 0.018% w/v of *clindamycin phosphate BPCRS* in the mobile phase. Solution (3) contains 0.012% w/v of *lincomycin hydrochloride EPCRS*, 0.024% w/v of *clindamycin phosphate BPCRS* and 0.0015% v/v of *benzyl alcohol* in the mobile phase.

The chromatographic procedure may be carried out using (a) a stainless steel column (20 cm × 4.6 mm) packed with *stationary phase B* (10 µm) (Zorbax C8 is suitable), (b) as the mobile phase a mixture of 25 volumes of *acetonitrile* and 75 volumes of a 1.36% w/v solution of *potassium dihydrogen orthophosphate* adjusted to pH 2.5 with *orthophosphoric acid* with a flow rate of 1 ml per minute and (c) a detection wavelength of 210 nm. Record the chromatograms for 3 times the retention time of the peak due to clindamycin.

The test is not valid unless the *resolution factor* between the peaks due to lincomycin hydrochloride and clindamycin phosphate is at least 7.7.

Calculate the content of $C_{18}H_{33}ClN_2O_5S$ in the injection using the declared content of $C_{18}H_{33}ClN_2O_5S$ in *clindamycin phosphate BPCRS*.

Storage Clindamycin Injection should be stored at a temperature of 8° to 30°.

Labelling The strength is stated as the equivalent amount of clindamycin in a suitable dose-volume.

Clioquinol Cream

Definition Clioquinol Cream contains 3% w/w of Clioquinol, in *microfine powder*, in a suitable basis.

Extemporaneous preparation The following formula and directions apply.

Clioquinol, in *microfine powder*,	30 g
Cetomacrogol Emulsifying Ointment	300 g
Chlorocresol	1 g
Purified Water, freshly boiled and cooled, sufficient to produce	1000 g

In a vessel that can be closed, heat about 650 g of Purified

Water to about 60°, add the Chlorocresol and when it melts shake vigorously to effect dissolution. Melt the Cetomacrogol Emulsifying Ointment, heat to about 60°, add the chlorocresol solution at the same temperature and mix. Stir gently until cool, add sufficient Purified Water to produce 970 g and incorporate the Clioquinol; mix.

The cream complies with the requirements stated under Topical Semi-solid Preparations and with the following requirements.

Content of clioquinol, C_9H_5ClINO 2.7 to 3.3% w/w.

Assay Disperse a quantity containing 15 mg of Clioquinol in 25 ml of *chloroform* in a stoppered centrifuge tube, shake vigorously and centrifuge. Add sufficient *anhydrous sodium sulphate* to absorb all the aqueous phase and dilute 15 ml of the clear chloroform solution to 50 ml with *chloroform*. Transfer 10 ml of this solution to a separating funnel, add 25 ml of *chloroform*, 10 ml of *water* and 10 ml of *weak copper sulphate solution*, shake vigorously and allow to separate. Dry the chloroform layer by shaking with *anhydrous sodium sulphate* and measure the *absorbance* of the clear solution at 430 nm, Appendix II B, using *chloroform* in the reference cell. Calculate the concentration of clioquinol in the preparation being examined by comparing the absorbance with that of a solution prepared in the following manner. Dissolve 90 mg of *clioquinol BPCRS* in sufficient *chloroform* to produce 100 ml , dilute 10 ml of this solution to 50 ml with *chloroform* and continue the procedure described above, beginning at the words 'Transfer 10 ml of this solution... '.

Storage Clioquinol Cream should be protected from light. If it is kept in aluminium tubes, their inner surfaces should be coated with a suitable lacquer.

Clobazam Capsules

Definition Clobazam Capsules contain Clobazam.

The capsules comply with the requirements stated under Capsules and with the following requirements.

Content of clobazam, $C_{16}H_{13}ClN_2O_2$ 95.0 to 105.0% of the prescribed or stated amount.

Identification

A. Shake a quantity of the contents of the capsules containing 20 mg of Clobazam with 10 ml of *dichloromethane*, filter and evaporate the filtrate to dryness. Dissolve the residue in the minimum amount of *methanol*, evaporate to dryness and dry the residue at 105° for 10 minutes. The *infrared absorption spectrum* of the residue, Appendix II A, is concordant with the *reference spectrum* of clobazam.

B. In the test for Related substances, the principal spot in the chromatogram obtained with solution (2) corresponds to that in the chromatogram obtained with solution (5).

Dissolution Comply with the *dissolution test for tablets and capsules*, Appendix XII D using Apparatus II. Use as the medium 500 ml of 0.1M *hydrochloric acid* and rotate the paddle at 75 revolutions per minute. Withdraw a sample of 10 ml of the medium and filter. Carry out the method for *liquid chromatography*, Appendix III D, using the following solutions. Use the filtered dissolution medium as solution (1). For solution (2) dissolve a sufficient quantity of *clobazam BPCRS* in 50 ml of *methanol* and dilute 2 ml of the resulting solution to 50 ml with 0.1M *hydrochloric acid*; the concentration of the final solution should be the same as that expected for solution (1).

The chromatographic procedure may be carried out using (a) a stainless steel column (12.5 cm × 4 mm) packed with *stationary phase* C (5 µm) (Superspher 100RP-18 is suitable), (b) a mixture of 470 volumes of *acetonitrile* and 530 volumes of *water* as the mobile phase with a flow rate of 0.7 ml per minute and (c) a detection wavelength of 230 nm.

Inject 50 µl of each solution. Calculate the total content of clobazam, $C_{16}H_{13}ClN_2O_2$, in the medium using the declared content of $C_{16}H_{13}ClN_2O_2$ in *clobazam BPCRS*.

Related substances Comply with the test described under Clobazam but preparing solutions (1), (2) and (3) in the following manner. For solution (1) shake a quantity of the contents of the capsules containing 40 mg of Clobazam with three 10-ml quantities of *dichloromethane*, combine the filtered extracts and evaporate to dryness; dissolve the residue in 2 ml of *methanol*. For solution (2) dilute 1 volume of solution (1) to 200 volumes. For solution (3) dilute 1 volume of solution (2) to 2.5 volumes.

Assay Carry out the method for *liquid chromatography*, Appendix III D, using the following solutions. For solution (1) weigh 20 capsules. Open the capsules without losing any part of the shell and transfer the contents as completely as possible to a 200-ml flask. Wash the shells with three 30-ml quantities of *methanol*, add the washings to the flask and dilute to volume. Allow the shells to dry at room temperature and weigh. The difference between the weights represents the weight of the total contents. Mix the contents of the flask with the aid of ultrasound for 10 minutes and stir magnetically for 20 minutes. Centrifuge a portion of the suspension and dilute a volume of the resulting supernatant liquid containing 5 mg of Clobazam to 100 ml with *methanol*. Solution (2) contains 0.005% w/v of *clobazam BPCRS* in *methanol*. Solution (3) contains 0.006% w/v of *7-chloro-1,5-dihydro-5-phenyl-1,5-benzodiazepine-2,4(3*H*)-dione BPCRS* (desmethylclobazam) and 0.0125% w/v of *clobazam BPCRS* in *methanol*.

The chromatographic procedure may be carried out using (a) a stainless steel column (20 cm × 4.6 mm) packed with *stationary phase C* (5 µm) (Nucleosil C18 is suitable), (b) a mixture of 470 volumes of *acetonitrile* and 530 volumes of *water* as the mobile phase with a flow rate of 0.7 ml per minute and (c) a detection wavelength of 230 nm. Adjust the composition of the mobile phase, if necessary, such that the *resolution factor* between the peaks corresponding to desmethylclobazam and clobazam in the chromatogram obtained with solution (3) is at least 3.

Calculate the content of $C_{16}H_{13}ClN_2O_2$ using the declared content of $C_{16}H_{13}ClN_2O_2$ in *clobazam BPCRS*.

Clobetasol Cream

Definition Clobetasol Cream contains Clobetasol Propionate in a suitable basis.

The cream complies with the requirements stated under Topical Semi-solid Preparations and with the following requirements.

Content of clobetasol propionate, $C_{25}H_{32}ClFO_5$ 90.0 to 115.0% of the prescribed or stated amount.

Identification

A. Carry out the method for *thin-layer chromatography*, Appendix III A, using *silica gel GF_{254}* as the coating substance and a mixture of 5 volumes of *absolute ethanol*, 10 volumes of *acetone* and 100 volumes of *dichloromethane* as the mobile phase. Apply separately to the plate 10 µl of each of the following solutions. Prepare solution (1) in the following manner. Transfer a quantity of the cream containing 0.75 mg of Clobetasol Propionate to a 25-ml centrifuge tube, add 10 ml of *methanol* and heat in a water bath at 60° for 4 minutes. Remove from the water bath and shake vigorously. Repeat the heating and shaking, cool to room temperature, add 3.5 ml of *water* and mix. Centrifuge for 10 minutes. Transfer 10 ml of the clear supernatant liquid to a 100-ml separating funnel, add 1 g of *sodium chloride* and 10 ml of *water* and mix. Add 5 ml of *dichloromethane* and shake for 1 minute. Evaporate the dichloromethane layer to dryness in a current of nitrogen with gentle heating and dissolve the residue in 0.5 ml of *dichloromethane*. Solution (2) contains 0.05% w/v of *clobetasol propionate BPCRS* in *dichloromethane*. Solution (3) is a mixture of equal volumes of solutions (1) and (2). After removal of the plate, allow it to dry in air and examine under *ultraviolet light (245 nm)*. The principal spot in the chromatogram obtained with solution (1) corresponds to that in the chromatogram obtained with solution (2). The principal spot in the chromatogram obtained with solution (3) appears as a single compact spot.

B. In the Assay, the chromatogram obtained with solution (2) shows a peak with the same retention time as the peak due to clobetasol propionate in the chromatogram obtained with solution (1).

Assay CAUTION *Carry out the preparation of solutions (2) and (3) with full facial protection and wearing heat-resistant gloves.*

Carry out the method for *liquid chromatography*, Appendix III D, using the following solutions. Solution (1) contains 0.005% w/v of *clobetasol propionate BPCRS* and 0.01% w/v of *beclomethasone dipropionate BPCRS* (internal standard) in *ethanol (50%)*. For solution (2) add 10 ml of *absolute ethanol* to a quantity of the cream containing 1 mg of Clobetasol Propionate, stopper firmly using a plastic stopper, heat on a water bath with intermittent shaking until the cream is completely dispersed. Cool the contents in ice for 30 minutes, centrifuge and dilute 5 ml of the supernatant liquid to 10 ml with *water*. Prepare solution (3) in the same manner as solution (2) but add 5 ml of a 0.04% w/v solution of *beclomethasone dipropionate BPCRS* in *absolute ethanol* and 5 ml of *absolute ethanol*. Solutions (2) and (3) may assume a gel-like appearance.

The chromatographic procedure may be carried out using (a) a stainless steel column (10 cm × 4.6 mm) packed with *stationary phase C* (5 µm) (Spherisorb ODS 1 is suitable) and maintained at 60°, (b) as the mobile phase with a flow rate of 2 ml per minute a mixture of 45 volumes of *absolute ethanol* and 55 volumes of *water* and (c) a detection wavelength of 240 nm.

Calculate the content of $C_{25}H_{32}ClFO_5$ using peak areas and the declared content of $C_{25}H_{32}ClFO_5$ in *clobetasol propionate BPCRS*.

Storage Clobetasol Cream should be stored at a temperature not exceeding 30°.

Clobetasol Ointment

Definition Clobetasol Ointment contains Clobetasol Propionate in a suitable basis.

The ointment complies with the requirements stated under Topical Semi-solid Preparations and with the following requirements.

Content of clobetasol propionate, $C_{25}H_{32}ClFO_5$ 90.0 to 115.0% of the prescribed or stated amount.

Identification

A. Carry out the method for *thin-layer chromatography*, Appendix III A, using *silica gel GF_{254}* as the coating substance and a mixture of 5 volumes of *absolute ethanol*, 10 volumes of *acetone* and 100 volumes of *dichloromethane* as the mobile phase. Apply separately to the plate 10 µl of each of the following solutions. Prepare solution (1) in the following manner. Transfer a quantity of the ointment containing 0.5 mg of Clobetasol Propionate to a 25-ml centrifuge tube, add 10 ml of *methanol* and heat in a water bath at 70° for 4 minutes. Remove from the water bath and shake vigorously. Repeat the heating and shaking, cool in ice for 5 minutes and centrifuge for 10 minutes. Transfer 5 ml of the clear supernatant liquid to a suitable vial, evaporate to dryness in a current of nitrogen and dissolve the residue in 0.5 ml of *dichloromethane*. Solution (2) contains 0.05% w/v of *clobetasol propionate BPCRS* in *dichloromethane*. Solution (3) is a mixture of equal volumes of solutions (1) and (2). After removal of the plate, allow it to dry in air and examine under *ultraviolet light (245 nm)*. The principal spot in the chromatogram obtained with solution (1) corresponds to that in the chromatogram obtained with solution (2). The principal spot in the chromatogram obtained with solution (3) appears as a single compact spot.

B. In the Assay, the chromatogram obtained with solution (2) shows a peak with the same retention time as the peak due to clobetasol propionate in the chromatogram obtained with solution (1).

Assay CAUTION *Carry out the preparation of solutions (2) and (3) with full facial protection and wearing heat-resistant gloves.*

Carry out the method for *liquid chromatography*, Appendix III D, using the following solutions. Solution (1) contains 0.005% w/v of *clobetasol propionate BPCRS* and 0.01% w/v of *beclomethasone dipropionate BPCRS* (internal standard) in *ethanol (50%)*. For solution (2) add 10 ml of *absolute ethanol* to a quantity of the ointment containing 1 mg of Clobetasol Propionate, stopper firmly using a plastic stopper, heat on a water bath with intermittent shaking until the ointment is completely dispersed. Cool the contents in ice for 30 minutes, centrifuge and dilute 5 ml of the supernatant liquid to 10 ml with *water*. Prepare solution (3) in the same manner as solution (2) but add 5 ml of a 0.04% w/v solution of *beclomethasone dipropionate BPCRS* in *absolute ethanol* and 5 ml of *absolute ethanol*. Solutions (2) and (3) may assume a gel-like appearance.

The chromatographic procedure may be carried out using (a) a stainless steel column (10 cm × 4.6 mm) packed with *stationary phase C* (5 µm) (Spherisorb ODS 1 is suitable) and maintained at 60°, (b) as the mobile phase with a flow rate of 2 ml per minute a mixture of 45 volumes of *absolute ethanol* and 55 volumes of *water* and (c) a detection wavelength of 240 nm.

Calculate the content of $C_{25}H_{32}ClFO_5$ using peak areas and the declared content of $C_{25}H_{32}ClFO_5$ in *clobetasol propionate BPCRS*.

Storage Clobetasol Ointment should be stored at a temperature not exceeding 30°.

Clobetasone Cream

Definition Clobetasone Cream contains Clobetasone Butyrate in a suitable basis.

The cream complies with the requirements stated under Topical Semi-solid Preparations and with the following requirements.

Content of clobetasone butyrate, $C_{26}H_{32}ClFO_5$ 90.0 to 110.0% of the prescribed or stated amount.

Identification

A. Carry out the method for *thin-layer chromatography*, Appendix III A, using *silica gel 60 GF_{254}* as the coating substance and a mixture of 5 volumes of *absolute ethanol*, 10 volumes of *acetone* and 100 volumes of *chloroform* as the mobile phase. Apply separately to the plate 10 µl of each of the following solutions. For solution (1) disperse a quantity of the cream containing 0.5 mg of Clobetasone Butyrate in a mixture of 5 volumes of *ethanol (80%)* and 10 volumes of n-*hexane*, taking 15 ml of the solvent mixture for each g of cream. Shake the mixture, allow to separate, filter the aqueous layer and add 1 ml of *water* for every 10 ml of n-*hexane* used. Cool the solution in ice for 30 minutes, centrifuge, filter the supernatant liquid and dilute with 10 ml of *water* for every 10 ml of n-*hexane* used. Add 1 g of *sodium chloride* for every 10 ml of *water* used and extract with 5 ml of *chloroform* for every 10 ml of *water* used. Evaporate the chloroform layer to dryness in a current of dry nitrogen with gentle heating and dissolve the residue in 0.5 ml of *chloroform*. Solution (2) contains 0.1% w/v of *clobetasone butyrate BPCRS* in *chloroform*. Solution (3) contains a mixture of equal volumes of solutions (1) and (2). After removal of the plate, allow it to dry in air and examine under *ultraviolet light (254 nm)*. The principal spot in the chromatogram obtained with solution (1) corresponds to that in the chromatogram obtained with solution (2). The principal spot in the chromatogram obtained with solution (3) appears as a single compact spot.

B. In the Assay, the chromatogram obtained with solution (2) shows a peak with the same retention time as the peak due to clobetasone butyrate in the chromatogram obtained with solution (1).

Assay CAUTION *Carry out the preparation of solutions (2) and (3) with full facial protection and wearing heat-resistant gloves.*

Carry out the method for *liquid chromatography*, Appendix III D, using the following solutions. Solution (1) contains 0.004% w/v of *clobetasone butyrate BPCRS* and 0.0028% w/v of *clobetasol propionate BPCRS* (internal standard) in *ethanol (50%)*. For solution (2) add 10 ml of *absolute ethanol* to a quantity of the cream containing 1 mg of Clobetasone Butyrate. Stopper firmly using a plastic stopper and heat on a water bath with intermittent shaking until the cream is completely dispersed. Cool the contents in ice for 30 minutes, centrifuge and dilute 5 ml of the supernatant liquid to 10 ml with *water*. Prepare solution (3) in the same manner as solution (2) but adding 5 ml of *absolute ethanol* and 5 ml of a 0.014% w/v solution of the internal standard in *absolute ethanol*. Solutions (2) and (3) may assume a gel-like appearance.

The chromatographic procedure may be carried out using (a) a stainless steel column (10 cm × 4.6 mm) packed with *stationary phase C* (5 µm) (Spherisorb ODS 1 is suitable) and maintained at 60°, (b) as the mobile phase with a flow rate of 2 ml per minute a mixture of 40 volumes of *absolute ethanol* and 60 volumes of *water* and (c) a detection wavelength of 241 nm. The proportions of the mobile phase may be adjusted to give a retention time for clobetasone butyrate of about 5.5 minutes.

Calculate the content of $C_{26}H_{32}ClFO_5$ in the cream using peak areas and the declared content of $C_{26}H_{32}ClFO_5$ in *clobetasone butyrate BPCRS*.

Storage Clobetasone Cream should be stored at a temperature not exceeding 30°.

Clobetasone Ointment

Definition Clobetasone Ointment contains Clobetasone Butyrate in a suitable basis.

The ointment complies with the requirements stated under Topical Semi-solid Preparations and with the following requirements.

Content of clobetasone butyrate, $C_{26}H_{32}ClFO_5$ 90.0 to 110.0% of the prescribed or stated amount.

Identification

A. Carry out the method for *thin-layer chromatography*, Appendix III A, using *silica gel 60 GF_{254}* as the coating substance and a mixture of 5 volumes of *absolute ethanol*, 10 volumes of *acetone* and 100 volumes of *chloroform* as the mobile phase. Apply separately to the plate 10 µl of each of the following solutions. For solution (1) disperse a quantity of the ointment containing 0.5 mg of Clobetasone Butyrate in a mixture of 5 volumes of *ethanol (80%)* and 10 volumes of n-*hexane*, taking 15 ml of the solvent mixture for each g of ointment. Shake the mixture, allow to separate, filter the aqueous layer and add 10 ml of *water* and 1 g of *sodium chloride* for every 15 ml of the solvent mixture used. Extract the resulting aqueous solution with 5 ml of *chloroform* for each g of *sodium chloride* used and evaporate the chloroform layer to dryness in a current of dry nitrogen with gentle heating. Dissolve the residue in 0.5 ml of *chloroform*. Solution (2) contains 0.1% w/v of *clobetasone butyrate BPCRS* in *chloroform*. Solution (3) contains a mixture of equal volumes of solutions (1) and (2). After removal of the plate, allow it to dry in air and examine under *ultraviolet light (254 nm)*. The principal spot in the chromatogram obtained with solution (1) corresponds to that in the chromatogram obtained with solution (2). The principal spot in the chromatogram obtained with solution (3) appears as a single compact spot.

B. In the Assay, the chromatogram obtained with solution (2) shows a peak with the same retention time as the peak due to clobetasone butyrate in the chromatogram obtained with solution (1).

Assay CAUTION *Carry out the preparation of solutions (2) and (3) with full facial protection and wearing heat-resistant gloves.*

Carry out the method for *liquid chromatography*, Appendix III D, using the following solutions. Solution (1) contains 0.004% w/v of *clobetasone butyrate BPCRS* and 0.0028% w/v of *clobetasol propionate BPCRS* (internal standard) in *ethanol (50%)*. For solution (2) add 10 ml of *absolute ethanol* to a quantity of the ointment containing 1 mg of Clobetasone Butyrate. Stopper firmly using a plastic stopper and heat on a water bath with intermittent shaking until the ointment is completely dispersed. Cool the contents in ice for 30 minutes, centrifuge and dilute 5 ml of the supernatant liquid to 10 ml with *water*. Prepare solution (3) in the same manner as solution (2) but adding 5 ml of *absolute ethanol* and 5 ml of a 0.014% w/v solution of the internal standard in *absolute ethanol*. Solutions (2) and (3) may assume a gel-like appearance.

The chromatographic procedure may be carried out using (a) a stainless steel column (10 cm × 4.6 mm) packed with *stationary phase C* (5 µm) (Spherisorb ODS 1 is suitable) and maintained at 60°, (b) as the mobile phase with a flow rate of 2 ml per minute a mixture of 40 volumes of *absolute ethanol* and 60 volumes of *water* and (c) a detection wavelength of 241 nm. The proportions of the mobile phase may be adjusted to give a retention time for clobetasone butyrate of about 5.5 minutes.

Calculate the content of $C_{26}H_{32}ClFO_5$ in the ointment using peak areas and the declared content of $C_{26}H_{32}ClFO_5$ in *clobetasone butyrate BPCRS*.

Storage Clobetasone Ointment should be stored at a temperature not exceeding 30°.

Clofazimine Capsules

Definition Clofazimine Capsules contain Clofazimine.

The capsules comply with the requirements stated under Capsules and with the following requirements.

Content of clofazimine, $C_{27}H_{22}Cl_2N_4$ 92.5 to 107.5% of the prescribed or stated amount.

Identification

A. The *light absorption*, Appendix II B, in the range 260 to 600 nm of the final solution obtained in the Assay, exhibits two maxima, at 289 nm and 491 nm.

B. Dissolve a quantity of the contents of the capsules containing 2 mg of Clofazimine in 3 ml of *acetone* and add 0.1 ml of *hydrochloric acid*; an intense violet colour is produced. Add 0.5 ml of 5M *sodium hydroxide*; the colour changes to orange-red.

Assay Dissolve a quantity of the mixed contents of the capsules containing 0.3 g of Clofazimine in 100 ml of *chloroform*, filter, dilute to 200 ml with *chloroform* and dilute 5 ml of this solution to 100 ml with *chloroform*. To 5 ml of this solution add 5 ml of 0.1M *methanolic hydrochloric acid*, dilute to 50 ml with *chloroform* and measure the *absorbance* of the resulting solution at the maximum at 491 nm, Appendix II B. Calculate the content of $C_{27}H_{22}Cl_2N_4$ taking 650 as the value of A(1%, 1 cm) at the maximum at 491 nm.

Clofibrate Capsules

Definition Clofibrate Capsules contain Clofibrate.

The capsules comply with the requirements stated under Capsules and with the following requirements.

Identification

The contents of the capsules comply with the following tests.

A. The *infrared absorption spectrum*, Appendix II A, is concordant with the spectrum of *clofibrate EPCRS*.

B. The *light absorption*, Appendix II B, in the range 220 to 250 nm of a 0.001% w/v solution in *methanol* exhibits a maximum only at 226 nm. The A(1%, 1 cm) at the maximum is about 460.

C. The *light absorption*, Appendix II B, in the range 250 to 350 nm of a 0.01% w/v solution in *methanol* exhibits two maxima, at 280 nm and 288 nm. The A(1%, 1 cm) at the maxima are about 44 and about 31, respectively.

Acidity Add 10 ml of the contents of the capsules to 100 ml of *ethanol (96%)* previously neutralised to *phenolphthalein solution R1* with 0.1M *sodium hydroxide VS* and titrate with 0.1M *sodium hydroxide VS*. Not more than 2.5 ml is required to change the colour of the solution.

Refractive index 1.500 to 1.505, determined on the contents of the capsules, Appendix V E.

Relative density 1.138 to 1.147, determined on the contents of the capsules, Appendix V G.

4-Chlorophenol Carry out the method for *gas chromatography*, Appendix III B, injecting 2 µl of each of the following solutions. Solution (1) contains 0.0025% w/v of *4-chlorophenol* in *chloroform*. For solution (2) extract a volume of the contents of the capsules containing 10.0 g of Clofibrate with 20 ml of 1M *sodium hydroxide*, wash the lower layer with 5 ml of *water*, add the washings to the aqueous layer and reserve the organic layer for the test for Volatile related substances. Extract the combined aqueous layer and washings with two 5-ml quantities of *chloroform*, discard the chloroform and acidify the aqueous layer by the dropwise addition of *hydrochloric acid*. Extract with three 3-ml quantities of *chloroform*, combine the organic extracts and dilute to 10 ml with *chloroform*.

The chromatographic procedure may be carried out using a column (1.5 m × 4 mm) maintained at 185° and packed with either *acid-washed, silanised diatomaceous support* (Gas Chrom Q or Chromosorb W/AW/DMCS are suitable) (40 to 60 mesh) impregnated with 30% w/w of dimethyl silicone fluid (E-301 and SE-30 are suitable) or *acid-washed, silanised diatomaceous support* (80 to 100 mesh) coated with 10% w/w of dimethyl silicone fluid.

The area of any peak corresponding to 4-chlorophenol in the chromatogram obtained with solution (2) is not greater than the area of the peak in the chromatogram obtained with solution (1) (25 ppm).

Volatile related substances Carry out the method for *gas chromatography*, Appendix III B, injecting 2 µl of each of the following solutions. For solution (1) dry the organic layer reserved in the test for 4-Chlorophenol with *anhydrous sodium sulphate*. For solution (2) use a solution of the contents of the capsules in *chloroform* containing 0.012% w/v of Clofibrate. Solution (3) is a 0.012% w/v solution of *methyl 2-(4-chlorophenoxy)-2-methylpropionate EPCRS* in the contents of the capsules.

The chromatographic procedure may be carried out as described in the test for 4-Chlorophenol.

In the chromatogram obtained with solution (3) measure from the baseline the height of the peak corresponding to methyl 2-(4-chlorophenoxy)-2-methylpropionate (*a*) and the height of the lowest part of the curve separating this peak from the peak corresponding to clofibrate (*b*). The test is not valid unless *a* is equal to at least 30% of full-scale deflection and *a* – *b* is greater than 75% of *a*.

The sum of the areas of any *secondary peaks* in the chromatogram obtained with solution (1) is not greater than 10 times the area of the peak due to clofibrate in the chromatogram obtained with solution (2) (0.1%).

Uniformity of weight Carry out the test for Uniformity of weight for Soft Capsules described under Capsules. The average weight of the contents of the 20 capsules is 95.0 to 105.0% of the prescribed or stated weight of Clofibrate.

Clofibrate, $C_{12}H_{15}ClO_3$ Not less than 97.0% w/w when determined by the following method. To a weighed quantity of the mixed contents of 10 capsules containing 1 g of Clofibrate add 25 ml of 0.5M *ethanolic potassium hydroxide* and heat under a reflux condenser fitted with a soda lime guard tube for 2 hours, rotating the flask frequently. Allow to cool, add 10 ml of *water* down the condenser and titrate the contents of the flask with 0.2M *hydrochloric acid VS* using 1 ml of *phenolphthalein solution R1* as indicator. Repeat the operation without the contents of the capsules. The difference between the titrations represents the amount of hydrochloric acid required. Each ml of 0.2M *hydrochloric acid VS* is equivalent to 48.54 mg of $C_{12}H_{15}ClO_3$.

Clomethiazole Capsules

Definition Clomethiazole Capsules contain a solution of Clomethiazole in a suitable fixed oil.

The capsules comply with the requirements stated under Capsules and with the following requirements.

Content of clomethiazole, C_6H_8ClNS 92.5 to 107.5% of the prescribed or stated amount.

Identification

A. Shake a quantity of the contents of the capsules containing 20 mg of Clomethiazole with 70 ml of 0.1M *hydrochloric acid* for 15 minutes and dilute to 100 ml with the same solvent. Filter and dilute 10 ml of the filtrate to 50 ml with 0.1M *hydrochloric acid.* The *light absorption* of the resulting solution, Appendix II B, in the range 230 to 350 nm exhibits a maximum only at 257 nm.

B. To a quantity of the contents of the capsules containing 0.3 g of Clomethiazole add 10 ml of 0.1M *hydrochloric acid* and shake. To the aqueous layer add 5 ml of 1M *sodium hydroxide*, mix and extract with 15 ml of *chloroform*. Dry the chloroform layer with *anhydrous sodium sulphate*, filter and evaporate to remove the solvent. The *infrared absorption spectrum* of a thin film of the residue, Appendix II A, is concordant with the *reference spectrum* of clomethiazole.

C. Mix a quantity of the contents of the capsules containing 0.1 g of Clomethiazole with 0.2 g of powdered *sodium hydroxide*, heat to fusion and continue heating for a further few seconds. Cool, add 0.5 ml of *water* and a slight excess of 2M *hydrochloric acid* and warm. Any fumes evolved do not turn moistened *starch iodate paper* blue (distinction from clomethiazole edisilate).

Related substances Carry out the method for *liquid chromatography*, Appendix III D, using the following solutions. For solution (1) add 100 ml of 1M *sulphuric acid* to whole capsules containing a total of 0.96 g of Clomethiazole, immerse in a water bath for 20 seconds, remove from the bath and shake vigorously. Repeat this treatment until the capsule shells have dissolved without exceeding a total heating time of 1 minute. Cool, centrifuge, filter the aqueous layer (Whatman GF/C paper is suitable) and dilute 5 ml of the filtrate to 50 ml with the mobile phase. For solution (2) dilute 1 volume of solution (1) to 200 volumes with the mobile phase. For solution (3) dilute 1 volume of a 0.030% w/v solution of *4-methyl-5-vinylthiazole edisilate BPCRS* in *methanol* (solution A) to 50 volumes with the mobile phase. For solution (4) dilute 1 volume of a 0.020% w/v solution of *5-(2-chloroethyl)-4-methyl-3-[2-(4-methylthiazol-5-yl)ethyl]thiazolium chloride BPCRS* (quaternary dimer) in *methanol* (solution B) to 50 volumes with the mobile phase. For solution (5) dilute 1 volume of a 0.020% w/v solution of *4-methyl-5-(2-hydroxyethyl)thiazole BPCRS* in *methanol* (solution C) to 50 volumes with the mobile phase. For solution (6) add 1 ml each of solutions A, B and C to 5 ml of the filtrate obtained in the preparation of solution (2) and dilute to 50 ml with the mobile phase.

The chromatographic procedure may be carried out using (a) a stainless steel column (20 cm × 4 mm) packed with *stationary phase C* (10 µm) (Lichrosorb RP18 is suitable), (b) as the mobile phase with a flow rate of 1 ml per minute a mixture of 70 volumes of a solution containing 0.13% w/v of *sodium hexanesulphonate* and 2.7% w/v of *tetramethylammonium hydrogen sulphate*, adjusted to pH 2.0 with 5M *sodium hydroxide*, and 30 volumes of *methanol* and (c) a detection wavelength of 257 nm.

The test is not valid unless in the chromatogram obtained with solution (6) baseline separation is achieved between the peaks due to the three specified impurities and also between each of these peaks and the principal peak.

Calculate the content of each of the specified impurities with reference to the stated content of Clomethiazole in the capsules expressing the content of 4-methyl-5-vinylthiazole as the base (1 mg of 4-methyl-5-vinylthiazole edisilate is equivalent to 0.568 mg of its base). Calculate the content of each of any other impurities from the areas of their peaks in the chromatogram obtained with solution (1) using the principal peak in the chromatogram obtained with solution (2) as reference and assuming the same response as clomethiazole. The content of each of the three specified impurities is not greater than 1.5% and the content of any other impurity is not greater than 0.5%. The total content of all the impurities is not greater than 3.0%.

Assay Carry out Method I for *non-aqueous titration*, Appendix VIII A, using a quantity of the mixed contents of 20 capsules containing 0.4 g of Clomethiazole and *crystal violet solution* as indicator. Each ml of 0.1M *perchloric acid VS* is equivalent to 16.16 mg of C_6H_8ClNS.

When chlormethiazole capsules are prescribed or demanded, Clomethiazole Capsules shall be dispensed or supplied.

Clomethiazole Intravenous Infusion

Definition Clomethiazole Intravenous Infusion is a sterile solution of Clomethiazole Edisilate in Water for Injections.

The intravenous infusion complies with the requirements stated under Parenteral Preparations and with the following requirements.

Content of clomethiazole edisilate, $(C_6H_8ClNS)_2$, $C_2H_6O_6S_2$ 92.5 to 107.5% of the prescribed or stated amount.

Identification

A. To a volume of the intravenous infusion containing 40 mg of Clomethiazole Edisilate add 4 ml of 2M *sodium hydroxide*, mix and extract with 25 ml of *dichloromethane*. Dry the extract with *anhydrous sodium sulphate*, filter and evaporate to dryness. The *infrared absorption spectrum* of the residue, Appendix II A, is concordant with the *reference spectrum* of clomethiazole.

B. Carry out the method for *thin-layer chromatography*, Appendix III A, using a silica gel G precoated plate (Merck silica gel 60 plates are suitable) and a mixture of 5 volumes of *water*, 10 volumes of 13.5M *ammonia*, 20 volumes of *butan-1-ol* and 65 volumes of *acetone* as the mobile phase. Apply separately to the plate 10 µl of each of the following solutions. For solution (1) add 90 ml of *acetone* to a volume of the preparation containing about 50 mg of Clomethiazole Edisilate, mix and centrifuge. Wash the oily residue with three 10-ml quantities of *acetone* and then with three 10-ml quantities of *ether*. Dry the residue with a current of warm air and then dry under reduced pressure at 35° for 30 minutes. Dissolve the residue in 1 ml of 1M *acetic acid*, dilute to 5 ml with *methanol*, mix and filter through a 0.45-µm membrane filter. For solution (2) dissolve 0.1 g of *disodium ethanedisulphonate* in 5 ml of 1M *acetic acid* and dilute to 25 ml with *methanol*. After removal of the plate, dry it in a current of air until the ammonia is removed and spray with a 0.1% w/v solution of *bromocresol purple* in *ethanol (96%)* previously adjusted to a purple colour with 2M *ammonia* and examine immediately. The principal spot in the chromatogram obtained with solution (1) corresponds to that in the chromatogram obtained with solution (2).

Acidity or alkalinity pH of the infusion, 5.0 to 7.5, Appendix V L.

Related substances Complies with the test described under Clomethiazole Capsules, calculating the content of each of the stated impurities with reference to the equivalent content of clomethiazole in the intravenous infusion (1 mg of clomethiazole edisilate is equivalent to 0.629 mg of base) and using the following solution as solution (1). Dilute a volume of the intravenous infusion with the mobile phase to produce a solution containing 0.04% w/v of Clomethiazole Edisilate.

Particulate contamination When supplied in a container with a nominal content of 100 ml or more, complies with the test for *sub-visible particles*, Appendix XIII A.

Assay Carry out the method for *liquid chromatography*, Appendix III D, using the following solutions. For solution (1) dilute a volume of the preparation with the mobile phase to produce a solution containing 0.01% w/v of Clomethiazole Edisilate. Solution (2) contains 0.01% w/v of *clomethiazole edisilate BPCRS* in the mobile phase.

The chromatographic procedure may be carried out using (a) stainless steel column (20 cm × 4 mm) packed with *stationary phase C* (10 µm) (Lichrosorb RP18 is suitable), (b) as the mobile phase with a flow rate of 1 ml per minute a mixture of 70 volumes of a solution containing 0.13% w/v of *sodium hexanesulphonate* and 2.7% w/v of *tetramethylammonium hydrogen sulphate* adjusted to pH 2.0 with 5M *sodium hydroxide* and 30 volumes of *methanol* and (c) a detection wavelength of 257 nm.

Calculate the content of $(C_6H_8ClNS)_2,C_2H_6O_6S_2$ from the declared content of $(C_6H_8ClNS)_2,C_2H_6O_6S_2$ in *clomethiazole edisilate BPCRS*.

Storage Clomethiazole Intravenous Infusion should be stored at a temperature of 2° to 8°.

When chlormethiazole intravenous infusion is prescribed or demanded, Clomethiazole Intravenous Infusion shall be dispensed or supplied.

Clomethiazole Oral Solution

Definition Clomethiazole Oral Solution is a solution of Clomethiazole Edisilate in a suitable flavoured vehicle.

The oral solution complies with the requirements stated under Oral Liquids and with the following requirements.

Content of clomethiazole edisilate, $(C_6H_8ClNS)_2$, $C_2H_6O_6S_2$ 92.5 to 107.5% of the prescribed or stated amount.

Identification

A. To a volume of the oral solution containing 0.1 g of Clomethiazole Edisilate add 4 ml of 2M *sodium hydroxide*, mix and extract with 25 ml of *dichloromethane*. Dry the extract with *anhydrous sodium sulphate*, filter and evaporate to dryness. The *infrared absorption spectrum* of the residue, Appendix II A, is concordant with the *reference spectrum* of clomethiazole.

B. Complies with test B for Identification described under Clomethiazole Intravenous Infusion.

Related substances Complies with the test prescribed under Clomethiazole Capsules, calculating the content of each of the stated impurities with reference to the equivalent content of clomethiazole in the oral solution (1 mg of clomethiazole edisilate is equivalent to 0.629 mg of base) and using the following solution as solution (1). Dilute a volume of the oral solution with the mobile phase to produce a solution containing 0.05% w/v of Clomethiazole Edisilate.

Assay Carry out the Assay described under Clomethiazole Intravenous Infusion.

Storage Clomethiazole Oral Solution should be stored at a temperature of 2° to 8°.

When chlormethiazole oral solution is prescribed or demanded, Clomethiazole Oral Solution shall be dispensed or supplied.

Clomifene Tablets

Definition Clomifene Tablets contain Clomifene Citrate.

The tablets comply with the requirements stated under Tablets and with the following requirements.

Content of clomifene citrate, $C_{26}H_{28}ClNO,C_6H_8O_7$ 92.5 to 107.5% of the prescribed or stated amount.

Identification

A. The *light absorption*, Appendix II B, in the range 220 to 350 nm of the solution obtained in the Assay exhibits two maxima, at 235 nm and 292 nm.

B. Dissolve a quantity of the powdered tablets containing 5 mg of Clomifene Citrate in 5 ml of a mixture of 1 volume of *acetic anhydride* and 5 volumes of *pyridine* and heat in a water bath. A dark red colour is produced.

Dissolution Comply with the *dissolution test for tablets and capsules*, Appendix XII D, using as the medium 900 ml of *water* and rotating the basket at 100 revolutions per minute. Withdraw a 10-ml sample of the medium and filter. Measure the *absorbance* of a layer of suitable thickness of the filtered sample, suitably diluted, if necessary, with 0.1M *hydrochloric acid*, at the maximum at 232 nm, Appendix II B. Calculate the total content of clomifene citrate, $C_{26}H_{28}ClNO,C_6H_8O_7$, in the medium taking 317 as the value of A(1%, 1 cm) at the maximum at 232 nm.

Z-Isomer 30.0 to 50.0% of the content of clomifene citrate as determined in the Assay when determined in the following manner. Carry out the method for *liquid chromatography*, Appendix III D, using the following solution. Shake a quantity of the powdered tablets containing 50 mg of Clomifene Citrate with 50 ml of 0.1M *hydrochloric acid* for 10 minutes and filter. To 25 ml of the filtrate add 5 ml of 1M *sodium hydroxide* and extract with three 25-ml quantities of *ethanol-free chloroform*. Wash the combined extracts with 10 ml of *water*, dry over *anhydrous sodium sulphate* and add sufficient *ethanol-free chloroform* to produce 100 ml. To 20 ml of the solution add 0.1 ml of *triethylamine* and sufficient *hexane* to produce 100 ml.

The chromatographic procedure may be carried out using (a) a stainless steel column (30 cm × 4 mm) packed with *stationary phase A* (10 µm) (Porasil is suitable), (b) a mixture of *ethanol-free chloroform* and *hexane*, each containing 0.10% v/v of *triethylamine*, adjusted so that baseline separation is obtained between *E*- and *Z*-clomifene as the mobile phase with a flow rate of 2 ml per minute (a mixture of 20 volumes of *ethanol-free chloroform* and 80 volumes of *hexane* is usually suitable) and (c) a detection wavelength of 302 nm. Pass the mobile phase through the system until stabilisation is achieved (about 250 ml).

In the chromatogram obtained with the solution being examined, a peak due to *E*-clomifene precedes the peak due to *Z*-clomifene. The test is not valid unless baseline separation is achieved between *E*- and *Z*-clomifene and the *column efficiency* is greater than 10,000 *theoretical plates* per metre determined using the peak due to the *E*-isomer.

Calculate the percentage of *Z*-isomer from the expression $100A_Z/(1.08A_D+A_Z)$ where A_Z and A_D are the areas of the peaks due to the *Z*- and *E*-isomers, respectively.

Assay Weigh and powder 20 tablets. Shake a quantity of the powder containing 50 mg of Clomifene Citrate for 30 minutes with 70 ml of 0.1M *hydrochloric acid* prepared using a 30% v/v solution of *propan-2-ol* as solvent, dilute to 100 ml with the propanolic hydrochloric acid and filter. Dilute 5 ml of the filtrate to 100 ml with 0.1M *hydrochloric acid* and measure the *absorbance* of the resulting solution at the maximum at 292 nm, Appendix II B, using in the reference cell a solution prepared by diluting 5 ml of the propanolic hydrochloric acid to 100 ml with 0.1M *hydrochloric acid*. Calculate the content of $C_{26}H_{28}ClNO,C_6H_8O_7$ taking 175 as the value of A(1%, 1 cm) at the maximum at 292 nm.

Storage Clomifene Tablets should be protected from light and stored at a temperature not exceeding 25°.

When clomiphene tablets are prescribed or demanded, Clomifene Tablets shall be dispnsed or supplied.

Clomipramine Capsules

Definition Clomipramine Capsules contain Clomipramine Hydrochloride.

The capsules comply with the requirements stated under Capsules and with the following requirements.

Content of clomipramine hydrochloride, $C_{19}H_{23}ClN_2,HCl$ 92.5 to 107.5% of the prescribed or stated amount.

Identification

A. The *light absorption*, Appendix II B, in the range 230 to 350 nm of the solution obtained in the Assay exhibits a maximum only at 252 nm and a shoulder at 270 nm.

B. Triturate a quantity of the contents of the capsules containing 0.15 g of Clomipramine Hydrochloride with 10 ml of *chloroform*, filter and evaporate the filtrate to dryness. The *infrared absorption spectrum* of the residue, Appendix II A, after recrystallisation from hot *acetone* and drying at 110° for 30 minutes, is concordant with the *reference spectrum* of clomipramine hydrochloride.

C. The residue obtained in test B yields the reactions characteristic of *chlorides*, Appendix VI.

Related substances Carry out the method for *thin-layer chromatography*, Appendix III A, using *silica gel G* as the coating substance and a mixture of 75 volumes of *ethyl acetate*, 25 volumes of *acetone* and 5 volumes of 13.5M *ammonia* as the mobile phase. Apply separately to the plate 5 µl of each of the following solutions. For solution (1) shake a quantity of the contents of the capsules containing 0.20 g of Clomipramine Hydrochloride with 10 ml of *methanol* and filter. Solution (2) contains 0.020% w/v of *imipramine hydrochloride EPCRS*. For solution (3) dilute 3 volumes of solution (1) to 100 volumes with *methanol* and dilute 1 volume of the resulting solution to 10 volumes with *methanol*. For solution (4) dilute 1 volume of solution (1) to 100 volumes with *methanol*. To 1 volume add 1 volume of solution (2) and dilute to 10 volumes with *methanol*. After removal of the plate allow it to dry in air and spray with a 0.5% w/v solution of *potassium dichromate* in *sulphuric acid (20%)*. Any spot corresponding to imipramine in the chromatogram obtained with solution (1) is not more intense than the spot in the chromatogram obtained with solution (2) and any other *secondary spot* is not more intense than the spot in the chromatogram obtained with solution (3). The test is not valid unless the chromatogram obtained with solution (4) shows two clearly separated principal spots.

Assay Shake a quantity of the mixed contents of 20 capsules containing 50 mg of Clomipramine Hydrochloride with 200 ml of 0.1M *hydrochloric acid* for 1 hour, dilute to 250 ml with 0.1M *hydrochloric acid* and filter. Dilute 15 ml of the filtrate to 100 ml with 0.1M *hydrochloric acid* and measure the *absorbance* of the resulting solution at the maximum at 252 nm, Appendix II B. Calculate the content of $C_{19}H_{23}ClN_2,HCl$ taking 226 as the value of A(1%, 1 cm) at the maximum at 252 nm.

Clonazepam Injection

Definition Clonazepam Injection is a sterile solution of Clonazepam. It is prepared immediately before use by diluting Sterile Clonazepam Concentrate with Water for Injections in accordance with the manufacturer's instructions.

The injection complies with the requirements stated under Parenteral Preparations.

STERILE CLONAZEPAM CONCENTRATE

Definition Sterile Clonazepam Concentrate is a sterile solution of Clonazepam in a suitable solvent.

The concentrate complies with the requirements for Concentrated Solutions for Injections stated under Parenteral Preparations and with the following requirements.

Content of clonazepam, $C_{15}H_{10}ClN_3O_3$ 95.0 to 105.0% of the stated amount.

Characteristics A clear, colourless or slightly greenish yellow solution.

Identification Carry out the method for *thin-layer chromatography*, Appendix III A, using a silica gel GF_{254} precoated plate (Merck silica gel 60 F_{254} plates are suitable) and a mixture of 2 volumes of 13.5M *ammonia*, 15 volumes of n-*heptane*, 30 volumes of *nitromethane* and 60 volumes of *ether* as the mobile phase but allowing the solvent front to ascend 10 cm above the line of application. Apply separately to the plate 10 µl of each of the following solutions. For solution (1) dilute 3 ml of a solution containing 3 mg of Clonazepam in a stoppered tube with an equal volume of *water*, shake with 1 ml of *chloroform*, allow to separate and use the chloroform layer. For solution (2) dissolve 3 mg of *clonazepam BPCRS* in 1 ml of *chloroform*. After removal of the plate, dry it in a current of cold air, spray with 2M *sodium hydroxide* and heat at 120° for 15 minutes. The yellow spot in the chromatogram obtained with solution (1) corresponds to that in the chromatogram obtained with solution (2). Spots due to excipients may also be observed.

Acidity pH, 3.4 to 4.3, Appendix V L.

Related substances Carry out the test protected from light. Carry out the method for *thin-layer chromatography*, Appendix III A, using *silica gel G* as the coating substance. For the first development use a mixture of 20 volumes of *chloroform* and 80 volumes of *ether* as the mobile phase. Apply separately to the plate 50 µl of each of the following solutions. For solution (1) dilute, if necessary, a volume of the solution containing 10 mg of Clonazepam to 20 ml with *water* and extract with three 3-ml quantities of *chloroform*. Wash each chloroform extract separately with the same 10-ml volume of *water*, combine the extracts and add sufficient *chloroform* to produce 10 ml. Solutions (2) and (3) contain 0.00050% w/v and 0.00020% w/v respectively of *2-amino-2′-chloro-5-nitrobenzophenone BPCRS* ('nitrobenzophenone') in *chloroform*. Solution (4) contains 0.00020% w/v of *3-amino-4-(2-chlorophenyl)-6-nitroquinolin-2-one BPCRS* ('carbostyril') in *chloroform*. After removal of the plate, allow it to dry in a current of cold air. For the second development use a mixture of 10 volumes of *ether* and 90 volumes of *nitromethane*. After removal of the plate, heat at a pressure of 2kPa at 120° for 3 hours, allow to cool and spray with a 10% w/v solution of *zinc chloride* in 0.1M *hydrochloric acid*. Allow the plate to dry in air and visualise by *Method I*, Appendix III A, beginning at the words 'expose to nitrous fumes...'. Any spots in the chromatogram obtained with solution (1) corresponding to the nitrobenzophenone and carbostyril impurities are not more intense than the spots in the chromatograms obtained with solutions (3) and (4) respectively (0.2%). Any other *secondary spot* in the chromatogram obtained with solution (1) is not more intense than the spot in the chromatogram obtained with solution (2) (0.5%).

Assay Protect the solutions from light throughout the assay. To a volume of the solution containing 20 mg of Clonazepam add sufficient *propan-2-ol* to produce 100 ml and dilute 10 ml to 100 ml with *propan-2-ol*. Measure the *absorbance* of the resulting solution at the maximum at 310 nm, Appendix II B. Calculate the content of $C_{15}H_{10}ClN_3O_3$ taking 364 as the value of A(1%, 1 cm) at the maximum at 310 nm.

Storage Clonazepam Injection should be protected from light.

Labelling The label states (1) 'Sterile Clonazepam Concentrate'; (2) that the diluted injection is to be given by intravenous injection.

Clonidine Injection

Definition Clonidine Injection is a sterile solution of Clonidine Hydrochloride in Water for Injections.

The injection complies with the requirements stated under Parenteral Preparations and with the following requirements.

Content of clonidine hydrochloride, $C_9H_9Cl_2N_3,HCl$ 90.0 to 110.0% of the prescribed or stated amount.

Characteristics A colourless solution.

Identification

A. Dilute a volume containing 0.3 mg of Clonidine Hydrochloride to 5 ml with 0.01M *hydrochloric acid*. The *light absorption* of the resulting solution, Appendix II B, in the range 245 to 350 nm exhibits maxima at 272 nm and 279 nm and an inflection at 265 nm.

B. To a volume containing 0.15 mg of Clonidine Hydrochloride add 1 ml of a 10% w/v solution of *ammonium reineckate* and allow to stand for 5 minutes. A pink precipitate is produced.

Acidity or alkalinity pH, 4.0 to 7.0, Appendix V L.

Related substances Carry out the method for *thin-layer chromatography*, Appendix III A, using *silica gel G* as the coating substance and as the mobile phase the filtered upper layer obtained by shaking together 10 volumes of *glacial acetic acid*, 40 volumes of *butan-1-ol* and 50 volumes of *water* and allowing the layers to separate. Apply separately to the plate 20 µl of each of the following solutions. For solution (1) add 10 ml of *methanol* to a volume containing 0.75 mg of Clonidine Hydrochloride, evaporate to dryness and dissolve the residue in 0.5 ml of *methanol*. For solution (2) dilute 1 volume of solution (1) to 100 volumes with *methanol*. After removal of the plate, allow it to dry in air and spray with *potassium iodobismuthate solution R2*. Allow to dry in air for 1 hour, spray again with the same reagent and immediately spray with a 5% w/v solution of *sodium nitrite*. Any *secondary spot* in the chromatogram obtained with solution (1) is not more intense than the spot in the chromatogram obtained with solution (2) (1%).

Assay To a volume containing 0.15 mg of Clonidine Hydrochloride add 25 ml of *citro-phosphate buffer pH 7.6*. Add 5 ml of *water* and 1 ml of a solution containing 0.15% w/v of *bromothymol blue* and 0.15% w/v of *anhydrous sodium carbonate*. Add 30 ml of *chloroform*, shake for 1 minute and centrifuge. To 15 ml of the chloroform layer add 10 ml of *boric acid solution* and measure the *absorbance* of the resulting solution at the maximum at 420 nm, Appendix II B, using in the reference cell a solution prepared by diluting 10 ml of *boric acid solution* to 25 ml with *chloroform*. Calculate the content of $C_9H_9Cl_2N_3$,HCl from the *absorbance* obtained by repeating the operation using 5 ml of a 0.003% w/v solution of *clonidine hydrochloride BPCRS*, previously dried to constant weight at 105°, adding 20 ml of *citro-phosphate buffer pH 7.6* and completing the procedure described above, beginning at the words 'Add 5 ml of *water*...'.

Clonidine Tablets

Definition Clonidine Tablets contain Clonidine Hydrochloride.

The tablets comply with the requirements stated under Tablets and with the following requirements.

Content of clonidine hydrochloride, $C_9H_9Cl_2N_3$,HCl 90.0 to 110.0% of the prescribed or stated amount.

Identification To a quantity of the powdered tablets containing 0.5 mg of Clonidine Hydrochloride add 30 ml of *water* and 5 ml of 1M *sodium hydroxide*. Swirl gently and extract with 20 ml of *chloroform*. Centrifuge the chloroform layer, dry with *anhydrous sodium sulphate*, filter and evaporate the filtrate to dryness. Dissolve the residue in 8 ml of 0.01M *hydrochloric acid*. The resulting solution complies with the following tests.

A. The *light absorption*, Appendix II B, in the range 245 to 350 nm exhibits maxima at 272 nm and 279 nm and an inflection at 265 nm.

B. Add 1 ml of a 10% w/v solution of *ammonium reineckate* and allow to stand for 5 minutes. A pink precipitate is produced.

Uniformity of content Tablets containing less than 2 mg of Clonidine Hydrochloride comply with the requirements stated under Tablets using the following method of analysis.

For tablets containing 0.3 mg or more of Clonidine Hydrochloride, add a suitable volume of *citro-phosphate buffer pH 7.6* to one tablet, shake until disintegrated and dilute with *citro-phosphate buffer pH 7.6*, if necessary, to give a solution containing about 0.0015% w/v of Clonidine Hydrochloride. To 5 ml of the supernatant liquid add 1 ml of a solution containing 0.15% w/v of *bromothymol blue* and 0.15% w/v of *anhydrous sodium carbonate*, add 10 ml of *chloroform*, shake and allow to separate. Filter the chloroform layer through absorbent cotton and dilute 5 ml of the filtrate to 10 ml with *boric acid solution*. Measure the *absorbance* of a 2-cm layer of the resulting solution at the maximum at 420 nm, Appendix II B, using 5 ml of *boric acid solution* diluted to 10 ml with *chloroform* in the reference cell. Calculate the content of $C_9H_9Cl_2N_3$, HCl from the *absorbance* obtained by repeating the procedure using a solution prepared by diluting 5 ml of a 0.030% w/v solution of *clonidine hydrochloride BPCRS* to 100 ml with *citro-phosphate buffer pH 7.6*, transferring 5 ml to a separating funnel and completing the procedure described above, beginning at the words 'add 1 ml of a solution...'.

For tablets containing less than 0.3 mg of Clonidine Hydrochloride, use the same procedure but with a concentration of 0.001% w/v or 0.0005% w/v of Clonidine Hydrochloride as appropriate and with correspondingly smaller concentrations of *clonidine hydrochloride BPCRS*.

Assay Weigh and powder 20 tablets. To a quantity of the powder containing 0.1 mg of Clonidine Hydrochloride add 25 ml of *citro-phosphate buffer pH 7.6* and shake for 15 minutes. Add 5 ml of *water* and 1 ml of a solution containing 0.15% w/v of *bromothymol blue* and 0.15% w/v of *anhydrous sodium carbonate* and shake to disperse. Add 30 ml of *chloroform*, shake continuously for 1 minute and centrifuge. To 15 ml of the chloroform layer add 10 ml of *boric acid solution* and measure the *absorbance* of the resulting solution at the maximum at 420 nm, Appendix II B, using in the reference cell a solution prepared by diluting 10 ml of *boric acid solution* to 25 ml with *chloroform*. Calculate the content of $C_9H_9Cl_2N_3$,HCl from the *absorbance* obtained by repeating the operation using 5 ml of a 0.002% w/v solution of *clonidine hydrochloride BPCRS* previously dried to constant weight at 105°, adding 20 ml of *citro-phosphate buffer pH 7.6* and completing the procedure described above beginning at the words 'Add 5 ml of *water*...'.

Clotrimazole Cream

Definition Clotrimazole Cream contains Clotrimazole in a suitable basis.

The cream complies with the requirements stated under Topical Semi-solid Preparations and with the following requirements.

Content of clotrimazole, $C_{22}H_{17}ClN_2$ 95.0 to 105.0% of the prescribed or stated amount.

Identification

A. Mix a quantity containing 40 mg of Clotrimazole with 20 ml of a mixture of 1 volume of 1M *sulphuric acid* and 4 volumes of *methanol* and shake with two 50-ml quantities of *carbon tetrachloride*, discarding the organic layers. Make the aqueous phase alkaline with 2M *ammonia*, add a further 5 ml of 2M *ammonia* and extract with two 40-ml quantities of *chloroform*. Combine the chloroform extracts, shake with 5 g of *anhydrous sodium sulphate*, filter and add sufficient *chloroform* to the filtrate to produce 100 ml. Evaporate 50 ml to dryness and dissolve the residue in 50 ml of a mixture of 1 volume of 0.1M *hydrochloric acid* and 9 volumes of *methanol*. The *light absorption* of the resulting solution, Appendix II B, in the range 230 to 350 nm exhibits two maxima, at 262 nm and 265 nm.

B. Carry out the method for *thin-layer chromatography*, Appendix III A, using a silica gel precoated plate (Merck silica gel 60 plates are suitable) and *di-isopropyl ether* as the mobile phase in a chromatography tank containing 25 ml of 13.5M *ammonia* in a beaker. Apply separately to the plate 10 µl of each of the following solutions. For solution (1) shake a quantity of the cream containing 20 mg of Clotrimazole with 4 ml of *dichloromethane* for 30 minutes, centrifuge and use the supernatant liquid. Solution (2) contains 0.5% w/v of *clotrimazole BPCRS* in *dichloromethane*. After removal of the plate, allow it to dry in a current of air and spray with *dilute potassium iodobismuthate solution*. The spot in the chromatogram obtained with solution (1) is reddish brown and corresponds to the spot in the chromatogram obtained with solution (2).

2-Chlorotritanol Carry out the method for *liquid chromatography*, Appendix III D, using the following solutions. Solution (1) contains 0.00020% w/v of *2-chlorotritanol BPCRS* in a mixture of 7 volumes of *methanol* and 3 volumes of 0.02M *orthophosphoric acid*. For solution (2) extract a quantity of the cream containing 20 mg of Clotrimazole by warming with 20 ml of *methanol* in a water bath at 50° for 5 minutes, shaking occasionally. Remove from the water bath, shake the mixture vigorously while cooling to room temperature, cool in ice for 15 minutes, centrifuge for 5 minutes and decant the supernatant liquid. Repeat the extraction with two further 20-ml quantities of *methanol*. To the combined methanol extracts add 10 ml of *methanol* and dilute to 100 ml with 0.02M *orthophosphoric acid*. Cool in ice and filter through a glass microfibre filter paper (Whatman GF/C is suitable). For solution (3) dilute 1 volume of solution (2) to 50 volumes with a mixture of 30 volumes of 0.02M *orthophosphoric acid* and 70 volumes of *methanol*.

The chromatographic procedure may be carried out using (a) a stainless steel column (20 cm × 4.6 mm) packed with *stationary phase C* (5 µm) (Lichrosorb RP-18 or Spherisorb ODS 1 is suitable), (b) as the mobile phase with a flow rate of 1.5 ml per minute a mixture of 30 volumes of 0.02M *orthophosphoric acid* and 70 volumes of *methanol*, the pH of the mixture being adjusted to 7.5 with a 10% v/v solution of *triethylamine* in *methanol* and (c) a detection wavelength of 215 nm.

The *column efficiency*, determined using the principal peak in the chromatogram obtained with solution (3), should be at least 9000 theoretical plates per metre.

Record the chromatogram for solution (2) for 1.5 times the retention time of the principal peak. The area of any peak corresponding to 2-chlorotritanol in the chromatogram obtained with solution (2) is not greater than the area of the peak in the chromatogram obtained with solution (1).

Assay Carry out the method for *liquid chromatography*, Appendix III D, using the following solutions. For solution (1) dissolve 20 mg of *clotrimazole BPCRS* in 70 ml of *methanol*, add sufficient 0.02M *orthophosphoric acid* to produce 100 ml and dilute 1 volume of the resulting solution to 5 volumes with a mixture of 70 volumes of *methanol* and 30 volumes of 0.02M *orthophosphoric acid*. For solution (2) treat a quantity of the cream containing 20 mg of Clotrimazole as described in the test for 2-Chlorotritanol and dilute 1 volume of the filtrate to 5 volumes with a mixture of 70 volumes of *methanol* and 30 volumes of 0.02M *orthophosphoric acid*.
The chromatographic procedure may be carried out using the conditions described in the test for 2-Chlorotritanol. The *column efficiency*, determined using the peak in the chromatogram obtained with solution (1), should be at least 9000 theoretical plates per metre.
Calculate the content of $C_{22}H_{17}ClN_2$ using the declared content of $C_{22}H_{17}ClN_2$ in *clotrimazole BPCRS*.

Clotrimazole Pessaries

Definition Clotrimazole Pessaries contain Clotrimazole in a suitable basis.

The pessaries comply with the requirements stated under Vaginal Preparations and with the following requirements.

Content of clotrimazole, $C_{22}H_{17}ClN_2$ 95.0 to 105.0% of the prescribed or stated amount.

Identification

A. Mix a quantity of the powdered pessaries containing 40 mg of Clotrimazole with 20 ml of a mixture of 1 volume of 1M *sulphuric acid* and 4 volumes of *methanol* and shake with two 50-ml quantities of *carbon tetrachloride*, discarding the organic layers. Make the aqueous phase alkaline with 2M *ammonia* and extract with two 40-ml quantities of *chloroform*. Combine the chloroform extracts, shake with 5 g of *anhydrous sodium sulphate*, filter and add sufficient *chloroform* to the filtrate to produce 100 ml. Evaporate 50 ml to dryness and dissolve the residue in 50 ml of a mixture of 1 volume of 0.1M *hydrochloric acid* and 9 volumes of *methanol*. The *light absorption* of the resulting solution, Appendix II B, in the range 230 to 350 nm exhibits two maxima, at 262 nm and 265 nm.

B. Carry out the method for *thin-layer chromatography*, Appendix III A, using a silica gel precoated plate (Merck silica gel 60 plates are suitable) and *di-isopropyl ether* as the mobile phase in a tank containing 25 ml of 13.5M *ammonia* in a beaker. Apply separately to the plate 10 µl of each of the following solutions. For solution (1) shake a quantity of the powdered pessaries containing 20 mg of Clotrimazole with 4 ml of *dichloromethane* for 30 minutes, centrifuge and use the supernatant liquid. Solution (2) contains 0.5% w/v of *clotrimazole BPCRS* in *dichloromethane*. After removal of the plate, allow it to dry in a current of air and spray with *dilute potassium iodobismuthate solution*. The spot in the chromatogram obtained with solution (1) is reddish brown and corresponds to the spot in the chromatogram obtained with solution (2).

Related substances Carry out the method for *liquid chromatography*, Appendix III D, using the following solutions. Solution (1) contains 0.00020% w/v of *2-chlorotritanol BPCRS* in a mixture of 70 volumes of *methanol* and 30 volumes of 0.02M *orthophosphoric acid*. For solution (2) add 50 ml of *methanol* to a quantity of the powdered pessaries containing 0.1 g of Clotrimazole and shake for 20 minutes. Dilute to 100 ml with *methanol* and filter. To 20 ml of the filtrate add 50 ml of *methanol* and sufficient 0.02M *orthophosphoric acid* to produce 100 ml. For solution (3) dilute 1 volume of solution (2) to 50 volumes with a mixture of 30 volumes of 0.02M *orthophosphoric acid* and 70 volumes of *methanol.*

The chromatographic procedure may be carried out using (a) a stainless steel column (20 cm × 4.6 mm) packed with *stationary phase C* (5 µm) (Lichrosorb RP-18 or Spherisorb ODS 1 is suitable), (b) as the mobile phase with a flow rate of 1.5 ml per minute a mixture of 30 volumes of 0.02M *orthophosphoric acid* and 70 volumes of *methanol,* the pH of the mixture being adjusted to 7.5 with a 10% v/v solution of *triethylamine* in *methanol* and (c) a detection wavelength of 215 nm.

The *column efficiency,* determined using the principal peak in the chromatogram obtained with solution (3), should be at least 9000 theoretical plates per metre. Record the chromatograms for solution (2) for 1.5 times the retention time of the principal peak. The area of any *secondary peak* in the chromatogram obtained with solution (2) is not greater than the area of the peak in the chromatogram obtained with solution (1).

Assay Carry out the method for *liquid chromatography,* Appendix III D, using the following solutions. For solution (1) dissolve 20 mg of *clotrimazole BPCRS* in 70 ml of *methanol,* add sufficient 0.02M *orthophosphoric acid* to produce 100 ml and dilute 1 volume of the resulting solution to 5 volumes with a mixture of 70 volumes of *methanol* and 30 volumes of 0.02M *orthophosphoric acid.* For solution (2) weigh and powder 20 pessaries. To a quantity of the powder containing 0.1 g of Clotrimazole add 50 ml of *methanol* and shake for 20 minutes. Dilute to 250 ml with *methanol,* filter and to 10 ml of the filtrate add 60 ml of *methanol* and sufficient 0.02M *orthophosphoric acid* to produce 100 ml.
The chromatographic procedure may be carried out using the conditions described in the test for Related substances. The *column efficiency,* determined using the peak in the chromatogram obtained with solution (1), should be at least 9000 theoretical plates per metre.
Calculate the content of $C_{22}H_{17}ClN_2$ using the declared content of $C_{22}H_{17}ClN_2$ in *clotrimazole BPCRS.*

Cloxacillin Capsules

Definition Cloxacillin Capsules contain Cloxacillin Sodium.

The capsules comply with the requirements stated under Capsules and with the following requirements.

Content of cloxacillin, $C_{19}H_{18}ClN_3O_5S$ 92.5 to 107.5% of the prescribed or stated amount.

Identification

A. The *infrared absorption spectrum* of the contents of the capsules, Appendix II A, is concordant with the *reference spectrum* of cloxacillin sodium.

B. The contents of the capsules yield the reactions characteristic of *sodium salts,* Appendix VI.

Assay To a quantity of the mixed contents of 20 capsules containing the equivalent of 0.25 g of cloxacillin add 70 ml of *water,* shake for 15 minutes and add sufficient *water* to produce 500 ml. Filter and dilute 10 ml of the filtrate to 100 ml with *water.* Place two 2-ml quantities of the resulting solution in separate stoppered tubes. To one tube add 10 ml of *imidazole—mercury reagent,* mix, stopper the tube and immerse in a water bath at 60° for exactly 25 minutes, swirling occasionally. Remove from the water bath and cool rapidly to 20° (solution A). To the second tube add 10 ml of *water* and mix (solution B). Without delay measure the *absorbances* of solutions A and B at the maximum at 346 nm, Appendix II B, using in the reference cell a mixture of 2 ml of *water* and 10 ml of *imidazole—mercury reagent* for solution A and *water* for solution B. Calculate the content of $C_{19}H_{18}ClN_3O_5S$ from the difference between the absorbances of solutions A and B, from the difference obtained by repeating the operation using a 0.0055% w/v solution of *cloxacillin sodium BPCRS* in place of the final solution obtained from the preparation being examined and from the declared content of $C_{19}H_{18}ClN_3O_5S$ in *cloxacillin sodium BPCRS.*

Labelling The quantity of active ingredient is stated in terms of the equivalent amount of cloxacillin.

Cloxacillin Injection

Definition Cloxacillin Injection is a sterile solution of cloxacillin sodium in Water for Injections. It is prepared by dissolving Cloxacillin Sodium for Injection in the requisite amount of Water for Injections.

The injection complies with the requirements stated under Parenteral Preparations.

Storage Cloxacillin Injection should be used immediately after preparation but, in any case, within the period recommended by the manufacturer when prepared and stored strictly in accordance with the manufacturer's instructions.

CLOXACILLIN SODIUM FOR INJECTION

Definition Cloxacillin Sodium for Injection is a sterile material prepared from Cloxacillin Sodium with or without excipients. It is supplied in a sealed container.

The contents of the sealed container comply with the requirements for Powders for Injections stated under Parenteral Preparations and with the following requirements.

Content of cloxacillin, $C_{19}H_{18}ClN_3O_5S$ 95.0 to 105.0% of the prescribed or stated amount.

Identification

A. The *infrared absorption spectrum,* Appendix II A, is concordant with the *reference spectrum* of cloxacillin sodium.

B. Yield the reactions characteristic of *sodium salts,* Appendix VI.

Acidity or alkalinity pH of a 10% w/v solution, 5.0 to 7.0, Appendix V L.

Iodine-absorbing substances Not more than 5%, calculated with reference to the anhydrous substance, when determined by the following method. Dissolve 0.125 g in sufficient *mixed phosphate buffer pH 7.0* to produce 25 ml. To 10 ml add 10 ml of *mixed phosphate buffer pH 4.0* and 10 ml of 0.01M *iodine VS* and titrate immediately with 0.01M *sodium thiosulphate VS* using *starch mucilage,* added towards the end of the titration, as indicator. Repeat the operation without the substance being examined. The difference between the titrations represents the amount of iodine-absorbing substances present. Each ml of 0.01M *sodium thiosulphate VS* is equivalent to 0.504 mg of iodine-absorbing substances.

Water Not more than 4.5% w/w, Appendix IX C. Use 0.3 g.

Bacterial endotoxins Carry out the *test for bacterial endotoxins*, Appendix XIV C. Dissolve the contents of the sealed container in *water BET* to give a solution containing 10 mg per ml (solution A). The endotoxin limit concentration of solution A is 4.0 IU per ml. Carry out the test using the maximum valid dilution of solution A calculated from the declared sensitivity of the lysate used in the test.

Assay Determine the weight of the contents of 10 containers as described in the test for Uniformity of weight under Parenteral Preparations, Powders for Injections.

Dissolve 0.1 g of the mixed contents of the 10 containers in sufficient *water* to produce 500 ml and dilute 25 ml to 100 ml with *water*. Place two 2-ml quantities of the resulting solution in separate stoppered tubes. To one tube add 10 ml of *imidazole—mercury reagent*, mix, stopper the tube and immerse in a water bath at 60° for exactly 25 minutes, swirling occasionally. Remove from the water bath and cool rapidly to 20° (solution A). To the second tube add 10 ml of *water* and mix (solution B). Without delay measure the *absorbances* of solutions A and B at the maximum at 346 nm, Appendix II B, using in the reference cell a mixture of 2 ml of *water* and 10 ml of *imidazole—mercury reagent* for solution A and *water* for solution B. Calculate the content of $C_{19}H_{18}ClN_3O_5S$ in a container of average content weight from the difference between the absorbances of solutions A and B, from the difference obtained by repeating the operation using a 0.0055% w/v solution of *cloxacillin sodium BPCRS* in place of the final solution obtained from the preparation being examined and from the declared content of $C_{19}H_{18}ClN_3O_5S$ in *cloxacillin sodium BPCRS*.

Storage The sealed container should be kept at a temperature not exceeding 25°.

Labelling The label of the sealed container states the quantity of Cloxacillin Sodium contained in it in terms of the equivalent amount of cloxacillin.

Cloxacillin Oral Solution

Definition Cloxacillin Oral Solution is a solution of Cloxacillin Sodium in a suitable flavoured vehicle. It is prepared by dissolving the dry ingredients in the specified volume of Water just before issue for use.

The dry ingredients comply with the requirements for Powders and Granules for the Preparation of Oral Liquids stated under Oral Liquids.

Storage The dry ingredients should be kept in a well-closed container and stored at a temperature not exceeding 25°.

For the following tests prepare the oral solution as directed on the label. The solution, examined immediately after preparation unless otherwise indicated, complies with the requirements stated under Oral Liquids and with the following requirements.

Content of cloxacillin, $C_{19}H_{18}ClN_3O_5S$ When freshly constituted, not more than 120.0% of the prescribed or stated amount. When stored at the temperature and for the period stated on the label during which the oral solution may be expected to be satisfactory for use, not less than 80.0% of the prescribed or stated amount.

Identification Carry out the method for *thin-layer chromatography*, Appendix III A, using a silanised silica gel F_{254} precoated plate (Merck silanised silica gel 60 F_{254} plates are suitable) and as the mobile phase a mixture of 70 volumes of 0.05M *potassium hydrogen phthalate*, 30 volumes of *acetone* and 1 volume of *formic acid*, the pH of the mixture having been adjusted first to 6.0 with 5M *sodium hydroxide* and then to 9.0 with 0.1M *sodium hydroxide*. Apply separately to the plate 1 µl of each of the following solutions. For solution (1) dilute a quantity of the oral solution containing the equivalent of 50 mg of cloxacillin to 20 ml with *phosphate buffer pH 7.0*. Solution (2) contains 0.25% w/v of *cloxacillin sodium BPCRS* in *phosphate buffer pH 7.0*. After removal of the plate, allow it to dry in air and spray with a mixture of 100 volumes of *starch mucilage*, 6 volumes of *glacial acetic acid* and 2 volumes of a 1% w/v solution of *iodine* in a 4% w/v solution of *potassium iodide*. The principal spot in the chromatogram obtained with solution (1) corresponds to that in the chromatogram obtained with solution (2).

Acidity or alkalinity pH, 4.0 to 7.0, Appendix V L.

Assay To a weighed quantity of the oral solution containing the equivalent of 0.25 g of cloxacillin add sufficient *water* to produce 500 ml and dilute 10 ml to 100 ml. Place two 2-ml quantities of the resulting solution in separate stoppered tubes. To one tube add 10 ml of *imidazole—mercury reagent*, mix, stopper the tube and immerse in a water bath at 60° for exactly 25 minutes, swirling occasionally. Remove from the water bath and cool rapidly to 20° (solution A). To the second tube add 10 ml of *water* and mix (solution B). Without delay measure the *absorbances* of solutions A and B at the maximum at 346 nm, Appendix II B, using in the reference cell a mixture of 2 ml of *water* and 10 ml of *imidazole—mercury reagent* for solution A and *water* for solution B. Calculate the content of $C_{19}H_{18}ClN_3O_5S$ from the difference between the absorbances of solutions A and B, from the difference obtained by repeating the operation using a 0.0055% w/v solution of *cloxacillin sodium BPCRS* in place of the solution obtained from the preparation being examined and from the declared content of $C_{19}H_{18}ClN_3O_5S$ in *cloxacillin sodium BPCRS*. Determine the *weight per ml* of the oral solution, Appendix V G, and calculate the content of $C_{19}H_{18}ClN_3O_5S$, weight in volume.

Repeat the procedure using a portion of the oral solution that has been stored at the temperature and for the period stated on the label during which it may be expected to be satisfactory for use.

Storage The Oral Solution should be stored at the temperature and used within the period stated on the label.

Labelling The quantity of active ingredient is stated in terms of the equivalent amount of cloxacillin.

Co-amilofruse Tablets

Amiloride and Furosemide
Frusemide Tablets

If the subsidiary title is used for the purposes of product labelling in the United Kingdom, the pair of names given above shall be used together (see Introduction, Changes in title).

Definition Co-amilofruse Tablets contain Amiloride Hydrochloride and Furosemide in the proportions one part of anhydrous amiloride hydrochloride to eight parts of Furosemide.

With the exception of the requirements for shape, the tablets comply with the requirements stated under Tablets and with the following requirements.

Content of anhydrous amiloride hydrochloride, $C_6H_8ClN_7O,HCl$ 95.0 to 105.0% of the prescribed or stated amount.

Content of furosemide, $C_{12}H_{11}ClN_2O_5S$ 95.0 to 105.0% of the prescribed or stated amount.

Identification

A. In the test for Related substances, the principal spots in the chromatogram obtained with solution (2) correspond to those in the chromatograms obtained with solutions (4) and (5) respectively.

B. In the Assay, the retention times of the two principal peaks in the chromatogram obtained with solution (1) are the same as those in the chromatogram obtained with solution (2).

Related substances Carry out the method for *thin-layer chromatography*, Appendix III A, using *silica gel GF_{254}* as the coating substance and a mixture of 5 volumes of *glacial acetic acid,* 5 volumes of *methanol* and 90 volumes of *chloroform* as the mobile phase. Apply separately to the plate 20 µl of each of the following solutions. For solution (1) mix with the aid of ultrasound a quantity of the powdered tablets containing 80 mg of Furosemide with 16 ml of *methanol* for 5 minutes, centrifuge and use the supernatant liquid. For solution (2) dilute 1 volume of solution (1) to 10 volumes with *methanol.* For solution (3) dilute 1 volume of solution (2) to 20 volumes with *methanol.* Solution (4) contains 0.05% w/v of *furosemide BPCRS* in *methanol.* Solution (5) contains 0.00625% w/v of *amiloride hydrochloride BPCRS* in *methanol.* Solution (6) contains 0.0025% w/v of *4-chloro-5-sulphamoylanthranilic acid BPCRS* in *methanol.* Solution (7) contains 0.00031% w/v of *methyl 3,5-diamino-6-chloropyrazine-2-carboxylate BPCRS* in *methanol.* After removal of the plate, dry it in a current of air and examine under *ultraviolet light (254 nm).* In the chromatogram obtained with solution (1) any *secondary spot* other than any spot remaining on the line of application or any spots corresponding to either of the named impurities is not more intense than the spot in the chromatogram obtained with solution (3) (0.5%, with reference to the content of furosemide). Examine under *ultraviolet light (365 nm)*. In the chromatogram obtained with solution (1) any spot corresponding to methyl 3,5-diamino-6-chloropyrazine-2-carboxylate is not more intense than the spot in the chromatogram obtained with solution (7) (0.5%, with reference to the content of anhydrous amiloride hydrochloride). Reveal the spots by *Method I.* In the chromatogram obtained with solution (1) any spot corresponding to 4-chloro-5-sulphamoylanthranilic acid is not more intense than the spot in the chromatogram obtained with solution (6) (0.5%, with reference to the content of furosemide).

Assay Weigh and powder 20 tablets. Carry out the method for *liquid chromatography*, Appendix III D, using the following solutions. For solution (1) disperse a quantity of the powdered tablets containing 40 mg of Furosemide in 70 ml of a mixture of 4 volumes of *water* and 6 volumes of *methanol* adjusted to pH 2.0 with *orthophosphoric acid,* mix with the aid of ultrasound for 20 minutes, dilute to 100 ml with the same solvent mixture, mix, filter and dilute 20 ml of the filtrate to 50 ml with the same solvent mixture. Solution (2) contains 0.002% w/v of *amiloride hydrochloride BPCRS* and 0.016% w/v of *furosemide BPCRS* in a mixture of 4 volumes of *water* and 6 volumes of *methanol* adjusted to pH 2.0 with *orthophosphoric acid.*

The chromatographic procedure may be carried out using (a) a stainless steel column (25 cm × 4.6 mm) packed with *stationary phase C* (10 µm) (Spherisorb ODS is suitable), (b) a 0.02M solution of *sodium hexanesulphonate* in a mixture of 4 volumes of *water* and 6 volumes of *methanol,* the pH of the solution adjusted to 4.0 with 1M *acetic acid,* as the mobile phase with a flow rate of 1.2 ml per minute and (c) a detection wavelength of 361 nm. The order of elution of the peaks is furosemide and then amiloride.

The method is not valid unless in the chromatogram obtained with solution (2) the *resolution factor* between the peaks due to furosemide and amiloride is at least 2.5.

Calculate the content of $C_6H_8ClN_7O,HCl$ and $C_{12}H_{11}ClN_2O_5S$ using the declared content of $C_6H_8ClN_7O,HCl$ and $C_{12}H_{11}ClN_2O_5S$ in *amiloride hydrochloride BPCRS* and *furosemide BPCRS,* respectively.

Storage Co-amilofruse Tablets should be protected from light.

Labelling The label states the quantities of Amiloride Hydrochloride, in terms of the equivalent amount of anhydrous amiloride hydrochloride, and of Furosemide (Frusemide) in each tablet.

Co-amilozide Oral Solution

Amiloride and Hydrochlorothiazide Oral Solution

Definition Co-amilozide Oral Solution is a solution containing Amiloride Hydrochloride and Hydrochlorothiazide in the proportions one part of anhydrous amiloride hydrochloride to ten parts of Hydrochlorothiazide in a suitable flavoured vehicle.

The oral solution complies with the requirements stated under Oral Liquids and with the following requirements.

Content of anhydrous amiloride hydrochloride, $C_6H_8ClN_7O,HCl$ 95.0 to 105.0% of the prescribed or stated amount.

Content of hydrochlorothiazide, $C_7H_8ClN_3O_4S_2$ 95.0 to 105.0% of the prescribed or stated amount.

Identification

A. Carry out the method for *thin-layer chromatography*, Appendix III A, using *silica gel GF_{254}* as the coating substance and a mixture of 88 volumes of *tetrahydrofuran* and 12 volumes of 3M *ammonia* as the mobile phase. Apply separately to the plate 10 µl of each of the following solutions. For solution (1) disperse a volume of the oral solution containing 0.1 g of Hydrochlorothiazide in *methanol*, dilute to 50 ml with *methanol* and mix. Solution (2) contains 0.2% w/v of *hydrochlorothiazide BPCRS* in *methanol*. Solution (3) contains 0.02% w/v of *amiloride hydrochloride BPCRS* in *methanol*. Solution (4) contains equal volumes of solutions (1), (2) and (3). After removal of the plate, allow it to dry in air and examine under *ultraviolet light (254 nm)*. The principal spots in the chromatogram obtained with solution (1) correspond to those in the chromatograms obtained with solutions (2) and (3). If the Rf values of the spots obtained with solution (1) do not correspond exactly with those of the principal spots in the chromatograms obtained with solutions (2) and (3), the chromatogram obtained with solution (4) exhibits only one compact spot at each of these Rf values.

B. In the Assay, the retention times of the two principal peaks in the chromatogram obtained with solution (3) correspond to those of the peaks in the chromatograms obtained with solutions (1) and (2).

Acidity pH, 2.8 to 3.2, Appendix V L.

4-Amino-6-chlorobenzene-1,3-disulphonamide Carry out the method for *liquid chromatography*, Appendix III D, using the following solutions. Solution (1) contains 0.00050% w/v of *4-amino-6-chlorobenzene-1,3-disulphonamide BPCRS* in the mobile phase. For solution (2) disperse a volume of the oral solution containing 50 mg of Hydrochlorothiazide in the mobile phase, dilute to 100 ml with the mobile phase and mix. Prepare solution (3) in the same manner as solution (2) but using solution (1) in place of the mobile phase.

The chromatographic procedure may be carried out using (a) a stainless steel column (20 cm × 4.6 mm) packed with *stationary phase C* (10 µm) (Nucleosil C18 is suitable), (b) a mixture of 76 volumes of *water*, 20 volumes of *methanol* and 4 volumes of *phosphate buffer pH 3.0* as the mobile phase with a flow rate of 2 ml per minute and (c) a detection wavelength of 265 nm.

The test is not valid unless a peak due to 4-amino-6-chlorobenzene-1,3-disulphonamide appears immediately before the principal peak in the chromatogram obtained with solution (3) and the height of the trough separating the two peaks is less than 5% of the height of the peak due to 4-amino-6-chlorobenzene-1,3-disulphonamide. The resolution between these two peaks may be improved by decreasing the methanol content in the mobile phase.

In the chromatogram obtained with solution (2) the area of any peak corresponding to 4-amino-6-chlorobenzene-1,3-disulphonamide is not greater than the area of the peak in the chromatogram obtained with solution (1).

Assay Carry out the method for *liquid chromatography*, Appendix III D, using the following solutions. For solution (1) dissolve 50 mg of *hydrochlorothiazide BPCRS* in a mixture of 20 ml of *methanol* and 4 ml of *phosphate buffer pH 3.0* and dilute to 100 ml with *water*. For solution (2) dissolve 50 mg of *amiloride hydrochloride BPCRS* in 200 ml of *methanol* and to 20 ml of the resulting solution add 4 ml of *phosphate buffer pH 3.0* and dilute to 100 ml with *methanol*. For solution (3) disperse a volume of the oral solution containing 50 mg of Hydrochlorothiazide in the mobile phase, dilute to 100 ml with the mobile phase and mix.

The chromatographic procedure may be carried out as described in the test for 4-Amino-6-chlorobenzene-1,3-disulphonamide but using a detection wavelength of 286 nm.

The assay is not valid unless the validity criteria of the test for 4-Amino-6-chlorobenzene-1,3-disulphonamide are met.

Determine the *weight per ml* of the oral solution, Appendix V G, and calculate the content of $C_6H_8ClN_7O$, HCl and $C_7H_8ClN_3O_4S_2$, weight in volume, using the declared content of $C_6H_8ClN_7O,HCl$ and $C_7H_8ClN_3O_4S_2$ in *amiloride hydrochloride BPCRS* and *hydrochlorothiazide BPCRS* respectively.

Labelling The label states the quantities of Amiloride Hydrochloride, in terms of anhydrous amiloride hydrochloride, and of Hydrochlorothiazide in a suitable dose-volume.

Co-amilozide Tablets

Amiloride and Hydrochlorothiazide Tablets

Definition Co-amilozide Tablets contain Amiloride Hydrochloride and Hydrochlorothiazide in the proportions one part of anhydrous amiloride hydrochloride to ten parts of Hydrochlorothiazide.

With the exception of the requirements for shape, the tablets comply with the requirements stated under Tablets and with the following requirements.

Content of anhydrous amiloride hydrochloride, $C_6H_8ClN_7O,HCl$ 95.0 to 105.0% of the prescribed or stated amount.

Content of hydrochlorothiazide, $C_7H_8ClN_3O_4S_2$ 95.0 to 105.0% of the prescribed or stated amount.

Identification

A. Shake a quantity of the powdered tablets containing 0.1 g of Hydrochlorothiazide with 50 ml of *acetone*, filter, evaporate the filtrate to dryness and dry the residue at 105° for 1 hour. The *infrared absorption spectrum* of the dried residue, Appendix II A, is concordant with the *reference spectrum* of hydrochlorothiazide.

B. In the test for Methyl 3,5-diamino-6-chloropyrazine-2-carboxylate, the principal spot in the chromatogram obtained with solution (3) corresponds to that in the chromatogram obtained with solution (4).

C. In the Assay, the retention times of the two principal peaks in the chromatogram obtained with solution (4) correspond to those in the chromatograms obtained with solutions (2) and (3).

Related substances Carry out the method for *thin-layer chromatography*, Appendix III A, using *silica gel G* as the coating substance and a mixture of 85 volumes of *ethyl acetate* and 15 volumes of *propan-2-ol* as the mobile phase. Apply separately to the plate 5 µl of each of the following solutions. For solution (1) shake vigorously a quantity of the powdered tablets containing 50 mg of Hydrochlorothiazide with 10 ml of *acetone* and filter. For solution (2) dilute 1 volume of solution (1) to 100 volumes with *acetone*. After removal of the plate, dry it in a current of air and reveal the spots by *Method I*. Any *secondary spot* in the chromatogram obtained with solution (1) is not more intense than the spot in the chromatogram obtained with solution (2). Disregard any spot remaining on the line of application.

Methyl 3,5-diamino-6-chloropyrazine-2-carboxylate Carry out the method for *thin-layer chromatography*,

Appendix III A, protected from light, using a silica gel precoated plate (Merck silica gel 60 plates are suitable) and a freshly prepared mixture of 90 volumes of *1,4-dioxan* and 12 volumes of 3M *ammonia* as the mobile phase. Apply separately to the plate 10 µl of each of the following solutions. For solution (1) shake a quantity of the powdered tablets containing the equivalent of 17.5 mg of anhydrous amiloride hydrochloride with 10 ml of *methanol* and centrifuge. Solution (2) contains 0.0010% w/v of *methyl 3,5-diamino-6-chloropyrazine-2-carboxylate BPCRS* in *methanol*. For solution (3) dilute 1 volume of solution (1) to 20 volumes with *methanol*. Solution (4) contains 0.010% w/v of *amiloride hydrochloride BPCRS* in *methanol*. After removal of the plate, allow it to dry in air and examine under *ultraviolet light (365 nm)*. Any spot corresponding to methyl 3,5-diamino-6-chloropyrazine-2-carboxylate in the chromatogram obtained with solution (1) is not more intense than the spot in the chromatogram obtained with solution (2).

Assay Weigh and powder 20 tablets. Carry out the method for *liquid chromatography*, Appendix III D, using the following solutions. Solution (1) contains 0.0010% w/v of *4-amino-6-chlorobenzene-1,3-disulphonamide BPCRS* in solution (3). For solution (2) dissolve 50 mg of *amiloride hydrochloride BPCRS* in sufficient *methanol* to produce 200 ml ; to 20 ml of the resulting solution add 4 ml of 0.1M *hydrochloric acid* and dilute to 100 ml with *water*. For solution (3) dissolve 50 mg of *hydrochlorothiazide BPCRS* in a mixture of 20 ml of *methanol* and 4 ml of 0.1M *hydrochloric acid* and dilute to 100 ml with *water*. For solution (4) add a mixture of 20 ml of *methanol* and 4 ml of 0.1M *hydrochloric acid* to a quantity of the powdered tablets containing 50 mg of Hydrochlorothiazide, mix with the aid of ultrasound for 15 minutes, dilute to 100 ml with *water*, mix and filter.

The chromatographic procedure may be carried out using (a) a stainless steel column (20 cm × 4.6 mm) packed with *stationary phase C* (10 µm) (Nucleosil C18 is suitable), (b) a mixture of 76 volumes of *water*, 20 volumes of *methanol* and 4 volumes of *phosphate buffer pH 3.0* as the mobile phase with a flow rate of 2 ml per minute and (c) a detection wavelength of 286 nm.

The assay is not valid unless a peak due to 4-amino-6-chlorobenzene-1,3-disulphonamide appears immediately before the principal peak in the chromatogram obtained with solution (1). Increase the sensitivity, if necessary, to obtain at least 10% of full-scale deflection on the chart paper for this peak. The assay is also not valid unless the height of the trough separating the two peaks is less than 10% of the height of the peak due to 4-amino-6-chlorobenzene-1,3-disulphonamide. The resolution between the two peaks may be improved by decreasing the methanol content of the mobile phase.

Calculate the content of $C_6H_8ClN_7O,HCl$ and $C_7H_8ClN_3O_4S_2$ using the declared content of $C_6H_8ClN_7O,HCl$ and $C_7H_8ClN_3O_4S_2$ in *amiloride hydrochloride BPCRS* and *hydrochlorothiazide BPCRS* respectively.

Storage Co-amilozide Tablets should be kept in a well-closed container, protected from light and stored at a temperature not exceeding 25°.

Labelling The label states the quantities of Amiloride Hydrochloride, in terms of the equivalent amount of anhydrous amiloride hydrochloride, and of Hydrochlorothiazide in each tablet.

Co-amoxiclav Tablets

Amoxicillin and Potassium Clavulanate Tablets

Definition Co-amoxiclav Tablets contain Amoxicillin Trihydrate and Potassium Clavulanate.

With the exception of the requirements for shape, the tablets comply with the requirements stated under Tablets and with the following requirements.

Content of amoxicillin, $C_{16}H_{19}O_5N_3S$ 90.0 to 105.0% of the prescribed or stated amount.

Content of clavulanic acid, $C_8H_9NO_5$ 90.0 to 105.0% of the prescribed or stated amount.

Identification Carry out the method for *thin-layer chromatography*, Appendix III A, using a silica gel pre-coated plate (Merck silica gel 60 F_{254} plates are suitable). Impregnate the plate by spraying it with a 0.1% w/v solution of *disodium edetate* in *mixed phosphate buffer pH 4.0* and allow to dry overnight. Activate the plate by heating at 105° for 1 hour just prior to use. Use as the mobile phase a mixture of 1 volume of *butan-1-ol*, 2 volumes of a 0.1% w/v solution of *disodium edetate* in *mixed phosphate buffer pH 4.0*, 6 volumes of *glacial acetic acid* and 10 volumes of *butyl acetate*. Apply separately to the plate 1 µl of each of the following solutions. For solution (1) shake a quantity of the powdered tablets containing the equivalent of 0.4 g of clavulanic acid in 100 ml of a mixture of 4 volumes of *methanol* and 6 volumes of *0.1M mixed phosphate buffer pH 7.0* and filter. Solution (2) contains 0.4% w/v of *lithium clavulanate BPCRS* and 0.8% w/v of *amoxicillin trihydrate BPCRS* in a mixture of 4 volumes of *methanol* and 6 volumes of *0.1M mixed phosphate buffer pH 7.0*. After removal of the plate, allow it to dry in air and examine under *ultraviolet light (254 nm)*. The principal spots in the chromatogram obtained with solution (1) are similar in position and colour to those in the chromatogram obtained with solution (2).

Amoxicillin degradation products Not more than 6.0% when determined by the following method. To a quantity of the powdered tablets containing the equivalent of 0.2 g of amoxicillin add 25 ml of *boric buffer pH 9.0* and 0.5 ml of *acetic anhydride*, stir for 3 minutes, add 10 ml of *acetate buffer pH 4.6* and titrate immediately with 0.02M *mercury(II) nitrate VS*. Determine the end point potentiometrically using a platinum or mercury indicator electrode and a mercury—mercury(I) sulphate reference electrode. Disregard any preliminary inflection of the titration curve. Each ml of 0.02M *mercury(II) nitrate VS* is equivalent to 7.308 mg of degradation products, calculated as $C_{16}H_{19}N_3O_5S$.

Assay Weigh and powder 20 tablets.

For amoxicillin Dissolve a quantity of the powdered tablets containing the equivalent of 0.1 g of amoxicillin in sufficient *water* to produce 100 ml, filter and dilute 2 ml to 100 ml with *buffered copper sulphate solution pH 5.2*. Transfer 10 ml of the solution to a stoppered test tube, heat in a water bath at 75° for 30 minutes and rapidly cool to room temperature, adjusting the volume if necessary to 10 ml with *water*. Measure the *absorbance* of the resulting solution at the maximum at 320 nm, Appendix II B, using in the reference cell the unheated buffered solution of the substance being examined. Repeat the procedure using 0.12 g of *amoxicillin trihydrate BPCRS* in place of the quantity of powdered tablets. Calculate the content of

$C_{16}H_{19}N_3O_5S$ using the declared content of $C_{16}H_{19}N_3O_5S$ in *amoxicillin trihydrate BPCRS*.

For clavulanic acid Dissolve a quantity of the powdered tablets containing the equivalent of 40 mg of clavulanic acid in 100 ml of *water*, filter and dilute 5 ml to 100 ml with *water*. Pipette two 2-ml quantities of this solution into separate stoppered tubes. To one tube add 10 ml of *imidazole solution*, mix, stopper the tube and immerse in a water bath at 30° for exactly 12 minutes, with occasional swirling. Remove the tubes and cool to 20° (solution A). To the second tube add 10 ml of *water* and mix (solution B) Without delay measure the *absorbances* of solutions A and B at the maximum at 313 nm, Appendix II B, using in the reference cell a mixture of 2 ml of *water* and 10 ml of *imidazole solution* for solution A and *water* for solution B. Calculate the content of $C_8H_9NO_5$ from the difference between the absorbances of solutions A and B, from the difference obtained by repeating the operation using 40 mg of *lithium clavulanate BPCRS* in place of the powdered tablets and from the declared content of $C_8H_9NO_5$ in *lithium clavulanate BPCRS*.

Storage Co-amoxiclav Tablets should be protected from light and stored at a temperature not exceeding 25° in an airtight container.

Labelling The label states the quantity of Amoxicillin Trihydrate, in terms of the equivalent amount of amoxicillin, and the quantity of Potassium Clavulanate, in terms of the equivalent amount of clavulanic acid, in each tablet.

Co-careldopa Tablets

Levodopa and Carbidopa Tablets

Definition Co-careldopa Tablets contain Carbidopa and Levodopa.

With the exception of the requirements for shape, the tablets comply with the requirements stated under Tablets and with the following requirements.

Content of anhydrous carbidopa, $C_{10}H_{14}N_2O_4$ 90.0 to 110.0% of the prescribed or stated amount.

Content of levodopa, $C_9H_{11}NO_4$ 95.0 to 105.0% of the prescribed or stated amount.

Identification

A. In the Assay, the chromatogram obtained with solution (3) exhibits two peaks with the same retention times as those due to carbidopa and levodopa in the chromatogram obtained with solution (1).

B. To a quantity of the powdered tablets containing the equivalent of 1 mg of anhydrous carbidopa add 5 ml of 0.05M *sulphuric acid*, shake for 2 minutes and filter. Add 5 ml of *dimethylaminobenzaldehyde reagent* to the filtrate. A yellow colour is produced.

C. To a quantity of the powdered tablets containing 50 mg of Levodopa add 4 ml of *ethanol (96%)* and 1 ml of 1M *sulphuric acid* and shake for 2 minutes. Add 2 ml of *cinnamaldehyde*, allow to stand for 20 minutes, add 50 ml of 0.1M *hydrochloric acid*, shake for 2 minutes and allow to stand. Filter the aqueous layer obtained and to 5 ml add 0.1 ml of *iron(III) chloride solution R1*. To half of the solution add an excess of 5M *ammonia*; a purple colour is produced. To the remainder add an excess of 2M *sodium hydroxide*; a deep red colour is produced.

Dissolution Comply with the *dissolution test for tablets and capsules*, Appendix XII D, using as the medium 750 ml of 0.1M *hydrochloric acid* and rotating the basket at 50 revolutions per minute. Carry out the method for *liquid chromatography*, Appendix III D, using the following solutions. Solution (1) contains 0.0050% w/v of *levodopa EPCRS* and 0.00054% w/v of *carbidopa BPCRS* in 0.1M *hydrochloric acid*. Use the filtered dissolution medium as solution (2).

The chromatographic procedure may be carried out using (a) a stainless steel column (20 cm × 4 mm) packed with *stationary phase B* (10 μm) (Lichrosorb RP8 is suitable), (b) 0.1M *potassium dihydrogen orthophosphate* adjusted to pH 3.0 with 1M *orthophosphoric acid* as the mobile phase with a flow rate of 1.5 ml per minute and (c) a detection wavelength of 282 nm.

Calculate the content of $C_{10}H_{14}N_2O_4$ and of $C_9H_{11}NO_4$ in the medium using the declared content of $C_{10}H_{14}N_2O_4$ in *carbidopa BPCRS* and taking 100% as the content of $C_9H_{11}NO_4$ in *levodopa EPCRS*.

Assay Carry out the method for *liquid chromatography*, Appendix III D, using the following solutions. Solution (1) contains 0.050% w/v of *levodopa EPCRS*, 0.0054% w/v of *carbidopa BPCRS* and 0.0050% w/v of *methyldopa BPCRS* (internal standard) in 0.1M *hydrochloric acid*. For solution (2) weigh and powder 20 tablets, shake a quantity of the powder containing 0.25 g of Levodopa with 60 ml of 0.1M *hydrochloric acid* for 15 minutes, add sufficient 0.1M *hydrochloric acid* to produce 100 ml and filter. Dilute 10 ml of the clear filtrate to 50 ml with 0.1M *hydrochloric acid*. For solution (3) add 5 ml of a 0.050% w/v solution of the internal standard in 0.1M *hydrochloric acid* to 10 ml of the clear filtrate obtained in the preparation of solution (2) and add sufficient 0.1M *hydrochloric acid* to produce 50 ml.

The chromatographic procedure may be carried out using (a) a stainless steel column (20 cm × 4 mm) packed with *stationary phase B* (10 μm) (Lichrosorb RP8 is suitable), (b) 0.1M *potassium dihydrogen orthophosphate* adjusted to pH 3.0 with 1M *orthophosphoric acid* as the mobile phase with a flow rate of 1.5 ml per minute and (c) a detection wavelength of 282 nm.

Calculate the content of $C_{10}H_{14}N_2O_4$ and of $C_9H_{11}NO_4$ using the declared content of $C_{10}H_{14}N_2O_4$ in *carbidopa BPCRS* and taking 100% as the content of $C_9H_{11}NO_4$ in *levodopa EPCRS*.

Labelling The label states the quantity of Carbidopa, in terms of the equivalent amount of anhydrous carbidopa, and the quantity of Levodopa in each tablet.

Co-codamol Tablets

Codeine Phosphate and Paracetamol Tablets

Definition Co-codamol Tablets contain Codeine Phosphate and Paracetamol.

The tablets comply with the requirements stated under Tablets and with the following requirements.

Content of codeine phosphate, $C_{18}H_{21}NO_3,H_3PO_4,\frac{1}{2}H_2O$ 95.0 to 105.0% of the prescribed or stated amount.

Content of paracetamol, $C_8H_9NO_2$ 95.0 to 105.0% of the prescribed or stated amount.

Identification

A. Shake a quantity of the powdered tablets containing 0.5 g of Paracetamol with 20 ml of *acetone*, filter and evaporate the filtrate to dryness. The *infrared absorption spectrum* of the residue, Appendix II A, is concordant with the *reference spectrum* of paracetamol.

B. Carry out the method for *thin-layer chromatography*, Appendix III A, using a silica gel F_{254} precoated plate (Merck silica gel 60 F_{254} plates are suitable) and a mixture of 90 volumes of *dichloromethane*, 10 volumes of *methanol* and 1 volume of 13.5M *ammonia* as the mobile phase. Apply separately to the plate 10 µl of each of the following solutions. For solution (1) shake a quantity of the powdered tablets containing 24 mg of Codeine Phosphate with 30 ml of *water* for 1 minute and centrifuge. Decant, add 10 ml of 1M *sodium hydroxide* and 30 ml of *chloroform* to the supernatant liquid, shake for 1 minute and filter the chloroform layer through glass-fibre paper (Whatman GF/C is suitable). Solution (2) contains 0.08% w/v of *codeine phosphate BPCRS* in *methanol (50%)*. Solution (3) contains 0.08% w/v each of *codeine phosphate BPCRS* and *dihydrocodeine tartrate BPCRS* in *methanol (50%)*. After removal of the plate, allow it to dry in air, spray with *ethanolic iron(III) chloride solution* and heat at 105° for 10 minutes. The principal spot in the chromatogram obtained with solution (1) corresponds in position and colour to that in the chromatogram obtained with solution (2). The test is not valid unless the chromatogram obtained with solution (3) shows two clearly separated spots of different colours.

C. In the Assay for codeine phosphate, the chromatogram obtained with solution (2) shows a peak with the same retention time as the principal peak in the chromatogram obtained with solution (1).

Dissolution Comply with the *dissolution test for tablets and capsules* with respect to the content of Paracetamol, Appendix XII D, using Apparatus II. Use as the medium 900 ml of *phosphate buffer pH 5.8* and rotate the paddle at 50 revolutions per minute. Withdraw a sample of 20 ml of the medium and filter. Dilute the filtrate with 0.1M *sodium hydroxide* to give a solution expected to contain about 0.00075% w/v of Paracetamol. Measure the *absorbance* of this solution, Appendix II B, at the maximum at 257 nm using 0.1M *sodium hydroxide* in the reference cell. Calculate the total content of paracetamol, $C_8H_9NO_2$ in the medium taking 715 as the value of A (1%, 1 cm) at the maximum at 257 nm.

4-Aminophenol Comply with the test described under Paracetamol Tablets but using the following solutions. Solution (1) contains 0.001% w/v of *4-aminophenol* in the mobile phase. For solution (2) shake a quantity of the powdered tablets containing 0.5 g of Paracetamol with 50 ml of the mobile phase for 10 minutes and filter.

Related substances

A. Carry out the method for *thin-layer chromatography*, Appendix III A, using *silica gel G* as the coating substance and a mixture of 6 volumes of 13.5M *ammonia*, 30 volumes of *cyclohexane* and 72 volumes of *absolute ethanol* as the mobile phase. Apply separately to the plate 20 µl of each of the following solutions. For solution (1) shake a quantity of the powdered tablets containing 50 mg of Codeine Phosphate with 50 ml of 0.1M *hydrochloric acid* for 10 minutes and filter. Make the filtrate alkaline with 5M *sodium hydroxide* and extract with two 40-ml quantities of *chloroform*. Wash the combined extracts with 10 ml of *water*, filter through a layer of *anhydrous sodium sulphate* on an absorbent cotton plug moistened with *chloroform*, evaporate the filtrate to dryness at a temperature not exceeding 45° using a rotary evaporator and dissolve the residue in 2 ml of *chloroform*. For solution (2) dilute 1.5 volumes of solution (1) to 100 volumes with *chloroform*. For solution (3) dilute 1 volume of solution (1) to 100 volumes with *chloroform*. After removal of the plate, allow it to dry in air and spray with *potassium iodobismuthate solution*. Any *secondary spot* in the chromatogram obtained with solution (1) is not more intense than the spot in the chromatogram obtained with solution (2) (1.5%) and not more than one such spot with an Rf value higher than that of the principal spot is more intense than the spot in the chromatogram obtained with solution (3) (1%).

B. Comply with the test for Related substances described under Paracetamol Tablets.

Uniformity of content Tablets containing less than 2% of Codeine Phosphate comply with the requirements stated under Tablets, with respect to the content of Codeine Phosphate, using the following method of analysis. Carry out the method for *liquid chromatography*, Appendix III D, using the following solutions. Solution (1) contains 0.004% w/v of *codeine phosphate BPCRS* in *methanol (25%)*. For solution (2) add 50 ml of *methanol* to one tablet and mix with the aid of ultrasound until completely dispersed. Add 100 ml of *water*, shake for 10 minutes, dilute to 200 ml with *water*, filter through glass-fibre paper (Whatman GF/C is suitable) and use the filtrate.

The chromatographic procedure may be carried out using (a) a stainless steel column (10 cm × 4.6 mm) packed with *stationary phase C* (5 µm) (Nucleosil C18 is suitable), (b) as the mobile phase with a flow rate of 1.5 ml per minute 0.01M *sodium pentanesulphonate* in a mixture of 78 volumes of *water* and 22 volumes of *methanol*, the pH of the solution being adjusted to 2.8 using 2M *hydrochloric acid*, and (c) a detection wavelength of 220 nm.

Calculate the content of $C_{18}H_{21}NO_3,H_3PO_4,\frac{1}{2}H_2O$ in each tablet using the declared content of $C_{18}H_{21}NO_3,H_3PO_4,\frac{1}{2}H_2O$ in *codeine phosphate BPCRS*.

Assay

For codeine phosphate Weigh and powder 20 tablets. Carry out the method for *liquid chromatography*, Appendix III D, using the following solutions. Solution (1) contains 0.004% w/v of *codeine phosphate BPCRS* in *methanol (25%)*. For solution (2) shake a quantity of the powdered tablets containing 8 mg of Codeine Phosphate with 50 ml of *methanol* for 1 minute, add 100 ml of *water*, shake for 10 minutes, dilute to 200 ml with *water*, filter through glass-fibre paper (Whatman GF/C is suitable) and use the filtrate.

The chromatographic conditions described under Uniformity of content may be used.

Calculate the content of $C_{18}H_{21}NO_3,H_3PO_4,\frac{1}{2}H_2O$ using the declared content of $C_{18}H_{21}NO_3,H_3PO_4,\frac{1}{2}H_2O$ in *codeine phosphate BPCRS*.

For paracetamol Carry out the method for *liquid chromatography*, Appendix III D, using the following solutions. Solution (1) contains 0.005% w/v of *paracetamol BPCRS* in *water*. For solution (2) shake a quantity of the powdered tablets containing 500 mg of Paracetamol with 50 ml of *methanol* for 1 minute, add 100 ml of *water*, shake for 10 minutes, dilute to 200 ml with water, filter through glass-fibre paper (Whatman GF/C is suitable) and dilute 5 ml of the filtrate to 250 ml with *water*.

The chromatographic conditions described under Uniformity of content may be used but with a detection wavelength of 243 nm.

Calculate the content of $C_8H_9NO_2$ using the declared content of $C_8H_9NO_2$ in *paracetamol BPCRS*.

Labelling The label states the quantities of Codeine Phosphate and of Paracetamol in each tablet.

When Co-codamol Tablets are prescribed or demanded no strength being stated, tablets containing 8 mg of Codeine Phosphate and 500 mg of Paracetamol shall be dispensed or supplied.

Co-codaprin Tablets

Aspirin and Codeine Tablets

Definition Co-codaprin Tablets contain Codeine Phosphate and Aspirin in the proportions, by weight, 1 part to 50 parts.

The tablets comply with the requirements stated under Tablets and with the following requirements.

Content of codeine phosphate, $C_{18}H_{21}NO_3,H_3PO_4,½H_2O$ 90.0 to 110.0% of the prescribed or stated amount.

Content of aspirin, $C_9H_8O_4$ 95.0 to 105.0% of the prescribed or stated amount.

Identification

A. Boil 1 g of the powdered tablets with 10 ml of 1M *sodium hydroxide*, cool and filter. Acidify the filtrate with 1M *sulphuric acid*; a white precipitate is produced. To a solution of the precipitate add *iron(III) chloride solution R1*; a deep violet colour is produced.

B. Shake 1 g of the powdered tablets with a mixture of 20 ml of *water* and 1 ml of 1M *sulphuric acid* for 5 minutes and filter. Reserve the residue for test C. The filtrate yields the reactions characteristic of *phosphates*, Appendix VI. Make the remainder of the filtrate alkaline with 5M *ammonia*, extract with *chloroform*, separate the chloroform layer and evaporate the chloroform. Place a small quantity of the residue on the surface of a drop of *nitric acid*; a yellow but no red colour is produced.

C. Dissolve 0.1 g of the residue obtained in test B in 1 ml of *sulphuric acid*, add 0.05 ml of *iron(III) chloride solution R1* or 0.05 ml of *ammonium molybdate—sulphuric acid solution* and warm gently. A bluish violet colour is produced which changes to red on the addition of 0.05 ml of 2M *nitric acid*.

Dissolution Comply with the *dissolution test for tablets and capsules* with respect to the content of Aspirin, Appendix XII D, using Apparatus II. Use as the medium 500 ml of a pH 4.5 buffer prepared by mixing 29.9 g of *sodium acetate* and 16.6 ml of *glacial acetic acid* with sufficient *water* to produce 10 litres and rotate the paddle at 50 revolutions per minute. Withdraw a sample of 20 ml of the medium and filter. Immediately measure the *absorbance* of the filtrate, Appendix II B, diluted with the dissolution medium if necessary, at 265 nm using dissolution medium in the reference cell. Measure the *absorbance* of a suitable solution of *aspirin BPCRS* in the dissolution medium and calculate the total content of aspirin, $C_9H_8O_4$, in the medium using the declared content of $C_9H_8O_4$ in *aspirin BPCRS*.

Foreign alkaloids Carry out the method for *thin-layer chromatography*, Appendix III A, using *silica gel G* as the coating substance and a mixture of 6 volumes of 13.5M *ammonia*, 30 volumes of *cyclohexane* and 72 volumes of *absolute ethanol* as the mobile phase. Apply separately to the plate 20 µl of each of the following solutions. For solution (1) shake a quantity of the powdered tablets containing 50 mg of Codeine Phosphate with 50 ml of 0.1M *hydrochloric acid*, filter and make the filtrate alkaline with 5M *sodium hydroxide*. Extract with two 40-ml quantities of *chloroform* and wash the combined extracts with 10 ml of *water*. Filter through a layer of *anhydrous sodium sulphate* on an absorbent cotton plug moistened with *chloroform*. Evaporate the filtrate to dryness and dissolve the residue in 2 ml of *chloroform*. For solution (2) dilute 1.5 volumes of solution (1) to 100 volumes with *chloroform*. For solution (3) dilute 1 volume of solution (1) to 100 volumes with *chloroform*. After removal of the plate, allow it to dry in air and spray with *potassium iodobismuthate solution*. Any *secondary spot* in the chromatogram obtained with solution (1) is not more intense than the spot in the chromatogram obtained with solution (2) (1.5%) and not more than one such spot with an Rf value higher than that of the principal spot is more intense than the spot in the chromatogram obtained with solution (3) (1%).

Salicylic acid To a quantity of the powdered tablets containing 0.50 g of Aspirin add 50 ml of *chloroform* and 10 ml of *water*, shake well and allow to separate. Filter the chloroform layer through a dry filter paper and evaporate 10 ml of the filtrate to dryness at room temperature using a rotary evaporator. To the residue add 4 ml of *ethanol (96%)*, stir well, dilute to 100 ml with *water* at a temperature not exceeding 10°, filter immediately and rapidly transfer 50 ml to a *Nessler cylinder*. Add 1 ml of freshly prepared *ammonium iron(III) sulphate solution R1*, mix and allow to stand for 1 minute. Any violet colour produced is not more intense than that obtained by adding 1 ml of freshly prepared *ammonium iron(III) sulphate solution R1* to a mixture of 3 ml of a freshly prepared 0.010% w/v solution of *salicylic acid*, 2 ml of *ethanol (96%)* and sufficient *water* to produce 50 ml contained in a second *Nessler cylinder* (0.6%).

Assay Weigh and powder 20 tablets.

For codeine phosphate To a quantity of the powder containing 24 mg of Codeine Phosphate add 5 ml of 5M *sodium hydroxide* and 15 ml of *water*, shake for 2 minutes and extract with three 50-ml quantities of *chloroform*. Wash each extract with the same 10 ml of *water*, filter through absorbent cotton previously moistened with *chloroform* and evaporate the combined extracts to about 60 ml on a water bath in a current of air. Cool, add 25 ml of *water*, 5 ml of *acetate buffer pH 2.8* and 5 ml of *dimethyl yellow—oracet blue B solution* and titrate with 0.01M *dioctyl sodium sulphosuccinate VS* with vigorous swirling until near the end point, then add the titrant dropwise and, after each addition, swirl vigorously, allow to separate and swirl gently for 5 seconds. The end point is indicated by the appearance of a permanent pinkish grey colour in the chloroform layer. Repeat the operation without the powdered tablets. The difference between the titrations represents the amount of dioctyl sodium sulphosuccinate required.

Calculate the content of $C_{18}H_{21}NO_3,H_3PO_4,½H_2O$ using the result obtained by dissolving 40 mg of *codeine phosphate BPCRS* in 25 ml of *water* and 5 ml of *acetate buffer pH 2.8*, adding 60 ml of *chloroform* and 5 ml of *dimethyl yellow—oracet blue B solution*, shaking well to dissolve the codeine phosphate and completing the method described above beginning at the words 'and titrate...'.

For aspirin To a quantity of the powder containing 0.8 g of Aspirin add 20 ml of *water* and 2 g of *sodium citrate* and boil under a reflux condenser for 30 minutes. Cool, wash the condenser with 30 ml of warm *water* and titrate with 0.5M *sodium hydroxide VS* using *phenolphthalein solution R1* as indicator. Each ml of 0.5M *sodium hydroxide VS* is equivalent to 45.04 mg of $C_9H_8O_4$.

Storage Co-codaprin Tablets should be protected from light.

Labelling The label states (1) that the tablets contain Aspirin, unless this word appears in the name of the tablets (this requirement does not apply in countries where exclusive proprietary rights in the name Aspirin are claimed); (2) the quantities of Codeine Phosphate and of Aspirin in each tablet.

Dispersible Co-codaprin Tablets

Dispersible Aspirin and Codeine Tablets

Definition Dispersible Co-codaprin Tablets contain Codeine Phosphate and Aspirin in the proportions, by weight, 1 part to 50 parts in a suitable dispersible basis.

The tablets comply with the requirements stated under Tablets and with the following requirements.

Content of codeine phosphate, $C_{18}H_{21}NO_3,H_3PO_4,½H_2O$ 90.0 to 110.0% of the prescribed or stated amount.

Content of aspirin, $C_9H_8O_4$ 95.0 to 105.0% of the prescribed or stated amount.

Identification

A. Effervesce on the addition of *water.*

B. Comply with the tests for Identification described under Co-codaprin Tablets.

Salicylic acid To a quantity of the powdered tablets containing 0.50 g of Aspirin add 50 ml of *chloroform* and a mixture of 2 ml of 1M *hydrochloric acid* and 8 ml of *water* and complete the test for Salicylic acid described under Co-codaprin Tablets beginning at the words 'shake well...'.

Assay Weigh and powder 20 tablets.

For codeine phosphate To a quantity of the powder containing 16 mg of Codeine Phosphate add 20 ml of *water* and 1 g of *disodium edetate*, swirl gently until effervescence ceases, shake to dissolve and carry out the Assay for codeine phosphate described under Co-codaprin Tablets beginning at the words 'add 5 ml of 5M *sodium hydroxide...*'.

For aspirin To a quantity of the powder containing 0.8 g of Aspirin add 15 ml of *water* and swirl until effervescence ceases. Add 5 ml of 0.5M *sulphuric acid* and extract with 50 ml of *ether* followed by three 30-ml quantities of *ether.* Wash the combined extracts with 10 ml of *water*, filter through absorbent cotton previously moistened with *ether*, washing the separating funnel and filter with *ether.* Evaporate the ether in a water bath at 30° in a current of air. Dissolve the residue in 5 ml of *acetone* and evaporate in a water bath at 30°; again dissolve the residue in 5 ml of *acetone* and evaporate in a water bath at 30°. Dissolve the residue in 25 ml of *ethanol (96%)* previously neutralised to *phenol red solution* and titrate with 0.1M *sodium hydroxide VS* using *phenol red solution* as indicator. Each ml of 0.1M *sodium hydroxide VS* is equivalent to 18.02 mg of $C_9H_8O_4$.

Storage Dispersible Co-codaprin Tablets should be protected from light.

Labelling The label states (1) that the tablets contain Aspirin, unless this word appears in the name of the tablets (this requirement does not apply in countries where exclusive proprietary rights in the name Aspirin are claimed); (2) the quantities of Codeine Phosphate and of Aspirin in each tablet; (3) that the tablets should be dispersed in water immediately before use.

Co-danthrusate Capsules

Dantron and Docusate Sodium Capsules

Definition Co-danthrusate Capsules contain Dantron and Docusate Sodium in the proportions, by weight, 5 parts to 6 parts.

The capsules comply with the requirements stated under Capsules and with the following requirements.

Content of dantron, $C_{14}H_8O_4$ 90.0 to 110.0% of the prescribed or stated amount.

Content of docusate sodium, $C_{20}H_{37}NaO_7S$ 90.0 to 110.0% of the prescribed or stated amount.

Identification

A. Carry out the method for *thin-layer chromatography*, Appendix III A, using a silica gel F_{254} precoated plate (Merck silica gel 60 F_{254} plates are suitable) and a mixture of 85 volumes of *ethyl acetate* and 15 volumes of *methanol* as the mobile phase. Apply separately to the plate 10 µl of each of the following solutions. For solution (1) shake a quantity of the contents of the capsules containing 50 mg of Dantron with 10 ml of *chloroform*, filter and dilute 2 ml of the filtrate to 20 ml with *chloroform.* Solution (2) contains 0.06% w/v of *docusate sodium BPCRS* in *chloroform.* Solution (3) contains 0.05% w/v of *dantron BPCRS* in *chloroform.* After removal of the plate, allow it to dry in air, spray with *ethanolic sulphuric acid (10%)* and heat at 120° for 15 minutes. The two principal spots in the chromatogram obtained with solution (1) correspond to the principal spots in the chromatograms obtained with solutions (2) and (3).

B. Shake a quantity of the contents of the capsules containing 60 mg of Docusate Sodium with 50 ml of *water.* To 5 ml of this mixture add 1 ml of 2M *sulphuric acid*, 10 ml of *chloroform* and 0.2 ml of *dimethyl yellow solution* and mix; a red colour is produced in the chloroform layer. Add 50 mg of *cetrimide* and mix; the chloroform layer is yellow.

C. To a quantity of the contents of the capsules containing 50 mg of Dantron add 10 ml of *chloroform* and 5 ml of 1M *ammonia* and mix. A red colour is produced in the aqueous layer.

Related substances Complies with the test described under Dantron but using the following solutions. For solution (1) dilute 1 volume of solution (2) to 50 volumes with the mobile phase. For solution (2) shake a quantity of the mixed contents of 20 capsules containing 50 mg of Dantron with 20 ml of *tetrahydrofuran* for 5 minutes and dilute to 100 ml with the mobile phase. For solution (3) dissolve 50 mg of *dantron impurity standard BPCRS* in 20 ml of *tetrahydrofuran* and dilute to 100 ml with the mobile phase. In the evaluation of the chromatogram obtained with solution (2) disregard any peak with a retention time less than one third of that of the principal peak.

Assay

For dantron To a quantity of the mixed contents of 20 capsules containing 35 mg of Dantron add 50 ml of *absolute ethanol*, heat on a water bath for 30 minutes and cool. Add sufficient *absolute ethanol* to produce 100 ml and filter through glass-fibre paper (Whatman GF/C is suitable). Dilute 5 ml of the filtrate to 100 ml with *absolute ethanol* and measure the *absorbance* of the resulting solution at the maximum at 430 nm, Appendix II B. Calculate the content of $C_{14}H_8O_4$ taking 458 as the value of A (1%, 1 cm) at the maximum at 430 nm.

For docusate sodium To a quantity of the mixed contents of 20 capsules containing 0.3 g of Docusate Sodium add 25 ml of *absolute ethanol*, heat to 60° for 5 minutes and cool. Add sufficient *water* to produce 200 ml and filter through glass-fibre paper (Whatman GF/C is suitable). To 25 ml of the filtrate add 10 ml of *water* and 15 ml of *chloroform* and titrate with *0.004M benzethonium chloride VS*, using *dimidium bromide—sulphan blue mixed solution* as indicator, to the first appearance of a green colour in the chloroform layer and shaking vigorously towards the end point. Each ml of *0.004M benzethonium chloride VS* is equivalent to 1.778 mg of $C_{20}H_{37}NaO_7S$.

Labelling The label states the quantities of Dantron and of Docusate Sodium in each capsule.

Codeine Linctus

Definition Codeine Linctus is an *oral solution* containing 0.3% w/v of Codeine Phosphate or an equivalent concentration of Codeine Phosphate Sesquihydrate in a suitable flavoured vehicle.

The title 'Diabetic Codeine Linctus' may be used for a preparation that complies with the requirements of this monograph and that is formulated with a vehicle appropriate for administration to diabetics.

The linctus complies with the requirements stated under Oral Liquids and with the following requirements.

Content of codeine phosphate $C_{18}H_{21}NO_3,H_3PO_4,$ ½H_2O 0.285 to 0.315% w/v.

Identification To 20 ml add 20 ml of *water* and 30 ml of *chloroform*, shake and discard the chloroform layer. To the aqueous layer add 10 ml of 1M *sodium hydroxide* and extract with 30 ml of *chloroform*. Wash the chloroform layer with two 10-ml quantities of 0.1M *sodium hydroxide* followed by 10 ml of *water*. Dry the chloroform layer with *anhydrous sodium sulphate*, filter, evaporate the filtrate to dryness and dry the residue at 60°. The *infrared absorption spectrum* of the residue, Appendix II A, is concordant with the *reference spectrum* of codeine.

Related substances Carry out the method for *thin-layer chromatography*, Appendix III A, using a silica gel precoated plate (Merck silica gel 60 plates are suitable) and a mixture of 72 volumes of *ethanol (96%)*, 30 volumes of *cyclohexane* and 6 volumes of 13.5M *ammonia* as the mobile phase. Apply separately to the plate 10 µl of each of the following solutions. For solution (1) add 20 ml of *water* and 2 ml of 13.5M *ammonia* to 20 ml of the preparation being examined and extract with two 20-ml quantities of *chloroform*. Dry the combined extracts with *anhydrous sodium sulphate*, filter, evaporate the filtrate to dryness and dissolve the residue in 1 ml of *chloroform*. For solution (2) dilute 1.5 volumes of solution (1) to 100 volumes with *chloroform*. For solution (3) dilute 1 volume of solution (1) to 100 volumes with *chloroform*. After removal of the plate, allow it to dry in air and spray with *potassium iodobismuthate solution*. Any *secondary spot* in the chromatogram obtained with solution (1) is not more intense than the spot in the chromatogram obtained with solution (2) and not more than one such spot with an Rf value higher than that of the principal spot is more intense than the spot in the chromatogram obtained with solution (3).

Assay Carry out the method for *liquid chromatography*, Appendix III D, using the following solutions. Solution (1) contains 0.06% w/v of *codeine phosphate BPCRS* in *water*. For solution (2) mix a quantity of the preparation being examined containing 15 mg of codeine phosphate with sufficient *water* to produce 25 ml.

The chromatographic procedure may be carried out using (a) a stainless steel column (20 cm × 4.6 mm) packed with *stationary phase C* (5 µm) (Nucleosil C18 is suitable), (b) as the mobile phase with a flow rate of 1 ml per minute 0.01M *sodium octanesulphonate* in a mixture of 55 volumes of *water*, 45 volumes of *methanol* and 1 volume of *glacial acetic acid* and (c) a detection wavelength of 285 nm.

A large peak due to sodium benzoate may be present. If this peak interferes with the peak due to codeine phosphate adjust the chromatographic conditions to achieve a satisfactory separation. An increase in the content of water in the mobile phase or an increase in the concentration of sodium octanesulphonate will increase the retention time of the peak due to codeine phosphate relative to that of the peak due to sodium benzoate.

Determine the *weight per ml* of the linctus, Appendix V G, and calculate the content of $C_{18}H_{21}NO_3,H_3PO_4,$ ½H_2O, weight in volume, using the declared content of $C_{18}H_{21}NO_3,H_3PO_4,$½$H_2O$ in *codeine phosphate BPCRS*.

Storage Codeine Linctus should be protected from light.

Labelling The label indicates the pharmaceutical form as 'oral solution'.

When Diabetic Codeine Linctus is prescribed or demanded, Codeine Linctus formulated with a vehicle appropriate for administration to diabetics, whether or not labelled 'Diabetic Codeine Linctus', shall be dispensed or supplied.

Paediatric Codeine Linctus

Definition Paediatric Codeine Linctus is an *oral solution* containing 0.06% w/v of Codeine Phosphate or an equivalent concentration of Codeine Phosphate Sesquihydrate in a suitable flavoured vehicle.

Extemporaneous preparation It may be prepared by diluting Codeine Linctus with a suitable vehicle in accordance with the manufacturer's instructions.

The linctus complies with the requirements stated under Oral Liquids and with the following requirements.

Content of codeine phosphate $C_{18}H_{21}NO_3,H_3PO_4,\frac{1}{2}H_2O$ 0.057 to 0.063% w/v.

Identification To 50 ml add 20 ml of *water* and 30 ml of *chloroform*, shake and discard the chloroform layer. To the aqueous layer add 10 ml of 1M *sodium hydroxide* and extract with 30 ml of *chloroform*. Wash the chloroform layer with two 10-ml quantities of 0.1M *sodium hydroxide* followed by 10 ml of *water*. Dry the chloroform layer with *anhydrous sodium sulphate*, filter, evaporate the filtrate to dryness and dry the residue at 60°. The *infrared absorption spectrum* of the residue, Appendix II A, is concordant with the *reference spectrum* of codeine.

Related substances Complies with the test described under Codeine Linctus, applying to the plate 20 µl of each of the following solutions. For solution (1) add 20 ml of *water* and 2 ml of 13.5M *ammonia* to 40 ml of the linctus and extract with two 20-ml quantities of *chloroform*. Dry the combined extracts with *anhydrous sodium sulphate*, filter, evaporate the filtrate to dryness and dissolve the residue in 1 ml of *chloroform*. For solution (2) dilute 1.5 volumes of solution (1) to 100 volumes with *chloroform*. For solution (3) dilute 1 volume of solution (1) to 100 volumes with *chloroform*.

Assay Carry out the Assay described under Codeine Linctus using the following solutions. Solution (1) contains 0.012% w/v of *codeine phosphate BPCRS* in *water*. For solution (2) mix a quantity of the linctus containing 3 mg of codeine phosphate with sufficient *water* to produce 25 ml.

Storage Paediatric Codeine Linctus should be protected from light.

Labelling The label indicates the pharmaceutical form as 'oral solution'.

Codeine Phosphate Oral Solution

Definition Codeine Phosphate Oral Solution is a solution containing 0.5% w/v of Codeine Phosphate or an equivalent concentration of Codeine Phosphate Sesquihydrate in a suitable flavoured vehicle.

Extemporaneous preparation The following formula and directions apply.

Codeine Phosphate	5 g
Water	15 ml
Chloroform Spirit	25 ml
Syrup	sufficient to produce 1000 ml

Dissolve the Codeine Phosphate in the Water, add 750 ml of the Syrup and mix. Add the Chloroform Spirit and sufficient of the Syrup to produce 1000 ml and mix. It should be recently prepared.

The oral solution complies with the requirements stated under Oral Liquids and with the following requirements.

Content of codeine phosphate $C_{18}H_{21}NO_3,H_3PO_4,\frac{1}{2}H_2O$ 0.475 to 0.525% w/v.

Identification; Related substances Complies with the requirements stated under Codeine Linctus.

Assay Carry out the Assay described under Codeine Linctus.

Storage Codeine Phosphate Oral Solution should be protected from light.

Codeine Phosphate Tablets

Definition Codeine Phosphate Tablets contain Codeine Phosphate or Codeine Phosphate Sesquihydrate.

The tablets comply with the requirements stated under Tablets and with the following requirements.

Content of codeine phosphate, $C_{18}H_{21}NO_3,H_3PO_4,\frac{1}{2}H_2O$ 92.5 to 107.5% of the prescribed or stated amount.

Identification

A. Macerate a quantity of the powdered tablets containing 50 mg of Codeine Phosphate or its equivalent with 5 ml of 1M *sulphuric acid* and 15 ml of *water*. Filter, make alkaline with 5M *ammonia*, extract with successive quantities of *chloroform* and evaporate the chloroform extracts on a water bath. Place a few mg of the residue, in powder, on the surface of a drop of *nitric acid*. A yellow but no red colour is produced (distinction from morphine).

B. Heat 10 mg of the residue obtained in test A on a water bath with 1 ml of *sulphuric acid* and 0.05 ml of *iron(III) chloride solution R1*. A blue colour is produced which changes to red on the addition of 0.05 ml of *nitric acid*.

C. Extract the powdered tablets with *water* and filter. The filtrate yields reaction B characteristic of *phosphates*, Appendix VI.

Foreign alkaloids Carry out the method for *thin-layer chromatography*, Appendix III A, using *silica gel G* as the coating substance and a mixture of 6 volumes of 13.5M *ammonia*, 30 volumes of *cyclohexane* and 72 volumes of *absolute ethanol* as the mobile phase. Apply separately to the plate 20 µl of each of the following solutions. For solution (1) shake a quantity of the powdered tablets containing 0.25 g of Codeine Phosphate or its equivalent with 10 ml of a mixture of 4 volumes of 0.01M *hydrochloric acid* and 1 volume of *absolute ethanol* for 15 minutes and filter. For solution (2) dilute 1.5 volumes of solution (1) to 100 volumes with a mixture of 4 volumes of 0.01M *hydrochloric acid* and 1 volume of *absolute ethanol*. For solution (3) dilute 1 volume of solution (1) to 100 volumes with a mixture of 4 volumes of 0.01M *hydrochloric acid* and 1 volume of *absolute ethanol*. After removal of the plate, allow it to dry in air and spray with *potassium iodobismuthate solution*. Any *secondary spot* in the chromatogram obtained with solution (1) is not more intense than the spot in the chromatogram obtained with solution (2) (1.5%) and not more than one such spot with an Rf value higher than that of the principal spot is more intense than the spot in the chromatogram obtained with solution (3) (1%).

Assay Weigh and powder 20 tablets. Dissolve a quantity of the powder containing 0.3 g of Codeine Phosphate or its equivalent as completely as possible in 20 ml of 0.25M *sulphuric acid*, filter and wash the residue on the filter with 0.25M *sulphuric acid* until *complete extraction* of the alkaloid is effected, Appendix XI G. Make alkaline with 5M *ammonia* and extract with successive quantities of *chloroform* until *complete extraction* of the alkaloid is effected. Wash each chloroform solution with the same 10 ml of *water* and evaporate the chloroform. To the residue add 5 ml of *ethanol (96%)* previously neutralised to *methyl red solution* and remove the ethanol by evaporation. Dissolve the residue in 1 ml of neutralised *ethanol (96%)*, add 10 ml of 0.1M *hydrochloric acid VS* and 10 ml of *water* and titrate with 0.1M *sodium hydroxide VS* using *methyl red solution* as indicator. Each ml of 0.1M *hydrochloric acid VS* is equivalent to 40.64 mg of $C_{18}H_{21}NO_3,H_3PO_4,\frac{1}{2}H_2O$.

Storage Codeine Phosphate Tablets should be protected from light.

Labelling When the active ingredient is Codeine Phosphate Sesquihydrate, the quantity is stated in terms of the equivalent amount of Codeine Phosphate.

Co-dergocrine Tablets

Definition Co-dergocrine Tablets contain Co-dergocrine Mesilate.

The tablets comply with the requirements stated under Tablets and with the following requirements.

Content of co-dergocrine mesilate 90.0 to 110.0% of the prescribed or stated amount.

Identification

A. In the Assay, the chromatogram obtained with solution (2) shows four major peaks with retention times corresponding to the peaks due to co-dergocrine mesilate in the chromatogram obtained with solution (1).

B. To a quantity of the powdered tablets containing 10 mg of Co-dergocrine Mesilate add 1 ml of *methanol* and 5 ml of a 1% w/v solution of *(+)-tartaric acid.* Stir for 15 minutes and filter through sintered glass (BS porosity No. 4). To 1 ml of the filtrate add slowly 2 ml of *dimethylaminobenzaldehyde solution R6* and mix. A deep blue colour is produced.

Related substances Carry out the method described under Co-dergocrine Mesilate, but applying 20 µl of each of the following solutions prepared immediately before use in a mixture of 9 volumes of *chloroform* and 1 volume of *methanol.* Solutions (1) and (2) contain 0.0040% w/v and 0.0010% w/v respectively of *dihydroergocristine mesilate BPCRS.* For solution (3) shake a sufficient quantity of the powdered tablets with the same solvent mixture to produce a solution containing 0.20% w/v of Co-dergocrine Mesilate, filter and use the filtrate. Any *secondary spot* in the chromatogram obtained with solution (3) is not more intense than the spot in the chromatogram obtained with solution (1) and not more than one such spot is more intense than the spot in the chromatogram obtained with solution (2). Disregard any spot remaining on the line of application.

Dissolution Carry out the *dissolution test for tablets and capsules*, Appendix XII D, protecting all solutions from light. Use as the medium 500 ml of 0.1M *hydrochloric acid* and rotate the basket at 120 revolutions per minute. Withdraw a sample of 20 ml of the medium and filter, discarding the first 10 ml of the filtrate. Measure the *fluorescence* of the solution, Appendix II E, using an excitation wavelength of 285 nm and an emission wavelength of 350 nm using 0.1M *hydrochloric acid* to set the instrument to zero. Measure the *fluorescence* of a solution of *co-dergocrine mesilate BPCRS* in 0.1M *hydrochloric acid* containing the equivalent amount of co-dergocrine mesilate as that expected in the test solution. Carry out the measurements as quickly as possible.

Calculate the total content of co-dergocrine mesilate in the medium from the absorbances obtained.

Uniformity of content Tablets containing less than 2 mg of Co-dergocrine Mesilate comply with the requirements stated under Tablets using the following method of analysis. Carry out the following procedure protected from light. Shake one tablet for 30 minutes with sufficient of a 1.0% w/v solution of *(+)-tartaric acid* to produce a solution containing 0.006% w/v of Co-dergocrine Mesilate and filter through sintered glass (BS porosity No. 4). To 3 ml of the filtrate add 6 ml of *dimethylaminobenzaldehyde solution R6*, mix, cool to room temperature and allow to stand for exactly 30 minutes. Measure the *absorbance* of the resulting solution at the maximum at 580 nm, Appendix II B, using in the reference cell a solution prepared by treating 3 ml of a 1.0% w/v solution of *(+)-tartaric acid* and 6 ml of *dimethylaminobenzaldehyde solution R6* in the same manner. Prepare a 0.006% w/v solution of *co-dergocrine mesilate BPCRS* in a 1.0% w/v solution of *(+)-tartaric acid*; to 3 ml of this solution add 6 ml of *dimethylaminobenzaldehyde solution R6* and complete the operation described above, beginning at the words 'mix, cool...'. From the absorbances so obtained calculate the content of co-dergocrine mesilate in the tablet.

Assay Carry out the method described under Co-dergocrine Mesilate, but prepare solution (2) as follows. Use a sufficient number of whole tablets to produce a final solution containing 0.06% w/v of Co-dergocrine Mesilate. Stir the tablets for 15 minutes with 50 ml of a mixture of 2 volumes of a 1.0% w/v solution of *(+)-tartaric acid* and 1 volume of *absolute ethanol*, filter through sintered glass (BS porosity No. 4), wash the filter with three 10-ml quantities of the solvent mixture and dilute the combined filtrate and washings to 100 ml with the same solvent mixture. Calculate the percentage content of the methanesulphonates of dihydroergocornine, of dihydroergocryptine (α- and β-forms) and of dihydroergocristine with reference to the sum of these components in solution (2), using the products of the molecular weights and peak area figures obtained as stated under Co-dergocrine Mesilate. Calculate the content of co-dergocrine mesilate, but defining w_s as the declared content of Co-dergocrine Mesilate in each tablet multiplied by the number of tablets used.

Storage Co-dergocrine Tablets should be protected from light.

Co-dydramol Tablets

Dihydrocodeine and Paracetamol Tablets

Definition Co-dydramol Tablets contain Dihydrocodeine Tartrate and Paracetamol in the proportions, by weight, 1 part to 50 parts.

The tablets comply with the requirements stated under Tablets and with the following requirements.

Content of dihydrocodeine tartrate, $C_{18}H_{23}NO_3,C_4H_6O_6$ 95.0 to 105.0% of the prescribed or stated amount.

Content of paracetamol, $C_8H_9NO_2$ 95.0 to 105.0% of the prescribed or stated amount.

Identification

A. Shake a quantity of the powdered tablets containing 0.5 g of Paracetamol with 20 ml of *acetone*, filter and evaporate the filtrate to dryness. The *infrared absorption spectrum* of the residue, Appendix II A, is concordant with the *reference spectrum* of paracetamol.

B. Carry out the method for *thin-layer chromatography*, Appendix III A, using a silica gel F_{254} precoated plate (Merck silica gel 60 F_{254} plates are suitable) and a mixture of 90 volumes of *dichloromethane*, 10 volumes of *methanol* and 1 volume of 13.5M *ammonia* as the mobile phase. Apply separately to the plate 10 µl of each of the following solutions. For solution (1) shake a quantity of the powdered tablets containing 30 mg of Dihydrocodeine Tartrate with 10 ml of *water* for 1 minute and centrifuge. Decant, add 10 ml of 1M *sodium hydroxide* and 30 ml of *chloroform* to the supernatant liquid, shake for 1 minute and filter the chloroform layer through glass-fibre paper (Whatman GF/C is suitable). Solution (2) contains 0.1% w/v of *dihydrocodeine tartrate BPCRS* in *methanol (50%)*. Solution (3) contains 0.1% w/v of *codeine phosphate BPCRS* in *methanol (50%)*. Solution (4) is a mixture of equal volumes of solutions (2) and (3). After removal of the plate, allow it to dry in air, spray with *ethanolic iron(III) chloride solution* and heat at 105° for 10 minutes. The principal spot in the chromatogram obtained with solution (1) corresponds in position and colour to that in the chromatogram obtained with solution (2). The test is not valid unless the chromatogram obtained with solution (4) shows two clearly separated spots of different colours.

C. In the Assay for dihydrocodeine tartrate, the chromatogram obtained with solution (2) shows a peak with the same retention time as the principal peak in the chromatogram obtained with solution (1).

Dissolution Comply with the *dissolution test for tablets and capsules* with respect to the content of Paracetamol, Appendix XII D, using Apparatus II. Use as the medium 900 ml of *phosphate buffer pH 5.8* and rotate the paddle at 50 revolutions per minute. Withdraw a sample of 20 ml of the medium and filter. Dilute the filtrate with 0.1M *sodium hydroxide* to give a solution expected to contain about 0.00075% w/v of Paracetamol. Measure the *absorbance* of this solution, Appendix II B, at the maximum at 257 nm using 0.1M *sodium hydroxide* in the reference cell. Calculate the total content of paracetamol, $C_8H_9NO_2$, in the medium taking 715 as the value of A(1%, 1 cm) at the maximum at 257 nm.

4-Aminophenol Comply with the test described under Paracetamol Tablets but using the following solutions. Solution (1) contains 0.001% w/v of *4-aminophenol* in the mobile phase. For solution (2) shake a quantity of the powdered tablets containing 0.5 g of Paracetamol with 50 ml of the mobile phase for 10 minutes and filter.

Related substances

A. Carry out the method for *thin-layer chromatography*, Appendix III A, using *silica gel GF_{254}* as the coating substance and a mixture of 1 volume of 13.5M *ammonia*, 10 volumes of *methanol* and 90 volumes of *dichloromethane* as the mobile phase. Apply separately to the plate 20 µl of each of the following solutions. For solution (1) shake a quantity of the powdered tablets containing 50 mg of Dihydrocodeine Tartrate with 0.5M *hydrochloric acid*, filter, make the filtrate alkaline with 5M *sodium hydroxide* and extract with four 25-ml quantities of *chloroform*. Wash each chloroform extract with 10 ml of each of 0.01M *sodium hydroxide* and *water*, filter the combined chloroform extracts, evaporate the filtrate to dryness at a temperature not exceeding 45° and dissolve the residue in 2 ml of *chloroform*. For solution (2) dilute 1 volume of solution (1) to 100 volumes with *chloroform*. For solution (3) dilute 1 volume of solution (1) to 200 volumes with *chloroform*. After removal of the plate, allow it to dry in air and spray with *dilute potassium iodobismuthate solution*. Any *secondary spot* in the chromatogram obtained with solution (1) is not more intense than the spot in the chromatogram obtained with solution (2) (1%) and not more than one such spot is more intense than the spot in the chromatogram obtained with solution (3) (0.5%).

B. Comply with the test for Related substances described under Paracetamol Tablets.

Uniformity of content Tablets containing 10 mg or less of Dihydrocodeine Tartrate comply with the requirements stated under Tablets, with respect to the content of dihydrocodeine tartrate, using the following method of analysis. Carry out the method for *liquid chromatography*, Appendix III D, using the following solutions. Solution (1) contains 0.005% w/v of *dihydrocodeine tartrate BPCRS* in *methanol (25%)*. For solution (2) add 50 ml of *methanol* to one tablet and mix with the aid of ultrasound until completely dispersed. Add 100 ml of *water*, shake for 10 minutes, dilute to 200 ml with *water*, filter through glass-fibre paper (Whatman GF/C is suitable) and use the filtrate.

The chromatographic procedure may be carried out using (a) a stainless steel column (10 cm × 4.6 mm) packed with *stationary phase C* (5 µm) (Nucleosil C18 is suitable), (b) as the mobile phase with a flow rate of 1.5 ml per minute 0.01M *sodium pentanesulphonate* in a mixture of 78 volumes of *water* and 22 volumes of *methanol*, the pH of the solution being adjusted to 2.8 using 2M *hydrochloric acid*, and (c) a detection wavelength of 225 nm.

Calculate the content of $C_{18}H_{23}NO_3,C_4H_6O_6$ in each tablet using the declared content of $C_{18}H_{23}NO_3,C_4H_6O_6$ in *dihydrocodeine tartrate BPCRS*.

Assay

For dihydrocodeine tartrate Weigh and powder 20 tablets. Carry out the method for *liquid chromatography*, Appendix III D, using the following solutions. Solution (1) contains 0.005% w/v of *dihydrocodeine tartrate BPCRS* in *methanol (25%)*. For solution (2) shake a quantity of the powdered tablets containing 10 mg of Dihydrocodeine Tartrate with 50 ml of *methanol* for 1 minute, add 100 ml of *water* and shake for a further 10 minutes. Dilute to 200 ml with *water*, filter through glass-fibre paper (Whatman GF/C is suitable) and use the filtrate.

The chromatographic conditions described under Uniformity of content may be used.

Calculate the content of $C_{18}H_{23}NO_3,C_4H_6O_6$ using the declared content of $C_{18}H_{23}NO_3,C_4H_6O_6$ in *dihydrocodeine tartrate BPCRS*.

For paracetamol Carry out the method for *liquid chromatography*, Appendix III D, using the following solutions. Solution (1) contains 0.005% w/v of *paracetamol BPCRS* in *water*. For solution (2) dilute 1 volume of solution (2) obtained in the Assay for dihydrocodeine tartrate to 50 volumes with *water*.

The chromatographic conditions described under Uniformity of content may be used but with a detection wavelength of 243 nm.

Calculate the content of $C_8H_9NO_2$ using the declared content of $C_8H_9NO_2$ in *paracetamol BPCRS*.

Labelling The label states the quantities of Dihydrocodeine Tartrate and of Paracetamol in each tablet.

Co-fluampicil Capsules

Flucloxacillin and Ampicillin Capsules

Definition Co-fluampicil Capsules contain Flucloxacillin Sodium and Ampicillin Trihydrate, in the proportions, by weight, 1 part flucloxacillin to 1 part ampicillin.

The capsules comply with the requirements stated under Capsules and with the following requirements.

Content of ampicillin, $C_{16}H_{19}N_3O_4S$ 92.5 to 107.5% of the prescribed or stated amount.

Content of flucloxacillin, $C_{19}H_{17}ClFN_3O_5S$ 92.5 to 107.5% of the prescribed or stated amount.

Identification

A. Carry out the method for *thin-layer chromatography*, Appendix III A, using a silanised silica gel precoated plate (Merck silanised silica gel 60 F_{254s} (RP-18) plates are suitable) and a mixture 10 volumes of *acetone* and 90 volumes of a 15.4% w/v solution of *ammonium acetate* adjusted to pH 5.0 with *glacial acetic acid* as the mobile phase. Apply separately to the plate 1 µl of each of the following solutions. For solution (1) shake a quantity of the contents of the capsules containing the equivalent of 0.125 g of each of ampicillin and flucloxacillin with 50 ml of *phosphate buffer pH 7.0* and filter through glass-fibre paper (Whatman GF/C is suitable). Solution (2) contains 0.28% w/v of *ampicillin trihydrate BPCRS* in *phosphate buffer pH 7.0*. Solution (3) contains 0.26% w/v of *flucloxacillin sodium BPCRS* in *phosphate buffer pH 7.0*. Solution (4) contains 0.28% w/v of each of *amoxicillin trihydrate BPCRS* and *ampicillin trihydrate BPCRS* in *phosphate buffer pH 7.0*. After removal of the plate, allow it to dry in air, expose to iodine vapour until the spots appear and examine in daylight. In the chromatogram obtained with solution (1) the spot with the lower Rf value corresponds to the principal spot in the chromatogram obtained with solution (3) and the spot with the higher Rf value corresponds to the principal spot in the chromatogram obtained with solution (2). The test is not valid unless the chromatogram obtained with solution (4) shows two clearly separated principal spots.

B. Carry out the method for *thin-layer chromatography*, Appendix III A, using a silanised silica gel precoated plate (Merck silanised silica gel 60 F_{254s} (RP-18) plates are suitable) and a mixture of 30 volumes of *acetone* and 70 volumes of a 15.4% w/v solution of *ammonium acetate* adjusted to pH 5.0 with *glacial acetic acid* as the mobile phase. Apply separately to the plate 1 µl of each of the following solutions. For solutions (1) to (3) use the solutions described under test A. Solution (4) contains 0.26% w/v of each of *cloxacillin sodium BPCRS*, *dicloxacillin sodium BPCRS* and *flucloxacillin sodium BPCRS* in *phosphate buffer pH 7.0*. After removal of the plate, allow it to dry in air, expose to iodine vapour until the spots appear and examine in daylight. In the chromatogram obtained with solution (1) the spot with the lower Rf value corresponds to the principal spot in the chromatogram obtained with solution (3) and the spot with the higher Rf value corresponds to the principal spot in the chromatogram obtained with solution (2). The test is not valid unless the chromatogram obtained with solution (4) shows three clearly separated principal spots.

C. In the Assay, the retention times of the two principal peaks in the chromatogram obtained with solution (1) correspond to those of the principal peaks in the chromatograms obtained with solutions (2) and (3).

Assay Carry out the method for *liquid chromatography*, Appendix III D, using the following freshly prepared solutions. For solution (1) add a quantity of the mixed contents of 20 capsules containing the equivalent of 0.25 g of each of ampicillin and flucloxacillin to 350 ml of *water*, mix with the aid of ultrasound for 15 minutes, cool and dilute to 500 ml with *water*, filter through glass-fibre paper (Whatman GF/C is suitable) and use the filtrate. Solution (2) contains 0.058% w/v of *ampicillin trihydrate BPCRS*. Solution (3) contains 0.056% w/v of *flucloxacillin sodium BPCRS*.

The chromatographic procedure may be carried out using (a) a stainless steel column (25 cm × 4.6 mm) packed with *stationary phase C* (5 µm) (Spherisorb ODS 1 is suitable), (b) as the mobile phase with a flow rate of 1.5 ml per minute a mixture of 50 volumes of *methanol* and 50 volumes of a buffer solution containing 0.01M *diammonium hydrogen orthophosphate* and 0.005M *tetrabutylammonium hydroxide*, the pH of the solution being adjusted to 7.0 with *orthophosphoric acid* and (c) a detection wavelength of 262 nm.

Calculate the content of $C_{16}H_{19}N_3O_4S$ and of $C_{19}H_{17}ClFN_3O_5S$ using the declared content of $C_{16}H_{19}N_3O_4S$ in *ampicillin trihydrate BPCRS* and the declared content of $C_{19}H_{17}ClFN_3O_5S$ in *flucloxacillin sodium BPCRS*.

Labelling The label states the quantity of Ampicillin Trihydrate in terms of the equivalent amount of ampicillin and the quantity of Flucloxacillin Sodium in terms of the equivalent amount of flucloxacillin.

Co-fluampicil Oral Suspension

Flucloxacillin and Ampicillin Oral Suspension

Definition Co-fluampicil Oral Suspension is a suspension containing equal amounts of Flucloxacillin Magnesium and Ampicillin Trihydrate in a suitable flavoured vehicle. It is prepared by dispersing the dry ingredients in the specified volume of Water just before issue for use.

The dry ingredients comply with the requirements for Powders and Granules for the Preparation of Oral Liquids stated under Oral Liquids.

Storage The dry ingredients should be kept in a well-closed container and stored at a temperature not exceeding 25°.

For the following tests prepare the oral suspension as directed on the label. The suspension examined immediately after preparation, unless otherwise indicated, complies with the requirements stated under Oral Liquids and with the following requirements.

Content of ampicillin, $C_{16}H_{19}N_3O_4S$ When freshly constituted, not more than 120.0% of the prescribed or stated amount. When stored at the temperature and for the period stated on the label during which the oral suspension may be expected to be satisfactory for use, not less than 80.0% of the prescribed or stated amount.

Content of flucloxacillin, $C_{19}H_{17}ClFN_3O_5S$ When freshly constituted, not more than 120.0% of the prescribed or stated amount. When stored at the temperature and for the period stated on the label during which the oral suspension may be expected to be satisfactory for use, not less than 80.0% of the prescribed or stated amount.

Identification

A. Carry out the method for *thin-layer chromatography*, Appendix III A, using a silanised silica gel precoated plate (Merck silanised silica gel 60 F_{254s} (RP-18) plates are suitable) and a mixture of 10 volumes of *acetone* and 90 volumes of a 15.4% w/v solution of *ammonium acetate* adjusted to pH 5.0 with *glacial acetic acid* as the mobile phase. Apply separately to the plate 1 µl of each of the following solutions. For solution (1) dilute a quantity of the oral suspension containing the equivalent of 0.125 g of each of ampicillin and flucloxacillin to 50 ml with *phosphate buffer pH 7.0*. Solution (2) contains 0.28% w/v of *ampicillin trihydrate BPCRS* in *phosphate buffer pH 7.0*. Solution (3) contains 0.26% w/v of *flucloxacillin sodium BPCRS* in *phosphate buffer pH 7.0*. Solution (4) contains 0.28% w/v of each of *amoxicillin trihydrate BPCRS* and *ampicillin trihydrate BPCRS* in *phosphate buffer pH 7.0*. After removal of the plate, allow it to dry in air, expose to iodine vapour until the spots appear and examine in daylight. In the chromatogram obtained with solution (1) the spot with the lower Rf value corresponds to the principal spot in the chromatogram obtained with solution (3) and the spot with the higher Rf value corresponds to the principal spot in the chromatogram obtained with solution (2). The test is not valid unless the chromatogram obtained with solution (4) shows two clearly separated principal spots.

B. Carry out the method for *thin-layer chromatography*, Appendix III A, using a silanised silica gel precoated plate (Merck silanised silica gel 60 F_{254s} (RP-18) plates are suitable) and a mixture of 30 volumes of *acetone* and 70 volumes of a 15.4% w/v solution of *ammonium acetate* adjusted to pH 5.0 with *glacial acetic acid* as the mobile phase. Apply separately to the plate 1 µl of each of the following solutions. For solutions (1) to (3) use the solutions described under test A. Solution (4) contains 0.26% w/v of each of *cloxacillin sodium BPCRS*, *dicloxacillin sodium BPCRS* and *flucloxacillin sodium BPCRS* in *phosphate buffer pH 7.0*. After removal of the plate, allow it to dry in air, expose to iodine vapour until the spots appear and examine in daylight. In the chromatogram obtained with solution (1) the spot with the lower Rf value corresponds to the principal spot in the chromatogram obtained with solution (3) and the spot with the higher Rf value corresponds to the principal spot in the chromatogram obtained with solution (2). The test is not valid unless the chromatogram obtained with solution (4) shows three clearly separated principal spots.

Acidity pH, 4.8 to 5.6, Appendix V L.

Assay To a weighed quantity of the oral suspension containing the equivalent of 0.1 g of each of ampicillin and flucloxacillin add sufficient *water* to produce 100 ml (solution A).

For ampicillin Dilute 2 ml of solution A to 50 ml with *buffered copper sulphate solution pH 5.2*, transfer 10 ml to a stoppered test tube and heat in a water bath at 75° for 30 minutes. Rapidly cool to room temperature, dilute to 20 ml with *buffered copper sulphate solution pH 5.2* and measure the *absorbance* of the resulting solution at the maximum at 320 nm, Appendix II B, using in the reference cell a solution prepared by diluting 2 ml of solution A to 100 ml with *buffered copper sulphate solution pH 5.2*. Calculate the content of $C_{16}H_{19}N_3O_4S$ from the *absorbance* obtained by carrying out the operation at the same time using 2 ml of a solution prepared by dissolving 0.12 g of *ampicillin trihydrate BPCRS* in 100 ml of *water*, diluting to 50 ml with *buffered copper sulphate solution pH 5.2* and beginning at the words 'transfer 10 ml...' and from the declared content of $C_{16}H_{19}N_3O_4S$ in *ampicillin trihydrate BPCRS*. Determine the *weight per ml* of the oral suspension, Appendix V G, and calculate the content of $C_{16}H_{19}N_3O_4S$, weight in volume.

Repeat the procedure using a portion of the oral suspension that has been stored at the temperature and for the period stated on the label during which it may be expected to be satisfactory for use.

For flucloxacillin Dilute 2 ml of solution A to 100 ml with 1M *hydrochloric acid*. Measure the *absorbance* of the resulting solution at the maximum at 352 nm, Appendix II B, after exactly 11 minutes using 1M *hydrochloric acid* in the reference cell. Calculate the content of $C_{19}H_{17}ClFN_3O_5S$ from the *absorbance* obtained by carrying out the operation at the same time using 2 ml of a solution prepared by dissolving 0.11 g of *flucloxacillin sodium BPCRS* in 100 ml of *water* and from the declared content of $C_{19}H_{17}ClFN_3O_5S$ in *flucloxacillin sodium BPCRS*. Determine the *weight per ml* of the oral suspension, Appendix V G, and calculate the content of $C_{19}H_{17}ClFN_3O_5S$, weight in volume.

Repeat the procedure using a portion of the oral suspension that has been stored at the temperature and for the period stated on the label during which it may be expected to be satisfactory for use.

Storage The Oral Suspension should be stored at the temperature and used within the period stated on the label.

Labelling The label states the quantity of Ampicillin Trihydrate in terms of the equivalent amount of ampicillin and the quantity of Flucloxacillin Magnesium in terms of the equivalent amount of flucloxacillin.

Colchicine Tablets

Definition Colchicine Tablets contain Colchicine.

The tablets comply with the requirements stated under Tablets and with the following requirements.

Content of colchicine, $C_{22}H_{25}NO_6$ 90.0 to 110.0% of the prescribed or stated amount.

Identification Mix a quantity of the powdered tablets containing 1 mg of Colchicine with 0.2 ml of *sulphuric acid* in a white dish; a lemon colour is produced. Add 0.05 ml of *nitric acid*; the colour changes to greenish blue and then rapidly becomes reddish and finally yellow or almost colourless. Add an excess of 5M *sodium hydroxide*; the colour changes to red.

Related substances Carry out the method for *thin-layer chromatography*, Appendix III A, protected from light using *silica gel HF_{254}* as the coating substance and a mixture of 1 volume of 13.5M *ammonia*, 25 volumes of *1,2-dichloroethane* and 50 volumes of *acetone* as the mobile phase. Apply separately to the plate 2 µl of each of the following solutions. For solution (1) extract a quantity of the powdered tablets containing 5 mg of Colchicine with 5 ml of *chloroform*, filter and evaporate the filtrate to dryness in a current of air. Dissolve the residue as completely as possible in 0.1 ml of *ethanol (96%)*, allow to settle and use the supernatant liquid. For solution (2) dilute 1 volume of solution (1) to 50 volumes with *ethanol (96%)*. For solution (3) dilute 1 volume of solution (2) to 2 volumes with *ethanol (96%)*. After removal of the plate, allow it to dry in air and examine under *ultraviolet light (254 nm)*. Any *secondary spot* in the chromatogram obtained with solution (1) is not more intense than the spot in the chromatogram obtained with solution (2) (2%) and not more than one such spot is more intense than the spot in the chromatogram obtained with solution (3) (1%).

Uniformity of content Tablets containing less than 2 mg of Colchicine comply with the requirements stated under Tablets using the following method of analysis. Carry out the following procedure in subdued light. Place one tablet in a centrifuge tube and add 10 ml of *absolute ethanol.* Crush the tablet to a fine powder, shake for 30 minutes, centrifuge and wash the residue with *absolute ethanol.* Combine the extract and washings and add sufficient *absolute ethanol* to produce a 0.001% w/v solution. Measure the *absorbance* of the resulting solution at the maximum at 350 nm, Appendix II B. Calculate the content of $C_{22}H_{25}NO_6$ taking 440 as the value of A(1%, 1 cm) at the maximum at 350 nm.

Assay Weigh and powder 20 tablets. Carry out the following procedure in subdued light. To a quantity of the powder containing 0.5 mg of Colchicine add 10 ml of *absolute ethanol* and shake for 30 minutes. Centrifuge, wash the residue with *absolute ethanol*, dilute the combined extract and washings to 50 ml with *absolute ethanol* and measure the *absorbance* of the resulting solution at the maximum at 350 nm, Appendix II B. Calculate the content of $C_{22}H_{25}NO_6$ taking 440 as the value of A(1%, 1 cm) at the maximum at 350 nm.

Storage Colchicine Tablets should be protected from light.

Colestipol Granules

Definition Colestipol Granules contain Colestipol Hydrochloride with or without suitable excipients.

The granules comply with the requirements stated under Granules and with the following requirements.

Identification Carry out the method for *gas chromatography*, Appendix III B, using a suitable gas chromatograph fitted with a pyrolysis unit.

To prepare the sample, mix 1 part of n-*eicosane* and 4 parts of the granules and grind the mixture in a mortar with *chloroform* until the preparation being examined is uniformly coated with the *n*-eicosane. Prepare the standard in the same manner but adding 4 parts of *colestipol hydrochloride BPCRS* in place of the preparation being examined. Load the sample and the standard separately into the pyrolysis unit.

The chromatographic procedure may be carried out using a glass column (1.8 m × 3 mm) packed with *acid-washed, silanised diatomaceous support* (80 to 100 mesh) (Chromosorb W is suitable) coated with 0.25% w/w of *potassium hydroxide* and 5% w/w of *polyethylene glycol 20,000* (Carbowax 20M is suitable) maintained at about 85° with the detector at about 270°. The pyrolysis unit is capable of attaining a temperature of about 1000° when fitted with a platinum ribbon probe and using *helium* as the carrier gas with a flow rate of 60 ml per minute. Operate the unit in accordance with the manufacturer's instructions to obtain a pyrogram for *colestipol hydrochloride BPCRS* that is similar to that supplied with the reference material.

The pyrogram obtained with the substance being examined is concordant with that obtained with *colestipol hydrochloride BPCRS.*

Acidity or alkalinity Shake a suspension containing 10% w/w of Colestipol Hydrochloride in a stoppered vial at approximately 10-minute intervals for 1 hour, and centrifuge. Transfer a portion of the clear supernatant liquid to a suitable container and record the pH as soon as the reading has stabilised. The pH is 5.3 to 7.5, Appendix V L.

Uniformity of weight Comply with the test for Uniformity of weight for Effervescent Granules described under Granules.

Water absorption capacity A quantity of the granules containing 1 g of Colestipol Hydrochloride absorbs not less than 3.3 g and not more than 5.3 g of *water* when determined in the following manner. Transfer a quantity of the granules containing 5 g of Colestipol Hydrochloride to a dry, plastic container and add 80 g of *water.* Cover the container and allow the resulting suspension to equilibrate for 72 hours. Filter the resulting slurry through a medium-porosity fritted-glass funnel (KIMAX 60-ml-40M is suitable) at a pressure of 2kPa; collect the filtrate in a tared, plastic container, disconnecting the vacuum 2 minutes after collection of the last portion of the filtrate. Immediately weigh the container and the filtrate and determine the weight, in g, of the filtrate. Calculate the weight of water absorbed from the difference between the weight of the filtrate and the original weight of *water* used in the test.

Cholate binding capacity A quantity of the granules containing 1 g of Colestipol Hydrochloride binds not less than 1.1 mEq and not more than 1.6 mEq of sodium cholate, determined by the following method. Prepare a solution containing 1.0% w/v of *sodium cholate* and 0.9% w/v of *sodium chloride* in *water* containing 1.8% v/v of 1M *sodium hydroxide* (solution A). Carry out the method for *liquid chromatography*, Appendix III D, using the following solutions. For solution (1) dilute 1 volume of solution A with 1 volume of the mobile phase. For solution (2) transfer a quantity of the granules containing 1 g of Colestipol Hydrochloride to a ground-glass-stoppered flask, add 100 ml of solution A and shake vigorously for 90 minutes with the flask positioned horizontally. Remove the flask from the shaker, allow the contents to settle for 5 minutes and filter through a 0.45-µm filter, discarding the first 5 ml of filtrate. Dilute 1 volume of the filtrate with 1 volume of the mobile phase. Solution (3) contains 0.45% w/v of *cholic acid BPCRS* in a solution prepared by mixing equal volumes of *acetonitrile* containing 2 ml per litre of *orthophosphoric acid* and *water*.

The chromatographic procedure may be carried out using (a) a stainless steel column (25 cm × 4.6 mm) packed with *stationary phase B* (5 mm) (Zorbax C8 is suitable), (b) as the mobile phase with a flow rate of 1.5 ml per minute a mixture of a solution containing 2.76 g of *anhydrous sodium dihydrogen orthophosphate* in 450 ml of *water* adjusted to pH 3.0 with *orthophosphoric acid*, 100 ml of *methanol* and 450 ml of *acetonitrile* and (c) a detection wavelength of 214 nm.

Inject 20 ml of each solution. The retention time of the peak due to cholic acid is about 6 minutes. From the chromatograms obtained determine the exact concentration of sodium cholate in solutions (1) and (2) in mg per ml using the declared content of cholic acid in *cholic acid BPCRS* and taking each g of cholic acid to be equivalent to 1.054 g of sodium cholate. The cholate binding capacity in mEq is determined by the expression:

(concentration of sodium cholate in solution (1) – concentration of sodium cholate in solution (2)) × 0.2325.

Colistimethate Injection

Definition Colistimethate Injection is a sterile solution of Colistimethate Sodium in Sodium Chloride Intravenous Infusion. It is prepared by dissolving Colistimethate Sodium for Injection in the requisite amount of Sodium Chloride Intravenous Infusion.

The injection complies with the requirements stated under Parenteral Preparations.

Storage Colistimethate Injection should be used immediately after preparation but, in any case, within the period recommended by the manufacturer when prepared and stored strictly in accordance with the manufacturer's instructions.

COLISTIMETHATE SODIUM FOR INJECTION

Colistimethate Sodium for Injection is a sterile material consisting of Colistimethate Sodium with or without excipients. It is supplied in a sealed container.

The contents of the sealed container comply with the requirements for Powders for Injections stated under Parenteral Preparations and with the following requirements.

Identification

A. Complies with test A for Identification described under Colistimethate Sodium.

B. Dissolve 10 mg in 5 ml of *water*. Heat 0.5 ml of the solution with 0.5 ml of *chromotropic acid solution* at 100° for 30 minutes. A purple colour is produced (distinction from colistin sulphate).

C. Dissolve 50 mg in 1 ml of 1M *hydrochloric acid* and add 0.5 ml of 0.01M *iodine*. The colour is discharged (distinction from colistin sulphate) and the resulting solution yields reaction A characteristic of *sulphates*, Appendix VI.

D. Yield reaction A characteristic of *sodium salts*, Appendix VI.

Acidity or alkalinity pH of a 1% w/v solution, 6.2 to 7.7, Appendix V L.

Free colistin Dissolve 80 mg in 3 ml of *water*, add 0.1 ml of a 10% w/v solution of *silicotungstic acid* and allow to stand for 10 to 20 seconds. The resulting solution is not more opalescent than *reference suspension II*, Appendix IV A.

Loss on drying When dried over *phosphorus pentoxide* at 60° at a pressure not exceeding 0.7kPa for 3 hours, lose not more than 5.0% of their weight. Use 1 g.

Pyrogens Comply with the *test for pyrogens*, Appendix XIV D. Use per kg of the rabbit's weight 1 ml of *water for injections* containing 2.5 mg per ml.

Assay Determine the weight of the contents of each of 10 containers as described in the test for Uniformity of weight under Parenteral Preparations, Powders for Injections.

Mix the contents of the 10 containers and carry out the *biological assay of antibiotics*, Appendix XIV A. The precision of the assay is such that the fiducial limits of error are not less than 95% and not more than 105% of the estimated potency. For a container of average content weight, the upper fiducial limit of error is not less than 95.0% and the lower fiducial limit of error is not more than 115.0% of the prescribed or stated number of IU.

Storage The sealed container should be protected from light.

Labelling The label of the sealed container states the total number of IU (Units) contained in it.

When colistin sulphomethate injection or colistin sulphomethate sodium for injection is prescribed or demanded, Colistimethate Injection or Colistimethate Sodium for Injection shall be dispensed or supplied.

Colistin Tablets

Definition Colistin Tablets contain Colistin Sulphate.

The tablets comply with the requirements stated under Tablets and with the following requirements.

Identification To a quantity of the powdered tablets containing 200,000 IU add 10 ml of *water*, shake and filter. Use the filtrate for the following tests.

A. Carry out the method for *thin-layer chromatography*, Appendix III A, protected from light using *silica gel G* as the coating substance and a mixture of 75 parts of *phenol* and 25 parts of *water* as the mobile phase but allowing the solvent front to ascend 12 cm above the line of application. Apply separately to the plate 5 ml of each of the following solutions as 10-mm bands. For solution (1) add 0.5 ml of *hydrochloric acid* to 0.5 ml of the filtrate, heat in a sealed tube at 135° for 5 hours, evaporate to dryness on a water bath, continue to heat until the odour of hydrogen chloride is no longer detectable, dissolve the residue in 0.5 ml of *water* and centrifuge, if necessary. Solutions (2) to (5) are solutions in *water* containing 0.2% w/v each of (2) *L-leucine*, (3) *L-threonine*, (4) *L-phenylalanine* and (5) *L-serine*. Place the plate in the tank so that it is not in contact with the mobile phase and expose it to the vapour of the mobile phase for at least 12 hours. Develop the chromatograms, remove the plate, heat it at 100° to 105°, spray with *ninhydrin solution R1* and heat the plate at 110° for 5 minutes. The bands in the chromatogram obtained with solution (1) correspond to those in the chromatograms obtained with solutions (2) and (3) and do not correspond to those in the chromatograms obtained with solutions (4) and (5). The chromatogram obtained with solution (1) also shows a band with a very low Rf value (2,4-diaminobutanoic acid).

B. Heat 0.5 ml of the filtrate with 0.5 ml of *chromotropic acid solution* at 100° for 30 minutes. No purple colour is produced (distinction from colistin sulphomethate).

C. The filtrate yields reaction A characteristic of *sulphates*, Appendix VI.

Assay Weigh and powder 20 tablets. Dissolve a suitable quantity of the powder in *phosphate buffer pH 6.0* and carry out the *biological assay of antibiotics*, Appendix XIV A. The precision of the assay is such that the fiducial limits of error are not less than 95% and not more than 105% of the estimated potency. The upper fiducial limit of error is not less than 97.0% and the lower fiducial limit of error is not more than 110.0% of the prescribed or stated number of IU.

Storage Colistin Tablets should be protected from light.

Labelling The strength is stated as the number of IU (Units) in each tablet.

Co-magaldrox Oral Suspension

Magnesium Hydroxide and Aluminium Hydroxide Oral Suspension

Definition Co-magaldrox Oral Suspension is a suspension containing Magnesium Hydroxide and Dried Aluminium Hydroxide in a suitable flavoured vehicle. The amount of Dried Aluminium Hydroxide is adjusted to give the required content of Al_2O_3.

The oral suspension complies with the requirements stated under Oral Liquids and with the following requirements.

Content of magnesium hydroxide, $Mg(OH)_2$ 90.0 to 110.0% of the prescribed or stated amount.

Content of Al_2O_3 45.4 to 58.8% of the prescribed or stated amount of Dried Aluminium Hydroxide.

Identification

A. Mix 5 ml with 10 ml of 2M *hydrochloric acid*, add 5 drops of *methyl red solution* and heat to boiling. Add 6M *ammonia* until the solution becomes yellow, continue boiling for 2 minutes and filter. To 1 ml of the filtrate add 1 ml of 6M *ammonia* and 1 ml of 2M *ammonium chloride*; no precipitate is produced. Add 0.25M *disodium hydrogen orthophosphate*; a white, crystalline precipitate is produced which is insoluble in 6M *ammonia*.

B. To 5 ml add 10 ml of 2M *hydrochloric acid*. The solution yields the reactions characteristic of *aluminium salts*, Appendix VI.

Heavy metals Not more than 10 ppm when determined by the following method. Dissolve 8.0 g in 20 ml of 3M *hydrochloric acid* with the aid of heat, filter if necessary and add sufficient *water* to produce 50 ml (solution A). Transfer 25 ml of solution A to a 50-ml *Nessler cylinder*, adjust the pH to between 3.0 and 4.0 using 6M *ammonia*, add sufficient *water* to produce 40 ml and mix. Add 10 ml of freshly prepared *hydrogen sulphide solution*, mix and allow to stand for 5 minutes. When viewed down the vertical axis of the tube against a white background the colour of the solution is not more intense than that of a solution prepared at the same time and in the same manner using a solution of 2 ml of *lead standard solution (20 ppm Pb)* diluted to 25 ml with *water* in place of solution A adjusted to a pH between 3.0 and 4.0 using either 1M *acetic acid* or 6M *ammonia* and beginning at the words 'add sufficient *water* to produce 40 ml...' (standard solution). The colour of the standard solution is not as intense as that of a solution prepared at the same time and in the same manner but using a mixture of 25 ml of solution A and 2 ml of *lead standard solution (20 ppm Pb)* adjusted to a pH between 3.0 and 4.0 using either 1M *acetic acid* or 6M *ammonia* and beginning at the words 'add sufficient *water* to produce 40 ml...'.

Microbial contamination Carry out a quantitative evaluation for Enterobacteriaceae and certain other Gram-negative bacteria, Appendix XVI B1. 0.01ml of the preparation gives a negative result, Table I (most probable number of bacteria per gram fewer than 10^2).

Assay

For Al_2O_3 To a weighed quantity containing 1.5 g of Dried Aluminium Hydroxide add 20 ml of *water*, stir and slowly add 10 ml of *hydrochloric acid*. Heat gently, if necessary, to aid solution, cool, filter, wash the filter well with *water*, dilute the combined filtrate and washings to 200 ml with *water* and mix. Reserve a portion of the solution for the Assay for magnesium hydroxide. To 10 ml add 20 ml of *water* and, with continuous stirring, 25 ml of 0.05M *disodium edetate VS* followed by 20 ml of a mixture of equal volumes of 2M *ammonium acetate* and 2M *acetic acid*. Heat near the boiling point for 5 minutes, cool, add 50 ml of *absolute ethanol* and 3 ml of a freshly prepared 0.025% w/v solution of *dithizone* in *absolute ethanol*. Titrate the excess of disodium edetate with 0.05M *zinc sulphate VS* until the colour of the solution changes from greenish blue to reddish violet. Each ml of 0.05M *disodium edetate VS* is equivalent to 2.549 mg of Al_2O_3. Determine the *weight per ml* of the suspension, Appendix V G, and calculate the percentage content of Al_2O_3, weight in volume.

For magnesium hydroxide To a volume of the solution reserved in the Assay for Al_2O_3 containing about 40 mg of Magnesium Hydroxide add 200 ml of *water* and 20 ml of *triethanolamine* and stir. Add 10 ml of *ammonia buffer pH 10.9* and cool the solution to between 3° and 4° by immersion in iced water. Titrate the cooled solution with 0.05M *disodium edetate VS* using *mordant black 11 solution* as indicator. Each ml of 0.05M *disodium edetate VS* is equivalent to 2.916 mg of $Mg(OH)_2$. Using the weight per ml of the suspension, calculate the percentage content of $Mg(OH)_2$, weight in volume.

Storage Co-magaldrox Oral Suspension should be kept in a well-closed container. It should not be allowed to freeze.

Co-magaldrox Tablets

Magnesium Hydroxide and Aluminium Hydroxide Tablets

Definition Co-magaldrox Tablets contain Magnesium Hydroxide and Dried Aluminium Hydroxide. The amount of Dried Aluminium Hydroxide is adjusted to give the required content of Al_2O_3.

The tablets comply with the requirements stated under Tablets and with the following requirements.

Content of magnesium hydroxide, $Mg(OH)_2$ 90.0 to 110.0% of the prescribed or stated amount.

Content of Al_2O_3 45.0 to 55.0% of the prescribed or stated amount of Dried Aluminium Hydroxide.

Identification

A. To a quantity of the powdered tablets containing about 0.2 g of Magnesium Hydroxide in 10 ml of 2M *hydrochloric acid* add 0.25 ml of *methyl red solution* and heat to boiling. Add 6M *ammonia* until the solution becomes yellow, continue boiling for 2 minutes and filter. To 1 ml of the filtrate add 1 ml of 6M *ammonia* and 1 ml of 2M *ammonium chloride*; no precipitate is produced. Add 0.25M *disodium hydrogen orthophosphate*; a white crystalline precipitate is produced which is insoluble in 6M *ammonia.*

B. Shake a quantity of the powdered tablets containing 0.25 g of Dried Aluminium Hydroxide with 25 ml of 2M *hydrochloric acid* and filter. The filtrate yields the reactions characteristic of *aluminium salts*, Appendix VI.

Assay

For Al_2O_3 Weigh and powder 20 tablets. To a quantity of the powdered tablets containing 1.5 g of Dried Aluminium Hydroxide add 20 ml of *water*, stir and slowly add 30 ml of 3M *hydrochloric acid.* Heat gently, if necessary, to aid solution, cool, filter, wash the filter well with *water*, dilute the combined filtrate and washings to 200 ml with *water* and mix. Reserve a portion of the solution for the Assay for magnesium hydroxide. To 10 ml add 20 ml of *water* and, with continuous stirring, 25 ml of 0.05M *disodium edetate VS* followed by 20 ml of a mixture of equal volumes of 2M *ammonium acetate* and 2M *acetic acid.* Heat near the boiling point for 5 minutes, cool, add 50 ml of *absolute ethanol* and 3 ml of a freshly prepared 0.025% w/v solution of *dithizone* in *absolute ethanol.* Titrate the excess of disodium edetate with 0.05M *zinc sulphate VS* until the colour of the solution changes from greenish blue to reddish violet. Each ml of 0.05M *disodium edetate VS* is equivalent to 2.549 mg of Al_2O_3.

For magnesium hydroxide To a volume of the solution reserved in the Assay for Al_2O_3 containing about 40 mg of Magnesium Hydroxide add 200 ml of *water* and 20 ml of *triethanolamine* and stir. Add 10 ml of *ammonia buffer pH 10.9* and cool the solution to between 3° and 4° by immersion in iced water. Titrate the cooled solution with 0.05M *disodium edetate VS* using *mordant black 11 solution* as indicator. Each ml of 0.05M *disodium edetate VS* is equivalent to 2.916 mg of $Mg(OH)_2$.

Co-proxamol Tablets

Dextropropoxyphene Hydrochloride and Paracetamol Tablets

Definition Co-proxamol Tablets contain Dextropropoxyphene Hydrochloride and Paracetamol in the proportions, by weight, 1 part to 10 parts.

With the exception of the requirements for shape, the tablets comply with the requirements stated under Tablets and with the following requirements.

Content of dextropropoxyphene hydrochloride, $C_{22}H_{29}NO_2,HCl$ 95.0 to 105.0% of the prescribed or stated amount.

Content of paracetamol, $C_8H_9NO_2$ 95.0 to 105.0% of the prescribed or stated amount.

Identification

A. Shake a quantity of the powdered tablets containing 0.1 g of Dextropropoxyphene Hydrochloride with 20 ml of 0.1M *hydrochloric acid* for 5 minutes and filter. To the filtrate add 5 ml of 2M *sodium hydroxide*, extract with two 25-ml quantities of *chloroform*, wash the combined extracts with 10 ml of *water*, shake with *anhydrous sodium sulphate*, filter and evaporate the filtrate to dryness. Dissolve the residue in 2 ml of *dichloromethane* and add 50 ml, dropwise, onto the surface of a disc prepared from about 0.3 g of *potassium bromide*, allowing the solvent to evaporate between applications; dry the disc at 50° for 2 minutes. The *infrared absorption spectrum* of the resulting thin film, Appendix II A, is concordant with the *reference spectrum* of dextropropoxyphene.

B. Shake a quantity of the powdered tablets containing 0.325 g of Paracetamol with 10 ml of *acetone* for 5 minutes, filter and evaporate the filtrate to dryness. The *infrared absorption spectrum* of the residue, Appendix II A, is concordant with the *reference spectrum* of paracetamol.

Dissolution Comply with the *dissolution test for tablets and capsules* with respect to the content of Paracetamol, Appendix XII D, using Apparatus II. Use as the medium 900 ml of *phosphate buffer pH 5.8* and rotate the paddle at 50 revolutions per minute. Withdraw a sample of 20 ml of the medium and filter. Dilute the filtrate with 0.1M *sodium hydroxide* to give a solution expected to contain about 0.00075% w/v of Paracetamol. Measure the *absorbance* of this solution, Appendix II B, at the maximum at 257 nm using 0.1M *sodium hydroxide* in the reference cell. Calculate the total content of paracetamol, $C_8H_9NO_2$, in the medium taking 715 as the value of A(1%, 1 cm) at the maximum at 257 nm.

4-Aminophenol Comply with the requirements stated under Paracetamol Tablets but using the following solutions. Solution (1) contains 0.001% w/v of *4-aminophenol* in the mobile phase. For solution (2) shake a quantity of the powdered tablets containing 0.5 g of Paracetamol with 50 ml of the mobile phase for 10 minutes and filter.

Related substances

A. Carry out the method for *liquid chromatography*,

Appendix III D, using the following solutions. Solution (1) contains 0.0005% w/v of *4 dimethylamino-3-methyl-1,2-diphenylbutan-2-ol hydrochloride BPCRS* and 0.0005% w/v of *(1S,2R)-1-benzyl-3-dimethylamino-2-methyl-1-phenylpropyl acetate BPCRS* in a mixture of 1 volume of *acetonitrile* and 4 volumes of *water*. For solution (2) shake a quantity of the powdered tablets containing 25 mg of Dextropropoxyphene Hydrochloride with 5 ml of *acetonitrile* for 2 minutes, add 5 ml of *water*, shake for a further 5 minutes, dilute to 25 ml with *water*, mix and filter (Whatman GF/F filter paper is suitable).

The chromatographic procedure may be carried out using (a) a stainless steel column (20 cm × 4.6 mm) packed with *stationary phase C* (5 μm) (Nucleosil C18 is suitable), (b) a mixture of 60 volumes of 0.2M *sodium perchlorate*, previously adjusted to pH 2.0 using 7M *hydrochloric acid*, and 40 volumes of *acetonitrile* as the mobile phase with a flow rate of 2 ml per minute and (c) a detection wavelength of 215 nm.

In the chromatogram obtained with solution (1) the peaks, in order of emergence, are due to 4-dimethylamino-3-methyl-1,2-diphenylbutan-2-ol hydrochloride and (1*S*,2*R*)-1-benzyl-3-dimethylamino-2-methyl-1-phenylpropyl acetate. The test is not valid unless the *resolution factor* between these two peaks is greater than 1.5. In the chromatogram obtained with solution (2) the areas of any peaks corresponding to 4-dimethylamino-3-methyl-1,2-diphenylbutan-2-ol hydrochloride and (1*S*,2*R*)-1-benzyl-3-dimethylamino-2-methyl-1-phenylpropyl acetate are not greater than the areas of the respective peaks in the chromatogram obtained with solution (1).

B. Comply with the test for Related substances described under Paracetamol Tablets.

Assay Weigh and powder 20 tablets.

For dextropropoxyphene hydrochloride Carry out the method for *liquid chromatography*, Appendix III D, using the following solutions. Solution (1) contains 0.0065% w/v of *dextropropoxyphene hydrochloride BPCRS* in a mixture of 40 volumes of *acetonitrile* and 60 volumes of 0.02M *hydrochloric acid*. For solution (2) disperse a quantity of the powdered tablets containing 32.5 mg of Dextropropoxyphene Hydrochloride in 100 ml of 0.02M *hydrochloric acid*, mix with the aid of ultrasound for 15 minutes, allow to cool, dilute to 500 ml with a mixture of equal volumes of *acetonitrile* and 0.02M *hydrochloric acid* and filter (Whatman GF/C filter paper is suitable).

The chromatographic conditions described in test A for Related substances may be used.

Calculate the content of $C_{22}H_{29}NO_2,HCl$ using the declared content of $C_{22}H_{29}NO_2,HCl$ in *dextropropoxyphene hydrochloride BPCRS*.

For paracetamol Disperse a quantity of the powdered tablets containing 0.325 g of Paracetamol in 5 ml of *water*, add 100 ml of *methanol* and shake. Add 300 ml of *water*, shake for 5 minutes, allow to cool, dilute to 500 ml with *water*, mix and filter. Dilute 5 ml of the filtrate to 250 ml with 0.01M *sodium hydroxide* and measure the *absorbance* of the resulting solution at the maximum at 257 nm, Appendix II B. Calculate the content of $C_8H_9NO_2$ taking 715 as the value of A(1%, 1 cm) at the maximum at 257 nm.

Storage Co-proxamol Tablets should be protected from light.

Labelling The label states the quantities of Dextropropoxyphene Hydrochloride and of Paracetamol in each tablet.

Cortisone Tablets

Definition Cortisone Tablets contain Cortisone Acetate in *fine powder*.

The tablets comply with the requirements stated under Tablets and with the following requirements.

Content of cortisone acetate, $C_{23}H_{30}O_6$ 90.0 to 110.0% of the prescribed or stated amount.

Identification

Extract a quantity of the powdered tablets containing 0.1 g of Cortisone Acetate with 5 ml of *chloroform*, filter and evaporate the chloroform. The residue complies with the following tests.

A. The *infrared absorption spectrum*, Appendix II A, is concordant with a spectrum prepared from the residue obtained by evaporating 5 ml of a 2% w/v solution of *cortisone acetate BPCRS* in *chloroform*. Use the same method of evaporation of the chloroform as that for the tablet extract. Prepare *potassium bromide* discs.

B. Complies with the test for *identification of steroids*, Appendix III A, using *impregnating solvent I* and *mobile phase B*.

Related substances Carry out the method for *thin-layer chromatography*, Appendix III A, using a silica gel F_{254} precoated plate (Merck silica gel 60 F_{254} plates are suitable) and a mixture of 77 volumes of *dichloromethane*, 15 volumes of *ether*, 8 volumes of *methanol* and 1.2 volumes of *water* as the mobile phase. Apply separately to the plate 10 μl of each of the following solutions. For solution (1) add 20 ml of *chloroform* to a quantity of the powdered tablets containing 20 mg of Cortisone Acetate, shake for 5 minutes, filter, evaporate the filtrate to dryness and dissolve the residue in 4 ml of *chloroform*. For solution (2) dilute 1 volume of solution (1) to 50 volumes with *chloroform*. For solution (3) dilute 1 volume of solution (1) to 100 volumes with *chloroform*. After removal of the plate, allow it to dry in air and examine under *ultraviolet light (254 nm)*. Any *secondary spot* in the chromatogram obtained with solution (1) is not more intense than the spot in the chromatogram obtained with solution (2) and not more than one such spot is more intense than the spot in the chromatogram obtained with solution (3).

Dissolution Comply with the *dissolution test for tablets and capsules*, Appendix XII D, using as the medium 900 ml of a mixture of 70 volumes of a 1% v/v solution of *hydrochloric acid* and 30 volumes of *propan-2-ol* and rotating the basket at 100 revolutions per minute. Withdraw a sample of 10 ml of the medium, filter and measure the *absorbance* of the filtrate, suitably diluted if necessary with the dissolution medium, at the maximum at 242 nm, Appendix II B, using in the reference cell the dissolution medium that has been subjected to the conditions of the test. Calculate the total content of cortisone acetate, $C_{23}H_{30}O_6$ in the medium taking 399 as the value of A(1%, 1 cm) at the maximum at 242 nm.

Assay Weigh and powder 20 tablets. Carry out the method for *liquid chromatography*, Appendix III D, using the following solutions. For solution (1) dilute 50 ml of a solution in *methanol* containing 0.02% w/v each of *cortisone acetate EPCRS* and *prednisolone* to 100 ml with *water*. For solution (2) add 50 ml of *methanol* to a quantity of the powdered tablets containing 10 mg of Cortisone Acetate, shake, mix with the aid of ultrasound for 2 minutes, dilute to 100 ml with *water*, shake, centrifuge and use the supernatant liquid.

The chromatographic procedure may be carried out using (a) a stainless steel column (15 cm × 4.6 mm) packed with *stationary phase C* (5 µm) (Hypersil ODS is suitable), (b) *methanol (60%)* as the mobile phase with a flow rate of 1.5 ml per minute and (c) a detection wavelength of 240 nm.

Calculate the content of $C_{23}H_{30}O_6$ taking 100.0% as the content of $C_{23}H_{30}O_6$ in *cortisone acetate EPCRS*. The assay is not valid unless the *resolution factor* between the peaks due to cortisone acetate and prednisolone in the chromatogram obtained with solution (1) is at least 5.0.

Storage Cortisone Tablets should be protected from light.

Co-tenidone Tablets

Atenolol and Chlorthalidone Tablets

Definition Co-tenidone Tablets contain Atenolol and Chlorthalidone in the proportions, by weight, 4 parts to 1 part.

The tablets comply with the requirements stated under Tablets and with the following requirements.

Content of atenolol, $C_{14}H_{22}N_2O_3$ 95.0 to 105.0% of the prescribed or stated amount.

Content of chlorthalidone, $C_{14}H_{11}ClN_2O_4S$ 92.5 to 107.5% of the prescribed or stated amount.

Identification

A. Carry out the method for *thin-layer chromatography*, Appendix III A, using *silica gel GF_{254}* as the coating substance and a mixture of 30 volumes of 18M *ammonia* and 150 volumes of *butan-1-ol* as the mobile phase. Apply separately to the plate 5 µl of each of the following solutions. For solution (1) remove any film coating from the tablets, powder and shake a quantity of the powdered tablets containing 0.1 g of Atenolol with 10 ml of *methanol* for 15 minutes and filter. Solution (2) contains 1.0% w/v of *atenolol BPCRS* in *methanol*. Solution (3) contains 0.25% w/v of *chlorthalidone BPCRS* in *methanol*. After removal of the plate, allow it to dry in air and examine under *ultraviolet light (254 nm)*. In the chromatogram obtained with solution (1) the two principal spots correspond in position, size and intensity to those of the principal spots in the chromatograms obtained with solutions (2) and (3).

B. In the Assay, the retention times of the two principal peaks in the chromatogram obtained with solution (1) correspond to those of the principal peaks in the chromatograms obtained with solutions (2) and (3).

Related substances Carry out the method for *liquid chromatography*, Appendix III D, using the following solutions. For solution (1) remove any film coating from the tablets, powder and shake a quantity of the powder containing 0.1 g of Atenolol (and 0.025 g of Chlorthalidone) with 25 ml of the mobile phase for 30 minutes with the aid of ultrasound. Filter through a suitable filter (Whatman No l is suitable) and use the filtrate. For solution (2) dilute 1 volume of solution (1) to 200 volumes with the mobile phase. For solution (3) dissolve 50 mg of *atenolol impurity standard BPCRS* in 0.1 ml of *dimethyl sulphoxide*, with the aid of gentle heat, and dilute to 100 ml with the mobile phase. Solution (4) contains 0.002% w/v of *2-(4-chloro-3-sulphamoylbenzoyl)benzoic acid EPCRS* in the mobile phase.

The chromatographic procedure may be carried out using (a) a stainless steel column (15 cm × 4.6 mm) packed with *stationary phase C* (5 µm) (Spherisorb ODS 2 is suitable), (b) as the mobile phase with a flow rate of 2 ml per minute a mixture of 20 volumes of *tetrahydrofuran*, 180 volumes of *methanol* and 800 volumes of 0.025M *potassium dihydrogen orthophosphate* containing 1.0 g of *sodium octanesulphonate* and 0.4 g of *tetrabutylammonium hydrogen sulphate* per litre and adjusted to pH 3.0 with *orthophosphoric acid* and (c) a detection wavelength of 226 nm.

The test is not valid unless the chromatogram obtained with solution (3) closely resembles the reference chromatogram supplied with *atenolol impurity standard BPCRS* and the peaks corresponding to tertiary amine, which is usually a doublet, and bis ether are clearly separated. If necessary, adjust the concentration of sodium octanesulphonate in the mobile phase; increasing the concentration increases the retention time of the tertiary amine.

In the chromatogram obtained with solution (1) the area of any peak corresponding to 2-(4-chloro-3-sulphamoylbenzoyl)benzoic acid is not greater than the area of the peak in the chromatogram obtained with solution (4) (2%, with reference to the content of chlorthalidone), the area of any peak corresponding to blocker acid is not greater than the area of the principal peak in the chromatogram obtained with solution (2) (0.5%, with reference to the content of atenolol), the area of any peak corresponding to either tertiary amine or bis ether is not greater than half of the area of the principal peak in the chromatogram obtained with solution (2) (0.25%, with reference to the content of atenolol).

Assay Carry out the method for *liquid chromatography*, Appendix III D, using the following solutions. For solution (1), weigh 20 tablets, remove the film coating, reweigh and powder. Extract a quantity of the powder containing 0.1 g of Atenolol with 70 ml of the mobile phase by shaking with the aid of ultrasound for 30 minutes, allow to cool, add sufficient of the mobile phase to produce 100 ml, filter and use the filtrate. Solution (2) contains 0.1% w/v of *atenolol BPCRS* in the mobile phase. Solution (3) contains 0.025% w/v of *chlorthalidone BPCRS* in the mobile phase.

The chromatographic procedure may be carried out using (a) a stainless steel column (20 cm× 4.6 mm) packed with *stationary phase C* (5 µm) (Nucleosil C18 is suitable), (b) as the mobile phase with a flow rate of 1.0 ml per minute a mixture of 10 volumes of *sulphuric acid (10%)*, 50 volumes of *propan-2-ol*, 200 volumes of *acetonitrile* and 740 volumes of *water* containing 0.5 g per litre of *sodium octanesulphonate* and adjusted to pH 3.0 with 2M *sodium hydroxide* and (c) a detection wavelength of 275 nm.

Calculate the content of $C_{14}H_{22}N_2O_3$ and of $C_{14}H_{11}ClN_2O_4S$ using the declared contents of $C_{14}H_{22}N_2O_3$ and of $C_{14}H_{11}ClN_2O_4S$ in *atenolol BPCRS* and in *chlorthalidone BPCRS*, respectively.

Co-triamterzide Tablets

Triamterene and Hydrochlorothiazide Tablets

Definition Co-triamterzide Tablets contain Triamterene and Hydrochlorothiazide in the proportions, by weight, 2 parts to 1 part.

The tablets comply with the requirements stated under Tablets and with the following requirements.

Content of triamterene, $C_{12}H_{11}N_7$ 95.0 to 105.0% of the prescribed or stated amount.

Content of hydrochlorothiazide, $C_7H_8ClN_3O_4S_2$ 95.0 to 105.0% of the prescribed or stated amount.

Identification

A. Shake a quantity of the powdered tablets containing 50 mg of hydrochlorothiazide with 25 ml of *acetone*, filter, evaporate the filtrate to dryness and dry the residue at 100° for 1 hour. The *infrared absorption spectrum* of the dried residue, Appendix II A, is concordant with the *reference spectrum* of hydrochlorothiazide.

B. In test A for Related substances, the principal spot in the chromatogram obtained with solution (1) corresponds to that in the chromatogram obtained with solution (3).

C. In the Assay, the two principal peaks in the chromatogram obtained with solution (3) have the same retention times as the peak due to triamterene in the chromatogram obtained with solution (1) and as the peak due to hydrochlorothiazide in the chromatogram obtained with solution (2).

5-Nitroso-2,4,6-triaminopyrimidine Carry out the method for *thin-layer chromatography*, Appendix III A, using *silica gel HF_{254}* as the coating substance. Apply separately to the plate, as 1.5-cm bands, two 10-µl applications of each of the following four freshly prepared solutions. For solution (1) shake a quantity of the powdered tablets containing 0.10 g of Triamterene with 10 ml of *anhydrous formic acid* for 5 minutes, centrifuge and use the clear supernatant liquid. For solution (2) dissolve 5 mg of *5-nitroso-2,4,6-triaminopyrimidine EPCRS* in 50 ml of *anhydrous formic acid* and dilute 1 volume of the solution to 10 volumes with the same solvent. Prepare solution (3) in the same manner as solution (1) but shaking with 10 ml of solution (2) in place of the formic acid. For solution (4) dissolve 5 mg of *hydrochlorothiazide BPCRS* in 1 ml of *acetone*.

Develop over a path of 5 cm using *ether* as the mobile phase, remove the plate, allow it to dry in air and develop over a path of 10 cm using a 0.05% w/v solution of *fluorescein sodium* in a mixture of 10 volumes of *glacial acetic acid*, 10 volumes of *methanol* and 80 volumes of *ethyl acetate* as the mobile phase. After removal of the plate, dry it in a current of air, expose to ammonia vapour for a few seconds and examine under *ultraviolet light (254* and *365 nm)*. Any band corresponding to 5-nitroso-2,4,6-triaminopyrimidine in the chromatogram obtained with solution (1) is not more intense than the band in the chromatogram obtained with solution (2) (0.1%). The test is not valid unless, in the chromatogram obtained with solution (3), a band corresponding to the band due to hydrochlorothiazide (obtained with solution (4)), appears above, and is clearly separated from, the band due to 5-nitroso-2,4,6-triaminopyrimidine.

Related substances

A. Carry out the method for *thin-layer chromatography*, Appendix III A, using *silica gel G* as the coating substance and a mixture of 10 volumes of 18M *ammonia*, 10 volumes of *methanol* and 90 volumes of *ethyl acetate* as the mobile phase. Apply separately to the plate 5 µl of each of the following solutions. For solution (1) shake a quantity of the powdered tablets containing 0.10 g of Triamterene with 20 ml of *dimethyl sulphoxide*, centrifuge and dilute 2 volumes of the supernatant liquid to 50 volumes with *methanol*. For solution (2) dilute 1 volume of solution (1) to 200 volumes with *methanol*. For solution (3) dissolve 20 mg of *triamterene BPCRS* in 4 ml of *dimethyl sulphoxide* and add sufficient *methanol* to produce 100 ml. After removal of the plate, allow it to dry in air until the odour of the solvent is no longer detectable and examine under *ultraviolet light (365 nm)*. Any *secondary spot* in the chromatogram obtained with solution (1) is not more intense than the spot in the chromatogram obtained with solution (2) (0.5%, with reference to the content of triamterene).

B. Carry out the method for *thin-layer chromatography*, Appendix III A, using *silica gel G* as the coating substance and a mixture of 15 volumes of *propan-2-ol* and 85 volumes of *ethyl acetate* as the mobile phase. Apply separately to the plate 5 µl of each of the following solutions. For solution (1) vigorously shake a quantity of the powdered tablets containing 50 mg of Hydrochlorothiazide with 50 ml of *acetone*, filter, evaporate the filtrate to dryness and dissolve the residue in 10 ml of *acetone*. For solution (2) dilute 1 volume of solution (1) to 100 volumes with *acetone*. After removal of the plate, dry it in a current of air and reveal the spots by *Method I*. Any *secondary spot* in the chromatogram obtained with solution (1) is not more intense than the spot in the chromatogram obtained with solution (2) (1%, with reference to the content of hydrochlorothiazide). Disregard any spot close to the line of application.

Assay Weigh and powder 20 tablets. Carry out the method for *liquid chromatography*, Appendix III D, using the following solutions. For solution (1) add 25 ml of *acetonitrile* and 4 ml of *glacial acetic acid* to a quantity of the powdered tablets containing 25 mg of Hydrochlorothiazide, mix, immediately add 20 ml of *water*, shake for 15 minutes, dilute to 100 ml with *water* and filter through glass-fibre paper (Whatman GF/A is suitable). Dilute 10 ml of the filtrate to 100 ml with *water*. For solution (2) dissolve 50 mg of *triamterene BPCRS* in 25 ml of *acetonitrile*, add 4 ml of *glacial acetic acid* and immediately add sufficient *water* to produce 100 ml. Dilute 10 ml to 100 ml with *water*. For solution (3) dissolve 25 mg of *hydrochlorothiazide BPCRS* in 25 ml of *acetonitrile*, add 4 ml of *glacial acetic acid* and immediately add sufficient *water* to produce 100 ml. Dilute 10 ml to 100 ml with *water*.

The chromatographic procedure may be carried out using (a) a stainless steel column (30 cm × 3.9 mm) packed with *stationary phase C* (10 µm) (µBondapak C18 is suitable), (b) a mixture of 2 volumes of *methanol*, 18 volumes of *acetonitrile*, 40 volumes of a 0.5% w/v solution of *ammonium chloride* and 40 volumes of 0.01M *sodium perchlorate* as the mobile phase with a flow rate of 2.0 ml per minute and (c) a detection wavelength of 273 nm.

Calculate the content of $C_{12}H_{11}N_7$ and $C_7H_8ClN_3O_4S_2$ using the declared contents of $C_{12}H_{11}N_7$ and $C_7H_8ClN_3O_4S_2$ in *triamterene BPCRS* and *hydrochlorothiazide BPCRS* respectively.

Storage Co-triamterzide Tablets should be stored at a temperature not exceeding 25° and protected from moisture.

Co-trimoxazole Intravenous Infusion

Trimethoprim and Sulfamethoxazole Intravenous Infusion

Definition Co-trimoxazole Intravenous Infusion is a sterile solution containing Trimethoprim and the sodium derivative of Sulfamethoxazole. It is prepared immediately before use by diluting Sterile Co-trimoxazole Concentrate with between 25 and 35 times its volume of Glucose Intravenous Infusion or Sodium Chloride Intravenous Infusion.

The intravenous infusion complies with the requirements stated under Parenteral Preparations.

STERILE CO-TRIMOXAZOLE CONCENTRATE

Definition Sterile Co-trimoxazole Concentrate is a sterile solution of Trimethoprim and sulfamethoxazole sodium, prepared by the interaction of Sulfamethoxazole and Sodium Hydroxide, in the proportion 1 part to 5 parts, in Water for Injections containing 40 to 45% v/v of Propylene Glycol.

The concentrate complies with the requirements for Concentrated Solutions for Injections stated under Parenteral Preparations and with the following requirements.

Content of trimethoprim, $C_{14}H_{18}N_4O_3$ 92.5 to 107.5% of the prescribed or stated amount of Trimethoprim.

Content of sulfamethoxazole, $C_{10}H_{11}N_3O_3S$ 92.5 to 107.5% of the prescribed or stated amount of Sulfamethoxazole.

Characteristics A colourless or slightly yellow solution.

Identification

A. Add dropwise to 75 ml of 0.1M *hydrochloric acid* a volume of the solution containing 0.8 g of Sulfamethoxazole, stirring continuously. Allow the suspension to stand for 5 minutes and filter through a sintered-glass filter. Wash the residue with 10 ml of *water*, recrystallise from *ethanol (96%)* and dry at 105°. Reserve part of the residue for test D and dissolve the remainder in the minimum volume of a 5% w/v solution of *sodium carbonate*, add 1M *hydrochloric acid* dropwise until precipitation is complete, filter, wash the residue sparingly with *water* and dry at 105°. The *infrared absorption spectrum* of the residue, Appendix II A, is concordant with the *reference spectrum* of sulfamethoxazole.

B. To a volume containing 80 mg of Trimethoprim add 30 ml of 0.1M *sodium hydroxide* and extract with two 50-ml quantities of *chloroform*. Wash the combined extracts with two 10-ml quantities of 0.1M *sodium hydroxide* and then with 10 ml of *water*, shake with 5 g of *anhydrous sodium sulphate*, filter and evaporate the filtrate to dryness using a rotary evaporator. The *infrared absorption spectrum* of the residue, Appendix II A, is concordant with the *reference spectrum* of trimethoprim.

C. Carry out the method for *thin-layer chromatography*, Appendix III A, using *silica gel G* as the coating substance and a mixture of 100 volumes of *chloroform*, 10 volumes of *methanol* and 5 volumes of *dimethylformamide* as the mobile phase. Apply separately to the plate 5 µl of each of the following solutions. For solution (1) evaporate to dryness a volume of the solution containing 0.16 g of Sulfamethoxazole, shake the residue with 8 ml of *methanol* and filter. Solution (2) contains 2.0% w/v of *sulfamethoxazole BPCRS* in *methanol*. Solution (3) contains 0.4% w/v of *trimethoprim BPCRS* in *methanol*. After removal of the plate, allow it to dry in air and spray with *dilute potassium iodobismuthate solution*. One of the principal spots in the chromatogram obtained with solution (1) corresponds to the spot in the chromatogram obtained with solution (2) and the other corresponds to that in the chromatogram obtained with solution (3).

Alkalinity pH, 9.5 to 11.0, Appendix V L.

Assay

For trimethoprim To a volume containing 48 mg of Trimethoprim add 30 ml of 0.1M *sodium hydroxide* and extract with four 50-ml quantities of *chloroform*, washing each extract with the same two 10-ml quantities of 0.1M *sodium hydroxide*. Combine the chloroform extracts, extract with four 50-ml quantities of 1M *acetic acid*, wash the combined extracts with 5 ml of *chloroform* and dilute the aqueous extracts to 250 ml with 1M *acetic acid*. To 10 ml of the resulting solution add 10 ml of 1M *acetic acid* and sufficient *water* to produce 100 ml and measure the *absorbance* of the resulting solution at the maximum at 271 nm, Appendix II B. Calculate the content of $C_{14}H_{18}N_4O_3$ taking 204 as the value of A(1%, 1 cm) at the maximum at 271 nm.

For sulfamethoxazole To a volume of the solution containing 0.4 g of Sulfamethoxazole add 60 ml of *water* and 10 ml of *hydrochloric acid*. Add 3 g of *potassium bromide*, cool in ice and titrate slowly with 0.1M *sodium nitrite VS*, stirring constantly and determining the end point electrometrically. Each ml of 0.1M *sodium nitrite VS* is equivalent to 25.33 mg of $C_{10}H_{11}N_3O_3S$.

Storage Sterile Co-trimoxazole Concentrate should be protected from light.

Labelling The label states (1) 'Sterile Co-trimoxazole Concentrate'; (2) the contents of Trimethoprim and of Sulfamethoxazole in a suitable volume; (3) that the solution should be protected from light; (4) that the solution must be diluted with between 25 and 35 times its volume of Glucose Intravenous Infusion or Sodium Chloride Intravenous Infusion immediately before use; (5) that the Co-trimoxazole Intravenous Infusion so prepared is to be administered intravenously; (6) that the intravenous infusion should be discarded if any visible particles appear.

Co-trimoxazole Oral Suspension

Trimethoprim and Sulfamethoxazole Oral Suspension

Definition Co-trimoxazole Oral Suspension is a suspension containing 1.6% w/v of Trimethoprim and 8.0% w/v of Sulfamethoxazole in a suitable flavoured vehicle.

The oral suspension complies with the requirements stated under Oral Liquids and with the following requirements.

Content of trimethoprim, $C_{14}H_{18}N_4O_3$ 1.44 to 1.76% w/v.

Content of sulfamethoxazole, $C_{10}H_{11}N_3O_3S$ 7.40 to 8.60% w/v.

Identification

A. To a quantity containing 50 mg of Trimethoprim add 30 ml of 0.1M *sodium hydroxide* and extract with four 50-ml quantities of *chloroform*. Wash the combined extracts with two 10-ml quantities of 0.1M *sodium hydroxide* and extract with two 50-ml quantities of *chloroform*. Wash the combined chloroform extracts with two 10-ml quantities of 0.1M *sodium hydroxide* and then with 10 ml of *water*. Shake with 5 g of *anhydrous sodium sulphate*, filter and evaporate to dryness using a rotary evaporator. The *infra-red absorption spectrum* of the residue, Appendix II A, is concordant with the *reference spectrum* of trimethoprim.

B. Carry out the method for *thin-layer chromatography*, Appendix III A, using *silica gel G* as the coating substance and a mixture of 100 volumes of *chloroform*, 10 volumes of *methanol* and 5 volumes of *dimethylformamide* as the mobile phase. Apply separately to the plate 5 µl of each of the following solutions. For solution (1) add 20 ml of *methanol* to 5 ml of the oral suspension, mix, shake with 10 g of *anhydrous sodium sulphate*, centrifuge and use the supernatant liquid. Solution (2) contains 2.0% w/v of *sulfamethoxazole BPCRS* in *methanol*. Solution (3) contains 0.4% w/v of *trimethoprim BPCRS* in *methanol*. After removal of the plate, allow it to dry in air and spray with *dilute potassium iodobismuthate solution*. One of the principal spots in the chromatogram obtained with solution (1) corresponds to the spot in the chromatogram obtained with solution (2) and the other corresponds to the spot in the chromatogram obtained with solution (3).

Acidity pH, 5.0 to 6.5, Appendix V L.

Assay

For trimethoprim Extract the chloroform solution reserved in the Assay for sulfamethoxazole with four 50-ml quantities of 1M *acetic acid*. Wash the combined extracts with 5 ml of *chloroform* and dilute the aqueous extracts to 250 ml with 1M *acetic acid*. To 10 ml of this solution add 10 ml of 1M *acetic acid* and sufficient *water* to produce 100 ml and measure the *absorbance* of the resulting solution at the maximum at 271 nm, Appendix II B. Calculate the content of $C_{14}H_{18}N_4O_3$ taking 204 as the value of A(1%, 1 cm) at the maximum at 271 nm. Using the weight per ml of the oral suspension, calculate the content of $C_{14}H_{18}N_4O_3$, weight in volume.

For sulfamethoxazole To 4 g of the oral suspension add 30 ml of 0.1M *sodium hydroxide*, shake and extract with four 50-ml quantities of *chloroform*, washing each extract with the same two 10-ml quantities of 0.1M *sodium hydroxide*. Reserve the combined chloroform extracts for the Assay for trimethoprim. Dilute the combined aqueous solution and washings to 250 ml with *water*, filter and dilute 5 ml of the filtrate to 200 ml with *water* (solution A). Carry out the following procedure protected from light using 2 ml of solution A. Add 0.5 ml of 4M *hydrochloric acid* and 1 ml of a 0.1% w/v solution of *sodium nitrite* and allow to stand for 2 minutes. Add 1 ml of a 0.5% w/v solution of *ammonium sulphamate* and allow to stand for 3 minutes. Add 1 ml of a 0.1% w/v solution of *N-(1-naphthyl)ethylenediamine dihydrochloride* and allow to stand for 10 minutes. Dilute the resulting solution to 25 ml with *water* and measure the *absorbance* at 538 nm, Appendix II B, using in the reference cell a solution prepared in the same manner but using 2 ml of *water* in place of solution A. Dissolve 0.25 g of *sulfamethoxazole BPCRS* in 50 ml of 0.1M *sodium hydroxide* and dilute to 250 ml with *water*. Dilute 5 ml of the resulting solution to 200 ml with *water* (solution B). Repeat the procedure using 2 ml of solution B and beginning at the words 'Add 0.5 ml of...'. Calculate the content of $C_{10}H_{11}N_3O_3S$ from the values of the absorbances obtained. Determine the *weight per ml* of the oral suspension, Appendix V G, and calculate the content of $C_{10}H_{11}N_3O_3S$, weight in volume.

Storage Co-trimoxazole Oral Suspension should be protected from light and stored at a temperature not exceeding 30°.

Co-trimoxazole Oral Suspension contains, in 5 ml, 80 mg of Trimethoprim and 400 mg of Sulfamethoxazole.

Paediatric Co-trimoxazole Oral Suspension

Paediatric Trimethoprim and Sulfamethoxazole Oral Suspension

Definition Paediatric Co-trimoxazole Oral Suspension is a suspension containing 0.8% w/v of Trimethoprim and 4% w/v of Sulfamethoxazole in a suitable flavoured vehicle.

The oral suspension complies with the requirements stated under Oral Liquids and with the following requirements.

Content of trimethoprim, $C_{14}H_{18}N_4O_3$ 0.72 to 0.88% w/v.

Content of sulfamethoxazole, $C_{10}H_{11}N_3O_3S$ 3.60 to 4.40% w/v.

Identification Complies with the tests described under Co-trimoxazole Oral Suspension but in test B for solution (2) use a 1.0% w/v solution of *sulfamethoxazole BPCRS* in *methanol* and for solution (3) use a 0.20% w/v solution of *trimethoprim BPCRS* in *methanol*. Apply to the plate 10 µl of each of the three solutions.

Acidity pH, 5.0 to 6.5, Appendix V L.

Assay Carry out the Assays for trimethoprim and sulfamethoxazole described under Co-trimoxazole Oral Suspension but using 8 g of the oral suspension.

Storage Paediatric Co-trimoxazole Oral Suspension should be protected from light and stored at a temperature not exceeding 30°.

Paediatric Co-trimoxazole Oral Suspension contains, in 5 ml, 40 mg of Trimethoprim and 200 mg of Sulfamethoxazole.

Co-trimoxazole Tablets

Trimethoprim and Sulfamethoxazole Tablets

Definition Co-trimoxazole Tablets contain Trimethoprim and Sulfamethoxazole in the proportions, by weight, 1 part to 5 parts.

With the exception of the requirements for shape, the tablets comply with the requirements stated under Tablets and with the following requirements.

Content of trimethoprim, $C_{14}H_{18}N_4O_3$ 92.5 to 107.5% of the prescribed or stated amount of Trimethoprim.

Content of sulfamethoxazole, $C_{10}H_{11}N_3O_3S$ 92.5 to 107.5% of the prescribed or stated amount of Sulfamethoxazole.

Identification

A. Filter the aqueous layer reserved in the Assay for trimethoprim. Add, dropwise, sufficient 2M *hydrochloric acid* to the filtrate to make it just acidic and extract with 50 ml of *ether*. Wash the ether layer with 10 ml of *water*, shake with 5 g of *anhydrous sodium sulphate*, filter and evaporate the filtrate to dryness using a rotary evaporator. Dissolve the residue in the minimum volume of a 5% w/v solution of *sodium carbonate*, add 1M *hydrochloric acid* dropwise until precipitation is complete and filter. Wash the residue sparingly with *water* and dry at 105°. The *infrared absorption spectrum* of the residue, Appendix II A, is concordant with the *reference spectrum* of sulfamethoxazole.

B. To a quantity of the powdered tablets containing 50 mg of Trimethoprim add 30 ml of 0.1M *sodium hydroxide* and extract with two 50-ml quantities of *chloroform*. Wash the combined chloroform extracts with two 10-ml quantities of 0.1M *sodium hydroxide* and then with 10 ml of *water*. Shake with 5 g of *anhydrous sodium sulphate*, filter and evaporate to dryness using a rotary evaporator. The *infrared absorption spectrum* of the residue, Appendix II A, is concordant with the *reference spectrum* of trimethoprim.

C. Carry out the method for *thin-layer chromatography*, Appendix III A, using *silica gel G* as the coating substance and a mixture of 100 volumes of *chloroform*, 10 volumes of *methanol* and 5 volumes of *dimethylformamide* as the mobile phase. Apply separately to the plate 5 µl of each of the following solutions. For solution (1) shake a quantity of the powdered tablets containing 0.4 g of Sulfamethoxazole with 20 ml of *methanol* and filter. Solution (2) contains 2.0% w/v of *sulfamethoxazole BPCRS* in *methanol*. Solution (3) contains 0.4% w/v of *trimethoprim BPCRS* in *methanol*. After removal of the plate, allow it to dry in air and spray with *dilute potassium iodobismuthate solution*. One of the principal spots in the chromatogram obtained with solution (1) corresponds to the spot in the chromatogram obtained with solution (2) and the other corresponds to the spot in the chromatogram obtained with solution (3).

Assay

For trimethoprim To a quantity of the powder containing 50 mg of Trimethoprim add 30 ml of 0.1M *sodium hydroxide* and extract with four 50-ml quantities of *chloroform*, washing each extract with the same two 10-ml quantities of 0.1M *sodium hydroxide*. Reserve the aqueous layer for test A for Identification. Combine the chloroform extracts and extract with four 50-ml quantities of 1M *acetic acid*. Wash the combined extracts with 5 ml of *chloroform* and dilute the aqueous extracts to 250 ml with 1M *acetic acid*. To 10 ml of the solution add 10 ml of 1M *acetic acid* and sufficient *water* to produce 100 ml and measure the *absorbance* of the resulting solution at the maximum at 271 nm, Appendix II B. Calculate the content of $C_{14}H_{18}N_4O_3$ taking 204 as the value of A(1%, 1 cm) at the maximum at 271 nm.

For sulfamethoxazole Weigh and powder 20 tablets. Dissolve, as completely as possible, a quantity of the powder containing 0.5 g of Sulfamethoxazole in 60 ml of *water* and 10 ml of *hydrochloric acid*. Add 3 g of *potassium bromide*, cool in ice and titrate slowly with 0.1M *sodium nitrite VS*, stirring constantly and determining the end point electrometrically. Each ml of 0.1M *sodium nitrite VS* is equivalent to 25.33 mg of $C_{10}H_{11}N_3O_3S$.

Labelling The label states the quantities of Trimethoprim and of Sulfamethoxazole in each tablet.

Dispersible Co-trimoxazole Tablets

Dispersible Trimethoprim and Sulfamethoxazole Tablets

Definition Dispersible Co-trimoxazole Tablets contain Trimethoprim and Sulfamethoxazole and in the proportions, by weight, 1 part to 5 parts in a suitable dispersible basis.

With the exception of the requirements for shape, the tablets comply with the requirements stated under Tablets and with the following requirements.

Content of trimethoprim, $C_{14}H_{18}N_4O_3$ 92.5 to 107.5% of the prescribed or stated amount of Trimethoprim.

Content of sulfamethoxazole, $C_{10}H_{11}N_3O_3S$ 92.5 to 107.5% of the prescribed or stated amount of Sulfamethoxazole.

Identification

A. Filter the aqueous layer reserved in the Assay for trimethoprim. Add, dropwise, sufficient 2M *hydrochloric acid* to the filtrate to make it just acidic and extract with 50 ml of *ether*. Wash the ether layer with 10 ml of *water*, shake with 5 g of *anhydrous sodium sulphate*, filter and evaporate the filtrate to dryness using a rotary evaporator. Dissolve the residue in the minimum volume of a 5% w/v solution of *sodium carbonate*, add 1M *hydrochloric acid* dropwise until precipitation is complete and filter. Wash the residue sparingly with *water* and dry at 105°. The *infrared absorption spectrum* of the residue, Appendix II A, is concordant with the *reference spectrum* of sulfamethoxazole.

B. To a quantity of the powdered tablets containing 50 mg of Trimethoprim add 30 ml of 0.1M *sodium hydroxide* and extract with two 50-ml quantities of *chloroform*. Wash the combined chloroform extracts with two 10-ml quantities of 0.1M *sodium hydroxide* and then with 10 ml of *water*. Shake with 5 g of *anhydrous sodium sulphate*, filter and evaporate to dryness using a rotary evaporator. The *infrared absorption spectrum* of the residue, Appendix II A, is concordant with the *reference spectrum* of trimethoprim.

C. Carry out the method for *thin-layer chromatography*, Appendix III A, using *silica gel G* as the coating substance and a mixture of 100 volumes of *chloroform*, 10 volumes of *methanol* and 5 volumes of *dimethylformamide* as the mobile phase. Apply separately to the plate 5 µl of each of the following solutions. For solution (1) shake a quantity of the powdered tablets containing 0.4 g of Sulfamethoxazole with 20 ml of *methanol* and filter. Solution (2) contains 2.0% w/v of *sulfamethoxazole BPCRS* in *methanol*. Solution (3) contains 0.4% w/v of *trimethoprim BPCRS* in *methanol*. After removal of the plate, allow it to dry in air and spray with *dilute potassium iodobismuthate solution*. One of the principal spots in the chromatogram obtained with solution (1) corresponds to the spot in the chromatogram obtained with solution (2) and the other corresponds to the spot in the chromatogram obtained with solution (3).

Disintegration The tablets disintegrate within 2 minutes when examined by the *disintegration test for tablets and capsules*, Appendix XII A, but using *water* at 19° to 21°.

Assay

For trimethoprim To a quantity of the powder containing 50 mg of Trimethoprim add 30 ml of 0.1M *sodium hydroxide* and extract with four 50-ml quantities of *chloroform*, washing each extract with the same two 10-ml quantities of 0.1M *sodium hydroxide*. Reserve the aqueous layer for test A for Identification. Combine the chloroform extracts and extract with four 50-ml quantities of 1M *acetic acid*. Wash the combined extracts with four 5-ml quantities of *chloroform* and dilute the aqueous extracts to 250 ml with 1M *acetic acid*. To 10 ml of the solution add 10 ml of 1M *acetic acid* and sufficient *water* to produce 100 ml and measure the *absorbance* of the resulting solution at the maximum at 271 nm, Appendix II B. Calculate the content of $C_{14}H_{18}N_4O_3$ taking 204 as the value of A(1%, 1 cm) at the maximum at 271 nm.

For sulfamethoxazole Weigh and powder 20 tablets. Dissolve, as completely as possible, a quantity of the powder containing 0.5 g of Sulfamethoxazole in 60 ml of *water* and 10 ml of *hydrochloric acid*. Add 3 g of *potassium bromide*, cool in ice and titrate slowly with 0.1M *sodium nitrite VS*, stirring constantly and determining the end point electrometrically. Each ml of 0.1M *sodium nitrite VS* is equivalent to 25.33 mg of $C_{10}H_{11}N_3O_3S$.

Labelling The label states (1) the quantities of Trimethoprim and of Sulfamethoxazole in each tablet; (2) that the tablets should be dispersed in water immediately before use.

Paediatric Co-trimoxazole Tablets

Paediatric Trimethoprim and Sulfamethoxazole Tablets

Definition Paediatric Co-trimoxazole Tablets contain, in each, 20 mg of Trimethoprim and 100 mg of Sulfamethoxazole.

With the exception of the requirements for shape, the tablets comply with the requirements stated under Tablets and with the following requirements.

Content of trimethoprim, $C_{14}H_{18}N_4O_3$ 0.0185 to 0.0215 g.

Content of sulfamethoxazole, $C_{10}H_{11}N_3O_3S$ 0.0925 to 0.1075 g.

Identification Comply with the tests described under Co-trimoxazole Tablets.

Assay Carry out the Assays for trimethoprim and for sulfamethoxazole described under Co-trimoxazole Tablets.

Labelling The label states the quantities of Trimethoprim and of Sulfamethoxazole in each tablet.

Crotamiton Cream

Definition Crotamiton Cream contains Crotamiton in a suitable basis.

The cream complies with the requirements stated under Topical Semi-solid Preparations and with the following requirements.

Content of crotamiton, $C_{13}H_{17}NO$ 93.0 to 107.0% of the prescribed or stated amount.

Identification

A. Mix a quantity of the cream containing 0.5 g of Crotamiton with 50 ml of *water* and then slowly add 50 ml of 1M *sodium hydroxide* while stirring vigorously. Filter the mixture, adjust the filtrate to pH 7 with 5M *hydrochloric acid* and extract with 50 ml of *ether*. Wash the ether layer with 10 ml of a saturated solution of *sodium chloride*, dry the organic layer over *anhydrous sodium sulphate*, filter and evaporate to an oily residue. The *light absorption*, Appendix II B, in the range 220 to 350 nm of a 0.003% w/v solution of the residue in *cyclohexane* exhibits a maximum only at 242 nm. The A(1%, 1 cm) at the maximum is about 315.

B. Carry out the method for *thin-layer chromatography*, Appendix III A, using *silica gel GF_{254}* as the coating substance and a mobile phase prepared in the following manner. Shake 98 volumes of *chloroform* with 2 volumes of 18M *ammonia*, dry over *anhydrous sodium sulphate*, filter and mix 97 volumes of the filtrate with 3 volumes of *propan-2-ol*. Apply separately to the plate 5 µl of each of the following solutions in *absolute ethanol*. Solution (1) contains 0.25% w/v of the residue obtained in test A. Solution (2) contains 0.25% w/v of *crotamiton BPCRS*. Solution (3) is a mixture of equal volumes of solutions (1) and (2). After removal of the plate, allow it to dry in air and examine under *ultraviolet light (254 nm)*. The principal spot in the chromatogram obtained with solution (1) corresponds to that in the chromatogram obtained with solution (2), but if not, the principal spot in the chromatogram obtained with solution (3) appears as a single compact spot.

C. In the Assay, the principal peak in the chromatogram obtained with solution (2) has the same retention time as the principal peak in the chromatogram obtained with solution (1).

Related substances Carry out the method for *liquid chromatography*, Appendix III D, using the following solutions. Solution (1) contains 0.0005% w/v of *crotamiton BPCRS* in *hexane*. Solution (2) contains 0.050% w/v of *crotamiton BPCRS* in *hexane*. For solution (3) add 2 ml of *water* and 100 ml of *hexane* to a quantity of the preparation being examined containing 0.1 g of Crotamiton, shake for 10 minutes and separate the lower, aqueous layer. Repeat the extraction using a further 10 ml of *hexane*, filter the combined hexane extracts and add sufficient *hexane* to produce 200 ml.

The chromatographic procedure may be carried out using (a) a stainless steel column (20 cm × 4.6 mm) packed with *stationary phase A* (10 µm) (Partisil is suitable), (b) a mixture of 200 volumes of *hexane* and 1.4 volumes of *absolute ethanol* as the mobile phase with a flow rate of 3 ml per minute and (c) a detection wavelength of 242 nm. For solution (3) allow the chromatography to proceed for at least twice the retention time of the peak due to crotamiton.

In the chromatogram obtained with solution (2) the principal peak, other than any peak due to solvent, is due to the *E*-isomer, the peak with a retention time of 0.6 relative to the principal peak is due to the *Z*-isomer and the peak with a retention time of 0.8 relative to the principal peak is due to *N*-ethyl-α-vinylaceto-*o*-toluidide. The content of *N*-ethyl-α-vinylaceto-*o*-toluidide in the preparation is not more than 3% of the total content of crotamiton calculated using the declared content of *N*-ethyl-α-vinylaceto-*o*-toluidide in *crotamiton BPCRS*. In the chromatogram obtained with solution (3) the sum of the areas of any peaks other than the solvent peak, the peaks due to the *E*- and *Z*-isomers and the peak due to *N*-ethyl-α-vinylaceto-*o*-toluidide is not greater than the sum of the areas of the peaks due to *E*- and *Z*-isomers in the chromatogram obtained with solution (1).

Z-Isomer Not more than 15% of the total content of *E*- and *Z*-isomers determined in the Assay.

Assay Carry out the method for *liquid chromatography*, Appendix III D, using the following solutions. Solution (1) contains 0.0025% w/v of *crotamiton BPCRS* in *hexane*. For solution (2) add 2 ml of *water* and 100 ml of *hexane* to a quantity of the preparation being examined containing 0.1 g of Crotamiton, shake for 10 minutes and separate the lower, aqueous layer. Repeat the extraction using two 10-ml quantities of *hexane*, filter the combined extracts and add sufficient *hexane* to produce 200 ml. Dilute 5 ml of this solution to 100 ml with *hexane*.

The chromatographic procedure described under Related substances may be used.

In the chromatogram obtained with solution (1) the principal peak is due to the *E*-isomer and the peak with a retention time of 0.6 relative to the principal peak is due to the *Z*-isomer. Calculate the contents of the *E*- and *Z*-isomers in the preparation being examined using the declared contents of *E*- and *Z*-crotamiton in *crotamiton BPCRS* and hence calculate the content of $C_{13}H_{17}NO$ in the preparation being examined.

Crotamiton Lotion

Definition Crotamiton Lotion is a *cutaneous suspension*. It contains Crotamiton in a suitable vehicle.

The lotion complies with the requirements stated under Liquids for Cutaneous Application and with the following requirements.

Content of crotamiton, $C_{13}H_{17}NO$ 93.0 to 107.0% of the prescribed or stated amount.

Identification

A. To a quantity of the lotion containing 0.5 g of Crotamiton add 30 ml of 1M *hydrochloric acid* and shake to produce a uniform suspension. Extract with 100 ml of *petroleum spirit (boiling range, 40° to 60°)*, wash the petroleum spirit layer with 10 ml of 1M *hydrochloric acid*, with two 10-ml quantities of 1M *sodium hydroxide* and then with 10 ml of a saturated solution of *sodium chloride*. Dry the organic layer over *anhydrous sodium sulphate*, filter and evaporate to an oily residue. The *light absorption*, Appendix II B, in the range 220 to 350 nm of a 0.003% w/v solution of the residue in *cyclohexane* exhibits a maximum only at 242 nm. The A(1%, 1 cm) at the maximum is about 315.

B. Carry out Identification test B described under Crotamiton Cream using the residue from test A above in the preparation of solution (1).

C. In the Assay, the principal peak in the chromatogram obtained with solution (2) has the same retention time as the principal peak in the chromatogram obtained with solution (1).

Related substances Complies with the test described under Crotamiton Cream using a quantity of the lotion containing 0.1 g of Crotamiton.

Z-Isomer Not more than 15% of the total content of *E*- and *Z*-isomers determined in the Assay.

Assay Carry out the Assay described under Crotamiton Cream using a quantity of the lotion containing 0.1 g of Crotamiton.

Labelling The label indicates the pharmaceutical form as 'cutaneous suspension'.

Cyanocobalamin Injection

Definition Cyanocobalamin Injection is a sterile solution of Cyanocobalamin in Water for Injections containing sufficient Acetic Acid or Hydrochloric Acid to adjust the pH to about 4.

The injection complies with the requirements stated under Parenteral Preparations and with the following requirements.

Content of anhydrous cyanocobalamin, $C_{63}H_{88}CoN_{14}O_{14}P$ 95.0 to 110.0% of the prescribed or stated amount.

In carrying out the test for Identification and the Assay, account must be taken of any added antimicrobial preservative.

Identification Measure the *absorbance* of the injection at 278, 361 and 550 nm, Appendix II B. The ratios of the absorbances at 278 nm and 550 nm to the absorbance at 361 nm are about 0.57 and 0.30, respectively.

Acidity pH, 3.8 to 5.5, Appendix V L.

Related substances Carry out the method for *liquid chromatography*, Appendix III D, injecting 20 µl of each of the following solutions. Solutions (1) to (3) are solutions of the injection, diluted if necessary, with the mobile phase containing (1) 0.10% w/v, (2) 0.0030% w/v and (3) 0.00010% w/v of Cyanocobalamin and must be used within 1 hour of preparation. For solution (4) add 1 ml of a 0.1% w/v solution of *chloramine T* and 0.1 ml of 0.05M *hydrochloric acid* to a volume of the injection containing 5 mg of Cyanocobalamin, dilute to 10 ml with *water*, shake and allow to stand for 5 minutes. Dilute 2 ml of this solution to 10 ml with the mobile phase and use immediately.

The chromatographic procedure may be carried out using (a) a stainless steel column (25 cm × 4 mm) packed with *stationary phase B* (5 µm) (Lichrosorb 100 CH8/11 is suitable), (b) a mixture of 53 volumes of *methanol* and 147 volumes of a 1.0% w/v solution of *disodium hydrogen orthophosphate* adjusted to pH 3.5 with *orthophosphoric acid* as the mobile phase with a flow rate of 0.8 ml per minute and (c) a detection wavelength of 361 nm. Use the mobile phase within 2 days of preparation. Record the chromatograms for three times the retention time of cyanocobalamin.

The test is not valid unless the chromatogram obtained with solution (4) exhibits two principal peaks, the *resolution factor* between those peaks is at least 2.5 and the chromatogram obtained with solution (3) exhibits one principal peak with a *signal-to-noise ratio* of at least 5.
In the chromatogram obtained with solution (1) the sum of the areas of any *secondary peaks* is not greater than twice the area of the principal peak in the chromatogram obtained with solution (2) (6%). Disregard any peak the area of which is less than that of the principal peak in the chromatogram obtained with solution (3) (0.1%).

Assay Carry out the following procedure protected from light. Dilute the injection, if necessary, with *water* to produce a solution containing not more than the equivalent of 0.0025% w/v of anhydrous cyanocobalamin and measure the *absorbance* at the maximum at 361 nm, Appendix II B, using *water* in the reference cell. Calculate the content of $C_{63}H_{88}CoN_{14}O_{14}P$ taking 207 as the value of A(1%, 1 cm) at the maximum at 361 nm.

Storage Cyanocobalamin Injection should be protected from light.

Cyclizine Injection

Definition Cyclizine Injection is a sterile solution in Water for Injections containing 5% w/v of cyclizine lactate prepared by the interaction of Cyclizine and Lactic Acid.

The injection complies with the requirements stated under Parenteral Preparations and with the following requirements.

Content of cyclizine lactate, $C_{18}H_{22}N_2,C_3H_6O_3$ 4.65 to 5.25% w/v.

Characteristics A clear, colourless solution.

Identification

A. To 0.5 ml add 10 ml of *water* followed by 5M *sodium hydroxide* until strongly alkaline to *litmus paper.* Extract with two 10-ml quantities of *chloroform* and reserve the aqueous layer for test B. Wash each chloroform extract with 5 ml of *water*, dry the combined extracts with *anhydrous sodium sulphate*, filter and evaporate the filtrate to dryness. Dissolve the residue in *ethanol (96%)* and evaporate to dryness. The *infrared absorption spectrum* of the final residue, Appendix II A, is concordant with the *reference spectrum* of cyclizine.

B. The aqueous solution reserved in test A, after acidification with 1M *sulphuric acid*, yields the reaction characteristic of *lactates*, Appendix VI.

Acidity pH, 3.3 to 3.7, Appendix V L.

Related substances Carry out the method for *thin-layer chromatography*, Appendix III A, using *silica gel G* as the coating substance and as the mobile phase the lower layer obtained after shaking together a mixture of 2 volumes of 13.5M *ammonia*, 8 volumes of *methanol* and 90 volumes of *dichloromethane* and allowing the layers to separate. Apply separately to the plate 20 µl of each of the following freshly prepared solutions. For solution (1) dilute 1 volume of the injection to 5 volumes with *methanol.* For solution (2) dilute 1 volume of solution (1) to 200 volumes with *methanol.* Solution (3) contains 0.020% w/v of N-*methylpiperazine* in *methanol.* For solution (4) dilute 1 volume of solution (1) to 10 volumes with a 0.10% w/v solution of *hydroxyzine hydrochloride EPCRS* in *methanol.* After removal of the plate, allow it to dry in air and expose to iodine vapour for 10 minutes. Any spot corresponding to N-*methylpiperazine* in the chromatogram obtained with solution (1) is not more intense than the spot in the chromatogram obtained with solution (3) (2%). Any other *secondary spot* in the chromatogram obtained with solution (1) is not more intense than the spot in the chromatogram obtained with solution (2) (0.5%). The test is not valid unless the chromatogram obtained with solution (4) shows two clearly separated spots.

Assay Dilute 5 ml to 100 ml with 1M *sulphuric acid.* To 20 ml of this solution add 2 g of *sodium chloride*, shake with two 50-ml quantities of *ether*, allow to separate and wash the ether with the same two 10-ml quantities of *water.* To the combined aqueous solution and washings add 20 ml of 5M *sodium hydroxide* and extract with three 50-ml quantities of *ether.* Combine the ether extracts and wash with two 10-ml quantities of a saturated solution of *sodium chloride.* Extract the ether layer with two 25-ml quantities of 0.05M *sulphuric acid* and then with two 10-ml quantities of *water.* Combine the acidic and aqueous extracts and dilute to 100 ml with *water.* Dilute 5 ml of this solution to 200 ml with 0.05M *sulphuric acid* and measure the *absorbance* of the resulting solution at the maximum at 225 nm, Appendix II B. Calculate the content of $C_{18}H_{22}N_2,C_3H_6O_3$ taking 331 as the value of A(1%, 1 cm) at the maximum at 225 nm.

Labelling The strength is stated in terms of the equivalent amount of cyclizine lactate in a suitable dose-volume.

Cyclizine Tablets

Definition Cyclizine Tablets contain Cyclizine Hydrochloride.

The tablets comply with the requirements stated under Tablets and with the following requirements.

Content of cyclizine hydrochloride, $C_{18}H_{22}N_2,HCl$ 92.5 to 107.5% of the prescribed or stated amount.

Identification

A. Extract a quantity of the powdered tablets containing 0.1 g of Cyclizine Hydrochloride with 10 ml of *ethanol (96%)*, filter and evaporate the filtrate to dryness. The *infrared absorption spectrum* of the residue, Appendix II A, is concordant with the *reference spectrum* of cyclizine hydrochloride.

B. Extract a quantity of the powdered tablets containing 0.5 g of Cyclizine Hydrochloride with 20 ml of *water* and filter. The filtrate yields reaction A characteristic of *chlorides*, Appendix VI.

Related substances Carry out the method for *thin-layer chromatography*, Appendix III A, using *silica gel G* as the coating substance and as the mobile phase the lower layer obtained after shaking together a mixture of 2 volumes of 13.5M *ammonia*, 8 volumes of *methanol* and 90 volumes of *dichloromethane* and allowing the layers to separate. Apply separately to the plate 20 µl of each of the following freshly prepared solutions. For solution (1) triturate a quantity of the powdered tablets containing 0.10 g of Cyclizine Hydrochloride with 10 ml of *methanol* and filter. For solution (2) dilute 1 volume of solution (1) to 200 volumes with *methanol.* Solution (3) contains 0.0050% w/v of N-*methylpiperazine* in *methanol.* For solution (4) dilute 1 volume of solution (1) to 10 volumes with a 0.10% w/v solution of *hydroxyzine hydrochloride EPCRS* in *methanol.* After removal of the plate, allow it to dry in air and expose to iodine vapour for 10 minutes. Any spot corresponding to N-*methylpiperazine* in the chromatogram obtained with solution (1) is not more intense than the spot in the chromatogram obtained with solution (3) (0.5%). Any other *secondary spot* in the chromatogram obtained with solution (1) is not more intense than the spot in the chromatogram obtained with solution (2) (0.5%). The test is not valid unless the chromatogram obtained with solution (4) shows two clearly separated spots.

Assay Weigh and powder 20 tablets. Shake a quantity of the powder containing 0.125 g of Cyclizine Hydrochloride with 400 ml of 0.05M *sulphuric acid* for 15 minutes. Add sufficient 0.05M *sulphuric acid* to produce 500 ml, filter, dilute 5 ml of the filtrate to 100 ml with 0.05M *sulphuric acid* and measure the *absorbance* of the resulting solution at the maximum at 225 nm, Appendix II B. Calculate the content of $C_{18}H_{22}N_2,HCl$ taking 390 as the value of A(1%, 1 cm) at the maximum at 225 nm.

Cyclopenthiazide Tablets

Definition Cyclopenthiazide Tablets contain Cyclopenthiazide.

The tablets comply with the requirements stated under Tablets and with the following requirements.

Content of cyclopenthiazide, $C_{13}H_{18}ClN_3O_4S_2$ 90.0 to 110.0% of the prescribed or stated amount.

Identification

Carry out the method for *thin-layer chromatography*, Appendix III A, using *silica gel GF_{254}* as the coating substance and *ethyl acetate* as the mobile phase. Apply separately to the plate 5 µl of each of the following solutions. For solution (1) shake a quantity of the powdered tablets containing 5 mg of Cyclopenthiazide with 5 ml of *acetone* and filter. Solution (2) contains 0.1% w/v of *cyclopenthiazide BPCRS* in *acetone*. After removal of the plate, dry it in a current of air, examine under *ultraviolet light (254 nm)* and then reveal the spots by *Method I*. By each method of visualisation the principal spot in the chromatogram obtained with solution (1) corresponds in colour and intensity to that in the chromatogram obtained with solution (2).

Related substances Carry out the method for *thin-layer chromatography*, Appendix III A, using *silica gel G* as the coating substance and *ethyl acetate* as the mobile phase. Apply separately to the plate 5 µl of each of the following solutions. For solution (1) shake a quantity of the powdered tablets containing 10 mg of Cyclopenthiazide with 50 ml of *acetone*, filter, evaporate the filtrate to dryness and dissolve the residue in 2 ml of *acetone*. For solution (2) dilute 1 volume of solution (1) to 100 volumes with *acetone*. After removal of the plate, dry it in a current of air and reveal the spots by *Method I*. Any *secondary spot* in the chromatogram obtained with solution (1) is not more intense than the spot in the chromatogram obtained with solution (2).

Uniformity of content Tablets containing less than 2 mg of Cyclopenthiazide comply with the requirements stated under Tablets using the following method of analysis. To one tablet add 50 ml of *methanol*, shake for 20 minutes, filter and measure the *absorbance* of the filtrate at the maximum at 273 nm, Appendix II B. Calculate the content of $C_{13}H_{18}ClN_3O_4S_2$ taking 585 as the value of A(1%, 1 cm) at the maximum at 273 nm.

Assay Weigh and powder 20 tablets. Shake a quantity of the powder containing 7.5 mg of Cyclopenthiazide with 50 ml of *methanol* for 10 minutes and dilute to 100 ml with *methanol*. Mix, filter, dilute 20 ml of the filtrate to 100 ml with *methanol* and measure the *absorbance* of the resulting solution at the maximum at 273 nm, Appendix II B. Calculate the content of $C_{13}H_{18}ClN_3O_4S_2$ taking 585 as the value of A(1%, 1 cm) at the maximum at 273 nm.

Cyclopentolate Eye Drops

Definition Cyclopentolate Eye Drops are a sterile solution of Cyclopentolate Hydrochloride in Purified Water.

The eye drops comply with the requirements stated under Eye Preparations and with the following requirements.

Content of cyclopentolate hydrochloride, $C_{17}H_{25}NO_3,HCl$ 90.0 to 110.0% of the prescribed or stated amount.

Identification

A. Add 2M *ammonia* to a volume of the eye drops containing 25 mg of Cyclopentolate Hydrochloride until alkaline and extract immediately with 50 ml of *ether*. Wash the extract with 5 ml of *water*, filter through *anhydrous sodium sulphate* and evaporate the filtrate to dryness. The *infrared absorption spectrum* of the oily residue, Appendix II A, is concordant with the *reference spectrum* of cyclopentolate.

B. To a volume containing 5 mg of Cyclopentolate Hydrochloride add 1 ml of 5M *sodium hydroxide*, mix, warm on a water bath for 1 minute and add 0.25 ml of *nitric acid*. A sweet odour resembling that of phenylacetic acid is produced.

Acidity pH, 3.0 to 5.5, Appendix V L.

Related substances Carry out the method for *thin-layer chromatography*, Appendix III A, using *silica gel G* as the coating substance and a mixture of 50 volumes of *propan-2-ol*, 30 volumes of *butyl acetate*, 15 volumes of *water* and 5 volumes of 13.5M *ammonia* as the mobile phase. Apply separately to the plate 20 µl of each of the following solutions. For solution (1) use the eye drops diluted, if necessary, to contain 0.5% w/v of Cyclopentolate Hydrochloride. For solution (2) dilute 1 volume of solution (1) to 50 volumes with *water*. For solution (3) dilute 1 volume of solution (1) to 200 volumes with *water*. After removal of the plate, dry it at 120° for 5 minutes, spray with *ethanolic sulphuric acid (10%)*, heat at 120° for 30 minutes and examine under *ultraviolet light (365 nm)*. Any *secondary spot* in the chromatogram obtained with solution (1) is not more intense than the spot in the chromatogram obtained with solution (2) and not more than one such spot is more intense than the spot in the chromatogram obtained with solution (3).

Assay Carry out the method for *liquid chromatography*, Appendix III D, using the following solutions. Prepare a solution containing 0.25% w/v of *4-chlorophenol* (internal standard) in *methanol* (solution A). For solution (1) add 4 ml of solution A to 4 ml of a 0.5% w/v solution of *cyclopentolate hydrochloride BPCRS* in *water* and dilute to 10 ml with the mobile phase. For solution (2) dilute a volume of the eye drops containing 20 mg of Cyclopentolate Hydrochloride to 10 ml with the mobile phase. For solution (3) add 4 ml of solution A to a volume of the eye drops containing 20 mg of Cyclopentolate Hydrochloride and dilute to 10 ml with the mobile phase.

The chromatographic procedure may be carried out using (a) a stainless steel column (20 cm × 4.6 mm) packed with *stationary phase C* (10 µm) (µNucleosil C18 is suitable), (b) a mixture of 55 volumes of *methanol* and 45 volumes of 0.2M *sodium dihydrogen orthophosphate*, the mixture adjusted to pH 3.0 with *orthophosphoric acid*, as the mobile phase with a flow rate of 2 ml per minute and (c) a detection wavelength of 254 nm.

The method is not valid unless the *resolution factor* between the peaks due to cyclopentolate hydrochloride and the internal standard is greater than 4.

Calculate the content of $C_{17}H_{25}NO_3,HCl$ using the declared content of $C_{17}H_{25}NO_3,HCl$ in *cyclopentolate hydrochloride BPCRS*.

Cyclophosphamide Injection

Definition Cyclophosphamide Injection is a sterile, isotonic solution of Cyclophosphamide in Water for Injections. It is prepared by dissolving Cyclophosphamide for Injection in the requisite amount of Water for Injections immediately before use.

The injection complies with the requirements stated under Parenteral Preparations.

Storage Cyclophosphamide Injection deteriorates on storage and should be used immediately after preparation.

CYCLOPHOSPHAMIDE FOR INJECTION

Definition Cyclophosphamide for Injection is a sterile material consisting of Cyclophosphamide with or without excipients. It is supplied in a sealed container.

The contents of the sealed container comply with the requirements for Powders for Injections stated under Parenteral Preparations and with the following requirements.

Content of cyclophosphamide, $C_7H_{15}Cl_2N_2O_2P$ 92.5 to 107.5% of the prescribed or stated amount of anhydrous cyclophosphamide.

Identification

A. Shake a quantity containing the equivalent of 0.2 g of anhydrous cyclophosphamide with 2 ml of *chloroform* and filter. The *infrared absorption spectrum* of the filtrate, Appendix II A, is concordant with the *reference spectrum* of cyclophosphamide.

B. Extract a quantity containing the equivalent of 0.1 g of anhydrous cyclophosphamide with *ether* and evaporate the extract to dryness. Dissolve the residue in 10 ml of *water* and add 5 ml of *silver nitrate solution*; no precipitate is produced. Boil; a white precipitate is produced which is insoluble in *nitric acid* but soluble in 5M *ammonia* from which it is reprecipitated on the addition of *nitric acid.*

Acidity pH of a freshly prepared 2% w/v solution, 4.0 to 6.0, Appendix V L.

Uniformity of content Sealed containers containing the equivalent of 1 g or less of anhydrous cyclophosphamide comply with the requirements stated under Parenteral Preparations, Powders for Injections. Use the individual results obtained in the Assay.

Related substances Carry out the method for *thin-layer chromatography*, Appendix III A, using *silica gel G* as the coating substance and a mixture of 2 volumes of *anhydrous formic acid*, 4 volumes of *acetone*, 12 volumes of *water* and 80 volumes of *butan-2-one* as the mobile phase. Apply separately to the plate 10 µl of each of the following solutions. For solution (1) dissolve a quantity of the contents of the sealed container containing the equivalent of 0.2 g of anhydrous cyclophosphamide in sufficient *ethanol (96%)* to produce 10 ml. For solution (2) dilute 1 volume of solution (1) to 100 volumes with *ethanol (96%).* After removal of the plate, dry it in a current of warm air and heat at 100° for 10 minutes. Place the plate while hot in a chromatography tank in which is placed an evaporating dish containing equal volumes of a 5% w/v solution of *potassium permanganate* and *hydrochloric acid*, close the tank and allow to stand for 2 minutes. Remove the plate and place it in a current of cold air until excess chlorine is removed and an area of coating below the line of application gives not more than a very faint blue colour with *potassium iodide and starch solution*; avoid prolonged exposure to cold air. Spray the plate with *potassium iodide and starch solution* and allow to stand for 5 minutes. Any *secondary spot* in the chromatogram obtained with solution (1) is not more intense than the spot in the chromatogram obtained with solution (2) (1%). Disregard any spot remaining on the line of application.

Assay Dissolve the contents of a sealed container containing the equivalent of 0.1 g of anhydrous cyclophosphamide in 30 ml of *chloroform*, shake vigorously for 15 minutes, filter (Whatman GF/F is suitable) and wash the filter with 15 ml of *chloroform*. Evaporate the combined filtrate and washings to dryness and dissolve the residue in 50 ml of a 0.1% w/v solution of *sodium hydroxide* in *ethane-1,2-diol*. Boil the solution under a reflux condenser for 30 minutes and allow to cool. Rinse the condenser with 25 ml of *water*, add 75 ml of *propan-2-ol*, 15 ml of 2M *nitric acid*, 10 ml of 0.1M *silver nitrate VS* and 2 ml of *ammonium iron(III) sulphate solution R2* and titrate with 0.1M *ammonium thiocyanate VS*. Each ml of 0.1M *silver nitrate VS* is equivalent to 13.05 mg of $C_7H_{15}Cl_2N_2O_2P$. Calculate the content of $C_7H_{15}Cl_2N_2O_2P$ in the sealed container.

Repeat the procedure with a further nine sealed containers. Calculate the content of $C_7H_{15}Cl_2N_2O_2P$ per container from the average of the 10 individual results thus obtained.

Labelling The label of the sealed container states (1) the weight of Cyclophosphamide contained in it; (2) the equivalent amount of anhydrous cyclophosphamide.

Cyclophosphamide Tablets

Definition Cyclophosphamide Tablets contain Cyclophosphamide. They are coated.

The tablets comply with the requirements stated under Tablets and with the following requirements.

Content of cyclophosphamide, $C_7H_{15}Cl_2N_2O_2P,H_2O$ 92.5 to 107.5% of the prescribed or stated amount.

Identification

A. Shake a quantity of the powdered tablets containing 0.2 g of Cyclophosphamide with 2 ml of *chloroform* and filter. The *infrared absorption spectrum* of the filtrate, Appendix II A, is concordant with the *reference spectrum* of cyclophosphamide.

B. Extract a quantity of the powdered tablets containing 0.1 g of Cyclophosphamide with *ether* and evaporate the extract to dryness. Dissolve the residue in 10 ml of *water* and add 5 ml of *silver nitrate solution*; no precipitate is produced. Boil; a white precipitate is produced which is insoluble in *nitric acid* but dissolves in 5M *ammonia* from which it is reprecipitated on the addition of *nitric acid.*

Acidity Shake a quantity of the powdered tablets containing 0.25 g of Cyclophosphamide with 20 ml of *carbon dioxide-free water*, filter and titrate the filtrate with 0.1M *sodium hydroxide VS* using *phenolphthalein solution R1* as indicator. Not more than 0.2 ml of 0.1M *sodium hydroxide VS* is required to change the colour of the solution.

Related substances Comply with the test described under Cyclophosphamide Injection but preparing solution (1) in the following manner. Shake vigorously a quantity of the powdered tablets containing 0.2 g of Cyclophosphamide with 50 ml of *chloroform* for 15 minutes, filter, evaporate the filtrate to dryness and dissolve the residue in 10 ml of *ethanol (96%)*.

Assay Weigh and powder 20 tablets. Dissolve a quantity of the powdered tablets containing 0.1 g of Cyclophosphamide in 30 ml of *chloroform*, shake vigorously for 15 minutes, filter (Whatman GF/F is suitable) and wash the filter with 15 ml of *chloroform*. Evaporate the combined filtrate and washings to dryness and dissolve the residue in 50 ml of a 0.1% w/v solution of *sodium hydroxide* in *ethane-1,2-diol*. Boil under a reflux condenser for 30 minutes and allow to cool. Rinse the condenser with 25 ml of *water*, add 75 ml of *propan-2-ol*, 15 ml of 2M *nitric acid*, 10 ml of 0.1M *silver nitrate VS* and 2 ml of *ammonium iron(III) sulphate solution R2* and titrate with 0.1M *ammonium thiocyanate VS*. Each ml of 0.1M *silver nitrate VS* is equivalent to 13.94 mg of $C_7H_{15}Cl_2N_2O_2P,H_2O$.

Cyproheptadine Tablets

Definition Cyproheptadine Tablets contain Cyproheptadine Hydrochloride.

The tablets comply with the requirements stated under Tablets and with the following requirements.

Content of cyproheptadine hydrochloride, $C_{21}H_{21}N,HCl$ 90.0 to 110.0% of the prescribed or stated amount of anhydrous cyproheptadine hydrochloride.

Identification

A. To a quantity of the powdered tablets containing the equivalent of 20 mg of anhydrous cyproheptadine hydrochloride add 10 ml of *water* and 2.5 ml of 0.1M *sodium hydroxide*, extract with 10 ml of *dichloromethane*, filter through *anhydrous sodium sulphate* moistened with *dichloromethane* on absorbent cotton and evaporate the filtrate to dryness. The *infrared absorption spectrum* of the residue, Appendix II A, is concordant with the *reference spectrum* of cyproheptadine.

B. In the test for Related substances, the principal spot in the chromatogram obtained with solution (3) corresponds to that in the chromatogram obtained with solution (5).

C. Extract a quantity of the powdered tablets containing the equivalent of 20 mg of anhydrous cyproheptadine hydrochloride with 7 ml of *water*, filter, add 0.3 ml of 5M *ammonia* to the filtrate and filter again. The filtrate yields reaction A characteristic of *chlorides*, Appendix VI.

Related substances Carry out the method for *thin-layer chromatography*, Appendix III A, using a silica gel precoated plate (Merck silica gel 60 plates are suitable) and as the mobile phase a mixture of 10 volumes of *methanol* and 90 volumes of *dichloromethane*. Apply separately to the plate 10 µl of each of the following solutions. For solution (1) add a quantity of the powdered tablets containing the equivalent of 50 mg of anhydrous cyproheptadine hydrochoride to 5 ml of the mobile phase, shake mechanically for 10 minutes and filter (Whatman GF/C filter paper is suitable). Solution (2) contains 0.002% w/v of *dibenzocycloheptene EPCRS* in the mobile phase. For solution (3) dilute 1 volume of solution (1) to 10 volumes with the mobile phase. For solution (4) dilute 1 volume of solution (1) to 100 volumes with the mobile phase and dilute 1 volume to 10 volumes with the mobile phase. Solution (5) contains 0.1% w/v of *cyproheptadine hydrochloride EPCRS* in the mobile phase. Allow the plate to dry in air and spray with *ethanolic sulphuric acid (20%)*. Heat at 110° for 30 minutes and examine under *ultraviolet light (365 nm)*. In the chromatogram obtained with solution (1) any spot corresponding to dibenzocycloheptene is not more intense than the spot in the chromatogram obtained with solution (2) (0.2%) and any other *secondary spot* is not more intense than the spot in the chromatogram obtained with solution (4) (0.1%).

Assay Weigh and powder 20 tablets. To a quantity of the powder containing the equivalent of 1.5 mg of anhydrous cyproheptadine hydrochloride add sufficient *ethanol (96%)* to produce 100 ml and filter if necessary. Measure the *absorbance* of the resulting solution at the maximum at 286 nm, Appendix II B. Calculate the content of $C_{21}H_{21}N,HCl$ taking 355 as the value of A(1%, 1 cm) at the maximum at 286 nm.

Labelling The quantity of active ingredient is stated in terms of the equivalent amount of anhydrous cyproheptadine hydrochloride.

Cytarabine Injection

Definition Cytarabine Injection is a sterile solution of Cytarabine in Water for Injections. It is supplied as a ready-to-use injection or it is prepared immediately before use by dissolving Cytarabine for Injection in the requisite amount of the liquid stated on the label.

The injection complies with the requirements stated under Parenteral Preparations.

When supplied as a ready-to-use injection, the injection complies with the following requirements.

Content of cytarabine, $C_9H_{13}N_3O_5$ 95.0 to 105.0% of the prescribed or stated amount.

Identification Evaporate a volume of the injection containing 0.1 g of Cytarabine to dryness at 60° at a pressure of 0.7 kPa, mix the residue with a minimum amount of hot *ethanol (96%)*, filter, allow the filtrate to cool and induce crystallisation if necessary. Filter, wash the crystals with 2 ml of *ethanol (96%)* and dry at 60° at a pressure of 0.7 kPa. The *infrared absorption spectrum* of the dried crystals, Appendix II A, is concordant with the *reference spectrum* of cytarabine.

Acidity or alkalinity pH, 7.0 to 9.5, Appendix V L.

Related substances Carry out the method for *thin-layer chromatography*, Appendix III A, using a silica gel 60 F_{254} precoated plate (Merck plates are suitable) and a mixture of 15 volumes of *water*, 20 volumes of *acetone* and 65 volumes of *butan-2-one* as the mobile phase. Apply separately to the plate 10 µl of each of the following solutions in *water*. For solution (1) dilute, if necessary, a volume of the injection to produce a solution containing 2% w/v of Cytarabine. For solution (2) dilute 1 volume of solution (1) to 200 volumes. Solution (3) contains 0.040% w/v of *uracil arabinoside EPCRS*. Solution (4) contains 0.020% w/v each of *uridine* and *uracil arabinoside EPCRS*. After removal of the plate, allow it to dry in air and examine under *ultraviolet light (254 nm)*. In the chromatogram obtained with solution (1) any spot corresponding to uracil arabinoside is not more intense than the spot in the chromatogram obtained with solution (3) (2%). Any other *secondary spot* in the chromatogram obtained with solution (1) is not more intense than the spot in the chromatogram obtained with solution (2) (0.5%). The test is not valid unless the chromatogram obtained with solution (4) shows two clearly separated spots.

Assay Carry out the method for *liquid chromatography*, Appendix III D, using the following solutions. For solution (1) dissolve 20 mg of *cytarabine BPCRS* in *water* and dilute to 100 ml with the same solvent. Dilute 10 ml to 100 ml with *water*. For solution (2) dilute a volume of the injection to produce a solution containing 0.002% w/v of Cytarabine.

The chromatographic procedure may be carried out using (a) a stainless steel column (25 cm × 4.6 mm) packed with *stationary phase C* (5 µm) (Spherisorb ODS 2 is suitable) and maintained at 30°, (b) a mixture of 7.5 volumes of *methanol* and 100 volumes of 0.005M *sodium pentanesulphonate* adjusted to pH 2.8 using *glacial acetic acid* as the mobile phase with a flow rate of 1 ml per minute and (c) a detection wavelength of 280 nm.

Calculate the content of $C_9H_{13}N_3O_5$ using the declared content of $C_9H_{13}N_3O_5$ in *cytarabine BPCRS*.

CYTARABINE FOR INJECTION

Definition Cytarabine for Injection is a sterile material consisting of Cytarabine with or without excipients. It is supplied in a sealed container.

The contents of the sealed container comply with the requirements for Powders for Injections stated under Parenteral Preparations and with the following requirements.

Content of cytarabine, $C_9H_{13}N_3O_5$ 95.0 to 105.0% of the prescribed or stated amount.

Identification Mix a quantity of the contents of the sealed container containing 0.1 g of Cytarabine with 10 ml of hot *ethanol (96%)*, filter, allow the filtrate to cool and induce crystallisation if necessary. Filter, wash the crystals with 2 ml of *ethanol (96%)* and dry at 60° at a pressure of 0.7 kPa. The *infrared absorption spectrum* of the crystals, Appendix II A, is concordant with the *reference spectrum* of cytarabine.

Acidity pH of a solution containing 2% w/v of Cytarabine in the solvent stated on the label, 4.0 to 6.0, Appendix V L.

Related substances Carry out the method for *thin-layer chromatography*, Appendix III A, using *silica gel GF_{254}* as the coating substance and a mixture of 15 volumes of *water*, 20 volumes of *acetone* and 65 volumes of *butan-2-one* as the mobile phase. Apply separately to the plate 10 µl of each of the following four solutions in *water*. For solution (1) dissolve the contents of the sealed container in a sufficient volume to produce a solution containing 2% w/v of Cytarabine. For solution (2) dilute 1 volume of solution (1) to 200 volumes. Solution (3) contains 0.020% w/v of *uracil arabinoside EPCRS*. Solution (4) contains 0.020% w/v each of *uridine* and *uracil arabinoside EPCRS*. After removal of the plate, allow it to dry in air and examine under *ultraviolet light (254 nm)*. In the chromatogram obtained with solution (1) any spot corresponding to uracil arabinoside is not more intense than the spot in the chromatogram obtained with solution (3) (1%). Any other *secondary spot* in the chromatogram obtained with solution (1) is not more intense than the spot in the chromatogram obtained with solution (2) (0.5%). The test is not valid unless the chromatogram obtained with solution (4) shows two clearly separated spots.

Water Not more than 3.0% w/w, Appendix IX C. Use 0.8 g.

Assay Determine the weight of the contents of each of 10 containers as described in the test for Uniformity of weight under Parenteral Preparations, Powders for Injections. Carry out the Assay described for the ready-to-use injection but using the following solution as solution (2). Dissolve sufficient of the mixed contents of the 10 containers in *water* to produce a solution containing 0.002% w/v of Cytarabine.

Calculate the content of $C_9H_{13}N_3O_5$ in a container of average content weight using the declared content of $C_9H_{13}N_3O_5$ in *cytarabine BPCRS*.

Dacarbazine Injection

Definition Dacarbazine Injection is a sterile solution of Dacarbazine in Water for Injections. It is prepared by dissolving Dacarbazine for Injection in the requisite amount of Water for Injections.

The injection complies with the requirements stated under Parenteral Preparations.

Storage Dacarbazine Injection should be used immediately after preparation but, in any case, within the period recommended by the manufacturer when prepared and stored strictly in accordance with the manufacturer's instructions.

DACARBAZINE FOR INJECTION

Definition Dacarbazine for Injection is a sterile material consisting of Dacarbazine with or without excipients. It is supplied in a sealed container.

The contents of the sealed container comply with the requirements for Powders for Injections stated under Parenteral Preparations and with the following requirements.

Content of dacarbazine, $C_6H_{10}N_6O$ 90.0 to 110.0% of the prescribed or stated amount.

Characteristics A white or very pale yellow powder.

Identification

A. Dissolve a quantity of the powder containing 0.1 g of Dacarbazine in 200 ml of *0.1M mixed phosphate buffer pH 7.0*, dilute with the buffer solution to 250 ml and dilute 3 ml to 200 ml with the same buffer solution. The *light absorption* of the resulting solution, Appendix II B, in the range 230 to 350 nm exhibits two maxima, at 237 nm and 330 nm.

B. Carry out the test for 5-Aminoimidazole-4-carboxamide hydrochloride described under Dacarbazine using the following solutions. For solution (1) dissolve a quantity of the powder containing 0.2 g of Dacarbazine in sufficient 0.1M *acetic acid* to produce 50 ml and dilute 1 ml of the resulting solution to 100 ml with the same solvent. Solution (2) contains 0.004% w/v of *dacarbazine BPCRS* in 0.1M *acetic acid*. The principal peak in the chromatogram obtained with solution (1) corresponds to that in the chromatogram obtained with solution (2).

5-Aminoimidazole-4-carboxamide hydrochloride; Related substances Comply with the tests described under Dacarbazine, but using as solution (2) in each test a solution prepared in the following manner. Dissolve a quantity of the powder containing 0.20 g of Dacarbazine in 40 ml of 0.1M *acetic acid* and add sufficient 0.1M *acetic acid* to produce 50 ml.

Uniformity of content Sealed containers containing 200 mg or less of Dacarbazine comply with the requirements stated under Parenteral Preparations, Powders for Injections. Use the individual results obtained in the Assay.

Assay Carry out the following procedure protected from light. Dissolve the contents of one container in 0.1M *hydrochloric acid* and dilute with sufficient 0.1M *hydrochloric acid* to produce a final solution containing 0.0008% w/v of Dacarbazine. Measure the *absorbance* of the resulting solution at the maximum at 323 nm, Appendix II B. Calculate the content of $C_6H_{10}N_6O$ in the sealed container taking 1090 as the value of A(1%, 1 cm) at the maximum at 323 nm.

Repeat the procedure with a further nine sealed containers and calculate the average content of $C_6H_{10}N_6O$ per container from the 10 individual results thus obtained.

Storage The sealed container should be protected from light and stored at a temperature of 2° to 8°.

Dapsone Tablets

Definition Dapsone Tablets contain Dapsone.

The tablets comply with the requirements stated under Tablets and with the following requirements.

Content of dapsone, $C_{12}H_{12}N_2O_2S$ 95.0 to 105.0% of the prescribed or stated amount.

Identification

A. Shake a quantity of the powdered tablets containing 0.1 g of Dapsone with 20 ml of *acetone*, filter and evaporate the filtrate to dryness. The *infrared absorption spectrum* of the residue, Appendix II A, is concordant with the *reference spectrum* of dapsone.

B. In the test for Related substances, the principal spot in the chromatogram obtained with solution (2) is similar in position, colour and size to that in the chromatogram obtained with solution (5).

Dissolution Comply with the *dissolution test for tablets and capsules*, Appendix XII D, using 900 ml of 0.1M *hydrochloric acid* as the medium and rotating the basket at 100 revolutions per minute. Withdraw a sample of 20 ml of the medium. To a volume of the filtered sample expected to contain 0.1 mg of Dapsone add 1 ml of a freshly prepared 0.5% w/v solution of *sodium nitrite*, allow to stand for 3 minutes, add 1.5 ml of a 1% w/v solution of *sulphamic acid*, allow to stand for 3 minutes, add 2.5 ml of a freshly prepared 0.2% w/v solution of N-*(1-naphthyl)-ethylenediamine dihydrochloride* in 0.1M *hydrochloric acid* and dilute to 20 ml with 1M *hydrochloric acid* (solution A). At the same time carry out the procedure using a volume of 0.1M *hydrochloric acid* equal to that of the filtered sample and beginning at the words 'add 1 ml of a freshly prepared 0.5% w/v solution of *sodium nitrite...*' (solution B). Allow solutions A and B to stand for at least 2 minutes and measure the *absorbance* of solution A at the maximum at 538 nm, Appendix II B, using solution B in the reference cell. Calculate the total content of dapsone, $C_{12}H_{12}N_2O_2S$, in the medium from the *absorbance* obtained by repeating the operation using a solution containing 0.1 mg of *dapsone BPCRS* in a volume of 0.1M *hydrochloric acid* equal to that of the filtered sample and beginning at the words 'add 1 ml of a freshly prepared 0.5% w/v solution of *sodium nitrite...*'.

Related substances Carry out the method for *thin-layer chromatography*, Appendix III A, using *silica gel G* as the coating substance, a mixture of 1 volume of 13.5M *ammonia*, 6 volumes of *methanol*, 20 volumes of *ethyl acetate* and 20 volumes of n-*heptane*, as the mobile phase and an unsaturated tank. Apply separately to the plate 10 µl of each of solutions (1), (3) and (4) and 1 µl of each of solutions (2) and (5). For solution (1) shake a quantity of the powdered tablets containing 0.1 g of Dapsone with 10 ml of *methanol* and filter. For solution (2) dilute 1 volume of solution (1) to 10 volumes with *methanol*. For solution (3) dilute 1 volume of solution (2) to 10 volumes with *methanol*. For solution (4) dilute 1 volume of solution (3) to 5 volumes with *methanol*. Solution (5) contains 0.1% w/v of *dapsone BPCRS*. After removal of the plate, allow it to dry in air, spray with a 0.1% w/v solution of *4-dimethylaminocinnamaldehyde* in a mixture of 1 volume of *hydrochloric acid* and 99 volumes of *ethanol (96%)* and examine in daylight. Any *secondary spot* in the chromatogram obtained with solution (1) is not more intense that the spot in the chromatogram obtained with solution (3) (1%) and not more than two such spots are more intense than the spot in the chromatogram obtained with solution (4) (0.2%).

Assay Weigh and powder 20 tablets. Dissolve a quantity of the powder containing 0.25 g of Dapsone in a mixture of 15 ml of *water* and 15 ml of 2M *hydrochloric acid*, add 3 g of *potassium bromide*, cool in ice and titrate slowly with 0.1M *sodium nitrite VS*, stirring constantly and determining the end point electrometrically. Each ml of 0.1M *sodium nitrite VS* is equivalent to 12.42 mg of $C_{12}H_{12}N_2O_2S$.

Debrisoquine Tablets

Definition Debrisoquine Tablets contain Debrisoquine Sulphate.

The tablets comply with the requirements stated under Tablets and with the following requirements.

Content of debrisoquine, $C_{10}H_{13}N_3$ 92.5 to 107.5% of the prescribed or stated amount.

Identification

A. Shake a quantity of the powdered tablets with sufficient 0.05M *sulphuric acid* to produce a solution containing the equivalent of 0.04% w/v of debrisoquine and centrifuge. The *light absorption* of the supernatant liquid, Appendix II B, in the range 230 to 350 nm exhibits two maxima, at 262 nm and 270 nm.

B. Carry out the method described under Related substances but applying separately to the plate 10 µl of each of the following solutions. For solution (1) use the supernatant liquid obtained by shaking a quantity of the powdered tablets with sufficient *water* to produce a solution containing the equivalent of 0.2% w/v of debrisoquine and centrifuging. Solution (2) contains 0.25% w/v of *debrisoquine sulphate BPCRS* in *water*. Solution (3) is a mixture of equal volumes of solutions (1) and (2). The principal spot in the chromatogram obtained with solution (1) corresponds to that in the chromatogram obtained with solution (2). The principal spot in the chromatogram obtained with solution (3) is a single, compact spot.

Related substances Carry out the method for *thin-layer chromatography*, Appendix III A, using *silica gel G* as the coating substance and a mixture of 60 volumes of *butan-1-ol*, 25 volumes of *water* and 15 volumes of *glacial acetic acid* as the mobile phase. Apply separately to the plate 10 µl of each of the following solutions. For solution (1) use the supernatant liquid obtained by shaking a quantity of the powdered tablets containing the equivalent of 80 mg of debrisoquine with 5 ml of *water* and centrifuging. Solution (2) contains 0.010% w/v of *debrisoquine sulphate BPCRS* in *water*. After removal of the plate, allow it to dry in air and spray with a solution prepared by adding 1 ml of *sulphuric acid* to 40 ml of a freshly prepared mixture of equal volumes of a 0.135% w/v solution of *chloroplatinic(IV) acid* and a 1.1% w/v solution of *potassium iodide*. Any *secondary spot* in the chromatogram obtained with solution (1) is not more intense than the spot in the chromatogram obtained with solution (2).

Assay Weigh and powder 20 tablets. To a quantity of the powder containing the equivalent of 0.13 g of debrisoquine add 150 ml of 0.05M *sulphuric acid* and heat in a water bath for 20 minutes, swirling occasionally. Cool, add sufficient 0.05M *sulphuric acid* to produce 500 ml, filter and dilute 10 ml of the filtrate to 100 ml with *water*. Transfer 5 ml of the resulting solution to a stoppered flask, add 5 ml of 0.01M *sodium hydroxide*, mix and add 5 ml of a solution prepared by triturating 0.1 g of *bromothymol blue* with 1.6 ml of 1M *sodium hydroxide* and diluting to 200 ml with *water*. Add 5 ml of *phosphate buffer pH 7.4* and 15 ml of *benzene* and shake for 20 minutes. Centrifuge and measure the *absorbance* of the upper layer at the maximum at 405 nm, Appendix II B, using in the reference cell the upper layer obtained by treating 5 ml of 0.005M *sulphuric acid* in the same manner beginning at the words 'add 5 ml of 0.01M *sodium hydroxide*...'. Calculate the content of $C_{10}H_{13}N_3$ from the *absorbance* obtained by repeating the operation using 5 ml of a solution of *debrisoquine sulphate BPCRS* in 0.005M *sulphuric acid* containing the equivalent of 0.0026% w/v of debrisoquine and beginning at the words 'add 5 ml of 0.01M *sodium hydroxide*...'.

Labelling The quantity of active ingredient is stated in terms of the equivalent amount of debrisoquine.

Demeclocycline Capsules

Definition Demeclocycline Capsules contain Demeclocycline Hydrochloride.

The capsules comply with the requirements stated under Capsules and with the following requirements.

Content of demeclocycline hydrochloride, $C_{21}H_{22}Cl_2N_2O_8$,HCl 90.0 to 107.0% of the prescribed or stated amount.

Identification

A. Carry out the method for *thin-layer chromatography*, Appendix III A, using *silica gel H* as the coating substance and a mixture of 6 volumes of *water*, 35 volumes of *methanol* and 59 volumes of *dichloromethane* as the mobile phase. Adjust the pH of a 10% w/v solution of *disodium edetate* to 7.0 with 10M *sodium hydroxide* and spray the solution evenly onto the plate (about 10 ml for a plate 100 mm × 200 mm). Allow the plate to dry in a horizontal position for at least 1 hour. At the time of use, dry the plate in an oven at 110° for 1 hour. Apply separately to the plate 1 µl of each of the following solutions. For solution (1) extract a quantity of the contents of the capsules containing 10 mg of Demeclocycline Hydrochloride with 20 ml of *methanol* and centrifuge. Solution (2) contains 0.05% w/v of *demeclocycline hydrochloride EPCRS* in *methanol*. Solution (3) contains 0.05% w/v each of *demeclocycline hydrochloride EPCRS*, *oxytetracycline hydrochloride EPCRS* and *metacycline hydrochloride EPCRS* in *methanol*. Allow the plate to dry in a stream of air and examine under *ultraviolet light (365 nm)*. The principal spot in the chromatogram obtained with solution (1) corresponds to that in the chromatogram obtained with solution (2). The test is not valid unless the chromatogram obtained with solution (3) shows three clearly separated spots.

B. Add 20 ml of warm *methanol* to a quantity of the contents of the capsules containing 10 mg of Demeclocycline Hydrochloride, allow to stand for 20 minutes, filter and evaporate the filtrate to dryness on a water bath. To 0.5 mg of the residue add 2 ml of *sulphuric acid*; a purple colour is produced. Add 1 ml of *water*; the colour changes to yellow.

C. To 1 mg of the residue obtained in test B add 7 ml of *water* and 7 ml of 2M *hydrochloric acid* and heat gently for 30 seconds. No colour is produced immediately.

Dissolution Comply with the *dissolution test for tablets and capsules*, Appendix XII D, using Apparatus II. Use as the medium 900 ml of 0.1M *hydrochloric acid* and rotate the paddle at 50 revolutions per minute. Withdraw a sample of 10 ml of the medium and filter. Carry out the method for *liquid chromatography*, Appendix III D, using the following solutions. For solution (1) dilute the filtered solution, if necessary, with 0.1M *hydrochloric acid* to give a solution expected to contain about 0.015% w/v of Demeclocycline Hydrochloride. Solution (2) contains 0.015% w/v of *demeclocycline hydrochloride EPCRS* in 0.1M *hydrochloric acid*.

The chromatographic procedure may be carried out using (a) a stainless steel column (25 cm × 4.6 mm) packed with *stationary phase C* (5 µm) (Lichrosorb RP18 is suitable) and maintained at 40°, (b) as the mobile phase with a flow rate of 2 ml per minute a mixture of 20 volumes of *dimethylformamide* and 80 volumes of 0.1M *oxalic acid* the pH of which has been adjusted to 2.2 with *triethylamine* and (c) a detection wavelength of 355 nm.

Calculate the total content of demeclocycline hydrochloride, $C_{21}H_{22}Cl_2N_2O_8$,HCl, in the medium using the declared content of $C_{21}H_{22}Cl_2N_2O_8$,HCl, in *demeclocycline hydrochloride EPCRS*.

Related substances Carry out the method for *liquid chromatography*, Appendix III D, using solutions (1) and (3) described under Assay.

The chromatographic conditions described under Dissolution may be used.

The area of any *secondary peak* in the chromatogram obtained with solution (1) is not greater than the area of the principal peak in the chromatogram obtained with solution (3) (10%) and the sum of the areas of any *secondary peaks* is not greater than 1.5 times the area of the principal peak in the chromatogram obtained with solution (3) (15%).

Loss on drying When dried at 60° at a pressure not exceeding 0.7 kPa for 3 hours, the contents of the capsules lose not more than 5.0% of their weight. Use 1 g.

Assay Carry out the method for *liquid chromatography*, Appendix III D, using the following solutions. For solution (1) mix a quantity of the mixed contents of 20 capsules containing 0.5 g of Demeclocycline Hydrochloride with 50 ml of 0.01M *hydrochloric acid*, add sufficient 0.01M *hydrochloric acid* to produce 100 ml, filter and dilute 1 volume of the filtrate to 5 volumes with 0.01M *hydrochloric acid*. Solution (2) contains 0.10% w/v of *demeclocycline hydrochloride EPCRS* in 0.01M *hydrochloric acid*. Solution (3) contains 0.010% w/v of *demeclocycline hydrochloride EPCRS* in 0.01M *hydrochloric acid*. Solution (4) contains 0.015% w/v each of *demeclocycline hydrochloride EPCRS* and *4-epidemeclocycline hydrochloride EPCRS* in 0.01M *hydrochloric acid*.

The chromatographic conditions described under Dissolution may be used.

The assay is not valid unless the *resolution factor* between the two principal peaks in the chromatogram obtained with solution (4) is at least 3.0.

Calculate the content of $C_{21}H_{22}Cl_2N_2O_8$,HCl in the capsules using the declared content of $C_{21}H_{22}Cl_2N_2O_8$, HCl in *demeclocycline hydrochloride EPCRS*.

Desferrioxamine Injection

Definition Desferrioxamine Injection is a sterile solution of Desferrioxamine Mesilate in Water for Injections. It is prepared by dissolving Desferrioxamine Mesilate for Injection in the requisite amount of Water for Injections immediately before use.

The injection complies with the requirements stated under Parenteral Preparations.

Storage Desferrioxamine Injection deteriorates on storage and should be used immediately after preparation. Cloudy solutions should be discarded.

DESFERRIOXAMINE MESILATE FOR INJECTION

Definition Desferrioxamine Mesilate for Injection is a sterile material consisting of Desferrioxamine Mesilate with or without excipients. It is supplied in a sealed container.

The contents of the sealed container comply with the requirements for Powders for Injections stated under Parenteral Preparations and with the following requirements.

Content of desferrioxamine mesilate, $C_{25}H_{48}N_6O_8$, CH_4SO_3 94.0 to 110.0% of the prescribed or stated amount.

Identification

A. Dissolve 40 mg of the contents of the sealed container in 2 ml of *absolute ethanol* by heating on a water bath at 60°, cool in ice until the substance begins to crystallise and evaporate to dryness at room temperature under a gentle current of *nitrogen*. The *infrared absorption spectrum* of the residue, Appendix II A, is concordant with the *reference spectrum* of desferrioxamine mesilate.

B. In the test for Related substances the chromatogram obtained with solution (1) shows a peak with the same retention time as the principal peak in the chromatogram obtained with solution (3).

Related substances Carry out the method for *liquid chromatography*, Appendix III D, using the following solutions. Prepare the solutions immediately before use and protect from light. For solution (1) dissolve a quantity of the contents of the sealed containers containing 75 mg of Desferrioxamine Mesilate in sufficient of the mobile phase to produce 50 ml. For solution (2) dilute 1 volume of solution (1) to 25 volumes with the mobile phase. Solution (3) contains 0.15% w/v of *deferoxamine mesilate EPCRS* in the mobile phase.

The chromatographic procedure may be carried out using (a) a stainless steel column (25 cm × 4.6 mm) packed with *stationary phase C* (10 µm) (Nucleosil C18 is suitable), (b) a mixture of 55 volumes of *tetrahydrofuran* and 950 volumes of a solution containing 0.039% w/v of *disodium edetate* and 0.139% w/v of *ammonium phosphate* adjusted to pH 2.8 with *orthophosphoric acid* in *water* as the mobile phase with a flow rate of 2 ml per minute and (c) a detection wavelength of 220 nm.

Inject 20 µl of solution (3). Adjust the sensitivity of the detector so that the height of the peak with a relative retention time of about 0.8 is not less than 15% of the full scale of the recorder. The test is not valid unless the *resolution factor* between the peak with the relative retention time of about 0.8 and the principal peak is at least 1.0.

Inject 20 µl of solutions (1) and (2). Continue the chromatography for three times the retention time of the principal peak. In the chromatogram obtained with solution (1) the area of any *secondary peak* is not greater than the area of the principal peak in the chromatogram obtained with solution (2) (4%) and the sum of the areas of any such peaks is not greater than 1.75 times the area of the principal peak in the chromatogram obtained with solution (2) (7%). Disregard any peak with an area less than 0.02 times the area of the principal peak in the chromatogram obtained with solution (2) (0.08%).

Assay Determine the weight of the contents of 10 containers as described in the test for Uniformity of weight under Parenteral Preparations, Powders for Injections.

Dissolve a quantity of the mixed contents of the 10 containers containing 0.3 g of Desferrioxamine Mesilate in 15 ml of *water* and add 2 ml of 0.05M *sulphuric acid*. Titrate slowly with 0.1M *ammonium iron(III) sulphate VS* determining the end point potentiometrically and using a platinum electrode and a calomel reference electrode. Each ml of 0.1M *ammonium iron(III) sulphate VS* is equivalent to 65.68 mg of $C_{25}H_{48}N_6O_8,CH_4SO_3$. Calculate the content of $C_{25}H_{48}N_6O_8,CH_4SO_3$ in a container of average content weight.

Desipramine Tablets

Definition Desipramine Tablets contain Desipramine Hydrochloride. They are coated.

The tablets comply with the requirements stated under Tablets and with the following requirements.

Content of desipramine hydrochloride, $C_{18}H_{22}N_2$, HCl 92.5 to 107.5% of the prescribed or stated amount.

Identification
Triturate a quantity of the powdered tablets containing 0.25 g of Desipramine Hydrochloride with 10 ml of *chloroform*, filter and evaporate the filtrate to 3 ml. Add *ether* until a slight turbidity is produced and allow to stand; filter, wash the crystals with a mixture of 1 volume of *chloroform* and 5 volumes of *ether* and dry at 100° at a pressure of 2 kPa for 90 minutes. The *infrared absorption spectrum* of the dried crystals, Appendix II A, is concordant with the *reference spectrum* of desipramine hydrochloride.

Related substances Carry out the method for *thin-layer chromatography*, Appendix III A, protected from light, using *silica gel G* as the coating substance and a mixture of 50 volumes of *glacial acetic acid*, 50 volumes of *toluene* and 5 volumes of *water* as the mobile phase but allowing the solvent front to ascend 7 cm above the line of application. Apply separately to the plate 5 µl of each of the following solutions. For solution (1) shake a quantity of the powdered tablets containing 0.2 g of Desipramine Hydrochloride with three 10-ml quantities of *chloroform* and filter; evaporate the combined filtrates to dryness and dissolve the residue in 10 ml of a mixture of equal volumes of *chloroform* and *absolute ethanol*. For solution (2) dilute 1 volume of solution (1) to 500 volumes with the same chloroform—ethanol mixture. After removal of the plate, dry it for 10 minutes in a current of air, spray with a 0.5% w/v solution of *potassium dichromate* in *sulphuric acid (20%)* and examine immediately. Any *secondary spot* in the chromatogram obtained with solution (1) is not more intense than the spot in the chromatogram obtained with solution (2).

Assay Weigh and powder 20 tablets. Shake a quantity of the powder containing 75 mg of Desipramine Hydrochloride with 100 ml of 0.1M *hydrochloric acid* for 30 minutes, add sufficient 0.1M *hydrochloric acid* to produce 250 ml and filter. Dilute 5 ml to 100 ml with 0.1M *hydrochloric acid* and measure the *absorbance* of the resulting solution at the maximum at 250 nm, Appendix II B. Calculate the content of $C_{18}H_{22}N_2$,HCl taking 270 as the value of A(1%, 1 cm) at the maximum at 250 nm.

Desmopressin Injection

Definition Desmopressin Injection is a sterile solution of Desmopressin in Water for Injections.

The injection complies with the requirements stated under Parenteral Preparations and with the following requirements.

Content of desmopressin, $C_{46}H_{64}N_{14}O_{12}S_2$ 90.0 to 110.0% of the prescribed or stated amount of the peptide.

Characteristics A colourless solution.

Identification In the Assay, the principal peak in the chromatogram obtained with solution (1) corresponds to that in the chromatogram obtained with solution (2).

Acidity pH, 3.5 to 5.0, Appendix V L.

Assay Carry out the method for *liquid chromatography*, Appendix III D, injecting 0.2 ml of the following two solutions. For solution (1) dilute the injection, if necessary, with *water* to give a final concentration of 0.0004% w/v of the peptide. For solution (2) dissolve a quantity of *desmopressin EPCRS* in sufficient *water* to produce a solution containing 0.0004% w/v of the peptide.

The chromatographic procedure may be carried out using (a) a stainless steel column (10 cm × 4.6 mm) packed with *stationary phase C* (10 µm) (Nucleosil C18 is suitable), (b) as the mobile phase with a flow rate of 2 ml per minute, a mixture of *0.067M mixed phosphate buffer pH 7.0* and *acetonitrile*, the mixture being adjusted so that the retention time of desmopressin is about 5 minutes (a mixture of 80 volumes of *0.067M mixed phosphate buffer pH 7.0* and 20 volumes of *acetonitrile* is usually suitable) and (c) a detection wavelength of 220 nm.

Calculate the content of $C_{46}H_{64}N_{14}O_{12}S_2$ using the declared content of $C_{46}H_{64}N_{14}O_{12}S_2$ in *desmopressin EPCRS*.

Storage Desmopressin Injection should be protected from light and stored at a temperature of 2° to 8°.

Labelling The strength is stated in terms of the equivalent amount of the peptide in micrograms per ml.

The label also states that the preparation is for intravenous infusion or intramuscular injection only.

Desmopressin Intranasal Solution

Definition Desmopressin Intranasal Solution is a solution of Desmopressin containing suitable buffering agents and preservatives.

The intranasal solution complies with the requirements stated under Nasal Preparations and with the following requirements.

Content of desmopressin, $C_{46}H_{64}N_{14}O_{12}S_2$ 90.0 to 110.0% of the prescribed or stated amount of the peptide.

Characteristics A colourless solution.

Identification In the Assay, the chromatogram obtained with solution (1) exhibits a peak with the same retention time as the principal peak in the chromatogram obtained with solution (2).

Acidity pH, 3.5 to 5.0, Appendix V L.

Assay Carry out the Assay described under Desmopressin Injection using the following solutions. For solution (1) dilute the intranasal solution, if necessary, with *water* to give a final concentration of 0.01% w/v of the peptide. For solution (2) dissolve a quantity of *desmopressin EPCRS* in sufficient *water* to produce a solution containing 0.01% w/v of the peptide.

The assay is not valid unless the peak due to desmopressin is clearly separated from the peak due to the antimicrobial preservative stated on the label. The proportion of acetonitrile in the mobile phase may be adjusted to achieve the separation. For example, for a preparation in which chlorbutol is used as an antimicrobial preservative, decrease the proportion of acetonitrile in order to increase the retention time of desmopressin relative to that of chlorbutol.

Storage Desmopressin Intranasal Solution should be protected from light and stored at a temperature of 2° to 8°.

Labelling The strength is stated in terms of the equivalent amount of the peptide in micrograms per ml.

The label also states (1) that the preparation is for intranasal administration; (2) the name and amount of any added substance.

Dexamethasone Tablets

Definition Dexamethasone Tablets contain Dexamethasone.

The tablets comply with the requirements stated under Tablets and with the following requirements.

Content of dexamethasone, $C_{22}H_{29}FO_5$ 90.0 to 110.0% of the prescribed or stated amount.

Identification Shake a quantity of the powdered tablets containing 20 mg of Dexamethasone with 50 ml of *chloroform* for 30 minutes, filter and evaporate to dryness. The residue, after drying at 105° for 2 hours, complies with the following tests.

A. The *infrared absorption spectrum*, Appendix II A, is concordant with the *reference spectrum* of dexamethasone.

B. To 2 ml of a 0.01% w/v solution in *ethanol (96%)* in a stoppered tube add 10 ml of *phenylhydrazine—sulphuric acid solution*, mix, place in a water bath at 60° for 20 minutes and cool immediately. The *absorbance* of the resulting solution at the maximum at 423 nm is not less than 0.40, Appendix II B.

Uniformity of content Tablets containing less than 2 mg of Dexamethasone comply with the requirements stated under Tablets using the following method of analysis. Carry out the method for *liquid chromatography*, Appendix III D, using the following solutions protected from light. Solution (1) contains 0.0025% w/v of *dexamethasone BPCRS* and 0.0020% w/v of *hydrocortisone* (internal standard) in *methanol (50%)*. For solution (2) finely crush one tablet, add sufficient internal standard solution to produce a solution containing 0.0025% w/v of Dexamethasone, shake for 10 minutes and filter through glass-fibre filter paper (Whatman GF/C is suitable).

The chromatographic procedure may be carried out using (a) a stainless steel column (20 cm × 5 mm) packed with *stationary phase C* (5 µm) (Spherisorb ODS 1 is suitable), (b) *methanol (47%)* as the mobile phase with a flow rate of 1.4 ml per minute and (c) a detection wavelength of 238 nm.

Calculate the content of $C_{22}H_{29}FO_5$ using the declared content of $C_{22}H_{29}FO_5$ in *dexamethasone BPCRS*.

Assay Carry out the method for *liquid chromatography*, Appendix III D, using the following solutions protected from light. Solution (1) contains 0.0125% w/v of *dexamethasone BPCRS* and 0.010% w/v of *hydrocortisone* (internal standard) in *methanol (50%)*. For solution (2) weigh and powder 20 tablets; to a quantity of the powder containing 2.5 mg of Dexamethasone add 20 ml of *methanol (50%)*, shake for 20 minutes and filter through glass-fibre filter paper (Whatman GF/C is suitable). Prepare solution (3) in the same manner as solution (2) but using 20 ml of a 0.010% w/v solution of *hydrocortisone* in *methanol (50%)* in place of the 20 ml of methanol (50%).

The chromatographic conditions described under Uniformity of content may be used.

Calculate the content of $C_{22}H_{29}FO_5$ using the declared content of $C_{22}H_{29}FO_5$ in *dexamethasone BPCRS.*

Storage Dexamethasone Tablets should be protected from light.

Dexamfetamine Tablets

Definition Dexamfetamine Tablets contain Dexamfetamine Sulphate.

The tablets comply with the requirements stated under Tablets and with the following requirements.

Content of dexamfetamine sulphate, $(C_9H_{13}N)_2,H_2SO_4$ 90.0 to 110.0% of the prescribed or stated amount.

Identification

A. Dissolve a quantity of the powdered tablets containing 0.1 g of Dexamfetamine Sulphate as completely as possible in 20 ml of *water*, filter, add 2 ml of 5M *sodium hydroxide* and extract with three 25-ml quantities of *ether*, washing the combined extracts with 5 ml of *water*. To the ether solution add 10 ml of 0.05M *sulphuric acid* and shake well. The acid layer, after warming to dispel residual ether and cooling to 20°, is dextrorotatory.

B. Extract a quantity of the powdered tablets containing 50 mg of Dexamfetamine Sulphate with 10 ml of *water*, filter, cool to about 15°, add 3 ml of 1M *sodium hydroxide* and shake for 2 minutes with 1 ml of a mixture of 1 volume of *benzoyl chloride* and 2 volumes of *ether*. Filter, wash the residue with 15 ml of *water* and recrystallise twice from *ethanol (50%)*. The *melting point* of the crystals, after drying at 105° for 1 hour, is about 156°, Appendix V A.

Assay Weigh and powder 20 tablets, or more if necessary. Dissolve a quantity of the powder containing 0.1 g of Dexamfetamine Sulphate as completely as possible in 20 ml of *water*, add 8 g of *sodium chloride* and 2 ml of 5M *sodium hydroxide* and extract with successive quantities of 50, 20, 20 and 20 ml of *ether*. Extract the combined ether extracts with four 10-ml quantities of 0.1M *hydrochloric acid* and make the combined acid extracts alkaline with 5M *sodium hydroxide*. Dilute to 120 ml with *water* and distil into 20 ml of 0.05M *hydrochloric acid VS* until only 5 ml of liquid remains in the distillation flask. Boil, cool and titrate the excess of acid with 0.05M *sodium hydroxide VS* using *methyl red solution* as indicator. Each ml of 0.05M *hydrochloric acid VS* is equivalent to 9.212 mg of $(C_9H_{13}N)_2,H_2SO_4$.

When dexamphetamine tablets are prescribed or demanded, Dexamfetamine Tablets shall be dispensed or supplied.

Dextran 40 Intravenous Infusion

Dextran 40 Injection

Definition Dextran 40 Intravenous Infusion is a sterile solution, in Glucose Intravenous Infusion or in Sodium Chloride Intravenous Infusion, of dextrans of weight average molecular weight about 40,000, derived from the dextrans produced by the fermentation of sucrose by means of a certain strain of *Leuconostoc mesenteroides* (National Collection of Type Cultures No. 10817). The dextrans are polymers of glucose in which the linkages between the glucose units are almost entirely of the α-1→6 type.

The intravenous infusion complies with the requirements stated under Parenteral Preparations and with the following requirements.

Content of dextrans 9.0 to 11.0% w/v.

Characteristics; Content of glucose; Heavy metals; Ethanol; Nitrogen; Sulphated ash; Foreign protein; Pyrogens Complies with the requirements stated under Dextran 110 Intravenous Infusion.

Acidity Titrate 25 ml with 0.01M *sodium hydroxide VS* using *phenol red solution* as indicator. Not more than 2.0 ml of 0.01M *sodium hydroxide VS* is required to neutralise the solution.

Molecular size For solutions in Glucose Intravenous Infusion, before proceeding with tests A, B and C add 4 volumes of *ethanol (96%)*, centrifuge and dissolve the residue in sufficient Sodium Chloride Intravenous Infusion to restore the original volume.

A. Carry out test A for Molecular size described under Dextran 110 Intravenous Infusion using solutions in *saline solution* containing about 3.5, 2.5, 1.5 and 0.75% w/v of dextrans. The intrinsic viscosity is 0.16 to 0.20.

B. Dilute the solution being examined with *saline solution* to contain 6% w/v of dextrans and carry out test B for Molecular size described under Dextran 110 Intravenous Infusion. The intrinsic viscosity is not more than 0.27.

C. Place in each of four stoppered flasks 100 ml of the diluted intravenous infusion in *saline solution* containing 6% w/v of dextrans and add slowly, with continuous stirring, 80, 90, 100 and 110 ml respectively of *absolute ethanol*. Stopper the flasks, transfer to a water bath maintained at 24.9° to 25.1° and allow to stand overnight or until two clear liquid phases are formed. Separate the supernatant solutions from the syrupy residues. Remove the ethanol from each supernatant solution separately by evaporation at a pressure of 2 kPa, dialyse in cellophane tubing against *water* to remove sodium chloride, adjust the volume to 25.0 ml with *water*, add sufficient *sodium chloride* to produce solutions containing 0.9% w/v and determine the *optical rotation*, Appendix V F. From the optical rotations calculate the amounts of dextrans present as described in the Assay under Dextran 110 Intravenous Infusion. Choose that fraction containing as nearly as possible but not more than 10% of the dextrans present in the infusion and determine the intrinsic viscosity by the method in test A above. The intrinsic viscosity is not less than 0.08.

Assay Carry out the Assay described under Dextran 110 Intravenous Infusion.

Storage Dextran 40 Intravenous Infusion should not be exposed to undue fluctuations of temperature.

Labelling The strength is stated as the percentage w/v of dextrans. The label states (1) the name of the solvent; (2) that the infusion should not be used if it is cloudy or if a deposit is present; (3) the strain of *Leuconostoc mesenteroides* used.

Action and use Plasma substitute.

Dextran 70 Intravenous Infusion

Dextran 70 Injection

Definition Dextran 70 Intravenous Infusion is a sterile solution, in Glucose Intravenous Infusion or in Sodium Chloride Intravenous Infusion, of dextrans of weight average molecular weight about 70,000, derived from the dextrans produced by the fermentation of sucrose by means of a certain strain of *Leuconostoc mesenteroides* (National Collection of Type Cultures No. 10817). The dextrans are polymers of glucose in which the linkages between the glucose units are almost entirely of the α-1→6 type.

The intravenous infusion complies with the requirements stated under Parenteral Preparations and with the following requirements.

Content of dextrans 5.5 to 6.5% w/v.

Characteristics; Acidity; Content of glucose; Heavy metals; Ethanol; Nitrogen; Sulphated ash; Foreign protein; Pyrogens Complies with the requirements stated under Dextran 110 Intravenous Infusion.

Molecular size For solutions in Glucose Intravenous Infusion, before proceeding with tests A, B and C add 4 volumes of *ethanol (96%)*, centrifuge and dissolve the residue in sufficient Sodium Chloride Intravenous Infusion to restore the original volume.

A. Carry out test A for Molecular size described under Dextran 110 Intravenous Infusion using solutions in *saline solution* containing about 3.5, 2.5, 1.5 and 0.75% w/v of dextrans. The intrinsic viscosity is 0.22 to 0.27.

B. Carry out test B for Molecular size described under Dextran 110 Intravenous Infusion. The intrinsic viscosity is not more than 0.36.

C. Dilute the solution being examined with *saline solution* to contain 6% w/v of dextrans. Place 100 ml in each of four stoppered flasks and add slowly, with continuous stirring, 80, 90, 100 and 110 ml respectively of *absolute ethanol*. Stopper the flasks, transfer to a water bath maintained at 24.9° to 25.1° and allow to stand overnight or until two clear liquid phases are formed. Separate the supernatant solutions from the syrupy residues. Remove the ethanol from each supernatant solution separately by evaporation at a pressure of 2 kPa, dialyse in cellophane tubing against *water* to remove sodium chloride, adjust the volume to 25.0 ml with *water*, add sufficient *sodium chloride* to produce solutions containing 0.9% w/v and determine the *optical rotation*, Appendix V F. From the optical rotations calculate the amounts of dextrans present as described in the Assay under Dextran 110 Intravenous Infusion. Choose that fraction containing as nearly as possible but not more than 10% of the dextrans present in the infusion and determine the intrinsic viscosity by the method in test A for Molecular size described under Dextran 110 Intravenous Infusion. The intrinsic viscosity is not less than 0.13.

Assay Carry out the procedure described under Dextran 110 Intravenous Infusion.

Storage Dextran 70 Intravenous Infusion should not be exposed to undue fluctuations in temperature.

Labelling The strength is stated as the percentage w/v of dextrans. The label states (1) the name of the solvent; (2) that the infusion should not be used if it is cloudy or if a deposit is present; (3) the strain of *Leuconostoc mesenteroides* used.

Action and use Plasma substitute.

Dextran 110 Intravenous Infusion

Dextran 110 Injection

Definition Dextran 110 Intravenous Infusion is a sterile solution, in Glucose Intravenous Infusion or in Sodium Chloride Intravenous Infusion, of dextrans of weight average molecular weight about 110,000, derived from the dextrans produced by the fermentation of sucrose by means of a certain strain of *Leuconostoc mesenteroides* (National Collection of Type Cultures No. 10817). The dextrans are polymers of glucose in which the linkages between the glucose units are almost entirely of the α-1→6 type.

The intravenous infusion complies with the requirements stated under Parenteral Preparations and with the following requirements.

Content of dextrans 5.5 to 6.5% w/v.

Characteristics An almost colourless, slightly viscous solution.

Acidity Titrate 25 ml with 0.01M *sodium hydroxide VS* using *phenol red solution* as indicator. Not more than 1.25 ml of 0.01M *sodium hydroxide VS* is required to neutralise the solution.

Molecular size For solutions in Glucose Intravenous Infusion, before proceeding with tests A, B and C, add 4 volumes of *ethanol (96%)*, centrifuge and dissolve the residue in sufficient Sodium Chloride Intravenous Infusion to restore the original volume.

A. Determine the viscosities, at 37°, of solutions in *saline solution* containing about 2.0, 1.0, 0.5 and 0.25% w/v of dextrans, accurately determined, Appendix V H, Method I, using a U-tube viscometer (size C). Calculate the viscosity ratio by dividing the time taken for the meniscus to fall from E to F using the liquid being examined by the time taken using *saline solution*. For each solution plot (viscosity ratio − 1.00)/concentration against concentration. The intercept on the viscosity ratio axis of a straight line through the points represents the intrinsic viscosity. The intrinsic viscosity is 0.27 to 0.32.

B. Place 100 ml in each of five stoppered flasks and adjust the temperature to 24.9° to 25.1°. Maintaining this temperature, add slowly with continuous stirring sufficient *absolute ethanol* to produce a faint cloudiness (about 45 ml). To the separate flasks add 0.5, 1.0, 1.5, 2.0 and 2.5 ml of *absolute ethanol*, stopper the flasks and immerse in a water bath at about 35°, shaking occasionally, until clear solutions are obtained. Transfer the flasks to a water bath maintained at 24.9° to 25.1° and allow to stand overnight or until two clear liquid phases are formed. Discard the supernatant liquids, dissolve separately the syrupy residues in sufficient *saline solution* to produce 25.0 ml, remove the ethanol by evaporation at a pressure of 2 kPa, dilute to 25.0 ml with *water* and determine the *optical rotation*, Appendix V F. From the optical rotations calculate the amounts of dextrans precipitated as described in the Assay. Choose that fraction containing as nearly as possible but not more than 10% of the dextrans present in the infusion and determine its intrinsic viscosity by the method described under test A using a U-tube viscometer (size A). The intrinsic viscosity is not more than 0.40.

C. Confirm that the weight average molecular weight is consistent with that stated under the Definition using a suitable method such as *size-exclusion chromatography*, Appendix III C.

Content of glucose For solutions in Glucose Intravenous Infusion, 4.5 to 5.5% w/v, when determined by the following method. Dilute 15 ml to 50 ml with *water*. To 5 ml in a stoppered flask add 25 ml of a buffer solution containing 14.3% w/v of *sodium carbonate* and 4.0% w/v of *potassium iodide* and 25 ml of 0.05M *iodine VS*. Stopper the flask, allow to stand for exactly 30 minutes at 20°, add 30 ml of 2M *hydrochloric acid* and titrate immediately with 0.1M *sodium thiosulphate VS*. Repeat the operation using 5 ml of *water* and beginning at the words 'add 25 ml...'. The difference between the titrations represents the amount of iodine required to oxidise the glucose. Each ml of 0.05M *iodine VS* is equivalent to 9.01 mg of glucose.

Heavy metals To 12 ml add 5 ml of 6M *acetic acid*, make alkaline with 5M *ammonia*, dilute to 50 ml with *water* and add 0.1 ml of *sodium sulphide solution*. Any colour produced is not more intense than that obtained by repeating the operation using a mixture of 2 ml of the liquid being examined and 2.5 ml of *lead standard solution (20 ppm Pb)*.

Ethanol Distil 100 ml, collecting the first 45 ml of distillate and dilute the distillate to 50 ml with *water*. Mix 10 ml of 0.0167M *potassium dichromate VS* and 10 ml of *sulphuric acid* in a stoppered boiling tube, immediately add 5 ml of the distillate, mix, stopper the tube and allow to stand for 5 minutes. Transfer to a 500-ml flask, dilute to about 300 ml with *carbon dioxide-free water*, add 2 g of *potassium iodide* and 1 ml of a 10% w/v solution of *potassium thiocyanate*, allow to stand for 5 minutes and titrate the liberated iodine with 0.1M *sodium thiosulphate VS* using *starch mucilage*, added towards the end of the titration, as indicator. Repeat the determination beginning at the words 'Mix 10 ml of 0.0167M *potassium dichromate VS*...' but using 5 ml of *water* in place of 5 ml of the distillate. The difference between the titrations is not more than 4.2 ml.

Nitrogen Carry out Method I for the *determination of nitrogen*, Appendix VIII H, using 50 ml. For solutions in Glucose Intravenous Infusion use 30 ml of *nitrogen-free sulphuric acid*. For solutions in Sodium Chloride Intravenous Infusion, use 20 ml of *nitrogen-free sulphuric acid*. Not more than 0.35 ml of 0.05M *sulphuric acid VS* is required.

Sulphated ash Not more than 0.05% w/v when determined by titrating 25 ml with 0.1M *silver nitrate VS* using *potassium chromate solution* as indicator and subtracting the theoretical value of the sulphated ash present due to the sodium chloride. Each ml of 0.1M *silver nitrate VS* is equivalent to 7.102 mg of sulphated ash.

Foreign protein Inject 0.5 ml on three occasions at intervals of 2 days into the peritoneal cavity of each of six guinea-pigs. Inject 0.2 ml intravenously into each of three of the guinea-pigs 14 days after the first intraperitoneal injection and into each of the other three guinea-pigs 21 days after the first intraperitoneal injection. Observe the guinea-pigs for 30 minutes after each intravenous injection and again 24 hours later. The animals exhibit no signs of anaphylaxis.

Pyrogens Complies with the *test for pyrogens*, Appendix XIV D. Use 10 ml per kg of the rabbit's weight.

Assay

For solutions in Glucose Intravenous Infusion Add 0.05 ml of 5M *ammonia* to the required volume and measure the *optical rotation*, Appendix V F. Calculate the content of dextrans from the expression

$$0.5076(\alpha-0.528D)$$

where α is the observed angular rotation and D is the content of glucose as a percentage w/v determined in the test for Content of glucose.

For solutions in Sodium Chloride Intravenous Infusion Measure the *optical rotation*, Appendix V F, and multiply the value obtained by 0.5076.

Storage Dextran 110 Intravenous Infusion should not be exposed to undue fluctuations of temperature.

Labelling The strength is stated as the percentage w/v of dextrans. The label states (1) the name of the solvent; (2) that the infusion should not be used if it is cloudy or if a deposit is present; (3) the strain of *Leuconostoc mesenteroides* used.

Action and use Plasma substitute.

Dextromoramide Injection

Definition Dextromoramide Injection is a sterile solution of Dextromoramide Tartrate in Water for Injections.

The injection complies with the requirements stated under Parenteral Preparations and with the following requirements.

Content of dextromoramide, $C_{25}H_{32}N_2O_2$ 95.0 to 105.0% of the prescribed or stated amount.

Identification Dilute a volume containing the equivalent of 25 mg of dextromoramide to 10 ml with *water*, make alkaline with 5M *ammonia* and extract with two 5-ml quantities of *ether*. Dry the combined ether extracts over *anhydrous sodium sulphate*, filter and evaporate to dryness. The *infrared absorption spectrum* of the residue, Appendix II A, is concordant with the *reference spectrum* of dextromoramide.

Related substances Carry out the method for *thin-layer chromatography*, Appendix III A, using *silica gel G* as the coating substance and *methanol* as the mobile phase. Apply separately to the plate 5 µl of each of the following solutions. For solution (1) evaporate a volume containing the equivalent of 20 mg of dextromoramide just to dryness on a water bath, add 1 ml of *methanol* to the residue and shake for 10 minutes. For solution (2) dilute 1 volume of solution (1) to 100 volumes with *methanol*. After removal of the plate, allow it to dry in air and spray with *dilute potassium iodobismuthate solution*. Any *secondary spot* in the chromatogram obtained with solution (1) is not more intense than the spot in the chromatogram obtained with solution (2).

Assay Evaporate a volume containing the equivalent of 50 mg of dextromoramide just to dryness on a water bath. Dissolve the residue, with the aid of gentle heat, in 30 ml of *anhydrous acetic acid* and carry out Method I for *non-aqueous titration*, Appendix VIII A, using 0.02M *perchloric acid VS* as titrant and 0.15 ml of *1-naphtholbenzein solution* as indicator. Each ml of 0.02M *perchloric acid VS* is equivalent to 7.851 mg of $C_{25}H_{32}N_2O_2$.

Labelling The quantity of active ingredient is stated in terms of the equivalent amount of dextromoramide.

Dextromoramide Tablets

Definition Dextromoramide Tablets contain Dextromoramide Tartrate.

The tablets comply with the requirements stated under Tablets and with the following requirements.

Content of dextromoramide, $C_{25}H_{32}N_2O_2$ 90.0 to 110.0% of the prescribed or stated amount.

Identification

A. Shake a quantity of the powdered tablets containing the equivalent of 30 mg of dextromoramide with 10 ml of *water* and filter. Make the filtrate alkaline with 5M *ammonia* and extract with two 5-ml quantities of *ether*. Dry the combined ether extracts over *anhydrous sodium sulphate*, filter and evaporate the filtrate to dryness. The *infrared absorption spectrum* of the residue, Appendix II A, is concordant with the *reference spectrum* of dextromoramide.

B. Shake a quantity of the powdered tablets containing the equivalent of 25 mg of dextromoramide with 25 ml of 1M *hydrochloric acid* and filter. The *light absorption* of the resulting solution, Appendix II B, in the range 230 to 350 nm exhibits maxima at 254, 259 and 264 nm.

Related substances Carry out the method for *thin-layer chromatography*, Appendix III A, using *silica gel G* as the coating substance and *methanol* as the mobile phase. Apply separately to the plate 10 µl of each of the following solutions. For solution (1) shake a quantity of the powdered tablets containing the equivalent of 20 mg of dextromoramide with 1 ml of *methanol* for 5 minutes, centrifuge and use the supernatant liquid. For solution (2) dilute 1 volume of solution (1) to 100 volumes with *methanol*. After removal of the plate, allow it to dry in air and spray with *dilute potassium iodobismuthate solution*. Any *secondary spot* in the chromatogram obtained with solution (1) is not more intense than the spot in the chromatogram obtained with solution (2).

Assay Weigh and powder 20 tablets. Shake a quantity of the powder containing the equivalent of 0.1 g of dextromoramide with 25 ml of 1M *hydrochloric acid* for 5 minutes. Add 25 ml of *water*, make alkaline with 5M *sodium hydroxide* and extract with four 25-ml quantities of *chloroform*. Wash the combined chloroform extracts with two 10-ml quantities of *water* and extract the combined washings with 10 ml of *chloroform*. Filter the combined chloroform extracts through absorbent cotton moistened with *chloroform* and wash the filter with a small quantity of *chloroform*. Heat on a water bath until the volume is reduced to about 25 ml, cool, add 50 ml of *anhydrous* *acetic acid*, previously neutralised to *crystal violet solution*, and titrate with 0.02M *perchloric acid VS* using *crystal violet solution* as indicator. Each ml of 0.02M *perchloric acid VS* is equivalent to 7.851 mg of $C_{25}H_{32}N_2O_2$.

Labelling The quantity of active ingredient is stated in terms of the equivalent amount of dextromoramide.

Dextropropoxyphene Capsules

Definition Dextropropoxyphene Capsules contain Dextropropoxyphene Napsylate.

The capsules comply with the requirements stated under Capsules and with the following requirements.

Content of dextropropoxyphene, $C_{22}H_{29}NO_2$ 92.5 to 107.5% of the prescribed or stated amount.

Identification Shake a quantity of the contents of the capsules containing the equivalent of 0.15 g of dextropropoxyphene with 5 ml of *chloroform* and filter. The filtrate complies with the following tests.

A. Evaporate 3 ml to dryness and dry the residue at 105° for 1 hour. The *infrared absorption spectrum* of the residue, Appendix II A, is concordant with the *reference spectrum* of dextropropoxyphene napsylate.

B. Evaporate 0.05 ml in a porcelain dish and streak the spot with *sulphuric acid* containing 0.05 ml of *formaldehyde solution* per ml. A purple colour is produced.

C. Evaporate 0.4 ml on a piece of filter paper and burn the residue by the method for *oxygen-flask combustion*, Appendix VIII C, using 5 ml of 1.25M *sodium hydroxide* as the absorbing liquid. When the process is complete, dilute the liquid to 25 ml with *water*. To 5 ml of the solution so obtained add 1 ml of *hydrogen peroxide solution (100 vol)* and 1 ml of 1M *hydrochloric acid*, mix and add 0.05 ml of *barium chloride solution*. The solution becomes turbid.

Assay Stir a quantity of the mixed contents of 20 capsules containing the equivalent of 0.5 g of dextropropoxyphene with 25 ml of *chloroform* and filter through absorbent cotton, washing the flask and filter with small quantities of *chloroform*. Add to the combined filtrates a mixture of 50 ml of *water* and 5 ml of 5M *sodium hydroxide*, shake, allow the layers to separate and wash the chloroform extract with 25 ml of *water*. Extract the aqueous layer with five 25-ml quantities of *chloroform*, washing each extract with the 25 ml of *water* and adding it to the original extract. Dry the combined extracts with *anhydrous sodium sulphate*, evaporate to about 3 ml on a water bath in a current of air, remove from the water bath and allow to evaporate to dryness at room temperature. Carry out Method I for *non-aqueous titration*, Appendix VIII A, on the residue using *crystal violet solution* as indicator. Each ml of 0.1M *perchloric acid VS* is equivalent to 33.95 mg of $C_{22}H_{29}NO_2$.

Labelling The quantity of active ingredient is stated in terms of the equivalent amount of dextropropoxyphene.

Diamorphine Injection

Definition Diamorphine Injection is a sterile solution of diamorphine hydrochloride in Water for Injections. It is prepared by dissolving Diamorphine Hydrochloride for Injection in the requisite amount of Water for Injections immediately before use.

The injection complies with the requirements stated under Parenteral Preparations.

Storage Diamorphine Injection deteriorates on storage and should be used immediately after preparation.

DIAMORPHINE HYDROCHLORIDE FOR INJECTION

Definition Diamorphine Hydrochloride for Injection is a sterile material prepared from Diamorphine Hydrochloride with or without excipients. It is supplied in a sealed container.

The contents of the sealed container comply with the requirements for Powders for Injections stated under Parenteral Preparations and with the following requirements.

Content of diamorphine hydrochloride, $C_{21}H_{23}NO_5,HCl,H_2O$ 95.0 to 105.0% of the prescribed or stated amount.

Identification Dissolve a sufficient quantity of the contents of the sealed container in the minimum volume of *dichloromethane* and evaporate to dryness. The *infrared absorption spectrum* of the residue, Appendix II A, is concordant with the *reference spectrum* of diamorphine hydrochloride.

Related substances Carry out the method for *liquid chromatography*, Appendix III D, using the following solutions. For solution (1) dissolve a quantity of the contents of the sealed container containing the equivalent of 0.2 g of diamorphine hydrochloride in 10 ml of *water*. For solution (2) dilute 1 volume of solution (1) to 20 volumes with *water*. For solution (3) dissolve a sufficient quantity of the contents of the sealed container to give a solution containing the equivalent of 1% w/v of diamorphine hydrochloride in 0.01M *sodium hydroxide*; the solution should be freshly prepared.

The chromatographic procedure may be carried out using (a) a stainless steel column (12.5 cm × 4.6 mm) packed with *stationary phase B* (5 µm) (Lichrosphere RP-select B 5µ is suitable), (b) as the mobile phase with a flow rate of 1 ml per minute a solution containing 0.11% w/v of *sodium octanesulphonate* in a mixture of 10 volumes of *glacial acetic acid*, 10 volumes of *methanol*, 115 volumes of *acetonitrile* and 365 volumes of *water* and (c) a detection wavelength of 283 nm.

The chromatogram obtained with solution (3) exhibits two *secondary peaks* with retention times relative to the principal peak of about 0.23 (morphine) and 0.43 (6-*O*-acetylmorphine). The test is not valid unless the *resolution factor* between the peaks due to morphine and 6-*O*-acetylmorphine is at least 2.

In the chromatogram obtained with solution (1) the area of any peak corresponding to 6-*O*-acetylmorphine is not greater than the area of the peak in the chromatogram obtained with solution (2) (5%).

Uniformity of content The content of $C_{21}H_{23}NO_5,HCl,H_2O$ in each of 10 individual containers as determined in the Assay is not less than 90.0% and not more than 110.0% of the average except that in one container the content may be not less than 80.0% and not more than 120.0% of the average.

Assay Dissolve the contents of a sealed container in a suitable volume of *water* and dilute with sufficient *water* to produce a solution containing 0.025% w/v of Diamorphine Hydrochloride. To 5 ml add 5 ml of 1M *hydrochloric acid* and boil vigorously under a reflux condenser for 15 minutes. Cool, add 5 ml of a freshly prepared 0.5% w/v solution of *sodium nitrite*, mix and add 2.5 ml of 5M *ammonia* and sufficient *water* to produce 25 ml. Repeat the operation with a further nine sealed containers. Measure the *absorbance* of each of the resulting solutions at the maximum at 435 nm, Appendix II B, and calculate the content of $C_{12}H_{23}NO_5,HCl,H_2O$ in each container by comparing the absorbances with that obtained by treating a mixture of 5 ml of a 0.015% w/v solution of *anhydrous morphine* in 1M *hydrochloric acid* and 5 ml of *water* in the same manner, beginning at the words 'add 5 ml of a freshly prepared...'. Each g of *anhydrous morphine* is equivalent to 1.486 g of $C_{21}H_{23}NO_5,HCl,H_2O$. Calculate the average content of $C_{21}H_{23}NO_5,HCl,H_2O$ per container from the 10 individual results thus obtained.

Storage The sealed container should be protected from light.

Diazepam Capsules

Definition Diazepam Capsules contain Diazepam.

The capsules comply with the requirements stated under Capsules and with the following requirements.

Content of diazepam, $C_{16}H_{13}ClN_2O$ 92.5 to 107.5% of the prescribed or stated amount.

Identification

A. The *light absorption*, Appendix II B, in the range 230 to 350 nm of the solution obtained in the Assay exhibits two maxima, at 242 nm and 284 nm.

B. Carry out the method for *thin-layer chromatography*, Appendix III A, using *silica gel G* as the coating substance and a mixture of 100 volumes of *chloroform* and 10 volumes of *methanol* as the mobile phase. Apply separately to the plate 2 µl of each of the following solutions. For solution (1) shake a quantity of the contents of the capsules with sufficient *methanol* to produce a solution containing 0.50% w/v of Diazepam, allow to settle and decant the supernatant liquid. Solution (2) contains 0.5% w/v of *diazepam BPCRS* in *methanol*. After removal of the plate, spray it with a 10% v/v solution of *sulphuric acid* in *absolute ethanol*, heat at 105° for 10 minutes and examine under *ultraviolet light (365 nm)*. The principal spot in the chromatogram obtained with solution (1) corresponds to that in the chromatogram obtained with solution (2).

Related substances and decomposition products Carry out in subdued light the method for *thin-layer chromatography*, Appendix III A, using *silica gel* GF_{254} as the coating substance and a mixture of equal volumes of *ethyl acetate* and *hexane* as the mobile phase, but allowing the solvent front to ascend 12 cm above the line of application. Apply separately to the plate 20 µl of solution (1) and 5 µl of solution (2) freshly prepared in the following manner. For solution (1) shake a quantity of the contents of the capsules containing 50 mg of Diazepam with 5 ml of *ethanol (96%)* and filter. For solution (2), dilute 1 volume of solution (1) to 50 volumes with *ethanol (96%)*. After removal of the plate, allow the solvent to evaporate and examine under *ultraviolet light (254 nm)*. Any *secondary spot* in the chromatogram obtained with solution (1) is not more intense than the spot in the chromatogram obtained with solution (2).

Uniformity of content Capsules containing 2 mg or less of Diazepam comply with the requirements stated under Capsules using the following method of analysis. Weigh an intact capsule. Open the capsule without losing any part of the shell and transfer the contents as completely as possible to a 100-ml graduated flask. Weigh the shell, remove any retained contents and reweigh the shell. To the flask add 1 ml of *water*, mix and allow to stand for 15 minutes. Add 80 ml of a 0.5% w/v solution of *sulphuric acid* in *methanol*, shake for 15 minutes, add sufficient of the methanolic sulphuric acid to produce 100 ml and filter. Measure the *absorbance* of the filtrate at the maximum at 284 nm, Appendix II B. Calculate the content of $C_{16}H_{13}ClN_2O$ taking 450 as the value of A(1%, 1 cm) at the maximum at 284 nm making an appropriate adjustment for any retained capsule content.

Assay To a quantity of the mixed contents of 20 capsules containing 10 mg of Diazepam add 5 ml of *water*, mix and allow to stand for 15 minutes. Add 90 ml of a 0.5% w/v solution of *sulphuric acid* in *methanol*, shake for 15 minutes, add sufficient of the methanolic sulphuric acid solution to produce 100 ml and filter. Dilute 10 ml of the filtrate to 50 ml with the same solvent and measure the *absorbance* of the resulting solution at the maximum at 284 nm, Appendix II B. Calculate the content of $C_{16}H_{13}ClN_2O$ taking 450 as the value of A(1%, 1 cm) at the maximum at 284 nm.

Storage Diazepam Capsules should be protected from light.

Diazepam Injection

Definition Diazepam Injection is a sterile solution of Diazepam in Water for Injections or other suitable solvent.

The injection complies with the requirements stated under Parenteral Preparations and with the following requirements.

Content of diazepam, $C_{16}H_{13}ClN_2O$ 90.0 to 110.0% of the prescribed or stated amount.

Identification

A. The *light absorption*, Appendix II B, of the solution obtained in the Assay exhibits a maximum at 368 nm.

B. Complies with test B for Identification described under Diazepam Capsules applying separately to the plate 10 µl of each of the following solutions. For solution (1) dilute a suitable volume of the injection with sufficient *methanol* to produce a solution containing 0.10% w/v of Diazepam. Solution (2) contains 0.10% w/v of *diazepam BPCRS* in *methanol*.

Acidity or alkalinity pH, 6.2 to 7.0, Appendix V L.

Assay To a volume containing 10 mg of Diazepam add 20 ml of *mixed phosphate buffer pH 7.0* and extract with four 20-ml quantities of *chloroform*, passing each extract through the same 5 g of *anhydrous sodium sulphate*. Combine the chloroform extracts, dilute to 100 ml with *chloroform* and mix. Evaporate 10 ml to dryness in a current of nitrogen, dissolve the residue in 25 ml of 0.05M *methanolic sulphuric acid*, mix and measure the *absorbance* of the resulting solution at the maximum at 368 nm, Appendix II B. Calculate the content of $C_{16}H_{13}ClN_2O$ taking 151 as the value of A(1%, 1 cm) at the maximum at 368 nm.

Storage Diazepam Injection should be protected from light.

Diazepam Oral Solution

Definition Diazepam Oral Solution is a solution of Diazepam in a suitable flavoured vehicle.

The oral solution complies with the requirements stated under Oral Liquids and with the following requirements.

Content of diazepam, $C_{16}H_{13}ClN_2O$ 95.0 to 115.0% of the prescribed or stated amount.

Identification

A. The *light absorption*, Appendix II B, in the range 320 to 400 nm of the final solution obtained in the Assay exhibits a maximum at 368 nm. The *light absorption* in the range 230 to 330 nm of a solution prepared by diluting 1 volume of the final solution obtained in the Assay to 5 volumes with 0.1M *methanolic sulphuric acid* exhibits two maxima, at 243 nm and 286 nm.

B. Carry out the method described under Related substances applying separately to the plate 10 µl of each of solution (1) and solution (2) and using as solution (2) a 0.4% w/v solution of *diazepam BPCRS* in *ethanol (96%)*. After removal of the plate, allow the solvent to evaporate and examine under *ultraviolet light (254 nm)*. The principal spot in the chromatogram obtained with solution (1) corresponds to that in the chromatogram obtained with solution (2).

Acidity pH, 4.7 to 5.4, Appendix V L.

Related substances Carry out in subdued light the method for *thin-layer chromatography*, Appendix III A, using *silica gel GF_{254}* as the coating substance and a mixture of equal volumes of *ethyl acetate* and *hexane* as the mobile phase but allowing the solvent front to ascend 12 cm above the line of application. Apply separately to the plate 25 µl of each of the following solutions. For solution (1) add 40 ml of *water* to a volume of the oral solution containing 8 mg of Diazepam and extract with three 50-ml quantities of *ether*. Wash the combined ether extracts with 30 ml of 1M *sodium hydroxide* followed by two 40-ml quantities of *water*. Shake the extract with *anhydrous sodium sulphate*, filter, evaporate to dryness and dissolve the residue in 2 ml of *ethanol (96%)*. Solution (2) contains 0.0080% w/v of *5-chloro-2-methylaminobenzophenone BPCRS* in *ethanol (96%)*. Solution (3) contains 0.0040% w/v of *3-amino-6-chloro-1-methyl-4-phenylquinolin-2-ol BPCRS* in *ethanol (96%)*. For solution (4) dilute 2 ml of solution (1) to 100 ml with *ethanol (96%)* and dilute 1 ml of the resulting solution to 10 ml with the same solvent. After removal of the plate, allow it to dry in air and examine under *ultraviolet light (254 nm)*. In the chromatogram obtained with solution (1) any spot corresponding to 5-chloro-2-methylaminobenzophenone is not more intense than the spot in the chromatogram obtained with solution (2) and any spot corresponding to 3-amino-6-chloro-1-methyl-4-phenylquinolin-2-ol is not more intense than the spot in the chromatogram obtained with solution (3). Any other *secondary spot* in the chromatogram obtained with solution (1) is not more intense than the spot in the chromatogram obtained with solution (4).

Assay To a weighed quantity containing 1 mg of Diazepam add 25 ml of a mixture of equal volumes of 1M *sodium hydroxide* and *methanol* and shake for 2 minutes. Extract with five 25-ml quantities of *chloroform*, shaking for 2 minutes each time. Combine the chloroform extracts, shake with 5 g of *anhydrous sodium sulphate* and filter. Evaporate to dryness, dissolve the residue in 25 ml of 0.1M *methanolic sulphuric acid* and filter. Measure the *absorbance* of the filtrate, Appendix II B, at the maximum at 368 nm. Calculate the content of $C_{16}H_{13}ClN_2O$ taking 151 as the value of A(1%, 1 cm) at the maximum at 368 nm. Determine the *weight per ml* of the oral solution, Appendix V G, and calculate the content of $C_{16}H_{13}ClN_2O$, weight in volume.

Storage Diazepam Oral Solution should be protected from light and stored at a temperature not exceeding 25°.

Diazepam Rectal Solution

Definition Diazepam Rectal Solution is a solution of Diazepam in a suitable vehicle.

The rectal solution complies with the requirements stated under Rectal Preparations and with the following requirements.

Content of diazepam, $C_{16}H_{13}ClN_2O$ 95.0 to 105.0% of the prescribed or stated amount.

Identification

A. The *light absorption*, Appendix II B, of the solution obtained in the Assay exhibits a maximum at 368 nm.

B. Carry out the method for *thin-layer chromatography*, Appendix III A, using *silica gel G* as the coating substance and a mixture of 10 volumes of *methanol* and 100 volumes of *chloroform* as the mobile phase. Apply separately to the plate 10 µl of each of the following solutions. For solution (1) dilute a suitable volume of the rectal solution with sufficient *methanol* to produce a solution containing 0.10% w/v of Diazepam. Solution (2) contains 0.10% w/v of *diazepam BPCRS* in *methanol*. After removal of the plate, spray it with a 10% v/v solution of *sulphuric acid* in *absolute ethanol*, heat at 105° for 10 minutes and examine under *ultraviolet light (365 nm)*. The principal spot in the chromatogram obtained with solution (1) corresponds to that in the chromatogram obtained with solution (2).

Acidity or alkalinity pH, 6.2 to 7.2, Appendix V L.

Assay To a volume containing 10 mg of Diazepam add 20 ml of *mixed phosphate buffer pH 7.0* and extract with four 20-ml quantities of *chloroform*, passing each extract through the same 5 g of *anhydrous sodium sulphate*. Combine the chloroform extracts, dilute to 100 ml with *chloroform* and mix. Evaporate 10 ml to dryness in a current of nitrogen, dissolve the residue in 25 ml of 0.05M *methanolic sulphuric acid*, mix and measure the *absorbance* of the resulting solution at the maximum at 368 nm, Appendix

II B. Calculate the content of $C_{16}H_{13}ClN_2O$ taking 151 as the value of A(1%, 1 cm) at the maximum at 368 nm.

Storage Diazepam Rectal Solution should be protected from light and stored at a temperature not exceeding 25°.

Diazepam Tablets

Definition Diazepam Tablets contain Diazepam.

The tablets comply with the requirements stated under Tablets and with the following requirements.

Content of diazepam, $C_{16}H_{13}ClN_2O$ 92.5 to 107.5% of the prescribed or stated amount.

Identification

A. The *light absorption*, Appendix II B, in the range 230 to 350 nm of the final solution obtained in the Assay exhibits two maxima, at 242 nm and 284 nm.

B. Comply with test B for Identification described under Diazepam Capsules, but using the powdered tablets to prepare solution (1).

Related substances and decomposition products Carry out in subdued light the method for *thin-layer chromatography*, Appendix III A, using *silica gel GF_{254}* as the coating substance and a mixture of equal volumes of *ethyl acetate* and *hexane* as the mobile phase but allowing the solvent front to ascend 12 cm above the line of application. Apply separately to the plate (1) 20 µl of a solution freshly prepared by shaking a quantity of the powdered tablets containing 50 mg of Diazepam with 5 ml of *ethanol (96%)* and filtering and (2) 5 µl of a solution freshly prepared by diluting 1 volume of solution (1) to 50 volumes with *ethanol (96%)*. After removal of the plate, allow the solvent to evaporate and examine under *ultraviolet light (254 nm)*. Any *secondary spot* in the chromatogram obtained with solution (1) is not more intense than the spot in the chromatogram obtained with solution (2).

Uniformity of content Tablets containing 2 mg or less of Diazepam comply with the requirement stated under Tablets using the following method of analysis. To one tablet add 1 ml of *water*, allow the tablet to disintegrate and stand for 15 minutes. Add 80 ml of a 0.5% w/v solution of *sulphuric acid* in *methanol*, shake for 15 minutes, add sufficient of the methanolic sulphuric acid to produce 100 ml and filter. Measure the *absorbance* of the filtrate at the maximum at 284 nm, Appendix II B. Calculate the content of $C_{10}H_{13}ClN_2O$ taking 450 as the value of A(1%, 1 cm) at the maximum at 284 nm.

Assay Weigh and powder 20 tablets. To a quantity of the powder containing 10 mg of Diazepam add 5 ml of *water*, mix and allow to stand for 15 minutes. Add 70 ml of a 0.5% w/v solution of *sulphuric acid* in *methanol*, shake for 15 minutes, add sufficient of the methanolic sulphuric acid to produce 100 ml and filter. Dilute 10 ml of the filtrate to 50 ml with the same solvent and measure the *absorbance* of the resulting solution at the maximum at 284 nm, Appendix II B. Calculate the content of $C_{16}H_{13}ClN_2O$ taking 450 as the value of A(1%, 1 cm) at the maximum at 284 nm.

Storage Diazepam Tablets should be protected from light.

Diazoxide Injection

Definition Diazoxide Injection is a sterile solution of Diazoxide in Water for Injections, prepared with the aid of Sodium Hydroxide.

The injection complies with the requirements stated under Parenteral Preparations and with the following requirements.

Content of diazoxide, $C_8H_7ClN_2O_2S$ 95.0 to 105.0% of the prescribed or stated amount.

Characteristics A colourless solution.

Identification To a volume containing 0.3 g of Diazoxide add 2 ml of *2M hydrochloric acid*, stir, filter the precipitate and wash the filter thoroughly with *water* until the filtrate is free from acid. The precipitate, after drying at 105°, complies with the following tests.

A. The *infrared absorption spectrum*, Appendix II A, is concordant with the *reference spectrum* of diazoxide.

B. The *light absorption*, Appendix II B, in the range 230 to 350 nm of a 0.001% w/v solution in *0.1M sodium hydroxide* exhibits a maximum only at 280 nm.

C. Carry out the method for *thin-layer chromatography*, Appendix III A, using *silica gel GF_{254}* as the coating substance and a mixture of 50 volumes of *toluene*, 30 volumes of *ether* and 20 volumes of *acetone* as the mobile phase. Apply separately to the plate 20 µl of each of two solutions in *methanol* containing (1) 0.02% w/v of the substance being examined and (2) 0.02% w/v of *diazoxide BPCRS*. After removal of the plate, allow it to dry in air until the odour of the solvent is no longer detectable, examine under *ultraviolet light (254 nm)* and then treat the plate by *Method I* and examine again. The principal spot in the chromatogram obtained with solution (1) corresponds in colour and intensity to that in the chromatogram obtained with solution (2).

Alkalinity pH, 11.2 to 11.9, Appendix V L.

Related substances Complies with the test described under Diazoxide. Use solutions (1) and (3) only. For solution (1) use a volume of the injection containing 0.75 g of Diazoxide. For solution (3) dilute 1 volume of solution (1) to 200 volumes with *0.1M sodium hydroxide*.

Assay To a volume containing 75 mg of Diazoxide add sufficient *0.1M sodium hydroxide* to produce 500 ml. Dilute 5 ml to 100 ml with *0.1M sodium hydroxide* and measure the *absorbance* of the resulting solution at the maximum at 280 nm, Appendix II B. Calculate the content of $C_8H_7ClN_2O_2S$ taking 585 as the value of A(1%, 1 cm) at the maximum at 280 nm.

Storage Diazoxide Injection should be protected from light.

Diazoxide Tablets

Definition Diazoxide Tablets contain Diazoxide.

The tablets comply with the requirements stated under Tablets and with the following requirements.

Content of diazoxide, $C_8H_7ClN_2O_2S$ 92.5 to 107.5% of the prescribed or stated amount.

Identification Shake a quantity of the powdered tablets containing 0.2 g of Diazoxide with 50 ml of *absolute ethanol*, filter and evaporate the filtrate to dryness at a pressure of 2 kPa. The residue complies with the following tests.

A. The *light absorption*, Appendix II B, in the range 230 to 350 nm of a 0.001% w/v solution in 0.1M *sodium hydroxide* exhibits a maximum only at 280 nm.

B. Carry out the method for *thin-layer chromatography*, Appendix III A, using *silica gel GF_{254}* as the coating substance and a mixture of 50 volumes of *toluene*, 30 volumes of *ether* and 20 volumes of *acetone* as the mobile phase. Apply separately to the plate 20 µl of each of two solutions in *methanol* containing (1) 0.02% w/v of the residue and (2) 0.02% w/v of *diazoxide BPCRS*. After removal of the plate, allow it to dry in air until the odour of the solvent is no longer detectable, examine under *ultraviolet light (254 nm)* and then treat the plate by *Method I* and examine again. The principal spot in the chromatogram obtained with solution (1) corresponds in colour and intensity to that in the chromatogram obtained with solution (2).

Related substances Comply with the test described under Diazoxide. Use solutions (1) and (3) only. For solution (1) shake a quantity of the powdered tablets containing 0.75 g of Diazoxide with 40 ml of 0.1M *sodium hydroxide* for 30 minutes, filter and dilute the filtrate to 50 ml with 0.1M *sodium hydroxide*. For solution (3) dilute 1 volume of solution (1) to 200 volumes with 0.1M *sodium hydroxide*.

Assay Weigh and powder 20 tablets. To a quantity of the powder containing 50 mg of Diazoxide add 70 ml of *methanol*, shake for 1 hour, add sufficient *methanol* to produce 100 ml, mix and filter. Dilute 5 ml of the filtrate to 250 ml with 0.1M *sodium hydroxide* and measure the *absorbance* of the resulting solution at the maximum at 280 nm, Appendix II B. Calculate the content of $C_8H_7ClN_2O_2S$ taking 585 as the value of A(1%, 1 cm) at the maximum at 280 nm.

Dichlorophen Tablets

Definition Dichlorophen Tablets contain Dichlorophen.

The tablets comply with the requirements stated under Tablets and with the following requirements.

Content of dichlorophen, $C_{13}H_{10}Cl_2O_2$ 95.0 to 105.0% of the prescribed or stated amount.

Identification

A. Shake a quantity of the powdered tablets containing 0.1 g of Dichlorophen with 50 ml of 0.1M *sodium hydroxide* for 15 minutes, add sufficient 0.1M *sodium hydroxide* to produce 100 ml, centrifuge and dilute a suitable volume of the supernatant liquid with 0.1M *sodium hydroxide* to produce a solution containing 0.002% w/v of Dichlorophen. The *light absorption* of the resulting solution, Appendix II B, in the range 220 to 350 nm exhibits two maxima, at 245 nm and 304 nm. The *absorbances* at the maxima are about 1.3 and about 0.54, respectively.

B. Shake a quantity of the powdered tablets containing 0.2 g of Dichlorophen with a mixture of 5 ml of *water* and 5 ml of 5M *sodium hydroxide*, filter, cool in ice and add a solution prepared by mixing 1 ml of *sodium nitrite solution* with a cold solution containing 0.15 ml of *aniline* in a mixture of 4 ml of *water* and 1 ml of *hydrochloric acid*. A reddish brown precipitate is produced.

C. Fuse a quantity of the powdered tablets containing 0.5 g of Dichlorophen with 2 g of *anhydrous sodium carbonate*, cool, extract the residue with *water* and filter. The filtrate yields reaction A characteristic of *chlorides*, Appendix VI.

Related substances Comply with the test for Related substances described under Dichlorophen using the following solutions. Solution (1) contains 1.0% w/v of *dichlorophen impurity standard BPRCS* in the mobile phase. For solution (2) shake a quantity of the powdered tablets containing 0.50 g of Dichlorophen with 20 ml of *methanol* for 10 minutes, filter, add 7 ml of *water* and dilute to 50 ml with the mobile phase. Solution (3) contains 0.0010% w/v of *4-chlorophenol* in the mobile phase.

Assay Weigh and powder 20 tablets. Shake a quantity of the powder containing 0.1 g of Dichlorophen with 50 ml of 0.1M *sodium hydroxide* for 15 minutes and add sufficient 0.1M *sodium hydroxide* to produce 100 ml. Centrifuge, dilute 10 ml of the clear supernatant liquid to 100 ml with 0.1M *sodium hydroxide*, dilute 20 ml of this solution to 100 ml with 0.1M *sodium hydroxide* and measure the *absorbance* of the resulting solution at the maximum at 304 nm, Appendix II B. Calculate the content of $C_{13}H_{10}Cl_2O_2$ taking 275 as the value of A(1%, 1 cm) at the maximum at 304 nm.

Diclofenac Tablets

Definition Diclofenac Tablets contain Diclofenac Sodium. They are made gastro-resistant by enteric-coating or by other means.

The tablets comply with the requirements stated under Tablets and with the following requirements.

Content of diclofenac sodium, $C_{14}H_{10}Cl_2NNaO_2$ 95.0 to 105.0% of the prescribed or stated amount.

Identification Remove the coating from 10 tablets and powder the cores. Add 0.5 ml of *glacial acetic acid* and 15 ml of *methanol* to a quantity of the powdered tablet cores containing 0.15 g of Diclofenac Sodium and mix with the aid of ultrasound. Shake gently for 1 minute, filter and collect the filtrate in 15 ml of *water*. Filter the precipitate under reduced pressure (Whatman GF/C filter paper is suitable), wash with four 5-ml quantities of *water* and dry at 105° for 2 to 3 hours. The *infrared absorption spectrum* of the dried precipitate, Appendix II A, is concordant with the *reference spectrum* of diclofenac.

Disintegration Tablets made gastro-resistant by enteric-coating comply with the *disintegration test for enteric-coated tablets*, Appendix XII B.

Related substances Carry out the method for *liquid chromatography*, Appendix III D, using the following solutions. For solution (1) shake a quantity of the powdered tablets containing 50 mg of Diclofenac Sodium with 70 ml of the mobile phase for 30 minutes, add sufficient of the mobile phase to produce 100 ml, mix, centrifuge an aliquot and filter the supernatant liquid through a 0.45-μm filter. For solution (2) dilute 1 volume of solution (1) to 100 volumes with the mobile phase and dilute 1 volume of this solution to 5 volumes with the mobile phase. Solution (3) contains 0.0005% w/v of *diclofenac sodium BPCRS* and 0.0005% w/v of *diclofenac impurity A EPCRS* in the mobile phase.

The chromatographic procedure may be carried out using (a) a stainless steel column (25 cm × 4.6 mm) packed with *octylsilyl silica gel for chromatography* (5 μm) (end-capped Zorbax C8 is suitable), (b) as mobile phase with a flow rate of 1 ml per minute a mixture of 34 volumes of a mixture of equal volumes of a 0.1% w/v solution of *orthophosphoric acid* and a 0.16% w/v solution of *sodium dihydrogen orthophosphate*, adjusted to pH 2.5, and 66 volumes of *methanol* and (c) a detection wavelength of 254 nm.

Inject solution (3). When the chromatograms are recorded in the prescribed conditions, the retention times are about 25 minutes for diclofenac and about 12 minutes for diclofenac impurity A. Continue the chromatography for 1.5 times the retention time of diclofenac. The test is not valid unless, in the chromatogram obtained with solution (3), the *resolution factor* between the peaks corresponding to diclofenac and diclofenac impurity A is at least 6.5.

Inject solution (1) and solution (2). In the chromatogram obtained with solution (1) the area of any *secondary peak* is not greater than the area of the principal peak in the chromatogram obtained with solution (2) (0.2%) and the sum of the areas of all the *secondary peaks* is not greater than 2.5 times the area of the principal peak in the chromatogram obtained with solution (2) (0.5%). Disregard any peak with an area less than 0.25 times the area of the principal peak in the chromatogram obtained with solution (2) (0.05%) and any peaks with retention times relative to the principal peak of 0.67 and 0.1.

Assay Weigh and powder 20 tablets. Carry out the method for *liquid chromatography*, Appendix III D, using the following solutions. For solution (1) shake a quantity of the powdered tablets containing 50 mg of Diclofenac Sodium with 70 ml of *methanol (50%)* for 30 minutes with the aid of ultrasound, add sufficient of the mobile phase to produce 100 ml, mix, centrifuge an aliquot and filter the supernatant liquid through a 0.45-μm filter. Dilute 1 volume of the resulting solution to 10 volumes with the mobile phase. Solution (2) contains 0.005% w/v of *diclofenac sodium BPCRS* in the mobile phase. Solution (3) contains 0.0005% w/v of *diclofenac sodium BPCRS* and 0.0005% w/v of *diclofenac impurity A EPCRS* in the mobile phase.

The chromatographic conditions described under Related substances may be used.

The Assay is not valid unless, in the chromatogram obtained with solution (3), the *resolution factor* between the peaks corresponding to diclofenac and diclofenac impurity A is at least 6.5.

Calculate the content of $C_{14}H_{10}Cl_2NNaO_2$ in the tablets from the chromatograms obtained and from the declared content of $C_{14}H_{10}Cl_2NNa0_2$ in *diclofenac sodium BPCRS*.

Storage Diclofenac Tablets should be protected from moisture.

IMPURITIES

The impurities limited by the requirements of this monograph include those listed in the monograph for Diclofenac Sodium.

Slow Diclofenac Tablets

Definition Slow Diclofenac Tablets contain Diclofenac Sodium. They are formulated so that the medicament is released over a period of several hours.

Production A suitable dissolution test is carried out to demonstrate the appropriate release of Diclofenac Sodium. The dissolution profile reflects the *in vivo* performance which in turn is compatible with the dosage schedule recommended by the manufacturer.

With the exception of the requirements for shape, the tablets comply with the requirements stated under Tablets and with the following requirements.

Content of diclofenac sodium, $C_{14}H_{10}Cl_2NNaO_2$ 95.0 to 105.0% of the prescribed or stated amount.

Identification Remove the coating from 10 tablets and powder the cores. Add 0.5 ml of *glacial acetic acid* and 15 ml of *methanol* to a quantity of the powdered tablet cores containing 0.15 g of Diclofenac Sodium and mix with the aid of ultrasound. Shake gently for 1 minute, filter and collect the filtrate in 15 ml of *water*. Filter the precipitate under reduced pressure (Whatman GF/C filter paper is suitable), wash with four 5-ml quantities of *water* and dry at 105° for 2 to 3 hours. The *infrared absorption spectrum* of the dried precipitate, Appendix II A, is concordant with the *reference spectrum* of diclofenac.

Related substances Carry out the method for *liquid chromatography*, Appendix III D, using the following solutions. For solution (1) shake a quantity of the powdered tablets containing 50 mg of Diclofenac Sodium with 70 ml of the mobile phase for 30 minutes, add sufficient of the mobile phase to produce 100 ml, mix, centrifuge an aliquot and filter the supernatant liquid through a 0.45-μm filter. For solution (2) dilute 1 volume of solution (1) to 100 volumes with the mobile phase and dilute 1 volume of this solution to 5 volumes with the mobile phase. Solution (3) contains 0.0005% w/v of *diclofenac sodium BPCRS* and 0.0005% w/v of *diclofenac impurity A EPCRS* in the mobile phase.

The chromatographic procedure may be carried out using (a) a stainless steel column (25 cm × 4.6 mm) packed with *octylsilyl silica gel for chromatography* (5 μm) (end-capped Zorbax C8 is suitable), (b) as mobile phase with a flow rate of 1 ml per minute a mixture of 34 volumes of a mixture of equal volumes of a 0.1% w/v solution of *orthophosphoric acid* and a 0.16% w/v solution of *sodium dihydrogen orthophosphate*, adjusted to pH 2.5, and 66 volumes of *methanol* and (c) a detection wavelength of 254 nm.

Inject solution (3). When the chromatograms are recorded in the prescribed conditions, the retention times are about 25 minutes for diclofenac and about 12 minutes for diclofenac impurity A. Continue the chromatography for 1.5 times the retention time of diclofenac. The test is not valid unless, in the chromatogram obtained with solution (3), the *resolution factor* between the peaks corresponding to diclofenac and diclofenac impurity A is at least 6.5.

Inject solution (1) and solution (2). In the chromatogram obtained with solution (1) the area of any *secondary peak* is not greater than the area of the principal peak in the chromatogram obtained with solution (2) (0.2%) and the sum of the areas of all the *secondary peaks* is not greater than 2.5 times the area of the principal peak in the chromatogram obtained with solution (2) (0.5%). Disregard any peak with an area less than 0.25 times the area of the principal peak in the chromatogram obtained with solution (2) (0.05%).

Assay Weigh and powder 20 tablets. Carry out the method for *liquid chromatography*, Appendix III D, using the following solutions. For solution (1) shake 10 tablets with 800 ml of *methanol (50%)* for 30 minutes, add sufficient of the mobile phase to produce 1000 ml, mix, centrifuge an aliquot and filter the supernatant liquid through a 0.45-µm filter. Dilute the resulting solution with the mobile phase to produce a solution containing 0.005% w/v of Diclofenac Sodium. Solution (2) contains 0.005% w/v of *diclofenac sodium BPCRS* in the mobile phase. Solution (3) contains 0.0005% w/v of *diclofenac sodium BPCRS* and 0.0005% w/v of *diclofenac impurity A EPCRS* in the mobile phase.

The chromatographic conditions described under Related substances may be used.

The Assay is not valid unless, in the chromatogram obtained with solution (3), the *resolution factor* between the peaks corresponding to diclofenac and diclofenac impurity A is at least 6.5.

Calculate the content of $C_{14}H_{10}Cl_2NNaO_2$ in the tablets from the chromatograms obtained and from the declared content of $C_{14}H_{10}Cl_2NNaO_2$ in *diclofenac sodium BPCRS*.

Storage Slow Diclofenac Tablets should be protected from moisture.

IMPURITIES

The impurities limited by the requirements of this monograph include those listed in the monograph for Diclofenac Sodium.

Dicycloverine Oral Solution
Dicyclomine Oral Solution

For the purposes of product labelling in the United Kingdom, the pair of names given above shall be used together (see Introduction, Changes in title).

Definition Dicycloverine Oral Solution is a solution of Dicycloverine Hydrochloride in a suitable flavoured vehicle.

The oral solution complies with the requirements stated under Oral Liquids and with the following requirements.

Content of dicycloverine hydrochloride, $C_{19}H_{35}NO_2$, HCl 90.0 to 110.0% of the prescribed or stated amount.

Identification

A. To a volume containing 0.1 g of Dicycloverine Hydrochloride add 10 ml of *water* and 1 ml of *hydrochloric acid*, shake with 30 ml of *ether* and allow to separate. Extract the aqueous layer with 30 ml of *chloroform*, wash the extract with two 10-ml quantities of *water* and filter the chloroform solution through *anhydrous sodium sulphate*. Evaporate the filtrate to dryness, recrystallise the residue from hot *acetone* and dry the precipitate at 105° for 30 minutes. The *infrared absorption spectrum* of the residue, Appendix II A, is concordant with the *reference spectrum* of dicycloverine hydrochloride.

B. Acidify the oral solution with 2M *nitric acid* and add *silver nitrate solution*. A white precipitate is produced.

Assay To a weighed quantity containing 5 mg of Dicycloverine Hydrochloride add 5 ml of *sulphuric acid (10%)* and 2 ml of 0.02M *potassium permanganate*, mix, allow to stand, add 20 ml of *water* and 20 ml of *chloroform* to the decolorised solution and titrate with 0.001M *sodium dodecyl sulphate VS* using 1 ml of *dimethyl yellow solution* as indicator. Each ml of 0.001M *sodium dodecyl sulphate VS* is equivalent to 0.3460 mg of $C_{19}H_{35}NO_2$,HCl. Determine the *weight per ml* of the oral solution, Appendix V G, and calculate the content of $C_{19}H_{35}NO_2$,HCl, weight in volume.

Storage Dicycloverine Oral Solution should be protected from light.

Labelling The label states 'Dicycloverine Oral Solution' and 'Dicyclomine Oral Solution'.

Dicycloverine Tablets
Dicyclomine Tablets

For the purposes of product labelling in the United Kingdom, the pair of names given above shall be used together (see Introduction, Changes in title)

Definition Dicycloverine Tablets contain Dicycloverine Hydrochloride.

The tablets comply with the requirements stated under Tablets and with the following requirements.

Content of dicycloverine hydrochloride, $C_{19}H_{35}NO_2$, HCl 92.5 to 107.5% of the prescribed or stated amount.

Identification

A. Extract a quantity of the powdered tablets containing 0.2 g of Dicycloverine Hydrochloride with 20 ml of *chloroform*, filter, evaporate the filtrate to dryness, recrystallise the residue from *acetone* and dry at 105° for 4 hours. The *infrared absorption spectrum* of the residue, Appendix II A, is concordant with the *reference spectrum* of dicycloverine hydrochloride.

B. Shake a quantity of the powdered tablets containing 10 mg of Dicycloverine Hydrochloride with 5 ml of *water* and 0.2 ml of 2M *nitric acid*, filter and add 0.5 ml of *silver nitrate solution* to the filtrate. A white precipitate is produced.

Related substances Carry out the method for *thin-layer chromatography*, Appendix III A, using *silica gel G* as the coating substance and a mixture of 50 volumes of *propan-1-ol*, 30 volumes of *ethyl acetate*, 15 volumes of *water* and 5 volumes of 13.5M *ammonia* as the mobile phase. Apply separately to the plate 10 µl of each of the following solutions. For solution (1) shake a quantity of the powdered tablets containing 0.2 g of Dicycloverine

Hydrochloride with 8 ml of *water* and 2 ml of 13.5M *ammonia*, extract with two 20-ml quantities of *chloroform*, shake with *anhydrous sodium sulphate*, filter, evaporate the filtrate to dryness and dissolve the residue in 4 ml of *chloroform*. For solution (2) dilute 1 volume of solution (1) to 500 volumes with *chloroform*. After removal of the plate, allow it to dry in air and spray with *dilute potassium iodobismuthate solution*. Any *secondary spot* in the chromatogram obtained with solution (1) is not more intense than the spot in the chromatogram obtained with solution (2).

Assay Weigh and powder 20 tablets. To a quantity of the powder containing 30 mg of Dicycloverine Hydrochloride add 20 ml of *water* and shake. Add 10 ml of 1M *sulphuric acid*, 1 ml of *dimethyl yellow solution* and 40 ml of *chloroform*, shake and titrate with 0.004M *sodium dodecyl sulphate VS*, shaking vigorously and allowing the layers to separate after each addition, until a permanent orange-pink colour is produced in the chloroform layer. Each ml of 0.004M *sodium dodecyl sulphate VS* is equivalent to 1.384 mg of $C_{19}H_{35}NO_2,HCl$.

Labelling The label states 'Dicycloverine Tablets' and 'Dicyclomine Tablets'.

Diethylamine Salicylate Cream

Definition Diethylamine Salicylate Cream is a dispersion of Diethylamine Salicylate in a suitable basis.

The cream complies with the requirements stated under Topical Semi-solid Preparations and with the following requirements.

Content of diethylamine salicylate, $C_{11}H_{17}NO_3$ 95.0 to 105.0% of the prescribed or stated amount.

Identification

A. To 5 g add 50 ml of 2M *sodium hydroxide*, shake well and filter. Acidify 30 ml of the filtrate with 2M *hydrochloric acid*, cool and allow to stand. The *infrared absorption spectrum* of the resulting precipitate, after recrystallisation from *water* and drying at 105°, Appendix II A, is concordant with the *reference spectrum* of salicylic acid.

B. To 5 ml of the filtrate obtained in test A, add 10 ml of *water* and 0.05 ml of *iron(III) chloride solution R1*. A deep violet colour is produced.

C. Mix 3 g with 25 ml of *chloroform* and shake with 20 ml of 0.1M *hydrochloric acid*. To the acidic layer add 10 ml of 2M *sodium hydroxide* and boil. Diethylamine, detectable by its ammoniacal odour, is produced.

Assay To a quantity containing 50 mg of Diethylamine Salicylate add 30 ml of 0.5M *sodium hydroxide* and 15 ml of *ethanol (96%)*, mix, heat under a reflux condenser for 30 minutes and cool. To the resulting mixture add 20 ml of 1M *hydrochloric acid*, mix, dilute to 250 ml with *water* and filter. Shake 15 ml of the filtrate with 25 ml of *chloroform* for 2 minutes. To 5 ml of the chloroform layer add 10 ml of *iron(III) nitrate solution* and shake for 5 minutes. Centrifuge the aqueous layer and measure the *absorbance* at the maximum at 530 nm, Appendix II B, using *iron(III) nitrate solution* in the reference cell. Calculate the content of salicylate as salicylic acid, $C_7H_6O_3$, from the *absorbance* obtained by repeating the operation using 15 ml of a 0.013% w/v solution of *salicylic acid* in 0.02M *hydrochloric acid*, beginning at the words 'Shake 15 ml...'. Each g of salicylic acid is equivalent to 1.530 g of $C_{11}H_{17}NO_3$.

Diethylstilbestrol Pessaries

Definition Diethylstilbestrol Pessaries contain Diethylstilbestrol and Propylene Glycol in a suitable basis.

The pessaries comply with the requirements stated under Vaginal Preparations and with the following requirements.

Content of diethylstilbestrol, $C_{18}H_{20}O_2$ 90.0 to 110.0% of the prescribed or stated amount.

Identification

A. The *light absorption*, Appendix II B, in the range 230 to 450 nm of the irradiated solution prepared as directed in the Assay exhibits maxima at 292 nm and 418 nm.

B. Carry out the method of extraction described under the Assay and dissolve the residue obtained in 0.2 ml of *glacial acetic acid*. Add 1 ml of *orthophosphoric acid* and heat in a water bath for 3 minutes. A deep yellow colour is produced, which almost disappears on dilution with 3 ml of *glacial acetic acid*.

Assay Weigh five pessaries, melt together by warming and allow to cool, stirring continuously. Dissolve a quantity of the mass containing 2.5 mg of Diethylstilbestrol in 25 ml of 2M *hydrochloric acid*, cool and dilute to 250 ml with *water*. Extract 50 ml with three 50-ml quantities of *chloroform*. Discard the aqueous layer and extract the combined chloroform extracts with three 15-ml quantities of 1M *sodium hydroxide*. Discard the chloroform layer and wash the combined aqueous extracts with two 10-ml quantities of *chloroform*. Adjust the pH of the aqueous layer to 9.5 with a 16% v/v solution of *orthophosphoric acid* and extract with four 20-ml quantities of *chloroform*. Filter the combined chloroform extracts through a layer of *anhydrous sodium sulphate*, wash the filter with *chloroform* and evaporate the combined chloroform extracts to dryness. Dissolve the residue in 25 ml of *absolute ethanol*, add 25 ml of a solution prepared by dissolving 1 g of *dipotassium hydrogen orthophosphate* in 55 ml of *water*, transfer a portion of the mixture to a 1-cm closed quartz cell, place the cell 10 cm from a 15-watt, short-wave ultraviolet lamp and irradiate for 10 minutes. Measure the *absorbance* of the irradiated solution at the maximum at 418 nm, Appendix II B, and calculate the content of $C_{18}H_{20}O_2$ from the *absorbance* obtained by repeating the operation using 25 ml of a 0.002% w/v solution of *diethylstilbestrol EPCRS* in *absolute ethanol* and beginning at the words 'add 25 ml of a solution...'.

Storage Diethylstilbestrol Pessaries should be stored at a temperature not exceeding 25°.

When stilboestrol pessaries are prescribed or demanded, Diethylstilbestrol Pessaries shall be dispensed or supplied.

Diethylstilbestrol Tablets

Definition Diethylstilbestrol Tablets contain Diethylstilbestrol.

The tablets comply with the requirements stated under Tablets and with the following requirements.

Content of diethylstilbestrol, $C_{18}H_{20}O_2$ 90.0 to 110.0% of the prescribed or stated amount.

Identification Extract a quantity of the powdered tablets containing 3 mg of Diethylstilbestrol with *ether*, filter and evaporate the filtrate to dryness. The residue complies with the following tests.

A. The *light absorption*, Appendix II B, in the range 230 to 350 nm of a 0.002% w/v solution in *absolute ethanol* exhibits a maximum only at 241 nm.

B. The *light absorption*, Appendix II B, in the range 230 to 450 nm of the irradiated solution prepared as directed in the Assay exhibits two maxima, at 292 nm and 418 nm.

C. Dissolve 0.5 mg in 0.2 ml of *glacial acetic acid*, add 1 ml of *orthophosphoric acid* and heat in a water bath for 3 minutes. A deep yellow colour is produced which almost disappears on dilution with 3 ml of *glacial acetic acid* (distinction from dienoestrol).

Assay Weigh and powder 20 tablets. To a quantity of the powder containing 5 mg of Diethylstilbestrol add 50 ml of *absolute ethanol*, shake for 15 minutes, add sufficient *absolute ethanol* to produce 100 ml and centrifuge. Dilute 20 ml of the clear supernatant liquid to 50 ml with *absolute ethanol* and to 25 ml of the resulting solution add 25 ml of a solution prepared by dissolving 1 g of *dipotassium hydrogen orthophosphate* in 55 ml of *water*. Transfer a portion of the mixture to a 1-cm, closed quartz cell, place the cell 10 cm from a 15-watt, short-wave, ultraviolet lamp and irradiate for 10 minutes. Measure the *absorbance* of the irradiated solution at the maximum at 418 nm, Appendix II B, and calculate the content of $C_{18}H_{20}O_2$ from the *absorbance* obtained by repeating the operation using *diethylstilbestrol EPCRS* in place of the powdered tablets.

Storage Diethylstilbestrol Tablets should be protected from light.

When stilboestrol tablets are prescribed or demanded, Diethylstilbestrol Tablets shall be dispensed or supplied.

Diflucortolone Cream

Definition Diflucortolone Cream contains Diflucortolone Valerate in a suitable non-oily basis.

The cream complies with the requirements stated under Topical Semi-solid Preparations and with the following requirements.

Content of diflucortolone valerate, $C_{27}H_{36}F_2O_5$ 90.0 to 110.0% of the prescribed or stated amount.

Identification

A. Carry out the method for *thin-layer chromatography*, Appendix III A, using a silica gel 60 F_{254} precoated plate (Merck silica gel 60 plates are suitable) and a mixture of 2 volumes of *diethylamine*, 50 volumes of *cyclohexane* and 50 volumes of *ethyl acetate* as the mobile phase. Apply separately to the plate 10 µl of each of the following solutions. For solution (1) disperse a quantity of the cream containing 1 mg of Diflucortolone Valerate in 5 ml of *dichloromethane* by heating on a water bath, shake vigorously for 15 seconds, cool in ice, filter the dispersion and use the filtrate. Solution (2) contains 0.02% w/v of *diflucortolone valerate BPCRS* in *dichloromethane*. Solution (3) contains a mixture of equal volumes of solutions (1) and (2). Develop the chromatogram twice drying the plate in air for 15 minutes between developments. After removal of the plate, allow it to dry in air for 15 minutes and examine under *ultraviolet light (254 nm)*. The principal spot in the chromatogram obtained with solution (1) corresponds to that in the chromatogram obtained with solution (2). The principal spot in the chromatogram obtained with solution (3) appears as a single compact spot.

B. In the Assay, the chromatogram obtained with solution (2) shows a peak with the same retention time as the peak due to diflucortolone valerate in the chromatogram obtained with solution (1).

Assay Carry out the method for *liquid chromatography*, Appendix III D, injecting 20 µl of each of the following solutions. For solution (1) dissolve 20 mg of *diflucortolone valerate BPCRS* in a 0.02% w/v solution of *clocortolone hexanoate BPCRS* (internal standard) in *methanol* and dilute to 200 ml with the internal standard solution. Add 30 ml of *methanol* to 10 ml of the resulting solution and dilute to 50 ml with *water*. For solution (2) add 40 ml of *methanol* to a quantity of the cream containing 1 mg of Diflucortolone Valerate, disperse by heating on a water bath at 60° for 5 minutes and shake for 30 seconds. Add 10 ml of *water*, cool in ice for 10 minutes and filter. Prepare solution (3) in the same manner as solution (2) but adding 10 ml of a 0.02% w/v solution of *clocortolone hexanoate BPCRS* in *methanol* and 30 ml of *methanol*.

The chromatographic procedure may be carried out using (a) a stainless steel column (30 cm × 3.9 mm) packed with *stationary phase C* (10 µm) (µBondapak C18 is suitable), (b) as the mobile phase with a flow rate of 2 ml per minute a mixture of 250 volumes of *water* and 750 volumes of *methanol* and (c) a detection wavelength of 254 nm.

Calculate the content of $C_{27}H_{36}F_2O_5$ in the cream using the declared content of $C_{27}H_{36}F_2O_5$ in *diflucortolone valerate BPCRS*.

Diflucortolone Oily Cream

Definition Diflucortolone Oily Cream contains Diflucortolone Valerate in a suitable oily basis.

The cream complies with the requirements stated under Topical Semi-solid Preparations and with the following requirements.

Content of diflucortolone valerate, $C_{27}H_{36}F_2O_5$ 90.0 to 110.0% of the prescribed or stated amount.

Identification

A. Carry out the method for *thin-layer chromatography*, Appendix III A, using a silica gel 60 F_{254} precoated plate (Merck silica gel 60 plates are suitable) and a mixture of 2 volumes of *diethylamine*, 50 volumes of *cyclohexane* and 50 volumes of *ethyl acetate* as the mobile phase. Apply separately to the plate 20 µl of each of the following solutions. For solution (1) disperse a quantity of the cream containing 1 mg of Diflucortolone Valerate in 10 ml of *dichloromethane* by heating on a water bath, shake vigorously for 1 minute, cool in ice, filter the dispersion and use the filtrate. Solution (2) contains 0.01% w/v of *diflucortolone valerate BPCRS* in *dichloromethane*. Solution (3) contains a mixture of equal volumes of solutions (1) and (2). Develop the chromatogram twice drying the plate in air for 15 minutes between developments. After removal of the plate, allow it to dry in air for 15 minutes and examine under *ultraviolet light (254 nm)*. The principal spot in the chromatogram obtained with solution (1) corresponds to that in the chromatogram obtained with solution (2). The principal spot in the chromatogram obtained with solution (3) appears as a single compact spot.

B. In the Assay, the chromatogram obtained with solution (2) shows a peak with the same retention time as the peak due to diflucortolone valerate in the chromatogram obtained with solution (1).

Assay Carry out the method for *liquid chromatography*, Appendix III D, injecting 20 µl of each of the following solutions. For solution (1) dissolve 20 mg of *diflucortolone valerate BPCRS* in a 0.02% w/v solution of *clocortolone hexanoate BPCRS* (internal standard) in *methanol* and dilute to 200 ml with the internal standard solution. Add 30 ml of *methanol* to 10 ml of the resulting solution and dilute to 50 ml with *water*. For solution (2) add 40 ml of *methanol* to a quantity of the cream containing 1 mg of Diflucortolone Valerate, disperse by heating on a water bath at 60° for 5 minutes and shake for 30 seconds. Add 10 ml of *water*, cool in ice for 10 minutes and filter. Prepare solution (3) in the same manner as solution (2) but adding 10 ml of a 0.02% w/v solution of *clocortolone hexanoate BPCRS* in *methanol* and 30 ml of *methanol*.

The chromatographic procedure described under Diflucortolone Cream may be used.

Calculate the content of $C_{27}H_{36}F_2O_5$ in the cream using the declared content of $C_{27}H_{36}F_2O_5$ in *diflucortolone valerate BPCRS*.

Diflucortolone Ointment

Definition Diflucortolone Ointment contains Diflucortolone Valerate in a suitable basis.

The ointment complies with the requirements stated under Topical Semi-solid Preparations and with the following requirements.

Content of diflucortolone valerate, $C_{27}H_{36}F_2O_5$ 90.0 to 110.0% of the prescribed or stated amount.

Identification

A. Carry out the method for *thin-layer chromatography*, Appendix III A, using a silica gel 60 F_{254} precoated plate (Merck silica gel 60 plates are suitable) and a mixture of 2 volumes of *diethylamine*, 50 volumes of *cyclohexane* and 50 volumes of *ethyl acetate* as the mobile phase. Apply separately to the plate 10 µl of each of the following solutions. For solution (1) disperse a quantity of the ointment containing 1 mg of Diflucortolone Valerate in 5 ml of *dichloromethane* by heating on a water bath, shake vigorously for 15 seconds, cool in ice, filter the dispersion and use the filtrate. Solution (2) contains 0.02% w/v of *diflucortolone valerate BPCRS* in *dichloromethane*. Solution (3) contains a mixture of equal volumes of solutions (1) and (2). Develop the chromatogram twice, drying the plate in air for 15 minutes between developments. After removal of the plate, allow it to dry in air for 15 minutes and examine under *ultraviolet light (254 nm)*. The principal spot in the chromatogram obtained with solution (1) corresponds to that in the chromatogram obtained with solution (2). The principal spot in the chromatogram obtained with solution (3) appears as a single compact spot.

B. In the Assay, the chromatogram obtained with solution (2) shows a peak with the same retention time as the peak due to diflucortolone valerate in the chromatogram obtained with solution (1).

Assay Carry out the method for *liquid chromatography*, Appendix III D, injecting 20 µl of each of the following solutions. For solution (1) dissolve 20 mg of *diflucortolone valerate BPCRS* in a 0.02% w/v solution of *clocortolone hexanoate BPCRS* (internal standard) in *methanol* and dilute to 200 ml with the internal standard solution. Add 30 ml of *methanol* to 10 ml of the resulting solution and dilute to 50 ml with *water*. For solution (2) shake a quantity of the ointment containing 1 mg of Diflucortolone Valerate with 10 ml of a 0.02% w/v solution of *clocortolone hexanoate BPCRS* in *methanol* and add 30 ml of *methanol*. Disperse by heating on a water bath at 60° for 5 minutes and shake for 30 seconds. Add 10 ml of *water*, cool in ice for 10 minutes and filter.

The chromatographic procedure described under Diflucortolone Cream may be used.

Calculate the content of $C_{27}H_{36}F_2O_5$ in the ointment using the declared content of $C_{27}H_{36}F_2O_5$ in *diflucortolone valerate BPCRS*.

Diflunisal Tablets

Definition Diflunisal Tablets contain Diflunisal. They are coated.

With the exception of the requirements for shape, the tablets comply with the requirements stated under Tablets and with the following requirements.

Content of diflunisal, $C_{13}H_8F_2O_3$ 95.0 to 105.0% of the prescribed or stated amount.

Identification Shake a quantity of the powdered tablets containing 0.5 g of Diflunisal with 20 ml of *ether* for 15 minutes, filter and evaporate the filtrate to dryness. The residue complies with the following tests.

A. The *infrared absorption spectrum*, Appendix II A, is concordant with the *reference spectrum* of diflunisal (form B).

B. The *light absorption*, Appendix II B, in the range 230 to 350 nm of a 0.002% w/v solution in 0.1M *methanolic hydrochloric acid* exhibits two maxima, at 251 nm and 315 nm.

C. Dissolve 2 mg in 10 ml of *ethanol (96%)* and add 0.1 ml of *iron(III) chloride solution*. A deep purple colour is produced.

Dissolution Comply with the *dissolution test for tablets and capsules*, Appendix XII D, using Apparatus II. Use as the medium 900 ml of a pH 7.2 buffer prepared as described below and rotate the paddle at 50 revolutions per minute. For the dissolution medium, dissolve 121 g of *tris(hydroxymethyl)methylamine* in 9 litres of *water*, adjust the pH to 7.45 at 25° with a 7.0% w/v solution of *anhydrous citric* acid, add sufficient *water* to produce 10 litres, allow to equilibrate at 37° and adjust the pH to 7.2 if necessary. Withdraw a sample of 20 ml of the medium and filter. Measure the *absorbance* of the filtrate, Appendix II B, diluted with the dissolution medium if necessary, at the maximum at 306 nm using dissolution medium in the reference cell. Calculate the total content of diflunisal, $C_{13}H_8F_2O_3$, in the medium taking 118 as the value of A(1%, 1 cm) at the maximum at 306 nm.

Related substances

A. Carry out the method for *thin-layer chromatography*, Appendix III A, using a silica gel F_{254} precoated plate

(Merck silica gel 60 F_{254} plates are suitable) and a mixture of 10 volumes of *glacial acetic acid*, 20 volumes of *acetone* and 70 volumes of *carbon tetrachloride* as the mobile phase. Apply separately to the plate 5 µl of each of the following solutions. Solution (1) contains 2.0% w/v of the residue obtained in the tests for Identification in *methanol*. Solution (2) contains 0.0030% w/v of *4-hydroxybiphenyl* in *methanol*. After removal of the plate, allow it to dry in a current of warm air and examine under *ultraviolet light (254 nm)*. Any *secondary spot* in the chromatogram obtained with solution (1) is not more intense than the spot in the chromatogram obtained with solution (2) (0.15%).

B. Carry out the method for *liquid chromatography*, Appendix III D, using the following solutions in a mixture of 4 volumes of *acetonitrile* and 1 volume of *water*. Solution (1) contains 0.00055% w/v of *fluoranthene* (internal standard). Solution (2) contains 0.50% w/v of the residue obtained in the tests for Identification and 0.00055% w/v of the internal standard.

The chromatographic procedure may be carried out using (a) a stainless steel column (30 cm × 4 mm) packed with *stationary phase C* (10 µm) (µBondapak C18 is suitable), (b) a mixture of 2 volumes of *glacial acetic acid*, 25 volumes of *methanol*, 55 volumes of *water* and 70 volumes of *acetonitrile* as the mobile phase with a flow rate of 2 ml per minute and (c) a detection wavelength of 254 nm.

In the chromatogram obtained with solution (2) the sum of the areas of any peaks with retention times greater than that of the internal standard is not greater than the area of the peak due to the internal standard.

Assay Weigh and powder 20 tablets. Shake a quantity of the powdered tablets containing 0.25 g of Diflunisal with 100 ml of 0.1M *methanolic hydrochloric acid* for 15 minutes, dilute to 250 ml with 0.1M *methanolic hydrochloric acid* and filter through a glass fibre filter (Whatman GF4 is suitable). Dilute 5 ml of the filtrate to 100 ml with 0.1M *methanolic hydrochloric acid* and measure the *absorbance* of the resulting solution at the maximum at 315 nm, Appendix II B. Calculate the content of $C_{13}H_8F_2O_3$ taking 130 as the value of A(1%, 1 cm) at the maximum at 315 nm.

Digitoxin Tablets

Definition Digitoxin Tablets contain Digitoxin.

The tablets comply with the requirements stated under Tablets and with the following requirements.

Content of digitoxin, $C_{41}H_{64}O_{13}$ 90.0 to 110.0% of the prescribed or stated amount.

Identification To a quantity of the powdered tablets containing 0.25 mg of Digitoxin add 1 ml of *glacial acetic acid* containing 0.01% w/v of *iron(III) chloride*, shake for a few minutes, filter through sintered glass and cautiously add 1 ml of *sulphuric acid* to the filtrate without mixing. A brown ring free from red colour is produced at the interface and, after a short time, an indigo colour is produced in the upper layer.

Uniformity of content Tablets containing less than 2 mg of Digitoxin comply with the requirements stated under Tablets using the following method of analysis. Shake one tablet with 15 ml of *methanol (50%)* for 30 minutes and dilute to 25 ml with the same solvent. Filter through a suitable membrane filter disc having an average pore diameter not greater than 0.8 µm, discarding the first few ml of the filtrate, and transfer 1 ml to a 10-ml graduated flask. Add 3 ml of a 0.1% w/v solution of *L-ascorbic acid* in *methanol* and 0.2 ml of a 0.009M solution of hydrogen peroxide prepared by accurately diluting *hydrogen peroxide solution (100 vol)* that has been standardised by titration with 0.02M *potassium permanganate VS*, mix and dilute to volume with *hydrochloric acid*. After exactly 30 minutes measure the *fluorescence* of the solution, Appendix II E, using an excitation wavelength of 400 nm and an emission wavelength of 570 nm and setting the instrument to zero with *water*. Calculate the content of digitoxin, $C_{41}H_{64}O_{13}$, from the *fluorescence* obtained by carrying out the operation at the same time using a 0.0004% w/v solution of *digitoxin EPCRS* in *methanol (50%)* and beginning at the words 'transfer 1 ml...'.

Assay Weigh and finely powder 20 tablets. To a quantity of the powder containing 1.25 mg of Digitoxin add 3 ml of *water*, swirl to disperse the powder and allow to stand for 10 minutes, swirling occasionally. Add 25 ml of *glacial acetic acid*, shake for 1 hour and filter (Whatman No. 1 paper is suitable), discarding the first few ml of filtrate. To 4 ml of the filtrate add 1 ml of *dimethyl sulphoxide*, dilute to 25 ml with *xanthydrol reagent*, mix well and allow to stand in the dark for 4.5 hours (solution A). At the same time prepare two further solutions in the same manner but using for solution B 4 ml of *digitoxin standard solution* and for solution C 4 ml of a mixture of 25 volumes of *glacial acetic acid* and 3 volumes of *water* and beginning at the words 'add 1 ml of *dimethyl sulphoxide*...'. Measure the *absorbances* of solutions A and B at the maximum at 550 nm, Appendix II B, using solution C in the reference cell.

Digoxin Injection

Definition

Digoxin	25 mg
Ethanol (80 per cent)	12.5 ml
Propylene Glycol	40 ml
Citric Acid Monohydrate	75 mg
Disodium Hydrogen Phosphate Dodecahydrate	0.45 g
Water for Injections	sufficient to produce 100 ml

Extemporaneous preparation The following directions apply.

Dissolve the Digoxin in the Ethanol (80 per cent) and add the Propylene Glycol, a solution of the Citric Acid Monohydrate and the Disodium Hydrogen Phosphate Dodecahydrate in Water for Injections and sufficient Water for Injections to produce 100 ml. Sterilise by *heating in an autoclave*.

The injection complies with the requirements stated under Parenteral Preparations and with the following requirements.

Content of digoxin, $C_{41}H_{64}O_{14}$ 0.0225 to 0.0275% w/v.

Identification Evaporate 2 ml to dryness, dissolve the residue in 1 ml of *glacial acetic acid* containing 0.01% w/v of *iron(III) chloride* and cautiously add 1 ml of *sulphuric acid* without mixing. A brown ring, free from red colour, is produced at the interface and, after a short time, an indigo colour is produced in the upper layer.

Acidity or alkalinity pH, 6.7 to 7.3, Appendix V L.

Assay Transfer 20 ml to a separating funnel containing 10 ml of *water*. Make alkaline with 5M *ammonia* and extract with four 25-ml quantities of *chloroform*. Wash each extract with the same 10 ml of *water*. Evaporate the combined chloroform extracts to dryness on a water bath, dry the residue at 105° for 15 minutes, cool, dissolve the residue in 5 ml of a mixture of 65 volumes of *chloroform* and 35 volumes of *methanol* and add 20 ml of *glacial acetic acid* (solution A). To 5 ml of a 0.2% w/v solution of *digoxin EPCRS* in *glacial acetic acid* add 10 ml of a mixture of 65 volumes of *chloroform* and 35 volumes of *methanol* and sufficient *glacial acetic acid* to produce 50 ml (solution B). Dilute 5 ml of solution A to 25 ml with *digoxin reagent*, mix, allow to stand for 1 hour and measure the *absorbance* of the resulting solution at 590 nm, Appendix II B, using *water* in the reference cell. Calculate the content of $C_{41}H_{64}O_{14}$ from the *absorbance* obtained by treating 5 ml of solution B at the same time and in the same manner.

Storage Digoxin Injection should be protected from light.

Paediatric Digoxin Injection

Definition

Digoxin	10 mg
Ethanol (80 per cent)	12.5 ml
Propylene Glycol	40 ml
Citric Acid Monohydrate	75 mg
Disodium Hydrogen Phosphate Dodecahydrate	0.45 g
Water for Injections	sufficient to produce 100 ml

Extemporaneous preparation The following directions apply.

Dissolve the Digoxin in the Ethanol (80 per cent) and add the Propylene Glycol, a solution of the Citric Acid Monohydrate and the Disodium Hydrogen Phosphate Dodecahydrate in Water for Injections and sufficient Water for Injections to produce 100 ml. Sterilise by *heating in an autoclave*.

The injection complies with the requirements stated under Parenteral Preparations and with the following requirements.

Content of digoxin, $C_{41}H_{64}O_{14}$ 0.0090 to 0.0110% w/v.

Identification Evaporate 5 ml to dryness, dissolve the residue in 1 ml of *glacial acetic acid* containing 0.01% w/v of *iron(III) chloride* and cautiously add 1 ml of *sulphuric acid* without mixing. A brown ring, free from red colour, is produced at the interface and, after a short time, an indigo colour is produced in the upper layer.

Acidity or alkalinity pH, 6.7 to 7.3, Appendix V L.

Assay Carry out the Assay described under Digoxin Injection, using 50 ml.

Storage Paediatric Digoxin Injection should be protected from light.

Paediatric Digoxin Oral Solution

Definition Paediatric Digoxin Oral Solution is a solution containing 0.005% w/v of Digoxin in a suitable flavoured vehicle.

Paediatric Digoxin Oral Solution should not be diluted.

The oral solution complies with the requirements stated under Oral Liquids and with the following requirements.

Content of digoxin, $C_{41}H_{64}O_{14}$ 0.0045 to 0.0055% w/v.

Identification Extract 5 ml with four 20-ml quantities of *chloroform*, washing each extract with the same 10 ml of *water*, evaporate the combined extracts to dryness and dissolve the residue in 1 ml of *glacial acetic acid* containing 0.01% w/v of *iron(III) chloride hexahydrate*. Cautiously add 1 ml of *sulphuric acid* without mixing. A brown ring, free from red colour, is produced at the interface and, after a short time, an indigo colour is produced in the upper layer.

Acidity or alkalinity pH, 6.8 to 7.2, Appendix V L.

Assay Extract 100 ml with four 25-ml quantities of *chloroform*, washing each extract with the same 5 ml of *water*, and evaporate the combined extracts to dryness. To the residue add 3 ml of *absolute ethanol* and carefully evaporate to dryness on a water bath with the aid of a gentle current of air. Repeat the evaporation using a further 3 ml of *absolute ethanol* and cool. Dissolve the residue in 5 ml of a mixture of 65 volumes of *chloroform* and 35 volumes of *methanol*, add 20 ml of *glacial acetic acid* and filter if necessary. Dilute 5 ml of the filtrate to 25 ml with *digoxin reagent*, allow to stand for 2 hours and measure the *absorbance* of the resulting solution at the maximum at 590 nm, Appendix II B. Calculate the content of $C_{41}H_{64}O_{14}$ from the *absorbance* obtained by carrying out the operation at the same time but using a solution prepared by mixing 5 ml of a 0.2% w/v solution of *digoxin EPCRS* in *glacial acetic acid* with 10 ml of a mixture of 65 volumes of *chloroform* and 35 volumes of *methanol* and adding sufficient *glacial acetic acid* to produce 50 ml, beginning at the words 'Dilute 5 ml of the filtrate...' and using *water* in the reference cell.

Storage Paediatric Digoxin Oral Solution should be protected from light and stored at a temperature not exceeding 25°.

Digoxin Tablets

Definition Digoxin Tablets contain Digoxin.

The tablets comply with the requirements stated under Tablets and with the following requirements.

Content of digoxin, $C_{41}H_{64}O_{14}$ 90.0 to 110.0% of the prescribed or stated amount.

Identification To a quantity of the powdered tablets containing 0.25 mg of Digoxin, add 1 ml of *glacial acetic acid* containing 0.01% w/v of *iron(III) chloride hexahydrate*, shake for a few minutes, filter through sintered glass and cautiously add 1 ml of *sulphuric acid* without mixing. A brown ring, free from red colour, is produced at the interface and, after a short time, an indigo colour is produced in the upper layer.

Dissolution Carry out the *dissolution test for tablets and capsules*, Appendix XII D, placing six tablets in the basket, using as the medium 600 ml of *water* freshly prepared by distillation and rotating the basket at 120 revolutions per minute for 60 minutes. Withdraw a sample of 5 ml of the medium. Filter the sample through a membrane filter disc with a nominal pore size not greater than 0.8 µm, discarding the first 1 ml of the filtrate, and transfer 1 ml to a 10-ml graduated flask. Add 3 ml of a 0.1% w/v solution of *L-ascorbic acid* in *methanol* and 0.2 ml of a 0.009M solution of hydrogen peroxide, prepared by accurately diluting *hydrogen peroxide solution (100 vol)* that has been standardised by titration with 0.02M *potassium permanganate VS*, mix and dilute to volume with *hydrochloric acid*. After exactly 2 hours measure the *fluorescence* of the solution, Appendix II E, using an excitation wavelength of 360 nm and an emission wavelength of 490 nm and setting the instrument to zero with *water* and to 100 with a solution prepared at the same time as the test solution in the following manner. Dilute 2.5 ml of a 0.100% w/v solution of *digoxin EPCRS* in *ethanol (80%)* to 100 ml with *water*, dilute the resulting solution further with *water* to produce a solution containing in 1 ml an amount of digoxin equal to one hundredth of the strength of the tablets being examined, transfer 1 ml of the solution to a 10-ml graduated flask and carry out the operation described above, beginning at the words 'Add 3 ml... '. The amount of digoxin, $C_{41}H_{64}O_{14}$, per tablet in solution is not less than 75% of the prescribed or stated amount.

Uniformity of content Tablets containing less than 2 mg of Digoxin comply with the requirements stated under Tablets using the following method of analysis. For tablets containing 0.125 mg of Digoxin, place one tablet in 5 ml of *water* at 37°, agitate to disintegrate, add 28 ml of *ethanol (96%)*, shake for 1 hour and add sufficient *ethanol (80%)* to produce 50 ml. For tablets containing more or less than 0.125 mg of Digoxin carry out the same procedure but using correspondingly greater or smaller quantities of *water*, *ethanol (96%)* and *ethanol (80%)*. Filter the resulting solution through a suitable membrane filter disc with a nominal pore size not greater than 0.8 µm, discarding the first few ml of the filtrate, and transfer 1.0 ml to a 10-ml graduated flask. Add 3 ml of a 0.1% w/v solution of *L-ascorbic acid* in *methanol*, 0.2 ml of a 0.009M solution of hydrogen peroxide prepared by accurately diluting *hydrogen peroxide solution (100 vol)* that has been standardised by titration with 0.02M *potassium permanganate VS*, mix and dilute to volume with *hydrochloric acid*. After exactly 2 hours measure the *fluorescence* of the solution, Appendix II E, using an excitation wavelength of 360 nm and an emission wavelength of 490 nm and setting the instrument to zero with *water*. Calculate the content of digoxin, $C_{41}H_{64}O_{14}$, from the *fluorescence* obtained by carrying out the operation at the same time using a solution containing 2.5 µg per ml of *digoxin EPCRS* in *ethanol (80%)* and beginning at the words 'transfer 1.0 ml...'.

Assay Weigh and finely powder 20 tablets. To a quantity of the powder containing 1.25 mg of Digoxin add 3 ml of *water*, swirl to disperse the powder and allow to stand for 10 minutes swirling occasionally. Add 25 ml of *glacial acetic acid*, shake for 1 hour and filter (Whatman No. 1 paper is suitable), discarding the first few ml. To 4 ml of the filtrate add 1 ml of *dimethyl sulphoxide*, dilute to 25 ml with *xanthydrol reagent*, mix well and allow to stand in the dark for 4 hours (solution A). At the same time prepare two further solutions in the same manner but using for solution B 4 ml of *digoxin standard solution* and for solution C 4 ml of a mixture of 25 volumes of *glacial acetic acid* and 3 volumes of *water* and beginning at the words 'add 1 ml of *dimethyl sulphoxide*...'. Measure the *absorbances* of solutions A and B at the maximum at 545 nm, Appendix II B, using solution C in the reference cell.

Dihydrocodeine Injection

Definition Dihydrocodeine Injection is a sterile solution of Dihydrocodeine Tartrate in Water for Injections.

The injection complies with the requirements stated under Parenteral Preparations and with the following requirements.

Content of dihydrocodeine tartrate, $C_{18}H_{23}NO_3,C_4H_6O_6$ 90.0 to 110.0% of the prescribed or stated amount.

Identification

A. Add 0.05 ml to a mixture of 5 ml of *sulphuric acid* and 0.05 ml of *formaldehyde solution*. A purple colour is produced (distinction from pholcodine).

B. To a volume containing 10 mg of Dihydrocodeine Tartrate add 0.05 ml of *nitric acid*. A yellow but no red colour is produced (distinction from morphine).

C. Evaporate a volume containing 0.1 g of Dihydrocodeine Tartrate to dryness on a water bath. Dissolve the residue in 1 ml of *sulphuric acid*, add 0.05 ml of *iron(III) chloride solution R1* and warm gently. A brownish yellow colour is produced which does not become red on the addition of 0.05 ml of 2M *nitric acid* (distinction from codeine and morphine).

D. Yields reaction B characteristic of *tartrates*, Appendix VI.

Acidity pH, 3.0 to 4.5, Appendix V L.

Assay Dilute a volume containing 50 mg of Dihydrocodeine Tartrate to 500 ml with *water* and measure the *absorbance* of the resulting solution at the maximum at 284 nm, Appendix II B. Calculate the content of $C_{18}H_{23}NO_3,C_4H_6O_6$ taking 35.7 as the value of A(1%, 1 cm) at the maximum at 284 nm.

Storage Dihydrocodeine Injection should be protected from light.

Dihydrocodeine Oral Solution

Definition Dihydrocodeine Oral Solution is a solution of Dihydrocodeine Tartrate in a suitable flavoured vehicle.

The oral solution complies with the requirements stated under Oral Liquids and with the following requirements.

Content of dihydrocodeine tartrate, $C_{18}H_{23}NO_3,C_4H_6O_6$ 95.0 to 105.0% of the prescribed or stated amount.

Identification To a volume of the oral solution containing 20 mg of Dihydrocodeine Tartrate add 10 ml of *water* and extract with two 25-ml quantities of *chloroform*. Discard the chloroform extracts, add 3 ml of 5M *sodium hydroxide* to the aqueous layer, mix and extract with 25 ml of *chloroform*. Wash the chloroform layer with 10 ml of *water*, shake with *anhydrous sodium sulphate* and filter. Wash the filter with *chloroform* and evaporate the combined filtrate and washings to dryness. Dissolve the residue in 1 ml of *dichloromethane* and apply 0.2 ml dropwise on to the surface of a disc prepared using 0.3 g of *potassium bromide*, allowing the solvent to evaporate between applications, and dry the disc at 50° for 2 minutes. The *infrared absorption spectrum*, Appendix II A, is concordant with the *reference spectrum* of dihydrocodeine.

Related substances Carry out the method for *thin-layer chromatography*, Appendix III A, using *silica gel GF_{254}* as the coating substance and a mixture of 90 volumes of *dichloromethane*, 10 volumes of *methanol* and 1 volume of 13.5M *ammonia* as the mobile phase. Apply separately to the plate 20 µl of each of solutions (1), (2), (3) and (4) and 40 µl of solution (5). For solution (1) add 10 ml of *water* and 3 ml of 5M *sodium hydroxide* to a quantity of the oral solution containing 20 mg of Dihydrocodeine Tartrate, mix, extract with two 30-ml quantities of *chloroform* and wash each extract successively with the same 10 ml of *water*. Filter each extract in turn through *anhydrous sodium sulphate* on a plug of absorbent cotton moistened with *chloroform*, wash the filter with *chloroform*, evaporate the combined filtrate and washings to dryness and dissolve the residue in 2 ml of *methanol*. For solution (2) dilute 1 volume of solution (1) to 100 volumes with *methanol*. For solution (3) dilute 1 volume of solution (2) to 2 volumes with *methanol*. Solution (4) contains 0.0050% w/v of *codeine phosphate BPCRS* in *methanol*. Solution (5) is a mixture of equal volumes of solution (1) and solution (4). After removal of the plate, allow it to dry in air and spray with *dilute potassium iodobismuthate solution*. Any spot in the chromatogram obtained with solution (1) corresponding to the spot due to codeine in the chromatogram obtained with solution (5) is not more intense than the spot in the chromatogram obtained with solution (4). Any other *secondary spot* in the chromatogram obtained with solution (1) is not more intense than the spot in the chromatogram obtained with solution (2) and not more than one such spot is more intense than the spot in the chromatogram obtained with solution (3). The method is not valid unless, in the chromatogram obtained with solution (5), the spot due to codeine is clearly separated from the principal spot.

Assay Carry out the method for *liquid chromatography*, Appendix III D, using the following solutions. Solution (1) contains 0.04% w/v of *dihydrocodeine tartrate BPCRS* in *water*. For solution (2) disperse a weighed quantity of the oral solution containing 10 mg of Dihydrocodeine Tartrate in *water*, dilute to 25 ml with *water* and mix.

The chromatographic procedure may be carried out using (a) a stainless steel column (10 cm × 4.6 mm) packed with *stationary phase C* (5 µm) (Nucleosil C18 is suitable), (b) as the mobile phase with a flow rate of 2 ml per minute, 0.01M *sodium acetate* and 0.005M *dioctyl sodium sulphosuccinate* in a mixture of 60 volumes of *methanol* and 40 volumes of *water*, the pH of the mixture being adjusted to 5.5 with *glacial acetic acid*, and (c) a detection wavelength of 284 nm.

Determine the *weight per ml* of the oral solution, Appendix V G, and calculate the content of $C_{18}H_{23}NO_3$,$C_4H_6O_6$, weight in volume, using the declared content of $C_{18}H_{23}NO_3$,$C_4H_6O_6$ in *dihydrocodeine tartrate BPCRS*.

Storage Dihydrocodeine Oral Solution should be protected from light and stored at a temperature not exceeding 25°.

Dihydrocodeine Tablets

Definition Dihydrocodeine Tablets contain Dihydrocodeine Tartrate.

The tablets comply with the requirements stated under Tablets and with the following requirements.

Content of dihydrocodeine tartrate, $C_{18}H_{23}NO_3$, $C_4H_6O_6$ 92.5 to 107.5% of the prescribed or stated amount.

Identification Shake a quantity of the powdered tablets containing 0.15 g of Dihydrocodeine Tartrate with 50 ml of *water*, filter and evaporate the filtrate to dryness on a water bath. The residue complies with the following tests.

A. Add 10 mg, in powder, to 1 ml of a mixture of *sulphuric acid* and 0.05 ml of *formaldehyde solution*. A purple colour is produced (distinction from pholcodine).

B. Dissolve 10 mg in 0.05 ml of *nitric acid*. A yellow but no red colour is produced (distinction from morphine).

C. Dissolve 0.1 g in 1 ml of *sulphuric acid*, add 0.05 ml of *iron(III) chloride solution R1* and warm gently. A brownish yellow colour is produced which does not become red on the addition of 0.05 ml of 2M *nitric acid* (distinction from codeine and morphine).

Assay Weigh and powder 20 tablets. Dissolve a quantity of the powder containing 0.15 g of Dihydrocodeine Tartrate as completely as possible in 30 ml of *water*, make alkaline with 5M *ammonia* and extract with five 20-ml quantities of *chloroform*, washing each extract with the same 10 ml of *water*. Filter the combined extracts through absorbent cotton moistened with *chloroform* and wash the filter with a small quantity of *chloroform*. Evaporate on a water bath until the volume is reduced to about 50 ml and titrate with 0.02M *perchloric acid VS* using *crystal violet solution* as indicator. Each ml of 0.02M *perchloric acid VS* is equivalent to 9.030 mg of $C_{18}H_{23}NO_3$,$C_4H_6O_6$.

Storage Dihydrocodeine Tablets should be protected from light.

Diloxanide Tablets

Definition Diloxanide Tablets contain Diloxanide Furoate.

The tablets comply with the requirements stated under Tablets and with the following requirements.

Content of diloxanide furoate, $C_{14}H_{11}Cl_2NO_4$ 95.0 to 105.0% of the prescribed or stated amount.

Identification Extract a quantity of the powdered tablets containing 0.2 g of Diloxanide Furoate with 20 ml of *chloroform*, filter and evaporate the filtrate to dryness. The dried residue complies with the following tests.

A. The *infrared absorption spectrum*, Appendix II A, is concordant with the *reference spectrum* of diloxanide furoate.

B. Burn 20 mg by the method for *oxygen-flask combustion*, Appendix VIII C, using 10 ml of 1M *sodium hydroxide* as the absorbing liquid. When the process is complete acidify the liquid with *nitric acid* and add *silver nitrate solution*. A white precipitate is produced.

C. *Melting point*, about 115°, Appendix V A.

Related substances Carry out the method for *thin-layer chromatography*, Appendix III A, using *silica gel HF_{254}* as the coating substance and a mixture of 96 volumes of *dichloromethane* and 4 volumes of *methanol* as the mobile phase. Apply separately to the plate 5 µl of each of the following solutions. For solution (1) shake a quantity of the powdered tablets containing 0.5 g of Diloxanide Furoate with 5 ml of *chloroform*, centrifuge and use the supernatant liquid. For solution (2) dilute 1 volume of solution (1) to 400 volumes with *chloroform*. After removal of the plate, allow it to dry in air and examine under *ultraviolet light (254 nm)*. Any *secondary spot* in the chromatogram obtained with solution (1) is not more intense than the spot in the chromatogram obtained with solution (2).

Assay Weigh and powder 20 tablets. Shake a quantity of the powder containing 40 mg of Diloxanide Furoate with 150 ml of *ethanol (96%)* for 30 minutes, add sufficient *ethanol (96%)* to produce 200 ml, mix and filter. Dilute 10 ml of the filtrate to 250 ml with *ethanol (96%)* and measure the *absorbance* of the resulting solution at the maximum at 258 nm, Appendix II B. Calculate the content of $C_{14}H_{11}Cl_2NO_4$ taking 705 as the value of A(1%, 1 cm) at the maximum at 258 nm.

Storage Diloxanide Tablets should be protected from light.

Dimenhydrinate Tablets

Definition Dimenhydrinate Tablets contain Dimenhydrinate.

The tablets comply with the requirements stated under Tablets and with the following requirements.

Content of dimenhydrinate, $C_{17}H_{21}NO,C_7H_7ClN_4O_2$ 95.0 to 105.0% of the prescribed or stated amount.

Identification Shake a quantity of the powdered tablets containing 0.1 g of Dimenhydrinate with 10 ml of a mixture of equal volumes of *chloroform* and *ether* for 5 minutes, filter and evaporate the filtrate to an oily residue on a water bath. Add 3 ml of *ether* to the residue and scratch the interface between the residue and the ether gently with a glass rod until crystals appear in the liquid. Transfer the suspension of crystalline material in ether to a watch glass, allow the solvent to evaporate in a current of air and dry the residue at 60°. The *infrared absorption spectrum* of the residue, Appendix II A, is concordant with the *reference spectrum* of dimenhydrinate.

Theophylline and substances related to diphenhydramine Carry out the method for *thin-layer chromatography*, Appendix III A, using *silica gel GF_{254}* as the coating substance and a mixture of 1 volume of 13.5M *ammonia*, 9 volumes of *methanol* and 90 volumes of *dichloromethane* as the mobile phase. Apply separately to the plate 10 µl of each of the following solutions. For solution (1) shake a quantity of the powdered tablets containing 0.1 g of Dimenhydrinate with three 10-ml quantities of *chloroform*, filter, evaporate the combined filtrates almost to dryness and dissolve the residue in 5 ml of *chloroform*. For solution (2) dilute 1 volume of solution (1) to 100 volumes with *chloroform*. Solution (3) contains 0.010% w/v of *theophylline* in *chloroform*. After removal of the plate, dry it in a current of cold air and examine under *ultraviolet light (254 nm)*. Any spot corresponding to theophylline in the chromatogram obtained with solution (1) is not more intense than the spot in the chromatogram obtained with solution (3) (0.5%). Spray the plate with *potassium iodobismuthate solution*, allow it to dry in air and spray with *hydrogen peroxide solution (10 vol)*. Any *secondary spot* in the chromatogram obtained with solution (1) is not more intense than the spot in the chromatogram obtained with solution (2) (1%). Disregard any spot extending from the line of application to an Rf value of about 0.1.

Assay Weigh and powder 20 tablets. Dissolve a quantity of the powder containing 0.1 g of Dimenhydrinate as completely as possible in 20 ml of *water*, add 10 ml of 5M *ammonia*, mix, extract with successive quantities of 15, 15, 15, 10 and 10 ml of *ether* and wash the combined extracts with 10 ml of *water*. Evaporate the ether, warm the residue with 10 ml of *ethanol (96%)* until dissolved, cool, add 50 ml of 0.01M *hydrochloric acid VS* and titrate the excess of acid with 0.01M *sodium hydroxide VS* using *methyl red mixed solution* as indicator. Each ml of 0.01M *hydrochloric acid VS* is equivalent to 4.700 mg of $C_{17}H_{21}NO,C_7H_7ClN_4O_2$.

Dimercaprol Injection

Definition

Dimercaprol	5 g
Benzyl Benzoate	9.6 ml
Arachis Oil	sufficient to produce 100 ml

Extemporaneous preparation The following directions apply.

Dissolve the Dimercaprol in the Benzyl Benzoate and add sufficient Arachis Oil to produce 100 ml. Add sufficient of a 35% v/v solution of Strong Ammonia Solution in Ethanol (96 per cent) until the acidity, when determined by the method described below, corresponds to a pH of 6.8 to 7.0. Add about 0.2 g of Activated Charcoal, stir, allow to stand for not less than 1 hour and filter. Distribute the solution in ampoules, the air in which is replaced by nitrogen or other suitable gas and seal immediately. Sterilise by *dry heat* at a minimum of 150° for not less than 1 hour.

The injection complies with the requirements stated under Parenteral Preparations and with the following requirements.

Content of dimercaprol, $C_3H_8OS_2$ 4.75 to 5.25% w/v.

Characteristics A bright, pale yellow solution.

Acidity Shake with an equal volume of *water* for 2 minutes and allow to separate. The pH of the aqueous layer, after filtration through neutral filter paper, is 4.5 to 6.5, Appendix V L.

Refractive index 1.482 to 1.486, Appendix V E.

Weight per ml 0.940 to 0.955 g, Appendix V G.

Assay To 1 g add 20 ml of 0.1M *hydrochloric acid* and titrate with 0.05M *iodine VS*. Each ml of 0.05M *iodine VS* is equivalent to 6.21 mg of $C_3H_8OS_2$. Use the *weight per ml* of the injection to calculate the percentage w/v of $C_3H_8OS_2$.

Storage Dimercaprol Injection should be protected from light.

Labelling The label states (1) the nature of the solvent; (2) that the preparation is intended for intramuscular injection only.

Dinoprost Injection

Definition Dinoprost Injection is a sterile solution of Dinoprost Trometamol in Water for Injections.

The injection complies with the requirements stated under Parenteral Preparations and with the following requirements.

Content of dinoprost, $C_{20}H_{34}O_5$ 90.0 to 105.0% of the prescribed or stated amount.

Characteristics A colourless or almost colourless solution.

Identification

A. In the Assay, the retention time of the principal peak in the chromatogram obtained with solution (1) corresponds to that of the principal peak in the chromatogram obtained with solution (2).

B. Carry out the method for *thin-layer chromatography,* Appendix III A, in subdued light, using *silica gel GF_{254}* as the coating substance and as the mobile phase the upper layer obtained by shaking together 25 volumes of *acetic acid,* 50 volumes of *2,2,4-trimethylpentane,* 90 volumes of *ethyl acetate* and 100 volumes of *water* and allowing to separate. Apply separately to the plate 20 µl of each of two solutions in *absolute ethanol* containing (1) a volume of the injection containing the equivalent of 0.015% w/v of dinoprost and (2) 0.020% w/v of *dinoprost trometamol BPCRS.* After removal of the plate, allow it to dry in air, spray with a 1% w/v solution of *vanillin* in a 50% v/v solution of *orthophosphoric acid* and heat at 105° for 20 minutes. The principal spot in the chromatogram obtained with solution (1) is similar in position to that in the chromatogram obtained with solution (2). Examine the plate under *ultraviolet light (365 nm).* The principal spot in the chromatogram obtained with solution (1) corresponds in colour and fluorescence to that in the chromatogram obtained with solution (2).

Acidity or alkalinity pH, 7.0 to 9.0, Appendix V L.

Assay Prepare a 0.075% w/v solution of *guaiphenesin* (internal standard) in the mobile phase (solution A). Carry out the method for *liquid chromatography,* Appendix III D, using the following solutions. For solution (1) dilute a volume of the injection containing the equivalent of 5 mg of dinoprost to 10 ml with *water for injections* containing 0.945% of *benzyl alcohol.* To 1 ml of the resulting solution add 1 ml of a citrate buffer prepared by dissolving 10.5 g of *citric acid* in 75 ml of *water,* adjusting the pH to 4.0 with 5M *sodium hydroxide* and diluting with sufficient *water* to produce 100 ml. Add 20 ml of *dichloromethane,* shake for 10 minutes and centrifuge for 5 minutes. Discard the upper aqueous layer and transfer 5 ml of the lower layer to a suitable container protected from light. Evaporate to dryness using a current of *nitrogen,* add 0.2 ml of a freshly prepared 1% w/v solution of *α-bromo-2′-acetonaphthone* in *acetonitrile* and swirl. Add 0.1 ml of a 0.5% v/v solution of *di-isopropylethylamine* in *acetonitrile* and swirl again. Allow to stand for 1 hour at room temperature, evaporate to dryness and add 4 ml of solution A. Prepare solution (2) in the same manner as solution (1) but using 6.7 mg of *dinoprost trometamol BPCRS* in place of the substance being examined.

The chromatographic procedure may be carried out using (a) a stainless steel column (30 cm × 3.9 mm) packed with *stationary phase A* (10 µm) (µ-Porasil is suitable), (b) a mixture of 0.25 volume of *water,* 3.5 volumes of *butane-1-3-diol* and 496 volumes of *dichloromethane* as the mobile phase with a flow rate of 1.5 ml per minute and (c) a detection wavelength of 254 nm. The relative retention times are about 0.4, 0.5, 1.0 and 1.2 for the internal standard, the 15*R*- epimer, dinoprost trometamol and the 5,6-*trans* isomer, respectively.

The test is not valid unless in the chromatogram obtained with solution (2) the *resolution factor* between the peak due to the derivatised guaiphenesin and dinoprost trometamol is at least 10.

Calculate the content of dinoprost, $C_{20}H_{34}O_5$, using the declared content of $C_{20}H_{34}O_5$ in *dinoprost trometamol BPCRS.*

Storage Dinoprost Injection should be stored at a temperature of 15° to 30°.

Labelling The strength is stated as the equivalent amount of dinoprost in a suitable dose-volume.

Diphenhydramine Oral Solution

Definition Diphenhydramine Oral Solution is a solution of Diphenhydramine Hydrochloride in a suitable flavoured vehicle.

The oral solution complies with the requirements stated under Oral Liquids and with the following requirements.

Content of diphenhydramine hydrochloride, $C_{17}H_{21}NO,HCl$ 90.0 to 110.0% of the prescribed or stated amount.

Identification

A. Carry out the method for *thin-layer chromatography,* Appendix III A, using *silica gel G* as the coating substance and a mixture of 50 volumes of *ethanol (96%),* 30 volumes of *glacial acetic acid* and 20 volumes of *water* as the mobile phase. Apply separately to the plate 5 µl of each of the following freshly prepared solutions. For solution (1) acidify a quantity of the oral solution containing 50 mg of Diphenhydramine Hydrochloride with 2M *hydrochloric acid,* shake with three 20-ml quantities of *ether,* discard the ether, extract with two 20-ml quantities of *chloroform,* dry the combined extracts over *anhydrous sodium sulphate,* filter, evaporate the chloroform and dissolve the cooled residue in 5 ml of *chloroform.* Solution (2) contains 1% w/v of *diphenhydramine hydrochloride EPCRS* in *chloroform.* After removal of the plate, allow it to dry in air and spray with a solution containing 0.25% w/v of *chloroplatinic(IV) acid* and 5% w/v of *potassium iodide.* The principal spot in the chromatogram obtained with solution (1) corresponds in colour and position to that in the chromatogram obtained with solution (2).

B. Evaporate to dryness 1 ml of solution (1) obtained in test A, dissolve the residue in 0.15 ml of *water* and add 2 ml of *sulphuric acid;* a yellow colour is produced which, on the addition of 0.5 ml of *nitric acid,* changes to red.

Add 15 ml of *water*, cool, add 5 ml of *chloroform*, shake and allow to separate; the chloroform layer is violet.

Related substances Carry out the method for *thin-layer chromatography*, Appendix III A, using *silica gel H* as the coating substance and a mixture of 80 volumes of *chloroform* and 20 volumes of *methanol* as the mobile phase. Apply separately to the plate 5 µl of each of the following solutions. For solution (1) use solution (1) described under test A for Identification. For solution (2) dilute 1 volume of solution (1) to 100 volumes with *chloroform*. After removal of the plate, allow it to dry in air and spray with *dilute potassium iodobismuthate solution*. Any *secondary spot* in the chromatogram obtained with solution (1) is not more intense than the spot in the chromatogram obtained with solution (2).

Assay Acidify a quantity containing 0.1 g of Diphenhydramine Hydrochloride with 2M *hydrochloric acid*, shake with three 20-ml quantities of *ether*, discard the ether, make the aqueous solution alkaline with 5M *sodium hydroxide* and extract with successive 15-ml quantities of *ether* until extraction is complete. Wash the combined ether extracts with two 5-ml quantities of *water*, extract the combined washings with 15 ml of *ether* and evaporate the combined ether extracts to dryness. Dissolve the residue in 15 ml of 0.05M *sulphuric acid VS* and titrate the excess of acid with 0.1M *sodium hydroxide VS* using *methyl red solution* as indicator. Each ml of 0.05M *sulphuric acid VS* is equivalent to 29.18 mg of $C_{17}H_{21}NO,HCl$.

Storage Diphenhydramine Oral Solution should be protected from light.

Dipipanone and Cyclizine Tablets

Definition Dipipanone and Cyclizine Tablets contain, in each, 10 mg of Dipipanone Hydrochloride and 30 mg of Cyclizine Hydrochloride.

The tablets comply with the requirements stated under Tablets and with the following requirements.

Content of dipipanone hydrochloride, $C_{24}H_{31}NO,HCl,H_2O$ 9.0 to 11.0 mg.

Content of cyclizine hydrochloride, $C_{18}H_{22}N_2,HCl$ 27.75 to 32.25 mg.

Identification

A. In the Assay, the chromatogram obtained with solution (3) exhibits two peaks having the same retention times as those due to dipipanone and cyclizine in the chromatogram obtained with solution (1).

B. Shake a quantity of the powdered tablets containing 60 mg of Cyclizine Hydrochloride with 10 ml of *acetone* and filter, reserving the filtrate for test C. Add 10 ml of *chloroform* to the residue, mix with the aid of ultrasound for 2 to 3 minutes, filter and evaporate to dryness. The residue yields reaction A characteristic of *chlorides*, Appendix VI.

C. Evaporate the filtrate reserved in test B to dryness. The residue yields reaction A characteristic of *chlorides*, Appendix VI.

Related substances Carry out the method for *thin-layer chromatography*, Appendix III A, using *silica gel G* as the coating substance and as the mobile phase the lower layer obtained after shaking together a mixture of 2 volumes of 13.5M *ammonia*, 8 volumes of *methanol* and 90 volumes of *dichloromethane* and allowing the layers to separate. Apply separately to the plate 20 µl of each of the following freshly prepared solutions. For solution (1) shake a quantity of the powdered tablets containing 30 mg of Cyclizine Hydrochloride with 50 ml of a mixture of equal volumes of *methanol* and *dichloromethane*, filter, evaporate the filtrate to dryness and dissolve the residue in 3 ml of the same solvent mixture. For solution (2) dilute 1 volume of solution (1) to 200 volumes with *methanol*. Solution (3) contains 0.0050% w/v of N-*methylpiperazine* in *methanol*. Solution (4) contains 0.10% w/v of each of *cyclizine hydrochloride BPCRS* and *hydroxyzine hydrochloride EPCRS* in *methanol*. After removal of the plate, allow it to dry in air and expose to iodine vapour for 10 minutes. Any spot corresponding to N-*methylpiperazine* in the chromatogram obtained with solution (1) is not more intense than the spot in the chromatogram obtained with solution (3) (0.5%). Any other *secondary spot* in the chromatogram obtained with solution (1) is not more intense than the spot in the chromatogram obtained with solution (2) (0.5%). The test is not valid unless the chromatogram obtained with solution (4) shows two clearly separated spots.

Assay Weigh and finely powder 20 tablets. Dissolve 0.5 g of *chlorcyclizine hydrochloride BPCRS* (internal standard) in sufficient *dichloromethane* to produce 100 ml (solution A). Carry out the method for *gas chromatography*, Appendix III B, using the following solutions. For solution (1) add 25 ml of solution A to 0.15 g of *cyclizine hydrochloride BPCRS* and 50 mg of *dipipanone hydrochloride BPCRS* and dilute to 50 ml with *dichloromethane*. For solution (2) add 40 ml of *dichloromethane* to a quantity of the powdered tablets containing 50 mg of Dipipanone Hydrochloride and mix with the aid of ultrasound for 20 minutes; dilute to 50 ml with *dichloromethane* and filter. Prepare solution (3) in the same manner as solution (2) but add 25 ml of solution A and 15 ml of *dichloromethane* in place of the 40 ml of dichloromethane.

The chromatographic procedure may be carried out using a glass column (1.5 m × 4 mm) packed with *acid-washed, silanised diatomaceous support* (80 to 100 mesh) coated with 3% w/w of silicone grease (Apiezon L is suitable) and 5% w/w of *potassium hydroxide* and maintained at 250°. In the chromatogram obtained with solution (2) the peaks, in order of emergence, are due to cyclizine, chlorcyclizine and dipipanone.

Calculate the content of $C_{24}H_{31}NO,HCl,H_2O$ using the declared content of $C_{24}H_{31}NO,HCl,H_2O$ in *dipipanone hydrochloride BPCRS* and the content of $C_{18}H_{22}N_2,HCl$ using the declared content of $C_{18}H_{22}N_2$, HCl in *cyclizine hydrochloride BPCRS*.

Dipyridamole Tablets

Definition Dipyridamole Tablets contain Dipyridamole. They are coated.

The tablets comply with the requirements stated under Tablets and with the following requirements.

Content of dipyridamole, $C_{24}H_{40}N_8O_4$ 92.5 to 107.5% of the prescribed or stated amount.

Identification

A. Shake a quantity of the powdered tablets containing 50 mg of Dipyridamole with 20 ml of *chloroform*, filter and evaporate to dryness. The *infrared absorption spectrum* of the residue, Appendix II A, is concordant with the *reference spectrum* of dipyridamole.

B. To a quantity of the powdered tablets containing 10 mg of Dipyridamole add 50 ml of *methanol*, warm slightly, shake for 15 minutes and allow to cool. Add sufficient *methanol* to produce 100 ml, filter and to 10 ml of the filtrate add 1 ml of 1M *hydrochloric acid* and sufficient *methanol* to produce 100 ml. The *light absorption* of the resulting solution, Appendix II B, in the range 220 to 450 nm exhibits three maxima, at 230, 285 and 405 nm.

Related substances Carry out the method for *thin-layer chromatography*, Appendix III A, using a silica gel precoated plate (Merck silica gel 60 plates are suitable) and *acetone* as the mobile phase. Apply separately to the plate 10 µl of each of the following freshly prepared solutions. For solution (1) shake a quantity of the powdered tablets containing 0.2 g of Dipyridamole with 10 ml of a mixture of equal volumes of *chloroform* and *methanol* for 20 minutes and centrifuge. For solution (2) dilute 1 volume of solution (1) to 200 volumes with the same solvent. After removal of the plate, allow it to dry in air and spray thoroughly with a solution prepared by dissolving a mixture of 1 g of *iodine* and 3 g of *potassium iodide* in 10 ml of *ethanol (96%)* and adding 20 ml of 1M *sulphuric acid* and sufficient *water* to produce 100 ml. Any *secondary spot* in the chromatogram obtained with solution (1) is not more intense than the spot in the chromatogram obtained with solution (2). Disregard any spot remaining on the line of application.

Assay To 10 whole tablets add 300 ml of 1M *hydrochloric acid*, heat at 40° for 20 minutes with shaking, allow to cool and add sufficient 1M *hydrochloric acid* to produce 500 ml. Filter and dilute, if necessary, with 1M *hydrochloric acid* to produce a solution containing 0.05% w/v of Dipyridamole. Dilute 1 volume to 50 volumes with *water* and measure the *absorbance* of the resulting solution at the maximum at 283 nm, Appendix II B. Calculate the content of $C_{24}H_{40}N_8O_4$ from the *absorbance* of a solution obtained by diluting 1 volume of a 0.05% w/v solution of *dipyridamole BPCRS* in 1M *hydrochloric acid* to 50 volumes with *water*.

Disodium Pamidronate Intravenous Infusion

Definition Disodium Pamidronate Intravenous Infusion is a sterile solution of disodium pamidronate in Water for Injections. It is prepared by dissolving Disodium Pamidronate for Intravenous Infusion in Water for Injections and then diluting with the requisite volume of a suitable diluent in accordance with the manufacturer's instructions.

The intravenous infusion complies with the requirements stated under Parenteral Preparations and with the following requirements.

Particulate contamination When the volume of the constituted intravenous infusion is 100 ml or more, it complies with the *test for sub-visible particles*, Appendix XIII A.

Bacterial endotoxins Carry out the *test for bacterial endotoxins*, Appendix XIV C. Dissolve the contents of the sealed container in *water BET* to give a solution containing the equivalent of 10 mg of anhydrous disodium pamidronate per ml (solution A). The endotoxin limit concentration of solution A is 30 IU of endotoxin per ml. Carry out the test using the maximum valid dilution of solution A calculated from the declared sensitivity of the lysate used in the test.

Storage Disodium Pamidronate Intravenous Infusion should be used immediately after preparation but, in any case, within the period recommended by the manufacturer when prepared and stored strictly in accordance with the manufacturer's instructions.

DISODIUM PAMIDRONATE FOR INTRAVENOUS INFUSION

Definition Disodium Pamidronate for Intravenous Infusion is a sterile material prepared from Disodium Pamidronate with or without excipients. It is supplied in a sealed container.

The contents of the sealed container comply with the requirements for Powders for Injections stated under Parenteral Preparations and with the following requirements.

Content of anhydrous disodium pamidronate, $C_3H_9NNa_2O_7P_2$ 95.0 to 105.0% of the prescribed or stated amount.

Identification In the Assay, the chromatogram obtained with solution (1) shows a peak with the same retention time as the peak due to disodium pamidronate in the chromatogram obtained with solution (2).

Acidity or alkalinity Dissolve the contents of a sealed container in sufficient *water* to produce a solution containing the equivalent of 0.3% w/v of anhydrous disodium pamidronate. The pH of the solution is 6.0 to 7.0, Appendix V L.

β-Alanine Carry out the method for *thin-layer chromatography* under subdued light, Appendix III A, using a silica gel precoated plate (Merck silica gel 60 plates are suitable) and a mixture of 4 volumes of 13.5M *ammonia*, 8 volumes of *di-isopropyl ether* and 9 volumes of *methanol* as the mobile phase but allowing the solvent front to ascend 7 cm above the line of application. Apply separately to the plate 10 µl of each of the following solutions. For solution (1) dissolve the contents of a sealed container in sufficient *water* to produce a solution containing the equivalent of 0.30% w/v of anhydrous disodium pamidronate. Solution (2) contains 0.0015% w/v of *3-aminopropionic acid*. After removal of the plate, allow it to dry in a current of warm air and spray with a 0.01% w/v solution of *fluorescamine* in *acetone*, immerse the plate for 2 seconds in a mixture of 1 volume of *liquid paraffin* and 2 volumes of n-*hexane*, allow to dry in air for 15 minutes and examine under *ultraviolet light (365 nm)*. In the chromatogram obtained with solution (1) any spot corresponding to β-alanine (3-aminopropionic acid) is not more intense than the spot in the chromatogram obtained with solution (2) (0.5%).

Phosphate and phosphite Carry out the method for *liquid chromatography*, Appendix III D, using the following solutions. For solution (1) dissolve the contents of a sealed container in sufficient *water* to produce a solution containing the equivalent of 0.20% w/v of anhydrous disodium pamidronate. For solution (2) dilute a mixture of 2 ml of a 0.030% w/v solution of *orthophosphoric acid* and 2 ml of a

0.025% w/v solution of *orthophosphorous acid* to 50 ml with *water*.

The chromatographic procedure may be carried out using (a) a stainless steel column (15 cm × 4.6 mm) packed with an anion-exchange stationary phase (5 µm) (Mitsubishi Kasai MCl Gel SCA 04 Polymer Anion is suitable) and maintained at 35°, (b) as the mobile phase with a flow rate of 1.2 ml per minute a solution prepared by adding 0.47 ml of *formic acid* to 2500 ml of *water* and adjusting the solution to pH 3.5 with 2M *sodium hydroxide* and (c) a refractive index detector. Inject 100 µl of each solution.

In the chromatogram obtained with solution (2) the peaks appear in the order orthophosphoric acid (retention time, 12 to 15 minutes) and orthophosphorous acid (retention time, 16 to 20 minutes).

In the chromatogram obtained with solution (1) the area of any peak corresponding to orthophosphoric acid (phosphate) or orthophosphorous acid (phosphite) is not greater than the area of the respective peak in the chromatogram obtained with solution (2) (0.5% of each).

Assay Determine the weight of the mixed contents of 10 containers as described in the test for Uniformity of weight under Parenteral Preparations, Powders for Injections.

Carry out the method for *liquid chromatography*, Appendix III D, using the following solutions. For solution (1) dissolve a quantity of the mixed contents of the 10 containers in *water* and dilute with the same solvent to produce a solution containing the equivalent of 0.20% w/v of anhydrous disodium pamidronate. Solution (2) contains 0.20% w/v of *disodium pamidronate BPCRS* in *water*.

The chromatographic conditions described under Phosphate and phosphite may be used.

Calculate the content of $C_3H_9NNa_2O_7P_2$ in a container of average content weight from the chromatograms obtained and using the declared content of $C_3H_9NNa_2O_7P_2$ in *disodium pamidronate BPCRS*.

Labelling The quantity of active ingredient is stated in terms of the equivalent amount of anhydrous disodium pamidronate.

IMPURITIES

The impurities limited by the requirements of this monograph include those listed under Disodium Pamidronate.

Disopyramide Capsules

Definition Disopyramide Capsules contain Disopyramide.

The capsules comply with the requirements stated under Capsules and with the following requirements.

Content of disopyramide, $C_{21}H_{29}N_3O$ 92.5 to 107.5% of the prescribed or stated amount.

Identification

A. Shake a quantity of the contents of the capsules containing 0.2 g of Disopyramide with 50 ml of *chloroform* for 15 minutes, filter, evaporate the filtrate to dryness using a rotary evaporator and dissolve the residue in 2 ml of *chloroform*. The *infrared absorption spectrum*, Appendix II A, is concordant with the *reference spectrum* of disopyramide.

B. The *light absorption*, Appendix II B, in the range 230 to 350 nm of the solution obtained in the Assay exhibits a maximum only at 269 nm.

Related substances Carry out the method for *thin-layer chromatography*, Appendix III A, using *silica gel GF₂₅₄* as the coating substance and a mixture of 1 volume of 18M *ammonia*, 30 volumes of *acetone* and 30 volumes of *cyclohexane* as the mobile phase. Apply separately to the plate 10 µl of the following solutions. For solution (1) shake a quantity of the contents of the capsules containing 0.20 g of Disopyramide with 20 ml of *methanol* for 30 minutes and filter. For solution (2) dilute 1 volume of solution (1) to 400 volumes with *methanol*. After removal of the plate, allow it to dry in a current of air and examine under *ultraviolet light (254 nm)*. Any *secondary spot* in the chromatogram obtained with solution (1) is not more intense than the spot in the chromatogram obtained with solution (2) (0.25%).

Assay To a quantity of the mixed contents of 20 capsules containing 40 mg of Disopyramide, add 40 ml of 0.05M *methanolic sulphuric acid*, shake for 15 minutes, dilute to 100 ml with the same solvent and filter. Dilute 5 ml of the filtrate to 100 ml with 0.05M *methanolic sulphuric acid* and measure the *absorbance* of the resulting solution at the maximum at 269 nm, Appendix II B. Calculate the content of $C_{21}H_{29}N_3O$ taking 198.5 as the value of A(1%, 1 cm) at the maximum at 269 nm.

Disopyramide Phosphate Capsules

Definition Disopyramide Phosphate Capsules contain Disopyramide Phosphate.

The capsules comply with the requirements stated under Capsules and with the following requirements.

Content of disopyramide, $C_{21}H_{29}N_3O$ 92.5 to 107.5% of the prescribed or stated amount.

Identification

A. Suspend a quantity of the contents of the capsules containing the equivalent of 0.2 g of disopyramide in 50 ml of *chloroform*, add 2 ml of 13.5M *ammonia*, shake and filter through *anhydrous sodium sulphate*. Evaporate the filtrate to dryness using a rotary evaporator and dissolve the residue in 2 ml of *chloroform*. The *infrared absorption spectrum*, Appendix II A, is concordant with the *reference spectrum* of disopyramide.

B. The *light absorption*, Appendix II B, in the range 230 to 350 nm of the solution obtained in the Assay exhibits a maximum only at 269 nm and a shoulder at 263 nm.

C. Shake a quantity of the contents of the capsules containing the equivalent of 0.4 g of disopyramide with 20 ml of *water* and filter. The filtrate yields the reactions characteristic of *phosphates*, Appendix VI.

Dissolution Comply with the *dissolution test for tablets and capsules*, Appendix XII D, using Apparatus II. Use as the medium 900 ml of *water* and rotate the paddle at 50 revolutions per minute. Withdraw a sample of 10 ml of the medium and measure the *absorbance* of the filtered sample, suitably diluted if necessary, at the maximum at 269 nm, Appendix II B. Calculate the total content of disopyramide phosphate, $C_{21}H_{29}N_3O,H_3PO_4$, in the medium taking 87 as the value of A(1%, 1 cm) at the maximum at 262 nm.

Related substances Carry out the method for *thin-layer chromatography*, Appendix III A, using *silica gel GF₂₅₄* as the coating substance and a mixture of 1 volume of 18M *ammonia*, 30 volumes of *acetone* and 30 volumes of *cyclohexane* as the mobile phase. Apply separately to the plate 10 µl of each of the following solutions. For solution (1) shake a quantity of the contents of the capsules containing 0.20 g of Disopyramide Phosphate with 20 ml of *methanol* for 30 minutes and filter. For solution (2) dilute 1 volume of solution (1) to 200 volumes with *methanol*. After removal of the plate, allow it to dry in a current of air and examine under *ultraviolet light (254 nm)*. Any *secondary spot* in the chromatogram obtained with solution (1) is not more intense than the spot in the chromatogram obtained with solution (2) (0.5%).

Assay To a quantity of the mixed contents of 20 capsules containing the equivalent of 40 mg of disopyramide, add 40 ml of 0.05M *methanolic sulphuric acid*, shake for 15 minutes, dilute to 100 ml with the same solvent and filter. Dilute 5 ml of the filtrate to 100 ml with 0.05M *methanolic sulphuric acid* and measure the *absorbance* of the resulting solution at the maximum at 269 nm, Appendix II B. Calculate the content of $C_{21}H_{29}N_3O$ taking 198.5 as the value of A(1%, 1 cm) at the maximum at 269 nm.

Labelling The quantity of active ingredient is stated in terms of the equivalent amount of disopyramide.

Disulfiram Tablets

Definition Disulfiram Tablets contain Disulfiram.

The tablets comply with the requirements stated under Tablets and with the following requirements.

Content of disulfiram, $C_{10}H_{20}N_2S_4$ 95.0 to 105.0% of the prescribed or stated amount.

Identification

A. Extract a quantity of the powdered tablets containing 0.2 g of Disulfiram by shaking with 5ml of *dichloromethane* and filter. Evaporate the filtrate to dryness and dry the residue at 40° at a pressure not exceeding 0.7 kPa. The *infrared absorption spectrum* of the residue, Appendix II A, is concordant with the *reference spectrum* of disulfiram.

B. In the test for Related substances, the principal spot in the chromatogram obtained with solution (2) corresponds to that in the chromatogram obtained with solution (3).

C. Extract a quantity of the powdered tablets containing 0.3 g of Disulfiram with *ethanol (96%)*, filter and evaporate the filtrate to dryness. Dissolve 50 mg of the residue in 5 ml of *ethanol (96%)* and add 1 ml of *potassium cyanide solution*. A yellow colour is produced which becomes green and then darkens to bluish green.

Diethyldithiocarbamate Shake a quantity of the powdered tablets containing 0.1 g of Disulfiram with 10 ml of *chloroform* and filter. Add 10 ml of 0.1M *sodium hydroxide* to the filtrate, shake, discard the chloroform layer and wash the aqueous layer with three 10-ml quantities of *chloroform*. To the aqueous layer add 0.25 ml of a 0.4% w/v solution of *copper(II) sulphate* and 2 ml of *dichloromethane*, shake and allow to separate. The lower layer is not more intensely coloured than a standard prepared at the same time and in the same manner by adding 10 ml of 0.1M *sodium hydroxide* to 0.2 ml of a freshly prepared 0.0075% w/v solution of *sodium diethyldithiocarbamate* and beginning at the words 'add 0.25 ml of a 0.4% w/v solution of *copper(II) sulphate*...' (0.01%, calculated as the acid).

Related substances Carry out the method for *thin-layer chromatography*, Appendix III A, using *silica gel GF_{254}* as the coating substance and a mixture of 30 volumes of *butyl acetate* and 70 volumes of *n-hexane* as the mobile phase. Apply separately to the plate 10 µl of each of the following solutions. For solution (1) extract a quantity of the powdered tablets containing 0.50 g of Disulfiram with 20 ml of *ethyl acetate* and filter. For solution (2) dilute 1 volume of solution (1) to 100 volumes with *ethyl acetate*. Solution (3) contains 0.025% w/v of *disulfiram BPCRS* in *ethyl acetate*. Solution (4) contains 0.050% w/v of *monosulfiram BPCRS* in *ethyl acetate*. After removal of the plate, allow it to dry in air and examine under *ultraviolet light (254 nm)*. In the chromatogram obtained with solution (1) any spot corresponding to monosulfiram is not more intense than the spot in the chromatogram obtained with solution (4) (2%) and any other *secondary spot* is not more intense than the spot in the chromatogram obtained with solution (2) (1%).

Assay Weigh and powder 20 tablets. To a quantity of the powder containing 0.4 g of Disulfiram add 75 ml of *methanol* and shake for 30 minutes. Add sufficient *methanol* to produce 100 ml, filter and dilute 5 ml of the filtrate to 100 ml with *methanol*. To 5 ml of this solution add sufficient of a 0.1% w/v solution of *copper(II) chloride* in *methanol* to produce 25 ml, mix and allow to stand for 1 hour. Measure the *absorbance* of the resulting solution at the maximum at 400 nm, Appendix II B, using in the reference cell a solution prepared by diluting 5 ml of *methanol* to 25 ml with the copper(II) chloride solution. Calculate the content of $C_{10}H_{20}N_2S_4$ from the *absorbance* obtained by repeating the operation using 5 ml of a 0.020% w/v solution of *disulfiram BPCRS* in *methanol* and beginning at the words 'add sufficient of a 0.1% w/v solution of *copper(II) chloride* ...'.

Storage Disulfiram Tablets should be kept in a well-closed container and protected from light.

Dithranol Cream

Definition Dithranol Cream contains Dithranol in a suitable oil-in-water emulsified basis.

The cream complies with the requirements stated under Topical Semi-solid Preparations and with the following requirements.

Content of dithranol, $C_{14}H_{10}O_3$ 85.0 to 110.0% of the prescribed or stated amount.

Identification

A. In the Assay the principal peak in the chromatogram obtained with solution (2) has the same retention time as that in the chromatogram obtained with solution (1).

B. Suspend a quantity containing 0.5 mg of dithranol in 5 ml of 1M *sodium hydroxide* and heat on a water bath for 1 minute while stirring. A pink colour is produced.

Dihydroxyanthraquinone and dithranol dimer Not more than 10.0% of the prescribed or stated amount of Dithranol, calculated as the sum of the amounts of dihydroxyanthraquinone and dithranol dimer when determined by the method for *liquid chromatography*, Appendix III D, using the following solutions. For creams containing more than 0.5% w/v of Dithranol, use as solution (1) solution A obtained in the Assay. For solution (2) add 4 ml of *glacial acetic acid* to 20 ml of a solution containing 0.005% w/v of *1,8-dihydroxyanthraquinone* and 0.005% w/v of *dithranol dimer BPCRS* in *dichloromethane* and add sufficient n-*hexane* to produce 100 ml. For creams containing 0.5% w/v or less of Dithranol, use as solution (1) solution B obtained in the Assay. For solution (2) add 20 ml of *glacial acetic acid* to 10 ml of a solution containing 0.005% w/v of *1,8-dihydroxyanthraquinone* and 0.005% w/v of *dithranol dimer BPCRS* in *dichloromethane* and add sufficient *dichloromethane* to produce 100 ml.

The chromatographic procedure described under Assay may be used but using a detection wavelength of 380 nm.

In the chromatogram obtained with solution (2) the peaks, other than the solvent peak, are, in order of emergence, due to dihydroxyanthraquinone and dithranol dimer. Calculate the amounts of dihydroxyanthraquinone and dithranol dimer in the cream with reference to the corresponding peaks in the chromatogram obtained with solution (2).

1-Hydroxy-9-anthrone Carry out the method for *liquid chromatography*, Appendix III D, in subdued light using the following freshly prepared solutions. For solution (1) disperse a quantity of the cream containing 10 mg of Dithranol in 30 ml of *water* at about 50°, add 30 ml of a warm, saturated solution of *sodium chloride*, cool and extract with three 40-ml quantities of *chloroform*. Filter the extract successively through *anhydrous sodium sulphate* on a suitable filter (Whatman GF/C is suitable). Evaporate the filtrate under reduced pressure to a volume of about 2 ml, add 25 ml of warm *methanol*, shake, cool in ice for 15 minutes and filter (Whatman GF/C paper is suitable). Evaporate the filtrate to dryness under reduced pressure and dissolve the residue in 10 ml of a mixture of 5 volumes of *glacial acetic acid* and 95 volumes of *acetonitrile*; filter if necessary. For solution (2) dissolve 25 mg of *1-hydroxy-9-anthrone BPCRS* in 0.5 ml of *glacial acetic acid* and add sufficient *acetonitrile* to produce 50 ml (solution A); dilute 1 ml of solution A to 20 ml with *acetonitrile*. For solution (3) dilute 1 volume of solution (1) to 40 ml with a mixture of 5 volumes of *glacial acetic acid* and 95 volumes of *acetonitrile*. For solution (4) dissolve 50 mg of *dithranol BPCRS* in 0.5 ml of *glacial acetic acid*, add 2 ml of solution A and sufficient *acetonitrile* to produce 50 ml.

The chromatographic procedure may be carried out using (a) a stainless steel column (20 cm × 4.6 mm) packed with *stationary phase C* (5 μm) (Nucleosil C18 and Spherisorb ODS 2 are suitable), (b) a mixture of 2.5 volumes of *glacial acetic acid*, 40 volumes of *tetrahydrofuran* and 60 volumes of *water* as the mobile phase with a flow rate of 1.5 ml per minute and (c) a detection wavelength of 254 nm.

The test is not valid unless the chromatogram obtained with solution (4) closely resembles the chromatogram supplied with *dithranol BPCRS*.

In the chromatogram obtained with solution (1) the area of any peak corresponding to the principal peak in the chromatogram obtained with solution (2) (1-hydroxy-9-anthrone) is not greater than the area of the principal peak in the chromatogram obtained with solution (3) (2.5%).

Assay Carry out the method for *liquid chromatography*, Appendix III D, using the following solutions. For creams containing more than 0.5% w/w of Dithranol prepare solution (1) in the following manner, protected from light. Disperse by shaking a quantity of the cream containing 50 mg of Dithranol in 10 ml of *glacial acetic acid* and 20 ml of *dichloromethane*, filter through a glass microfibre filter paper (Whatman GF/C is suitable) into a 100-ml graduated flask, wash the filter with *dichloromethane* and add sufficient *dichloromethane* to produce 100 ml. Shake the flask vigorously and allow to stand until two layers are obtained, add *dichloromethane* until the dichloromethane and water interface is level with the calibration mark, shake vigorously and again allow to stand until two layers are obtained. Dilute 20 volumes of the lower layer to 50 volumes with n-*hexane* (solution A). Dilute a suitable volume of solution A with n-*hexane* to contain 0.002% w/v of Dithranol. For creams containing 0.5% w/w or less of Dithranol prepare solution (1) in the following manner, protected from light. Disperse, by shaking, a quantity of the cream containing 5 mg of Dithranol in 10 ml of *glacial acetic acid* and 20 ml of *dichloromethane*, filter through a glass microfibre filter paper (Whatman GF/C is suitable) into a 50-ml graduated flask, wash the filter with *dichloromethane* and add sufficient *dichloromethane* to produce 50 ml. Shake the flask vigorously and allow to stand until two layers are obtained, add *dichloromethane* until the dichloromethane and water interface is level with the calibration mark, shake vigorously and again allow to stand until two layers are obtained (solution B). Dilute a suitable volume of solution B with n-*hexane* to contain 0.002% w/v of Dithranol. For solution (2) add 1 ml of *glacial acetic acid* to 10 ml of a 0.02% w/v solution of *dithranol BPCRS* in *dichloromethane* and add sufficient of the mobile phase to produce 100 ml.

The chromatographic procedure may be carried out using (a) a stainless steel column (25 cm × 4.6 mm) packed with *stationary phase A* (5 μm) (Lichrosorb Si 60 is suitable), (b) a mixture of 1 volume of *glacial acetic acid*, 5 volumes of *dichloromethane* and 82 volumes of n-*hexane* as the mobile phase with a flow rate of 2 ml per minute and (c) a detection wavelength of 354 nm.

Calculate the content of $C_{14}H_{10}O_3$ in the cream using the declared content of $C_{14}H_{10}O_3$ in *dithranol BPCRS*.

Storage Dithranol Cream should be kept in a well-closed container, protected from light and stored at a temperature not exceeding 25°.

Dithranol Ointment

Definition Dithranol Ointment contains Dithranol, in *fine powder*, in a suitable hydrophobic basis.

Extemporaneous preparation The following directions apply.

Triturate Dithranol, in *fine powder*, with Yellow Soft Paraffin, add sufficient Yellow Soft Paraffin to produce an ointment of the required strength and mix thoroughly. Part of the Yellow Soft Paraffin may be replaced by Hard Paraffin to produce an ointment of stiffer consistency.

The ointment complies with the requirements stated under Topical Semi-solid Preparations and with the following requirements.

Content of dithranol, $C_{14}H_{10}O_3$ 85.0 to 110.0% of the prescribed or stated amount.

Identification

A. In the Assay, the principal peak in the chromatogram obtained with solution (2) corresponds to the principal peak in the chromatogram obtained with solution (1).

B. Heat a quantity containing 0.5 mg of Dithranol with 5 ml of 1M *sodium hydroxide* on a water bath with constant stirring. A pink colour is produced in the aqueous layer.

Dihydroxyanthraquinone and dithranol dimer Not more than 10.0% of the prescribed or stated amount of Dithranol, calculated as the sum of the amounts of dihydroxyanthraquinone and dithranol dimer, when determined by the method for *liquid chromatography*, Appendix III D, using the following solutions. For solution (1) add 1 ml of *glacial acetic acid* to 20 ml of a solution containing 0.0050% w/v of *1,8-dihydroxyanthraquinone* and 0.0050% w/v of *dithranol dimer BPCRS* in *dichloromethane* and add sufficient *hexane* to produce 100 ml. For solution (2) disperse a quantity of the ointment containing 20 mg of Dithranol in 20 ml of *dichloromethane*, add 1 ml of *glacial acetic acid*, dilute to 100 ml with *hexane* and filter through a fine glass microfibre filter paper (Whatman GF/C is suitable).

The chromatographic procedure may be carried out using (a) a stainless steel column (25 cm × 4.6 mm) packed with *stationary phase A* (5 µm) (Lichrosorb Si 60 is suitable), (b) a mixture of 82 volumes of *hexane*, 5 volumes of *dichloromethane* and 1 volume of *glacial acetic acid* as the mobile phase with a flow rate of 2 ml per minute and (c) a detection wavelength of 380 nm.

In the chromatogram obtained with solution (1) the peaks, other than the solvent peak, in order of emergence are due to dihydroxyanthraquinone and dithranol dimer. Calculate the amounts of dihydroxyanthraquinone and dithranol dimer in the ointment with reference to the corresponding peaks in the chromatogram obtained with solution (1).

1-Hydroxy-9-anthrone Carry out the method for *liquid chromatography*, Appendix III D, in subdued light using the following freshly prepared solutions. For solution (1) disperse a quantity of the ointment containing 10 mg of Dithranol in 25 ml of *chloroform*, evaporate under reduced pressure to a volume of about 2 ml, add 25 ml of warm *methanol*, shake, cool in ice for 15 minutes and filter (Whatman GF/C paper is suitable). Evaporate the filtrate to dryness under reduced pressure and dissolve the residue in 10 ml of a mixture of 5 volumes of *glacial acetic acid* and 95 volumes of *acetonitrile*; filter if necessary. For solution (2) dissolve 25 mg of *1-hydroxy-9-anthrone BPCRS* in 0.5 ml of *glacial acetic acid* and add sufficient *acetonitrile* to produce 50 ml (solution A); dilute 1 ml of solution A to 20 ml with *acetonitrile*. For solution (3) dilute 1 volume of solution (1) to 40 ml with a mixture of 5 volumes of *glacial acetic acid* and 95 volumes of *acetonitrile*. For solution (4) dissolve 50 mg of *dithranol BPCRS* in 0.5 ml of *glacial acetic acid*, add 2 ml of solution A and sufficient *acetonitrile* to produce 50 ml.

The chromatographic procedure may be carried out using (a) a stainless steel column (20 cm × 4.6 mm) packed with *stationary phase C* (5 µm) (Nucleosil C18 and Spherisorb ODS 2 are suitable), (b) a mixture of 2.5 volumes of *glacial acetic acid*, 40 volumes of *tetrahydrofuran* and 60 volumes of *water* as the mobile phase with a flow rate of 1.5 ml per minute and (c) a detection wavelength of 254 nm.

The test is not valid unless the chromatogram obtained with solution (4) closely resembles the chromatogram supplied with *dithranol BPCRS*.

In the chromatogram obtained with solution (1) the area of any peak corresponding to the principal peak in the chromatogram obtained with solution (2) (1-hydroxy-9-anthrone) is not greater than the area of the principal peak in the chromatogram obtained with solution (3) (2.5%).

Assay Carry out the method for *liquid chromatography*, Appendix III D, using the following solutions. For solution (1) add 1 ml of *glacial acetic acid* to 20 ml of a 0.025% w/v solution of *dithranol BPCRS* in *dichloromethane* and add sufficient *hexane* to produce 100 ml. For solution (2) disperse a quantity of the ointment containing 5 mg of Dithranol in 20 ml of *dichloromethane*, add 1 ml of *glacial acetic acid*, dilute to 100 ml with *hexane* and filter through a fine glass microfibre filter paper (Whatman GF/C is suitable).

The chromatographic procedure described under Dihydroxyanthraquinone and dithranol dimer may be used but using a detection wavelength of 354 nm.

Calculate the content of $C_{14}H_{10}O_3$ in the ointment using the declared content of $C_{14}H_{10}O_3$ in *dithranol BPCRS*.

Storage Dithranol Ointment should be protected from light.

Dithranol Paste

Definition Dithranol Paste contains Dithranol in a suitable hydrophobic basis containing 24% w/w each of Zinc Oxide and Starch and 2% w/w of Salicylic Acid.

Extemporaneous preparation The following formula and directions apply.

Dithranol	1 g, or a sufficient quantity
Zinc and Salicylic Acid Paste	sufficient to produce 1000 g

Mix the Dithranol with a portion of the Zinc and Salicylic Acid Paste until a smooth, even dispersion is obtained and gradually incorporate the remainder of the Zinc and Salicylic Acid Paste.

The paste complies with the requirements stated under Topical Semi-solid Preparations and with the following requirements.

Content of dithranol, $C_{14}H_{10}O_3$ 85.0 to 110.0% of the prescribed or stated amount.

Content of salicylic acid, $C_7H_6O_3$ 1.9 to 2.1% w/w.

Content of zinc oxide, ZnO 22.5 to 25.5% w/w.

Identification

A. In the Assay for dithranol, the principal peak in the chromatogram obtained with solution (2) corresponds to the principal peak in the chromatogram obtained with solution (1).

B. Suspend a quantity containing 0.5 mg of Dithranol in 5 ml of 1M *sodium hydroxide* and heat on a water bath for 1 minute while stirring. A pink colour is produced.

C. Disperse 0.5 g in 10 ml of *chloroform*, filter, extract the filtrate with 10 ml of a 1% w/v solution of *sodium hydrogen carbonate* and wash the extract with 5 ml of *chloroform*. To

5 ml add 3 ml of *iron(III) chloride solution R1.* A violet colour is produced which persists after the addition of 0.5 ml of 5M *acetic acid.*

Dihydroxyanthraquinone and dithranol dimer Not more than 10.0% of the prescribed or stated amount of Dithranol, calculated as the sum of the amounts of dihydroxyanthraquinone and dithranol dimer, when determined by the method for *liquid chromatography*, Appendix III D, using the following solutions. For solution (1) add 1 ml of *glacial acetic acid* to 20 ml of a solution containing 0.0050% w/v of *1,8-dihydroxyanthraquinone* and 0.0050% w/v of *dithranol dimer BPCRS* in *dichloromethane* and add sufficient *hexane* to produce 100 ml. For solution (2) disperse a quantity of the paste containing 20 mg of Dithranol in 20 ml of *dichloromethane* with warming and stirring, centrifuge and decant the supernatant layer into a 100-ml flask. Disperse the residue in 20 ml of *hexane*, centrifuge, decant the supernatant layer into the 100-ml flask and repeat the procedure with a further two 20-ml quantities of *hexane*. Add 1 ml of *glacial acetic acid* to the combined extracts, dilute to 100 ml with *hexane* and filter through a fine glass microfibre filter paper (Whatman GF/C paper is suitable).

The chromatographic procedure may be carried out using (a) a stainless steel column (25 cm × 4.6 mm) packed with *stationary phase A* (5 µm) (Lichrosorb Si 60 is suitable), (b) a mixture of 82 volumes of *hexane*, 5 volumes of *dichloromethane* and 1 volume of *glacial acetic acid* as the mobile phase with a flow rate of 2 ml per minute and (c) a detection wavelength of 380 nm.

In the chromatogram obtained with solution (1) the peaks, other than the solvent peak, in order of emergence are due to dihydroxyanthraquinone and dithranol dimer. Calculate the amounts of dihydroxyanthraquinone and dithranol dimer in the paste with reference to the corresponding peaks in the chromatogram obtained with solution (1).

Assay

For dithranol Carry out the method for *liquid chromatography*, Appendix III D, using the following solutions. For solution (1) add 1 ml of *glacial acetic acid* to 20 ml of a 0.025% w/v solution of *dithranol BPCRS* in *dichloromethane* and add sufficient *hexane* to produce 100 ml. For solution (2) disperse a quantity of the paste containing 5 mg of Dithranol in 20 ml of *dichloromethane* with warming and stirring, centrifuge and decant the supernatant layer into a 100-ml flask. Disperse the residue in 20 ml of *hexane*, centrifuge, decant the supernatant layer into the 100-ml flask and repeat the procedure with a further two 20-ml quantities of *hexane*. Add 1 ml of *glacial acetic acid* to the combined extracts, dilute to 100 ml with *hexane* and filter through a fine glass microfibre filter paper (Whatman GF/C paper is suitable).

The chromatographic procedure described under Dihydroxyanthraquinone and dithranol dimer may be used but using a detection wavelength of 354 nm.

Calculate the content of $C_{14}H_{10}O_3$ in the paste using the declared content of $C_{14}H_{10}O_3$ in *dithranol BPCRS*.

For salicylic acid Shake 0.5 g with 10 ml of 1M *hydrochloric acid* and 10 ml of *ether* until fully dispersed. Decant and reserve the aqueous layer. Extract the ether layer with two further 10-ml quantities of 1M *hydrochloric acid*, combine the aqueous extracts with the reserved aqueous layer, wash with 10 ml of *ether* and reserve for the Assay for zinc oxide. Combine the ether extracts and washings, add 15 ml of *petroleum spirit (boiling range, 40° to 60°)* and extract with successive quantities of 20 ml, 10 ml and 10 ml of *borate buffer pH 9.0.* Dilute the combined extracts to 100 ml with 2M *hydrochloric acid*, dilute 15 ml of the resulting solution to 50 ml with the same solvent and measure the *absorbance* of the final solution at the maximum at 302 nm. Calculate the content of $C_7H_6O_3$ taking 260 as the value of A(1%, 1 cm) at the maximum at 302 nm.

For zinc oxide To the combined aqueous extracts obtained in the Assay for salicylic acid add 20 ml of 1M *sodium hydroxide* and 50 mg of *xylenol orange triturate.* To the resulting solution add sufficient *hexamine* to change the colour of the solution to red, and then a further 3 g of *hexamine,* and titrate with 0.1M *disodium edetate VS.* Each ml of 0.1M *disodium edetate VS* is equivalent to 8.137 mg of ZnO.

Storage Dithranol Paste should be protected from light.

Docusate Tablets

Dioctyl Sodium Sulphosuccinate Tablets

Definition Docusate Tablets contain Docusate Sodium.

The tablets comply with the requirements stated under Tablets and with the following requirements.

Content of docusate sodium, $C_{20}H_{37}NaO_7S$ 90.0 to 110.0% of the prescribed or stated amount.

Identification

A. Shake a quantity of the powdered tablets containing 0.1 g of Docusate Sodium with 50 ml of n-*hexane* for 30 minutes, centrifuge and filter the supernatant liquid. Evaporate the filtrate to dryness. The *infrared absorption spectrum* of the residue, Appendix II A, is concordant with the *reference spectrum* of docusate sodium.

B. To 5 mg of the residue obtained in test A add 5 ml of *water* and shake. Add 1 ml of 1M *sulphuric acid,* 10 ml of *chloroform* and 0.2 ml of *dimethyl yellow solution* and shake; a red colour is produced in the chloroform layer. Add 50 mg of *cetrimide* and shake; the chloroform layer is yellow.

Related non-ionic substances Comply with the test described under Docusate Sodium, but for the preparation of each of solutions (1) and (2) use the total residue obtained as follows in place of the substance being examined. Shake a quantity of the powdered tablets containing 0.1 g of Docusate Sodium for 30 minutes with 50 ml of n-*hexane*, centrifuge, filter the supernatant liquid and evaporate the filtrate to dryness.

Assay Weigh and powder 20 tablets. To a quantity of the powder containing 50 mg of Docusate Sodium add 8 ml of *propan-2-ol,* mix with the aid of ultrasound for 5 minutes and add sufficient *propan-2-ol* to produce 10 ml. Centrifuge and dilute 5 ml of the supernatant liquid to 250 ml with *water.* To 4 ml add 20 ml of a 1.6% w/v solution of *sodium sulphate* in 0.1M *sulphuric acid* and 4 ml of *basic fuchsin solution.* Mix and extract immediately with four 20-ml quantities of *chloroform,* filtering each extract successively through absorbent cotton moistened with *chloroform.* Wash the cotton with *chloroform* and dilute the combined washings and extracts to 100 ml with *chloroform.* Measure the *absorbance* of the resulting solution at the maximum at 557 nm, Appendix II B, using in the reference cell a solution prepared using 4 ml of *water* and beginning at the words 'add 20 ml of ...'. Calculate the content of $C_{20}H_{37}NaO_7S$ from the *absorbance* of a solution obtained by repeating the procedure, using 4 ml of a solution prepared by dissolving 50 mg of *docusate sodium BPCRS* in sufficient *propan-2-ol* to produce 10 ml and diluting 5 ml to 250 ml with *water*, and beginning at the words 'add 20 ml of ...'.

Dopamine Intravenous Infusion

Definition Dopamine Intravenous Infusion is a sterile solution of Dopamine Hydrochloride. It is supplied as a ready-to-use solution in Glucose Intravenous Infusion (50 g per litre) or it is prepared immediately before use in accordance with the manufacturer's instructions either from Sterile Dopamine Concentrate or from Dopamine Hydrochloride for Injection.

The intravenous infusion complies with the requirements stated under Parenteral Preparations and with the following requirements.

Particulate contamination When the ready-to-use solution is supplied in a container with a nominal content of 100 ml or more, or when the volume of the constituted intravenous infusion is 100 ml or more, it complies with the test for *sub-visible particles*, Appendix XIII A.

When supplied as a ready-to-use solution, the intravenous infusion complies with the following requirements.

Content of dopamine hydrochloride, $C_8H_{11}NO_2$,HCl 95.0% to 105.0% of the prescribed or stated amount.

Content of glucose, $C_6H_{12}O_6$ 4.75 to 5.25% w/v.

Characteristics A colourless liquid.

Identification

A. Saturate a volume containing 0.1 g of Dopamine Hydrochloride with *sodium chloride* and extract with three 20-ml quantities of *butan-1-ol*. Filter the combined extracts through *anhydrous sodium sulphate* and evaporate the filtrate to dryness. The *infrared absorption spectrum* of the residue, Appendix II A, is concordant with the *reference spectrum* of dopamine hydrochloride.

B. To a volume containing 10 mg of Dopamine Hydrochloride add 0.1 ml of *iron(III) chloride solution R1*. An intense green colour is produced.

Acidity pH, 3.0 to 4.5, Appendix V L.

5-Hydroxymethylfurfural Carry out the method for *liquid chromatography*, Appendix III D, using the following solutions. For solution (1) use the intravenous infusion. Solution (2) contains 0.0025% w/v of *5-hydroxymethylfurfural* in *water*.

The chromatographic procedure may be carried out using (a) a stainless steel column (10 cm × 4.6 mm) packed with *stationary phase C* (5 µm) (Nucleosil C18 is suitable), (b) 0.05M *disodium hydrogen orthophosphate* adjusted to pH 7.0 with *orthophosphoric acid* as the mobile phase with a flow rate of 2.0 ml per minute and (c) a detection wavelength of 284 nm.

The area of any peak corresponding to 5-hydroxymethylfurfural in the chromatogram obtained with solution (1) is not greater than the area of the peak in the chromatogram obtained with solution (2) (1%).

Related substances Carry out the method for *liquid chromatography*, Appendix III D, using the following solutions. For solution (1) dilute 1 volume of solution (2) to 50 volumes with the mobile phase. For solution (2) dilute the infusion with the mobile phase to produce a solution containing 0.032% w/v of Dopamine Hydrochloride. For solution (3) dilute 1 volume of solution (2) and 1 volume of a solution containing 0.030% w/v each of *4-ethylcatechol* and *3,4-dimethoxyphenethylamine* to 50 volumes with the mobile phase.

The chromatographic conditions described under the Assay for dopamine hydrochloride may be used.

Examine the chromatogram obtained with solution (3). The test is not valid unless the retention time of the peak due to 4-ethylcatechol is about 3.5 minutes, that due to dopamine is about 5.5 minutes and that due to 3,4 dimethoxyphenethylamine is about 12 minutes. If necessary, adjust the amount of acetonitrile used in the mobile phase to achieve the required retention times.

The area of any *secondary peak* in the chromatogram obtained with solution (2) is not greater than the area of the principal peak in the chromatogram obtained with solution (1).

Assay

For dopamine hydrochloride Carry out the method for *liquid chromatography*, Appendix III D, using the following solutions. Solution (1) contains 0.0032% w/v of *dopamine hydrochloride BPCRS* in the mobile phase. For solution (2) dilute a suitable volume of the infusion with the mobile phase to produce a solution containing 0.0032% w/v of Dopamine Hydrochloride.

The chromatographic procedure may be carried out using (a) a stainless steel column (10 cm × 4.6 mm) packed with *stationary phase C* (5 µm) (Nucleosil C18 is suitable), (b) a mixture of 700 volumes of 0.005M *sodium dodecyl sulphate*, 300 volumes of *acetonitrile*, 10 volumes of *glacial acetic acid* and 2 volumes of 0.1M *disodium edetate* as the mobile phase with a flow rate of 2 ml per minute and (c) a detection wavelength of 280 nm.

Calculate the content of $C_8H_{11}NO_2$,HCl using the declared content of $C_8H_{11}NO_2$,HCl in *dopamine hydrochloride BPCRS*.

For glucose To 50 ml add 0.2 ml of 5M *ammonia* and sufficient *water* to produce 100 ml. Mix well, allow to stand for 30 minutes and determine the *optical rotation* in a 2-dm tube, Appendix V F. The observed rotation in degrees multiplied by 0.9477 represents the weight in g of glucose, $C_6H_{12}O_6$, in the volume taken for assay.

STERILE DOPAMINE CONCENTRATE

Definition Sterile Dopamine Concentrate is a sterile solution of Dopamine Hydrochloride in Water for Injections.

The concentrate complies with the requirements for Concentrated Solutions for Injections stated under Parenteral Preparations and with the following requirements.

Content of dopamine hydrochloride, $C_8H_{11}NO_2$,HCl 95.0 to 105.0% of the prescribed or stated amount.

Characteristics A colourless or pale yellow solution.

Identification

A. Extract a volume containing 0.1 g of Dopamine Hydrochloride with 10 ml of *butan-1-ol*. Filter the extract through *anhydrous sodium sulphate* and evaporate the filtrate to dryness. The *infrared absorption spectrum* of the residue, Appendix II A, is concordant with the *reference spectrum* of dopamine hydrochloride.

B. To a volume containing 10 mg of Dopamine Hydrochloride add 0.05 ml of *iron(III) chloride solution R1*. An intense green colour is produced.

Acidity pH, 2.5 to 5.5, Appendix V L.

Related substances Carry out the method for *thin-layer chromatography*, Appendix III A, using *silica gel G* as the coating substance and a mixture of 2 volumes of *anhydrous formic acid*, 7 volumes of *water*, 36 volumes of *methanol* and 52 volumes of *chloroform* as the mobile phase. Apply separately to the plate 10 µl of each of the following solutions. For solution (1) dilute a volume of the concentrate containing 0.15 g of Dopamine Hydrochloride to 5 ml with *methanol*. Solution (2) contains 0.0075% w/v of *4-O-methyldopamine hydrochloride* in *methanol*. Solution (3) contains 0.0075% w/v each of *3-O-methyldopamine hydrochloride* and *4-O-methyldopamine hydrochloride* in *methanol*. After removal of the plate, allow it to dry in air for 15 minutes and spray evenly and abundantly with a mixture, prepared immediately before use, of equal volumes of *iron(III) chloride solution R1* and *potassium hexacyanoferrate(III) solution*. In the chromatogram obtained with solution (1) any spot with an Rf value higher than that of the principal spot is not more intense than the spot in the chromatogram obtained with solution (2) (0.25%). The test is not valid unless the chromatogram obtained with solution (3) shows two clearly separated spots.

Assay Carry out the method for Assay of dopamine hydrochloride described in the requirements for the ready-to-use infusion.

Storage Sterile Dopamine Concentrate should be protected from light.

Labelling The label states that the solution must not be diluted with alkaline solutions.

DOPAMINE HYDROCHLORIDE FOR INJECTION

Definition Dopamine Hydrochloride for Injection is a sterile material consisting of Dopamine Hydrochloride with or without excipients. It is supplied in a sealed container.

The contents of the sealed container comply with the requirements for Powders for Injections stated under Parenteral Preparations and with the following requirements.

Content of dopamine hydrochloride, $C_8H_{11}NO_2,HCl$ 95.0 to 105.0% of the prescribed or stated amount.

Characteristics A white or almost white, crystalline powder.

Identification

A. The *infrared absorption spectrum*, Appendix II A, is concordant with the *reference spectrum* of dopamine hydrochloride.

B. Dissolve 10 mg in 2 ml of *water* and add 0.05 ml of *iron(III) chloride solution R1*. An intense green colour is produced.

Acidity pH of a 4% w/v solution in a 1.0% w/v solution of *sodium metabisulphite*, 2.5 to 5.5, Appendix V L.

Related substances Carry out the method for *thin-layer chromatography*, Appendix III A, using *silica gel G* as the coating substance and a mixture of 2 volumes of *anhydrous formic acid*, 7 volumes of *water*, 36 volumes of *methanol* and 52 volumes of *chloroform* as the mobile phase. Apply separately to the plate 10 µl of each of three solutions in *methanol* containing (1) 3.0% w/v of the substance being examined, (2) 0.0075% w/v of *4-O-methyldopamine hydrochloride* and (3) 0.0075% w/v each of *3-O-methyldopamine hydrochloride* and *4-O-methyldopamine hydrochloride*. After removal of the plate, allow it to dry in air for 15 minutes and spray evenly and abundantly with a mixture, prepared immediately before use, of equal volumes of *iron(III) chloride solution R1* and *potassium hexacyanoferrate(III) solution*. In the chromatogram obtained with solution (1) any spot with an Rf value higher than that of the principal spot is not more intense than the spot in the chromatogram obtained with solution (2) (0.25%). The test is not valid unless the chromatogram obtained with solution (3) shows two clearly separated spots.

Assay Determine the weight of the contents of 10 containers as described in the test for Uniformity of weight under Parenteral Preparations, Powders for Injections. Carry out the method for *liquid chromatography*, Appendix III D, using the following solutions. Solution (1) contains 0.0032% w/v of *dopamine hydrochloride BPCRS* in the mobile phase. For solution (2) dissolve sufficient of the mixed contents of the 10 containers in the mobile phase to produce a solution containing 0.0032% w/v of dopamine hydrochloride.

The chromatographic procedure described under Assay for dopamine hydrochloride in the requirements for the ready-to-use infusion may be used.

Calculate the content of $C_8H_{11}NO_2,HCl$ in a container of average content weight using the declared content of $C_8H_{11}NO_2,HCl$ in *dopamine hydrochloride BPCRS*.

Dosulepin Capsules
Dothiepin Capsules

For the purposes of product labelling in the United Kingdom, the pair of names given above shall be used together (see Introduction, Changes in title).

Definition Dosulepin Capsules contain Dosulepin Hydrochloride.

The capsules comply with the requirements stated under Capsules and with the following requirements.

Content of dosulepin hydrochloride, $C_{19}H_{21}NS,HCl$ 92.5 to 107.5% of the prescribed or stated amount.

Identification Extract a quantity of the contents of the capsules containing 0.1 g of Dosulepin Hydrochloride with 20 ml of *absolute ethanol*, filter and remove the ethanol from the filtrate by evaporation. The *infrared absorption spectrum* of the residue, Appendix II A, is concordant with the *reference spectrum* of dosulepin hydrochloride.

Related compounds Comply with the test for Related substances described under Dosulepin Hydrochloride but using a silica gel F_{254} precoated plate (Merck silica gel 60 F_{254} plates are suitable) and using the following solutions. For solution (1) extract a quantity of the contents of the capsules containing 0.25 g of Dosulepin Hydrochloride by shaking for 2 minutes with 5 ml of *chloroform*, centrifuge and use the supernatant liquid. For solution (2) dilute 2 ml of solution (1) to 5 ml with *chloroform*.

***Z*-Isomer** Comply with the test described under Dosulepin Hydrochloride but using as solution (2) the supernatant liquid obtained by extracting a quantity of the mixed contents of 20 capsules containing 25 mg of Dosulepin Hydrochloride with 5 ml of *methanol* and centrifuging.

Assay Extract a quantity of the mixed contents of 20 capsules containing 0.5 g of Dosulepin Hydrochloride with 20 ml followed by four 10-ml quantities of *chloroform*, filtering each extract through the same filter. Evaporate the combined extracts to dryness, dissolve the residue in 100 ml of *acetone*, add 10 ml of *mercury(II) acetate solution* and carry out Method I for *non-aqueous titration*, Appendix VIII A, using 3 ml of a saturated solution of *methyl orange* in *acetone* as indicator. Each ml of 0.1M *perchloric acid VS* is equivalent to 33.19 mg of $C_{19}H_{21}NS,HCl$.

Labelling The label states 'Dosulepin Capsules' and 'Dothiepin Capsules'.

Dosulepin Tablets
Dothiepin Tablets

For the purposes of product labelling in the United Kingdom, the pair of names given above shall be used together (see Introduction, Changes in title).

Definition Dosulepin Tablets contain Dosulepin Hydrochloride. They are coated.

The tablets comply with the requirements stated under Tablets and with the following requirements.

Content of dosulepin hydrochloride, $C_{19}H_{21}NS,HCl$ 95.0 to 105.0% of the prescribed or stated amount.

Identification Remove the coating. Shake a quantity of the powdered tablet cores containing 0.2 g of Dosulepin Hydrochloride with 20 ml of *dichloromethane*, centrifuge, filter the supernatant liquid and evaporate the filtrate to dryness. Dissolve the residue in the minimum quantity of *ethanol (70%)* and add an excess of *ether*. Filter the precipitate, wash with *ether* and dry at 60° at a pressure of 2 kPa for 5 minutes. The *infrared absorption spectrum* of the residue, Appendix II A, is concordant with the *reference spectrum* of dosulepin hydrochloride. Examine the substance as a dispersion in *liquid paraffin*.

Related substances Carry out the test described under Dosulepin Hydrochloride but using a silica gel 60 F_{254} precoated plate (Merck silica gel 60 F_{254} plates are suitable) and using the following solutions. For solution (1) shake a quantity of the powdered tablets containing 0.25 g of Dosulepin Hydrochloride for 2 minutes with 5 ml of *dichloromethane*, centrifuge and use the supernatant liquid. For solution (2) dilute 2 ml of solution (1) to 5 ml with *dichloromethane*. Solution (3) contains 0.010% w/v each of *11-(3-dimethylaminopropylidene)-6H-dibenzo*[b,e]*thiepin 5-oxide BPCRS* and *6H-dibenzo*[b,e]*thiepin-11-one BPCRS* in *chloroform*.

In the chromatogram obtained with solution (3) the spot with the lower Rf value is more intense than any corresponding spot in the chromatogram obtained with solution (2) (0.5%). In the chromatogram obtained with solution (1) any *secondary spot* other than any spot corresponding to the spot with the lower Rf value in the chromatogram obtained with solution (3) is not more intense than the proximate spot in the chromatogram obtained with solution (3) (0.2%).

***Z*-Isomer** Carry out the test described under Dosulepin Hydrochloride but using as solution (2) the supernatant liquid obtained by shaking a quantity of the powdered tablets containing 25 mg of Dosulepin Hydrochloride with 5 ml of *methanol* for 15 minutes and centrifuging.

In the chromatogram obtained with solution (1) a peak due to *Z*-dosulepin is present with a retention time of approximately 0.83 relative to the retention time of the principal peak which is due to *E*-dosulepin. In the chromatogram obtained with solution (2) the area of any peak corresponding to *Z*-dosulepin is not greater than 7.5% of the sum of the areas of the peaks due to *Z*-dosulepin and *E*-dosulepin.

Assay Weigh and powder 20 tablets. Carry out the method for *liquid chromatography*, Appendix III D, using the following solutions. For solution (1) shake a quantity of the powdered tablets containing 50 mg of Dosulepin Hydrochloride with 60 ml of 0.1M *hydrochloric acid* for 30 minutes, dilute to 100 ml with 0.1M *hydrochloric acid* and filter. Discard the first 25 ml of the filtrate. Dilute 25 ml of the remaining filtrate to 100 ml with 0.1M *hydrochloric acid*. Solution (2) contains 0.0125% w/v of *dosulepin hydrochloride BPCRS* in 0.1M *hydrochloric acid*.

The chromatographic procedure may be carried out using (a) a stainless steel column (25 cm × 4.6 mm) packed with *stationary phase C* (5 µm) (Spherisorb ODS 1 is suitable), (b) as the mobile phase with a flow rate of 1.5 ml per minute a mixture of 10 volumes of *tetrahydrofuran*, 40 volumes of *acetonitrile* and 50 volumes of a 0.5% w/v solution of *potassium dihydrogen orthophosphate*, the pH of the mixture being adjusted to 3.0 with *orthophosphoric acid* and (c) a detection wavelength of 231 nm.

Calculate the content of $C_{19}H_{21}NS,HCl$ using the declared content of $C_{19}H_{21}NS,HCl$ in *dosulepin hydrochloride BPCRS*.

Labelling The label states 'Dosulepin Tablets' and 'Dothiepin Tablets'.

Doxapram Injection

Definition Doxapram Injection is a sterile solution of Doxapram Hydrochloride in Water for Injections.

The injection complies with the requirements stated under Parenteral Preparations and with the following requirements.

Content of doxapram hydrochloride, $C_{24}H_{30}N_2O_2,HCl,H_2O$ 90.0 to 110.0% of the prescribed or stated amount.

Identification

A. To a volume containing 50 mg of Doxapram Hydrochloride add 10 ml of *water* and 2 ml of 1M *sodium hydroxide* and extract with two 10-ml quantities of *ether*. Wash the combined extracts with 5 ml of *water*, dry over *anhydrous sodium sulphate*, filter and evaporate to dryness. Recrystallise the residue from 10 ml of 0.01M *methanolic hydrochloric acid*. The *infrared absorption spectrum* of the dried residue, Appendix II A, is concordant with the *reference spectrum* of doxapram hydrochloride.

B. The *light absorption*, Appendix II B, in the range 230 to 350 nm of the solution obtained in the Assay exhibits maxima at 253, 258 and 265 nm.

C. Yields the reactions characteristic of *chlorides*, Appendix VI.

Acidity pH of a solution containing 1% w/v of Doxapram Hydrochloride, 3.5 to 5.0, Appendix V L.

Assay Dilute a volume containing 0.2 g of Doxapram Hydrochloride to 250 ml with *water*. Measure the *absorbance* of the resulting solution at the maximum at 258 nm, Appendix II B. Calculate the content of $C_{24}H_{30}N_2O_2$, HCl,H_2O from the *absorbance* of a 0.08% w/v solution of *doxapram hydrochloride BPCRS*.

Storage Doxapram Injection should be stored at a temperature not exceeding 25°. It should not be allowed to freeze.

Doxepin Capsules

Definition Doxepin Capsules contain Doxepin Hydrochloride.

The capsules comply with the requirements stated under Capsules and with the following requirements.

Content of doxepin, $C_{19}H_{21}NO$ 90.0 to 110.0% of the prescribed or stated amount.

Identification Wash a quantity of the contents of the capsules containing the equivalent of 0.1 g of doxepin with three 5-ml quantities of *petroleum spirit (boiling range, 40° to 60°)*. Dry in air, extract the residue with three 10-ml quantities of *chloroform*, evaporate the combined extracts to dryness and dry the residue at 105°. The residue complies with the following tests.

A. The *infrared absorption spectrum*, Appendix II A, is concordant with the *reference spectrum* of doxepin hydrochloride.

B. Yields reaction A characteristic of *chlorides*, Appendix VI.

Z-Isomer 13.0 to 18.5% when determined by the following method. Carry out the method for *gas chromatography*, Appendix III B, using the following solutions. For solution (1) extract a quantity of the mixed contents of 20 capsules containing the equivalent of 25 mg of doxepin with 5 ml of *methanol*, centrifuge and use the supernatant liquid. Solution (2) contains 0.5% w/v of *doxepin hydrochloride BPCRS* in *methanol*.

The chromatographic procedure may be carried out using a glass column (1.5 m × 4 mm) packed with *acid-washed, silanised diatomaceous support* (100 to 120 mesh) coated with 3% w/w of cyanopropylmethyl phenyl methyl silicone fluid (OV-225 is suitable) and maintained at 200°.

In the chromatogram obtained with solution (2) a peak due to *Z*-doxepin immediately precedes, and is adequately separated from, the principal peak which is due to *E*-doxepin. Measure the areas or heights of the peaks due to *Z*- and *E*-isomers in the chromatograms obtained with solutions (1) and (2) and calculate the content of *Z*-isomer in the substance being examined using the declared content of *Z*-isomer in *doxepin hydrochloride BPCRS*.

Assay To a quantity of the mixed contents of 20 capsules containing the equivalent of 30 mg of doxepin add 50 ml of 0.01M *methanolic hydrochloric acid*, shake for 30 minutes and add sufficient 0.01M *methanolic hydrochloric acid* to produce 100 ml. Centrifuge 40 ml, dilute 10 ml of the clear solution to 100 ml with 0.01M *methanolic hydrochloric acid* and measure the *absorbance* of the resulting solution at the maximum at 297 nm, Appendix II B. Calculate the content of $C_{19}H_{21}NO$ taking 150 as the value of A(1%, 1 cm) at the maximum at 297 nm.

Labelling The quantity of active ingredient is stated in terms of the equivalent amount of doxepin.

Doxorubicin Injection

Definition Doxorubicin Injection is a sterile solution of Doxorubicin Hydrochloride in Water for Injections or Sodium Chloride Injection. It is either supplied as a ready-to-use solution or it is prepared by dissolving Doxorubicin Hydrochloride for Injection in the requisite amount of Water for Injections or Sodium Chloride Injection.

The injection complies with the requirements stated under Parenteral Preparations and, when supplied as a ready-to-use solution, with the following requirements.

Characteristics A red solution.

Content of doxorubicin hydrochloride, $C_{27}H_{29}NO_{11}$, HCl 95.0 to 110.0% of the prescribed or stated amount.

Identification

A. Dilute the injection with sufficient *ethanol (96%)* to produce a solution containing 0.001% w/v of Doxorubicin Hydrochloride. The *light absorption* of the resulting solution, Appendix II B, in the range 220 to 550 nm exhibits two maxima, at 234 and 252 nm, and four less clearly defined maxima at 288, 475, 495 and 530 nm.

B. In the test for Related substances, the principal spot in the chromatogram obtained with solution (1) is similar in position, colour and size to that in the chromatogram obtained with solution (2) and differs in position from that in the chromatogram obtained with solution (3).

C. In the Assay, the retention time of the principal peak in the chromatogram obtained with solution (1) corresponds to that of the principal peak in the chromatogram obtained with solution (2).

Acidity pH, 2.5 to 3.5, Appendix V L.

Related substances Carry out the method for *thin-layer chromatography*, Appendix III A, using a silica gel precoated plate (Merck silica gel 60 plates are suitable) and a mixture of 1 volume of *water*, 2 volumes of *anhydrous formic acid*, 15 volumes of *methanol* and 82 volumes of *dichloromethane* as the mobile phase in an unsaturated tank. Apply separately to the plate, as 5 mm bands, 25 µl of each of the following solutions. For solution (1) dilute the injection, if necessary, with *methanol (90%)* to produce a solution containing 0.2% w/v of Doxorubicin Hydrochloride. Solution (2) contains 0.20% w/v of *doxorubicin hydrochloride EPCRS* in *methanol (90%)*. Solution (3) contains 0.20% w/v of *daunorubicin hydrochloride EPCRS* in *methanol (90%)*. Solution (4) contains 0.0010% w/v of *doxorubicin aglycone EPCRS* in *dichloromethane*. Solution (5) contains 0.0040% w/v of *doxorubicin hydrochloride EPCRS* in *methanol*. After removal of the plate, allow it to dry in air and examine immediately. In the chromatogram obtained with solution (1) any spot corresponding to doxorubicin aglycone is not more intense than the principal spot in the chromatogram obtained with solution (4) (0.5%) and any other *secondary spot* is not more intense than the principal spot in the chromatogram obtained with solution (5) (2%).

Bacterial endotoxins Carry out the *test for bacterial endotoxins*, Appendix XIV C. Dilute the injection, if necessary, with *water BET* to give a solution containing 2 mg of Doxorubicin Hydrochloride per ml (solution A). The endotoxin limit concentration of solution A is 4.4 IU of endotoxin per ml. Carry out the test using the maximum valid dilution of solution A calculated from the declared sensitivity of the lysate used in the test.

Assay Carry out the method for *liquid chromatography*, Appendix III D, injecting 20 µl of each of the following solutions in the mobile phase. For solution (1) dilute a volume of the injection to produce a solution containing 0.05% w/v of Doxorubicin Hydrochloride. Solution (2) contains 0.05% w/v of *doxorubicin hydrochloride EPCRS*. Solution (3) contains 0.002% w/v each of *doxorubicin hydrochloride EPCRS* and *epirubicin EPCRS*.

The chromatographic procedure may be carried out using (a) a stainless steel column (25 cm × 4.6 mm) packed with *stationary phase C* (5 µm) (Hypersil ODS and Partisil 5 ODS 3 are suitable), (b) as the mobile phase with a flow rate of 0.8 ml per minute a mixture of 5 volumes of *methanol R1*, 45 volumes of *acetonitrile* and 50 volumes of a solution containing 0.288% w/v of *sodium dodecyl sulphate* and 0.230% w/v of *orthophosphoric acid* and (c) a detection wavelength of 254 nm.

The assay is not valid unless, in the chromatogram obtained with solution (3), the *resolution factor* between the peaks due to doxorubicin and epirubicin is at least 2.0. If necessary, adjust the operating conditions.

Calculate the content of $C_{27}H_{29}NO_{11},HCl$ in the injection using the declared content of $C_{27}H_{29}NO_{11},HCl$ in *doxorubicin hydrochloride EPCRS*.

Storage When supplied as a ready-to-use solution, Doxorubicin Injection should be stored at a temperature of 2° to 8°.

Doxorubicin Injection prepared by dissolving the contents of a sealed container in the liquid stated on the label should be used immediately after preparation but, in any case, within the period recommended by the manufacturer when prepared and stored strictly in accordance with the manufacturer's instructions.

DOXORUBICIN HYDROCHLORIDE FOR INJECTION

Definition Doxorubicin Hydrochloride for Injection is a sterile material consisting of Doxorubicin Hydrochloride with or without excipients. It is supplied in a sealed container.

The contents of the sealed container comply with the requirements for Powders for Injections stated under Parenteral Preparations and with the following requirements.

Content of doxorubicin hydrochloride, $C_{27}H_{29}NO_{11}$, HCl 90.0 to 110.0% of the prescribed or stated amount.

Identification

A. Shake a quantity of the powder containing 10 mg of Doxorubicin Hydrochloride with 5 ml of 0.01M *hydrochloric acid*, extract 2 ml of the resulting solution with two 5-ml quantities of *ether* and discard the ether layer. Dilute the aqueous solution with *ethanol (96%)* to contain 0.001% w/v of Doxorubicin Hydrochloride. The *light absorption* of the resulting solution, Appendix II B, in the range 220 to 550 nm exhibits two maxima, at 234 and 252 nm, and four less clearly defined maxima at 288, 475, 495 and 530 nm.

B. In the test for Related substances, the principal spot in the chromatogram obtained with solution (2) is similar in position, colour and size to that in the chromatogram obtained with solution (3) and differs in position from that in the chromatogram obtained with solution (4).

C. In the Assay, the retention time of the principal peak in the chromatogram obtained with solution (1) corresponds to that of the principal peak in the chromatogram obtained with solution (2).

Acidity pH of a 0.2% w/v solution in *water for injections*, 4.5 to 6.5, Appendix V L.

Related substances Carry out the method for *thin-layer chromatography*, Appendix III A, using a silica gel precoated plate (Merck silica gel 60 plates are suitable) and a mixture of 1 volume of *water*, 2 volumes of *anhydrous formic acid*, 15 volumes of *methanol* and 82 volumes of *dichloromethane* as the mobile phase in an unsaturated tank. Apply separately to the plate 10 µl of each of the following solutions. For solution (1) shake a quantity of the powder containing 20 mg of Doxorubicin Hydrochloride with 2 ml of *methanol (90%)*, allow to stand and use the supernatant liquid. For solution (2) dilute 1 ml of solution (1) to 5 ml with *methanol (90%)*. Solution (3) contains 0.20% w/v of *doxorubicin hydrochloride EPCRS* in *methanol (90%)*. Solution (4) contains 0.20% w/v of *daunorubicin hydrochloride EPCRS* in *methanol (90%)*. Solution (5) contains 0.0050% w/v of *doxorubicin aglycone EPCRS* in *dichloromethane*. Solution (6) contains 0.0050% w/v of *doxorubicin hydrochloride EPCRS* in *methanol*. After removal of the plate, allow it to dry in air and examine immediately. In the chromatogram obtained with solution (1) any spot corresponding to doxorubicin aglycone is not more intense than the principal spot in the chromatogram obtained with solution (5) (0.5%) and any other *secondary spot* is not more intense than the principal spot in the chromatogram obtained with solution (6) (0.5%).

Water Not more than 4.0% w/w, Appendix IX C. Use 0.1 g.

Bacterial endotoxins Carry out the *test for bacterial endotoxins*, Appendix XIV C. Dissolve the contents of the sealed container in *water BET* to give a solution containing 10 mg of Doxorubicin Hydrochloride per ml (solution A). The endotoxin limit concentration of solution A is 22 IU of endotoxin per ml. Carry out the test using the maximum valid dilution of solution A calculated from the declared sensitivity of the lysate used in the test.

Assay Determine the weight of the contents of 10 containers as described in the test for Uniformity of weight under Parenteral Preparations, Powders for Injections. Carry out the method for *liquid chromatography*, Appendix III D, injecting 20 µl of each of three solutions in the mobile phase. For solution (1) dissolve a sufficient quantity of the mixed contents of the 10 containers to produce a solution containing 0.05% w/v of Doxorubicin Hydrochloride. Solution (2) contains 0.05% w/v of *doxorubicin hydrochloride EPCRS*. Solution (3) contains 0.002% w/v each of *doxorubicin hydrochloride EPCRS* and *epirubicin hydrochloride EPCRS*.

The chromatographic procedure described under the Assay for the ready-to-use solution may be used.

The assay is not valid unless in the chromatogram obtained with solution (3) the *resolution factor* between the peaks due to doxorubicin and epirubicin is at least 2.0. If necessary, adjust the operating conditions.

Calculate the content of $C_{27}H_{29}NO_{11}$,HCl using the declared content of $C_{27}H_{29}NO_{11}$,HCl in *doxorubicin hydrochloride EPCRS*.

Storage The sealed container should be stored at a temperature not exceeding 25°.

Doxycycline Capsules

Definition Doxycycline Capsules contain Doxycycline Hyclate.

The capsules comply with the requirements stated under Capsules and with the following requirements.

Content of anhydrous doxycycline, $C_{22}H_{24}N_2O_8$ 95.0 to 105.0% of the prescribed or stated amount.

Identification

A. Carry out the method for *thin-layer chromatography*, Appendix III A, using *silica gel H* as the coating substance and a mixture of 6 volumes of *water*, 35 volumes of *methanol* and 59 volumes of *dichloromethane* as the mobile phase. Spray the plate evenly with a 10% w/v solution of *disodium edetate* the pH of which has been adjusted to 9.0 with 10M *sodium hydroxide* (about 10 ml for a 100 mm × 200 mm plate). Allow the plate to dry in a horizontal position for at least 1 hour. Immediately before use dry it at 110° for 1 hour. Apply separately to the plate 1 µl of each of the following solutions. For solution (1) shake a quantity of the contents of the capsules containing the equivalent of 50 mg of anhydrous doxycycline with 100 ml of *methanol* for 1 to 2 minutes, centrifuge and use the supernatant liquid. Solution (2) contains 0.05% w/v of *doxycycline hyclate EPCRS* in *methanol*. Solution (3) contains 0.05% w/v each of *doxycycline hyclate EPCRS* and *tetracycline hydrochloride EPCRS* in *methanol*. After removal of the plate, dry it in a current of air and examine under *ultraviolet light (365 nm)*. The principal spot in the chromatogram obtained with solution (1) is similar in position, colour and size to that in the chromatogram obtained with solution (2). The test is not valid unless the chromatogram obtained with solution (3) shows two clearly separated spots.

B. To 0.5 mg of the contents of the capsules add 2 ml of *sulphuric acid*. A yellow colour is produced.

C. The contents of the capsules yield the reactions characteristic of *chlorides*, Appendix VI.

Light-absorbing impurities Dissolve the contents of five capsules as completely as possible in sufficient of a mixture of 1 volume of 1M *hydrochloric acid* and 99 volumes of *methanol* to produce a solution containing the equivalent of 1.0% w/v of anhydrous doxycycline and filter. The *absorbance* of the filtrate at 490 nm is not more than 0.20, calculated with reference to the dried capsule contents, Appendix II B.

Related substances Carry out the method for *liquid chromatography*, Appendix III D, using the following solutions. For solution (1) dissolve a quantity of the contents of the capsules containing the equivalent of 7.0 mg of anhydrous doxycycline in 10 ml of 0.01M *hydrochloric acid*, filter and use the filtrate. Solutions (2) to (5) are solutions in 0.01M *hydrochloric acid* containing (2) 0.080% w/v of *doxycycline hyclate EPCRS*, (3) 0.080% w/v of *6-epidoxycycline hydrochloride EPCRS*, (4) 0.080% w/v of *metacycline hydrochloride EPCRS* and (5) 0.0016% w/v each of *6-epidoxycycline hydrochloride EPCRS* and *metacycline hydrochloride EPCRS*. For solution (6) dilute a mixture of 4 volumes of solution (2), 1.5 volumes of solution (3) and 1 volume of solution (4) to 25 volumes with 0.01M *hydrochloric acid*.

The chromatographic procedure may be carried out using (a) a column (25 cm × 4.6 mm) packed with styrene—divinylbenzene co-polymer (8 µm) with a pore size of 10 nm (PLRP-S from Polymer Laboratories is suitable) and maintained at 60°, (b) as the mobile phase with a flow rate of 1 ml per minute a solution prepared as described below and (c) a detection wavelength of 254 nm. For the mobile phase add 60 g of *2-methylpropan-2-ol* to a graduated flask with the aid of 200 ml of *water*, add 400 ml of *phosphate buffer pH 8.0*, 50 ml of a 1% w/v solution of *tetrabutylammonium hydrogen sulphate* previously adjusted to pH 8.0 with 2M *sodium hydroxide* and 10 ml of a 4% w/v solution of *disodium edetate* previously adjusted to pH 8.0 with 2M *sodium hydroxide* and dilute to 1 litre with *water*. Inject 20 µl of each solution.

Using solution (6) adjust the attenuation to obtain peaks with a height corresponding to at least 50% of full-scale deflection of the recorder. The test is not valid unless (a) the *resolution factor* between the first peak (methacycline) and the second peak (6-epidoxycycline) is at least 1.25 and (b) the *resolution factor* between the second peak and the third peak (doxycycline) is at least 2.0 (adjust the content of 2-methylpropan-2-ol in the mobile phase if necessary).

In the chromatogram obtained with solution (1) the area of any peak corresponding to methacycline or 6-epidoxycycline is not greater than the area of the corresponding peak in the chromatogram obtained with solution (5) (2%, with reference to doxycycline hyclate); the area of any peak appearing between the solvent peak and the peak corresponding to methacycline and the area of any peak appearing on the tail of the main peak is not greater than 25% of that of the peak corresponding to 6-epidoxycycline in the chromatogram obtained with solution (5) (0.5%, with reference to doxycycline hyclate).

Loss on drying When dried at 105° for 2 hours, the contents of the capsules lose not more than 8.5% of their weight. Use 1 g.

Assay Carry out the method for *liquid chromatography*, Appendix III D, using the following solutions. For solution (1) dissolve the mixed contents of 20 capsules containing the equivalent of 17.5 mg of anhydrous doxycycline in sufficient 0.01M *hydrochloric acid* to produce 25 ml and dilute 4 ml of the solution to 25 ml with the same solvent. Solution (2) contains 0.0128% w/v of *doxycycline hyclate EPCRS* in 0.01M *hydrochloric acid*.

The chromatographic conditions described under Related substances may be used.

Calculate the content of $C_{22}H_{24}N_2O_8$ using the declared content of $C_{22}H_{24}N_2O_8$ in *doxycycline hyclate EPCRS*.

Labelling The quantity of active ingredient is stated in terms of the equivalent amount of anhydrous doxycycline.

Dydrogesterone Tablets

Definition Dydrogesterone Tablets contain Dydrogesterone.

The tablets comply with the requirements stated under Tablets and with the following requirements.

Content of dydrogesterone, $C_{21}H_{28}O_2$ 92.5 to 107.5% of the prescribed or stated amount.

Identification Extract a quantity of the powdered tablets containing 60 mg of Dydrogesterone with 20 ml of *methanol,* filter and evaporate the filtrate to dryness. The residue complies with the following tests.

A. The *infrared absorption spectrum,* Appendix II A, is concordant with the *reference spectrum* of dydrogesterone.

B. Complies with the test for *identification of steroids,* Appendix III A, using *impregnating solvent II* and *mobile phase E.*

Related substances Comply with the test described under Dydrogesterone using the following solutions. For solution (1) extract a quantity of the powdered tablets containing 20 mg of Dydrogesterone with 50 ml of a 0.020% w/v solution of *1,2,3,4-tetraphenylcyclopenta-1,3-diene* (internal standard) in *chloroform* and filter. For solution (2) extract a quantity of the powdered tablets containing 20 mg of Dydrogesterone with 20 ml of *chloroform,* filter, evaporate to dryness using a rotary evaporator and dissolve the residue in 1 ml of *chloroform.* Prepare solution (3) in the same manner as solution (2) but extracting the powdered tablets with 20 ml of a 0.0010% w/v solution of the internal standard in *chloroform.*

Assay Weigh and powder 20 tablets. Shake a quantity of the powder containing 10 mg of Dydrogesterone for 15 minutes with 70 ml of *methanol,* dilute to 200 ml with *methanol* and filter. Dilute 5 ml of the filtrate to 100 ml with *methanol* and measure the *absorbance* of the resulting solution at the maximum at 286 nm, Appendix II B. Calculate the content of $C_{21}H_{28}O_2$ taking 845 as the value of A(1%, 1 cm) at the maximum at 286 nm.

Storage Dydrogesterone Tablets should be protected from light.

Econazole Cream

Definition Econazole Cream contains Econazole Nitrate in a suitable basis.

The cream complies with the requirements stated under Topical Semi-solid Preparations and with the following requirements.

Content of econazole nitrate, $C_{18}H_{15}Cl_3N_2O,HNO_3$ 90.0 to 110.0% of the prescribed or stated amount.

Identification

A. Mix a quantity of the cream containing 40 mg of Econazole Nitrate with 20 ml of a mixture of 1 volume of 1M *sulphuric acid* and 4 volumes of *methanol* and shake with two 50-ml quantities of *carbon tetrachloride,* discarding the organic layers. Make the aqueous phase alkaline with 2M *ammonia* and extract with two 40-ml quantities of *chloroform.* Combine the chloroform extracts, shake with 5 g of *anhydrous sodium sulphate,* filter and dilute the filtrate to 100 ml with *chloroform.* Evaporate 50 ml to dryness and dissolve the residue in 50 ml of a mixture of 1 volume of 0.1M *hydrochloric acid* and 9 volumes of *propan-2-ol.* The *light absorption* of the resulting solution, Appendix II B, in the range 240 to 350 nm exhibits maxima at 265, 271 and 280 nm. The ratio of the *absorbance* at the maximum at 271 nm to that at the maximum at 280 nm is 1.55 to 1.77. The test is not valid unless the ratio of the *absorbance* in the test for *resolution* is at least 2.

B. In the Assay, the principal peak in the chromatogram obtained with solution (4) has the same retention time as the peak due to econazole in the chromatogram obtained with solution (2).

Assay Carry out the method for *liquid chromatography,* Appendix III D, using the following solutions. Solution (1) is a 0.05% w/v solution of miconazole nitrate (internal standard) in *methanol.* Solution (2) is a 0.1% w/v solution of *econazole nitrate BPCRS* in *methanol.* For solution (3) mix 1 g of the cream with 20 ml of solution (1) and 55 ml of *methanol, warm* on a water bath for 30 seconds and shake for 1 minute, repeat the process twice and add 25 ml of a solution prepared by dissolving 2.5 g of *potassium dihydrogen orthophosphate* and 2.5 g of *dipotassium hydrogen orthophosphate* in 1000 ml of *water* (solution A), cool in an ice bath for 15 minutes and centrifuge for 10 minutes; use the supernatant liquid, filtered if necessary. Prepare solution (4) in the same manner as solution (2) but replace solution (1) with 20 ml of *methanol.*

The chromatographic procedure may be carried out using (a) a stainless steel column (5 cm × 4.6 mm) packed with *stationary phase C* (3 μm) (Hypersil ODS is suitable) (alternatively use a 20 cm × 4.6 mm Hypersil ODS 5 μm column), (b) as the mobile phase with a flow rate of 2.0 ml per minute a mixture of 1 volume of solution A and 3 volumes of *methanol* and (c) a detection wavelength of 232 nm.

Calculate the content of $C_{18}H_{15}Cl_3N_2O,HNO_3$ using the declared content of $C_{18}H_{15}Cl_3N_2O,HNO_3$ in *econazole nitrate BPCRS.*

Storage If Econazole Cream is kept in aluminium tubes, their inner surfaces should be coated with a suitable lacquer.

Econazole Pessaries

Definition Econazole Pessaries contain Econazole Nitrate in a suitable basis.

The pessaries comply with the requirements stated under Vaginal Preparations and with the following requirements.

Content of econazole nitrate, $C_{18}H_{15}Cl_3N_2O,HNO_3$ 90.0 to 110.0% of the prescribed or stated amount.

Identification

A. Mix a quantity of the crushed pessaries containing 40 mg of Econazole Nitrate with 20 ml of a mixture of 1 volume of 1M *sulphuric acid* and 4 volumes of *methanol* and shake with two 50-ml quantities of *hexane,* discarding the organic layers. Make the aqueous phase alkaline with 2M *ammonia* and extract with two 40-ml quantities of *chloroform.* Combine the chloroform extracts, shake with 5 g of *anhydrous sodium sulphate,* filter and dilute the filtrate to 100 ml with *chloroform.* Evaporate 50 ml to dryness and dissolve the residue in 50 ml of a mixture of 1 volume of

0.1M *hydrochloric acid* and 9 volumes of *propanol-2-ol*. The *light absorption* of the resulting solution, Appendix II B, in the range 240 to 350 nm exhibits maxima at 265, 271 and 280 nm. The ratio of the *absorbance* at the maximum at 271 nm to that at the maximum at 280 nm is 1.55 to 1.77. The test is not valid unless the ratio of the *absorbance* in the test for *resolution* is at least 2.

B. In the test for Related substances, the principal spot in the chromatogram obtained with solution (1) corresponds to that in the chromatogram obtained with solution (3).

Related substances Carry out the method for *thin-layer chromatography*, Appendix III A, using a silica gel pre-coated plate (Merck silica gel 60 plates are suitable) and a mixture of 70 volumes of *chloroform*, 20 volumes of *methanol* and 10 volumes of an 85% w/v solution of *formic acid* as the mobile phase. Apply separately to the plate 20 µl of each of the following solutions. For solution (1) mix a quantity of the crushed pessaries containing 40 mg of Econazole Nitrate with 40 ml of *methanol* and heat under a reflux condenser for 15 minutes. Allow to cool, filter (Whatman No. 1 paper is suitable), wash the filter paper with *methanol* and evaporate the filtrate and washings to a volume of about 5 ml. Filter (Whatman No. 50 paper is suitable), wash the paper with *methanol*, evaporate the filtrate and washings to dryness and dissolve the residue in 2 ml of *methanol*. For solution (2) dilute 0.5 ml of solution (1) to 100 ml with *methanol*. Solution (3) contains 2% w/v of *econazole nitrate BPCRS* in *methanol*. After removal of the plate, allow it to dry in air and expose to iodine vapour for 1 hour. Any *secondary spot* in the chromatogram obtained with solution (1) is not more intense than the spot in the chromatogram obtained with solution (2). Disregard any spot with an Rf value higher than 0.9.

Assay Dissolve five pessaries in 250 ml of *anhydrous acetic acid* with the aid of gentle heat, allow to cool and carry out Method I for *non-aqueous titration*, Appendix VIII A, using a quantity of the solution containing 0.3 g of Econazole Nitrate and determining the end point potentiometrically. Each ml of 0.1M *perchloric acid VS* is equivalent to 44.47 mg of $C_{18}H_{15}Cl_3N_2O,HNO_3$.

Edrophonium Injection

Definition Edrophonium Injection is a sterile solution of Edrophonium Chloride in Water for Injections.

The injection complies with the requirements stated under Parenteral Preparations and with the following requirements.

Content of edrophonium chloride, $C_{10}H_{16}ClNO$ 95.0 to 105.0% of the prescribed or stated amount.

Identification

A. Dilute a sufficient volume of the injection with 0.1M *sodium hydroxide* to give a solution containing 0.001% w/v of Edrophonium Chloride. The *light absorption* of the resulting solution, Appendix II B, in the range 220 to 350 nm exhibits two maxima, at 240 nm and 294 nm. The *absorbances* at the maxima are about 1.1 and about 0.34 respectively.

B. To a volume containing 20 mg of Edrophonium Chloride add 0.05 ml of *iron(III) chloride solution R1*. A reddish violet colour is produced.

C. Yields reaction A characteristic of *chlorides*, Appendix VI.

Acidity pH, 5.0 to 6.0, Appendix V L.

Dimethylaminophenol To a volume containing 50 mg of Edrophonium Chloride add 10 ml of *phosphate buffer pH 8.0* and extract with two 20-ml quantities of *chloroform*. Wash the extracts successively with two 10-ml quantities of *water*, extract with 10 ml of 0.1M *sodium hydroxide* and discard the chloroform. The *absorbance* of the resulting solution at 293 nm is not more than 0.125, Appendix II B.

Assay To a volume containing 50 mg of Edrophonium Chloride add sufficient *water* to produce 100 ml. Dilute 10 ml of this solution to 100 ml with *water* and measure the *absorbance* of the resulting solution at the maximum at 273 nm, Appendix II B. Calculate the content of $C_{10}H_{16}ClNO$ taking 110 as the value of A(1%, 1 cm) at the maximum at 273 nm.

Storage Edrophonium Injection should be protected from light.

Emulsifying Ointment

Definition

Emulsifying Wax	300 g
White Soft Paraffin	500 g
Liquid Paraffin	200 g

Extemporaneous preparation The following directions apply.

Melt together and stir until cold.

The ointment complies with the requirements stated under Topical Semi-solid Preparations.

Emulsifying Wax

Anionic Emulsifying Wax

Definition Emulsifying Wax contains Cetostearyl Alcohol and either Sodium Laurilsulfate or sodium salts of similar sulphated higher primary aliphatic alcohols.

Extemporaneous preparation The following formula and directions may be used.

Cetostearyl Alcohol	90 g
Sodium Laurilsulfate	10 g
Purified Water	4 ml

Melt the Cetostearyl Alcohol and heat to about 95°. Add the Sodium Laurilsulfate , mix, add the Purified Water, heat to 115° and maintain at this temperature, stirring vigorously, until frothing ceases and the product is translucent. Cool quickly.

Characteristics An almost white or pale yellow, waxy solid or flakes, becoming plastic when warmed; odour, faint and characteristic.

Practically insoluble in *water*, forming an emulsion; partly soluble in *ethanol (96%)*.

Identification

A. *Melting point* of the residue obtained in the test for Unsaponifiable matter, about 52°, Appendix V A.

B. Complies with the test for Sulphated ash.

Acidity To 20 g add a mixture of 40 ml of *ether* and 75 ml of *ethanol (96%)* previously neutralised to *phenolphthalein solution R1* and warm gently until solution is effected. Titrate with 0.1M *sodium hydroxide VS* using *phenolphthalein solution R1* as indicator until a pink colour which persists for at least 15 seconds is obtained. Not more than 1.0 ml of 0.1M *sodium hydroxide VS* is required.

Alkalinity Disperse 5.0 g in 25 ml of warm *ethanol (96%)* previously neutralised to *phenolphthalein solution R1* and cool. No colour is produced on the addition of 0.5 ml of *phenolphthalein solution R1*.

Alcohols To 3.5 g of the residue obtained in the test for Unsaponifiable matter add 12 g of *stearic anhydride* and 10 ml of *xylene* and heat gently under a reflux condenser for 30 minutes. Cool, add a mixture of 40 ml of *pyridine* and 4 ml of *water*, heat under a reflux condenser for a further 30 minutes and titrate the hot solution with 1M *sodium hydroxide VS* using *phenolphthalein solution R1* as indicator. Repeat the operation without the residue. The difference between the titrations is 12.8 to 14.2 ml.

Iodine value Not more than 3.0 *(iodine monochloride method)*, Appendix X E.

Saponification value Not more than 2.0, Appendix X G. Use 20 g.

Sodium alkyl sulphates Not less than 8.7%, calculated as $C_{12}H_{25}O_4SNa$ with reference to the anhydrous substance, when determined by the following method. Dissolve 0.25 g as completely as possible in 15 ml of *chloroform*, add 30 ml of *water*, 10 ml of 1M *sulphuric acid* and 1 ml of *dimethyl yellow—oracet blue B solution* and titrate with *0.004M benzethonium chloride VS*, shaking vigorously and allowing the layers to separate after each addition, until the chloroform layer acquires a permanent clear green colour. Each ml of *0.004M benzethonium chloride VS* is equivalent to 1.154 mg of $C_{12}H_{25}O_4SNa$.

Sulphated ash 2.5 to 4.0%, Appendix IX A.

Unsaponifiable matter Not less than 86.0%, calculated with reference to the anhydrous substance, Appendix X H. Use 5 g and omit the titration of the residue.

Water Not more than 4.0% w/w, Appendix IX C. Use 0.6 g.

Ephedrine Elixir

Ephedrine Oral Solution

Definition Ephedrine Elixir is an *oral solution* containing 0.3% w/v of Ephedrine Hydrochloride in a suitable flavoured vehicle containing a sufficient volume of Ethanol (96 per cent) or of an appropriate Dilute Ethanol to give a final concentration of 12% v/v of ethanol.

The elixir complies with the requirements stated under Oral Liquids and with the following requirements.

Content of ephedrine hydrochloride, $C_{10}H_{15}NO,HCl$
0.27 to 0.33% w/v.

Identification

A. To 30 ml of the elixir add 2 ml of 2M *hydrochloric acid*, extract with two 20-ml quantities of *ether* and discard the ether. Add sufficient 5M *ammonia* to the aqueous phase to make it alkaline, extract with two 30-ml quantities of *ether*, wash the combined ether extracts with three 15-ml quantities of *water*, dry with *anhydrous sodium sulphate*, filter and evaporate the filtrate to dryness. The *infrared absorption spectrum* of the residue, Appendix II A, is concordant with the *reference spectrum* of ephedrine.

B. In the test for Related substances, the principal spot in the chromatogram obtained with solution (2) corresponds to that in the chromatogram obtained with solution (4).

Ethanol content 11 to 13% v/v, Appendix VIII F.

Related substances Carry out the method for *thin-layer chromatography*, Appendix III A, using a silica gel precoated plate (Merck silica gel 60 plates are suitable) and a mixture of 80 volumes of *propan-2-ol*, 15 volumes of 13.5M *ammonia* and 5 volumes of *chloroform* as the mobile phase. Apply separately to the plate 10 µl of each of the following solutions. For solution (1) add sufficient 5M *ammonia* to 50 ml of the elixir to make it alkaline, extract with two 100-ml quantities of *ether*, wash the combined extracts with 10 ml of *water*, dry with *anhydrous sodium sulphate*, filter and evaporate the filtrate to dryness. Dissolve the oily residue in sufficient *methanol* to produce 5 ml. For solution (2) dilute 1 volume of solution (1) to 10 volumes with *methanol*. For solution (3) dilute 1 volume of solution (1) to 200 volumes with *methanol*. Solution (4) contains 0.30% w/v of *ephedrine hydrochloride BPCRS* in *methanol*. After removal of the plate, allow it to dry in air, spray with *ninhydrin solution* and heat at 100° for 5 minutes. Any *secondary spot* in the chromatogram obtained with solution (1) is not more intense than the spot in the chromatogram obtained with solution (3). Disregard any spot of lighter colour than the background.

Assay Carry out the method for *liquid chromatography*, Appendix III D, using the following solutions. For solution (1) dilute a weighed quantity of the elixir containing 60 mg of Ephedrine Hydrochloride to 50 ml with *methanol (65%)*. Solution (2) contains 0.12% w/v of *ephedrine hydrochloride BPCRS* in *methanol*.

The chromatographic procedure may be carried out using (a) a stainless steel column (20 cm × 4.6 mm) packed with *stationary phase C* (10 µm) (Nucleosil C18 is suitable), (b) 0.005M *dioctyl sodium sulphosuccinate* in a mixture of 65 volumes of *methanol*, 35 volumes of *water* and 1 volume of *glacial acetic acid* as the mobile phase with a flow rate of 1.5 ml per minute and (c) a detection wavelength of 263 nm.

Determine the *weight per ml* of the elixir, Appendix V G, and calculate the content of $C_{10}H_{15}NO,HCl$, weight in volume, using the declared content of $C_{10}H_{15}NO,HCl$ in *ephedrine hydrochloride BPCRS*.

Labelling The label indicates the pharmaceutical form as 'oral solution'.

Ephedrine Nasal Drops

Definition Ephedrine Nasal Drops are a solution of Ephedrine Hydrochloride in a suitable aqueous vehicle.

The nasal drops comply with the requirements stated under Nasal Preparations and with the following requirements.

Content of ephedrine hydrochloride, $C_{10}H_{15}NO,HCl$
95.0 to 105.0% of the prescribed or stated amount.

Identification
A. To a quantity of the nasal drops containing 0.1 g of Ephedrine Hydrochloride add 2 ml of 2M *hydrochloric acid*, shake with two 20-ml quantities of *chloroform* and discard the chloroform. Add 5M *ammonia* until the aqueous layer is alkaline, extract with two 30-ml quantities of a mixture of 3 volumes of *chloroform* and 1 volume of *ethanol*, dry the combined extracts over *anhydrous sodium sulphate*, filter and evaporate to dryness at a pressure of 2 kPa, heating gently to remove the last traces of solvent. The *infrared absorption spectrum* of the residue, Appendix II A, is concordant with the *reference spectrum* of ephedrine.

B. In the test for Related substances, the principal spot in the chromatogram obtained with solution (2) corresponds to that in the chromatogram obtained with solution (4).

Acidity or alkalinity pH 4.0 to 7.0, Appendix V L.

Related substances Carry out the method for *thin-layer chromatography*, Appendix III A, using a silica gel pre-coated plate (Merck silica gel 60 plates are suitable) and a mixture of 80 volumes of *propan-2-ol*, 15 volumes of 13.5M *ammonia* and 5 volumes of *chloroform* as the mobile phase. Apply separately to the plate 20 µl of each of the following solutions. For solution (1) use the nasal drops diluted, if necessary, with *water* to contain 0.5% w/v of Ephedrine Hydrochloride. For solution (2) dilute 1 volume of solution (1) to 5 volumes with *methanol*. For solution (3) dilute 1 volume of solution (1) to 200 volumes with *water*. Solution (4) contains 0.1% w/v of *ephedrine hydrochloride BPCRS* in *methanol*. After removal of the plate, allow it to dry in air, spray with *ninhydrin solution* and heat at 100° for 5 minutes. Any *secondary spot* in the chromatogram obtained with solution (1) is not more intense than the spot in the chromatogram obtained with solution (3). Disregard any spot of lighter colour than the background and any spot remaining on the line of application.

Assay Carry out the method for *liquid chromatography*, Appendix III D, using the following solutions. Solution (1) is a 0.1% w/v solution of *ephedrine hydrochloride BPCRS* in *methanol (65%)*. For solution (2) dilute the nasal drops with *methanol (80%)* to contain 0.1% w/v of Ephedrine Hydrochloride.

The chromatographic procedure may be carried out using (a) a stainless steel column (20 cm × 4.6 mm) packed with *stationary phase C* (10 µm) (Nucleosil C18 is suitable), (b) 0.005M *dioctyl sodium sulphosuccinate* in a mixture of 65 volumes of *methanol*, 35 volumes of *water* and 1 volume of *glacial acetic acid* as the mobile phase with a flow rate of 2 ml per minute and (c) a detection wavelength of 263 nm.

Calculate the content of $C_{10}H_{15}NO,HCl$ in the nasal drops using the declared content of $C_{10}H_{15}NO,HCl$ in *ephedrine hydrochloride BPCRS*.

When Ephedrine Nasal Drops are prescribed or demanded no strength being stated, Nasal Drops containing 0.5% w/v of Ephedrine Hydrochloride shall be dispensed or supplied.

Ephedrine Hydrochloride Tablets

Definition Ephedrine Hydrochloride Tablets contain Ephedrine Hydrochloride.

The tablets comply with the requirements stated under Tablets and with the following requirements.

Content of ephedrine hydrochloride, $C_{10}H_{15}NO,HCl$
92.5 to 107.5% of the prescribed or stated amount.

Identification
A. Shake a quantity of the tablets containing 0.1 g of Ephedrine Hydrochloride with 20 ml of 0.1M *hydrochloric acid*, filter, wash the filtrate with two 20-ml quantities of *chloroform* and discard the chloroform. Make the aqueous layer alkaline with 5M *ammonia* and extract with two 30-ml quantities of a mixture of 3 volumes of *chloroform* and 1 volume of *ethanol (96%)*. Dry the combined extracts over *anhydrous sodium sulphate*, filter and evaporate to a low volume at a pressure of 2 kPa. Prepare a disc using 0.3 g of *potassium bromide*, apply the chloroform solution to the surface of the disc and heat at 50° for 2 minutes. The *infrared absorption spectrum*, Appendix II A, is concordant with the *reference spectrum* of ephedrine.

B. In the test for Related substances, the principal spot in the chromatogram obtained with solution (2) corresponds to that in the chromatogram obtained with solution (3).

C. Triturate a quantity of the powdered tablets containing 0.4 g of Ephedrine Hydrochloride with two 10-ml quantities of *chloroform* and discard the chloroform. Macerate the residue with 30 ml of warm *ethanol (96%)* for 20 minutes, filter, evaporate the filtrate to dryness on a water bath and dry the residue at 80°. Dissolve 10 mg of the residue in 1 ml of *water* and add 0.1 ml of *weak copper sulphate solution* followed by 1 ml of 5M *sodium hydroxide*; a violet colour is produced. Add 1 ml of *ether* and shake; the ether layer is purple and the aqueous layer is blue.

Related substances Carry out the method for *thin-layer chromatography*, Appendix III A, using *silica gel G* as the coating substance and a mixture of 80 volumes of *propan-2-ol*, 15 volumes of 13.5M *ammonia* and 5 volumes of *chloroform* as the mobile phase. Apply separately to the plate 10 µl of each of the following solutions. For solution (1) extract a quantity of the powdered tablets containing 0.10 g of Ephedrine Hydrochloride with 5 ml of *methanol* and filter. For solution (2) dilute 1 volume of solution (1) to 10 volumes with *methanol*. Solution (3) contains 0.20% w/v of *ephedrine hydrochoride BPCRS* in *methanol*. For solution (4) dilute 1 volume of solution (1) to 200 volumes with *methanol*. After removal of the plate, allow it to dry in air, spray with *ninhydrin solution* and heat at 110° for 5 minutes. Any *secondary spot* in the chromatogram obtained with solution (1) is not more intense than the spot in the chromatogram obtained with solution (4). Disregard any spot of lighter colour than the background.

Assay Weigh and powder 20 tablets. Carry out the method for *liquid chromatography*, Appendix III D, using the following solutions. For solution (1) shake a quantity of the powdered tablets containing 50 mg of Ephedrine Hydrochloride with 30 ml of *methanol* for 10 minutes, add sufficient *water* to produce 50 ml, filter through glass-fibre paper (Whatman GF/C is suitable) and use the filtrate. Solution (2) contains 0.1% w/v of *ephedrine hydrochloride BPCRS* in *methanol (60%)*.

The chromatographic procedure may be carried out using (a) a stainless steel column (20 cm × 4.6 mm) packed with *stationary phase C* (10 µm) (Nucleosil C18 is suitable), (b) 0.005M *dioctyl sodium sulphosuccinate* in a mixture of 65 volumes of *methanol*, 35 volumes of *water* and 1 volume of *glacial acetic acid* as the mobile phase with a flow rate of 2 ml per minute and (c) a detection wavelength of 263 nm.

Calculate the content of $C_{10}H_{15}NO,HCl$ using the declared content of $C_{10}H_{15}NO,HCl$ in *ephedrine hydrochloride BPCRS*.

Ergometrine Injection

Definition Ergometrine Injection is a sterile solution of Ergometrine Maleate in Water for Injections. The acidity of the solution is adjusted to pH 3 by the addition of Maleic Acid.

The injection complies with the requirements stated under Parenteral Preparations and with the following requirements.

Content of ergometrine maleate, $C_{19}H_{23}N_3O_2$, $C_4H_4O_4$ 90.0 to 110.0% of the prescribed or stated amount.

Characteristics A colourless or faintly yellow solution.

Identification

A. In the test for Related substances, the principal spot in the chromatogram obtained with solution (1) corresponds to that in the chromatogram obtained with solution (5).

B. Exhibits a blue fluorescence.

C. To a volume containing 0.1 mg of Ergometrine Maleate, add 0.5 ml of *water* and 2 ml of *dimethylaminobenzaldehyde solution R6*. A deep blue colour is produced after about 5 minutes.

Acidity pH, 2.7 to 3.5, Appendix V L.

Related substances Carry out the following procedure in subdued light and protect from light any solutions not used immediately. Carry out the method for *thin-layer chromatography*, Appendix III A, using a suspension of *silica gel G* in 0.1M *sodium hydroxide* to prepare the plate and a mixture of 90 volumes of *chloroform* and 10 volumes of *methanol* as the mobile phase. Apply separately to the plate 5 µl of each of the following solutions. For solution (1) evaporate a volume of the injection containing 1 mg of Ergometrine Maleate to dryness at 20° at a pressure of 2 kPa and dissolve the residue in 0.25 ml of *methanol*. Solutions (2), (3), (4) and (5) are solutions of *ergometrine maleate EPCRS* in *methanol* containing 0.010% w/v, 0.020% w/v, 0.040% w/v and 0.40% w/v respectively. After removal of the plate, allow it to dry in air and examine under *ultraviolet light (365 nm)*. Assess the intensities of any *secondary spots* in the chromatogram obtained with solution (1) by reference to the spots in the chromatograms obtained with solutions (2), (3) and (4). The total of the intensities so assessed does not exceed 10% of the intensity of the principal spot.

Assay Carry out the following procedure protected from light. Dilute a suitable volume with sufficient *water* to produce a solution containing 0.004% w/v of Ergometrine Maleate. To 3 ml add 6 ml of *dimethylaminobenzaldehyde solution R6*, mix, cool to room temperature and allow to stand for 30 minutes (solution A). At the same time prepare solution B in the same manner but using 3 ml of a 0.004% w/v solution of *ergometrine maleate EPCRS* and beginning at the words 'add 6 ml ...'. Measure the *absorbance* of solution B at the maximum at 545 nm, Appendix II B, using in the reference cell a solution prepared by mixing 6 ml of *dimethylaminobenzaldehyde solution R6* and 3 ml of *water*. Without delay replace solution B with solution A, using the same cell, and measure the *absorbance* of solution A at the same wavelength. Calculate the content of $C_{19}H_{23}N_3O_2,C_4H_4O_4$ taking 100.0% as the content of $C_{19}H_{23}N_3O_2,C_4H_4O_4$ in *ergometrine maleate EPCRS*.

Storage Ergometrine Injection should be protected from light and stored at a temperature of 2° to 8°.

Ergometrine and Oxytocin Injection

Definition Ergometrine and Oxytocin Injection is a sterile solution containing Ergometrine Maleate and either Oxytocin or Oxytocin Concentrated Solution in Water for Injections. The acidity of the solution is adjusted to pH 3.3 by the addition of Maleic Acid.

The injection complies with the requirements stated under Parenteral Preparations and with the following requirements.

Content of ergometrine maleate, $C_{19}H_{23}N_3O_2$, $C_4H_4O_4$ 90.0 to 110.0% of the prescribed or stated amount.

Content of oxytocin, $C_{43}H_{66}N_{12}O_{12}S_2$ 90.0 to 110.0% of the prescribed or stated amount.

Characteristics A colourless solution.

Identification

A. In the test for Substances related to ergometrine, the principal spot in the chromatogram obtained with solution (1) corresponds to that in the chromatogram obtained with solution (2).

B. To a volume containing 0.1 mg of Ergometrine Maleate, add 0.5 ml of *water* and 2 ml of *dimethylaminobenzaldehyde solution R6*. After about 5 minutes a deep blue colour is produced.

C. In the Assay for oxytocin a peak in the chromatogram obtained with solution (2) corresponds to the peak due to oxytocin in the chromatogram obtained with solution (1).

Acidity pH, 2.9 to 3.5, Appendix V L.

Substances related to ergometrine Carry out in subdued light the method for *thin-layer chromatography*, Appendix III A, using *silica gel G* as the coating substance and a mixture of 75 volumes of *chloroform*, 25 volumes of *methanol* and 3 volumes of *water* as the mobile phase but allowing the solvent front to ascend 14 cm above the line of application. Apply separately to the plate 5 µl of each of the following solutions. For solution (1) add 10 ml of *absolute ethanol* to a volume of the injection containing 0.5 mg of Ergometrine Maleate and evaporate to dryness at a temperature not exceeding 30° at a pressure of 2 kPa; to the residue add 0.2 ml of a mixture of 1 volume of 13.5M *ammonia* and 9 volumes of *ethanol (80%)*, mix, centrifuge and use the supernatant liquid. Solutions (2), (3), (4), (5) and (6) contain 0.250% w/v, 0.0250% w/v, 0.0125% w/v, 0.0050% w/v and 0.00250% w/v of *ergometrine maleate EPCRS* respectively in a mixture of 1 volume of 3.5M *ammonia* and 9 volumes of *ethanol (80%)*. After removal of the plate, dry it in a current of cold air, spray with *dimethylaminobenzaldehyde solution R7* and dry the plate at 105° for 2 minutes. Assess the intensities of any *secondary spots* in the chromatogram obtained with solution (1) by reference to the spots in the chromatograms obtained with solutions (3) to (6), making allowance for area in assessing the intensities of spots of different Rf values. The sum of the intensities so assessed does not exceed 10% of the intensity of the principal spot.

Assay

For ergometrine maleate Carry out the method for *liquid chromatography*, Appendix III D, using the following solutions. Solution (1) contains 0.05% w/v of *ergometrine maleate BPCRS*. Solution (2) is the injection diluted, if necessary, to give a solution containing 0.05% w/v of Ergometrine Maleate.

The chromatographic procedure may be carried out using (a) a stainless steel column (10 cm × 4.6 mm) packed with *stationary phase C* (5 µm) (Nucleosil C18 is suitable) and maintained at 40°, (b) a mixture of 92 volumes of a 0.2% v/v solution of *orthophosphoric acid* and 8 volumes of *acetonitrile* as the mobile phase with a flow rate of 1 ml per minute and (c) a detection wavelength of 320 nm.

Calculate the content of $C_{19}H_{23}N_3O_2,C_4H_4O_4$ from the declared content of $C_{19}H_{23}N_3O_2,C_4H_4O_4$ in *ergometrine maleate BPCRS*.

For oxytocin Carry out the method for *liquid chromatography*, Appendix III D, injecting 0.2 ml of each of the following solutions. Solution (1) contains 8 µg of *oxytocin EPCRS* per ml. Solution (2) is the injection diluted, if necessary, to give a solution containing about 8 µg of oxytocin per ml.

The chromatographic procedure may be carried out using a stainless steel column (10 cm × 4.6 mm) packed with *stationary phase C* (5 µm) (Nucleosil C18 is suitable) and maintained at 40°, (b) a mixture of 85 volumes of a 0.2% v/v solution of *orthophosphoric acid* and 15 volumes of *acetonitrile* as the mobile phase with a flow rate of 1 ml per minute and (c) a detection wavelength of 220 nm. If necessary adjust the content of *acetonitrile* in the mobile phase so that the retention time of oxytocin is about 14 minutes. Record the chromatogram for sufficient time to ensure elution of any preservatives.

The *column efficiency*, determined using the peak due to oxytocin in the chromatogram obtained with solution (1), should be not less than 50,000 theoretical plates per metre.

Calculate the content of $C_{43}H_{66}N_{12}O_{12}S_2$ from the declared content of peptide in *oxytocin EPCRS*..

Storage Ergometrine and Oxytocin Injection should be protected from light and stored at a temperature of 2° to 8°. Under these conditions it may be expected to retain its potency for not less than 3 years.

Labelling The strength with respect to Oxytocin is stated as the number of IU (Units) per ml. The label also states the equivalent number of micrograms of oxytocin per ml.

Ergometrine Tablets

Definition Ergometrine Tablets contain Ergometrine Maleate.

The tablets comply with the requirements stated under Tablets and with the following requirements.

Content of ergometrine maleate, $C_{19}H_{23}N_3O_2,C_4H_4O_4$ 90.0 to 110.0% of the prescribed or stated amount.

Identification

A. In the test for Related substances the principal spot in the chromatogram obtained with solution (1) corresponds to that in the chromatogram obtained with solution (5).

B. Extract a quantity of the powdered tablets containing 2 mg of Ergometrine Maleate with 20 ml of *water*, filter and wash the residue with sufficient *water* to produce 20 ml. The solution exhibits a blue fluorescence.

C. To 2 ml of the solution obtained in test B add 4 ml of *dimethylaminobenzaldehyde solution R6*. A deep blue colour is produced after a few minutes.

Related substances Carry out the method for *thin-layer chromatography* protected from light, Appendix III A, using a suspension of *silica gel G* in 0.1M *sodium hydroxide* to prepare the plate and a mixture of 90 volumes of *chloroform* and 10 volumes of *methanol* as the mobile phase. Apply separately to the plate 5 µl of each of the following solutions. For solution (1) triturate a quantity of the powdered tablets containing 1 mg of Ergometrine Maleate with 0.2 ml of a 1% w/v solution of *domiphen bromide*, add 2 ml of *methanol*, centrifuge and remove the supernatant liquid. Extract the residue with two 1-ml quantities of *methanol*, evaporate the combined extracts to dryness at 20° at a pressure of 2 kPa and dissolve the residue in 0.25 ml of *methanol*; centrifuge if necessary. Solutions (2), (3), (4) and (5) are solutions of *ergometrine maleate EPCRS* in *methanol* containing 0.010% w/v, 0.020% w/v, 0.040% w/v and 0.40% w/v respectively. After removal of the plate, allow it to dry in air and examine under *ultraviolet light (365 nm)*. Assess the intensities of any *secondary spots* in the chromatogram obtained with solution (1) by reference to the spots in the chromatograms obtained with solutions (2), (3) and (4). The sum of the intensities so assessed does not exceed 10% of the intensity of the principal spot. In addition, no single *secondary spot* in the chromatogram obtained with solution (1) is more intense than the spot in the chromatogram obtained with solution (2).

Uniformity of content Tablets containing less than 2 mg of Ergometrine Maleate comply with the requirements stated under Tablets using the following method of analysis. Carry out the following procedure protected from light. To one tablet add 10 ml of a 1% w/v solution of *(+)-tartaric acid*, shake for 30 minutes and centrifuge. Carry out the Assay described under Ergometrine Injection, beginning at the words 'Dilute a suitable volume ...' and calculate the content of $C_{19}H_{23}N_3O_2,C_4H_4O_4$.

Assay Weigh and powder 20 tablets. Shake a quantity of the powder containing 2 mg of Ergometrine Maleate with 50 ml of a 1% w/v solution of *(+)-tartaric acid* for 30 minutes, centrifuge and use the supernatant liquid. Carry out the Assay described under Ergometrine Injection, beginning at the words 'To 3 ml ...'.

Storage Ergometrine Tablets should be protected from light.

Ergotamine Injection

Definition Ergotamine Injection is a sterile solution prepared by dissolving Ergotamine Tartrate in Water for Injections containing Ethanol (96%), Glycerol and sufficient Tartaric Acid to adjust the acidity of the solution to pH 3.3.

The injection complies with the requirements stated under Parenteral Preparations and with the following requirements.

Content of total alkaloids, calculated as $(C_{33}H_{35}N_5O_5)_2,C_4H_6O_6$ 90.0 to 110.0% of the prescribed or stated amount of Ergotamine Tartrate, of which 50 to 70% is present as ergotamine tartrate.

Characteristics A colourless or almost colourless solution.

Identification

A. In the test for Ergot alkaloids and related substances, the spot due to ergotamine in the chromatogram obtained with solution (1) corresponds in position to those due to ergotamine in the chromatograms obtained with solution (2).

B. To a volume containing 0.2 mg of Ergotamine Tartrate add 1 ml of *dimethylaminobenzaldehyde solution R6*. A deep blue colour is produced.

C. Mix a volume containing 2 mg of Ergotamine Tartrate with 2 ml of 1M *sulphuric acid*, dissolve a few mg of *magnesium*, in powder, in the solution, add 25 mg of *resorcinol*, shake to dissolve, carefully pour 2 ml of *sulphuric acid* down the inside of the tube and warm gently. A red ring is produced at the interface of the two liquid layers and diffuses throughout the lower layer.

Acidity pH, 2.8 to 3.8, Appendix V L.

Ergot alkaloids and related substances Carry out the method for *thin-layer chromatography*, Appendix III A, using a suspension of *silica gel G* in 0.1M *sodium hydroxide* to prepare the plate and a mixture of 90 volumes of *chloroform* and 10 volumes of *methanol* as the mobile phase. Prepare the following solutions. For solution (1) add sufficient of a 10% w/v solution of *sodium hydrogen carbonate* to a volume of the injection containing 5.0 mg of Ergotamine Tartrate to make it distinctly alkaline to *litmus paper*. Extract with five 10-ml quantities of *chloroform*, filter the extracts through a small double filter paper, wash the filter with *chloroform*, evaporate the combined filtrates and washings to dryness at 20° at 2 kPa and dissolve the residue in 1 ml of a mixture of equal volumes of *methanol* and *chloroform*. For solution (2) dissolve 5.0 mg of *ergotamine tartrate EPCRS* in 10 ml of a 1% w/v solution of *(+)-tartaric acid* and complete the preparation as described for solution (1) beginning at the words 'Extract with five 10-ml quantities ...'. Without delay, apply separately to the plate 20 µl of solution (1) and 14, 10, 7 and 2 µl of solution (2).

After removal of the plate, allow it to dry in air and examine under *ultraviolet light (365 nm)*. The chromatogram obtained with solution (1) shows two principal spots, corresponding to ergotamine and, of higher Rf value, ergotaminine. A spot between the two principal spots and a number of spots of lower Rf values may also be observed.

Compare the chromatogram obtained from solution (1) with the chromatograms obtained from solution (2). The spot corresponding to ergotaminine is not larger or more intense than the spot corresponding to ergotamine in the chromatogram obtained from 7 µl of solution (2). The spot corresponding to ergotamine is not smaller or less intense than the spot corresponding to ergotamine in the chromatogram obtained from 10 µl of solution (2) and is not larger or more intense than the spot corresponding to ergotamine in the chromatogram obtained from 14 µl of solution (2), corresponding to not less than 50% and not more than 70% of ergotamine tartrate. Any other spots are not larger or more intense than the spot corresponding to ergotamine obtained from 2 µl of solution (2); the total of the intensities so assessed does not exceed 10%.

Assay Dilute a suitable volume of the injection with sufficient of a 0.25% w/v solution of *(+)-tartaric acid* to produce a solution containing 0.005% w/v of Ergotamine Tartrate. To 3 ml add 6 ml of *dimethylaminobenzaldehyde solution R6*, mix, cool to room temperature and allow to stand for 30 minutes (solution A). At the same time mix 3 ml of a 0.003% w/v solution of *ergometrine maleate EPCRS* in a 0.25% w/v solution of *(+)-tartaric acid* with 6 ml of *dimethylaminobenzaldehyde solution R6*, cool to room temperature and allow to stand for 30 minutes (solution B). Prepare solution C by mixing 3 ml of a 0.25% w/v solution of *(+)-tartaric acid* with 6 ml of *dimethylaminobenzaldehyde solution R6*. Measure the *absorbance* of solution B at the maximum at 545 nm, Appendix II B, using solution C in the reference cell. Without delay replace solution B with solution A, using the same cell, and measure the *absorbance* of solution A at the same wavelength. Calculate the content of total alkaloids as $(C_{33}H_{35}N_5O_5)_2,C_4H_6O_6$ from the absorbances obtained. Each mg of *ergometrine maleate EPCRS* is equivalent to 1.488 mg of $(C_{33}H_{35}N_5O_5)_2,C_4H_6O_6$.

Storage Ergotamine Injection should be protected from light.

Erythromycin Estolate Capsules

Definition Erythromycin Estolate Capsules contain Erythromycin Estolate.

The capsules comply with the requirements stated under Capsules and with the following requirements.

Identification

A. The *infrared absorption spectrum* of the contents of the capsules, Appendix II A, is concordant with the *reference spectrum* of erythromycin estolate.

B. In the test for Related substances, the principal spot in the chromatogram obtained with solution (2) is similar in position and colour to that in the chromatogram obtained with solution (3).

Disintegration Maximum time, 30 minutes, Appendix XII A. Use a 0.6% v/v solution of *hydrochloric acid* in place of *water*.

Water The contents of the capsules contain not more than 5.0% w/w of water, Appendix IX C. Use 0.5 g.

Related substances Carry out the method for *thin-layer chromatography*, Appendix III A, using a silica gel precoated plate (Merck silica gel 60 plates are suitable) and as the mobile phase a mixture of 1 volume of a 15% w/v solution of *ammonium acetate* previously adjusted to pH 7.0, 15 volumes of *ethanol (96%)* and 85 volumes of *chloroform*. Apply separately to the plate 10 µl of each of the following solutions. For solution (1) shake a quantity of the contents of the capsules containing the equivalent of 0.4 g of erythromycin with 100 ml of *acetone*, filter and use the filtrate. For solution (2) dilute 1 volume of solution (1) to 4 volumes with *acetone*. Solution (3) contains 0.13% w/v of *erythromycin estolate EPCRS* in *acetone*. Solution (4) contains 0.1% w/v each of *erythromycin estolate EPCRS* and *erythromycin ethylsuccinate EPCRS* in *acetone*. Solution (5) contains 0.01% w/v of *erythromycin EPCRS* in *acetone*. After removal of the plate, allow it to dry in air, spray with *anisaldehyde solution*, heat at 110° for 5 minutes and allow to cool. Any *secondary spot* in the chromatogram obtained with solution (1) is not more intense than the spot in the chromatogram obtained with solution (5) (2.5%, with respect to erythromycin). The test is not valid unless the chromatogram obtained with solution (4) shows two clearly separated spots.

Assay Dissolve a quantity of the mixed contents of 20 capsules containing the equivalent of 0.25 g of erythromycin in 400 ml of *methanol* and add 200 ml of sterile *phosphate buffer pH 7.0* and sufficient *water for injections* to produce 1000 ml. Maintain the solution at 60° for 3 hours, cool, filter and carry out the *biological assay of antibiotics* for erythromycin, Appendix XIV A. The precision of the assay is such that the fiducial limits of error are not less than 95% and not more than 105% of the estimated potency.

Calculate the content of erythromycin in a capsule of average content weight, taking each 1000 IU found to be equivalent to 1 mg of erythromycin. The upper fiducial limit of error is not less than 95.0% and the lower fiducial limit of error is not more than 110.0% of the prescribed or stated content.

Labelling The quantity of active ingredient is stated in terms of the equivalent amount of erythromycin.

Erythromycin Lactobionate Intravenous Infusion

Definition Erythromycin Lactobionate Intravenous Infusion is a sterile solution of Erythromycin Lactobionate in Sodium Chloride Intravenous Infusion. It is prepared immediately before use by dissolving Erythromycin Lactobionate for Intravenous Infusion in the requisite amount of Water for Injections and diluting the resulting solution with the requisite amount of Sodium Chloride Intravenous Infusion.

The intravenous infusion complies with the requirements stated under Parenteral Preparations and with the following requirements.

Storage Erythromycin Lactobionate Intravenous Infusion should be used immediately after preparation but, in any case, within the period recommended by the manufacturer when prepared and stored strictly in accordance with the manufacturer's instructions.

Particulate contamination When the volume of the constituted intravenous infusion is 100 ml or more, it complies with the *test for sub-visible particles*, Appendix XIII A.

ERYTHROMYCIN LACTOBIONATE FOR INTRAVENOUS INFUSION

Definition Erythromycin Lactobionate for Intravenous Infusion is a sterile material consisting of Erythromycin Lactobionate with or without excipients. It is supplied in a sealed container.

The contents of the sealed container comply with the requirements for Powders for Injections stated under Parenteral Preparations and with the following requirements.

Content of erythromycins, calculated as the sum of erythromycin A ($C_{37}H_{67}NO_{13}$), erythromycin B ($C_{37}H_{67}NO_{12}$) and erythromycin C ($C_{36}H_{65}NO_{13}$) 90.0 to 110.0% of the prescribed or stated amount of erythromycin.

Identification

A. The *infrared absorption spectrum*, Appendix II A, is concordant with the *reference spectrum* of erythromycin lactobionate.

B. Carry out the method for *thin-layer chromatography*, Appendix III A, using *silica gel H* as the coating substance and a mixture of 3 volumes of *glacial acetic acid*, 10 volumes of *water* and 90 volumes of *methanol* as the mobile phase. Apply separately to the plate 5 µl of each of the following solutions. For solution (1) dissolve a quantity of the contents of a sealed container in sufficient *methanol* to produce a solution containing the equivalent of 0.2% w/v of erythromycin. Solution (2) contains 0.2% w/v of *erythromycin A EPCRS* in *methanol*. Solution (3) contains 0.1% w/v of *lactobionic acid* in *water*. After removal of the plate, allow it to dry in air and spray with a 0.5% w/v solution of *potassium permanganate* in 1M *sodium hydroxide* and heat at 110° for 5 minutes. The chromatogram obtained with solution (1) shows two spots, one of which corresponds in position, colour and size to the principal spot in the chromatogram obtained with solution (2) and the other to the principal spot in the chromatogram obtained with solution (3).

C. To a quantity of the contents of a sealed container containing the equivalent of 5 mg of erythromycin add 5 ml of a 0.02% w/v solution of *xanthydrol* in a mixture of 1 volume of *hydrochloric acid* and 99 volumes of 5M *acetic acid*. A red colour develops.

Acidity or alkalinity pH of a 2.0% w/v solution, 6.5 to 7.5, Appendix V L.

Related substances Carry out the method for *liquid chromatography*, Appendix III D, using solutions (1) and (3) described under Assay.

The chromatographic conditions described under Assay may be used.

Inject 100 µl of each solution. For solution (1) allow the chromatography to proceed for 5 times the retention time of the peak corresponding to erythromycin A. In the chromatogram obtained with solution (1) the area of any peak other than those peaks corresponding to erythromycin A, erythromycin B or erythromycin C is not greater than 1.5 times the area of the principal peak in the chromatogram obtained with solution (3) (3%).

The content of each of erythromycin B and erythromycin C, as determined in the Assay, is not more than 5%.

Pyrogens Complies with the *test for pyrogens*, Appendix XIV D, administering the intravenous infusion over not more than 30 seconds. Use per kg of the rabbit's weight

1 ml of a solution in *water for injections* containing a quantity equivalent to 5 mg of erythromycin per ml.

Assay Determine the weight of the contents of each of 10 containers as described in the test for Uniformity of weight under Parenteral Preparations, Powders for Injections.

Carry out the method for *liquid chromatography*, Appendix III D, using the following solutions. For solution (1) dissolve a quantity of the mixed contents of the 10 containers containing the equivalent of 60 mg of erythromycin in a mixture of 1 volume of *methanol* and 3 volumes of *citro-phosphate buffer pH 7.0* and dilute to 10 ml with the same mixture of solvents. Solution (2) contains 0.4% w/v of *erythromycin A EPCRS* in a mixture of 1 volume of *methanol* and 3 volumes of *citro-phosphate buffer pH 7.0*. Solution (3) contains 0.012% w/v of *erythromycin A EPCRS* in a mixture of 1 volume of *methanol* and 3 volumes of *citro-phosphate buffer pH 7.0*. Solution (4) contains 0.02% w/v of each of *erythromycin B EPCRS* and *erythromycin C EPCRS* in a mixture of 1 volume of *methanol* and 3 volumes of *citro-phosphate buffer pH 7.0*. For solution (5) dissolve 5 mg of N-*demethylerythromycin A EPCRS* in solution (4), add 1 ml of solution (2) and sufficient of solution (4) to produce 25 ml. The solutions can be used within one day if stored at 5°.

The chromatographic procedure may be carried out using (a) a column (25 cm × 4.6 mm) packed with *styrene—divinylbenzene copolymer* (8 to 10 µm) with a pore size of 100 nm (PLRP-S is suitable), (b) as mobile phase with a flow rate of 2.0 ml per minute a solution prepared in the following manner: to 50 ml of a 3.5% w/v solution of *dipotassium hydrogen orthophosphate*, adjusted to pH 9.0 with 1M *orthophosphoric acid*, add 400 ml of *water*, 165 ml of *2-methylpropan-2-ol* and 30 ml of *acetonitrile*, and dilute to 1000 ml with *water* and (c) a detection wavelength of 215 nm. Maintain the temperature of the column at 70°.

Inject 100 µl of solution (5). Adjust the sensitivity of the system so that the height of the peaks is at least 25% of the full-scale of the recorder. The substances are eluted in the following order: *N*-demethylerythromycin A, erythromycin C, erythromycin A and erythromycin B. The test is not valid unless the *resolution factor* between the peaks corresponding to *N*-demethylerythromycin A and erythromycin C is at least 0.8 and the *resolution factor* between the peaks corresponding to *N*-demethylerythromycin A and erythromycin A is at least 5.5. If necessary, adjust the concentration of 2-methylpropan-2-ol in the mobile phase or reduce the flow rate to 1.5 or 1.0 ml per minute.

Inject alternately 100 µl of solutions (1), (2) and (4). Calculate the percentage content of erythromycin A using the chromatograms obtained with solutions (1) and (2) and from the declared content of $C_{37}H_{67}NO_{13}$ in *erythromycin A EPCRS*. Calculate the percentage contents of erythromycin B and erythromycin C using the chromatograms obtained with solutions (1) and (4) and from the declared contents of $C_{37}H_{67}NO_{12}$ and $C_{36}H_{65}NO_{13}$ in *erythromycin B EPCRS* and *erythromycin C EPCRS* respectively.

Storage The sealed container should be stored at a temperature not exceeding 25°.

Labelling The quantity of active ingredient is stated in terms of the equivalent amount of erythromycin.

Erythromycin Ethyl Succinate Oral Suspension

Definition Erythromycin Ethyl Succinate Oral Suspension is a suspension of Erythromycin Ethyl Succinate in a suitable flavoured vehicle. It is prepared by dispersing the dry ingredients in the specified volume of Water just before issue for use.

The dry ingredients comply with the requirements for Powders and Granules for the Preparation of Oral Liquids stated under Oral Liquids.

Storage The dry ingredients should be kept in a well-closed container and stored at a temperature not exceeding 25°.

For the following tests prepare the oral suspension as directed on the label. The suspension examined immediately after preparation, unless otherwise indicated, complies with the requirements stated under Oral Liquids and with the following requirements.

Identification Dilute a quantity of the oral suspension containing the equivalent of 0.1 g of erythromycin to 25 ml with *water* and extract with two 10-ml quantities of *dichloromethane*. Wash the combined extracts with five 10-ml quantities of *water*, filter using silicone-treated filter paper (Phase Separator paper is suitable) and evaporate to dryness. The residue, after drying at 105° for 15 minutes complies with the following tests.

A. The *infrared absorption spectrum*, Appendix II A, is concordant with the *reference spectrum* of erythromycin ethyl succinate.

B. Carry out the method for *thin-layer chromatography*, Appendix III A, using *silica gel G* as the coating substance and a mixture of 1 volume of a 15% w/v solution of *ammonium acetate* previously adjusted to pH 7.0, 15 volumes of *ethanol (96%)* and 85 volumes of *chloroform* as the mobile phase. Apply separately to the plate 10 µl of each of the following solutions. For solution (1) dissolve a quantity of the residue in *acetone* to produce a solution containing the equivalent of 0.1% w/v of erythromycin. Solution (2) contains 0.1% w/v of *erythromycin ethylsuccinate EPCRS* in *acetone*. Solution (3) contains 0.1% w/v of *erythromycin ethylsuccinate EPCRS* and 0.1% w/v of *erythromycin estolate EPCRS* in *acetone*. After removal of the plate, allow it to dry in air, spray with *anisaldehyde solution*, heat at 110° for 5 minutes and allow to cool. The principal spot in the chromatogram obtained with solution (1) is similar in position and colour to that in the chromatogram obtained with solution (2). The test is not valid unless the chromatogram obtained with solution (3) shows two clearly separated spots.

Acidity or alkalinity pH, 6.5 to 9.5, Appendix V L.

Assay To a weighed quantity of the oral suspension containing the equivalent of 0.25 g of erythromycin add 10 ml of *water* and swirl to mix. Add 200 ml of *methanol*, shake for 1 hour and dilute to 500 ml with *methanol*. Dilute 10 ml to 100 ml with *phosphate buffer pH 8.0*, stand at room temperature for 16 hours and carry out the *biological assay of antibiotics* for erythromycin, Appendix XIV A. The precision of the assay is such that the fiducial limits of error are not less than 95% and not more than 105% of the estimated potency.

Repeat the procedure using a portion of the oral suspension that has been stored at the temperature and for the period stated on the label during which it may be expected to be satisfactory for use.

Calculate the content of erythromycin in the oral suspension taking each 1000 IU found to be equivalent to 1 mg of erythromycin. When freshly constituted the lower fiducial limit of error is not more than 120.0% of the prescribed or stated amount and when stored at the temperature and for the period stated on the label during which the Oral Suspension may be expected to be satisfactory for use, the upper fiducial limit of error is not less than 90.0% of the prescribed or stated content.

Storage The oral suspension should be stored at the temperature and used within the period stated on the label.

Labelling The quantity of the active ingredient is stated in terms of the equivalent amount of erythromycin.

Erythromycin Tablets

Definition Erythromycin Tablets contain Erythromycin. They are made gastro-resistant by enteric-coating or by other means.

The tablets comply with the requirements stated under Tablets and with the following requirements.

Content of erythromycins, calculated as the sum of erythromycin A ($C_{37}H_{67}NO_{13}$), erythromycin B ($C_{37}H_{67}NO_{12}$) and erythromycin C ($C_{36}H_{65}NO_{13}$) 90.0 to 110.0% of the prescribed or stated amount of Erythromycin.

Identification

A. Shake a quantity of the powdered tablets containing 0.1 g of Erythromycin with 5 ml of *chloroform*, decolorise, if necessary, with *activated charcoal*, filter and evaporate the filtrate to dryness. The *infrared absorption spectrum* of the residue, Appendix II A, after drying at a pressure not exceeding 0.7 kPa, is concordant with the *reference spectrum* of erythromycin.

B. Dissolve a quantity of the powdered tablets containing 3 mg of Erythromycin as completely as possible in 2 ml of *acetone* and add 2 ml of *hydrochloric acid*; an orange colour is produced which changes to red and then to deep purplish red. Add 2 ml of *chloroform* and shake; the chloroform layer becomes purple.

Disintegration Tablets made gastro-resistant by enteric-coating comply with the *disintegration test for enteric-coated tablets*, Appendix XII B, but operating the apparatus for 1 hour in 0.1M *hydrochloric acid*.

Related substances Carry out the method for *liquid chromatography*, Appendix III D, using solutions (1) to (4) described under Assay.

The chromatographic conditions described under Assay may be used.

Inject 0.1 ml of each solution. For solution (1), allow the chromatography to proceed for 5 times the retention time of the peak corresponding to erythromycin A. In the chromatogram obtained with solution (1) the area of any peak other than those peaks corresponding to erythromycin A, erythromycin B and erythromycin C, identified from the peaks in the chromatograms obtained with solutions (2) and (3), is not greater than the area of the principal peak in the chromatogram obtained with solution (4) (3%).

The content of each of erythromycin B and erythromycin C, as determined under Assay, is not more than 5%.

Assay Carry out the method for *liquid chromatography*, Appendix III D, using the following solutions. Weigh and powder 20 tablets (if necessary, remove the coating from 20 tablets using a sharp blade, taking care not to damage the cores, weigh the cores and powder). For solution (1) dissolve a quantity of the powdered tablets containing 40 mg of Erythromycin in 10 ml of a mixture of 1 volume of *methanol* and 3 volumes of *citro-phosphate buffer pH 7.0*, filter and use the filtrate. Solution (2) contains 0.4% w/v of *erythromycin A EPCRS* in a mixture of 1 volume of *methanol* and 3 volumes of *citro-phosphate buffer pH 7.0* (solvent A). Solution (3) contains 0.02% w/v of each of *erythromycin B EPCRS* and *erythromycin C EPCRS* in solvent A. Solution (4) contains 0.012% w/v of *erythromycin A EPCRS* in solvent A. For solution (5) dissolve 5 mg of N-*demethylerythromycin A EPCRS* in solution (3), add 1 ml of solution (2) and sufficient of solution (3) to produce 25 ml. The solutions can be used within one day if stored at 5°.

The chromatographic procedure may be carried out using (a) a column (25 cm × 4.6 mm) packed with *styrene—divinylbenzene copolymer* (8 µm) with a pore size of 100 nm (PLRP-S is suitable), (b) as mobile phase at a flow rate of 2.0 ml per minute a solution prepared in the following manner: to 50 ml of a 3.5% w/v solution of *dipotassium hydrogen orthophosphate* adjusted to pH 9.0 with 1M *orthophosphoric acid* add 400 ml of *water*, 165 ml of *2-methylpropan-2-ol* and 30 ml of *acetonitrile* and dilute to 1000 ml with *water* and (c) a detection wavelength of 215 nm. Maintain the temperature of the column at 70°.

Inject 0.1 ml of solution (5). Adjust the sensitivity of the detector so that the height of the peaks is at least 25% of the full scale of the recorder. The substances are eluted in the following order: *N*-demethylerythromycin A, erythromycin C, erythromycin A and erythromycin B. The test is not valid unless the *resolution factor* between the peaks corresponding to *N*-demethylerythromycin A and erythromycin C is at least 0.8 and the *resolution factor* between the peaks corresponding to *N*-demethylerythromycin A and erythromycin A is at least 5.5. If necessary, adjust the concentration of 2-methylpropan-2-ol in the mobile phase (180 ml has been found to be suitable) or reduce the flow rate to 1.5 or 1.0 ml per minute.

Inject alternately 0.1 ml of solutions (1), (2) and (3). Calculate the content of erythromycin A using the chromatograms obtained with solutions (1) and (2) and from the declared content of $C_{37}H_{67}NO_{13}$ in *erythromycin A EPCRS*. Calculate the contents of erythromycin B and erythromycin C using the chromatograms obtained with solutions (1) and (3) and from the declared contents of $C_{37}H_{67}NO_{12}$ and $C_{36}H_{65}NO_{13}$ in *erythromycin B EPCRS* and *erythromycin C EPCRS* respectively.

Storage Erythromycin Tablets should be kept in a well-closed container, protected from light and stored at a temperature not exceeding 25°.

Erythromycin Ethyl Succinate Tablets

Definition Erythromycin Ethyl Succinate Tablets contain Erythromycin Ethyl Succinate.

With the exception of the requirements for shape, the tablets comply with the requirements stated under Tablets and with the following requirements.

Identification

A. Shake a quantity of the powdered tablets containing the equivalent of 0.1 g of erythromycin with 20 ml of a mixture of equal volumes of *chloroform* and *methanol* for 15 minutes. Centrifuge and evaporate the upper layer to dryness. Dissolve the residue in a minimum volume of *dichloromethane,* evaporate to dryness and dry at 105° for 15 minutes. The *infrared absorption spectrum* of the residue, Appendix II A, is concordant with the *reference spectrum* of erythromycin ethyl succinate.

B. In the test for Related substances, the principal spot in the chromatogram obtained with solution (2) is similar in position and colour to that in the chromatogram obtained with solution (3). The test is not valid unless the chromatogram obtained with solution (4) shows two clearly separated spots.

Related substances Carry out the method for *thin-layer chromatography,* Appendix III A, using *silica gel G* as the coating substance and a mixture of 1 volume of a 15% w/v solution of *ammonium acetate* previously adjusted to pH 7.0, 15 volumes of *ethanol (96%)* and 85 volumes of *chloroform* as the mobile phase. Apply separately to the plate 10 µl of each of the following solutions. For solution (1) shake a quantity of the powdered tablets containing the equivalent of 0.1 g of erythromycin with 25 ml of a mixture of equal volumes of *chloroform* and *methanol* for 15 minutes, centrifuge and use the supernatant liquid. For solution (2) dilute 1 volume of solution (1) to 4 volumes with the same solvent. Solution (3) contains 0.1% w/v of *erythromycin ethylsuccinate EPCRS* in *acetone.* Solution (4) contains 0.1% w/v of *erythromycin ethylsuccinate EPCRS* and 0.1% w/v of *erythromycin estolate EPCRS* in *acetone.* Solution (5) contains 0.020% w/v of *erythromycin EPCRS* in *acetone.* After removal of the plate, allow it to dry in air, spray with *anisaldehyde solution,* heat at 110° for 5 minutes and allow to cool. Any *secondary spot* in the chromatogram obtained with solution (1) is not more intense than the spot in the chromatogram obtained with solution (5) (5%).

Assay Weigh and powder 20 tablets. To a quantity of the powdered tablets containing the equivalent of 0.25 g of erythromycin add 200 ml of *methanol,* shake for 1 hour and dilute to 500 ml with *methanol.* Dilute 10 ml to 100 ml with *phosphate buffer pH 8.0,* stand at room temperature for 16 hours and carry out the *biological assay of antibiotics* for erythromycin, Appendix XIV A. The precision of the assay is such that the fiducial limits of error are not less than 95% and not more than 105% of the estimated potency.

Calculate the content of erythromycin in the tablets taking each 1000 IU found to be equivalent to 1 mg of erythromycin. The upper fiducial limit of error is not less than 97.0% and the lower fiducial limit of error is not more than 110.0% of the prescribed or stated content.

Storage Erythromycin Ethyl Succinate Tablets should be kept in a well-closed container and protected from light.

Labelling The quantity of active ingredient is stated in terms of the equivalent amount of erythromycin.

Erythromycin Stearate Tablets

Definition Erythromycin Stearate Tablets contain Erythromycin Stearate.

The tablets comply with the requirements stated under Tablets and with the following requirements.

Identification

A. To a quantity of the powdered tablets containing the equivalent of 0.1 g of erythromycin add 10 ml of *water* and shake well. Decant the supernatant liquid and discard. Extract the residue by shaking with 10 ml of *methanol,* filter the extract and evaporate to dryness. The *infrared absorption spectrum,* Appendix II A, of the residue after drying at a pressure not exceeding 0.7 kPa is concordant with the *reference spectrum* of erythromycin stearate.

B. Dissolve a quantity of the powdered tablets containing the equivalent of 3 mg of erythromycin in 2 ml of *acetone* and add 2 ml of *hydrochloric acid*; an orange colour is produced which changes to red and then to deep violet-red. Add 2 ml of *chloroform* and shake; the chloroform layer becomes violet.

C. Extract a quantity of the powdered tablets containing the equivalent of 50 mg of erythromycin with 10 ml of *chloroform,* filter and evaporate to dryness. Heat 0.1 g of the residue gently with 5 ml of 2M *hydrochloric acid* and 10 ml of *water* until the solution boils; oily globules rise to the surface. Cool, remove the fatty layer, heat it with 3 ml of 0.1M *sodium hydroxide* and allow to cool; the solution sets to a gel. Add 10 ml of hot *water* and shake; the solution froths. To 1 ml add a 10% w/v solution of *calcium chloride*; a granular precipitate is produced which is insoluble in *hydrochloric acid.*

Dissolution Comply with the *dissolution test for tablets and capsules,* Appendix XII D, using Apparatus II. Use as the medium 900 ml of a 2.722% w/v solution of *sodium acetate,* the pH of which has been adjusted to 5.0 with *glacial acetic acid* and rotate the paddle at 50 revolutions per minute. Transfer 5 ml of a filtered sample to a graduated flask, add 40 ml of *glacial acetic acid* and 10 ml of a 0.5% w/v solution of *4-dimethylaminobenzaldehyde* in *glacial acetic acid* and dilute to 100 ml with a mixture of 35 volumes of *glacial acetic acid* and 70 volumes of *hydrochloric acid.* Allow to stand for 15 minutes and measure the *absorbance* of the resulting solution at the maximum at 485 nm, Appendix II B, using the reference cell dissolution medium that has been subjected to the conditions of the test. Calculate the total content of $C_{37}H_{67}NO_{13}$ in the medium using the *absorbance* of a range of suitable solutions of *erythromycin stearate BPCRS,* filtered if necessary, and using the declared content of $C_{37}H_{67}NO_{13}$ in *erythromycin stearate BPCRS.*

Assay Weigh and powder 20 tablets. Dissolve a quantity of the powder containing the equivalent of 25 mg of erythromycin as completely as possible in sufficient *methanol* to produce 100 ml and carry out the *biological assay of antibiotics* for erythromycin, Appendix XIV A. The precision of the assay is such that the fiducial limits of error are not less than 95% and not more than 105% of the estimated potency.

Calculate the content of erythromycin in the tablets, taking each 1000 IU found to be equivalent to 1 mg of erythromycin. The upper fiducial limit of error is not less than 97.0% and the lower fiducial limit of error is not more than 110.0% of the prescribed or stated content.

Storage Erythromycin Stearate Tablets should be protected from light.

Labelling The quantity of active ingredient is stated in terms of the equivalent amount of erythromycin.

Estradiol Injection

Definition Estradiol Injection is a sterile solution of Estradiol Benzoate in Ethyl Oleate or other suitable ester, in a suitable fixed oil or in any mixture of these. It may contain suitable alcohols.

The injection complies with the requirements stated under Parenteral Preparations and with the following requirements.

Content of estradiol benzoate, $C_{25}H_{28}O_3$ 90.0 to 110.0% of the prescribed or stated amount.

Identification Carry out the method for *thin-layer chromatography*, Appendix III A, using *silica gel G* as the coating substance and a mixture of 20 volumes of *ethyl acetate* and 80 volumes of *toluene* as the mobile phase. Apply separately to the plate 5 µl of each of the following solutions. For solution (1) add 10 ml of *2,2,4-trimethylpentane* to a volume of the injection containing 2 mg of Estradiol Benzoate and extract with three 10-ml quantities of *ethanol (70%)*. Wash the combined extracts with 15 ml of *2,2,4-trimethylpentane*, evaporate the ethanolic extract to dryness using a rotary evaporator and dissolve the residue in 2 ml of *chloroform*. Solution (2) contains 0.1% w/v of *estradiol benzoate BPCRS* in *chloroform*. After removal of the plate, allow it to dry in air, spray with *ethanolic sulphuric acid (20%)*, heat at 105° for 10 minutes and examine under *ultraviolet light (365 nm)*. The principal spot in the chromatogram obtained with solution (1) corresponds to that in the chromatogram obtained with solution (2).

Assay Carry out the method for *liquid chromatography*, Appendix III D.

For injections containing 0.2% w/v or more of Estradiol Benzoate Dissolve 15 mg of *4-hydroxybenzaldehyde* (internal standard) in 5 ml of *1,4-dioxan*, add sufficient *cyclohexane* to produce 10 ml (solution A) and use the following solutions. For solution (1) add 1.0 ml of solution A to 10 mg of *estradiol benzoate BPCRS* and add sufficient of a mixture of 9 volumes of *cyclohexane* and 1 volume of *1,4-dioxan* to produce 10 ml. Prepare solution (2) in the same manner as solution (1) using a quantity of the injection containing 10 mg of Estradiol Benzoate but omitting the addition of solution A. Prepare solution (3) in the same manner as solution (1) using a quantity of the injection containing 10 mg of Estradiol Benzoate.

For injections containing less than 0.2% w/v of Estradiol Benzoate Dissolve 15 mg of the internal standard in 10 ml of *1,4-dioxan*, add sufficient *cyclohexane* to produce 100 ml (solution B) and use the following solutions. For solution (1) add 10 ml of solution B to 10 mg of *estradiol benzoate BPCRS* and add sufficient of a mixture of 9 volumes of *cyclohexane* and 1 volume of *1,4-dioxan* to produce 100 ml. For solution (2) dilute a quantity of the injection containing 1 mg of Estradiol Benzoate to 10 ml with a mixture of 9 volumes of *cyclohexane* and 1 volume of *1,4-dioxan*. For solution (3) add 1 ml of solution B to a quantity of the injection containing 1 mg of Estradiol Benzoate and dilute to 10 ml with the same solvent mixture.

The chromatographic procedure may be carried out using (a) a stainless steel column (30 cm × 4 mm) packed with *stationary phase A* (10 µm) (µPorasil is suitable), (b) a mixture of 1 volume of *1,4-dioxan* and 9 volumes of *cyclohexane* as the mobile phase with a flow rate of 2 ml per minute and (c) a detection wavelength of 254 nm.

The assay is not valid unless the *resolution factor* between the peaks due to benzyl alcohol (if present) and estradiol benzoate and between the peaks due to estradiol benzoate and the internal standard is more than 1.5.

Calculate the content of $C_{25}H_{28}O_3$ using the declared content of $C_{25}H_{28}O_3$ in *estradiol benzoate BPCRS*.

Storage Estradiol Injection should be protected from light. If solid matter separates on standing it should be redissolved by warming before use.

Labelling The label states (1) that the preparation is for intramuscular injection only; (2) that any solid matter that has separated on standing should be redissolved by warming before use.

When oestradiol injection is prescribed or demanded, Estradiol Injection shall be dispensed or supplied.

Estramustine Phosphate Capsules

Definition Estramustine Phosphate Capsules contain Estramustine Sodium Phosphate.

The capsules comply with the requirements stated under Capsules and with the following requirements.

Content of estramustine phosphate, $C_{23}H_{32}Cl_2NO_6P$ 92.5 to 107.5% of the prescribed or stated amount.

Identification

A. Shake a quantity of the contents of the capsules containing the equivalent of 0.2 g of estramustine phosphate with 10 ml of *methanol*, filter and evaporate the filtrate to dryness. The *infrared absorption spectrum* of the residue, Appendix II A, is concordant with the *reference spectrum* of estramustine sodium phosphate. In preparing the potassium bromide disc precautions should be taken to exclude moisture and avoid excessive grinding; if necessary heat the prepared disc at 90° for 2 minutes.

B. A 1% w/v solution of the residue obtained in test A yields the reactions characteristic of *sodium salts*, Appendix VI.

Related substances Comply with the test described under Estramustine Sodium Phosphate using for solutions (1) and (2) the residue obtained in test A for Identification in place of the substance being examined.

Assay Shake a quantity of the mixed contents of 20 capsules containing the equivalent of 0.28 g of estramustine phosphate with 20 ml of *water*, dilute to 50 ml with *water* and filter. Dilute 5 ml of the filtrate to 100 ml with *ethanol (50%)* and measure the *absorbance* of the resulting solution at the maximum at 275 nm, Appendix II B. Calculate the content of $C_{23}H_{32}Cl_2NO_6P$ taking 15.4 as the value of A(1%, 1 cm) at the maximum at 275 nm.

Labelling The quantity of active ingredient is stated in terms of the equivalent amount of estramustine phosphate.

Estropipate Tablets

Definition Estropipate Tablets contain Estropipate.

With the exception of the requirements for shape, the tablets comply with the requirements stated under Tablets and with the following requirements.

Content of estropipate, $C_{18}H_{22}O_5S,C_4H_{10}N_2$ 95.0 to 105.0% of the prescribed or stated amount.

Identification In the Assay, the chromatogram obtained with solution (1) shows a peak with the same retention time as the principal peak in the chromatogram obtained with solution (2).

Free estrone Carry out the method for *liquid chromatography*, Appendix III D, using the following solutions. For solution (1) shake a quantity of the powdered tablets containing 5 mg of Estropipate with 20 ml of *methanol (50%)* for 30 minutes, centrifuge and filter the supernatant liquid. Solution (2) contains 0.0005% w/v of *estrone BPCRS* in *methanol (50%)*.

The chromatographic procedure may be carried out using (a) a stainless steel column (30 cm × 3.9 mm) packed with *stationary phase C* (10 µm) (µBondapak C18 is suitable), (b) a mixture of 35 volumes of *acetonitrile* and 65 volumes of 0.025M *potassium dihydrogen orthophosphate* as the mobile phase with a flow rate of 1.5 ml per minute and (c) a detection wavelength of 213 nm. The peak due to estrone has a retention time, relative to the peak due to estropipate, of about 5.

In the chromatogram obtained with solution (1), the area of any peak corresponding to estrone is not greater than the area of the peak in the chromatogram obtained with solution (2) (2%).

Uniformity of content Tablets containing less than 2 mg of Estropipate comply with the requirements stated under Tablets using the following method of analysis. Carry out the method for *liquid chromatography*, Appendix III D, using the following solutions. For solution (1) add 20 ml of *water* to one tablet and shake for 30 minutes, add 20 ml of *methanol* to the mixture and shake for a further 30 minutes, dilute to 50 ml with *methanol (50%)* and filter. Dilute 10 ml of the filtrate to 20 ml with *methanol (50%)*. Solution (2) contains 0.0015% w/v of *estropipate BPCRS* in *methanol (50%)*.

The chromatographic procedure described under Free estrone may be used.

Calculate the content of $C_{18}H_{22}O_5S,C_4H_{10}N_2$ in each tablet using the declared content of $C_{18}H_{22}O_5S,C_4H_{10}N_2$ in *estropipate BPCRS*.

Assay Weigh and powder 20 tablets. Carry out the method for *liquid chromatography*, Appendix III D, using the following solutions. For solution (1) shake a quantity of the powdered tablets containing 3 mg of Estropipate with 40 ml of *methanol (50%)* for 30 minutes, dilute to 100 ml with the same solvent and filter. Solution (2) contains 0.003% w/v of *estropipate BPCRS* in *methanol (50%)*.

The chromatographic procedure described under Free estrone may be used.

Calculate the content of $C_{18}H_{22}O_5S,C_4H_{10}N_2$ in the tablets using the declared content of $C_{18}H_{22}O_5S,C_4H_{10}N_2$ in *estropipate BPCRS*.

Etacrynic Acid Tablets

Definition Etacrynic Acid Tablets contain Etacrynic Acid.

The tablets comply with the requirements stated under Tablets and with the following requirements.

Content of etacrynic acid, $C_{13}H_{12}Cl_2O_4$ 92.5 to 107.5% of the prescribed or stated amount.

Identification Mix a quantity of the powdered tablets containing 50 mg of Etacrynic Acid with 25 ml of 0.1M *hydrochloric acid* and extract with two 40-ml quantities of *dichloromethane*. Dry the combined extracts with *anhydrous sodium sulphate*, filter and evaporate to dryness using a rotary evaporator. The residue complies with the following tests.

A. The *infrared absorption spectrum*, Appendix II A, is concordant with the *reference spectrum* of etacrynic acid.

B. The *light absorption*, Appendix II B, in the range 230 to 350 nm of a 0.005% w/v solution in 0.01M *methanolic hydrochloric acid* exhibits a maximum only at 270 nm and may exhibit a shoulder at 285 nm.

C. Dissolve 25 mg in 2 ml of 1M *sodium hydroxide* and heat on a water bath for 5 minutes. Cool, add 0.25 ml of a 50% v/v solution of *sulphuric acid*, 0.5 ml of a 10% w/v solution of *chromotropic acid sodium salt* and, carefully, 2 ml of *sulphuric acid*. An intense violet colour is produced.

Dissolution Comply with the *dissolution test for tablets and capsules*, Appendix XII D, using Apparatus II. Use as the dissolution medium 900 ml of a buffer solution prepared by dissolving 13.6 g of *potassium dihydrogen orthophosphate* in *water*, adding 72 ml of a 50% w/v solution of *sodium hydroxide* and 800 ml of *water*, adjusting the pH to 8.0 with 1M *sodium hydroxide*, and adding sufficient *water* to produce 1000 ml, and rotate the paddle at 50 revolutions per minute. Withdraw a sample of 10 ml of the medium and filter. Measure the *absorbance* of the filtrate, Appendix II B, at 279 nm using dissolution medium in the reference cell. Calculate the total content of etacrynic acid, $C_{13}H_{12}Cl_2O_4$ in the medium taking 132 as the value of A(1%, 1 cm) at the maximum at 270 nm.

Related substances Carry out the method for *thin-layer chromatography*, Appendix III A, using *silica gel GF_{254}* as the coating substance and a mixture of 20 volumes of *glacial acetic acid*, 50 volumes of *ethyl acetate* and 60 volumes of *chloroform* as the mobile phase. Apply separately to the plate 10 µl of each of the following solutions. For solution (1) shake a quantity of the powdered tablets containing 0.2 g of Etacrynic Acid with 10 ml of *ethanol (96%)* and filter. For solution (2) dilute 10 volumes of solution (1) to 200 volumes with *ethanol (96%)*. For solution (3) dilute 1 volume of solution (2) to 10 volumes with *ethanol (96%)*. After removal of the plate, allow it to dry in air and examine under *ultraviolet light (254 nm)*. Any *secondary spot* occurring at an Rf value of 0.6 in the chromatogram obtained with solution (1) is not more intense than the spot in the chromatogram obtained with solution (2) (5%) and any other *secondary spot* is not more intense than the spot in the chromatogram obtained with solution (3) (0.5%).

Assay Weigh and powder 20 tablets. Carry out the method for *liquid chromatography*, Appendix III D, using the following solutions. For solution (1) dissolve 50 mg of *etacrynic acid BPCRS* in 5 ml of a 0.15% w/v solution of *propyl hydroxybenzoate* (internal standard) in *acetonitrile* and dilute to 50 ml with a mixture of 70 volumes of *acetonitrile* and 30 volumes of *water*. For solution (2) shake a quantity of the powdered tablets containing 50 mg of Etacrynic Acid with 0.5 ml of *glacial acetic acid* and 50 ml of *acetonitrile* for 15 minutes and filter. Prepare solution (3) in the same manner as solution (2) but using 0.5 ml of *glacial acetic acid*, 45 ml of *acetonitrile* and 5 ml of the internal standard solution.

The chromatographic procedure may be carried out using a stainless steel column (20 cm × 4 mm) packed with *stationary phase C* (10 µm) (Spherisorb ODS 1 is suitable), (b) a mixture of 1 volume of *glacial acetic acid*, 40 volumes of *acetonitrile* and 60 volumes of *water* as the mobile phase with a flow rate of 2 ml per minute and (c) a detection wavelength of 270 nm.

Calculate the content of $C_{13}H_{12}Cl_2O_4$ using the declared content of $C_{13}H_{12}Cl_2O_4$ in *etacrynic acid BPCRS*.

When ethacrynic acid tablets are prescribed or demanded, Etacrynic Acid Tablets shall be dispensed or supplied.

Etamiphylline Injection

Definition Etamiphylline Injection is a sterile solution of Etamiphylline Camsilate in Water for Injections.

The injection complies with the requirements stated under Parenteral Preparations and with the following requirements.

Content of etamiphylline camsilate, $C_{13}H_{21}N_5O_2$, $C_{10}H_{16}O_4S$ 95.0 to 105.0% of the prescribed or stated amount.

Identification Prepare a quantity of the residue as described in the Assay. The residue complies with the following tests.

A. The *infrared absorption spectrum*, Appendix II A, is concordant with the *reference spectrum* of etamiphylline.

B. Yields the reactions characteristic of *xanthines*, Appendix VI.

Acidity pH, 3.9 to 5.4, Appendix V L.

Related substances Carry out the method for *thin-layer chromatography*, Appendix III A, using *silica gel HF_{254}* as the coating substance and a mixture of 80 volumes of *chloroform*, 20 volumes of *ethanol (96%)* and 1 volume of 13.5M *ammonia* as the mobile phase. Apply separately to the plate 10 µl of each of the following solutions. For solution (1) dilute the injection with sufficient *water* to produce a solution containing 3.5% w/v of Etamiphylline Camsilate. For solution (2) dilute 1 volume of solution (1) to 500 volumes with *water*. After removal of the plate, allow it to dry in air and examine under *ultraviolet light (254 nm)*. Any *secondary spot* in the chromatogram obtained with solution (1) is not more intense than the spot in the chromatogram obtained with solution (2).

Assay To a volume containing 0.7 g of Etamiphylline Camsilate add 15 ml of *water*, make alkaline with 5M *ammonia* and extract with three 25-ml quantities of *chloroform*, washing each extract with the same 5-ml quantity of *water*. Evaporate the combined extracts to dryness, dissolve the residue in 25 ml of *water* and titrate with 0.05M *sulphuric acid VS* using *bromocresol green solution* as indicator. Each ml of 0.05M *sulphuric acid VS* is equivalent to 51.16 mg of $C_{13}H_{21}N_5O_2,C_{10}H_{16}O_4S$.

Etamiphylline Suppositories

Definition Etamiphylline Suppositories contain Etamiphylline Camsilate in a suitable suppository basis.

The suppositories comply with the requirements stated under Rectal Preparations and with the following requirements.

Content of etamiphylline camsilate, $C_{13}H_{21}N_5O_2$, $C_{10}H_{16}O_4S$ 95.0 to 105.0% of the prescribed or stated amount.

Identification Prepare a quantity of the residue as described in the Assay. The residue complies with the following tests.

A. The *infrared absorption spectrum*, Appendix II A, is concordant with the *reference spectrum* of etamiphylline.

B. Yields the reactions characteristic of *xanthines*, Appendix VI.

Related substances Carry out the method for *thin-layer chromatography*, Appendix III A, using *silica gel HF_{254}* as the coating substance and a mixture of 80 volumes of *chloroform*, 20 volumes of *ethanol (96%)* and 1 volume of 13.5M *ammonia* as the mobile phase. Apply separately to the plate 10 µl of each of the following solutions. For solution (1) add 5 ml of *water* to a quantity of the frozen and powdered suppositories containing 0.2 g of Etamiphylline Camsilate, warm to melt the basis, mix thoroughly, cool in ice and filter through absorbent cotton. For solution (2) dilute 1 volume of solution (1) to 500 volumes with *water*. After removal of the plate, allow it to dry in air and examine under *ultraviolet light (254 nm)*. Any *secondary spot* in the chromatogram obtained with solution (1) is not more intense than the spot in the chromatogram obtained with solution (2).

Assay Weigh, freeze and powder five suppositories. Dissolve a quantity of the powder containing 0.5 g of Etamiphylline Camsilate in 70 ml of *petroleum spirit (boiling range, 40° to 60°)* and extract with three 15-ml quantities of *ethanol (60%)*. Combine the ethanolic solutions, make alkaline with 5M *ammonia* and extract with successive quantities of 50, 25 and 25 ml of *chloroform*, washing each chloroform extract with the same 5-ml quantity of *water*. Evaporate the combined chloroform extracts to dryness, dissolve the residue in 25 ml of *water* and titrate with 0.05M *sulphuric acid VS* using *bromocresol green solution* as indicator. Each ml of 0.05M *sulphuric acid VS* is equivalent to 51.16 mg of $C_{13}H_{21}N_5O_2$, $C_{10}H_{16}O_4S$.

Etamivan Oral Solution

Definition Etamivan Oral Solution is a solution containing 5% w/v of Etamivan and 25% v/v of Ethanol in Purified Water.

Etamivan Oral Solution should not be diluted.

The oral solution complies with the requirements stated under Oral Liquids and with the following requirements.

Content of etamivan, $C_{12}H_{17}NO_3$ 4.75 to 5.25% w/v.

Identification To 20 ml add 4 ml of 2M *hydrochloric acid*, mix and extract with two 40-ml quantities of *chloroform*. Wash the combined chloroform extracts with two 10-ml quantities of *water*, shake the extracts with 10 g of *anhydrous sodium sulphate*, filter and evaporate to dryness using a rotary evaporator. The *infrared absorption spectrum* of the residue, Appendix II A, is concordant with the *reference spectrum* of etamivan.

Ethanol content 24.0 to 26.0% v/v, Appendix VIII F, Method I.

Related substances Carry out the method for *thin-layer chromatography*, Appendix III A, using *silica gel G* as the coating substance and a mixture of 80 volumes of *chloroform* and 20 volumes of *methanol* as the mobile phase. Apply separately to the plate 20 µl of each of the following solutions. For solution (1) mix a quantity containing 0.40 g of Etamivan with 2 ml of 2M *hydrochloric acid*, extract with two 20-ml quantities of *chloroform*, filter the extracts through absorbent cotton and combine the filtrates. Solution (2) is a 0.0025% w/v solution of *vanillic acid* in *chloroform*. After removal of the plate, dry it in a current of air, spray with *diazotised sulphanilic acid*, allow to dry and spray with *dilute sodium carbonate solution*. Any *secondary spot* in the chromatogram obtained with solution (1) is not more intense than the spot in the chromatogram obtained with solution (2).

Assay Dilute 5 ml to 250 ml with *water*. Dilute 5 ml of the solution to 250 ml with 0.01M *hydrochloric acid* and measure the *absorbance* of the resulting solution at the maximum at 280 nm, Appendix II B. Calculate the content of $C_{12}H_{17}NO_3$ taking 155 as the value of A(1%, 1 cm) at the maximum at 280 nm.

Storage Etamivan Oral Solution should be stored at a temperature not exceeding 15°.

When ethamivan oral solution is prescribed or demanded, Etamivan Oral Solution shall be dispensed or supplied.

Ethambutol Tablets

Definition Ethambutol Tablets contain Ethambutol Hydrochloride.

The tablets comply with the requirements stated under Tablets and with the following requirements.

Content of ethambutol hydrochloride, $C_{10}H_{24}N_2O_2$, 2HCl 95.0 to 105.0% of the prescribed or stated amount.

Identification

A. Extract a quantity of the powdered tablets containing 50 mg of Ethambutol Hydrochloride with 5 ml of *methanol*, filter and evaporate the filtrate to dryness. The *infrared absorption spectrum* of the residue, Appendix II A, is concordant with the *reference spectrum* of ethambutol hydrochloride.

B. Shake a quantity of the powdered tablets containing 0.1 g of Ethambutol Hydrochloride with 10 ml of *water*, filter and add to the filtrate 2 ml of a 1% w/v solution of *copper(II) sulphate* followed by 1 ml of 1M *sodium hydroxide*. A blue colour is produced.

2-Aminobutanol Carry out the method for *thin-layer chromatography*, Appendix III A, using *silica gel G* as the coating substance and a mixture of 10 volumes of 13.5M *ammonia*, 15 volumes of *water* and 75 volumes of *methanol* as the mobile phase. Apply separately to the plate 2 µl of each of the following solutions. For solution (1) shake a quantity of the powdered tablets containing 0.50 g of Ethambutol Hydrochloride for 5 minutes with sufficient *methanol* to produce 10 ml. Solution (2) contains 0.050% w/v of *2-aminobutan-1-ol* in *methanol*. After removal of the plate, allow it to dry in air, heat at 110° for 10 minutes, cool, spray with *ninhydrin solution R1* and heat at 110° for 5 minutes. Any spot corresponding to 2-aminobutanol in the chromatogram obtained with solution (1) is not more intense than the spot in the chromatogram obtained with solution (2) (1%).

Assay Weigh and powder 20 tablets. Dissolve a quantity of the powder containing 0.2 g of Ethambutol Hydrochloride in 10 ml of 2M *sodium hydroxide* and extract with five successive 25-ml quantities of *chloroform*. Evaporate the combined extracts to about 25 ml, filter, add 100 ml of *anhydrous acetic acid* and carry out Method I for *non-aqueous titration*, Appendix VIII A, using *1-naphtholbenzein solution* as indicator. Each ml of 0.1M *perchloric acid VS* is equivalent to 13.86 mg of $C_{10}H_{24}N_2O_2$,2HCl.

Ethanolamine Oleate Injection

Definition Ethanolamine Oleate Injection is a sterile solution containing 5% w/v of ethanolamine oleate, prepared by the interaction of Ethanolamine and Oleic Acid, in Water for Injections.

The injection complies with the requirements stated under Parenteral Preparations and with the following requirements.

Content of oleic acid, $C_{18}H_{34}O_2$ 3.9 to 4.5% w/v.

Content of ethanolamine, C_2H_7NO 0.85 to 0.95% w/v.

Alkalinity pH, 8.0 to 9.0, Appendix V L.

Assay

For oleic acid To 10 ml add 20 ml of 0.05M *sulphuric acid VS* and extract with three 25-ml volumes of *chloroform*, washing each extract with the same 10 ml of *water*. Reserve the aqueous solution and washings for the Assay for ethanolamine. Evaporate the combined extracts to dryness, dissolve the residue in *ethanol (96%)* previously neutralised to *phenolphthalein solution R1* and titrate with 0.1M *sodium hydroxide VS* using *phenolphthalein solution R1* as indicator. Each ml of 0.1M *sodium hydroxide VS* is equivalent to 28.25 mg of $C_{18}H_{34}O_2$.

For ethanolamine Titrate the excess of acid in the combined aqueous solution and washings reserved in the Assay for oleic acid with 0.1M *sodium hydroxide VS* using *methyl orange solution* as indicator. Each ml of 0.05M *sulphuric acid VS* is equivalent to 6.108 mg of C_2H_7NO.

Storage Ethanolamine Oleate Injection should be protected from light.

Labelling The label states (1) that the preparation contains 5% of ethanolamine oleate; (2) that the preparation is intended for intravenous injection.

Ethinylestradiol Tablets

Definition Ethinylestradiol Tablets contain Ethinylestradiol.

The tablets comply with the requirements stated under Tablets and with the following requirements.

Content of ethinylestradiol, $C_{20}H_{24}O_2$ 90.0 to 110.0% of the prescribed or stated amount.

Identification

A. Carry out the method for *thin-layer chromatography*, Appendix III A, using *silica gel G* as the coating substance and a mixture of 90 volumes of *toluene* and 10 volumes of *ethanol (96%)* as the mobile phase. Apply separately to the plate 20 µl of each of the following solutions. For solution (1) shake a quantity of the powdered tablets containing 0.25 mg of Ethinylestradiol with four 20-ml quantities of *acetone*, filter each extract in turn, evaporate the combined filtrates to dryness on a water bath in a current of *nitrogen* and dissolve the residue in 0.25 ml of *acetone*. Solution (2) contains 0.1% w/v of *ethinylestradiol BPCRS* in *acetone*. After removal of the plate, allow it to dry in air, spray with *ethanolic sulphuric acid (20%)*, heat at 110° for 10 minutes and examine under *ultraviolet light (365 nm)* and in daylight. By each method of visualisation the principal spot in the chromatogram obtained with solution (1) corresponds to that in the chromatogram obtained with solution (2).

B. Triturate a quantity of the powdered tablets containing 0.1 mg of Ethinylestradiol with 0.5 ml of 0.1M *sodium hydroxide* and 5 ml of *water*, allow to stand for 5 minutes, filter, acidify the filtrate with 0.15 ml of *sulphuric acid*, add 3 ml of *ether*, shake and allow to separate. Evaporate the ether layer to dryness and heat the residue on a water bath for 5 minutes with 0.2 ml of *glacial acetic acid* and 2 ml of *orthophosphoric acid*. A pink colour with an intense orange fluorescence is produced.

Uniformity of content Tablets containing less than 2 mg of Ethinylestradiol comply with the requirements stated under Tablets using the following method of analysis. Carry out the method for *liquid chromatography*, Appendix III D, using the following solutions. Solution (1) contains 0.0025% w/v of *ethinylestradiol BPCRS* in the mobile phase. For tablets containing less than 50 µg of Ethinylestradiol, solution (1) contains 0.0005% w/v of *ethinylestradiol BPCRS* in the mobile phase. For solution (2) add 2 ml of the mobile phase to one tablet, allow to stand for 5 minutes, mix with the aid of ultrasound for 5 minutes, centrifuge and use the clear supernatant liquid.

The chromatographic procedure may be carried out using (a) a stainless steel column (20 cm × 4.6 mm) packed with *stationary phase C* (5 µm) (Zorbax ODS is suitable), (b) a mixture of 40 volumes of *water* and 60 volumes of *acetonitrile* as the mobile phase with a flow rate of 1.5 ml per minute and (c) a detection wavelength of 280 nm.

Calculate the content of $C_{20}H_{24}O_2$ using the declared content of $C_{20}H_{24}O_2$ in *ethinylestradiol BPCRS*.

Assay Use the average of the 10 individual results obtained in the test for Uniformity of content.

Storage Ethinylestradiol Tablets should be protected from light.

When ethinyloestradiol tablets are prescribed or demanded, Ethinylestradiol Tablets shall be dispensed or supplied.

Ethosuximide Capsules

Definition Ethosuximide Capsules contain Ethosuximide.

The capsules comply with the requirements stated under Capsules and with the following requirements.

Content of ethosuximide, $C_7H_{11}NO_2$ 95.0 to 105.0% of the prescribed or stated amount.

Identification

A. Heat a quantity of the contents of the capsules containing 0.1 g of Ethosuximide with 0.2 g of *resorcinol* and 0.1 ml of *sulphuric acid* at 140° for 5 minutes, add 5 ml of *water*, make alkaline with 5M *sodium hydroxide* and add 0.2 ml to a large volume of *water*. A bright green fluorescence is produced.

B. To a quantity of the contents of the capsules containing 0.5 g of Ethosuximide add 15 ml of a 40% w/v solution of *sodium hydroxide*. Boil under a reflux condenser for 30 minutes, cool, acidify with *hydrochloric acid* and extract with three 30-ml quantities of *ether*. Wash the combined extracts with 5 ml of *water* and evaporate to dryness. The *melting point* of the residue, after recrystallisation from *toluene* and *petroleum spirit (boiling range, 40° to 60°)*, is about 102°, Appendix V A.

Assay Weigh 20 capsules. Open the capsules carefully without loss of shell material, express as much of the contents as possible and reserve the expressed material. Wash the shells with *ether*, discard the washings, allow the shells to stand at room temperature until the odour of the ether is no longer detectable and weigh. The difference between the weights represents the weight of the total contents. Dissolve a quantity of the contents containing 0.2 g of Ethosuximide in 30 ml of *dimethylformamide* and carry out Method II for *non-aqueous titration*, Appendix VIII A, using *magneson solution* as indicator and 0.1M *tetrabutylammonium hydroxide VS* as titrant. Each ml of 0.1M *tetrabutylammonium hydroxide VS* is equivalent to 14.12 mg of $C_7H_{11}NO_2$.

Ethosuximide Oral Solution

Definition Ethosuximide Oral Solution is a solution of Ethosuximide in a suitable flavoured vehicle.

The oral solution complies with the requirements stated under Oral Liquids and with the following requirements.

Content of ethosuximide, $C_7H_{11}NO_2$ 95.0 to 105.0% of the prescribed or stated amount.

Identification
A. Extract a quantity containing 0.5 g of Ethosuximide with two 30-ml quantities of *chloroform*, filter the combined extracts through absorbent cotton and evaporate the filtrate to dryness. Heat 0.1 g of the residue with 0.2 g of *resorcinol* and 0.1 ml of *sulphuric acid* at 140° for 5 minutes, cool, add 5 ml of *water*, make alkaline with 5M *sodium hydroxide* and add 0.2 ml to a large volume of *water*. A bright green fluorescence is produced.

B. In the Assay, the chromatogram obtained with solution (2) shows a peak with the same retention time as that due to *ethosuximide BPCRS* in the chromatogram obtained with solution (1).

Assay Carry out the method for *gas chromatography*, Appendix III B, using the following solutions. For solution (1) add 2 ml of a 3.0% w/v solution of *dimethyl phthalate* (internal standard) in *chloroform* to 25 ml of a 0.2% w/v solution of *ethosuximide BPCRS* in *chloroform*. Prepare solution (2) in the same manner as solution (3) but omit the internal standard. For solution (3) add 10 ml of *water* and 2 g of *sodium hydrogen carbonate* to a weighed quantity of the oral solution containing 0.25 g of Ethosuximide and extract with five 25-ml quantities of *chloroform*, washing each extract with the same 10 ml of *water*. To the combined extracts add 10 ml of the internal standard solution, shake with 10 g of *anhydrous sodium sulphate* and filter.

The chromatographic procedure may be carried out using a glass column (1.5 m × 4 mm) packed with *acid-washed, silanised diatomaceous support* (80 to 100 mesh) coated with 3% w/w of cyanopropylmethyl phenyl methyl silicone fluid (OV-225 is suitable) and maintained at 165°.

Determine the *weight per ml* of the oral solution, Appendix V G, and calculate the content of $C_7H_{11}NO_2$, weight in volume, using the declared content of $C_7H_{11}NO_2$ in *ethosuximide BPCRS*.

Storage Ethosuximide Oral Solution should be stored at a temperature not exceeding 25°.

Ethylestrenol Tablets

Definition Ethylestrenol Tablets contain Ethylestrenol.

The tablets comply with the requirements stated under Tablets and with the following requirements.

Content of ethylestrenol, $C_{20}H_{32}O$ 90.0 to 110.0% of the prescribed or stated amount.

Identification
A. Carry out the method for *thin-layer chromatography*, Appendix III A, using *silica gel G* as the coating substance and a mixture of 80 volumes of n-*heptane* and 20 volumes of *acetone* as the mobile phase but allowing the solvent front to ascend 10 cm above the line of application. Apply separately to the plate 2 µl of each of the following solutions. For solution (1) extract a quantity of the powdered tablets containing 1 mg of Ethylestrenol with *chloroform*, filter, evaporate the filtrate to dryness at 20° at a pressure of 2 kPa and dissolve the residue in 0.4 ml of a mixture of 9 volumes of *chloroform* and 1 volume of *methanol*. Solution (2) contains 0.25% w/v of *ethylestrenol BPCRS* in a mixture of 9 volumes of *chloroform* and 1 volume of *methanol*. Solution (3) is a mixture of equal volumes of solutions (1) and (2). After removal of the plate, heat it at 105° for 10 minutes, spray with *ethanolic sulphuric acid (20%)*, heat at 105° for a further 10 minutes, allow to cool and examine in daylight and under *ultraviolet light (365 nm)*. The principal spot in the chromatogram obtained with solution (1) corresponds in colour, size and fluorescence to that in the chromatogram obtained with solution (2).

B. In the Assay, the chromatogram obtained with solution (2) shows a peak with the same retention time as the peak due to ethylestrenol in the chromatogram obtained with solution (1).

17α-Ethylestran-17β-ol Comply with the test described under Ethylestrenol using the following solutions. For solution (1) dissolve 20 mg of the residue obtained in the test for Related substances in 0.5 ml of a mixture of 9 volumes of *chloroform* and 1 volume of *methanol*. Solution (2) contains 0.080% w/v of *17α-ethylestran-17β-ol BPCRS* in a mixture of 9 volumes of *chloroform* and 1 volume of *methanol*.

Related substances Comply with the test described under Ethylestrenol using the following solutions. For solution (1) extract a quantity of the powdered tablets containing 40 mg of Ethylestrenol with *chloroform*, filter, evaporate the filtrate to dryness and dissolve 10 mg of the residue in 1 ml of a mixture of 9 volumes of *chloroform* and 1 volume of *methanol*. For solution (2) dilute 1 volume of solution (1) to 100 volumes with the same solvent. For solution (3) dilute 1 volume of solution (2) to 2 volumes with the same solvent.

Assay Weigh and powder 20 tablets. Carry out the method for *gas chromatography*, Appendix III B, using the following solutions. Solution (1) contains 0.1% w/v of *arachidic alcohol* (internal standard) and 0.2% w/v of *ethylestrenol BPCRS* in *chloroform*. For solution (2) extract a quantity of the powdered tablets containing 8 mg of Ethylestrenol with 20 ml of *acetone*, filter, evaporate the filtrate to dryness on a water bath and dissolve the residue in 4 ml of *chloroform*. Prepare solution (3) in the same manner as solution (2) but extract with 20 ml of a 0.02% w/v solution of *arachidic alcohol* in *acetone*.

The chromatographic procedure may be carried out using a glass column (1.0 m × 4 mm) packed with *acid-washed, silanised diatomaceous support* (80 to 100 mesh) and coated with 3% w/w of phenyl methyl silicone fluid (50% phenyl) (OV-17 is suitable) and maintained at 200°.

Calculate the content of $C_{20}H_{32}O$ using the declared content of $C_{20}H_{32}O$ in *ethylestrenol BPCRS*.

Storage Ethylestrenol Tablets should be protected from light and stored at a temperature not exceeding 15°.

When ethyloestrenol tablets are prescribed or demanded, Ethylestrenol Tablets shall be dispensed or supplied.

Etodolac Capsules

Definition Etodolac Capsules contain Etodolac.

The capsules comply with the requirements stated under Capsules and with the following requirements.

Content of etodolac $C_{17}H_{21}NO_3$ 95.0 to 105.0% of the prescribed or stated amount.

Identification
A. To a quantity of the contents of the capsules containing about 0.1 g of Etodolac add 4 ml of 0.01M *hydrochloric*

acid and mix with the aid of ultrasound for 5 minutes, shaking occasionally, centrifuge for 10 minutes, discard the supernatant liquid and wash the residue with 4 ml of *water*. Shake to disperse, centrifuge for 10 minutes and discard the supernatant liquid. Add 4 ml of 0.01M *sodium hydroxide* to the residue and mix with the aid of ultrasound for 5 minutes, shaking occasionally and centrifuge for 10 minutes. Transfer the supernatant liquid to a second centrifuge tube, add about 1 ml of 0.1M *hydrochloric acid* (the pH of the supernatant liquid should be 2 or less). Centrifuge for 10 minutes, discard the supernatant liquid and wash the residue with 4 ml of *water*, shake to disperse and centrifuge for 10 minutes. Discard the supernatant liquid and dry the residue at 105° for 1 hour. The *infrared absorption spectrum* of the residue, Appendix II A, is concordant with the *reference spectrum* of etodolac.

B. In the Assay, the chromatogram obtained with solution (1) shows a peak with the same retention time as the peak due to etodolac in the chromatogram obtained with solution (2).

Dissolution Comply with the *dissolution test for tablets and capsules*, Appendix XII D, using as the medium 900 ml of *phosphate buffer pH 7.5* and rotating the basket at 100 revolutions per minute. Withdraw a 10-ml sample of the medium and measure the *absorbance* of the filtered sample, suitably diluted if necessary, at the maximum at 278 nm, Appendix II B. Measure the *absorbance* of a suitable solution of *etodolac BPCRS* prepared by dissolving 30 mg in 100 ml of the dissolution medium and diluting to a suitable volume with the dissolution medium and using dissolution medium in the reference cell. Calculate the total content of etodolac, $C_{17}H_{21}NO_3$ in the medium from the absorbances obtained and from the declared content of $C_{17}H_{21}NO_3$ in *etodolac BPCRS*.

Related substances Carry out the method for *thin-layer chromatography*, Appendix III A, using a silica gel F_{254} precoated plate (Merck silica gel 60 F_{254} plates are suitable), previously activated by heating at 105° for 1 hour, and a mixture of 0.5 volumes of *glacial acetic acid*, 30 volumes of *absolute ethanol* and 70 volumes of *toluene* as the mobile phase. Place the plate in an unlined tank containing a solution prepared by dissolving 0.5 g of *L-ascorbic acid* in 20 ml of *water* and adding 80 ml of *methanol*. Allow the solution to ascend 1 cm above the line of application on the plate, remove the plate and allow it to dry for at least 30 minutes. Apply separately to the plate 10 µl of each of the following solutions in *acetone*. For solution (1) shake a quantity of the contents of the capsules containing 0.2 g of Etodolac with 20 ml of *acetone*, mix with the aid of ultrasound for 5 minutes and filter. For solution (2) dilute 1 volume of solution (1) to 200 volumes with *acetone* and for solution (3) dilute 1 volume of solution (2) to 2 volumes with *acetone*. After removal of the plate, allow it to dry in air and examine under *ultraviolet light (254 nm)*. Any *secondary spot* in the chromatogram obtained with solution (1) is not more intense than the spot in the chromatogram obtained with solution (2) (0.5%) and not more than one such spot is more intense than the spot in the chromatogram obtained with solution (3) (0.25%).

Etodolac acid dimer Carry out the method for *thin-layer chromatography*, Appendix III A, using a silica gel F_{254} precoated plate (Merck silica gel 60 F_{254} plates are suitable), previously activated by heating at 105° for 1 hour, and a mixture of 3 volumes of *glacial acetic acid*, 17 volumes of *1,4-dioxan* and 60 volumes of *toluene* as the mobile phase. Place the plate in an unlined tank containing a solution prepared by dissolving 0.5 g of *L-ascorbic acid* in 20 ml of *water* and adding 80 ml of *methanol*. Allow the solution to ascend 1 cm above the line of application on the plate, remove the plate and allow it to dry for at least 30 minutes. Apply separately to the plate 20 µl of each of the following solutions. For solution (1) shake a quantity of the contents of the capsules containing 0.2 g of Etodolac with 20 ml of *methanol*, mix with the aid of ultrasound for 5 minutes and filter. Solution (2) contains 0.001% w/v of *etodolac acid dimer BPCRS* in *methanol*. After removal of the plate, allow it to dry in air and examine under *ultraviolet light (254 nm)*. Any *secondary spot* in the chromatogram obtained with solution (1) corresponding to the acid dimer is not more intense than the spot in the chromatogram obtained with solution (2) (0.1%).

Total methyl analogue impurities Comply with the test described under Etodolac but preparing solution (1) in the following manner. Shake a quantity of the contents of the capsules containing 0.1 g of Etodolac with 40 ml of *methanol*, mix with the aid of ultrasound for 5 minutes, filter and dilute 10 ml of the filtrate to 25 ml with *water*.

Assay Carry out the method for *liquid chromatography*, Appendix III D, using the following solutions. For solution (1) shake a quantity of the mixed contents of 20 capsules containing 50 mg of Etodolac with about 70 ml of 0.1M *sodium hydroxide* for 30 minutes, dilute to 100 ml with 0.1M *sodium hydroxide*, mix and filter through a glass-fibre filter (Whatman GF/C is suitable) and dilute 2 ml of the filtrate to 100 ml with the mobile phase. For solution (2) dilute 2 ml of a 0.05% w/v solution of *etodolac BPCRS* in 0.1M *sodium hydroxide* to 100 ml with the mobile phase. For solution (3) add 2 ml of a 0.05% w/v solution of *etodolac 1-methyl analogue BPCRS* to 2 ml of a 0.05% w/v solution of *etodolac BPCRS* in 0.1M *sodium hydroxide* and dilute to 100 ml with the mobile phase.

The chromatographic procedure may be carried out using (a) a stainless steel column (12.5 cm × 4.6 mm) packed with *stationary phase C* (5 µm) (Spherisorb ODS1 is suitable), (b) a mixture of 45 volumes of *acetonitrile* and 55 volumes of *phosphate buffer pH 4.75* as the mobile phase with a flow rate of 1 ml per minute and (c) a detection wavelength of 225 nm.

The test is not valid unless the *resolution factor* between etodolac and etodolac 1-methyl analogue in the chromatogram obtained with solution (3) is at least 1.5.

Calculate the content of $C_{17}H_{21}NO_3$ using the declared content of $C_{17}H_{21}NO_3$ in *etodolac BPCRS*.

Etodolac Tablets

Definition Etodolac Tablets contain Etodolac.

With the exception of the requirements for shape, the tablets comply with the requirements stated under Tablets and with the following requirements.

Content of etodolac $C_{17}H_{21}NO_3$ 95.0 to 105.0% of the prescribed or stated amount.

Identification

A. Shake a quantity of the powdered tablets containing 0.5 g of Etodolac with 30 ml of *hexane* for 5 minutes, centrifuge, discard the clear hexane layer and add about 40 ml of *ether* to the residue; shake for 5 minutes, centrifuge for 5 minutes, decant the ether layer and filter if necessary. Evaporate the solution to dryness under nitrogen and add about 5 ml of 0.1M *hydrochloric acid* to the residue. Warm on a water bath until the residue begins to crystallise and triturate with a glass rod to promote crystallisation. Cool the mixture in an ice bath, filter through a glass-fibre filter (Whatman GF/C is suitable) and dry the crystals at a pressure of 2 kPa at 60° for 1 hour. The *infrared absorption spectrum* of the residue, Appendix II A, is concordant with the *reference spectrum* of etodolac.

B. In the Assay, the chromatogram obtained with solution (1) shows a peak with the same retention time as the peak due to etodolac in the chromatogram obtained with solution (2).

Dissolution Comply with the *dissolution test for tablets and capsules*, Appendix XII D, using as the medium 900 ml of *phosphate buffer pH 7.5* and rotating the basket at 100 revolutions per minute. Withdraw a 10-ml sample of the medium and measure the *absorbance* of the filtered sample, suitably diluted if necessary, at the maximum at 278 nm, Appendix II B. Measure the *absorbance* of a suitable solution of *etodolac BPCRS* prepared by dissolving 20 mg in 100 ml of the dissolution medium and diluting to a suitable volume with the dissolution medium and using dissolution medium in the reference cell. Calculate the total content of etodolac, $C_{17}H_{21}NO_3$ in the medium from the absorbances obtained and from the declared content of $C_{17}H_{21}NO_3$ in *etodolac BPCRS*.

Related substances Comply with the test described under Etodolac Capsules using a quantity of the powdered tablets containing 0.2 g of Etodolac in place of the contents of the capsules.

Etodolac acid dimer Comply with the test described under Etodolac Capsules using a quantity of the powdered tablets containing 0.2 g of Etodolac in place of the contents of the capsules.

Total methyl analogue impurities Comply with the test described under Etodolac but preparing solution (1) in the following manner. Shake a quantity of the powdered tablets containing 0.1 g of Etodolac with 40 ml of *methanol*, mix with the aid of ultrasound for 5 minutes, filter and dilute 10 ml of the filtrate to 25 ml with *water*.

Assay Weigh and powder 20 tablets. Carry out the method for *liquid chromatography*, Appendix III D, using the following solutions. For solution (1) shake a quantity of the powdered tablets containing 50 mg of Etodolac with about 70 ml of 0.1M *sodium hydroxide* for 30 minutes, dilute to 100 ml with 0.1M *sodium hydroxide*, mix, filter through a glass-fibre filter (Whatman GF/C is suitable) and dilute 2 ml of the resulting solution to 100 ml with the mobile phase. For solution (2) dilute 2 ml of a 0.05% w/v solution of *etodolac BPCRS* in 0.1M *sodium hydroxide* to 100 ml with the mobile phase. For solution (3) add 2 ml of a 0.05% w/v solution of *etodolac 1-methyl analogue BPCRS* to 2 ml of a 0.05% w/v solution of *etodolac BPCRS* in 0.1M *sodium hydroxide* and dilute to 100 ml with the mobile phase.

The chromatographic procedure may be carried out using (a) a stainless steel column (12.5 cm × 4.6 mm) packed with *stationary phase C* (5 μm) (Spherisorb ODS 1 is suitable), (b) a mixture of 45 volumes of *acetonitrile* and 55 volumes of *phosphate buffer pH 4.75* as the mobile phase with a flow rate of 1 ml per minute and (c) a detection wavelength of 225 nm.

The test is not valid unless the *resolution factor* between etodolac and etodolac 1-methyl analogue in the chromatogram obtained with solution (3) is at least 1.5.

Calculate the content of $C_{17}H_{21}NO_3$ using the declared content of $C_{17}H_{21}NO_3$ in *etodolac BPCRS*.

Fenbufen Capsules

Definition Fenbufen Capsules contain Fenbufen.

The capsules comply with the requirements stated under Capsules and with the following requirements.

Content of fenbufen, $C_{16}H_{14}O_3$ 95.0 to 105.0% of the prescribed or stated amount.

Identification

A. To a quantity of the contents of the capsules containing 0.9 g of Fenbufen add 10 ml of *acetone*, triturate using a glass pestle, filter through filter paper wetted with *acetone* into 100 ml of *petroleum spirit (boiling point, 40° to 60°)*, stir rapidly with a glass rod to induce crystallisation and allow to stand for 15 minutes. Filter through a fine porosity sintered-glass funnel, rinse the crystals with 25 ml of *petroleum spirit (boiling point, 40° to 60°)*, remove the solvent under reduced pressure and dry the crystals at 105° for 15 minutes. The *infrared absorption spectrum* of the dried crystals, Appendix II A, is concordant with the *reference spectrum* of fenbufen.

B. In the Assay, the retention time of the principal peak in the chromatogram obtained with solution (1) is the same as that of the peak in the chromatogram obtained with solution (2).

Dissolution Comply with the *dissolution test for tablets and capsules*, Appendix XII D, using Apparatus II. Use as the medium 900 ml of a phosphate buffer prepared by dissolving 6.69 g of *potassium dihydrogen orthophosphate* and 1.63 g of *sodium hydroxide* in sufficient *water* to produce 1000 ml, adjusting the pH to 7.5 with 5M *sodium hydroxide* if necessary, and rotate the paddle at 100 revolutions per minute. Withdraw a sample of 10 ml of the medium, filter (Whatman 541 paper is suitable) and dilute 1 ml of the filtrate to 50 ml with the dissolution medium. Measure the *absorbance* of this solution, Appendix II B, at 285 nm using dissolution medium in the reference cell. Measure the *absorbance* of a suitable solution of *fenbufen BPCRS* prepared by dissolving 50 mg in 50 ml of *methanol* and diluting to a suitable volume with the dissolution medium and using dissolution medium in the reference cell. Calculate the total content of fenbufen, $C_{16}H_{14}O_3$ in the medium from the absorbances obtained and from the declared content of $C_{16}H_{14}O_3$ in *fenbufen BPCRS*.

Related substances Carry out the method for *liquid chromatography*, Appendix III D, using the following solutions. For solution (1) add to a quantity of the contents of the capsules containing 0.25 g of Fenbufen 20 ml of *dimethylformamide*, mix with the aid of ultrasound for 20 minutes, dilute to 50 ml with the initial mobile phase and filter (Whatman GF/F paper is suitable). For solution (2) dilute 1 volume of solution (1) to 100 volumes with the initial mobile phase and further dilute 1 volume of this solution to 10 volumes with the initial mobile phase. Solution (3) contains 0.0025% w/v of *fenbufen BPCRS* and 0.0006% w/v of *3-(4-chlorobenzoyl)propionic acid.*

The chromatographic procedure may be carried out using a stainless steel column (10 cm × 4.6 mm) packed with *stationary phase C* (5 µm) (Spherisorb ODS 2 is suitable). Use as the initial mobile phase a mixture of 32 volumes of *acetonitrile* and 68 volumes of a solution consisting of 1 volume of *glacial acetic acid* and 55 volumes of *water* and as the final mobile phase a mixture of 45 volumes of *acetonitrile* and 55 volumes of a solution consisting of 1 volume of *glacial acetic acid* and 55 volumes of *water*. Maintain the initial mobile phase for 15 minutes, carry out a linear gradient elution with a flow rate of 2 ml per minute for 5 minutes and maintain the final mobile phase for 15 minutes with the same flow rate. Use a detection wavelength of 254 nm.

The test is not valid unless in the chromatogram obtained with solution (3) the *resolution factor* between the two principal peaks is at least 10.

In the chromatogram obtained with solution (1) the area of any *secondary peak* is not greater than the area of the principal peak in the chromatogram obtained with solution (2) (0.1%) and the sum of the areas of any such peaks is not greater than five times the area of the principal peak in the chromatogram obtained with solution (2) (0.5%).

Assay Carry out the method for *liquid chromatography*, Appendix III D, using the following solutions. For solution (1) add to a quantity of the mixed contents of 20 capsules containing 0.25 g of Fenbufen 20 ml of *acetonitrile*, mix with the aid of ultrasound for 15 minutes, add sufficient mobile phase to produce 250 ml and dilute 1 volume of this solution to 10 volumes with the mobile phase. Solution (2) contains 0.01% w/v of *fenbufen BPCRS* in the mobile phase.

The chromatographic procedure may be carried out using (a) a stainless steel column (30 cm × 3.9 mm) packed with *stationary phase C* (10 µm) (µBondapak C18 is suitable), maintained about 40°, (b) a mixture of 1 volume of *glacial acetic acid*, 44 volumes of *acetonitrile* and 55 volumes of *water* as the mobile phase with a flow rate of 1.5 ml per minute and (c) a detection wavelength of 280 nm.

Calculate the content of $C_{16}H_{14}O_3$ in the capsules using the declared content of $C_{16}H_{14}O_3$ in *fenbufen BPCRS*.

Fenbufen Tablets

Definition Fenbufen Tablets contain Fenbufen.

With the exception of the requirements for shape, the tablets comply with the requirements stated under Tablets and with the following requirements.

Content of fenbufen, $C_{16}H_{14}O_3$ 95.0 to 105.0% of the prescribed or stated amount.

Identification

A. To a quantity of the powdered tablets containing 0.9 g of Fenbufen add 10 ml of *acetone*, triturate using a glass pestle, filter through filter paper wetted with *acetone* into 100 ml of *petroleum spirit (boiling point, 40° to 60°)*, stir rapidly with a glass rod to induce crystallisation and allow to stand for 15 minutes. Filter through a fine porosity sintered-glass funnel, rinse the crystals with 25 ml of *petroleum spirit (boiling point, 40° to 60°)*, remove the solvent under reduced pressure and dry the crystals at 105° for 15 minutes. The *infrared absorption spectrum* of the dried crystals, Appendix II A, is concordant with the *reference spectrum* of fenbufen.

B. In the Assay, the retention time of the principal peak in the chromatogram obtained with solution (1) is the same as that of the peak in the chromatogram obtained with solution (2).

Dissolution Comply with the *dissolution test for tablets and capsules*, Appendix XII D, using Apparatus II. Use as the medium 900 ml of a phosphate buffer prepared by dissolving 6.69 g of *potassium dihydrogen orthophosphate* and 1.63 g of *sodium hydroxide* in sufficient *water* to produce 1000 ml, adjusting the pH to 7.5 with 5M *sodium hydroxide* if necessary, and rotate the paddle at 100 revolutions per minute. Withdraw a sample of 10 ml of the medium, filter (Whatman 541 paper is suitable) and dilute 1 ml of the filtrate to 50 ml with the dissolution medium. Measure the *absorbance* of this solution, Appendix II B, at 285 nm using dissolution medium in the reference cell. Measure the *absorbance* of a suitable solution of *fenbufen BPCRS* prepared by dissolving 50 mg in 50 ml of *methanol* and diluting to volume with the dissolution medium and using dissolution medium in the reference cell. Calculate the total content of fenbufen, $C_{16}H_{14}O_3$ in the medium from the absorbances obtained and from the declared content of $C_{16}H_{14}O_3$ in *fenbufen BPCRS*.

Related substances Comply with the test described under Fenbufen Capsules but using as solution (1) a solution prepared in the following manner. To a quantity of the powdered tablets containing 0.25 g of Fenbufen add 20 ml of *dimethylformamide*, mix with the aid of ultrasound for 20 minutes, add sufficient of the initial mobile phase to produce 50 ml and filter (Whatman GF/F paper is suitable).

Assay Weigh and powder 20 tablets. Carry out the Assay described under Fenbufen Capsules but using as solution (1) a solution prepared in the following manner. To a quantity of the powdered tablets containing 0.25 g of Fenbufen add 20 ml of *acetonitrile*, mix with the aid of ultrasound for 20 minutes, add sufficient of the mobile phase to produce 50 ml, filter through a 0.45-µm filter (Whatman GF/C is suitable) and dilute 1 volume to 50 volumes with the mobile phase.

Fenoprofen Tablets

Definition Fenoprofen Tablets contain Fenoprofen Calcium. They are coated.

With the exception of the requirements for shape, the tablets comply with the requirements stated under Tablets and with the following requirements.

Content of fenoprofen, $C_{15}H_{14}O_3$ 95.0 to 105.0% of the prescribed or stated amount.

Identification

A. The *light absorption*, Appendix II B, in the range 230 to 350 nm of the final solution obtained in the Assay exhibits two maxima, at 272 nm and 278 nm, and a shoulder at 266 nm.

B. Suspend a quantity of the powdered tablets containing the equivalent of 0.3 g of fenoprofen in 10 ml of 0.1M *hydrochloric acid*. Extract with 20 ml of *chloroform*, filter the extract through *anhydrous sodium sulphate* and evaporate the filtrate to dryness. The *infrared absorption spectrum* of a thin film of the residue, Appendix II A, is concordant with the *reference spectrum* of fenoprofen.

C. Ignite a quantity of the powdered tablets. The residue yields the reactions characteristic of *calcium salts*, Appendix VI.

Related substances Carry out the method for *liquid chromatography*, Appendix III D, using the following solutions. For solution (1) add 80 ml of the mobile phase to a quantity of the powdered tablets containing the equivalent of 0.5 g of fenoprofen, mix with the aid of ultrasound, allow to cool, add sufficient mobile phase to produce 100 ml and filter. For solution (2) dilute 1 volume of solution (1) to 200 volumes with the mobile phase. Solution (3) contains 0.04% w/v of *fenoprofen calcium* and 0.0015% w/v of *4,4′-dimethoxybenzophenone*.

The chromatographic procedure may be carried out using (a) a stainless steel column (25 cm × 4.6 mm) packed with *stationary phase C* (7 to 8 µm) (Zorbax ODS is suitable), (b) a mixture of 61 volumes of *water*, 30 volumes of *acetonitrile*, 7 volumes of *tetrahydrofuran* and 2 volumes of *glacial acetic acid* as the mobile phase with a flow rate of 2 ml per minute and (c) a detection wavelength of 270 nm. For solution (1) allow the chromatography to proceed for 3 times the retention time of the peak due to fenoprofen.

The test is not valid unless the *resolution factor* between the peaks corresponding to fenoprofen calcium and 4,4′-dimethoxybenzophenone in the chromatogram obtained with solution (3) is at least 3.0.

In the chromatogram obtained with solution (1) the area of any *secondary peak* is not greater than twice the area of the peak in the chromatogram obtained with solution (2), not more than one such peak has an area greater than the area of the peak in the chromatogram obtained with solution (2) and the sum of the areas of all such peaks is not greater than four times the area of the peak in the chromatogram obtained with solution (2).

Assay Weigh and powder 20 tablets. To a quantity of the powder containing the equivalent of 0.2 g of fenoprofen add 5 ml of *glacial acetic acid* and shake for 1 minute. Add 100 ml of *methanol*, shake for 5 minutes, dilute to 200 ml with *methanol* and filter. Dilute 10 ml of the filtrate to 200 ml with *methanol* and measure the *absorbance* of the resulting solution at the maximum at 272 nm, Appendix II B. Calculate the content of $C_{15}H_{14}O_3$ taking 80.7 as the value of A(1%, 1 cm) at the maximum at 272 nm.

Labelling The quantity of active ingredient is stated in terms of the equivalent amount of fenoprofen.

Ferrous Fumarate Oral Suspension

Definition Ferrous Fumarate Oral Suspension is a suspension of Ferrous Fumarate in a suitable flavoured vehicle.

The oral suspension complies with the requirements stated under Oral Liquids and with the following requirements.

Content of ferrous iron, Fe(II) 90.0 to 110.0% of the prescribed or stated amount.

Identification

A. Mix a volume of the oral suspension containing about 0.6 g of Ferrous Fumarate with 20 ml of *water*, centrifuge and discard the supernatant liquid. Repeat with a further 20 ml of *water*. Add 15 ml of 3M *hydrochloric acid* to the residue, dissolve with minimum warming, cool and extract with two 50-ml quantities of *ether*. Wash the combined ether extracts with two 20-ml quantities of *water*, shake with *anhydrous sodium sulphate*, filter and evaporate to dryness. The *infrared absorption spectrum* of the residue, Appendix II A, is concordant with the *reference spectrum* of fumaric acid.

B. Mix a volume of the oral suspension containing about 0.3 g of Ferrous Fumarate in 10 ml of *water*, centrifuge and discard the supernatant liquid. To 0.2 g of the residue add 10 ml of a mixture of equal volumes of *hydrochloric acid* and *water*, dissolve with minimum warming, cool and filter. The filtrate yields reaction A characteristic of *iron salts*, Appendix VI.

Ferric iron Disperse a quantity of the oral suspension containing 0.28 g of Ferrous Fumarate in 20 ml of *water*, centrifuge and decant the supernatant liquid into a 500-ml graduated flask. Dissolve the residue in 20 ml of 1M *sulphuric acid* with minimum warming, cool and transfer the resulting solution to the same graduated flask, dilute to 500 ml with *water* and filter. To 5 ml of the filtrate in a *Nessler cylinder* add 40 ml of *water* and 5 ml of a 10% w/v solution of *ammonium thiocyanate* and mix. Any red colour produced is not more intense than that obtained by treating in the same manner a mixture of 42 ml of *water*, 0.2 ml of 1M *sulphuric acid* and 3 ml of a 0.0173% w/v solution of *ammonium iron(III) sulphate* in 0.01M *hydrochloric acid* [6.0%, with respect to the content of Fe(II)].

Assay Mix a quantity of the oral suspension containing 0.28 g of Ferrous Fumarate with 10 ml of *water* and 25 ml of *nitric acid*, carefully warm until the vigorous reaction subsides, add a further 25 ml of *nitric acid*, evaporate to about 10 ml and allow to cool. Carefully add 10 ml of *sulphuric acid* to the cooled solution, evaporate until white fumes are evolved, cool, add 10 ml of *nitric acid* and again evaporate until white fumes are evolved. Repeat the evaporation with 10-ml quantities of *nitric acid* until all of the organic matter has been destroyed. To the resulting solution add 10 ml of *water* and 0.5 g of *ammonium oxalate*, evaporate until white fumes are evolved, add 50 ml of *water*, boil until a clear solution is obtained, cool, dilute to 100 ml with *water* and add *dilute potassium permanganate solution*, dropwise, until a faint pink colour persists for 10 seconds. Add 10 ml of *hydrochloric acid* and 3 g of *potassium iodide*, allow to stand for 15 minutes protected from light, add 10 ml of *chloroform* and titrate the liberated iodine with 0.1M *sodium thiosulphate VS*, with vigorous shaking, until the chloroform layer becomes colourless. Repeat the procedure without the preparation being examined. The difference between the titrations represents the amount of sodium thiosulphate required. Each ml of 0.1M *sodium thiosulphate VS* is equivalent to 5.585 mg of Fe(II).

Storage Ferrous Fumarate Oral Suspension should be protected from light.

Labelling The quantity of the active ingredient is stated both as the amount of Ferrous Fumarate and in terms of the equivalent amount of ferrous iron.

Ferrous Fumarate Tablets

Definition Ferrous Fumarate Tablets contain Ferrous Fumarate.

The tablets comply with the requirements stated under Tablets and with the following requirements.

Content of ferrous iron, Fe(II) 90.0 to 105.0% of the prescribed or stated amount.

Identification

A. Heat 1 g of the powdered tablets with 25 ml of a mixture of equal volumes of *hydrochloric acid* and *water* on a water bath for 15 minutes, cool and filter. Retain the residue for test B. The filtrate yields reaction A characteristic of *iron salts*, Appendix VI.

B. Wash the residue reserved in Test A with a mixture of 1 volume of 2M *hydrochloric acid* and 9 volumes of *water* and dry at 105°. Suspend 0.1 g of the residue in 2 ml of *dilute sodium carbonate solution* and add *dilute potassium permanganate solution* dropwise. The permanganate is decolorised and a brownish solution is produced.

C. Mix a quantity of the powdered tablets containing 0.5 g of Ferrous Fumarate with 1 g of *resorcinol*. To 0.5 g of the mixture in a crucible add 0.15 ml of *sulphuric acid* and heat gently; a deep red, semi-solid mass is produced. Add the mass to a large volume of *water*; an orange-yellow solution is produced which exhibits no fluorescence.

Dissolution Comply with the *dissolution test for tablets and capsules*, Appendix XII D, using Apparatus II. Use as the medium 900 ml of 0.1M *hydrochloric acid* and rotate the paddle at 75 revolutions per minute. Withdraw a sample of 100 ml of the medium and filter. Titrate the filtrate with 0.01M *ammonium cerium(IV) sulphate VS* using *ferroin solution* as indicator. Calculate the total content of Fe(II) in the medium taking each ml of 0.01M *ammonium cerium(IV) sulphate VS* to be equivalent to 0.5585 mg of Fe(II).

Ferric iron In a flask with a ground-glass stopper dissolve a quantity of the powder prepared for the Assay containing 1.5 g of Ferrous Fumarate in a mixture of 10 ml of *hydrochloric acid* and 100 ml of *water* by heating rapidly to boiling. Boil for 15 seconds. Cool rapidly, add 3 g of *potassium iodide*, stopper the flask and allow to stand protected from light for 15 minutes. Add 2 ml of *starch solution* as indicator. Titrate the liberated iodine with 0.1M *sodium thiosulphate VS*. Carry out a blank test. The difference between the volumes used in the two titrations corresponds to the amount of iodine liberated by ferric ion. The difference between the titrations is not more than 13.4 ml (5%).

Assay Weigh and powder 20 tablets. Dissolve a quantity of the powder containing 0.3 g of Ferrous Fumarate in 7.5 ml of 1M *sulphuric acid* with gentle heating. Cool, add 25 ml of *water* and titrate immediately with 0.1M *ammonium cerium(IV) sulphate VS* using *ferroin solution* as indicator. Each ml of 0.1M *ammonium cerium(IV) sulphate VS* is equivalent to 5.585 mg of Fe(II).

Labelling The quantity of the active ingredient is stated both as the amount of Ferrous Fumarate and in terms of the equivalent amount of ferrous iron.

Ferrous Fumarate and Folic Acid Tablets

Definition Ferrous Fumarate and Folic Acid Tablets contain Ferrous Fumarate and Folic Acid. They are coated.

The tablets comply with the requirements stated under Tablets and with the following requirements.

Content of ferrous fumarate, $C_4H_2FeO_4$ 90.0 to 105.0% of the prescribed or stated amount.

Content of folic acid, $C_{19}H_{19}N_7O_6$ 90.0 to 115.0% of the prescribed or stated amount.

Identification

A. In the Assay for folic acid, the chromatogram obtained with solution (2) shows a peak with the same retention time as the principal peak in the chromatogram obtained with solution (1).

B. Heat a quantity of the powdered tablets containing 0.77 g of Ferrous Fumarate with 25 ml of a mixture of equal volumes of *hydrochloric acid* and *water* on a water bath for 15 minutes, cool and filter. Retain the residue for test C. The filtrate yields reaction A characteristic of *iron salts*, Appendix VI.

C. Wash the residue reserved in test B with a mixture of 1 volume of 2M *hydrochloric acid* and 9 volumes of *water* and dry at 105°. Suspend 0.1 g of the residue in 2 ml of *sodium carbonate solution* and add *potassium permanganate solution* dropwise. The permanganate is decolorised and a brownish solution is produced.

Ferric iron Dissolve a quantity of the powder prepared for the Assay for ferrous fumarate containing 1.5 g of Ferrous Fumarate in a mixture of 100 ml of *water* and 10 ml of *hydrochloric acid* by heating rapidly to the boiling point. Boil for 15 seconds, cool rapidly, add 3 g of *potassium iodide*, stopper, allow to stand in the dark for 15 minutes and titrate the liberated iodine with 0.1M *sodium thiosulphate VS* using *starch mucilage* as indicator. Repeat the operation without the substance being examined. The difference between the titrations is not more than 13.4 ml.

Assay Weigh and powder 20 tablets.

For ferrous fumarate Dissolve a quantity of the powder containing 0.3 g of Ferrous Fumarate in 7.5 ml of 1M *sulphuric acid* with gentle heating. Cool, add 25 ml of *water* and titrate immediately with 0.1M *ammonium cerium(IV) sulphate VS* using *ferroin solution* as indicator. Each ml of 0.1M *ammonium cerium(IV) sulphate VS* is equivalent to 16.99 mg of $C_4H_2FeO_4$.

For folic acid Carry out the method for *liquid chromatography*, Appendix III D, using the following solutions. Solution (1) contains 0.0006% w/v of *folic acid EPCRS* in a 0.57% w/v solution of *dipotassium hydrogen orthophosphate*. For solution (2) mix a quantity of the powdered tablets containing 0.3 mg of Folic Acid with 25 ml of a 0.57% w/v solution of *dipotassium hydrogen orthophosphate* for 30 minutes with the aid of ultrasound, centrifuge and decant the supernatant liquid. Shake the residue with 10 ml of the solvent for 15 minutes with the aid of ultrasound, centrifuge and decant the supernatant liquid. Repeat the procedure with a further 10 ml of solvent. Combine the supernatant liquids, dilute to 50 ml and filter (Whatman GF/C is suitable).

The chromatographic procedure may be carried out using (a) a stainless steel column (25 cm × 4.6 mm) packed with *stationary phase C* (5 µm) (Spherisorb ODS 1 is suitable), (b) as the mobile phase with a flow rate of 1 ml per minute a mixture of 135 volumes of *methanol* and 800 volumes of a solution containing 0.938% w/v of *sodium perchlorate* and 0.075% w/v of *potassium dihydrogen orthophosphate* adjusted to pH 7.2 with 0.1M *potassium hydroxide* and diluted to 1000 volumes with *water* and (c) a detection wavelength of 277 nm.

Calculate the content of $C_{19}H_{19}N_7O_6$ using the declared content of $C_{19}H_{19}N_7O_6$ in *folic acid EPCRS*.

Storage Ferrous Fumarate and Folic Acid Tablets should be protected from light.

308 mg of ferrous fumarate is equivalent to 100 mg of ferrous iron.

Ferrous Gluconate Tablets

Definition Ferrous Gluconate Tablets contain Ferrous Gluconate. They are coated.

The tablets comply with the requirements stated under Tablets and with the following requirements.

Content of ferrous iron, Fe(II) 90.0 to 105.0% of the stated amount.

Identification

A. Shake a quantity of the powdered tablets containing 0.5 g of Ferrous Gluconate with 10 ml of 2M *hydrochloric acid*, filter and add to the filtrate 1 ml of *barium chloride solution*. An opalescence may be produced but no precipitate is produced.

B. The powdered tablets yield reaction A characteristic of *iron salts*, Appendix VI.

Ferric iron Dissolve a quantity of the powder prepared for the Assay containing 5 g of Ferrous Gluconate as completely as possible without heating in a mixture of 100 ml of freshly boiled and cooled *water* and 10 ml of *hydrochloric acid* and add 3 g of *potassium iodide*. Close the vessel, allow to stand in the dark for 5 minutes and titrate the liberated iodine with 0.1M *sodium thiosulphate VS* using *starch mucilage* as indicator. Repeat the operation without the powder. The difference between the titrations represents the amount of iodine liberated by the ferric iron. Not more than 11.2 ml of 0.1M *sodium thiosulphate VS* is required.

Assay Weigh and powder 20 tablets. Dissolve a quantity of the powder containing 1 g of Ferrous Gluconate as completely as possible in a mixture of 30 ml of *water* and 20 ml of 1M *sulphuric acid* and titrate with 0.1M *ammonium cerium(IV) sulphate VS* using *ferroin solution* as indicator. Each ml of 0.1M *ammonium cerium(IV) sulphate VS* is equivalent to 5.585 mg of Fe(II).

Labelling The quantity of active ingredient is stated both as the amount of Ferrous Gluconate and in terms of the equivalent amount of ferrous iron.

Paediatric Ferrous Sulphate Oral Solution

Definition Paediatric Ferrous Sulphate Oral Solution is a solution containing 1.2% w/v of Ferrous Sulphate and a suitable antioxidant in a suitable vehicle with an orange flavour. It is intended to be diluted well with water before use.

Extemporaneous preparation The following formula and directions apply.

Ferrous Sulphate	12 g
Ascorbic Acid	2 g
Orange Syrup	100 ml
Double-strength Chloroform Water	500 ml
Water	sufficient to produce 1000 ml

Dissolve the Ascorbic Acid in the Double-strength Chloroform Water and use this solution to dissolve the Ferrous Sulphate. Add the Orange Syrup and sufficient Water to produce 1000 ml and mix. The oral solution should be recently prepared.

The oral solution complies with the requirements stated under Oral Liquids and with the following requirements.

Content of ferrous sulphate, $FeSO_4,7H_2O$ 1.10 to 1.30% w/v.

Assay To 20 ml add 45 ml of *water*, 0.2 ml of *hydrochloric acid* and *dilute potassium permanganate solution* dropwise until a permanent pink colour is produced. Add 10 ml of *hydrochloric acid* and 3 ml of a 10% w/v solution of *ammonium thiocyanate* and titrate with 0.1M *titanium(III) chloride VS* maintaining a steady flow of *carbon dioxide* through the flask. Each ml of 0.1M *titanium(III) chloride VS* is equivalent to 27.80 mg of $FeSO_4,7H_2O$.

Labelling The label states that the oral solution should be diluted well with water before use.

Paediatric Ferrous Sulphate Oral Solution contains in 5 ml about 12 mg of ferrous iron.

Ferrous Sulphate Tablets

Definition Ferrous Sulphate Tablets contain Dried Ferrous Sulphate. They are coated.

The tablets comply with the requirements stated under Tablets and with the following requirements.

Content of ferrous iron, Fe(II) 95.0 to 105.0% of the stated amount.

Identification

A. The powdered tablets yield reaction A characteristic of *iron salts*, Appendix VI.

B. Extract the powdered tablets with 2M *hydrochloric acid* and filter. The filtrate yields reaction A characteristic of *sulphates*, Appendix VI.

Assay Weigh and powder 20 tablets. Dissolve a quantity of the powder containing 0.5 g of Dried Ferrous Sulphate as completely as possible in a mixture of 30 ml of *water* and 20 ml of 1M *sulphuric acid* and titrate with 0.1M *ammonium cerium(IV) sulphate VS* using *ferroin solution* as indicator. Each ml of 0.1M *ammonium cerium(IV) sulphate VS* is equivalent to 5.585 mg of Fe(II).

Labelling The quantity of active ingredient is stated both as the amount of Dried Ferrous Sulphate and in terms of the equivalent amount of ferrous iron.

Flavoxate Tablets

Definition Flavoxate Tablets contain Flavoxate Hydrochloride. They are coated.

The tablets comply with the requirements stated under Tablets and with the following requirements.

Content of flavoxate hydrochloride, $C_{24}H_{25}NO_4,HCl$ 95.0 to 105.0% of the prescribed or stated amount.

Identification

A. Extract a quantity of the powdered tablets containing 0.2 g of Flavoxate Hydrochloride with 10 ml of *dichloromethane*, filter and evaporate the filtrate to dryness. The *infrared absorption spectrum* of the residue, Appendix II A, is concordant with the *reference spectrum* of flavoxate hydrochloride.

B. In the test for Related substances, the principal spot in the chromatogram obtained with solution (5) corresponds to that in the chromatogram obtained with solution (6).

Related substances Carry out the method for *thin-layer chromatography*, Appendix III A, using *silica gel GF_{254}* as the coating substance and a mixture of 1 volume of 18M *ammonia*, 80 volumes of *propan-2-ol* and 200 volumes of *ethyl acetate* as the mobile phase. Apply separately to the plate (1) 50 µl of a solution prepared by shaking a quantity of the powdered tablets containing 0.2 g of Flavoxate Hydrochloride with 10 ml of *chloroform* and filtering, (2) 10 µl of a 0.030% w/v solution of *3-methylflavone-8-carboxylic acid BPCRS* in *chloroform*, (3) 10 µl of a 0.015% w/v solution of *3-methylflavone-8-carboxylic acid ethyl ester BPCRS* in *chloroform*, (4) 25 µl of a solution obtained by diluting one volume of solution (1) to 500 volumes with *chloroform*, (5) 10 µl of a solution obtained by diluting 1 volume of solution (1) to 20 volumes with *chloroform* and (6) 10 µl of a 0.1% w/v solution of *flavoxate hydrochloride BPCRS* in *chloroform*. After removal of the plate, allow it to dry in air and examine under *ultraviolet light (254 nm)*. Any spot corresponding to 3-methylflavone-8-carboxylic acid ethyl ester in the chromatogram obtained with solution (1) is not more intense than the spot in the chromatogram obtained with solution (3) (0.15%) and any other *secondary spot* in the chromatogram obtained with solution (1), other than the spot corresponding to 3-methyflavone-8-carboxylic acid, is not more intense than the spot in the chromatogram obtained with solution (4) (0.1%).

3-Methylflavone-8-carboxylic acid Carry out the method for *thin-layer chromatography*, Appendix III A, using *silica gel GF_{254}* as the coating substance and a mixture of 4 volumes of *glacial acetic acid*, 25 volumes of *ethyl acetate* and 70 volumes of *cyclohexane* as the mobile phase. Apply separately to the plate (1) 50 µl of a solution prepared by shaking a quantity of the powdered tablets containing 0.2 g of Flavoxate Hydrochloride with 10 ml of *chloroform* and filtering and (2) 10 µl of a 0.030% w/v solution of *3-methylflavone-8-carboxylic acid BPCRS*. After removal of the plate, allow it to dry in air and spray with *dilute potassium iodobismuthate solution*. Any spot corresponding to 3-methylflavone-8-carboxylic acid in the chromatogram obtained with solution (1) is not more intense than the spot in the chromatogram obtained with solution (2) (0.3%).

Assay Weigh and finely powder 20 tablets. To a quantity of the powdered tablets containing 1 g of Flavoxate Hydrochloride add 600 ml of 0.1M *hydrochloric acid* and disperse with the aid of ultrasound for 10 minutes. Place in a water bath at 70° for 90 minutes, cool, add sufficient 0.1M *hydrochloric acid* to produce 1 litre and filter. Dilute 5 ml to 250 ml with 0.1M *hydrochloric acid* and measure the *absorbance* of the resulting solution at 293 nm, Appendix II B. Calculate the content of $C_{24}H_{25}NO_4,HCl$ from the absorbance obtained by repeating the measurement using a 0.002% w/v solution of *flavoxate hydrochloride BPCRS* in 0.1M *hydrochloric acid and* from the declared content of $C_{24}H_{25}NO_4,HCl$ in *flavoxate hydrochloride BPCRS*.

Storage Flavoxate Tablets should be protected from light.

Flexible Collodion

Definition Flexible Collodion is a solution of Colophony in a mixture of Castor Oil and Collodion.

Extemporaneous preparation The following formula and directions apply.

Colophony	25 g
Castor Oil	25 g
Collodion	sufficient to produce 1000 ml

Mix the ingredients and stir until the Colophony has dissolved; allow any deposit to settle and decant the clear liquid.

Flexible Collodion complies with the requirements stated under Liquids for Cutaneous Application and with the following requirements.

Identification

A. Expose a thin layer to the air. A thin, tenacious film is left which, when ignited, burns rapidly with a yellow flame.

B. Mix with an equal volume of *water*. A white, viscid, stringy mass is obtained.

Ethanol content 20 to 23% v/v when determined by the following method. Carry out the method for *gas chromatography*, Appendix III B, using the following solutions in *ether*. Solution (1) contains 5% v/v of *absolute ethanol* and 5% v/v of *acetonitrile* (internal standard). Solution (2) contains 20% v/v of the substance being examined. Solution (3) contains 20% v/v of the substance being examined and 5% v/v of the internal standard.

The chromatographic procedure may be carried out using a glass column (1.5 m × 4 mm) packed with porous polymer beads (100 to 120 mesh) (Porapak Q is suitable) and maintained at 120° with a flow rate of 40 ml per minute for the carrier gas.

Calculate the content of C_2H_6O from the areas of the peaks due to ethanol and acetonitrile in the chromatograms obtained with solution (1) and solution (3).

For preparations in which Industrial Methylated Spirit has been used, determine the content of ethanol as described above.

Determine the concentration of methanol in the following manner. Carry out the chromatographic procedure described above but using the following solutions. Solution (1) contains 0.25% v/v of *methanol* and 0.25% v/v of *acetonitrile* (internal standard). For solution (2) dilute a volume of the preparation being examined with *ether* to contain between 0.2% and 0.3% v/v of *methanol.* Prepare solution (3) in the same manner as solution (2) but adding sufficient of the internal standard to produce a final concentration of 0.25% v/v.

The sum of the contents of ethanol and methanol is 20 to 23% v/v and the ratio of the content of methanol to that of ethanol is commensurate with Industrial Methylated Spirit having been used.

Action and use Skin protective.

COLLODION FOR THE PREPARATION OF FLEXIBLE COLLODION

Definition Collodion is a solution of Pyroxylin in a mixture of Solvent Ether and Ethanol (90 per cent).

Production It may be prepared by adding 100 g of Pyroxylin to 900 ml of a mixture of 3 volumes of Solvent Ether and 1 volume of Ethanol (90 per cent) and agitating continuously until dissolved. The viscosity of the resulting solution is determined and the solution is diluted with the solvent mixture until it complies with the requirement for Kinematic viscosity.

In making Collodion the Ethanol (90 per cent) may be replaced by Industrial Methylated Spirit diluted so as to be of equivalent alcoholic strength, provided that the law and the statutory regulations governing the use of Industrial Methylated Spirit are observed.

Characteristics A clear, viscid, colourless or pale straw-coloured liquid; odour, characteristic of ether.

Weight per ml 0.785 to 0.795 g, Appendix V G.

Kinematic viscosity 405 to 700 mm^2s^{-1} determined on the collodion being examined using the method described under Pyroxylin.

When Collodion is prescribed or demanded, Flexible Collodion shall be dispensed or supplied.

Flucloxacillin Capsules

Definition Flucloxacillin Capsules contain Flucloxacillin Sodium.

The capsules comply with the requirements stated under Capsules and with the following requirements.

Content of flucloxacillin, $C_{19}H_{17}ClFN_3O_5S$ 92.5 to 110.0% of the prescribed or stated amount.

Identification The *infrared absorption spectrum* of the contents of the capsules, Appendix II A, is concordant with the *reference spectrum* of flucloxacillin sodium.

Assay To a quantity of the mixed contents of 20 capsules containing the equivalent of 0.25 g of flucloxacillin add 70 ml of *water*, shake for 15 minutes and add sufficient *water* to produce 500 ml. Filter and dilute 10 ml of the filtrate to 100 ml with *water.* Place two 2-ml quantities of the resulting solution in separate stoppered tubes. To one tube add 10 ml of *imidazole—mercury reagent*, mix, stopper the tube and immerse in a water bath at 60° for exactly 25 minutes, swirling occasionally. Remove from the water bath and cool rapidly to 20° (solution A). To the second tube add 10 ml of *water* and mix (solution B). Without delay measure the *absorbances* of solutions A and B at the maximum at 346 nm, Appendix II B, using in the reference cell a mixture of 2 ml of *water* and 10 ml of *imidazole—mercury reagent* for solution A and *water* for solution B. Calculate the content of $C_{19}H_{17}ClFN_3O_5S$ from the difference between the absorbances of solutions A and B, from the difference obtained by repeating the operation using a 0.0055% w/v solution of *flucloxacillin sodium BPCRS* in place of the final solution obtained from the preparation being examined and from the declared content of $C_{19}H_{17}ClFN_3O_5S$ in *flucloxacillin sodium BPCRS.*

Labelling The quantity of active ingredient is stated in terms of the equivalent amount of flucloxacillin.

Flucloxacillin Injection

Definition Flucloxacillin Injection is a sterile solution of flucloxacillin sodium in Water for Injections. It is prepared by dissolving Flucloxacillin Sodium for Injection in the requisite amount of Water for Injections immediately before use.

The injection complies with the requirements stated under Parenteral Preparations.

Storage Flucloxacillin Injection should be used immediately after preparation but, in any case, within the period recommended by the manufacturer when prepared and stored strictly in accordance with the manufacturer's instructions.

FLUCLOXACILLIN SODIUM FOR INJECTION

Definition Flucloxacillin Sodium for Injection is a sterile material prepared from Flucloxacillin Sodium with or without excipients. It is supplied in a sealed container.

The contents of the sealed container comply with the requirements for Powders for Injections stated under Parenteral Preparations and with the following requirements.

Content of flucloxacillin, $C_{19}H_{17}ClFN_3O_5S$ 95.0 to 105.0% of the prescribed or stated amount.

Identification

A. The *infrared absorption spectrum*, Appendix II A, is concordant with the *reference spectrum* of flucloxacillin sodium.

B. Yield reaction B characteristic of *sodium salts*, Appendix VI.

Acidity or alkalinity pH of a 10% w/v solution, 5.0 to 7.0, Appendix V L.

Iodine-absorbing substances Not more than 5.0%, calculated with reference to the anhydrous substance, when determined by the following method. Dissolve 0.125 g in sufficient *mixed phosphate buffer pH 7.0* to produce 25 ml. To 10 ml add 10 ml of *mixed phosphate buffer pH 4.0* and 10 ml of 0.01M *iodine VS* and titrate immediately with 0.01M *sodium thiosulphate VS* using *starch mucilage*, added towards the end of the titration, as indicator. Repeat the operation without the substance being examined. The difference between the titrations represents the amount of iodine-absorbing substances present. Each ml of 0.01M *sodium thiosulphate VS* is equivalent to 0.524 mg of iodine-absorbing substances.

Water Not more than 4.3% w/w, Appendix IX C. Use 0.3 g.

Bacterial endotoxins Carry out the *test for bacterial endotoxins*, Appendix XIV C. Dissolve the contents of the sealed container in *water BET* to give a solution containing 10 mg per ml (solution A). The endotoxin limit concentration of solution A is 3.5 IU per ml. Carry out the test using the maximum valid dilution of solution A calculated from the declared sensitivity of the lysate used in the test.

Assay Determine the weight of the contents of 10 containers as described in the test for Uniformity of weight under Parenteral Preparations, Powders for Injections.

Dissolve 0.1 g of the mixed contents of the 10 containers in sufficient *water* to produce 500 ml and dilute 25 ml to 100 ml with *water*. Place two 2-ml quantities of the resulting solution in separate stoppered tubes. To one tube add 10 ml of *imidazole—mercury reagent*, mix, stopper the tube and immerse in a water bath at 60° for exactly 25 minutes, swirling occasionally. Remove from the water bath and cool rapidly to 20° (solution A). To the second tube add 10 ml of *water* and mix (solution B). Without delay measure the *absorbances* of solutions A and B at the maximum at 346 nm, Appendix II B, using in the reference cell a mixture of 2 ml of *water* and 10 ml of *imidazole—mercury reagent* for solution A and *water* for solution B. Calculate the content of $C_{19}H_{17}ClFN_3O_5S$ in a container of average content weight from the difference between the absorbances of solutions A and B, from the difference obtained by repeating the operation using a 0.0055% w/v solution of *flucloxacillin sodium BPCRS* in place of the final solution obtained from the preparation being examined and from the declared content of $C_{19}H_{17}ClFN_3O_5S$ in *flucloxacillin sodium BPCRS*.

Storage The sealed container should be stored at a temperature not exceeding 25°.

Labelling The label of the sealed container states the quantity of Flucloxacillin Sodium contained in it in terms of the equivalent amount of flucloxacillin.

Flucloxacillin Oral Solution

Definition Flucloxacillin Oral Solution is a solution of Flucloxacillin Sodium in a suitable flavoured vehicle. It is prepared by dissolving the dry ingredients in the specified volume of Water just before issue for use.

The dry ingredients comply with the requirements for Powders and Granules for the Preparation of Oral Liquids stated under Oral Liquids.

Storage The dry ingredients should be kept in a well-closed container and stored at a temperature not exceeding 25°.

For the following tests prepare the oral solution as directed on the label. The solution, examined immediately after preparation unless otherwise indicated, complies with the requirements stated under Oral Liquids and with the following requirements.

Content of flucloxacillin, $C_{19}H_{17}ClFN_3O_5S$ When freshly constituted, not more than 120.0% of the prescribed or stated amount. When stored at the temperature and for the period stated on the label during which the oral solution may be expected to be satisfactory for use, not less than 80.0% of the prescribed or stated amount.

Identification Carry out the method for *thin-layer chromatography*, Appendix III A, using a silanised silica gel F_{254} precoated plate (Merck silanised silica gel 60 F_{254} plates are suitable) and as the mobile phase a mixture of 70 volumes of 0.05M *potassium hydrogen phthalate*, 30 volumes of *acetone* and 1 volume of *formic acid* that has been adjusted first to pH 6.0 with 5M *sodium hydroxide* and then to pH 9.0 with 0.1M *sodium hydroxide*. Apply separately to the plate 1 µl of each of the following solutions. For solution (1) dilute a quantity of the oral solution containing the equivalent of 50 mg of flucloxacillin to 20 ml with *phosphate buffer pH 7.0*. Solution (2) contains 0.25% w/v of *flucloxacillin sodium BPCRS* in *phosphate buffer pH 7.0*. After removal of the plate, allow it to dry in air and spray with a mixture of 100 volumes of *starch mucilage*, 6 volumes of *glacial acetic acid* and 2 volumes of a 1% w/v solution of *iodine* in a 4% w/v solution of *potassium iodide*. The principal spot in the chromatogram obtained with solution (1) corresponds to that in the chromatogram obtained with solution (2).

Acidity or alkalinity pH, 4.0 to 7.0, Appendix V L.

Assay To a weighed quantity of the oral solution containing the equivalent of 0.25 g of flucloxacillin add sufficient *water* to produce 500 ml and dilute 10 ml to 100 ml. Place two 2-ml aliquots of the resulting solution in separate stoppered tubes. To one tube add 10 ml of *imidazole—mercury reagent*, mix, stopper the tube and immerse in a water bath at 60° for exactly 25 minutes, swirling occasionally. Remove from the water bath and cool rapidly to 20° (solution A). To the second tube add 10 ml of *water* and mix (solution B). Without delay measure the *absorbances* of solutions A and B at the maximum at 346 nm, Appendix II B, using in the reference cell a mixture of 2 ml of *water* and 10 ml of *imidazole—mercury reagent* for solution A and *water* for solution B. Calculate the content of $C_{19}H_{17}ClFN_3O_5S$ from the difference between the absorbances of solutions A and B, from the difference obtained by repeating the procedure using a 0.0055% w/v solution of *flucloxacillin sodium BPCRS* in place of the solution obtained from the preparation being examined and from the declared content of $C_{19}H_{17}ClFN_3O_5S$ in *flucloxacillin sodium BPCRS*. Determine the *weight per ml* of the oral solution, Appendix V G, and calculate the content of $C_{19}H_{17}ClFN_3O_5S$, weight in volume.

Repeat the procedure using a portion of the oral solution that has been stored at the temperature and for the period stated on the label during which it may be expected to be satisfactory for use.

Storage The Oral Solution should be stored at the temperature and used within the period stated on the label.

Labelling The quantity of active ingredient is stated in terms of the equivalent amount of flucloxacillin.

Flucloxacillin Oral Suspension

Definition Flucloxacillin Oral Suspension is a suspension of Flucloxacillin Magnesium in a suitable flavoured vehicle. It is prepared by dispersing the dry ingredients in the specified volume of Water just before issue for use.

The dry ingredients comply with the requirements for Powders and Granules for the Preparation of Oral Liquids stated under Oral Liquids.

Storage The dry ingredients should be kept in a well-closed container and stored at a temperature not exceeding 25°.

For the following tests prepare the oral suspension as directed on the label. The suspension examined immediately after preparation, unless otherwise indicated, complies with the requirements stated under Oral Liquids and with the following requirements.

Content of flucloxacillin, $C_{19}H_{17}ClFN_3O_5S$ When freshly constituted, not more than 120.0% of the prescribed or stated amount. When stored at the temperature and for the period stated on the label during which the oral suspension may be expected to be satisfactory for use, not less than 80.0% of the prescribed or stated amount.

Identification

A. Carry out the method for *thin-layer chromatography*, Appendix III A, using a silanised silica gel F_{254} precoated plate (Merck silanised silica gel 60 F_{254} plates are suitable) and as the mobile phase a mixture of 70 volumes of 0.05M *potassium hydrogen phthalate*, 30 volumes of *acetone* and 1 volume of *formic acid*, the mixture having been adjusted first to pH 6.0 with 5M *sodium hydroxide* and then to pH 9.0 with 0.1M *sodium hydroxide*. Apply separately to the plate 1 µl of each of the following solutions. For solution (1) dilute a quantity of the oral suspension containing the equivalent of 50 mg of flucloxacillin to 20 ml with *phosphate buffer pH 7.0*. Solution (2) contains 0.25% w/v of *flucloxacillin sodium BPCRS* in *phosphate buffer pH 7.0*. After removal of the plate, allow it to dry in air and spray with a mixture of 100 volumes of *starch mucilage*, 6 volumes of *glacial acetic acid* and 2 volumes of a 1% w/v solution of *iodine* in a 4% w/v solution of *potassium iodide*. The principal spot in the chromatogram obtained with solution (1) corresponds to that in the chromatogram obtained with solution (2).

B. Dilute a quantity of the oral suspension containing the equivalent of 50 mg of flucloxacillin to 20 ml with *water*, shake to dissolve and filter if necessary. The filtrate yields reaction B characteristic of *magnesium salts*, Appendix VI.

Acidity pH, 4.8 to 5.8, Appendix V L.

Assay To a weighed quantity of the oral suspension containing the equivalent of 0.25 g of flucloxacillin add sufficient *buffered sodium acetate solution pH 6.0* to produce 500 ml. Dilute 10 ml to 100 ml with the same buffered solution and complete the Assay described under Flucloxacillin Oral Solution beginning at the words 'Place two 2 ml aliquots ...'. Determine the *weight per ml* of the oral suspension, Appendix V G, and calculate the content of $C_{19}H_{17}ClFN_3O_5S$, weight in volume.

Repeat the procedure using a portion of the oral suspension that has been stored at the temperature and for the period stated on the label during which it may be expected to be satisfactory for use.

Storage The Oral Suspension should be stored at the temperature and used within the period stated on the label.

Labelling The quantity of active ingredient is stated in terms of the equivalent amount of flucloxacillin.

Flucytosine Tablets

Definition Flucytosine Tablets contain Flucytosine.

The tablets comply with the requirements stated under Tablets and with the following requirements.

Content of flucytosine, $C_4H_4FN_3O$ 92.5 to 107.5% of the prescribed or stated amount.

Identification

A. Shake a quantity of the powdered tablets containing 0.5 g of Flucytosine with 100 ml of *methanol* for 30 minutes, filter and evaporate the filtrate to dryness. The *infrared absorption spectrum* of the residue, Appendix II A, is concordant with the *reference spectrum* of flucytosine.

B. The *light absorption*, Appendix II B, in the range 230 to 350 nm of the solution used in the Assay exhibits a maximum only at 286 nm.

Related substances Carry out the method for *thin-layer chromatography*, Appendix III A, using a suitable silica gel as the coating substance and a mixture of 1 volume of *anhydrous formic acid*, 15 volumes of *water*, 25 volumes of *methanol* and 60 volumes of *ethyl acetate* as the mobile phase in an unsaturated tank but allowing the solvent front to ascend 12 cm above the line of application. Apply separately to the plate 10 µl of each of the following solutions. For solution (1) shake a quantity of the powdered tablets containing 0.10 g of Flucytosine with 10 ml of a mixture of equal volumes of 13.5M *ammonia* and *methanol* and filter. For solution (2) dilute 1 volume of solution (1) to 10 volumes with *methanol (60%)* and dilute 1 volume of the resulting solution to 100 volumes with *methanol (60%)*. For solution (3) dilute 1 volume of solution (1) to 10 volumes and dissolve 5 mg of *fluorouracil EPCRS* in 5 ml of the resulting solution. After removal of the plate, allow the solvent to evaporate, stand the plate in a tank of chlorine vapour prepared by the addition of *hydrochloric acid* to a 5% w/v solution of *potassium permanganate* contained in a beaker placed in the tank and allow to stand for 15 minutes. Remove the plate and place it in a current of cold air until the excess of chlorine is removed and an area of the coating substance below the line of application does not give a blue colour with a drop of *potassium iodide and starch solution*. Spray the plate with *potassium iodide and starch solution* and examine the plate in daylight. Any *secondary spot* in the chromatogram obtained with solution (1) is not more intense than the spot in the chromatogram obtained with solution (2) (0.1%). The test is not valid unless the chromatogram obtained with solution (3) shows two clearly separated spots.

Assay Weigh and powder 20 tablets. To a quantity of the powder containing 0.1 g of Flucytosine add 80 ml of 0.1M *hydrochloric acid* and shake for 15 minutes. Dilute to 100 ml with 0.1M *hydrochloric acid* and filter. Dilute 10 ml of the filtrate to 100 ml with 0.1M *hydrochloric acid* and further dilute 10 ml of the solution to 100 ml with 0.1M *hydrochloric acid*. Measure the *absorbance* of the resulting solution at the maximum at 286 nm, Appendix II B. Calculate the content of $C_4H_4FN_3O$ taking 709 as the value of A(1%, 1 cm) at the maximum at 286 nm.

Storage Flucytosine Tablets should be protected from light.

Fludrocortisone Tablets

Definition Fludrocortisone Tablets contain Fludrocortisone Acetate.

The tablets comply with the requirements stated under Tablets and with the following requirements.

Content of fludrocortisone acetate, $C_{23}H_{31}FO_6$ 90.0 to 110.0% of the prescribed or stated amount.

Identification

A. Complies with the test for *identification of steroids,* Appendix III A, using *impregnating solvent I* and *mobile phase B.* Apply separately to the plate 20 µl of each of the following solutions. For solution (1) shake a quantity of the powdered tablets containing 1 mg of Fludrocortisone Acetate with 20 ml of *chloroform* for 5 minutes, filter, evaporate the filtrate to dryness and dissolve the residue in 4 ml of a mixture of 9 volumes of *chloroform* and 1 volume of *methanol.* Solution (2) contains 0.025% w/v of *fludrocortisone acetate BPCRS* in a mixture of 9 volumes of *chloroform* and 1 volume of *methanol.*

B. In the Assay, the chromatogram obtained with solution (2) shows a peak with the same retention time as the peak due to fludrocortisone acetate in the chromatogram obtained with solution (1).

Uniformity of content Tablets containing less than 2 mg of Fludrocortisone Acetate comply with the requirement stated under Tablets using the following method of analysis. Carry out the method for *liquid chromatography,* Appendix III D, using the following solutions protected from light. Solution A contains 0.002% w/v of *norethisterone BPCRS* in *acetonitrile.* Solution (1) is a mixture of 4 volumes of a 0.0025% w/v solution of *fludrocortisone acetate BPCRS* in solution A and 1 volume of *water.* For solution (2) place a single tablet in a centrifuge tube, add 1 ml of *water,* shake on a vortex-type mixer for 1 minute, add 4.0 ml of solution A and shake again for 1 minute. Shake for a further 40 minutes on a mechanical shaker, centrifuge and use the clear supernatant solution.

The chromatographic procedure may be carried out using (a) a stainless steel column (20 cm × 4.6 mm) packed with *stationary phase C* (10 µm) (Spherisorb ODS 1 is suitable), (b) a mixture of 40 volumes of *acetonitrile* and 60 volumes of *water* as the mobile phase with a flow rate of 2 ml per minute and (c) a detection wavelength of 240 nm.

Assay Weigh and powder 20 tablets. Carry out the method for *liquid chromatography,* Appendix III D, using the following solutions. Solution A contains 0.01% w/v of *norethisterone BPCRS* (internal standard) in *acetonitrile.* Solution (1) is a mixture of 20 ml of solution A, 25 ml of a 0.01% w/v solution of *fludrocortisone acetate BPCRS* in *acetonitrile* and 10 ml of *water* diluted to 100 ml with *acetonitrile.* Prepare solution (2) in the same manner as solution (3) but using 8 ml of *acetonitrile* in place of 4 ml of solution A and 4 ml of acetonitrile. For solution (3) shake a quantity of the powdered tablets containing 0.5 mg of Fludrocortisone Acetate with 2 ml of *water* for 1 minute, add 4 ml of solution A and 4 ml of *acetonitrile* and shake on a mechanical shaker for 40 minutes. Dilute the mixture to 20 ml with *acetonitrile,* centrifuge and use the supernatant liquid.

The chromatographic conditions prescribed under the test for Uniformity of content may be used.

Calculate the content of $C_{23}H_{31}FO_6$ using the declared content of $C_{23}H_{31}FO_6$ in *fludrocortisone acetate BPCRS.*

Fluocinolone Cream

Definition Fluocinolone Cream contains Fluocinolone Acetonide or Fluocinolone Acetonide Dihydrate in a suitable basis.

The cream complies with the requirements stated under Topical Semi-solid Preparations and with the following requirements.

Content of fluocinolone acetonide, $C_{24}H_{30}F_2O_6$ 90.0 to 110.0% of the prescribed or stated amount.

Identification

A. Complies with test A for Identification described under Fluocinolone Ointment.

B. In the Assay, the chromatogram obtained with solution (2) shows a peak with the same retention time as the peak due to fluocinolone acetonide in the chromatogram obtained with solution (1).

Assay Carry out the method for *liquid chromatography,* Appendix III D, using the following solutions.

For creams containing 0.025% to 0.2% w/w of fluocinolone acetonide, solution (1) contains 0.025% w/v of *fluocinolone acetonide BPCRS* and 0.005% w/v of *phenacetin* (internal standard) in *chloroform.* Prepare solution (2) in the following manner. To a quantity of the cream containing 2.5 mg of fluocinolone acetonide add 60 ml of a solution prepared by adding 80 ml of *methanol* to 20 ml of a 25% w/v solution of *lithium chloride* and disperse by shaking vigorously. Add 100 ml of *cyclohexane,* shake gently for 2 minutes and separate the lower, aqueous methanolic layer, taking care to exclude any solid matter that separates at the interface. Repeat the extraction using a further 25 ml of the lithium chloride solution. To the combined extracts add a solution of 11 g of *aluminium potassium sulphate* in 214 ml of *water* followed by 50 ml of *chloroform,* shake vigorously for about 3 minutes, allow the layers to separate and filter the chloroform extract through filter paper (Whatman No. 1 is suitable), previously moistened with *chloroform,* again excluding any solid matter at the interface. Repeat the extraction with 50- and 10-ml quantities of *chloroform,* filtering the extracts as before. Evaporate the combined extracts to dryness on a water bath in a current of nitrogen, dissolve the residue in 5 ml of *chloroform,* transfer to a 10-ml graduated flask with the aid of *chloroform* and add sufficient *chloroform* to produce 10 ml. Prepare solution (3) in the same manner as solution (2) but adding 1.0 ml of a 0.050% w/v solution of *phenacetin* to the chloroform solution before dilution to 10 ml.

For creams containing 0.01% w/w of fluocinolone acetonide, solution (1) contains 0.01% w/v of *fluocinolone acetonide BPCRS* and 0.002% w/v of *phenacetin* (internal standard) in *chloroform*. Prepare solution (2) as described above but using a quantity of the cream containing 1 mg of fluocinolone acetonide. Prepare solution (3) in the same manner as solution (2) but adding 1 ml of a 0.02% w/v solution of *phenacetin* to the chloroform solution before diluting to 10 ml.

For creams containing 0.00625% w/w of fluocinolone acetonide, solution (1) contains 0.00625% w/v of *fluocinolone acetonide BPCRS* and 0.00125% w/v of *phenacetin* (internal standard) in *chloroform*. Prepare solution (2) as described above but using a quantity of the cream containing 0.62 mg of fluocinolone acetonide. Prepare solution (3) in the same manner as solution (2) but adding 1 ml of a 0.0125% w/v solution of *phenacetin* to the chloroform solution before diluting to 10 ml.

For creams containing 0.0025% w/w of fluocinolone acetonide, solution (1) contains 0.0025% w/v of *fluocinolone acetonide BPCRS* and 0.0005% w/v of *phenacetin* (internal standard) in *chloroform*. Prepare solution (2) as described above but using a quantity of the cream containing 0.25 mg of fluocinolone acetonide. Prepare solution (3) in the same manner as solution (2) but adding 1 ml of a 0.005% w/v solution of *phenacetin* to the chloroform solution before diluting to 10 ml.

The chromatographic procedure may be carried out using (a) a stainless steel column (20 cm × 5 mm) packed with *stationary phase C* (5 µm) (Spherisorb ODS 1 is suitable), (b) a mixture of 58 volumes of *hexane*, 40 volumes of *chloroform*, 2 volumes of *methanol* and 0.1 volume of *glacial acetic acid* as the mobile phase with a flow rate of 1.8 ml per minute and (c) a detection wavelength of 243 nm.

The assay is not valid unless the *resolution factor* (R_s) between the peaks due to fluocinolone acetonide and phenacetin is more than 2, and the *capacity factors* (k') of fluocinolone acetonide and phenacetin are about 3 and 2, respectively. If these conditions are not achieved, adjust the concentration of *methanol* in the mobile phase, increasing its concentration to reduce the value of k' and reducing its concentration to increase the value of k'. If the correct values cannot be obtained by this means, the column is faulty and must be repacked. If, when the correct k' values have been obtained, the value of R_s is less than 2, reduce the concentration of *chloroform* in the mobile phase by 5% to obtain an increased retention time for both fluocinolone acetonide and phenacetin and re-adjust the k' values to the specified values by increasing the concentration of *methanol*. Repeat the adjustment of chloroform and methanol concentrations until correct values for both R_s and k' have been obtained.

Calculate the content of $C_{24}H_{30}F_2O_6$ in the cream using the declared content of $C_{24}H_{30}F_2O_6$ in *fluocinolone acetonide BPCRS*.

Labelling When the active ingredient is Fluocinolone Acetonide Dihydrate, the quantity is stated in terms of the equivalent amount of fluocinolone acetonide.

Fluocinolone Ointment

Definition Fluocinolone Ointment contains Fluocinolone Acetonide or Fluocinolone Acetonide Dihydrate in a suitable basis.

The ointment complies with the requirements stated under Topical Semi-solid Preparations and with the following requirements.

Content of fluocinolone acetonide, $C_{24}H_{30}F_2O_6$ 90.0 to 110.0% of the prescribed or stated amount.

Identification

A. Carry out the method for *thin-layer chromatography*, Appendix III A, using *silica gel G* as the coating substance and a mixture of 60 volumes of n-*hexane*, 40 volumes of *chloroform*, 10 volumes of *methanol* and 1 volume of *triethylamine* as the mobile phase. Apply separately to the plate 5 µl of each of the following solutions. For solution (1) disperse, by shaking, a quantity of the preparation being examined containing 0.25 mg of fluocinolone acetonide in 2 ml of *chloroform*, add 10 ml of *methanol*, shake vigorously, cool in ice for 15 minutes, centrifuge at 3000 revolutions per minute for 15 minutes, decant the clear, supernatant liquid, evaporate to dryness on a water bath in a current of nitrogen and dissolve the residue in 1 ml of *chloroform*. Solution (2) contains 0.025% w/v solution of *fluocinolone acetonide BPCRS* in *chloroform*. After removal of the plate, allow it to dry in air until the odour of solvent is no longer detectable, heat at 105° for 5 minutes and spray whilst hot with *alkaline tetrazolium blue solution*. The principal spot in the chromatogram obtained with solution (1) corresponds to that in the chromatogram obtained with solution (2).

B. In the Assay the chromatogram obtained with solution (3) shows a peak with the same retention time as the peak due to fluocinolone acetonide in the chromatogram obtained with solution (1).

Assay Carry out the method for *liquid chromatography*, Appendix III D, using the following solutions. Solution (1) contains 0.0050% w/v of *fluocinolone acetonide BPCRS* and 0.40% v/v of *toluene* (internal standard) in *methanol (80%)*.

For ointments containing 0.01% w/w or less of fluocinolone acetonide prepare solution (2) in the following manner. To a quantity of the ointment containing 0.5 mg of fluocinolone acetonide add 50 ml of *2,2,4-trimethylpentane* and 8 ml of *methanol (80%)*, warm gently on a water bath until the preparation is dispersed and shake vigorously for 2 minutes. Separate the lower, aqueous methanolic layer and wash the upper layer with 1 ml of *methanol (80%)*, adding the washing to the previous extract. To the combined extracts add sufficient *methanol (80%)* to produce 10 ml. Prepare solution (3) in the same manner as solution (2) but adding 1 ml of a 4% v/v solution of the internal standard in *methanol* to the combined extracts before dilution to 10 ml.

For ointments containing 0.025% w/w of fluocinolone acetonide, prepare solution (2) in the following manner. To a quantity of the ointment containing 1.25 mg of fluocinolone acetonide add 50 ml of *2,2,4-trimethylpentane* and 20 ml of *methanol (80%)*, warm gently on a water bath until the preparation is dispersed and shake vigorously for 2 minutes. Separate the lower, aqueous methanolic layer and wash the upper layer with 2 ml of *methanol (80%)*, adding the washing to the previous extract. To the combined extracts add sufficient *methanol (80%)* to produce 25 ml. Prepare solution (3) in the same manner as solution (2) but adding 1 ml of a 10% v/v solution of the internal standard in *methanol* to the combined extracts before dilution to 25 ml.

The chromatographic procedure may be carried out using (a) a stainless steel column (20 cm × 5 mm) packed with *stationary phase C* (5 µm) (Spherisorb ODS 1 is suitable), (b) a mixture of 55 volumes of *water*, 45 volumes of *acetonitrile* and 0.1 volume of *glacial acetic acid* as the mobile phase with a flow rate of 1 ml per minute and (c) a detection wavelength of 238 nm.

Calculate the content of $C_{24}H_{30}F_2O_6$ in the ointment using the declared content of $C_{24}H_{30}F_2O_6$ in *fluocinolone acetonide BPCRS*.

Labelling When the active ingredient is Fluocinolone Acetonide Dihydrate, the quantity is stated in terms of the equivalent amount of fluocinolone acetonide.

Fluocinonide Cream

Definition Fluocinonide Cream contains Fluocinonide in a suitable basis.

The cream complies with the requirements stated under Topical Semi-solid Preparations and with the following requirements.

Content of fluocinonide, $C_{26}H_{32}F_2O_7$ 90.0 to 110.0% of the prescribed or stated amount.

Identification

A. Carry out the method for *thin-layer chromatography*, Appendix III A, using *silica gel F_{254}* as the coating substance and a mixture of 12 volumes of *water*, 80 volumes of *methanol*, 150 volumes of *ether* and 770 volumes of *dichloromethane* as the mobile phase. Mix the water and the methanol before adding to the remaining solvents of the mobile phase. Apply separately to the plate 10 µl of each of the following two solutions. For solution (1) disperse a quantity of the cream containing 2.5 mg of Fluocinonide in 25 ml of *methanol (80%)*, add 50 ml of *ether* and shake vigorously to produce a clear, homogeneous solution. Add 15 ml of *water*, shake and transfer the lower layer to a second separating funnel. Add 100 ml of *water*, extract with 10 ml of *chloroform*, filter the chloroform layer through filter paper and evaporate to a volume of about 1 ml in a current of air on a water bath. Solution (2) contains 0.1% w/v of *fluocinonide BPCRS* in a mixture of 1 volume of *methanol* and 9 volumes of *dichloromethane*. After removal of the plate, allow it to dry in air and examine under *ultraviolet light (254 nm)*. The principal spot in the chromatogram obtained with solution (1) corresponds to that in the chromatogram obtained with solution (2).

B. In the Assay the retention time of the principal peak in the chromatogram obtained with solution (1) is similar to that of the principal peak in the chromatogram obtained with solution (2).

Assay Carry out the method for *liquid chromatography*, Appendix III D, using the following solutions. For solution (1) disperse a quantity of the cream containing 1.5 mg of Fluocinonide in 20 ml of *methanol (80%)*, warming gently over a water bath if necessary. Add 50 ml of *2,2,4-trimethylpentane*, shake for 2 minutes and transfer the lower aqueous methanol layer to a 50-ml flask. Repeat the extraction with a further 20 ml of *methanol (80%)*. Dilute the combined extracts to volume with the same solvent. Solution (2) contains 0.003% w/v of *fluocinonide BPCRS* in *methanol (80%)*.

The chromatographic procedure may be carried out using (a) a stainless steel column (20 cm × 4.6 mm) packed with *stationary phase C* (5 µm) (Spherisorb ODS 1 is suitable), (b) a mixture of 0.1 volume of *glacial acetic acid*, 45 volumes of *acetonitrile* and 55 volumes of *water* as the mobile phase with a flow rate of 2 ml per minute and (c) a detection wavelength of 238 nm.

Calculate the content of $C_{26}H_{32}F_2O_7$ in the cream using the declared content of $C_{26}H_{32}F_2O_7$ in *fluocinonide BPCRS*.

Fluocinonide Ointment

Definition Fluocinonide Ointment contains Fluocinonide in a suitable basis.

The ointment complies with the requirements stated under Topical Semi-solid Preparations and with the following requirements.

Content of fluocinonide, $C_{26}H_{32}F_2O_7$ 90.0 to 110.0% of the prescribed or stated amount.

Identification

A. Carry out the method for *thin-layer chromatography*, Appendix III A, using *silica gel F_{254}* as the coating substance and a mixture of 12 volumes of *water*, 80 volumes of *methanol*, 150 volumes of *ether* and 770 volumes of *dichloromethane* as the mobile phase. Mix the water and the methanol before adding to the remaining components of the mobile phase. Apply separately to the plate 10 µl of each of the following solutions. For solution (1) disperse a quantity of the ointment containing 2 mg of Fluocinonide in 20 ml of *methanol (80%)* in a 100-ml separating funnel containing 50 ml of *2,2,4-trimethylpentane*. Warm the contents over a water bath and shake gently. Allow the layers to separate and transfer the lower layer to a 250-ml separating funnel containing 100 ml of *water*. Add 10 ml of *chloroform* and shake for 3 minutes. Allow the layers to separate, evaporate the lower layer to dryness on a water bath in a current of air and dissolve the residue in 1 ml of *chloroform*. Solution (2) contains 0.2% w/v of *fluocinonide BPCRS* in *chloroform*. After removal of the plate, allow it to dry in air until the odour of solvent is no longer detectable. Heat at 105° for 5 minutes and spray while hot with *alkaline tetrazolium blue solution*. The principal spot in the chromatogram obtained with solution (1) corresponds to that in the chromatogram obtained with solution (2).

B. In the Assay, the retention time of the principal peak in the chromatogram obtained with solution (1) is similar to that of the principal peak in the chromatogram obtained with solution (2).

Assay Carry out the method for *liquid chromatography*, Appendix III D, using the following solutions. For solution (1) disperse a quantity of the ointment containing 1.5 mg of Fluocinonide in 20 ml of *methanol (80%)* in a 100-ml separating funnel containing 50 ml of *2,2,4-trimethylpentane*. Warm the contents over a water bath and shake gently for 2 minutes. Allow the layers to separate and transfer the lower layer to a 50-ml flask. Repeat the extraction with a further 20 ml of *methanol (80%)*. Dilute the combined extracts to 50 ml with the same solvent. Solution (2) contains 0.003% w/v of *fluocinonide BPCRS* in *methanol (80%)*.

The chromatographic procedure may be carried out using (a) a stainless steel column (20 cm × 4.6 mm) packed with *stationary phase C* (5 μm) (Spherisorb ODS 1 is suitable), (b) a mixture of 0.1 volume of *glacial acetic acid*, 45 volumes of *acetonitrile* and 55 volumes of *water* as the mobile phase with a flow rate of 2 ml per minute and (c) a detection wavelength of 238 nm.

Calculate the content of $C_{26}H_{32}F_2O_7$ in the ointment using the declared content of $C_{26}H_{32}F_2O_7$ in *fluocinonide BPCRS*.

Fluocortolone Cream

Definition Fluocortolone Cream contains Fluocortolone Pivalate and Fluocortolone Hexanoate in a suitable basis.

The cream complies with the requirements stated under Topical Semi-solid Preparations and with the following requirements.

Content of fluocortolone pivalate, $C_{27}H_{37}FO_5$ 90.0 to 110.0% of the prescribed or stated amount.

Content of fluocortolone hexanoate, $C_{28}H_{39}FO_5$ 90.0 to 110.0% of the prescribed or stated amount.

Identification

A. Carry out the method for *thin-layer chromatography*, Appendix III A, using a silanised silica gel precoated plate the surface of which has been modified by chemically-bonded octadecylsilyl groups. (Whatman KC18F plates are suitable) and a mixture of 65 volumes of *acetonitrile* and 35 volumes of *water* as the mobile phase. Apply separately to the plate 10 μl of each of the following solutions. For solution (1) transfer a quantity of the preparation being examined containing 1 mg of Fluocortolone Pivalate to a separating funnel with the aid of 10 ml of *methanol*, add 50 ml of *2,2,4-trimethylpentane* and shake vigorously for 1 minute. Allow to stand, separate the lower methanol layer, add 100 ml of *water* and 50 ml of *chloroform*, shake vigorously for 1 minute and centrifuge at 1500 revolutions per minute for 5 minutes. Evaporate 25 ml of the chloroform layer to dryness on a water bath in a current of nitrogen and dissolve the residue in 1 ml of a mixture of 9 volumes of *chloroform* and 1 volume of *methanol*. For solution (2) mix 0.5 ml of a 0.2% w/v solution of *fluocortolone pivalate BPCRS* in a mixture of 9 volumes of *chloroform* and 1 volume of *methanol* with 0.5 ml of a 0.2% w/v solution of *fluocortolone hexanoate BPCRS* in the same solvent. Solution (3) is a mixture of equal volumes of solutions (1) and (2). After removal of the plate, allow it to dry in air for 10 minutes and examine under *ultraviolet light (254 nm)*. The two principal spots in the chromatogram obtained with solution (1) correspond to those in the chromatogram obtained with solution (2). The test is not valid unless the chromatogram obtained with solution (3) shows two compact spots.

B. In the Assay, the chromatogram obtained with solution (3) shows two peaks with the same retention times as the peaks due to fluocortolone pivalate and fluocortolone hexanoate in the chromatogram obtained with solution (1).

Assay Carry out the method for *liquid chromatography*, Appendix III D, using the following solutions. Solution (1) contains 0.004% w/v each of *fluocortolone pivalate BPCRS*, *fluocortolone hexanoate BPCRS* and *benzyl benzoate* (internal standard) in a mixture of 4 volumes of *acetonitrile* and 1 volume of *water*. For solution (2) add 20 ml of a mixture of 4 volumes of *acetonitrile* and 1 volume of *water* followed by 50 ml of *2,2,4-trimethylpentane* to a quantity of the preparation being examined containing 2 mg of Fluocortolone Pivalate and heat on a water bath, shaking intermittently, until the preparation is completely dispersed. Remove from the water bath, shake vigorously for 3 minutes, allow to separate and transfer the lower, aqueous acetonitrile layer to a flask. Repeat the extraction of the 2,2,4-trimethylpentane solution with a further 20 ml of the acetonitrile—water mixture and again transfer the lower, aqueous acetonitrile layer to the flask. Dilute the combined extracts to 50 ml with a mixture of 4 volumes of *acetonitrile* and 1 volume of *water* and filter a portion using a pressure filter (a Swinnex filter holder prepared with a double thickness of Whatman No. 42 filter paper is suitable). Prepare solution (3) in the same manner as solution (2) but adding 2 ml of a 0.100% v/v solution of *benzyl benzoate* in a mixture of 4 volumes of *acetonitrile* and 1 volume of *water* to the combined extracts before dilution to 50 ml.

The chromatographic procedure may be carried out using (a) a stainless steel column (20 cm × 5 mm) packed with *stationary phase C* (5 μm) (Spherisorb ODS 1 is suitable), (b) as the mobile phase with a flow rate of 1 ml per minute, a mixture of *acetonitrile* and *water* each containing 1% v/v of *glacial acetic acid* adjusted so that the retention time of fluocortolone pivalate is about 9 minutes and baseline separation is obtained from benzyl benzoate and fluocortolone hexanoate (retention time, about 11 minutes) (a mixture of 53 volumes of *acetonitrile*, 47 volumes of *water* and 1 volume of *glacial acetic acid* is usually suitable) and (c) a detection wavelength of 238 nm.

Calculate the contents of $C_{27}H_{37}FO_5$ and $C_{28}H_{39}FO_5$ in the preparation being examined using the declared contents of $C_{27}H_{37}FO_5$ in *fluocortolone pivalate BPCRS* and $C_{28}H_{39}FO_5$ in *fluocortolone hexanoate BPCRS* respectively.

Storage Fluocortolone Cream should be stored at a temperature not exceeding 30°.

Labelling The strength is stated as the percentages w/w of Fluocortolone Pivalate and Fluocortolone Hexanoate.

Fluocortolone Ointment

Definition Fluocortolone Ointment contains Fluocortolone Pivalate and Fluocortolone Hexanoate in a suitable basis.

The ointment complies with the requirements stated under Topical Semi-solid Preparations and with the following requirements.

Content of fluocortolone pivalate, $C_{27}H_{37}FO_5$ 90.0 to 110.0% of the prescribed or stated amount.

Content of fluocortolone hexanoate, $C_{28}H_{39}FO_5$ 90.0 to 110.0% of the prescribed or stated amount.

Identification

A. Complies with test A for Identification described under Fluocortolone Cream but preparing solution (1) as follows. Transfer a quantity of the ointment containing 1 mg of Fluocortolone Pivalate to a separating funnel with the aid of 10 ml of *methanol*, add 2 ml of *water* and 50 ml of *2,2,4-trimethylpentane*, shake vigorously for 1 minute and allow to separate. Separation of the layers may be aided by warming the separating funnel under a jet of hot water. To the lower, aqueous methanol layer add 100 ml of *water*, extract with 50 ml of *chloroform*, filter the chloroform layer (Whatman No. 1 filter paper is suitable), evaporate to dryness on a water bath in a current of nitrogen and dissolve the residue in 1 ml of a mixture of 9 volumes of *chloroform* and 1 volume of *methanol*.

B. In the Assay, the chromatogram obtained with solution (3) shows two peaks with the same retention times as the peaks due to fluocortolone pivalate and fluocortolone hexanoate in the chromatogram obtained with solution (1).

Assay Carry out the Assay described under Fluocortolone Cream, but omitting the final filtration of the extract in the preparation of solutions (2) and (3).

Storage Fluocortolone Ointment should be stored at a temperature not exceeding 30°.

Labelling The strength is stated as the percentages w/w of Fluocortolone Pivalate and Fluocortolone Hexanoate.

Fluorescein Eye Drops

Definition Fluorescein Eye Drops are a sterile solution of Fluorescein Sodium in Purified Water.

The eye drops comply with the requirements stated under Eye Preparations and with the following requirements.

Content of fluorescein sodium, $C_{20}H_{10}Na_2O_5$ 90.0 to 110.0% of the prescribed or stated amount.

Identification

A. Evaporate a volume containing 20 mg of Fluorescein Sodium and dry at 105° for 30 minutes. The *infrared absorption spectrum* of the residue, Appendix II A, is concordant with the *reference spectrum* of fluorescein sodium.

B. The eye drops are strongly fluorescent, even in extreme dilution; the fluorescence disappears when the solution is made acidic and reappears when it is made alkaline.

C. Dilute with *water* to produce a solution containing 0.05% w/v of Fluorescein Sodium. One drop of the solution, absorbed by a piece of filter paper, colours the paper yellow. On exposing the moist paper to bromine vapour for 1 minute and then to ammonia vapour the yellow colour becomes deep pink.

Acidity or alkalinity pH, 7.0 to 9.0, Appendix V L.

Chloroform-soluble matter To a volume containing 0.1 g of Fluorescein Sodium add 1 ml of 2M *sodium hydroxide*, extract with 10 ml of *chloroform* and dry the chloroform layer with *anhydrous sodium sulphate*. The *absorbance* of the resulting solution at 480 nm is not more than 0.05, Appendix II B, using *chloroform* in the reference cell.

Dimethylformamide Carry out the method for *gas chromatography*, Appendix III B, using the following solutions. Solution (1) contains 0.0020% v/v of *dimethylformamide* and 0.0020% v/v of *dimethylacetamide* (internal standard). For solution (2) dilute the eye drops with *water*, if necessary, to produce a solution containing 1.0% w/v of Fluorescein Sodium. To 5 ml of this solution add, with stirring, 0.3 ml of 1M *hydrochloric acid*, allow to stand for 15 minutes and centrifuge; dissolve 10 mg of *trisodium orthophosphate* in 2 ml of the supernatant liquid. Prepare solution (3) in the same manner as solution (2) but adding 1 ml of a 0.010% v/v solution of *dimethylacetamide* before the hydrochloric acid.

The chromatographic procedure may be carried out using a glass column (1.5 m × 4 mm) packed with *acid-washed, silanised diatomaceous support* (80 to 100 mesh) coated with 10% w/w of *polyethylene glycol 1000* and maintained at 120°.

In the chromatogram obtained with solution (3) the ratio of the area of any peak corresponding to dimethylformamide to the area of the peak due to the internal standard is not greater than the corresponding ratio in the chromatogram obtained with solution (1) (0.2%).

Resorcinol Carry out the method for *thin-layer chromatography*, Appendix III A, using a silica gel F_{254} precoated plate (Merck silica gel 60 F_{254} plates are suitable) and a mixture of 40 volumes of *ethyl acetate* and 60 volumes of *hexane* as the mobile phase. Apply separately to the plate 5 µl of each of the following solutions. For solution (1) dilute the eye drops with *water*, if necessary, to produce a solution containing 1.0% w/v of Fluorescein Sodium and to 10 ml of this solution add, with stirring, 2.5 ml of 0.25M *hydrochloric acid*. Allow to stand for 15 minutes, centrifuge and dissolve 0.1 g of *trisodium orthophosphate* in 5 ml of the supernatant liquid. Solution (2) contains 0.0040% w/v of *resorcinol*. After removal of the plate, allow it to dry in air and expose to iodine vapour for 30 minutes. Any spot corresponding to resorcinol in the chromatogram obtained with solution (1) is not more intense than the spot in the chromatogram obtained with solution (2) (0.5%).

Related substances Carry out the method for *thin-layer chromatography*, Appendix III A, using a silica gel F_{254} precoated plate (Merck silica gel 60 F_{254} plates are suitable) and a mixture of 20 volumes of *methanol* and 80 volumes of *chloroform* as the mobile phase. Apply separately to the plate 5 µl of each of the following solutions. For solution (1) dilute a suitable volume of the eye drops with an equal volume of 0.1M *methanolic hydrochloric acid*. For solution (2) dilute 1 volume of solution (1) to 500 volumes with 0.1M *methanolic hydrochloric acid*. After removal of the plate, allow it to dry in air and examine under *ultraviolet light (365 nm)*. Expose the plate to iodine vapour for 30 minutes and re-examine. By each method of visualisation, any *secondary spot* in the chromatogram obtained with solution (1) is not more intense than the spot in the chromatogram obtained with solution (2) (0.2%).

Assay Dilute a volume containing 0.1 g of Fluorescein Sodium to 20 ml with *water*, add 5 ml of 2M *hydrochloric acid* and extract with four 20-ml quantities of a mixture of equal volumes of *2-methylpropan-1-ol* and *chloroform*. Wash the combined extracts with 10 ml of *water*, extract the washings with 5 ml of the solvent mixture and add to the combined extracts. Evaporate the combined extracts to dryness on a water bath in a current of air, dissolve the residue in 10 ml of *ethanol (96%)*, evaporate to dryness on a water bath and dry to constant weight at 105°. Each g of residue is equivalent to 1.132 g of $C_{20}H_{10}Na_2O_5$.

Storage Fluorescein Eye Drops should be protected from light.

Labelling The label states that the eye drops should be discarded after use on a single occasion.

Fluorescein Injection

Definition Fluorescein Injection is a sterile solution of Fluorescein Sodium in Water for Injections.

The injection complies with the requirements stated under Parenteral Preparations and with the following requirements.

Content of fluorescein sodium, $C_{20}H_{10}Na_2O_5$ 95.0 to 105.0% of the prescribed or stated amount.

Identification

A. Evaporate 1 ml to dryness on a water bath and dry the residue at 105° for 30 minutes. The *infrared absorption spectrum* of the residue, Appendix II A, is concordant with the *reference spectrum* of fluorescein sodium.

B. The injection is strongly fluorescent, even in extreme dilution; the fluorescence disappears when the solution is made acidic and reappears when it is made alkaline.

C. Dilute with *water* to produce a solution containing 0.05% w/v of Fluorescein Sodium. One drop of the solution, absorbed by a piece of filter paper, colours the paper yellow. On exposing the moist paper to bromine vapour for 1 minute and then to ammonia vapour the yellow colour becomes deep pink.

Alkalinity pH, 8.0 to 9.8, Appendix V L.

Chloroform-soluble matter Dilute the injection with *water*, if necessary, to produce a solution containing 5% w/v of Fluorescein Sodium. To 4 ml add 1 ml of 1M *sodium hydroxide*, dilute to 10 ml with *water*, extract with 10 ml of *chloroform* and dry the chloroform layer over *anhydrous sodium sulphate*. The *absorbance* of the resulting solution at 480 nm is not more than 0.10, Appendix II B, using *chloroform* in the reference cell.

Dimethylformamide Complies with the test described under Fluorescein Eye Drops using the following solutions in place of solutions (2) and (3). For solution (2) dilute the injection with *water*, if necessary, to produce a solution containing 5.0% w/v of Fluorescein Sodium. To 10 ml of this solution add, with stirring, 1 ml of 3M *hydrochloric acid*, allow to stand for 15 minutes and centrifuge; dissolve 0.1 g of *trisodium orthophosphate* in 5 ml of the supernatant liquid. Prepare solution (3) in the same manner as solution (2) but adding 1.0 ml of a 0.10% v/v solution of *dimethylacetamide* (internal standard) before the hydrochloric acid.

Resorcinol Complies with the test described under Fluorescein Eye Drops using the following solutions. For solution (1) dilute the injection with *water*, if necessary, to produce a solution containing 5.0% w/v of Fluorescein Sodium. To 20 ml of this solution, add, with stirring, 2 ml of 3M *hydrochloric acid*, dilute to 25 ml with *water* and allow to stand for 15 minutes, centrifuge and dissolve 0.1 g of *trisodium orthophosphate* in 5 ml of the supernatant liquid. Solution (2) contains 0.020% w/v of *resorcinol*.

Related substances Complies with the test described under Fluorescein Eye Drops using the following solutions. For solution (1) dilute the injection with *water*, if necessary, to produce a solution containing 5.0% w/v of Fluorescein Sodium and dilute 5 volumes of this solution to 25 volumes with 0.1M *methanolic hydrochloric acid*. For solution (2) dilute 1 volume of solution (1) to 500 volumes with 0.1M *methanolic hydrochloric acid*.

Assay Dilute a suitable volume of the injection with sufficient *water* to produce a solution containing 2.5% w/v of Fluorescein Sodium, add 5 ml of 2M *hydrochloric acid* and extract with four 20-ml quantities of a mixture of equal volumes of *2-methylpropan-1-ol* and *chloroform*. Wash the combined extracts with 10 ml of *water*, extract the washings with 5 ml of the solvent mixture and add to the combined extracts. Evaporate the combined extracts and washings to dryness on a water bath in a current of air, dissolve the residue in 10 ml of *ethanol (96%)*, evaporate to dryness on a water bath and dry to constant weight at 105°. Each g of residue is equivalent to 1.132 g of $C_{20}H_{10}Na_2O_5$.

Storage Fluorescein Injection should be protected from light.

Fluorometholone Eye Drops

Definition Fluorometholone Eye Drops are a sterile suspension of Fluorometholone in Purified Water.

The eye drops comply with the requirements stated under Eye Preparations and with the following requirements.

Content of fluorometholone, $C_{22}H_{29}FO_4$ 95.0 to 105.0% of the prescribed or stated amount.

Identification

A. Shake a quantity of the eye drops containing 5 mg of Fluorometholone with 20 ml of *acetone*, filter and evaporate the filtrate to dryness. Dissolve the residue in 10 ml of *acetone* , filter and evaporate the filtrate to dryness. The *infrared absorption spectrum* of the residue, Appendix II A, is concordant with the *reference spectrum* of fluorometholone.

B. In the Assay, the principal peak in the chromatogram obtained with solution (1) has the same retention time as the principal peak in the chromatogram obtained with solution (2).

Acidity or alkalinity pH, 6.0 to 7.5, Appendix V L.

Related substances Carry out the method for *liquid chromatography*, Appendix III D, using the following solutions. For solution (1) dilute a quantity of the eye drops containing 1 mg of Fluorometholone to 10 ml with a mixture of equal volumes of *methanol* and *water*. Solution contains (2) 0.00005% w/v of the substance being examined in *methanol* and solution (3) contains 0.00005% w/v each of *deltamedrane BPCRS* and *fluorometholone BPCRS*.

The chromatographic procedure may be carried out using (a) a stainless steel column (30 cm × 3.9 mm) packed with *stationary phase C* (10 μm) (μBondapak C18 is suitable), (b) a mixture of 40 volumes of *water* and 60 volumes of *methanol* as the mobile phase with a flow rate of 2 ml per minute and.(c) a detection wavelength of 254 nm.

The test is not valid unless, in the chromatogram obtained with solution (3), the *resolution factor* between the peaks due to deltamedrane and fluorometholone is at least 2.0.

In the chromatogram obtained with solution (1), the area of any *secondary peak* is not greater than the area of the principal peak in the chromatogram obtained with solution (2) (0.5%) and the sum of the areas of any *secondary peaks* is not greater than twice the area of the principal peak in the chromatogram obtained with solution (2) (1%).

Assay Carry out the method for *liquid chromatography*, Appendix III D, using the following solutions. For solution (1) mix the eye drops thoroughly and dilute a quantity containing 1 mg of Fluorometholone to 25 ml with a mixture of equal volumes of *methanol* and *water*. For solution (2) prepare a 0.05% w/v solution of *fluorometholone BPCRS* in *methanol* and dilute 4 ml of the solution to 50 ml with a mixture of equal volumes of *methanol* and *water*. Solution (3) contains 0.00005% w/v each of *deltamedrane BPCRS* and *fluorometholone BPCRS*.

The chromatographic procedure described under Related substances may be used.

The test is not valid unless, in the chromatogram obtained with solution (3), the *resolution factor* between the peaks due to deltamedrane and fluorometholone is at least 2.0.

Calculate the content of $C_{22}H_{29}FO_4$ in the eye drops using the declared content of $C_{22}H_{29}FO_4$ in *fluorometholone BPCRS*.

Fluorouracil Cream

Definition Fluorouracil Cream contains Fluorouracil in a suitable basis.

The cream complies with the requirements stated under Topical Semi-solid Preparations and with the following requirements.

Content of fluorouracil, $C_4H_3FN_2O_2$ 90.0 to 110.0% of the prescribed or stated amount.

Identification

A. Dry a quantity containing 50 mg of Fluorouracil at a pressure not exceeding 0.7 kPa, mix with 100 ml of *ether*, decant, wash the white, crystalline residue with 50 ml of *ether* and dry in air. The *infrared absorption spectrum* of the residue, Appendix II A, is concordant with the *reference spectrum* of fluorouracil.

B. The *light absorption*, Appendix II B, in the range 230 to 350 nm of the final solution obtained in the Assay exhibits a maximum only at 266 nm.

5-Hydroxyuracil Carry out the method for *thin-layer chromatography*, Appendix III A, using a silica gel precoated plate (Merck silica gel 60 plates are suitable) and a mixture of 70 volumes of *ethyl acetate*, 40 volumes of *acetone* and 10 volumes of *water* as the mobile phase. Apply separately to the plate 20 µl of each of the following solutions. For solution (1) shake a quantity of the cream containing 0.10 g of Fluorouracil with 10 ml of *water* for 5 minutes, add 10 ml of *ethanol (96%)*, mix and filter through glass fibre paper. Solution (2) contains 0.00125% w/v of *5-hydroxyuracil* in *methanol (50%)*. After removal of the plate, allow it to dry in air, spray with a freshly prepared 0.5% w/v solution of *fast blue B salt* and then with 0.1M *sodium hydroxide*. Any spot corresponding to 5-hydroxyuracil in the chromatogram obtained with solution (1) is not more intense than the spot in the chromatogram obtained with solution (2).

Urea Carry out the method described under 5-Hydroxyuracil applying separately to the plate 20 µl of each of the following solutions. For solution (1) shake a quantity of the cream containing 0.10 g of Fluorouracil with 10 ml of *water* for 5 minutes, add 10 ml of *ethanol (96%)*, mix and filter through glass fibre paper. Solution (2) contains 0.0050% w/v of *urea* in *water*. After removal of the plate, allow it to dry in air, spray with a mixture of 10 volumes of a 1% w/v solution of *4-dimethylaminobenzaldehyde* in *ethanol (96%)* and 1 volume of *hydrochloric acid* and heat at 100° until maximum intensity of the spots is obtained. Any spot corresponding to urea in the chromatogram obtained with solution (1) is not more intense than the spot in the chromatogram obtained with solution (2).

Assay To a quantity containing 50 mg of Fluorouracil add 50 ml of 0.1M *hydrochloric acid* and shake for 5 minutes. Extract with three 25-ml quantities of *chloroform*, discard the chloroform, dilute the aqueous solution to 250 ml with 0.1M *hydrochloric acid* and filter (Whatman No. 42 paper is suitable). Dilute 5 ml to 100 ml with 0.1M *hydrochloric acid* and measure the *absorbance* of the resulting solution at the maximum at 266 nm, Appendix II B. Calculate the content of $C_4H_3FN_2O_2$ taking 552 as the value of A(1%, 1 cm) at the maximum at 266 nm.

Fluorouracil Injection

Definition Fluorouracil Injection is a sterile solution in Water for Injections of fluorouracil sodium, prepared by the interaction of Fluorouracil and Sodium Hydroxide.

The injection complies with the requirements stated under Parenteral Preparations and with the following requirements.

Content of fluorouracil, $C_4H_3FN_2O_2$ 90.0 to 110.0% of the prescribed or stated amount.

Characteristics A colourless or almost colourless solution.

Identification

A. Carefully acidify a volume containing the equivalent of 0.1 g of Fluorouracil with *glacial acetic acid*, stir, cool and filter. Wash the precipitate with 1 ml of *water* and dry over *phosphorus pentoxide* at 80° at a pressure of 2 kPa for 4 hours. The *infrared absorption spectrum* of the residue, Appendix II A, is concordant with the *reference spectrum* of fluorouracil.

B. The *light absorption*, Appendix II B, in the range 230 to 350 nm of the solution obtained in the Assay exhibits a maximum only at 266 nm.

Alkalinity pH, 8.5 to 9.1, Appendix V L.

Urea Carry out the method described under Related substances applying separately to the plate 20 µl of each of the following solutions. For solution (1) dilute a suitable quantity of the injection with *water* to produce a solution containing the equivalent of 0.50% w/v of Fluorouracil. Solution (2) contains 0.020% w/v of *urea* in *water*. After removal of the plate, allow it to dry in air, spray with a mixture of 10 volumes of a 1% w/v solution of *4-dimethylaminobenzaldehyde* in *ethanol (96%)* and 1 volume of *hydrochloric acid* and heat at 100° until maximum intensity of the spots is obtained. Any spot corresponding to urea in the chromatogram obtained with solution (1) is not more intense than the spot in the chromatogram obtained with solution (2).

Related substances Carry out the method for *thin-layer chromatography*, Appendix III A, using a silica gel F_{254} precoated plate (Merck silica gel 60 F_{254} plates are suitable) and a mixture of 70 volumes of *ethyl acetate*, 15 volumes of *methanol* and 15 volumes of *water* as the mobile phase. Apply separately to the plate 10 µl of each of the following solutions. For solution (1) dilute a suitable quantity of the injection with *water* to produce a solution containing the equivalent of 2.0% w/v of Fluorouracil. For solution (2) dilute 1 volume of solution (1) to 400 volumes with *methanol (50%)*. Solution (3) contains 0.0050% w/v of *5-hydroxyuracil* in *methanol (50%)*. After removal of the plate, allow it to dry in a current of air and examine under *ultraviolet light (254 nm)*. Any *secondary spot* in the chromatogram obtained with solution (1) is not more intense than the spot in the chromatogram obtained with solution (2). Spray with a freshly prepared 0.5% w/v solution of *fast blue B salt* and then with 0.1M *sodium hydroxide*. Any spot corresponding to 5-hydroxyuracil in the chromatogram obtained with solution (1) is not more intense than the spot in the chromatogram obtained with solution (3).

Assay To a volume containing the equivalent of 75 mg of Fluorouracil add 20 ml of 1M *hydrochloric acid* and sufficient *water* to produce 200 ml. Dilute 3 ml to 100 ml with 0.1M *hydrochloric acid* and measure the *absorbance* of the resulting solution at the maximum at 266 nm, Appendix II B. Calculate the content of $C_4H_3FN_2O_2$ taking 552 as the value of A(1%,1 cm) at the maximum at 266 nm.

Storage Fluorouracil Injection should be protected from light and stored at a temperature of 15° to 25°.

Labelling The strength is stated in terms of the equivalent amount of Fluorouracil in a suitable dose-volume.

Flupentixol Injection

Definition Flupentixol Injection is a sterile solution of Flupentixol Decanoate in a suitable vegetable oil.

The injection complies with the requirements stated under Parenteral Preparations and with the following requirements.

Content of Flupentixol decanoate, $C_{33}H_{43}F_3N_2O_2S$ 95.0 to 105.0% of the prescribed or stated amount.

Identification

A. Dilute 1 volume of solution A obtained in the Assay to 2 volumes with *ethanol (96%)*. The *light absorption*, Appendix II B, in the range 205 to 300 nm of the resulting solution exhibits two maxima at 230 nm and 264 nm.

B. Carry out the method for *thin-layer chromatography*, Appendix III A, using a silica gel F_{254} precoated plate (Merck silica gel 60 F_{254} plates are suitable) and a mixture of 3 volumes of *diethylamine* and 90 volumes of *cyclohexane* as the mobile phase and an unsaturated tank. Apply separately to the plate 5 µl of each of the following solutions. For solution (1) dilute the injection with *ethanol (96%)* to contain 0.4% w/v of Flupentixol Decanoate. Solution (2) contains 0.4% w/v of *flupentixol decanoate BPCRS* in *ethanol (96%)*. After removal of the plate, allow it to dry in air, spray with a 1% w/v solution of *sodium molybdate* in *sulphuric acid*, heat at 110° for 20 minutes and examine in daylight. The principal spot in the chromatogram obtained with solution (1) is similar in colour, position and size to that in the chromatogram obtained with solution (2).

Free alcohol Carry out the method for *thin-layer chromatography*, Appendix III A, using a silica gel F_{254} precoated plate (Merck silica gel 60 F_{254} plates are suitable) and a mixture of 10 volumes of *diethylamine*, 40 volumes of *dichloromethane* and 50 volumes of *cyclohexane* as the mobile phase and an unsaturated tank. Apply separately to the plate 10 µl of each of the following solutions. For solution (1) dissolve a quantity of the injection containing 20 mg of Flupentixol Decanoate in *dichloromethane* and dilute to 10 ml with the same solvent. For solution (2) dilute 3 volumes of solution (1) to 100 volumes with *dichloromethane*. After removal of the plate, allow it to dry in air, spray with a mixture of equal volumes of *sulphuric acid* and *absolute ethanol*, heat at 110° for 5 minutes and examine under *ultraviolet light (365 nm)*. In the chromatogram obtained with solution (1) any *secondary spot* of the same colour as the principal spot is not more intense than the spot in the chromatogram obtained with solution (2) (3%).

2-Trifluoromethylthioxanthone Carry out the method for *thin-layer chromatography*, Appendix III A, protected from light, using a silica gel F_{254} precoated plate (Merck silica gel 60 F_{254} plates are suitable) and a mixture of 30 volumes of *dichloromethane* and 70 volumes of *toluene* as the mobile phase and an unsaturated tank. Apply separately to the plate 10 µl of each of the following solutions. For solution (1) dissolve a quantity of the injection containing 20 mg of Flupentixol Decanoate in *dichloromethane* and dilute to 10 ml with the same solvent. Solution (2) contains 0.001% w/v of *2-trifluoromethylthioxanthone BPCRS* in *dichloromethane*. After removal of the plate, allow it to dry in air, spray with a mixture of equal volumes of *sulphuric acid* and *absolute ethanol*, heat at 110° for 5 minutes and examine under *ultraviolet light (365 nm)*. Any *secondary spot* in the chromatogram obtained with solution (1) corresponding to 2-trifluoromethylthioxanthone is not more intense than the spot in the chromatogram obtained with solution (2) (0.5%).

***trans*-Flupentixol decanoate** Carry out the method for *liquid chromatography*, Appendix III D, using the following solutions. For solution (1) dilute the injection with *dichloromethane* to contain 0.10% w/v of Flupentixol Decanoate. Solution (2) contains 0.0010% w/v of *trans-flupentixol dihydrochloride BPCRS* in *dichloromethane*. Solution (3) contains 0.0010% w/v of *trans-flupentixol decanoate dihydrochloride BPCRS* in solution (1).

The chromatographic procedure may be carried out using (a) a stainless steel column (25 cm × 4.6 mm) packed with *stationary phase A* (5 µm) (Spherisorb S 5W is suitable), (b) a mixture of 0.005 volume of 13.5M *ammonia*, 15 volumes of *acetonitrile*, 42.5 volumes of *dichloromethane* and 42.5 volumes of *n-heptane* as the mobile phase with a flow rate of 2.3 ml per minute and (c) a detection wavelength of 254 nm.

The test is not valid unless the chromatogram obtained with solution (3) shows clearly separated peaks.

In the chromatogram obtained with solution (1) the area of any peak corresponding to *trans*-flupentixol decanoate is not greater than the area of the peak in the chromatograms obtained with solution (2) (1%).

Assay Shake a quantity of the injection containing 20 mg of Flupentixol Decanoate with 90 ml of a mixture of 45 volumes of 0.5M *acetic acid* and 55 volumes of *ethanol (96%)* for 15 minutes and dilute to 100 ml with the same solvent mixture; centrifuge a portion of the extract until a clear supernatant liquid is obtained and dilute 15 ml of the supernatant liquid to 100 ml with *ethanol (96%)* (solution A). Prepare a reference standard in the following manner. Dissolve 20 mg of *Flupentixol dihydrochloride BPCRS* in 50 ml of a mixture of 45 volumes of 0.5M *acetic acid* and 55 volumes of *ethanol (96%)* by heating gently on a water bath. Cool and dilute to 100 ml with the same solvent mixture. Dilute 15 ml of the resulting solution to 100 ml with *ethanol (96%)* (solution B). Measure the *absorbance* of solutions A and B respectively at the maximum at 264 nm, Appendix II B, using 20 ml of the solvent mixture diluted to 100 ml with *ethanol (96%)* in the reference cell. Determine the *weight per ml* of the injection, Appendix V G, and calculate the content of $C_{33}H_{43}F_3N_2O_2S$, weight in volume, using the declared content of $C_{23}H_{25}F_3N_2OS,2HCl$ in *Flupentixol dihydrochloride BPCRS*. Each mg of Flupentixol dihydrochloride is equivalent to 1.160 mg of Flupentixol decanoate.

Storage Flupentixol Injection should be protected from light and stored at a temperature of 15° to 25°.

Labelling When flupenthixol injection is prescribed or demanded Flupentixol Injection shall be dispensed or supplied.

Fluphenazine Decanoate Injection

Definition Fluphenazine Decanoate Injection is a sterile solution of Fluphenazine Decanoate in Sesame Oil.

The injection complies with the requirements stated under Parenteral Preparations and with the following requirements.

Content of fluphenazine decanoate, $C_{32}H_{44}F_3N_3O_2S$ 90.0 to 110.0% of the prescribed or stated amount.

Identification

A. Carry out in subdued light the method for *thin-layer chromatography*, Appendix III A, using a plate 200 mm × 200 mm in size and *silica gel GF_{254}* as the coating substance. For the first development use *chloroform* as the mobile phase. Apply to the bottom right-hand corner of the plate a volume of the injection containing 25 µg of Fluphenazine Decanoate and develop over a path of 12 cm. After removal of the plate, allow it to dry in air, turn the plate through 90° in a clockwise direction, impregnate the coating with a 5% v/v solution of n-*tetradecane* in n-*hexane* and allow it to dry in air. Apply to the bottom right-hand corner of the plate, to the right of the solvent front of the first development, 1 µl of a 2.0% w/v solution of *fluphenazine decanoate BPCRS* in *ethanol (96%)*. For the second development use *methanol (90%)* as the mobile phase. After removal of the plate, allow it to dry in air and examine under *ultraviolet light (254 nm)*. The principal spot in the chromatogram obtained with the injection corresponds to that in the chromatogram obtained with the reference substance.

B. Shake a volume containing 5 mg of Fluphenazine Decanoate with 1 ml of a 1% w/v solution of *sucrose* in *hydrochloric acid* and allow to stand for 5 minutes. A red colour is produced in the acid layer.

Related substances Protect the solutions from light. Carry out the method for *liquid chromatography*, Appendix III D, using the following solutions. For solution (1) dilute a volume of the injection with sufficient *chloroform* to produce a solution containing 0.50% w/v of Fluphenazine Decanoate, dilute 1 volume of this solution to 25 volumes with *acetonitrile* and mix. For solution (2) dilute 1 volume of solution (1) to 100 volumes with *acetonitrile*. For solution (3) add 0.05 ml of 10M *sodium hydroxide* to 2 ml of solution (1) and allow to stand for 48 hours before use (generation of fluphenazine impurity). For solution (4) add 0.05 ml of *hydrogen peroxide solution (200 vol)* to 5 mg of *fluphenazine decanoate BPCRS*, allow to stand for 10 minutes, add sufficient *chloroform* to produce 1 ml, mix and dilute to 100 ml with *acetonitrile* (generation of mono- and di-*N*-oxide impurities).

The chromatographic procedure may be carried out using (a) a stainless steel column (25 cm × 4.6 mm) packed with *stationary phase C* (5 µm) (Hypersil ODS is suitable), (b) as the mobile phase with a flow rate of 1 ml per minute a solution prepared by adding 450 volumes of *acetonitrile* to a mixture of 75 volumes of a 1% w/v solution of *ammonium carbonate* and 450 volumes of *methanol* and (c) a detection wavelength of 260 nm. Inject separately 20 µl of each solution.

The test is not valid unless, in the chromatogram obtained with solution (4), the *resolution factor* between the peaks corresponding to the two fluphenazine mono-*N*-oxides is at least 2.

In the chromatogram obtained with solution (1) the area of any peak corresponding to the peak due to fluphenazine in the chromatogram obtained with solution (3) is not greater than 4 times the area of the peak in the chromatogram obtained with solution (2) (4%), the area of any other *secondary peak* is not greater than the area of the peak in the chromatogram obtained with solution (2) (1%) and the sum of the areas of any *secondary peaks* other than any peak corresponding to fluphenazine is not greater than twice the area of the peak in the chromatogram obtained with solution (2) (2%). Disregard any peak with a retention time relative to Fluphenazine Decanoate of 0.2 or less.

Assay Carry out Method I for *non-aqueous titration*, Appendix VIII A, using a volume containing 0.15 g of Fluphenazine Decanoate diluted with 75 ml of *anhydrous acetic acid* and *crystal violet solution* as indicator. Each ml of 0.1M *perchloric acid VS* is equivalent to 29.59 mg of $C_{32}H_{44}F_3N_3O_2S$.

Storage Fluphenazine Decanoate Injection should be protected from light.

Labelling The label states that the injection is for intramuscular injection only.

Fluphenazine Tablets

Definition Fluphenazine Tablets contain Fluphenazine Hydrochloride. They are coated.

The tablets comply with the requirements stated under Tablets and with the following requirements.

Content of fluphenazine hydrochloride, $C_{22}H_{26}F_3N_3OS,2HCl$ 90.0 to 110.0% of the prescribed or stated amount.

Identification

A. Carry out in subdued light the method for *thin-layer chromatography*, Appendix III A, using *kieselguhr G* as the coating substance. Impregnate the dry plate by placing it in a tank containing a shallow layer of a mixture of 5 volumes of *2-phenoxyethanol*, 15 volumes of *formamide* and 180 volumes of *acetone*, allowing the impregnating solvent to ascend to the top, removing the plate from the tank and using it immediately. Use a mixture of 2 volumes of *diethylamine* and 100 volumes of *petroleum spirit (boiling range, 40° to 60°)* saturated with *2-phenoxyethanol* as the mobile phase. Apply separately to the plate 2 µl of each of the following solutions. For solution (1) shake a quantity of the powdered tablets with sufficient *methanol* to produce a solution containing 0.2% w/v of Fluphenazine Hydrochloride, centrifuge and use the supernatant liquid. Solution (2) contains 0.2% w/v of *fluphenazine hydrochloride BPCRS* in *methanol*. After removal of the plate, allow it to dry in air, examine under *ultraviolet light (365 nm)* and observe the fluorescence produced after about 2 minutes. Heat the plate at 120° for 20 minutes, cool, spray with *ethanolic sulphuric acid (20%)* and observe the colour produced. The principal spot in the chromatogram obtained with solution (1) corresponds in position, fluorescence and colour to that in the chromatogram obtained with solution (2).

B. Extract a quantity of the powdered tablets containing 5 mg of Fluphenazine Hydrochloride with 5 ml of *acetone*, filter and evaporate the filtrate to dryness. Add 2 ml of *sulphuric acid* to the residue and allow to stand for 5 minutes. An orange colour is produced.

C. Extract a quantity of the powdered tablets containing 10 mg of Fluphenazine Hydrochloride with 10 ml of *absolute ethanol* containing 0.2% v/v of 13.5M *ammonia* and evaporate the extract to dryness. Heat 0.5 ml of *chromic—sulphuric acid mixture* in a small test tube in a water bath for 5 minutes; the solution wets the side of the tube readily and there is no greasiness. Add 2 or 3 mg of the residue and again heat in a water bath for 5 minutes; the solution does not wet the side of the tube and does not pour easily from the tube.

Related substances Carry out in subdued light the method for *thin-layer chromatography*, Appendix III A, using *silica gel GF_{254}* as the coating substance and a mixture of 5 volumes of 13.5M *ammonia*, 30 volumes of *cyclohexane* and 80 volumes of *acetone* as the mobile phase. Apply separately to the plate 50 µl of solution (1) and 25 µl of each of solutions (2) and (3). For solution (1) remove the coating from a suitable number of tablets; shake a quantity of the powdered tablet cores containing 20 mg of Fluphenazine Hydrochloride with 10 ml of 0.1M *methanolic sodium hydroxide* for 5 minutes, centrifuge and use the supernatant liquid. For solution (2) dilute 1 volume of solution (1) to 50 volumes with 0.1M *methanolic sodium hydroxide*. For solution (3) dilute 1 volume of solution (1) to 100 volumes with 0.1M *methanolic sodium hydroxide*. After removal of the plate, allow it to dry in air and examine under *ultraviolet light (254 nm)*. Any *secondary spot* in the chromatogram obtained with solution (1) is not more intense than the spot in the chromatogram obtained with solution (2) (1%) and not more than two such spots are more intense than the spot in the chromatogram obtained with solution (3) (0.5%). Disregard any spot remaining on the line of application.

Uniformity of content Tablets containing less than 2 mg of Fluphenazine Hydrochloride comply with the requirements stated under Tablets using the following method of analysis. Carry out the following procedure protected from light. Record *second-derivative ultraviolet absorption spectra* of the following solutions in the range 230 to 300 nm, Appendix II B. For solution (1) add 2 ml of 0.1M *hydrochloric acid* to one tablet and mix with the aid of ultrasound until the tablet is dispersed. Add 60 ml of a mixture of 1 volume of 1M *hydrochloric acid* and 99 volumes of *ethanol (80%)*, shake for 20 minutes, dilute to 100 ml with the same solvent mixture, mix and filter. Solution (2) contains 0.001% w/v of *fluphenazine hydrochloride BPCRS*.

For each solution measure the amplitude from the peak at about 266 nm to the trough at about 258 nm. Calculate the content of $C_{22}H_{26}F_3N_3OS,2HCl$ in each tablet using the declared content of $C_{22}H_{26}F_3N_3OS,2HCl$ in *fluphenazine hydrochloride BPCRS*.

Assay

For tablets containing 2 mg or more of Fluphenazine Hydrochloride Carry out the following procedure protected from light. Record *second-derivative ultraviolet absorption spectra* of the following solutions in the range 230 to 300 nm, Appendix II B. For solution (1) add 20 ml of 0.1M *hydrochloric acid* to 10 tablets, mix with the aid of ultrasound until the tablets are dispersed, add 600 ml of a mixture of 1 volume of 1M *hydrochloric acid* and 99 volumes of *ethanol (80%)*, shake for 20 minutes, dilute to 1000 ml with the same solvent mixture, mix and filter. Solution (2) contains 0.001% w/v of *fluphenazine hydrochloride BPCRS*.

For each solution measure the amplitude from the peak at about 266 nm to the trough at about 258 nm. Calculate the content of $C_{22}H_{26}F_3N_3OS,2HCl$ in the tablets using the declared content of $C_{22}H_{26}F_3N_3OS, 2HCl$ in *fluphenazine hydrochloride BPCRS*.

For tablets containing less than 2 mg of Fluphenazine Hydrochloride Use the average of the 10 individual results obtained in the test for Uniformity of content.

Flurazepam Capsules

Definition Flurazepam Capsules contain Flurazepam Monohydrochloride.

The capsules comply with the requirements stated under Capsules and with the following requirements.

Content of flurazepam, $C_{21}H_{23}ClFN_3O$ 90.0 to 110.0% of the prescribed or stated amount.

Identification

A. Shake a quantity of the contents of the capsules containing the equivalent of 0.15 g of flurazepam with 3 ml of *chloroform IR* and filter. The *infrared absorption spectrum* of the filtrate, Appendix II A, is concordant with the *reference spectrum* of flurazepam monohydrochloride.

B. The *light absorption*, Appendix II B, in the range 220 to 350 nm of the final solution obtained in the Assay exhibits two maxima, at 240 nm and 284 nm.

Related substances Carry out the method for *thin-layer chromatography*, Appendix III A, using *silica gel GF_{254}* as the coating substance and a mixture of 2.5 volumes of *diethylamine* and 97.5 volumes of *ether* as the mobile phase. Apply separately to the plate 10 µl of each of the following solutions. For solution (1) shake vigorously a quantity of the contents of the capsules containing the equivalent of 0.1 g of flurazepam with 2 ml of a mixture of 2 volumes of 13.5M *ammonia* and 98 volumes of *methanol* and centrifuge. For solution (2) dilute 1 volume of solution (1) to 200 volumes with the same solvent mixture. After removal of the plate, dry it in a current of air and examine under *ultraviolet light (254 nm)*. Any *secondary spot* in the chromatogram obtained with solution (1) is not more intense than the spot in the chromatogram obtained with solution (2) (0.5%).

Assay Carry out the following procedure protected from light. Transfer a quantity of the capsule contents containing the equivalent of 0.1 g of flurazepam into about 150 ml of 1M *methanolic sulphuric acid*, washing the inner surfaces of the capsule shells, shake for 10 minutes and add sufficient 1M *methanolic sulphuric acid* to produce 250 ml. Further dilute this solution with 1M *methanolic sulphuric acid* to produce a solution containing the equivalent of about 0.002% w/v of flurazepam and measure the *absorbance* of the resulting solution at the maximum at 284 nm, Appendix II B. Calculate the content of $C_{21}H_{23}ClFN_3O$ taking 319 as the value of A(1%, 1 cm) at the maximum at 284 nm.

Labelling The quantity of active ingredient is stated in terms of the equivalent amount of flurazepam.

Flurbiprofen Eye Drops

Definition Flurbiprofen Eye Drops are a sterile solution of Flurbiprofen Sodium in Purified Water.

The eye drops comply with the requirements stated under Eye Preparations and with the following requirements.

Content of flurbiprofen sodium dihydrate, $C_{15}H_{12}FNaO_2,2H_2O$ 90.0 to 110.0% of the prescribed or stated amount.

Identification

A. Carry out the method for *thin-layer chromatography*, Appendix III A, using *silica gel GF_{254}* as the coating substance and a mixture of 5 volumes of *propan-2-ol* and 95 volumes of *dichloromethane* as the mobile phase. Apply separately to the plate 5 µl of each of the following solutions. For solution (1) dilute the eye drops, if necessary, with a mixture of 25 volumes of *water* and 50 volumes of *methanol* to produce a solution containing 0.01% w/v of Flurbiprofen Sodium. Solution (2) contains 0.01% w/v of *flurbiprofen sodium BPCRS* in a mixture of 25 volumes of *water* and 50 volumes of *methanol*. After removal of the plate, allow it to dry in air and examine under *ultraviolet light (254 nm)*. The principal spot in the chromatogram obtained with solution (1) corresponds to that in the chromatogram obtained with solution (2).

B. In the Assay, the principal peak in the chromatogram obtained with solution (1) has the same retention time as the principal peak in the chromatogram obtained with solution (2).

Acidity or alkalinity pH, 6.0 to 7.0, Appendix V L.

2-(Biphenyl-4-yl)propionic acid Carry out the method for *liquid chromatography*, Appendix III D, using the following solutions. For solution (1) dilute the eye drops, if necessary, with a mixture of 25 volumes of *water* and 50 volumes of *methanol* to produce a solution containing 0.030% w/v of Flurbiprofen Sodium. Solution (2) contains 0.00015% w/v of *2-(biphenyl-4-yl)propionic acid BPCRS* in a mixture of 25 volumes of *water* and 50 volumes of *methanol*. Solution (3) contains 0.00050% w/v of *flurbiprofen sodium BPCRS* and 0.00050% w/v of *2-(biphenyl-4-yl)propionic acid BPCRS* in a mixture of 25 volumes of *water* and 50 volumes of *methanol*.

The chromatographic procedure may be carried out using (a) a stainless steel column (15 cm × 3.9 mm) packed with *stationary phase C* (5 µm) (Resolve 5µ is suitable), (b) a mixture of 5 volumes of *glacial acetic acid*, 35 volumes of *acetonitrile* and 60 volumes of *water* as the mobile phase with a flow rate of 1 ml per minute and (c) a detection wavelength of 254 nm. Adjust the sensitivity so that the heights of the principal peaks in the chromatogram obtained with solution (3) are about 40% of full-scale deflection on the chart paper.

The test is not valid unless the *resolution factor* between the two principal peaks in the chromatogram obtained with solution (3) is at least 1.5.

In the chromatogram obtained with solution (1) the area of any peak corresponding to 2-(biphenyl-4-yl)propionic acid is not greater than the area of the peak in the chromatogram obtained with solution (2) (0.5%).

Assay Carry out the method for *liquid chromatography*, Appendix III D, using the following solutions. For solution (1) dilute the eye drops, if necessary, with a mixture of 25 volumes of *water* and 50 volumes of *methanol* to produce a solution containing 0.015% w/v of Flurbiprofen Sodium. Solution (2) contains 0.015% w/v of *flurbiprofen sodium BPCRS* in a mixture of 25 volumes of *water* and 50 volumes of *methanol*. Solution (3) contains 0.0005% w/v of *flurbiprofen sodium BPCRS* and 0.0005% w/v of *2-(biphenyl-4-yl)propionic acid BPCRS* in a mixture of 25 volumes of *water* and 50 volumes of *methanol*.

The chromatographic procedure described under the test for 2-(Biphenyl-4-yl)propionic acid may be used.

The assay is not valid unless the *resolution factor* between the two principal peaks in the chromatogram obtained with solution (3) is at least 1.5.

Calculate the content of $C_{15}H_{12}FNaO_2,2H_2O$ in the eye drops using the declared content of $C_{15}H_{12}FNaO_2,2H_2O$ in *flurbiprofen sodium BPCRS*.

Flurbiprofen Tablets

Definition Flurbiprofen Tablets contain Flurbiprofen. They are coated.

The tablets comply with the requirements stated under Tablets and with the following requirements.

Content of flurbiprofen, $C_{15}H_{13}FO_2$ 92.5 to 107.5% of the prescribed or stated amount.

Identification Extract a quantity of the powdered tablets containing 0.5 g of Flurbiprofen with 25 ml of *acetone*, filter, evaporate the filtrate to dryness with the aid of a current of air without heating and dry at 60° at a pressure of 2 kPa. The residue complies with the following tests.

A. The *infrared absorption spectrum*, Appendix II A, is concordant with the *reference spectrum* of flurbiprofen.

B. Heat 0.5 ml of *chromic—sulphuric acid mixture* in a small test tube in a water bath for 5 minutes; the solution wets the side of the tube readily and there is no greasiness. Add 2 or 3 mg of the residue and heat in a water bath for 5 minutes; the solution does not wet the side of the tube and does not pour easily from the tube.

C. *Melting point*, about 114°, Appendix V A.

Related substances Carry out the method for *liquid chromatography*, Appendix III D, using the following solutions. For solution (1) disperse a quantity of the powdered tablets containing 0.5 g of Flurbiprofen in 50 ml of *water*, add 200 ml of *acetonitrile*, mix, centrifuge and use the supernatant liquid. For solution (2) dilute 1 volume of solution (1) to 100 volumes with a mixture of 45 volumes of *acetonitrile* and 55 volumes of *water* and further dilute 1 volume to 5 volumes with the same solvent mixture. Solution (3) contains 0.0010% w/v of *2-(biphenyl-4-yl)propionic acid BPCRS* in a mixture of 45 volumes of *acetonitrile* and 55 volumes of *water*. For solution (4) dilute 1 volume of solution (1) to 200 volumes with solution (3).

The chromatographic procedure may be carried out using (a) a stainless steel column (15 cm × 3.9 mm) packed with *stationary phase C* (5 µm) (Resolve 5µ is suitable), (b) a mixture of 5 volumes of *glacial acetic acid*, 35 volumes of *acetonitrile* and 60 volumes of *water* as the mobile phase with a flow rate of 1 ml per minute and (c) a detection wavelength of 254 nm.

Adjust the sensitivity so that the heights of the principal peaks in the chromatogram obtained with solution (4) are about 40% of full-scale deflection on the chart paper.

The test is not valid unless the *resolution factor* between the two principal peaks in the chromatogram obtained with solution (4) is at least 1.5.

In the chromatogram obtained with solution (1) the area of any peak corresponding to 2-(biphenyl-4-yl)-propionic acid is not greater than the area of the peak in the chromatogram obtained with solution (3) (0.5%), the area of any other *secondary peak* is not greater than the area of the peak in the chromatogram obtained with solution (2) (0.2%) and the sum of the areas of any *secondary peaks* is not greater than five times the area of the peak in the chromatogram obtained with solution (2) (1%).

Assay Weigh and powder 20 tablets. Shake a quantity of the powder containing 0.1 g of Flurbiprofen with 60 ml of 0.1M *sodium hydroxide* for 5 minutes, dilute to 100 ml with 0.1M *sodium hydroxide*, filter if necessary and dilute 10 ml of the filtrate to 100 ml with the same solvent. Further dilute 10 ml to 100 ml with the same solvent and measure the *absorbance* of the resulting solution at the maximum at 247 nm, Appendix II B. Calculate the content of $C_{15}H_{13}FO_2$ taking 802 as the value of A(1%, 1 cm) at the maximum at 247 nm.

Fluticasone Cream

Definition Fluticasone Cream contains Fluticasone Propionate in a suitable basis.

The cream complies with the requirements stated under Topical Semi-solid Preparations and with the following requirements.

Content of fluticasone propionate, $C_{25}H_{31}F_3O_5S$ 95.0 to 105.0% of the prescribed or stated amount.

Identification

A. Carry out the method for *thin-layer chromatography*, Appendix III A, using a silica gel F_{254} precoated plate (Merck silica gel 60 F_{254} plates are suitable) and a mixture of 1 volume of *glacial acetic acid*, 8 volumes of *ethyl acetate* and 30 volumes of *dichloromethane* as the mobile phase but allowing the solvent front to ascend 12 cm above the line of application. Apply separately to the plate 40 µl of each of the following solutions. For solution (1) transfer a quantity of the cream containing 1 mg of Fluticasone Propionate to a separating funnel, add 25 ml of *acetonitrile* and 25 ml of n-*hexane*, shake for 3 minutes and allow to separate. Filter the lower layer through an absorbent cotton plug, previously washed with *acetonitrile*, into a 50-ml graduated flask, repeat the extraction with one 5-ml and one 2-ml quantities of *acetonitrile*, filter and add the extracts to the filtered layer; wash the absorbent cotton plug with 1 to 2 ml of *acetonitrile*, add the washings to the filtered layer and dilute the combined extracts to 50 ml with *acetonitrile*. Evaporate 4 ml of the resulting solution to dryness using a rotary evaporator at a temperature of 40° and dissolve the residue in 0.2 ml of *acetonitrile*. Solution (2) contains 0.04% w/v of *fluticasone propionate BPCRS* in *acetonitrile*. After removal of the plate, allow it to dry in a current of air and examine under *ultraviolet light (254 nm)*. The principal spot in the chromatogram obtained with solution (1) corresponds to that in the chromatogram obtained with solution (2).

B. In the Assay, the principal peak in the chromatogram obtained with solution (1) shows a peak with the same retention time as that in the chromatogram obtained with solution (2).

Assay Carry out the method for *liquid chromatography*, Appendix III D, using the following solutions, protected from light. For solution (1) transfer a quantity of the cream containing 1 mg of Fluticasone Propionate to a separating funnel, add 25 ml of *ethanol (65%)*, stopper and shake until the cream is completely dispersed. Add 25 ml of n-*hexane*, shake for 3 minutes and allow to separate, filter the lower aqueous layer through an absorbent cotton plug, previously washed with *ethanol (65%)*, into a graduated flask and repeat the extraction with one 5-ml and then one 2-ml quantity of *ethanol (65%)*, filtering the aqueous ethanol extracts into the same graduated flask. Wash the absorbent cotton plug with *ethanol (65%)*, collecting the washings in the flask and dilute the combined extracts to 50 ml with *ethanol (65%)*. For solution (2) dilute 2 ml of a 0.05% w/v solution of *fluticasone propionate BPCRS* in *methanol (80%)* to 50 ml with *ethanol (65%)*. Solution (3) contains 0.0004% w/v of *fluticasone S-methyl impurity BPCRS* and 0.002% w/v of *fluticasone propionate BPCRS* in the mobile phase.

The chromatographic procedure may be carried out using (a) a stainless steel column (25 cm × 4.6 mm) packed with *stationary phase C* (5 µm) (Spherisorb ODS 1 is suitable) and maintained at a temperature of 50°, (b) as the mobile phase with a flow rate of 2 ml per minute a mixture of 15 volumes of *acetonitrile*, 35 volumes of 0.01M *ammonium dihydrogen orthophosphate* previously adjusted to pH 3.5 with *orthophosphoric acid* and 50 volumes of *methanol* and (c) a detection wavelength of 240 nm.

The assay is not valid unless, in the chromatogram obtained with solution (3), the *resolution factor* between the peaks due to fluticasone *S*-methyl impurity and fluticasone propionate is at least 1.6. If necessary, adjust the proportion of acetonitrile in the mobile phase.

Calculate the content of $C_{25}H_{31}F_3O_5S$ in the cream using the declared content of $C_{25}H_{31}F_3O_5S$ in *fluticasone propionate BPCRS*.

Fluticasone Ointment

Definition Fluticasone Ointment contains Fluticasone Propionate in a suitable basis.

The ointment complies with the requirements stated under Topical Semi-solid Preparations and with the following requirements.

Content of fluticasone propionate, $C_{25}H_{31}F_3O_5S$ 95.0 to 105.0% of the prescribed or stated amount.

Identification

A. Carry out the method for *thin-layer chromatography*, Appendix III A, using a silica gel F_{254} precoated plate (Merck silica gel 60 F_{254} plates are suitable) and a mixture of 1 volume of *glacial acetic acid*, 8 volumes of *ethyl acetate* and 30 volumes of *dichloromethane* as the mobile phase but allowing the solvent front to ascend 12 cm above the line of application. Apply separately to the plate 20 µl of each of the following solutions. For solution (1) transfer a quantity of the ointment containing 0.1 mg of Fluticasone Propionate to a separating funnel, add 10 ml of *acetonitrile* and 50 ml of n-*hexane*, shake for 5 minutes and allow to separate. Filter the lower layer through an absorbent cotton plug previously washed with *acetonitrile*, extract the hexane layer with two 5-ml quantities of *acetonitrile*, filter each extract through the absorbent cotton plug and wash the absorbent cotton plug with 2 ml of *acetonitrile*. Add the washings to the combined filtrates, evaporate the resulting solution to dryness using a rotary evaporator at a temperature of 40° and dissolve the residue in 0.5 ml of *acetonitrile*. Solution (2) contains 0.020% w/v of *fluticasone propionate BPCRS* in *acetonitrile*. After removal of the plate, allow it to dry in a current of air and examine under *ultraviolet light (254 nm)*. The principal spot in the chromatogram obtained with solution (1) corresponds to that in the chromatogram obtained with solution (2).

B. In the Assay, the chromatogram obtained with solution (2) shows a peak with the same retention time as the principal peak in the chromatogram obtained with solution (1).

Assay Carry out the method for *liquid chromatography*, Appendix III D, using the following solutions, protected from light. For solution (1) transfer a quantity of the ointment containing 0.1 mg of Fluticasone Propionate to a separating funnel, add 45 ml of n-*hexane*, previously heated to 60° in a water bath, stopper the funnel and shake until the ointment is dispersed, venting frequently. Wash the stopper and neck of the funnel with 5 ml of n-*hexane* collecting the washings in the funnel, allow the funnel to cool to room temperature, add 10 ml of *methanol (80%)*, stopper, shake for 1 minute and allow to separate. Filter the lower aqueous layer through an absorbent cotton plug, previously washed with *methanol (80%)*, into a graduated flask; repeat the extraction with two 5-ml quantities of *methanol (80%)*, filtering the aqueous methanol extracts into the same graduated flask. Wash the absorbent cotton plug with 2 ml of *methanol (80%)*, collecting the washings in the flask and dilute the extract to 25 ml with *methanol (80%)*. For solution (2) dilute 2 ml of a 0.005% w/v solution of *fluticasone propionate BPCRS* in *methanol (80%)* to 25 ml with the same solvent. Solution (3) contains 0.0004% w/v of *fluticasone S-methyl impurity BPCRS* and 0.002% w/v of *fluticasone propionate BPCRS* in *methanol (80%)*.

The chromatographic procedure may be carried out using (a) a stainless steel column (25 cm × 4.6 mm) packed with *stationary phase C* (5 µm) (Spherisorb ODS 1 is suitable) and maintained at a temperature of 50°, (b) as the mobile phase with a flow rate of 2 ml per minute a mixture of 15 volumes of *acetonitrile*, 35 volumes of 0.01M *ammonium dihydrogen orthophosphate* previously adjusted to pH 3.5 with *orthophosphoric acid* and 50 volumes of *methanol* and (c) a detection wavelength of 240 nm.

The assay is not valid unless, in the chromatogram obtained with solution (3), the *resolution factor* between the peaks due to fluticasone *S*-methyl impurity and fluticasone propionate is at least 1.6. If necessary, adjust the proportion of acetonitrile in the mobile phase.

Calculate the content of $C_{25}H_{31}F_3O_5S$ in the ointment using the declared content of $C_{25}H_{31}F_3O_5S$ in *fluticasone propionate BPCRS*.

Fluvoxamine Tablets

Definition Fluvoxamine Tablets contain Fluvoxamine Maleate.

With the exception of the requirements for shape, the tablets comply with the requirements stated under Tablets and with the following requirements.

Content of fluvoxamine maleate, $C_{15}H_{21}F_3N_2O_2,C_4H_4O_4$ 92.5 to 105.0% of the prescribed or stated amount.

Identification

A. Shake a quantity of the powdered tablets containing 50 mg of Fluvoxamine Maleate with 10 ml of *acetonitrile* for 10 minutes, centrifuge and evaporate the supernatant liquid to dryness using a rotary evaporator. The *infrared absorption spectrum* of the residue, Appendix II A, is concordant with the *reference spectrum* of fluvoxamine maleate.

B. Carry out the method for *thin-layer chromatography*, Appendix III A, using a silica gel HF precoated plate (Analtech Uniplates are suitable) and a mixture of 5 volumes of 13.5M *ammonia* and 95 volumes of *ethanol (96%)* as the mobile phase. Apply separately to the plate 5 µl of each of the following solutions. For solution (1) shake a quantity of the powdered tablets containing 50 mg of Fluvoxamine Maleate with 5 ml of *methanol* for 10 minutes, centrifuge and use the supernatant liquid. Solution (2) contains 1.0% w/v of *fluvoxamine maleate BPCRS* in *methanol*. After removal of the plate, allow it to dry in air and examine under *ultraviolet light (254 nm)*. The two principal spots in the chromatogram obtained with solution (1) correspond to those in the chromatogram obtained with solution (2).

Dissolution Carry out the *dissolution test for tablets and capsules*, Appendix XII D, using Apparatus II. Use as the medium 900 ml of *water* and rotate the paddle at 50 revolutions per minute. After 20 minutes, withdraw a sample of 10 ml of the medium and centrifuge. Measure the *absorbance* of the clear supernatant liquid, Appendix II B, suitably diluted with *water* if necessary, at 244 nm using *water* in the reference cell. Calculate the total content of fluvoxamine maleate, $C_{15}H_{21}F_3N_2O_2,C_4H_4O_4$, in the medium taking 270 as the value of A(1%, 1 cm) at the maximum at 244 nm. The amount is not less than 70% of the prescribed or stated amount.

Related substances Carry out the method for *liquid chromatography*, Appendix III D, using the following solutions. For solution (1) shake a quantity of the powdered tablets containing 0.25 g of Fluvoxamine Maleate with 125 ml of the mobile phase for 10 minutes, add sufficient mobile phase to produce 250 ml, mix, centrifuge and use the supernatant liquid. For solution (2) dilute 1 volume of solution (1) to 100 volumes with the mobile phase. For solution (3) heat a 0.20% w/v solution of *fluvoxamine maleate BPCRS* in 0.1M *hydrochloric acid* on a water bath for 10 minutes. Cool, shake vigorously for 1 minute and dilute 1 volume to 5 volumes with the mobile phase.

The chromatographic procedure may be carried out using (a) a stainless steel column (25 cm × 4.6 mm) packed with *stationary phase B* (7 µm) (Zorbax C8 is suitable) and maintained at 35°, (b) as the mobile phase with a flow rate of 2 ml per minute a mixture of 40 volumes of a solution containing 1.25% w/v of *diammonium hydrogen orthophosphate* and 0.275% w/v of *sodium heptanesulphonate monohydrate* and 60 volumes of *methanol*, adjusting the pH of the mixture to 3.5 with *orthophosphoric acid* and (c) a detection wavelength of 254 nm.

When the chromatograms are recorded under the conditions described above, the retention time of fluvoxamine maleate is 7 to 9 minutes. If necessary, adjust the composition of the mobile phase (increasing the methanol content decreases the retention time, increasing the water content increases the retention time).

The test is not valid unless, in the chromatogram obtained with solution (3), the *resolution factor* between the principal peak and the peak immediately preceding the principal peak (the *Z*-isomer) is at least 1.0.

In the chromatogram obtained with solution (1) the area of any peak with a retention time of about 0.7 relative to the principal peak is not greater than 3 times the area of the principal peak in the chromatogram obtained with solution (2) (3% of the addition product), and the area of any other *secondary peak* is not greater than half the area of the principal peak in the chromatogram obtained with solution (2) (0.5%). Disregard the peak corresponding to maleic acid (which elutes immediately after the solvent front) and any peak with an area less than one twentieth of the area of the principal peak in the chromatogram obtained with solution (2) (0.05%).

Assay Weigh and powder 20 tablets. Carry out the method for *liquid chromatography*, Appendix III D, using the following solutions. For solution (1) shake a quantity of the powdered tablets containing 0.25 g of Fluvoxamine Maleate with 125 ml of the mobile phase for 10 minutes, add sufficient of the mobile phase to produce 250 ml, mix, centrifuge and dilute 1 volume of the supernatant liquid to 10 volumes with the mobile phase. Solution (2) contains 0.010% w/v of *fluvoxamine maleate BPCRS* in the mobile phase.

The chromatographic conditions described under Related substances may be used.

Calculate the content of $C_{15}H_{21}F_3N_2O_2,C_4H_4O_4$ in the tablets using the declared content of $C_{15}H_{21}F_3N_2O_2$, $C_4H_4O_4$ in *fluvoxamine maleate BPCRS*.

Storage Fluvoxamine Tablets should be protected from light.

IMPURITIES

The impurities limited by the requirements of this monograph include those listed under Fluvoxamine Maleate.

Folic Acid Tablets

Definition Folic Acid Tablets contain Folic Acid.

The tablets comply with the requirements stated under Tablets and with the following requirements.

Content of folic acid, $C_{19}H_{19}N_7O_6$ 90.0 to 110.0% of the prescribed or stated amount.

Identification Carry out the method for *thin-layer chromatography*, Appendix III A, using *silica gel G* as the coating substance and a mixture of 20 volumes of 13.5M *ammonia*, 20 volumes of *propan-1-ol* and 60 volumes of *ethanol (96%)* as the mobile phase. Apply separately to the plate 2 µl of each of the following solutions. For solution (1) extract a quantity of the powdered tablets containing 0.5 mg of Folic Acid with 1 ml of a mixture of 1 volume of 13.5M *ammonia* and 9 volumes of *methanol*, centrifuge and use the supernatant liquid. Solution (2) contains 0.05% w/v of *folic acid EPCRS* in a mixture of 2 volumes of 13.5M *ammonia* and 9 volumes of *methanol*. After removal of the plate, allow it to dry in air and examine under *ultraviolet light (365 nm)*. The principal spot in the chromatogram obtained with solution (1) is similar in position, fluorescence and size to that in the chromatogram obtained with solution (2).

Hydrolysis products Carry out the method for *liquid chromatography*, Appendix III D, using the following solutions and protecting solutions (1) and (2) from light. Solution (1) is a solution in the mobile phase containing 0.5 µg of *4-aminobenzoic acid* and 2.0 µg of N-*(4-aminobenzoyl)-*L*-glutamic acid* per ml. For solution (2) shake a quantity of the powdered tablets containing 5.0 mg of Folic Acid with 50 ml of the mobile phase, centrifuge and use the supernatant liquid.

The chromatographic procedure may be carried out using (a) a stainless steel column (20 cm × 4.6 mm) packed with *stationary phase C* (10 µm) (Spherisorb ODS 1 is suitable), (b) 0.05M *potassium dihydrogen orthophosphate*, adjusted to pH 5.5 with 5M *sodium hydroxide*, as the mobile phase with a flow rate of 2 ml per minute and (c) a detection wavelength of 269 nm.

In the chromatogram obtained with solution (1) two peaks, due to *N*-(4-aminobenzoyl)-L-glutamic acid and 4-aminobenzoic acid, are obtained in order of their emergence. The test is not valid unless the *resolution factor* between the two peaks is at least 3.

The areas of the peaks due to 4-aminobenzoic acid and *N*-(4-aminobenzoyl)-L-glutamic acid in the chromatogram obtained with solution (1) are greater than the areas of any corresponding peaks in the chromatogram obtained with solution (2).

Uniformity of content Tablets containing less than 2 mg of Folic Acid comply with the requirements stated under Tablets using the following method of analysis. Carry out the method for *liquid chromatography*, Appendix III D, using the following solutions. For solution (1) add 1 ml of 0.5M *hydrochloric acid* to 5 ml of a 0.0020% w/v solution of *folic acid EPCRS* in 0.1M *sodium hydroxide* and dilute to 10 ml with the mobile phase. For solution (2) shake one tablet with 5 ml of 0.1M *sodium hydroxide*, add sufficient mobile phase to produce a solution containing 0.001% w/v of Folic Acid, centrifuge and use the supernatant liquid.

The chromatographic procedure may be carried out using (a) a stainless steel column (20 cm × 4.6 mm) packed with *stationary phase C* (10 µm) (Spherisorb ODS 1 is suitable), (b) a mixture of 93 volumes of 0.05M *potassium dihydrogen orthophosphate* and 7 volumes of *acetonitrile* adjusted to pH 6.0 with 5M *sodium hydroxide* as the mobile phase with a flow rate of 2 ml per minute and (c) a detection wavelength of 283 nm.

Calculate the content of $C_{19}H_{19}N_7O_6$ in each tablet using the declared content of $C_{19}H_{19}N_7O_6$ in *folic acid EPCRS*.

Assay

For tablets containing 2 mg or more of Folic Acid Weigh and powder 20 tablets. Carry out the method for *liquid chromatography*, Appendix III D, using the following solutions, protected from light. For solution (1) dilute 5 ml of a 0.020% w/v solution of *folic acid EPCRS* in 0.1M *sodium hydroxide* to 100 ml with the mobile phase. For solution (2) shake a quantity of the powdered tablets containing 20 mg of Folic Acid with 50 ml of 0.1M *sodium hydroxide*, dilute to 100 ml with the same solvent, centrifuge and dilute 5 ml of the supernatant liquid to 100 ml with the mobile phase.

The chromatographic procedure described under Uniformity of content may be used.

Calculate the content of $C_{19}H_{19}N_7O_6$ in the tablets using the declared content of $C_{19}H_{19}N_7O_6$ in *folic acid EPCRS*.

For tablets containing less than 2 mg of Folic Acid Use the average of the 10 individual results obtained in the test for Uniformity of content.

Storage Folic Acid Tablets should be protected from light.

Foscarnet Intravenous Infusion

Definition Foscarnet Intravenous Infusion is a sterile solution of Foscarnet Sodium in Water for Injections.

The intravenous infusion complies with the requirements stated under Parenteral Preparations and with the following requirements.

Content of foscarnet sodium, $CNa_3O_5P,6H_2O$ 95.0 to 105.0% of the prescribed or stated amount.

Characteristics A clear, colourless solution.

Identification A. Dry a quantity containing 48 mg of Foscarnet Sodium over *phosphorus pentoxide* at a pressure not exceeding 0.7 kPa for 16 hours. The *infrared absorption spectrum* of the residue, Appendix II A, is concordant with the *reference spectrum* of foscarnet sodium. Disregard any peak occurring at 902 cm^{-1} or any shoulder at 1179 cm^{-1}.

B. In the Assay, the chromatogram obtained with solution (1) shows a peak with the same retention time as the principal peak in the chromatogram obtained with solution (2).

Alkalinity pH, 7.2 to 7.6, Appendix V L.

Particulate contamination When supplied in a container with a nominal content of 100 ml or more, complies with the *test for sub-visible particles*, Appendix XIII A.

Phosphate and phosphite Carry out the method for *liquid chromatography*, Appendix III D, using the following solutions. Prepare a solution containing 0.04% w/v of *sodium dihydrogen orthophosphate monohydrate* and 0.06% w/v of *sodium phosphite* (solution A). For solution (1) add 6 ml of solution A to 60 mg of *foscarnet sodium BPCRS* and dilute to 25 ml with *water*. For solution (2) dilute a volume of the intravenous infusion with sufficent *water* to produce a solution containing 0.24% w/v of Foscarnet Sodium.

The chromatographic procedure may be carried out using (a) a stainless steel column (5 cm × 4.6 mm) packed with an anion exchange resin (Waters IC PAK is suitable) at a temperature of 25°, (b) as the mobile phase with a flow rate of 1.4 ml per minute a solution prepared by dissolving 0.204 g of *potassium hydrogen phthalate* in *water*, adding 5 ml of 1M *nitric acid VS* and sufficient *water* to produce 2000 ml and (c) a detection wavelength of 290 nm. Inject 20 µl of each solution.

Allow the column to stabilise by passing mobile phase through it for at least 2 hours before starting the chromatography. The test is not valid unless, in the chromatogram obtained with solution (1), the peak due to phosphate (which elutes first) shows baseline separation from the peak due to phosphite.

In the chromatogram obtained with solution (2) the area of any peak corresponding to phosphate is not greater than 0.7 times the area of the corresponding peak in the chromatogram obtained with solution (1) and the area of any peak corresponding to phosphite is not greater than half the area of the corresponding peak in the chromatogram obtained with solution (1) (2.0% of phosphate and 1.0% of phosphite).

Related esters Carry out the method for *liquid chromatography*, Appendix III D, using the following solutions in the mobile phase. Solutions (1) and (2) are solutions of the intravenous infusion diluted to contain (1) 1.0% w/v and (2) 0.0020% w/v respectively of Foscarnet Sodium. Solution (3) contains 0.02% w/v of *foscarnet sodium BPCRS* and 0.02% w/v of *disodium ethoxyphosphonatoformate BPCRS*.

The chromatographic procedure may be carried out using (a) a stainless steel column (10 cm × 4.6 mm) packed with *stationary phase C* (3 µm) (Microsphere C18 is suitable), (b) as the mobile phase at a flow rate of 1 ml per minute a solution prepared as described below and (c) a detection wavelength of 230 nm. Prepare two solutions containing (A) 100 ml of 0.5M *acetic acid*, 6 ml of 0.1M *sodium pyrophosphate* and 3.22 g of *sodium sulphate* in sufficient *water* to produce 1000 ml and (B) 6.8 g of *sodium acetate*, 6 ml of 0.1M *sodium pyrophosphate* and 3.22 g of *sodium sulphate* in sufficient *water* to produce 1000 ml. Mix solution A and solution B to produce a solution of pH 4.4 and to 1000 ml of this solution add 0.25 g of *tetrahexylammonium hydrogen sulphate* and 100 ml of *methanol*. Inject 5 µl of each solution.

The test is not valid unless, in the chromatogram obtained with solution (3), the *resolution factor* between the peaks due to foscarnet sodium and disodium ethoxyphosphonatoformate is at least 7.

For solution (1) allow the chromatography to proceed for at least 2.5 times the retention time of the principal peak. In the chromatogram obtained with solution (1) the area of any *secondary peak* is not greater than the area of the principal peak in the chromatogram obtained with solution (2) (0.2%) and the sum of the areas of any such peaks is not greater than 2.5 times the area of the principal peak in the chromatogram obtained with solution (2) (0.5%).

Bacterial endotoxins The endotoxin limit concentration is 2 IU per ml, Appendix XIV C.

Assay Carry out the method for *liquid chromatography*, Appendix III D, using the following solutions in the mobile phase containing (1) a solution of the intravenous infusion diluted to contain 0.10% w/v of Foscarnet Sodium and (2) 0.10% w/v of *foscarnet sodium BPCRS*.

The chromatographic procedure described under Related esters may be used injecting 5 µl of each solution.

Calculate the content of $CNa_3O_5P,6H_2O$ in the intravenous infusion using the declared content of $CNa_3O_5P,6H_2O$ in *foscarnet sodium BPCRS*.

Storage Foscarnet Intravenous Infusion should be stored at a temperature not exceeding 30°. It should not be refrigerated.

Labelling The label states that Foscarnet Intravenous Infusion may be administered as supplied via a central venous line or via a peripheral vein after dilution with Glucose Intravenous Infusion (50 g per litre) or Sodium Chloride Intravenous Infusion (0.9% w/v).

IMPURITIES

The impurities limited by the requirements of this monograph include those listed in the monograph for Foscarnet Sodium with the exception of disodium ethoxycarbonyl phosphonate and sodium ethyl phosphonate.

Standardised Frangula Bark Dry Extract

Standardised Frangula Dry Extract complies with the requirements of the 3rd edition of the European Pharmacopoeia [1214]. These requirements are reproduced after the heading 'Definition' below.

Ph Eur

DEFINITION

Standardised frangula bark dry extract is produced from *Frangula bark (25)*. It contains not less than 15.0 per cent and not more than 30.0 per cent of glucofrangulins, expressed as glucofrangulin A ($C_{27}H_{30}O_{14}$; M_r 578.5) and calculated with reference to the dried extract. The measured content does not deviate from that stated on the label by more than 10 per cent.

PRODUCTION

The extract is produced from the drug and ethanol (50 to 80 per cent *V/V*) by an appropriate procedure according to the monograph on *Extracts (765)*.

CHARACTERS

A yellowish-brown, fine powder.

IDENTIFICATION

A. Examine by thin-layer chromatography (*2.2.27*), using a suitable silica gel as the coating substance.

Test solution. To 0.05 g add 5 ml of *alcohol (70 per cent V/V) R* and heat to boiling. Cool and centrifuge. Decant the supernatant solution immediately and use within 30 min.

Reference solution. Dissolve 20 mg of *barbaloin R* in *alcohol (70 per cent V/V) R* and dilute to 10 ml with the same solvent.

Apply separately to the plate, as bands, 10 µl of each solution. Develop over a path of 10 cm using a mixture of 13 volumes of *water R*, 17 volumes of *methanol R* and 100 volumes of *ethyl acetate R*. Allow the plate to dry for 5 min, then spray with a 50 g/l solution of *potassium hydroxide R* in *alcohol (50 per cent V/V) R* and heat at 100°C to 105°C for 15 min. Examine immediately after heating. The chromatogram obtained with the reference solution shows a reddish-brown zone in the median third corresponding to barbaloin. The chromatogram obtained with the test solution shows two orange-brown zones (glucofrangulins) in the lower third and two to four red zones (frangulins, not always clearly separated, and above them frangula-emodine) in the upper third.

B. To about 25 mg add 25 ml of *dilute hydrochloric acid R* and heat the mixture on a water-bath for 15 min. Allow to cool, shake with 20 ml of *ether R* and discard the aqueous layer. Shake the ether layer with 10 ml of *dilute ammonia R1*. The aqueous layer becomes reddish-violet.

TESTS

Loss on drying Not more than 5.0 per cent. The test is carried out as described for dry extracts in the monograph on *Extracts (765)*.

Microbial contamination Total viable aerobic count (*2.6.12*) not more than 10^4 per gram of which not more than 10^2 fungi per gram, determined by plate count. It complies with the test for *Escherichia coli* and *Salmonella* (*2.6.13*).

ASSAY

Carry out the assay protected from bright light.

In a tared round-bottomed flask with a ground-glass neck, weigh 0.100 g of the preparation to be examined. Add 25.0 ml of a 70 per cent *V/V* solution of *methanol R* mix and weigh again. Heat the flask in a water-bath under a reflux condenser at 70°C for 15 min. Allow to cool, weigh and adjust to the original mass with a 70 per cent *V/V* solution of *methanol R*. Filter and transfer 5.0 ml of the filtrate to a separating funnel. Add 50 ml of *water R* and 0.1 ml of *hydrochloric acid R*. Shake with five quantities, each of 20 ml, of *light petroleum R1*. Allow the layers to separate and transfer the aqueous layer to a 100 ml volumetric flask. Combine the light petroleum layers and wash with two quantities, each of 15 ml, of *water R*. Use this water for washing the separating funnel and add it to the aqueous solution in the volumetric flask. Add 5 ml of a 50 g/l solution of *sodium carbonate R* and dilute to 100.0 ml with *water R*. Discard the light petroleum layer. Transfer 40.0 ml of the aqueous solution to a 200 ml round-bottomed flask with a ground-glass neck. Add 20 ml of a 200 g/l solution of *ferric chloride R* and heat under a reflux condenser for 20 min in a water-bath with the water level above that of the liquid in the flask. Add

2 ml of *hydrochloric acid R* and continue heating for 20 min, shaking frequently, until the precipitate is dissolved. Allow to cool, transfer the mixture to a separating funnel and shake with three quantities, each of 25 ml, of *ether R*, previously used to rinse the flask. Combine the ether extracts and wash with two quantities, each of 15 ml, of *water R*. Transfer the ether layer to a volumetric flask and dilute to 100.0 ml with *ether R*. Evaporate 20.0 ml carefully to dryness and dissolve the residue in 10.0 ml of a 5 g/l solution of *magnesium acetate* R in *methanol R*. Measure the absorbance (2.2.25) at 515 nm using *methanol R* as the compensation liquid.

Calculate the percentage of glucofrangulins, expressed as glucofrangulin A from the expression:

$$\frac{A \times 3.06}{m}$$

i.e. taking the specific absorbance of glucofrangulin A to be 204, calculated on the basis of the specific absorbance of barbaloin,

A = absorbance at 515 nm,

m = mass of the preparation to be examined in grams.

STORAGE

Store in an airtight container, protected from light.

LABELLING

The labelling complies with the requirements in the monograph on *Extracts (765)*.

The label states the content of glucofrangulins.

Ph Eur

Fructose Intravenous Infusion

Definition Fructose Intravenous Infusion is a sterile solution of Fructose in Water for Injections.

The intravenous infusion complies with the requirements stated under Parenteral Preparations and with the following requirements.

Content of fructose, $C_6H_{12}O_6$ 95.0 to 105.0% of the prescribed or stated amount.

Characteristics A colourless or pale yellow solution.

Identification

A. Heat with *cupri-tartaric solution R1*. A copious red precipitate is produced.

B. The solution prepared in the Assay is laevorotatory.

Acidity pH, 3.0 to 5.5, Appendix V L, when determined on a solution diluted if necessary with *water for injections* to contain 5% w/v of Fructose and to which 0.30 ml of a saturated solution of *potassium chloride* has been added for each 100 ml of solution.

5-Hydroxymethylfurfural and related substances Dilute a volume containing 1.0 g of Fructose to 500 ml with *water*. The *absorbance* of the resulting solution at the maximum at 284 nm is not more than 0.50, Appendix II B.

Particulate contamination When supplied in a container with a nominal content of 100 ml or more, complies with the *test for sub-visible particles*, Appendix XIII A.

Pyrogens Complies with the *test for pyrogens*, Appendix XIV D. Use per kg of the rabbit's weight a volume containing 0.5 g of Fructose.

Assay To a volume containing 5 g of Fructose add 0.2 ml of 5M *ammonia* and sufficient *water* to produce 100 ml. Mix well, allow to stand for 30 minutes and determine the *optical rotation* in a 2-dm tube, Appendix V F. The observed rotation in degrees multiplied by 0.5427 represents the weight in g of fructose, $C_6H_{12}O_6$, in the volume taken for assay.

Storage Fructose Intravenous Infusion should be stored at a temperature not exceeding 25°.

Labelling The strength is stated as the number of grams of Fructose per litre.

Furosemide Injection
Frusemide Injection

For the purposes of product labelling in the United Kingdom, the pair of names given above shall be used together (see Introduction, Changes in title).

Definition Furosemide Injection is a sterile solution of furosemide sodium, prepared by the interaction of Furosemide with Sodium Hydroxide, in Water for Injections.

The injection complies with the requirements stated under Parenteral Preparations and with the following requirements.

Content of furosemide, $C_{12}H_{11}ClN_2O_5S$ 95.0 to 105.0% of the prescribed or stated amount.

Characteristics A colourless or almost colourless solution.

Identification

A. The *light absorption*, Appendix II B, in the range 220 to 320 nm of the final solution obtained in the Assay exhibits two maxima, at 228 nm and 271 nm.

B. In the test for Related substances, the chromatogram obtained with solution (2) shows a peak with the same retention time as that of the principal peak in the chromatogram obtained with solution (3).

Alkalinity pH, 8.0 to 9.3, Appendix V L.

Related substances Carry out the method for *liquid chromatography*, Appendix III D, using the following solutions. Prepare the solutions immediately before use and protect from light. For solution (1) dilute a quantity of the injection with sufficient of the mobile phase to produce a solution containing 0.1% w/v of Furosemide. For solution (2) dilute 1 volume of solution (1) to 400 volumes with the mobile phase. Solution (3) contains 0.00025% w/v of *furosemide BPCRS* in the mobile phase. Solution (4) contains 0.00025% w/v of each of *furosemide BPCRS* and *furosemide impurity A EPCRS* in the mobile phase. Solution (5) contains 0.001% w/v of *4-chloro-2-sulphamoylanthranilic acid BPCRS* in the mobile phase.

The chromatographic procedure may be carried out using (a) a stainless steel column (25 cm × 4.6 mm) packed with *stationary phase B* (5 µm) (Chromosphere C8 is suitable), (b) as the mobile phase with a flow rate of 1 ml per minute a mixture prepared in the following manner: dissolve 0.2 g of *potassium dihydrogen orthophosphate* and 0.25 g of *cetrimide* in 70 ml of *water*, adjust the pH to 7.0 with 6M *ammonia* and add 30 ml of *propan-1-ol*, and (c) a detection wavelength of 238 nm.

Inject 100 µl of solution (4). Adjust the sensitivity of the system so that the heights of the two peaks in the chromatogram obtained are not less than 20% of the full-scale of the recorder. The test is not valid unless the *resolution factor* between the first peak (furosemide impurity A) and the second peak (furosemide) is at least 4.

Inject 100 µl of solution (1) and allow the chromatography to proceed for three times the retention time of the principal peak. The area of any peak corresponding to 4-chloro-2-sulphamoylanthranilic acid is not greater than the area of the peak in the chromatogram obtained with solution (5) (1%) and the sum of the areas of any other *secondary peaks* is not greater than twice the area of the first peak in the chromatogram obtained with solution (4) (0.5%). Disregard any peak with an area less than 0.1 times the area of the first peak in the chromatogram obtained with solution (4) (0.025%).

Bacterial endotoxins Carry out the *test for bacterial endotoxins*, Appendix XIV C. Dilute the injection with *water BET*, if necessary, to contain the equivalent of 10 mg of Furosemide per ml (solution A). The endotoxin limit concentration of this solution is 35 IU of endotoxin per ml. Carry out the test using the maximum valid dilution of solution A calculated from the declared sensitivity of the lysate used in the test.

Assay To a volume containing the equivalent of 20 mg of Furosemide add sufficient *water* to produce 100 ml. Dilute 5 ml to 100 ml with 0.1M *sodium hydroxide* and measure the *absorbance* of the resulting solution at the maximum at 271 nm, Appendix II B. Calculate the content of $C_{12}H_{11}ClN_2O_5S$ taking 580 as the value of A(1%, 1 cm) at the maximum at 271 nm.

Storage Furosemide Injection should be protected from light.

Labelling The label states 'Furosemide Injection' and 'Frusemide Injection'.

The strength is stated in terms of the equivalent amount of Furosemide (Frusemide) in a suitable dose-volume.

Furosemide Tablets
Frusemide Tablets

For the purposes of product labelling in the United Kingdom, the pair of names given above shall be used together (see Introduction, Changes in title)

Definition Furosemide Tablets contain Furosemide.

The tablets comply with the requirements stated under Tablets and with the following requirements.

Content of furosemide, $C_{12}H_{11}ClN_2O_5S$ 95.0 to 105.0% of the prescribed or stated amount.

Identification

A. The *light absorption*, Appendix II B, in the range 220 to 320 nm of the final solution obtained in the Assay exhibits two maxima, at 228 nm and 271 nm.

B. In the test for Related substances, the principal peak in the chromatogram obtained with solution (2) shows a peak with the same retention time as the principal peak in the chromatogram obtained with solution (3).

Dissolution Tablets containing less than 100 mg of Furosemide comply with the *dissolution test for tablets and capsules*, Appendix XII D, using Apparatus II. Use as the medium 900 ml of *phosphate buffer pH 5.8* and rotate the paddle at 50 revolutions per minute. Withdraw a sample of 10 ml of the medium, filter and dilute the filtrate with sufficient of the dissolution medium to give a solution expected to contain about 0.001% w/v of Furosemide. Measure the *absorbance* of this solution, Appendix II B, at 277 nm using dissolution medium in the reference cell. Calculate the total content of furosemide, $C_{12}H_{11}ClN_2O_5S$, in the medium from the *absorbance* obtained from a 0.001% w/v solution of *furosemide BPCRS* in the dissolution medium and using the declared content of $C_{12}H_{11}ClN_2O_5S$ in *furosemide BPCRS*.

Related substances Carry out the method for *liquid chromatography*, Appendix III D, using the following solutions. Prepare the solutions immediately before use and protect from light. Dissolve 1.92 g of *sodium pentanesulphonate* in 22 ml of *glacial acetic acid* and add sufficient of a mixture of equal volumes of *acetonitrile* and *water* to produce 1000 ml (solution A). For solution (1) dissolve a quantity of the powdered tablets containing 20 mg of Furosemide in 50 ml of solution A and mix with the aid of ultrasound for 15 minutes. For solution (2) dilute 1 volume of solution (1) to 500 volumes with the mobile phase. Solution (3) contains 0.00008% w/v of *furosemide BPCRS* in the mobile phase. Solution (4) contains 0.00008% w/v of each of *furosemide BPCRS* and *furosemide impurity A EPCRS* in the mobile phase. Solution (5) contains 0.00032% w/v of *4-chloro-2-sulphamoylanthranilic acid BPCRS* in the mobile phase.

The chromatographic procedure may be carried out using (a) a stainless steel column (25 cm × 4.6 mm) packed with *stationary phase B* (5 µm) (Chromosphere C8 is suitable), (b) as the mobile phase with a flow rate of 1 ml per minute a mixture prepared in the following manner: dissolve 0.2 g of *potassium dihydrogen orthophosphate* and 0.25 g of *cetrimide* in 70 ml of *water*, adjust the pH to 7.0 with 6M *ammonia* and add 30 ml of *propan-1-ol*, and (c) a detection wavelength of 238 nm.

Inject 100 µl of solution (4). Adjust the sensitivity of the system so that the heights of the two peaks in the chromatogram obtained are not less than 20% of the full-scale of the recorder. The test is not valid unless the *resolution factor* between the first peak (furosemide impurity A) and the second peak (furosemide) is at least 4.

Inject 100 µl of solution A. Inject 100 µl of solution (1) and allow the chromatography to proceed for three times the retention time of the principal peak. In the chromatogram obtained with solution (1) the area of any peak corresponding to 4-chloro-2-sulphamoylanthranilic acid is not greater than the area of the peak in the chromatogram obtained with solution (5) (0.8%) and the sum of the areas of any other *secondary peaks* is not greater than 2.5 times the area of the first peak in the chromatogram obtained with solution (4) (0.5%). Disregard any peak with an area less than 0.1 times the area of the first peak in the chromatogram obtained with solution (4) (0.02%) and any peaks corresponding to those in the chromatogram obtained with solution A.

Assay Weigh and powder 20 tablets. Shake a quantity of the powder containing 0.2 g of Furosemide with 300 ml of 0.1M *sodium hydroxide* for 10 minutes, add sufficient 0.1M *sodium hydroxide* to produce 500 ml and filter. Dilute 5 ml to 250 ml with 0.1M *sodium hydroxide* and measure the *absorbance* of the resulting solution at the maximum at 271 nm, Appendix II B. Calculate the content of $C_{12}H_{11}ClN_2O_5S$ taking 580 as the value of A(1%, 1 cm) at the maximum at 271 nm.

Labelling The label states 'Furosemide Tablets' and 'Frusemide Tablets'.

Fusidic Acid Oral Suspension

Definition Fusidic Acid Oral Suspension is a suspension of Fusidic Acid in powder of suitable fineness in a suitable flavoured vehicle.

Fusidic Acid Oral Suspension should not be diluted.

The oral suspension complies with the requirements stated under Oral Liquids and with the following requirements.

Content of fusidic acid, $C_{31}H_{48}O_6$ 92.5 to 107.5% of the prescribed or stated amount.

Identification

A. To a quantity containing the equivalent of 0.1 g of anhydrous fusidic acid add 5 ml of *water* and extract with three 10-ml quantities of *chloroform*. Wash the combined extracts with two 10-ml quantities of *water*, dry with *anhydrous sodium sulphate*, evaporate to dryness and dissolve the residue in 1 ml of *chloroform IR*. The *infrared absorption spectrum* of the resulting solution, Appendix II A, is concordant with the *reference spectrum* of fusidic acid.

B. In the Assay, the principal peak in the chromatogram obtained with solution (2) has the same retention time as the peak due to fusidic acid in the chromatogram obtained with solution (1).

Acidity pH, 4.8 to 5.2, Appendix V L.

Related substances Carry out the method for *liquid chromatography*, Appendix III D, using the following three solutions. For solution (1) extract a quantity of the oral suspension containing the equivalent of 0.10 g of anhydrous fusidic acid with two 20-ml quantities of *chloroform*, evaporate the combined extracts to dryness and dissolve the residue in 20 ml of the mobile phase. For solution (2) mix 1 ml of a 0.10% w/v solution of *3-ketofusidic acid EPCRS* in the mobile phase with 0.2 ml of solution (1) and dilute to 20 ml with the mobile phase. For solution (3) dilute 20 µl of solution (1) to 100 ml with the mobile phase.

The chromatographic procedure may be carried out using (a) a stainless steel column (12.5 to 15 cm × 4 to 5 mm) packed with *stationary phase C* (5 µm) (Lichrosphere 100 RP18 is suitable) (b) a mixture of 10 volumes of *methanol*, 20 volumes of a 1% w/v solution of *orthophosphoric acid*, 20 volumes of *water* and 50 volumes of *acetonitrile* as the mobile phase with a flow rate of 2 ml per minute and (c) a detection wavelength of 235 nm.

Inject separately 20 µl of each solution. Continue the chromatography for at least 3.5 times the retention time of the principal peak. The test is not valid unless the *resolution factor* between the peaks corresponding to 3-ketofusidic acid and fusidic acid in the chromatogram obtained with solution (2) is at least 2.5 and unless the principal peak in the chromatogram obtained with solution (3) has a *signal-to-noise ratio* of at least 3.

In the chromatogram obtained with solution (1) the sum of the areas of any *secondary peaks* is not greater than three times the area of the peak corresponding to fusidic acid in the chromatogram obtained with solution (2) (3%). Disregard any peak with an area less than that of the principal peak in the chromatogram obtained with solution (3) (0.02%).

Assay Carry out the method for *liquid chromatography*, Appendix III D, using the following solutions. Solution (1) contains 0.07% w/v of *diethanolamine fusidate BPCRS* in the mobile phase. For solution (2) shake thoroughly a weighed quantity of the oral suspension containing the equivalent of 30 mg of anhydrous fusidic acid with 25 ml of the mobile phase, dilute to 50 ml with the mobile phase, filter and use the clear filtrate.

The chromatographic procedure may be carried out using (a) a stainless steel column (20 cm × 4.6 mm) packed with *stationary phase C* (5 µm) (LiChrosorb RP-18 is suitable), (b) a mixture of 60 volumes of *acetonitrile*, 30 volumes of a 1% v/v solution of *glacial acetic acid* and 10 volumes of *methanol* as the mobile phase with a flow rate of 1.5 ml per minute and (c) a detection wavelength of 235 nm.

The *column efficiency*, determined using the principal peak in the chromatogram obtained with solution (1), should be at least 14,000 theoretical plates per metre.

Determine the *weight per ml* of the oral suspension, Appendix V G, and calculate the content of $C_{31}H_{48}O_6$, weight in volume, using the equivalent declared content of $C_{31}H_{48}O_6$ in *diethanolamine fusidate BPCRS*.

Storage Fusidic Acid Oral Suspension should be protected from light and stored at a temperature not exceeding 25°.

Labelling The quantity of active ingredient is stated in terms of the equivalent amount of anhydrous fusidic acid.

When Fusidic Acid Oral Suspension is prescribed or demanded, no strength being stated, an Oral Suspension containing the equivalent of 250 mg of anhydrous fusidic acid in 5 ml shall be dispensed or supplied.

Gallamine Injection

Definition Gallamine Injection is a sterile solution of Gallamine Triethiodide in Water for Injections.

The injection complies with the requirements stated under Parenteral Preparations and with the following requirements.

Content of gallamine triethiodide, $C_{30}H_{60}I_3N_3O_3$ 95.0 to 105.0% of the prescribed or stated amount.

Characteristics A colourless or almost colourless solution.

Identification

A. The *light absorption*, Appendix II B, in the range 220 to 350 nm of the final solution obtained in the Assay exhibits a maximum only at 225 nm.

B. To 1 ml add 1 ml of *iodinated potassium iodide solution*. A brown precipitate is produced.

C. To 1 ml add 1 ml of *potassium tetraiodomercurate solution*. A yellow precipitate is produced.

Acidity or alkalinity pH, 5.5 to 7.5, Appendix V L.

Related substances Carry out the method for *liquid chromatography*, Appendix III D, using the following solutions. For solution (1) dilute a volume of the injection with sufficient of the mobile phase to produce a solution containing 0.060% w/v of Gallamine Triethiodide. For solution (2) dilute 1 volume of solution (1) to 100 volumes with the mobile phase.

The chromatographic procedure may be carried out using (a) a stainless steel column (25 cm × 4.6 mm) packed with particles of silica the surface of which has been modified with a mixture of chemically-bonded octylsilyl and octadecylsilyl groups and treated to reduce the level of residual silanol groups (5 μm) (HiChrom RPB is suitable), (b) as the mobile phase with a flow rate of 1.5 ml per minute a solution prepared as described below, (c) a detection wavelength of 205 nm and (d) a column temperature of 40°. For the mobile phase dissolve 14 g of *sodium perchlorate* in 850 ml of a solution prepared by diluting 0.7 ml of *orthophosphoric acid* to 900 ml with *water*, adjusting to pH 3.0 with 10M *sodium hydroxide* and diluting to 1000 ml with *water*, and add 130 ml of *methanol*.

Inject separately 20 μl of each solution. For solution (1) allow the chromatography to proceed for 1.5 times the retention time of gallamine as perchlorate.

In the chromatogram obtained with solution (1) the area of any *secondary peak* is not greater than the area of the principal peak in the chromatogram obtained with solution (2) (1%) and the sum of the areas of all the *secondary peaks* is not greater than twice the area of the principal peak in the chromatogram obtained with solution (2) (2%). Disregard the peak due to iodide (retention time, 0).

Assay Dilute a volume containing 40 mg of Gallamine Triethiodide with sufficient 0.01M *hydrochloric acid* to produce 200 ml. Dilute 5 ml of this solution to 100 ml with 0.01M *hydrochloric acid* and measure the *absorbance* of the resulting solution at the maximum at 225 nm, Appendix II B. Calculate the content of $C_{30}H_{60}I_3N_3O_3$ taking 525 as the value of A(1%, 1 cm) at the maximum at 225 nm.

Storage Gallamine Injection should be protected from light.

IMPURITIES

The impurities limited by this monograph include those listed in the monograph for Gallamine Triethiodide.

Gemfibrozil Capsules

Definition Gemfibrozil Capsules contain Gemfibrozil.

The capsules comply with the requirements stated under Capsules and with the following requirements.

Content of gemfibrozil, $C_{15}H_{22}O_3$ 95.0 to 105.0% of the prescribed or stated amount.

Identification Shake a quantity of the contents of the capsules containing about 0.5 g of Gemfibrozil with 10 ml of n-*hexane* for 10 minutes, filter through a filter paper previously washed with 20 ml of n-*hexane*, evaporate the filtrate to dryness on a water bath and then dry over *silica gel* at a pressure of 2 kPa for 2 hours or until a waxy solid is obtained. The *infrared absorption spectrum* of the residue, Appendix II A, is concordant with the *reference spectrum* of gemfibrozil.

Related substances Carry out the method for *liquid chromatography*, Appendix III D, using the following solutions. For solution (1) shake a quantity of the contents of the capsules containing 0.4 g of Gemfibrozil with 100 ml of *methanol* and filter. For solution (2) dilute 1 volume of solution (1) to 100 volumes with the mobile phase and further dilute 1 volume of this solution to 5 volumes with the mobile phase. Solution (3) contains 0.0004% w/v of *gemfibrozil impurity A BPCRS* in the mobile phase. Solution (4) contains 0.001% w/v of *gemfibrozil methyl ester BPCRS* and 0.0004% w/v of *gemfibrozil impurity A BPCRS* in solution (2).

The chromatographic procedure described under Assay may be used. For solution (1) allow the chromatography to proceed for twice the retention time of the principal peak.

The test is not valid unless, in the chromatogram obtained with solution (4), the *resolution factor* between the peaks due to gemfibrozil and gemfibrozil methyl ester is at least 4.0 and the *resolution factor* between the peaks due to gemfibrozil methyl ester and gemfibrozil impurity A is at least 1.2.

In the chromatogram obtained with solution (1) the area of any peak corresponding to gemfibrozil impurity A is not greater than the area of the peak in the chromatogram obtained with solution (3) (0.1%), the area of any other *secondary peak* is not greater than the area of the peak in the chromatogram obtained with solution (2) (0.2%) and the sum of the areas of any secondary peaks other than any peak corresponding to gemfibrozil impurity A is not greater than 2.5 times the area of the peak in the chromatogram obtained with solution (2) (0.5%).

Dissolution Comply with the *dissolution test for tablets and capsules*, Appendix XII D, using Apparatus II. Use as the medium 900 ml of 0.2M *phosphate buffer pH 7.5* and rotate the paddle at 50 revolutions per minute. Withdraw a 10-ml sample of the medium and measure the *absorbance* of the filtered sample, suitably diluted with the dissolution medium if necessary, at the maximum at 276 nm, Appendix II B. At the same time measure the *absorbance* at the maximum at 276 nm of a suitable solution of *gemfibrozil BPCRS* in the dissolution medium, adding the minimum volume of 0.1M *sodium hydroxide*, if necessary, to complete dissolution. Calculate the total content of gemfibrozil, $C_{15}H_{22}O_3$, in the medium from the absorbances obtained and from the declared content of $C_{15}H_{22}O_3$ in *gemfibrozil BPCRS*.

Assay Carry out the method for *liquid chromatography*, Appendix III D, using the following solutions. For solution (1) add 50 ml of *methanol* to a quantity of the mixed contents of 20 capsules containing 0.15 g of Gemfibrozil, shake on a mechanical shaker for 10 minutes, add 20 ml of *water*, 1 ml of *glacial acetic acid* and sufficient *methanol* to produce 100 ml, mix and filter (Whatman GF/C paper is suitable), discarding the first 20 ml of filtrate. Dilute 1 volume of the filtrate to 5 volumes with the mobile phase. For solution (2) dissolve 30 mg of *gemfibrozil BPCRS* in 80 ml of *methanol*, add 1 ml of *glacial acetic acid* and dilute to 100 ml with *water*. Solution (3) contains 0.01% w/v of *gemfibrozil methyl ester BPCRS* in a solution prepared by diluting 1 volume of solution (1) to 3 volumes with the mobile phase.

The chromatographic procedure may be carried out using (a) a stainless steel column (10 cm × 4.6 mm) packed with *stationary phase C* (3 µm) (Spherisorb ODS 2 or Regis C18 are suitable), (b) a mixture of 1 volume of *glacial acetic acid*, 19 volumes of *water* and 80 volumes of *methanol* as the mobile phase with a flow rate of 1 ml per minute and (c) a detection wavelength of 276 nm.

Inject 20 µl of each solution. The test is not valid unless in the chromatogram obtained with solution (3) the *resolution factor* between the peaks due to gemfibrozil and gemfibrozil methyl ester is at least 4.0.

Calculate the content of $C_{15}H_{22}O_3$ in the capsules from the declared content of $C_{15}H_{22}O_3$ in *gemfibrozil BPCRS.*

Gemfibrozil Tablets

Definition Gemfibrozil Tablets contain Gemfibrozil.

With the exception of the requirements for shape, the tablets comply with the requirements stated under Tablets and with the following requirements.

Content of gemfibrozil, $C_{15}H_{22}O_3$ 95.0 to 105.0% of the prescribed or stated amount.

Identification Mix a quantity of the powdered tablets containing 0.3 g of Gemfibrozil with 10 ml of 0.1M *sodium hydroxide*, filter (Whatman 541 paper is suitable), acidify with a few drops of 2M *sulphuric acid*, shake and centrifuge. Wash the precipitate with *water*, allow to dry in air and dry over *anhydrous silica gel* at a pressure of 2 kPa for 4 hours. The *infrared absorption spectrum* of the dried residue, Appendix II A, is concordant with the *reference spectrum* of gemfibrozil.

Related substances Carry out the method for *liquid chromatography*, Appendix III D, using the following solutions. For solution (1) shake a quantity of the powdered tablets containing 0.6 g of Gemfibrozil with 70 ml of *methanol* for 15 minutes, add sufficient *methanol* to produce 100 ml and filter. For solution (2) dilute 1 volume of solution (1) to 100 volumes with the mobile phase and further dilute 1 volume of this solution to 5 volumes with the mobile phase. Solution (3) contains 0.0006% w/v of *gemfibrozil impurity A BPCRS* in the mobile phase. Solution (4) contains 0.001% w/v of *gemfibrozil methyl ester BPCRS* and 0.0004% w/v of *gemfibrozil impurity A BPCRS* in solution (2).

The chromatographic procedure described under Assay may be used. For solution (1) allow the chromatography to proceed for twice the retention time of the principal peak.

The test is not valid unless, in the chromatogram obtained with solution (4), the *resolution factor* between the peaks due to gemfibrozil and gemfibrozil methyl ester is at least 4.0 and the *resolution factor* between the peaks due to gemfibrozil methyl ester and gemfibrozil impurity A is at least 1.2.

In the chromatogram obtained with solution (1) the area of any peak corresponding to gemfibrozil impurity A is not greater than the area of the peak in the chromatogram obtained with solution (3) (0.1%), the area of any other *secondary peak* is not greater than the area of the peak in the chromatogram obtained with solution (2) (0.2%) and the sum of the areas of any secondary peaks other than the peak corresponding to gemfibrozil impurity A is not greater than 2.5 times the area of the peak in the chromatogram obtained with solution (2) (0.5%).

Dissolution Comply with the *dissolution test for tablets and capsules*, Appendix XII D, using Apparatus II. Use as the medium 900 ml of 0.2M *phosphate buffer pH 7.5* and rotate the paddle at 50 revolutions per minute. Withdraw a 10-ml sample of the medium and measure the *absorbance* of the filtered sample, suitably diluted with the dissolution medium if necessary, at the maximum at 276 nm, Appendix II B. At the same time measure the *absorbance* at the maximum at 276 nm of a suitable solution of *gemfibrozil BPCRS* prepared by dissolving the substance in the minimum volume of *methanol* and diluting with 0.2M *phosphate buffer pH 7.5*. Calculate the total content of gemfibrozil, $C_{15}H_{22}O_3$, in the medium from the absorbances obtained and from the declared content of $C_{15}H_{22}O_3$ in *gemfibrozil BPCRS.*

Assay Weigh and powder 20 tablets. Carry out the method for *liquid chromatography*, Appendix III D, using the following solutions. For solution (1) shake a quantity of the powdered tablets containing 84 mg of Gemfibrozil with 80 ml of *methanol (80%)* on a mechanical shaker for 15 minutes, add sufficient *methanol (80%)* to produce 100 ml, mix and filter (Whatman 542 paper is suitable), discarding the first 20 ml of filtrate. Solution (2) contains 0.084% w/v of *gemfibrozil BPCRS* prepared by dissolving the substance in the minimum volume of *methanol* and diluting with *methanol (80%)*. Solution (3) contains 0.01% w/v of *gemfibrozil methyl ester BPCRS* in a solution prepared by diluting 1 volume of solution (1) to 10 volumes with a mixture of 2 volumes of *methanol* and 3 volumes of the mobile phase.

The chromatographic procedure may be carried out using (a) a stainless steel column (10 cm × 4.6 mm) packed with *stationary phase C* (3 µm) (Spherisorb ODS 2 or Regis C18 are suitable), (b) a mixture of 1 volume of *glacial acetic acid*, 19 volumes of *water* and 80 volumes of *methanol* as the mobile phase with a flow rate of 1 ml per minute and (c) a detection wavelength of 276 nm.

Inject 20 µl of each solution. The test is not valid unless the *resolution factor* between the peaks due to gemfibrozil and gemfibrozil methyl ester in the chromatogram obtained with solution (3) is at least 4.0.

Calculate the content of $C_{15}H_{22}O_3$ in the tablets from the declared content of $C_{15}H_{22}O_3$ in *gemfibrozil BPCRS.*

Storage Gemfibrozil Tablets should be protected from light.

Gentamicin Cream

Definition Gentamicin Cream is a viscous oil-in-water emulsion containing Gentamicin Sulphate dissolved in the aqueous phase.

The cream complies with the requirements stated under Topical Semi-solid Preparations and with the following requirements.

Identification

A. Carry out the method for *thin-layer chromatography*, Appendix III A, using a silica gel precoated plate (Merck silica gel 60 plates are suitable) and as the mobile phase the lower layer obtained by shaking together equal volumes of 13.5M *ammonia*, *chloroform* and *methanol* and allowing to separate. Apply separately to the plate 20 µl of each of the following solutions. For solution (1) disperse a quantity of the cream containing the equivalent of 7.5 mg of gentamicin in 20 ml of *chloroform*, extract with 10 ml of *water* and use the aqueous layer. Solution (2) is a solution of *gentamicin sulphate EPCRS* in *water* containing the equivalent of 0.075% w/v of gentamicin. After removal of the plate, allow it to dry in air, spray with *ninhydrin solution R1* and heat at 105° for 2 minutes. The three principal spots in the chromatogram obtained with solution (1) correspond to the three principal spots in the chromatogram obtained with solution (2).

B. In the test for Composition of gentamicin sulphate, the retention times of the four principal peaks in the chromatogram obtained with solution (2) correspond to those of the four principal peaks in the chromatogram obtained with solution (1)

Composition of gentamicin sulphate Complies with the test described under Gentamicin Injection but preparing solution (2) in the following manner. Disperse a quantity of the cream containing the equivalent of 15 mg of gentamicin in 10 ml of *chloroform*, add 10 ml of a 0.25% w/v solution of *sodium tetraborate*, shake vigorously, centrifuge and separate the aqueous layer. Repeat the extraction with two 5-ml quantities of the sodium tetraborate solution, dilute the combined aqueous extracts to 25 ml with the same solution and filter. To 10 ml of the clear filtrate add 5 ml of *methanol*, swirl, add 4 ml of *phthalaldehyde reagent*, mix, add sufficient *methanol* to produce 25 ml, heat in a water bath at 60° for 15 minutes and cool.

Assay Dissolve as completely as possible a quantity containing the equivalent of 3 mg of gentamicin in 20 ml of *chloroform* and shake vigorously with 75 ml of *phosphate buffer pH 8.0*. Dilute 10 ml of the aqueous extract to 50 ml with *phosphate buffer pH 8.0*. Carry out the *biological assay of antibiotics*, Appendix XIV A. The precision of the assay is such that the fiducial limits of error are not less than 95% and not more than 105% of the estimated potency.

Calculate the content of gentamicin in the cream, taking each 1000 IU found to be equivalent to 1 mg of gentamicin. The upper fiducial limit of error is not less than 90.0% and the lower fiducial limit of error is not more than 120.0% of the prescribed or stated content.

Labelling The quantity of active ingredient is stated in terms of the equivalent amount of gentamicin.

Gentamicin Eye Drops

Definition Gentamicin Eye Drops are a sterile solution of Gentamicin Sulphate in Purified Water.

The eye drops comply with the requirements stated under Eye Preparations and with the following requirements.

Identification

A. Carry out the method for *thin-layer chromatography*, Appendix III A, using a silica gel precoated plate (Merck silica gel 60 plates are suitable) and as the mobile phase the lower layer obtained by shaking together equal volumes of 13.5M *ammonia*, *chloroform* and *methanol* and allowing to separate. Apply separately to the plate (1) a volume of the eye drops containing the equivalent of 30 µg of gentamicin and (2) 0.1 mg of *gentamicin sulphate EPCRS* dissolved in a volume of *water* equal to the volume of the eye drops used. After removal of the plate, allow it to dry in air, spray with *ninhydrin solution R1* and heat at 105° for 2 minutes. The three principal spots in the chromatogram obtained with solution (1) correspond to the three principal spots in the chromatogram obtained with solution (2).

B. In the test for Composition of gentamicin sulphate, the retention times of the four principal peaks in the chromatogram obtained with solution (2) correspond to those of the four principal peaks in the chromatogram obtained with solution (1).

Composition of gentamicin sulphate Comply with the test described under Gentamicin Injection, using for solution (2) a solution prepared in the same manner as solution (1) but using 10 ml of a solution prepared by diluting a suitable volume of the eye drops with *water* to contain the equivalent of 0.045% w/v of gentamicin.

Assay Dilute a volume of the eye drops containing the equivalent of 15 mg of gentamicin to 50 ml with sterile *phosphate buffer pH 8.0* and dilute 10 ml of the resulting solution to 50 ml with the same solvent. Carry out the *biological assay of antibiotics*, Appendix XIV A. The precision of the assay is such that the fiducial limits of error are not less than 95% and not more than 105% of the estimated potency.

Calculate the content of gentamicin in the eye drops, taking each 1000 IU found to be equivalent to 1 mg of gentamicin. The upper fiducial limit of error is not less than 90.0% and the lower fiducial limit of error is not more than 120.0% of the prescribed or stated content.

Labelling The quantity of active ingredient is stated in terms of the equivalent amount of gentamicin.

Gentamicin Injection

Definition Gentamicin Injection is a sterile solution of Gentamicin Sulphate in Water for Injections.

The injection complies with the requirements stated under Parenteral Preparations and with the following requirements.

Identification

A. Carry out the method for *thin-layer chromatography*, Appendix III A, using a silica gel precoated plate (Merck silica gel 60 plates are suitable) and as the mobile phase the lower layer obtained by shaking together equal volumes of 13.5M *ammonia*, *chloroform* and *methanol* and allowing to separate. Apply separately to the plate (1) a volume of the injection containing the equivalent of 30 µg of gentamicin and (2) 0.1 mg of *gentamicin sulphate EPCRS* dissolved in a volume of *water* equal to the volume of the injection used. After removal of the plate, allow it to dry in air, spray with *ninhydrin solution R1* and heat at 105° for 2 minutes. The three principal spots in the chromatogram obtained with solution (1) correspond to the three principal spots in the chromatogram obtained with solution (2).

B. In the test for Composition of gentamicin sulphate, the retention times of the four principal peaks in the chromatogram obtained with solution (2) correspond to those of the four principal peaks in the chromatogram obtained with solution (1).

Acidity pH, 3.0 to 5.5, Appendix V L.

Composition of gentamicin sulphate Carry out the method for *liquid chromatography*, Appendix III D, using the following solutions. For solution (1) add 5 ml of *methanol* to 10 ml of a 0.065% w/v solution of *gentamicin sulphate EPCRS,* swirl and add 4 ml of *phthalaldehyde reagent*, mix, add sufficient *methanol* to produce 25 ml, heat in a water bath at 60° for 15 minutes and cool. If the solution is not used immediately, cool to 0° and use within 4 hours. Prepare solution (2) in the same manner as solution (1) but using 10 ml of a solution prepared by diluting a suitable volume of the injection with *water* to contain the equivalent of 0.045% of gentamicin.

The chromatographic procedure may be carried out using (a) a stainless steel column (10 to 12.5 cm × 4.6 to 5 mm) packed with *stationary phase C* (5 µm) (Hypersil ODS is suitable), (b) 0.025M *sodium heptanesulphonate monohydrate* in a mixture of 70 volumes of *methanol,* 25 volumes of *water* and 5 volumes of *glacial acetic acid* as the mobile phase with a flow rate of 1.5 ml per minute and (c) a detection wavelength of 330 nm. When the chromatograms are recorded under the operating conditions described above, in the chromatogram obtained with solution (1) the retention time of component C_2 is 10 to 20 minutes and the peaks are well separated with relative retention times of about 0.13 (reagent), 0.27 (component C_1), 0.65 (component C_{1a}), 0.85 (component C_{2a}) and 1.00 (component C_2).

Adjust the sensitivity and the volume of solution (1) injected so that the height of the peak due to component C_1 is about 75% of full-scale deflection. Plot a horizontal baseline on the chromatogram from the horizontal portion of the curve immediately before the reagent peak. Measure the peak height above this baseline for each component. Repeat the procedure with solution (2). The test is not valid unless the *resolution factor* between the peaks due to components C_{2a} and C_2 is at least 1.3.

From the peak heights in the chromatogram obtained with solution (1) and the proportions of the components declared for *gentamicin sulphate EPCRS*, calculate the response factors for components C_1, C_{1a}, C_{2a} and C_2. From these response factors and the peak heights in the chromatogram obtained with solution (2), calculate the proportions of components C_1, C_{1a}, C_{2a} and C_2 in the injection. The proportions are within the following limits: C_1, 25.0 to 50.0%; C_{1a}, 10.0 to 35.0%; C_2 plus C_{2a}, 25.0 to 55.0%.

Bacterial endotoxins Carry out the *test for bacterial endotoxins*, Appendix XIV C. Dilute the injection, if necessary, with *water BET* to give a solution containing the equivalent of 10 mg of gentamicin per ml (solution A). The endotoxin limit concentration of solution A is 16.7 IU per ml. Carry out the test using the maximum valid dilution of solution A calculated from the declared sensitivity of the lysate used in the test.

Assay Carry out the *biological assay of antibiotics*, Appendix XIV A. The precision of the assay is such that the fiducial limits of error are not less than 95% and not more than 105% of the estimated potency.

Calculate the content of gentamicin in the injection, taking each 1000 IU found to be equivalent to 1 mg of gentamicin. The upper fiducial limit of error is not less than 97.0% and the lower fiducial limit of error is not more than 110.0% of the prescribed or stated content.

Labelling The strength is stated in terms of the equivalent amount of gentamicin in a suitable dose-volume.

Gentamicin Ointment

Definition Gentamicin Ointment is a dispersion of Gentamicin Sulphate in *microfine powder* in White Soft Paraffin or other suitable anhydrous greasy basis.

The ointment complies with the requirements stated under Topical Semi-solid Preparations and with the following requirements.

Identification

A. Carry out the method for *thin-layer chromatography*, Appendix III A, using a silica gel precoated plate (Merck silica gel 60 plates are suitable) and as the mobile phase the lower layer obtained by shaking together equal volumes of 13.5M *ammonia, chloroform* and *methanol* and allowing to separate. Apply separately to the plate 20 µl of each of the following solutions. For solution (1) disperse a quantity of the ointment containing the equivalent of 7.5 mg of gentamicin in 20 ml of *chloroform*, extract with 10 ml of *water* and use the aqueous layer. Solution (2) is a solution of *gentamicin sulphate EPCRS* in *water* containing the equivalent of 0.075% w/v of gentamicin. After removal of the plate, allow it to dry in air, spray with *ninhydrin solution R1* and heat at 105° for 2 minutes. The three principal spots in the chromatogram obtained with solution (1) correspond to the three principal spots in the chromatogram obtained with solution (2).

B. In the test for Composition of gentamicin sulphate, the retention times of the four principal peaks in the chromatogram obtained with solution (2) correspond to those of the four principal peaks in the chromatogram obtained with solution (1).

Composition of gentamicin sulphate Complies with the test described under Gentamicin Injection but preparing solution (2) in the following manner. Disperse a quantity of the ointment containing the equivalent of 20 mg of gentamicin in 10 ml of *chloroform,* add 20 ml of a 0.25% w/v solution of *sodium tetraborate*, shake vigorously, centrifuge and separate the aqueous layer. Filter and dilute to 50 ml with *water.* To 10 ml add 5 ml of *methanol*, swirl, add 4 ml of *phthalaldehyde reagent*, mix, add sufficient *methanol* to produce 25 ml, heat in a water bath at 60° for 15 minutes and cool.

Assay Dissolve as completely as possible a quantity containing the equivalent of 4 mg of gentamicin in 50 ml of *chloroform*, extract with three 20-ml quantities of *phosphate buffer pH 8.0* and dilute the combined extracts to 100 ml with *phosphate buffer pH 8.0*. Dilute 10 ml of the resulting solution to 50 ml with *phosphate buffer pH 8.0*. Carry out the *biological assay of antibiotics*, Appendix XIV A. The precision of the assay is such that the fiducial limits of error are not less than 95% and not more than 105% of the estimated potency.

Calculate the content of gentamicin in the ointment, taking each 1000 IU found to be equivalent to 1 mg of gentamicin. The upper fiducial limit of error is not less than 90.0% and the lower fiducial limit of error is not more than 120.0% of the prescribed or stated content.

Labelling The quantity of active ingredient is stated in terms of the equivalent amount of gentamicin.

Compound Gentian Infusion

Definition

Concentrated Compound Gentian Infusion	100 ml
Water	sufficient to produce 1000 ml

The infusion complies with the requirements stated under Infusions.

CONCENTRATED COMPOUND GENTIAN INFUSION

Definition

Gentian, cut small and bruised	125 g
Dried Bitter-Orange Peel, cut small	125 g
Dried Lemon Peel, cut small	125 g
Ethanol (25 per cent)	1200 ml

Extemporaneous preparation The following directions apply.

Macerate the Gentian, the Dried Bitter-Orange Peel and the Dried Lemon Peel in a covered vessel for 48 hours with 1000 ml of the Ethanol (25 per cent); express the liquid. To the pressed marc add 200 ml of the Ethanol (25 per cent), macerate for 24 hours, press and add the liquid to the product of the first pressing. Allow to stand for not less than 14 days; filter.

Ethanol content 20 to 24% v/v, Appendix VIII F.

Total solids Not less than 9.5% w/v, Appendix XI A.

Acid Gentian Mixture

Acid Gentian Oral Solution

Definition Acid Gentian Mixture is an *oral solution* containing 10% v/v of Concentrated Compound Gentian Infusion and 5% v/v of Dilute Hydrochloric Acid in a suitable vehicle.

Extemporaneous preparation It is recently prepared according to the following formula.

Concentrated Compound Gentian Infusion	100 ml
Dilute Hydrochloric Acid	50 ml
Double-strength Chloroform Water	500 ml
Water	sufficient to produce 1000 ml

The mixture complies with the requirements stated under Oral Liquids and with the following requirements.

Content of hydrochloric acid, HCl 0.48 to 0.56% w/v.

Assay To 10 ml add 10 ml of *water*, adjust the pH to between 5.0 and 6.0 with 2M *sodium hydroxide* and dilute to 25 ml with *water*. Add 75 ml of *acetate buffer pH 5.0* and titrate with 0.1M *silver nitrate VS* determining the end point potentiometrically using a silver indicator electrode and a glass reference electrode and stirring throughout the titration. Each ml of 0.1M *silver nitrate VS* is equivalent to 3.646 mg of HCl.

Labelling The label indicates the pharmaceutical form as 'oral solution'.

Alkaline Gentian Mixture

Alkaline Gentian Oral Solution

Definition Alkaline Gentian Mixture is an *oral solution* containing 10% v/v of Concentrated Compound Gentian Infusion and 5% w/v of Sodium Bicarbonate in a suitable vehicle.

Extemporaneous preparation It is recently prepared according to the following formula.

Concentrated Compound Gentian Infusion	100 ml
Sodium Bicarbonate	50 g
Double-strength Chloroform Water	500 ml
Water	sufficient to produce 1000 ml

The mixture complies with the requirements stated under Oral Liquids and with the following requirements.

Content of sodium bicarbonate, $NaHCO_3$ 4.75 to 5.25% w/v.

Assay To 10 ml of the mixture add 100 ml of *water* and 25 ml of 0.5M *hydrochloric acid VS*, boil for 10 minutes and titrate the excess of hydrochloric acid with 0.5M *sodium hydroxide VS* using 0.5 ml of *methyl red solution* as indicator. Each ml of 0.5M *hydrochloric acid VS* is equivalent to 42.00 mg of $NaHCO_3$.

Labelling The label indicates the pharmaceutical form as 'oral solution'.

Strong Ginger Tincture

Ginger Essence

Definition

Ginger, in moderately coarse powder	500 g
Ethanol (90 per cent)	sufficient to produce 1000 ml

Extemporaneous preparation The following directions apply.

Prepare by *percolation*, Appendix XI F.

The tincture complies with the requirements stated under Tinctures and with the following requirements.

Ethanol content 80 to 88% v/v, Appendix VIII F, Method III.

Dry residue 2.0 to 3.0% w/v.

Relative density 0.832 to 0.846, Appendix V G.

Weak Ginger Tincture

Definition

Strong Ginger Tincture	200 ml
Ethanol (90 per cent)	sufficient to produce 1000 ml

The tincture complies with the requirements stated under Tinctures and with the following requirements.

Ethanol content 86 to 90% v/v, Appendix VIII F, Method III.

Dry residue Not less than 0.4% w/v. Use 10 ml.

Relative density 0.825 to 0.835, Appendix V G.

Glibenclamide Tablets

Definition Glibenclamide Tablets contain Glibenclamide.

With the exception of the requirements for shape, the tablets comply with the requirements stated under Tablets and with the following requirements.

Content of glibenclamide, $C_{23}H_{28}ClN_3O_5S$ 95.0 to 105.0% of the prescribed or stated amount.

Identification

A. In the Assay, the principal peak in the chromatogram obtained with solution (1) has the same retention time as that of the principal peak in the chromatogram obtained with solution (2).

B. In the test for Related substances, the principal spot in the chromatogram obtained with solution (1) corresponds to that in the chromatogram obtained with solution (4).

Related substances Carry out the method for *thin-layer chromatography*, Appendix III A, using *silica gel GF_{254}* as the coating substance and a mixture of 45 volumes of *chloroform*, 45 volumes of *cyclohexane*, 5 volumes of *ethanol (96%)* and 5 volumes of *glacial acetic acid* as the mobile phase. Apply separately to the plate 10 µl of each of the following solutions. For solution (1) extract a quantity of the powdered tablets containing 20 mg of Glibenclamide with four 5-ml quantities of a mixture of 20 volumes of *dichloromethane* and 10 volumes of *acetone*, evaporate the combined extracts to dryness at a temperature not exceeding 40° at a pressure of 2 kPa and dissolve the residue in 4 ml of a mixture of equal volumes of *chloroform* and *methanol*. Solution (2) contains 0.012% w/v of *4-[2-(5-chloro-2-methoxybenzamido)ethyl]benzenesulphonamide BPCRS* in a mixture of equal volumes of *chloroform* and *methanol*. Solution (3) contains 0.0020% w/v of *methyl* N-*4-[2-(5-chloro-2-methoxybenzamido)ethyl]benzenesulphonylcarbamate BPCRS* in a mixture of equal volumes of *chloroform* and *methanol*. Solution (4) contains 0.5% w/v of *glibenclamide BPCRS* in a mixture of equal volumes of *chloroform* and *methanol*. After removal of the plate, allow it to dry in air and examine under *ultraviolet light (254 nm)*. Any spots corresponding to 4-[2-(5-chloro-2-methoxybenzamido)ethyl]benzenesulphonamide and methyl *N*-4-[2-(5-chloro-2-methoxybenzamido)ethyl]-benzenesulphonylcarbamate in the chromatogram obtained with solution (1) are not more intense than the spots in the chromatograms obtained with solutions (2) and (3) respectively.

Uniformity of content Tablets containing 5 mg or less of Glibenclamide comply with the requirements stated under Tablets using the following method of analysis. Carry out the method for *liquid chromatography*, Appendix III D, using the following solutions. For solution (1) powder one tablet, add a mixture of 2 ml of *water* and 20 ml of *methanol*, mix with the aid of ultrasound until fully dispersed and filter through a 0.2-µm membrane filter (Anatop LC is suitable). For solution (2) add 2 ml of *water* to 20 ml of a 0.025% w/v solution of *glibenclamide BPCRS* in *methanol*, mix with the aid of ultrasound until fully dispersed and filter (0.2-µm Anatop LC is suitable).

The chromatographic procedure described under Assay may be used.

Calculate the content of $C_{23}H_{28}ClN_3O_5S$ in each tablet using the declared content of $C_{23}H_{28}ClN_3O_5S$ in *glibenclamide BPCRS*.

Assay Weigh and powder 20 tablets. Carry out the method for *liquid chromatography*, Appendix III D, using the following solutions. For solution (1) mix, with the aid of ultrasound, a quantity of the powdered tablets containing 5 mg of Glibenclamide with a mixture of 2 ml of *water* and 20 ml of *methanol* until fully dispersed and filter through a 0.2-µm membrane filter (Anatop LC is suitable). For solution (2) dissolve 50 mg of *glibenclamide BPCRS* in 10 ml of *methanol* with the aid of ultrasound for 20 minutes, add sufficient *methanol* to produce 50 ml and dilute 1 volume of this solution to 4 volumes with *methanol*. To 20 ml of this solution add 2 ml of *water* and mix.

The chromatographic procedure may be carried out using (a) a stainless steel column (10 cm × 4.6 mm) packed with *stationary phase C* (5 µm) (Spherisorb ODS 1 is suitable), (b) as the mobile phase with a flow rate of 1.5 ml per minute a mixture of 47 volumes of *acetonitrile* and 53 volumes of a 1.36% w/v solution of *potassium dihydrogen orthophosphate* previously adjusted to pH 3.0 with *orthophosphoric acid* and (c) a detection wavelength of 300 nm. Inject 20 µl of each solution.

Calculate the content of $C_{23}H_{28}ClN_3O_5S$ using the declared content of $C_{23}H_{28}ClN_3O_5S$ in *glibenclamide BPCRS*.

Gliclazide Tablets

Definition Gliclazide Tablets contain Gliclazide.

The tablets comply with the requirements stated under Tablets and with the following requirements.

Content of gliclazide, $C_{15}H_{21}N_3O_3S$ 95.0 to 105.0% of the prescribed or stated amount.

Identification Shake a quantity of the powdered tablets containing 0.16 g of Gliclazide with 20 ml of *dichloromethane*, centrifuge and evaporate the supernatant liquid to dryness. The *infrared absorption spectrum* of the residue, Appendix II A, is concordant with the *reference spectrum* of gliclazide.

Related substances Carry out the method for *liquid chromatography*, Appendix III D, using the following solutions without delay. For solution (1) shake a quantity of the powdered tablets containing 0.8 g of Gliclazide for 1 hour with 200 ml of *acetonitrile*, filter and dilute 10 ml of the filtrate to 50 ml with a mixture of 1 volume of *acetonitrile* and 2 volumes of *water*. For solution (2) dilute 1 volume of solution (1) to 500 volumes with a mixture of 45 volumes of *acetonitrile* and 55 volumes of *water*. For solution (3) dissolve 5 mg of *gliclazide BPCRS* and 15 mg of *1-(3-azabicyclo[3.3.0]oct-3-yl)-3-*o*-tolylsulphonylurea BPCRS* in 25 ml of *acetonitrile*, dilute to 50 ml with *water* and dilute 1 volume of the resulting solution to 20 volumes with a mixture of 45 volumes of *acetonitrile* and 55 volumes of *water*. For solution (4) dissolve 8 mg of *1-(3-azabicyclo[3.3.0]oct-3-yl)-3-*o*-tolylsulphonylurea BPCRS* in 25 ml of *acetonitrile*, dilute to 50 ml with *water* and dilute 1 volume of the resulting solution to 100 volumes with a mixture of 45 volumes of *acetonitrile* and 55 volumes of *water*.

The chromatographic procedure may be carried out using (a) a stainless steel column (25 cm × 4 mm) packed with *stationary phase B* (4 µm) (Superspher 60RP8 is suitable), (b) a mixture of 0.1 volume of *triethylamine*, 0.1 volume of *trifluoroacetic acid*, 45 volumes of *acetonitrile* and 55 volumes of *water* as the mobile phase with a flow rate of 0.9 ml per minute and (c) a detection wavelength of 235 nm. Inject separately 20 µl of each solution. For solution (1) allow the chromatography to proceed for twice the retention time of the principal peak.

The test is not valid unless the *resolution factor* between the peaks in the chromatogram obtained with solution (3) is at least 1.8.

In the chromatogram obtained with solution (1) the area of any peak corresponding to 1-(3-azabicyclo[3.3.0]-oct-3-yl)-3-*o*-tolylsulphonylurea is not greater than the area of the principal peak in the chromatogram obtained with solution (4) (0.2%), the area of any other *secondary peak* is not greater than the area of the principal peak in the chromatogram obtained with solution (2) (0.2%) and the sum of the areas of any other *secondary peaks* is not greater than twice the area of the principal peak in the chromatogram obtained with solution (2) (0.4%). Disregard any peak with an area less than one quarter of the area of the peak corresponding to gliclazide in the chromatogram obtained with solution (2) (0.05%).

Assay Weigh and powder 20 tablets. Carry out the method for *liquid chromatography*, Appendix III D, using the following solutions. For solution (1) shake a quantity of the powdered tablets containing 0.8 g of Gliclazide for 1 hour with 200 ml of *acetonitrile*, filter and dilute 10 ml of the filtrate to 200 ml with a mixture of 2 volumes of *acetonitrile* and 3 volumes of *water*. For solution (2) dissolve 40 mg of *gliclazide BPCRS* in 10 ml of *acetonitrile* and dilute to 200 ml with a mixture of 2 volumes of *acetonitrile* and 3 volumes of *water*. For solution (3) dissolve 5 mg of *gliclazide BPCRS* and 15 mg of *1-(3-azabicyclo[3.3.0]oct-3-yl)-3-*o*-tolylsulphonylurea BPCRS* in 25 ml of *acetonitrile*, dilute to 50 ml with *water* and dilute 1 volume of the resulting solution to 20 volumes with a mixture of 45 volumes of *acetonitrile* and 55 volumes of *water*.

The chromatographic procedure described under Related substances may be used.

The test is not valid unless the *resolution factor* between the peaks in the chromatogram obtained with solution (3) is at least 1.8.

Calculate the content of $C_{15}H_{21}N_3O_3S$ in the tablets using the declared content of $C_{15}H_{21}N_3O_3S$ in *gliclazide BPCRS*.

Glipizide Tablets

Definition Glipizide Tablets contain Glipizide.

The tablets comply with the requirements stated under Tablets and with the following requirements.

Content of glipizide $C_{21}H_{27}N_5O_4S$ 90.0 to 110.0% of the prescribed or stated amount.

Identification

A. The *light absorption*, Appendix II B, in the range 210 to 320 nm of the final solution obtained in the Assay exhibits maxima at 226 nm and 274 nm.

B. Shake a quantity of the powdered tablets containing 25 mg of Glipizide with 10 ml of *dichloromethane* for 5 minutes, filter, dry the filtrate with *anhydrous sodium sulphate*, filter again and evaporate the filtrate to dryness. The *infrared absorption spectrum* of the residue, Appendix II A, is concordant with the *reference spectrum* of glipizide.

Related substances Carry out the method for *thin-layer chromatography*, Appendix III A, using a silica gel GF_{254} precoated plate (Merck silica gel 60 F_{254} plates are suitable) and a mixture of 20 volumes of *ethyl acetate*, 20 volumes of *anhydrous formic acid* and 40 volumes of *dichloromethane* as the mobile phase. Apply separately to the plate 20 µl of each of the following solutions. For solution (1) extract a quantity of the powdered tablets containing 0.1 g of Glipizide with four 10-ml quantities of *acetone*, evaporate the combined extracts to dryness under reduced pressure at a temperature not exceeding 30° and dissolve the residue in sufficient of a mixture of equal volumes of *dichloromethane* and *methanol* to produce 5 ml. For solution (2) dilute 1 volume of solution (1) to 200 volumes with a mixture of equal volumes of *dichloromethane* and *methanol*. For solution (3) dilute 1 volume of solution (1) to 500 volumes with the same solvent mixture. Solution (4) contains 0.010% w/v of *4-[2-(5-methylpyrazine-2-carboxamido)ethyl]benzenesulphonamide BPCRS* in a mixture of equal volumes of *dichloromethane* and *methanol*. After removal of the plate, allow it to dry in air and examine under *ultraviolet light (254 nm)*. Any spot corresponding to 4-[2-(5-methylpyrazine-2-carboxamido)ethyl]-benzenesulphonamide in the chromatogram obtained with solution (1) is not more intense than the spot in the chromatogram obtained with solution (4) (0.5%). Any other *secondary spot* is not more intense than the spot in the chromatogram obtained with solution (2) (0.5%) and not more than two such spots are more intense than the spot in the chromatogram obtained with solution (3) (0.2%).

Assay Weigh and powder 20 tablets. To a quantity of the powder containing 15 mg of Glipizide add 30 ml of *methanol*, heat gently on a water bath whilst shaking, cool and add sufficient *methanol* to produce 50 ml. Filter and dilute 5 ml of the filtrate to 50 ml with *methanol*. Measure the *absorbance* of the resulting solution at the maximum at 274 nm, Appendix II B, using *methanol* in the reference cell. Calculate the content of $C_{21}H_{27}N_5O_4S$ taking 237 as the value of A(1%, 1 cm) at the maximum at 274 nm.

Gliquidone Tablets

Definition Gliquidone Tablets contain Gliquidone.

The tablets comply with the requirements stated under Tablets and with the following requirements.

Content of gliquidone, $C_{27}H_{33}N_3O_6S$ 95.0 to 105.0% of the prescribed or stated amount.

Identification

A. Extract a quantity of the powdered tablets containing 30 mg of Gliquidone in 10 ml of *methanol* with the aid of ultrasound, filter, evaporate the filtrate to dryness using a rotary evaporator and dry the residue at a temperature of 50° at a pressure of 2 kPa for 1 hour. The *infrared absorption spectrum* of the dried residue, Appendix II A, is concordant with the *reference spectrum* of gliquidone.

B. In the test for Related substances, the principal spot in the chromatogram obtained with solution (1) corresponds to that in the chromatogram obtained with solution (2).

Dissolution Comply with the *dissolution test for tablets and capsules*, Appendix XII D, using Apparatus II. Use as the medium 900 ml of a citro-phosphate buffer prepared by dissolving 35.6 g of *disodium hydrogen orthophosphate dihydrate* in sufficient *water* to produce 1000 ml, adjusting the pH to 8.5 with *citric acid*, and rotate the paddle at 75 revolutions per minute. Withdraw a sample of 50 ml of the medium and filter (Whatman No 1 filter paper is suitable), discarding the first 15 ml of filtrate. Measure the *absorbance* of the filtered solution, Appendix II B, at the maximum at 314 nm using a filtered solution of the dissolution medium in the reference cell. Measure the *absorbance* of a solution of *gliquidone BPCRS* prepared in the following manner. Dissolve about 30 mg of *gliquidone BPCRS* in 10 ml of *dimethylformamide*, add sufficient dissolution medium to produce 100 ml and mix. Dilute 10 ml of this solution to 100 ml with dissolution medium, mix and filter (Whatman No 1 filter paper is suitable), discarding the first 15 ml of filtrate. Calculate the total content of gliquidone, $C_{27}H_{33}N_3O_6S$, in the medium from the absorbances obtained and from the declared content of $C_{27}H_{33}N_3O_6S$ in *gliquidone BPCRS*.

Related substances Carry out the method for *thin-layer chromatography*, Appendix III A, using *silica gel GF_{254}* as the coating substance and a mixture of 5 volumes of *glacial acetic acid*, 5 volumes of *ethanol (96%)*, 45 volumes of *chloroform* and 45 volumes of *cyclohexane* as the mobile phase but allowing the solvent front to ascend 10 cm above the line of application. Apply separately to the plate 10 µl of each of the following five solutions. For solution (1) mix a quantity of the powdered tablets containing 0.1 g of Gliquidone with 8 ml of a mixture of 50 volumes of *dichloromethane* and 50 volumes of *methanol*, mix with the aid of ultrasound for 10 minutes, add sufficient of the same solvent mixture to produce 10 ml, filter (Whatman GF/C filter paper is suitable) and use the filtrate. Solution (2) contains 1.0% w/v of *gliquidone BPCRS* in a mixture of 50 volumes of *dichloromethane* and 50 volumes of *methanol*. Solution (3) contains 0.0030% w/v of *gliquidone BPCRS* in a mixture of 50 volumes of *dichloromethane* and 50 volumes of *methanol*. Solution (4) contains 0.010% w/v of *gliquidone sulphonamide BPCRS* in a mixture of 50 volumes of *dichloromethane* and 50 volumes of *methanol*. For solution (5) mix 1 volume of solution (3) and 1 volume of solution (4). After removal of the plate, allow it to dry in air and examine under *ultraviolet light (254 nm)*. In the chromatogram obtained with solution (1) any spot corresponding to gliquidone sulphonamide is not more intense than the spot in the chromatogram obtained with solution (4) (1%) and any other *secondary spot* is not more intense than the spot in the chromatogram obtained with solution (3) (0.3%). The test is not valid unless the chromatogram obtained with solution (5) shows two clearly separated principal spots.

Assay Weigh and powder 20 tablets. To a quantity of the powdered tablets containing 0.1 g of Gliquidone add 50 ml of *methanol*, mix with the aid of ultrasound for 10 minutes, allow to cool, add sufficient *methanol* to produce 100 ml and filter. Dilute 15 ml of the filtrate to 100 ml with *methanol* and measure the *absorbance* of the resulting solution at the maximum at 310 nm, Appendix II B. Calculate the content of $C_{27}H_{33}N_3O_6S$ in the tablets from the *absorbance* of a 0.015% w/v solution of *gliquidone BPCRS* in *methanol* and using the declared content of $C_{27}H_{33}N_3O_6S$ in *gliquidone BPCRS*.

Glucagon Injection

Definition Glucagon Injection is a sterile solution of Glucagon with Hydrochloric Acid and Lactose in a suitable liquid. It is prepared by dissolving Glucagon for Injection in the liquid stated on the label.

The injection complies with the requirements stated under Parenteral Preparations.

Storage Glucagon Injection should be used immediately after preparation but, in any case, within the period recommended by the manufacturer when prepared and stored strictly in accordance with the manufacturer's instructions. If it shows any signs of gel formation or insoluble matter it should be discarded.

GLUCAGON FOR INJECTION

Definition Glucagon for Injection is a sterile material consisting of Glucagon with or without excipients. It is supplied in a sealed container.

The contents of the sealed container comply with the requirements for Powders for Injections stated under Parenteral Preparations and with the following requirements.

Identification

A. In the test for Related peptides, the principal band in the gel obtained with solution (4) corresponds to that in the gel obtained with solution (3).

B. When heated with *cupri-tartaric solution R1* a copious precipitate of copper(I) oxide is produced.

Acidity pH of a solution containing 1 IU per ml, 2.5 to 4.0, Appendix V L.

Light absorption Dissolve the contents of a sealed container in sufficient *water* to produce a solution containing 1 IU in 10 ml (solution A). Add 2 ml of 0.5M *hydrochloric acid* to 4 ml of solution A and add sufficient *water* to produce 10 ml (solution B). Add 2 ml of 0.5M *sodium hydroxide* to 4 ml of solution A and add sufficient *water* to produce 10 ml (solution C). Measure the *absorbances* of solutions B and C at 244 nm, Appendix II B, using *water* in the reference cell and subtract the *absorbance* of solution B from that of solution C (ΔA_u).

Repeat the entire operation using a solution prepared by dissolving an amount of the Standard Preparation of glucagon containing 1.49 IU in sufficient *water* to produce 10 ml in place of solution A (ΔA_s).

The ratio $\Delta A_u/\Delta A_s$ for sealed containers containing 1 IU is 0.634 to 0.833 and for sealed containers containing 10 IU is 0.620 to 0.753.

Related peptides Carry out the method for *polyacrylamide gel electrophoresis*, Appendix III F, using *rod gels* 75 mm long and 5 mm in diameter and, as buffer, *tris-glycine buffer solution pH 8.3*. The electrode in the upper reservoir is the cathode and that in the lower reservoir the anode. Use a gel mixture prepared in the following manner. Mix 1 volume of a solution containing 36.6 mg of *tris(hydroxymethyl)methylamine*, 0.23 ml of *tetramethylethylenediamine* and 48 ml of 1M *hydrochloric acid* in sufficient *water* to produce 100 ml and 2 volumes of a solution containing 0.735 g of *N,N′-methylenebisacrylamide* and 30.0 g of *acrylamide* in sufficient *water* to produce 100 ml. Apply 100 µl of each of the following solutions separately to the surface of a gel. Solutions (1), (2) and (3) contain 6 × 10^{-3}, 8 × 10^{-3} and 10 × 10^{-3} IU respectively of the Standard Preparation of glucagon in 50 ml of 0.01M *sodium hydroxide*. Solutions (4) and (5) contain 10×10^{-3} and 50×10^{-3} IU respectively of the preparation being examined in 50 ml of 0.01M *sodium hydroxide*. After the addition of the buffer, add 0.2 ml of *bromophenol blue solution*. Allow electrophoresis to take place with a constant current of 1 mA per tube for 30 minutes and then increase the current to 3 mA per tube. Immerse the gels for 1 hour in *naphthalene black solution* in test tubes, transfer to stoppered plastic containers with perforated walls and stir in 1M *acetic acid* overnight to remove the excess of dye. Evaluate the gels on a cold-light illuminator. In the gel prepared with solution (5) the intensity of any band that migrates immediately ahead of the principal band does not exceed that of the principal band in the gel prepared with solution (3). The test is not valid unless a gradation is observed in the intensity of staining of the gels prepared with solutions (1) to (3).

Water Not more than 7.5% w/w, Appendix IX C. Use 0.3 g.

Bacterial endotoxins Carry out the *test for bacterial endotoxins*, Appendix XIV C. Dissolve the contents of the sealed container in *water BET* to give a solution containing 1 IU of Glucagon per ml (solution A). The endotoxin limit concentration of solution A is 116.67 IU of endotoxin per ml. Carry out the test using the maximum valid dilution of solution A calculated from the declared sensitivity of the lysate used in the test.

Assay Carry out the Assay described under Glucagon. The estimated potency is not less than 80% and not more than 125% of the stated potency. The fiducial limits of error are not less than 64% and not more than 156% of the stated potency.

Storage The sealed container should be protected from light and stored at a temperature not exceeding 25°.

Labelling The label of the sealed container states the number of IU (Units) contained in it.

Glucose Intravenous Infusion

Definition Glucose Intravenous Infusion is a sterile solution of Anhydrous Glucose or Glucose in Water for Injections.

The intravenous infusion complies with the requirements stated under Parenteral Preparations and with the following requirements.

Content of glucose, $C_6H_{12}O_6$ 95.0 to 105.0% of the prescribed or stated amount.

Characteristics A colourless solution. Solutions containing the equivalent of 200 g per litre or more of glucose, $C_6H_{12}O_6$, may be not more than faintly straw coloured.

Identification

A. Heat with *cupri-tartaric solution R1*. A red precipitate is produced.

B. The solution prepared as directed in the Assay is dextrorotatory.

Acidity pH, 3.5 to 6.5, Appendix V L, when determined on a solution diluted, if necessary, with *water for injections*, to contain not more than the equivalent of 5% w/v of glucose, $C_6H_{12}O_6$, and to which 0.30 ml of a saturated solution of *potassium chloride* has been added for each 100 ml of solution.

5-Hydroxymethylfurfural and related substances Dilute a volume containing the equivalent of 1.0 g of glucose, $C_6H_{12}O_6$, to 250 ml with *water*. The *absorbance* of the resulting solution at the maximum at 284 nm is not more than 0.25, Appendix II B.

Particulate contamination When supplied in a container with a nominal content of 100 ml or more, complies with the *test for sub-visible particles*, Appendix XIII A.

Bacterial endotoxins The endotoxin limit concentration is 0.25 IU per ml, Appendix XIV C. Dilute infusions containing more than 5% w/v (50 g per litre) of Glucose with *water BET* to contain 5% w/v.

Assay To a volume containing the equivalent of 2 g to 5 g of glucose, $C_6H_{12}O_6$, add 0.2 ml of 5M *ammonia* and sufficient *water* to produce 100 ml. Mix well, allow to stand for 30 minutes and determine the *optical rotation* in a 2-dm tube, Appendix V F. The observed rotation in degrees multiplied by 0.9477 represents the weight in g of glucose, $C_6H_{12}O_6$, in the volume taken for assay.

Storage Glucose Intravenous Infusion should be stored at a temperature not exceeding 25°.

Labelling The strength is stated as the equivalent number of grams of glucose, $C_6H_{12}O_6$, per litre.

When Glucose Intravenous Infusion is required as a diluent for Injections or Intravenous Infusions of the Pharmacopoeia, Glucose Intravenous Infusion (50 g per litre) shall be used.

Glucose Irrigation Solution

Definition Glucose Irrigation Solution is a sterile, aqueous solution of Anhydrous Glucose or Glucose.

Production Glucose Irrigation Solution intended to be used for the irrigation of body cavities, for the flushing of wounds or operation cavities or for the irrigation of the urogenital system is prepared using Water for Irrigation.

The irrigation solution complies with the requirements stated under Preparations for Irrigation and with the following requirements.

Content of glucose, $C_6H_{12}O_6$ 95.0 to 105.0% of the prescribed or stated amount.

Characteristics A colourless solution. Solutions containing the equivalent of 200 g per litre or more of glucose, $C_6H_{12}O_6$, may be not more than faintly straw coloured.

Identification

A. Heat with *cupri-tartaric solution R1*. A red precipitate is produced.

B. The solution prepared in the Assay is dextrorotatory.

Acidity pH, 3.5 to 6.5, Appendix V L, when determined in a solution diluted, if necessary, with *water* to contain not more than the equivalent of 5% w/v of glucose, $C_6H_{12}O_6$, and to which 0.30 ml of a saturated solution of *potassium chloride* has been added for each 100 ml of solution.

5-Hydroxymethylfurfural and related substances Dilute a volume containing the equivalent of 1.0 g of glucose, $C_6H_{12}O_6$, to 250 ml with *water*. The *absorbance* of the resulting solution at the maximum at 284 nm is not more than 0.25, Appendix II B.

Assay To a volume containing the equivalent of 2 to 5 g of glucose, $C_6H_{12}O_6$, add 0.2 ml of 5M *ammonia* and sufficient *water* to produce 100 ml. Mix well, allow to stand for 30 minutes and determine the *optical rotation* in a 2-dm tube, Appendix V F. The observed rotation in degrees multiplied by 0.9477 represents the weight, in g, of glucose, $C_6H_{12}O_6$, in the volume taken for assay.

Storage Glucose Irrigation Solution should be stored at a temperature not exceeding 25°.

Labelling The strength is stated in terms of the equivalent amount of glucose, $C_6H_{12}O_6$.

Glutaraldehyde Solution

Definition Glutaraldehyde Solution is a dilution of Strong Glutaraldehyde Solution in a mixture of Purified Water and Ethanol (96 per cent).

In making Glutaraldehyde Solution, Ethanol (96 per cent) may be replaced by Industrial Methylated Spirit[1].

Content of glutaraldehyde, $C_5H_8O_2$ 9.2 to 10.5% w/v.

Identification

A. Heat 5 ml with 10 ml of a solution containing 1 g of *hydroxylamine hydrochloride* and 2 g of *sodium acetate* on a water bath for 10 minutes, allow to cool and filter. The *melting point* of the residue, after washing with *water* and drying at 105°, is about 178°, Appendix V A.

B. To 1 ml add 2 ml of *ammoniacal silver nitrate solution* and mix gently for a few minutes. Silver is deposited.

Ethanol content 50.0 to 60.0% v/v, Appendix VIII F.

Assay Mix 10 ml with 100 ml of a 7% w/v solution of *hydroxylamine hydrochloride* previously neutralised to *bromophenol blue solution* with 1M *sodium hydroxide VS* and allow to stand for 30 minutes. Add 20 ml of *petroleum spirit (boiling range, 40° to 60°)* and titrate with 1M *sodium hydroxide VS* until the colour of the aqueous phase matches that of a 7% w/v solution of *hydroxylamine hydrochloride* previously neutralised to *bromophenol blue solution* with 1M *sodium hydroxide VS*. Each ml of 1M *sodium hydroxide VS* is equivalent to 50.05 mg of $C_5H_8O_2$.

Storage Glutaraldehyde Solution should be kept in a well-closed container and stored at a temperature not exceeding 15°.

Labelling The label states (1) the date after which the solution is not intended to be used; (2) the conditions under which it should be stored.

[1]The law and the statutory regulations governing the use of Industrial Methylated Spirit must be observed.

Glycerol Suppositories

Glycerin Suppositories

Definition

Gelatin	14 g
Glycerol	70 g
Purified Water	a sufficient quantity

In tropical and subtropical countries the quantity of Gelatin may be increased to an amount not exceeding 18 g.

Extemporaneous preparation The following directions apply.

Add the Gelatin to about 30 ml of Purified Water heated nearly to boiling, then add the Glycerol previously heated to 100° and heat the mixture on a water bath for 15 minutes or until solution is complete. Adjust the weight of the product to 100 g by the addition of hot Purified Water or by evaporation on a water bath and pour into suitable moulds.

The suppositories comply with the requirements stated under Rectal Preparations and with the following requirements.

Content of glycerol, $C_3H_8O_3$ 66.5 to 73.5% w/w.

Disintegration Maximum time, 1 hour, Appendix XII C.

Assay Dissolve a number of suppositories containing 8 g of Glycerol in 50 ml of *water* and add sufficient *water* to produce 250 ml. To 5 ml add 150 ml of *water* and 0.25 ml of *bromocresol purple solution* and neutralise with 0.1M *sodium hydroxide VS* to the blue colour of the indicator. Add 1.6 g of *sodium periodate* and allow to stand for 15 minutes. Add 3 ml of *propan-1,2-diol*, shake, allow to stand for 5 minutes and titrate with 0.1M *sodium hydroxide VS* to the same blue colour. Each ml of 0.1M *sodium hydroxide VS* is equivalent to 9.210 mg of $C_3H_8O_3$.

Glyceryl Trinitrate Tablets

Trinitrin Tablets; Nitroglycerin Tablets

Definition Glyceryl Trinitrate Tablets are made with Mannitol as the basis and may be prepared by adding Concentrated Glyceryl Trinitrate Solution to dried granules of Mannitol, mixing intimately, drying at a temperature not exceeding 50° or without heating for not more than 4 hours and compressing.

CAUTION *Undiluted glyceryl trinitrate can be exploded by percussion or excessive heat. Appropriate precautions should be exercised and only exceedingly small amounts should be isolated.*

The tablets comply with the requirements stated under Tablets and with the following requirements.

Content of glyceryl trinitrate, $C_3H_5N_3O_9$ 85.0 to 115.0% of the prescribed or stated amount.

Identification

A. Carry out the method for *thin-layer chromatography*, Appendix III A, using *silica gel G* as the coating substance and *toluene* as the mobile phase. Apply separately to the plate 20 µl of each of the following solutions. For solution (1) extract a quantity of the powdered tablets containing 0.5 mg of glyceryl trinitrate with 1 ml of *acetone* and centrifuge. For solution (2) extract one powdered *glyceryl trinitrate tablet 0.5 mg BPCRS* with 1 ml of *acetone* and centrifuge. After removal of the plate, dry it in a stream of air, spray with *diphenylamine solution R1* and irradiate for 15 minutes with *ultraviolet light (365 nm)*. Examine the plate in daylight. The spot in the chromatogram obtained with solution (1) corresponds to that in the chromatogram obtained with solution (2).

B. Extract a quantity of the powdered tablets containing 3 mg of glyceryl trinitrate with 5 ml of *ether* and filter. Evaporate the ether and dissolve the residue in 0.2 ml of *sulphuric acid* containing a trace of *diphenylamine*. An intense blue colour is produced.

Distintegration The requirement for Disintegration does not apply to Glyceryl Trinitrate Tablets.

Uniformity of content Tablets containing less than 2 mg of glyceryl trinitrate comply with the requirements stated under Tablets using the following method of analysis. Place one tablet in a centrifuge tube containing a few glass beads, add 5.0 ml of a 90% v/v solution of *glacial acetic acid*, shake for 1 hour and centrifuge. Carry out the Assay described under Concentrated Glyceryl Trinitrate Solution beginning at the words 'To 1 ml of the resulting solution ...'.

For tablets containing 0.4 to 0.6 mg of glyceryl trinitrate Use 1 ml of a mixture of equal volumes of the potassium nitrate solution and *glacial acetic acid* in the repeat procedure.

For tablets containing 0.2 to 0.3 mg of glyceryl trinitrate Use 2.0 ml of the resulting solution, prepare the blank with 2 ml of a 90% v/v solution of *glacial acetic acid* and use 2.0 ml of a mixture of 3 volumes of *glacial acetic acid* and 1 volume of the potassium nitrate solution in the repeat procedure.

For tablets containing less than 0.2 mg of glyceryl trinitrate Use 2 ml of the resulting solution, measure the *absorbance* of 2-cm layers, prepare the blank with 2 ml of a 90% v/v solution of *glacial acetic acid* and use 2 ml of a mixture of 7 volumes of *glacial acetic acid* and 1 volume of the potassium nitrate solution in the repeat procedure.

Assay Weigh and powder 20 tablets. To a quantity of the powder containing 1 mg of glyceryl trinitrate add 5 ml of a 90% v/v solution of *glacial acetic acid*, shake for 1 hour and centrifuge. To 1 ml of the resulting solution add 2 ml of *phenoldisulphonic acid solution*, mix and allow to stand for 15 minutes. Add 8 ml of *water*, mix well, allow to cool and add slowly, with swirling, 10 ml of 13.5M *ammonia*. Cool and dilute to 20 ml with *water*. Measure the *absorbance* of the resulting solution at 405 nm, Appendix II B, using in the reference cell 1 ml of a 90% v/v solution of *glacial acetic acid* treated in the same manner, beginning at the words 'add 2 ml of *phenoldisulphonic acid solution* ...'. Dissolve 0.1335 g of *potassium nitrate* previously dried at 105° in sufficient *water* to produce 50 ml; to 10 ml add sufficient *glacial acetic acid* to produce 100 ml. Using 1 ml of this solution, repeat the procedure beginning at the words 'add 2 ml of *phenoldisulphonic acid solution* ...'. Calculate the content of $C_3H_5N_3O_9$ from the values of the absorbances so obtained. Each ml of the potassium nitrate solution is equivalent to 0.2000 mg of $C_3H_5N_3O_9$.

Storage Glyceryl Trinitrate Tablets should be protected from light and stored at a temperature not exceeding 25° in a glass container closed by means of a screw closure lined with aluminium or tin foil; additional packing that absorbs glyceryl trinitrate should be avoided. Glyceryl Trinitrate Tablets should be issued for patients in containers of not more than 100 tablets.

Labelling The label states that the tablets should be allowed to dissolve slowly in the mouth.

Glycine Irrigation Solution

Definition Glycine Irrigation Solution is a sterile, apyrogenic solution of Glycine in Water for Irrigation.

The irrigation solution complies with the requirements stated under Preparations for Irrigation and with the following requirements.

Content of glycine, $C_2H_5NO_2$ 95.0 to 105.0% of the prescribed or stated amount.

Characteristics A colourless solution.

Identification

A. Evaporate 5 ml to dryness on a water bath and dry at 105° for 1 hour. The *infrared absorption spectrum*, Appendix II A, is concordant with the *reference spectrum* of glycine.

B. Carry out the method for *thin-layer chromatography*, Appendix III A, using *silica gel G* as the coating substance and a mixture of 30 volumes of 13.5M *ammonia* and 70 volumes of *propan-1-ol* as the mobile phase. Apply separately to the plate 2 µl of each of the following solutions. For solution (1) dilute the irrigation solution with *water* to contain 0.25% w/v of Glycine. Solution (2) contains 0.25% w/v of *glycine* in *water*. After removal of the plate, dry it at 100° to 105° for 10 minutes, spray with *ninhydrin solution* and heat at 100° to 105° for 2 minutes. The principal spot in the chromatogram obtained with solution (1) corresponds to that in the chromatogram obtained with solution (2).

Acidity pH, 4.5 to 6.5, Appendix V L.

Ammonium compounds Dilute a volume containing 0.2 g of Glycine to 70 ml with *water* in an ammonia-distillation apparatus, add 25 ml of a solution prepared by boiling 25 ml of 5M *sodium hydroxide* with 50 ml of *water* and 50 mg of *aluminium* until the volume is reduced to 25 ml and distil into 2 ml of a saturated solution of *boric acid* until 50 ml is obtained. Add 2 ml of a solution prepared by boiling 25 ml of 5M *sodium hydroxide* with 50 ml of *water* until the volume is reduced to 25 ml and 2 ml of *alkaline potassium tetraiodomercurate solution*. Any colour produced is not more intense than that obtained by treating 70 ml of *water* containing 4 ml of *ammonia standard solution (10 ppm NH_4)* in the same manner, beginning at the words 'add 25 ml of ...' (200 ppm, calculated with reference to the content of glycine).

Assay Dilute a volume containing 0.15 g of Glycine to 25 ml with *water* and add 10 ml of *formaldehyde solution* previously adjusted to pH 9.0 and 0.25 ml of a mixed indicator solution prepared by dissolving 75 mg of *phenolphthalein* and 25 mg of *thymol blue* in 100 ml of *ethanol (50%)*. Titrate with 0.1M *sodium hydroxide VS* until the yellow colour disappears and a faint violet colour is produced. Each ml of 0.1M *sodium hydroxide VS* is equivalent to 7.507 mg of $C_2H_5NO_2$.

Labelling The label states that the Irrigation Solution is apyrogenic.

Gonadorelin Injection

Definition Gonadorelin Injection is a sterile solution of Gonadorelin Acetate or Gonadorelin Hydrochloride in Water for Injections. It is either supplied as a ready-to-use solution or it is prepared by dissolving Gonadorelin for Injection in the liquid stated on the label.

The injection complies with the requirements stated under Parenteral Preparations and, when supplied as a ready-to-use solution, with the following requirements.

Content of gonadorelin, $C_{55}H_{75}N_{17}O_{13}$ 90.0 to 110.0% of the prescribed or stated amount of the peptide.

Characteristics A colourless solution.

Identification

A. Carry out the method for *thin-layer chromatography*, Appendix III A, using *silica gel H* as the coating substance and a mixture of 6 volumes of *glacial acetic acid*, 14 volumes of *water*, 45 volumes of *methanol* and 60 volumes of *chloroform* as the mobile phase. Apply separately to the plate 10 µl of each of the following solutions. For solution (1) freeze dry a volume of the injection containing the equivalent of 20 mg of the peptide and dissolve the residue in 0.2 ml of *water*. Solution (2) contains a quantity of *gonadorelin EPCRS* in sufficient *water* to produce a solution containing the equivalent of 0.01% w/v of the peptide. For solution (3) mix equal volumes of solutions (1) and (2). After removal of the plate, allow it to dry in air for 5 minutes. Place the plate in a closed tank of chlorine gas, prepared by the addition of *hydrochloric acid* to a 5% w/v solution of *potassium permanganate* in a container placed at the bottom of the tank, and allow to stand for 2 minutes. Dry in a current of cold air until a sprayed area of the plate below the line of application gives at most a very faint blue colour with 0.05 ml of a 0.5% w/v solution of *potassium iodide* in *starch mucilage*; avoid prolonged exposure to cold air. Spray the plate with a 0.5% w/v solution of *potassium iodide* in *starch mucilage*. The principal spot in the chromatogram obtained with solution (1) corresponds to that in the chromatogram obtained with solution (2). If it does not, the principal spot in the chromatogram obtained with solution (3) appears as a single, compact spot.

B. In the Assay, the principal peak in the chromatogram obtained with solution (1) corresponds to that in the chromatogram obtained with solution (2).

Acidity or alkalinity pH, 4.5 to 8.0, Appendix V L.

Assay Carry out the method for *liquid chromatography*, Appendix III D, using the following solutions. For solution (1) dilute the injection with a mixture of 85 volumes of 0.1M *orthophosphoric acid* adjusted to pH 3.0 with *triethylamine* and 15 volumes of *acetonitrile* to give a final concentration of 0.01% w/v of the peptide. For solution (2) dissolve a quantity of *gonadorelin EPCRS* in sufficient of the above solvent mixture to produce a solution containing 0.01% w/v of the peptide.

The chromatographic procedure may be carried out using (a) a stainless steel column (15 cm × 4.6 mm) packed with *stationary phase* C (5 µm) (Spherisorb ODS 1 is suitable), (b) as the mobile phase with a flow rate of 1 ml per minute, a mixture of a 1% w/v solution of *orthophosphoric acid* adjusted to pH 3.0 with *triethylamine* and *acetonitrile*, the mixture being adjusted so that the retention time of gonadorelin is about 10 minutes (a mixture of 75 volumes of a 1% w/v solution of *orthophosphoric acid* adjusted to pH 3.0 with *triethylamine* and 25 volumes of *acetonitrile* is usually suitable) and (c) a detection wavelength of 220 nm.

The assay is not valid unless the *column efficiency* is at least 20,000 theoretical plates per metre.

Storage When supplied as a ready-to-use solution, Gonadorelin Injection should be protected from light and stored at a temperature not exceeding 25°.

Gonadorelin Injection prepared by dissolving the contents of a sealed container in the liquid stated on the label should be used immediately after preparation but, in any case, within the period recommended by the manufacturer when prepared and stored strictly in accordance with the manufacturer's instructions.

Labelling The label states whether the contents are Gonadorelin Acetate or Gonadorelin Hydrochloride.

The strength is stated in terms of the equivalent number of micrograms of the peptide in a suitable dose-volume.

GONADORELIN FOR INJECTION

Definition Gonadorelin for Injection is a sterile material consisting of Gonadorelin Acetate or Gonadorelin Hydrochloride with or without excipients. It is supplied in a sealed container.

The contents of the sealed container comply with the requirements for Powders for Injections stated under Parenteral Preparations and with the following requirements.

Content of gonadorelin, $C_{55}H_{75}N_{17}O_{13}$ 90.0 to 110.0% of the prescribed or stated amount of the peptide.

Identification

A. Comply with test A described for the ready-to-use solution preparing solution (1) by dissolving a quantity containing the equivalent of 20 mg of the peptide in 0.2 ml of *water*.

B. In the Assay the principal peak in the chromatogram obtained with solution (1) corresponds to that in the chromatogram obtained with solution (2).

Assay Carry out the Assay described for the ready-to-use solution using the following solutions. For solution (1) dissolve the contents of a sealed container in sufficient of a mixture of 85 volumes of 0.1M *orthophosphoric acid* adjusted to pH 3.0 with *triethylamine* and 15 volumes of *acetonitrile* to give a final concentration of 0.01% w/v of the peptide. For solution (2) dissolve a quantity of *gonadorelin EPCRS* in sufficient of the above solvent mixture to produce a solution containing 0.01% w/v of the peptide.

Storage The contents of the sealed container should be stored at a temperature not exceeding 25°.

Labelling The label of the sealed container states (1) the total equivalent number of micrograms of the peptide in it; (2) whether the contents are Gonadorelin Acetate or Gonadorelin Hydrochloride.

Griseofulvin Tablets

Definition Griseofulvin Tablets contain Griseofulvin.

The tablets comply with the requirements stated under Tablets and with the following requirements.

Content of griseofulvin, $C_{17}H_{17}ClO_6$ 95.0 to 105.0% of the prescribed or stated amount.

Identification

A. Extract a quantity of the powdered tablets containing 0.125 g of Griseofulvin with 20 ml of *chloroform*, add 1 g of *anhydrous sodium sulphate*, shake and filter. Evaporate the filtrate to dryness and dry at a pressure not exceeding 0.7 kPa for 1 hour. The *infrared absorption spectrum* of the residue, Appendix II A, is concordant with the *reference spectrum* of griseofulvin.

B. Shake a quantity of the powdered tablets containing 80 mg of Griseofulvin with 150 ml of *ethanol (96%)* for 20 minutes. Dilute to 200 ml with *ethanol (96%)* and filter. Dilute 2 ml of the filtrate to 100 ml with *ethanol (96%)*. The *light absorption* of the resulting solution, Appendix II B, in the range 240 to 400 nm exhibits two maxima, at 291 nm and 325 nm, and a shoulder at 250 nm.

C. Dissolve 5 mg of the powdered tablets in 1 ml of *sulphuric acid* and add 5 mg of powdered *potassium dichromate*. A red colour is produced.

Dissolution Comply with the *dissolution test for tablets and capsules*, Appendix XII D, using Apparatus II. Use as the medium 1000 ml of a 1.5% w/v solution of *sodium dodecyl sulphate* and rotate the paddle at 100 revolutions per minute. Withdraw a sample of 10 ml of the medium and filter. Measure the *absorbance* of the filtrate, suitably diluted if necessary with *methanol (80%)*, at the maximum at 291 nm, Appendix II B. Calculate the total content of $C_{17}H_{17}ClO_6$ in the medium taking 725 as the value of A(1%, 1 cm) at the maximum at 291 nm.

Related substances Dissolve 50 mg of *9,10-diphenylanthracene* (internal standard) in sufficient *chloroform* to produce 50 ml (solution A). Carry out the method for *gas chromatography*, Appendix III B, using the following solutions. For solution (1) dissolve 5 mg of *griseofulvin BPCRS* in *chloroform* and add 2 ml of solution A and sufficient *chloroform* to produce 200 ml. Evaporate 20 ml of the solution to about 1 ml. For solution (2) add 60 ml of *chloroform* to a quantity of the powdered tablets containing 50 mg of Griseofulvin, heat at 60° with shaking for 20 minutes, cool and dilute to 100 ml with *chloroform*. Centrifuge and evaporate 20 ml of the clear supernatant liquid to about 1 ml. Prepare solution (3) in the same manner as solution (2) but adding 1 ml of solution A before diluting to 100 ml with *chloroform*.

The chromatographic procedure may be carried out using a glass column (1.0 m × 4 mm) packed with *acid-washed, silanised diatomaceous support* (100 to 120 mesh) coated with 1% w/w of cyanopropylmethyl phenyl methyl silicone fluid (OV-225 is suitable) and maintained at 250°.

In the chromatogram obtained with solution (3) the ratios of the areas of any peak corresponding to dechlorogriseofulvin (retention time about 0.6 times that of griseofulvin) and of any peak corresponding to dehydrogriseofulvin (retention time about 1.4 times that of griseofulvin) to the area of the peak due to the internal standard are, respectively, not greater than 0.6 times and not greater than 0.15 times the ratio of the area of the peak due to griseofulvin to that of the internal standard in the chromatogram obtained with solution (1).

Assay Weigh and powder 20 tablets. To a quantity of the powder containing 35 mg of Griseofulvin add 60 ml of *ethyl acetate*, mix and heat to 60° with shaking for 20 minutes. Allow to cool and dilute to 100 ml with *ethyl acetate*. Centrifuge and transfer two 5-ml aliquots of the clear supernatant liquid into separate 100-ml graduated flasks. Add 5 ml of 2M *methanolic methanesulphonic acid* to the first flask, allow to stand at 20° for 30 minutes and dilute to 100 ml with *methanol* (solution A). Dilute the contents of the second flask to 100 ml with *methanol* (solution B). To a third flask add 5 ml of 2M *methanolic methanesulphonic acid* and dilute to 100 ml with *methanol* (solution C). Measure the *absorbance* of each solution at 266 nm, Appendix II B. Calculate the content of $C_{17}H_{17}ClO_6$ from the difference between the absorbance obtained with solution A and the sum of the absorbances obtained with solutions B and C and from the difference obtained by repeating the operation using 35 mg of *griseofulvin BPCRS* in place of the powdered tablets and from the declared content of $C_{17}H_{17}ClO_6$ in *griseofulvin BPCRS.*

Guanethidine Tablets

Definition Guanethidine Tablets contain Guanethidine Monosulphate.

The tablets comply with the requirements stated under Tablets and with the following requirements.

Content of guanethidine monosulphate, $C_{10}H_{22}N_4,H_2SO_4$ 90.0 to 110.0% of the prescribed or stated amount.

Identification Extract a quantity of the powdered tablets containing 50 mg of Guanethidine Monosulphate with a mixture of 5 ml of *hydrochloric acid* and 45 ml of *water*, filter, neutralise 25 ml of the filtrate with 5M *sodium hydroxide* and add 20 ml of *picric acid solution R1*. The *melting point* of the precipitate, after washing with *water*, is about 153°, Appendix V A.

Assay Weigh and powder 20 tablets. Shake a quantity of the powder containing 30 mg of Guanethidine Monosulphate for 15 minutes with 50 ml of *water*, dilute to 100 ml with *water* and filter. To 5 ml of the filtrate add 10 ml of a solution prepared by dissolving 1 g of *sodium nitroprusside* and 1 g of *potassium hexacyanoferrate(II)* in 50 ml of a 0.5% w/v solution of *sodium hydroxide*, adding 5 ml of *hydrogen peroxide solution (100 vol)*, swirling gently and diluting to 100 ml with the solution of sodium hydroxide. Mix, allow to stand for 20 minutes, add sufficient *water* to produce 25 ml and measure the *absorbance* of the resulting solution at 520 nm, Appendix II B, using in the reference cell a solution prepared by treating 5 ml of *water* in the same manner, beginning at the words 'add 10 ml of a solution ...'. Calculate the content of $C_{10}H_{22}N_4,H_2SO_4$ from the *absorbance* obtained by repeating the operation using 5 ml of a 0.03% w/v solution of *guanethidine monosulphate BPCRS* and beginning at the words 'add 10 ml of a solution ...'.

Storage Guanethidine Tablets should be protected from light.

Haemodialysis Solutions

Haemodialysis Solutions comply with the requirements of the 3rd edition of the European Pharmacopoeia for Solutions for Haemodialysis [0128]. These requirements are reproduced after the heading 'Definition' below.

Ph Eur

DEFINITION

Solutions for haemodialysis are solutions of electrolytes with a concentration close to the electrolytic composition of plasma. Glucose may be included in the formulation.

Because of the large volumes used, haemodialysis solutions are usually prepared by diluting a concentrated solution with water of suitable quality (see the monograph on *Haemodialysis solutions concentrated, water for diluting (1167)*), using for example an automatic, dosing device.

Concentrated Solutions for Haemodialysis

Concentrated haemodialysis solutions are prepared and stored using materials and methods designed to produce solutions having as low a degree of microbial contamination as possible. In certain circumstances, it may be necessary to use sterile solutions.

During dilution and use, precautions are taken to avoid microbial contamination. Diluted solutions are to be used immediately after preparation.

Concentrated solutions for haemodialysis are supplied in:
— rigid, semi-rigid or flexible plastic containers,
— glass containers.

Two types of concentrated solutions are used.

1 Concentrated solutions with acetate or lactate

Several formulations of concentrated solutions are used. The concentrations of the components in the solutions are such that after dilution to the stated volume the concentrations of the components per litre are usually in the following ranges.

Table 128-1

	Expression in mmol	Expression in mEq
Sodium	130–145	130–145
Potassium	0–3.0	0–3.0
Calcium	0–2.0	0–4.0
Magnesium	0–1.2	0–2.4
Acetate or lactate	32–45	32–45
Chloride	90–120	90–120
Glucose	0–12.0	

Concentrated solutions with acetate or lactate are diluted before use.

2 Concentrated acidic solutions

Several formulations of concentrated solutions are used. The concentrations of the components in the solutions are such that after dilution to the stated volume and before neutralisation with sodium hydrogen carbonate the concentrations of the components per litre are usually in the following ranges.

Table 128-2

Volume of *0.1M sodium thiosulphate* (millilitres)	Anhydrous glucose (milligrams)
8	19.8
9	22.4
10	25.0
11	27.6
12	30.3
13	33.0
14	35.7
15	38.5
16	41.3

Solutions of sodium hydrogen carbonate or solid sodium hydrogen carbonate may be added immediately before use to a final concentration of not more 45 mmol per litre. The concentrated solution of sodium hydrogen carbonate is supplied in a separate container. The concentrated acidic solutions and the concentrated solution of sodium hydrogen carbonate are diluted and mixed immediately before use using a suitable device. Alternatively, solid sodium hydrogen carbonate may be added to the diluted solution.

IDENTIFICATION

According to the stated composition, the solution to be examined gives the following identification reactions (*2.3.1*):
— potassium: reaction (b);
— calcium: reaction (a);
— sodium: reaction (b);
— chlorides: reaction (a);
— lactates;
— carbonates and bicarbonates;
— acetates:
if the solution is free from glucose, use reaction (b),
if the solution contains glucose, use the following method: to 5 ml of the solution to be examined add 1 ml of *hydrochloric acid R* in a test tube fitted with a stopper and a bent tube, heat and collect a few millilitres of distillate; carry out reaction (b) of acetates on the distillate;
— magnesium: to 0.1 ml of *titan yellow solution R* add 10 ml of *water R*, 2 ml of the solution to be examined and 1 ml of *1M sodium hydroxide*; a pink colour is produced;
— glucose: to 5 ml of the solution to be examined, add 2 ml of *dilute sodium hydroxide solution R* and 0.05 ml of *copper sulphate solution R*; the solution is blue and clear; heat to boiling; an abundant red precipitate is formed.

TESTS

Appearance of solution The solution is clear (*2.2.1*). If it does not contain glucose, it is colourless (*Method I, 2.2.2*). If it contains glucose, it is not more intensely coloured than reference solution Y_7 (*Method I, 2.2.2*).

Aluminium (*2.4.17*). Take 20 ml, adjust to pH 6.0 and add 10 ml of *acetate buffer solution pH 6.0 R*. The solution complies with the limit test for aluminium (0.1 mg/l). Use as the reference solution a mixture of 1 ml of *aluminium standard solution (2 ppm Al) R*, 10 ml of *acetate buffer solution pH 6.0 R* and 9 ml of *water R*. To prepare the blank use a mixture of 10 ml of *acetate buffer solution pH 6.0 R* and 10 ml of *water R*.

Extractable volume (*2.9.17*). The volume measured is not less than the nominal volume stated on the label.

Sterility (*2.6.1*). If the label states that the concentrated haemodialysis solution is sterile, it complies with the test for sterility.

Bacterial endotoxins (*2.6.14*). In the solution diluted for use, not more than 0.5 IU of endotoxin per millilitre.

Pyrogens (*2.6.8*). Solutions for which a validated test for bacterial endotoxins cannot be carried out comply with the test for pyrogens. Dilute the solution to be examined with *water for injections R* to the concentration prescribed for use. Inject 10 ml of the solution per kilogram of the rabbit's mass.

ASSAY

Determine the relative density (2.2.5) of the solution and calculate the content in grams per litre and in millimoles per litre.

Sodium 97.5 per cent to 102.5 per cent of the content of sodium (Na) stated on the label, determined by atomic absorption spectrometry (*Method II, 2.2.23*).

Test solution. Dilute with *water R* an accurately weighed quantity of the solution to be examined to a concentration suitable for the instrument to be used.

Reference solutions. Prepare the reference solutions using *sodium standard solution (200 ppm Na) R.*

Measure the absorbance at 589.0 nm using a sodium hollow-cathode lamp as source of radiation and an air-acetylene or an air-propane flame.

Potassium 95.0 per cent to 105.0 per cent of the content of potassium (K) stated on the label, determined by atomic absorption spectrometry (*Method I, 2.2.23*).

Test solution. Dilute with *water R* an accurately weighed quantity of the solution to be examined to a concentration suitable for the instrument to be used. To 100 ml of the solution add 10 ml of a 22 g/l solution of *sodium chloride R*.

Reference solutions. Prepare the reference solutions using *potassium standard solution (100 ppm K) R*. To 100 ml of each reference solution add 10 ml of a 22 g/l solution of *sodium chloride R*.

Measure the absorbance at 766.5 nm, using a potassium hollow-cathode lamp as source of radiation and an air-acetylene or an air-propane flame.

Calcium 95.0 per cent to 105.0 per cent of the content of calcium (Ca) stated on the label, determined by atomic absorption spectrometry (*Method I, 2.2.23*).

Test solution. Dilute with *water R* an accurately weighed quantity of the solution to be examined to a concentration suitable for the instrument to be used.

Reference solutions. Prepare the reference solutions using *calcium standard solution (400 ppm Ca) R.*

Measure the absorbance at 422.7 nm using a calcium hollow-cathode lamp as source of radiation and an air-acetylene or an air-propane flame.

Magnesium 95.0 per cent to 105.0 per cent of the content of magnesium (Mg) stated on the label, determined by atomic absorption spectrometry (*Method I, 2.2.23*).

Test solution. Dilute with *water R* an accurately weighed quantity of the solution to be examined to a concentration suitable for the instrument to be used.

Reference solutions. Prepare the reference solutions using *magnesium standard solution (100 ppm Mg) R.*

Measure the absorbance at 285.2 nm using a magnesium hollow-cathode lamp as source of radiation and an air-acetylene or an air-propane flame.

Total chloride 95.0 per cent to 105.0 per cent of the content of chloride (Cl) stated on the label. Dilute to 50 ml with *water R* an accurately weighed quantity of the solution to be examined containing the equivalent of about 60 mg of chloride ion. Add 5 ml of *dilute nitric acid R*, 25.0 ml of *0.1M silver nitrate* and 2 ml of *dibutyl phthalate R*. Shake. Using 2 ml of *ferric ammonium sulphate solution R2* as indicator, titrate with *0.1M ammonium thiocyanate* until a reddish-yellow colour is obtained.

1 ml of *0.1M silver nitrate* is equivalent to 3.545 mg of Cl.

Acetate 95.0 per cent to 105.0 per cent of the content of acetate stated on the label. To a volume of the solution to be examined, corresponding to about 0.7 mmol of acetate, add 10.0 ml of *0.1M hydrochloric acid.* Carry out a potentiometric titration (*2.2.20*), using *0.1M sodium hydroxide*. Read the volume added between the two points of inflexion.

1 ml of *0.1M sodium hydroxide* is equivalent to 0.1 mmol of acetate.

Lactate 95.0 per cent to 105.0 per cent of the content stated on the label. To a volume of the solution to be examined, corresponding to about 0.7 mmol of lactate, add 10.0 ml of *0.1M hydrochloric acid.* Then add 50 ml of *acetonitrile R*. Carry out a potentiometric titration (*2.2.20*), using *0.1M sodium hydroxide*. Read the volume added between the two points of inflexion.

1 ml of *0.1M sodium hydroxide* is equivalent to 0.1 mmol of lactate.

Hydrogen carbonate 95.0 per cent to 105.0 per cent of the content of sodium hydrogen carbonate stated on the label. Titrate with *0.1M hydrochloric acid* a volume of the solution to be examined corresponding to about 0.1 g of sodium hydrogen carbonate, determining the end-point potentiometrically (*2.2.20*).

1 ml of *0.1M hydrochloric acid* is equivalent to 8.40 mg of $NaHCO_3$.

Reducing sugars (expressed as anhydrous glucose). 95.0 per cent to 105.0 per cent of the content of glucose stated on the label. Transfer a volume of solution to be examined containing the equivalent of 25 mg of glucose to a 250 ml ground-glass conical flask and add 25.0 ml of *cupri-citric solution R*. Add a few grains of pumice, fit a reflux condenser, heat so that boiling occurs within 2 min and maintain ebullition for exactly 10 min. Cool and add 3 g of *potassium iodide R* dissolved in 3 ml of *water R*. Carefully add, in small amounts, 25 ml of a 25 per cent *m/m* solution of *sulphuric acid R*. Titrate with *0.1M sodium thiosulphate* using *starch solution R*, added towards at the end of the titration, as indicator. Carry out a blank titration using 25.0 ml of *water R*.

Calculate the content of glucose, expressed as anhydrous glucose ($C_6H_{12}O_6$), using Table 128-3.

Table 128-3

Volume of *0.1M sodium thiosulphate* (millilitres)	Anhydrous glucose (milligrams)
8	19.8
9	22.4
10	25.0
11	27.6
12	30.3
13	33.0
14	35.7
15	38.5
16	41.3

STORAGE

Store at a temperature not below 4°C.

LABELLING

The label of the concentrated solution states:

— the formula of the solution expressed in grams per litre and in millimoles per litre,
— the nominal volume of the solution in the container,
— where applicable, that the concentrated solution is sterile,
— the storage conditions,
— that the concentrated solution is to be diluted immediately before use,
— the dilution to be made,
— that the volume taken for use is to be measured accurately,
— the ionic formula for the diluted solution ready for use in millimoles per litre,
— that any unused portion of solution is to be discarded,
— where applicable, that sodium hydrogen carbonate is to be added before use.

Ph Eur

Water for Diluting Concentrated Haemodialysis Solutions

Information and guidance concerning Water for Diluting Concentrated Haemodialysis Solutions is provided in the 3rd edition of the European Pharmacopoeia [1167]. This information and guidance is reproduced after the heading 'Definition' below.

Ph Eur

The following monograph is given for information and guidance; it does not form a mandatory part of the Pharmacopoeia.

The analytical methods described and the limits proposed are intended to be used for validating the procedure for obtaining the water.

DEFINITION

Water for diluting concentrated haemodialysis solutions is obtained from potable water by distillation, by reverse osmosis, by ion exchange or by any other suitable method. The conditions of preparation, transfer and storage are designed to minimise the risk of chemical and microbial contamination.

When water obtained by one of the methods described above is not available, potable water may be used for home dialysis. Because the chemical composition of potable water varies considerably from one locality to another, consideration must be given to its chemical composition to enable adjustments to be made to the content of ions so that the concentrations in the diluted solution correspond to the intended use.

Attention has also to be paid to the possible presence of residues from water treatment (for example, chloramines) and volatile halogenated hydrocarbons.

For the surveillance of the quality of water for diluting concentrated haemodialysis solutions, the following methods may be used to determine the chemical composition and/or to detect the presence of the possible contaminants together with suggested limits to be obtained.

CHARACTERS

A clear, colourless, tasteless liquid.

TESTS

Acidity or alkalinity To 10 ml of the water to be examined, freshly boiled and cooled in a borosilicate glass flask, add 0.05 ml of *methyl red solution R*. The solution is not red. To 10 ml of the water to be examined add 0.1 ml of *bromothymol blue solution R1*. The solution is not blue.

Oxidisable substances To 100 ml of the water to be examined add 10 ml of *dilute sulphuric acid R* and 0.1 ml of *0.02M potassium permanganate* and boil for 5 min. The solution remains faintly pink.

Total available chlorine In a 125 ml test-tube (*A*), place successively 5 ml of *buffer solution pH 6.5 R*, 5 ml of *diethylphenylenediamine sulphate solution R* and 1 g of *potassium iodide R*. In a second 125 ml test-tube (*B*), place successively 5 ml of *buffer solution pH 6.5 R* and 5 ml of *diethylphenylenediamine sulphate solution R*. Add as simultaneously as possible to tube *A* 100 ml of the water to be examined and to tube *B* a reference solution prepared as follows: to 1 ml of a 10 mg/l solution of *potassium iodate R*, add 1 g of *potassium iodide R* and 1 ml of *dilute sulphuric acid R*; allow to stand for 1 min, add 1 ml of *dilute sodium hydroxide solution R* and dilute to 100 ml with *water R*. Any colour in the mixture obtained with the water to be examined is not more intense than that in the mixture obtained with the reference solution (0.1 ppm).

Chlorides (*2.4.4*). Dilute 1 ml of the water to be examined to 15 ml with *water R*. The solution complies with the limit test for chlorides (50 ppm).

Fluorides To 50 ml of the water to be examined add, mixing after each addition, 10 ml of *succinate buffer solution pH 4.6 R*, 10 ml of *aminomethylalizarindiacetic acid solution R*, 5 ml of a 0.4 g/l solution of *lanthanum nitrate R* and 20 ml of *acetone R*. Dilute to 100 ml with *water R*. Allow to stand in the dark for 1 h. Any colour in the solution is not more intense than that in a standard prepared at the same time and in the same manner using a mixture of 1 ml of *fluoride standard solution (10 ppm F) R* and 49 ml of *water R* (0.2 ppm).

Nitrates Dilute 2 ml of the water to be examined to 100 ml with *nitrate-free water R*. Place 5 ml of the dilution in a test-tube immersed in iced water, add 0.4 ml of a 100 g/l solution of *potassium chloride R* and 0.1 ml of *diphenylamine solution R* and then, dropwise and with shaking, 5 ml of *sulphuric acid R*. Transfer the tube to a water-bath at 50°C. Allow to stand for 15 min. Any blue colour in the solution is not more intense than that in a standard prepared at the same time and in the same manner using a mixture of 0.1 ml of *nitrate standard solution (2 ppm NO_3) R* and 4.9 ml of *nitrate-free water R* (2 ppm).

Sulphates (*2.4.13*). Dilute 3 ml of the water to be examined to 15 ml with *distilled water R*. The solution complies with the limit test for sulphates (50 ppm).

Aluminium (*2.4.17*). To 400 ml of the water to be examined add 10 ml of *acetate buffer solution pH 6.0 R* and 100 ml of *water R*. The solution complies with the limit test for aluminium (10 µg/l). Use as the reference solution a mixture of 2 ml of *aluminium standard solution (2 ppm Al) R*, 10 ml of *acetate buffer solution pH 6.0 R* and 98 ml of *water R*. To prepare the blank, use a mixture of 10 ml of *acetate buffer solution pH 6.0 R* and 100 ml of *water R*.

Ammonium To 20 ml of the water to be examined in a flat-bottomed and transparent tube, add 1 ml of *alkaline potassium tetraiodomercurate solution R*. Allow to stand for 5 min. The solution is not more intensely coloured than a standard prepared at the same time and in the same manner using a mixture of 4 ml of *ammonium standard solution (1 ppm NH_4) R* and 16 ml of *ammonium-free water R* (0.2 ppm). Examine the solutions along the vertical axis of the tube.

Calcium Not more than 2 ppm of Ca, determined by atomic absorption spectrometry (*Method I, 2.2.23*).

Test solution. Use the water to be examined.

Reference solutions. Prepare reference solutions (1 ppm to 5 ppm) using *calcium standard solution (400 ppm Ca) R*.

Measure the absorbance at 422.7 nm using a calcium hollow-cathode lamp as the radiation source and an oxidising air-acetylene flame.

Magnesium Not more than 2 ppm of Mg, determined by atomic absorption spectrometry (*Method I, 2.2.23*).

Test solution. Dilute 10 ml of the water to be examined to 100 ml with *distilled water R*.

Reference solutions. Prepare reference solutions (0.1 ppm to 0.5 ppm) using *magnesium standard solution (100 ppm Mg) R*.

Measure the absorbance at 285.2 nm using a magnesium hollow-cathode lamp as the radiation source and an oxidising air-acetylene flame.

Mercury Not more than 0.001 ppm of Hg, determined by atomic absorption spectrometry (*Method I, 2.2.23*).

Test solution. Add 5 ml of *nitric acid R per* litre of the water to be examined. In a 50 ml borosilicate glass flask with a ground-glass-stopper, place 20 ml of the water to be examined and add 1 ml of *dilute nitric acid R* and shake. Add 0.3 ml of *bromine water R1*. Stopper the flask, shake and heat the stoppered flask at 45°C for 4 h. Allow to cool. If the solution does not become yellow, add 0.3 ml of *bromine water R1* and re-heat at 45°C for 4 h. Add 0.5 ml of a freshly prepared 10 g/l solution of *hydroxylamine* hydro*chloride R*. Shake. Allow to stand for 20 min.

Reference solutions. Prepare reference solutions by treating as described under test solution for the water to be examined, freshly prepared solutions (0.0005 ppm to 0.002 ppm of mercury) obtained by diluting *mercury standard solution (1000 ppm Hg) R* with a 5 per cent *V/V* solution of *dilute nitric acid R*.

To a volume of solution suitable for the instrument to be used, add *stannous chloride solution R2* equal to 1/5 of this volume. Fit immediately the device for the entrainment of the mercury vapour. Wait 20 s and pass through the device a stream of *nitrogen R* as the carrier gas.

Measure the absorbance at 253.7 nm using a mercury hollow-cathode tube or a discharge lamp as the radiation source and as the atomisation device, a flameless system whereby the mercury can be entrained in the form of cold vapour.

Heavy metals (*2.4.8*). Heat 150 ml of the water to be examined in a glass evaporating dish on a water-bath until the volume is reduced to 15 ml. 12 ml of the solution complies with limit test A for heavy metals (0.1 ppm). Prepare the standard using *lead standard solution (1 ppm Pb) R*.

Potassium Not more than 2 ppm of K, determined by atomic emission spectrometry (*Method I, 2.2.22*).

Test solution (a). Dilute 50.0 ml of the water to be examined to 100 ml with *distilled water R*. Carry out a determination using this solution. If the potassium content is more than 0.75 mg per litre, further dilute the water to be examined with *distilled water R*.

Test solution (b). Take 50.0 ml of the water to be examined or, if necessary, the water to be examined diluted as described in the preparation of test solution (a). Add 1.25 ml of *potassium standard solution (20 ppm K) R* and dilute to 100.0 ml with *distilled water R*.

Reference solutions. Prepare reference solutions (0, 0.25, 0.50, 0.75 and 1 ppm) using *potassium standard solution (20 ppm K) R*.

Measure the emission intensity at 766 nm.

Calculate the potassium content of the water to be examined in parts per million from the expression:

$$\frac{\rho \times n_1 \times 0.5}{n_2 - n_1}$$

ρ = dilution factor used for the preparation of test solution (a),

n_1 = measured value of test solution (a),

n_2 = measured value of test solution (b).

Sodium Not more than 50 ppm of Na, determined by atomic emission spectrometry (*Method I, 2.2.22*).

Test solution. Use the water to be examined. If the sodium content is more than 10 mg per litre, dilute with *distilled water R* to obtain a concentration suitable for the apparatus used.

Reference solutions. Prepare reference solutions (0, 2.5, 5.0, 7.5 and 10 ppm) using *sodium standard solution (200 ppm Na) R*.

Measure the emission intensity at 589 nm.

Zinc Not more than 0.1 ppm of Zn, determined by atomic absorption spectrometry (*Method I, 2.2.23*). Use sampling and analytical equipment free from zinc or not liable to yield zinc under the conditions of use.

Test solution. Use the water to be examined.

Reference solutions. Prepare reference solutions (0.05 ppm to 0.15 ppm of zinc) using *zinc standard solution (100 ppm Zn) R*.

Measure the absorbance at 213.9 nm, using a zinc hollow-cathode lamp as the radiation source and an oxidising air-acetylene flame.

Microbial contamination Total viable aerobic count (*2.6.12*) not more than 10^2 micro-organisms per millilitre, determined by plate-count.

Bacterial endotoxins (*2.6.14*). Not more than 0.25 IU of endotoxin per millilitre.

Ph Eur

Haemofiltration Solutions

Haemofiltration Solutions comply with the requirements of the 3rd edition of the European Pharmacopoeia for Solutions for Haemofiltration [0861]. These requirements are reproduced after the heading 'Definition' below.

Ph Eur

DEFINITION

Solutions for haemofiltration are preparations for parenteral use containing electrolytes with a concentration close to the electrolytic composition of plasma. Glucose may be included in the formulation.

Solutions for haemodiafiltration also comply with the requirements of this monograph.

Solutions for haemofiltration are supplied in:
— rigid or semi-rigid plastic containers,
— flexible plastic containers inside sealed protective envelopes,
— glass containers.

The containers and closures comply with the requirements for containers for preparations for parenteral use (*3.2. Containers*).

Several formulations are used. The concentrations of the components per litre of solution are usually in the following range:

Table 861-1

	Expression in mmol	Expression in mEq
Sodium	125–150	125–150
Potassium	0–4.5	0–4.5
Calcium	1.0–2.5	2.0–5.0
Magnesium	0.25–1.5	0.50–3.0
Acetate or lactate	30–60	30–60
Chloride	90–120	90–120
Glucose	0–25	

Antioxidants such as metabisulphite are not added to the solutions.

IDENTIFICATION

According to the stated composition, the solution to be examined gives the following identification reactions (*2.3.1*):
— potassium: reaction (b);
— calcium: reaction (a);
— sodium: reaction (b);
— chlorides: reaction (a);
— acetates:
if the solution is free from glucose, use reaction (b), if the solution contains glucose, use the following method: to 5 ml of the solution to be examined add 1 ml of *hydrochloric acid R* in a test-tube fitted with a stopper and a bent tube, heat and collect a few millilitres of distillate; carry out reaction (b) of acetates on the distillate;
— lactates;
— magnesium: to 0.1 ml of *titan yellow solution R* add 10 ml of *water R*, 2 ml of the solution to be examined and 1 ml of *1M sodium hydroxide*; a pink colour is produced;
— glucose: to 5 ml of the solution to be examined, add 2 ml of *dilute sodium hydroxide solution R* and 0.05 ml of *copper sulphate solution R*; the solution is blue and clear; heat to boiling; an abundant red precipitate is formed.

TESTS

Appearance of solution The solution is clear (*2.2.1*). If it does not contain glucose, it is colourless (*Method I, 2.2.2*). If it contains glucose, it is not more intensely coloured than reference solution Y_7 (*Method I, 2.2.2*).

pH (*2.2.3*). The pH of the solution is 5.0 to 7.5. If the solution contains glucose, the pH is 4.5 to 6.5.

Hydroxymethylfurfural To a volume of the solution containing the equivalent of 25 mg of glucose, add 5.0 ml of a 100 g/l solution of *p- toluidine R* in *2-propanol R* containing 10 per cent *V/V* of *glacial acetic acid R* and 1.0 ml of a 5 g/l solution of *barbituric acid R*. The absorbance (*2.2.25*), determined at 550 nm after allowing the mixture to stand for 2 min to 3 min, is not greater than that of a standard prepared at the same time in the same manner using a solution containing 10 µg of *hydroxymethylfurfural R* in the same volume as the solution to be examined.

Aluminium (*2.4.17*). Take 200 ml, adjust to pH 6.0 and add 10 ml of *acetate buffer solution pH 6.0 R*. The solution complies with the limit test for aluminium (10 µg/l). Use as the reference solution a mixture of 1 ml of *aluminium standard solution (2 ppm Al) R*, 10 ml of *acetate buffer solution pH 6.0 R* and 9 ml of *water R*. To prepare the blank use a mixture of 10 ml of *acetate buffer solution pH 6.0 R* and 10 ml of *water R*.

Particulate contamination Carry out the test for sub-visible particles (*2.9.19*) using 50 ml of solution.

Particles larger than	5 µm	25 µm
Maximum number of particles per millilitre	100	5

Extractable volume (*2.9.17*). The solution complies with the test described for parenteral infusions.

Sterility (*2.6.1*). The solution complies with the test for sterility.

Bacterial endotoxins (*2.6.14*). Not more than 0.25 I.U. of endotoxin per millilitre.

Pyrogens (*2.6.8*). Solutions for which a validated test for bacterial endotoxins cannot be carried out comply with the test for pyrogens. Inject per kilogram of the rabbit's mass 10 ml of the solution.

ASSAY

Sodium 97.5 per cent to 102.5 per cent of the content of sodium (Na) stated on the label, determined by atomic absorption spectrometry (*Method II, 2.2.23*).

Test solution. If necessary, dilute the solution to be examined with *water R* to a concentration suitable for the instrument to be used.

Reference solutions. Prepare the reference solutions using *sodium standard solution (200 ppm Na) R.*

Measure the absorbance at 589.0 nm using a sodium hollow-cathode lamp as source of radiation and an air-acetylene or an air-propane flame.

Potassium 95.0 per cent to 105.0 per cent of the content of potassium (K) stated on the label, determined by atomic absorption spectrometry (*Method I, 2.2.23*).

Test solution. If necessary, dilute the solution to be examined with *water R* to a concentration suitable for the instrument to be used. To 100 ml of the solution add 10 ml of a 22 g/l solution of *sodium chloride R.*

Reference solutions. Prepare the reference solutions using *potassium standard solution (100 ppm K) R.* To 100 ml of each reference solution add 10 ml of a 22 g/l solution of *sodium chloride R.*

Measure the absorbance at 766.5 nm using a potassium hollow-cathode lamp as source of radiation and an air-acetylene or an air-propane flame.

Calcium 95.0 per cent to 105.0 per cent of the content of calcium (Ca) stated on the label, determined by atomic absorption spectrometry (*Method I, 2.2.23*).

Test solution. If necessary, dilute the solution to be examined with *water R* to a concentration suitable for the instrument to be used.

Reference solutions. Prepare the reference solutions using *calcium standard solution (400 ppm Ca) R.*

Measure the absorbance at 422.7 nm using a calcium hollow-cathode lamp as source of radiation and an air-acetylene or an air-propane flame.

Magnesium 95.0 per cent to 105.0 per cent of the content of magnesium (Mg) stated on the label, determined by atomic absorption spectrometry (*Method I, 2.2.23*).

Test solution. If necessary, dilute the solution to be examined with *water R* to a concentration suitable for the instrument to be used.

Reference solutions. Prepare the reference solutions using *magnesium standard solution (100 ppm Mg) R.*

Measure the absorbance at 285.2 nm using a magnesium hollow-cathode lamp as source of radiation and an air-acetylene or an air-propane flame.

Total chloride 95.0 per cent to 105.0 per cent of the content of chloride (Cl) stated on the label. Dilute to 50 ml with *water R* an accurately measured volume of the solution to be examined containing the equivalent of about 60 mg of chloride ion. Add 5 ml of *dilute nitric acid R,* 25.0 ml of *0.1M silver nitrate* and 2 ml of *dibutyl phthalate R.* Shake. Using 2 ml of *ferric ammonium sulphate solution R2* as indicator, titrate with *0.1M ammonium thiocyanate* until a reddish-yellow colour is obtained.

1 ml of *0.1M silver nitrate* is equivalent to 3.545 mg of Cl.

Acetate 95.0 per cent to 105.0 per cent of the content of acetate stated on the label. To a volume of the solution to be examined, corresponding to about 0.7 mmol of acetate, add 10.0 ml of *0.1M hydrochloric acid.* Carry out a potentiometric titration (*2.2.20*), using *0.1M sodium hydroxide.* Read the volume added between the two points of inflexion.

1 ml of *0.1M sodium hydroxide* is equivalent to 0.1 mmol of acetate.

Lactate 95.0 per cent to 105.0 per cent of the content of lactate stated on the label. To a volume of the solution to be examined, corresponding to about 0.7 mmol of lactate, add 10.0 ml of *0.1M hydrochloric acid.* Add 50 ml of *acetonitrile R.* Carry out a potentiometric titration (*2.2.20*), using *0.1M sodium hydroxide.* Read the volume added between the two points of inflexion.

1 ml of *0.1M sodium hydroxide* is equivalent to 0.1 mmol of lactate.

Reducing sugars (expressed as anhydrous glucose). 95.0 per cent to 105.0 per cent of the content of glucose stated on the label. Transfer a volume of the solution to be examined containing the equivalent of 25 mg of glucose to a 250 ml ground-glass conical flask and add 25.0 ml of *cupri-citric solution R.* Add a few grains of pumice, fit a reflux condenser, heat so that boiling occurs within 2 min and boil for exactly 10 min. Cool and add 3 g of *potassium iodide R* dissolved in 3 ml of *water R.* Carefully add, in small amounts, 25 ml of a 25 per cent *m/m* solution of *sulphuric acid R.* Titrate with *0.1M sodium thiosulphate* using *starch solution R,* added towards the end of titration, as indicator. Carry out a blank titration using 25.0 ml of *water R.*

Calculate the content of reducing sugars expressed as anhydrous glucose ($C_6H_{12}O_6$), using Table 861-2.

Table 861-2

Volume of *0.1M sodium thiosulphate* (millilitres)	Anhydrous glucose (milligrams)
8	19.8
9	22.4
10	25.0
11	27.6
12	30.3
13	33.0
14	35.7
15	38.5
16	41.3

STORAGE

Store at a temperature not lower than 4°C.

LABELLING

The label states:

— the formula of the solution for haemofiltration expressed in grams per litre and in millimoles per litre,
— the calculated osmolarity expressed in milliosmoles per litre,
— the nominal volume of the solution for haemofiltration in the container,
— that the solution is free from bacterial endotoxins, or where applicable, that it is apyrogenic,
— the storage conditions.

Ph Eur

Halibut-liver Oil Capsules

Definition Halibut-liver Oil Capsules are soft capsules containing Halibut-liver Oil diluted, if necessary, with a suitable fixed oil to a volume of 0.12 to 0.18 ml in each capsule.

The capsules comply with the requirements stated under Capsules and with the following requirements.

Content of vitamin A 3500 to 4700 IU.

Assay Weigh 10 capsules. Open the capsules carefully without loss of shell material, express as much of the contents as possible and reserve the expressed material. Wash the shells with *ether*, discard the washings, allow the shells to stand at room temperature until the odour of ether is no longer detectable and weigh. The difference between the weights represents the weight of the total contents. Determine the content of vitamin A in the reserved portion of the contents by the *assay of vitamin A*, Appendix VIII K, and calculate the content in a capsule of average content weight.

Storage Halibut-liver Oil Capsules should be protected from light and stored at a temperature not exceeding 20°. When stored under these conditions, they may be expected to retain their potency for at least 3 years after the date of preparation.

Labelling The label states that each capsule contains 4000 IU (Units) of vitamin A activity.

Haloperidol Capsules

Definition Haloperidol Capsules contain Haloperidol.

The capsules comply with the requirements stated under Capsules and with the following requirements.

Content of haloperidol, $C_{21}H_{23}ClFNO_2$ 95.0 to 105.0% of the prescribed or stated amount.

Identification

A. To a quantity of the contents of the capsules containing 10 mg of Haloperidol add 10 ml of *water* and 1 ml of 1M *sodium hydroxide* and extract with 10 ml of *ether*. Filter the ether extract through absorbent cotton, evaporate the filtrate to dryness and dry the residue at 60° at a pressure not exceeding 0.7 kPa. The *infrared absorption spectrum* of the residue, Appendix II A, is concordant with the *reference spectrum* of haloperidol.

B. In the Assay, the principal peak in the chromatogram obtained with solution (1) has the same retention time as the principal peak in the chromatogram obtained with solution (2).

Related substances Carry out the method described under Haloperidol applying to the plate 10 µl of each of the following solutions. For solution (1) shake a quantity of the contents of the capsules containing 10 mg of Haloperidol with 30 ml of *chloroform*, disperse with the aid of ultrasound for 15 minutes, filter, evaporate the filtrate to dryness and dissolve the residue in 1 ml of *chloroform*. For solution (2) dilute 1 volume of solution (1) to 200 volumes with *chloroform*. Any *secondary spot* in the chromatogram obtained with solution (1) is not more intense than the spot in the chromatogram obtained with solution (2) (0.5%). The test is not valid unless the chromatogram obtained with solution (2) shows a distinct and clearly visible spot.

Uniformity of content Capsules containing less than 2 mg of Haloperidol comply with the requirements stated under Capsules using the following method of analysis. Carry out the method for *liquid chromatography*, Appendix III D, using the following solutions. For solution (1) add sufficient of the mobile phase to the contents of one capsule to produce a solution containing 0.005% w/v of Haloperidol, disperse with the aid of ultrasound for 2 minutes, centrifuge and use the supernatant solution. Solution (2) contains 0.005% w/v of *haloperidol BPCRS* in the mobile phase.

The chromatographic procedure may be carried out using (a) a stainless steel column (15 cm × 5 mm) packed with *stationary phase C* (5 µm) (Hypersil ODS is suitable), (b) a mixture of 45 volumes of *acetonitrile* and 55 volumes of a 1% w/v solution of *ammonium acetate* as the mobile phase with a flow rate of 2 ml per minute and (c) a detection wavelength of 247 nm.

Calculate the content of $C_{21}H_{23}ClFNO_2$ in each capsule using the declared content of $C_{21}H_{23}ClFNO_2$ in *haloperidol BPCRS*.

Assay Use the average of the 10 individual results obtained in the test for Uniformity of content.

Haloperidol Injection

Definition Haloperidol Injection is a sterile solution of Haloperidol in Lactic Acid diluted with Water for Injections.

The injection complies with the requirements stated under Parenteral Preparations and with the following requirements.

Content of haloperidol, $C_{21}H_{23}ClFNO_2$ 90.0 to 110.0% of the prescribed or stated amount.

Identification

A. To a volume containing 20 mg of Haloperidol add 5 ml of *water* and 1 ml of 1M *sodium hydroxide* and extract with 10 ml of *chloroform*. Filter the chloroform extract through absorbent cotton, evaporate the filtrate to dryness and dry the residue at 60° at a pressure not exceeding 0.7 kPa. The *infrared absorption spectrum* of the residue, Appendix II A, is concordant with the *reference spectrum* of haloperidol.

B. The *light absorption*, Appendix II B, in the range 230 to 350 nm of the final solution obtained in the Assay exhibits a maximum only at 245 nm.

Acidity pH, 2.8 to 3.6, Appendix V L.

Related substances Carry out the method for *thin-layer chromatography*, Appendix III A, using a silica gel precoated plate (Merck silica gel 60 plates are suitable) and a mixture of 92 volumes of *chloroform*, 8 volumes of *methanol* and 1 volume of 13.5M *ammonia* as the mobile phase. Apply separately to the plate (1) a volume of the injection containing 0.1 mg of Haloperidol, (2) the same volume of a solution prepared by diluting 1 volume of the injection to 100 volumes with *methanol* and (3) the same volume of a solution prepared by diluting 1 volume of the injection to 200 volumes with *methanol*. After removal of the plate, allow it to dry in air and spray with *dilute potassium iodobismuthate solution*. Any *secondary spot* in the chromatogram obtained with solution (1) is not more intense than the spot in the chromatogram obtained with solution (2) and not more than one such spot is more intense than the spot in the chromatogram obtained with solution (3).

Assay To a quantity containing 10 mg of Haloperidol add 8 ml of *water* and 10 ml of 1M *hydrochloric acid.* Extract with successive quantities of 25, 25, 10 and 10 ml of *ether.* Wash the combined ether extracts with 10 ml of *water,* combine the aqueous layers and remove the ether using a rotary evaporator. Add sufficient *water* to produce 100 ml and dilute 10 ml to 100 ml with *methanol.* Measure the *absorbance* of the resulting solution at the maximum at 245 nm, Appendix II B. Calculate the content of $C_{21}H_{23}ClFNO_2$ taking 346 as the value of A(1%, 1 cm) at the maximum at 245 nm.

Storage Haloperidol Injection should be protected from light.

Haloperidol Oral Solution

Haloperidol Oral Drops

Definition Haloperidol Oral Solution is an aqueous solution containing not more than 0.2% w/v of Haloperidol.

The oral solution complies with the requirements stated under Oral Liquids and with the following requirements.

Content of haloperidol, $C_{21}H_{23}ClFNO_2$ 95.0 to 105.0% of the prescribed or stated amount.

Characteristics A clear, colourless solution.

Identification

A. To a volume containing 20 mg of Haloperidol add 1 ml of 1M *sodium hydroxide,* extract with 10 ml of *chloroform,* filter and evaporate the filtrate to dryness. The *infrared absorption spectrum* of the residue, Appendix II A, is concordant with the *reference spectrum* of haloperidol.

B. The *light absorption,* Appendix II B, in the range 230 to 350 nm of the final solution obtained in the Assay exhibits a maximum only at 245 nm.

Acidity pH, 2.5 to 3.5, Appendix V L.

Related substances Carry out the method for *thin-layer chromatography,* Appendix III A, using a silica gel precoated plate (Merck silica gel 60 plates are suitable) and a mixture of 92 volumes of *dichloromethane,* 8 volumes of *methanol* and 1 volume of 13.5M *ammonia* as the mobile phase. Apply separately to the plate 50 µl of each of the following solutions. For solution (1) dilute the oral solution if necessary with *methanol* to contain 0.1% w/v of Haloperidol. For solution (2) dilute 1 volume of solution (1) to 100 volumes with *methanol.* For solution (3) dilute 1 volume of solution (1) to 200 volumes with *methanol.* After removal of the plate, allow it to dry in air and spray with *dilute potassium iodobismuthate solution.* Any *secondary spot* in the chromatogram obtained with solution (1) is not more intense than the spot in the chromatogram obtained with solution (2) and not more than one such spot is more intense than the spot in the chromatogram obtained with solution (3).

Assay To a volume containing 10 mg of Haloperidol add 8 ml of *water* and 10 ml of 1M *hydrochloric acid* and extract with two 10-ml quantities of *ether.* Wash the combined ether extracts with 10 ml of *water,* combine the aqueous solutions and remove the ether using a rotary evaporator. Add sufficient *water* to produce 100 ml and dilute 10 ml to 100 ml with *methanol.* Measure the *absorbance* of the resulting solution at the maximum at 245 nm, Appendix II B. Calculate the content of $C_{21}H_{23}ClFNO_2$ taking 346 as the value of A(1%, 1 cm) at the maximum at 245 nm.

Storage Haloperidol Oral Solution should be protected from light and stored at a temperature of 15° to 25°.

When Haloperidol Oral Solution or Haloperidol Oral Drops is prescribed or demanded and no strength is stated, an Oral Solution containing 0.2% w/v of Haloperidol shall be dispensed or supplied.

Strong Haloperidol Oral Solution

Strong Haloperidol Oral Drops

Definition Strong Haloperidol Oral Solution is an aqueous solution containing 1% w/v of Haloperidol. It is intended to be diluted before use.

The oral solution complies with the requirements stated under Oral Liquids and with the following requirements.

Content of haloperidol, $C_{21}H_{23}ClFNO_2$ 0.95 to 1.05% w/v.

Characteristics A clear, colourless solution.

Identification

A. To 2 ml add 10 ml of *water* and 1 ml of 1M *sodium hydroxide,* extract with 10 ml of *chloroform,* filter and evaporate the filtrate to dryness. The *infrared absorption spectrum* of the residue, Appendix II A, is concordant with the *reference spectrum* of haloperidol.

B. The *light absorption,* Appendix II B, in the range 230 to 350 nm of the final solution obtained in the Assay exhibits a maximum only at 245 nm.

Acidity pH, 3.5 to 4.5, Appendix V L.

Related substances Carry out the method for *thin-layer chromatography,* Appendix III A, using a silica gel precoated plate (Merck silica gel 60 plates are suitable) and a mixture of 92 volumes of *dichloromethane,* 8 volumes of *methanol* and 1 volume of 13.5M *ammonia* as the mobile phase. Apply separately to the plate 5 µl of each of the following solutions. Solution (1) is the preparation being examined. For solution (2) dilute 1 volume of solution (1) to 100 volumes with *water.* For solution (3) dilute 1 volume of solution (1) to 200 volumes with *water.* After removal of the plate, allow it to dry in air and spray with *dilute potassium iodobismuthate solution.* Any *secondary spot* in the chromatogram obtained with solution (1) is not more intense than the spot in the chromatogram obtained with solution (2) and not more than one such spot is more intense than the spot in the chromatogram obtained with solution (3).

Assay To 1 ml add 10 ml of *water* and 10 ml of 1M *hydrochloric acid* and extract with two 10-ml quantities of *ether.* Wash the combined ether extracts with 10 ml of *water,* combine the aqueous solutions and remove the ether using a rotary evaporator. Add sufficient *water* to produce 100 ml and dilute 10 ml to 100 ml with *methanol.* Measure the *absorbance* of the resulting solution at the maximum at 245 nm, Appendix II B. Calculate the content of $C_{21}H_{23}ClFNO_2$ taking 346 as the value of A(1%, 1 cm) at the maximum at 245 nm.

Storage Strong Haloperidol Oral Solution should be protected from light and stored at a temperature of 15° to 25°.

Labelling The label states that the preparation is to be diluted before use.

Haloperidol Tablets

Definition Haloperidol Tablets contain Haloperidol.

The tablets comply with the requirements stated under Tablets and with the following requirements.

Content of haloperidol, $C_{21}H_{23}ClFNO_2$ 90.0 to 110.0% of the prescribed or stated amount.

Identification To a quantity of the powdered tablets containing 10 mg of Haloperidol add 10 ml of *water* and 1 ml of 1M *sodium hydroxide* and extract with 10 ml of *ether*. Filter the ether extract through absorbent cotton, evaporate the filtrate to dryness and dry the residue at 60° at a pressure not exceeding 0.7 kPa. The *infrared absorption spectrum* of the residue, Appendix II A, is concordant with the *reference spectrum* of haloperidol.

Related substances Carry out the method described under Haloperidol applying to the plate 10 µl of each of the following solutions. For solution (1) shake a quantity of the powdered tablets containing 10 mg of Haloperidol with 10 ml of *chloroform*, filter, evaporate the filtrate to dryness and dissolve the residue in 1 ml of *chloroform*. For solution (2) dilute 1 volume of solution (1) to 200 volumes with *chloroform*. Any *secondary spot* in the chromatogram obtained with solution (1) is not more intense than the spot in the chromatogram obtained with solution (2) (0.5%). The test is not valid unless the chromatogram obtained with solution (2) shows a distinct and clearly visible spot.

Uniformity of content Tablets containing less than 2 mg of Haloperidol comply with the requirements stated under Tablets using the following method of analysis. Carry out the method for *liquid chromatography*, Appendix III D, using the following solutions. Solution (1) contains 0.005% w/v of *haloperidol BPCRS* in the mobile phase. For solution (2) place one tablet in 10 ml of the mobile phase, disperse with the aid of ultrasound for 2 minutes and centrifuge. If necessary, dilute the supernatant liquid with the mobile phase to produce a solution containing 0.005% w/v of Haloperidol.

The chromatographic procedure may be carried out using (a) a stainless steel column (15 cm × 5 mm) packed with *stationary phase C* (5 µm) (Hypersil ODS is suitable), (b) a mixture of 55 volumes of a 1% w/v solution of *ammonium acetate* and 45 volumes of *acetonitrile* as the mobile phase with a flow rate of 2 ml per minute and (c) a detection wavelength of 247 nm.

Calculate the content of $C_{21}H_{23}ClFNO_2$ using the declared content of $C_{21}H_{23}ClFNO_2$ in *haloperidol BPCRS*.

Assay

For tablets containing 2 mg or more of Haloperidol Weigh and powder 20 tablets and carry out the method for *liquid chromatography*, Appendix III D, using the following solutions. Solution (1) contains 0.020% w/v of *haloperidol BPCRS* in the mobile phase. For solution (2) add 60 ml of the mobile phase to a quantity of the powdered tablets containing 20 mg of Haloperidol, disperse with the aid of ultrasound for 2 minutes, add sufficient mobile phase to produce 100 ml, mix and filter.

The chromatographic procedure described under Uniformity of content may be used.

Calculate the content of $C_{21}H_{23}ClFNO_2$ using the declared content of $C_{21}H_{23}ClFNO_2$ in *haloperidol BPCRS*.

For tablets containing less than 2 mg of Haloperidol Use the average of the 10 individual results obtained in the test for Uniformity of content.

Heparin Injection

Definition Heparin Injection is a sterile solution of Heparin Calcium or Heparin Sodium in Water for Injections. The pH of the solution may be adjusted by the addition of a suitable alkali.

The injection complies with the requirements stated under Parenteral Preparations and with the following requirements.

Characteristics A colourless or straw-coloured liquid, free from turbidity and from matter that deposits on standing.

Identification

A. It delays the clotting of freshly shed blood.

B. Carry out the method for *zone electrophoresis*, Appendix III F, using *agarose for electrophoresis* as the supporting medium. To equilibrate the agarose and as electrolyte solution use a mixture of 50 ml of *glacial acetic acid* and 800 ml of *water* adjusted to pH 3 by the addition of *lithium hydroxide* and diluted to 1000 ml with *water*. Apply separately to the strip 2 µl to 3 µl of each of the following solutions. For solution (1) dilute a volume of the injection with *water* to give a solution containing 375 IU per ml. For solution (2), dilute *heparin sodium EPBRP* with an equal volume of *water*. Pass a current of 1 mA to 2 mA per centimetre of strip width at a potential difference of 300 volts for about 10 minutes. Stain the strips using a 0.1% w/v solution of *toluidine blue* and remove the excess by washing. The ratio of the distance migrated by the principal band or bands in the gel obtained with solution (1) to the distance migrated by the principal band in the gel obtained with solution (2) is 0.9 to 1.1.

C. When the injection contains Heparin Calcium, it yields reactions A and B characteristic of *calcium salts*, Appendix VI. When the injection contains Heparin Sodium, it yields reaction A characteristic of *sodium salts*, Appendix VI.

Acidity or alkalinity pH, 5.5 to 8.0, Appendix V L.

Bacterial endotoxins Carry out the *test for bacterial endotoxins*, Appendix XIV C.

For a preparation supplied in a container with a nominal content of less than 100 ml, dilute the injection if necessary with *water BET* to give a solution containing 1000 IU of heparin activity per ml (solution A). The endotoxin limit concentration of solution A is 10 IU of endotoxin per ml. Carry out the test using a lysate with a declared sensitivity not less sensitive than 0.0625 IU of endotoxin per ml and using the maximum valid dilution of solution A calculated from the declared sensitivity of the lysate used in the test.

For a preparation supplied in a container with a nominal content of 100 ml or more, the endotoxin limit concentration is 0.25 IU of endotoxin per ml.

For Heparin Injection prepared from Heparin Calcium it may be necessary to add divalent cations in order to achieve the validation criteria.

Assay Carry out the *assay of heparin*, Appendix XIV K. The estimated potency is not less than 90% and not more than 111% of the stated potency. The fiducial limits of error are not less than 80% and not more than 125% of the stated potency.

Storage Heparin Injection should be stored at a temperature not exceeding 25° and should preferably be kept in a container sealed by fusion of the glass.

Labelling The strength is stated as the number of IU (Units) in a suitable dose-volume except that for multidose containers the strength is stated as the number of IU (Units) per ml.

The label states (1) the source of the material (lung or mucosal) and whether it is the calcium or sodium salt; (2) when no antimicrobial preservative is present that the preparation contains no antimicrobial preservative and that any portion of the contents not used at once should be discarded.

Hexachlorophene Dusting Powder

Zinc and Hexachlorophene Dusting Powder

Definition Hexachlorophene Dusting Powder is a *cutaneous powder*. It is a mixture of Hexachlorophene and Zinc Oxide with a suitable inert diluent.

The dusting powder complies with the requirements stated under Topical Powders and with the following requirements.

Content of hexachlorophene, $C_{13}H_6Cl_6O_2$ 90.0 to 110.0% of the prescribed or stated amount.

Content of zinc oxide, ZnO 90.0 to 110.0% of the prescribed or stated amount.

Identification

A. Shake a quantity of the powder containing 30 mg of Hexachlorophene with 25 ml of *ether* for 15 minutes, filter, wash the filtrate with 10 ml of *water*, dry the ether layer over *anhydrous sodium sulphate*, filter and evaporate to dryness. The *infrared absorption spectrum* of the residue, Appendix II A, is concordant with the *reference spectrum* of hexachlorophene.

B. Shake a quantity of the powder containing 30 mg of Zinc Oxide with 10 ml of 2M *hydrochloric acid* for 15 minutes and filter. 5 ml of the filtrate yields the reaction characteristic of *zinc salts*, Appendix VI.

Assay

For hexachlorophene Shake a quantity of the powder containing 15 mg of Hexachlorophene with 50 ml of *methanolic tris(hydroxymethyl)methylamine solution* for 10 minutes, filter through a sintered-glass crucible (BS porosity No. 3), wash the filter with two 10-ml quantities of the tris(hydroxymethyl)methylamine solution and dilute the combined filtrate and washings to 100 ml with the same solution. Dilute 10 ml of the resulting solution to 50 ml with *methanolic tris(hydroxymethyl)methylamine solution* and measure the *absorbance* at the maximum at 312 nm, Appendix II B, using in the reference cell a solution prepared by diluting a further 10 ml of the solution to 50 ml with *acidified methanol*. An absorbance of 0.432 is equivalent to 15 mg of $C_{13}H_6Cl_6O_2$ in the weight of powder taken.

For zinc oxide To a quantity of the powder containing 90 mg of Zinc Oxide add 10 ml of 2M *nitric acid* and 20 ml of *water*, boil for 2 minutes, cool, filter and wash the filter with two 25-ml quantities of *water*. To the combined filtrate and washings add 3 g of *hexamine* and titrate with 0.05M *disodium edetate VS* using 2 ml of *xylenol orange solution* as indicator. Each ml of 0.05M *disodium edetate VS* is equivalent to 4.068 mg of ZnO.

Labelling The label states that the preparation should not be applied to infants or to large areas of skin except in accordance with medical advice.

The label indicates the pharmaceutical form as 'cutaneous powder'.

When hexachlorophane dusting powder or zinc and hexachlorophane dusting powder is prescribed or demanded, Hexachlorophene Dusting Powder or Zinc and Hexachlorophene Dusting Powder shall be dispensed or supplied.

Homatropine Eye Drops

Definition Homatropine Eye Drops are a sterile solution of Homatropine Hydrobromide in Purified Water.

The eye drops comply with the requirements stated under Eye Preparations and with the following requirements.

Content of homatropine hydrobromide, $C_{16}H_{21}NO_3$, HBr 90.0 to 110.0% of the prescribed or stated amount.

Identification

A. To a volume containing 60 mg of Homatropine Hydrobromide add 3 ml of 5M *ammonia*, extract with 15 ml of *chloroform*, dry the chloroform over *anhydrous sodium sulphate*, filter and evaporate the filtrate to dryness. The *infrared absorption spectrum* of the residue, Appendix II A, is concordant with the *reference spectrum* of homatropine.

B. In the Assay, the chromatogram obtained with solution (2) shows a peak with the same retention time as the peak derived from homatropine hydrobromide in the chromatogram obtained with solution (1).

C. To 1 ml of the eye drops, diluted with *water* if necessary to give a solution containing 1% w/v of Homatropine Hydrobromide, add 1 ml of 5M *ammonia*, shake with *chloroform* and evaporate the chloroform solution to dryness on a water bath. To the residue add 1.5 ml of a 2% w/v solution of *mercury(II) chloride* in *ethanol (60%)*. A yellow colour is produced which becomes red on gentle warming (distinction from most other alkaloids except atropine and hyoscyamine).

Tropine Carry out the method for *thin-layer chromatography*, Appendix III A, using *silica gel G* as the coating substance and a mixture of 33 volumes of *anhydrous formic acid*, 33 volumes of *water* and 134 volumes of *ethyl acetate* as the mobile phase. Apply separately to the plate 40 µl of each of the following solutions. For solution (1) use the eye drops diluted, if necessary, with *water* to contain 1% w/v of Homatropine Hydrobromide. Solution (2) contains 0.0050% w/v of *tropine*. After removal of the plate, dry it at 100° to 105° until the odour of the solvent is no longer detectable, allow to cool and spray with *dilute potassium iodobismuthate solution* until spots appear. Any spot corresponding to tropine in the chromatogram obtained with solution (1) is not more intense than the spot in the chromatogram obtained with solution (2) (0.5%).

Assay Carry out the method for *gas chromatography*, Appendix III B, using the following solutions. For solution

(1) add 1 ml of a 2% w/v solution of *atropine sulphate BPCRS* (internal standard) in *methanol* (solution A) and 1 ml of 5M *ammonia* to 5 ml of a 0.4% w/v solution of *homatropine hydrobromide BPCRS*. Extract with two 5-ml quantities of *chloroform*, shake the combined extracts with 1 g of *anhydrous sodium sulphate*, filter and evaporate the filtrate to dryness. Dissolve the residue in 10 ml of *dichloromethane*. To 1 ml of this solution add 0.2 ml of a mixture of 4 volumes of N,O-*bis(trimethylsilyl)acetamide* and 1 volume of *trimethylchlorosilane*, mix and allow to stand for 30 minutes. Prepare solution (2) in the same manner as solution (3) but omitting the addition of solution A. For solution (3) add 1 ml of solution A and 1 ml of 5M *ammonia* to a volume of the eye drops containing 20 mg of Homatropine Hydrobromide, diluted if necessary to 5 ml with *water*, and complete the procedure described under solution (1), beginning at the words 'Extract with two 5-ml quantities of *chloroform* ...'.

The chromatographic procedure may be carried out using a glass column (1.5 m × 4 mm) packed with *acid-washed, silanised diatomaceous support* (80 to 100 mesh) coated with 3% w/w of phenyl methyl silicone fluid (50% phenyl) (OV-17 is suitable) and maintained at 220°.

Calculate the content of $C_{16}H_{21}NO_3,HBr$ using the declared content of $C_{16}H_{21}NO_3,HBr$ in *homatropine hydrobromide BPCRS*.

Hyaluronidase Injection

Definition Hyaluronidase Injection is a sterile solution of Hyaluronidase in Water for Injections. It is prepared by dissolving Hyaluronidase for Injection in the requisite amount of Water for Injections immediately before use.

The injection complies with the requirements stated under Parenteral Preparations.

Storage Hyaluronidase Injection should be used immediately after preparation.

HYALURONIDASE FOR INJECTION

Definition Hyaluronidase for Injection is a sterile material consisting of Hyaluronidase with or without excipients. It is supplied in a sealed container.

The contents of the sealed container comply with the requirements for Powders for Injections stated under Parenteral Preparations and with the following requirements.

Identification A solution containing 100 IU in 1 ml of a 0.9% w/v solution of *sodium chloride* depolymerises an equal volume of a 1% w/v solution of *sodium hyaluronate EPBRP* at 20° in 1 minute, as shown by a pronounced decrease in viscosity. This action is destroyed by heating the initial solution at 100° for 30 minutes.

Acidity or alkalinity pH of a 0.3% w/v solution in *carbon dioxide-free water*, 4.5 to 7.5, Appendix V L.

Clarity and colour of solution A 1.0% w/v solution in *carbon dioxide-free water* is *clear*, Appendix IV A, and not more than faintly yellow.

Bacterial endotoxins Carry out the *test for bacterial endotoxins*, Appendix XIV C. Dissolve the contents of the sealed container in *water BET* to give a solution containing 150 IU of Hyaluronidase per ml (solution A). The endotoxin limit concentration of solution A is 30 IU per ml. Carry out the test using the maximum valid dilution of solution A calculated from the declared sensitivity of the lysate used in the test.

Assay Carry out the Assay described under Hyaluronidase. The estimated potency is not less than 90% and not more than 115% of the stated potency.

Storage The contents of the sealed container should be stored at a temperature not exceeding 25°.

Labelling The label of the sealed container states (1) the total number of IU (Units) contained in it; (2) that the preparation is not intended for intravenous injection.

Hydralazine Injection

Definition Hydralazine Injection is a sterile solution of Hydralazine Hydrochloride in Water for Injections. It is prepared by dissolving Hydralazine Hydrochloride for Injection in the requisite amount of Water for Injections immediately before use. For intravenous infusion, the Hydralazine Hydrochloride for Injection should be dissolved in, and then diluted with, an appropriate volume of a suitable diluent.

The injection complies with the requirements stated under Parenteral Preparations.

Storage Hydralazine Injection deteriorates on storage and should be used immediately after preparation.

HYDRALAZINE HYDROCHLORIDE FOR INJECTION

Definition Hydralazine Hydrochloride for Injection is a sterile material consisting of Hydralazine Hydrochloride with or without excipients. It is supplied in a sealed container.

The contents of the sealed container comply with the requirements for Powders for Injections stated under Parenteral Preparations and with the following requirements.

Content of hydralazine hydrochloride, $C_8H_8N_4,HCl$ 98.0 to 114.0% of the prescribed or stated amount.

Identification

A. The *infrared absorption spectrum*, Appendix II A, is concordant with the *reference spectrum* of hydralazine hydrochloride.

B. The *light absorption*, Appendix II B, in the range 230 to 350 nm of a 0.002% w/v solution exhibits four maxima, at 240, 260, 305 and 315 nm.

C. Yield the reactions characteristic of *chlorides*, Appendix VI.

Acidity pH of a 2% w/v solution, 3.5 to 4.2, Appendix V L.

Clarity of solution A 2.0% w/v solution is not more opalescent than *reference suspension II*, Appendix IV A.

Colour of solution A 2.0% w/v solution in 0.01M *hydrochloric acid* is not more intensely coloured than *reference solution GY_6*, Appendix IV B, Method II.

Hydrazine Carry out the method for *thin-layer chromatography*, Appendix III A, using a silica gel precoated plate (Merck silica gel 60 plates are suitable) and as the mobile phase the upper layer of the mixture obtained by shaking together 80 volumes of *hexane*, 20 volumes of 13.5M *ammonia* and 20 volumes of *ethyl acetate* and allowing to stand. Apply separately to the plate 40 µl of each of the following solutions. For solution (1) dissolve the contents of a sealed container in sufficient 0.1M *methanolic hydrochloric acid* to produce a solution containing 0.5% w/v of Hydralazine Hydrochloride. To 2 ml add 1 ml of a 2% w/v solution of *salicylaldehyde* in *methanol* and 0.1 ml of *hydrochloric acid*, centrifuge and decant the supernatant liquid. Prepare solution (2) in the same manner, but use 2 ml of a 0.00025% w/v solution of *hydrazine sulphate* in 0.1M *methanolic hydrochloric acid* in place of the solution of the material being examined. After removal of the plate, allow it to dry in air and spray with *dimethylaminobenzaldehyde solution R1*. Any spot corresponding to hydrazine in the chromatogram obtained with solution (1) is not more intense than the spot in the chromatogram obtained with solution (2).

Uniformity of content Sealed containers each containing 20 mg or less of Hydralazine Hydrochloride comply with the requirements stated under Parenteral Preparations, Powders for Injections using the following method of analysis. Dissolve the contents of a sealed container in sufficient *water* to produce 100 ml and dilute a volume containing 1 mg of Hydralazine Hydrochloride to 100 ml with *water*. Measure the *absorbance* of the resulting solution at the maximum at 260 nm, Appendix II B. Calculate the content of $C_8H_8N_4$,HCl taking 535 as the value of A(1%, 1 cm) at the maximum at 260 nm.

Assay Determine the weight of the contents of 10 containers as described in the test for Uniformity of weight under Parenteral Preparations, Powders for Injections.

Dissolve 0.1 g of the mixed contents of the 10 containers in a mixture of 25 ml of *water* and 35 ml of *hydrochloric acid* and titrate with 0.025M *potassium iodate VS* determining the end point potentiometrically using a platinum indicator electrode and a calomel reference electrode. Each ml of 0.025M *potassium iodate VS* is equivalent to 4.916 mg of $C_8H_8N_4$,HCl. Calculate the content of $C_8H_8N_4$,HCl in a container of average content weight.

Storage The sealed container should be protected from light and stored at a temperature not exceeding 25°.

Labelling The label of the sealed container states that solutions containing glucose should not be used in the preparation of the intravenous infusion.

Hydralazine Tablets

Definition Hydralazine Tablets contain Hydralazine Hydrochloride.

The tablets comply with the requirements stated under Tablets and with the following requirements.

Content of hydralazine hydrochloride, $C_8H_8N_4$,HCl 95.0 to 105.0% of the prescribed or stated amount.

Identification

A. Dissolve a quantity of the powdered tablets containing 0.1 g of Hydralazine Hydrochloride in 10 ml of *water*, make alkaline with 2 ml of 5M *ammonia* and extract with two 10-ml quantities of *chloroform*. Combine the chloroform extracts and evaporate to dryness. The *infrared absorption spectrum* of the residue, Appendix II A, is concordant with the *reference spectrum* of hydralazine.

B. Shake a quantity of the powdered tablets containing 25 mg of Hydralazine Hydrochloride with 30 ml of *methanol* for 15 minutes, add sufficient *methanol* to produce 50 ml and filter. Dilute 1 volume of the filtrate to 50 volumes with *water*. The *light absorption* of the resulting solution, Appendix II B, in the range 230 to 350 nm exhibits four maxima, at 240, 260, 305 and 315 nm.

C. Extract a quantity of the powdered tablets containing 0.1 g of Hydralazine Hydrochloride with two 25-ml quantities of *methanol*, filter the combined extracts and evaporate to dryness. To 5 ml of a 1% w/v solution of the residue in *methanol* add 5 ml of a 2% w/v solution of *2-nitrobenzaldehyde* in *ethanol (96%)*. An orange precipitate is produced.

Hydrazine Carry out the method for *thin-layer chromatography*, Appendix III A, using a silica gel precoated plate (Merck silica gel 60 plates are suitable) and as the mobile phase the upper layer obtained by shaking together 20 volumes of 13.5M *ammonia*, 20 volumes of *ethyl acetate* and 80 volumes of *hexane* and allowing to separate. Apply separately to the plate 40 µl of each of the following solutions. For solution (1) extract a quantity of the powdered tablets containing 50 mg of Hydralazine Hydrochloride with 10 ml of 0.1M *methanolic hydrochloric acid*; to 2 ml add 1 ml of a 2% w/v solution of *salicylaldehyde* in *methanol* and 0.1 ml of *hydrochloric acid*, centrifuge and use the supernatant liquid. Prepare solution (2) in the same manner, but using 2 ml of a 0.00025% w/v solution of *hydrazine sulphate* in 0.1M *methanolic hydrochloric acid* in place of the solution of the substance being examined. After removal of the plate, allow it to dry in air and spray with *dimethylaminobenzaldehyde solution R1*. Any spot corresponding to hydrazine in the chromatogram obtained with solution (1) is not more intense than the spot in the chromatogram obtained with solution (2) (0.05%).

Assay Weigh and powder 20 tablets. To a quantity of the powder containing 50 mg of Hydralazine Hydrochloride add 50 ml of *water* and shake for 20 minutes. Add 60 ml of *hydrochloric acid* and titrate with 0.025M *potassium iodate VS* determining the end point potentiometrically using platinum and calomel electrodes. Each ml of 0.025M *potassium iodate VS* is equivalent to 4.916 mg of $C_8H_8N_4$,HCl.

Storage Hydralazine Tablets should be protected from light and stored at a temperature not exceeding 25°.

Hydrochlorothiazide Tablets

Definition Hydrochlorothiazide Tablets contain Hydrochlorothiazide.

The tablets comply with the requirements stated under Tablets and with the following requirements.

Content of hydrochlorothiazide, $C_7H_8ClN_3O_4S_2$ 92.5 to 107.5% of the prescribed or stated amount.

Identification Carry out the method for *thin-layer chromatography*, Appendix III A, using *silica gel GF_{254}* as the coating substance and *ethyl acetate* as the mobile phase. Apply separately to the plate 5 µl of each of the following solutions. For solution (1) triturate a quantity of the powdered tablets containing 10 mg of Hydrochlorothiazide with 10 ml of *acetone* and filter. Solution (2) contains 0.1% w/v of *hydrochlorothiazide EPCRS* in *acetone*. After removal of the plate, dry it in a current of air, examine under *ultraviolet light (254 nm)* and then treat the plate by *Method I* and examine again. By each method of visualisation the principal spot in the chromatogram obtained with solution (1) corresponds in colour and intensity to that in the chromatogram obtained with solution (2).

Related substances Carry out the method for *thin-layer chromatography*, Appendix III A, using *silica gel G* as the coating substance and a mixture of 85 volumes of *ethyl acetate* and 15 volumes of *propan-2-ol* as the mobile phase. Apply separately to the plate 5 µl of each of the following solutions. For solution (1) shake vigorously a quantity of the powdered tablets containing 50 mg of Hydrochlorothiazide with 50 ml of *acetone*, filter, evaporate the filtrate to dryness and dissolve the residue in 10 ml of *acetone*. For solution (2) dilute 1 volume of solution (1) to 100 volumes with *acetone*. After removal of the plate, dry it in a current of air and reveal the spots by *Method I*. Any *secondary spot* in the chromatogram obtained with solution (1) is not more intense than the spot in the chromatogram obtained with solution (2).

Assay Weigh and powder 20 tablets. To a quantity of the powder containing 30 mg of Hydrochlorothiazide add 50 ml of 0.1M *sodium hydroxide*, shake for 20 minutes and dilute to 100 ml with 0.1M *sodium hydroxide*. Mix, filter, dilute 5 ml of the filtrate to 100 ml with *water* and measure the *absorbance* of the resulting solution at the maximum at 273 nm, Appendix II B. Calculate the content of $C_7H_8ClN_3O_4S_2$ taking 520 as the value of A(1%, 1 cm) at the maximum at 273 nm.

Hydrocortisone Cream

Definition Hydrocortisone Cream contains Hydrocortisone in a suitable basis.

The cream complies with the requirements stated under Topical Semi-solid Preparations and with the following requirements.

Content of hydrocortisone, $C_{21}H_{30}O_5$ 90.0 to 110.0% of the prescribed or stated amount.

Identification

A. Carry out the method for *thin-layer chromatography*, Appendix III A, using *silica gel G* as the coating substance and a mixture of 77 volumes of *dichloromethane*, 15 volumes of *ether*, 8 volumes of *methanol* and 1.2 volumes of *water* as the mobile phase. Apply separately to the plate 5 µl of each of the following solutions.

For creams containing more than 0.5% w/w of Hydrocortisone, prepare three solutions in the following manner. For solution (1) mix a quantity containing 25 mg of Hydrocortisone with 10 ml of *methanol (90%)*, add 50 ml of hot *hexane* and shake. Separate the lower layer, add 5 g of *anhydrous sodium sulphate*, mix and filter through a glass microfibre filter (Whatman GF/C is suitable). Solution (2) contains 0.25% w/v of *hydrocortisone BPCRS* in *methanol*. Solution (3) is a mixture of equal volumes of solutions (1) and (2).

For creams containing 0.5% w/w or less of Hydrocortisone, prepare solution (1) in the same manner as solution (1) above but use a quantity containing 5 mg of Hydrocortisone. Solution (2) contains 0.05% w/v of *hydrocortisone BPCRS* in *methanol*. Solution (3) is a mixture of equal volumes of solutions (1) and (2).

After removal of the plate, allow it to dry in air and spray with *alkaline tetrazolium blue solution*. The principal spot in the chromatogram obtained with solution (1) corresponds to that in the chromatogram obtained with solution (2); if it does not, the principal spot in the chromatogram obtained with solution (3) appears as a single, compact spot.

B. In the Assay, the chromatogram obtained with solution (2) shows a peak with the same retention time as the peak due to hydrocortisone in the chromatogram obtained with solution (1).

Assay Carry out the method for *liquid chromatography*, Appendix III D, using the following solutions.

For creams containing more than 0.5% w/w of Hydrocortisone, prepare solutions (1) and (2) in the following manner. For solution (1) dissolve 25 mg of *hydrocortisone BPCRS* in 45 ml of *methanol*, add 5 ml of a 0.5% w/v solution of *betamethasone* (internal standard) in *methanol* and add sufficient *water* to produce 100 ml. For solution (2) disperse, by shaking, a quantity of the cream containing 25 mg of Hydrocortisone in 40 ml of a mixture of 3 volumes of *methanol* and 1 volume of a 15% w/v solution of *sodium chloride*. Add 50 ml of hot *hexane*, shake and separate the lower layer. Repeat the extraction using a further two 10-ml quantities of the methanolic sodium chloride solution. To the combined extracts add 5 ml of *methanol* and sufficient *water* to produce 100 ml, mix and filter through a glass microfibre paper (Whatman GF/C is suitable).

For creams containing 0.5% or less of Hydrocortisone, prepare solutions (1) and (2) in the following manner. For solution (1) dissolve 5 mg of *hydrocortisone BPCRS* in 45 ml of *methanol* and add 5 ml of a 0.110% w/v solution of *betamethasone* (internal standard) in *methanol* and sufficient *water* to produce 100 ml. Prepare solution (2) in the same manner as solution (2) above but use a quantity of the cream containing 5 mg of Hydrocortisone.

For all preparations prepare solution (3) in the same manner as solution (2) but add 5 ml of the appropriate internal standard solution in place of the 5 ml of methanol before diluting to volume.

The chromatographic procedure may be carried out using (a) a stainless steel column (10 cm × 5 mm) packed with *stationary phase C* (5 µm) (Spherisorb ODS 1 is suitable), (b) *methanol (50%)* as the mobile phase with a flow rate of 2 ml per minute and (c) a detection wavelength of 240 nm.

Calculate the content of $C_{21}H_{30}O_5$ in the preparation being examined using the declared content of $C_{21}H_{30}O_5$ in *hydrocortisone BPCRS*.

Hydrocortisone Acetate Cream

Definition Hydrocortisone Acetate Cream contains Hydrocortisone Acetate in a suitable basis.

The cream complies with the requirements stated under Topical Semi-solid Preparations and with the following requirements.

Content of hydrocortisone acetate, $C_{23}H_{32}O_6$ 90.0 to 110.0% of the prescribed or stated amount.

Identification

A. Carry out the method for *thin-layer chromatography*, Appendix III A, using *silica gel G* as the coating substance and a mixture of 77 volumes of *dichloromethane*, 15 volumes of *ether*, 8 volumes of *methanol* and 1.2 volumes of *water* as the mobile phase. Apply separately to the plate 5 µl of each of the following solutions.

For creams containing more than 0.5% w/w of Hydrocortisone Acetate, prepare two solutions in the following manner. For solution (1) mix a quantity of the cream containing 25 mg of Hydrocortisone Acetate with 10 ml of *methanol (90%)*, add 50 ml of hot *hexane* and shake. Discard the upper layer, add 5 g of *anhydrous sodium sulphate* to the lower layer, mix and filter through a glass microfibre filter (Whatman GF/C is suitable). Solution (2) is a mixture of equal volumes of solution (1) and a 0.25% w/v solution of *hydrocortisone acetate BPCRS* in *methanol*.

For creams containing 0.5% w/w or less of Hydrocortisone Acetate, prepare solution (1) in the same manner as solution (1) described above but using a quantity of the cream containing 5 mg of Hydrocortisone Acetate. Solution (2) is a mixture of equal volumes of solution (1) and a 0.05% w/v solution of *hydrocortisone acetate BPCRS* in *methanol*.

After removal of the plate, allow it to dry in air and spray with *alkaline tetrazolium blue solution*. The principal spot in the chromatogram obtained with solution (1) corresponds to that in the chromatogram obtained with solution (2), which appears as a single, compact spot.

B. In the Assay, the chromatogram obtained with solution (2) shows a peak with the same retention time as the peak due to hydrocortisone acetate in the chromatogram obtained with solution (1).

Assay Carry out the method for *liquid chromatography*, Appendix III D, using the following solutions.

For creams containing more than 0.5% w/w of Hydrocortisone Acetate, prepare solutions (1) and (2) in the following manner. For solution (1) dissolve 25 mg of *hydrocortisone acetate BPCRS* in 45 ml of *methanol*, add 5 ml of a 0.5% w/v solution of *betamethasone* (internal standard) in *methanol* and add sufficient *water* to produce 100 ml. For solution (2) disperse, by shaking, a quantity containing 25 mg of Hydrocortisone Acetate in 40 ml of a solution prepared by mixing 75 ml of *methanol* with 25 ml of a 15% w/v solution of *sodium chloride*. Add 50 ml of hot *hexane*, shake and separate the lower layer. Repeat the extraction using two 10-ml quantities of the methanolic sodium chloride solution. Add 5 ml of *methanol* to the combined extracts and sufficient *water* to produce 100 ml, mix and filter through a glass microfibre filter paper (Whatman GF/C is suitable).

For creams containing 0.5% w/w or less of Hydrocortisone Acetate, prepare solutions (1) and (2) in the following manner. For solution (1) dissolve 5 mg of *hydrocortisone acetate BPCRS* in 45 ml of *methanol* and add 5 ml of a 0.110% w/v solution of *betamethasone* (internal standard) in *methanol* and sufficient *water* to produce 100 ml. Prepare solution (2) in the same manner as solution (2) above but use a quantity containing 5 mg of Hydrocortisone Acetate.

For all creams prepare solution (3) in the same manner as solution (2) but adding 5 ml of the appropriate internal standard solution in place of the 5 ml of methanol before diluting to volume.

The chromatographic procedure may be carried out using (a) a stainless steel column (10 cm × 5 mm) packed with *stationary phase C* (5 µm) (Spherisorb ODS 1 is suitable), (b) *methanol (50%)* as the mobile phase with a flow rate of 2 ml per minute and (c) a detection wavelength of 240 nm.

Calculate the content of $C_{23}H_{32}O_6$ in the preparation being examined using the declared content of $C_{23}H_{32}O_6$ in *hydrocortisone acetate BPCRS*.

Hydrocortisone and Clioquinol Cream

Definition Hydrocortisone and Clioquinol Cream contains Hydrocortisone and Clioquinol, the latter in *very fine powder*, in a suitable basis.

The cream complies with the requirements stated under Topical Semi-solid Preparations and with the following requirements.

Content of hydrocortisone, $C_{21}H_{30}O_5$ 92.5 to 107.5% of the prescribed or stated amount.

Content of clioquinol, C_9H_5ClINO 90.0 to 110.0% of the prescribed or stated amount.

Identification

A. Carry out the method for *thin-layer chromatography*, Appendix III A, using *silica gel G* as the coating substance and a mixture of 1.2 volumes of *water*, 8 volumes of *methanol*, 15 volumes of *ether* and 77 volumes of *dichloromethane* as the mobile phase. Apply separately to the plate 5 µl of each of the following solutions. For solution (1) disperse, by warming and shaking, a quantity of the cream containing 2.5 g of Hydrocortisone in 10 ml of *ethanol (96%)*, cool, allow to stand at 0° for 30 minutes, filter and use the filtrate. Solution (2) contains 0.25% w/v of *hydrocortisone BPCRS* in *ethanol (96%)*. For solution (3) dissolve 12.5 mg of *hydrocortisone BPCRS* in 5 ml of solution (1). After removal of the plate, allow it to dry in air and spray with *alkaline tetrazolium blue solution*. The principal spot in the chromatogram obtained with solution (1) corresponds to that in the chromatogram obtained with solution (2). The principal spot in the chromatogram obtained with solution (3) appears as a single, compact spot.

B. In the Assay for hydrocortisone, the chromatogram obtained with solution (3) shows a peak with the same retention time as the peak due to hydrocortisone in the chromatogram obtained with solution (1).

C. Fuse a quantity of the cream containing 0.1 g of Clioquinol with *anhydrous sodium carbonate*, dissolve the fused mass in *water* and acidify with 2M *nitric acid*. Add *silver nitrate solution*; a pale yellow precipitate is produced which is insoluble in 5M *ammonia*. Add 5M *ammonia* until the solution becomes alkaline, boil gently, filter and acidify the filtrate with 2M *nitric acid*; a white precipitate is produced which darkens on exposure to light.

Assay

For hydrocortisone Carry out the method for *liquid chromatography*, Appendix III D, using the following solutions. For solution (1) dissolve 5 mg of *hydrocortisone BPCRS* in 5 ml of a 4% v/v solution of *bromobenzene* (internal standard) in *methanol* and dilute to 50 ml with *methanol (80%)*. For solution (2) add 30 ml of *2,2,4-trimethylpentane* to a quantity of the cream containing 10 mg of Hydrocortisone and warm on a water bath until the preparation has melted. Extract the warm mixture with successive quantities of 30, 20 and 20 ml of *methanol (80%)*, combine the aqueous methanolic layers, cool to about 20° and dilute to 100 ml with the same solvent. Prepare solution (3) in the same manner as solution (2) but adding 10 ml of a 4% v/v solution of *bromobenzene* in *methanol* to the cooled methanolic extract.

The chromatographic procedure may be carried out using (a) a stainless steel column (25 cm × 5 mm) packed with *stationary phase C* (5 µm) (Spherisorb ODS 1 is suitable), (b) *methanol (65%)* as the mobile phase with a flow rate of 1 ml per minute and (c) a detection wavelength of 242 nm.

Calculate the content of $C_{21}H_{30}O_5$ in the cream taking 100.0% as the content of $C_{21}H_{30}O_5$ in *hydrocortisone BPCRS*.

For clioquinol To a quantity of the cream containing 25 mg of Clioquinol add 80 ml of a hot mixture of 6 volumes of *water* and 24 volumes of *2-methoxyethanol* and heat on a water bath for 5 minutes. Cool in ice for 10 minutes, allow to warm to room temperature, dilute to 100 ml with the aqueous methoxyethanol, mix and filter. To 10 ml of the filtrate add 10 ml of *2-methoxyethanol* and 2 ml of a solution prepared by dissolving 0.5 g of *iron(III) chloride hexahydrate* in 80 ml of *2-methoxyethanol* and adding 0.1 ml of *hydrochloric acid* and sufficient *2-methoxyethanol* to produce 100 ml. Dilute the solution to 25 ml with *2-methoxyethanol* and measure the *absorbance* of the resulting solution at the maximum at 650 nm, Appendix II B, using in the reference cell a solution prepared by treating 10 ml of the aqueous methoxyethanol in the same manner beginning at the words 'add 10 ml of *2-methoxyethanol...*'.

Calculate the content of C_9H_5ClINO from the *absorbance* obtained by repeating the operation beginning at the words 'add 10 ml of *2-methoxyethanol...*' and using 10 ml of a solution prepared in the following manner. Dissolve 0.125 g of *clioquinol BPCRS* in sufficient *2-methoxyethanol* to produce 50 ml, warming to effect solution; add 1 ml of *water* to 5 ml of the solution and add sufficient of a mixture of 6 volumes of *water* and 24 volumes of *2-methoxyethanol* to produce 50 ml.

Storage Hydrocortisone and Clioquinol Cream should be protected from light.

Hydrocortisone and Neomycin Cream

Definition Hydrocortisone and Neomycin Cream contains Hydrocortisone and Neomycin Sulphate in a suitable basis.

The cream complies with the requirements stated under Topical Semi-solid Preparations and with the following requirements.

Content of hydrocortisone, $C_{21}H_{30}O_5$ 90.0 to 110.0% of the prescribed or stated amount.

Identification

A. Carry out the method for *thin-layer chromatography*, Appendix III A, using *silica gel GF_{254}* as the coating substance and a mixture of 90 volumes of *dichloromethane* and 8 volumes of *methanol* as the mobile phase. Apply separately to the plate 10 µl of each of the following solutions. For solution (1) add 10 ml of *hexane* saturated with *acetonitrile* to a quantity of the preparation being examined containing 5 mg of Hydrocortisone and shake for 2 to 3 minutes. Add 10 ml of *acetonitrile* saturated with *hexane*, shake for 10 minutes and allow the layers to separate. Centrifuge, filter the acetonitrile layer if necessary, evaporate 5 ml to dryness and dissolve the residue in 5 ml of a mixture of equal volumes of *chloroform* and *ethanol (96%)*. Solution (2) contains 0.05% w/v of *hydrocortisone BPCRS* in a mixture of equal volumes of *chloroform* and *ethanol (96%)*. After removal of the plate, allow it to dry in air and spray with *alkaline tetrazolium blue solution*. The principal spot in the chromatogram obtained with solution (1) corresponds to that in the chromatogram obtained with solution (2).

B. In the Assay for hydrocortisone the chromatogram obtained with solution (2) shows a peak with the same retention time as the peak due to hydrocortisone in the chromatogram obtained with solution (1).

C. Carry out the method for *thin-layer chromatography*, Appendix III A, using a silica gel precoated plate (Merck silica gel 60 plates are suitable) and a mixture of 60 volumes of *methanol*, 40 volumes of 13.5M *ammonia* and 20 volumes of *chloroform* as the mobile phase. Apply separately to the plate 5 µl of each of the following solutions. For solution (1) disperse a quantity containing 7000 IU of Neomycin Sulphate with 10 ml of *chloroform*, add 5 ml of *water*, shake, centrifuge and use the clear, upper layer. Solution (2) contains 0.2% w/v of *neomycin sulphate EPCRS* in *water*. After removal of the plate, allow it to dry in air, spray with a 1% w/v solution of *ninhydrin* in *butan-1-ol* and heat at 105° for 2 minutes. The principal red spot in the chromatogram obtained with solution (1) corresponds to that in the chromatogram obtained with solution (2).

Neamine Carry out the method for *thin-layer chromatography*, Appendix III A, using *silica gel H* as the coating substance and a freshly prepared 3.85% w/v solution of *ammonium acetate* as the mobile phase. Apply separately to the plate 2 µl of each of the following solutions. For solution (1) dissolve a quantity containing 7000 IU of Neomycin Sulphate in 10 ml of *chloroform*, shake gently with 5 ml of *water*, centrifuge and use the aqueous layer. Solution (2) contains 0.004% w/v of *neamine EPCRS* in *water*. After removal of the plate, dry it in a current of warm air, heat at 110° for 10 minutes and spray the hot plate with a solution prepared immediately before use by diluting *sodium hypochlorite solution* with *water* to contain 0.5% of available chlorine. Dry in a current of cold air until a sprayed area of the plate below the line of application gives at most a very faint blue colour with a drop of a 0.5% w/v solution of *potassium iodide* in *starch mucilage*; avoid prolonged exposure to the cold air. Spray the plate with a 0.5% w/v solution of *potassium iodide* in *starch mucilage*. Any spot corresponding to neamine in the chromatogram obtained with solution (1) is not more intense than the spot in the chromatogram obtained with solution (2).

Neomycin C Carry out the method for *liquid chromatography*, Appendix III D, injecting 10 µl of each of the following solutions. For solution (1) add 1.5 ml of a freshly prepared 2% w/v solution of *1-fluoro-2,4-dinitrobenzene* in *methanol* to 0.5 ml of a 0.10% w/v solution of *framycetin sulphate BPCRS* in 0.02M *sodium tetraborate*, heat in a water bath at 60° for 1 hour and cool; dilute the solution to 25 ml with the mobile phase, allow to stand and use the clear lower layer. For solution (2) shake a quantity containing 3500 IU of Neomycin Sulphate with 10 ml of *chloroform*, add 5 ml of 0.02M *sodium tetraborate*, mix, allow to separate and centrifuge the upper layer. Proceed as for solution (1) but using 0.5 ml of the clear supernatant liquid in place of 0.5 ml of the framycetin sulphate solution.

The chromatographic procedure may be carried out using (a) a stainless steel column (20 cm × 4.6 mm) packed with *stationary phase A* (5 μm) (Nucleosil 100-5 is suitable), (b) as the mobile phase with a flow rate of 1.6 ml per minute a solution prepared by mixing 97 ml of *tetrahydrofuran*, 1.0 ml of *water* and 0.5 ml of *glacial acetic acid* with sufficient of a 2.0% v/v solution of *absolute ethanol* in *ethanol-free chloroform* to produce 250 ml and (c) a detection wavelength of 350 nm. If necessary adjust the tetrahydrofuran and water content of the mobile phase so that the chromatogram obtained with solution (1) shows resolution similar to that in the specimen chromatogram supplied with *framycetin sulphate BPCRS*. Pass the mobile phase through the column for several hours before starting the analysis. Record the chromatogram for 1.4 times the retention time of the peak due to neomycin B.

The *column efficiency*, determined using the peak due to neomycin B in the chromatogram obtained with solution (1), should be at least 13,000 *theoretical plates* per metre.

In the chromatogram obtained with solution (2) the area of the peak corresponding to neomycin C is 3 to 15% of the sum of the areas of the peaks corresponding to neomycin B and neomycin C.

Assay

For hydrocortisone Carry out the method for *liquid chromatography*, Appendix III D, using the following solutions. Solution (1) contains 0.010% w/v of *hydrocortisone BPCRS* and 0.018% w/v of *fluoxymesterone BPCRS* (internal standard) in *chloroform*. For solution (2) shake together a quantity of the preparation being examined containing 25 mg of Hydrocortisone, several small glass beads and 25 ml of a 0.036% w/v solution of *fluoxymesterone BPCRS* in *chloroform* for 15 minutes, add sufficient *chloroform* to produce 50 ml, mix and centrifuge. Remove any excipient material present at the interface and use the clear supernatant liquid.

The chromatographic procedure may be carried out using (a) a stainless steel column (30 cm × 3.9 mm) packed with *stationary phase A* (10 μm) (μPorasil is suitable), (b) a mixture of 425 volumes of *butyl chloride*, 425 volumes of *butyl chloride* saturated with *water*, 70 volumes of *tetrahydrofuran*, 35 volumes of *methanol* and 30 volumes of *glacial acetic acid* as the mobile phase with a flow rate of 1 ml per minute and (c) a detection wavelength of 254 nm.

Calculate the content of $C_{21}H_{30}O_5$ in the cream using the declared content of $C_{21}H_{30}O_5$ in *hydrocortisone BPCRS*.

For neomycin sulphate Stir a quantity containing 4200 IU with 15 ml of *chloroform* until the emulsion is completely broken. Transfer to a separating funnel with 25 ml of *phosphate buffer pH 8.0* and 5 ml of *chloroform*, shake vigorously, allow to separate and reserve the aqueous phase. Extract the chloroform layer with two 25-ml quantities of *phosphate buffer pH 8.0* and discard the chloroform layer. Pass *nitrogen* through the combined aqueous solutions to remove dissolved chloroform and dilute to 100 ml with sterile *phosphate buffer pH 8.0*. Dilute 10 ml of the resulting solution to 50 ml with the same solvent and carry out the *biological assay of antibiotics*, Appendix XIV A. The precision of the assay is such that the fiducial limits of error are not less than 95% and not more than 105% of the estimated potency. The upper fiducial limit of error is not less than 90.0% and the lower fiducial limit of error is not more than 115.0% of the prescribed or stated amount.

Labelling The strength with respect to Neomycin Sulphate is stated as the number of IU (Units) per g.

Hydrocortisone Acetate and Neomycin Ear Drops

Hydrocortisone and Neomycin Ear Drops

Definition Hydrocortisone Acetate and Neomycin Ear Drops are a suspension of Hydrocortisone Acetate in a solution of Neomycin Sulphate in Purified Water.

The ear drops comply with the requirements stated under Ear Preparations and with the following requirements.

Content of hydrocortisone acetate, $C_{23}H_{32}O_6$ 90.0 to 110.0% w/v of the prescribed or stated amount.

Identification

A. Comply with test A for Identification described under Hydrocortisone and Neomycin Cream using the following solutions. For solution (1) add 10 ml of *chloroform* to a quantity of the ear drops containing 5 mg of Hydrocortisone Acetate in a separating funnel, shake for 2 to 3 minutes and allow the layers to separate. Filter if necessary and use the chloroform layer. Solution (2) contains 0.05% w/v of *hydrocortisone acetate BPCRS* in *chloroform*.

B. In the Assay for hydrocortisone acetate the chromatogram obtained with solution (3) shows a peak with the same retention time as the peak due to hydrocortisone acetate in the chromatogram obtained with solution (1).

C. Comply with test C for Identification described under Hydrocortisone and Neomycin Cream. For solution (1) dilute a volume containing 3500 IU of Neomycin Sulphate with *water* to 2.5 ml, shake with 3 ml of *chloroform*, centrifuge and use the clear, upper layer.

Acidity or alkalinity pH, 6.5 to 8.0, Appendix V L.

Neamine Comply with the test described under Hydrocortisone and Neomycin Cream. For solution (1) dilute a volume containing 3500 IU of Neomycin Sulphate with 2.5 ml of *water*, shake gently with 3 ml of *chloroform*, centrifuge and use the aqueous layer.

Neomycin C Comply with the test described under Hydrocortisone and Neomycin Cream but using as solution (2) a solution prepared in the following manner. Dilute the ear drops with 0.02M *sodium tetraborate* to contain 700 IU per ml. To 0.5 ml of the resulting solution add 1.5 ml of a freshly prepared 2% w/v solution of *1-fluoro-2,4-dinitrobenzene* in *methanol*, heat in a water bath at 60° for 1 hour, cool and dilute the solution to 25 ml with the mobile phase; allow to stand and use the clear, lower layer.

Assay

For hydrocortisone acetate Carry out the method for *liquid chromatography*, Appendix III D, using the following solutions. Solution (1) contains 0.020% w/v of *hydrocortisone acetate BPCRS* and 0.016% w/v of *fluoxymesterone*

BPCRS (internal standard) in *chloroform*. For solution (2) shake a quantity of the ear drops containing 10 mg of Hydrocortisone Acetate with 25 ml of a 0.032% w/v solution of *fluoxymesterone BPCRS* in *chloroform*, add 25 ml of *chloroform*, mix and filter through *anhydrous sodium sulphate*.

The chromatographic procedure may be carried out using (a) a stainless steel column (30 cm × 3.9 mm) packed with *stationary phase A* (10 μm) (μPorasil is suitable), (b) a mixture of 425 volumes of *butyl chloride*, 425 volumes of *butyl chloride* saturated with *water*, 70 volumes of *tetrahydrofuran*, 35 volumes of *methanol* and 30 volumes of *glacial acetic acid* as the mobile phase with a flow rate of 1 ml per minute and (c) a detection wavelength of 254 nm.

Calculate the content of $C_{23}H_{32}O_6$ in the ear drops using the declared content of $C_{23}H_{32}O_6$ in *hydrocortisone acetate BPCRS*.

For neomycin sulphate Dilute a volume containing 3500 IU to 50 ml with sterile *phosphate buffer pH 8.0*, dilute 10 ml of the resulting solution to 100 ml with the same solvent and carry out the *biological assay of antibiotics*, Appendix XIV A. The precision of the assay is such that the fiducial limits of error are not less than 95% and not more than 105% of the estimated potency. The upper fiducial limit of error is not less than 90.0% and the lower fiducial limit of error is not more than 115.0% of the prescribed or stated number of IU per ml.

Labelling The strength with respect to Neomycin Sulphate is stated as the number of IU (Units) per ml.

Hydrocortisone Acetate and Neomycin Eye Drops

Hydrocortisone and Neomycin Eye Drops

Definition Hydrocortisone Acetate and Neomycin Eye Drops are a sterile suspension of Hydrocortisone Acetate in a solution of Neomycin Sulphate in Purified Water.

The eye drops comply with the requirements stated under Eye Drops and with the following requirements.

Content of hydrocortisone acetate, $C_{23}H_{32}O_6$ 90.0 to 110.0% w/v of the prescribed or stated amount.

Identification

A. Comply with test A for Identification described under Hydrocortisone and Neomycin Cream using the following solutions. For solution (1) add 10 ml of *chloroform* to a quantity of the eye drops containing 5 mg of Hydrocortisone Acetate in a separating funnel, shake for 2 to 3 minutes and allow the layers to separate. Filter if necessary and use the chloroform layer. Solution (2) contains 0.05% w/v of *hydrocortisone acetate BPCRS* in *chloroform*.

B. In the Assay for hydrocortisone acetate the chromatogram obtained with solution (2) shows a peak with the same retention time as the peak due to hydrocortisone acetate in the chromatogram obtained with solution (1).

C. Comply with test C for Identification described under Hydrocortisone and Neomycin Cream. For solution (1) dilute a volume containing 3500 IU of Neomycin Sulphate with *water* to 2.5 ml, shake with 3 ml of *chloroform*, centrifuge and use the clear, upper layer.

Acidity or alkalinity pH, 6.5 to 8.0, Appendix V L.

Neamine Comply with the test described under Hydrocortisone and Neomycin Cream. For solution (1) dilute a volume containing 3500 IU of Neomycin Sulphate with 2.5 ml of *water*, shake gently with 3 ml of *chloroform*, centrifuge and use the aqueous layer.

Neomycin C Comply with the test described under Hydrocortisone and Neomycin Cream but using as solution (2) a solution prepared in the following manner. Dilute the eye drops with 0.02M *sodium tetraborate* to contain 700 IU per ml. To 0.5 ml of the resulting solution add 1.5 ml of a freshly prepared 2% w/v solution of *1-fluoro-2,4-dinitrobenzene* in *methanol*, heat in a water bath at 60° for 1 hour, cool and dilute the solution to 25 ml with the mobile phase; allow to stand and use the clear, lower layer.

Assay

For hydrocortisone acetate Carry out the method for *liquid chromatography*, Appendix III D, using the following solutions. Solution (1) contains 0.020% w/v of *hydrocortisone acetate BPCRS* and 0.016% w/v of *fluoxymesterone BPCRS* (internal standard) in *chloroform*. For solution (2) shake a quantity of the eye drops containing 10 mg of Hydrocortisone Acetate with 25 ml of a 0.032% w/v solution of *fluoxymesterone BPCRS* in *chloroform*, add 25 ml of *chloroform*, mix and filter through *anhydrous sodium sulphate*.

The chromatographic procedure may be carried out using (a) a stainless steel column (30 cm × 3.9 mm) packed with *stationary phase A* (10 μm) (μPorasil is suitable), (b) a mixture of 425 volumes of *butyl chloride*, 425 volumes of *butyl chloride* saturated with *water*, 70 volumes of *tetrahydrofuran*, 35 volumes of *methanol* and 30 volumes of *glacial acetic acid* as the mobile phase with a flow rate of 1 ml per minute and (c) a detection wavelength of 254 nm.

Calculate the content of $C_{23}H_{32}O_6$ in the eye drops using the declared content of $C_{23}H_{32}O_6$ in *hydrocortisone acetate BPCRS*.

For neomycin sulphate Dilute a volume containing 3500 IU to 50 ml with sterile *phosphate buffer pH 8.0*, dilute 10 ml of the resulting solution to 100 ml with the same solvent and carry out the *biological assay of antibiotics*, Appendix XIV A. The precision of the assay is such that the fiducial limits of error are not less than 95% and not more than 105% of the estimated potency. The upper fiducial limit of error is not less than 90.0% and the lower fiducial limit of error is not more than 115.0% of the prescribed or stated number of IU per ml.

Labelling The strength with respect to Neomycin Sulphate is stated as the number of IU (Units) per ml.

Hydrocortisone Acetate and Neomycin Eye Ointment

Definition Hydrocortisone Acetate and Neomycin Eye Ointment is a sterile preparation containing Hydrocortisone Acetate and Neomycin Sulphate in a suitable basis.

The eye ointment complies with the requirements stated under Eye Ointments and with the following requirements.

Content of hydrocortisone acetate, $C_{23}H_{32}O_6$ 92.5 to 107.5% of the prescribed or stated amount.

Identification

A. Complies with test A for Identification described under Hydrocortisone and Neomycin Cream using the following solutions. For solution (1) add 10 ml of *hexane* saturated with *acetonitrile* to a quantity of the ointment containing 5 mg of Hydrocortisone Acetate and shake for 2 to 3 minutes. Add 10 ml of *acetonitrile* saturated with *hexane*, shake for 10 minutes and allow the layers to separate. Centrifuge, filter the acetonitrile layer if necessary, evaporate 5 ml to dryness and dissolve the residue in 5 ml of a mixture of equal volumes of *chloroform* and *ethanol (96%)*. Solution (2) contains 0.05% w/v of *hydrocortisone acetate BPCRS* in a mixture of equal volumes of *chloroform* and *ethanol (96%)*.

B. In the Assay for hydrocortisone acetate the chromatogram obtained with solution (3) shows a peak with the same retention time as the peak due to hydrocortisone acetate in the chromatogram obtained with solution (1).

C. Complies with test C for Identification described under Hydrocortisone and Neomycin Cream. For solution (1) shake a quantity containing 7000 IU of Neomycin Sulphate with 10 ml of *chloroform*, add 5 ml of *water*, shake, centrifuge and use the clear, upper layer.

Neamine Complies with the test described under Hydrocortisone and Neomycin Cream. For solution (1) disperse a quantity containing 7000 IU of Neomycin Sulphate in 10 ml of *chloroform*, shake gently with 5 ml of *water*, centrifuge and use the aqueous layer.

Neomycin C Complies with the test described under Hydrocortisone and Neomycin Cream.

Assay

For hydrocortisone acetate Carry out the method for *liquid chromatography*, Appendix III D, using the following solutions. Solution (1) contains 0.025% w/v of *hydrocortisone acetate BPCRS* and 0.050% w/v of *fluoxymesterone BPCRS* (internal standard) in *chloroform*. For solution (2) shake a quantity of the ointment containing 25 mg of Hydrocortisone Acetate with 20 ml of a 0.25% w/v solution of *fluoxymesterone BPCRS* in *chloroform* and several glass beads for 30 minutes. Centrifuge; to 10 ml of the clear, supernatant layer add sufficient *chloroform* to produce 50 ml.

The chromatographic procedure may be carried out using (a) a stainless steel column (30 cm × 3.9 mm) packed with *stationary phase A* (10 μm) (μPorasil is suitable), (b) a mixture of 425 volumes of *butyl chloride*, 425 volumes of *butyl chloride* saturated with *water*, 70 volumes of *tetrahydrofuran*, 35 volumes of *methanol* and 30 volumes of *glacial acetic acid* as the mobile phase with a flow rate of 1 ml per minute and (c) a detection wavelength of 254 nm.

Calculate the content of $C_{23}H_{32}O_6$ in the ointment using the declared content of $C_{23}H_{32}O_6$ in *hydrocortisone acetate BPCRS*.

For neomycin sulphate Dissolve a quantity containing 3500 IU in 50 ml of *ether*, extract the solution with three 30-ml quantities of sterile *phosphate buffer pH 8.0* and discard the ether phase. Pass *nitrogen* through the combined aqueous extracts to remove dissolved ether, dilute to 100 ml with sterile *phosphate buffer pH 8.0* and carry out the *biological assay of antibiotics*, Appendix XIV A. The precision of the assay is such that the fiducial limits of error are not less than 95% and not more than 105% of the estimated potency. The upper fiducial limit of error is not less than 90.0% and the lower fiducial limit of error is not more than 115.0% of the prescribed or stated number of IU per g.

Labelling The strength with respect to Neomycin Sulphate is stated as the number of IU (Units) per g.

Hydrocortisone Acetate Injection

Definition Hydrocortisone Acetate Injection is a sterile suspension of Hydrocortisone Acetate in Water for Injections. It is prepared using aseptic technique.

The injection complies with the requirements stated under Parenteral Preparations and with the following requirements.

Content of hydrocortisone acetate, $C_{23}H_{32}O_6$ 90.0 to 110.0% of the prescribed or stated amount.

Characteristics A white suspension that settles on standing but readily disperses on shaking. On examination under a microscope, the particles are seen to be crystalline and rarely exceed 30 μm in diameter.

Identification Filter a volume containing 50 mg of Hydrocortisone Acetate through a sintered-glass filter, wash the residue with four 5-ml quantities of *water*, dissolve in 20 ml of *chloroform*, wash the chloroform solution with four 10-ml quantities of *water*, discard the washings, filter the chloroform solution through absorbent cotton and evaporate the filtrate to dryness. The residue complies with the following tests.

A. The *infrared absorption spectrum*, Appendix II A, is concordant with the *reference spectrum* of hydrocortisone acetate.

B. Complies with the test for *identification of steroids*, Appendix III A, using *impregnating solvent I* and *mobile phase B*.

C. Yields the reaction characteristic of *acetyl groups*, Appendix VI.

Assay To a quantity containing 50 mg of Hydrocortisone Acetate add 20 ml of *water* and extract with three 30-ml quantities of *chloroform*. Filter the extracts through absorbent cotton and add sufficient *chloroform* to produce 100 ml. Dilute 10 ml to 50 ml with *chloroform*, transfer 4 ml of the resulting solution to a 25-ml graduated flask and remove the chloroform in a current of air. Dissolve the residue in 10 ml of *aldehyde-free ethanol (96%)* and complete the *tetrazolium assay of steroids*, Appendix VIII J, beginning at the words 'add 2 ml of *triphenyltetrazolium chloride solution* ...'. Transfer 10 ml of a solution containing 390 to 410 μg of *hydrocortisone acetate BPCRS* in *aldehyde-free ethanol (96%)* to a 25-ml graduated flask and repeat the assay beginning at the words 'and complete the *tetrazolium assay of steroids* ...'. From the *absorbances* obtained calculate the content of $C_{23}H_{32}O_6$ in the injection.

Storage Hydrocortisone Acetate Injection should be protected from light.

Labelling The label states (1) that it is intended for local action; (2) that the container should be gently shaken before a dose is withdrawn.

Hydrocortisone Sodium Phosphate Injection

Definition Hydrocortisone Sodium Phosphate Injection is a sterile solution of Hydrocortisone Sodium Phosphate in Water for Injections.

The injection complies with the requirements stated under Parenteral Preparations and with the following requirements.

Content of hydrocortisone, $C_{21}H_{30}O_5$ 92.5 to 107.5% of the prescribed or stated amount.

Characteristics A colourless or very pale yellow solution.

Identification

A. Carry out the method for *thin-layer chromatography*, Appendix III A, using *silica gel G* as the coating substance and a freshly prepared mixture of 60 volumes of *butan-1-ol*, 20 volumes of *acetic anhydride* and 20 volumes of *water* as the mobile phase. Apply separately to the plate 5 µl of each of the following solutions. For solution (1) dilute a volume of the injection containing the equivalent of 0.25 g of hydrocortisone to 100 ml with *water*. Solution (2) contains 0.34% w/v of *hydrocortisone sodium phosphate BPCRS* in *methanol*. Solution (3) is a mixture of equal volumes of solutions (1) and (2). Solution (4) is a mixture of equal volumes of solution (1) and a 0.25% w/v solution of *betamethasone sodium phosphate BPCRS* in *methanol*. After removal of the plate, allow it to dry in air until the odour of solvent is no longer detectable, spray with *ethanolic sulphuric acid (20%)*, heat at 120° for 10 minutes and examine under *ultraviolet light (365 nm)*. The principal spot in the chromatogram obtained with solution (1) corresponds to that in the chromatogram obtained with solution (2). The principal spot in the chromatogram obtained with solution (3) appears as a single compact spot and the chromatogram obtained with solution (4) exhibits two principal spots with almost identical Rf values.

B. Evaporate 0.1 ml to dryness on a water bath and dissolve the residue in 2 ml of *sulphuric acid*. A yellowish green fluorescence is produced immediately (distinction from betamethasone sodium phosphate, dexamethasone sodium phosphate and prednisolone sodium phosphate).

Alkalinity pH, 7.5 to 8.5, Appendix V L.

Related substances Carry out the method for *thin-layer chromatography*, Appendix III A, using *silica gel GF_{254}* as the coating substance and a mixture of 77 volumes of *dichloromethane*, 15 volumes of *ether*, 8 volumes of *methanol* and 1.2 volumes of *water* as the mobile phase. Apply separately to the plate 2 µl of each of the following solutions. For solution (1) dilute a volume of the injection with *water* to contain the equivalent of 0.75% w/v of hydrocortisone. Solutions (2) and (3) contain 1.0% w/v of *hydrocortisone sodium phosphate BPCRS* and 0.020% w/v of *hydrocortisone BPCRS* in *methanol*, respectively. After removal of the plate, allow it to dry in air for 5 minutes and examine under *ultraviolet light (254 nm)*. Any *secondary spot* in the chromatogram obtained with solution (1) is not more intense than the spot in the chromatogram obtained with solution (3).

Assay Dilute a volume containing the equivalent of 0.2 g of hydrocortisone to 1000 ml with *water*. To 5 ml add 15 ml of *water*, 2.5 g of *sodium chloride* and 0.5 ml of *hydrochloric acid* and extract with three 25-ml quantities of *chloroform*. Wash each chloroform layer with the same 1-ml quantity of 0.1M *hydrochloric acid*, add the washings to the aqueous solution and discard the chloroform. Extract the aqueous solution with two 10-ml quantities of *tributyl orthophosphate*, discard the aqueous phase and extract the combined tributyl phosphate solutions with two 25-ml quantities of a solution containing 10% w/v of *sodium chloride* and 1% w/v of *anhydrous disodium hydrogen orthophosphate*. Filter the extracts successively through absorbent cotton and wash the filter with 10 ml of the chloride—phosphate solution. Dilute the combined filtrates to 100 ml with the chloride—phosphate solution and measure the *absorbance* of the resulting solution at the maximum at 248 nm, Appendix II B, using in the reference cell a solution prepared in the same manner but using 20 ml of a solution containing 2.5 g of *sodium chloride* and 0.5 ml of *hydrochloric acid* and beginning at the words 'Extract the aqueous solution ...'. Calculate the content of hydrocortisone sodium phosphate as $C_{21}H_{30}O_5$ taking 447 as the value of A(1%, 1 cm) at the maximum at 248 nm.

Storage Hydrocortisone Sodium Phosphate Injection should be protected from light and stored at a temperature not exceeding 25°. The injection should not be allowed to freeze.

Labelling The strength is stated in terms of the equivalent amount of hydrocortisone in a suitable dose-volume.

Hydrocortisone Sodium Succinate Injection

Definition Hydrocortisone Sodium Succinate Injection is a sterile solution of hydrocortisone sodium succinate in Water for Injections. It is prepared by dissolving Hydrocortisone Sodium Succinate for Injection in the requisite amount of Water for Injections immediately before use.

The injection complies with the requirements stated under Parenteral Preparations.

Storage Hydrocortisone Sodium Succinate Injection deteriorates on storage and should be used immediately after preparation.

HYDROCORTISONE SODIUM SUCCINATE FOR INJECTION

Definition Hydrocortisone Sodium Succinate for Injection is a sterile material prepared from Hydrocortisone Hydrogen Succinate with the aid of a suitable alkali. It may contain excipients. It is supplied in a sealed container.

The contents of the sealed container comply with the requirements for Powders for Injections stated under Parenteral Preparations and with the following requirements.

Content of hydrocortisone, $C_{21}H_{30}O_5$ 95.0 to 105.0% of the prescribed or stated amount.

Identification

A. The *infrared absorption spectrum*, Appendix II A, is concordant with the *reference spectrum* of hydrocortisone sodium succinate.

B. Carry out the method for *thin-layer chromatography*, Appendix III A, using *silica gel GF_{254}* as the coating substance and a mixture of 1 volume of *anhydrous formic acid*, 10 volumes of *absolute ethanol* and 150 volumes of *dichloromethane* as the mobile phase. Apply separately to the plate 5 µl of each of the following solutions in a mixture of 1 volume of *methanol* and 9 volumes of *dichloromethane*. Solution (1) contains 0.1% w/v of the contents of the sealed container. Solution (2) contains 0.1% w/v of *hydrocortisone hydrogen succinate EPCRS*. Solution (3) contains 0.1% w/v each of *hydrocortisone hydrogen succinate EPCRS* and *methylprednisolone hydrogen succinate EPCRS*. After removal of the plate, allow it to dry in air and examine in daylight and under *ultraviolet light (365 nm)*. By each method of visualisation the principal spot in the chromatogram obtained with solution (1) is similar in position to the spot in the chromatogram obtained with solution (2). The test is not valid unless the chromatogram obtained with solution (3) shows two spots which may not be completely separated.

Acidity or alkalinity pH of a solution containing the equivalent of 5% w/v of hydrocortisone, 6.5 to 8.0, Appendix V L.

Related substances Carry out the method for *liquid chromatography*, Appendix III D, using the following solutions. For solution (1) dissolve a sufficient quantity of the contents of the sealed container in a mixture of equal volumes of *acetonitrile* and *water* to produce a solution containing the equivalent of 0.25% w/v of hydrocortisone. For solution (2) dilute 2 volumes of solution (1) to 100 volumes with a mixture of equal volumes of *acetonitrile* and *water*. For solution (3) dilute a 0.035% w/v solution of *hydrocortisone BPCRS* in *acetonitrile* with an equal volume of *water*. For solution (4) dilute a solution containing 0.04% w/v each of *hydrocortisone hydrogen succinate EPCRS* and *dexamethasone EPCRS* in *acetonitrile* with an equal volume of *water*.

The chromatographic procedure may be carried out using (a) a stainless steel column (25 cm × 4.6 mm) packed with *stationary phase C* (5 µm) (Hypersil ODS is suitable), (b) a mixture of 330 volumes of *acetonitrile*, 600 volumes of *water* and 1 volume of *orthophosphoric acid* which is allowed to equilibrate and then diluted to 1000 volumes with *water* as the mobile phase with a flow rate of 1 ml per minute and (c) a detection wavelength of 254 nm.

The test is not valid unless in the chromatogram obtained with solution (4) the *resolution factor* between the peaks corresponding to dexamethasone and hydrocortisone hydrogen succinate is at least 5.0.

For solution (1) allow the chromatography to proceed for twice the retention time of the principal peak. In the chromatogram obtained with solution (1) the area of any peak corresponding to hydrocortisone is not greater than the area of the peak in the chromatogram obtained with solution (3) (7%) and the area of any other *secondary peak* is not greater than the area of the peak in the chromatogram obtained with solution (2) (2%).

Uniformity of content The content of hydrocortisone in each of 10 individual containers as determined in the Assay is not less than 92.5% and not more than 107.5% of the content of hydrocortisone stated on the label, except that in one container the weight may be not less than 85.0% and not more than 115.0% of the stated content.

Assay Dissolve the contents of a sealed container in sufficient *water* to produce a solution containing the equivalent of 0.001% w/v of hydrocortisone. Measure the *absorbance* of the resulting solution at the maximum at 248 nm, Appendix II B, and calculate the content of $C_{21}H_{30}O_5$ taking 449 as the value of A(1%, 1 cm) at the maximum at 248 nm. Repeat the procedure with a further nine sealed containers and calculate the average content of $C_{21}H_{30}O_5$ per container from the ten individual results thus obtained.

Labelling The label of the sealed container states the quantity of hydrocortisone sodium succinate contained in it in terms of the equivalent amount of hydrocortisone.

Hydrocortisone Ointment

Definition Hydrocortisone Ointment contains Hydrocortisone in a suitable basis.

The ointment complies with the requirements stated under Topical Semi-solid Preparations and with the following requirements.

Content of hydrocortisone, $C_{21}H_{30}O_5$ 90.0 to 110.0% of the prescribed or stated amount.

Identification

A. Complies with test A for Identification described under Hydrocortisone Cream but preparing solution (1) in the following manner. For ointments containing more than 0.5% w/w of Hydrocortisone, disperse a quantity containing 25 mg of Hydrocortisone in 5 ml of hot *hexane*, cool, extract with 10 ml of *methanol (90%)* and filter. For ointments containing 0.5% w/w or less of Hydrocortisone, disperse a quantity containing 5 mg of Hydrocortisone in 50 ml of hot *hexane*, cool, extract with 10 ml of *methanol (90%)* and filter.

B. In the Assay, the chromatogram obtained with solution (2) shows a peak with the same retention time as the peak due to hydrocortisone in the chromatogram obtained with solution (1).

Assay Carry out the Assay described under Hydrocortisone Cream but prepare solution (2) in the following manner. For ointments containing more than 0.5% w/w of Hydrocortisone, disperse a quantity containing 25 mg of Hydrocortisone in 100 ml of hot *hexane*, cool and extract with 20 ml of a solution prepared by mixing 3 volumes of *methanol* with 1 volume of a 15% w/v solution of *sodium chloride*. Repeat the extraction using a further two 10-ml quantities of the methanolic sodium chloride solution. To the combined extracts add 5 ml of *methanol* and sufficient *water* to produce 100 ml, mix and filter through a glass microfibre filter (Whatman GF/C is suitable). For ointments containing 0.5% w/w or less of Hydrocortisone, prepare solution (2) in the same manner as solution (2) above but use a quantity containing 5 mg of Hydrocortisone.

Storage Hydrocortisone Ointment should be protected from light.

Hydrocortisone Acetate Ointment

Definition Hydrocortisone Acetate Ointment contains Hydrocortisone Acetate in a suitable basis.

The ointment complies with the requirements stated under Topical Semi-solid Preparations and with the following requirements.

Content of hydrocortisone acetate, $C_{23}H_{32}O_6$ 90.0 to 110.0% of the prescribed or stated amount.

Identification

A. Carry out the method for *thin-layer chromatography*, Appendix III A, using *silica gel G* as the coating substance and a mixture of 77 volumes of *dichloromethane*, 15 volumes of *ether*, 8 volumes of *methanol* and 1.2 volumes of *water* as the mobile phase. Apply separately to the plate 5 µl of each of the following solutions.

For ointments containing more than 0.5% w/w of Hydrocortisone Acetate, prepare two solutions in the following manner. For solution (1) disperse a quantity containing 25 mg of Hydrocortisone Acetate in 5 ml of hot *hexane*, cool, extract with 10 ml of *methanol (90%)* and filter. Solution (2) is a mixture of equal volumes of solution (1) and a 0.25% w/v solution of *hydrocortisone acetate BPCRS* in *methanol*.

For ointments containing 0.5% w/w or less of Hydrocortisone Acetate, prepare solution (1) in the same manner as solution (1) above but use a quantity containing 5 mg of Hydrocortisone Acetate. Solution (2) is a mixture of equal volumes of solution (1) and a 0.05% w/v solution of *hydrocortisone acetate BPCRS* in *methanol*.

After removal of the plate, allow it to dry in air and spray with *alkaline tetrazolium blue solution*. The principal spot in the chromatogram obtained with solution (1) corresponds to that in the chromatogram obtained with solution (2) which appears as a single, compact spot.

B. In the Assay, the chromatogram obtained with solution (2) shows a peak with the same retention time as the peak due to hydrocortisone acetate in the chromatogram obtained with solution (1).

Assay Carry out the method for *liquid chromatography*, Appendix III D, using the following solutions.

For ointments containing more than 0.5% w/w of Hydrocortisone Acetate, prepare solutions (1) and (2) in the following manner. For solution (1) dissolve 25 mg of *hydrocortisone acetate BPCRS* in 45 ml of *methanol*, add 5 ml of a 0.5% w/v solution of *betamethasone* (internal standard) in *methanol* and sufficient *water* to produce 100 ml. For solution (2) disperse a quantity of the ointment containing 25 mg of Hydrocortisone Acetate in 100 ml of hot *hexane*, cool and extract with 20 ml of a solution prepared by mixing 3 volumes of *methanol* and 1 volume of a 15% w/v solution of *sodium chloride*. Repeat the extraction using two 10-ml quantities of the methanolic sodium chloride solution. Add 5 ml of *methanol* to the combined extracts and sufficient *water* to produce 100 ml, mix and filter through a glass microfibre filter (Whatman GF/C is suitable).

For ointments containing 0.5% w/w or less of Hydrocortisone Acetate, prepare solutions (1) and (2) in the following manner. For solution (1) dissolve 5 mg of *hydrocortisone acetate BPCRS* in 45 ml of *methanol*, add 5 ml of a 0.110% w/v solution of *betamethasone* (internal standard) in *methanol* and add sufficient *water* to produce 100 ml. Prepare solution (2) in the same manner as solution (2) above but use a quantity containing 5 mg of Hydrocortisone Acetate.

In each case prepare solution (3) in the same manner as solution (2) but add 5 ml of the internal standard solution in place of the 5 ml of methanol before diluting to volume.

The chromatographic procedure may be carried out using (a) a stainless steel column (10 cm × 5 mm) packed with *stationary phase C* (5 µm) (Spherisorb ODS 1 is suitable), (b) *methanol (50%)* as the mobile phase with a flow rate of 2 ml per minute and (c) a detection wavelength of 240 nm.

Calculate the content of $C_{23}H_{32}O_6$ in the ointment using the declared content of $C_{23}H_{32}O_6$ in *hydrocortisone acetate BPCRS*.

Storage Hydrocortisone Acetate Ointment should be protected from light.

Hydrocortisone and Clioquinol Ointment

Definition Hydrocortisone and Clioquinol Ointment contains Hydrocortisone and Clioquinol, the latter in *very fine powder*, in a suitable basis.

The ointment complies with the requirements stated under Topical Semi-solid Preparations and with the following requirements.

Content of hydrocortisone, $C_{21}H_{30}O_5$ 92.5 to 107.5% of the prescribed or stated amount.

Content of clioquinol, C_9H_5ClINO 90.0 to 110.0% of the prescribed or stated amount.

Identification

A. Carry out the method for *thin-layer chromatography*, Appendix III A, using *silica gel G* as the coating substance and a mixture of 77 volumes of *dichloromethane*, 15 volumes of *ether*, 8 volumes of *methanol* and 1.2 volumes of *water* as the mobile phase. Apply separately to the plate 5 µl of each of the following solutions. For solution (1) disperse, by warming and shaking, a quantity of the ointment containing 2.5 g of Hydrocortisone in 10 ml of *ethanol (96%)*, cool, allow to stand at 0° for 30 minutes, filter and use the filtrate. Solution (2) contains 0.25% w/v of *hydrocortisone BPCRS* in *ethanol (96%)*. For solution (3) dissolve 12.5 mg of *hydrocortisone BPCRS* in 5 ml of solution (1). After removal of the plate, allow it to dry in air and spray with *alkaline tetrazolium blue solution*. The principal spot in the chromatogram obtained with solution (1) corresponds to that in the chromatogram obtained with solution (2). The principal spot in the chromatogram obtained with solution (3) appears as a single, compact spot.

B. In the Assay for hydrocortisone the chromatogram obtained with solution (3) shows a peak with the same retention time as the peak due to hydrocortisone in the chromatogram obtained with solution (1).

C. Fuse a quantity of the ointment containing 0.1 g of Clioquinol with *anhydrous sodium carbonate*, dissolve the fused mass in *water* and acidify with 2M *nitric acid*. Add *silver nitrate solution*; a pale yellow precipitate is produced which is insoluble in 5M *ammonia*. Add 5M *ammonia* until the solution becomes alkaline, boil gently, filter and acidify the filtrate with 2M *nitric acid*; a white precipitate is produced which darkens on exposure to light.

Assay

For hydrocortisone Carry out the method for *liquid chromatography*, Appendix III D, using the following solutions. For solution (1) dissolve 5 mg of *hydrocortisone BPCRS* in 5 ml of a 4% v/v solution of *bromobenzene* (internal standard) in *methanol* and dilute to 50 ml with *methanol (80%)*. For solution (2) add 30 ml of *2,2,4-trimethylpentane* to a quantity of the ointment containing 10 mg of Hydrocortisone and warm on a water bath until the preparation has melted. Extract the warm mixture with successive quantities of 30, 20 and 20 ml of *methanol (80%)*, combine the aqueous methanolic layers, cool to about 20° and dilute to 100 ml with the same solvent. Prepare solution (3) in the same manner as solution (2) but adding 10 ml of a 4% v/v solution of *bromobenzene* in *methanol* to the cooled methanolic extract.

The chromatographic procedure may be carried out using (a) a stainless steel column (25 cm × 5 mm) packed with *stationary phase C* (Spherisorb ODS 1 is suitable), (b) *methanol (65%)* as the mobile phase with a flow rate of 1 ml per minute and (c) a detection wavelength of 242 nm.

Calculate the content of $C_{21}H_{30}O_5$ in the ointment taking 100.0% as the content of $C_{21}H_{30}O_5$ in *hydrocortisone BPCRS*.

For clioquinol To a quantity containing 25 mg of Clioquinol add 80 ml of a hot mixture of 24 volumes of *2-methoxyethanol* and 6 volumes of *water* and heat on a water bath for 5 minutes. Cool in ice for 10 minutes, allow to warm to room temperature, dilute to 100 ml with the aqueous methoxyethanol, mix and filter. To 10 ml of the filtrate add 10 ml of *2-methoxyethanol* and 2 ml of a solution prepared by dissolving 0.5 g of *iron(III) chloride hexahydrate* in 80 ml of *2-methoxyethanol* and adding 0.1 ml of *hydrochloric acid* and sufficient *2-methoxyethanol* to produce 100 ml. Dilute the solution to 25 ml with *2-methoxyethanol* and measure the *absorbance* of the resulting solution at the maximum at 650 nm, Appendix II B, using in the reference cell a solution prepared by treating 10 ml of the aqueous methoxyethanol in the same manner beginning at the words 'add 10 ml of *2-methoxyethanol* ...'.

Calculate the content of C_9H_5ClINO from the *absorbance* obtained by repeating the operation beginning at the words 'add 10 ml of *2-methoxyethanol* ...' and using 10 ml of a solution prepared in the following manner. Dissolve 0.125 g of *clioquinol BPCRS* in sufficient *2-methoxyethanol* to produce 50 ml, warming to effect solution; add 1 ml of *water* to 5 ml of the solution and add sufficient of a mixture of 24 volumes of *2-methoxyethanol* and 6 volumes of *water* to produce 50 ml.

Storage Hydrocortisone and Clioquinol Ointment should be protected from light.

Hydroflumethiazide Tablets

Definition Hydroflumethiazide Tablets contain Hydroflumethiazide.

The tablets comply with the requirements stated under Tablets and with the following requirements.

Content of hydroflumethiazide, $C_8H_8F_3N_3O_4S_2$ 92.5 to 107.5% of the prescribed or stated amount.

Identification Carry out the method for *thin-layer chromatography*, Appendix III A, using *silica gel GF_{254}* as the coating substance and *ethyl acetate* as the mobile phase. Apply separately to the plate 5 µl of each of the following solutions. For solution (1) shake a quantity of the powdered tablets containing 10 mg of Hydroflumethiazide with 10 ml of *acetone* for 10 minutes and filter. Solution (2) contains 0.1% w/v of *hydroflumethiazide BPCRS* in *acetone*. After removal of the plate, dry it in a current of air, examine under *ultraviolet light (254 nm)* and then treat the plate by *Method I* and examine again. By each method of visualisation the principal spot in the chromatogram obtained with solution (1) corresponds in colour and intensity to that in the chromatogram obtained with solution (2).

Related substances Carry out the method for *thin-layer chromatography*, Appendix III A, using *silica gel G* as the coating substance and *ethyl acetate* as the mobile phase. Apply separately to the plate 10 µl of each of the following solutions. For solution (1) shake a quantity of the powdered tablets containing 25 mg of Hydroflumethiazide with 25 ml of *acetone* for 10 minutes, filter, evaporate the filtrate to dryness and dissolve the residue in 2.5 ml of *acetone*. For solution (2) dilute 1 volume of solution (1) to 100 volumes with *acetone*. After removal of the plate, dry it in a current of air and reveal the spots by *Method I*. Any *secondary spot* in the chromatogram obtained with solution (1) is not more intense than the spot in the chromatogram obtained with solution (2) (1%).

Assay Weigh and powder 20 tablets. Shake a quantity of the powder containing 15 mg of Hydroflumethiazide with 50 ml of *methanol* for 10 minutes and dilute to 100 ml with *methanol*. Mix, filter, dilute 10 ml of the filtrate to 100 ml with *methanol* and measure the *absorbance* of the resulting solution at the maximum at 273 nm, Appendix II B. Calculate the content of $C_8H_8F_3N_3O_4S_2$ taking 595 as the value of A(1%, 1 cm) at the maximum at 273 nm.

Hydrogen Peroxide Mouthwash

Definition Hydrogen Peroxide Mouthwash is Hydrogen Peroxide Solution (6 per cent).

The mouthwash complies with the requirements stated under Mouthwashes and with the following requirements.

Content of hydrogen peroxide, H_2O_2 5.0 to 7.0% w/v.

Identification; Acidity; Non-volatile matter; Organic stabilisers Complies with the requirements stated under Hydrogen Peroxide Solution (6 per cent).

Assay Dilute 10 ml to 100 ml with *water*. To 10 ml of the resulting solution add 20 ml of 1M *sulphuric acid* and titrate with 0.02M *potassium permanganate VS*. Each ml of 0.02M *potassium permanganate VS* is equivalent to 1.701 mg of H_2O_2.

Storage Hydrogen Peroxide Mouthwash should be protected from light.

Labelling The label states, where applicable, that the Mouthwash contains a stabilising agent.

Hydrotalcite Tablets

Definition Hydrotalcite Tablets contain Hydrotalcite.

The tablets comply with the requirements stated under Tablets and with the following requirements.

Content of hydrotalcite, $Al_2Mg_6(OH)_{16}CO_3,4H_2O$ 90.0 to 110.0% of the prescribed or stated amount.

Identification Add 20 ml of 2M *hydrochloric acid* to a quantity of the powdered tablets containing 1.0 g of Hydrotalcite, shake and filter. Add 30 ml of *water* to the filtrate and boil. Add 2M *ammonia* until just alkaline to *methyl red*, continue boiling for 2 minutes and filter. Wash the precipitate with 50 ml of a hot 2% w/v solution of *ammonium chloride* and dissolve in 15 ml of 2M *hydrochloric acid*. The resulting solution yields the reactions characteristic of *aluminium salts*, Appendix VI.

Neutralising capacity Weigh and powder 20 tablets, pass the powder as completely as possible through a sieve of nominal mesh aperture about 225 µm and remix the sifted powder. Mix a quantity equivalent to one tablet with a small quantity of *water*, added slowly with stirring, to give a smooth paste and add gradually sufficient further quantities of *water* to produce 100 ml. Warm to 37°, add 100 ml of 0.1M *hydrochloric acid VS* previously heated to 37° and stir continuously using a paddle stirrer at a rate of about 200 revolutions per minute, maintaining the temperature at 37°. The pH of the solution at 37°, after 10 minutes and after 20 minutes, is 3.0 to 4.2, Appendix V L. Add 12 ml of 0.5M *hydrochloric acid VS* at 37°, stir continuously for 1 hour, maintaining the temperature at 37°, and titrate with 0.1M *sodium hydroxide VS* to pH 3.5. Subtract the number of ml of 0.1M *sodium hydroxide VS* from 160 ml to obtain the number of ml of 0.1M *hydrochloric acid VS* required for neutralisation. Not less than 130 ml of 0.1M *hydrochloric acid VS* is required to neutralise one tablet.

Assay Weigh and powder 20 tablets. To a quantity of the powder containing 0.3 g of Hydrotalcite add 2 ml of 7M *hydrochloric acid* and heat on a water bath for 15 minutes. Allow to cool, add 250 ml of *water* and 50 ml of 0.05M *disodium edetate VS* and neutralise with 1M *sodium hydroxide* using *methyl red solution* as indicator. Heat the solution on a water bath for 30 minutes and allow to cool. Add 3 g of *hexamine* and titrate the excess of disodium edetate with 0.05M *lead nitrate VS* using *xylenol orange solution* as indicator. Each ml of 0.05M *disodium edetate VS* is equivalent to 15.09 mg of $Al_2Mg_6(OH)_{16}CO_3,4H_2O$.

Hydrous Ointment

Oily Cream

Definition

Wool Alcohols Ointment	500 g
Phenoxyethanol	10 g
Dried Magnesium Sulphate	5 g
Purified Water, freshly boiled and cooled,	sufficient to produce 1000 g

In preparing Hydrous Ointment the proportions of Hard Paraffin, Soft Paraffin and Liquid Paraffin used to make the Wool Alcohols Ointment may be varied to produce Hydrous Ointment having suitable properties.

When Hydrous Ointment is used in a white ointment, it should be prepared from Wool Alcohols Ointment made with White Soft Paraffin; when used in a coloured ointment, it should be prepared from Wool Alcohols Ointment made with Yellow Soft Paraffin.

Extemporaneous preparation The following directions apply.

Dissolve the Phenoxyethanol and the Dried Magnesium Sulphate in sufficient warm Purified Water to produce about 500 g. Melt the Wool Alcohols Ointment and heat to about 60°; gradually add the aqueous solution at about 60° with vigorous stirring until a smooth cream is obtained. Stir until cool, add sufficient Purified Water to produce 1000 g and mix.

The ointment complies with the requirements stated under Topical Semi-solid Preparations.

Storage Hydrous Ointment should be kept in a container made from non-absorbent material. If, on storage, some aqueous liquid separates, it is readily reincorporated by stirring.

Hydroxocobalamin Injection

Definition Hydroxocobalamin Injection is a sterile solution of Hydroxocobalamin Acetate, Hydroxocobalamin Chloride or Hydroxocobalamin Sulphate in Water for Injections containing sufficient Acetic Acid, Hydrochloric Acid or Sulphuric Acid respectively to adjust the pH to about 4.

The injection complies with the requirements stated under Parenteral Preparations and with the following requirements.

Content of hydroxocobalamin, $C_{62}H_{89}CoN_{13}O_{15}P$ 95.0 to 110.0% of the prescribed or stated amount of anhydrous hydroxocobalamin.

Identification Measure the *absorbance* at 351 nm and at 361 nm, Appendix II B. The ratio of the absorbance at 361 nm to that at 351 nm is about 0.65.

Acidity pH, 3.8 to 5.5, Appendix V L.

Related substances Carry out the method for *liquid chromatography*, Appendix III D, injecting 20 µl of each of the following solutions. Solutions (1) to (3) are freshly prepared solutions of the injection, diluted if necessary with the mobile phase, containing the equivalent of (1) 0.10% w/v, (2) 0.005% w/v and (3) 0.00010% w/v of hydroxocobalamin. For solution (4) add 0.2 ml of a freshly prepared 2% w/v solution of *chloramine T* and 0.1 ml of 0.05M *hydrochloric acid* to a volume containing the equivalent of 5 mg of hydroxocobalamin, dilute to 10 ml with *water*, shake, allow to stand for 5 minutes and inject immediately. Protect the solutions from bright light.

The chromatographic procedure may be carried out using (a) a stainless steel column (25 cm × 4 mm) packed with *stationary phase B* (5 µm) (Lichrosorb 100 CH8/11 is suitable), (b) a mixture of 19.5 volumes of *methanol* and 80.5 volumes of a solution containing 1.5% w/v of *citric acid* and 0.81% w/v of *disodium hydrogen orthophosphate* as the mobile phase with a flow rate of 1.5 ml per minute and (c) a detection wavelength of 351 nm.

The test is not valid unless the chromatogram obtained with solution (4) shows three principal peaks, the *resolution factor* between each pair of adjacent peaks is not less than

3.0 and the chromatogram obtained with solution (3) shows one principal peak with a *signal-to-noise ratio* of not less than 5.

In the chromatogram obtained with solution (1) the sum of the areas of any *secondary peaks* is not greater than twice the area of the principal peak in the chromatogram obtained with solution (2) (10%). Disregard any peak the area of which is less than that of the principal peak in the chromatogram obtained with solution (3) (0.1%).

Assay Carry out the following procedure protected from light. Dilute a quantity containing the equivalent of 2.5 mg of anhydrous hydroxocobalamin to 100 ml with a solution containing 0.8% v/v of *glacial acetic acid* and 1.09% w/v of *sodium acetate* and measure the *absorbance* of the resulting solution at the maximum at 351 nm, Appendix II B. Calculate the content of $C_{62}H_{89}CoN_{13}O_{15}P$ taking 195 as the value of A(1%, 1 cm) at the maximum at 351 nm.

Storage Hydroxocobalamin Injection should be protected from light.

Labelling The strength is stated in terms of the equivalent amount of anhydrous hydroxocobalamin in a suitable dose-volume.

When vitamin B_{12} injection is prescribed or demanded, Hydroxocobalamin Injection shall be dispensed or supplied.

Hydroxycarbamide Capsules

Definition Hydroxycarbamide Capsules contain Hydroxycarbamide.

The capsules comply with the requirements stated under Capsules and with the following requirements.

Content of hydroxycarbamide, $CH_4N_2O_2$ 95.0 to 105.0% of the prescribed or stated amount.

Identification

A. Shake a quantity of the contents of the capsules containing 30 mg of Hydroxycarbamide with 10 ml of *methanol* and filter. Evaporate the filtrate to dryness and dry the residue at 60° at a pressure of 2 kPa for 3 hours. The *infrared absorption spectrum* of the residue, Appendix II A, is concordant with the *reference spectrum* of hydroxycarbamide.

B. In the test for Urea and related substances the principal spot in the chromatogram obtained with solution (3) corresponds to that in the chromatogram obtained with solution (4).

Urea and related substances Comply with the test described under Hydroxycarbamide but using the following solutions. For solution (1) use the supernatant liquid obtained by shaking a quantity of the contents of the capsules containing 1 g of Hydroxycarbamide for 15 minutes with 10 ml of *water* and centrifuging the solution for 5 minutes. Solution (2) contains 0.050% w/v of *urea* in *water*. For solution (3) dilute 1 ml of solution (1) to 10 ml with *water*. Solution (4) contains 1.0% w/v of *hydroxycarbamide BPCRS* in *water*.

Assay To a quantity of the powdered contents of five capsules containing 0.1 g of Hydroxycarbamide add 30 ml of *water* and shake for 5 minutes. Dilute to 100 ml with *water* and centrifuge a portion for 5 minutes. To 2 ml of the supernatant solution add 5 ml of a 10% w/v solution of *sodium hydrogen carbonate*, mix and allow to stand for 15 minutes. Add 20 ml of 0.005M *iodine VS* and allow to stand for 5 minutes. Add 5 ml of a 20% w/v solution of *sodium dihydrogen orthophosphate*, mix, allow to stand until effervescence ceases and titrate with 0.01M *sodium thiosulphate VS* using *starch mucilage* as indicator. Repeat the operation using 2 ml of *water* in place of the supernatant solution and beginning at the words 'add 5 ml...'. Repeat the assay using *hydroxycarbamide BPCRS* in place of the substance being examined. Calculate the content of $CH_4N_2O_2$ using the declared content of $CH_4N_2O_2$ in *hydroxycarbamide BPCRS*.

Storage Hydroxycarbamide Capsules should be kept in a well-closed container and protected from moisture.

When hydroxyurea capsules are prescribed or demanded, Hydroxycarbamide Capsules shall be dispensed or supplied.

Hydroxychloroquine Tablets

Definition Hydroxychloroquine Tablets contain Hydroxychloroquine Sulphate. They are coated.

The tablets comply with the requirements stated under Tablets and with the following requirements.

Content of hydroxychloroquine sulphate, $C_{18}H_{26}ClN_3O,H_2SO_4$ 92.5 to 107.5% of the prescribed or stated amount.

Identification

A. Dissolve a quantity of the powdered tablets containing 0.1 g of Hydroxychloroquine Sulphate in a mixture of 10 ml of *water* and 2 ml of 2M *sodium hydroxide* and extract with two 20-ml quantities of *chloroform*. Wash the chloroform extracts with *water*, dry with *anhydrous sodium sulphate*, evaporate to dryness and dissolve the residue in 2 ml of *chloroform IR*. The *infrared absorption spectrum* of the resulting solution, Appendix II A, is concordant with the *reference spectrum* of hydroxychloroquine.

B. Extract a quantity of the powdered tablets containing 0.2 g of Hydroxychloroquine Sulphate with 10 ml of *water* and filter. To the filtrate add 30 ml of hot *picric acid solution R1* and allow to cool. The *melting point* of the precipitate, after washing with 10 ml of *water*, is about 189°, Appendix V A.

C. Shake a quantity of the powdered tablets containing 0.1 g of Hydroxychloroquine Sulphate with 10 ml of *water* and filter. To the filtrate add 1 ml of 2M *hydrochloric acid* and 1 ml of *barium chloride solution*. A white precipitate is produced.

Disintegration Maximum time, 45 minutes, Appendix XII A.

Assay Weigh and powder 20 tablets. Dissolve a quantity of the powder containing 0.5 g of Hydroxychloroquine Sulphate in 20 ml of 1M *sodium hydroxide* and extract with four 25-ml quantities of *chloroform*. Combine the chloroform extracts and evaporate to a volume of about 10 ml. Add 40 ml of *anhydrous acetic acid* and carry out Method I for *non-aqueous titration*, Appendix VIII A, determining the end point potentiometrically. Each ml of 0.1M *perchloric* *acid VS* is equivalent to 21.70 mg of $C_{18}H_{26}ClN_3O,H_2SO_4$.

200 mg of Hydroxychloroquine Sulphate is approximately equivalent to 156 mg of hydroxychloroquine.

Hydroxyprogesterone Injection

Definition Hydroxyprogesterone Injection is a sterile solution of Hydroxyprogesterone Caproate in a suitable ester, in a suitable fixed oil or in any mixture of these.

The injection complies with the requirements stated under Parenteral Preparations and with the following requirements.

Content of hydroxyprogesterone caproate, $C_{27}H_{40}O_4$ 92.5 to 107.5% of the prescribed or stated amount.

Identification

A. Carry out the method for *thin-layer chromatography*, Appendix III A, using *silica gel HF_{254}* as the coating substance and a mixture of equal volumes of *cyclohexane* and *ethyl acetate* as the mobile phase. Apply separately to the plate 1 µl of each of the following solutions. For solution (1) dilute the injection with *chloroform* to give a solution containing 1.0% w/v of Hydroxyprogesterone Caproate. Solution (2) contains 1.0% w/v of *hydroxyprogesterone caproate BPCRS* in *chloroform*. After removal of the plate, allow it to dry in air and examine under *ultraviolet light (254 nm)*. The principal spot in the chromatogram obtained with solution (1) corresponds to the principal spot in the chromatogram obtained with solution (2). Secondary spots due to the vehicle may also be observed.

B. Dissolve a volume containing 0.1 g of Hydroxyprogesterone Caproate in 10 ml of *petroleum spirit (boiling range, 40° to 60°)* and extract with three 10-ml quantities of a mixture of 7 volumes of *glacial acetic acid* and 3 volumes of *water*. Wash the combined extracts with 10 ml of *petroleum spirit (boiling range, 40° to 60°)*, dilute with *water* until the solution becomes turbid and allow to stand in ice for about 2 hours until a white precipitate is produced. The *melting point* of the precipitate, after washing with *water*, is about 120°, Appendix V A.

Assay To a quantity containing 0.125 g of Hydroxyprogesterone Caproate add sufficient *chloroform* to produce 100 ml. Dilute 5 ml to 100 ml with *chloroform*; to 5 ml add 10 ml of *isoniazid solution* and sufficient *methanol* to produce 20 ml. Allow to stand for 45 minutes and measure the *absorbance* of the resulting solution at the maximum at 380 nm, Appendix II B, using in the reference cell 5 ml of *chloroform* treated in the same manner and beginning at the words 'add 10 ml of...'. Calculate the content of $C_{27}H_{40}O_4$ from the *absorbance* obtained by repeating the operation using a 0.00625% w/v solution of *hydroxyprogesterone caproate BPCRS* in *chloroform* and beginning at the words 'to 5 ml...'.

Storage Hydroxyprogesterone Injection should be protected from light.

Labelling The label states that the preparation is for intramuscular injection only.

Hyoscine Butylbromide Injection

Definition Hyoscine Butylbromide Injection is a sterile solution of Hyoscine Butylbromide in Water for Injections.

The injection complies with the requirements stated under Parenteral Preparations and with the following requirements.

Content of hyoscine butylbromide, $C_{21}H_{30}BrNO_4$ 92.5 to 107.5% of the prescribed or stated amount.

Identification

A. Evaporate to dryness a volume containing 0.1 g of Hyoscine Butylbromide, shake the residue with *chloroform*, filter, evaporate the filtrate to dryness and triturate the residue with 5 ml of *acetonitrile*. Evaporate to dryness and dry the residue at 50° at a pressure not exceeding 0.7 kPa for 1 hour. The *infrared absorption spectrum* of the residue, Appendix II A, is concordant with the *reference spectrum* of hyoscine butylbromide. Retain the residue for use in test C.

B. The *light absorption*, Appendix II B, in the range 230 to 350 nm of the solution obtained in the Assay exhibits maxima at 252, 257 and 264 nm and a less well-defined maximum at 247 nm.

C. To 1 mg of the residue obtained in test A add 0.2 ml of *fuming nitric acid* and evaporate to dryness on a water bath. Dissolve the residue in 2 ml of *acetone* and add 0.1 ml of a 3% w/v solution of *potassium hydroxide* in *methanol*. A violet colour is produced.

Acidity pH, 3.7 to 5.5, Appendix V L.

Hyoscine Carry out the method for *liquid chromatography*, Appendix III D, using the following solutions. For solution (1) use the injection diluted, if necessary, with 0.001M *hydrochloric acid* to contain 1.0% w/v of Hyoscine Butylbromide. Solution (2) contains 0.0010% w/v of *hyoscine hydrobromide BPCRS* in 0.001M *hydrochloric acid*. For solution (3) add 10 µl of solution (1) to 10 ml of solution (2).

The chromatographic procedure may be carried out using (a) a stainless steel column (25 cm × 4.6 mm) packed with *stationary phase B* (10 µm) (Lichrosorb 10µ C8 is suitable), (b) a solution of 2.0 g of *sodium dodecyl sulphate* in a mixture of 370 ml of 0.001M *hydrochloric acid* and 680 ml of *methanol* as the mobile phase with a flow rate of 2 ml per minute and (c) a detection wavelength of 210 nm.

Inject 20 µl of solution (3). The test is not valid unless the *resolution factor* between the peaks corresponding to hyoscine and butylhyoscine is at least 5.

Inject 20 µl of each of solutions (1) and (2). The area of any peak corresponding to hyoscine in the chromatogram obtained with solution (1) is not greater than the area of the principal peak in the chromatogram obtained with solution (2) (0.1%).

Related substances Carry out the method for *thin-layer chromatography*, Appendix III A, using a silica gel F_{254} high-performance precoated plate (Merck silica gel 60 F_{254} HPTLC plates are suitable) and a mixture of 0.5 volume of *anhydrous formic acid*, 1.5 volumes of *water*, 9 volumes of *absolute ethanol* and 9 volumes of *dichloromethane* as the mobile phase but allowing the solvent front to ascend 4 cm above the line of application. Apply separately to the plate 2 µl of each of the following solutions.

For solution (1) dilute the injection with 0.01M *hydrochloric acid* to contain 0.2% w/v of Hyoscine Butylbromide and centrifuge. For solution (2) dilute 3 volumes of solution (1) to 100 volumes with 0.01M *hydrochloric acid.* For solution (3) dilute 1 volume of solution (1) to 50 volumes with 0.01M *hydrochloric acid.* For solution (4) dilute 1 volume of solution (1) to 400 volumes with 0.01M *hydrochloric acid.* After removal of the plate, dry it at 60° for 15 minutes, spray with a solution prepared by mixing equal volumes of a 40% w/v solution of *potassium iodide* in *water* and a solution prepared by dissolving 0.85 g of *bismuth oxynitrate* in a mixture of 10 ml of *glacial acetic acid* and 40 ml of *water* and diluting 1 volume of the mixture with 2 volumes of *glacial acetic acid* and 10 volumes of *water* immediately before use. Allow the plate to dry in air, spray well with a 5% w/v solution of *sodium nitrite* and examine immediately. In the chromatogram obtained with solution (1) the principal spot has an Rf value of about 0.45. In the chromatogram obtained with solution (1) any *secondary spot* with an Rf value less than that of the principal spot is not more intense than the spot in the chromatogram obtained with solution (2) (3%) and not more than two such spots are more intense than the spot in the chromatogram obtained with solution (4) (0.25%); any *secondary spot* with an Rf value greater than that of the principal spot is not more intense than the spot in the chromatogram obtained with solution (3) (2%) and not more than one such spot is more intense than the spot in the chromatogram obtained with solution (4) (0.25%).

Assay Carry out the method for *liquid chromatography*, Appendix III D, using the following solutions. For solution (1) dilute the injection to contain 0.04% w/v of Hyoscine Butylbromide with 0.001M *hydrochloric acid.* Solution (2) contains 0.04% w/v of *hyoscine butylbromide BPCRS* in 0.001M *hydrochloric acid.*

The chromatographic procedure described under the test for Hyoscine may be used.

Calculate the content of $C_{21}H_{30}BrNO_4$ using the declared content of $C_{21}H_{30}BrNO_4$ in *hyoscine butylbromide BPCRS.*

Storage Hyoscine Butylbromide Injection should be protected from light.

Hyoscine Butylbromide Tablets

Definition Hyoscine Butylbromide Tablets contain Hyoscine Butylbromide.

The tablets comply with the requirements stated under Tablets and with the following requirements.

Content of hyoscine butylbromide, $C_{21}H_{30}BrNO_4$
92.5 to 107.5% of the prescribed or stated amount.

Identification

A. Shake a quantity of the powdered tablets containing 50 mg of Hyoscine Butylbromide with 20 ml of *chloroform*, filter, evaporate the filtrate to dryness and triturate the residue with 5 ml of *acetonitrile.* Evaporate to dryness and dry the residue at 50° at a pressure not exceeding 0.7 kPa for 1 hour. The *infrared absorption spectrum* of the residue, Appendix II A, is concordant with the *reference spectrum* of hyoscine butylbromide.

B. To 1 mg of the residue obtained in test A add 0.2 ml of *fuming nitric acid* and evaporate to dryness on a water bath. Dissolve the residue in 2 ml of *acetone* and add 0.1 ml of a 3% w/v solution of *potassium hydroxide* in *methanol.* A violet colour is produced.

C. Shake a quantity of the powdered tablets containing 50 mg of Hyoscine Butylbromide with 20 ml of *chloroform*, filter, evaporate the filtrate to dryness, shake the residue with 50 ml of *water* and filter. The *light absorption* of the filtrate, Appendix II B, in the range 230 to 350 nm exhibits maxima at 252, 257 and 264 nm and a less well-defined maximum at 247 nm.

Hyoscine Carry out the method for *liquid chromatography*, Appendix III D, using the following solutions. For solution (1) shake a quantity of the powdered tablets containing 0.1 g of Hyoscine Butylbromide with 10 ml of 0.001M *hydrochloric acid* with the aid of ultrasound for 15 minutes, centrifuge and filter. Solution (2) contains 0.0010% w/v of *hyoscine hydrobromide BPCRS* in 0.001M *hydrochloric acid.* For solution (3) add 10 µl of solution (1) to 10 ml of solution (2).

The chromatographic procedure may be carried out using (a) a stainless steel column (25 cm × 4.6 mm) packed with *stationary phase B* (10 µm) (Lichrosorb 10µ C8 is suitable), (b) a solution of 2.0 g of *sodium dodecyl sulphate* in a mixture of 370 ml of 0.001M *hydrochloric acid* and 680 ml of *methanol* as the mobile phase with a flow rate of 2 ml per minute and (c) a detection wavelength of 210 nm.

Inject 20 µl of solution (3). The test is not valid unless the *resolution factor* between the peaks corresponding to hyoscine and butylhyoscine is at least 5.

Inject 20 µl of each of solutions (1) and (2). The area of any peak corresponding to hyoscine in the chromatogram obtained with solution (1) is not greater than the area of the principal peak in the chromatogram obtained with solution (2) (0.1%).

Related substances Carry out the method for *thin-layer chromatography*, Appendix III A, using a silica gel F_{254} high-performance precoated plate (Merck silica gel 60 F_{254} HPTLC plates are suitable) and a mixture of 0.5 volume of *anhydrous formic acid*, 1.5 volumes of *water*, 9 volumes of *absolute ethanol* and 9 volumes of *dichloromethane* as the mobile phase but allowing the solvent front to ascend 4 cm above the line of application. Apply separately to the plate 2 µl of each of the following solutions. For solution (1) shake a quantity of the powdered tablets containing 20 mg of Hyoscine Butylbromide with 5 ml of 0.01M *hydrochloric acid* and centrifuge. For solution (2) dilute 3 volumes of solution (1) to 100 volumes with 0.01M *hydrochloric acid.* For solution (3) dilute 1 volume of solution (1) to 50 volumes with 0.01M *hydrochloric acid.* For solution (4) dilute 1 volume of solution (1) to 400 volumes with 0.01M *hydrochloric acid.* After removal of the plate, dry it at 60° for 15 minutes, spray with a solution prepared by mixing equal volumes of a 40% w/v solution of *potassium iodide* in *water* and a solution prepared by dissolving 0.85 g of *bismuth oxynitrate* in a mixture of 10 ml of *glacial acetic acid* and 40 ml of *water* and diluting 1 volume of the mixture with 2 volumes of *glacial acetic acid* and 10 volumes of *water* immediately before use. Allow the plate to dry in air, spray well with a 5% w/v solution of *sodium nitrite* and examine immediately. In the chromatogram obtained with solution (1) the principal spot has an Rf value of about 0.45. In the chromatogram obtained with solution (1) any *secondary spot* with an Rf value less than that of the principal spot is not more intense than the spot in the chromatogram obtained with solution (2) (3%) and not more than two such spots are more intense than the spot in the chromatogram obtained with solution (4) (0.25%); any *secondary spot* with an Rf value greater than that of the principal spot is not more intense than the spot in the chromatogram obtained with solution (3) (2%) and not more than one such spot is more intense than the spot in the chromatogram obtained with solution (4) (0.25%).

Assay Weigh and powder 20 tablets. Carry out the method for *liquid chromatography*, Appendix III D, using the following solutions. For solution (1) shake a quantity of the powdered tablets containing 40 mg of Hyoscine Butylbromide with 60 ml of 0.001M *hydrochloric acid* with the aid of ultrasound for 15 minutes, dilute to 100 ml with the same solvent, centrifuge and filter to obtain a clear filtrate. Solution (2) contains 0.04% w/v of *hyoscine butylbromide BPCRS* in 0.001M *hydrochloric acid.*

The chromatographic procedure described under the test for Hyoscine may be used.

Calculate the content of $C_{21}H_{30}BrNO_4$ in the tablets using the declared content of $C_{21}H_{30}BrNO_4$ in *hyoscine butylbromide BPCRS.*

Hyoscine Eye Drops

Definition Hyoscine Eye Drops are a sterile solution of Hyoscine Hydrobromide in Purified Water.

The eye drops comply with the requirements stated under Eye Preparations and with the following requirements.

Content of hyoscine hydrobromide, $C_{17}H_{23}NO_4$, $HBr,3H_2O$ 90.0 to 110.0% of the prescribed or stated amount.

Identification

A. In the Assay, the chromatogram obtained with solution (2) shows a peak with the same retention time as the peak derived from hyoscine hydrobromide in the chromatogram obtained with solution (1).

B. To a volume containing 3 mg of Hyoscine Hydrobromide add an equal volume of *chloroauric acid solution.* The *melting point* of the precipitate, after recrystallisation from *water* and drying at 105°, is about 202°, Appendix V A.

Assay Carry out the method for *gas chromatography*, Appendix III B, using the following solutions. For solution (1) add 1 ml of a 0.3% w/v solution of *atropine sulphate BPCRS* (internal standard) in *methanol* (solution A) and 1 ml of 5M *ammonia* to 5 ml of a 0.1% w/v solution of *hyoscine hydrobromide BPCRS*. Extract with two 5-ml quantities of *chloroform*, shake the combined extracts with 1 g of *anhydrous sodium sulphate*, filter and evaporate the filtrate to dryness. Dissolve the residue in 2 ml of *dichloromethane*. To 1 ml of the solution add 0.2 ml of a mixture of 4 volumes of N,O-*bis(trimethylsilyl)acetamide* and 1 volume of *trimethylchlorosilane*, mix and allow to stand for 30 minutes. Prepare solution (2) in the same manner as solution (3) but omitting the addition of solution A. For solution (3) add 1 ml of solution A and 1 ml of 5M *ammonia* to a volume of the eye drops containing 5 mg of Hyoscine Hydrobromide, diluted if necessary to 5 ml with *water*, and complete the procedure described under solution (1), beginning at the words 'Extract with two 5-ml quantities of *chloroform*...'.

The chromatographic procedure may be carried out using a glass column (1.5 m × 4 mm) packed with *acid-washed, silanised diatomaceous support* (80 to 100 mesh) coated with 3% w/w of phenyl methyl silicone fluid (50% phenyl) (OV-17 is suitable) and maintained at 230°.

Calculate the content of $C_{17}H_{21}NO_4,HBr,3H_2O$ using the declared content of $C_{17}H_{21}NO_4,HBr,1\frac{1}{2}H_2O$ in *hyoscine hydrobromide BPCRS*. Each mg of $C_{17}H_{21}NO_4$, $HBr,1\frac{1}{2}H_2O$ is equivalent to 1.066 mg of $C_{17}H_{21}NO_4$, $HBr,3H_2O$.

Hyoscine Injection

Definition Hyoscine Injection is a sterile solution of Hyoscine Hydrobromide in Water for Injections.

The injection complies with the requirements stated under Parenteral Preparations and with the following requirements.

Content of hyoscine hydrobromide, $C_{17}H_{21}NO_4$, $HBr,3H_2O$ 90.0 to 110.0% of the prescribed or stated amount.

Identification

A. Carry out the method for *thin-layer chromatography*, Appendix III A, using *silica gel G* as the coating substance and a mixture of 10 volumes of *diethylamine*, 40 volumes of *acetone* and 50 volumes of *chloroform* as the mobile phase. Apply separately to the plate 5 µl of each of the following solutions. For solution (1) evaporate a volume of the injection containing 5 mg of Hyoscine Hydrobromide to dryness on a water bath, triturate the residue with 1 ml of *ethanol (96%)*, allow to stand and use the supernatant liquid. Solution (2) contains 0.5% w/v of *hyoscine hydrobromide BPCRS* in *ethanol (96%)*. After removal of the plate, heat it at 105° for 20 minutes, allow to cool and spray with *potassium iodobismuthate solution R1*. The spot in the chromatogram obtained with solution (1) corresponds to that in the chromatogram obtained with solution (2).

B. In the Assay, the chromatogram obtained with solution (2) shows a peak with the same retention time as the peak derived from hyoscine hydrobromide in the chromatogram obtained with solution (1).

C. To 0.2 ml of *fuming nitric acid* add 1 mg of the residue obtained by evaporating a suitable quantity to dryness and again evaporate to dryness on a water bath; a yellow residue is obtained. To the cooled residue add 2 ml of *acetone* and 0.2 ml of a 3% w/v solution of *potassium hydroxide* in *methanol*; a deep violet colour is produced. (Atropine and hyoscyamine yield the same reaction; the reaction is masked by the presence of other alkaloids.)

D. Evaporate a suitable volume to dryness. To 1 ml of a 1% w/v solution of the residue add 1 ml of 5M *ammonia*, shake with *chloroform* and evaporate the chloroform solution to dryness on a water bath. To the residue add 1.5 ml of a 2% w/v solution of *mercury(II) chloride* in *ethanol (60%)*. A white precipitate is produced which dissolves on warming (distinction from atropine and hyoscyamine).

E. Yields reaction A characteristic of *bromides*, Appendix VI.

Assay Carry out the method for *gas chromatography*, Appendix III B, using the following solutions. For solution (1) add 1 ml of a 0.30% w/v solution of *atropine sulphate BPCRS* (internal standard) in *methanol* (solution A) and

1 ml of 5M *ammonia* to 15 ml of a 0.033% w/v solution of *hyoscine hydrobromide BPCRS*. Extract with two 10-ml quantities of *chloroform*, shake the combined extracts with 2 g of *anhydrous sodium sulphate*, filter and evaporate the filtrate to dryness. Dissolve the residue in 2 ml of *dichloromethane*. To 1 ml of this solution add 0.2 ml of a mixture of 4 volumes of N,O-*bis(trimethylsilyl)acetamide* and 1 volume of *trimethylchlorosilane*, mix and allow to stand for 30 minutes. Prepare solution (2) in the same manner as solution (3) but omitting the addition of solution A. For solution (3) add 1 ml of solution A and 1 ml of 5M *ammonia* to a volume of the injection containing 5 mg of Hyoscine Hydrobromide, diluted if necessary to 15 ml with *water*, and complete the procedure described under solution (1), beginning at the words 'Extract with two 10-ml quantities of *chloroform*...'.

The chromatographic procedure may be carried out using a glass column (1.5 m × 4 mm) packed with *acid-washed, silanised diatomaceous support* (80 to 100 mesh) coated with 3% w/w of phenyl methyl silicone fluid (50% phenyl) (OV-17 is suitable) and maintained at 230°.

Calculate the content of $C_{17}H_{21}NO_4,HBr,3H_2O$ using the declared content of $C_{17}H_{21}NO_4,HBr,1\frac{1}{2}H_2O$ in *hyoscine hydrobromide BPCRS*. Each mg of $C_{17}H_{21}NO_4,HBr,1\frac{1}{2}H_2O$ is equivalent to 1.066 mg of $C_{17}H_{21}NO_4,HBr,3H_2O$.

Storage Hyoscine Injection should be protected from light.

Hyoscine Tablets

Definition Hyoscine Tablets contain Hyoscine Hydrobromide.

The tablets comply with the requirements stated under Tablets and with the following requirements.

Content of hyoscine hydrobromide, $C_{17}H_{21}NO_4,HBr,3H_2O$ 90.0 to 110.0% of the prescribed or stated amount.

Identification

A. Carry out the method for *thin-layer chromatography*, Appendix III A, using *silica gel G* as the coating substance and a mixture of 10 volumes of *diethylamine*, 40 volumes of *acetone* and 50 volumes of *chloroform* as the mobile phase. Apply separately to the plate 5 µl of each of the following solutions. For solution (1) shake a quantity of the powdered tablets containing 10 mg of Hyoscine Hydrobromide with 2 ml of *ethanol (96%)* and centrifuge. Solution (2) contains 0.5% w/v of *hyoscine hydrobromide BPCRS* in *ethanol (96%)*. After removal of the plate, heat it at 105° for 20 minutes, allow to cool and spray with *potassium iodobismuthate solution R1*. The spot in the chromatogram obtained with solution (1) corresponds to that in the chromatogram obtained with solution (2).

B. In the Assay, the chromatogram obtained with solution (2) shows a peak with the same retention time as the peak derived from hyoscine hydrobromide in the chromatogram obtained with solution (1).

C. Extract a quantity of the powdered tablets containing 1 mg of Hyoscine Hydrobromide with 5 ml of *ethanol (96%)*, filter and evaporate the filtrate to dryness on a water bath. Cool, add 0.2 ml of *fuming nitric acid* and again evaporate to dryness on a water bath; a yellow residue is produced. To the cooled residue add 2 ml of *acetone* and 0.2 ml of a 3% w/v solution of *potassium hydroxide* in *methanol*; a deep violet colour is produced.

D. The powdered tablets yield reaction A characteristic of *bromides*, Appendix VI.

Uniformity of content Tablets containing less than 2 mg of Hyoscine Hydrobromide comply with the requirements given under Tablets using the following method of analysis. Carry out the method for *gas chromatography*, Appendix III B.

For tablets containing 600 µg of Hyoscine Hydrobromide use the following solutions. For solution (1) add 1 ml of a 0.0375% w/v solution of *atropine sulphate BPCRS* (internal standard) in *methanol* (solution A) and 1 ml of 5M *ammonia* to 5 ml of a 0.012% w/v solution of *hyoscine hydrobromide BPCRS*. Extract with two 5-ml quantities of *chloroform*, shake the combined extracts with 1 g of *anhydrous sodium sulphate*, filter and evaporate the filtrate to dryness. Dissolve the residue in 0.5 ml of a mixture of 20 volumes of *dichloromethane*, 4 volumes of N,O-*bis(trimethylsilyl)acetamide* and 1 volume of *trimethylchlorosilane*, mix and allow to stand for 30 minutes. Prepare solution (2) in the same manner as solution (3) but omitting the addition of solution A. For solution (3) powder one tablet and triturate with 5 ml of 0.1M *hydrochloric acid*. Add 1 ml of solution A, extract with two 5-ml quantities of *chloroform* and discard the chloroform extracts. Add 1 ml of 5M *ammonia* and complete the procedure described under solution (1) beginning at the words 'Extract with two 5-ml quantities of *chloroform*...'.

For tablets containing less than 600 µg of Hyoscine Hydrobromide use the same procedure but with correspondingly smaller concentrations of *hyoscine hydrobromide BPCRS* and *atropine sulphate BPCRS*.

The chromatographic procedure may be carried out using a glass column (1.5 m × 4 mm) packed with *acid-washed, silanised diatomaceous support* (80 to 100 mesh) coated with 3% w/w of phenyl methyl silicone fluid (50% phenyl) (OV-17 is suitable) and maintained at 230°.

Calculate the content of $C_{17}H_{21}NO_4,HBr,3H_2O$ using the declared content of $C_{17}H_{21}NO_4,HBr,1\frac{1}{2}H_2O$ in *hyoscine hydrobromide BPCRS*. Each mg of $C_{17}H_{21}NO_4,HBr,1\frac{1}{2}H_2O$ is equivalent to 1.066 mg of $C_{17}H_{21}NO_4,HBr,3H_2O$.

Assay Weigh and powder 20 tablets. Carry out the method for *gas chromatography*, Appendix III B, using the following solutions. For solution (1) add 1 ml of a 0.3% w/v solution of *atropine sulphate BPCRS* (internal standard) in *methanol* (solution B) and 1 ml of 5M *ammonia* to 15 ml of a 0.033% w/v solution of *hyoscine hydrobromide BPCRS*. Extract with two 10-ml quantities of *chloroform*, shake the combined extracts with 2 g of *anhydrous sodium sulphate*, filter and evaporate to dryness. Dissolve the residue in 2 ml of *dichloromethane*. To 1 ml of this solution add 0.2 ml of a mixture of 4 volumes of N,O-*bis(trimethylsilyl)acetamide* and 1 volume of *trimethylchlorosilane*, mix and allow to stand for 30 minutes. Prepare solution (2) in the same manner as solution (3) but omitting the addition of solution B. For solution (3) shake a quantity of the powdered tablets containing 5 mg of Hyoscine Hydrobromide with 10 ml of 0.1M *hydrochloric acid*. Add 1 ml of solution B, extract with two 10-ml quantities of *chloroform* and discard the chloroform extracts. Add 1 ml of 5M *ammonia* and complete the procedure described under solution (1) beginning at the words 'Extract with two 10-ml quantities of *chloroform*...'.

The chromatographic conditions described under Uniformity of content may be used.

Calculate the content of $C_{17}H_{21}NO_4,HBr,3H_2O$ using the declared content of $C_{17}H_{21}NO_4,HBr,1\frac{1}{2}H_2O$ in *hyoscine hydrobromide BPCRS*. Each mg of $C_{17}H_{21}NO_4,HBr,1\frac{1}{2}H_2O$ is equivalent to 1.066 mg of $C_{17}H_{21}NO_4,HBr,3H_2O$.

Hyoscyamus Dry Extract

Definition Hyoscyamus Dry Extract is prepared by extracting Hyoscyamus Leaf with Ethanol (70 per cent) and removing the solvent. It contains not less than 0.27% and not more than 0.33% w/w of alkaloids calculated as hyoscyamine.

In making Hyoscyamus Dry Extract, Ethanol (70 per cent) may be replaced by Industrial Methylated Spirit[1] diluted so as to be of equivalent ethanolic strength.

Extemporaneous preparation The following formula and directions apply.

Hyoscyamus Leaf, in *moderately coarse powder*	1000 g
Hyoscyamus Leaf, in *fine powder*, dried at 80°	a sufficient quantity
Ethanol (70 per cent)	a sufficient quantity

Percolate the Hyoscyamus Leaf in *moderately coarse powder* with Ethanol (70 per cent) until 4000 ml of percolate has been obtained.

Determine the proportion of total solids in the percolate by evaporating 20 ml, drying the residue at 80° and weighing. Determine also the proportion of alkaloids in the percolate by the Assay, using 100 ml, and the proportion of alkaloids in the Hyoscyamus Leaf in *fine powder*. From the results of the three determinations, calculate the amount of Hyoscyamus Leaf in *fine powder* that must be added to the percolate to produce a dry extract containing 0.3% w/w of alkaloids.

Add to the percolate a slightly smaller amount of Hyoscyamus Leaf in *fine powder* than calculation has shown to be necessary, remove the ethanol, evaporate to dryness under reduced pressure at a temperature not exceeding 60° and dry in a current of air at 80°. Powder the residue, add the final necessary amount of Hyoscyamus Leaf in *fine powder* and triturate in a dry, slightly warmed mortar until thoroughly mixed. Pass the powdered extract through a sieve with a nominal mesh aperture of 710 µm and mix.

The extract complies with the requirements stated under Extracts and with the following requirements.

Loss on drying Not more than 5.0%.

Assay Mix 10 g with 50 ml of *ethanol (70%)*, warm on a water bath, allow to stand for 30 minutes, shaking frequently, transfer the mixture to a percolator and percolate slowly with successive portions of *ethanol (70%)* until *complete extraction* of the alkaloids is effected, Appendix XI G. Evaporate the percolate at as low a temperature as possible to about 10 ml, transfer to a separating funnel with the aid of 40 ml of *chloroform* and add a mixture of 10 ml of *water* and 5 ml of 5M *ammonia*. Shake well, allow to separate and filter the chloroform layer into a second separating funnel through a plug of absorbent cotton previously moistened with *chloroform*. Continue the extraction with further 25-ml quantities of *chloroform* until *complete extraction* of the alkaloids is effected, filtering each chloroform solution through the same plug of absorbent cotton. Extract the combined chloroform solutions with successive quantities of a mixture of 3 volumes of 0.1M *sulphuric acid* and 1 volume of *ethanol (96%)* until *complete extraction* of the alkaloids is effected, filtering each extract through absorbent cotton previously moistened with *water*. Wash the mixed acid solutions with successive quantities of 10, 5 and 5 ml of *chloroform*, extracting each chloroform solution with the same 20 ml of 0.05M *sulphuric acid*, and discard the chloroform. Combine the acid solutions, neutralise with 5M *ammonia*, add 5 ml in excess and shake with successive 25-ml quantities of *chloroform* until *complete extraction* of the alkaloids is effected. Wash each chloroform solution with the same 10 ml of *water* and filter into a flask through absorbent cotton previously moistened with *chloroform*. Distil most of the chloroform from the combined extracts and transfer the remainder of the solution to a shallow, open dish. Evaporate the remainder of the chloroform without the aid of a current of air, heat the residue in an oven at 100° for 15 minutes, dissolve in a little *chloroform*, evaporate to dryness without the aid of a current of air and again heat in an oven at 100° for 15 minutes. Dissolve the residue in 2 ml of *chloroform*, add 5 ml of 0.025M *sulphuric acid VS*, warm to remove the chloroform, cool and titrate the excess of acid with 0.05M *sodium hydroxide VS* using *methyl red solution* as indicator. Each ml of 0.025M *sulphuric acid VS* is equivalent to 14.47 mg of alkaloids, calculated as hyoscyamine.

Storage Hyoscyamus Dry Extract should be kept in a small, wide-mouthed, airtight container.

[1]The law and the statutory regulations governing the use of Industrial Methylated Spirit must be observed.

Hypromellose Eye Drops

Alkaline Eye Drops; Artificial Tears

Definition Hypromellose Eye Drops are a sterile solution of Hypromellose 4000, Hypromellose 4500 or Hypromellose 5000 in Purified Water. They are isotonic with tear secretions.

The eye drops comply with the requirements stated under Eye Preparations and with the following requirements.

Identification

A. Heat 5 ml in a water bath, with stirring. Above 50° the solution becomes cloudy or a flocculent precipitate is produced. The solution becomes clear on cooling.

B. To 5 ml add 0.15 ml of 2M *acetic acid* and 1.2 ml of a 10% w/v solution of *tannic acid*. A yellowish white, flocculent precipitate is produced which dissolves in 6M *ammonia*.

Alkalinity pH, 8.2 to 8.6, Appendix V L.

Viscosity 70 to 130% of the declared value when determined by Appendix V H, Method I, at 20° and using a viscometer of a size appropriate to the nominal viscosity.

Clarity of solution The eye drops are not more opalescent than *reference suspension IV*, Appendix IV A.

Labelling The label states the nominal viscosity in millipascal seconds.

When methylcellulose eye drops are prescribed or demanded, Hypromellose Eye Drops shall be dispensed or supplied.

Ibuprofen Cream

Definition Ibuprofen Cream contains Ibuprofen in a suitable basis.

The cream complies with the requirements stated under Topical Semi-solid Preparations and with the following requirements.

Content of ibuprofen, $C_{13}H_{18}O_2$ 95.0 to 105.0% of the prescribed or stated amount.

Identification

A. Carry out the method for *thin-layer chromatography*, Appendix III A, using *silica gel H* as the coating substance and a mixture of 5 volumes of *anhydrous acetic acid*, 25 volumes of *ethyl acetate* and 75 volumes of *n-hexane* as the mobile phase but allowing the solvent front to ascend 10 cm above the line of application. Apply separately to the plate 5 µl of each of the following solutions. For solution (1) shake vigorously a quantity of the cream containing 50 mg of Ibuprofen with 10 ml of *dichloromethane* for 5 minutes and filter (Whatman GF/C paper is suitable). Solution (2) contains 0.5% w/v of *ibuprofen BPCRS* in *dichloromethane*. After removal of the plate, dry it at 120° for 30 minutes, lightly spray the plate with a 1% w/v solution of *potassium permanganate* in 1M *sulphuric acid*, heat at 120° for 20 minutes and examine under *ultraviolet light (365 nm)*. The principal spot in the chromatogram obtained with solution (1) is similar in position, colour and size to that in the chromatogram obtained with solution (2).

B. In the Assay the retention time of the principal peak in the chromatogram obtained with solution (1) corresponds to that of the principal peak in the chromatogram obtained with solution (2).

Related substances Carry out the method for *liquid chromatography*, Appendix III D, using 20 µl of each of the following solutions. For solution (1) shake vigorously a quantity of the cream containing 0.1 g of Ibuprofen with 25 ml of *methanol* for 10 minutes, decant the solution into a 50-ml graduated flask, rinse the original flask with two 10-ml quantities of *methanol*, dilute the combined solution and rinsings to 50 ml with *methanol* and filter (Whatman GF/C paper is suitable). For solution (2) dilute 1 volume of solution (1) to 100 volumes with *methanol*. For solution (3) dissolve 0.1 g of *ibuprofen BPCRS* in 5 ml of a 0.006% w/v solution of *2-(4-butylphenyl)propionic acid EPCRS* in *methanol* and add sufficient *methanol* to produce 50 ml.

The chromatographic procedure may be carried out using (a) a stainless steel column (15 cm × 4.6 mm) packed with *stationary phase C* (5 µm) (Spherisorb ODS 2 is suitable), (b) as the mobile phase with a flow rate of 2 ml per minute a mixture of 0.5 volume of *orthophosphoric acid*, 340 volumes of *acetonitrile* and 600 volumes of *water* diluted to 1000 volumes with *water* after equilibration and (c) a detection wavelength of 214 nm. Adjust the sensitivity so that the height of the principal peak in the chromatogram obtained with solution (1) is 70 to 90% of full-scale deflection on the chart paper. Record the chromatogram for 1.5 times the retention time of the principal peak.

Equilibrate the column with the mobile phase for about 45 minutes before starting the chromatography.

When the chromatograms are recorded under the conditions described above, the retention time of ibuprofen is about 20 minutes. In the chromatogram obtained with solution (3) measure the height (*a*) of the peak due to 2-(4-butylphenyl)propionic acid and the height (*b*) of the lowest point of the curve separating this peak from that due to ibuprofen. The test is not valid unless *a* is greater than 1.5*b*. If necessary, adjust the concentration of acetonitrile in the mobile phase to obtain the required resolution.

In the chromatogram obtained with solution (1) the area of any peak corresponding to 2-(4-butylphenyl)propionic acid is not greater than that of the peak due to 2-(4-butylphenyl)propionic acid in the chromatogram obtained with solution (3) (0.3%), the area of any other *secondary peak* is not greater than 0.3 times the area of the principal peak in the chromatogram obtained with solution (2) (0.3%) and the sum of the areas of any such peaks is not greater than 0.7 times the area of the principal peak in the chromatogram obtained with solution (2) (0.7%). Disregard any peak the area of which is less than 0.1 times the area of the principal peak in the chromatogram obtained with solution (2) (0.1%).

Assay Carry out the method for *liquid chromatography*, Appendix III D, using the following solutions. For solution (1) shake vigorously a quantity of the cream containing 50 mg of Ibuprofen with 25 ml of the mobile phase for 10 minutes, decant the solution into a 50-ml graduated flask, rinse the original flask with two 10-ml quantities of the mobile phase, dilute the combined solution and rinsings to 50 ml with the mobile phase and filter (Whatman GF/C paper is suitable). Solution (2) contains 0.1% w/v of *ibuprofen BPCRS* in the mobile phase.

The chromatographic procedure may be carried out using (a) a stainless steel column (25 cm × 4.6 mm) packed with *stationary phase C* (10 µm) (Nucleosil C18 is suitable), (b) a mixture of 3 volumes of *orthophosphoric acid*, 247 volumes of *water* and 750 volumes of *methanol* as the mobile phase with a flow rate of 1.5 ml per minute and (c) a detection wavelength of 264 nm.

Calculate the content of $C_{13}H_{18}O_2$ using the declared content of $C_{13}H_{18}O_2$ in *ibuprofen BPCRS*.

Ibuprofen Gel

Definition Ibuprofen Gel is a solution of Ibuprofen in a suitable water-miscible basis.

The gel complies with the requirements stated under Topical Semi-solid Preparations and with the following requirements.

Content of ibuprofen, $C_{13}H_{18}O_2$ 95.0 to 105.0% of the prescribed or stated amount.

Identification

A. Carry out the method for *thin-layer chromatography*, Appendix III A, using *silica gel H* as the coating substance and a mixture of 5 volumes of *anhydrous acetic acid*, 25 volumes of *ethyl acetate* and 75 volumes of *n-hexane* as the mobile phase but allowing the solvent front to ascend 10 cm above the line of application. Apply separately to the plate 5 µl of each of the following solutions. For solution (1) shake vigorously a quantity of the gel containing 0.125 g of Ibuprofen with 25 ml of *dichloromethane* for 5 minutes and use the upper layer. Solution (2) contains 0.5% w/v of *ibuprofen BPCRS* in *dichloromethane*. After removal of the plate, dry it at 120° for 30 minutes, lightly spray the plate with a 1% w/v solution of *potassium permanganate* in 1M *sulphuric acid*, heat at 120° for 20 minutes and examine under *ultraviolet light (365 nm)*. The principal spot in the chromatogram obtained with solution (1) corresponds to that in the chromatogram obtained with solution (2).

B. In the Assay the retention time of the principal peak in the chromatogram obtained with solution (1) is the same as that of the principal peak in the chromatogram obtained with solution (2).

Related substances Carry out the method for *liquid chromatography*, Appendix III D, using 20 µl of each of the following solutions. For solution (1) disperse a quantity of the gel containing 0.1 g of Ibuprofen in 25 ml of warm *methanol*, cool and dilute to 50 ml with *methanol*. For solution (2) dilute 1 volume of solution (1) to 100 volumes with *methanol*. For solution (3) dissolve 0.1 g of *ibuprofen BPCRS* in 5 ml of a 0.006% w/v solution of *2-(4-butylphenyl)propionic acid EPCRS* in *methanol* and add sufficient *methanol* to produce 50 ml.

The chromatographic procedure may be carried out using (a) a stainless steel column (15 cm × 4.6 mm) packed with *stationary phase C* (5 µm) (Spherisorb ODS 2 is suitable), (b) as the mobile phase with a flow rate of 2 ml per minute a mixture of 0.5 volume of *orthophosphoric acid*, 340 volumes of *acetonitrile* and 600 volumes of *water* diluted to 1000 volumes with *water* after equilibration and (c) a detection wavelength of 214 nm. Adjust the sensitivity so that the height of the principal peak in the chromatogram obtained with solution (1) is 70 to 90% of full-scale deflection on the chart paper. Record the chromatogram for 1.5 times the retention time of the principal peak.

Equilibrate the column with the mobile phase for about 45 minutes before starting the chromatography.

When the chromatograms are recorded under the conditions described above, the retention time of ibuprofen is about 20 minutes. In the chromatogram obtained with solution (3) measure the height (*a*) of the peak due to 2-(4-butylphenyl)propionic acid and the height (*b*) of the lowest point of the curve separating this peak from that due to ibuprofen. The test is not valid unless *a* is greater than 1.5*b*. If necessary, adjust the concentration of acetonitrile in the mobile phase to obtain the required resolution.

In the chromatogram obtained with solution (1) the area of any peak corresponding to 2-(4-butylphenyl)-propionic acid is not greater than that of the peak due to 2-(4-butylphenyl)propionic acid in the chromatogram obtained with solution (3) (0.3%), the area of any other *secondary peak* is not greater than 0.3 times the area of the principal peak in the chromatogram obtained with solution (2) (0.3%) and the sum of the areas of any such peaks is not greater than 0.7 times the area of the principal peak in the chromatogram obtained with solution (2) (0.7%). Disregard any peak the area of which is less than 0.1 times the area of the principal peak in the chromatogram obtained with solution (2) (0.1%).

Assay Carry out the method for *liquid chromatography*, Appendix III D, using the following solutions. For solution (1) disperse a quantity of the gel containing 50 mg of Ibuprofen with 50 ml of warm *methanol* for 10 minutes, cool and add sufficient *methanol* to produce 100 ml. Dilute 10 volumes of this solution to 20 volumes with the mobile phase. For solution (2) dilute 10 volumes of a solution containing 0.05% w/v of *ibuprofen BPCRS* in *methanol* to 20 volumes with the mobile phase.

The chromatographic procedure may be carried out using (a) a stainless steel column (25 cm × 4.6 mm) packed with *stationary phase C* (10 µm) (Nucleosil C18 is suitable), (b) a mixture of 3 volumes of *orthophosphoric acid*, 247 volumes of *water* and 750 volumes of *methanol* as the mobile phase with a flow rate of 1.5 ml per minute and (c) a detection wavelength of 264 nm.

Calculate the content of $C_{13}H_{18}O_2$ using the declared content of $C_{13}H_{18}O_2$ in *ibuprofen BPCRS*.

Storage Ibuprofen Gel should be kept in a well-closed container and stored at a temperature not exceeding 25°.

Ibuprofen Oral Suspension

Definition Ibuprofen Oral Suspension is a suspension of Ibuprofen in a suitable flavoured vehicle.

The oral suspension complies with the requirements stated under Oral Liquids and with the following requirements.

Content of ibuprofen, $C_{13}H_{18}O_2$ 95.0 to 105.0% of the prescribed or stated amount.

Identification

A. Shake a quantity of the oral suspension containing 0.5 g of Ibuprofen with 20 ml of *chloroform*, allow to stand until the layers have separated, filter and evaporate the filtrate to dryness in a current of air without heating. The *infrared absorption spectrum* of the residue, Appendix II A, is concordant with the *reference spectrum* of ibuprofen.

B. Carry out the method for *thin-layer chromatography*, Appendix III A, using *silica gel H* as the coating substance and a mixture of 1 volume of *anhydrous acetic acid*, 5 volumes of *ethyl acetate* and 15 volumes of *n-hexane* as the mobile phase but allowing the solvent front to ascend 10 cm above the line of application. Apply separately to the plate 10 µl of each of the following solutions. For solution (1) dilute a quantity of the oral suspension containing 0.1 g of Ibuprofen to 100 ml with *absolute ethanol*, shake vigorously for 5 minutes, filter (Whatman GF/C paper is suitable) and use the filtrate. Solution (2) contains 0.1% w/v of *ibuprofen BPCRS* in *absolute ethanol*. After removal of the plate dry it at 120° for 30 minutes, lightly spray the plate with a 1% w/v solution of *potassium permanganate* in 1M *sulphuric acid*, heat at 120° for 20 minutes and examine under *ultraviolet light (365 nm)*. The principal spot in the chromatogram obtained with solution (1) is similar in position, colour and size to that in the chromatogram obtained with solution (2). Disregard any spot remaining on the line of application.

4′-Isobutylacetophenone Carry out the method for *liquid chromatography*, Appendix III D, using the following solutions immediately after preparation. For solution (1) mix a quantity of the oral suspension containing 0.2 g of Ibuprofen with 30 ml of *acetonitrile*, add a further 10 ml of acetonitrile and 10 ml of 0.01M *orthophosphoric acid*, shake vigorously, dilute to 100 ml with 0.01M *orthophosphoric acid* and filter (Whatman GF/C paper is suitable). For solution

(2) dilute 0.0006% w/v of *4′-isobutylacetophenone BPCRS* in *acetonitrile*. Solution (3) contains 0.0006% w/v of *4′-isobutylacetophenone BPCRS* and 0.2% w/v of *ibuprofen BPCRS* in the mobile phase.

The chromatographic procedure described under Assay may be used.

The test is not valid unless, in the chromatogram obtained with solution (3), the *resolution factor* between the peaks corresponding to ibuprofen and 4′-isobutylacetophenone is at least 1.0.

In the chromatogram obtained with solution (1) the area of any peak corresponding to 4′-isobutylacetophenone is not greater than the area of the principal peak in the chromatogram obtained with solution (2) (0.3%).

Assay Carry out the method for *liquid chromatography*, Appendix III D, using the following solutions immediately after preparation. For solution (1) mix a quantity of the oral suspension containing 0.1 g of Ibuprofen with 30 ml of *acetonitrile*, add a further 10 ml of *acetonitrile* and 10 ml of 0.01M *orthophosphoric acid*, shake vigorously, dilute to 100 ml with 0.01M *orthophosphoric acid* and filter (Whatman GF/C paper is suitable). For solution (2) prepare a 0.1% w/v of *ibuprofen BPCRS* by dissolving a suitable quantity in 40 volumes of *acetonitrile* and adding 60 volumes of 0.01M *orthophosphoric acid*.

The chromatographic procedure may be carried out using (a) a stainless steel column (30 cm × 3.9 mm) packed with *stationary phase C* (10 μm) (μBondapak C18 is suitable), (b) a mixture of 400 volumes of *acetonitrile* and 600 volumes of 0.01M *orthophosphoric acid* as the mobile phase with a flow rate of 2 ml per minute and (c) a detection wavelength of 220 nm. Inject 10 μl of each solution.

Determine the *weight per ml* of the oral suspension, Appendix V G, and calculate the content of $C_{13}H_{18}O_2$, weight in volume, from the declared content of $C_{13}H_{18}O_2$ in *ibuprofen BPCRS*.

Storage Ibuprofen Oral Suspension should be protected from light and stored at a temperature not exceeding 25°.

Ibuprofen Tablets

Definition Ibuprofen Tablets contain Ibuprofen. They are coated.

With the exception of the requirements for shape, the tablets comply with the requirements stated under Tablets and with the following requirements.

Content of ibuprofen, $C_{13}H_{18}O_2$ 95.0 to 105.0% of the prescribed or stated amount.

Identification

A. Extract a quantity of the powdered tablets containing 0.5 g of Ibuprofen with 20 ml of *acetone*, filter and evaporate the filtrate to dryness in a current of air without heating. The *infrared absorption spectrum* of the residue, Appendix II A, is concordant with the *reference spectrum* of ibuprofen.

B. *Melting point* of the residue obtained in test A, after recrystallisation from *petroleum spirit (boiling range, 40° to 60°)*, about 75°, Appendix V A.

Related substances Carry out the method for *liquid chromatography*, Appendix III D, using 20 μl of each of the following solutions. For solution (1) add 30 ml of *methanol* to a quantity of the powdered tablets containing 0.2 g of Ibuprofen, shake for 30 minutes, add 30 ml of *methanol* and sufficient *water* to produce 100 ml, mix and filter through a glass microfibre filter paper (Whatman GF/C is suitable). For solution (2) dilute 1 volume of solution (1) to 100 volumes with the mobile phase. For solution (3) dissolve 0.1 g of *ibuprofen BPCRS* in 5 ml of a 0.006% w/v solution of *2-(4-butylphenyl)propionic acid EPCRS* in *methanol* and add sufficient *methanol* to produce 50 ml.

The chromatographic procedure may be carried out using (a) a stainless steel column (15 cm × 4.6 mm) packed with *stationary phase C* (5 μm) (Spherisorb ODS 2 is suitable), (b) as the mobile phase with a flow rate of 2 ml per minute a mixture of 0.5 volume of *orthophosphoric acid*, 340 volumes of *acetonitrile* and 600 volumes of *water* diluted to 1000 volumes with *water* after equilibration and (c) a detection wavelength of 214 nm. Adjust the sensitivity so that the height of the principal peak in the chromatogram obtained with solution (2) is 70 to 90% of full-scale deflection on the chart paper. Record the chromatogram for 1.5 times the retention time of the principal peak.

Equilibrate the column with the mobile phase for about 45 minutes before starting the chromatography.

When the chromatograms are recorded under the conditions described above, the retention time of ibuprofen is about 20 minutes. In the chromatogram obtained with solution (3) measure the height (*a*) of the peak due to 2-(4-butylphenyl)propionic acid and the height (*b*) of the lowest point of the curve separating this peak from that due to ibuprofen. The test is not valid unless *a* is greater than 1.5*b*. If necessary, adjust the concentration of acetonitrile in the mobile phase to obtain the required resolution.

In the chromatogram obtained with solution (1) the area of any peak corresponding to 2-(4-butylphenyl)-propionic acid is not greater than that of the peak due to 2-(4-butylphenyl)propionic acid in the chromatogram obtained with solution (3) (0.3%), the area of any other *secondary peak* is not greater than 0.3 times the area of the principal peak in the chromatogram obtained with solution (2) (0.3%) and the sum of the areas of any such peaks is not greater than 0.7 times the area of the principal peak in the chromatogram obtained with solution (2) (0.7%). Disregard any peak the area of which is less than 0.1 times the area of the principal peak in the chromatogram obtained with solution (2) (0.1%).

Assay Weigh and powder 20 tablets. Carry out the method for *liquid chromatography*, Appendix III D, using the following solutions. For solution (1) shake a quantity of the powdered tablets containing 0.2 g of Ibuprofen with 30 ml of the mobile phase for 30 minutes, add sufficient of the mobile phase to produce 100 ml and mix thoroughly. Centrifuge 25 ml of the solution at 2500 *g* for 5 minutes and use the supernatant liquid. Solution (2) contains 0.2% w/v of *ibuprofen BPCRS* in the mobile phase.

The chromatographic procedure may be carried out using (a) a stainless steel column (25 cm × 4.6 mm) packed with *stationary phase C* (10 μm) (Nucleosil C18 is suitable), (b) a mixture of 3 volumes of *orthophosphoric acid*, 247 volumes of *water* and 750 volumes of *methanol* as the mobile phase with a flow rate of 1.5 ml per minute and (c) a detection wavelength of 264 nm.

Calculate the content of $C_{13}H_{18}O_2$ using the declared content of $C_{13}H_{18}O_2$ in *ibuprofen BPCRS*.

Idoxuridine Eye Drops

Definition Idoxuridine Eye Drops are a sterile solution of Idoxuridine in Purified Water.

Except that they may be supplied in containers not exceeding 15 ml capacity, the eye drops comply with the requirements stated under Eye Preparations and with the following requirements.

Content of idoxuridine, $C_9H_{11}IN_2O_5$ 90.0 to 110.0% of the prescribed or stated amount.

Identification

A. Dilute a suitable volume of the eye drops with 0.01M *sodium hydroxide* to produce a solution containing 0.004% w/v of Idoxuridine. The *light absorption* of the resulting solution, Appendix II B, in the range 230 to 350 nm exhibits a maximum only at 279 nm.

B. In the Assay, the chromatogram obtained with solution (2) shows a peak having the same retention time as the peak due to idoxuridine in the chromatogram obtained with solution (1).

Related substances Carry out the method for *liquid chromatography*, Appendix III D, using the following solutions. Solution (1) contains 0.00040% w/v of *2′-deoxyuridine*, 0.00080% w/v of *5-iodouracil*, 0.00040% w/v of *5-bromo-2′-deoxyuridine* and 0.00010% w/v of *sulphanilamide* (internal standard). For solution (2) dilute a suitable volume of the eye drops with *water* to give a final concentration of 0.080% w/v of Idoxuridine. For solution (3) dilute a suitable volume of the eye drops with sufficient of a suitable solution of *sulphanilamide* to give a final concentration of 0.080% w/v of Idoxuridine and 0.00010% w/v of the internal standard.

The chromatographic conditions described under the Assay may be used but using as the mobile phase a mixture of 4 volumes of *methanol* and 96 volumes of *water*. The order of elution of the peaks following the internal standard is deoxyuridine, iodouracil, bromodeoxyuridine and idoxuridine. Several peaks due to excipients may appear in the chromatogram obtained with solution (3) before the peak due to the internal standard.

In the chromatogram obtained with solution (3) the ratios of the areas of any peaks due to 2′-deoxyuridine, 5-iodouracil and 5-bromo-2′-deoxyuridine to the area of the peak due to sulphanilamide are not greater than the ratios of the areas of the corresponding peaks in the chromatogram obtained with solution (1).

Assay Prepare a solution containing 0.12 g of *sulphathiazole* (internal standard) in 10 ml of *ethanol (96%)*, warming if necessary, and dilute to 100 ml with *water* (solution A). Prepare a solution by diluting a suitable volume of the eye drops with *water* if necessary to give a final concentration of 0.10% w/v of Idoxuridine (solution B). Carry out the method for *liquid chromatography*, Appendix III D, using the following solutions. For solution (1) shake 0.1 g of *idoxuridine BPCRS* with 50 ml of *water* until dissolved and then dilute to 100 ml with *water*; to 15 ml of this solution add 2 ml of solution A and dilute to 20 ml with *water*. For solution (2) add 2 ml of a 10% v/v solution of *ethanol (96%)* to 15 ml of solution B and dilute to 20 ml with *water*. For solution (3) add 2 ml of solution A to 15 ml of solution B and dilute to 20 ml with *water*.

The chromatographic procedure may be carried out using (a) a stainless steel column (30 cm × 4 mm) packed with *stationary phase C* (10 µm) (µBondapak C18 is suitable), (b) a mixture of 13 volumes of *methanol* and 87 volumes of *water* as the mobile phase with a flow rate of 1.7 ml per minute and (c) a detection wavelength of 254 nm.

Calculate the content of $C_9H_{11}IN_2O_5$ using the declared content of $C_9H_{11}IN_2O_5$ in *idoxuridine BPCRS*.

Storage Idoxuridine Eye Drops should be stored at a temperature not exceeding 8° but should not be allowed to freeze.

Labelling The label states that the Eye Drops should not be used for continuous periods of treatment exceeding 21 days.

Imipramine Tablets

Definition Imipramine Tablets contain Imipramine Hydrochloride. They are coated.

The tablets comply with the requirements stated under Tablets and with the following requirements.

Content of imipramine hydrochloride, $C_{19}H_{24}N_2$, HCl 92.5 to 107.5% of the prescribed or stated amount.

Identification

Triturate a quantity of the powdered tablets containing 0.25 g of Imipramine Hydrochloride with 10 ml of *chloroform*, filter, evaporate the filtrate to low volume, add *ether* until a turbidity is produced and allow to stand. The precipitate complies with the following tests.

A. *Melting point*, after recrystallisation from *acetone*, about 172°, Appendix V A.

B. Dissolve 5 mg in 2 ml of *nitric acid*. An intense blue colour is produced.

C. Yields the reactions characteristic of *chlorides*, Appendix VI.

Related substances Carry out the method for *thin-layer chromatography*, Appendix III A, using *silica gel G* as the coating substance and a mixture of 5 volumes of *hydrochloric acid*, 5 volumes of *water*, 35 volumes of *glacial acetic acid* and 55 volumes of *ethyl acetate* as the mobile phase but allowing the solvent front to ascend 12 cm above the line of application. Apply separately to the plate 10 µl of each of the following solutions prepared immediately before use. For solution (1) shake a quantity of the powdered tablets containing 0.20 g of Imipramine Hydrochloride with three 10-ml quantities of *chloroform*, filter the combined chloroform extracts, evaporate to dryness and dissolve the residue in 10 ml of *methanol*. For solution (2) dilute 3 volumes of solution (1) to 100 volumes with *methanol* and dilute 1 volume of the resulting solution to 10 volumes with *methanol*. Solution (3) contains 0.0060% w/v of *iminodibenzyl* in *methanol*. After removal of the plate, allow it to dry for 5 minutes, spray with a 0.5% w/v solution of *potassium dichromate* in *sulphuric acid (20%)* and examine immediately. In the chromatogram obtained with solution (1) any spot corresponding to iminodibenzyl is not more intense than the spot in the chromatogram obtained with solution (3) (0.3%) and any other *secondary spot* is not more intense than the spot in the chromatogram obtained with solution (2) (0.3%).

Assay Powder 10 tablets and transfer quantitatively without loss into 300 ml of 0.1M *hydrochloric acid*. Shake for 30 minutes, add sufficient 0.1M *hydrochloric acid* to produce 500 ml and filter through a fine glass microfibre filter (GF/C paper is suitable). Dilute a suitable volume of the filtrate with 0.1M *hydrochloric acid* to produce a solution containing 0.0025% w/v of Imipramine Hydrochloride and measure the *absorbance* of the resulting solution at the maximum at 250 nm, Appendix II B. Calculate the content of $C_{19}H_{24}N_2,HCl$ taking 264 as the value of A(1%, 1 cm) at the maximum at 250 nm.

Indometacin Capsules

Definition Indometacin Capsules contain Indometacin.

The capsules comply with the requirements stated under Capsules and with the following requirements.

Content of indometacin, $C_{19}H_{16}ClNO_4$ 90.0 to 110.0% of the prescribed or stated amount.

Identification

A. Shake a quantity of the contents of the capsules containing 0.1 g of Indometacin with 5 ml of *chloroform*, filter and evaporate the filtrate to dryness. Dry the residue at 60° at a pressure not exceeding 0.7 kPa for 1 hour. The *infrared absorption spectrum* of the residue, Appendix II A, is concordant with the *reference spectrum* of indometacin.

B. The *light absorption*, Appendix II B, in the range 300 to 350 nm of the solution obtained in the Assay exhibits a maximum only at 320 nm.

C. Mix a quantity of the contents of the capsules containing 25 mg of Indometacin with 2 ml of *water* and add 2 ml of 2M *sodium hydroxide*. A bright yellow colour is produced which fades rapidly.

Dissolution Comply with the *dissolution test for tablets and capsules*, Appendix XII D, using Apparatus II. Use as the medium 900 ml of *phosphate buffer pH 7.2* and rotate the paddle at 50 revolutions per minute. Withdraw a 10-ml sample of the medium and measure the *absorbance* of the filtered sample, suitably diluted if necessary, at the maximum at 320 nm, Appendix II B, using *phosphate buffer pH 7.2* in the reference cell. Calculate the total content of indometacin, $C_{19}H_{16}ClNO_4$, in the medium taking 196 as the value of A(1%, 1 cm) at the maximum at 320 nm.

Related substances Carry out the method for *thin-layer chromatography*, Appendix III A, using a suspension of *silica gel HF_{254}* in a 4.68% w/v solution of *sodium dihydrogen orthophosphate* to coat the plate and a mixture of 70 volumes of *ether* and 30 volumes of *petroleum spirit (boiling range, 60° to 80°)* as the mobile phase. Apply separately to the plate 5 µl of each of the following solutions. For solution (1) shake a quantity of the contents of the capsules containing 0.10 g of Indometacin with 5 ml of *chloroform*, filter and use the filtrate. For solution (2) dilute 1 volume of solution (1) to 200 volumes with *chloroform*. After removal of the plate, allow it to dry in air and examine under *ultraviolet light (254 nm)*. Any *secondary spot* in the chromatogram obtained with solution (1) is not more intense than the spot in the chromatogram obtained with solution (2).

Assay To a quantity of the mixed contents of 20 capsules containing 50 mg of Indometacin add 10 ml of *water* and allow to stand for 10 minutes, swirling occasionally. Add 75 ml of *methanol*, shake well, add sufficient *methanol* to produce 100 ml and filter if necessary. To 5 ml of the filtrate add sufficient of a mixture of equal volumes of *methanol* and *phosphate buffer pH 7.2* to produce 100 ml. Measure the *absorbance* of the resulting solution at the maximum at 320 nm, Appendix II B. Calculate the content of $C_{19}H_{16}ClNO_4$ taking 193 as the value of A(1%, 1 cm) at the maximum at 320 nm.

When indomethacin capsules are prescribed or demanded, Indometacin Capsules shall be dispensed or supplied.

Indometacin Suppositories

Definition Indometacin Suppositories contain Indometacin in a suitable suppository basis.

The suppositories comply with the requirements stated under Rectal Preparations and with the following requirements.

Content of indometacin, $C_{19}H_{16}ClNO_4$ 90.0 to 110.0% of the prescribed or stated amount.

Identification

A. Dissolve a quantity of the suppositories containing 0.1 g of Indometacin as completely as possible in 50 ml of hot *water*, filter, wash the residue with hot *water* and allow to dry in air. Dissolve the residue in 5 ml of *chloroform* and evaporate to dryness. The *infrared absorption spectrum* of the final residue, Appendix II A, is concordant with the *reference spectrum* of indometacin.

B. Shake a quantity of the suppositories containing 25 mg of Indometacin with 5 ml of *water* until the basis dissolves; a white suspension is produced. Add 2 ml of 2M *sodium hydroxide*; a bright yellow colour is produced which fades rapidly.

Disintegration Carry out the *disintegration test for suppositories and pessaries*, Appendix XII C, using a weighed suppository and *phosphate buffer pH 6.8* in place of *water* and operating the apparatus for 90 minutes. At the end of this period remove the suppository, dry with filter paper and weigh. Repeat the operation with two further weighed suppositories. Not less than 75% of each suppository is dissolved.

Related substances Carry out the method for *liquid chromatography*, Appendix III D, using the following freshly prepared solutions. For solution (1) dilute 3 volumes of solution (2) to 100 volumes with the mobile phase. For solution (2) powder or cut into small pieces a suitable number of the suppositories, dissolve a quantity containing 0.1 g of Indometacin in sufficient *methanol* to produce 50 ml.

The chromatographic procedure may be carried out using (a) a stainless steel column (30 cm × 4 mm) packed with *stationary phase C* (10 µm) (µBondapak C18 is suitable), (b) a mixture of 40 volumes of 0.2% v/v solution of *orthophosphoric acid* and 60 volumes of *methanol* as the mobile phase with a flow rate of 2 ml per minute and (c) a detection wavelength of 320 nm.

The *column efficiency*, determined using the principal peak in the chromatogram obtained with solution (1), should be not less than 7500 theoretical plates per metre.

The sum of the areas of any *secondary peaks* that elute before the principal peak in the chromatogram obtained with solution (2) is not greater than the area of the peak in the chromatogram obtained with solution (1).

Repeat the procedure but using the following freshly prepared solutions and a detection wavelength of 240 nm. For solution (3) dilute 10 volumes of solution (2) to 20 volumes with the mobile phase. Solution (4) contains 0.001% w/v of *4-chlorobenzoic acid* in the mobile phase. In the chromatogram obtained with solution (3) the sum of the areas of any *secondary peaks* that elute before the principal peak, other than those determined in solution (2), is not greater than the area of the peak in the chromatogram obtained with solution (4).

Assay Weigh 10 suppositories and powder or cut into small pieces. To a quantity containing 0.1 g of Indometacin add 50 ml of *methanol*, shake until dispersion is complete and, if necessary, filter. To 2 ml add sufficient of a mixture of equal volumes of *methanol* and *phosphate buffer pH 7.2* to produce 100 ml. Measure the *absorbance* of the resulting solution at the maximum at 318 nm, Appendix II B. Calculate the content of $C_{19}H_{16}ClNO_4$ taking 193 as the value of A(1%, 1 cm) at the maximum at 318 nm.

When indomethacin suppositories are prescribed or demanded, Indometacin Suppositories shall be dispensed or supplied.

Indoramin Tablets

Definition Indoramin Tablets contain Indoramin Hydrochloride. They are coated.

With the exception of the requirements for shape, the tablets comply with the requirements stated under Tablets and with the following requirements.

Content of indoramin, $C_{22}H_{25}N_3O$ 95.0 to 105.0% of the prescribed or stated amount.

Identification Shake a quantity of the powdered tablets containing the equivalent of 0.1 g of indoramin with 25 ml of *water* for 5 minutes, filter (Whatman GF/C paper is suitable), make the filtrate alkaline with 2M *sodium hydroxide* and extract with 20 ml of *dichloromethane*. Wash the extracts with two 10-ml quantities of *water*, dry by shaking with *anhydrous sodium sulphate* and evaporate to dryness using a rotary evaporator. The *infrared absorption spectrum* of the residue, Appendix II A, is concordant with the *reference spectrum* of indoramin.

Related substances Carry out the method for *thin-layer chromatography*, Appendix III A, using a silica gel F_{254} precoated plate (Merck silica gel 60 F_{254} plates are suitable) and a mixture of 1 volume of 18M *ammonia*, 20 volumes of *absolute ethanol* and 79 volumes of *toluene* as the mobile phase. Apply separately to the plate 10 µl of each of the following solutions. For solution (1) add 10 ml of *ethanol (96%)* to a quantity of the powdered tablets containing the equivalent of 0.1 g of indoramin, shake for 30 minutes and filter. For solution (2) dilute 1 volume of solution (1) to 200 volumes with *ethanol (96%)*. For solution (3) dilute 1 volume of solution (2) to 5 volumes with *ethanol (96%)*. After removal of the plate, allow it to dry in a current of warm air and examine it under *ultraviolet light (254 nm)*. Any *secondary spot* in the chromatogram obtained with solution (1) is not more intense than the spot in the chromatogram obtained with solution (2) (0.5%) and not more than one such spot is more intense than the spot in the chromatogram obtained with solution (3) (0.1%). Disregard any spot remaining on the line of application.

Dissolution Comply with the *dissolution test for tablets and capsules*, Appendix XII D, using Apparatus II. Use 900 ml of 0.1M *hydrochloric acid* as the medium and rotate the paddle at 50 revolutions per minute. Withdraw a sample of 10 ml of the medium. Measure the *absorbance* of a layer of suitable thickness of the filtered sample, suitably diluted if necessary, at the maximum at 280 nm, Appendix II B. Calculate the total content of indoramin, $C_{22}H_{25}N_3O$, in the medium taking 172 as the value of A(1%, 1 cm) at the maximum at 280 nm.

Assay Shake 10 whole tablets with 50 ml of 0.1M *hydrochloric acid* until the tablets have disintegrated, add 300 ml of *ethanol (96%)* and mix with the aid of ultrasound for 10 minutes, shaking occasionally. Add sufficient *ethanol (96%)* to produce 500 ml, filter (Whatman GF/C paper is suitable), dilute the filtrate with *ethanol (96%)* to contain 0.005% w/v of indoramin and measure the *absorbance* of the resulting solution at the maximum at 280 nm, Appendix II B. Calculate the content of $C_{22}H_{25}N_3O$ taking 172 as the value of A(1%, 1 cm) at the maximum at 280 nm.

Storage Indoramin Tablets should be protected from light and stored at a temperature not exceeding 25°.

Labelling The quantity of active ingredient is stated in terms of the equivalent amount of indoramin.

Inositol Nicotinate Tablets

Definition Inositol Nicotinate Tablets contain Inositol Nicotinate.

The tablets comply with the requirements stated under Tablets and with the following requirements.

Content of inositol nicotinate, $C_{42}H_{30}N_6O_{12}$ 95.0 to 105.0% of the prescribed or stated amount.

Identification

A. Shake a quantity of the powdered tablets containing 1 g of Inositol Nicotinate with 30 ml of a mixture of 9 volumes of *chloroform* and 1 volume of *methanol*, filter and evaporate to dryness. The *infrared absorption spectrum* of the residue, Appendix II A, is concordant with the *reference spectrum* of inositol nicotinate. Retain the remainder of the residue for use in test B and in the Related substances test.

B. Heat a small quantity of the residue obtained in test A with four times its weight of *anhydrous sodium carbonate*. Pyridine, recognisable by its odour, is evolved.

Dissolution Comply with the *dissolution test for tablets and capsules*, Appendix XII D, using Apparatus II. Use as the medium 900 ml of 1M *hydrochloric acid* and rotate the paddle at 50 revolutions per minute. Withdraw a sample of 20 ml of the medium and filter. Measure the *absorbance* of the filtrate, Appendix II B, diluted with 1M *hydrochloric acid* if necessary, at the maximum at 262 nm using 1M *hydrochloric acid* in the reference cell. Calculate the total content of inositol nicotinate, $C_{42}H_{30}N_6O_{12}$, in the medium taking 398 as the value of A(1%, 1 cm) at the maximum at 262 nm.

Free nicotinic acid To a quantity of the powdered tablets containing 1 g of Inositol Nicotinate add 75 ml of water, shake for 15 minutes and titrate with 0.02M *sodium hydroxide VS* using *phenolphthalein solution R1* as indicator. Not more than 1.0 ml of 0.02M *sodium hydroxide VS* is required to produce the first pink colour.

Related substances Carry out the test described under Inositol Nicotinate using three solutions of the residue obtained in test A for Identification in a mixture of 9 volumes of *chloroform* and 1 volume of *methanol* containing (1) 5.0% w/v, (2) 0.075% w/v and (3) 0.050% w/v. Any *secondary spot* in the chromatogram obtained with solution (1) is not more intense than the spot in the chromatogram obtained with solution (2) (1.5%) and not more than one such spot is more intense than the spot in the chromatogram obtained with solution (3) (1%).

Assay Weigh and powder 20 tablets. To a quantity of the powdered tablets containing 0.25 g of Inositol Nicotinate add 50 ml of *anhydrous acetic acid*, heat to boiling and allow to cool. Carry out Method I for *non-aqueous titration*, Appendix VIII A, using *1-naphtholbenzein solution* as indicator. Each ml of 0.1M *perchloric acid VS* is equivalent to 13.51 mg of $C_{42}H_{30}N_6O_{12}$.

INSULIN PREPARATIONS

Insulin Preparations comply with the requirements of the 3rd edition of the European Pharmacopoeia for Injectable Insulin Preparations [0854]. These requirements are reproduced under the heading 'Definition' below.

For preparations of Human Insulin, the label states the approved code in lower case letters indicative of the method of production.

The provisions of this monograph apply to the following Insulin Preparations:

Biphasic Insulin Injection

Biphasic Isophane Insulin Injection

Insulin Injection

Insulin Zinc Suspension

Insulin Zinc Suspension (Amorphous)

Insulin Zinc Suspension (Crystalline)

Isophane Insulin Injection

Ph Eur

DEFINITION

Injectable insulin preparations comply with the requirements for Injections prescribed in the monograph on Parenteral preparations (520).

Injectable insulin preparations are sterile preparations of *Insulin, human (838)* or *Insulin (276)* containing, unless otherwise stated, either beef insulin or pork insulin. They contain not less than 90.0 per cent and not more than the equivalent of 110.0 per cent of the amount of insulin stated on the label. They are either solutions or suspensions or they are prepared by combining solutions and suspensions.

PRODUCTION

The methods of preparation are designed to confer suitable properties with respect to the onset and duration of therapeutic action.

The following procedures are carried out in a suitable sequence, depending on the method of preparation:

- addition of suitable antimicrobial preservatives,
- addition of a suitable substance or substances to render the preparation isotonic with blood,
- addition of a suitable substance or substances to adjust the pH to the appropriate value,
- determination of the strength of the insulin-containing component or components followed, where necessary, by adjustment so that the final preparation contains the requisite number of International Units per millilitre,
- sterilisation by filtration of the insulin-containing component or components; once this procedure has been carried out, all subsequent procedures are carried out aseptically using materials that have been sterilised by a suitable method.

In addition, where appropriate, suitable substances are added and suitable procedures carried out to confer the appropriate physical form on the insulin-containing component or components. The final preparation is distributed aseptically into sterile containers which are closed so as to exclude microbial contamination.

TESTS

pH (*2.2.3*). The pH of the solution or suspension is 6.9 to 7.8, unless otherwise prescribed in the specific monograph.

Insulin in the supernatant For injectable insulin preparations that are suspensions, not more than 2.5 per cent of the total insulin content, unless otherwise stated. Centrifuge 10 ml of the suspension at 1500 g for 10 min and carefully separate the supernatant liquid from the residue. Determine the insulin content of the supernatant liquid (*S*) by a suitable method. Calculate the percentage of insulin in solution from the expression:

$$\frac{100S}{T}$$

where *T* is the total insulin content determined as described under Assay.

Related proteins Examine by liquid chromatography (*2.2.29*).

Test solution. Use the test solution prepared for the assay.

Reference solution (a). Use either reference solution (a) prepared for the assay or reference solution (b) prepared for the assay, as appropriate

Reference solution (b). Use reference solution (c) prepared for the assay.

The chromatographic procedure may be carried out using:

- a stainless steel column 0.25 m long and 4.6 mm in internal diameter packed with *octadecylsilyl silica gel for chromatography R* (5 µm),
- as mobile phases at a flow rate of 1 ml per minute the following solutions, prepared and maintained at a temperature not lower than 20°C:

  Mobile phase A. Dissolve 28.4 g of *anhydrous sodium sulphate R* in *water R* and dilute to 1000 ml with *water R*, add 2.7 ml of *phosphoric acid R*, adjust to pH 2.3, if necessary, with *ethanolamine R*, filter and degas by passing *helium for chromatography R* through the solution,

Mobile phase B. Mix 500 ml of mobile phase A with 500 ml of *acetonitrile R*; filter and degas by passing *helium for chromatography R* through the solution,

Interval (min)	Mobile phase A (per cent *V/V*)	Mobile phase B (per cent *V/V*)	Comment
0–30	48	52	Isocratic
30–44	48→20	52→80	Linear gradient
44–50	20	80	Isocratic

— as detector a spectrophotometer set at 214 nm, maintaining the temperature of the column at 40°C.

Inject 20 µl of reference solution (b). Record the chromatogram. The test is not valid unless the resolution between the peaks corresponding to human insulin and porcine insulin is at least 1.2. If necessary, adjust the concentration of acetonitrile in the mobile phase by slight decrease or increase until this resolution is achieved. In the chromatogram obtained with reference solution (b), the two principal peaks, in order of elution, are due to human insulin and porcine insulin and any smaller peaks appearing immediately following each of the principal peaks are due to the corresponding monodesamido derivatives.

Inject separately 20 µl of the test solution and 20 µl of reference solution (a). If necessary, make further adjustments to the mobile phase in order to ensure that the antimicrobial preservatives present in the test solution are well separated from the insulin and have a shorter retention time. A small reduction in the concentration of acetonitrile increases the retention time of the insulin peaks relatively more than those of the preservatives.

Inject separately 20 µl of reference solution (a) and 20 µl of the test solution. In the chromatogram obtained with the reference solution, desamido insulin appears as a small peak after the principal peak and has a retention time of about 1.3 relative to the principal peak, due to insulin. In the chromatogram obtained with the test solution: the area of any peak corresponding to desamido insulin is not greater than 5.0 per cent of the total area of the peaks other than those due to preservatives; the sum of the areas of any other peaks, apart from that corresponding to insulin, that corresponding to desamido insulin, and those due to preservatives, is not greater than 3.0 per cent of the total area of the peaks other than those due to the preservatives.

Total zinc Not more than the amount stated in the individual monograph, determined by atomic absorption spectrometry (*Method I, 2.2.23*).

Use the following method, unless otherwise prescribed in the specific monograph.

Test solution. Dilute a volume of the gently shaken preparation containing 200 International Units to 25.0 ml with *0.01M hydrochloric acid.* Dilute if necessary to a suitable concentration (for example, 0.4 µg to 1.6 µg of Zn per millilitre) with *0.01M hydrochloric acid.*

Reference solutions. Use solutions containing 0.40 µg, 0.80 µg, 1.00 µg, 1.20 µg and 1.60 µg of Zn per millilitre, freshly prepared by dilution of *zinc standard solution (5 mg/ml Zn) R* with *0.01M hydrochloric acid.*

Measure the absorbance at 213.9 nm using a zinc hollow-cathode lamp as source of radiation and an air-acetylene flame of suitable composition (for example 11 litres of air and 2 litres of acetylene per minute).

Zinc in solution Where applicable, not more than the amount stated in the individual monograph, determined by atomic absorption spectrometry (*Method I, 2.2.23*).

Test solution. Dilute 1 ml of the clear supernatant liquid obtained by centrifuging the preparation to be examined to 25.0 ml with *water R*. Dilute if necessary to a suitable concentration (for example, 0.4 µg to 1.6 µg of Zn per millilitre) with *water R*.

Reference solutions. Use solutions containing 0.40 µg, 0.80 µg, 1.00 µg, 1.20 µg and 1.60 µg of Zn per millilitre, freshly prepared by diluting *zinc standard solution (5 mg/ml Zn) R* with *0.01M hydrochloric acid.*

Measure the absorbance at 213.9 nm using a zinc hollow-cathode lamp as source of radiation and an air-acetylene flame of suitable composition (for example 11 litres of air and 2 litres of acetylene per minute).

ASSAY

Examine by liquid chromatography (*2.2.29*).

Test solution. Add 4 µl of *6M hydrochloric acid* per millilitre of the preparation to be examined, whether a suspension or a solution, to obtain a clear acid insulin solution.

Reference solution (a). For a preparation containing a single species of insulin, dissolve in *0.01M hydrochloric acid*, as appropriate, the contents of a vial of *human insulin CRS* or *porcine insulin CRS*, or a defined quantity of *bovine insulin CRS* to obtain a concentration of 4.0 mg/ml. For a preparation containing both bovine and porcine insulins, mix 1.0 ml of a solution containing 4.0 mg of *bovine insulin CRS* per millilitre of *0.01M hydrochloric acid* and 1.0 ml of a solution containing 4.0 mg of *porcine insulin CRS* per millilitre *of 0.01M hydrochloric acid. Reference solution (a) is used for the assay of insulin preparations containing 100 International Units per millilitre.*

Reference solution (b). Dilute 4.0 ml of reference solution (a) to 10.0 ml with *0.01M hydrochloric acid. Reference solution (b) is used for the assay of insulin preparations containing 40 I.U.* per *millilitre.*

Reference solution (c). Mix 1.0 ml of a solution containing 4.0 mg of *human insulin CRS* per millilitre of *0.01M hydrochloric acid* with 1.0 ml of a solution containing 4.0 mg *of porcine insulin CRS* per millilitre of *0.01M hydrochloric acid.*

The chromatographic procedure may be carried out using:

— a stainless steel column 0.25 m long and 4.6 mm in internal diameter packed with *octadecylsilyl silica gel for chromatography R* (5 µm),

— as mobile phase at a flow rate of 1 ml per minute the following solutions, prepared and maintained at a temperature not lower than 20°C:

Mobile phase A. Dissolve 28.4 g of *anhydrous sodium sulphate R* in *water R* and dilute to 1000 ml with the same solvent. Add 2.7 ml of *phosphoric acid R.* Adjust to pH 2.3, if necessary, with *ethanolamine R.* Filter and degas by passing *helium for chromatography R* through the solution,

Mobile phase B. Mix 500 ml of mobile phase A with 500 ml of *acetonitrile R.* Filter and degas by passing *helium for chromatography R* through the solution,

— as detector a spectrophotometer set at 214 nm, maintaining the temperature of the column at 40°C.

Record the chromatograms eluting with a mobile phase consisting of a mixture of 48 volumes of mobile phase A and 52 volumes of mobile phase B, adjusted if necessary.

Inject 10 µl of reference solution (c). Record the chromatogram. The test is not valid unless the resolution between the peaks corresponding to human insulin and porcine insulin is at least 1.2. If necessary, adjust the concentration of acetonitrile in the mobile phase by slight decrease or increase until the required resolution is obtained. In the chromatogram obtained with reference solution (c), the two principal peaks, in order of elution, are due to human insulin and porcine insulin and any smaller peaks appearing immediately following each of the principal peaks are due to the corresponding monodesamido derivatives.

Inject separately 10 µl of the test solution and 10 µl of either reference solution (a), for insulin preparations containing 100 International Units per millilitre, or 10 µl of reference solution (b), for insulin preparations containing 40 International Units per millilitre. If necessary, make further adjustments of the mobile phase in order to ensure that the antimicrobial preservatives present in the test solution are well separated from the insulin and have shorter retention times. A small reduction in the concentration of acetonitrile increases the retention time of the insulin peaks relatively more than those of the preservatives. If necessary, after having carried out the chromatography of a solution wash the column with a mixture of equal volumes of *acetonitrile R* and *water R* for a sufficient time to ensure elution of any interfering substances before injecting the next solution.

Calculate the content of insulin from the area of the peak due to the bovine, porcine or human insulin and that of any peak due to the monodesamido derivative of the insulin using the declared content of insulin in *bovine insulin CRS*, *porcine insulin CRS* or *human insulin CRS*, as appropriate. For preparations containing both bovine or porcine insulin use the sum of the areas of both the bovine and porcine insulin peaks and of any peak due to the desamido derivative of either insulin(1).

STORAGE

Unless otherwise prescribed, store in a sterile, airtight, tamper-proof container, protected from light, at a temperature of 2°C to 8°C. Insulin preparations are not to be frozen.

LABELLING

The label states:
- the potency in International Units per millilitre,
- the concentration in terms of the number of milligrams of insulin per millilitre (for preparations containing both bovine insulin and porcine insulin the concentration is stated as the combined amount of both insulins),
- where applicable, that the substance is produced by enzymatic modification of porcine insulin,
- where applicable, that the substance is produced by recombinant DNA technology,
- where applicable, the animal species of origin,
- that the preparation must not be frozen,
- where applicable, that the preparation must be resuspended before use.

[1] 100 I.U. corresponds to 3.5 mg of insulin peptide. 40 I.U. corresponds to 1.4 mg of insulin peptide.

Ph Eur

Biphasic Insulin Injection

Biphasic Insulin

Biphasic Insulin Injection complies with the requirements of the 3rd edition of the European Pharmacopoeia [0831]. These requirements are reproduced below.

Ph Eur

Biphasic insulin injection complies with the monograph on Insulin preparations, injectable (854) with the amendments prescribed below.

DEFINITION

Biphasic insulin injection is a sterile suspension of crystals containing bovine insulin in a solution of porcine insulin.

CHARACTERS

A white suspension. When examined under a microscope, the majority of the particles are seen to be rhombohedral crystals, with a maximum dimension measured from corner to corner through the crystal greater than 10 µm but rarely exceeding 40 µm.

IDENTIFICATION

Examine the chromatograms obtained in the assay. The position of the peaks due to the two insulins in the chromatogram obtained with the test solution correspond to those of the principal peaks in the chromatogram obtained with the appropriate reference solution.

TESTS

pH (*2.2.3*). The pH of the suspension to be examined is 6.6 to 7.2.

Insulin in the supernatant 22.0 per cent to 28.0 per cent of insulin in solution. Determine by the method described in the test for insulin in the supernatant in the monograph on *Insulin preparations, injectable (854)*.

Total zinc 26.0 µg to 37.5 µg per 100 I.U. of insulin. Determine by the method described in the monograph on *Insulin preparations, injectable (854)*.

Ph Eur

Biphasic Isophane Insulin Injection

Biphasic Isophane Insulin

Biphasic Isophane Insulin Injection complies with the requirements of the 3rd edition of the European Pharmacopoeia [0832]. These requirements are reproduced below.

Ph Eur

Biphasic isophane insulin injection complies with the monograph on Insulin preparations, injectable (854) with the exception of the test for Insulin in the supernatant and with the amendments prescribed below for the other tests.

DEFINITION

Biphasic isophane insulin injection is a sterile, buffered suspension of either porcine or human insulin, complexed with protamine sulphate or another suitable protamine, in a solution of insulin of the same species.

PRODUCTION

Biphasic isophane insulin injection is prepared by carrying

out the procedures described in the monograph on *Insulin preparations, injectable (854)*.

Biphasic isophane insulin injection is produced by mixing, in defined ratios, soluble insulin injection and isophane insulin injection.

The amount of protamine corresponds to the isophane ratio and is not less than the equivalent of 0.3 mg and not more than the equivalent of 0.6 mg of protamine sulphate for each 100 I.U. of insulin in the insulin-protamine complex.

CHARACTERS

A white suspension which on standing deposits a white sediment and leaves a colourless or almost colourless supernatant liquid; the sediment is readily resuspended by gently shaking. When examined under a microscope, the particles are seen to be rod-shaped crystals, the majority with a maximum dimension greater than 1 μm but rarely exceeding 60 μm, free from large aggregates.

IDENTIFICATION

Examine the chromatograms obtained in the assay. The position of the peak due to insulin in the chromatogram obtained with the test solution corresponds to that of the principal peak obtained with the appropriate reference solution.

TESTS

Total zinc Not more than 40.0 μg per 100 I.U. of insulin. Determine by the method described in the monograph on *Insulin preparations, injectable (854)*.

LABELLING

The label states in addition to the indications mentioned in the monograph on *Insulin preparations, injectable (854)*:

— the ratio of soluble insulin injection to isophane insulin injection used in the manufacturing process of biphasic isophane insulin injection.

Ph Eur

Insulin Injection

Neutral Insulin; Neutral Insulin Injection;

Soluble Insulin

Insulin Injection complies with the requirements of the 3rd edition of the European Pharmacopoeia for Soluble Insulin Injection [0834]. These requirements are reproduced below.

Ph Eur

Soluble insulin injection complies with the monograph on Insulin preparations, injectable (854) with the amendments prescribed below.

DEFINITION

Soluble insulin injection is a neutral, sterile solution of bovine, porcine or human insulin.

CHARACTERS

A colourless liquid, free from turbidity and foreign matter; during storage, traces of a very fine sediment may be deposited.

IDENTIFICATION

Examine the chromatograms obtained in the assay. The position of the peak due to insulin in the chromatogram obtained with the test solution corresponds to that of the principal peak obtained with the appropriate reference solution.

TESTS

Total zinc Not more than 40.0 μg per 100 International Units of insulin.

Determine by the method described in the monograph on *Insulin preparations, injectable (854)*.

Use the following test solution.

Test solution. Dilute a volume of the gently shaken preparation containing 200 I.U. to 25.0 ml with *water R*. Dilute if necessary to a suitable concentration (for example, 0.4 μg to 1.6 μg of Zn per millilitre) with *water R*.

Ph Eur

Insulin Zinc Suspension

I.Z.S.; Insulin Zinc Suspension (Mixed);

I.Z.S. (Mixed)

Insulin Zinc Suspension complies with the requirements of the 3rd edition of the European Pharmacopoeia for Insulin Zinc Injectable Suspension [0837]. These requirements are reproduced below.

Ph Eur

Insulin zinc injectable suspension complies with the monograph on Insulin preparations, injectable (854) with the amendments prescribed below.

DEFINITION

Insulin zinc injectable suspension is a sterile, neutral suspension of insulin (bovine, porcine or bovine and porcine) or human insulin with a suitable zinc salt; the insulin is in a form insoluble in water.

PRODUCTION

Insulin zinc injectable suspension is prepared by carrying out the procedures described in the monograph on *Insulin preparations, injectable (854)*.

Insulin zinc injectable suspension is produced by mixing in the ratio 7 to 3 insulin zinc injectable suspension (crystalline) and insulin zinc injectable suspension (amorphous).

CHARACTERS

A white suspension which on standing deposits a white sediment and leaves a colourless or almost colourless supernatant liquid; the sediment is readily resuspended by gently shaking. When examined under a microscope, the majority of the particles are seen to be rhombohedral crystals with a maximum dimension measured from corner to corner through the crystal greater than 10 μm but rarely exceeding 40 μm; a considerable proportion of the particles can be seen under high power magnification to have no uniform shape and not to exceed 2 μm in maximum dimension.

IDENTIFICATION

Examine the chromatograms obtained in the assay.

For preparations made from a single species of insulin (bovine, porcine or human), the position of the peak due to insulin in the chromatogram obtained with the test solution corresponds to that of the principal peak in the chromatogram obtained with the appropriate reference solution. For preparations made from a mixture of bovine and porcine insulin, the positions of the peaks due to the two insulins in the chromatogram obtained with the test solution correspond to those of the principal peaks in the chromatogram obtained with the appropriate reference solution.

TESTS

Insulin not extractable with buffered acetone solution 63 per cent to 77 per cent of the total insulin content. Centrifuge a volume of the substance to be examined containing 200 I.U. of insulin and discard the supernatant liquid. Thoroughly suspend the residue in 1.65 ml of *water R*, add 3.3 ml of *buffered acetone solution R*, stir for 3 min, again centrifuge, discard the supernatant liquid and repeat all the operations with the residue. Dissolve the residue in *0.1M hydrochloric acid* to give a final volume of 2.0 ml. Determine the insulin content (*R*) of the residue and determine the total insulin content *(T)* of an equal volume of the suspension by a suitable method. Calculate the percentage of insulin not extractable with buffered acetone solution from the expression:

Total zinc Not more than 0.095 g/l for preparations containing 40 I.U. of insulin per millilitre, not more than 0.140 g/l for preparations containing 80 I.U. of insulin per millilitre and not more than 0.20 g/l for preparations containing 100 I.U. of insulin per millilitre. Determine by the method described in the monograph on *Insulin preparations, injectable (854)*.

Zinc in solution Not more than 70 per cent of the total zinc is in the form of zinc in solution for preparations containing 40 I.U. of insulin per millilitre, not more than 55 per cent of the total zinc is in the form of zinc in solution for preparations containing 80 I.U. of insulin per millilitre and not more than 50 per cent of the total zinc is in the form of zinc in solution for preparations containing 100 I.U. of insulin per millilitre. Determine by the method described in the monograph on *Insulin preparations, injectable (854)*.

Ph Eur

Insulin Zinc Suspension (Amorphous)

Amorph. I.Z.S.

Insulin Zinc Suspension (Amorphous) complies with the requirements of the 3rd edition of the European Pharmacopoeia for Insulin Zinc Injectable Suspension (Amorphous) [0835]. These requirements are reproduced below.

Ph Eur

Insulin zinc injectable suspension (amorphous) complies with the monograph on Insulin preparations, injectable (854) with the amendments prescribed below.

DEFINITION

Insulin zinc injectable suspension (amorphous) is a sterile neutral suspension of insulin (bovine or porcine) complexed with a suitable zinc salt; the insulin is in a form insoluble in water.

CHARACTERS

A white suspension which on standing deposits a white sediment and leaves a colourless or almost colourless supernatant liquid; the sediment is readily resuspended by gently shaking. When examined under a microscope, the particles are seen to have no uniform shape and a maximum dimension rarely exceeding 2 µm.

IDENTIFICATION

Examine the chromatograms obtained in the assay. The position of the peak due to insulin in the chromatogram obtained with the test solution corresponds to that of the principal peak in the chromatogram obtained with the appropriate reference solution.

TESTS

Total zinc Not more than 0.095 g/l for preparations containing 40 I.U. of insulin per millilitre, not more than 0.140 g/l for preparations containing 80 I.U. of insulin per millilitre and not more than 0.20 g/l for preparations containing 100 I.U. of insulin per millilitre. Determine by the method described in the monograph on *Insulin preparations, injectable (854)*.

Zinc in solution Not more than 70 per cent of the total zinc is in the form of zinc in solution for preparations containing 40 I.U. of insulin per millilitre, not more than 55 per cent of the total zinc is in the form of zinc in solution for preparations containing 80 I.U. of insulin per millilitre and not more than 50 per cent of the total zinc is in the form of zinc in solution for preparations containing 100 I.U. of insulin per millilitre. Determine by the method described in the monograph on *Insulin preparations, injectable (854)*.

Ph Eur

Insulin Zinc Suspension (Crystalline)

Cryst. I.Z.S.

Insulin Zinc Suspension (Crystalline) complies with the requirements of the 3rd edition of the European Pharmacopoeia for Insulin Zinc Injectable Suspension (Crystalline) [0836]. These requirements are reproduced below.

Ph Eur

Insulin zinc injectable suspension (crystalline) complies with the monograph on Insulin preparations, injectable (0854) with the amendments prescribed below.

DEFINITION

Insulin zinc injectable suspension (crystalline) is a sterile neutral suspension of insulin (porcine or bovine) or human insulin, complexed with a suitable zinc salt; the insulin is in the form of crystals insoluble in water.

CHARACTERS

A white suspension which on standing deposits a white sediment and leaves a colourless or almost colourless supernatant liquid; the sediment is readily resuspended by gently shaking. When examined under a microscope, the particles are seen to be rhombohedral crystals, the majority having a maximum dimension measured from corner to corner through the crystal greater than 10 µm but rarely exceeding 40 µm.

IDENTIFICATION
Examine the chromatograms obtained in the assay. The position of the peak due to insulin in the chromatogram obtained with the test solution corresponds to that of the principal peak in the chromatogram obtained with the appropriate reference solution.

TESTS
Insulin not extractable with buffered acetone solution Not less than 90 per cent of the total insulin content. Centrifuge a volume of the substance to be examined containing 200 I.U. of insulin and discard the supernatant liquid. Thoroughly suspend the residue in 1.65 ml of *water R*, add 3.3 ml of *buffered acetone solution R*, stir for 3 min, again centrifuge, discard the supernatant liquid and repeat all the operations with the residue. Dissolve the residue in *0.1M hydrochloric acid* to give a final volume of 2.0 ml. Determine the insulin content (*R*) of the residue and determine the total insulin content *(T)* of an equal volume of the suspension by a suitable method. Calculate the percentage of insulin not extractable with buffered acetone solution from the expression:

Total zinc Not more than 0.095 g/l for preparations containing 40 I.U. of insulin per millilitre, not more than 0.140 g/l for preparations containing 80 I.U. of insulin per millilitre and not more than 0.20 g/l for preparations containing 100 I.U. of insulin per millilitre. Determine by the method described in the monograph on *Insulin preparations, injectable (854)*.

Zinc in solution Not more than 70 per cent of the total zinc is in the form of zinc in solution for preparations containing 40 I.U. of insulin per millilitre, not more than 55 per cent of the total zinc is in the form of zinc in solution for preparations containing 80 I.U. of insulin per millilitre and not more than 50 per cent of the total zinc is in the form of zinc in solution for preparations containing 100 I.U. of insulin per millilitre. Determine by the method described in the monograph on *Insulin preparations, injectable (854)*.

Ph Eur

Isophane Insulin Injection

Isophane Insulin; Isophane Insulin (NPH)

Isophane Insulin Injection complies with the requirements of the 3rd edition of the European Pharmacopoeia [0833]. These requirements are reproduced below.

Ph Eur

Isophane insulin injection complies with the monograph on Insulin preparations, injectable (854) with the amendments prescribed below.

DEFINITION
Isophane insulin injection is a sterile suspension of bovine, porcine or human insulin, complexed with protamine sulphate or another suitable protamine.

PRODUCTION
Isophane insulin injection is prepared by carrying out the procedures described in the monograph on *Insulin preparations, injectable (854)*.

The amount of protamine corresponds to the isophane ratio and is not less than 0.3 mg and not more than 0.6 mg of protamine sulphate for each 100 International Units of insulin in the complex.

CHARACTERS
A white suspension which on standing deposits a white sediment and leaves a colourless or almost colourless supernatant liquid; the sediment is readily resuspended by gently shaking. When examined under a microscope, the particles are seen to be rod-shaped crystals, the majority with a maximum dimension greater than 1 µm but rarely exceeding 60 µm, free from large aggregates.

IDENTIFICATION
Examine the chromatograms obtained in the assay. The position of the peak due to insulin in the chromatogram obtained with the test solution corresponds to that of the principal peak in the chromatogram obtained with the appropriate reference solution.

TESTS
Total zinc Not more than 40.0 µg per 100 I.U. of insulin. Determine by the method described in the monograph on *Insulin preparations, injectable (854)*.

Ph Eur

Inulin Injection

Definition Inulin Injection is a sterile solution containing 10% w/v of Inulin and 0.8% w/v of Sodium Chloride in Water for Injections.

The injection complies with the requirements stated under Parenteral Preparations and with the following requirements.

Content of inulin 9.5 to 10.5% w/v.

Content of sodium chloride, NaCl 0.75 to 0.85% w/v.

Before carrying out the following tests dissolve any solid matter by heating in a water bath.

Identification
A. Complies with test A for Identification described under Inulin using as solution (1) a mixture of 1 volume of the injection and 3 volumes of *water* and as solution (2) a mixture of 1 volume of the injection and 3 volumes of a 12.5% w/v solution of *oxalic acid*, the mixture being boiled for 10 minutes and cooled before application.

B. Dilute 1 ml to 20 ml with *water*. To 2 ml of the diluted solution add 3 ml of a 0.15% w/v solution of *resorcinol* in *ethanol (96%)* followed by 3 ml of *hydrochloric acid*, mix and heat at 80°. A red colour is produced.

C. Yields the *reactions* characteristic of *sodium salts* and reaction A characteristic of *chlorides*, Appendix VI.

Acidity or alkalinity pH, 5.0 to 7.0, Appendix V L.

Reducing sugars Heat 5.0 ml of *cupri-tartaric solution R1* and titrate with the injection adding a few ml at a time and boiling for 10 to 15 seconds between each addition. When the solution becomes greenish yellow, add 0.25 ml of a 1% w/v solution of *methylene blue* and continue the titration until the solution becomes orange. Repeat the operation using a 0.50% w/v solution of *D-fructose* in place of the injection. The volume of the fructose solution used is not greater than that of the injection.

Pyrogens Complies with the *test for pyrogens*, Appendix XIV D. Use 10 ml per kg of the rabbit's weight.

Assay

For inulin Dilute 50 ml with sufficient *water* to produce 100 ml. Mix well, allow to stand for 30 minutes and measure the *optical rotation* using a 2-dm tube, Appendix V F. The observed rotation in degrees multiplied by 1.299 represents the weight in g of inulin in the volume of the injection taken for assay.

For NaCl Titrate 10 ml with 0.1M *silver nitrate VS* using *potassium chromate solution* as indicator. Each ml of 0.1M *silver nitrate VS* is equivalent to 5.845 mg of NaCl.

Storage Inulin Injection deposits solid matter on storage. Before use, solid matter should be completely redissolved by heating for not more than 15 minutes; the solution should be cooled to a suitable temperature before administration and should not be reheated.

Invert Syrup

Definition Invert Syrup is a mixture of glucose and fructose prepared by hydrolysing a 66.7% w/w solution of Sucrose with a suitable mineral acid, such as hydrochloric acid, and neutralising the resulting solution using, for example, calcium carbonate or sodium carbonate. The degree of inversion is at least 95%.

The syrup complies with the requirements stated under Syrups and with the following requirements.

Content of reducing sugars, expressed as invert sugar Not less than 67.0% w/w.

Characteristics A clear, colourless to pale straw-coloured syrupy liquid; odourless or almost odourless; taste, sweet.

Miscible with *water*, producing a clear solution; it dissolves in *ethanol (96%)* with the formation of an insoluble residue.

Identification

A. Heat 1 g with 10 ml of *water* and 5 ml of *cupri-tartaric solution.* A red precipitate is produced.

B. A solution in *water* is laevorotatory.

Acidity pH, 5.0 to 6.0, Appendix V L.

Arsenic To 4.0 g add 50 ml of *water* and 10 ml of *brominated hydrochloric acid*, allow to stand for 5 minutes and remove the excess of bromine by adding *tin(II) chloride solution AsT* and dilute to 100 ml with *water*. 25 ml of the resulting solution complies with the *limit test for arsenic*, Appendix VII (1 ppm).

Lead Prepare two solutions as follows. For solution (1) add 5 ml of 6M *acetic acid* to 12 g of the syrup. For solution (2) add 5 ml of 6M *acetic acid* and 2 ml of *lead standard solution (10 ppm Pb)* to 2.0 g of the syrup. Make solutions (1) and (2) alkaline with 5M *ammonia*, if necessary, and to each add 1 ml of *potassium cyanide solution PbT*. The solutions should not be more than faintly opalescent. If the colours of the solutions differ, equalise by the addition of a few drops of a highly diluted solution of burnt sugar or other non-reactive substance. Dilute each solution to 50 ml with *water*, add 0.1 ml of a 10% w/v solution of *sodium sulphide* to each and mix thoroughly. When viewed against a white background, the colour produced in solution (1) is not more intense than that produced in solution (2) (2 ppm).

Refractive index 1.4608 to 1.4630, Appendix V E.

Sulphur dioxide Not more than 70 ppm, Appendix IX B.

Quantity of prepared solution required ml	Invert sugar factor*	Quantity of invert sugar per 100 ml mg	Quantity of prepared solution required ml	Invert sugar factor*	Quantity of invert sugar per 100 ml mg
15	50.5	336.0	33	51.7	156.6
16	50.6	316.0	34	51.7	152.2
17	50.7	298.0	35	51.8	147.9
18	50.8	282.0	36	51.8	143.9
19	50.8	267.0	37	51.9	140.2
20	50.9	254.5	38	51.9	136.6
21	51.0	242.9	39	52.0	133.3
22	51.0	231.8	40	52.0	130.1
23	51.1	222.2	41	52.1	127.1
24	51.2	213.3	42	52.1	124.2
25	51.2	204.8	43	52.2	121.4
26	51.3	197.4	44	52.2	118.7
27	51.4	190.4	45	52.3	116.1
28	51.4	183.7	46	52.3	113.7
29	51.5	177.6	47	52.4	111.4
30	51.5	171.7	48	52.4	109.2
31	51.6	166.3	49	52.5	107.1
32	51.6	161.2	50	52.5	105.1

* mg of invert sugar corresponding to 10.00 ml of *cupri-tartaric solution R1*.

Weight per ml 1.338 to 1.344 g, Appendix V G.

Sulphated ash Not more than 0.1%, Appendix IX A.

Assay Dilute the syrup so that the volume of the diluted solution required in the following method is between 15 and 50 ml. Add 10.00 ml of *cupri-tartaric solution R1* to a 300-ml conical flask, add from a burette 15 ml of the diluted solution, heat to boiling over wire gauze covered with insulating material and continue adding the diluted solution in quantities of about 5 ml at 15-second intervals until the colour of the mixture indicates that the reduction appears to be almost complete. Boil for 2 minutes, add 0.2 ml of a 1% w/v solution of *methylene blue* and continue the titration until the blue colour is discharged. Repeat the operation, but, before heating, add almost the full quantity of the diluted solution required to reduce all the copper and then boil moderately for 2 minutes. Without removing the flask from either the gauze or the flame during the remainder of the titration, add 0.2 ml of the methylene blue solution and continue the titration so that it is just complete in a total boiling time of exactly 3 minutes; the end point is indicated by the disappearance of the blue colour, the solution becoming orange. From the Table calculate the content of reducing sugars (expressed as invert sugar) in 100 ml of the diluted solution and hence the percentage weight in weight in the substance being examined.

Storage Invert Syrup should be stored at a temperature of 35° to 45°.

Aqueous Iodine Oral Solution

Definition

Iodine	50 g
Potassium Iodide	100 g
Purified Water, freshly boiled and cooled	sufficient to produce 1000 ml

Extemporaneous preparation The following directions apply.

Dissolve the Potassium Iodide and the Iodine in 100 ml of the Purified Water and add sufficient of the Purified Water to produce 1000 ml.

The oral solution complies with the requirements stated under Oral Liquids and with the following requirements.

Content of iodine, I 4.75 to 5.25% w/v.

Content of potassium iodide, KI 9.5 to 10.5% w/v.

Assay Dilute 25 ml to 100 ml with *water.*

For iodine To 20 ml of the diluted solution add 10 ml of *water* and titrate with 0.1M *sodium thiosulphate VS*. Each ml of 0.1M *sodium thiosulphate VS* is equivalent to 12.69 mg of I.

For potassium iodide To 10 ml of the diluted solution add 20 ml of *water* and 40 ml of *hydrochloric acid* and titrate with 0.05M *potassium iodate VS* until the dark brown solution which is produced becomes pale brown. Add 1 ml of *amaranth solution* and continue the titration until the red colour just changes to pale yellow. From the number of ml of 0.05M *potassium iodate VS* required subtract one quarter of the number of ml of 0.1M *sodium thiosulphate VS* required in the Assay for iodine. Each ml of the remainder is equivalent to 16.60 mg of KI.

Storage Aqueous Iodine Oral Solution should be kept in a well-closed container, the materials of which are resistant to iodine.

Labelling The label states that the solution should be well diluted before use.

Aqueous Iodine Oral Solution contains in 1 ml 50 mg of Iodine and about 130 mg of total iodine, free and combined.

Aqueous Iodine Oral Solution is intended to be diluted before use.

When aqueous iodine solution is prescribed or demanded, Aqueous Iodine Oral Solution shall be dispensed or supplied.

Alcoholic Iodine Solution

Definition Alcoholic Iodine Solution is a *cutaneous solution.*

Iodine	25 g
Potassium Iodide	25 g
Purified Water	25 ml
Ethanol (90 per cent)	sufficient to produce 1000 ml

Extemporaneous preparation The following directions apply.

Dissolve the Potassium Iodide and the Iodine in the Purified Water and add sufficient Ethanol (90 per cent) to produce 1000 ml.

The solution complies with the requirements stated under Liquids for Cutaneous Application and with the following requirements.

Content of iodine, I 2.4 to 2.7% w/v.

Content of potassium iodide, KI 2.4 to 2.7% w/v.

Ethanol content 83 to 88% v/v, Appendix VIII F.

Assay

For iodine Dilute 10 ml with 20 ml of *water* and titrate with 0.1M *sodium thiosulphate VS*. Each ml of 0.1M *sodium thiosulphate VS* is equivalent to 12.69 mg of I.

For potassium iodide To 10 ml add 30 ml of *water* and 50 ml of *hydrochloric acid* and titrate with 0.05M *potassium iodate VS* until the dark brown solution which is produced becomes pale brown. Add 1 ml of *amaranth solution* and continue the titration until the red colour just changes to pale yellow. From the number of ml of 0.05M *potassium iodate VS* required subtract half the number of ml of 0.1M *sodium thiosulphate VS* required in the Assay for iodine. Each ml of the remainder is equivalent to 16.60 mg of KI.

Storage Alcoholic Iodine Solution should be kept in a well-closed container, the materials of which are resistant to iodine.

Labelling The label states (1) the date after which the solution is not intended to be used; (2) the conditions under which it should be stored.

The label indicates the pharmaceutical form as 'cutaneous solution'.

When iodine tinture is prescribed or demanded Alcoholic Iodine Solution shall be dispensed or supplied.

Iodised Oil Fluid Injection

Definition Iodised Oil Fluid Injection is a sterile iodine addition product of the ethyl esters of the fatty acids obtained from poppy-seed oil.

The injection complies with the requirements stated under Parenteral Preparations and with the following requirements.

Content of combined iodine 37.0 to 39.0% w/w.

Characteristics A straw-coloured or yellow, oily liquid; odour, not more than slightly alliaceous.

Practically insoluble in *water*; soluble in *chloroform*, in *ether* and in *petroleum spirit (boiling range, 40° to 60°)*.

Identification Boil 0.05 ml with 2 ml of *glacial acetic acid* and 0.1 g of *zinc powder* for 2 minutes, add 5 ml of *water*, shake, decant from any undissolved zinc and add 1 ml of *hydrogen peroxide solution (20 vol)*. Iodine vapour is evolved.

Acidity To 5 ml of *chloroform* add 5 ml of *ethanol (96%)* previously neutralised to *phenolphthalein solution R1* with 0.1M *ethanolic sodium hydroxide VS*, add 5 g of the injection, shake and titrate with 0.1M *ethanolic sodium hydroxide VS* using *phenolphthalein solution R1* as indicator. Not more than 1.0 ml is required to change the colour of the solution.

Weight per ml 1.28 to 1.30 g, Appendix V G.

Free iodine Shake 1 g with 1 ml of *starch mucilage* and 1 ml of *cadmium iodide solution*. Any blue colour disappears on the addition of 0.4 ml of 0.01M *sodium thiosulphate*.

Assay Boil 1 g with 10 ml of *glacial acetic acid* and 1 g of *zinc powder* under a reflux condenser for 1 hour. Add through the condenser 30 ml of hot *water*, filter through absorbent cotton, wash the flask with two 20-ml quantities of hot *water* and pass the washings through the filter. Cool the filtrate, add 25 ml of *hydrochloric acid* and 8 ml of *potassium cyanide solution* and titrate with 0.05M *potassium iodate VS* until the dark brown solution which is produced becomes light brown; add 5 ml of *starch mucilage* and continue the titration until the blue colour disappears. Each ml of 0.05M *potassium iodate VS* is equivalent to 12.69 mg of combined iodine.

Storage Iodised Oil Fluid Injection should be kept in an atmosphere of carbon dioxide or nitrogen and protected from light.

Action and use Radio-opaque injection.

Iofendylate Injection

Definition Iofendylate Injection is a sterile mixture of stereoisomers of ethyl 10-(4-iodophenyl)undecanoate ($C_{19}H_{29}IO_2$).

The injection complies with the requirements stated under Parenteral Preparations and with the following requirements.

Content of iofendylate, $C_{19}H_{29}IO_2$ 98.0 to 101.0% w/w.

Characteristics Almost colourless to pale yellow, viscous liquid.

Very slightly soluble in *water*; freely soluble in *ethanol (96%)*; miscible with *chloroform* and with *ether*.

Identification

A. When heated with *sulphuric acid*, violet vapours of iodine are evolved.

B. To 1 ml add 15 ml of *water* and 7 g of *potassium dichromate*, cool and carefully add 10 ml of *sulphuric acid*. Allow to stand until the reaction ceases, heat under a reflux condenser for 2 hours, cool, pour into 25 ml of *water* and filter. Wash the residue with a little *water*, recrystallise from 10 ml of aqueous ethanol and sublime the crystals. The *melting point* of the sublimate is about 270°, Appendix V A.

Acid value Not more than 1.5, Appendix X B.

Refractive index 1.525 to 1.527, Appendix V E.

Saponification value 132 to 142, Appendix X G. Use 1 g.

Weight per ml 1.245 to 1.260 g, Appendix V G.

Aliphatic iodine Mix 0.5 g with 10 ml of 1M *ethanolic potassium hydroxide* and boil vigorously under a reflux condenser in a water bath for 1 hour. Add 40 ml of *water* and 15 ml of *hydrochloric acid*, cool, filter and wash the residue with 10 ml of *water*. To the combined filtrate and washings add 10 ml of *potassium cyanide solution*, 5 ml of *starch mucilage* and 0.2 ml of 0.05M *potassium iodate*. A blue colour is not produced.

Free iodine *Absorbance* of a 4-cm layer at 485 nm, not more than 0.20, Appendix II B.

Assay Carry out the method for *oxygen-flask combustion for iodine*, Appendix VIII C, using 20 mg absorbed on filter paper surrounded by greaseproof paper. Each ml of 0.02M *sodium thiosulphate VS* is equivalent to 1.388 mg of $C_{19}H_{29}IO_2$.

Storage Iophendylate Injection should be protected from light.

Action and use Radio-opaque injection.

When iophendylate injection is prescribed or demanded Iofendylate Injection shal be dispensed or supplied.

Iopanoic Acid Tablets

Definition Iopanoic Acid Tablets contain Iopanoic Acid.

The tablets comply with the requirements stated under Tablets and with the following requirements.

Content of iopanoic acid, $C_{11}H_{12}I_3NO_2$ 95.0 to 105.0% of the prescribed or stated amount.

Identification

A. Shake a quantity of the powdered tablets containing 30 mg of Iopanoic Acid with 10 ml of *ethanol (96%)*, filter, evaporate the filtrate to dryness and dry the residue at 105°. The *infrared absorption spectrum* of the residue, Appendix II A, is concordant with the *reference spectrum* of iopanoic acid.

B. Spray the chromatograms obtained in the test for Related substances with a 0.1% w/v solution of *dimethylaminocinnamaldehyde* in a mixture of 1 volume of *hydrochloric acid* and 99 volumes of *ethanol (96%)*. The principal spot in the chromatogram obtained with solution (2) is similar in position, colour and size to that in the chromatogram obtained with solution (4).

Halide To a quantity of the powdered tablets containing 0.8 g of Iopanoic Acid add just sufficient 0.2M *sodium hydroxide* to dissolve the iopanoic acid, dilute to 10 ml with *water*, add sufficient 2M *nitric acid* dropwise to ensure complete precipitation of the iodinated acid and add 3 ml in excess. Filter (Whatman GF/C filter paper is suitable), wash the precipitate with 5 ml of *water* and combine the solutions. 15 ml of the resulting solution complies with the *limit test for chlorides*, Appendix VII (180 ppm, calculated as chloride).

Related substances Carry out the method for *thin-layer chromatography*, Appendix III A, using *silica gel* GF_{254} as the coating substance and a mixture of 10 volumes of 13.5M *ammonia*, 20 volumes of *methanol*, 20 volumes of *toluene* and 50 volumes of *1,4-dioxan* as the mobile phase but allowing the solvent front to ascend 10 cm above the line of application. Apply separately to the plate 5 µl of each of the following solutions. For solution (1) extract a quantity of the powdered tablets containing 1.0 g of Iopanoic Acid with five 10-ml quantities of *ethanol (96%)*, filter, evaporate the combined filtrates to dryness using a rotary evaporator and dissolve the residue in 10 ml of a mixture of 3 volumes of 10M *ammonia* and 97 volumes of *methanol*. For solution (2) dilute 1 volume of solution (1) to 10 volumes with a mixture of 3 volumes of 10M *ammonia* and 97 volumes of *methanol*. For solution (3) dilute 1 volume of solution (1) to 500 volumes with a mixture of 3 volumes of 10M *ammonia* and 97 volumes of *methanol*. Solution (4) contains 1.0% w/v of *iopanoic acid EPCRS* in a mixture of 3 volumes of 10M *ammonia* and 97 volumes of *methanol*. After removal of the plate, allow it to dry in air and examine under *ultraviolet light (254 nm)*. Any *secondary spot* in the chromatogram obtained with solution (1) is not more intense that the spot in the chromatogram obtained with solution (3) (0.2%).

Assay Weigh and powder 20 tablets. Triturate a quantity of the powder containing 0.4 g of Iopanoic Acid with five 10-ml quantities of *ethanol (96%)*, decanting and filtering each extract through the same filter. Evaporate the combined filtrates almost to dryness on a water bath, cool, add 20 ml of *water*, 12 ml of 5M *sodium hydroxide* and 1 g of *zinc powder* and boil under a reflux condenser for 30 minutes. Cool, rinse the condenser with 30 ml of *water*, filter through absorbent cotton and wash the flask and filter with two 20-ml quantities of *water*. To the combined filtrate and washings add 80 ml of *hydrochloric acid*, cool and titrate with 0.05M *potassium iodate VS* until the dark brown solution becomes light brown. Add 5 ml of *chloroform* and continue the titration, shaking well after each addition, until the chloroform becomes colourless. Each ml of 0.05M *potassium iodate VS* is equivalent to 19.03 mg of $C_{11}H_{12}I_3NO_2$.

Storage Iopanoic Acid Tablets should be protected from light.

Ipecacuanha Liquid Extract

Definition Ipecacuanha Liquid Extract is prepared by extracting Ipecacuanha with Ethanol (80 per cent). It contains not less than 1.90% and not more than 2.10% of total alkaloids, calculated as emetine, $C_{29}H_{40}N_2O_4$.

Extemporaneous preparation The following formula and directions apply.

Ipecacuanha, in *fine powder*	1000 g
Ethanol (80 per cent)	a sufficient quantity

Exhaust the Ipecacuanha by *percolation*, Appendix XI F, with Ethanol (80 per cent), reserving the first 750 ml of the percolate. Remove the ethanol from the remainder of the percolate by evaporation under reduced pressure at a temperature not exceeding 60° and dissolve the residual extract in the reserved portion. Determine the proportion of alkaloids in the liquid thus obtained by the Assay described below. To the remainder of the liquid add sufficient Ethanol (80%) to produce an Ipecacuanha Liquid Extract containing 2% w/v of total alkaloids calculated as emetine. Allow to stand for not less than 24 hours; filter.

The extract complies with the requirements stated under Extracts and with the following requirements.

Ethanol content 63 to 69% v/v, Appendix VIII F, Method III.

Relative density 0.910 to 0.940, Appendix V G.

Dry residue The requirement for Dry residue does not apply to Ipecacuanha Liquid Extract.

Assay To 5 ml in a separating funnel add 20 ml of *water*, 5 ml of 1M *sulphuric acid* and 10 ml of *chloroform* and shake well. Transfer the chloroform extract to a second separating funnel containing a mixture of 4 ml of *ethanol (96%)* and 20 ml of 0.05M *sulphuric acid*, shake, allow to separate and discard the chloroform layer. Continue the extraction of the liquid in the first separating funnel with two further 10-ml quantities of *chloroform*, transferring the chloroform solution each time to the second separating funnel and washing as before. Transfer the acidic liquid from the second separating funnel to the first separating funnel, make distinctly alkaline with 5M *ammonia* and shake with successive quantities of *chloroform* until *complete extraction* of the alkaloids is effected, Appendix XI G, washing each chloroform solution with the same 10 ml of *water* contained in a third separating funnel. Remove the chloroform, add to the residue 2 ml of *ethanol (96%)*, evaporate to dryness and dry for 5 minutes at 80° in a current of air. Dissolve the residue in 2 ml of *ethanol (96%)*, previously neutralised to *methyl red solution*, add 10 ml of 0.05M *sulphuric acid VS* and titrate with 0.1M *sodium hydroxide VS* using *methyl red mixed solution* as indicator. Each ml of 0.05M *sulphuric acid VS* is equivalent to 24.03 mg of total alkaloids, calculated as emetine, $C_{29}H_{40}N_2O_4$.

Preparation
Ipecacuanha Tincture

Action and use Expectorant.

Paediatric Ipecacuanha Emetic Mixture

Paediatric Ipecacuanha Emetic; Paediatric Ipecacuanha Oral Solution

Definition Paediatric Ipecacuanha Emetic Mixture is an *oral solution*.

Ipecacuanha Liquid Extract	70 ml
Hydrochloric Acid	2.5 ml
Glycerol	100 ml
Syrup	sufficient to produce 1000 ml

The mixture complies with the requirements stated under Oral Liquids and with the following requirements.

Content of total alkaloids 0.12 to 0.16% w/v, calculated as emetine, $C_{29}H_{40}N_2O_4$.

Identification Carry out the method for *thin-layer chromatography*, Appendix III A, using *silica gel G* as the coating substance and a mixture of 90 volumes of *chloroform* and 10 volumes of *diethylamine* as the mobile phase. Apply separately to the plate 2 µl of each of the following solutions. For solution (1) mix 5 ml with 10 ml of 1M *sulphuric acid*, shake with two 10-ml quantities of *chloroform* and discard the chloroform. Add sufficient 5M *ammonia* to make the aqueous solution distinctly alkaline to *litmus paper*, extract with four 10-ml quantities of *chloroform*, evaporate the combined extracts to dryness, cool the residue and dissolve it in 0.5 ml of *ethanol (96%)*. Solution (2) contains 0.1% w/v of *cephaeline hydrochloride EPCRS* in *ethanol (96%)*. Solution (3) contains 0.1% w/v of *emetine hydrochloride EPCRS* in *ethanol (96%)*. After removal of the plate, dry it at 105° to 110° for 30 minutes, allow to cool and spray with *dilute potassium iodobismuthate solution*. The principal spots in the chromatogram obtained with solution (1) correspond in colour and position to the spots in the chromatograms obtained with solutions (2) and (3). Disregard any *secondary spots*.

Assay To 25 ml in a separating funnel add 20 ml of *water* and 5 ml of 1M *sulphuric acid*, shake with three 10-ml quantities of *chloroform* and wash each chloroform extract with a mixture of 20 ml of 0.05M *sulphuric acid* and 4 ml of *ethanol (96%)* contained in a second separating funnel. Transfer the acid—ethanol mixture from the second separating funnel to the first, make the combined liquids distinctly alkaline to *litmus paper* with 5M *ammonia* and extract with successive quantities of *chloroform* until *complete extraction* of the alkaloids is effected, Appendix XI G. Wash each chloroform extract with the same 10 ml of *water*, combine the chloroform extracts, evaporate the chloroform, add 2 ml of *ethanol (96%)* to the residue, evaporate to dryness and dry the residue at 80° in a current of air for 5 minutes. Dissolve the residue in 2 ml of *ethanol (96%)* previously neutralised to *methyl red solution*, add 10 ml of 0.01M *sulphuric acid VS* and titrate the excess of acid with 0.02M *sodium hydroxide VS* using *methyl red solution* as indicator. Each ml of 0.01M *sulphuric acid VS* is equivalent to 4.806 mg of $C_{29}H_{40}N_2O_4$.

Labelling The label indicates the pharmaceutical form as 'oral solution'.

Ipecacuanha Tincture

Definition

Ipecacuanha Liquid Extract	100 ml
Acetic Acid (6 per cent)	16.5 ml
Ethanol (90 per cent)	210 ml
Glycerol	200 ml
Purified Water	sufficient to produce 1000 ml

Extemporaneous preparation The following directions apply.

Mix the Ethanol (90 per cent) and the Acetic Acid (6 per cent) with the Glycerol and 450 ml of Purified Water and add the Ipecacuanha Liquid Extract and sufficient Purified Water to produce 1000 ml. Allow to stand for not less than 24 hours; filter.

The tincture complies with the requirements stated under Tinctures and with the following requirements.

Content of total alkaloids 0.190 to 0.210% w/v, calculated as emetine, $C_{29}H_{40}N_2O_4$.

Ethanol content 24 to 28% v/v, Appendix VIII F, Method III.

Relative density 1.01 to 1.04, Appendix V G.

Assay To 50 ml in a separating funnel add 5 ml of 1M *sulphuric acid*, shake with three 10-ml quantities of *chloroform* and wash each chloroform solution with a mixture of 20 ml of 0.05M *sulphuric acid* and 4 ml of *ethanol (96%)* contained in a second separating funnel. Transfer the acid—ethanol mixture from the second separating funnel to the first, make the combined liquids distinctly alkaline to *litmus paper* with 5M *ammonia* and extract with successive quantities of *chloroform* until *complete extraction* of the alkaloids is effected, Appendix XI G. Wash each chloroform extract with the same 10 ml of *water*, combine the chloroform extracts, evaporate the chloroform, add 2 ml of *ethanol (96%)* to the residue, evaporate to dryness and dry the residue at 80° in a current of air for 5 minutes. Dissolve the residue in 2 ml of *ethanol (96%)* previously neutralised to *methyl red solution*, add 10 ml of 0.05M *sulphuric acid VS* and titrate the excess acid with 0.1M *sodium hydroxide VS* using *methyl red mixed solution* as indicator. Each ml of 0.05M *sulphuric acid VS* is equivalent to 24.03 mg of total alkaloids calculated as $C_{29}H_{40}N_2O_4$.

When ipecacuanha wine is prescribed or demanded, Ipecacuanha Tincture shall be dispensed or supplied.

Ipratropium Pressurised Inhalation

Definition Ipratropium Pressurised Inhalation is a suspension of Ipratropium Bromide in a suitable liquid in a suitable pressurised container.

The pressurised inhalation complies with the requirements stated under Preparations for Inhalations and with the following requirements.

Content of ipratropium bromide, $C_{20}H_{30}NO_3Br,H_2O$ 85.0 to 115.0% of the amount stated to be delivered by actuation of the valve.

Identification

A. In the test for Related substances, the principal spot in the chromatogram obtained with solution (2) corresponds to that in the chromatogram obtained with solution (6).

B. In the Assay, the chromatogram obtained with solution (1) shows a peak with the same retention time as the peak due to ipratropium bromide in the chromatogram obtained with solution (2).

Related substances Carry out the method for *thin-layer chromatography*, Appendix III A, using a high performance silica gel precoated plate (Merck silica gel 60 HPTLC plates are suitable) and a mixture of 5 volumes of *water*, 8 volumes of *anhydrous formic acid*, 28 volumes of *methanol* and 70 volumes of *dichloromethane* as the mobile phase but allowing the solvent front to ascend 6 cm above the line of application. Apply separately to the plate 5 µl of each of the following solutions. For solution (1) punch a small hole in the ferrule of each of three cooled containers, allow the propellant to evaporate for about 1 minute and transfer the contents of the containers, through the punched holes, to a beaker. Stir, using a magnetic stirrer, for about 10 minutes, add 3.5 ml of 0.01M *hydrochloric acid* and continue stirring for about 1 hour, until the propellant has completely evaporated, filter, add 10 ml of *chloroform* to the filtrate and shake vigorously for 1 minute. Allow the phases to separate and use the upper layer. For solution (2) dilute 1 volume of solution (1) to 50 volumes with 0.01M *hydrochloric acid.* For solution (3) dilute 1 volume of solution (2) to 4 volumes with 0.01M *hydrochloric acid.* For solution (4) dilute 2 volumes of solution (3) to 5 volumes with 0.01M *hydrochloric acid.* Solution (5) contains 0.008% w/v of *8s-isopropyl-3β-hydroxytropanium bromide BPCRS* in 0.01M *hydrochloric acid.* Solution (6) contains 0.008% w/v of *ipratropium bromide BPCRS* in 0.01M *hydrochloric acid.* After removal of the plate, dry it in a current of warm air for about 30 minutes. Spray the plate with a mixture of 1 volume of *potassium iodobismuthate solution*, 2 volumes of *glacial acetic acid* and 10 volumes of *water*, allow to dry briefly, spray with a 5% w/v solution of *sodium nitrite* and immediately examine the plate. In the chromatogram obtained with solution (1) any spot corresponding to 8*s*-isopropyl-3β-hydroxytropanium bromide is not more intense than the spot in the chromatogram obtained with solution (2) (2%), any other *secondary spot* is not more intense than the spot in the chromatogram obtained with solution (3) (0.5%) and not more than two such spots are more intense than the spot in the chromatogram obtained with solution (4) (0.2%).

Deposition of the emitted dose Carry out the test for *aerodynamic assessment of fine particles*, Appendix XII F, but determining the content of active ingredient as described below. Use Apparatus A with 7 ml of 0.001M *hydrochloric acid* in the upper impingement chamber and 40 ml of a mixture of equal volumes of 0.001M *hydrochloric acid* and *methanol* in the lower impingement chamber. Use the same solvent mixture to wash the coupling tube, E, and transfer the combined solution and washings in the lower impingement chamber to a 100-ml graduated flask, rinsing the chamber with the solvent mixture and dilute the combined solution to 100 ml with the solvent mixture.

Carry out the method for *liquid chromatography*, Appendix III D, using the following solutions. Solution (1) contains 0.00007% w/v of *ipratropium bromide BPCRS* in a mixture of equal volumes of 0.001M *hydrochloric acid* and *methanol.* For solution (2) use the diluted solution from the lower impingement chamber.

The chromatographic procedure may be carried out using (a) a stainless steel column (12.5 cm × 4 mm) packed with *stationary phase B* (Lichrosphere RP8 select B is suitable), (b) a mixture of 345 volumes of *acetonitrile* and 750 volumes of 0.012M *sodium heptanesulphonate* previously adjusted to pH 3.2 with 0.05M *orthophosphoric acid* as the mobile phase with a flow rate of 2 ml per minute and (c) a detection wavelength of 210 nm.

The test is not valid unless in the chromatogram obtained with solution (1) the *symmetry factor* of the peak due to ipratropium bromide is less than 3.0 and unless the *signal-to-noise ratio* of the peak is at least 3.0.

Calculate the amount of ipratropium bromide, $C_{20}H_{30}BrNO_3,H_2O$, delivered to the lower impingement chamber per actuation of the valve using the declared content of $C_{20}H_{30}BrNO_3,H_2O$ in *ipratropium bromide BPCRS.* Not less than 25% of the average amount of ipratropium bromide delivered per actuation of the valve, calculated as the average of the three results determined in the Assay, is deposited in the lower impingement chamber.

Assay Determine the content of active ingredient delivered by the first 10 successive combined actuations of the valve after priming. Carry out the procedure for content of active ingredient delivered by actuation of the valve described under Pressurised Inhalations, Preparations for Inhalation, beginning at the words 'Remove the pressurised container from the actuator...' and ending at the words '.... to the volume specified in the monograph' using 20 ml of a mixture of equal volumes of 0.001M *hydrochloric acid* and *methanol* in the vessel. Use the same solvent mixture to wash the pressurised container and to dilute the combined solution and washings obtained from the set of 10 combined actuations to 50 ml (solution A). Determine the amount of active ingredient in the 10 combined actuations using the following method of analysis.

Carry out the method for *liquid chromatography*, Appendix III D, using the following solutions. Solution (1) contains 0.00040% w/v of *ipratropium bromide BPCRS* in a mixture of equal volumes of 0.001M *hydrochloric acid* and *methanol.* For solution (2) use solution A.

The chromatographic conditions described under Deposition of the emitted dose may be used. In the chromatogram obtained with solution (1) long-running peaks due to excipients may appear.

The test is not valid unless in the chromatogram obtained with solution (1) the *symmetry factor* for the peak due to ipratropium bromide is less than 3.0.

Calculate the average content of $C_{20}H_{30}BrNO_3,H_2O$ delivered by a single actuation of the valve using the declared content of $C_{20}H_{30}BrNO_3,H_2O$ in *ipratropium bromide BPCRS.*

Determine the content of active ingredient a second and a third time by repeating the procedure on the middle 10 and the last 10 successive combined actuations of the valve, as estimated from the number of deliveries available from the container as stated on the label. For each of the three determinations the average content of $C_{20}H_{30}BrNO_3,H_2O$ delivered by a single actuation of the valve is within the limits stated under Content of ipratropium bromide.

IMPURITIES

In addition to the impurities shown in the monograph for Ipratropium Bromide the degradation impurities limited by the requirements of this monograph include:

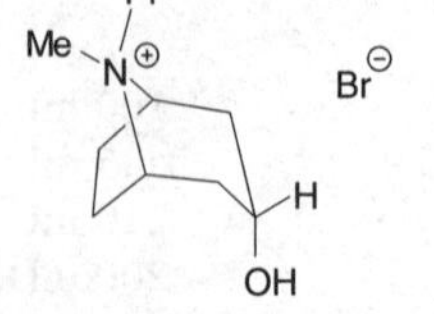

8*s*-isopropyl-3β-hydroxytropanium bromide

Iron Dextran Injection

Definition Iron Dextran Injection is a sterile colloidal solution containing a complex of iron(III) hydroxide with dextrans of weight average molecular weight between 5000 and 7500.

Production Iron Dextran Injection is produced by a method of manufacture designed to provide an iron—dextran complex with appropriate iron absorption characteristics. This may be confirmed for routine control purposes by the use of an appropriate combination of physicochemical tests, subject to the agreement of the competent authority.

The method of manufacture is validated to demonstrate that, if tested, the injection would comply with the following test.

Undue toxicity Inject 0.10 ml into a tail vein of each of 10 mice; not more than three mice die within 5 days of injection. If more than three mice die within 5 days, repeat the test on another group of 20 mice. Not more than 10 of the 30 mice used in the combined tests die within 5 days of injection.

The injection complies with the requirements stated under Parenteral Preparations and with the following requirements.

Content of iron, Fe 4.75 to 5.25% w/v.

Content of dextrans 17.0 to 23.0% w/v.

Characteristics A dark brown solution.

Identification

A. Add 5M *ammonia* to 0.2 ml of the injection previously diluted to 5 ml with *water*. No precipitate is produced.

B. Mix 1 ml with 100 ml of *water*. To 10 ml of this solution add 0.2 ml of *hydrochloric acid*, boil for 30 seconds, cool rapidly, add 4 ml of 13.5M *ammonia* and 10 ml of *hydrogen sulphide solution*, boil for at least 4 minutes to remove hydrogen sulphide, cool and filter. Boil 5 ml of the filtrate with 5 ml of *cupri-tartaric solution R1*; the solution remains greenish in colour and no precipitate is produced. Boil a further 5 ml of the filtrate with 0.5 ml of *hydrochloric acid* for 5 minutes, cool, add 2.5 ml of 5M *sodium hydroxide* and 5 ml of *cupri-tartaric solution R1* and boil again; a reddish precipitate is produced.

C. To 1 ml add 20 ml of *water* and 5 ml of *hydrochloric acid* and boil for 5 minutes. Cool, add an excess of 13.5M *ammonia* and filter. Wash the precipitate with *water*, dissolve in the minimum volume of 2M *hydrochloric acid* and add sufficient *water* to produce 20 ml. The resulting solution yields reaction B characteristic of *iron salts*, Appendix VI.

Acidity pH, 5.2 to 6.5, Appendix V L.

Arsenic To 5.0 ml in a Kjeldahl flask add 10 ml of *water* and 10 ml of *nitric acid* and heat until the vigorous evolution of brown fumes ceases. Cool, add 10 ml of *sulphuric acid* and heat again until fumes are evolved, adding *nitric acid* dropwise at intervals until oxidation is complete. Cool, add 30 ml of *water*, bring to the boil and continue boiling until the volume of liquid is reduced to about 20 ml. Cool and dilute to 50 ml with *water*. Reserve a portion of the solution for the test for Lead. To 5 ml of the solution add 10 ml of *water*, 15 ml of *stannated hydrochloric acid* and 3 ml of *tin(II) chloride solution AsT*. Connect to a condenser and distil 15 ml into 10 ml of *water*. To the distillate add 0.2 ml of *bromine water* and remove the excess of bromine with *tin(II) chloride solution AsT*. The solution complies with the *limit test for arsenic*, Appendix VII (2 µg per ml).

Copper To 5.0 ml add 5 ml of *nitric acid* and heat until the vigorous evolution of brown fumes ceases. Cool, add 2 ml of *sulphuric acid* and heat again until fumes are evolved, adding *nitric acid* dropwise at intervals until oxidation is complete. Cool, add 25 ml of *hydrochloric acid*, warm to dissolve, cool and extract with four 25-ml quantities of *isobutyl acetate*, discarding the extracts. Evaporate the acid solution to dryness, adding *nitric acid* dropwise if charring occurs. Dissolve the residue in 10 ml of 1M *hydrochloric acid*, reserving a portion of the solution for the test for Zinc. To 1 ml add 25 ml of *water* and 1 g of *citric acid*, make alkaline to *litmus paper* with 5M *ammonia*, dilute to 50 ml with *water*, add 1 ml of *sodium diethyldithiocarbamate solution* and allow to stand for 5 minutes. Any colour produced is not more intense than that produced by treating in the same manner a mixture of 3 ml of *copper standard solution (10 ppm Cu)* and 1 ml of 1M *hydrochloric acid* beginning at the words 'add 25 ml of *water*...' (60 µg per ml).

Lead To 16.0 ml of the solution reserved in the test for Arsenic add 50 ml of *hydrochloric acid* and extract with four 20-ml quantities of *isobutyl acetate*, discarding the extracts. Evaporate the acid solution to dryness and dissolve the residue in 20 ml of *water*. 12 ml of the solution complies with *limit test A for heavy metals*, Appendix VII. Use *lead standard solution (2 ppm Pb)* to prepare the standard (25 µg per ml).

Zinc To 5.0 ml of the solution reserved in the test for Copper add 15 ml of 1M *sodium hydroxide*, boil, filter, wash the residue with *water* and dilute the combined filtrate and washings to 25 ml with *water*. To 5 ml add 5 ml of 1M *hydrochloric acid* and 2 g of *ammonium chloride*, dilute to 50 ml with *water*, add 1 ml of freshly prepared *dilute potassium hexacyanoferrate(II) solution* and allow to stand for 20 minutes. Any opalescence produced is not more than that produced when 1 ml of freshly prepared *dilute potassium hexacyanoferrate(II) solution* is added to a solution prepared from 3 ml of *zinc standard solution (25 ppm Zn)*, 3 ml of 1M *sodium hydroxide*, 6 ml of 1M *hydrochloric acid* and 2 g of *ammonium chloride* diluted to 50 ml with *water* and allowed to stand for 20 minutes (150 µg per ml).

Chloride To 5 ml add 75 ml of *water* and 0.05 ml of *nitric acid* and titrate immediately with 0.1M *silver nitrate VS* determining the end point potentiometrically. 6.8 to 9.6 ml of 0.1M *silver nitrate VS* is required.

Iron absorption Using at least two rabbits, each weighing between 1.5 and 2.5 kg, clip the right hind leg free from hair over the injection site and swab the area with a bactericidal solution. Inject into each rabbit 0.4 ml of the injection per kg of the rabbit's weight using a 2-ml syringe fitted with a No. 12 hypodermic needle [22 gauge × 1.25 inch (0.7 × 32 mm approx.)]. Insert the needle at the distal end of the semitendinosus muscle, passing through the sartorius and entering the vastus medialis; the angle of the needle must be such that the full length is used. After 7 days, kill the rabbits and remove the legs into which the injections were made. Carefully cut open the muscles and examine the site of injection; it should be only very lightly stained and should show no dark brown deposits and no evidence of leakage along fascial planes. Skin the leg, dissect the flesh from the bone and cut into small pieces. Transfer the pieces to a 1000-ml beaker, add 75 ml of 2M *sodium hydroxide* and sufficient *water* to cover the flesh, cover the beaker with a watch glass and boil until most of the solid matter has disintegrated. Cool, cautiously add 50 ml of *sulphuric acid,* heat the mixture almost to boiling and add carefully ten 1-ml quantities of *fuming nitric acid* until no charring occurs when the excess of nitric acid has been boiled off. Cool, add 170 ml of *water,* boil until solution is complete, cool and dilute to 250 ml with *water.* To 5 ml of this solution add 3 ml of *sulphuric acid,* heat to fuming and complete the oxidation by the addition of small quantities of *nitric acid* until the solution is colourless. Cool, add 20 ml of *water,* boil for 3 minutes and add 10 ml of *ammonium citrate solution,* 10 ml of *ammonium mercaptoacetate solution,* 5M *ammonia* dropwise until the iron colour is fully developed, 1 ml of 5M *ammonia* in excess and sufficient *water* to produce 100 ml. Measure the *absorbance* of the resulting solution at 530 nm, Appendix II B.

Prepare a reference solution by adding 20 ml of *water* the same quantities of *ammonium citrate solution, ammonium mercaptoacetate solution* and 5M *ammonia* as used above, dilute to 100 ml with *water* and measure the *absorbance* at 530 nm. From the difference between the absorbances, calculate the amount of Fe present in the legs from a reference curve prepared by treating suitable aliquots of a solution of *ammonium iron(III) sulphate* containing 0.01% w/v of Fe by the procedure described above beginning at the words 'add 10 ml of *ammonium citrate solution...*'. Repeat the determination of Fe on the corresponding legs into which no injection was made, beginning at the words 'Carefully cut open the muscles...'. From the difference between the two amounts of iron, calculate the proportion of injected iron, as Fe, remaining in the leg tissues. Not more than 20% of the injected iron remains.

Pyrogens Complies with the *test for pyrogens,* Appendix XIV D. Use 0.5 ml per kg of the rabbit's weight, the rate of injection being 1 ml in 15 seconds.

Assay

For iron To 2 g add 10 ml of *water* and 5 ml of *sulphuric acid* and stir for several minutes. Allow to stand for 5 minutes, cool and dilute to 50 ml with *water.* Prepare a suitable zinc amalgam by covering 300 g of *zinc shot* with a 2% w/v solution of *mercury(II) chloride* and stir for 10 minutes. Decant the solution, wash the residue three times with *water* and transfer it to a column (30 cm × 18 mm) fitted with a sintered-glass disc (BS porosity No. 0). Activate the zinc amalgam by passing through the column 200 ml of *sulphuric acid (5%).* Pass the prepared solution slowly through the column and wash successively with 50 ml of *water,* four 25-ml quantities of *sulphuric acid (5%)* and 50 ml of *water.* Titrate the combined eluates with 0.1M *ammonium cerium(IV) sulphate VS* using *ferroin solution* as indicator. Each ml of 0.1M *ammonium cerium(IV) sulphate VS* is equivalent to 5.585 mg of Fe. Determine the *weight per ml* of the injection, Appendix V G, and calculate the percentage w/v of Fe.

For dextrans Dilute 1 g to 500 ml with *water,* dilute 10 ml of the solution to 100 ml with *water,* transfer 3 ml of the resulting solution to a test tube and cool to 0°. Add, to form a lower layer, 6 ml of a solution prepared and maintained at 0° containing 0.2% w/v of *anthrone* in a mixture of 19 volumes of *sulphuric acid* and 1 volume of *water,* mix and immediately heat on a water bath for 5 minutes. Cool and measure the *absorbance* of the resulting solution at the maximum at 625 nm, Appendix II B. Repeat the operation using 3 ml of *water* in place of the dilution of the injection. From the difference between the absorbances calculate the content of glucose present using a calibration curve prepared by treating suitable amounts of *D-glucose* in the same manner. Each g of *D-glucose* is equivalent to 0.94 g of dextrans. Determine the *weight per ml* of the injection, Appendix V G, and calculate the percentage w/v of dextrans.

Labelling The strength is stated as the equivalent amount of iron, Fe, in a suitable dose-volume.

Action and use Used in prevention and treatment of anaemia.

Iron Sorbitol Injection

Definition Iron Sorbitol Injection is a sterile colloidal solution of a complex of iron(III), Sorbitol and Citric Acid, stabilised with Dextrin and Sorbitol.

Production Iron Sorbitol Injection is produced by a method of manufacture designed to provide an iron—sorbitol complex with appropriate iron absorption characteristics. This may be confirmed for routine control purposes by the use of an appropriate combination of physico-chemical tests, subject to the agreement of the competent authority.

The method of manufacture is validated to demonstrate that, if tested, the injection would comply with the following test.

Undue toxicity Inject 20 µl mixed with 0.2 ml of *sodium chloride injection* into a tail vein of each of 10 mice; not more than three mice die within 5 days of injection. If more than three mice die within 5 days, repeat the test on another group of 20 mice. Not more than 10 of the 30 mice used in the combined tests die within 5 days of injection.

The injection complies with the requirements stated under Parenteral Preparations and with the following requirements.

Content of Fe 4.75 to 5.25% w/v.

Characteristics A brown solution.

Identification

A. Add 5M *ammonia* to 0.15 ml of the injection previously diluted to 5 ml with *water.* No precipitate is produced.

B. To 1 ml add 4 ml of *water* and 10 ml of *hydrochloric acid,* extract with three 15-ml quantities of *di-isopropyl ether* and dilute the aqueous layer to 25 ml with *water.* To 0.5 ml add 10 ml of *water,* 2 ml of 1M *sulphuric acid* and 10 mg of *sodium periodate,* allow to stand for 10 minutes and add 10 ml of 0.05M *sodium arsenite VS.* When the solution is colourless add 10 ml of a 0.4% w/v solution of *phenylhydrazine hydrochloride* in 0.5M *hydrochloric acid,* allow to stand for 10 minutes, add 1 ml of *dilute potassium hexacyanoferrate(III) solution,* allow to stand for 15 minutes and add 3 ml of *hydrochloric acid.* A red colour is produced.

C. Dilute 0.2 ml to 50 ml with *water.* To 5 ml add 1.5 ml of *sulphuric acid* and 1 ml of *bromine water,* heat on a water bath for 10 minutes and cool in ice. Add 4 ml of 0.025M *bromine* followed by 50 mg of *potassium permanganate*, shake well and allow to stand for 30 minutes. Decolorise the solution by the dropwise addition of a 10% w/v solution of *hydrazine hydrate* and shake with 15 ml of n-*heptane* for 10 minutes. Separate the heptane layer, wash with 10 ml of *water* and shake with 10 ml of a solution containing 4% w/v of *thiourea* and 2% w/v of *sodium tetraborate*. A yellow colour is produced in the aqueous layer.

D. Heat 0.15 ml of the injection with 2 ml of *sulphuric acid* until a charred residue is produced, extract the residue with 2M *hydrochloric acid* and filter. Reserve a sufficient quantity of the filtrate for test E. The filtrate yields a brown, flocculent precipitate with 5M *ammonia*.

E. The filtrate reserved in test D yields reaction B characteristic of *iron salts*, Appendix VI.

Alkalinity pH, 7.2 to 7.9, Appendix V L.

Viscosity At 20°, 7.0 to 11.0 $mm^2 s^{-1}$, Appendix V H, Method I, using a U-tube viscometer (size C).

Weight per ml 1.17 to 1.19 g, Appendix V G.

Arsenic To 5.0 ml in a Kjeldahl flask add 10 ml of *water* and 10 ml of *nitric acid* and heat until the vigorous evolution of brown fumes ceases. Cool, add 10 ml of *sulphuric acid* and heat again until fumes are evolved, adding *nitric acid* dropwise at intervals until oxidation is complete. Cool, add 30 ml of *water*, bring to the boil and continue boiling until the volume of liquid is reduced to about 20 ml; cool and dilute to 50 ml with *water*. Reserve a portion of the solution for the test for Lead. To 5 ml of the solution add 10 ml of *water*, 15 ml of *stannated hydrochloric acid* and 3 ml of *tin(II) chloride solution AsT*. Connect to a condenser and distil 15 ml into 10 ml of *water*. To the distillate add 0.2 ml of *bromine water* and remove the excess of bromine with *tin(II) chloride solution AsT*. The solution complies with the *limit test for arsenic*, Appendix VII (2 µg per ml).

Copper To 5.0 ml add 5 ml of *nitric acid* and heat until the vigorous evolution of brown fumes ceases. Cool, add 2 ml of *sulphuric acid* and heat again until fumes are evolved, adding *nitric acid* dropwise at intervals until oxidation is complete. Cool, add 25 ml of *hydrochloric acid*, warm to dissolve, cool and extract with four 25-ml quantities of *isobutyl acetate*, discarding the extracts. Evaporate the acid solution to dryness, adding *nitric acid* dropwise if charring occurs. Dissolve the residue in 10 ml of 1M *hydrochloric acid*, reserving a portion of the solution for the test for Zinc. To 1 ml add 25 ml of *water* and 1 g of *citric acid*, make alkaline to *litmus paper* with 5M *ammonia*, dilute to 50 ml with *water*, add 1 ml of *sodium diethyldithiocarbamate solution* and allow to stand for 5 minutes. Any colour obtained is not more intense than that produced by treating in the same manner a mixture of 3 ml of *copper standard solution (10 ppm Cu)* and 1 ml of 1M *hydrochloric acid* beginning at the words 'add 25 ml of *water*...' (60 µg per ml).

Lead To 16.0 ml of the solution prepared in the test for Arsenic add 50 ml of *hydrochloric acid* and extract with four 20-ml quantities of *isobutyl acetate*, discarding the extracts. Evaporate the acid solution to dryness and dissolve the residue in 20 ml of *water*. 12 ml of the solution complies with *limit test A for heavy metals*, Appendix VII. Use *lead standard solution (2 ppm Pb)* to prepare the standard (25 µg per ml).

Zinc To 5.0 ml of the solution reserved in the test for Copper add 15 ml of 1M *sodium hydroxide*, boil, filter, wash the residue with *water* and dilute the combined filtrate and washings to 25 ml with *water*. To 5 ml add 5 ml of 1M *hydrochloric acid* and 2 g of *ammonium chloride*, dilute to 50 ml with *water*, add 1 ml of freshly prepared *dilute potassium hexacyanoferrate(II) solution* and allow to stand for 20 minutes. Any opalescence produced is not greater than that obtained when 1 ml of freshly prepared *dilute potassium hexacyanoferrate(II) solution* is added to a solution prepared from 3 ml of *zinc standard solution (25 ppm Zn)*, 3 ml of 1M *sodium hydroxide*, 6 ml of 1M *hydrochloric acid* and 2 g of *ammonium chloride* diluted to 50 ml with *water* and allowed to stand for 20 minutes (150 µg per ml).

Iron absorption Complies with the test described under Iron Dextran Injection.

Bacterial endotoxins The endotoxin limit concentration is 0.50 IU per mg of iron, Appendix XIV C.

Assay To 2 g add 10 ml of *water* and 5 ml of *sulphuric acid* and stir for several minutes. Allow to stand for 5 minutes, cool and dilute to 50 ml with *water*. Prepare a suitable zinc amalgam by covering 300 g of *zinc shot* with a 2% w/v solution of *mercury(II) chloride* and stirring for 10 minutes. Decant the solution, wash the residue three times with *water* and transfer it to a column (30 cm × 18 mm) fitted with a sintered-glass disc (BS porosity No. 0). Activate the zinc amalgam by passing through the column 200 ml of 0.5M *sulphuric acid*. Pass the prepared solution slowly through the column and wash successively with 50 ml of *water*, four 25-ml quantities of 0.5M *sulphuric acid* and 50 ml of *water*. Titrate the combined washings with 0.1M *ammonium cerium(IV) sulphate VS* using *ferroin solution* as indicator. Each ml of 0.1M *ammonium cerium(IV) sulphate VS* is equivalent to 5.585 mg of Fe. Using the weight per ml of the injection calculate the percentage w/v of Fe.

Storage Iron Sorbitol Injection should be stored at a temperature of 15° to 30°. It should not be stored at a low temperature and should not be allowed to freeze.

Labelling The strength is stated as the equivalent amount of iron, Fe, in a suitable dose-volume.

Action and use Used in the treatment of anaemia.

Isoniazid Injection

Definition Isoniazid Injection is a sterile solution of Isoniazid in Water for Injections.

The injection complies with the requirements stated under Parenteral Preparations and with the following requirements.

Content of isoniazid, $C_6H_7N_3O$ 95.0 to 105.0% of the prescribed or stated amount.

Identification

A. Using a rotary evaporator, evaporate a volume of the injection containing 50 mg of Isoniazid to dryness, extract the residue with two 10-ml quantities of *ethanol (96%)*, filter and evaporate the combined ethanol extracts to dryness. The *infrared absorption spectrum* of the residue, Appendix II A, is concordant with the *reference spectrum* of isoniazid.

B. To a volume containing 25 mg of Isoniazid add 5 ml of *ethanol (96%)*, 0.1 g of *sodium tetraborate* and 5 ml of a

5.0% w/v solution of *1-chloro-2,4-dinitrobenzene* in *ethanol (96%)*, evaporate to dryness on a water bath, heat for a further 10 minutes and dissolve the residue in 10 ml of *methanol*. A reddish purple colour is produced.

Acidity pH, 5.6 to 6.0, Appendix V L.

Assay Dilute a quantity containing 0.4 g of Isoniazid to 250 ml with *water*. To 25 ml of the solution in a glass-stoppered flask add 25 ml of 0.05M *bromine VS* and 5 ml of *hydrochloric acid*, shake for 1 minute, allow to stand for 15 minutes, add 1 g of *potassium iodide* and titrate with 0.1M *sodium thiosulphate VS* using *starch mucilage* as indicator. Repeat the operation without the injection. The difference between the titrations represents the amount of bromine required. Each ml of 0.05M *bromine VS* is equivalent to 3.429 mg of $C_6H_7N_3O$.

Storage Isoniazid Injection should be protected from light.

Isoniazid Tablets

Definition Isoniazid Tablets contain Isoniazid.

The tablets comply with the requirements stated under Tablets and with the following requirements.

Content of isoniazid, $C_6H_7N_3O$ 95.0 to 105.0% of the prescribed or stated amount.

Identification

A. Shake a quantity of the powdered tablets containing 0.1 g of Isoniazid with 10 ml of *ethanol (96%)* for 15 minutes, centrifuge and decant the supernatant liquid. Extract the residue with two further 10-ml quantities of *ethanol (96%)* and evaporate the combined extracts to dryness. The *infrared absorption spectrum* of the residue, Appendix II A, is concordant with the *reference spectrum* of isoniazid.

B. Shake a quantity of the powdered tablets containing 1 mg of Isoniazid with 50 ml of *ethanol (96%)* and filter. To 5 ml of the filtrate add 0.1 g of *sodium tetraborate* and 5 ml of a 5% w/v solution of *1-chloro-2,4-dinitrobenzene* in *ethanol (96%)*, evaporate to dryness on a water bath and continue heating for a further 10 minutes. To the residue add 10 ml of *methanol* and mix. A reddish purple colour is produced.

Dissolution Comply with the *dissolution test for tablets and capsules*, Appendix XII D, using as the medium 900 ml of *water* and rotating the basket at 100 revolutions per minute. Withdraw a sample of 10 ml of the medium. Measure the *absorbance* of the filtered sample, suitably diluted if necessary, at the maximum at 263 nm, Appendix II B. Calculate the total content of isoniazid, $C_6H_7N_3O$, in the medium taking 307 as the value of A(1%, 1 cm) at the maximum at 263 nm.

Assay Weigh and powder 20 tablets. Dissolve a quantity of the powder containing 0.4 g of Isoniazid as completely as possible in *water*, filter and wash the residue with sufficient *water* to produce 250 ml. To 50 ml of the resulting solution add 50 ml of *water*, 20 ml of *hydrochloric acid* and 0.2 g of *potassium bromide* and titrate with 0.0167M *potassium bromate VS* determining the end point electrometrically. Each ml of 0.0167M *potassium bromate VS* is equivalent to 3.429 mg of $C_6H_7N_3O$.

Storage Isoniazid Tablets should be protected from light.

Isoprenaline Injection

Definition Isoprenaline Injection is a sterile solution of Isoprenaline Hydrochloride in Water for Injections.

The injection complies with the requirements stated under Parenteral Preparations and with the following requirements.

Content of isoprenaline hydrochloride, $C_{11}H_{17}NO_3$, HCl 95.0 to 105.0% of the prescribed or stated amount.

Characteristics A colourless or very pale yellow solution.

Identification

A. Record *second-derivative ultraviolet absorption spectra* of the following solutions, Appendix II B, in the range 250 to 330 nm. For solution (1) dilute the injection, if necessary, with *methanol* to contain 0.002% w/v of Isoprenaline Hydrochloride. Solution (2) is a 0.002% w/v solution of *isoprenaline hydrochloride BPCRS* in *methanol*. The spectrum obtained with solution (1) exhibits a maximum at 294 nm and a trough at 289 nm and is similar to the spectrum obtained with solution (2) in the range 280 to 298 nm.

B. Carry out the method for *thin-layer chromatography*, Appendix III A, using a reversed-phase high performance plate (Merck plates are suitable) and a mixture of 0.1 volume of *glacial acetic acid*, 40 volumes of *water* and 60 volumes of *methanol* as the mobile phase. Apply separately to the plate 20 µl of each of the following solutions. Prepare solution (1) in the following manner. For injections containing 0.1% w/v or more of Isoprenaline Hydrochloride, dilute the injection with *methanol* to produce a solution containing 0.01% w/v of Isoprenaline Hydrochloride. For injections containing less than 0.1% w/v of Isoprenaline Hydrochloride, evaporate a suitable quantity of the injection just to dryness and dissolve the residue in sufficient *methanol* to produce a 0.01% w/v solution. Solution (2) contains 0.01% w/v of *isoprenaline hydrochloride BPCRS* in *methanol*. After removal of the plate, allow it to dry in air, heat at 105° for 15 minutes and examine under *ultraviolet light (254 nm)*. The principal spot in the chromatogram obtained with solution (1) corresponds to that in the chromatogram obtained with solution (2).

C. To 2 ml add 0.1 ml of *iron(III) chloride solution R1*. An emerald green colour is produced which, on the gradual addition of *sodium hydrogen carbonate solution*, changes first to blue and then to red.

Acidity pH, 2.5 to 3.0, Appendix V L.

Assay To a quantity containing 5 mg of Isoprenaline Hydrochloride add sufficient *water* to produce 50 ml. To 20 ml add 0.5 ml of *iron(II) sulphate—citrate solution* and 2 ml of *glycine buffer solution*, mix and allow to stand for 20 minutes. Add sufficient *water* to produce 25 ml, mix and measure the *absorbance* of the resulting solution at 540 nm, Appendix II B. Calculate the content of $C_{11}H_{17}NO_3$,HCl from the *absorbance* obtained by repeating the determination using 5 ml of a 0.1% w/v solution of *isoprenaline hydrochloride BPCRS* in place of the injection and using the declared content of $C_{11}H_{17}NO_3$, HCl in *isoprenaline hydrochloride BPCRS*.

Storage Isoprenaline Injection should be protected from light and stored at a temperature not exceeding 25°.

Isosorbide Dinitrate Tablets

Definition Isosorbide Dinitrate Tablets contain Diluted Isosorbide Dinitrate.

CAUTION *Undiluted isosorbide dinitrate can be exploded by percussion or excessive heat. Appropriate precautions should be exercised and only exceedingly small amounts should be isolated.*

With the exception of the requirements for shape, the tablets comply with the requirements stated under Tablets and with the following requirements.

Content of isosorbide dinitrate, $C_6H_8N_2O_8$ 90.0 to 110.0% of the prescribed or stated amount.

Identification

A. Carry out the method for *thin-layer chromatography*, Appendix III A, using *silica gel G* as the coating substance and *toluene* as the mobile phase. Apply separately to the plate 20 µl of each of the following solutions. For solution (1) extract a quantity of the powdered tablets containing 2 mg of isosorbide dinitrate with 1 ml of *ether* and centrifuge. Prepare solution (2) in the same manner but use *diluted isosorbide dinitrate BPCRS* in place of the powdered tablets. After removal of the plate, dry it in a current of air, spray with *diphenylamine solution R1* and irradiate for 15 minutes with *ultraviolet light (254* and *365 nm)*. The principal spot in the chromatogram obtained with solution (1) corresponds to that in the chromatogram obtained with solution (2).

B. Shake a quantity of the powdered tablets containing 50 mg of isosorbide dinitrate with warm *sulphuric acid (50%)* containing a trace of *diphenylamine*. An intense blue colour is produced.

Dissolution Tablets intended to be swallowed whole comply with the *dissolution test for tablets and capsules*, Appendix XII D, using Apparatus II. Use as the medium 900 ml of 0.1M *hydrochloric acid* and rotate the paddle at 50 revolutions per minute. Withdraw a sample of 10 ml of the medium and filter through a membrane filter with a nominal pore size not greater than 0.45 µm. Carry out the method for *liquid chromatography*, Appendix III D, using the following solutions. Solution (1) is a solution of *isosorbide dinitrate EPCRS* in the dissolution medium containing the same concentration of isosorbide dinitrate as that expected in the dissolution vessel. Solution (2) is the filtrate from the dissolution vessel.

The chromatographic procedure may be carried out using (a) a stainless steel column (20 cm × 4.6 mm) packed with *stationary phase C* (5 µm) (Hypersil ODS is suitable), (b) as the mobile phase with a flow rate of 1 ml per minute, a mixture of equal volumes of *methanol* and *water* and (c) a detection wavelength of 222 nm. Inject 100 µl of each solution.

Calculate the total content of isosorbide dinitrate, $C_6H_8N_2O_8$, in the medium using the declared content of $C_6H_8N_2O_8$ in *isosorbide dinitrate EPCRS*.

Inorganic nitrate Carry out the method for *thin-layer chromatography*, Appendix III A, using *silica gel H* as the coating substance and a mixture of 15 volumes of *glacial acetic acid*, 30 volumes of *acetone* and 60 volumes of *toluene* as the mobile phase. Apply separately to the plate 20 µl of each of the following solutions. For solution (1) extract a quantity of the powdered tablets with sufficient *ethanol (96%)* to produce a solution containing 2.5% w/v of isosorbide dinitrate. For solution (2) dissolve 12.5 mg of *potassium nitrate* in 5 ml of *water* and dilute to 50 ml with *absolute ethanol*; this solution should be freshly prepared. After removal of the plate, dry it in a current of air and spray with *diphenylamine solution R1*. Any spot corresponding to potassium nitrate in the chromatogram obtained with solution (1) is not more intense than the spot in the chromatogram obtained with solution (2) (1%).

Related substances Carry out the method for *thin-layer chromatography*, Appendix III A, using *silica gel G* as the coating substance and a mixture of 80 volumes of *toluene* and 20 volumes of *ethyl acetate* as the mobile phase. Apply separately to the plate 20 µl of each of the following solutions. For solution (1) shake a quantity of the powdered tablets containing 0.2 g of isosorbide dinitrate with 5 ml of *acetone* and filter. For solution (2) dilute 1 volume of solution (1) to 200 volumes with *acetone*. After removal of the plate, dry it in a current of air and spray with *diphenylamine solution R1*. Any *secondary spot* in the chromatogram obtained with solution (1) is not more intense than the spot in the chromatogram obtained with solution (2).

Disintegration The requirement for Disintegration does not apply to Isosorbide Dinitrate Tablets intended to be chewed before swallowing or intended to be allowed to dissolve in the mouth.

Assay Weigh and powder 20 tablets. To a quantity of the powder containing 5 mg of isosorbide dinitrate add 5 ml of *glacial acetic acid*, shake for 1 hour, centrifuge and carry out the Assay described under Diluted Isosorbide Dinitrate, using 1 ml of the clear solution and beginning at the words 'add 2 ml of *phenoldisulphonic acid solution...*'.

Labelling The label states whether the tablets are to be swallowed whole, chewed before swallowing or allowed to dissolve in the mouth.

Kanamycin Injection

Definition Kanamycin Injection is either a sterile solution of Kanamycin Sulphate in Water for Injections containing Sulphuric Acid or a sterile solution prepared by dissolving Kanamycin Acid Sulphate for Injection in Water for Injections.

The injection complies with the requirements stated under Parenteral Preparations and with the following requirements.

Characteristics A colourless to pale yellow solution.

Identification

Carry out the method for *thin-layer chromatography*, Appendix III A, using a plate coated with a 0.75-mm layer of the following mixture. Mix 0.3 g of *carbomer* (Carbopol 934 is suitable) with 240 ml of *water* and allow to stand, with moderate shaking, for 1 hour. Adjust to pH 7 by the gradual addition, with continuous shaking, of 2M *sodium hydroxide* and add 30 g of *silica gel H*. Heat the plate at 110° for 1 hour, allow to cool and use immediately. Use a 7% w/v solution of *potassium dihydrogen orthophosphate* as the mobile phase and allow the solvent front to ascend 12 cm above the line of application. Apply separately to the plate 10 µl of each of the following solutions. For solution (1) use a suitable volume of the injection diluted with *water* to contain 800 IU per ml. Solution (2) contains 0.1% w/v of *kanamycin monosulphate EPCRS* in *water*. Solution (3) contains 0.1% w/v each of *kanamycin mono-*

sulphate EPCRS, *neomycin sulphate EPCRS* and *streptomycin sulphate EPCRS* in *water*. After removal of the plate, dry it in a current of warm air, spray with a mixture of equal volumes of a 0.2% w/v solution of *naphthalene-1,3-diol* in *ethanol (96%)* and *sulphuric acid (46% v/v)* and heat at 150° for 5 to 10 minutes. The principal spot in the chromatogram obtained with solution (1) is similar in position, colour and size to that in the chromatogram obtained with solution (2). The test is not valid unless the chromatogram obtained with solution (3) shows three clearly separated spots.

Pyrogens Dilute the injection with *water for injections* to contain 10,000 IU per ml. The resulting solution complies with the *test for pyrogens*, Appendix XIV D. Use 1 ml per kg of the rabbit's weight.

Storage Kanamycin Injection prepared by dissolving the contents of a sealed container in Water for Injections should be used immediately after preparation but, in any case, within the period recommended by the manufacturer when prepared and stored strictly in accordance with the manufacturer's instructions.

Labelling The strength of the injection is stated as the number of IU (Units) in a suitable dose-volume.

When supplied as a ready-to-use solution, the injection also complies with the following requirements.

Acidity pH, 4.0 to 6.0, Appendix V L.

Kanamycin B Carry out the method for *thin-layer chromatography*, Appendix III A, using a plate prepared immediately before use as described under Identification. Use a 7% w/v solution of *potassium dihydrogen orthophosphate* as the mobile phase and allow the solvent front to ascend 12 cm above the line of application. Apply separately to the plate 4 µl of each of the following solutions. For solution (1) use a suitable volume of the injection diluted with *water* to contain 3750 IU per ml. Solution (2) contains 0.020% w/v of *kanamycin B sulphate EPCRS* in *water*. After removal of the plate, dry it in a current of warm air, spray with *ninhydrin and stannous chloride reagent* and heat at 110° for 15 minutes. Any spot corresponding to kanamycin B in the chromatogram obtained with solution (1) is not more intense than the spot in the chromatogram obtained with solution (2) (4%).

Assay Carry out the *biological assay of antibiotics*, Appendix XIV A. The precision of the assay is such that the fiducial limits of error are not less than 95% and not more than 105% of the estimated potency. The upper fiducial limit of error is not less than 97.0% and the lower fiducial limit of error is not more than 110.0% of the prescribed or stated number of IU.

KANAMYCIN ACID SULPHATE FOR INJECTION

Definition Kanamycin Acid Sulphate for Injection is a sterile material consisting of Kanamycin Acid Sulphate with or without excipients. It is supplied in a sealed container.

The contents of the sealed container comply with the requirements for Powders for Injections stated under Parenteral Preparations and with the following requirements.

Identification Carry out the test described under Kanamycin Injection but using as solution (1) sufficient of the contents of the sealed container to produce a solution containing 800 IU per ml in *water*.

Acidity or alkalinity When dissolved in the volume of *water for injections* stated on the label, pH, 5.5 to 7.5, Appendix V L.

Kanamycin B Comply with the test described under Kanamycin Injection but using as solution (1) a suitable quantity dissolved in sufficient *water* to contain 3750 IU per ml.

Assay Determine the weight of the contents of each of 10 containers as described in the test for Uniformity of weight under Parenteral Preparations, Powders for Injections.

Mix the contents of the 10 containers and carry out the *biological assay of antibiotics*, Appendix XIV A. The precision of the assay is such that the fiducial limits of error are not less than 95% and not more than 105% of the estimated potency. For a container of average content weight, the upper fiducial limit of error is not less than 95.0% and the lower fiducial limit of error is not more than 115.0% of the prescribed or stated number of IU.

Storage The contents of the sealed container should be protected from light.

Labelling The label of the sealed container states the total number of IU (Units) contained in it.

Kaolin Mixture

Kaolin Oral Suspension

Definition Kaolin Mixture is an *oral suspension* containing 20% w/v of Light Kaolin or Light Kaolin (Natural) and 5% w/v each of Light Magnesium Carbonate and Sodium Bicarbonate in a suitable vehicle with a peppermint flavour.

It should be recently prepared unless the kaolin has been sterilised.

Extemporaneous preparation The following formula applies.

Light Kaolin or Light Kaolin (Natural)	200 g
Light Magnesium Carbonate	50 g
Sodium Bicarbonate	50 g
Concentrated Peppermint Emulsion	25 ml
Double-strength Chloroform Water	500 ml
Water sufficient to produce	1000 ml

The mixture complies with the requirements stated under Oral Liquids and with the following requirements.

Content of magnesium, Mg 1.04 to 1.25% w/w.

Content of sodium bicarbonate, $NaHCO_3$ 4.05 to 4.65% w/w.

Acid-insoluble matter 13.8 to 18.4% w/w when determined by the following method. Dry and ignite the residue reserved in the Assay for magnesium to constant weight at red heat.

Assay

For magnesium To 3 g add 15 ml of *water*, make acidic to *litmus paper* by the cautious addition of 2M *hydrochloric acid*, boil for 5 minutes, replacing the water lost by evaporation, cool and filter the supernatant liquid. Boil the residue with 20 ml of *water* and 10 ml of 2M *hydrochloric acid*, cool, filter through the same filter and wash the residue with *water* until the washings are free from chloride. Reserve the residue for the test for Acid-insoluble matter. Dilute the combined filtrate and washings to

100 ml with *water*. To 20 ml add 0.1 g of *L-ascorbic acid*, make slightly alkaline to *litmus paper* with 5M *ammonia* and add 10 ml of *triethanolamine*, 10 ml of *ammonia buffer pH 10.9* and 1 ml of a 10% w/v solution of *potassium cyanide*. Titrate with 0.05M *disodium edetate VS*, using *mordant black 11 solution* as indicator, to a full blue colour. Each ml of 0.05M *disodium edetate VS* is equivalent to 1.215 mg of Mg.

For sodium bicarbonate Boil 10 g with 100 ml of *water* for 5 minutes, filter, boil the residue with 100 ml of *water* for 5 minutes and filter. Combine the filtrates, cool and titrate with 0.5M *hydrochloric acid VS* using *methyl orange—xylene cyanol FF solution* as indicator. Add 10 ml of *ammonia buffer pH 10.9* and titrate with 0.05M *disodium edetate VS* using *mordant black 11 solution* as indicator. After subtracting one fifth of the volume of 0.05M *disodium edetate VS*, each ml of 0.5M *hydrochloric acid VS* is equivalent to 42.00 mg of $NaHCO_3$.

Labelling The label indicates the pharmaceutical form as 'oral suspension'.

Kaolin and Morphine Mixture

Kaolin and Morphine Oral Suspension

Definition Kaolin and Morphine Mixture is an *oral suspension* containing 20% w/v of Light Kaolin or Light Kaolin (Natural), 5% w/v of Sodium Bicarbonate and 4% v/v of Chloroform and Morphine Tincture in a suitable vehicle.

It should be recently prepared unless the kaolin has been sterilised.

Extemporaneous preparation The following formula applies.

Light Kaolin or Light Kaolin (Natural)	200 g
Sodium Bicarbonate	50 g
Chloroform and Morphine Tincture	40 ml
Water	sufficient to produce 1000 ml

The mixture complies with the requirements stated under Oral Liquids and with the following requirements.

Content of sodium bicarbonate, $NaHCO_3$ 4.65 to 5.35% w/v.

Content of anhydrous morphine, $C_{17}H_{19}NO_3$ 0.0055 to 0.0080% w/v.

Identification Carry out the method for *thin-layer chromatography*, Appendix III A, using *silica gel G* as the coating substance and a mixture of 70 volumes of *toluene*, 20 volumes of *ethyl acetate* and 10 volumes of *diethylamine* as the mobile phase. Apply separately to the plate 10 µl of each of the following solutions. For solution (1) centrifuge 10 ml of the preparation, reserving the supernatant liquid. Extract the residue with four 10-ml quantities of a mixture of 38 ml of *acetone* and 2 ml of 5M *ammonia*, centrifuging between each extraction, and evaporate the combined extracts on a water bath to about 5 ml. Mix with the reserved supernatant liquid, add 10 ml of 1M *sulphuric acid*, shake with two 10-ml quantities of *chloroform* and discard the chloroform. Add sufficient 5M *ammonia* to make the aqueous solution alkaline to *litmus paper*, extract with three 10-ml quantities of a mixture of equal volumes of *chloroform* and *ethanol (96%)*, evaporate to dryness and dissolve the residue in 0.5 ml of *ethanol (96%)*. Solution (2) contains 0.10% w/v of *morphine hydrochloride*. After removal of the plate, heat it at 105° to 110° for 30 minutes, allow to cool and spray with *dilute potassium iodobismuthate solution*. The principal spot in the chromatogram obtained with solution (1) corresponds in colour and position to that in the chromatogram obtained with solution (2).

Acid-insoluble matter 13.8 to 18.4% w/w when determined by the following method. To 3 g add 15 ml of *water*, cautiously add sufficient 2M *hydrochloric acid* to make the suspension acidic to *litmus paper*, boil for 5 minutes, replacing the water lost by evaporation, cool and filter the supernatant liquid. Boil the residue with 20 ml of *water* and 10 ml of 2M *hydrochloric acid*, cool, filter through the same filter and wash the residue with *water* until the washings are free from chloride. Dry and ignite the residue to constant weight at red heat.

Assay

For sodium bicarbonate Boil 20 ml with 40 ml of *water* for 5 minutes, replacing the water lost by evaporation, add 50 ml of *ethanol (96%)* previously neutralised to *methyl red solution* and allow to stand for 1 hour. Filter and wash the residue with 100 ml of a mixture of equal volumes of the neutralised ethanol and *water*. Add 50 ml of 0.5M *hydrochloric acid VS* to the combined filtrate and washings, boil, cool and titrate the excess of hydrochloric acid with 0.5M *sodium hydroxide VS* using *methyl red solution* as indicator. Each ml of 0.5M *hydrochloric acid VS* is equivalent to 42.00 mg of $NaHCO_3$.

For anhydrous morphine Centrifuge 25 ml, reserving the supernatant liquid, and extract the residue with three 25-ml quantities of *ethanol (96%)*, centrifuging between each extraction and reserving each supernatant liquid. Add 40 ml of *water* and 7 ml of 5M *ammonia* to the combined supernatant liquids and extract the mixture with three 30-ml quantities of *chloroform*. Gently shake each extract with the same 15 ml of a mixture of 2 volumes of *water* and 1 volume of *ethanol (96%)* and discard the aqueous ethanol. Evaporate the combined chloroform solutions just to dryness, warm the residue with 10 ml of 1M *hydrochloric acid*, cool the solution, which may be slightly cloudy, add sufficient *water* to produce 50 ml and filter (Whatman No. 42 paper is suitable). To 20 ml of the filtrate add 8 ml of a freshly prepared 1% w/v solution of *sodium nitrite*, allow to stand in the dark for 15 minutes, add 12 ml of 5M *ammonia* and sufficient *water* to produce 50 ml and measure the *absorbance* of a 4-cm layer at 442 nm without delay, Appendix II B. Use in the reference cell a solution prepared in the same manner but using *water* in place of the sodium nitrite solution. Calculate the content of anhydrous morphine taking 124 as the value of A(1%, 1 cm) at the maximum at 442 nm.

Storage Kaolin and Morphine Mixture should be kept in well-filled, well-closed glass containers.

Labelling The label indicates the pharmaceutical form as 'oral suspension'.

Kaolin Poultice

Definition

Heavy Kaolin[1], finely sifted	527 g
Boric Acid, finely sifted	45 g
Methyl Salicylate	2 ml
Thymol	500 mg
Peppermint Oil	0.5 ml
Glycerol	425 g

Extemporaneous preparation The following directions apply.

Mix the Heavy Kaolin, previously dried at 100°, and the Boric Acid with the Glycerol, heat at 120° for 1 hour, stirring occasionally, and allow to cool. Separately, dissolve the Thymol in the Methyl Salicylate, add to the cooled mixture, add the Peppermint Oil and mix thoroughly.

The heating step may be omitted if some other satisfactory means of mixing the solid ingredients with the Glycerol is used but in this case Heavy Kaolin that has been sterilised is used.

Content of boric acid, H_3BO_3 4.25 to 4.75% w/w.

Assay Mix 20 g with a solution containing 10 g of *D-mannitol* in 40 ml of *water*, warm and stir until completely dispersed and titrate with 1M *sodium hydroxide VS* using *phenolphthalein solution R1* as indicator. Each ml of 1M *sodium hydroxide VS* is equivalent to 61.83 mg of H_3BO_3.

Storage Kaolin Poultice should be kept in suitable containers that minimise absorption, diffusion or evaporation of the ingredients.

[1]If an appropriate heating step, such as that described under Extemporaneous preparation, is not included in the manufacturing process, Heavy Kaolin that has been sterilised is used.

Ketamine Injection

Definition Ketamine Injection is a sterile solution of Ketamine Hydrochloride in Water for Injections.

The injection complies with the requirements stated under Parenteral Preparations and with the following requirements.

Content of ketamine, $C_{13}H_{16}ClNO$ 95.0 to 105.0% of the prescribed or stated amount.

Identification

A. Dilute a volume of the injection with a mixture of 1 volume of 1M *sodium hydroxide* and 49 volumes of *methanol* to produce a solution containing the equivalent of 0.07% w/v of ketamine. The *light absorption*, Appendix II B, in the range 230 to 350 nm of this solution exhibits a maximum at 301 nm and shoulders at 274, 268 and 261 nm.

B. Dilute a volume of the injection with 0.1M *hydrochloric acid* to produce a solution containing the equivalent of 0.025% w/v of ketamine. The *light absorption*, Appendix II B, in the range 230 to 350 nm of this solution exhibits two maxima at 276 nm and at 269 nm and a shoulder at 260 nm.

Acidity pH, 3.5 to 5.5, Appendix V L.

Foreign amines Carry out the method for *thin-layer chromatography*, Appendix III A, using a silica gel precoated plate (Merck silica gel 60 plates are suitable) and a mixture of 0.5 volume of 13.5M *ammonia*, 19.5 volumes of *propan-2-ol* and 80 volumes of *toluene* as the mobile phase. For injections containing the equivalent of 5% w/v or more of ketamine, apply to the plate 10 µl of each of the following solutions. For solution (1) use the injection diluted, if necessary, to contain the equivalent of 5% w/v of ketamine. For solution (2) dilute 1 volume of solution (1) to 200 volumes with *methanol.* For injections containing less than the equivalent of 5% w/v of ketamine, apply to the plate 50 µl of each of the following solutions. For solution (1) use the injection diluted, if necessary, to contain the equivalent of 1% w/v of ketamine. For solution (2) dilute 1 volume of solution (1) to 200 volumes with *methanol.* Pour the mobile phase into an unlined tank, immediately place the prepared plate in the tank and close the tank. After removal of the plate, allow it to dry in air and spray with freshly prepared *acid potassium iodobismuthate solution.* Any *secondary spot* in the chromatogram obtained with solution (1) is not more intense than the spot in the chromatogram obtained with solution (2) (0.5%).

Related substances Carry out the method for *thin-layer chromatography*, Appendix III A, using a silica gel precoated plate (Merck silica gel 60 plates are suitable) and a mixture of 0.5 volume of 13.5M *ammonia*, 19.5 volumes of *propan-2-ol* and 80 volumes of *toluene* as the mobile phase in an unsaturated tank. For injections containing the equivalent of 5% w/v or more of ketamine, apply to the plate 10 µl of each of the following solutions. For solution (1) use the injection diluted, if necessary, to contain the equivalent of 5% w/v of ketamine. For solution (2) dilute 1 volume of solution (1) to 250 volumes with *methanol.* For solution (3) dilute 25 volumes of solution (2) to 40 volumes with *methanol.* For injections containing less than the equivalent of 5% w/v of ketamine, apply to the plate 50 µl of each of the following solutions. For solution (1) use the injection diluted, if necessary, to contain the equivalent of 1% w/v of ketamine. For solution (2) dilute 1 volume of solution (1) to 250 volumes with *methanol.* For solution (3) dilute 25 volumes of solution (2) to 40 volumes with *methanol.* Pour the mobile phase into an unlined tank, immediately place the prepared plate in the tank and close the tank. After removal of the plate, allow it to dry in air, expose to iodine vapour for 1 hour and re-examine. Any *secondary spot* in the chromatogram obtained with solution (1) is not more intense than the spot in the chromatogram obtained with solution (2) (0.4%) and not more than one such spot is more intense than the spot in the chromatogram obtained with solution (3) (0.25%).

Assay Dilute a volume of the injection containing the equivalent of 0.5 g of ketamine to 200 ml with *water* and mix. To 20 ml of the resulting solution add 3 ml of 0.1M *sodium hydroxide* and extract with three 15-ml quantities of *chloroform.* Combine the chloroform extracts and extract with three 30-ml quantities of 0.05M *sulphuric acid,* add sufficient 0.05M *sulphuric acid* (saturated with *chloroform*) to produce 200 ml, mix and measure the *absorbance* of the resulting solution at the maximum at 269 nm, Appendix II B. Calculate the content of $C_{13}H_{16}ClNO$ taking 22.4 as the value of A(1%, 1 cm) at the maximum at 269 nm.

Storage Ketamine Injection should be protected from light and stored at a temperature not exceeding 30°.

Labelling The quantity of active ingredient is stated in terms of the equivalent amount of ketamine in a suitable dose-volume.

Ketoprofen Capsules

Definition Ketoprofen Capsules contain Ketoprofen.

The capsules comply with the requirements stated under Capsules and with the following requirements.

Content of ketoprofen, $C_{16}H_{14}O_3$ 92.5 to 107.5% of the prescribed or stated amount.

Identification Shake a quantity of the contents of the capsules containing 0.5 g of Ketoprofen with 50 ml of *chloroform* for 5 minutes, filter, evaporate to dryness using a rotary evaporator and induce crystallisation by prolonged scratching of the side of the container with a glass rod. The *infrared absorption spectrum* of the crystals, Appendix II A, is concordant with the *reference spectrum* of ketoprofen.

Dissolution Comply with the *dissolution test for tablets and capsules*, Appendix XII D, using Apparatus II. Use as the medium 900 ml of a phosphate buffer prepared by dissolving 1.46 g of *potassium dihydrogen orthophosphate* and 20.06 g of *disodium hydrogen orthophosphate* in sufficient *water* to produce 1000 ml, adjusting the pH to 7.5 if necessary with *orthophosphoric acid*, and rotate the paddle at 50 revolutions per minute. Withdraw a sample of 10 ml of the medium, filter and dilute the filtrate with sufficient of the dissolution medium to give a solution expected to contain about 0.001% w/v of Ketoprofen. Measure the *absorbance* of this solution, Appendix II B, at the maximum at 260 nm using dissolution medium in the reference cell. Calculate the total content of ketoprofen, $C_{16}H_{14}O_3$, in the medium taking 662 as the value of A(1%, 1 cm) at the maximum at 260 nm.

Related substances Protect the solutions from light. Carry out the method for *liquid chromatography*, Appendix III D, using the following freshly prepared solutions. For solution (1) shake a quantity of the contents of the capsules containing 0.1 g of Ketoprofen with 100 ml of a mixture of 40 volumes of *acetonitrile* and 60 volumes of *water* (solvent A), filter and use the filtrate. For solution (2) dilute 1 volume of solution (1) to 50 volumes with solvent A and further dilute 1 volume to 10 volumes with solvent A. Solution (3) contains 0.0002% w/v of *2-(3-carboxyphenyl)propionic acid EPCRS* in solvent A. Solution (4) contains 0.0003% w/v of *3-acetylbenzophenone EPCRS* in solvent A. For solution (5) dilute 1 volume of solution (1) to 100 volumes with solvent A; to 1 ml add 1 ml of solution (4).

The chromatographic procedure may be carried out using (a) a stainless steel column (15 cm × 4.6 mm) packed with *stationary phase C* (5 µm) (Nucleosil C18 is suitable), (b) a mixture of 2 volumes of freshly prepared *phosphate buffer pH 3.5*, 43 volumes of *acetonitrile* and 55 volumes of *water* as the mobile phase with a flow rate of 1 ml per minute and (c) a detection wavelength of 233 nm.

Inject 20 µl of solution (5). The test is not valid unless the *resolution factor* between the peaks due to ketoprofen and 3-acetylbenzophenone is at least 7.

Inject separately 20 µl of solutions (1) to (4). Allow the chromatography to proceed for seven times the retention time of ketoprofen. In the chromatogram obtained with solution (1) the area of any peak corresponding to 2-(3-carboxyphenyl)propionic acid is not greater than the area of the principal peak in the chromatogram obtained with solution (3) (0.2%), the area of any peak corresponding to 3-acetylbenzophenone is not greater than the area of the principal peak in the chromatogram obtained with solution (4) (0.3%), the area of any other *secondary peak* is not greater than the area of the principal peak in the chromatogram obtained with solution (2) (0.2%) and the sum of the areas of all the *secondary peaks* other than those due to the two named impurities is not greater than 2.5 times the area of the principal peak in the chromatogram obtained with solution (2) (0.5%). Disregard any peak with an area less than 0.1 times the area of the principal peak in the chromatogram obtained with solution (2) (0.02%).

Assay Shake a quantity of the mixed contents of 20 capsules containing 50 mg of Ketoprofen for 10 minutes with 300 ml of *methanol (75%)*, mix and dilute to 500 ml with *methanol (75%)*. Allow to stand, dilute 5 ml of the supernatant liquid to 100 ml with *methanol (75%)* and measure the *absorbance* of the resulting solution at the maximum at 258 nm, Appendix II B. Calculate the content of $C_{16}H_{14}O_3$ taking 662 as the value of A(1%, 1 cm) at the maximum at 258 nm.

Labetalol Injection

Definition Labetalol Injection is a sterile solution of Labetalol Hydrochloride in Water for Injections.

The injection complies with the requirements stated under Parenteral Preparations and with the following requirements.

Content of labetalol hydrochloride, $C_{19}H_{24}N_2O_3$,HCl 90.0 to 110.0% of the prescribed or stated amount.

Characteristics A colourless or very pale yellow solution.

Identification

A. Mix a volume containing 50 mg of Labetalol Hydrochloride with 50 ml of 0.1M *hydrochloric acid* and heat on a water bath for 30 minutes. Cool, filter, add 10 ml of *ammonia buffer pH 10.0* and extract with three 15-ml quantities of *dichloromethane*. Shake the combined extracts with 5 g of *anhydrous sodium sulphate*, filter and evaporate the filtrate to dryness. The *infrared absorption spectrum* of the residue, Appendix II A, is concordant with the *reference spectrum* of labetalol.

B. The *light absorption*, Appendix II B, in the range 250 to 400 nm of a 0.004% w/v solution of the residue obtained in test A in 0.1M *sodium hydroxide* exhibits a maximum only at 333 nm.

Acidity pH, 3.5 to 4.5, Appendix V L.

Diastereoisomer ratio Examine by *gas chromatography*, Appendix III B, using a solution prepared in the following manner. Dilute a volume of the injection containing 20 mg of Labetalol Hydrochloride with *ethanol (96%)* to about 10 ml and evaporate to dryness using a rotary evaporator. Dissolve 2.0 mg of the residue in 1 ml of a 1.2% w/v solution of *1-butaneboronic acid* in *anhydrous* *pyridine* and allow to stand for 20 minutes.

The chromatographic procedure may be carried out using (a) a glass column (1.5 m × 4 mm) packed with *silanised diatomaceous support* (125 µm to 150 µm) impregnated with 3% w/w of *polymethylphenylsiloxane*, (b) *nitrogen for chromatography* as the carrier gas, (c) a flame-ionisation detector, maintaining the temperature of the column, the injection port and the detector at 300°. Inject 2 µl of the solution.

Two peaks each corresponding to a pair of diastereoisomers appear in the chromatogram. Adjust the sensitivity of the detector so that in the chromatogram obtained, the height of the taller of the diastereoisomer peaks is about 80% of the full scale of the recorder. The test is not valid unless the height of the trough separating these peaks is less than 5% of the full scale of the recorder. The area of each peak is not less than 45% and not more than 55% of the total area of both peaks.

Free carboxylic acid and other related substances Carry out the method for *thin-layer chromatography*, Appendix III A, using *silica gel* GF_{254} as the coating substance and a mixture of 5 volumes of 13.5M *ammonia*, 25 volumes of *methanol* and 75 volumes of *dichloromethane* as the mobile phase. Apply separately to the plate 20 µl of each of the following solutions. For solution (1) dilute a volume of the injection containing 80 mg of Labetalol Hydrochloride to about 50 ml with *ethanol (96%)*, evaporate to dryness using a rotary evaporator and dissolve the residue in 1 ml of *methanol*. For solution (2) dilute 1 volume of solution (1) to 200 volumes with *methanol*. Solution (3) contains 0.160% w/v of *5-[1-hydroxy-2-(1-methyl-3-phenylpropylamino)ethyl]salicylic acid hydrochloride BPCRS* in *methanol*. After removal of the plate, dry it in a current of warm air, heat at 105° for 30 minutes, cool and examine under *ultraviolet light (254 nm)*. In the chromatogram obtained with solution (1) any spot corresponding to 5-[1-hydroxy-2-(1-methyl-3-phenylpropylamino)ethyl]-salicylic acid is not more intense that the spot in the chromatogram obtained with solution (3) (2%) and any other *secondary spot* is not more intense than the spot in the chromatogram obtained with solution (2) (0.5%).

Assay Dilute a volume containing 50 mg of Labetalol Hydrochloride to 100 ml with *water*. To 10 ml of the solution add 10 ml of 0.05M *sulphuric acid* and dilute to 100 ml with *water*. Measure the *absorbance* of the resulting solution at the maximum at 302 nm, Appendix II B. Calculate the content of $C_{19}H_{24}N_2O_3$,HCl taking 86 as the value of A(1%, 1 cm) at the maximum at 302 nm.

Storage Labetalol Injection should be protected from light.

Labetalol Tablets

Definition Labetalol Tablets contain Labetalol Hydrochloride.

The tablets comply with the requirements stated under Tablets and with the following requirements.

Content of labetalol hydrochloride, $C_{19}H_{24}N_2O_3$,HCl 95.0 to 105.0% of the prescribed or stated amount.

Identification

A. To a quantity of the powdered tablets containing 50 mg of Labetalol Hydrochloride add 50 ml of 0.1M *hydrochloric acid* and heat on a water bath for 30 minutes. Cool, filter, add 10 ml of *ammonia buffer pH 10.0* and extract with three 15-ml quantities of *dichloromethane*. Shake the combined extracts with 5 g of *anhydrous sodium sulphate*, filter and evaporate the filtrate to dryness. The *infrared absorption spectrum* of the residue, Appendix II A, is concordant with the *reference spectrum* of labetalol.

B. The *light absorption*, Appendix II B, in the range 250 to 400 nm of a 0.004% w/v solution in 0.1M *sodium hydroxide* of the residue obtained in test A exhibits a maximum only at 333 nm.

Diastereoisomer ratio Comply with the test described under Labetalol Injection using 2 mg of the residue prepared in the following manner. Shake a quantity of the powdered tablets containing 0.5 g of Labetalol Hydrochloride with 10 ml of *methanol*, filter and evaporate the filtrate to dryness using a rotary evaporator.

Related substances Carry out the method for *thin-layer chromatography*, Appendix III A, using *silica gel* GF_{254} as the coating substance and a mixture of 5 volumes of 13.5M *ammonia*, 25 volumes of *methanol* and 75 volumes of *dichloromethane* as the mobile phase. Apply separately to the plate 20 µl of each of the following solutions. For solution (1) shake a quantity of the powdered tablets containing 0.5 g of Labetalol Hydrochloride with 10 ml of *methanol*, filter and use the filtrate. For solution (2) dilute 1 volume of solution (1) to 100 volumes with *methanol*. For solution (3) dilute 1 volume of solution (2) to 2 volumes with *methanol*. After removal of the plate, dry it in a current of warm air, heat at 105° for 30 minutes, cool and examine under *ultraviolet light (254 nm)*. Any *secondary spot* in the chromatogram obtained with solution (1) is not more intense than the spot in the chromatogram obtained with solution (2) (1%) and not more than one such spot is more intense than the spot in the chromatogram obtained with solution (3) (0.5%).

Assay Weigh and powder 20 tablets. Shake a quantity of the powdered tablets containing 1 g of Labetalol Hydrochloride with 250 ml of 0.05M *sulphuric acid* for 30 minutes. Dilute the mixture to 500 ml with 0.05M *sulphuric acid*, mix, filter and dilute 10 ml of the filtrate to 250 ml with 0.05M *sulphuric acid*. Measure the *absorbance* of the resulting solution at the maximum at 302 nm, Appendix II B. Calculate the content of $C_{19}H_{24}N_2O_3$, HCl taking 86 as the value of A(1%, 1 cm) at the maximum at 302 nm.

Lactic Acid Pessaries

Definition Lactic Acid Pessaries contain Lactic Acid in a suitable basis.

The pessaries comply with the requirements stated under Vaginal Preparations and with the following requirements.

Content of lactic acid, $C_3H_6O_3$ 95.0 to 105.0% of the prescribed or stated amount.

Assay Weigh five pessaries, melt together by warming and allow to cool, stirring continuously. Dissolve a quantity of the mass containing 1 g of Lactic Acid in 50 ml of *water*, add 50 ml of 0.5M *sodium hydroxide VS*, boil gently for 5 minutes, cool and titrate the excess of alkali with 0.5M *hydrochloric acid VS* using *phenolphthalein solution R1* as indicator. Each ml of 0.5M *sodium hydroxide VS* is equivalent to 45.04 mg of $C_3H_6O_3$.

Lemon Spirit

Definition

Terpeneless Lemon Oil	100 ml
Ethanol (96 per cent)	sufficient to produce 1000 ml

The spirit complies with the requirements stated under Spirits and with the following requirements.

Content of aldehydes 3.45 to 4.60% w/v, calculated as citral, $C_{10}H_{16}O$.

Ethanol content 84 to 88% v/v, Appendix VIII F.

Weight per ml 0.814 to 0.823 g, Appendix V G.

Assay Carry out the method for the *determination of aldehydes*, Appendix X K, using 10 ml, omitting the *toluene* and using a volume, not less than 7 ml, of *alcoholic hydroxylamine solution* that exceeds by 1 to 2 ml the volume of 0.5M *potassium hydroxide in ethanol (60%) VS* required. Each ml of 0.5M *potassium hydroxide in ethanol (60%) VS* is equivalent to 76.73 mg of $C_{10}H_{16}O$.

Lemon Syrup

Definition

Lemon Spirit	5 ml
Citric Acid Monohydrate	25 g
Invert Syrup	100 ml
Syrup	sufficient to produce 1000 ml

Extemporaneous preparation The following directions apply.

Dissolve the Citric Acid Monohydrate in some of the Syrup, add the Invert Syrup, the Lemon Spirit and sufficient Syrup to produce 1000 ml and mix.

Characteristics Lemon Syrup has a weight per ml of about 1.33 g.

The syrup complies with the requirements stated under Syrups and with the following requirements.

Content of citric acid monohydrate, $C_6H_8O_7,H_2O$ 2.2 to 2.6% w/v.

Assay Mix 8 g with 100 ml of *water* and titrate with 0.1M *sodium hydroxide VS* using *phenolphthalein solution R1* as indicator. Each ml of 0.1M *sodium hydroxide VS* is equivalent to 7.005 mg of $C_6H_8O_7,H_2O$. Determine the *weight per ml*, Appendix V G, and calculate the content of $C_6H_8O_7,H_2O$, weight in volume.

Storage Lemon Syrup should be stored at a temperature not exceeding 25°.

Levobunolol Eye Drops

Definition Levobunolol Eye Drops are a sterile solution of Levobunolol Hydrochloride in Purified Water.

The eye drops comply with the requirements stated under Eye Preparations and with the following requirements.

Content of levobunolol hydrochloride, $C_{17}H_{25}NO_3$, HCl 90.0 to 110.0% of the prescribed or stated amount.

Identification

A. The *light absorption*, Appendix II B, in the range 210 to 350 nm of a solution prepared by diluting the eye drops with *ethanol (96%)* to contain 0.001% w/v of Levobunolol Hydrochloride exhibits two maxima, at 223 nm and at 255 nm and a broad peak at 315 nm.

B. In the Assay, the retention time of the principal peak in the chromatogram obtained with solution (1) is the same as that of the peak in the chromatogram obtained with solution (2).

Acidity or alkalinity pH, 5.5 to 7.5, Appendix V L.

Related substances The nominal total amount of related substances determined by tests A and B below is not more than 1.0% of the stated content of Levobunolol Hydrochloride.

A. Carry out the method for *liquid chromatography*, Appendix III D, using 20 µl of the following solutions. For solution (1) dilute a suitable volume of the eye drops with the mobile phase to produce a solution containing 0.10% w/v of Levobunolol Hydrochloride. For solution (2) dilute 1 volume of solution (1) to 200 volumes with the mobile phase. Solution (3) contains 0.0010% w/v of *disodium edetate* in the mobile phase.

The chromatographic procedure described under Assay may be used.

In the chromatogram obtained with solution (1) the area of any *secondary peak* is not greater than the area of the principal peak in the chromatogram obtained with solution (2) (0.5%). Determine the sum of the areas of any *secondary peaks*. Disregard any peak corresponding to the principal peak in the chromatogram obtained with solution (3).

B. Carry out test A as described above but using a detection wavelength of 400 nm and injecting solution (1). The area of any peak with a retention time corresponding to that of the principal peak in the chromatogram obtained with solution (2) in test A is not greater than one fifth of the area of that peak (0.5%, assuming a response factor of 5). Calculate the nominal percentage content of this impurity from the area of the peak in the chromatogram obtained with solution (1) taking one fifth of the area of the peak in the chromatogram obtained with solution (2) in test A to be equivalent to 0.5%.

Assay Carry out the method for *liquid chromatography*, Appendix III D, using 20 µl of the following solutions. For solution (1) dilute a suitable volume of the eye drops with the mobile phase to produce a solution containing 0.005% w/v of Levobunolol Hydrochloride. Solution (2) contains 0.005% w/v of *levobunolol hydrochloride BPCRS* in the mobile phase.

The chromatographic procedure may be carried out using (a) a stainless steel column (30 cm × 3.9 mm) packed with *stationary phase C* (10 µm) (µBondapak is suitable), (b) as the mobile phase a mixture of 5 volumes of *glacial acetic acid*, 450 volumes of 0.005M *sodium heptanesulphonate* and 550 volumes of *methanol* with a flow rate of 1.5 ml per minute and (c) a detection wavelength of 254 nm.

Calculate the content of $C_{17}H_{25}NO_3$,HCl in the eye drops from the declared content of $C_{17}H_{25}NO_3$,HCl in *levobunolol hydrochloride BPCRS*.

Storage Levobunolol Eye Drops should be protected from light.

Levodopa Capsules

Definition Levodopa Capsules contain Levodopa.

The capsules comply with the requirements stated under Capsules and with the following requirements.

Content of levodopa, $C_9H_{11}NO_4$ 95.0 to 105.0% of the prescribed or stated amount.

Identification

A. Dissolve as completely as possible a quantity of the contents of the capsules containing 0.5 g of Levodopa in 25 ml of 1M *hydrochloric acid* and filter. Adjust to pH 3 with 5M *ammonia*, added dropwise with stirring, and allow to stand for several hours, protected from light. Filter, wash the precipitate and dry it at 105°. The *infrared absorption spectrum* of the residue, Appendix II A, is concordant with the *reference spectrum* of levodopa.

B. Carry out the method for *thin-layer chromatography*, Appendix III A, using *microcrystalline cellulose* as the coating substance and a mixture of 25 volumes of *glacial acetic acid*, 25 volumes of *water* and 50 volumes of *butan-1-ol* as the mobile phase. Apply separately to the plate 5 µl of each of the following solutions. For solution (1) shake a quantity of the contents of the capsules containing 0.1 g of Levodopa with 10 ml of 1M *hydrochloric acid* and filter. Solution (2) contains 1% w/v of *levodopa EPCRS* in 1M *hydrochloric acid*. After removal of the plate, dry it in a current of warm air and spray with a freshly prepared mixture of equal volumes of a 10% w/v solution of *iron(III) chloride hexahydrate* and a 5% w/v solution of *potassium hexacyanoferrate(III)*. The principal spot in the chromatogram obtained with solution (1) corresponds to that in the chromatogram obtained with solution (2).

C. Shake a quantity of the contents of the capsules containing 20 mg of Levodopa with 5 ml of 0.1M *hydrochloric acid*. Add 0.1 ml of *iron(III) chloride solution R1*; a green colour is produced. To half of the solution add an excess of 5M *ammonia*; a purple colour is produced. To the remainder of the solution add an excess of 5M *sodium hydroxide*; a red colour is produced.

Dissolution Comply with the *dissolution test for tablets and capsules*, Appendix XII D, using Apparatus II. Use as the medium 900 ml of 0.1M *hydrochloric acid* and rotate the paddle at 50 revolutions per minute. Withdraw a sample of 10 ml of the medium. For capsules containing 0.25 g of Levodopa or less, filter and dilute 2 ml of the filtrate to 10 ml with 0.1M *hydrochloric acid*. For capsules containing more than 0.25 g of Levodopa, filter and dilute 1 ml of the filtrate to 10 ml with 0.1M *hydrochloric acid*. Measure the *absorbance* of the solution, Appendix II B, at 280 nm using 0.1M *hydrochloric acid* in the reference cell. Calculate the total content of $C_9H_{11}NO_4$ in the medium taking 142 as the value of A(1%, 1 cm) at the maximum at 280 nm.

Specific optical rotation −38.5° to −41.5°, Appendix V F, when determined in the following manner. Shake a quantity of the contents of the capsules containing 1.25 g of Levodopa with 25 ml of 0.5M *hydrochloric acid* for 30 minutes, centrifuge and filter the supernatant liquid (Whatman No. 42 filter paper is suitable). To 10 ml of the filtrate add 10 ml of a 21.5% w/v solution of *aluminium sulphate*, 20 ml of a 21.8% w/v solution of *sodium acetate* and sufficient *water* to produce 50 ml and measure the *optical rotation*. Separately dilute 5 ml of the filtrate to 200 ml with 0.1M *hydrochloric acid*, mix well and dilute 10 ml to 200 ml with 0.1M *hydrochloric acid*. Measure the *absorbance* of the resulting solution at the maximum at 280 nm, Appendix II B. Calculate the content of levodopa, $C_9H_{11}NO_4$, in the filtrate taking 142 as the value of A(1%, 1 cm) at the maximum at 280 nm and hence calculate the *specific optical rotation*.

Related substances Carry out the method for *thin-layer chromatography*, Appendix III A, using *cellulose* as the coating substance and a mixture of 25 volumes of *glacial acetic acid*, 25 volumes of *water* and 50 volumes of *butan-1-ol* as the mobile phase. Apply separately to the plate, as bands 20 mm long, 10 µl of each of solutions (1) and (2) and 20 µl of solution (3) and dry in a current of air. For solution (1) shake a quantity of the contents of the capsules containing 0.1 g of Levodopa with 10 ml of a mixture of equal volumes of *anhydrous formic acid* and *methanol*; prepare immediately before use. For solution (2) dilute 1 volume of solution (1) to 200 volumes with *methanol*. Solution (3) is a mixture of equal volumes of solution (1) and a solution prepared by dissolving 30 mg of *L-tyrosine* in 1 ml of *anhydrous formic acid* and diluting to 100 ml with *methanol*. After removal of the plate, dry it in a current of warm air, spray with a freshly prepared mixture of equal volumes of a 10% w/v solution of *iron(III) chloride hexahydrate* and a 5% w/v solution of *potassium hexacyanoferrate(III)* and examine the plate immediately. Any *secondary band* in the chromatogram obtained with solution (1) is not more intense than the band in the chromatogram obtained with solution (2) (0.5%). The test is not valid unless the chromatogram obtained with solution (3) shows a distinct band, at a higher Rf value than the principal band, which is more intense than the band in the chromatogram obtained with solution (2).

Assay Dissolve as completely as possible a quantity of the mixed contents of 20 capsules containing 0.6 g of Levodopa in 10 ml of *anhydrous formic acid*, add 80 ml of *glacial acetic acid* and carry out Method I for *non-aqueous titration*, Appendix VIII A, using *oracet blue B solution* as indicator. Each ml of 0.1M *perchloric acid VS* is equivalent to 19.72 mg of $C_9H_{11}NO_4$.

When L-dopa capsules are prescribed or demanded, Levodopa Capsules shall be dispensed or supplied.

Levodopa Tablets

Definition Levodopa Tablets contain Levodopa.

The tablets comply with the requirements stated under Tablets and with the following requirements.

Content of levodopa, $C_9H_{11}NO_4$ 95.0 to 105.0% of the prescribed or stated amount.

Identification

A. Dissolve as completely as possible a quantity of the powdered tablets containing 0.5 g of Levodopa in 25 ml of 1M *hydrochloric acid* and filter. Adjust to pH 3 with 5M *ammonia*, added dropwise with stirring, and allow to stand for several hours, protected from light. Filter, wash the precipitate with *water* and dry it at 105°. The *infrared absorption spectrum* of the residue, Appendix II A, is concordant with the *reference spectrum* of levodopa.

B. Comply with test B for Identification described under Levodopa Capsules, but using as solution (1) a solution obtained by shaking a quantity of the powdered tablets containing 0.1 g of Levodopa with 10 ml of 1M *hydrochloric acid* and filtering.

C. Shake a quantity of the powdered tablets containing 20 mg of Levodopa with 5 ml of 0.1M *hydrochloric acid.* Add 0.1 ml of *iron(III) chloride solution R1*; a green colour is produced. To half of the solution add an excess of 5M *ammonia*; a purple colour is produced. To the remainder of the solution add an excess of 5M *sodium hydroxide*; a red colour is produced.

Specific optical rotation −38.5° to −41.5°, Appendix V F, when determined in the following manner. Shake a quantity of the finely powdered tablets containing 1.25 g of Levodopa with 25 ml of 0.5M *hydrochloric acid* for 30 minutes, centrifuge and filter the supernatant liquid (Whatman No. 42 filter paper is suitable). To 10 ml of the filtrate add 10 ml of a 21.5% w/v solution of *aluminium sulphate*, 20 ml of a 21.8% w/v solution of *sodium acetate* and sufficient *water* to produce 50 ml and measure the *optical rotation*. Further dilute 5 ml of the filtrate to 200 ml with 0.1M *hydrochloric acid*, mix well and dilute 10 ml to 200 ml with 0.1M *hydrochloric acid*. Measure the *absorbance* of the resulting solution at the maximum at 280 nm, Appendix II B. Calculate the concentration of levodopa, $C_9H_{11}NO_4$, in the filtrate taking 142 as the value of A(1%, 1 cm) at the maximum at 280 nm and hence calculate the *specific optical rotation*.

Related substances Comply with the test described under Levodopa Capsules using as solution (1) a solution prepared immediately before use by shaking a quantity of the powdered tablets containing 0.1 g of Levodopa with 10 ml of a mixture of equal volumes of *anhydrous formic acid* and *methanol*.

Assay Weigh and powder 20 tablets. Dissolve as completely as possible a quantity of the powder containing 0.6 g of Levodopa in 10 ml of *anhydrous formic acid*, add 80 ml of *anhydrous acetic acid* and carry out Method I for *non-aqueous titration*, Appendix VIII A, using *oracet blue B solution* as indicator. Each ml of 0.1M *perchloric acid VS* is equivalent to 19.72 mg of $C_9H_{11}NO_4$.

When L-dopa tablets are prescribed or demanded, Levodopa Tablets shall be dispensed or supplied.

Levonorgestrel and Ethinylestradiol Tablets

Definition Levonorgestrel and Ethinylestradiol Tablets contain Levonorgestrel and Ethinylestradiol. They are coated.

The tablets comply with the requirements stated under Tablets and with the following requirements. For Levonorgestrel and Ethinylestradiol Tablets presented in 21-day or 28-day calendar packs, apply the requirements separately to tablets of each combination of different proportions, by weight, of the active ingredients. Where applicable, disregard any tablets that contain no active ingredient (placebo tablets).

Content of levonorgestrel, $C_{21}H_{28}O_2$ 90.0 to 110.0% of the prescribed or stated amount.

Content of ethinylestradiol, $C_{20}H_{24}O_2$ 90.0 to 110.0% of the prescribed or stated amount.

Identification Carry out the method for *thin-layer chromatography*, Appendix III A, using *silica gel GF_{254}* as the coating substance and a mixture of 1 volume of *methanol* and 99 volumes of *chloroform* as the mobile phase. Apply separately to the plate 20 µl of each of the following solutions. For solution (1) extract 15 powdered tablets with 30 ml of *acetone*, filter, evaporate to dryness and dissolve the residue in 1 ml of *chloroform*. Solution (2) contains 0.075% w/v of *levonorgestrel BPCRS* in *chloroform*. Solution (3) contains 0.045% w/v of *ethinylestradiol BPCRS* in *chloroform*. Develop the chromatograms twice, drying the plates between developments. After removal of the plate, allow it to dry in air and examine under *ultraviolet light (254 nm)*. One of the principal spots in the chromatogram obtained with solution (1) corresponds to that in the chromatogram obtained with solution (2) and the other principal spot corresponds to that in the chromatogram obtained with solution (3). Spray the plate with a 2% w/v solution of *toluene-p-sulphonic acid* in *water* and heat at 110° for 10 minutes and examine under *ultraviolet light (365 nm)*. The spots corresponding to levonorgestrel and ethinylestradiol appear as blue spots.

Uniformity of content Comply with the requirements stated under Tablets using the following method of analysis. Carry out the method for *liquid chromatography*, Appendix III D, using the following solutions.

Prepare the following stock solutions using a mixture of 40 volumes of *water* and 60 volumes of *acetonitrile*. Solution A contains 0.0625% w/v of *levonorgestrel BPCRS*. Solution B contains 0.025% of *ethinylestradiol BPCRS*. Solution C contains 0.020% w/v of *2-hydroxybiphenyl* (internal standard). For solution D dilute solution C with sufficient of the solvent mixture to produce a solution containing 0.0010% of 2-hydroxybiphenyl.

For solution (1) mix the volumes of solutions A and B specified in the table with 5 ml of solution C and dilute to 100 ml with a mixture of 40 volumes of *water* and 60 volumes of *acetonitrile*. For solution (2) add 4 ml of solution D to one tablet, and heat at 60° in an ultrasonic bath for 25 minutes, shake and repeat the ultrasound treatment. Cool, centrifuge and use the clear supernatant liquid.

Content of		Volume of	
Levonorgestrel µg	Ethinyloestradiol µg	Solution A ml	Solution B ml
250	50	10.0	5.0
250	30	10.0	3.0
150	30	6.0	3.0
125	30	5.0	3.0
75	40	3.0	4.0
50	30	2.0	3.0

The chromatographic procedure may be carried out using (a) a stainless steel column (15 cm × 4.6 mm) packed with *stationary phase C* (5 µm) (Hypersil ODS is suitable), (b) a mixture of 49 volumes of *acetonitrile* and 51 volumes of *water* as the mobile phase with a flow rate of 1.5 ml per minute and (c) a detection wavelength of 215 nm.

Calculate the content of $C_{21}H_{28}O_2$ and of $C_{20}H_{24}O_2$ in each tablet using the declared content of $C_{21}H_{28}O_2$ in *levonorgestrel BPCRS* and the declared content of $C_{20}H_{24}O_2$ in *ethinylestradiol BPCRS*.

Assay For both levonorgestrel and ethinylestradiol use the average of the 10 individual results obtained in the test for Uniformity of content.

When levonorgestrel and ethinyloestradiol tablets are prescribed or demanded, Levonorgestrel and Ethinylestradiol Tablets shall be dispensed or supplied.

Levothyroxine Tablets

Definition Levothyroxine Tablets contain Levothyroxine Sodium.

The tablets comply with the requirements stated under Tablets and with the following requirements.

Content of anhydrous levothyroxine sodium, $C_{15}H_{10}I_4NNaO_4$ 90.0 to 110.0% of the prescribed or stated amount.

Identification

A. In the Assay, the retention time of the principal peak in the chromatogram obtained with solution (1) is the same as that of the peak in the chromatogram obtained with solution (2).

B. To a quantity of the powdered tablets containing the equivalent of 0.5 mg of anhydrous levothyroxine sodium add a mixture of 3 ml of *ethanol (50%)* and 0.2 ml of *hydrochloric acid*, boil gently for 30 seconds, cool, filter, add 0.1 ml of a 10% w/v solution of *sodium nitrite* and boil; a yellow colour is produced. Cool and make alkaline with 5M *ammonia*; the solution becomes orange.

Uniformity of content Comply with the requirements stated under Tablets using the following method of analysis. Carry out the method for *liquid chromatography*, Appendix III D, using the following solutions. For solution (1) add sufficient 0.05M *sodium hydroxide* to one tablet to produce a solution containing the equivalent of about 6 µg per ml of anhydrous levothyroxine sodium, mix with the aid of ultrasound until the tablet is fully dispersed, cool and shake for 2 minutes. Add sufficient 0.05M *sodium hydroxide* to produce a solution containing the equivalent of 0.0004% w/v of anhydrous levothyroxine sodium, filter through glass microfibre filter paper (Whatman GF/C is suitable) and use the filtrate. Solution (2) contains 0.0004% w/v of *levothyroxine sodium EPCRS* in 0.05M *sodium hydroxide*.

The chromatographic procedure may be carried out using (a) a stainless steel column (25 cm × 4.6 mm) packed with *nitrile silica gel for chromatography* (5 µm) (Nucleosil 5 CN is suitable), (b) a mixture of 5 volumes of *orthophosphoric acid*, 300 volumes of *acetonitrile* and 700 volumes of *water* as the mobile phase with a flow rate of 1 ml per minute and (c) a detection wavelength of 225 nm. Inject 20 µl of each solution.

Calculate the content of $C_{15}H_{10}I_4NNaO_4$ in each tablet using the declared content of $C_{15}H_{10}I_4NNaO_4$ in *levothyroxine sodium EPCRS*.

Assay Weigh and powder 20 tablets. Carry out the method for *liquid chromatography*, Appendix III D.

For tablets containing the equivalent of less than 50 µg of anhydrous levothyroxine sodium, use the following solutions. For solution (1) disperse with the aid of ultrasound for 10 minutes a quantity of the powdered tablets containing the equivalent of 50 µg of anhydrous levothyroxine sodium with 8 ml of a mixture of equal volumes of *methanol* and 0.1M *sodium hydroxide* (solvent A). Shake for 2 minutes, cool, add sufficient solvent A to produce 10 ml, mix, filter through glass microfibre filter paper (Whatman GF/C is suitable) and use the filtrate. Solution (2) contains 0.0005% w/v of *levothyroxine sodium EPCRS* in solvent A. Solution (3) contains 0.0005% w/v of *liothyronine sodium EPCRS* and 0.0005% w/v of *levothyroxine sodium EPCRS* in solvent A.

For tablets containing the equivalent of 50 µg of anhydrous levothyroxine sodium or more, use the following solutions. For solution (1) disperse with the aid of ultrasound for 10 minutes a quantity of the powdered tablets containing the equivalent of 0.1 mg of anhydrous levothyroxine sodium with 8 ml of a mixture of equal volumes of *methanol* and 0.1M *sodium hydroxide* (solvent A). Shake for 2 minutes, cool, add sufficient solvent A to produce 10 ml, mix, filter through glass microfibre filter paper (Whatman GF/C is suitable) and use the filtrate. Solution (2) contains 0.001% w/v of *levothyroxine sodium EPCRS* in solvent A. Solution (3) contains 0.0005% w/v of *liothyronine sodium EPCRS* and 0.0005% w/v of *levothyroxine sodium EPCRS* in solvent A.

The chromatographic procedure may be carried out using the conditions described under the test for Uniformity of content.

The assay is not valid unless the *resolution factor* between the two principal peaks in the chromatogram obtained with solution (3) is at least 4.

Calculate the content of $C_{15}H_{10}I_4NNaO_4$ in the tablets using peak areas and the declared content of $C_{15}H_{10}I_4NNaO_4$ in *levothyroxine sodium EPCRS*.

Storage Levothyroxine Tablets should be protected from light.

Labelling The quantity of active ingredient is stated in terms of the equivalent amount of anhydrous levothyroxine sodium.

When thyroxine tablets are prescribed or demanded, Levothyroxine Tablets shall be dispensed or supplied.

Lidocaine Gel

Definition Lidocaine Gel is a sterile solution of Lidocaine Hydrochloride in a suitable water-miscible basis.

The gel complies with the requirements stated under Topical Semi-solid Preparations and with the following requirements.

Content of anhydrous lidocaine hydrochloride, $C_{14}H_{22}N_2O,HCl$ 95.0 to 105.0% of the prescribed or stated amount.

Identification To a quantity of the gel containing the equivalent of 80 mg of anhydrous lidocaine hydrochloride add 4 ml of *hydrochloric acid* and heat on a water bath for 10 minutes. Allow to cool, transfer to a separating funnel with the aid of 20 ml of *water*, add 5M *sodium hydroxide* until precipitation is complete and extract with two 20-ml quantities of *chloroform*. Filter the chloroform extracts through *anhydrous sodium sulphate* and evaporate the filtrate to dryness on a water bath using a current of nitrogen. The residue complies with the following tests.

A. The *infrared absorption spectrum*, Appendix II A, is concordant with the *reference spectrum* of lidocaine.

B. Dissolve 20 mg in 1 ml of *ethanol (96%)*, add 0.5 ml of a 10% w/v solution of *cobalt(II) chloride* and 0.5 ml of 5M *sodium hydroxide* and shake for 2 minutes. A bluish green precipitate is produced.

C. Dissolve 40 mg in 5 ml of a 1% w/v solution of *cetrimide* and add 1 ml of 5M *sodium hydroxide* and 1 ml of *bromine water*. A yellow colour is produced.

2,6-Dimethylaniline Mix a quantity of the gel containing the equivalent of 15 mg of anhydrous lidocaine hydrochloride with sufficient *water* to produce 3 ml using a rotary vortex mixer. To 2 ml of the resulting solution add 1 ml of a freshly prepared 1% w/v solution of *4-dimethylaminobenzaldehyde* in *methanol*, mix thoroughly using a rotary vortex mixer, add 2 ml of *glacial acetic acid* and allow to stand for 10 minutes. The yellow colour produced is not more intense than that obtained using a mixture of 2 ml of a solution of *2,6-dimethylaniline* in *methanol* containing 2 µg per ml in place of the solution of the gel.

Sterility Complies with the *test for sterility*, Appendix XVI A.

Assay Disperse a quantity containing the equivalent of 10 mg of anhydrous lidocaine hydrochloride in 20 ml of *water*. Add 5 ml of *acetate buffer pH 2.8*, 120 ml of *chloroform* and 5 ml of *dimethyl yellow—oracet blue B solution* and titrate with 0.005M *dioctyl sodium sulphosuccinate VS*, swirling vigorously. Near the end point add the titrant dropwise and, after each addition, swirl vigorously, allow to separate and swirl gently for 5 seconds. The end point is indicated when the colour of the chloroform layer changes from green to pinkish grey. Repeat the operation without the preparation being examined. The difference between the titrations represents the amount of dioctyl sodium sulphosuccinate required. Each ml of 0.005M *dioctyl sodium sulphosuccinate VS* is equivalent to 1.354 mg of $C_{14}H_{22}N_2O,HCl$. Determine the *weight per ml* of the gel, Appendix V G, and calculate the percentage of $C_{14}H_{22}N_2O,HCl$, weight in volume.

Storage Lidocaine Gel should be stored in accordance with the manufacturer's instructions.

Labelling The label on the container states (1) the strength in terms of the equivalent amount of anhydrous lidocaine hydrochloride; (2) that any of the gel not used in a single application should be discarded.

When lignocaine gel is prescribed or demanded, Lidocaine Gel shall be dispensed or supplied.

Lidocaine and Chlorhexidine Gel

Definition Lidocaine and Chlorhexidine Gel is a sterile solution of Lidocaine Hydrochloride containing 0.25% v/v of Chlorhexidine Gluconate Solution in a suitable water-miscible basis.

The gel complies with the requirements stated under Topical Semi-solid Preparations and with the following requirements.

Content of anhydrous lidocaine hydrochloride, $C_{14}H_{22}N_2O,HCl$ 95.0 to 105.0% of the prescribed or stated amount.

Content of chlorhexidine gluconate solution 0.225 to 0.275% v/v.

Identification

A. Carry out the extraction procedure described under Lidocaine Gel. The residue complies with tests A and B described under Lidocaine Gel, except that in test B an orange colour is produced.

B. In the Assay for chlorhexidine gluconate solution, the chromatogram obtained with solution (2) shows a peak with the same retention time as the peak due to chlorhexidine acetate in the chromatogram obtained with solution (1).

Aromatic amines Mix a quantity of the gel containing the equivalent of 15 mg of anhydrous lidocaine hydrochloride with sufficient *water* to produce 3 ml using a rotary vortex mixer. To 2 ml of the resulting solution add 1 ml of a freshly prepared 1% w/v solution of *4-dimethylaminobenzaldehyde* in *methanol*, mix thoroughly using a rotary vortex mixer, add 2 ml of *glacial acetic acid* and allow to stand for 10 minutes. The yellow colour produced is not more intense than that obtained using 2 ml of a solution of *2,6-dimethylaniline* in *methanol* containing 2 µg per ml in place of the solution of the gel.

Sterility Complies with the *test for sterility*, Appendix XVI A.

Assay

For lidocaine hydrochloride Carry out the Assay described under Lidocaine Gel.

For chlorhexidine gluconate solution Carry out the method for *liquid chromatography*, Appendix III D, using the following solutions. For solution (1) add 5 ml of a 0.080% w/v solution of *diphenylamine* (internal standard) in the mobile phase to 5 ml of a 0.070% w/v solution of *chlorhexidine acetate BPCRS* in the mobile phase and dilute to 100 ml with the mobile phase. For solution (2) mix 10 g of the gel with sufficient of the mobile phase to produce 100 ml. Prepare solution (3) in the same manner as solution (2) but adding 5 ml of the internal standard solution before diluting to 100 ml.

The chromatographic procedure may be carried out using (a) a stainless steel column (20 cm × 4.6 mm) packed with *stationary phase C* (10 µm) (Nucleosil C18 is suitable), (b) as the mobile phase with a flow rate of 1.5 ml per minute 0.01M *sodium octanesulphonate* in *methanol (73%)* adjusted to pH 3.0 with *glacial acetic acid* and (c) a detection wavelength of 254 nm.

Calculate the content of $C_{22}H_{30}Cl_2N_{10},2C_6H_{12}O_7$ from the declared content of $C_{22}H_{30}Cl_2N_{10}$ in *chlorhexidine acetate BPCRS*. Each mg of $C_{22}H_{30}Cl_2N_{10}$ is equivalent to 1.775 mg of $C_{22}H_{30}Cl_2N_{10},2C_6H_{12}O_7$. Determine the *weight per ml* of the gel, Appendix V G, and express the result as the percentage volume in volume of Chlorhexidine Gluconate Solution, which contains 20% w/v of $C_{22}H_{30}Cl_2N_{10},2C_6H_{12}O_7$.

Storage Lidocaine and Chlorhexidine Gel should be stored in accordance with the manufacturer's instructions.

Labelling The label states (1) the strength with respect to Lidocaine Hydrochloride in terms of the equivalent amount of anhydrous lidocaine hydrochloride; (2) that any of the gel not used in a single application should be discarded.

When lignocaine and chlorhexidine gel is prescribed or demanded, Lidocaine and Chlorhexidine Gel shall be dispensed or supplied.

Lidocaine Injection

Definition Lidocaine Injection is a sterile solution of Lidocaine Hydrochloride in Water for Injections.

The injection complies with the requirements stated under Parenteral Preparations and with the following requirements.

Content of lidocaine hydrochloride, $C_{14}H_{22}N_2O,HCl,H_2O$ 95.0 to 105.0% of the prescribed or stated amount.

Identification

A. Make a volume containing 0.1 g of Lidocaine Hydrochloride alkaline with 5M *sodium hydroxide*, filter, wash the residue with *water*, dissolve it in 1 ml of *ethanol (96%)*, add 0.5 ml of a 10% w/v solution of *cobalt(II) chloride* and shake for 2 minutes. A bluish green precipitate is produced.

B. To a volume containing 0.1 g of Lidocaine Hydrochloride add 10 ml of *picric acid solution R1*. The *melting point* of the precipitate, after washing with *water* and drying at 105°, is about 229°, Appendix V A.

C. Yields the reactions characteristic of *chlorides*, Appendix VI.

2,6-Dimethylaniline To a volume of the injection containing 25 mg of Lidocaine Hydrochloride add *water* if necessary to produce 10 ml, add 2M *sodium hydroxide* until the solution is just alkaline and extract with three 5-ml quantities of *chloroform*. Dry the combined chloroform extracts over *anhydrous sodium sulphate*, filter, wash with a further 5 ml of *chloroform* and evaporate the filtrate to dryness at a pressure of 2 kPa. Dissolve the residue in 2 ml of *methanol*, add 1 ml of a 1% w/v solution of *4-dimethylaminobenzaldehyde* in *methanol* and 2 ml of *glacial acetic acid* and allow to stand at room temperature for 10 minutes. Any yellow colour produced is not more intense than the colour obtained by repeating the operation using 10 ml of a solution of *2,6-dimethylaniline* in *water* containing 1 µg per ml in place of the injection (400 ppm).

Assay Make a quantity containing 0.1 g of Lidocaine Hydrochloride alkaline with 2M *sodium hydroxide* and extract with three 20-ml quantities of *chloroform*, washing each extract with the same 10 ml of *water*. Filter the washed extracts through a filter paper moistened with *chloroform* and wash the filter with 10 ml of *chloroform*. Add the washings to the filtrate and carry out Method I for *non-aqueous titration*, Appendix VIII A, using 0.02M *perchloric acid VS* as titrant and *crystal violet solution* as indicator. Each ml of 0.02M *perchloric acid VS* is equivalent to 5.776 mg of $C_{14}H_{22}N_2O,HCl,H_2O$.

When lignocaine injection is prescribed or demanded, Lidocaine Injection shall be dispensed or supplied.

Lidocaine and Adrenaline Injection
Lidocaine and Epinephrine Injection

For the purposes of product labelling in the United Kingdom, the pair of names given above shall be used together (see Introduction, Changes in title).

Definition Lidocaine and Adrenaline Injection is a sterile solution of Lidocaine Hydrochloride and Adrenaline Acid Tartrate in Water for Injections.

The injection complies with the requirements stated under Parenteral Preparations and with the following requirements.

Content of lidocaine hydrochloride, $C_{14}H_{22}N_2O,HCl,H_2O$ 95.0 to 105.0% of the prescribed or stated amount.

Content of adrenaline, $C_9H_{13}NO_3$ 87.5 to 112.5% of the prescribed or stated amount.

Characteristics A colourless solution.

Identification

A. Carry out the method for *thin-layer chromatography*, Appendix III A, using a silica gel precoated plate (Merck silica gel G60 plates are suitable) and a mixture of 5 volumes of *methanol* and 95 volumes of *dichloromethane* as the mobile phase. Apply separately to the plate 5 µl of each of the following solutions. For solution (1) dilute a quantity of the injection, if necessary, with *water* to produce a solution containing 0.2% w/v of Lidocaine Hydrochloride. Solution (2) contains 0.2% w/v of *lidocaine hydrochloride BPCRS* in *water*. Solution (3) contains 0.2% w/v of *lidocaine hydrochloride BPCRS* and 0.2% w/v of *bupivacaine hydrochloride BPCRS* in *water*. After removal of the plate, dry it in a current of cold air, heat at 110° for 1 hour, place the hot plate in a tank of chlorine gas prepared by the addition of *hydrochloric acid* to a 5% w/v solution of *potassium permanganate* contained in a beaker placed in the tank and allow to stand for 2 minutes. Dry the plate in a current of cold air until an area of the plate below the line of application gives at most a very faint blue colour with a 0.5% w/v solution of *potassium iodide* in *starch mucilage*; avoid prolonged exposure to cold air. Spray the plate with a 0.5% w/v solution of *potassium iodide* in *starch mucilage*. The principal spot in the chromatogram obtained with solution (1) corresponds to that in the chromatogram obtained with solution (2). The test is not valid unless the chromatogram obtained with solution (3) shows two clearly separated principal spots.

B. In the Assay for adrenaline, the chromatogram obtained with solution (2) shows a peak with the same retention time as the principal peak in the chromatogram obtained with solution (1).

Acidity pH, 3.0 to 4.5, Appendix V L.

Assay

For lidocaine hydrochloride Carry out the assay described under Lidocaine Injection.

For adrenaline Prepare a solution by adding 8.0 g of *tetramethylammonium hydrogen sulphate*, 2.2 g of *sodium heptanesulphonate* and 2 ml of 0.1M *disodium edetate* to a mixture of 900 ml of *water* and 100 ml of *methanol*, adjust the pH to 3.5 using 1M *sodium hydroxide* and filter through glass microfibre paper under reduced pressure (solution A). Carry out the method for *liquid chromatography*, Appendix III D, using the following solutions. For solution (1) dilute 5 ml of a 0.001% w/v solution of *adrenaline acid tartrate BPCRS* to 10 ml with solution A. For solution (2) dilute the injection, if necessary, to contain 0.0005% w/v of adrenaline and dilute 5 ml of the resulting solution to 10 ml with solution A. For solution (3) mix 5 ml of solution (1) with 5 ml of a 0.001% w/v solution of *noradrenaline acid tartrate* in the mobile phase.

The chromatographic procedure may be carried out using (a) a stainless steel column (10 cm × 4.6 mm) packed with *stationary phase C* (5 µm) (Nucleosil C18 is

suitable), (b) as the mobile phase with a flow rate of 2 ml per minute a solution prepared by adding 4.0 g of *tetramethylammonium hydrogen sulphate*, 1.1 g of *sodium heptanesulphonate* and 2 ml of 0.1M *disodium edetate* to a mixture of 950 ml of *water* and 50 ml of *methanol* and adjusting the pH to 3.5 with 1M *sodium hydroxide* and (c) a detection wavelength of 205 nm.

The test is not valid unless the *resolution factor* between the two principal peaks in the chromatogram obtained with solution (3) is at least 2.0.

Calculate the content of $C_9H_{13}NO_3$ in the injection using the declared content of $C_9H_{13}NO_3$ in *adrenaline acid tartrate BPCRS*.

Storage Lidocaine and Adrenaline Injection should be protected from light.

Labelling The label states 'Lidocaine and Adrenaline Injection' and 'Lidocaine and Epinephrine Injection'.

The quantity of Adrenaline Acid Tartrate is stated in terms of the equivalent amount of adrenaline (epinephrine).

Sterile Lidocaine Solution

Definition Sterile Lidocaine Solution is a sterile *cutaneous solution*. It contains Lidocaine Hydrochloride in Purified Water.

The solution complies with the requirements stated under Liquids for Cutaneous Application and with the following requirements.

Content of lidocaine hydrochloride, $C_{14}H_{22}N_2O$, HCl,H_2O 95.0 to 105.0% of the prescribed or stated amount.

Identification

A. Make a volume containing 0.1 g of Lidocaine Hydrochloride alkaline with 5M *sodium hydroxide*, filter, wash the residue with *water*, dissolve it in 1 ml of *ethanol (96%)*, add 0.5 ml of a 10% w/v solution of *cobalt(II) chloride* and shake for 2 minutes. A bluish green precipitate is produced.

B. To a volume containing 0.1 g of Lidocaine Hydrochloride add 10 ml of *picric acid solution R1*. The *melting point* of the precipitate, after washing with *water* and drying at 105°, is about 229°, Appendix V A.

C. Yields the reactions characteristic of *chlorides*, Appendix VI.

2,6-Dimethylaniline Dilute the solution to contain 0.25% w/v of Lidocaine Hydrochloride. To 10 ml of this solution add 2M *sodium hydroxide* until the solution is just alkaline and extract with three 5-ml quantities of *chloroform*, dry the combined chloroform extracts over *anhydrous sodium sulphate*, filter, wash with a further 5 ml of *chloroform* and evaporate the filtrate to dryness at a pressure of 2 kPa. Dissolve the residue in 2 ml of *methanol*, add 1 ml of a 1% w/v solution of *4-dimethylaminobenzaldehyde* in *methanol* and 2 ml of *glacial acetic acid* and allow to stand at room temperature for 10 minutes. Any yellow colour produced is not more intense than the colour obtained by repeating the operation using 10 ml of a solution of *2,6-dimethylaniline* in *water* containing 1 µg per ml in place of the solution being examined (400 ppm).

Assay Make a quantity containing 0.1 g of Lidocaine Hydrochloride alkaline with 2M *sodium hydroxide* and extract with three 20-ml quantities of *chloroform*, washing each extract with the same 10 ml of *water*. Filter the washed extracts through a filter paper moistened with *chloroform* and wash the filter with 10 ml of *chloroform*. Add the washings to the filtrate and carry out Method I for *non-aqueous titration*, Appendix VIII A, using 0.02M *perchloric acid VS* as titrant and *crystal violet solution* as indicator. Each ml of 0.02M *perchloric acid VS* is equivalent to 5.776 mg of $C_{14}H_{22}N_2O,HCl,H_2O$.

Sterility Complies with the *test for sterility*, Appendix XVI A.

Labelling The label states (1) 'Sterile Lidocaine Solution'; (2) that the solution is not intended for injection; (3) that the solution should be used on one occasion only and that any remainder should be discarded; (4) the date after which the solution is not intended to be used; (5) the conditions under which it should be stored.

The label indicates the pharmaceutical form as 'cutaneous solution'.

When sterile lignocaine solution is prescribed or demanded, Sterile Lidocaine Solution shall be dispensed or supplied.

Lincomycin Capsules

Definition Lincomycin Capsules contain Lincomycin Hydrochloride.

The capsules comply with the requirements stated under Capsules and with the following requirements.

Content of lincomycin, $C_{18}H_{34}N_2O_6S$ 90.0 to 105.0% of the prescribed or stated amount.

Identification

A. Extract a quantity of the capsules contents containing 0.2 g of Lincomycin Hydrochloride with 5 ml of a mixture of 4 volumes of *chloroform* and 1 volume of *methanol*, filter and evaporate the filtrate. Dissolve the oily residue in 1 ml of *water*, add *acetone* until precipitation begins and add a further 20 ml of *acetone*. Filter the precipitate, wash with two 10-ml quantities of *acetone*, dissolve the residue in a little of the chloroform—methanol mixture, evaporate to dryness and dry at 60° at a pressure not exceeding 2 kPa for 4 hours. The *infrared absorption spectrum* of the dried precipitate, Appendix II A, is concordant with the *reference spectrum* of lincomycin hydrochloride.

B. In the Assay, the retention time of the principal peak derived from lincomycin hydrochloride relative to that of the internal standard in solution (3) is the same as the retention time of the principal peak derived from *lincomycin hydrochloride EPCRS* relative to that of the internal standard in solution (1).

Lincomycin B Examine solution (3) as described under the Assay but increasing the sensitivity by 8 to 10 times while recording the peak derived from lincomycin B, which is eluted immediately before that derived from lincomycin. The area of the peak derived from lincomycin B, when corrected for the sensitivity factor, is not more than 5% of the area of the peak derived from lincomycin.

Water The contents of the capsules contain not more than 7.0% w/w of water, Appendix IX C. Use 0.3 g.

Assay Carry out the method for *gas chromatography*, Appendix III B, using the following solutions. For solution (1) add 10 ml of a 0.8% w/w solution of *dotriacontane* (internal standard) in *chloroform* to 0.1 g of *lincomycin hydrochloride EPCRS*, dilute to 100 ml with a 2% w/v solution of *imidazole* in *chloroform* and shake to dissolve. Place 4 ml of the resulting solution in a 15-ml ground-glass-stoppered centrifuge tube, add 1 ml of a mixture of 99 volumes of N,O-*bis(trimethylsilyl)acetamide* and 1 volume of *trimethylchlorosilane* and swirl gently. Loosen the glass stopper and heat at 65° for 30 minutes. Prepare solution (2) in the same manner as solution (1) but omitting the internal standard and using a quantity of the mixed contents of 20 capsules containing the equivalent of 90 mg of lincomycin in place of the *lincomycin hydrochloride EPCRS*. Prepare solution (3) in the same manner as solution (1) but using a quantity of the mixed contents of 20 capsules containing the equivalent of 90 mg of lincomycin in place of the *lincomycin hydrochloride EPCRS*.

The chromatographic procedure may be carried out using a glass column (1.5 m × 3 mm) packed with *acid-washed silanised diatomaceous support* impregnated with 3% w/w of phenyl methyl silicone fluid (50% phenyl) (OV-17 is suitable) and maintained at 260° with both the inlet port and the detector at 260° to 290° and using *helium* as the carrier gas with a flow rate of about 45 ml per minute.

Labelling The quantity of active ingredient is stated in terms of the equivalent amount of lincomycin.

Lincomycin Injection

Definition Lincomycin Injection is a sterile solution of Lincomycin Hydrochloride in Water for Injections.

The injection complies with the requirements stated under Parenteral Preparations and with the following requirements.

Content of lincomycin, $C_{18}H_{34}N_2O_6S$ 92.5 to 107.5% of the prescribed or stated amount.

Characteristics A colourless or almost colourless solution.

Identification

A. Add *acetone* to a volume of the injection containing 0.2 g of Lincomycin Hydrochloride until precipitation begins and add a further 20 ml of *acetone*. Filter the precipitate, wash with two 10-ml quantities of *acetone*, dissolve the residue in the minimum of a mixture of 4 volumes of *chloroform* and 1 volume of *methanol*, evaporate to dryness and dry at 60° at a pressure not exceeding 2 kPa for 4 hours. The *infrared absorption spectrum* of the dried precipitate, Appendix II A, is concordant with the *reference spectrum* of lincomycin hydrochloride.

B. In the Assay the retention time of the principal peak derived from lincomycin hydrochloride relative to that of the internal standard in solution (3) is the same as the retention time of the principal peak derived from *lincomycin hydrochloride EPCRS* relative to that of the internal standard in solution (1).

Acidity pH, 3.0 to 5.5, Appendix V L.

Lincomycin B Examine solution (3) as described under the Assay but increase the sensitivity by 8 to 10 times while recording the peak derived from lincomycin B, which is eluted immediately before that derived from lincomycin. The area of the peak derived from lincomycin B, when corrected for the sensitivity factor, is not more than 5% of the area of the peak derived from lincomycin.

Bacterial endotoxins Carry out the *test for bacterial endotoxins*, Appendix XIV C. Dilute the injection if necessary with *water BET* to give a solution containing the equivalent of 10 mg of lincomycin per ml (solution A). The endotoxin limit concentration of solution A is 5.0 Units per ml. Carry out the test using the maximum valid dilution of solution A calculated from the declared sensitivity of the lysate used in the test.

Assay Carry out the method for *gas chromatography*, Appendix III B, using the following solutions. For solution (1) add 10 ml of a 0.8% w/w solution of *dotriacontane* (internal standard) in *chloroform* to 0.1 g of *lincomycin hydrochloride EPCRS*, dilute to 100 ml with a 2% w/v solution of *imidazole* in *chloroform* and shake to dissolve. Place 4 ml of the resulting solution in a 15-ml ground-glass-stoppered centrifuge tube, add 1 ml of a mixture of 99 volumes of N,O-*bis(trimethylsilyl)acetamide* and 1 volume of *trimethylchlorosilane* and swirl gently. Loosen the glass stopper and heat at 65° for 30 minutes. Prepare solution (2) in the same manner as solution (1) but omitting the internal standard and using the residue obtained by evaporating to dryness 1 ml of a solution prepared by diluting a volume of the injection containing the equivalent of 0.9 g of lincomycin to 10 ml with *methanol* in place of the lincomycin hydrochloride EPCRS. Prepare solution (3) in the same manner as solution (1) but using the residue obtained by evaporating to dryness 1 ml of a solution prepared by diluting a volume of the injection containing the equivalent of 0.9 g of lincomycin to 10 ml with *methanol* in place of the lincomycin hydrochloride EPCRS.

The chromatographic procedure may be carried out using a glass column (1.5 m × 3 mm) packed with *acid-washed silanised diatomaceous support* impregnated with 3% w/w of phenyl methyl silicone fluid (50% phenyl) (OV-17 is suitable) and maintained at 260° with both the inlet port and the detector at 260° to 290° and using *helium* as the carrier gas with a flow rate of about 45 ml per minute.

Storage Lincomycin Injection should be protected from light and stored at a temperature not exceeding 30°.

Labelling The strength is stated as the equivalent amount of lincomycin in a suitable dose-volume.

Liothyronine Tablets

Definition Liothyronine Tablets contain Liothyronine Sodium.

The tablets comply with the requirements stated under Tablets and with the following requirements.

Content of liothyronine sodium, $C_{15}H_{11}I_3NNaO_4$ 90.0 to 110.0% of the prescribed or stated amount.

Identification In the Assay, the retention time of the principal peak in the chromatogram obtained with solution (1) is the same as that of the peak in the chromatogram obtained with solution (2).

Uniformity of content Comply with the requirements stated under Tablets using the following method of analysis. Carry out the method for *liquid chromatography*,

Appendix III D, using the following solutions. For solution (1) add sufficient 0.05M *sodium hydroxide* to one tablet to produce a solution containing about 6 µg per ml of Liothyronine Sodium, mix with the aid of ultrasound until the tablet is fully dispersed, cool and shake for 2 minutes. Add sufficient 0.05M *sodium hydroxide* to produce a solution containing 0.0004% w/v of Liothryonine Sodium, filter through glass microfibre filter paper (Whatman GF/C is suitable) and use the filtrate. Solution (2) contains 0.0004% w/v of *liothyronine sodium EPCRS* in 0.05M *sodium hydroxide*.

The chromatographic procedure may be carried out using (a) a stainless steel column (25 cm × 4.6 mm) packed with *nitrile silica gel for chromatography* (5 µm) (Nucleosil 5 CN is suitable), (b) a mixture of 5 volumes of *orthophosphoric acid*, 300 volumes of *acetonitrile* and 700 volumes of *water* as the mobile phase with a flow rate of 1 ml per minute and (c) a detection wavelength of 225 nm. Inject 20 µl of each solution.

Calculate the content of $C_{15}H_{11}I_3NNaO_4$ in each tablet using the declared content of $C_{15}H_{11}I_3NNaO_4$ in *liothyronine sodium EPCRS*.

Assay Weigh and powder 20 tablets. Carry out the method for *liquid chromatography*, Appendix III D, using the following solutions. For solution (1) disperse with the aid of ultrasound for 10 minutes a quantity of the powdered tablets containing 0.1 mg of Liothyronine Sodium with 8 ml of a mixture of equal volumes of *methanol* and 0.1M *sodium hydroxide* (solvent A). Shake for 2 minutes, cool, add sufficient solvent A to produce 10 ml, mix, filter through glass microfibre filter paper (Whatman GF/C is suitable) and use the filtrate. Solution (2) contains 0.001% w/v of *liothyronine sodium EPCRS* in solvent A. Solution (3) contains 0.0005% w/v of *liothyronine sodium EPCRS* and 0.0005% w/v of *levothyroxine sodium EPCRS* in solvent A.

The chromatographic procedure may be carried out using the conditions described under the test for Uniformity of content.

The assay is not valid unless the *resolution factor* between the two principal peaks in the chromatogram obtained with solution (3) is at least 4.

Calculate the content of $C_{15}H_{11}I_3NNaO_4$ in the tablets using peak areas and the declared content of $C_{15}H_{11}I_3NNaO_4$ in *liothyronine sodium EPCRS*.

Storage Liothyronine Tablets should be protected from light.

Liquorice Liquid Extract

Definition Liquorice Liquid Extract is prepared by extracting Liquorice with Purified Water and adding sufficient Ethanol (90 per cent) to give an ethanol content of 18% v/v in the final extract.

Extemporaneous preparation The following formula and directions apply.

Liquorice, unpeeled, in *coarse powder*	1000 g
Purified Water	a sufficient quantity
Ethanol (90 per cent)	a sufficient quantity

Exhaust the Liquorice with Purified Water by *percolation*, Appendix XI F. Boil the percolate for 5 minutes and set aside for not less than 12 hours. Decant the clear liquid, filter the remainder, mix the two liquids and evaporate until the *weight per ml* of the liquid is 1.198 g, Appendix V G. Add to this liquid, when cold, one quarter of its volume of Ethanol (90 per cent). Allow to stand for not less than 4 weeks; filter.

The extract complies with the requirements stated under Extracts and with the following requirements.

Identification Carry out the method for *thin-layer chromatography*, Appendix III A, using a suspension of *silica gel GF_{254}* in a 0.25% v/v solution of *orthophosphoric acid* to prepare the plate and a mixture of 5 volumes of *methanol* and 95 volumes of *chloroform* as the mobile phase. Apply separately to the plate 10 µl of solution (1) and 5 µl of solution (2). For solution (1) extract 5 ml of the liquid extract with 20 ml of *chloroform*. Heat 2.5 ml of the aqueous layer with 30 ml of 0.5M *sulphuric acid* under a reflux condenser for 1 hour, cool and extract with two 20-ml quantities of *chloroform*. Dry the combined chloroform extracts over *anhydrous sodium sulphate*, filter and evaporate the filtrate to dryness; dissolve the residue in 4 ml of a mixture of equal volumes of *chloroform* and *methanol*. For solution (2) dissolve 10 mg of *glycyrrhetinic acid* in 2 ml of a mixture of equal volumes of *chloroform* and *methanol*. After removal of the plate, examine it under *ultraviolet light (254 nm)*. The chromatogram obtained with solution (1) exhibits a dark spot corresponding to the principal spot in the chromatogram obtained with solution (2).

Ethanol content 16 to 20% v/v, Appendix VIII F, Method III.

Ammonia Place 5 ml in a distillation apparatus of about 500 ml capacity fitted with an efficient splash-head and a delivery tube that dips below the surface of a mixture of 10 ml of 0.05M *sulphuric acid VS* and 50 ml of *water* contained in the receiver. Add 200 ml of *water*, a little *pumice powder* and 30 ml of a solution prepared by dissolving 1.43 g of *potassium dihydrogen orthophosphate* and 9.1 g of *dipotassium hydrogen orthophosphate* in 100 ml of *water* and distil until about 175 ml of distillate has been collected. Titrate the excess of acid with 0.1M *sodium hydroxide VS* using *methyl red solution* as indicator. Not less than 5 ml of 0.1M *sodium hydroxide VS* is required.

Dry residue 40 to 45% w/v.

Relative density 1.125 to 1.140, Appendix V G.

Lithium Carbonate Tablets

Definition Lithium Carbonate Tablets contain Lithium Carbonate.

The tablets comply with the requirements stated under Tablets and with the following requirements.

Content of lithium carbonate, Li_2CO_3 95.0 to 105.0% of the prescribed or stated amount.

Identification A small quantity of the powdered tablets, when moistened with *hydrochloric acid* and introduced on a platinum wire into a flame, imparts a carmine red colour to the flame.

Assay Weigh and powder 20 tablets. Add a quantity of the powder containing 1 g of Lithium Carbonate to 100 ml of *water*, add 50 ml of 1M *hydrochloric acid VS* and boil for 1 minute to remove the carbon dioxide. Cool and titrate the excess of acid with 1M *sodium hydroxide VS* using *methyl orange solution* as indicator. Each ml of 1M *hydrochloric acid VS* is equivalent to 36.95 mg of Li_2CO_3.

Slow Lithium Carbonate Tablets

Definition Slow Lithium Carbonate Tablets contain Lithium Carbonate and are formulated so as to release the medicament over a period of several hours.

Production A suitable dissolution test is carried out to demonstrate the appropriate release of lithium carbonate. The dissolution profile reflects the *in vivo* performance which in turn is compatible with the dosage schedule recommended by the manufacturer.

With the exception of the requirements for shape, the tablets comply with the requirements stated under Tablets and with the following requirements.

Content of lithium carbonate, Li_2CO_3 95.0 to 105.0% of the prescribed or stated amount.

Identification A small quantity of the powdered tablets, when moistened with *hydrochloric acid* and introduced on a platinum wire into a flame, imparts a carmine red colour to the flame.

Assay Weigh and powder 20 tablets. Add a quantity of the powder containing 1 g of Lithium Carbonate to 100 ml of *water*, add 50 ml of 1M *hydrochloric acid VS* and boil for 1 minute to remove the carbon dioxide. Cool and titrate the excess of acid with 1M *sodium hydroxide VS* using *methyl orange solution* as indicator. Each ml of 1M *hydrochloric acid VS* is equivalent to 36.95 mg of Li_2CO_3.

Lomustine Capsules

Definition Lomustine Capsules contain Lomustine.

The capsules comply with the requirements stated under Capsules and with the following requirements.

Content of lomustine, $C_9H_{16}ClN_3O_2$ 90.0 to 110.0% of the prescribed or stated amount.

Identification Carry out the following procedure in subdued light. Shake a quantity of the contents of the capsules containing 0.2 g of Lomustine with 10 ml of *methanol*, filter and evaporate the filtrate to dryness using a rotary evaporator on a water bath maintained at not more than 60°. The residue, after drying at 60° at a pressure not exceeding 0.7 kPa for 30 minutes, complies with the following tests.

A. The *infrared absorption spectrum*, Appendix II A, is concordant with the *reference spectrum* of lomustine.

B. *Melting point*, about 88°, Appendix V A.

Related substances

A. Examine by *thin-layer chromatography*, Appendix III A, using *silica gel G* as the coating substance and a mixture of 20 volumes of *glacial acetic acid* and 80 volumes of *toluene* as the mobile phase. Apply separately to the plate 5 µl of each of the following solutions. For solution (1) shake a quantity of the contents of the capsules containing 0.20 g of Lomustine with 10 ml of *methanol* and filter. For solution (2) dilute 1 volume of solution (1) to 25 volumes with *methanol*. For solution (3) dilute 1 volume of solution (2) with 1 volume of *methanol*. For solution (4) dilute 1 volume of solution (2) to 10 volumes with *methanol*. For solution (5) dilute 1 volume of solution (2) to 20 volumes with *methanol*. For solution (6) dissolve 10 mg of *lomustine EPCRS* and 10 mg of *1,3-dicyclohexylurea* in *methanol* and dilute to 10 ml with the same solvent. After removal of the plate, dry it at 110° for 1 hour. At the bottom of a chromatography tank, place an evaporating dish containing a mixture of 1 volume of 7M *hydrochloric acid*, 1 volume of *water* and 2 volumes of a 1.5% w/v solution of *potassium permanganate*, close the tank and allow to stand for 15 minutes. Place the dried plate in the tank and close the tank. Leave the plate in contact with the chlorine vapour for 5 minutes. Withdraw the plate and place it in a current of cold air until the excess of chlorine is removed and an area of coating below the line of application does not give a blue colour with a drop of *potassium iodide and starch solution*. Spray with *potassium iodide and starch solution*. Any *secondary spot* in the chromatogram obtained with solution (1) is not more intense than the spot in the chromatogram obtained with solution (4) (0.4%) and at most one such spot is more intense than the spot in the chromatogram obtained with solution (5) (0.2%). The test is not valid unless the chromatogram obtained with solution (6) shows two clearly separated principal spots.

B. Examine by *liquid chromatography*, Appendix III D. For solution (1) shake a quantity of the contents of the capsules containing 0.20 g of Lomustine with 10 ml of *methanol* and filter. For solution (2) dilute 2 volumes of solution (2) to 100 volumes with *methanol*.

The chromatographic procedure may be carried out using (a) a stainless steel column (25 cm × 4 mm) packed with *stationary phase C* (5 to 10 µm) (Nucleosil C18 is suitable), (b) as mobile phase with a flow rate of 2 ml per minute a mixture of 50 volumes of *methanol* and 50 volumes of *water*, (c) a detection wavelength of 230 nm and (d) a loop injector.

Inject 20 µl of solution (1). When the chromatograms are recorded in the prescribed conditions, the retention time of lomustine is about 25 minutes. When using a recorder, adjust the sensitivity of the system so that the height of the principal peak in the chromatogram obtained with solution (1) is not less than 50% of the full scale of the recorder.

Inject separately 20 µl of each solution. In the chromatogram obtained with solution (1) the sum of the areas of any *secondary peaks* is not greater than the area of the principal peak in the chromatogram obtained with solution (2) (2%). Disregard any peak with an area less than 0.05 times that of the principal peak in the chromatogram obtained with solution (2) (0.1%).

Assay Carry out the following procedure in subdued light. Shake a quantity of the mixed contents of 20 capsules containing 40 mg of Lomustine with 70 ml of *ethanol (96%)* for 20 minutes, dilute to 100 ml with the same solvent and filter. Dilute 5 ml of the filtrate to 100 ml with *ethanol (96%)* and measure the *absorbance* of the resulting solution at the maximum at 230 nm, Appendix II B. Calculate the content of $C_9H_{16}ClN_3O_2$ taking 260 as the value of A(1%, 1 cm) at the maximum at 230 nm.

Loprazolam Tablets

Definition Loprazolam Tablets contain Loprazolam Mesilate.

The tablets comply with the requirements stated under Tablets and with the following requirements.

Content of loprazolam, $C_{23}H_{21}ClN_6O_3$ 90.0 to 110.0% of the prescribed or stated amount.

Identification

A. The *light absorption,* Appendix II B, in the range 210 to 370 nm of the filtrate obtained in the Assay exhibits a maximum at 330 nm and a shoulder at 240 nm.

B. Carry out the method for *thin-layer chromatography,* Appendix III A, using a silica gel F_{254} precoated plate (Merck silica gel 60 F_{254} plates are suitable) and a mixture of 80 volumes of *chloroform* and 20 volumes of *methanol* as the mobile phase. Apply separately to the plate 10 µl of each of the following solutions. For solution (1) shake a quantity of the powdered tablets containing the equivalent of 2 mg of loprazolam with 10 ml of a mixture of 46 volumes of *chloroform,* 46 volumes of *methanol* and 8 volumes of *water,* centrifuge and use the clear supernatant liquid. Solution (2) contains 0.02% w/v of *loprazolam mesilate BPCRS* in the same solvent mixture. After removal of the plate, allow it to dry in air and examine under *ultraviolet light (254 nm).* The principal spot in the chromatogram obtained with solution (1) corresponds to that in the chromatogram obtained with solution (2).

Related substances Complies with the test described under Loprazolam Mesilate, using 40 µl of each of the following solutions. For solution (1) shake a quantity of the powdered tablets containing the equivalent of 10 mg of loprazolam with 4 ml of a mixture of 46 volumes of *chloroform,* 46 volumes of *methanol* and 8 volumes of *water,* mix the suspension with the aid of ultrasound for 5 minutes, centrifuge and use the clear supernatant liquid. Solution (2) contains 0.00025% w/v of *loprazolam mesilate BPCRS* and solution (3) contains 0.00125% w/v of *6-(2-chlorophenyl)-2,4-dihydro-2-[(dimethylamino)methylene]-8-nitroimidazo[1,2-a][1,4]benzodiazepin-1-one BPCRS* (dimethylamino analogue), both in the same solvent mixture. Any spot corresponding to the dimethylamino analogue in the chromatogram obtained with solution (1) is not more intense than the spot in the chromatogram obtained with solution (3) and any other *secondary spot* is not more intense than the spot in the chromatogram obtained with solution (2).

Uniformity of content Tablets containing less than the equivalent of 2 mg of loprazolam comply with the requirements stated under Tablets using the following method of analysis. Shake one tablet with 8 ml of *water,* add 80 ml of *absolute ethanol,* mix with the aid of ultrasound for 10 minutes, cool and dilute to 200 ml with *absolute ethanol.* Mix, filter, discarding the first 20 ml of filtrate, and measure the *absorbance* of the resulting solution at the maximum at 330 nm, Appendix II B. Calculate the content of $C_{23}H_{21}ClN_6O_3$ taking 890 as the value of A(1%, 1 cm) at the maximum at 330 nm.

Assay Use the average of the 10 individual results obtained in the test for Uniformity of content.

Labelling The quantity of active ingredient is stated in terms of the equivalent amount of loprazolam.

Lorazepam Injection

Definition Lorazepam Injection is a sterile solution of Lorazepam in a suitable solvent.

The injection complies with the requirements stated under Parenteral Preparations and with the following requirements.

Content of lorazepam, $C_{15}H_{10}Cl_2N_2O_2$ 92.5 to 105.0% of the prescribed or stated amount.

Identification

A. Carry out the method for *thin-layer chromatography,* Appendix III A, using a silica gel precoated plate (Merck silica gel 60 plates are suitable) and *toluene* as the mobile phase. Apply separately to the plate 10 µl of each of the following solutions. For solution (1) add 5 ml of *hydrochloric acid* to a volume of the injection containing 10 mg of Lorazepam, heat in a water bath for 20 minutes and cool. Transfer the cooled solution to a separating funnel, add 8 ml of 10M *sodium hydroxide,* extract with two 25-ml quantities of *ether* and filter the combined extracts through absorbent cotton. Evaporate the filtrate to about 2 ml and dilute to 10 ml with *methanol.* For solution (2) add 5 ml of *hydrochloric acid* to 10 ml of a 0.1% w/v solution of *lorazepam BPCRS* in *absolute ethanol* and treat in the same manner as for solution (1) beginning at the words 'heat in a water bath ...'. After removal of the plate, allow it to dry and spray with a freshly prepared 1.25% w/v solution of *sodium nitrite* in 0.5M *hydrochloric acid.* Heat the plate at 100° for 5 minutes, allow to cool and spray with a 0.1% w/v solution of N-*(1-naphthyl)ethylenediamine dihydrochloride* in *absolute ethanol.* The principal spot in the chromatogram obtained with solution (1) corresponds to that in the chromatogram obtained with solution (2).

B. In the Assay, the principal peak in the chromatogram obtained with solution (2) has the same retention time as the principal peak in the chromatogram obtained with solution (1).

Related substances Carry out the method for *thin-layer chromatography,* Appendix III A, using a silica gel precoated plate (Merck silica gel 60 F_{254} plates are suitable) and a mixture of 100 volumes of *chloroform* and 10 volumes of *methanol* as the mobile phase. Before use, stand the plate in *methanol* and allow the solvent front to ascend 17 cm. Allow the plate to dry in air, heat it at 100° to 105° for 1 hour and use with the flow of mobile phase in the same direction as that used for the pretreatment. Apply separately to the plate 40 µl of each of the following solutions. For solution (1) add 10 ml of *water* to a volume of the injection containing 4 mg of Lorazepam, extract with two 10-ml quantities of *dichloromethane,* wash the combined extracts with 10 ml of *water* and evaporate the washed extract to dryness at 20° in a current of nitrogen. Dissolve the residue in 2 ml of *acetone.* Solution (2) contains 0.010% w/v of *6-chloro-4-(2-chlorophenyl)quinazoline-2-carboxaldehyde BPCRS* in *acetone.* For solution (3) dilute 1 volume of solution (1) to 100 volumes with *acetone.* For solution (4) dilute 1 volume of solution (1) to 200 volumes with *acetone.* Solution (5) contains 0.1% v/v of *benzyl alcohol* in *acetone.* After removal of the plate, allow it to dry in air and examine under *ultraviolet light (254 nm).* Any spot corresponding to 6-chloro-4-(2-chlorophenyl)-quinazoline-2-carboxaldehyde in the chromatogram obtained with solution (1) is not more intense than the spot in the chromatogram obtained with solution (2). Any other *secondary spot* in the chromatogram obtained with solution (1) is not more intense than the spot in the chromatogram obtained with solution (3) and not more than one such spot is more intense than the spot in the chromatogram obtained with solution (4). Disregard any spot with an Rf value similar to that of the spot in the chromatogram obtained with solution (5).

Assay Carry out the method for *liquid chromatography*, Appendix III D, using the following solutions. Solution (1) contains 0.008% w/v of *lorazepam BPCRS* in the mobile phase. For solution (2) dilute a suitable volume of the injection with sufficient mobile phase to produce a solution containing 0.008% w/v of Lorazepam.

The chromatographic procedure may be carried out using (a) a stainless steel column (12.5 cm × 4.6 mm) packed with *stationary phase C* (5 µm) (Hypersil ODS is suitable), (b) a mixture of 70 volumes of *methanol* and 30 volumes of *water* as the mobile phase with a flow rate of 1.5 ml per minute and (c) a detection wavelength of 254 nm.

Calculate the content of $C_{15}H_{10}Cl_2N_2O_2$ from the declared content of $C_{15}H_{10}Cl_2N_2O_2$ in *lorazepam BPCRS*.

Storage Lorazepam Injection should be protected from light and stored at a temperature of 2° to 8°.

Lorazepam Tablets

Definition Lorazepam Tablets contain Lorazepam.

The tablets comply with the requirements stated under Tablets and with the following requirements.

Content of lorazepam, $C_{15}H_{10}Cl_2N_2O_2$ 90.0 to 110.0% of the prescribed or stated amount.

Identification

A. The *light absorption*, Appendix II B, in the range 210 to 350 nm of the solution obtained in the Assay exhibits two maxima, at 230 nm and 316 nm.

B. Extract a quantity of the powdered tablets containing 20 mg of Lorazepam with 25 ml of *chloroform*, filter, evaporate to dryness and dry the residue at 60° at a pressure not exceeding 0.7 kPa. The *infrared absorption spectrum* of the residue, Appendix II A, is concordant with the *reference spectrum* of lorazepam.

C. Carry out the method for *thin-layer chromatography*, Appendix III A, using a silica gel precoated plate (Merck silica gel 60 plates are suitable) and *toluene* as the mobile phase. Apply separately to the plate 10 ml of each of the following solutions. For solution (1) shake a quantity of the powdered tablets containing 10 mg of Lorazepam with 10 ml of *acetone* for 20 minutes, filter and evaporate the filtrate to dryness. Dissolve the residue in 10 ml of *absolute ethanol*, add 5 ml of *hydrochloric acid*, heat on a water bath for 20 minutes and cool. Transfer the cooled solution to a separating funnel, add 8 ml of 10M *sodium hydroxide*, extract with two 25-ml quantities of *ether* and filter the combined extracts through absorbent cotton. Evaporate the filtrate to about 2 ml and dilute to 10 ml with *methanol*. For solution (2) treat 10 ml of a 0.1% w/v solution of *lorazepam BPCRS* in *absolute ethanol* in the same manner as described for solution (1) beginning at the words 'add 5 ml of *hydrochloric acid* ...'. After removal of the plate, allow it to dry and spray with a freshly prepared 1.25% w/v solution of *sodium nitrite* in 0.5M *hydrochloric acid*. Heat the plate at 100° for 5 minutes, allow to cool and spray with a 0.1% w/v solution of N-*(1-naphthyl)ethylenediamine dihydrochloride* in *absolute ethanol*. The principal spot in the chromatogram obtained with solution (1) corresponds to that in the chromatogram obtained with solution (2).

Related substances Carry out the method for *thin-layer chromatography*, Appendix III A, using a silica gel F_{254} precoated plate (Merck silica gel 60 F_{254} plates are suitable) and a mixture of 100 volumes of *chloroform* and 10 volumes of *methanol* as the mobile phase. Before use, stand the plate in *methanol*, allowing the solvent front to ascend 17 cm, heat the plate at 100° to 105° for 1 hour. Use with the flow of mobile phase in the same direction as that used for the prewash. Apply separately to the plate 40 µl of each of the following solutions. For solution (1) shake a quantity of powdered tablets containing 10 mg of Lorazepam with 4 ml of *acetone*, centrifuge and use the supernatant liquid. Solution (2) contains 0.0025% w/v of *6-chloro-4-(2-chlorophenyl)quinazoline-2-carboxaldehyde BPCRS* in *acetone*. For solution (3) dilute 1 volume of solution (1) to 100 volumes with *acetone*. For solution (4) dilute 1 volume of solution (1) to 200 volumes with *acetone*. After removal of the plate, allow it to dry in air and examine under *ultraviolet light (254 nm)*. Any spot corresponding to 6-chloro-4-(2-chlorophenyl)quinazoline-2-carboxaldehyde in the chromatogram obtained with solution (1) is not more intense than the spot in the chromatogram obtained with solution (2). Any other *secondary spot* in the chromatogram obtained with solution (1) is not more intense than the spot in the chromatogram obtained with solution (3) and not more than one such spot is more intense than the spot in the chromatogram obtained with solution (4).

Uniformity of content Tablets containing less than 2 mg of Lorazepam comply with the requirements stated under Tablets using the following method of analysis. Crush one tablet to a fine powder, add 40 ml of *ethanol (96%)* and shake for 1 hour. Add sufficient *ethanol (96%)* to produce 50 ml, centrifuge and dilute the supernatant liquid with sufficient *ethanol (96%)* to produce a solution containing 0.0005% w/v of Lorazepam. Measure the *absorbance* of the resulting solution at the maximum at 230 nm, Appendix II B, and calculate the content of $C_{15}H_{10}Cl_2N_2O_2$ taking 1150 as the value of A(1%, 1 cm) at the maximum at 230 nm.

Assay Weigh and powder 20 tablets. To a quantity of the powdered tablets containing 5 mg of Lorazepam add 40 ml of *ethanol (96%)* and shake for 1 hour. Add sufficient *ethanol (96%)* to produce 50 ml, centrifuge, dilute 5 ml to 100 ml with the same solvent and measure the *absorbance* of the resulting solution at the maximum at 230 nm, Appendix II B. Calculate the content of $C_{15}H_{10}Cl_2N_2O_2$ taking 1150 as the value of A(1%, 1 cm) at the maximum at 230 nm.

Storage Lorazepam Tablets should be protected from light and stored at a temperature not exceeding 25°.

Lormetazepam Tablets

Definition Lormetazepam Tablets contain Lormetazepam.

The tablets comply with the requirements stated under Tablets and with the following requirements.

Content of lormetazepam, $C_{16}H_{12}Cl_2N_2O_2$ 95.0 to 105.0% of the prescribed or stated amount.

Identification

A. Shake a quantity of the powdered tablets containing 10 mg of Lormetazepam with 5 ml of *acetone*, filter, wash the residue with a further 5 ml of *acetone*, combine the acetone extracts and evaporate to dryness on a water bath using a current of *nitrogen*. The *infrared absorption spectrum* of the dried residue, Appendix II A, is concordant with the *reference spectrum* of lormetazepam.

B. Carry out the method for *thin-layer chromatography*, Appendix III A, using *silica gel GF_{254}* as the coating substance and a mixture of 10 volumes of *chloroform* and 1 volume of *methanol* as the mobile phase. Apply separately to the plate 10 µl of each of the following solutions. For solution (1) shake a quantity of the powdered tablets containing 10 mg of Lormetazepam with 5 ml of *acetone* for 15 minutes and filter. Solution (2) contains 0.2% w/v of *lormetazepam BPCRS* in *acetone*. After removal of the plate, allow it to dry in air and examine under *ultraviolet light (254 nm)*. The principal spot in the chromatogram obtained with solution (1) corresponds to that in the chromatogram obtained with solution (2).

Related substances Carry out the method for *liquid chromatography*, Appendix III D, using the following solutions. For solution (1) dissolve a quantity of the powdered tablets containing 10 mg of Lormetazepam in 100 ml of *methanol (60%)*, centrifuge and use the clear supernatant liquid. Solution (2) contains 0.00010% w/v of *lormetazepam BPCRS* in *methanol*. Solution (3) contains 0.0010% w/v each of *lormetazepam BPCRS* and *lorazepam BPCRS* in *methanol*.

The chromatographic procedure may be carried out using (a) a column (20 cm × 4.6 mm) packed with *stationary phase C* (5 µm) (Hypersil ODS is suitable), (b) as the mobile phase with a flow rate of 2 ml per minute a mixture of 48 volumes of *methanol* and 52 volumes of a phosphate buffer prepared by dissolving 4.91 g of *sodium dihydrogen orthophosphate* and 0.633 g of *disodium hydrogen orthophosphate* in sufficient *water* to produce 1000 ml and (c) a detection wavelength of 230 nm.

The test is not valid unless the *resolution factor* between the two principal peaks in the chromatogram obtained with solution (3) is at least 4.

In the chromatogram obtained with solution (1) the area of any *secondary peak* is not greater than 0.5 times the area of the principal peak in the chromatogram obtained with solution (2) (0.5%) and the sum of the areas of any *secondary peaks* is not greater than the area of the peak in the chromatogram obtained with solution (2) (1%). Disregard any peaks with a retention time of less than half that of lormetazepam.

Uniformity of content Tablets containing less than 2 mg of Lormetazepam comply with the requirements stated under Tablets using the following method of analysis.

Carry out the method for *liquid chromatography*, Appendix III D, using the following solutions. For solution (1) add 3 ml of *water* to one tablet, allow to stand for 20 minutes with occasional shaking, mix with the aid of ultrasound for 2 minutes, add 35 ml of *methanol*, mix with the aid of ultrasound for 5 minutes and then shake for a further 15 minutes; cool and dilute with sufficient *methanol* to produce a solution containing 0.001% w/v of Lormetazepam, centrifuge for 10 minutes and use the clear supernatant liquid. Solution (2) contains 0.001% w/v of *lormetazepam BPCRS* in *methanol*.

The chromatographic conditions described under Related substances may be used.

Calculate the content of $C_{16}H_{12}Cl_2N_2O_2$ in each tablet using the declared content of $C_{16}H_{12}Cl_2N_2O_2$ in *lormetazepam BPCRS*.

Assay Weigh and powder 20 tablets. Carry out the method for *liquid chromatography*, Appendix III D, using the following solutions. For solution (1) disperse a quantity of the powdered tablets containing 10 mg of Lormetazepam in 500 ml of *methanol (60%)*, centrifuge for 15 minutes and use the clear supernatant liquid. Solution (2) contains 0.002% w/v of *lormetazepam BPCRS* in *methanol*.

The chromatographic conditions described under Related substances may be used.

Calculate the content of $C_{16}H_{12}Cl_2N_2O_2$ in the tablets from the declared content of $C_{16}H_{12}Cl_2N_2O_2$ in *lormetazepam BPCRS*.

Lymecycline Capsules

Definition Lymecycline Capsules contain Lymecycline.

The capsules comply with the requirements stated under Capsules and with the following requirements.

Identification The contents of the capsules comply with the following tests.

A. Carry out the method for *thin-layer chromatography*, Appendix III A, using *silica gel H* as the coating substance and a mixture of 6 volumes of *water*, 35 volumes of *methanol* and 59 volumes of *dichloromethane* as the mobile phase. Adjust the pH of a 10% w/v solution of *disodium edetate* to 8.0 with 10M *sodium hydroxide* and spray the solution evenly onto the plate (about 10 ml for a plate 100 mm × 200 mm). Allow the plate to dry in a horizontal position for at least 1 hour. Before use, dry the plate in an oven at 110° for 1 hour. Apply separately to the plate 1 µl of each of the following solutions. For solution (1) shake a quantity of the contents of the capsules containing 5 mg of Lymecycline with 10 ml of *methanol*, centrifuge and use the supernatant liquid. Solution (2) contains 0.05% w/v of *lymecycline BPCRS* in *methanol*. Solution (3) contains 0.05% w/v each of *tetracycline hydrochloride EPCRS*, *chlortetracycline hydrochloride EPCRS* and *doxycycline hyclate EPCRS* in *methanol*. After removal of the plate, allow it to dry in a current of air and examine under *ultraviolet light (365 nm)*. The principal spot in the chromatogram obtained with solution (1) is similar in position, colour and size to the principal spot in the chromatogram obtained with solution (2). The test is not valid unless the chromatogram obtained with solution (3) shows three clearly separated spots.

B. To 0.5 mg add 2 ml of *sulphuric acid*. A purplish red colour is produced.

C. Dissolve 50 mg in 5 ml of *water*, add 50 mg of *ninhydrin*, boil and add 15 ml of *water*. A bluish violet colour is produced.

D. Dissolve 0.2 g in 5 ml of *water*, add 0.3 ml of *orthophosphoric acid* and distil. To 1 ml of the distillate add 10 ml of *chromotropic acid solution*. A violet colour is produced.

Light-absorbing impurities Dissolve the contents of five capsules as completely as possible in sufficient 0.1M *hydrochloric acid* to produce a solution containing 0.15% w/v of Lymecycline and filter. The *absorbance* of the filtrate at 430 nm, when measured within 1 hour of preparing the solution, is not more than 0.60, calculated with reference to the anhydrous capsule contents, Appendix II B.

Water The contents of the capsules contain not more than 7.0% w/w of water, Appendix IX C. Use 0.3 g.

Assay To a quantity of the mixed contents of 20 capsules containing 0.3 g of Lymecycline add 500 ml of 0.05M *hydrochloric acid*, mix and carry out the *biological assay of antibiotics*, Appendix XIV A. The precision of the assay is such that the fiducial limits of error are not less than 95% and not more than 105% of the estimated potency.

Calculate the content of lymecycline in a capsule of average content weight taking each 1000 IU found to be equivalent to 1 mg of lymecycline. The upper fiducial limit of error is not less than 95.0% and the lower fiducial limit of error is not more than 110.0% of the prescribed or stated content.

204 mg of Lymecycline is equivalent to approximately 150 mg of tetracycline.

Lypressin Injection

Cys-Tyr-Phe-Gln-Asn-Cys-Pro-Lys-Gly-NH_2

Lypressin Injection complies with the requirements of the 3rd edition of the European Pharmacopoeia [0506]. These requirements are reproduced after the heading 'Definition' below.

Ph Eur

DEFINITION

Lypressin injection is a sterile solution in water for injections of the cyclic nonapeptide lypressin. It may contain a suitable buffer and a suitable antimicrobial preservative and may be made isotonic with blood by the addition of *Sodium chloride (193)*. It is distributed aseptically into sterile containers of glass type I (*3.2.1*) which are then sealed.

Lypressin injection complies with the monograph on *Parenteral preparations (520)*.

CHARACTERS

A clear, colourless liquid.

IDENTIFICATION

A. It causes a rise in arterial blood pressure when injected intravenously into an anaesthetised rat as prescribed in the assay.

B. When injected subcutaneously into a mammal at the same time as a volume of water is given orally, it delays the excretion of water.

TESTS

pH (*2.2.3*). The pH of the preparation to be examined is 3.7 to 4.3.

Amino acids Examine by means of an amino-acid analyser, using *DL-norleucine R* as the internal standard. Standardise the apparatus with a mixture containing equimolar amounts of ammonia, glycine and the L-form of the following amino acids:

Lysine	Serine	Methionine
Histidine	Glutamic acid	Isoleucine
Arginine	Proline	Leucine
Aspartic acid	Alanine	Tyrosine
Threonine	Valine	Phenylalanine

together with half the equimolar amount of L-cystine.

Internal standard solution. Dissolve 0.25 g of *DL-norleucine R* in a mixture of equal volumes of hydro*chloric acid R* and *water R* and dilute to 100.0 ml with the same mixture of solvents.

Test solution. Prepare a column about 10 mm in diameter using 5 ml of *weak cationic resin R*. Treat the resin with a 500 g/l solution of *glacial acetic acid R* and wash with *water R* until the eluate is neutral to methyl red. Pass through the column a quantity of the preparation to be examined equivalent to 1000 I.U. Pass through the column six quantities, each of 5 ml, of a 1 g/l solution of *glacial acetic acid R* to elute the non-peptide constituents. Pass through the column ten quantities, each of 5 ml, of a 500 g/l solution of *glacial acetic acid R* to elute lypressin. Combine these latter eluates, evaporate to dryness under reduced pressure at 30°C, add to the residue an accurately measured volume of the internal standard solution containing an amount of *DL-norleucine R* corresponding approximately to the expected number of moles of lypressin and transfer the solution to a rigorously cleaned hard-glass tube 100 mm long and 6 mm in internal diameter with the aid of four quantities, each of 0.3 ml, of a mixture of equal volumes of hydro*chloric acid R* and *water R*. Immerse the tube in a freezing mixture at –5°C, reduce the pressure to below 133 Pa and seal the tube. Heat at 110°C to 115°C for 16 h. Cool, open the tube, transfer the contents to a 10 ml flask with the aid of five quantities, each of 0.2 ml, of *water R* and evaporate to dryness over *potassium hydroxide R* under reduced pressure. Take up the residue in a suitable buffer solution (pH 2.2) and dilute to a suitable volume with the same buffer solution.

Apply to the amino-acid analyser a suitable, accurately measured volume of the test solution such that the peak given by the amino acid present in the largest amount occupies most of the available chart height. Express the content of each amino acid in moles. Calculate the relative proportions of the amino acids taking one-sixth of the sum of the number of moles of aspartic acid, glutamic acid, proline, glycine, phenylalanine and lysine as equal to one. The values fall within the following limits : aspartic acid 0.95 to 1.05; glutamic acid 0.95 to 1.05; proline 0.95 to 1.05; glycine 0.95 to 1.05; lysine 0.95 to 1.05; phenylalanine 0.95 to 1.05; tyrosine 0.7 to 1.05; half-cystine 1.4 to 2.1. Arginine, isoleucine and leucine are absent; not more than traces of other amino acids are present.

Peptide content The quantity of amino acids determined as prescribed in the test for amino acids corresponds to a content of 3.7 ± 0.4 µg of lypressin per International Unit of estimated pressor activity. The determination is not valid unless the number of moles of norleucine, corrected for the volume of test solution applied, is within ±5 per cent of the amount taken for hydrolysis.

ASSAY

The potency of the preparation to be examined is determined by comparing its blood pressor activity in the rat with that of the International Standard for lysine vasopressin or of a reference preparation of lysine vasopressin, calibrated in International Units.

The International Unit is the vasopressor activity contained in a specified quantity of the International Standard which consists of synthetic lysine vasopressin with albumin and citric acid. The equivalence in International Units of the International standard is stated by the World Health Organisation.

Inject slowly into the tail vein of a male albino rat weighing about 300 g a solution of a suitable α-adrenergic blocking agent, for example 10 ml per kilogram of body mass of a solution prepared by dissolving 5 mg of *phenoxybenzamine* hydro*chloride R* in 0.1 ml of *alcohol R* adding 0.05 ml of *1M* hydro*chloric acid* and diluting to 5 ml with a 9 g/l solution of *sodium chloride R*. After 18 h, anaesthetise the rat using an anaesthetic favourable to the maintenance of uniform blood pressure. After 45 min to 60 min, tie the rat on its back by its hind legs on an operating table. Introduce a cannula consisting of a short glass or polyethylene tube of 2.5 mm external diameter into the trachea and dissect a carotid artery ready for cannulation. Cannulate the femoral vein close to the inguinal ligament, retract the abdominal muscles to expose the inguinal ligament, retract the superficial pudendal vein to one side and dissect the femoral vein towards the inguinal ligament from the corresponding artery. When dissecting, locate and tie off a deep branch reaching the femoral vein to prevent bleeding during cannulation. Tie a short polyethylene cannula of about 1 mm external diameter into the femoral vein by two ligatures and join by a short piece of flexible tubing to a 1 ml burette with an attached thistle funnel containing a 9 g/l solution of *sodium chloride R* at about 37°C. Fix a wet cotton swab firmly to the thigh so as to cover the incision and cannula. At this stage, 200 I.U. of heparin per 100 g of body mass, dissolved in a 9 g/l solution of *sodium chloride R*, may be injected through the venous cannula. Tie in a carotid cannula, about 1 mm in external diameter, and connect it via a tube containing a 9 g/l solution of *sodium chloride R* to which heparin has been added, to a suitable pressure-measuring device such as a mercury manometer about 2 mm to 3 mm in internal diameter. Leave intact the central and peripheral nervous system, including both vagi and associated sympathetic nerves. No artificial respiration is necessary. Inject all solutions through the venous cannula using a 1 ml syringe graduated in 0.01 ml and after each injection inject 0.2 ml of the 9 g/l solution of *sodium chloride R* from the burette. Care should be taken that no air is injected.

Dilute the solution of the reference preparation and the preparation to be examined with a 9 g/l solution of *sodium chloride R* so that the volume to be injected is 0.1 ml to 0.5 ml. Choose two doses of the reference preparation such that the elevation of the blood pressure is about 4 kPa for the lower dose and about 6.67 kPa, but always submaximal, for the higher dose; the ratio of low to high dose is determined by the response and is usually three to five. As an initial approximation, doses of 3 milliunits and 5 milliunits may be tried. Choose two doses of the preparation to be examined such that responses as close as possible to those produced by the reference preparation are obtained and the ratio between the two doses is the same as for the reference preparation. Inject doses at intervals of 10 min to 15 min, the two doses of the reference preparation and the two doses of the preparation to be examined constituting one group of four doses and the order in which they are given being varied at random in successive groups to a total of four or five groups (i.e. sixteen to twenty injections in all). Record the maximum rise in blood pressure in response to each dose. Calculate the results of the assay by the usual statistical methods.

The estimated potency is not less than 90 per cent and not more than 111 per cent of the stated potency. The fiducial limits of error of the estimated potency ($P = 0.95$) are not less than 80 per cent and not more than 125 per cent of the stated potency.

STORAGE

Store at a temperature of 2°C to 15°C.

LABELLING

The label states:

— the potency in International Units per millilitre,
— the name and quantity of any added substance.

Ph Eur

Macrogol Ointment

Definition

Macrogol 4000	350 g
Macrogol 300	650 g

Extemporaneous preparation The following directions apply.

Add the Macrogol 4000 to the Macrogol 300, warm until homogeneous and stir continuously until cold.

The ointment complies with the requirements stated under Topical Semi-solid Preparations.

Magaldrate Oral Suspension

Definition Magaldrate Oral Suspension contains Magaldrate in a suitable flavoured vehicle.

The oral suspension complies with the requirements stated under Oral Liquids and with the following requirements.

Content of anhydrous magaldrate, $Al_5Mg_{10}(OH)_{31}(SO_4)_2$ 90.0 to 110.0% of the prescribed or stated amount.

Identification

A. Dissolve a quantity of the oral suspension containing the equivalent of 0.8 g of anhydrous magaldrate in 20 ml of 3M *hydrochloric acid*, add 30 ml of *water* and heat to boiling. Add 6M *ammonia* until a pH of 6.2 is obtained, continue boiling for a further 2 minutes, filter and retain the precipitate and the filtrate. To 2 ml of the filtrate add 2 ml of *ammonium chloride solution* and neutralise with a solution prepared by dissolving 2 g of *ammonium carbonate* and 2 ml of 6M *ammonia* in sufficient *water* to produce 20 ml; no precipitate is produced. Add *disodium hydrogen phosphate solution*; a white, crystalline precipitate is produced which is insoluble in 6M *ammonia*.

B. The precipitate retained in test A yields the reaction characteristic of *aluminium salts*, Appendix VI.

C. The filtrate obtained in test A yields the reactions characteristic of *sulphates*, Appendix VI.

Neutralising capacity Disperse a quantity containing the equivalent of 0.8 g of anhydrous magaldrate in 70 ml of water, heat to 37° and mix for 1 minute. Maintain the temperature at 37° and, while stirring continuously, add from a pipette 30 ml of 1M *hydrochloric acid VS*. Stir for 15 minutes and, over a period not exceeding 5 minutes, titrate the excess acid with 1M *sodium hydroxide VS* to a pH of 3.5 which is stable for a period of 10 to 15 seconds. Not more than 12 ml of 1M *sodium hydroxide VS* is required.

Magnesium hydroxide Not less than 49.2% and not more than 66.6% of the content of anhydrous magaldrate when determined by the following method. Mix a quantity of the oral suspension containing the equivalent of 1 g of magaldrate in 30 ml of 2M *hydrochloric acid* and add sufficient *water* to produce 100 ml (solution A). Dilute 10 ml of this solution to 200 ml with *water*. Add, while stirring, 1 g of *ammonium chloride*, 20 ml of *triethanolamine*, 10 ml of *ammonia buffer pH 10.9* and 0.4 ml of *mordant black 11 solution*. Titrate with 0.05M *disodium edetate VS* until a blue colour is obtained. Repeat the procedure without the substance being examined. The difference between the titrations represents the amount of disodium edetate required. Each ml of 0.05M *disodium edetate VS* is equivalent to 2.916 g of $Mg(OH)_2$.

Aluminium hydroxide Not less than 32.1% and not more than 45.9% of the stated content of anhydrous magaldrate when determined by the following method. Dilute 10 ml of solution A obtained in the test for Magnesium hydroxide with 20 ml of *water*. Add 25 ml of 0.05M *disodium edetate VS*, mix, allow to stand for 5 minutes and add 20 ml of *acetate buffer pH 4.4*, 60 ml of *ethanol (96%)* and 2 ml of a 0.026% w/v solution of *dithizone* in *ethanol (96%)*. Titrate with 0.05M *zinc sulphate VS* until a bright pink colour is obtained. Repeat the procedure without the substance being examined. The difference between the titrations represents the amount of disodium edetate required. Each ml of 0.05M *disodium edetate VS* is equivalent to 3.90 g of $Al(OH)_3$.

Microbial contamination Carry out a quantitative evaluation for Enterobacteriaceae and certain other Gram-negative bacteria, Appendix XVI B1. 0.01 ml of the preparation gives a negative result, Table 1 (most probable number of bacteria per gram fewer than 10^2).

Assay To a quantity of the oral suspension containing the equivalent of 3 g of anhydrous magaldrate add 100 ml of 1M *hydrochloric acid VS* and mix using a magnetic stirrer to achieve dissolution. Titrate the excess acid with 1M *sodium hydroxide VS* to pH 3, determined potentiometrically. Repeat the procedure without the preparation being examined. The difference between the titrations represents the amount of hydrochloric acid required. Each ml of 1M *hydrochloric acid VS* is equivalent to 35.40 mg of $Al_5Mg_{10}(OH)_{31}(SO_4)_2$.

Labelling The quantity of the active ingredient is stated in terms of the equivalent amount of anhydrous magaldrate.

Aromatic Magnesium Carbonate Mixture

Aromatic Magnesium Carbonate Oral Suspension

Definition Aromatic Magnesium Carbonate Mixture is an *oral suspension* containing 3% w/v of Light Magnesium Carbonate and 5% w/v of Sodium Bicarbonate in a suitable vehicle containing Aromatic Cardamom Tincture.

Extemporaneous preparation It is recently prepared according to the following formula.

Light Magnesium Carbonate	30 g
Sodium Bicarbonate	50 g
Aromatic Cardamom Tincture	30 ml
Double-strength Chloroform Water	500 ml
Water	sufficient to produce 1000 ml

The mixture complies with the requirements stated under Oral Liquids and with the following requirements.

Content of sodium bicarbonate, $NaHCO_3$ 4.7 to 5.3% w/v.

Content of magnesium, Mg 0.70 to 0.86% w/v.

Assay

For sodium bicarbonate Boil 10 g with 100 ml of *water* for 5 minutes, filter, boil the residue with 100 ml of *water* for 5 minutes and filter. Combine the filtrates, cool and titrate with 0.5M *hydrochloric acid VS* using *methyl orange–xylene cyanol FF solution* as indicator. Add 10 ml of *ammonia buffer pH 10.9* and titrate with 0.05M *disodium edetate VS* using *mordant black 11 solution* as indicator. After subtracting one fifth of the volume of 0.05M *disodium edetate VS*, each ml of 0.5M *hydrochloric acid VS* is equivalent to 42.00 mg of $NaHCO_3$. Determine the *weight per ml* of the mixture, Appendix V G, and calculate the percentage of $NaHCO_3$, weight in volume.

For magnesium Dissolve 30 g in the minimum quantity of 2M *hydrochloric acid* and dilute to 200 ml with *water*. To 20 ml of this solution add 200 ml of *water* and 10 ml of *ammonia buffer pH 10.9* and titrate with 0.05M *disodium edetate VS* using *mordant black 11 solution* as indicator. Each ml of 0.05M *disodium edetate VS* is equivalent to 1.215 mg of Mg. Use the *weight per ml* of the mixture to calculate the percentage of Mg, weight in volume.

Labelling The label indicates the pharmaceutical form as 'oral suspension'.

Magnesium Hydroxide Mixture

Magnesium Hydroxide Oral Suspension

Definition Magnesium Hydroxide Mixture is an aqueous *oral suspension* of hydrated magnesium oxide. It may be prepared from a suitable grade of Light Magnesium Oxide.

Extemporaneous preparation The following formula and directions apply.

Magnesium Sulphate	47.5 g
Sodium Hydroxide	15 g
Light Magnesium Oxide	52.5 g
Chloroform	2.5 ml
Purified Water, freshly boiled and cooled	sufficient to produce 1000 ml

Dissolve the Sodium Hydroxide in 150 ml of Purified Water, add the Light Magnesium Oxide, mix to form a smooth cream and then add sufficient Purified Water to produce 2500 ml. Pour this suspension in a thin stream into a solution of the Magnesium Sulphate in 2500 ml of Purified Water, stirring continuously during the mixing. Allow the precipitate to subside, remove the clear liquid, transfer the residue to a calico strainer, allow to drain and wash the precipitate with Purified Water until the washings give only a slight reaction for *sulphates*, Appendix VI. Mix the washed precipitate with Purified Water, dissolve the Chloroform in the mixture and add sufficient Purified Water to produce 1000 ml.

The mixture complies with the requirements stated under Oral Liquids and with the following requirements.

Content of hydrated magnesium oxide, calculated as $Mg(OH)_2$ 7.45 to 8.35% w/w.

Characteristics A white, uniform suspension which does not separate readily on standing.

Heavy metals Dissolve 12.5 g in 10 ml of *hydrochloric acid* and 20 ml of *water*, add 0.5 ml of *nitric acid*, boil to remove any carbon dioxide and filter. To the cooled filtrate add 2 g of *ammonium chloride* and 2 g of *ammonium thiocyanate* and extract with two successive 10-ml quantities of a mixture of equal volumes of *amyl alcohol* and *ether*. To the aqueous layer add 2 g of *citric acid* and sufficient *water* to produce 50 ml. 12 ml of the resulting solution complies with *limit test A for heavy metals*, Appendix VII. Use *lead standard solution (1 ppm Pb)* to prepare the standard (4 ppm).

Sulphate Dissolve 2.5 ml in 20 ml of *hydrochloric acid* and dilute to 500 ml with *water*. 15 ml of the solution, filtered if necessary, complies with the *limit test for sulphates*, Appendix VII (0.2%).

Assay Mix 10 g with 50 ml of *water*, add 50 ml of 0.5M *sulphuric acid VS* and titrate the excess of acid with 1M *sodium hydroxide VS* using *methyl orange solution* as indicator. Each ml of 0.5M *sulphuric acid VS* is equivalent to 29.16 mg of hydrated magnesium oxide calculated as $Mg(OH)_2$.

Storage Magnesium Hydroxide Mixture should not be kept in a cold place.

Labelling The label indicates the pharmaceutical form as 'oral suspension'.

Magnesium Sulphate Injection

Definition Magnesium Sulphate Injection is a sterile solution of Magnesium Sulphate in Water for Injections.

The injection complies with the requirements stated under Parenteral Preparations and with the following requirements.

Content of magnesium sulphate, $MgSO_4,7H_2O$ 95.0 to 105.0% of the prescribed or stated amount.

Characteristics A clear, colourless solution.

Identification Yields the reactions characteristic of *magnesium salts* and of *sulphates*, Appendix VI.

Acidity or alkalinity pH, 5.5 to 7.0, Appendix V L.

Assay Dilute a volume containing 1.25 g of Magnesium Sulphate to 100 ml with *water*. To 20 ml of this solution add 10 ml of *ammonia buffer pH 10.9* and titrate with 0.05M *disodium edetate VS* using 0.1 g of *mordant black 11 triturate* as indicator, until the pink tint is discharged from the blue colour. Each ml of 0.05M *disodium edetate VS* is equivalent to 12.32 mg of $MgSO_4,7H_2O$.

Labelling The strength is stated as the percentage w/v of Magnesium Sulphate.

Magnesium Sulphate Mixture

Magnesium Sulphate Oral Suspension

Definition Magnesium Sulphate Mixture is an *oral suspension* containing 40% w/v of Magnesium Sulphate and 5% w/v of Light Magnesium Carbonate in a suitable vehicle with a peppermint flavour.

Extemporaneous preparation It is recently prepared according to the following formula.

Magnesium Sulphate	400 g
Light Magnesium Carbonate	50 g
Concentrated Peppermint Emulsion	25 ml
Double-strength Chloroform Water	300 ml
Water	sufficient to produce 1000 ml

The mixture complies with the requirements stated under Oral Liquids and with the following requirements.

Content of magnesium sulphate, $MgSO_4,7H_2O$ 36.0 to 44.0% w/v.

Content of magnesium carbonate, calculated as Mg 1.14 to 1.49% w/v.

Identification

A. Filter 10 ml of the mixture and reserve the residue. The filtrate yields reaction A characteristic of *magnesium salts*, Appendix VI. Wash the residue with 10 ml of *water*, dissolve 25 mg in 1 ml of 1M *hydrochloric acid* and adjust the pH to 6 to 7 with 1M *sodium hydroxide*. The resulting solution yields reaction A characteristic of *magnesium salts*, Appendix VI.

B. The residue obtained in test A yields reaction A characteristic of *carbonates*, Appendix VI.

C. The filtrate obtained in test A yields reaction A characteristic of *sulphates*, Appendix VI.

Assay

For magnesium sulphate Boil 0.7 g with 50 ml of a mixture of equal volumes of *ethanol (96%)* and *water*, cool, filter and wash the residue with successive small quantities of the diluted ethanol until the washings are free from sulphate. Reserve the residue for the Assay for magnesium carbonate. To the combined filtrate and washings add 10 ml of *ammonia buffer pH 10.9* and titrate with 0.05M *disodium edetate VS* using *mordant black 11 solution* as indicator. Each ml of 0.05M *disodium edetate VS* is equivalent to 12.32 mg of $MgSO_4,7H_2O$. Determine the *weight per ml* of the mixture, Appendix V G, and calculate the percentage of $MgSO_4,7H_2O$, weight in volume.

For magnesium carbonate Dissolve the residue obtained in the Assay for magnesium sulphate in 10 ml of 1M *hydrochloric acid* and wash the filter with successive small quantities of *water* until the washings are free from chloride. To the combined filtrate and washings add 10 ml of *ammonia buffer pH 10.9* and titrate with 0.05M *disodium edetate VS* using *mordant black 11 solution* as indicator. Each ml of 0.05M *disodium edetate VS* is equivalent to 1.215 mg of Mg. Using the *weight per ml*, calculate the percentage of Mg, weight in volume.

Labelling The label indicates the pharmaceutical form as 'oral suspension'.

Magnesium Sulphate Paste

Morison's Paste

Definition

Dried Magnesium Sulphate	a sufficient quantity
Phenol	0.5 g
Glycerol, previously heated at 120° for 1 hour and cooled	55 g

Extemporaneous preparation The following directions apply.

Dry about 70 g of Dried Magnesium Sulphate at 150° for 1.5 hours or at 130° for 4 hours and allow to cool in a desiccator. Mix 45 g of the dried material in a warm mortar with the Phenol dissolved in the Glycerol.

In preparing larger quantities of the paste the period of heating the Dried Magnesium Sulphate should be increased, if necessary, to ensure that the dried material contains not less than 85% of magnesium sulphate, calculated as $MgSO_4$.

The paste complies with the requirements stated under Topical Semi-solid Preparations and with the following requirements.

Content of magnesium sulphate, $MgSO_4$ 36.0 to 41.0% w/w.

Content of phenol, C_6H_6O 0.45 to 0.55% w/w.

Assay

For magnesium sulphate Dissolve 5 g in sufficient *water* to produce 100 ml. To 10 ml of the resulting solution add 150 ml of *water* and 10 ml of *ammonia buffer pH 10.9* and titrate with 0.05M *disodium edetate VS*, using *mordant black 11 solution* as indicator, to a full blue colour. Each ml of 0.05M *disodium edetate VS* is equivalent to 6.018 mg of $MgSO_4$.

For phenol Dissolve 5 g in 25 ml of *water*, add 25 ml of 0.05M *bromine VS* and 5 ml of *hydrochloric acid*, stopper the flask, allow to stand for 30 minutes with occasional swirling and then allow to stand for a further 15 minutes. Add 5 ml of a 20% w/v solution of *potassium iodide*, shake thoroughly, titrate with 0.1M *sodium thiosulphate VS* until only a faint yellow colour remains, add 0.25 ml of *starch mucilage* and 10 ml of *chloroform* and complete the titration with vigorous shaking. Repeat the operation without the substance being examined. The difference between the titrations represents the amount of bromine required. Each ml of 0.05M *bromine VS* is equivalent to 1.569 mg of C_6H_6O.

Storage Magnesium Sulphate Paste should be kept in a well-closed container.

Labelling The label states that the Paste should be stirred before use.

Magnesium Trisilicate Mixture

Magnesium Trisilicate Oral Suspension; Compound Magnesium Trisilicate Mixture

Definition Magnesium Trisilicate Mixture is an *oral suspension* containing 5% w/v each of Magnesium Trisilicate, Light Magnesium Carbonate and Sodium Bicarbonate in a suitable vehicle with a peppermint flavour.

Extemporaneous preparation It is recently prepared according to the following formula.

Magnesium Trisilicate	50 g
Light Magnesium Carbonate	50 g
Sodium Bicarbonate	50 g
Concentrated Peppermint Emulsion	25 ml
Double-strength Chloroform Water	500 ml
Water	sufficient to produce 1000 ml

The mixture complies with the requirements stated under Oral Liquids and with the following requirements.

Content of magnesium, Mg 1.70 to 2.20% w/v.

Content of sodium bicarbonate, $NaHCO_3$ 4.60 to 5.40% w/v.

Identification

A. Filter 50 ml of the mixture using a Buchner funnel, reserving the filtrate, wash the filter with 50 ml of *water* and dry the residue at 100° to 105° for 1 hour. The filtrate yields reaction B characteristic of *sodium salts* and reaction A characteristic of *bicarbonates*, Appendix VI.

B. Shake 0.5 g of the residue obtained in test A with 5 ml of 1M *hydrochloric acid* for 5 minutes, add 5 ml of 1M *sodium hydroxide* and centrifuge. The supernatant liquid yields reaction B characteristic of *magnesium salts*, Appendix VI.

C. The residue obtained in test A yields reaction A characteristic of *carbonates*, Appendix VI.

D. 30 mg of the residue obtained in test A yields the reaction characteristic of *silicates*, Appendix VI.

Neutralising capacity To 5 g add 100 ml of *water* and heat to 37°. Add 100 ml of 0.1M *hydrochloric acid VS* previously heated to 37° and stir continuously using a suitable paddle stirrer rotating at a rate of about 200 revolutions per minute, maintaining the temperature at 37°. The pH of the suspension at 37° after 10 and 20 minutes is not less than 2.0 and not less than 2.4 respectively and at no time is it more than 4.0. Add 10 ml of 0.5M *hydrochloric acid VS* previously heated to 37°, stir continuously for 1 hour, maintaining the temperature at 37°, and titrate with 0.1M *sodium hydroxide VS* to pH 3.5. Subtract the volume of 0.1M *sodium hydroxide VS* from 150 to obtain the number of ml of 0.1M *hydrochloric acid VS* required for the neutralisation. Determine the *weight per ml* of the mixture, Appendix V G, and hence the volume of 0.1M *hydrochloric acid VS* required to neutralise 5 ml of the mixture. Not less than 100 ml of 0.1M *hydrochloric acid VS* is required.

Assay

For magnesium To 5 g add 7 ml of *hydrochloric acid* and 7 ml of *water*, stir and heat on a water bath for 15 minutes. Add 30 ml of hot *water*, mix, filter while still hot and wash the filter with hot *water*. Cool the combined filtrate and washings and dilute to 100 ml with *water*. To 25 ml of the resulting solution add 150 ml of *water* and 5 ml of *ammonia buffer pH 10.9* and titrate with 0.05M *disodium edetate VS* using *mordant black 11 solution* as indicator. Each ml of 0.05M *disodium edetate VS* is equivalent to 1.215 mg of Mg. Using the weight per ml of the mixture calculate the percentage of Mg, weight in volume.

For sodium bicarbonate Boil 20 g with 100 ml of *water* for 5 minutes, filter, boil the residue with 100 ml of *water* for 5 minutes and filter. Combine the filtrates, cool and titrate with 0.5M *hydrochloric acid VS* using *methyl orange—xylene cyanol FF solution* as indicator. Add 10 ml of *ammonia buffer pH 10.9* and titrate with 0.05M *disodium edetate VS* using *mordant black 11 solution* as indicator. After subtracting one fifth of the volume of 0.05M *disodium edetate VS*, each ml of 0.5M *hydrochloric acid VS* is equivalent to 42.00 mg of $NaHCO_3$. Using the weight per ml of the mixture calculate the percentage of $NaHCO_3$, weight in volume.

Labelling The label indicates the pharmaceutical form as 'oral suspension'.

Compound Magnesium Trisilicate Oral Powder

Definition

Magnesium Trisilicate	250 g
Chalk, *in powder*	250 g
Sodium Bicarbonate	250 g
Heavy Magnesium Carbonate	250 g

The oral powder complies with the requirements stated under Powders and with the following requirements.

Content of magnesium trisilicate, calculated as silica, SiO_2 11.0 to 15.2% w/w.

Content of sodium bicarbonate, $NaHCO_3$ 23.7 to 26.9% w/w.

Identification Shake 0.5 g with 5 ml of 2M *hydrochloric acid* and filter. The filtrate complies with the following tests.

A. To 0.05 ml add 0.2 ml of a 1% w/v solution of *glyoxal bis(2-hydroxyanil)* in *ethanol (96%)* and 0.05 ml of a 10% w/v solution of *sodium hydroxide*; a reddish brown precipitate is produced. Add *chloroform*; the precipitate dissolves to produce a red solution.

B. Add to the filtrate an excess of a 2.5% w/v solution of *ammonium oxalate*, filter and to the filtrate add 5M *sodium hydroxide* followed by *diphenylcarbazide solution*. A violet-red precipitate is produced.

Assay

For silica Mix 1.5 g with 5 ml of *water* and 10 ml of 9M *perchloric acid* in a beaker, heat until dense white fumes are evolved, cover the beaker with a watch glass, continue heating for a further 3 hours and allow to cool. Add 30 ml of *water*, filter, wash the filter with 200 ml of hot *water*, discard the filtrate and washings, dry the filter paper and its contents, ignite at 1000°, cool and weigh. To the residue add 0.25 ml of *sulphuric acid* followed by 15 ml of *hydrofluoric acid*, heat cautiously on a sand bath until all the acid has evaporated, ignite at 1000°, cool and weigh. Subtract the weight of any residue so obtained from the weight of the residue obtained above and calculate the content of SiO_2 from the corrected weight of residue.

For sodium bicarbonate Boil 2.5 g with 100 ml of *water* for 5 minutes, filter, boil the residue with 100 ml of *water* for 5 minutes and filter. Combine the filtrates, cool and titrate with 0.5M *hydrochloric acid VS* using *methyl orange—xylene cyanol FF solution* as indicator. Add 10 ml of *ammonia buffer pH 10.9* and titrate with 0.05M *disodium edetate VS* using *mordant black 11 solution* as indicator. After subtracting one fifth of the volume of 0.05M *disodium edetate VS*, each ml of 0.5M *hydrochloric acid VS* is equivalent to 42.00 mg of $NaHCO_3$.

Compound Magnesium Trisilicate Tablets

Aluminium Hydroxide and Magnesium Trisilicate Tablets

Definition Compound Magnesium Trisilicate Tablets contain, in each, 250 mg of Magnesium Trisilicate and 120 mg of Dried Aluminium Hydroxide. They have a peppermint flavour.

The tablets comply with the requirements stated under Tablets and with the following requirements.

Content of aluminium, Al 28 to 40 mg.

Content of magnesium, Mg 30 to 41 mg.

Disintegration The requirement for Disintegration does not apply to Compound Magnesium Trisilicate Tablets.

Neutralising capacity Weigh and powder 20 tablets. Pass the powder as completely as possible, regrinding if necessary, through a sieve of nominal mesh aperture about 75 µm and remix the sifted powder. Mix a quantity equivalent to two tablets with a small quantity of *water*, added slowly with stirring, to give a smooth paste and slowly add further quantities of *water*, with stirring, to a total volume of 100 ml. Warm to 37°, add 100 ml of 0.1M *hydrochloric acid VS* previously heated to 37° and stir continuously, using a suitable paddle stirrer at a rate of about 200 revolutions per minute, maintaining the temperature at 37°. The pH of the suspension at 37°, after 10, 15 and 20 minutes, is not less than 2.0, 2.4 and 2.7 respectively and at no time during this period is it more than 4.0. Add 10 ml of 0.5M *hydrochloric acid VS* previously heated to 37°, stir continuously for 1 hour maintaining the temperature at 37° and titrate with 0.1M *sodium hydroxide VS* to pH 3.5. Subtract the volume of 0.1M *sodium hydroxide VS* from 150 ml to obtain the number of ml of 0.1M *hydrochloric acid VS* required for the neutralisation. Not less than 50 ml of 0.1M *hydrochloric acid VS* is required to neutralise one tablet.

Assay

For aluminium Weigh and powder 20 tablets. To a quantity of the powder equivalent to two tablets add 7 ml of *hydrochloric acid* and 7 ml of *water*, stir and heat on a water bath for 15 minutes, stirring occasionally. Add 30 ml of hot *water*, mix and filter whilst hot, washing the filter well with hot *water*. Cool the combined filtrate and washings and dilute to 100 ml with *water*. Reserve 25 ml for the Assay for magnesium. To 30 ml add 70 ml of *water* and 40 ml of 0.05M *disodium edetate VS*. Add 0.2 ml of *methyl red solution*, neutralise to the orange colour of the indicator with 1M *sodium hydroxide* and heat on a water bath for 30 minutes. Cool, add 3 g of *hexamine* and titrate the excess of disodium edetate with 0.05M *lead nitrate VS* using *xylenol orange solution* as indicator. Each ml of 0.05M *disodium edetate VS* is equivalent to 1.349 mg of Al.

For magnesium To 25 ml of the solution reserved in the Assay for aluminium add 1 g of *ammonium chloride* and 10 ml, or a quantity sufficient to redissolve the precipitate that is produced, of *triethanolamine*. Add 150 ml of *water* and 5 ml of *ammonia buffer pH 10.9* and titrate immediately with 0.05M *disodium edetate VS* using *mordant black 11 solution* as indicator. Each ml of 0.05M *disodium edetate VS* is equivalent to 1.215 mg of Mg.

Labelling The label states that the tablets should be chewed before being swallowed.

Mannitol Intravenous Infusion

Definition Mannitol Intravenous Infusion is a sterile solution of Mannitol in Water for Injections.

The intravenous infusion complies with the requirements stated under Parenteral Preparations and with the following requirements.

Content of mannitol, $C_6H_{12}O_6$ 95.0 to 105.0% of the prescribed or stated amount.

Characteristics A colourless or almost colourless solution.

Identification

A. Evaporate to dryness on a water bath a volume containing 0.2 g of Mannitol. The *melting point* of the residue, Appendix V A, is about 167°.

B. Carry out the method for *thin-layer chromatography*, Appendix III A, using *silica gel G* as the coating substance and a mixture of 10 volumes of *water*, 70 volumes of *propan-1-ol* and 20 volumes of *ethyl acetate* as the mobile phase but allowing the solvent front to ascend 17 cm above the line of application. Apply separately to the plate 2 µl of each of the following solutions. For solution (1) dilute a volume of the intravenous infusion with *water* to contain 0.25% w/v of Mannitol. Solution (2) contains 0.25% w/v of *mannitol EPCRS* in *water*. After removal of the plate, allow it to dry in air and spray with a 0.2% w/v solution of *sodium periodate*. Allow the plate to dry in air for 15 minutes and spray with a 2% w/v solution of *4,4′-methylenebis-*N,N*-dimethylaniline* in a mixture of 1 volume of *glacial acetic acid* and 4 volumes of *acetone*. The principal spot in the chromatogram obtained with solution (1) is similar in position, colour and size to that in the chromatogram obtained with solution (2).

C. Add 0.3 ml of a solution containing 10% w/v of Mannitol to 3 ml of a cooled mixture prepared by adding 6 ml of *sulphuric acid* to 3 ml of a freshly prepared 10% w/v solution of *catechol* while cooling in ice. Heat gently over a naked flame for about 30 seconds. A pink colour develops.

Acidity or alkalinity pH, 4.5 to 7.0, Appendix V L, when determined on solutions diluted, if necessary, with *water for injections* to contain 10% w/v of Mannitol and to which 0.30 ml of a saturated solution of *potassium chloride* has been added for each 100 ml of solution.

Reducing sugars Add 20 ml of *cupri-citric solution* and a few glass beads to a volume of the intravenous infusion containing 5 g of Mannitol. Heat so that boiling begins after 4 minutes and continue boiling for 3 minutes. Cool rapidly and add 100 ml of a 2.4% v/v solution of *glacial acetic acid* and 20 ml of 0.025M *iodine VS*. With continuous shaking add 25 ml of a mixture of 6 volumes of *hydrochloric acid* and 94 volumes of *water* and, when the precipitate has dissolved, titrate the excess of iodine with 0.05M *sodium thiosulphate VS* using 1 ml of *starch solution*, added towards the end of the titration, as indicator. Not less than 12.8 ml of 0.05M *sodium thiosulphate VS* is required.

Particulate contamination When supplied in a container with a nominal content of 100 ml or more, complies with the *test for sub-visible particles*, Appendix XIII A.

Pyrogens Complies with the *test for pyrogens*, Appendix XIV D. Use per kg of the rabbit's weight a volume containing 0.5 g of Mannitol.

Assay Dilute a quantity containing 0.4 g of Mannitol to 100 ml with *water*, transfer 10 ml to a stoppered flask, add 20 ml of 0.1M *sodium periodate* and 2 ml of 1M *sulphuric acid* and heat on a water bath for 15 minutes. Cool, add 3 g of *sodium hydrogen carbonate* and 25 ml of 0.1M *sodium arsenite VS*, mix, add 5 ml of a 20% w/v solution of *potassium iodide*, allow to stand for 15 minutes and titrate with 0.05M *iodine VS* until the first trace of yellow colour appears. Repeat the operation without the substance being examined. The difference between the titrations represents the amount of iodine required. Each ml of 0.05M *iodine VS* is equivalent to 1.822 mg of $C_6H_{12}O_6$.

Storage Mannitol Intravenous Infusion should be stored at a temperature of 20° to 30°. Exposure to lower temperatures may cause the deposition of crystals, which should be dissolved by warming before use.

Labelling The strength is stated as the percentage w/v of Mannitol.

Mebeverine Tablets

Definition Mebeverine Tablets contain Mebeverine Hydrochloride. They are coated.

The tablets comply with the requirements stated under Tablets and with the following requirements.

Content of mebeverine hydrochloride, $C_{25}H_{35}NO_5$,HCl 95.0 to 105.0% of the prescribed or stated amount.

Identification

A. Suspend a quantity of the powdered tablets containing 0.2 g of Mebeverine Hydrochloride in 20 ml of *water*, add 5 ml of 5M *sodium hydroxide* and extract with two 25-ml quantities of *chloroform*. Dry the combined extracts over *anhydrous sodium sulphate* and evaporate to dryness using a rotary evaporator. The *infrared absorption spectrum* of the residue, Appendix II A, is concordant with the *reference spectrum* of mebeverine.

B. The *light absorption*, Appendix II B, in the range 230 to 350 nm of the final solution obtained in the Assay exhibits a maximum at 263 nm and a less well-defined maximum at 292 nm.

Related substances Comply with the requirement stated under Mebeverine Hydrochloride using the following solutions. For solution (1) shake a quantity of the powdered tablets containing 0.2 g of Mebeverine Hydrochloride with 10 ml of *acetone* and filter. For solution (2) dilute 1 volume of solution (1) to 200 volumes with *acetone*. Solution (3) contains 0.01% w/v of *veratric acid* in *acetone*.

Assay Weigh and powder 20 tablets. Heat a quantity of the powdered tablets containing 0.5 g of Mebeverine Hydrochloride with 100 ml of 0.1M *hydrochloric acid* for 10 minutes on a water bath, shaking occasionally. Cool, add sufficient 0.1M *hydrochloric acid* to produce 250 ml and filter. To 10 ml of the filtrate add sufficient 0.1M *hydrochloric acid* to produce 100 ml and dilute 15 ml of the resulting solution to 100 ml with the same solvent. Measure the *absorbance* of the solution at the maximum at 263 nm, Appendix II B. Calculate the content of $C_{25}H_{35}NO_5$,HCl taking 263 as the value of A(1%, 1 cm) at the maximum at 263 nm.

Storage Mebeverine Tablets should be kept in an airtight container, protected from light and stored at a temperature not exceeding 30°.

Mefenamic Acid Capsules

Definition Mefenamic Acid Capsules contain Mefenamic Acid.

The capsules comply with the requirements stated under Capsules and with the following requirements.

Content of mefenamic acid, $C_{15}H_{15}NO_2$ 95.0 to 105.0% of the prescribed or stated amount.

Identification

Extract a quantity of the contents of the capsules containing 0.25 g of Mefenamic Acid with two 30-ml quantities of *ether*. Wash the combined extracts with *water* and evaporate to dryness on a water bath. The residue, after drying at 105°, complies with the following tests.

A. Dissolve a sufficient quantity in the minimum volume of *absolute ethanol* and evaporate to dryness on a water bath. The *infrared absorption spectrum*, Appendix II A, is concordant with the *reference spectrum* of mefenamic acid.

B. Dissolve 25 mg in 15 ml of *chloroform* and examine under ultraviolet light (365 nm); the solution exhibits a strong greenish yellow fluorescence. Carefully add 0.5 ml of a saturated solution of *trichloroacetic acid* dropwise and examine under ultraviolet light (365 nm); the solution does not exhibit fluorescence.

C. Dissolve 5 mg in 2 ml of *sulphuric acid* and add 0.05 ml of 0.0167M *potassium dichromate*. An intense blue colour is produced immediately, fading rapidly to brownish green.

Disintegration Maximum time, 15 minutes, Appendix XII A.

2,3-Dimethylaniline Carry out the method for *thin-layer chromatography*, Appendix III A, using *silica gel G* as the coating substance and a mixture of 1 volume of 18M *ammonia*, 25 volumes of *1,4-dioxan* and 90 volumes of *toluene* as the mobile phase. Apply separately to the plate 40 µl of each of the following solutions. For solution (1) shake a quantity of the contents of the capsules containing 0.25 g of Mefenamic Acid with a mixture of 7.5 ml of *chloroform* and 2.5 ml of *methanol*, allow the insoluble matter to settle and use the supernatant liquid. Solution (2) contains 0.00025% w/v of *2,3-dimethylaniline* in a mixture of 3 volumes of *chloroform* and 1 volume of *methanol*. After removal of the plate, dry it in a current of warm air and visualise by *Method I*. Any spot corresponding to 2,3-dimethylaniline in the chromatogram obtained with solution (1) is not more intense than the spot in the chromatogram obtained with solution (2) (100 ppm).

Related substances Carry out the method for *thin-layer chromatography*, Appendix III A, using *silica gel GF_{254}* as the coating substance and a mixture of 1 volume of *glacial acetic acid*, 25 volumes of *1,4-dioxan* and 90 volumes of *toluene* as the mobile phase. Apply separately to the plate 20 µl of each of the following solutions. For solution (1) use the supernatant liquid obtained in the test for 2,3-Dimethylaniline. For solution (2) dilute 1 volume of solution (1) to 500 volumes with a mixture of 3 volumes of *chloroform* and 1 volume of *methanol*. After removal of the plate, allow it to dry in air, expose to iodine vapour for 5 minutes and examine under *ultraviolet light (254 nm)*. Any *secondary spot* in the chromatogram obtained with solution (1) is not more intense than the spot in the chromatogram obtained with solution (2) (0.2%).

Assay Dissolve a quantity of the mixed contents of 20 capsules containing 0.5 g of Mefenamic Acid in 100 ml of warm *absolute ethanol* previously neutralised to *phenol red solution* and titrate with 0.1M *sodium hydroxide VS* using *phenol red solution* as indicator. Each ml of 0.1M *sodium hydroxide VS* is equivalent to 24.13 mg of $C_{15}H_{15}NO_2$.

Megestrol Tablets

Definition Megestrol Tablets contain Megestrol Acetate.

With the exception of the requirements for shape, the tablets comply with the requirements stated under Tablets and with the following requirements.

Content of megestrol acetate, $C_{24}H_{32}O_4$ 92.5 to 107.5% of the prescribed or stated amount.

Identification

Shake a quantity of the powdered tablets containing 40 mg of Megestrol Acetate with 250 ml of *chloroform* for 30 minutes, filter into a separating funnel, wash the filtrate with 20 ml of *water* and evaporate the chloroform. The residue, after drying at 60° at a pressure not exceeding 0.7 kPa for 2 hours, complies with the following tests.

A. The *infrared absorption spectrum*, Appendix II A, is concordant with the *reference spectrum* of megestrol acetate.

B. Complies with the test for *identification of steroids*, Appendix III A, using *impregnating solvent II* and *mobile phase D*.

Disintegration Maximum time, 30 minutes, Appendix XII A.

Related foreign steroids Carry out the method for *thin-layer chromatography*, Appendix III A, using a silica gel precoated plate (Merck silica gel 60 plates are suitable) and a mixture of 0.5 volume of *water*, 8 volumes of *methanol* and 92 volumes of *1,2-dichloroethane* as the mobile phase. Apply separately to the plate 5 µl of each of the following solutions. For solution (1) shake a quantity of the powdered tablets containing 0.1 g of Megestrol Acetate with 10 ml of a mixture of 1 volume of *methanol* and 9 volumes of *chloroform* for 10 minutes, centrifuge and use the clear supernatant liquid. Solution (2) contains 0.005% w/v of *megestrol BPCRS* in a mixture of 1 volume of *methanol* and 9 volumes of *chloroform*. After removal of the plate, allow it to dry in air, spray with *ethanolic sulphuric acid (20%)*, heat at 110° for 10 minutes and examine under *ultraviolet light (365 nm)*. Any *secondary spot* in the chromatogram obtained with solution (1) is not more intense that the spot in the chromatogram obtained with solution (2) (0.5%).

Assay Weigh and powder 20 tablets. Prepare a 0.016% w/v solution of *propyl 4-hydroxybenzoate* (internal standard) in *acetonitrile* (solution A) and carry out the method for *liquid chromatography*, Appendix III D, using the following solutions. For solution (1) mix 4 ml of a 0.02% w/v solution of *megestrol acetate BPCRS* in *acetonitrile* with 10 ml of solution A and dilute to 50 ml with a 40% v/v solution of *acetonitrile*. For solution (2) shake a quantity of the powdered tablets containing 0.08 g of Megestrol Acetate with 10 ml of *water* for 10 minutes, add 75 ml of *acetonitrile*, shake for 30 minutes, dilute to 100 ml with *acetonitrile*, centrifuge and dilute 10 ml of the clear supernatant liquid to 50 ml with a 40% v/v solution of *acetonitrile*; to 5 ml of this solution add 10 ml of *acetonitrile* and dilute to 50 ml with a 40% v/v solution of *acetonitrile*. Prepare solution (3) in the same manner as solution (2) but adding 10 ml of solution A in place of the 10 ml of acetonitrile.

The chromatographic procedure may be carried out using (a) a stainless steel column (25 cm × 4.6 mm) packed with *stationary phase* C (5 µm) (Spherisorb ODS 1 is suitable), (b) a mixture of 32 volumes of *water* and 68 volumes of *acetonitrile* as the mobile phase with a flow rate of 1 ml per minute and (c) a detection wavelength of 280 nm.

The assay is not valid unless in the chromatogram obtained with solution (1) the *resolution factor* between the peaks due to propyl 4-hydroxybenzoate and megestrol acetate is at least 8.

Calculate the content of $C_{24}H_{32}O_4$ using the declared content of $C_{24}H_{32}O_4$ in *megestrol acetate BPCRS*.

Meglumine Amidotrizoate Injection

Definition Meglumine Amidotrizoate Injection is a sterile solution of the Meglumine salt of Amidotrizoic Acid Dihydrate in Water for Injections.

The injection complies with the requirements stated under Parenteral Preparations and with the following requirements.

Content of meglumine amidotrizoate, $C_{11}H_9I_3N_2O_4$, $C_7H_{17}NO_5$ 97.0 to 103.0% of the prescribed or stated amount.

Characteristics A colourless to pale yellow, slightly viscous liquid.

Identification

A. Evaporate 2 ml of the injection to dryness and heat 50 mg of the residue. Violet vapours of iodine are evolved.

B. To 20 mg of the residue obtained by evaporating the injection to dryness add 5 ml of 1M *sodium hydroxide* and boil gently under a reflux condenser for 10 minutes. Cool, add 5 ml of 2M *hydrochloric acid* and cool in ice for 5 minutes. Add 4 ml of a 1% w/v solution of *sodium nitrite*, cool in ice for 5 minutes, add 0.3 g of *sulphamic acid*, swirl gently until effervescence ceases and add 2 ml of a 0.4% w/v solution of N-*(1-naphthyl)ethylenediamine dihydrochloride*. An orange-red colour is produced.

C. To 0.5 g of the residue obtained by evaporating the injection to dryness, add 1 ml of *sulphuric acid*, heat on a water bath until a pale violet solution is obtained, add 2 ml of *ethanol (96%)* and again heat. Ethyl acetate, recognisable by its odour, is produced.

D. To a quantity containing 1 g of meglumine amidotrizoate add 50 ml of *water* and a slight excess of 2M *hydrochloric acid* and filter. Evaporate the filtrate to dryness on a water bath, dissolve the residue in a small quantity of boiling *ethanol (90%)*, filter and cool the filtrate in ice. The *melting point* of the dried precipitate is about 146°, Appendix V A.

Acidity or alkalinity pH, 6.0 to 7.0, Appendix V L.

Meglumine 22.9 to 25.3% of the stated content of meglumine amidotrizoate when determined by the following method. Measure the *optical rotation* of the injection, Appendix V F, using a 2-dm tube. Calculate the percentage content of meglumine using the expression $2.104R$ where R is the numerical value of the rotation.

Free amine To a quantity containing 1 g of meglumine amidotrizoate in a 50-ml glass-stoppered graduated flask add sufficient *water* to produce 5 ml, 10 ml of 0.1M *sodium hydroxide* and 25 ml of *dimethyl sulphoxide*. Stopper the flask, mix the contents by gentle swirling and cool in ice, protected from light. After 5 minutes add slowly 2 ml of *hydrochloric acid*, mix and allow to stand for 5 minutes. Add 2 ml of a 2% w/v solution of *sodium nitrite*, mix and allow to stand for 5 minutes. Add 1 ml of an 8% w/v solution of *sulphamic acid*, mix and allow to stand for 5 minutes. Add 2 ml of a 0.1% w/v solution of N-*(1-naphthyl)ethylenediamine dihydrochloride* in a 70% v/v solution of *propane-1,2-diol* and mix. Remove the flask from the ice and allow to stand in water at 22° to 25° for 10 minutes, occasionally shaking gently. Add sufficient *dimethyl sulphoxide* to produce 50 ml and mix. Within 5 minutes of diluting to 50 ml measure the *absorbance* of the resulting solution at the maximum at 470 nm, Appendix II B, using in the reference cell a solution prepared by treating 5 ml of *water* in the same manner. The absorbance is not more than 0.40.

Inorganic iodide Dilute a quantity containing 0.80 g of meglumine amidotrizoate to 10 ml with *water*, add sufficient 2M *nitric acid* dropwise to ensure complete precipitation of the iodinated acid and add 3 ml in excess. Filter, wash the precipitate with 5 ml of *water*, add to the filtrate 1 ml of *hydrogen peroxide solution (100 vol)* and 1 ml of *chloroform* and shake. Any purple colour in the chloroform layer is not more intense than that obtained by adding 2 ml of *iodide standard solution (20 ppm I)* to a mixture of 3 ml of 2M *nitric acid* and sufficient *water* to equal the volume of the test solution, adding 1 ml of *hydrogen peroxide solution (100 vol)* and 1 ml of *chloroform* and shaking (50 ppm).

Pyrogens Complies with the *test for pyrogens*, Appendix XIV D. Use per kg of the rabbit's weight a quantity containing 2.5 g of meglumine amidotrizoate.

Assay Mix a quantity containing 0.5 g of meglumine amidotrizoate with 12 ml of 5M *sodium hydroxide* and 20 ml of *water*, add 1 g of *zinc powder* and boil under a reflux condenser for 30 minutes. Cool, rinse the condenser with 30 ml of *water*, filter through absorbent cotton and wash the flask and filter with two 20-ml quantities of *water*. To the combined filtrate and washings add 80 ml of *hydrochloric acid*, cool and titrate with 0.05M *potassium iodate VS* until the dark brown solution becomes light brown. Add 5 ml of *chloroform* and continue the titration, shaking well after each addition, until the chloroform becomes colourless. Each ml of 0.05M *potassium iodate VS* is equivalent to 26.97 mg of $C_{11}H_9I_3N_2O_4,C_7H_{17}NO_5$. Determine the *weight per ml* of the injection, Appendix V G, and calculate the percentage w/v of $C_{11}H_9I_3N_2O_4,C_7H_{17}NO_5$.

Storage Meglumine Amidotrizoate Injection should be protected from light.

Labelling The strength is stated as the percentage w/v of meglumine amidotrizoate.

Action and use Contrast medium used in angiography and urography.

When meglumine diatrizoate injection is prescribed or demanded, Meglumine Amidotrizoate Injection shall be dispensed or supplied.

Meglumine Iodipamide Injection

Definition Meglumine Iodipamide Injection is a sterile solution of the Meglumine salt of 3,3′-adipoyldiamino-bis(2,4,6-tri-iodobenzoic acid) (2:1) in Water for Injections.

The injection complies with the requirements stated under Parenteral Preparations and with the following requirements.

Content of meglumine iodipamide, $C_{20}H_{14}I_6N_2O_6$, $2C_7H_{17}NO_5$ 97.0 to 103.0% of the prescribed or stated amount.

Characteristics A colourless to pale yellow solution.

Identification

A. To a volume of the injection containing 0.6 g of meglumine iodipamide add 1 ml of 1M *hydrochloric acid*, stir until the precipitate becomes crystalline, add 5 ml of 1M *hydrochloric acid*, stir, filter and reserve the filtrate for test C. Wash the residue with 1M *hydrochloric acid* and then with *water* and dry at 105°. The *infrared absorption spectrum* of the residue, Appendix II A, is concordant with the *reference spectrum* of iodipamide.

B. Heat 50 mg of the residue obtained in test A. Violet vapours of iodine are evolved.

C. Evaporate the filtrate reserved in test A to dryness on a water bath, dissolve the residue in a small quantity of boiling *ethanol (90%)*, filter and cool the filtrate in ice. The *melting point* of the dried precipitate is about 146°, Appendix V A.

Acidity or alkalinity pH, 6.0 to 7.1, Appendix V L.

Meglumine 11.8 to 13.7% of the stated content of meglumine iodipamide when determined by the following method. Measure the *optical rotation* of the injection, Appendix V G, using a 2-dm tube. Calculate the percentage content of meglumine using the expression 2.104*R* where *R* is the numerical value of the rotation.

Free amine To a quantity containing 0.25 g of meglumine iodipamide add 25 ml of *water*, 8 ml of 1M *hydrochloric acid* and 4 ml of a 1.0% w/v solution of *sodium nitrite* and shake for 2 minutes. Add 6 ml of a 2% w/v solution of *ammonium sulphamate* and swirl gently until effervescence ceases. Add 0.4 ml of a 10% w/v solution of *1-naphthol* in *ethanol (96%)*, shake and add 3 ml of 5M *sodium hydroxide*. Dilute the solution to 50 ml with *water* and measure the *absorbance* at the maximum at 485 nm, Appendix II B, using in the reference cell a solution prepared in the same manner but omitting the injection. The absorbance is not more than 0.17.

Inorganic iodide Dilute a quantity containing 0.80 g of meglumine iodipamide to 10 ml with *water*, add sufficient 2M *nitric acid* dropwise to ensure complete precipitation of the iodinated acid and add 3 ml in excess. Filter, wash the precipitate with 5 ml of *water*, add to the filtrate 1 ml of *hydrogen peroxide solution (100 vol)* and 1 ml of *chloroform* and shake. Any purple colour in the chloroform layer is not more intense than that obtained by adding 2 ml of *iodide standard solution (20 ppm I)* to a mixture of 3 ml of 2M *nitric acid* and sufficient *water* to equal the volume of the test solution, adding 1 ml of *hydrogen peroxide solution (100 vol)* and 1 ml of *chloroform* and shaking (50 ppm).

Pyrogens Complies with the *test for pyrogens*, Appendix XIV D. Use per kg of the rabbit's weight a quantity containing 1.25 g of meglumine iodipamide.

Assay Mix 0.4 g with 12 ml of 5M *sodium hydroxide* and 20 ml of *water*, add 1 g of *zinc powder* and boil under a reflux condenser for 30 minutes. Cool, rinse the condenser with 30 ml of *water*, filter through absorbent cotton and wash the flask and filter with two 20-ml quantities of *water*. To the combined filtrate and washings add 80 ml of *hydrochloric acid*, cool and titrate with 0.05M *potassium iodate VS* until the dark brown solution becomes light brown. Add 5 ml of *chloroform* and continue the titration, shaking well after each addition, until the chloroform becomes colourless. Each ml of 0.05M *potassium iodate VS* is equivalent to 25.50 mg of $C_{20}H_{14}I_6N_2O_6,2C_7H_{17}NO_5$. Determine the *weight per ml* of the injection, Appendix V G, and calculate the percentage w/v of $C_{20}H_{14}I_6N_2O_6,2C_7H_{17}NO_5$.

Labelling The strength is stated as the percentage w/v of meglumine iodipamide.

Action and use Contrast medium used in intravenous cholangiography.

Meglumine Iotalamate Injection

Definition Meglumine Iotalamate Injection is a sterile solution of the Meglumine salt of Iotalamic Acid in Water for Injections.

The injection complies with the requirements stated under Parenteral Preparations and with the following requirements.

Content of meglumine iotalamate, $C_{11}H_9I_3N_2O_4$, $C_7H_{17}NO_5$ 97.0 to 103.0% of the prescribed or stated amount.

Characteristics An almost colourless to pale yellow liquid.

Identification

A. To a quantity containing 1 g of meglumine iotalamate add 50 ml of *water* and a slight excess of 2M *hydrochloric acid*, filter, reserve the filtrate for test B, wash the residue with *water* and dry at 105°. The *infrared absorption spectrum* of the residue, Appendix II A, is concordant with the *reference spectrum* of iotalamic acid.

B. Evaporate the filtrate reserved in test A to dryness on a water bath, dissolve the residue in a small volume of boiling *ethanol (90%)*, filter and cool the filtrate in ice. The *melting point* of the dried precipitate is about 146°, Appendix V A.

Acidity or alkalinity pH, 6.5 to 7.5, Appendix V L. Take the first measurement 5 minutes after inserting the electrodes and repeat every 30 seconds until constant.

Meglumine 22.3 to 25.9% of the stated content of meglumine iotalamate when determined by the following method. Measure the *optical rotation* of the injection, Appendix V F, using a 2-dm tube. Calculate the percentage content of meglumine using the expression 2.104R where R is the numerical value of the rotation.

Halide Mix a quantity of the injection containing 0.73 g of meglumine iotalamate with 4 ml of 2M *sodium hydroxide* and 5 ml of *water*, mix, add 6 ml of 2M *nitric acid*, shake, dilute to 25 ml with *water* and filter. 15 ml of the filtrate complies with the *limit test for chlorides*, Appendix VII (100 ppm expressed as chloride).

Related substances Carry out the method for *thin-layer chromatography*, Appendix III A, using *silica gel GF_{254}* as the coating substance and a mixture of 1 volume of *glacial acetic acid*, 1 volume of *anhydrous formic acid*, 1 volume of *methanol*, 5 volumes of *ether* and 10 volumes of *dichloromethane* as the mobile phase but allowing the solvent front to ascend 10 cm above the line of application. Apply separately to the plate 5 µl of each of the following solutions. For solution (1) dilute the injection being examined with *methanol* containing 3% v/v of 10M *ammonia* to contain 10% w/v of meglumine iotalamate. For solution (2) dilute 1 volume of solution (1) to 50 volumes with *methanol* and dilute 1 volume of this solution to 10 volumes with *methanol*. Solution (3) contains 0.05% w/v of *5-amino-2,4,6-tri-iodo-*N*-methylisophthalamic acid EPCRS* in *methanol* containing 3% v/v of 10M *ammonia*. For solution (4) dissolve 1 mg of *5-amino-2,4,6-tri-iodo-*N*-methylisophthalamic acid EPCRS* in 5 ml of solution (2). After removal of the plate, allow it to dry until the solvents have evaporated and examine under *ultraviolet light (254 nm)*. Any spot in the chromatogram obtained with solution (1) corresponding to 5-amino-2,4,6-tri-iodo-*N*-methylisophthalamic acid is not more intense than the spot in the chromatogram obtained with solution (3) (0.5%) and any other *secondary spot* is not more intense than the spot in the chromatogram obtained with solution (2) (0.2%). The test is not valid unless the chromatogram obtained with solution (3) shows two clearly separated spots.

Pyrogens Complies with the *test for pyrogens*, Appendix XIV D. Use per kg of the rabbit's weight a quantity containing 2.5 g of meglumine iotalamate.

Assay Mix a quantity containing 0.5 g of meglumine iotalamate with 12 ml of 5M *sodium hydroxide* and 20 ml of *water*, add 1 g of *zinc powder* and boil under a reflux condenser for 30 minutes. Cool, rinse the condenser with 30 ml of *water*, filter through absorbent cotton and wash the flask and filter with two 20-ml quantities of *water*. To the combined filtrate and washings add 80 ml of *hydrochloric acid*, cool and titrate with 0.05M *potassium iodate VS* until the dark brown solution becomes light brown. Add 5 ml of *chloroform* and continue the titration, shaking well after each addition, until the chloroform becomes colourless. Each ml of 0.05M *potassium iodate VS* is equivalent to 26.97 mg of $C_{11}H_9I_3N_2O_4,C_7H_{17}NO_5$. Determine the *weight per ml* of the injection, Appendix V G, and calculate the content of $C_{11}H_9I_3N_2O_4,C_7H_{17}NO_5$, weight in volume.

Storage Meglumine Iotalamate Injection should be protected from light.

Labelling The strength is stated as the percentage w/v of meglumine iotalamate.

Action and use Contrast medium used in angiography and urography.

When meglumine iothalamate injection is prescribed or demanded, Meglumine Iotalamate Injection shall be dispensed or supplied.

Melphalan Injection

Definition Melphalan Injection is a sterile solution of melphalan hydrochloride. It is prepared immediately before use by dissolving Melphalan for Injection in a suitable solvent and then diluting with the requisite volume of a suitable diluent in accordance with the manufacturer's instructions.

The injection complies with the requirements stated under Parenteral Preparations and with the following requirements.

Acidity or alkalinity 6.0 to 7.0, Appendix V L.

Clarity of solution Not more more opalescent than *reference suspension II*, Appendix IV A.

Storage Melphalan Injection deteriorates on storage and should be used immediately after preparation.

MELPHALAN FOR INJECTION

Definition Melphalan for Injection is a sterile material consisting of Melphalan with or without excipients. It is supplied in a sealed container.

The contents of the sealed container comply with the requirements for Powders for Injections stated under Parenteral Preparations and with the following requirements.

Content of melphalan, $C_{13}H_{18}Cl_2N_2O_2$ 90.0 to 110.0% of the prescribed or stated amount of anhydrous melphalan.

Identification

A. The *light absorption*, Appendix II B, in the range 230 to 350 nm of a 0.001% w/v solution in *methanol* exhibits a maximum at 260 nm and a less well-defined maximum at 310 nm.

B. In the Assay, the principal peak in the chromatogram obtained with solution (2) has the same retention time as the principal peak in the chromatogram obtained with solution (1).

C. Dissolve a quantity containing the equivalent of 20 mg of anhydrous melphalan in 50 ml of *methanol* with the aid of gentle heat, add 1 ml of a 5% w/v solution of *4-(4-nitrobenzyl)pyridine* in *acetone* and evaporate to dryness. Dissolve the residue in 1 ml of hot *methanol* and add 0.1 ml of 13.5M *ammonia*. A red colour is produced.

D. Heat a quantity of the powder containing 0.1 g of anhydrous melphalan with 10 ml of 0.1M *sodium hydroxide* for 10 minutes on a water bath. The resulting solution, after acidification with 2M *nitric acid*, yields reaction A characteristic of *chlorides*, Appendix VI.

Ionisable chlorine Dissolve a quantity containing the equivalent of 0.1 g of anhydrous melphalan in a mixture of 15 ml of *water* and 0.5 ml of *nitric acid*, allow to stand for 2 minutes and titrate with 0.02M *silver nitrate VS* determining the end point potentiometrically. Not more than 1.7 ml is required.

Uniformity of content Sealed containers containing the equivalent of 100 mg or less of anhydrous melphalan comply with the requirements stated under Parenteral Preparations, Powders for Injections. Use the individual results obtained in the Assay.

Assay Carry out the method for *liquid chromatography*, Appendix III D, using the following solutions. Solution (1) contains 0.01% w/v of *melphalan BPCRS* in a mixture of 4 volumes of *acetonitrile* and 1 volume of 0.1M *hydrochloric acid*. For solution (2) dissolve the contents of one container in a mixture of 4 volumes of *acetonitrile* and 1 volume of 0.1M *hydrochloric acid* and dilute with sufficient of the same solvent mixture to produce a final solution containing the equivalent of 0.01% w/v of anhydrous melphalan.

The chromatographic procedure may be carried out using (a) a stainless steel column (20 cm × 4.6 mm) packed with *stationary phase C* (10 µm) (Spherisorb ODS 1 is suitable), (b) a mixture of 200 volumes of a 0.375% w/v solution of *ammonium carbonate*, 180 volumes of *methanol* and 2.7 volumes of *glacial acetic acid* as the mobile phase with a flow rate of 2 ml per minute and (c) a detection wavelength of 254 nm.

Calculate the amount of $C_{13}H_{18}Cl_2N_2O_2$ in the sealed container using the declared content of $C_{13}H_{18}Cl_2N_2O_2$ in *melphalan BPCRS*.

Repeat the procedure with a further nine sealed containers and calculate the average content of $C_{13}H_{18}Cl_2N_2O_2$ per container from the 10 individual results thus obtained.

Labelling The label of the sealed container states the equivalent amount of anhydrous melphalan contained in it.

Melphalan Tablets

Definition Melphalan Tablets contain Melphalan. They are coated.

The tablets comply with the requirements stated under Tablets and with the following requirements.

Content of melphalan, $C_{13}H_{18}Cl_2N_2O_2$ 90.0 to 110.0% of the prescribed or stated amount.

Identification

A. Extract a quantity of the powdered tablets containing 25 mg of Melphalan with 50 ml of hot *methanol*, filter and dilute 5 ml of the filtrate to 500 ml with *methanol*. The *light absorption* of the resulting solution, Appendix II B, exhibits a maximum at 260 nm and a less well-defined maximum at 301 nm.

B. To the remainder of the filtrate obtained in test A add 1 ml of a 5% w/v solution of *4-(4-nitrobenzyl)pyridine* in *acetone* and evaporate to dryness. Dissolve the residue in 1 ml of hot *methanol* and add 0.1 ml of 13.5M *ammonia*. A red colour is produced.

Dissolution Comply with the *dissolution test for tablets and capsules*, Appendix XII D, using as the medium 900 ml of 0.1M *hydrochloric acid* and rotating the basket at 100 revolutions per minute. Withdraw a sample of 10 ml of the medium and filter. Carry out the method for *liquid chromatography*, Appendix III D, using the following solutions. For solution (1) dilute a suitable volume of a 0.10% w/v solution of *melphalan BPCRS* in a mixture of 4 volumes of *acetonitrile* and 1 volume of 0.1M *hydrochloric acid* with sufficient 0.1M *hydrochloric acid* to produce a solution containing 0.0002% w/v. For solution (2) dilute the filtered solution, if necessary, with 0.1M *hydrochloric acid* to give a solution expected to contain about 0.0002% w/v of Melphalan.

The chromatographic procedure may be carried out using (a) a stainless steel column (20 cm × 4.6 mm) packed with *stationary phase C* (10 µm) (Spherisorb ODS 1 is suitable), (b) a mixture of 2.7 volumes of *glacial acetic acid*, 180 volumes of *methanol* and 200 volumes of a 0.375% w/v solution of *ammonium carbonate* as the mobile phase with a flow rate of 2 ml per minute, (c) a detection wavelength of 254 nm and (d) a 100-µl loop injector.

Calculate the content of melphalan, $C_{13}H_{18}Cl_2N_2O_2$ in the medium using the declared content of $C_{13}H_{18}Cl_2N_2O_2$ in *melphalan BPCRS*.

Uniformity of content Tablets containing 2 mg or less of Melphalan comply with the requirements stated under Tablets using the following method of analysis. Carry out the method for *liquid chromatography*, Appendix III D, using the following solutions. Solution (1) contains 0.01% w/v of *melphalan BPCRS* in a mixture of 4 volumes of *acetonitrile* and 1 volume of 0.1M *hydrochloric acid*. For solution (2) add 20 ml of a mixture of 4 volumes of *acetonitrile* and 1 volume of 0.1M *hydrochloric acid* to one tablet, mix with the aid of ultrasound for 10 minutes or until the tablet has disintegrated, filter, discarding the first 5 ml of filtrate, and use the filtrate.

The chromatographic procedure may be carried out using (a) a stainless steel column (20 cm × 4.6 mm) packed with *stationary phase C* (10 µm) (Spherisorb ODS 1 is suitable), (b) a mixture of 200 volumes of a 0.375% w/v solution of *ammonium carbonate*, 180 volumes of *methanol* and 2.7 volumes of *glacial acetic acid* as the mobile phase with a flow rate of 2 ml per minute and (c) a detection wavelength of 254 nm.

Calculate the content of $C_{13}H_{18}Cl_2N_2O_2$ using the declared content of $C_{13}H_{18}Cl_2N_2O_2$ in *melphalan BPCRS*.

Assay

For tablets containing more than 2 mg of Melphalan Carry out the method for *liquid chromatography*, Appendix III D, using the following solutions. Solution (1) contains 0.01% w/v of *melphalan BPCRS* in a mixture of 4 volumes of *acetonitrile* and 1 volume of 0.1M *hydrochloric acid*. For solution (2) add about 300 ml of a mixture of 4 volumes of *acetonitrile* and 1 volume of 0.1M *hydrochloric acid* to 10 tablets, shake until the tablets have disintegrated (about 30 minutes), mix with the aid of ultrasound for 5 minutes, dilute to 500 ml with the same solvent mixture, filter, discarding the first 20 ml of filtrate, and use the filtrate.

The chromatographic procedure described under Uniformity of content may be used.

Calculate the content of $C_{13}H_{18}Cl_2N_2O_2$ in the tablets using the declared content of $C_{13}H_{18}Cl_2N_2O_2$ in *melphalan BPCRS*.

For tablets containing 2 mg or less of Melphalan Use the average of the 10 individual results determined in the test for Uniformity of content.

Storage Melphalan Tablets should be stored at a temperature not exceeding 25°.

Menadiol Phosphate Injection

Definition Menadiol Phosphate Injection is a sterile solution of Menadiol Sodium Phosphate in Water for Injections.

The injection complies with the requirements stated under Parenteral Preparations and with the following requirements.

Content of menadiol phosphate, $C_{11}H_{12}O_8P_2$ 90.0 to 110.0% of the prescribed or stated amount.

Identification

A. Dilute a volume of the injection containing the equivalent of 0.2 g of menadiol phosphate to 20 ml with *water* and add 20 ml of 1M *sulphuric acid*, 20 ml of 0.1M *cerium(IV) sulphate* and 2 ml of *hydrogen peroxide solution (20 vol)*. Extract with two 20-ml quantities of *chloroform*, evaporate the combined chloroform extracts to dryness on a water bath and dry the residue at 40° at a pressure not exceeding 0.7 kPa. The *infrared absorption spectrum* of the residue, Appendix II A, is concordant with the *reference spectrum* of menadione.

B. To 50 mg of the residue obtained in test A add 5 ml of *water* followed by 75 mg of *sodium metabisulphite* and heat in a water bath, shaking vigorously, until an almost colourless solution is obtained. Dilute to 50 ml with *water*. To 2 ml of the resulting solution add 2 ml of a mixture of equal volumes of *ethanol (96%)* and 13.5M *ammonia*, shake and add 0.15 ml of *ethyl cyanoacetate*. A deep purplish blue colour is produced which changes to green on the addition of 1 ml of 10M *sodium hydroxide*.

Acidity or alkalinity pH, 7.0 to 8.0, Appendix V L.

Related substances

A. Carry out in subdued light the method for *thin-layer chromatography*, Appendix III A, using *silica gel GF_{254}* as the coating substance and a mixture of 50 volumes of *propan-1-ol*, 50 volumes of a 2% w/v solution of *ammonium chloride*, 5 volumes of *butan-1-ol* and 1.5 volumes of *diethylamine* as the mobile phase. Apply separately to the plate 5 µl of each of the following solutions. For solution (1) evaporate a volume of the injection containing the equivalent of 0.5 g of menadiol phosphate to dryness and dissolve the residue in 10 ml of *methanol (50%)*. For solution (2) dilute 1 volume of solution (1) to 200 volumes with *methanol (50%)*. Solutions (3) and (4) contain 0.0025% w/v of *methyl 4-hydroxybenzoate* and 0.0025% w/v *of propyl 4-hydroxybenzoate* respectively in *methanol (50%)*. After removal of the plate, allow it to dry in air and examine under *ultraviolet light (254 nm)*. Any *secondary spot* in the chromatogram obtained with solution (1) is not more intense than the spot in the chromatogram obtained with solution (2). Disregard any spots corresponding to those in the chromatograms obtained with solutions (3) and (4).

B. Carry out the method for *thin-layer chromatography*, Appendix III A, using *silica gel GF_{254}* as the coating substance and a mixture of 80 volumes of *cyclohexane*, 20 volumes of *ether* and 1 volume of *methanol* as the mobile phase. Apply separately to the plate 5 µl of each of the following solutions. Solution (1) is the injection diluted, if necessary, with *methanol* to contain the equivalent of 1.0% w/v of menadiol phosphate. Solution (2) contains 0.0050% w/v of *2-methyl-1,4-naphthoquinone* in *methanol*. After removal of the plate, allow it to dry in air and examine under *ultraviolet light (254 nm)*. Any spot corresponding to 2-methyl-1,4-naphthoquinone (menadione) in the chromatogram obtained with solution (1) is not more intense than the spot in the chromatogram obtained with solution (2).

Assay Dilute, if necessary, a volume of the injection containing the equivalent of 50 mg of menadiol phosphate to 50 ml with *water*. Dilute 5 ml of the solution to 10 ml with 0.1M *hydrochloric acid* and measure the *absorbance* of the resulting solution at the maximum at 290 nm, Appendix II B. Calculate the content of $C_{11}H_{12}O_8P_2$ taking 138 as the value of A(1%, 1 cm) at the maximum at 290 nm.

Labelling The strength is stated in terms of the equivalent amount of menadiol phosphate in a suitable dose-volume.

Menadiol Phosphate Tablets

Definition Menadiol Phosphate Tablets contain Menadiol Sodium Phosphate.

The tablets comply with the requirements stated under Tablets and with the following requirements.

Content of menadiol phosphate, $C_{11}H_{12}O_8P_2$ 92.5 to 107.5% of the prescribed or stated amount.

Identification

A. Shake a quantity of the powdered tablets containing the equivalent of 0.15 g of menadiol phosphate with 15 ml of *water*, centrifuge and filter the supernatant liquid. To 10 ml of the filtrate add 10 ml of 1M *sulphuric acid*, 10 ml of 0.1M *cerium(IV) sulphate* and 1 ml of *hydrogen peroxide solution (20 vol)* and extract with two 10-ml quantities of *chloroform*. Evaporate the combined chloroform extracts to dryness in a water bath and dry the residue at 40° at a pressure not exceeding 0.7 kPa. The *infrared absorption spectrum* of the residue, Appendix II A, is concordant with the *reference spectrum* of menadione.

B. To 50 mg of the residue obtained in test A add 5 ml of *water* followed by 75 mg of *sodium metabisulphite*, heat in a water bath, shaking vigorously, until an almost colourless solution is obtained and dilute to 50 ml with *water*. To 2 ml of the resulting solution add 2 ml of a mixture of equal volumes of 13.5M *ammonia* and *ethanol (96%)*, shake and add 0.15 ml of *ethyl cyanoacetate*. A deep purplish blue colour is produced which changes to green on the addition of 1 ml of 10M *sodium hydroxide*.

Related substances Carry out in subdued light the method for *thin-layer chromatography*, Appendix III A, using *silica gel GF_{254}* as the coating substance and a mixture of 50 volumes of *propan-1-ol*, 50 volumes of a 2% w/v solution of *ammonium chloride*, 5 volumes of *butan-1-ol* and 1.5 volumes of *diethylamine* as the mobile phase. Apply separately to the plate 5 µl of each of the following solutions. For solution (1) shake a quantity of the powdered tablets containing the equivalent of 0.25 g of menadiol phosphate with 10 ml of *methanol (50%)* and filter. For solution (2) dilute 1 volume of solution (1) to 200 volumes with *methanol (50%)*. Solution (3) contains 0.0080% w/v of *2-methyl-1,4-naphthoquinone* in *methanol*. After removal of the plate, allow it to dry in air and examine under *ultraviolet light (254 nm)*. Any *secondary spot* in the chromatogram obtained with solution (1) is not more intense than the spot in the chromatogram obtained with solution (3). Examine the plate under *ultraviolet light (365 nm)*. Any *secondary spot* in the chromatogram obtained with solution (1) is not more intense than the spot in the chromatogram obtained with solution (2).

Assay Weigh and powder 20 tablets. Shake a quantity of the powder containing the equivalent of 10 mg of menadiol phosphate with 100 ml of 0.1M *hydrochloric acid* for 30 minutes. Dilute to 250 ml with 0.1M *hydrochloric acid*, filter and measure the *absorbance* of the filtrate at the maximum at 290 nm, Appendix II B. Calculate the content of $C_{11}H_{12}O_8P_2$ taking 138 as the value of A(1%, 1 cm) at the maximum at 290 nm.

Labelling The quantity of active ingredient is stated in terms of the equivalent amount of menadiol phosphate.

Menotrophin Injection

Definition Menotrophin Injection is a sterile solution of Menotrophin in Water for Injections. It is prepared by dissolving Menotrophin for Injection in the requisite amount of Water for Injections immediately before use.

The injection complies with the requirements stated under Parenteral Preparations.

Storage Menotrophin Injection should be used immediately after preparation.

MENOTROPHIN FOR INJECTION

Definition Menotrophin for Injection is a sterile material consisting of Menotrophin with or without excipients. It is supplied in a sealed container.

The contents of the sealed container comply with the requirements for Powders for Injections stated under Parenteral Preparations and with the following requirements.

Identification Cause enlargement of the ovaries of immature female rats and increase the weight of the seminal vesicles and prostate gland of immature male rats when administered as directed in the Assay.

Acidity or alkalinity Dissolve the contents of the sealed container in 3 ml of *water* (solution A). The pH is 6.0 to 8.0, Appendix V L.

Clarity and colour of solution Solution A is *clear*, Appendix IV A, and *colourless*, Appendix IV B, Method I.

Water Comply with the test described under Menotrophin.

Pyrogens Comply with the *test for pyrogens*, Appendix XIV D. Use per kg of the rabbit's weight 1 ml of a solution in *sodium chloride injection* containing 5 IU of follicle stimulating hormone activity per ml.

Assay Carry out the *biological assay of menotrophin* described under Menotrophin. The estimated potency for each component is not less than 80% and not more than 125% of the stated potency. The fiducial limits of error are not less than 64% and not more than 156% of the stated potency.

Storage The sealed container should be protected from light and stored at a temperature not exceeding 25°. Under these conditions, the contents may be expected to retain their potency for not less than 3 years.

Labelling The label of the sealed container states the number of IU (Units) of follicle stimulating-hormone activity, the number of IU (Units) of luteinising hormone activity and, where applicable, the number of IU (Units) of chorionic gonadotrophin activity contained in it.

Menthol and Benzoin Inhalation

Definition Menthol and Benzoin Inhalation is an *inhalation vapour, solution*.

Racementhol or Levomenthol	20 g
Benzoin Inhalation	sufficient to produce 1000 ml

Extemporaneous preparation The following directions apply.

Dissolve the Racementhol or the Levomenthol in a portion of the Benzoin Inhalation, add sufficient Benzoin Inhalation to produce 1000 ml and mix.

The inhalation complies with the requirements stated under Preparations for Inhalation and with the following requirements.

Content of total balsamic acids Not less than 2.8% w/v, calculated as cinnamic acid, $C_9H_8O_2$.

Total solids 9.0 to 12.0% w/v when determined by

drying at 105° for 4 hours, Appendix XI A. Use 2 ml.

Assay Carry out the Assay described under Sumatra Benzoin using 10 ml of the inhalation. Each ml of 0.1M *sodium hydroxide VS* is equivalent to 14.82 mg of total balsamic acids, calculated as cinnamic acid, $C_9H_8O_2$.

Labelling The label indicates the pharmaceutical form as 'inhalation vapour'.

Meptazinol Injection

Definition Meptazinol Injection is a sterile solution of Meptazinol Hydrochloride in Water for Injections.

The injection complies with the requirements stated under Parenteral Preparations and with the following requirements.

Content of meptazinol, $C_{15}H_{23}NO$ 95.0 to 105.0% of the prescribed or stated amount.

Identification

A. The *light absorption*, Appendix II B, in the range 220 to 330 nm of the solution obtained in the Assay exhibits a maximum at 273 nm.

B. Carry out the method for *thin-layer chromatography*, Appendix III A, using a silica gel F_{254} precoated plate (Merck silica gel 60 F_{254} plates are suitable) and a mixture of 1 volume of 18M *ammonia*, 20 volumes of *absolute ethanol* and 79 volumes of *toluene* as the mobile phase. Apply separately to the plate 10 µl of each of the following two solutions. For solution (1) dilute the injection, if necessary, with *ethanol (96%)* to contain the equivalent of 0.05% w/v of meptazinol. Solution (2) contains 0.05% w/v of *meptazinol hydrochloride BPCRS* in *ethanol (96%)*. After removal of the plate, allow it to dry in air and examine under *ultraviolet light (254 nm)*. The principal spot in the chromatogram obtained with solution (1) corresponds in intensity, position and size to that in the chromatogram obtained with solution (2).

Acidity pH, 3.5 to 6.0, Appendix V L.

Colour of solution The injection is not more intensely coloured than *reference solution* Y_5, Appendix IV B, Method II.

Related substances Carry out the method for *thin-layer chromatography*, Appendix III A, using a silica gel precoated plate (Merck silica gel 60 F_{254} plates are suitable) and a mixture of 1 volume of 18M *ammonia*, 30 volumes of *chloroform* and 70 volumes of *ethyl acetate* as the mobile phase. Apply separately to the plate 10 µl of each of the following solutions. For solution (1) dilute a volume of the injection with *water* to produce a solution containing the equivalent of 1.0% w/v of meptazinol. For solution (2) dilute 1 volume of solution (1) to 100 volumes with *water*. For solution (3) dilute a volume of solution (2) with an equal volume of *water*. After removal of the plate, allow it to dry in air, examine under *ultraviolet light (254 nm)*, expose to iodine vapour for 2 hours and examine again. By each method of visualisation, any *secondary spot* in the chromatogram obtained with solution (1) is not more intense than the spot in the chromatogram obtained with solution (2) (1%) and not more than one such spot is more intense than the spot in the chromatogram obtained with solution (3) (0.5%).

Assay Dilute a suitable volume of the injection with sufficient *water* to produce a solution containing the equivalent of 0.01% w/v of meptazinol and measure the *absorbance* at the maximum at 273 nm, Appendix II B. Calculate the content of $C_{15}H_{23}NO$ from the *absorbance* obtained using a 0.01% w/v solution of *meptazinol hydrochloride BPCRS* and from the declared content of $C_{15}H_{23}NO$ in *meptazinol hydrochloride BPCRS*.

Storage Meptazinol Injection should be stored at a temperature not exceeding 25°.

Labelling The label of the sealed container states the quantity of active ingredient contained in it in terms of the equivalent amount of meptazinol.

Meptazinol Tablets

Definition Meptazinol Tablets contain Meptazinol Hydrochloride.

With the exception of the requirements for shape, the tablets comply with the requirements stated under Tablets and with the following requirements.

Content of meptazinol, $C_{15}H_{23}NO$ 95.0 to 105.0% of the prescribed or stated amount.

Identification

A. The *light absorption*, Appendix II B, in the range 220 to 330 nm of the solution obtained in the Assay exhibits a maximum at 273 nm.

B. Comply with the test described under Meptazinol Injection but preparing solution (1) and solution (2) in the following manner. For solution (1) shake a quantity of the powdered tablets containing the equivalent of 50 mg of meptazinol with 5 ml of *ethanol (96%)*, centrifuge and dilute 1 volume of the supernatant liquid to 50 volumes with *ethanol (96%)*. Solution (2) contains 0.02% w/v of *meptazinol hydrochloride BPCRS* in *ethanol (96%)*.

Related substances Comply with the test described under Meptazinol Injection but using the following solutions. For solution (1) shake a quantity of the powdered tablets containing the equivalent of 0.2 g of meptazinol with 20 ml of *ethanol (96%)*, centrifuge and use the supernatant liquid. For solution (2) dilute 1 volume of solution (1) to 100 volumes with *ethanol (96%)*. For solution (3) dilute a volume of solution (2) with an equal volume of *ethanol (96%)*.

Assay To a quantity of the powdered tablets containing the equivalent of 0.2 g of meptazinol add 40 ml of 0.06M *hydrochloric acid*, shake, dilute to 50 ml with the same solvent, filter through a glass-fibre paper (Whatman GF/C paper is suitable); dilute 5 ml of the filtrate to 250 ml with 0.06M *hydrochloric acid* and measure the *absorbance* of the resulting solution at the maximum at 273 nm, Appendix II B. Calculate the content of $C_{15}H_{23}NO$ from the *absorbance* obtained using a 0.0080% w/v solution of *meptazinol hydrochloride BPCRS* in 0.06M *hydrochloric acid* and from the declared content of $C_{15}H_{23}NO$ in *meptazinol hydrochloride BPCRS*.

Storage Meptazinol Tablets should be stored at a temperature not exceeding 25°.

Labelling The label states the quantity of active ingredient in terms of the equivalent amount of meptazinol.

Mepyramine Tablets

Definition Mepyramine Tablets contain Mepyramine Maleate.

The tablets comply with the requirements stated under Tablets and with the following requirements.

Content of mepyramine maleate, $C_{17}H_{23}N_3O$, $C_4H_4O_4$ 95.0 to 105.0% of the prescribed or stated amount.

Identification

A. Shake a quantity of the powdered tablets containing 0.1 g of Mepyramine Maleate with 10 ml of *dichloromethane*, filter and evaporate the filtrate to dryness. The *infrared absorption spectrum* of the residue, Appendix II A, is concordant with the *reference spectrum* of mepyramine maleate.

B. In the test for Related substances, the principal spot in the chromatogram obtained with solution (2) is similar in position and size to that in the chromatogram obtained with solution (4).

C. Dissolve a quantity of the powdered tablets containing 0.2 g of Mepyramine Maleate, freed as far as possible from any sugar coating, in 3 ml of *water*, add 2 ml of 5M *sodium hydroxide* and shake with three 3-ml quantities of *ether*. Warm the aqueous layer in a water bath for 10 minutes with 2 ml of *bromine solution*, heat to boiling, cool and add 0.2 ml to a solution of 10 mg of *resorcinol* in 3 ml of *sulphuric acid*. A bluish black colour is produced on heating for 15 minutes in a water bath.

Related substances Carry out the method for *thin-layer chromatography*, Appendix III A, using *silica gel GF_{254}* as the coating substance and a mixture of 2 volumes of *diethylamine* and 100 volumes of *ethyl acetate* as the mobile phase. Apply separately to the plate 5 µl of each of the following solutions prepared immediately before use. For solution (1) shake a quantity of the powdered tablets containing 0.4 g of Mepyramine Maleate with 10 ml of *chloroform* and filter. For solution (2) dilute 1 volume of solution (1) to 10 volumes with *chloroform*. Solutions (3), (4), (5) and (6) contain 4% w/v, 0.4% w/v, 0.008% w/v and 0.004% w/v of *mepyramine maleate EPCRS* in *chloroform* respectively. After removal of the plate, allow it to dry in air and examine under *ultraviolet light (254 nm)*. Any *secondary spot* in the chromatogram obtained with solution (1) is not more intense than the spot in the chromatogram obtained with solution (5) (0.2%). The test is not valid unless the Rf values of the principal spots in the chromatograms obtained with solutions (1) and (3) are at least 0.2 and unless the spot in the chromatogram obtained with solution (6) is clearly visible. Disregard the spot due to maleic acid on the line of application.

Assay Weigh and powder 20 tablets. To a quantity of the powder containing 0.1 g of Mepyramine Maleate add 75 ml of *water* and 5 ml of 2M *hydrochloric acid*, shake vigorously for 15 minutes and dilute to 100 ml with *water*. Centrifuge and dilute 10 ml of the clear, supernatant liquid to 100 ml with *water*. To 10 ml add 10 ml of 0.1M *hydrochloric acid* and dilute to 100 ml with *water*. Measure the *absorbance* of the resulting solution at the maximum at 316 nm, Appendix II B. Calculate the content of $C_{17}H_{23}N_3O$, $C_4H_4O_4$ taking 206 as the value of A(1%, 1 cm) at the maximum at 316 nm.

Mercaptopurine Tablets

Definition Mercaptopurine Tablets contain Mercaptopurine.

The tablets comply with the requirements stated under Tablets and with the following requirements.

Content of mercaptopurine, $C_5H_4N_4S,H_2O$ 90.0 to 110.0% of the prescribed or stated amount.

Identification Shake a quantity of the powdered tablets containing 50 mg of Mercaptopurine with a mixture of 20 ml of *water* and 0.5 ml of 5M *sodium hydroxide* for not more than 5 minutes, add sufficient *water* to produce 100 ml, mix and filter. Dilute a portion of the filtrate with sufficient 0.1M *hydrochloric acid* to give a final concentration of 0.0005% w/v of Mercaptopurine. The *light absorption* of the resulting solution, Appendix II B, exhibits a maximum at 325 nm.

Assay Weigh and powder 20 tablets. Dissolve a quantity of the powder containing 50 mg of Mercaptopurine as completely as possible in 5 ml of *dimethyl sulphoxide* and add sufficient 0.1M *hydrochloric acid* to produce 500 ml. Dilute 25 ml to 1000 ml with 0.1M *hydrochloric acid*, filter if necessary and measure the *absorbance* of the resulting solution at the maximum at 325 nm, Appendix II B. Calculate the content of $C_5H_4N_4S,H_2O$ taking 1165 as the value of A(1%, 1 cm) at the maximum at 325 nm.

Storage Mercaptopurine Tablets should be protected from light.

Metaraminol Injection

Definition Metaraminol Injection is a sterile solution of Metaraminol Tartrate in Water for Injections.

The injection complies with the requirements stated under Parenteral Preparations and with the following requirements.

Content of metaraminol, $C_9H_{13}NO_2$ 90.0 to 110.0% of the prescribed or stated amount.

Identification

A. In the test for Related substances, the principal spot in the chromatogram obtained with solution (2) corresponds to that in the chromatogram obtained with solution (5).

B. Dilute a volume containing the equivalent of 5 mg of metaraminol to 10 ml with *water* and extract with four 15-ml quantities of *chloroform*. To 0.5 ml of the aqueous layer add 0.5 ml of *lithium and sodium molybdotungstophosphate solution* and 5 ml of *dilute sodium carbonate solution* and allow to stand for 5 minutes. An intense blue colour is produced.

C. To 4 ml of the aqueous layer obtained in test B add 5 ml of *borate buffer pH 9.6* and 1 ml of a freshly prepared 0.5% w/v solution of *sodium 1,2-naphthoquinone-4-sulphonate* and allow to stand for 1 minute. Add 0.2 ml of a 2% v/v solution of *benzalkonium chloride solution* and 5 ml of *toluene* and shake. A mauve colour is produced immediately in the toluene layer (distinction from phenylephrine).

Acidity pH, 3.2 to 4.5, Appendix V L.

Related substances Carry out the test described under Metaraminol Tartrate using the following solutions. For solution (1) evaporate a volume of the injection containing the equivalent of 20 mg of metaraminol to dryness, dissolve the residue as completely as possible in 2 ml of *methanol* and filter. For solution (2) dilute 1 volume of solution (1) to 20 volumes with *methanol*. For solution (3) dilute 1 volume of solution (1) to 100 volumes with *methanol*. Solution (4) contains 0.1% w/v of *methyl 4-hydroxybenzoate* in *methanol*. Solution (5) contains 0.050% w/v of *metaraminol tartrate BPCRS* in *methanol*. Any *secondary spot* in the chromatogram obtained with solution (1), other than any spot corresponding to methyl 4-hydroxybenzoate, is not more intense than the spot in the chromatogram obtained with solution (3).

Assay To a quantity containing the equivalent of 10 mg of metaraminol add sufficient *water* to produce 200 ml. Wash 25 ml with four 25-ml quantities of *chloroform*, discard the washings and filter the aqueous solution. Measure the *absorbance* of the filtrate at the maximum at 272 nm, Appendix II B. Calculate the content of $C_9H_{13}NO_2$ taking 111 as the value of A(1%, 1 cm) at the maximum at 272 nm.

Storage Metaraminol Injection should be protected from light.

Labelling The strength is stated in terms of the equivalent amount of metaraminol in a suitable dose-volume.

Metformin Tablets

Definition Metformin Tablets contain Metformin Hydrochloride. They are coated.

The tablets comply with the requirements stated under Tablets and with the following requirements.

Content of metformin hydrochloride, $C_4H_{11}N_5$,HCl 95.0 to 105.0% of the prescribed or stated amount.

Identification

A. Shake a quantity of the powdered tablets containing 20 mg of Metformin Hydrochloride with 20 ml of *absolute ethanol*, filter, evaporate the filtrate to dryness on a water bath and dry the residue at 105° for 1 hour. The *infrared absorption spectrum* of the residue, Appendix II A, is concordant with the *reference spectrum* of metformin hydrochloride.

B. Triturate a quantity of the powdered tablets containing 50 mg of Metformin Hydrochloride with 10 ml of *water* and filter. To 5 ml of the filtrate add 1.5 ml of 5M *sodium hydroxide*, 1 ml of *strong 1-naphthol solution* and, dropwise with shaking, 0.5 ml of *dilute sodium hypochlorite solution*. An orange-red colour is produced which darkens on standing.

C. Triturate a quantity of the powdered tablets containing 50 mg of Metformin Hydrochloride with 10 ml of *water* and filter. The filtrate yields reaction A characteristic of *chlorides*, Appendix VI.

Dissolution Comply with the *dissolution test for tablets and capsules*, Appendix XII D, using as the medium 900 ml of a 0.68% w/v solution of *potassium dihydrogen orthophosphate* adjusted to pH 6.8 by the addition of 1M *sodium hydroxide* and rotating the basket at 100 revolutions per minute. Withdraw a sample of 10 ml of the medium. Filter, dilute 10 ml of the filtrate to 100 ml with *water* and dilute 10 ml of the resulting solution to 100 ml with *water*. Measure the *absorbance* of a layer of suitable thickness of the filtered sample, suitably diluted if necessary, at the maximum at 233 nm, Appendix II B. Calculate the total content of metformin hydrochloride, $C_4H_{11}N_5$,HCl, in the medium taking 806 as the value of A(1%, 1 cm) at the maximum at 233 nm.

Related substances Carry out the method for *liquid chromatography*, Appendix III D, using the following solutions. For solution (1) shake a quantity of the powdered tablets containing 0.50 g of Metformin Hydrochloride with 100 ml of the mobile phase, filter and use the filtrate. For solution (2) dissolve 20 mg of *1-cyanoguanidine* in *water*, dilute to 100 ml with *water* and dilute 1 ml of the resulting solution to 200 ml with the mobile phase. For solution (3) dilute 1 ml of solution (1) to 50 ml with the mobile phase and dilute 1 ml of the resulting solution to 20 ml with the mobile phase. For solution (4) dissolve 10 mg of *melamine* in about 90 ml of *water*, add 5 ml of solution (1) and dilute to 100 ml with *water*; dilute 1 ml of the solution to 50 ml with the mobile phase.

The chromatographic procedure may be carried out using (a) a stainless steel column (0.125 m × 4.7 mm) packed with a regular, porous silica gel to which benzenesulphonic acid groups have been chemically bonded (5 μm) (Partisphere 5μ SCX is suitable), (b) a 1.7% w/v solution of *ammonium dihydrogen orthophosphate* adjusted to pH 3.0 with *orthophosphoric acid* as the mobile phase with a flow rate of 1 ml per minute and (c) a detection wavelength of 218 nm.

Inject 20 μl of solution (2). Adjust the sensitivity of the system so that the height of the principal peak in the chromatogram obtained is not less than 50% of the full scale of the recorder. Inject 20 μl of solution (4). The test is not valid unless the *resolution factor* between the peaks corresponding to melamine and metformin hydrochloride is at least 10.

Inject separately 20 μl of solutions (1), (2) and (3). Continue the chromatography for twice the retention time of metformin hydrochloride. In the chromatogram obtained with solution (1) the area of any peak corresponding to cyanoguanidine is not greater than the area of the peak in the chromatogram obtained with solution (2) (0.02%) and the area of any other *secondary peak* is not greater than the area of the principal peak in the chromatogram obtained with solution (3) (0.1%).

Assay Weigh and powder 20 tablets. Shake a quantity of the powder containing 0.1 g of Metformin Hydrochloride with 70 ml of *water* for 15 minutes, dilute to 100 ml with *water* and filter, discarding the first 20 ml. Dilute 10 ml of the filtrate to 100 ml with *water* and dilute 10 ml of the resulting solution to 100 ml with *water*. Measure the *absorbance* of the resulting solution at the maximum at 232 nm, Appendix II B. Calculate the content of the $C_4H_{11}N_5$,HCl taking 798 as the value of A(1%, 1 cm) at the maximum at 232 nm.

Methadone Injection

Definition Methadone Injection is a sterile solution of Methadone Hydrochloride in Water for Injections.

The injection complies with the requirements stated under Parenteral Preparations and with the following requirements.

Content of methadone hydrochloride, $C_{21}H_{27}NO$,

HCl 92.5 to 107.5% of the prescribed or stated amount.

Identification Make a volume containing 0.1 g of Methadone Hydrochloride alkaline with 5M *sodium hydroxide*, stir with a glass rod until the precipitate solidifies, filter, wash with *water* and dry over *phosphorus pentoxide* at room temperature at a pressure of 2 kPa. The residue complies with the following tests.

A. The *infrared absorption spectrum*, Appendix II A, is concordant with the *reference spectrum* of methadone.

B. To 5 mg add 0.05 ml of *dinitrobenzene solution* and 0.05 ml of a 50% w/v solution of *sodium hydroxide*. A purple colour is produced which changes slowly to dark brown.

Assay To a volume containing 10 mg of Methadone Hydrochloride add 1 ml of *glacial acetic acid* and dilute to 100 ml with *water*. To 10 ml of this solution add 10 ml of a 0.4% w/v solution of *picric acid* and 10 ml of *phosphate buffer pH 4.9*, extract with three 15-ml quantities of *chloroform* and dilute the combined chloroform extracts to 50 ml with *chloroform*. To 10 ml add sufficient *chloroform* to produce 20 ml and measure the *absorbance* of the resulting solution at the maximum at 350 nm, Appendix II B, using in the reference cell a solution prepared in the same manner but omitting the injection. Calculate the content of $C_{21}H_{27}NO,HCl$ taking 448 as the value of A(1%, 1 cm) at the maximum at 350 nm.

Methadone Linctus

Definition Methadone Linctus is an *oral solution* containing 0.04% w/v of Methadone Hydrochloride in a suitable vehicle with a tolu flavour.

The linctus complies with the requirements stated under Oral Liquids and with the following requirements.

Content of methadone hydrochloride, $C_{21}H_{27}NO$, HCl 0.036 to 0.044% w/v.

Identification To 50 ml add 30 ml of *water* and add 1M *sulphuric acid* until the solution is acidic to *litmus paper*. Extract with two 20-ml quantities of *petroleum spirit (boiling range, 40° to 60°)*, discarding the extracts, and add 5M *sodium hydroxide* until the solution is alkaline to *litmus paper*. Add 4 g of *sodium chloride*, shake to dissolve, extract with two 25-ml quantities of *ether* and wash the combined ether extracts with five 20-ml quantities of *water*. Dry with *anhydrous sodium sulphate*, filter, evaporate to dryness and dry the residue over *phosphorus pentoxide* at a pressure of 2 kPa. The residue complies with the following tests.

A. The *infrared absorption spectrum*, Appendix II A, is concordant with the *reference spectrum* of methadone.

B. To 5 mg add 0.05 ml of *dinitrobenzene solution* and 0.05 ml of a 50% w/v solution of *sodium hydroxide*. A purple colour is produced which changes slowly to dark brown.

Assay To 30 g add 1 ml of *glacial acetic acid* and dilute to 100 ml with *water*. To 10 ml of the resulting solution add 10 ml of a 0.4% w/v solution of *picric acid* and 10 ml of *phosphate buffer pH 4.9*, extract with three 15-ml quantities of *chloroform* and dilute the combined chloroform extracts to 50 ml with *chloroform*. To 10 ml add sufficient *chloroform* to produce 20 ml and measure the *absorbance* of the resulting solution, Appendix II B, at the maximum at 350 nm using in the reference cell a solution prepared in the same manner but using 10 ml of a 1% v/v solution of *glacial acetic acid* and beginning at the words 'add 10 ml ...'. Calculate the content of $C_{21}H_{27}NO,HCl$ taking 448 as the value of A(1%, 1 cm) at the maximum at 350 nm. Determine the *weight per ml*, Appendix V G, and calculate the content of $C_{21}H_{27}NO,HCl$, weight in volume.

Labelling The label indicates the pharmaceutical form as 'oral solution'.

Methadone Tablets

Definition Methadone Tablets contain Methadone Hydrochloride.

The tablets comply with the requirements stated under Tablets and with the following requirements.

Content of methadone hydrochloride, $C_{21}H_{27}NO$, HCl 92.5 to 107.5% of the prescribed or stated amount.

Identification

A. Shake a quantity of the powdered tablets containing 0.1 g of Methadone Hydrochloride with 20 ml of *water* and centrifuge. Make the supernatant liquid alkaline with 5M *sodium hydroxide*, stir with a glass rod until the precipitate solidifies, filter, wash with *water* and dry over *phosphorus pentoxide* at room temperature at a pressure of 2 kPa. The *infrared absorption spectrum* of the residue, Appendix II A, is concordant with the *reference spectrum* of methadone.

B. Extract a quantity of the powdered tablets containing 0.1 g of Methadone Hydrochloride with 10 ml of *water*, filter and wash the residue with sufficient *water* to bring the volume of the filtrate to 10 ml. Add to the filtrate 0.125 g of *picrolonic acid* dissolved in 50 ml of boiling *water*, stir and allow to stand for 2 hours. The *melting point* of the residue, after recrystallisation from *ethanol (20%)*, washing with *ethanol (20%)* and drying at 105°, is about 160° or about 180°, Appendix V A.

C. Extract a quantity of the powdered tablets containing 5 mg of Methadone Hydrochloride with 5 ml of *ethanol (96%)*, filter and evaporate the filtrate to dryness. To the residue add 0.05 ml of *dinitrobenzene solution* and 0.05 ml of a 50% w/v solution of *sodium hydroxide*. A purple colour is produced which changes slowly to dark brown.

Assay Weigh and powder 20 tablets. To a quantity of the powder containing 50 mg of Methadone Hydrochloride add 60 ml of *water* and 5 ml of *glacial acetic acid*, heat on a water bath for 5 minutes, mix with the aid of ultrasound for 10 minutes and dilute to 100 ml with water. Filter through a glass fibre paper, discarding the first 10 ml of filtrate, and dilute 20 ml to 100 ml with *water*. To 10 ml of the resulting solution add 10 ml of *phosphate buffer pH 4.9* and 5 ml of a 0.4% w/v solution of *picric acid*. Extract with three 15-ml quantities of *chloroform* and dilute the combined chloroform extracts to 50 ml with *chloroform*. To 10 ml add sufficient *chloroform* to produce 20 ml and measure the *absorbance* of the resulting solution, Appendix II B, at the maximum at 350 nm using in the reference cell a solution prepared in the same manner but using a 5% v/v solution of *glacial acetic acid* and beginning at the words 'Filter through a glass fibre paper ...'. Calculate the content of $C_{21}H_{27}NO,HCl$ taking 448 as the value of A(1%, 1 cm) at the maximum at 350 nm.

Methohexital Injection

Definition Methohexital Injection is a sterile solution of methohexital sodium in Water for Injections free from carbon dioxide. It is prepared by dissolving Methohexital Sodium for Injection in the requisite amount of Water for Injections free from carbon dioxide.

The injection complies with the requirements stated under Parenteral Preparations.

Storage Methohexital Injection should be used immediately after preparation but, in any case, within the period recommended by the manufacturer when prepared and stored strictly in accordance with the manufacturer's instructions.

METHOHEXITAL SODIUM FOR INJECTION

Definition Methohexital Sodium for Injection is a sterile mixture of 100 parts by weight of the monosodium salt of methohexital [5-allyl-1-methyl-5-(1-methylpent-2-ynyl)barbituric acid] (a-form) and 6 parts by weight of dried sodium carbonate with or without excipients. It is supplied in a sealed container.

The contents of the sealed container comply with the requirements for Powders for Injections stated under Parenteral Preparations and with the following requirements.

Content of methohexital sodium, $C_{14}H_{17}N_2NaO_3$ 90.0 to 95.0%, calculated with reference to the dried material, and 95.0 to 105.0% of the prescribed or stated amount.

Content of Na 9.5 to 10.5%, calculated with reference to the dried material.

Identification

A. Dissolve 0.5 g in 10 ml of *water*, add 10 ml of 0.1M *hydrochloric acid*, filter, wash the precipitate with *water* and dry at 70° at a pressure not exceeding 0.7 kPa. The *infrared absorption spectrum* of the residue, Appendix II A, is concordant with the *reference spectrum* of methohexital.

B. The residue on incineration yields the reactions characteristic of *sodium salts*, Appendix VI.

C. Yield the reactions characteristic of *carbonates*, Appendix VI.

Melting point of methohexital Heat 0.3 g of the residue obtained in the Assay for methohexital sodium on a water bath with 10 ml of *ethanol (70%)* until dissolved, allow to cool, filter through sintered glass, wash the crystals with a small quantity of *ethanol (70%)* and dry at 70° at a pressure not exceeding 0.7 kPa. The *melting point* of the crystals is 92° to 96°, Appendix V A.

Alkalinity pH of a 5% w/v solution, 10.6 to 11.6, Appendix V L.

Clarity of solution A 5.0% w/v solution in *carbon dioxide-free water* is *clear*, Appendix IV A.

Chloride Dissolve 0.24 g in 40 ml of *water*, add 10 ml of 2M *nitric acid* and extract with three 25-ml quantities of *ether*. The aqueous layer complies with the *limit test for chlorides*, Appendix VII (700 ppm).

Related substances Carry out the method for *thin-layer chromatography*, Appendix III A, using *silica gel GF_{254}* as the coating substance and a mixture of 75 volumes of *chloroform* and 25 volumes of *ether* as the mobile phase. Apply separately to the plate 10 µl of each of the following solutions. For solution (1) dissolve a quantity of the contents of a sealed container in sufficient *water* to produce a solution containing 1% w/v of methohexital sodium. For solution (2) dilute 1 volume of solution (1) to 100 volumes with *water*. After removal of the plate, allow it to dry in air and examine under *ultraviolet light (254 nm)*. Any *secondary spot* in the chromatogram obtained with solution (1) is not more intense than the spot in the chromatogram obtained with solution (2).

Loss on drying When dried to constant weight at 70° at a pressure not exceeding 0.7 kPa, lose not more than 3.0% of their weight. Use 0.5 g.

Assay Determine the weight of the contents of 10 containers as described in the test for Uniformity of weight under Parenteral Preparations, Powders for Injections.

For Na Dissolve 0.6 g of the mixed contents of the 10 containers in 20 ml of *water* and titrate with 0.1M *hydrochloric acid VS*, using *methyl red solution* as indicator, until the yellow colour changes to pink; boil gently for 1 to 2 minutes, cool and if necessary continue the titration with 0.1M *hydrochloric acid VS* until the pink colour is restored. Each ml of 0.1M *hydrochloric acid VS* is equivalent to 2.299 mg of Na.

For methohexital sodium To the liquid from the completed Assay for Na add a further 5 ml of 0.1M *hydrochloric acid* and extract with successive quantities of 25, 25, 20, 15, 15 and 10 ml of *chloroform*, washing each extract with the same 5 ml of *water*. Remove the chloroform from the mixed extracts by evaporation and dry the residue to constant weight at 70° at a pressure not exceeding 0.7 kPa. Each g of residue is equivalent to 1.084 g of $C_{14}H_{17}N_2NaO_3$. Calculate the content of $C_{14}H_{17}N_2NaO_3$ in a container of average content weight.

Labelling The label of the sealed container states the equivalent amount of methohexital sodium contained in it.

Action and use Anaesthetic.

When methohexitone injection is prescribed or demanded, Methohexital Injection shall be dispensed or supplied.

Methotrexate Injection

Definition Methotrexate Injection is a sterile solution of Methotrexate in Water for Injections containing Sodium Hydroxide.

The injection complies with the requirements stated under Parenteral Preparations and with the following requirements.

Content of methotrexate, $C_{20}H_{22}N_8O_5$ 95.0 to 110.0% of the prescribed or stated amount.

Characteristics A yellowish solution.

Identification The *light absorption*, Appendix II B, of the final solution obtained in the Assay exhibits maxima at 242 nm and 306 nm.

Alkalinity pH, 7.5 to 9.0, Appendix V L.

Assay Carry out the method for *liquid chromatography*, Appendix III D, using the following solutions. Solution (1) contains 0.0025% w/v of *methotrexate EPCRS* in the mobile phase. For solution (2) dilute a volume of the injection with the mobile phase to produce a solution containing 0.0025% w/v of Methotrexate. Solution (3) contains 0.0025% w/v each of *methotrexate EPCRS* and *folic acid* in the mobile phase.

The chromatographic procedure may be carried out using (a) a stainless steel column (20 cm × 4.6 mm), packed with *stationary phase C* (5 μm) (Spherisorb ODS 1 is suitable), (b) a mixture of 92 volumes of *phosphate buffer pH 6.0* and 8 volumes of *acetonitrile* as the mobile phase with a flow rate of 1.4 ml per minute and (c) a detection wavelength of 303 nm.

The assay is not valid unless the *resolution factor* between the peaks due to methotrexate and folic acid in the chromatogram obtained with solution (3) is at least 5.0.

Calculate the content of $C_{20}H_{22}N_8O_5$ using the declared content of $C_{20}H_{22}N_8O_5$ in *methotrexate EPCRS*.

Storage Methotrexate Injection should be protected from light.

Labelling When an antimicrobial preservative is present the label states that the contents are not intended for intrathecal injection.

Methotrexate Tablets

Definition Methotrexate Tablets contain Methotrexate or methotrexate sodium prepared by the interaction of Methotrexate with Sodium Hydroxide.

The tablets comply with the requirements stated under Tablets and with the following requirements.

Content of methotrexate, $C_{20}H_{22}N_8O_5$ 90.0 to 110.0% of the prescribed or stated amount.

Identification Extract a quantity of the powdered tablets containing 10 mg of Methotrexate with sufficient 0.1M *sodium hydroxide* to produce 100 ml, filter and dilute 10 ml of the filtrate to 100 ml with 0.1M *sodium hydroxide*. The *light absorption* of the resulting solution, Appendix II B, exhibits three maxima, at 258, 303 and 371 nm.

Disintegration Maximum time, 30 minutes, Appendix XII A.

Dissolution Comply with the *dissolution test for tablets and capsules*, Appendix XII D, using Apparatus II. Use as the medium 900 ml of 0.1M *hydrochloric acid* and rotate the paddle at 50 revolutions per minute. Withdraw a 10-ml sample of the medium and measure the *absorbance* of the filtered sample, suitably diluted if necessary with 0.1M *hydrochloric acid*, at the maximum at 303 nm, Appendix II B. At the same time measure the *absorbance* at the maximum at 303 nm of a suitable solution of *methotrexate EPCRS* in the dissolution medium. Calculate the total content of methotrexate, $C_{20}H_{22}N_8O_5$, in the medium from the *absorbances* obtained and from the declared content of $C_{20}H_{22}N_8O_5$ in *methotrexate EPCRS*.

Assay Weigh and powder 20 tablets. Carry out the method for *liquid chromatography*, Appendix III D, using the following solutions. Solution (1) contains 0.0025% w/v of *methotrexate EPCRS* in the mobile phase. For solution (2) mix a quantity of the powdered tablets containing 2.5 mg of Methotrexate with 100 ml of the mobile phase with the aid of ultrasound, centrifuge and use the supernatant liquid. Solution (3) contains 0.0025% w/v each of *methotrexate EPCRS* and *folic acid* in the mobile phase.

The chromatographic procedure may be carried out using (a) a stainless steel column (20 cm × 4.6 mm), packed with *stationary phase C* (5 μm) (Spherisorb ODS 1 is suitable), (b) a mixture of 92 volumes of *phosphate buffer pH 6.0* and 8 volumes of *acetonitrile* as the mobile phase with a flow rate of 1.4 ml per minute and (c) a detection wavelength of 303 nm.

The assay is not valid unless the *resolution factor* between the peaks due to methotrexate and folic acid in the chromatogram obtained with solution (3) is at least 5.0.

Calculate the content of $C_{20}H_{22}N_8O_5$ using the declared content of $C_{20}H_{22}N_8O_5$ in *methotrexate EPCRS*.

Storage Methotrexate Tablets should be protected from light.

Labelling When the active ingredient is methotrexate sodium, the quantity is expressed in terms of the equivalent amount of Methotrexate.

Methoxamine Injection

Definition Methoxamine Injection is a sterile solution containing 2% w/v of Methoxamine Hydrochloride in Water for Injections.

The injection complies with the requirements stated under Parenteral Preparations and with the following requirements.

Content of methoxamine hydrochloride, $C_{11}H_{17}NO_3$,HCl 1.90 to 2.10% w/v.

Characteristics A colourless or almost colourless solution.

Identification

A. The *light absorption* of the solution obtained in the Assay, Appendix II B, in the range 230 to 350 nm exhibits a maximum only at 290 nm.

B. Dilute 1 ml with 1 ml of *water*, add 5 ml of *diazotised nitroaniline solution* and 1 ml of *dilute sodium carbonate solution*, allow to stand for 2 minutes and add 1 ml of 1M *sodium hydroxide*. A deep red colour is produced which is extractable with *butan-1-ol*.

Related substances Carry out the method for *thin-layer chromatography*, Appendix III A, using *silica gel GF_{254}* as the coating substance and a mixture of 86 volumes of *chloroform*, 12 volumes of *methanol* and 2 volumes of 13.5M *ammonia* as the mobile phase. Apply separately to the plate 5 μl of each of the following solutions. For solution (1) use the injection being examined. Solution (2) contains 0.010% w/v of *2,5-dimethoxybenzaldehyde* in *methanol*. For solution (3) dilute 1 volume of the injection to 100 volumes with *water*. After removal of the plate, allow it to dry in air and examine under *ultraviolet light (365 nm)*. Any spot corresponding to 2,5-dimethoxybenzaldehyde in the chromatogram obtained with solution (1) is not more intense than the spot in the chromatogram obtained with solution (2). Spray the plate with a 0.3% w/v solution of *ninhydrin* in *butan-1-ol* containing 3% v/v of *glacial acetic acid* and heat at 105° for 5 minutes. Any other *secondary spot* in the chromatogram obtained with solution (1) is not more intense than the spot in the chromatogram obtained with solution (3).

Assay Dilute 1 ml to 100 ml with *water*, further dilute 20 ml of this solution to 100 ml with *water* and measure the *absorbance* of the resulting solution at the maximum at 290 nm, Appendix II B. Calculate the content of $C_{11}H_{17}NO_3$,HCl taking 137 as the value of A(1%, 1 cm) at the maximum at 290 nm.

Methyl Salicylate Liniment

Definition Methyl Salicylate is a *cutaneous emulsion*. It contains 25% v/v of Methyl Salicylate in Arachis Oil or other suitable fixed oil.

The liniment complies with the requirements stated under Liquids for Cutaneous Application and with the following requirements.

Content of methyl salicylate, $C_8H_8O_3$ 23.0 to 26.5% v/v.

Identification

A. In the Assay, the chromatogram obtained with solution (2) shows a peak with the same retention time as that due to methyl salicylate in the chromatogram obtained with solution (1).

B. The liniment has a characteristic odour.

Assay Carry out the method for *gas chromatography*, Appendix III B, using three solutions in *petroleum spirit (boiling range, 80° to 100°)* containing (1) 1% w/v of *benzyl alcohol* (internal standard) and 1% w/v of *methyl salicylate*, (2) 4% w/v of the liniment and (3) 4% w/v of the liniment and 1% w/v of the internal standard.

The chromatographic procedure may be carried out using a glass column (1.5 m × 4 mm) packed with *diatomaceous support* (60 to 80 mesh) coated with 10% w/w of polyethylene glycol 1540 and maintained at 110°.

Determine the *weight per ml* of the liniment, Appendix V G, and calculate the content of $C_8H_8O_3$, volume in volume, taking the content of $C_8H_8O_3$ in *methyl salicylate* to be 100.0% and its *weight per ml* to be 1.18 g.

Labelling The label indicates the pharmaceutical form as 'cutaneous emulsion'.

Methyl Salicylate Ointment

Strong Methyl Salicylate Ointment

Definition Methyl Salicylate Ointment contains 50% w/w of Methyl Salicylate in a suitable water-emulsifying basis.

Extemporaneous preparation The following formula and directions apply.

Methyl Salicylate	500 g
White Beeswax	250 g
Hydrous Wool Fat	250 g

Melt together the White Beeswax and the Hydrous Wool Fat, cool, add the Methyl Salicylate and stir until cold.

The ointment complies with the requirements stated under Topical Semi-solid Preparations and with the following requirements.

Content of methyl salicylate, $C_8H_8O_3$ 45.0 to 52.5% w/w.

Identification

A. In the Assay, the chromatogram obtained with solution (2) shows a peak with the same retention time as that due to methyl salicylate in the chromatogram obtained with solution (1).

B. The ointment has a characteristic odour.

Assay Carry out the method for *gas chromatography*, Appendix III B, using three solutions in *petroleum spirit (boiling range, 80° to 100°)* containing (1) 1% w/v of *benzyl alcohol* (internal standard) and 1% w/v of *methyl salicylate*, (2) 2% w/v of the ointment and (3) 2% w/v of the ointment and 1% w/v of the internal standard.

The chromatographic procedure may be carried out using a glass column (1.5 m × 4 mm) packed with *diatomaceous support* (60 to 80 mesh) coated with 10% w/w of polyethylene glycol 1540 and maintained at 110°.

Calculate the content of $C_8H_8O_3$ taking 100.0% as the content of $C_8H_8O_3$ in *methyl salicylate*.

Storage Certain plastic containers, such as those made from polystyrene, are unsuitable for Methyl Salicylate Ointment.

Methylcellulose Granules

Definition

Methylcellulose	64 g
Amaranth, food grade of commerce	20 mg
Saccharin Sodium	100 mg
Vanillin	200 mg
Acacia	4 g
Lactose	sufficient to produce 100 g

Extemporaneous preparation The following directions apply.

Mix the ingredients, in powder, add sufficient Water to form a coherent mass suitable for granulation, pass the mass through a sieve with a nominal mesh aperture of 2.8 mm, place the granules on a sieve with a nominal mesh aperture of 710 µm, discard the material passing through the sieve and dry the granules at a temperature not exceeding 60°.

The granules comply with the requirements stated under Granules and with the following requirements.

Kinematic viscosity of aqueous solution Not less than 2000 $mm^2 s^{-1}$ when determined by the following method. To 3.25 g in a wide-necked bottle add 100 ml of *water* previously heated to 85° to 90°, close the bottle with a device fitted with a stirrer, stir for 10 minutes, place the bottle in ice, continue stirring until the solution is of uniform consistency, remove the bottle from the ice and allow the solution to attain ambient temperature. Determine the *kinematic viscosity* of the solution, Appendix V H, Method II, using a suspended-level viscometer (size 4).

Storage Methylcellulose Granules should be kept in a wide-mouthed, airtight container.

Methylcellulose Tablets

Definition Methylcellulose Tablets contain Methylcellulose 450 in a suitable flavoured basis.

The tablets comply with the requirements stated under Tablets and with the following requirements.

Identification

A. Whilst stirring, introduce a quantity of the powdered tablets containing 1.0 g of Methylcellulose 450 into 50 ml of *carbon dioxide-free water* heated at 90°. Allow to cool, dilute to 100 ml with the same solvent and continue stirring until solution is complete (solution A). Heat 10 ml of solution A in a water bath, with stirring. At temperatures above 50° either the solution becomes cloudy or a flocculent precipitate is produced. The solution becomes clear on cooling.

B. Mix thoroughly a quantity of the powdered tablets containing 1 g of Methylcellulose 450 with 2 g of finely powdered *manganese(II) sulphate* in a test tube about 16 cm long. Impregnate a strip of filter paper with a freshly prepared mixture of 1 volume of a 20% v/v solution of *diethanolamine* and 11 volumes of a 5% w/v solution of *sodium nitroprusside* adjusted to pH 9.8 with 1M *hydrochloric acid*. Insert the strip to a depth of 2 cm into the upper part of the tube, immerse the tube to a depth of 8 cm in a silicone oil bath and heat at 190° to 200°. The filter paper does not become blue within 10 minutes. Carry out a blank test.

Kinematic viscosity For tablets containing 500 mg of Methylcellulose 450, at 20°, 350 to 550 $mm^2\ s^{-1}$, when determined by the following method. Place 2.6 g of the powdered tablets in a wide-mouthed bottle, add 100 ml of *water* heated to 85° to 90°, close the bottle with a stopper fitted with a stirrer and stir for 10 minutes. Cool in ice and continue stirring until the solution is of uniform consistence. Remove the ice and allow the solution to attain room temperature. Determine the *kinematic viscosity* of the solution, Appendix V H, Method II, using a suspended-level viscometer (size 3).

Disintegration The requirement for Disintegration does not apply to Methylcellulose Tablets.

Labelling The label states that the tablets should be broken in the mouth before swallowing.

Methyldopa Tablets

Definition Methyldopa Tablets contain Methyldopa. They are coated.

The tablets comply with the requirements stated under Tablets and with the following requirements.

Content of anhydrous methyldopa, $C_{10}H_{13}NO_4$ 95.0 to 105.0% of the prescribed or stated amount.

Identification Remove the coating from a suitable number of tablets by washing with *chloroform*. To a quantity of the powdered tablet cores containing the equivalent of 5 g of anhydrous methyldopa add 35 ml of a mixture of equal volumes of *chloroform* and *methanol* and shake for 3 minutes. Centrifuge and discard the supernatant liquid. Repeat the operation with a further 35 ml of a mixture of equal volumes of *chloroform* and *methanol*. Dry the residue in a current of nitrogen, add 20 ml of *methanol* and 15 ml of 2M *hydrochloric acid*, shake for 2 minutes and filter. Adjust the pH of the filtrate to 4.9 with 5M *ammonia*, allow to stand for several hours at 2° to 8° and filter. Wash the precipitate with 15 ml of *water* and dry it at 50° at a pressure not exceeding 0.7 kPa for 3 hours. Reserve a portion of the residue for the test for Optical rotation. The remainder of the residue complies with the following tests.

A. The *infrared absorption spectrum*, Appendix II A, is concordant with the *reference spectrum* of methyldopa.

B. Carry out the method for *thin-layer chromatography*, Appendix III A, using *microcrystalline cellulose* as the coating substance and a mixture of 50 volumes of *butan-1-ol*, 25 volumes of *glacial acetic acid* and 25 volumes of *water* as the mobile phase. Apply separately to the plate 5 µl of each of two solutions in 1M *hydrochloric acid* containing (1) 1% w/v of the residue and (2) 1% w/v of *methyldopa BPCRS*. After removal of the plate, dry it in a current of warm air and spray with a freshly prepared mixture of equal volumes of a 10% w/v solution of *iron(III) chloride hexahydrate* and a 5% w/v solution of *potassium hexacyanoferrate(III)*. The principal spot in the chromatogram obtained with solution (1) corresponds to that in the chromatogram obtained with solution (2).

C. Add 0.1 ml of *iron(III) chloride solution R1* to 5 ml of a 0.4% w/v solution in 0.1M *hydrochloric acid*; a green colour is produced. To half of the solution add an excess of 5M *ammonia*; a purple colour is produced. To the remainder of the solution add an excess of 5M *sodium hydroxide*; a red colour is produced.

Optical rotation Determine the content of $C_{10}H_{13}NO_4$ in the residue reserved in the test for Identification by carrying out Method I for *non-aqueous titration*, Appendix VIII A, using 0.2 g of the residue and *crystal violet solution* as indicator. Each ml of 0.1M *perchloric acid VS* is equivalent to 21.12 mg of $C_{10}H_{13}NO_4$. Dissolve a quantity of the residue containing 0.39 g of $C_{10}H_{13}NO_4$ in sufficient *aluminium chloride solution* to produce 10 ml. The *optical rotation* of the resulting solution at 25° is –0.98° to –1.09°, Appendix V F.

Assay Weigh and powder 20 tablets. Dissolve a quantity of the powder containing the equivalent of 0.1 g of anhydrous methyldopa as completely as possible in sufficient 0.05M *sulphuric acid* to produce 100 ml and filter. To 5 ml of the filtrate add 2 ml of *iron(II) sulphate—citrate solution*, 8 ml of *glycine buffer solution* and sufficient *water* to produce 100 ml. Measure the *absorbance* of the resulting solution at the maximum at 545 nm, Appendix II B. Repeat the procedure using 5 ml of a 0.10% w/v solution of *methyldopa BPCRS* in place of 5 ml of the filtrate, beginning at the words 'add 2 ml of ...'. Calculate the content of $C_{10}H_{13}NO_4$ using the declared content of $C_{10}H_{13}NO_4$ in *methyldopa BPCRS*.

Storage Methyldopa Tablets should be protected from light.

Labelling The quantity of active ingredient is expressed in terms of the equivalent amount of anhydrous methyldopa.

Methyldopate Injection

Definition Methyldopate Injection is a sterile solution prepared by dissolving Methyldopate Hydrochloride in Water for Injections.

The injection complies with the requirements stated under Parenteral Preparations and with the following requirements.

Content of methyldopate hydrochloride and methyldopa calculated as $C_{12}H_{17}NO_4,HCl$ The equivalent of 92.5 to 107.5% of the prescribed or stated amount of Methyldopate Hydrochloride.

Identification

A. Dilute with 0.1M *hydrochloric acid* to produce a solution containing 0.004% w/v of Methyldopate Hydrochloride.

The *light absorption* of the resulting solution, Appendix II B, exhibits a maximum only at 280 nm.

B. Dilute with 0.1M *hydrochloric acid* to produce a solution containing 2% w/v of Methyldopate Hydrochloride. The *optical rotation* of the resulting solution, measured at 25° in a 2-dm tube, is –0.28° to –0.35°, Appendix V F.

C. Yields reaction A characteristic of *chlorides*, Appendix VI.

Acidity pH, 3.0 to 4.2, Appendix V L.

Methyldopa Not more than 10% of the declared content of Methyldopate Hydrochloride when determined as described in the Assay and calculated as $C_{12}H_{17}NO_4,HCl$.

Assay Carry out the method for *liquid chromatography*, Appendix III D, using the following solutions. Solution (1) contains 0.1% w/v of *methyldopate hydrochloride BPCRS* and 0.01% w/v of *methyldopa BPCRS* in the mobile phase. For solution (2) dilute a volume of the injection being examined with the mobile phase to contain 0.1% w/v of Methyldopate Hydrochloride.

The chromatographic procedure may be carried out using (a) a stainless steel column (20 cm × 4.6 mm) packed with *stationary phase C* (10 µm) (Nucleosil C18 is suitable), (b) a 0.3% w/v solution of *sodium dihydrogen orthophosphate* in a mixture of 155 volumes of *water* and 45 volumes of *methanol*, the mixture containing 0.1% v/v of *orthophosphoric acid* as the mobile phase with a flow rate of 1 ml per minute and (c) a detection wavelength of 280 nm.

Determine the content of methyldopa, expressed as methyldopate hydrochloride, $C_{12}H_{17}NO_4,HCl$, using the declared content of $C_{10}H_{13}NO_4$ in *methyldopa BPCRS* and taking each mg of $C_{10}H_{13}NO_4$ as equivalent to 1.305 mg of $C_{12}H_{17}NO_4,HCl$. Determine the content of $C_{12}H_{17}NO_4,HCl$ from the declared content of $C_{12}H_{17}NO_4,HCl$ in *methyldopate hydrochloride BPCRS*. Calculate the total content of methyldopate hydrochloride and methyldopa as $C_{12}H_{17}NO_4,HCl$ as the sum of the two determinations.

Storage Methyldopate Injection should be protected from light.

Methylprednisolone Acetate Injection

Definition Methylprednisolone Acetate Injection is a sterile suspension of Methylprednisolone Acetate in Water for Injections. It is prepared using aseptic technique.

The injection complies with the requirements stated under Parenteral Preparations and with the following requirements.

Content of methylprednisolone acetate, $C_{24}H_{32}O_6$ 90.0 to 110.0% of the prescribed or stated amount.

Characteristics A white suspension which settles on standing but readily disperses on shaking. On examination under a microscope, the particles are seen to be crystalline and rarely exceed 20 µm in diameter.

Identification Dilute a volume containing 0.1 g of Methylprednisolone Acetate to 5 ml with *water*, centrifuge and discard the supernatant liquid. Wash the residue with five 5-ml quantities of *water*, resuspending the residue in the *water* each time, centrifuging and discarding the washings. The residue, after drying at 105° for 3 hours, complies with the following tests.

A. The *infrared absorption spectrum*, Appendix II A, is concordant with the *reference spectrum* of methylprednisolone acetate.

B. Complies with the test for *identification of steroids*, Appendix III A, using *impregnating solvent I* and *mobile phase A*.

Acidity or alkalinity pH, 3.5 to 7.0, Appendix V L.

Assay Carry out the method for *liquid chromatography*, Appendix III D, using the following solutions. Mix 0.12 g of *prednisone BPCRS* (internal standard) with 0.6 ml of *glacial acetic acid*, slowly add *chloroform* with the aid of ultrasound, shake to dissolve and dilute with sufficient *chloroform* to produce 20 ml (solution A). For solution (1) add 10 ml of solution A to a quantity of the injection containing 40 mg of Methylprednisolone Acetate, add sufficient *chloroform* to produce 25 ml and shake for 15 minutes or until the aqueous layer is clear; to 4 ml of the chloroform layer, add 30 ml of *chloroform* and 0.4 g of *anhydrous sodium sulphate*, shake for 5 minutes and use the clear solution. For solution (2) dissolve 20 mg of *methylprednisolone acetate BPCRS* in 5 ml of solution A and add sufficient *chloroform* to produce 100 ml.

The chromatographic procedure may be carried out using (a) a column (25 cm × 4 mm) packed with *stationary phase A* (5 to 10 µm), (b) a mixture of 30 volumes of *glacial acetic acid*, 35 volumes of *methanol*, 70 volumes of *tetrahydrofuran*, 475 volumes of water-saturated *1-chlorobutane* and 475 volumes of *1-chlorobutane* as the mobile phase with a flow rate of 1 ml per minute and (c) a detection wavelength of 254 nm.

The assay is not valid unless the *resolution factor* between the peaks due to methylprednisolone acetate and the internal standard is at least 2.5.

Calculate the content of $C_{24}H_{32}O_6$ from the declared content of $C_{24}H_{32}O_6$ in *methylprednisolone acetate BPCRS*.

Storage Methylprednisolone Acetate Injection should be protected from light and stored at a temperature not exceeding 30°. It should not be allowed to freeze.

Labelling The label states (1) that the preparation is not to be given by intravenous injection; (2) that the container should be shaken gently before a dose is withdrawn.

Methylprednisolone Tablets

Definition Methylprednisolone Tablets contain Methylprednisolone.

With the exception of the requirements for shape, the tablets comply with the requirements stated under Tablets and with the following requirements.

Content of methylprednisolone, $C_{22}H_{30}O_5$ 90.0 to 110.0% of the prescribed or stated amount.

Identification

Extract a quantity of the powdered tablets containing 50 mg with 100 ml of *chloroform*, filter and evaporate the filtrate to dryness. The residue complies with the following tests.

A. The *infrared absorption spectrum*, Appendix II A, is concordant with the *reference spectrum* of methylprednisolone.

B. Complies with test B described under Methylprednisolone.

Dissolution Comply with the *dissolution test for tablets and capsules*, Appendix XII D, using as the medium 900 ml of *water* and rotating the basket at 100 revolutions per minute. Withdraw a sample of 5 ml of the medium. Measure the *absorbance* of a layer of suitable thickness of the filtered sample at the maximum at 256 nm, Appendix II B. Calculate the total content of methylprednisolone, $C_{22}H_{30}O_5$, in the medium taking 400 as the value of A(1%, 1 cm) at the maximum at 256 nm.

Related substances Carry out the method for *thin-layer chromatography*, Appendix III A, using as the coating substance a suitable silica gel containing a fluorescent indicator with an optimal intensity at 254 nm and a mixture of 1.2 volumes of *water*, 8 volumes of *methanol*, 15 volumes of *ether* and 77 volumes of *dichloromethane* as the mobile phase. Apply separately to the plate 5 µl of each of the following solutions. For solution (1) shake a quantity of the powdered tablets containing 20 mg of Methylprednisolone for 15 minutes with 2 ml of a mixture of 1 volume of *methanol* and 9 volumes of *chloroform*, centrifuge and use the supernatant liquid. For solution (2) dilute 1 volume of the supernatant liquid to 50 volumes with the same solvent mixture. For solution (3) dilute 1 volume of solution (2) to 4 volumes with the same solvent mixture. For solution (4) dissolve 1 mg of *hydrocortisone* in a mixture of 0.1 ml of solution (1) and 0.9 ml of *methanol.* After removal of the plate, allow it to dry in air and examine under *ultraviolet light (254 nm)*. Any *secondary spot* in the chromatogram obtained with solution (1) is not more intense than the spot in the chromatogram obtained with solution (2) (2%) and not more than one such spot is more intense than the spot in the chromatogram obtained with solution (3) (0.5%). The test is not valid unless the chromatogram obtained with solution (4) shows two principal spots that are close together but separated.

Assay Weigh and powder 20 tablets. Suspend a quantity of the powder containing 10 mg of Methylprednisolone in 10 ml of *water* and extract with successive quantities of 100, 50, 50 and 40 ml of *chloroform*. Wash each extract with the same 10-ml quantity of *water*, filter and dilute the combined filtrates to 250 ml with *chloroform*. Evaporate 25 ml just to dryness, dissolve the residue in sufficient *aldehyde-free ethanol (96%)* to produce a solution containing between 390 and 410 µg of Methylprednisolone in 10 ml and complete the *tetrazolium assay of steroids*, Appendix VIII J, beginning at the words 'Transfer 10 ml ...'.

Dissolve a quantity of *methylprednisolone BPCRS* in sufficient *aldehyde-free ethanol (96%)* to produce a solution containing between 390 and 410 µg in 10 ml and complete the tetrazolium assay beginning at the words 'Transfer 10 ml ...'. From the *absorbances* so obtained, and using the declared content of $C_{22}H_{30}O_5$ in *methylprednisolone BPCRS*, calculate the content of $C_{22}H_{30}O_5$ in the tablets.

Storage Methylprednisolone Tablets should be protected from light.

Methysergide Tablets

Definition Methysergide Tablets contain Methysergide Maleate. They are coated.

The tablets comply with the requirements stated under Tablets and with the following requirements.

Content of methysergide, $C_{21}H_{27}N_3O_2$ 90.0 to 110.0% of the prescribed or stated amount.

Identification

A. In the test for Related substances, the principal spot in the chromatogram obtained with solution (1) corresponds to that in the chromatogram obtained with solution (8).

B. To 5 ml of solution A obtained in the Assay add 10 ml of *dimethylaminobenzaldehyde solution R6*. A violet-blue colour is produced.

Dissolution Carry out the following procedure protected from light. The tablets comply with the *dissolution test for tablets and capsules*, Appendix XII D, using as the medium 500 ml of 0.1M *hydrochloric acid* and rotating the basket at 120 revolutions per minute. Withdraw a sample of 20 ml of the medium and filter through a membrane filter having a nominal pore size not greater than 0.45 µm, discarding the first 10 ml of filtrate. Carry out the method for *liquid chromatography*, Appendix III D, using the following solutions protected from light. For solution (1) dissolve 15 mg of *methysergide maleate BPCRS* in 500 ml of 0.1M *hydrochloric acid* and dilute 10 ml to 100 ml with 0.1M *hydrochloric acid.* Solution (2) is the filtrate from the dissolution vessel.

The chromatographic procedure may be carried out using (a) a stainless steel column (20 cm × 4.6 mm) packed with *stationary phase B* (5 µm) (Spherisorb C8 is suitable), (b) a mixture of 65 volumes of 0.01M *diammonium hydrogen orthophosphate* and 35 volumes of *acetonitrile* as the mobile phase with a flow rate of 2 ml per minute and (c) a fluorimetric detector with an excitation wavelength of 325 nm and an emission wavelength of 430 nm.

Calculate the total content of methysergide, $C_{21}H_{27}N_3O_2$, in the medium using the declared content of $C_{21}H_{27}N_3O_2$ in *methysergide maleate BPCRS*.

Related substances Carry out in subdued light the method for *thin-layer chromatography*, Appendix III A, using a suspension of *silica gel G* in 0.1M *sodium hydroxide* to prepare the plate and a mixture of 90 volumes of *chloroform* and 10 volumes of *methanol* as the mobile phase. Apply separately to the plate 10 µl of each of the following solutions. For solution (1) place a quantity of the powdered tablets containing the equivalent of 5.0 mg of methysergide in a sintered-glass filter, add 10 ml of *petroleum spirit (boiling range, 40° to 60°)*, stir for 2 minutes and filter. Repeat the washing with two further 10-ml quantities of the petroleum spirit and discard the washings. Extract with four 20-ml quantities of a solution prepared by shaking 100 ml of *chloroform* vigorously with 0.15 ml of 13.5M *ammonia*. Evaporate the filtrate to dryness at room temperature at a pressure of 2 kPa and dissolve the residue in 1 ml of a mixture of 1 volume of 13.5M *ammonia* and 100 volumes of *methanol.* Solutions (2), (3), (4), (5), (6) and (7) contain the equivalent of 0.0025% w/v, 0.005% w/v, 0.01% w/v, 0.015% w/v, 0.02% w/v and 0.025% w/v respectively of methysergide and are prepared by diluting appropriate volumes of solution (8) with a mixture of 1 volume of 13.5M *ammonia* and 100 volumes of *methanol*. For solution (8) dissolve 14 mg of *methysergide maleate BPCRS* in a mixture of 1 ml of *ethanol (96%)* and 19 ml of a 1% w/v solution of *(+)-tartaric acid*. Make alkaline by the addition of 0.15 ml of 13.5M *ammonia* and extract with successive quantities of 20, 10, 10 and 10 ml of *chloroform*. Filter the combined extracts and evaporate to dryness at room temperature at a pressure of 2 kPa. Dissolve the residue in 2 ml of a mixture of 1 volume of 13.5M *ammonia* and 100 volumes of *methanol*.

After removal of the plate, allow it to dry in air and examine under *ultraviolet light (365 nm)*. Assess the intensities of any *secondary spots* in the chromatogram obtained with solution (1) by reference to the spots in the chromatograms obtained with solutions (2) to (7), making allowance for area in assessing the intensities of spots with different Rf values and disregarding any spots less intense than the spot in the chromatogram obtained with solution (2). The sum of the intensities so assessed does not exceed 5% of the intensity of the principal spot in the chromatogram obtained with solution (1).

Uniformity of content Tablets containing less than the equivalent of 2 mg of methysergide comply with the requirements stated under Tablets using the following method of analysis protected from light. To one tablet add 50 ml of a 1% w/v solution of *(+)-tartaric acid*, shake for 30 minutes and centrifuge. Measure the *absorbance* of the supernatant liquid at the maximum at 322 nm, Appendix II B. Calculate the content of $C_{21}H_{27}N_3O_2$ taking 227 as the value of A(1%, 1 cm) at the maximum at 322 nm.

Assay Carry out the following procedure protected from light. Weigh and powder 20 tablets. To a quantity of the powder containing the equivalent of 20 mg of methysergide add 50 ml of a 1% w/v solution of *(+)-tartaric acid* and 0.2 ml of a 20% w/v solution of *benzalkonium chloride* and shake for 30 minutes. Dilute with the tartaric acid solution to 100 ml, mix and filter, discarding the first few ml. To 10 ml of the filtrate add sufficient of the tartaric acid solution to produce 100 ml and measure the *absorbance* at the maximum at 322 nm, Appendix II B. Calculate the content of $C_{21}H_{27}N_3O_2$ taking 227 as the value of A(1%, 1 cm) at the maximum at 322 nm.

Storage Methysergide Tablets should be protected from light.

Labelling The quantity of active ingredient is stated in terms of the equivalent amount of methysergide.

Metoclopramide Injection

Definition Metoclopramide Injection is a sterile solution of Metoclopramide Hydrochloride in Water for Injections free from dissolved air.

The injection complies with the requirements stated under Parenteral Preparations and with the following requirements.

Content of anhydrous metoclopramide hydrochloride, $C_{14}H_{22}ClN_3O_2$,HCl 90.0 to 110.0% of the prescribed or stated amount.

Characteristics A colourless solution.

Identification

A. In the test for Related substances the chromatogram obtained with solution (2) shows a peak with the same retention time as the principal peak in the chromatogram obtained with solution (3).

B. To a volume containing the equivalent of 50 mg of anhydrous metoclopramide hydrochloride add 5 ml of *water* and 5 ml of a 1% w/v solution of *4-dimethylaminobenzaldehyde* in 1M *hydrochloric acid*. A yellowish orange colour is produced.

Acidity pH, 3.0 to 5.0, Appendix V L.

Related substances Protect the solutions from light. Carry out the method for *liquid chromatography*, Appendix III D, using the following solutions. For solution (1) dilute a volume of the injection with sufficient of the mobile phase to produce a solution containing the equivalent of 0.1% w/v of anhydrous metoclopramide hydrochloride. For solution (2) dilute 1 volume of solution (1) to 200 volumes with the mobile phase. Solution (3) contains 0.0005% w/v of *metoclopramide hydrochloride BPCRS* in the mobile phase.

The chromatographic procedure may be carried out using (a) a stainless steel column (20 cm × 4.6 mm) packed with *stationary phase C* (10 μm) (Spherisorb ODS 1 is suitable), (b) 0.01M *sodium hexanesulphonate* in a mixture of 40 volumes of *water* and 60 volumes of *acetonitrile*, adjusted to pH 4.0 with *glacial acetic acid*, as the mobile phase with a flow rate such that the retention time of the principal peak is about 8 minutes (1.8 ml per minute may be suitable) and (c) a detection wavelength of 265 nm.

The area of any *secondary peak* in the chromatogram obtained with solution (1) is not greater than the area of the principal peak in the chromatogram obtained with solution (2) (0.5%). Disregard any peaks with a retention time relative to the principal peak of 0.5 or less.

Assay To a volume containing the equivalent of 10 mg of anhydrous metoclopramide hydrochloride add sufficient *water* to produce 100 ml. To 20 ml add 15 ml of 1.25M *sodium hydroxide*, extract with three 30-ml quantities of *chloroform*, dry each extract with *anhydrous sodium sulphate* and filter. To the combined extracts add sufficient *chloroform* to produce 100 ml and measure the *absorbance* of the resulting solution at the maximum at 305 nm, Appendix II B. Calculate the content of $C_{14}H_{22}ClN_3O_2$,HCl taking 265 as the value of A(1%, 1 cm) at the maximum at 305 nm.

Storage Metoclopramide Injection should be protected from light.

Labelling The quantity of active ingredient is stated in terms of the equivalent amount of anhydrous metoclopramide hydrochloride.

Metoclopramide Oral Solution

Definition Metoclopramide Oral Solution is a solution of Metoclopramide Hydrochloride in a suitable flavoured vehicle.

The oral solution complies with the requirements stated under Oral Liquids and with the following requirements.

Content of anhydrous metoclopramide hydrochloride, $C_{14}H_{22}ClN_3O_2$,HCl 90.0 to 110.0% of the prescribed or stated amount.

Identification

A. The *light absorption*, Appendix II B, of the final solution obtained in the Assay exhibits a maximum at 534 nm.

B. In the test for Related substances the retention time of the principal peak in the chromatogram obtained with solution (2) is similar to the retention time of the principal peak in the chromatogram obtained with solution (3).

Related substances Protect the solutions from light. Carry out the method for *liquid chromatography*, Appendix III D, using the following solutions. For solution (1) mix a quantity of the oral solution containing the equivalent of 10 mg of anhydrous metoclopramide hydrochloride with sufficient of the mobile phase to produce 10 ml and filter (Whatman GF/C filter paper is suitable). For solution (2) dilute 1 volume of solution (1) to 200 volumes with the mobile phase. Solution (3) contains 0.0005% w/v of *metoclopramide hydrochloride BPCRS* in the mobile phase.

The chromatographic procedure may be carried out using (a) a stainless steel column (20 cm × 4.6 mm) packed with *stationary phase C* (10 μm) (Spherisorb ODS 1 is suitable), (b) 0.01M *sodium hexanesulphonate* in a mixture of 40 volumes of *water* and 60 volumes of *acetonitrile*, adjusted to pH 4.0 with *glacial acetic acid*, as the mobile phase with a flow rate such that the retention time of the principal peak is about 8 minutes (1.8 ml per minute may be suitable) and (c) a detection wavelength of 265 nm.

The area of any *secondary peak* in the chromatogram obtained with solution (1) is not greater than the area of the principal peak in the chromatogram obtained with solution (2) (0.5%). Disregard any peaks with a retention time relative to the principal peak of 0.5 or less.

Assay Protect the solutions from light. Dilute a quantity of the oral solution containing the equivalent of 10 mg of anhydrous metoclopramide hydrochloride to 100 ml with *water*. To 5 ml of this solution add 5 ml of 1M *hydrochloric acid*, mix, add 5 ml of a freshly prepared solution containing 1% w/v of *sodium nitrite*, mix and allow to stand for 10 minutes. Add 5 ml of a freshly prepared solution containing 5% w/v of *ammonium sulphamate*, mix and allow to stand for 25 minutes. Add 5 ml of a freshly prepared solution containing 0.5% w/v of N-*(1-naphthyl)ethylenediamine dihydrochloride* in 1M *hydrochloric acid*, mix, add sufficient *water* to produce 100 ml, mix and allow to stand for 5 minutes. Measure the *absorbance* of the resulting solution at the maximum at 534 nm, Appendix II B, using *water* in the reference cell. Calculate the content of $C_{14}H_{22}ClN_3O_2,HCl$ from the *absorbance* obtained by repeating the procedure using 5 ml of a 0.01% w/v solution of *metoclopramide hydrochloride BPCRS* in place of the solution being examined, beginning at the words 'add 5 ml of 1M *hydrochloric acid*... ', and using the declared content of $C_{14}H_{22}ClN_3O_2,HCl$ in *metoclopramide hydrochloride BPCRS*.

Storage Metoclopramide Oral Solution should be protected from light.

Labelling The quantity of active ingredient is stated in terms of the equivalent amount of anhydrous metoclopramide hydrochloride.

Metoclopramide Tablets

Definition Metoclopramide Tablets contain Metoclopramide Hydrochloride.

The tablets comply with the requirements stated under Tablets and with the following requirements.

Content of anhydrous metoclopramide hydrochloride, $C_{14}H_{22}ClN_3O_2,HCl$ 90.0 to 110.0% of the prescribed or stated amount.

Identification

A. In the test for Related substances the chromatogram obtained with solution (2) shows a peak with the same retention time as the principal peak in the chromatogram obtained with solution (3).

B. Shake a quantity of the powdered tablets containing the equivalent of 50 mg of anhydrous metoclopramide hydrochloride with 5 ml of *water*, filter and add to the filtrate 5 ml of a 1% w/v solution of *4-dimethylaminobenzaldehyde* in 1M *hydrochloric acid*. A yellowish orange colour is produced.

Related substances Protect the solutions from light. Carry out the method for *liquid chromatography*, Appendix III D, using the following solutions. For solution (1) shake a quantity of the powdered tablets containing the equivalent of 0.1 g of anhydrous metoclopramide hydrochloride with 20 ml of *methanol* for 5 minutes, filter (Whatman GF/C filter paper is suitable) and add sufficient of the mobile phase to produce 100 ml. For solution (2) dilute 1 volume of solution (1) to 200 volumes with the mobile phase. Solution (3) contains 0.0005% w/v of *metoclopramide hydrochloride BPCRS* in the mobile phase.

The chromatographic procedure may be carried out using (a) a stainless steel column (20 cm × 4.6 mm) packed with *stationary phase C* (10 μm) (Spherisorb ODS 1 is suitable), (b) 0.01M *sodium hexanesulphonate* in a mixture of 40 volumes of *water* and 60 volumes of *acetonitrile*, adjusted to pH 4.0 with *glacial acetic acid*, as the mobile phase with a flow rate such that the retention time of the principal peak is about 8 minutes (1.8 ml per minute may be suitable) and (c) a detection wavelength of 265 nm.

The area of any *secondary peak* in the chromatogram obtained with solution (1) is not greater than the area of the principal peak in the chromatogram obtained with solution (2) (0.5%).

Assay Weigh and powder 20 tablets. To a quantity of the powder containing the equivalent of 10 mg of anhydrous metoclopramide hydrochloride add 50 ml of 0.1M *hydrochloric acid*, heat on a water bath at 70° for 15 minutes, cool, add sufficient *water* to produce 100 ml and filter. To 20 ml of the filtrate add 10 ml of 2M *sodium hydroxide*, extract with three 30-ml quantities of *chloroform*, filter each extract through *anhydrous sodium sulphate* supported on absorbent cotton previously moistened with *chloroform* and wash the filter with 5 ml of *chloroform*. To the combined extracts and washings add sufficient *chloroform* to produce 100 ml and measure the *absorbance* of the resulting solution at the maximum at 305 nm, Appendix II B. Calculate the content of $C_{14}H_{22}ClN_3O_2,HCl$ taking 265 as the value of A(1%, 1 cm) at the maximum at 305 nm.

Storage Metoclopramide Tablets should be protected from light.

Labelling The quantity of active ingredient is stated in terms of the equivalent amount of anhydrous metoclopramide hydrochloride.

Metoprolol Injection

Definition Metoprolol Injection is a sterile solution of Metoprolol Tartrate in Water for Injections.

The injection complies with the requirements stated under Parenteral Preparations and with the following requirements.

Content of metoprolol tartrate, $(C_{15}H_{25}NO_3)_2$, $C_4H_6O_6$ 95.0 to 105.0% of the prescribed or stated amount.

Identification

A. To a volume of the injection containing 20 mg of Metoprolol Tartrate add 2 ml of 5M *ammonia*, mix, extract with 30 ml of *dichloromethane*, filter the dichloromethane layer through *anhydrous sodium sulphate* and evaporate the filtrate to dryness using a rotary evaporator with gentle heating if necessary. Cool the residue to −18° for 30 minutes and allow to warm to room temperature. The *infrared absorption spectrum* of the residue, Appendix II A, is concordant with the *reference spectrum* of metoprolol.

B. In the test for Related substances, the chromatogram obtained with solution (2) shows a peak with the same retention time as that of the principal peak in the chromatogram obtained with solution (4).

Acidity or alkalinity pH, 5.5 to 7.5, Appendix V L.

Related substances Carry out the method for *liquid chromatography*, Appendix III D, using the following solutions. For solution (1) evaporate a volume of the injection containing 10 mg of Metoprolol Tartrate to dryness at a temperature not exceeding 40° and dissolve the residue in 2 ml of the mobile phase. For solution (2) dilute 6 volumes of solution (1) to 100 volumes with the mobile phase and further dilute 10 volumes of this solution to 100 volumes with the mobile phase. For solution (3) dilute 10 volumes of solution (2) to 20 volumes with the mobile phase. Solution (4) contains 0.0030% w/v of *metoprolol tartrate EPCRS* in the mobile phase. Solution (5) contains 0.0025% w/v of *metoprolol tartrate EPCRS* and 0.0015% w/v of *metoprolol impurity D EPCRS* in the mobile phase.

The chromatographic procedure may be carried out using (a) a stainless steel column (25 cm × 4.6 mm) packed with *stationary phase C* (10 μm) (Nucleosil C18 is suitable) maintained at a temperature of 40°, (b) as the *mobile phase* with a flow rate of 1 ml per minute a mixture of 2 volumes of *triethylamine*, 3 volumes of *orthophosphoric acid*, 10 volumes of *glacial acetic acid*, 190 volumes of *acetonitrile* and 810 volumes of a 0.48% w/v solution of *ammonium acetate* and (c) a detection wavelength of 275 nm. Equilibrate the column with the mobile phase with a flow rate of 1 ml per minute until a stable baseline is obtained (at least 20 minutes).

Adjust the sensitivity of the system so that the height of the principal peak in the chromatogram obtained with 10 μl of solution (3) is not less than 50% of the full scale of the recorder.

Inject 10 μl of solution (5). When the chromatograms are recorded under the prescribed conditions, the retention times are metoprolol, about 10 minutes and metoprolol impurity D, about 13.5 minutes. The test is not valid unless the *resolution factor* between the peaks corresponding to metoprolol impurity D and metoprolol is at least 4.0. If necessary, adjust the concentration of acetonitrile in the mobile phase.

Inject separately 10 μl of solution (1) and 10 μl of solution (3). Continue the chromatography for three times the retention time of the principal peak. In the chromatogram obtained with solution (1) the area of any *secondary peak* is not greater than the area of the principal peak in the chromatogram obtained with solution (3) (0.3%) and the sum of the areas of any such peaks is not greater than 1.7 times the area of the principal peak in the chromatogram obtained with solution (3) (0.5%). If any of the above limits are exceeded and if a secondary peak occurs with a retention time of about 5 minutes (metoprolol impurity C), prepare solution (6) in a fume cupboard in the following manner. Place an evaporating dish 10 cm in diameter containing 10 ml of a 0.1% w/v solution of *metoprolol tartrate EPCRS* in 0.1M *hydrochloric acid* so that the surface of the solution is 5 cm from a lamp emitting ultraviolet light at 254 nm for 6 hours. Dilute 1 volume of this solution to 50 volumes with the mobile phase (solution (6)).

In the chromatogram obtained with solution (1): divide the area of the peak corresponding to the principal peak in the chromatogram obtained with solution (6) (metoprolol impurity C) by 10: this divided area is not greater than the area of the principal peak in the chromatogram obtained with solution (3) (0.3%); the sum of this divided area and the areas of any other *secondary peaks* is not greater than 1.7 times the area of the principal peak in the chromatogram obtained with solution (3) (0.5%). Disregard any peak with an area less than 0.2 times the area of the principal peak in the chromatogram obtained with solution (3) (0.06%).

Assay Dilute a volume of the injection containing 3 mg of Metoprolol Tartrate to 20 ml with *water* and measure the *absorbance* of the resulting solution at the maximum at 274 nm, Appendix II B. Calculate the content of $(C_{15}H_{25}NO_3)_2,C_4H_6O_6$ from the *absorbance* obtained with a 0.015% w/v solution of *metoprolol tartrate BPCRS* and from the declared content of $(C_{15}H_{25}NO_3)_2,C_4H_6O_6$ in *metoprolol tartrate BPCRS*.

Metoprolol Tartrate Tablets

Definition Metoprolol Tartrate Tablets contain Metoprolol Tartrate.

The tablets comply with the requirements stated under Tablets and with the following requirements.

Content of metoprolol tartrate, $(C_{15}H_{25}NO_3)_2$, $C_4H_6O_6$ 95.0 to 105.0% of the prescribed or stated amount.

Identification

A. Mix a quantity of the powdered tablets containing 50 mg of Metoprolol Tartrate with 25 ml of *water*, add 2 ml of 5M *ammonia*, extract with 20 ml of *dichloromethane*, filter the dichloromethane layer through *anhydrous sodium sulphate*, wash the filter with 10 ml of *dichloromethane* and evaporate the combined filtrate and washings to dryness using a rotary evaporator, using gentle heat if necessary. Cool the residue to −18° for 30 minutes and allow to warm to room temperature. The *infrared absorption spectrum* of the residue, Appendix II A, is concordant with the *reference spectrum* of metoprolol.

B. Carry out the method for *thin-layer chromatography*, Appendix III A, using a silica gel H precoated plate (Analtech Uniplate plates are suitable) and a mixture of 40 volumes of *anhydrous formic acid* and 140 volumes of *ether* as the mobile phase, but allowing the solvent front to ascend 5 cm above the line of application. Pre-wash the plate with the mobile phase and allow to dry in air for at least 1 hour before use. Apply separately to the plate 10 µl of each of the following solutions. For solution (1) shake a quantity of the powdered tablets containing 0.5 g of Metoprolol Tartrate with 15 ml of *methanol* for 1 hour, add sufficient *methanol* to produce 25 ml and mix. Filter through a glass microfibre filter (Whatman GF/F is suitable) and use the filtrate. Solution (2) contains 2.0% w/v of *metoprolol tartrate BPCRS* in *methanol*. Solution (3) contains 0.5% w/v of *(+)-tartaric acid* in *methanol*. For solution (4) mix 1 volume of solution (1) with 1 volume of solution (3). After removal of the plate, allow it to dry in air for about 10 minutes, dry in an oven at 100° for 20 minutes and spray the plate with a solution prepared in the following manner. Dissolve 75 mg of *bromocresol green* and 25 mg of *bromophenol blue* in 100 ml of *absolute ethanol* (solution A); dissolve 0.25 g of *potassium permanganate* and 0.5 g of *sodium carbonate* in 100 ml of *water* (solution B); mix 9 volumes of solution A and 1 volume of solution B and use immediately. The chromatogram obtained with solution (1) closely resembles the chromatogram obtained with solution (2). In the chromatogram obtained with solution (1) the spot with the higher Rf value corresponds to the spot in the chromatogram obtained with solution (3). The test is not valid unless the chromatogram obtained with solution (4) shows two clearly separated principal spots; the spot of low Rf value is purple and the spot of high Rf value, which is a single, compact spot, is yellow.

Related substances Carry out the method for *liquid chromatography*, Appendix III D, using the following solutions. For solution (1) shake a quantity of the powdered tablets containing 0.25 g of Metoprolol Tartrate with 10 ml of *chloroform* for 10 minutes, centrifuge, remove and retain the supernatant layer. Extract the residue with a further 10-ml quantity of *chloroform*, centrifuge and remove the supernatant layer. Evaporate the combined chloroform extracts to dryness at a temperature not exceeding 40°, add sufficient mobile phase to produce 50 ml, mix and filter. Solution (2) contains 0.0025% w/v of *metoprolol tartrate EPCRS* and 0.0015% w/v of *metoprolol impurity D EPCRS* in the mobile phase. For solution (3) dilute 3 volumes of solution (1) to 100 volumes with the mobile phase and further dilute 10 volumes of this solution to 100 volumes with the mobile phase.

The chromatographic procedure may be carried out using (a) a stainless steel column (25 cm × 4.6 mm) packed with *stationary phase C* (10 µm) (Nucleosil C18 is suitable) maintained at a temperature of 40°, (b) as the mobile phase with a flow rate of 1 ml per minute a mixture of 2 volumes of *triethylamine*, 3 volumes of *orthophosphoric acid*, 10 volumes of *glacial acetic acid*, 190 volumes of *acetonitrile* and 810 volumes of a 0.48% w/v solution of *ammonium acetate* and (c) a detection wavelength of 275 nm. Equilibrate the column with the mobile phase at a flow rate of 1 ml per minute until a stable baseline is obtained (at least 20 minutes).

Adjust the sensitivity of the system so that the height of the principal peak in the chromatogram obtained with 10 µl of solution (3) is not less than 50% of the full scale of the recorder.

Inject 10 µl of solution (2). When the chromatograms are recorded under the prescribed conditions, the retention times are metoprolol, about 10 minutes and metoprolol impurity D, about 13.5 minutes. The test is not valid unless the *resolution factor* between the peaks corresponding to metoprolol impurity D and metoprolol is at least 4.0. If necessary, adjust the concentration of acetonitrile in the mobile phase.

Inject separately 10 µl of solution (1) and 10 µl of solution (3). Continue the chromatography for three times the retention time of the principal peak. In the chromatogram obtained with solution (1) the area of any *secondary peak* is not greater than the area of the principal peak in the chromatogram obtained with solution (3) (0.3%) and the sum of the areas of any such peaks is not greater than 1.7 times the area of the principal peak in the chromatogram obtained with solution (3) (0.5%). If any of the above limits are exceeded and if a secondary peak occurs with a retention time of about 5 minutes (metoprolol impurity C), prepare solution (4) in a fume cupboard in the following manner. Place an evaporating dish 10 cm in diameter containing 10 ml of a 0.1% w/v solution of *metoprolol tartrate EPCRS* in 0.1M *hydrochloric acid* so that the surface of the solution is 5 cm from a lamp emitting ultraviolet light at 254 nm for 6 hours. Dilute 1 volume of this solution to 50 volumes with the mobile phase (solution (4)).

In the chromatogram obtained with solution (1): divide the area of the peak corresponding to the principal peak in the chromatogram obtained with solution (4) (metoprolol impurity C) by 10: this divided area is not greater than the area of the principal peak in the chromatogram obtained with solution (3) (0.3%); the sum of this divided area and the areas of any other *secondary peaks* is not greater than 1.7 times the area of the principal peak in the chromatogram obtained with solution (3) (0.5%). Disregard any peak with an area less than 0.2 times the area of the principal peak in the chromatogram obtained with solution (3) (0.06%).

Assay Weigh and powder 20 tablets. Add to a quantity of the powdered tablets containing 75 mg of Metoprolol Tartrate 150 ml of *absolute ethanol*, shake with the aid of ultrasound for 15 minutes, allow to cool, add sufficient *absolute ethanol* to produce 200 ml and filter (Whatman GF/C paper is suitable). To 20 ml of the filtrate add sufficient *absolute ethanol* to produce 50 ml and measure the *absorbance* of the resulting solution at the maximum at 274 nm, Appendix II B. Calculate the content of $(C_{15}H_{25}NO_3)_2,C_4H_6O_6$ from the *absorbance* obtained with a 0.015% w/v solution of *metoprolol tartrate BPCRS* in *absolute ethanol* and from the declared content of $(C_{15}H_{25}NO_3)_2,C_4H_6O_6$ in *metoprolol tartrate BPCRS*.

Metronidazole Gel

Definition Metronidazole Gel contains Metronidazole in a suitable water-soluble basis.

The gel complies with the requirements stated under Topical Semi-solid Preparations and with the following requirements.

Content of metronidazole, $C_6H_9N_3O_3$ 92.5 to 107.5% of the prescribed or stated amount.

Identification In the Assay, the retention time of the principal peak in the chromatogram obtained with solution (1) corresponds to that in the chromatogram obtained with solution (2).

Acidity pH, 4.5 to 6.0, Appendix V L.

Nitrite Disperse 1.0 g of the gel in sufficient *water* to produce 100 ml. To 40 ml of the solution add 2 ml of *sulphanilic acid solution*, 2 ml of *aminonaphthalenesulphonic acid solution* and sufficient *water* to produce 50 ml. Allow to stand at room temperature for 1 hour. Measure the *absorbance* of the resulting solution at the maximum at 524 nm, Appendix II B, using in the reference cell a solution prepared by treating 40 ml of *water* in the same manner, beginning at the words 'add 2 ml of *sulphanilic acid solution...*'. The *absorbance* is not greater than that obtained by repeating the procedure using 1 ml of *nitrite standard solution (20 ppm)* diluted to 40 ml with *water* and treated at the same time and in the same manner, beginning at the words 'add 2 ml of *sulphanilic acid solution...*' (50 ppm, calculated with reference to the gel).

2-Methyl-5-nitroimidazole Carry out the method for *thin-layer chromatography*, Appendix III A, using a silica gel F_{254} precoated plate (Merck silica gel 60 F_{254} plates are suitable) and as the mobile phase a mixture of 1 volume of *water*, 10 volumes of *ethanol (96%)*, 10 volumes of *diethylamine* and 80 volumes of *dichloromethane*. Apply separately to the plate 20 µl of each of the following solutions. For solution (1) shake for 1 hour a quantity of the gel containing 45 mg of Metronidazole with 150 ml of *methanol*, filter, evaporate the filtrate to dryness and dissolve the residue in 10 ml of a mixture of equal volumes of *dichloromethane* and *methanol*. Solution (2) contains 0.0023% w/v of *2-methyl-5-nitroimidazole* in a mixture of equal volumes of *dichloromethane* and *methanol*. After removal of the plate, allow it to dry in air and examine under *ultraviolet light (254 nm)*. Spray with *titanium(III) chloride solution* and heat at 110° until the blue grey colour disappears, cool and spray with a 1% w/v solution of *fast blue B salt* followed by a mixture of 5 volumes of *ethanol (96%)*, 3 volumes of *water* and 2 volumes of 18M *ammonia*. Any *secondary spot* corresponding to 2-methyl-5-nitroimidazole in the chromatogram obtained with solution (1) is not more intense than the spot in the chromatogram obtained with solution (2) (0.5%).

Assay Carry out the method for *liquid chromatography*, Appendix III D, using the following solutions. For solution (1) dissolve a quantity of the gel in 10 ml of *methanol (8%)* to produce a solution containing 0.030% w/v of Metronidazole. For solution (2) dissolve 37.5 mg of *metronidazole BPCRS* in 10 ml of *methanol (8%)* and dilute 2 ml of this solution to 25 ml with *water*.

The chromatographic procedure may be carried out using (a) a stainless steel column (5 cm × 4.6 mm) packed with *stationary phase C* (3 µm) (Spherisorb ODS 2) is suitable, (b) as the mobile phase with a flow rate of 1.5 ml per minute a mixture of 3 volumes of *methanol* and 97 volumes of 0.005M *potassium dihydrogen orthophosphate*, the pH of the mixture being adjusted to 4.0 with *orthophosphoric acid*, and (c) a detection wavelength of 240 nm.

Calculate the content of $C_6H_9N_3O_3$ in the gel using the declared content of $C_6H_9N_3O_3$ in *metronidazole BPCRS*.

Storage Metronidazole Gel should be kept in a well-closed container and stored at a temperature not exceeding 25°.

Metronidazole Intravenous Infusion

Definition Metronidazole Intravenous Infusion is a sterile solution of Metronidazole in Water for Injections.

The intravenous infusion complies with the requirements stated under Parenteral Preparations and with the following requirements.

Content of metronidazole, $C_6H_9N_3O_3$ 95.0 to 110.0% of the prescribed or stated amount.

Characteristics An almost colourless to pale yellow solution.

Identification Shake a volume of the intravenous infusion containing 0.1 g of Metronidazole with 9 g of *sodium chloride* for 5 minutes, add 20 ml of *acetone*, shake for a further 5 minutes and allow to separate. Evaporate the upper layer to dryness. The *infrared absorption spectrum* of the residue, Appendix II A, is concordant with the *reference spectrum* of metronidazole.

Acidity pH, 4.5 to 6.0, Appendix V L.

Related substances Carry out the test described under Metronidazole Tablets but preparing solution (2) in the following manner. Dilute a suitable volume of the intravenous infusion with sufficient mobile phase to produce a solution containing 0.1% w/v of Metronidazole.

In the chromatogram obtained with solution (2) the area of any *secondary peak* is not greater than the area of the peak due to 2-methyl-5-nitroimidazole in the chromatogram obtained with solution (1) (0.5%).

Nitrite To a volume of the infusion containing 2.5 mg of Metronidazole add 40 ml of *water*, 2 ml of *sulphanilic acid solution*, 2 ml of *aminonaphthalenesulphonic acid solution* and sufficient *water* to produce 50 ml. Allow to stand at room temperature for 1 hour. Measure the *absorbance* of the resulting solution at the maximum at 524 nm, Appendix II B, using in the reference cell a solution prepared by treating 1 ml of *water* in the same manner, beginning at the words 'add 40 ml ...'. The *absorbance* is not greater than that obtained by repeating the procedure using 1 ml of *nitrite standard solution (20 ppm)* treated at the same time and in the same manner, beginning at the words 'add 40 ml ...' (40 ppm).

Particulate contamination When supplied in a container with a nominal content of 100 ml or more, complies with the test for *sub-visible particles*, Appendix XIII A.

Assay Dilute a volume of the infusion containing 50 mg of Metronidazole to 100 ml with 0.1M *hydrochloric acid*. Dilute 10 ml of the resulting solution to 250 ml with 0.1M *hydrochloric acid* and measure the *absorbance* of the resulting solution at the maximum at 277 nm, Appendix II B. Calculate the content of $C_6H_9N_3O_3$ taking 375 as the value of A(1%, 1 cm) at the maximum at 277 nm.

Storage Metronidazole Intravenous Infusion should be protected from light.

Labelling The label states that solutions containing visible solid particles must not be used.

Metronidazole Suppositories

Definition Metronidazole Suppositories contain Metronidazole in a suitable suppository basis.

The suppositories comply with the requirements stated under Rectal Preparations and with the following requirements.

Content of metronidazole, $C_6H_9N_3O_3$ 92.5 to 107.5% of the prescribed or stated amount.

Identification Dissolve a quantity of the suppositories containing 0.5 g of Metronidazole as completely as possible by heating with 30 ml of *petroleum spirit (boiling range, 40° to 60°)* on a water bath. Filter, wash the residue with the same solvent and dry at 100°. The *infrared absorption spectrum* of the residue, Appendix II A, is concordant with the *reference spectrum* of metronidazole.

Related substances Carry out the method for *liquid chromatography*, Appendix III D, using the following solutions. For solution (1) melt a quantity of the suppositories containing 0.25 g of Metronidazole using gentle heat, allow to cool and dissolve as completely as possible in 20 ml of *petroleum spirit (boiling range, 40° to 60°)* by warming on a water bath. Filter, wash the residue with *petroleum spirit (boiling range, 40° to 60°)*, dry in a current of air and dissolve in 250 ml of the mobile phase. Solutions (2) and (3) contain 0.00050% w/v of *2-methyl-5-nitroimidazole BPCRS* in the mobile phase and in solution (1) respectively.

The chromatographic procedure may be carried out using (a) a stainless steel column (25 cm × 4.6 mm) packed with *stationary phase C* (10 µm) (Spherisorb ODS 1 is suitable), (b) a mixture of 30 volumes of *methanol* and 70 volumes of 0.01M *potassium dihydrogen orthophosphate* as the mobile phase with a flow rate of 1 ml per minute and (c) a detection wavelength of 315 nm. Record the chromatogram for 3 times the retention time of the principal peak in the chromatogram obtained with solution (2).

Adjust the sensitivity so that the height of the peak due to 2-methyl-5-nitroimidazole in the chromatogram obtained with solution (3) is about 50% of full-scale deflection on the chart paper. Measure the height *(a)* of the peak due to 2-methyl-5-nitroimidazole and the height *(b)* of the lowest part of the curve separating this peak from the principal peak. The test is not valid unless *a* is greater than 10*b*.

The area of any *secondary peak* in the chromatogram obtained with solution (1) is not greater than the area of the peak due to 2-methyl-5-nitroimidazole in the chromatogram obtained with solution (2) (0.5%).

Assay Weigh five suppositories, melt together by warming and allow to cool, stirring continuously until the mass is set. To a quantity containing 0.5 g of Metronidazole add 60 ml of *anhydrous acetic acid*, previously neutralised to *1-naphtholbenzein solution* with 0.1M *perchloric acid VS*, warm at 30° for 30 minutes and shake for 5 minutes. Cool and carry out Method I for *non-aqueous titration*, Appendix VIII A, using *1-naphtholbenzein solution* as indicator. Each ml of 0.1M *perchloric acid VS* is equivalent to 17.12 mg of $C_6H_9N_3O_3$.

Storage Metronidazole Suppositories should be protected from light.

Metronidazole Tablets

Definition Metronidazole Tablets contain Metronidazole.

With the exception of the requirements for shape, the tablets comply with the requirements stated under Tablets and with the following requirements.

Content of metronidazole, $C_6H_9N_3O_3$ 95.0 to 105.0% of the prescribed or stated amount.

Identification

A. Shake a quantity of the powdered tablets containing 0.1 g of Metronidazole with 40 ml of *chloroform* for 15 minutes, filter and evaporate the filtrate to dryness. The *infrared absorption spectrum* of the residue, Appendix II A, is concordant with the *reference spectrum* of metronidazole.

B. Shake a quantity of the powdered tablets containing 0.2 g of Metronidazole with 4 ml of 0.5M *sulphuric acid* and filter. To the filtrate add 10 ml of *picric acid solution R1* and allow to stand. The *melting point* of the precipitate, after washing with *water* and drying at 105°, is about 150°, Appendix V A.

C. Heat a quantity of the powdered tablets containing 10 mg of Metronidazole on a water bath with 10 mg of *zinc powder*, 1 ml of *water* and 0.25 ml of *hydrochloric acid* for 5 minutes, cool in ice, add 0.5 ml of *sodium nitrite solution* and remove the excess of nitrite with *sulphamic acid*. Add 0.5 ml of *2-naphthol solution* and 2 ml of 5M *sodium hydroxide*. An orange-red colour is produced.

Related substances Carry out the method for *liquid chromatography*, Appendix III D, using the following solutions. Solution (1) contains 0.00050% w/v of *2-methyl-5-nitroimidazole BPCRS* in the mobile phase. For solution (2) shake a quantity of the powdered tablets containing 0.2 g of Metronidazole with 100 ml of the mobile phase for 5 minutes, dilute to 200 ml with the mobile phase, filter and use the filtrate. Solution (3) contains 0.00050% w/v of *2-methyl-5-nitroimidazole BPCRS* in solution (2).

The chromatographic procedure may be carried out using (a) a stainless steel column (20 cm × 4.6 mm) packed with *stationary phase C* (10 µm) (Spherisorb ODS 1 is suitable), (b) a mixture of 30 volumes of *methanol* and 70 volumes of 0.01M *potassium dihydrogen orthophosphate* as the mobile phase with a flow rate of 1 ml per minute and (c) a detection wavelength of 315 nm. Record the chromatograms for 3 times the retention time of the principal peak in the chromatogram obtained with solution (2).

Adjust the sensitivity so that the height of the peak due to 2-methyl-5-nitroimidazole in the chromatogram obtained with solution (3) is about 50% of full-scale deflection. Measure the height (*a*) of the peak due to 2-methyl-5-nitroimidazole and the height (*b*) of the lowest part of the curve separating this peak from the principal peak. The test is not valid unless *a* is greater than 10*b*.

The area of any *secondary peak* in the chromatogram obtained with solution (2) is not greater than the area of the peak due to 2-methyl-5-nitroimidazole in the chromatogram obtained with solution (1).

Assay Weigh and powder 20 tablets. Transfer a quantity of the powder containing 0.2 g of Metronidazole to a sintered-glass crucible and extract with six 10-ml quantities of hot *acetone*. Cool, add to the combined extracts 50 ml of *acetic anhydride* and 0.1 ml of a 1% w/v solution of *brilliant green* in *anhydrous acetic acid* and titrate with 0.1M *perchloric acid VS* to a yellowish green end point. Repeat the operation without the powdered tablets. The difference between the titrations represents the amount of perchloric acid required. Each ml of 0.1M *perchloric acid VS* is equivalent to 17.12 mg of $C_6H_9N_3O_3$.

Metyrapone Capsules

Definition Metyrapone Capsules contain Metyrapone.

The capsules comply with the requirements stated under Capsules and with the following requirements.

Content of metyrapone, $C_{14}H_{14}N_2O$ 95.0 to 105.0% of the prescribed or stated amount.

Identification

A. The *infrared absorption spectrum* of the contents of the capsules, Appendix II A, is concordant with *reference spectrum 2* of metyrapone.

B. To a quantity of the contents of the capsules containing 50 mg of Metyrapone add 5 ml of 0.5M *sulphuric acid* and 0.2 ml of *potassium tetraiodomercurate solution.* A cream precipitate is produced.

Related substances Carry out in subdued light the method for *thin-layer chromatography*, Appendix III A, using *silica gel GF_{254}* as the coating substance and a mixture of 5 volumes of 13.5M *ammonia*, 5 volumes of *water* and 90 volumes of *propan-2-ol* as the mobile phase. Apply separately to the plate 10 µl of each of the following solutions. For solution (1) dissolve a quantity of the contents of the capsules containing 0.5 g of Metyrapone in 10 ml of *chloroform*. For solution (2) dilute 1 volume of solution (1) to 500 volumes with *chloroform*. After removal of the plate, allow it to dry in air and examine under *ultraviolet light (254 nm)*. Any *secondary spot* in the chromatogram obtained with solution (1) is not more intense than the spot in the chromatogram obtained with solution (2) (0.2%).

Assay Weigh 10 capsules. Open the capsules carefully without loss of shell material, express as much of the contents as possible and reserve the expressed material. Wash the shells with *ether*, discard the washings, allow the shells to stand at room temperature until the odour of ether is no longer detectable and weigh. The difference between the weights represents the weight of the total contents. Dissolve a quantity of the contents containing 0.1 g of Metyrapone in 40 ml of 0.1M *hydrochloric acid* and add sufficient 0.1M *hydrochloric acid* to produce 100 ml. Dilute 5 ml to 50 ml with 0.1M *hydrochloric acid* and dilute 5 ml of this solution to 50 ml with 0.1M *hydrochloric acid.* Measure the *absorbance* of the resulting solution at the maximum at 260 nm, Appendix II B. Calculate the content of $C_{14}H_{14}N_2O$ taking 500 as the value of A(1%, 1 cm) at the maximum at 260 nm.

Storage Metyrapone Capsules should be protected from light.

Mexenone Cream

Definition Mexenone Cream is a dispersion of Mexenone in a suitable basis.

The cream complies with the requirements stated under Topical Semi-solid Preparations and with the following requirements.

Content of mexenone, $C_{15}H_{14}O_3$ 95.0 to 105.0% of the prescribed or stated amount.

Identification Carry out the method for *thin-layer chromatography*, Appendix III A, using *silica gel GF_{254}* as the coating substance and a mixture of 10 volumes of *butan-2-one* and 100 volumes of *toluene* as the mobile phase. Apply separately to the plate 5 µl of each of the following solutions. For solution (1) disperse a quantity of the cream containing 0.1 g of Mexenone in 50 ml of *water*, add 5 g of *sodium chloride*, extract with two 25-ml quantities of *chloroform*, wash the combined extracts with 50 ml of *water* and filter the chloroform solution through *kieselguhr*. Solution (2) contains 0.2% w/v of *mexenone BPCRS* in *chloroform*. After removal of the plate, allow it to dry in air and examine under *ultraviolet light (254 nm)*. The principal spot in the chromatogram obtained with solution (1) corresponds to that in the chromatogram obtained with solution (2).

Acidity pH of a dispersion prepared by mixing 4 g with 20 ml of *carbon dioxide-free water*, 4.0 to 5.0, Appendix V L.

Assay To a quantity containing 20 mg of Mexenone add 20 ml of *methanol*, warm to disperse, dilute to 100 ml with *methanol* and filter, discarding the first portion of the filtrate. Dilute 20 ml of the clear filtrate to 100 ml with *methanol*, further dilute 20 ml of this solution to 100 ml with the same solvent and measure the *absorbance* of the resulting solution at the maximum at 287 nm, Appendix II B. Calculate the content of $C_{15}H_{14}O_3$ taking 640 as the value of A(1%, 1 cm) at the maximum at 287 nm.

Mexiletine Capsules

Definition Mexiletine Capsules contain Mexiletine Hydrochloride.

The capsules comply with the requirements stated under Capsules and with the following requirements.

Content of mexiletine hydrochloride, $C_{11}H_{17}NO,HCl$ 92.5 to 107.5% of the prescribed or stated amount.

Identification

A. Shake a quantity of the contents of the capsules containing 50 mg of Mexiletine Hydrochloride with 10 ml of *methanol* for 15 minutes, filter (Whatman GF/C filter paper is suitable), evaporate to dryness on a rotary evaporator and dry the residue at 105° for 2 hours. The *infrared absorption spectrum* of the dried residue, Appendix II A, is concordant with the *reference spectrum* of mexiletine hydrochloride.

B. In the test for Related substances, the principal peak in the chromatogram obtained with solution (2) has the same retention time as that of the principal peak in the chromatogram obtained with solution (3).

Related substances Carry out the method for *liquid chromatography*, Appendix III D, using the following solutions. For solution (1) mix, with the aid of ultrasound for 15 minutes, a quantity of the contents of the capsules containing 20 mg of Mexiletine Hydrochloride with 8 ml of the mobile phase, add sufficient of the mobile phase to produce 10 ml and filter (Whatman GF/C filter paper is suitable). For solution (2) dilute 1 volume of solution (1) to 200 volumes with the mobile phase. Solution (3) contains 0.001% w/v of *mexiletine hydrochloride EPCRS* in the mobile phase. For solution (4) mix a suitable volume of a 0.005% w/v solution of *2,6-dimethylphenoxyacetone EPCRS* in the mobile phase with an equal volume of solution (2). Solution (5) contains 0.0004% w/v of *2,6-dimethylphenol* in the mobile phase.

The chromatographic procedure may be carried out using (a) a stainless steel column (25 cm × 4.6 mm) packed with *stationary phase C* (5 µm) (Kromasil C18 is suitable), (b) as mobile phase with a flow rate of 1 ml per minute a mixture of 40 volumes of *water* and 60 volumes of *acetonitrile* containing 0.6% w/v of *potassium dihydrogen orthophosphate* and 0.29% w/v of *sodium dodecyl sulphate* and (c) a detection wavelength of 262 nm. For solution (1) allow the chromatography to proceed for twice the retention time of the principal peak (about 8 minutes).

Inject 20 µl of solution (4). Adjust the sensitivity of the system so that the heights of the two principal peaks are not less than 50% of the full-scale of the recorder. The test is not valid unless in the chromatogram obtained the *resolution factor* between the peaks corresponding to 2,6-dimethylphenoxyacetone and mexiletine is at least 2.

In the chromatogram obtained with solution (1) the area of any peak corresponding to 2,6-dimethylphenol is not greater than the area of the principal peak in the chromatogram obtained with solution (5) (0.2%) and the area of any other *secondary peak* is not greater than the area of the principal peak in the chromatogram obtained with solution (2) (0.5%). Disregard any peak with an area less than 0.1 times the area of the principal peak in the chromatogram obtained with solution (2) (0.05%).

Assay Shake a quantity of the mixed contents of 20 capsules containing 50 mg of Mexiletine Hydrochloride with 50 ml of 0.01M *hydrochloric acid* for 30 minutes. Dilute to 100 ml with 0.01M *hydrochloric acid* and centrifuge. Measure the *absorbance* of the supernatant liquid at the maximum at 260 nm, Appendix II B. Calculate the content of $C_{11}H_{17}NO,HCl$ taking 11.6 as the value of A(1%, 1 cm) at the maximum at 260 nm.

Mexiletine Injection

Definition Mexiletine Injection is a sterile solution of Mexiletine Hydrochloride in Water for Injections.

The injection complies with the requirements stated under Parenteral Preparations and with the following requirements.

Content of mexiletine hydrochloride, $C_{11}H_{17}NO, HCl$ 92.5 to 107.5% of the prescribed or stated amount.

Identification

A. In the test for Related substances, the principal peak in the chromatogram obtained with solution (2) has the same retention time as that of the principal peak in the chromatogram obtained with solution (3).

B. A volume containing 2.5 mg of Mexiletine Hydrochloride diluted to 2 ml yields reaction A characteristic of *chlorides*, Appendix VI.

Acidity pH, 5.0 to 6.0, Appendix V L.

Related substances Complies with the test described under Mexiletine Capsules but using a solution prepared in the following manner as solution (1). Dilute a volume of the injection with sufficient of the mobile phase to produce a solution containing 0.2% w/v of Mexiletine Hydrochloride.

Assay Dilute a volume containing 0.125 g of Mexiletine Hydrochloride to 250 ml with 0.01M *hydrochloric acid*. Measure the *absorbance* of the resulting solution at the maximum at 260 nm, Appendix II B. Calculate the content of $C_{11}H_{17}NO,HCl$ taking 11.6 as the value of A(1%, 1 cm) at the maximum at 260 nm.

Mianserin Tablets

Definition Mianserin Tablets contain Mianserin Hydrochloride.

The tablets comply with the requirements stated under Tablets and with the following requirements.

Content of mianserin hydrochloride, $C_{18}H_{20}N_2,HCl$ 90.0 to 110.0% of the prescribed or stated amount.

Identification

A. Shake a quantity of the powdered tablets containing 20 mg of Mianserin Hydrochloride with 10 ml of *methanol*, filter and evaporate the filtrate to dryness. The *infrared absorption spectrum* of the residue, Appendix II A, is concordant with the *reference spectrum* of mianserin hydrochloride.

B. In the Assay, the chromatogram obtained with solution (2) shows a peak with the same retention time as that due to mianserin in the chromatogram obtained with solution (1).

C. The residue obtained in test A yields the reactions characteristic of *chlorides*, Appendix VI.

Related substances Carry out the method for *thin-layer chromatography*, Appendix III A, using *silica gel G* as the coating substance and a mixture of 10 volumes of *methanol* and 90 volumes of *dichloromethane* as the mobile phase. Apply separately to the plate 5 µl of each of the following solutions. For solution (1) triturate a quantity of the powdered tablets containing 40 mg of Mianserin Hydrochloride with 2 ml of a mixture of 4 volumes of *methanol* and 1 volume of 13.5M *ammonia* and centrifuge. For solution (2) dilute 1 volume of solution (1) to 200 volumes with the same solvent mixture. For solution (3) dilute 1 volume of solution (1) to 500 volumes with the same solvent mixture. After removal of the plate, allow it to dry in a current of cold air for 5 minutes and then expose to iodine vapour for 20 minutes. Any *secondary spot* in the chromatogram obtained with solution (1) is not more intense than the spot in the chromatogram obtained with solution (2) (0.5%) and not more than two such spots are more intense than the spot in the chromatogram obtained with solution (3) (0.2%). Disregard any spot with an Rf value lower than 0.15.

Assay Weigh and powder 20 tablets. Carry out the method for *gas chromatography*, Appendix III B, using the following solutions. For solution (1) add 3 ml of 1M *sodium hydroxide* and 10 ml of *toluene* containing 0.2% w/v of *triphenylamine* (internal standard) to 10 ml of a solution containing 0.2% w/v of *mianserin hydrochloride BPCRS* in 0.2M *hydrochloric acid*, mix for 5 minutes with a vortex mixer, centrifuge and use the clear upper layer. For solution (2) shake a quantity of the powdered tablets containing 60 mg of Mianserin Hydrochloride with 30 ml of 0.2M *hydrochloric acid* for 1 hour and filter. To 10 ml of the filtrate add 3 ml of 1M *sodium hydroxide* and 10 ml of *toluene*, mix for 5 minutes with a vortex mixer, centrifuge and use the clear upper layer. For solution (3) treat a further 10 ml of the filtrate obtained under solution (2) in the same manner as for solution (1) beginning at the words 'add 3 ml of 1M *sodium hydroxide* ...'.

The chromatographic procedure may be carried out using a glass column (1.0 m × 4 mm) packed with *acid-washed, silanised diatomaceous support* (80 to 100 mesh) coated with 3% w/w of phenylmethyl silicone fluid (50% phenyl) (OV-17 is suitable) and maintained at 255°.

Calculate the content of $C_{18}H_{20}N_2,HCl$ using the declared content of $C_{18}H_{20}N_2,HCl$ in *mianserin hydrochloride BPCRS*.

Storage Mianserin Tablets should be protected from light.

Miconazole Cream

Definition Miconazole Cream contains Miconazole Nitrate in a suitable basis.

The cream complies with the requirements stated under Topical Semi-solid Preparations and with the following requirements.

Content of miconazole nitrate, $C_{18}H_{14}Cl_4N_2O,HNO_3$ 90.0 to 110.0% of the prescribed or stated amount.

Identification

A. Mix a quantity containing 40 mg of Miconazole Nitrate with 20 ml of a mixture of 1 volume of 1M *sulphuric acid* and 4 volumes of *methanol* and shake with two 50-ml quantities of *hexane*, discarding the organic layers. Make the aqueous phase alkaline with 2M *ammonia* and extract with two 40-ml quantities of *chloroform*. Combine the chloroform extracts, shake with 5 g of *anhydrous sodium sulphate*, filter and dilute the filtrate to 100 ml with *chloroform*. Evaporate 50 ml to dryness and dissolve the residue in 50 ml of a mixture of 1 volume of 0.1M *hydrochloric acid* and 9 volumes of *methanol*. The *light absorption* of the resulting solution, Appendix II B, in the range 230 to 350 nm exhibits maxima at 264, 272 and 280 nm.

B. In the Assay, the principal peak in the chromatogram obtained with solution (2) has the same retention time as the peak due to miconazole in the chromatogram obtained with solution (1).

Assay Carry out the method for *gas chromatography*, Appendix III B, using the following solutions. For solution (1) shake 40 mg of *miconazole nitrate BPCRS* with 10 ml of a 0.3% w/v solution of *1,2,3,4-tetraphenylcyclopenta-1,3-dienone* (internal standard) in *chloroform* and 0.2 ml of 13.5M *ammonia*, add 1 g of *anhydrous sodium sulphate*, shake again and filter. Prepare solution (2) in the same manner as solution (3) but omitting the addition of the internal standard solution. For solution (3) mix a quantity of the cream containing 40 mg of Miconazole Nitrate with 20 ml of a mixture of 1 volume of 0.5M *sulphuric acid* and 4 volumes of *methanol* and shake with two 50-ml quantities of *carbon tetrachloride*. Wash each organic layer in turn with the same 10-ml quantity of a mixture of 1 volume of 0.5M *sulphuric acid* and 4 volumes of *methanol*. Combine the aqueous phase and the washings, make alkaline with 2M *ammonia* and extract with two 50-ml quantities of *chloroform*. To the combined extracts add 10 ml of a 0.3% w/v solution of the internal standard in *chloroform* and 5 g of *anhydrous sodium sulphate*, shake, filter, evaporate the filtrate to a low volume and add sufficient *chloroform* to produce 10 ml.

The chromatographic procedure may be carried out using a glass column (1.5 m × 2 mm) packed with *acid-washed, silanised diatomaceous support* (80 to 100 mesh) coated with 3% w/w of phenyl methyl silicone fluid (50% phenyl) (OV-17 is suitable) and maintained at 270°.

Calculate the content of $C_{18}H_{14}Cl_4N_2O,HNO_3$ using the declared content of $C_{18}H_{14}Cl_4N_2O,HNO_3$ in *miconazole nitrate BPCRS*.

Storage If Miconazole Cream is kept in aluminium tubes, their inner surfaces should be coated with a suitable lacquer.

Midazolam Injection

Definition Midazolam Injection is a sterile solution of Midazolam in Water for Injections containing Hydrochloric Acid.

The injection complies with the requirements stated under Parenteral Preparations and with the following requirements.

Content of midazolam, $C_{18}H_{13}ClFN_3$ 95.0% to 105.0% of the prescribed or stated amount.

Identification

A. To a volume of the injection containing 20 mg of Midazolam add sufficient 5M *ammonia* to make the solution just alkaline, extract with two 10-ml quantities of *dichloromethane*, dry the combined extracts over *anhydrous sodium sulphate*, filter and evaporate the filtrate to dryness. The *infrared absorption spectrum* of the residue, Appendix II A, is concordant with the *reference spectrum* of midazolam.

B. In the test for Related substances, the principal spot in the chromatogram obtained with solution (1) corresponds to that in the chromatogram obtained with solution (3).

Acidity pH, 2.9 to 3.7, Appendix V L.

Related substances Carry out the method for *thin-layer chromatography*, Appendix III A, using a silica gel F_{254} precoated plate (Merck silica gel 60 F_{254} plates are suitable) and a mixture of 2 volumes of *glacial acetic acid*, 15 volumes of *water*, 20 volumes of *methanol* and 80 volumes of *ethyl acetate* as the mobile phase and allowing the solvent front to ascend 12 cm above the line of application. Apply separately to the plate 50 µl of each of the following solutions. For solution (1) mix a volume of the injection containing 20 mg of Midazolam with 4 ml of *methanol* and 0.1 ml of 5M *ammonia* and dilute to 10 ml with *methanol*; allow the solution to stand in the dark for 1 hour. For solution (2) dilute 1 volume of solution (1) to 200 volumes with *methanol*. Solution (3) contains 0.2% w/v of *midazolam EPCRS* in *methanol*. For solution (4) dissolve 8 mg of each of *midazolam EPCRS* and *chlordiazepoxide EPCRS* in sufficient *ethanol (96%)* to produce 10 ml. After removal of the plate, dry it in a current of warm air and examine under *ultraviolet light (254 nm)*. Any *secondary spot* in the chromatogram obtained with solution (1) is not more intense than the spot in the chromatogram obtained with solution (2) (0.5%). The test is not valid unless the chromatogram obtained with solution (4) shows two clearly separated spots.

Assay To a volume of the injection containing 25 mg of Midazolam add sufficient 0.1M *hydrochloric acid* to produce 100 ml. Dilute 10 ml of the solution to 100 ml with 0.1M *hydrochloric acid*, allow to stand for 35 minutes and measure the *absorbance* of the resulting solution at the maximum at 258 nm, Appendix II B. Calculate the content of $C_{18}H_{13}ClFN_3$ taking 369 as the value of A(1%, 1 cm) at the maximum at 258 nm.

Storage Midazolam Injection should be protected from light.

Minocycline Tablets

Definition Minocycline Tablets contain Minocycline Hydrochloride.

The tablets comply with the requirements stated under Tablets and with the following requirements.

Content of minocycline, $C_{23}H_{27}N_3O_7$ 92.5 to 107.5% of the prescribed or stated amount.

Identification

A. Carry out the method for *thin-layer chromatography*, Appendix III A, using *silica gel GF_{254}* as the coating substance and a mixture of 6 volumes of *water*, 35 volumes of *methanol* and 59 volumes of *dichloromethane* as the mobile phase. Adjust the pH of a 10.0% w/v solution of *disodium edetate* to 9.0 with 10M *sodium hydroxide* and spray the solution evenly onto the plate (about 10 ml for a plate 100 mm × 200 mm). Allow the plate to dry in a horizontal position for at least 1 hour. Dry the plate at 110° for 1 hour immediately before use.

Apply separately to the plate 2 µl of each of the following solutions. For solution (1) extract a quantity of the powdered tablets containing the equivalent of 10 mg of minocycline with 20 ml of *methanol*, centrifuge and use the supernatant liquid. Solution (2) contains 0.05% w/v of *minocycline hydrochloride EPCRS* in *methanol*. Solution (3) contains 0.05% w/v of each of *minocycline hydrochloride EPCRS* and *doxycycline hyclate EPCRS* in *methanol*. After removal of the plate, dry it in a current of air and examine under *ultraviolet light (254 nm)*. The principal spot in the chromatogram obtained with solution (1) is similar in position and size to that in the chromatogram obtained with solution (2). The test is not valid unless the chromatogram obtained with solution (3) shows two clearly separated principal spots.

B. In the Assay, the principal peak in the chromatogram obtained with solution (2) has the same retention time as the principal peak in the chromatogram obtained with solution (1).

C. Shake a quantity of the powdered tablets containing the equivalent of 50 mg of minocycline with 5 ml of *water* and filter. The filtrate yields reaction A characteristic of *chlorides*, Appendix VI.

Related substances Carry out the method for *liquid chromatography*, Appendix III D, protected from light. Store the solutions at a temperature of 2° to 8° and use within 3 hours of preparation. For solution (1) shake a quantity of the powdered tablets containing the equivalent of 25 mg of minocycline with 50 ml of *water*, dilute to 100 ml with the same solvent and filter. For solution (2) dilute 1 volume of solution (1) to 50 volumes with *water*. For solution (3) dilute 1.2 volumes of solution (1) to 100 volumes with *water*. For solution (4) heat 5 ml of a 0.20% w/v solution of *minocycline hydrochloride EPCRS* on a water bath for 60 minutes, evaporate to dryness and dissolve the residue in sufficient *water* to produce 25 ml.

The chromatographic procedure may be carried out using (a) a stainless steel column (20 cm × 4.6 mm) packed with *stationary phase B* (5 µm) (Nucleosil C8 is suitable), (b) as the mobile phase with a flow rate of 1 ml per minute a mixture of 25 volumes of 0.01M *disodium edetate*, 27 volumes of *dimethylformamide*, and 50 volumes of a 2.84% w/v solution of *ammonium oxalate*, adjusted to a pH of 6.2 to 7.0 with 0.4M *tetrabutylammonium hydroxide* (pH 7.0 is suitable with a Nucleosil C8 column) and (c) a detection wavelength of 280 nm. Record the chromatograms for 1.5 times the retention time of the principal peak of the substance being examined. After use, the apparatus should be flushed thoroughly with *water*.

The test is not valid unless the *resolution factor* between the two principal peaks in the chromatogram obtained with solution (4) is at least 2.0.

In the chromatogram obtained with solution (1) the area of any peak corresponding to epi-minocycline, which is identified by reference to the principal peak in the chromatogram obtained with solution (4), is not greater than the area of the peak in the chromatogram obtained with solution (2) (2%), the area of any other *secondary peak* is not greater than the area of the peak in the chromatogram obtained with solution (3) (1.2%) and the sum of the areas of all the *secondary peaks*, excluding the peak corresponding to epi-minocycline, is not greater than the area of the peak in the chromatogram obtained with solution (2) (2%).

Dissolution Comply with the *dissolution test for tablets and capsules*, Appendix XII D, using Apparatus II. Use as the medium 900 ml of 0.1M *hydrochloric acid* and rotate the paddle at 50 revolutions per minute. Withdraw a sample of 10 ml of the medium and filter, discarding the first few ml of filtrate. Dilute the filtered solution, if necessary, with 0.1M *hydrochloric acid* to give a solution expected to contain the equivalent of about 0.001% w/v of minocycline Measure the *absorbance* of the solution at the maximum at 348 nm, Appendix II B, using 0.1M *hydrochloric acid* in the reference cell. Calculate the total content of minocycline, $C_{23}H_{27}N_3O_7$, in the medium from the *absorbance* obtained from a 0.0012% w/v solution of *minocycline hydrochloride EPCRS* in 0.1M *hydrochloric acid* and using the declared content of $C_{23}H_{27}N_3O_7$ in *minocycline hydrochloride EPCRS*.

Assay Weigh and powder 20 tablets. Carry out the method for *liquid chromatography*, Appendix III D, protected from light. Store the solutions at a temperature of 2° to 8° and use within 3 hours of preparation. Solution (1) contains 0.0125% w/v of *minocycline hydrochloride EPCRS* in *water*. For solution (2) shake a quantity of the powdered tablets containing the equivalent of 25 mg of minocycline with 50 ml of *water*, dilute to 100 ml with the same solvent, filter and dilute 10 ml of the filtrate to 20 ml with *water*.

The chromatographic procedure may be carried out using the conditions described in the test for Related substances.

The *column efficiency*, determined using the peak in the chromatogram obtained with solution (1), should be at least 15,000 *theoretical plates* per metre.

Calculate the content of $C_{23}H_{27}N_3O_7$ using the declared content of $C_{23}H_{27}N_3O_7$ in *minocycline hydrochloride EPCRS*.

Labelling The quantity of active ingredient is stated in terms of the equivalent amount of minocycline.

Mitobronitol Tablets

Definition Mitobronitol Tablets contain Mitobronitol.

The tablets comply with the requirements stated under Tablets and with the following requirements.

Content of mitobronitol, $C_6H_{12}Br_2O_4$ 92.5 to 107.5% of the prescribed or stated amount.

Identification Extract a quantity of the powdered tablets containing 0.5 g of Mitobronitol with 10 ml of hot *methanol*, filter and allow the filtrate to cool. The crystalline precipitate, after filtering and drying at 105° for 2 hours, complies with the following tests.

A. The *infrared absorption spectrum*, Appendix II A, is concordant with the *reference spectrum* of mitobronitol.

B. Dissolve 0.1 g in 10 ml of 1M *sodium hydroxide*, boil, cool, acidify with 2M *nitric acid* and add 1 ml of *silver nitrate solution*. A pale yellow, curdy precipitate is produced.

Ionic halide Shake a quantity of powdered tablets containing 1 g of Mitobronitol with 50 ml of *water* for 15 minutes, dilute to 100 ml with *water* and filter. To 50 ml of the filtrate add 10 ml of 2M *nitric acid* and 5 ml of 0.01M *silver nitrate VS* and mix. Titrate the excess of silver nitrate with 0.01M *ammonium thiocyanate VS* using *ammonium iron(III) sulphate solution R2* as indicator. Not more than 3.2 ml of 0.01M *silver nitrate VS* is required.

Assay Weigh and powder 20 tablets. To a quantity of the powder containing 0.2 g of Mitobronitol add 40 ml of 0.5M *sodium hydroxide*, heat to boiling, cool, add 25 ml of 0.1M *silver nitrate VS*, acidify with 5 ml of 5M *nitric acid* and titrate the excess of silver nitrate with 0.1M *ammonium thiocyanate VS* determining the end point potentiometrically. Each ml of 0.1M *silver nitrate VS* is equivalent to 15.40 mg of $C_6H_{12}Br_2O_4$.

Storage Mitobronitol Tablets should be protected from light.

Morphine Sulphate Injection

Definition Morphine Sulphate Injection is a sterile solution of Morphine Sulphate in Water for Injections.

The injection complies with the requirements stated under Parenteral Preparations and with the following requirements.

Content of morphine sulphate, $(C_{17}H_{19}NO_3)_2,H_2SO_4,5H_2O$ 92.5 to 107.5% of the prescribed or stated amount.

Characteristics A colourless or almost colourless solution.

Identification

A. In the Assay, the retention time of the principal peak in the chromatogram obtained with solution (1) is the same as that of the peak in the chromatogram obtained with solution (2).

B. Evaporate a volume containing 5 mg of Morphine Sulphate to dryness on a water bath. Dissolve the residue in 5 ml of *water* and add 0.15 ml of *dilute potassium hexacyanoferrate(III) solution* and 0.05 ml of *iron(III) chloride solution R1*. A bluish green colour is produced immediately, which changes rapidly to blue.

C. Yields reaction A characteristic of *sulphates*, Appendix VI.

Assay Carry out the method for *liquid chromatography*, Appendix III D, using the following solutions. For solution (1) dilute the injection to contain 0.1% w/v of Morphine Sulphate with *methanol (60%)*. Solution (2) contains 0.1% w/v of *morphine hydrochloride BPCRS* in *methanol (60%)*.

The chromatographic procedure may be carried out using (a) a stainless steel column (10 cm × 4.6 mm) packed with *stationary phase C* (5 μm) (Nucleosil C18 is suitable), (b) as the mobile phase with a flow rate of 2 ml per minute a solution containing 0.01M *sodium acetate* and 0.005M *dioctyl sodium sulphosuccinate* in *methanol (60%)* adjusted to pH 5.5 with *glacial acetic acid* and (c) a detection wavelength of 285 nm.

Calculate the content of $(C_{17}H_{19}NO_3)_2,H_2SO_4,5H_2O$ using the declared content of $C_{17}H_{19}NO_3$ in *morphine hydrochloride BPCRS*. Each mg of $C_{17}H_{19}NO_3$ is equivalent to 1.33 mg of $(C_{17}H_{19}NO_3)_2,H_2SO_4,5H_2O$.

Storage Morphine Sulphate Injection should be protected from light.

Morphine and Atropine Injection

Definition Morphine and Atropine Injection is a sterile isotonic solution containing 1.0% w/v of Morphine Sulphate and 0.06% w/v of Atropine Sulphate in Water for Injections.

The injection complies with the requirements stated under Parenteral Preparations and with the following requirements.

Content of atropine sulphate, $(C_{17}H_{23}NO_3)_2,H_2SO_4,H_2O$ 0.054 to 0.066% w/v.

Content of morphine sulphate, $(C_{17}H_{19}NO_3)_2,H_2SO_4,5H_2O$ 0.92 to 1.07% w/v.

Identification

A. Carry out the method for *thin-layer chromatography*, Appendix III A, using *silica gel G* as the coating substance and a mixture of 3 volumes of 13.5M *ammonia* and 200 volumes of *methanol* as the mobile phase. Apply separately to the plate 10 μl of each of the following solutions. For solution (1) add 1 ml of 5M *ammonia* to 1 ml of the injection, extract with two 5-ml quantities of *chloroform*, filter the combined extracts through *anhydrous sodium sulphate*, evaporate to dryness in a current of warm air and dissolve the residue in 0.5 ml of *chloroform*. For solution (2) treat 1 ml of a 0.06% w/v solution of *atropine sulphate*

BPCRS in the same manner as for solution (1). For solution (3) treat 1 ml of a 1% w/v solution of *morphine hydrochloride BPCRS* in the same manner as for solution (1). After removal of the plate, allow it to dry in a current of air and spray with *dilute potassium iodobismuthate solution*. The spots in the chromatogram obtained with solution (1) correspond to the spots in the chromatograms obtained with solutions (2) and (3).

B. In the Assay for atropine sulphate, the retention time of the principal peak in the chromatogram obtained with solution (1) is the same as that of the peak in the chromatogram obtained with solution (2).

C. In the Assay for morphine sulphate, the retention time of the principal peak in the chromatogram obtained with solution (1) is the same as that of the peak in the chromatogram obtained with solution (2).

Assay

For atropine sulphate Carry out the method for *liquid chromatography*, Appendix III D, using the following solutions. For solution (1) use the injection being examined. Solution (2) contains 0.06% w/v of *atropine sulphate BPCRS* in *methanol (60%)*.

The chromatographic procedure may be carried out using (a) a stainless steel column (10 cm × 4.6 mm) packed with *stationary phase C* (5 µm) (Nucleosil C18 is suitable), (b) as the mobile phase with a flow rate of 2 ml per minute a solution containing 0.01M *sodium acetate* and 0.005M *dioctyl sodium sulphosuccinate* in *methanol (60%)* adjusted to pH 5.5 with *glacial acetic acid* and (c) a detection wavelength of 257 nm.

Calculate the content of $(C_{17}H_{23}NO_3)_2,H_2SO_4,H_2O$ using the declared content of $(C_{17}H_{23}NO_3)_2,H_2SO_4,H_2O$ in *atropine sulphate BPCRS*.

For morphine sulphate Carry out the method for *liquid chromatography*, Appendix III D, using the following solutions. For solution (1) dilute 1 volume of the injection to 10 volumes with *methanol (60%)*. Solution (2) contains 0.1% w/v of *morphine hydrochloride BPCRS* in *methanol (60%)*.

The chromatographic procedure described under Assay for atropine sulphate may be used but with a detection wavelength of 285 nm.

Calculate the content of $(C_{17}H_{19}NO_3)_2,H_2SO_4,5H_2O$ using the declared content of $C_{17}H_{19}NO_3$ in *morphine hydrochloride BPCRS*. Each mg of $C_{17}H_{19}NO_3$ is equivalent to 1.33 mg of $(C_{17}H_{19}NO_3)_2,H_2SO_4,5H_2O$.

Morphine Suppositories

Definition Morphine Suppositories contain Morphine Hydrochloride or Morphine Sulphate in a suitable suppository basis.

The suppositories comply with the requirements stated under Rectal Preparations and with the following requirements.

Content of morphine As the hydrochloride, $C_{17}H_{19}NO_3,HCl,3H_2O$, or as the sulphate, $(C_{17}H_{19}NO_3)_2,H_2SO_4,5H_2O$, 95.0 to 105.0% of the prescribed or stated amount.

Identification Dissolve a quantity of the suppositories containing 90 mg of Morphine Hydrochloride or Morphine Sulphate in 25 ml of *chloroform*, extract with 50 ml of 0.01M *hydrochloric acid* and wash the aqueous layer with two 20-ml quantities of *chloroform*. Make the aqueous layer alkaline with *ammonia buffer pH 10.0* and extract with two 40-ml quantities of a mixture of 3 volumes of *chloroform* and 1 volume of *propan-2-ol*. Dry the combined extracts with *anhydrous sodium sulphate*, filter and evaporate the filtrate to dryness. The *infrared absorption spectrum* of the residue, Appendix II A, is concordant with the *reference spectrum* of morphine.

Related substances Carry out the method for *thin-layer chromatography*, Appendix III A, using *silica gel G* as the coating substance and a mixture of 2.5 volumes of 13.5M *ammonia*, 32.5 volumes of *acetone*, 35 volumes of *ethanol (70%)* and 35 volumes of *toluene* as the mobile phase. Apply separately to the plate 10 µl of each of the following solutions. For solution (1) disperse a quantity of the mixed suppositories prepared for the assay containing 0.1 g of Morphine Hydrochloride or Morphine Sulphate in 10 ml of hot *water*, mix vigorously, allow to cool until the mass sets and filter the lower, aqueous layer. For solution (2) dissolve 50 mg of *codeine phosphate* in 5 ml of solution (1) and dilute 1 volume of the resulting solution to 100 volumes with *water*. After removal of the plate, dry it in a current of air, spray with *potassium iodobismuthate solution*, dry for 15 minutes in a current of air and spray with *hydrogen peroxide solution (10 vol)*. The spot due to codeine is bluish grey and the spot due to morphine is pinkish. In the chromatogram obtained with solution (1) any spot corresponding to codeine is not more intense than the spot due to codeine in the chromatogram obtained with solution (2) (1%) and any other *secondary spot* is not more intense than the spot due to morphine in the chromatogram obtained with solution (2) (1%). The test is not valid unless the chromatogram obtained with solution (2) shows two clearly separated spots.

Assay Carry out the method for *liquid chromatography*, Appendix III D, using the following solutions. For solution (1) dissolve 30 mg of *morphine hydrochloride BPCRS* in 60 ml of 0.01M *hydrochloric acid*, add 20 ml of 0.3M *dipotassium hydrogen orthophosphate* and dilute to 100 ml with *water*. For solution (2) weigh 10 suppositories, melt together by warming and allow to cool, stirring continuously until the mass has set. Dissolve a quantity containing 30 mg of Morphine Hydrochloride or Morphine Sulphate in 25 ml of *chloroform*, extract with two quantities of 40 ml and 20 ml of 0.01M *hydrochloric acid*, wash the combined aqueous layers with two 20-ml quantities of *chloroform*, add 20 ml of 0.3M *dipotassium hydrogen orthophosphate* and dilute to 100 ml with *water*. Solution (3) contains 0.03% w/v of *morphine hydrochloride BPCRS* and 0.04% w/v of *codeine phosphate BPCRS* in the mobile phase.

The chromatographic procedure may be carried out using (a) a stainless steel column (10 cm × 4.6 mm) packed with *stationary phase C* (5 µm) (Nucleosil C18 is suitable), (b) as the mobile phase with a flow rate of 2 ml per minute, a solution containing 0.22% w/v of *dioctyl sodium sulphosuccinate* and 0.14% w/v of *sodium acetate* in a mixture of 60 volumes of *methanol* and 40 volumes of *water*, the pH of the solution being adjusted to 5.5 with *glacial acetic acid*, and (c) a detection wavelength of 285 nm.

The test is not valid unless in the chromatogram obtained with solution (3) the *resolution factor* between the peaks due to morphine and codeine is at least 2.0.

Calculate the content of $C_{17}H_{19}NO_3,HCl,3H_2O$ or $(C_{17}H_{19}NO_3)_2,H_2SO_4,5H_2O$, as appropriate, using the declared content of $C_{17}H_{19}NO_3$ in *morphine hydrochloride BPCRS*. Each g of $C_{17}H_{19}NO_3$ is equivalent to 1.317 g of $C_{17}H_{19}NO_3,HCl,3H_2O$ or 1.330 g of $(C_{17}H_{19}NO_3)_2,H_2SO_4,5H_2O$.

Labelling The label states the quantity of Morphine Hydrochloride or of Morphine Sulphate in each suppository.

Morphine Tablets

Definition Morphine Tablets contain Morphine Sulphate.

The tablets comply with the requirements stated under Tablets and with the following requirements.

Content of morphine sulphate, $(C_{17}H_{19}NO_3)_2,H_2SO_4,5H_2O$ 92.5 to 107.5% of the prescribed or stated amount.

Identification

A. Extract a quantity of the powdered tablets containing 20 mg of Morphine Sulphate with 5 ml of *water*, filter and add to the filtrate 0.05 ml of *iron(III) chloride solution R1*. A blue colour is produced.

B. Extract a quantity of the powdered tablets containing 10 mg of Morphine Sulphate with 10 ml of *water*, filter and to 5 ml of the filtrate add 0.15 ml of *dilute potassium hexacyanoferrate(III) solution* and 0.05 ml of *iron(III) chloride solution R1*. A bluish green colour is produced immediately which changes rapidly to blue.

C. The powdered tablets yield the reactions characteristic of *sulphates*, Appendix VI.

Dissolution Comply with the *dissolution test for tablets and capsules*, Appendix XII D, using Apparatus II. Use as the medium 900 ml of *phosphate buffer pH 6.5* and rotate the paddle at 50 revolutions per minute. Withdraw a sample of 10 ml of the medium and filter. Carry out the method for *liquid chromatography*, Appendix III D, using the following solutions. Solution (1) contains 0.001% w/v of *morphine hydrochloride BPCRS* in *phosphate buffer pH 6.5*. Solution (2) is the filtered dissolution medium, diluted with *phosphate buffer pH 6.5*, if necessary, to produce a solution containing about 0.001% w/v of Morphine Sulphate.

The chromatographic procedure may be carried out using (a) a stainless steel column (10 cm × 4.6 mm) packed with *stationary phase C* (5 μm) (Spherisorb ODS 2 is suitable), (b) a mixture of 50 volumes of *methanol* and 50 volumes of 0.01M *sodium heptanesulphonate* in 0.1M *acetic acid* as the mobile phase with a flow rate of 2.0 ml per minute and (c) a detection wavelength of 211 nm.

Inject 50 μl of each solution. Calculate the total content of morphine sulphate, $(C_{17}H_{19}NO_3)_2,H_2SO_4,5H_2O$, in the medium using the declared content of $C_{17}H_{19}NO_3$ in *morphine hydrochloride BPCRS*. Each g of $C_{17}H_{19}NO_3$ is equivalent to 1.330 g of $(C_{17}H_{19}NO_3)_2,H_2SO_4,5H_2O$.

Assay Weigh and powder 20 tablets. Shake a quantity of the powder containing 0.1 g of Morphine Sulphate with 25 ml of *water* and 5 ml of 1M *sodium hydroxide*, add 1 g of *ammonium sulphate*, shake to dissolve, add 20 ml of *ethanol (96%)* and extract with successive quantities of 40, 20, 20 and 20 ml of a mixture of 3 volumes of *chloroform* and 1 volume of *ethanol (96%)*. Wash each extract with the same 5 ml of *water*, filter and evaporate the solvent. Dissolve the residue in 10 ml of 0.05M *hydrochloric acid VS*, boil, cool, add 15 ml of *water* and titrate the excess of acid with 0.05M *sodium hydroxide VS* using *methyl red solution* as indicator. Each ml of 0.05M *hydrochloric acid VS* is equivalent to 18.97 mg of $(C_{17}H_{19}NO_3)_2,H_2SO_4,5H_2O$.

Storage Morphine Tablets should be protected from light.

Moxisylyte Tablets
Thymoxamine Tablets

For the purposes of product labelling in the United Kingdom, the pair of names given above shall be used together (see Introduction, Changes in title).

Definition Moxisylyte Tablets contain Moxisylyte Hydrochloride.

The tablets comply with the requirements stated under Tablets and with the following requirements.

Content of moxisylyte, $C_{16}H_{25}NO_3$ 92.5 to 107.5% of the prescribed or stated amount.

Identification Shake a quantity of the powdered tablets containing the equivalent of 20 mg of moxisylyte with 10 ml of *chloroform*, filter and evaporate the filtrate to dryness. The residue complies with the following tests.

A. The *infrared absorption spectrum*, Appendix II A, is concordant with the *reference spectrum* of moxisylyte hydrochloride.

B. Dilute 20 ml of a 0.03% w/v solution to 100 ml with *water* (solution A). Dilute a further 20 ml of the same solution to 100 ml with 0.1M *sodium hydroxide* (solution B). The ratio of the *absorbance* of solution B at 302 nm, measured 30 minutes after preparation, to that of solution A at 275 nm is about 1.7, Appendix II B.

Related substances Carry out the test described under Moxisylyte Hydrochloride using the following solutions. Solution (1) contains 0.040% w/v of *2-(6-hydroxythymoxy)ethyldimethylamine hydrochloride BPCRS*, 0.0050% w/v of *2-thymoxyethyldimethylamine hydrochloride BPCRS* and 0.020% w/v of *2-(6-chlorothymoxy)ethyldimethylamine hydrochloride BPCRS* in the mobile phase. For solution (2) shake a quantity of the powdered tablets containing the equivalent of 0.18 g of moxisylyte with 10 ml of the mobile phase for 15 minutes, centrifuge and use the clear supernatant liquid.

Assay Weigh and powder 20 tablets. Shake a quantity of the powder containing the equivalent of 13 mg of moxisylyte with 150 ml of 0.1M *hydrochloric acid*, add sufficient 0.1M *hydrochloric acid* to produce 250 ml and filter. Measure the *absorbance* of the filtrate at the maximum at 275 nm, Appendix II B. Calculate the content of $C_{16}H_{25}NO_3$ taking 79.7 as the value of A(1%, 1 cm) at the maximum at 275 nm.

Storage Moxisylyte Tablets should be protected from light.

Labelling The label states 'Moxisylyte Tablets' and 'Thymoxamine Tablets'.

The quantity of active ingredient is stated in terms of the equivalent amount of the free base.

40 mg of the free base is equivalent to 45.2 mg of Moxisylyte Hydrochloride (Thymoxamine Hydrochloride).

Nabumetone Oral Suspension

Definition Nabumetone Oral Suspension contains Nabumetone in a suitable flavoured vehicle.

The oral suspension complies with the requirements stated under Oral Liquids and with the following requirements.

Content of nabumetone, $C_{15}H_{16}O_2$ 95.0 to 105.0% of the prescribed or stated amount.

Identification

A. Carry out the method for *thin-layer chromatography*, Appendix III A, using a silica gel GF_{254} precoated plate (Merck 5715 plates are suitable) and *chloroform* as the mobile phase. Apply separately to the plate 2 µl of each of the following solutions. For solution (1) add a volume of the well-shaken suspension containing 0.1 g of Nabumetone to 10 ml of *chloroform*, shake, allow to separate and use the lower layer. Solution (2) contains 1.0% w/v of *nabumetone BPCRS* in *chloroform*. Solution (3) is a mixture of equal volumes of solutions (1) and (2). After removal of the plate, allow it to dry in air and examine under *ultraviolet light (254 nm)*. The principal spot in the chromatogram obtained with solution (1) is similar in position to the spot in the chromatogram obtained with solution (2) and the chromatogram obtained with solution (3) shows a single, compact spot at the same Rf value as the spot in the chromatogram obtained with solution (2).

B. In the Assay the retention time of the principal peak in the chromatogram obtained with solution (1) is the same as that of the peak in the chromatogram obtained with solution (2).

Related substances Carry out the method for *liquid chromatography*, Appendix III D, using the following solutions. For solution (1) add a volume of the well-shaken suspension containing 0.5 g of Nabumetone to 10 ml of *1,2-dichloroethane*, shake, allow to separate and dilute 1 volume of the dichloroethane layer to 10 volumes with *1,2-dichloroethane*. For solution (2) dilute 1 volume of solution (1) to 200 volumes with *1,2-dichloroethane*. Solution (3) contains 0.0015% w/v of *6,6-dimethoxy-2,2-binaphthyl BPCRS* in *1,2-dichloroethane*. Solution (4) contains 0.005% w/v of *nabumetone BPCRS* and 0.005% w/v of *5-(6-methoxy-2-naphthyl)-3-methylcyclohexan-1-one BPCRS* in *1,2-dichloroethane*.

The chromatographic procedure may be carried out using (a) a stainless steel column (25 cm × 4.6 mm) packed with *stationary phase A* (5 µm) (Spherisorb S5W is suitable), (b) *1,2-dichloroethane* as the mobile phase at a flow rate such that the retention time of the principal peak in the chromatogram obtained with solution (2) is about 10 minutes (0.8 ml per minute may be suitable) and (c) a detection wavelength of 254 nm.

The test is not valid unless, in the chromatogram obtained with solution (3), the retention time of the principal peak is at least 3 minutes and, in the chromatogram obtained with solution (4), the *resolution factor* between the peaks corresponding to nabumetone and 5-(6-methoxy-2-naphthyl)-3-methylcyclohexan-1-one is at least 3.

In the chromatogram obtained with solution (1) the area of any peak corresponding to 6,6-dimethoxy-2,2-binaphthyl is not greater than the area of the peak in the chromatogram obtained with solution (3) (0.3%) and the sum of the areas of any other *secondary peaks* is not greater than the area of the principal peak in the chromatogram obtained with solution (2) (0.5%). Allow the chromatography to proceed for 6 times the retention time of the principal peak.

Assay Carry out the method for *liquid chromatography*, Appendix III D, using the following solutions. For solution (1) add to a weighed quantity of the suspension containing 1 g of Nabumetone 70 ml of *ethanol (96%)*, mix with the aid of ultrasound for 45 minutes, and add sufficient *ethanol (96%)* to produce 100 ml and filter (Whatman GF/C paper is suitable). Dilute 1 volume of the filtrate to 25 volumes with the mobile phase and further dilute 2 volumes of this solution to 25 volumes with the mobile phase. Solution (2) contains 0.0035% w/v of *nabumetone BPCRS* in the mobile phase. Solution (3) contains 0.005% w/v of *nabumetone BPCRS* and 0.005% w/v of *5-(6-methoxy-2-naphthyl)-3-methylcyclohexan-1-one BPCRS* in the mobile phase.

The chromatographic procedure may be carried out using (a) a stainless steel column (15 cm × 3.9 mm) packed with *stationary phase C* (Nova-pak C18 is suitable), (b) a mixture of 2 volumes of *glacial acetic acid*, 88 volumes of *acetonitrile* and 110 volumes of *water* as the mobile phase at a flow rate of 1.4 ml per minute and (c) a detection wavelength of 254 nm.

The assay is not valid unless, in the chromatogram obtained with solution (3), the *resolution factor* between the peaks due to nabumetone and 5-(6-methoxy-2-naphthyl)-3-methylcyclohexan-1-one is at least 14.

Determine the *weight per ml* of the oral suspension, Appendix V G, adding 0.05 ml of *octanoic acid* if necessary to suppress froth, and calculate the content of $C_{15}H_{16}O_2$, weight in volume, in the oral suspension using the declared content of $C_{15}H_{16}O_2$ in *nabumetone BPCRS*.

Nabumetone Tablets

Definition Nabumetone Tablets contain Nabumetone.

The tablets comply with the requirements stated under Tablets and with the following requirements.

Content of nabumetone, $C_{15}H_{16}O_2$ 95.0 to 105.0% of the prescribed or stated amount.

Identification The *infrared absorption spectrum* of the powdered tablets, Appendix II A, is concordant with the *reference spectrum* of nabumetone.

Related substances Comply with the test described under Nabumetone Oral Suspension but using as solution (1) a solution prepared in the following manner. Extract a quantity of the powdered tablets containing 2 g of Nabumetone with 50 ml of *1,2-dichloroethane* for 15 minutes with the aid of ultrasound, add sufficient *1,2-dichloroethane* to produce 100 ml and filter (Whatman GF/C paper is suitable). Dilute 1 volume of the filtrate to 4 volumes with *1,2-dichloroethane*.

Assay Carry out the method for *liquid chromatography*, Appendix III D, using the following solutions. For solution (1) finely powder a quantity of whole tablets containing 5 g of Nabumetone, add 450 ml of *1,2-di-chloroethane*, mix with the aid of ultrasound for 15 minutes, add sufficient *1,2-dichloroethane* to produce 500 ml and filter (Whatman GF/C paper is suitable). Dilute 5 volumes of the filtrate to 250 volumes with *1,2-dichloroethane*. Solution (2) contains 0.02% w/v of *nabumetone BPCRS* in *1,2-dichloroethane*. Solution (3) contains 0.002% w/v each of *nabumetone BPCRS* and *5-(6-methoxy-2-naphthyl)-3-methylcyclohexan-1-one BPCRS* in *1,2-dichloroethane*.

The chromatographic procedure may be carried out using (a) a stainless steel column (25 cm × 4.6 mm) packed with *stationary phase A* (5 µm) (Spherisorb S5W is suitable), (b) *1,2-dichloroethane* as the mobile phase at a flow rate such that the retention time of the principal peak in the chromatogram obtained with solution (2) is about 5 minutes (2 ml per minute may be suitable) and (c) a detection wavelength of 254 nm.

The assay is not valid unless, in the chromatogram obtained with solution (3), the *resolution factor* between the peaks due to nabumetone and 5-(6-methoxy-2-naphthyl)-3-methylcyclohexan-1-one is at least 3.

Calculate the content of $C_{15}H_{16}O_2$ in the tablets using the declared content of $C_{15}H_{16}O_2$ in *nabumetone BPCRS*.

Naftidrofuryl Capsules

Definition Naftidrofuryl Capsules contain Naftidrofuryl Oxalate.

The capsules comply with the requirements stated under Capsules and with the following requirements.

Content of naftidrofuryl oxalate, $C_{26}H_{35}NO_7$ 95.0 to 105.0% of the prescribed or stated amount.

Identification

A. Shake, with the aid of ultrasound, a quantity of the powdered contents of the capsules containing 0.1 g of Naftidrofuryl Oxalate with 5 ml of *water* and filter (Whatman GF/C filter paper is suitable). Add 5 ml of 2M *sodium hydroxide* to the filtrate, extract with two 10-ml quantities of *chloroform*, wash the combined chloroform extracts with two 10-ml quantities of *water*, evaporate to dryness using a rotary evaporator and dry the oily residue over *phosphorus pentoxide* at a pressure of 2 kPa for 18 hours. The *infrared absorption spectrum* of the oily residue, Appendix II A, is concordant with the *reference spectrum* of naftidrofuryl.

B. Mix a quantity of the powdered contents of the capsules containing 0.25 g of Naftidrofuryl Oxalate with 5 ml of *water*, shake for 10 minutes and filter. Add *calcium chloride solution* to the filtrate; a white precipitate is produced. The residue dissolves in mineral acids but is practically insoluble in 2M *acetic acid* and in 6M *ammonia*.

Related substances Carry out the method for *liquid chromatography*, Appendix III D, using 20 µl of the following solutions. For solution (1) mix with the aid of ultrasound a quantity of the powdered contents of the capsules with sufficient of the mobile phase to produce a solution containing 0.1% w/v of Naftidrofuryl Oxalate and filter (Whatman GF/C filter paper is suitable). Solution (2) contains 0.001% w/v of *3-(1-naphthyl)-2-tetrahydrofurfurylpropionic acid BPCRS* in the mobile phase. Solution (3) contains 0.0002% w/v of *2-diethylaminoethyl-3-(1-naphthyl)-2-(1-naphthylmethyl)propionate oxalate BPCRS* in the mobile phase. Solution (4) contains 0.01% w/v of *naftidrofuryl oxalate BPCRS* and 0.005% w/v of *2-diethylaminoethyl-3-(1-naphthyl)-2-(1-naphthylmethyl)propionate oxalate BPCRS* in the mobile phase.

The chromatographic conditions described under Assay may be used.

The test is not valid unless in the chromatogram obtained with solution (4) the *resolution factor* between the two principal peaks is at least 4.

Inject solution (1) and record the chromatography for twice the retention time of the principal peak. In the chromatogram obtained with solution (1) the area of any peak corresponding to 3-(1-naphthyl)-2-tetrahydrofurfurylpropionic acid is not greater than the area of the peak in the chromatogram obtained with solution (2) (1%), the area of any peak corresponding to 2-diethylaminoethyl-3-(1-naphthyl)-2-(1-naphthylmethyl)propionate oxalate is not greater than the area of the peak in the chromatogram obtained with solution (3) (0.2%), the area of any other *secondary peak* is not greater than half the area of the peak in the chromatogram obtained with solution (3) (0.1%) and the sum of the areas of all the *secondary peaks* other than those corresponding to the named impurities is not greater than 1.5 times the area of the peak in the chromatogram obtained with solution (3) (0.3%).

Assay Carry out the method for *liquid chromatography*, Appendix III D, using 20 µl of the following solutions. For solution (1) finely powder the contents of 10 capsules, mix with the aid of a spatula, dissolve with the aid of ultrasound in sufficient of the mobile phase to produce a solution containing 1% w/v of Naftidrofuryl Oxalate, filter (Whatman GF/C filter paper is suitable) and dilute 1 volume of the filtrate to 10 volumes with the mobile phase. Solution (2) contains 0.1% w/v of *naftidrofuryl oxalate BPCRS* in the mobile phase.

The chromatographic procedure may be carried out using (a) a stainless steel column (25 cm × 4.6 mm) packed with particles of silica the surface of which has been modified by chemically-bonded phenyl groups (5 µm) (Spherisorb Phenyl is suitable), (b) a mixture of 40 volumes of 0.05M *sodium acetate*, adjusted to pH 4.0 with an 85% v/v solution of *orthophosphoric acid*, and 60 volumes of *acetonitrile* as the mobile phase with a flow rate of 1 ml per minute and (c) a detection wavelength of 283 nm.

Calculate the content of $C_{26}H_{35}NO_7$ in the capsules using the declared content of $C_{26}H_{35}NO_7$ in *naftidrofuryl oxalate BPCRS*.

Nalidixic Acid Oral Suspension

Definition Nalidixic Acid Oral Suspension is a suspension of Nalidixic Acid in a suitable flavoured vehicle.

The oral suspension complies with the requirements stated under Oral Liquids and with the following requirements.

Content of nalidixic acid, $C_{12}H_{12}N_2O_3$ 92.5 to 107.5% of the prescribed or stated amount.

Identification To 5 ml add 30 ml of *water* and 20 ml of *dilute sodium carbonate solution*, mix and shake with two

30-ml quantities of *chloroform*; discard the chloroform layers. Acidify the aqueous solution with 5M *hydrochloric acid*, shake with 40 ml of *chloroform*, wash the chloroform layer with 10 ml of *water* to which has been added 0.5 ml of 5M *hydrochloric acid*, filter the chloroform layer through absorbent cotton and evaporate the filtrate to dryness. Dissolve the residue in sufficient 0.1M *sodium hydroxide* to produce a solution containing 0.0008% w/v of Nalidixic Acid. The *light absorption* of the solution, Appendix II B, in the range 230 to 350 nm exhibits two maxima, at 258 nm and 334 nm.

Assay Dilute a weighed quantity containing 0.12 g of Nalidixic Acid to 100 ml with 0.01M *sodium hydroxide*, dilute 2 ml to 250 ml with 0.01M *sodium hydroxide* and measure the *absorbance* of the resulting solution at the maximum at 334 nm, Appendix II B. Determine the *weight per ml* of the oral suspension, Appendix V G, and calculate the content of $C_{12}H_{12}N_2O_3$, weight in volume, taking 494 as the value of A(1%, 1 cm) at the maximum at 334 nm.

Nalidixic Acid Tablets

Definition Nalidixic Acid Tablets contain Nalidixic Acid.

The tablets comply with the requirements stated under Tablets and with the following requirements.

Content of nalidixic acid, $C_{12}H_{12}N_2O_3$ 95.0 to 105.0% of the prescribed or stated amount.

Identification To a quantity of the powdered tablets containing 1 g of Nalidixic Acid add 50 ml of *chloroform*, shake for 15 minutes, filter and evaporate the filtrate to dryness. The residue, after drying at 105°, complies with the following tests.

A. The *infrared absorption spectrum*, Appendix II A, is concordant with the *reference spectrum* of nalidixic acid.

B. The *light absorption*, Appendix II B, in the range 230 to 350 nm of a 0.0008% w/v solution in 0.1M *sodium hydroxide* exhibits maxima at 258 nm and 334 nm.

C. *Melting point*, about 228°, Appendix V A.

Dissolution Comply with the *dissolution test for tablets and capsules*, Appendix XII D, using Apparatus II. Rotate the paddle at 50 revolutions per minute and use as the medium 900 ml of a methanolic phosphate buffer prepared in the following manner: mix 2.3 volumes of 0.2M *sodium hydroxide* with 2.5 volumes of 0.2M *potassium dihydrogen orthophosphate* and 2.0 volumes of *methanol*, dilute to 10 volumes with *water* and, if necessary, adjust the pH to 8.6 using 1M *sodium hydroxide*. Withdraw a sample of 10 ml of the medium, filter and measure the *absorbance* of the solution, suitably diluted if necessary, at the maximum at 351 nm, Appendix II B. Calculate the total content of nalidixic acid, $C_{12}H_{12}N_2O_3$, in the medium taking 175 as the value of A(1%, 1 cm) at the maximum at 351 nm.

Related substances Carry out the method for *thin-layer chromatography*, Appendix III A, using *silica gel GF_{254}* as the coating substance and a mixture of 10 volumes of 5M *ammonia*, 20 volumes of *dichloromethane* and 70 volumes of *ethanol (96%)* as the mobile phase. Apply separately to the plate 10 µl of each of the following solutions. For solution (1) shake a quantity of the powdered tablets containing 0.10 g of Nalidixic Acid with 50 ml of *dichloromethane* for 15 minutes, filter, evaporate to dryness and dissolve the residue in 5 ml of *dichloromethane*. For solution (2) dilute 1 volume of solution (1) to 200 volumes with *dichloromethane* and further dilute 1 volume of the resulting solution to 2 volumes with *dichloromethane*. For solution (3) dilute 1 volume of solution (2) to 2.5 volumes with *dichloromethane*. After removal of the plate, allow it to dry in air and examine under *ultraviolet light (254 nm)*. Any *secondary spot* in the chromatogram obtained with solution (1) is not more intense than the spot in the chromatogram obtained with solution (2) (0.25%) and not more than one such spot is more intense than the spot in the chromatogram obtained with solution (3) (0.1%).

Assay Weigh and powder 20 tablets. To a quantity of the powdered tablets containing 0.1 g of Nalidixic Acid add 150 ml of 1M *sodium hydroxide*, shake for 3 minutes, dilute to 200 ml with 1M *sodium hydroxide*, mix and allow to stand for 15 minutes. Dilute 2 ml to 200 ml with *water* and measure the *absorbance* of the resulting solution at the maximum at 334 nm, Appendix II B, using 0.01M *sodium hydroxide* in the reference cell. Calculate the content of $C_{12}H_{12}N_2O_3$ taking 494 as the value of A(1%, 1 cm) at the maximum at 334 nm.

Storage Nalidixic Acid Tablets should be protected from light.

Naloxone Injection

Definition Naloxone Injection is a sterile solution of Naloxone Hydrochloride in Water for Injections.

The injection complies with the requirements stated under Parenteral Preparations and with the following requirements.

Content of naloxone hydrochloride, $C_{19}H_{21}NO_4,HCl$ 95.0 to 105.0% of the prescribed or stated amount.

Identification

A. In the Assay, the retention time of the principal peak in the chromatogram obtained with solution (1) has the same retention time as the principal peak in the chromatogram obtained with solution (2).

B. Carry out the method for *thin-layer chromatography*, Appendix III A, using *silica gel G* as the coating substance. Heat the plate at 105° for 15 minutes immediately before use. Use a mixture of 5 volumes of *methanol* and 95 volumes of the upper layer from a mixture of 60 ml of 2M *ammonia* and 100 ml of *butan-1-ol* as the mobile phase but allowing the solvent front to ascend 10 cm above the line of application. Apply separately to the plate 20 µl of each of the following solutions. For solution (1) add to a volume of the injection containing 2 mg of Naloxone Hydrochloride 1 ml of *ammonia buffer pH 10.0*, extract with three 20-ml quantities of a mixture of 1 volume of *propan-2-ol* and 3 volumes of *chloroform*, dry the combined extracts over *anhydrous sodium sulphate*, filter, evaporate the filtrate to dryness and dissolve the residue in 1 ml of *methanol*. Dilute 1 volume of this solution to 20 volumes with *methanol*. Solution (2) contains 0.010% w/v of *naloxone hydrochloride BPCRS* in *methanol*. Protect the plate from light during development. After removal of the plate, dry it in a current of air, spray with a freshly prepared 0.5% w/v solution of *potassium hexacyanoferrate(III)* in *iron(III) chloride solution R1* and examine in daylight. The principal spot in the chromatogram obtained with solution (1) corresponds to that in the chromatogram obtained with solution (2).

Acidity pH, 3.0 to 4.5, Appendix V L.

Related substances Carry out the method for *thin-layer chromatography*, Appendix III A, using *silica gel G* as the coating substance. Heat the plate at 105° for 15 minutes immediately before use. Use a mixture of 5 volumes of *methanol* and 95 volumes of the upper layer from a mixture of 60 ml of 2M *ammonia* and 100 ml of *butan-1-ol* as the mobile phase but allowing the solvent front to ascend 10 cm above the line of application. Apply separately to the plate 20 µl of each of the following solutions. For solution (1) add to a volume of the injection containing 2 mg of Naloxone Hydrochloride 1 ml of *ammonia buffer pH 10.0*, extract with three 20-ml quantities of a mixture of 1 volume of *propan-2-ol* and 3 volumes of *chloroform*, dry the combined extracts over *anhydrous sodium sulphate*, filter, evaporate the filtrate to dryness and dissolve the residue in 1 ml of *methanol*. For solution (2) dilute 1 volume of solution (1) to 200 volumes with *methanol*. Protect the plate from light during development. After removal of the plate, dry it in a current of air, spray with a freshly prepared 0.5% w/v solution of *potassium hexacyanoferrate(III)* in *iron(III) chloride solution R1* and examine in daylight. Any *secondary spot* in the chromatogram obtained with solution (1) is not more intense than the spot in the chromatogram obtained with solution (2) (0.5%). Disregard any spot remaining on the line of application.

Bacterial endotoxins Carry out the *test for bacterial endotoxins*, Appendix XIV C. The endotoxin limit concentration of the injection, diluted if necessary with *water BET* to give a solution containing 0.04% w/v of Naloxone Hydrochloride per ml, is 70 IU of endotoxin per ml. Carry out the test using the maximum valid dilution of the above defined solution calculated from the declared sensitivity of the lysate used in the test.

Assay Carry out the method for *liquid chromatography*, Appendix III D, using the following solutions. For solution (1) dilute the injection to contain 0.001% w/v of Naloxone Hydrochloride with a mixture of 1 volume of *orthophosphoric acid*, 450 volumes of *methanol* and 550 volumes of *water*. Solution (2) contains 0.001% w/v of *naloxone hydrochloride BPCRS* in a mixture of 1 volume of *orthophosphoric acid*, 450 volumes of *methanol* and 550 volumes of *water*. Solution (3) contains 0.001% w/v of *naloxone hydrochloride BPCRS* and 0.0005% w/v of *noroxymorphone* in a mixture of 1 volume of *orthophosphoric acid*, 450 volumes of *methanol* and 550 volumes of *water*.

The chromatographic procedure may be carried out using (a) a stainless steel column (25 cm × 4.6 mm) packed with *stationary phase C* (5 to 10 µm) (Zorbax C18 7 to 8 µm is suitable), (b) as the mobile phase with a flow rate of 1 ml per minute a solution containing 0.068% w/v of *sodium octanesulphonate* and 0.1% w/v of *sodium chloride* in a mixture of 1 volume of *orthophosphoric acid*, 450 volumes of *methanol* and 550 volumes of *water* and (c) a detection wavelength of 229 nm.

The test is not valid unless the *resolution factor* between the peaks due to naloxone and noroxymorphone in the chromatogram obtained with solution (3) is at least 1.3.

Calculate the content of $C_{19}H_{21}NO_4,HCl$ in the injection using the declared content of $C_{19}H_{21}NO_4,HCl$ in *naloxone hydrochloride BPCRS*.

Storage Naloxone Injection should be protected from light.

When naloxone is prescribed for neonatal use, Neonatal Naloxone Injection (containing 20 micrograms per ml of Naloxone Hydrochloride) shall be dispensed.

Neonatal Naloxone Injection

Definition Neonatal Naloxone Injection is a sterile solution containing 20 micrograms per ml of Naloxone Hydrochloride in Water for Injections.

The injection complies with the requirements stated under Parenteral Preparations and with the following requirements.

Content of naloxone hydrochloride, $C_{19}H_{21}NO_4,HCl$
0.0185 to 0.0215% w/v.

Identification

A. In the Assay, the retention time of the principal peak in the chromatogram obtained with solution (1) has the same retention time as the principal peak in the chromatogram obtained with solution (2).

B. Carry out the method for *thin-layer chromatography*, Appendix III A, using *silica gel G* as the coating substance. Heat the plate at 105° for 15 minutes immediately before use. Use a mixture of 5 volumes of *methanol* and 95 volumes of the upper layer from a mixture of 60 ml of 2M *ammonia* and 100 ml of *butan-1-ol* as the mobile phase but allowing the solvent front to ascend 10 cm above the line of application. Apply separately to the plate 20 µl of each of the following solutions. For solution (1) add to a volume of the injection containing 0.1 mg of Naloxone Hydrochloride 1 ml of *ammonia buffer pH 10.0*, extract with three 20-ml quantities of a mixture of 1 volume of *propan-2-ol* and 3 volumes of *chloroform*, dry the combined extracts over *anhydrous sodium sulphate*, filter, evaporate the filtrate to dryness and dissolve the residue in 1 ml of *methanol*. Solution (2) contains 0.010% w/v of *naloxone hydrochloride BPCRS* in *methanol*. Protect the plate from light during development. After removal of the plate, dry it in a current of air, spray with a freshly prepared 0.5% w/v solution of *potassium hexacyanoferrate(III)* in *iron(III) chloride solution R1* and examine in daylight. The principal spot in the chromatogram obtained with solution (1) corresponds to that in the chromatogram obtained with solution (2).

Acidity pH, 3.0 to 4.5, Appendix V L.

Bacterial endotoxins Carry out the *test for bacterial endotoxins*, Appendix XIV C. The endotoxin limit concentration is 3.5 IU per ml.Carry out the test using the maximum valid dilution of the injection calculated from the declared sensitivity of the lysate used in the test.

Assay Carry out the method for *liquid chromatography*, Appendix III D, using the following solutions. For solution (1) dilute the injection to contain 0.001% w/v of Naloxone Hydrochloride with a mixture of 1 volume of *orthophosphoric acid*, 450 volumes of *methanol* and 550 volumes of *water*. Solution (2) contains 0.001% w/v of *naloxone hydrochloride BPCRS* in a mixture of 1 volume of *orthophosphoric acid*, 450 volumes of *methanol* and 550 volumes of *water*. Solution (3) contains 0.001% w/v of *naloxone hydrochloride BPCRS* and 0.0005% w/v of *noroxymorphone* in a mixture of 1 volume of *orthophosphoric* *acid*, 450 volumes of *methanol* and 550 volumes of *water*.

The chromatographic procedure may be carried out using (a) a stainless steel column (25 cm × 4.6 mm) packed with *stationary phase C* (5 to 10 µm) (Zorbax C18 7 to 8 µm is suitable), (b) as the mobile phase with a flow rate of 1 ml per minute a solution containing 0.068% w/v of *sodium octanesulphonate* and 0.1% w/v of *sodium chloride* in a mixture of 1 volume of *orthophosphoric acid*, 450 volumes of *methanol* and 550 volumes of *water* and (c) a detection wavelength of 229 nm.

The test is not valid unless the *resolution factor* between the peaks due to naloxone and noroxymorphone in the chromatogram obtained with solution (3) is at least 1.3.

Calculate the content of $C_{19}H_{21}NO_4,HCl$ in the injection using the declared content of $C_{19}H_{21}NO_4,HCl$ in *naloxone hydrochloride BPCRS*.

Storage Neonatal Naloxone Injection should be protected from light.

Labelling The label states that the injection is intended for neonatal use.

Nandrolone Decanoate Injection

Definition Nandrolone Decanoate Injection is a sterile solution of Nandrolone Decanoate in Ethyl Oleate or other suitable ester, in a suitable fixed oil or in any mixture of these.

The injection complies with the requirements stated under Parenteral Preparations and with the following requirements.

Content of nandrolone decanoate, $C_{28}H_{44}O_3$ 92.5 to 107.5% of the prescribed or stated amount.

Identification Carry out the method for *thin-layer chromatography*, Appendix III A, using a silica gel F_{254} precoated plate the surface of which has been modified by chemically-bonded octadecylsilyl groups (Whatman KC 18F plates are suitable) and a mixture of 20 volumes of *water*, 40 volumes of *acetonitrile* and 60 volumes of *propan-2-ol* as the mobile phase. Apply separately to the plate 5 µl of each of the following three solutions. For solution (1) dilute the injection with *chloroform* to give a solution containing 0.5% w/v of Nandrolone Decanoate. Solution (2) contains 0.5% w/v of *nandrolone decanoate BPCRS* in *chloroform*. Solution (3) is a mixture of equal volumes of solutions (1) and (2). After removal of the plate, allow it to dry in air until the odour of solvent is no longer detectable and heat at 100° for 10 minutes. Allow to cool and examine under *ultraviolet light (254 nm)*. The principal spot in the chromatogram obtained with solution (1) corresponds to that in the chromatogram obtained with solution (2). The principal spot in the chromatogram obtained with solution (3) appears as a single, compact spot.

Assay To a quantity containing 0.1 g of Nandrolone Decanoate add sufficient *chloroform* to produce 100 ml. Dilute 3 ml to 50 ml with *chloroform* and to 5 ml of this solution add 10 ml of *isoniazid solution* and sufficient *methanol* to produce 20 ml. Allow to stand for 45 minutes and measure the *absorbance* of the resulting solution at the maximum at 380 nm, Appendix II B, using in the reference cell 5 ml of *chloroform* treated in the same manner. Calculate the content of $C_{28}H_{44}O_3$ from the *absorbance* obtained by repeating the operation using a suitable quantity of *nandrolone BPCRS* and from the declared content of $C_{18}H_{26}O_2$ in *nandrolone BPCRS*. Each mg of $C_{18}H_{26}O_2$ is equivalent to 1.562 mg of $C_{28}H_{44}O_3$.

Storage Nandrolone Decanoate Injection should be protected from light.

Labelling The label states that the preparation is for intramuscular injection only.

Nandrolone Phenylpropionate Injection

Definition Nandrolone Phenylpropionate Injection is a sterile solution of Nandrolone Phenylpropionate in Ethyl Oleate or other suitable ester, in a suitable fixed oil or in any mixture of these.

The injection complies with the requirements stated under Parenteral Preparations and with the following requirements.

Content of nandrolone phenylpropionate, $C_{27}H_{34}O_3$ 92.5 to 107.5% of the prescribed or stated amount.

Identification Dissolve a volume containing 50 mg of Nandrolone Phenylpropionate in 8 ml of *petroleum spirit (boiling range, 40° to 60°)* and extract with three 8-ml quantities of a mixture of 7 volumes of *glacial acetic acid* and 3 volumes of *water*. Wash the combined extracts with 10 ml of *petroleum spirit (boiling range, 40° to 60°)*, dilute with *water* until the solution becomes turbid, allow to stand for 2 hours in ice and filter. The precipitate, after washing with *water* and drying over *phosphorus pentoxide* at a pressure not exceeding 0.7 kPa, complies with the following tests.

A. Carry out the method for *thin-layer chromatography*, Appendix III A, using a silica gel F_{254} precoated plate the surface of which has been modified by chemically-bonded octadecylsilyl groups (Whatman KC 18F plates are suitable) and a mixture of 20 volumes of *water*, 40 volumes of *acetonitrile* and 60 volumes of *propan-2-ol* as the mobile phase. Apply separately to the plate 5 µl of each of the following three solutions. Solution (1) contains 0.5% w/v of the dried precipitate in *chloroform*. Solution (2) contains 0.5% w/v of *nandrolone phenylpropionate BPCRS* in *chloroform*. Solution (3) is a mixture of equal volumes of solutions (1) and (2). After removal of the plate, allow it to dry in air until the odour of solvent is no longer detectable and heat at 100° for 10 minutes. Allow to cool and examine under *ultraviolet light (254 nm)*. The principal spot in the chromatogram obtained with solution (1) corresponds to that in the chromatogram obtained with solution (2). The principal spot in the chromatogram obtained with solution (3) appears as a single, compact spot.

B. *Melting point*, about 97°, Appendix V A.

Assay To a quantity containing 0.1 g of Nandrolone Phenylpropionate add sufficient *chloroform* to produce 100 ml. Dilute 3 ml to 50 ml with *chloroform* and to 5 ml of the solution add 10 ml of *isoniazid solution* and sufficient *methanol* to produce 20 ml. Allow to stand for 45 minutes and measure the *absorbance* of the resulting solution at the maximum at 380 nm, Appendix II B, using in the reference cell 5 ml of *chloroform* treated in the same manner. Calculate the content of $C_{27}H_{34}O_3$ from the *absorbance* obtained by repeating the operation using a

0.006% w/v solution of *nandrolone phenylpropionate BPCRS* in *chloroform* and beginning at the words 'to 5 ml ...' and using the declared content of $C_{27}H_{34}O_3$ in *nandrolone phenylpropionate BPCRS*.

Storage Nandrolone Phenylpropionate Injection should be protected from light.

Labelling The label states that the preparation is for intramuscular injection only.

Naproxen Oral Suspension

Definition Naproxen Oral Suspension is an aqueous suspension of Naproxen in a suitable flavoured vehicle.

The oral suspension complies with the requirements stated under Oral Liquids and with the following requirements.

Content of naproxen, $C_{14}H_{14}O_3$ 90.0 to 110.0% of the prescribed or stated amount.

Identification Evaporate 50 ml of solution A obtained in the Assay to dryness using a rotary evaporator. The residue complies with the following tests.

A. The *infrared absorption spectrum*, Appendix II A, is concordant with the *reference spectrum* of naproxen.

B. The *light absorption*, Appendix II B, in the range 230 to 350 nm of a 0.004% w/v solution in *methanol* exhibits four maxima, at 262, 271, 316 and 331 nm.

Acidity pH, 2.1 to 4.0, Appendix V L.

Related substances Carry out the method for *thin-layer chromatography*, Appendix III A, using *silica gel GF_{254}* as the coating substance and a mixture of 3 volumes of *glacial acetic acid*, 9 volumes of *tetrahydrofuran* and 90 volumes of *toluene* as the mobile phase. Apply separately to the plate 10 µl of each of the following solutions. For solution (1) evaporate solution A obtained in the Assay to dryness on a rotary evaporator and dissolve the residue in sufficient *methanol* to produce a solution containing 5.0% w/v of Naproxen. For solution (2) dilute 1 volume of solution (1) to 200 volumes with *methanol*. After removal of the plate, allow it to dry in air and examine under *ultraviolet light (254 nm)*. Any *secondary spot* in the chromatogram obtained with solution (1) is not more intense than the spot in the chromatogram obtained with solution (2) (0.5%).

Assay To a quantity of the oral suspension containing 0.5 g of Naproxen add 20 ml of 3.5M *hydrochloric acid*, mix, extract with three 50-ml quantities of *chloroform*, filter each extract through *anhydrous sodium sulphate*, combine the filtrates and add sufficient *chloroform* to produce 200 ml (solution A). To 5 ml of solution A add sufficient *methanol* to produce 250 ml and measure the *absorbance* of the resulting solution at the maximum at 331 nm, Appendix II B. Calculate the content of $C_{14}H_{14}O_3$ taking 81.0 as the value of A(1%, 1 cm) at the maximum at 331 nm.

Naproxen Suppositories

Definition Naproxen Suppositories contain Naproxen in a suitable suppository basis.

The suppositories comply with the requirements stated under Rectal Preparations and with the following requirements.

Content of naproxen $C_{14}H_{14}O_3$ 95.0 to 105.0% of the prescribed or stated amount.

Identification Dissolve a quantity of the suppositories containing 0.5 g of Naproxen in 50 ml of *2,2,4-trimethylpentane* and extract with four 25-ml quantities of *methanol (80%)*. To the combined extracts add 100 ml of a 2% w/v solution of *sodium chloride*, extract with four 25-ml quantities of *chloroform*, dry the combined extracts over *anhydrous sodium sulphate*, filter and add sufficient *chloroform* to produce 200 ml (solution A). Evaporate 100 ml of solution A to dryness using a rotary evaporator. The residue complies with the following tests.

A. The *infrared absorption spectrum*, Appendix II A, is concordant with the *reference spectrum* of naproxen.

B. The *light absorption*, Appendix II B, in the range 230 to 350 nm of a 0.004% w/v solution in *methanol* exhibits four maxima, at 262, 271, 316 and 331 nm.

Related substances Comply with the test described under Naproxen Oral Suspension using the following solutions. For solution (1) weigh 20 suppositories and cut into small pieces. Dissolve a quantity of the suppositories containing 0.5 g of Naproxen in 50 ml of *2,2,4-trimethylpentane* and extract with four 25-ml quantities of *methanol (80%)*. Combine the extracts, add 100 ml of a 2% w/v solution of *sodium chloride*, extract with four 25-ml quantities of *chloroform* filtering each extract through a layer of *anhydrous sodium sulphate* on an absorbent cotton plug moistened with *chloroform*. Evaporate the combined filtrates to dryness using a rotary evaporator with the aid of gentle heat. Shake the residue with 10 ml of *methanol*, centrifuge and use the supernatant liquid. For solution (2) dilute 1 volume of solution (1) to 200 volumes with *methanol*.

Assay Carry out the method for *liquid chromatography*, Appendix III D, using the following solutions. Solution (1) is a 0.01% w/v solution of *naproxen BPCRS* in the mobile phase. For solution (2) disperse ten suppositories in 500 ml of *methanol* on a water bath for 40 minutes with the aid of ultrasound and by swirling the flask. Cool at 5° for 1 hour, centrifuge and use the clear, supernatant liquid; if the solution is still cloudy filter through glass-fibre paper (Whatman GF/C is suitable). To 5 ml of the filtrate add sufficient of the mobile phase to produce a solution containing 0.01% w/v of naproxen. Solution (3) contains 0.01% w/v each of *naproxen BPCRS* and *2-naphthylacetic acid* in the mobile phase.

The chromatographic procedure may be carried out using (a) a stainless steel column (20 cm × 4 mm) packed with *stationary phase C* (5 µm) (Nucleosil C18 is suitable), (b) as the mobile phase with a flow rate of 2 ml per minute a mixture of 1 volume of a 0.52% w/v solution of *sodium acetate*, adjusted to pH 5.8 using *glacial acetic acid*, and 1 volume of *methanol* and (c) a detection wavelength of 254 nm.

The assay is not valid unless the *resolution factor* between the peaks due to naproxen and 2-naphthylacetic acid in the chromatogram obtained with solution (3) is greater than 3.0.

Calculate the content of $C_{14}H_{14}O_3$ using the declared content of $C_{14}H_{14}O_3$ in *naproxen BPCRS*.

Storage Naproxen Suppositories should be protected from light.

Naproxen Tablets

Definition Naproxen Tablets contain Naproxen.

The tablets comply with the requirements stated under Tablets and with the following requirements.

Content of naproxen, $C_{14}H_{14}O_3$ 95.0 to 105.0% of the prescribed or stated amount.

Identification

A. Extract a quantity of the powdered tablets containing 20 mg of Naproxen with sufficient *methanol* to produce 100 ml and filter. Reserve 10 ml of the filtrate for test B, evaporate the remainder and dry the residue at 105°. The *infrared absorption spectrum* of the residue, Appendix II A, is concordant with the *reference spectrum* of naproxen.

B. Dilute the 10-ml portion of the filtrate reserved in test A to 100 ml with *methanol*. The *light absorption* of the resulting solution, Appendix II B, in the range 230 to 350 nm exhibits maxima at 262, 271, 316 and 331 nm.

Related substances Comply with the test described under Naproxen Oral Suspension using the following solutions. For solution (1) shake a quantity of the powdered tablets containing 0.5 g of Naproxen with 10 ml of *methanol* for 15 minutes, centrifuge and use the supernatant liquid. For solution (2) dilute 1 volume of solution (1) to 200 volumes with *methanol*.

Assay Weigh and powder 20 tablets. Shake a quantity of the powder containing 50 mg of Naproxen with 70 ml of *methanol* for 30 minutes, add sufficient *methanol* to produce 100 ml and filter. Dilute 10 ml of the filtrate to 50 ml with *methanol* and measure the *absorbance* at the maximum at 331 nm, Appendix II B. Calculate the content of $C_{14}H_{14}O_3$ from the *absorbance* obtained by repeating the operation using a 0.01% w/v solution of *naproxen BPCRS* in *methanol* and using the declared content of $C_{14}H_{14}O_3$ in *naproxen BPCRS*.

Storage Naproxen Tablets should be protected from light.

Neomycin Eye Drops

Definition Neomycin Eye Drops are a sterile solution of Neomycin Sulphate in Purified Water.

The eye drops comply with the requirements stated under Eye Preparations and with the following requirements.

Identification

A. Carry out the method for *thin-layer chromatography*, Appendix III A, using a silica gel precoated plate (Merck silica gel 60 plates are suitable) and a mixture of 20 volumes of *chloroform*, 40 volumes of 13.5M *ammonia* and 60 volumes of *methanol* as the mobile phase. Apply separately to the plate (1) a volume of the eye drops containing 3.5 IU, (2) 1 µl of a 0.5% w/v solution of *neomycin sulphate EPCRS* in *water* and (3) 1 µl of a mixture of equal volumes of the eye drops and solution (2). After removal of the plate, allow it to dry in air, spray with a 1% w/v solution of *ninhydrin* in *butan-1-ol* and heat at 105° for 2 minutes. The principal red spot in the chromatogram obtained with solution (1) corresponds to that in the chromatogram obtained with solution (2) and the principal red spot in the chromatogram obtained with solution (3) appears as a single spot.

B. Yield the reactions characteristic of *sulphates*, Appendix VI.

Neamine Carry out the method for *thin-layer chromatography*, Appendix III A, using *silica gel H* as the coating substance and a freshly prepared 3.85% w/v solution of *ammonium acetate* as the mobile phase. Apply separately to the plate (1) a volume of the eye drops containing 3.5 IU and (2) the same volume of *water* containing 0.1 µg of *neamine EPCRS*. After removal of the plate, dry it in a current of warm air, heat at 110° for 10 minutes and spray the hot plate with a solution prepared immediately before use by diluting *sodium hypochlorite solution* with *water* to contain 0.5% w/v of available chlorine. Dry in a current of cold air until a sprayed area of the plate below the line of application gives not more than a very faint blue colour with one drop of a 0.5% w/v solution of *potassium iodide* in *starch mucilage*. Avoid prolonged exposure to the cold air. Spray the plate with a 0.5% w/v solution of *potassium iodide* in *starch mucilage*. Any spot corresponding to neamine in the chromatogram obtained with solution (1) is not more intense than the spot in the chromatogram obtained with solution (2).

Neomycin C Carry out the method for *liquid chromatography*, Appendix III D, injecting 10 µl of each of the following solutions. For solution (1) add 1.5 ml of a freshly prepared 2% w/v solution of *1-fluoro-2,4-dinitrobenzene* in *methanol* to 0.5 ml of a 0.10% w/v solution of *framycetin sulphate BPCRS* in 0.02M *sodium tetraborate*, heat in a water bath at 60° for 1 hour and cool; dilute the solution to 25 ml with the mobile phase, allow to stand and use the clear lower layer. For solution (2) dilute the eye drops with 0.02M *sodium tetraborate* to contain 700 IU per ml; proceed as for solution (1) but using 0.5 ml of the diluted solution in place of 0.5 ml of the framycetin sulphate solution.

The chromatographic procedure may be carried out using (a) a stainless steel column (20 cm × 4.6 mm) packed with *stationary phase A* (5 µm) (Nucleosil 100-5 is suitable), (b) as the mobile phase with a flow rate of 1.6 ml per minute a solution prepared by mixing 97 ml of *tetrahydrofuran*, 1.0 ml of *water* and 0.5 ml of *glacial acetic acid* with sufficient of a 2.0% v/v solution of *absolute ethanol* in *ethanol-free chloroform* to produce 250 ml and (c) a detection wavelength of 350 nm. If necessary adjust the tetrahydrofuran and water content of the mobile phase so that the chromatogram obtained with solution (1) shows resolution similar to that in the specimen chromatogram supplied with *framycetin sulphate BPCRS*.

Pass the mobile phase through the column for several hours before injecting the solutions. Record the chromatograms for 1.4 times the retention time of the peak due to neomycin B.

The *column efficiency*, determined using the peak due to neomycin B in the chromatogram obtained with solution (1), should be not less than 13,000 theoretical plates per metre.

In the chromatogram obtained with solution (2) the area of the peak corresponding to neomycin C is not less than 3% and not more than 15% of the sum of the areas of the peaks corresponding to neomycin B and neomycin C.

Assay Dilute a quantity containing 3500 IU to 50 ml with sterile *phosphate buffer pH 8.0*; dilute 10 ml of the resulting solution to 100 ml with the same solvent and carry out the *biological assay of antibiotics*, Appendix XIV A. The precision of the assay is such that the fiducial limits of error are not less than 95% and not more than 105% of the estimated potency. The upper fiducial limit of error is not less than 90.0% and the lower fiducial limit of error is not more than 115.0% of the prescribed or stated number of IU per ml.

Storage Neomycin Eye Drops should be protected from light.

Labelling The strength is stated as the number of IU (Units) per ml.

Neomycin Eye Ointment

Definition Neomycin Eye Ointment is a sterile preparation containing Neomycin Sulphate in a suitable basis.

The eye ointment complies with the requirements stated under Eye Preparations and with the following requirements.

Identification Carry out the method for *thin-layer chromatography*, Appendix III A, using a silica gel precoated plate (Merck silica gel 60 plates are suitable) and a mixture of 20 volumes of *chloroform*, 40 volumes of 13.5M *ammonia* and 60 volumes of *methanol* as the mobile phase. Apply separately to the plate 1 µl of each of the following solutions. For solution (1) disperse a quantity of the eye ointment containing 14,000 IU in 100 ml of *chloroform*, extract with 5 ml of *water* and use the aqueous extract. Solution (2) contains 0.4% w/v of *neomycin sulphate EPCRS* in *water*. Solution (3) is a mixture of equal volumes of solutions (1) and (2). After removal of the plate, allow it to dry in air, spray with a 1% w/v solution of *ninhydrin* in *butan-1-ol* and heat at 105° for 2 minutes. The principal red spot in the chromatogram obtained with solution (1) corresponds to that in the chromatogram obtained with solution (2) and the principal red spot in the chromatogram obtained with solution (3) appears as a single spot.

Neamine Carry out the method for *thin-layer chromatography*, Appendix III A, using *silica gel H* as the coating substance and a freshly prepared 3.85% w/v solution of *ammonium acetate* as the mobile phase. Apply separately to the plate 2 µl of each of the following solutions. For solution (1) disperse a quantity containing 14,000 IU in 20 ml of *chloroform*, shake gently with 8 ml of *water*, allow the layers to separate and use the aqueous layer. Solution (2) contains 0.005% w/v of *neamine EPCRS*. After removal of the plate, dry it in a current of warm air, heat at 110° for 10 minutes and spray the hot plate with a solution prepared immediately before use by diluting *sodium hypochlorite solution* with *water* to contain 0.5% w/v of available chlorine. Dry in a current of cold air until a sprayed area of the plate below the line of application gives not more than a very faint blue colour with one drop of a 0.5% w/v solution of *potassium iodide* in *starch mucilage*; avoid prolonged exposure to cold air. Spray the plate with a 0.5% w/v solution of *potassium iodide* in *starch mucilage*. Any spot corresponding to neamine in the chromatogram obtained with solution (1) is not more intense than the spot in the chromatogram obtained with solution (2).

Neomycin C Complies with the test described under Neomycin Eye Drops but preparing solution (2) in the following manner. Disperse a quantity of the eye ointment containing 3500 IU in 20 ml of *petroleum spirit (boiling range, 120° to 160°)*, add 5 ml of 0.02M *sodium tetraborate*, shake, separate the aqueous layer and centrifuge; proceed as for solution (1) but using 0.5 ml of the separated aqueous layer in place of 0.5 ml of the framycetin sulphate solution.

Assay Dissolve a quantity containing 3500 IU in 25 ml of *chloroform*, extract with four 20-ml quantities of sterile *phosphate buffer pH 8.0*, combine the extracts and add sufficient of the buffer solution to produce 100 ml. Carry out the *biological assay of antibiotics*, Appendix XIV A. The precision of the assay is such that the fiducial limits of error are not less than 95% and not more than 105% of the estimated potency. The upper fiducial limit of error is not less than 90.0% and the lower fiducial limit of error is not more than 115.0% of the prescribed or stated number of IU per g.

Labelling The strength is stated as the number of IU (Units) per g.

Neomycin Oral Solution

Definition Neomycin Oral Solution is a solution of Neomycin Sulphate in a suitable flavoured vehicle.

The oral solution complies with the requirements stated under Oral Liquids and with the following requirements.

Identification Carry out the method for *thin-layer chromatography*, Appendix III A, using a silica gel precoated plate (Merck silica gel 60 plates are suitable) and a mixture of 20 volumes of *chloroform*, 40 volumes of 13.5M *ammonia* and 60 volumes of *methanol* as the mobile phase. Apply separately to the plate 2 µl of each of the following solutions. For solution (1) dilute a suitable volume of the oral solution with *water* to contain 1750 IU per ml. Solution (2) contains 0.25% w/v of *neomycin sulphate EPCRS* in *water*. Solution (3) is a mixture of equal volumes of solutions (1) and (2). After removal of the plate, allow it to dry in air, spray with a 1% w/v solution of *ninhydrin* in *butan-1-ol* and heat at 105° for 2 minutes. The principal red spot in the chromatogram obtained with solution (1) corresponds to that in the chromatogram obtained with solution (2) and the principal red spot in the chromatogram obtained with solution (3) appears as a single compact spot.

Acidity pH, 4.0 to 5.0, Appendix V L.

Neamine Complies with the test described under Neomycin Eye Ointment but preparing solution (1) in the following manner. Dilute a suitable volume of the oral solution with sufficient *water* to produce a solution containing 1750 IU per ml.

Neomycin C Complies with the test described under Neomycin Eye Drops but preparing solution (2) in the following manner. Dilute the oral solution with 0.02M *sodium tetraborate* to contain 700 IU per ml; proceed as for solution (1) but using 0.5 ml of the diluted solution in place of 0.5 ml of the framycetin sulphate solution.

Assay Carry out the *biological assay of antibiotics*, Appendix XIV A. The precision of the assay is such that the fiducial limits of error are not less than 95% and not more than 105% of the estimated potency. The upper fiducial limit of error is not less than 90.0% and the lower fiducial limit of error is not more than 115.0% of the prescribed or stated number of IU per ml.

Storage Neomycin Oral Solution should be protected from light and stored at a temperature not exceeding 15°.

Labelling The strength is stated as the number of IU (Units) per ml.

Neomycin Tablets

Definition Neomycin Tablets contain Neomycin Sulphate.

The tablets comply with the requirements stated under Tablets and with the following requirements.

Identification

A. Carry out the method for *thin-layer chromatography*, Appendix III A, using a silica gel precoated plate (Merck silica gel 60 plates are suitable) and a mixture of 20 volumes of *chloroform*, 40 volumes of 13.5M *ammonia* and 60 volumes of *methanol* as the mobile phase. Apply separately to the plate 2 µl of each of the following solutions. For solution (1) shake a quantity of the powdered tablets containing 70,000 IU with 25 ml of *water* and filter. Solution (2) contains 0.4% w/v of *neomycin sulphate EPCRS* in *water*. Solution (3) is a mixture of equal volumes of solutions (1) and (2). After removal of the plate, allow it to dry in air, spray with a 1% w/v solution of *ninhydrin* in *butan-1-ol* and heat at 105° for 2 minutes. The principal red spot in the chromatogram obtained with solution (1) corresponds to that in the chromatogram obtained with solution (2) and the principal red spot in the chromatogram obtained with solution (3) appears as a single compact spot.

B. The powdered tablets yield the reactions characteristic of *sulphates*, Appendix VI.

Neamine Comply with the test described under Neomycin Eye Drops but applying separately to the plate 2 µl of each of the following solutions. For solution (1) add 5 ml of *water* to a quantity of the powdered tablets containing 7000 IU, shake for 5 minutes and filter. Solution (2) contains 0.004% w/v of *neamine EPCRS*.

Neomycin C Comply with the test described under Neomycin Eye Drops but preparing solution (2) in the following manner. Shake a quantity of the powdered tablets containing 17,500 IU with 20 ml of 0.02M *sodium tetraborate*, dilute to 25 ml with the same solvent, mix and centrifuge; proceed as for solution (1) but using 0.5 ml of the separated aqueous layer in place of the 0.5 ml of framycetin sulphate solution.

Assay Weigh and powder 20 tablets. Transfer an accurately weighed quantity of the powder containing 15,000 IU to a flask containing 150 ml of sterile *phosphate buffer pH 8.0* and add sufficient of the buffer solution to produce 250 ml. Allow to stand, dilute 10 ml of the clear supernatant liquid to 100 ml with the buffer solution and carry out the *biological assay of antibiotics*, Appendix XIV A. The precision of the assay is such that the fiducial limits of error are not less than 95% and not more than 105% of the estimated potency. The upper fiducial limit of error is not less than 97.0% and the lower fiducial limit of error is not more than 110.0% of the prescribed or stated number of IU.

Storage Neomycin Tablets should be protected from light and stored at a temperature not exceeding 30°.

Labelling The quantity of active ingredient is stated in terms of the number of IU (Units).

Neostigmine Injection

Definition Neostigmine Injection is a sterile solution of Neostigmine Metilsulfate in Water for Injections.

The injection complies with the requirements stated under Parenteral Preparations and with the following requirements.

Content of neostigmine metilsulfate, $C_{13}H_{22}N_2O_6S$ 90.0 to 110.0% of the prescribed or stated amount.

Identification

A. Dilute, if necessary, a volume of the injection containing 2.5 mg of Neostigmine Metilsulfate to 5 ml with *water*, shake with three 10-ml quantities of *ether* and discard the ether extracts. The *light absorption* of the aqueous solution, Appendix II B, in the range 230 to 350 nm exhibits two maxima, at 260 nm and 266 nm.

B. Carry out the method for *thin-layer chromatography*, Appendix III A, using *silica gel G* as the coating substance and a mixture of 5 volumes of *water*, 10 volumes of *formic acid*, 35 volumes of *methanol* and 50 volumes of *chloroform* as the mobile phase. Apply separately to the plate 10 µl of each of the following solutions. For solution (1) use the injection diluted, if necessary, with *water* to produce a solution containing 0.05% w/v of Neostigmine Metilsulfate. Solution (2) contains 0.05% w/v of *neostigmine metilsulfate BPCRS*. Solution (3) is a mixture of equal volumes of solutions (1) and (2). After removal of the plate, allow it to dry in air and spray with *dilute potassium iodobismuthate solution*. The principal spot in the chromatogram obtained with solution (1) corresponds to that in the chromatogram obtained with solution (2). The principal spot in the chromatogram obtained with solution (3) appears as a single, compact spot.

C. To 1 ml add 0.5 ml of 5M *sodium hydroxide* and evaporate to dryness on a water bath. Heat rapidly on an oil bath to about 250° and maintain at this temperature for about 30 seconds. Cool, dissolve the residue in 1 ml of *water*, cool in ice and add 1 ml of *diazobenzenesulphonic acid solution*. An orange-red colour is produced.

Acidity pH, 4.5 to 6.5, Appendix V L.

(3-Hydroxy)trimethylanilinium methyl sulphate Carry out the method for *liquid chromatography*, Appendix III D, using the following solutions. Solution (1) is the injection diluted, if necessary, with *water* to contain 0.05% w/v of Neostigmine Metilsulfate. For solution (2) dilute 1 volume of solution (1) to 100 volumes with *water*. For solution (3) add 0.05 ml of 5M *sodium hydroxide* to 1 ml of solution (1) and allow to stand for 5 minutes. Add 0.1 ml of 5M *hydrochloric acid* and use immediately.

The chromatographic procedure may be carried out using (a) a stainless steel column (25 cm × 4.6 mm) packed with *stationary phase C* (5 µm) (Lichrosphere 60

RP-select B is suitable), (b) as the mobile phase at a flow rate of 1.1 ml per minute a 0.0015M solution of *sodium heptanesulphonate* in a mixture of 15 volumes of *acetonitrile* and 85 volumes of 0.05M *potassium dihydrogen orthophosphate* adjusted to pH 3.0 with *orthophosphoric acid* and (c) a detection wavelength of 215 nm.

In the chromatogram obtained with solution (3) the principal peak has a retention time of about 6.8 minutes (neostigmine metilsulfate) and there is a peak with a relative retention time of about 0.5 ((3-hydroxy)trimethylanilinium methylsulphate). In the chromatogram obtained with solution (1), the area of any *secondary peak* with a retention time corresponding to that of the peak due to (3hydroxy)trimethylanilinium methylsulphate in the chromatogram obtained with solution (3) is not greater than the area of the principal peak in the chromatogram obtained with solution (2) (1%).

Assay Dilute a quantity containing 25 mg of Neostigmine Metilsulfate to 50 ml with *water*. Measure the *absorbance* of the resulting solution at the maximum at 260 nm, Appendix II B. Calculate the content of $C_{13}H_{22}N_2O_6S$ taking 14.35 as the value of A(1%, 1 cm) at the maximum at 260 nm.

Storage Neostigmine Injection should be protected from light.

Neostigmine Tablets

Definition Neostigmine Tablets contain Neostigmine Bromide.

The tablets comply with the requirements stated under Tablets and with the following requirements.

Content of neostigmine bromide, $C_{12}H_{19}BrN_2O_2$ 92.5 to 107.5% of the prescribed or stated amount.

Identification

A. Triturate a quantity of the powdered tablets containing 60 mg of Neostigmine Bromide with two 5-ml quantities of hot *chloroform* and filter. Evaporate the filtrate to dryness on a water bath, extract the residue with 5 ml of hot *water*, cool and filter. To 0.1 ml of the filtrate add 0.5 ml of 5M *sodium hydroxide* and evaporate to dryness on a water bath. Heat quickly in an oil bath to about 250° and maintain at this temperature for about 30 seconds. Cool, dissolve the residue in 1 ml of *water*, cool in ice and add 1 ml of *diazobenzenesulphonic acid solution*. A cherry-red colour is produced.

B. The aqueous filtrate obtained in text A yields the reactions characteristic of *bromides*, Appendix VI.

Assay Weigh and powder 20 tablets. Transfer a quantity of the powder containing 0.15 g of Neostigmine Bromide to a semi-micro ammonia-distillation apparatus, add 20 ml of a 50% w/v solution of *sodium hydroxide* and 0.5 ml of a 2% solution of *octan-2-ol* in *liquid paraffin*. Pass a current of steam through the mixture, collect the distillate in 50 ml of 0.01M *sulphuric acid VS* until the total volume is about 200 ml and titrate the excess of acid with 0.02M *sodium hydroxide VS* using *methyl red solution* as indicator. Repeat the operation without the powdered tablets. The difference between the titrations represents the amount of acid required to neutralise the dimethylamine produced. Each ml of 0.01M *sulphuric acid VS* is equivalent to 6.064 mg of $C_{12}H_{19}BrN_2O_2$.

Storage Neostigmine Tablets should be protected from light.

Niclosamide Tablets

Definition Niclosamide Tablets contain Anhydrous Niclosamide or Niclosamide Monohydrate.

The tablets comply with the requirements stated under Tablets and with the following requirements.

Content of anhydrous niclosamide, $C_{13}H_8Cl_2N_2O_4$ 95.0 to 105.0% of the prescribed or stated amount.

Identification Heat a quantity of the powdered tablets containing 0.5 g of anhydrous niclosamide with 25 ml of hot *ethanol (96%)*, filter while hot and evaporate the filtrate to dryness on a water bath. The residue complies with the following tests.

A. The *infrared absorption spectrum*, Appendix II A, is concordant with the *reference spectrum* of niclosamide. If the spectra are not concordant heat a suitable quantity of the residue at 120° for 1 hour and prepare a new spectrum.

B. Burn 20 mg by the method for *oxygen-flask combustion*, Appendix VIII C, using 5 ml of 2M *sodium hydroxide* as the absorbing liquid. The resulting solution yields a white precipitate with *silver nitrate solution* which is insoluble in 2M *nitric acid* but soluble in 5M *ammonia*.

C. Heat 50 mg with 5 ml of 1M *hydrochloric acid* and 0.1 g of *zinc powder* in a water bath for 10 minutes, cool and filter. To the filtrate add 0.5 ml of a 1% w/v solution of *sodium nitrite* and allow to stand for 10 minutes. Add 2 ml of a 2% w/v solution of *ammonium sulphamate*, shake, allow to stand for 10 minutes and add 2 ml of a 0.5% w/v solution of N-*(1-naphthyl)ethylenediamine dihydrochloride*. A deep red colour is produced.

Disintegration The requirement for Disintegration does not apply to Niclosamide Tablets.

2-Chloro-4-nitroaniline Boil a quantity of the powdered tablets containing 0.10 g of anhydrous niclosamide with 20 ml of *methanol* for 2 minutes, cool, add sufficient 1M *hydrochloric acid* to produce 50 ml and filter. To 10 ml of the filtrate add 0.5 ml of a 0.5% w/v solution of *sodium nitrite* and allow to stand for 10 minutes. Add 1 ml of a 2% w/v solution of *ammonium sulphamate*, shake, allow to stand for 10 minutes and add 1 ml of a 0.5% w/v solution of N-*(1-naphthyl)ethylenediamine dihydrochloride*. Any colour produced is not more intense than that obtained by treating 20 ml of a solution in *methanol* containing 10 µg of *2-chloro-4-nitroaniline* in the same manner and at the same time, beginning at the words 'add sufficient 1M *hydrochloric acid* ...'.

5-Chlorosalicylic acid Boil a quantity of the powdered tablets containing 0.50 g of anhydrous niclosamide with 10 ml of *water* for 2 minutes, cool, filter and to the filtrate add 0.2 ml of *iron(III) chloride solution R1*. No red or violet colour is produced.

Related substances Carry out the method for *liquid chromatography*, Appendix III D, using the following solutions. For solution (1) dilute 1 volume of solution (2) to 100 volumes with *acetonitrile* and further dilute 1 volume of this solution to 20 volumes with *acetonitrile*. For solution (2) shake a quantity of the powdered tablets containing 0.1 g of anhydrous niclosamide with 80 ml of *methanol* for 15 minutes, add sufficient *methanol* to produce 100 ml and filter.

The chromatographic procedure may be carried out using (a) a stainless steel column (10 cm × 4.6 mm) packed with *stationary phase C* (5 μm) (Nucleosil C18 is suitable), (b) a mixture of 50 volumes of *acetonitrile* and 50 volumes of a solution containing 0.2% w/v of *potassium dihydrogen orthophosphate*, 0.2% w/v of *tetrabutylammonium hydrogen sulphate* and 0.1% w/v of *disodium hydrogen orthophosphate* as the mobile phase with a flow rate of 1 ml per minute and (c) a detection wavelength of 230 nm. Adjust the sensitivity so that the height of the peak corresponding to niclosamide in the chromatogram obtained with solution (1) is not less than 20% of full-scale deflection. Record the chromatogram for twice the retention time of niclosamide.

The sum of the areas of any *secondary peaks* in the chromatogram obtained with solution (2) is not greater than 4 times the area of the principal peak in the chromatogram obtained with solution (1). Disregard any peak with an area less than 10% of the area of the area of the principal peak in the chromatogram obtained with solution (1).

Assay Weigh and powder 20 tablets. Carry out Method II for *non-aqueous titration*, Appendix VIII A, using a quantity of the powdered tablets containing 0.3 g of anhydrous niclosamide dissolved in 60 ml of *dimethylformamide*, 0.1M *tetrabutylammonium hydroxide VS* as titrant and determining the end point potentiometrically. Each ml of 0.1M *tetrabutylammonium hydroxide VS* is equivalent to 32.71 mg of $C_{13}H_8Cl_2N_2O_4$.

Storage Niclosamide Tablets should be protected from light.

Labelling The label states that the tablets should be chewed before swallowing.

When the active ingredient is Niclosamide Monohydrate the quantity is stated in terms of the equivalent amount of anhydrous niclosamide.

Nicotinamide Tablets

Definition Nicotinamide Tablets contain Nicotinamide.

The tablets comply with the requirements stated under Tablets and with the following requirements.

Content of nicotinamide, $C_6H_6N_2O$ 92.5 to 107.5% of the prescribed or stated amount.

Identification

A. Shake a quantity of the powdered tablets containing 0.1 g of Nicotinamide with 25 ml of *absolute ethanol* for 15 minutes, filter and evaporate the filtrate to dryness on a water bath. The *infrared absorption spectrum* of the residue, Appendix II A, is concordant with the *reference spectrum* of nicotinamide.

B. The *light absorption* of the solution obtained in the Assay, Appendix II B, in the range 230 to 350 nm exhibits a maximum only at 262 nm and two shoulders, at 258 nm and 269 nm.

C. Shake a quantity of the powdered tablets containing 50 mg of Nicotinamide with 50 ml of *water* and filter. To 2 ml of the filtrate add 2 ml of *cyanogen bromide solution* and 3 ml of a 2.5% v/v solution of *aniline* and shake. A yellow colour is produced.

Related substances Carry out the method for *thin-layer chromatography*, Appendix III A, using a silica gel F_{254} precoated plate (Merck silica gel 60 F_{254} plates are suitable) and a mixture of 10 volumes of *water*, 45 volumes of *ethanol (96%)* and 48 volumes of *chloroform* as the mobile phase but allowing the solvent front to ascend 10 cm above the line of application. Apply separately to the plate 5 μl of each of the following solutions. For solution (1) shake a quantity of the powdered tablets containing 0.1 g of Nicotinamide with 15 ml of *absolute ethanol* for 15 minutes, filter, evaporate to dryness on a water bath and dissolve the residue as completely as possible in 1 ml of *absolute ethanol*. For solution (2) dilute 1 volume of solution (1) to 400 volumes with *absolute ethanol*. After removal of the plate, allow it to dry in air and examine under *ultraviolet light (254 nm)*. Any *secondary spot* in the chromatogram obtained with solution (1) is not more intense than the spot in the chromatogram obtained with solution (2) (0.25%).

Assay Weigh and powder 20 tablets. Shake a quantity of the powder containing 50 mg of Nicotinamide with 50 ml of *ethanol (96%)* for 15 minutes and dilute to 100 ml with *ethanol (96%)*. Mix, filter, dilute 5 ml of the filtrate to 100 ml with *ethanol (96%)* and measure the *absorbance* of the resulting solution at the maximum at 262 nm, Appendix II B. Calculate the content of $C_6H_6N_2O$ taking 241 as the value of A(1%, 1 cm) at the maximum at 262 nm.

Storage Nicotinamide Tablets should be protected from light.

Nicotinic Acid Tablets

Definition Nicotinic Acid Tablets contain Nicotinic Acid.

The tablets comply with the requirements stated under Tablets and with the following requirements.

Content of nicotinic acid, $C_6H_5NO_2$ 92.5 to 107.5% of the prescribed or stated amount.

Identification

A. Carry out the method for *thin-layer chromatography*, Appendix III A, using *silica gel GF_{254}* as the coating substance and a mixture of 8 volumes of *water*, 45 volumes of *ethanol (96%)* and 48 volumes of *chloroform* as the mobile phase. Apply separately to the plate 5 μl of each of the following solutions. For solution (1) shake a quantity of the powdered tablets containing 50 mg of Nicotinic Acid with 50 ml of hot *ethanol (96%)*, filter and allow the filtrate to cool. Solution (2) contains 0.1% w/v of *nicotinic acid* in *ethanol (96%)*. After removal of the plate, allow it to dry in air and examine under *ultraviolet light (254 nm)*. The spot in the chromatogram obtained with solution (1) corresponds to that in the chromatogram obtained with solution (2).

B. Shake a quantity of the powdered tablets containing 0.1 g of Nicotinic Acid with *ethanol (96%)*, filter and evaporate the filtrate to dryness. To the residue add 10 mg of *citric acid* and 0.15 ml of *acetic anhydride* and heat on a water bath. A reddish violet colour is produced.

C. Triturate a quantity of the powdered tablets containing 50 mg of Nicotinic Acid with 10 ml of *water* and filter. To 2 ml of the filtrate add 6 ml of *cyanogen bromide solution* and 1 ml of a 2.5% v/v solution of *aniline*. A golden yellow colour is produced.

Assay Weigh and powder 20 tablets. To a quantity of the powder containing 0.3 g of Nicotinic Acid add 40 ml of hot *ethanol (96%)*, previously neutralised to *phenolphthalein solution R1*, and shake. Allow to stand for 15 minutes, swirling occasionally, and then shake for 10 minutes. Filter through absorbent cotton and wash the filter with *ethanol (96%)*. Add 50 ml of *carbon dioxide-free water* and titrate with 0.1M *sodium hydroxide VS* using *phenol red solution* as indicator. Each ml of 0.1M *sodium hydroxide VS* is equivalent to 12.31 mg of $C_6H_5NO_2$.

Nicotinyl Alcohol Tablets

Definition Nicotinyl Alcohol Tablets contain Nicotinyl Alcohol Tartrate.

The tablets comply with the requirements stated under Tablets and with the following requirements.

Content of nicotinyl alcohol tartrate, C_6H_7NO, $C_4H_6O_6$ 92.5 to 107.5% of the prescribed or stated amount.

Identification In the test for Related substances, the principal spot in the chromatogram obtained with solution (2) corresponds to that in the chromatogram obtained with solution (4).

Related substances Comply with the test described under Nicotinyl Alcohol Tartrate using 10 µl of each of the following solutions. For solution (1) shake a quantity of the powdered tablets containing 0.25 g of Nicotinyl Alcohol Tartrate with 50 ml of *methanol*, filter and evaporate the filtrate to dryness at about 30° at a pressure of 2 kPa. Add 2 ml of *water* to the residue, shake, filter and add 0.1 ml of 13.5M *ammonia* to the filtrate. For solution (2) dilute 1 volume of solution (1) to 500 volumes with 0.1M *ammonia*. Solution (3) contains 0.025% w/v of *3(aminomethyl)-pyridine* in 0.1M *ammonia*. Solution (4) contains 0.025% w/v of *nicotinyl alcohol tartrate BPCRS* in 0.1M *ammonia*.

Assay Weigh and powder 20 tablets. Shake a quantity of the powder containing 50 mg of Nicotinyl Alcohol Tartrate with 150 ml of 0.1M *hydrochloric acid* for 10 minutes, dilute to 250 ml with the same solvent, mix and filter. Dilute 10 ml of the filtrate to 100 ml with 0.1M *hydrochloric acid* and measure the *absorbance* of the resulting solution at the maximum at 261 nm, Appendix II B. Calculate the content of $C_6H_7NO,C_4H_6O_6$ taking 210 as the value of A(1%, 1 cm) at the maximum at 261 nm.

Nifedipine Capsules

Definition Nifedipine Capsules contain Nifedipine.

The capsules comply with the requirements stated under Capsules and with the following requirements.

Content of nifedipine, $C_{17}H_{18}N_2O_6$ 95.0 to 105.0% of the prescribed or stated amount.

Carry out all the following procedures in the dark or under long-wavelength light (greater than 420 nm). Prepare solutions immediately before use and protect them from light.

Identification

A. Add a quantity of the contents of the capsules containing 50 mg of Nifedipine to 10 ml of *water* and mix with the aid of ultrasound for 5 minutes, filter (Whatman GF/C paper is suitable), wash the residue with *water* and dry at 110°. The *infrared absorption spectrum* of the residue, Appendix II A, is concordant with the *reference spectrum* of nifedipine.

B. Carry out the method for *thin-layer chromatography*, Appendix III A, using *silica gel GF_{254}* as the coating substance and a mixture of 40 volumes of *ethyl acetate* and 60 volumes of *cyclohexane* as the mobile phase in an unsaturated tank. Apply separately to the plate 5 µl of each of the following solutions in a mixture of equal volumes of *dichloromethane* and *methanol*. For solution (1) shake a quantity of the contents of the capsules containing 20 mg of Nifedipine with 10 ml of the solvent mixture and filter. Solution (2) contains 0.2% w/v of *nifedipine BPCRS* in the solvent mixture. After removal of the plate, allow it to dry in air and examine under *ultraviolet light (254 nm)*. The principal spot in the chromatogram obtained with solution (1) is similar in position, appearance under ultraviolet light and size to that in the chromatogram obtained with solution (2).

Nitro- and nitroso-phenylpyridine analogues Carry out the method for *liquid chromatography*, Appendix III D, using the following solutions. For solution (1) dissolve a quantity of the contents of the capsules containing 20 mg of Nifedipine in 8 ml of *methanol* and dilute to 20 ml with a mixture of 9 volumes of *acetonitrile*, 36 volumes of *methanol* and 55 volumes of *water*. Solution (2) contains 0.0010% w/v of *dimethyl-2,6-dimethyl-4-(2-nitrophenyl)pyridine-3,5-dicarboxylate EPCRS* (nitrophenylpyridine analogue) in a mixture of 5 volumes of *acetonitrile*, 33 volumes of *water* and 62 volumes of *methanol*. Solution (3) contains 0.00050% w/v of *dimethyl-2,6-dimethyl-4-(2-nitrosophenyl)pyridine-3,5-dicarboxylate EPCRS* (nitrosophenylpyridine analogue) in a mixture of 5 volumes of *acetonitrile*, 33 volumes of *water* and 62 volumes of *methanol*. For solution (4) dilute 2 volumes of a solution in *methanol* containing 0.25% w/v of *nifedipine BPCRS*, 0.0025% w/v each of the nitrophenylpyridine analogue and nitrosophenylpyridine analogue and 0.0050% w/v of *propyl hydroxybenzoate* to 5 volumes with a mixture of 9 volumes of *acetonitrile*, 36 volumes of *methanol* and 55 volumes of *water*.

The chromatographic procedure may be carried out using (a) a stainless steel column (25 cm × 4.6 mm) packed with *stationary phase C* (5 µm) (Lichrosorb RP18 is suitable), (b) a mixture of 9 volumes of *acetonitrile*, 36 volumes of *methanol* and 55 volumes of *borate buffer pH 8.0* as the mobile phase with a flow rate of 2.0 ml per minute and (c) a detection wavelength of 220 nm.

The test is not valid unless the chromatogram obtained with solution (4) closely resembles the reference chromatogram supplied with *nifedipine BPCRS*.

In the chromatogram obtained with solution (1) the areas of any peaks corresponding to the nitrophenylpyridine analogue and the nitrosophenylpyridine analogue are not greater than the areas of the corresponding peaks in the chromatograms obtained with solution (2) (1%) and solution (3) (0.5%), respectively.

Dissolution Comply with the *dissolution test for tablets and capsules*, Appendix XII D, using Apparatus II. Use as the medium 900 ml of 0.1M *hydrochloric acid* and rotate the paddle at 50 revolutions per minute. Withdraw a sample of 10 ml of the medium and measure the *absorbance* of a 2-cm layer of the solution, suitably diluted if necessary, at the maximum at 340 nm, Appendix II B. Measure the *absorbance* of a 2-cm layer of a suitable solution of *nifedipine BPCRS* prepared by dissolving 20 mg in 100 ml of the dissolution medium and diluting to a suitable volume with the dissolution medium and using dissolution medium in the reference cell. Calculate the total content of nifedipine, $C_{17}H_{18}N_2O_6$, in the medium from the absorbances obtained and from the declared content of $C_{17}H_{18}N_2O_6$ in *nifedipine BPCRS*.

Assay Carry out the method for *liquid chromatography*, Appendix III D, using the following solutions. For solution (1) take ten capsules and break them beneath the surface of 30 ml of *acetonitrile*. Stir to dissolve the capsule contents. Transfer the resulting solution to a 250-ml graduated flask. Wash the capsule shells with several portions of the mobile phase, transferring the washings to the flask, add sufficient of the mobile phase to produce 250 ml and mix. If necessary, further dilute a portion of the solution with the mobile phase to give a solution containing 0.02% w/v of nifedipine. For solution (2) dissolve 50 mg of *nifedipine BPCRS* in 30 ml of *acetonitrile* and dilute to 250 ml with the mobile phase.

The chromatographic procedure may be carried out using (a) a stainless steel column (10 cm × 4.6 mm) packed with *stationary phase C* (5 µm) (Hypersil C18 is suitable), (b) a mixture of 40 volumes of *acetonitrile* and 60 volumes of a 0.03% v/v solution of *orthophosphoric acid* as the mobile phase with a flow rate of 1 ml per minute and (c) a detection wavelength of 235 nm.

Calculate the content of $C_{17}H_{18}N_2O_6$ in the capsules using the declared content of $C_{17}H_{18}N_2O_6$ in *nifedipine BPCRS*.

Nikethamide Injection

Definition Nikethamide Injection is a sterile solution containing 25% w/v of Nikethamide in Water for Injections.

The injection complies with the requirements stated under Parenteral Preparations and with the following requirements.

Content of nikethamide, $C_{10}H_{14}N_2O$ 24.0 to 26.0% w/v.

Characteristics A colourless solution.

Identification Make 1 ml alkaline with 5M *sodium hydroxide*, extract with 5 ml of *dichloromethane* and evaporate the solvent. The *infrared absorption spectrum* of the oily residue, Appendix II A, is concordant with the *reference spectrum* of nikethamide.

Acidity or alkalinity pH, 6.0 to 8.0, Appendix V L.

Related substances Carry out the method for *thin-layer chromatography*, Appendix III A, using *silica gel GF_{254}* as the coating substance and a mixture of 25 volumes of *propan-1-ol* and 75 volumes of *chloroform* as the mobile phase. Apply separately to the plate 10 µl of each of the following solutions. For solution (1) dilute 1 ml of the injection to 5 ml with *methanol*. Solutions (2) and (3) contain 0.05% w/v and 0.005% w/v respectively of *ethylnicotinamide EPCRS* in *methanol*. After removal of the plate, allow it to dry in air and examine under *ultraviolet light (254 nm)*. Any spot corresponding to ethylnicotinamide in the chromatogram obtained with solution (1) is not more intense than the spot in the chromatogram obtained with solution (2) (1%) and any other *secondary spot* is not more intense than the spot in the chromatogram obtained with solution (3) (0.1%).

Assay Dilute 5 ml to 500 ml with *water*. To 5 ml of the solution add 5 ml of 1M *hydrochloric acid* and dilute to 500 ml with *water*. Measure the *absorbance* of the resulting solution at the maximum at 263 nm, Appendix II B. Calculate the content of $C_{10}H_{14}N_2O$ taking 282 as the value of A(1%, 1 cm) at the maximum at 263 nm.

Nitrazepam Capsules

Definition Nitrazepam Capsules contain Nitrazepam.

The capsules comply with the requirements stated under Capsules and with the following requirements.

Content of nitrazepam, $C_{15}H_{11}N_3O_3$ 90.0 to 110.0% of the prescribed or stated amount.

Identification

A. The *light absorption*, Appendix II B, in the range 230 to 350 nm of the final solution obtained in the Assay exhibits a maximum only at 280 nm.

B. Carry out the method for *thin-layer chromatography*, Appendix III A, using *silica gel G* as the coating substance and a mixture of 10 volumes of *methanol* and 100 volumes of *chloroform* as the mobile phase. Apply separately to the plate 2 µl of each of the following solutions. For solution (1) shake a quantity of the contents of the capsules with sufficient *methanol* to produce a solution containing 0.5% w/v of Nitrazepam, allow to settle and decant the supernatant liquid. Solution (2) contains 0.5% w/v of *nitrazepam BPCRS* in *methanol*. After removal of the plate, spray it with a 10% v/v solution of *sulphuric acid* in *absolute ethanol*, heat at 105° for 10 minutes and examine under *ultraviolet light (365 nm)*. The principal spot in the chromatogram obtained with solution (1) corresponds to that in the chromatogram obtained with solution (2).

C. To a quantity of the contents of the capsules containing 5 mg of Nitrazepam add 5 ml of *hydrochloric acid* and 10 ml of *water*, heat on a water bath for 15 minutes and filter. To the clear filtrate add 1 ml of a 0.1% w/v solution of *sodium nitrite*, allow to stand for 3 minutes and add 1 ml of a 0.5% w/v solution of *sulphamic acid*. Allow to stand for 3 minutes and add 1 ml of a 0.1% w/v solution of *N-(1-naphthyl)ethylenediamine dihydrochloride*. A red colour is produced.

Related substances and decomposition products Carry out the method for *thin-layer chromatography*, Appendix III A, protected from light, using *silica gel GF₂₅₄* as the coating substance and a mixture of 20 volumes of *chloroform*, 40 volumes of *nitromethane* and 40 volumes of *toluene* as the mobile phase. Apply separately to the plate 20 µl of each of the following freshly prepared solutions. For solution (1) shake a quantity of the contents of the capsules containing 20 mg of Nitrazepam with 4 ml of a mixture of equal volumes of *chloroform* and *methanol* for 5 minutes, centrifuge and use the clear supernatant liquid. For solution (2) dilute 1 volume of solution (1) to 100 volumes with a mixture of equal volumes of *chloroform* and *methanol*. After removal of the plate, allow it to dry in air until the odour of the solvent is no longer detectable and examine under *ultraviolet light (254 nm)*. Any *secondary spot* in the chromatogram obtained with solution (1) with an Rf value of 0.5 or lower is not more intense than the spot in the chromatogram obtained with solution (2) (1%). Treat the plate by *Method I* and examine again. Any *secondary spot* in the chromatogram obtained with solution (1) having an Rf value higher than 0.5 is not more intense than the spot in the chromatogram obtained with solution (2) (1%).

Assay To a quantity of the mixed contents of 20 capsules containing 5 mg of Nitrazepam add 5 ml of *water*, mix and allow to stand for 15 minutes, protected from light. Add 90 ml of a 0.5% v/v solution of *hydrochloric acid* in *methanol*, shake for 15 minutes protected from light, add sufficient of the hydrochloric acid solution to produce 100 ml and filter. Dilute 10 ml of the filtrate to 100 ml with the same solution and measure the *absorbance* of the resulting solution immediately at the maximum at 280 nm, Appendix II B. Calculate the content of $C_{15}H_{11}N_3O_3$ taking 910 as the value of A(1%, 1 cm) at the maximum at 280 nm.

Nitrazepam Oral Suspension

Definition Nitrazepam Oral Suspension is a suspension of Nitrazepam in a suitable flavoured vehicle, which may be coloured.

The oral suspension complies with the requirements stated under Oral Liquids and with the following requirements.

Content of nitrazepam, $C_{15}H_{11}N_3O_3$ 90.0 to 110.0% of the prescribed or stated amount.

Identification

A. Carry out the method for *thin-layer chromatography*, Appendix III A, using *silica gel GF_{254}* as the coating substance and a mixture of 15 volumes of *ethyl acetate* and 85 volumes of *nitromethane* as the mobile phase. Apply separately to the plate 10 µl of each of the following solutions. For solution (1) add a quantity of the oral suspension containing 20 mg of Nitrazepam to 40 ml of *water*, extract with successive quantities of 50, 20 and 20 ml of *chloroform*, filtering each extract through phase-separating paper, and add sufficient *chloroform* to the combined extracts to produce 100 ml. Solution (2) contains 0.02% w/v of *nitrazepam BPCRS* in *chloroform*. After removal of the plate, allow it to dry in air and visualise the spots by *Method I*. A spot in the chromatogram obtained with solution (1) corresponds to the principal spot in the chromatogram obtained with solution (2).

B. In the Assay, the principal peak in the chromatogram obtained with solution (2) has a similar retention time to the peak due to nitrazepam in the chromatogram obtained with solution (1).

Assay Carry out the method for *liquid chromatography*, Appendix III D, using the following solutions. Solution (1) contains 0.00625% w/v of *nitrazepam BPCRS* in *chloroform*. For solution (2) add a quantity of the oral suspension containing 12.5 mg of Nitrazepam to 25 ml of *water*, extract with three 50-ml quantities of *chloroform*, filtering each extract through phase-separating paper, and add sufficient *chloroform* to produce 200 ml.

The chromatographic procedure may be carried out using (a) a stainless steel column (20 cm × 4.6 mm) packed with *stationary phase A* (5 µm) (Lichrosorb or Partisil is suitable), (b) a mixture of 10 volumes of *absolute ethanol* and 90 volumes of *n-hexane* as the mobile phase with a flow rate of 2 ml per minute and (c) a detection wavelength of 254 nm.

Determine the *weight per ml* of the oral suspension, Appendix V G, and calculate the content of $C_{15}H_{11}N_3O_3$, weight in volume, using the declared content of $C_{15}H_{11}N_3O_3$ in *nitrazepam BPCRS*.

Storage Nitrazepam Oral Suspension should be protected from light and stored at a temperature not exceeding 25°.

Nitrazepam Tablets

Definition Nitrazepam Tablets contain Nitrazepam.

The tablets comply with the requirements stated under Tablets and with the following requirements.

Content of nitrazepam, $C_{15}H_{11}N_3O_3$ 90.0 to 110.0% of the prescribed or stated amount.

Identification

A. The *light absorption*, Appendix II B, in the range 230 to 350 nm of the final solution obtained in the Assay exhibits a maximum only at 280 nm.

B. Carry out the method for *thin-layer chromatography*, Appendix III A, using *silica gel G* as the coating substance and a mixture of 10 volumes of *methanol* and 100 volumes of *chloroform* as the mobile phase. Apply separately to the plate 2 µl of each of the following solutions. For solution (1) shake a quantity of the powdered tablets with sufficient *methanol* to produce a solution containing 0.5% w/v of Nitrazepam, allow to settle and decant the supernatant liquid. Solution (2) contains 0.5% w/v of *nitrazepam BPCRS* in *methanol*. After removal of the plate, spray it with a 10% v/v solution of *sulphuric acid* in *absolute ethanol*, heat at 105° for 10 minutes and examine under *ultraviolet light (365 nm)*. The principal spot in the chromatogram obtained with solution (1) corresponds to that in the chromatogram obtained with solution (2).

C. To a quantity of the powdered tablets containing 5 mg of Nitrazepam add 5 ml of *hydrochloric acid* and 10 ml of *water*, heat on a water bath for 15 minutes and filter. To the clear filtrate add 1 ml of a 0.1% w/v solution of *sodium nitrite*, allow to stand for 3 minutes and add 1 ml of a 0.5% w/v solution of *sulphamic acid*. Allow to stand for 3 minutes and add 1 ml of a 0.1% w/v solution of *N-(1-naphthyl)ethylenediamine dihydrochloride*. A red colour is produced.

Related substances and decomposition products Carry out the method for *thin-layer chromatography*, Appendix III A, protected from light, using *silica gel GF_{254}* as the coating substance and a mixture of 20 volumes of *chloroform*, 40 volumes of *nitromethane* and 40 volumes of *toluene* as the mobile phase. Apply separately to the plate 20 µl of each of the following freshly prepared solutions. For solution (1) shake a quantity of the powdered tablets containing 20 mg of Nitrazepam with 4 ml of a mixture of equal volumes of *chloroform* and *methanol* for 5 minutes, centrifuge and use the clear supernatant liquid. For solution (2) dilute 1 volume of solution (1) to 100 volumes with a mixture of equal volumes of *chloroform* and *methanol*. After removal of the plate, allow it to dry in air until the odour of the solvent is no longer detectable and examine under *ultraviolet light (254 nm)*. Any *secondary spot* in the chromatogram obtained with solution (1) with an Rf value of 0.5 or lower is not more intense than the spot in the chromatogram obtained with solution (2) (1%). Treat the plate by *Method I* and examine again. Any *secondary spot* in the chromatogram obtained with solution (1) with an Rf higher than 0.5 is not more intense than the spot in the chromatogram obtained with solution (2) (1%).

Assay Weigh and powder 20 tablets. To a quantity of the powder containing 5 mg of Nitrazepam add 5 ml of *water*, mix and allow to stand for 15 minutes, protected from light. Add 70 ml of a 0.5% v/v solution of *hydrochloric acid* in *methanol*, shake for 15 minutes protected from light, add sufficient of the hydrochloric acid solution to produce 100 ml and filter. Dilute 10 ml of the filtrate to 50 ml with the same solution and measure the *absorbance* of the resulting solution immediately at the maximum at 280 nm, Appendix II B. Calculate the content of $C_{15}H_{11}N_3O_3$ taking 910 as the value of A(1%, 1 cm) at the maximum at 280 nm.

Storage Nitrazepam Tablets should be protected from light.

Nitrofurantoin Oral Suspension

Definition Nitrofurantoin Oral Suspension is a suspension of Nitrofurantoin in a suitable flavoured vehicle.

Nitrofurantoin Oral Suspension should not be diluted.

The oral suspension complies with the requirements stated under Oral Liquids and with the following requirements.

Content of nitrofurantoin, $C_8H_6N_4O_5$ 90.0 to 110.0% of the prescribed or stated amount.

Identification

A. The *light absorption*, Appendix II B, in the range 220 to 400 nm of the final solution obtained in the Assay exhibits two maxima, at 266 nm and 367 nm.

B. Dissolve 5 mg of the residue obtained by centrifuging a quantity of the oral suspension containing 50 mg of Nitrofurantoin in 5 ml of 0.1M *sodium hydroxide*. A deep yellow solution is produced, which changes to deep orange-red.

Assay Carry out the following procedure in subdued light. To a weighed quantity containing 30 mg of Nitrofurantoin add, in successive small volumes, 50 ml of *dimethylformamide*, stirring well between each addition. Continue stirring until the sample is completely dissolved and dilute to 500 ml with an aqueous solution containing 1.8% w/v of *sodium acetate* and 0.14% v/v of *glacial acetic acid*. Dilute 10 ml of this solution to 100 ml with the sodium acetate—acetic acid solution and measure the *absorbance* of the resulting solution at the maximum at 367 nm, Appendix II B, using in the reference cell a 1% v/v solution of *dimethylformamide* in the sodium acetate—acetic acid solution. Calculate the content of $C_8H_6N_4O_5$ taking 765 as the value of A(1%, 1 cm) at the maximum at 367 nm. Determine the *weight per ml* of the oral suspension, Appendix V G, and calculate the content of $C_8H_6N_4O_5$, weight in volume.

Storage Nitrofurantoin Oral Suspension should be protected from light and stored at a temperature not exceeding 25°.

Nitrofurantoin Tablets

Definition Nitrofurantoin Tablets contain Nitrofurantoin.

With the exception of the requirements for shape, the tablets comply with the requirements stated under Tablets and with the following requirements.

Content of nitrofurantoin, $C_8H_6N_4O_5$ 90.0 to 110.0% of the prescribed or stated amount.

Identification The *light absorption*, Appendix II B, in the range 220 to 400 nm of the final solution obtained in the Assay exhibits two maxima, at 266 nm and 367 nm.

Related substances Carry out the method for *thin-layer chromatography*, Appendix III A, using *silica gel HF_{254}* as the coating substance and a mixture of 10 volumes of *methanol* and 90 volumes of *nitromethane* as the mobile phase. Apply separately to the plate 10 µl of each of the following solutions. For solution (1) shake a quantity of the powdered tablets containing 0.1 g of Nitrofurantoin with 10 ml of a mixture of 1 volume of *dimethylformamide* and 9 volumes of *acetone* and filter. For solution (2) dilute 1 volume of solution (1) to 100 volumes with *acetone*. After removal of the plate, allow it to dry in air, heat at 100° to 105° for 5 minutes and examine under *ultraviolet light (254 nm)*. Spray the plate with *phenylhydrazine hydrochloride solution* and heat it at 100° to 105° for a further 10 minutes. By each method of visualisation, any *secondary spot* in the chromatogram obtained with solution (1) is not more intense than the spot in the chromatogram obtained with solution (2) (1%).

Assay Carry out the following procedure in subdued light. Weigh and powder 20 tablets. To a quantity of the powder containing 0.12 g of Nitrofurantoin add 50 ml of *dimethylformamide*, shake for 5 minutes, add sufficient *water* to produce 1000 ml and mix. Dilute 5 ml to 100 ml with a solution containing 1.8% w/v of *sodium acetate* and 0.14% v/v of *glacial acetic acid* and filter. Measure the *absorbance* of the filtrate at the maximum at 367 nm, Appendix II B, using the sodium acetate—acetic acid solution in the reference cell. Calculate the content of $C_8H_6N_4O_5$ taking 765 as the value of A(1%, 1 cm) at 367 nm.

Storage Nitrofurantoin Tablets should be protected from light and stored at a temperature not exceeding 25°.

Noradrenaline Injection
Norepinephrine Injection

For the purposes of product labelling in the United Kingdom, the pair of names given above shall be used together (see Introduction, Changes in title).

Definition Noradrenaline Injection is a sterile solution of Noradrenaline Acid Tartrate. It is prepared immediately before use by diluting Sterile Noradrenaline Concentrate to 250 times its volume with Sodium Chloride and Glucose Intravenous Infusion or with Glucose Intravenous Infusion (5.0% w/v). Noradrenaline Injection contains in 1 ml 8 micrograms of Noradrenaline Acid Tartrate equivalent to approximately 4 micrograms of noradrenaline.

The injection complies with the requirements stated under Parenteral Preparations.

Storage Noradrenaline Injection should be used immediately after preparation but, in any case, within the period rcommended by the manufacturer when prepared and stored strictly in accordance with the manufacturer's instructions.

Labelling The label states 'Noradrenaline Injection' and 'Norepinephrine Injection'.

STERILE NORADRENALINE CONCENTRATE
STERILE NOREPINEPHRINE CONCENTRATE

For the purposes of product labelling in the United Kingdom, the pair of names given above shall be used together (see Introduction, Changes in title).

Definition Sterile Noradrenaline Concentrate is a sterile, isotonic solution containing 0.2% w/v of Noradrenaline Acid Tartrate in Water for Injections.

The concentrate complies with the requirements for Concentrated Solutions for Injections stated under Parenteral Preparations and with the following requirements.

Content of noradrenaline acid tartrate, $C_8H_{11}NO_3,C_4H_6O_6,H_2O$ 0.18 to 0.23% w/v.

Identification

A. In the Assay, the principal peak in the chromatogram obtained with solution (1) has the same retention time as that in the chromatogram obtained with solution (2).

B. Mix 0.5 ml with 10 ml of *phthalate buffer pH 3.6*, add 1 ml of 0.05M *iodine*, allow to stand for 5 minutes and add 2 ml of 0.1M *sodium thiosulphate*; not more than a very faint red colour is produced. Repeat the test using *phosphate buffer pH 6.6*; a strong reddish violet colour is produced.

Acidity pH, 3.0 to 4.6, Appendix V L.

Adrenaline Carry out the method for *liquid chromatography*, Appendix III D, using the following solutions. For solution (1) use the concentrate being examined. Solution (2) contains 0.002% w/v of *adrenaline acid tartrate BPCRS* in the mobile phase. Solution (3) contains 0.002% w/v of *adrenaline acid tartrate BPCRS* and 0.002% w/v of *noradrenaline acid tartrate BPCRS* in the mobile phase.

The chromatographic procedure may be carried out using (a) a stainless steel column (10 cm × 4.6 mm) packed with *stationary phase C* (5 µm) (Nucleosil C18 is suitable), (b) as the mobile phase with a flow rate of 2 ml per minute a solution containing 4.0 g of *tetramethylammonium hydrogen sulphate*, 1.1 g of *sodium heptanesulphonate* and 2 ml of 0.1M *disodium edetate* in a mixture of 50 ml of *methanol* and 950 ml of *water* and adjusting the pH to 3.5 with 1M *sodium hydroxide* and (c) a detection wavelength of 205 nm.

The test is not valid unless the *resolution factor* between the two principal peaks in the chromatogram obtained with solution (3) is at least 5.0.

In the chromatogram obtained with solution (1) the area of any peak corresponding to adrenaline is not greater than the area of the principal peak in the chromatogram obtained with solution (2) (1%).

Assay Carry out the method for *liquid chromatography*, Appendix III D, using the following solutions. For solution (1) dilute one volume of the concentrate being examined to 100 volumes with the mobile phase. Solution (2) contains 0.002% w/v of *noradrenaline acid tartrate BPCRS* in the mobile phase. Solution (3) contains 0.002% w/v of *adrenaline acid tartrate BPCRS* and 0.002% w/v of *noradrenaline acid tartrate BPCRS* in the mobile phase.

The chromatographic procedure described under Adrenaline may be used.

The test is not valid unless the *resolution factor* between the two principal peaks in the chromatogram obtained with solution (3) is at least 5.0.

Calculate the content of $C_8H_{11}NO_3,C_4H_6O_6,H_2O$ using the declared content of $C_8H_{11}NO_3,C_4H_6O_6,H_2O$ in *noradrenaline acid tartrate BPCRS.*

Storage Sterile Noradrenaline Concentrate should be protected from light. If the solution is brown it should be discarded.

Labelling The label states (1) 'Sterile Noradrenaline Concentrate' and 'Sterile Norepinephrine Concentrate'; (2) that 1 volume of the solution diluted to 250 volumes with Sodium Chloride and Glucose Intravenous Infusion or with Glucose Intravenous Infusion (5.0% w/v) produces an injection which must be used immediately after preparation.

Norethisterone Tablets

Definition Norethisterone Tablets contain Norethisterone.

The tablets comply with the requirements stated under Tablets and with the following requirements.

Content of norethisterone, $C_{20}H_{26}O_2$ 90.0 to 110.0% of the prescribed or stated amount.

Identification Carry out the method for *thin-layer chromatography*, Appendix III A, using a silica gel precoated plate (Merck silica gel 60 plates are suitable) and a mixture of 20 volumes of *ethyl acetate* and 80 volumes of *toluene* as the mobile phase but allowing the solvent front to ascend 10 cm above the line of application. Apply separately to the plate 20 µl of each of the following solutions. For solution (1) crush one tablet in sufficient *ethanol (96%)* to produce a final solution containing approximately 0.035% w/v of Norethisterone, warm to 50° for 10 minutes, mix with the aid of ultrasound, allow to cool and centrifuge to obtain a clear supernatant liquid. Solution (2) contains 0.035% w/v of *norethisterone BPCRS* in *ethanol (96%)*. After removal of the plate, allow it to dry in air and spray with a mixture of 30 volumes of *methanol* and 70 volumes of *sulphuric acid* and examine under *ultraviolet light (365 nm)*. The Rf value of the principal spot in the chromatogram obtained with solution (1) is the same as that of the spot in the chromatogram obtained with solution (2).

Uniformity of content Tablets containing less than 2 mg of Norethisterone comply with the requirements stated under Tablets using the following method of analysis. Carry out the method for *liquid chromatography*, Appendix III D, using the following solutions. Solution (1) contains 0.007% w/v of *norethisterone BPCRS* in *methanol (60%)*. For solution (2) disperse one tablet in 2 ml of *water* with the aid of ultrasound for 15 minutes, add sufficient *methanol* to produce 5 ml, centrifuge for 10 minutes and use the clear supernatant liquid.

The chromatographic procedure may be carried out using (a) a stainless steel column (25 cm × 4.6 mm) packed with *stationary phase C* (10 µm) (Spherisorb ODS 1 is suitable), (b) a mixture of 28 volumes of *water* and 72 volumes of *methanol* as the mobile phase with a flow rate of 1 ml per minute and (c) a detection wavelength of 254 nm.

Calculate the content of $C_{20}H_{26}O_2$ in each tablet using the declared content of $C_{20}H_{26}O_2$ in *norethisterone BPCRS*.

Assay

For tablets containing less than 2 mg of norethisterone Calculate the average of the 10 individual results obtained in the test for Uniformity of content.

For tablets containing 2 mg or more of norethisterone Weigh and powder 20 tablets. Carry out the method for *liquid chromatography*, Appendix III D, using the conditions described in the test for Uniformity of content and using the following solutions. Solution (1) contains 0.02% w/v of *norethisterone BPCRS* in *methanol (60%)*. For solution (2) mix a quantity of the powdered tablets containing 5 mg of Norethisterone in 10 ml of *water* with the aid of ultrasound for 15 minutes, add sufficient *methanol* to produce 25 ml, centrifuge for 10 minutes and use the supernatant liquid.

The chromatographic procedure described under Uniformity of content may be used.

Calculate the content of $C_{20}H_{26}O_2$ using the declared content of $C_{20}H_{26}O_2$ in *norethisterone BPCRS*.

Storage Norethisterone Tablets should be protected from light.

Nortriptyline Capsules

Definition Nortriptyline Capsules contain Nortriptyline Hydrochloride.

The capsules comply with the requirements stated under Capsules and with the following requirements.

Content of nortriptyline, $C_{19}H_{21}N$ 92.5 to 107.5% of the prescribed or stated amount.

Identification

A. Shake a quantity of the contents of the capsules containing the equivalent of 5 mg of nortriptyline with 20 ml of *methanol* and filter. To 1 ml of the filtrate add 1 ml of a 2.5% w/v solution of *sodium hydrogen carbonate*, 1 ml of a 2% w/v solution of *sodium periodate* and 1 ml of a 0.3% w/v solution of *potassium permanganate*. Allow to stand for 15 minutes, acidify with 1M *sulphuric acid* and extract with 10 ml of *2,2,4-trimethylpentane*. The *light absorption* of the resulting solution, Appendix II B, in the range 230 to 350 nm exhibits a maximum only at 265 nm.

B. Triturate a quantity of the contents of the capsules containing the equivalent of 0.1 g of nortriptyline with 10 ml of *chloroform*, filter and evaporate the chloroform. Dissolve 50 mg of the residue in 3 ml of warm *water*, cool and add 0.05 ml of a 2.5% w/v solution of *quinhydrone* in *methanol*. A red colour develops (distinction from amitriptyline).

C. The residue obtained in test B yields reaction A characteristic of *chlorides*, Appendix VI.

Dibenzosuberone Carry out the method for *thin-layer chromatography*, Appendix III A, using *silica gel G* as the coating substance and a mixture of 3 volumes of *diethylamine*, 15 volumes of *ethyl acetate* and 85 volumes of *cyclohexane* as the mobile phase but allowing the solvent front to ascend 12 cm above the line of application. Apply separately to the plate 5 µl of each of the following solutions. For solution (1) extract a quantity of the contents of the capsules containing the equivalent of 20 mg of nortriptyline with 5 ml of a mixture of 1 volume of 2M *hydrochloric acid* and 9 volumes of *ethanol (96%)*, centrifuge and use the supernatant liquid. Solution (2) contains 0.0010% w/v of *dibenzosuberone* in *ethanol (96%)*. After removal of the plate, allow it to dry in air until the odour of solvent is no longer detectable, spray with *sulphuric acid* containing 4% v/v of *formaldehyde solution* and examine immediately under *ultraviolet light (365 nm)*. Any spot corresponding to dibenzosuberone in the chromatogram obtained with solution (1) is not more intense than the spot in the chromatogram obtained with solution (2) (0.5%).

Assay Carry out Method I for *non-aqueous titration*, Appendix VIII A, using a quantity of the mixed contents of 20 capsules containing the equivalent of 0.1 g of nortriptyline, adding 3 ml of *mercury(II) acetate solution* and using 0.02M *perchloric acid VS* as titrant and *crystal violet solution* as indicator. Each ml of 0.02M *perchloric acid VS* is equivalent to 5.268 mg of $C_{19}H_{21}N$.

Labelling The quantity of active ingredient is stated in terms of the equivalent amount of nortriptyline.

Nortriptyline Tablets

Definition Nortriptyline Tablets contain Nortriptyline Hydrochloride. They are coated.

The tablets comply with the requirements stated under Tablets and with the following requirements.

Content of nortriptyline, $C_{19}H_{21}N$ 90.0 to 110.0% of the prescribed or stated amount.

Identification

A. Shake a quantity of the powdered tablets containing the equivalent of 5 mg of nortriptyline with 20 ml of *methanol* and filter. To 1 ml of the filtrate add 1 ml of a 2.5% w/v solution of *sodium hydrogen carbonate*, 1 ml of a 2% w/v solution of *sodium periodate* and 1 ml of a 0.3% w/v solution of *potassium permanganate*. Allow to stand for 15 minutes, acidify with 1M *sulphuric acid* and extract with 10 ml of *2,2,4-trimethylpentane*. The *light absorption* of the resulting trimethylpentane solution, Appendix II B, in the range 230 to 350 nm exhibits a maximum only at 265 nm.

B. Triturate a quantity of the powdered tablets containing the equivalent of 0.1 g of nortriptyline with 10 ml of *chloroform*, filter and evaporate the filtrate to a low volume. Add *ether* until a turbidity is produced and allow to stand. Dissolve 50 mg of the precipitate in 3 ml of warm *water*, cool and add 0.05 ml of a 2.5% w/v solution of *quinhydrone* in *methanol*. A red colour develops (distinction from amitriptyline).

C. The precipitate obtained in test B yields reaction A characteristic of *chlorides*, Appendix VI.

Dibenzosuberone Carry out the method for *thin-layer chromatography*, Appendix III A, using *silica gel G* as the coating substance and a mixture of 3 volumes of *diethylamine*, 15 volumes of *ethyl acetate* and 85 volumes of *cyclohexane* as the mobile phase but allowing the solvent front to ascend 12 cm above the line of application. Apply separately to the plate 5 µl each of the following solutions. For solution (1) extract a quantity of the powdered tablets containing the equivalent of 20 mg of nortriptyline with 5 ml of a mixture of 1 volume of 2M *hydrochloric acid* and 9 volumes of *ethanol (96%)*, centrifuge and use the supernatant liquid. Solution (2) contains 0.0010% w/v of *dibenzosuberone* in *ethanol (96%)*. After removal of the plate, allow it to dry in air until the odour of the solvent is no longer detectable, spray with *sulphuric acid* containing 4% v/v of *formaldehyde solution* and examine immediately under *ultraviolet light (365 nm)*. Any spot corresponding to dibenzosuberone in the chromatogram obtained with solution (1) is not more intense than the spot in the chromatogram obtained with solution (2) (0.25%).

Assay Carry out the method for *liquid chromatography*, Appendix III D, using as solution (1) a 0.025% w/v solution of *nortriptyline hydrochloride BPCRS* in *methanol (50%)*. For solution (2) add 50 ml of *water* to 20 tablets, shake vigorously until the tablets have completely disintegrated, add 100 ml of *methanol* and shake for 30 minutes. Add sufficient *water* to produce 200 ml, filter and dilute a volume of the filtrate containing the equivalent of 25 mg of nortriptyline to 100 ml with *methanol (50%)*.

The chromatographic procedure may be carried out using (a) a stainless steel column (20 cm × 4.6 mm) packed with *stationary phase C* (10 µm) (Nucleosil C18 is suitable), (b) a 0.56% w/v solution of *sodium hexanesulphonate* in a mixture of equal volumes of *water* and *acetonitrile* adjusted to pH 4.5 with *glacial acetic acid* as the mobile phase with a flow rate of 2 ml per minute and (c) a detection wavelength of 239 nm.

Calculate the content of $C_{19}H_{21}N$ using the declared content of $C_{19}H_{21}N$ in *nortriptyline hydrochloride BPCRS*.

Labelling The quantity of active ingredient is stated in terms of the equivalent amount of nortriptyline.

Nystatin Ointment

Definition Nystatin Ointment is a dispersion of Nystatin in *microfine powder* in a suitable basis.

The ointment complies with the requirements stated under Topical Semi-solid Preparations and with the following requirements.

Identification Disperse a quantity containing 25,000 IU in 10 ml of *chloroform*, add 40 ml of *methanol* and shake. Filter and dilute 1 ml of the filtrate to 25 ml with *methanol*. The *light absorption* of the resulting solution, Appendix II B, in the range 250 to 350 nm exhibits three maxima, at 291, 305 and 319 nm. The ratios of the *absorbances* at the maxima at 291 nm and 319 nm to the *absorbance* at the maximum at 305 nm are 0.61 to 0.73 and 0.83 to 0.96, respectively. Use in the reference cell a solution prepared in exactly the same manner but omitting the preparation being examined.

Assay Carry out the following procedure protected from light. Disperse a quantity containing 400,000 IU in 20 ml of *ether* in a stoppered flask, add 70 ml of *dimethylformamide* and shake for 15 minutes. Add 10 ml of *water*, shake vigorously for 2 minutes and filter. Dilute 10 ml of the filtrate to 100 ml with a solution containing 9.56% w/v of *potassium dihydrogen orthophosphate* and 11.5% v/v of 1M *potassium hydroxide* and carry out the *biological assay of antibiotics*, Appendix XIV A. The precision of the assay is such that the fiducial limits of error are not less than 95% and not more than 105% of the estimated potency. The upper fiducial limit of error is not less than 90.0% and the lower fiducial limit of error is not more than 115.0% of the prescribed or stated number of IU.

Labelling The strength is stated as the number of IU (Units) per g.

Nystatin Oral Suspension

Nystatin Oral Drops

Definition Nystatin Oral Suspension is a suspension of Nystatin in a suitable flavoured vehicle.

Nystatin Oral Suspension should not be diluted.

The oral suspension complies with the requirements stated under Oral Liquids and with the following requirements.

Identification To a quantity containing 300,000 IU add a mixture of 5.00 ml of *glacial acetic acid* and 50 ml of *methanol* and shake. Add sufficient *methanol* to produce 100 ml, filter and dilute 1 ml of the filtrate to 100 ml with *methanol*. The *light absorption* of the resulting solution, Appendix II B, in the range 250 to 350 nm exhibits three maxima, at 291, 305 and 319 nm. The ratios of the *absorbances* at the maxima at 291 nm and 319 nm to the *absorbance* at the maximum at 305 nm are 0.61 to 0.73 and 0.83 to 0.96, respectively. Use in the reference cell a solution prepared in exactly the same manner but omitting the preparation being examined.

Assay Carry out the following procedure protected from light. Dissolve a quantity containing 200,000 IU in sufficient *dimethylformamide* to produce 50 ml, dilute 10 ml to 200 ml with a solution containing 9.56% w/v of *potassium dihydrogen orthophosphate* and 11.5% v/v of 1M *potassium hydroxide* and carry out the *biological assay of antibiotics*, Appendix XIV A. The precision of the assay is such that the fiducial limits of error are not less than 95% and not more than 105% of the estimated potency. The upper fiducial limit of error is not less than 95.0% and the lower fiducial limit of error is not more than 120.0% of the prescribed or stated number of IU.

Storage Nystatin Oral Suspension should be protected from light and stored at a temperature not exceeding 15°.

Labelling The strength is stated as the number of IU (Units) per ml.

Nystatin Pessaries

Definition Nystatin Pessaries contain Nystatin.

The pessaries comply with the requirements stated under Vaginal Preparations and with the following requirements.

Identification To a quantity of the powdered pessaries containing 300,000 IU add a mixture of 5.00 ml of *glacial acetic acid* and 50 ml of *methanol* and shake. Add sufficient *methanol* to produce 100 ml, filter and dilute 1 ml of the filtrate to 100 ml with *methanol*. The *light absorption* of the resulting solution, Appendix II B, in the range 250 to 350 nm exhibits three maxima, at 291, 305 and 319 nm. The ratios of the *absorbances* at the maxima at 291 nm and 319 nm to the *absorbance* at the maximum at 305 nm are 0.61 to 0.73 and 0.83 to 0.96, respectively. Use in the reference cell a solution prepared in exactly the same manner but omitting the preparation being examined.

Loss on drying When dried to constant weight at 105°, the powdered pessaries lose not more than 5.0% of their weight. Use 1 g.

Assay Carry out the following procedure protected from light. Weigh and powder 20 pessaries. Shake a quantity of the powder containing 200,000 IU with 50 ml of *dimethylformamide* for 1 hour. Centrifuge, dilute 10 ml of the clear supernatant liquid to 200 ml with a solution containing 9.56% w/v of *potassium dihydrogen orthophosphate* and 11.5% v/v of 1M *potassium hydroxide* and carry out the *biological assay of antibiotics*, Appendix XIV A. The precision of the assay is such that the fiducial limits of error are not less than 95% and not more than 105% of the estimated potency. The upper fiducial limit of error is not less than 95.0% and the lower fiducial limit of error is not more than 125.0% of the prescribed or stated number of IU.

Storage Nystatin Pessaries should be stored at a temperature not exceeding 25°.

Labelling The quantity of active ingredient is stated as the number of IU (Units).

Nystatin Tablets

Definition Nystatin Tablets contain Nystatin. They are coated.

The tablets comply with the requirements stated under Tablets and with the following requirements.

Identification Extract a quantity of the powdered tablets containing 300,000 IU with a mixture of 5.00 ml of *glacial acetic acid* and 50 ml of *methanol*, add sufficient *methanol* to produce 100 ml and filter. Dilute 1 ml of the filtrate to 100 ml with *methanol*. The *light absorption* of the resulting solution, Appendix II B, in the range 250 to 350 nm exhibits three maxima, at 291, 305 and 319 nm. The ratios of the *absorbances* at the maxima at 291 nm and 319 nm to the *absorbance* at the maximum at 305 nm are 0.61 to 0.73 and 0.83 to 0.96, respectively. Use in the reference cell a solution prepared in exactly the same manner but omitting the preparation being examined.

Disintegration Maximum time, 30 minutes, Appendix XII A, but using a 0.6% v/v solution of *hydrochloric acid* in place of *water*. If the tablets fail to disintegrate, wash them rapidly by immersion in *water* and continue the test using *phosphate buffer pH 6.8*; the tablets then disintegrate within a further 30 minutes.

Loss on drying When dried at 60° at a pressure not exceeding 0.7 kPa for 3 hours, the powdered tablets lose not more than 5.0% of their weight. Use 1 g.

Assay Carry out the following procedure protected from light. Weigh and powder 20 tablets. Shake a quantity of the powder containing 200,000 IU with 50 ml of *dimethylformamide* for 1 hour. Centrifuge, dilute 10 ml of the clear, supernatant liquid to 200 ml with a solution containing 9.56% w/v of *potassium dihydrogen orthophosphate* and 11.5% v/v of 1M *potassium hydroxide* and carry out the *biological assay of antibiotics*, Appendix XIV A. The precision of the assay is such that the fiducial limits of error are not less than 95% and not more than 105% of the estimated potency. The upper fiducial limit of error is not less than 97.0% and the lower fiducial limit of error is not more than 110.0% of the prescribed or stated number of IU.

Storage Nystatin Tablets should be stored at a temperature not exceeding 25°.

Labelling The quantity of active ingredient is stated as the number of IU (Units).

Olive Oil Ear Drops

Definition Olive Oil Ear Drops are Olive Oil in a suitable container.

The ear drops comply with the requirements stated under Ear Preparations and with the following requirements.

Identification Carry out the test for the *identification of fixed oils by thin-layer chromatography*, Appendix X N. The chromatogram obtained from the oil being examined shows spots corresponding to those in the *typical chromatogram* for olive oil. For certain types of olive oil the difference in the sizes of spots E and F is less pronounced than in the figure.

Acid value Not more than 2.0, Appendix X B. Use 5 g.

Light absorption The *absorbance* of a 1% w/v solution in *cyclohexane* at the maximum at 270 nm is not more than 0.20, Appendix II B. The ratio of the *absorbance* at 232 nm to that at 270 nm is greater than 8.

Peroxide value Not more than 15, Appendix X F.

Relative density 0.910 to 0.916, Appendix V G.

Unsaponifiable matter Not more than 1.5% w/w when determined by the following method. To 5 g of the oil in a 150-ml flask add 50 ml of 2M *ethanolic potassium hydroxide* and heat under a reflux condenser on a water bath for 1 hour, shaking frequently. Add 50 ml of *water* through the condenser, shake, allow to cool and transfer the contents of the flask to a separating funnel, rinsing the flask with 50 ml of *petroleum spirit (boiling range, 40° to 60°)* in portions and adding the rinsings to the separating funnel. Shake vigorously for 1 minute, allow to separate and transfer the aqueous layer to a second separating funnel. If an emulsion forms add small quantities of *ethanol (96%)* or a concentrated solution of *potassium hydroxide*. Extract the aqueous layer with two 50-ml quantities of *petroleum spirit (boiling range, 40° to 60°)* and combine the organic layers in a third separating funnel. Wash with three 50-ml quantities of *ethanol (50%)*, transfer the petroleum spirit layer to a weighed 250-ml flask, rinse the separating funnel with small quantities of *petroleum spirit (boiling range, 40° to 60°)* and add the rinsings to the flask. Evaporate the solvent on a water bath, dry at 100° to 105° for 15 minutes with the flask in a horizontal position, allow to cool and weigh. Repeat the drying for successive 15-minute periods until the loss in weight between two successive weighings does not exceed 0.1%. Dissolve the residue in 20 ml of *ethanol (96%)* previously neutralised to 0.1 ml of *bromophenol blue solution* and, if necessary, titrate with 0.1M *hydrochloric acid VS*. Calculate the percentage content of unsaponifiable matter from the expression

$$100(a - 0.032b)/w$$

where a is the weight, in g, of the residue, b is the volume, in ml, of 0.1M *hydrochloric acid VS* required and w is the weight, in g, of oil taken. The test is not valid if $0.032b$ is greater than 5% of a and must be repeated.

Foreign fixed oils Carry out the test for *foreign oils by gas chromatography*, Appendix X N. The fatty-acid fraction of the oil has the following composition.

Saturated fatty acids of chain length less than C_{16} Not more than 0.1%.

Palmitic acid 7.5 to 20.0%.

Palmitoleic acid (equivalent chain length on polyethylene glycol adipate, 16.3) Not more than 3.5%.

Stearic acid 0.5 to 5.0%.

Oleic acid (equivalent chain length on polyethylene glycol adipate, 18.3) 56.0 to 85.0%.

Linoleic acid (equivalent chain length on polyethylene glycol adipate, 18.9) 3.5 to 20.0%.

Linolenic acid (equivalent chain length on polyethylene glycol adipate, 19.7) Not more than 1.5%.

Arachidic acid Not more than 0.5%.

Gadoleic acid (equivalent chain length on polyethylene glycol adipate, 20.3) Not more than 0.2%.

Behenic acid Not more than 0.2%.

Erucic acid (equivalent chain length on polyethylene glycol adipate, 22.3) Not more than 0.1%.

Sterols Carry out the test for the *determination of sterols*, Appendix X N. The sterol fraction of the oil contains more than 93% of β-sitosterol, less than 0.5% of cholesterol, less than 0.5% of Δ^7-stigmasterol and less than 4% of campesterol. The content of stigmasterol is less than the content of campesterol. Any other sterols present at relative retention times identical with those of β-sitosterol and Δ^7-stigmasterol are to be calculated as β-sitosterol and Δ^7-stigmasterol respectively.

Sesame oil Shake 10 ml for about 1 minute with a mixture of 0.5 ml of a 0.35% v/v solution of *furfuraldehyde* in *acetic anhydride* and 4.5 ml of *acetic anhydride* in a cylinder closed with a ground-glass stopper, filter through paper impregnated with *acetic anhydride* and add 0.2 ml of *sulphuric acid* to the filtrate. No bluish green colour develops.

Storage Olive Oil Ear Drops should be kept in a well-filled, well-closed container and protected from light.

Opium Tincture

Definition

Opium, sliced	200 g
Ethanol (90 per cent)	a sufficient quantity
Purified Water	a sufficient quantity

Extemporaneous preparation The following directions apply.

Pour 500 ml of boiling Purified Water on to the Opium and allow to stand for 6 hours; add 500 ml of Ethanol (90 per cent), mix thoroughly and allow to stand in a covered vessel for 24 hours; strain, press the marc, mix the liquids and allow to stand for not less than 24 hours; filter.

Determine the concentration of morphine, calculated as anhydrous morphine, in the tincture so prepared by the Assay. To the remainder of the liquid add sufficient of a mixture of equal volumes of Ethanol (90 per cent) and Purified Water to produce an Opium Tincture containing 1% w/v of anhydrous morphine.

The tincture complies with the requirements stated under Tinctures and with the following requirements.

Content of anhydrous morphine, $C_{17}H_{19}NO_3$ 0.925 to 1.075% w/v.

Ethanol content 41 to 46% v/v, Appendix VIII F, Method III.

Relative density 0.898 to 0.969, Appendix V G.

Assay Dilute 5 ml to 100 ml with *ethanol (45%)*. To 10 ml of the resulting solution add 5 ml of *water* and 1 ml of 5M *ammonia* and extract with 30 ml of a mixture of equal volumes of *ethanol (96%)* and *chloroform* and then with two 22.5-ml quantities of a mixture of 2 volumes of *chloroform* and 1 volume of *ethanol (96%)*, washing each extract with the same 20 ml of a mixture of equal volumes of *ethanol (96%)* and *water*. Evaporate the combined extracts just to dryness, extract the residue with two 5-ml quantities of *calcium hydroxide solution*, filter and wash the filter with 10 ml of *calcium hydroxide solution*. To the combined filtrate and washings add 0.1 g of *ammonium sulphate*, extract with two 10-ml quantities of *ethanol-free chloroform*, wash the combined extracts with 10 ml of *water* and discard the chloroform solution. To the combined alkaline liquid and aqueous washings add 10 ml of 1M *hydrochloric acid*, heat on a water bath to remove any chloroform, cool and dilute to 100 ml with *water*. To 10 ml of this solution add 10 ml of 0.1M *hydrochloric acid* and 8 ml of a freshly prepared 1.0% w/v solution of *sodium nitrite*, allow to stand for 15 minutes, add 12 ml of 5M *ammonia*, dilute to 50 ml with *water* and measure the *absorbance* of a 4-cm layer of the resulting solution at the maximum at 442 nm, Appendix II B, using in the reference cell a solution prepared at the same time and in the same manner but using 8 ml of *water* in place of the solution of sodium nitrite. Calculate the content of $C_{17}H_{19}NO_3$ taking 124 as the value of A(1%, 1 cm) at the maximum at 442 nm.

Camphorated Opium Tincture

Paregoric

Definition

Opium Tincture	50 ml
Benzoic Acid	5 g
Racemic Camphor	3 g
Anise Oil	3 ml
Ethanol (60 per cent)	sufficient to produce 1000 ml

Extemporaneous preparation The following directions apply.

Dissolve the Benzoic Acid, the Racemic Camphor and the Anise Oil in 900 ml of Ethanol (60 per cent), add the Opium Tincture and sufficient Ethanol (60 per cent) to produce 1000 ml and mix. Filter, if necessary.

The tincture complies with the requirements stated under Tinctures and with the following requirements.

Content of anhydrous morphine, $C_{17}H_{19}NO_3$ 0.045 to 0.055% w/v.

Ethanol content 56 to 60% v/v, Appendix VIII F, Method III.

Relative density 0.90 to 0.92, Appendix V G.

Assay To 10 ml add 5 ml of *water* and 1 ml of 5M *ammonia* and extract with 30 ml of a mixture of equal volumes of *ethanol* (96%) and *chloroform* and then with two 22.5-ml quantities of a mixture of 2 volumes of *chloroform* and 1 volume of *ethanol (96%)*, washing each extract with the same 20 ml of a mixture of equal volumes of *ethanol (96%)* and *water*. Evaporate the combined extracts almost to dryness, extract the residue with 10 ml of *calcium hydroxide solution*, filter and wash the filter with 10 ml of *calcium hydroxide solution*. To the combined filtrate and washings add 0.1 g of *ammonium sulphate*, extract with two 10-ml quantities of *ethanol-free chloroform*, wash the combined extracts with 10 ml of *water* and discard the chloroform solution. To the combined alkaline liquid and aqueous washings add 10 ml of 1M *hydrochloric acid*, heat on a water bath to remove any chloroform, cool and dilute to 100 ml with *water*. To 10 ml of this solution add 10 ml of 0.1M *hydrochloric acid* and 8 ml of a freshly prepared 1.0% w/v solution of *sodium nitrite*, allow to stand for 15 minutes, add 12 ml of 5M *ammonia*, dilute to 50 ml with *water* and measure the *absorbance* of a 4-cm layer of the resulting solution at the maximum at 442 nm, Appendix II B, using in the reference cell a solution prepared at the same time and in the same manner but using 8 ml of *water* in place of the solution of sodium nitrite. Calculate the content of $C_{17}H_{19}NO_3$ taking 124 as the value of A(1%, 1 cm) at the maximum at 442 nm.

Concentrated Camphorated Opium Tincture

Definition

Opium Tincture	400 ml
Benzoic Acid	40 g
Racemic Camphor	24 g
Anise Oil	24 ml
Ethanol (96 per cent)	400 ml
Water	sufficient to produce 1000 ml

Extemporaneous preparation The following directions apply.

Dissolve the Benzoic Acid, the Racemic Camphor and the Anise Oil in the Ethanol (96 per cent), add the Opium Tincture and sufficient Water to produce 1000 ml, mix and filter if necessary.

The tincture complies with the requirement stated under Tinctures and with the following requirements.

Content of anhydrous morphine, $C_{17}H_{19}NO_3$ 0.36 to 0.44% w/v.

Ethanol content 54 to 59% v/v, Appendix VIII F, Method III.

Relative density 0.912 to 0.930, Appendix V G.

Assay Dilute 10 ml to 100 ml with *ethanol (50%)* and carry out the Assay described under Camphorated Opium Tincture using 10 ml of the diluted solution.

Oral Rehydration Salts

Definition Oral Rehydration Salts are *oral powders* containing either Anhydrous Glucose or Glucose, Sodium Chloride, Potassium Chloride and either Sodium Citrate or Sodium Bicarbonate. After being dissolved in the requisite volume of Water they are intended for the prevention and treatment of dehydration due to diarrhoea, including maintenance therapy. Oral Rehydration Salts may contain suitable flavouring agents. Where necessary they may also contain suitable flow agents in the minimum quantity required to achieve a satisfactory product.

The composition of one of the formulations in use is described below in terms of the amount in grams to be dissolved in sufficient Water to produce 1000 ml. It is that recommended by the Diarrhoeal Diseases Control Programme of the World Health Organization (WHO) and the United Nations Childrens Fund (UNICEF).

Sodium Chloride	3.5 g
Potassium Chloride	1.5 g
Sodium Citrate	2.9 g
Anhydrous Glucose	20.0 g

The oral powders comply with the requirements stated under Powders and with the following requirements.

Content of potassium, K, sodium, Na, bicarbonate, HCO_3, chloride, Cl, and citrate, $C_6H_5O_7$, as appropriate 90.0 to 110.0% of the requisite amount, the latter being calculated from the stated amounts of the relevant constituents.

Content of anhydrous glucose, $C_6H_{12}O_6$, or of glucose monohydrate $C_6H_{12}O_6,H_2O$, as appropriate 90.0 to 110.0% of the stated amount.

Identification

A. When heated with *cupri-tartaric solution R1* a copious precipitate of copper(I) oxide is produced.

B. Yield reaction B characteristic of *potassium salts*, Appendix VI.

C. Yield reaction A characteristic of *sodium salts*, Appendix VI.

D. Yield reaction A characteristic of *chlorides*, Appendix VI.

E. For preparations containing Sodium Citrate a quantity of the oral powder containing the equivalent of 50 mg of citric acid yields reactions A and B characteristic of *citrates*, Appendix VI.

F. For preparations containing Sodium Bicarbonate add 2 ml of *hydrochloric acid*. A vigorous effervescence is produced.

Assay Carry out the following assays on the well-mixed contents of an individual sachet or on a suitable sample from the well-mixed contents of a bulk container. Where the amount in an individual sachet is insufficient to carry out all the assays, take a separate sachet for the Assay for citrate and for the Assay for glucose.

For the Assays for potassium, for sodium, for chloride and for bicarbonate dissolve 8 g in sufficient *water* to produce 500 ml (solution A).

For potassium Dilute a suitable volume of solution A with a solution of *strontium chloride* such that there is a 1500- to 2000-fold excess of strontium ions in the final solution and determine by Method I for *atomic emission spectrophotometry*, Appendix II D, measuring at 767 nm. Use *potassium standard solution (600 ppm K)*, suitably diluted with the strontium chloride solution, for the standard solutions. Each mg of Potassium Chloride is equivalent to 0.5245 mg of K.

For sodium Dilute a suitable volume of solution A with a solution of *strontium chloride* such that there is a 1500- to 2000-fold excess of strontium ions in the final solution and determine by Method I for *atomic emission spectrophotometry*, Appendix II D, measuring at 589 nm. Use *sodium standard solution (200 ppm Na)*, suitably diluted with the strontium chloride solution, for the standard solutions. Each mg of Sodium Chloride, of Sodium Bicarbonate and of Sodium Citrate is equivalent to 0.3934, 0.2737 and 0.2345 mg of Na respectively.

For chloride Titrate a suitable volume (50 ml for the formula stated above) of solution A with 0.1M *silver nitrate VS* using a 5% w/v solution of *potassium chromate* as indicator. Each ml of 0.1M *silver nitrate VS* is equivalent to 3.545 mg of Cl. Each mg of Potassium Chloride and of Sodium Chloride is equivalent to 0.4756 mg and 0.6066 mg of Cl respectively.

For citrate Disperse 2.8 g in 80 ml of *anhydrous acetic acid*, heat to about 50°, cool, dilute to 100 ml with *anhydrous acetic acid*, allow to stand for 10 minutes and carry out Method I for *non-aqueous titration*, Appendix VIII A, using 20 ml of the supernatant liquid and *1-naphtholbenzein solution* as indicator. Each ml of 0.1M *perchloric acid VS* is equivalent to 6.303 mg of $C_6H_5O_7$. Each mg of Sodium Citrate is equivalent to 0.6430 mg of $C_6H_5O_7$.

For bicarbonate Titrate 200 ml of solution A with 0.1M *hydrochloric acid VS* using *methyl orange solution* as indicator. Each ml of 0.1M *hydrochloric acid VS* is equivalent to 6.101 mg of HCO_3. Each mg of Sodium Bicarbonate is equivalent to 0.7263 mg of HCO_3.

For glucose Dissolve 7.5 g in 40 ml of *water*, add 0.5 ml of 1M *ammonia*, dilute to 50 ml with *water*, mix well and allow to stand for 30 minutes. If necessary use a suitable method of filtration to obtain a clear solution. Determine the *optical rotation* of the solution, Appendix V F. The observed rotation in degrees multiplied by 0.9477 represents the weight, in g, of $C_6H_{12}O_6$ in the weight taken for the Assay.

Storage Oral Rehydration Salts should be protected from moisture. They should be kept in sachets, preferably made of aluminium foil, containing sufficient for a single dose or for a single day's treatment. Powders for use in hospitals may be presented in bulk containers containing sufficient to produce a volume of solution appropriate to the daily requirements of the establishment concerned.

Labelling The label states (1) for sachets the total weights, in grams, of each of the constituents; (2) for bulk containers the weights, in grams, of each of the constituents in a stated quantity, in grams, of the oral powder; (3) the directions for use; (4) that any portion of the solution prepared using the oral powder that remains unused 24 hours after preparation should be discarded.

The label indicates the pharmaceutical form as 'oral powder'.

Orange Peel Infusion

Definition

Concentrated Orange Peel Infusion	100 ml
Water	sufficient to produce 1000 ml

The infusion complies with the requirements stated under Infusions.

CONCENTRATED ORANGE PEEL INFUSION

Definition

Dried Bitter-Orange Peel, cut small	500 g
Ethanol (25 per cent)	1350 ml

Extemporaneous preparation The following directions apply.

Macerate the Dried Bitter-Orange Peel in a covered vessel for 48 hours with 1000 ml of the Ethanol (25 per cent) and press out the liquid. To the pressed marc add 350 ml of the Ethanol (25 per cent), macerate for 24 hours, press and add the liquid to the product of the first pressing. Allow to stand for not less than 14 days and filter.

Ethanol content 18 to 23% v/v, Appendix VIII F.

Total solids 10 to 15% w/v, Appendix XI A. Use 1 ml.

Weight per ml 1.01 to 1.04 g, Appendix V G.

Compound Orange Spirit

Definition

Terpeneless Orange Oil	2.5 ml
Terpeneless Lemon Oil	1.3 ml
Anise Oil	4.25 ml
Coriander Oil	6.25 ml
Ethanol (90 per cent)	sufficient to produce 1000 ml

The spirit complies with the requirements stated under Spirits and with the following requirements.

Ethanol content 86 to 90% v/v, Appendix VIII F.

Weight per ml 0.828 to 0.841 g, Appendix V G.

Orange Syrup

Definition

Orange Tincture	60 ml
Syrup	sufficient to produce 1000 ml

The syrup complies with the requirements stated under Syrups and with the following requirement.

Weight per ml 1.29 to 1.31 g, Appendix V G.

Orange Tincture

Definition

Dried Bitter-Orange Peel, in *moderately fine powder*	110 g
Ethanol (70 per cent)	a sufficient quantity

Extemporaneous preparation The following directions apply.

Prepare 1000 ml of tincture by *percolation*, Appendix XI F.

The tincture complies with the requirements stated under Tinctures and with the following requirements.

Ethanol content 62 to 69% v/v, Appendix VIII F, Method III.

Dry residue 3.5 to 4.5% w/v.

Relative density 0.895 to 0.920, Appendix V G.

Orciprenaline Oral Solution

Definition Orciprenaline Oral Solution is a solution of Orciprenaline Sulphate in a suitable flavoured vehicle.

The oral solution complies with the requirements stated under Oral Liquids and with the following requirements.

Content of orciprenaline sulphate, $(C_{11}H_{17}NO_3)_2$, H_2SO_4 95.0 to 105.0% of the prescribed or stated amount.

Identification

A. In the test for Related substances, the principal spot in the chromatogram obtained with solution (2) corresponds in position, colour and size to that in the chromatogram obtained with solution (5). The test is not valid unless the chromatogram obtained with solution (6) shows a single, compact spot.

B. To 2 ml add 2 ml of a 0.1% w/v solution of *2,6-dichloroquinone-4-chloroimide* in *ethanol (96%)* and 1 ml of *sodium carbonate solution*; a violet colour is produced immediately changing to greenish brown and then light brown over a period of 5 minutes. The final colour is not more intense than that of a blank prepared at the same time and in the same manner but using 2 ml of *ethanol (96%)* in place of the preparation being examined.

Related substances Carry out the method for *thin-layer chromatography*, Appendix III A, using a silica gel G precoated plate (Merck plates are suitable) and a mixture of 4 volumes of 13.5M *ammonia*, 16 volumes of *water*, 30 volumes of *propan-2-ol* and 50 volumes of *ethyl acetate* as the mobile phase. Apply separately to the plate 20 µl of each of the following solutions. For solution (1) dilute the oral solution, if necessary, with a mixture of 5 volumes of *methanol* and 1 volume of *water* to produce a solution containing 0.20% w/v of Orciprenaline Sulphate. For solution (2) dilute 1 volume of solution (1) to 10 volumes with the same solvent. For solution (3) dilute 1 volume of solution (1) to 200 volumes with the same solvent. Solution (4) contains 0.1% w/v of *methyl 4-hydroxybenzoate* in a mixture of 5 volumes of *methanol* and 1 volume of *water*. Solution (5) contains 0.020% w/v of *orciprenaline sulphate BPCRS* in a mixture of 5 volumes of *methanol* and 1 volume of *water*. For solution (6) mix 1 volume of solution (2) and 1 volume of solution (5). After removal of the plate, allow it to dry in air and expose to iodine vapour until spots appear. Any *secondary spot* in the chromatogram obtained with solution (1) is not more intense than the spot in the chromatogram obtained with solution (3) (0.5%). Disregard any spot with an Rf value equal to or higher than that of the principal spot in the chromatogram obtained with solution (4). The test is not valid unless the spot in the chromatogram obtained with solution (3) is clearly visible.

Assay To a weighed quantity of the oral solution containing 20 mg of Orciprenaline Sulphate add 5 ml of *water*, extract with 15 ml of *ether*, wash the ether layer with 20 ml of *water*, discard the ether and combine the aqueous layers. To the resulting solution add 10 ml of 0.0167M *potassium bromate VS*, 1 g of *potassium bromide* and 5 ml of *hydrochloric acid*, shake gently for 1 minute, add 0.5 g of *potassium iodide* and titrate with 0.1M *sodium thiosulphate VS* using *starch mucilage* as indicator. Repeat the procedure without the oral solution. The difference between the titrations represents the amount of potassium bromate required. Each ml of 0.0167M *potassium bromate VS* is equivalent to 4.337 mg of $(C_{11}H_{17}NO_3)_2,H_2SO_4$. Determine the *weight per ml* of the oral solution, Appendix V G, and calculate the content of $(C_{11}H_{17}NO_3)_2,H_2SO_4$, weight in volume.

Storage Orciprenaline Oral Solution should be protected from light.

When Orciprenaline Oral Solution is prescribed or demanded, no strength being stated, an Oral Solution containing 10 mg in 5 ml shall be dispensed or supplied.

Orciprenaline Tablets

Definition Orciprenaline Tablets contain Orciprenaline Sulphate.

The tablets comply with the requirements stated under Tablets and with the following requirements.

Content of orciprenaline sulphate, $(C_{11}H_{17}NO_3)_2$, H_2SO_4 90.0 to 110.0% of the prescribed or stated amount.

Identification

A. Extract a quantity of the powdered tablets containing 0.1 g of Orciprenaline Sulphate with *methanol*, filter and evaporate the filtrate to dryness. The *light absorption*, Appendix II B, in the range 230 to 350 nm of a 0.015% w/v solution of the residue in 0.01M *hydrochloric acid* exhibits a broad maximum at 278 nm. The *absorbance* over the range 276 to 280 nm is about 1.0.

B. Carry out the method for *thin-layer chromatography*, Appendix III A, using *silica gel G* as the coating substance and a mixture of 1.5 volumes of 13.5M *ammonia*, 10 volumes of *water* and 90 volumes of *aldehyde-free methanol* as the mobile phase. Apply separately to the plate 2 µl of each of the following solutions. For solution (1) shake a quantity of the powdered tablets containing 10 mg of Orciprenaline Sulphate with 10 ml of *ethanol (80%)* for 10 minutes with the aid of ultrasound and filter (Whatman GF/C filter paper is suitable). Solution (2) contains 0.1% w/v of *orciprenaline sulphate BPCRS* in *ethanol (80%)*. Solution (3) contains 0.1% w/v of each of *orciprenaline sulphate BPCRS* and *salbutamol sulphate BPCRS* in *ethanol (80%)*. Allow the plate to dry in air and spray with a 1% w/v solution of *potassium permanganate*. The principal spot in the chromatogram obtained with solution (1) corresponds to that in the chromatogram obtained with solution (2). The test is not valid unless the chromatogram obtained with solution (3) shows two clearly separated principal spots.

C. The residue obtained in test A yields the reactions characteristic of *sulphates*, Appendix VI.

Related substances Carry out the method for *thin-layer chromatography*, Appendix III A, using *silica gel G* as the coating substance and a mixture of 4 volumes of 13.5M *ammonia*, 16 volumes of *water*, 30 volumes of *propan-2-ol* and 50 volumes of *ethyl acetate* as the mobile phase. Apply separately to the plate 10 µl of each of the following solutions. For solution (1) shake a quantity of the powdered tablets containing 0.1 g of Orciprenaline Sulphate with 10 ml of *ethanol (80%)* for 10 minutes with the aid of ultrasound and filter (Whatman GF/C filter paper is suitable). For solution (2) dilute 1 volume of solution (1) to 100 volumes with *ethanol (80%)*. For solution (3) dilute 1 volume of solution (1) to 200 volumes with *ethanol (80%)*. Allow the plate to dry in air and expose the plate to iodine vapour. Any *secondary spot* in the chromatogram obtained with solution (1) is not more intense than the principal spot in the chromatogram obtained with solution (2) (1%) and at most one such spot is more intense than the principal spot in the chromatogram obtained with solution (3) (0.5%). Disregard any spot with an Rf value lower than that of the principal spot in the chromatogram obtained with solution (1). The test is not valid unless the spot in the chromatogram obtained with solution (3) is clearly visible.

Assay Weigh and powder 20 tablets. Shake a quantity of the powder containing 80 mg of Orciprenaline Sulphate with 50 ml of 0.01M *hydrochloric acid*, filter and add sufficient 0.01M *hydrochloric acid* to the filtrate to produce 100 ml. Dilute 10 ml to 100 ml with 0.01M *hydrochloric acid* and measure the *absorbance* of the resulting solution at the maximum at 276 nm, Appendix II B. Calculate the content of $(C_{11}H_{17}NO_3)_2,H_2SO_4$ taking 72.3 as the value of A(1%, 1 cm) at the maximum at 276 nm.

Storage Orciprenaline Tablets should be protected from light.

Organ Preservation Solutions

Organ Preservation Solutions comply with the requirements of the 3rd edition of the European Pharmacopoeia for Solutions for Organ Preservation [1264]. These requirements are reproduced after the heading 'Definition' below.

Ph Eur

DEFINITION

Solutions for organ preservation are sterile, aqueous preparations, intended for storage, protection and/or perfusion of mammalian body organs that are, in particular, destined for transplantation.

They contain electrolytes that are typically at a concentration close to the intracellular electrolyte composition.

They may contain carbohydrates (such as glucose or mannitol), amino acids, calcium-complexing agents (such as citrate or phosphate), hydrocolloids (such as starch or gelatin derivatives) and other auxiliary substances, intended, for example, to make the preparation isotonic with blood, to adjust or buffer the pH and to prevent deterioration of the ingredients, but without adversely affecting the intended action of the preparation or, at the concentration used, causing toxicity or undue local irritation. Solutions for organ preservation may also contain active ingredients or these drugs may be added immediately before use.

Before use, the solutions for organ preservation are cooled below room temperature, typically to 2°C to 6°C to reduce the temperature of the organ and its metabolism.

Solutions for organ preservation, examined under suitable conditions of visibility, are clear and practically free from particles.

Solutions for organ preservation may also be presented as concentrated solutions. They are diluted to the prescribed volume with a prescribed liquid immediately before use. After dilution, they comply with the requirements for solutions for organ preservation.

Where applicable, the containers for solutions for organ preservation comply with the requirements for *Materials used for the manufacture of containers* (*3.1* and subsections) and *Containers and closures* (*3.2* and subsections). Solutions for organ preservation are supplied in glass containers (*3.2.1*) or in other containers such as plastic containers (*3.2.2* and *3.2.8*). The tightness of the container is ensured by suitable means. Closures ensure a good seal, prevent the access of micro-organisms and other contaminants and usually permit the withdrawal of a part or the whole of the contents without removal of the closure. The plastic materials or elastomers (*3.2.10*) of which the closure is composed are sufficiently firm and elastic to allow the passage of a needle with the least possible shedding of particles.

PRODUCTION

Solutions for organ preservation are prepared using materials and methods designed to ensure their sterility and to avoid the introduction of contaminants and the growth of micro-organisms; recommendations on this aspect are provided in *Methods for preparation of sterile products (5.1.1)*.

Unless otherwise justified and authorised, solutions for

organ preservation are prepared using *Water for injections (169)* and do not contain antimicrobial preservatives.

TESTS

pH (*2.2.3*). *Carry out the test at room temperature.* The pH of the solution is 5.0 to 8.0.

Osmolality (*2.2.35*). The osmolality of the solution is 250 mosmol/kg to 380 mosmol/kg.

Hydroxymethylfurfural If the solution contains glucose, it complies with the following test: to a volume of the solution containing the equivalent of 25 mg of glucose, add 5.0 ml of a 100 g/l solution of *p-toluidine R* in *2-propanol R* containing 10 per cent *V/V* of *glacial acetic acid R* and 1.0 ml of a 5 g/l solution of *barbituric acid R*. The absorbance (*2.2.25*), determined at 550 nm after allowing the mixture to stand for 2 min to 3 min, is not greater than that of a standard prepared at the same time in the same manner using a solution containing 10 µg of *hydroxymethylfurfural R* in the same volume as the solution to be examined.

Particulate contamination Carry out the test for sub-visible particles (*2.9.19*) using 50 ml of solution. The solution contains not more than 50 particles per millilitre larger than 10 µm and not more than 5 particles per millilitre larger than 25 µm.

Sterility (*2.6.1*). The solution complies with the test for sterility.

Bacterial endotoxins (*2.6.14*). Not more than 0.5 IU of endotoxin per millilitre.

Pyrogens (*2.6.8*). Solutions for which a validated test for bacterial endotoxins cannot be carried out comply with the test for pyrogens. Inject per kilogram of rabbit's mass 10 ml of the solution, unless otherwise justified and authorised.

LABELLING

The label states:

— that the solution is not to be used for injection,
— the formula of the solution for organ preservation expressed in grams per litre and in millimoles per litre,
— the nominal volume of the solution for organ preservation in the container,
— the osmolality expressed in milliosmoles per kilogram,
— that any unused portion of the ready-to-use solution, concentrated or diluted solution must be discarded,
— the storage conditions.

In addition, for concentrated solutions the label states:

— that the solution must be diluted with a suitable liquid immediately before use.

Ph Eur

Orphenadrine Hydrochloride Tablets

Definition Orphenadrine Hydrochloride Tablets contain Orphenadrine Hydrochloride.

The tablets comply with the requirements stated under Tablets and with the following requirements.

Content of orphenadrine hydrochloride, $C_{18}H_{23}NO,HCl$ 92.5 to 107.5% of the prescribed or stated amount.

Identification Extract a quantity of the powdered tablets containing 0.15 g of Orphenadrine Hydrochloride with *chloroform*, filter and evaporate the filtrate to dryness. The residue complies with the following tests.

A. Dissolve 5 mg in 2 ml of *sulphuric acid*. An orange-red colour is produced.

B. Dissolve 50 mg in 10 ml of *ethanol (50%)*, add 10 ml of *picric acid solution R1* and allow to stand. The *melting point* of the precipitate, after recrystallisation from *ethanol (96%)*, is about 89° or about 107°, Appendix V A.

C. Yields reaction A characteristic of *chlorides*, Appendix VI.

Assay Weigh and powder 20 tablets. Dissolve a quantity of the powder containing 70 mg of Orphenadrine Hydrochloride as completely as possible in a mixture of 5 ml of *water* and 5 ml of 2M *hydrochloric acid*. Without delay extract with four 15-ml quantities of *chloroform*, filter the combined extracts and evaporate to about 20 ml. Carry out Method I for *non-aqueous titration*, Appendix VIII A, using 0.02M *perchloric acid VS*, adding 2 ml of *mercury(II) acetate solution* and determining the end point potentiometrically. Each ml of 0.02M *perchloric acid VS* is equivalent to 6.118 mg of $C_{18}H_{23}NO,HCl$.

Oxazepam Tablets

Definition Oxazepam Tablets contain Oxazepam.

The tablets comply with the requirements stated under Tablets and with the following requirements.

Content of oxazepam, $C_{15}H_{11}ClN_2O_2$ 90.0 to 110.0% of the prescribed or stated amount.

Identification

A. Extract a quantity of the powdered tablets containing 20 mg of Oxazepam with 25 ml of *chloroform*, filter, evaporate to dryness and dry the residue at 60° at a pressure not exceeding 0.7 kPa. The *infrared absorption spectrum* of the residue, Appendix II A, is concordant with the *reference spectrum* of oxazepam.

B. The *light absorption*, Appendix II B, in the range 210 to 350 nm of the solution obtained in the Assay exhibits two maxima, at 230 nm and 316 nm.

Related substances Carry out the test protected from light. Carry out the method for *thin-layer chromatography*, Appendix III A, using as the coating substance a suitable silica gel containing a fluorescent indicator with an optimal intensity at 254 nm (Merck silica gel 60 F_{254} is suitable) and a mixture of 10 volumes of *methanol* and 100 volumes of *dichloromethane* as the mobile phase. Before use, wash the plate with *methanol* allowing the solvent front to ascend 17 cm above the line of application. Develop the plate in the same direction as the washing with methanol. Apply separately to the plate 20 µl of each of the following solutions. For solution (1) shake a quantity of the powdered tablets containing 30 mg of Oxazepam with 6 ml of *acetone* and centrifuge. For solution (2) dilute 1 volume of solution (1) to 100 volumes with *acetone*. For solution (3) dilute 1 volume of solution (1) to 500 volumes with *acetone*. Solution (4) contains 0.10% w/v of each of *oxazepam EPCRS* and *bromazepam EPCRS* in *acetone*. After removal of the plate, allow it to dry in air and examine under *ultraviolet light (254 nm)*. Any *secondary spot* in the chromatogram obtained with solution (1) is not more intense than the spot in the chromatogram obtained with solution (2) (1%) and not more than one such spot is more intense than the spot in the chromatogram obtained with solution (3) (0.2%). The test is not valid unless the chromatogram obtained with solution (4) shows two clearly separated spots.

Assay Weigh and powder 20 tablets. To a quantity of the powder containing 25 mg of Oxazepam add 150 ml of *ethanol (96%)* and shake for 30 minutes. Add sufficient *ethanol (96%)* to produce 250 ml, centrifuge, dilute 5 ml of the supernatant liquid to 100 ml with the same solvent and measure the *absorbance* of the resulting solution at the maximum at 230 nm, Appendix II B. Calculate the content of $C_{15}H_{11}ClN_2O_2$ taking 1250 as the value of A(1%, 1 cm) at the maximum at 230 nm.

Storage Oxazepam Tablets should be protected from light and stored at a temperature not exceeding 25°.

Oxprenolol Tablets

Definition Oxprenolol Tablets contain Oxprenolol Hydrochloride. They are coated.

The tablets comply with the requirements stated under Tablets and with the following requirements.

Content of oxprenolol hydrochloride, $C_{15}H_{23}NO_3$, HCl 95.0 to 105.0% of the prescribed or stated amount.

Identification

A. To a quantity of the powdered tablets containing 50 mg of Oxprenolol Hydrochloride add 10 ml of *water* and 2 ml of 1.25M *sodium hydroxide*, extract with 10 ml of *chloroform* and reserve the aqueous layer for test D. Dry the chloroform extract over *anhydrous sodium sulphate*, filter and evaporate the filtrate to dryness. The *infrared absorption spectrum* of the residue, Appendix II A, is concordant with the *reference spectrum* of oxprenolol.

B. The aqueous layer obtained in test A yields reaction A characteristic of *chlorides*, Appendix VI.

Related substances Carry out the method for *thin-layer chromatography*, Appendix III A, using *silica gel G* as the coating substance and a mixture of 2 volumes of 13.5M *ammonia*, 12 volumes of *methanol* and 88 volumes of *chloroform* as the mobile phase, but allowing the solvent front to ascend 13 cm above the line of application. Apply separately to the plate 2 µl of each of the following solutions. For solution (1) shake a quantity of the powdered tablets containing 0.25 g of Oxprenolol Hydrochloride with 5 ml of *water*, centrifuge and use the supernatant liquid. For solution (2) dilute 1 volume of solution (1) to 200 volumes with *water*. Allow the spots to dry in air for 15 minutes before development. After removal of the plate, dry it in a current of warm air for 10 minutes, allow to cool, spray with *anisaldehyde solution*, heat at 100° to 105° for 5 to 10 minutes and examine in daylight. Any *secondary spot* in the chromatogram obtained with solution (1) is not more intense than the spot in the chromatogram obtained with solution (2) (0.5%).

Assay Weigh and powder 20 tablets. Mix a quantity of the powder containing 20 mg of Oxprenolol Hydrochloride with 25 ml of 0.1M *hydrochloric acid* and add sufficient *water* to produce 250 ml. Mix with the aid of ultrasound for 5 minutes, shake for 15 minutes and filter. Measure the *absorbance* of the solution at the maximum at 273 nm, Appendix II B. Calculate the content of $C_{15}H_{23}NO_3$,HCl taking 74.5 as the value of A(1%, 1 cm) at the maximum at 273 nm.

Oxymetholone Tablets

Definition Oxymetholone Tablets contain Oxymetholone.

The tablets comply with the requirements stated under Tablets and with the following requirements.

Content of oxymetholone, $C_{21}H_{32}O_3$ 90.0 to 110.0% of the prescribed or stated amount.

Identification

To a quantity of the powdered tablets containing 50 mg of Oxymetholone add 10 ml of *water*, extract with two 10-ml quantities of *chloroform* and evaporate the chloroform extract to dryness. The residue, after drying over *phosphorus pentoxide* at a pressure not exceeding 0.7 kPa, complies with the following tests.

A. The *infrared absorption spectrum*, Appendix II A, is concordant with the *reference spectrum* of oxymetholone.

B. Complies with the test for *identification of steroids*, Appendix III A, using *impregnating solvent II* and *mobile phase D*.

Assay Weigh and powder 20 tablets. Extract a quantity of the powder containing 25 mg of Oxymetholone with 0.01M *ethanolic sodium hydroxide* and add sufficient 0.01M *ethanolic sodium hydroxide* to produce 250 ml. Filter if necessary, dilute 5 ml of the filtrate to 50 ml with 0.01M *ethanolic sodium hydroxide* and measure the *absorbance* of the resulting solution at the maximum at 315 nm, Appendix II B. Calculate the content of $C_{21}H_{32}O_3$ taking 547 as the value of A(1%, 1 cm) at the maximum at 315 nm.

Storage Oxymetholone Tablets should be kept free from contact with ferrous metals and protected from light.

Oxyphenbutazone Eye Ointment

Definition Oxyphenbutazone Eye Ointment is a sterile preparation containing Oxyphenbutazone in a suitable basis.

The eye ointment complies with the requirements stated under Eye Preparations and with the following requirements.

Content of oxyphenbutazone, $C_{19}H_{20}N_2O_3,H_2O$ 95.0 to 105.0% of the prescribed or stated amount.

Identification Dissolve a quantity containing 0.15 g of Oxyphenbutazone in 20 ml of *dichloromethane* and shake with a mixture of 6 ml of 1M *sodium hydroxide* and 10 ml of *water*. Shake the aqueous layer with 10 ml of *dichloromethane* and discard the dichloromethane. To the aqueous phase add 10 ml of 1M *hydrochloric acid* and extract with 3 ml of *dichloromethane*. Separate the dichloromethane extract and filter through *anhydrous sodium sulphate*. The filtrate complies with the following tests.

A. The *infrared absorption spectrum*, Appendix II A, is concordant with the *reference spectrum* of oxyphenbutazone.

B. Evaporate the remainder of the filtrate to dryness, add 1 ml of *glacial acetic acid* and 2 ml of *hydrochloric acid* and heat on a water bath for 30 minutes. Cool, add 10 ml of *water* and filter. To the filtrate add 3 ml of 0.1M *sodium nitrite*; a yellow colour is produced. Add 1 ml of the solution to 5 ml of *2-naphthol solution*; a pinkish red precipitate is produced which is soluble in *ethanol (96%)*, giving a brownish red solution.

Related substances Carry out the method for *thin-layer chromatography*, Appendix III A, using *silica gel HF_{254}* as the coating substance and a 0.02% w/v solution of *butylated hydroxytoluene* in a mixture of 20 volumes of *glacial acetic acid* and 80 volumes of *chloroform* as the mobile phase. To prepare the plate allow the solvent front to ascend 4 cm, remove the plate and dry it in a current of cold air for 1 minute. Without delay and under a current of nitrogen, apply separately to the plate 5 µl of each of the following solutions prepared immediately before use. For solution (1) add 5 ml of a freshly prepared 0.02% w/v solution of *butylated hydroxytoluene* in *ethanol (96%)* to a quantity of the eye ointment containing 0.10 g of Oxyphenbutazone, warm gently on a water bath until molten, shake, cool in ice, filter and use the filtrate. For solution (2) dilute 3 volumes of solution (1) to 200 volumes with the ethanolic butylated hydroxytoluene solution. Develop immediately, allowing the solvent front to ascend 10 cm above the line of application. After removal of the plate, dry it in a current of cold air for 15 minutes and examine under *ultraviolet light (254 nm)*. Any *secondary spot* in the chromatogram obtained with solution (1) is not more intense than the spot in the chromatogram obtained with solution (2) (1.5%). Disregard any spot with an Rf value higher than 0.75.

Assay Disperse a quantity containing 0.1 g of Oxyphenbutazone by shaking with 40 ml of *petroleum spirit (boiling range, 60° to 80°)* and extract the petroleum spirit layer with four 40-ml quantities of 0.1M *sodium carbonate*. Combine the aqueous extracts and wash with three 40-ml quantities of *ether*, freshly purified before use by passing it through a column of *basic aluminium oxide*. Discard the ethereal extracts, dilute the combined aqueous extracts to 250 ml with 0.1M *sodium carbonate* and mix. Filter the solution (Whatman No. 42 filter paper is suitable) and dilute 10 ml to 500 ml with *water*. Measure the *absorbance* of the resulting solution at the maximum at 254 nm, Appendix II B, using *water* in the reference cell. Calculate the content of $C_{19}H_{20}N_2O_3,H_2O$ from the *absorbance* of the solution obtained by dissolving 0.1 g of *oxyphenbutazone BPCRS* in sufficient 0.1M *sodium carbonate* to produce 250 ml and diluting 10 ml to 500 ml with water.

Oxytetracycline Capsules

Definition Oxytetracycline Capsules contain Oxytetracycline Hydrochloride.

The capsules comply with the requirements stated under Capsules and with the following requirements.

Content of oxytetracycline hydrochloride, $C_{22}H_{24}N_2O_9,HCl$ 95.0 to 110.0% of the prescribed or stated amount.

A. Carry out the method for *thin-layer chromatography*, Appendix III A, using a suitable silica gel precoated plate (Merck silica gel 60 plates are suitable) and a mixture of 6 volumes of *water*, 35 volumes of *methanol* and 59 volumes of *dichloromethane* as the mobile phase. Adjust the pH of a 10% w/v solution of *disodium edetate* to 7.0 with 10M *sodium hydroxide* and spray the solution evenly onto the plate (about 10 ml for a plate 100 mm × 200 mm). Allow the plate to dry in a horizontal position for at least 1 hour. Before use, dry the plate at 110° for 1 hour. Apply separately to the plate 1 µl of each of the following solutions. For solution (1) extract a quantity of the contents of the capsules containing 10 mg of Oxytetracycline Hydrochloride with 20 ml of *methanol*, centrifuge and use the supernatant liquid. For solution (2) dissolve 5 mg of *oxytetracycline hydrochloride EPCRS* in sufficient *methanol* to produce 10 ml. For solution (3) dissolve 5 mg of *oxytetracycline hydrochloride EPCRS* and 5 mg of *demeclocycline hydrochloride EPCRS* in sufficient *methanol* to produce 10 ml. After removal of the plate, dry it in a current of air and examine under *ultraviolet light (365 nm)*. The principal spot in the chromatogram obtained with solution (1) is similar in position, colour and size to that in the chromatogram obtained with solution (2). The test is not valid unless the chromatogram obtained with solution (3) shows two clearly separated spots.

B. To 0.5 mg of the contents of the capsules add 2 ml of *sulphuric acid*; a deep crimson colour is produced. Add 1 ml of *water*; the colour changes to yellow.

C. The contents of the capsules yield the reactions characteristic of *chlorides*, Appendix VI.

Dissolution Comply with the *dissolution test for tablets and capsules*, Appendix XII D, using as the medium 900 ml of 0.1M hydrochloric acid and rotating the basket at 100 revolutions per minute. Withdraw a sample of 10 ml of the medium. Measure the *absorbance* of the filtered sample, suitably diluted if necessary, at the maximum at 353 nm, Appendix II B. Calculate the total content of oxytetracycline hydrochloride, $C_{22}H_{24}N_2O_9,HCl$, in the medium taking 282 as the value of A(1%, 1 cm) at the maximum at 353 nm.

Light-absorbing impurities Dissolve a portion of the mixed contents of five capsules as completely as possible in sufficient of a mixture of 1 volume of 1M *hydrochloric acid* and 99 volumes of *methanol* to produce two solutions of Oxytetracycline Hydrochloride containing (1) 0.20% w/v and (2) 1.0% w/v and filter each solution. The *absorbance* of the filtrate obtained from solution (1) at 430 nm is not more than 0.75, Appendix II B, calculated with reference to the dried capsule contents. The *absorbance* of the filtrate obtained from solution (2) at 490 nm is not more than 0.40, calculated with reference to the dried capsule contents.

Loss on drying When dried at 60° at a pressure not exceeding 0.7 kPa for 3 hours, the contents of the capsules lose not more than 5.0% of their weight. Use 1 g.

Assay Carry out the method for *liquid chromatography*, Appendix III D, using the following solutions. For solution (1) shake with the aid of ultrasound a quantity of the mixed contents of 20 capsules containing 0.1 g of Oxytetracycline Hydrochloride with 80 ml of 0.1M methanolic hydrochloric acid prepared by diluting 1 volume of 1M *hydrochloric acid* to 10 volumes with *methanol*. Add sufficient of the methanolic hydrochloric acid to produce 100 ml. Centrifuge and use the supernatant solution. Solution (2) contains 0.1% w/v of *oxytetracycline hydrochloride BPCRS* in the same solvent. Solution (3) contains 0.1% w/v each of *oxytetracycline hydrochloride BPCRS* and *tetracycline* in the same solvent.

The chromatographic procedure may be carried out using (a) a stainless steel column (25 cm × 4.6 mm) packed with a silanised cation-exchange silica (5 µm) (Bio-Sil SP 90-5S for oxytetracycline is suitable), (b) as the mobile phase with a flow rate of 1 ml per minute a mixture of 0.2 volume of *diethylamine*, 35 volumes of *methanol* and 65 volumes of a buffer solution consisting of a 0.035 molar solution of each of *potassium dihydrogen orthophosphate* and *disodium edetate*, the pH of the mixture being adjusted to 6.0 with *orthophosphoric acid*, and (c) a detection wavelength of 263 nm.

The assay is not valid unless the *resolution factor* between the two principal peaks in the chromatogram obtained with solution (3) is at least 4.5.

Calculate the content of $C_{22}H_{24}N_2O_9,HCl$ using the declared content of $C_{22}H_{24}N_2O_9,HCl$ in *oxytetracycline hydrochloride BPCRS*.

Oxytetracycline Tablets

Definition Oxytetracycline Tablets contain Oxytetracycline. They are coated.

The tablets comply with the requirements stated under Tablets and with the following requirements.

Content of oxytetracycline dihydrate, $C_{22}H_{24}N_2O_9$, $2H_2O$ 95.0 to 110.0% of the prescribed or stated amount.

Identification

A. Carry out the method for *thin-layer chromatography*, Appendix III A, using a suitable silica gel precoated plate (Merck silica gel 60 plates are suitable) and a mixture of 6 volumes of *water*, 35 volumes of *methanol* and 59 volumes of *dichloromethane* as the mobile phase. Adjust the pH of a 10% w/v solution of *disodium edetate* to 7.0 with 10M *sodium hydroxide* and spray the solution evenly onto the plate (about 10 ml for a plate 100 mm × 200 mm). Allow the plate to dry in a horizontal position for at least 1 hour. Before use, dry the plate at 110° for 1 hour. Apply separately to the plate 1 µl of each of the following solutions. For solution (1) extract a quantity of the powdered tablets containing the equivalent of 10 mg of oxytetracycline dihydrate with 20 ml of *methanol*, centrifuge and use the supernatant liquid. For solution (2) dissolve 5 mg of *oxytetracycline hydrochloride EPCRS* in sufficient *methanol* to produce 10 ml. For solution (3) dissolve 5 mg of *oxytetracycline hydrochloride EPCRS* and 5 mg of *demeclocycline hydrochloride EPCRS* in sufficient *methanol* to produce 10 ml. After removal of the plate, dry it in a current of air and examine under *ultraviolet light (365 nm)*. The principal spot in the chromatogram obtained with solution (1) is similar in position, colour and size to that in the chromatogram obtained with solution (2). The test is not valid unless the chromatogram obtained with solution (3) shows two clearly separated spots.

B. To 2 mg of the powdered tablets add 2 ml of *sulphuric acid*; a deep crimson colour is produced. Add 1 ml of *water*; the colour changes to yellow.

C. Shake 4 mg of the powdered tablets with 5 ml of a 1% w/v solution of *sodium carbonate* and add 2 ml of *diazobenzenesulphonic acid solution*. A light brown colour is produced.

Dissolution Comply with the *dissolution test for tablets and capsules*, Appendix XII D, using as the medium 900 ml of 0.1M *hydrochloric acid* and rotating the basket at 100 revolutions per minute. Withdraw a sample of 10 ml of the medium. Measure the *absorbance* of the filtered sample, suitably diluted if necessary, at the maximum at 353 nm, Appendix II B. Calculate the total content of oxytetracycline dihydrate, $C_{22}H_{24}N_2O_9,2H_2O$, in the medium taking 282 as the value of A(1%, 1 cm) at the maximum at 353 nm.

Light-absorbing impurities Wash five tablets with *water* or *chloroform* until any coloured coating is removed, dry with filter paper and powder. Dissolve portions of the powder as completely as possible in sufficient of a mixture of 1 volume of 1M *hydrochloric acid* and 99 volumes of *methanol* to produce two solutions containing the equivalent of (1) 0.20% w/v of oxytetracycline dihydrate and (2) 1.0% w/v of oxytetracycline dihydrate and filter each solution. The *absorbance* of the filtrate obtained from solution (1) at 430 nm is not more than 0.50 and the *absorbance* of the filtrate obtained from solution (2) at 490 nm is not more than 0.40, Appendix II B.

Assay Weigh and powder 20 tablets. Carry out the method for *liquid chromatography*, Appendix III D, using the following solutions. For solution (1) shake with the aid of ultrasound a quantity of the powdered tablets containing the equivalent of 0.1 g of oxytetracycline dihydrate with 80 ml of 0.1M methanolic hydrochloric acid prepared by diluting 1 volume of 1M *hydrochloric acid* to 10 volumes with *methanol*. Add sufficient of the methanolic hydrochloric acid to produce 100 ml. Centrifuge and use the supernatant solution. Solution (2) contains 0.1% w/v of oxytetracycline hydrochloride BPCRS in the same solvent. Solution (3) contains 0.1% w/v each of *oxytetracycline hydrochloride BPCRS* and *tetracycline* in the same solvent.

The chromatographic procedure may be carried out using (a) a stainless steel column (25 cm × 4.6 mm) packed with a silanised cation-exchange silica (5 µm) (Bio-Sil SP 90-5S for oxytetracycline is suitable), (b) as the mobile phase with a flow rate of 1 ml per minute, a mixture of 0.2 volume of *diethylamine*, 35 volumes of *methanol* and 65 volumes of a buffer solution consisting of a 0.035 molar solution of each of *potassium dihydrogen orthophosphate* and *disodium edetate*, the pH of the mixture being adjusted to 6.0 with *orthophosphoric acid*, and (c) a detection wavelength of 263 nm.

The assay is not valid unless the *resolution factor* between the two principal peaks in the chromatogram obtained with solution (3) is at least 4.5.

Calculate the content of $C_{22}H_{24}N_2O_9,2H_2O$ using the declared content of $C_{22}H_{24}N_2O_9$ in *oxytetracycline hydrochloride BPCRS*. Each mg of $C_{22}H_{24}N_2O_9$ is equivalent to 1.078 mg of $C_{22}H_{24}N_2O_9,2H_2O$.

Labelling The quantity of active ingredient is stated in terms of the equivalent amount of oxytetracycline dihydrate.

Oxytocin Injection

Definition Oxytocin Injection is a sterile solution of Oxytocin or a sterile dilution of Oxytocin Concentrated Solution in Water for Injections.

Content of oxytocin, $C_{43}H_{66}N_{12}O_{12}S_2$ 90.0 to 110.0% of the prescribed or stated amount of the peptide.

The injection complies with the requirements stated under Parenteral Preparations and with the following requirements.

Characteristics A clear, colourless liquid.

Identification

A. Carry out the method for *thin-layer chromatography*, Appendix III A, using a high performance *silica gel G* precoated plate (Merck 5631 plates are suitable) and a mixture of 1 volume of *glacial acetic acid,* 6 volumes of *water*, 30 volumes of *methanol* and 70 volumes of *dichloromethane* as the mobile phase but allowing the solvent front to ascend 8 cm above the line of application. Prepare a solution containing 17 µg per ml of *oxytocin EPCRS* by dissolving the contents of one vial in the requisite volume of a 1.56% w/v solution of *sodium dihydrogen orthophosphate* (solution A). For solution (1) evaporate 5 ml of the injection on a rotary evaporator at 30° and dissolve the residue in 0.5 ml of *water.*

For injections containing 10 IU per ml prepare solution (2) by evaporating 5 ml of solution A on a rotary evaporator at 30° and dissolving the residue in 0.5 ml of *water.* Apply separately to the plate 1 µl of solutions (1) and (2), dry in a stream of cold air and develop immediately.

For injections containing 5 IU per ml prepare solution (2) by evaporating 2.5 ml of solution A on a rotary evaporator at 30° and dissolving the residue in 0.5 ml of *water.* Apply separately to the plate 2 µl of solutions (1) and (2), dry in a stream of cold air and develop immediately.

For injections containing 1 IU per ml use solution A as solution (2). Apply separately to the plate 10 µl of solutions (1) and (2), dry in a stream of cold air and develop immediately.

After removal of the plate, allow it to dry in a stream of cold air for 10 minutes and develop again in a tank, previously equilibrated for 30 minutes with fresh mobile phase. After removal of the plate, allow it to dry in a stream of warm air for 10 minutes, cool and spray with *lithium and sodium molybdotungstophosphate solution* until the plate appears translucent. Immediately place the plate in a tank, previously equilibrated for 30 minutes with 13.5M *ammonia,* for 5 minutes, remove and dry in a stream of warm air. The principal spot in the chromatogram obtained with solution (1) corresponds in position, size and intensity to that in the chromatogram obtained with solution (2).

B. In the Assay, the chromatogram obtained with solution (1) exhibits a peak with the same retention time as the principal peak in the chromatogram obtained with solution (2).

Acidity pH, 3.5 to 4.5, Appendix V L.

Assay Carry out the Assay described under Oxytocin. For solution (1) use the injection being examined. For solution (2) dissolve the contents of one vial of *oxytocin EPCRS* in a 1.56% w/v solution of *sodium dihydrogen orthophosphate* to produce a solution containing the same concentration in µg per ml of oxytocin as that stated on the label of the injection. Inject 200 µl of each solution.

Calculate the content of $C_{43}H_{66}N_{12}O_{12}S_2$ from the declared content of peptide in *oxytocin EPCRS* and using peak areas.

Storage Oxytocin Injection should be stored at a temperature of 2° to 15°.

Labelling The strength is stated as the number of IU (Units) per ml. The label also states the equivalent number of micrograms of oxytocin per ml.

Pancreatin Granules

Definition Pancreatin Granules contain Pancreatin and may also contain suitable gastro-resistant substances.

The granules comply with the requirements stated under Granules and with the following requirements.

Content of pancreatin Not less than 90.0% of the stated minimum number of Units of free protease activity, of lipase activity and of amylase activity.

Identification Triturate a quantity of powdered granules containing 2.5 g of Pancreatin with 100 ml of *water.* The liquid complies with the tests described under Pancreatin.

Assay Carry out the *assay of pancreatin* described under Pancreatin using in the determination of each activity a quantity of the powdered granules estimated to contain the number of Units specified in the method.

Storage Pancreatin Granules should be kept in a well-closed container and stored at a temperature not exceeding 15°.

Labelling The label states (1) the minimum number of Units of free protease activity, of lipase activity and of amylase activity per g; (2) where applicable, that the granules contain gastro-resistant substances.

Pancreatin Tablets

Definition Pancreatin Tablets contain Pancreatin. They are made gastro-resistant by enteric-coating or by other means.

The tablets comply with the requirements stated under Tablets and with the following requirements.

Content of pancreatin Not less than 90.0% of the stated minimum numbers of Units of free protease activity, of lipase activity and of amylase activity.

Identification Triturate a quantity of powdered tablets containing 2.5 g of Pancreatin with 100 ml of *water* and filter. The filtrate complies with the tests described under Pancreatin.

Disintegration Tablets made gastro-resistant by enteric-coating comply with the *disintegration test for enteric-coated tablets,* Appendix XII B.

Assay Weigh and powder 20 tablets. Carry out the *assay of pancreatin* described under Pancreatin using in the determination of each activity a quantity of powder estimated to contain the number of Units specified in the method.

Storage Pancreatin Tablets should be stored at a temperature not exceeding 15°.

Labelling The label states the minimum number of Units of free protease activity, of lipase activity and of amylase activity in each tablet.

Pancuronium Injection

Definition Pancuronium Injection is a sterile solution of Pancuronium Bromide in Sodium Chloride Intravenous Infusion.

The injection complies with the requirements stated under Parenteral Preparations and with the following requirements.

Content of pancuronium bromide, $C_{35}H_{60}Br_2N_2O_4$ 95.0 to 105.0% of the prescribed or stated amount.

Characteristics A colourless liquid.

Identification

A. In the test for Related substances, the principal spot in the chromatogram obtained with solution (1) is similar in position, colour and size to the principal spot in the chromatogram obtained with solution (2).

B. To a volume containing 5 mg of Pancuronium Bromide, diluted if necessary to 10 ml with *water*, add 10 ml of *1,2-dichloroethane* followed by 1 ml of *methyl orange solution*. Shake, centrifuge, allow the layers to separate and acidify the organic layer with 1M *sulphuric acid*. A red colour is produced.

C. Yields reaction A characteristic of *bromides*, Appendix VI.

Acidity pH, 3.8 to 4.2, Appendix V L.

Related substances Carry out the method for *thin-layer chromatography*, Appendix III A, using a suitable silica gel as the coating substance and a mixture of 5 volumes of a 20% w/v solution of *sodium iodide*, 10 volumes of *acetonitrile* and 85 volumes of *propan-2-ol* as the mobile phase. Use an unlined, unsaturated tank and allow the solvent front to ascend 12 cm above the line of application. Apply separately to the plate 2 µl of each of the following solutions prepared immediately before use. For solution (1) evaporate a volume of the injection containing 2 mg of Pancuronium Bromide to dryness in a current of *nitrogen*, add 0.2 ml of *acetonitrile* to the residue and mix with the aid of ultrasound for 1 minute. Solution (2) contains 1.0% w/v of *pancuronium bromide BPCRS* in *acetonitrile*. For solution (3) dilute 1 volume of solution (1) to 50 volumes with *acetonitrile*. For solution (4) dilute 1 volume of solution (3) to 2 volumes with *acetonitrile*. Solution (5) contains 0.030% w/v of *dacuronium bromide EPCRS* in *acetonitrile*. Solution (6) contains 1.0% w/v of *pancuronium bromide BPCRS* and 0.030% w/v of *dacuronium bromide EPCRS* in *acetonitrile*. After removal of the plate, dry it in a current of cold air and spray with a 1% w/v solution of *sodium nitrite* in *methanol*. Allow to stand for 2 minutes, spray the plate with *potassium iodobismuthate solution* and dry in a current of cold air. In the chromatogram obtained with solution (1) any spot corresponding to dacuronium bromide is not more intense than the spot in the chromatogram obtained with solution (5) (3%), any other *secondary spot* is not more intense than the spot in the chromatogram obtained with solution (3) (2%) and not more than one such spot is more intense than the spot in the chromatogram obtained with solution (4) (1%). The test is not valid unless the chromatogram obtained with solution (6) shows two distinct spots and the Rf value of the spot due to dacuronium bromide relative to that due to pancuronium bromide is at least 1.2.

Assay To a volume containing 4 mg of Pancuronium Bromide add 1 ml of a 13.9% w/v solution of *hydroxylamine hydrochloride* followed by 1 ml of a 15% w/v solution of *sodium hydroxide*. Allow to stand for 10 minutes and then add 1 ml of a solution prepared by diluting *hydrochloric acid* with *water* to contain 12.76% w/v of HCl. Add 1 ml of a 10% w/v solution of *iron(III) chloride* in 0.1M *hydrochloric acid*, add sufficient *water* to produce 25 ml, centrifuge and measure the *absorbance* of the clear, supernatant liquid at the maximum at 510 nm, Appendix II B, using in the reference cell a solution prepared by carrying out the operation using an equal volume of *water* in place of the injection. Calculate the content of $C_{35}H_{60}Br_2N_2O_4$ from the *absorbance* obtained by repeating the operation using a suitable quantity of *pancuronium bromide BPCRS* dissolved in *water* and using the declared content of $C_{35}H_{60}Br_2N_2O_4$ in *pancuronium bromide BPCRS*.

Storage Pancuronium Injection should be stored at a temperature of 2° to 8°.

Papaveretum Injection

Definition Papaveretum Injection is a sterile solution of Papaveretum in Water for Injections.

The injection complies with the requirements stated under Parenteral Preparations and with the following requirements.

Content of morphine, $C_{17}H_{19}NO_3$ 59.7 to 69.3% of the prescribed or stated amount of Papaveretum.

Content of papaverine, $C_{20}H_{21}NO_4$ 6.2 to 7.7% of the prescribed or stated amount of Papaveretum.

Content of codeine, $C_{18}H_{21}NO_3$ 4.9 to 5.9% of the prescribed or stated amount of Papaveretum.

Characteristics A clear, colourless to yellowish brown solution.

Identification Carry out the method for *thin-layer chromatography*, Appendix III A, using a silica gel precoated plate (Merck silica gel 60 plates are suitable) and a mixture of 2 volumes of 13.5M *ammonia*, 6 volumes of *ethanol (96%)*, 40 volumes of *acetone* and 40 volumes of *toluene* as the mobile phase. Apply separately to the plate 10 µl of each of the following solutions. Solution (1) is the injection diluted, if necessary, to contain 1.6% w/v of Papaveretum. Solutions (2), (3) and (4) are solutions in *water* containing (2) 1.28% w/v of *morphine hydrochloride BPCRS*, (3) 0.115% w/v of *papaverine hydrochloride BPCRS* and (4) 0.10% w/v of *codeine hydrochloride BPCRS*. After removal of the plate, dry it at 100° to 105° for 15 minutes, allow to cool and spray with *potassium iodobismuthate solution* and then with a 0.4% v/v solution of *sulphuric acid*. The chromatogram obtained with solution (1) shows three principal spots corresponding to the principal spots in the chromatograms obtained with solutions (2), (3) and (4).

Acidity pH, 2.5 to 4.0, Appendix V L.

Assay Carry out the method for *liquid chromatography*, Appendix III D, using the following solutions. Solution

(1) contains 0.128% w/v of *morphine hydrochloride BPCRS*, 0.0115% w/v of *papaverine hydrochloride BPCRS* and 0.010% w/v of *codeine hydrochloride BPCRS* in *methanol (60%)*. Solution (2) contains 0.128% w/v of *morphine hydrochloride BPCRS* in *methanol (60%)*. For solution (3) dilute a volume of the injection containing 80 mg of Papaveretum to 50 ml with *methanol (60%)*.

The chromatographic procedure may be carried out using a stainless steel column (10 cm × 4.6 mm) packed with *stationary phase C* (5 μm) (Nucleosil C18 is suitable), (b) as the mobile phase with a flow rate of 2 ml per minute a solution containing 0.01M *sodium acetate* and 0.005M *dioctyl sodium sulphosuccinate* in *methanol (60%)* adjusted to pH 5.5 with *glacial acetic acid* and (c) a detection wavelength of 285 nm. If necessary, adjust the proportion of methanol in the mobile phase in the range 55% v/v to 65% v/v so that the retention time of morphine in solution (2) is 4 to 5 minutes. Adjust the pH of the mobile phase with either *glacial acetic acid* or 2M *sodium hydroxide* in order to obtain optimum separation of the three principal components in solution (1). The retention times of codeine and papaverine relative to that of morphine are about 1.3 and 1.7 respectively.

For morphine Calculate the content of $C_{17}H_{19}NO_3$ using the declared content of $C_{17}H_{19}NO_3$ in *morphine hydrochloride BPCRS*.

For papaverine Calculate the content of $C_{20}H_{21}NO_4$ using the declared content of $C_{20}H_{21}NO_4$ in *papaverine hydrochloride BPCRS*.

For codeine Calculate the content of $C_{18}H_{21}NO_3$ using the declared content of $C_{18}H_{21}NO_3$ in *codeine hydrochloride BPCRS*.

Storage Papaveretum Injection should be protected from light.

Labelling The label states (1) the amount of Papaveretum in a suitable dose-volume; (2) the content of morphine in a suitable dose-volume.

Papaveretum Injection contains the three alkaloids morphine, papaverine and codeine. In reformulating the injection to remove noscapine, the amounts of the other three alkaloids have been maintained. Thus the total amount of material per ml has decreased.

Before reformulation the lower strength injection (which provides the equivalent of 5 mg of the major component, morphine) contained 10 mg per ml of the four-component material. It now contains 7.7 mg of Papaveretum per ml.

Likewise, before reformulation the higher strength injection (which provides the equivalent of 10 mg of morphine) contained 20 mg per ml of the four-component material. It now contains 15.4 mg of Papaveretum per ml.

Paediatric Paracetamol Oral Solution

Definition Paediatric Paracetamol Oral Solution is a solution containing 2.4% w/v of Paracetamol in a suitable flavoured vehicle.

Paediatric Paracetamol Oral Solution should not be diluted.

The oral solution complies with the requirements stated under Oral Liquids and with the following requirements.

Content of paracetamol, $C_8H_9NO_2$ 2.28 to 2.52% w/v.

Identification

A. Carry out the method for *thin-layer chromatography*, Appendix III A, using *silica gel GF_{254}* as the coating substance and a mixture of 65 volumes of *chloroform* 0.5 volume of *glacial acetic acid*, 10 volumes of *toluene*, 25 volumes of *acetone* and 65 volumes of *chloroform* as the mobile phase. Apply separately to the plate 10 μl of each of the following solutions. For solution (1) dilute 1 ml of the preparation being examined to 10 ml with *methanol* and filter if necessary. Solution (2) contains 0.24% w/v of *paracetamol BPCRS* in *methanol*. After removal of the plate, dry it in a current of warm air, examine under *ultraviolet light (254 nm)* and also reveal the spots using *Method I*. By each method of visualisation the principal spot in the chromatogram obtained with solution (1) corresponds to that in the chromatogram obtained with solution (2).

B. In the Assay, the chromatogram obtained with solution (2) shows a peak with the same retention time as the peak due to paracetamol in the chromatogram obtained with solution (1).

4-Aminophenol Carry out the method for *liquid chromatography*, Appendix III D, using the following solutions. Solution (1) contains 0.0024% w/v of *4-aminophenol* in the mobile phase. For solution (2) shake 5 ml of the preparation being examined with 15 ml of the mobile phase, dilute to 25 ml with the mobile phase and filter if necessary.

The chromatographic procedure may be carried out using (a) a stainless steel column (20 cm × 4.6 mm) packed with *stationary phase C* (10 μm) (Nucleosil C18 is suitable), (b) 0.01M *sodium butanesulphonate* in a mixture of 0.4 volume of *formic acid*, 15 volumes of *methanol* and 85 volumes of *water* as the mobile phase with a flow rate of 2 ml per minute and (c) a detection wavelength of 272 nm.

In the chromatogram obtained with solution (2) the area of any peak corresponding to 4-aminophenol is not greater than the area of the peak in the chromatogram obtained with solution (1). In the chromatogram obtained with solution (2) peaks with a long retention time may occur due to preservatives in the preparation (0.5%).

Assay Carry out the method for *liquid chromatography*, Appendix III D, using the following solutions. Solution (1) contains 0.012% w/v of *paracetamol BPCRS* in the mobile phase. For solution (2) mix a weighed quantity of the preparation being examined containing 24 mg of Paracetamol with 100 ml of the mobile phase, dilute to 200 ml with the mobile phase and filter if necessary.

The chromatographic procedure may be carried out using the conditions described in the test for 4-Aminophenol but using a detection wavelength of 243 nm.

Determine the *weight per ml* of the preparation, Appendix V G, and calculate the percentage content of $C_8H_9NO_2$, weight in volume, using the declared content of $C_8H_9NO_2$ in *paracetamol BPCRS*.

Storage Paediatric Paracetamol Oral Solution should be protected from light.

Labelling The label states that Paediatric Paracetamol Oral Solution should not be refrigerated.

Paracetamol Oral Suspension

Definition Paracetamol Oral Suspension is a suspension of Paracetamol in a suitable flavoured vehicle.

The oral suspension complies with the requirements stated under Oral Liquids and with the following requirements.

Content of paracetamol 95.0 to 105.0% of the prescribed or stated amount.

Identification; 4-Aminophenol Complies with the requirements stated under Paediatric Paracetamol Oral Solution using a volume of the oral suspension diluted, if necessary, to contain 2.4% w/v of Paracetamol.

Assay Carry out the Assay described under Paediatric Paracetamol Oral Solution.

Storage Paracetamol Oral Suspension should be protected from light.

When paediatric paracetamol oral suspension or paediatric paracetamol mixture is prescribed or demanded, Paracetamol Oral Suspension containing 2.4% w/v of Paracetamol shall be dispensed or supplied.

Paracetamol Tablets

Definition Paracetamol Tablets contain Paracetamol.

With the exception of the requirements for shape, the tablets comply with the requirements stated under Tablets and with the following requirements.

Content of paracetamol, $C_8H_9NO_2$ 95.0 to 105.0% of the prescribed or stated amount.

Identification Extract a quantity of the powdered tablets containing 0.5 g of Paracetamol with 20 ml of *acetone*, filter, evaporate the filtrate to dryness and dry at 105°. The residue complies with the following tests.

A. The *infrared absorption spectrum*, Appendix II A, is concordant with the *reference spectrum* of paracetamol.

B. Boil 0.1 g with 1 ml of *hydrochloric acid* for 3 minutes, add 10 ml of *water* and cool; no precipitate is produced. Add 0.05 ml of 0.0167M *potassium dichromate*; a violet colour is produced slowly which does not turn red.

C. *Melting point*, about 169°, Appendix V A.

Dissolution Comply with the *dissolution test for tablets and capsules*, Appendix XII D, using Apparatus II. Use as the medium 900 ml of *phosphate buffer pH 5.8* and rotate the paddle at 50 revolutions per minute. Withdraw a sample of 20 ml of the medium and filter. Dilute the filtrate with 0.1M *sodium hydroxide* to give a solution expected to contain about 0.00075% w/v of Paracetamol. Measure the *absorbance* of this solution, Appendix II B, at the maximum at 257 nm using 0.1M *sodium hydroxide* in the reference cell. Calculate the total content of paracetamol, $C_8H_9NO_2$, in the medium taking 715 as the value of A(1%, 1 cm) at the maximum at 257 nm.

4-Aminophenol Carry out the method for *liquid chromatography*, Appendix III D, using the following solutions. Solution (1) contains 0.001% w/v of *4-aminophenol* in *methanol (15%)*. For solution (2) shake a quantity of the powdered tablets containing 1.0 g of Paracetamol with 15 ml of *methanol*, dilute to 100 ml with *water* and filter.

The chromatographic procedure may be carried out using (a) a stainless steel column (20 cm × 4.6 mm) packed with *stationary phase C* (10 µm) (Nucleosil C18 is suitable), (b) 0.01M *sodium butanesulphonate* in a mixture of 0.4 volume of *formic acid*, 15 volumes of *methanol* and 85 volumes of *water* as the mobile phase with a flow rate of 2 ml per minute and (c) a detection wavelength of 272 nm.

In the chromatogram obtained with solution (2) the area of any peak corresponding to 4-aminophenol is not greater than the area of the peak in the chromatogram obtained with solution (1). In the chromatogram obtained with solution (2) peaks with a long retention time may occur due to excipients (0.1%).

Related substances Carry out the method for *thin-layer chromatography*, Appendix III A, using *silica gel GF_{254}* as the coating substance and a mixture of 10 volumes of *toluene*, 25 volumes of *acetone* and 65 volumes of *chloroform* as the mobile phase. Pour the mobile phase into an unlined tank, immediately place the prepared plate in the tank, close the tank and allow the solvent front to ascend 14 cm above the line of application. Apply separately to the plate 200 µl of solution (1) and 40 µl of each of solutions (2), (3) and (4). For solution (1) transfer a quantity of the finely-powdered tablets containing 1.0 g of Paracetamol to a ground-glass-stoppered 15-ml centrifuge tube, add 5 ml of *peroxide-free ether*, shake mechanically for 30 minutes, centrifuge at 1000 revolutions per minute for 15 minutes or until a clear supernatant liquid is obtained and use the supernatant liquid. For solution (2) dilute 1 ml of solution (1) to 10 ml with *ethanol (96%)*. Solution (3) contains 0.0050% w/v of *4′-chloroacetanilide* in *ethanol (96%)*. For solution (4) dissolve 0.25 g of *4′-chloroacetanilide* and 0.10 g of *paracetamol* in sufficient *ethanol (96%)* to produce 100 ml. After removal of the plate, dry it in a current of warm air and examine under *ultraviolet light (254 nm)*. Any spot corresponding to 4′-chloroacetanilide in the chromatogram obtained with solution (1) is not more intense than the spot in the chromatogram obtained with solution (3). Any *secondary spot* in the chromatogram obtained with solution (2) with an Rf value lower than than that of 4′-chloroacetanilide is not more intense than the spot in the chromatogram obtained with solution (3). The test is not valid unless the chromatogram obtained with solution (4) shows two clearly separated principal spots, the spot corresponding to 4′-chloroacetanilide having the higher Rf value.

Assay Weigh and powder 20 tablets. Add a quantity of the powder containing 0.15 g of Paracetamol to 50 ml of 0.1M *sodium hydroxide*, dilute with 100 ml of *water*, shake for 15 minutes and add sufficient *water* to produce 200 ml. Mix, filter and dilute 10 ml of the filtrate to 100 ml with *water*. Add 10 ml of the resulting solution to 10 ml of 0.1M *sodium hydroxide*, dilute to 100 ml with *water* and measure the *absorbance* of the resulting solution at the maximum at 257 nm, Appendix II B. Calculate the content of $C_8H_9NO_2$ taking 715 as the value of A(1%, 1 cm) at the maximum at 257 nm.

Storage Paracetamol Tablets should be protected from light.

Dispersible Paracetamol Tablets

Definition Dispersible Paracetamol Tablets contain Paracetamol in a suitable dispersible basis.

With the exception of the requirements for shape, the tablets comply with the requirements stated under Tablets and with the following requirements.

Content of paracetamol, $C_8H_9NO_2$ 95.0 to 105.0% of the prescribed or stated amount.

Identification

A. Disperse in *water* to form a uniform suspension.

B. The *light absorption*, Appendix II B, in the range 230 to 350 nm of the final solution obtained in the Assay exhibits a maximum only at 257 nm.

C. In the test for Related substances the principal spot in the chromatogram obtained with solution (5) corresponds to that in the chromatogram obtained with solution (6).

Disintegration Comply with the requirements for Dispersible Tablets.

4-Aminophenol Carry out the method for *liquid chromatography*, Appendix III D, using the following solutions. Solution (1) contains 0.001% w/v of *4-aminophenol* in *methanol (15%)*. For solution (2) shake a quantity of the powdered tablets, containing 1.0 g of Paracetamol with 15 ml of *methanol*, dilute to 100 ml with *water* and filter.

The chromatographic procedure may be carried out using (a) a stainless steel column (20 cm × 4.6 mm) packed with *stationary phase C* (10 μm) (Nucleosil C18 is suitable), (b) 0.01M *sodium butanesulphonate* in a mixture of 0.4 volume of *formic acid*, 15 volumes of *methanol* and 85 volumes of *water* as the mobile phase with a flow rate of 2 ml per minute and (c) a detection wavelength of 272 nm.

In the chromatogram obtained with solution (2) the area of any peak corresponding to 4-aminophenol is not greater than the area of the peak in the chromatogram obtained with solution (1) (0.1%). In the chromatogram obtained with solution (2) peaks with long retention times may occur due to excipients.

Related substances Carry out the method for *thin-layer chromatography*, Appendix III A, using *silica gel GF_{254}* as the coating substance and a mixture of 10 volumes of *toluene*, 25 volumes of *acetone* and 65 volumes of *chloroform* as the mobile phase but allowing the solvent front to ascend 14 cm above the line of application. Apply separately to the plate 200 μl of solution (1) and 40 μl of each of solutions (2) to (6). Pour the mobile phase into the unlined tank, immediately place the prepared plate in the tank and close the tank. For solution (1) transfer a quantity of the finely-powdered tablets containing 1.0 g of Paracetamol to a ground-glass-stoppered 15-ml centrifuge tube, add 10 ml of *peroxide-free ether*, shake mechanically for 30 minutes, centrifuge at 1000 revolutions per minute for 15 minutes or until a clear supernatant liquid is obtained and use the supernatant liquid. For solution (2) dilute 1 ml of solution (1) to 10 ml with *ethanol (96%)*. Solution (3) contains 0.0025% w/v of *4′-chloroacetanilide* in *ethanol (96%)*. For solution (4) dissolve 0.25 g of *4′-chloroacetanilide* and 0.10 g of *paracetamol* in sufficient *ethanol (96%)* to produce 100 ml. For solution (5) add 50 ml of *ethanol (96%)* to a quantity of the powdered tablets containing 0.10 g of Paracetamol, shake for 10 minutes, add sufficient *ethanol (96%)* to produce 100 ml and filter. Solution (6) contains 0.10% w/v of *paracetamol BPCRS* in *ethanol (96%)*. After removal of the plate, dry it in a current of warm air and examine under *ultraviolet light (254 nm)*. Any spot corresponding to 4′-chloroacetanilide in the chromatogram obtained with solution (1) is not more intense than the spot in the chromatogram obtained with solution (3) (0.005%). Any *secondary spot* in the chromatogram obtained with solution (2) with an Rf value lower than that of 4′-chloroacetanilide is not more intense than the spot in the chromatogram obtained with solution (3) (0.25%). Disregard any *secondary spot* on or just above the line of application. The test is not valid unless the chromatogram obtained with solution (4) shows two clearly separated principal spots, the spot corresponding to 4′-chloroacetanilide having the higher Rf value.

Assay Weigh and powder 20 tablets. Add 50 ml of 0.1M *sodium hydroxide* slowly to a quantity of the powder containing 0.2 g of Paracetamol, dilute with 100 ml of *water*, shake for 15 minutes and add sufficient *water* to produce 250 ml. Mix, filter and dilute 10 ml of the filtrate to 100 ml with *water*. Add 10 ml of the resulting solution to 10 ml of 0.1M *sodium hydroxide*, dilute to 100 ml with *water* and measure the *absorbance* of the resulting solution at the maximum at 257 nm, Appendix II B. Calculate the content of $C_8H_9NO_2$ taking 715 as the value of A(1%, 1 cm) at the maximum at 257 nm.

Storage Dispersible Paracetamol Tablets should be protected from light.

Soluble Paracetamol Tablets

Definition Soluble Paracetamol Tablets contain Paracetamol in either a suitable soluble basis or a suitable soluble, effervescent basis.

With the exception of the requirements for shape, the tablets comply with the requirements stated under Tablets and with the following requirements.

Content of paracetamol, $C_8H_9NO_2$ 95.0 to 105.0% of the prescribed or stated amount.

Identification

A. Dissolve, with or without vigorous effervescence as appropriate, on the addition of warm *water* to produce a slightly opalescent solution.

B. The *light absorption*, Appendix II B, in the range 230 to 350 nm of the final solution obtained in the Assay exhibits a maximum only at 257 nm.

C. In the test for Related substances the principal spot in the chromatogram obtained with solution (5) corresponds to that in the chromatogram obtained with solution (6).

Disintegration Comply with the requirements for Soluble Tablets or with the requirement for Effervescent Tablets, as appropriate.

4-Aminophenol Carry out the method for *liquid chromatography*, Appendix III D, using the following solutions. Solution (1) contains 0.001% w/v of *4-aminophenol* in *methanol (15%)*. For solution (2) shake a quantity of the powdered tablets, containing 1.0 g of Paracetamol with 15 ml of *methanol*, dilute to 100 ml with *water* and filter.

The chromatographic procedure may be carried out using (a) a stainless steel column (20 cm × 4.6 mm) packed with *stationary phase C* (10 μm) (Nucleosil C18 is

suitable), (b) 0.01M *sodium butanesulphonate* in a mixture of 0.4 volume of *formic acid*, 15 volumes of *methanol* and 85 volumes of *water* as the mobile phase with a flow rate of 2 ml per minute and (c) a detection wavelength of 272 nm.

In the chromatogram obtained with solution (2) the area of any peak corresponding to 4-aminophenol is not greater than the area of the peak in the chromatogram obtained with solution (1) (0.1%). In the chromatogram obtained with solution (2) peaks with long retention times may occur due to excipients.

Related substances Carry out the method for *thin-layer chromatography*, Appendix III A, using *silica gel* GF_{254} as the coating substance and a mixture of 10 volumes of *toluene*, 25 volumes of *acetone* and 65 volumes of *chloroform* as the mobile phase but allowing the solvent front to ascend 14 cm above the line of application. Apply separately to the plate 200 µl of solution (1) and 40 µl of each of solutions (2) to (6). Pour the mobile phase into the unlined tank, immediately place the prepared plate in the tank and close the tank. For solution (1) transfer a quantity of the finely-powdered tablets containing 1.0 g of Paracetamol to a ground-glass-stoppered 15-ml centrifuge tube, add 10 ml of *peroxide-free ether*, shake mechanically for 30 minutes, centrifuge at 1000 revolutions per minute for 15 minutes or until a clear supernatant liquid is obtained and use the supernatant liquid. For solution (2) dilute 1 ml of solution (1) to 10 ml with *ethanol (96%)*. Solution (3) contains 0.0025% w/v of *4′-chloroacetanilide* in *ethanol (96%)*. For solution (4) dissolve 0.25 g of *4′-chloroacetanilide* and 0.10 g of *paracetamol* in sufficient *ethanol (96%)* to produce 100 ml. For solution (5) add 50 ml of *ethanol (96%)* to a quantity of the powdered tablets containing 0.10 g of Paracetamol, shake for 10 minutes, add sufficient *ethanol (96%)* to produce 100 ml and filter. Solution (6) contains 0.10% w/v of *paracetamol BPCRS* in *ethanol (96%)*. After removal of the plate, dry it in a current of warm air and examine under *ultraviolet light (254 nm)*. Any spot corresponding to 4′-chloroacetanilide in the chromatogram obtained with solution (1) is not more intense than the spot in the chromatogram obtained with solution (3) (0.005%). Any *secondary spot* in the chromatogram obtained with solution (2) with an Rf value lower than that of 4′-chloroacetanilide is not more intense than the spot in the chromatogram obtained with solution (3) (0.25%). Disregard any *secondary spot* on or just above the line of application. The test is not valid unless the chromatogram obtained with solution (4) shows two clearly separated principal spots, the spot corresponding to 4′-chloroacetanilide having the higher Rf value.

Assay Weigh and powder 20 tablets. Add 50 ml of 0.1M *sodium hydroxide* slowly to a quantity of the powdered tablets containing 0.2 g of Paracetamol. If necessary, wait until effervescence has ceased, dilute with 100 ml of *water*, shake for 15 minutes and add sufficient *water* to produce 250 ml. Mix, filter and dilute 10 ml of the filtrate to 100 ml with *water*. Add 10 ml of the resulting solution to 10 ml of 0.1M *sodium hydroxide*, dilute to 100 ml with *water* and measure the *absorbance* of the resulting solution at the maximum at 257 nm, Appendix II B. Calculate the content of $C_8H_9NO_2$ taking 715 as the value of A(1%, 1 cm) at the maximum at 257 nm.

Storage Soluble Paracetamol Tablets should be protected from light.

Labelling The label states, where applicable, that the tablets are effervescent.

Paraffin Ointment

Definition

White Beeswax	20 g
Hard Paraffin	30 g
Cetostearyl Alcohol	50 g
White Soft Paraffin	900 g

Extemporaneous preparation The following directions apply.

Mix the ingredients, heat gently with stirring until homogeneous and stir until cold.

The ointment complies with the requirements stated under Topical Semi-solid Preparations.

Liquid Paraffin Oral Emulsion

Liquid Paraffin Emulsion

Definition

Liquid Paraffin	500 ml
Vanillin	500 mg
Chloroform	2.5 ml
Benzoic Acid Solution	20 ml
Methylcellulose 20	20 g
Saccharin Sodium	50 mg
Water	a sufficient quantity

Extemporaneous preparation The following directions apply.

Heat about 120 ml of Water until it boils and add the Methylcellulose; when thoroughly hydrated add sufficient Water in the form of ice to produce 350 ml and stir until homogeneous. Mix the Chloroform and the Benzoic Acid Solution, dissolve the Vanillin in the mixture and add to the methylcellulose dispersion while stirring vigorously for 5 minutes. Add the Saccharin Sodium dissolved in Water and dilute to 500 ml with Water. Add the Liquid Paraffin, stirring constantly, and pass through a homogeniser.

The oral emulsion complies with the requirements stated under Oral Liquids and with the following requirements.

Content of liquid paraffin 44.0 to 49.0% w/w.

Assay To 5 g add 10 ml of *water*, extract with two 40-ml quantities of a mixture of 2 volumes of *ethanol (96%)*, 3 volumes of *petroleum spirit (boiling range, 40° to 60°)* and 3 volumes of *ether* and then with 30 ml of a mixture of equal volumes of *petroleum spirit (boiling range, 40° to 60°)* and *ether*. Wash the combined extracts with 15 ml of 0.5M *sodium hydroxide* and then with 15 ml of *water*, evaporate the solvent, add 5 ml of *acetone* and evaporate again. Repeat the addition and evaporation of *acetone* until the residue is free from water, dry at 105° for 15 minutes and weigh.

Liquid Paraffin and Magnesium Hydroxide Oral Emulsion

Definition Liquid Paraffin and Magnesium Hydroxide Oral Emulsion is a 25% v/v dispersion of Liquid Paraffin in an aqueous suspension containing 6% w/w of hydrated magnesium oxide prepared from a suitable grade of Light Magnesium Oxide.

Extemporaneous preparation The following formula and directions apply.

Liquid Paraffin	250 ml
Chloroform Spirit	15 ml
Magnesium Hydroxide Mixture sufficient to produce	1000 ml

Mix the Chloroform Spirit with 650 ml of Magnesium Hydroxide Mixture, add to the Liquid Paraffin, add sufficient Magnesium Hydroxide Mixture to produce 1000 ml and pass through a homogeniser.

The oral emulsion complies with the requirements stated under Oral Liquids and with the following requirements.

Content of magnesium hydroxide, Mg(OH)2 5.1 to 7.0% w/w.

Content of liquid paraffin 19.7 to 24.0% w/w.

Assay

For magnesium hydroxide Dilute 4 g with 50 ml of *water*, shake with 25 ml of 0.5M *hydrochloric acid VS* and titrate with 0.5M *sodium hydroxide VS* using *methyl orange solution* as indicator. Each ml of 0.5M *hydrochloric acid VS* is equivalent to 14.58 mg of Mg(OH)2

For liquid paraffin Extract the neutralised liquid obtained in the Assay for magnesium hydroxide with three 25-ml quantities of a mixture of equal volumes of *petroleum spirit (boiling range, 40° to 60°)* and *ether*, wash the combined extracts with two 10-ml quantities of *water*, discard the washings, evaporate the solvent, add 5 ml of *acetone* and again evaporate. Repeat the addition and evaporation of *acetone* until the residue is free from water, dry at 105° for 15 minutes and weigh.

Paraldehyde Injection

Definition Paraldehyde Injection is Paraldehyde that has been sterilised. It does not contain any added antimicrobial preservatives.

The injection complies with the requirements stated under Parenteral Preparations and with the following requirements.

Identification

A. A 10.0% v/v solution in *carbon dioxide-free water* (solution A) is *clear*, Appendix IV A, but becomes turbid on warming.

B. Heat 5 ml with 0.1 ml of 1M *sulphuric acid.* Acetaldehyde, recognisable by its odour, is evolved.

C. To 5 ml of solution A in a test tube add 5 ml of *ammoniacal silver nitrate solution* and heat on a water bath. Silver is deposited as a mirror on the side of the tube.

Acidity Titrate 50 ml of solution A with 0.1M *sodium hydroxide VS* using 0.05 ml of *phenolphthalein solution* as indicator. Not more than 1.5 ml of 0.1M *sodium hydroxide VS* is required to change the colour of the solution.

Distillation range Not more than 10% distils below 123° and not less than 95% distils below 126°, Appendix V C.

Freezing point 10° to 13°, Appendix V B.

Refractive index 1.403 to 1.406, Appendix V E.

Relative density 0.991 to 0.996, Appendix V G.

Acetaldehyde Shake 5 ml with a mixture of 5 ml of *ethanol (60%)*, 5 ml of *alcoholic hydroxylamine solution* and 0.2 ml of *methyl orange solution*. Not more than 0.8 ml of 0.5M *sodium hydroxide VS* is required to change the colour of the solution to pure yellow.

Peroxides To 50 ml of solution A in a ground-glass-stoppered flask add 5 ml of 1M *sulphuric acid* and 10 ml of *potassium iodide solution*, close the flask and allow to stand in the dark for 15 minutes. Titrate with 0.1M *sodium thiosulphate VS* using 1 ml of *starch solution* as indicator; allow to stand for 5 minutes and, if necessary, complete the titration. Not more than 2.0 ml of 0.1M *sodium thiosulphate VS* is required.

Storage Paraldehyde Injection is supplied in single-dose glass ampoules sealed by fusion of the glass. It should be kept in complete darkness and stored at a temperature not exceeding 25°.

Labelling The label states that plastic syringes should not be used for the administration of the injection.

Penicillamine Tablets

Definition Penicillamine Tablets contain Penicillamine. They are coated.

The tablets comply with the requirements stated under Tablets and with the following requirements.

Content of penicillamine, $C_5H_{11}NO_2S$ 95.0 to 105.0% of the prescribed or stated amount.

Identification

A. Shake a quantity of the powdered tablets containing 20 mg of Penicillamine with 4 ml of *water* and filter. Add to the filtrate 2 ml of *phosphotungstic acid solution* and allow to stand for a few minutes. A deep blue colour is produced.

B. Dissolve a quantity of the powdered tablets containing 10 mg of Penicillamine in 5 ml of *water* and add 0.3 ml of 5M *sodium hydroxide* and 20 mg of *ninhydrin*. An intense blue or violet-blue colour is produced immediately.

Mercuric salts Not more than 40 ppm, calculated with reference to the content of penicillamine, when determined by the following method. Disperse a quantity of the powdered tablets containing 1 g of Penicillamine in 10 ml of *water* in a stoppered flask, add 0.2 ml of 9M *perchloric acid* and swirl to dissolve. Add 1 ml of *ammonium pyrrolidinedithiocarbamate solution*, mix, add 2 ml of *4-methylpentan-2-one*, shake well for 1 minute and add sufficient *water* to produce 25 ml. Determine by *atomic absorption spectrophotometry*, Appendix II D, introducing the methylpentanone layer into the flame, measuring at 254 nm and using *4-methylpentan-2-one* in place of *water*. Use *mercury standard solution (100 ppm Hg)*, suitably diluted with *water*, for the standard solutions, adjusted to contain the same concentrations of 9M perchloric acid, ammonium pyrrolidinedithiocarbamate solution and 4-methylpentan-2-one as the solution being examined.

Penicillamine disulphide Carry out the method for *liquid chromatography*, Appendix III D, using the following solutions. The solutions should be prepared with degassed mobile phase and used immediately. For solution (1) shake a quantity of the powdered tablets containing 40 mg of Penicillamine with 10 ml of the mobile phase, filter and use the filtrate. Solution (2) contains 0.004% w/v of *penicillamine disulphide EPCRS* in the mobile phase.

The chromatographic procedure may be carried out using (a) a stainless steel column (25 cm × 5 mm) packed with *stationary phase B* (5 µm) (Lichrosphere 5 C8 is suitable), (b) a solution containing 0.2% w/v of *methane sulphonic acid* and 0.01% w/v of *disodium edetate* as the mobile phase with a flow rate of 2 ml per minute and (c) a detection wavelength of 220 nm.

In the chromatogram obtained with solution (1) the area of any peak corresponding to penicillamine disulphide is not greater than the area of the principal peak in the chromatogram obtained with solution (2) (1.0%).

Assay Weigh and powder 20 tablets. Dissolve a quantity of the powder containing 0.1 g of Penicillamine as completely as possible in 50 ml of *water* and filter. Add to the filtrate 5 ml of 1M *sodium hydroxide* and 0.2 ml of a 0.1% w/v solution of *dithizone in ethanol (96%)* and titrate with 0.02M *mercury(II) nitrate VS*. Each ml of 0.02M *mercury(II) nitrate VS* is equivalent to 5.968 mg of $C_5H_{11}NO_2S$.

Storage Penicillamine Tablets should be stored at a temperature not exceeding 25°.

Pentaerythritol Tetranitrate Tablets

Pentaerythritol Tablets

Definition Pentaerythritol Tetranitrate Tablets contain pentaerythritol tetranitrate [2,2-bis(hydroxymethyl)-propane-1,3-diol tetranitrate].

CAUTION *Undiluted pentaerythritol tetranitrate can be exploded by percussion or excessive heat. Appropriate precautions should be exercised and only exceedingly small amounts should be isolated.*

The tablets comply with the requirements stated under Tablets and with the following requirements.

Content of pentaerythritol tetranitrate, $C_5H_8N_4O_{12}$ 90.0 to 110.0% of the prescribed or stated amount.

Identification Extract a portion of the powdered tablets obtained in the Assay with *acetone*, filter and evaporate the filtrate to dryness. The *melting point* of the residue is about 141°, Appendix V A.

Assay Weigh and powder 20 tablets. To a quantity containing 50 mg of pentaerythritol tetranitrate add 50 ml of *glacial acetic acid*, heat on a water bath for 15 minutes, cool and add sufficient *glacial acetic acid* to produce 100 ml. To 1 ml add 2 ml of *phenoldisulphonic acid solution*, allow to stand for 5 minutes, add 25 ml of *water* and 20 ml of 5M *ammonia*, cool and add sufficient *water* to produce 100 ml. Measure the *absorbance* of the resulting solution at 405 nm, Appendix II B, using in the reference cell a solution obtained by treating 1 ml of *glacial acetic acid* in the same manner, beginning at the words 'add 2 ml of *phenoldisulphonic acid solution*...'.

Dissolve 0.1279 g of *potassium nitrate* previously dried at 105° in 3 ml of *water* and add sufficient *glacial acetic acid* to produce 200 ml. Repeat the operation using 1 ml of this solution beginning at the words 'add 2 ml of *phenoldisulphonic acid solution* ...'.

Calculate the content of pentaerythritol tetranitrate from the values of the absorbances so obtained. Each ml of the potassium nitrate solution is equivalent to 0.5 mg of $C_5H_8N_4O_{12}$.

Storage Pentaerythritol Tetranitrate Tablets should be stored at a temperature not exceeding 25° and protected from light.

Pentagastrin Injection

Definition Pentagastrin Injection is a sterile isotonic solution of Pentagastrin in Water for Injections.

The injection complies with the requirements stated under Parenteral Preparations and with the following requirements.

Content of pentagastrin, $C_{37}H_{49}N_7O_9S$ 90.0 to 110.0% of the prescribed or stated amount.

Identification Complies with test B described under Pentagastrin applying separately to each plate (1) a volume of the injection containing 5 µg of Pentagastrin and (2) 1 µl of a solution of *pentagastrin BPCRS* in 0.1M *ammonia* containing 0.5% w/v of pentagastrin.

Related substances Complies with the requirement stated under Pentagastrin applying separately to the plate (1) four successive 5-µl quantities of the injection diluted if necessary with *water* to contain 0.025% w/v of Pentagastrin and (2) 5 µl of the injection diluted with *water* to contain 0.005% w/v of Pentagastrin. Dry the plate in a current of nitrogen after each application.

Acidity or alkalinity pH, 7.0 to 8.5, Appendix V L.

Assay Dilute a volume containing 0.75 mg of Pentagastrin to 10 ml with 0.01M *ammonia* and measure the *absorbance* at the maximum at about 280 nm, Appendix II B. Calculate the content of $C_{37}H_{49}N_7O_9S$ taking 70.0 as the value of A(1%, 1 cm) at the maximum at 280 nm.

Storage Pentagastrin Injection should be protected from light and stored at a temperature of 2° to 8°. It should not be allowed to freeze.

Pentamidine Injection

Definition Pentamidine Injection is a sterile solution of Pentamidine Isetionate in Water for Injections. It is prepared by dissolving Pentamidine Isetionate for Injection in the requisite amount of Water for Injections immediately before use.

The injection complies with the requirements stated under Parenteral Preparations.

Storage Pentamidine Injection deteriorates on storage and should be used immediately after preparation.

PENTAMIDINE ISETHIONATE FOR INJECTION

Definition Pentamidine Isetionate for Injection is a sterile material consisting of Pentamidine Isetionate with or without excipients. It is supplied in a sealed container.

The contents of the sealed container comply with the requirements for Powders for Injections stated under Parenteral Preparations and with the following requirements.

Content of pentamidine isetionate, $C_{19}H_{24}N_4O_2$, $2C_2H_6O_4S$ 95.0 to 105.0% of the prescribed or stated amount.

Identification

A. The *infrared absorption spectrum*, Appendix II A, is concordant with the *reference spectrum* of pentamidine isetionate.

B. The *light absorption*, Appendix II B, in the range 230 to 350 nm of a 0.002% w/v solution in 0.01M *hydrochloric acid* exhibits a maximum only at 262 nm. The *absorbance* at 262 nm is about 0.95.

C. To 10 ml of a 0.05% w/v solution add 1 ml of a 0.1% w/v solution of *glyoxal sodium bisulphite* and 1 ml of a solution prepared by dissolving 4 g of *boric acid* in a mixture of 27 ml of 1M *sodium hydroxide* and sufficient *water* to produce 100 ml. Heat on a water bath for 10 minutes. A magenta colour is produced.

Acidity pH of a 5% w/v solution, 4.5 to 6.5, Appendix V L.

Ammonium isetionate To a quantity of the powder containing 1 g of Pentamidine Isetionate in a test tube about 4 cm in diameter add 10 ml of *water* and 20 ml of 1M *sodium hydroxide*. Immediately insert a stopper fitted with a splash head and an aspirator tube about 0.5 cm in diameter. Connect the splash head to two test tubes in series, each containing 20 ml of 0.01M *sulphuric acid VS*. Heat the tube containing the substance being examined in a water bath at 45° to 50° and, maintaining this temperature, draw a current of air, previously passed through 1M *sulphuric acid*, through the liquids in the series of tubes for 3 hours at such a rate that the bubbles are just too rapid to count. Titrate the combined solutions from the two absorption tubes with 0.02M *sodium hydroxide VS* using *methyl red mixed solution* as indicator. Not less than 36.5 ml is required.

Related substances Carry out the method for *liquid chromatography*, Appendix III D, using the following solutions. For solution (1) dilute 1 volume of solution (2) to 100 volumes with the mobile phase. Solution (2) contains 0.1% w/v of the contents of the sealed container in the mobile phase.

The chromatographic procedure may be carried out using (a) a stainless steel column (25 cm × 4.6 mm) packed with *stationary phase C* (5 μm) (Spherisorb ODS 1 is suitable), (b) as the mobile phase with a flow rate of 1 ml per minute a mixture of 7 volumes of a 3% w/v solution of *ammonium acetate* and 13 volumes of *methanol*, the pH of the mixture being adjusted to 7.5 with *triethylamine*, and (c) a detection wavelength of 265 nm.

In the chromatogram obtained with solution (2) the area of any *secondary peak* is not greater than one fifth of the area of the peak in the chromatogram obtained with solution (1) (0.2%) and the sum of the areas of all such peaks is not greater than two fifths of the area of the peak in the chromatogram obtained with solution (1) (0.4%).

Assay Determine the weight of the contents of 10 containers as described in the test for Uniformity of weight under Parenteral Preparations, Powders for Injections.

Dissolve 0.25 g of the mixed contents of the 10 containers in 50 ml of *dimethylformamide* and carry out Method II for *non-aqueous titration*, Appendix VIII A, using 0.1M *tetrabutylammonium hydroxide VS* as titrant and determining the end point potentiometrically. Each ml of 0.1M *tetrabutylammonium hydroxide VS* is equivalent to 29.63 mg of $C_{19}H_{24}N_4O_2,2C_2H_6O_4S$. Calculate the content of pentamidine isetionate, $C_{19}H_{24}N_4O_2$, $2C_2H_6O_4S$, in a container of average content weight.

Pentazocine Capsules

Definition Pentazocine Capsules contain Pentazocine Hydrochloride.

The capsules comply with the requirements stated under Capsules and with the following requirements.

Content of pentazocine hydrochloride, $C_{19}H_{27}NO$, HCl 95.0 to 105.0% of the prescribed or stated amount.

Identification

A. To a quantity of the contents of the capsules containing 50 mg of Pentazocine Hydrochloride add 70 ml of *water*, shake for 15 minutes, add sufficient *water* to produce 100 ml and filter. To 10 ml of the filtrate add 10 ml of 1M *sodium hydroxide* and sufficient *water* to produce 100 ml. The *light absorption* of the resulting solution, Appendix II B, in the range 225 to 350 nm exhibits maxima at 238 and 298 nm. The *light absorption* of the filtrate obtained in the Assay, Appendix II B, in the range 225 to 350 nm exhibits a maximum only at 278 nm.

B. Shake a quantity of the contents of the capsules containing 50 mg of Pentazocine Hydrochloride with 3 ml of 0.1M *sodium hydroxide* and 3 ml of *chloroform* and allow to separate. Evaporate 0.1 ml of the chloroform extract to dryness in a porcelain crucible. To the residue add 0.5 ml of a 1% w/v solution of *ammonium molybdate* in *sulphuric acid*. An intense blue colour is produced which changes to bluish green, green and finally, on standing, yellow.

Dissolution Comply with the *dissolution test for tablets and capsules*, Appendix XII D, using as the medium 900 ml of *water* and rotating the basket at 100 revolutions per minute. Withdraw a sample of 10 ml of the medium and filter. Measure the *absorbance* of the filtered solution, suitably diluted if necessary, at the maximum at 278 nm, Appendix II B. Calculate the total content of pentazocine hydrochloride, $C_{19}H_{27}NO,HCl$, in the medium taking 61.2 as the value of A(1%, 1 cm) at the maximum at 278 nm.

Related substances Comply with the test described under Pentazocine Tablets, but preparing solution (1) in the following manner. For solution (1) shake a quantity of the contents of the capsules containing 0.2 g of Pentazocine Hydrochloride with 10 ml of 0.1M *methanolic ammonia*, centrifuge and use the clear supernatant liquid.

Assay Shake a quantity of the mixed contents of 20 capsules containing 50 mg of Pentazocine Hydrochloride with 200 ml of *water* for 15 minutes, add 5 ml of 1M *hydrochloric acid* and sufficient *water* to produce 500 ml, mix and filter. Measure the *absorbance* of the filtrate at the maximum at 278 nm, Appendix II B. Calculate the content of $C_{19}H_{27}NO,HCl$ taking 61.2 as the value of A(1%, 1 cm) at the maximum at 278 nm.

Pentazocine Injection

Definition Pentazocine Injection is a sterile solution in Water for Injections of either Pentazocine Lactate or pentazocine lactate prepared by the interaction of Pentazocine and Lactic Acid.

The injection complies with the requirements stated under Parenteral Preparations and with the following requirements.

Content of pentazocine, $C_{19}H_{27}NO$ 95.0 to 105.0% of the prescribed or stated amount.

Characteristics A colourless or almost colourless solution; odour, faint and characteristic of lactic acid.

Identification

A. To a volume containing the equivalent of 90 mg of pentazocine add 5 ml of 0.1M *sodium hydroxide* and shake the resulting solution with 5 ml of *chloroform*. Wash the chloroform extract with 2 ml of *water*, dry over *anhydrous sodium sulphate* and filter. Evaporate the chloroform using a rotary evaporator and dry the oily residue at a temperature not exceeding 25° at a pressure of 2 kPa for 1 hour. The *infrared absorption spectrum* of the residue, Appendix II A, is concordant with the *reference spectrum* of pentazocine (form B).

B. To a volume containing the equivalent of 60 mg of pentazocine add 2 ml of *water*, make alkaline with *dilute sodium carbonate solution* and shake with two 10-ml quantities of *chloroform*. Acidify the aqueous solution with 1M *sulphuric acid* and add a few crystals of *potassium permanganate*. On warming, the odour of acetaldehyde is produced.

Acidity pH, 4.0 to 5.0, Appendix V L.

Related substances Carry out the method for *thin-layer chromatography*, Appendix III A, using a silica gel F_{254} precoated plate (Merck silica gel 60 F_{254} plates are suitable) and a mixture of 3 volumes of *methanol*, 3 volumes of *isopropylamine* and 94 volumes of *chloroform* as the mobile phase. Apply separately to the plate 10 µl of each of the following solutions. For solution (1) dilute a quantity of the injection with sufficient *ethanol (96%)* to produce a solution containing the equivalent of 2.0% w/v of pentazocine. For solution (2) dilute 1 volume of solution (1) to 100 volumes with *ethanol (96%)*. For solution (3) dilute 1 volume of solution (1) to 200 volumes with *ethanol (96%)*. For solution (4) dilute 1 volume of solution (1) to 400 volumes with *ethanol (96%)*. After removal of the plate, allow it to dry in air and examine under *ultraviolet light (254 nm)*. Heat the plate at 105° for 15 minutes, allow to cool, expose to iodine vapour and re-examine under *ultraviolet light (254 nm)*. By each method of visualisation any *secondary spot* in the chromatogram obtained with solution (1) is not more intense than the spot in the chromatogram obtained with solution (2) (1%), not more than one such spot is more intense than the spot in the chromatogram obtained with solution (3) (0.5%) and not more than four such spots are more intense than the spot in the chromatogram obtained with solution (4) (0.25%). Disregard any spot remaining on the line of application.

Assay To a quantity containing the equivalent of 0.15 g of pentazocine add sufficient *water* to produce 100 ml. To 5 ml add 1 ml of 1M *hydrochloric acid*, dilute to 100 ml with *water* and measure the *absorbance* of the resulting solution at the maximum at 278.5 nm, Appendix II B. Calculate the content of $C_{19}H_{27}NO$ taking 69.0 as the value of A(1%, 1 cm) at the maximum at 278.5 nm.

Storage Pentazocine Injection should be protected from light.

Labelling The strength is stated in terms of the equivalent amount of pentazocine in a suitable dose-volume.

Pentazocine Suppositories

Definition Pentazocine Suppositories contain Pentazocine Lactate in a suitable suppository basis.

The suppositories comply with the requirements stated under Rectal Preparations and with the following requirements.

Content of pentazocine, $C_{19}H_{27}NO$ 95.0 to 105.0% of the prescribed or stated amount.

Identification

A. To a volume of the filtrate obtained in the Assay containing the equivalent of 0.1 g of pentazocine add sufficient 1M *sodium hydroxide* to make alkaline and extract with three 10-ml quantities of *dichloromethane*. Wash the combined extracts with 5 ml of *water*, dry over *anhydrous sodium sulphate* and filter. Evaporate the dichloromethane using a rotary evaporator and dry the oily residue at a temperature not exceeding 25° over *phosphorus pentoxide* at a pressure of 1.5 to 2.5 kPa for 16 hours. The *infrared absorption spectrum* of the residue, Appendix II A, is concordant with the *reference spectrum* of pentazocine (form B).

B. Disperse a suppository containing the equivalent of 50 mg of pentazocine in 5 ml of *petroleum spirit (boiling range, 40° to 60°)* and extract with 2 ml of 0.1M *sodium hydroxide*. Add 25 ml of *methanol* to the aqueous layer, evaporate to dryness using a rotary evaporator and dry the residue at 60° under reduced pressure for 16 hours. To the residue add 0.2 ml of *methanol* and 2 ml of *sulphuric acid* and heat the resulting solution at 85° for 2 minutes. Allow to cool and add a few mg of *4-hydroxybiphenyl*. A violet-red colour is produced within 5 minutes.

Related substances Carry out the method for *thin-layer chromatography*, Appendix III A, using a silica gel F_{254} precoated plate (Merck silica gel 60 F_{254} plates are suitable) and a mixture of 3 volumes of *isopropylamine*, 3 volumes of *methanol* and 94 volumes of *chloroform* as the mobile phase. Apply separately to the plate 20 µl of each of the following solutions. For solution (1) disperse two suppositories in 10 ml of *chloroform* with the aid of ultrasound and filter (Whatman GF/A is suitable). For solution (2) dilute 1 volume of solution (1) to 100 volumes with *chloroform*. For solution (3) dilute 5 volumes of solution (2) to 10 volumes with *chloroform*. For solution (4) dilute 5 volumes of solution (3) to 10 volumes with *chloroform*. After removal of the plate, allow it to dry in air and examine under *ultraviolet light (254 nm)*. Heat the plate at 105° for 15 minutes, allow to cool, expose to iodine vapour and re-examine under *ultraviolet light (254 nm)*. In the chromatogram obtained with solution (1) any *secondary spot* is not more intense than the spot in the chromatogram obtained with solution (2) (1%), not more than one such spot is more intense than the spot in the chromatogram obtained with solution (3) (0.5%) and not more than four such spots are more intense than the spot in the chromatogram obtained with solution (4) (0.25% each).

Assay Dissolve a quantity of the suppositories containing the equivalent of 0.5 g of pentazocine in 50 ml of *petroleum spirit (boiling range, 40° to 60°)* and extract with six 50-ml quantities of 0.01M *hydrochloric acid.* Wash the combined extracts with two 10-ml quantities of *chloroform* and dilute to 500 ml with 0.01M *hydrochloric acid,* mix and filter (Whatman No. 1 is suitable). Dilute 10 ml of the clear filtrate to 100 ml with 0.01M *hydrochloric acid.* Measure the *absorbance* of the resulting solution at the maximum at 278 nm, Appendix II B, using 0.01M *hydrochloric acid* in the reference cell. Calculate the content of $C_{19}H_{27}NO$ taking 69.0 as the value of A(1%, 1 cm) at the maximum at 278 nm.

Labelling The quantity of active ingredient is stated in terms of the equivalent amount of pentazocine.

Pentazocine Tablets

Definition Pentazocine Tablets contain Pentazocine Hydrochloride.

The tablets comply with the requirements stated under Tablets and with the following requirements.

Content of pentazocine hydrochloride, $C_{19}H_{27}NO,HCl$ 92.5 to 107.5% of the prescribed or stated amount.

Identification Shake a quantity of the powdered tablets containing 0.1 g of Pentazocine Hydrochloride with 10 ml of *water,* filter (Whatman GF/C is suitable), add 1 ml of 1M *sodium hydroxide* and shake the resulting solution with 20 ml of *chloroform.* Wash the chloroform extract with 5 ml of *water,* dry over *anhydrous sodium sulphate* and filter. Evaporate the chloroform using a rotary evaporator and dry the oily residue at 60° at a pressure of 2 kPa for 1 hour. The *infrared absorption spectrum* of the powdered residue, Appendix II A, is concordant with the *reference spectrum* of pentazocine (form B). If the spectra are not concordant, dissolve the residue in *chloroform,* evaporate to dryness and prepare a new spectrum of the residue.

Related substances Carry out the method for *thin-layer chromatography,* Appendix III A, using a silica gel F_{254} precoated plate (Merck silica gel 60 F_{254} plates are suitable) and a mixture of 94 volumes of *chloroform,* 3 volumes of *methanol* and 3 volumes of *isopropylamine* as the mobile phase. Apply separately to the plate 10 µl of each of the following solutions. For solution (1) shake a quantity of the powdered tablets containing 0.2 g of Pentazocine Hydrochloride with 10 ml of 0.1M *methanolic ammonia* for 10 minutes, centrifuge and use the supernatant liquid. For solution (2) dilute 1 volume of solution (1) to 100 volumes with the same solvent. For solution (3) dilute 1 volume of solution (1) to 200 volumes with the same solvent. For solution (4) dilute 1 volume of solution (1) to 400 volumes with the same solvent. After removal of the plate, allow it to dry in air and examine under *ultraviolet light (254 nm)*. Heat the plate at 105° for 15 minutes, allow to cool, expose to iodine vapour and re-examine under *ultraviolet light (254 nm)*. By each method of visualisation any *secondary spot* in the chromatogram obtained with solution (1) is not more intense than the spot in the chromatogram obtained with solution (2), not more than one such spot is more intense than the spot in the chromatogram obtained with solution (3) and not more than four such spots are more intense than the spot in the chromatogram obtained with solution (4). Disregard any spot remaining on the line of application.

Assay Weigh and powder 20 tablets. Shake a quantity of the powder containing 25 mg of Pentazocine Hydrochloride with 100 ml of *water* for 15 minutes, add 2.5 ml of 1M *hydrochloric acid* and sufficient *water* to produce 250 ml and filter. Measure the *absorbance* of the filtrate at the maximum at 278 nm, Appendix II B. Calculate the content of $C_{19}H_{27}NO,HCl$ taking 61.2 as the value of A(1%, 1 cm) at the maximum at 278 nm.

Pentobarbital Tablets

Definition Pentobarbital Tablets contain Pentobarbital Sodium.

The tablets comply with the requirements stated under Tablets and with the following requirements.

Content of pentobarbital sodium, $C_{11}H_{17}N_2NaO_3$ 92.5 to 107.5% of the prescribed or stated amount.

Identification

A. The *infrared absorption spectrum* of the crystals obtained in test A, Appendix II A, is concordant with the *reference spectrum* of pentobarbital.

B. The powdered tablets yield the reactions characteristic of *sodium salts,* Appendix VI.

Isomer Dissolve a quantity of the powdered tablets containing 0.3 g of Pentobarbital Sodium in 5 ml of a 5% w/v solution of *anhydrous sodium carbonate,* heating gently if necessary. Add 10 ml of a 3% w/v solution of *4-nitrobenzyl chloride* in *ethanol (96%)* and heat under a reflux condenser for 30 minutes. Cool to 25°, filter and wash the precipitate with five 5-ml quantities of *water.* Heat the precipitate with 25 ml of *ethanol (96%)* in a small flask under a reflux condenser until dissolved (about 10 minutes). Filter the hot solution, cool to 25° and, if necessary, scratch the side of the flask with a glass rod to induce crystallisation. Filter, wash the precipitate with two 5-ml quantities of *water* and dry at 100° to 105° for 30 minutes. The *melting point* of the dried precipitate is 136° to 148°, Appendix V A, Method I.

Assay Weigh and powder 20 tablets. Dissolve a quantity of the powder containing 0.3 g of Pentobarbital Sodium as completely as possible in 10 ml of a 2% w/v solution of *sodium hydroxide,* saturate with *sodium chloride,* acidify with *hydrochloric acid* and extract with successive 15-ml quantities of *ether* until complete extraction is effected. Wash the combined extracts with two 2-ml quantities of *water* and extract the combined washings with 10 ml of *ether.* Add the ether to the main ether layer, filter and wash the filter with *ether.* Evaporate the solvent and dry the residue to constant weight at 105°. Each g of residue is equivalent to 1.097 g of $C_{11}H_{17}N_2NaO_3$.

When pentobarbitone tablets are prescribed or demanded, Pentobarbital Tablets shall be dispensed or supplied.

Concentrated Peppermint Emulsion

Definition Concentrated Peppermint Emulsion is a 2% v/v dispersion of Peppermint Oil in a suitable vehicle containing a non-ionic surface-active agent.

Extemporaneous preparation The following formula and directions apply.

Peppermint Oil	20 ml
Polysorbate 20	1 ml
Double-strength Chloroform Water	500 ml
Purified Water, freshly boiled and cooled	sufficient to produce 1000 ml

Shake the Peppermint Oil with the Polysorbate 20 and add gradually, shaking well after each addition, the Double-strength Chloroform Water and sufficient Purified Water to produce 1000 ml.

Peppermint Spirit

Peppermint Essence

Definition

Peppermint Oil	100 ml
Ethanol (90 per cent)	sufficient to produce 1000 ml

Extemporaneous preparation The following directions apply.

Dissolve the Peppermint Oil in Ethanol (90 per cent) and add sufficient Ethanol (90 per cent) to produce 1000 ml. If the solution is not clear, shake with previously sterilised Purified Talc and filter.

The spirit complies with the requirements stated under Spirits and with the following requirements.

Ethanol content 78 to 82% v/v, Appendix VIII F.

Weight per ml 0.830 to 0.840 g, Appendix V G.

Content of oil 9.0 to 11.0% v/v when determined by the following method. Add 25 ml of the spirit and 5 ml of *xylene* to 90 ml of a 10% w/v solution of *sodium chloride* containing 1.0% v/v of *hydrochloric acid* in a flask of about 150-ml capacity with a long neck graduated in 0.1-ml increments and of such a diameter that a 15-cm length has a capacity of 10 ml. Shake the mixture for about 30 minutes, allow to separate and raise the undissolved oily layer into the graduated part of the neck of the flask by the gradual addition of more of the acidified sodium chloride solution, allow to stand for 2 hours or until there is no further change in volume of the oily layer and measure the volume of the oily layer. The volume of the oily layer, after the subtraction of 5 ml, is taken to be the volume of oil.

Peritoneal Dialysis Solutions

Solutions for Peritoneal Dialysis comply with the requirements of the 3rd edition of the European Pharmacopoeia for Solutions for Peritoneal Dialysis [0862]. These requirements are reproduced after the heading 'Definition' below.

Ph Eur

DEFINITION

Solutions for peritoneal dialysis are preparations for intraperitoneal use containing electrolytes with a concentration close to the electrolytic composition of plasma. They contain glucose in varying concentrations.

Solutions for peritoneal dialysis are supplied in:

— rigid or semi-rigid plastic containers,
— flexible plastic containers fitted with a special connecting device; these are generally filled to a volume below their nominal capacity and presented in sealed protective envelopes,
— glass containers.

The containers and closures comply with the requirements for containers for preparations for parenteral use (*3.2.1 and 3.2.2*).

Several formulations are used. The concentrations of the components per litre of solution are usually in the following range:

Table 862-1

	Expression in mmol	Expression in mEq
Sodium	125–150	125–150
Potassium	0–4.5	0–4.5
Calcium	0–2.5	0–5.0
Magnesium	0.25–1.5	0.50–3.0
Acetate ot lactate	30–60	30–60
Chloride	90–120	90–120
Glucose	25–250	

Unless otherwise justified and authorised, antioxidants such as metabisulphite are not added to the solutions.

IDENTIFICATION

According to the stated composition, the solution to be examined gives the following identification reactions (*2.3.1*):

— potassium: reaction (b);
— calcium: reaction (a);
— sodium: reaction (b);
— chlorides: reaction (a);
— acetates: to 5 ml of the solution to be examined add 1 ml of *hydrochloric acid R* in a test-tube fitted with a stopper and a bent tube, heat and collect a few millilitres of distillate; carry out reaction (b) of acetates on the distillate;
— lactates;
— magnesium: to 0.1 ml of *titan yellow solution R* add 10 ml of *water R*, 2 ml of the solution to be examined and 1 ml of *1M sodium hydroxide*; a pink colour is produced;
— glucose: to 5 ml of the solution to be examined, add 2 ml of *dilute sodium hydroxide solution R* and 0.05 ml of *copper sulphate solution R*; the solution is blue and clear; heat to boiling; an abundant red precipitate is formed.

TESTS

Appearance of the solution The solution is clear (*2.2.1*) and not more intensely coloured than reference solution Y_4 (*Method I, 2.2.2*).

pH (*2.2.3*). The pH of the solution is 5.0 to 6.5.

Hydroxymethylfurfural To a volume of the solution containing the equivalent of 25 mg of glucose, add 5.0 ml of a 100 g/l solution of *p- toluidine R* in *2-propanol R* containing 10 per cent *V/V* of *glacial acetic acid R* and 1.0 ml of a 5 g/l solution of *barbituric acid R*. The absorbance (*2.2.25*) determined at 550 nm after allowing the mixture to stand for 2 min to 3 min is not greater than that of a standard prepared at the same time in the same manner using a solution containing 10 µg of *hydroxymethylfurfural R* in the same volume as the solution to be examined.

Aluminium (*2.4.17*). Take 400 ml, adjust to pH 6.0 and add 10 ml of *acetate buffer solution pH 6.0 R*. The solution complies with the limit test for aluminium (15 µg/l). Use as the reference solution a mixture of 3 ml of *aluminium standard solution (2 ppm Al) R,* 10 ml of *acetate buffer solution pH 6.0 R* and 9 ml of *water R*. To prepare the blank use a mixture of 10 ml of *acetate buffer solution pH 6.0 R* and 10 ml of *water R*.

Particulate contamination Carry out the test for subvisible particles (*2.9.19*) using 50 ml of solution.

Table 862-2

Particles larger than	5 µm	25 µm
Maximum number of particles per millilitre	100	5

Extractable volume (*2.9.17*). The solution complies with the test described for parenteral infusions.

Sterility (*2.6.1*). The solution complies with the test for sterility.

Bacterial endotoxins (*2.6.14*). Not more than 0.25 I.U. of endotoxin per millilitre.

Pyrogens (*2.6.8*). Solutions for which a validated test for bacterial endotoxins cannot be carried out comply with the test for pyrogens. Inject per kilogram of the rabbit's mass 10 ml of the solution.

ASSAY

Sodium 97.5 per cent to 102.5 per cent of the content of sodium (Na) stated on the label, determined by atomic absorption spectrometry (*Method II, 2.2.23*).

Test solution. If necessary, dilute the solution to be examined with *water R* to a concentration suitable for the instrument to be used.

Reference solutions. Prepare the reference solutions using *sodium standard solution (200 ppm Na) R*.

Measure the absorbance at 589.0 nm using a sodium hollow-cathode lamp as source of radiation and an air-acetylene or an air-propane flame.

Potassium 95.0 per cent to 105.0 per cent of the content of potassium (K) stated on the label, determined by atomic absorption spectrometry (*Method I, 2.2.23*).

Test solution. If necessary, dilute the solution to be examined with *water R* to a concentration suitable for the instrument to be used. To 100 ml of the solution add 10 ml of a 22 g/l solution of *sodium chloride R*.

Reference solutions. Prepare the reference solutions using *potassium standard solution (100 ppm K) R*. To 100 ml of each reference solution add 10 ml of a 22 g/l solution of *sodium chloride R*.

Measure the absorbance at 766.5 nm, using a potassium hollow-cathode lamp as source of radiation and an air-acetylene or an air-propane flame.

Calcium 95.0 per cent to 105.0 per cent of the content of calcium (Ca) stated on the label, determined by atomic absorption spectrometry (*Method I, 2.2.23*).

Test solution. If necessary, dilute the solution to be examined with *water R* to a concentration suitable for the instrument to be used.

Reference solutions. Prepare the reference solutions using *calcium standard solution (400 ppm Ca) R*.

Measure the absorbance at 422.7 nm using a calcium hollow-cathode lamp as source of radiation and an air-acetylene or an air-propane flame.

Magnesium 95.0 per cent to 105.0 per cent of the content of magnesium (Mg) stated on the label, determined by atomic absorption spectrometry (*Method I, 2.2.23*).

Test solution. If necessary, dilute the solution to be examined with *water R* to a concentration suitable for the instrument to be used.

Reference solutions. Prepare the reference solutions using *magnesium standard solution (100 ppm Mg) R*.

Measure the absorbance at 285.2 nm using a magnesium hollow-cathode lamp as source of radiation and an air-acetylene or an air-propane flame.

Total chloride 95.0 per cent to 105.0 per cent of the content of chloride (Cl) stated on the label. Dilute to 50 ml with *water R* an accurately measured volume of the solution to be examined containing the equivalent of about 60 mg of chloride ion. Add 5 ml of *dilute nitric acid R*, 25.0 ml of *0.1M silver nitrate* and 2 ml of *dibutyl phthalate R*. Shake. Using 2 ml of *ferric ammonium sulphate solution R2* as indicator, titrate with *0.1M ammonium thiocyanate* until a reddish-yellow colour is obtained.

1 ml of *0.1M silver nitrate* is equivalent to 3.545 mg of Cl.

Acetate 95.0 per cent to 105.0 per cent of the content of acetate stated on the label. To a volume of the solution to be examined, corresponding to about 0.7 mmol of acetate, add 10.0 ml of *0.1M hydrochloric acid*. Carry out a potentiometric titration (*2.2.20*), using *0.1M sodium hydroxide*. Read the volume added between the two points of inflexion.

1 ml of *0.1M sodium hydroxide* is equivalent to 0.1 mmol of acetate.

Lactate 95.0 per cent to 105.0 per cent of the content of lactate stated on the label. To a volume of the solution to be examined, corresponding to about 0.7 mmol of lactate, add 10.0 ml of *0.1M hydrochloric acid*. Then add 50 ml of *acetonitrile R*. Carry out a potentiometric titration (*2.2.20*), using *0.1M sodium hydroxide*. Read the volume added between the two points of inflexion.

1 ml of *0.1M sodium hydroxide* is equivalent to 0.1 mmol of lactate.

Reducing sugars (expressed as anhydrous glucose) 95.0 per cent to 105.0 per cent of the content of glucose stated on the label. Transfer a volume of solution to be examined containing the equivalent of 25 mg of glucose to a 250 ml ground-glass conical flask and add 25.0 ml of *cupri-citric solution R*. Add a few grains of pumice, fit a reflux condenser, heat so that boiling occurs within 2 min and boil for exactly 10 min. Cool and add 3 g of *potassium iodide R* dissolved in 3 ml of *water R*. Carefully add, in small amounts, 25 ml of a 25 per cent *m/m* solution of *sulphuric acid R*. Titrate with *0.1M sodium thiosulphate* using *starch solution R*, added towards the end of the titration, as indicator. Carry out a blank titration using 25.0 ml of *water R*.

Calculate the content of reducing sugars expressed as anhydrous glucose ($C_6H_{12}O_6$), by means of the Table 862-3 below.

Table 862-3

Volume of *0.1M sodium thiosulphate* (millilitres)	Anhydrous glucose (milligrams)
8	19.8
9	22.4
10	25.0
11	27.6
12	30.3
13	33.0
14	35.7
15	38.5
16	41.3

STORAGE

Store at a temperature not below 4°C.

LABELLING

The label states:

— the formula of the solution for peritoneal dialysis expressed in grams per litre and in millimoles per litre,
— the calculated osmolarity expressed in milliosmoles per litre,
— the nominal volume of the solution for peritoneal dialysis in the container,
— that the solution is free from bacterial endotoxins, or where applicable, that it is apyrogenic,
— the storage conditions,
— that the solution is not to be used for intravenous infusion,
— that any unused portion of solution is to be discarded.

Ph Eur

Perphenazine Tablets

Definition Perphenazine Tablets contain Perphenazine. They are coated.

The tablets comply with the requirements stated under Tablets and with the following requirements.

Content of perphenazine, $C_{21}H_{26}ClN_3OS$ 92.5 to 107.5% of the prescribed or stated amount.

Identification

A. To a quantity of the powdered tablets containing 40 mg of Perphenazine add 10 ml of *water* and 2 ml of 1M *sodium hydroxide*, shake and extract with 15 ml of *ether*. Wash the ether layer with 5 ml of *water*, dry with *anhydrous sodium sulphate* and evaporate the ether to dryness. The *infrared absorption spectrum* of the residue, Appendix II A, is concordant with the *reference spectrum* of perphenazine.

B. Extract a quantity of the powdered tablets containing 20 mg of Perphenazine with 10 ml of *chloroform*, filter and evaporate the filtrate to dryness. Dissolve the residue in 2 ml of *methanol*, pour into a solution of 0.4 g of *picric acid* in 10 ml of *methanol* at 50°, cool and allow to stand for 4 hours. The *melting point* of the precipitate, after recrystallisation from *methanol*, is about 248°, with decomposition, Appendix V A.

C. To a quantity of the powdered tablets containing 5 mg of Perphenazine add 5 ml of *sulphuric acid* and allow to stand for 5 minutes. A red colour is produced.

Related substances Comply with the test for *related substances in phenothiazines*, Appendix III A, using *mobile phase C* and applying separately to the plate 50 µl of each of the following freshly prepared solutions. For solution (1) extract a quantity of the powdered tablets containing 20 mg of Perphenazine with 10 ml of *ethanol (96%)* and filter. For solution (2) dilute 1 volume of solution (1) to 200 volumes with *ethanol (96%)*.

Uniformity of content Tablets containing 2 mg or less of Perphenazine comply with the requirements stated under Tablets using the following method of analysis. Carry out the following procedure protected from light. Record *second-derivative ultraviolet absorption spectra* of the following solutions, Appendix II B, in the range 210 to 290 nm. For solution (1) add 5 ml of *water* to one tablet, mix with the aid of ultrasound for 15 minutes or until the tablet has completely disintegrated, heat on a water bath for 3 minutes, swirling continuously and cool. Add 50 ml of *ethanol (96%)*, mix with the aid of ultrasound for 2 minutes, shake for 5 minutes, dilute to 100 ml with *ethanol (96%)* and filter through a glass microfibre filter paper. Dilute the filtrate, if necessary, with *ethanol (96%)* to produce a solution containing 0.001% w/v of Perphenazine. Solution (2) contains 0.001% w/v of *perphenazine BPCRS* in *ethanol (96%)*.

For each solution measure the amplitude from the peak at 265 nm to the trough at 255 nm. Calculate the content of $C_{21}H_{26}N_3OS$ in each tablet using the declared content of $C_{21}H_{26}N_3OS$ in *perphenazine BPCRS*.

Assay

For tablets containing more than 2 mg of Perphenazine Carry out the following procedure protected from light. Record *second-derivative ultraviolet absorption spectra* of the following solutions, Appendix II B, in the range 210 to 290 nm. For solution (1) add 50 ml of *water* to 10 tablets, mix with the aid of ultrasound for 15 minutes or until the tablets have completely disintegrated, heat on a water bath for 3 minutes, swirling continuously, cool, add 400 ml of *ethanol (96%)*, mix with the aid of ultrasound for 2 minutes, shake for 5 minutes, dilute to 500 ml with *ethanol (96%)* and filter through a glass microfibre filter paper. Dilute the filtrate with *ethanol (96%)* to produce a solution containing 0.001% w/v of Perphenazine. Solution (2) contains 0.001% w/v of *perphenazine BPCRS* in *ethanol (96%)*. Measure the amplitude from the peak at 265 nm to the trough at 255 nm. Calculate the content of $C_{21}H_{26}N_3OS$ using the declared content of $C_{21}H_{26}N_3OS$ in *perphenazine BPCRS*.

For tablets containing 2 mg or less of Perphenazine Use the average of the 10 individual results obtained in the test for Uniformity of content.

Pethidine Injection

Definition Pethidine Injection is a sterile solution of Pethidine Hydrochloride in Water for Injections.

The injection complies with the requirements stated under Parenteral Preparations and with the following requirements.

Content of pethidine hydrochloride, $C_{15}H_{21}NO_2,HCl$ 95.0 to 105.0% of the prescribed or stated amount.

Identification

A. To a volume containing 50 mg of Pethidine Hydrochloride add sufficient 1M *sodium hydroxide* to make strongly alkaline to *litmus paper* and extract with two 10-ml quantities of *chloroform*. Wash the combined extracts with 5 ml of *water*, dry over *anhydrous sodium sulphate*, filter and evaporate the filtrate to dryness. Remove the last traces of chloroform by drying the residual oil at 60° at a pressure not exceeding 0.7 kPa. The *infrared absorption spectrum* of the oily residue, Appendix II A, is concordant with the *reference spectrum* of pethidine.

B. Yields the reactions characteristic of *chlorides*, Appendix VI.

Related substances Complies with the requirements stated under Pethidine Hydrochloride, using as solution (1) the upper layer obtained by shaking a volume of the injection containing 0.1 g of Pethidine Hydrochloride, diluted if necessary to 5 ml with *water*, with 0.5 ml of 5M *sodium hydroxide* and 2 ml of *ether* and allowing the layers to separate.

Assay Dilute a volume containing 0.15 g of Pethidine Hydrochloride with 40 ml of *water*, add 1 ml of 5M *sodium hydroxide* and extract immediately with successive quantities of 25, 10 and 10 ml of *chloroform*. Wash each extract with the same 15 ml of *water* and filter into a dry flask. Titrate the combined extracts, which should be clear and free from droplets of water, with 0.02M *perchloric acid VS* using 0.15 ml of *1-naphtholbenzein solution* as indicator. Each ml of 0.02M *perchloric acid VS* is equivalent to 5.676 mg of $C_{15}H_{21}NO_2,HCl$.

Pethidine Tablets

Definition Pethidine Tablets contain Pethidine Hydrochloride.

The tablets comply with the requirements stated under Tablets and with the following requirements.

Content of pethidine hydrochloride, $C_{15}H_{21}NO_2,HCl$ 92.5 to 107.5% of the prescribed or stated amount.

Identification

A. Shake a quantity of the powdered tablets containing 50 mg of Pethidine Hydrochloride with 20 ml of *chloroform*, filter, evaporate the filtrate to dryness and dry the residue at a pressure of 2 kPa. The *infrared absorption spectrum* of the residue, Appendix II A, is concordant with the *reference spectrum* of pethidine hydrochloride.

B. Shake a quantity of the powdered tablets containing 0.2 g of Pethidine Hydrochloride with 20 ml of *water* and filter. To 5 ml of the filtrate add 10 ml of *picric acid solution R1*. The *melting point* of the crystals so obtained, after washing with *water*, is about 190°, Appendix V A.

Related substances Comply with the test described under Pethidine Hydrochloride, using as solution (1) the upper layer obtained by shaking a quantity of the powdered tablets containing 0.1 g of Pethidine Hydrochloride with 5 ml of *water*, filtering, shaking the filtrate with 0.5 ml of 5M *sodium hydroxide* and 2 ml of *ether* and allowing the layers to separate.

Assay Weigh and powder 20 tablets. Dissolve a quantity of the powder containing 0.5 g of Pethidine Hydrochloride in 40 ml of *water*, add 2 ml of 5M *sodium hydroxide* and extract immediately with quantities of 25, 10 and 10 ml of *chloroform*. Wash each extract with the same 15 ml of *water* and filter into a dry flask. Titrate the combined extracts, which should be clear and free from droplets of *water*, with 0.05M *perchloric acid VS* using 0.15 ml of *1-naphtholbenzein solution* as indicator. Each ml of 0.05M *perchloric acid VS* is equivalent to 14.19 mg of $C_{15}H_{21}NO_2,HCl$.

Phenelzine Tablets

Definition Phenelzine Tablets contain Phenelzine Sulphate. They are coated.

The tablets comply with the requirements stated under Tablets and with the following requirements.

Content of phenelzine, $C_8H_{12}N_2$ 90.0 to 110.0% of the prescribed or stated amount.

Identification

A. Shake a quantity of the powdered tablets containing the equivalent of 30 mg of phenelzine with 25 ml of *water* for 5 minutes and filter. Make the filtrate alkaline with 5M *sodium hydroxide* and extract with two 25-ml quantities of *chloroform*. Extract the combined chloroform layers with two 25-ml quantities of 0.05M *sulphuric acid* and dilute the combined extracts to 100 ml with 0.05M *sulphuric acid*. The *light absorption* of the resulting solution, Appendix II B, in the range 230 to 350 nm exhibits three well-defined maxima, at 252, 258 and 263 nm.

B. Extract a quantity of the powdered tablets containing the equivalent of 30 mg of phenelzine with 10 ml of *water* and filter. Make 5 ml of the filtrate alkaline with 5M *sodium hydroxide* and add 1 ml of *cupri-tartaric solution R1*. A red precipitate is produced.

C. Extract a quantity of the powdered tablets containing the equivalent of 45 mg of phenelzine with 5 ml of *water* and filter. The filtrate yields the reactions characteristic of *sulphates*, Appendix VI.

Assay Weigh and powder 20 tablets. To a quantity of the powder containing the equivalent of 0.1 g of phenelzine add 20 ml of *water* and 2 ml of 2M *hydrochloric acid*, heat to boiling and boil for 30 seconds, stirring constantly. Add 25 ml of *water*, cool, add 2 g of *sodium hydrogen carbonate* and 50 ml of 0.05M *iodine VS*, stopper the flask and allow to stand for 90 minutes. Add 15 ml of 2M *hydrochloric acid* and titrate with 0.1M *sodium thiosulphate VS* using *starch mucilage*, added towards the end of the titration, as indicator. Repeat the operation without the powder. The difference between the titrations represents the amount of iodine required. Each ml of 0.05M *iodine VS* is equivalent to 3.405 mg of $C_8H_{12}N_2$.

Labelling The quantity of active ingredient is stated in terms of the equivalent amount of phenelzine.

Phenindamine Tablets

Definition Phenindamine Tablets contain Phenindamine Tartrate. They are coated.

The tablets comply with the requirements stated under Tablets and with the following requirements.

Content of phenindamine tartrate, $C_{19}H_{19}N,C_4H_6O_6$ 92.5 to 107.5% of the prescribed or stated amount.

Identification

A. Shake a quantity of the powdered tablets containing 20 mg of Phenindamine Tartrate with 100 ml of *water*, dilute 10 ml of the mixture to 50 ml with *water* and filter. The *light absorption* of the filtrate, Appendix II B, exhibits a maximum only at 259 nm.

B. To a quantity of the powdered tablets containing 50 mg of Phenindamine Tartrate add 5 ml of *water* and 3 ml of 5M *ammonia* and extract with two 10-ml quantities of *ether*. Wash the combined extracts with 2 ml of *water*, evaporate to dryness and dissolve the residue in 5 ml of *sulphuric acid*. An orange-brown colour is produced which is discharged when the solution is carefully diluted with 20 ml of *water*.

Assay Digest 20 tablets with 70 ml of *water* and 5 ml of 2M *hydrochloric acid* until completely disintegrated, filter into a tared flask and wash the residue with about 20 ml of *water*. Dilute the combined filtrate and washings to 100 ml with *water*. To a quantity of the combined filtrate and washings containing 0.2 g of Phenindamine Tartrate add 10 ml of 5M *sodium hydroxide* and extract with successive quantities of 25, 10, 10 and 10 ml of *chloroform*. Wash each extract with the same 15 ml of *water* and filter into a dry flask. Titrate the combined extracts, which should be clear and free from droplets of water, with 0.02M *perchloric acid VS* using *oracet blue B solution* as indicator. Each ml of 0.02M *perchloric acid VS* is equivalent to 8.229 mg of $C_{19}H_{19}N,C_4H_6O_6$.

Phenindione Tablets

Definition Phenindione Tablets contain Phenindione.

The tablets comply with the requirements stated under Tablets and with the following requirements.

Content of phenindione, $C_{15}H_{10}O_2$ 92.5 to 107.5% of the prescribed or stated amount.

Identification

A. Shake a quantity of the powdered tablets containing 0.2 g of Phenindione with 50 ml of *chloroform*, filter and evaporate the filtrate to dryness. The *infrared absorption spectrum* of the residue, Appendix II A, is concordant with the *reference spectrum* of phenindione.

B. Recrystallise the residue obtained in test A from *ethanol (96%)*, dissolve 20 mg in 10 ml of *ethanol (96%)* with the aid of heat, cool, dilute to 250 ml with 0.1M *sodium hydroxide* and dilute 5 ml to 100 ml with 0.1M *sodium hydroxide*. The *absorbance* of the resulting solution at 278 nm is about 1.1 and at 330 nm is about 0.32, Appendix II B.

Related substances Comply with the test described under Phenindione using the following solutions. For solution (1) shake a quantity of the powdered tablets containing 50 mg of Phenindione with 15 ml of *dichloromethane*, filter, evaporate the filtrate to dryness and dissolve the residue in 5 ml of *dichloromethane*. For solution (2) dilute 1 volume of solution (1) to 50 volumes with *dichloromethane*. For solution (3) dilute 1 volume of solution (1) to 200 volumes with *dichloromethane*.

Uniformity of content Tablets containing 50 mg or less of Phenindione comply with the requirements stated under Tablets using the following method of analysis. Place one tablet in 50 ml of 0.1M *sodium hydroxide*, dissolve the tablet completely by shaking gently, add a further 100 ml of 0.1M *sodium hydroxide* and shake for 1 hour. Dilute to 250 ml with 0.1M *sodium hydroxide*, filter and dilute a portion of the filtrate with sufficient 0.1M *sodium hydroxide* to produce a solution containing 4 µg of Phenindione per ml. Measure the *absorbance* of the resulting solution at the maximum at 278 nm, Appendix II B. Calculate the content of $C_{15}H_{10}O_2$ taking 1310 as the value of A(1%, 1 cm) at the maximum at 278 nm.

Assay Weigh and powder 20 tablets. Shake a quantity of the powder containing 50 mg of Phenindione with 150 ml of 0.1M *sodium hydroxide* for 1 hour, add sufficient 0.1M *sodium hydroxide* to produce 250 ml, filter and dilute 5 ml of the filtrate to 250 ml with 0.1M *sodium hydroxide*. Measure the *absorbance* of the resulting solution at the maximum at 278 nm, Appendix II B. Calculate the content of $C_{15}H_{10}O_2$ taking 1310 as the value of A(1%, 1 cm) at the maximum at 278 nm.

Phenobarbital Elixir

Phenobarbital Oral Solution

Definition Phenobarbital Elixir is an *oral solution* containing 0.3% w/v of Phenobarbital in a suitable flavoured vehicle containing a sufficient volume of Ethanol (96 per cent) or of an appropriate Dilute Ethanol to give a final concentration of 38% v/v of ethanol.

The elixir complies with the requirements stated under Oral Liquids and with the following requirements.

Content of phenobarbital, $C_{12}H_{12}N_2O_3$ 0.27 to 0.33% w/v.

Identification The residue obtained in the Assay complies with the following tests.

A. The *infrared absorption spectrum*, Appendix II A, is concordant with the *reference spectrum* of Phenobarbital.

B. *Melting point*, about 175°, Appendix V A.

Ethanol content 36 to 40% v/v, Appendix VIII F.

Assay Extract 50 ml with three 50-ml quantities of *ether*, wash the combined ether extracts with 20 ml of *water*, discard the washings, extract the ether solution with a mixture of 5 ml of 2M *sodium hydroxide* and 25 ml of *water* and then with two 5-ml quantities of *water*. Acidify the combined aqueous extracts to *litmus paper* with 2M *hydrochloric acid*, extract with four 25-ml quantities of *ether*, wash the combined ether extracts with two 2-ml quantities of *water*, wash the combined aqueous washings with 10 ml of *ether*, add the ether washings to the combined ether extracts, evaporate the ether and dry the residue of phenobarbital to constant weight at 105°.

Storage Phenobarbital Elixir should be protected from light.

Labelling The label indicates the pharmaceutical form as 'oral solution'.

When phenobarbitone elixir is prescribed or demanded, Phenobarbital Elixir shall be dispensed or supplied.

Phenobarbital Injection

Definition Phenobarbital Injection is a sterile solution containing 20% w/v of Phenobarbital Sodium in a mixture of nine volumes of Propylene Glycol and one volume of Water for Injections.

The injection complies with the requirements stated under Parenteral Preparations and with the following requirements.

Content of phenobarbital sodium, $C_{12}H_{11}N_2NaO_3$ 19.0 to 21.0% w/v.

Identification To 5 ml add 15 ml of *water*, make slightly acidic with 1M *sulphuric acid* and filter. The residue, after washing with *water* and drying at 105°, complies with the following tests.

A. The *infrared absorption spectrum*, Appendix II A, is concordant with the reference spectrum of phenobarbital.

B. *Melting point*, about 175°, Appendix V A.

C. Dissolve 50 mg in 2 ml of a 0.2% w/v solution of *cobalt(II) acetate* in *methanol*, warm, add 50 mg of powdered *sodium tetraborate* and heat to boiling. A bluish violet colour is produced.

Alkalinity pH, 10.0 to 11.0, Appendix V L.

Weight per ml 1.090 to 1.100 g, Appendix V G.

Assay To 2 g add 30 ml of *water* and 3 g of *sodium carbonate*, stir to dissolve and titrate with 0.1M *silver nitrate VS* until a distinct turbidity is observed when viewed against a black background, the solution being stirred vigorously throughout the titration. Each ml of 0.1M *silver nitrate VS* is equivalent to 25.42 mg of $C_{12}H_{11}N_2NaO_3$. Use the *weight per ml* of the injection to calculate the percentage w/v of phenobarbital sodium, $C_{12}H_{11}N_2NaO_3$.

When phenobarbitone injection is prescribed or demanded, Phenobarbital Injection shall be dispensed or supplied.

Phenobarbital Tablets

Definition Phenobarbital Tablets contain Phenobarbital.

The tablets comply with the requirements stated under Tablets and with the following requirements.

Content of phenobarbital, $C_{12}H_{12}N_2O_3$ 92.5 to 107.5% of the prescribed or stated amount.

Identification Heat 0.2 g of the residue obtained in the Assay on a water bath with 15 ml of *ethanol (25%)* until dissolved, filter while hot and allow the filtrate to cool. Filter, wash the crystals with a small quantity of *ethanol (25%)* and dry at 105°. The residue complies with the following tests.

A. *Melting point*, about 175°, Appendix V A.

B. The *infrared absorption spectrum*, Appendix II A, is concordant with the *reference spectrum* of phenobarbital. If the spectra obtained are not concordant, heat the residue in a sealed tube at 105° for 1 hour and prepare a new spectrum of the residue.

C. Dissolve 50 mg in 2 ml of a 0.2% w/v solution of *cobalt(II) acetate* in *methanol*, warm, add 50 mg of powdered *sodium tetraborate* and heat to boiling. A bluish violet colour is produced.

Disintegration Maximum time, 30 minutes, Appendix XII A.

Assay Weigh and powder 20 tablets. Extract a quantity of the powder containing 0.3 g of Phenobarbital in a continuous extraction apparatus with *ether* until complete extraction is effected. Remove the ether and dry the residue of $C_{12}H_{12}N_2O_3$ to constant weight at 105°.

When phenobarbitone tablets are prescribed or demanded, Phenobarbital Tablets shall be dispensed or supplied.

Phenobarbital Sodium Tablets

Definition Phenobarbital Sodium Tablets contain Phenobarbital Sodium.

The tablets comply with the requirements stated under Tablets and with the following requirements.

Content of phenobarbital sodium, $C_{12}H_{11}N_2NaO_3$ 92.5 to 107.5% of the prescribed or stated amount.

Identification

A. The *infrared absorption spectrum* of the residue obtained in test A, Appendix II A, is concordant with the *reference spectrum* of phenobarbital.

B. The powdered tablets yield the reactions characteristic of *sodium salts*, Appendix VI.

Assay Weigh and powder 20 tablets. Dissolve a quantity of the powdered tablets containing 0.3 g of Phenobarbital Sodium as completely as possible in 10 ml of a 2% w/v solution of *sodium hydroxide*, saturate with *sodium chloride*, acidify with *hydrochloric acid* and extract with successive 15-ml quantities of *ether* until complete extraction is effected. Wash the combined extracts with two 2-ml quantities of *water* and extract the combined washings with 10 ml of *ether*. Add the ether to the main ether layer, filter and wash the filter with *ether*. Evaporate the solvent and dry the residue to constant weight at 105°. Each g of residue is equivalent to 1.095 g of $C_{12}H_{11}N_2NaO_3$.

When phenobarbitone sodium tablets are prescribed or demanded, Phenobarbital Sodium Tablets shall be dispensed or supplied.

Oily Phenol Injection

Definition Oily Phenol Injection is a sterile solution containing 5% w/v of Phenol in a suitable fixed oil.

The injection complies with the requirements stated under Parenteral Preparations and with the following requirements.

Content of phenol, C_6H_6O 4.75 to 5.25% w/v.

Assay Dissolve 8 g in 50 ml of *ether* and extract with successive 10-ml quantities of 2M *sodium hydroxide* until extraction is complete, boil the combined extracts for 2 minutes, cool and dilute to 250 ml with *water*. To 20 ml of this solution in a glass-stoppered flask add 30 ml of 0.05M *bromine VS* and 6 ml of *hydrochloric acid*, stopper, shake repeatedly during 15 minutes and allow to stand for a further 15 minutes. Add 30 ml of *dilute potassium iodide solution*, taking care to avoid loss of bromine, and titrate the liberated iodine with 0.1M *sodium thiosulphate VS*. Repeat the operation without the injection. The difference between the titrations represents the amount of bromine required. Each ml of 0.05M *bromine VS* is equivalent to 1.569 mg of C_6H_6O. Determine the *weight per ml*, Appendix V G, and calculate the percentage w/v of C_6H_6O.

Action and use Rectal soothing agent.

Phenol and Glycerol Injection

Definition Phenol and Glycerol Injection is a sterile solution containing 5% w/v of Phenol in Glycerol that has been previously dried at 120° for 1 hour.

The injection complies with the requirements stated under Parenteral Preparations and with the following requirements.

Content of phenol, C_6H_6O 4.75 to 5.25% w/v.

Characteristics A pale straw-coloured, viscous solution.

Identification

A. Add *bromine water* to a 1% w/v solution. A white precipitate is produced, which, on the continued addition of *bromine water*, at first dissolves then reappears and becomes permanent.

B. To 0.5 ml add 5 ml of *water* and 0.05 ml of *sodium nitrite solution* and carefully pour on to the surface of *sulphuric acid*. A coloured zone, red above and green below, appears at the junction of the two layers.

C. When heated on a borax bead in a naked flame, it imparts a green colour to the flame.

Assay Dissolve 2 g in sufficient *water* to produce 50 ml, transfer 25 ml to a 500-ml glass-stoppered flask and add 50 ml of 0.05M *bromine VS* and 5 ml of *hydrochloric acid*, stopper, swirl occasionally during 30 minutes and allow to stand for a further 15 minutes. Add 5 ml of a 20% w/v solution of *potassium iodide*, taking care to avoid loss of bromine, shake thoroughly and titrate with 0.1M *sodium thiosulphate VS* until only a faint yellow colour remains. Add 0.1 ml of *starch mucilage* and 10 ml of *chloroform* and complete the titration with vigorous shaking. Repeat the operation without the injection. The difference between the titrations represents the amount of bromine required. Each ml of 0.05M *bromine VS* is equivalent to 1.569 mg of C_6H_6O. Determine the *weight per ml* of the injection, Appendix V G, and calculate the percentage w/v of C_6H_6O.

Storage Phenol and Glycerol Injection should be protected from light.

Labelling The strength is stated as the percentage w/v of Phenol.

Action and use Sclerosant used in relief of pain and spasticity.

Phenoxybenzamine Capsules

Definition Phenoxybenzamine Capsules contain Phenoxybenzamine Hydrochloride.

The capsules comply with the requirements stated under Capsules and with the following requirements.

Content of phenoxybenzamine hydrochloride, $C_{18}H_{22}ClNO,HCl$ 92.5 to 107.5% of the prescribed or stated amount.

Identification

A. Dissolve a quantity of the contents of the capsules containing 40 mg of Phenoxybenzamine Hydrochloride in 50 ml of *ethanol-free chloroform*, wash the solution with three 20-ml quantities of 0.01M *hydrochloric acid*, filter the chloroform solution and dilute 10 ml of the filtrate to 50 ml with *ethanol-free chloroform*. The *light absorption* of the resulting solution, Appendix II B, exhibits two maxima, at 272 nm and 279 nm.

B. The contents of the capsules yield reaction A characteristic of *chlorides*, Appendix VI.

Assay Weigh 20 capsules. Open the capsules carefully without loss of shell material, remove the contents, wash the shells with three 10-ml quantities of *chloroform* and add the washings to the capsule contents. Allow the shells to stand at room temperature until the odour of chloroform is no longer detectable and weigh. The difference between the weights represents the weight of the total contents. Evaporate the mixed capsule contents and washings to dryness, stirring continuously, and carry out Method I for *non-aqueous titration*, Appendix VIII A, adding 10 ml of *mercury(II) acetate solution* and using *oracet blue B solution* as indicator. Each ml of 0.1M *perchloric acid VS* is equivalent to 34.03 mg of $C_{18}H_{22}ClNO,HCl$.

Phenoxymethylpenicillin Oral Solution

Definition Phenoxymethylpenicillin Oral Solution is a solution of Phenoxymethylpenicillin Potassium in a suitable flavoured vehicle. It is prepared by dissolving the dry ingredients in the specified volume of Water just before issue for use.

The dry ingredients comply with the requirements for Powders and Granules for the Preparation of Oral Liquids stated under Oral Liquids.

Storage The dry ingredients should be kept in a well-closed container.

For the following tests prepare the Oral Solution as directed on the label. The solution, examined immediately after preparation unless otherwise indicated, complies with the requirements stated under Oral Liquids and with the following requirements.

Content of phenoxymethylpenicillin, $C_{16}H_{18}N_2O_5S$ When freshly constituted, not more than 120.0% of the prescribed or stated amount. When stored at the temperature and for the period stated on the label during which the Oral Solution may be expected to be satisfactory for use, not less than 80.0% of the prescribed or stated amount.

Identification

A. Carry out the method for *thin-layer chromatography*, Appendix III A, using *silanised silica gel H* as the coating substance and a mixture of 20 volumes of *acetone* and 80 volumes of *mixed phosphate buffer pH 5.4* as the mobile phase. Apply separately to the plate 1 µl of each of the following solutions. For solution (1) dilute a volume of the oral solution containing the equivalent of 0.1 g of phenoxymethylpenicillin to 100 ml with *mixed phosphate buffer pH 5.4*. Solution (2) contains 0.11% w/v of *phenoxymethylpenicillin potassium BPCRS* in *mixed phosphate buffer pH 5.4*. After removal of the plate, allow it to dry in air, spray with 0.1M *sodium hydroxide*, heat at 50° for 10 minutes, allow to cool and spray with a mixture of 100 volumes of *starch mucilage*, 6 volumes of *glacial acetic acid* and 2 volumes of a 1% w/v solution of *iodine* in a 4% w/v solution of *potassium iodide*. The principal spot in the chromatogram obtained with solution (1) corresponds to that in the chromatogram obtained with solution (2).

B. Dilute a volume containing the equivalent of 25 mg of phenoxymethylpenicillin to 20 ml with *water*. To 10 ml add 0.5 ml of *neutral red solution* and sufficient 0.01M *sodium hydroxide* to produce a permanent orange colour and then add 1.0 ml of *penicillinase solution*. The colour changes rapidly to red.

Assay To a weighed quantity of the oral solution containing the equivalent of 0.125 g of phenoxymethylpenicillin add sufficient *water* to produce 500 ml and dilute 25 ml to 100 ml with *water*. Place two 2-ml aliquots of the resulting solution into separate stoppered tubes. To one tube add 10 ml of *imidazole—mercury reagent*, mix, stopper the tube and immerse in a water bath at 60° for exactly 25 minutes, swirling occasionally. Remove from the water bath and cool rapidly to 20° (solution A). To the second tube add 10 ml of *water* and mix (solution B). Without delay measure the *absorbances* of solutions A and B at the maximum at 325 nm, Appendix II B, using in the reference cell a mixture of 2 ml of *water* and 10 ml of *imidazole—mercury reagent* for solution A and *water* for solution B. Calculate the content of $C_{16}H_{18}N_2O_5S$ from the difference between the absorbances of solutions A and B, from the difference obtained by repeating the operation using 0.14 g of *phenoxymethylpenicillin potassium BPCRS* in place of the oral solution and from the declared content of $C_{16}H_{18}N_2O_5S$ in *phenoxymethylpenicillin potassium BPCRS*. Determine the *weight per ml* of the oral solution, Appendix V G, and calculate the content of $C_{16}H_{18}N_2O_5S$, weight in volume.

Repeat the procedure using a portion of the oral solution that has been stored at the temperature and for the period stated on the label during which it may be expected to be satisfactory for use.

Storage The Oral Solution should be stored at the temperature and used within the period stated on the label.

Labelling The quantity of active ingredient is stated in terms of the equivalent amount of phenoxymethylpenicillin.

Phenoxymethylpenicillin Tablets

Definition Phenoxymethylpenicillin Tablets contain Phenoxymethylpenicillin Potassium.

The tablets comply with the requirements stated under Tablets and with the following requirements.

Content of phenoxymethylpenicillin, $C_{16}H_{18}N_2O_5S$ 92.5 to 107.5% of the prescribed or stated amount.

Identification

A. Shake a quantity of the powdered tablets containing the equivalent of 80 mg of phenoxymethylpenicillin with *water*, dilute to 250 ml with *water* and filter. The *light absorption* of the filtrate, Appendix II B, exhibits maxima at 268 nm and 274 nm and a minimum at 272 nm.

B. Shake a quantity of the powdered tablets containing the equivalent of 10 mg of phenoxymethylpenicillin with 10 ml of *water*, filter and add 0.5 ml of *neutral red solution*. Add sufficient 0.01M *sodium hydroxide* to produce a permanent orange colour and then add 1.0 ml of *penicillinase solution*. The colour changes rapidly to red.

C. Ignite 0.5 g of the powdered tablets, add 5 ml of 2M *hydrochloric acid*, boil, cool and filter. The filtrate yields reaction B characteristic of *potassium salts*, Appendix VI.

Dissolution Comply with the *dissolution test for tablets and capsules*, Appendix XII D, using as the medium 900 ml of a 0.68% w/v solution of *potassium dihydrogen orthophosphate* adjusted to pH 6.8 by the addition of 1M *sodium hydroxide* and rotating the basket at 100 revolutions per minute. Withdraw a sample of 10 ml of the medium. Measure the *absorbance* of the filtered sample, suitably diluted if necessary, at the maximum at 268 nm, Appendix II B. At the same time measure the *absorbance* at the maximum at 268 nm of a suitable solution of *phenoxymethylpenicillin potassium BPCRS* in a solution containing 0.68% w/v of *potassium dihydrogen orthophosphate* adjusted to pH 6.8 by the addition of 1M *sodium hydroxide*. Calculate the total content of phenoxymethylpenicillin, $C_{16}H_{18}N_2O_5S$, in the medium from the absorbances obtained and from the declared content of $C_{16}H_{18}N_2O_5S$ in *phenoxymethylpenicillin potassium BPCRS*.

Assay Weigh and powder 20 tablets. Shake a quantity of the powder containing the equivalent of 0.125 g of phenoxymethylpenicillin with 300 ml of *water* for 30 minutes, add sufficient *water* to produce 500 ml, dilute 25 ml to 100 ml with *water* and filter. Place two 2-ml aliquots of the filtrate in separate stoppered tubes. To one tube add 10 ml of *imidazole—mercury reagent*, mix, stopper the tube and immerse in a water bath at 60° for exactly 25 minutes, swirling occasionally. Remove from the water bath and cool rapidly to 20° (solution A). To the second tube add 10 ml of *water* and mix (solution B). Without delay measure the *absorbances* of solutions A and B at the maximum at 325 nm, Appendix II B, using in the reference cell a mixture of 2 ml of *water* and 10 ml of *imidazole—mercury reagent* for solution A and *water* for solution B. Calculate the content of $C_{16}H_{18}N_2O_5S$ from the difference between the absorbances of solutions A and B, from the difference obtained by repeating the operation using 0.14 g of *phenoxymethylpenicillin potassium BPCRS* in place of the preparation being examined and from the declared content of $C_{16}H_{18}N_2O_5S$ in *phenoxymethylpenicillin potassium BPCRS*.

Labelling The quantity of active ingredient is stated in terms of the equivalent amount of phenoxymethylpenicillin.

Phentolamine Injection

Definition Phentolamine Injection is a sterile solution of Phentolamine Mesilate in Water for Injections containing Anhydrous Glucose.

The injection complies with the requirements stated under Parenteral Preparations and with the following requirements.

Content of phentolamine mesilate, $C_{17}H_{19}N_3O$, CH_4SO_3 95.0 to 105.0% of the prescribed or stated amount.

Identification In the test for Related substances, the principal spot in the chromatogram obtained with solution (2) corresponds to that in the chromatogram obtained with solution (4).

Acidity pH, 3.5 to 5.0, Appendix V L.

Related substances Carry out the method for *thin-layer chromatography*, Appendix III A, using *silica gel G* as the coating substance and a mixture of 5 volumes of 13.5M *ammonia*, 15 volumes of *acetone* and 85 volumes of *butan-2-one* as the mobile phase. Apply separately to the plate 20 µl of each of the following solutions. For solution (1) dilute the injection, if necessary, with *ethanol (96%)* to give a solution containing 1% w/v of Phentolamine Mesilate. For solution (2) dilute 1 volume of solution (1) to 20 volumes with *ethanol (96%)*. For solution (3) dilute 1 volume of solution (1) to 200 volumes with *ethanol (96%)*. Solution (4) contains 0.05% w/v of *phentolamine mesilate BPCRS* in *ethanol (96%)*. After removal of the plate, allow it to dry in air and spray with *dilute potassium iodobismuthate solution*. Any *secondary spot* in the chromatogram obtained with solution (1) is not more intense than the spot in the chromatogram obtained with solution (3) (0.5%).

Assay Dilute a volume of the injection with *methanol* to produce a solution containing of 0.004% w/v of Phentolamine Mesilate. Measure the *absorbance* at the maximum at 278 nm, Appendix II B. Calculate the content of $C_{17}H_{19}N_3O,CH_4O_3S$ taking 204 as the value of A(1%, 1 cm) at the maximum at 278 nm.

Storage Phentolamine Injection should be protected from light.

Phenylephrine Eye Drops

Definition Phenylephrine Eye Drops are a sterile solution of Phenylephrine Hydrochloride in Purified Water.

The eye drops comply with the requirements stated under Eye Preparations and with the following requirements.

Content of phenylephrine hydrochloride $C_9H_{13}NO_2$, HCl 90.0 to 110.0% of the prescribed or stated amount.

Identification

A. In the test for Related substances, the principal spot in the chromatogram obtained with solution (2) corresponds to that in the chromatogram obtained with solution (4).

B. To a volume containing 10 mg of Phenylephrine Hydrochloride diluted with *water* if necessary to produce 1 ml add 0.05 ml of *copper sulphate solution* and 1 ml of 5M *sodium hydroxide*; a violet colour is produced. Add 1 ml of *ether* and shake; the ether layer remains colourless.

Acidity or alkalinity pH, 3.0 to 7.5, Appendix V L.

Related substances Carry out the method for *thin-layer chromatography*, Appendix III A, using *silica gel H* as the coating substance and a mixture of 5 volumes of *chloroform*, 15 volumes of 10M *ammonia* and 80 volumes of *propan-2-ol* as the mobile phase. Apply separately to the plate 5 µl of each of the following solutions. For solution (1) dilute the eye drops with sufficient *methanol* to give a solution containing 2% w/v of Phenylephrine Hydrochloride. For solution (2) dilute 1 volume of solution (1) to 40 volumes with *methanol*. For solution (3) dilute 1 volume of solution (1) to 100 volumes with *methanol*. Solution (4) contains 0.05% w/v of *phenylephrine hydrochloride BPCRS* in *methanol*. After removal of the plate, dry it in a current of cold air, spray with *ninhydrin solution*, heat at 100° to 105° for 5 to 10 minutes and examine in daylight. Any *secondary spot* in the chromatogram obtained with solution (1) is not more intense than the spot in the chromatogram obtained with solution (3) (1%).

Assay Carry out the method for *liquid chromatography*, Appendix III D, using the following solutions. Solution (1) contains 0.1% w/v of *phenylephrine hydrochloride BPCRS* in *water*. For solution (2) dilute the eye drops with sufficient *water* to give a solution containing 0.1% w/v of Phenylephrine Hydrochloride.

The chromatographic procedure may be carried out using (a) a stainless steel column (15 cm × 4.6 mm) packed with *stationary phase C* (5 µm) (Hypersil C18 is suitable) (b) a solution of 0.10% w/v *sodium heptanesulphonate* in a mixture of 2 volumes of *glacial acetic acid*, 400 volumes of *methanol* and 600 volumes of *water* as the mobile phase with a flow rate of 1.5 ml per minute and (c) a detection wavelength of 273 nm.

Calculate the content of $C_9H_{13}NO_2$,HCl using the declared content of $C_9H_{13}NO_2$,HCl in *phenylephrine hydrochloride BPCRS*.

Storage Phenylephrine Eye Drops should be protected from light.

Phenylephrine Injection

Definition Phenylephrine Injection is a sterile solution of Phenylephrine Hydrochloride in Water for Injections.

The injection complies with the requirements stated under Parenteral Preparations and with the following requirements.

Content of phenylephrine hydrochloride, $C_9H_{13}NO_2$, HCl 95.0 to 105.0% of the prescribed or stated amount.

Identification

A. In the test for Related substances, the principal spot in the chromatogram obtained with solution (2) corresponds to that in the chromatogram obtained with solution (4).

B. To a volume containing 10 mg of Phenylephrine Hydrochloride add, if necessary, sufficient *water* to produce 1 ml and then add 0.05 ml of *weak copper sulphate solution* and 1 ml of 5M *sodium hydroxide*; a violet colour is produced. Add 1 ml of *ether* and shake; the ether layer remains colourless.

C. Yields reaction A characteristic of *chlorides*, Appendix VI.

Acidity pH, 4.5 to 6.5, Appendix V L.

Related substances Carry out the method for *thin-layer chromatography*, Appendix III A, using *silica gel H* as the coating substance and a mixture of 5 volumes of *chloroform*, 15 volumes of 10M *ammonia* and 80 volumes of *propan-2-ol* as the mobile phase. Apply separately to the plate 5 µl of each of the following solutions. For solution (1) evaporate a volume of the injection containing 20 mg of Phenylephrine Hydrochloride to dryness and dissolve the residue in 1 ml of *methanol*. For solution (2) dilute 1 volume of solution (1) to 200 volumes with *methanol*. For solution (3) dilute 1 volume of solution (2) to 2.5 volumes with *methanol*. Solution (4) contains 0.01% w/v of *phenylephrine hydrochloride BPCRS* in *methanol*. After removal of the plate, dry it in a current of cold air, spray with *ninhydrin solution*, heat at 100° to 105° for 10 minutes and examine in daylight. Any *secondary spot* in the chromatogram obtained with solution (1) is not more intense than the spot in the chromatogram obtained with solution (2) (0.5%) and not more than two such spots are more intense than the spot in the chromatogram obtained with solution (3) (0.2%).

Assay To a quantity containing 50 mg of Phenylephrine Hydrochloride add sufficient 0.5M *sulphuric acid* to produce 100 ml. Dilute 10 ml to 100 ml with 0.5M *sulphuric acid* and measure the *absorbance* of the resulting solution at the maximum at 273 nm, Appendix II B. Calculate the content of $C_9H_{13}NO_2$,HCl taking 90 as the value of A(1%, 1 cm) at the maximum at 273 nm.

Storage Phenylephrine Injection should be protected from light.

Phenytoin Capsules

Definition Phenytoin Capsules contain Phenytoin Sodium.

The capsules comply with the requirements stated under Capsules and with the following requirements.

Content of phenytoin sodium, $C_{15}H_{11}N_2NaO_2$ 92.5 to 107.5% of the prescribed or stated amount.

Identification

A. Centrifuge the precipitated mixture obtained in test B, dissolve the residue in *methanol*, evaporate and dry at 105° for 30 minutes. The *infrared absorption spectrum* of the residue, Appendix II A, is concordant with the *reference spectrum* of phenytoin.

B. Shake a quantity of the contents of the capsules containing 0.5 g of Phenytoin Sodium with 10 ml of *water* and filter. The filtrate yields a white precipitate on the addition of 2M *hydrochloric acid*.

C. To 0.1 g of the residue obtained in test A add 0.5 ml of 1M *sodium hydroxide*, 10 ml of a 10% w/v solution of *pyridine* and 1 ml of *copper sulphate—pyridine reagent* and allow to stand for 10 minutes. A blue precipitate is produced.

Related substances Carry out the method for *thin-layer chromatography*, Appendix III A, using as the coating substance a suitable silica gel containing a fluorescent indicator with an optimal intensity at 254 nm (Merck silica gel 60 F_{254} is suitable) and a mixture of 10 volumes of 13.5M *ammonia*, 45 volumes of *chloroform* and 45 volumes of *propan-2-ol* as the mobile phase. Apply separately to the plate 10 µl of each of the following solutions. For solution (1) shake a quantity of the contents of the capsules containing 0.20 g of Phenytoin Sodium with 5 ml of *methanol*, warm on a water bath with shaking and filter. For solution (2) dilute 1 volume of solution (1) to 200 volumes with *methanol*. Solution (3) contains 0.020% w/v of *benzophenone* in *methanol*. Allow the plate to dry in a current of cold air for 2 minutes before development of the chromatograms. After removal of the plate, dry it at 80° for 5 minutes and examine under *ultraviolet light (254 nm)*. In the chromatogram obtained with solution (1) any spot corresponding to benzophenone is not more intense than the spot in the chromatogram obtained with solution (3) (0.5%) and any other *secondary spot* is not more intense than the spot in the chromatogram obtained with solution (2) (0.5%).

Assay Shake a quantity of the mixed contents of 20 capsules containing 0.25 g of Phenytoin Sodium with 40 ml of 0.01M *sodium hydroxide* for 5 minutes and dilute to 50 ml with 0.01M *sodium hydroxide*. Centrifuge, acidify 25 ml of the clear liquid with 10 ml of 0.1M *hydrochloric acid* and extract with successive quantities of 50, 40 and 25 ml of *ether*. Wash the combined extracts with 10 ml of *water*, evaporate to dryness and dry the residue at 105°. Dissolve in 50 ml of *anhydrous pyridine* and carry out Method II for *non-aqueous titration*, Appendix VIII A, using 0.1M *tetrabutylammonium hydroxide VS* as titrant and a 0.3% w/v solution of *thymol blue* in *anhydrous pyridine* as indicator. Each ml of 0.1M *tetrabutylammonium hydroxide VS* is equivalent to 27.43 mg of $C_{15}H_{11}N_2NaO_2$.

Phenytoin Injection

Definition Phenytoin Injection is a sterile solution containing 5% w/v of Phenytoin Sodium in a mixture of 40% v/v of Propylene Glycol and 10% v/v of Ethanol in Water for Injections.

The injection complies with the requirements stated under Parenteral Preparations and with the following requirements.

Content of phenytoin sodium, $C_{15}H_{11}N_2NaO_2$ 4.75 to 5.25% w/v.

Characteristics A colourless solution.

Identification

A. The *infrared absorption spectrum*, Appendix II A, of the residue obtained in the Assay for phenytoin sodium is concordant with the *reference spectrum* of phenytoin.

B. Evaporate to a small volume the aqueous solution obtained in the Assay for phenytoin sodium. Gently heat a small portion of the residue with *potassium hydrogen sulphate*. A pleasant fruity odour is produced and, on evaporation to dryness, no odour of acrolein is detectable.

C. Mix 0.2 g of the residue obtained in the Assay for phenytoin sodium with 1.4 g of *chlorotriphenylmethane* and 2 ml of *pyridine* and heat under a reflux condenser on a water bath for 1 hour. Cool, dissolve the mixture in 40 ml of warm *acetone*, add 50 mg of *activated charcoal*, mix well and filter. Evaporate the filtrate to about 20 ml and allow to stand overnight at about 4°. The *melting point* of the crystalline precipitate, after drying in a current of air, is about 176°, Appendix V A.

Alkalinity pH, 11.5 to 12.1, Appendix V L.

Weight per ml 1.025 to 1.035 g, Appendix V G.

Benzil and benzophenone Carry out the method for *thin-layer chromatography*, Appendix III A, using *silica gel* GF_{254} as the coating substance and a mixture of 30 volumes of *1,4-dioxan* and 75 volumes of *hexane* as the mobile phase but allowing the solvent front to ascend 12 cm above the line of application. Apply separately to the plate 5 µl of each of the following solutions. For solution (1) dilute 1 ml of the injection to 2.5 ml with *methanol*. Solution (2) contains 0.0010% w/v of *benzophenone* in *ethanol (96%)*. Solution (3) contains 0.0010% w/v of *benzil* in *ethanol (96%)*. After removal of the plate, allow the solvent to evaporate and examine under *ultraviolet light (254 nm)*. In the chromatogram obtained with solution (1) any spots corresponding to benzophenone and benzil are not more intense than the spots in the chromatograms obtained with solutions (2) and (3) respectively (0.5% of each).

Ethanol 9.0 to 11.0% v/v, when determined by the following method. Carry out the method for *gas chromatography*, Appendix III B, using three solutions containing (1) 2% v/v of *propan-1-ol* (internal standard) and 2% v/v of *absolute ethanol*, (2) the injection diluted with *water* to contain 2% v/v of Ethanol and (3) the injection diluted with a solution of the internal standard to contain 2% v/v of Ethanol and 2% v/v of propan-1-ol.

The chromatographic procedure may be carried out using a column (1.8 m × 2 mm) packed with porous polymer beads (Chromosorb 102 is suitable) (80 to 100 mesh) and maintained at 120°.

Propylene glycol 37.0 to 43.0% v/v, when determined by the following method. Carry out the method for *gas chromatography*, Appendix III B, using solutions containing (1) 4% w/v of *ethane-1,2-diol* (internal standard) and 4% w/v of *propane-1,2-diol*, (2) the injection diluted with *water* to contain 4% w/v of Propylene Glycol and (3) the injection diluted with a solution of the internal standard to contain 4% w/v of Propylene Glycol and 4% w/v of the ethane-1,2-diol.

The chromatographic procedure may be carried out using the conditions described under Ethanol but maintaining the column at 175°.

Calculate the content of $C_3H_8O_2$, volume in volume, taking 1.036 g as its weight per ml.

Assay To 6 g add 25 ml of *water* and extract with successive quantities of 50, 30 and 30 ml of *ethyl acetate*, shaking each extract thoroughly for 1 minute, allowing to stand for 5 minutes and again shaking for 1 minute before separating the solvent. Wash each extract by shaking thoroughly for 1 minute with the same 15 ml of *water*, filter the extracts successively and wash the filter with 10 ml of *ethyl acetate*. Evaporate the solvent from the combined filtrates and washing and dry the residue to constant weight at 105°. Each g of residue is equivalent to 1.087 g of $C_{15}H_{11}N_2NaO_2$. Using the *weight per ml* of the injection, calculate the content of $C_{15}H_{11}N_2NaO_2$, weight in volume.

Storage Phenytoin Injection should be protected from light and stored at a temperature not exceeding 25°. Solutions in which a haziness or precipitate develops should not be used.

Phenytoin Oral Suspension

Definition Phenytoin Oral Suspension is a suspension of Phenytoin in a suitable flavoured vehicle.

The oral suspension complies with the requirements stated under Oral Liquids and with the following requirements.

Content of phenytoin, $C_{15}H_{12}N_2O_2$ 90.0 to 110.0% of the prescribed or stated amount.

Identification The *infrared absorption spectrum*, Appendix II A, of the final residue obtained in the Assay is concordant with the *reference spectrum* of phenytoin.

Acidity pH, 4.5 to 5.5, Appendix V L.

Benzil and benzophenone Carry out the method for *thin-layer chromatography*, Appendix III A, using *silica gel* GF_{254} as the coating substance and a mixture of 30 volumes of *1,4-dioxan* and 75 volumes of *hexane* as the mobile phase but allowing the solvent front to ascend 12 cm above the line of application. Apply separately to the plate 5 µl of each of the following solutions. For solution (1) add 5 ml of *water* and 2 ml of 2M *hydrochloric acid* to a quantity of the oral suspension containing 30 mg of Phenytoin, mix well and extract with five 20-ml quantities of *ether*. Combine the ether extracts, wash with three 10-ml quantities of *water*, evaporate to dryness and dissolve the residue in 1.5 ml of a mixture of 1 volume of *glacial acetic acid* and 9 volumes of *acetone*. Solution (2) contains 0.0040% w/v of *benzophenone* in *ethanol (96%)*. Solution (3) contains 0.0040% w/v of *benzil* in *ethanol (96%)*. After removal of the plate, allow the solvent to evaporate and examine under *ultraviolet light (254 nm)*. Any spots corresponding to benzophenone and benzil in the chromatogram obtained with solution (1) are not more intense than the spots in the chromatograms obtained with solutions (2) and (3) respectively (0.2% of each).

Assay To a weighed quantity containing 0.2 g of Phenytoin add 10 ml of 2M *hydrochloric acid* and 15 ml of *water*, extract with three 50-ml quantities of a mixture of 3 volumes of *chloroform* and 1 volume of *propan-2-ol* and evaporate the combined extracts to dryness. Dry the residue at 105° for 1 hour, cool and dissolve in a mixture of 3 ml of 1M *sodium hydroxide* and 50 ml of *water* with the aid of gentle heat. Cool and pass a current of *carbon dioxide* through the solution until precipitation of phenytoin is complete. Filter through a sintered-glass filter (BS porosity No. 4), wash the residue with two 10-ml quantities of *water* and dry at 105° for 2 hours. Determine the *weight per ml* of the oral suspension, Appendix V G, and calculate the content of $C_{15}H_{12}N_2O_2$, weight in volume.

Phenytoin Tablets

Definition Phenytoin Tablets contain Phenytoin Sodium. They are coated.

The tablets comply with the requirements stated under Tablets and with the following requirements.

Content of phenytoin sodium, $C_{15}H_{11}N_2NaO_2$ 95.0 to 105.0% of the prescribed or stated amount.

Identification

A. Shake a quantity of the powdered tablets containing 0.1 g of Phenytoin Sodium with 20 ml of *water*, filter, acidify with 2M *hydrochloric acid* and extract with *chloroform*. Wash the chloroform extract with *water*, dry with *anhydrous sodium sulphate* and evaporate to dryness. The *infrared absorption spectrum* of the residue, Appendix II A, is concordant with the *reference spectrum* of phenytoin.

B. Triturate a quantity of the powdered tablets containing 0.5 g of Phenytoin Sodium with 10 ml of *water* and filter. Add 2M *hydrochloric acid*; a white precipitate is produced.

C. The powdered tablets, when moistened with *hydrochloric acid* and introduced on a platinum wire into a flame, impart a yellow colour to the flame.

Related substances Complies with the test described under Phenytoin Capsules but using a quantity of the powdered tablets containing 0.2 g of Phenytoin Sodium to prepare solution (1).

Assay Weigh and powder 20 tablets. Shake a quantity of the powder containing 0.25 g of Phenytoin Sodium with 40 ml of 0.01M *sodium hydroxide* for 5 minutes and dilute to 50 ml with 0.01M *sodium hydroxide*. Centrifuge, acidify 25 ml of the clear liquid with 10 ml of 0.1M *hydrochloric acid* and extract with successive quantities of 50, 40 and 25 ml of *ether*. Wash the combined extracts with 10 ml of *water*, evaporate to dryness and dry the residue at 105°. Dissolve the residue in 50 ml of *anhydrous pyridine* and carry out Method II for *non-aqueous titration*, Appendix VIII A, using 0.1M *tetrabutylammonium hydroxide VS* as titrant and a 0.3% w/v solution of *thymol blue* in *pyridine* as indicator. Each ml of 0.1M *tetrabutylammonium hydroxide VS* is equivalent to 27.43 mg of $C_{15}H_{11}N_2NaO_2$.

Pholcodine Linctus

Definition Pholcodine Linctus is an *oral solution* containing 0.1% w/v of Pholcodine and 1% w/v of Citric Acid Monohydrate in a suitable flavoured vehicle.

The linctus complies with the requirements stated under Oral Liquids and with the following requirements.

Content of pholcodine, $C_{23}H_{30}N_2O_4,H_2O$ 0.090 to 0.110% w/v.

Identification To 20 ml add 20 ml of *water*, make alkaline to *litmus paper* with 5M *ammonia*, extract with two 20-ml quantities of *chloroform*, washing each extract with 5 ml of *water*, dry the combined extracts with *anhydrous sodium sulphate*, filter and evaporate to dryness. If necessary add 0.1 ml of *ether* and scratch the side of the vessel with a glass rod to induce crystallisation. The crystals, dried at a pressure not exceeding 2 kPa, comply with the following tests.

A. The *infrared absorption spectrum*, Appendix II A, is concordant with the *reference spectrum* of pholcodine.

B. The *light absorption*, Appendix II B, in the range 230 to 350 nm of a 0.01% w/v solution in 0.01M *sodium hydroxide* exhibits a maximum only at 284 nm.

C. Dissolve the remainder of the crystals in 1 ml of *sulphuric acid* and add 0.05 ml of *ammonium molybdate—sulphuric acid solution*; a pale blue colour is produced. Warm gently; the colour changes to deep blue. Add 0.05 ml of 2M *nitric acid*; the colour changes to brownish red.

Assay To 50 g add sufficient 5M *ammonia* to make the solution alkaline to *litmus paper* and extract with four 25-ml quantities of *chloroform*, washing each extract with the same 5 ml of *water*. Combine the extracts and evaporate until the volume is reduced to 15 ml. Carry out Method I for *non-aqueous titration*, Appendix VIII A, using 0.02M *perchloric acid VS* as titrant and *quinaldine red solution* as indicator. Each ml of 0.02M *perchloric acid VS* is equivalent to 4.165 mg of $C_{23}H_{30}N_2O_4,H_2O$. Determine the *weight per ml* of the linctus, Appendix V G, and calculate the content of $C_{23}H_{30}N_2O_4,H_2O$, weight in volume.

Storage Pholcodine Linctus should be protected from light.

Labelling The label indicates the pharmaceutical form as 'oral solution.'

Strong Pholcodine Linctus

Definition Strong Pholcodine Linctus is an *oral solution* containing 0.2% w/v of Pholcodine and 2% w/v of Citric Acid Monohydrate in a suitable flavoured vehicle.

The linctus complies with the requirements stated under Oral Liquids and with the following requirements.

Content of pholcodine, $C_{23}H_{30}N_2O_4,H_2O$ 0.180 to 0.220% w/v.

Identification To 10 ml add 20 ml of *water*, make alkaline to *litmus paper* with 5M *ammonia*, extract with two 15-ml quantities of *chloroform*, washing each extract with 5 ml of *water*, dry the combined extracts with *anhydrous sodium sulphate*, filter and evaporate to dryness. If necessary add 0.1 ml of *ether* and scratch the side of the vessel with a glass rod to induce crystallisation. The crystals, dried at a pressure not exceeding 2 kPa, comply with the following tests.

A. The *infrared absorption spectrum*, Appendix II A, is concordant with the *reference spectrum* of pholcodine.

B. The *light absorption*, Appendix II B, in the range 230 to 350 nm of a 0.01% w/v solution in 0.01M *sodium hydroxide* exhibits a maximum only at 284 nm.

C. Dissolve the remainder of the crystals in 1 ml of *sulphuric acid* and add 0.05 ml of *ammonium molybdate—sulphuric acid solution*; a pale blue colour is produced. Warm gently; the colour changes to deep blue. Add 0.05 ml of 2M *nitric acid*; the colour changes to brownish red.

Assay To 25 g add sufficient 5M *ammonia* to make the solution alkaline to *litmus paper* and extract with four 25-ml quantities of *chloroform*, washing each extract with the same 5 ml of *water*. Combine the extracts and evaporate until the volume is reduced to 15 ml. Carry out Method I for *non-aqueous titration*, Appendix VIII A, using 0.02M *perchloric acid VS* as titrant and *quinaldine red solution* as indicator. Each ml of 0.02M *perchloric acid VS* is equivalent to 4.165 mg of $C_{23}H_{30}N_2O_4,H_2O$. Determine the *weight per ml* of the linctus, Appendix V G, and calculate the content of $C_{23}H_{30}N_2O_4,H_2O$, weight in volume.

Storage Strong Pholcodine Linctus should be protected from light.

Labelling The label indicates the pharmaceutical form as 'oral solution.'

Phosphates Enema

Sodium Phosphates Enema

Definition Phosphates Enema is a *rectal solution* containing suitable quantities of either Anhydrous Sodium Dihydrogen Phosphate, Sodium Dihydrogen Phosphate Monohydrate, Sodium Dihydrogen Phosphate Dihydrate or Phosphoric Acid and either Anhydrous Disodium Hydrogen Phosphate, Disodium Hydrogen Phosphate Dodecahydrate or Disodium Hydrogen Phosphate Dihydrate in freshly boiled and cooled Purified Water. A suitable antimicrobial preservative may be included.

The composition of two established formulations is described below.

Formula A

Sodium Dihydrogen Phosphate Dihydrate	160 g
Disodium Hydrogen Phosphate Dodecahydrate	60 g
Purified Water, freshly boiled and cooled sufficient to produce	1000 ml

A suitable antimicrobial preservative may be included.

Formula B

Sodium Dihydrogen Phosphate Dihydrate	100 g
Disodium Hydrogen Phosphate Dodecahydrate	80 g
Purified Water, freshly boiled and cooled sufficient to produce	1000 ml

A suitable antimicrobial preservative may be included.

The enema complies with the requirements stated under Rectal Preparations and with the following requirements.

Content of sodium dihydrogen phosphate dihydrate, $NaH_2PO_4,2H_2O$ *Formula A*: 15.2 to 16.8% w/v; *Formula B*: 9.5 to 10.5% w/v; *any other formulation*: 95.0 to 105.0% of the prescribed or stated amount.

Content of disodium hydrogen phosphate dodecahydrate, $Na_2HPO_4,12H_2O$ *Formula A*: 5.6 to 6.4% w/v; *Formula B*: 7.5 to 8.5% w/v; *any other formulation*: 95.0 to 105.0% of the prescribed or stated amount.

Identification

A. Yields the reactions characteristic of *sodium salts*, Appendix VI.

B. Yields the reactions characteristic of *phosphates*, Appendix VI.

Clarity and colour of solution The enema being examined is *clear*, Appendix IV A, and *colourless*, Appendix IV B, Method II.

Acidity pH, 5.0 to 6.2, Appendix V L.

Assay

For sodium dihydrogen phosphate dihydrate To 20 ml add 80 ml of *water* and 25 g of *sodium chloride* and titrate with 0.5M *sodium hydroxide VS* using *phenolphthalein solution R1* as indicator. Each ml of 0.5M *sodium hydroxide VS* is equivalent to 78.00 mg of NaH_2PO_4, $2H_2O$.

For disodium hydrogen phosphate dodecahydrate Titrate 50 ml with 0.5M *hydrochloric acid VS* using 2 ml of a mixture of 4 volumes of *bromocresol green solution* and 1 volume of *methyl red solution* as indicator and titrating to the colour indicative of pH 4.4. Each ml of 0.5M *hydrochloric acid VS* is equivalent to 179.0 mg of Na_2HPO_4, $12H_2O$.

Labelling The label states (1) where appropriate, that the enema is Formula A or Formula B; (2) for any formulation other than Formula A or B, the content in terms of the amount or equivalent of Sodium Dihydrogen Phosphate Dihydrate and Disodium Hydrogen Phosphate Dodecahydrate; (3) the date after which the enema is not intended to be used; (4) the conditions under which it should be stored.

The label states the pharmaceutical form as 'rectal solution'.

Phytomenadione Injection

Definition Phytomenadione Injection is a sterile preparation of Phytomenadione in Water for Injections.

The injection complies with the requirements stated under Parenteral Preparations and with the following requirements.

Content of phytomenadione, $C_{31}H_{46}O_2$ 90.0 to 115.0% of the prescribed or stated amount.

Characteristics A clear to slightly opalescent liquid when maintained at a temperature below 25°.

Identification

A. Dilute with *absolute ethanol* to produce a solution containing 0.01% w/v of Phytomenadione. The *light absorption* of the solution, Appendix II B, in the range 230 to 350 nm exhibits a maximum at 328 nm and a minimum at 292 nm.

B. Dilute a quantity of the solution used in test A with *absolute ethanol* to produce a solution containing 0.001% w/v of Phytomenadione. The *light absorption* of the solution, Appendix II B, in the range 230 to 350 nm exhibits maxima at 245, 249, 263 and 271 nm and minima at 256 nm and 266 nm.

Acidity or alkalinity pH, 5.0 to 7.5, Appendix V L.

Assay Carry out the method for *liquid chromatography*, Appendix III D, using the following solutions. Solution (1) contains 0.01% w/v of *phytomenadione BPCRS* in the mobile phase. For solution (2) dilute a volume of the injection containing 10 mg of Phytomenadione with sufficient of the mobile phase to produce 100 ml.

The chromatographic procedure may be carried out using (a) a stainless steel column (20 cm × 4 mm) packed with *stationary phase C* (5 μm) (Spherisorb ODS 1 is suitable), (b) a mixture of 95 volumes of *ethanol (96%)* and 5 volumes of *water* as the mobile phase with a flow rate of 1.5 ml per minute and (c) a detection wavelength of 254 nm.

Calculate the content of $C_{31}H_{46}O_2$ using the declared content of $C_{31}H_{46}O_2$ in *phytomenadione BPCRS*.

Storage Phytomenadione Injection deteriorates on exposure to light and should be stored in the dark. It should not be allowed to freeze.

Labelling The label states that the injection should not be used if separation has occurred or if oil droplets have appeared.

When vitamin K_1 injection is prescribed or demanded, Phytomenadione Injection shall be dispensed or supplied.

Phytomenadione Tablets

Definition Phytomenadione Tablets contain Phytomenadione.

The tablets comply with the requirements stated under Tablets and with the following requirements.

Content of phytomenadione, $C_{31}H_{46}O_2$ 90.0 to 110.0% of the prescribed or stated amount.

Identification Shake a quantity of the powdered tablets containing 50 mg of Phytomenadione with 50 ml of *absolute ethanol* for 1 hour, allow to stand and dilute 5 ml of the clear supernatant liquid to 50 ml with *absolute ethanol*. The *light absorption* of the resulting solution, Appendix II B, in the range 230 to 350 nm exhibits a maximum at 328 nm and a minimum at 292 nm. Dilute a suitable volume of the solution with sufficient *absolute ethanol* to produce a solution containing 0.001% w/v of Phytomenadione. The *light absorption* of this solution, in the range 230 to 350 nm, exhibits maxima at 245, 249, 263 and 271 nm and minima at 256 nm and 266 nm.

Disintegration The requirement for Disintegration does not apply to Phytomenadione Tablets.

Related substances Carry out in subdued light the method for *thin-layer chromatography*, Appendix III A, using *silica gel GF_{254}* as the coating substance and a mixture of 1 volume of *methanol*, 20 volumes of *ether* and 80 volumes of *cyclohexane* as the mobile phase. Apply separately to the plate 20 µl of each of the following solutions. For solution (1) disperse a quantity of the powdered tablets containing 50 mg of Phytomenadione in 5 ml of *water* and extract with two 10-ml quantities of *2,2,4-trimethylpentane*. Shake the combined trimethylpentane extracts with 2 g of *anhydrous sodium sulphate* and filter. Solution (2) contains 0.0050% w/v of *2-methyl-1,4-naphthoquinone* in *2,4,4-trimethylpentane*. After removal of the plate, allow it to dry in air and examine under *ultraviolet light (254 nm)*. Any *secondary spot* in the chromatogram obtained with solution (1) is not more intense than the spot in the chromatogram obtained with solution (2) (1%).

Assay Weigh and powder 20 tablets. Carry out in subdued light the method for *liquid chromatography*, Appendix III D, using the following solutions. Solution (1) contains 0.01% w/v of *phytomenadione BPCRS* in the mobile phase. For solution (2) add 5 ml of 0.5M *ammonia* to a quantity of the powdered tablets containing 10 mg of Phytomenadione and mix with the aid of ultrasound for 5 minutes. Add 90 ml of *ethanol (96%)* and mix with the aid of ultrasound for 10 minutes. Shake for 10 minutes, add sufficient *ethanol (96%)* to produce 100 ml, centrifuge and use the clear supernatant layer.

The chromatographic procedure may be carried out using (a) a stainless steel column (20 cm × 4 mm) packed with *stationary phase C* (5 µm) (Spherisorb ODS 1 is suitable), (b) a mixture of 5 volumes of *water* and 95 volumes of *ethanol (96%)* as the mobile phase with a flow rate of 1.5 ml per minute and (c) a detection wavelength of 254 nm.

Calculate the content of $C_{31}H_{46}O_2$ using the declared content of $C_{31}H_{46}O_2$ in *phytomenadione BPCRS*.

Labelling The label states that the tablets should be chewed before swallowing or allowed to dissolve slowly in the mouth.

When vitamin K_1 tablets are prescribed or demanded, Phytomenadione Tablets shall be dispensed or supplied.

Pilocarpine Hydrochloride Eye Drops

Definition Pilocarpine Hydrochloride Eye Drops are a sterile solution of Pilocarpine Hydrochloride in Purified Water.

The eye drops comply with the requirements stated under Eye Preparations and with the following requirements.

Content of pilocarpine hydrochloride, $C_{11}H_{16}N_2O_2$, HCl 90.0 to 110.0% of the prescribed or stated amount.

Identification To a volume containing 10 mg of Pilocarpine Hydrochloride add 0.1 ml of 1M *sulphuric acid*, 1 ml of *hydrogen peroxide solution (20 vol)*, 1 ml of *toluene* and 0.05 ml of *potassium chromate solution*, shake well and allow to separate. The toluene layer is bluish violet and the aqueous layer remains yellow.

Acidity pH, 3.0 to 5.0, Appendix V L.

Pilocarpic acid Carry out the method for *liquid chromatography*, Appendix III D, using 20 µl of each of the following solutions. For solution (1) dilute a suitable volume with *water* to produce a solution containing 0.080% w/v of Pilocarpine Hydrochloride. For solution (2) dilute 1 volume of solution (1) to 25 volumes with *water*. For solution (3) dissolve 8.0 mg of *pilocarpine nitrate BPCRS* in 10 ml of 0.0025M *sodium hydroxide*, heat in a boiling water bath for 30 minutes and cool.

The chromatographic procedure may be carried out using (a) a stainless steel column (15 cm × 4.6 mm) packed with *stationary phase C* (5 µm) (Hypersil ODS is suitable), (b) as the mobile phase a mixture of 55 volumes of *methanol*, 60 volumes of *acetonitrile* and 885 volumes of 0.002M *tetrabutylammonium dihydrogen orthophosphate*, the pH of the mixture being adjusted to 7.75 using 6M *ammonia*, with a flow rate of 1.2 ml per minute and (c) a detection wavelength of 220 nm. Record the chromatogram of solution (1) for twice the retention time of the main peak.

The test is not valid unless the chromatogram obtained with solution (3) closely resembles the reference chromatogram supplied with *pilocarpine nitrate BPCRS*.

In the chromatogram obtained with solution (1) the area of any peak corresponding to pilocarpic acid is not greater than the area of the principal peak in the chromatogram obtained with solution (2) (4.0%).

Assay Use Method A for eye drops that contain less than 1% w/v of Pilocarpine Hydrochloride and in which benzalkonium chloride is used as an antimicrobial preservative. For other eye drops use Method B.

A. To 2 ml in a stoppered flask add 5 ml of *mixed phosphate buffer pH 10*, 5 ml of *chloroform* and 0.1 ml of *bromophenol blue solution*. Titrate slowly with 0.01M *sodium tetraphenylborate VS*, shaking well between successive small additions, until the chloroform layer becomes colourless. Using a further 2 ml of the eye drops, carry out the procedure described under Method B beginning at the words 'add 5 ml of *acetate buffer pH 3.7* ...'. The difference between the titrations at pH 3.7 and pH 10 represents the amount of sodium tetraphenylborate required.

B. Dilute if necessary with *water* to produce a solution containing 1% w/v of Pilocarpine Hydrochloride. To 2 ml add 5 ml of *acetate buffer pH 3.7* and 15 ml of 0.01M *sodium tetraphenylborate VS*, mix and allow to stand for 10 minutes. Filter, wash the container and filter with 5 ml of *water*, combine the filtrate and washings and titrate with

0.005M *cetylpyridinium chloride VS* using 0.5 ml of *bromophenol blue solution* as indicator. Repeat the operation without the preparation being examined. The difference between the titrations represents the amount of sodium tetraphenylborate required.

Each ml of 0.01M *sodium tetraphenylborate VS* is equivalent to 2.447 mg of $C_{11}H_{16}N_2O_2$,HCl.

Pilocarpine Nitrate Eye Drops

Definition Pilocarpine Nitrate Eye Drops are a sterile solution of Pilocarpine Nitrate in Purified Water.

The eye drops comply with the requirements stated under Eye Preparations and with the following requirements.

Content of pilocarpine nitrate, $C_{11}H_{16}N_2O_2$,HNO_3 90.0 to 110.0% of the prescribed or stated amount.

Identification Evaporate to dryness a volume containing 20 mg of Pilocarpine Nitrate on a water bath and heat for 1 hour at 105°. The *infrared absorption spectrum* of the residue, Appendix II A, is concordant with the *reference spectrum* of pilocarpine nitrate.

Acidity pH 2.5 to 4.2, Appendix V L.

Pilocarpic acid Carry out the method for *liquid chromatography*, Appendix III D, using 20 µl of each of the following solutions. For solution (1) dilute a suitable volume with *water* to produce a solution containing 0.080% w/v of Pilocarpine Nitrate. For solution (2) dilute 1 volume of solution (1) to 25 volumes with *water*. For solution (3) dissolve 8.0 mg of *pilocarpine nitrate BPCRS* in 10 ml of 0.0025M *sodium hydroxide*, heat in a boiling water bath for 30 minutes and cool.

The chromatographic procedure may be carried out using (a) a stainless steel column (15 cm × 4.6 mm) packed with *stationary phase C* (5 µm) (Hypersil ODS is suitable), (b) as the mobile phase a mixture of 55 volumes of *methanol*, 60 volumes of *acetonitrile* and 885 volumes of 0.002M *tetrabutylammonium dihydrogen orthophosphate*, the pH of the mixture being adjusted to 7.75 using 6M *ammonia*, with a flow rate of 1.2 ml per minute and (c) a detection wavelength of 220 nm. Record the chromatogram of solution (1) for twice the retention time of the main peak.

The test is not valid unless the chromatogram obtained with solution (3) closely resembles the reference chromatogram supplied with *pilocarpine nitrate BPCRS*.

In the chromatogram obtained with solution (1) the area of any peak corresponding to pilocarpic acid is not greater than the area of the principal peak in the chromatogram obtained with solution (2) (4.0%).

Assay Carry out the method for *liquid chromatography*, Appendix III D, using 20 µl of each of the following solutions. For solution (1) dilute a suitable volume of the eye drops with *water* to produce a solution containing 0.08% w/v of Pilocarpine Nitrate. Solution (2) contains 0.08% w/v of *pilocarpine nitrate BPCRS*.

The chromatographic procedure may be carried out using (a) a stainless steel column (15 cm × 4.6 mm) packed with *stationary phase C* (5 µm) (Hypersil ODS is suitable), (b) as the mobile phase a mixture of 55 volumes of *methanol*, 60 volumes of *acetonitrile* and 885 volumes of 0.002M *tetrabutylammonium dihydrogen orthophosphate*, the pH of the mixture being adjusted to 7.75 using 6M *ammonia*, with a flow rate of 1.2 ml per minute and (c) a detection wavelength of 220 nm. Two major peaks are obtained with both solutions. Disregard the peak that is due to nitric acid and has the shorter retention time. Record the chromatogram of solution (1) for twice the retention time of the principal peak.

Calculate the content of $C_{11}H_{16}N_2O_2$,HNO_3 using the declared content of $C_{11}H_{16}N_2O_2$,HNO_3 in *pilocarpine nitrate BPCRS*.

Pindolol Tablets

Definition Pindolol Tablets contain Pindolol.

The tablets comply with the requirements stated under Tablets and with the following requirements.

Content of pindolol, $C_{14}H_{20}N_2O_2$ 90.0 to 110.0% of the prescribed or stated amount.

Identification

A. Shake a quantity of the powdered tablets containing 50 mg of Pindolol with 80 ml of *ether* for 30 minutes, filter and dry the extract with *anhydrous sodium sulphate*. Filter the dried extract, remove the ether using a rotary evaporator and dry the residue over *phosphorus pentoxide* at 110° at a pressure not exceeding 2 kPa for 1 hour. The *infrared absorption spectrum* of the dried residue, Appendix II A, is concordant with the *reference spectrum* of pindolol.

B. The *light absorption*, Appendix II B, in the range 230 to 350 nm of the final solution obtained in the Assay exhibits two maxima, at 264 nm and 287 nm.

C. Shake a quantity of the powdered tablets containing 20 mg of Pindolol with 5 ml of a mixture of 1 volume of *glacial acetic acid* and 99 volumes of *methanol* for 45 minutes. Centrifuge and dilute 1 ml of the supernatant liquid to 50 ml with the acetic acid—methanol mixture. To 2 ml of this solution add 1 ml of *dimethylaminobenzaldehyde solution R7*. A violet-blue colour is produced.

Related substances Carry out the following procedure as rapidly as possible protected from light. Carry out the method for *thin-layer chromatography*, Appendix III A, using *silica gel GF_{254}* as the coating substance and a freshly prepared mixture of 4 volumes of 13.5M *ammonia*, 50 volumes of *ethyl acetate* and 50 volumes of *methanol* as the mobile phase but allowing the solvent front to ascend 10 cm above the line of application. Apply separately to the plate 10 µl of each of the following solutions. For solution (1) shake a quantity of the powdered tablets containing 20 mg of Pindolol with 5 ml of a mixture of 1 volume of *glacial acetic acid* and 99 volumes of *methanol* for 15 minutes, centrifuge and use the supernatant liquid; apply to the plate as the last solution. For solution (2) dilute 1 volume of solution (1) to 10 volumes with the acetic acid—methanol mixture and further dilute 7 volumes of this solution to 100 volumes with the same solvent mixture. For solution (3) dilute 1 volume of solution (1) to 10 volumes with the acetic acid—methanol mixture and further dilute 3 volumes of this solution to 100 volumes with the same solvent mixture. Develop the chromatograms without delay. After removal of the plate, spray immediately with *dimethylaminobenzaldehyde solution R7* and warm at 50° for 20 minutes. Any spot with an Rf value of about 0.1 in the chromatogram obtained with solution (1) is not more intense than the spot in the chromatogram obtained with solution (2) (0.7%). Any other *secondary spot* in the chromatogram obtained with solution (1) is not more intense than the spot in the chromatogram obtained with solution (3) (0.3%). Disregard any spot remaining on the line of application.

Assay Shake a quantity of whole tablets containing 90 mg of Pindolol with 90 ml of *methanol* for 45 minutes. Centrifuge and dilute 15 ml of the supernatant liquid to 100 ml with *methanol.* Dilute 5 ml of this solution to 50 ml with *methanol* and measure the *absorbance* of the resulting solution at the maximum at 264 nm, Appendix II B. Calculate the content of $C_{14}H_{20}N_2O_2$ taking 338 as the value of A(1%, 1 cm) at the maximum at 264 nm. Make no allowance for the fact that fewer than 20 tablets may have been taken.

Storage Pindolol Tablets should be protected from light.

Piperazine Citrate Elixir

Piperazine Citrate Oral Solution

Definition Piperazine Citrate Elixir is an *oral solution* containing 18.75% w/v of Piperazine Citrate in a suitable flavoured vehicle.

The elixir complies with the requirements stated under Oral Liquids and with the following requirements.

Content of piperazine citrate, $(C_4H_{10}N_2)_3$,$2C_6H_8O_7$ 15.3 to 17.7% w/v.

Identification

A. To 1 ml add 5 ml of 2M *hydrochloric acid* and, with stirring, 1 ml of a freshly prepared 50% w/v solution of *sodium nitrite*, cool in ice for 15 minutes, induce crystallisation, wash the crystalline precipitate with *water* and dry at 105°. The *melting point* is about 159°, Appendix V A.

B. Warm 10 ml with *activated charcoal* and filter. Boil a portion of the filtrate with an excess of *mercury(II) sulphate solution*, filter, boil the filtrate and add 0.25 ml of *dilute potassium permanganate solution*. The potassium permanganate solution is decolorised and a white precipitate is produced.

C. Acidify a portion of the filtrate obtained in test B with 1M *sulphuric acid*, add 0.25 ml of *dilute potassium permanganate solution*, warm until the colour is discharged and add an excess of *bromine water*. A white precipitate is produced either immediately or on cooling.

Weight per ml 1.24 to 1.26 g, Appendix V G.

Assay To 1.5 g add 3.5 ml of 0.5M *sulphuric acid* and 10 ml of *water*, add 100 ml of *picric acid solution R1*, heat on a water bath for 15 minutes, allow to stand for 1 hour and filter through a sintered-glass filter (BS porosity No. 4). Wash the residue with successive 10-ml quantities of a mixture of equal volumes of a saturated solution of *picric acid* and *water* until the washings are free from sulphate, then wash the residue with five 10-ml quantities of *absolute ethanol* and dry to constant weight at 105°. Each g of residue is equivalent to 0.3935 g of $(C_4H_{10}N_2)_3$,$2C_6H_8O_7$. Use the weight per ml of the elixir to calculate the percentage weight in volume of $(C_4H_{10}N_2)_3$, $2C_6H_8O_7$.

Storage Piperazine Citrate Elixir should be protected from light and stored at a temperature not exceeding 25°.

Labelling The label indicates the pharmaceutical form as 'oral solution'.

Piperazine Citrate Elixir contains, in 5 ml, the equivalent of about 750 mg of piperazine hydrate.

Piperazine Phosphate Tablets

Definition Piperazine Phosphate Tablets contain Piperazine Phosphate. If the tablets are intended to be chewed before swallowing they may contain suitable flavouring agents.

The tablets comply with the requirements stated under Tablets and with the following requirements.

Content of piperazine phosphate, $C_4H_{10}N_2$,H_3PO_4,H_2O 92.5 to 107.5% of the prescribed or stated amount.

Identification Extract a quantity of the powdered tablets containing 1 g of Piperazine Phosphate with 20 ml of *water* and filter. The filtrate complies with the following tests.

A. Dilute 1 ml to 5 ml with *water*, add 0.5 g of *sodium hydrogen carbonate*, 0.5 ml of a freshly prepared 5% w/v solution of *potassium hexacyanoferrate(III)* and 0.1 ml of *mercury*, shake vigorously for 1 minute and allow to stand for 20 minutes. A reddish colour is produced slowly.

B. To 4 ml add 1 ml of *hydrochloric acid* and, with stirring, 1 ml of a 50% w/v solution of *sodium nitrite* and cool in ice for 15 minutes, stirring if necessary to induce crystallisation. The *melting point* of the crystals, after washing with 10 ml of cold *water* and drying at 105°, is about 159°, Appendix V A.

C. Yields the reactions characteristic of *phosphates*, Appendix VI.

Disintegration The requirement for Disintegration does not apply to Piperazine Phosphate Tablets intended to be chewed before swallowing.

Assay Weigh and powder 20 tablets. Shake a quantity of the powder containing 0.15 g of Piperazine Phosphate with 10 ml of *water* for 1 hour, filter and wash the residue with two 10-ml quantities of *water*. To the combined extract and washings add 5 ml of 1M *sulphuric acid* and 50 ml of *picric acid solution R1*, bring to the boil, allow to stand for several hours, filter through a sintered-glass crucible (BS porosity No. 4) and wash the residue with successive 10-ml quantities of a mixture of equal volumes of a saturated solution of *picric acid* and *water* until the washings are free from sulphate. Wash the residue with five 10-ml quantities of *absolute ethanol* and dry to constant weight at 100° to 105°. Each g of residue is equivalent to 0.3714 g of $C_4H_{10}N_2$,H_3PO_4,H_2O.

Labelling The label states, where applicable, that the tablets are to be chewed before swallowing.

520 mg of Piperazine Phosphate is approximately equivalent to 500 mg of piperazine hydrate.

Piroxicam Capsules

Definition Piroxicam Capsules contain Piroxicam.

The capsules comply with the requirements stated under Capsules and with the following requirements.

Content of piroxicam, $C_{15}H_{13}N_3O_4S$ 95.0 to 105.0% of the prescribed or stated amount.

Identification

A. In the test for Related substances the spot in the chromatogram obtained with solution (2) corresponds to that in the chromatogram obtained with solution (3).

B. In the Assay, the retention time of the principal peak in the chromatogram obtained with solution (1) corresponds to that of the principal peak in the chromatogram obtained with solution (2).

2-Pyridylamine Carry out the method for *thin-layer chromatography*, Appendix III A, using *silica gel GF_{254}* as the coating substance and a mixture of 1 volume of *diethylamine* and 8 volumes of *dichloromethane* as the mobile phase. Apply separately to the plate 20 µl of each of the following solutions. For solution (1) shake a quantity of the contents of the capsules containing 80 mg of Piroxicam with 25 ml of *dichloromethane*, filter, evaporate the filtrate to dryness using a rotary evaporator and dissolve the residue in 2 ml of *dichloromethane*. Solution (2) contains 0.010% w/v of *2-pyridylamine* in *dichloromethane*. After removal of the plate, allow it to dry in air and examine under *ultraviolet light (254 nm)*. Any spot corresponding to 2-pyridylamine in the chromatogram obtained with solution (1) is not more intense than the spot in the chromatogram obtained with solution (2) (0.25%).

Related substances Carry out the method for *thin-layer chromatography*, Appendix III A, using *silica gel GF_{254}* as the coating substance and a mixture of 10 volumes of *glacial acetic acid* and 90 volumes of *toluene* as the mobile phase. Apply separately to the plate 7.5 µl of each of the following solutions. For solution (1) shake a quantity of the contents of the capsules containing 80 mg of Piroxicam with 25 ml of *dichloromethane*, filter, evaporate the filtrate to dryness using a rotary evaporator and dissolve the residue in 2 ml of *dichloromethane*. For solution (2) dilute 1 ml of solution (1) to 20 ml with *dichloromethane*. Solution (3) contains 0.20% w/v of *piroxicam BPCRS* in *dichloromethane*. For solution (4) dilute 2 ml of solution (2) to 50 ml with *dichloromethane*. After removal of the plate, allow it to dry in air and examine under *ultraviolet light (254 nm)*. Any *secondary spot* in the chromatogram obtained with solution (1) is not more intense than the spot in the chromatogram obtained with solution (4) (0.2%). Disregard any spot remaining on the line of application.

Dissolution Comply with the *dissolution test for tablets and capsules*, Appendix XII D, using as the medium 900 ml of 0.1M *hydrochloric acid* and rotating the basket at 100 revolutions per minute. Withdraw a 10-ml sample of the medium and measure the *absorbance* of the filtered sample, suitably diluted if necessary, at the maximum at 242 nm, Appendix II B. Calculate the total content of piroxicam, $C_{15}H_{13}N_3O_4S$, in the medium taking 386 as the value of A(1%, 1 cm) at the maximum at 242 nm.

Assay Carry out the method for *liquid chromatography*, Appendix III D, using the following solutions. For solution (1) add a quantity of the mixed contents of 20 capsules containing 10 mg of Piroxicam to 150 ml of 0.01M *methanolic hydrochloric acid*, mix with the aid of ultrasound for 30 minutes, cool and dilute to 200 ml with the same solvent, filter through glass-fibre paper (Whatman GF/C is suitable) and use the filtrate. Solution (2) contains 0.005% w/v of *piroxicam BPCRS* in 0.01M *methanolic hydrochloric acid*.

The chromatographic procedure may be carried out using (a) a stainless steel column (30 cm × 3.9 mm) packed with *octadecylsilyl silica gel for chromatography* (10 µm) (µBondapak C18 is suitable), (b) as the mobile phase with a flow rate of 2 ml per minute a mixture of 60 volumes of *methanol* and 40 volumes of a buffer solution prepared by adding a solution containing 5.35 g of *disodium hydrogen orthophosphate* in 100 ml of *water* to a solution containing 7.72 g of *citric acid* in 400 ml of *water* and diluting to 1000 ml and (c) a detection wavelength of 242 nm.

Calculate the content $C_{15}H_{13}N_3O_4S$ using the declared content of $C_{15}H_{13}N_3O_4S$ in *piroxicam BPCRS*.

Piroxicam Gel

Definition Piroxicam Gel contains Piroxicam.

The gel complies with the requirements stated under Topical Semi-solid Preparations and with the following requirements.

Content of piroxicam, $C_{15}H_{13}N_3O_4S$ 95.0 to 105.0% of the prescribed or stated amount.

Identification

A. Carry out the method for *thin-layer chromatography*, Appendix III A, using *silica gel GF_{254}* as the coating substance and a mixture of 1 volume of *glacial acetic acid*, 10 volumes of *methanol* and 80 volumes of *ethyl acetate* as the mobile phase. Apply separately to the plate 5 µl of each of the following solutions. For solution (1) mix a quantity of the gel containing 10 mg of Piroxicam with 0.1 ml of a saturated solution of *sodium chloride* until the mixture becomes turbid. Dilute to 5 ml with 0.01M *methanolic hydrochloric acid*, shake well, centrifuge and use the clear supernatant solution. Filter the supernatant solution if necessary. Solution (2) contains 0.2% w/v of *piroxicam BPCRS* in 0.01M *methanolic hydrochloric acid*. After removal of the plate, dry it in a current of air and examine under *ultraviolet light (254 nm)*. The principal spot in the chromatogram obtained with solution (1) is similar in position and size to that in the chromatogram obtained with solution (2).

B. In the Assay, the retention time of the principal peak in the chromatogram obtained with solution (1) corresponds to that in the chromatogram obtained with solution (2).

Alkalinity pH of a 10% w/v solution of the gel, 7.2 to 8.2, Appendix V L.

2-Pyridylamine Carry out the method for *liquid chromatography*, Appendix III D, using the following solutions. For solution (1) add 5 ml of 0.01M *methanolic hydrochloric acid* to a quantity of the gel containing 5 mg of Piroxicam, shake gently for 30 minutes, add 50 ml of the mobile phase and shake vigorously for 30 minutes. Dilute to 100 ml with the mobile phase, mix and filter through a glass fibre membrane filter (1-µm). For solution (2) dilute 5 volumes of a 0.00050% w/v solution of *2-pyridylamine* in

0.01M *methanolic hydrochloric acid* to 100 volumes with the mobile phase.

The chromatographic procedure may be carried out using (a) a stainless steel column (25 cm × 4.6 mm) packed with *stationary phase B* (5 μm) (Zorbax stablebond C8 is suitable) and a stainless steel guard column (10 cm × 4.6 mm) packed with *stationary phase B* (5 μm), both columns maintained at 40°, (b) a mixture of 15 volumes of *methanol*, 30 volumes of *acetonitrile* and 55 volumes of 0.05M *sodium dihydrogen orthophosphate* previously adjusted to pH 3.5 with 5M *orthophosphoric acid* as the mobile phase with a flow rate of 1.0 ml per minute and (c) a fluorimetric detector with an excitation wavelength of 313 nm and an emission wavelength of 380 nm.

In the chromatogram obtained with solution (1) the area of any peak corresponding to 2-pyridylamine is not greater than that of the principal peak in the chromatogram obtained with solution (2) (0.5%).

Assay Carry out the method for *liquid chromatography*, Appendix III D, using the following solutions. For solution (1) add 5 ml of 0.01M *methanolic hydrochloric acid* to a quantity of the gel containing 5 mg of Piroxicam, shake gently for 30 minutes, add 50 ml of the mobile phase and shake vigorously for 30 minutes. Dilute to 100 ml with the mobile phase, mix and filter through a glass fibre membrane filter (1 μm). For solution (2) prepare a 0.10% w/v solution of *piroxicam BPCRS* in 0.01M *methanolic hydrochloric acid*, with the aid of ultrasound if necessary, and dilute 5 volumes of this solution to 100 volumes with the mobile phase.

The chromatographic procedure described under 2-Pyridylamine may be used but use an ultraviolet spectrophotometer detector at a wavelength of 248 nm.

Calculate the content of $C_{15}H_{13}N_3O_4S$ in the gel using the declared content of $C_{15}H_{13}N_3O_4S$ in *piroxicam BPCRS*.

Pizotifen Tablets

Definition Pizotifen Tablets contain Pizotifen Malate.

The tablets comply with the requirements stated under Tablets and with the following requirements.

Content of pizotifen, $C_{19}H_{21}NS$ 90.0 to 110.0% of the prescribed or stated amount.

Identification

A. To a quantity of the powdered tablets containing the equivalent of 10 mg of pizotifen add 50 ml of *water*, mix with the aid of ultrasound for 15 minutes and centrifuge. Make the clear supernatant liquid alkaline with 5M *sodium hydroxide* and extract with three 25-ml quantities of *ether*, washing each extract with the same 20 ml of *water*. Combine the ether extracts, dry with *anhydrous sodium sulphate*, filter and evaporate the filtrate to dryness. The *infrared absorption spectrum* of the residue, Appendix II A, is concordant with the *reference spectrum* of pizotifen.

B. In the test for Related substances, the principal spot in the chromatogram obtained with solution (1) corresponds to the spot in the chromatogram obtained with solution (2).

C. In the test for Uniformity of content, the chromatogram obtained with solution (1) shows a peak with the same retention time as the peak due to pizotifen in the chromatogram obtained with solution (2).

Related substances Carry out the method for *thin-layer chromatography*, Appendix III A, using a silica gel precoated plate (Merck silica gel 60 plates are suitable) and a mixture of 1 volume of 13.5M *ammonia*, 15 volumes of *absolute ethanol* and 85 volumes of *toluene* as the mobile phase. Apply separately to the plate 20 μl of each of the following solutions prepared using a mixture of 200 volumes of *methanol*, 100 volumes of *chloroform* and 3 volumes of 13.5M *ammonia* (solvent A). For solution (1) mix a quantity of the powdered tablets containing the equivalent of 6 mg of pizotifen with 60 ml of solvent A for 20 minutes, centrifuge, evaporate 50 ml of the clear supernatant liquid to dryness at 40° at a pressure of 2 kPa and dissolve the residue in 2 ml of solvent A. Centrifuge and use the supernatant liquid. Solution (2) contains 0.36% w/v of *pizotifen malate BPCRS* in solvent A. For solution (3) dilute 1 volume of solution (1) to 100 volumes with solvent A. For solution (4) dilute 1 volume of solution (3) to 2 volumes with solvent A. After removal of the plate, dry it in a current of warm air for 5 minutes, spray with a mixture of 1 volume of *potassium iodobismuthate solution* and 10 volumes of 2M *acetic acid* and then with *hydrogen peroxide solution (10 vol)*, cover immediately with a glass plate and examine in daylight. Any *secondary spot* in the chromatogram obtained with solution (1) is not more intense than the spot in the chromatogram obtained with solution (3) (1%) and not more than two such spots are more intense than the spot in the chromatogram obtained with solution (4) (0.5%). Disregard any spots with Rf values lower than 0.1.

Uniformity of content Tablets containing less than the equivalent of 2 mg of pizotifen comply with the requirements stated under Tablets using the following method of analysis. Carry out the method for *liquid chromatography*, Appendix III D, using the following solutions. Solution (1) contains 0.0073% w/v of *pizotifen malate BPCRS* in the mobile phase. For solution (2) add sufficient mobile phase to one tablet to produce a solution containing the equivalent of 0.0050% w/v of pizotifen, mix with the aid of ultrasound until the tablet has disintegrated, stir for 15 minutes and centrifuge.

The chromatographic procedure may be carried out using (a) a stainless steel column (10 cm × 5 mm) packed with *stationary phase C* (5 μm) (Hypersil ODS is suitable), (b) a mixture of 0.3 volume of *triethylamine*, 45 volumes of *water* and 55 volumes of *acetonitrile* as the mobile phase with a flow rate of 2 ml per minute and (c) a detection wavelength of 256 nm.

Calculate the content of pizotifen, $C_{19}H_{21}NS$, using the declared content of $C_{19}H_{21}NS$ in *pizotifen malate BPCRS*.

Assay Calculate the content of $C_{19}H_{21}NS$ using the average of the 10 results obtained in the test for Uniformity of content.

Storage Pizotifen Tablets should be protected from light.

Labelling The quantity of active ingredient is stated in terms of the equivalent amount of pizotifen.

Compound Podophyllin Paint

Definition Compound Podophyllin Paint is a *cutaneous solution.*

Podophyllum Resin 150 g
Compound Benzoin Tincture
sufficient to produce 1000 ml

In making the Compound Benzoin Tincture used to prepare Compound Podophyllin Paint, the Ethanol (90 per cent) may be replaced by Industrial Methylated Spirit[1] diluted so as to be of equivalent ethanolic strength.

The paint complies with the requirements stated under Liquids for Cutaneous Application and with the following requirements.

Identification Carry out the method for *thin-layer chromatography,* Appendix III A, using a silica gel pre-coated plate (Merck silica gel 60 plates are suitable) and a mixture of 1 volume of *methanol* and 25 volumes of *chloroform* as the mobile phase, but allowing the solvent front to ascend 10 cm above the line of application. Apply separately to the plate, as bands 15 mm long and not more than 3 mm wide, 10 µl of each of the following solutions. For solution (1) dilute 1 volume of the paint to 15 volumes with *absolute ethanol.* Solution (2) is a 0.5% w/v solution of *podophyllotoxin* in *absolute ethanol.* After removal of the plate, allow it to dry in air, spray with *methanolic sulphuric acid (50%)* and heat at 130° for 10 minutes. The chromatogram obtained with solution (1) exhibits a band corresponding in position and colour to the principal band in the chromatogram obtained with solution (2). It does not show greyish pink bands at Rf values higher than that of podophyllotoxin (*P. peltatum*).

Weight per ml 0.925 to 0.975 g, Appendix V G.

Total solids 27.0 to 33.0% w/v when determined by evaporating 1 ml to dryness on a water bath and drying the residue at 105° for 4 hours.

Labelling The label indicates the pharmaceutical form as 'cutaneous solution'.

---

[1]The law and the statutory regulations governing the use of Industrial Methylated Spirit must be observed.

Poldine Tablets

Definition Poldine Tablets contain Poldine Metilsulfate.

The tablets comply with the requirements stated under Tablets and with the following requirements.

Content of poldine metilsulfate, $C_{22}H_{29}NO_7S$ 90.0 to 110.0% of the prescribed or stated amount.

Identification Shake a quantity of the powdered tablets containing 2 mg of Poldine Metilsulfate with 10 ml of *water* and allow to stand. Decant the supernatant liquid, add 20 ml of *ammonium cobaltothiocyanate solution* and 5 ml of *chloroform* and shake well. The chloroform layer becomes blue.

Related substances Carry out the method for *thin-layer chromatography,* Appendix III A, using a silica gel precoated plate (Merck silica gel 60 plates are suitable) and a mixture of 5 volumes of *formic acid,* 5 volumes of *water,* 30 volumes of *methanol* and 60 volumes of *chloroform* as the mobile phase. Apply separately to the plate 50 µl of each of the following solutions. For solution (1) add 4 ml of *methanol* to a quantity of the powdered tablets containing 20 mg of Poldine Metilsulfate, mix with the aid of ultrasound for 5 minutes, centrifuge and to 1 ml of the supernatant liquid add 0.2 ml of *formic acid.* For solution (2) dilute 1 volume of solution (1) to 100 volumes with a mixture of 5 volumes of *methanol* and 1 volume of *formic acid.* After removal of the plate, allow it to dry in air, spray with a 50% v/v solution of *sulphuric acid* and heat at 110° for 20 minutes. Any pink *secondary spot* in the chromatogram obtained with solution (1) is not more intense than the spot in the chromatogram obtained with solution (2) (1%). Disregard any brown spots due to excipients in the chromatogram obtained with solution (1).

Assay Weigh and powder 20 tablets. Shake a quantity of the powder containing 2 mg of Poldine Metilsulfate with 10 ml of *water* for 10 minutes and allow to stand. To 5 ml of the supernatant liquid add 20 ml of *ammonium cobaltothiocyanate solution,* shake vigorously for 1 minute and allow to stand for 5 minutes. Extract with four 5-ml quantities of *chloroform,* add to the combined extracts sufficient *chloroform* to produce 25 ml and centrifuge. Measure the *absorbance* of the clear, chloroform solution at the maximum at 322 nm, Appendix II B. Calculate the content of $C_{22}H_{29}NO_7S$ from the *absorbance* obtained by repeating the operation using 5 ml of a 0.02% w/v solution of *poldine metilsulfate BPCRS* and beginning at the words 'add 20 ml...'.

Polymyxin and Bacitracin Eye Ointment

Definition Polymyxin and Bacitracin Eye Ointment is a sterile preparation containing Polymyxin B Sulphate and Bacitracin Zinc in a suitable basis.

The eye ointment complies with the requirements stated under Eye Preparations and with the following requirements.

Identification Carry out the method for *thin-layer chromatography,* Appendix III A, using *silica gel G* as the coating substance and a mixture of 60 volumes of *propan-2-ol,* 40 volumes of *water* and 10 volumes of 13.5M *ammonia* as the mobile phase. Apply separately to the plate 10 µl of each of the following solutions. For solution (1) add 20 ml of *chloroform* to a quantity of the eye ointment containing 2500 IU of Bacitracin Zinc, shake, add 5 ml of 0.1M *hydrochloric acid,* shake vigorously, centrifuge and use the aqueous layer. Solution (2) contains 0.13% w/v of *polymyxin B sulphate EPCRS* in 0.1M *hydrochloric acid.* Solution (3) contains 0.75% w/v of *bacitracin zinc EPCRS* in 0.1M *hydrochloric acid.* After removal of the plate, dry it at 105°, spray with a 0.5% w/v solution of *ninhydrin* in *butan-1-ol* and heat at 105° for 15 minutes. The two principal spots in the chromatogram obtained with solution (1) correspond to those in the chromatograms obtained with solutions (2) and (3).

Assay

For polymyxin B sulphate To a quantity containing 10,000 IU of Polymyxin B Sulphate add 15 ml of *chloroform* and 40 ml of sterile *phosphate buffer pH 6.0,* mix thoroughly, centrifuge and discard the chloroform layer. Using the aqueous layer, carry out the *biological assay of* *antibiotics*, Appendix XIV A. The precision of the assay is such that the fiducial limits of error are not less than 95% and not more than 105% of the estimated potency. The upper fiducial limit of error is not less than 90.0% and the lower fiducial limit of error is not more than 120.0% of the prescribed or stated number of IU of Polymyxin B Sulphate.

For bacitracin zinc To a quantity containing 500 IU of Bacitracin Zinc add 15 ml of *chloroform* and 40 ml of 0.01M *hydrochloric acid*, mix thoroughly, centrifuge and discard the chloroform layer. Using the aqueous layer, carry out the *biological assay of antibiotics*, Appendix XIV A. The precision of the assay is such that the fiducial limits of error are not less than 95% and not more than 105% of the estimated potency. The upper fiducial limit of error is not less than 90.0% and the lower fiducial limit of error is not more than 120.0% of the prescribed or stated number of IU of Bacitracin Zinc.

Labelling The strength is stated as the number of IU (Units) of Polymyxin B Sulphate per g and the number of IU (Units) of Bacitracin Zinc per g.

Polythiazide Tablets

Definition Polythiazide Tablets contain Polythiazide.

The tablets comply with the requirements stated under Tablets and with the following requirements.

Content of polythiazide, $C_{11}H_{13}ClF_3N_3O_4S_3$ 92.5 to 107.5% of the prescribed or stated amount.

Identification Comply with test C for Identification described under Polythiazide, but using for solution (1) the supernatant liquid obtained by extracting a quantity of the powdered tablets containing 4 mg of Polythiazide with 20 ml of *methanol* and centrifuging.

Related substances Comply with the test described under Polythiazide but applying separately to the plate 10 µl of solution (1) and quantities of 2, 4, 6, 8 and 10 µl of solution (2). For solution (1) use the supernatant liquid obtained by shaking a quantity of the powdered tablets containing 10 mg of Polythiazide with 2 ml of *acetone* and centrifuging. For solution (2) dilute 1 volume of solution (1) to 50 volumes with *acetone*. Assess the intensity of each *secondary spot* in the chromatogram obtained with solution (1) by reference to the spots in the chromatograms obtained with the applications of solution (2). The sum of the intensities so assessed does not exceed 3% of that of the spot in the chromatogram obtained with solution (1) and no such spot is more intense than the spot in the chromatogram obtained with 10 µl of solution (2). Disregard any brown spot.

Uniformity of content Tablets containing less than 2 mg of Polythiazide comply with the requirements stated under Tablets using the following method of analysis. Carry out the method for *liquid chromatography*, Appendix III D, using the following solutions. For solution (1) mix a 0.004% w/v solution of *polythiazide BPCRS* in *methanol* with an equal volume of 0.1M *potassium dihydrogen orthophosphate* adjusted to pH 3.5 with *orthophosphoric acid* (buffer solution). For solution (2) shake one tablet with 25 ml of the buffer solution for 10 minutes, add 25 ml of *methanol* and shake for a further 20 minutes. Centrifuge 5 ml of the resulting solution for 5 minutes at 2000 revolutions per minute and use the supernatant liquid.

The chromatographic procedure may be carried out using (a) a stainless steel column (20 cm × 4.6 mm) packed with *stationary phase C* (5 µm) (Spherisorb ODS 1 is suitable), (b) a mixture of 55 volumes of 0.1M *potassium dihydrogen orthophosphate* adjusted to pH 3.5 with *orthophosphoric acid* and 45 volumes of *methanol* as the mobile phase with a flow rate of 1.5 ml per minute and (c) a detection wavelength of 268 nm.

Calculate the content of $C_{11}H_{13}ClF_3N_3O_4S_3$ using the declared content of $C_{11}H_{13}ClF_3N_3O_4S_3$ in *polythiazide BPCRS*.

Assay Weigh and powder 20 tablets. Carry out the method for *liquid chromatography*, Appendix III D, using the following solutions. For solution (1) mix a 0.004% w/v solution of *polythiazide BPCRS* in *methanol* with an equal volume of 0.1M *potassium dihydrogen orthophosphate* adjusted to pH 3.5 with *orthophosphoric acid* (buffer solution). For solution (2) shake a quantity of the powdered tablets containing 4 mg of Polythiazide with 100 ml of *methanol* for 20 minutes, filter and mix equal volumes of the filtrate and the buffer solution.

The chromatographic procedure may be carried out using the conditions described under Uniformity of content.

Calculate the content of $C_{11}H_{13}ClF_3N_3O_4S_3$ using the declared content of $C_{11}H_{13}ClF_3N_3O_4S_3$ in *polythiazide BPCRS*.

Storage Polythiazide Tablets should be protected from light.

Sterile Potassium Chloride Concentrate

Definition Sterile Potassium Chloride Concentrate is a sterile solution of Potassium Chloride in Water for Injections.

The concentrate complies with the requirements for Concentrated Solutions for Injections stated under Parenteral Preparations and with the following requirements.

Content of potassium chloride, KCl 95.0 to 105.0% of the stated amount.

Identification The residue on evaporation yields the reactions characteristic of *potassium salts* and the reactions characteristic of *chlorides*, Appendix VI.

Acidity or alkalinity pH, 4.5 to 7.5, Appendix V L.

Bacterial endotoxins Carry out the test for *bacterial endotoxins*, Appendix XIV C. Dilute the concentrate being examined with *water BET* to contain 0.5% w/v of Potassium Chloride and adjust the pH, if necessary, to 7 (solution A). The endotoxin limit concentration of solution A is 3.0 IU of endotoxin per ml. Carry out the test using a lysate with a declared sensitivity not less sensitive than 0.0625 IU of endotoxin per ml, and using the maximum valid dilution of solution A calculated from the declared sensitivity of the lysate used in the test.

Assay Dilute 5 ml to 100 ml with *water*. To a volume of the solution containing 0.15 g of Potassium Chloride add 30 ml of *water* and titrate with 0.1M *silver nitrate VS* using *potassium chromate solution* as indicator. Each ml of 0.1M *silver nitrate VS* is equivalent to 7.456 mg of KCl.

Labelling The label states (1) 'Sterile Potassium Chloride Concentrate'; (2) the strength as a percentage w/v of Potassium Chloride; (3) the approximate concentration of the potassium ions and the chloride ions in mmol in a suitable volume; (4) the volume of Sodium Chloride Intravenous Infusion (0.9% w/v) or other suitable diluent with which the concentrate must be diluted and mixed well before use.

Potassium Chloride and Glucose Intravenous Infusion

Potassium Chloride and Dextrose Injection; Potassium Chloride and Glucose Injection; Potassium Chloride and Dextrose Intravenous Infusion

Definition Potassium Chloride and Glucose Intravenous Infusion is a sterile solution of Potassium Chloride and either Anhydrous Glucose or Glucose in Water for Injections.

The intravenous infusion complies with the requirements stated under Parenteral Preparations and with the following requirements.

Content of potassium chloride, KCl 95.0 to 105.0% of the prescribed or stated amount.

Content of glucose, $C_6H_{12}O_6$ 95.0 to 105.0% of the prescribed or stated amount.

Characteristics A colourless or faintly straw-coloured solution.

Identification

A. When heated with *cupri-tartaric solution R1* a copious precipitate of copper(I) oxide is produced.

B. The residue on evaporation yields the reactions characteristic of *potassium salts* and of *chlorides*, Appendix VI.

Acidity pH, 3.5 to 6.5, Appendix V L.

5-Hydroxymethylfurfural and related substances Dilute a volume containing 1.0 g of glucose, $C_6H_{12}O_6$, to 500 ml with *water*. The *absorbance* of the resulting solution at the maximum at 284 nm is not more than 0.25, Appendix II B.

Sodium The content of Na is not more than 1.0% of the content of K, calculated from the content of potassium chloride determined in the Assay. Determine the content of Na by Method II for *atomic emission spectrophotometry*, Appendix II D, measuring at 589 nm and using *sodium standard solution (200 ppm Na)*, diluted if necessary with *water*, to prepare the standard solutions.

Particulate contamination When supplied in a container with a nominal content of 100 ml or more, complies with the test for *sub-visible particles*, Appendix XIII A.

Pyrogens Dilute with an equal volume of *sodium chloride injection*. The solution complies with the *test for pyrogens*, Appendix XIV D. Use 10 ml per kg of the rabbit's weight.

Assay

For potassium chloride Dilute appropriately with *water* and determine by *atomic emission spectrophotometry*, Appendix II D, measuring at 767 nm and using *potassium standard solution (600 ppm K)*, suitably diluted with *water*, to prepare the standard solutions.

For glucose To a quantity containing 2 to 5 g of glucose, $C_6H_{12}O_6$, add 0.2 ml of 5M *ammonia* and sufficient *water* to produce 100 ml. Mix well, allow to stand for 30 minutes and measure the *optical rotation* in a 2-dm tube, Appendix V F. The observed rotation in degrees multiplied by 0.9477 represents the weight in g of glucose, $C_6H_{12}O_6$, in the quantity of the intravenous infusion taken for assay.

Storage Potassium Chloride and Glucose Intravenous Infusion should be stored at a temperature not exceeding 25°.

Labelling The strength is stated as the percentages w/v of Potassium Chloride and of glucose, $C_6H_{12}O_6$.

When the preparation is intended for intravenous infusion, the label also states (1) that rapid infusion may be harmful; (2) the approximate concentrations, in millimoles per litre, of the potassium ions and the chloride ions and the number of grams per litre of glucose, $C_6H_{12}O_6$.

For a preparation containing 0.3% w/v of Potassium Chloride, the concentration of each ion is stated as 40 millimoles per litre.

Potassium Chloride and Sodium Chloride Intravenous Infusion

Potassium Chloride and Sodium Chloride Injection

Definition Potassium Chloride and Sodium Chloride Intravenous Infusion is a sterile solution of Potassium Chloride and Sodium Chloride in Water for Injections.

The intravenous infusion complies with the requirements stated under Parenteral Preparations and with the following requirements.

Content of potassium chloride, KCl 95.0 to 105.0% of the prescribed or stated amount.

Content of sodium chloride, NaCl 95.0 to 105.0% of the prescribed or stated amount.

Characteristics A colourless solution.

Identification The residue on evaporation yields the reactions characteristic of *potassium salts*, the reactions characteristic of *sodium salts* and the reactions characteristic of *chlorides*, Appendix VI.

Particulate contamination When supplied in a container with a nominal content of 100 ml or more, complies with the test for *sub-visible particles*, Appendix XIII A.

Pyrogens Dilute with an equal volume of *sodium chloride injection*. The solution complies with the *test for pyrogens*, Appendix XIV D. Use 10 ml per kg of the rabbit's weight.

Assay

For potassium chloride Dilute appropriately with *water* and determine by *atomic emission spectrophotometry*, Appendix II D, measuring at 767 nm and using *potassium standard solution (600 ppm K)*, suitably diluted with *water*, to prepare the standard solutions.

For sodium chloride Dilute appropriately with *water* and determine by *atomic emission spectrophotometry*, Appendix II D, measuring at 589 nm and using *sodium standard solution (200 ppm Na)*, suitably diluted with *water*, to prepare the standard solutions.

Labelling The strength is stated as the percentages w/v of Potassium Chloride and of Sodium Chloride.

When the preparation is intended for intravenous infusion, the label also states (1) that rapid infusion may be harmful; (2) the approximate concentrations, in millimoles per litre, of the potassium ions, the sodium ions and the chloride ions.

For a preparation containing 0.3% w/v of Potassium Chloride and 0.9% w/v of Sodium Chloride, the concentrations of the ions are stated as 40 millimoles of potassium, 150 millimoles of sodium and 190 millimoles of chloride per litre.

Potassium Chloride, Sodium Chloride and Glucose Intravenous Infusion

Potassium Chloride, Sodium Chloride and Dextrose Injection; Potassium Chloride, Sodium Chloride and Glucose Injection; Potassium Chloride, Sodium Chloride and Dextrose Intravenous Infusion

Definition Potassium Chloride, Sodium Chloride and Glucose Intravenous Infusion is a sterile solution of Potassium Chloride, Sodium Chloride and either Anhydrous Glucose or Glucose in Water for Injections.

The intravenous infusion complies with the requirements stated under Parenteral Preparations and with the following requirements.

Content of potassium chloride, KCl 95.0 to 105.0% of the prescribed or stated amount.

Content of sodium chloride, NaCl 0.17 to 0.19% w/v.

Content of glucose, $C_6H_{12}O_6$ 3.8 to 4.2% w/v.

Characteristics A colourless or faintly straw-coloured solution.

Identification

A. When heated with *cupri-tartaric solution R1* a copious precipitate of copper(I) oxide is produced.

B. The residue on evaporation and ignition yields reaction B characteristic of *potassium salts*, reaction B characteristic of *sodium salts* and reaction A characteristic of *chlorides*, Appendix VI.

Acidity pH, 3.5 to 6.5, Appendix V L.

5-Hydroxymethylfurfural and related substances Dilute 25 ml to 500 ml with *water*. The *absorbance* of the resulting solution at the maximum at 284 nm is not more than 0.25, Appendix II B.

Particulate contamination When supplied in a container with a nominal content of 100 ml or more, complies with the test for *sub-visible particles*, Appendix XIII A.

Pyrogens Dilute with an equal volume of *sodium chloride injection*. The solution complies with the *test for pyrogens*, Appendix XIV D. Use 10 ml per kg of the rabbit's weight.

Assay

For potassium chloride Dilute appropriately with *water* and determine by *atomic emission spectrophotometry*, Appendix II D, measuring at 767 nm and using *potassium standard solution (600 ppm K)*, suitably diluted with *water*, to prepare the standard solutions.

For sodium chloride Dilute appropriately with *water* and determine by *atomic emission spectrophotometry*, Appendix II D, measuring at 589 nm and using *sodium standard solution (200 ppm Na)*, suitably diluted with *water*, to prepare the standard solutions.

For glucose To a quantity containing 2 to 5 g of glucose, $C_6H_{12}O_6$, add 0.2 ml of 5M *ammonia* and sufficient *water* to produce 100 ml. Mix well, allow to stand for 30 minutes and measure the *optical rotation* in a 2-dm tube, Appendix V F. The observed rotation in degrees multiplied by 0.9477 represents the weight in g of glucose, $C_6H_{12}O_6$, in the quantity of the intravenous infusion taken for assay.

Storage Potassium Chloride, Sodium Chloride and Glucose Intravenous Infusion should be stored at a temperature not exceeding 25°. The separation of small solid particles from a glass container may occur. A solution containing such particles must not be used.

Labelling The label states (1) the content of Potassium Chloride as a percentage w/v and that the preparation contains 0.18% w/v of Sodium Chloride and 4.0% w/v of glucose, $C_6H_{12}O_6$; (2) the concentration of Potassium Chloride in grams per litre and the approximate concentration of potassium ions in millimoles per litre; (3) that the preparation contains 1.8 grams per litre of Sodium Chloride, equivalent to approximately 30 millimoles of sodium ions per litre; (4) the approximate quantity of chloride ions present, in millimoles per litre; (5) that the preparation contains 40 grams per litre of glucose, $C_6H_{12}O_6$; (6) that rapid infusion may be harmful; (7) that solutions containing visible solid particles must not be used.

Effervescent Potassium Chloride Tablets

Definition Effervescent Potassium Chloride Tablets contain potassium ions and chloride ions in an effervescent basis. The proportion of chloride ions to potassium ions may vary, but the stated molar proportion of chloride ions should be not less than 66% of that of potassium ions.

The tablets comply with the requirements stated under Tablets and with the following requirements.

Content of potassium ions, K^+ 95.0 to 105.0% of the prescribed or stated amount.

Content of chloride ions, Cl^- 95.0 to 105.0% of the prescribed or stated amount.

Identification

A. The powdered tablets yield the reactions characteristic of *potassium salts* and of *chlorides*, Appendix VI.

B. Effervesce on the addition of *water*.

Disintegration The requirement for Disintegration does not apply to Effervescent Potassium Chloride Tablets.

Solution One tablet dissolves in 100 ml of *water* at 20° with brisk effervescence in not more than 3 minutes. The resulting solution is not more than faintly opalescent.

Assay Weigh and powder 20 tablets.

For potassium ions Dissolve a quantity of the powder containing 35 mg of potassium ions in sufficient *water* to produce 500 ml. Dilute 5 ml of the resulting solution to 100 ml with a 0.6% w/v solution of *strontium chloride* and determine the content of potassium by Method I for *atomic emission spectrophotometry*, Appendix II D, measuring at 767 nm and using *potassium standard solution (600 ppm K)*, suitably diluted with a 0.6% w/v solution of *strontium chloride*, to prepare the standard solutions.

For chloride ions Dissolve a quantity of the powder containing 0.12 g of chloride ions in *water*, dilute to 50 ml with *water* and titrate with 0.1M *silver nitrate VS* using *potassium chromate solution* as indicator. Each ml of 0.1M *silver nitrate VS* is equivalent to 3.545 mg of Cl.

Storage Effervescent Potassium Chloride Tablets should be stored at a temperature not exceeding 25°.

Labelling The label states (1) the content of potassium ions and the content of chloride ions in terms of the weight and the number of millimoles of ion present in each tablet; (2) that the tablets must be dissolved before administration; (3) directions for dissolving the tablets before administration.

When Effervescent Potassium Chloride Tablets are prescribed or demanded, the amount of potassium required in each tablet must be specified.

Slow Potassium Chloride Tablets

Definition Slow Potassium Chloride Tablets contain Potassium Chloride and are formulated so as to release the medicament over a period of several hours. They are coated.

With the exception of the requirements for shape, the tablets comply with the requirements stated under Tablets and with the following requirements.

Content of potassium chloride, KCl 95.0 to 105.0% of the prescribed or stated amount.

Identification Stir 3 tablets in successive 20-ml portions of *water* until the outer coating is removed and separate the cores from the water. The powdered cores comply with the following tests.

A. Yield reaction A characteristic of *chlorides*, Appendix VI.

B. Yield the reactions characteristic of *potassium salts*, Appendix VI.

Dissolution Carry out the *dissolution test for tablets and capsules*, Appendix XII D, using Apparatus II. Use as the medium 900 ml of *water* and rotate the paddle at 50 revolutions per minute. Withdraw a sample of 10 ml of the medium after 1, 2 and 6 hours and treat each sample in the following manner. Add 25 ml of *water*, 5 ml of a 25% v/v solution of *glacial acetic acid* and 0.1 ml of a saturated solution of *potassium sulphate* and titrate with 0.01M *silver nitrate VS* determining the end point potentiometrically. Each ml of 0.01M *silver nitrate VS* is equivalent to 0.7455 mg of KCl. The amount of potassium chloride released after 1 hour is not more than 50%, after 2 hours is not less than 25% and not more than 75%, and after 6 hours is not less than 75%, calculated with reference to the declared content of Potassium Chloride.

Assay Shake 10 whole tablets with 400 ml of *water* for 30 minutes then heat on a water bath for 45 minutes. Cool, add sufficient *water* to produce 500 ml and allow to stand for 24 hours. Filter and dilute to give a suitable concentration. Carry out the method for *atomic emission spectrophotometry*, Appendix II D, measuring at 766.5 nm and using *potassium standard solution (600 ppm K)*, suitably diluted with *water*, to prepare the standard solutions. Each mg of potassium is equivalent to 1.908 mg of KCl.

Potassium Citrate Mixture

Potassium Citrate Oral Solution

Definition Potassium Citrate Mixture is an *oral solution* containing 30% w/v of Potassium Citrate and 5% w/v of Citric Acid Monohydrate in a suitable vehicle with a lemon flavour. It is intended to be diluted with water before use.

Extemporaneous preparation It is recently prepared according to the following formula.

Potassium Citrate	300 g
Citric Acid Monohydrate	50 g
Lemon Spirit	5 ml
Quillaia Tincture	10 ml
Syrup	250 ml
Double-strength Chloroform Water	300 ml
Water	sufficient to produce 1000 ml

The mixture complies with the requirements stated under Oral Liquids and with the following requirements.

Content of citric acid monohydrate, $C_6H_8O_7,H_2O$ 4.75 to 5.25% w/v.

Content of potassium citrate, $C_6H_5K_3O_7,H_2O$ 28.5 to 31.5% w/v.

Identification

A. Yields reaction A characteristic of *potassium salts*, Appendix VI.

B. Yields reaction B characteristic of *citrates*, Appendix VI.

Assay

For citric acid monohydrate To 5 ml add 100 ml of *water*, boil, cool and titrate with carbonate-free 0.1M *sodium hydroxide VS* using *thymol blue solution* as indicator. Each ml of carbonate-free 0.1M *sodium hydroxide VS* is equivalent to 7.005 mg of $C_6H_8O_7,H_2O$.

For potassium citrate To 1 g add 5 ml of *acetic anhydride* and 20 ml of *anhydrous acetic acid*, heat on a water bath for 20 minutes, allow to cool and carry out Method I for *non-aqueous titration*, Appendix VIII A, using *1-naphtholbenzein solution* as indicator. Each ml of 0.1M *perchloric acid VS* is equivalent to 10.81 mg of $C_6H_5K_3O_7,H_2O$. Determine the *weight per ml* of the mixture, Appendix V G, and calculate the content of $C_6H_5K_3O_7,H_2O$, weight in volume.

Labelling The label states that the mixture should be well diluted with water before use.

The label indicates the pharmaceutical form as 'oral solution'.

Potassium Hydroxide Solution

Potash Solution

Definition Potassium Hydroxide Solution is a solution of Potassium Hydroxide in Purified Water.

Content of total alkali, calculated as KOH 4.9 to 5.1% w/v.

Characteristics A colourless solution.

Identification Strongly alkaline and when neutralised with 2M *hydrochloric acid* yields the reactions characteristic of *potassium salts*, Appendix VI.

Weight per ml 1.040 to 1.050 g, Appendix V G.

Assay Titrate 20 ml with 1M *hydrochloric acid VS* using *methyl orange solution* as indicator. Each ml of 1M *hydrochloric acid VS* is equivalent to 56.11 mg of total alkali, calculated as KOH.

Storage Potassium Hydroxide Solution should be kept in a well-closed container of lead-free glass or of a suitable plastic.

Labelling The label states (1) the date after which the solution is not intended to be used; (2) the conditions under which it should be stored.

Potassium Hydroxyquinoline Sulphate and Benzoyl Peroxide Cream

Definition Potassium Hydroxyquinoline Sulphate and Benzoyl Peroxide Cream contains Potassium Hydroxyquinoline Sulphate and Hydrous Benzoyl Peroxide in a suitable astringent basis.

The cream complies with the requirements stated under Topical Semi-solid Preparations and with the following requirements.

Content of potassium hydroxyquinoline sulphate, $(C_9H_7NO)_2,H_2SO_4:K_2SO_4$ 90.0 to 110.0% of the prescribed or stated amount.

Content of anhydrous benzoyl peroxide, $C_{14}H_{10}O_4$ 90.0 to 110.0% of the prescribed or stated amount.

Identification

A. Carry out the method for *thin-layer chromatography*, Appendix III A, using *silica gel GF_{254}* as the coating substance and a mixture of 2 volumes of *glacial acetic acid*, 4 volumes of *dichloromethane* and 100 volumes of *toluene* as the mobile phase. Apply separately to the plate 5 µl of each of the following solutions. For solution (1) shake a quantity of the cream containing the equivalent of 50 mg of anhydrous benzoyl peroxide with 10 ml of *chloroform* and filter. Solution (2) contains 0.5% w/v of *benzoyl peroxide* in *chloroform*. After removal of the plate, allow it to dry in air and examine under *ultraviolet light (254 nm)*. The principal spot in the chromatogram obtained with solution (1) corresponds to that in the chromatogram obtained with solution (2).

B. Add 20 ml of *methanol* to a quantity of the cream containing 10 mg of Potassium Hydroxyquinoline Sulphate, heat in a water bath, shaking occasionally, cool and filter through *anhydrous sodium sulphate*. To 10 ml of the filtrate add 5 ml of a 0.5% w/v solution of *iron(II) sulphate* in *methanol (70%)*. A dark blue or green colour is produced immediately.

Related substances Carry out the method for *liquid chromatography*, Appendix III D, using the following solutions. For solution (1) dilute 2 volumes of solution (2) to 100 volumes with the mobile phase. For solution (2) disperse a quantity of the cream containing the equivalent of 0.10 g of anhydrous benzoyl peroxide with 25 ml of *acetonitrile* by shaking vigorously, add sufficient *water* to produce 50 ml, mix and filter. Solution (3) contains 0.020% w/v of *benzoic acid* in the mobile phase. Solution (4) contains 0.0020% w/v of *ethyl benzoate* in the mobile phase. Solution (5) contains 0.0020% w/v of *benzaldehyde* in the mobile phase.

The chromatographic procedure may be carried out using (a) a stainless steel column (20 cm × 4.6 mm) packed with *stationary phase C* (10 µm) (Spherisorb ODS 1 is suitable), (b) a mixture of 1 volume of *glacial acetic acid*, 500 volumes of *acetonitrile and* 500 volumes of *water* as the mobile phase with a flow rate of 1 ml per minute and (c) a detection wavelength of 235 nm.

In the chromatogram obtained with solution (2) the areas of any peaks corresponding to benzoic acid, ethyl benzoate and benzaldehyde are not greater than the areas of the principal peaks in the chromatograms obtained with solutions (3) (10%), (4) (1%) and (5) (1%) respectively. The area of any other *secondary peak* is not greater than half of the area of the principal peak in the chromatogram obtained with solution (1) (0.5%).

Assay

For potassium hydroxyquinoline sulphate Shake vigorously a quantity of the cream containing 35 mg of Potassium Hydroxyquinoline Sulphate with 50 ml of *chloroform* and 10 ml of 13.5M *ammonia* for 5 minutes. Separate and reserve the chloroform layer and extract the aqueous layer with a further 50 ml of *chloroform*. Extract the combined chloroform layers with two 50-ml quantities of 3.5M *hydrochloric acid*, combine the extracts, wash gently with three 50-ml quantities of *chloroform* and discard the chloroform layers. Add 50 ml of 0.01M *bromine VS*, stopper the flask, shake for 20 minutes and allow to stand for 20 minutes. Add 10 ml of *dilute potassium iodide solution* and titrate with 0.02M *sodium thiosulphate VS* using *starch solution*, added towards the end of the titration, as indicator. Repeat the titration using 100 ml of 3.5M *hydrochloric acid* and beginning at the words 'Add 50 ml ...'. The difference between the titrations represents the amount of bromine required. Each ml of 0.01M *bromine VS* is equivalent to 1.107 mg of $(C_9H_7NO)_2,H_2SO_4.K_2SO_4$.

For benzoyl peroxide Shake gently a quantity of the cream containing the equivalent of 0.4 g of anhydrous benzoyl peroxide with 50 ml of *chloroform* until the cream has dispersed and filter the lower layer excluding any solid matter that separates at the interface. Repeat the extraction with two further 50-ml quantities of *chloroform*, wash the filter with *chloroform*, combine the extracts and washings and dilute to 250 ml with *chloroform*. To 25 ml of the chloroform extract add 40 ml of a 0.0005% w/v solution of *iron(III) chloride hexahydrate* in *glacial acetic acid* and 10 ml of *dilute potassium iodide solution* and shake for 20 minutes protected from light. Add 60 ml of *water* and titrate with 0.0125M *sodium thiosulphate VS* using *starch solution*, added towards the end of the titration, as indicator. Repeat the titration using 25 ml of *chloroform* in place of the chloroform extract. The difference between the titrations represents the amount of sodium thiosulphate required. Each ml of 0.0125M *sodium thiosulphate VS* is equivalent to 1.514 mg of $C_{14}H_{10}O_4$.

Labelling The content of Hydrous Benzoyl Peroxide is stated in terms of the equivalent amount of anhydrous benzoyl peroxide.

Potassium Iodate Tablets

Definition Potassium Iodate Tablets contain Potassium Iodate.

The tablets comply with the requirements stated under Tablets and with the following requirements.

Content of potassium iodate, KIO_3 95.0 to 105.0% of the prescribed or stated amount.

Identification

A. Shake a quantity of the powdered tablets containing 0.4 g of Potassium Iodate with 10 ml of *water* and filter (solution A). 1 ml of solution A yields reaction B characteristic of *potassium salts*, Appendix VI.

B. Add 1 g of *potassium iodide* and 1 ml of *hydrochloric acid* to 5 ml of solution A and shake. A brown colour is produced.

Dissolution Comply with the *dissolution test for tablets and capsules*, Appendix XII D, using as the medium 900 ml of *water* and rotating the basket at 100 revolutions per minute. Filter the medium after first wetting the filter paper with *water* and note the volume of filtrate. Treat the filtrate as described under Assay beginning at the words 'To 50 ml of the filtrate...'. Repeat the assay procedure without the dissolution medium. Calculate the total content of potassium iodate, KIO_3, in the dissolution medium from the difference between the titrations.

Iodide Shake a quantity of the powdered tablets containing 2.5 g of Potassium Iodate with 50 ml *water* and filter (solution B). Add 1 ml of 1.8M *sulphuric acid* and 1 ml of *chloroform* to 25 ml of solution B and shake. Any violet colour produced is not more intense than that of a solution prepared at the same time and in the same manner but using 5 ml of solution B and 2 ml of a solution containing 1.31% w/v of *potassium iodide* (0.002%).

Assay Weigh and powder 20 tablets. Transfer a quantity of the powdered tablets containing 0.3 g of Potassium Iodate to an iodine flask, add 100 ml of *water*, shake and filter. To 50 ml of the filtrate add 3 g of *potassium iodide* followed by 50 ml of 2M *hydrochloric acid*. Stopper the flask, mix and stand in the dark for 5 minutes. Titrate the resulting solution with 0.1M *sodium thiosulphate VS* to a light straw colour and then complete the titration to a colourless end point using *starch solution* as indicator. Repeat the titration without the powdered tablets. The difference between the titrations represents the amount of sodium thiosulphate required. Each ml of 0.1M *sodium thiosulphate VS* is equivalent to 3.567 mg of KIO_3.

Povidone—Iodine Solution

Definition Povidone—Iodine Solution is either an aqueous solution of Iodinated Povidone or it is prepared by the interaction between Iodine and Povidone. It is a *cutaneous solution.*

The solution complies with the requirements stated under Liquids for Cutaneous Application and with the following requirements.

Content of available iodine, I 0.85 to 1.20% w/v.

Characteristics A deep brown liquid; odour, characteristic of iodine.

Identification

A. Dilute 1 ml to 20 ml with *water* and add 1 ml of the resulting solution to a mixture of 1 ml of *starch mucilage* and 9 ml of *water*. A deep blue colour is produced.

B. Transfer 10 ml to a small flask and cover the mouth of the flask with filter paper moistened with 0.05 ml of *starch mucilage*. No blue colour is produced on the paper within 60 seconds.

C. Dilute 20 ml to 100 ml with *water*. To 10 ml add dropwise 0.1M *sodium thiosulphate* until the colour of the iodine is just discharged. Reserve 5 ml of the resulting solution for test D. To 5 ml of the solution add 10 ml of 1M *hydrochloric acid* and 5 ml of a 7.0% w/v solution of *potassium dichromate*. A red precipitate is produced.

D. To 5 ml of the solution reserved in test C add 2 ml of *ammonium cobaltothiocyanate solution* previously acidified with 5M *hydrochloric acid*. A blue precipitate is produced.

Acidity pH, 3.0 to 6.5, Appendix V L.

Iodide Not more than 0.6% w/v when determined by the following method. Dilute 5 ml of the solution being examined to 100 ml with *water* and add *sodium metabisulphite* until the colour of iodine has disappeared. Add 25 ml of 0.1M *silver nitrate VS*, 10 ml of *nitric acid* and 5 ml of *ferric ammonium sulphate solution R2*. Titrate with 0.1M *ammonium thiocyanate VS*. Repeat the procedure without the solution being examined. Each ml of 0.1M *silver nitrate VS* is equivalent to 12.69 mg of total iodine. Calculate the percentage content of total iodine and subtract the percentage content of available iodine determined in the Assay to obtain the percentage content of iodide.

Assay To 10 ml add 10 ml of 0.1M *hydrochloric acid* and sufficient *water* to produce 150 ml and titrate with 0.02M *sodium thiosulphate VS* determining the end point potentiometrically. Each ml of 0.02M *sodium thiosulphate VS* is equivalent to 2.538 mg of I.

Storage Povidone—Iodine Solution should be kept in a well-closed container.

Labelling The label states (1) the date after which the solution is not intended to be used; (2) the conditions under which it should be stored.

The label states the pharmaceutical form as 'cutaneous solution'.

Prazosin Tablets

Definition Prazosin Tablets contain Prazosin Hydrochloride.

The tablets comply with the requirements stated under Tablets and with the following requirements.

Content of prazosin, $C_{19}H_{21}N_5O_4$ 90.0 to 110% of the prescribed or stated amount.

Identification Shake a quantity of the powdered tablets containing the equivalent of 10 mg of prazosin with a mixture of 10 ml of *dichloromethane* and 10 ml of 0.05M *potassium hydroxide*, filter the organic layer through absorbent cotton, evaporate to dryness and dry the residue at 60° at a pressure not exceeding 2 kPa for 2 hours. The *infrared absorption spectrum* of the residue, Appendix II A, is concordant with the reference spectrum of prazosin.

Uniformity of content Tablets containing less than the equivalent of 2 mg of prazosin comply with the requirements stated under Tablets using the following method of analysis. Carry out the method for *liquid chromatography*, Appendix III D, using the following solutions in a mixture of 96 volumes of *methanol*, 2 volumes of *glacial acetic acid* and 2 volumes of *water*. Solution (1) contains 0.00220% w/v of *prazosin hydrochloride BPCRS*. For solution (2) shake one tablet for 1 hour in a suitable volume of the solvent to produce a solution containing the equivalent of 0.002% w/v of prazosin, centrifuge and use the supernatant liquid.

The chromatographic procedure may be carried out using (a) a stainless steel column (20 cm × 4 mm) packed with *stationary phase A* (5 µm) (Zorbax Sil is suitable), (b) 0.01% w/v of *diethylamine* in a mixture of 96 volumes of *methanol*, 2 volumes of *glacial acetic acid* and 2 volumes of *water* as the mobile phase with a flow rate of 1 ml per minute and (c) a detection wavelength of 254 nm.

Calculate the content of $C_{19}H_{21}N_5O_4$ using the declared content of $C_{19}H_{21}N_5O_4$ in prazosin hydrochloride BPCRS.

Related substances Carry out the method for *thin-layer chromatography*, Appendix III A, using a silica gel GF_{254} precoated plate (Analtech Uniplates are suitable) and a mixture of 95 volumes of *ethyl acetate* and 5 volumes of *diethylamine* as the mobile phase. Apply separately to the plate 20 µl of each of the following solutions. For solution (1) shake a quantity of the powdered tablets containing the equivalent of 5 mg of prazosin with 2 ml of a mixture of 95 volumes of *chloroform* and 5 volumes of *diethylamine*, centrifuge and pass the supernatant liquid through a 0.5 µm PTFE filter. For solution (2) dilute 1 volume of solution (1) to 200 volumes with the same solvent. For solution (3) dilute 2 volumes of solution (2) to 5 volumes with the same solvent. After removal of the plate, allow it to dry in air and examine under *ultraviolet light (254 nm)*. Any secondary spot in the chromatogram obtained with solution (1) is not more intense than the spot in the chromatogram obtained with solution (2) and not more than two such spots are more intense than the spot in the chromatogram obtained with solution (3).

Assay Weigh and powder 20 tablets. Carry out the method for *liquid chromatography*, Appendix III D, using the following solutions in a mixture of 96 volumes of *methanol*, 2 volumes of *glacial acetic acid* and 2 volumes of *water*. Solution (1) contains 0.00220% of *prazosin hydrochloride BPCRS*. For solution (2) shake a quantity of the powdered tablets containing the equivalent of 2 mg of prazosin with 100 ml of the solvent mixture for 30 minutes, centrifuge and use the supernatant liquid.

The chromatographic procedure described under Uniformity of content may be used.

Calculate the content of $C_{19}H_{21}N_5O_4$ using the declared content of $C_{19}H_{21}N_5O_4$ in *prazosin hydrochloride BPCRS*.

Labelling The quantity of active ingredient is stated in terms of the equivalent amount of prazosin.

Prednisolone Enema

Definition Prednisolone Enema is a solution of Prednisolone Sodium Phosphate in Purified Water. It contains suitable buffering and stabilising agents and a suitable antimicrobial preservative.

The enema complies with the requirements stated under Rectal Preparations and with the following requirements.

Content of prednisolone, $C_{21}H_{28}O_5$ 90.0 to 115.0% of the prescribed or stated amount.

Identification

A. In the Assay, the chromatogram obtained with solution (1) shows a peak having the same retention time as the peak due to prednisolone sodium phosphate in the chromatogram obtained with solution (2).

B. Evaporate 5 ml to dryness on a water bath, cool and dissolve the residue in 0.5 ml of *sulphuric acid*. A dark red colour is produced.

Acidity or alkalinity pH, 5.5 to 7.5, Appendix V L.

Free prednisolone Carry out the method for *thin-layer chromatography*, Appendix III A, using *silica gel GF_{254}* as the coating substance and a mixture of equal volumes of *acetone* and *toluene* as the mobile phase. Apply separately to the plate 25 µl of each of the following solutions. For solution (1) dilute a volume of the enema containing the equivalent of 2.0 mg of prednisolone with sufficient *water* to produce 25 ml, add 2.5 g of *sodium chloride* and 1 ml of *hydrochloric acid*, extract with three 25-ml quantities of *chloroform* and wash each extract with the same 1-ml quantity of 0.1M *hydrochloric acid* in a second separating funnel. Evaporate the combined chloroform extracts to about 5 ml using a rotary evaporator, transfer to a 15-ml stoppered tube and rinse the rotary evaporator flask with a few millilitres of *chloroform*, adding the rinsings to the tube. Evaporate in a gentle current of nitrogen and dissolve the residue in 1 ml of *chloroform*. Solution (2) contains 0.0134% w/v of *prednisolone BPCRS* in *chloroform*. After removal of the plate, allow it to dry and examine under *ultraviolet light (254 nm)*. Any spot in the chromatogram obtained with solution (1) corresponding to prednisolone is not more intense than the spot in the chromatogram obtained with solution (2).

Assay Carry out the method for *liquid chromatography*, Appendix III D, using the following solutions. For solution (1) dilute, if necessary, a quantity of the enema containing the equivalent of 2 mg of prednisolone to 10 ml with *water*, add 10 ml of *water*, extract with three 20-ml quantities of *chloroform* and discard the lower layer. For solution (2) dissolve 55 mg of *prednisolone sodium* *phosphate BPCRS* in *water* and dilute to 200 ml (solution A); to 10 ml of solution A add 10 ml of a 0.035% w/v solution of *betamethasone sodium phosphate* in *water* (internal standard), extract with three 20-ml quantities of *chloroform* and discard the lower layer. Prepare solution (3) in the same manner as solution (1) but add 10 ml of a 0.035% w/v solution of *betamethasone sodium phosphate* in *water* in place of the 10 ml of water.

The chromatographic procedure may be carried out using (a) a stainless steel column (20 cm × 5 mm) packed with *stationary phase C* (10 µm) (Spherisorb ODS 1 is suitable) and maintained at 60°, (b) a mixture of 45 volumes of *methanol* and 55 volumes of *citro-phosphate buffer pH 5.0* as the mobile phase with a flow rate of 2 ml per minute and (c) a detection wavelength of 247 nm.

Calculate the content of $C_{21}H_{28}O_5$ in solution A by measuring the *absorbance*, Appendix II B, of a solution obtained by diluting 1 volume of solution A to 10 volumes with *water* at the maximum at 247 nm and taking 419 as the value of A(1%, 1 cm) at the maximum at 247 nm. Calculate the content of $C_{21}H_{28}O_5$ in the enema using peak areas.

Storage Prednisolone Enema should be protected from light and stored at a temperature not exceeding 25°.

Labelling The content of Prednisolone Sodium Phosphate is stated in terms of the equivalent amount of prednisolone.

The label states (1) the date after which the enema is not intended to be used; (2) the conditions under which it should be stored.

The label states the pharmaceutical form as 'rectal solution'.

Prednisolone Sodium Phosphate Eye Drops

Definition Prednisolone Sodium Phosphate Eye Drops are a sterile solution of Prednisolone Sodium Phosphate in Purified Water.

The eye drops comply with the requirements stated under Eye Preparations and with the following requirements.

Content of prednisolone sodium phosphate, $C_{21}H_{27}Na_2O_8P$ 90.0 to 115.0% of the prescribed or stated amount.

Identification *For eye drops containing less than 0.1% w/v of Prednisolone Sodium Phosphate carry out test B only.*

A. Carry out the method for *thin-layer chromatography*, Appendix III A, using *silica gel GF_{254}* as the coating substance and a mixture of 20 volumes of *acetic anhydride*, 20 volumes of *water* and 60 volumes of *butan-1-ol*, prepared immediately before use, as the mobile phase. Apply separately to the plate 10 µl of each of the following solutions. For solution (1) use the eye drops diluted, if necessary, with *water* to contain 0.1% w/v of Prednisolone Sodium Phosphate. Solution (2) contains 0.1% w/v of *prednisolone sodium phosphate BPCRS* in *water*. Solution (3) is a mixture of equal volumes of solutions (1) and (2). Solution (4) is a mixture of equal volumes of solution (2) and a 0.1% w/v solution of *betamethasone sodium phosphate BPCRS* in *water*. After removal of the plate, allow it to dry in air, heat at 110° for 10 minutes and examine under *ultraviolet light (254 nm)*. The chromatograms obtained with solutions (1), (2) and (3) show single principal spots with similar Rf values. The chromatogram obtained with solution (4) shows two principal spots with almost identical Rf values.

B. In the Assay, the chromatogram obtained with solution (1) shows a peak with the same retention time as the peak due to prednisolone sodium phosphate in the chromatogram obtained with solution (2).

C. To a volume containing 0.2 mg of Prednisolone Sodium Phosphate slowly add 1 ml of *sulphuric acid* and allow to stand for 2 minutes. A deep red colour is produced.

Acidity or alkalinity pH, 7.0 to 8.5, Appendix V L.

Free prednisolone Carry out the method for *liquid chromatography*, Appendix III D. For eye drops containing 0.010% w/v or more of Prednisolone Sodium Phosphate use 50 µl of the following solutions. Solution (1) contains 0.00040% w/v of *prednisolone BPCRS* in the mobile phase. Prepare solution (2) in the following manner. Dilute the eye drops, if necessary, with the mobile phase to produce a solution containing 0.010% w/v of Prednisolone Sodium Phosphate. For eye drops containing less than 0.010% w/v of Prednisolone Sodium Phosphate, use 0.2 ml of the following solutions. Solution (1) contains 0.00004% w/v of *prednisolone BPCRS* in the mobile phase. For solution (2) dilute the eye drops, if necessary, with the mobile phase to produce a solution containing 0.0010% w/v of Prednisolone Sodium Phosphate.

The chromatographic procedure may be carried out using (a) a stainless steel column (20 cm × 4.6 mm) packed with *stationary phase C* (10 µm) (Spherisorb ODS 1 is suitable), (b) a mixture of 45 volumes of *methanol* and 55 volumes of *citro-phosphate buffer pH 5.0* as the mobile phase with a flow rate of 2 ml per minute and (c) a detection wavelength of 247 nm.

In the chromatogram obtained with solution (2) the area of any peak corresponding to prednisolone is not greater than the area of the principal peak in the chromatogram obtained with solution (1) (4%).

Assay Carry out the method for *liquid chromatography*, Appendix III D, using 50 µl of the following solutions. For solution (1) dilute a quantity of the eye drops, if necessary, to contain 0.001% w/v of Prednisolone Sodium Phosphate. For solution (2) dissolve 10 mg of *prednisolone sodium phosphate BPCRS* in sufficient *water* to produce 100 ml (solution A) and dilute 10 ml of the solution to 100 ml. For solution (3) add 10 ml of a 0.01% w/v solution of *betamethasone sodium phosphate BPCRS* in *water* to 10 ml of solution A and dilute to 100 ml with *water*.

The chromatographic procedure may be carried out using (a) a stainless steel column (20 cm × 4.6 mm) packed with *stationary phase C* (10 µm) (Spherisorb ODS 1 is suitable), (b) a mixture of 45 volumes of *methanol* and 55 volumes of *citro-phosphate buffer pH 5.0* as the mobile phase with a flow rate of 2 ml per minute and (c) a detection wavelength of 247 nm.

The assay is not valid unless the *resolution factor* between the peaks due to betamethasone sodium phosphate and prednisolone sodium phosphate in the chromatogram obtained with solution (3) is at least 3.

Calculate the content of $C_{21}H_{27}Na_2O_8P$ in solution A by measuring the *absorbance*, Appendix II B, of a solution obtained by diluting 1 volume of solution A to 4 volumes with *water* at the maximum at 247 nm and taking 312 as the value of A(1%, 1 cm) at the maximum at 247 nm. Calculate the content of $C_{21}H_{27}Na_2O_8P$ in the eye drops using peak areas.

Storage Prednisolone Sodium Phosphate Eye Drops should be protected from light and stored at a temperature not exceeding 25°.

Prednisolone Tablets

Definition Prednisolone Tablets contain Prednisolone.

The tablets comply with the requirements stated under Tablets and with the following requirements.

Content of prednisolone, $C_{21}H_{28}O_5$ 90.0 to 110.0% of the prescribed or stated amount.

Identification Extract a quantity of the powdered tablets with *acetone*, filter and evaporate the filtrate to dryness. The residue complies with the following tests.

A. The *infrared absorption spectrum*, Appendix II A, is concordant with the *reference spectrum* of prednisolone.

B. Complies with the test for the Identification of steroids, Appendix III A, using *impregnating solvent I* and *mobile phase A*.

Related substances Carry out the method for *thin-layer chromatography*, Appendix III A, using *silica gel GF_{254}* as the coating substance and a mixture of 1.2 volumes of *water*, 8 volumes of *methanol*, 15 volumes of *ether* and 77 volumes of *dichloromethane* as the mobile phase. Apply separately to the plate 5 µl of each of the following solutions. For solution (1) shake a quantity of the powdered tablets containing 50 mg of Prednisolone with 25 ml of *chloroform*, filter and evaporate the filtrate to a volume of about 10 ml. For solution (2) dilute 1 volume of solution (1) to 50 volumes with a mixture of equal volumes of *chloroform* and *methanol*. After removal of the plate, allow it to dry in air and examine under *ultraviolet light (254 nm)*. Heat at 105° for 10 minutes, cool and spray with *alkaline tetrazolium blue solution*. By each method of visualisation, any *secondary spot* in the chromatogram obtained with solution (1) is not more intense than the spot in the chromatogram obtained with solution (2) (2%).

Uniformity of content Tablets containing less than 2 mg of Prednisolone comply with the requirements stated under Tablets using the following method of analysis. Carry out the method for *liquid chromatography*, Appendix III D, using the following solutions. Solution (1) contains 0.0050% w/v of *prednisolone EPCRS* and 0.0075% w/v of *dexamethasone* (internal standard) in the mobile phase. For solution (2) add 20 ml of the mobile phase to one tablet, mix with the aid of ultrasound for at least 10 minutes, mix thoroughly, centrifuge and use the supernatant liquid. Prepare solution (3) in the same manner as solution (2) but using a 0.0075% w/v solution of the internal standard in the mobile phase in place of the mobile phase.

The chromatographic procedure may be carried out using (a) a stainless steel column (20 cm × 4.6 mm) packed with *stationary phase C* (5 µm) (Spherisorb ODS 1 is suitable), (b) a mixture of 58 volumes of *methanol* and 42 volumes of *water* as the mobile phase with a flow rate of 1.5 ml per minute and (c) a detection wavelength of 254 nm.

The test is not valid unless the *resolution factor* between the peaks due to prednisolone and dexamethasone is greater than 2.5 and the *column efficiency*, determined using the peak due to prednisolone in the chromatogram obtained with solution (1), is greater than 15,000 theoretical plates per metre.

Calculate the content of $C_{21}H_{28}O_5$ taking 100.0% as the content of $C_{21}H_{28}O_5$ in *prednisolone EPCRS*.

Dissolution Tablets containing less than 2 mg of Prednisolone comply with the *dissolution test for tablets and capsules*, Appendix XII D, using as the medium 900 ml of *water* and rotating the basket at 100 revolutions per minute.

Carry out the method for *liquid chromatography*, Appendix III D, injecting 0.2 ml of each of the following solutions. For solution (1) prepare a 0.1% w/v solution of *prednisolone EPCRS* in *methanol* and dilute with *water* to contain 0.0001% w/v. For solution (2) use the dissolution medium diluted, if necessary, with *water* to contain 0.0001% w/v of prednisolone.

The chromatographic procedure described under Uniformity of content may be used.

The test is not valid unless the *column efficiency*, determined using the peak due to prednisolone in the chromatogram obtained with solution (1), is greater than 15,000 theoretical plates per metre.

Calculate the total content of $C_{21}H_{28}O_5$ in the medium taking 100.0% as the content of $C_{21}H_{28}O_5$ in *prednisolone EPCRS*.

Assay Weigh and powder 20 tablets. Carry out the method for *liquid chromatography*, Appendix III D, using the following solutions. Solution (1) contains 0.005% w/v of *prednisolone EPCRS* and 0.0075% w/v of *dexamethasone* (internal standard) in a mixture of 58 volumes of *methanol* and 42 volumes of *water*. For solution (2) add 58 ml of *methanol* to a quantity of the powder containing 5 mg of Prednisolone, shake for 10 minutes, add sufficient *water* to produce 100 ml, mix and filter. Prepare solution (3) in the same manner as solution (2) but add 10 ml of a 0.075% w/v solution of *dexamethasone* in *methanol* and 48 ml of *methanol* in place of the 58 ml of methanol.

The chromatographic procedure may be carried out using (a) a stainless steel column (20 cm × 4.6 mm) packed with *stationary phase C* (5 µm) (Spherisorb ODS 1 is suitable), (b) a mixture of 42 volumes of *water* and 58 volumes of *methanol* as the mobile phase with a flow rate of about 1 ml per minute and (c) a detection wavelength of 254 nm.

The assay is not valid unless the *resolution factor* between the peaks due to prednisolone and dexamethasone is greater than 2.5 and the *column efficiency*, determined using the peak due to prednisolone in the chromatogram obtained with solution (1), is greater than 15,000 *theoretical plates* per metre.

Calculate the content of $C_{21}H_{28}O_5$ in the tablets using the declared content of $C_{21}H_{28}O_5$ in *prednisolone EPCRS*.

Storage Prednisolone Tablets should be protected from light.

Enteric-coated Prednisolone Tablets

Gastro-resistant Prednisolone Tablets

Definition Enteric-coated Prednisolone Tablets contain Prednisolone. They are enteric-coated.

The tablets comply with the requirements stated under Tablets and with the following requirements.

Content of prednisolone, $C_{21}H_{28}O_5$ 95.0 to 105.0% of the prescribed or stated amount.

Identification

A. Extract a quantity of the powdered tablets with *dichloromethane*, filter and evaporate the filtrate to dryness. The residue complies with the test for *identification of steroids*, Appendix III A, using *impregnating solvent I* and *mobile phase A*.

B. In the Assay, the chromatogram obtained with solution (2) shows a peak having the same retention time as the peak due to prednisolone in the chromatogram obtained with solution (1).

Related substances Carry out the method for *thin-layer chromatography*, Appendix III A, using a silica gel F_{254} precoated plate (Merck plates are suitable) and as the mobile phase a mixture of 1.2 volumes of *water*, 8 volumes of *methanol*, 15 volumes of *ether* and 77 volumes of *dichloromethane*. Apply separately to the plate 10 µl of each of the following solutions. For solution (1) shake a quantity of the powdered tablets containing 50 mg of Prednisolone with 25 ml of *dichloromethane*, filter and evaporate the filtrate to a volume of about 10 ml. For solution (2) dilute 1 volume of solution (1) to 50 volumes with a mixture of equal volumes of *dichloromethane* and *methanol*. After removal of the plate, allow it to dry in air and examine under *ultraviolet light (254 nm)*. Heat at 105° for 10 minutes, cool and spray with *alkaline tetrazolium blue solution*. By each method of visualisation, any *secondary spot* in the chromatogram obtained with solution (1) is not more intense than the spot in the chromatogram obtained with solution (2) (2%).

Dissolution Comply with the *dissolution test for tablets and capsules*, Appendix XII D. Using the apparatus described in the *disintegration test for enteric-coated tablets*, Appendix XII B, introduce one tablet into each of six tubes and operate the apparatus without the discs for 60 minutes in 0.1M *hydrochloric acid*. Remove the tablets and use these tablets to carry out the dissolution test using 900 ml of *mixed phosphate buffer pH 6.8* and rotating the basket at 100 revolutions per minute. Withdraw a sample of 20 ml of the medium and filter through a membrane filter having a nominal pore size not greater than 0.45 µm, discarding the first 10 ml of filtrate.

Carry out the method for *liquid chromatography*, Appendix III D, injecting 20 µl of each of the following solutions. For solution (1) prepare a 0.05% w/v solution of *prednisolone EPCRS* in a mixture of 42 volumes of *water* and 58 volumes of *methanol* and dilute with the dissolution medium to contain 0.00025% w/v. For solution (2) use the filtered sample diluted, if necessary, with the dissolution medium to contain 0.00025% w/v of prednisolone.

The chromatographic procedure may be carried out using (a) a stainless steel column (20 cm × 4.6 mm) packed with *stationary phase C* (10 µm) (Spherisorb ODS 1 is suitable), (b) a mixture of 42 volumes of *water* and 58 volumes of *methanol* as the mobile phase with a flow rate of 1 ml per minute and (c) a detection wavelength of 254 nm.

The test is not valid unless the *column efficiency*, determined using the peak due to prednisolone in the chromatogram obtained with solution (1), is greater than 15,000 theoretical plates per metre.

Calculate the content of $C_{21}H_{28}O_5$ in the medium using the declared content of $C_{21}H_{28}O_5$ in *prednisolone EPCRS*.

Assay Weigh and powder 20 tablets. Carry out the method for *liquid chromatography*, Appendix III D, using the following solutions. Solution (1) contains 0.005% w/v of *prednisolone EPCRS* and 0.0075% w/v of *dexamethasone* (internal standard) in a mixture of 42 volumes of *water* and 58 volumes of *methanol*. For solution (2) add 58 ml of *methanol* to a quantity of the powder containing 5 mg of Prednisolone, shake for 10 minutes, add sufficient *water* to produce 100 ml, mix and filter. Prepare solution (3) in the same manner as solution (2) but add 10 ml of a 0.075% w/v solution of *dexamethasone* in *methanol* and 48 ml of *methanol* in place of the 58 ml of methanol.

The chromatographic procedure described under Dissolution may be used.

The assay is not valid unless the *resolution factor* between the peaks due to prednisolone and dexamethasone is greater than 2.5 and the *column efficiency*, determined using the peak due to prednisolone in the chromatogram obtained with solution (1), is greater than 15,000 theoretical plates per metre.

Calculate the content of $C_{21}H_{28}O_5$ in the tablets using the declared content of $C_{21}H_{28}O_5$ in *prednisolone EPCRS*.

Labelling The label states that the tablets should be swallowed whole and not chewed.

Prednisone Tablets

Definition Prednisone Tablets contain Prednisone.

The tablets comply with the requirements stated under Tablets and with the following requirements.

Content of prednisone, $C_{21}H_{26}O_5$ 90.0 to 110.0% of the prescribed or stated amount.

Identification Extract a quantity of the powdered tablets with *chloroform*, filter and evaporate the filtrate to dryness. The residue complies with the following tests.

A. The *infrared absorption spectrum*, Appendix II A, is concordant with the *reference spectrum* of prednisone.

B. Complies with the test for *identification of steroids*, Appendix III A, using *impregnating solvent I* and *mobile phase A*.

Related substances Carry out the method for *thin-layer chromatography*, Appendix III A, using *silica gel GF_{254}* as the coating substance and a mixture of 1.2 volumes of *water*, 8 volumes of *methanol*, 15 volumes of *ether* and 77 volumes of *dichloromethane* as the mobile phase. Apply separately to the plate 5 µl of each of the following solutions. For solution (1) shake a quantity of the powdered tablets containing 50 mg of Prednisone with 25 ml of *chloroform*, filter and evaporate the filtrate to a volume of about 10 ml. For solution (2) dilute 1 volume of solution (1) to 50 volumes with a mixture of equal volumes of *chloroform* and *methanol*. After removal of the plate, allow it to dry in air and examine under *ultraviolet light (254 nm)*. Heat at 105° for 10 minutes, cool and spray with *alkaline tetrazolium blue solution*. By each method of visualisation, any *secondary spot* in the chromatogram obtained with solution (1) is not more intense than the spot in the chromatogram obtained with solution (2) (2%).

Uniformity of content Tablets containing less than 2 mg of Prednisone comply with the requirements stated under Tablets using the following method of analysis. Carry out the method for *liquid chromatography*, Appendix III D, using the following solutions. Solution (1) contains 0.005% w/v of *prednisone BPCRS* and 0.0075% w/v of *dexamethasone* (internal standard) in the mobile phase. For solution (2) shake one tablet with 20 ml of the mobile phase for at least 10 minutes, mix with the aid of ultrasound for 2 minutes, centrifuge and use the supernatant liquid. Prepare solution (3) in the same manner as solution (2) but using 20 ml of a 0.0075% w/v solution of *dexamethasone* in the mobile phase in place of the mobile phase.

The chromatographic procedure may be carried out using (a) a stainless steel column (20 cm × 4.6 mm) packed with *stationary phase C* (5 µm) (Spherisorb ODS 1 is suitable), (b) a mixture of 42 volumes of *water* and 58 volumes of *methanol* as the mobile phase with a flow rate of 1.5 ml per minute and (c) a detection wavelength of 254 nm.

The test is not valid unless the *resolution factor* between the peaks due to prednisone and dexamethasone is greater than 3.0 and the *column efficiency*, determined using the peak due to prednisone in the chromatogram obtained with solution (1), is greater than 15,000 *theoretical plates* per metre.

Calculate the content of $C_{21}H_{26}O_5$ taking 100.0% as the content of $C_{21}H_{26}O_5$ in *prednisone BPCRS*.

Dissolution Tablets containing less than 2 mg of Prednisone comply with the *dissolution test for tablets and capsules*, Appendix XII D, using as the medium 900 ml of *water* and rotating the basket at 100 revolutions per minute.

Carry out the method for *liquid chromatography*, Appendix III D, injecting 0.2 ml of each of the following solutions. For solution (1) prepare a 0.1% w/v solution of *prednisone BPCRS* in *methanol* and dilute with *water* to contain 0.0001% w/v. For solution (2) use the dissolution medium diluted, if necessary, with *water* to contain 0.0001% w/v of prednisone.

The chromatographic procedure described under Uniformity of content may be used.

The test is not valid unless the *column efficiency*, determined using the peak due to prednisone in the chromatogram obtained with solution (1), is greater than 15,000 theoretical plates per metre.

Calculate the total content of $C_{21}H_{26}O_5$ in the medium taking 100.0% as the content of $C_{21}H_{26}O_5$ in *prednisone BPCRS*.

Assay Carry out the method for *liquid chromatography*, Appendix III D, using the following solutions. Solution (1) contains 0.005% w/v of *prednisone BPCRS* and 0.0075% w/v of *dexamethasone* (internal standard) in a mixture of 58 volumes of *methanol* and 42 volumes of *water*. For solution (2) weigh and powder 20 tablets; to a quantity of the powder containing 5 mg of Prednisone add 58 ml of *methanol*, shake for 10 minutes, add sufficient *water* to produce 100 ml, mix and filter. Prepare solution (3) in the same manner as solution (2) but add 10 ml of a 0.0075% w/v solution of *dexamethasone* in *methanol* and 48 ml of *methanol* in place of the 58 ml of methanol.

The chromatographic procedure may be carried out using (a) a stainless steel column (20 cm × 4.6 mm) packed with *stationary phase C* (5 µm) (Spherisorb ODS 1 is suitable), (b) a mixture of 42 volumes of *water* and 58 volumes of *methanol* as the mobile phase with a flow rate of about 1 ml per minute and (c) a detection wavelength of 254 nm.

The assay is not valid unless the *resolution factor* between the peaks due to prednisone and dexamethasone is greater than 3.0 and the *column efficiency*, determined using the peak due to prednisone in the chromatogram obtained with solution (1), is greater than 15,000 theoretical plates per metre.

Calculate the content of $C_{21}H_{26}O_5$ using the declared content of $C_{21}H_{26}O_5$ in *prednisone BPCRS*.

Storage Prednisone Tablets should be protected from light.

Prilocaine Injection

Definition Prilocaine Injection is a sterile solution of Prilocaine Hydrochloride in Water for Injections.

The injection complies with the requirements stated under Parenteral Preparations and with the following requirements.

Content of prilocaine hydrochloride, $C_{13}H_{20}N_2O$, HCl 95.0 to 105.0% of the prescribed or stated amount.

Characteristics A colourless solution.

Identification

A. To a volume containing 0.1 g of Prilocaine Hydrochloride add 2M *sodium hydroxide* until the solution is about pH 11. Add 20 ml of *ethyl acetate*, shake, allow the layers to separate, dry the organic layer over *anhydrous calcium chloride* at a pressure of 2 kPa, filter and evaporate the filtrate to dryness under reduced pressure. The *infrared absorption spectrum* of the oily residue, Appendix II A, is concordant with the *reference spectrum* of prilocaine.

B. In the Assay, the principal peak in the chromatogram obtained with solution (3) has the same retention time as the peak due to prilocaine in the chromatogram obtained with solution (1).

Acidity pH, 5.0 to 7.0, Appendix V L.

Aromatic amines To 1 ml of the injection, diluted if necessary to contain 0.05% w/v of Prilocaine Hydrochloride, add 1 ml of a 1% w/v solution of *4-dimethylaminobenzaldehyde* in *methanol* and 2 ml of *glacial acetic acid*. Shake and allow to stand for 10 minutes. Measure the *absorbance* of the solution at 430 nm, Appendix II B, using *water* in the reference cell. The absorbance is not more intense than that produced in a solution prepared at the same time and in the same manner but using 1 ml of a solution in *water* containing 6.7 µg per ml of *o-toluidine hydrochloride* (1%, calculated as *o*-toluidine).

Assay Carry out the method for *liquid chromatography*, Appendix III D, using the following solutions. Solution (1) contains 0.01% w/v of *prilocaine hydrochloride BPCRS* in the mobile phase. For solution (2) dilute the injection with the mobile phase to produce a solution containing 0.01% w/v of Prilocaine Hydrochloride.

The chromatographic procedure may be carried out using (a) a stainless steel column (15 cm × 4.6 mm) packed with *stationary phase C* (5 µm) (Spherisorb ODS 2 is suitable), (b) a mixture of 30 volumes of 0.05M *mixed phosphate buffer pH 8* and 70 volumes of *methanol* as the mobile phase with a flow rate of 1 ml per minute and (c) a detection wavelength of 240 nm.

Calculate the content of $C_{13}H_{20}N_2O,HCl$ in the injection using the declared content of $C_{13}H_{20}N_2O,HCl$ in *prilocaine hydrochloride BPCRS*.

Primidone Oral Suspension

Definition Primidone Oral Suspension is a suspension of Primidone in a suitable flavoured vehicle.

The oral suspension complies with the requirements stated under Oral Liquids and with the following requirements.

Content of primidone, $C_{12}H_{14}N_2O_2$ 95.0 to 105.0% of the prescribed or stated amount.

Identification

A. In the Assay, the chromatogram obtained with solution (2) shows a peak with the same retention time as the peak due to primidone in the chromatogram obtained with solution (1).

B. To a quantity containing 0.5 g of Primidone add 100 ml of *methanol*, boil gently for 10 minutes, stirring constantly, centrifuge, evaporate the clear supernatant liquid almost to dryness on a water bath, add 40 ml of *water* at about 60°, stir for 3 minutes, filter under reduced pressure, wash the residue with three 5-ml quantities of hot *water* and dry at 100° to 105° for 30 minutes. Dissolve 0.1 g of the residue in 5 ml of *chromotropic acid solution* and heat in a water bath for 30 minutes. A pinkish blue colour is produced.

Assay Carry out the method for *gas chromatography*, Appendix III B, using the following solutions. Dissolve 0.24 g of N-*phenylcarbazole* (internal standard) in sufficient *methanol* to produce 100 ml (solution A). For solution (1) add 25 ml of solution A to 0.15 g of *primidone BPCRS* and add sufficient *methanol* to produce 50 ml, warming to dissolve if necessary. For solution (2) add 100 ml of *methanol* to a weighed quantity of the oral suspension containing 0.3 g of Primidone and heat on a water bath for 5 minutes, shaking occasionally, cool, allow any undissolved material to settle and use the supernatant liquid. Prepare solution (3) in the same manner as solution (2) but add 50 ml of solution A and 50 ml of *methanol* in place of the 100 ml of methanol.

The chromatographic procedure may be carried out using a glass column (1.5 m × 4 mm) packed with *acid-washed, silanised diatomaceous support* (100 to 200 mesh) coated with 3% w/w of phenyl methyl silicone fluid (50% phenyl) (OV-17 is suitable) and maintained at 260°.

Calculate the content of $C_{12}H_{14}N_2O_2$ using the declared content of $C_{12}H_{14}N_2O_2$ in *primidone BPCRS*. Determine the *weight per ml* of the oral suspension, Appendix V G, and calculate the content of $C_{12}H_{14}N_2O_2$, weight in volume.

Primidone Tablets

Definition Primidone Tablets contain Primidone.

The tablets comply with the requirements stated under Tablets and with the following requirements.

Content of primidone, $C_{12}H_{14}N_2O_2$ 95.0 to 105.0% of the prescribed or stated amount.

Identification Extract a quantity of the powdered tablets containing 0.5 g of Primidone with 50 ml of hot *ethanol (96%)*, filter and evaporate the filtrate to dryness. The residue complies with the following tests.

A. The *infrared absorption spectrum*, Appendix II A, is concordant with the *reference spectrum* of primidone.

B. Dissolve 0.1 g in 5 ml of *chromotropic acid solution* and heat in a water bath for 30 minutes. A pinkish blue colour is produced.

2-Ethyl-2-phenylmalondiamide Dissolve 25 mg of *octadecan-1-ol* (internal standard) in sufficient *pyridine* to produce 50 ml (solution A). Carry out the method for *gas chromatography*, Appendix III B, using the following solutions. For solution (1) add 2 ml of solution A and 1 ml of N,O-*bis(trimethylsilyl)acetamide* to 2 ml of a 0.050% w/v solution of *2-ethyl-2-phenylmalondiamide* in *pyridine*. For solution (2) mix of a quantity of the powdered tablets containing 0.1 g of Primidone with 2 ml of *pyridine*, add 2 ml of solution A and 1 ml of N,O-*bis-(trimethylsilyl)acetamide*, allow to stand at 100° for 5 minutes, cool and dilute to 10 ml with *pyridine*. Prepare solution (3) in the same manner as solution (2) but use 4 ml of *pyridine* and omit the addition of solution A.

The chromatographic procedure may be carried out using a glass column (1.5 m × 4 mm) packed with *acid-washed, silanised diatomaceous support* (100 to 120 mesh) coated with 3% w/w of phenyl methyl silicone fluid (50% phenyl)(OV-17 is suitable) and maintained at 170°.

In the chromatogram obtained with solution (2) the ratio of the area of any peak derived from 2-ethyl-2-phenylmalondiamide to the area of the peak derived from the internal standard is not greater than the corresponding ratio in the chromatogram obtained with solution (1).

Assay Weigh and powder 20 tablets. Dissolve 0.24 g of N-*phenylcarbazole* (internal standard) in sufficient *methanol* to produce 100 ml (solution A). Carry out the method for *gas chromatography*, Appendix III B, using the following solutions. For solution (1) add 25 ml of solution A to 0.15 g of *primidone BPCRS* and dilute to 50 ml with *methanol*, warming to dissolve if necessary. For solution (2) add 100 ml of *methanol* to a quantity of the powdered tablets containing 0.3 g of Primidone, heat on a water bath for 5 minutes, shaking occasionally, cool, allow any undissolved material to settle and use the clear supernatant liquid. Prepare solution (3) in the same manner as solution (2) but add 50 ml of solution A and 50 ml of *methanol* in place of 100 ml of *methanol*.

The chromatographic procedure may be carried out using (a) a glass column (1.5 m × 4 mm) packed with *acid-washed, silanised diatomaceous support* (100 to 120 mesh) coated with 3% w/w of phenyl methyl silicone fluid (50% phenyl) (OV-17 is suitable) and maintained at 260°.

Calculate the content of $C_{12}H_{14}N_2O_2$ using the declared content of $C_{12}H_{14}N_2O_2$ in *primidone BPCRS*.

Probenecid Tablets

Definition Probenecid Tablets contain Probenecid.

The tablets comply with the requirements stated under Tablets and with the following requirements.

Content of probenecid, $C_{13}H_{19}NO_4S$ 95.0 to 105.0% of the prescribed or stated amount.

Identification

A. Triturate a quantity of the powdered tablets containing 0.5 g of Probenecid with *ethanol (96%)*, filter, concentrate the filtrate by evaporation on a water bath, cool, filter and recrystallise the residue from *ethanol (50%)*. The *infrared absorption spectrum* of the residue, Appendix II A, is concordant with the *reference spectrum* of probenecid.

B. The *light absorption* of the final solution obtained in the Assay, Appendix II B, exhibits maxima at 225 nm and 248 nm.

C. *Melting point* of the residue obtained in test A, about 199°, Appendix V A.

Disintegration Maximum time, 30 minutes, Appendix XII A.

Related substances Carry out the method for *thin-layer chromatography*, Appendix III A, using *silica gel GF_{254}* as the coating substance and a mixture of 10 volumes of *glacial acetic acid*, 15 volumes of *chloroform*, 20 volumes of *di-isopropyl ether* and 55 volumes of *toluene* as the mobile phase. Apply separately to the plate 20 µl of each of the following solutions. For solution (1) extract a quantity of the powdered tablets containing 0.2 g of Probenecid with 20 ml of *acetone*, filter and use the filtrate. For solution (2) dilute 1 volume of solution (1) to 200 volumes with *acetone*. After removal of the plate, allow it to dry in air and examine under *ultraviolet light (254 nm)*. Any *secondary spot* in the chromatogram obtained with solution (1) is not more intense than the spot in the chromatogram obtained with solution (2) (0.5%).

Dissolution Comply with the *dissolution test for tablets and capsules*, Appendix XII D, using Apparatus II. Rotate the paddle at 50 revolutions per minute and use as the medium 900 ml of a phosphate buffer prepared in the following manner. Dissolve 6.8 g of *potassium dihydrogen orthophosphate* in 250 ml of *water*, add 190 ml of 0.2M *sodium hydroxide* and 400 ml of *water*, adjust the pH to 7.5 with 0.2M *sodium hydroxide* and add sufficient *water* to produce 1000 ml. Withdraw a sample of 10 ml of the medium, filter and dilute 4 ml of the filtrate to 100 ml with 0.1M *sodium hydroxide*. Measure the *absorbance* of this solution, Appendix II B, at 244 nm using in the reference cell a solution prepared by diluting 4 ml of the phosphate buffer to 100 ml with 0.1M *sodium hydroxide*. Calculate the total content of $C_{13}H_{19}NO_4S$ in the medium taking 359 as the value of A(1%, 1 cm) at the maximum at 244 nm.

Assay Weigh and powder 20 tablets. To a quantity of the powder containing 0.2 g of Probenecid add 200 ml of *ethanol (96%)* and 5 ml of 1M *hydrochloric acid*, heat on a water bath at 70° for 30 minutes, shaking occasionally, cool, add sufficient *ethanol (96%)* to produce 250 ml and filter. To 5 ml of the filtrate add 5 ml of 0.1M *hydrochloric acid*, dilute to 250 ml with *ethanol (96%)* and measure the *absorbance* of the resulting solution at the maximum at 248 nm, Appendix II B. Calculate the content of $C_{13}H_{19}NO_4S$ taking 332 as the value of A(1%, 1 cm) at the maximum at 248 nm.

Procainamide Injection

Definition Procainamide Injection is a sterile solution of Procainamide Hydrochloride in Water for Injections.

The injection complies with the requirements stated under Parenteral Preparations and with the following requirements.

Content of procainamide hydrochloride, $C_{13}H_{21}N_3O,HCl$ 95.0 to 105.0% of the prescribed or stated amount.

Characteristics A colourless or almost colourless solution.

Identification

A. Dilute a volume containing 0.25 g of Procainamide Hydrochloride to 25 ml with *water*, make alkaline with 5M *sodium hydroxide* and extract with two 10-ml quantities of *chloroform*. Filter the combined extracts through *anhydrous sodium sulphate*, evaporate the filtrate to dryness using a rotary evaporator and dissolve the residue in 5 ml of *chloroform*. The *infrared absorption spectrum* of the resulting solution, Appendix II A, is concordant with the *reference spectrum* of procainamide.

B. Dilute with *water* to produce a solution containing 0.0005% w/v of Procainamide Hydrochloride. The *absorbance* at 280 nm is about 0.30, Appendix II B.

C. Yields reaction A characteristic of *chlorides*, Appendix VI.

Acidity pH, 4.0 to 5.5, Appendix V L.

Related substances Carry out the method for *thin-layer chromatography*, Appendix III A, using *silica gel G* as the coating substance and a mixture of 0.7 volumes of 13.5M ammonia, 30 volumes of *methanol* and 70 volumes of *chloroform* as the mobile phase. Apply separately to the plate 10 µl of each of two solutions prepared in the following manner. For solution (1) dilute a volume of the injection containing 0.10 g of Procainamide Hydrochloride to 5 ml with *methanol*. For solution (2) dilute 1 volume of solution (1) to 100 volumes with *methanol*. To each point of application apply 10 µl of a 20% v/v solution of 13.5M *ammonia* in *methanol*. After removal of the plate, allow it to dry in air and spray with *alcoholic dimethylaminobenzaldehyde solution*. Any *secondary spot* in the chromatogram obtained with solution (1) is not more intense than the spot in the chromatogram obtained with solution (2) (1%).

Assay To a volume containing 0.5 g of Procainamide Hydrochloride add 45 ml of 6M *hydrochloric acid* and boil for 1 minute. Cool and titrate with 0.1M *sodium nitrite VS*, using 1 ml of *ferrocyphen solution* as indicator, until a violet colour is produced that is stable for not less than 3 minutes. Repeat the operation without the injection. The difference between the titrations represents the amount of sodium nitrite required. Each ml of 0.1M *sodium nitrite VS* is equivalent to 27.18 mg of $C_{13}H_{21}N_3O,HCl$.

Procainamide Tablets

Definition Procainamide Tablets contain Procainamide Hydrochloride.

The tablets comply with the requirements stated under Tablets and with the following requirements.

Content of procainamide hydrochloride, $C_{13}H_{21}N_3O,HCl$ 95.0 to 105.0% of the prescribed or stated amount.

Identification

A. Shake a quantity of the powdered tablets containing 0.25 g of Procainamide Hydrochloride with 25 ml of *water*, make alkaline with 5M *sodium hydroxide* and extract with two 5-ml quantities of *chloroform*. Filter the combined extracts through *anhydrous sodium sulphate*, evaporate the filtrate to dryness using a rotary evaporator and dissolve the residue in 5 ml of *chloroform*. The *infrared absorption spectrum* of the resulting solution, Appendix II A, is concordant with the *reference spectrum* of procainamide.

B. Triturate a quantity of the powdered tablets containing 2 g of Procainamide Hydrochloride with 20 ml of *water* and filter. Reserve 10 ml of the filtrate for test C. To the remainder add 10 ml of 5M *sodium hydroxide* and extract with 10 ml of *chloroform*. Add 10 ml of *toluene* to the extract, dry over *anhydrous sodium sulphate* and filter. Mix the filtrate with 5 ml of dry *pyridine*, add 1 ml of *benzoyl chloride* dropwise, heat on a water bath for 30 minutes and pour into 100 ml of 2.5M *sodium hydroxide*. Extract with 10 ml of *ether*, wash the extract with 20 ml of *water*, dilute with 30 ml of *ether* and allow to crystallise. The *melting point* of the crystals, after recrystallisation from *ethanol (45%)*, is about 186°, Appendix V A.

C. 10 ml of the filtrate reserved in test B yields the reactions characteristic of *chlorides*, Appendix VI.

Related substances Comply with the test described under Procainamide Injection using the following solutions. For solution (1) shake a quantity of the powdered tablets containing 0.4 g of Procainamide Hydrochloride with 20 ml of *methanol (90%)* for 15 minutes and filter. For solution (2) dilute 1 volume of solution (1) to 100 volumes with *methanol*.

Assay Weigh and powder 20 tablets. To a quantity of the powder containing 0.5 g of Procainamide Hydrochloride in a stoppered flask add 100 ml of 6M *hydrochloric acid*, shake for 15 minutes and titrate with 0.1M *sodium nitrite VS*, using *ferrocyphen solution* as indicator, until a violet colour is produced that is stable for not less than 3 minutes. Repeat the operation without the powdered tablets. The difference between the titrations represents the amount of sodium nitrite required. Each ml of 0.1M *sodium nitrite VS* is equivalent to 27.18 mg of $C_{13}H_{21}N_3O,HCl$.

Procaine Benzylpenicillin Injection
Procaine Penicillin Injection

For the purposes of product labelling in the United Kingdom, the pair of names given above shall be used together (see Introduction, Changes in title).

Definition Procaine Benzylpenicillin Injection is a sterile suspension of procaine benzylpenicillin in Water for Injections. It is either supplied as a ready-to-use suspension of Procaine Benzylpenicillin or prepared by suspending Procaine Benzylpenicillin for Injection in Water for Injections.

The injection complies with the requirements stated under Parenteral Preparations and, when supplied as a ready-to-use suspension, with the following requirements.

Content of total penicillins, calculated as $C_{13}H_{20}N_2O_2,C_{16}H_{18}N_2O_4,H_2O$ 90.0 to 110.0% of the prescribed or stated amount of Procaine Benzylpenicillin.

Content of procaine, $C_{13}H_{20}N_2O_2$ 36.0 to 44.0% of the prescribed or stated amount of Procaine Benzylpenicillin.

Characteristics A white suspension.

Identification

A. Dilute a volume of the well-shaken suspension containing 10 mg of Procaine Benzylpenicillin to 10 ml with *water* and add 0.5 ml of *neutral red solution*. Add sufficient 0.01M *sodium hydroxide* to produce a permanent orange colour and then add 1 ml of *penicillinase solution*. A red colour is produced rapidly.

B. Carry out the method for *thin-layer chromatography*, Appendix III A, using *silanised silica gel H* as the coating substance and a mixture of 30 volumes of *acetone* and 70 volumes of a 15.4% w/v solution of *ammonium acetate* adjusted to pH 7.0 with 10M *ammonia* as the mobile phase. Apply separately to the plate 1 µl of each of the following solutions. For solution (1) shake a volume of the well-shaken suspension containing 50 mg of Procaine Benzylpenicillin with 5 ml of *methanol*, add a small quantity of *water* to dissolve any residue and dilute to 10 ml with *water*. Solution (2) contains 0.5% w/v of *procaine benzylpenicillin BPCRS* in *acetone*. After removal of the plate, allow it to dry in air, expose to iodine vapour until spots appear and examine in daylight. The two principal spots in the chromatogram obtained with solution (1) are similar in position, colour and size to those in the chromatogram obtained with solution (2). The test is not valid unless the chromatogram obtained with solution (2) shows two clearly separated spots.

C. Yields the reaction characteristic of *primary aromatic amines*, Appendix VI, producing a bright orange-red precipitate.

Pyrogens Complies with the *test for pyrogens*, Appendix XIV D. Use per kg of the rabbit's weight a volume of the suspension containing 2.4 mg of Procaine Benzylpenicillin.

Assay

For total penicillins To a volume of the well-shaken suspension containing 0.2 g of Procaine Benzylpenicillin add 5 ml of *methanol* and dilute to 250 ml with *water*. Dilute 10 ml of the resulting solution to 100 ml with *water*. Place two 2-ml quantities of the resulting solution in separate stoppered tubes. To one tube add 10 ml of *imidazole—mercury reagent*, mix, stopper the tube and place in a water bath at 60° for 35 minutes, swirling occasionally. Remove from the water bath and cool rapidly to 20° (solution A). Add 10 ml of *imidazole solution* to the second tube and allow to stand at 20° for 35 minutes swirling occasionally (solution B). Without delay measure the *absorbances* of solutions A and B at 325 nm, Appendix II B, using in the reference cell a mixture of 2 ml of *water* and 10 ml of *imidazole—mercury reagent* for solution A and a mixture of 2 ml of *water* and 10 ml of *imidazole solution* for solution B. Calculate the content of total penicillins, as $C_{13}H_{20}N_2O_2,C_{16}H_{18}N_2O_4S,H_2O$, from the difference between the absorbances of solutions A and B, from the difference obtained by repeating the operation using a 0.008% w/v solution of *procaine benzylpenicillin BPCRS* in place of the dilution of the preparation being examined and from the declared content of $C_{13}H_{20}N_2O_2,C_{16}H_{18}N_2O_4S,H_2O$ in *procaine benzylpenicillin BPCRS*.

For procaine To a volume of the well-shaken suspension containing 0.1 g of Procaine Benzylpenicillin add 20 ml of *water* and 5 ml of 1M *sodium carbonate* and extract with successive 25-ml quantities of *chloroform* until complete extraction of the procaine is effected, washing each chloroform extract with the same 5 ml of *water*. Shake the combined chloroform extracts in succession with 20 ml of 0.005M *sulphuric acid VS* and 5 ml of *water*. Titrate the excess of acid in the combined acid and aqueous layers with 0.01M *sodium hydroxide VS* using *methyl red solution* as indicator. Each ml of 0.005M *sulphuric acid VS* is equivalent to 2.363 mg of $C_{13}H_{20}N_2O_2$.

Storage When supplied as a ready-to-use suspension, Procaine Benzylpenicillin Injection should be protected from light and stored at a temperature of 8° to 15°.

When prepared by suspending the contents of a sealed container in Water for Injections, Procaine Benzylpenicillin Injection should be used immediately after preparation but, in any case, within the period recommended by the manufacturer when prepared and stored strictly in accordance with the manufacturer's instructions.

Labelling The label states (1) 'Procaine Benzylpenicillin Injection' and 'Procaine Penicillin Injection'; (2) that the contents are to be used for intramuscular injection only.

PROCAINE BENZYLPENICILLIN FOR INJECTION
PROCAINE PENICILLIN FOR INJECTION

For the purposes of product labelling in the United Kingdom, the pair of names given above shall be used together (see Introduction, Changes in title).

Definition Procaine Benzylpenicillin for Injection is a sterile material prepared from Procaine Benzylpenicillin with or without excipients. It is supplied in a sealed container.

The contents of the sealed container comply with the requirements for Powders for Injections stated under Parenteral Preparations and with the following requirements.

Content of total penicillins, calculated as $C_{13}H_{20}N_2O_2,C_{16}H_{18}N_2O_4S,H_2O$ 90.0 to 110.0% of the prescribed or stated amount of Procaine Benzylpenicillin.

Content of procaine, $C_{13}H_{20}N_2O_2$ 36.0 to 44.0% of the prescribed or stated amount of Procaine Benzylpenicillin.

Assay Determine the weight of the contents of 10 containers as described in the test for Uniformity of weight under Parenteral Preparations, Powders for Injections.

For total penicillins To a quantity of the mixed contents of the 10 containers containing 0.2 g of Procaine Benzylpenicillin add 5 ml of *methanol*, shake, dilute to 250 ml with *water* and carry out the procedure described above beginning at the words 'Dilute 10 ml ...'. Calculate the content of total penicillins, as $C_{13}H_{20}N_2O_2$, $C_{16}H_{18}N_2O_4S,H_2O$, in a container of average content weight.

For procaine To a quantity of the mixed contents of the 10 containers containing 0.1 g of Procaine Benzylpenicillin add 20 ml of *water* and 5 ml of 1M *sodium carbonate* and complete the assay described above beginning at the words 'extract with successive 25-ml quantities...'.

Labelling The label of the sealed container states 'Procaine Benzylpenicillin for Injection' and 'Procaine Penicillin for Injection'.

The contents of the sealed container suspended in the volume of water for injections *stated on the label comply with the requirements for Characteristics, Identification and Pyrogens stated above for the ready-to-use suspension.*

3 g of Procaine Benzylpenicillin (procaine penicillin) is approximately equivalent to 2 g of benzylpenicillin.

Fortified Procaine Benzylpenicillin Injection
Fortified Procaine Penicillin Injection

For the purposes of product labelling in the United Kingdom, the pair of names given above shall be used together (see Introduction, Changes in title).

Definition Fortified Procaine Benzylpenicillin Injection is a sterile suspension of procaine benzylpenicillin in Water for Injections containing Benzylpenicillin Potassium or Benzylpenicillin Sodium in solution. It is prepared by adding the requisite amount of Water for Injections to Fortified Procaine Benzylpenicillin for Injection immediately before use.

The injection complies with the requirements stated under Parenteral Preparations.

Storage Fortified Procaine Benzylpenicillin Injection should be used immediately after preparation but, in any case, within the period recommended by the manufacturer when prepared and stored strictly in accordance with the manufacturer's instructions.

Labelling The label states (1) 'Fortified Procaine Benzylpenicillin Injection' and 'Fortified Procaine Penicillin Injection'; (2) that the preparation is to be used for intramuscular injection only.

FORTIFIED PROCAINE BENZYLPENICILLIN FOR INJECTION
FORTIFIED PROCAINE PENICILLIN INJECTION

For the purposes of product labelling in the United Kingdom, the pair of names given above shall be used together (see Introduction, Changes in title).

Definition Fortified Procaine Benzylpenicillin for Injection is a sterile material prepared from a mixture of 5 parts of Procaine Benzylpenicillin and 1 part of Benzylpenicillin Potassium or Benzylpenicillin Sodium with or without excipients. It is supplied in a sealed container.

The contents of the sealed container comply with the requirements for Powders for Injections stated under Parenteral Preparations and with the following requirements.

Content of total penicillins, calculated as $C_{16}H_{17}N_2NaO_4S$ 60.0 to 74.0% of the total content of Procaine Benzylpenicillin and Benzylpenicillin Potassium or Benzylpenicillin Sodium stated on the label.

Content of procaine, $C_{13}H_{20}N_2O_2$ 36.0 to 44.0% of the content of Procaine Benzylpenicillin stated on the label.

Identification

A. Dissolve 10 mg in 10 ml of *water* and add 0.5 ml of *neutral red solution*. Add sufficient 0.01M *sodium hydroxide* to give a permanent orange colour and then add 1 ml of *penicillinase solution*. A red colour is produced rapidly.

B. Carry out the method for *thin-layer chromatography*, Appendix III A, using *silanised silica gel H* as the coating substance and a mixture of 30 volumes of *acetone* and 70 volumes of a 15.4% w/v solution of *ammonium acetate* adjusted to pH 7.0 with 10M *ammonia* as the mobile phase. Apply separately to the plate 1 µl of each of the following solutions. Solution (1) is a solution of the contents of the sealed container in *acetone* containing the equivalent of 0.5% w/v of total penicillins. Solution (2) contains 0.5% w/v of *procaine benzylpenicillin BPCRS* in *acetone*. After removal of the plate, allow it to dry in air, expose to iodine vapour until spots appear and examine in daylight. The two principal spots in the chromatogram obtained with solution (1) are similar in position, colour and size to those in the chromatogram obtained with solution (2). The test is not valid unless the chromatogram obtained with solution (2) shows two clearly separated spots.

C. Yield the reaction characteristic of *primary aromatic amines*, Appendix VI, producing a bright, orange-red precipitate.

Water Not more than 3.5% w/w, Appendix IX C. Use 0.5 g.

Assay Determine the weight of the contents of 10 containers as described in the test for Uniformity of weight under Parenteral Preparations, Powders for Injections.

For total penicillins To a quantity of the mixed contents of the 10 containers containing 0.2 g of Procaine Benzylpenicillin add 5 ml of *methanol*, shake and dilute to 250 ml with *water*. Dilute 10 ml of the resulting solution to 100 ml with *water*. Place two 2-ml quantities of the resulting solution in separate stoppered tubes. To one tube add 10 ml of *imidazole—mercury reagent*, mix, stopper the tube and place in a water bath at 60° for 35 minutes, swirling occasionally. Remove from the water bath and cool rapidly to 20° (solution A). Add 10 ml of *imidazole solution* to the second tube, mix, stopper the tube and allow to stand at about 20° for 35 minutes swirling occasionally (solution B). Without delay measure the *absorbances* of solutions A and B at 325 nm, Appendix II B, using in the reference cell a mixture of 2 ml of *water* and 10 ml of *imidazole—mercury reagent* for solution A and a mixture of 2 ml of *water* and 10 ml of *imidazole solution* for solution B. Calculate the content of total penicillins, as $C_{16}H_{17}N_2NaO_4S$, in a container of average content weight from the difference between the absorbances of solutions A and B, from the difference obtained by repeating the operation using a 0.005% w/v solution of *benzylpenicillin sodium EPCRS* in place of the contents of the sealed containers and from the declared content of $C_{16}H_{17}N_2NaO_4S$ in *benzylpenicillin sodium EPCRS*.

For procaine To a quantity of the mixed contents of the 10 containers containing 0.1 g of Procaine Benzylpenicillin add 20 ml of *water* and 5 ml of 1M *sodium carbonate* and extract with successive 25-ml quantities of *chloroform* until complete extraction of the procaine is effected, washing each chloroform extract with the same 5 ml of *water*. Shake the mixed chloroform extracts in succession with 20 ml of 0.005M *sulphuric acid VS* and 5 ml of *water* and titrate the excess of acid in the combined acid and aqueous layers with 0.01M *sodium hydroxide VS* using *methyl red solution* as indicator. Each ml of 0.005M *sulphuric acid VS* is equivalent to 2.363 mg of $C_{13}H_{20}N_2O_2$.

Storage The sealed container should be stored at a temperature not exceeding 15°.

Labelling The label of the sealed container states (1) 'Fortified Procaine Benzylpenicillin for Injection' and 'Fortified Procaine Penicillin for Injection'; (2) the quantities of Procaine Benzylpenicillin (Procaine Penicillin) and of Benzylpenicillin Potassium or Benzylpenicillin Sodium contained in it.

Prochlorperazine Injection

Definition Prochlorperazine Injection is a sterile solution of Prochlorperazine Mesilate in Water for Injections free from dissolved air.

The injection complies with the requirements stated under Parenteral Preparations and with the following requirements.

Content of prochlorperazine mesilate, $C_{20}H_{24}ClN_3S,2CH_4SO_3$ 95.0 to 105.0% of the prescribed or stated amount.

Characteristics A colourless or almost colourless solution.

Identification

A. To a volume containing 0.1 g of Prochlorperazine Mesilate add 20 ml of *water* and 2 ml of 10M *sodium hydroxide*. Shake and extract the mixture with 25 ml of *ether*. Wash the ether layer with two 5-ml quantities of *water*, dry with *anhydrous sodium sulphate* and evaporate to dryness. Dissolve the residue in 1 ml of *chloroform*. The *infrared absorption spectrum* of the resulting solution, Appendix II A, is concordant with the *reference spectrum* of prochlorperazine.

B. To a volume containing 5 mg of Prochlorperazine Mesilate add carefully 2 ml of *sulphuric acid* and allow to stand for 5 minutes. A red colour is produced.

C. To a volume containing 0.2 g of Prochlorperazine Mesilate add 1.5 ml of 5M *sodium hydroxide* and extract with 10 ml of *ether*. Wash the ether layer with two 5-ml quantities of *water*, evaporate the ether layer to dryness, dissolve the residue in 10 ml of *methanol* and add a solution of 0.3 g of *picric acid* in a mixture of 5 ml of *methanol* and 5 ml of *water*. The *melting point* of the precipitate, after washing with 15 ml of *methanol*, is about 255°, with decomposition, Appendix V A.

Acidity pH, 5.5 to 6.5, Appendix V L.

Related substances Carry out the test for *related substances in phenothiazines*, Appendix III A, using *mobile phase A* and the following solutions. For solution (1) use the injection being examined. For solution (2) dilute 1 volume of solution (1) to 40 volumes with *methanol* containing 0.5% v/v of 13.5M *ammonia* immediately before use. For solution (3) dilute 1 volume of solution (1) to 200 volumes with the methanol—ammonia mixture immediately before use. Any *secondary spot* in the chromatogram obtained with solution (1) is not more intense than the principal spot in the chromatogram obtained with solution (2) (2.5%) and not more than one such spot is more intense than the spot in the chromatogram obtained with solution (3) (0.5%).

Assay Carry out the following procedure protected from light. To a quantity containing 12.5 mg of Prochlorperazine Mesilate add sufficient *absolute ethanol* containing 0.01% v/v of 13.5M *ammonia* to produce 100 ml. Dilute 5 ml of the solution to 100 ml with the ammoniacal ethanol and measure the *absorbance* of the resulting solution at the maximum at 258 nm, Appendix II B. Calculate the content of $C_{20}H_{24}ClN_3S,2CH_4SO_3$ taking 635 as the value of A(1%, 1 cm) at the maximum at 258 nm.

Storage Prochlorperazine Injection should be protected from light.

Prochlorperazine Oral Solution

Definition Prochlorperazine Oral Solution contains Prochlorperazine Mesilate in a suitable aqueous vehicle.

The oral solution complies with the requirements stated under Oral Liquids and with the following requirements.

Content of prochlorperazine mesilate, $C_{20}H_{24}ClN_3S,2CH_4SO_3$ 90.0 to 110.0% of the prescribed or stated amount.

Identification

A. To a volume of the oral solution containing 50 mg of Prochlorperazine Mesilate add 50 ml of *water* and 2 ml of 10M *sodium hydroxide*, add *sodium chloride* and extract with two 50-ml quantities of *ether*. Wash the combined ether extracts with two 5-ml quantities of *water*, filter through *anhydrous sodium sulphate* and evaporate to dryness. Dissolve the residue in 10 ml of *methanol* and add a solution prepared by dissolving 0.1 g of *picric acid* in a mixture of 5 ml of *methanol* and 5 ml of *water*, wash the resulting precipitate with 15 ml of *methanol* and dry at 100° for 40 minutes. The *melting point* of the dried precipitate is about 255°, with decomposition, Appendix V A.

B. In the test for Prochlorperazine sulphoxide, the principal spot in the chromatogram obtained with solution (2) is similar in position, size and intensity to that in the chromatogram obtained with solution (3).

Prochlorperazine sulphoxide Carry out the method for *thin-layer chromatography*, Appendix III A, protected from light, using a precoated silica gel F_{254} plate activated by drying at 105° for 1 hour and a mixture of 5 volumes of *diethylamine*, 45 volumes of *acetone* and 50 volumes of *hexane* as the mobile phase. Apply separately to the plate 2 µl of each of the following solutions. For solution (1) mix a quantity of the oral solution containing 10 mg of Prochlorperazine Mesilate with 35 ml of *water* and 5 ml of a 20% w/v solution of *sodium hydroxide*, extract with four 40-ml quantities of *chloroform*, shaking for 2 minutes each time, and filter each extract through *anhydrous sodium sulphate* washing the sodium sulphate with 5 ml of *chloroform*. Evaporate the combined chloroform extracts and washings to dryness at 30° under reduced pressure using a current of *nitrogen* to remove the last of the solvent and dissolve the residue in 1 ml of a mixture of equal volumes of *chloroform* and *methanol*. For solution (2) dilute 1 volume of solution (1) to 10 volumes with a mixture of equal volumes of *chloroform* and *methanol*. Solution (3) contains 0.1% w/v of *prochlorperazine mesilate BPCRS* in a mixture of equal volumes of *chloroform* and *methanol*. Solution (4) contains 0.03% w/v of *prochlorperazine sulphoxide BPCRS* in a mixture of equal volumes of *chloroform* and *methanol*. After removal of the plate, allow it to dry in air and examine under *ultraviolet light (254 nm)*. Any spot corresponding to prochlorperazine sulphoxide in the chromatogram obtained with solution (1) is not more intense than the spot in the chromatogram obtained with solution (4) (3%).

Assay Carry out the following procedure protected from light. To a weighed quantity containing 10 mg of Prochlorperazine Mesilate add 25 ml of *water* and 5 ml of a 10% w/v solution of *sodium hydroxide*. Extract the mixture with three 50-ml quantities of *chloroform*, shaking vigorously for 1 minute, allowing to separate and shaking vigorously for two further 1-minute intervals each time. Evaporate the combined extracts to dryness at about 30° under reduced pressure and dissolve the residue in sufficient 0.1M *hydrochloric acid* to produce 25 ml (solution A). Dilute 10 ml of solution A to 50 ml with *water* (solution B). To a further 10 ml of solution A add 5 ml of *peroxyacetic acid solution*, allow to stand for 10 minutes and add sufficient *water* to produce 50 ml (solution C). Measure the *absorbance* of solution C at the maximum at 343 nm, Appendix II B, using solution B in the reference cell. Repeat the procedure using a 0.04% w/v solution of *prochlorperazine mesilate BPCRS* in 0.1M *hydrochloric acid* in place of solution A and beginning at the words 'Dilute 10 ml of...'. Determine the *weight per ml* of the oral solution, Appendix V G, and calculate the content of $C_{20}H_{24}ClN_3S,2CH_4SO_3$, weight in volume, using the declared content of $C_{20}H_{24}ClN_3S,2CH_4SO_3$ in *prochlorperazine mesilate BPCRS*.

Storage Prochlorperazine Oral Solution should be protected from light.

Prochlorperazine Tablets

Definition Prochlorperazine Tablets contain Prochlorperazine Maleate.

The tablets comply with the requirements stated under Tablets and with the following requirements.

Content of prochlorperazine maleate, $C_{20}H_{24}ClN_3S,2C_4H_4O_4$ 92.5 to 107.5% of the prescribed or stated amount.

Identification

A. To a quantity of the powdered tablets containing 40 mg of Prochlorperazine Maleate add 10 ml of *water* and 2 ml of 1M *sodium hydroxide*, shake and extract with

15 ml of *ether*. Wash the ether with 5 ml of *water*, dry with *anhydrous sodium sulphate*, evaporate to dryness and dissolve the residue in 0.4 ml of *chloroform*. The *infrared absorption spectrum* of the resulting solution, Appendix II A, is concordant with the *reference spectrum* of prochlorperazine.

B. To a quantity of the powdered tablets containing 5 mg of Prochlorperazine Maleate add 5 ml of *sulphuric acid* and allow to stand for 5 minutes. A red colour is produced.

C. To a quantity of the powdered tablets containing 0.2 g of Prochlorperazine Maleate add 2 ml of *water* and 1 ml of 5M *sodium hydroxide*, mix and extract with three 10-ml quantities of *ether*. Dry the combined extracts with *anhydrous sodium sulphate*, filter, evaporate to dryness, dissolve the residue in 10 ml of *methanol* and add a solution of 0.15 g of *picric acid* in 10 ml of *methanol*. The *melting point* of the precipitate, after washing with a small quantity of *methanol*, is about 255°, with decomposition, Appendix V A.

Related substances Comply with the test for *related substances in phenothiazines*, Appendix III A, using *mobile phase A* and applying separately to the plate 20 µl of each of the following freshly prepared solutions. For solution (1) extract a quantity of the powdered tablets containing 0.1 g of Prochlorperazine Maleate with 10 ml of *methanol* containing 0.5% v/v of 13.5M *ammonia* and filter. For solution (2) dilute 1 volume of solution (1) to 200 volumes with the same solvent.

Assay Carry out the following procedure protected from light. Weigh and powder 20 tablets. Extract a quantity of the powder containing 25 mg of Prochlorperazine Maleate with 10 ml of *absolute ethanol* containing 1% v/v of 13.5M *ammonia* and successive 10-ml quantities of *absolute ethanol*. Combine the extracts, filter and to the filtrate add sufficient *absolute ethanol* to produce 100 ml. Dilute 10 ml to 50 ml with *absolute ethanol*, dilute 10 ml of this solution to 50 ml with *absolute ethanol* and measure the *absorbance* of the resulting solution at the maximum at 258 nm, Appendix II B. Calculate the content of $C_{20}H_{24}ClN_3S,2C_4H_4O_4$ taking 620 as the value of A(1%, 1 cm) at the maximum at 258 nm.

Storage Prochlorperazine Tablets should be protected from light.

Procyclidine Injection

Definition Procyclidine Injection is a sterile solution of Procyclidine Hydrochloride in Water for Injections.

The injection complies with the requirements stated under Parenteral Preparations and with the following requirements.

Content of procyclidine hydrochloride, $C_{19}H_{29}NO$, HCl 95.0 to 105.0% of the prescribed or stated amount.

Characteristics A colourless solution.

Identification

A. Extract a volume of the injection containing 30 mg of Procyclidine Hydrochloride with three 5-ml quantities of *dichloromethane*, dry the combined extracts with *anhydrous sodium sulphate*, filter and evaporate to dryness. The *infrared absorption spectrum* of the residue, Appendix II A, is concordant with the *reference spectrum* of procyclidine hydrochloride.

B. Carry out the method described in the test for Related substances under Procyclidine Tablets but applying 2 µl of each of the following solutions. For solution (1) dilute the injection, if necessary, with *water* to give a solution containing 0.50% w/v of Procyclidine Hydrochloride. Solution (2) contains 0.50% w/v of *procyclidine hydrochloride BPCRS*. By each method of visualisation the principal spot in the chromatogram obtained with solution (1) corresponds to that in the chromatogram obtained with solution (2).

Acidity pH, 4.0 to 6.8, Appendix V L.

Related substances Complies with the test for Related substances described under Procyclidine Tablets but applying 20 µl of each of the following solutions. For solution (1) dilute the injection, if necessary, with *water* to give a solution containing 0.50% w/v of Procyclidine Hydrochloride. Solution (2) contains 0.0010% w/v of *1-phenyl-3-pyrrolidinopropan-1-one hydrochloride BPCRS* in *chloroform*. For solution (3) dilute 1 volume of solution (1) to 200 volumes with *water*.

Assay Record *second-derivative ultraviolet absorption spectra*, Appendix II B, of the following solutions in the range 220 to 280 nm. For solution (1) dilute a volume of the injection containing 25 mg of Procyclidine Hydrochloride to 100 ml with 0.1M *hydrochloric acid*. Solution (2) contains 0.025% w/v of *procyclidine hydrochloride BPCRS* in 0.1M *hydrochloric acid*.

For each solution measure the amplitude from the largest trough at about 257 nm to the largest peak at about 254 nm. Calculate the content of $C_{19}H_{29}NO,HCl$ using the declared content of $C_{19}H_{29}NO,HCl$ in *procyclidine hydrochloride BPCRS*.

Procyclidine Tablets

Definition Procyclidine Tablets contain Procyclidine Hydrochloride.

The tablets comply with the requirements stated under Tablets and with the following requirements.

Content of procyclidine hydrochloride, $C_{19}H_{29}NO$, HCl 90.0 to 110.0% of the prescribed or stated amount.

Identification

A. Disperse a quantity of the powdered tablets containing 25 mg of Procyclidine Hydrochloride in 10 ml of *water*, shake with 20 ml of *ether* and discard the ether layer. Make the aqueous layer alkaline with 2M *sodium hydroxide* and extract with two 20-ml quantities of *ether*. Wash the combined ether extracts with two 10-ml quantities of *water*, dry by shaking with *anhydrous sodium sulphate*, filter and evaporate the filtrate to dryness. If necessary, induce crystallisation by scratching with a glass rod. The *infrared absorption spectrum* of the residue, Appendix II A, is concordant with the *reference spectrum* of procyclidine.

B. The powdered tablets yield the reactions characteristic of *chlorides*, Appendix VI.

Related substances Carry out the method for *thin-layer chromatography*, Appendix III A, using *silica gel GF_{254}* as the coating substance and a mixture of 1 volume of 13.5M *ammonia* and 100 volumes of *ether* as the mobile phase. Apply separately to the plate 20 µl of each of the following solutions. For solution (1) shake a quantity of the powdered tablets containing 25 mg of Procyclidine Hydrochloride with 5 ml of *chloroform* and filter. Solution (2) contains 0.001% w/v of *1-phenyl-3-pyrrolidinopropan-1-one hydrochloride BPCRS* in *chloroform*. For solution (3) dilute 1 volume of solution (1) to 200 volumes with *chloroform*. After removal of the plate, dry it at 105° for 15 minutes and examine under *ultraviolet light (254 nm)*. Any spot corresponding to 1-phenyl-3-pyrrolidinopropan-1-one in the chromatogram obtained with solution (1) is not more intense than the spot in the chromatogram obtained with solution (2) (0.2%). Spray the plate with *dilute potassium iodobismuthate solution*. Any *secondary spot* in the chromatogram obtained with solution (1) is not more intense than the spot in the chromatogram obtained with solution (3) (0.5%). Disregard any spot due to excipient on the line of application.

Assay Weigh and finely powder 20 tablets. Record *second-derivative ultraviolet absorption spectra* of the following solutions, Appendix II B, in the range 220 to 280 nm. For solution (1) add 80 ml of 0.1M *hydrochloric acid* to a quantity of the powdered tablets containing 25 mg of Procyclidine Hydrochloride, mix with the aid of ultrasound for 15 minutes, cool, dilute to 100 ml with 0.1M *hydrochloric acid* and filter through a glass fibre paper having a maximum pore size of 0.7 µm (Whatman GF/F paper is suitable) discarding the first 10 ml of filtrate. Solution (2) contains 0.025% w/v of *procyclidine hydrochloride BPCRS* in 0.1M *hydrochloric acid*.

For each solution measure the amplitude from the largest trough at about 257 nm to the largest peak at about 254 nm. Calculate the content of $C_{19}H_{29}NO,HCl$ using the declared content of $C_{19}H_{29}NO,HCl$ in *procyclidine hydrochloride BPCRS*.

Progesterone Injection

Definition Progesterone Injection is a sterile solution of Progesterone in Ethyl Oleate or other suitable ester, in a suitable fixed oil or in any mixture of these. It may contain suitable alcohols.

The injection complies with the requirements stated under Parenteral Preparations and with the following requirements.

Content of progesterone, $C_{21}H_{30}O_2$ 92.5 to 107.5% of the prescribed or stated amount.

Identification Dissolve a volume containing 50 mg of Progesterone in 8 ml of *petroleum spirit (boiling range, 40° to 60°)* and extract with three 8-ml quantities of a mixture of 7 volumes of *glacial acetic acid* and 3 volumes of *water*. Wash the combined extracts with 10 ml of *petroleum spirit (boiling range, 40° to 60°)*, dilute with *water* until the solution becomes turbid, allow to stand in ice for 2 hours and filter. The precipitate, after washing with *water* and drying at 105°, complies with the following tests.

A. The *infrared absorption spectrum*, Appendix II A, is concordant with the *reference spectrum* of progesterone.

B. Complies with the test for *identification of steroids*, Appendix III A, using *impregnating solvent II* and *mobile phase E*.

Assay To a quantity containing 50 mg of Progesterone add sufficient *chloroform* to produce 100 ml. Dilute 3 ml to 50 ml with *chloroform* and to 5 ml of the solution add 10 ml of *isoniazid solution* and sufficient *methanol* to produce 20 ml. Allow to stand for 45 minutes and measure the *absorbance* of the resulting solution at the maximum at 380 nm, Appendix II B, using in the reference cell 5 ml of *chloroform* treated in the same manner. Calculate the content of $C_{21}H_{30}O_2$ from the *absorbance* obtained by repeating the operation using a 0.003% w/v solution of *progesterone BPCRS* in *chloroform* and beginning at the words 'to 5 ml...'.

Storage Progesterone Injection should be protected from light. On standing, solid matter may separate; it should be redissolved by heating before use.

Labelling The label states that the preparation is intended for intramuscular injection only.

Proguanil Tablets

Definition Proguanil Tablets contain Proguanil Hydrochloride.

The tablets comply with the requirements stated under Tablets and with the following requirements.

Content of proguanil hydrochloride, $C_{11}H_{16}ClN_5$, HCl 95.0 to 105.0% of the prescribed or stated amount.

Identification

A. To a quantity of the powdered tablets containing 0.2 g of Proguanil Hydrochloride add 25 ml of *methanol*, shake for 10 minutes, filter, evaporate the filtrate to dryness and dry the residue at 105°. The *infrared absorption spectrum* of the residue, Appendix II A, is concordant with the *reference spectrum* of proguanil hydrochloride.

B. Boil a quantity of the powdered tablets containing 0.5 g of Proguanil Hydrochloride with 5 ml of 2M *hydrochloric acid*, cool and filter. To the filtrate add a slight excess of 5M *sodium hydroxide*, extract with 30 ml of *ether*, evaporate the ether and dry the residue at 105°. The *melting point* of the residue is about 131°, Appendix V A.

4-Chloroaniline To a quantity of the powdered tablets containing 0.1 g of Proguanil Hydrochloride add 5 ml of *ethanol (96%)* and shake for 10 minutes. Add 2.5 ml of 2M *hydrochloric acid* and 15 ml of *water*, mix and filter through a moistened filter paper, washing the filter with 5 ml of *water*. The filtrate complies with the test described under Proguanil Hydrochloride, beginning at the words 'cool to 5°... '.

Related substances Carry out the method for *liquid chromatography*, Appendix III D, using the following solutions. For solution (1) dilute 1 volume of solution (2) to 100 volumes with the mobile phase. For solution (2) add 50 ml of *methanol* to a quantity of the powdered tablets containing 0.1 g of Proguanil Hydrochloride, shake for 10 minutes, dilute to 100 ml with *methanol*, mix, filter and dilute 5 ml of the filtrate to 50 ml with the mobile phase.

The chromatographic procedure may be carried out using (a) a stainless steel column (10 cm × 5 mm) packed with *stationary phase C* (5 µm) (Nucleosil C18 is suitable), (b) 0.01M *sodium hexanesulphonate* in a mixture of 1 volume of *glacial acetic acid*, 80 volumes of *water* and 120 volumes of *methanol* as the mobile phase with a flow rate of 1 ml per minute and (c) a detection wavelength of 254 nm.

The sum of the areas of any *secondary peaks* in the chromatogram obtained with solution (2) is not greater than the area of the principal peak in the chromatogram obtained with solution (1) (1%).

Dissolution Comply with the *dissolution test for tablets and capsules*, Appendix XII D, using Apparatus II. Use as the medium 900 ml of 0.2M *hydrochloric acid* containing 0.2% w/v of *sodium chloride* and rotate the paddle at 50 revolutions per minute. Withdraw a sample of 10 ml of the medium, filter and dilute 2 ml of the filtrate to 10 ml with dissolution medium. Measure the *absorbance* of this solution, Appendix II B, at 242 nm using dissolution medium in the reference cell. Measure the *absorbance* of a 0.001% w/v solution of *proguanil hydrochloride BPCRS* in dissolution medium using dissolution medium in the reference cell. Calculate the total content of proguanil hydrochloride, $C_{11}H_{16}ClN_5,HCl$, in the medium from the absorbances obtained and from the declared content of $C_{11}H_{16}ClN_5,HCl$ in *proguanil hydrochloride BPCRS*.

Assay Carry out the method for *liquid chromatography*, Appendix III D, using the following solutions. Solution (1) contains 0.002% w/v of *proguanil hydrochloride BPCRS* in the mobile phase. For solution (2) weigh and powder 20 tablets, add 50 ml of *methanol* to a quantity of the powdered tablets containing 0.1 g of Proguanil Hydrochloride, shake for 10 minutes, dilute to 100 ml with *methanol*, mix and filter. To 5 ml of the filtrate add sufficient *methanol* to produce 50 ml and dilute 10 ml of the resulting solution to 50 ml with the mobile phase.

The chromatographic procedure described under Related substances may be used.

Calculate the content of $C_{11}H_{16}ClN_5,HCl$ using the declared content of $C_{11}H_{16}ClN_5,HCl$ in *proguanil hydrochloride BPCRS*.

Promazine Injection

Definition Promazine Injection is a sterile solution of Promazine Hydrochloride in Water for Injections free from dissolved air.

The injection complies with the requirements stated under Parenteral Preparations and with the following requirements.

Content of promazine hydrochloride, $C_{17}H_{20}N_2S,HCl$ 95.0 to 105.0% of the prescribed or stated amount.

Characteristics A colourless or almost colourless solution.

Identification

A. To a volume containing 0.1 g of Promazine Hydrochloride add 20 ml of *water* and 2 ml of 10M *sodium hydroxide*. Shake and extract the mixture with 25 ml of *ether*. Wash the ether with two 5-ml quantities of *water*, dry with *anhydrous sodium sulphate* and evaporate the ether to dryness. Dissolve the residue in 1 ml of *chloroform*. The *infrared absorption spectrum* of the resulting solution, Appendix II A, is concordant with the *reference spectrum* of promazine.

B. To a volume containing 5 mg of Promazine Hydrochloride carefully add 2 ml of *sulphuric acid* and allow to stand for 5 minutes. An orange colour is produced.

C. To a volume containing 0.2 g of Promazine Hydrochloride add 1 ml of 1M *sodium hydroxide* and extract with four 10-ml quantities of *ether*. Wash the combined extracts with 10 ml of *water*, remove the ether and dissolve the residue in 4 ml of *methanol*. Heat on a water bath almost to boiling, immediately add 2 ml of a boiling 3.5% w/v solution of *picric acid* in *methanol* and boil for 2 minutes. Cool in ice, filter, wash the crystals with three quantities of *methanol*, dissolve in 10 ml of hot *methanol* and repeat the crystallisation and washing. The *melting point* of the rust-red crystals so obtained, after drying at 105° for 1 hour, is about 144°, Appendix V A.

Acidity pH, 4.4 to 5.2, Appendix V L.

Related substances Carry out the test for *related substances in phenothiazines*, Appendix III A, using *mobile phase A* and applying separately to the plate 10 µl of each of the following freshly prepared solutions. For solution (1) dilute a volume of the injection with sufficient *methanol* to produce a solution containing 1.0% w/v of Promazine Hydrochloride. For solution (2) dilute 1 volume of solution (1) to 40 volumes with *methanol*. For solution (3) dilute 1 volume of solution (1) to 200 volumes with *methanol*. Any *secondary spot* in the chromatogram obtained with solution (1) is not more intense than the spot in the chromatogram obtained with solution (2) (2.5%) and not more than one such spot is more intense than the spot in the chromatogram obtained with solution (3) (0.5%).

Assay Carry out the following procedure protected from light. To a quantity containing 50 mg of Promazine Hydrochloride add 5 ml of 2M *hydrochloric acid* and sufficient *water* to produce 1000 ml. To 10 ml add 10 ml of 0.1M *hydrochloric acid*, dilute to 100 ml with *water* and measure the *absorbance* of the resulting solution at the maximum at 251 nm, Appendix II B. Calculate the content of $C_{17}H_{20}N_2S,HCl$ taking 935 as the value of A(1%, 1 cm) at the maximum at 251 nm.

Storage Promazine Injection should be protected from light.

Promazine Tablets

Definition Promazine Tablets contain Promazine Hydrochloride. They are coated.

The tablets comply with the requirements stated under Tablets and with the following requirements.

Content of promazine hydrochloride, $C_{17}H_{20}N_2S,HCl$ 92.5 to 107.5% of the prescribed or stated amount.

Identification

A. To a quantity of the powdered tablets containing 40 mg of Promazine Hydrochloride add 10 ml of *water* and 2 ml of 1M *sodium hydroxide*, shake and extract with 15 ml of *ether*. Wash the extract with 5 ml of *water*, dry with *anhydrous sodium sulphate*, evaporate to dryness and dissolve the residue in 0.4 ml of *chloroform*. The *infrared absorption spectrum* of the resulting solution, Appendix II A, is concordant with the *reference spectrum* of promazine.

B. To a quantity of the powdered tablets containing 5 mg of Promazine Hydrochloride add 5 ml of *sulphuric acid* and allow to stand for 5 minutes. An orange colour is produced.

C. Triturate a quantity of the powdered tablets containing 0.2 g of Promazine Hydrochloride with 4 ml of *methanol*, centrifuge, filter the supernatant liquid, heat almost to boiling, immediately add 2 ml of a boiling 3.5% w/v solution of *picric acid* in *methanol* and boil for 2 minutes. Cool in ice, filter, wash the crystals with three quantities of *methanol*, dissolve in 10 ml of hot *methanol* and repeat the crystallisation and washing. The *melting point* of the rust red crystals so obtained, after drying at 105° for 1 hour, is about 144°, Appendix V A.

Related substances Comply with the test for *related substances in phenothiazines*, Appendix III A, using *mobile phase A* and the following freshly prepared solutions. For solution (1) extract a quantity of the powdered tablets containing 0.1 g of Promazine Hydrochloride with 10 ml of *methanol* and filter. For solution (2) dilute 1 volume of solution (1) to 200 volumes with *methanol*.

Assay Carry out the following procedure protected from light. Weigh and powder 20 tablets. Triturate a quantity of the powder containing 50 mg of Promazine Hydrochloride with 10 ml of 2M *hydrochloric acid* and then add 200 ml of *water*. Shake for 15 minutes, add sufficient *water* to produce 500 ml and centrifuge about 50 ml of the mixture. To 5 ml of the clear, supernatant liquid add 10 ml of 0.1M *hydrochloric acid* and sufficient *water* to produce 100 ml. Measure the *absorbance* of the resulting solution at the maximum at 251 nm, Appendix II B. Calculate the content of $C_{17}H_{20}N_2S,HCl$ taking 935 as the value of A(1%, 1 cm) at the maximum at 251 nm.

Promethazine Injection

Definition Promethazine Injection is a sterile solution of Promethazine Hydrochloride in Water for Injections free from dissolved air.

The injection complies with the requirements stated under Parenteral Preparations and with the following requirements.

Content of promethazine hydrochloride, $C_{17}H_{20}N_2S$, HCl 95.0 to 105.0% of the prescribed or stated amount.

Characteristics A colourless or almost colourless solution.

Identification

A. To a volume containing 0.1 g of Promethazine Hydrochloride add 20 ml of *water* and 2 ml of 10M *sodium hydroxide*. Shake and extract the mixture with 25 ml of *ether*. Wash the ether layer with two 5-ml quantities of *water*, dry with *anhydrous sodium sulphate* and evaporate the ether. Dissolve the residue in 1 ml of *chloroform*. The *infrared absorption spectrum* of the resulting solution, Appendix II A, is concordant with the *reference spectrum* of promethazine.

B. To a volume containing 5 mg of Promethazine Hydrochloride carefully add 2 ml of *sulphuric acid* and allow to stand for 5 minutes. A red colour is produced.

C. To a volume containing 0.2 g of Promethazine Hydrochloride add sufficient *potassium carbonate sesquihydrate* to saturate the solution, extract with two 10-ml quantities of *ether* and evaporate the combined extracts to dryness. Dissolve the residue in 2 ml of *methanol* and pour into a solution of 0.4 g of *picric acid* in 10 ml of *methanol*, previously warmed to about 50°. Cool, scratch the side of the tube to induce crystallisation, allow to stand for 3 to 4 hours and filter. The *melting point* of the residue, after washing with *methanol* and drying, is about 160°, Appendix V A.

Acidity pH, 5.0 to 6.0, Appendix V L.

Related substances Carry out the method for *thin-layer chromatography*, Appendix III A, protected from light under an atmosphere of nitrogen using *silica gel GF_{254}* as the coating substance (Merck silica gel 60 F_{254} plates are suitable) and a mixture of 15 volumes of *diethylamine*, 45 volumes of *hexane* and 50 volumes of *acetone* as the mobile phase but allowing the solvent front to ascend 12 cm above the line of application. Apply separately to the plate 10 µl of each of the following freshly prepared solutions. For solution (1) use a volume of the injection diluted, if necessary, with a mixture of 5 volumes of *diethylamine* and 95 volumes of *methanol* to contain 1.0% w/v of Promethazine Hydrochloride. For solution (2) dilute 1 volume of solution (1) to 200 volumes with a mixture of 5 volumes of *diethylamine* and 95 volumes of *methanol*. Solution (3) contains 0.01% w/v of *isopromethazine hydrochloride EPCRS* in a mixture of 5 volumes of *diethylamine* and 95 volumes of *methanol*. Solution (4) contains 0.025% w/v of *promethazine sulphoxide BPCRS* in a mixture of 5 volumes of *diethylamine* and 95 volumes of *methanol*. After removal of the plate, allow it to dry in air, spray with a 20% w/v solution of *perchloric acid* and heat at 100° for 5 minutes. In the chromatogram obtained with solution (1) any spot corresponding to isopromethazine is not more intense than the principal spot in the chromatogram obtained with solution (3) (1%), any spot corresponding to promethazine sulphoxide is not more intense than the spot in the chromatogram obtained with solution (4) (2.5%) and any other *secondary spot* is not more intense than the spot in the chromatogram obtained with solution (2) (0.5%). Disregard any spot remaining on the line of application.

Assay Carry out the following procedure protected from light. To a volume containing 25 mg of Promethazine Hydrochloride add sufficient 0.01M *hydrochloric acid* to produce 100 ml. Dilute 10 ml to 100 ml with 0.01M *hydrochloric acid*, dilute 10 ml of this solution to 50 ml with 0.01M *hydrochloric acid* and measure the *absorbance* of the resulting solution at the maximum at 249 nm, Appendix II B. Calculate the content of $C_{17}H_{20}N_2S,HCl$ taking 910 as the value of A(1%, 1 cm) at the maximum at 249 nm.

Storage Promethazine Injection should be protected from light.

Promethazine Oral Solution

Definition Promethazine Oral Solution is a solution containing Promethazine Hydrochloride in a suitable flavoured vehicle.

The oral solution complies with the requirements stated under Oral Liquids and with the following requirements.

Content of promethazine hydrochloride, $C_{17}H_{20}N_2S$, HCl 90.0 to 110.0% of the prescribed or stated amount.

Identification Carry out the method for *identification of phenothiazines*, Appendix III A, but applying as solution (1) 5 µl of a solution prepared by diluting a suitable volume of the oral solution with *water* to contain 0.08% w/v of Promethazine Hydrochloride.

Related substances Carry out the method for *thin-layer chromatography*, Appendix III A, protected from light under an atmosphere of nitrogen using *silica gel GF_{254}* as the coating substance (Merck silica gel 60 F_{254} plates are suitable) and a mixture of 15 volumes of *diethylamine*, 45 volumes of *hexane* and 50 volumes of *acetone* as the mobile phase but allowing the solvent front to ascend 12 cm above the line of application. Apply separately to the plate 10 µl of each of the following freshly prepared solutions. For solution (1) add 50 ml of *water* and 10 ml of a 5% w/v solution of *sodium hydroxide* to a quantity of the oral solution containing 20 mg of Promethazine Hydrochloride in a separating funnel and swirl to mix. Extract with two 100-ml quantities of *chloroform*, shaking vigorously for 1 minute each time, and filter successively through *anhydrous sodium sulphate*, washing the sodium sulphate with 50 ml of *chloroform*. Evaporate the combined extracts and washings to dryness at 30° using a rotary evaporator and dissolve the residue in 2 ml of a mixture of 5 volumes of *diethylamine* and 95 volumes of *methanol*. For solution (2) dilute 1 volume of solution (1) to 200 volumes with the same solvent. Solution (3) contains 0.01% w/v of *isopromethazine hydrochloride EPCRS* in the same solvent. Solution (4) contains 0.025% w/v of *promethazine sulphoxide BPCRS* in the same solvent. After removal of the plate, allow it to dry in air, spray with a 20% w/v solution of *perchloric acid* and heat at 100° for 5 minutes. In the chromatogram obtained with solution (1) any spot corresponding to isopromethazine is not more intense than the principal spot in the chromatogram obtained with solution (3) (1%), any spot corresponding to promethazine sulphoxide is not more intense than the principal spot in the chromatogram obtained with solution (4) (2.5%) and any other *secondary spot* is not more intense than the spot in the chromatogram obtained with solution (2) (0.5%). Disregard any spot remaining on the line of application.

Assay Carry out the following procedure protected from light. To a weighed quantity containing 10 mg of Promethazine Hydrochloride add 25 ml of *water* and 5 ml of a 5% w/v solution of *sodium hydroxide*. Extract the mixture with two 50-ml quantities of *chloroform*, shaking vigorously for 1 minute each time, evaporate the combined extracts to dryness at about 30° at a pressure of 2 kPa and dissolve the residue in sufficient 0.1M *hydrochloric acid* to produce 50 ml (solution A). Dilute 10 ml of solution A to 50 ml with *water* (solution B). To a further 10 ml of solution A add 5 ml of *peroxyacetic acid solution*, allow to stand for 10 minutes and add sufficient *water* to produce 50 ml (solution C). Measure the *absorbance* of solution C at the maximum at 336 nm, Appendix II B, using solution B in the reference cell and measure the *absorbance* of solution B at the same wavelength using *water* in the reference cell. Repeat the procedure using a 0.02% w/v solution of *promethazine hydrochloride BPCRS* in 0.1M *hydrochloric acid* in place of solution A and beginning at the words 'Dilute 10 ml of ...'. Determine the *weight per ml* of the oral solution, Appendix V G, and calculate the content of $C_{17}H_{20}N_2S,HCl$, weight in volume, using the declared content of $C_{17}H_{20}N_2S,HCl$ in *promethazine hydrochloride BPCRS*. The result is not valid if the absorbance of solution B is more than 0.10.

Storage Promethazine Oral Solution should be protected from light and stored at a temperature not exceeding 25°.

Promethazine Hydrochloride Tablets

Definition Promethazine Hydrochloride Tablets contain Promethazine Hydrochloride. They are coated.

The tablets comply with the requirements stated under Tablets and with the following requirements.

Content of promethazine hydrochloride, $C_{17}H_{20}N_2S$, HCl 95.0 to 105.0% of the prescribed or stated amount.

Identification

A. To a quantity of the powdered tablets containing 40 mg of Promethazine Hydrochloride add 10 ml of *water* and 2 ml of 1M *sodium hydroxide*, shake and extract with 15 ml of *ether*. Wash the ether with 5 ml of *water*, dry with *anhydrous sodium sulphate*, evaporate to dryness and dissolve the residue in 0.4 ml of *chloroform*. The *infrared absorption spectrum* of the resulting solution, Appendix II A, is concordant with the *reference spectrum* of promethazine.

B. To a quantity of the powdered tablets containing 5 mg of Promethazine Hydrochloride add 5 ml of *sulphuric acid* and allow to stand for 5 minutes. A red colour is produced.

C. Dissolve a quantity of the powdered tablets containing 0.2 g of Promethazine Hydrochloride in 2 ml of *water*, filter, saturate with *potassium carbonate sesquihydrate*, extract with two 10-ml quantities of *ether* and evaporate the combined extracts to dryness. Dissolve the residue in 2 ml of *methanol* and pour into a solution of 0.4 g of *picric acid* in 10 ml of *methanol* at about 50°. Cool, scratch the side of the tube to induce crystallisation, allow to stand for 3 to 4 hours and filter. The *melting point* of the crystals, after washing with *methanol* and drying, is about 160°, Appendix V A.

Related substances Carry out the test for *related substances in phenothiazines*, Appendix III A, using *mobile phase B* and applying separately to the plate 20 µl of each of the following freshly prepared solutions. For solution (1) extract a quantity of the powdered tablets containing 0.1 g of Promethazine Hydrochloride with 10 ml of a mixture of 95 volumes of *methanol* and 5 volumes of *diethylamine* and filter. Solution (2) contains 0.010% w/v of *isopromethazine hydrochloride EPCRS* in the same solvent. For solution (3) dilute 1 volume of solution (1) to 200 volumes with the same solvent. Any spot corresponding to isopromethazine in the chromatogram obtained with solution (1) is not more intense than the spot in the chromatogram obtained with solution (2) (1%) and any other *secondary spot* is not more intense than the spot in the chromatogram obtained with solution (3) (0.5%).

Assay Carry out the following procedure protected from light. Weigh and powder 20 tablets. Triturate a quantity of the powder containing 50 mg of Promethazine Hydrochloride with 10 ml of 2M *hydrochloric acid* and add 200 ml of *water*. Shake for 15 minutes, add sufficient *water* to produce 500 ml and centrifuge about 50 ml of the mixture. To 5 ml of the clear, supernatant liquid add 10 ml of 0.1M *hydrochloric acid* and sufficient *water* to produce 100 ml. Measure the *absorbance* of the resulting solution at the maximum at 249 nm, Appendix II B. Calculate the content of $C_{17}H_{20}N_2S,HCl$ taking 910 as the value of A(1%, 1 cm) at the maximum at 249 nm.

Promethazine Teoclate Tablets

Definition Promethazine Teoclate Tablets contain Promethazine Teoclate.

The tablets comply with the requirements stated under Tablets and with the following requirements.

Content of promethazine teoclate, $C_{17}H_{20}N_2S,C_7H_7ClN_4O_2$ 92.5 to 107.5% of the prescribed or stated amount.

Identification

A. To a quantity of the powdered tablets containing 60 mg of Promethazine Teoclate add 10 ml of *water* and 2 ml of 1M *sodium hydroxide*, shake and extract with 15 ml of *ether*. Wash the extract with 5 ml of *water*, dry with *anhydrous sodium sulphate*, evaporate to dryness and dissolve the residue in 0.4 ml of *chloroform*. The *infrared absorption spectrum* of the resulting solution, Appendix II A, is concordant with the *reference spectrum* of promethazine.

B. To a quantity of the powdered tablets containing 5 mg of Promethazine Teoclate add 5 ml of *sulphuric acid* and allow to stand for 5 minutes. A red colour is produced.

C. Extract a quantity of the powdered tablets containing 0.2 g of Promethazine Teoclate with *chloroform*, filter and evaporate the filtrate to dryness. Shake the residue with 10 ml of *water*, add 4 ml of 5M *ammonia* and extract with two 30-ml quantities of *ether*. Wash the combined extracts with 10 ml of *water* and reserve the aqueous layer and washings. To the combined aqueous layer and washings add 4 ml of *hydrochloric acid*; a white precipitate is produced. Filter, wash the residue with *water* and dry at 105°. Dissolve 10 mg of the residue in 1 ml of *hydrochloric acid*, add 0.1 g of *potassium chlorate* and evaporate to dryness. A reddish residue remains which becomes purple on exposure to the vapour of 5M *ammonia*.

Related substances Carry out the test for *related substances in phenothiazines*, Appendix III A, using *mobile phase B* and applying separately to the plate 10 µl of each of the following freshly prepared solutions. For solution (1) extract a quantity of the powdered tablets containing 0.2 g of Promethazine Teoclate with 10 ml of a mixture of 95 volumes of *methanol* and 5 volumes of *diethylamine* and filter. Solution (2) contains 0.020% w/v of *isopromethazine hydrochloride EPCRS* in the same solvent. For solution (3) dilute 1 volume of solution (1) to 200 volumes with the same solvent. Any spot corresponding to isopromethazine in the chromatogram obtained with solution (1) is not more intense than the spot in the chromatogram obtained with solution (2) (1%) and any other *secondary spot* is not more intense than the spot in the chromatogram obtained with solution (3) (0.5%).

Assay Carry out the following procedure protected from light. Weigh and powder 20 tablets. To a quantity of the powder containing 50 mg of Promethazine Teoclate add 5 ml of *water* and 1 ml of 13.5M *ammonia* and allow to stand for 5 minutes. Add 50 ml of *absolute ethanol*, shake for 5 minutes and filter, washing the residue with five 5-ml quantities of *absolute ethanol*. Add sufficient *absolute ethanol* to the filtrate to produce 100 ml. Dilute 10 ml to 100 ml with *absolute ethanol* and dilute 10 ml of this dilution to 100 ml with *absolute ethanol*. Measure the *absorbance* of the resulting solution at the maximum at 255 nm, Appendix II B. Calculate the content of $C_{17}H_{20}N_2S,C_7H_7ClN_4O_2$ taking 755 as the value of A(1%, 1 cm) at the maximum at 255 nm.

Storage Promethazine Teoclate Tablets should be protected from light.

When promethazine theoclate tablets are prescribed or demanded, Promethazine Teoclate Tablets shall be dispensed or supplied.

Propantheline Tablets

Definition Propantheline Tablets contain Propantheline Bromide. They are coated.

The tablets comply with the requirements stated under Tablets and with the following requirements.

Content of propantheline bromide, $C_{23}H_{30}BrNO_3$ 95.0 to 105.0% of the prescribed or stated amount.

Identification Triturate a quantity of the powdered tablets containing 75 mg of Propantheline Bromide with 10 ml of *chloroform*, filter, evaporate the chloroform and stir the residue with 5 ml of *ether* until it solidifies. The solid complies with the following tests.

A. Dissolve 60 mg in 2 ml of *water*, add 2 ml of 5M *sodium hydroxide*, boil for 2 minutes, cool slightly, acidify with 2M *hydrochloric acid*, heat to boiling, add *ethanol (96%)* dropwise until the precipitate just dissolves, cool and filter. The *melting point* of the residue, after washing with *water*, recrystallising from *ethanol (50%)* and drying at 105° for 1 hour, is about 215°, Appendix V A. The crystals dissolve in *sulphuric acid* to produce a bright yellow solution which fluoresces strongly in ultraviolet light (365 nm).

B. Yields the reactions characteristic of *bromides*, Appendix VI.

Xanthanoic acid Shake the combined ether extracts reserved in the Assay with two 30-ml quantities of 0.1M *sodium hydroxide* containing 1.5% w/v of *sodium chloride*. Remove the ether from the combined aqueous extracts by heating on a water bath, add sufficient 0.1M *sodium hydroxide* to produce 100 ml and dilute 25 ml to 100 ml with 0.1M *sodium hydroxide*. The *absorbance* of the resulting solution at the maximum at 248 nm is not more than 0.31, Appendix II B.

Assay Weigh and powder 20 tablets or more if necessary. Place a quantity of the powder containing 0.5 g of Propantheline Bromide on a sintered-glass filter, add 10 ml of *peroxide-free ether*, dried over sodium and distilled before use, stir and filter. Repeat the extraction with four 10-ml quantities of the ether and reserve the combined ether extracts for the test for Xanthanoic acid. Extract the residue on the filter with four 10-ml quantities of *chloroform*, evaporate the combined chloroform extracts to about 10 ml, add 10 ml of *mercury(II) acetate solution* and carry out Method I for *non-aqueous titration*, Appendix VIII A, using *crystal violet solution* as indicator. Each ml of 0.1M *perchloric acid VS* is equivalent to 44.84 mg of $C_{23}H_{30}BrNO_3$.

Propranolol Injection

Definition Propranolol Injection is a sterile solution of Propranolol Hydrochloride in Water for Injections containing Anhydrous Citric Acid or Citric Acid Monohydrate.

The injection complies with the requirements stated under Parenteral Preparations and with the following requirements.

Content of propranolol hydrochloride, $C_{16}H_{21}NO_2$, HCl 90.0 to 110.0% of the prescribed or stated amount.

Identification

A. Make alkaline with 1M *sodium hydroxide* a volume containing 10 mg of Propranolol Hydrochloride and extract with three 5-ml quantities of *ether*. Wash the combined extracts with *water* until the washings are free from alkali, dry with *anhydrous sodium sulphate*, filter, evaporate the filtrate to dryness and dry the residue at 50° at a pressure of 2 kPa for 1 hour. The *infrared absorption spectrum* of the residue, Appendix II A, is concordant with the *reference spectrum* of propranolol.

B. The *light absorption* of the solution obtained in the Assay, Appendix II B, exhibits maxima at 290, 306 and 319 nm.

Acidity pH, 3.0 to 3.5, Appendix V L.

Related substances Carry out the method for *liquid chromatography*, Appendix III D, injecting 10 µl of each of the following solutions. Solution (1) contains 0.1% w/v of *propranolol hydrochloride for performance test EPCRS* and 0.002% w/v of *phenanthrene* in the mobile phase. For solution (2) dilute the injection being examined with *acetonitrile*, if necessary, to contain 0.10% w/v of Propranolol Hydrochloride. For solution (3) dilute 1 volume of solution (1) to 500 volumes with the mobile phase.

The chromatographic procedure may be carried out using (a) a stainless steel column (20 cm × 5 mm) packed with *stationary phase C* (5 µm) (Hypersil ODS 5µ is suitable), (b) as the mobile phase with a flow rate of 1.8 ml per minute a mixture of 1.15 g of *sodium dodecyl sulphate*, 10 ml of a mixture of 1 volume of *sulphuric acid* and 9 volumes of *water*, 20 ml of a 1.7% w/v solution of *tetrabutylammonium dihydrogen orthophosphate*, 370 ml of *water* and 600 ml of *acetonitrile*, the mixture adjusted to pH 3.3 with 2M *sodium hydroxide*, and (c) a detection wavelength of 292 nm.

The chromatogram obtained with solution (1) should exhibit well-separated peaks with retention times of about 1.8 minutes (3-(1-naphthyloxy)propane-1,2-diol) (diol impurity), about 2.5 minutes (propranolol), about 8 minutes (1,1′-isopropyliminobis[3-(1-naphthyloxy)-propan-2-ol]) (tertiary amine impurity) and about 10 minutes (phenanthrene). If this pattern is not obtained, adjust the composition of the mobile phase in the following manner. Adjust the concentration of acetonitrile to obtain a retention time of 10 minutes for phenanthrene (increasing the concentration to decrease the retention time and decreasing the concentration to increase the retention time); then adjust the concentration of sodium dodecyl sulphate to obtain a retention time of 8 minutes for the tertiary amine impurity (increasing the concentration to increase the retention time and decreasing the concentration to decrease the retention time); if the peaks due to the diol impurity and propranolol are not separated make small adjustments in the concentration of acetonitrile to achieve separation. Adjust the sensitivity so that the deflection (A) for the diol impurity measured from the base line is at least 50% of full-scale deflection. Measure the height (B) above the base line of the lowest point of the curve separating this peak from that due to propranolol. The test is not valid unless B is less than 25% of A.

For solutions (2) and (3) record the chromatograms for twice the retention time of phenanthrene. In the chromatogram obtained with solution (2) the area of any *secondary peak* is not greater than the area of the principal peak in the chromatogram obtained with solution (3) (0.2%) and the sum of the areas of any *secondary peaks* is not greater than four times the area of the principal peak in the chromatogram obtained with solution (3) (0.8%).

Assay To a volume containing 2 mg of Propranolol Hydrochloride add sufficient *methanol* to produce 100 ml and measure the *absorbance* of the resulting solution at the maximum at 290 nm, Appendix II B. Calculate the content of $C_{16}H_{21}NO_2$,HCl taking 206 as the value of A(1%, 1 cm) at the maximum at 290 nm.

Propranolol Tablets

Definition Propranolol Tablets contain Propranolol Hydrochloride.

The tablets comply with the requirements stated under Tablets and with the following requirements.

Content of propranolol hydrochloride, $C_{16}H_{21}NO_2$, HCl 92.5 to 107.5% of the prescribed or stated amount.

Identification

A. Suspend a quantity of the powdered tablets containing 0.1 g of Propranolol Hydrochloride in 20 ml of *water*, filter, make the filtrate alkaline with 1M *sodium hydroxide* and extract with three 10-ml quantities of *ether*. Wash the combined extracts with *water* until the washings are free from alkali, dry with *anhydrous sodium sulphate*, filter, evaporate the filtrate to dryness and dry the residue at 50° at a pressure of 2 kPa for 1 hour. The *infrared absorption spectrum* of the residue, Appendix II A, is concordant with the *reference spectrum* of propranolol.

B. The *light absorption* of the solution obtained in the Assay, Appendix II B, exhibits maxima at 290, 306 and 319 nm.

C. *Melting point* of the residue obtained in test A, about 94°, Appendix V A.

Related substances Carry out the method for *liquid chromatography*, Appendix III D, injecting 10 µl of each of the following solutions. Solution (1) contains 0.1% w/v of *propranolol hydrochloride for performance test EPCRS* and 0.002% w/v of *phenanthrene* in the mobile phase. For solution (2) add 100 ml of *methanol* to a quantity of the powdered tablets containing 0.1 g of Propranolol Hydrochloride, shake, filter through glass-microfibre paper (Whatman GF/C is suitable) and use the filtrate. For solution (3) dilute 1 volume of solution (1) to 500 volumes with the mobile phase.

The chromatographic procedure may be carried out using (a) a stainless steel column (20 cm × 5 mm) packed with *stationary phase C* (5 µm) (Hypersil ODS 5µ is suitable), (b) as the mobile phase with a flow rate of 1.8 ml per minute a mixture of 1.15 g of *sodium dodecyl sulphate*,

10 ml of a mixture of 1 volume of *sulphuric acid* and 9 volumes of *water*, 20 ml of a 1.7% w/v solution of *tetrabutylammonium dihydrogen orthophosphate*, 370 ml of *water* and 600 ml of *acetonitrile*, the mixture adjusted to pH 3.3 with 2M *sodium hydroxide*, and (c) a detection wavelength of 292 nm.

The chromatogram obtained with solution (1) should exhibit well-separated peaks with retention times of about 1.8 minutes (3-(1-naphthyloxy)propane-1,2-diol) (diol impurity), about 2.5 minutes (propranolol), about 8 minutes (1,1′-isopropyliminobis[3-(1-naphthyloxy)-propan-2-ol]) (tertiary amine impurity) and about 10 minutes (phenanthrene). If this pattern is not obtained, adjust the composition of the mobile phase in the following manner. Adjust the concentration of acetonitrile to obtain a retention time of 10 minutes for phenanthrene (increasing the concentration to decrease the retention time and decreasing the concentration to increase the retention time); then adjust the concentration of sodium dodecyl sulphate to obtain a retention time of 8 minutes for the tertiary amine impurity (increasing the concentration to increase the retention time and decreasing the concentration to decrease the retention time); if the peaks due to the diol impurity and propranolol are not separated make small adjustments in the concentration of acetonitrile to achieve separation. Adjust the sensitivity so that the deflection (A) for the diol impurity measured from the base line is at least 50% of full-scale deflection. Measure the height (B) above the base line of the lowest point of the curve separating this peak from that due to propranolol. The test is not valid unless B is less than 25% of A.

For solutions (2) and (3) record the chromatograms for twice the retention time of phenanthrene. In the chromatogram obtained with solution (2) the area of any *secondary peak* is not greater than the area of the principal peak in the chromatogram obtained with solution (3) (0.2%) and the sum of the areas of any *secondary peaks* is not greater than four times the area of the principal peak in the chromatogram obtained with solution (3) (0.8%).

Assay Weigh and powder 20 tablets. Shake a quantity of the powder containing 20 mg of Propranolol Hydrochloride with 20 ml of *water* for 10 minutes. Add 50 ml of *methanol*, shake for a further 10 minutes, add sufficient *methanol* to produce 100 ml and filter. Dilute 10 ml of the filtrate to 50 ml with *methanol* and measure the *absorbance* of the resulting solution at the maximum at 290 nm, Appendix II B. Calculate the content of $C_{16}H_{21}NO_2,HCl$ taking 206 as the value of A(1%, 1 cm) at the maximum at 290 nm.

Propyliodone Injection

Propyliodone Suspension

Definition Propyliodone Injection is a sterile suspension of Propyliodone in Water for Injections.

The injection complies with the requirements stated under Parenteral Preparations and with the following requirements.

Content of propyliodone, $C_{10}H_{11}I_2NO_3$ 47.5 to 52.5% w/v.

Identification

A. Mix 1 g with 25 ml of *water*, filter through a sintered-glass filter and wash with three 25-ml quantities of *water*. The *melting point* of the residue, after drying at 105°, is about 188°, Appendix V A.

B. Heat the residue obtained in test A with *sulphuric acid*. Violet vapours of iodine are evolved.

Acidity or alkalinity pH, 6.0 to 7.5, Appendix V L.

Weight per ml At 20°, 1.260 to 1.295 g when determined by the following method. To 10 g in a tared, 50-ml density bottle add about 30 ml of *water* and swirl to disperse. Dilute almost to volume with *water*, add 0.1 ml of *ether* and remove the ether by passing a gentle current of air over the surface. Adjust the temperature of the mixture to between 19.8° and 20.2°, dilute to 50 ml with *water* at the same temperature and weigh. Calculate the weight per ml at 20° from the expression

$$[0.9972(w_1-w)]/[(w_3-w)-(w_2-w_1)]$$

where w = the weight of the density bottle,

w_1 = the combined weight of the bottle and injection,

w_2 = the combined weight of the bottle and its total contents and

w_3 = the weight of the bottle filled with *water* at a temperature between 19.8° and 20.2°.

3,5-Di-iodo-4-oxo-1-pyridylacetic acid Not more than 0.5% w/v when determined by the following method. To 6.4 g of the well-shaken injection add 100 ml of a solution containing 0.6% w/v of *sodium chloride* and 1% w/v of *sodium citrate*, shake continuously at 20° for 1 hour, filter, dilute 10 ml of the filtrate to 50 ml with the extracting solution and measure the *absorbance* of a 0.5-cm layer of the resulting solution at the maximum at 284 nm, Appendix II B. Calculate the content of 3,5-di-iodo-4-oxo-1-pyridylacetic acid, $C_7H_5I_2NO_3$, from the expression $(5.025A/w)-0.10$, where A is the observed absorbance and w is the weight, in g, of injection taken.

Inorganic iodide Mix 8.8 ml of *water* with 1.2 ml of the supernatant liquid obtained by centrifuging the injection, add 1 ml of 2M *nitric acid*, 1 ml of a 0.2% w/v solution of *sodium nitrite* and 1 ml of *chloroform*, shake and centrifuge. Any purple colour in the chloroform layer is not more intense than that obtained when a mixture of 2 ml of *iodide standard solution (20 ppm I)* and 8 ml of *water* is treated in the same manner.

Assay Carry out the method for *oxygen-flask combustion for iodine*, Appendix VIII C. Use 30 mg enclosed in a suitable filter paper capsule containing a small plug of absorbent cotton, allow the capsule and contents to stand for 30 minutes before combustion and use a 1000-ml flask. Each ml of 0.02M *sodium thiosulphate VS* is equivalent to 0.7450 mg of $C_{10}H_{11}I_2NO_3$. Using the weight per ml of the injection, calculate the percentage w/v of $C_{10}H_{11}I_2NO_3$.

Storage Propyliodone Injection should be protected from light and stored at a temperature of 10° to 30°.

Propyliodone Oily Injection

Propyliodone Oily Suspension

Definition Propyliodone Oily Injection is a sterile suspension of Propyliodone in Arachis Oil.

The injection complies with the requirements stated under Parenteral Preparations and with the following requirements.

Content of propyliodone, $C_{10}H_{11}I_2NO_3$ 57.0 to 63.0% w/v.

Characteristics A white or almost white suspension.

Identification

A. Mix 1 g with 20 ml of *petroleum spirit (boiling range, 40° to 60°)*, filter through a sintered-glass filter and wash free from arachis oil with *petroleum spirit (boiling range, 40° to 60°)*. The *melting point* of the residue, after drying at 105°, is about 188°, Appendix V A.

B. Heat the residue obtained in test A with *sulphuric acid.* Violet vapours of iodine are evolved.

Weight per ml 1.235 to 1.280 g when determined by the following method. Transfer 60 to 70 ml of the well-shaken injection to a 250-ml beaker, place in a vacuum desiccator and cautiously reduce the pressure. When vigorous frothing ceases, reduce the pressure to about 1.4 kPa and allow to stand for 15 minutes. Remove from the desiccator, mix gently taking care not to introduce air bubbles and transfer to a tared, 50-ml density bottle. Adjust the temperature to 20°, remove any excess of the injection and weigh.

Inorganic iodide Disperse 3.3 ml in 125 ml of *ethanol-free chloroform*, add 25 ml of 0.01M *sodium hydroxide* and shake. Extract the aqueous layer with 125 ml of *ethanol-free chloroform*, discard the chloroform layer and neutralise the aqueous layer to *litmus paper* with 2M *nitric acid.* To 10 ml add 1 ml of 2M *nitric acid*, 1 ml of a 0.2% w/v solution of *sodium nitrite* and 1 ml of *chloroform*, shake and centrifuge. Any purple colour in the chloroform layer is not more intense than that obtained when a mixture of 2 ml of *iodide standard solution (20 ppm I)* and 8 ml of *water* is treated in the same manner.

Assay Carry out the method for *oxygen-flask combustion for iodine*, Appendix VIII C, using 30 mg enclosed in a suitable filter paper capsule containing a small plug of absorbent cotton and a 1000-ml flask. Each ml of 0.02M *sodium thiosulphate VS* is equivalent to 0.7450 mg of $C_{10}H_{11}I_2NO_3$. Using the weight per ml of the suspension, calculate the percentage w/v of $C_{10}H_{11}I_2NO_3$.

Storage Propyliodone Oily Injection should be protected from light and stored at a temperature not exceeding 30°.

Propylthiouracil Tablets

Definition Propylthiouracil Tablets contain Propylthiouracil.

The tablets comply with the requirements stated under Tablets and with the following requirements.

Content of propylthiouracil, $C_7H_{10}N_2OS$ 92.5 to 107.5% of the prescribed or stated amount.

Identification

A. Shake a quantity of the powdered tablets containing 50 mg of Propylthiouracil with 20 ml of *methanol* for 10 minutes, filter and evaporate to dryness. The *infrared absorption spectrum* of the residue, Appendix II A, is concordant with the *reference spectrum* of propylthiouracil.

B. Shake a quantity of the powdered tablets containing 50 mg of Propylthiouracil with 60 ml of *methanol* for 20 minutes, dilute to 100 ml with *methanol* and filter. Dilute 5 ml of this solution to 250 ml with *methanol.* The *light absorption* of the resulting solution, Appendix II B, in the range 230 to 350 nm exhibits a maximum only at 274 nm.

C. Extract a quantity of the powdered tablets in a continuous extraction apparatus with *ether* and evaporate the solution to dryness. The *melting point* of the residue, after drying at 105°, is about 219°, Appendix V A.

Related substances Carry out the method for *thin-layer chromatography*, Appendix III A, using *silica gel GF_{254}* as the coating substance and a mixture of 0.2 volume of *glacial acetic acid*, 12 volumes of *propan-2-ol* and 100 volumes of *chloroform* as the mobile phase. Apply separately to the plate 10 µl of each of the following solutions. For solution (1) shake a quantity of the powdered tablets containing 50 mg of Propylthiouracil with 5 ml of *methanol* for 15 minutes, filter and use the filtrate. For solution (2) dilute 1 volume of solution (1) to 100 volumes with *methanol.* Solution (3) contains 0.0010% w/v of *thiourea* in *methanol.* After removal of the plate, allow it to dry in air, examine under *ultraviolet light (254 nm)* and expose to iodine vapour for 10 minutes. Any spot corresponding to thiourea in the chromatogram obtained with solution (1) is not more intense than the spot in the chromatogram obtained with solution (3) (0.1%) and any other *secondary spot* is not more intense than the spot in the chromatogram obtained with solution (2) (1%). Disregard any spot remaining on the line of application.

Assay Weigh and powder 20 tablets. Dissolve a quantity of the powder containing 0.15 g of Propylthiouracil in a mixture of 20 ml of 0.1M *sodium hydroxide VS* and 75 ml of *water* with the aid of gentle heat. Cool, add 4 g of *sodium acetate*, just acidify the solution to *litmus paper* with 6M *acetic acid*, add 0.5 ml of a freshly prepared 0.5% w/v solution of *1,5-diphenylcarbazone* in *ethanol (96%)* and titrate with 0.02M *mercury nitrate VS* until a pinkish violet colour persists for 2 to 3 minutes. Each ml of 0.02M *mercury nitrate VS* is equivalent to 6.808 mg of $C_7H_{10}N_2OS$.

Protamine Sulphate Injection

Definition Protamine Sulphate Injection is a sterile solution of Protamine Sulphate in Water for Injections.

The injection complies with the requirements stated under Parenteral Preparations and with the following requirements.

Content of protamine sulphate Not less than 80.0% of the prescribed or stated amount.

Identification

A. Produces a precipitate under the conditions of the Assay.

B. Dilute the injection with *water* to give a solution containing 0.2% w/v of Protamine Sulphate. To 5 ml add 1 ml of a 10% w/v solution of *sodium hydroxide* and 1 ml of a 0.02% w/v solution of *1-naphthol* and mix. Cool to 5°

and add 0.5 ml of *sodium hypobromite solution.* An intense pink colour is produced.

C. Heat 2 ml in a water bath at 60° and add 0.1 ml of *mercury(II) sulphate solution*; no precipitate is produced. Cool the mixture in ice; a white precipitate is produced.

D. Yields reaction A characteristic of *sulphates*, Appendix VI.

Acidity pH, 2.5 to 3.5, Appendix V L.

Optical rotation Dilute the injection with 0.5M *hydrochloric acid* to produce a solution containing 0.8% w/v of Protamine Sulphate. The *optical rotation* of the resulting solution is –0.52° to –0.68°, Appendix V F.

Light absorption Dilute the injection, if necessary, with *water* to produce a solution containing 1% w/v of Protamine Sulphate. The *absorbance* at 260 to 280 nm is not more than 0.1, Appendix II B.

Bacterial endotoxins Carry out the *test for bacterial endotoxins*, Appendix XIV C. Dilute the injection, if necessary, with *water BET* to give a solution containing 10 mg of Protamine Sulphate per ml (solution A). The endotoxin limit concentration of solution A is 70 IU of endotoxin per ml. Carry out the test using the maximum allowable concentration of solution A calculated from the declared sensitivity of the lysate used in the test.

Assay Carry out the Assay described under Protamine Sulphate using solutions prepared by diluting the injection with *water* to contain (1) 0.015% w/v, (2) 0.010% w/v and (3) 0.005% w/v of Protamine Sulphate.

Labelling The label states that the dose is calculated from the results of determinations of the amount required to produce an acceptable blood clotting time in the patient.

Protriptyline Tablets

Definition Protriptyline Tablets contain Protriptyline Hydrochloride. They are coated.

The tablets comply with the requirements stated under Tablets and with the following requirements.

Content of protriptyline hydrochloride, $C_{19}H_{21}N$, HCl 90.0 to 110.0% of the prescribed or stated amount.

Identification

A. The *light absorption*, Appendix II B, in the range 230 to 350 nm of the solution obtained in the Assay exhibits a maximum only at 292 nm.

B. Shake a quantity of the powdered tablets containing 5 mg of Protriptyline Hydrochloride with 20 ml of *methanol* and filter. To 1 ml of the filtrate add 1 ml of a 2.5% w/v solution of *sodium hydrogen carbonate*, 1 ml of a 2% w/v solution of *sodium periodate* and 1 ml of a 0.3% w/v solution of *potassium permanganate*. Allow to stand for 15 minutes, acidify with 1M *sulphuric acid* and extract with 10 ml of *2,2,4-trimethylpentane*, washing the extract with 10 ml of 0.25M *sulphuric acid*. The *light absorption* of the resulting trimethylpentane solution, Appendix II B, does not exhibit a maximum at 265 nm (distinction from amitriptyline and nortriptyline).

C. Triturate a quantity of the powdered tablets containing 0.1 g of Protriptyline Hydrochloride with 10 ml of *chloroform*, filter and evaporate the filtrate to dryness. Dissolve part of the residue in 3 ml of *water* and add 0.05 ml of a 2.5% w/v solution of *quinhydrone* in *methanol*. A red colour develops.

Assay Triturate 10 tablets for 15 minutes with 100 ml of a solution prepared by mixing 1 volume of 1M *hydrochloric acid* and 9 volumes of *methanol*, transfer to a graduated flask using sufficient of the solvent mixture to produce 250 ml, mix and filter through a fine filter paper. Dilute a volume of the filtrate containing 1 mg of Protriptyline Hydrochloride to 100 ml with the solvent mixture and measure the *absorbance* of the resulting solution at the maximum at 292 nm, Appendix II B. Calculate the content of $C_{19}H_{21}N$,HCl taking 465 as the value of A(1%, 1 cm) at the maximum at 292 nm.

Proxymetacaine Eye Drops

Definition Proxymetacaine Eye Drops are a sterile solution of Proxymetacaine Hydrochloride in Purified Water. They may contain Glycerol.

With the exception that they may be supplied in containers not exceeding 15 ml in capacity, the eye drops comply with the requirements stated under Eye Preparations and with the following requirements.

Content of proxymetacaine hydrochloride, $C_{16}H_{26}N_2O_3$,HCl 90.0 to 110.0% of the prescribed or stated amount.

Identification

A. The *light absorption*, Appendix II B, in the range 250 to 350 nm of the solution used in the Assay exhibits two maxima, at 268 nm and 310 nm.

B. To a volume containing 50 mg of Proxymetacaine Hydrochloride add 2 ml of 2M *hydrochloric acid* and extract with 25 ml of *chloroform*. Discard the chloroform layer, make alkaline with 5M *sodium hydroxide* and extract with two 25-ml quantities of *chloroform*. Filter the combined extracts through *anhydrous sodium sulphate* and evaporate the filtrate to dryness using a rotary evaporator. The *infrared absorption spectrum* of the oily residue, Appendix II A, is concordant with the *reference spectrum* of proxymetacaine.

C. A volume containing 5 mg of Proxymetacaine Hydrochloride yields the reaction characteristic of *primary aromatic amines*, Appendix VI.

Related substances

A. Comply with test A described under Proxymetacaine Hydrochloride using the following solutions. For solution (1) use the eye drops, diluted if necessary to contain 0.5% w/v of Proxymetacaine Hydrochloride. For solution (2) dilute 1 volume of solution (1) to 100 volumes with *methanol*. For solution (3) dilute 1 volume of solution (2) with an equal volume of *methanol*.

B. Carry out test B described under Proxymetacaine Hydrochloride using 10 µl of solution (1) described in test A above and 10 µl of each of two solutions of *3-amino-4-propoxybenzoic acid BPCRS* in *methanol* containing (2) 0.020% w/v and (3) 0.0050% w/v. Any *secondary spot* in the chromatogram obtained with solution (1) is not more intense than the spot in the chromatogram obtained with solution (2) (4%) and not more than one such spot is more intense than the spot in the chromatogram obtained with solution (3) (1%). The principal spot in the chromatogram obtained with solution (1) remains on the line of application.

Assay Dilute a volume containing 10 mg of Proxymetacaine Hydrochloride to 200 ml with *water* and measure the *absorbance* of the resulting solution at the maximum at 310 nm, Appendix II B. Calculate the content of $C_{16}H_{26}N_2O_3$,HCl taking 162 as the value of A(1%, 1 cm) at the maximum at 310 nm.

Storage Proxymetacaine Eye Drops should be protected from light, stored at a temperature of 2° to 8° and should not be allowed to freeze.

Pseudoephedrine Tablets

Definition Pseudoephedrine Tablets contain Pseudoephedrine Hydrochloride.

The tablets comply with the requirements stated under Tablets and with the following requirements.

Content of pseudoephedrine hydrochloride, $C_{10}H_{15}NO$,HCl 95.0 to 105.0% of the prescribed or stated amount.

Identification

A. Shake a quantity of the powdered tablets containing 60 mg of Pseudoephedrine Hydrochloride with 10 ml of *water* and filter. Shake the filtrate with 10 ml of *ether*, discard the ether, add 1 ml of 1M *sodium hydroxide* to the aqueous layer and extract with two 10-ml quantities of *ether*. Dry the combined ether extracts with *anhydrous sodium sulphate*, filter and evaporate the filtrate to dryness. The *infrared absorption spectrum* of the residue, Appendix II A, is concordant with the *reference spectrum* of pseudoephedrine.

B. In the test for Related substances, the principal spot in the chromatogram obtained with solution (2) corresponds to that in the chromatogram obtained with solution (4).

Related substances Comply with the requirements stated under Pseudoephedrine Hydrochloride but using a solution prepared in the following manner as solution (1). Remove any film coating from the tablets before proceeding. Add 25 ml of *methanol* to a quantity of the powdered tablets containing 0.5 g of Pseudoephedrine Hydrochloride, shake for 5 minutes, filter, wash the filter with *methanol* and evaporate the combined filtrate and washings to dryness. Dissolve the residue as completely as possible in 5 ml of *methanol*, centrifuge and dilute 1 ml of the supernatant liquid to 50 ml with the mobile phase.

Assay Weigh and powder 20 tablets. Carry out the method for *liquid chromatography*, Appendix III D, using the following solutions. Solution (1) is a 0.12% w/v solution of *pseudoephedrine hydrochloride BPCRS* in *methanol (50%)*. For solution (2) add 50 ml of 0.1M *hydrochloric acid* to a quantity of the powdered tablets containing 0.12 g of Pseudoephedrine Hydrochloride, mix with the aid of ultrasound for 15 minutes, add sufficient *methanol* to produce 100 ml, filter and use the filtrate.

The chromatographic procedure may be carried out using (a) a stainless steel column (20 cm × 4.6 mm) packed with *stationary phase C* (10 μm) (Nucleosil C18 is suitable), (b) 0.005M *dioctyl sodium sulphosuccinate* in a mixture of 65 volumes of *methanol*, 35 volumes of *water* and 1 volume of *glacial acetic acid* as the mobile phase with a flow rate of 1.5 ml per minute and (c) a detection wavelength of 258 nm.

Calculate the content of $C_{10}H_{15}NO$,HCl using the declared content of $C_{10}H_{15}NO$,HCl in *pseudoephedrine hydrochloride BPCRS*.

Pyrazinamide Tablets

Definition Pyrazinamide Tablets contain Pyrazinamide.

The tablets comply with the requirements stated under Tablets and with the following requirements.

Content of pyrazinamide, $C_5H_5N_3O$ 95.0 to 105.0% of the prescribed or stated amount.

Identification

A. Shake a quantity of the powdered tablets containing 0.25 g of Pyrazinamide with 20 ml of *absolute ethanol*, filter, evaporate the filtrate to dryness and dry the residue at 105° for 30 minutes. The *infrared absorption spectrum* of the residue, Appendix II A, is concordant with the *reference spectrum* of pyrazinamide.

B. Shake a quantity of the powdered tablets containing 50 mg of Pyrazinamide with 50 ml of *water* and filter. Dilute 1 ml of the filtrate to 100 ml with *water*. The *light absorption* of the resulting solution, Appendix II B, in the range 230 to 350 nm exhibits two maxima, at 268 nm and 310 nm.

C. Boil a quantity of the powdered tablets containing 20 mg of Pyrazinamide with 5 ml of 5M *sodium hydroxide*. Ammonia, recognisable by its odour, is evolved.

Related substances Carry out the method for *thin-layer chromatography*, Appendix III A, using *silica gel GF_{254}* as the coating substance and a mixture of 20 volumes of *glacial acetic acid*, 20 volumes of *water* and 60 volumes of *butan-1-ol* as the mobile phase but allowing the solvent front to ascend 10 cm above the line of application. Apply separately to the plate 20 μl of each of the following solutions. For solution (1) shake a quantity of the powdered tablets containing 0.10 g of Pyrazinamide with 50 ml of a mixture of 9 volumes of *chloroform* and 1 volume of *methanol*, filter, evaporate to dryness and dissolve the residue in sufficient of the same solvent mixture to produce 10 ml. For solution (2) dilute 1 volume of solution (1) to 500 volumes with a mixture of 9 volumes of *chloroform* and 1 volume of *methanol*. After removal of the plate, allow it to dry in air and examine immediately under *ultraviolet light (254 nm)*. Any *secondary spot* in the chromatogram obtained with solution (1) is not more intense than the spot in the chromatogram obtained with solution (2) (0.2%).

Assay Weigh and powder 20 tablets. To a quantity of the powder containing 0.1 g of Pyrazinamide add 200 ml of *water*, allow to stand for 10 minutes, swirling occasionally, mix with the aid of ultrasound for 10 minutes and dilute to 500 ml with *water*. Filter and discard the first 20 ml of filtrate. Dilute 5 ml of the filtrate to 100 ml with *water* and measure the *absorbance* of the resulting solution at the maximum at 268 nm, Appendix II B. Calculate the content of $C_5H_5N_3O$ taking 650 as the value of A(1%, 1 cm) at the maximum at 268 nm.

Pyridostigmine Injection

Definition Pyridostigmine Injection is a sterile solution of Pyridostigmine Bromide in Water for Injections.

The injection complies with the requirements stated under Parenteral Preparations and with the following requirements.

Content of pyridostigmine bromide, $C_9H_{13}BrN_2O_2$
95.0 to 105.0% of the prescribed or stated amount.

Identification

A. The *light absorption*, Appendix II B, of the solution obtained in the Assay exhibits a maximum at 270 nm.

B. Carry out the method for *thin-layer chromatography*, Appendix III A, using *silica gel G* as the coating substance and a mixture of 5 volumes of *water*, 10 volumes of *formic acid*, 35 volumes of *methanol* and 50 volumes of *chloroform* as the mobile phase. Apply separately to the plate 10 µl of each of the following solutions. For solution (1) use the injection being examined, diluted if necessary with *water* to produce a solution containing 0.05% w/v of Pyridostigmine Bromide. Solution (2) contains 0.05% w/v of *neostigmine methylsulphate BPCRS* in *water*. After removal of the plate, allow it to dry in air and spray with *dilute potassium iodobismuthate solution*. The principal spot in the chromatogram obtained with solution (1) has an Rf value of about 1.3 relative to the spot in the chromatogram obtained with solution (2).

C. Yields the reactions characteristic of *bromides*, Appendix VI.

Acidity pH, 5.7 to 6.3, Appendix V L.

Light absorption Extract a volume containing 5 mg of Pyridostigmine Bromide with five 10-ml quantities of *ether*. Separate the aqueous layer, rinsing the separating funnel with 2 ml of *phosphate buffer pH 7.0*, and dilute the combined aqueous layers to 10 ml with *water*. The *absorbance* of the resulting solution at 320 nm is not more than 0.50, Appendix II B.

Assay To a volume containing 5 mg of Pyridostigmine Bromide add 20 ml of 0.01M *hydrochloric acid* and extract with three 20-ml quantities of *ether*. Wash the combined ether extracts with the same two 10-ml quantities of 0.01M *hydrochloric acid*, combine the aqueous solutions, remove any residual ether by passing *nitrogen* through the solution and dilute to 200 ml with *water*. Measure the *absorbance* of the resulting solution at the maximum at 270 nm, Appendix II B. Calculate the content of $C_9H_{13}BrN_2O_2$ taking 186 as the value of A(1%, 1 cm) at the maximum at 270 nm.

Storage Pyridostigmine Injection should be protected from light.

Pyridostigmine Tablets

Definition Pyridostigmine Tablets contain Pyridostigmine Bromide.

The tablets comply with the requirements stated under Tablets and with the following requirements.

Content of pyridostigmine bromide, $C_9H_{13}BrN_2O_2$
92.5 to 107.5% of the prescribed or stated amount.

Identification

A. Triturate a quantity of the powdered tablets containing 0.1 g of Pyridostigmine Bromide with two 5-ml quantities of *water* and filter. Dilute the filtrate with *water* to contain 0.005% w/v of Pyridostigmine Bromide. The *light absorption* of the resulting solution, Appendix II B, exhibits a maximum at 270 nm. Reserve the filtrate for use in tests B and C.

B. Carry out the method for *thin-layer chromatography*, Appendix III A, using *silica gel G* as the coating substance and a mixture of 5 volumes of *water*, 10 volumes of *formic acid*, 35 volumes of *methanol* and 50 volumes of *chloroform* as the mobile phase. Apply separately to the plate 10 µl of each of the following solutions. For solution (1) dilute 1 volume of the filtrate obtained in test A to 10 volumes with *methanol*. Solution (2) contains 0.1% w/v of *neostigmine methylsulphate BPCRS* in *methanol*. After removal of the plate, allow it to dry in air and spray with *dilute potassium iodobismuthate solution*. The principal spot in the chromatogram obtained with solution (1) has an Rf value of about 1.3 relative to the spot in the chromatogram obtained with solution (2).

C. The filtrate obtained in test A yields the reactions characteristic of *bromides*, Appendix VI.

Related substances Carry out the method for *thin-layer chromatography*, Appendix III A, using *silica gel G* as the coating substance and a mixture of 3 volumes of *diethylamine*, 30 volumes of *methanol* and 67 volumes of *water* as the mobile phase. Apply separately to the plate 20 µl of each of the following solutions. For solution (1) shake a quantity of the powdered tablets containing 0.2 g of Pyridostigmine Bromide with 20 ml of *methanol (80%)* and filter. For solution (2) dilute 1 volume of solution (1) to 20 volumes with *methanol (80%)*. After removal of the plate, dry it in a current of warm air, spray with *diazotised nitroaniline solution* and then with 0.1M *sodium hydroxide*. Dry the plate in a current of warm air and spray with *dilute potassium iodobismuthate solution*. Any *secondary spot* in the chromatogram obtained with solution (1) is not more intense than the spot in the chromatogram obtained with solution (2) (5%).

Assay Weigh and powder 20 tablets. Shake a quantity of the powdered tablets containing 0.15 g of Pyridostigmine Bromide with 50 ml of *water* for 30 minutes, filter, wash the residue with *water* and add sufficient *water* to produce 250 ml. Dilute 5 ml to 100 ml with *water* and measure the *absorbance* of the resulting solution at the maximum at 270 nm, Appendix II B. Calculate the content of $C_9H_{13}BrN_2O_2$ taking 186 as the value of A(1%, 1 cm) at the maximum at 270 nm.

Storage Pyridostigmine Tablets should be protected from light.

Pyridoxine Tablets

Definition Pyridoxine Tablets contain Pyridoxine Hydrochloride.

The tablets comply with the requirements stated under Tablets and with the following requirements.

Content of pyridoxine hydrochloride, $C_8H_{11}NO_3$,HCl 90.0 to 110.0% of the prescribed or stated amount.

Identification

A. Shake a quantity of the powdered tablets containing 0.1 g of Pyridoxine Hydrochloride with 50 ml of *methanol* for 15 minutes, warming occasionally, filter and add sufficient 13.5M *ammonia* to make the filtrate alkaline. Evaporate the resulting solution to dryness, dissolve the residue as completely as possible in 15 ml of *chloroform* and filter. To the filtrate add 2 ml of a solution prepared by carefully adding 2 ml of *acetyl chloride* dropwise to 8 ml of cooled *methanol* and evaporate the resulting solution to dryness. The *infrared absorption spectrum* of the residue, Appendix II A, is concordant with the *reference spectrum* of pyridoxine hydrochloride.

B. Shake a quantity of the powdered tablets containing 20 mg of Pyridoxine Hydrochloride with 50 ml of *0.025M standard phosphate buffer* for 15 minutes and dilute to 100 ml with the same solvent. Mix, filter and dilute 5 ml of the filtrate to 100 ml with the same solvent. The *light absorption* of the resulting solution, Appendix II B, in the range 230 to 350 nm exhibits two maxima, at 254 nm and 324 nm.

C. Triturate a quantity of the powdered tablets containing 20 mg of Pyridoxine Hydrochloride with 50 ml of *water* and allow to stand. To 1 ml of the supernatant liquid add 10 ml of a 5% w/v solution of *sodium acetate*, 1 ml of *water* and 1 ml of a 0.5% w/v solution of *2-6-dichloroquinone-4-chloroimide* in *ethanol (96%)* and shake; a blue colour is produced which fades rapidly and becomes brown. Repeat the operation but adding 1 ml of a 0.3% w/v solution of *boric acid* in place of the 1 ml of *water*; no blue colour is produced.

Related substances Carry out the method for *thin-layer chromatography*, Appendix III A, using *silica gel G* as the coating substance and a mixture of 9 volumes of 13.5M *ammonia*, 13 volumes of *tetrahydrofuran*, 13 volumes of *dichloromethane* and 65 volumes of *acetone* as the mobile phase. Apply separately to the plate 10 µl of each of the following solutions. For solution (1) shake a quantity of the powdered tablets containing 40 mg of Pyridoxine Hydrochloride with 10 ml of *water* for 15 minutes, filter and use the filtrate. For solution (2) dilute 1 ml of solution (1) to 200 ml with *water*. After removal of the plate, allow it to dry in air and spray with a 5% w/v solution of *sodium carbonate* in *ethanol (30%)*. Allow the plate to dry in air, spray with a 0.1% w/v solution of *2,6-dichloroquinone-4-chloroimide* in *ethanol (96%)* and examine immediately. Any *secondary spot* in the chromatogram obtained with solution (1) is not more intense than the spot in the chromatogram obtained with solution (2) (0.5%). Disregard any spot remaining on the line of application.

Assay Weigh and powder 20 tablets. To a quantity of the powdered tablets containing 25 mg of Pyridoxine Hydrochloride add 50 ml of 0.1M *hydrochloric acid* and heat on a water bath for 15 minutes, swirling occasionally. Cool, dilute to 100 ml with 0.1M *hydrochloric acid* and filter, discarding the first 20 ml of filtrate. Dilute 5 ml of the filtrate to 100 ml with 0.1M *hydrochloric acid* and measure the *absorbance* of the resulting solution at the maximum at 290 nm, Appendix II B. Calculate the content of $C_8H_{11}NO_3$,HCl taking 430 as the value of A(1%, 1 cm) at the maximum at 290 nm.

Storage Pyridoxine Tablets should be protected from light and stored at a temperature not exceeding 30°.

When vitamin B_6 tablets are prescribed or demanded, Pyridoxine Tablets shall be dispensed or supplied.

Pyrimethamine Tablets

Definition Pyrimethamine Tablets contain Pyrimethamine.

The tablets comply with the requirements stated under Tablets and with the following requirements.

Content of pyrimethamine, $C_{12}H_{13}ClN_4$ 92.5 to 107.5% of the prescribed or stated amount.

Identification

A. Shake a quantity of the powdered tablets containing 50 mg of Pyrimethamine with 50 ml of *ethanol (96%)* for 20 minutes, filter and evaporate the filtrate to dryness. The *infrared absorption spectrum* of the residue, Appendix II A, is concordant with the *reference spectrum* of pyrimethamine.

B. Extract the powdered tablets with 1M *sulphuric acid*, filter and add *potassium tetraiodomercurate solution* to the filtrate. A creamy white precipitate is produced.

C. Extract a quantity of the powdered tablets containing 50 mg of Pyrimethamine with two 10-ml quantities of *chloroform* and evaporate the combined extracts to dryness. The *melting point* of the residue is about 240°, Appendix V A.

Related substances Carry out the method for *thin-layer chromatography*, Appendix III A, using *silica gel GF_{254}* as the coating substance and a mixture of 4 volumes of *chloroform*, 8 volumes of *propan-1-ol*, 12 volumes of *glacial acetic acid* and 76 volumes of *toluene* as the mobile phase but allowing the solvent front to ascend 10 cm above the line of application. Apply separately to the plate 20 µl of each of the following freshly prepared solutions. For solution (1) shake a quantity of the powdered tablets containing 50 mg of Pyrimethamine with 5 ml of a mixture of 9 volumes of *chloroform* and 1 volume of *methanol* and filter. For solution (2) dilute 1 volume of solution (1) to 400 volumes with the same solvent mixture. After removal of the plate, allow it to dry in air and examine under *ultraviolet light (254 nm)*. Any *secondary spot* in the chromatogram obtained with solution (1) is not more intense than the spot in the chromatogram obtained with solution (2) (0.25%).

Assay Weigh and powder 20 tablets. To a quantity of the powdered tablets containing 25 mg of Pyrimethamine add 50 ml of hot 0.1M *hydrochloric acid* and heat on a water bath for 10 minutes, swirling occasionally. Mix with the aid of ultrasound for 30 minutes, remove and cool to room temperature. Add sufficient 0.1M *hydrochloric acid* to produce 100 ml, filter and dilute 5 ml of the filtrate to 100 ml with 0.1M *hydrochloric acid*. Measure the *absorbance* of the resulting solution at the maximum at 272 nm, Appendix II B, using 0.1M *hydrochloric acid* in the reference cell. Calculate the content of $C_{12}H_{13}ClN_4$ taking 316 as the value of A(1%, 1 cm) at the maximum at 272 nm.

Quillaia Liquid Extract

Definition Quillaia Liquid Extract is prepared by extracting Quillaia with Ethanol (45 per cent).

Extemporaneous preparation The following formula and directions apply.

Quillaia, in *moderately fine powder*	1000 g
Ethanol (45 per cent)	a sufficient quantity

Exhaust the Quillaia in *moderately fine powder* with Ethanol (45 per cent) by *percolation*, Appendix XI F, and reserve the first 850 ml of percolate. Evaporate the subsequent percolate to the consistence of a soft extract, dissolve it in the reserved portion and add sufficient Ethanol (45 per cent) to produce 1000 ml. Allow to stand for not less than 24 hours; filter.

The extract complies with the requirements stated under Extracts and with the following requirements.

Ethanol content 28 to 34% v/v, Appendix VIII F, Method III.

Dry residue 20 to 30% w/v.

Relative density 1.02 to 1.06, Appendix V G.

Quillaia Tincture

Definition

Quillaia Liquid Extract	50 ml
Ethanol (45 per cent)	sufficient to produce 1000 ml

Extemporaneous preparation The following directions apply.

Mix, allow to stand for not less than 12 hours and filter.

The tincture complies with the requirements stated under Tinctures and with the following requirements.

Ethanol content 43 to 45% v/v, Appendix VIII F, Method III.

Dry residue 1.0 to 1.5% w/v. Use 10 ml.

Relative density 0.940 to 0.955, Appendix V G.

Quinidine Sulphate Tablets

Definition Quinidine Sulphate Tablets contain Quinidine Sulphate.

The tablets comply with the requirements stated under Tablets and with the following requirements.

Content of quinidine sulphate, $(C_{20}H_{24}N_2O_2)_2$, H_2SO_4,$2H_2O$ 95.0 to 105.0% of the prescribed or stated amount.

Identification

A. Carry out the method for *thin-layer chromatography*, Appendix III A, using *silica gel G* as the coating substance and a mixture of 10 volumes of *diethylamine*, 20 volumes of *acetone* and 80 volumes of *toluene* as the mobile phase. Apply separately to the plate 2 µl of each of the following solutions. For solution (1) extract a quantity of the powdered tablets containing 0.1 g of Quinidine Sulphate with 10 ml of a mixture of 2 volumes of *chloroform* and 1 volume of *ethanol (96%)* and filter. Solution (2) contains 1.0% w/v of *quinidine sulphate EPCRS* in a mixture of 2 volumes of *chloroform* and 1 volume of *ethanol (96%)*. Solution (3) contains 1.0% w/v each of *quinidine sulphate EPCRS* and *quinine sulphate EPCRS*. After removal of the plate, allow it to dry in air and spray with 0.05M *ethanolic sulphuric acid* and then with *dilute potassium iodobismuthate solution*. The principal spot in the chromatogram obtained with solution (1) corresponds to that in the chromatogram obtained with solution (2). The test is not valid unless the chromatogram obtained with solution (3) shows two clearly separated spots.

B. Shake a quantity of the powdered tablets containing 0.25 g of Quinidine Sulphate with 25 ml of a mixture of 2 volumes of *chloroform* and 1 volume of *ethanol (96%)* and filter. Evaporate the filtrate to dryness and wash the residue with 10 ml of *ether*. Filter, wash the residue with 10 ml of *ether* and dry the residue at 60° at a pressure not exceeding 15 Pa for 2 hours. The pH of a 1% w/v solution of the residue is 6.0 to 6.8, Appendix V L.

C. Extract a quantity of the powdered tablets containing 0.1 g of Quinidine Sulphate with 20 ml of *water* and filter. The filtrate yields the reactions characteristic of *sulphates*, Appendix VI.

Other cinchona alkaloids Carry out the method for *liquid chromatography*, Appendix III D, using the following solutions. For solution (1) mix a quantity of the powdered tablets containing 50 mg of Quinidine Sulphate with 20 ml of the mobile phase. Heat gently to dissolve the powder as completely as possible, cool, dilute to 25 ml with the mobile phase and filter, discarding the first few ml of filtrate. For solution (2) dissolve 20 mg of *quinine sulphate EPCRS*, with gentle heating if necessary, in 5 ml of the mobile phase and dilute to 10 ml with the mobile phase. Prepare solution (3) in the same manner as solution (2) but using *quinidine sulphate EPCRS* in place of *quinine sulphate EPCRS*. Solution (4) is a mixture of equal volumes of solutions (2) and (3). For solution (5) dilute 1 volume of solution (2) to 10 volumes with the mobile phase and dilute 1 volume of the resulting solution to 50 volumes with the mobile phase. Solution (6) contains 0.10% w/v of *thiourea* in the mobile phase.

The chromatographic procedure may be carried out using (a) a stainless steel column (15 to 25 cm × 4.6 mm) packed with *stationary phase C* (5 µm or 10 µm) (Hypersil ODS 5 µm is suitable), (b) as the mobile phase with a flow rate of 1.5 ml per minute a solution prepared by dissolving 6.8 g of *potassium dihydrogen orthophosphate* and 3.0 g of *hexylamine* in 700 ml of *water*, adjusting the pH to 2.8 with 1M *orthophosphoric acid*, adding 60 ml of *acetonitrile* and diluting to 1000 ml with *water* and (c) a detection wavelength of 250 nm for recording the chromatogram obtained with solution (6) and 316 nm for the other solutions.

Inject separately 10 µl of each of solutions (3) and (6). If necessary, adjust the concentration of acetonitrile in the mobile phase so that in the chromatogram obtained with solution (3) the *capacity factor* of the peak due to quinidine is 3.5 to 4.5, V_0 being calculated from the peak due to thiourea in the chromatogram obtained with solution (6). Inject 10 µl of each of solutions (2), (3), (4) and (5). The chromatogram obtained with solution (2) shows a principal peak due to quinine and a peak due to dihydroquinine with a retention time relative to quinine of about 1.4. The chromatogram obtained with solution (3) shows a principal peak due to quinidine and a peak due to dihydroquinidine, with a retention time relative to quinine of about 1.2. The chromatogram obtained with solution (4) shows four peaks due to quinine, dihydroquinine, quinidine and dihydroquinidine which are identified by comparison of their retention times with those of the corresponding peaks in the chromatograms obtained with solutions (2) and (3).

The test is not valid unless (a) in the chromatogram obtained with solution (4) the *resolution factor* between the peaks due to quinine and quinidine is at least 1.5 and the *resolution factor* between the peaks due to dihydroquinidine and quinine is at least 1.0 and (b) the *signal-to-noise ratio* of the principal peak in the chromatogram obtained with solution (5) is at least 5.

Inject 10 µl of solution (1) and allow the chromatography to proceed for 2.5 times the retention time of the principal peak. Calculate the percentage content of related substances by *normalisation*, disregarding any peaks the areas of which are less than that of the peak in the chromatogram obtained with solution (5) (0.2%). The content of dihydroquinidine is not greater than 15%, the content of any related substance eluting before quinidine is not greater than 5% and the content of any other related substance is not greater than 2.5%.

Assay Weigh and powder 20 tablets. Dissolve as completely as possible using heat a quantity of the powdered tablets containing 0.4 g of Quinidine Sulphate in 40 ml of *acetic anhydride* and carry out Method I for *non-aqueous titration*, Appendix VIII A, using *crystal violet solution* as indicator. Each ml of 0.1M *perchloric acid VS* is equivalent to 26.10 mg of $(C_{20}H_{24}N_2O_2)_2,H_2SO_4,2H_2O$.

Storage Quinidine Sulphate Tablets should be protected from light.

Quinine Bisulphate Tablets

Definition Quinine Bisulphate Tablets contain Quinine Bisulphate. They are coated.

The tablets comply with the requirements stated under Tablets and with the following requirements.

Content of quinine bisulphate, $C_{20}H_{24}N_2O_2,H_2SO_4,7H_2O$ 95.0 to 105.0% of the prescribed or stated amount.

Identification

A. Carry out the method for *thin-layer chromatography*, Appendix III A, using *silica gel G* as the coating substance and a mixture of 10 volumes of *diethylamine*, 20 volumes of *acetone* and 80 volumes of *toluene* as the mobile phase. Apply separately to the plate 2 µl of each of the following solutions. For solution (1) extract a quantity of the powdered tablets containing 0.1 g of Quinine Bisulphate with 10 ml of a mixture of 2 volumes of *chloroform* and 1 volume of *ethanol (96%)* and filter. Solution (2) contains 1.0% w/v of *quinine sulphate EPCRS* in a mixture of 2 volumes of *chloroform* and 1 volume of *ethanol (96%)*. Solution (3) contains 1.0% w/v each of *quinidine sulphate EPCRS* and *quinine sulphate EPCRS*. After removal of the plate, allow it to dry in air and spray with 0.05M *ethanolic sulphuric acid* and then with *dilute potassium iodobismuthate solution*. The principal spot in the chromatogram obtained with solution (1) corresponds to that in the chromatogram obtained with solution (2). The test is not valid unless the chromatogram obtained with solution (3) shows two clearly separated spots.

B. Shake a quantity of the powdered tablets containing 0.25 g of Quinine Bisulphate with 25 ml of a mixture of 2 volumes of *chloroform* and 1 volume of *ethanol (65%)* and filter. Evaporate the filtrate to dryness and wash the residue with 10 ml of *ether*. Filter, wash the residue with 10 ml of *ether* and dry at 60° at a pressure not exceeding 15 Pa for 2 hours. The pH of a 1% w/v solution is 2.8 to 3.4, Appendix V L.

C. Extract a quantity of the powdered tablets containing 0.5 g of Quinine Bisulphate with 10 ml of *water* and filter. The filtrate yields the reactions characteristic of *sulphates*, Appendix VI.

D. Solution A yields the reactions characteristic of *sulphates*, Appendix VI.

Dissolution Comply with the *dissolution test for tablets and capsules*, Appendix XII D, using as the medium 900 ml of 0.1M *hydrochloric acid* and rotating the basket at 100 revolutions per minute. Withdraw a sample of 10 ml of the medium. Measure the *absorbance* of a layer of suitable thickness of the filtered sample, suitably diluted if necessary, at the maximum at 348 nm, Appendix II B. Calculate the total content of quinine bisulphate, $C_{20}H_{24}N_2O_2,H_2SO_4,7H_2O$, in the medium taking 99 as the value of A(1%, 1 cm) at the maximum at 348 nm.

Other cinchona alkaloids Carry out the method for *liquid chromatography*, Appendix III D, using the following solutions. For solution (1) mix a quantity of the powdered tablets containing 50 mg of Quinine Bisulphate with 20 ml of the mobile phase. Heat gently to dissolve the powder as completely as possible, cool, dilute to 25 ml with the mobile phase and filter, discarding the first few ml of the filtrate. For solution (2) dissolve 20 mg of *quinine sulphate EPCRS*, with gentle heating if necessary, in 5 ml of the mobile phase and dilute to 10 ml with the mobile phase. Prepare solution (3) in the same manner as solution (2) using *quinidine sulphate EPCRS* in place of *quinine sulphate EPCRS*. Solution (4) is a mixture of equal volumes of solutions (2) and (3). For solution (5) dilute 1 volume of solution (2) to 10 volumes with the mobile phase and dilute 1 volume of the resulting solution to 50 volumes with the mobile phase. Solution (6) contains 0.10% w/v of *thiourea* in the mobile phase.

The chromatographic procedure may be carried out using (a) a stainless steel column (15 to 25 cm × 4.6 mm) packed with *stationary phase C* (5 µm or 10 µm) (Hypersil ODS 5 µm is suitable), (b) as the mobile phase with a flow rate of 1.5 ml per minute a solution prepared by dissolving 6.8 g of *potassium dihydrogen orthophosphate* and 3.0 g of *hexylamine* in 700 ml of *water*, adjusting the pH to 2.8 with 1M *orthophosphoric acid*, adding 60 ml of *acetonitrile* and diluting to 1000 ml with *water* and (c) a detection wavelength of 250 nm for recording the chromatogram obtained with solution (6) and 316 nm for the other solutions.

Inject separately 10 µl of each of solutions (3) and (6). If necessary adjust the concentration of acetonitrile in the mobile phase so that in the chromatogram obtained with solution (3) the *capacity factor* of the peak due to quinidine is 3.5 to 4.5, V_0 being calculated from the peak due to thiourea in the chromatogram obtained with solution (6). Inject 10 µl of each of solutions (2), (3), (4) and (5). The chromatogram obtained with solution (2) shows a principal peak due to quinine and a peak due to dihydroquinine with a retention time relative to quinine of about 1.4. The chromatogram obtained with solution (3) shows a principal peak due to quinidine and a peak due to dihydroquinidine, with a retention time relative to quinine of about 1.2. The chromatogram obtained with solution (4) shows four peaks due to quinine, dihydroquinine, quinidine and dihydroquinidine which are identified by comparison of their retention times with those of the corresponding peaks in the chromatograms obtained with solutions (2) and (3).

The test is not valid unless (a) in the chromatogram obtained with solution (4) the *resolution factor* between the peaks due to quinine and quinidine is at least 1.5 and the *resolution factor* between the peaks due to dihydroquinidine and quinine is at least 1.0 and (b) the *signal-to-noise ratio* of the principal peak in the chromatogram obtained with solution (5) is at least 5.

Inject 10 µl of solution (1) and allow the chromatography to proceed for 2.5 times the retention time of the principal peak. Calculate the percentage content of related substances by *normalisation*, disregarding any peaks the areas of which are less than that of the peak in the chromatogram obtained with solution (5) (0.2%). The content of dihydroquinidine is not greater than 10%, the content of any related substance eluting before quinine is not greater than 5% and the content of any other related substance is not greater than 2.5%.

Assay Weigh and powder 20 tablets. Dissolve as completely as possible a quantity of the powdered tablets containing 0.6 g of Quinine Bisulphate in 40 ml of *acetic anhydride* using heat. Carry out Method I for *non-aqueous titration*, Appendix VIII A, using *crystal violet solution* as indicator. Each ml of 0.1M *perchloric acid VS* is equivalent to 54.86 mg of $C_{20}H_{24}N_2O_2,H_2SO_4,7H_2O$.

Storage Quinine Bisulphate Tablets that are not sugar-coated should be protected from light.

300 mg of Quinine Bisulphate is approximately equivalent to 177.5 mg of anhydrous quinine.

Quinine Sulphate Tablets

Definition Quinine Sulphate Tablets contain Quinine Sulphate. They are coated.

The tablets comply with the requirements stated under Tablets and with the following requirements.

Content of quinine sulphate, $(C_{20}H_{24}N_2O_2)_2,H_2SO_4,2H_2O$ 95.0 to 105.0% of the prescribed or stated amount.

Identification

A. Carry out the method for *thin-layer chromatography*, Appendix III A, using *silica gel G* as the coating substance and a mixture of 10 volumes of *diethylamine*, 20 volumes of *acetone* and 80 volumes of *toluene* as the mobile phase. Apply separately to the plate 2 µl of each of the following solutions. For solution (1) extract a quantity of the powdered tablets containing 0.1 g of Quinine Sulphate with 10 ml of a mixture of 2 volumes of *chloroform* and 1 volume of *ethanol (96%)* and filter. Solution (2) contains 1.0% w/v of *quinine sulphate EPCRS* in a mixture of 2 volumes of *chloroform* and 1 volume of *ethanol (96%)*. Solution (3) contains 1.0% w/v each of *quinidine sulphate EPCRS* and *quinine sulphate EPCRS*. After removal of the plate, allow it to dry in air and spray with 0.05M *ethanolic sulphuric acid* and then with *dilute potassium iodobismuthate solution*. The principal spot in the chromatogram obtained with solution (1) corresponds to that in the chromatogram obtained with solution (2). The test is not valid unless the chromatogram obtained with solution (3) shows two clearly separated spots.

B. Extract a quantity of the powdered tablets containing 0.25 g of Quinine Sulphate with 25 ml of a mixture of 2 volumes of *chloroform* and 1 volume of *ethanol (96%)* and filter. Evaporate the filtrate to dryness and wash the residue with 10 ml of *ether*. Filter and wash the residue with 10 ml of *ether*. Dry the residue at 60° at a pressure not exceeding 15 Pa for 2 hours. The pH of a 1% w/v suspension of the residue is 5.7 to 6.6, Appendix V L.

C. Extract a quantity of the powdered tablets containing 0.1 g of Quinine Sulphate with 20 ml of *water* and filter. The filtrate yields the reactions characteristic of *sulphates*, Appendix VI.

Dissolution Comply with the *dissolution test for tablets and capsules*, Appendix XII D, using as the medium 900 ml of 0.1M *hydrochloric acid* and rotating the basket at 100 revolutions per minute. Withdraw a sample of 10 ml of the medium. Measure the *absorbance* of a layer of suitable thickness of the filtered sample, suitably diluted if necessary, at the maximum at 348 nm, Appendix II B. Calculate the total content of quinine sulphate, $(C_{20}H_{24}N_2O_2)_2, H_2SO_4,2H_2O$, in the medium taking 136 as the value of A(1%, 1 cm) at the maximum at 348 nm.

Other cinchona alkaloids Carry out the method for *liquid chromatography*, Appendix III D, using the following solutions. For solution (1) mix a quantity of the powdered tablets containing 50 mg of Quinine Sulphate with 20 ml of the mobile phase. Heat gently to dissolve the powder as completely as possible, cool, dilute to 25 ml with the mobile phase and filter, discarding the first few ml of the filtrate. For solution (2) dissolve 20 mg of *quinine sulphate EPCRS*, with gentle heating if necessary, in 5 ml of the mobile phase and dilute to 10 ml with the mobile phase. Prepare solution (3) in the same manner as solution (2) using *quinidine sulphate EPCRS* in place of *quinine sulphate EPCRS*. Solution (4) is a mixture of equal volumes of solution (2) and solution (3). For solution (5) dilute 1 volume of solution (2) to 10 volumes with the mobile phase and dilute 1 volume of the resulting solution to 50 volumes with the mobile phase. Solution (6) contains 0.10% w/v of *thiourea* in the mobile phase.

The chromatographic procedure may be carried out using (a) a stainless steel column (15 to 25 cm × 4.6 mm) packed with *stationary phase* C (5 or 10 µm) (Hypersil ODS 5 µm is suitable), (b) as the mobile phase with a flow rate of 1.5 ml per minute a solution prepared by dissolving 6.8 g of *potassium dihydrogen orthophosphate* and 3.0 g of *hexylamine* in 700 ml of *water*, adjusting the pH to 2.8 with 1M *orthophosphoric acid*, adding 60 ml of *acetonitrile* and diluting to 1000 ml with *water* and (c) a detection wavelength of 250 nm for recording the chromatogram obtained with solution (6) and 316 nm for the other solutions.

Inject 10 µl of each of solutions (3) and (6). If necessary adjust the concentration of acetonitrile in the mobile phase so that in the chromatogram obtained with solution (3) the *capacity factor* of the peak due to quinidine is 3.5 to 4.5, V_0 being calculated from the peak due to thiourea in the chromatogram obtained with solution (6). Inject 10 µl of each of solutions (2), (3), (4) and (5). The chromatogram obtained with solution (2) shows a principal peak due to quinine and a peak due to dihydroquinidine, with a retention time relative to quinine of about 1.4. The chromatogram obtained with solution (3) shows a principal peak due to quinidine and a peak due to dihydroquinidine, with a retention time relative to quinine of about 1.2. The chromatogram obtained with solution (4) shows four peaks due to quinine, dihydroquinine, quinidine and dihydroquinidine which are identified by comparison of their retention times with those of the corresponding peaks in the chromatogram obtained with solutions (2) and (3).

The test is not valid unless (a) in the chromatogram obtained with solution (4) the *resolution factor* between the peaks due to quinine and quinidine is at least 1.5 and the *resolution factor* between the peaks due to dihydroquinidine and quinine is at least 1.0 and (b) the *signal-to-noise ratio* of the principal peak in the chromatogram obtained with solution (5) is at least 5.

Inject 10 µl of solution (1) and record the chromatogram for 2.5 times the retention time of the principal peak. Calculate the percentage content of related substances by *normalisation*, disregarding any peaks the areas of which are less than that of the peak in the chromatogram obtained with solution (5) (0.5%). The content of dihydroquinine is not greater than 10%, the content of any related substance eluted before quinine is not greater than 5% and the content of any other related substance is not greater than 2.5%.

Assay Weigh and powder 20 tablets and dissolve as completely as possible, using heat, a quantity of the powdered tablets containing 0.4 g of Quinine Sulphate in 40 ml of *acetic anhydride*. Carry out Method I for *non-aqueous titration*, Appendix VIII A, using *crystal violet solution* as indicator. Each ml of 0.1M *perchloric acid VS* is equivalent to 26.10 mg of $(C_{20}H_{24}N_2O_2)_2,H_2SO_4,2H_2O$.

Storage Quinine Sulphate Tablets that are not sugar-coated should be protected from light.

300 mg of Quinine Sulphate is approximately equivalent to 248.6 mg of anhydrous quinine.

Ranitidine Injection

Definition Ranitidine Injection is a sterile solution of Ranitidine Hydrochloride in Water for Injections.

The injection complies with the requirements stated under Parenteral Preparations and with the following requirements.

Content of ranitidine, $C_{13}H_{22}N_4O_3S$ 92.5 to 105.0% of the prescribed or stated amount.

Identification

A. To a volume of the injection containing the equivalent of 25 mg of ranitidine add 20 ml of *methanol*, mix and evaporate to dryness. Add 1 ml of *petroleum spirit (boiling range, 60° to 80°)* to the resulting residue, scratch the side of the vessel with a glass rod to induce crystallisation, evaporate to dryness and dry the residue at 60° for 10 minutes. The *infrared absorption spectrum* of the dried residue, Appendix II A, is concordant with the *reference spectrum* of ranitidine hydrochloride.

B. In the Assay, the retention time of the principal peak in the chromatogram obtained with solution (1) is the same as that of the principal peak in the chromatogram obtained with solution (2).

Acidity or alkalinity Buffered formulations, pH 6.7 to 7.3; unbuffered formulations, pH 4.5 to 7.0, Appendix V L.

Related substances Carry out the method *for thin-layer chromatography*, Appendix III A, using *silica gel GF_{254}* as the coating substance and a mixture of 2 volumes of *water*, 4 volumes of 18M *ammonia*, 15 volumes of *propan-2-ol* and 25 volumes of *ethyl acetate* as the mobile phase. For injections containing the equivalent of 1% w/v or less of ranitidine apply 25 µl of each solution. For injections containing more than the equivalent of 1% w/v of ranitidine apply 10 µl of each solution. For solution (1) dilute, if necessary, a volume of the injection with *water* to contain the equivalent of 2.5% w/v of ranitidine or, for an injection containing 1% w/v or less of ranitidine, use the injection undiluted. For solution (2) dilute 1 volume of solution (1) to 50 volumes with *water*. For solution (3) dilute 1 volume of solution (1) to 100 volumes with *water*. For solution (4) dilute 0.5 volume of solution (1) to 100 volumes with *water*. For solution (5) dilute 1 volume of solution (3) to 5 volumes with *water*. Solution (6) contains 0.10% w/v of *ranitidine impurity B BPCRS* in *methanol*. Solution (7) contains 0.10% w/v of *ranitidine impurity B BPCRS* in solution (1). After removal of the plate, allow it to dry thoroughly in air and expose to iodine vapour in a closed chamber until the spots are visible. Any *secondary spot* in the chromatogram obtained with solution (1) is not more intense than the spot in the chromatogram obtained with solution (2) (2%), not more than one such spot is more intense than the spot in the chromatogram obtained with solution (3) (1%), not more than two other such spots are more intense than the spot in the chromatogram obtained with solution (4) (0.5%) and not more than two further such spots are more intense than the spot in the chromatogram obtained with solution (5) (0.2%). The test is not valid unless the chromatogram obtained with solution (7) shows two clearly separated spots corresponding to ranitidine impurity B and ranitidine.

Assay Carry out the method for *liquid chromatography*, Appendix III D, using the following solutions in the mobile phase. For solution (1) dilute a volume of the injection to contain the equivalent of 0.01% w/v of ranitidine. Solution (2) contains 0.0112% w/v of *ranitidine hydrochloride BPCRS*. Solution (3) contains 0.0112% w/v of *ranitidine hydrochloride BPCRS* and 0.0002% w/v of *dimethyl{5-[2-(1-methylamino-2-nitrovinylamino)ethylsulphinylmethyl]furfuryl}amine BPCRS*.

The chromatographic procedure may be carried out using (a) a stainless steel column (20 cm × 4.6 mm) packed with *stationary phase C* (10 µm) (Partisil ODS is suitable), (b) a mixture of 15 volumes of 0.1M *ammonium acetate* and 85 volumes of *methanol* as the mobile phase with a flow rate of 2 ml per minute and (c) a detection wavelength of 322 nm.

The assay is not valid unless the peak due to ranitidine in the chromatogram obtained with solution (3) shows baseline separation from the peak due to dimethyl{5-[2-(1-methylamino-2-nitrovinylamino)ethylsulphinylmethyl]-furfuryl}amine.

Calculate the content of $C_{13}H_{22}N_4O_3S$ using the declared content of $C_{13}H_{22}N_4O_3S$ in *ranitidine hydrochloride BPCRS*.

Storage Ranitidine Injection should be protected from light.

Labelling The label states (1) the quantity of active ingredient in terms of the equivalent amount of ranitidine; (2) where appropriate, that the injection is buffered.

Ranitidine Oral Solution

Definition Ranitidine Oral Solution is a solution of Ranitidine Hydrochloride in a suitable vehicle.

The oral solution complies with the requirements stated under Oral Liquids and with the following requirements.

Content of ranitidine, $C_{13}H_{22}N_4O_3S$ 90.0 to 105.0% of the prescribed or stated amount.

Identification

A. In the test for Related substances, the principal spot in the chromatogram obtained with solution (2) corresponds in position to that in the chromatogram obtained with solution (3).

B. In the Assay, the retention time of the principal peak in the chromatogram obtained with solution (1) is the same as that of the principal peak in the chromatogram obtained with solution (2).

Acidity or alkalinity pH, 6.7 to 7.5, Appendix V L.

Related substances Carry out the method for *thin-layer chromatography*, Appendix III A, using *silica gel GF_{254}* as the coating substance and a mixture of 4 volumes of *water*, 8 volumes of 18M *ammonia*, 30 volumes of *propan-2-ol* and 50 volumes of *ethyl acetate* as the mobile phase. Apply separately to the plate 20 µl of each of the following solutions. For solution (1) prepare a solid phase extraction cartridge containing a C_{18} sorbent (Sep-Pak C_{18} cartridges are suitable) by passing 10 ml of *methanol* followed by 20 ml of 0.5M *ammonia* through the cartridge; attach the tip of a suitable syringe to the cartridge; transfer a weighed quantity of the oral solution containing the equivalent of 10 mg of ranitidine to the barrel of the syringe; add 2 ml of 0.5M *ammonia* to the syringe, insert the plunger and slowly force the mixture through the cartridge, discarding the eluant; repeat with two 4-ml quantities of 0.5M *ammonia* discarding the eluant; pass two 5-ml quantities of a mixture of 25 volumes of 0.1M *hydrochloric acid* and 75 volumes of *methanol* through the cartridge and collect the eluant; add 40 ml of *absolute ethanol* to the collected eluant, evaporate the resulting solution to dryness at a temperature not exceeding 30° under reduced pressure and dissolve the residue in 1 ml of *methanol*. For solution (2) dilute 1 volume of solution (1) to 50 volumes with *methanol*. Solution (3) contains 0.0223% w/v of *ranitidine hydrochloride BPCRS* in *methanol*. Solution (4) contains 0.0112% w/v of *ranitidine hydrochloride BPCRS* in *methanol*. Solution (5) contains 0.0056% w/v of *ranitidine hydrochloride BPCRS* in *methanol*. Solution (6) contains 0.1% w/v of *ranitidine impurity B BPCRS* in solution (1).

Prepare a further solution in *water* containing 1.12% w/v of *ranitidine hydrochloride BPCRS* and 0.01% w/v of *ranitidine impurity B BPCRS* and repeat the sample preparation procedure applying 1 ml of the solution to the barrel of the syringe. Apply 20 µl of the resulting solution (solution A) to the plate.

After removal of the plate, allow it to dry thoroughly in air and expose to iodine vapour in a closed chamber until the spots are visible. The test is not valid unless (a) the chromatogram obtained with solution A shows two clearly separated spots and the spot due to ranitidine impurity B is of equal intensity to that of the spot in the chromatogram obtained with solution (4) and (b) the chromatogram obtained with solution (6) shows two clearly separated spots.

Any *secondary spot* in the chromatogram obtained with solution (1) is not more intense than the spot in the chromatogram obtained with solution (3) (2%), not more than one such spot is more intense than the spot in the chromatogram obtained with solution (4) (1%) and not more than two other such spots are more intense than the spot in the chromatogram obtained with solution (5) (0.5%).

Assay Carry out the method for *liquid chromatography*, Appendix III D, using the following solutions in the mobile phase. For solution (1) dilute a weighed quantity of the oral solution containing the equivalent of 10 mg of ranitidine with sufficient of the mobile phase to produce 100 ml. Solution (2) contains 0.0112% w/v of *ranitidine hydrochloride BPCRS*. Solution (3) contains 0.0112% w/v of *ranitidine hydrochloride BPCRS* and 0.0002% w/v of *dimethyl{5-[2-(1-methylamino-2-nitrovinylamino)ethyl-sulphinylmethyl]furfuryl}amine BPCRS*.

The chromatographic procedure may be carried out using (a) a stainless steel column (20 cm × 4.6 mm) packed with *stationary phase C* (10 µm) (Partisil ODS is suitable), (b) a mixture of 15 volumes of 0.1M *ammonium acetate* and 85 volumes of *methanol* as the mobile phase with a flow rate of 2 ml per minute and (c) a detection wavelength of 322 nm.

The assay is not valid unless the peak due to ranitidine in the chromatogram obtained with solution (3) shows baseline separation from the peak due to dimethyl{5-[2-(1-methylamino-2-nitrovinylamino)ethylsulphinyl-methyl]furfuryl}amine.

Determine the *weight per ml* of the oral solution, Appendix V G, and calculate the content of $C_{13}H_{22}N_4O_3S$, weight in volume, using the declared content of $C_{13}H_{22}N_4O_3S$ in *ranitidine hydrochloride BPCRS*.

Storage Ranitidine Oral Solution should be protected from light and stored at a temperature not exceeding 25°.

Labelling The label states the quantity of active ingredient in terms of the equivalent amount of ranitidine.

Ranitidine Tablets

Definition Ranitidine Tablets contain Ranitidine Hydrochloride. They are coated.

The tablets comply with the requirements stated under Tablets and with the following requirements.

Content of ranitidine, $C_{13}H_{22}N_4O_3S$ 95.0 to 105.0% of the prescribed or stated amount.

Identification

A. Shake a quantity of the powdered tablets containing the equivalent of 25 mg of ranitidine with 5 ml of *methanol* for 5 minutes, filter and evaporate the filtrate to dryness. Add 1 ml of *petroleum spirit (boiling range, 60° to 80°)* to the residue, scratch the side of the vessel to induce crystallisation, evaporate to dryness and dry the residue at 60° for 10 minutes. The *infrared absorption spectrum* of the dried residue, Appendix II A, is concordant with the *reference spectrum* of ranitidine hydrochloride.

B. In the Assay, the retention time of the principal peak in the chromatogram obtained with solution (1) is the same as that of the principal peak in the chromatogram obtained with solution (2).

Related substances Carry out the method described under Ranitidine Injection but applying 10 µl of the following solutions. For solution (1) shake a quantity of the powdered tablets containing the equivalent of 0.45 g of ranitidine with 20 ml of *methanol* and filter (Whatman No 1 paper is suitable). For solution (2) dilute 1 volume of solution (1) to 200 volumes with *methanol.* For solution (3) dilute 1 volume of solution (1) to 20 volumes with *methanol* and dilute 3 volumes of this solution to 50 volumes with *methanol.* For solution (4) dilute 1 volume of solution (1) to 20 volumes with *methanol* and dilute 1 volume of this solution to 50 volumes with *methanol.* Solution (5) contains 0.10% w/v of *ranitidine impurity B BPCRS* in *methanol.* Solution (6) contains 0.10% w/v of *ranitidine impurity B BPCRS* in solution (1). Any *secondary* spot in the chromatogram obtained with solution (1) is not more intense than the spot in the chromatogram obtained with solution (2) (0.5%), not more than one such spot is more intense than the spot in the chromatogram obtained with solution (3) (0.3%) and not more than three other such spots are more intense than the spot in the chromatogram obtained with solution (4) (0.1%). The test is not valid unless the chromatogram obtained with solution (6) shows two clearly separated spots corresponding to ranitidine impurity B and ranitidine.

Assay Carry out the Assay described under Ranitidine Injection using the following solutions. For solution (1) shake 10 tablets with 400 ml of the mobile phase until the tablets have completely disintegrated (about 15 minutes), dilute to 500 ml with the mobile phase, filter (Whatman GF/C paper is suitable) and dilute the filtrate with the mobile phase to produce a solution containing the equivalent of 0.01% w/v of ranitidine. Solution (2) contains 0.0112% w/v of *ranitidine hydrochloride BPCRS.* Solution (3) contains 0.0112% w/v of *ranitidine hydrochloride BPCRS* and 0.0002% w/v of *dimethyl{5-[2-(1-methylamino-2-nitrovinylamino)ethylsulphinylmethyl]furfuryl}amine BPCRS.*

Calculate the content of $C_{13}H_{22}N_4O_3S$ using the declared content of $C_{13}H_{22}N_4O_3S$ in *ranitidine hydrochloride BPCRS.*

Storage Ranitidine Tablets should be protected from light.

Labelling The label states the quantity of active ingredient in terms of the equivalent amount of ranitidine.

Compound Rhubarb Tincture

Definition

Rhubarb, in *moderately coarse powder*		100 g
Cardamom Oil		0.40 ml
Coriander Oil		0.03 ml
Glycerol		100 ml
Ethanol (60 per cent)	sufficient to produce	1000 ml

Extemporaneous preparation The following directions apply.

Moisten the Rhubarb with a sufficient quantity of Ethanol (60 per cent) and prepare 850 ml of tincture by *percolation,* Appendix XI F. Add the Cardamom Oil, the Coriander Oil and the Glycerol and sufficient Ethanol (60 per cent) to produce 1000 ml. Mix and filter, if necessary.

The tincture complies with the requirements stated under Tinctures and with the following requirements.

Ethanol content 48 to 53% v/v, Appendix VIII F, Method III.

Glycerol 9.0 to 11.0% v/v when determined by the following method. Dilute 20 ml to 100 ml with *water;* to 10 ml of this solution add 100 ml of *water* and 1 g of *activated charcoal* and boil under a reflux condenser for 15 minutes. Filter, wash the filter and charcoal with sufficient *water* to produce 150 ml, add 0.25 ml of *bromocresol purple solution* and neutralise with 0.1M *sodium hydroxide* or 0.05M *sulphuric acid* to the blue colour of the indicator. Add 1.4 g of *sodium periodate,* allow to stand for 15 minutes, add 3 ml of *propane-1,2-diol,* shake and allow to stand for 5 minutes. Add 0.25 ml of *bromocresol purple solution* and titrate with 0.1M *sodium hydroxide VS* to the same blue colour. Each ml of 0.1M *sodium hydroxide VS* is equivalent to 9.210 mg of glycerol. Calculate the percentage v/v of glycerol, taking 1.260 g as its weight per ml.

Relative density 0.958 to 0.977, Appendix V G.

Rifampicin Capsules

Definition Rifampicin Capsules contain Rifampicin.

The capsules comply with the requirements stated under Capsules and with the following requirements.

Content of rifampicin, $C_{43}H_{58}N_4O_{12}$ 92.5 to 107.5% of the prescribed or stated amount.

Identification

A. Shake a quantity of the contents of the capsules containing 0.15 g of Rifampicin with 5 ml of *chloroform,* filter and evaporate the filtrate to dryness. The *infrared absorption spectrum* of the residue, Appendix II A, is concordant with the *reference spectrum* of rifampicin.

B. The *light absorption,* Appendix II B, in the range 220 to 500 nm of the final solution obtained in the Assay exhibits four maxima, at 237, 254, 334 and 475 nm.

Related substances Carry out the method for *liquid chromatography*, Appendix III D, using solutions prepared in the solvent mixture described below. To 10 volumes of a 21.01% w/v solution of *citric acid* add 23 volumes of a 13.61% w/v solution of *potassium dihydrogen orthophosphate*, 77 volumes of a 17.42% w/v solution of *dipotassium hydrogen orthophosphate*, 250 volumes of *acetonitrile* and 640 volumes of *water* and mix. Prepare the solutions immediately before use. For solution (1) shake a quantity of the contents of the capsules containing 20 mg of Rifampicin with 10 ml of *acetonitrile*, centrifuge and dilute 5 ml of the clear supernatant liquid to 50 ml with the solvent mixture. For solution (2) dilute 1 volume of solution (1) to 100 volumes. Solution (3) contains 0.00080% w/v of *rifampicin quinone EPCRS*. Solution (4) contains 0.00030% w/v of *rifampicin* N-*oxide BPCRS*. Solution (5) contains 0.00010% w/v of *3-formylrifamycin SV BPCRS*. For solution (6) dilute 1 volume of solution (3) to 4 volumes and mix 1 volume of the resulting solution with 1 volume of solution (2).

The chromatographic procedure may be carried out using (a) a stainless steel column (10 cm × 4.6 mm) packed with *stationary phase B* (5 μm) (Partisil C8 is suitable), (b) as mobile phase with a flow rate of 1.5 ml per minute a mixture of 35 volumes of *acetonitrile* and 65 volumes of a solution containing 0.1% v/v of *orthophosphoric acid*, 0.19% w/v of *sodium perchlorate*, 0.59% w/v of *citric acid* and 2.09% w/v of *potassium dihydrogen orthophosphate* and (c) a detection wavelength of 254 nm. Inject 20 μl of each solution.

Inject solution (6). Adjust the sensitivity of the detector so that the height of the two principal peaks is not less than half the full-scale of the recorder. The test is not valid unless the *resolution factor* between the two principal peaks is at least 4.0. If necessary, adjust the concentration of acetonitrile in the mobile phase.

Inject solution (1) and allow the chromatography to proceed for at least 3 times the retention time of the peak due to rifampicin. The area of any peak corresponding to rifampicin quinone is not greater than the area of the peak in the chromatogram obtained with solution (3) (4%); the area of any peak corresponding to rifampicin *N*-oxide is not greater than the area of the peak in the chromatogram obtained with solution (4) (1.5%); the area of any peak corresponding to 3-formylrifamycin SV is not greater than the area of the peak in the chromatogram obtained with solution (5) (0.5%) and the area of any other *secondary peak* is not greater than the area of the peak in the chromatogram obtained with solution (2) (1%).

Dissolution Comply with the *dissolution test for tablets and capsules*, Appendix XII D, using as the medium 900 ml of 0.1M *hydrochloric acid* and rotating the basket at 100 revolutions per minute. Withdraw a sample of 10 ml of the medium and filter. Measure the *absorbance* of the filtered sample, diluted if necessary with 0.1M *hydrochloric acid*, at the maximum at 336 nm, Appendix II B, using 0.1M *hydrochloric acid* in the reference cell. Calculate the total content of rifampicin, $C_{43}H_{58}N_4O_{12}$, in the medium taking 263 as the value of A(1%, 1 cm) at the maximum at 336 nm.

Assay Shake a quantity of the mixed contents of 20 capsules containing 0.1 g of Rifampicin with 80 ml of *methanol*, add sufficient *methanol* to produce 100 ml and filter. Dilute 2 ml of the filtrate to 100 ml with *phosphate buffer pH 7.4* and measure the *absorbance* of the resulting solution at the maximum at 475 nm, Appendix II B. Calculate the content of $C_{43}H_{58}N_4O_{12}$ taking 187 as the value of A(1%, 1 cm) at 475 nm.

Rifampicin Oral Suspension

Definition Rifampicin Oral Suspension is a suspension of Rifampicin in powder of suitable fineness in a suitable flavoured vehicle.

The oral suspension complies with the requirements stated under Oral Liquids and with the following requirements.

Content of rifampicin, $C_{43}H_{58}N_4O_{12}$ 90.0 to 110.0% of the prescribed or stated amount.

Identification To a quantity containing 0.1 g of Rifampicin add 30 ml of *water* and shake with two 50-ml quantities of *chloroform*. Dry the combined extracts with *anhydrous sodium sulphate*, filter and evaporate the filtrate to dryness at a temperature not exceeding 70°. The residue, after washing with 1 ml of *ether* and drying at 70°, complies with the following tests.

A. The *infrared absorption spectrum*, Appendix II A, is concordant with the *reference spectrum* of rifampicin.

B. Dissolve 10 mg of the residue in 10 ml of *methanol* and dilute 2 ml to 100 ml with *phosphate buffer pH 7.4*. The *light absorption* of the resulting solution, Appendix II B, in the range 240 to 500 nm exhibits three maxima, at 254, 334 and 475 nm.

Related substances Carry out the method for *liquid chromatography*, Appendix III D, using solutions prepared in the solvent mixture described below. To 10 volumes of a 21.01% w/v solution of *citric acid* add 23 volumes of a 13.61% w/v solution of *potassium dihydrogen orthophosphate*, 77 volumes of a 17.42% w/v solution of *dipotassium hydrogen orthophosphate*, 250 volumes of *acetonitrile* and 640 volumes of *water* and mix. Prepare the solutions immediately before use. For solution (1) add 5 ml of *water* to a quantity of the oral suspension containing 20 mg of Rifampicin and extract with four 10-ml quantities of *dichloromethane*, filter the combined extracts and evaporate to dryness at a temperature not exceeding 40°. Dissolve the residue in 10 ml of *acetonitrile* and dilute 5 ml of the solution to 50 ml with the solvent mixture. For solution (2) dilute 1 volume of solution (1) to 100 volumes. Solution (3) contains 0.00030% w/v of *rifampicin quinone EPCRS*. Solution (4) contains 0.00020% w/v of *rifampicin* N-*oxide BPCRS*. Solution (5) contains 0.0010% w/v of *3-formylrifamycin SV BPCRS*. For solution (6) dilute 1 volume of solution (3) to 1.5 volumes and mix 1 volume of the resulting solution with 1 volume of solution (2).

The chromatographic procedure may be carried out using (a) a stainless steel column (10 cm × 4.6 mm) packed with *stationary phase B* (5 μm) (Partisil C8 is suitable), (b) as mobile phase with a flow rate of 1.5 ml per minute a mixture of 35 volumes of *acetonitrile* and 65 volumes of a solution containing 0.1% v/v of *orthophosphoric acid*, 0.19% w/v of *sodium perchlorate*, 0.59% w/v of *citric acid* and 2.09% w/v of *potassium dihydrogen orthophosphate* and (c) a detection wavelength of 254 nm. Inject 20 μl of each solution.

Inject solution (6). Adjust the sensitivity of the detector so that the height of the two principal peaks is not less than half the full-scale of the recorder. The test is not valid unless the *resolution factor* between the two principal peaks is at least 4.0. If necessary, adjust the concentration of acetonitrile in the mobile phase.

Inject solution (1) and allow the chromatography to proceed for at least 3 times the retention time of the peak due to rifampicin. The area of any peak corresponding to rifampicin quinone is not greater than the area of the peak in the chromatogram obtained with solution (3) (1.5%); the area of any peak corresponding to rifampicin *N*-oxide is not greater than the area of the peak in the chromatogram obtained with solution (4) (1%); the area of any peak corresponding to 3-formylrifamycin SV is not greater than the area of the peak in the chromatogram obtained with solution (5) (5%) and the area of any other *secondary peak* is not greater than the area of the peak in the chromatogram obtained with solution (2) (1%). Disregard any peaks with retention times lower than that of the peak due to rifampicin quinone.

Acidity pH, 4.2 to 4.8, Appendix V L.

Assay Dilute a weighed quantity containing 0.4 g of Rifampicin to 500 ml with *methanol*, mix thoroughly, dilute 2 ml to 100 ml with *phosphate buffer pH 7.4* and measure the *absorbance* of the resulting solution at the maximum at 475 nm, Appendix II B. Calculate the content of $C_{43}H_{58}N_4O_{12}$ taking 187 as the value of A(1%, 1 cm) at 475 nm. Determine the *weight per ml* of the oral suspension, Appendix V G, and calculate the content of $C_{43}H_{58}N_4O_{12}$, weight in volume.

Ritodrine Injection

Definition Ritodrine Injection is a sterile solution of Ritodrine Hydrochloride in Water for Injections.

The injection complies with the requirements stated under Parenteral Preparations and with the following requirements.

Content of ritodrine hydrochloride, $C_{17}H_{21}NO_3$,HCl
93.0 to 105.0% of the prescribed or stated amount.

Identification

A. Dilute a suitable volume of the injection with sufficient *methanol (30%)* to produce a solution containing 0.010% w/v of Ritodrine Hydrochloride. The *light absorption* of the resulting solution, Appendix II B, in the range 230 to 350 nm exhibits a maximum at 275 nm and a shoulder at about 280 nm.

B. In the Assay, the retention time of the principal peak in the chromatogram obtained with solution (1) is the same as that of the principal peak in the chromatogram obtained with solution (2).

Related substances Carry out the method for *liquid chromatography*, Appendix III D, using the following solutions. For solution (1) dilute, if necessary, a volume of the injection with sufficient of the mobile phase to produce a solution containing 0.10% w/v of Ritodrine Hydrochloride. For solution (2) dilute 1 volume of solution (1) to 50 volumes with the mobile phase. For solution (3) heat a solution containing 0.10% w/v of *ritodrine hydrochloride BPCRS* in the mobile phase containing 5.6% v/v of *sulphuric acid* for 2 hours at 85°. Cool and mix 10 volumes of this solution with 8 volumes of a 10% w/v solution of *sodium hydroxide* (generation of *threo*-diastereoisomer).

The chromatographic procedure may be carried out using (a) a stainless steel column (25 cm × 4.6 mm) packed with *stationary phase B* (7 μm) (Zorbax C8 is suitable), (b) as the mobile phase with a flow rate of 2 ml per minute a mixture of a solution containing 6.6 g of *diammonium hydrogen orthophosphate* and 1.1 g of *sodium heptanesulphonate* in 700 ml of *water* and 300 ml of *methanol* adjusted to pH 3.0 with an 85% v/v solution of *orthophosphoric acid* and (c) a detection wavelength of 275 nm.

The test is not valid unless, in the chromatogram obtained with solution (3), the *resolution factor* between the two principal peaks (ritodrine and the *threo*-diastereoisomer) is at least 1.5.

In the chromatogram obtained with solution (1), the area of any *secondary peak* is not greater than twice the area of the principal peak in the chromatogram obtained with solution (2) (4%), not more than one such peak has an area greater than 0.5 times the area of the principal peak in the chromatogram obtained with solution (2) (1%), not more than one such peak has an area greater than 0.25 times the area of the principal peak in the chromatogram obtained with solution (2) (0.5%) and the sum of the areas of all such peaks is not greater than 2.5 times the area of the peak in the chromatogram obtained with solution (2) (5%).

Assay Carry out the method for *liquid chromatography*, Appendix III D, using the following solutions. For solution (1) dilute a volume of the injection with sufficient of the mobile phase to produce a solution containing 0.02% w/v of Ritodrine Hydrochloride. Solution (2) contains 0.02% w/v of *ritodrine hydrochloride BPCRS* in the mobile phase. For solution (3) heat a solution containing 0.1% w/v of *ritodrine hydrochloride BPCRS* in the mobile phase containing 5.6% v/v of *sulphuric acid* for 2 hours at 85°. Cool and mix 10 volumes with 8 volumes of a 10% w/v solution of *sodium hydroxide* (generation of *threo*-diastereoisomer).

The chromatographic procedure described under Related substances may be used.

The test is not valid unless, in the chromatogram obtained with solution (3), the *resolution factor* between the two principal peaks (ritodrine and the *threo*-diastereoisomer) is at least 1.5.

Calculate the content of $C_{17}H_{21}NO_3$,HCl in the injection from the chromatograms obtained and from the declared content of $C_{17}H_{21}NO_3$,HCl in *ritodrine hydrochloride BPCRS*.

Storage Ritodrine Injection should be protected from light and stored at a temperature not exceeding 25°.

Ritodrine Tablets

Definition Ritodrine Tablets contain Ritodrine Hydrochloride.

The tablets comply with the requirements stated under Tablets and with the following requirements.

Content of ritodrine hydrochloride, $C_{17}H_{21}NO_3$,HCl
93.0 to 105.0% of the prescribed or stated amount.

Identification In the Assay, the retention time of the principal peak in the chromatogram obtained with solution (1) is the same as that of the principal peak in the chromatogram obtained with solution (2).

Related substances Carry out the method for *liquid chromatography*, Appendix III D, using the following solutions. For solution (1) shake a quantity of the powdered tablets containing 20 mg of Ritodrine Hydrochloride in 50 ml of the mobile phase for 5 minutes, add sufficient mobile phase to produce 100 ml, mix and filter. For solution (2) dilute 1 volume of solution (1) to 100 volumes with the mobile phase. For solution (3) dissolve about 20 mg of *ritodrine hydrochloride BPCRS* in 50 ml of the mobile phase, add 5.6 ml of *sulphuric acid* and sufficient of the mobile phase to produce 100 ml, mix and heat at a temperature of 85° for 2 hours. Cool to room temperature, carefully mix 10 ml of the cooled solution with 8 ml of a 10% w/v solution of *sodium hydroxide* and allow to cool (generation of *threo*-diastereoisomer).

The chromatographic procedure may be carried out using (a) a stainless steel column (25 cm × 4.6 mm) packed with *stationary phase B* (7 µm) (Zorbax C8 is suitable), (b) as the mobile phase with a flow rate of 2 ml per minute a mixture of a solution containing 6.6 g of *diammonium hydrogen orthophosphate* and 1.1 g of *sodium heptanesulphonate* in 700 ml of *water* and 300 ml of *methanol* adjusted to pH 3.0 with an 85% v/v solution of *orthophosphoric acid* and (c) a detection wavelength of 275 nm.

The test is not valid unless, in the chromatogram obtained with solution (3), the *resolution factor* between the two principal peaks (ritodrine and the *threo*-diastereoisomer) is at least 1.5.

In the chromatogram obtained with solution (1), identify any peaks corresponding to tyramine (relative retention time to ritodrine, 0.3), *threo*-diastereoisomer (1.15) and 'aminoketone' (2.3). In the chromatogram obtained with solution (1) the area of any peaks corresponding to tyramine and the *threo*-diastereoisomer is not greater than the area of the principal peak in the chromatogram obtained with solution (2) (1% of each), the area of any peak corresponding to 'aminoketone' is not greater than 5 times the area of the principal peak in the chromatogram obtained with solution (2) (1% [relative response to ritodrine, 5]). The degradation products 4-hydroxybenzoic acid and 4-hydroxybenzaldehyde are formed in equimolar amounts with tyramine.

Assay Weigh and powder 20 tablets. Carry out the method for *liquid chromatography*, Appendix III D, using the following solutions. For solution (1) shake a quantity of the powdered tablets containing 20 mg of Ritodrine Hydrochloride in 50 ml of the mobile phase for 5 minutes, add sufficient of the mobile phase to produce 100 ml, mix and filter. Solution (2) contains 0.02% w/v of *ritodrine hydrochloride BPCRS* in the mobile phase. For solution (3) dissolve about 20 mg of *ritodrine hydrochloride BPCRS* in 50 ml of the mobile phase, add 5.6 ml of *sulphuric acid* and sufficient of the mobile phase to produce 100 ml, mix and heat at a temperature of 85° for 2 hours. Cool to room temperature, carefully mix 10 ml of the cooled solution with 8 ml of a 10% w/v solution of *sodium hydroxide* and allow to cool (generation of *threo*-diastereoisomer).

The chromatographic procedure described under Related substances may be used.

The test is not valid unless, in the chromatogram obtained with solution (3), the *resolution factor* between the two principal peaks (ritodrine and the *threo*-diastereoisomer) is at least 1.5.

Calculate the content of $C_{17}H_{21}NO_3,HCl$ in the tablets from the chromatograms obtained and from the declared content of $C_{17}H_{21}NO_3,HCl$ in *ritodrine hydrochloride BPCRS*.

Storage Ritodrine Tablets should be protected from light and stored at a temperature not exceeding 25°.

Salbutamol Injection

Definition Salbutamol Injection is a sterile solution of Salbutamol Sulphate in Water for Injections.

The injection complies with the requirements stated under Parenteral Preparations and with the following requirements.

Content of salbutamol, $C_{13}H_{21}NO_3$ 90.0 to 110.0% of the prescribed or stated amount.

Characteristics A colourless or very pale yellow solution.

Identification

A. Dilute a volume of the injection with sufficient 0.1M *hydrochloric acid* to produce a solution containing the equivalent of 0.004% w/v of salbutamol. The *light absorption* of the resulting solution, Appendix II B, in the range 230 to 350 nm exhibits a maximum only at 276 nm.

B. Carry out the method for *thin-layer chromatography*, Appendix III A, using *silica gel G* as the coating substance and a mixture of 50 volumes of *ethyl acetate*, 30 volumes of *propan-2-ol*, 16 volumes of *water* and 4 volumes of 13.5M *ammonia* as the mobile phase. Apply separately to the plate 2 µl of each of the following solutions. For solution (1) evaporate a suitable volume of the injection to dryness using a rotary evaporator, wash the residue with four 5-ml quantities of *absolute ethanol*, filter, evaporate the filtrate to dryness and dissolve the residue in sufficient *water* to produce a solution containing the equivalent of 0.1% w/v of salbutamol. Solution (2) contains 0.12% w/v of *salbutamol sulphate BPCRS*. After removal of the plate, allow it to dry in air until the odour of the solvent is no longer detectable, place it in an atmosphere saturated with *diethylamine* for a few minutes and spray with *diazotised nitroaniline solution*. The spot in the chromatogram obtained with solution (1) corresponds to that in the chromatogram obtained with solution (2).

C. Dilute a volume containing the equivalent of 0.5 mg of salbutamol to 50 ml with *water*, add 1 ml of 5M *ammonia*, 1 ml of a 3% w/v solution of *4-aminophenazone*, 10 ml of a 2% w/v solution of *potassium hexacyanoferrate(III)* and 10 ml of *chloroform*, shake and allow to separate. An orange-red colour is produced in the chloroform layer.

D. A volume containing the equivalent of 1 mg of salbutamol yields the reactions characteristic of *sulphates*, Appendix VI.

Acidity pH, 3.4 to 5.0, Appendix V L.

Assay Carry out the method for *liquid chromatography*, Appendix III D, using the following solutions. For solution (1) dilute the injection with the mobile phase to produce a solution containing the equivalent of 0.0025% w/v of salbutamol. Solution (2) contains 0.003% w/v of *salbutamol sulphate BPCRS* in the mobile phase. Solution (3) contains 0.003% w/v of *salbutamol sulphate BPCRS* and 0.003% w/v of *2-tert-butylamino-1-(4-hydroxy-3-methylphenyl)ethanol sulphate BPCRS* in the mobile phase.

The chromatographic procedure may be carried out using (a) a stainless steel column (20 cm × 5 mm) packed with spherical particles of silica, 5 µm in diameter, the surface of which has been modified with chemically-bonded nitrile groups (Spherisorb CN is suitable), (b) as the mobile phase with a flow rate of 2.0 ml per minute a mixture of 15 volumes of *propan-2-ol*, 300 volumes of 0.05M *ammonium acetate* and 685 volumes of *water* the pH of the mixture being adjusted to 4.5 with *glacial acetic acid* and (c) a detection wavelength of 276 nm.

The test is not valid unless the *resolution factor* between the two principal peaks in the chromatogram obtained with solution (3) is at least 1.5.

Calculate the content of $C_{13}H_{21}NO_3$ using the declared content of $C_{13}H_{21}NO_3$ in *salbutamol sulphate BPCRS.*

Labelling The quantity of active ingredient is stated in terms of the equivalent amount of salbutamol.

Salbutamol Pressurised Inhalation

Definition Salbutamol Pressurised Inhalation is a suspension of either Salbutamol or Salbutamol Sulphate in a suitable liquid in a suitable pressurised container.

The pressurised inhalation complies with the requirements stated under Preparations for Inhalation and with the following requirements.

Content of salbutamol, $C_{13}H_{21}NO_3$ 80.0 to 120.0% of the amount stated to be delivered by actuation of the valve.

Identification

A. The *infrared absorption spectrum*, Appendix II A, in the range 1650 to 400 cm^{-1} is concordant with the *reference spectrum* of either salbutamol or salbutamol sulphate, as appropriate. Examine the substance as a dispersion in *potassium bromide* prepared in the following manner. Discharge the inhaler a sufficient number of times into a mortar to obtain 2 mg of Salbutamol, grind the residue thoroughly with 0.1 g of *potassium bromide*, add a further 0.2 g of *potassium bromide* and mix thoroughly.

B. In the test for Related substances, the principal spot in the chromatogram obtained with solution (2) corresponds in position and colour to that in the chromatogram obtained with solution (3).

Related substances Carry out the method for *thin-layer chromatography*, Appendix III A, using *silica gel G* as the coating substance and a mixture of 4 volumes of 13.5M *ammonia*, 16 volumes of *water*, 30 volumes of *propan-2-ol* and 50 volumes of *ethyl acetate* as the mobile phase. Apply separately to the plate 5 µl of each of the following solutions.

For pressurised inhalations containing Salbutamol use the following solution as solution (1). Discharge the inhaler a sufficient number of times into a small, dry beaker to obtain 10 mg of Salbutamol and dissolve the residue in 0.5 ml of *methanol.*

For pressurised inhalations containing Salbutamol Sulphate use the following solution as solution (1). Discharge the inhaler a sufficient number of times into a small, dry beaker to obtain the equivalent of 10 mg of Salbutamol, dissolve the residue in 0.5 ml of *water*, dry at 50° at a pressure of 2 kPa for 1 hour and dissolve the dried residue in 0.5 ml of *water.*

For solution (2) dilute 1 volume of solution (1) to 200 volumes with *methanol.* Solution (3) contains 0.010% w/v of *salbutamol BPCRS* in *methanol.* After removal of the plate, allow it to dry in air, spray with a 0.1% w/v solution of *3-methylbenzothiazolin-2-one hydrazone hydrochloride* in *methanol (90%)* and dry in air for 10 minutes. Spray the plate with a 2% w/v solution of *potassium hexacyanoferrate(III)* in a mixture of 1 volume of 18M *ammonia* and 3 volumes of *water* and spray again with the solution of 3-methylbenzothiazolin-2-one hydrazone hydrochloride. Any *secondary spot* in the chromatogram obtained with solution (1) is not more intense than the spot in the chromatogram obtained with solution (2) (0.5%). Disregard any spot with an Rf value higher than 0.85.

Deposition of the emitted dose Carry out the test for *aerodynamic assessment of fine particles*, Appendix XII F, using Apparatus A but determining the content of active ingredient as described below.

For pressurised inhalations containing Salbutamol use 7 ml of *methanol* in the upper impingement chamber and 30 ml of *methanol* in the lower impingement chamber. Use *methanol* to wash the coupling tube, E, and transfer the combined solution and washings in the lower impingement chamber to a 100-ml graduated flask containing 22.5 ml of a 0.1% w/v solution of *ammonium acetate*, rinsing the chamber with *methanol*, and dilute the combined solution and washings to 100 ml with *methanol.*

For pressurised inhalations containing Salbutamol Sulphate use 7 ml of *water* in the upper impingement chamber and 30 ml of *water* in the lower impingement chamber. Use a mixture of equal volumes of *methanol* and *water* to wash the coupling tube, E, and transfer the combined solution and washings in the lower impingement chamber to a 100-ml graduated flask containing 22.5 ml of a 0.1% w/v solution of *ammonium acetate*, rinsing the chamber with a mixture of equal volumes of *methanol* and *water*, and dilute the combined solution and washings to 100 ml with *water.*

Carry out the method for *liquid chromatography*, Appendix III D, using the following solutions. Solution (1) contains 0.0006% w/v of *2-tert-butylamino-1-(4-hydroxy-3-methylphenyl)ethanol sulphate BPCRS* and 0.0005% w/v of *salbutamol BPCRS* in the mobile phase. Solution (2) is a 0.0005% w/v solution of *salbutamol BPCRS* in the mobile phase. For solution (3) use the diluted solution from the lower impingement chamber.

The chromatographic procedure may be carried out using (a) a stainless steel column (10 cm × 5 mm) packed with *stationary phase C* (5 µm) (Spherisorb ODS 1 is suitable), (b) a mixture of 225 volumes of a 0.1% w/v solution of *ammonium acetate* and 800 volumes of *methanol* as the mobile phase with a flow rate of 2 ml per minute and (c) a detection wavelength of 276 nm.

The test is not valid unless the *resolution factor* between the two principal peaks in the chromatogram obtained with solution (1) is at least 1.5.

Calculate the amount of salbutamol, $C_{13}H_{21}NO_3$, delivered to the lower impingement chamber per actuation of the valve using the declared content of $C_{13}H_{21}NO_3$ in *salbutamol BPCRS.* Not less than 35% of the average amount of salbutamol delivered per actuation of the valve, calculated as the average of the three results determined in the Assay, is deposited in the lower impingement chamber.

Assay Determine the content of active ingredient delivered by the first 10 successive combined actuations of the valve after priming.

For pressurised inhalations containing Salbutamol carry out the procedure for Content of active ingredient delivered by actuation of the valve described under Pressurised Inhalations, beginning at the words 'Remove the pressurised container from the actuator...' and ending at the words '... to the volume specified in the monograph', using 35 ml of *methanol* in the vessel. Add 22.5 ml of a 0.1% w/v solution of *ammonium acetate* to the combined solution and washings obtained from the set of 10 combined actuations and dilute to 100 ml with *methanol* (solution A).

For pressurised inhalations containing Salbutamol Sulphate carry out the procedure for Content of active ingredient delivered by actuation of the valve described under Pressurised Inhalations, beginning at the words 'Remove the pressurised container from the actuator...' and ending at the words '... to the volume specified in the monograph', using 35 ml of a mixture of equal volumes of *methanol* and *water* in the vessel. Add 22.5 ml of a 0.1% w/v solution of *ammonium acetate* to the combined solution and washings obtained from the set of 10 combined actuations and dilute to 100 ml with *water* (solution A).

Determine the amount of active ingredient in the 10 combined actuations using the following method of analysis. Carry out the method for *liquid chromatography*, Appendix III D, using the following solutions. Solution (1) contains 0.0012% w/v of *2-tert-butylamino-1-(4-hydroxy-3-methylphenyl)ethanol sulphate BPCRS* and 0.001% w/v of *salbutamol BPCRS* in the mobile phase. Solution (2) contains 0.001% w/v of *salbutamol BPCRS* in the mobile phase. For solution (3) use solution A.

The chromatographic conditions described under Deposition of the emitted dose may be used.

The test is not valid unless the *resolution factor* between the two principal peaks in the chromatogram obtained with solution (1) is at least 1.5.

Calculate the average content of $C_{13}H_{21}NO_3$ delivered by a single actuation of the valve using the declared content of $C_{13}H_{21}NO_3$ in *salbutamol BPCRS*.

Determine the content of active ingredient a second and a third time by repeating the procedure on the middle 10 and on the last 10 successive combined actuations of the valve, as estimated from the number of deliveries available from the container as stated on the label. For each of the three determinations the average content of $C_{13}H_{21}NO_3$ delivered by a single actuation of the valve is within the limits stated under Content of salbutamol.

Labelling The label on the container states (1) whether the preparation contains Salbutamol or Salbutamol Sulphate; (2) where applicable, that the preparation does not contain chlorofluorocarbon propellants (CFCs).

When the active ingredient is Salbutamol Sulphate, the quantity is stated in terms of the equivalent amount of Salbutamol.

Salbutamol Tablets

Definition Salbutamol Tablets contain Salbutamol Sulphate.

The tablets comply with the requirements stated under Tablets and with the following requirements.

Content of salbutamol, $C_{13}H_{21}NO_3$ 92.5 to 107.5% of the prescribed or stated amount.

Identification

A. Carry out the method described under Related substances applying separately to the plate 2 µl of each of the following solutions. For solution (1) shake a quantity of the powdered tablets containing the equivalent of 10 mg of salbutamol with 10 ml of *methanol (80%)* and filter. Solution (2) contains 0.12% w/v of *salbutamol sulphate BPCRS*. The principal spot in the chromatogram obtained with solution (1) corresponds to that in the chromatogram obtained with solution (2).

B. Shake a quantity of the powdered tablets containing the equivalent of 2.5 mg of salbutamol with 50 ml of a 2% w/v solution of *sodium tetraborate*, add 1 ml of a 3% w/v solution of *4-aminophenazone*, 10 ml of a 2% w/v solution of *potassium hexacyanoferrate(III)* and 10 ml of *chloroform*, shake and allow to separate. An orange-red colour is produced in the chloroform layer.

C. Shake a quantity of the powdered tablets containing the equivalent of 4 mg of salbutamol with 10 ml of *water* and filter. The filtrate yields the reactions characteristic of *sulphates*, Appendix VI.

Related substances Carry out the method for *thin-layer chromatography*, Appendix III A, using *silica gel G* as the coating substance and a mixture of 3 volumes of 13.5M *ammonia*, 18 volumes of *water*, 35 volumes of *ethyl acetate*, 45 volumes of *propan-2-ol* and 50 volumes of *4-methylpentan-2-one* as the mobile phase but allowing the solvent front to ascend 18 cm above the line of application. Apply separately to the plate 10 µl of each of the following solutions. For solution (1) shake a quantity of the tablets containing the equivalent of 48 mg of salbutamol with 60 ml of *ethanol (50%)* for 30 minutes, filter, evaporate to dryness using a rotary evaporator and gentle heat and dissolve the residue in 2 ml of *water*; if the residue is coloured, pass the final solution through a column (3 cm × 6 mm) packed with *activated acid aluminium oxide* (Brockmann Grade I is suitable). Solution (2) contains 0.058% w/v of *salbutamol sulphate BPCRS* in *water*. Solution (3) contains 0.022% w/v of *salbutamol sulphate BPCRS* in *water*. After removal of the plate, allow it to dry in air until the odour of the solvent is no longer perceptible and spray with a 0.1% w/v solution of *3-methylbenzothiazolin-2-one hydrazone hydrochloride* in *methanol (90%)* followed by a 2% w/v solution of *potassium hexacyanoferrate(III)* in a mixture of 1 volume of 18M *ammonia* and 3 volumes of *water* and spray again with the solution of methylbenzothiazolinone hydrazone hydrochloride. Any *secondary spot* in the chromatogram obtained with solution (1) is not more intense than the spot in the chromatogram obtained with solution (2) (2%) and not more than one such spot is more intense than the spot in the chromatogram obtained with solution (3) (0.75%).

Uniformity of content Tablets containing the equivalent of 2 mg or less of Salbutamol comply with the requirements stated under Tablets using the following method of analysis. Carry out the method for *liquid chromatography*, Appendix III A, using the following solutions. Solution (1) contains 0.060% w/v of *2-tert-butylamino-1-(4-hydroxy-3-methylphenyl)ethanol sulphate BPCRS* and 0.060% w/v of *salbutamol sulphate BPCRS* in the mobile phase. Solution (2) contains 0.0024% w/v of *salbutamol sulphate BPCRS* in *water*. For solution (3) add 50 ml of *water* to one tablet, shake for 1 hour, add sufficient *water* to produce 100 ml, mix and filter.

The chromatographic procedure may be carried out using (a) a stainless steel column (20 cm × 5 mm) packed with spherical particles of silica, 5 µm in diameter, the surface of which has been modified with chemically-bonded nitrile groups (Spherisorb CN is suitable), (b) as the mobile phase with a flow rate of 2.0 ml per minute a mixture of 65 volumes of *water*, 30 volumes of 0.05M *ammonium acetate* and 5 volumes of *propan-2-ol*, the pH of the mixture being adjusted to 4.5 with *glacial acetic acid*, and (c) a detection wavelength of 276 nm.

Calculate the content of $C_{13}H_{21}NO_3$ in each tablet using the declared content of $C_{13}H_{21}NO_3$ in *salbutamol sulphate BPCRS*. The test is not valid unless the *resolution factor* between the two principal peaks in the chromatogram obtained with solution (1) is at least 1.5.

Assay

For tablets containing the equivalent of more than 2 mg of salbutamol Carry out the method for *liquid chromatography*, Appendix III D, using the following solutions. Solution (1) contains 0.048% w/v of *2-tert-butylamino-1-(4-hydroxy-3-methylphenyl)ethanol sulphate BPCRS* and 0.048% w/v of *salbutamol sulphate BPCRS* in *methanol (10%)*. Solution (2) contains 0.048% w/v of *salbutamol sulphate BPCRS* in *water*. For solution (3) shake 10 tablets with 100 ml of *water* for 1 hour, add sufficient *water* to produce a solution containing the equivalent of 0.040% w/v of salbutamol, mix and filter.

The chromatographic procedure described under Uniformity of content may be used.

The test is not valid unless the *resolution factor* between the two principal peaks in the chromatogram obtained with solution (1) is at least 1.5.

Calculate the content of $C_{13}H_{21}NO_3$ using the declared content of $C_{13}H_{21}NO_3$ in *salbutamol sulphate BPCRS*.

For tablets containing the equivalent of 2 mg or less of salbutamol Use the average of the 10 individual results obtained in the test for Uniformity of content.

Labelling The quantity of active ingredient is stated in terms of the equivalent amount of salbutamol.

Salicylic Acid Collodion

Definition

Salicylic Acid	120 g
Flexible Collodion	sufficient to produce 1000 ml

The collodion complies with the requirements stated under Liquids for Cutaneous Application and with the following requirements.

Content of salicylic acid, $C_7H_6O_3$ 13.0 to 15.8% w/w.

Assay Dilute 2 g to 200 ml with *acetone* and to 2 ml of this solution add 35 ml of *acetate buffer pH 2.45* and 4 ml of a freshly prepared 0.5% w/v solution of *iron(III) chloride hexahydrate*. Dilute to 50 ml with *acetate buffer pH 2.45*, filter, discarding the first 10 ml of the filtrate, and measure the *absorbance* of the resulting solution at the maximum at 525 nm, Appendix II B. Calculate the content of $C_7H_6O_3$ from the *absorbance* obtained by repeating the operation using 2 ml of a 0.12% w/v solution of *salicylic acid* in *ethanol (96%)* and beginning at the words 'add 35 ml of *acetate buffer pH 2.45* ...'.

Salicylic Acid Ointment

Definition Salicylic Acid Ointment contains 2% w/w of Salicylic Acid in a suitable water-emulsifying basis.

Extemporaneous preparation The following formula and directions apply.

Salicylic Acid, finely sifted	20 g
Wool Alcohols Ointment	980 g

Melt the Wool Alcohols Ointment, gradually add the Salicylic Acid and stir until cold.

The ointment complies with the requirements stated under Topical Semi-solid Preparations and with the following requirements.

Content of salicylic acid, $C_7H_6O_3$ 1.9 to 2.1% w/w.

Identification Shake 1 g with 10 ml of *water*, filter and add to the filtrate *iron(III) chloride solution R1*; an intense reddish violet colour is produced which persists on the addition of 6M *acetic acid*. Add 2M *hydrochloric acid*; the colour disappears and a white, crystalline precipitate is produced.

Assay Dissolve 10 g in a mixture of 20 ml of *ethanol (96%)*, previously neutralised to *phenol red solution*, and 20 ml of *ether* and titrate with 0.1M *sodium hydroxide VS* using *phenol red solution* as indicator. Each ml of 0.1M *sodium hydroxide VS* is equivalent to 13.81 mg of $C_7H_6O_3$.

Selenium Sulphide Scalp Application

Selenium Sulphide Application

Definition Selenium Sulphide Scalp Application is a *cutaneous suspension* of Selenium Sulphide in a suitable liquid basis.

The scalp application complies with the requirements stated under Liquids for Cutaneous Application and with the following requirements.

Content of selenium sulphide, SeS_2 90.0 to 110.0% of the prescribed or stated amount.

Identification

A. Gently boil a quantity containing 50 mg of Selenium Sulphide with 5 ml of *nitric acid* for 1 hour, dilute to 50 ml with *water* and filter. To 5 ml of the filtrate add 10 ml of *water* and 5 g of *urea*, boil, cool and add 2 ml of *dilute potassium iodide solution*. A yellow to orange colour is produced, which darkens rapidly on standing.

B. Allow the coloured solution obtained in test A to stand for 10 minutes and filter through *kieselguhr*. The filtrate yields the reactions characteristic of *sulphates*, Appendix VI.

Acidity pH, 4.0 to 5.5, Appendix V L.

Assay To a quantity containing 0.15 g of Selenium Sulphide add 25 ml of *fuming nitric acid*, heat on a water bath for 2 hours, cool and dilute to 250 ml with *water*. To 25 ml of the solution add 10 g of *urea* and 25 ml of *water*, boil, cool, add 10 ml of *dilute potassium iodide solution* and 10 ml of *chloroform* and titrate immediately with 0.05M *sodium thiosulphate VS* using *starch mucilage*, added towards the end of the titration, as indicator. Shake vigorously as the end point is approached. Each ml of 0.05M *sodium thiosulphate VS* is equivalent to 1.789 mg of SeS_2.

Labelling The label indicates the pharmaceutical form as 'cutaneous suspension'.

Standardised Senna Leaf Dry Extract

Standardised Senna Leaf Dry Extract complies with the requirements of the 3rd edition of the European Pharmacopoeia [1261]. These requirements are reproduced after the heading 'Definition' below.

Ph Eur

DEFINITION

Standardised senna leaf dry extract is produced from *Senna leaf (206)*. It contains not less than 5.5 per cent and not more than 8.0 per cent of hydroxyanthracene glycosides, calculated as sennoside B ($C_{42}O_{20}H_{36}$; M_r 863) with reference to the dried extract.

The measured content does not deviate from the value stated on the label by more than ± 10 per cent.

PRODUCTION

The extract is produced from the drug and ethanol 50 to 80 per cent *V/V* with an appropriate procedure according to the monograph *Extracts (765)*.

CHARACTERS

Brownish or brown powder.

IDENTIFICATION

A. Examine by thin-layer chromatography (*2.2.27*), using a suitable silica gel as the coating substance.

Test solution. To 0.1 g of the extract add 5 ml of a mixture of equal volumes of *alcohol R* and *water R* and heat to boiling. Cool and centrifuge. Use the supernatant liquid.

Reference solution. Dissolve 10 mg of *senna extract CRS* in 1 ml of a mixture of equal volumes of *alcohol R* and *water R* (a slight residue remains).

Apply separately to the plate, as bands, 10 µl of each solution. Develop over a path of 10 cm using a mixture of 1 volume of *glacial acetic acid R*, 30 volumes of *water R*, 40 volumes of *ethyl acetate R* and 40 volumes of *propanol R*. Allow the plate to dry in air, spray with a 20 per cent *V/V* solution of *nitric acid R* and heat at 120°C for 10 min. Allow to cool and spray with a 50 g/l solution of *potassium hydroxide* in *alcohol (50 per cent V/V)* R until the zones appear. The principal zones in the chromatogram obtained with the test solution are similar in position, colour and size to the principal zones in the chromatogram obtained with the reference solution. The chromatograms show in the lower third a prominent brown zone corresponding to sennoside B and above it a yellow zone followed by another prominent brown zone corresponding to sennoside A. In the upper half of the chromatograms are visible, in increasing R_f, value, a prominent reddish-brown band and an orange-brown zone followed by a faint pink band and two yellow bands. Close to the solvent front a dark pink zone appears, which may be followed by several faint bands.

B. Place about 25 mg of the extract in a conical flask and add 50 ml of *water R* and 2 ml of *hydrochloric acid R*. Heat in a water-bath for 15 min, cool and shake with 40 ml of *ether R*. Separate the ether, dry over *anhydrous sodium sulphate R*, evaporate 5 ml to dryness and to the cooled residue add 5 ml of *dilute ammonia R1*. A yellow or orange colour develops. Heat on a water-bath for 2 min. A reddish-violet colour develops.

TESTS

Loss on drying Not more than 5.0 per cent. The test is carried out as described for dry extracts in the monograph *Extracts (765)*.

Microbial contamination Total viable aerobic count not more than 10^4 microorganisms per gram of which not more than 10^2 fungi per gram, determined by plate-count (*2.6.12*). It complies with the tests for *Escherichia coli* and for *Salmonella* (*2.6.13*).

ASSAY

Carry out the assay protected from bright light.

Place 0.150 g of the extract in a 100 ml flask, dissolve in *water R* and dilute to 100.0 ml with the same solvent. Filter the solution, discard the first 10 ml of the filtrate. Transfer 20.0 ml of the filtrate to a 150 ml separating funnel. Add 0.1 ml of *dilute hydrochloric acid R* and shake with three quantities, each of 15 ml, of *ether R*. Allow the layers to separate and discard the ether layer. Add 0.10 g of *sodium hydrogen carbonate R* to the aqueous layer and shake for 3 min. Centrifuge and transfer 10.0 ml of the supernatant liquid to a 100 ml round-bottomed flask with a ground-glass neck. Add 20 ml of *ferric chloride solution R1* and mix. Heat for 20 min under a reflux condenser in a water-bath with the water level above that of the liquid in the flask; add 3 ml of *hydrochloric acid R* and heat for a further 30 min with frequent shaking to dissolve the precipitate. Cool, transfer the mixture to a separating funnel and shake with three quantities, each of 25 ml, of *ether R* previously used to rinse the flask. Combine the ether layers and wash with two quantities, each of 15 ml, of *water R*. Transfer the ether layers to a volumetric flask and dilute to 100.0 ml with *ether R*. Evaporate 10.0 ml carefully to dryness and dissolve the residue in 10.0 ml of a 5.0 g/l solution of *magnesium acetate R* in *methanol R*. Measure the absorbance (*2.2.25*) at 515 nm using *methanol R* as the compensation liquid.

Calculate the percentage of hydroxyanthracene glycosides expressed as sennoside B from the expression:

$$\frac{a \times 4.167}{m}$$

i.e. taking the specific absorbance of sennoside B to be 240.

A = absorbance at 515 nm,

m = mass of the substance to be examined in grams.

STORAGE

Store in an airtight container protected from light.

LABELLING

See *Extracts (765)*.

The label states the content of hydroxyanthracene glycosides.

Ph Eur

Senna Liquid Extract

Definition

Senna Fruit, Alexandrian or Tinnevelly, crushed	1000 g
Coriander Oil	6 ml
Ethanol (90 per cent)	250 ml
Purified Water, freshly boiled and cooled	a sufficient quantity

Extemporaneous preparation The following directions apply.

Macerate the crushed Senna Fruit in 5 litres of Purified Water for 8 hours, decant the clear liquid and strain; repeat the process twice using 2 litres of Purified Water for each maceration. Lightly press the marc, strain the expressed liquid, mix the strained liquid with the previously decanted liquid and heat the combined liquids at 80° for 3 minutes in a covered vessel. Allow to stand for not less than 24 hours; filter.

Evaporate the filtrate to 750 ml under reduced pressure at a temperature not exceeding 60°. Separately, dissolve the Coriander Oil in the Ethanol (90 per cent), add the solution to the evaporated filtrate and add sufficient Purified Water to produce 1000 ml. Allow to stand for not less than 24 hours; filter.

The extract complies with the requirements stated under Extracts and with the following requirements.

Ethanol content 21 to 24% v/v, Appendix VIII F, Method III.

Dry residue 17 to 25% w/v.

Relative density 1.02 to 1.09, Appendix V G.

Standardised Senna Granules

Definition Standardised Senna Granules contain Alexandrian Senna Fruit in powder form with suitable excipients. The granules contain 0.55% w/w of sennosides, calculated as sennoside B.

The granules comply with the requirements stated under Granules and with the following requirements.

Content of sennosides calculated as sennoside B 0.467 to 0.633% w/w.

Identification

A. To 25 mg, in *No. 180 powder*, add 50 ml of *water* and 2 ml of *hydrochloric acid*, heat in a water bath for 15 minutes, allow to cool and shake with 40 ml of *ether*. Dry the ether layer over *anhydrous sodium sulphate*, filter, evaporate 5 ml of the filtrate to dryness, cool and add 5 ml of 6M *ammonia* to the residue; a yellow or orange colour is produced. Heat on a water bath for 2 minutes; a reddish violet colour is produced.

B. In the Assay, the chromatogram obtained with solution (1) exhibits two peaks corresponding to the peaks due to sennoside A and sennoside B in the chromatogram obtained with solution (2).

Loss on drying When dried at 105° for 5 hours, lose not more than 2.0% of their weight. Use 5 g.

Assay Carry out the method for *liquid chromatography*, Appendix III D, using the following solutions. For solution (1) shake 2 g of the granules with 50 ml of a 0.3% v/v solution of *acetic acid* adjusted to pH 5.9 with 1M *sodium hydroxide* for 30 minutes, centrifuge, filter through a glass fibre paper (Whatman GF/C is suitable) and use the filtrate. Prepare solution (2) in the same manner as solution (1) but using a quantity of *senna powder BPCRS* containing the equivalent of 11 mg of sennoside B.

The chromatographic procedure may be carried out using (a) a stainless steel column (15 cm × 4.6 mm) packed with *stationary phase C* (5 μm) (Spherisorb ODS 2 is suitable), (b) a mixture of 83 volumes of a 1% v/v solution of *glacial acetic acid* and 17 volumes of *acetonitrile* as the mobile phase with a flow rate of 2 ml per minute and (c) a detection wavelength of 350 nm.

Calculate the total content of sennosides A and B as sennoside B from the sum of the areas of the peaks corresponding to sennoside A and sennoside B and from the declared content of sennosides in *senna powder BPCRS.*

Storage Standardised Senna Granules should be kept in an airtight container at a temperature of 8° to 15°.

Labelling The quantity of active ingredient is stated in terms of the equivalent amount of sennoside B.

Senna Tablets

Definition Senna Tablets contain the powdered pericarp of Senna Fruit, Alexandrian or Tinnevelly.

The tablets comply with the requirements stated under Tablets and with the following requirements.

Content of total sennosides, calculated as sennoside B 85.0 to 115.0% of the prescribed or stated amount.

Identification The powdered tablets exhibit diagnostic structures of senna pericarp. External epidermis of isodiametric cells with very thick outer walls. Occasional stomata. Trichomes few, unicellular, conical and warty. Parenchymatous cells from inner part of a two- to five-layered zone subjacent to the epidermis, each containing a single prism of calcium oxalate. Thick-walled fibres in two to four layers, the fibres of the outer and inner zones respectively with their long axes at right angles to each other. Sutural vascular strands sheathed by cells containing prisms of calcium oxalate; elements of seed tissue may also be present.

Disintegration Maximum time, 30 minutes, Appendix XII A.

Loss on drying The powdered tablets, when dried to constant weight at 105°, lose not more than 6.0% of their weight. Use 1 g.

Assay Weigh and powder 20 tablets. Carry out the following procedure protected from light. To a quantity of the powder containing 7.5 mg of total sennosides add 30 ml of *water*, weigh, heat under a reflux condenser on a water bath for 15 minutes, allow to cool, weigh and restore the original weight with *water*. Centrifuge, transfer 20 ml of the supernatant liquid to a separating funnel, add 0.1 ml of 2M *hydrochloric acid*, shake with two 15-ml quantities of *chloroform*, allow to separate and discard the chloroform layers. Add 0.10 g of *sodium hydrogen carbonate* and shake for 3 minutes; centrifuge and transfer 10 ml of the liquid to a round-bottomed flask fitted with a ground-glass neck. Add a mixture of 8 ml of *iron(III) chloride solution* and 12 ml of *water* and mix. Heat under a reflux condenser on a water bath for 20 minutes, add 1 ml of *hydrochloric acid* and continue heating for a further 20 minutes, shaking frequently, until the precipitate is dissolved. Allow to cool, transfer the mixture to a separating funnel and extract with three 25-ml quantities of *ether* previously used to rinse the flask. Wash the combined ether extracts with two 15-ml quantities of *water* and add sufficient *ether* to produce 100 ml. Evaporate 10 ml just to dryness on a water bath and dissolve the residue in 10 ml of 1M *potassium hydroxide*, filtering if necessary through a sintered glass filter (BS porosity No. 3). Measure the *absorbance* of the resulting solution without delay at the maximum at 500 nm, Appendix II B. Calculate the content of total sennosides, as sennoside B, taking 200 as the value of A(1%, 1 cm) at the maximum at 500 nm.

Labelling The quantity of active ingredient is stated in terms of total sennosides.

Simple Eye Ointment

Eye Ointment Basis

Definition

Wool Fat	100 g
Yellow Soft Paraffin	800 g
Liquid Paraffin	sufficient to produce 1000 g

Extemporaneous preparation The following directions apply.

Melt together the Wool Fat and the Yellow Soft Paraffin, add the Liquid Paraffin, filter the hot mixture through coarse filter paper placed in a heated funnel, sterilise the filtrate by *dry heat* at a minimum of 150° for not less than 1 hour and allow to cool.

The eye ointment complies with the requirements stated under Eye Preparations.

Simple Linctus

Definition Simple Linctus is an *oral solution* containing 2.5% w/v of Citric Acid Monohydrate in a suitable vehicle with an anise flavour.

The linctus complies with the requirements stated under Oral Liquids and with the following requirements.

Content of free acid, calculated as citric acid monohydrate, $C_6H_8O_7,H_2O$ 2.00 to 2.65% w/v.

Identification Dilute 5 ml to 50 ml with *water*, add 2 g of *activated charcoal*, mix and filter. To 1 ml of the filtrate add 1 ml of *pyridine*, swirl to mix, add 5 ml of *acetic anhydride* and mix using, for example, a rotary vortex mixer. Immediately place in a water bath at about 30° for 5 minutes. A yellow colour is produced.

Assay Dilute 15 g with 50 ml of *water* and titrate with 0.5M *sodium hydroxide VS* using 2 ml of *thymol blue solution* as indicator. Each ml of 0.5M *sodium hydroxide VS* is equivalent to 35.02 mg of $C_6H_8O_7,H_2O$. Determine the *weight per ml* of the linctus, Appendix V G, and calculate the content of $C_6H_8O_7,H_2O$, weight in volume.

Storage Simple Linctus should be stored at a temperature not exceeding 25°.

Labelling The label indicates the pharmaceutical form as 'oral solution.'

Paediatric Simple Linctus

Definition Paediatric Simple Linctus is an *oral solution* containing 0.625% w/v of Citric Acid Monohydrate in a suitable vehicle with an anise flavour.

Extemporaneous preparation It may be prepared extemporaneously by diluting Simple Linctus with a suitable vehicle in accordance with the manufacturer's instructions.

The linctus complies with the requirements stated under Oral Liquids and with the following requirements.

Content of free acid, calculated as citric acid monohydrate, $C_6H_8O_7,H_2O$ 0.53 to 0.69% w/v.

Identification Dilute 20 ml to 50 ml with *water*, add 2 g of *activated charcoal*, mix and filter. To 1 ml of the filtrate add 1 ml of *pyridine*, swirl to mix, add 5 ml of *acetic anhydride* and mix using, for example, a rotary vortex mixer. Immediately place in a water bath at about 30° for 5 minutes. A yellow colour is produced.

Assay Dilute 15 g with 50 ml of *water* and titrate with 0.1M *sodium hydroxide VS* using 2 ml of *thymol blue solution* as indicator. Each ml of 0.1M *sodium hydroxide VS* is equivalent to 7.005 mg of $C_6H_8O_7,H_2O$. Determine the *weight per ml* of the linctus, Appendix V G, and calculate the content of $C_6H_8O_7,H_2O$, weight in volume.

Storage Paediatric Simple Linctus should be stored at a temperature not exceeding 25°.

Labelling The label indicates the pharmaceutical form as 'oral solution.'

Simple Ointment

Definition

Wool Fat	50 g
Hard Paraffin	50 g
Cetostearyl Alcohol	50 g
White Soft Paraffin or Yellow Soft Paraffin	850 g

Unless otherwise directed in the monograph, when Simple Ointment is used in a white ointment, it should be prepared with White Soft Paraffin; when used in a coloured ointment it should be prepared with Yellow Soft Paraffin.

Extemporaneous preparation The following directions apply.

Mix the ingredients, heat gently with stirring until homogeneous and stir until cold.

The ointment complies with the requirements stated under Topical Semi-solid Preparations.

Soap Spirit

Definition

Soft Soap	650 g
Ethanol (90 per cent)	sufficient to produce 1000 ml

In making Soap Spirit, the Ethanol (90 per cent) may be replaced by Industrial Methylated Spirit[1] diluted so as to be of equivalent ethanolic strength.

Extemporaneous preparation The following directions apply.

Dissolve the Soft Soap in 300 ml of Ethanol (90 per cent), add sufficient Ethanol (90 per cent) to produce 1000 ml, mix, allow to stand and decant.

The spirit complies with the requirements stated under Spirits and with the following requirements.

Acidity or alkalinity 10 ml requires for neutralisation not more than 1.0 ml of 0.1M *sodium hydroxide VS* or 0.2 ml of 0.1M *hydrochloric acid VS* using *phenolphthalein solution R1* as indicator.

Weight per ml 0.945 to 0.970 g, Appendix V G.

Ethanol content 28 to 32% v/v, Appendix VIII F.

Content of fatty acids Not less than 27.0% w/v when determined by the following method. To 10 ml add 20 ml of *water* and 20 ml of 1M *hydrochloric acid*, extract with two 20-ml quantities of *petroleum spirit (boiling range, 40° to 60°)*, wash the combined extracts with two 10-ml quantities of *water*, evaporate the petroleum spirit, add 5 ml of *acetone*, again evaporate and dry the residue at 80° for 2 hours.

[1]The law and the statutory regulations governing the use of Industrial Methylated Spirit must be observed.

Sodium Amidotrizoate Injection

Definition Sodium Amidotrizoate Injection is a sterile solution of Sodium Amidotrizoate in Water for Injections.

The injection complies with the requirements stated under Parenteral Preparations and with the following requirements.

Content of sodium amidotrizoate, $C_{11}H_8I_3N_2NaO_4$ 97.0 to 103.0% of the prescribed or stated amount.

Characteristics An almost colourless to pale yellow solution.

Identification

A. Dry 1 ml of the injection over *phosphorus pentoxide* at a pressure of 2 kPa for 16 hours. The *infrared absorption spectrum* of the dried residue, Appendix II A, is concordant with the *reference spectrum* of sodium amidotrizoate.

B. In the test for Related substances, the principal spot in the chromatogram obtained with solution (2) is similar in position and size to the principal spot in the chromatogram obtained with solution (4).

Acidity or alkalinity pH, 6.6 to 7.6, Appendix V L. Take the first measurement 3 minutes after inserting the electrodes and repeat every 30 seconds until constant.

Free amine Carry out the test described under Sodium Amidotrizoate using a volume containing 1.0 g of Sodium Amidotrizoate. The absorbance is not more than 0.30.

Inorganic iodide Dilute a quantity containing 0.80 g of Sodium Amidotrizoate to 10 ml with *water*, add sufficient 2M *nitric acid* dropwise to ensure complete precipitation of the iodinated acid and 3 ml in excess. Filter, wash the precipitate with 5 ml of *water*, add to the filtrate 1 ml of *hydrogen peroxide solution (100 vol)* and 1 ml of *chloroform* and shake. Any purple colour in the chloroform is not more intense than that obtained by adding 2 ml of *iodide standard solution (20 ppm I)* to a mixture of 3 ml of 2M *nitric acid* and sufficient *water* to equal the volume of the test solution, adding 1 ml of *hydrogen peroxide solution (100 vol)* and 1 ml of *chloroform* and shaking (50 ppm).

Related substances *Prepare the solutions in subdued light and develop the chromatograms protected from light.* Carry out the method for *thin-layer chromatography*, Appendix III A, using *silica gel GF_{254}* as the coating substance and a mixture of 20 volumes of *anhydrous formic acid*, 25 volumes of *butan-2-one* and 60 volumes of *toluene* as the mobile phase. Apply separately to the plate 2 µl of each of the following solutions. Solutions (1), (2) and (3) are solutions of the injection diluted with a 3% v/v solution of 13.5M *ammonia* in *methanol* to contain (1) 5.0% w/v, (2) 0.50% w/v and (3) 0.010% w/v of Sodium Amidotrizoate respectively. Solution (4) contains 0.50% w/v of *sodium amidotrizoate EPCRS* in a 3% v/v solution of 13.5M *ammonia* in *methanol*. After removal of the plate, allow it to dry in air and examine under *ultraviolet light (254 nm)*. Any *secondary spot* in the chromatogram obtained with solution (1) is not more intense than the principal spot in the chromatogram obtained with solution (3) (0.2%).

Pyrogens Complies with the *test for pyrogens*, Appendix XIV D. Use per kg of the rabbit's weight a quantity containing 2.5 g of Sodium Amidotrizoate.

Assay Mix a quantity containing 0.7 g of Sodium Amidotrizoate with 12 ml of 5M *sodium hydroxide* and 20 ml of *water*, add 1 g of *zinc powder* and boil under a reflux condenser for 30 minutes. Cool, rinse the condenser with 30 ml of *water*, filter through absorbent cotton and wash the flask and the filter with two 20-ml quantities of *water*. To the combined filtrate and washings add 80 ml of *hydrochloric acid*, cool and titrate with 0.05M *potassium iodate VS* until the dark brown solution becomes light brown. Add 5 ml of *chloroform* and continue the titration, shaking well after each addition, until the chloroform becomes colourless. Each ml of 0.05M *potassium iodate VS* is equivalent to 21.20 mg of $C_{11}H_8I_3N_2NaO_4$. Determine the *weight per ml* of the injection, Appendix V G, and calculate the percentage w/v of sodium amidotrizoate, $C_{11}H_8I_3N_2NaO_4$.

Storage Sodium Amidotrizoate Injection should be protected from light.

Labelling The strength is stated as the percentage w/v of Sodium Amidotrizoate.

When sodium diatrizoate injection is prescribed or demanded, Sodium Amidotrizoate Injection shall be dispensed or supplied.

Sodium Aurothiomalate Injection

Definition Sodium Aurothiomalate Injection is a sterile solution of Sodium Aurothiomalate in Water for Injections.

The injection complies with the requirements stated under Parenteral Preparations and with the following requirements.

Content of gold, Au 42.3 to 48.3% of the prescribed or stated amount of Sodium Aurothiomalate.

Characteristics A pale yellow solution.

Identification

A. To a volume containing 20 mg of Sodium Aurothiomalate add 2 ml of *hydrogen peroxide solution (100 vol)* and 1 ml of 5M *sodium hydroxide* and boil for 30 seconds. A colloidal precipitate of gold is produced which appears bluish green by transmitted light.

B. To a volume containing 10 mg of Sodium Aurothiomalate add 0.1 ml of *potassium cyanide solution* and 0.1 ml of a 1.0% w/v solution of *sodium nitroprusside*. A deep magenta colour is produced.

Colour of solution Dilute, if necessary, with *water* to give a solution containing 1.0% w/v of Sodium Aurothiomalate. The colour of the solution is not more intense than that of a 0.020% w/v solution of *potassium hexacyanoferrate(III)*.

Assay To a volume containing 0.1 g of Sodium Aurothiomalate, add 0.4 g of *potassium bromide* and 5 ml of *nitric acid*. Slowly evaporate the solution to dryness and continue heating until fumes cease to be evolved. Allow to cool, add 50 ml of *water*, warm, filter, wash the filter with hot *water*, dry and ignite the residue of gold, Au, for 3 hours at a temperature not lower than 600°.

Storage Sodium Aurothiomalate Injection should be protected from light.

Sodium Bicarbonate Ear Drops

Definition

Sodium Bicarbonate	5 g
Glycerol	30 ml
Purified Water, freshly boiled and cooled	sufficient to produce 100 ml

Extemporaneous preparation The following directions apply.

Dissolve the Sodium Bicarbonate in about 60 ml of Purified Water, add the Glycerol and sufficient Purified Water to produce 100 ml and mix.

Sodium Bicarbonate Ear Drops should be recently prepared.

The ear drops comply with the requirements stated under Ear Preparations and with the following requirements.

Content of sodium bicarbonate, $NaHCO_3$ 4.75 to 5.25% w/v.

Weight per ml 1.10 to 1.12 g, Appendix V G.

Assay To 5 ml add 20 ml of *water* and titrate with 0.1M *hydrochloric acid VS* using *methyl orange—xylene cyanol FF solution* as indicator. Each ml of 0.1M *hydrochloric acid VS* is equivalent to 8.401 mg of $NaHCO_3$.

Sodium Bicarbonate Eye Lotion

Definition Sodium Bicarbonate Eye Lotion is a sterile aqueous solution of Sodium Bicarbonate.

Extemporaneous preparation The following directions apply.

Dissolve the Sodium Bicarbonate in sufficient Purified Water, clarify by filtration, transfer the filtered solution into the final container, close the container so as to exclude micro-organisms and sterilise by *heating in an autoclave*.

The eye lotion complies with the requirements stated under Eye Preparations and with the following requirements.

Content of sodium bicarbonate, $NaHCO_3$ 90.0 to 110.0% of the prescribed or stated amount.

Identification

A. The residue on evaporation, when moistened with *hydrochloric acid* and introduced on a platinum wire into a flame, imparts a yellow colour to the flame.

B. Yields reaction A characteristic of *sodium salts* and the reactions characteristic of *bicarbonates*, Appendix VI.

Assay Titrate a volume containing 1 g of Sodium Bicarbonate with 0.5M *hydrochloric acid VS* using *methyl orange solution* as indicator. Each ml of 0.5M *hydrochloric acid VS* is equivalent to 42.00 mg of $NaHCO_3$.

Containers Sodium Bicarbonate Eye Lotion is supplied in suitable containers with a nominal volume of not more than 1 litre.

Storage Sodium Bicarbonate Eye Lotion should not be kept in containers that have previously been subjected to heating in an autoclave.

Labelling The label states that any Eye Lotion not used within 24 hours of opening the container should be discarded.

When Sodium Bicarbonate Eye Lotion is prescribed or demanded no strength being stated, a lotion containing 2% w/v of Sodium Bicarbonate shall be dispensed or supplied.

Sodium Bicarbonate Intravenous Infusion

Sodium Bicarbonate Injection

Definition Sodium Bicarbonate Intravenous Infusion is a sterile solution of Sodium Bicarbonate in Water for Injections.

The intravenous infusion complies with the requirements stated under Parenteral Preparations and with the following requirements.

Content of sodium bicarbonate, $NaHCO_3$ 94.0 to 106.0% of the prescribed or stated amount.

Identification

A. The residue on evaporation, when moistened with *hydrochloric acid* and introduced on a platinum wire into a flame, imparts a yellow colour to the flame.

B. Yields reaction A characteristic of *sodium salts* and the reactions characteristic of *bicarbonates*, Appendix VI.

Particulate contamination When supplied in a container with a nominal content of 100 ml or more, complies with the *test for sub-visible particles*, Appendix XIII A.

Pyrogens Complies with the *test for pyrogens*, Appendix XIV D. For intravenous infusions containing 2.5% w/v or less of Sodium Bicarbonate slowly inject 10 ml per kg of the rabbit's weight. For intravenous infusions containing more than 2.5% w/v of Sodium Bicarbonate dilute to contain 2.5% w/v of Sodium Bicarbonate and slowly inject 10 ml per kg of the rabbit's weight.

Assay Titrate a volume containing 1 g of Sodium Bicarbonate with 0.5M *hydrochloric acid VS* using *methyl orange solution* as indicator. Each ml of 0.5M *hydrochloric acid VS* is equivalent to 42.00 mg of $NaHCO_3$.

Storage Sodium Bicarbonate Intravenous Infusion should not be kept in containers that have previously been subjected to heating in an autoclave.

Labelling The strength is stated as the percentage w/v of Sodium Bicarbonate.

The label states (1) that containers containing visible particles must not be used; (2) the approximate concentrations, in millimoles per litre, of the sodium ions and the bicarbonate ions.

For a preparation containing 1.4% w/v of Sodium Bicarbonate the concentration of each ion is stated as 167 millimoles per litre.

Compound Sodium Bicarbonate Tablets

Soda Mint Tablets

Definition Compound Sodium Bicarbonate Tablets contain, in each, 300 mg of Sodium Bicarbonate. They have a peppermint flavour.

The tablets comply with the requirements stated under Tablets and with the following requirements.

Content of total carbonate 275 to 325 mg, calculated as $NaHCO_3$.

Identification

A. The powdered tablets, when moistened with *hydrochloric acid* and introduced on a platinum wire into a flame, impart a yellow colour to the flame.

B. The powdered tablets yield the reactions characteristic of *bicarbonates*, Appendix VI.

C. The tablets have the odour of peppermint.

Carbonate Dissolve 2.5 g of the powder prepared for use in the Assay in 50 ml of *carbon dioxide-free water*. The pH of the resulting solution is not more than 8.6, Appendix V L.

Disintegration The requirement for Disintegration does not apply to Compound Sodium Bicarbonate Tablets.

Assay Weigh and powder 20 tablets. Dissolve 1 g of the powder in 20 ml of *water* and titrate with 0.5M *hydrochloric acid VS* using *methyl orange solution* as indicator. Each ml of 0.5M *hydrochloric acid VS* is equivalent to 42.00 mg of $NaHCO_3$.

Storage Compound Sodium Bicarbonate Tablets should be stored at a temperature not exceeding 25°.

Labelling The label states that the tablets should be allowed to dissolve slowly in the mouth.

Sodium Calcium Edetate Intravenous Infusion

Sodium Calcium Edetate Injection

Definition Sodium Calcium Edetate Intravenous Infusion is a sterile solution of Sodium Calcium Edetate. It is prepared immediately before use by diluting Sterile Sodium Calcium Edetate Concentrate with a suitable diluent in accordance with the manufacturer's instructions.

The intravenous infusion complies with the requirements stated under Parenteral Preparations and with the following requirements.

Particulate contamination When the volume of the diluted intravenous infusion is 100 ml or more, it complies with the *test for sub-visible particles*, Appendix XIII A.

Labelling The strength is stated as the equivalent amount of anhydrous sodium calcium edetate in a suitable dose-volume.

STERILE SODIUM CALCIUM EDETATE CONCENTRATE

Definition Sterile Sodium Calcium Edetate Concentrate is a sterile solution of Sodium Calcium Edetate in Water for Injections containing the equivalent of 20% w/v of anhydrous sodium calcium edetate.

The concentrate complies with the requirements for Concentrated Solutions for Injections stated under Parenteral Preparations and with the following requirements.

Content of anhydrous sodium calcium edetate, $C_{10}H_{12}CaN_2Na_2O_8$ 19.0 to 21.0% w/v.

Characteristics A colourless solution.

Identification

A. Dilute 2.5 ml with 7.5 ml of *water*, make alkaline to *litmus paper* with 5M *ammonia* and add 5 ml of a 2.5% w/v solution of *ammonium oxalate*. Not more than a trace of precipitate is produced.

B. To 10 ml add 2 ml of a 10% w/v solution of *lead(II) nitrate*, shake and add 5 ml of *dilute potassium iodide solution*; no yellow precipitate is produced. Make alkaline to *litmus paper* with 5M *ammonia* and add 5 ml of a 2.5% w/v solution of *ammonium oxalate*; a white precipitate is produced.

C. Evaporate to dryness and ignite. The residue yields the reactions characteristic of *sodium salts* and *calcium salts*, Appendix VI.

Acidity or alkalinity pH, 6.5 to 8.0, Appendix V L.

Pyrogens Complies with the *test for pyrogens*, Appendix XIV D. Use 2 ml per kg of the rabbit's weight.

Assay To 2.5 ml add 90 ml of *water*, 7 g of *hexamine* and 5 ml of 2M *hydrochloric acid* and titrate with 0.05M *lead nitrate VS* using *xylenol orange solution* as indicator. Each ml of 0.05M *lead nitrate VS* is equivalent to 18.71 mg of $C_{10}H_{12}CaN_2Na_2O_8$.

Storage Sterile Sodium Calcium Edetate Concentrate should be kept in containers made from lead-free glass.

Labelling The label states (1) 'Sterile Sodium Calcium Edetate Concentrate'; (2) that the solution must be diluted with Sodium Chloride Intravenous Infusion or Glucose Intravenous Infusion before administration.

When sodium calciumedetate intravenous infusion or sodium calciumedetate injection is prescribed or demanded, Sodium Calcium Edetate Intravenous Infusion shall be dispensed or supplied.

Sodium Chloride Eye Drops

Definition Sodium Chloride Eye Drops are a sterile solution of Sodium Chloride in Purified Water.

The eye drops comply with the requirements stated under Eye Preparations and with the following requirements.

Content of sodium chloride, NaCl 90.0 to 110.0% of the prescribed or stated amount.

Identification

A. Yield the reactions characteristic of *sodium salts*, Appendix VI.

B. Yields reaction A characteristic of *chlorides*, Appendix VI.

Assay Titrate a volume containing 0.1 g of Sodium Chloride with 0.1M *silver nitrate VS* using *potassium chromate solution* as indicator. Each ml of 0.1M *silver nitrate VS* is equivalent to 5.844 mg of NaCl.

When Sodium Chloride Eye Drops are prescribed or demanded no strength being stated, eye drops containing 0.9% w/v of Sodium Chloride shall be dispensed or supplied.

Sodium Chloride Eye Lotion

Definition Sodium Chloride Eye Lotion is a sterile aqueous solution containing 0.9% w/v of Sodium Chloride.

Extemporaneous preparation The following directions apply.

Dissolve the Sodium Chloride in sufficient Purified Water, clarify by filtration, transfer the filtered solution into the final container, close the container so as to exclude micro-organisms and sterilise by *heating in an autoclave*.

The eye lotion complies with the requirements stated under Eye Preparations and with the following requirements.

Content of sodium chloride, NaCl 0.85 to 0.95% w/v.

Identification Yields the reactions characteristic of *sodium salts* and reaction A characteristic of *chlorides*, Appendix VI.

Sterility Complies with the *test for sterility*, Appendix XVI A.

Assay To 25 ml add 75 ml of *acetate buffer pH 5.0* and titrate with 0.1M *silver nitrate VS*, stirring constantly and determining the end point potentiometrically. Each ml of 0.1M *silver nitrate VS* is equivalent to 5.844 mg of NaCl.

Containers Sodium Chloride Eye Lotion is supplied in suitable containers with a nominal volume of not more than 1 litre.

Labelling The label states that any Eye Lotion not used within 24 hours of opening the container should be discarded.

Sodium Chloride Intravenous Infusion

Sodium Chloride Injection

Definition Sodium Chloride Intravenous Infusion is a sterile solution of Sodium Chloride in Water for Injections.

The intravenous infusion complies with the requirements stated under Parenteral Preparations and with the following requirements.

Content of sodium chloride, NaCl 95.0 to 105.0% of the prescribed or stated amount.

Identification Yields the reactions characteristic of *sodium salts* and reaction A characteristic of *chlorides*, Appendix VI.

Particulate contamination When supplied in a container with a nominal content of 100 ml or more, complies with the *test for sub-visible particles*, Appendix XIII A.

Bacterial endotoxins The endotoxin limit concentration is 0.25 IU per ml, Appendix XIV C. Dilute infusions containing more than 0.9% w/v of Sodium Chloride with *water BET* to contain 0.9% w/v.

Assay Titrate a volume containing 0.2 g of Sodium Chloride with 0.1M *silver nitrate VS* using *potassium chromate solution* as indicator. Each ml of 0.1M *silver nitrate VS* is equivalent to 5.844 mg of NaCl.

Storage Sodium Chloride Intravenous Infusion should be stored at a temperature not exceeding 25°.

Labelling The strength is stated as the percentage w/v of Sodium Chloride. The label states that solutions containing visible solid particles must not be used.

When the preparation is intended for intravenous infusion, the label states the approximate concentrations, in millimoles per litre, of the sodium ions and the chloride ions. For a preparation containing 0.9% w/v of Sodium Chloride the concentration of each ion is stated as 150 millimoles per litre.

For concentrated solutions supplied for the preparation of Sodium Chloride Intravenous Infusion by dilution, the label states 'Sterile Sodium Chloride Concentrate' as the title of the preparation.

When Sodium Chloride Intravenous Infusion or Sodium Chloride Injection is prescribed or demanded and no strength is stated, Sodium Chloride Intravenous Infusion (0.9% w/v) shall be dispensed or supplied.

When Sodium Chloride Injection is required as a diluent for Parenteral Preparations of the Pharmacopoeia, Sodium Chloride Intravenous Infusion (0.9% w/v) shall be used.

When normal saline solution for injection is prescribed or demanded, Sodium Chloride Intravenous Infusion (0.9% w/v) shall be dispensed or supplied.

Sodium Chloride and Glucose Intravenous Infusion

Sodium Chloride and Dextrose Injection; Sodium Chloride and Glucose Injection; Sodium Chloride and Dextrose Intravenous Infusion

Definition Sodium Chloride and Glucose Intravenous Infusion is a sterile solution of Sodium Chloride and either Anhydrous Glucose or Glucose in Water for Injections.

The intravenous infusion complies with the requirements stated under Parenteral Preparations and with the following requirements.

Content of sodium chloride, NaCl 95.0 to 105.0% of the prescribed or stated amount.

Content of glucose, $C_6H_{12}O_6$ 95.0 to 105.0% of the prescribed or stated amount.

Characteristics A colourless or faintly straw-coloured solution.

Identification

A. When heated with *cupri-tartaric solution R1*, a copious precipitate of copper(I) oxide is produced.

B. Yields reaction B characteristic of *sodium salts* and reaction A characteristic of *chlorides*, Appendix VI.

Acidity pH, 3.5 to 6.5, Appendix V L.

5-Hydroxymethylfurfural and related substances Dilute a volume containing 1.0 g of glucose, $C_6H_{12}O_6$, to 500 ml with *water* and measure the *absorbance* of the resulting solution at the maximum at 284 nm, Appendix II B. The *absorbance* is not more than 0.25.

Particulate contamination When supplied in a container with a nominal volume of 100 ml or more, complies with the test for *sub-visible particles*, Appendix XIII A.

Bacterial endotoxins The endotoxin limit concentration is 0.25 IU per ml, Appendix XIV C. Dilute infusions containing more than 0.9% w/v of Sodium Chloride with *water BET* to contain 0.9% w/v.

Assay

For sodium chloride Titrate a quantity containing 0.1 g of Sodium Chloride with 0.1M *silver nitrate VS* using *potassium chromate solution* as indicator. Each ml of 0.1M *silver nitrate VS* is equivalent to 5.844 mg of NaCl.

For glucose To a quantity containing 2 to 5 g of glucose, $C_6H_{12}O_6$, add 0.2 ml of 5M *ammonia* and sufficient *water* to produce 100 ml. Mix well, allow to stand for 30 minutes and measure the *optical rotation* in a 2-dm tube, Appendix V F. The observed rotation in degrees multiplied by 0.9477 represents the weight in g of glucose, $C_6H_{12}O_6$, in the volume of the injection taken for assay.

Storage Sodium Chloride and Glucose Intravenous Infusion should be stored at a temperature not exceeding 25°.

Labelling The strength is stated as the percentages w/v of Sodium Chloride and of glucose, $C_6H_{12}O_6$. The label states that solutions containing visible particles must not be used.

When the preparation is intended for intravenous infusion, the label states the approximate concentrations, in millimoles per litre, of the sodium ions and the chloride ions and the number of grams per litre of glucose, $C_6H_{12}O_6$. For a preparation containing 0.18% w/v of Sodium Chloride, the concentration of each ion is stated as 30 millimoles per litre.

Compound Sodium Chloride Mouthwash

Definition Compound Sodium Chloride Mouthwash contains 1% w/v of Sodium Bicarbonate and 1.5% w/v of Sodium Chloride in a suitable vehicle with a flavour of peppermint.

Extemporaneous preparation The following formula applies.

Sodium Bicarbonate	10 g
Sodium Chloride	15 g
Concentrated Peppermint Emulsion	25 ml
Double-strength Chloroform Water	500 ml
Water	sufficient to produce 1000 ml

The mouthwash complies with the requirements stated under Mouthwashes and with the following requirements.

Content of sodium bicarbonate, $NaHCO_3$ 0.95 to 1.05% w/v.

Content of sodium chloride, NaCl 1.42 to 1.58% w/v.

Assay

For sodium bicarbonate Titrate 20 ml with 0.1M *hydrochloric acid VS* using *methyl orange—xylene cyanol FF solution* as indicator. Each ml of 0.1M *hydrochloric acid VS* is equivalent to 8.401 mg of $NaHCO_3$.

For sodium chloride To 10 ml add 10 ml of *water* and carry out the method for *ion-selective potentiometry*, Appendix VIII E, using 0.1M *silver nitrate VS*. Each ml of 0.1M *silver nitrate VS* is equivalent to 5.844 mg of NaCl.

Compound Sodium Chloride Mouthwash should be diluted with an equal volume of warm water before use.

Sodium Chloride Irrigation Solution

Definition Sodium Chloride Irrigation Solution is a sterile aqueous solution of Sodium Chloride.

Production Sodium Chloride Irrigation Solution intended to be used for the irrigation of body cavities, for the flushing of wounds or operation cavities or for the irrigation of the urogenital system is prepared using Water for Irrigation.

The irrigation solution complies with the requirements stated under Irrigation Solutions and with the following requirements.

Content of sodium chloride, NaCl 95.0 to 105.0% of the prescribed or stated amount.

Identification A. Yields the reactions characteristic of *sodium salts*, Appendix VI.

B. Yields reaction A characteristic of *chlorides*, Appendix VI.

Assay Titrate a volume containing 0.2 g of Sodium Chloride with 0.1M *silver nitrate VS* using *potassium chromate solution* as indicator. Each ml of 0.1M *silver nitrate VS* is equivalent to 5.844 mg of NaCl.

Sodium Chloride Solution

Definition Sodium Chloride Solution is a 0.9% w/v *cutaneous solution* of Sodium Chloride in Purified Water. The solution may be clarified by filtration.

The solution complies with the requirements stated under Liquids for Cutaneous Application and with the following requirements.

Content of sodium chloride, NaCl 0.85 to 0.95% w/v.

Identification

A. When introduced on a platinum wire into a flame, imparts a yellow colour to the flame.

B. Yields reaction A characteristic of *chlorides*, Appendix VI.

Assay Titrate 20 ml with 0.1M *silver nitrate VS* using *potassium chromate solution* as indicator. Each ml of 0.1M *silver nitrate VS* is equivalent to 5.844 mg of NaCl.

Labelling The label states, where applicable, that the contents of the container are sterile.

The label indicates the pharmaceutical form as 'cutaneous solution'.

When normal saline is prescribed or demanded, Sodium Chloride Solution shall be dispensed or supplied.

If the label states that the contents of the container are sterile, the solution complies with the following additional requirements.

Sterility Complies with the *test for sterility*, Appendix XVI A.

Labelling The label states (1) 'Sterile Sodium Chloride Solution'; (2) that the solution is not intended for injection; (3) the date after which the solution is not intended to be used; (4) the conditions under which it should be stored.

Sodium Chloride Tablets

Definition Sodium Chloride Tablets contain Sodium Chloride.

The tablets comply with the requirements stated under Tablets and with the following requirements.

Content of sodium chloride, NaCl 95.0 to 105.0% of the prescribed or stated amount.

Identification The powdered tablets yield the reactions characteristic of *sodium salts* and the reactions characteristic of *chlorides*, Appendix VI.

Clarity of solution Dissolve a quantity of the tablets containing 0.6 g of Sodium Chloride in 100 ml of *water*. The solution is *clear*, Appendix IV A.

Disintegration The tablets dissolve completely within 15 minutes when examined by the *disintegration test for tablets and capsules*, Appendix XII A, but using *water* at 19° to 21°.

Assay Weigh and powder 20 tablets. Dissolve a quantity of the powder containing 0.2 g of Sodium Chloride in 35 ml of *water*, add 15 ml of 2M *nitric acid*, 5 ml of *dibutyl phthalate* and 50 ml of 0.1M *silver nitrate VS* and shake vigorously for about 1 minute. Add 5 ml of *ammonium iron(III) sulphate solution R2* and titrate with 0.1M *ammonium thiocyanate VS* until a reddish brown colour is obtained which, after shaking, does not fade within 5 minutes. Each ml of 0.1M *silver nitrate VS* is equivalent to 5.844 mg of NaCl.

Labelling The label states that the tablets should be dissolved in water before administration.

Sodium Citrate Eye Drops

Definition Sodium Citrate Eye Drops are a sterile solution of Sodium Citrate in Purified Water.

The eye drops comply with the requirements stated under Eye Preparations and with the following requirements.

Content of sodium citrate, C6H5Na3O7,2H2O 95.0 to 105.0% of the prescribed or stated amount.

Characteristics A colourless solution.

Identification A. Yield reaction A characteristic of *sodium salts*, Appendix VI.

B. Yield reaction A characteristic of *citrates*, Appendix VI.

Acidity or alkalinity pH, 7.0 to 7.5, Appendix V L.

Assay Evaporate a volume containing 0.15 g of Sodium Citrate to dryness and dissolve the residue in *anhydrous acetic acid*, warming to about 50°. Allow to cool and carry out Method I for *non-aqueous titration*, Appendix VIII A, using 0.25 ml of *1-naphtholbenzein solution* as indicator. Each ml of 0.1M *perchloric acid VS* is equivalent to 9.803 mg of $C_6H_5Na_3O_7,2H_2O$.

Sodium Citrate Irrigation Solution

Sterile Sodium Citrate Solution for Bladder Irrigation

Definition Sodium Citrate Irrigation Solution is a sterile, apyrogenic solution of Sodium Citrate in Water for Irrigation containing Anhydrous Citric Acid or Citric Acid Monohydrate.

The irrigation solution complies with the requirements stated under Preparations for Irrigation and with the following requirements.

Content of sodium citrate, $C_6H_5Na_3O_7,2H_2O$ 95.0 to 105.0% of the prescribed or stated amount.

Characteristics A colourless solution.

Identification Yields reaction A characteristic of *sodium salts* and reaction A characteristic of *citrates*, Appendix VI.

Acidity or alkalinity pH, 6.0 to 7.5, Appendix V L.

Assay Evaporate a volume containing 0.15 g of Sodium Citrate to dryness and dissolve the residue in *anhydrous acetic acid*, warming to about 50°. Allow to cool and carry out Method I for *non-aqueous titration*, Appendix VIII A, using 0.25 ml of *1-naphtholbenzein solution* as indicator. Each ml of 0.1M *perchloric acid VS* is equivalent to 9.803 mg of $C_6H_5Na_3O_7,2H_2O$.

Labelling The label states that Sodium Citrate Irrigation Solution is apyrogenic.

When Sodium Citrate Irrigation Solution is prescribed or demanded, no strength being stated, a solution containing 3.0% w/v of Sodium Citrate shall be dispensed or supplied.

Sodium Citrate Tablets

Definition Sodium Citrate Tablets contain Sodium Citrate.

The tablets comply with the requirements stated under Tablets and with the following requirements.

Content of sodium citrate, $C_6H_5Na_3O_7,2H_2O$ 95.0 to 105.0% of the prescribed or stated amount.

Identification A. Boil a quantity of the powdered tablets with an excess of *mercury(II) sulphate solution* and filter if necessary. Boil and add 0.15 ml of *dilute potassium permanganate solution*. The reagent is decolorised and a white precipitate is produced.

B. The powdered tablets yield the reactions characteristic of *sodium salts*, Appendix VI.

Disintegration Comply with the requirements for Soluble Tablets stated under Tablets.

Assay Weigh and powder 20 tablets. Heat a quantity of the powder containing 2 g of Sodium Citrate until carbonised, cool and boil the residue with 50 ml of *water* and 50 ml of 0.5M *hydrochloric acid VS*. Filter, wash the filter with *water* and titrate the excess of acid in the filtrate and washings with 0.5M *sodium hydroxide VS* using *methyl orange solution* as indicator. Each ml of 0.5M *hydrochloric acid VS* is equivalent to 49.02 mg of $C_6H_5Na_3O_7,2H_2O$.

Labelling The label states that the tablets should be dissolved in water before use.

Sodium Citrate Tablets are intended for use in feeding infants. They should be dissolved in water and the solution added to the feed.

Sodium Cromoglicate Powder for Inhalation

Definition Sodium Cromoglicate Powder for Inhalation consists of hard gelatin capsules containing either Sodium Cromoglicate appropriately treated or Sodium Cromoglicate admixed with an approximately equal amount of Lactose. The contents of the capsules are in powder of a suitable fineness.

The powder for inhalation complies with the requirements stated under Preparations for Inhalation and the contents of the capsules comply with the following requirements.

Content of sodium cromoglicate, $C_{23}H_{14}Na_2O_{11}$ 20.0 to 24.4 mg per capsule.

Characteristics A white powder; hygroscopic. When examined microscopically immediately after dispersion in *pentan-1-ol* by exposure for 20 seconds to low intensity ultrasonic waves, exhibit small, rounded particles of maximum dimension 10 µm, often present as loose agglomerates up to 30 µm. The contents of capsules containing Lactose also exhibit larger angular particles, usually axe-head in shape, of length 10 to 150 µm but mostly within the range 20 to 80 µm.

Identification

A. Dissolve a suitable quantity in sufficient *phosphate buffer pH 7.4* to produce a solution containing 0.001% w/v of Sodium Cromoglicate. The *light absorption* of the resulting solution, Appendix II B, in the range 230 to 350 nm exhibits two maxima, at 238 nm and 326 nm.

B. To a quantity containing 0.1 g of Sodium Cromoglicate add 2 ml of *water* and 2 ml of 1.25M *sodium hydroxide* and boil for 1 minute; a yellow colour is produced. Add 0.5 ml of *diazobenzenesulphonic acid solution*; a blood-red colour is produced.

C. Yield reaction A characteristic of *sodium salts*, Appendix VI.

D. For capsules containing Lactose the contents when heated with *cupri-tartaric solution R1* produce a copious precipitate of copper(I) oxide.

Related substances Carry out the method for *thin-layer chromatography*, Appendix III A, using *silica gel GF_{254}* as the coating substance and a mixture of 5 volumes of *glacial acetic acid*, 50 volumes of *ethyl acetate* and 50 volumes of *toluene* as the mobile phase but allowing the solvent front to ascend 10 cm above the line of application. Apply separately to the plate 5 µl of each of the following solutions. For solution (1) dissolve a quantity containing 0.1 g of Sodium Cromoglicate in sufficient of a mixture of 1 volume of *acetone*, 4 volumes of *tetrahydrofuran* that has been freed from stabiliser by passage through a column of suitable alumina and 6 volumes of *water* to produce 5 ml and filter. For solution (2) dilute 1 volume of solution (1) to 200 volumes with the same solvent. After removal of the plate, allow it to dry in air and examine under *ultraviolet light (254 nm)*. Any *secondary spot* in the chromatogram obtained with solution (1) is not more intense than the spot in the chromatogram obtained with solution (2) (0.5%). The principal spot remains on the line of application.

Uniformity of weight Weigh one capsule. Open without loss of shell material, remove the contents and weigh all parts of the shell; the difference between the weights represents the weight of the contents. Repeat the operation with a further 19 capsules and calculate the average weight of the contents of the 20 capsules.

For preparations containing no Lactose the weight of the contents of each capsule does not deviate from the average by more than 25%. For preparations containing Lactose the weight of the contents of each capsule does not deviate from the average weight by more than 15% except that, for two capsules, the weight of the contents may deviate by not more than 25%.

Loss on drying When dried to constant weight at 100° at a pressure not exceeding 0.7 kPa, the contents of the capsules containing no Lactose lose 9.0 to 18.0% of their weight and the contents of capsules containing Lactose lose 5.5 to 10.0% of their weight.

Assay Dissolve a quantity of the mixed contents of 20 capsules containing 0.1 g of Sodium Cromoglicate in sufficient *phosphate buffer pH 7.4* to produce 1000 ml, dilute 25 ml to 100 ml with *phosphate buffer pH 7.4* and measure the *absorbance* of the resulting solution at the maximum at 326 nm, Appendix II B. Calculate the content of $C_{23}H_{14}Na_2O_{11}$ in a capsule of average content weight taking 164 as the value of A(1%, 1 cm) at the maximum at 326 nm.

Storage Sodium Cromoglicate Powder for Inhalation should be protected from moisture and stored at a temperature not exceeding 30°.

Labelling The label states (1) that each capsule contains 20 mg of Sodium Cromoglicate; (2) that the capsules are intended for use in an inhaler and are not to be swallowed; (3) where applicable, that the capsules contain Lactose.

When sodium cromoglycate powder for inhalation is prescribed or demanded, Sodium Cromoglicate Powder for Inhalation shall be dispensed or supplied.

Sodium Etacrynate Injection

Definition Sodium Etacrynate Injection is a sterile solution of sodium etacrynate in Water for Injections. It is prepared by dissolving Sodium Etacrynate for Injection in the requisite amount of the liquid stated on the label.

The injection complies with the requirements stated under Parenteral Preparations.

Storage Sodium Etacrynate Injection should be protected from light and used immediately after preparation but, in any case, within the period recommended by the manufacturer when prepared and stored strictly in accordance with the manufacturer's instructions.

SODIUM ETACRYNATE FOR INJECTION

Definition Sodium Etacrynate for Injection is a sterile material consisting of the sodium salt of Etacrynic Acid with or without excipients.

The contents of the sealed container comply with the requirements for Powders for Injections stated under Parenteral Preparations and with the following requirements.

Content of sodium etacrynate, calculated as etacrynic acid, $C_{13}H_{12}Cl_2O_4$ 90.0 to 105.0% of the prescribed or stated amount of Etacrynic Acid.

Identification Suspend a quantity containing the equivalent of 50 mg of Etacrynic Acid in 25 ml of 0.1M *hydrochloric acid* and extract with two 40-ml quantities of *dichloromethane*. Dry the combined extracts with *anhydrous sodium sulphate*, filter and evaporate to dryness using a rotary evaporator. The residue complies with the following tests.

A. The *infrared absorption spectrum*, Appendix II A, is concordant with the *reference spectrum* of etacrynic acid.

B. The *light absorption*, Appendix II B in the range 230 to 350 nm of a 0.005% w/v solution in 0.01M *methanolic hydrochloric acid* exhibits a maximum only at 270 nm and may exhibit a shoulder at 285 nm.

C. Dissolve a quantity containing the equivalent of 25 mg of Etacrynic Acid in 2 ml of 1M *sodium hydroxide* and heat on a water bath for 5 minutes. Cool, add 0.25 ml of a 50% v/v solution of *sulphuric acid*, 0.5 ml of a 10% w/v solution of *chromotropic acid sodium salt* and, carefully, 2 ml of *sulphuric acid*. An intense violet colour is produced.

Acidity or alkalinity pH of a solution containing the equivalent of 0.1% w/v of Etacrynic Acid, 6.3 to 7.7, Appendix V L.

Related substances Carry out the method for *liquid chromatography*, Appendix III D, using the following solutions. For solution (1) dissolve the contents of a sealed container in sufficient of a mixture of 32 volumes of 0.05M *hydrochloric acid* and 70 volumes of *acetonitrile* to produce a solution containing the equivalent of 0.5% w/v of Etacrynic Acid. For solution (2) dilute 1 volume of solution (1) to 40 volumes with a mixture of 7 volumes of *acetonitrile* and 3 volumes of *water*.

The chromatographic procedure may be carried out using (a) a stainless steel column (20 cm × 4 mm) packed with *stationary phase C* (10 μm) (Spherisorb ODS 1 is suitable), (b) a mixture of 57 volumes of *acetonitrile*, 43 volumes of *water* and 1 volume of *glacial acetic acid* as the mobile phase with a flow rate of 2 ml per minute and (c) a detection wavelength of 270 nm.

In the chromatogram obtained with solution (1) the sum of the areas of all the peaks appearing after the principal peak is not more than twice the area of the principal peak in the chromatogram obtained with solution (2).

Assay Determine the weight of the contents of 10 containers as described in the test for Uniformity of weight under Parenteral Preparations, Powders for Injections with the following modification. Instead of emptying the containers as completely as possible by gently tapping, dissolve the contents and use in the preparation of solutions (2) and (3) below.

Prepare a 0.15% w/v solution of *propyl 4-hydroxybenzoate* (internal standard) in *acetonitrile* (solution A). Carry out the method for *liquid chromatography*, Appendix III D, using the following solutions. For solution (1) dissolve 50 mg of *etacrynic acid BPCRS* in 5 ml of solution A and dilute to 50 ml with a mixture of 70 volumes of *acetonitrile* and 30 volumes of *water*. For solutions (2) and (3) add 3.2 ml of 0.05M *hydrochloric acid* to each of 10 containers and shake to dissolve. Combine the resulting solutions and wash each container with a mixture of 70 volumes of *acetonitrile* and 30 volumes of *water* and dilute the combined solutions and washings to 100 ml with the same solvent mixture (solution B). For solution (2) dilute 10 ml of solution B to 50 ml with the same solvent mixture. For solution (3) add 5 ml of solution A to 10 ml of solution B and dilute to 50 ml with the same solvent mixture.

The chromatographic procedure described under Related substances may be used but using as the mobile phase a mixture of 1 volume of *glacial acetic acid*, 40 volumes of *acetonitrile* and 60 volumes of *water*.

Calculate the content of $C_{13}H_{12}Cl_2O_4$ in a container of average content weight using the declared content of $C_{13}H_{12}Cl_2O_4$ in *etacrynic acid BPCRS*.

Storage The sealed container should be protected from light.

Labelling The label of the sealed container states the quantity of sodium etacrynate contained in it in terms of the equivalent amount of Etacrynic Acid.

When sodium ethacrynate injection or sodium ethacrynate for injection is prescribed or demanded, Sodium Etacrynate Injection or Sodium Etacrynate for Injection shall be dispensed or supplied.

Sodium Fusidate Ointment

Definition Sodium Fusidate Ointment contains Sodium Fusidate in a suitable basis.

The ointment complies with the requirements stated under Topical Semi-solid Preparations and with the following requirements.

Content of sodium fusidate, $C_{31}H_{47}NaO_6$ 92.5 to 107.5% of the prescribed or stated amount.

Identification

A. Disperse a quantity of the ointment containing 60 mg of Sodium Fusidate in 30 ml of n-*hexane* and shake with 6 ml of *water.* Allow to separate, remove the aqueous layer and add to it 5 ml of 0.2M *orthophosphoric acid.* Extract with two 10-ml quantities of *chloroform,* dry the combined chloroform extracts with *anhydrous sodium sulphate,* evaporate to dryness and dissolve the residue in 0.6 ml of *chloroform IR.* The *infrared absorption spectrum* of the resulting solution, Appendix II A, is concordant with the *reference spectrum* of fusidic acid.

B. In the Assay, the principal peak in the chromatogram obtained with solution (2) has the same retention time as the peak due to fusidic acid in the chromatogram obtained with solution (1).

Related substances Carry out the method for *liquid chromatography,* Appendix III D, using the following three solutions. For solution (1) add 25 ml of n-*hexane* to a quantity of the ointment containing 50 mg of Sodium Fusidate, stir, extract with 10 ml of *ethanol (70%)* and allow the layers to separate. Use the ethanol layer and filter if necessary. For solution (2) mix 1 ml of a 0.10% w/v solution of *3-ketofusidic acid EPCRS* in the mobile phase with 0.2 ml of solution (1) and dilute to 20 ml with the mobile phase. For solution (3) dilute 20 µl of solution (1) to 100 ml with the mobile phase.

The chromatographic procedure may be carried out using (a) a stainless steel column (12.5 to 15 cm × 4 to 5 mm) packed with *stationary phase C* (5 µm) (Lichrosphere 100 RP18 is suitable) (b) a mixture of 10 volumes of *methanol,* 20 volumes of a 1% w/v solution of *orthophosphoric acid,* 20 volumes of *water* and 50 volumes of *acetonitrile* as the mobile phase with a flow rate of 2 ml per minute and (c) a detection wavelength of 235 nm.

Inject separately 20 µl of each solution. Continue the chromatography for at least 3.5 times the retention time of the principal peak. The test is not valid unless the *resolution factor* between the peaks corresponding to 3-ketofusidic acid and sodium fusidate in the chromatogram obtained with solution (2) is at least 2.5 and unless the principal peak in the chromatogram obtained with solution (3) has a *signal-to-noise ratio* of at least 3.

In the chromatogram obtained with solution (1) the sum of the areas of any *secondary peaks* is not greater than 4 times the area of the peak corresponding to sodium fusidate in the chromatogram obtained with solution (2) (4%). Disregard any peak with an area less than that of the principal peak in the chromatogram obtained with solution (3) (0.02%).

Assay Carry out the method for *liquid chromatography,* Appendix III D, using the following solutions. Solution (1) contains 0.07% w/v of *diethanolamine fusidate BPCRS* in the mobile phase. For solution (2) add 10 ml of n-*hexane* and 25 ml of the mobile phase to a quantity of the ointment containing 30 mg of Sodium Fusidate, shake vigorously for 15 minutes and allow the layers to separate. Remove all of the lower layer, dilute to 50 ml with the mobile phase and filter through glass-fibre paper (Whatman GF/C is suitable).

The chromatographic procedure may be carried out using (a) a stainless steel column (20 cm × 4.6 mm) packed with *stationary phase C* (5 µm) (LiChrosorb RP-18 is suitable), (b) a mixture of 60 volumes of *acetonitrile,* 30 volumes of a 1% v/v solution of *glacial acetic acid* and 10 volumes of *methanol* as the mobile phase with a flow rate of 1.5 ml per minute and (c) a detection wavelength of 235 nm.

The *column efficiency,* determined using the principal peak in the chromatogram obtained with solution (1), should be not less than 14,000 theoretical plates per metre.

Calculate the content of $C_{31}H_{47}NaO_6$ from the declared equivalent content of $C_{31}H_{47}NaO_6$ in *diethanolamine fusidate BPCRS.*

Strong Sodium Hypochlorite Solution

Definition Strong Sodium Hypochlorite Solution is an aqueous solution of sodium hypochlorite containing not less than 8% of available chlorine. It may contain suitable stabilising agents.

Content of available chlorine, Cl Not less than 8.0% w/w.

Total alkalinity Not more than 1.8% w/w, calculated as NaOH, when determined by the following method. To 25 ml add 50 ml of *water* and 35 ml of *hydrogen peroxide solution (20 vol)* and titrate with 0.5M *hydrochloric acid VS* using *methyl orange solution* as indicator. Each ml of 0.5M *hydrochloric acid VS* is equivalent to 20 mg of NaOH. Determine the *weight per ml* of the solution, Appendix V G, and calculate the total alkalinity as a percentage weight in weight.

Assay Dilute 10 ml to 250 ml with *water.* To 10 ml of the resulting solution add 50 ml of 0.05M *sodium arsenite VS* and then 5 g of *sodium hydrogen carbonate,* swirl to dissolve and titrate the excess of sodium arsenite with 0.05M *iodine VS* using *starch mucilage* as indicator. Each ml of 0.05M *sodium arsenite VS* is equivalent to 3.545 mg of Cl. Determine the *weight per ml* of the solution, Appendix V G, and calculate the percentage w/w of available chlorine.

Storage Strong Sodium Hypochlorite Solution should be kept in a well-filled, well-closed container fitted with a glass stopper or a suitable plastic cap and protected from light. It should be stored at a temperature not exceeding 20° and away from acids.

Labelling The label states (1) that the solution must be diluted before use; (2) the date after which it is not intended to be used; (3) the conditions under which it should be stored.

Dilute Sodium Hypochlorite Solution

Definition Dilute Sodium Hypochlorite Solution is an aqueous *cutaneous solution* of sodium hypochlorite containing 1% of available chlorine. It may contain suitable stabilising agents and Sodium Chloride.

The solution complies with the requirements stated under Liquids for Cutaneous Application and with the following requirements.

Content of available chlorine, Cl 0.90 to 1.10% w/w.

Assay To 10 ml add 50 ml of 0.05M *sodium arsenite VS* and then 5 g of *sodium hydrogen carbonate*, swirl to dissolve and titrate the excess of sodium arsenite with 0.05M *iodine VS* using *starch mucilage* as indicator. Each ml of 0.05M *sodium arsenite VS* is equivalent to 3.545 mg of Cl. Determine the *weight per ml* of the solution, Appendix V G, and calculate the percentage w/w of available chlorine.

Storage Dilute Sodium Hypochlorite Solution should be kept in a well-filled, well-closed container and protected from light. It should be stored at a temperature not exceeding 20° and away from acids.

Labelling The label states (1) the date after which the solution is not intended to be used; (2) the conditions under which it should be stored.

The label indicates the pharmaceutical form as 'cutaneous solution'.

Sodium Iodide Injection

Definition Sodium Iodide Injection is a sterile solution of Sodium Iodide in Water for Injections. It contains not more than 0.1% w/v of Sodium Thiosulphate or other suitable reducing agent.

The injection complies with the requirements stated under Parenteral Preparations and with the following requirements.

Content of sodium iodide, NaI 95.0 to 105.0% of the prescribed or stated amount.

Characteristics A clear, colourless solution.

Identification

A. Yields the reactions characteristic of *sodium salts*, Appendix VI.

B. Yields the reactions characteristic of *iodides*, Appendix VI.

Assay Dilute a volume containing 0.3 g of Sodium Iodide to 10 ml with *water*, and add 10 ml of a mixture of 0.05 ml of a 1% w/v solution of *iodine* in *ethanol (96%)* and 100 ml of *iodide-free starch solution*. Titrate with 0.1M *silver nitrate VS* until only a pale yellow colour remains. Each ml of 0.1M *silver nitrate VS* is equivalent to 14.99 mg of NaI.

Storage Sodium Iodide Injection should be kept free from contact with metals.

Sodium Iotalamate Injection

Definition Sodium Iotalamate Injection is a sterile solution of the sodium salt of Iotalamic Acid in Water for Injections.

The injection complies with the requirements stated under Parenteral Preparations and with the following requirements.

Content of sodium iotalamate, $C_{11}H_8I_3N_2NaO_4$ 97.0 to 103.0% of the prescribed or stated amount.

Characteristics An almost colourless to pale yellow liquid.

Identification

A. To a volume containing 1 g of sodium iotalamate add 100 ml of *water* and a slight excess of 2M *hydrochloric acid*, wash the residue with *water* and dry at 105°. The *infrared absorption spectrum* of the residue, Appendix II A, is concordant with the *reference spectrum* of iotalamic acid.

B. Ignite 0.5 g of the residue obtained by evaporating the injection to dryness. The residue yields the reactions characteristic of *sodium salts*, Appendix VI.

Acidity or alkalinity pH, 6.5 to 7.5, Appendix V L. Using separate glass and calomel electrodes, take the first measurement 3 minutes after inserting the electrodes and repeat every 30 seconds until constant.

Halide Mix a quantity of the injection containing 0.55 g of sodium iotalamate with 4 ml of 2M *sodium hydroxide* and 5 ml of *water*, mix, add 6 ml of 2M *nitric acid*, shake, dilute to 25 ml with *water* and filter. 15 ml of the filtrate complies with the *limit test for chlorides*, Appendix VII (150 ppm, expressed as chloride).

Related substances Carry out the method for *thin-layer chromatography*, Appendix III A, using *silica gel GF_{254}* as the coating substance and a mixture of 1 volume of *glacial acetic acid*, 1 volume of *anhydrous formic acid*, 1 volume of *methanol*, 5 volumes of *ether* and 10 volumes of *dichloromethane* as the mobile phase but allowing the solvent front to ascend 10 cm above the line of application. Apply separately to the plate 5 µl of each of the following solutions. For solution (1) dilute the injection being examined with *methanol* containing 3% v/v of 10M *ammonia* to contain 10% w/v of sodium iotalamate. For solution (2) dilute 1 volume of solution (1) to 50 volumes with *methanol* and dilute 1 volume of this solution to 10 volumes with *methanol*. Solution (3) contains 0.05% w/v of *5-amino-2,4,6-tri-iodo-*N*-methylisophthalamic acid EPCRS* in *methanol* containing 3% v/v of 10M *ammonia*. For solution (4) dissolve 1 mg of *5-amino-2,4,6-tri-iodo-*N*-methylisophthalamic acid EPCRS* in 5 ml of solution (2). After removal of the plate, allow it to dry until the solvents have evaporated and examine under *ultraviolet light (254 nm)*. Any spot in the chromatogram obtained with solution (1) corresponding to 5-amino-2,4,6-tri-iodo-*N*-methylisophthalamic acid is not more intense than the spot in the chromatogram obtained with solution (3) (0.5%) and any other *secondary spot* is not more intense than the spot in the chromatogram obtained with solution (2) (0.2%). The test is not valid unless the chromatogram obtained with solution (3) shows two clearly separated spots.

Pyrogens Complies with the *test for pyrogens*, Appendix XIV D. Use per kg of the rabbit's weight a quantity containing 2.5 g of sodium iotalamate.

Assay Mix a quantity containing 0.5 g of sodium iotalamate with 12 ml of 5M *sodium hydroxide* and 20 ml of *water*, add 1 g of *zinc powder* and boil under a reflux condenser for 30 minutes. Cool, rinse the condenser with 30 ml of *water*, filter through absorbent cotton and wash the flask and filter with two 20-ml quantities of *water*. To the combined filtrate and washings add 80 ml of *hydrochloric acid*, cool and titrate with 0.05M *potassium iodate VS* until the dark brown solution becomes light brown. Add 5 ml of *chloroform* and continue the titration, shaking well after each addition, until the chloroform becomes colourless. Each ml of 0.05M *potassium iodate VS* is equivalent to 21.20 mg of $C_{11}H_8I_3N_2NaO_4$. Determine the *weight per ml* of the injection, Appendix V G, and calculate the percentage content of $C_{11}H_8I_3N_2NaO_4$, weight in volume.

Storage Sodium Iotalamate Injection should be protected from light.

Labelling The strength is stated as the percentage w/v of sodium iotalamate.

Action and use Contrast medium used in urography.

When sodium iothalamate injection is prescribed or demanded, Sodium Iotalamate Injection shall be dispensed or supplied.

Sodium Lactate Intravenous Infusion

Sodium Lactate Injection

Definition Sodium Lactate Intravenous Infusion is a sterile solution containing 1.85% w/v of sodium lactate in Water for Injections. It may be prepared from Sodium Lactate Solution or from Lactic Acid.

The intravenous infusion complies with the requirements stated under Parenteral Preparations and with the following requirements.

Content of sodium lactate, $C_3H_5NaO_3$ 1.75 to 1.95% w/v.

Characteristics A colourless solution.

Identification

A. When warmed with *potassium permanganate*, yields acetaldehyde, recognisable by its odour.

B. The residue on evaporation, when moistened with *hydrochloric acid* and introduced on a platinum wire into a flame, imparts a yellow colour to the flame.

C. Carry out reaction C characteristic of *calcium salts*, Appendix VI. No white precipitate is produced.

Acidity or alkalinity pH, 5.0 to 7.0, Appendix V L.

Particulate contamination When supplied in a container with a nominal content of 100 ml or more, complies with the test for *sub-visible particles*, Appendix XIII A.

Bacterial endotoxins The endotoxin limit concentration is 0.25 IU per ml, Appendix XIV C.

Assay Carry out the method for *liquid chromatography*, Appendix III D, using the following solutions. Solution (1) contains 0.30% w/v of *lithium lactate BPCRS* in the mobile phase. For solution (2) dilute 1 volume of the infusion to 5 volumes with the mobile phase.

The chromatographic procedure may be carried out using (a) a stainless steel column (20 cm × 4.6 mm) packed with *stationary phase C* (10 µm) (Nucleosil C18 is suitable), (b) as the mobile phase with a flow rate of 2 ml per minute a mixture of 90 volumes of *water* and 10 volumes of a 2% v/v solution of *octylamine* in *acetonitrile*, the pH of the final mixture being adjusted to 7.0 with a 10% v/v solution of *orthophosphoric acid*, and (c) a detection wavelength of 210 nm.

Calculate the content of $C_3H_5NaO_3$ in the infusion using the declared equivalent content of $C_3H_5NaO_3$ in *lithium lactate BPCRS*.

Storage Sodium Lactate Intravenous Infusion should be stored at a temperature not exceeding 25°.

Labelling The label states (1) that solutions containing visible solid particles should not be used; (2) that the Intravenous Infusion is one-sixth molar and contains, in one litre, approximately 167 millimoles of sodium ions and of bicarbonate ions (as lactate).

Compound Sodium Lactate Intravenous Infusion

Compound Sodium Lactate Injection; Hartmann's Solution for Injection; Ringer-Lactate Solution for Injection

Definition Compound Sodium Lactate Intravenous Infusion is a sterile solution containing 0.32% w/v of sodium lactate with 0.6% w/v of Sodium Chloride, 0.04% w/v of Potassium Chloride and 0.027% w/v of Calcium Chloride in Water for Injections. It may be prepared from Sodium Lactate Solution or from Lactic Acid.

The intravenous infusion complies with the requirements stated under Parenteral Preparations and with the following requirements.

Content of sodium, Na 0.27 to 0.32% w/v.

Content of potassium, K 0.019 to 0.022% w/v.

Content of total chloride, Cl 0.37 to 0.42% w/v.

Content of calcium chloride, $CaCl_2,2H_2O$ 0.025 to 0.029% w/v.

Content of lactate, calculated as $C_3H_6O_3$ 0.23 to 0.28% w/v.

Characteristics A colourless solution.

Identification

A. When warmed with *potassium permanganate*, yields acetaldehyde, recognisable by its odour.

B. The residue obtained by evaporation, when moistened with *hydrochloric acid* and introduced on a platinum wire into a flame, imparts a yellow colour to the flame. When viewed through a suitable blue glass, the flame is tinged with reddish purple.

C. Yields reaction C characteristic of *calcium salts*, Appendix VI.

Acidity or alkalinity pH, 5.0 to 7.0, Appendix V L.

Particulate contamination When supplied in a container with a nominal content of 100 ml or more, complies with the test for *sub-visible particles*, Appendix XIII A.

Bacterial endotoxins The endotoxin limit concentration is 0.25 IU per ml, Appendix XIV C.

Assay ***For Na*** Prepare a suitable dilution in *water* and determine by *atomic emission spectrophotometry*, Appendix II D, measuring at 589 nm and using *sodium standard solution (200 ppm Na)*, suitably diluted with *water*, for the standard solutions.

For K Prepare a suitable dilution in *water* and determine by *atomic emission spectrophotometry*, Appendix II D, measuring at 767 nm and using *potassium standard solution (600 ppm K)*, suitably diluted with *water*, for the standard solutions.

For total chloride To 20 ml add 30 ml of *water*, 50 ml of 0.1M *silver nitrate VS* and 2 ml of *nitric acid*, filter, wash the precipitate with *water* slightly acidified with *nitric acid* and titrate the excess of silver nitrate with 0.1M *ammonium thiocyanate VS* using *ammonium iron(III) sulphate solution R2* as indicator. Each ml of 0.1M *silver nitrate VS* is equivalent to 3.545 mg of total Cl.

For calcium chloride To 50 ml add 5 ml of 0.01M *magnesium sulphate VS* and 5 ml of *ammonia buffer pH 10.9* and titrate with 0.01M *disodium edetate VS* using *mordant black 11 triturate* as indicator. From the volume of 0.01M *disodium edetate VS* required subtract the volume of 0.01M *magnesium sulphate VS* added. Each ml of the remainder is equivalent to 1.470 mg of $CaCl_2,2H_2O$.

For lactate, calculated as $C_3H_6O_3$ Carry out the method for *liquid chromatography*, Appendix III D, using the following solutions. Solution (1) contains 0.28% w/v of *lithium lactate BPCRS* in the mobile phase. For solution (2) use the infusion.

The chromatographic procedure may be carried out using (a) a stainless steel column (20 cm × 4.6 mm) packed with *stationary phase C* (Nucleosil C18 is suitable), (b) as the mobile phase with a flow rate of 2 ml per minute a mixture of 90 volumes of *water* and 10 volumes of a 2% v/v solution of *octylamine* in *acetonitrile*, the pH of the final mixture being adjusted to 7.0 with a 10% v/v solution of *orthophosphoric acid*, and (c) a detection wavelength of 210 nm.

Calculate the content of lactate as $C_3H_6O_3$ in the infusion using the declared equivalent content of $C_3H_6O_3$ in *lithium lactate BPCRS*.

Storage Compound Sodium Lactate Intravenous Infusion should be stored at a temperature not exceeding 25°.

Labelling The label states (1) that solutions containing visible solid particles must not be used; (2) that the Intravenous Infusion contains, in millimoles per litre, the following approximate amounts of the ions present: sodium, 131; potassium, 5; calcium, 2; bicarbonate (as lactate), 29 and chloride, 111.

Sodium Nitroprusside Intravenous Infusion

Definition Sodium Nitroprusside Intravenous Infusion is a sterile solution of sodium nitroprusside in Glucose Intravenous Infusion containing 50 g of anhydrous glucose per litre. It is prepared immediately before use by dissolving Sodium Nitroprusside for Injection in the requisite amount of Glucose Intravenous Infusion (50 g per litre) and diluting the resulting solution with 250 to 500 times its volume of Glucose Intravenous Infusion (50 g per litre).

The intravenous infusion complies with the requirements stated under Parenteral Preparations.

Storage Sodium Nitroprusside Intravenous Infusion should be used immediately after preparation.

SODIUM NITROPRUSSIDE FOR INJECTION

Definition Sodium Nitroprusside for Injection is a sterile material obtained from a solution of Sodium Nitroprusside by freeze drying. It is supplied in a sealed container and may contain excipients.

The contents of the sealed container comply with the requirements for Powders for Injections stated under Parenteral Preparations and with the following requirements.

Content of sodium nitroprusside The equivalent of 90.0 to 110.0% of the stated amount of sodium nitroprusside dihydrate, $Na_2Fe(CN)_5NO,2H_2O$.

Identification

A. The *light absorption*, Appendix II B, in the range 350 to 600 nm of a 1.6% w/v solution exhibits a maximum only at 395 nm. The *absorbance* at 395 nm is about 1.1.

B. Dissolve 20 mg in 2 ml of *water* and add 0.1 ml of *sodium sulphide solution*. A deep purple colour is produced.

C. Yields the reactions characteristic of *sodium salts*, Appendix VI.

Uniformity of content Sealed containers containing the equivalent of 50 mg or less of sodium nitroprusside dihydrate comply with the requirements stated under Parenteral Preparations, Powders for Injections. Use the individual results obtained in the Assay.

Assay Carry out the method for *liquid chromatography*, Appendix III D, protected from light, using the following solutions. Solution (1) contains 0.15% w/v of *sodium nitroprusside BPCRS* in *water*. For solution (2) dissolve the contents of a sealed container in 5 ml of *water* and dilute the resulting solution with *water* to produce a solution containing the equivalent of 0.15% w/v of sodium nitroprusside dihydrate. Solution (3) contains 0.015% w/v of *sodium nitroprusside BPCRS* and 0.015% w/v of *potassium hexacyanoferrate(III)* in *water*.

The chromatographic procedure may be carried out using (a) a stainless steel column (30 cm × 3.9 mm) packed with particles of silica 10 μm in diameter the surface of which has been modified with chemically-bonded phenyl groups (μBondapak phenyl is suitable), (b) as the mobile phase with a flow rate of 1.2 ml per minute a mixture of 9 volumes of a solution containing 0.34% w/v of *tetrabutylammonium hydrogen sulphate* and 0.284% w/v of *anhydrous disodium hydrogen orthophosphate* adjusted to pH 6.0 with *orthophosphoric acid* and 6 volumes of *methanol* and (c) a detection wavelength of 254 nm.

Calculate the content of $Na_2Fe(CN)_5NO,2H_2O$ in the sealed container using the declared content of $Na_2Fe(CN)_5NO,2H_2O$ in *sodium nitroprusside BPCRS*. The Assay is not valid unless, in the chromatogram obtained with solution (3), the *resolution factor* between the peaks corresponding to ferricyanide and nitroprusside is at least 3.0.

Repeat the procedure with a further nine sealed containers and calculate the average content of $Na_2Fe(CN)_5NO,2H_2O$ from the individual results thus obtained.

Labelling The label states (1) the content of sodium nitroprusside in terms of the equivalent of sodium nitroprusside dihydrate contained in it; (2) that the contents of the sealed container should be dissolved in, and immediately diluted with, the stated volume of Glucose Intravenous Infusion (50 g per litre); (3) that Sodium Nitroprusside Intravenous Infusion must be used immediately after preparation; (4) that highly coloured solutions must not be used; (5) that the diluted solution must be protected from light during infusion.

Sodium Picosulfate Oral Powder

Definition Sodium Picosulfate Oral Powder contains Sodium Picosulfate, Light Magnesium Oxide and Anhydrous Citric Acid.

The oral powder complies with the requirements stated under Powders and with the following requirements.

Content of sodium picosulfate, $C_{18}H_{13}NNa_2O_8S_2$ 90.0 to 110.0% of the prescribed or stated amount.

Content of light magnesium oxide, MgO 90.0 to 110.0% of the stated amount.

Content of anhydrous citric acid, $C_6H_8O_7$ 90.0 to 110.0% of the stated amount.

Identification

A. In the test for Uniformity of content, the chromatogram obtained with solution (1) shows a peak with the same retention time as the peak in the chromatogram obtained with solution (2).

B. Dissolve the contents of one sachet in *water*; the solution becomes hot.

C. Add 100 ml of *water* to the contents of one sachet and allow to cool. Centrifuge and dilute 10 ml of the supernatant liquid to 100 ml with *water*. 5 ml of the resulting solution yields reaction A characteristic of *citrates*, Appendix VI.

D. Place about 1 g of the oral powder in a silica crucible, moisten with *sulphuric acid*, ignite gently, again moisten with *sulphuric acid* and ignite at 800° until a carbon-free residue is obtained. Disperse about 0.1 g of the residue obtained in 10 ml of *water*, adjust the pH to about 3 with 2M *sulphuric acid*, shake and filter. The filtrate yields the reactions characteristic of *magnesium salts*, Appendix VI.

Uniformity of content Complies with the requirements stated under Powders with respect to the content of Sodium Picosulfate using the following method of analysis. Carry out the method for *liquid chromatography*, Appendix III D, using the following solutions. For solution (1) dissolve the contents of one sachet in about 70 ml of *water*, allow to stand until effervescence has ceased, cool to room temperature, add sufficient *water* to produce 100 ml, mix and centrifuge; use the clear supernatant liquid. Solution (2) contains 0.01% w/v of *sodium picosulfate BPCRS* in *water*.

The chromatographic procedure may be carried out using (a) a stainless steel column (10 cm × 4.6 mm) packed with *stationary phase C* (5 μm) (Nucleosil C18 is suitable), (b) a guard column (4.5 mm × 2.5 cm) packed with *stationary phase C*, (c) as the mobile phase with a flow rate of 1.5 ml per minute a mixture of 15 volumes of *acetonitrile* and 85 volumes of *0.067M mixed phosphate buffer pH 7.0* and (d) a detection wavelength of 263 nm.

Calculate the content of $C_{18}H_{13}NNa_2O_8S_2$ using the declared content of $C_{18}H_{13}NNa_2O_8S_2$ in *sodium picosulfate BPCRS*.

Assay *For sodium picosulfate* Use the average of the 10 individual results obtained in the test for Uniformity of content.

For light magnesium oxide To a quantity of the powder containing 30 mg of Light Magnesium Oxide add 4 ml of 3M *hydrochloric acid*, dissolve by warming on a water bath, cool and add 50 ml of *water*. Carry out the *complexometric titration of magnesium*, Appendix VIII D, beginning at the words 'To the resulting solution ... ', but using 0.05M *disodium edetate VS* as titrant. Each ml of 0.05M *disodium edetate VS* is equivalent to 2.015 mg of MgO.

For anhydrous citric acid Dissolve a quantity of the powder containing 0.1 g of anhydrous citric acid in 60 ml of *dimethylformamide* and carry out Method II for *non-aqueous titration*, Appendix VIII A, using 0.1M *tetrabutylammonium hydroxide VS* as titrant, determining the end point potentiometrically and taking the second inflection as the end point. Each ml of 0.1M *tetrabutylammonium hydroxide VS* is equivalent to 96.05 mg of $C_6H_8O_7$. The 0.1M *tetrabutylammonium hydroxide VS* is standardised before use by titrating with it 0.1 g, accurately weighed, of *citric acid* previously dried at 105° and dissolved in 60 ml of *dimethylformamide*. During the titration care is taken to exclude carbon dioxide.

Labelling The label states (1) the total weights, in grams, of the constituents in each sachet; (2) that heat is evolved when the contents of the sachet are added to water.

When sodium picosulphate oral powder is prescribed or demanded, Sodium Picosulfate Oral Powder shall be dispensed or supplied.

Sodium Stibogluconate Injection

Definition Sodium Stibogluconate Injection is a sterile solution of Sodium Stibogluconate in Water for Injections.

The injection complies with the requirements stated under Parenteral Preparations and with the following requirements.

Content of pentavalent antimony, Sb(V) 9.5 to 10.5% w/v.

Characteristics A colourless or faintly straw-coloured solution.

Identification

A. It is dextrorotatory.

B. Dilute 2 ml to 10 ml with *water* and pass *hydrogen sulphide* through the solution; no immediate precipitate is produced. Continue to pass *hydrogen sulphide* through the solution for several minutes; an orange precipitate is produced.

C. The residue after evaporation to dryness and incineration yields the reactions characteristic of *antimony compounds* and the reactions characteristic of *sodium salts*, Appendix VI.

Acidity pH, 5.0 to 5.6, Appendix V L.

Assay To 0.5 ml add 30 ml of *hydrochloric acid*, mix, add

70 ml of *orthophosphoric acid* and stir carefully until completely mixed. Titrate with 0.05M *ammonium iron(II) sulphate VS* prepared with *water* containing, in each litre, 20 ml of *sulphuric acid (50%)*, determining the end point potentiometrically using a platinum electrode and a silver—silver chloride reference electrode. Each ml of 0.05M *ammonium iron(II) sulphate VS* is equivalent to 3.044 mg of Sb(V).

Storage Sodium Stibogluconate Injection should be protected from light.

Labelling The strength is stated in terms of the equivalent amount of pentavalent antimony per ml.

Sodium Stibogluconate Injection contains, in 6 ml, the equivalent of 600 mg of pentavalent antimony or 2 g of Sodium Stibogluconate.

Sodium Tetradecyl Sulphate Injection

Definition Sodium Tetradecyl Sulphate Injection is a sterile solution of Sodium Tetradecyl Sulphate Concentrate in Water for Injections.

The injection complies with the requirements stated under Parenteral Preparations and with the following requirements.

Content of sodium tetradecyl sulphate, $C_{14}H_{29}NaO_4S$ 95.0 to 105.0% of the prescribed or stated amount.

Identification

A. Complies with test A for Identification described under Sodium Tetradecyl Sulphate Concentrate using a volume of the injection containing 0.1 g of sodium tetradecyl sulphate to prepare solution (1). A peak due to benzyl alcohol with a retention time less than that of the peak due to decan-1-ol may also be seen.

B. Mix 0.1 ml with 0.1 ml of a 0.1% w/v solution of *methylene blue* and 2 ml of 1M *sulphuric acid*, add 2 ml of *chloroform* and shake. The chloroform layer is intensely blue.

C. Dilute 0.5 ml with 10 ml of *ethanol (96%)* and heat to boiling on a water bath, shaking frequently. Filter immediately and evaporate the ethanol. Dissolve the residue in 8 ml of *water*, add 3 ml of 2M *hydrochloric acid*, evaporate the solution to half its volume and cool. Filter to remove the congealed fatty alcohols and add 1 ml of 0.25M *barium chloride* to the filtrate. A white crystalline precipitate is produced.

Alkalinity pH, 7.5 to 7.9, Appendix V L.

Assay Dilute a volume containing 0.12 g of sodium tetradecyl sulphate to 100 ml with *water*. To 20 ml add 15 ml of *chloroform* and 10 ml of *dimidium bromide—sulphan blue mixed solution* and titrate with *0.004M benzethonium bromide VS*, shaking vigorously and allowing the layers to separate after each addition, until the pink colour of the chloroform layer is completely discharged and a greyish blue colour is produced. Each ml of *0.004M benzethonium chloride VS* is equivalent to 1.266 mg of $C_{14}H_{29}NaO_4S$.

Storage Sodium Tetradecyl Sulphate Injection should be protected from light and stored at a temperature not exceeding 25°.

Labelling The label states (1) that the injection is for the treatment of varicose veins only; (2) the strength as the amount of sodium tetradecyl sulphate in a suitable dose-volume.

Sodium Thiosulphate Injection

Definition Sodium Thiosulphate Injection is a sterile solution of Sodium Thiosulphate in Water for Injections.

The injection complies with the requirements stated under Parenteral Preparations and with the following requirements.

Content of sodium thiosulphate, $Na_2S_2O_3,5H_2O$ 95.0 to 105.0% of the prescribed or stated amount.

Characteristics A clear, colourless solution.

Identification

A. Yields the reactions characteristic of *sodium salts*, Appendix VI.

B. To 5 ml add *iodine solution* dropwise. The reagent is decolorised and the mixture does not yield the reactions characteristic of *sulphates*, Appendix VI.

C. To 5 ml add 1 ml of *hydrochloric acid*. A white precipitate which quickly changes to yellow is formed, and a gas is evolved which turns *starch iodate paper* blue.

Acidity or alkalinity pH, 7.0 to 9.0, Appendix V L.

Assay Dilute a volume containing 0.5 g of Sodium Thiosulphate to about 20 ml with *water* and titrate with 0.05M *iodine VS* using 1 ml of *starch solution*, added towards the end of the titration, as indicator. Each ml of 0.05M *iodine VS* is equivalent to 24.82 mg of $Na_2S_2O_3$, $5H_2O$.

Sodium Valproate Oral Solution

Definition Sodium Valproate Oral Solution is a solution of Sodium Valproate in a suitable flavoured vehicle.

The oral solution complies with the requirements stated under Oral Liquids and with the following requirements.

Content of sodium valproate, $C_8H_{15}NaO_2$ 95.0 to 105.0% of the prescribed or stated amount.

Identification

A. Shake a quantity of the oral solution containing 0.25 g of Sodium Valproate with two 25-ml quantities of *chloroform* and discard the chloroform extracts. Add 10 ml of a saturated solution of *sodium chloride* and 10 ml of 2M *hydrochloric acid*, mix and shake with 25 ml of *chloroform*. Wash the chloroform layer with 5 ml of *water*, shake with *anhydrous sodium sulphate*, filter and evaporate to dryness. The *infrared absorption spectrum* of a thin film of the residue, Appendix II A, is concordant with the *reference spectrum* of valproic acid.

B. In the Assay, the chromatogram obtained with solution (2) exhibits a peak with the same retention time as the peak due to sodium valproate in the chromatogram obtained with solution (1).

Related substances Carry out the method for *gas chromatography*, Appendix III B, using the following solutions. Solution (1) contains 0.020% w/v of *octanoic acid* (internal standard) in *dichloromethane*. For solution (2) shake a quantity of the oral solution containing 0.50 g of Sodium Valproate with 10 ml of *water*, acidify with 2M *sulphuric* *acid* and shake with three 20-ml quantities of *dichloromethane*. Wash the combined dichloromethane extracts with 10 ml of *water*, shake with *anhydrous sodium sulphate*, filter and evaporate the filtrate to a volume of about 10 ml at a temperature not exceeding 30° using a rotary evaporator. For solution (3) shake a quantity of the oral solution containing 0.50 g of Sodium Valproate with 10 ml of a 0.020% w/v solution of the internal standard in 0.1M *sodium hydroxide* and continue as described for solution (2), beginning at the words 'acidify with 2M *sulphuric acid* ...'.

The chromatographic procedure may be carried out using a glass column (1.5 m × 4 mm) packed with *acid-washed, silanised diatomaceous support* (80 to 100 mesh) coated with 15% w/w of free fatty acid phase (Supelco FFAP 2-1063 is suitable) and 1% w/w of *orthophosphoric acid* and maintained at 170°.

In the chromatogram obtained with solution (3) the sum of the areas of any *secondary peaks* is not greater than the area of the peak due to the internal standard.

Assay Carry out the method for *liquid chromatography*, Appendix III D, using the following freshly prepared solutions. For solution (1) dissolve 0.16 g of *sodium valproate BPCRS* in 15 ml of the mobile phase, add 1 ml of a 10% v/v solution of *orthophosphoric acid*, mix and dilute to 50 ml with the mobile phase. For solution (2) add 1 ml of a 10% v/v solution of *orthophosphoric acid* to a weighed quantity of the oral solution containing 0.16 g of Sodium Valproate and dilute to 50 ml with the mobile phase. Solution (3) contains 0.002% w/v of *propyl* p-*hydroxybenzoate* in solution (1).

The chromatographic procedure may be carried out using (a) a stainless steel column (20 cm × 4.6 mm) packed with *stationary phase C* (10 μm) (Spherisorb ODS 1 is suitable), (b) as the mobile phase with a flow rate of 1 ml per minute a mixture of 65 volumes of *methanol* and 35 volumes of 0.05M *potassium dihydrogen orthophosphate*, the pH of the final mixture being adjusted to 5.0 with a 10% v/v solution of *orthophosphoric acid*, and (c) a detection wavelength of 210 nm.

The method is not valid unless the *resolution factor* between the two peaks in the chromatogram obtained with solution (3) is at least 2.0.

Determine the *weight per ml* of the oral solution, Appendix V G, and calculate the content of $C_8H_{15}NaO_2$, weight in volume, from the declared content of $C_8H_{15}NaO_2$ in *sodium valproate BPCRS*.

Sodium Valproate Tablets

Definition Sodium Valproate Tablets contain Sodium Valproate.

The tablets comply with the requirements stated under Tablets and with the following requirements.

Content of sodium valproate, $C_8H_{15}NaO_2$ 95.0 to 105.0% of the prescribed or stated amount.

Identification

A. Shake a quantity of the powdered tablets containing 0.5 g of Sodium Valproate with 10 ml of *water* and centrifuge. Acidify 5 ml of the supernatant liquid with 2M *sulphuric acid*, shake with 25 ml of *chloroform* and wash the chloroform layer with 5 ml of *water*. Dry by shaking with *anhydrous sodium sulphate*, filter and evaporate the chloroform. The *infrared absorption spectrum* of a thin film of the residue, Appendix II A, is concordant with the *reference spectrum* of valproic acid.

B. Shake a quantity of the powdered tablets containing 0.25 g of Sodium Valproate with 3 ml of *water* and centrifuge. To 2 ml of the supernatant liquid add 0.5 ml of a 10% w/v solution of *cobalt(II) nitrate*. A purple precipitate is produced which is soluble in *dichloromethane*.

Dissolution Comply with the *dissolution test for tablets and capsules*, Appendix XII D, using Apparatus II. Use as the medium 900 ml of *phosphate buffer pH 6.8* and rotate the paddle at 50 revolutions per minute. Withdraw a sample of 20 ml of the medium and filter. Carry out the method for *liquid chromatography*, Appendix III D, using the following solutions. For solution (1) use the filtrate from the dissolution vessel diluted, if necessary, to give a solution expected to contain 0.002% w/v of sodium valproate. Solution (2) contains 0.002% w/v of *sodium valproate BPCRS* in *phosphate buffer pH 6.8*.

The chromatographic procedure may be carried out using (a) a stainless steel column (25 cm × 4.6 mm) packed with *stationary phase C* (5 μm) (μBondapak C18 is suitable), (b) a mixture of 45 volumes of a 0.32% w/v solution of *potassium dihydrogen orthophosphate* adjusted to pH 3.0 with *orthophosphoric acid* and 55 volumes of *acetonitrile* as the mobile phase with a flow rate of 2 ml per minute and (c) a detection wavelength of 220 nm.

Inject 50 μl of each solution. Calculate the content of sodium valproate, $C_8H_{15}NaO_2$, in the medium from the chromatogram obtained and using the declared content of $C_8H_{15}NaO_2$ in *sodium valproate BPCRS*.

Related substances Carry out the method for *gas chromatography*, Appendix III B, using the following solutions. Solution (1) contains 0.020% w/v of *octanoic acid* (internal standard) in *dichloromethane*. For solution (2) shake a quantity of the powdered tablets containing 0.50 g of Sodium Valproate with 10 ml of *water*, acidify with 2M *sulphuric acid* and shake with three 20-ml quantities of *dichloromethane*. Wash the combined dichloromethane extracts with 10 ml of *water*, shake with *anhydrous sodium sulphate*, filter and evaporate the filtrate to a volume of about 10 ml at a temperature not exceeding 30° using a rotary evaporator. For solution (3) shake a quantity of the powdered tablets containing 0.50 g of Sodium Valproate with 10 ml of a 0.020% w/v solution of the internal standard in 0.1M *sodium hydroxide* and continue as described for solution (2), beginning at the words 'acidify with 2M *sulphuric acid* ...'.

The chromatographic procedure may be carried out using a glass column (1.5 m × 4 mm) packed with *acid-washed, silanised diatomaceous support* (80 to 100 mesh) coated with 15% w/w of free fatty acid phase (Supelco FFAP 2-1063 is suitable) and 1% w/w of *orthophosphoric acid* and maintained at 170°.

In the chromatogram obtained with solution (3) the sum of the areas of any *secondary peaks* is not greater than the area of the peak due to the internal standard.

Assay Weigh and powder 20 tablets. To a quantity of the powder containing 0.3 g of Sodium Valproate add 70 ml of *water*, shake for 10 minutes, dilute to 100 ml with *water* and filter. To 50 ml of the filtrate add 10 ml of a 30% w/v solution of *sodium chloride* and 10 ml of 2M *hydrochloric acid*. Extract with 40 ml of a mixture of 2 volumes of *ether* and 1 volume of *petroleum spirit (boiling range, 40° to 60°)*

and allow to separate. Shake the aqueous layer with a further 40 ml of the ether—petroleum spirit mixture. Shake each of the ether extracts with the same three 10-ml quantities of a saturated solution of *sodium chloride*, combine the ether extracts and evaporate to a volume of about 1 ml at a temperature not exceeding 30°. Add 50 ml of *ethanol (96%)*, previously neutralised with 0.1M *sodium hydroxide VS*, using *phenolphthalein solution R1* as indicator, and titrate with 0.1M *sodium hydroxide VS*. Each ml of 0.1M *sodium hydroxide VS* is equivalent to 16.62 mg of $C_8H_{15}NaO_2$.

Sodium Valproate Enteric-coated Tablets

Definition Sodium Valproate Enteric-coated Tablets contain Sodium Valproate. They are enteric-coated.

The tablets comply with the requirements stated under Tablets and with the following requirements.

Content of sodium valproate, $C_8H_{15}NaO_2$ 95.0 to 105.0% of the prescribed or stated amount.

Identification Shake a quantity of the powdered tablets containing 0.5 g of Sodium Valproate with 10 ml of *water* and centrifuge. Acidify 5 ml of the supernatant liquid with 2M *sulphuric acid*, shake with 25 ml of *chloroform* and wash the chloroform layer with 5 ml of *water*. Dry by shaking with *anhydrous sodium sulphate*, filter and evaporate the chloroform to dryness. The *infrared absorption spectrum* of a thin film of the residue, Appendix II A, is concordant with the *reference spectrum* of valproic acid.

Disintegration Comply with the *disintegration test for enteric-coated tablets*, Appendix XII B.

Related substances Carry out the method for *gas chromatography*, Appendix III B, using the following solutions. Solution (1) contains 0.020% w/v of *octanoic acid* (internal standard) in *dichloromethane*. For solution (2) shake a quantity of the powdered tablets containing 0.50 g of Sodium Valproate with 10 ml of *water*, acidify with 2M *sulphuric acid* and shake with three 20-ml quantities of *dichloromethane*. Wash the combined dichloromethane extracts with 10 ml of *water*, shake with *anhydrous sodium sulphate*, filter and evaporate the filtrate to a volume of about 10 ml at a temperature not exceeding 30° using a rotary evaporator. For solution (3) shake a quantity of the powdered tablets containing 0.50 g of Sodium Valproate with 10 ml of a 0.020% w/v solution of the internal standard in 0.1M *sodium hydroxide* and continue as described for solution (2), beginning at the words 'acidify with 2M *sulphuric acid* ... '.

The chromatographic procedure may be carried out using a glass column (1.5 m × 4 mm) packed with *acid-washed, silanised diatomaceous support* (80 to 100 mesh) coated with 15% w/w of free fatty acid phase (Supelco FFAP 2-1063 is suitable) and 1% w/w of *orthophosphoric acid* and maintained at 170°.

In the chromatogram obtained with solution (3) the sum of the areas of any *secondary peaks* is not greater than the area of the peak due to the internal standard.

Assay Weigh and powder 20 tablets. Carry out the method for *gas chromatography*, Appendix III B, using the following solutions. For solution (1) shake 0.1 g of *sodium valproate BPCRS* with 10 ml of a 1% w/v solution of *octanoic acid* (internal standard) in 0.1M *sodium hydroxide*, acidify with 2M *sulphuric acid* and shake with three 20-ml quantities of *dichloromethane*. Wash the combined dichloromethane extracts with 10 ml of *water*, shake with *anhydrous sodium sulphate*, filter and wash the filter paper with 20 ml of *dichloromethane*. To 50 ml of the filtrate add sufficient *dichloromethane* to produce 100 ml. Prepare solution (2) in the same manner as solution (3) but using 10 ml of a solution of 0.1M *sodium hydroxide* in place of the internal standard solution. For solution (3) shake a quantity of the powdered tablets containing 0.1 g of Sodium Valproate with 10 ml of a 1% w/v solution of the internal standard in 0.1M *sodium hydroxide* and continue as described for solution (1) beginning at the words 'acidify with 2M *sulphuric acid* ... '.

The chromatographic conditions described under the test for Related substances may be carried out.

Calculate the content of $C_8H_{15}NaO_2$ in the sample using the declared content of $C_8H_{15}NaO_2$ in *sodium valproate BPCRS*.

Storage Sodium Valproate Enteric-coated Tablets should be kept in an airtight container at a temperature not exceeding 30°.

Labelling The label states that the tablets should be swallowed whole and not chewed.

Somatropin Injection

Definition Somatropin Injection is a sterile solution of somatropin in a suitable liquid. It is prepared by dissolving Somatropin for Injection in the liquid stated on the label.

The injection complies with the requirements stated under Parenteral Preparations.

Storage Somatropin Injection should be used within the period recommended by the manufacturer when prepared and stored strictly in accordance with the manufacturer's instructions.

SOMATROPIN FOR INJECTION

Somatropin for Injection complies with the requirements of the 3rd edition of the European Pharmacopoeia [0952]. These requirements are reproduced after the heading 'Definition' below.

Ph Eur

DEFINITION

Somatropin for injection is a freeze-dried, sterile preparation of a protein having the structure (191 amino-acid residues) of the major component of growth hormone produced by the human pituitary. It contains not less than 89.0 per cent and not more than 105.0 per cent of the amount of somatropin[1] ($C_{990}H_{1528}N_{262}O_{300}S_7$) stated on the label. It complies with the requirements of the monographs on *Preparations for parenteral use (520)* and *Recombinant DNA technology, products of (784)*.

PRODUCTION

Somatropin for injection is prepared either from somatropin or from somatropin bulk solution, or by a method based on recombinant DNA (rDNA) technology in which the injectable preparation is produced without the isolation of an intermediate solid or liquid bulk. In the latter case, during the course of product development, it must be demonstrated that the manufacturing process produces a product having a biological activity of at least 2.5 I.U. per milligram, using a suitable, validated bioassay, based on growth promotion and approved by the competent authority. The purified preparation, to which buffers and stabilisers may be added, is filtered through a bacteria-retentive filter, aseptically distributed in sterile containers of glass type I (*3.2.1*) and freeze-dried. The containers are immediately sealed so as to exclude microbial contamination and moisture.

Prior to release, the following tests are carried out on each batch, unless exemption has been granted by the competent authority.

Host-cell-derived proteins The limit is approved by the competent authority.

Host-cell-and vector-derived DNA The limit is approved by the competent authority.

Where somatropin for injection is prepared from somatropin or from somatropin bulk solution and provided exemption has been granted by the competent authority, identification test C need not be performed by the manufacturer on somatropin for injection.

CHARACTERS

A white or almost white powder.

IDENTIFICATION

A. Examine the electrophoretograms obtained in the test for isoelectric focusing. In the electrophoretogram obtained with test solution (a), the major band corresponds in position to that in the electrophoretogram obtained with the reference solution. In the electrophoretogram obtained with test solution (c), there is a single major band.

B. Examine the chromatograms obtained in the test for related proteins. The retention time of the principal peak in the chromatogram obtained with test solution (a) is similar to that of the principal peak in the chromatogram obtained with reference solution (a).

C. Examine by peptide mapping.

Test solution. Prepare a solution of the substance to be examined in *tris acetate buffer solution pH 8.5 R* containing per millilitre 2.0 mg of somatropin and transfer about 1.0 ml to a tube made from suitable material such as polypropylene. Freshly prepare a 1 g/l solution of *trypsin for peptide mapping R* in a suitable acetate buffer at about pH 5.0 and add 30 µl to the solution of the substance to be examined. Cap the tube and place in a water-bath at 37°C for 4 h. Remove from the water-bath and stop the reaction immediately by the addition of 200 µl of *glacial acetic acid R*.

Reference solution. Prepare at the same time and in the same manner as for the test solution but using *somatropin CRS* instead of the substance to be examined.

Examine by liquid chromatography (*2.2.29*).

The chromatographic procedure may be carried out using:
- a stainless steel column 0.25 m long and 4.6 mm in internal diameter packed with *octylsilyl silica gel for chromatography R* (5 µm to 10 µm),
- as mobile phase at a flow rate of 1 ml per minute a mixture of mobile phases A and B prepared as follows: dilute 1 ml of *trifluoroacetic acid R* to 1000 ml with *water R* (mobile phase A). To 100 ml of *water R* add 1 ml of *trifluoroacetic acid R* and dilute to 1000 ml with *acetonitrile R* (mobile phase B). Use the following gradient:

Time (min)	Mobile phase A (per cent *V/V*)	Mobile phase B (per cent *V/V*)
0	100	0
20	80	20
40	75	25
60	50	50

- as detector a spectrophotometer set at 214 nm.

Equilibrate the column with mobile phase A for at least 15 min. Carry out a blank run using the above-mentioned gradient and continue elution for 5 min, increasing progressively the content of mobile phase B to 80 per cent. Then equilibrate the column again with mobile phase A for 15 min. Inject separately 100 µl of each solution. At the end of the gradient and before the next injection, increase the content of mobile phase B to 80 per cent over 5 min and equilibrate the column with mobile phase A for 15 min.

The profile of the chromatogram obtained with the test solution corresponds to that of the chromatogram obtained with the reference solution. The test is not valid unless the chromatogram obtained with each solution is qualitatively similar to the reference chromatogram provided with *somatropin CRS*.

D. Examine the chromatograms obtained in the Assay. The retention time of the principal peak in the chromatogram obtained with the test solution is similar to that of the principal peak in the chromatogram obtained with reference solution (b).

TESTS

Related proteins Examine by liquid chromatography (*2.2.29*).

Test solution (a). Prepare a solution of the substance to be examined in *tris(hydroxymethyl)aminomethane buffer solution pH 7.5 R1* containing per millilitre 2.0 mg of somatropin.

Test solution (b). Dilute 100 µl of test solution (a) to 1.5 ml with *tris(hydroxymethyl)aminomethane buffer solution pH 7.5 R1*.

Reference solution (a). Prepare a solution of *somatropin CRS* in *tris(hydroxymethyl)aminomethane buffer solution pH 7.5 R1* containing per millilitre 2.0 mg of somatropin.

Reference solution (b). Prepare a solution of *somatropin CRS* in *tris(hydroxymethyl)aminomethane buffer solution pH 7.5 R1* containing per millilitre 2.0 mg of somatropin. Add a freshly prepared solution of *strong hydrogen peroxide solution R* to give a final concentration of 0.01 per cent *V/V* and allow to stand at 4°C for 5 h. Add 4.5 mg *L-methionine R* per millilitre of solution.

Maintain the solutions at 2°C to 8°C and use within 24 h. If an automatic injector is used, maintain the temperature at 2°C to 8°C.

The chromatographic procedure may be carried out using:
- a stainless steel column 0.25 m long and 4.6 mm in internal diameter packed with *butylsilyl silica gel for chromatography R* (5 µm to 10 µm),
- as mobile phase at a flow rate of 0.5 ml per minute a mixture of 29 volumes of *propanol R* and 71 volumes

of *tris(hydroxymethyl)aminomethane buffer solution pH 7.5 R1*,
— as detector a spectrophotometer set at 220 nm,

maintaining the temperature of the column at 45°C.

Inject 20 μl of reference solution (a). If necessary, adjust the concentration of propanol in the mobile phase so that the retention time of the principal peak is 33 ± 3 min. Inject 20 μl of reference solution (b). Identify the peaks with the aid of the reference chromatogram supplied with *somatropin CRS*. The test is not valid unless the resolution between the peaks corresponding to somatropin and oxidised somatropin is at least 1.0.

Inject 20 μl of each solution and record the chromatograms for at least 50 min. In the chromatogram obtained with test solution (a): the area of any peak, apart from the principal peak is not greater than the area of the principal peak in the chromatogram obtained with test solution (b) (6.67 per cent); the sum of the areas of all the peaks, apart from the principal peak is not greater than twice the area of the principal peak in the chromatogram obtained with test solution (b) (13 per cent). Disregard any peak due to the solvent.

Dimer and related substances of higher molecular mass Examine by size-exclusion chromatography (*2.2.30*) as described under Assay.

Inject 50 μl of reference solution (a). Adjust the sensitivity of the detector so that the height of the principal peak in the chromatogram obtained is 50 per cent to 70 per cent of the full scale of the recorder. The resolution defined by the ratio of the height above the baseline of the valley separating the monomer and dimer peaks to the height of the dimer peak is less than 0.6 (the retention times relative to monomer are approximately 0.94 for the dimer and 0.87 for polymers). Inject reference solution (a) a sufficient number of times (at least three times); the test is not valid unless the relative standard deviation of the area of the principal peak is at most 2.5 per cent.

Inject 50 μl each of the test solution and reference solution (a). In the chromatogram obtained with the test solution, the sum of the areas of any peaks with a retention time less than that of the principal peak is not greater than the area of the principal peak in the chromatogram obtained with reference solution (a) (6.0 per cent).

Isoelectric focusing Examine by isoelectric focusing.

Test solution (a). Prepare a solution of the substance to be examined in a 3.95 g/l solution of *ammonium hydrogen carbonate R* containing per millilitre, 2.0 mg of somatropin.

Test solution (b) Add 0.1 ml of test solution (a) to 1.5 ml of a 3.95 g/l solution of *ammonium hydrogen carbonate R*.

Test solution (c). Mix 0.1 ml of test solution (a) and 0.1 ml of the reference solution.

Reference solution. Prepare a solution of *somatropin CRS* in *water R* containing per millilitre 2.0 mg of somatropin.

Isoelectric point calibration solution pH range 2.5 to 6.5, prepared and used according to the manufacturer's instructions.

Operate the apparatus in accordance with the manufacturer's instructions. The isoelectric focusing procedure may be carried out using a pre-cast gel 245 mm × 110 mm × 1 mm, with a pH in the range 4.0 to 6.5. Apply separately to the gel 15 μl of each solution. Use as the anode solution a 147.1 g/l solution of *glutamic acid R* in phosphoric acid (50 g/l H_3PO_4) and as the cathode solution an 89.1 g/l solution of *β-alanine R*. Adjust the operating conditions to 2000 V and 25 mA. Allow focusing to take place for 2.5 h at a constant voltage. Immerse the gel for 30 min in a solution containing 115 g/l of *trichloroacetic acid R* and 34.5 g/l of *sulphosalicylic acid R*, and then for 5 min in a mixture of 8 volumes of *acetic acid R*, 25 volumes of *ethanol R* and 67 volumes of deionised *water R* (de-stain solution). Stain the gel by immersion in a 1.15 g/l solution of *acid blue 83 R* in de-stain solution at 60°C for 10 min, and then place the gel in de-stain solution until excess stain is removed. The test is not valid unless the distribution of bands in the isoelectric point calibration solution corresponds to the manufacturer's indications. The electrophoretogram obtained with the reference solution contains a major band with an isoelectric point of approximately five and a slightly more acidic minor band at approximately 4.8. In the electrophoretogram obtained with test solution (a), no band is more intense than the major band in the electrophoretogram obtained with test solution (b) (6.25 per cent).

Water Not more than 3.0 per cent *m/m*, determined by gas chromatography (*2.2.28*), using *anhydrous methanol R* as the internal standard.

Use dry glassware which may be silicone-treated.

Internal standard solution. Dilute 15 μl of *anhydrous methanol R* to 100 ml with *2-propanol R1*.

Test solution (a). Suspend 1.0 mg of the preparation to be examined in 0.1 ml of *2-propanol R1*. Shake for 30 min and clarify by centrifugation; use the supernatant liquid.

Test solution (b). Suspend 1.0 mg of the preparation to be examined in 0.1 ml of the internal standard solution. Shake for 30 min and clarify by centrifugation; use the supernatant liquid.

Reference solution. Add 10 μl of *water R* to 50 ml of the internal standard solution.

The chromatographic procedure may be carried out using:
— a stainless steel column 1 m long and 2 mm in internal diameter packed with *styrene-divinylbenzene copolymer R* (180 μm to 250 μm),
— *helium for chromatography R* as the carrier gas,
— a thermal-conductivity detector,

maintaining the temperature of the column at 120°C and that of the detector at 150°C. Inject the chosen volume of each solution. Calculate the content of water assuming its density (*2.2.5*) at 20°C to be 0.997 g/ml and taking into account any water detectable in the internal standard solution.

Bacterial endotoxins (*2.6.14*). Not more than 5 I.U. of endotoxin per milligram of somatropin.

ASSAY

Examine by size-exclusion chromatography (*2.2.30*).

Test solution. Prepare a solution of the substance to be examined in a 3.95 g/l solution of *ammonium hydrogen carbonate R* containing per millilitre, 1.0 mg of somatropin.

Reference solution (a). Dilute 300 μl of test solution to 5.0 ml with a 3.95 g/l solution of *ammonium hydrogen carbonate R*.

Reference solution (b). Prepare a solution of *somatropin CRS* in a 3.95 g/l solution of *ammonium hydrogen carbonate R* containing per millilitre, 1.0 mg of somatropin.

The chromatographic procedure may be carried out using:
- a stainless steel column about 0.25 m long and 9.4 mm in internal diameter packed with *hydrophilic silica gel for chromatography R* of a grade suitable for fractionation of globular proteins in the molecular mass range 5000 to 60,000,
- as mobile phase at a flow rate of 0.6 ml per minute a 3.95 g/l solution of *ammonium hydrogen carbonate R* that has been filtered and degassed,
- as detector a spectrophotometer set at 214 nm.

Inject 50 µl of reference solution (b). Adjust the sensitivity of the detector so that the height of the principal peak corresponds to at least half of the full scale of the recorder. Inject reference solution (b) a sufficient number of times (at least three times). The test is not valid unless the relative standard deviation of the peak area for somatropin is at most 2.5 per cent. Inject alternately 50 µl of the test solution and reference solution (b).

Calculate the content of somatropin ($C_{990}H_{1528}N_{262}O_{300}S_7$) from the peak areas in the chromatogram obtained with the test solution and the reference solution (b) and the declared content of $C_{990}H_{1528}N_{262}O_{300}S_7$ in *somatropin CRS*.

STORAGE

Store in a sterile, tamper-proof container, at a temperature of 2°C to 8°C.

LABELLING

The label states:
- the content of somatropin in milligrams.
- the composition and volume of the liquid to be added for reconstitution,
- the time within which the reconstituted solution shall be used and the storage conditions during this period,
- the name and quantity of any added substance,
- the storage temperature,
- that the preparation shall not be shaken during reconstitution,
- the equivalent in International Units.

[1] 1 mg of anhydrous somatropin ($C_{990}H_{1528}N_{262}O_{300}S_7$) is equivalent to 3.0 I.U. of biological activity.

Ph Eur

Sorbitol Intravenous Infusion

Sorbitol Injection

Definition Sorbitol Intravenous Infusion is a sterile solution of Sorbitol in Water for Injections.

The intravenous infusion complies with the requirements stated under Parenteral Preparations and with the following requirements.

Content of sorbitol, $C_6H_{14}O_6$ 95.0 to 105.0% of the prescribed or stated amount.

Characteristics A colourless or almost colourless solution.

Identification

A. To a volume containing 50 mg of Sorbitol add 3 ml of a freshly prepared 10% w/v solution of *catechol* and pour the mixture cautiously into 6 ml of *sulphuric acid*. A pink colour is produced.

B. Evaporate a volume containing 5 g of Sorbitol using a rotary evaporator until the liquid becomes viscous, cool, add 7 ml of *methanol*, 1 ml of *benzaldehyde* and 1 ml of *hydrochloric acid*, mix and shake continuously for 2 hours. Filter, dissolve the crystals in 20 ml of boiling *sodium hydrogen carbonate solution* and allow to crystallise. The *melting point* of the residue, after washing rapidly with 5 ml of *methanol (50%)* and drying in a current of air, is about 175°, Appendix V A.

Acidity To a volume containing 2.5 g of Sorbitol add 0.1 ml of *phenolphthalein solution* and titrate with 0.02M *sodium hydroxide VS*. Not more than 0.25 ml is required to change the colour of the solution.

Reducing sugars Evaporate a volume containing 5 g of Sorbitol using a rotary evaporator until the volume is reduced to about 10 ml, cool, add 20 ml of *cupri-citric solution* and a few glass beads, heat in such a manner that the solution boils in 4 minutes and continue boiling for a further 3 minutes. Cool rapidly and add 100 ml of a 2.4% v/v solution of *glacial acetic acid* followed by 20 ml of 0.025M *iodine VS*. Add, shaking continuously, 25 ml of a 6% v/v solution of *hydrochloric acid* and, when any precipitate has redissolved, titrate the excess iodine with 0.05M *sodium thiosulphate VS* using *starch solution*, added towards the end of the titration, as indicator. Not less than 12.8 ml of 0.05M *sodium thiosulphate VS* is required.

Particulate contamination When supplied in a container with a nominal content of 100 ml or more, complies with the *test for sub-visible particles*, Appendix XIII A.

Pyrogens Complies with the *test for pyrogens*, Appendix XIV D. Use per kg of the rabbit's weight a volume containing 0.5 g of Sorbitol.

Assay Dilute a volume containing 0.4 g of Sorbitol to 100 ml with *water*. Transfer 10 ml to a stoppered flask, add 20 ml of a 2.14% w/v solution of *sodium periodate* and 2 ml of 1M *sulphuric acid* and heat on a water bath for 15 minutes. Cool, add 3 g of *sodium hydrogen carbonate* and 25 ml of 0.1M *sodium arsenite VS*, mix, add 5 ml of a 20% w/v solution of *potassium iodide*, allow to stand for 15 minutes and titrate with 0.05M *iodine VS* until the first trace of yellow appears. Repeat the operation without the substance being examined. The difference between the titrations represents the amount of iodine required. Each ml of 0.05M *iodine VS* is equivalent to 18.22 mg of $C_6H_{14}O_6$.

Labelling The strength is stated as the percentage w/v of Sorbitol.

Sorbitol Intravenous Infusion should be administered through a plastic catheter.

Sotalol Injection

Definition Sotalol Injection is a sterile solution of Sotalol Hydrochloride in Water for Injections.

The injection complies with the requirements stated under Parenteral Preparations and with the following requirements.

Content of sotalol hydrochloride, $C_{12}H_{20}N_2O_3S,HCl$ 95.0 to 105.0% of the prescribed or stated amount.

Characteristics A clear, colourless solution.

Identification
A. The *light absorption*, Appendix II B, in the range 230 to 350 nm, of the final solution obtained in the Assay exhibits a maximum only at 249 nm.

B. Carry out the method for *thin-layer chromatography*, Appendix III A, using *silica gel GF$_{254}$* as the coating substance and a mixture of 30 volumes of *methanol* and 70 volumes of *chloroform* as the mobile phase in a tank saturated with ammonia vapour. Allow the mobile phase to ascend 10 cm above the line of application. Apply separately to the plate 2 µl of each of the following solutions. For solution (1) dilute the injection with *water* to produce a solution containing 0.2% w/v of Sotalol Hydrochloride. Solution (2) contains 0.2% w/v of *sotalol hydrochloride BPCRS* in *water*. After removal of the plate, dry it in a current of air for at least 5 minutes and examine under *ultraviolet light (254 nm)*. The principal spot in the chromatogram obtained with solution (1) corresponds in position, size and intensity to that in the chromatogram obtained with solution (2).

Acidity pH, 4.0 to 5.5, Appendix V L.

Related substances Complies with the test described under Sotalol Hydrochloride but using as solution (1) a solution prepared in the following manner. Dilute the injection with the mobile phase to produce a solution containing 0.2% w/v of Sotalol Hydrochloride.

Assay Dilute a volume of the injection containing 20 mg of Sotalol Hydrochloride to 100 ml with *water*. To 10 ml of this solution add 20 ml of 1M *sodium hydroxide* and sufficient *water* to produce 200 ml. Measure the *absorbance* of the resulting solution at the maximum at 249 nm, Appendix II B, using 0.1M *sodium hydroxide* in the reference cell. Calculate the content of $C_{12}H_{20}N_2O_3S,HCl$ taking 480 as the value of A(1%, 1 cm) at the maximum at 249 nm.

Sotalol Tablets

Definition Sotalol Tablets contain Sotalol Hydrochloride.

The tablets comply with the requirements stated under Tablets and with the following requirements.

Content of sotalol hydrochloride, $C_{12}H_{20}N_2O_3S,HCl$ 95.0 to 105.0% of the prescribed or stated amount.

Identification
A. The *light absorption*, Appendix II B, in the range 230 to 350 nm, of the final solution obtained in the Assay exhibits a maximum only at 249 nm.

B. Carry out the method for *thin-layer chromatography*, Appendix III A, using *silica gel GF$_{254}$* as the coating substance and a mixture of 30 volumes of *methanol* and 70 volumes of *chloroform* as the mobile phase in a tank saturated with ammonia vapour. Allow the mobile phase to ascend 10 cm above the line of application. Apply separately to the plate 2 µl of each of the following solutions. For solution (1) shake a quantity of the powdered tablets containing 50 mg of Sotalol Hydrochloride with 25 ml of *methanol* for 15 minutes, centrifuge and use the supernatant liquid. Solution (2) contains 0.2% w/v of *sotalol hydrochloride BPCRS* in *water*. After removal of the plate, dry it in a current of air for at least 5 minutes and examine under *ultraviolet light (254 nm)*. The principal spot in the chromatogram obtained with solution (1) corresponds in position, size and intensity to that in the chromatogram obtained with solution (2).

Related substances Comply with the test described under Sotalol Hydrochloride but preparing solution (1) in the following manner. Shake a quantity of the powdered tablets containing 50 mg of Sotalol Hydrochloride with 25 ml of the mobile phase for 15 minutes, centrifuge and use the supernatant liquid.

Assay Weigh and powder 20 tablets. Shake a quantity of the powdered tablets containing 50 mg of Sotalol Hydrochloride with 175 ml of *water* for 15 minutes, add sufficient *water* to produce 250 ml and centrifuge. To 10 ml of the supernatant liquid add 20 ml of 1M *sodium hydroxide* and sufficient *water* to produce 200 ml. Measure the *absorbance* of the resulting solution at the maximum at 249 nm, Appendix II B, using 0.1M *sodium hydroxide* in the reference cell. Calculate the content of $C_{12}H_{20}N_2O_3S$, HCl taking 480 as the value of A(1%, 1 cm) at the maximum at 249 nm.

Storage Sotalol Tablets should be protected from light.

Spectinomycin Injection

Definition Spectinomycin Injection is a sterile suspension of Spectinomycin Hydrochloride in a suitable liquid. It is prepared by suspending Spectinomycin Hydrochloride for Injection in the requisite amount of the liquid stated on the label.

The injection complies with the requirements stated under Parenteral Preparations.

Storage Spectinomycin Injection should be used immediately after preparation but, in any case, within the period recommended by the manufacturer when prepared and stored strictly in accordance with the manufacturer's instructions.

SPECTINOMYCIN HYDROCHLORIDE FOR INJECTION

Definition Spectinomycin Hydrochloride for Injection is a sterile material consisting of Spectinomycin Hydrochloride, with or without excipients.

The contents of the sealed container comply with the requirements for Powders for Injections stated under Parenteral Preparations and with the following requirements.

Content of spectinomycin, $C_{14}H_{24}N_2O_7$ 90.0 to 105.0% of the prescribed or stated amount.

Identification
A. The *infrared absorption spectrum*, Appendix II A, is concordant with the *reference spectrum* of spectinomycin hydrochloride.

B. A 1% w/v solution yields reaction A characteristic of *chlorides*, Appendix VI.

Acidity or alkalinity Suspend the contents of a sealed container in the stated volume of the liquid stated on the label. The pH of the resulting suspension is 4.0 to 7.0, Appendix V L.

Related substances Carry out the method for *thin-layer chromatography*, Appendix III A, using *silica gel G* as the coating substance and a mixture of 5 volumes of *glacial acetic acid*, 5 volumes of *pyridine*, 40 volumes of *water* and 50 volumes of *propan-1-ol* as the mobile phase but allowing the solvent front to ascend 12 cm above the line of application. Apply separately to the plate 10 µl of each of two solutions of the contents of a sealed container in *water* containing the equivalent of (1) 1.4% w/v and (2) 0.014% w/v of spectinomycin. After removal of the plate, allow it to dry in air, spray with a 5% w/v solution of *potassium permanganate* and allow to stand for 2 to 3 minutes. Any *secondary spot* in the chromatogram obtained with solution (1) is not more intense than the spot in the chromatogram obtained with solution (2) (1%).

Water Not more than 20.0% w/w, Appendix IX C. Use 0.2 g.

Bacterial endotoxins Carry out the *test for bacterial endotoxins*, Appendix XIV C. Dissolve the contents of the sealed container in a solution containing 0.05M *sodium hydrogen carbonate* in *water BET* to give a solution containing 1 mg of spectinomycin per ml (solution A). The endotoxin limit concentration of solution A is 0.09 IU per ml. Carry out the test using the maximum valid dilution of solution A calculated from the declared sensitivity of the lysate used in the test.

Assay Prepare a 0.15% w/v solution of *phenazone* (internal standard) in *dimethylformamide* (solution A). Carry out the method for *gas chromatography*, Appendix III B, using the following solutions which have been allowed to stand for 1 hour before use. For solution (1) add 10 ml of solution A and 2 ml of *hexamethyldisilazane* to 60 mg of *spectinomycin hydrochloride EPCRS*, shake to dissolve and add sufficient *dimethylformamide* to produce 20 ml. For solution (2) suspend the contents of a sealed container in sufficient of the liquid stated on the label to produce a suspension containing the equivalent of 400 mg of spectinomycin per ml and dilute 5 ml of this suspension to 100 ml with *water* (solution B). Add 15 ml of *acetone* to 2 ml of solution B and evaporate to dryness. Add 10 ml of *dimethylformamide* and 2 ml of *hexamethyldisilazane* to the residue, shake to dissolve and add sufficient *dimethylformamide* to produce 20 ml. For solution (3) add 15 ml of *acetone* to 2 ml of solution B and evaporate to dryness. Add 10 ml of solution A and 2 ml of *hexamethyldisilazane* to the residue, shake to dissolve and add sufficient *dimethylformamide* to produce 20 ml.

The chromatographic procedure may be carried out using a glass column (1.5 m × 4 mm) packed with *silanised diatomaceous earth for gas chromatography* (100-120 mesh) coated with 3% w/w of phenylmethyl silicone fluid (50% phenyl) (OV-17 is suitable) and maintained at 200° with both the inlet port and the detector between 200° and 230° and a flow rate of 45 ml per minute for the carrier gas.

The test is not valid unless, in the chromatogram obtained with solution (3), the *resolution factor* between the principal peak and the peak corresponding to the internal standard is at least 8.0.

Calculate the content of $C_{14}H_{24}N_2O_7$ using the declared content of $C_{14}H_{24}N_2O_7,2HCl$ in *spectinomycin hydrochloride EPCRS*. Each mg of $C_{14}H_{24}N_2O_7,2HCl$ is equivalent to 0.8528 mg of $C_{14}H_{24}N_2O_7$.

Labelling The quantity of active ingredient is stated in terms of the equivalent amount of spectinomycin.

Spironolactone Tablets

Definition Spironolactone Tablets contain Spironolactone.

The tablets comply with the requirements stated under Tablets and with the following requirements.

Content of spironolactone, $C_{24}H_{32}O_4S$ 95.0 to 105.0% of the prescribed or stated amount.

Identification

A. Extract a quantity of the powdered tablets containing 0.125 g of Spironolactone with two 10-ml quantities of *chloroform*, filter, evaporate the combined filtrates to dryness and dissolve the residue in 2.5 ml of *chloroform*. The *infrared absorption spectrum* of the resulting solution, Appendix II A, is concordant with the *reference spectrum* of spironolactone.

B. Carry out the method for *thin-layer chromatography*, Appendix III A, using *silica gel GF_{254}* as the coating substance and a mixture of 1 volume of *water*, 24 volumes of *cyclohexane* and 75 volumes of *ethyl acetate* as the mobile phase. Apply separately to the plate 5 µl of each of the following solutions. For solution (1) extract a quantity of the powdered tablets containing 20 mg of Spironolactone with 10 ml of *dichloromethane*. Solution (2) contains 0.2% w/v of *spironolactone EPCRS* in *dichloromethane*. After removal of the plate, allow it to dry in air and examine under *ultraviolet light (254 nm)*. The principal spot in the chromatogram obtained with solution (1) is similar in position and size to that in the chromatogram obtained with solution (2).

Dissolution Comply with the *dissolution test for tablets and capsules*, Appendix XII D, using Apparatus II. Use as the medium 1000 ml of 0.1M *hydrochloric acid* containing 0.1% w/v *sodium dodecyl sulphate* and rotate the paddle at 75 revolutions per minute. Withdraw a sample of 10 ml of the medium, filter and measure the *absorbance* of the filtrate, suitably diluted if necessary, at the maximum at 242 nm, Appendix II B. Calculate the total content of $C_{24}H_{32}O_4S$ in the medium taking 445 as the value of A(1%, 1 cm) at the maximum at 242 nm.

Related substances Carry out the method for *liquid chromatography*, Appendix III D, using the following solutions. For solution (1) disperse a quantity of the powdered tablets containing 62.5 mg of Spironolactone with 25 ml of *chloroform*, place in an ultrasonic bath for 5 minutes, shake for 10 to 15 minutes, centrifuge and filter the supernatant liquid through glass fibre paper (Whatman GF/C is suitable). Repeat the procedure on the residue with a further 25 ml of *chloroform*. Combine the chloroform extracts and evaporate to dryness using a rotary evaporator. Add 2.5 ml of *tetrahydrofuran* and 22.5 ml of the mobile phase to the residue. For solution (2) dilute 1 ml of solution (1) to 100 ml with the mobile phase. For solution (3) dissolve 25 mg of *canrenone EPCRS* in 1 ml of *tetrahydrofuran* and dilute to 10 ml with the mobile phase. For solution (4) dilute 1 ml of solution (3) to 100 ml with the mobile phase. For solution (5) mix 1 ml each of solutions (1) and (3) and dilute to 100 ml with the mobile phase. For solution (6) dilute 0.5 ml of solution (2) to 10 ml with the mobile phase.

The chromatographic procedure may be carried out using (a) a stainless steel column (15 cm × 4.6 mm) packed with *stationary phase B* (5 µm) (Spherisorb C8 is suitable), (b) a mixture of 8 volumes of *acetonitrile*, 18 volumes of *tetrahydrofuran* and 74 volumes of *water* as the mobile phase with a flow rate of 1.8 ml per minute and (c) detection wavelengths of 254 nm and 283 nm as directed below.

Inject separately 20 µl of each of solutions (1), (2), (5) and (6) and record the chromatograms for twice the retention time of spironolactone using a detection wavelength of 254 nm. In the chromatogram obtained with solution (1) the sum of the areas of any *secondary peaks*, other than any peak corresponding to canrenone, is not greater than the area of the peak due to spironolactone in the chromatogram obtained with solution (2) (1%). Disregard any peak the area of which is less than that of the principal peak in the chromatogram obtained with solution (6).

Inject 20 µl of each of solutions (1) and (4) and record the chromatograms using a detection wavelength of 283 nm. The test is not valid unless (a) the chromatogram obtained with solution (5) shows two peaks due to canrenone and spironolactone with a *resolution factor* greater than 1.4 and (b) the principal peak in the chromatogram obtained with solution (6) has a *signal-to-noise ratio* of at least 6.

In the chromatogram obtained with solution (1) the area of any peak corresponding to canrenone is not greater than that of the peak due to canrenone in the chromatogram obtained with solution (4) (1%). Calculate the percentage content of canrenone found when recording at 283 nm and the percentage content of the other related substances found when recording at 254 nm. The sum is not greater than 1.0%.

Assay Weigh and powder 20 tablets. To a quantity of the powder containing 25 mg of Spironolactone add 100 ml of *methanol* and heat just to boiling, with swirling. Cool, add sufficient *methanol* to produce 250 ml, dilute 10 ml to 100 ml with *methanol* and measure the *absorbance* of the resulting solution at the maximum at 238 nm, Appendix II B. Calculate the content of $C_{24}H_{32}O_4S$ taking 470 as the value of A(1%, 1 cm) at the maximum at 238 nm.

Storage Spironolactone Tablets should be protected from light.

Squill Liquid Extract

Definition Squill Liquid Extract is prepared by extracting Squill with Ethanol (70 per cent).

Extemporaneous preparation The following formula and directions apply.

Squill, in *coarse powder*	1000 g
Ethanol (70 per cent)	a sufficient quantity

Exhaust the Squill, in *coarse powder*, with Ethanol (70 per cent) by *percolation*, Appendix XI F. Reserve the first 850 ml of the percolate; evaporate the subsequent percolate to the consistence of a soft extract and dissolve it in the reserved portion. Add sufficient Ethanol (70 per cent) to produce 1000 ml and filter.

The extract complies with the requirements stated under Extracts and with the following requirements.

Ethanol content 34 to 50% v/v, Appendix VIII F, Method III.

Dry residue 40 to 55% w/v.

Relative density 1.00 to 1.14, Appendix V G.

Opiate Squill Linctus

Compound Squill Linctus; Gee's Linctus

Definition Opiate Squill Linctus is an opalescent *oral solution* containing 33% v/v each of Squill Oxymel and Camphorated Opium Tincture in a suitable vehicle with a tolu flavour.

Extemporaneous preparation The following formula applies.

Squill Oxymel	300 ml
Camphorated Opium Tincture	300 ml
Tolu Syrup	300 ml

The linctus complies with the requirements stated under Oral Liquids and with the following requirements.

Content of anhydrous morphine, $C_{17}H_{19}NO_3$ 0.013 to 0.020% w/v.

Ethanol content 18.0 to 22.0% v/v, Appendix VIII F.

Assay To 12 g add 5 ml of *water* and 1 ml of 5M *ammonia* and extract with 30 ml of a mixture of equal volumes of *ethanol (96%)* and *chloroform* and then with two 22.5-ml quantities of a mixture of 2 volumes of *chloroform* and 1 volume of *ethanol (96%)*, washing each extract with the same 20 ml of a mixture of equal volumes of *ethanol (96%)* and *water*. Evaporate the combined extracts, extract the residue with 10 ml of *calcium hydroxide solution*, filter and wash the filter with 10 ml of *calcium hydroxide solution*. To the combined filtrate and washings add 0.1 g of *ammonium sulphate*, extract with two 10-ml quantities of *ethanol-free chloroform*, wash the combined extracts with 10 ml of *water* and discard the chloroform solution. To the combined alkaline liquid and aqueous washings add 10 ml of 1M *hydrochloric acid*, heat on a water bath to remove any chloroform, cool and dilute to 100 ml with *water*. To 20 ml of this solution add 8 ml of a freshly prepared 1.0% w/v solution of *sodium nitrite*, allow to stand for 15 minutes, add 12 ml of 5M *ammonia*, dilute to 50 ml with *water* and measure the *absorbance* of a 4-cm layer of the resulting solution at the maximum at 442 nm, Appendix II B, using in the reference cell a solution prepared in the same manner and at the same time but using 8 ml of *water* in place of the solution of sodium nitrite. Calculate the content of $C_{17}H_{19}NO_3$ from a calibration curve prepared using quantities of 2, 4, 6 and 8 ml of a 0.008% w/v solution of *anhydrous morphine* in 0.1M *hydrochloric acid*, each diluted to 20 ml with 0.1M *hydrochloric acid* and using the method described above beginning at the words 'add 8 ml ...'. Determine the *weight per ml* of the linctus, Appendix V G, and calculate the content of $C_{17}H_{19}NO_3$, weight in volume.

Labelling The label indicates the pharmaceutical form as 'oral solution.'

Paediatric Opiate Squill Linctus

Opiate Linctus for Infants

Definition Paediatric Opiate Squill Linctus is an *oral solution* containing 6% v/v each of Squill Oxymel and Camphorated Opium Tincture in a suitable vehicle with a tolu flavour.

Extemporaneous preparation The following formula applies.

Squill Oxymel	60 ml
Camphorated Opium Tincture	60 ml
Tolu Syrup	60 ml
Glycerol	200 ml
Syrup	sufficient to produce 1000 ml

The linctus complies with the requirements stated under Oral Liquids and with the following requirements.

Content of anhydrous morphine, $C_{17}H_{19}NO_3$ 0.0024 to 0.0036% w/v.

Assay Carry out the Assay described under Opiate Squill Linctus with the following modifications. Use 32 g, add 5 ml of 1M *hydrochloric acid* to the combined alkaline liquid and aqueous washings and after heating and cooling dilute to 50 ml with *water.*

Labelling The label indicates the pharmaceutical form as 'oral solution'.

Squill Oxymel

Definition

Squill, bruised *or* Indian Squill, bruised	50 g
Acetic Acid (33 per cent)	90 ml or a sufficient quantity
Purified Water, freshly boiled and cooled	250 ml
Purified Honey	a sufficient quantity

Extemporaneous preparation The following directions apply.

Macerate the Squill or the Indian Squill with the Acetic Acid (33 per cent) and the Purified Water for 7 days with occasional agitation, strain, press out the liquid, heat the mixed liquids to boiling, filter whilst hot, cool, determine the content of acetic acid, add sufficient Acetic Acid (33 per cent) to the remainder of the filtrate to produce a solution containing about 8.5% w/v of acetic acid and mix. To every three volumes of the resulting solution add seven volumes of Purified Honey and mix thoroughly.

Content of acetic acid, $C_2H_4O_2$ 2.2 to 2.7% w/v.

Optical rotation +0.6° to –3.0°, Appendix V F, when measured in a 25% w/v solution in *water* decolorised, if necessary, with *activated charcoal.*

Weight per ml 1.260 to 1.270 g, Appendix V G.

Assay Dilute 20 ml with 20 ml of *carbon dioxide-free water* and titrate with 1M *sodium hydroxide VS* using *phenolphthalein solution R1* as indicator. Each ml of 1M *sodium hydroxide VS* is equivalent to 60.05 mg of $C_2H_4O_2$.

Stanozolol Tablets

Definition Stanozolol Tablets contain Stanozolol.

The tablets comply with the requirements stated under Tablets and with the following requirements.

Content of stanozolol, $C_{21}H_{32}N_2O$ 90.0 to 110.0% of the prescribed or stated amount.

Identification

A. Shake a quantity of the powdered tablets containing 15 mg of Stanozolol with 10 ml of *chloroform* for 10 minutes, filter, wash the filtrate with 10 ml of *water,* dry the chloroform layer over *anhydrous sodium sulphate,* filter and evaporate to dryness in a current of nitrogen at room temperature. The *infrared absorption spectrum* of the residue, Appendix II A, is concordant with the *reference spectrum* of stanozolol.

B. Shake a quantity of the powdered tablets containing 10 mg of Stanozolol with 50 ml of a mixture of equal volumes of 0.2M *hydrochloric acid* and *methanol,* add sufficient of the same solvent mixture to produce 100 ml, filter and dilute 10 ml of the filtrate to 25 ml with the same solvent mixture. The *light absorption* of the resulting solution, Appendix II B, in the range 220 to 350 nm exhibits a maximum only at 230 nm.

C. Boil a quantity of the powdered tablets containing 2 mg of Stanozolol with 5 ml of *toluene,* filter and evaporate the filtrate to dryness. To the residue add 3 ml of *dimethylaminobenzaldehyde reagent.* A yellow colour is produced which exhibits a green fluorescence when viewed under ultraviolet light (365 nm).

Related substances Comply with the test described under Stanozolol using 10 µl of each of the following solutions. For solution (1) shake a quantity of the powdered tablets containing 10 mg of Stanozolol with 1 ml of *chloroform* for 10 minutes, centrifuge and use the clear supernatant liquid. For solution (2) dilute 1 volume of solution (1) to 200 volumes with *chloroform.*

Assay Weigh and powder 20 tablets. To a quantity of the powder containing 4 mg of Stanozolol add 25 ml of *ethanol (96%)* and heat on a water bath for 15 minutes, while stirring. Cool, add sufficient *ethanol (96%)* to produce 50 ml and filter. Dilute 5 ml of the filtrate to 10 ml with 0.15M *ethanolic hydrochloric acid* and measure the *absorbance* of the resulting solution at the maximum at 235 nm, Appendix II B, using in the reference cell a solution prepared by diluting 5 ml of the filtrate to 10 ml with *ethanol (96%).* An absorbance of 0.504 at the maximum at 235 nm is equivalent to 4 mg of $C_{21}H_{32}N_2O$ in the weight of powder taken.

Storage Stanozolol Tablets should be protected from light.

Sterculia Granules

Definition Sterculia Granules are Sterculia in granule form.

The granules comply with the requirements stated under Granules and with the following requirements.

Characteristics White or buff with a distinct odour of acetic acid; transparent, irregular shaped granules of about 1 to 4 mm which swell when treated with water.

Identification

A. Irregular or vermiform pieces, about 5 to 20 mm thick; greyish white with a brown or pink tinge; surface striated.

B. When powdered and mounted in *ethanol (96%)* it appears as small, transparent, angular particles of various sizes and shapes; the particles lose their sharp edges when *water* is added and each gradually swells until a large, indefinite, almost structureless mass results; when mounted in *ruthenium red solution* the particles are stained red; no blue coloured particles (starch) are visible when mounted in *iodine solution R1*.

C. Add 1 g to 80 ml of *water* and allow to stand for 24 hours, shaking occasionally. A tacky and viscous granular mucilage is produced. Retain the mucilage for use in test D.

D. Boil 4 ml of the mucilage obtained in test C with 0.5 ml of *hydrochloric acid*, add 1 ml of 5M *sodium hydroxide*, filter, add 3 ml of *cupri-tartaric solution R1* to the filtrate and heat. A red precipitate is produced.

Acid-insoluble ash Not more than 1.0%, Appendix XI K.

Ash Not more than 7.0%, Appendix XI J.

Volatile acid Not less than 13.0%, calculated as acetic acid, $C_2H_4O_2$, when determined by the following method. To 1 g contained in a 700-ml Kjeldahl flask add 100 ml of *water* and 5 ml of *orthophosphoric acid*, allow to stand for several hours, or until the granules are completely swollen, and boil gently under a reflux condenser for 2 hours. Steam distil until 800 ml of the distillate is obtained and the acid residue measures about 20 ml and titrate the distillate with 0.1M *sodium hydroxide VS* using *phenolphthalein solution R1* as indicator. Repeat the operation without the substance being examined. The difference between the titrations represents the amount of alkali required to neutralise the volatile acid. Each ml of 0.1M *sodium hydroxide VS* is equivalent to 6.005 mg of volatile acid, calculated as $C_2H_4O_2$.

Loss on drying The powdered granules, when dried to constant weight at 105°, lose not more than 20.0% of their weight. Use 1 g.

Microbial contamination 1.0 g is free from *Escherichia coli*, Appendix XVI B1.

Storage Sterculia Granules should be stored in a dry place at a temperature not exceeding 25°.

Streptokinase Injection

Definition Streptokinase Injection is a sterile solution of Streptokinase in Water for Injections. It is prepared by dissolving Streptokinase for Injection in the requisite amount of Water for Injections immediately before use.

The injection complies with the requirements stated under Parenteral Preparations.

Storage Streptokinase Injection should be used immediately after preparation.

STREPTOKINASE FOR INJECTION

Definition Streptokinase for Injection is a sterile material consisting of Streptokinase with or without excipients. It is supplied in a sealed container.

The contents of the sealed container comply with the requirements for Powders for Injections stated under Parenteral Preparations and with the following requirements.

Characteristics A white powder or a white friable solid; hygroscopic.

Freely soluble in *water*.

Identification

A. Place 0.5 ml of citrated human, canine or rabbit plasma in a haemolysis tube maintained in a water bath at 37°. Add 0.1 ml of a solution of the preparation being examined containing 10,000 IU of streptokinase activity per ml in *citro-phosphate buffer pH 7.2* and 0.1 ml of a solution of *thrombin* containing 20 IU per ml in *citro-phosphate buffer pH 7.2* and shake immediately. A clot forms and lyses within 30 minutes. Repeat the procedure using citrated bovine plasma. Lysis does not occur within 60 minutes.

B. Comply with test B for Identification described under Streptokinase.

Acidity or alkalinity pH of a solution in freshly boiled and cooled *water* containing 5,000 IU per ml, 6.8 to 7.5, Appendix V L.

Streptodornase Comply with the test described under Streptokinase.

Streptolysin Comply with the test described under Streptokinase.

Bacterial endotoxins Carry out the *test for bacterial endotoxins*, Appendix XIV C. Dissolve the contents of the sealed container in *water BET* to give a solution containing 100,000 IU of Streptokinase per ml (solution A). The endotoxin limit concentration of solution A is 23.33 IU of endotoxin per ml. Carry out the test using the maximum valid dilution of solution A calculated from the declared sensitivity of the lysate used in the test.

Assay Carry out the Assay described under Streptokinase. The estimated potency is not less than 90% and not more than 111% of the stated potency. The fiducial limits of error are not less than 80% and not more than 125% of the stated potency.

Storage The sealed container should be protected from light and stored at a temperature of 2° to 8°. Under these conditions the contents may be expected to retain their potency for 2 years.

Labelling The label of the sealed container states (1) the total number of IU (Units) contained in it; (2) that the preparation is antigenic.

Streptomycin Injection

Definition Streptomycin Injection is a sterile solution of Streptomycin Sulphate in Water for Injections. It is either supplied as a ready-to-use solution or it is prepared by dissolving Streptomycin Sulphate for Injection in Water for Injections.

The injection complies with the requirements stated under Parenteral Preparations and with the following requirements.

Characteristics A colourless to yellow solution.

Bacterial endotoxins Carry out the *test for bacterial endotoxins*, Appendix XIV C. Dilute the injection, if necessary, with *water BET* to give a solution containing the equivalent of 10 mg of streptomycin per ml (solution A). The endotoxin limit concentration of solution A is 2.5 IU per ml. Carry out the test using the maximum valid dilution of solution A calculated from the declared sensitivity of the lysate used in the test.

Storage Streptomycin Injection prepared by dissolving the contents of a sealed container in Water for Injections should be used immediately after preparation but, in any case, within the period recommended by the manufacturer when prepared and stored strictly in accordance with the manufacturer's instructions.

Labelling The strength is stated in terms of the equivalent amount of streptomycin in a suitable dose-volume.

When supplied as a ready-to-use solution, the injection also complies with the following requirements.

Identification

A. Carry out the method for *thin-layer chromatography*, Appendix III A, using a 7% w/v solution of *potassium dihydrogen orthophosphate* as the mobile phase and a plate prepared in the following manner. Mix 0.3 g of *carbomer* (Carbopol 934 is suitable) with 240 ml of *water*, allow to stand with moderate shaking for 1 hour, adjust to pH 7 by the gradual addition, with constant shaking, of 2M *sodium hydroxide* and add 30 g of *silica gel H.* Spread a uniform layer of the resulting suspension 0.75 mm thick. Heat the plate at 110° for 1 hour, allow to cool and use immediately. Apply separately to the plate 10 µl of each of the following solutions. For solution (1) dilute a suitable volume of the injection with sufficient *water* to produce a solution containing the equivalent of 0.08% w/v of streptomycin. Solution (2) contains 0.1% w/v of *streptomycin sulphate EPCRS* in *water.* Solution (3) contains 0.1% w/v of *streptomycin sulphate EPCRS*, 0.1% w/v of *neomycin sulphate EPCRS* and 0.1% w/v of *kanamycin monosulphate EPCRS* in *water.* Allow the solvent front to ascend 12 cm above the line of application. After removal of the plate, dry it in a current of warm air, spray with a mixture of equal volumes of a 0.2% w/v solution of *naphthalene-1,3-diol* in *ethanol (96%)* and a 46% w/v solution of *sulphuric acid* and heat at 150° for 5 to 10 minutes. The principal spot in the chromatogram obtained with solution (1) corresponds to that in the chromatogram obtained with solution (2). The test is not valid unless the chromatogram obtained with solution (3) shows three clearly separated principal spots.

B. Mix 0.05 ml with 4 ml of *water*, add 1 ml of 1M *sodium hydroxide* and heat in a water bath for 4 minutes. Add a slight excess of *hydrochloric acid* and 0.1 ml of *iron(III) chloride solution R1.* A violet colour is produced.

Acidity pH, 5.0 to 6.5, Appendix V L.

Streptomycin B Carry out the method for *thin-layer chromatography*, Appendix III A, using *silica gel G* as the coating substance and a mixture of 25 volumes of *glacial acetic acid*, 25 volumes of *methanol* and 50 volumes of *toluene* as the mobile phase but allowing the solvent front to ascend 13 to 15 cm above the line of application. Apply separately to the plate 10 µl of each of the following solutions. For solution (1) dilute a volume of the injection containing the equivalent of 0.16 g of streptomycin in sufficient of a freshly prepared mixture of 3 volumes of *sulphuric acid* and 97 volumes of *methanol* to produce 5 ml, heat under a reflux condenser for 1 hour, cool, rinse the condenser with *methanol* and add sufficient *methanol* to produce 20 ml (1% w/v solution). For solution (2) dissolve 36 mg of *D-mannose* in sufficient of a freshly prepared mixture of 3 volumes of *sulphuric acid* and 97 volumes of *methanol* to produce 5 ml, heat under a reflux condenser for 1 hour, cool, rinse the condenser with *methanol* and add sufficient *methanol* to produce 50 ml. Dilute 5 ml of the resulting solution to 50 ml with *methanol*; this solution contains the equivalent of 0.03% w/v of streptomycin B (1 mg of D-mannose is equivalent to 4.13 mg of streptomycin B). After removal of the plate, allow it to dry in air and spray with a freshly prepared mixture of equal volumes of a 0.2% w/v solution of *naphthalene-1,3-diol* in *ethanol (96%)* and a 20% v/v solution of *sulphuric acid* and heat at 110° for 5 minutes. Any spot corresponding to streptomycin B in the chromatogram obtained with solution (1) is not more intense than the spot in the chromatogram obtained with solution (2) (3%).

Assay Dilute a quantity containing the equivalent of 0.33 g of streptomycin to 100 ml with *water for injections* and carry out the *biological assay of antibiotics*, Appendix XIV A. The precision of the assay is such that the fiducial limits of error are not less than 95% and not more than 105% of the estimated potency.

Calculate the content of streptomycin in the injection, taking each 1000 IU found to be equivalent to 1 mg of streptomycin. The upper fiducial limit of error is not less than 97.0% and the lower fiducial limit of error is not more than 110.0% of the prescribed or stated content.

Storage Streptomycin Injection should be protected from light and stored at a temperature of 2° to 8°.

STREPTOMYCIN SULPHATE FOR INJECTION

Definition Streptomycin Sulphate for Injection is a sterile material consisting of Streptomycin Sulphate with or without excipients. It is supplied in a sealed container.

The contents of the sealed container comply with the requirements for Powders for Injections stated under Parenteral Preparations and with the following requirements.

Identification

A. Comply with test A for Identification described in the requirements for the ready-to-use solution but using as solution (1) a solution prepared by dissolving a quantity of the contents of the sealed container in sufficient *water* to produce a solution containing the equivalent of 0.08% w/v of streptomycin.

B. Dissolve 5 to 10 mg in 4 ml of *water* and add 1 ml of 1M *sodium hydroxide.* Heat in a water bath for 4 minutes.

Add a slight excess of 2M *hydrochloric acid* and 0.1 ml of *iron(III) chloride solution R1*. A violet colour develops.

C. Yield the reactions characteristic of *sulphates*, Appendix VI.

Acidity or alkalinity pH of a solution containing the equivalent of 25% w/v of streptomycin, 4.5 to 7.0, Appendix V L.

Streptomycin B Comply with the test described in the requirements for the ready-to-use solution but using as solution (1) a solution prepared in the following manner. Dissolve a quantity containing the equivalent of 0.16 g of streptomycin in sufficient of a freshly prepared mixture of 3 volumes of *sulphuric acid* and 97 volumes of *methanol* to produce 5 ml, heat under a reflux condenser for 1 hour, cool, rinse the condenser with *methanol* and add sufficient *methanol* to produce 20 ml (1% w/v solution).

Loss on drying When dried over *phosphorus pentoxide* at 60° at a pressure not exceeding 0.1 kPa for 24 hours, lose not more than 7.0% of their weight. Use 1 g.

Assay Determine the weight of the contents of 10 containers as described in the test for Uniformity of weight under Parenteral Preparations, Powders for Injections.

Dissolve a quantity of the mixed contents of the 10 containers containing the equivalent of 0.33 g of streptomycin in sufficient *water for injections* to produce 100 ml and carry out the *biological assay of antibiotics*, Appendix XIV A. The precision of the assay is such that the fiducial limits of error are not less than 95% and not more than 105% of the estimated potency. Calculate the content of streptomycin in the injection, taking each 1000 IU found to be equivalent to 1 mg of streptomycin. For a container of average content weight, the upper fiducial limit of error is not less than 95.0% and the lower fiducial limit of error is not more than 115.0% of the prescribed or stated content.

Labelling The label on the sealed container states the quantity of streptomycin sulphate contained in it in terms of the equivalent amount of streptomycin.

Sulindac Tablets

Definition Sulindac Tablets contain Sulindac.

With the exception of the requirements for shape, the tablets comply with the requirements stated under Tablets and with the following requirements.

Content of sulindac, $C_{20}H_{17}FO_3S$ 95.0 to 105.0% of the prescribed or stated amount.

Identification

A. Shake a quantity of the powdered tablets containing 0.1 g of Sulindac with 10 ml of a mixture of equal volumes of *chloroform* and *methanol* for 10 minutes, filter and evaporate the filtrate to dryness. The *infrared absorption spectrum* of the residue, Appendix II A, is concordant with the *reference spectrum* of sulindac.

B. The *light absorption*, Appendix II B, in the range 230 to 350 nm of the solution obtained in the Assay exhibits two maxima, at 284 nm and 327 nm, and a less well-defined maximum at 258 nm.

Dissolution Comply with the *dissolution test for tablets and capsules*, Appendix XII D, using Apparatus II. Use as the medium 900 ml of *phosphate buffer pH 7.2* and rotate the paddle at 50 revolutions per minute. Withdraw a sample of 10 ml of the medium, filter and dilute with *phosphate buffer pH 7.2* to give a solution expected to contain 0.001% w/v of Sulindac. Measure the *absorbance* of this solution, Appendix II B, at 327 nm using *phosphate buffer pH 7.2* in the reference cell. Calculate the total content of $C_{20}H_{17}FO_3S$ in the medium taking 373 as the value of A(1%, 1 cm) at the maximum at 327 nm.

Related substances Carry out the method for *liquid chromatography*, Appendix III D, using the following solutions. For solution (1) shake a quantity of the powdered tablets containing 0.1 g of Sulindac with 10 ml of a mixture of equal volumes of *chloroform* and *methanol* for 10 minutes, filter (Whatman GF/C filter paper is suitable), evaporate the filtrate to dryness using a rotary evaporator at a temperature not exceeding 40° and dissolve the residue in 50 ml of the mobile phase. For solution (2) dilute 1 volume of solution (1) to 100 volumes with the mobile phase and further dilute 5 volumes of this solution to 10 volumes with the mobile phase. Solution (3) contains 0.2% w/v of *sulindac EPCRS* (which contains 0.5% w/w of the *E*-isomer) in the mobile phase.

The chromatographic procedure may be carried out using (a) a stainless steel column (30 cm × 3.9 mm) packed with *stationary phase A* (10 µm) (µPorasil is suitable), (b) a mixture of 1 volume of *glacial acetic acid*, 4 volumes of *ethanol (96%)*, 100 volumes of *ethyl acetate* and 400 volumes of *ethanol-free chloroform* as the mobile phase with a flow rate of 2 ml per minute and (c) a detection wavelength of 280 nm.

Equilibrate the column by passage of the mobile phase for several hours before use.

Inject 20 µl of solution (2) and adjust the sensitivity of the detector so that the height of the principal peak in the chromatogram obtained is not less than 50% of the full scale deflection of the recorder. Inject 20 µl of solution (3) and continue the chromatography for twice the retention time of the principal peak. The chromatogram obtained shows a principal peak corresponding to sulindac and a peak corresponding to the *E*-isomer with a retention time relative to sulindac of about 1.75.

Inject separately 20 µl of solutions (1), (2) and (3). In the chromatogram obtained with solution (1) the area of any peak corresponding to the *E*-isomer is not greater than the area of the corresponding peak in the chromatogram obtained with solution (3) (0.5%), the area of any other *secondary peak* is not greater than the area of the principal peak in the chromatogram obtained with solution (2) (0.5%) and the sum of the areas of all the *secondary peaks* is not greater than twice the area of the principal peak in the chromatogram obtained with solution (2) (1%).

Assay Weigh and powder 20 tablets. Shake a quantity of the powdered tablets containing 0.1 g of Sulindac with 80 ml of 0.1M *methanolic hydrochloric acid* for 10 minutes and dilute to 100 ml with the same solvent. Filter and dilute 3 ml of the filtrate to 200 ml with the same solvent. Measure the *absorbance* of the resulting solution at the maximum at 327 nm, Appendix II B, and calculate the content of $C_{20}H_{17}FO_3S$ taking 373 as the value of A(1%, 1 cm) at the maximum at 327 nm.

Storage Sulindac Tablets should be protected from light.

Sulfacetamide Eye Drops

Definition Sulfacetamide Eye Drops are a sterile solution of Sulfacetamide Sodium in Purified Water.

The eye drops comply with the requirements stated under Eye Preparations and with the following requirements.

Content of sulfacetamide sodium, $C_8H_9N_2NaO_3S,H_2O$ 95.0 to 105.0% of the prescribed or stated amount.

Identification To a volume containing 0.5 g of Sulfacetamide Sodium add 6 ml of 5M *acetic acid*, stirring constantly. Filter the precipitate, wash with *water* and dry at 105° for 4 hours. The residue complies with the following tests.

A. The *infrared absorption spectrum*, Appendix II A, is concordant with the *reference spectrum* of sulfacetamide.

B. The *light absorption*, Appendix II B, in the range 230 to 350 nm of a 0.001% w/v solution in *citro-phosphate buffer pH 7.0* exhibits a maximum only at 255 nm.

C. Dissolve 10 mg in 2 ml of 2M *hydrochloric acid*. The solution yields the reaction characteristic of *primary aromatic amines*, Appendix VI.

Colour of solution Dilute the eye drops, if necessary, to contain 10% w/v of Sulfacetamide Sodium. The solution is not more intensely coloured than *reference solution BY_4*, Appendix IV B, Method II.

Acidity or alkalinity pH 6.6 to 8.6, Appendix V L.

Related substances Carry out the method for *thin-layer chromatography*, Appendix III A, using *silica gel GF_{254}* as the coating substance and a mixture of 10 volumes of 13.5M *ammonia*, 25 volumes of *absolute ethanol*, 25 volumes of *water* and 50 volumes of *butan-1-ol* as the mobile phase. Apply separately to the plate 10 µl of each of the following solutions. For solution (1) dilute the eye drops with *water* to contain 4.0% w/v of Sulfacetamide Sodium. Solution (2) contains 0.20% w/v of *sulfanilamide* in *water*. After removal of the plate, heat it at 105° for 10 minutes, allow to cool and spray with *dimethylaminobenzaldehyde solution R2*. Any *secondary spot* in the chromatogram obtained with solution (1) is not more intense than the spot in the chromatogram obtained with solution (2) (5%).

Assay To a volume containing 0.5 g of Sulfacetamide Sodium add 75 ml of *water* and 10 ml of *hydrochloric acid*. Add 3 g of *potassium bromide*, cool in ice and titrate slowly with 0.1M *sodium nitrite VS*, stirring constantly and determining the end point electrometrically. Each ml of 0.1M *sodium nitrite VS* is equivalent to 25.42 mg of $C_8H_9N_2NaO_3S,H_2O$.

Storage Sulfacetamide Eye Drops should be protected from light and stored at a temperature not exceeding 25°. The Eye Drops should not be allowed to freeze.

When sulphacetamide eye drops are prescribed or demanded, Sulfacetamide Eye Drops shall be dispensed or supplied.

Sulfacetamide Eye Ointment

Definition Sulfacetamide Eye Ointment is a sterile preparation containing Sulfacetamide Sodium in a suitable hydrophobic basis.

The eye ointment complies with the requirements stated under Eye Preparations and with the following requirements.

Content of sulfacetamide sodium, $C_8H_9N_2NaO_3S,H_2O$ 90.0 to 110.0% of the prescribed or stated amount.

Identification Mix a quantity of the eye ointment containing 0.1 g of Sulfacetamide Sodium with 10 ml of *chloroform* and extract with 10 ml of 0.1M *sodium hydroxide*. Wash the aqueous layer with two 20-ml quantities of *chloroform* and add 2 ml of 2M *hydrochloric acid* and 10 ml of *acetone*. Extract with two 10-ml quantities of *ether*, filter the combined ether extracts through *anhydrous sodium sulphate* and evaporate to dryness. The residue, after drying at 105° for 4 hours, complies with the following tests.

A. The *infrared absorption spectrum*, Appendix II A, is concordant with the *reference spectrum* of sulfacetamide.

B. The *light absorption*, Appendix II B, in the range 230 to 350 nm of a 0.001% w/v solution in *citro-phosphate buffer pH 7.0* exhibits a maximum only at 255 nm.

C. Dissolve 10 mg in 2 ml of 2M *hydrochloric acid*. The solution yields the reaction characteristic of *primary aromatic amines*, Appendix VI.

Assay Transfer a quantity of the eye ointment containing 0.25 g of Sulfacetamide Sodium to a separating funnel using 20 ml of *petroleum spirit (boiling range, 40° to 60°)*, 30 ml of *ether* and two 5-ml quantities of 2M *hydrochloric acid*. Shake well, allow to separate, remove and retain the acid layer and extract with two further 30-ml quantities of 2M *hydrochloric acid*. Add 3 g of *potassium bromide* to the combined extracts, cool in ice and titrate slowly with 0.1M *sodium nitrite VS*, stirring constantly and determining the end point electrometrically. Each ml of 0.1M *sodium nitrite VS* is equivalent to 25.42 mg of $C_8H_9N_2NaO_3S,H_2O$.

When sulphacetamide eye ointment is prescribed or demanded, Sulfacetamide Eye Ointment shall be dispensed or supplied.

Sulfadiazine Injection

Definition Sulfadiazine Injection is a sterile solution of the sodium derivative of Sulfadiazine in Water for Injections free from dissolved air.

The injection complies with the requirements stated under Parenteral Preparations and with the following requirements.

Content of sulfadiazine, $C_{10}H_{10}N_4O_2S$ 95.0 to 105.0% of the prescribed or stated amount.

Identification Acidify a volume containing the equivalent of 0.5 g of Sulfadiazine with 6M *acetic acid* and filter. The residue, after washing with *water* and drying at 105°, complies with the following tests.

A. The *infrared absorption spectrum*, Appendix II A, is concordant with the *reference spectrum* of sulfadiazine.

B. In the test for Related substances, the principal spot in the chromatogram obtained with solution (2) corresponds to that in the chromatogram obtained with solution (4).

C. Yields the reaction characteristic of *primary aromatic amines*, Appendix VI, producing a bright orange-red precipitate.

Alkalinity pH, 10.0 to 11.0, Appendix V L.

Colour of solution An injection containing the equivalent of 1 g of Sulfadiazine in 4 ml is not more intensely coloured than *reference solution* BY_5, Appendix IV B, Method II.

Related substances Carry out the method for *thin-layer chromatography*, Appendix III A, using *silica gel* GF_{254} as the coating substance and a mixture of 3 volumes of 6M *ammonia*, 5 volumes of *water*, 40 volumes of *nitromethane* and 50 volumes of *1,4-dioxan* as the mobile phase. Apply separately to the plate 5 µl of each of the following solutions. For solution (1) dilute a volume of the injection containing the equivalent of 0.5 g of Sulfadiazine with sufficient of a mixture of 1 volume of 13.5M *ammonia* and 9 volumes of *methanol* to produce 25 ml. For solution (2) dilute 1 volume of solution (1) to 5 volumes with a mixture of 1 volume of 13.5M *ammonia* and 24 volumes of *methanol*. For solution (3) dilute 1 volume of solution (1) to 200 volumes with a mixture of 1 volume of 13.5M *ammonia* and 24 volumes of *methanol*. Solution (4) contains 0.40% w/v of *sulfadiazine EPCRS* in a mixture of 1 volume of 13.5M *ammonia* and 24 volumes of *methanol*. After removal of the plate, dry it at 100° to 105° and examine under *ultraviolet light (254 nm)*. Any *secondary spot* in the chromatogram obtained with solution (1) is not more intense than the spot in the chromatogram obtained with solution (3) (0.5%).

Assay To a volume containing the equivalent of 0.5 g of Sulfadiazine add a mixture of 75 ml of *water* and 10 ml of *hydrochloric acid*, add 3 g of *potassium bromide*, cool in ice and titrate slowly with 0.1M *sodium nitrite VS*, stirring constantly and determining the end point electrometrically. Each ml of 0.1M *sodium nitrite VS* is equivalent to 25.03 mg of $C_{10}H_{10}N_4O_2S$.

Storage Sulfadiazine Injection should be protected from light.

Labelling The strength is stated in terms of the equivalent amount of Sulfadiazine in a suitable dose-volume.

When sulphadiazine injection is prescribed or demanded, Sulfadiazine Injection shall be dispensed or supplied.

Sulfadimidine Injection

Definition Sulfadimidine Injection is a sterile solution of sulfadimidine sodium in Water for Injections free from dissolved air. It is prepared either from Sulfadimidine Sodium or by the interaction of Sulfadimidine and Sodium Hydroxide.

The injection complies with the requirements stated under Parenteral Preparations and with the following requirements.

Content of sulfadimidine sodium, $C_{12}H_{13}N_4NaO_2S$ 95.0 to 105.0% of the prescribed or stated amount.

Identification

A. Acidify a volume containing 0.1 g of sulfadimidine sodium with 6M *acetic acid*, filter, reserving the filtrate, wash the residue with *water* and dry at 105°. The *infrared absorption spectrum* of the residue, Appendix II A, is concordant with the *reference spectrum* of sulfadimidine.

B. The residue obtained in test A yields the reaction characteristic of *primary aromatic amines*, Appendix VI, producing a bright orange-red precipitate.

Alkalinity pH, 10.0 to 11.0, Appendix V L.

Colour of solution An injection containing 1 g of sulfadimidine sodium in 3 ml is not more intensely coloured than *reference solution* Y_4, Appendix IV B, Method I.

Related substances Carry out the method for *thin-layer chromatography*, Appendix III A, using *silica gel H* as the coating substance and a mixture of 18 volumes of 10M *ammonia* and 90 volumes of *butan-1-ol* as the mobile phase. Apply separately to the plate 10 µl of each of the following solutions. For solution (1) use the injection being examined diluted with *water* to contain 0.20% w/v of sulfadimidine sodium. Solution (2) contains 0.0020% w/v of *sulfanilamide* in a mixture of 1 volume of 13.5M *ammonia* and 9 volumes of *ethanol (96%)*. After removal of the plate, heat it at 105° for 10 minutes and spray with a 0.1% w/v solution of *4-dimethylaminobenzaldehyde* in *ethanol (96%)* containing 1% v/v of *hydrochloric acid*. Any *secondary spot* in the chromatogram obtained with solution (1) is not more intense than the spot in the chromatogram obtained with solution (2) (1%).

Assay Dilute a volume containing 0.5 g of sulfadimidine sodium to 75 ml with *water*, add 10 ml of *hydrochloric acid* and pass air slowly through the solution until the odour of sulphur dioxide is no longer detectable and the vapours do not turn moistened *starch iodate paper* blue. Add 3 g of *potassium bromide*, cool in ice and titrate slowly with 0.1M *sodium nitrite VS*, stirring constantly and determining the end point electrometrically. Each ml of 0.1M *sodium nitrite VS* is equivalent to 30.03 mg of $C_{12}H_{13}N_4NaO_2S$.

Storage Sulfadimidine Injection should be protected from light.

Labelling When the injection is prepared from Sulfadimidine the strength is stated as the amount of sulfadimidine sodium in a suitable dose-volume.

When sulphadimidine injection is prescribed or demanded, Sulfadimidine Injection shall be dispensed or supplied.

Paediatric Sulfadimidine Oral Suspension

Definition Paediatric Sulfadimidine Oral Suspension is a suspension containing 10% w/v of Sulfadimidine in a suitable flavoured vehicle.

The oral suspension complies with the requirements stated under Oral Liquids and with the following requirements.

Content of sulfadimidine, $C_{12}H_{14}N_4O_2S$ 9.50 to 10.50% w/v.

Identification

A. Mix 10 ml with 10 ml of *water*, centrifuge and discard the supernatant liquid. Repeat the extraction with two 20-ml quantities of *water*. Dissolve the residue as completely as possible in 20 ml of 0.5M *sodium hydroxide* and filter. To the filtrate add *glacial acetic acid* dropwise until the solution is acidic, filter, wash the precipitate with *water* and dry at 105°. The *infrared absorption spectrum* of the residue, Appendix II A, is concordant with the *reference spectrum* of sulfadimidine.

B. In the test for Related substances, the principal spot in the chromatogram obtained with solution (2) corresponds to that in the chromatogram obtained with solution (4).

C. The residue obtained in test A yields the reaction characteristic of *primary aromatic amines*, Appendix VI, producing a bright orange-red precipitate.

Related substances Carry out the method for *thin-layer chromatography*, Appendix III A, using *silica gel GF_{254}* as the coating substance and a mixture of 3 volumes of 6M *ammonia*, 5 volumes of *water*, 40 volumes of *nitromethane* and 50 volumes of *1,4-dioxan* as the mobile phase. Apply separately to the plate 5 µl of each of the following solutions. For solution (1) dilute 5 ml of the oral suspension with sufficient of a mixture of 1 volume of 13.5M *ammonia* and 9 volumes of *methanol* to produce 25 ml, filter and use the filtrate. For solution (2) dilute 1 volume of solution (1) to 5 volumes with a mixture of 1 volume of 13.5M *ammonia* and 24 volumes of *methanol*. For solution (3) dilute 1 volume of solution (1) to 200 volumes with a mixture of 1 volume of 13.5M *ammonia* and 24 volumes of *methanol*. Solution (4) contains 0.40% w/v of *sulfadimidine EPCRS* in a mixture of 1 volume of 13.5M *ammonia* and 24 volumes of *methanol*. After removal of the plate, dry it at 100° to 105° and examine under *ultraviolet light (254 nm)*. Any *secondary spot* in the chromatogram obtained with solution (1) is not more intense than the spot in the chromatogram obtained with solution (3) (0.5%).

Assay Dissolve 6 g in a mixture of 75 ml of *water* and 10 ml of *hydrochloric acid* by warming gently, add 3 g of *potassium bromide*, cool in ice and titrate slowly with 0.1M *sodium nitrite VS*, stirring constantly and determining the end point electrometrically. Each ml of 0.1M *sodium nitrite VS* is equivalent to 27.83 mg of $C_{12}H_{14}N_4O_2S$. Determine the *weight per ml* of the oral suspension, Appendix V G, and calculate the content of $C_{12}H_{14}N_4O_2S$, weight in volume.

When paediatric sulphadimidine oral suspension is prescribed or demanded, Paediatric Sulfadimidine Oral Suspension shall be dispensed or supplied.

Sulfadimidine Tablets

Definition Sulfadimidine Tablets contain Sulfadimidine.

The tablets comply with the requirements stated under Tablets and with the following requirements.

Content of sulfadimidine, $C_{12}H_{14}N_4O_2S$ 95.0 to 105.0% of the prescribed or stated amount.

Identification

A. Triturate a quantity of the powdered tablets containing 0.5 g of Sulfadimidine with two 5-ml quantities of *chloroform* and discard the chloroform. Triturate the residue with 10 ml of 5M *ammonia* for 5 minutes, add 10 ml of *water* and filter. Warm the filtrate until most of the ammonia has been removed, cool, acidify with 6M *acetic acid*, wash the precipitate with *water* and dry at 105°. The *infrared absorption spectrum* of the residue, Appendix II A, is concordant with the *reference spectrum* of sulfadimidine.

B. In the test for Related substances, the principal spot in the chromatogram obtained with solution (2) corresponds to that in the chromatogram obtained with solution (4).

C. The residue obtained in test A yields the reaction characteristic of *primary aromatic amines*, Appendix VI, producing a bright orange-red precipitate.

Related substances Carry out the method for *thin-layer chromatography*, Appendix III A, using *silica gel GF_{254}* as the coating substance and a mixture of 3 volumes of 6M *ammonia*, 5 volumes of *water*, 40 volumes of *nitromethane* and 50 volumes of *1,4-dioxan* as the mobile phase. Apply separately to the plate 5 µl of each of the following solutions. For solution (1) extract a quantity of the powdered tablets containing 0.5 g of Sulfadimidine with 25 ml of a mixture of 1 volume of 13.5M *ammonia* and 9 volumes of *methanol* by shaking for 10 minutes, filter and use the filtrate. For solution (2) dilute 1 volume of solution (1) to 5 volumes with a mixture of 1 volume of 13.5M *ammonia* and 24 volumes of *methanol*. For solution (3) dilute 1 volume of solution (1) to 200 volumes with a mixture of 1 volume of 13.5M *ammonia* and 24 volumes of *methanol*. Solution (4) contains 0.40% w/v of *sulfadimidine EPCRS* in a mixture of 1 volume of 13.5M *ammonia* and 24 volumes of *methanol*. After removal of the plate, dry it at 100° to 105° and examine under *ultraviolet light (254 nm)*. Any *secondary spot* in the chromatogram obtained with solution (1) is not more intense than the spot in the chromatogram obtained with solution (3) (0.5%).

Assay Weigh and powder 20 tablets. Dissolve a quantity of the powder containing 0.5 g of Sulfadimidine as completely as possible in a mixture of 50 ml of *water* and 10 ml of *hydrochloric acid*, add 3 g of *potassium bromide*, cool in ice and titrate slowly with 0.1M *sodium nitrite VS*, stirring constantly and determining the end point electrometrically. Each ml of 0.1M *sodium nitrite VS* is equivalent to 27.83 mg of $C_{12}H_{14}N_4O_2S$.

Storage Sulfadimidine Tablets should be protected from light.

When sulphadimidine tablets are prescribed or demanded, Sulfadimidine Tablets shall be dispensed or supplied.

Sulfinpyrazone Tablets

Definition Sulfinpyrazone Tablets contain Sulfinpyrazone. They are coated.

The tablets comply with the requirements stated under Tablets and with the following requirements.

Content of sulfinpyrazone, $C_{23}H_{20}N_2O_3S$ 92.5 to 107.5% of the prescribed or stated amount.

Identification

Extract a quantity of the powdered tablets containing 0.2 g of Sulfinpyrazone with *chloroform*, filter and evaporate the filtrate to dryness on a water bath. The residue complies with the following tests.

A. The *light absorption*, Appendix II B, in the range 230 to 350 nm of a 0.002% w/v solution in 0.01M *sodium hydroxide* exhibits a maximum only at 260 nm.

B. Dissolve 10 mg in 3 ml of *acetone* and add 0.05 ml of *iron(III) chloride solution R2* and 3 ml of *water*. A red colour is produced.

Related substances Carry out the method for *thin-layer chromatography*, Appendix III A, using as the coating substance a suitable silica gel containing a fluorescent indicator with an optimal intensity at 254 nm (Merck silica gel 60 F_{254} plates are suitable) and a mixture of 20 volumes of *glacial acetic acid* and 80 volumes of *chloroform* as the mobile phase. Place the plate in a tank containing a beaker of *glacial acetic acid* and allow it to stand for 10 minutes. Heat the plate at 60° for 40 minutes, cool and pass a current of nitrogen over the plate for 10 minutes. Apply separately to the plate, under an atmosphere of nitrogen, 2 µl of each of the following solutions. For solution (1) shake a quantity of the powdered tablets containing 0.2 g of Sulfinpyrazone with 10 ml of *chloroform*, filter and use the filtrate. For solution (2) dilute 2 volumes of solution (1) to 100 volumes with *acetone* and dilute 1 volume of the resulting solution to 10 volumes with *acetone*. For solution (3) dissolve 10 mg of *1,2-diphenyl-4-(2-phenylsulphonylethyl)pyrazolidine-3,5-dione EPCRS* (impurity A) in 10 ml of *acetone*. For solution (4) dilute 5 volumes of solution (3) to 10 volumes with *acetone*. For solution (5) dissolve 10 mg of *1,2-diphenyl-4-(2-phenylthioethyl)pyrazolidine-3,5-dione EPCRS* (impurity B) in 10 ml of *acetone*. For solution (6) dilute 5 volumes of solution (5) to 10 volumes with *acetone*. After removal of the plate, allow it to dry in air and examine under *ultraviolet light (254 nm)*. In the chromatogram obtained with solution (1) any spots corresponding to impurity A and impurity B are not more intense than the spots in the chromatograms obtained with solutions (3) and (5) respectively (5% of each), not more than one such spot is more intense than the corresponding spot in the chromatogram obtained with solution (4) or (6) (2.5%) and any other *secondary spot* is not more intense than the spot in the chromatogram obtained with solution (2) (0.2%).

Assay Weigh and powder 20 tablets. Stir a quantity of the powder containing 0.5 g of Sulfinpyrazone with 10 ml of *petroleum spirit (boiling range, 40° to 60°)* for 10 minutes in a glass-stoppered flask. Decant through a sintered-glass filter, wash with two 7-ml quantities of *petroleum spirit (boiling range, 40° to 60°)* and discard the petroleum spirit. Warm to 80° to remove the solvent and extract the residue with six 20-ml quantities of hot *acetone* previously neutralised to *bromothymol blue solution R3*, decanting each solution and filtering through the sintered-glass filter. Titrate the combined extracts with 0.1M *sodium hydroxide VS* using *bromothymol blue solution R3* as indicator. Each ml of 0.1M *sodium hydroxide VS* is equivalent to 40.45 mg of $C_{23}H_{20}N_2O_3S$.

When sulphinpyrazone tablets are prescribed or demanded, Sulfinpyrazone Tablets shall be dispensed or supplied.

Surgical Spirit

Definition

Methyl Salicylate	5 ml
Diethyl Phthalate	20 ml
Castor Oil	25 ml
Industrial Methylated Spirit	sufficient to produce 1000 ml

The spirit complies with the requirements stated under Spirits and with the following requirements.

Content of methyl salicylate, $C_8H_8O_3$ 0.45 to 0.55% v/v.

Content of diethyl phthalate, $C_{12}H_{14}O_4$ 1.80 to 2.20% v/v.

Identification

A. To 1 ml add 0.5 ml of 0.4M *iron(III) chloride hexahydrate*. A violet colour is produced.

B. To 1 ml add 50 mg of *resorcinol* and 1 ml of *sulphuric acid*, heat for 1 minute, cool, pour into *water* and make alkaline with 5M *sodium hydroxide*. A distinct green fluorescence is produced which disappears when the solution is made acidic and reappears when it is made alkaline.

Weight per ml 0.817 to 0.827 g, Appendix V G.

Assay

For methyl salicylate Dilute 5 ml to 100 ml with *absolute ethanol*, further dilute 10 ml of this solution to 100 ml with *absolute ethanol* and measure the *absorbance* of the resulting solution at the maximum at 306 nm, Appendix II B. Calculate the content of $C_8H_8O_3$ taking 335 as the value of the *absorbance* of a 1% v/v solution of methyl salicylate at the maximum at 306 nm using a 1-cm cell.

For diethyl phthalate Further dilute 10 ml of the final solution prepared in the Assay for methyl salicylate to 50 ml with *absolute ethanol* and measure the *absorbance* of the resulting solution at 227 nm, Appendix II B. Subtract from the observed absorbance the absorbance due to the methyl salicylate present, as determined above, taking 432 as the value of the *absorbance* of a 1% v/v solution of methyl salicylate using a 1-cm cell. For the purposes of calculation take 419 as the value of the *absorbance* of a 1% v/v solution of diethyl phthalate at 227 nm using a 1-cm cell.

Labelling The label states that the preparation is flammable and should be kept away from a naked flame.

Suxamethonium Chloride Injection

Definition Suxamethonium Chloride Injection is a sterile solution of Suxamethonium Chloride in Water for Injections.

The injection complies with the requirements stated under Parenteral Preparations and with the following requirements.

Content of suxamethonium chloride, $C_{14}H_{30}Cl_2N_2O_4,2H_2O$ 90.0 to 107.5% of the prescribed or stated amount.

Identification Dilute a volume containing 20 mg of Suxamethonium Chloride to 50 ml with *water*. To 0.5 ml add 2 ml of *chloroform*, 2 ml of a solution containing 0.16% w/v of *citric acid* and 6.6% w/v of *disodium hydrogen orthophosphate* and 0.1 ml of a solution containing 0.15% w/v of *bromothymol blue* and 0.15% w/v of *anhydrous sodium carbonate*. Shake for 2 minutes and allow to separate. The chloroform layer is yellow.

Acidity pH, 3.0 to 5.0, Appendix V L.

Hydrolysis products The volume of 0.1M *sodium hydroxide VS* required for the preliminary neutralisation in the Assay is not more than one tenth of the total volume of 0.1M *sodium hydroxide VS* required for the preliminary neutralisation and the hydrolysis.

Assay To a volume containing 0.2 g of Suxamethonium Chloride add 30 ml of *carbon dioxide-free water* and shake with five 20-ml quantities of *ether*. Wash the combined ether solutions with two 10-ml quantities of *water* and discard the ether. Shake the combined washings with two 10-ml quantities of *ether*, add the washings to the original aqueous solution and neutralise with 0.1M *sodium hydroxide VS* using *bromothymol blue solution R3* as indicator. Add 25 ml of 0.1M *sodium hydroxide VS*, heat under a reflux condenser for 40 minutes, allow to cool and titrate the excess of alkali with 0.1M *hydrochloric acid VS* using *bromothymol blue solution R3* as indicator. Repeat the operation using 40 ml of *carbon dioxide-free water* and beginning at the words 'Add 25 ml ...'. The difference between the titrations represents the amount of sodium hydroxide required. Each ml of 0.1M *sodium hydroxide VS* is equivalent to 19.87 mg of $C_{14}H_{30}Cl_2N_2O_4,2H_2O$.

Storage Suxamethonium Chloride Injection should be stored at a temperature of 2° to 8°. It should not be allowed to freeze. Under these conditions it may be expected to continue to meet the requirements of the monograph for not less than 18 months after the date of preparation.

Syrup

Definition

Sucrose	667 g
Purified Water	sufficient to produce 1000 g

One or more suitable antimicrobial preservatives may be added.

Extemporaneous preparation The following directions apply.

Heat together until dissolved and add sufficient boiling Purified Water to produce 1000 g.

The syrup complies with the requirements stated under Syrups and with the following requirements.

Optical rotation +56° to +60°, Appendix V F.

Weight per ml 1.315 to 1.333 g, Appendix V G.

Storage Syrup should not be exposed to undue fluctuations in temperature.

Labelling The label states the names and proportions of any added antimicrobial preservatives.

When antimicrobial preservatives are added the suitability of the Syrup as a vehicle or diluent should be confirmed before use. The pH of Syrup may affect the solubility of basic or acidic materials.

Talc Dusting Powder

Definition Talc Dusting Powder is a sterile *cutaneous powder* of suitable fineness consisting of 10% of starch[1] and 90% of Purified Talc.

Production The starch is triturated with the Purified Talc and passed through a sieve of suitable mesh size (250 µm may be suitable). Either the Purified Talc is sterilised before use or the final product is subjected to a suitable sterilisation procedure.

The dusting powder complies with the requirements stated under Powders and with the following requirement.

Acid-insoluble matter 86.0 to 91.0% when determined by the following method. Boil 0.5 g with 10 ml of 2M *hydrochloric acid* for 5 minutes, cool, filter through a tared sintered-glass crucible (BS porosity No. 4), wash the residue with *water* until the washings are free from acid and dry to constant weight at 105°.

Labelling The label indicates the pharmaceutical form as 'cutaneous powder'.

[1]Maize Starch, Potato Starch, Rice Starch, Wheat Starch or, in tropical and subtropical countries where these are not available, Tapioca Starch may be used.

Tamoxifen Tablets

Definition Tamoxifen Tablets contain Tamoxifen Citrate.

With the exception of the requirements for shape, the tablets comply with the requirements stated under Tablets and with the following requirements.

Content of tamoxifen, $C_{26}H_{29}NO$ 90.0 to 110.0% of the prescribed or stated amount.

Identification

A. To a quantity of the powdered tablets containing the equivalent of 0.1 g of tamoxifen add 20 ml of *water*, warm, add 2 ml of 5M *sodium hydroxide* and cool. Extract with two 10-ml quantities of *ether*, filtering each extract in turn. Combine the ether extracts and evaporate to dryness in a current of nitrogen at room temperature. Dry the residue at a pressure not exceeding 0.7 kPa for 30 minutes. The *infrared absorption spectrum* of the dried residue, Appendix II A, is concordant with the *reference spectrum* of tamoxifen.

B. Shake a quantity of the powdered tablets containing the equivalent of 0.1 g of tamoxifen with 10 ml of *methanol*, filter, evaporate the filtrate to dryness on a water bath and dry the residue at 100° for 30 minutes. Dissolve 10 mg of the dried residue in 4 ml of *pyridine*, add 2 ml of *acetic anhydride* and heat on a water bath. A rose-pink to red colour is produced.

***E*-Isomer and other related substances** Carry out the method for *liquid chromatography*, Appendix III D, using the following solutions. For solution (1) mix a quantity of the powdered tablets containing the equivalent of 65 mg of tamoxifen with 60 ml of a mixture of 12 volumes of *acetonitrile*, 5 volumes of *water* and 3 volumes of *tetrahydrofuran* with the aid of ultrasound for 5 minutes, dilute to 100 ml with the same solvent mixture and filter (Whatman No. 1 is suitable). Solution (2) contains 0.1% w/v of *tamoxifen citrate impurity standard BPCRS* in the same solvent mixture. For solution (3) dilute 1 volume of solution (1) to 100 volumes with the same solvent mixture.

The chromatographic procedure may be carried out using (a) a stainless steel column (20 cm × 5 mm) packed with *stationary phase C* (5 µm) (Spherisorb ODS 1 is suitable), (b) a mixture of 2 volumes of 18M *ammonia*, 75 volumes of *tetrahydrofuran*, 125 volumes of *water* and 300 volumes of *acetonitrile* as the mobile phase with a flow rate of 1.5 ml per minute and (c) a detection wavelength of 240 nm.

In the chromatogram obtained with solution (2) a peak due to the *E*-isomer immediately follows the peak due to *Z*-tamoxifen. Adjust the sensitivity of the instrument so that the height of the peak due to *E*-tamoxifen is about 15% of full-scale deflection on the recorder. Measure the height of the peak due to *E*-tamoxifen by dropping a perpendicular from the apex of the peak to a line drawn tangentially between the troughs on each side of the *E*-isomer peak or the trough between the *E*- and *Z*-isomer peaks and the baseline, whichever is appropriate.

The test is not valid unless the height of the trough separating the peaks due to *E*- and *Z*-tamoxifen in the chromatogram obtained with solution (2) is less than 7% of full-scale deflection on the recorder and the retention time of the principal peak is less than 30 minutes. The retention time decreases with increasing concentration of ammonia in the mobile phase.

The content of *E*-isomer in the substance being examined is not more than 1% when calculated using the declared content of *E*-isomer in *tamoxifen citrate impurity standard BPCRS*. The area of any *secondary peak* in the chromatogram obtained with solution (1), other than a peak due to the *E*-isomer, is not greater than half that of the peak due to tamoxifen in the chromatogram obtained with solution (3) (0.5%) and the sum of the areas of all such peaks is not greater than the area of the peak due to tamoxifen in the chromatogram obtained with solution (3) (1%).

Dissolution Comply with the *dissolution test for tablets and capsules*, Appendix XII D, using as the medium 1000 ml of 0.02M *hydrochloric acid* and rotating the basket at 150 revolutions per minute. Withdraw a sample of 5 ml of the medium. Measure the *absorbance* of the filtered sample, suitably diluted if necessary, at 275 nm, Appendix II B. Calculate the total content of $C_{26}H_{29}NO$ in the medium taking 305 as the value of A(1%, 1 cm) at 275 nm.

Assay Weigh and powder 20 tablets. To a quantity of the powder containing the equivalent of 25 mg of tamoxifen add 100 ml of *methanol*, shake for 15 minutes and add sufficient *methanol* to produce 250 ml. Filter, dilute 10 ml of the filtrate to 100 ml with *methanol* and measure the *absorbance* of the resulting solution at 275 nm, Appendix II B. Calculate the content of $C_{26}H_{29}NO$ taking 325 as the value of A(1%, 1 cm) at 275 nm.

Storage Tamoxifen Tablets should be protected from light.

Labelling The quantity of active ingredient is stated in terms of the equivalent amount of tamoxifen.

Coal Tar and Salicylic Acid Ointment

Definition Coal Tar and Salicylic Acid Ointment contains 2% w/v of each of Coal Tar and Salicylic Acid in a suitable emulsifying basis.

Extemporaneous preparation The following formula and directions apply.

Coal Tar	20 g
Polysorbate 80	40 g
Salicylic Acid	20 g
Emulsifying Wax	114 g
White Soft Paraffin	190 g
Coconut Oil	540 g
Liquid Paraffin	76 g

Disperse the Coal Tar in the Polysorbate 80, incorporate the Salicylic Acid and mix with the previously melted Emulsifying Wax. Separately, melt the White Soft Paraffin and the Coconut Oil, incorporate the Liquid Paraffin warmed to the same temperature and add, with stirring, the resulting solution to the Coal Tar dispersion. Mix thoroughly and stir until cold.

The ointment complies with the requirements stated under Topical Semi-solid Preparations and with the following requirements.

Content of salicylic acid, $C_7H_6O_3$ 1.90 to 2.10% w/w.

Identification Disperse 2 g of the ointment in 20 ml of *water* with the aid of gentle heat, cool and filter. The filtrate yields reaction A characteristic of *salicylates*, Appendix VI.

Assay To 2 g add 50 ml of *water*, warm until melted, cool and decant the supernatant liquid through moistened absorbent cotton. Repeat the operation with a further three 50-ml quantities of *water*. Dilute the combined aqueous extracts to 250 ml with *water*, filter and dilute 10 ml of the filtrate to 50 ml with *iron(III) nitrate solution*. Filter if necessary and measure the *absorbance* of the resulting solution at the maximum at 530 nm, Appendix II B, using in the reference cell a solution prepared by diluting 10 ml of the filtered extract to 50 ml with *water*. Calculate the content of $C_7H_6O_3$ from the *absorbance* of the solution obtained by diluting 10 ml of a 0.016% w/v solution of *salicylic acid* to 50 ml with *iron(III) nitrate solution*, filtering if necessary, and using *water* in the reference cell.

Coal Tar and Zinc Ointment

Definition Coal Tar and Zinc Ointment contains 30% w/w of Zinc Oxide and 10% w/w of Strong Coal Tar Solution in a suitable hydrophobic basis.

Extemporaneous preparation The following formula and directions apply.

Strong Coal Tar Solution	100 g
Zinc Oxide, finely sifted	300 g
Yellow Soft Paraffin	600 g

Mix the Zinc Oxide with the Strong Coal Tar Solution, triturate with a portion of the Yellow Soft Paraffin until smooth, gradually incorporate the remainder of the Yellow Soft Paraffin and mix.

The ointment complies with the requirements stated under Topical Semi-solid Preparations and with the following requirements.

Content of zinc oxide, ZnO 28.5 to 31.5% w/w.

Identification The residue obtained in the Assay is yellow when hot and white when cool.

Assay Heat 0.5 g of the ointment gently in a porcelain dish over a small flame until the basis is completely volatilised or charred. Increase the heat until all the carbon is removed. Dissolve the residue in 10 ml of 2M *acetic acid* and add sufficient *water* to produce 50 ml. To the resulting solution add 50 mg of *xylenol orange triturate* and sufficient *hexamine* to produce a violet-pink colour. Add a further 2 g of *hexamine* and titrate with 0.1M *disodium edetate VS* until the solution becomes yellow. Each ml of 0.1M *disodium edetate VS* is equivalent to 8.138 mg of ZnO.

Coal Tar Paste

Definition

Strong Coal Tar Solution	75 g
Compound Zinc Paste	925 g

Extemporaneous preparation The following directions apply.

Triturate the Strong Coal Tar Solution with a portion of the Compound Zinc Paste until smooth and gradually incorporate the remainder of the Compound Zinc Paste.

The paste complies with the requirements stated under Topical Semi-solid Preparations and with the following requirements.

Content of zinc oxide, ZnO 21.0 to 25.0% w/w.

Identification The residue obtained in the Assay is yellow when hot and white when cool.

Assay Heat 0.5 g of the paste gently in a porcelain dish over a small flame until the basis is completely volatilised or charred. Increase the heat until all the carbon is removed. Dissolve the residue in 10 ml of 2M *acetic acid* and add sufficient *water* to produce 50 ml. To the resulting solution add 50 mg of *xylenol orange triturate* and sufficient *hexamine* to produce a violet-pink colour. Add a further 2 g of *hexamine* and titrate with 0.1M *disodium edetate VS* until the solution becomes yellow. Each ml of 0.1M *disodium edetate VS* is equivalent to 8.138 mg of ZnO.

Coal Tar Solution

Definition

Coal Tar	200 g
Polysorbate 80	50 g
Ethanol (96 per cent)	sufficient to produce 1000 ml

In making Coal Tar Solution, the Ethanol (96 per cent) may be replaced by Industrial Methylated Spirit[1].

Extemporaneous preparation The following directions apply.

Mix the Coal Tar, warmed if necessary to render it fluid, with the Polysorbate 80, pour this mixture in a thin stream into 800 ml of Ethanol (96 per cent) in a closed vessel fitted with an agitator; continue agitation throughout the addition of the mixture and for 1 hour thereafter. Allow the mixture to stand for not less than 24 hours, decant and filter the supernatant liquid, wash the vessel and filter with Ethanol (96 per cent), combine the filtrate and washings and add sufficient Ethanol (96 per cent) to produce 1000 ml.

Ethanol content 80 to 90% v/v, Appendix VIII F.

Storage Coal Tar Solution should be kept in a well-closed container.

Labelling The label states (1) the date after which the solution is not intended to be used; (2) the conditions under which it should be stored.

[1]The law and the statutory regulations governing the use of Industrial Methylated Spirit must be observed.

Strong Coal Tar Solution

Definition

Coal Tar	400 g
Polysorbate 80	50 g
Ethanol (96 per cent)	sufficient to produce 1000 ml

In making Strong Coal Tar Solution the Ethanol (96 per cent) may be replaced by Industrial Methylated Spirit[1].

Extemporaneous preparation The following directions apply.

Mix the Coal Tar, warmed if necessary to render it fluid, with the Polysorbate 80, pour this mixture in a thin stream into 700 ml of Ethanol (96 per cent) in a closed vessel fitted with an agitator; continue agitation throughout the addition of the mixture and for 1 hour thereafter. Allow the mixture to stand for not less than 24 hours, decant and filter the supernatant liquid, wash the vessel and filter with Ethanol (96 per cent), combine the filtrate and washings and add sufficient Ethanol (96 per cent) to produce 1000 ml.

Ethanol content 70 to 80% v/v, Appendix VIII F.

Storage Strong Coal Tar Solution should be kept in a well-closed container.

Labelling The label states (1) the date after which the solution is not intended to be used; (2) the conditions under which it should be stored.

[1]The law and the statutory regulations governing the use of Industrial Methylated Spirit must be observed.

Temazepam Oral Solution

Definition Temazepam Oral Solution is a solution of Temazepam in a suitable flavoured vehicle.

The oral solution complies with the requirements stated under Oral Liquids and with the following requirements.

Content of temazepam, $C_{16}H_{13}ClN_2O_2$ 90.0 to 110.0% of the prescribed or stated amount.

Identification

A. Dilute a quantity of the oral solution with sufficient 0.1M *methanolic hydrochloric acid* to produce a solution containing 0.001% w/v of Temazepam. The *light absorption* of the resulting solution, Appendix II B, in the range

210 to 400 nm exhibits three maxima, at 238 nm, 283 nm and 358 nm.

B. Carry out the method for *thin-layer chromatography*, Appendix III A, using a silica gel F_{254} precoated plate (Merck silica gel 60 F_{254} plates are suitable) and a mixture of 50 volumes of *cyclohexane*, 40 volumes of *chloroform* and 10 volumes of *diethylamine* as the mobile phase. Apply separately to the plate 2 µl of each of the following solutions. For solution (1) add 5 ml of *water* to a quantity of the oral solution containing 10 mg of Temazepam and extract with two 10-ml quantities of *ether*. Evaporate the combined ether extracts almost to dryness and dissolve the residue in 2 ml of *acetone*. Solution (2) contains 0.5% w/v of *temazepam BPCRS* in *acetone*. After removal of the plate, allow it to dry in air and examine under *ultraviolet light (254 nm)*. The principal spot in the chromatogram obtained with solution (1) corresponds to that in the chromatogram obtained with solution (2).

C. In the Assay, the chromatogram obtained with solution (2) exhibits a peak with the same retention time as that due to temazepam in the chromatogram obtained with solution (1).

Alkalinity pH, 7.3 to 8.3, Appendix V L.

6-Chloro-1,4-dihydro-1-methyl-4-phenylquinazolin-4-ol Carry out the method for *thin-layer chromatography*, Appendix III A, using a silica gel precoated plate (Merck silica gel 60 F_{254} plates are suitable) and a mixture of 92.5 volumes of *chloroform* and 7.5 volumes of *methanol* as the mobile phase but allowing the solvent front to ascend 12 cm above the line of application. Apply separately to the plate 10 µl of each of the following solutions. For solution (1) add 5 ml of *water* to a quantity of the oral solution containing 10 mg of Temazepam and extract with two 10-ml quantities of *ether*. Evaporate the combined ether extracts almost to dryness and dissolve the residue in 1 ml of *acetone*. Solution (2) contains 0.010% w/v of *6-chloro-1,4-dihydro-1-methyl-4-phenylquinazolin-4-ol BPCRS*. After removal of the plate, allow it to dry in a current of warm air and examine under *ultraviolet light (365 nm)*. In the chromatogram obtained with solution (1) any spot corresponding to 6-chloro-1,4-dihydro-1-methyl-4-phenylquinazolin-4-ol is not more intense than the spot in the chromatogram obtained with solution (2).

5-Chloro-2-methylaminobenzophenone Carry out the method for *liquid chromatography*, Appendix III D, using the following solutions. Solution (1) contains 0.00050% w/v of *5-chloro-2-methylaminobenzophenone BPCRS* in *methanol (50%)*. For solution (2) dilute a quantity of the oral solution with sufficient *methanol (50%)* to produce a solution containing 0.020% w/v of Temazepam.

The chromatographic procedure may be carried out using (a) a stainless steel column (25 cm × 5 mm) packed with *stationary phase C* (5 µm) (Lichrosorb RP-18 is suitable), (b) a mixture of 75 volumes of *methanol*, 25 volumes of *water* and 0.03 volume of *diethylamine* as the mobile phase with a flow rate of 1.5 ml per minute and (c) a detection wavelength of 254 nm.

In the chromatogram obtained with solution (2) the area of any peak corresponding to 5-chloro-2-methylaminobenzophenone is not greater than the area of the peak in the chromatogram obtained with solution (1).

Assay Carry out the method for *liquid chromatography*, Appendix III D, using the following solutions. Solution (1) contains 0.02% w/v of *temazepam BPCRS* in *methanol (50%)*. For solution (2) add sufficient *methanol (50%)* to a weighed quantity of the oral solution containing 20 mg of Temazepam to produce 100 ml.

The chromatographic procedure may be carried out using (a) a stainless steel column (20 cm × 4.6 mm) packed with *stationary phase C* (5 µm) (Hypersil ODS is suitable), (b) a mixture of 60 volumes of *methanol*, 40 volumes of *water* and 0.03 volumes of *diethylamine* as the mobile phase with a flow rate of 2 ml per minute and (c) a detection wavelength of 254 nm.

Determine the *weight per ml* of the oral solution, Appendix V G, and calculate the content of $C_{16}H_{13}ClN_2O_2$, weight in volume, using the declared content of $C_{16}H_{13}ClN_2O_2$ in *temazepam BPCRS*.

Storage Temazepam Oral Solution should be protected from light.

Terbutaline Tablets

Definition Terbutaline Tablets contain Terbutaline Sulphate.

The tablets comply with the requirements stated under Tablets and with the following requirements.

Content of terbutaline sulphate ($(C_{12}H_{19}NO_3)_2, H_2SO_4$) 90.0 to 110.0% of the prescribed or stated amount.

Identification

A. Shake a quantity of the powdered tablets containing 20 mg of Terbutaline Sulphate with 50 ml of 0.1M *sodium hydroxide* for 10 minutes, dilute to 100 ml with 0.1M *sodium hydroxide* and filter. Dilute 20 ml of the filtrate to 50 ml with 0.1M *sodium hydroxide*. The *light absorption* of the resulting solution, Appendix II B, in the range 230 to 350 nm exhibits a maximum only at 296 nm.

B. Carry out the method for *thin-layer chromatography*, Appendix III A, using a silica gel precoated plate (Merck silica gel 60 plates are suitable) and a mixture of 65 volumes of *propan-2-ol*, 25 volumes of *cyclohexane* and 5 volumes of *formic acid* as the mobile phase. Apply separately to the plate 2 µl of each of the following solutions. For solution (1) shake a quantity of the powdered tablets containing 10 mg of Terbutaline Sulphate with 4 ml of a mixture of equal volumes of *ethanol (96%)* and *water* for 10 minutes, centrifuge and use the clear solution. Solution (2) contains 0.25% w/v of *terbutaline sulphate BPCRS* in *water*. Solution (3) is a mixture of equal volumes of solutions (1) and (2). After removal of the plate, allow it to dry in air, allow to stand for a few minutes in an atmosphere saturated with *diethylamine* and spray with *diazotised nitroaniline solution*. The spot in the chromatogram obtained with solution (1) corresponds to that in the chromatogram obtained with solution (2) and the principal spot in the chromatogram obtained with solution (3) appears as a single compact spot.

Assay Weigh and powder 20 tablets. Carry out the method for *liquid chromatography*, Appendix III D, using the following solutions. For solution (1) dissolve 30 mg of *terbutaline sulphate BPCRS* in 50 ml of a 0.05% w/v solution of *orciprenaline sulphate BPCRS* (internal standard) in 0.05M *sulphuric acid* and add 4 ml of 1.5M *sodium acetate*. For solution (2) mix a quantity of the powdered tablets containing 15 mg of Terbutaline Sulphate with 25 ml of

0.05M *sulphuric acid,* shake for 15 minutes, add 2 ml of 1.5M *sodium acetate,* filter and use the filtrate. Prepare solution (3) in the same manner as solution (2) but using 25 ml of the internal standard solution in place of the sulphuric acid.

The chromatographic procedure may be carried out using (a) a stainless steel column (20 cm × 4 mm) packed with *stationary phase C* (10 µm) (Nucleosil C18 is suitable), (b) a mixture of *acetonitrile* and 0.005M *sodium octanesulphonate* adjusted to pH 3.4 with *glacial acetic acid* (21 volumes of *acetonitrile* and 79 volumes of the sodium octanesulphonate solution are usually suitable) as the mobile phase with a flow rate of 2 ml per minute and (c) a detection wavelength of 280 nm.

The assay is not valid unless baseline separation is obtained between the terbutaline sulphate peak and the internal standard peak.

Determine the areas of the peaks and calculate the content of $(C_{12}H_{19}NO_3)_2,H_2SO_4$ using the declared content of $(C_{12}H_{19}NO_3)_2,H_2SO_4$ in *terbutaline sulphate BPCRS.*

Testosterone Implants

Definition Testosterone Implants are sterile cylinders prepared by the fusion or heavy compression of Testosterone without the addition of any other substance.

The implants comply with the requirements stated under Parenteral Preparations and with the following requirements.

Content of testosterone, $C_{19}H_{28}O_2$ 97 to 103%, calculated with reference to the dried substance, and 90 to 110% of the prescribed or stated amount.

Diameter Implants containing less than 50 mg, 2.0 to 2.5 mm; implants containing 50 mg or more, 4.25 to 4.75 mm.

Where appropriate, powder the implants before carrying out the following tests.

Identification

A. The *infrared absorption spectrum,* Appendix II A, is concordant with the *reference spectrum* of testosterone.

B. Comply with the test for *identification of steroids,* Appendix III A, using *impregnating solvent II* and *mobile phase D.*

C. To 0.1 g in a stoppered tube add 3 ml of *anhydrous pyridine* and 0.6 ml of *acetic anhydride.* Heat on a water bath for 3 hours, add *water* dropwise until crystals begin to form, then add slowly a further 15 ml of *water* and allow to stand until precipitation is complete. Filter the precipitate using a sintered-glass crucible and wash with *water* until the washings are neutral to *methyl red solution.* Recrystallise from *ethanol (96%),* adding a few drops of *water* if necessary to aid crystallisation, and dry at 105°. The *melting point* of the crystals is about 140°, Appendix V A.

Melting point 152° to 156°, Appendix V A.

Specific optical rotation In a 1% w/v solution in *absolute ethanol,* +106° to +112°, Appendix V F, calculated with reference to the dried substance.

Carbonisation A 1% w/v solution in *ethanol (96%)* is *clear,* Appendix IV A, and *colourless,* Appendix IV B, Method I.

Loss on drying When dried to constant weight at 105°, lose not more than 1.0% of their weight. Use 1 g.

Sulphated ash Not more than 0.1%, Appendix IX A.

Assay Weigh and powder a single implant. Dissolve 10 mg of the powdered implant in sufficient *absolute ethanol* to produce 100 ml, dilute 5 ml to 50 ml with *absolute ethanol* and measure the *absorbance* of the resulting solution at the maximum at 240 nm, Appendix II B. Calculate the content of $C_{19}H_{28}O_2$ taking 560 as the value of A(1%, 1 cm) at the maximum at 240 nm.

Storage Testosterone Implants should be protected from light.

Testosterone Propionate Injection

Definition Testosterone Propionate Injection is a sterile solution of Testosterone Propionate in Ethyl Oleate or other suitable ester, in a suitable fixed oil or in any mixture of these.

The injection complies with the requirements stated under Parenteral Preparations and with the following requirements.

Content of testosterone propionate, $C_{22}H_{32}O_3$ 92.5 to 107.5% of the prescribed or stated amount.

Identification Dissolve a volume containing 50 mg of Testosterone Propionate in 8 ml of *petroleum spirit (boiling range, 40° to 60°)* and extract with three 8-ml quantities of a mixture of 7 volumes of *glacial acetic acid* and 3 volumes of *water.* Wash the combined extracts with 10 ml of *petroleum spirit (boiling range, 40° to 60°),* dilute with *water* until the solution becomes turbid, allow to stand for 2 hours in ice and filter. The precipitate, after washing with *water* and drying at 105°, complies with the following tests.

A. The *infrared absorption spectrum,* Appendix II A, is concordant with the *reference spectrum* of testosterone propionate.

B. Complies with the test for *identification of steroids,* Appendix III A, using *impregnating solvent III* and *mobile phase F.*

Assay To a volume containing 0.1 g of Testosterone Propionate add sufficient *chloroform* to produce 100 ml. Dilute 3 ml to 50 ml with *chloroform* and to 5 ml of the solution add 10 ml of *isoniazid solution* and sufficient *methanol* to produce 20 ml. Allow to stand for 45 minutes and measure the *absorbance* of the resulting solution at the maximum at 380 nm, Appendix II B, using in the reference cell a solution prepared by treating 5 ml of *chloroform* in the same manner. Calculate the content of $C_{22}H_{32}O_3$ from the *absorbance* obtained by repeating the operation using a 0.006% w/v solution of *testosterone propionate EPCRS* in *chloroform* and beginning at the words 'to 5 ml ... '.

Storage Testosterone Propionate Injection should be protected from light.

Labelling The label states that the preparation is intended for intramuscular injection only.

Tetracaine Eye Drops
Amethocaine Eye Drops

For the purposes of product labelling in the United Kingdom, the pair of names given above shall be used together (see Introduction, Changes in title).

Definition Tetracaine Eye Drops are a sterile solution of Tetracaine Hydrochloride in Purified Water.

The eye drops comply with the requirements stated under Eye Preparations and with the following requirements.

Content of tetracaine hydrochloride, $C_{15}H_{24}N_2O_2$, HCl 90.0 to 110.0% of the prescribed or stated amount.

Identification To a volume containing 10 mg of Tetracaine Hydrochloride add 1 ml of a 5% w/v solution of *sodium acetate* and 1 ml of a 25% w/v solution of *ammonium thiocyanate* and mix. A white precipitate is produced which, after recrystallisation from *water* and drying at 80° for 2 hours, has a *melting point* of about 131°, Appendix V A.

Related substances Carry out the method for *thin-layer chromatography*, Appendix III A, using *silica gel GF_{254}* as the coating substance and a mixture of 80 volumes of *dibutyl ether*, 16 volumes of *n-hexane* and 4 volumes of *glacial acetic acid* as the mobile phase. Place the plate in the tank, allow to stand until the solvent front has ascended about 12 cm, remove the plate and dry for a few minutes in a current of warm air. Allow to cool and apply separately to the plate 20 µl of solution (1) and 5 µl of solution (2). For solution (1) use the eye drops, diluted if necessary to contain 0.25% w/v of Tetracaine Hydrochloride. Solution (2) contains 0.0050% w/v of *4-aminobenzoic acid*. Allow the solvent front to ascend 10 cm above the line of application. After removal of the plate, dry it at 100° to 105° for 10 minutes and examine under *ultraviolet light (254 nm)*. Any *secondary spot* in the chromatogram obtained with solution (1) is not more intense than the spot in the chromatogram obtained with solution (2). The principal spot in the chromatogram obtained with solution (1) remains on the line of application.

Assay To a volume of the eye drops containing 20 mg of Tetracaine Hydrochloride add 5 ml of *acetate buffer pH 3.7* and 15 ml of 0.01M *sodium tetraphenylborate VS*, mix well, allow to stand for 10 minutes, filter through a sintered-glass filter (BS porosity No. 4), wash the filter with 5 ml of *water* and titrate the excess of sodium tetraphenylborate with 0.005M *cetylpyridinium chloride VS* using 0.5 ml of *bromophenol blue solution* as indicator. Repeat the operation without the eye drops. The difference between the titrations represents the amount of sodium tetraphenylborate required. Each ml of 0.01M *sodium tetraphenylborate VS* is equivalent to 3.008 mg of $C_{15}H_{24}N_2O_2$,HCl.

Storage Tetracaine Eye Drops should be protected from light.

Labelling The label states 'Tetracaine Eye Drops' and 'Amethocaine Eye Drops'.

Tetracosactide Injection

Definition Tetracosactide Injection is a sterile solution of Tetracosactide in Water for Injections.

The injection complies with the requirements stated under Parenteral Preparations and with the following requirements.

Content of tetracosactide, $C_{136}H_{210}N_{40}O_{31}$ 80.0 to 110.0% of the prescribed or stated amount of the peptide.

Characteristics A colourless solution.

Identification Mix 24 ml of *pyridine* and 16 ml of *glacial acetic acid* and add sufficient *water* to produce 100 ml (solution A). Carry out the method for *zone electrophoresis*, Appendix III F, using cellulose acetate foil as the support medium and an electrolyte solution containing 8% v/v of *glacial acetic acid* and 2% v/v of *pyridine*. Immerse the cellulose acetate foil in the electrolyte solution for 5 minutes and press dry between sheets of filter paper. Apply separately to the foil at points 1 cm from the anode edge and 2.5 cm apart 2 µl of each of the following solutions. For solution (1) evaporate to dryness a volume of the injection containing 0.5 mg of the peptide and dissolve the residue in 0.1 ml of solution A with the aid of gentle heat. For solution (2) dissolve 3.5 mg of *tetracosactide EPCRS* in 10 ml of *water* containing 10 µl of *glacial acetic acid*, 8.2 mg of *sodium acetate* and 81 mg of *sodium chloride*, evaporate 2 ml of the solution and dissolve the residue in 0.1 ml of solution A with the aid of gentle heat. Apply a voltage of 100 volts and allowing electrophoresis to proceed for 2 hours. Press the strips dry and immerse in a solution prepared by dissolving 1 g of *potassium hexacyanoferrate(III)* in 50 ml of *water* and adding 2 ml of a saturated solution of *iron(III) chloride hexahydrate*. Wash with a 5% v/v solution of *orthophosphoric acid* until the background is as pale as possible and finally wash with *water*. Examine the electrophoretograms while still moist. The principal spot in the electrophoretogram obtained with solution (1) corresponds to that in the electrophoretogram obtained with solution (2).

Acidity pH, 3.8 to 4.5, Appendix V L.

Tetracosactide sulphoxide Carry out the method for *liquid chromatography*, Appendix III D, using the following solutions prepared with de-aerated solvents. For solution (1) dilute the injection, if necessary, with *water* to give a final concentration of 0.025% w/v of the peptide. For solution (2) add 10 µl of a solution prepared by diluting 1 volume of *hydrogen peroxide solution (20 vol)* to 200 volumes with *water* to 1 ml of solution (1) and allow to stand for 2 hours.

The chromatographic conditions described under Assay may be used. Take care to ensure that the syringe used to inject solution (1) is not contaminated with peroxide.

The chromatogram obtained with solution (2) exhibits a peak due to tetracosactide corresponding to the principal peak in the chromatogram obtained with solution (1) and a peak with a shorter retention time, due to tetracosactide sulphoxide, of significantly greater area than any corresponding peak in the chromatogram obtained with solution (1). In the chromatogram obtained with solution (1) the relative amount of tetracosactide sulphoxide is not more than 10% by *normalisation*.

Assay Carry out the method for *liquid chromatography*, Appendix III D, using the following solutions. For solution (1) dilute the injection, if necessary, with *water* to give a final concentration of 0.025% w/v of the peptide. For solution (2) dissolve an amount of *tetracosactide EPCRS* in sufficient *water* to produce a solution containing 0.025% w/v of the peptide.

The chromatographic procedure may be carried out using (a) a stainless steel column (25 cm × 4.6 mm) packed with *stationary phase C* (10 µm) (Nucleosil C18 is suitable), (b) a mixture of 10 ml of *glacial acetic acid*, 365 ml of *acetonitrile* and 10 g of *ammonium sulphate* diluted to 2000 ml with *water* as the mobile phase with a flow rate of 2 ml per minute and (c) a detection wavelength of 280 nm.

Calculate the content of the peptide $C_{136}H_{210}N_{140}O_{31}S$ from the chromatograms obtained and using the declared content of $C_{136}H_{210}N_{140}O_{31}S$ in *tetracosactide EPCRS*.

The result obtained is not valid unless the *resolution factor* between the peaks due to tetracosactide and tetracosactide sulphoxide in the chromatogram obtained with solution (1) in the test for Tetracosactide sulphoxide is at least 7.

Storage Tetracosactide Injection should be protected from light and stored at a temperature of 2° to 8°.

Labelling The strength is stated in terms of the equivalent amount of the peptide in micrograms per ml.

The label also states that the preparation is for intravenous infusion or intramuscular injection only.

When tetracosactrin injection is prescribed or demanded, Tetracosactide Injection shall be dispensed or supplied.

Tetracosactide Zinc Injection

Definition Tetracosactide Zinc Injection is a sterile aqueous suspension of Tetracosactide with zinc hydroxide.

The injection complies with the requirements stated under Parenteral Preparations and with the following requirements.

Content of tetracosactide, $C_{136}H_{210}N_{40}O_{31}$ 80.0 to 110.0% of the prescribed or stated amount of the peptide.

Characteristics A white, flocculent suspension which settles slowly and is readily resuspended. On examination under a microscope the majority of the particles are seen as amorphous or microcrystalline particles or aggregates thereof. The maximum dimension of single particles rarely exceeds 50 µm. Under high power magnification a considerable proportion of the particles can be seen to have no uniform shape.

Identification

A. Carry out the test for Identification described under Tetracosactide Injection using the following solutions. For solution (1) freeze dry a quantity of the well-shaken suspension containing 2 mg of the peptide and dissolve the residue in a mixture of 0.1 ml of *formic acid* and 0.1 ml of *water* with the aid of gentle heat. For solution (2) dissolve 10.45 g of *zinc chloride* in 20 ml of *water*, add 95 ml of *formic acid* followed by 4.2 g of *disodium hydrogen orthophosphate* and 4.0 g of *sodium chloride*. Dissolve 6.04 g of *sodium hydroxide* in 40 ml of *water*. Mix the two solutions carefully with cooling and add sufficient *water* to produce 200 ml. Dissolve 2.8 mg of *tetracosactide EPCRS* in 0.2 ml of the resulting solution. The principal spot in the electrophoretogram obtained with solution (1) corresponds to that in the electrophoretogram obtained with solution (2).

B. Evaporate 1 ml of the well-shaken suspension to dryness in a crucible and heat strongly until combustion of the organic material is complete. The residue is yellow while hot and becomes white on cooling.

Alkalinity pH, 7.8 to 9.2, Appendix V L.

Light absorption Centrifuge 7 ml of the well-shaken suspension for 10 minutes at about 2000 *g*. Shake the clear, supernatant liquid with five 5-ml quantities of *chloroform*, previously washed with *water*. Discard the chloroform and centrifuge the aqueous phase for 5 minutes at about 2000 *g*. The *absorbance* of the clear, supernatant liquid at 276 nm, Appendix II B, is not more than 0.38 for preparations containing 1 mg of the peptide per ml and not more than 0.19 for preparations containing 0.5 mg of the peptide per ml.

Sediment volume Transfer 3.0 ml of the well-shaken suspension to a cuvette 10 mm × 10 mm in cross section. Allow to stand for 5 hours. The depth of the sediment is between 8 and 25 mm and the supernatant liquid is clear.

Zinc To a volume of the well-shaken suspension containing 1 mg of the peptide add 5 ml of 0.1M *hydrochloric acid* and sufficient *water* to produce 1000 ml. Carry out the method for *atomic absorption spectrophotometry*, Appendix II D, measuring at 214 nm and using *zinc standard solution (5 mg/ml Zn)*, diluted if necessary with *water*, to prepare the standard solution. Preparations containing 1 mg of the peptide per ml contain 2.25 to 2.75 mg of zinc per ml; preparations containing 0.5 mg of the peptide per ml contain 1.35 to 1.65 mg of zinc per ml.

Tetracosactide sulphoxide Carry out the test described under Tetracosactide Injection using the following solutions. For solution (1) mix a volume of the well-shaken suspension containing 1 mg of the peptide with 15 µl of *glacial acetic acid*. For solution (2) add 50 µl of a solution prepared by diluting 1 volume of *hydrogen peroxide solution (20 vol)* to 200 volumes to 1 ml of a 0.1% w/v solution of *tetracosactide EPCRS* in a 1% v/v solution of *glacial acetic acid* and allow to stand for 2 hours. The chromatogram obtained with solution (2) exhibits a peak due to tetracosactide and a significant peak with a shorter retention time, due to tetracosactide sulphoxide. In the chromatogram obtained with solution (1) the area of the peak due to tetracosactide sulphoxide is not more than 18% of the area of the peak due to tetracosactide. The peaks due to associated substances may be identified from the chromatogram obtained with solution (2) in the Assay.

Assay Carry out the Assay described under Tetracosactide Injection using the following solutions. For solution (1) mix 1 ml of the well-shaken suspension with 15 µl of *glacial acetic acid*. For preparations containing 1 mg of the peptide per ml prepare solution (2) by dissolving quantities of *tetracosactide EPCRS* and *benzyl alcohol* in sufficient *water* to produce a solution containing the equivalent of 0.10% w/v of the peptide and 1.0% w/v of *benzyl alcohol* and adding 15 µl of *glacial acetic acid* per ml. For preparations containing 0.5 mg of the peptide per ml prepare solution (2) by dissolving quantities of *tetracosactide EPCRS* and *benzyl alcohol* in sufficient *water* to produce a solution containing the equivalent of 0.05% w/v of the peptide and 1.0% w/v of *benzyl alcohol* and adding 15 µl of *glacial acetic acid* per ml. If necessary, adjust the ratio of the volumes of *acetonitrile* and *water* in the mobile phase so that in the chromatogram obtained with solution (2) the *resolution factor* between the peaks due to benzyl alcohol (eluted before tetracosactide) and tetracosactide is between 1.5 and 2.0.

Storage Tetracosactide Zinc Injection should be protected from light and stored at a temperature of 2° to 8°. It should not be allowed to freeze.

Labelling The strength is stated in terms of the equivalent amount of the peptide in mg per ml.

The label also states (1) that the preparation is for intramuscular injection only; (2) that the container should be gently shaken before a dose is withdrawn.

When tetracosactrin zinc injection is prescribed or demanded, Tetracosactide Zinc Injection shall be dispensed or supplied.

Tetracycline Capsules

Definition Tetracycline Capsules contain Tetracycline Hydrochloride.

The capsules comply with the requirements stated under Capsules and with the following requirements.

Content of tetracycline hydrochloride, $C_{22}H_{24}N_2O_8$, HCl 95.0 to 105.0% of the prescribed or stated amount.

Identification

A. Carry out the method for *thin-layer chromatography*, Appendix III A, using *silica gel H* as the coating substance. Adjust the pH of a 10% w/v solution of *disodium edetate* to 8.0 with 10M *sodium hydroxide* and spray the solution evenly onto the plate (about 10 ml for a plate 100 mm × 200 mm). Allow the plate to dry in a horizontal position at room temperature for at least 1 hour. Before use, dry the plate in an oven at 110° for 1 hour. Use a mixture of 6 volumes of *water*, 35 volumes of *methanol* and 59 volumes of *dichloromethane* as the mobile phase. Apply separately to the plate 1 µl of each of the following solutions. For solution (1) extract a quantity of the contents of the capsules containing 10 mg of Tetracycline Hydrochloride with 20 ml of *methanol* and centrifuge. Solution (2) contains 0.05% w/v of *tetracycline hydrochloride EPCRS* in *methanol*. Solution (3) contains 0.05% w/v of each of *tetracycline hydrochloride EPCRS*, *chlortetracycline hydrochloride EPCRS* and *doxycycline hyclate EPCRS* in *methanol*. Dry the plate in a current of air and examine under *ultraviolet light (365 nm)*. The principal spot in the chromatogram obtained with solution (1) is similar in position, colour and size to the principal spot in the chromatogram obtained with solution (2). The test is not valid unless the chromatogram obtained with solution (3) shows three clearly separated spots.

B. To a quantity of the contents of the capsules containing 10 mg of Tetracycline Hydrochloride add 20 ml of warm *ethanol (96%)*, allow to stand for 20 minutes, filter and evaporate the filtrate to dryness on a water bath. To 0.5 mg of the residue add 2 ml of *sulphuric acid*; a deep crimson colour is produced. Add 1 ml of *water*; the colour changes to deep yellow.

C. The residue obtained in test B yields the reactions characteristic of *chlorides*, Appendix VI.

Dissolution Comply with the *dissolution test for tablets and capsules*, Appendix XII D, using as the medium 900 ml of 0.1M *hydrochloric acid* and rotating the basket at 100 revolutions per minute. Withdraw a sample of 10 ml of the medium. Measure the *absorbance* of the filtered sample, suitably diluted if necessary, at the maximum at 353 nm, Appendix II B. Calculate the total content of tetracycline hydrochloride, $C_{22}H_{24}N_2O_8$,HCl, in the medium taking 310 as the value of A(1%, 1 cm) at the maximum at 353 nm.

4-Epitetracycline hydrochloride Carry out the method for *liquid chromatography*, Appendix III D, using the following solutions. For solution (1) shake a quantity of the mixed contents of 20 capsules containing 25 mg of Tetracycline Hydrochloride in 80 ml of 0.01M *methanolic hydrochloric acid* for 10 minutes, dilute to 100 ml with the same solvent, mix and filter if necessary. Solution (2) contains 0.0020% w/v of *4- epitetracycline hydrochloride EPCRS* in 0.01M *methanolic hydrochloric acid*. Solution (3) contains 0.0015% w/v each of *4-epitetracycline hydrochloride EPCRS* and *tetracycline hydrochloride EPCRS* in 0.01M *methanolic hydrochloric acid*.

The chromatographic procedure may be carried out using (a) a stainless steel column (20 cm × 4.6 mm) packed with *stationary phase B* or *C* (10 µm) (Nucleosil C18 is suitable) and maintained at 40°, (b) as the mobile phase with a flow rate of 2 ml per minute a mixture of 5 volumes of *dimethylformamide* and 95 volumes of 0.1M *oxalic acid* the pH of which has been adjusted to 3.9 with *triethylamine* and (c) a detection wavelength of 280 nm.

The test is not valid unless the resolution factor between the two principal peaks in the chromatogram obtained with solution (3) is at least 2.0.

In the chromatogram obtained with solution (1) the area of any peak corresponding to 4-epitetracycline is not greater than the area of the principal peak in the chromatogram obtained with solution (2).

Anhydrotetracycline hydrochloride and 4-epianhydrotetracycline hydrochloride Carry out the method for *liquid chromatography*, Appendix III D, using the following solutions. For solution (1) shake a quantity of the mixed contents of 20 capsules containing 25 mg of Tetracycline Hydrochloride in 20 ml of 0.01M *methanolic hydrochloric acid* for 10 minutes, dilute to 25 ml with the same solvent, mix and filter if necessary. Solution (2) contains 0.0010% w/v each of *anhydrotetracycline hydrochloride EPCRS* and *4-epianhydrotetracycline hydrochloride EPCRS* in 0.01M *methanolic hydrochloric acid*. Solution (3) contains 0.0010% w/v each of *4-epianhydrotetracycline hydrochloride EPCRS* and *tetracycline hydrochloride EPCRS*.

The chromatographic conditions described under Epitetracycline hydrochloride may be used but use as the mobile phase a mixture of 10 volumes of *dimethylformamide*, 12 volumes of *acetonitrile* and 78 volumes of 0.1M *oxalic acid* the pH of which has been adjusted to 3.9 with *triethylamine*. The order of emergence of the peaks is tetracycline, 4-epianhydrotetracycline and anhydrotetracycline.

The test is not valid unless the *resolution factor* between the two principal peaks in the chromatogram obtained with solution (3) is at least 6.0.

In the chromatogram obtained with solution (1) the area of any peaks corresponding to anhydrotetracycline hydrochloride and 4-epianhydrotetracycline hydrochloride is not greater than the area of the respective principal peak in the chromatogram obtained with solution (2).

Loss on drying When dried at 60° at a pressure not exceeding 0.7 kPa for 3 hours, the contents of the capsules lose not more than 3.0% of their weight. Use 1 g.

Assay Carry out the method for *liquid chromatography*, Appendix III D, using the following solutions. For solution (1) shake a quantity of the mixed contents of 20 capsules containing 25 mg of Tetracycline Hydrochloride in 80 ml of 0.01M *methanolic hydrochloric acid* for 10 minutes, dilute to 100 ml with the same solvent, mix and filter if necessary. Solution (2) contains 0.025% w/v of *tetracycline hydrochloride EPCRS* in 0.01M *methanolic hydrochloric acid*. Solution (3) contains 0.025% w/v each of *4-epitetracycline hydrochloride EPCRS* and *tetracycline hydrochloride EPCRS* in 0.01M *methanolic hydrochloric acid*.

The chromatographic conditions described under 4-Epitetracycline hydrochloride may be used.

The assay is not valid unless the *resolution factor* between the two principal peaks in the chromatogram obtained with solution (3) is at least 2.0.

Calculate the content of $C_{22}H_{24}N_2O_8$,HCl in the capsules using the declared content of $C_{22}H_{24}N_2O_8$,HCl in *tetracycline hydrochloride EPCRS*.

Tetracycline Intravenous Infusion

Tetracycline Injection

Definition Tetracycline Intravenous Infusion is a sterile solution of Tetracycline Hydrochloride in Water for Injections. It is prepared by dissolving Tetracycline Hydrochloride for Intravenous Infusion in the requisite amount of Water for Injections and diluting the resulting solution with a suitable diluent in accordance with the manufacturer's instructions immediately before use.

The intravenous infusion complies with the requirements stated under Parenteral Preparations.

Storage Tetracycline Intravenous Infusion deteriorates on storage and should be used immediately after preparation.

TETRACYCLINE HYDROCHLORIDE FOR INTRAVENOUS INFUSION

Definition Tetracycline Hydrochloride for Intravenous Infusion is a sterile material consisting of Tetracycline Hydrochloride with or without auxiliary substances. It is supplied in a sealed container.

The contents of the sealed container comply with the requirements for Powders for Injections stated under Parenteral Preparations and with the following requirements.

Content of tetracycline hydrochloride, $C_{22}H_{24}N_2O_8$, HCl 95.0 to 105.0% of the prescribed or stated amount.

Characteristics A pale yellow solid.

Identification

A. Comply with test A described under Tetracycline Capsules using a 0.05% w/v solution of the preparation being examined as solution (1).

B. To 0.5 mg add 2 ml of *sulphuric acid*; a purplish red colour is produced. Add 1 ml of *water*; the colour changes to deep yellow.

C. Yield reaction A characteristic of *chlorides*, Appendix VI.

Acidity pH of a 10% w/v solution, 2.0 to 3.0, Appendix V L.

Clarity and colour of solution A 10.0% w/v solution is *clear*, Appendix IV A, and yellow.

4-Epitetracycline hydrochloride Complies with test described under Tetracycline Capsules. For solution (1) dissolve a quantity of the mixed contents of 10 containers containing 25 mg of Tetracycline Hydrochloride in sufficient 0.01M *methanolic hydrochloric acid* to produce 100 ml.

Anhydrotetracycline hydrochloride and 4-epi-anhydrotetracycline hydrochloride Complies with the test described under Tetracycline Capsules. For solution (1) dissolve a quantity of the mixed contents of 10 containers containing 25 mg of Tetracycline Hydrochloride in sufficient 0.01M *methanolic hydrochloric acid* to produce 25 ml.

Bacterial endotoxins Carry out the *test for bacterial endotoxins*, Appendix XIV C. Dissolve the contents of the sealed container in *water BET* to give a solution containing 10 mg of Tetracycline Hydrochloride per ml (solution A). The endotoxin limit concentration of solution A is 5 IU of endotoxin per ml. Carry out the test using the maximum valid dilution of solution A calculated from the declared sensitivity of the lysate used in the test.

Assay Determine the weight of the contents of 10 containers as described in the test for Uniformity of weight under Parenteral Preparations, Powders for Injections.

Carry out the Assay described under Tetracycline Capsules. For solution (1) dissolve a quantity of the mixed contents of 10 containers containing 25 mg of Tetracycline Hydrochloride in sufficent 0.01M *methanolic hydrochloric acid* to produce 100 ml.

Calculate the content of $C_{22}H_{24}N_2O_8$,HCl in a container of average content weight using the declared content of $C_{22}H_{24}N_2O_8$,HCl in *tetracycline hydrochloride EPCRS*.

Storage The sealed container should be protected from light.

Labelling The label of the sealed container states (1) the weight of Tetracycline Hydrochloride contained in it; (2) that the contents are to be used for intravenous infusion only, in a well-diluted solution.

Tetracycline Tablets

Definition Tetracycline Tablets contain Tetracycline Hydrochloride. They are coated.

The tablets comply with the requirements stated under Tablets and with the following requirements.

Content of tetracycline hydrochloride, $C_{22}H_{24}N_2O_8$, HCl 95.0 to 105.0% of the prescribed or stated amount.

Identification

A. Comply with test A described under Tetracycline Capsules using the following solution as solution (1). Extract a quantity of the powdered tablets containing 10 mg of Tetracycline Hydrochloride with 20 ml of *methanol*, centrifuge and use the supernatant liquid.

B. Extract a quantity of the powdered tablets containing 25 mg of Tetracycline Hydrochloride with 25 ml of *methanol* for 20 minutes, filter and evaporate the filtrate to dryness on a water bath. To 0.5 mg of the residue add 2 ml of *sulphuric acid*; a purplish red colour is produced. Add 1 ml of *water*; the colour changes to deep yellow.

C. The residue obtained in test B yields the reactions characteristic of *chlorides*, Appendix VI.

Dissolution Comply with the *dissolution test for tablets and capsules*, Appendix XII D, using as the medium 900 ml of 0.1M *hydrochloric acid* and rotating the basket at 100 revolutions per minute. Withdraw a sample of 10 ml of the medium. Measure the *absorbance* of the filtered sample, suitably diluted if necessary, at the maximum at 353 nm, Appendix II B. Calculate the total content of tetracycline hydrochloride, $C_{22}H_{24}N_2O_8$,HCl, in the medium taking 310 as the value of A(1%, 1 cm) at the maximum at 353 nm.

4-Epitetracycline hydrochloride Complies with test described under Tetracycline Capsules. For solution (1) shake a quantity of the powdered tablets containing 25 mg of Tetracycline Hydrochloride with 80 ml of 0.01M *methanolic hydrochloric acid*, dilute to 100 ml with the same solvent, mix and filter if necessary.

Anhydrotetracycline hydrochloride and 4-epianhydrotetracycline hydrochloride Complies with the test described under Tetracycline Capsules. For solution (1) shake a quantity of the powdered tablets containing 25 mg of Tetracycline Hydrochloride with 20 ml of 0.01M *methanolic hydrochloric acid*, dilute to 25 ml with the same solvent, mix and filter if necessary.

Loss on drying When dried at 60° at a pressure not exceeding 0.7 kPa for 3 hours, the powdered tablets lose not more than 3.0% of their weight. Use 1 g.

Assay Weigh and powder 20 tablets and carry out the Assay described under Tetracycline Capsules. For solution (1) shake a quantity of the powdered tablets containing 25 mg of Tetracycline Hydrochloride with 80 ml of 0.01M *methanolic hydrochloric acid*, dilute to 100 ml with the same solvent, mix and filter if necessary.

Calculate the content of $C_{22}H_{24}N_2O_8$,HCl in the tablets using the declared content of $C_{22}H_{24}N_2O_8$,HCl in *tetracycline hydrochloride EPCRS*.

Thiamine Injection

Definition Thiamine Injection is a sterile solution of Thiamine Hydrochloride in Water for Injections.

The injection complies with the requirements stated under Parenteral Preparations and with the following requirements.

Content of thiamine hydrochloride, $C_{12}H_{17}ClN_4OS$, HCl 95.0 to 105.0% of the prescribed or stated amount.

Characteristics A colourless or almost colourless solution.

Identification

A. Carry out the method for *thin-layer chromatography*, Appendix III A, using *cellulose F_{254}* as the coating substance and a mixture of 60 volumes of *butan-1-ol*, 25 volumes of *water* and 15 volumes of *glacial acetic acid* as the mobile phase. Apply separately to the plate 2 µl of each of the following solutions. For solution (1) use the injection diluted if necessary with *water* to contain 0.1% w/v of Thiamine Hydrochloride. Solution (2) contains 0.1% w/v of *thiamine mononitrate BPCRS* in *water*. After removal of the plate, allow it to dry in air, heat at 105° for 30 minutes, spray with a mixture of equal volumes of a 0.3% w/v solution of *potassium hexacyanoferrate(III)* and a 10% w/v solution of *sodium hydroxide* and examine under *ultraviolet light (365 nm)*. The principal spot in the chromatogram obtained with solution (1) corresponds to that in the chromatogram obtained with solution (2).

B. To a volume containing 20 mg of Thiamine Hydrochloride diluted, if necessary, to 10 ml with *water*, add 2 ml of 1M *acetic acid* and 1.6 ml of 1M *sodium hydroxide*, heat in a water bath for 30 minutes and cool. Add 5 ml of 5M *sodium hydroxide*, 10 ml of *dilute potassium hexacyanoferrate(III) solution* and 10 ml of *butan-1-ol* and shake vigorously for 2 minutes. The upper layer shows an intense light blue fluorescence on exposure to ultraviolet light. Repeat the test but adding 0.9 ml of 1M *sodium hydroxide* and 0.2 g of *sodium sulphite* in place of the 1.6 ml of 1M *sodium hydroxide*. Not more than a slight fluorescence is produced.

C. To a mixture of 0.1 ml of *nitrobenzene* and 0.2 ml of *sulphuric acid* add a volume of the injection containing 5 mg of Thiamine Hydrochloride. Allow to stand for 10 minutes, cool in ice and add slowly with stirring 5 ml of *water* followed by 5 ml of 10M *sodium hydroxide*. Add 5 ml of *acetone* and allow to stand. No violet colour is produced in the upper layer.

Acidity pH, 2.8 to 3.4, Appendix V L.

Assay Carry out the method for *liquid chromatography*, Appendix III D, using the following solutions. Solution (1) contains 0.005% w/v of *thiamine mononitrate BPCRS* in 0.005M *hydrochloric acid*. For solution (2) dilute a volume of the injection containing 0.1 g of Thiamine Hydrochloride to 100 ml with 0.1M *hydrochloric acid* and further dilute 5 ml to 100 ml with *water*.

The chromatographic procedure may be carried out using (a) a stainless steel column (10 cm × 4.6 mm) packed with *stationary phase C* (5 µm) (Nucleosil C18 is suitable), (b) as the mobile phase with a flow rate of 2 ml per minute a solution prepared by dissolving 1 g of *sodium heptanesulphonate* in a mixture of 180 ml of *methanol* and 10 ml of *triethylamine*, diluting to 1000 ml with *water* and adjusting the pH to 3.2 with *orthophosphoric acid* and (c) a detection wavelength of 244 nm.

Calculate the content of $C_{12}H_{17}ClN_4OS$,HCl using the declared content of $C_{12}H_{17}N_5O_4S$ in *thiamine mononitrate BPCRS*. Each mg of $C_{12}H_{17}N_5O_4S$ is equivalent to 1.030 mg of $C_{12}H_{17}ClN_4OS$,HCl.

Storage Thiamine Injection should be protected from light.

When vitamin B_1 injection is prescribed or demanded, Thiamine Injection shall be dispensed or supplied.

Thiamine Tablets

Definition Thiamine Tablets contain Thiamine Hydrochloride.

The tablets comply with the requirements stated under Tablets and with the following requirements.

Content of thiamine hydrochloride, $C_{12}H_{17}ClN_4OS$, HCl 92.5 to 107.5% of the prescribed or stated amount.

Identification

A. Carry out the method for *thin-layer chromatography*,

Appendix III A, using *cellulose F_{254}* as the coating substance and a mixture of 60 volumes of *butan-1-ol*, 25 volumes of *water* and 15 volumes of *glacial acetic acid* as the mobile phase. Apply separately to the plate 2 µl of each of the following solutions. For solution (1) shake a quantity of the powdered tablets containing 20 mg of Thiamine Hydrochloride with 20 ml of *water* and filter. Solution (2) contains 0.1% w/v of *thiamine mononitrate BPCRS*. After removal of the plate, allow it to dry in air, heat at 105° for 30 minutes, spray with a mixture of equal volumes of a 0.3% w/v solution of *potassium hexacyanoferrate(III)* and a 10% w/v solution of *sodium hydroxide* and examine under *ultraviolet light (365 nm)*. The principal spot in the chromatogram obtained with solution (1) corresponds to that in the chromatogram obtained with solution (2).

B. Dissolve a quantity of the powdered tablets containing 20 mg of Thiamine Hydrochloride as completely as possible in 10 ml of *water* and 2 ml of 1M *acetic acid*, filter, add 1.6 ml of 1M *sodium hydroxide*, heat in a water bath for 30 minutes and cool. Add 5 ml of 5M *sodium hydroxide*, 10 ml of *dilute potassium hexacyanoferrate(III) solution* and 10 ml of *butan-1-ol* and shake vigorously for 2 minutes. The alcohol layer shows an intense light blue fluorescence on exposure to ultraviolet light. Repeat the test but adding 0.9 ml of 1M *sodium hydroxide* and 0.2 g of *sodium sulphite* in place of the 1.6 ml of 1M sodium hydroxide; not more than a slight fluorescence is produced.

Assay Weigh and powder 20 tablets. Carry out the Assay described under Thiamine Injection using the following solutions. Solution (1) contains 0.006% w/v of *thiamine mononitrate BPCRS* in 0.005M *hydrochloric acid*. Prepare solution (2) in the following manner. For tablets containing less than 10 mg of thiamine hydrochloride, add 5 ml of 0.1M *hydrochloric acid* and 50 ml of *water* to a quantity of the powdered tablets containing 6 mg of Thiamine Hydrochloride, shake for 20 minutes, dilute to 100 ml with *water* and filter. For tablets containing 10 mg or more of Thiamine Hydrochloride, add 50 ml of 0.1M *hydrochloric acid* and 500 ml of *water* to a quantity of the powdered tablets containing 60 mg of Thiamine Hydrochloride, shake for 20 minutes, dilute to 1000 ml with *water* and filter.

Storage Thiamine Tablets should be kept free from contact with metal and protected from light.

When vitamin B_1 tablets are prescribed or demanded, Thiamine Tablets shall be dispensed or supplied.

Thiopental Injection

Definition Thiopental Injection is a sterile solution of Thiopental Sodium in Water for Injections. It is prepared by dissolving Thiopental Sodium for Injection in the requisite amount of Water for Injections.

The injection complies with the requirements stated under Parenteral Preparations.

Storage Thiopental Injection should be used immediately after preparation but, in any case, within the period recommended by the manufacturer when prepared and stored strictly in accordance with the manufacturer's instructions.

THIOPENTAL SODIUM FOR INJECTION

Definition Thiopental Sodium for Injection is a sterile material consisting of Thiopental Sodium with or without excipients. It is supplied in a sealed container.

The contents of the sealed container comply with the requirements for Powders for Injections stated under Parenteral Preparations and with the following requirements.

Content of $C_{11}H_{18}N_2O_2S$ 77.0 to 92.0% of the prescribed or stated amount of Thiopental Sodium.

Content of Na 9.4 to 11.8% of the prescribed or stated amount of Thiopental Sodium.

Identification

A. Dissolve 0.1 g in 5 ml of *water*, add 1 ml of 2M *hydrochloric acid* and extract with two 25-ml quantities of *chloroform*. Wash the extracts with *water*, dry with *anhydrous sodium sulphate*, evaporate to dryness and dry the residue at 50° at a pressure of 2 kPa. The *infrared absorption spectrum* of the residue, Appendix II A, is concordant with the *reference spectrum* of thiopental.

B. Yield the reaction characteristic of *non-nitrogen substituted barbiturates*, Appendix VI.

C. Yield reaction A characteristic of *sodium salts*, Appendix VI.

Clarity and colour of solution A 10.0% w/v solution in *carbon dioxide-free water* is *clear*, Appendix IV A, and not more intensely coloured than *reference solution GY_3*, Appendix IV B, Method II.

Related substances Carry out the method for *thin-layer chromatography*, Appendix III A, using *silica gel GF_{254}* as the coating substance and the lower layer of a mixture of 5 volumes of 13.5M *ammonia*, 15 volumes of *ethanol (96%)* and 80 volumes of *chloroform* as the mobile phase. Apply separately to the plate 20 µl of each of two solutions of the substance being examined in *water* containing (1) 1.0% w/v and (2) 0.005% w/v. Disregard any slight residue in solution (1). After removal of the plate, examine it immediately under *ultraviolet light (254 nm)*. Any *secondary spot* in the chromatogram obtained with solution (1) is not more intense than the spot in the chromatogram obtained with solution (2) (0.5%). Disregard any spot remaining on the line of application.

Loss on drying When dried at 100° at a pressure not exceeding 2.7 kPa for 4 hours, lose not more than 2.5% of their weight. Use 0.5 g.

Assay Determine the weight of the contents of 10 containers as described in the test for Uniformity of weight under Parenteral Preparations, Powders for Injections. Carry out the following procedures using the mixed contents of the 10 containers.

For Na Dissolve 0.6 g in 20 ml of *water* and titrate with 0.1M *hydrochloric acid VS*, using *methyl red solution* as indicator, until the yellow colour changes to pink; boil gently for 1 or 2 minutes, cool and if necessary continue the titration with 0.1M *hydrochloric acid VS* until the pink colour is restored. Each ml of 0.1M *hydrochloric acid VS* is equivalent to 2.299 mg of Na.

For $C_{11}H_{18}N_2O_2S$ To the liquid from the completed Assay for Na add a further 5 ml of 0.1M *hydrochloric acid* and extract with successive quantities of 25, 25, 20, 15, 15 and 10 ml of *chloroform*, washing each extract with the same 5 ml of *water*. Evaporate the chloroform from the mixed extracts and dry the residue of $C_{11}H_{18}N_2O_2S$ to constant weight at 105°. Calculate the content of $C_{11}H_{18}N_2O_2S$ in a container of average content weight.

Labelling The label of the sealed container states the weight of Thiopental Sodium contained in it.

When thiopentone injection or thiopentone sodium for injection is prescribed or demanded, Thiopental Injection or Thiopental Sodium for Injection shall be dispensed or supplied.

Thioridazine Oral Solution

Definition Thioridazine Oral Solution contains Thioridazine Hydrochloride in a suitable aqueous vehicle.

The oral solution complies with the requirements stated under Oral Liquids and with the following requirements.

Content of thioridazine, $C_{21}H_{26}N_2S_2$ 90.0 to 110.0% of the prescribed or stated amount.

Identification

A. In the test for Related substances, the principal spot in the chromatogram obtained with solution (1) corresponds in position, colour and size to that in the chromatogram obtained with solution (2).

B. In the Assay, the retention time of the principal peak in the chromatogram obtained with solution (1) is the same as that of the principal peak in the chromatogram obtained with solution (2).

Related substances Carry out the method for *thin-layer chromatography*, Appendix III A, protected from light and as quickly as possible using *silica gel G* as the coating substance and a mixture of 1 volume of 13.5M *ammonia*, 25 volumes of *propan-2-ol* and 74 volumes of *chloroform* as the mobile phase. Apply separately to the plate 5 µl of each of the following solutions in a mixture of equal volumes of *chloroform* and *methanol*. For solution (1) add to a quantity of the oral solution containing the equivalent of 5 mg of thioridazine 5 ml of *water* and 5 ml of 13.5M *ammonia*, extract with four 20-ml quantities of *chloroform*, filtering each extract successively through *anhydrous sodium sulphate*, evaporate the combined extracts to dryness at about 30° under reduced pressure and dissolve the residue in 1 ml of a mixture of equal volumes of *chloroform* and *methanol*. Solution (2) contains 0.5% w/v of *thioridazine BPCRS*. Solution (3) contains 0.015% w/v of *mesoridazine besylate BPCRS*. Solution (4) contains 0.0037% w/v of *mesoridazine besylate BPCRS*. After removal of the plate, allow it to dry in air and spray with a mixture of 1 volume of *potassium iodobismuthate solution* and 10 volumes of 2M *acetic acid*, immediately spray with freshly prepared *hydrogen peroxide solution (10 vol)* and cover with a glass plate of the same size. Any *secondary spot* in the chromatogram obtained with solution (1) is not more intense than the spot in the chromatogram obtained with solution (3) (2%, with reference to thioridazine) and not more than one such spot is more intense than the spot in the chromatogram obtained with solution (4) (0.5%, with reference to thioridazine).

Assay Carry out the method for *liquid chromatography*, Appendix III D, protected from light, using the following solutions. For solution (1) dilute a weighed quantity of the oral solution with a mixture of equal volumes of *acetonitrile* and *water* to give a solution containing the equivalent of 0.0025% w/v of thioridazine. Solution (2) contains 0.0025% w/v of *thioridazine BPCRS* in a mixture of equal volumes of *acetonitrile* and *water*. Solution (3) contains 0.0025% w/v of *thioridazine BPCRS* and 0.0035% w/v of *mesoridazine besylate BPCRS* in a mixture of equal volumes of *acetonitrile* and *water*.

The chromatographic procedure may be carried out using (a) a stainless steel column (15 cm × 4.6 mm) packed with *stationary phase C* (5 µm) (Hypersil ODS is suitable), (b) a mixture of 10 volumes of a 10% w/v solution of *ammonium carbonate* and 90 volumes of *methanol* as the mobile phase with a flow rate of 1.5 ml per minute and (c) a detection wavelength of 263 nm.

The assay is not valid unless the *resolution factor* between the two principal peaks in the chromatogram obtained with solution (3) is at least 3.0. If necessary, adjust the concentration of methanol in the mobile phase to achieve the required resolution; decreasing the concentration increases the resolution.

Determine the *weight per ml* of the oral solution, Appendix V G, and calculate the content of $C_{21}H_{26}N_2S_2$, weight in volume, using the declared content of $C_{21}H_{26}N_2S_2$ in *thioridazine BPCRS*.

Storage Thioridazine Oral Solution should be protected from light.

Labelling The quantity of active ingredient is stated in terms of the equivalent amount of thioridazine.

Thioridazine Oral Suspension

Definition Thioridazine Oral Suspension is a suspension of Thioridazine in a suitable aqueous vehicle.

The oral suspension complies with the requirements stated under Oral Liquids and with the following requirements.

Content of thioridazine, $C_{21}H_{26}N_2S_2$ 90.0 to 110.0% of the prescribed or stated amount.

Identification Complies with the tests described under Thioridazine Oral Solution.

Alkalinity pH, 8.0 to 10.0, Appendix V L.

Related substances Complies with the test described under Thioridazine Oral Solution but using as solution (1) a solution prepared in the following manner. To a quantity of the oral suspension containing 25 mg of Thioridazine add 5 ml of *water* and extract with three 20-ml quantities of *chloroform* filtering each extract through *anhydrous sodium sulphate*. Evaporate the combined extracts to dryness at 30° under reduced pressure and dissolve the residue in 5 ml of a mixture of equal volumes of *chloroform* and *methanol*. Disregard any *secondary spot* with an Rf value of 0.15 or less.

Assay Carry out the Assay described under Thioridazine Oral Solution but using as solution (1) a solution prepared by diluting a weighed quantity of the oral suspension with the mobile phase to give a solution containing 0.0025% w/v of Thioridazine.

Storage Thioridazine Oral Suspension should be protected from light.

Thioridazine Tablets

Definition Thioridazine Tablets contain Thioridazine Hydrochloride. They are coated.

The tablets comply with the requirements stated under Tablets and with the following requirements.

Content of thioridazine hydrochloride, $C_{21}H_{26}N_2S_2$, HCl 92.5 to 107.5% of the prescribed or stated amount.

Identification

A. If the tablets are film-coated, remove the coating. To a quantity of the powdered tablets containing 40 mg of Thioridazine Hydrochloride add 10 ml of *water* and 2 ml of 1M *sodium hydroxide*, shake and extract with 15 ml of *ether*. Wash the ether with 5 ml of *water*, dry with *anhydrous sodium sulphate* and evaporate to dryness. The *infrared absorption spectrum* of the residue, Appendix II A, is concordant with *reference spectrum 2* of thioridazine.

B. To a quantity of the powdered tablets containing 5 mg of Thioridazine Hydrochloride add 5 ml of *sulphuric acid* and allow to stand for 5 minutes. A deep blue colour is produced.

Related substances Carry out in subdued light the method for *thin-layer chromatography*, Appendix III A, using a silica gel F_{254} precoated plate (Merck silica gel 60 F_{254} plates are suitable) and a mixture of 74 volumes of *chloroform*, 25 volumes of *propan-2-ol* and 1 volume of 13.5M *ammonia* as the mobile phase. Apply separately to the plate 5 µl of each of the following solutions. For solution (1) extract a quantity of the powdered tablets containing 50 mg of Thioridazine Hydrochloride with 5 ml of a mixture of 2 volumes of 13.5M *ammonia* and 98 volumes of *methanol*, centrifuge and use the supernatant liquid. For solution (2) dilute 1 volume of solution (1) to 200 volumes with the same solvent. For solution (3) dilute 1 volume of solution (1) to 500 volumes with the same solvent. After removal of the plate, allow it to dry in air and spray with a freshly prepared mixture of 1 volume of *potassium iodobismuthate solution* and 10 volumes of 2M *acetic acid* and then with freshly prepared *hydrogen peroxide solution (10 vol)* and immediately cover the plate with a clear glass plate of the same size. Any *secondary spot* in the chromatogram obtained with solution (1) is not more intense than the spot in the chromatogram obtained with solution (2) and not more than one such spot is more intense than the spot in the chromatogram obtained with solution (3). Disregard any spot with an Rf value lower than 0.1. The test is not valid unless the spot in the chromatogram obtained with solution (3) is clearly visible.

Assay Carry out the following procedure protected from light. Weigh and powder 20 tablets. To a quantity of the powder containing 50 mg of Thioridazine Hydrochloride add 80 ml of *ethanol (96%)*, shake for 20 minutes and filter through a sintered-glass filter. Wash the residue with *ethanol (96%)* and add to the filtrate and washings sufficient *ethanol (96%)* to produce 100 ml. Dilute 10 ml to 100 ml with *ethanol (96%)* and dilute 5 ml of this solution to 50 ml with *ethanol (96%)*. Measure the *absorbance* of the resulting solution at the maximum at 264 nm, Appendix II B. Calculate the content of $C_{21}H_{26}N_2S_2$,HCl taking 950 as the value of A(1%, 1 cm) at the maximum at 264 nm.

Thiotepa Injection

Definition Thiotepa Injection is a sterile solution of Thiotepa in Water for Injections. It is prepared by dissolving Thiotepa for Injection in Water for Injections.

The injection complies with the requirements stated under Parenteral Preparations.

Storage Thiotepa Injection should be used immediately after preparation but, in any case, within the period recommended by the manufacturer when prepared and stored strictly in accordance with the manufacturer's instructions. If solid matter separates, the solution should not be used.

THIOTEPA FOR INJECTION

Definition Thiotepa for Injection is a sterile material consisting of Thiotepa with or without excipients. It is supplied in a sealed container.

The contents of the sealed container comply with the requirements for Powders for Injections stated under Parenteral Preparations and with the following requirements.

Content of thiotepa, $C_6H_{12}N_3PS$ 95.0 to 110.0% of the prescribed or stated amount.

Characteristics A white powder.

Identification Burn 20 mg by the method for *oxygen-flask combustion*, Appendix VIII C, using 5 ml of 1.25M *sodium hydroxide* as the absorbing liquid. When the process is complete, dilute to 25 ml with *water*. The resulting solution complies with the following tests.

A. To 5 ml add 0.1 ml of *hydrogen peroxide solution (100 vol)* and 1 ml of 1M *hydrochloric acid*, mix and add 0.05 ml of *barium chloride solution*. The solution becomes turbid.

B. To 2 ml add 40 ml of *water* and 4 ml of *ammonium molybdate—sulphuric acid solution*, mix, add 0.1 g of *L-ascorbic acid* and boil for 1 minute. A blue colour is produced.

Acidity or alkalinity Dissolve a quantity containing 20 mg of Thiotepa in 2 ml of *carbon dioxide-free water*. The pH of the resulting solution is 5.5 to 7.5, Appendix V L.

Clarity of solution Dissolve a quantity containing 15 mg of Thiotepa in 4 ml of *water*. The solution is *clear*, Appendix IV A.

Related substances Carry out the method for *liquid chromatography*, Appendix III D, using the following freshly prepared solutions. For solution (1) dissolve, with shaking, a quantity of the contents of the sealed container containing 15 mg of Thiotepa in 4 ml of *water*, filter and use the filtrate. For solution (2) dilute 1 volume of solution (1) to 100 volumes with *water* and further dilute 1 volume to 10 volumes with *water*. For solution (3) dissolve 10 mg of *thiotepa BPCRS* in 2 ml of *methanol* in a ground-glass-stoppered tube, add 50 µl of a 0.1% v/v solution of *orthophosphoric acid*, stopper the tube and heat in a water bath at 65° for 50 seconds (generation of methoxythiotepa). Allow the solution to cool and add 1 ml of *methanol*. For solution (4) dissolve 15 mg of *thiotepa BPCRS* in 10 ml of *water*, add 1 g of *sodium chloride*, boil in a water bath for 10 minutes and cool (generation of chloro-adduct).

The chromatographic procedure may be carried out using (a) a stainless steel column (15 cm × 4.6 mm) packed with *stationary phase C* (5 µm) (Nucleosil C18 is suitable), (b) 15 volumes of *acetonitrile* and 85 volumes of 0.1M *mixed phosphate buffer pH 7.0* as the mobile phase with a flow rate of 1 ml per minute and (c) a detection wavelength of 215 nm.

The chromatogram obtained with solution (3) shows a peak corresponding to methoxy-thiotepa with a retention time relative to thiotepa of about 1.3 and the chromatogram obtained with solution (4) shows a peak corresponding to the chloro-adduct with a retention time relative to thiotepa of about 3.75. The test is not valid unless the *resolution factor* between the two principal peaks in the chromatogram obtained with solution (3) is at least 3.

For solution (1) allow the chromatography to proceed for 4 times the retention time of the principal peak. In the chromatogram obtained with solution (1) the area of any peak corresponding to the 'chloro-adduct' (identified from the peak in the chromatogram obtained with solution (4)) is not greater than 1.5 times the area of the principal peak in the chromatogram obtained with solution (2) (0.15%), the area of any other *secondary peak* is not greater than twice the area of the principal peak in the chromatogram obtained with solution (2) (0.2%), the area of not more than two such peaks is greater than the area of the principal peak in the chromatogram obtained with solution (2) (0.1%) and the sum of the areas of all the *secondary peaks* is not greater than four times the area of the principal peak in the chromatogram obtained with solution (2) (0.4%).

Assay Carry out the method for *liquid chromatography*, Appendix III D, using the following solutions. For solution (1) dissolve the contents of a sealed container in sufficient *water* to produce a solution containing 0.15% w/v of Thiotepa. Solution (2) contains 0.15% w/v of *thiotepa BPCRS*. For solution (3) dissolve 10 mg of *thiotepa BPCRS* in 2 ml of *methanol* in a ground-glass-stoppered tube, add 50 µl of a 0.1% v/v solution of *orthophosphoric acid*, stopper the tube and heat in a water bath at 65° for 50 seconds (to produce a sufficient quantity of methoxy-thiotepa). Allow the solution to cool and add 1 ml of *methanol*.

The chromatographic procedure may be carried out using (a) a stainless steel column (15 cm × 4.6 mm) packed with *stationary phase C* (5 µm) (Nucleosil C18 is suitable), (b) 15 volumes of *acetonitrile* and 85 volumes of *0.1M mixed phosphate buffer pH 7.0* as the mobile phase with a flow rate of 1 ml per minute and (c) a detection wavelength of 215 nm.

The chromatogram obtained with solution (3) shows a peak corresponding to methoxy-thiotepa with a retention time relative to thiotepa of about 1.3. The assay is not valid unless the *resolution factor* between the two principal peaks in the chromatogram obtained with solution (3) is at least 3.

Calculate the amount of $C_6H_{12}N_3PS$ in the sealed container using the declared content of $C_6H_{12}N_3PS$ in *thiotepa BPCRS*.

Repeat the procedure with a further nine sealed containers. Calculate the average content of $C_6H_{12}N_3PS$ per container from the 10 individual results thus obtained.

Storage The sealed container should be stored at a temperature of 2° to 8°.

Labelling The label of the sealed container states the amount of Thiotepa contained in it.

Tiabendazole Tablets

Definition Tiabendazole Tablets contain Tiabendazole.

The tablets comply with the requirements stated under Tablets and with the following requirements.

Content of tiabendazole, $C_{10}H_7N_3S$ 95.0 to 105.0% of the prescribed or stated amount.

Identification Dissolve a quantity of the powdered tablets containing 20 mg of Tiabendazole in 5 ml of 0.1M *hydrochloric acid*, add 3 mg of *p-phenylenediamine dihydrochloride* and shake until dissolved. Add 0.1 g of *zinc powder*, mix, allow to stand for 2 minutes and add 10 ml of *ammonium iron(III) sulphate solution R2*. A deep blue or bluish violet colour is produced.

Disintegration The requirement for Disintegration does not apply to Tiabendazole Tablets.

Related substances Carry out the method for *thin-layer chromatography*, Appendix III A, using *silica gel HF_{254}* as the coating substance and a mixture of 2.5 volumes of *water*, 10 volumes of *acetone*, 25 volumes of *glacial acetic acid* and 62.5 volumes of *toluene* as the mobile phase. Apply separately to the plate 20 µl of each of the following solutions. For solution (1) shake a quantity of the powdered tablets containing 0.5 g of Tiabendazole with 50 ml of 0.1M *methanolic hydrochloric acid*, adjust the pH to 12 with 1M *methanolic sodium hydroxide solution* and filter (Whatman GF/C filter paper is suitable). For solution (2) dilute 1 volume of solution (1) to 100 volumes with *methanol*. For solution (3) dilute 1 volume of solution (1) to 250 volumes with *methanol*. After removal of the plate, allow it to dry in air and examine under *ultraviolet light (254 nm)*. Any *secondary spot* in the chromatogram obtained with solution (1) is not more intense than the spot in the chromatogram obtained with solution (2) (1%) and not more than one such spot is more intense than the spot in the chromatogram obtained with solution (3) (0.4%). Disregard any spot remaining on the line of application.

Assay Weigh and powder 20 tablets. To a quantity of the powder containing 0.1 g of Tiabendazole add 75 ml of 0.1M *hydrochloric acid*, warm on a water bath for 15 minutes, shaking occasionally, cool, dilute to 100 ml with 0.1M *hydrochloric acid* and filter. Dilute 5 ml of the filtrate to 1000 ml with 0.1M *hydrochloric acid* and measure the *absorbance* of the resulting solution at the maximum at 302 nm, Appendix II B. Calculate the content of $C_{10}H_7N_3S$ taking 1230 as the value of A(1%, 1 cm) at the maximum at 302 nm.

Labelling The label states that the tablets should be chewed before swallowing.

When thiabendazole tablets are prescribed or demanded, Tiabendazole Tablets shall be dispensed or supplied.

Timolol Eye Drops

Definition Timolol Eye Drops are a sterile solution of Timolol Maleate in Purified Water.

The eye drops comply with the requirements stated under Eye Preparations and with the following requirements.

Content of timolol, $C_{13}H_{24}N_4O_3S$ 90.0 to 110.0% of the prescribed or stated amount.

Identification

A. Add a volume of the eye drops containing the equivalent of 50 mg of timolol to an equal volume of *carbonate buffer pH 9.7* and extract with two 40-ml quantities of *dichloromethane*. Reserve the aqueous layer for test B, dry the extracts with *anhydrous sodium sulphate*, evaporate to dryness using a rotary evaporator and dry at 60° under reduced pressure for 15 minutes. The *infrared absorption spectrum* of the residue, Appendix II A, is concordant with the *reference spectrum* of timolol.

B. Evaporate the aqueous solution reserved in test A to about 1 ml. Add 1 ml of *bromine solution*, heat in a water bath for 10 minutes, boil, cool and add 0.1 ml of the solution to a solution of 10 mg of *resorcinol* in 3 ml of *sulphuric acid*. A bluish black colour is produced on heating in a water bath for 15 minutes.

Acidity or alkalinity pH, 6.5 to 7.5, Appendix V L.

Related substances Carry out the method for *liquid chromatography*, Appendix III D, using 20 µl of each of the following solutions. For solution (1) dilute 1 volume of the eye drops to 250 volumes with the mobile phase. For solution (2) use the eye drops undiluted. For solution (3) dilute 1 volume of the eye drops to 500 volumes with the mobile phase. Solution (4) contains 0.30% w/v of *maleic acid* in the mobile phase.

The chromatographic procedure may be carried out using (a) a stainless steel column (20 cm × 4 mm) packed with *stationary phase C* (10 µm) (Nucleosil C18 is suitable), (b) as the mobile phase a mixture of 42.5 volumes of 0.02M *sodium octanesulphonate* and 57.5 volumes of *methanol*, adjusted to pH 3.0 using *glacial acetic acid*, with a flow rate of 2 ml per minute and (c) a detection wavelength of 295 nm. For solution (2) record the chromatogram for 4 times the retention time of the principal peak.

In the chromatogram obtained with solution (2) the area of any *secondary peak*, other than the peak corresponding to maleic acid, is not greater than the area of the peak obtained with solution (1) (0.4%) and not more than two such peaks have an area greater than that of the peak obtained with solution (3) (0.2%).

Assay Dilute a volume containing the equivalent of 25 mg of timolol to 50 ml with *water*. To 5 ml add 15 ml of *carbonate buffer pH 9.7* and extract with three 20-ml quantities and one 10-ml quantity of *toluene*. Wash each extract successively with the same 10-ml volume of *carbonate buffer pH 9.7*, combine the toluene extracts and extract with four 20-ml quantities of 0.05M *sulphuric acid*. Combine the extracts, dilute to 100 ml, filter and measure the *absorbance* at the maximum at 295 nm, Appendix II B, using in the reference cell a solution prepared by treating 5 ml of *water* in the same manner, beginning at the words 'add 15 ml ...'. Calculate the content of $C_{13}H_{24}N_4O_3S$ taking 279 as the value of A(1%, 1 cm) at the maximum at 295 nm.

Labelling The quantity of active ingredient is stated in terms of the equivalent amount of timolol.

Timolol Tablets

Definition Timolol Tablets contain Timolol Maleate.

The tablets comply with the requirements stated under Tablets and with the following requirements.

Content of timolol maleate, $C_{13}H_{24}N_4O_3S,C_4H_4O_4$ 90.0 to 110.0% of the prescribed or stated amount.

Identification

A. To a quantity of the powdered tablets containing 70 mg of Timolol Maleate add 20 ml of *carbonate buffer pH 9.7* and extract with two 40-ml quantities of *dichloromethane*. Reserve the aqueous layer for test B, dry the extracts with *anhydrous sodium sulphate*, evaporate to dryness using a rotary evaporator and dry at 60° under reduced pressure for 15 minutes. The *infrared absorption spectrum* of the residue, Appendix II A, is concordant with the *reference spectrum* of timolol.

B. Filter the aqueous layer reserved in test A and evaporate to about 1 ml. Add 1 ml of *bromine solution*, heat in a water bath for 10 minutes, boil, cool and add 0.1 ml of the solution to a solution of 10 mg of *resorcinol* in 3 ml of *sulphuric acid*. A bluish black colour is produced on heating in a water bath for 15 minutes.

Related substances Comply with the test described under Timolol Eye Drops, but preparing solutions (1), (2) and (3) in the following manner. For solution (1) dilute 1 volume of solution (2) to 250 volumes with the mobile phase. For solution (2) shake a quantity of the powdered tablets containing 0.1 g of Timolol Maleate with 10 ml of the mobile phase for 10 minutes and filter. For solution (3) dilute 1 volume of solution (2) to 500 volumes with the mobile phase.

Assay Weigh and powder 20 tablets. To a quantity of the powder containing 15 mg of Timolol Maleate add 25 ml of 0.05M *sulphuric acid*, shake for 20 minutes and centrifuge until clear. Add 5 ml of the resulting supernatant liquid to 15 ml of *carbonate buffer pH 9.7* and extract with three 20-ml quantities and one 10-ml quantity of *toluene*. Wash each extract successively with the same 10-ml volume of *carbonate buffer pH 9.7*, combine the toluene extracts and extract with four 20-ml quantities of 0.05M *sulphuric acid*. Combine the acid extracts, dilute to 100 ml, filter and measure the *absorbance* at the maximum at 295 nm, Appendix II B, using in the reference cell a solution prepared by treating a mixture of 5 ml of *water* and 15 ml of *carbonate buffer pH 9.7* in the same manner. Calculate the content of $C_{13}H_{24}N_4O_3S,C_4H_4O_4$ taking 204 as the value of A(1%, 1 cm) at the maximum at 295 nm.

Tioguanine Tablets

Definition Tioguanine Tablets contain Tioguanine.

The tablets comply with the requirements stated under Tablets and with the following requirements.

Content of tioguanine, $C_5H_5N_5S$ 92.5 to 107.5% of the prescribed or stated amount.

Identification

A. Shake a quantity of the powdered tablets containing 0.5 g of Tioguanine with 10 ml of 1M *sodium hydroxide* and filter. Acidify the filtrate with *hydrochloric acid*, filter, dissolve the precipitate in 13.5M *ammonia*, evaporate to dryness and dry the residue at 105° at a pressure not exceeding 0.7 kPa for 5 hours. The *infrared absorption spectrum* of the residue, Appendix II A, is concordant with the *reference spectrum* of tioguanine.

B. Mix a quantity of the powdered tablets containing 5 mg of Tioguanine with 5 mg of *sodium formate* in a test tube and heat gently until melted. A gas is evolved which turns *lead acetate paper* black.

Guanine Carry out the method for *thin-layer chromatography*, Appendix III A, using *silica gel GF_{254}* as the coating substance and a mixture of 90 volumes of *methanol* and 15 volumes of 13.5M *ammonia* as the mobile phase. Apply separately to the plate 5 µl of each of the following solutions. For solution (1) add sufficient 0.1M *sodium hydroxide* to a quantity of the powdered tablets containing 0.50 g of Tioguanine to produce 50 ml. Solution (2) contains 0.025% w/v of *guanine* in 0.1M *sodium hydroxide*. After removal of the plate, allow it to dry in air and examine under *ultraviolet light (254 nm)*. Any spot corresponding to guanine in the chromatogram obtained with solution (1) is not more intense than the spot in the chromatogram obtained with solution (2).

Assay Weigh and powder 20 tablets. To a quantity of the powder containing 40 mg of Tioguanine add 20 ml of 0.1M *sodium hydroxide* and shake for 15 minutes. Add sufficient 0.1M *hydrochloric acid* to produce 200 ml, mix and filter through glass wool. Dilute 5 ml of the filtrate to 200 ml with 0.1M *hydrochloric acid*, mix and measure the *absorbance* of the resulting solution at the maximum at 348 nm, Appendix II B. Calculate the content of $C_5H_5N_5S$ taking 1240 as the value of A(1%, 1 cm) at the maximum at 348 nm.

When thioguanine tablets are prescribed or demanded, Tioguanine Tablets shall be dispensed or supplied.

Tobramycin Injection

Definition Tobramycin Injection is a sterile solution of Tobramycin in Water for Injections containing Sulphuric Acid.

The injection complies with the requirements stated under Parenteral Preparations and with the following requirements.

Characteristics A colourless solution.

Identification

A. Carry out the method for *thin-layer chromatography*, Appendix III A, using a silica gel precoated plate (Merck silica gel 60 plates are suitable) and a mixture of 60 volumes of *methanol*, 40 volumes of 13.5M *ammonia* and 20 volumes of *chloroform* as the mobile phase. Apply separately to the plate 5 µl of each of the following solutions. For solution (1) dilute a suitable volume of the injection with *water* to produce a solution containing 0.4% w/v of Tobramycin. Solution (2) contains 0.4% w/v of *tobramycin EPCRS* in *water*. Solution (3) contains 0.4% w/v each of of *kanamycin sulphate EPCRS*, *neomycin sulphate EPCRS* and *tobramycin EPCRS*. After removal of the plate, dry it in a current of warm air, spray with a mixture of equal volumes of a 0.2% w/v solution of *naphthalene-1,3-diol* in *ethanol (96%)* and a 46% w/v solution of *sulphuric acid* and heat at 105° for 5 to 10 minutes. The principal spot in the chromatogram obtained with solution (1) is similar in position, colour and size to that in the chromatogram obtained with solution (2). The test is not valid unless the chromatogram obtained with solution (3) shows three clearly separated principal spots.

B. Yields the reactions characteristic of *sulphates*, Appendix VI.

Acidity pH, 3.5 to 6.0, Appendix V L.

Related substances Carry out the method for *thin-layer chromatography*, Appendix III A, using *silica gel H* as the coating substance and a mixture of equal volumes of 13.5M *ammonia*, *butan-2-one* and *ethanol (96%)* as the mobile phase. Apply separately to the plate 4 µl of each of the following solutions. For solution (1) dilute a suitable volume of the injection with 0.01M *ammonia* to give a solution containing 40 mg of Tobramycin in 4 ml, shake with 10 ml of *ether* and use the aqueous layer. For solution (2) dilute 1 volume of solution (1) to 50 volumes with 0.01M *ammonia*. After removal of the plate, allow it to dry in air, heat at 110° for 10 minutes and spray the hot plate with a solution prepared immediately before use by diluting *sodium hypochlorite solution (3% Cl)* with *water* to contain 0.5% w/v of available chlorine. Dry in a current of cold air until a sprayed area of the plate below the line of application gives at most a very faint blue colour with a drop of *potassium iodide and starch solution*; avoid prolonged exposure to cold air. Spray the plate with *potassium iodide and starch solution*. Any *secondary spot* in the chromatogram obtained with solution (1) is not more intense than the spot in the chromatogram obtained with solution (2) (2%).

Bacterial endotoxins Carry out the *test for bacterial endotoxins*, Appendix XIV C. Dilute the injection, if necessary, with *water BET* to give a solution containing 10 mg of Tobramycin per ml (solution A). The endotoxin limit concentration of solution A is 20 IU per ml. Carry out the test using the maximum valid dilution of solution A calculated from the declared sensitivity of the lysate used in the test.

Assay Carry out the *biological assay of antibiotics*, Appendix XIV A. The precision of the assay is such that the fiducial limits of error are not less than 95% and not more than 105% of the estimated potency.

Calculate the content of tobramycin in the injection, taking each 1000 IU found to be equivalent to 1 mg of tobramycin. The upper fiducial limit of error is not less than 97.0% and the lower fiducial limit is not more than 110.0% of the prescribed or stated potency.

Labelling The strength is stated as the weight of Tobramycin in a suitable dose-volume.

Alpha Tocopheryl Succinate Tablets

Definition Alpha Tocopheryl Succinate Tablets contain Alpha Tocopheryl Succinate. They are coated.

The tablets comply with the requirements stated under Tablets and with the following requirements.

Content of α-tocopherol, $C_{29}H_{50}O_2$ 95.0 to 105.0% of the prescribed or stated amount.

Identification

A. Carry out the method for *thin-layer chromatography*, Appendix III A, using *silica gel HF_{254}* as the coating substance and a mixture of 20 volumes of *ether* and 80 volumes of *cyclohexane* as the mobile phase. Apply separately to the plate 10 µl of each of the following solutions. For solution (1) shake a quantity of the powdered tablets containing the equivalent of 0.134 g of α-tocopherol with three 10-ml quantities of *ether*, filter, evaporate the combined filtrates to 2 ml and then evaporate the solution to dryness under a current of nitrogen. Prepare a 0.5% w/v solution from a portion of the resulting residue in *cyclohexane*. For solution (2) dissolve 10 mg of the residue obtained in the preparation of solution (1) in 2 ml of 5M *ethanolic sulphuric acid*, heat in a water bath for 1 minute, cool, add 2 ml each of *water* and *cyclohexane* and shake for 1 minute; use the upper layer. Solution (3) contains 0.5% w/v of *α-tocopheryl succinate BPCRS* in *cyclohexane*. Prepare solution (4) in the same manner as solution (2) but using 10 mg of *α-tocopheryl succinate BPCRS* in place of the substance being examined.

After removal of the plate, allow it to dry in air and examine under *ultraviolet light (254 nm)*. The principal spot in the chromatogram obtained with solution (1) is similar in position and size to that in the chromatogram obtained with solution (3). There are two spots in each of the chromatograms obtained with solutions (2) and (4). Spray the plate with a mixture of 1 volume of *hydrochloric acid*, 4 volumes of a 0.25% w/v solution of *iron(III) chloride hexahydrate* in *ethanol (96%)* and 4 volumes of a 1% w/v solution of *1,10-phenanthroline hydrochloride* in *ethanol (96%)*. In the chromatograms obtained with solutions (2) and (4) the spot of higher Rf value, due to α-tocopherol, is orange.

B. In the Assay the principal peak in the chromatogram obtained with solution (1) shows a peak with the same retention time as the peak due to the methylated alpha tocopheryl succinate in the chromatogram obtained with solution (2).

Free tocopherol Carry out the method for *thin-layer chromatography*, Appendix III A, using *silica gel HF_{254}* as the coating substance and a mixture of 20 volumes of *ether* and 80 volumes of *cyclohexane* as the mobile phase. Apply separately to the plate 10 µl of each of the following solutions. For solution (1) shake a quantity of the powdered tablets containing the equivalent of 134 mg of α-tocopherol with three 10-ml quantities of *ether*, filter and evaporate the combined filtrates to 2 ml, evaporate the final solution to dryness under a current of nitrogen and prepare a 0.5% w/v solution from the resulting residue in *cyclohexane*. Solution (2) contains 0.005% w/v of *α-tocopherol EPCRS* in *cyclohexane*. After removal of the plate, allow it to dry in air and examine under *ultraviolet light (254 nm)*. Any *secondary spot* in the chromatogram obtained with solution (1) is not more intense than the principal spot in the chromatogram obtained with solution (2) (1%).

Assay Carry out the method for *gas chromatography*, Appendix III B, using the following solutions. Dissolve 0.15 g of *dotriacontane* (internal standard) in sufficient *hexane* to produce 100 ml (solution A). For solution (1) mix a quantity of the powdered tablets containing the equivalent of 134 mg of α-tocopherol with 20 ml of *methanol*, mix with the aid of ultrasound for 5 minutes and centrifuge for 15 minutes. To 4 ml of the clear supernatant liquid add 2 ml of *2,2-dimethoxypropane* and 0.2 ml of *hydrochloric acid* and allow to stand in the dark at room temperature for 1 hour. Evaporate to dryness on a water bath with the aid of a current of nitrogen and dissolve the residue in 10 ml of solution A. For solution (2) dissolve 0.165 g of *α-tocopheryl succinate BPCRS* in 20 ml of *methanol* and continue in the same manner as solution (1) using 4 ml and beginning at the words 'add 2 ml of *2,2-dimethoxypropane* ...'.

The chromatographic procedure may be carried out using a borosilicate glass column (2 m × 4 mm) packed with *acid-washed, silanised diatomaceous support* (100 to 120 mesh) (Chromosorb W/AW is suitable) coated with 2 to 5% of polymethylsiloxane. Set the temperature of the column and the rate of flow of carrier gas at values such that the required resolution is achieved (a column temperature of 280° and a rate of flow of carrier gas of 40 ml per minute are suitable). Maintain the temperature of the injection port at 290° and the detector at 350°. The retention times of dotriacontane and methyl α-tocopheryl succinate (obtained in solution (1)) are about 8 minutes and 20 minutes, respectively.

Calculate the content of $C_{29}H_{50}O_2$ from the areas of the peaks due to dotriacontane and methyl α-tocopheryl succinate in the chromatograms obtained with solution (1) and solution (2) and from the declared content of $C_{29}H_{50}O_2$ in *α-tocopheryl succinate BPCRS*.

Storage Alpha Tocopheryl Succinate Tablets should be protected from light.

Labelling The quantity of active ingredient is stated in terms of the equivalent amount of α-tocopherol.

Tolazamide Tablets

Definition Tolazamide Tablets contain Tolazamide.

The tablets comply with the requirements stated under Tablets and with the following requirements.

Content of tolazamide, $C_{14}H_{21}N_3O_3S$ 95.0 to 105.0% of the prescribed or stated amount.

Identification Triturate a quantity of the powdered tablets containing 0.25 g of Tolazamide with 50 ml of *acetone* and filter. Evaporate the filtrate to dryness and dry at 60° at a pressure of 2 kPa for 3 hours. The *infrared absorption spectrum* of the residue, Appendix II A, is concordant with the *reference spectrum* of tolazamide.

Related substances Comply with the requirement stated under Tolazamide but preparing solution (1) as follows. Shake a quantity of the powdered tablets containing 0.20 g of Tolazamide with 10 ml of *acetone* and filter.

Assay Weigh and powder 20 tablets. Shake a quantity of the powdered tablets containing 0.5 g of Tolazamide with

50 ml of *chloroform*, filter, wash the residue with *chloroform* and evaporate the combined filtrate and washings to dryness. Dissolve the residue in 20 ml of *butan-2-one* with the aid of gentle heat. Allow to cool, add 30 ml of *ethanol (96%)* and titrate the resulting solution with 0.1M *sodium hydroxide VS* using *phenolphthalein solution R1* as indicator. Each ml of 0.1M *sodium hydroxide VS* is equivalent to 31.14 mg of $C_{14}H_{21}N_3O_3S$.

Tolbutamide Tablets

Definition Tolbutamide Tablets contain Tolbutamide.

The tablets comply with the requirements stated under Tablets and with the following requirements.

Content of tolbutamide, $C_{12}H_{18}N_2O_3S$ 95.0 to 105.0% of the prescribed or stated amount.

Identification Extract a quantity of the powdered tablets containing 1 g of Tolbutamide with 10 ml of *chloroform*, filter, evaporate the filtrate to dryness, scratching the side of the container, if necessary, to induce crystallisation, and dry the residue at 100° to 105° for 30 minutes. The *infrared absorption spectrum* of the residue, Appendix II A, is concordant with the *reference spectrum* of tolbutamide.

Dissolution Comply with the *dissolution test for tablets and capsules*, Appendix XII D, using as the medium 900 ml of a solution containing 2.04% w/v of *disodium hydrogen orthophosphate* and 0.135% w/v of *potassium dihydrogen orthophosphate* and rotating the basket at 100 revolutions per minute. Withdraw a sample of 10 ml of the medium. Measure the *absorbance* of the filtered sample, suitably diluted if necessary, at the maximum at 228 nm, Appendix II B. Calculate the total content of tolbutamide, $C_{12}H_{18}N_2O_3S$, in the medium taking 417 as the value of A(1%, 1 cm) at the maximum at 228 nm.

Related substances Carry out the method for *thin-layer chromatography*, Appendix III A, using *silica gel G* as the coating substance and a mixture of 2 volumes of *anhydrous formic acid*, 8 volumes of *methanol* and 90 volumes of *chloroform* as the mobile phase. Apply separately to the plate 5 µl of each of solutions (1) and (2) and 10 µl of solution (3). For solution (1) shake a quantity of the powdered tablets containing 0.50 g of Tolbutamide with 10 ml of *acetone* and filter. Solution (2) contains 0.015% w/v of *toluene-*p*-sulphonamide* in *acetone*. Solution (3) is a mixture of equal volumes of solutions (1) and (2). After removal of the plate, dry it in a current of warm air and heat at 110° for 10 minutes. While still hot, place the plate in a chromatography tank with an evaporating dish containing a 5% w/v solution of *potassium permanganate*, add an equal volume of *hydrochloric acid* and close the tank. Leave the plate in the tank for 2 minutes, then place it in a current of cold air until the excess of chlorine is removed and an area of coating below the line of application gives at most a very faint blue colour with *potassium iodide and starch solution*; avoid prolonged exposure to cold air. Spray the plate with *potassium iodide and starch solution* and allow to stand for 5 minutes. Any *secondary spot* in the chromatogram obtained with solution (1) is not more intense than the spot in the chromatogram obtained with solution (2) (0.3%). The test is not valid unless the chromatogram obtained with solution (3) shows two clearly separated spots.

Assay Weigh and powder 20 tablets. To a quantity of the powder containing 0.5 g of Tolbutamide add 50 ml of *ethanol (96%)* previously neutralised to *phenolphthalein solution R1*, warm to dissolve, add 25 ml of *water* and titrate with 0.1M *sodium hydroxide VS* using *phenolphthalein solution R1* as indicator. Each ml of 0.1M *sodium hydroxide VS* is equivalent to 27.04 mg of $C_{12}H_{18}N_2O_3S$.

Paediatric Compound Tolu Linctus

Definition Paediatric Compound Tolu Linctus is an *oral solution* containing 0.6% w/v of Citric Acid Monohydrate in a suitable vehicle with a tolu flavour.

The linctus complies with the requirements stated under Oral Liquids and with the following requirements.

Content of total acid, calculated as citric acid monohydrate, $C_6H_8O_7,H_2O$ 0.60 to 0.66% w/v.

Assay To 15 g add 100 ml of *water* and titrate with 0.1M *sodium hydroxide VS* using *phenolphthalein solution R1* as indicator. Each ml of 0.1M *sodium hydroxide VS* is equivalent to 7.005 mg of $C_6H_8O_7,H_2O$. Determine the *weight per ml* of the linctus, Appendix V G, and calculate the content of $C_6H_8O_7,H_2O$, weight in volume.

Storage Paediatric Compound Tolu Linctus should be stored at a temperature not exceeding 25°.

Labelling The label indicates the pharmaceutical form as 'oral solution'.

Tolu-flavour Solution

Definition

Cinnamic Acid	5.0 g
Benzoic Acid	2.5 g
Ethyl Cinnamate	0.3 g
Vanillin	0.1 g
Cinnamon Oil	0.02 ml
Sucrose	500 g
Ethanol (96 per cent)	350 ml
Water	sufficient to produce 1000 ml

Extemporaneous preparation The following directions apply.

Dissolve the Sucrose in 320 ml of Water. Add 250 ml of the Ethanol (96 per cent), with mixing. Dissolve the Cinnamic Acid, Benzoic Acid, Ethyl Cinnamate, Vanillin and Cinnamon Oil in the remaining 100 ml of Ethanol (96 per cent), add this solution to the sucrose solution with mixing, dilute to 1000 ml with Water and mix. Allow to stand for a few hours before use.

Identification Carry out the method for *thin-layer chromatography*, Appendix III A, using *silica gel GF_{254}* as the coating substance and a mixture of 75 volumes of *n-pentane*, 25 volumes of *hexane* and 15 volumes of *glacial acetic acid* as the mobile phase. Apply separately to the plate 5 µl of each of the following solutions. For solution (1) use the solution being examined. Solution (2) contains 0.5% w/v of *cinnamic acid*, 0.25% w/v of *benzoic acid* and 0.03% v/v of *ethyl cinnamate* in *ethanol (90%)*. After removal of the plate, allow it to dry in air for 15 minutes and repeat the development using the same mobile phase. Remove the plate, allow the solvent to evaporate and examine under *ultraviolet light (254 nm)*. The spots in the chromatogram obtained with solution (1) are similar in size and correspond in position to those in the chromatogram obtained with solution (2).

Ethanol content 31 to 36% v/v, Appendix VIII F.

Weight per ml 1.125 to 1.155 g, Appendix V G.

Storage Tolu-flavour Solution should be kept in a well-closed container.

Labelling The label states (1) the date after which the solution is not intended to be used; (2) the conditions under which it should be stored.

Tolu Syrup

Definition

Tolu-flavour Solution	100 ml
Syrup	sufficient to produce 1000 ml

The syrup complies with the requirements stated under Syrups and with the following requirement.

Weight per ml 1.29 to 1.32 g, Appendix V G.

Tranexamic Acid Injection

Definition Tranexamic Acid Injection is a sterile solution of Tranexamic Acid in Water for Injections.

The injection complies with the requirements stated under Parenteral Preparations and with the following requirements.

Content of tranexamic acid, $C_8H_{15}NO_2$ 95.0 to 105.0% of the prescribed or stated amount.

Identification To a volume containing 0.4 g of Tranexamic Acid add 2 ml of *ether*, stir, add 5 ml of *methanol*, stir again and allow to crystallise. The crystals, after drying, comply with the following tests.

A. The *infrared absorption spectrum*, Appendix II A, is concordant with the *reference spectrum* of tranexamic acid.

B. To 1 ml of a 1% w/v solution add 1 ml of a 0.2% w/v solution of *ninhydrin* in *ethanol (96%)* and heat on a water bath for 2 minutes. A dark bluish violet colour is produced.

C. Dissolve 0.2 g in 10 ml of 5M *sodium hydroxide*, add 0.2 ml of *benzoyl chloride* and shake vigorously for 10 minutes. Acidify to pH 4 with 2M *hydrochloric acid*, filter, wash the residue with 5 ml of *ether* and dry at 50° at a pressure of 2 kPa. The *melting point* of the residue is about 186°, Appendix V A.

Acidity or alkalinity pH, 6.5 to 7.5, Appendix V L.

Iminodi-acid Carry out the method for *thin-layer chromatography*, Appendix III A, using *silica gel G* as the coating substance and a mixture of 20 volumes of *glacial acetic acid*, 20 volumes of *water* and 80 volumes of *butan-1-ol* as the mobile phase. Apply separately to the plate 2 µl of each of the following solutions. For solution (1) dilute the injection, if necessary, to contain 10.0% w/v of Tranexamic Acid. Solution (2) contains 0.10% w/v of *tranexamic acid impurity EPCRS*. After removal of the plate, allow it to dry in air, spray with a 0.25% w/v solution of *ninhydrin* in a mixture of equal volumes of *methanol* and *pyridine* and heat at 130° for 15 minutes. Any spot corresponding to the iminodi-acid in the chromatogram obtained with solution (1) is not more intense than the spot in the chromatogram obtained with solution (2) (1%).

***cis*-Isomer** Carry out the method for *liquid chromatography*, Appendix III D, using the following solutions. For solution (1) evaporate a volume of the injection containing 20 mg of Tranexamic Acid to dryness, dissolve the residue in 1 ml of 0.1M *boric acid*, add 4 ml of a 10% w/v solution of *1-fluoro-2-nitro-4-trifluoromethylbenzene* in *dimethyl sulphoxide* and shake for 10 minutes. Add 50 ml of 0.1M *hydrochloric acid* and extract with two 10-ml quantities of *chloroform*. Evaporate the chloroform extract to dryness and dissolve the residue in 2 ml of *ethanol-free chloroform*. For solution (2) dilute 1 volume of solution (1) to 200 volumes with *ethanol-free chloroform*.

The chromatographic procedure may be carried out using (a) a stainless steel column (30 cm × 4 mm) packed with *stationary phase A* (10 µm) (µPorasil is suitable), (b) a mixture of 1 volume of *glacial acetic acid*, 80 volumes of *ethanol-free chloroform* and 120 volumes of *hexane* as the mobile phase with a flow rate of 2 ml per minute and (c) a detection wavelength of 420 nm.

In the chromatogram obtained with solution (1) the area of any peak eluting immediately before the principal peak is not greater than the area of the principal peak in the chromatogram obtained with solution (2) (0.5%).

Pyrogens Complies with the *test for pyrogens*, Appendix XIV D, using 3 ml per kg of the rabbit's weight.

Assay To a volume containing 0.1 g of Tranexamic Acid add 50 ml of *water* and adjust the solution to pH 7.0 with 0.1M *sodium hydroxide* or 0.1M *hydrochloric acid*. Add 25 ml of *formaldehyde solution*, previously adjusted to pH 7.0, and 20 ml of 0.1M *sodium hydroxide VS* and titrate with 0.1M *hydrochloric acid VS* determining the end point potentiometrically. Repeat the operation without the injection. The difference between the titrations represents the amount of sodium hydroxide required. Each ml of 0.1M *sodium hydroxide VS* is equivalent to 15.72 mg of $C_8H_{15}NO_2$.

Tranexamic Acid Tablets

Definition Tranexamic Acid Tablets contain Tranexamic Acid.

The tablets comply with the requirements stated under Tablets and with the following requirements.

Content of tranexamic acid, $C_8H_{15}NO_2$ 95.0 to 105.0% of the prescribed or stated amount.

Identification Shake a quantity of the powdered tablets containing 0.5 g of Tranexamic Acid with 5 ml of *water* for 15 minutes, filter and add 2 ml of *ether* to the filtrate. Stir, add 10 ml of *methanol*, stir again and allow to crystallise. The crystals, after drying, comply with the following tests.

A. The *infrared absorption spectrum*, Appendix II A, is concordant with the *reference spectrum* of tranexamic acid.

B. To 1 ml of a 1% w/v solution add 1 ml of a 0.2% w/v solution of *ninhydrin* in *ethanol (96%)* and heat on a water bath for 2 minutes. A dark bluish violet colour is produced.

C. Dissolve 0.2 g in 10 ml of 5M *sodium hydroxide*, add 0.2 ml of *benzoyl chloride* and shake vigorously for 10 minutes. Acidify to pH 4 with 2M *hydrochloric acid*, filter, wash the residue with 5 ml of *ether* and dry at 50° at a pressure of 2 kPa. The *melting point* of the residue is about 186°, Appendix V A.

Iminodi-acid Carry out the method for *thin-layer chromatography*, Appendix III A, using *silica gel G* as the coating substance and a mixture of 20 volumes of *glacial acetic acid*, 20 volumes of *water* and 80 volumes of *butan-1-ol* as the mobile phase. Apply separately to the plate 2 µl of each of the following solutions. For solution (1) shake a quantity of the powdered tablets containing 0.5 g of Tranexamic Acid with 10 ml of *water* for 10 minutes, filter and use the filtrate. Solution (2) contains 0.10% w/v of *tranexamic acid impurity EPCRS*. After removal of the plate, allow it to dry in air, spray with a 0.25% w/v solution of *ninhydrin* in a mixture of equal volumes of *methanol* and *pyridine* and heat at 130° for 15 minutes. Any spot corresponding to the iminodi-acid in the chromatogram obtained with solution (1) is not more intense than the spot in the chromatogram obtained with solution (2) (2%).

***cis*-Isomer** Carry out the method for *liquid chromatography*, Appendix III D, using the following solutions. For solution (1) shake a quantity of the powdered tablets containing 0.5 g of Tranexamic Acid with 10 ml of *water* for 10 minutes and filter. To 0.2 ml of the filtrate add 1 ml of 0.1M *boric acid*, add 4 ml of a 10% w/v solution of *1-fluoro-2-nitro-4-trifluoromethylbenzene* in *dimethyl sulphoxide* and shake for 10 minutes. Add 50 ml of 0.1M *hydrochloric acid* and extract with two 10-ml quantities of *chloroform*. Evaporate the chloroform extract to dryness and dissolve the residue in 2 ml of *ethanol-free chloroform*. For solution (2) dilute 1 volume of solution (1) to 200 volumes with *ethanol-free chloroform*.

The chromatographic procedure may be carried out using (a) a stainless steel column (30 cm × 4 mm) packed with *stationary phase A* (10 µm) (µPorasil is suitable), (b) a mixture of 1 volume of *glacial acetic acid*, 80 volumes of *ethanol-free chloroform* and 120 volumes of *hexane* as the mobile phase with a flow rate of 2 ml per minute and (c) a detection wavelength of 420 nm.

In the chromatogram obtained with solution (1) the area of any peak eluting immediately before the principal peak is not greater than the area of the principal peak in the chromatogram obtained with solution (2) (0.5%).

Assay Weigh and powder 20 tablets. Dissolve a quantity of the powdered tablets containing 0.25 g of Tranexamic Acid in 50 ml of *anhydrous acetic acid* and carry out Method I for *non-aqueous titration*, Appendix VIII A, using *crystal violet solution* as indicator. Each ml of 0.1M *perchloric acid VS* is equivalent to 15.72 mg of $C_8H_{15}NO_2$.

Tranylcypromine Tablets

Definition Tranylcypromine Tablets contain Tranylcypromine Sulphate. They are coated.

The tablets comply with the requirements stated under Tablets and with the following requirements.

Content of tranylcypromine, $C_9H_{11}N$ 95.0 to 105.0% of the prescribed or stated amount.

Identification

A. The *light absorption*, Appendix II B, in the range 230 to 350 nm of the solution obtained in the Assay exhibits three maxima, at 258, 264 and 271 nm. The *absorbances* at the maxima are about 1.2, about 1.3 and about 0.96, respectively.

B. Suspend a quantity of the powdered tablets containing the equivalent of 5 mg of tranylcypromine in 0.5 ml of *ethanol (96%)* and add 5 mg of *ninhydrin*. A purple colour is produced within 15 minutes.

C. The powdered tablets yield the reactions characteristic of *sulphates*, Appendix VI.

Related substances Comply with the test described under Tranylcypromine Sulphate using as solutions (2) and (3) solutions prepared in the following manner. For solution (2) add 10 ml of 0.05M *sulphuric acid* to a quantity of the powdered tablets containing the equivalent of 75 mg of tranylcypromine, shake for 15 minutes, filter and wash the filter with two 5-ml quantities of 0.05M *sulphuric acid*. To the combined filtrate and washings add 1 ml of 5M *sodium hydroxide* and extract with 10 ml of *dichloromethane*. Dry the dichloromethane extract with *anhydrous sodium sulphate*, evaporate to about 5 ml without heating, add 1 ml of *trifluoroacetic anhydride* and allow to stand for 10 minutes. Evaporate the solvent at a pressure of 2 kPa using a rotary evaporator and a water bath at 20° and dissolve the residue in 2 ml of *dichloromethane*. For solution (3) add 10 ml of 0.05M *sulphuric acid* and 1 ml of solution A to a quantity of the powdered tablets containing the equivalent of 75 mg of tranylcypromine and complete the procedure described above, beginning at the words 'shake for 15 minutes ... '.

Assay Weigh and powder 20 tablets. To a quantity of the powder containing the equivalent of 30 mg of tranylcypromine add 60 ml of 0.1M *sulphuric acid*, shake for 30 minutes, add sufficient 0.1M *sulphuric acid* to produce 100 ml and filter. Measure the *absorbance* of the resulting solution at the maximum at 271 nm and at 282 nm, Appendix II B. Calculate the content of $C_9H_{11}N$ from the difference between the absorbances taking 14.6 as the value of A(1%, 1 cm).

Labelling The quantity of active ingredient is stated in terms of the equivalent amount of tranylcypromine.

Tretinoin Gel

Definition Tretinoin Gel is a solution of Tretinoin in a suitable basis.

The gel complies with the requirements stated under Topical Semi-solid Preparations and with the following requirements.

Content of tretinoin, $C_{20}H_{28}O_2$ 90.0 to 120.0% of the prescribed or stated amount.

Identification Carry out in subdued light the method for *thin-layer chromatography*, Appendix III A, using *silica gel GF_{254}* as the coating substance and a mixture of 70 volumes of *cyclohexane* and 30 volumes of *propan-2-ol* as the mobile phase. Apply separately to the plate 10 µl of each of the following solutions. For solution (1) disperse a quantity of the gel containing 1.25 mg of Tretinoin as completely as possible in 25 ml of warm *methanol*, allow to cool to room temperature and extract with three 50-ml quantities of *hexane*. Wash the combined extracts with 20 ml of *water*, filter through *anhydrous sodium sulphate* and evaporate the filtrate to dryness using a rotary evaporator at a temperature not exceeding 60°. Dissolve the residue in 5 ml of *methanol*. Solution (2) contains 0.025% w/v of *tretinoin EPCRS* in *methanol*. After removal of the plate, allow it to dry in air and examine under *ultraviolet light (254 nm)*. The principal spot in the chromatogram obtained with solution (1) corresponds to that in the chromatogram obtained with solution (2).

Related substances Carry out the method for *liquid chromatography*, Appendix III D, using the following solutions. For solution (1) use solution (1) from the test for Identification. For solution (2) dilute 3 volumes of solution (1) to 100 volumes with *methanol*.

The chromatographic procedure may be carried out using (a) a stainless steel column (20 cm × 4.6 mm) packed with *stationary phase C* (10 μm) (Spherisorb ODS 1 is suitable), (b) as the mobile phase with a flow rate of 1.4 ml per minute a solution containing 0.5% v/v of *glacial acetic acid* in a mixture of *methanol* and *water* the proportions being adjusted to give a retention time for tretinoin of about 15 minutes (a mixture of 77 volumes of *methanol* and 23 volumes of *water* is usually suitable) and (c) a detection wavelength of 353 nm. Adjust the sensitivity of the instrument so that the height of the principal peak in the chromatogram obtained with solution (2) is about 70% of full-scale deflection.

In the chromatogram obtained with solution (1) the sum of the areas of any *secondary peaks* is not greater than the area of the peak in the chromatogram obtained with solution (2).

Assay Dissolve a quantity of the gel containing 0.5 mg of Tretinoin in sufficient *chloroform* to produce 100 ml and measure the *absorbance* of the resulting solution at the maximum at 365 nm, Appendix II B. Calculate the content of $C_{20}H_{28}O_2$ taking 1430 as the value of A(1%, 1 cm) at the maximum at 365 nm.

Tretinoin Solution

Definition Tretinoin Solution is a *cutaneous solution* of Tretinoin in a suitable ethanolic solvent. It contains a suitable antioxidant.

The solution complies with the requirements stated under Liquids for Cutaneous Application and with the following requirements.

Content of tretinoin, $C_{20}H_{28}O_2$ 90.0 to 120.0% of the prescribed or stated amount.

Characteristics A clear, yellow liquid with the odour of ethanol.

Identification Complies with the test described under Tretinoin Gel but preparing solution (1) in the following manner. Add 5 ml of *water* to a quantity containing 1.25 mg of Tretinoin and extract with two 20-ml quantities of *hexane*. Wash the combined extracts with two 10-ml quantities of *water*, filter through *anhydrous sodium sulphate*, evaporate the filtrate to dryness using a rotary evaporator at a temperature not exceeding 60° and dissolve the residue in 5 ml of *methanol*.

Ethanol content 50 to 60% v/v, Appendix VIII F, Method II.

Related substances Carry out the test described under Tretinoin Gel using as solution (1) the solution being examined and as solution (2) 3 volumes of the solution being examined diluted to 100 volumes with *methanol*. The sum of the areas of any *secondary peaks* in the chromatogram obtained with solution (1) is not greater than the area of the principal peak in the chromatogram obtained with solution (2).

Assay To a quantity containing 0.5 mg of Tretinoin add 1 ml of 1M *hydrochloric acid*, dilute to 100 ml with *propan-2-ol* and measure the *absorbance* of the resulting solution at the maximum at 353 nm, Appendix II B. Determine the *weight per ml*, Appendix V G, and calculate the percentage w/w of $C_{20}H_{28}O_2$ taking 1520 as the value of A(1%, 1 cm) at the maximum at 353 nm.

Storage Tretinoin Solution should be protected from light and stored at a temperature below 15°.

Labelling The label states (1) the date after which the solution is not intended to be used; (2) the conditions under which it should be stored.

The label indicates the pharmaceutical form as 'cutaneous solution'.

Triamcinolone Cream

Definition Triamcinolone Cream contains Triamcinolone Acetonide in a suitable basis.

The cream complies with the requirements stated under Topical Semi-solid Preparations and with the following requirements.

Content of triamcinolone acetonide, $C_{24}H_{31}FO_6$ 90.0 to 110.0% of the prescribed or stated amount.

Identification

A. Carry out the method for *thin-layer chromatography*, Appendix III A, using *silica gel G* as the coating substance and *ethyl acetate* as the mobile phase. Apply separately to the plate 10 μl of each of the following solutions. For solution (1) add 25 ml of *methanol* and 5 g of *anhydrous sodium sulphate* to a quantity of the preparation being examined containing 5 mg of Triamcinolone Acetonide, shake for 10 minutes and filter through a sintered-glass crucible (BS porosity No. 4) containing a 2-cm layer of *washed, flux-calcined diatomaceous filter-aid*, rinsing the flask and crucible with 10 ml of *methanol*; evaporate the combined filtrate and washings to dryness on a water bath and dissolve the residue in 10 ml of *chloroform*. Solution (2) contains 0.05% w/v of *triamcinolone acetonide BPCRS* in *chloroform*. Solution (3) is a mixture of equal volumes of solutions (1) and (2). After removal of the plate, allow it to dry in air and spray with *alkaline tetrazolium blue solution*. The principal spot in the chromatogram obtained with solution (1) corresponds to the spot in the chromatogram obtained with solution (2) and the chromatogram obtained with solution (3) shows a single, compact principal spot.

B. In the Assay, the chromatogram obtained with solution (3) shows a peak with the same retention time as the peak due to triamcinolone acetonide in the chromatogram obtained with solution (1).

Assay Carry out the method for *liquid chromatography*, Appendix III D, using the following solutions. For solution (1) add 1 ml of a 0.1% w/v solution of *fluoxymesterone BPCRS* (internal standard) in *methanol* to 1 ml of a 0.1% w/v solution of *triamcinolone acetonide BPCRS* in *methanol* and add sufficient *methanol* to produce 10 ml. For solution (2) add 10 ml of *methanol* to a quantity of the preparation being examined containing 1 mg of Triamcinolone Acetonide, heat on a water bath at 60° to 70° until the preparation has melted, shake vigorously for 2 minutes, cool in ice and centrifuge; filter the supernatant liquid, if necessary. Prepare solution (3) in the same manner as solution (2) but use 1 ml of the internal standard solution and 9 ml of *methanol* in place of the 10 ml of methanol.

The chromatographic procedure may be carried out using (a) a stainless steel column (20 cm × 4 mm) packed with *stationary phase C* (10 µm) (Spherisorb ODS 1 is suitable), (b) a mixture of 65 volumes of *methanol*, 35 volumes of *water* and 0.025 volume of *triethylamine* as the mobile phase with a flow rate of 1 ml per minute and (c) a detection wavelength of 254 nm.

Calculate the content of $C_{24}H_{31}FO_6$ in the preparation being examined using the declared content of $C_{24}H_{31}FO_6$ in *triamcinolone acetonide BPCRS*.

Triamcinolone Acetonide Injection

Definition Triamcinolone Acetonide Injection is a sterile suspension of Triamcinolone Acetonide, in very fine particles, in Water for Injections containing suitable dispersing agents.

The injection complies with the requirements stated under Parenteral Preparations and with the following requirements.

Content of triamcinolone acetonide, $C_{24}H_{31}FO_6$ 90.0 to 110.0% of the prescribed or stated amount.

Characteristics A white suspension which settles on standing but readily disperses on shaking. On examination under a microscope, the particles are seen to be crystalline and rarely exceed 40 µm in diameter.

Identification Extract a volume containing 50 mg of Triamcinolone Acetonide with two 10-ml quantities of *ether* and discard the ether extracts. Filter the aqueous layer through a sintered-glass filter, wash the residue with four 5-ml quantities of *water* and dry at 105° for 1 hour. The residue complies with the following tests.

A. The *infrared absorption spectrum*, Appendix II A, is concordant with the *reference spectrum* of triamcinolone acetonide.

B. Complies with the test for *identification of steroids*, Appendix III A, using *impregnating solvent I* and *mobile phase B*.

Acidity or alkalinity pH, 5.0 to 7.5, Appendix V L.

Assay Carry out the method for *liquid chromatography*, Appendix III D, using the following two solutions in *methanol*. Solution (1) contains 0.01% w/v of *prednisolone EPCRS* (internal standard) and 0.02% w/v of *triamcinolone acetonide BPCRS*. Solution (2) is the clear supernatant liquid obtained by mixing a volume of the injection, diluted with *methanol*, with sufficient of a solution of *prednisolone EPCRS* in *methanol* to give a final concentration of 0.01% w/v of prednisolone and 0.02% w/v of triamcinolone acetonide and centrifuging. Prepare solution (3) in the same manner as solution (2) but omitting the internal standard.

The chromatographic procedure may be carried out using (a) a stainless steel column (25 cm × 4 mm) packed with *stationary phase C* (10 µm) (Spherisorb ODS 1 is suitable), (b) a mixture of 56 volumes of *methanol* and 44 volumes of *water* as the mobile with a flow rate of 1.4 ml per minute and (c) a detection wavelength of 254 nm.

Calculate the content of $C_{24}H_{31}FO_6$ in the preparation being examined using peak heights and the declared content of $C_{24}H_{31}FO_6$ in *triamcinolone acetonide BPCRS*.

Storage Triamcinolone Acetonide Injection should be protected from light and stored at a temperature below 15°.

Triamcinolone Ointment

Definition Triamcinolone Ointment contains Triamcinolone Acetonide in a suitable basis.

The ointment complies with the requirements stated under Topical Semi-solid Preparations and with the following requirements.

Content of triamcinolone acetonide, $C_{24}H_{31}FO_6$ 90.0 to 110.0% of the prescribed or stated amount.

Identification

A. Complies with test A for Identification described under Triamcinolone Cream but preparing solution (1) in the following manner. To a quantity of the ointment containing 5 mg of Triamcinolone Acetonide add 10 ml of *chloroform* and shake for 10 minutes. Add 25 ml of *methanol* and shake for a further 10 minutes. Filter through a sintered-glass crucible (BS porosity No. 4) containing a 2-cm layer of *washed, flux-calcined diatomaceous filter-aid*, rinsing the flask and crucible with 10 ml of *methanol*. Evaporate the combined filtrate and washings to dryness on a water bath and dissolve the residue in 10 ml of *chloroform*.

B. In the Assay, the chromatogram obtained with solution (3) shows a peak with the same retention time as the peak due to triamcinolone acetonide in the chromatogram obtained with solution (1).

Assay Carry out the method for *liquid chromatography*, Appendix III D, using the following solutions. For solution (1) add 1 ml of a 0.1% w/v solution of *fluoxymesterone BPCRS* (internal standard) in *methanol*, 2 ml of *chloroform* and 8 ml of *methanol* to 1 ml of a 0.1% w/v solution of *triamcinolone acetonide BPCRS* in *methanol*. For solution (2) add 2 ml of *chloroform* to a quantity of the preparation being examined containing 1 mg of Triamcinolone Acetonide, shake vigorously until it is completely dispersed, add 10 ml of *methanol* and shake vigorously for 1 minute. Cool in ice and centrifuge; use the supernatant liquid or the liquid beneath the crust, filtered if necessary. Prepare solution (3) in the same manner as solution (2) but add 1 ml of the internal standard solution, 2 ml of *chloroform* and 9 ml of *methanol* in place of the 10 ml of methanol.

The chromatographic procedure may be carried out using (a) a stainless steel column (20 cm × 4 mm) packed with *stationary phase C* (10 µm) (Spherisorb ODS 1 is suitable), (b) a mixture of 65 volumes of *methanol*, 35 volumes of *water* and 0.025 volume of *triethylamine* as the mobile phase with a flow rate of 1 ml per minute and (c) a detection wavelength of 254 nm.

Calculate the content of $C_{24}H_{31}FO_6$ in the preparation being examined using the declared content of $C_{24}H_{31}FO_6$ in *triamcinolone acetonide BPCRS*.

Triamcinolone Dental Paste

Definition Triamcinolone Dental Paste contains Triamcinolone Acetonide in a suitable basis.

The dental paste complies with the requirements stated under Topical Semi-solid Preparations and with the following requirements.

Content of triamcinolone acetonide, $C_{24}H_{31}FO_6$ 90.0 to 110.0% of the prescribed or stated amount.

Identification

A. Complies with test A for Identification described under Triamcinolone Cream but preparing solution (1) in the following manner. To a quantity of the paste containing 5 mg of Triamcinolone Acetonide add 25 ml of *methanol* and shake for 10 minutes. Filter through a sintered-glass crucible (BS porosity No. 4) containing a 2-cm layer of *washed, flux-calcined diatomaceous filter-aid*, rinsing the flask and crucible with 10 ml of *methanol*. Evaporate the combined filtrate and washings to dryness on a water bath and dissolve the residue in 10 ml of *chloroform*.

B. In the Assay, the chromatogram obtained with solution (3) shows a peak with the same retention time as the peak due to triamcinolone acetonide in the chromatogram obtained with solution (1).

Assay Carry out the Assay described under Triamcinolone Ointment.

Triamcinolone Tablets

Definition Triamcinolone Tablets contain Triamcinolone.

With the exception of the requirements for shape, the tablets comply with the requirements stated under Tablets and with the following requirements.

Content of triamcinolone, $C_{21}H_{27}FO_6$ 90.0 to 110.0% of the prescribed or stated amount.

Identification

A. Dissolve 1 mg of the residue obtained in the test for Related substances in 6 ml of *ethanol (96%)*, add 5 ml of a 1% w/v solution of *butylated hydroxytoluene* in ethanol *(96%)* and 5 ml of 1M *sodium hydroxide* and heat on a water bath under a reflux condenser for 20 minutes. A pinkish lavender colour is produced.

B. In the Assay, the chromatogram obtained with solution (2) shows a peak with the same retention time as the peak due to triamcinolone in the chromatogram obtained with solution (1).

Related substances Comply with the test described under Triamcinolone using the following solutions. For solution (1) shake a quantity of the powdered tablets containing 15 mg of Triamcinolone with 15 ml of *absolute ethanol* for 15 minutes, filter under reduced pressure through fine filter paper (Whatman No. 42 is suitable) and evaporate to dryness using a rotary evaporator. Reserve 1 mg of the residue for test A for Identification. Dissolve the remainder of the residue in 15 ml of *methanol* (solution A). Dilute 5 ml to 50 ml with *methanol* and dilute 5 ml of the resulting solution to 50 ml with the same solvent. For solution (2) dilute 4 ml of solution A to 100 ml with *methanol*. For solution (3) use solution A.

Uniformity of content Tablets containing 2 mg or less of Triamcinolone comply with the requirements stated under Tablets using the following method of analysis. Crush one tablet to a fine powder, add 10 ml of *ethanol (96%)* and shake for 10 minutes. Filter, dilute 2 ml of the filtrate with sufficient *ethanol (96%)* to produce a solution containing 0.0008% w/v of Triamcinolone and measure the *absorbance* of the resulting solution at the maximum at 238 nm, Appendix II B. Calculate the content of $C_{21}H_{27}FO_6$ taking 380 as the value of A(1%, 1 cm) at the maximum at 238 nm.

Assay Weigh and powder 20 tablets. Prepare a 0.06% w/v solution of *testosterone* (internal standard) in *methanol* (solution B) and carry out the method for *liquid chromatography*, Appendix III D, using the following solutions. For solution (1) add 5 ml of solution B to 5 ml of a 0.08% w/v solution of *triamcinolone BPCRS* in *methanol* and add 15 ml of *methanol (50%)*. For solution (2) shake a quantity of the powdered tablets containing 2.5 mg of Triamcinolone with 5 ml of *methanol* and 20 ml of a mixture of 5 volumes of *methanol* and 3 volumes of *water*. Shake for 15 minutes, mix with the aid of ultrasound for 10 minutes, centrifuge and use the supernatant liquid. Prepare solution (3) in the same manner as solution (2) but add 5 ml of solution B in place of the 5 ml of methanol.

The chromatographic procedure may be carried out using (a) a stainless steel column (20 cm × 4 mm) packed with *stationary phase C* (10 µm) (Spherisorb ODS 1 is suitable), (b) a mixture of 70 volumes of *methanol*, 30 volumes of *water* and 0.1 volume of *glacial acetic acid* as the mobile phase with a flow rate of 2 ml per minute and (c) a detection wavelength of 238 nm.

Calculate the content of $C_{21}H_{27}FO_6$ using the declared content of $C_{21}H_{27}FO_6$ in *triamcinolone BPCRS*.

Triamterene Capsules

Definition Triamterene Capsules contain Triamterene.

The capsules comply with the requirements stated under Capsules and with the following requirements.

Content of triamterene, $C_{12}H_{11}N_7$ 95.0 to 105.0% of the prescribed or stated amount.

Identification The final solution obtained in the Assay has a bluish fluorescence and the *light absorption*, Appendix II B, in the range 230 to 365 nm exhibits a maximum only at 360 nm.

Related substances Carry out the method for *thin-layer chromatography*, Appendix III A, using *silica gel G* as the coating substance and a mixture of 90 volumes of *ethyl acetate*, 10 volumes of *methanol* and 10 volumes of 18M *ammonia* as the mobile phase. Apply separately to the plate 5 µl of each of the following solutions. For solution (1) dissolve a quantity of the contents of the capsules containing 0.10 g of Triamterene in sufficient *dimethyl sulphoxide* to produce 20 ml and dilute 2 ml to 50 ml with *methanol*. For solution (2) dilute 1 volume of solution (1) to 200 volumes with *methanol*. After removal of the plate, allow it to dry in air until the odour of solvent is no longer detectable and examine under *ultraviolet light (365 nm)*. Any *secondary spot* in the chromatogram obtained with solution (1) is not more intense than the spot in the chromatogram obtained with solution (2).

Assay Dissolve a quantity of the mixed contents of 20 capsules containing 0.1 g of Triamterene in 50 ml of a mixture of equal volumes of *glacial acetic acid* and *water* with the aid of gentle heat, cool and add sufficient *water* to produce 500 ml. Dilute 5 ml to 200 ml with 1M *acetic acid* and measure the *absorbance* of the resulting solution at the maximum at 360 nm, Appendix II B. Calculate the content of $C_{12}H_{11}N_7$ from a calibration curve prepared by treating suitable quantities of a solution of *triamterene BPCRS* in 1M *acetic acid* in the same manner and using the declared content of $C_{12}H_{11}N_7$ in *triamterene BPCRS*.

Tribavirin Solution for Nebulisation

Definition Tribavirin Solution for Nebulisation is a sterile solution of Tribavirin in Water for Injections. It is prepared by dissolving Tribavirin for Nebulisation in the requisite amount of Water for Injections.

Storage Tribavirin Solution for Nebulisation should be used immediately after preparation but, in any case, within the period recommended by the manufacturer when prepared and stored strictly in accordance with the manufacturer's instructions.

The contents of the sealed container when reconstituted comply with the requirements stated under Preparations for Inhalation.

TRIBAVIRIN FOR NEBULISATION

Definition Tribavirin for Nebulisation is a sterile material consisting of Tribavirin with or without excipients. It is supplied in a sealed container.

Content of tribavirin, $C_8H_{12}N_4O_5$ 95.0 to 105.0% of the prescribed or stated amount.

Identification

A. Carry out the method for *thin-layer chromatography*, Appendix III A, using *silica gel G* as the coating substance and a mixture of 20 volumes of 0.1M *ammonium chloride* and 90 volumes of *acetonitrile* as the mobile phase. Apply separately to the plate 10 µl of each of two solutions in *water* containing (1) 1% w/v tribavirin and (2) 1% w/v of *tribavirin BPCRS*. After removal of the plate, allow the spots to dry in air for 15 minutes and spray the plate with mixture of 0.5 ml of *anisaldehyde*, 0.5 ml of *sulphuric acid*, 0.1 ml of *glacial acetic acid* and 9 ml of *ethanol (96%)*. Heat the plate at 105° for 40 minutes. The principal spot in the chromatogram obtained with solution (1) is similar in position, colour and size to that in the chromatogram obtained with solution (2).

B. In the Assay the retention time of the principal peak in the chromatogram obtained with solution (1) is similar to that of the principal peak in the chromatogram obtained with solution (2).

Related substances Carry out the method for *liquid chromatography*, Appendix III D, using two solutions of the contents of the container in the mobile phase containing (1) 0.050% w/v and (2) 0.000125% w/v of Tribavirin respectively. Solution (3) contains 0.050% w/v of *tribavirin impurity standard BPCRS* in the mobile phase.

The chromatographic procedure may be carried out using (a) a stainless steel column (10 cm × 7.8 mm) packed with a strong cation-exchange resin of sulphonated, cross-linked *styrene—divinylbenzene co-polymer* in the hydrogen form (7 to 11 µm) (Aminex HPAH is suitable) and maintained at 40°, (b) *water* adjusted to pH 2.5 with *sulphuric acid* as the mobile phase with a flow rate of 1 ml per minute and (c) a detection wavelength of 207 nm. Inject separately 10 µl of each solution. For solution (1) allow the chromatography to proceed for ten times the retention time of the principal peak.

The test is not valid unless the *symmetry factor* for the principal peak in the chromatogram obtained with solution (1) is at least 0.7 and not more than 1.5 and unless the chromatogram obtained with solution (3) closely resembles the reference chromatogram supplied with *tribavirin impurity standard BPCRS*.

In the chromatogram obtained with solution (1) the area of any *secondary peak* is not greater than that of the principal peak in the chromatogram obtained with solution (2) (0.25%) and the sum of the areas of any such peaks is not greater than 4 times the area of the principal peak in the chromatogram obtained with solution (2) (1%).

Assay Carry out the method for *liquid chromatography*, Appendix III D, using the following solutions in the mobile phase. For solution (1) reconstitute the contents of 1 container as instructed on the label using an accurately measured volume of diluent, dilute a suitable volume of the solution to 200 volumes with the mobile phase to produce a solution containing 0.10% w/v of Tribavirin; mix and dilute 5 volumes of the resulting solution to 20 volumes with the mobile phase. Solution (2) contains 0.0025% w/v of *tribavirin BPCRS*.

The chromatographic procedure described under Related substances may be used.

Calculate the content of $C_8H_{12}N_4O_5$ in the container using the declared content of $C_8H_{12}N_4O_5$ in *tribavirin BPCRS*.

Storage The sealed container should be stored at a temperature not exceeding 25°.

Labelling The label of the sealed container states (1) the procedure for preparing the solution; (2) the delivery system to be used for the constituted solution; (3) the conditions under which it should be stored.

Triclofos Oral Solution

Definition Triclofos Oral Solution is a solution of Triclofos Sodium in a suitable flavoured vehicle.

The oral solution complies with the requirements stated under Oral Liquids and with the following requirements.

Content of triclofos sodium, $C_2H_3Cl_3NaO_4P$ 95.0 to 105.0% of the prescribed or stated amount.

Identification Mix a quantity of the oral solution containing 0.25 g of Triclofos Sodium with 40 ml of *water*, add 5 ml of 1M *sulphuric acid* and extract with 25 ml of *amyl alcohol*. The extract complies with the following tests.

A. Evaporate 5 ml to dryness, heat the residue with 1 ml of a 50% v/v solution of *sulphuric acid* and 1 ml of a 5% w/v solution of *potassium permanganate* in a water bath for 5 minutes, add 7 ml of *water* and decolorise the solution with 1 ml of a 5% w/v solution of *oxalic acid*. To 1 ml add 1 ml of *pyridine* and 1 ml of 2M *sodium hydroxide*, heat in a water bath for 1 minute, stirring continuously. A pink colour is produced in the pyridine layer.

B. Evaporate 10 ml to dryness, heat the residue with 1 g of *anhydrous sodium carbonate* at a dull red heat for 10 minutes, cool, extract the residue with *water* and filter. The residue yields the reactions characteristic of *chlorides* and of *phosphates*, Appendix VI.

Assay To a quantity containing 0.13 g of Triclofos Sodium add 15 ml of *water*, 1 ml of 1M *sodium hydroxide* and 15 ml of *ether*, shake for 1 minute, allow to separate, wash the ether layer with 1 ml of *water* and discard the ether solution. Add 2.5 ml of 1M *sulphuric acid* to the combined aqueous layer and washings, extract with four 10-ml quantities of *amyl alcohol*, allowing each extract to stand until good separation is achieved, combine the amyl alcohol extracts, remove any further water that separates and dilute to 50 ml with *amyl alcohol*. Transfer 10 ml of this solution to a 20-ml glass ampoule, add 10 ml of *alcoholic potassium hydroxide solution*, seal the ampoule, mix well and heat in an autoclave at 120° for 2 hours. Allow the ampoule to cool, transfer the contents to a flask with the aid of 20 ml of 2M *nitric acid* and add 25 ml of 0.02M *silver nitrate VS*. Titrate with 0.02M *ammonium thiocyanate VS* using *ammonium iron(III) sulphate solution R2* as indicator. Repeat the titration using 10 ml of *alcoholic potassium hydroxide solution* in place of the contents of the ampoule. The difference between the titrations represents the amount of silver nitrate required. Each ml of 0.02M *silver nitrate VS* is equivalent to 1.676 mg of $C_2H_3Cl_3NaO_4P$. Determine the *weight per ml* of the oral solution, Appendix V G, and calculate the content of $C_2H_3Cl_3NaO_4P$, weight in volume.

Storage Triclofos Oral Solution should be stored at a temperature not exceeding 25°.

Trifluoperazine Tablets

Definition Trifluoperazine Tablets contain Trifluoperazine Hydrochloride. They are coated.

The tablets comply with the requirements stated under Tablets and with the following requirements.

Content of trifluoperazine, $C_{21}H_{24}F_3N_3S$ 92.5 to 107.5% of the prescribed or stated amount.

Identification

A. Shake a quantity of the powdered tablets containing the equivalent of 20 mg of trifluoperazine with 30 ml of 1M *hydrochloric acid* for 10 minutes, filter, make the filtrate alkaline to *litmus paper* with 5M *sodium hydroxide* and extract with two 20-ml quantities of *petroleum spirit (boiling range, 60° to 80°)*. Combine the extracts, wash with 10 ml of *water*, shake with 5 g of *anhydrous sodium sulphate*, filter and evaporate the filtrate carefully to dryness. The *infrared absorption spectrum* of the residue, Appendix II A, is concordant with the *reference spectrum* of trifluoperazine.

B. Extract a quantity of the powdered tablets containing the equivalent of 5 mg of trifluoperazine with 5 ml of *acetone*, filter and evaporate the filtrate to dryness. Add 2 ml of *sulphuric acid* to the residue and allow to stand for 5 minutes. An orange colour is produced.

C. Extract a quantity of the powdered tablets containing the equivalent of 7 mg of trifluoperazine with 5 ml of *acetone*, filter and evaporate the filtrate to dryness. Separately, heat 0.5 ml of *chromic—sulphuric acid mixture* in a small test tube in a water bath for 5 minutes; the solution readily wets the sides of the tube and there is no greasiness. Add the residue to the acid mixture and heat again on a water bath for 5 minutes; the solution does not wet the sides of the tube and does not pour easily from the tube.

Uniformity of content Tablets containing the equivalent of less than 2 mg of Trifluoperazine comply with the requirements stated under Tablets using the following method of analysis. Carry out the following procedure protected from light. Place one tablet in a 100-ml graduated flask, add 50 ml of a mixture of 5 volumes of *hydrochloric acid* and 95 volumes of *water*, shake until the tablet has completely disintegrated, dilute to volume with the same solvent, mix and filter, discarding the first 10 ml of filtrate. Measure the *absorbance* of the filtrate at the maximum at 256 nm, Appendix II B. Calculate the content of $C_{21}H_{24}F_3N_3S$ taking 743 as the value of A(1%, 1 cm) at the maximum at 256 nm.

Assay Carry out the following procedure protected from light. Weigh and powder 20 tablets. Shake a quantity of the powder containing the equivalent of 5 mg of trifluoperazine for 15 minutes with 400 ml of a mixture of 5 volumes of *hydrochloric acid* and 95 volumes of *water*, dilute to 500 ml with the same mixture, mix and filter. Measure the *absorbance* of the filtrate at the maximum at 256 nm, Appendix II B. Calculate the content of $C_{21}H_{24}F_3N_3S$ taking 743 as the value of A(1%, 1 cm) at the maximum at 256 nm.

Labelling The quantity of active ingredient is stated in terms of the equivalent amount of trifluoperazine.

Trihexyphenidyl Tablets
Benzhexol Tablets

For the purposes of product labelling in the United Kingdom, the pair of names given above shall be used together (see Introduction, Changes in title).

Definition Trihexyphenidyl Tablets contain Trihexyphenidyl Hydrochloride.

The tablets comply with the requirements stated under Tablets and with the following requirements.

Content of trihexyphenidyl hydrochloride, $C_{20}H_{31}NO,HCl$ 90.0 to 110.0% of the prescribed or stated amount.

Identification

A. Shake a quantity of the powdered tablets containing Trihexyphenidyl Hydrochloride with 20 ml of *water* and filter. The filtrate yields a yellow precipitate with *picric acid solution R1* and a white precipitate with 5M *sodium hydroxide.*

B. Carry out the method for *thin-layer chromatography*, Appendix III A, using *silica gel G* as the coating substance and a mixture of 90 volumes of *chloroform* and 10 volumes of *methanol* as the mobile phase. Apply separately to the plate 10 µl of each of the following solutions. For solution (1) shake a quantity of the powdered tablets with sufficient *chloroform* to produce a solution containing 0.2% w/v of Trihexyphenidyl Hydrochloride and filter. Solution (2) contains 0.2% w/v of *trihexyphenidyl hydrochloride BPCRS* in *chloroform*. After removal of the plate, allow it to dry in air and spray with *dilute potassium iodobismuthate solution*. The principal spot in the chromatogram obtained with solution (1) corresponds to that in the chromatogram obtained with solution (2).

Uniformity of content Tablets containing 2 mg or less of Trihexyphenidyl Hydrochloride comply with the requirements stated under Tablets using the following method of analysis. Carry out the method for *liquid chromatography*, Appendix III D, using the following solutions. Solution (1) contains 0.008% w/v of *trihexyphenidyl hydrochloride BPCRS* and 0.004% w/v of *3-piperidylpropiophenone hydrochloride BPCRS* in the mobile phase. For solution (2) add 5 ml of *water* to one tablet and mix with the aid of ultrasound for 5 minutes or until the tablet is dispersed. Add 10 ml of *methanol*, shake for 15 minutes, dilute to 25 ml with *methanol*, mix and filter through a filter with a maximum pore size of 0.2 µm.

The chromatographic procedure may be carried out using (a) a stainless steel column (15 cm × 3.9 mm) packed with *stationary phase C* (5 µm) (Resolve C18 is suitable), (b) as the mobile phase with a flow rate of 2 ml per minute, a mixture of 800 volumes of *acetonitrile*, 200 volumes of *water* and 0.2 volume of *triethylamine*, the pH of the mixture being adjusted to 4.0 with *orthophosphoric acid* and (c) a detection wavelength of 210 nm.

The test is not valid unless the *resolution factor* between the two principal peaks in the chromatogram obtained with solution (1) is greater than 4.0.

Calculate the content of $C_{20}H_{31}NO,HCl$ in each tablet using the declared content of $C_{20}H_{31}NO,HCl$ in *trihexyphenidyl hydrochloride BPCRS*.

Related substances Carry out the method for *liquid chromatography*, Appendix III D, using the following solutions. For solution (1) mix a quantity of the powdered tablets containing 50 mg of Trihexyphenidyl Hydrochloride with 10 ml of *water*, add 10 ml of *methanol*, disperse with the aid of ultrasound for 5 minutes, shake for 15 minutes, add sufficient *methanol* to produce 25 ml and filter. For solution (2) dilute 1 volume of solution (1) to 100 volumes with *methanol (60%)*. Solution (3) contains 0.01% w/v of *3-piperidylpropiophenone hydrochloride BPCRS* in solution (1).

The chromatographic procedure described under Uniformity of content may be used.

The test is not valid unless the *resolution factor* between the two principal peaks in the chromatogram obtained with solution (3) is greater than 4.0.

The area of any *secondary peak* in the chromatogram obtained with solution (1) is not greater than the area of the peak in the chromatogram obtained with solution (2) (1%) and the total area of any *secondary peaks* is not greater than twice the area of the peak in the chromatogram obtained with solution (2) (2%).

Assay

For tablets containing more than 2 mg of Trihexyphenidyl hydrochloride Weigh and powder 20 tablets. Carry out the method for *liquid chromatography*, Appendix III D, using the following solutions. Solution (1) contains 0.02% w/v of *trihexyphenidyl hydrochloride BPCRS* and 0.01% w/v of *3-piperidylpropiophenone hydrochloride BPCRS* in the mobile phase. For solution (2) add 5 ml of *water* to a quantity of the powdered tablets containing 5 mg of Trihexyphenidyl Hydrochloride and mix with the aid of ultrasound for 5 minutes. Add 10 ml of *methanol*, shake for 15 minutes, dilute to 25 ml with *methanol* and filter through a filter with a maximum pore size of 0.2 µm.

The chromatographic procedure described under Uniformity of content may be used.

The assay is not valid unless the *resolution factor* between the two principal peaks in the chromatogram obtained with solution (1) is greater than 4.0.

Calculate the content of $C_{20}H_{31}NO,HCl$ using the declared content of $C_{20}H_{31}NO,HCl$ in *trihexyphenidyl hydrochloride BPCRS*.

For tablets containing 2 mg or less of Trihexyphenidyl Hydrochloride Use the average of the 10 individual results obtained in the test for Uniformity of content.

Labelling The label states 'Trihexyphenidyl Tablets' and 'Benzhexol Tablets'.

Trimethoprim Tablets

Definition Trimethoprim Tablets contain Trimethoprim.

The tablets comply with the requirements stated under Tablets and with the following requirements.

Content of trimethoprim, $C_{14}H_{18}N_4O_3$ 95.0 to 105.0% of the prescribed or stated amount.

Identification

A. Shake a quantity of the powdered tablets containing 0.1 g of Trimethoprim with 10 ml of *chloroform*, filter and evaporate the filtrate to dryness. The *infrared absorption spectrum* of the residue, Appendix II A, is concordant with the *reference spectrum* of trimethoprim.

B. Shake a quantity of the powdered tablets containing 0.1 g of Trimethoprim with 60 ml of 0.1M *hydrochloric acid* for 20 minutes, add sufficient 0.1M *hydrochloric acid* to produce 100 ml, filter and dilute 5 ml of the filtrate to 250 ml with 0.1M *sodium hydroxide*. The *light absorption* of the resulting solution, Appendix II B, in the range 230 to 350 nm exhibits a maximum only at 287 nm.

Related substances Carry out the method for *liquid chromatography*, Appendix III D, using the following solutions. Shake a quantity of the powdered tablets containing 0.2 g of Trimethoprim with 50 ml of the mobile phase and filter. For solution (1) dilute 1 volume of the filtrate to 100 volumes with the mobile phase. For solution (2) use the filtrate undiluted.

The chromatographic procedure may be carried out using (a) a stainless steel column (20 cm × 5 mm) packed with *stationary phase C* (5 µm) (Spherisorb ODS 1 is suitable), (b) as the mobile phase with a flow rate of 1.3 ml per minute a 0.14% w/v solution of *sodium perchlorate* in *methanol (60%)* adjusted to pH 3.1 with 0.1M *hydrochloric acid* and (c) a detection wavelength of 280 nm.

The *column efficiency*, determined using the peak due to trimethoprim in the chromatogram obtained with solution (1), should be at least 8,000 theoretical plates per metre.

In the chromatogram obtained with solution (2) the sum of the areas of any *secondary peaks* is not greater than the area of the principal peak in the chromatogram obtained with solution (1).

Assay Weigh and powder 20 tablets. To a quantity of the powder containing 0.1 g of Trimethoprim add 100 ml of *glacial acetic acid*, shake for 20 minutes, dilute to 200 ml with *glacial acetic acid* and filter. To 5 ml of the filtrate add 15 ml of *glacial acetic acid* and dilute to 100 ml with *water*. Measure the *absorbance* of the resulting solution at the maximum at 271 nm, Appendix II B. Calculate the content of $C_{14}H_{18}N_4O_3$ taking 204 as the value of A(1%, 1 cm) at the maximum at 271 nm.

Trimipramine Tablets

Definition Trimipramine Tablets contain Trimipramine Maleate. They are coated.

The tablets comply with the requirements stated under Tablets and with the following requirements.

Content of trimipramine, $C_{20}H_{26}N_2$ 92.5 to 107.5% of the prescribed or stated amount.

Identification Triturate a quantity of the powdered tablets containing the equivalent of 0.25 g of trimipramine with 10 ml of *chloroform*, filter and evaporate the filtrate to low volume. Add *ether* until a turbidity is produced and allow to stand. The *infrared absorption spectrum*, Appendix II A, of the precipitate, after recrystallisation from *acetone*, is concordant with the *reference spectrum* of trimipramine maleate.

Related substances Carry out the method for *thin-layer chromatography*, Appendix III A, using *silica gel G* as the coating substance and a mixture of 0.7 volume of 13.5M *ammonia*, 10 volumes of *ethanol (96%)* and 90 volumes of *toluene* as the mobile phase. Apply separately to the plate 5 µl of each of the following solutions prepared immediately before use. For solution (1) shake a quantity of the powdered tablets containing the equivalent of 0.18 g of trimipramine with three 10-ml quantities of *chloroform* and filter. Evaporate the combined filtrates to dryness and dissolve the residue in 10 ml of *methanol*. For solution (2) dilute 1 volume of solution (1) to 200 volumes with *methanol*. For solution (3) dilute 2 volumes of solution (2) to 5 volumes with *methanol*. Solution (4) contains 0.0125% w/v of *iminodibenzyl* in *methanol*. After removal of the plate, allow it to dry in air for 15 minutes and spray with a 0.5% w/v solution of *potassium dichromate* in *sulphuric acid (20% v/v)*. Examine the plate immediately. Any spot corresponding to iminodibenzyl in the chromatogram obtained with solution (1) is not more intense than the spot in the chromatogram obtained with solution (4) (0.7%, with reference to trimipramine). Any other *secondary spot* is not more intense than the spot in the chromatogram obtained with solution (2) (0.5%) and not more than three such spots are more intense than the spot in the chromatogram obtained with solution (3) (0.2%). Disregard any spot remaining on the line of application.

Assay Weigh and powder 20 tablets. Shake a quantity of the powder containing the equivalent of 50 mg of trimipramine with 190 ml of a mixture of equal volumes of *acetonitrile* and *water* for 1 minute, mix with the aid of ultrasound for 5 minutes, shake for 1 minute and mix again with the aid of ultrasound for 5 minutes. Add sufficient of a mixture of equal volumes of *acetonitrile* and *water* to produce 200 ml, filter and dilute 10 ml of the filtrate to 100 ml with the same solvent. Measure the *absorbance* of the resulting solution at the maximum at 250 nm, Appendix II B. Calculate the content of $C_{20}H_{26}N_2$ taking 320 as the value of A(1%, 1 cm) at the maximum at 250 nm.

Labelling The quantity of active ingredient is stated in terms of the equivalent amount of trimipramine.

Triprolidine Tablets

Definition Triprolidine Tablets contain Triprolidine Hydrochloride.

The tablets comply with the requirements stated under Tablets and with the following requirements.

Content of triprolidine hydrochloride, $C_{19}H_{22}N_2,HCl,H_2O$ 90.0 to 110.0% of the prescribed or stated amount.

Identification

A. Extract a quantity of the powdered tablets containing 10 mg of Triprolidine Hydrochloride with *ether*, filter, discard the ether and dry the residue. Extract the residue with *chloroform* and evaporate to dryness. Add 0.1 ml of *ether*, stir and allow to evaporate. The *infrared absorption spectrum* of the residue, Appendix II A, is concordant with the *reference spectrum* of triprolidine hydrochloride.

B. In the test for Related substances, the principal spot in the chromatogram obtained with solution (1) corresponds to that in the chromatogram obtained with solution (4).

Related substances Carry out the method for *thin-layer chromatography*, Appendix III A, using a silica gel F_{254} precoated plate (Merck silica gel 60 F_{254} plates are suitable) and a mixture of equal volumes of *butan-2-one* and *dimethylformamide* as the mobile phase. Apply separately to the plate 5 µl of each of the following solutions. For solution (1) extract a quantity of the powdered tablets containing 10 mg of Triprolidine Hydrochloride with *methanol*, filter, evaporate to dryness and dissolve the residue in 1 ml of *methanol*. Solution (2) contains 0.020% w/v of *Z-triprolidine BPCRS* in *methanol*. Solutions (3) and (4) contain 0.010% w/v and 1.0% w/v respectively of *triprolidine hydrochloride BPCRS* in *methanol*. After removal of the plate, allow it to dry in air and examine under *ultraviolet light (254 nm)*. In the chromatogram obtained with solution (1) any spot corresponding to *Z*-triprolidine is not more intense than the spot in the chromatogram obtained with solution (2) and any other *secondary spot* is not more intense than the spot in the chromatogram obtained with solution (3).

Assay Weigh and powder 20 tablets. To a quantity of the powder containing 7.5 mg of Triprolidine Hydrochloride, add 15 ml of *water* and 1 g of *sodium chloride*, shake for 2 to 3 minutes and make alkaline with 5M *sodium hydroxide*. Extract with four 20-ml quantities of *ether* and wash the combined extracts with two 5-ml quantities of a mixture of equal volumes of a saturated solution of *sodium chloride* and *water*. Extract the ether solution with 20 ml of 0.1M *hydrochloric acid*, wash the ether with two 5-ml quantities of *water* and add the washings to the acid extract. Heat on a water bath for 30 minutes, cool and add sufficient *water* to produce 50 ml. Dilute 10 ml to 100 ml with 0.1M *hydrochloric acid* and measure the *absorbance* of the resulting solution at the maximum at 290 nm, Appendix II B. Calculate the content of $C_{19}H_{22}N_2,HCl,H_2O$ taking 290 as the value of A(1%, 1 cm) at the maximum at 290 nm.

Trisodium Edetate Intravenous Infusion

Trisodium Edetate Injection

Definition Trisodium Edetate Intravenous Infusion is a sterile solution of trisodium edetate. It is prepared immediately before use by diluting Sterile Trisodium Edetate Concentrate with a suitable diluent in accordance with the manufacturer's instructions.

The intravenous infusion complies with the requirements stated under Parenteral Preparations and with the following requirements.

Particulate contamination When the volume of the diluted intravenous infusion is 100 ml or more, it complies with the test for *sub-visible particles*, Appendix XIII A.

Labelling The strength is stated as the amount of trisodium edetate in a suitable dose-volume.

STERILE TRISODIUM EDETATE CONCENTRATE

Definition Sterile Trisodium Edetate Concentrate is a sterile solution in Water for Injections containing 20% w/v of trisodium edetate prepared by the interaction of Disodium Edetate and Sodium Hydroxide.

The concentrate complies with the requirements for Concentrated Solutions for Injections stated under Parenteral Preparations and with the following requirements.

Content of trisodium edetate, $C_{10}H_{13}N_2Na_3O_8$ 19.0 to 21.0% w/v.

Characteristics A colourless solution.

Identification

A. Dilute 2.5 ml with 7.5 ml of *water* and add 0.5 ml of a 10% w/v solution of *calcium chloride*; make alkaline to *litmus paper* with 5M *ammonia* and add 5 ml of a 2.5% w/v solution of *ammonium oxalate*. No precipitate is produced.

B. Dilute 10 ml with 15 ml of *water*, add 2 ml of a 10% w/v solution of *lead(II) nitrate*, shake and add 5 ml of *dilute potassium iodide solution*; no yellow precipitate is produced. Make alkaline to *litmus paper* with 5M *ammonia* and add 5 ml of a 2.5% w/v solution of *ammonium oxalate*; no precipitate is produced.

C. Evaporate to dryness and ignite. The residue yields the reactions characteristic of *sodium salts*, Appendix VI.

Acidity or alkalinity pH, 7.0 to 8.0, Appendix V L.

Pyrogens Complies with the *test for pyrogens*, Appendix XIV D, using per kg of the rabbit's weight 5 ml of a solution prepared as follows. To 1 volume of the solution being examined add 2.5 volumes of *calcium gluconate solution*. Dilute the resulting solution with sufficient *water for injections* to give a final concentration of 5.0% w/v of trisodium edetate.

Assay Dilute 10 ml to 100 ml with *water* and use this solution to titrate a mixture of 25 ml of 0.05M *magnesium sulphate VS* and 10 ml of *ammonia buffer pH 10.9* using *mordant black 11 mixed triturate* as indicator. Each ml of 0.05M *magnesium sulphate VS* is equivalent to 17.91 mg of trisodium edetate, $C_{10}H_{13}N_2Na_3O_8$.

Storage Sterile Trisodium Edetate Concentrate should be kept in containers made from lead-free glass.

Labelling The label states (1) 'Sterile Trisodium Edetate Concentrate'; (2) that the solution must be diluted with either Sodium Chloride Intravenous Infusion or Glucose Intravenous Infusion before administration.

Action and use Used in treatment of hypercalcaemia.

Tropicamide Eye Drops

Definition Tropicamide Eye Drops are a sterile solution of Tropicamide in Purified Water.

The eye drops comply with the requirements stated under Eye Preparations and with the following requirements.

Content of tropicamide, $C_{17}H_{20}N_2O_2$ 95.0 to 110.0% of the prescribed or stated amount.

Identification

A. Shake a volume of the eye drops containing 20 mg of Tropicamide with 10 ml of *chloroform*, dry the chloroform layer over *anhydrous sodium sulphate*, filter and evaporate the filtrate to dryness. Dissolve the residue in the minimum quantity of *chloroform*, add dropwise to finely powdered *potassium bromide*, mix and dry at 60°. The *infrared absorption spectrum*, Appendix II A, of the dispersion examined as a disc is concordant with the *reference spectrum* of tropicamide.

B. The *light absorption*, Appendix II B, in the range 230 to 350 nm of the final solution obtained in the Assay exhibits a maximum only at 254 nm.

Acidity pH, 4.0 to 5.8, Appendix V L.

Related substances Carry out the method for *thin-layer chromatography*, Appendix III A, using *silica gel GF_{254}* as the coating substance and a mixture of 1 volume of 13.5M *ammonia*, 10 volumes of *methanol* and 190 volumes of *chloroform* as the mobile phase. Apply separately to the plate (1) a volume of the eye drops containing 0.2 mg of Tropicamide, (2) the same volume of a solution prepared by diluting 1 volume of the eye drops to 200 volumes and (3) the same volume of a solution prepared by diluting 1 volume of the eye drops to 500 volumes. After removal of the plate, allow it to dry in air and examine under *ultraviolet light (254 nm)*. Any *secondary spot* in the chromatogram obtained with solution (1) is not more intense than the spot in the chromatogram obtained with solution (2) (0.5%) and not more than one such spot is more intense than the spot in the chromatogram obtained with solution (3) (0.2%).

Assay To a quantity containing 30 mg of Tropicamide add sufficient *water* to produce 100 ml and mix. To 10 ml of the resulting solution add 2 ml of a 10% w/v solution of *anhydrous sodium carbonate* and extract with four 20-ml quantities of *chloroform*. Wash the combined chloroform extracts with 25 ml of a solution containing 0.0176% w/v of *disodium hydrogen orthophosphate* and 0.243% w/v of *sodium dihydrogen orthophosphate*. Wash the aqueous layer with 10 ml of *chloroform*, combine the chloroform extracts and shake with four 20-ml quantities of 0.5M *sulphuric acid*. Combine the acid extracts and add sufficient 0.5M *sulphuric acid* to produce 100 ml. Measure the *absorbance* of the resulting solution at the maximum at 254 nm, Appendix II B. Calculate the content of $C_{17}H_{20}N_2O_2$ in the eye drops taking 172 as the value of A(1%, 1 cm) at the maximum at 254 nm.

Storage Tropicamide Eye Drops should be stored at a temperature of 8° to 15°.

Urea Cream

Definition Urea Cream contains Urea in a suitable basis.

The cream complies with the requirements stated under Topical Semi-solid Preparations and with the following requirements.

Content of urea, CH_4N_2O 90.0 to 110.0% of the prescribed or stated amount.

Identification

A. Carry out the method for *thin-layer chromatography*, Appendix III A, using a silica gel precoated plate (Merck silica gel 60 plates are suitable). Apply separately to the plate 10 µl of each of the following solutions. For solution (1) disperse with heating a quantity of the cream containing 50 mg of Urea in 1 ml of *water*, cool, add 4 ml of *acetone*, mix and filter. For solution (2) dissolve 50 mg of *urea* in 1 ml of *water* and add 4 ml of *acetone*. Solution (3) is a mixture of equal volumes of solutions (1) and (2). For the first development use *2,2,4-trimethylpentane* as the mobile phase. Remove the plate and allow it to dry in air. For the second development use as the mobile phase a mixture of 99 volumes of *absolute ethanol* and 1 volume of 13.5M *ammonia*. After removal of the plate, allow it to dry in air and spray with a solution containing 0.5% w/v of *4-dimethylaminobenzaldehyde* and 0.5% v/v of *sulphuric acid* in *absolute ethanol*. The principal spot in the chromatogram obtained with solution (1) corresponds to that in the chromatogram obtained with solution (2). The test is not valid unless the chromatogram obtained with solution (3) shows a single, compact principal spot.

B. To a quantity containing 0.1 g of Urea add 50 ml of *water* and heat until dispersed, cool in ice and filter through glass wool. Adjust the pH of the filtrate, which may not be clear, to between 6.0 and 7.0 using 0.1M *hydrochloric acid* or 0.1M *sodium hydroxide* as necessary. To 5 ml add 5 ml of a 0.1% w/v suspension of *urease-active meal* and allow to stand for 30 minutes in a stoppered flask at 37°. When the resulting solution is heated in a water bath, a vapour is produced that turns moist *red litmus paper* blue.

Ammonia Not more than 2.0% with respect to the content of urea, CH_4N_2O (determined in the Assay) when determined by the following method. Prepare a 0.035% w/v solution of *ammonium sulphate* in 1M *sulphuric acid* (solution A). Carry out the method for *ion-selective potentiometry*, Appendix VIII E, using an ammonia-selective electrode. Determine the response slope of the electrode using standard ammonia solutions and measure the emf in the following solutions. For solution (1) shake a quantity of the cream (w_1 g) containing 40 mg of Urea with 5 ml of 1M *sulphuric acid* to disperse, warming if necessary, add 10 ml of *2,2,4-trimethylpentane*, shake for 2 minutes and centrifuge. Dilute 3 ml of the aqueous layer to 50 ml with *water* and to 20 ml of the resulting solution add 4 ml of 1M *sodium hydroxide*. Prepare solution (2) in the same manner but shaking a quantity of the cream (w_2 g) containing 40 mg of Urea with 5 ml of solution A in place of 5 ml of 1M *sulphuric acid*.

Calculate C_1 and hence the concentration of ammonia in the cream from the expression

$$\Delta E = a \log(w_2/w_1 + C_2/C_1)$$

where ΔE = the difference in the emf, in mV, obtained with the two solutions,

a = the response slope in mV per decade,

C_1 = the concentration of ammonia in solution (1) as % w/v,

C_2 = the concentration of standard added ammonia in solution (2) as % w/v (this is 0.0129 times the concentration of ammonium sulphate in solution A as % w/v), namely 0.000451% w/v.

Assay Shake a quantity containing 42 mg of Urea with 150 ml of hot *water* for 20 minutes, allow to cool and dilute to 500 ml with *water*. Filter through a fine glass microfibre filter paper (Whatman GF/C is suitable), transfer 1 ml of the filtrate to a 100-ml graduated flask, add 2 ml of a 0.1% w/v suspension of *urease-active meal*, stopper the flask and allow to stand for 15 minutes at 37°. Immediately add 25 ml of a solution containing 12 g of *sodium salicylate* and 0.24 g of *sodium nitroprusside* in 200 ml and 25 ml of a solution prepared by diluting a volume of *sodium hypochlorite solution* containing the equivalent of 0.66 g of available chlorine with 0.2M *sodium hydroxide* to 1000 ml. Mix well, allow to stand at 37° for 5 minutes and dilute to 100 ml with *water*. Measure the *absorbance* of the resulting solution at the maximum at 665 nm, Appendix II B, using in the reference cell a solution prepared in the same manner but using 1 ml of *water* in place of 1 ml of the filtrate. Calculate the content of CH_4N_2O from the *absorbance* obtained using 42 mg of *urea BPCRS* in place of the cream being examined.

Storage Urea Cream should be stored in accordance with the manufacturer's instructions.

Urofollitropin Injection

Definition Urofollitropin Injection is a sterile solution of Urofollitropin in Sodium Chloride Intravenous Infusion. It is prepared by dissolving Urofollitropin for Injection in the requisite amount of Sodium Chloride Intravenous Infusion immediately before use.

The injection complies with the requirements stated under Parenteral Preparations.

Storage Urofollitropin Injection should be used immediately after preparation.

UROFOLLITROPIN FOR INJECTION

Definition Urofollitropin for Injection is a sterile material consisting of Urofollitropin with or without excipients. It is supplied in a sealed container.

The contents of the sealed container comply with the requirements for Powders for Injections stated under Parenteral Preparations and with the following requirements.

Characteristics An almost white or slightly yellow powder.

Identification Cause enlargement of the ovaries of immature female rats when administered as directed in the Assay.

Acidity or alkalinity Dissolve the contents of the sealed container in 3 ml of *water* (solution A). The pH is 6.0 to 8.0, Appendix V L.

Clarity and colour of solution Solution A is *clear*, Appendix IV A, and *colourless*, Appendix IV B, Method I.

Residual luteinising activity Comply with the test described under Urofollitropin.

Water Comply with the test described under Urofollitropin.

Pyrogens Comply with the *test for pyrogens*, Appendix XIV D. Use per kg of the rabbit's weight 1 ml of a solution in *sodium chloride injection* containing 5 IU of follicle-stimulating hormone activity per ml.

Assay Carry out the Assay described under Urofollitropin. The estimated potency for each component is not less than 80% and not more than 125% of the stated potency. The fiducial limits of error are not less than 64% and not more than 156% of the stated potency.

Storage The sealed container should be protected from light and stored at a temperature not exceeding 25°. Under these conditions, the contents may be expected to retain their potency for not less than 3 years.

Labelling The label of the sealed container states the number of IU (Units) of follicle-stimulating hormone activity contained in it.

When urofollitrophin injection or urofollitrophin for injection is prescribed or demanded, Urofollitropin Injection or Urofollitropin for Injection shall be dispensed or supplied.

Vancomycin Injection

Definition Vancomycin Injection is a sterile solution of Vancomycin Hydrochloride in Water for Injections. It is prepared by dissolving Vancomycin Hydrochloride for Injection in the requisite amount of Water for Injections.

The injection complies with the requirements stated under Parenteral Preparations.

Storage Vancomycin Injection should be used immediately after preparation but, in any case, within the period recommended by the manufacturer when prepared and stored strictly in accordance with the manufacturer's instructions.

VANCOMYCIN HYDROCHLORIDE FOR INJECTION

Definition Vancomycin Hydrochloride for Injection is a sterile material consisting of Vancomycin Hydrochloride with or without excipients. It is supplied in a sealed container.

The contents of the sealed container comply with the requirements for Powders for Injections stated under Parenteral Preparations and with the following requirements.

Identification

A. In the test for Vancomycin B, the retention time of the principal peak in the chromatogram obtained with solution (1) is similar to that of the principal peak in the chromatogram obtained with solution (4).

B. Yield reaction A characteristic of *chlorides*, Appendix VI.

Acidity pH of a 5% w/v solution, 2.5 to 4.5, Appendix V L.

Clarity of solution A 10.0% w/v solution in *water* is *clear*, Appendix IV A. The *absorbance* of the solution at 450 nm is not greater than 0.10, Appendix II B.

Vancomycin B Not less than 88.0% when determined by the following method. Carry out the method for *liquid chromatography*, Appendix III D, using the following solutions in mobile phase A. For solution (1) dissolve a quantity of the contents of the sealed container in sufficient of mobile phase A to produce a solution containing 2,000 IU of vancomycin per ml. For solution (2) dilute 2 volumes of solution (1) to 50 volumes with mobile phase A. For solution (3) dilute 0.5 volume of solution (2) to 20 volumes with mobile phase A. For solution (4) heat a 0.050% w/v solution of *vancomycin hydrochloride EPCRS* in *water* at 65° for 24 hours and allow to cool. Use the solutions within 4 hours of preparation.

The chromatographic procedure may be carried out using (a) a stainless steel column (25 cm × 4.6 mm) packed with *stationary phase C* (5 µm) (Hypersil ODS is suitable), (b) as mobile phases A and B at a flow rate of 1 ml per minute the solutions described below and (c) a detection wavelength of 280 nm.

Mobile phase A To 4 ml of *triethylamine* add 1996 ml of *water* and adjust to pH 3.2 with *orthophosphoric acid* (solution A); to 920 ml of solution A add 10 ml of *tetrahydrofuran* and 70 ml of *acetonitrile*.

Mobile phase B To 700 ml of solution A add 10 ml of *tetrahydrofuran* and 290 ml of *acetonitrile*.

Inject 20 µl of each solution and record the chromatograms under the following conditions. Elute initially with mobile phase A. After 13 minutes, use linear gradient elution increasing the concentration of mobile phase B by 11% v/v per minute. Finally, elute for 4 minutes using mobile phase B.

Inject solution (3). The test is not valid unless the principal peak in the chromatogram obtained has a *signal-to-noise ratio* of at least 5. Inject solution (2). The test is not valid unless the *symmetry factor* of the vancomycin peak is not greater than 1.6. Inject solution (4). The test is not valid unless the *resolution factor* between the two principal peaks is at least 5.0. Inject solution (1).

Using the chromatograms obtained with solutions (1) and (2), calculate the percentage content of vancomycin B.

Related substances Carry out the method for *liquid chromatography*, Appendix III D, using solutions (1), (2) and (3) as described under Vancomycin B.

Using the chromatograms obtained with solutions (1) and (2), calculate the percentage content of each impurity. The content of any impurity is not greater than 4.0% and the sum of the contents of any such impurities is not greater than 12.0%. Disregard any peak with an area less than that of the principal peak in the chromatogram obtained with solution (3) (0.1%).

Water Not more than 5.0% w/w, Appendix IX C. Use 0.5 g.

Bacterial endotoxins Carry out the *test for bacterial endotoxins*, Appendix XIV C. Dissolve the contents of the sealed container in *tris-chloride buffer pH 7.4* to give a solution containing 9000 IU of vancomycin per ml (solution A). The endotoxin limit concentration of solution A is 2.5 IU of endotoxin per ml. Carry out the test using the maximum valid dilution of solution A calculated from the declared sensitivity of the lysate used in the test.

Assay Determine the weight of the contents of 10 containers as described in the test for Uniformity of weight under Parenteral Preparations, Powders for Injections.

Mix the contents of the 10 containers and carry out the *biological assay of antibiotics*, Appendix XIV A. The precision of the assay is such that the fiducial limits of error are not less than 95% and not more than 105% of the estimated potency.

For a container of average content weight, the upper fiducial limit of error is not less than 95.0% and the lower fiducial limit of error is not more than 115.0% of the prescribed or stated number of IU.

Labelling The label of the sealed container states (1) the total number of IU (Units) contained in it and (2) the number of IU (Units) per mg.

Verapamil Injection

Definition Verapamil Injection is a sterile solution of Verapamil Hydrochloride in Water for Injections.

The injection complies with the requirements stated under Parenteral Preparations and with the following requirements.

Content of verapamil hydrochloride, $C_{27}H_{38}N_2O_4$, HCl 90.0 to 110.0% of the prescribed or stated amount.

Identification

A. Dilute a volume containing 10 mg of Verapamil Hydrochloride to 5 ml with 0.1M *hydrochloric acid*, extract with 5 ml of *ether*, discard the extract and make the aqueous layer just alkaline with 2M *potassium carbonate sesquihydrate*. Extract with 5 ml of *ether*, filter the ether layer through *anhydrous sodium sulphate* and evaporate to dryness. The *infrared absorption spectrum* of the residue, Appendix II A, is concordant with the *reference spectrum* of verapamil.

B. To a volume containing 5 mg of Verapamil Hydrochloride add 0.2 ml of a 5% w/v solution of *mercury(II) chloride*. A white precipitate is produced.

C. To a volume containing 5 mg of Verapamil Hydrochloride add 0.5 ml of 3M *sulphuric acid* and 0.2 ml of *dilute potassium permanganate solution*. A violet precipitate is produced which quickly dissolves to produce a very pale yellow solution.

Acidity pH, 4.5 to 6.0, Appendix V L.

Related substances

A. Carry out the method for *thin-layer chromatography*, Appendix III A, using a suitable silica gel as the coating substance (Merck silica gel 60 is suitable) and a mixture of 5 volumes of *glacial acetic acid*, 5 volumes of *acetone*, 20 volumes of *methanol* and 70 volumes of *toluene* as the mobile phase. Apply separately to the plate 30 µl of each of the following solutions. For solution (1) evaporate a volume containing 5 mg of Verapamil Hydrochloride carefully to dryness on a water bath in a current of nitrogen and dissolve the residue as completely as possible in 0.25 ml of *chloroform*. For solution (2) dilute 1 volume of solution (1) to 100 volumes with *chloroform* and dilute 1 volume of the resulting solution to 10 volumes with *chloroform*. Remove the plate, allow it to dry in air for 10 minutes and repeat the development. After removal of the plate, heat it at 110° for 30 minutes and allow to stand until the odour of the solvent is no longer detectable. Spray with a solution prepared by dissolving 5 g of *iron(III) chloride hexahydrate* and 2 g of *iodine* in sufficient of a mixture of equal volumes of *acetone* and a 20% w/v solution of *(+)-tartaric acid* to produce 100 ml, applying a total of 15 to 20 ml of the reagent for a plate 200 mm × 200 mm, and examine immediately. Any *secondary spot* in the chromatogram obtained with solution (1) is not more intense than the spot in the chromatogram obtained with solution (2) (0.1%). Disregard any spot remaining on the line of application.

B. Carry out test A but with the following modifications. Use a mixture of 15 volumes of *diethylamine* and 85 volumes of *cyclohexane* as the mobile phase and heat at 110° for 90 minutes after the second development.

Assay Dilute a volume containing 5 mg of Verapamil Hydrochloride to 100 ml with 0.01M *hydrochloric acid*. Measure the *absorbance* of the resulting solution at the maximum at 278 nm, Appendix II B. Calculate the content of $C_{27}H_{38}N_2O_4$,HCl taking 118 as the value of A(1%, 1 cm) at the maximum at 278 nm.

Storage Verapamil Injection should be protected from light.

Verapamil Tablets

Definition Verapamil Tablets contain Verapamil Hydrochloride. They are coated.

The tablets comply with the requirements stated under Tablets and with the following requirements.

Content of verapamil hydrochloride, $C_{27}H_{38}N_2O_4$, HCl 92.5 to 107.5% of the prescribed or stated amount.

Identification

A. Shake a quantity of the powdered tablets containing 0.1 g of Verapamil Hydrochloride with 25 ml of 0.1M *hydrochloric acid*, filter, extract the filtrate with 25 ml of *ether*, discard the extract and make the aqueous solution just alkaline with 2M *potassium carbonate sesquihydrate*. Extract with 25 ml of *ether*, filter the ether layer through *anhydrous sodium sulphate* and evaporate to dryness. The *infrared absorption spectrum* of a thin film of the oily residue, Appendix II A, is concordant with the *reference spectrum* of verapamil.

B. Shake a quantity of the powdered tablets containing 0.1 g of Verapamil Hydrochloride with 10 ml of *dichloromethane*, filter, evaporate the filtrate to dryness and dissolve the residue in 10 ml of *water*. To 2 ml of the resulting solution add 0.2 ml of a 5% w/v solution of *mercury(II) chloride*. A white precipitate is produced.

C. To 2 ml of the solution obtained in test B add 0.5 ml of 3M *sulphuric acid* and 0.2 ml of *dilute potassium permanganate solution*. A violet precipitate is produced which quickly dissolves to produce a very pale yellow solution.

Related substances Comply with the tests described under Verapamil Injection using 10 µl of each of the following solutions. For solution (1) shake a quantity of the powdered tablets containing 0.1 g of Verapamil Hydrochloride with 10 ml of *dichloromethane*, filter, wash the filter with a further 5 ml of *dichloromethane*, evaporate the combined filtrate and washings to dryness and dissolve the residue in 2 ml of *chloroform*. For solution (2) dilute 1 volume of solution (1) to 100 volumes with *chloroform* and dilute 1 volume of the resulting solution to 10 volumes with *chloroform*.

Assay Weigh and powder 20 tablets. Shake a quantity of the powder containing 0.1 g of Verapamil Hydrochloride with 150 ml of 0.1M *hydrochloric acid* for 10 minutes, add sufficient 0.1M *hydrochloric acid* to produce 200 ml and filter. Dilute 10 ml of the filtrate to 100 ml with *water* and measure the *absorbance* of the resulting solution at the maximum at 278 nm, Appendix II B. Calculate the content of $C_{27}H_{38}N_2O_4$,HCl taking 118 as the value of A(1%, 1 cm) at the maximum at 278 nm.

Vigabatrin Oral Powder

Definition Vigabatrin Oral Powder contains Vigabatrin.

The oral powder complies with the requirements stated under Oral Powders and with the following requirements.

Content of vigabatrin, $C_6H_{11}NO_2$ 95.0 to 105.0% of the prescribed or stated amount.

Identification

A. The *infrared absorption spectrum*, Appendix II A, is concordant with the *reference spectrum* of vigabatrin.

B. In the Assay, the retention time of the principal peak in the chromatogram obtained with solution (1) is the same as that of the principal peak in the chromatogram obtained with solution (2).

5-Vinyl-2-pyrrolidone In the Assay, the area of any peak corresponding to 5-vinyl-2-pyrrolidone in the chromatogram obtained with solution (1) is not greater than the area of the peak in the chromatogram obtained with solution (3) (0.5%).

Assay Carry out the method for *liquid chromatography*, Appendix III D, using the following solutions. For solution (1) dissolve a quantity of the mixed contents of 20 sachets containing 0.2 g of Vigabatrin in sufficient of the mobile phase to produce 100 ml. Solution (2) contains 0.2% w/v of *vigabatrin BPCRS* in the mobile phase. Solution (3) contains 0.001% w/v of *5-vinyl-2-pyrrolidone BPCRS*. Solution (4) contains 0.002% w/v of *5-vinyl-2-pyrrolidone BPCRS*, 0.2% w/v of *povidone* and 0.2% w/v of *vigabatrin BPCRS* in the mobile phase.

The chromatographic procedure may be carried out using (a) a stainless steel column (25 cm × 4.6 mm) packed with cation exchange resin (10 µm) (Whatman Partisil 10 SCX is suitable), (b) as the mobile phase with a flow rate of 1.5 ml per minute a mixture of 4 volumes of *acetonitrile*, 40 volumes of *methanol* and 1000 volumes of a 0.34% w/v solution of *potassium dihydrogen orthophosphate*, adjusted to pH 2.8 with *orthophosphoric acid* and (c) a detection wavelength of 210 nm.

Inject 20 µl of solution (4). When the chromatogram is recorded under the prescribed conditions, the retention times are povidone, about 4 minutes, 5-vinyl-2-pyrrolidone, about 5 minutes and vigabatrin, about 8 minutes. The test is not valid unless the *resolution factor* between the peaks corresponding to 5-vinyl-2-pyrrolidone and vigabatrin is at least 1.5 and the *resolution factor* between the peaks corresponding to povidone and 5-vinyl-2-pyrrolidone is at least 1.5.

Inject separately 20 µl of solutions (1) and (2). Calculate the content of $C_6H_{11}NO_2$ in one sachet from the areas of the peaks and using the declared content of $C_6H_{11}NO_2$ in *vigabatrin BPCRS*.

Vigabatrin Tablets

Definition Vigabatrin Tablets contain Vigabatrin.

With the exception of the requirements for shape, the tablets comply with the requirements stated under Tablets and with the following requirements.

Content of vigabatrin, $C_6H_{11}NO_2$ 95.0 to 105.0% of the prescribed or stated amount.

Identification To a quantity of the powdered tablets containing 0.5 g of Vigabatrin add 10 ml of *water*, shake and filter through a 0.7 µm filter (Whatman GF/F is suitable). To 0.2 ml of the filtrate add 5 ml of *acetone* and allow the solvent to evaporate in a current of nitrogen. The *infrared absorption spectrum* of the residue, Appendix II A, is concordant with the *reference spectrum* of vigabatrin.

5-Vinyl-2-pyrrolidone In the Assay, the area of any peak corresponding to 5-vinyl-2-pyrrolidone in the chromatogram obtained with solution (1) is not greater than the area of the peak in the chromatogram obtained with solution (3) (0.5%).

Assay Carry out the method for *liquid chromatography*, Appendix III D, injecting 20 µl of each of the following solutions. For solution (1) add 800 ml of the mobile phase to 10 whole tablets, stir vigorously until all of the tablets are uniformly dispersed into fine particles, add sufficient of the mobile phase to produce 1000 ml, mix well and filter through a 0.2 µm nylon-66 filter. Dilute 10 ml of the filtrate to 50 ml with the mobile phase. Solution (2) contains 0.10% w/v of *vigabatrin BPCRS* in the mobile phase. Solution (3) contains 0.0005% w/v of *5-vinyl-2-pyrrolidone* in the mobile phase. Solution (4) contains 0.0005% w/v of *5-vinyl-2-pyrrolidone*, 0.1% w/v of *povidone* and 0.1% w/v of *vigabatrin BPCRS* in the mobile phase.

The chromatographic procedure may be carried out using (a) a stainless steel column (25 cm × 4.6 mm) packed with cation exchange resin (10 µm) (Whatman Partisil 10 SCX is suitable), (b) as the mobile phase with a flow rate of 1.5 ml per minute, a mixture of 4 volumes of *acetonitrile*, 40 volumes of *methanol* and 1000 volumes of a 0.34% w/v solution of *potassium dihydrogen orthophosphate*, adjusting the pH to 2.8 with *orthophosphoric acid* and (c) a detection wavelength of 210 nm.

In the chromatogram obtained with solution (4), the retention times are about 4 minutes for povidone, about 5 minutes for 5-vinyl-2-pyrrolidone and about 8 minutes for vigabatrin. The test is not valid unless the *resolution factor* between the peaks corresponding to 5-vinyl-2-pyrrolidone and vigabatrin in the chromatogram obtained with solution (4) is at least 1.5 and the *resolution factor* between the peaks corresponding to povidone and 5-vinyl-2-pyrrolidone is at least 1.5.

Calculate the percentage content of $C_6H_{11}NO_2$ in the tablets from the areas of the peaks for vigabatrin in the chromatograms obtained with solutions (1) and (2) and from the declared content of $C_6H_{11}NO_2$ in *vigabatrin BPCRS.*

Vinblastine Injection

Definition Vinblastine Injection is a sterile solution of Vinblastine Sulphate in Water for Injections. It is prepared by dissolving Vinblastine Sulphate for Injection in the requisite amount of Sodium Chloride Intravenous Infusion containing 0.9% w/v of Sodium Chloride.

The injection complies with the requirements stated under Parenteral Preparations.

Storage Vinblastine Injection should be used immediately after preparation but, in any case, within the period recommended by the manufacturer when prepared and stored strictly in accordance with the manufacturer's instructions.

VINBLASTINE SULPHATE FOR INJECTION

Definition Vinblastine Sulphate for Injection is a sterile material prepared from Vinblastine Sulphate. It may contain excipients. It is supplied in a sealed container.

The contents of the sealed container comply with the requirements for Powders for Injections stated under Parenteral Preparations and with the following requirements.

Content of vinblastine sulphate, $C_{46}H_{58}N_4O_9,H_2SO_4$ 92.5 to 107.5% of the prescribed or stated amount of anhydrous vinblastine sulphate.

Identification

A. In the test for Related substances the principal peak in the chromatogram obtained with solution (1) has the same retention time as the principal peak in the chromatogram obtained with solution (3).

B. To 1 mg add 0.2 ml of a freshly prepared 1% w/v solution of *vanillin* in *hydrochloric acid.* A pink colour is produced in about 1 minute (distinction from vincristine sulphate).

C. Yield the reactions characteristic of *sulphates*, Appendix VI.

Acidity pH of a solution containing the equivalent of 0.15% w/v of anhydrous vinblastine sulphate, 3.5 to 5.0, Appendix V L.

Clarity of solution Dissolve the contents of a sealed container in 10 ml of *carbon dioxide-free water*. The resulting solution is *clear*, Appendix IV A.

Related substances Carry out the method for *liquid chromatography*, Appendix III D, using the following solutions. For solution (1) dissolve the contents of a sealed container in sufficient *water* to produce a solution containing the equivalent of 0.10% w/v of anhydrous vinblastine sulphate. Solution (2) contains 0.10% w/v each of *vinblastine sulphate EPCRS* and *vincristine sulphate EPCRS* in *water*. Solutions (3), (4) and (5) contain 0.10% w/v, 0.0020% w/v and 0.00010% w/v, respectively, of *vinblastine sulphate EPCRS* in *water*. Keep the solutions in ice before use.

The chromatographic procedure may be carried out using (a) a stainless steel column (25 cm × 4.6 mm) packed with *stationary phase B* (5 µm) (Zorbax C8 is suitable), (b) a guard column packed with a suitable silica gel placed between the pump and the injection device, (c) as the mobile phase with a flow rate of 1.0 ml per minute a mixture of 12 volumes of *acetonitrile*, 38 volumes of a 1.5% v/v solution of *diethylamine* adjusted to pH 7.5 with *orthophosphoric acid* and 50 volumes of *methanol* and (d) a detection wavelength of 262 nm. Inject 10 µl of each solution using a loop injector and record the chromatograms for 3 times the retention time of the peak due to vinblastine.

The test is not valid unless the *resolution factor* between the peaks due to vinblastine and vincristine in the chromatogram obtained with solution (2) is at least 4 and unless the *signal-to-noise ratio* in the peak in the chromatogram obtained with solution (5) is at least 5.

In the chromatogram obtained with solution (1) the area of any *secondary peak* is not greater than the area of the principal peak in the chromatogram obtained with solution (4) (2%) and the sum of the areas of any such peaks is not greater than 2.5 times the area of the principal peak in the chromatogram obtained with solution (4) (5%). Disregard any peak with an area less than that of the peak in the chromatogram obtained with solution (5) (0.1%).

Loss on drying When dried at 60° at a pressure not exceeding 0.7 kPa for 16 hours, lose not more than 17.0% of their weight.

Uniformity of content The content of anhydrous vinblastine sulphate in each of 10 individual containers as determined in the Assay is not less than 90.0% and not more than 110.0% of the average except that in one container the content may be not less than 80.0% and not more than 120.0% of the average.

Assay Dissolve the contents of a sealed container in a suitable volume of *methanol* and dilute with sufficient *methanol* to produce a solution containing 0.004% w/v of anhydrous vinblastine sulphate. Measure the *absorbance* of the resulting solution at the maximum at 267 nm, Appendix II B. Calculate the content of $C_{46}H_{58}N_4O_9$, H_2SO_4 in the sealed container taking 185 as the value of A(1%, 1 cm) at the maximum at 267 nm. Repeat the procedure with a further nine sealed containers. Calculate the average content of $C_{46}H_{58}N_4O_9,H_2SO_4$ per container from the 10 individual results thus obtained.

Storage Vinblastine Sulphate for Injection should be stored at a temperature of 2° to 8°.

Labelling The label of the sealed container states the weight of anhydrous vinblastine sulphate contained in it.

Vincristine Injection

Definition Vincristine Injection is a sterile solution prepared by dissolving Vincristine Sulphate for Injection in the requisite amount of Sodium Chloride Intravenous

Infusion containing 0.9% w/v of Sodium Chloride.

The injection complies with the requirements stated under Parenteral Preparations.

Storage Vincristine Injection should be used immediately after preparation but, in any case, within the period recommended by the manufacturer when prepared and stored strictly in accordance with the manufacturer's instructions.

VINCRISTINE SULPHATE FOR INJECTION

Definition Vincristine Sulphate for Injection is a sterile material consisting of a mixture of one part by weight of Vincristine Sulphate and ten parts by weight of Lactose with or without other excipients. It is supplied in a sealed container.

The contents of the sealed container comply with the requirements for Powders for Injections stated under Parenteral Preparations and with the following requirements.

Content of vincristine sulphate, $C_{46}H_{56}N_4O_{10},H_2SO_4$ 92.5 to 107.5% of the prescribed or stated amount of anhydrous vincristine sulphate.

Identification

A. In the test for Related substances the principal peak in the chromatogram obtained with solution (1) has the same retention time as the principal peak in the chromatogram obtained with solution (3).

B. Shake a quantity containing the equivalent of 1 mg of anhydrous vincristine sulphate with 3 ml of *chloroform*, filter and wash the filter with 2 ml of *chloroform*. Evaporate the combined chloroform solutions to dryness at 40°. Add 0.2 ml of a freshly prepared 1% w/v solution of *vanillin* in *hydrochloric acid* to the residue. An orange colour is produced in about 1 minute (distinction from vinblastine sulphate).

Clarity of solution Dissolve the contents of a sealed container in 10 ml of *carbon dioxide-free water*. The solution is *clear*, Appendix IV A.

Related substances Carry out the method for *liquid chromatography*, Appendix III D, using the following solutions. For solution (1) dissolve the contents of a sealed container in sufficient *water* to produce a solution containing the equivalent of 0.10% w/v of anhydrous vincristine sulphate. Solution (2) contains 0.10% w/v each of *vincristine sulphate EPCRS* and *vinblastine sulphate EPCRS* in *water*. Solutions (3), (4) and (5) contain 0.10% w/v, 0.0020% w/v and 0.00010% w/v, respectively, of *vincristine sulphate EPCRS* in *water*. Keep the solutions in ice before use.

The chromatographic procedure may be carried out using (a) a stainless steel column (25 cm × 4.6 mm) packed with *stationary phase B* (5 µm) (Zorbax C8 is suitable), (b) a guard column packed with a suitable silica gel placed between the pump and the injection device, (c) as the mobile phase with a flow rate of 1.0 ml per minute a mixture of 30 volumes of a 1.5% v/v solution of *diethylamine* adjusted to pH 7.5 with *orthophosphoric acid* and 70 volumes of *methanol* and (d) a detection wavelength of 297 nm. Inject 10 µl of each solution using a loop injector and record the chromatograms for 3 times the retention time of the peak due to vincristine.

The test is not valid unless the *resolution factor* between the peaks due to vincristine and vinblastine in the chromatogram obtained with solution (2) is at least 4 and unless the *signal-to-noise ratio* in the peak in the chromatogram obtained with solution (5) is at least 5.

In the chromatogram obtained with solution (1) the area of any *secondary peak* is not greater than the area of the principal peak in the chromatogram obtained with solution (4) (2%) and the sum of the areas of any such peaks is not greater than 2.5 times the area of the principal peak in the chromatogram obtained with solution (4) (5%). Disregard any peak with an area less than that of the peak in the chromatogram obtained with solution (5) (0.1%).

Uniformity of content The content of anhydrous vincristine sulphate in each of 10 individual containers as determined in the Assay is not less than 90.0% and not more than 110.0% of the average except that in one container the content may be not less than 80.0% and not more than 120.0% of the average.

Assay Dissolve the contents of a sealed container in a suitable volume of *methanol* and dilute with sufficient *methanol* to produce a solution containing the equivalent of 0.005% w/v of anhydrous vincristine sulphate. Measure the *absorbance* of the resulting solution at the maximum at 297 nm, Appendix II B. Calculate the content of $C_{46}H_{56}N_4O_{10},H_2SO_4$ in the sealed container taking 177 as the value of A(1%, 1 cm) at the maximum at 297 nm. Repeat the procedure with a further nine containers. Calculate the average content of $C_{46}H_{56}N_4O_{10},H_2SO_4$ per container from the 10 individual results thus obtained.

Storage Vincristine Sulphate for Injection should be stored at a temperature of 2° to 8°.

Labelling The label of the sealed container states the weight of anhydrous vincristine sulphate contained in it.

Vitamins B and C Injection

Definition Vitamins B and C Injection is a sterile solution of Thiamine Hydrochloride, Pyridoxine Hydrochloride, Riboflavin Sodium Phosphate, Nicotinamide and Ascorbic Acid (as the sodium salt) in Water for Injections, containing Anhydrous Glucose for the intravenous injection or Benzyl Alcohol for the intramuscular injection.

Vitamins B and C Injection is prepared immediately before use by mixing the contents of two ampoules, (1) and (2). Ampoule (1) contains Thiamine Hydrochloride, Pyridoxine Hydrochloride, Riboflavin Sodium Phosphate and, where appropriate, Benzyl Alcohol. Ampoule (2) contains Nicotinamide and Ascorbic Acid and, where appropriate, Anhydrous Glucose. The air in ampoule (2) is replaced by nitrogen or other suitable inert gas.

The injection complies with the requirements stated under Parenteral Preparations and the contents of ampoules (1) and (2) comply with the following requirements, as appropriate.

Content of thiamine hydrochloride, $C_{12}H_{17}ClN_4OS,HCl$ 92.0 to 106.0% of the stated amount.

Content of pyridoxine hydrochloride, $C_8H_{11}NO_3,HCl$ 90.0 to 110.0% of the stated amount.

Content of riboflavin, $C_{17}H_{20}N_4O_6$ 90.0 to 110.0% of the stated amount.

Content of nicotinamide, $C_6H_6N_2O$ 95.0 to 105.0% of the stated amount.

Content of ascorbic acid, $C_6H_8O_6$ 95.0 to 105.0% of the stated amount.

Content of glucose, $C_6H_{12}O_6$ Where appropriate, 90.0 to 110.0% of the stated amount.

Identification

A. Carry out the method for *thin-layer chromatography*, Appendix III A, using a silica gel F_{254} precoated plate (Merck silica gel 60 F_{254} plates are suitable) and a mixture of 60 volumes of *methanol* and 40 volumes of a solution containing 0.14% w/v of *potassium dihydrogen orthophosphate* and 0.5% w/v of *disodium edetate* as the mobile phase. Apply separately to the plate 2 µl of each of the following solutions in *water*. For solution (1) use a volume of the contents of ampoule (1) diluted, if necessary, with *water* to contain 0.2% w/v of Pyridoxine Hydrochloride. For solution (2) use a volume of the injection in ampoule (2) diluted, if necessary, with *water* to contain 2% w/v of Ascorbic Acid. Solutions (3) and (4) contain 1% w/v and 0.4% w/v respectively of *thiamine mononitrate BPCRS*. Solution (5) contains 0.2% w/v of *pyridoxine hydrochloride BPCRS*. Solution (6) contains 0.022% w/v of *riboflavin sodium phosphate BPCRS*. Solution (7) contains 0.64% w/v of *nicotinamide BPCRS*. Solution (8) contains 2% w/v of *ascorbic acid BPCRS*. After removal of the plate, allow it to dry in air and examine under *ultraviolet light (254 nm and 365 nm)*. The principal spots in the chromatogram obtained with solution (1) correspond to those in the chromatograms obtained with either solutions (3), (5) and (6) or solutions (4), (5) and (6). The principal spots in the chromatogram obtained with solution (2) correspond to those in the chromatograms obtained with solutions (7) and (8).

B. For injections containing Benzyl Alcohol, add 1 ml of the contents of ampoule (1) to 10 ml of a 3% w/v solution of *potassium permanganate* acidified with 1 ml of 1M *sulphuric acid*. Benzaldehyde, recognisable by its odour, is produced.

C. For injections containing Anhydrous Glucose, heat 1 ml of the contents of ampoule (2) with *cupri-tartaric solution R1*. A copious precipitate of copper(I) oxide is produced.

Assay

For thiamine hydrochloride, pyridoxine hydrochloride and nicotinamide Carry out the method for *liquid chromatography*, Appendix III D, using the following solutions in *water*. Solution (1) contains 0.01% w/v of *thiamine mononitrate BPCRS* and 0.002% w/v of *pyridoxine hydrochloride BPCRS*. Solution (2) contains 0.01% w/v of *thiamine mononitrate BPCRS* and 0.005% w/v of *pyridoxine hydrochloride BPCRS*. Solution (3) contains 0.016% w/v of *nicotinamide BPCRS*. For solution (4) dilute a suitable volume of the contents of ampoule (1) with *water* to contain 0.01% w/v of Thiamine Hydrochloride. For solution (5) dilute a suitable volume of the contents of ampoule (2) to contain 0.016% w/v of Nicotinamide.

The chromatographic procedure may be carried out using (a) a stainless steel column (30 cm × 3.9 mm) packed with *stationary phase C* (10 µm) (µBondapak C18 is suitable), (b) as the mobile phase with a flow rate of 1 ml per minute, 0.22% w/v of *sodium heptanesulphonate* in a mixture of 75 volumes of a 1.36% w/v solution of *potassium dihydrogen orthophosphate* and 25 volumes of *methanol*, the pH of the final mixture being adjusted to 3.0 with *orthophosphoric acid*, and (c) a detection wavelength of 280 nm.

Calculate the content of $C_{12}H_{17}ClN_4OS,HCl$ using the declared content of $C_{12}H_{17}N_5O_4S$ in *thiamine mononitrate BPCRS*. Each mg of $C_{12}H_{17}N_5O_4S$ is equivalent to 1.030 mg of $C_{12}H_{17}ClN_4OS,HCl$. Calculate the content of $C_8H_{11}NO_3,HCl$ using the declared content of $C_8H_{11}NO_3,HCl$ in *pyridoxine hydrochloride BPCRS*. Calculate the content of $C_6H_6N_2O$ using the declared content of $C_6H_6N_2O$ in *nicotinamide BPCRS*.

For riboflavin Dilute a volume of the contents of ampoule (1) containing the equivalent of 4 mg of riboflavine with sufficient *phthalate buffer pH 4.0* to produce 200 ml and measure the *absorbance* of the resulting solution at the maximum at 446 nm, Appendix II B. Calculate the content of $C_{17}H_{20}N_4O_6$ taking 323 as the value of A(1%, 1 cm) at the maximum at 446 nm.

For ascorbic acid Dilute a volume of the contents of ampoule (2) with *water* to produce a solution containing 1% w/v of Ascorbic Acid. To 20 ml of the resulting solution add 5 ml of 1M *sulphuric acid* and 50 ml of 0.05M *iodine VS* and titrate the excess iodine with 0.1M *sodium thiosulphate VS* using *starch mucilage* as indicator. Each ml of 0.05M *iodine VS* is equivalent to 8.806 mg of $C_6H_8O_6$.

For anhydrous glucose For injections containing Anhydrous Glucose, dilute a volume of the contents of ampoule (2) containing 0.8 g of Anhydrous Glucose to 500 ml with *water* and dilute 2 ml of the resulting solution to 100 ml with *water*. Transfer 3 ml of this solution to a boiling tube previously cleaned with *chromic—sulphuric acid mixture* and rinsed with *water*. In two similar tubes place separately 3 ml of *glucose standard solution* and 3 ml of *water*. Add 6 ml of *anthrone reagent* in such a manner as to ensure rapid mixing, allow to stand for 10 minutes, cool quickly and measure the *absorbance*, Appendix II B, of the test solution and of the standard solution at the maximum at 625 nm using the solution prepared with *water* in the reference cell. Calculate the concentration of $C_6H_{12}O_6$ in the test solution.

Storage Ampoules (1) and (2) for Vitamins B and C Injection should be protected from light.

Labelling For each ampoule the label states (1) the directions for the preparation of the injection; (2) whether the final injection is for intravenous or intramuscular use; (2) that the final injection is a high potency injection.

For ampoule (1) the label states the quantity of Riboflavin Sodium Phosphate in terms of the equivalent amount of riboflavin.

Warfarin Tablets

Definition Warfarin Tablets contain Warfarin Sodium or Warfarin Sodium Clathrate.

The tablets comply with the requirements stated under Tablets and with the following requirements.

Content of warfarin sodium, $C_{19}H_{15}NaO_4$ 92.5 to 107.5% of the prescribed or stated amount.

Identification

A. Extract a quantity of the powdered tablets containing 0.1 g of warfarin sodium with 30 ml of *water*, add 0.1 ml of 2M *hydrochloric acid*, filter, wash the precipitate with *water* and dry. Warm the residue gently with 3 ml of *ethanol (96%)*, filter and add the filtrate to 25 ml of *water* containing 0.1 ml of 2M *hydrochloric acid*. Filter, wash the precipitate with *water* and dry it at 105°. The *infrared absorption spectrum* of the residue, Appendix II A, is concordant with the *reference spectrum* of warfarin.

B. The *melting point* of the residue obtained in test A is about 159°, Appendix V A.

Dissolution Comply with the *dissolution test for tablets and capsules*, Appendix XII D, using as the medium 900 ml of a 0.68% w/v solution of *potassium dihydrogen orthophosphate* adjusted to pH 6.8 by the addition of 1M *sodium hydroxide* and rotating the basket at 100 revolutions per minute. For tablets containing 2 mg or less of warfarin sodium, place three tablets in the basket for each test; for tablets containing more than 2 mg of warfarin sodium, place a single tablet in the basket for each test. Withdraw a sample of 10 ml of the medium. Measure the *absorbance* of a layer of suitable thickness of the filtered sample, suitably diluted if necessary, at the maxima at 307 nm and 360 nm, Appendix II B, and calculate the difference between the two readings (ΔA). Calculate the total content of warfarin sodium, $C_{19}H_{15}NaO_4$, in the medium taking 428 as the value of ΔA(1%, 1 cm).

Related substances Carry out the method for *thin-layer chromatography*, Appendix III A, using *silica gel* GF_{254} as the coating substance and a mixture of 50 volumes of *chloroform*, 50 volumes of *cyclohexane* and 20 volumes of *glacial acetic acid* as the mobile phase. Apply separately to the plate 20 µl of each of the following solutions. For solution (1) shake a quantity of the powdered tablets containing 40 mg of warfarin sodium with 30 ml of *water* for 15 minutes, add 0.1 ml of *hydrochloric acid* and extract with three 10-ml quantities of *chloroform*, drying each extract with *anhydrous sodium sulphate*; evaporate the combined extracts using a rotary evaporator at a temperature not exceeding 40° and dissolve the residue in 2 ml of *acetone*. Solution (2) contains 0.0020% w/v of (E)-*4-phenylbut-3-en-2-one* in *acetone*. Solution (3) contains 0.0020% w/v of *4-hydroxycoumarin* in *acetone*. For solution (4) dilute 1 volume of solution (1) to 200 volumes with *acetone*. After removal of the plate, allow it to dry in air, examine immediately in visible light noting the position of any coloured spots and then examine under *ultraviolet light (254 nm)*, disregarding any spot that was noted in visible light. Any spots corresponding to (*E*)-4-phenylbut-3-en-2-one and 4-hydroxycoumarin in the chromatogram obtained with solution (1) are not more intense than the spots in the chromatograms obtained with solutions (2) and (3) respectively and any other *secondary spot* is not more intense than the spot in the chromatogram obtained with solution (4).

Uniformity of content Tablets containing less than 2 mg of warfarin sodium comply with the requirements stated under Tablets but using in place of the content of active ingredient the individual peak areas obtained by the following method of analysis. Carry out the method for *liquid chromatography*, Appendix III D, using the following solution. Shake one tablet with 10 ml of 0.01M *sodium hydroxide* for 15 minutes, add 10 ml of a 2% v/v solution of *glacial acetic acid* in *acetonitrile*, centrifuge for 10 minutes and use the clear supernatant liquid.

The chromatographic procedure may be carried out using (a) a stainless steel column (10 cm × 4.6 mm) packed with *stationary phase C* (5 µm) (Hypersil ODS is suitable), (b) a mixture of 55 volumes of *acetonitrile*, 45 volumes of *water* and 1 volume of *glacial acetic acid* as the mobile phase with a flow rate of 2 ml per minute and (c) a detection wavelength of 283 nm.

Assay Weigh and powder 20 tablets. Carry out the method for *liquid chromatography*, Appendix III D, using the following solutions. For solution (1) shake a quantity of the powdered tablets containing 5 mg of Warfarin Sodium with 50 ml of 0.01M *sodium hydroxide* for 15 minutes, add 50 ml of a 2% v/v solution of *glacial acetic acid* in *acetonitrile*, centrifuge for 10 minutes and use the clear supernatant liquid. For solution (2) dilute 5 ml of a 0.010% w/v solution of *warfarin sodium BPCRS* in 0.01M *sodium hydroxide* to 10 ml with the mobile phase.

The chromatographic procedure may be carried out using the conditions described under Uniformity of content.

Calculate the content of $C_{19}H_{15}NaO_4$ in the tablets from the chromatograms obtained and using the declared content of $C_{19}H_{15}NaO_4$ in *warfarin sodium BPCRS*.

Storage Warfarin Tablets should be protected from light.

Labelling When the active ingredient is Warfarin Sodium Clathrate the quantity is stated in terms of the equivalent amount of warfarin sodium.

Water for Irrigation

Definition Water for Irrigation is sterilised, apyrogenic, distilled water.

Water for Irrigation is intended to be used for the irrigation of body cavities, for the flushing of wounds or operation cavities or for the irrigation of the urogenital system. It is supplied in containers holding sufficient of the water for use on one occasion only. Where water is required for use in the manufacture of an Irrigation Solution intended to be used for the above purposes, water prepared by the process described under Production is used. However the sterilisation at this stage may be omitted provided that the final product is sterilised immediately.

Production Water for Irrigation is obtained by distilling potable water or Purified Water from a neutral glass, quartz or suitable metal still fitted with an efficient device for preventing the entrainment of droplets. The first portion of the distillate is discarded and the remainder is collected in suitable containers, previously rinsed with freshly distilled water obtained under the same conditions from the apparatus. The containers are sealed and sterilised by *heating in an autoclave*.

Water for Irrigation complies with the requirements stated under Preparations for Irrigation and with the following requirements.

Characteristics A clear, colourless liquid; odourless and tasteless.

Acidity or alkalinity To 20 ml add 0.05 ml of *phenol red solution*. If the solution is yellow, not more than 0.1 ml of 0.01M *sodium hydroxide VS* is required to change it to red; if the solution is red, not more than 0.15 ml of 0.01M *hydrochloric acid VS* is required to change it to yellow.

Clarity and colour When examined in suitable conditions of visibility, it is clear, colourless and practically free from suspended particles.

Ammonium To 20 ml add 1 ml of *alkaline potassium tetraiodomercurate solution* and allow to stand for 5 minutes. When viewed vertically the solution is not more intensely coloured than a solution prepared at the same time by adding 1 ml of *alkaline potassium tetraiodomercurate solution* to a mixture of 4 ml of *ammonium standard solution (1 ppm NH_4)* and 16 ml of *ammonia-free water* (0.2 ppm).

Calcium and magnesium To 100 ml add 2 ml of *ammonia buffer pH 10.0*, 50 mg of *mordant black 11 triturate* and 0.5 ml of 0.01M *disodium edetate*. A pure blue colour is produced.

Heavy metals In a glass evaporating dish evaporate 200 ml to 20 ml on a water bath. 12 ml of the resulting solution complies with *limit test A for heavy metals*, Appendix VII. Use *lead standard solution (1 ppm Pb)* to prepare the standard (0.1 ppm).

Chloride To 10 ml add 1 ml of 2M *nitric acid* and 0.2 ml of 0.1M *silver nitrate*. The appearance of the solution does not change within 15 minutes.

When the volume in the final container is 100 ml or less, 15 ml complies with the *limit test for chlorides*, Appendix VII (0.5 ppm). Use a mixture of 1.5 ml of *chloride standard solution (5 ppm Cl)* and 13.5 ml of *water* to prepare the standard. Examine the solutions down the vertical axes of the tubes.

Nitrate To 5 ml in a test tube immersed in ice add 0.4 ml of a 10% w/v solution of *potassium chloride*, 0.1 ml of *diphenylamine solution* and, dropwise with shaking, 5 ml of *sulphuric acid*. Transfer the tube to a water bath at 50° and allow to stand for 15 minutes. Any blue colour in the solution is not more intense than that in a solution prepared at the same time and in the same manner using a mixture of 4.5 ml of *nitrate-free water* and 0.5 ml of *nitrate standard solution (2 ppm NO_3)* (0.2 ppm).

Sulphate To 10 ml add 0.1 ml of 2M *hydrochloric acid* and 0.1 ml of *barium chloride solution R1*. The solution shows no change in appearance for at least 1 hour.

Oxidisable substances Boil 100 ml with 10 ml of 1M *sulphuric acid*, add 0.2 ml of 0.02M *potassium permanganate* and boil for 5 minutes. The pink colour is not completely discharged.

Residue on evaporation When evaporated on a water bath and dried to constant weight at 100° to 105°, leaves not more than 0.003% of residue. Use 100 ml.

Labelling The label states that Water for Irrigation is apyrogenic.

White Liniment

White Embrocation

Definition White Liniment is a *cutaneous emulsion*.

Oleic Acid	85 ml
Turpentine Oil	250 ml
Dilute Ammonia Solution	45 ml
Ammonium Chloride	12.5 g
Purified Water	625 ml

Extemporaneous preparation The following directions apply.

Mix the Oleic Acid with the Turpentine Oil. Dilute the Dilute Ammonia Solution with 45 ml of the Purified Water, previously warmed, add to the oily solution and shake to form an emulsion. Separately dissolve the Ammonium Chloride in the remainder of the Purified Water, add to the emulsion and mix.

The liniment complies with the requirements stated under Liquids for Cutaneous Application and with the following requirements.

Content of volatile oil 24.5 to 27.5% v/w.

Refractive index Of the oily liquid obtained in the Assay, 1.465 to 1.477, Appendix V E.

Assay Acidify 100 g with 1M *sulphuric acid* using *methyl orange solution* as indicator, distil in steam and collect the distillate in a separating funnel; occasionally separate the aqueous portion of the distillate and return it to the flask. When all the volatile matter has been distilled, remove the aqueous portion of the distillate and measure the volume of the oily liquid.

Labelling The label indicates the pharmaceutical form as 'cutaneous emulsion'.

Wool Alcohols Ointment

Definition

Wool Alcohols	60 g
Hard Paraffin	240 g
White Soft Paraffin or Yellow Soft Paraffin	100 g
Liquid Paraffin	600 g

In preparing Wool Alcohols Ointment, the proportions of Hard Paraffin, Soft Paraffin and Liquid Paraffin may be varied to produce Wool Alcohols Ointment having suitable properties.

When Wool Alcohols Ointment is used in a white ointment, it should be prepared with White Soft Paraffin; when used in a coloured ointment it should be prepared with Yellow Soft Paraffin.

Extemporaneous preparation The following directions apply.

Melt together with the aid of gentle heat and stir until cold.

The ointment complies with the requirements stated under Topical Semi-solid Preparations.

Xylometazoline Nasal Drops

Definition Xylometazoline Nasal Drops are a solution of Xylometazoline Hydrochloride in Purified Water.

The nasal drops comply with the requirements stated under Nasal Preparations and with the following requirements.

Content of xylometazoline hydrochloride, $C_{16}H_{24}N_2$, HCl 90.0 to 110.0% of the prescribed or stated amount.

Identification

A. To a volume of the nasal drops containing 50 mg of Xylometazoline Hydrochloride add 5 ml of 1M *sodium hydroxide*, extract with 10 ml of *dichloromethane IR*, evaporate to dryness and dissolve the residue in 0.5 ml of *dichloromethane IR*. The *infrared absorption spectrum* of the resulting solution, Appendix II A, is concordant with the *reference spectrum* of xylometazoline.

B. To a volume containing 0.5 mg of Xylometazoline Hydrochloride add 0.2 ml of a 5% w/v solution of *sodium nitroprusside* and 0.1 ml of 5M *sodium hydroxide* and allow to stand for 10 minutes. Add 1 ml of a 10% w/v solution of *sodium hydrogen carbonate*. A violet colour is produced.

Acidity pH, 5.6 to 6.6, Appendix V L.

***N*-(2-Aminoethyl)-4-*tert*-butyl-2,6-xylylacetamide** Carry out the method for *thin-layer chromatography*, Appendix III A, using *silica gel* HF_{254} as the coating substance and a mixture of 200 volumes of *methanol* and 3 volumes of 13.5M *ammonia* as the mobile phase. Apply separately to the plate 5 µl of each of the following solutions. For solution (1) add a volume of the nasal drops containing 10 mg of Xylometazoline Hydrochloride to 30 ml of *water*, add 5 ml of 5M *sodium hydroxide*, mix, extract with three 20-ml quantities of *dichloromethane*, evaporate the combined extracts to dryness and dissolve the residue in 1 ml of *dichloromethane*. Solution (2) contains 0.03% w/v of N-*(2-aminoethyl)-4-*tert-*butyl-2,6-xylylacetamide BPCRS* in *dichloromethane*. After removal of the plate, allow it to dry in air and spray with a solution prepared by dissolving 0.3 g of *ninhydrin* in a mixture of 100 ml of *butan-1-ol* and 3 ml of *glacial acetic acid*. Heat at 100° for 10 minutes, allow to cool, and spray with *dilute potassium iodobismuthate solution*. Any spot corresponding to *N*-(2-aminoethyl)-4-*tert*-butyl-2,6-xylylacetamide in the chromatogram obtained with solution (1) is not more intense than the spot in the chromatogram obtained with solution (2).

Assay To a volume of the nasal drops containing 10 mg of Xylometazoline Hydrochloride add 5 ml of *water*, 10 ml of 2M *hydrochloric acid* and 10 ml of *dichloromethane* and shake for 1 minute. Discard the dichloromethane layer and repeat the extraction with two further 10-ml quantities of *dichloromethane*. Add to the aqueous extract 10 ml of 5M *sodium hydroxide* and 10 ml of *dichloromethane*, shake for 1 minute and allow to separate. Filter the dichloromethane extract through glass wool and repeat the extraction with four further 10-ml quantities of *dichloromethane*. Evaporate the combined dichloromethane extracts almost to dryness on a water bath, removing the final traces of solvent in a current of air, and dissolve the residue in 10 ml of 0.01M *hydrochloric acid*. To 2 ml of this solution add 3 ml of *water*, 2.5 ml of 1M *sodium hydroxide* and 2.5 ml of a 5% w/v solution of *sodium nitroprusside*, mix and allow to stand protected from light for 10 minutes. Add 10 ml of a freshly prepared 8.3% w/v solution of *sodium hydrogen carbonate*, dilute to 100 ml with *water*, allow to stand protected from light for 10 minutes and measure the *absorbance* of the resulting solution at the maximum at 560 nm, Appendix II B, using in the reference cell a solution prepared by treating 5 ml of *water* and 2.5 ml of 1M *sodium hydroxide* in the same manner, beginning at the words 'and 2.5 ml of a 5% w/v solution of *sodium nitroprusside* ...'. Calculate the content of $C_{12}H_{24}N_2$,HCl from the *absorbance* obtained by repeating the operation using a 0.1% w/v solution of *xylometazoline hydrochloride BPCRS*, diluted if necessary with *water*, in place of the nasal drops.

Storage Xylometazoline Nasal Drops should be protected from light.

Zinc Cream

Definition Zinc Cream contains 32% w/w of Zinc Oxide in a suitable water-in-oil emulsified basis.

Extemporaneous preparation The following formula and directions apply.

Zinc Oxide, finely sifted	320 g
Calcium Hydroxide	0.45 g
Oleic Acid	5 ml
Arachis Oil	320 ml
Wool Fat	80 g
Purified Water, freshly boiled and cooled	sufficient to produce 1000 g

Mix the Zinc Oxide and the Calcium Hydroxide, triturate to a smooth paste with a mixture of the Oleic Acid and Arachis Oil, incorporate the Wool Fat and add gradually with continuous stirring sufficient Purified Water to produce 1000 g.

The suitability of the Cream for use as a diluent should be confirmed before use.

The cream complies with the requirements stated under Topical Semi-solid Preparations and with the following requirements.

Content of zinc oxide, ZnO 30.0 to 34.0% w/w.

Identification The residue obtained in the Assay is yellow when hot and white when cool.

Assay Heat 0.5 g of the cream gently in a porcelain dish over a small flame until the basis is completely volatilised or charred. Increase the heat until all the carbon is removed. Dissolve the residue in 10 ml of 2M *acetic acid* and add sufficient *water* to produce 50 ml. To the resulting solution add 50 mg of *xylenol orange triturate* and sufficient *hexamine* to produce a violet-pink colour. Add a further 2 g of *hexamine* and titrate with 0.1M *disodium edetate VS* until the solution becomes yellow. Each ml of 0.1M *disodium edetate VS* is equivalent to 8.138 mg of ZnO.

Zinc and Ichthammol Cream

Definition Zinc and Ichthammol Cream contains 5% w/w of Ichthammol dispersed in a suitable basis of which about 82% w/w is Zinc Cream.

Extemporaneous preparation The following formula and directions apply.

Ichthammol	50 g
Cetostearyl Alcohol	30 g
Wool Fat	100 g
Zinc Cream	sufficient to produce 1000 g

Melt together the Wool Fat and the Cetostearyl Alcohol with the aid of gentle heat, triturate the mixture with 800 g of Zinc Cream until smooth, incorporate the Ichthammol, add sufficient Zinc Cream to produce 1000 g and mix.

The cream complies with the requirements stated under Topical Semi-solid Preparations and with the following requirements.

Content of zinc oxide, ZnO 23.4 to 29.3% w/w.

Assay Gently heat 0.4 g, taking precautions to avoid loss caused by spitting, until the basis is completely volatilised or charred, cool, dissolve the residue in 10 ml of 2M *sulphuric acid*, add 40 ml of *water*, adjust the solution to about pH 10 with 5M *ammonia*, add 10 ml of *ammonia buffer pH 10.9* and titrate with 0.05M *disodium edetate VS* using *mordant black 11 solution* as indicator. Each ml of 0.05M *disodium edetate VS* is equivalent to 4.069 mg of ZnO.

Zinc Ointment

Definition Zinc Ointment contains 15% w/w of Zinc Oxide in a suitable water-emulsifying basis.

Extemporaneous preparation The following formula and directions apply.

Zinc Oxide, finely sifted	150 g
Simple Ointment	850 g

Triturate the Zinc Oxide with a portion of the Simple Ointment until smooth, gradually add the remainder of the Simple Ointment and mix thoroughly.

The ointment complies with the requirements stated under Topical Semi-solid Preparations and with the following requirements.

Content of zinc oxide, ZnO 14.0 to 16.0% w/w.

Identification The residue obtained in the Assay is yellow when hot and white when cool.

Assay Heat 0.5 g of the ointment gently in a porcelain dish over a small flame until the basis is completely volatilised or charred. Increase the heat until all the carbon is removed. Dissolve the residue in 10 ml of 2M *acetic acid* and add sufficient *water* to produce 50 ml. To the resulting solution add 50 mg of *xylenol orange triturate* and sufficient *hexamine* to produce a violet-pink colour. Add a further 2 g of *hexamine* and titrate with 0.05M *disodium edetate VS* until the solution becomes yellow. Each ml of 0.05M *disodium edetate VS* is equivalent to 4.069 mg of ZnO.

Zinc and Castor Oil Ointment

Zinc and Castor Oil Cream

Definition

Zinc Oxide, finely sifted	75 g
Castor Oil	500 g
Cetostearyl Alcohol	20 g
White Beeswax	100 g
Arachis Oil	305 g

Extemporaneous preparation The following directions apply.

Triturate the Zinc Oxide with a portion of the Castor Oil until smooth and add the mixture to the remainder of the ingredients previously melted together. Stir while cooling until the temperature is about 40°.

The ointment complies with the requirements stated under Topical Semi-solid Preparations and with the following requirements.

Content of zinc oxide, ZnO 7.0 to 8.0% w/w.

Identification

A. Heat 1.3 g of the ointment gently in a porcelain dish over a small flame until the basis is completely volatilised or charred. Increase the heat until all the carbon is removed. The residue obtained is yellow when hot and white when cold.

B. Dissolve the cooled residue obtained in test A in 5 ml of 1M *hydrochloric acid*. The resulting solution yields the reaction characteristic of *zinc salts*, Appendix VI.

Assay Heat 1 g of the ointment gently in a porcelain dish over a small flame until the basis is completely volatilised or charred. Increase the heat until all the carbon is removed. Dissolve the residue in 10 ml of 2M *acetic acid* and add sufficient *water* to produce 50 ml. To the resulting solution add 50 mg of *xylenol orange triturate* and sufficient *hexamine* to produce a violet-pink colour. Add a further 2 g of *hexamine* and titrate with 0.05M *disodium edetate VS* until the solution becomes yellow. Each ml of 0.05M *disodium edetate VS* is equivalent to 4.069 mg of ZnO.

Compound Zinc Paste

Definition Compound Zinc Paste contains 25% w/w each of Zinc Oxide and Starch in a suitable hydrophobic basis.

Extemporaneous preparation The following formula and directions apply.

Zinc Oxide, finely sifted	250 g
Starch, finely sifted	250 g
White Soft Paraffin	500 g

Melt the White Soft Paraffin, incorporate the Zinc Oxide and the Starch and stir until cold.

The paste complies with the requirements stated under Topical Semi-solid Preparations and with the following requirements.

Content of zinc oxide, ZnO 23.5 to 26.5% w/w.

Identification The residue obtained in the Assay is yellow when hot and white when cool.

Assay Heat 0.5 g of the paste gently in a porcelain dish over a small flame until the basis is completely volatilised or charred. Increase the heat until all the carbon is removed. Dissolve the residue in 10 ml of 2M *acetic acid* and add sufficient *water* to produce 50 ml. To the resulting solution add 50 mg of *xylenol orange triturate* and sufficient *hexamine* to produce a violet-pink colour. Add a further 2 g of *hexamine* and titrate with 0.1M *disodium edetate VS* until the solution becomes yellow. Each ml of 0.1M *disodium edetate VS* is equivalent to 8.138 mg of ZnO.

Zinc and Coal Tar Paste

White's Tar Paste

Definition Zinc and Coal Tar Paste contains 6% w/w each of Zinc Oxide and Coal Tar with 38% w/w of Starch in a suitable hydrophobic basis.

Extemporaneous preparation The following formula and directions apply.

Emulsifying Wax	50 g
Coal Tar	60 g
Zinc Oxide, finely sifted	60 g
Starch	380 g
Yellow Soft Paraffin	450 g

Melt the Emulsifying Wax at 70°, add the Coal Tar and 225 g of the Yellow Soft Paraffin, stir at 70° until completely melted, add the remainder of the Yellow Soft Paraffin, cool to 30°, add the Zinc Oxide and the Starch, stirring constantly, and stir until cold.

The paste complies with the requirements stated under Topical Semi-solid Preparations and with the following requirements.

Content of zinc oxide, ZnO 5.7 to 6.3% w/w.

Identification The residue obtained in the Assay is yellow when hot and white when cool.

Assay Heat 1.0 g of the paste gently in a porcelain dish over a small flame until the basis is completely volatilised or charred. Increase the heat until all the carbon is removed. Dissolve the residue in 10 ml of 2M *acetic acid* and add sufficient *water* to produce 50 ml. To the resulting solution add 50 mg of *xylenol orange triturate* and sufficient *hexamine* to produce a violet-pink colour. Add a further 2 g of *hexamine* and titrate with 0.05M *disodium edetate VS* until the solution becomes yellow. Each ml of 0.05M *disodium edetate VS* is equivalent to 4.069 mg of ZnO.

Zinc and Salicylic Acid Paste

Lassar's Paste

Definition

Zinc Oxide, finely sifted	240 g
Salicylic Acid, finely sifted	20 g
Starch, finely sifted	240 g
White Soft Paraffin	500 g

Extemporaneous preparation The following directions apply.

Melt the White Soft Paraffin, incorporate the Zinc Oxide, the Salicylic Acid and the Starch and stir until cold.

The paste complies with the requirements stated under Topical Semi-solid Preparations and with the following requirements.

Content of zinc oxide, ZnO 22.5 to 25.5% w/w.

Content of salicylic acid, $C_7H_6O_3$ 1.9 to 2.1% w/w.

Identification

A. Shake 1 g with 10 ml of *water*, filter and add *iron(III) chloride solution R1* to the filtrate. An intense reddish violet colour is produced which remains on the addition of 5M *acetic acid* but disappears on the addition of 2M *hydrochloric acid* with the separation of a white, crystalline precipitate.

B. Heat 0.5 g gently in a porcelain dish over a very small flame until the basis is completely volatilised or charred. Increase the heat until all the carbon is removed. The residue is yellow when hot and white when cool.

Assay

For salicylic acid Shake 0.5 g with 10 ml of 1M *hydrochloric acid* and 10 ml of *ether* until fully dispersed. Decant and reserve the aqueous layer. Extract the ether layer with two further 10-ml quantities of 1M *hydrochloric acid*, combine the aqueous extracts with the reserved aqueous layer, wash with 10 ml of *ether* and reserve for the Assay for zinc oxide. Combine the ether extracts, add 15 ml of *petroleum spirit (boiling range, 40° to 60°)* and extract with successive quantities of 20 ml, 10 ml and 10 ml of a mixture of equal volumes of *ethanol (90%)* and 1M *sodium hydroxide*. Dilute the combined extracts to 100 ml with 2M *hydrochloric acid*, further dilute 15 ml of the resulting solution to 50 ml with the same solvent and measure the *absorbance* of the final solution at the maximum at 302 nm, Appendix II B. Calculate the content of $C_7H_6O_3$ taking 260 as the value of A(1%, 1 cm) at the maximum at 302 nm.

For zinc oxide To the combined aqueous extracts obtained in the Assay for salicylic acid add 20 ml of 1M *sodium hydroxide* and 50 mg of *xylenol orange triturate*. To the resulting solution add sufficient *hexamine* to change the colour of the solution to red and then a further 3 g of *hexamine* and titrate with 0.1M *disodium edetate VS*. Each ml of 0.1M *disodium edetate VS* is equivalent to 8.139 mg of ZnO.

Zinc Sulphate Eye Drops

Definition Zinc Sulphate Eye Drops are a sterile solution containing 0.25% w/v of Zinc Sulphate in Purified Water.

The eye drops comply with the requirements stated under Eye Preparations and with the following requirements.

Content of zinc sulphate, $ZnSO_4,7H_2O$ 0.22 to 0.28% w/v.

Assay To 5 ml add 50 ml of *water* and 5 ml of *ammonia buffer pH 10.9* and titrate with 0.01M *disodium edetate VS* using *mordant black 11 solution* as indicator. Each ml of 0.01M *disodium edetate VS* is equivalent to 2.875 mg of $ZnSO_4,7H_2O$.

Zinc Sulphate Lotion

Definition Zinc Sulphate Lotion is a *cutaneous solution*. It contains 1% w/v of Zinc Sulphate in a suitable aqueous vehicle.

The lotion complies with the requirements stated under Liquids for Cutaneous Application and with the following requirements.

Content of zinc sulphate, $ZnSO_4,7H_2O$ 0.95 to 1.05% w/v.

Assay To 20 ml add 25 ml of 0.1M *hydrochloric acid* and 0.1 g of *activated charcoal*, shake, filter and wash the residue with 100 ml of 0.01M *hydrochloric acid*. To the combined filtrate and washings add 5 ml of *ammonia buffer pH 10.9* and titrate with 0.05M *disodium edetate VS* using *mordant black 11 solution* as indicator. Repeat the procedure using 20 ml of *water* in place of the preparation being examined. The difference between the titrations represents the amount of disodium edetate required. Each ml of 0.05M *disodium edetate VS* is equivalent to 14.38 mg of $ZnSO_4,7H_2O$.

Labelling The label indicates the pharmaceutical form as 'cutaneous solution'.

Zuclopenthixol Acetate Injection

Definition Zuclopenthixol Acetate Injection is a sterile solution of Zuclopenthixol Acetate in a suitable vegetable oil.

The injection complies with the requirements stated under Parenteral Preparations and with the following requirements.

Content of zuclopenthixol acetate, $C_{24}H_{27}ClN_2O_2S$ 95.0 to 105.0% of the prescribed or stated amount.

Identification

A. Carry out the method for *thin-layer chromatography*, Appendix III A, protected from light, using a silica gel F_{254} precoated plate (Merck silica gel 60 F_{254} plates are suitable) and a mixture of 3 volumes of *diethylamine* and 90 volumes of *cyclohexane* as the mobile phase but using an unlined tank. Apply separately to the plate 5 µl of each of the following solutions. For solution (1) dilute a volume of the injection with *ethanol (96%)* to contain 0.5% w/v of Zuclopenthixol Acetate. Solution (2) contains 0.5% w/v of *zuclopenthixol acetate dihydrochloride BPCRS* in *ethanol (96%)*. Solution (3) contains 0.5% w/v each of *zuclopenthixol acetate dihydrochloride BPCRS* and *zuclopenthixol decanoate dihydrochloride BPCRS*. After removal of the plate, allow it to dry in air, spray with a 1% w/v solution of *sodium molybdate* in *sulphuric acid*, heat at 110° for 20 minutes and examine in daylight. The principal spot in the chromatogram obtained with solution (1) corresponds to that in the chromatogram obtained with solution (2). The test is not valid unless the chromatogram obtained with solution (3) shows two clearly separated spots.

B. In the Assay, the chromatogram obtained with solution (1) shows a peak with the same retention time as the principal peak in the chromatogram obtained with solution (2).

Related substances Carry out the method for *thin-layer chromatography*, Appendix III A, protected from light, using a silica gel F_{254} precoated plate (Merck silica gel 60 F_{254} plates are suitable), a mixture of 10 volumes of *diethylamine*, 40 volumes of *dichloromethane* and 50 volumes of *cyclohexane* as the mobile phase and an unlined tank. Apply separately to the plate 5 µl of each of the following solutions. For solution (1) dissolve a quantity of the injection containing 0.10 g of Zuclopenthixol Acetate in sufficient *dichloromethane* to produce 50 ml. Solution (2) contains 0.0010% w/v of *2-chlorothioxanthone BPCRS* in *dichloromethane*. Solutions (3) to (5) contain (3) 0.0020% w/v, (4) 0.00040% w/v and (5) 0.00020% w/v respectively of *zuclopenthixol hydrochloride BPCRS* in *dichloromethane* containing a few drops of *diethylamine*. After removal of the plate, allow it to dry in air, spray with a mixture of equal volumes of *sulphuric acid* and *absolute ethanol*, heat at 110° for 5 minutes and examine under *ultraviolet light (365 nm)*. In the chromatogram obtained with solution (1) any spot corresponding to 2-chlorothioxanthone is not more intense than the spot in the chromatogram obtained with solution (2) (0.5%) and any spot corresponding to zuclopenthixol is not more intense than the spot in the chromatogram obtained with solution (3) (1%). Any other *secondary spot* in the chromatogram obtained with solution (1) is not more intense than the spot in the chromatogram obtained with solution (4) (0.2%) and not more than one such spot is more intense than the spot in the chromatogram obtained with solution (5) (0.1%).

***trans*-Isomer** Carry out the method for *liquid chromatography*, Appendix III D, protected from light, using the following solutions. For solution (1) dissolve a quantity of the injection containing 20 mg of Zuclopenthixol Acetate in 25 ml of *dichloromethane* and dilute to 50 ml with *dichloromethane*. For solution (2) dissolve 23 mg of *trans-clopenthixol acetate dihydrochloride BPCRS* (equivalent to 20 mg of *trans*-clopenthixol acetate) in sufficient *dichloromethane* containing a few drops of *diethylamine* to produce 50 ml; dilute 1 ml of the resulting solution to 100 ml with *dichloromethane*. For solution (3) mix equal volumes of solution (1) and undiluted solution (2).

The chromatographic procedure may be carried out using (a) a stainless steel column (25 cm × 4.6 mm) packed with *stationary phase A* (5 µm) (Spherisorb S 5W is suitable), (b) a mixture of 0.08 volume of 13.5M *ammonia*, 45 volumes of n-*heptane*, 45 volumes of *dichloromethane* and 50 volumes of *acetonitrile* as the mobile phase with a flow rate of 2 ml per minute and (c) a detection wavelength of 254 nm.

Inject 50 µl of each solution. The test is not valid unless the *resolution factor* between the principal peaks in the chromatogram obtained with solution (3) is at least 2.6.

In the chromatogram obtained with solution (1) the area of any peak corresponding to *trans*-clopenthixol acetate is not greater than the area of the peak in the chromatogram obtained with solution (2) (1%).

Assay Carry out the method for *liquid chromatography*, Appendix III D, using the following solutions. Prepare a 0.2% w/v solution of cis-*flupenthixol propionate dihydrochloride BPCRS* (internal standard) in *dichloromethane*. For solution (1) dissolve a quantity of the injection containing 20 mg of Zuclopenthixol Acetate in 25 ml of *dichloromethane*, add 5 ml of the internal standard solution and dilute to 50 ml with *dichloromethane*. For solution (2) dissolve 20 mg of *zuclopenthixol acetate dihydrochloride BPCRS* in 25 ml of *dichloromethane* containing a few drops of *diethylamine*, add 5 ml of the internal standard solution and dilute to 50 ml with *dichloromethane*.

The chromatographic conditions described under *trans*-Isomer may be used. Inject 50 µl of each solution.

Determine the *weight per ml* of the injection, Appendix V G, and calculate the content of $C_{24}H_{27}ClN_2O_2S$ using the declared content of $C_{24}H_{27}ClN_2O_2S$ in *zuclopenthixol acetate dihydrochloride BPCRS*.

Storage Zuclopenthixol Acetate Injection should be protected from light and stored at a temperature not exceeding 25°.

Zuclopenthixol Decanoate Injection

Definition Zuclopenthixol Decanoate Injection is a sterile solution of Zuclopenthixol Decanoate in a suitable vegetable oil.

The injection complies with the requirements stated under Parenteral Preparations and with the following requirements.

Content of zuclopenthixol decanoate, $C_{32}H_{43}ClN_3O_2S$ 95.0 to 105.0% of the prescribed or stated amount.

Identification Carry out the method for *thin-layer chromatography*, Appendix III A, protected from light, using a silica gel F_{254} precoated plate (Merck silica gel 60

F_{254} plates are suitable) and a mixture of 3 volumes of *diethylamine* and 90 volumes of *cyclohexane* as the mobile phase but using an unlined tank. Before use, heat the plate at 110° for 30 minutes. Apply separately to the plate 5 µl of each of the following solutions. For solution (1) dilute a volume of the injection with *ethanol (96%)* to contain 0.5% w/v of Zuclopenthixol Decanoate. Solution (2) contains 0.5% w/v of *zuclopenthixol decanoate dihydrochloride BPCRS* in *ethanol (96%)*. Solution (3) contains 0.5% w/v each of *zuclopenthixol decanoate dihydrochloride BPCRS* and *zuclopenthixol acetate dihydrochloride BPCRS*. After removal of the plate, allow it to dry in air, spray with a 1% w/v solution of *sodium molybdate* in *sulphuric acid*, heat at 110° for 20 minutes and examine in daylight. The principal spot in the chromatogram obtained with solution (1) corresponds to that in the chromatogram obtained with solution (2). The test is not valid unless the chromatogram obtained with solution (3) shows two clearly separated spots.

Related substances Carry out the method for *thin-layer chromatography*, Appendix III A, protected from light, using a silica gel F_{254} precoated plate (Merck silica gel 60 F_{254} plates are suitable, a mixture of 10 volumes of *diethylamine*, 40 volumes of *dichloromethane* and 50 volumes of *cyclohexane* as the mobile phase and an unlined tank. Apply separately to the plate 5 µl of each of the following solutions. For solution (1) dissolve a quantity of the injection containing 0.50 g of Zuclopenthixol Decanoate in 100 ml of *dichloromethane*. Solution (2) contains 0.0025% w/v of *2-chlorothioxanthone BPCRS* in *dichloromethane*. Solutions (3) to (5) contain (3) 0.015% w/v, (4) 0.00040% w/v and (5) 0.00020% w/v respectively of *zuclopenthixol hydrochloride BPCRS* in *dichloromethane* containing a few drops of *diethylamine*. After removal of the plate, allow it to dry in air, spray with a mixture of equal volumes of *sulphuric acid* and *absolute ethanol*, heat at 110° for 5 minutes and examine under *ultraviolet light (365 nm)*. In the chromatogram obtained with solution (1) any spot corresponding to 2-chlorothioxanthone is not more intense than the spot in the chromatogram obtained with solution (2) (0.5%) and any spot corresponding to zuclopenthixol is not more intense than the spot in the chromatogram obtained with solution (3) (3%). Any other *secondary spot* in the chromatogram obtained with solution (1) is not more intense than the spot in the chromatogram obtained with solution (4) (0.2%) and not more than one such spot is more intense than the spot in the chromatogram obtained with solution (5) (0.1%).

***trans*-Isomer** Carry out the method for *thin-layer chromatography*, Appendix III A, protected from light, using a silica gel F_{254} precoated plate (Merck silica gel 60 F_{254} plates are suitable) and a mixture of 30 volumes of *acetone* and 80 volumes of *toluene* as the mobile phase but using an unlined tank. Apply separately to the plate 5 µl of each of the following solutions. For solution (1) dissolve a quantity of the injection containing 0.5 g of Zuclopenthixol Decanoate in 100 ml of *dichloromethane*. Dilute 1 ml of the resulting solution to 50 ml with *dichloromethane*. Solution (2) contains 0.000115% w/v of *trans-clopenthixol decanoate dihydrochloride BPCRS* in *dichloromethane* (equivalent to 0.00010% w/v of *trans*-clopenthixol decanoate). After removal of the plate, allow it to dry in air, spray with a mixture of equal volumes of *sulphuric acid* and *absolute ethanol*, heat at 110° for 5 minutes and examine under *ultraviolet light (365 nm)*. Any spot in the chromatogram obtained with solution (1) corresponding to the *trans*-isomer is not more intense than the spot in the chromatogram obtained with solution (2) (1%).

Assay Dissolve a weighed quantity of the injection containing 0.25 g of Zuclopenthixol Decanoate in 50 ml of *glacial acetic acid* and carry out Method I for *non-aqueous titration*, Appendix VIII A, determining the end point potentiometrically. Each ml of 0.1M *perchloric acid VS* is equivalent to 27.76 mg of $C_{32}H_{43}ClN_3O_2S$. Determine the *weight per ml* of the injection, Appendix V G, and calculate the percentage content of $C_{32}H_{43}ClN_3O_2S$, weight in volume.

Storage Zuclopenthixol Decanoate Injection should be protected from light and stored at a temperature not exceeding 25°.

Zuclopenthixol Tablets

Definition Zuclopenthixol Tablets contain Zuclopenthixol Hydrochloride.

The tablets comply with the requirements stated under Tablets and with the following requirements.

Content of zuclopenthixol, $C_{22}H_{25}ClN_2OS$ 95.0 to 105% of the prescribed or stated amount.

Identification

A. The *light absorption*, Appendix II B, in the range 205 to 350 nm of solution A prepared in the Assay exhibits maxima at 230, 268 and 325 nm.

B. Carry out the method for *thin-layer chromatography*, Appendix III A, using a silica gel F_{254} precoated plate (Merck silica gel 60 F_{254} plates are suitable) and a mixture of 2 volumes of 13.5M *ammonia*, 2 volumes of *propan-1-ol*, 40 volumes of *toluene* and 60 volumes of *acetone* as the mobile phase and an unsaturated tank. Apply separately to the plate 10 µl of each of the following solutions. For solution (1) shake a quantity of the tablets containing the equivalent of 10 mg of zuclopenthixol with 10 ml of *methanol*, centrifuge and use the supernatant liquid. Solution (2) contains 0.1% w/v of *zuclopenthixol hydrochloride BPCRS* in *methanol*. Solution (3) contains 0.1% w/v each of *zuclopenthixol hydrochloride BPCRS* and *trans-clopenthixol BPCRS*. After removal of the plate, allow it to dry in air, spray with a 1% w/v solution of *sodium molybdate* in *sulphuric acid*, heat at 110° for 20 minutes and examine in daylight. The principal spot in the chromatogram obtained with solution (1) corresponds to that in the chromatogram obtained with solution (2). The test is not valid unless the chromatogram obtained with solution (3) shows two clearly separated spots.

2-Chlorothioxanthone Carry out the method for *thin-layer chromatography*, Appendix III A, protected from light, using a silica gel F_{254} precoated plate (Merck silica gel 60 F_{254} plates are suitable) and a mixture of 30 volumes of *dichloromethane* and 70 volumes of *toluene* as the mobile phase but using an unsaturated tank and allowing the solvent front to ascend 10 cm above the line of application. Apply separately to the plate 5 µl of each of the following solutions. For solution (1) shake a quantity of the powdered tablets containing the equivalent of 20 mg of zuclopenthixol with 10 ml of *dichloromethane* and filter. For tablets containing the equivalent of 2 mg of zuclopenthixol or less, solution (2) contains 0.004% w/v of *2-chlorothioxanthone BPCRS* in *dichloromethane*. For tablets containing the equivalent of more than 2 mg of zuclopenthixol, solution (2) contains 0.001% w/v of *2-chlorothioxanthone BPCRS* in *dichloromethane*. After removal of the plate, allow it to dry in air, spray with a mixture of equal volumes of *sulphuric acid* and *absolute ethanol,* heat at 110° for 5 minutes and examine under *ultraviolet light (365 nm)* immediately. Any *secondary spot* in the chromatogram obtained with solution (1) corresponding to 2-chlorothioxanthone is not more intense than the spot in the chromatogram obtained with solution (2) (2.0% for tablets containing the equivalent of 2 mg or less of zuclopenthixol and 0.5% for tablets containing the equivalent of more than 2 mg of zuclopenthixol).

Free amine Carry out the method for *thin-layer chromatography*, Appendix III A, protected from light, using a silica gel F_{254} precoated plate (Merck silica gel 60 F_{254} plates are suitable) and a mixture of 2 volumes of *water*, 10 volumes of 13.5M *ammonia*, 20 volumes of *butan-1-ol* and 65 volumes of *acetone* as the mobile phase. Apply separately to the plate 4 µl of each of the following solutions. For solution (1) use the filtrate prepared in the test for 2-Chlorothioxanthone. For solution (2) dilute 1 volume of solution (1) to 300 volumes with dichloromethane. After removal of the plate, allow it to dry in air, spray with a mixture of equal volumes of *sulphuric acid* and *absolute ethanol,* heat at 110° for 5 minutes and examine under *ultraviolet light (365 nm)* immediately. Any *secondary spot* in the chromatogram obtained with solution (1) is not more intense than the spot in the chromatogram obtained with solution (2) (0.3%).

Assay Weigh and powder 20 tablets. To a quantity of the powder containing the equivalent of 20 mg of zuclopenthixol add 40 ml of 0.1M *hydrochloric acid,* heat on a water bath for 30 minutes, shaking occasionally, cool, dilute to 200 ml with *water* and shake thoroughly. Centrifuge some of the resulting solution and dilute 20 ml of the supernatant liquid to 200 ml with *water* and mix (solution A). Prepare a reference standard in the following manner. Dissolve 25 mg of *zuclopenthixol hydrochloride BPCRS*, in 40 ml of 0.1M *hydrochloric acid,* dilute to 200 ml with *water* and shake thoroughly. Dilute 20 ml of the resulting solution to 200 ml with *water* and mix (solution B). Measure the *absorbance*, Appendix II B, of solution B and solution A at 230 nm using 0.002M *hydrochloric acid* in the reference cell. Calculate the content of $C_{22}H_{25}ClN_2OS$ using the *absorbances* at the maximum at 230 nm and the declared content of $C_{22}H_{25}ClN_2OS$ in *zuclopenthixol hydrochloride BPCRS.*

Labelling The quantity of active ingredient is stated in terms of the equivalent amount of zuclopenthixol.

IMPURITIES

The impurities limited by the requirements of this monograph include those shown under Zuclopenthixol Hydrochoride and the following:

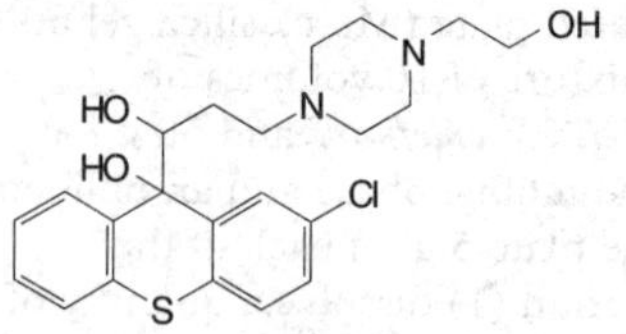

A. 2-chloro-9-(1-hydroxy-3-{(4-(2-hydroxyethyl)]piperazin-1-yl}propyl)thioxanthen-9-ol

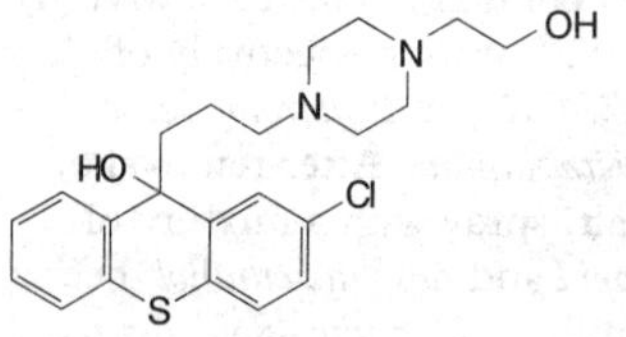

B. 2-chloro-9-(3-{[4-(2-hydroxyethyl)]-piperazin-1-yl}propyl)thioxanthen-9-ol

Monographs

Blood Products

BLOOD PRODUCTS

Anticoagulant and Preservative Solutions for Blood

Anticoagulant and Preservative Solutions for Blood comply with the requirements of the 3rd edition of the European Pharmacopoeia for Anticoagulant and Preservative Solutions for Human Blood [0209]. These requirements are reproduced after the heading 'Definition' below.

Ph Eur

DEFINITION

Anticoagulant and preservative solutions for human blood are sterile and pyrogen-free solutions prepared with water for injections, filtered, distributed in the final containers and sterilised. The content of sodium citrate ($C_6H_5Na_3O_7,2H_2O$), glucose monohydrate ($C_6H_{12}O_6,H_2O$) or anhydrous glucose ($C_6H_{12}O_6$) and sodium dihydrogen phosphate dihydrate ($NaH_2PO_4,2H_2O$) is not less than 95.0 per cent and not more than 105.0 per cent of that stated in the formulae below. The content of citric acid monohydrate ($C_6H_8O_7,H_2O$) or anhydrous citric acid ($C_6H_8O_7$) is not less than 90.0 per cent and not more than 110.0 per cent of that stated in the formulae below. Subject to agreement by the competent authority, other substances, such as red-cell preservatives, may be included in the formula provided that their name and concentration are stated on the label.

Anticoagulant and preservative solutions for human blood are presented in airtight, tamper-proof containers of glass (*3.2.1*) or plastic (*3.2.3*).

ANTICOAGULANT ACID-CITRATE-GLUCOSE SOLUTIONS (ACD)

	A	B
Sodium citrate (412)	22.0 g	13.2 g
Citric acid monohydrate (456)	8.0 g	4.8 g
or *Anhydrous citric acid (455)*	7.3 g	4.4 g
*Glucose monohydrate (178)**	24.5 g	14.7 g
or *Glucose, anhydrous (177)**	22.3 g	13.4 g
Water for injections (169) to	1000.0 ml	1000.0 ml
Volume to be used per 100 ml of blood	15.0 ml	25.0 ml

*The competent authority may require that the substance comply with the test for pyrogens given in the monographs on *Glucose monohydrate (178)* and *Glucose, anhydrous (177)*, respectively.

CHARACTERS

A colourless or faintly yellow, clear liquid, practically free from particles.

IDENTIFICATION

A. Examine by thin-layer chromatography (*2.2.27*), using *silica gel G R* as the coating substance.

Test Solution. Dilute 2 ml of the solution to be examined (for formula A) or 3 ml (for formula B) to 100 ml with a mixture of 2 volumes of *water R* and 3 volumes of *methanol R*.

Reference solution (a). Dissolve 10 mg of *glucose CRS* in a mixture of 2 volumes of *water R* and 3 volumes of *methanol R* and dilute to 20 ml with the same mixture of solvents.

Reference solution (b). Dissolve 10 mg each of *glucose CRS, lactose CRS, fructose CRS* and *sucrose CRS* in a mixture of 2 volumes of *water R* and 3 volumes of *methanol R* and dilute to 20 ml with the same mixture of solvents.

Apply separately to the plate 2 µl of each solution and thoroughly dry the starting points. Develop over a path of 15 cm using a mixture of 10 volumes of *water R*, 15 volumes of *methanol R*, 25 volumes of *anhydrous acetic acid R* and 50 volumes of *ethylene chloride R*. The volumes of solvents have to be measured accurately since a slight excess of water produces cloudiness. Dry the plate in a current of warm air. Repeat the development immediately, after renewing the mobile phase. Dry the plate in a current of warm air and spray evenly with a solution of 0.5 g of *thymol R* in a mixture of 5 ml of *sulphuric acid R* and 95 ml of *alcohol R*. Heat at 130°C for 10 min. The principal spot in the chromatogram obtained with the test solution is similar in position, colour and size to the principal spot in the chromatogram obtained with reference solution (a). The test is not valid unless the chromatogram obtained with reference solution (b) shows four clearly separated spots.

B. To 2 ml add 5 ml of *cupri-citric solution R*. Heat to boiling. An orange precipitate is formed and the solution becomes yellow.

C. To 2 ml (for formula A) add 3 ml of *water R* or to 4 ml (for formula B) add 1 ml of *water R*. The solution gives the reaction of citrates (*2.3.1*).

D. 0.5 ml gives reaction (b) of sodium (*2.3.1*).

TESTS

pH (*2.2.3*). The pH of the solution to be examined is 4.7 to 5.3.

Hydroxymethylfurfural To 2.0 ml add 5.0 ml of a 100 g/l solution of *p- toluidine R* in *2-propanol R* containing 10 per cent *V/V* of *glacial acetic acid R* and 1.0 ml of a 5 g/l solution of *barbituric acid R*. The absorbance (*2.2.25*), determined at 550 nm after allowing the mixture to stand for 2 min to 3 min, is not greater than that of a standard prepared at the same time in the same manner using 2.0 ml of a solution containing 5 ppm of *hydroxymethylfurfural R* for formula A or 3 ppm of *hydroxymethylfurfural R* for formula B.

Sterility (*2.6.1*). They comply with the test for sterility.

Pyrogens (*2.6.8*). They comply with the test for pyrogens. Dilute with a pyrogen-free, 9 g/l solution of *sodium chloride R* to obtain a solution containing approximately 5 g/l of *sodium citrate R*. Inject 10 ml of the diluted solution per kilogram of the rabbit's mass.

ASSAY

Citric acid To 10.0 ml (for formula A) or to 20.0 ml (for formula B) add 0.1 ml of *phenolphthalein solution R1*. Titrate with *0.2M sodium hydroxide* until a pink colour is obtained.

1 ml of *0.2M sodium hydroxide* is equivalent to 14.01 mg of $C_6H_8O_7,H_2O$ or to 12.81 mg of $C_6H_8O_7$.

Sodium citrate Prepare a chromatography column 0.1 m long and 10 mm in internal diameter and filled with *strongly acidic ion exchange resin R* (300 µm to 840 µm). Maintain a 1 cm layer of liquid above the resin at all times. Wash the column with 50 ml of de-ionised *water R* at a flow rate of 12 ml to 14 ml per minute.

Dilute 10.0 ml of the solution to be examined (for formula A) or 15.0 ml (for formula B) to about 40 ml with de-ionised *water R* in a beaker and transfer to the column reservoir, washing the beaker three times with a few millilitres of de-ionised *water R*. Allow the solution to run through the column at a flow rate of 12 ml to 14 ml per minute and collect the eluate. Wash the column with two quantities, each of 30 ml, and with one quantity of 50 ml, of de-ionised *water R*. The column can be used for three successive determinations before regeneration with three times its volume of *dilute hydrochloric acid R*. Titrate the combined eluate and washings (about 150 ml) with *0.2M sodium hydroxide*, using 0.1 ml of *phenolphthalein solution R1* as indicator.

Calculate the content of sodium citrate in grams per litre from the following expressions:

For formula A: $1.961n - 1.40C$ or $1.961n - 1.53C'$

For formula B: $1.307n - 1.40C$ or $1.307n - 1.53C'$

n = number of millilitres of *0.2M sodium hydroxide* used in the titration,

C = content of citric acid monohydrate in grams per litre determined as prescribed above,

C' = content of anhydrous citric acid in grams per litre determined as prescribed above.

Reducing sugars Dilute 5.0 ml (for formula A) or 10.0 ml (for formula B) to 100.0 ml with *water R*. Introduce 25.0 ml of the solution into a 250 ml conical flask with ground-glass neck and add 25.0 ml of *cupri-citric solution R1*. Add a few pieces of porous material, attach a reflux condenser, heat so that boiling begins within 2 min and boil for exactly 10 min. Cool and add 3 g of *potassium iodide R* dissolved in 3 ml of *water R*. Add 25 ml of a 25 per cent *m/m* solution of *sulphuric acid R* with caution and in small quantities. Titrate with *0.1M sodium thiosulphate* using 0.5 ml of *starch solution R*, added towards the end of the titration, as indicator (n_1 ml). Carry out a blank titration using 25.0 ml of *water R* (n_2 ml).

Calculate the content of reducing sugars as anhydrous glucose or as glucose monohydrate, as appropriate, from the Table 209-1.

Table 209-1

Volume of 0.1M sodium thiosulphate ($n_2 - n_1$ ml)	Anhydrous glucose in milligrams	Glucose monohydrate in milligrams
8	19.8	21.6
9	22.4	24.5
10	25.0	27.4
11	27.6	30.2
12	30.3	33.1
13	33.0	36.1
14	35.7	39.0
15	38.5	42.1
16	41.3	45.2

STORAGE

Store in an airtight, tamper-proof container, protected from light.

LABELLING

The label states:

— the composition and volume of the solution,

— the maximum amount of blood to be collected in the container.

ANTICOAGULANT CITRATE-PHOSPHATE-GLUCOSE SOLUTION (CPD)

Sodium citrate (412)	26.3g
Citric acid monohydrate (456)	3.27 g
or *Anhydrous citric acid (455)*	2.99 g
Glucose monohydrate (178) *	25.5 g
or *Glucose, anhydrous (177)* *	23.2 g
Sodium dihydrogen phosphate dihydrate (194)	2.51 g
Water for injections (169) to	1000.0 ml
Volume to be used per 100 ml of blood	14.0 ml

*The competent authority may require that the substance comply with the test for pyrogens given in the monographs on *Glucose monohydrate (178)* and *Glucose, anhydrous (177)*, respectively.

CHARACTERS

A colourless or faintly yellow, clear liquid, practically free from particles.

IDENTIFICATION

A. Examine by thin-layer chromatography (*2.2.27*), using *silica gel G R* as the coating substance.

Test Solution. Dilute 2 ml of the solution to be examined to 100 ml with a mixture of 2 volumes of *water R* and 3 volumes of *methanol R*.

Reference solution (a). Dissolve 10 mg of *glucose CRS* in a mixture of 2 volumes of *water R* and 3 volumes of *methanol R* and dilute to 20 ml with the same mixture of solvents.

Reference solution (b). Dissolve 10 mg each of *glucose CRS, lactose CRS, fructose CRS* and *sucrose CRS* in a mixture of 2 volumes of *water R* and 3 volumes of *methanol R* and dilute to 20 ml with the same mixture of solvents.

Apply separately to the plate 2 µl of each solution and thoroughly dry the starting points. Develop over a path of 15 cm using a mixture of 10 volumes of *water R*, 15 volumes of *methanol R*, 25 volumes of *anhydrous acetic acid R* and 50 volumes of *ethylene chloride R*. The volumes of solvents have to be measured accurately since a slight excess of water produces cloudiness. Dry the plate in a current of warm air. Repeat the development immediately, after renewing the mobile phase. Dry the plate in a current of warm air and spray evenly with a solution of 0.5 g of *thymol R* in a mixture of 5 ml of *sulphuric acid R* and 95 ml of *alcohol R*. Heat at 130°C for 10 min. The principal spot in the chromatogram obtained with the test solution is similar in position, colour and size to the principal spot in the chromatogram obtained with reference solution (a). The test is not valid unless the chromatogram obtained with reference solution (b) shows four clearly separated spots.

B. To 2 ml add 5 ml of *cupri-citric solution R*. Heat to boiling. An orange precipitate is formed and the solution becomes yellow.

C. To 2 ml add 3 ml of *water R*. The solution gives the reaction of citrates (*2.3.1*).

D. 1 ml gives reaction (b) of phosphates (*2.3.1*).

E. 0.5 ml gives reaction (b) of sodium (*2.3.1*).

TESTS

pH (*2.2.3*). The pH of the solution is 5.3 to 5.9.

Hydroxymethylfurfural To 2.0 ml add 5.0 ml of a 100 g/l solution of *p- toluidine R* in *2-propanol R* containing 10 per cent *V/V* of *glacial acetic acid R* and 1.0 ml of a 5 g/l solution of *barbituric acid R*. The absorbance (*2.2.25*), determined at 550 nm after allowing the mixture to stand for 2 min to 3 min, is not greater than that of a standard prepared at the same time in the same manner using 2.0 ml of a solution containing 5 ppm of *hydroxymethylfurfural R*.

Sterility (*2.6.1*). They comply with the test for sterility.

Pyrogens (*2.6.8*). They comply with the test for pyrogens. Dilute with a pyrogen-free, 9 g/l solution of *sodium chloride R* to obtain a solution containing approximately 5 g/l of *sodium citrate R*. Inject 10 ml of the diluted solution per kilogram of the rabbit's mass.

ASSAY

Sodium dihydrogen phosphate Dilute 10.0 ml to 100.0 ml with *water R*. To 10.0 ml of this solution add 10.0 ml of *nitro-vanado-molybdic reagent R*. Mix and allow to stand at 20°C to 25°C for 30 min. At the same time and in the same manner, prepare a reference solution using 10.0 ml of a standard solution containing 0.219 g of *potassium dihydrogen phosphate R* per litre. Measure the absorbance (*2.2.25*) of the two solutions at 450 nm using as the compensation liquid a solution prepared in the same manner using 10 ml of *water R*. Calculate the content of sodium dihydrogen phosphate dihydrate (*P*) in grams per litre from the expression:

$$\frac{11.46 \times C \times A_1}{A_2}$$

C = concentration of *potassium dihydrogen phos-phate R* in the standard solution in grams per litre,

A_1 = absorbance of the test solution,

A_2 = absorbance of the reference solution.

Citric acid To 20.0 ml add 0.1 ml of *phenolphthalein solution R1* and titrate with *0.2M sodium hydroxide*.

Calculate the content of citric acid monohydrate (*C*), or anhydrous citric acid (*C′*), in grams per litre from the equations:

$$C = 0.7005n - 0.4490P$$

$$C' = 0.6404n - 0.4105P$$

n = number of millilitres of *0.2M sodium hydroxide* used in the titration,

P = content of sodium dihydrogen phosphate dihydrate in grams per litre determined as prescribed above.

Sodium citrate Prepare a chromatography column 100 mm long and 10 mm in internal diameter and filled with *strongly acidic ion exchange resin R* (300 µm to 840 µm). Maintain a 1 cm layer of liquid above the resin at all times. Wash the column with 50 ml of de-ionised *water R* at a flow rate of 12 ml to 14 ml per minute.

Dilute 10.0 ml of the solution to be examined to about 40 ml with de-ionised *water R* in a beaker and transfer to the column reservoir, washing the beaker three times with a few millilitres of de-ionised *water R*. Allow the solution to run through the column at a flow rate of 12 ml to 14 ml per minute and collect the eluate. Wash the column with two quantities, each of 30 ml, and with one quantity of 50 ml, of de-ionised *water R*. The column can be used for three successive determinations before regeneration with three times its volume of *dilute hydrochloric acid R*. Titrate the combined eluate and washings (about 150 ml) with *0.2M sodium hydroxide*, using 0.1 ml of *phenolphthalein solution R1* as indicator.

Calculate the content of sodium citrate in grams per litre from the following expressions:

$$1.961n - 1.257P - 1.40C$$

$$1.961n - 1.257P - 1.53C'$$

n = number of millilitres of *0.2M sodium hydroxide* used in the titration,

P = content of sodium dihydrogen phosphate dihydrate in grams per litre determined as prescribed above,

C = content of citric acid monohydrate in grams per litre determined as prescribed above,

C' = content of anhydrous citric acid in grams per litre determined as prescribed above.

Reducing sugars Dilute 5.0 ml to 100.0 ml with *water R*. Introduce 25.0 ml of the solution into a 250 ml conical flask with ground-glass neck and add 25.0 ml of *cupri-citric solution R1*. Add a few pieces of porous material, attach a reflux condenser, heat so that boiling begins within 2 min and boil for exactly 10 min. Cool and add 3 g of *potassium iodide R* dissolved in 3 ml of *water R*. Add 25 ml of a 25 per cent *m/m* solution of *sulphuric acid R* with caution and in small quantities. Titrate with *0.1M sodium thiosulphate* using 0.5 ml of *starch solution R*, added towards the end of the titration, as indicator (n_1 ml). Carry out a blank titration using 25.0 ml of *water R* (n_2 ml).

Calculate the content of reducing sugars as anhydrous glucose or as glucose monohydrate, as appropriate, from the Table 209-1.

STORAGE

Store in an airtight, tamper-proof container, protected from light.

LABELLING

The label states:

— the composition and volume of the solution,

— the maximum amount of blood to be collected in the container.

Ph Eur

Plasma for Fractionation

Plasma for Fractionation complies with the requirements of the 3rd edition of the European Pharmacopoeia for Human Plasma for Fractionation [0853]. These requirements are reproduced after the heading 'Definition' below.

Ph Eur

DEFINITION

Human plasma for fractionation is the liquid part of human blood remaining after separation of the cellular elements from blood collected in a receptacle containing an anticoagulant, or separated by continuous filtration or centrifugation of anticoagulated blood in an apheresis procedure; it is intended for the manufacture of plasma-derived products.

PRODUCTION

DONORS

Only a carefully selected, healthy donor who, as far as can be ascertained after medical examination, laboratory blood tests and a study of the donor's medical history, is free from detectable agents of infection transmissible by plasma-derived products may be used in the collection of plasma for fractionation. Recommendations in this field are made by the Council of Europe (*Recommendation No R (95) 15 on the preparation, use and quality assurance of blood components*, or subsequent revision).

Persons who have been treated with substances of human pituitary origin such as growth hormone, gonadotropin or thyroid-stimulating hormone (thyrotropin) are not acceptable as donors.

Immunisation of donors Deliberate immunisation of donors to obtain immunoglobulins with specified activities may be carried out when sufficient supplies of material of suitable quality cannot be obtained from naturally immunised donors. Recommendations for such immunisation are formulated by the World Health Organisation (*Requirements for the collection, processing and quality control of blood, blood components and plasma derivatives*, WHO Technical Report Series, No. 840, 1994 or subsequent revision).

Records Records of donors and donations made are kept in such a way that, while maintaining the required degree of confidentiality concerning the donor's identity, the origin of each donation in a plasma pool, and the results of the corresponding acceptance procedures and laboratory tests can be traced.

Laboratory tests Laboratory tests are carried out for each donation to detect the following viral markers:

1. antibodies against human immunodeficiency virus 1 (anti-HIV-1),
2. antibodies against human immunodeficiency virus 2 (anti-HIV-2),
3. the surface antigen of hepatitis B virus (HBsAg),
4. antibodies against hepatitis C virus (anti-HCV).

Pending complete harmonisation of the laboratory tests to be carried out, the competent authority may require that a test for alanine-lysine-aminotransferase (ALT) be also carried out.

The test methods used are of suitable sensitivity and specificity and are approved by the competent authority. If a repeat-reactive result is found in any of these tests, the donation is not accepted.

INDIVIDUAL PLASMA UNITS

The plasma is prepared by a method that removes cells and cell debris as completely as possible. Whether prepared from human blood or by plasmapheresis, the plasma is separated from the cells by a method designed to prevent the introduction of micro-organisms. No antibacterial or antifungal agent is added to the plasma at any stage, including the subsequent processing to obtain plasma derivatives. The containers comply with the requirements for glass containers (*3.2.1*) or for plastic containers for blood (*3.2.3*). The containers are closed so as to prevent contamination.

If two or more units are pooled prior to freezing, the operations are carried out using sterile connecting devices or under aseptic conditions and using containers that have not previously been used.

Plasma intended for the manufacture of coagulation factors and other labile derivatives is either processed shortly after separation or collection or it is frozen by cooling rapidly at −30°C or below. Plasma obtained from whole blood and intended for the manufacture of coagulation factors and other labile derivatives is separated from cellular elements and frozen as soon as possible and at the latest within 24 h of donation. Plasma intended for the manufacture of non-labile derivatives is separated within 5 days of the expiry date of the whole blood.

It is not intended that the determination of total protein and factor VIII shown below be carried out on each unit of plasma. They are rather given as guidelines for good manufacturing practice, the test for factor VIII being relevant for plasma intended for use in the preparation of concentrates of labile components.

The total protein content of a unit of plasma depends on the serum protein content of the donor and the degree of dilution inherent in the donation procedure. When plasma is obtained from a suitable donor and using the intended proportion of anticoagulant solution, a total protein content complying with the limit of 50 g per litre is obtained. If a volume of blood or plasma smaller than intended is collected into the anticoagulant solution, the resulting plasma is not necessarily unsuitable for pooling for fractionation. The aim of good manufacturing practice must be to achieve the prescribed limit for all normal donations.

Preservation of factor VIII in the donation depends on the collection procedure and the subsequent handling of the blood and plasma. With good practice, 0.7 I.U. per millilitre can usually be achieved, but units of plasma with a lower content may still be suitable for use in the production of blood coagulation factor concentrates. The aim of good manufacturing practice is to conserve labile components as much as possible.

Total protein Carry out the test using a pool of not fewer than ten units. Dilute the pool with a 9 g/l solution of *sodium chloride R* to obtain a solution containing about 15 mg of protein in 2 ml. To 2.0 ml of this solution in a round-bottomed centrifuge tube add 2 ml of a 75 g/l solution of *sodium molybdate R* and 2 ml of a mixture of 1 volume of *nitrogen-free sulphuric acid R* and 30 volumes of *water R*. Shake, centrifuge for 5 min, decant the supernatant liquid and allow the inverted tube to drain on filter paper. Determine the nitrogen in the residue by the method of sulphuric acid digestion (*2.5.9*) and calculate the quantity of protein by multiplying by 6.25. The total protein content is not less than 50 g/l.

Factor VIII Carry out the test using a pool of not fewer than ten units. Thaw the samples to be examined, if necessary, at a temperature not exceeding 37°C. Carry out the assay of factor VIII (*2.7.4*), using a reference plasma calibrated against the International Standard for blood coagulation factor VIII in plasma. The activity is not less than 0.7 I.U. per millilitre.

POOLED PLASMA

During the manufacture of plasma products, the first homogeneous pool of plasma (for example, after removal of cryo-precipitate) is tested for hepatitis B surface antigen, for hepatitis C virus antibodies and for HIV antibodies using test methods of suitable sensitivity and specificity: the pool must give negative results in these tests.

CHARACTERS

Before freezing, a clear or slightly turbid liquid without visible signs of haemolysis; it may vary in colour from light yellow to green.

STORAGE

Store frozen plasma at or below −20°C; the plasma may still be used for fractionation if a temperature of −20°C is exceeded on at most one occasion for not more than 72 h and if the plasma is at all times maintained at a temperature of −5°C or lower.

LABELLING

The label enables each individual unit to be traced to a specific donor.

Ph Eur

Albumin Solution

Albumin; Human Albumin

Albumin Solution complies with the requirements of the 3rd edition of the European Pharmacopoeia for Human Albumin Solution [0255]. These requirements are reproduced after the heading 'Definition' below.

Ph Eur

DEFINITION

Human albumin solution is an aqueous solution of protein obtained from plasma that complies with the requirements of the monograph on *Plasma for fractionation, human (853)*.

PRODUCTION

Separation of the albumin is carried out under controlled conditions, particularly of pH, ionic strength and temperature so that in the final product not less than 95 per cent of the total protein is albumin. Human albumin solution is prepared as a concentrated solution containing 150 g/l to 250 g/l of total protein or as an isotonic solution containing 35 g/l to 50 g/l of total protein. A suitable stabiliser against the effects of heat, such as sodium caprylate (sodium octanoate) or *N*-acetyltryptophan or a combination of these two, at a suitable concentration, may be added but no antimicrobial preservative is added at any stage during preparation. The solution is passed through a bacteria-retentive filter and distributed aseptically into sterile containers which are then closed so as to prevent contamination. The solution in its final container is heated to 60 ± 0.5°C and maintained at this temperature for not less than 10 h. The containers are then incubated at 30°C to 32°C for not less than 14 days or at 20°C to 25°C for not less than 4 weeks and examined visually for evidence of microbial contamination.

CHARACTERS

A clear, slightly viscous liquid; it is almost colourless, yellow or green.

IDENTIFICATION

A. Using a suitable range of species-specific antisera, carry out precipitation tests on the preparation to be examined. It is recommended that the test be carried out using antisera specific to the plasma proteins of each species of domestic animal commonly used in the preparation of materials of biological origin in the country concerned. The preparation is shown to contain proteins of human origin and gives negative results with antisera specific to plasma proteins of other species.

B. Examine by a suitable immunoelectrophoresis technique. Using antiserum to normal human serum, compare normal human serum and the preparation to be examined, both diluted to contain 10 g/l of protein. The main component of the preparation to be examined corresponds to the main component of normal human serum. The preparation may show the presence of small quantities of other plasma proteins.

TESTS

pH (*2.2.3*). Dilute the preparation to be examined with a 9 g/l solution of *sodium chloride R* to obtain a solution containing 10 g/l of protein. The pH of the solution is 6.7 to 7.3.

Total protein Dilute the preparation to be examined with a 9 g/l solution of *sodium chloride R* to obtain a solution containing about 15 mg of protein in 2 ml. To 2.0 ml of this solution in a round-bottomed centrifuge tube add 2 ml of a 75 g/l solution of *sodium molybdate R* and 2 ml of a mixture of 1 volume of *nitrogen-free sulphuric acid R* and 30 volumes of *water R*. Shake, centrifuge for 5 min, decant the supernatant liquid and allow the inverted tube to drain on filter paper. Determine the nitrogen in the residue by the method of sulphuric acid digestion (*2.5.9*) and calculate the quantity of protein by multiplying by 6.25. The preparation contains not less than 95 per cent and not more than 105 per cent of the quantity of protein stated on the label.

Protein composition Examine by zone electrophoresis (*2.2.31*), using strips of suitable cellulose acetate gel as the supporting medium and *barbital buffer solution pH 8.6 R1* as the electrolyte solution.

Test solution. Dilute the preparation to be examined with a 9 g/l solution of *sodium chloride R* to a protein concentration of 20 g/l.

Reference solution. Dilute *human albumin for electrophoresis BRP* with a 9 g/l solution of *sodium chloride R* to a protein concentration of 20 g/l.

To a strip apply 2.5 µl of the test solution as a 10 mm

band or apply 0.25 µl per millimetre if a narrower strip is used. To another strip apply in the same manner the same volume of the reference solution. Apply a suitable electric field such that the most rapid band migrates at least 30 mm. Treat the strips with *amido black 10B solution R* for 5 min. Decolorise with a mixture of 10 volumes of *glacial acetic acid R* and 90 volumes of *methanol R* until the background is just free of colour. Develop the transparency of the strips with a mixture of 19 volumes of *glacial acetic acid R* and 81 volumes of *methanol R*. Measure the absorbance of the bands at 600 nm in an instrument having a linear response over the range of measurement. Calculate the result as the mean of three measurements of each strip. In the electrophoretogram obtained with the test solution, not more than 5 per cent of the protein has a mobility different from that of the principal band. The test is not valid unless, in the electrophoretogram obtained with the reference preparation, the proportion of protein in the principal band is within the limits stated in the leaflet accompanying the reference preparation.

Polymers and aggregates Examine by liquid chromatography (*2.2.29*).

Test solution. Dilute the preparation to be examined with a 9 g/l solution of *sodium chloride R* to a concentration suitable for the chromatographic system used. A concentration in the range 4 g/l to 12 g/l and injection of 50 µg to 600 µg of protein are usually suitable.

The chromatographic procedure may be carried out using:
— a column 0.6 m long and 7.5 mm in internal diameter packed with *hydrophilic silica gel for chromatography R*,
— as mobile phase at a flow rate of 0.5 ml per minute a solution containing per litre: 4.873 g of *disodium hydrogen phosphate dihydrate R*, 1.741 g of *sodium dihydrogen phosphate monohydrate R*, 11.688 g of *sodium chloride R* and 50 mg of *sodium azide R*,
— a detector set at 280 nm.

The peak corresponding to polymers and aggregates is located in the part of the chromatogram representing the void volume. The area of this peak divided by 2 is not greater than 5 per cent of the total area of the chromatogram.

Haem Dilute the preparation to be examined using a 9 g/l solution of *sodium chloride R* to obtain a solution containing 10 g/l of protein. The absorbance (*2.2.25*) of the solution measured at 403 nm using *water R* as the compensation liquid is not greater than 0.15.

Prekallikrein activator (*2.6.15*). Not more than 35 I.U. per millilitre.

Aluminium If intended for administration to patients undergoing dialysis or to premature infants, it complies with the test for aluminium. Not more than 200 µg of Al per litre, determined by atomic absorption spectrometry (*Method I, 2.2.23*), using a furnace as atomic generator.

Use plastic containers for preparation of the solutions. Wash equipment in nitric acid (200 g/l HNO_3) before use.

Test solution. Use the preparation to be examined.

Validation solution. Use *human albumin for aluminium validation BRP*.

Reference solutions. Prepare a suitable range of reference solutions by adding suitable volumes of *aluminium standard solution (10 ppm Al) R* to known volumes of *water R*.

Dilute the solutions as necessary using nitric acid (10 g/l HNO_3) containing 1.7 g/l of *magnesium nitrate R* and 0.05 per cent *V/V* of *octoxinol 10 R*. Measure the absorbance at 309.3 nm. The test is not valid unless the aluminium content determined for *human albumin for aluminium validation BRP* is within 20 per cent of the value stated in the leaflet accompanying the reference preparation.

Potassium Not more than 0.05 mmol of K per gram of protein, determined by atomic emission spectrometry (*Method I, 2.2.22*). Measure the emission intensity at 766 nm.

Sodium Not more than 160 mmol of Na per litre and not less than 95 per cent and not more than 105 per cent of the content of Na stated on the label, determined by atomic emission spectrometry (*Method I, 2.2.22*). Measure the emission intensity at 589 nm.

Sterility (*2.6.1*). It complies with the test for sterility.

Pyrogens (*2.6.8*). It complies with the test for pyrogens. For a solution containing 35 g/l to 50 g/l of protein, inject per kilogram of the rabbit's mass 10 ml of the preparation to be examined. For a solution containing 150 g/l to 250 g/l of protein, inject per kilogram of the rabbit's mass 3 ml of the preparation to be examined.

STORAGE

Store protected from light.

LABELLING

The label states:
— the name of the preparation,
— the volume of the preparation,
— the content of protein expressed in grams per litre,
— the content of sodium expressed in millimoles per litre,
— the storage conditions,
— the expiry date,
— that the product is not to be used if it is cloudy or if a deposit has formed,
— the name and concentration of any added substance (for example stabiliser),
— where applicable, that the preparation is suitable for administration to patients undergoing dialysis and to premature infants.

Ph Eur

Antithrombin III Concentrate

Antithrombin III Concentrate complies with the requirements of the 3rd edition of the European Pharmacopoeia for Freeze-dried Human Antithrombin III Concentrate [0878]. These requirements are reproduced after the heading 'Definition' below.

Action and use Used to correct deficiencies of antithrombin III.

Ph Eur

DEFINITION

Freeze-dried human antithrombin III concentrate is a preparation of a glycoprotein fraction obtained from human plasma that inactivates thrombin in the presence of an excess of heparin. It is obtained from plasma that complies with the requirements of the monograph on *Human plasma for fractionation (853)*.

When reconstituted in the volume of solvent stated on the label or on the leaflet, the potency is not less than 25 I.U. of antithrombin III per millilitre.

PRODUCTION

The method of preparation includes a step or steps that have been shown to remove or to inactivate known agents of infection; if substances are used for inactivation of viruses during production, the subsequent purification procedure must be validated to demonstrate that the concentration of these substances is reduced to a suitable level and any residues are such as not to compromise the safety of the preparation for patients.

The antithrombin III is purified and concentrated and a suitable stabiliser may be added. The specific activity is not less than 3 I.U. of antithrombin III per milligram of total protein, excluding albumin. The antithrombin III concentrate is passed through a bacteria-retentive filter, distributed aseptically into its final, sterile containers and immediately frozen. It is then freeze-dried and the containers are closed under vacuum or in an atmosphere of inert gas. No antimicrobial preservative is added at any stage of production.

VALIDATION TEST

It shall be demonstrated that the manufacturing process yields a product that consistently complies with the following test:

Heparin-binding fraction. Examine by agarose gel electrophoresis (*2.2.31*). Prepare a 10 g/l solution of *agarose for electrophoresis R* containing 15 I.U. of *heparin R* per millilitre in *barbital buffer solution pH 8.4 R*. Pour 5 ml of this solution onto a glass plate 5 cm square. Cool at 4°C for 30 min. Cut two wells 2 mm in diameter 1 cm and 4 cm from the side of the plate and 1 cm from the cathode. Introduce into one well 5 µl of the preparation to be examined, diluted to an activity of about 1 I.U. of antithrombin III per millilitre. Introduce into the other well 5 µl of a solution of a marker dye such as *bromophenol blue R*. Allow the electrophoresis to proceed at 4°C, using a constant electric field of 7 V per centimetre, until the dye reaches the anode.

Cut across the agarose gel 1.5 cm from that side of the plate on which the preparation to be examined was applied and remove the larger portion of the gel leaving a band 1.5 cm wide containing the material to be examined. Replace the removed portion with an even layer consisting of 3.5 ml of a 10 g/l solution of *agarose for electrophoresis R* in *barbital buffer solution pH 8.4 R*, containing a rabbit anti-human antithrombin III antiserum at a suitable concentration, previously determined, to give adequate peak heights of at least 1.5 cm. Place the plate with the original gel at the cathode so that a second electrophoretic migration can occur at right angles to the first. Allow this second electrophoresis to proceed using a constant electric field of 2 V per centimetre for 16 h. Cover the plates with filter paper and several layers of thick lint soaked in a 9 g/l solution of *sodium chloride R* and compress for 2 h, renewing the saline several times. Rinse with *water R*, dry the plates and stain with *acid blue 92 solution R*.

Calculate the fraction of antithrombin III bound to heparin, which is the peak closest to the anode, with respect to the total amount of antithrombin III, by measuring the area defined by the two precipitation peaks.

The fraction of antithrombin III able to bind to heparin is not less than 60 per cent.

CHARACTERS

A white, friable solid or a powder.

Reconstitute the preparation to be examined as stated on the label or on the leaflet immediately before carrying out the identification, the tests (except those for solubility, total protein and water), and the assay.

IDENTIFICATION

A. Using a suitable range of species-specific antisera, carry out precipitation tests on the preparation to be examined and stain the gels with *acid blue 92 R*. It is recommended that the tests be carried out using antisera specific to the plasma proteins of each species of domestic animal commonly used in the preparation of materials of biological origin in the country concerned. The preparation is shown to contain proteins of human origin and gives negative results with antisera specific to plasma proteins of other species.

B. The assay for antithrombin III activity contributes to the identification of the preparation.

TESTS

pH (*2.2.3*). The pH of the preparation to be examined is 6.0 to 7.5.

Solubility It dissolves completely under gentle swirling within 10 min in the volume of the solvent stated on the label or the leaflet, forming a clear or slightly turbid, colourless solution.

Osmolality (*2.2.35*). Not less than 240 milliosmoles per kilogram.

Total protein If necessary, dilute an accurately measured volume of the preparation to be examined with *water R* to obtain a solution containing about 15 mg of protein in 2 ml. To 2.0 ml of the solution in a round-bottomed centrifuge tube add 2 ml of a 75 g/l solution of *sodium molybdate R* and 2 ml of a mixture of 1 volume of *nitrogen-free sulphuric acid R* and 30 volumes of *water R*. Shake, centrifuge for 5 min, decant the supernatant liquid and allow the inverted tube to drain on filter paper. Determine the nitrogen in the residue by the method of sulphuric acid digestion (*2.5.9*) and calculate the amount of protein by multiplying the result by 6.25.

Heparin (*2.7.5*). Not more than 0.1 I.U. of heparin activity per International Unit of antithrombin III activity. It is necessary to validate the method for assay of heparin for each specific preparation to be examined to allow for interference by antithrombin III.

Water (*2.5.12*). Not more than 3.0 per cent, determined on not less than 0.500 g by the semi-micro determination of water.

Sterility (*2.6.1*). It complies with the test for sterility.

Pyrogens (*2.6.8*). It complies with the test for pyrogens. Inject per kilogram of the rabbit's mass a volume of the preparation to be examined equivalent to 50 I.U. of antithrombin III, calculated from the activity stated on the label.

ASSAY

The antithrombin III content of the preparation to be examined is determined by comparing its ability to inactivate thrombin in the presence of an excess of heparin with the same ability of a reference preparation of human anti-thrombin III concentrate calibrated in International Units. Varying quantities of the preparation to be examined are mixed with a given quantity of thrombin and the remaining thrombin activity is determined using a suitable chromogenic substrate.

The International Unit is the activity of a stated amount of the International Standard for human antithrombin III concentrate. The equivalence in International Units of the International Standard is stated by the World Health Organisation.

Method. Prepare two independent series of three or four dilutions in the range 1/75 to 1/200 from 1 I.U. per millilitre, for both the preparation to be examined and the reference preparation, using *tris-EDTA BSA buffer solution pH 8.4 R* containing 15 I.U. of heparin per millilitre.

Warm 200 µl of each dilution at 37°C for 1 min to 2 min. Add to each dilution 200 µl of a solution of *bovine thrombin R* containing 2 I.U. per millilitre in *tris-EDTA BSA buffer solution pH 8.4 R*. Mix and maintain at 37°C for exactly 1 min. Add 500 µl of a suitable chromogenic substrate (for example, D-phenylalanyl-L-pipecolyl-L-arginyl 4-nitroanilide, reconstituted in *water R* to give a solution containing 4 mmol per litre and further diluted for the assay using *tris-EDTA BSA buffer solution pH 8.4 R without albumin*). Immediately start measurement of the change in absorbance at 405 nm, continuing the measurement for at least 30 s. Calculate the rate of change of absorbance (ΔA/min). (Alternatively, an end-point assay may be used by stopping the reaction with acetic acid and measuring the absorbance at 405 nm.)

The rate of change of absorbance (ΔA/min) is inversely proportional to antithrombin III activity. Plot the regression of absorbance or ΔA/min against concentration on a linear scale and determine the potency by comparing the slopes for the reference preparation and the preparation to be examined.

Check the validity of the assay and calculate the potency of the test preparation by the usual statistical methods for a slope-ratio assay (for example, *5.3. Statistical Analysis of Results of Biological Assays and Tests*).

The estimated potency is not less than 90 per cent and not greater than 110 per cent of the potency stated on the label. The confidence interval ($P = 0.95$) is not greater than 90 per cent to 110 per cent of the estimated potency.

STORAGE

Store protected from light.

LABELLING

The label states:
— the content of antithrombin III expressed in International Units per container.
— the name and volume of solvent to be used to reconstitute the preparation,
— where applicable, the amount of albumin present as a stabiliser.

Ph Eur

Dried Factor VII Fraction

Dried Factor VII Fraction complies with the requirements of the 3rd edition of the European Pharmacopoeia for Freeze-dried Human Coagulation Factor VII [1224]. These requirements are reproduced after the heading 'Definition' below.

Action and use Used to correct deficiencies of coagulation factor VII.

Ph Eur

DEFINITION

Freeze-dried human coagulation factor VII is a plasma protein fraction that contains the single-chain glycoprotein factor VII and may also contain small amounts of the activated form, the two-chain derivative factor VIIa, as well as coagulation factors II, IX and X and protein C and protein S. It is obtained from human plasma that complies with the monograph on *Human plasma for fractionation (853)*.

The potency of the preparation, reconstituted as stated on the label, is not less than 15 I.U. of factor VII per millilitre.

PRODUCTION

The method of preparation is designed to minimise activation of any coagulation factor (to minimise potential thrombogenicity) and includes a step or steps that have been shown to remove or to inactivate known agents of infection; if substances are used for inactivation of viruses during production, the subsequent purification procedure must be validated to demonstrate that the concentration of these substances is reduced to a suitable level and that any residues are such as not to compromishe safety of the preparation for patients.

The specific activity is not less than 2 I.U. of factor VII per milligram of protein, before the addition of any protein stabiliser.

The factor VII fraction is dissolved in a suitable liquid. Heparin, antithrombin and other auxiliary substances such as a stabiliser may be added. No antimicrobial preservative is added. The solution is passed through a bacteria-retentive filter, distributed aseptically into the final containers and immediately frozen. It is subsequently freeze-dried and the containers are closed under vacuum or under an inert gas.

CONSISTENCY OF THE METHOD OF PRODUCTION

The consistency of the method of production with respect to the activities of factors II, IX and X of the preparation, expressed in International Units relative to the activity of factor VII, shall be demonstrated.

The consistency of the method of production with respect to the activity of factor VIIa of the preparation shall be demonstrated. The activity of factor VIIa may be determined, for example, using a recombinant soluble tissue factor that does not activate factor VII but possesses a cofactor function specific for factor VIIa; after incubation of a mixture of the recombinant soluble tissue factor with phospholipids reagent and the dilution of the test sample in factor VII-deficient plasma, calcium chloride is added and the clotting time determined; the clotting time is inversely related to the factor VIIa activity of the test sample.

CHARACTERS

A powder or friable solid that may be white, pale yellow, green or blue.

Reconstitute the preparation to be examined as stated on the label immediately before carrying out the identification, tests (except those for solubility and water) and assay

IDENTIFICATION

A. Using a suitable range of species-specific antisera, carry out precipitation tests on the preparation to be examined. It is recommended that the tests be carried out using antisera specific to the plasma proteins of each species of domestic animal commonly used in the preparation of materials of biological origin in the country concerned. The preparation is shown to contain proteins of human origin and gives negative results with antisera specific to plasma proteins of other species.

B. The assay for factor VII contributes to the identification of the preparation.

TESTS

pH (*2.2.3*). 6.5 to 7.5.

Solubility To a container of the preparation to be examined add the volume of liquid stated on the label at the recommended temperature. The preparation dissolves completely with gentle swirling within 10 min, giving a clear or slightly opalescent solution that may be coloured.

Osmolality (*2.2.35*). Not less than 240 mosmol/kg.

Total protein If necessary, dilute an accurately measured volume of the reconstituted preparation with a 9 g/l solution of *sodium chloride R* to obtain a solution expected to contain about 15 mg of protein in 2 ml. To 2.0 ml of the solution in a round-bottomed centrifuge tube add 2 ml of a 75 g/l solution of *sodium molybdate R* and 2 ml of a mixture of 1 volume of *nitrogen-free sulphuric acid R* and 30 volumes of *water R*. Shake, centrifuge for 5 min, decant the supernatant liquid and allow the inverted tube to drain on filter paper. Determine the nitrogen in the residue by the method of sulphuric acid digestion (*2.5.9*) and calculate the amount of protein by multiplying the result by 6.25.

Water (*2.5.12*). Not more than 3.0 per cent. Add a suitable volume of *anhydrous methanol R* to the container of the preparation to be examined, shake, allow to stand and carry out the determination on a known volume of the supernatant liquid.

Activated coagulation factors If the preparation to be examined contains heparin, determine the amount present as described in the test for heparin and neutralise the heparin by addition of *protamine sulphate R* (10 µg of protamine sulphate neutralises 1 I.U. of heparin). Prepare 1 in 10 and 1 in 100 dilutions of the reconstituted preparation to be examined using *tris(hydroxymethyl)aminomethane buffer solution pH 7.5 R*. Place a series of polystyrene tubes in a water-bath at 37°C and add to each tube 0.1 ml of *platelet-poor plasma R* and 0.1 ml of a suitable dilution of *cephalin R* or *platelet substitute R*. Allow to stand for 60 s. Add to each tube either 0.1 ml of one of the dilutions or 0.1 ml of the buffer solution (control tube). To each tube, add immediately 0.1 ml of a 3.7 g/l solution of *calcium chloride R*, previously heated to 37°C, and measure within 30 min of the original dilution the time that elapses between addition of the calcium chloride solution and formation of a clot. For each of the dilutions, the coagulation time is not less than 150 s. The test is not valid unless the coagulation time measured for the control tube is 200 s to 350 s.

Heparin If heparin has been added during preparation, determine the amount present by the assay of heparin in coagulation factor concentrates (*2.7.12*). The preparation to be examined contains not more than the amount of heparin stated on the label and in any case not more than 0.5 I.U. of heparin per International Unit of factor VII.

Thrombin If the preparation to be examined contains heparin, determine the amount present as described in the test for heparin and neutralise the heparin by addition of *protamine sulphate R* (10 µg of protamine sulphate neutralises 1 I.U. of heparin). In each of two test-tubes, mix equal volumes of the reconstituted preparation and a 3 g/l solution of *fibrinogen R*. Keep one of the tubes at 37°C for 6 h and the other at room temperature for 24 h. In a third tube, mix a volume of the fibrinogen solution with an equal volume of a solution of *human thrombin R* (1 I.U./ml) and place the tube in a water-bath at 37°C. No coagulation occurs in the tubes containing the preparation to be examined. Coagulation occurs within 30 s in the tube containing thrombin.

Sterility (*2.6.1*). It complies with the test for sterility.

Pyrogens (*2.6.8*). It complies with the test for pyrogens. Inject per kilogram of the rabbit's mass a volume equivalent to not less than 30 I.U. of factor VII.

ASSAY

Carry out the assay of human blood coagulation factor VII (*2.7.10*).

The estimated potency is not less than 80 per cent and not more than 120 per cent of the stated potency. The confidence interval ($P = 0.95$) of the estimated potency is not greater than 80 per cent to 120 per cent.

STORAGE

Store protected from light.

LABELLING

The label states:

— the number of International Units of factor VII per container,

— the amount of protein per container,

— the name and quantity of any added substances, including where applicable, heparin,

— the name and volume of the liquid to be used for reconstitution,

— the storage conditions,

— the expiry date,

— that the transmission of infectious agents cannot be totally excluded when medicinal products prepared from human blood or plasma are administered.

Ph Eur

Dried Factor VIII Fraction

Dried Human Antihaemophilic Fraction

Dried Factor VIII Fraction complies with the requirements of the 3rd edition of the European Pharmacopoeia for Freeze-dried Human Coagulation Factor VIII [0275]. These requirements are reproduced after the heading 'Definition' below.

Action and use Used to correct deficiencies of coagulation factor VIII.

Ph Eur

DEFINITION

Freeze-dried human coagulation factor VIII is a plasma protein fraction that contains the glycoprotein coagulation factor VIII together with varying amounts of von Willebrand factor, depending on the method of preparation. It is prepared from human plasma that complies with the monograph on *Human plasma for fractionation (853)*.

The potency of the preparation, reconstituted as stated on the label, is not less than 20 I.U. of factor VIII:C per millilitre.

PRODUCTION

The method of preparation includes a step or steps that have been shown to remove or to inactivate known agents of infection; if substances are used for the inactivation of viruses during production, the subsequent purification procedure must be validated to demonstrate that the concentration of these substances is reduced to a suitable level and that any residues are such as not to compromise the safety of the preparation for patients.

The specific activity is not less than 1 I.U. of factor VIII:C per milligram of total protein before the addition of protein stabiliser.

The factor VIII fraction is dissolved in a suitable liquid. Auxiliary substances such as a stabiliser may be added. No anti-microbial preservative is added. The solution is passed through a bacteria-retentive filter, distributed aseptically into the final containers and immediately frozen. It is subsequently freeze-dried and the containers are closed under vacuum or under an inert gas.

Validation test applied to products stated to have von Willebrand factor activity For products intended for treatment of von Willebrand's disease it shall be demonstrated that the manufacturing process yields a product with a consistent composition with respect to von Willebrand factor. This composition may be characterised in a number of ways. For example, the number and the relative amount of the different multimers may be determined by sodium dodecyl sulphate (SDS) agarose gel electrophoresis (≈ 1 per cent agarose) with or without Western blot analysis on nitrocellulose, using a normal human plasma pool as reference; visualisation of the multimeric pattern may be performed using an immunoenzymatic technique and quantitative evaluation may be carried out by densitometric analysis or by other suitable methods.

von Willebrand factor activity For products intended for treatment of von Willebrand's disease the von Willebrand factor activity is determined by a suitable method using a reference preparation of the same type as the preparation to be examined, calibrated against the International Standard for von Willebrand factor in plasma. Suitable methods include determination of ristocetin cofactor activity and determination of collagen-binding activity. The following method for determination of ristocetin cofactor activity is given as an example of a suitable method.

Ristocetin cofactor activity. Carry out appropriate dilutions of the preparation to be examined and of the reference preparation using as diluent a solution containing 9 g/l of *sodium chloride R* and 50 g/l of human albumin. Add to each dilution suitable amounts of a von Willebrand reagent containing stabilised human platelets and ristocetin A. Mix on a glass plate by moving it gently in circles for 1 min. Allow to stand for a further 1 min and read the result against a dark background with side lighting. The last dilution which shows clearly visible agglutination indicates the ristocetin cofactor titre of the sample. Use diluent as a negative control.

The estimated potency is not less than 60 per cent and not more than 140 per cent of the potency approved for the particular product.

CHARACTERS

A white or pale yellow powder or friable solid.

Reconstitute the preparation to be examined as stated on the label immediately before carrying out the identification, tests (except those for solubility and water) and assay.

IDENTIFICATION

A. Using a suitable range of species-specific antisera, carry out precipitation tests on the preparation to be examined. It is recommended that the test be carried out using antisera specific to the plasma proteins of each species of domestic animal commonly used in the preparation of materials of biological origin in the country concerned. The preparation is shown to contain proteins of human origin and gives negative results with antisera specific to plasma proteins of other species.

B. The assays for factor VIII:C and von Willebrand factor activity (where applicable) contribute to the identification of the preparation.

TESTS

pH (*2.2.3*). 6.5 to 7.5.

Solubility To a container of the preparation to be examined add the volume of the solvent stated on the label at the recommended temperature. The preparation dissolves completely with gentle swirling within 10 min, giving a clear or slightly opalescent, colourless or slightly yellow solution.

Osmolality (*2.2.35*). Not less than 240 mosmol/kg.

Total protein If necessary, dilute an accurately measured volume of the preparation to be examined with a 9 g/l solution of *sodium chloride R* to obtain a solution containing about 15 mg of protein in 2 ml. To 2.0 ml of the solution in a round-bottomed centrifuge tube add 2 ml of a 75 g/l solution of *sodium molybdate R* and 2 ml of a mixture of 1 volume of *nitrogen-free sulphuric acid R* and 30 volumes of *water R*. Shake, centrifuge for 5 min, decant the supernatant liquid and allow the inverted tube to drain on filter paper. Determine the nitrogen in the residue by the method of sulphuric acid digestion (*2.5.9*) and calculate the amount of protein by multiplying the result by 6.25.

For some products, especially those without a protein stabiliser such as albumin, this method may not be applicable and another validated method for protein determination must therefore be performed.

Haemagglutinins anti-A and anti-B Dilute the preparation with a 9 g/l solution of *sodium chloride R* to contain 3 I.U. of factor VIII:C per millilitre. Carry out the indirect determination of haemagglutinins A and B (*2.6.20*). The 1 to 64 dilutions do not show agglutination.

Hepatitis B surface antigen Examine the reconstituted preparation by a suitably sensitive method such as enzyme immunoassay (*2.7.1*). Hepatitis B surface antigen is not detected.

Water (*2.5.12*). Not more than 3.0 per cent. Add a suitable volume of *anhydrous methanol R* to the container of the preparation to be examined, shake, allow to stand and carry out the determination on a known volume of the supernatant liquid.

Sterility (*2.6.1*). It complies with the test for sterility.

Pyrogens (*2.6.8*). It complies with the test for pyrogens. Inject per kilogram of the rabbit's mass a volume of the preparation to be examined equivalent to not less than 30 I.U. of factor VIII:C.

ASSAY

Carry out the assay of human coagulation factor VIII (*2.7.4*).

The estimated potency is not less than 80 per cent and not more than 120 per cent of the stated potency. The confidence interval ($P = 0.95$) of the estimated potency is not greater than 80 per cent to 120 per cent.

STORAGE

Store protected from light.

LABELLING

The label states:
- the number of International Units of factor VIII:C and, where applicable, of von Willebrand factor in the container,
- the amount of protein in the container,
- the name and quantity of any added substance,
- the name and volume of the liquid to be used for reconstitution,
- the storage conditions,
- the expiry date,
- that the transmission of infectious agents cannot be totally excluded when medicinal products prepared from human blood or plasma are administered.

Ph Eur

Dried Factor IX Fraction

Dried Factor IX Fraction complies with the requirements of the 3rd edition of the European Pharmacopoeia for Freeze-dried Human Coagulation Factor IX [1223]. These requirements are reproduced after the heading 'Definition' below.

Action and use Used to correct deficiencies of coagulation factor IX (Christmas disease).

Ph Eur

DEFINITION

Freeze-dried human coagulation factor IX is a plasma protein fraction containing coagulation factor IX, prepared by a method that effectively separates factor IX from other prothrombin complex factors (factors II, VII and X). It is obtained from human plasma that complies with the monograph on *Human plasma for fractionation (853)*.

The potency of the preparation, reconstituted as stated on the label, is not less than 20 I.U. of factor IX per millilitre.

PRODUCTION

The method of preparation is designed to maintain functional integrity of factor IX, to minimise activation of any coagulation factor (to minimise potential thrombogenicity) and includes a step or steps that have been shown to remove or to inactivate known agents of infection; if substances are used for inactivation of viruses during production, the subsequent purification procedure must be validated to demonstrate that the concentration of these substances is reduced to a suitable level and that any residues are such as not to compromise the safety of the aration for patients.

The specific activity is not less than 50 I.U. of factor IX per milligram of total protein, before the addition of any protein stabiliser.

The factor IX fraction is dissolved in a suitable liquid. Heparin, antithrombin and other auxiliary substances such as a stabiliser may be included. No antimicrobial preservative is added. The solution is passed through a bacteria-retentive filter, distributed aseptically into the final containers and immediately frozen. It is subsequently freeze-dried and the containers are closed under vacuum or under an inert gas.

CONSISTENCY OF THE METHOD OF PRODUCTION

The consistency of the method of production is evaluated by suitable analytical procedures that are determined during process development and which normally include:
- assay of factor IX,
- determination of activated coagulation factors,
- determination of activities of factors II, VII and X which shall be shown to be not more than 5 per cent of the activity of factor IX.

CHARACTERS

A white, or pale yellow powder or friable solid.

Reconstitute the preparation to be examined as stated on the label, immediately before carrying out the identification, tests (except those for solubility and water) and assay.

IDENTIFICATION

A. Using a suitable range of species-specific antisera, carry out precipitation tests on the preparation to be examined. It is recommended that the tests be carried out using antisera specific to the plasma proteins of each species of domestic animal commonly used in the preparation of materials of biological origin in the country concerned. The preparation is shown to contain proteins of human origin and gives negative results with antisera specific to plasma proteins of other species.

B. The assay for coagulation factor IX contributes to the identification of the preparation.

TESTS

pH (*2.2.3*). 6.5 to 7.5.

Solubility To a container of the preparation to be examined add the volume of the liquid stated on the label at the recommended temperature. The preparation dissolves completely with gentle swirling within 10 min, giving a clear or slightly opalescent, colourless solution.

Osmolality (*2.2.35*). Not less than 240 mosmol/kg.

Total protein If necessary, dilute an accurately measured volume of the preparation to be examined with a 9 g/l solution of *sodium chloride R*, to obtain a solution which may be expected to contain about 15 mg of protein in 2 ml. To 2.0 ml of that solution, in a round-bottomed centrifuge tube, add 2 ml of a 75 g/l solution of *sodium molybdate R* and 2 ml of a mixture of 1 volume of *nitrogen-free sulphuric acid R* and 30 volumes of *water R*. Shake, centrifuge for 5 min, decant the supernatant liquid and allow the inverted tube to drain on filter paper. Determine the nitrogen in the residue by the method of sulphuric acid digestion (*2.5.9*) and calculate the amount of protein by multiplying the result by 6.25.

For some products, especially those without a protein stabiliser such as albumin, this method may not be applicable. Another validated method for protein determination must therefore be performed.

Activated coagulation factors Where applicable, determine the amount of heparin present as described below and neutralise the heparin by addition of *protamine sulphate R* (10 µg of protamine sulphate neutralises 1 I.U. of heparin). If necessary, dilute the preparation to be examined to contain 20 I.U. of factor IX per millilitre. Prepare 1 to 10 and 1 to 100 dilutions using *tris(hydroxymethyl)aminomethane buffer solution pH 7.5 R*. Place a series of polystyrene tubes in a water-bath at 37°C and add to each tube 0.1 ml of *platelet-poor plasma R* and 0.1 ml of a suitable dilution of *cephalin R* or *platelet substitute R*. Allow to stand for 60 s. Add to each tube either 0.1 ml of one of the dilutions or 0.1 ml of the buffer solution (control tube). To each tube add immediately 0.1 ml of a 3.7 g/l solution of *calcium chloride R* (previously warmed to 37°C) and measure, within 30 min of the original dilution, the time that elapses between addition of the calcium chloride solution and the formation of a clot. For each of the dilutions the coagulation time is not less than 150 s. The test is not valid unless the coagulation time measured for the control tube is 200 s to 350 s.

Heparin If heparin has been added during preparation, determine the amount by the assay of heparin in coagulation factor concentrates (*2.7.12*). The preparation to be examined contains not more than the amount of heparin stated on the label and in any case not more than 0.5 I.U. of heparin per International Unit of factor IX.

Water (*2.5.12*). Not more than 3.0 per cent. Add a suitable volume of *anhydrous methanol R* to the container of the preparation to be examined, shake, allow to stand and carry out the determination on a known volume of the supernatant liquid.

Sterility (*2.6.1*). It complies with the test for sterility.

Pyrogens (*2.6.8*). It complies with the test for pyrogens. Inject per kilogram of the rabbit's mass a volume equivalent to not less than 30 I.U. of factor IX.

ASSAY

Carry out the assay of human blood coagulation factor IX (*2.7.11*).

The estimated potency is not less than 80 per cent and not more than 125 per cent of the stated potency. The confidence interval ($P = 0.95$) of the estimated potency is not greater than 80 per cent to 125 per cent.

STORAGE

Store protected from light.

LABELLING

The label states:

— the number of International Units of factor IX per container,

— the amount of protein per container,

— the name and quantity of any added substances, including where applicable heparin,

— the name and volume of the liquid to be used for reconstitution,

— the storage conditions,

— the expiry date,

— that the transmission of infectious agents cannot be totally excluded when medicinal products prepared from human blood or plasma are administered.

Ph Eur

Dried Prothrombin Complex

Dried Prothrombin Complex complies with the requirements of the 3rd edition of the European Pharmacopoeia for Freeze-dried Human Prothrombin Complex [0554]. These requirements are reproduced after the heading 'Definition' below.

Action and use Used to correct deficiencies of coagulation factor IX (Christmas disease). Preparations with appropriate activity may be used to correct deficiencies of coagulation factors II or X.

Ph Eur

DEFINITION

Freeze-dried human prothrombin complex is a plasma protein fraction containing blood coagulation factor IX together with variable amounts of coagulation factors II, VII and X; the presence and proportion of these additional factors depends on the method of fractionation. It is obtained from human plasma that complies with the monograph on *Human plasma for fractionation (853)*.

The potency of the preparation, reconstituted as stated on the label, is not less than 20 I.U. of factor IX per millilitre.

PRODUCTION

The method of preparation is designed to minimise activation of any coagulation factor (to minimise potential thrombogenicity) and includes a step or steps that have been shown to remove or to inactivate known agents of infection; if substances are used for inactivation of viruses during production, the subsequent purification procedure must be validated to demonstrate that the concentration of these substances is reduced to a suitable level and that any residues are such as not to compromise the safety of the preparation for patients.

The specific activity is not less than 0.6 I.U. of factor IX per milligram of total protein, before the addition of any protein stabiliser.

The prothrombin complex fraction is dissolved in a suitable liquid. Heparin, antithrombin and other auxiliary substances such as a stabiliser may be added. No antimicrobial preservative is added. The solution is passed through a bacteria-retentive filter, distributed aseptically into the final containers and immediately frozen. It is subsequently freeze-dried and the containers are closed under vacuum or under an inert gas.

CHARACTERS

A white or slightly coloured powder or friable solid, very hygroscopic.

Reconstitute the preparation to be examined as stated on the label immediately before carrying out the identification, tests (except those for solubility and water) and assay.

IDENTIFICATION

A. Using a suitable range of species-specific antisera, carry out precipitation tests on the preparation to be examined. It is recommended that the test be carried out using antisera specific to the plasma proteins of each species of domestic animal commonly used in the preparation of materials of biological origin in the country concerned. The preparation is shown to contain proteins of human origin and gives negative results with antisera specific to plasma proteins of other species.

B. The assay for coagulation factor IX activity and, where applicable, those for factors II, VII and X contribute to the identification of the preparation.

TESTS

pH (*2.2.3*). 6.5 to 7.5.

Solubility To a container of the preparation to be examined add the volume of the liquid stated on the label at the recommended temperature. The preparation dissolves completely with gentle swirling within 10 min, giving a clear solution that may be coloured.

Osmolality (*2.2.35*). Not less than 240 mosmol/kg.

Total protein If necessary, dilute an accurately measured volume of the reconstituted preparation with a 9 g/l solution of *sodium chloride R* to obtain a solution expected to contain about 15 mg of protein in 2 ml. To 2.0 ml of the solution in a round-bottomed centrifuge tube add 2 ml of a 75 g/l solution of *sodium molybdate R* and 2 ml of a mixture of 1 volume of *nitrogen-free sulphuric acid R* and 30 volumes of *water R*. Shake, centrifuge for 5 min, decant the supernatant liquid and allow the inverted tube to drain on filter paper. Determine the nitrogen in the residue by the method of sulphuric acid digestion (*2.5.9*) and calculate the amount of protein by multiplying the result by 6.25.

Activated coagulation factors Where applicable, determine the amount of heparin present as described in the test for heparin and neutralise it by addition of *protamine sulphate R* (10 µg of protamine sulphate neutralises 1 I.U. of heparin). Prepare 1 in 10 and 1 in 100 dilutions of the reconstituted preparation to be examined using *tris-(hydroxymethyl)aminomethane buffer solution pH 7.5 R*. Place a series of polystyrene tubes in a water-bath at 37°C and add to each tube 0.1 ml of *platelet-poor plasma R* and 0.1 ml of a suitable dilution of *cephalin R* or *platelet substitute R*. Allow to stand for 60 s. Add to each tube either 0.1 ml of one of the dilutions or 0.1 ml of the buffer solution (control tube). To each tube, add immediately 0.1 ml of a 3.7 g/l solution of *calcium chloride R*, previously heated to 37°C, and measure within 30 min of the original dilution the time that elapses between addition of the calcium chloride solution and formation of a clot. For each of the dilutions, the coagulation time is not less than 150 s. The test is not valid unless the coagulation time measured for the control tube is 200 s to 350 s.

Heparin If heparin has been added during preparation, determine the amount present by the assay of heparin in coagulation factor concentrates (*2.7.12*). The preparation to be examined contains not more than the amount of heparin stated on the label and in any case not more than 0.5 I.U. of heparin per International Unit of factor IX.

Thrombin If the preparation to be examined contains heparin, determine the amount present as described in the test for heparin and neutralise it by addition of *protamine sulphate R* (10 µg of protamine sulphate neutralises 1 I.U. of heparin). In each of two test-tubes, mix equal volumes of the reconstituted preparation and a 3 g/l solution of *fibrinogen R*. Keep one of the tubes at 37°C for 6 h and the other at room temperature for 24 h. In a third tube, mix a volume of the fibrinogen solution with an equal volume of a solution of *human thrombin R* (1 I.U./ml) and place the tube in a water-bath at 37°C. No coagulation occurs in the tubes containing the preparation to be examined. Coagulation occurs within 30 s in the tube containing thrombin.

Water (*2.5.12*). Not more than 3.0 per cent. Add a suitable volume of *anhydrous methanol R* to the container of the preparation to be examined, shake, allow to stand and carry out the determination on a known volume of the supernatant liquid.

Sterility (*2.6.1*). It complies with the test for sterility.

Pyrogens (*2.6.8*). It complies with the test for pyrogens. Inject per kilogram of the rabbit's mass a volume of the reconstituted preparation equivalent to not less than 30 I.U. of factor IX.

ASSAY

Factor IX Carry out the assay of coagulation factor IX (*2.7.11*).

The estimated potency is not less than 80 per cent and not more than 125 per cent of the stated potency. The confidence interval of the estimated potency ($P = 0.95$) is not greater than 80 per cent to 125 per cent.

Factor VII If the label states that the preparation contains factor VII, carry out the assay of coagulation factor VII (*2.7.10*).

The estimated potency is not less than 80 per cent and not more than 125 per cent of the stated potency. The confidence interval of the estimated potency ($P = 0.95$) is not greater than 80 per cent to 125 per cent.

Factors II and X If the label states that the preparation contains factors II and X, carry out validated assays for these components.

The estimated potency is not less than 80 per cent and not more than 125 per cent of the stated potency. The confidence interval of the estimated potency ($P = 0.95$) is not greater than 80 per cent to 125 per cent.

STORAGE

Store protected from light.

LABELLING

The label states:

— the number of International Units of factor IX and, where applicable, of factors II, VII and X per container,
— where applicable, that the preparation contains protein C and/or protein S,
— the amount of protein per container,
— the name and quantity of any added substances, including where applicable heparin,
— the name and quantity of the liquid to be used for reconstitution,
— the storage conditions,
— the expiry date,
— that the transmission of infectious agents cannot be totally excluded when medicinal products prepared from human blood or plasma are administered.

Ph Eur

Dried Fibrinogen

Dried Fibrinogen complies with the requirements of the 3rd edition of the European Pharmacopoeia for Freeze-dried Human Fibrinogen [0024]. These requirements are reproduced after the heading 'Definition' below.

Ph Eur

DEFINITION

Freeze-dried human fibrinogen contains the soluble constituent of human plasma that is transformed to fibrin on the addition of thrombin. It is obtained from *Human plasma for fractionation (853)*. The preparation may contain auxiliary substances such as salts, buffers and stabilisers.

When dissolved in the volume of the solvent stated on the label, the solution contains not less than 10 g/l of fibrinogen.

PRODUCTION

The method of preparation includes a step or steps that have been shown to remove or to inactivate known agents of infection; if substances are used for inactivation of viruses during production, the subsequent purification procedure must be validated to demonstrate that the concentration of these substances is reduced to a suitable level and any residues are such as not to compromise the safety of the preparation for patients.

No antibiotic is added to the plasma used and no antimicrobial preservative is included in the preparation.

The method of preparation is such as to obtain fibrinogen with a specific activity (fibrinogen content with respect to total protein content) not less than 80 per cent. The fibrinogen content is determined by a suitable method such as that described under Assay and the total protein content is determined by a suitable method such as that described under Total protein in *Human Albumin Solution (255)*. If a protein stabiliser (for example, human albumin) is added to the preparation, the requirement for specific activity applies to the fibrinogen before addition of the stabiliser. Albumin may also be obtained with fibrinogen during fractionation and a specific determination of albumin is then carried out by a suitable immunochemical method (*2.7.1*) and the quantity of albumin determined is subtracted from the total protein content for the calculation of the specific activity.

CHARACTERS

A white or pale yellow powder or friable solid.

IDENTIFICATION

A. Using a suitable range of species-specific antisera, carry out precipitation tests on the preparation to be examined, reconstituted as stated on the label immediately before use. It is recommended that the tests be carried out using antisera specific to the plasma proteins of each species of domestic animal commonly used in the preparation of materials of biological origin in the country concerned. The preparation is shown to contain proteins of human origin and gives negative results with antisera specific to plasma proteins of other species.

B. The assay contributes to the identification of the preparation.

TESTS

pH (*2.2.3*). The pH of the reconstituted preparation is 6.5 to 7.5.

Osmolality (*2.2.35*). The osmolality of the reconstituted preparation is not less than 240 mosm/kg.

Solubility Add the volume of solvent stated on the label to the contents of a container. The preparation dissolves within 30 min at 20°C to 25°C, forming an almost colourless, slightly opalescent solution.

Stability of solution Allow the reconstituted solution to stand at 20°C to 25°C. No gel formation appears within 60 min of reconstitution.

Hepatitis B surface antigen Examine the reconstituted preparation by an immunochemical method (*2.7.1*) of suitable sensitivity, such as radio-immunoassay. Hepatitis B surface antigen is not detected.

Water (*2.5.12*). Not more than 3.0 per cent, determined by the semi-micro determination of water.

Sterility (*2.6.1*). The reconstituted preparation complies with the test for sterility.

Pyrogens (*2.6.8*). The reconstituted preparation complies with the test for pyrogens. Inject per kilogram of the rabbit's mass a volume of the reconstituted preparation equivalent to not less than 30 mg of fibrinogen, calculated from the quantity stated on the label.

ASSAY

Mix 0.2 ml of the reconstituted preparation with 2 ml of a suitable buffer solution (pH 6.6 to 6.8) containing sufficient thrombin (approximately 3 I.U./ml) and calcium (0.05 mol/l). Maintain at 37°C for 20 min, separate the precipitate by centrifugation (5000 *g*, 20 min), wash thoroughly with a 9 g/l solution of *sodium chloride R*. Determine the nitrogen content by sulphuric acid digestion (*2.5.9*) and calculate the fibrinogen (clottable protein) content by multiplying the result by 6.0. The content is not less than 70 per cent and not more than 130 per cent of the amount of fibrinogen stated on the label.

STORAGE

Store protected from light.

LABELLING

The label states:
— the amount of fibrinogen in the container,
— the name and volume of the solvent to be used to reconstitute the preparation,
— where applicable, the name and quantity of protein stabiliser in the preparation.

Ph Eur

Fibrin Sealant Kit

Fibrin Sealant Kit complies with the requirements of the 3rd edition of the European Pharmacopoeia [0903]. These requirements are reproduced after the heading 'Definition' below.

Ph Eur

DEFINITION

Fibrin sealant kit is essentially composed of two components, namely component 1 (fibrinogen concentrate), a protein fraction containing human fibrinogen and human factor XIII, and component 2, a preparation containing human thrombin; the latter component converts the former to fibrin after reconstitution and combining in the presence of calcium ions. Other ingredients (for example, human fibronectin and a plasmin inhibitor such as aprotinin) and stabilisers (for example, human albumin) may be added before or during the thrombin-induced generation of fibrin. No antimicrobial preservative is added.

Human constituents are obtained from plasma that complies with the requirements of the monograph on *Human plasma for fractionation (853)*. No antibiotic is added to the plasma used.

When thawed or reconstituted in the volume of solvent stated on the label, component 1 contains not less than 60 g/litre of clottable protein and not less than 10 units of factor XIII per millilitre; the thrombin activity of component 2 varies over a wide range (approximately 4 to 500 I.U./ml).

PRODUCTION

The method of preparation includes a step or steps that have been shown to remove or to inactivate known agents of infection; if substances are used for inactivation of viruses during production, the subsequent purification procedure must be validated to demonstrate that the concentration of these substances is reduced to a suitable level and any residues are such as not to compromise the safety of the preparation for patients.

Constituents or mixtures of constituents are passed through a bacteria-retentive filter and distributed aseptically into sterile containers. Containers of freeze-dried constituents are closed under vacuum or filled with oxygen-free nitrogen or other suitable inert gas before being closed. In either case, they are closed so as to exclude micro-organisms.

CHARACTERS

Freeze-dried constituents are white or pale yellow powders or friable solids. Frozen constituents are colourless or pale yellow, opaque solids. Liquid constituents are colourless or pale yellow.

For the freeze-dried and frozen constituents, reconstitute or thaw as stated on the label immediately before carrying out the identification and the tests, except those for solubility and water.

I Component 1 (Fibrinogen concentrate)

IDENTIFICATION

A. Using a suitable range of species-specific antisera, carry out precipitation tests on the preparation to be examined. It is recommended that the test be carried out using antisera specific to the plasma proteins of each species of domestic animal commonly used in the preparation of materials of biological origin in the country concerned. The preparation is shown to contain proteins of human origin and gives negative reactions with antisera specific to plasma proteins of other species.

B. The assay for fibrinogen contributes to the identification of component 1.

C. The assay for factor XIII contributes to the identification of component 1.

TESTS

pH (*2.2.3*). The pH is 6.5 to 8.0.

Solubility Freeze-dried concentrates dissolve within 20 min in the volume of solvent for reconstitution and at the temperature stated on the label, forming an almost colourless, clear or slightly turbid solution.

Stability of solution No gel formation appears within 120 min of reconstitution or thawing.

Water (*2.5.12*). For a freeze-dried preparation, not more than 3.0 per cent *m/m*, determined by the semi-micro determination of water.

Sterility (2.6.1). It complies with the test for sterility.

ASSAY

Fibrinogen (clottable protein) *Use method A or method B.*

The estimated content in milligrams of clottable protein is not less than 70 per cent and not more than 130 per cent of the stated amount.

A. *Clottable protein (determination of nitrogen by sulphuric acid digestion).* Mix 0.2 ml of the reconstituted preparation with 2 ml of a suitable buffer solution (pH 6.6 to 6.8) containing sufficient *human thrombin R* (approximately 3 I.U./ml) and calcium (0.05 mol/litre). Maintain at 37°C for 20 min, separate the precipitate by centrifugation (5000 g, 20 min), wash thoroughly with a 9 g/l solution of *sodium chloride R* and determine the protein as nitrogen by sulphuric acid digestion (*2.5.9*). Calculate the protein content by multiplying the result by 6.0.

B. *Clotting assay.* Dilute the reconstituted preparation with a 9 g/l solution of *sodium chloride R* to a fibrinogen content in the range 0.1 to 1 mg/ml. Take 0.2 ml of the dilution, maintain at 37°C for 60 s and add 0.2 ml of a suitable solution of *human thrombin R* (approximately 20 I.U./ml and containing at least 1 mmol/litre of calcium). Determine the clotting time by a suitable method. Repeat the procedure with each of at least three different dilutions, in the range stated above, of a suitable fibrinogen standard (for example, standard human plasma). Standard human plasma is calibrated against a pool of fresh plasma (>100 donors) by means of the assay. Draw a calibration curve on log-log graph paper using the measured clotting times for the standard dilutions and the fibrinogen content; use the curve obtained to determine the fibrinogen content of the preparation to be examined.

Factor XIII For determination of potency (functional factor XIII), make appropriate dilutions of the reconstituted component 1 and of standard human plasma (reference preparation) using as diluent a solution containing 9 g/l of *sodium chloride R* and 4 g/l of human albumin. Add to each dilution suitable amounts of a solution of bovine fibrinogen free from factor XIII activity ($A_{F\ XIII}$) and an excess of calcium and thrombin, to coagulate the fibrinogen. Allow to stand at 37°C for 1 h. Add to each tube a suitable amount of a 10 g/l solution of *chloroacetic acid R*, shake every 10 min and after 30 min note for each sample the highest dilution factor (*D*) at which the clot has not yet been dissolved. Calculate the factor XIII activity in units per millilitre from the expression:

$$A_{F\ XIII} = \frac{D_{comp\ 1}}{D_{ref}} \times A_{F\ XIII\ (ref)}$$

The estimated potency given in units is not less than 60 per cent and not more than 140 per cent of the stated potency.

II Component 2 (Thrombin preparation)

IDENTIFICATION

A. Using a suitable range of species-specific antisera, carry out precipitation tests on the preparation to be examined. It is recommended that the test be carried out using antisera specific to the plasma proteins of each species of domestic animal commonly used in the preparation of materials of biological origin in the country concerned. The preparation is shown to contain proteins of human origin and gives negative reactions with antisera specific to plasma proteins of other species.

B. The assay for thrombin contributes to the identification of component 2.

TESTS

pH (*2.2.3*). The pH is 6.0 to 8.0.

Solubility Freeze-dried preparations dissolve within 5 min in the volume of solvent for reconstitution stated on the label, forming a colourless, clear to slightly turbid solution.

Water (*2.5.12*). For a freeze-dried preparation, not more than 3.0 per cent *m/m*, determined by the semi-micro determination of water.

Sterility (*2.6.1*). It complies with the test for sterility.

ASSAY

Thrombin Dilute the reconstituted preparation to be examined with a solution containing 9 g/l of *sodium chloride R* and 10 g/l of *bovine albumin R* to approximately 4 to 10 I.U. of thrombin per millilitre. To 0.1 ml of the dilution add 0.9 ml of fibrinogen solution (1 g/l of clottable protein) warmed to 30°C and start measurement of the clotting time immediately. Repeat the procedure with each of at least three dilutions, in the range stated above, of a reference preparation of thrombin, calibrated in International Units. Draw a calibration curve on log-log graph paper using the measured clotting times for the dilutions of the reference preparation and the content in thrombin units; use the curve obtained to determine the content in International Units of thrombin in the preparation to be examined.

The estimated potency is not less than 80 per cent and not more than 125 per cent of the stated potency.

STORAGE

Store protected from light.

LABELLING

The label states:

— the amount of fibrinogen (milligrams of clottable protein), factor XIII (units) and thrombin (International Units) per respective container,
— where applicable, the volume of solvent to be used to reconstitute the preparation.

Ph Eur

Normal Immunoglobulin

Normal Immunoglobulin Injection

Normal Immunoglobulin complies with the requirements of the 3rd edition of the European Pharmacopoeia for Human Normal Immunoglobulin [0338]. These requirements are reproduced after the heading 'Definition' below.

Ph Eur

DEFINITION

Human normal immunoglobulin is a liquid or freeze-dried preparation containing immunoglobulins, mainly immunoglobulin G (IgG). Other proteins may be present. Human normal immunoglobulin contains the IgG antibodies of normal subjects. It is intended for intramuscular injection.

Human normal immunoglobulin is obtained from plasma that complies with the requirements of the monograph on *Human plasma for fractionation (853)*. No antibiotic is added to the plasma used.

PRODUCTION

The method of preparation includes a step or steps that have been shown to remove or to inactivate known agents of infection; if substances are used for inactivation of viruses, it shall have been shown that any residues present in the final product have no adverse effects on the patients treated with the immunoglobulin.

The product shall have been shown, by suitable tests in animals and evaluation during clinical trials, to be well tolerated when administered intramuscularly.

Human normal immunoglobulin is prepared from pooled material from at least 1000 donors by a method that has been shown to yield a product that:

— does not transmit infection;
— at a protein concentration of 160 g/l, contains antibodies for at least two of which (one viral and one bacterial) an International Standard or Reference Preparation is available, the concentration of such antibodies being at least ten times that in the initial pooled material.

Human normal immunoglobulin is prepared as a stabilised solution, for example in a 9 g/l solution of sodium chloride, a 22.5 g/l solution of glycine or, if the preparation is to be freeze-dried, a 60 g/l solution of glycine. Multidose preparations contain an antimicrobial preservative. Single-dose preparations do not contain an antimicrobial preservative. Any antimicrobial preservative or stabilising agent used shall have been shown to have no deleterious effect on the final product in the amount present. The solution is passed through a bacteria-retentive filter.

The stability of the preparation is demonstrated by suitable tests carried out during development studies.

CHARACTERS

The liquid preparation is clear and pale-yellow to light-brown; during storage it may show formation of slight turbidity or a small amount of particulate matter. The freeze-dried preparation is a white or slightly yellow powder or solid, friable mass.

For the freeze-dried preparation, reconstitute as stated on the label immediately before carrying out the identification and the tests, except those for solubility and water.

IDENTIFICATION

A. Using a suitable range of species-specific antisera carry out precipitation tests on the preparation to be examined. It is recommended that the test be carried out using antisera specific to the plasma proteins of each species of domestic animal commonly used in the preparation of materials of biological origin in the country concerned. The preparation is shown to contain proteins of human origin and gives negative reactions with antisera specific to plasma proteins of other species.

B. Examine by a suitable immunoelectrophoresis technique. Using antiserum to normal human serum, compare normal human serum and the preparation to be examined, both diluted to contain 10 g/l of protein. The main component of the preparation to be examined corresponds to the IgG component of normal human serum. The solution may show the presence of small quantities of other plasma proteins.

TESTS

Solubility For the freeze-dried preparation, add the volume of the liquid stated on the label. The preparation dissolves completely within 20 min at 20°C to 25°C.

pH (*2.2.3*). Dilute the preparation to be examined with a 9 g/l solution of *sodium chloride R* to obtain a solution containing 10 g/l of protein. The pH of the solution is 6.4 to 7.2.

Total protein Dilute the preparation to be examined with a 9 g/l solution of *sodium chloride R* to obtain a solution containing about 15 mg of protein in 2 ml. To 2.0 ml of this solution in a round-bottomed centrifuge tube add 2 ml of a 75 g/l solution of *sodium molybdate R* and 2 ml of a mixture of 1 volume of *nitrogen-free sulphuric acid R* and 30 volumes of *water R*. Shake, centrifuge for 5 min, decant the supernatant liquid and allow the inverted tube to drain on filter paper. Determine the nitrogen in the residue by the method of sulphuric acid digestion (*2.5.9*) and calculate the content of protein by multiplying by 6.25. The preparation contains not less than 100 g/l and not more than 180 g/l of protein and not less than 90 per cent and not more than 110 per cent of the quantity of protein stated on the label.

Protein composition Examine by zone electrophoresis (*2.2.31*), using strips of suitable cellulose acetate gel as the supporting medium and *barbital buffer solution pH 8.6 R1* as the electrolyte solution.

Test solution. Dilute the preparation to be examined with a 9 g/l solution of *sodium chloride R* to a protein concentration of 50 g/l.

Reference solution. Reconstitute *human immunoglobulin for electrophoresis BRP* and dilute with a 9 g/l solution of *sodium chloride R* to a protein concentration of 50 g/l.

To a strip apply 2.5 µl of the test solution as a 10 mm band or apply 0.25 µl per millimetre if a narrower strip is used. To another strip apply in the same manner the same volume of the reference solution. Apply a suitable electric field such that the albumin band of normal human serum applied on a control strip migrates at least 30 mm. Stain the strip with *amido black 10B solution R* for 5 min. Decolorise with a mixture of 10 volumes of *glacial acetic acid R* and 90 volumes of *methanol R* so that the background is just free of colour. Develop the transparency of the strips with a mixture of 19 volumes of *glacial acetic acid R* and 81 volumes of *methanol R*. Measure the absorbance of the bands at 600 nm in an instrument having a linear response over the range of measurement. Calculate the result as the mean of three measurements of each strip. In the electrophoretogram obtained with the test solution, not more than 10 per cent of the protein has a mobility different from that of the principal band. The test is not valid unless, in the electrophoretogram obtained with the reference preparation, the proportion of protein in the principal band is within the limits stated in the leaflet accompanying the reference preparation.

Distribution of molecular size Examine by liquid chromatography (*2.2.29*).

Test solution. Dilute the preparation to be examined with a 9 g/l solution of *sodium chloride R* to a concentration suitable for the chromatographic system used. A concentration in the range 4 g/litre to 12 g/litre and injection of 50 µg to 600 µg of protein are usually suitable.

Reference solution. Dilute *human immunoglobulin BRP* with a 9 g/l solution of *sodium chloride R* to the same protein concentration as the test solution.

The chromatographic procedure may be carried out using:

— a column 0.6 m long and 7.5 mm in internal diameter packed with *hydrophilic silica gel for* chromatography *R*,

— as mobile phase at a flow rate of 0.5 ml per minute a solution containing per litre: 4.873 g of *disodium hydrogen phosphate dihydrate R*, 1.741 g of *sodium dihydrogen phosphate* mono*hydrate R*, 11.688 g of *sodium chloride R* and 50 mg of *sodium azide R*,

— as detector a spectrophotometer set at 280 nm.

In the chromatogram obtained with the reference solution, the principal peak corresponds to IgG monomer and there is a peak corresponding to dimer with a retention time relative to monomer of about 0.85. Identify the peaks in the chromatogram obtained with the test solution by comparison with the chromatogram obtained with the reference solution; any peak with a retention time shorter than that of dimer corresponds to polymers and aggregates. The preparation to be examined complies with the test if, in the chromatogram obtained with the test solution: for monomer and dimer, the retention time relative to the corresponding peak in the chromatogram obtained with the reference solution is 1 ± 0.02; the sum of monomer and dimer represents not less than 85 per cent of the total area of the chromatogram and polymers and aggregates represent not more than 10 per cent of the total area of the chromatogram.

Water (*2.5.12*). For a freeze-dried preparation, not more than 3.0 per cent, determined on 0.500 g by the semi-micro determination of water.

Sterility (*2.6.1*). It complies with the test for sterility.

Pyrogens (*2.6.8*). It complies with the test for pyrogens. Inject 1 ml per kilogram of the rabbit's mass.

Antibody to hepatitis B surface antigen Not less than 0.5 I.U. per gram of immunoglobulin, determined by a suitable immunochemical method (*2.7.1*).

Antibody to hepatitis A virus If intended for use in the prophylaxis of hepatitis A, it complies with the following additional requirement. Determine the antibody content by comparison with a reference preparation calibrated in International Units, using an immunoassay of suitable sensitivity and specificity (*2.7.1*).

The International Unit is the activity contained in a stated amount of the International Reference Preparation of hepatitis A immunoglobulin. The equivalence in International Units of the International Reference Preparation is stated by the World Health Organisation.

The stated potency is not less than 100 I.U. per millilitre. The estimated potency is not less than the stated potency. The fiducial limits of error ($P = 0.95$) of the estimated potency are not less than 80 per cent and not more than 125 per cent.

STORAGE

For the liquid preparation, store in a colourless glass container, protected from light. For the freeze-dried preparation, store in a colourless glass container, under vacuum or under an inert gas, protected from light.

LABELLING

The label states:

— for liquid preparations, the volume of the preparation in the container and the protein content expressed in grams per litre,
— for freeze-dried preparations, the quantity of protein in the container,
— the route of administration,
— the storage conditions,
— the expiry date,
— for freeze-dried preparations, the name or composition and the volume of the reconstituting liquid to be added,
— where applicable, that the preparation is suitable for use in the prophylaxis of hepatitis A infection,
— where applicable, the anti-hepatitis A virus activity in International Units per millilitre,
— where applicable, the name and amount of antimicrobial preservative in the preparation.

Ph Eur

Normal Immunoglobulin for Intravenous Use

Normal Immunoglobulin for Intravenous Use complies with the requirements of the 3rd edition of the European Pharmacopoeia for Human Normal Immunoglobulin for Intravenous Administration [1016]. These requirements are reproduced after the heading 'Definition' below.

Ph Eur

DEFINITION

Human normal immunoglobulin for intravenous administration is a liquid or freeze-dried preparation containing immunoglobulins, mainly immunoglobulin G (IgG). Other proteins may be present. Human normal immunoglobulin for intravenous administration contains the IgG antibodies of normal subjects. This monograph does not apply to products intentionally prepared to contain fragments or chemically modified IgG.

Human normal immunoglobulin for intravenous administration is obtained from plasma that complies with the requirements of the monograph on *Human plasma for fractionation (853)*. No antibiotic is added to the plasma used.

PRODUCTION

The method of preparation includes a step or steps that have been shown to remove or to inactivate known agents of infection; if substances are used for inactivation of viruses, it shall have been shown that any residues present in the final product have no adverse effects on the patients treated with the immunoglobulin.

The product shall have been shown, by suitable tests in animals and evaluation during clinical trials, to be well tolerated when administered intravenously.

Human normal immunoglobulin is prepared from pooled material from not fewer than 1000 donors by a method that has been shown to yield a product that:

— does not transmit infection,
— at an immunoglobulin concentration of 50 g/l, contains antibodies for at least two of which (one viral and one bacterial) an International Standard or Reference Preparation is available, the concentration of such antibodies being at least three times that in the initial pooled material,
— has a defined distribution of immunoglobulin G subclasses,
— complies with the test for Fc function of immunoglobulin (*2.7.9*).

Human normal immunoglobulin for intravenous administration is prepared as a stabilised solution or as a freeze-dried preparation. A stabiliser may be added. In both cases the preparation is passed through a bacteria-retentive filter. No antimicrobial preservative is added either during fractionation or at the stage of the final bulk solution.

The stability of the preparation is demonstrated by suitable tests carried out during development studies.

CHARACTERS

The liquid preparation is clear or slightly opalescent and colourless or pale yellow. The freeze-dried preparation is a white or slightly yellow powder or solid friable mass.

For the freeze-dried preparation, reconstitute as stated on the label immediately before carrying out the identification and the tests, except those for solubility and water.

IDENTIFICATION

A. Using a suitable range of species-specific antisera, carry out precipitation tests on the preparation to be examined. It is recommended that the tests be carried out using antisera specific to the plasma proteins of each species of domestic animal commonly used in the preparation of materials of biological origin in the country concerned. The preparation is shown to contain proteins of human origin and gives negative reactions with antisera specific to plasma proteins of other species.

B. Examine by a suitable immunoelectrophoresis technique. Using antiserum to normal human serum, compare normal human serum and the preparation to be examined, both diluted to contain 10 g/l of protein. The main component of the preparation to be examined corresponds to the IgG component of normal human serum. The solution may show the presence of small quantities of other plasma proteins; if human albumin has been added as a stabiliser, it may be seen as a major component.

TESTS

Solubility For the freeze-dried preparation, add the volume of the liquid stated on the label. The preparation dissolves completely within 30 min at 20°C to 25°C.

pH (*2.2.3*). Dilute the preparation to be examined with a 9 g/l solution of *sodium chloride R* to obtain a solution containing 10 g/l of protein. The pH of the solution is 4.0 to 7.4.

Osmolality (*2.2.35*). Not less than 240 mosmol/kg.

Total protein Dilute the preparation to be examined with a 9 g/l solution of *sodium chloride R* to obtain a solution containing about 15 mg of protein in 2 ml. To 2.0 ml of this solution in a round-bottomed centrifuge tube add 2 ml of a 75 g/l solution of *sodium molybdate R* and 2 ml of a mixture of 1 volume of *nitrogen-free sulphuric acid R* and 30 volumes of *water R*. Shake, centrifuge for 5 min, decant the supernatant liquid and allow the inverted tube to drain on filter paper. Determine the nitrogen in the residue by the method of sulphuric acid digestion (*2.5.9*) and calculate the content of protein by multiplying by 6.25. The preparation contains not less than 30 g/l of protein and not less than 90 per cent and not more than 110 per cent of the quantity of protein stated on the label.

Protein composition Examine by zone electrophoresis (*2.2.31*), using strips of suitable cellulose acetate gel as the supporting medium and *barbital buffer solution pH 8.6 R1* as the electrolyte solution.

Test solution. Dilute the preparation to be examined with a 9 g/l solution of *sodium chloride R* to an immunoglobulin concentration of 30 g/l.

Reference solution. Reconstitute *human immunoglobulin for electrophoresis BRP* and dilute with a 9 g/l solution of *sodium chloride R* to a protein concentration of 30 g/l.

To a strip apply 4.0 µl of the test solution as a 10 mm band or apply 0.4 µl per millimetre if a narrower strip is used. To another strip apply in the same manner the same volume of the reference solution. Apply a suitable electric field such that the albumin band of normal human serum applied on a control strip migrates at least 30 mm. Stain the strips with *amido black 10B solution R* for 5 min. Decolorise with a mixture of 10 volumes of *glacial acetic acid R* and 90 volumes of *methanol R* so that the background is just free of colour. Develop the transparency of the strips with a mixture of 19 volumes of *glacial acetic acid R* and 81 volumes of *methanol R*. Measure the absorbance of the bands at 600 nm in an instrument having a linear response over the range of measurement. Calculate the result as the mean of three measurements of each strip. In the electrophoretogram obtained with the test solution, not more than 5 per cent of protein has a mobility different from that of the principal band. This limit is not applicable if albumin has been added to the preparation as a stabiliser; for such preparations, a test for protein composition is carried out during manufacture before addition of the stabiliser. The test is not valid unless, in the electrophoretogram obtained with the reference preparation, the proportion of protein in the principal band is within the limits stated in the leaflet accompanying the reference preparation.

Distribution of molecular size Examine by liquid chromatography (*2.2.29*).

Test solution. Dilute the preparation to be examined with a 9 g/l solution of *sodium chloride R* to a concentration suitable for the chromatographic system used. A concentration in the range 4 g/litre to 12 g/litre and injection of 50 µg to 600 µg of protein are usually suitable.

Reference solution. Dilute *human immunoglobulin BRP* with a 9 g/l solution of *sodium chloride R* to the same protein concentration as the test solution.

The chromatographic procedure may be carried out using:

— a column 0.6 m long and 7.5 mm in internal diameter packed with *hydrophilic silica gel for chromatography R*,

— as mobile phase at a flow-rate of 0.5 ml per minute a solution containing per litre: 4.873 g of *disodium hydrogen phosphate dihydrate R*, 1.741 g of *sodium dihydrogen phosphate monohydrate R*, 11.688 g of *sodium chloride R* and 50 mg of *sodium azide R*,

— as detector a spectrophotometer set at 280 nm.

In the chromatogram obtained with the reference solution, the principal peak corresponds to IgG monomer and there is a peak corresponding to dimer with a retention time relative to monomer of about 0.85. Identify the peaks in the chromatogram obtained with the test solution by comparison with the chromatogram obtained with the reference solution; any peak with a retention time shorter than that of dimer corresponds to polymers and aggregates. The preparation to be examined complies with the test if, in the chromatogram obtained with the test solution: for monomer and dimer, the retention time relative to the corresponding peak in the chromatogram obtained with the reference solution is 1 ± 0.02; the sum of monomer and dimer represents not less than 90 per cent of the total area of the chromatogram and polymers and aggregates represent not more than 3 per cent of the total area of the chromatogram. This requirement does not apply to products where albumin has been added as a stabiliser; for products stabilised with albumin, a test for distribution of molecular size is carried out during manufacture before addition of the stabiliser.

Anticomplementary activity (*2.6.17*). The consumption of complement is not greater than 50 per cent (1 CH_{50} per milligram of immunoglobulin).

Prekallikrein activator (*2.6.15*). Not more than 35 I.U. per millilitre, calculated with reference to a solution containing 30 g/l of immunoglobulin.

Anti-A and anti-B haemagglutinins (*2.6.20*). Carry out the tests for anti-A and anti-B haemagglutinins. If the preparation to be examined contains more than 30 g/l of immunoglobulin, dilute to this concentration before preparing the dilutions to be used in the test. The 1:64 dilutions do not show agglutination.

Water (*2.5.12*). For a freeze-dried preparation, not more than 3.0 per cent, determined on not less than 0.500 g by the semi-micro determination of water.

Sterility (*2.6.1*). It complies with the test for sterility.

Pyrogens (*2.6.8*). It complies with the test for pyrogens. Inject per kilogram of the rabbit's mass a volume equivalent to 0.5 g of immunoglobulin but not more than 10 ml per kilogram of body mass.

Antibody to hepatitis B surface antigen Not less than 0.5 I.U. per gram of immunoglobulin, determined by a suitable immunochemical method (*2.7.1*).

STORAGE

For the liquid preparation, store in a colourless glass container, protected from light, at the temperature stated on the label. For the freeze-dried preparation, store in a colourless glass container, under vacuum or under an inert gas, protected from light, at a temperature not exceeding 25°C.

LABELLING

The label states:

- for liquid preparations, the volume of the preparation in the container and the protein content expressed in grams per litre,
- for freeze-dried preparations, the quantity of protein in the container,
- the amount of immunoglobulin in the container,
- the route of administration,
- the storage conditions,
- the expiry date,
- for freeze-dried preparations, the name or composition and the volume of the reconstituting liquid to be added.
- the distribution of subclasses of immunoglobulin G present in the preparation,
- where applicable, the amount of albumin added as a stabiliser,
- the maximum content of immunoglobulin A.

Ph Eur

Anti-D (Rh_0) Immunoglobulin

Anti-D (Rh_0) Immunoglobulin complies with the requirements of the 3rd edition of the European Pharmacopoeia for Human Anti-D Immunoglobulin [0557]. These requirements are reproduced after the heading 'Definition' below.

Ph Eur

DEFINITION

Human anti-D immunoglobulin is a liquid or freeze-dried preparation containing immunoglobulins, mainly immunoglobulin G. The preparation is intended for intramuscular administration. It is obtained from plasma from D-negative donors who have been immunised against D antigen. It contains specific antibodies against erythrocyte D antigen and may also contain small quantities of other blood-group antibodies, for example anti-C, anti-E, anti-A or anti-B. *Human normal immunoglobulin (338)* may be added. It is presented in containers containing not less than 1 ml, after reconstitution if necessary.

It complies with the monograph on *Human normal immunoglobulin (338)* except for the minimum number of donors and the minimum total protein content.

For the liquid preparation, an accelerated degradation test is carried out on the final product by heating it at 37°C for 4 weeks; the loss of anti-D activity after heating does not exceed 20 per cent of the initial value.

POTENCY

The potency of human anti-D immunoglobulin is determined by comparing the quantity necessary to produce agglutination of D-positive red blood cells with the quantity of a reference preparation, calibrated in International Units, required to produce the same effect.

The International Unit is the activity of a stated amount of the International Reference Preparation. The equivalence in International Units of the International Reference Preparation is stated by the World Health Organisation.

Use pooled D-positive red blood cells, less than 7 days old and suitably stored, obtained from not fewer than four R_1R_1 donors. To a suitable volume of the cells, previously washed three times with a 9 g/l solution of *sodium chloride R*, add an equal volume of *bromelains solution R*, allow to stand at 37°C for 10 min, centrifuge, remove the supernatant liquid and wash three times with a 9 g/l solution of *sodium chloride R*. Suspend 20 volumes of the red blood cells in a mixture of 15 volumes of inert group AB serum, 20 volumes of a 300 g/l solution of *bovine albumin R* and 45 volumes of a 9 g/l of *sodium chloride R*. Stand the resulting suspension in iced water, stirring continuously.

Using a calibrated automated dilutor, prepare suitable dilutions of the preparation to be examined and of the reference preparation using as diluent a solution containing 5 g/l of *bovine albumin R* and 9 g/l of *sodium chloride R*.

Use a suitable apparatus for automatic continuous analysis: maintain the temperature in the manifold, except for the incubation coils, at 15.0°C. Pump the red blood cell suspension into the manifold of the apparatus at a rate of 0.1 ml per minute and a 3 g/l solution of *methylcellulose 450 R* at a rate of 0.05 ml per minute. Introduce the dilutions of the preparation to be examined and the reference preparation at a rate of 0.1 ml per minute for 2 min followed by the diluent solution at 0.1 ml per minute for 4 min before the next dilution is introduced.

Introduce air at a rate of 0.6 ml per minute. Incubate at 37°C for 18 min and then disperse the rouleaux by introducing at a rate of 1.6 ml per minute a 9 g/l solution of *sodium chloride R* containing a suitable wetting agent (for example, polysorbate 20 at a final concentration of 0.02 per cent *V/V*) to prevent disruption of the bubble pattern. Allow the agglutinates to settle and decant twice, first at 0.4 ml per minute and then at 0.6 ml per minute. Lyse the unagglutinated red blood cells with a solution containing 0.5 per cent *V/V* of *octoxinol 10 R*, 0.2 g/l of *potassium ferricyanide R*, 1 g/l of *sodium hydrogen carbonate*

R and 0.05 g/l of *potassium cyanide R* at 2.5 ml per minute. A ten-minute delay coil is introduced to allow for conversion of the haemoglobin. Continuously record the absorbance (*2.2.25*) of the haemolysate at a wavelength between 540 nm and 550 nm. Determine the range of antibody concentrations over which there is a linear relationship between concentration and the resultant change in absorbance (ΔA). From the results, prepare a standard curve and use the linear portion of the curve to determine the activity of the preparation to be examined.

Calculate the potency of the preparation to be examined in International Units per millilitre from the expression:

$$\frac{a \times d}{D}$$

d = dilution factor of the preparation to be examined at which a given value of ΔA was found,

D = dilution factor of the reference preparation at which the same value of ΔA was found,

a = activity in International Units per millilitre of a 1 in D dilution of the reference preparation.

For a freeze-dried preparation, the estimated activity in International Units per container is not less than 90 per cent and not more than 111 per cent of the stated activity and the fiducial limits of error ($P = 0.95$) of the estimated activity are not less than 80 per cent and not more than 125 per cent of the stated activity. For a liquid preparation, the estimated activity in International Units per container is not less than 90 per cent and not more than 133 per cent of the stated activity and the fiducial limits of error ($P = 0.95$) of the estimated activity are not less than 80 per cent and not more than 148 per cent of the stated activity.

STORAGE

See *Human normal immunoglobulin (338)*.

LABELLING

See *Human normal immunoglobulin (338)*.

The label states the number of International Units per container.

Ph Eur

Hepatitis A Immunoglobulin

Hepatitis A Immunoglobulin complies with the requirements of the 3rd edition of the European Pharmacopoeia for Human Hepatitis A Immunoglobulin [0769]. These requirements are reproduced after the heading 'Definition' below.

Ph Eur

DEFINITION

Human hepatitis A immunoglobulin is a liquid or freeze-dried preparation containing immunoglobulins, mainly immunoglobulin G. The preparation is intended for intramuscular administration. It is obtained from plasma from selected donors having antibodies against hepatitis A virus. *Human normal immunoglobulin (338)* may be added.

It complies with the monograph on *Human normal immunoglobulin (338)*, except for the minimum number of donors and the minimum total protein content.

POTENCY

The potency is determined by comparing the antibody titre of the immunoglobulin to be examined with that of a reference preparation calibrated in International Units, using an immunoassay of suitable sensitivity and specificity (*2.7.1. Immunochemical Methods*).

The International Unit is the activity contained in a stated amount of the International Reference Preparation of hepatitis A immunoglobulin. The equivalence in International Units of the International Standard is stated by the World Health Organisation.

The stated potency is not less than 600 I.U. per millilitre. The estimated potency is not less than the stated potency. The fiducial limits of error ($P = 0.95$) of the estimated potency are not less than 80 per cent and not more than 125 per cent.

STORAGE

See *Human normal immunoglobulin (338)*.

LABELLING

The label states the number of International Units per container.

Ph Eur

Hepatitis B Immunoglobulin

Hepatitis B Immunoglobulin complies with the requirements of the 3rd edition of the European Pharmacopoeia for Human Hepatitis B Immunoglobulin [0722]. These requirements are reproduced after the heading 'Definition' below.

Ph Eur

DEFINITION

Human hepatitis B immunoglobulin is a liquid or freeze-dried preparation containing immunoglobulins, mainly immunoglobulin G. The preparation is intended for intramuscular administration. It is obtained from plasma from selected and/or immunised donors having antibodies against hepatitis B surface antigen. *Human normal immunoglobulin (338)* may be added.

It complies with the monograph on *Human normal immunoglobulin (338)*, except for the minimum number of donors and the minimum total protein content.

POTENCY

The potency is determined by comparing the antibody titre of the immunoglobulin to be examined with that of a reference preparation calibrated in International Units, using an immunoassay of suitable sensitivity and specificity (*2.7.1. Immunochemical Methods*).

The International Unit is the activity contained in a stated amount of the International Reference Preparation of hepatitis B immunoglobulin. The equivalence in International Units of the International Reference Preparation is stated by the World Health Organisation.

The stated potency is not less than 100 I.U. per millilitre. The estimated potency is not less than the stated potency. The fiducial limits of error ($P = 0.95$) of the estimated potency are not less than 80 per cent and not more than 125 per cent.

STORAGE

See *Human normal immunoglobulin (338)*.

LABELLING

See *Human normal immunoglobulin (338)*.

The label states the number of International Units per container.

Ph Eur

Hepatitis B Immunoglobulin for Intravenous Use

Hepatitis B Immunoglobulin for Intravenous Use complies with the requirements of the 3rd edition of the European Pharmacopoeia for Human Hepatitis B Immunoglobulin for Intravenous Use [1016]. These requirements are reproduced after the heading 'Definition' below.

Ph Eur

DEFINITION

Human hepatitis B immunoglobulin for intravenous use is a liquid or freeze-dried preparation containing immunoglobulins, mainly immunoglobulin G. It is obtained from plasma from selected and/or immunised donors having antibodies against hepatitis B surface antigen. *Human normal immunoglobulin for intravenous use (918)* may be added.

It complies with the monograph on *Human normal immunoglobulin for intravenous administration (918)*, except for the minimum number of donors, the minimum total protein content and the limit for osmolality.

POTENCY

The potency is determined by comparing the antibody titre of the immunoglobulin to be examined with that of a reference preparation calibrated in International Units, using an immunoassay (*2.7.1*) of suitable sensitivity and specificity.

The International Unit is the activity contained in a stated amount of the International Reference Preparation of hepatitis B immunoglobulin. The equivalence in International Units of the International Reference Preparation is stated by the World Health Organisation.

The stated potency is not less than 50 I.U. per millilitre. The estimated potency is not less than the stated potency. The confidence interval ($P = 0.95$) of the estimated potency is not greater than 80 per cent to 125 per cent.

STORAGE

See *Human normal immunoglobulin for intravenous administration (918)*.

LABELLING

See *Human normal immunoglobulin for intravenous administration (918)*.

The label states the minimum number of International Units of hepatitis B immunoglobulin per container.

Ph Eur

Measles Immunoglobulin

Measles Immunoglobulin complies with the requirements of the 3rd edition of the European Pharmacopoeia for Human Measles Immunoglobulin [0397]. These requirements are reproduced after the heading 'Definition' below.

Ph Eur

DEFINITION

Human measles immunoglobulin is a liquid or freeze-dried preparation containing immunoglobulins, mainly immunoglobulin G. The preparation is intended for intramuscular administration. It is obtained from plasma containing specific antibodies against the measles virus. *Human normal immunoglobulin (338)* may be added.

It complies with the monograph on *Human normal immunoglobulin (338)*, except for the minimum number of donors and the minimum total protein content.

POTENCY

The potency of the liquid preparation and of the freeze-dried preparation after reconstitution as stated on the label is not less than 50 I.U. per millilitre of neutralising antibody against measles virus.

The potency is determined by comparing the antibody titres of the immunoglobulin to be examined and of a reference preparation calibrated in International Units, using a challenge dose of measles virus in a suitable cell culture system. A method of equal sensitivity and precision may be used providing that the competent authority is satisfied that it correlates with neutralising activity for the measles virus by comparison with the reference preparation.

The International Unit is the specific neutralising activity for measles virus contained in a stated amount of the International Reference Preparation of human anti-measles serum. The equivalence in International Units of the International Reference Preparation is stated by the World Health Organisation.

Prepare serial two-fold dilutions of the immunoglobulin to be examined and of the reference preparation. Mix each dilution with an equal volume of a suspension of measles virus containing about 100 $CCID_{50}$ in 0.1 ml and incubate protected from light at 37°C for 2 h. Using not fewer than six cell cultures per mixture, inoculate 0.2 ml of each mixture into each of the cell cultures allocated to that mixture and incubate for not less than 10 days. Examine the cultures for viral activity and compare the dilution containing the smallest quantity of the immunoglobulin which neutralises the virus with that of the corresponding dilution of the reference preparation.

Calculate the potency of the immunoglobulin to be examined in International Units per millilitre of neutralising antibody against measles virus.

STORAGE

See *Human normal immunoglobulin (338)*.

LABELLING

See *Human normal immunoglobulin (338)*.

The label states the number of International Units per container.

Ph Eur

Rabies Immunoglobulin

Rabies Immunoglobulin complies with the requirements of the 3rd edition of the European Pharmacopoeia for Human Rabies Immunoglobulin [0723]. These requirements are reproduced after the heading 'Definition' below.

Ph Eur

DEFINITION

Human rabies immunoglobulin is a liquid or freeze-dried preparation containing immunoglobulins, mainly immunoglobulin G. The preparation is intended for intramuscular administration. It is obtained from plasma from donors immunised against rabies. It contains specific antibodies neutralising the rabies virus. *Human normal immunoglobulin (338)* may be added.

It complies with the monograph on *Human normal immunoglobulin (338)*, except for the minimum number of donors and the minimum total protein content.

POTENCY

The potency is determined by comparing the dose of immunoglobulin required to neutralise the infectivity of a rabies virus suspension with the dose of a reference preparation, calibrated in International Units, required to produce the same degree of neutralisation *(2.7.1. Immunochemical Methods)*. The test is performed in sensitive cell cultures and the presence of unneutralised virus is revealed by immunofluorescence.

The International Unit is the specific neutralising activity for rabies virus in a stated amount of the International Standard of human rabies immunoglobulin. The equivalence in International Units of the International Standard is stated by the World Health Organisation.

Carry out the test in suitable sensitive cells. It is usual to use the BHK 21 cell line, grown in the medium described below, between the 18th and 30th passage levels counted from the ATCC seed lot. Harvest the cells after 2 to 4 days of growth, treat with trypsin and prepare a suspension containing 500,000 cells per millilitre (cell suspension). 10 min before using this suspension add 10 µg of *diethylaminoethyldextran R* per millilitre, if necessary, to increase the sensitivity of the cells.

Use a fixed virus strain grown in sensitive cells, such as the CVS strain of rabies virus adapted to growth in the BHK 21 cell line (seed virus suspension). Estimate the titre of the seed virus suspension as follows.

Prepare a series of dilutions of the viral suspension. In the chambers of cell-culture slides (8 chambers per slide), place 0.1 ml of each dilution and 0.1 ml of medium and add 0.2 ml of the cell suspension. Incubate in an atmosphere of carbon dioxide at 37°C for 24 h. Carry out fixation, immunofluorescence staining and evaluation as described below. Determine the end-point titre of the seed virus suspension and prepare the working virus dilution corresponding to 100 $CCID_{50}$ per 0.1 ml.

For each assay, check the amount of virus used by performing a control titration: from the dilution corresponding to 100 $CCID_{50}$ per 0.1 ml, make three tenfold dilutions. Add 0.1 ml of each dilution to four chambers containing 0.1 ml of medium and add 0.2 ml of the cell suspension. The test is not valid unless the titre lies between 30 $CCID_{50}$ and 300 $CCID_{50}$.

Dilute the reference preparation to a concentration of 2 I.U. per millilitre using non-supplemented culture medium (stock reference dilution, stored below –80°C). Prepare two suitable predilutions (1:8 and 1:10) of the stock reference dilution so that the dilution of the reference preparation that reduces the number of fluorescent fields by 50 per cent lies within the four dilutions of the cell-culture slide. Add 0.1 ml of the medium to each chamber, except the first in each of two rows, to which add respectively 0.2 ml of the two predilutions of the stock reference dilution transferring successively 0.1 ml to the other chambers.

Dilute the preparation to be examined 1 in 100 using non-supplemented medium (stock immunoglobulin dilution) – to reduce to a minimum errors due to viscosity of the undiluted preparation – and make three suitable predilutions so that the dilution of the preparation to be examined that reduces the number of fluorescent fields by 50 per cent lies within the four dilutions of the cell-culture slide. Add 0.1 ml of the medium to all the chambers except the first in each of three rows, to which add respectively 0.2 ml of the three predilutions of the stock immunoglobulin dilution. Prepare a series of twofold dilutions transferring successively 0.1 ml to the other chambers.

To all the chambers containing the dilutions of the reference preparation and the dilutions of the preparation to be examined, add 0.1 ml of the virus suspension corresponding to 100 $CCID_{50}$ per 0.1 ml (working virus dilution), shake manually, allow to stand in an atmosphere of carbon dioxide at 37°C for 90 min, add 0.2 ml of the cell suspension, shake manually and allow to stand in an atmosphere of carbon dioxide at 37°C for 24 h.

After 24 h, discard the medium and remove the plastic walls. Wash the cell monolayer with *phosphate buffered saline pH 7.4 R* and then with a mixture of 20 volumes of *water R* and 80 volumes of *acetone R* and fix in a mixture of 20 volumes of *water R* and 80 volumes of *acetone R* at –20°C for 3 min. Spread on the slides *fluorescein-conjugated rabies antiserum R* ready for use. Allow to stand in an atmosphere with a high level of moisture at 37°C for 30 min. Wash with *phosphate buffered saline pH 7.4 R* and dry. Examine twenty fields in each chamber at a magnification of ×250, using a microscope equipped for fluorescence readings. Note the number of fields with at least one fluorescent cell. Check the test dose used in the virus titration slide and determine the dilution of the reference preparation and the dilution of the preparation to be examined that reduce the number of fluorescent fields by 50 per cent, calculating the two or three dilutions together using probit analysis. The test is not valid unless the statistical analysis shows a significant slope of the dose-response curve and no evidence of deviation from linearity or parallelism.

The stated potency is not less than 150 I.U. per millilitre. The estimated potency is not less than the stated potency and is not greater than two times the stated potency. The fiducial limits of error ($P = 0.95$) of the estimated potency are not less than 80 per cent and not more than 125 per cent.

CULTURE MEDIUM FOR GROWTH OF BHK 21 CELLS

Commercially available media that have a slightly different composition from that shown below may also be used.

Sodium chloride	6.4 g
Potassium chloride	0.40 g
Calcium chloride, anhydrous	0.20 g
Magnesium sulphate, heptahydrate	0.20 g
Sodium dihydrogen phosphate, monohydrate	0.124 g
Glucose monohydrate	4.5 g
Ferric nitrate, nonahydrate	0.10 mg
L-Arginine hydrochloride	42.0 mg
L-Cystine	24.0 mg
L-Histidine	16.0 mg
L-Isoleucine	52.0 mg
L-Leucine	52.0 mg
L-Lysine hydrochloride	74.0 mg
L -Phenylalanine	33.0 mg
L -Threonine	48.0 mg
L -Tryptophan	8.0 mg
L-Tyrosine	36.0 mg
L-Valine	47.0 mg
L -Methionine	15.0 mg
L-Glutamine	0.292 g
i-Inositol	3.60 mg
Choline chloride	2.0 mg
Folic acid	2.0 mg
Nicotinamide	2.0 mg
Calcium pantothenate	2.0 mg
Pyridoxal hydrochloride	2.0 mg
Thiamine hydrochloride	2.0 mg
Riboflavine	0.2 mg
Phenol red	15.0 mg
Sodium hydrogen carbonate	2.75 g
Water	to 1000 ml

The medium is supplemented with:

Foetal calf serum (heated at 56°C for 30 min)	10 per cent
Tryptose phosphate broth	10 per cent
Benzylpenicillin sodium	60 mg/litre
Streptomycin	0.1 g/litre

STORAGE

See *Human normal immunoglobulin (338)*.

LABELLING

See *Human normal immunoglobulin (338)*.

The label states the number of International Units per container.

Ph Eur

Rubella Immunoglobulin

Rubella Immunoglobulin complies with the requirements of the 3rd edition of the European Pharmacopoeia for Human Rubella Immunoglobulin [0617]. These requirements are reproduced after the heading 'Definition' below.

Ph Eur

DEFINITION

Human rubella immunoglobulin is a liquid or freeze-dried preparation containing immunoglobulins, mainly immunoglobulin G. The preparation is intended for intramuscular administration. It is obtained from plasma containing specific antibodies against rubella virus. *Human normal immunoglobulin (338)* may be added.

It complies with the monograph on *Human normal immunoglobulin (338)*, except for the minimum number of donors and the minimum total protein content.

POTENCY

The potency is determined by comparing the activity of the preparation to be examined in a suitable haemagglutination–inhibition test with that of a reference preparation calibrated in International Units.

The International Unit is the activity contained in a stated amount of the International Reference Preparation of human anti-rubella serum. The equivalence in International Units of the International Reference Preparation is stated by the World Health Organisation.

The estimated potency is not less than 4500 I.U. per millilitre. The fiducial limits of error ($P = 0.95$) of the estimate of potency are not less than 50 per cent and not more than 200 per cent of the stated potency.

STORAGE

See *Human normal immunoglobulin (338)*.

LABELLING

See *Human normal immunoglobulin (338)*.

The label states the number of International Units per millilitre.

Ph Eur

Tetanus Immunoglobulin

Tetanus Immunoglobulin complies with the requirements of the 3rd edition of the European Pharmacopoeia for Human Tetanus Immunoglobulin [0398]. These requirements are reproduced after the heading 'Definition' below.

Ph Eur

DEFINITION

Human tetanus immunoglobulin is a liquid or freeze-dried preparation containing immunoglobulins, mainly immunoglobulin G. It is obtained from plasma containing specific antibodies against the toxin of *Clostridium tetani*. *Human normal immunoglobulin (338)* may be added.

It complies with the monograph on *Human normal immunoglobulin (338)*, except for the minimum number of donors and the minimum total protein content.

PRODUCTION

During development, a satisfactory relationship shall be established between the potency determined by immunoassay as described under Potency and that determined by means of the following test for toxin-neutralising capacity in mice.

Toxin-neutralising capacity in mice. The potency is determined by comparing the quantity necessary to protect mice against the paralytic effects of a fixed quantity of tetanus toxin with the quantity of a reference preparation of human tetanus immunoglobulin, calibrated in International Units, necessary to give the same protection.

The International Unit of antitoxin is the specific neutralising activity for tetanus toxin contained in a stated amount of the International Standard, which consists of freeze-dried human immunoglobulin. The equivalence in International Units of the International Standard is stated by the World Health Organisation.

Human tetanus immunoglobulin BRP is calibrated in International Units by comparison with the International Standard.

Selection of animals. Use mice weighing 16 g to 20 g.

Preparation of the test toxin. Prepare the test toxin by a suitable method from the sterile filtrate of a culture in liquid medium of *C. tetani.* The two methods shown below are given as examples and any other suitable method may be used.

(1) To the filtrate of an approximately 9-day culture add 1 to 2 volumes of *glycerol R* and store the mixture in the liquid state at a temperature slightly below 0°C.

(2) Precipitate the toxin by addition to the filtrate of *ammonium sulphate R*, dry the precipitate *in vacuo* over *diphosphorus pentoxide R*, reduce to a powder and store dry, either in sealed ampoules or *in vacuo* over *diphosphorus pentoxide R*.

Determination of test dose of toxin (Lp/10 dose). Prepare a solution of the reference preparation in a suitable liquid such that it contains 0.5 I.U. of antitoxin per millilitre. If the test toxin is stored dry, reconstitute it using a suitable liquid. Prepare mixtures of the solution of the reference preparation and the test toxin such that each contains 2.0 ml of the solution of the reference preparation, one of a graded series of volumes of the test toxin and sufficient of a suitable liquid to bring the volume to 5.0 ml. Allow the mixtures to stand, protected from light, for 60 min. Using six mice for each mixture, inject a dose of 0.5 ml subcutaneously into each mouse. Observe the mice for 96 h. Mice that become paralysed may be killed. The test dose of toxin is the quantity in 0.5 ml of the mixture made with the smallest amount of toxin capable of causing, despite partial neutralisation by the reference preparation, paralysis in all six mice injected with the mixture, within the observation period.

Determination of potency of the immunoglobulin. Prepare a solution of the reference preparation in a suitable liquid such that it contains 0.5 I.U. of antitoxin per millilitre. Prepare a solution of the test toxin in a suitable liquid such that it contains five test doses per millilitre. Prepare mixtures of the solution of the test toxin and the immunoglobulin to be examined such that each contains 2.0 ml of the solution of the test toxin, one of a graded series of volumes of the immunoglobulin to be examined and sufficient of a suitable liquid to bring the total volume to 5.0 ml. Also prepare mixtures of the solution of the test toxin and the solution of the reference preparation such that each contains 2.0 ml of the solution of the test toxin, one of a graded series of volumes of the solution of the reference preparation centred on that volume (2.0 ml) that contains 1 I.U. and sufficient of a suitable liquid to bring the total volume to 5.0 ml. Allow the mixtures to stand, protected from light, for 60 min. Using six mice for each mixture, inject subcutaneously a dose of 0.5 ml into each mouse. Observe the mice for 96 h. Mice that become paralysed may be killed. The mixture that contains the largest volume of immunoglobulin that fails to protect the mice from paralysis contains 1 I.U. This quantity is used to calculate the potency of the immunoglobulin in International Units per millilitre.

The test is not valid unless all the mice injected with mixtures containing 2.0 ml or less of the solution of the reference preparation show paralysis and all those injected with mixtures containing more do not.

POTENCY

The potency is determined by comparing the antibody titre of the immunoglobulin to be examined with that of a reference preparation calibrated in International Units, using an immunoassay of suitable sensitivity and specificity (*2.7.1*).

Human tetanus immunoglobulin BRP is calibrated in International Units by comparison with the International Standard.

The stated potency is not less than 100 I.U. of tetanus antitoxin per millilitre. The estimated potency is not less than the stated potency. The fiducial limits of error ($P = 0.95$) of the estimated potency are not less than 80 per cent and not more than 125 per cent.

STORAGE

See *Human normal immunoglobulin (338)*.

LABELLING

See *Human normal immunoglobulin (338)*.

The label states the number of International Units per container.

Ph Eur

Varicella Immunoglobulin

Varicella Immunoglobulin complies with the requirements of the 3rd edition of the European Pharmacopoeia for Human Varicella Immunoglobulin [0724]. These requirements are reproduced after the heading 'Definition' below.

Ph Eur

DEFINITION

Human varicella immunoglobulin is a liquid or freeze-dried preparation containing immunoglobulins, mainly immunoglobulin G. The preparation is intended for intramuscular administration. It is obtained from plasma from selected donors having antibodies against *Herpesvirus varicellae*. *Human normal immunoglobulin (338)* may be added.

It complies with the monograph on *Human normal immunoglobulin (338)* except for the minimum number of donors, the minimum total protein content and, where authorised, the test for antibody to hepatitis B surface antigen.

POTENCY

The potency is determined by comparing the antibody titre of the immunoglobulin to be examined with that of a reference preparation calibrated in International Units, using an immunoassay of suitable sensitivity and specificity (*2.7.1. Immunochemical Methods*).

The International Unit is the activity contained in a stated amount of the International Standard for human varicella immunoglobulin. The equivalence in International Units of the International Standard is stated by the World Health Organisation.

The stated potency is not less than 100 I.U. per millilitre. The estimated potency is not less than the stated potency. The fiducial limits of error ($P = 0.95$) of the estimated potency are not less than 80 per cent and not more than 125 per cent.

STORAGE

See *Human normal immunoglobulin (338)*.

LABELLING

See *Human normal immunoglobulin (338)*.

The label states the number of International Units per container.

Ph Eur

Monographs

Immunological Products

ANTISERA

An antiserum for human use that is the subject of an individual monograph in the European Pharmacopoeia or in the British Pharmacopoeia complies with the requirements of the 3rd edition of the European Pharmacopoeia for Immunosera for Human Use [0084]. These requirements are reproduced after the heading 'Definition' below.

The provisions of this monograph apply to the following antisera:

Botulinum Antitoxin
Diphtheria Antitoxin
European Viper Venom Antiserum
Gas-gangrene Antitoxin (Novyi)
Gas-gangrene Antitoxin (Perfringens)
Gas-gangrene Antitoxin (Septicum)
Mixed Gas-gangrene Antitoxin
Scorpion Venom Antiserum
Tetanus Antitoxin

Ph Eur

The statements in this monograph are intended to be read in conjunction with the monographs on immunosera for human use in the Pharmacopoeia. The requirements do not necessarily apply to immunosera which are not the subject of such monographs.

DEFINITION

Immunosera for human use are purified preparations containing immunoglobulins obtained from serum of immunised animals. The immunoglobulins have the power of specifically neutralising venins or the toxins formed by bacteria or of specifically combining with the bacteria, viruses or other antigens.

PRODUCTION

Immunosera are obtained from healthy animals immunised by injections of the appropriate toxins or toxoids, venins, suspensions of micro-organisms or other antigens. During the immunisation the animals must not be treated with penicillin. The globulins containing the immunising substances may be obtained from the serum by enzyme treatment and fractional precipitation or by other chemical or physical methods.

A suitable antimicrobial preservative may be added and is invariably added if the preparations are issued in multidose containers. The final sterile products are distributed aseptically into sterile containers which are then closed so as to exclude contamination.

The products may be freeze-dried by a procedure which reduces the water content of the finished product to not more than 1.0 per cent *m/m*.

Immunosera prepared by enzyme treatment and fractional precipitation are most stable at about pH 6. The method of preparation of immunosera is such that the products lose not more than 5 per cent of their activity per year at this pH when stored at 20°C and not more than 20 per cent per year when stored at 37°C.

The production method is validated to demonstrate that the product, if tested, would comply with the test for abnormal toxicity for immunosera and vaccines for human use (*2.6.9*).

CHARACTERS

Immunosera are almost colourless or very faintly yellow liquids free from turbidity. Freeze-dried immunosera consist of white or pale-yellow crusts or powders, freely soluble in water to form colourless or pale-yellow solutions having the same characters as the corresponding liquid preparations.

TESTS

The following requirements refer to liquid immunosera and to the reconstituted freeze-dried preparations.

pH (*2.2.3*). The pH is 6.0 to 7.0.

Foreign proteins When examined by precipitation tests with specific antisera, only protein from the declared animal species is shown to be present.

Total protein Not more than 170 g/l. Carry out the determination of nitrogen by sulphuric acid digestion (*2.5.9*) and multiply the result by 6.25.

Albumins Unless otherwise prescribed in the monograph, when examined electrophoretically, they show not more than traces of albumins.

Phenol (*2.5.15*). When the immunosera contain phenol, the concentration is not more than 2.5 g/l.

Sterility (*2.6.1*). They comply with the test for sterility.

POTENCY

Carry out a biological assay as indicated in the monograph and express the result in International Units per millilitre, where appropriate.

STORAGE

Store at a temperature of 5 ± 3°C. Liquid immunosera should not be allowed to freeze.

Expiry date. The expiry date is calculated from the beginning of the test for Potency. It applies to immunosera stored in the prescribed conditions.

LABELLING

The label states:

— the name of the preparation,
— the number of International Units per millilitre where applicable,
— the batch number or other reference,
— the route of administration,
— the storage conditions,
— the expiry date, except that for containers of 1 ml or less which are individually packed, the expiry date may be omitted from the label on the container provided it is shown on the package and the label on the package states that the container must be kept in the package until required for use,
— the name of the animal species of origin,
— the name and amount of any antimicrobial preservative or other substance added to the immunoserum,
— a declaration of any substance likely to cause any adverse reaction and any contra-indications to the use of the product,
— for freeze-dried immunosera:
— the name or composition and the volume of the reconstituting liquid to be added,
— that the immunoserum should be used immediately after reconstitution,
— the name and address of the manufacturer.

Ph Eur

Botulinum Antitoxin

Botulinum Antitoxin complies with the requirements of the 3rd edition of the European Pharmacopoeia [0085]. These requirements are reproduced after the heading 'Definition' below.

The label may state 'Bot/Ser' followed by a letter or letters indicating the type or types present.

When Mixed Botulinum Antitoxin or Botulinum Antitoxin is prescribed or demanded and the types to be present are not stated, Botulinum Antitoxin prepared from types A, B and E shall be dispensed or supplied.

Ph Eur

DEFINITION

Botulinum antitoxin is a preparation containing antitoxic globulins that have the power of specifically neutralising the toxins formed by *Clostridium botulinum* type A, type B or type E, or any mixture of these types.

PRODUCTION

It is obtained by fractionation from the serum of horses, or other mammals, that have been immunised against *Cl. botulinum* type A, type B and type E toxins.

IDENTIFICATION

It specifically neutralises the types of *Cl. botulinum* toxins stated on the label, rendering them harmless to susceptible animals.

TESTS

It complies with the tests prescribed in the monograph on *Immunosera for human use (84)*.

POTENCY

Not less than 500 I.U. of antitoxin per millilitre for each of types A and B and not less than 50 I.U. of antitoxin per millilitre for type E.

The potency of botulinum antitoxin is determined by comparing the dose necessary to protect mice against the lethal effects of a fixed dose of botulinum toxin with the quantity of the standard preparation of botulinum antitoxin necessary to give the same protection. For this comparison a reference preparation of each type of botulinum antitoxin, calibrated in International Units, and suitable preparations of botulinum toxins, for use as test toxins, are required. The potency of each test toxin is determined in relation to the specific reference preparation; the potency of the botulinum antitoxin to be examined is determined in relation to the potency of the test toxins by the same method.

International Units of the antitoxin are the specific neutralising activity for botulinum toxin type A, type B and type E contained in stated amounts of the International Standards which consist of dried immune horse sera of types A, B and E. The equivalence in International Units of the International Standard is stated from time to time by the World Health Organisation.

Selection of animals. Use mice having body masses such that the difference between the lightest and the heaviest does not exceed 5 g.

Preparation of test toxins. Warning: Botulinum toxin is extremely toxic: exceptional care must be taken in any procedure in which it is employed. Prepare type A, B and E toxins from sterile filtrates of approximately 7-day cultures in liquid medium of *Cl. botulinum* types A, B and E. To the filtrates, add 2 volumes of glycerol, concentrate, if necessary, by dialysis against glycerol and store at or slightly below 0°C.

Selection of test toxins. Select toxins of each type for use as test toxins by determining for mice the L+/10 dose and the LD_{50}, the observation period being 96 h. The test toxins contain at least 1000 LD_{50} in an L+/10 dose.

Determination of test doses of the toxins (L+/10 dose). Prepare solutions of the reference preparations in a suitable liquid such that each contains 0.25 I.U. of antitoxin per millilitre. Using each solution in turn, determine the test dose of the corresponding test toxin.

Prepare mixtures of the solution of the reference preparation and the test toxin such that each contains 2.0 ml of the solution of the reference preparation, one of a graded series of volumes of the test toxin and sufficient of a suitable liquid to bring the total volume to 5.0 ml. Allow the mixtures to stand at room temperature, protected from light, for 60 min. Using four mice for each mixture, inject a dose of 1.0 ml intraperitoneally into each mouse. Observe the mice for 96 h.

The test dose of toxin is the quantity in 1.0 ml of the mixture made with the smallest amount of toxin capable of causing, despite partial neutralisation by the reference preparation, the death of all four mice injected with the mixture within the observation period.

Determination of potency of the antitoxin

Prepare solutions of each reference preparation in a suitable liquid such that each contains 0.25 I.U. of antitoxin per millilitre.

Prepare solutions of each test toxin in a suitable liquid such that each contains 2.5 test doses per millilitre.

Using each toxin solution and the corresponding reference preparation in turn, determine the potency of the antitoxin. Prepare mixtures of the solution of the test toxin and the antitoxin to be examined such that each contains 2.0 ml of the solution of the test toxin, one of a graded series of volumes of the antitoxin to be examined, and sufficient of a suitable liquid to bring the total volume to 5.0 ml. Also prepare mixtures of the solution of the test toxin and the solution of the reference preparation such that each contains 2.0 ml of the solution of the test toxin, one of a graded series of volumes of the solution of the reference preparation centred on that volume (2.0 ml) that contains 0.5 I.U., and sufficient of a suitable liquid to bring the total volume to 5.0 ml. Allow the mixtures to stand at room temperature, protected from light, for 60 min. Using four mice for each mixture, inject a dose of 1.0 ml intraperitoneally into each mouse. Observe the mice for 96 h.

The mixture that contains the largest volume of antitoxin that fails to protect the mice from death contains 0.5 I.U. This quantity is used to calculate the potency of the antitoxin in International Units per millilitre.

The test is not valid unless all the mice injected with mixtures containing 2.0 ml or less of the solution of the reference preparation die and all those injected with mixtures containing more survive.

STORAGE

See *Immunosera for human use (84)*.

LABELLING

See *Immunosera for human use (84)*.

The label states the types of *Cl. botulinum* toxin neutralised by the preparation.

Ph Eur

Diphtheria Antitoxin

Diphtheria Antitoxin complies with the requirements of the 3rd edition of the European Pharmacopoeia [0086]. These requirements are reproduced after the heading 'Definition' below.

The label may state 'Dip/Ser'.

Ph Eur

DEFINITION

Diphtheria antitoxin is a preparation containing antitoxic globulins that have the power of specifically neutralising the toxin formed by *Corynebacterium diphtheriae*.

PRODUCTION

It is obtained by fractionation from the serum of horses, or other mammals, that have been immunised against diphtheria toxin.

IDENTIFICATION

It specifically neutralises the toxin formed by *C. diphtheriae*, rendering it harmless to susceptible animals.

TESTS

It complies with the tests prescribed in the monograph on *Immunosera for human use (84)*.

ASSAY

Not less than 1000 I.U. of antitoxin per millilitre for antitoxin obtained from horse serum. Not less than 500 I.U. of antitoxin per millilitre for antitoxin obtained from the serum of other mammals.

The potency of diphtheria antitoxin is determined by comparing the dose necessary to protect guinea-pigs or rabbits against the erythrogenic effects of a fixed dose of diphtheria toxin with the quantity of the standard preparation of diphtheria antitoxin necessary to give the same protection. For this comparison a reference preparation of diphtheria antitoxin, calibrated in International Units, and a suitable preparation of diphtheria toxin, for use as a test toxin, are required. The potency of the test toxin is determined in relation to the reference preparation; the potency of the diphtheria antitoxin to be examined is determined in relation to the potency of the test toxin by the same method.

The International Unit of antitoxin is the specific neutralising activity for diphtheria toxin contained in a stated amount of the International Standard, which consists of a quantity of dried immune horse serum. The equivalence in International Units of the International Standard is stated by the World Health Organisation.

Preparation of test toxin. Prepare diphtheria toxin from cultures of *C. diphtheriae* in a liquid medium. Filter the culture to obtain a sterile toxic filtrate and store at 4°C.

Selection of test toxin. Select a toxin for use as a test toxin by determining for guinea-pigs or rabbits the lr/100 dose and the minimal reacting dose, the observation period being 48 h. The test toxin has at least 200 minimal reacting doses in the lr/100 dose.

Minimal reacting dose. This is the smallest quantity of toxin which, when injected intracutaneously into guinea-pigs or rabbits, causes a small, characteristic reaction at the site of injection within 48 h.

The test toxin is allowed to stand for some months before being used for the assay of antitoxin. During this time its toxicity declines and the lr/100 dose may be increased. Determine the minimal reacting dose and the lr/100 dose at frequent intervals. When experiment shows that the lr/100 dose is constant, the test toxin is ready for use and may be used for a long period. Store the test toxin in the dark at 0°C to 5°C. Maintain its sterility by the addition of toluene or other antimicrobial preservative that does not cause a rapid decline in specific toxicity.

Determination of test dose of toxin (lr/100 dose). Prepare a solution of the reference preparation in a suitable liquid such that it contains 0.1 I.U. of antitoxin per millilitre.

Prepare mixtures of the solution of the reference preparation and of the test toxin such that each contains 1.0 ml of the solution of the reference preparation, one of a graded series of volumes of the test toxin and sufficient of a suitable liquid to bring the total volume to 2.0 ml. Allow the mixtures to stand at room temperature, protected from light, for 15 min to 60 min. Using two animals for each mixture, inject a dose of 0.2 ml intracutaneously into the shaven or depilated flanks of each animal. Observe the animals for 48 h.

The test dose of toxin is the quantity in 0.2 ml of the mixture made with the smallest amount of toxin capable of causing, despite partial neutralisation by the reference preparation, a small but characteristic erythematous lesion at the site of injection.

Determination of potency of the antitoxin.

Prepare a solution of the reference preparation in a suitable liquid such that it contains 0.125 I.U. of antitoxin per millilitre.

Prepare a solution of the test toxin in a suitable liquid such that it contains 12.5 test doses per millilitre.

Prepare mixtures of the solution of the test toxin and of the antitoxin to be examined such that each contains 0.8 ml of the solution of the test toxin, one of a graded series of volumes of the antitoxin to be examined and sufficient of a suitable liquid to bring the total volume to 2.0 ml. Also prepare mixtures of the solution of the test toxin and the solution of the reference preparation such that each contains 0.8 ml of the solution of the test toxin, one of a graded series of volumes of the solution of the reference preparation centred on that volume (0.8 ml) that contains 0.1 I.U. and sufficient of a suitable liquid to bring the total volume to 2.0 ml. Allow the mixtures to stand at room temperature, protected from light, for 15 min to 60 min. Using two animals for each mixture, inject a dose of 0.2 ml intracutaneously into the shaven or depilated flanks of each animal. Observe the animals for 48 h.

The mixture that contains the largest volume of antitoxin that fails to protect the guinea-pigs from the erythematous effects of the toxin contains 0.1 I.U. This quantity is used to calculate the potency of the antitoxin in International Units per millilitre.

The test is not valid unless all the sites injected with mixtures containing 0.8 ml or less of the solution of the reference preparation show erythematous lesions and at all those injected with mixtures containing more there are no lesions.

STORAGE

See *Immunosera for human use (84)*.

LABELLING

See *Immunosera for human use (84)*.

Ph Eur

European Viper Venom Antiserum

European Viper Venom Antiserum complies with the requirements of the 3rd edition of the European Pharmacopoeia [0145]. These requirements are reproduced after the heading 'Definition' below.

The only poisonous snake native to the British Isles is the adder or common viper, *Vipera berus*. In a geographical region where other species of snake (including elapids) are found, antisera able to neutralise the venoms of the species of snake indigenous to the region should be used. When the preparation is intended to neutralise the venom or venoms of one or more snakes other than vipers, the title Snake Venom Antiserum is used.

Ph Eur

DEFINITION

European viper venom antiserum is a preparation containing antitoxic globulins that have the power of neutralising the venom of one or more species of viper. The globulins are obtained by fractionation of the serum of animals that have been immunised against the venom or venoms.

IDENTIFICATION

It neutralises the venom of *Vipera ammodytes*, or *Vipera aspis*, or *Vipera berus*, or *Vipera ursinii* or the mixture of these venoms stated on the label, rendering them harmless to susceptible animals.

TESTS

It complies with the tests prescribed in the monograph on *Immunosera for human use (84)*.

ASSAY

Each millilitre of the preparation to be examined contains sufficient antitoxic globulins to neutralise not less than 100 mouse LD_{50} of *Vipera ammodytes* venom or *Vipera aspis* venom and not less than 50 mouse LD_{50} of the venoms of other species of viper.

The potency of European viper venom antiserum is determined by estimating the dose necessary to protect mice against the lethal effects of a fixed dose of venom of the relevant species of viper.

Selection of test venoms†. Use venoms which have the normal physicochemical, toxicological and immunological characteristics of venoms from the particular species of vipers. They are preferably freeze-dried and stored in the dark at 5 ± 3°C.

Select a venom for use as a test venom by determining the LD_{50} for mice, the observation period being 48 h.

Determination of the test dose of venom. Prepare graded dilutions of the reconstituted venom in a 9 g/l solution of *sodium chloride R* or other isotonic diluent in such a manner that the middle dilution contains in 0.25 ml the dose expected to be the LD_{50}. Dilute with an equal volume of the same diluent. Using at least four mice, each weighing 18 g to 20 g, for each dilution, inject 0.5 ml intravenously into each mouse. Observe the mice for 48 h and record the number of deaths. Calculate the LD_{50} using the usual statistical methods.

Determination of the potency of the antiserum to be examined. Dilute the reconstituted test venom so that 0.25 ml contains the test dose of 5 LD_{50} (test venom solution).

Prepare serial dilutions of the antiserum to be examined in a 9 g/l solution of *sodium chloride R* or other isotonic diluent, the dilution factor being 1.5 to 2.5. Use a sufficient number and range of dilutions to enable a mortality curve between 20 per cent and 80 per cent mortality to be established and to permit an estimation of the statistical variation.

Prepare mixtures such that 5 ml of each mixture contains 2.5 ml of one of the dilutions of the antiserum to be examined and 2.5 ml of the test venom solution. Allow the mixtures to stand in a water-bath at 37°C for 30 min. Using not fewer than six mice, each weighing 18 g to 20 g, for each mixture, inject 0.5 ml intravenously into each mouse. Observe the mice for 48 h and record the number of deaths. Calculate the PD_{50}, using the usual statistical methods. At the same time verify the number of LD_{50} in the test dose of venom, using the method described above. Calculate the potency of the antiserum from the expression:

$$\frac{T_v - 1}{PD_{50}}$$

T_v = number of LD_{50} in the test dose of venom.

In each mouse dose of the venom-antiserum mixture at the end point there is one LD_{50} of venom remaining unneutralised by the antiserum and it is this unneutralised venom that is responsible for the deaths of 50 per cent of the mice inoculated with the mixture. The amount of venom neutralised by the antiserum is thus one LD_{50} less than the total amount contained in each mouse dose. Therefore, as the potency of the antiserum is defined in terms of the number of LD_{50} of venom that are neutralised rather than the number of LD_{50} in each mouse dose, the expression required in the calculation of potency is T_v-1 rather than T_v.

Alternatively, the quantity of test venom in milligrams that is neutralised by 1 ml or some other defined volume of the antiserum to be examined may be calculated.

STORAGE

See *Immunosera for human use (84)*.

LABELLING

See *Immunosera for human use (84)*.

The label states the venom or venoms against which the antiserum is effective.

†*Warning: Because of the allergenic properties of viper venoms, inhalation of venom dust should be avoided by suitable precautions.*

Ph Eur

Gas-gangrene Antitoxin (Novyi)

Gas-gangrene Antitoxin (Oedematiens)

Gas-gangrene Antitoxin (Novyi) complies with the requirements of the 3rd edition of the European Pharmacopoeia [0087]. These requirements are reproduced after the heading 'Definition' below.

The label may state 'Nov/Ser'.

Preparation

Mixed Gas-gangrene Antiserum

Ph Eur

DEFINITION

Gas-gangrene antitoxin (novyi) is a preparation containing antitoxic globulins that have the power of neutralising the alpha toxin formed by *Clostridium novyi* (Former nomenclature: *Clostridium oedematiens*). It is obtained by fractionation from the serum of horses, or other mammals, that have been immunised against *Cl. novyi* alpha toxin.

IDENTIFICATION

It specifically neutralises the alpha toxin formed by *Cl. novyi*, rendering it harmless to susceptible animals.

TESTS

It complies with the tests prescribed in the monograph on *Immunosera for human use (84)*.

ASSAY

Not less than 3750 I.U. of antitoxin per millilitre.

The potency of gas-gangrene antitoxin (novyi) is determined by comparing the dose necessary to protect mice or other suitable animals against the lethal effects of a fixed dose of *Cl. novyi* toxin with the quantity of the standard preparation of gas-gangrene antitoxin (novyi) necessary to give the same protection. For this comparison a reference preparation of gas-gangrene antitoxin (novyi), calibrated in International Units, and a suitable preparation of *Cl. novyi* toxin for use as a test toxin are required. The potency of the test toxin is determined in relation to the reference preparation; the potency of the gas-gangrene antitoxin (novyi) to be examined is determined in relation to the potency of the test toxin by the same method.

The International Unit of antitoxin is the specific neutralising activity for *Cl. novyi* toxin contained in a stated amount of the International Standard, which consists of a quantity of dried immune horse serum. The equivalence in International Units of the International Standard is stated by the World Health Organisation.

Selection of animals. Use mice having body masses such that the difference between the lightest and the heaviest does not exceed 5 g.

Preparation of test toxin. Prepare the test toxin from a sterile filtrate of an approximately 5-day culture in liquid medium of *Cl. novyi.* Treat the filtrate with ammonium sulphate, collect the precipitate, which contains the toxin, dry *in vacuo* over *diphosphorus pentoxide R*, powder and store dry.

Selection of test toxin. Select a toxin for use as a test toxin by determining for mice the L+ dose and the LD_{50}, the observation period being 72 h. The test toxin has an L+ dose of 0.5 mg or less and contains not less than 25 LD_{50} in each L+ dose.

Determination of test dose of toxin (L+ dose). Prepare a solution of the reference preparation in a suitable liquid such that it contains 12.5 I.U. of antitoxin per millilitre.

Prepare a solution of the test toxin in a suitable liquid such that 1 ml contains a precisely known amount such as 10 mg.

Prepare mixtures of the solution of the reference preparation and the solution of the test toxin such that each contains 0.8 ml of the solution of the reference preparation, one of a graded series of volumes of the solution of the test toxin and sufficient of a suitable liquid to bring the total volume to 2.0 ml. Allow the mixtures to stand at room temperature, protected from light, for 60 min. Using six mice for each mixture, inject a dose of 0.2 ml intramuscularly into each mouse. Observe the mice for 72 h.

The test dose of toxin is the quantity in 0.2 ml of the mixture made with the smallest amount of toxin capable of causing, despite partial neutralisation by the reference preparation, the death of all six mice injected with the mixture within the observation period.

Determination of potency of the antitoxin.

Prepare a solution of the reference preparation in a suitable liquid such that it contains 12.5 I.U. of antitoxin per millilitre.

Prepare a solution of the test toxin in a suitable liquid such that it contains 12.5 test doses per millilitre.

Prepare mixtures of the solution of the test toxin and the antitoxin to be examined such that each contains 0.8 ml of the solution of the test toxin, one of a graded series of volumes of the antitoxin to be examined and sufficient of a suitable liquid to bring the total volume to 2.0 ml. Also prepare mixtures of the solution of the test toxin and the solution of the reference preparation such that each contains 0.8 ml of the solution of the test toxin, one of a graded series of volumes of the solution of the reference preparation centred on that volume (0.8 ml) that contains 10 I.U. and sufficient of a suitable liquid to bring the total volume to 2.0 ml. Allow the mixtures to stand at room temperature, protected from light, for 60 min. Using six mice for each mixture, inject a dose of 0.2 ml intramuscularly into each mouse. Observe the mice for 72 h.

The mixture that contains the largest volume of antitoxin that fails to protect the mice from death contains 10 I.U. This quantity is used to calculate the potency of the antitoxin in International Units per millilitre.

The test is not valid unless all the mice injected with mixtures containing 0.8 ml or less of the solution of the reference preparation die and all those injected with mixtures containing a larger volume survive.

STORAGE

See the monograph on *Immunosera for human use (84)*.

LABELLING

See the monograph on *Immunosera for human use (84)*.

Ph Eur

Gas-gangrene Antitoxin (Perfringens)

Gas-gangrene Antitoxin (Perfringens) complies with the requirements of the 3rd edition of the European Pharmacopoeia [0088]. These requirements are reproduced after the heading 'Definition' below.

The label may state 'Perf/Ser'.

Preparation

Mixed Gas-gangrene Antiserum

Ph Eur

DEFINITION

Gas-gangrene antitoxin (perfringens) is a preparation containing antitoxic globulins that have the power of specifically neutralising the alpha toxin formed by *Clostridium perfringens*. It is obtained by fractionation from the serum of horses, or other mammals, that have been immunised against *Cl. perfringens* alpha toxin.

IDENTIFICATION

It specifically neutralises the alpha toxin formed by *Cl. perfringens*, rendering it harmless to susceptible animals.

TESTS

It complies with the tests prescribed in the monograph on *Immunosera for human use (84)*.

ASSAY

Not less than 1500 I.U. of antitoxin per millilitre.

The potency of gas-gangrene antitoxin (perfringens) is determined by comparing the dose necessary to protect mice or other suitable animals against the lethal effects of a fixed dose of *Cl. perfringens* toxin with the quantity of the standard preparation of gas-gangrene antitoxin (perfringens) necessary to give the same protection. For this comparison a reference preparation of gas-gangrene antitoxin (perfringens), calibrated in International Units, and a suitable preparation of *Cl. perfringens* toxin for use as a test toxin are required. The potency of the test toxin is determined in relation to the reference preparation; the potency of the gas-gangrene antitoxin (perfringens) to be examined is determined in relation to the potency of the test toxin by the same method.

The International Unit of antitoxin is the specific neutralising activity for *Cl. perfringens* toxin contained in a stated amount of the International Standard, which consists of a quantity of dried immune horse serum. The equivalence in International Units of the International Standard is stated by the World Health Organisation.

Selection of animals. Use mice having body masses such that the difference between the lightest and the heaviest does not exceed 5 g.

Preparation of test toxin. Prepare the test toxin from a sterile filtrate of an approximately 5-day culture in liquid medium of *Cl. perfringens*. Treat the filtrate with ammonium sulphate, collect the precipitate, which contains the toxin, dry *in vacuo* over *diphosphorus pentoxide R*, powder and store dry.

Selection of test toxin. Select a toxin for use as a test toxin by determining for mice the L+ dose and the LD_{50}, the observation period being 48 h. The test toxin has an L+ dose of 4 mg or less and contains not less than 20 LD_{50} in each L+ dose.

Determination of test dose of toxin (L+ dose). Prepare a solution of the reference preparation in a suitable liquid such that it contains 5 I.U. of antitoxin per millilitre.

Prepare a solution of the test toxin in a suitable liquid such that 1 ml contains a precisely known amount such as 10 mg.

Prepare mixtures of the solution of the reference preparation and the solution of the test toxin such that each contains 2.0 ml of the solution of the reference preparation, one of a graded series of volumes of the solution of the test toxin and sufficient of a suitable liquid to bring the total volume to 5.0 ml. Allow the mixtures to stand at room temperature, protected from light, for 60 min. Using six mice for each mixture, inject a dose of 0.5 ml intravenously into each mouse. Observe the mice for 48 h.

The test dose of toxin is the quantity in 0.5 ml of the mixture made with the smallest amount of toxin capable of causing, despite partial neutralisation by the reference preparation, the death of all six mice injected with the mixture within the observation period.

Determination of potency of the antitoxin.

Prepare a solution of the reference preparation in a suitable liquid such that it contains 5 I.U. of antitoxin per millilitre.

Prepare a solution of the test toxin in a suitable liquid such that it contains five test doses per millilitre.

Prepare mixtures of the solution of the test toxin and the antitoxin to be examined such that each contains 2.0 ml of the solution of the test toxin, one of a graded series of volumes of the antitoxin to be examined and sufficient of a suitable liquid to bring the total volume to 5.0 ml. Also prepare mixtures of the solution of the test toxin and the solution of the reference preparation such that each contains 2.0 ml of the solution of the test toxin, one of a graded series of volumes of the solution of the reference preparation centred on that volume (2.0 ml) that contains 10 I.U. and sufficient of a suitable liquid to bring the total volume to 5.0 ml. Allow the mixtures to stand at room temperature, protected from light, for 60 min. Using six mice for each mixture, inject a dose of 0.5 ml intravenously into each mouse. Observe the mice for 48 h.

The mixture that contains the largest volume of antitoxin that fails to protect the mice from death contains 10 I.U. This quantity is used to calculate the potency of the antitoxin in International Units per millilitre.

The test is not valid unless all the mice injected with mixtures containing 2.0 ml or less of the solution of the reference preparation die and all those injected with mixtures containing a larger volume survive.

STORAGE

See the monograph on *Immunosera for human use (84)*.

LABELLING

See the monograph on *Immunosera for human use (84)*.

Ph Eur

Gas-gangrene Antitoxin (Septicum)

Gas-gangrene Antitoxin (Septicum) complies with the requirements of the 3rd edition of the European Pharmacopoeia [0089]. These requirements are reproduced after the heading 'Definition' below.

The label may state 'Sep/Ser'.

Preparation

Mixed Gas-gangrene Antiserum

Ph Eur

DEFINITION

Gas-gangrene antitoxin (septicum) is a preparation containing antitoxic globulins that have the power of specifically neutralising the alpha toxin formed by *Clostridium septicum*. It is obtained by fractionation from the serum of horses, or other mammals, that have been immunised against *Cl. septicum* alpha toxin.

IDENTIFICATION

It specifically neutralises the alpha toxin formed by *Cl. septicum*, rendering it harmless to susceptible animals.

TESTS

It complies with the tests prescribed in the monograph on *Immunosera for human use (84)*.

ASSAY

Not less than 1500 I.U. of antitoxin per millilitre.

The potency of gas-gangrene antitoxin (septicum) is determined by comparing the dose necessary to protect mice or other suitable animals against the lethal effects of a fixed dose of *Cl. septicum* toxin with the quantity of the standard preparation of gas-gangrene antitoxin (septicum) necessary to give the same protection. For this comparison a reference preparation of gas-gangrene antitoxin (septicum), calibrated in International Units, and a suitable preparation of *Cl. septicum* toxin for use as a test toxin are required. The potency of the test toxin is determined in relation to the reference preparation; the potency of the gas-gangrene antitoxin (septicum) to be examined is determined in relation to the potency of the test toxin by the same method.

The International Unit of antitoxin is the specific neutralising activity for *Cl. septicum* toxin contained in a stated amount of the International Standard, which consists of a quantity of dried immune horse serum. The equivalence in International Units of the International Standard is stated by the World Health Organisation.

Selection of animals. Use mice having body masses such that the difference between the lightest and the heaviest does not exceed 5 g.

Preparation of test toxin. Prepare the test toxin from a sterile filtrate of an approximately 5-day culture in liquid medium of *Cl. septicum*. Treat the filtrate with ammonium sulphate, collect the precipitate, which contains the toxin, dry *in vacuo* over *diphosphorus pentoxide R*, powder and store dry.

Selection of test toxin. Select a toxin for use as a test toxin by determining for mice the L+ dose and the LD_{50}, the observation period being 72 h. The test toxin has an L+ dose of 0.5 mg or less and contains not less than 25 LD_{50} in each L+ dose.

Determination of test dose of toxin (L+ dose). Prepare a solution of the reference preparation in a suitable liquid such that it contains 5 I.U. of antitoxin per millilitre.

Prepare a solution of the test toxin in a suitable liquid such that 1 ml contains a precisely known amount such as 20 mg.

Prepare mixtures of the solution of the reference preparation and the solution of the test toxin such that each contains 2.0 ml of the solution of the reference preparation, one of a graded series of volumes of the solution of the test toxin and sufficient of a suitable liquid to bring the total volume to 5.0 ml. Allow the mixtures to stand at room temperature, protected from light, for 60 min. Using six mice for each mixture, inject a dose of 0.5 ml intravenously into each mouse. Observe the mice for 72 h.

The test dose of toxin is the quantity in 0.5 ml of the mixture made with the smallest amount of toxin capable of causing, despite partial neutralisation by the reference preparation, the death of all six mice injected with the mixture within the observation period.

Determination of potency of the antitoxin.

Prepare a solution of the reference preparation in a suitable liquid such that it contains 5 I.U. of antitoxin per millilitre.

Prepare a solution of the test toxin in a suitable liquid such that it contains five test doses per millilitre.

Prepare mixtures of the solution of the test toxin and the antitoxin to be examined such that each contains 2.0 ml of the solution of the test toxin, one of a graded series of volumes of the antitoxin to be examined and sufficient of a suitable liquid to bring the total volume to 5.0 ml. Also prepare mixtures of the solution of the test toxin and the solution of the reference preparation such that each contains 2.0 ml of the solution of the test toxin, one of a graded series of volumes of the solution of the reference preparation centred on that volume (2.0 ml) that contains 10 I.U. and sufficient of a suitable liquid to bring the total volume to 5.0 ml. Allow the mixtures to stand at room temperature, protected from light, for 60 min. Using six mice for each mixture, inject a dose of 0.5 ml intravenously into each mouse. Observe the mice for 72 h.

The mixture that contains the largest volume of antitoxin that fails to protect the mice from death contains 10 I.U. This quantity is used to calculate the potency of the antitoxin in International Units per millilitre.

The test is not valid unless all the mice injected with mixtures containing 2.0 ml or less of the solution of the reference preparation die and all those injected with mixtures containing more survive.

STORAGE

See the monograph on *Immunosera for human use (84)*.

LABELLING

See the monograph on *Immunosera for human use (84)*.

Ph Eur

Mixed Gas-gangrene Antitoxin

Mixed Gas-gangrene Antitoxin complies with the requirements of the 3rd edition of the European Pharmacopoeia [0090]. These requirements are reproduced after the heading 'Definition' below.

The label may state 'Gas/Ser'.

Ph Eur

DEFINITION

Mixed gas-gangrene antitoxin is prepared by mixing gas-gangrene antitoxin (novyi), gas-gangrene antitoxin (perfringens) and gas-gangrene antitoxin (septicum) in appropriate quantities.

IDENTIFICATION

It specifically neutralises the alpha toxins formed by *Clostridium novyi* (former nomenclature: *Clostridium oedematiens*), *Clostridium perfringens* and *Clostridium septicum*, rendering them harmless to susceptible animals.

TESTS

It complies with the tests prescribed in the monograph on *Immunosera for human use (84)*.

ASSAY

Gas-gangrene antitoxin (novyi), not less than 1000 I.U. of antitoxin per millilitre; gas-gangrene antitoxin (perfringens), not less than 1000 I.U. of antitoxin per millilitre; gas-gangrene antitoxin (septicum) not less than 500 I.U. of antitoxin per millilitre.

Carry out the assay for each component, as prescribed in the monographs on *Gas-gangrene antitoxin (novyi) (87)*, *Gas-gangrene antitoxin (perfringens) (88)* and *Gas-gangrene antitoxin (septicum) (89)*.

STORAGE

See the monograph on *Immunosera for human use (84)*.

LABELLING

See the monograph on *Immunosera for human use (84)*.

Ph Eur

Scorpion Venom Antiserum

Definition Scorpion Venom Antiserum is a preparation containing antitoxic globulins that have the power of specifically neutralising the venom of one or more species of scorpion. The species of scorpion the venom or venoms of which the antiserum neutralises vary according to the geographical region in which the antiserum is intended to be used and for any particular region should include those species prevalent in that region.

The antiserum complies with the requirements stated under Antisera, with the following modifications.

Identification Specifically neutralises the venom or venoms of the one or more species of scorpion stated on the label, rendering them harmless to susceptible animals.

Total protein Not more than 17.0% w/v when determined by the method for *determination of protein in blood products*, Appendix VIII H, Method VI.

Abnormal toxicity Inject 0.5 ml intraperitoneally into each of two guinea-pigs. Neither of the animals dies or shows a significant local or systemic reaction within 7 days. If one of the animals dies or shows signs of ill-health during this time, repeat the test. Neither of the animals dies or shows a significant local or systemic reaction.

Potency In view of the numerous toxic fractions and venoms and the various requirements of different localities, no standard for potency is included.

The potency of scorpion venom antiserum should be such that the dose stated on the label will completely neutralise the maximum amount of venom likely to be delivered by a single sting. This is determined either by estimating the ability of the antiserum being examined to protect mice, or other suitable animals, against the lethal effect of a fixed dose of a standard venom of the relevant scorpion species or by comparing its ability to do so with that of a standard preparation of antiserum of established potency.

Labelling The label states (1) the nominal volume in the container; (2) the species of scorpion against the venom or venoms of which the antiserum is effective.

Tetanus Antitoxin

Tetanus Antitoxin complies with the requirements of the 3rd edition of the European Pharmacopoeia for Tetanus Antitoxin for Human Use [0091]. These requirements are reproduced after the heading 'Definition' below.

The label may state 'Tet/Ser'.

Ph Eur

DEFINITION

Tetanus antitoxin for human use is a preparation containing antitoxic globulins that have the power of specifically neutralising the toxin formed by *Clostridium tetani*.

PRODUCTION

It is obtained by fractionation from the serum of horses, or other mammals, that have been immunised against tetanus toxin.

IDENTIFICATION

It specifically neutralises the toxin formed by *Cl. tetani*, rendering it harmless to susceptible animals.

TESTS

It complies with the tests prescribed in the monograph on *Immunosera for human use (84)*.

POTENCY

Not less than 1000 I.U. of antitoxin per millilitre when intended for prophylactic use. Not less than 3000 I.U. of antitoxin per millilitre when intended for therapeutic use.

The potency of tetanus antitoxin is determined by comparing the dose necessary to protect guinea-pigs or mice against the paralytic effects of a fixed dose of tetanus toxin with the quantity of the standard preparation of tetanus antitoxin necessary to give the same protection. In countries where the paralysis method is not obligatory the lethal method may be used. For this method the number of animals and the procedure are identical with those described for the paralysis method but the end-point is the death of the animal rather than the onset of paralysis and the L+/10 dose is used instead of the Lp/10 dose. For this comparison a reference preparation of tetanus antitoxin, calibrated in International Units, and a suitable preparation of tetanus toxin, for use as a test toxin, are required. The potency of the test toxin is determined in relation to the reference preparation; the potency of the tetanus antitoxin to be examined is determined in relation to the potency of the test toxin by the same method.

The International Unit of antitoxin is the specific neutralising activity for tetanus toxin contained in a stated amount of the International Standard which consists of a quantity of dried immune horse serum. The equivalence in International Units of the International Standard is stated by the World Health Organisation.

Selection of animals. If mice are used, the body masses should be such that the difference between the lightest and the heaviest does not exceed 5 g.

Preparation of test toxin. Prepare the test toxin from a sterile filtrate of an approximately 9-day culture in liquid medium of *Cl. tetani*. To the filtrate add 1 to 2 volumes of glycerol and store slightly below 0°C. Alternatively, treat the filtrate with ammonium sulphate, collect the precipitate, which contains the toxin, dry *in vacuo* over *diphosphorus pentoxide R*, powder and store dry, either in sealed ampoules or *in vacuo* over *diphosphorus pentoxide R*.

Determination of test dose of toxin (Lp/10 dose). Prepare a solution of the reference preparation in a suitable liquid such that it contains 0.5 I.U. of antitoxin per millilitre.

If the test toxin is stored dry, reconstitute it using a suitable liquid.

Prepare mixtures of the solution of the reference preparation and the test toxin such that each contains 2.0 ml of the solution of the reference preparation, one of a graded series of volumes of the test toxin and sufficient of a suitable liquid to bring the volume to 5.0 ml. Allow the mixtures to stand at room temperature, protected from light, for 60 min. Using six mice for each mixture, inject a dose of 0.5 ml subcutaneously into each mouse. Observe the mice for 96 h. Mice that become paralysed may be killed.

The test dose of toxin is the quantity in 0.5 ml of the mixture made with the smallest amount of toxin capable of causing, despite partial neutralisation by the reference preparation, paralysis in all six mice injected with the mixture within the observation period.

Determination of potency of the antitoxin

Prepare a solution of the reference preparation in a suitable liquid such that it contains 0.5 I.U. of antitoxin per millilitre.

Prepare a solution of the test toxin in a suitable liquid such that it contains five test doses per millilitre.

Prepare mixtures of the solution of the test toxin and the antitoxin to be examined such that each contains 2.0 ml of the solution of the test toxin, one of a graded series of volumes of the antitoxin to be examined and sufficient of a suitable liquid to bring the total volume to 5.0 ml. Also prepare mixtures of the solution of the test toxin and the solution of the reference preparation such that each contains 2.0 ml of the solution of the test toxin, one of a graded series of volumes of the solution of the reference preparation centred on that volume (2.0 ml) that contains 1 I.U. and sufficient of a suitable liquid to bring the total volume to 5.0 ml. Allow the mixtures to stand at room temperature, protected from light, for 60 min. Using six mice for each mixture, inject into each mouse subcutaneously a dose of 0.5 ml. Observe the mice for 96 h. Mice that become paralysed may be killed.

The mixture that contains the largest volume of antitoxin that fails to protect the mice from paralysis contains 1 I.U. This quantity is used to calculate the potency of the antitoxin in International Units per millilitre.

The test is not valid unless all the mice injected with mixtures containing 2.0 ml or less of the solution of the reference preparation show paralysis and all those injected with mixtures containing more do not.

STORAGE

See *Immunosera for human use (84)*.

LABELLING

See *Immunosera for human use (84)*.

Ph Eur

VACCINES

A vaccine for human use that is the subject of an individual monograph in the European Pharmacopoeia or in the British Pharmacopoeia complies with the requirements of the 3rd edition of the European Pharmacopoeia for Vaccines for Human Use [0153]. These requirements are reproduced after the heading 'Definition' below.

The provisions of this monograph apply to the following vaccines:

Bacterial vaccines
Bacillus Calmette-Guérin Vaccine
Percutaneous Calmette-Guérin Vaccine
Cholera Vaccine
Haemophilus Type B Conjugate Vaccine
Meningococcal Polysaccharide Vaccine
Pertussis Vaccine
Pneumococcal Polysaccharide Vaccine
Tetanus Vaccine
Typhoid (Strain Ty 21a) Vaccine, Live (Oral)
Typhoid Polysaccharide Vaccine
Typhoid Vaccine

Bacterial toxoids
Adsorbed Diphtheria Vaccine
Adsorbed Diphtheria Vaccine for Adults and Adolescents
Adsorbed Tetanus Vaccine

Rickettsial vaccine
Typhus Vaccine

Viral vaccines
Inactivated Hepatitis A Vaccine
Hepatitis B Vaccine (rDNA)
Inactivated Influenza Vaccine (Whole Virion)
Inactivated Influenza Vaccine (Split Virion)
Inactivated Influenza Vaccine (Surface Antigen)
Measles Vaccine, Live
Mumps Vaccine, Live
Inactivated Poliomyelitis Vaccine
Poliomyelitis Vaccine, Live (Oral)
Rabies Vaccine
Rubella Vaccine, Live
Varicella Vaccine Live
Yellow Fever Vaccine

Mixed Vaccines
Adsorbed Diphtheria and Tetanus Vaccine
Adsorbed Diphtheria and Tetanus Vaccine for Adults and Adolescents
Adsorbed Diphtheria, Tetanus and Pertussis Vaccine
Measles, Mumps and Rubella Vaccine, Live
Typhoid and Tetanus Vaccine

Ph Eur

The statements in this monograph are intended to be read in conjunction with the monographs on vaccines for human use in the Pharmacopoeia. The requirements do not necessarily apply to vaccines which are not the subject of such monographs. For a combined vaccine, where there is no monograph to cover a particular combination, the vaccine complies with the monograph for each individual component, with any necessary modifications approved by the competent authority.

DEFINITION

Vaccines for human use are preparations containing antigenic substances capable of inducing a specific and active immunity in man against an infecting agent or the toxin or the antigen elaborated by it. They shall have been shown to have acceptable immunogenic activity in man with the intended vaccination schedule.

Vaccines for human use may contain: organisms inactivated by chemical or physical means that maintain adequate immunogenic properties; living organisms that are naturally avirulent or that have been treated to attenuate their virulence whilst retaining adequate immunogenic properties; antigens extracted from the organisms or secreted by them or produced by recombinant DNA technology; the antigens may be used in their native state or may be detoxified by chemical or physical means and may be aggregated, polymerised or conjugated to a carrier to increase their immunogenicity.

Terminology used in monographs on vaccines for human use is defined in chapter *5.2.1*.

Bacterial vaccines are suspensions of various degrees of opacity in colourless or almost colourless liquids, or may be freeze-dried. The concentration of living or inactivated bacteria is expressed in terms of International Units of Opacity or, where appropriate, is determined by direct cell count or, for living bacteria, by viable count.

Bacterial toxoids are prepared from toxins by diminishing their toxicity to a non-detectable level or by completely eliminating it by physical or chemical procedures whilst retaining adequate immunogenic properties. The toxins are obtained from selected strains of micro-organisms. The method of production is such that the toxoid does not revert to toxin.

Toxoids may be liquid or freeze-dried. They may be purified and adsorbed. Adsorbed toxoids are suspensions of white or grey particles dispersed in colourless or pale yellow liquids and may form a sediment at the bottom of the container.

Viral vaccines are prepared from viruses grown in animals, in fertilised eggs, in suitable cell cultures or in suitable tissues or by culture of genetically engineered cells. They are liquids that vary in opacity according to the type of preparation or may be freeze-dried. Liquid preparations and freeze-dried preparations after reconstitution may be coloured if a pH indicator such as phenol red has been used in the culture medium.

PRODUCTION

General provisions Requirements for production including in-process testing are included in individual monographs. Where justified and authorised, certain tests may be omitted where it can be demonstrated, for example by validation studies, that the production process consistently ensures compliance with the test.

Unless otherwise justified and authorised, vaccines are produced using a seed-lot system. The methods of preparation are designed to maintain adequate immunogenic properties, to render the preparation harmless and to prevent contamination with extraneous agents.

Vaccines produced by recombinant DNA technology comply with the monograph *Products of recombinant DNA technology (784)*.

Unless otherwise justified and authorised, in the production of a final lot of vaccine, the number of passages of a virus, or the number of subcultures of a bacterium, from the master seed lot shall not exceed that used for production of the vaccine shown in clinical studies to be satisfactory with respect to safety and efficacy.

Vaccines are as far as possible free from ingredients known to cause toxic, allergic or other undesirable reactions in man. Suitable additives, including stabilisers and adjuvants may be incorporated. Penicillin and streptomycin are not used at any stage of production nor added to the final product; however, master seed lots prepared with media containing penicillin or streptomycin may, where justified and authorised, be used for production.

Measures must be taken to avoid contamination of vaccines with the causal agents of spongiform encephalopathies, for example bovine spongiform encephalopathy. If material of bovine origin or from sheep is used for production, the source animals shall be free from spongiform encephalopathy and shall not have been exposed to risk factors such as feeding with ruminant protein. To achieve this objective, the animals shall come from certified sources. The relative infectivity and hence the potential risk associated with different tissues shall be taken into account in choosing the source of animal tissue to be used.

Substrates for propagation Substrates for propagation comply with the relevant requirements of the Pharmacopoeia (*5.2.2, 5.2.3*) or in the absence of such requirements with those of the competent authority. Processing of cell banks and subsequent cell cultures is done under aseptic conditions in an area where no other cells are being handled. Serum and trypsin used in the preparation of cell suspensions shall be shown to be free from extraneous agents.

Seed lots The strain of bacterium or virus used in a master seed lot is identified by historical records that include information on the origin of the strain and its subsequent manipulation. No micro-organism other than the seed strain shall be present in a seed lot.

Culture media Culture media are as far as possible free from ingredients known to cause toxic, allergic or other undesirable reactions in man; if inclusion of such ingredients is necessary, it shall be demonstrated that the amount present in the final lot is reduced to such a level as to render the product safe. Approved animal (but not human) serum may be used in the growth medium for cell cultures but the medium used for maintaining cell growth during virus multiplication shall not contain serum, unless otherwise stated. Cell culture media may contain a pH indicator such as phenol red and approved antibiotics at the lowest effective concentration although it is preferable to have a medium free from antibiotics during production.

Propagation and harvest The seed cultures are propagated and harvested under defined conditions. The purity of the harvest is verified by suitable tests as defined in the monograph.

Control cells For vaccines produced in cell cultures, control cells are maintained and tested as prescribed. In order to provide a valid control, these cells must be maintained in conditions that are rigorously identical with those used for the production cell cultures, including use of the same batches of media and media changes.

Control eggs For live vaccines produced in eggs, control eggs are incubated and tested as prescribed in the monograph.

Purification Where applicable, validated purification procedures may be applied.

Inactivation Inactivated vaccines are produced using a validated inactivation process whose effectiveness and consistency have been demonstrated. Where there are recognised potential contaminants of a harvest, for example in vaccines produced in eggs from healthy, non-SPF flocks, the inactivation process is also validated with respect to the potential contaminants. A test for inactivation is carried out as soon as possible after the inactivation process, unless otherwise justified and authorised.

Intermediates Where applicable, the stability of intermediates in given storage conditions shall be evaluated and a period of validity established.

Final bulk The final bulk is prepared by aseptically blending the ingredients of the vaccine.

Adsorbents. Vaccines may be adsorbed on aluminium hydroxide, aluminium phosphate, calcium phosphate or other suitable adsorbent; the adsorbents are prepared in special conditions which confer the appropriate physical form and adsorptive properties.

Antimicrobial preservative. A suitable antimicrobial preservative may be included in sterile and inactivated vaccines and is invariably added if these preparations are issued in multidose containers, unless otherwise stated. If an antimicrobial preservative is used, it shall be shown that it does not impair the safety or efficacy of the vaccine and its effectiveness throughout the period of validity shall be demonstrated.

Final lot For vaccines for parenteral administration, the final lot is prepared by aseptically distributing the final bulk into sterile tamper-proof containers which, after freeze-drying where applicable, are closed so as to exclude contamination. For vaccines for administration by a non-parenteral route, the final lot is prepared by distributing the final bulk under suitable conditions into sterile, tamper-proof containers.

Stability. Maintenance of potency of the final lot throughout the period of validity shall be demonstrated by validation studies; the loss of potency in the recommended storage conditions is assessed and excessive loss even within the limits of acceptable potency may indicate that the vaccine is unacceptable.

Degree of adsorption. During development of an adsorbed vaccine, the degree of adsorption is evaluated as part of the consistency testing. A release specification for the degree of adsorption is established in the light of results found for batches used in clinical testing. From the stability data generated for the vaccine it must be shown that at the end of the period of validity the degree of adsorption will not be less than for batches used in clinical testing.

TESTS

Vaccines comply with the tests prescribed in the particular monograph including, where applicable, the following:

Aluminium (*2.5.13*). Where an aluminium adsorbent has been used in the vaccine, not more than 1.25 mg of aluminium (Al) per single human dose, unless otherwise stated.

Calcium (*2.5.14*). Where a calcium adsorbent has been used in the vaccine, not more than 1.3 mg of calcium (Ca) per single human dose, unless otherwise stated.

Formaldehyde (*2.4.18*). Where formaldehyde has been used in the preparation of the vaccine, not more than 0.2 g/l of free formaldehyde is present in the final product, unless otherwise stated.

Phenol (*2.5.15*). Where phenol has been used in the preparation of the vaccine, not more than 2.5 g/l is present in the final product, unless otherwise stated.

Water (*2.5.12*). For freeze-dried vaccines, not more than 3.0 per cent *m/m*, unless otherwise stated.

STORAGE

Store protected from light. Unless otherwise stated, the storage temperature is 5 ± 3°C; liquid adsorbed vaccines must not be allowed to freeze.

Expiry date. Unless otherwise stated, the expiry date is calculated from the beginning of the assay. It applies to vaccines stored in the prescribed conditions.

LABELLING

The label states:
— the name of the preparation,
— a reference identifying the final lot,
— the recommended human dose and route of administration,
— the storage conditions,
— the expiry date,
— the name and amount of any antimicrobial preservative,
— the name of any antibiotic, adjuvant, flavour or stabiliser present in the vaccine,
— the name of any constituent that may cause adverse reactions and any contra-indications to the use of the vaccine,
— for freeze-dried vaccines:
— the name or composition and the volume of the reconstituting liquid to be added,
— the time within which the vaccine is to be used after reconstitution.

Ph Eur

Bacillus Calmette-Guérin Vaccine

BCG Vaccine

Bacillus Calmette-Guérin Vaccine complies with the requirements of the 3rd edition of the European Pharmacopoeia for Freeze-dried BCG Vaccine [0163]. These requirements are reproduced after the heading 'Definition' below.

The label may state 'Dried/Tub/Vac/BCG'.

Ph Eur

DEFINITION

Freeze-dried BCG vaccine is a preparation of live bacteria derived from a culture of the bacillus of Calmette and Guérin (*Mycobacterium bovis* BCG) whose capacity to protect against tuberculosis has been established.

PRODUCTION

BCG vaccine shall be produced by a staff consisting of healthy persons who do not work with other infectious agents; in particular they shall not work with virulent strains of *Mycobacterium tuberculosis,* nor shall they be exposed to a known risk of tuberculosis infection. BCG vaccine is susceptible to sunlight: the procedures for the preparation of the vaccine shall be so designed that all cultures and vaccines are protected from direct sunlight and from ultraviolet light at all stages of manufacture, testing and storage.

Production of the vaccine is based on a seed-lot system. The production method shall have been shown to yield consistently BCG vaccines that induce adequate sensitivity to tuberculin in man, that have acceptable protective potency in animals and are safe. The vaccine is prepared from cultures which are separated from the master seed lot by as few subcultures as possible and in any case not more than eight subcultures. During the course of these subcultures the preparation is not freeze-dried more than once.

BACTERIAL SEED LOTS

The strain used to establish the master seed lot is chosen for and maintained to preserve its stability, its capacity to sensitise man and guinea-pigs to tuberculin and to protect animals against tuberculosis, and its relative absence of pathogenicity for man and laboratory animals. The strain used shall be identified by historical records that include information on its origin and subsequent manipulation.

A suitable batch of vaccine is prepared from the first working seed lot and is reserved for use as the comparison vaccine. When a new working seed lot is established, a suitable test for delayed hypersensitivity in guinea-pigs is carried out on a batch of vaccine prepared from the new working seed lot; the vaccine is shown to be not significantly different in activity from the comparison vaccine.

Only a working seed lot that complies with the following requirements may be used for propagation.

Identification The bacteria in the working seed lot are identified as *Mycobacterium bovis* BCG.

Bacterial and fungal contamination Carry out the test for sterility (*2.6.1*), using 10 ml for each medium. The working seed lot complies with the test for sterility except for the presence of mycobacteria.

Virulent mycobacteria Examine the working seed lot as prescribed under Tests, using ten guinea-pigs.

Sensitisation of guinea-pigs The capacity of the working seed lot to induce sensitivity to tuberculin in guinea-pigs is demonstrated.

PROPAGATION AND HARVEST

The bacteria are grown in a suitable medium for not more than 21 days by surface or submerged culture. The culture medium shall contain no substances known to cause toxic or allergic reactions in human beings or to cause the bacteria to become virulent for guinea-pigs. The culture is harvested and suspended in a sterile liquid medium that protects the viability of the vaccine as determined by a suitable method of viable count.

FINAL BULK VACCINE

The final bulk vaccine is prepared from a single harvest or by pooling a number of single harvests. A stabiliser may be added; if the stabiliser interferes with the determination of bacterial concentration on the final bulk vaccine, the determination is carried out before addition of the stabiliser.

Only final bulk vaccine that complies with the following requirements may be used in the preparation of the final lot.

Virulent mycobacteria Examine as prescribed under Tests.

Bacterial and fungal contamination. Carry out the test for sterility (*2.6.1*), using 10 ml for each medium. The final bulk vaccine complies with the test for sterility except for the presence of mycobacteria.

Count of viable units Determine the number of viable units per millilitre by viable count on solid medium using a method suitable for the vaccine to be examined or by determination of adenosine triphosphate by a bioluminescence reaction. Carry out the test in parallel on a reference preparation of the same strain.

Bacterial concentration Determine the total bacterial concentration by a suitable method, either directly by determining the mass of the micro-organisms, or indirectly by an opacity method that has been calibrated in relation to the mass of the organisms; if the bacterial concentration is determined before addition of a stabiliser, the concentration in the final bulk vaccine is established by calculation. The total bacterial concentration is within the limits approved for the particular product.

The ratio of the count of viable units to the total bacterial concentration is not less than that approved for the particular product.

FINAL LOT

The final bulk vaccine is distributed into sterile containers and freeze-dried to a moisture content favourable to the stability of the vaccine; the containers are closed either under vacuum or under a gas that is not deleterious to the vaccine.

Except where the filled and closed containers are stored at a temperature of −20°C or lower, the expiry date is not later than 4 years from the date of harvest.

Only a final lot that complies with the following requirement for count of viable units and with each of the requirements given below under Identification, Tests and Assay may be released for use. Provided the test for virulent mycobacteria has been carried out with satisfactory results on the final bulk vaccine, it may be omitted on the final lot. Provided the test for excessive dermal reactivity has been carried out with satisfactory results on the working seed lot and on five consecutive final lots produced from it, the test may be omitted on the final lot.

Count of viable units Determine the number of viable units per millilitre of the reconstituted vaccine by viable count on solid medium using a method suitable for the vaccine to be examined or by determination of adenosine triphosphate by a bioluminescence reaction. The ratio of the count of viable units after freeze-drying to that before is not less than that approved for the particular product.

IDENTIFICATION

BCG vaccine is identified by microscopic examination of the bacilli in stained smears demonstrating their acid-fast property and by the characteristic appearance of colonies grown on solid medium.

TESTS

Virulent mycobacteria Inject subcutaneously or intramuscularly into each of six guinea-pigs, each weighing 250 g to 400 g and having received no treatment likely to interfere with the test, a quantity of vaccine equivalent to at least fifty human doses. Observe the animals for at least 42 days. At the end of this period, kill the guinea-pigs and examine by autopsy for signs of infection with tuberculosis, ignoring any minor reactions at the site of injection. Animals that die during the observation period are also examined for signs of tuberculosis. The vaccine complies with the test if none of the guinea-pigs shows signs of tuberculosis and if not more than one animal dies during the observation period. If two animals die during this period and autopsy does not reveal signs of tuberculosis repeat the test on six other guinea-pigs. The vaccine complies with the test if not more than one animal dies during the 42 days following the injection and autopsy does not reveal any sign of tuberculosis.

Bacterial and fungal contamination The reconstituted vaccine complies with the test for sterility (*2.6.1*) except for the presence of mycobacteria.

Excessive dermal reactivity Use six healthy white or pale-coloured guinea-pigs, each weighing not less than 250 g and having received no treatment likely to interfere with the test. Inject intradermally into each guinea-pig, according to a randomised plan, 0.1 ml of the reconstituted vaccine and of two tenfold serial dilutions of the vaccine and identical doses of the comparison vaccine. Observe the lesions formed at the site of the injection for 4 weeks. The vaccine complies with the test if the reaction it produces is not markedly different from that produced by the comparison vaccine.

Temperature stability Maintain samples of the freeze-dried vaccine at 37°C for 4 weeks. Determine the number of viable units in the heated vaccine and in unheated vaccine as described below. The number of viable units in the heated vaccine is not less than 20 per cent that in unheated vaccine.

Water (*2.5.12*). Not more than 3.0 per cent, determined by the semi-micro determination of water.

ASSAY

Determine the number of viable units in the reconstituted vaccine by viable count on solid medium using a method suitable for the vaccine to be examined. The number is within the range stated on the label. Determine the number of viable units in the comparison vaccine in parallel.

STORAGE

See *Vaccines for human use (153)*.

LABELLING

See *Vaccines for human use (153)*.

The label states:

- the minimum and maximum number of viable units per millilitre in the reconstituted vaccine,
- that the vaccine must be protected from direct sunlight,
- that the vaccine is to be used immediately after broaching the container and any residue is to be discarded,
- the age group for which the vaccine is intended,
- the dose for each age group.

Ph Eur

Percutaneous Bacillus Calmette-Guérin Vaccine

Percut. BCG Vaccine

Definition Percutaneous Bacillus Calmette-Guérin Vaccine is a suspension of living cells of an authentic strain of the bacillus of Calmette and Guérin with a higher viable bacterial count than Bacillus Calmette-Guérin Vaccine. It is prepared immediately before use by reconstitution from the dried vaccine with an appropriate volume of a suitable sterile liquid.

Production Production is based on an approved seed-lot system. The strain is chosen for and maintained to preserve its stability, its capacity to sensitise man and guinea-pigs to tuberculin and to protect animals against tuberculosis and its relative absence of pathogenicity for man and laboratory animals. A suitable batch of vaccine is prepared from the seed lot and is reserved for use as the comparison vaccine in the tests prescribed below.

The dried vaccine is prepared by the following method. The bacilli are grown in or on a suitable medium for not more than 14 days. The harvested growth, diluted if necessary to a suitable concentration, is suspended in a sterile liquid medium designed to preserve the antigenicity and viability of the vaccine and freeze dried.

The vaccine, reconstituted as stated on the label, complies with the requirements stated under Vaccines, with the following modifications.

Identification

A. When examined microscopically in stained smears, the bacilli exhibit the characteristics of an authentic strain of the bacillus of Calmette and Guérin.

B. Colonies grown on a suitable solid culture medium have a characteristic appearance.

Skin-sensitising potency Prepare a 25-fold dilution of the vaccine using an appropriate sterile liquid. Inject 0.5 ml subcutaneously or intramuscularly into each of two guinea-pigs. Within 4 weeks of injection, inject intracutaneously into each guinea-pig 10 Units of Old Tuberculin, or of Tuberculin Purified Protein Derivative, in a volume of 0.1 ml. An inflammatory area of induration and oedema not less than 5 mm in diameter, irrespective of the area of erythema, is induced within 24 hours.

Excessive reactivity Inject intracutaneously into each of two guinea-pigs, in a volume of 0.1 ml, 1, 0.1, 0.01 and 0.001 doses of the vaccine being tested and of the comparison vaccine. Use an appropriate sterile liquid as diluent. The vaccine passes the test if the skin reactions produced within 3 weeks do not differ markedly from those produced by the comparison vaccine.

Sterility Complies with the *test for sterility*, Appendix XVI A, except for the presence of mycobacteria.

Virulent mycobacteria Prepare a 5-fold dilution of the vaccine using an appropriate sterile liquid. Inject 1 ml intramuscularly into each of six guinea-pigs weighing 250 to 400 g. None of the animals dies within 42 days or if one dies, a post-mortem examination establishes that it is free from tuberculosis. If two of the animals die within this period and a post-mortem examination establishes that both are free from tuberculosis, repeat the test on six further guinea-pigs. None of the second group of animals dies within 42 days or, if one dies, a post mortem examination establishes that it is free from tuberculosis.

Storage When stored under the prescribed conditions the dried vaccine may be expected to retain its potency for at least 2 years. When reconstituted the vaccine should be used immediately.

Labelling The label states (1) 'Tub/Vac/BCG(Perc)'; (2) that the vaccine is a living culture of the bacillus of Calmette and Guérin; (3) that any portion of the reconstituted vaccine not used at once should be discarded; (4) that the vaccine is for percutaneous administration and must not be given by the intradermal route.

Cholera Vaccine

When Cholera Vaccine is issued as a liquid, it complies with the requirements of the 3rd edition of the European Pharmacopoeia for Cholera Vaccine [0154]. These requirements are reproduced after the heading 'Liquid Vaccine' below.

When Cholera Vaccine is prepared immediately before use by reconstitution from the dried vaccine, the dried vaccine complies with the requirements of the 3rd edition of the European Pharmacopoeia for Freeze-dried Cholera Vaccine [0155]. These requirements are reproduced after the heading 'Dried Vaccine' below.

The label may state 'Cho/Vac' or 'Dried/Cho/Vac', as appropriate.

Ph Eur

LIQUID VACCINE [0154]

DEFINITION

Cholera vaccine is a homogeneous suspension of a suitable strain or strains of *Vibrio cholerae* containing not less than 8×10^9 bacteria in each human dose. The human dose does not exceed 1.0 ml.

PRODUCTION

The vaccine is prepared using a seed-lot system.

The vaccine consists of a mixture of equal parts of vaccines prepared from smooth strains of the two main serological types, Inaba and Ogawa. These may be of the classical biotype with or without the El-Tor biotype. A single strain or several strains of each type may be included. All strains must contain, in addition to their type O antigens, the heat-stable O antigen common to Inaba and Ogawa. If more than one strain each of Inaba and Ogawa are used, these may be selected so as to contain other O antigens in addition. The World Health Organisation recommends new strains which may be used if necessary, in accordance with the regulations in force in the signatory States of the Convention on the Elaboration of a European Pharmacopoeia. In order to comply with the requirements for vaccination certificates required for international travel, the vaccine must contain not less than 8×10^9 organisms of the classical biotype.

Each strain is grown separately. The bacteria are inactivated either by heating the suspensions (for example, at 56°C for 1 h) or by treatment with formaldehyde or phenol or by a combination of the physical and chemical methods.

The production method is validated to demonstrate that the product, if tested, would comply with the test for abnormal toxicity for immunosera and vaccines for human use (*2.6.9*) modified as follows: inject 0.5 ml of the vaccine into each mouse and 1.0 ml into each guinea-pig.

IDENTIFICATION

It is identified by specific agglutination tests.

TESTS

Phenol (*2.5.15*). If phenol has been used in the preparation, the concentration is not more than 5 g/l.

Antibody production Test the ability of the vaccine to induce antibodies (such as agglutinating, vibriocidal or haemagglutinating antibodies) in the guinea-pig, the rabbit or the mouse. Administer the vaccine to a group of at least six animals. At the end of the interval of time necessary for maximum antibody formation, determined in preliminary tests, collect sera from the animals and titrate them individually for the appropriate antibody using a suitable method. The vaccine to be examined passes the test if each serotype has elicited a significant antibody response.

Sterility (*2.6.1*). It complies with the test for sterility.

STORAGE

See *Vaccines for human use (153)*.

LABELLING

See *Vaccines for human use (153)*.

The label states:
— the method used to inactivate the bacteria,
— the number of bacteria in each human dose.

DRIED VACCINE [0155]

DEFINITION

Freeze-dried cholera vaccine is a preparation of a suitable strain or strains of *Vibrio cholerae*. The vaccine is reconstituted as stated on the label to give a uniform suspension containing not less than 8×10^9 bacteria in each human dose. The human dose does not exceed 1.0 ml of the reconstituted vaccine.

PRODUCTION

The vaccine is prepared using a seed-lot system.

The vaccine consists of a mixture of equal parts of vaccines prepared from smooth strains of the two main serological types, Inaba and Ogawa. These may be of the classical biotype with or without the El-Tor biotype. A single strain or several strains of each type may be included. All strains must contain, in addition to their type O antigens, the heat-stable O antigen common to Inaba and Ogawa. If more than one strain each of Inaba and Ogawa are used, these may be selected so as to contain other O antigens in addition. The World Health Organisation recommends new strains which may be used if necessary in accordance with the regulations in force in the signatory States of the Convention on the Elaboration of a European Pharmacopoeia. In order to comply with the requirements for vaccination certificates required for international travel, the vaccine must contain not less than 8×10^9 organisms of the classical biotype.

Each strain is grown separately. The bacteria are inactivated either by heating the suspensions (for example, at 56°C for 1 h) or by treatment with formaldehyde or by a combination of the physical and chemical methods. Phenol is not used in the preparation. The vaccine is distributed into sterile containers and freeze-dried to a moisture content favourable to the stability of the vaccine. The containers are then closed so as to exclude contamination.

The production method is validated to demonstrate that the product, if tested, would comply with the test for abnormal toxicity for immunosera and vaccines for human use (*2.6.9*) modified as follows: inject 0.5 ml of the vaccine into each mouse and 1.0 ml into each guinea-pig.

IDENTIFICATION

The vaccine reconstituted as stated on the label is identified by specific agglutination tests.

TESTS

The reconstituted vaccine complies with the tests prescribed in the monograph on *Cholera vaccine (154)*.

STORAGE

See *Vaccines for human use (153)*.

LABELLING

See *Vaccines for human use (153)*.

The label states:
— the method used to inactivate the bacteria,
— the number of bacteria in each human dose.

Adsorbed Diphtheria Vaccine

Adsorbed Diphtheria Prophylactic

Adsorbed Diphtheria Vaccine complies with the requirements of the 3rd edition of the European Pharmacopoeia for Diphtheria Vaccine (Adsorbed) [0443]. These requirements are reproduced after the heading 'Definition' below.

The label may state 'Dip/Vac/Ads(Child)'.

Ph Eur

DEFINITION

Diphtheria vaccine (adsorbed) is a preparation of diphtheria formol toxoid adsorbed on a mineral carrier. The formol toxoid is prepared from the toxin produced by the growth of *Corynebacterium diphtheriae*.

PRODUCTION

BULK PURIFIED TOXOID

For the production of diphtheria toxin, from which toxoid is prepared, seed cultures are managed in a defined seed-lot system in which toxinogenicity is conserved and, where necessary, restored by deliberate reselection. A highly toxinogenic strain of *Corynebacterium diphtheriae* with known origin and history is grown in a suitable liquid medium. At the end of cultivation, the purity of each culture is tested and contaminated cultures are discarded. Toxin-containing culture medium is separated aseptically from the bacterial mass as soon as possible. The toxin content (Lf per millilitre) is checked to monitor consistency of production. Single harvests may be pooled to prepare the bulk purified toxoid. The toxin is purified to remove components likely to cause adverse reactions in humans. The purified toxin is detoxified with formaldehyde by a method that avoids destruction of the immunogenic potency of the toxoid and reversion of the toxoid to toxin, particularly on exposure to heat. Alternatively, purification may be carried out after detoxification.

Only bulk purified toxoid that complies with the following requirements may be used in the preparation of the final bulk vaccine.

Sterility (*2.6.1*). Carry out the test for sterility using 10 ml for each medium.

Absence of diphtheria toxin Inject subcutaneously at least 500 Lf of purified toxoid in a volume of 1 ml into each of five healthy guinea-pigs, each weighing 250 g to 350 g, that have not previously been treated with any material that will interfere with the test. If within 42 days of the injection any of the animals shows signs of or dies from diphtheria toxaemia, the toxoid does not comply with the test. If more than one animal dies from non-specific causes, repeat the test once; if more than one animal dies in the second test, the toxoid does not comply with the test.

Irreversibility of toxoid Using the buffer for the final vaccine without adsorbent, prepare a dilution of the bulk purified toxoid containing the same toxoid concentration as the final vaccine. Divide the dilution into two equal parts. Keep one of them at 5 ± 3°C and the other at 37°C for 6 weeks. Test both samples by a suitable sensitive assay for active diphtheria toxin such as inoculation on to cell cultures or intradermal injection into guinea-pigs. The toxoid complies with the test if neither sample produces any sign of a toxic reaction attributable to diphtheria toxin.

Antigenic purity Not less than 1500 Lf per milligram of protein nitrogen.

FINAL BULK VACCINE

The final bulk vaccine is prepared by adsorption of a suitable quantity of bulk purified toxoid onto hydrated aluminium phosphate, aluminium hydroxide or calcium phosphate; the resulting mixture is approximately isotonic with blood. Suitable antimicrobial preservatives may be added. Certain antimicrobial preservatives, particularly those of the phenolic type, adversely affect the antigenic activity and must not be used.

Only final bulk vaccine that complies with the following requirements may be used in the preparation of the final lot.

Antimicrobial preservative Where applicable, determine the amount of antimicrobial preservative by a suitable chemical method. The amount is not less than 85 per cent and not greater than 115 per cent of the intended amount.

Sterility (*2.6.1*). Carry out the test for sterility using 10 ml for each medium.

Potency Carry out the test described under Assay.

FINAL LOT

The final bulk vaccine is distributed aseptically into sterile, tamper-proof containers. The containers are closed so as to prevent contamination.

Only a final lot that is satisfactory with respect to each of the requirements given below under Identification, Tests and Assay may be released for use. Provided the tests for specific toxicity, free formaldehyde and antimicrobial preservative and the assay have been carried out with satisfactory results on the final bulk vaccine, they may be omitted on the final lot.

IDENTIFICATION

Dissolve in the vaccine to be examined sufficient *sodium citrate R* to give a 100 g/l solution. Maintain at 37°C for about 16 h and centrifuge until a clear supernatant liquid is obtained. The clear supernatant liquid reacts with a suitable diphtheria antitoxin, giving a precipitate.

TESTS

Specific toxicity Inject subcutaneously five times the single human dose stated on the label into each of five healthy guinea-pigs, each weighing 250 g to 350 g, that have not previously been treated with any material that will interfere with the test. If within 42 days of the injection any of the animals shows signs of or dies from diphtheria toxaemia, the vaccine does not comply with the test. If more than one animal dies from non-specific causes, repeat the test once; if more than one animal dies in the second test, the vaccine does not comply with the test.

Aluminium When hydrated aluminium phosphate or aluminium hydroxide is used as the adsorbent, the vaccine complies with the test prescribed in the monograph on *Vaccines for human use (153)*.

Calcium When calcium phosphate is used as the adsorbent, the vaccine complies with the test prescribed in the monograph on *Vaccines for human use (153)*.

Free formaldehyde The vaccine complies with the test prescribed in the monograph on *Vaccines for human use (153)*.

Antimicrobial preservative Where applicable, determine the amount of antimicrobial preservative by a suitable chemical method. The content is not less than the minimum amount shown to be effective and is not greater than 115 per cent of the quantity stated on the label.

Sterility (*2.6.1*). The vaccine complies with the test for sterility.

ASSAY

Carry out one of the prescribed methods for the assay of diphtheria vaccine (adsorbed) (*2.7.6*).

The lower confidence limit ($P = 0.95$) of the estimated potency is not less than 30 I.U. per single human dose.

STORAGE

See *Vaccines for human use (153)*.

LABELLING

See *Vaccines for human use (153)*.

The label states:

- the minimum number of International Units per single human dose,
- where applicable, that the vaccine is intended for primary vaccination of children and is not necessarily suitable for reinforcing doses or for administration to adults,
- the name and the amount of the adsorbent,
- that the vaccine must be shaken before use,
- that the vaccine is not to be frozen.

Ph Eur

Adsorbed Diphtheria Vaccine for Adults and Adolescents

Adsorbed Diphtheria Vaccine for Adults and Adolescents complies with the requirements of the 3rd edition of the European Pharmacopoeia for Diphtheria Vaccine (Adsorbed) for Adults and Adolescents [0646]. These requirements are reproduced after the heading 'Definition' below..

The label may state 'Dip/Vac/Ads(Adult)'.

For a vaccine for use in the United Kingdom, the amount of toxoid used is adjusted so that the final vaccine contains not more than 2.0 flocculation equivalents (2.0 Lf) per dose.

Ph Eur

DEFINITION

Diphtheria vaccine (adsorbed) for adults and adolescents is a preparation of diphtheria formol toxoid adsorbed on a mineral carrier. The formol toxoid is prepared from the toxin produced by the growth of *Corynebacterium diphtheriae*. It shall have been demonstrated to the competent authority that the quantity of diphtheria toxoid used does not produce adverse reactions in subjects from the age groups for which the vaccine is intended.

PRODUCTION

BULK PURIFIED TOXOID

For the production of diphtheria toxin, from which toxoid is prepared, seed cultures are managed in a defined seed-lot system in which toxinogenicity is conserved and, where necessary, restored by deliberate reselection. A highly toxinogenic strain of *Corynebacterium diphtheriae* with known origin and history is grown in a suitable liquid medium. At the end of cultivation, the purity of each culture is tested and contaminated cultures are discarded. Toxin-containing culture medium is separated aseptically from the bacterial mass as soon as possible. The toxin content (Lf per millilitre) is checked to monitor consistency of production. Single harvests may be pooled to prepare the bulk purified toxoid. The toxin is purified to remove components likely to cause adverse reactions in humans. The purified toxin is detoxified with formaldehyde by a method that avoids destruction of the immunogenic potency of the toxoid and reversion of the toxoid to toxin, particularly on exposure to heat. Alternatively, purification may be carried out after detoxification.

Only bulk purified toxoid that complies with the following requirements may be used in the preparation of the final bulk vaccine.

Sterility (*2.6.1*). Carry out the test for sterility using 10 ml for each medium.

Absence of diphtheria toxin Inject subcutaneously at least 500 Lf of purified toxoid in a volume of 1 ml into each of five healthy guinea-pigs, each weighing 250 g to 350 g, that have not previously been treated with any material that will interfere with the test. If within 42 days of the injection any of the animals shows signs of or dies from diphtheria toxaemia, the toxoid does not comply with the test. If more than one animal dies from non-specific causes, repeat the test once; if more than one animal dies in the second test, the toxoid does not comply with the test.

Irreversibility of toxoid Using the buffer for the final vaccine without adsorbent, prepare a dilution of the bulk purified toxoid containing the same toxoid concentration as the final vaccine. Divide the dilution into two equal parts. Keep one of them at 5 ± 3°C and the other at 37°C for 6 weeks. Test both samples by a suitable sensitive assay for active diphtheria toxin such as inoculation on to cell cultures or intradermal injection into guinea-pigs. The toxoid complies with the test if neither sample produces any sign of a toxic reaction attributable to diphtheria toxin.

Antigenic purity Not less than 1500 Lf per milligram of protein nitrogen.

FINAL BULK VACCINE

The final bulk vaccine is prepared by adsorption of a suitable quantity of bulk purified toxoid onto hydrated aluminium phosphate, aluminium hydroxide or calcium phosphate; the resulting mixture is approximately isotonic with blood. Suitable antimicrobial preservatives may be added. Certain antimicrobial preservatives, particularly those of the phenolic type, adversely affect the antigenic activity and must not be used.

Only final bulk vaccine that complies with the following requirements may be used in the preparation of the final lot.

Antimicrobial preservative Where applicable, determine the amount of antimicrobial preservative by a suitable chemical method. The amount is not less than 85 per cent and not greater than 115 per cent of the intended amount.

Sterility (*2.6.1*). Carry out the test for sterility using 10 ml for each medium.

Potency Carry out the test described under Potency.

FINAL LOT

The final bulk vaccine is distributed aseptically into sterile, tamper-proof containers. The containers are closed so as to prevent contamination.

Only a final lot that is satisfactory with respect to each of the requirements given below under Identification, Tests and Potency may be released for use. Provided the tests for specific toxicity, free formaldehyde and antimicrobial preservative and the determination of potency have been carried out with satisfactory results on the final bulk vaccine, they may be omitted on the final lot.

IDENTIFICATION

Dissolve in the vaccine to be examined sufficient *sodium citrate R* to give a 100 g/l solution. Maintain at 37°C for about 16 h and centrifuge until a clear supernatant liquid is obtained. The clear supernatant liquid reacts with a suitable diphtheria antitoxin, giving a precipitate. If a satisfactory result is not obtained with a vaccine adsorbed on aluminium hydroxide, carry out the test as follows. Centrifuge 15 ml of the vaccine to be examined and suspend the residue in 5 ml of a freshly prepared mixture of 1 volume of a 56 g/l solution of *sodium edetate R* and 49 volumes of a 90 g/l solution of *disodium hydrogen phosphate R*. Maintain at 37°C for not less than 6 h and centrifuge. The clear supernatant liquid reacts with a suitable diphtheria antitoxin, giving a precipitate.

TESTS

Specific toxicity Inject subcutaneously five times the single human dose stated on the label into each of five healthy guinea-pigs, each weighing 250 g to 350 g, that have not previously been treated with any material that will interfere with the test. If within 42 days of the injection any of the animals shows signs of or dies from diphtheria toxaemia, the vaccine does not comply with the test. If more than one animal dies from non-specific causes, repeat the test once; if more than one animal dies in the second test, the vaccine does not comply with the test.

Aluminium When hydrated aluminium phosphate or aluminium hydroxide is used as the adsorbent, the vaccine complies with the test prescribed in the monograph on *Vaccines for human use (153)*.

Calcium When calcium phosphate is used as the adsorbent, the vaccine complies with the test prescribed in the monograph on *Vaccines for human use (153)*.

Free formaldehyde The vaccine complies with the test prescribed in the monograph on *Vaccines for human use (153)*.

Antimicrobial preservative Where applicable, determine the amount of antimicrobial preservative by a suitable chemical method. The content is not less than the minimum amount shown to be effective and is not greater than 115 per cent of the quantity stated on the label.

Sterility (*2.6.1*). The vaccine complies with the test for sterility.

ASSAY

Carry out one of the prescribed methods for the assay of diphtheria vaccine (adsorbed) (*2.7.6*).

The lower confidence limit ($P = 0.95$) of the estimated potency is not less than 2 I.U. per single human dose.

STORAGE

See *Vaccines for human use (153)*.

LABELLING

See *Vaccines for human use (153)*.

The label states:
- the minimum number of International Units per single human dose,
- the name and the amount of the adsorbent,
- that the vaccine must be shaken before use,
- that the vaccine is not to be frozen.

Adsorbed Diphtheria and Tetanus Vaccine

Adsorbed Diphtheril—Tetanus Prophylactic

Adsorbed Diphtheria and Tetanus Vaccine complies with the requirements of the 3rd edition of the European Pharmacopoeia for Diphtheria and Tetanus Vaccine (Adsorbed).[0444]. These requirements are reproduced after the heading 'Definition' below.

The label may state 'DT/Vac/Ads(Child)'.

Ph Eur

DEFINITION

Diphtheria and tetanus vaccine (adsorbed) is a preparation of diphtheria formol toxoid and tetanus formol toxoid adsorbed on a mineral carrier. The formol toxoids are prepared from the toxins produced by the growth of *Corynebacterium diphtheriae* and *Clostridium tetani*, respectively.

PRODUCTION

BULK PURIFIED DIPHTHERIA TOXOID

For the production of diphtheria toxin, from which toxoid is prepared, seed cultures are managed in a defined seed-lot system in which toxinogenicity is conserved and, where necessary, restored by deliberate reselection. A highly toxinogenic strain of *Corynebacterium diphtheriae* with known origin and history is grown in a suitable liquid medium. At the end of cultivation, the purity of each culture is tested and contaminated cultures are discarded. Toxin-containing culture medium is separated aseptically from the bacterial mass as soon as possible. The toxin content (Lf per millilitre) is checked to monitor consistency of production. Single harvests may be pooled to prepare the bulk purified toxoid. The toxin is purified to remove components likely to cause adverse reactions in humans. The purified toxin is detoxified with formaldehyde by a method that avoids destruction of the immunogenic potency of the toxoid and reversion of the toxoid to toxin, particularly on exposure to heat. Alternatively, purification may be carried out after detoxification.

Only bulk purified toxoid that complies with the following requirements may be used in the preparation of the final bulk vaccine.

Sterility (*2.6.1*). Carry out the test for sterility using 10 ml for each medium.

Absence of diphtheria toxin Inject subcutaneously at least 500 Lf of purified toxoid in a volume of 1 ml into each of five healthy guinea-pigs, each weighing 250 g to 350 g, that have not previously been treated with any material that will interfere with the test. If within 42 days of the injection any of the animals shows signs of or dies from diphtheria toxaemia, the toxoid does not comply with the test. If more than one animal dies from non-specific causes, repeat the test once; if more than one animal dies in the second test, the toxoid does not comply with the test.

Irreversibility of toxoid Using the buffer for the final vaccine without adsorbent, prepare a dilution of the bulk purified toxoid containing the same toxoid concentration as the final vaccine. Divide the dilution into two equal parts. Keep one of them at 5 ± 3°C and the other at 37°C for 6 weeks. Test both samples by a suitable sensitive assay for active diphtheria toxin such as inoculation on to cell cultures or intradermal injection into guinea-pigs. The toxoid complies with the test if neither sample produces any sign of a toxic reaction attributable to diphtheria toxin.

Antigenic purity Not less than 1500 Lf per milligram of protein nitrogen.

BULK PURIFIED TETANUS TOXOID

For the production of tetanus toxin, from which toxoid is prepared, seed cultures are managed in a defined seed-lot system in which toxinogenicity is conserved and, where necessary, restored by deliberate reselection. A highly toxinogenic strain of *Clostridium tetani* with known origin and history is grown in a suitable liquid medium. At the end of cultivation, the purity of each culture is tested and contaminated cultures are discarded. Toxin-containing culture medium is collected aseptically. The toxin content (Lf per millilitre) is checked to monitor consistency of production. Single harvests may be pooled to prepare the bulk purified toxoid. The toxin is purified to remove components likely to cause adverse reactions in humans. The purified toxin is detoxified with formaldehyde by a method that avoids destruction of the immunogenic potency of the toxoid and reversion of toxoid to toxin, particularly on exposure to heat. Alternatively, purification may be carried out after detoxification.

Only bulk purified toxoid that complies with the following requirements may be used in the preparation of the final bulk vaccine.

Sterility (*2.6.1*). Carry out the test for sterility using 10 ml for each medium.

Absence of tetanus toxin Inject subcutaneously at least 500 Lf of purified toxoid in a volume of 1 ml into each of five healthy guinea-pigs, each weighing 250 g to 350 g, that have not previously been treated with any material that will interfere with the test. If within 21 days of the injection any of the animals shows signs of or dies from tetanus, the toxoid does not comply with the test. If more than one animal dies from non-specific causes, repeat the test once; if more than one animal dies in the second test, the toxoid does not comply with the test.

Irreversibility of toxoid Using the buffer for the final vaccine without adsorbent, prepare a dilution of the bulk purified toxoid containing the same toxoid concentration as the final vaccine. Divide the dilution into two equal parts. Keep one of them at 5 ± 3°C and the other at 37°C for 6 weeks. Test both dilutions by a suitable sensitive assay for active tetanus toxin, such as inoculation into mice or guinea-pigs. The toxoid complies with the test if neither sample produces any sign of a toxic reaction attributable to tetanus toxin.

Antigenic purity Not less than 1000 Lf per milligram of protein nitrogen.

FINAL BULK VACCINE

The final bulk vaccine is prepared by adsorption of suitable quantities of bulk purified diphtheria toxoid and tetanus toxoid onto hydrated aluminium phosphate, aluminium hydroxide or calcium phosphate; the resulting mixture is approximately isotonic with blood. Suitable antimicrobial preservatives may be added. Certain antimicrobial preservatives, particularly those of the phenolic type, adversely affect the antigenic activity and must not be used.

Only final bulk vaccine that complies with the following requirements may be used in the preparation of the final lot.

Antimicrobial preservative Where applicable, determine the amount of antimicrobial preservative by a suitable chemical method. The amount is not less than 85 per cent and not greater than 115 per cent of the intended amount.

Sterility (*2.6.1*). Carry out the test for sterility using 10 ml for each medium.

Potency Carry out the tests described under Assay.

FINAL LOT

The final bulk vaccine is distributed aseptically into sterile, tamper-proof containers. The containers are closed so as to prevent contamination.

Only a final lot that is satisfactory with respect to each of the requirements given below under Identification, Tests and Assay may be released for use. Provided the tests for specific toxicity, free formaldehyde and antimicrobial preservative and the assay have been carried out with satisfactory results on the final bulk vaccine, they may be omitted on the final lot.

IDENTIFICATION

A. Dissolve in the vaccine to be examined sufficient *sodium citrate R* to give a 100 g/l solution. Maintain at 37°C for about 16 h and centrifuge until a clear supernatant liquid is obtained. The clear supernatant liquid reacts with a suitable diphtheria antitoxin, giving a precipitate.

B. The clear supernatant liquid obtained during test A reacts with a suitable tetanus antitoxin, giving a precipitate.

TESTS

Specific toxicity Inject subcutaneously five times the single human dose stated on the label into each of five healthy guinea-pigs, each weighing 250 g to 350 g, that have not previously been treated with any material that will interfere with the test. If within 42 days of the injection any of the animals shows signs of or dies from diphtheria toxaemia or tetanus, the vaccine does not comply with the test. If more than one animal dies from non-specific causes, repeat the test once; if more than one animal dies in the second test, the vaccine does not comply with the test.

Aluminium When hydrated aluminium phosphate or aluminium hydroxide is used as the adsorbent, the vaccine complies with the test prescribed in the monograph on *Vaccines for human use (153)*.

Calcium When calcium phosphate is used as the adsorbent, the vaccine complies with the test prescribed in the monograph on *Vaccines for human use (153)*.

Free formaldehyde The vaccine complies with the test prescribed in the monograph on *Vaccines for human use (153)*.

Antimicrobial preservative Where applicable, determine the amount of antimicrobial preservative by a suitable chemical method. The content is not less than the minimum amount shown to be effective and is not greater than 115 per cent of the quantity stated on the label.

Sterility (*2.6.1*). The vaccine complies with the test for sterility.

ASSAY

Diphtheria component Carry out one of the prescribed methods for the assay of diphtheria vaccine (adsorbed) (*2.7.6*).

The lower confidence limit ($P = 0.95$) of the estimated potency is not less than 30 I.U. per single human dose.

Tetanus component Carry out one of the prescribed methods for the assay of tetanus vaccine (adsorbed) (*2.7.8*).

The lower confidence limit ($P = 0.95$) of the estimated potency is not less than 40 I.U. per single human dose.

STORAGE

See *Vaccines for human use (153)*.

LABELLING

See *Vaccines for human use (153)*.

The label states:

— the minimum number of International Units of each component per single human dose,

— where applicable, that the vaccine is intended for primary vaccination of children and is not necessarily suitable for reinforcing doses or for administration to adults,

— the name and the amount of the adsorbent,

— that the vaccine must be shaken before use,

— that the vaccine is not to be frozen.

Ph Eur

Adsorbed Diphtheria and Tetanus Vaccine for Adults and Adolescents

Adsorbed Diphtheria and Tetanus Vaccine for Adults and Adolescents complies with the requirements of the 3rd edition of the European Pharmacopoeia for Diphtheria and Tetanus Vaccine (Adsorbed) for Adults and Adolescents [0647]. These requirements are reproduced after the heading 'Definition' below..

The label may state 'DT/Vac/Ads(Adult)'.

For a vaccine for use in the United Kingdom, the amount of diphtheria toxoid used is adjusted so that the final vaccine contains not more than 2.0 flocculation equivalents (2.0 Lf) of diphtheria toxoid per dose.

Ph Eur

DEFINITION

Diphtheria and tetanus vaccine (adsorbed) for adults and adolescents is a preparation of diphtheria formol toxoid and tetanus formol toxoid adsorbed on a mineral carrier. The formol toxoids are prepared from the toxins produced by the growth of *Corynebacterium diphtheriae* and *Clostridium tetani*, respectively. It shall have been demonstrated to the competent authority that the quantity of diphtheria toxoid used does not produce adverse reactions in subjects from the age groups for which the vaccine is intended.

PRODUCTION

BULK PURIFIED DIPHTHERIA TOXOID

For the production of diphtheria toxin, from which toxoid is prepared, seed cultures are managed in a defined seed-lot system in which toxinogenicity is conserved and, where necessary, restored by deliberate reselection. A highly toxinogenic strain of *Corynebacterium diphtheriae* with known origin and history is grown in a suitable liquid medium. At the end of cultivation, the purity of each culture is tested and contaminated cultures are discarded. Toxin-containing culture medium is separated aseptically from the bacterial mass as soon as possible. The toxin content (Lf per millilitre) is checked to monitor consistency of production. Single harvests may be pooled to prepare the bulk purified toxoid. The toxin is purified to remove components likely to cause adverse reactions in humans. The purified toxin is detoxified with formaldehyde by a method that avoids destruction of the immunogenic potency of the toxoid and reversion of the toxoid to toxin, particularly on exposure to heat. Alternatively, purification may be carried out after detoxification.

Only bulk purified toxoid that complies with the following requirements may be used in the preparation of the final bulk vaccine.

Sterility (*2.6.1*). Carry out the test for sterility using 10 ml for each medium.

Absence of diphtheria toxin Inject subcutaneously at least 500 Lf of purified toxoid in a volume of 1 ml into each of five healthy guinea-pigs, each weighing 250 g to 350 g, that have not previously been treated with any material that will interfere with the test. If within 42 days of the injection any of the animals shows signs of or dies from diphtheria toxaemia, the toxoid does not comply with the test. If more than one animal dies from non-specific causes, repeat the test once; if more than one animal dies in the second test, the toxoid does not comply with the test.

Irreversibility of toxoid Using the buffer for the final vaccine without adsorbent, prepare a dilution of the bulk purified toxoid containing the same toxoid concentration as the final vaccine. Divide the dilution into two equal parts. Keep one of them at 5 ± 3°C and the other at 37°C for 6 weeks. Test both samples by a suitable sensitive assay for active diphtheria toxin such as inoculation on to cell cultures or intradermal injection into guinea-pigs. The toxoid complies with the test if neither sample produces any sign of a toxic reaction attributable to diphtheria toxin.

Antigenic purity Not less than 1500 Lf per milligram of protein nitrogen.

BULK PURIFIED TETANUS TOXOID

For the production of tetanus toxin, from which toxoid is prepared, seed cultures are managed in a defined seed-lot system in which toxinogenicity is conserved and, where necessary, restored by deliberate reselection. A highly toxinogenic strain of *Clostridium tetani* with known origin and history is grown in a suitable liquid medium. At the end of cultivation, the purity of each culture is tested and contaminated cultures are discarded. Toxin-containing culture medium is collected aseptically. The toxin content (Lf per millilitre) is checked to monitor consistency of production. Single harvests may be pooled to prepare the bulk purified toxoid. The toxin is purified to remove components likely to cause adverse reactions in humans. The purified toxin is detoxified with formaldehyde by a method that avoids destruction of the immunogenic potency of the toxoid and reversion of toxoid to toxin, particularly on exposure to heat. Alternatively, purification may be carried out after detoxification.

Only bulk purified toxoid that complies with the following requirements may be used in the preparation of the final bulk vaccine.

Sterility (*2.6.1*). Carry out the test for sterility using 10 ml for each medium.

Absence of tetanus toxin Inject subcutaneously at least 500 Lf of purified toxoid in a volume of 1 ml into each of five healthy guinea-pigs, each weighing 250 g to 350 g, that have not previously been treated with any material that will interfere with the test. If within 21 days of the injection any of the animals shows signs of or dies from tetanus, the toxoid does not comply with the test. If more than one animal dies from non-specific causes, repeat the test once; if more than one animal dies in the second test, the toxoid does not comply with the test.

Irreversibility of toxoid Using the buffer for the final vaccine without adsorbent, prepare a dilution of the bulk purified toxoid containing the same toxoid concentration as the final vaccine. Divide the dilution into two equal parts. Keep one of them at 5 ± 3°C and the other at 37°C for 6 weeks. Test both dilutions by a suitable sensitive assay for active tetanus toxin, such as inoculation into mice or guinea-pigs. The toxoid complies with the test if neither sample produces any sign of a toxic reaction attributable to tetanus toxin.

Antigenic purity Not less than 1000 Lf per milligram of protein nitrogen.

FINAL BULK VACCINE

The vaccine is prepared by adsorption of suitable quantities of bulk purified diphtheria toxoid and tetanus toxoid onto hydrated aluminium phosphate, aluminium hydroxide or calcium phosphate; the resulting mixture is approximately isotonic with blood. Suitable antimicrobial preservatives may be added. Certain antimicrobial preservatives, particularly those of the phenolic type, adversely affect the antigenic activity and must not be used.

Only final bulk vaccine that complies with the following requirements may be used in the preparation of the final lot.

Antimicrobial preservative Where applicable, determine the amount of antimicrobial preservative by a suitable chemical method. The amount is not less than 85 per cent and not greater than 115 per cent of the intended amount.

Sterility (*2.6.1*). Carry out the test for sterility using 10 ml for each medium.

Potency Carry out the tests described under Assay.

FINAL LOT

The final bulk vaccine is distributed aseptically into sterile, tamper-proof containers. The containers are closed so as to prevent contamination.

Only a final lot that is satisfactory with respect to each of the requirements given below under Identification, Tests and Assay may be released for use. Provided the tests for specific toxicity, free formaldehyde and antimicrobial preservative and the assay have been carried out with satisfactory results on the final bulk vaccine, they may be omitted on the final lot.

IDENTIFICATION

A. Dissolve in the vaccine to be examined sufficient *sodium citrate R* to give a 100 g/l solution. Maintain at 37°C for about 16 h and centrifuge until a clear supernatant liquid is obtained. The clear supernatant liquid reacts with a suitable diphtheria antitoxin, giving a precipitate. If a satisfactory result is not obtained with a vaccine adsorbed on aluminium hydroxide, carry out the test as follows. Centrifuge 15 ml of the vaccine to be examined and suspend the residue in 5 ml of a freshly prepared mixture of 1 volume of a 56 g/l solution of *sodium edetate R* and 49 volumes of a 90 g/l solution of *disodium hydrogen phosphate R*. Maintain at 37°C for not less than 6 h and centrifuge. The clear supernatant liquid reacts with a suitable diphtheria antitoxin, giving a precipitate.

B. The clear supernatant liquid obtained during test A reacts with a suitable tetanus antitoxin, giving a precipitate.

TESTS

Specific toxicity Inject subcutaneously five times the single human dose stated on the label into each of five healthy guinea-pigs, each weighing 250 g to 350 g, that have not previously been treated with any material that will interfere with the test. If within 42 days of the injection any of the animals shows signs of or dies from diphtheria toxaemia or tetanus, the vaccine does not comply with the test. If more than one animal dies from non-specific causes, repeat the test once; if more than one animal dies in the second test, the vaccine does not comply with the test.

Aluminium When hydrated aluminium phosphate or aluminium hydroxide is used as the adsorbent, the vaccine complies with the test prescribed in the monograph on *Vaccines for human use (153)*.

Calcium When calcium phosphate is used as the adsorbent, the vaccine complies with the test prescribed in the monograph on *Vaccines for human use (153)*.

Free formaldehyde The vaccine complies with the test prescribed in the monograph on *Vaccines for human use (153)*.

Antimicrobial preservative Where applicable, determine the amount of antimicrobial preservative by a suitable chemical method. The content is not less than the minimum amount shown to be effective and is not greater than 115 per cent of the quantity stated on the label.

Sterility (*2.6.1*). The vaccine complies with the test for sterility.

ASSAY

Diphtheria component Carry out one of the prescribed methods for the assay of diphtheria vaccine (adsorbed) (*2.7.6*).

The lower confidence limit ($P = 0.95$) of the estimated potency is not less than 2 I.U. per single human dose.

Tetanus component Carry out one of the prescribed methods for the assay of tetanus vaccine (adsorbed) (*2.7.8*).

The lower confidence limit ($P = 0.95$) of the estimated potency is not less than 20 I.U. per single human dose.

STORAGE

See *Vaccines for human use (153)*.

LABELLING

See *Vaccines for human use (153)*.

The label states:

- the minimum number of International Units of each component per single human dose,
- the name and the amount of the adsorbent,
- that the vaccine must be shaken before use,
- that the vaccine is not to be frozen.

Ph Eur

Adsorbed Diphtheria, Tetanus and Pertussis Vaccine

Adsorbed Diphtheria—Tetanus—Whooping-cough Prophylactic

Adsorbed Diphtheria, Tetanus and Pertussis Vaccine complies with the requirements of the 3rd edition of the European Pharmacopoeia for Diphtheria, Tetanus and Pertussis Vaccine (Adsorbed) [0445]. These requirements are reproduced after the heading 'Definition' below..

The label may state 'DTPer/Vac/Ads'.

Ph Eur

DEFINITION

Diphtheria, tetanus and pertussis vaccine (adsorbed) is a preparation of diphtheria formol toxoid and tetanus formol toxoid adsorbed on a mineral carrier to which a suspension of inactivated *Bordetella pertussis* has been added. The formol toxoids are prepared from the toxins produced by the growth of *Corynebacterium diphtheriae* and *Clostridium tetani*, respectively.

PRODUCTION

BULK PURIFIED DIPHTHERIA TOXOID

For the production of diphtheria toxin, from which toxoid is prepared, seed cultures are managed in a defined seed-lot system in which toxinogenicity is conserved and, where necessary, restored by deliberate reselection. A highly toxinogenic strain of *Corynebacterium diphtheriae* with known origin and history is grown in a suitable liquid medium. At the end of cultivation, the purity of each culture is tested and contaminated cultures are discarded. Toxin-containing culture medium is separated aseptically from the bacterial mass as soon as possible. The toxin content (Lf per millilitre) is checked to monitor consistency of production. Single harvests may be pooled to prepare the bulk purified toxoid. The toxin is purified to remove components likely to cause adverse reactions in humans. The purified toxin is detoxified with formaldehyde by a method that avoids destruction of the immunogenic potency of the toxoid and reversion of the toxoid to toxin, particularly on exposure to heat. Alternatively, purification may be carried out after detoxification.

Only bulk purified toxoid that complies with the following requirements may be used in the preparation of the final bulk vaccine.

Sterility (*2.6.1*). Carry out the test for sterility using 10 ml for each medium.

Absence of diphtheria toxin Inject subcutaneously at least 500 Lf of purified toxoid in a volume of 1 ml into each of five healthy guinea-pigs, each weighing 250 g to 350 g, that have not previously been treated with any material that will interfere with the test. If within 42 days of the injection any of the animals shows signs of or dies from diphtheria toxaemia, the toxoid does not comply with the test. If more than one animal dies from non-specific causes, repeat the test once; if more than one animal dies in the second test, the toxoid does not comply with the test.

Irreversibility of toxoid Using the buffer for the final vaccine without adsorbent, prepare a dilution of the bulk purified toxoid containing the same toxoid concentration as the final vaccine. Divide the dilution into two equal parts. Keep one of them at 5 ± 3°C and the other at 37°C for 6 weeks. Test both samples by a suitable sensitive assay for active diphtheria toxin such as inoculation on to cell cultures or intradermal injection into guinea-pigs. The toxoid complies with the test if neither sample produces any sign of a toxic reaction attributable to diphtheria toxin.

Antigenic purity Not less than 1500 Lf per milligram of protein nitrogen.

BULK PURIFIED TETANUS TOXOID

For the production of tetanus toxin, from which toxoid is prepared, seed cultures are managed in a defined seed-lot system in which toxinogenicity is conserved and, where necessary, restored by deliberate reselection. A highly toxinogenic strain of *Clostridium tetani* with known origin and history is grown in a suitable liquid medium. At the end of cultivation, the purity of each culture is tested and contaminated cultures are discarded. Toxin-containing culture medium is collected aseptically. The toxin content (Lf per millilitre) is checked to monitor consistency of production. Single harvests may be pooled to prepare the bulk purified toxoid. The toxin is purified to remove components likely to cause adverse reactions in humans. The purified toxin is detoxified with formaldehyde by a method that avoids destruction of the immunogenic potency of the toxoid and reversion of toxoid to toxin, particularly on exposure to heat. Alternatively, purification may be carried out after detoxification.

Only bulk purified toxoid that complies with the following requirements may be used in the preparation of the final bulk vaccine.

Sterility (*2.6.1*). Carry out the test for sterility using 10 ml for each medium.

Absence of tetanus toxin Inject subcutaneously at least 500 Lf of purified toxoid in a volume of 1 ml into each of five healthy guinea-pigs, each weighing 250 g to 350 g, that have not previously been treated with any material that will interfere with the test. If within 21 days of the injection any of the animals shows signs of or dies from tetanus, the toxoid does not comply with the test. If more than one animal dies from non-specific causes, repeat the test once; if more than one animal dies in the second test, the toxoid does not comply with the test.

Irreversibility of toxoid Using the buffer for the final vaccine without adsorbent, prepare a dilution of the bulk purified toxoid containing the same toxoid concentration as the final vaccine. Divide the dilution into two equal parts. Keep one of them at 5 ± 3°C and the other at 37°C for 6 weeks. Test both dilutions by a suitable sensitive assay for active tetanus toxin, such as inoculation into mice or guinea-pigs. The toxoid complies with the test if neither sample produces any sign of a toxic reaction attributable to tetanus toxin.

Antigenic purity Not less than 1000 Lf per milligram of protein nitrogen.

INACTIVATED B. PERTUSSIS *SUSPENSION*

Production of the vaccine is based on a seed-lot system. One or more strains of *B. pertussis* with known origin and history are used. Strains, culture medium and cultivation method are chosen in such a way that agglutinogens 1, 2 and 3 are present in the final vaccine. Each strain is grown for 24 h to 72 h in a liquid medium or on a solid medium; the medium used in the final cultivation stage does not contain blood or blood products. Human blood or blood products are not used in any culture media. The bacteria are harvested, washed to remove substances derived from the medium and suspended in a 9 g/l solution of sodium chloride or other suitable isotonic solution. The opacity of the suspension is determined not later than 2 weeks after harvest by comparison with the International Reference Preparation of Opacity and used as the basis of calculation for subsequent stages in vaccine preparation. The equivalence in International Units of the International Reference Preparation is stated by the World Health Organisation.

Single harvests are not used for the final bulk vaccine unless they have been shown to contain *B. pertussis* cells with the same characteristics, with regard to growth and agglutinogens, as the parent strain and to be free from contaminating bacteria and fungi. The bacteria are killed and detoxified in controlled conditions by means of a suitable chemical agent or by heating or by a combination of these two methods. Freedom from live *B. pertussis* is tested using a suitable culture medium. The suspension is maintained at 5 ± 3°C for a suitable period to diminish its toxicity.

FINAL BULK VACCINE

The final bulk vaccine is prepared by adsorption of suitable quantities of bulk purified diphtheria toxoid and tetanus toxoid onto hydrated aluminium phosphate, aluminium hydroxide or calcium phosphate and admixture of an appropriate quantity of a suspension of inactivated *B. pertussis*; the resulting mixture is approximately isotonic with blood. The *B. pertussis* concentration of the final bulk vaccine does not exceed that corresponding to an opacity of 20 I.U. per single human dose. If two or more strains of *B. pertussis* are used, the composition of consecutive lots of the final bulk vaccine shall be consistent with respect to the proportion of each strain as measured in opacity units. Suitable antimicrobial preservatives may be added to the bulk vaccine. Certain antimicrobial preservatives, particularly those of the phenolic type, adversely affect the antigenic activity and must not be used.

Only final bulk vaccine that complies with the following requirements may be used in the preparation of the final lot.

Antimicrobial preservative Where applicable, determine the amount of antimicrobial preservative by a suitable chemical method. The amount is not less than 85 per cent and not greater than 115 per cent of the intended amount.

Sterility (*2.6.1*). Carry out the test for sterility using 10 ml for each medium.

Potency Carry out the tests described under Assay.

FINAL LOT

The final bulk vaccine is distributed aseptically into sterile, tamper-proof containers. The containers are closed so as to prevent contamination.

Only a final lot that is satisfactory with respect to each of the requirements given below under Identification, Tests and Assay may be released for use. Provided the tests for specific toxicity, free formaldehyde and antimicrobial preservative and the assay have been carried out with satisfactory results on the final bulk vaccine, they may be omitted on the final lot.

IDENTIFICATION

A. Dissolve in the vaccine to be examined sufficient *sodium citrate R* to give a 100 g/l solution. Maintain at 37°C for about 16 h and centrifuge until a clear supernatant liquid is obtained; reserve the precipitate for identification test C. The clear supernatant liquid reacts with a suitable diphtheria antitoxin, giving a precipitate.

B. The clear supernatant liquid obtained during identification test A reacts with a suitable tetanus antitoxin, giving a precipitate.

C. The pertussis component is identified by agglutination of the bacteria from the resuspended centrifugation residue (see identification test A; other suitable methods for separating the bacteria from the adsorbent may also be used) by antisera specific to *B. pertussis* or by the assay of the pertussis component.

TESTS

Specific toxicity *Diphtheria and tetanus components* Inject subcutaneously five times the single human dose stated on the label into each of five healthy guinea-pigs, each weighing 250 g to 350 g, that have not previously been treated with any material that will interfere with the test. If within 42 days of the injection any of the animals shows signs of or dies from diphtheria toxaemia or tetanus, the vaccine does not comply with the test. If more than one animal dies from non-specific causes, repeat the test once; if more than one animal dies in the second test, the vaccine does not comply with the test.

Pertussis component. Use not fewer than ten healthy mice each weighing 14 g to 16 g for the vaccine group and for the saline control. Use mice of the same sex or distribute males and females equally between the groups. Allow the animals access to food and water for at least 2 h before injection and during the test. Inject each mouse of the vaccine group intraperitoneally with 0.5 ml, containing a quantity of the vaccine equivalent to not less than half the single human dose. Inject each mouse of the control group with 0.5 ml of a 9 g/l sterile solution of *sodium chloride R*, preferably containing the same amount of antimicrobial preservative as that injected with the vaccine. Weigh the groups of mice immediately before the injection and 72 h and 7 days after the injection. The vaccine complies with the test if: (a) at the end of 72 h the total mass of the group of vaccinated mice is not less than that preceding the injection; (b) at the end of 7 days the average increase in mass per vaccinated mouse is not less than 60 per cent of that per control mouse; and (c) not more than 5 per cent of the vaccinated mice die during the test.

Aluminium When hydrated aluminium phosphate or aluminium hydroxide is used as the adsorbent, the vaccine complies with the test prescribed in the monograph on *Vaccines for human use (153)*.

Calcium When calcium phosphate is used as the adsorbent, the vaccine complies with the test prescribed in the monograph on *Vaccines for human use (153)*.

Free formaldehyde The vaccine complies with the test prescribed in the monograph on *Vaccines for human use (153)*.

Antimicrobial preservative Where applicable, determine the amount of antimicrobial preservative by a suitable chemical method. The content is not less than the minimum amount shown to be effective and is not greater than 115 per cent of the quantity stated on the label.

Sterility (*2.6.1*). The vaccine complies with the test for sterility.

ASSAY

Diphtheria component Carry out one of the prescribed methods for the assay of diphtheria vaccine (adsorbed) (*2.7.6*).

The lower confidence limit ($P = 0.95$) of the estimated potency is not less than 30 I.U. per single human dose.

Tetanus component Carry out one of the prescribed methods for the assay of tetanus vaccine (adsorbed) (*2.7.8*).

If the test is carried out in guinea-pigs, the lower confidence limit ($P = 0.95$) of the estimated potency is not less than 40 I.U. per single human dose; if the test is carried out in mice, the lower confidence limit ($P = 0.95$) of the estimated potency is not less than 60 I.U. per single human dose.

Pertussis component Carry out the assay of pertussis vaccine (*2.7.7*).

The estimated potency is not less than 4 I.U. per single human dose and the lower confidence limit ($P = 0.95$) of the estimated potency is not less than 2 I.U. per single human dose.

STORAGE

See *Vaccines for human use (153)*.

LABELLING

See *Vaccines for human use (153)*.

The label states:

— the minimum number of International Units of each component per single human dose,
— where applicable, that the vaccine is intended for primary vaccination of children and is not necessarily suitable for reinforcing doses or for administration to adults,
— the name and the amount of the adsorbent,
— that the vaccine must be shaken before use,
— that the vaccine is not to be frozen.

Ph Eur

Haemophilus Type B Conjugate Vaccine

Haemophilus Type B Conjugate Vaccine complies with the requirements of the 3rd edition of the European Pharmacopoeia [1219]. These requirements are reproduced after the heading 'Definition' below.

The lable may state 'Hib/Vac'.

Ph Eur

DEFINITION

Haemophilus type B conjugate vaccine is a liquid or freeze-dried preparation of a polysaccharide, derived from a suitable strain of *Haemophilus influenzae* type B, covalently bound to a carrier protein. The polysaccharide, polyribosylribitol phosphate, referred to as PRP, is a linear copolymer composed of repeated units of 3-β-D-ribofuranosyl-(1→1)-ribitol-5-phosphate [$(C_{10}H_{19}O_{12}P)_n$], with a defined molecular size. The carrier protein, when conjugated to PRP, is capable of inducing a T-cell-dependent B-cell immune response to the polysaccharide.

The vaccine complies with the monograph on *Vaccines for human use (153)*.

PRODUCTION

GENERAL PROVISIONS

The production method shall have been shown to yield consistently haemophilus type b conjugate vaccines of adequate safety and immunogenicity in man. The production of PRP and of the carrier are based on seed-lot systems.

The production method is validated to demonstrate that the product, if tested, would comply with the test for abnormal toxicity for immunosera and vaccines for human use (*2.6.9*).

The stability of the final lot and relevant intermediates is evaluated using one or more indicator tests. Such tests may include determination of molecular size, determination of free PRP in the conjugate and the immunogenicity test in mice. Taking account of the results of the stability testing, release requirements are set for these indicator tests to ensure that the vaccine will be satisfactory at the end of the period of validity.

BACTERIAL SEED LOTS

The seed lots of *H. influenzae* type b are shown to be free from contamination by examination of Gram-stained smears and by inoculation on suitable media. Several microscopic fields are examined at high magnification so that at least 10,000 organisms are inspected.

H. INFLUENZAE TYPE B POLYSACCHARIDE (PRP)

H. influenzae type b is grown in a liquid medium that does not contain high-molecular-mass polysaccharides; if any ingredient of the medium contains blood-group substances, the process shall be validated to demonstrate that after the purification step they are no longer detectable. The bacterial purity of the culture is verified by suitable methods. The culture may be inactivated. PRP is separated from the culture liquid and purified by a suitable method. Volatile matter, including water, in the purified polysaccharide is determined by a suitable method such as thermogravimetry (*2.2.34*); the result is used to calculate the results of certain tests with reference to the dried substance, as prescribed below.

Only PRP that complies with the following requirements may be used in the preparation of the conjugate.

Identification PRP is identified by an immunochemical method (*2.7.1*) or other suitable method.

Molecular-size distribution The percentage of PRP eluted before a given K_D value or within a range of K_D values, is determined by size-exclusion chromatography (*2.2.30*); an acceptable value is established for the particular product and each batch of PRP must be shown to comply with this limit. Limits for currently approved products, using the indicated stationary phases, are shown for information in Table 1219.-1. Where applicable, the molecular-size distribution is also determined after chemical modification of the polysaccharide.

A validated determination of the degree of polymerisation or of the weight-average molecular weight and the dispersion of molecular masses may be used instead of the determination of molecular size distribution.

Ribose (*2.5.31*). Not less than 32 per cent, calculated with reference to the dried substance.

Table 1219–1. – *Product characteristics and specifications for PRP and carrier protein in currently approved products*

Carrier			Haemophilus material		Conjugation	
Type	Purity	Nominal amount per dose (micrograms)	Type of PRP	Nominal amount per dose (micrograms)	Coupling method	Procedure
Diphtheria toxoid	>1500 Lf per milligram of nitrogen	18 µg	Polysaccharide (size reduced) K_D: 0.6–0.7, using *cross-linked agarose for chromatography R*	25 µg	cyanogen bromide activation of PRP	activated diphtheria toxoid (D-AH$^+$, cyanogen bromide-activated PRP, conjugated vaccine
Tetanus toxoid	>1500 Lf per milligram of nitrogen	20 µg	Polysaccharide ≥50 per cent ≤ K_D 0.30, using *cross-linked agarose for chromatography R*	10 µg	carbodi-imide mediated	ADH-activated PRP (PRP-cov.-AH) + conc. tetanus protein + EDAC – conjugated vaccine
CRM 197 diphtheria protein	>90 per cent diphtheria protein	25 µg	Polysaccharide (size reduced) Dp = 15–35 *or* 10–35	10 µg	reductive amination (one-step method) *or* N-hydroxy-succinimide activation	direct coupling of oligo-saccharide to CRM 197 (cyanoborohydride activated)
Meningo-coccal group membrane B outer protein (OMP)	outer membrane protein vesicles; ≤6 per cent of lipopolysaccha-ride	250 µg	Polysaccharide (size reduced) K_D > 0.6, using *cross-linked agarose for chromatography R* or $M_w > 50 \times 10^3$	15 µg	thioether bond	PRP activation by CDI PRP-IM + BuA2 + BrAc = PRP-BuA2-BrAc + thio-activated OMP conjugated vaccine

Legend

ADH = adipic acid dihydrazide

BrAc = bromoacetyl chloride

BuA2 = butane-1,4-diamide

CDI = carbonyldi-imidazole

Dp = degree of polymerisation

EDAC = 1-ethyl-3-(3-dimethylaminopropyl)carbodiimide

M_w = weight-average molecular weight

IM = imidazolium

Phosphorus (*2.5.18*). 6.8 per cent to 9.0 per cent, calculated with reference to the dried substance.

Protein (*2.5.16*). Not more than 1.0 per cent, calculated with reference to the dried substance. Use sufficient PRP to allow detection of 1 per cent of protein.

Nucleic acid (*2.5.17*). Not more than 1.0 per cent, calculated with reference to the dried substance.

Bacterial endotoxins (*2.6.14*). Not more than 25 I.U. of endotoxin per microgram of PRP.

Residual reagents Where applicable, tests are carried out to determine residues of reagents used during inactivation and purification. An acceptable value for each reagent is established for the particular product and each batch of PRP must be shown to comply with this limit. Where validation studies have demonstrated removal of a residual reagent, the test on PRP may be omitted.

CARRIER PROTEIN

The carrier protein is chosen so that when the PRP is conjugated it is able to induce a T-cell-dependent immune response. Currently approved carrier proteins and coupling methods are listed for information in Table 1219–1. The carrier proteins are produced by culture of suitable micro-organisms; the bacterial purity of the culture is verified; the culture may be inactivated; the carrier protein is purified by a suitable method.

Only a carrier protein that complies with the following requirements may be used in preparation of the conjugate.

Identification The carrier protein is identified by a suitable immunochemical method (*2.7.1*).

Sterility (*2.6.1*). Carry out the test using for each medium 10 ml or the equivalent of one hundred doses, whichever is the less.

Diphtheria toxoid Diphtheria toxoid is produced as described in *Diphtheria vaccine (adsorbed) (443)* and complies with the requirements prescribed there for bulk purified toxoid.

Tetanus toxoid Tetanus toxoid is produced as described in *Tetanus vaccine (adsorbed) (452)* and complies with the requirements prescribed there for bulk purified toxoid except that the antigenic purity is not less than 1500 Lf per milligram of protein nitrogen.

Diphtheria protein CRM 197 It contains not less than 90 per cent of diphtheria CRM 197 protein, determined by a suitable method. Suitable tests are carried out, for

Table 1219-2. — Bulk conjugate requirements for currently approved products

Test	Protein carrier			
	Diphtheria toxoid	Tetanus toxoid	CRM 197	OMP
Free PRP	<37 %	<20 %	<25 %	<15 %
Free protein	<4%	<1%, where applicable	<1% or <2%, depending on the coupling method	not applicable
PRP to protein ratio	1.25–1.8	0.30–0.55	0.3–0.7	0.05–0.1
Molecular size (K_D)				
cross-linked agarose for chromatography R	95% <0.75	60% <0.2	50% 0.3–0.6	85% <0.3
cross-linked agarose for chromatography R1	0.6–0.7	85% <0.5		

validation or routinely, to demonstrate that the product is non-toxic.

OMP (meningococcal group B outer membrane protein complex) OMP complies with the following requirements for lipopolysaccharide and pyrogens.

Lipopolysaccharide. Not more than 8 per cent of lipopolysaccharide, determined by a suitable method.

Pyrogens (*2.6.8*). Inject into each rabbit 0.25 µg of OMP per kilogram of body mass.

BULK CONJUGATE

PRP is chemically modified to enable conjugation; it is usually partly depolymerised either before or during this procedure. Reactive functional groups or spacers may be introduced into the carrier protein or PRP prior to conjugation. The conjugate is obtained by the covalent binding of PRP and carrier protein. Where applicable, unreacted but potentially reactogenic functional groups are made unreactive by means of capping agents; the conjugate is purified to remove reagents.

Only a bulk conjugate that complies with the following requirements may be used in preparation of the final bulk vaccine. For each test and for each particular product, limits of acceptance are established and each batch of conjugate must be shown to comply with these limits. Limits applied to currently approved products for some of these tests are listed for information in Table 1219–2. For a freeze-dried vaccine, some of the tests may be carried out on the final lot rather than on the bulk conjugate where the freeze-drying process may affect the component being tested.

PRP The PRP content is determined by assay of phosphorus (*2.5.18*) or by assay of ribose (*2.5.31*) or by an immunochemical method (*2.7.1*).

Protein The protein content is determined by a suitable chemical method (for example, *2.5.16*).

PRP to protein ratio Determine the ratio by calculation.

Molecular-size distribution Molecular-size distribution is determined by size-exclusion chromatography (*2.2.30*).

Free PRP Unbound PRP is determined after removal of the conjugate, for example by size-exclusion or hydrophobic chromatography, ultrafiltration or other validated methods.

Free carrier protein Determine by a suitable method (which may include deriving the content by calculation from the results of other tests). The amount is within the limits approved for the particular product.

Unreacted functional groups No unreacted functional groups are detectable in the bulk conjugate unless process validation has shown that unreacted functional groups detectable at this stage are removed during the subsequent manufacturing process (for example, owing to short half-life).

Residual reagents Removal of residual reagents such as cyanide, EDAC (ethyldimethylaminopropylcarbodi-imide) and phenol is confirmed by suitable tests or by validation of the process.

Sterility (*2.6.1*). Carry out the test using for each medium 10 ml or the equivalent of one hundred doses, whichever is the less.

FINAL BULK VACCINE

An adjuvant, an antimicrobial preservative and a stabiliser may be added to the bulk conjugate before dilution to the final concentration with a suitable diluent.

Only a final bulk vaccine that complies with the following requirements may be used in preparation of the final lot.

Antimicrobial preservative Where applicable, determine the amount of antimicrobial preservative by a suitable chemical or physico-chemical method. The content is not less than 85 per cent and not greater than 115 per cent of the intended amount.

Sterility (*2.6.1*). It complies with the test for sterility, carried out using 10 ml for each medium.

FINAL LOT

Only a final lot that is satisfactory with respect to each of the requirements given below under Identification, Tests and Assay may be released for use. Provided the test for antimicrobial preservative and, for liquid vaccines, the assay have been carried out on the final bulk vaccine, they may be omitted on the final lot.

pH (*2.2.3*). The pH of the vaccine, reconstituted if necessary, is within the range approved for the product.

IDENTIFICATION

The vaccine is identified by a suitable immunochemical method (*2.7.1*) for PRP or the assay serves also to identify the vaccine.

TESTS

PRP content Not less than 80 per cent of the amount of PRP stated on the label. Determine either ribose (*2.5.31*) or phosphorus (*2.5.18*) or apply an immunochemical method (*2.7.1*).

Aluminium When aluminium hydroxide is used as the adsorbent, the vaccine complies with the test prescribed in *Vaccines for human use (153)*.

Antimicrobial preservative Where applicable, determine the amount of antimicrobial preservative by a suitable chemical or physico-chemical method. The content is not less than the minimum amount shown to be effective and not greater than 115 per cent of the quantity stated on the label.

Water (*2.5.12*). For freeze-dried vaccines, not more than 3.0 per cent.

Sterility (*2.6.1*). It complies with the test for sterility.

Pyrogens (*2.6.8*). It complies with the test for pyrogens. Inject per kilogram of the rabbit's mass a quantity of the vaccine equivalent to: 1 mg of PRP for a vaccine with diphtheria toxoid or CRM 197 diphtheria protein as carrier; 0.1 mg of PRP for a vaccine with tetanus toxoid as carrier; 0.025 mg of PRP for a vaccine with OMP as a carrier.

ASSAY

Unless otherwise justified and authorised, carry out a suitable test for immunogenicity in mice to demonstrate the ability to induce a T-cell dependent immune response. The following is cited as an example of a test that may be used after validation.

Use in the test two groups of not fewer than eight healthy mice about 6 to 8 weeks old and from the same stock. Inject subcutaneously into each animal of one of the groups on days 0 and 14 a suitable quantity of the vaccine. Maintain the other group as controls. Bleed the animals on day 21. Pool the sera from the control group. Assay the individual sera from the treated group and the pooled sera from the control group for anti-PRP antibodies using a suitable immunochemical method, for example enzyme-linked immunosorbent assay for IgG (*2.7.1*). Not less than half the vaccinated mice show seroconversion, that is they have a titre not less than four times that of the pooled control serum.

STORAGE

See Vaccines for human use (153).

LABELLING

See Vaccines for human use (153).

The label states:
— the number of micrograms of PRP per human dose,
— the type and nominal amount of carrier protein per single human dose.

Ph Eur

Inactivated Hepatitis A Vaccine

Inactivated Hepatitis A Vaccine complies with the requirements of the 3rd edition of the European Pharmacopoeia for Hepatitis A Vaccine (Inactivated, Adsorbed) [1107]. These requirements are reproduced after the heading 'Definition' below.

The label may state 'Hep A/Vac'.

Ph Eur

DEFINITION

Hepatitis A vaccine (inactivated, adsorbed) is a liquid preparation of a suitable strain of hepatitis A virus grown in cell cultures, inactivated by a validated method and adsorbed on a mineral carrier. The vaccine is an opalescent suspension.

The vaccine complies with the monograph on *Vaccines for human use (153)*.

PRODUCTION

Production of the vaccine is based on a virus seed-lot system and a cell-bank system. The production method shall have been shown to yield consistently vaccines that comply with the requirements for immunogenicity, safety and stability.

The production method is validated to demonstrate that the product, if tested, would comply with the test for abnormal toxicity for immunosera and vaccines for human use (*2.6.9*).

Unless otherwise justified and authorised, the virus in the final vaccine shall not have undergone more passages from the master seed lot than were used to prepare the vaccine shown in clinical studies to be satisfactory with respect to safety and efficacy.

Reference preparation. A part of a batch shown to be at least as immunogenic as a batch that, in clinical studies in young healthy adults, produced not less than 95 per cent seroconversion, corresponding to a level of neutralising antibody accepted to be protective, after a full-course primary immunisation is used as a reference preparation. An antibody level of 20 mI.U./ml determined by enzyme-linked immunosorbent assay is recognised as being protective.

SUBSTRATE FOR VIRUS PROPAGATION

The virus is propagated in a human diploid cell line (*5.2.3*) or in a continuous cell line approved by the competent authority.

SEED LOTS

The strain of hepatitis A virus used to prepare the master seed lot shall be identified by historical records that include information on the origin of the strain and its subsequent manipulation.

Only a seed lot that complies with the following requirements may be used for virus propagation.

identification Each master and working seed lot is identified as hepatitis A virus using specific antibodies.

Virus concentration The virus concentration of each master and working seed lot is determined to monitor consistency of production.

Extraneous agents The master and working seed lots comply with the requirements for seed lots for virus vaccines (*2.6.16*). In addition, if primary monkey cells have been used for isolation of the strain, measures are taken to ensure that the strain is not contaminated with simian viruses such as simian immunodeficiency virus and filoviruses.

VIRUS PROPAGATION AND HARVEST

All processing of the cell bank and subsequent cell cultures is done under aseptic conditions in an area where no other cells are being handled. Approved animal serum (but not human serum) may be used in the cell culture media. Serum and trypsin used in the preparation of cell suspensions and media are shown to be free from extraneous agents. The cell culture media may contain a pH indicator such as phenol red and approved antibiotics at the lowest effective concentration. Not less than 500 ml of the cell cultures employed for vaccine production is set aside as uninfected cell cultures (control cells). Multiple harvests from the same production cell culture may be pooled and considered as a single harvest.

Only a single harvest that complies with the following requirements may be used in the preparation of the vaccine. When the determination of the ratio of virus concentration to antigen content has been carried out on a suitable number of single harvests to demonstrate consistency, it may subsequently be omitted as a routine test.

Identification The test for antigen content also serves to identify the single harvest.

Bacterial and fungal contamination (*2.6.1*). The single harvest complies with the test for sterility, carried out using 10 ml for each medium.

Mycoplasmas (*2.6.7*). The single harvest complies with the test for mycoplasmas carried out using 1 ml for each medium.

Control cells The control cells of the production cell culture comply with a test for identity and the requirements for extraneous agents (*2.6.16*).

Antigen content Determine the hepatitis A antigen content by a suitable immunochemical method (*2.7.1*) to monitor production consistency; the content is within the limits approved for the particular product.

Ratio of virus concentration to antigen content The consistency of the ratio of the concentration of infectious virus, as determined by a suitable cell culture method, to antigen content is established by validation on a suitable number of single harvests.

PURIFICATION AND PURIFIED HARVEST

The harvest, which may be a pool of several single harvests, is purified by validated methods. If continuous cell lines are used for production, the purification process shall have been shown to reduce consistently the level of host-cell DNA. Only a purified harvest that complies with the following requirements may be used in the preparation of the inactivated harvest.

Virus concentration The concentration of infective virus in the purified harvest is determined by a suitable cell culture method to monitor production consistency and as a starting point for monitoring the inactivation curve.

Antigen:total protein ratio Determine the hepatitis A virus antigen content by a suitable immunochemical method (*2.7.1*). Determine the total protein by a validated method. The ratio of hepatitis A virus antigen content to total protein content is within the limits approved for the particular product.

Bovine serum albumin Not more than 50 ng in the equivalent of a single human dose, determined by a suitable immunochemical method (*2.7.1*). Where appropriate in view of the manufacturing process, other suitable protein markers may be used to demonstrate effective purification.

Residual host-cell DNA If a continuous cell line is used for virus propagation, the content of residual host-cell DNA, determined using a suitable method as described in *Products of recombinant DNA technology* (*784*), is not greater than 100 pg in the equivalent of a single human dose.

Residual chemicals If chemical substances are used during the purification process, tests for these substances are carried out on the purified harvest (or on the inactivated harvest), unless validation of the process has demonstrated total clearance. The concentration must not exceed the limits approved for the particular product.

INACTIVATION AND INACTIVATED HARVEST

Several purified harvests may be pooled before inactivation. In order to avoid interference with the inactivation process, virus aggregation must be prevented or aggregates must be removed immediately before and/or during the inactivation process. The virus suspension is inactivated by a validated method; the method shall have been shown to be consistently capable of inactivating hepatitis A virus without destroying the antigenic and immunogenic activity; as part of the validation studies, an inactivation curve is plotted representing residual live virus concentration measured on at least three occasions (for example, on days 0, 1 and 2 of the inactivation process). If formaldehyde is used for inactivation, the presence of excess free formaldehyde is verified at the end of the inactivation process.

Only an inactivated harvest that complies with the following requirements may be used in the preparation of the final bulk vaccine.

Inactivation. Carry out an amplification test for residual infectious hepatitis A virus by inoculating a quantity of the inactivated harvest equivalent to 5 per cent of the batch but not more than 1500 doses of vaccine into cell cultures of the same type as those used for production of the vaccine and incubating the cells for at least 28 days. Make two passages and carry out a test of suitable sensitivity for residual infectious virus. No evidence of hepatitis A virus multiplication is found in the samples taken at the end of the inactivation process. Use infective virus inocula concurrently as positive controls to demonstrate cellular susceptibility and absence of interference.

Sterility (*2.6.1*). The inactivated viral harvest complies with the test for sterility, carried out using 10 ml for each medium.

Bacterial endotoxins (*2.6.14*). Not more than 2 I.U. of endotoxin in the equivalent of a single human dose.

Antigen content. Determine the hepatitis A virus antigen content by a suitable immunochemical method (*2.7.1*).

Residual chemicals See under Purification and purified harvest.

FINAL BULK VACCINE

The final bulk vaccine is prepared from one or more inactivated harvests. Approved adjuvants, stabilisers and antimicrobial preservatives may be added.

Only a final bulk vaccine that complies with the following requirements may be used in the preparation of the final lot.

Sterility (*2.6.1*). The final bulk vaccine complies with the test for sterility, carried out using 10 ml for each medium.

Antimicrobial preservative Where applicable, determine the amount of antimicrobial preservative by a suitable chemical or physico-chemical method. The amount is not less than 85 per cent and not greater than 115 per cent of the intended amount.

FINAL LOT

The final bulk vaccine is distributed aseptically into sterile containers. The containers are then closed so as to avoid contamination.

Only a final lot that complies with each of the requirements given below under Identification, Tests and Assay may be released for use. Provided that the tests for free formaldehyde (where applicable) and antimicrobial preservative content (where applicable) and the assay have been carried out on the final bulk vaccine with satisfactory results, these tests may be omitted on the final lot.

IDENTIFICATION

The vaccine is shown to contain hepatitis A virus antigen by a suitable immunochemical method (*2.7.1*) using specific antibodies or by the mouse immunogenicity test described under Assay.

TESTS

Aluminium When hydrated aluminium phosphate or aluminium hydroxide is used as the adsorbent, the vaccine complies with the test prescribed in *Vaccines for human use* (*153*).

Free formaldehyde When formaldehyde has been used for inactivation, the vaccine complies with the test prescribed in *Vaccines for human use* (*153*).

Antimicrobial preservative Where applicable, determine the amount of antimicrobial preservative by a suitable chemical or physico-chemical method. The amount is not less than the minimum amount shown to be effective and is not greater than 115 per cent of that stated on the label.

Sterility (*2.6.1*). The vaccine complies with the test for sterility.

ASSAY

Either the potency of the vaccine is determined by comparing the quantity necessary to induce specific antibodies in mice with the quantity of a reference preparation required to produce the same effect, or a validated *in vitro* determination of antigen content is carried out.

The test in mice shown below is given as an example of a method that has been found suitable for a given vaccine; other validated methods may also be used.

Selection and distribution of the test animals. Use in the test healthy mice from the same stock, about 5 weeks old and from a strain shown to be suitable. Use animals of the same sex. Distribute the animals in at least seven equal groups of a number suitable for the requirements of the assay.

Determination of potency of the vaccine to be examined. Using a 9 g/l solution of *sodium chloride R* containing the aluminium adjuvant used for the vaccine, prepare at least three dilutions of the vaccine to be examined and matching dilutions of the reference preparation. Allocate the dilutions one to each of the groups of animals and inject subcutaneously not more than 1.0 ml of each dilution into each animal in the group to which that dilution is allocated. Maintain a group of unvaccinated controls, injected subcutaneously with the same volume of diluent. After 28 to 32 days, anaesthetise and bleed all animals, keeping the individual sera separate. Assay the individual sera for specific antibodies against hepatitis A virus by a suitable immunochemical method (*2.7.1*).

Calculations. Carry out the calculations by the usual statistical methods for an assay with a quantal response (for example, *5.3. Statistical analysis of results of biological assays and tests, section 4*).

From the distribution of reaction levels measured on all the sera in the unvaccinated group, determine the maximum reaction level that can be expected to occur in an unvaccinated animal for that particular assay. Any response in vaccinated animals that exceeds this level is by definition a seroconversion.

Make a suitable transformation of the percentage of animals showing seroconversion in each group (for example, a probit transformation) and analyse the data according to a parallel-line log dose-response model. Determine the potency of the test preparation relative to the reference preparation.

Validity conditions. The test is not valid unless:

— for both the test and the reference vaccine, the ED_{50} lies between the smallest and the largest doses given to the animals,

— the statistical analysis shows no significant deviation from linearity or parallelism,

— the fiducial limits of the estimated relative potency fall between 33 and 300 per cent of the estimated potency.

Potency requirement. The upper fiducial limit ($P = 0.95$) of the estimated relative potency is not less than 1.0.

STORAGE

See *Vaccines for human use* (*153*).

LABELLING

See *Vaccines for human use* (*153*).

The label states the biological origin of the cells and the adjuvant used for the preparation of the vaccine.

Ph Eur

Hepatitis B Vaccine (rDNA)

Hepatitis B Vaccine (rDNA) complies with the requirements of the 3rd edition of the European Pharmacopoeia [1056]. These requirements are reproduced after the heading 'Definition' below.

The label may state 'Hep B/Vac'.

Ph Eur

DEFINITION

Hepatitis B vaccine (rDNA) is a preparation of hepatitis B surface antigen, a component protein of hepatitis B virus. The antigen is obtained by recombinant DNA technology.

Hepatitis B vaccine (rDNA) complies with the requirements of the monographs on *Recombinant DNA technology, products of (784)* and on *Vaccines for human use (153)*.

PRODUCTION

See the monograph on *Recombinant DNA technology, products of (784)*, particularly the sections Cloning and expression, Cell-bank system, Validation of the cell banks, Validation of the production process and Production consistency.

The vaccine shall have been shown to induce specific, protective antibodies in man. The production method shall have been shown to yield consistently vaccines that comply with the requirements for immunogenicity and safety.

The production method is validated to demonstrate that the product, if tested, would comply with the test for abnormal toxicity for immunosera and vaccines for human use (*2.6.9*).

Hepatitis B vaccine (rDNA) is produced by the expression of the viral gene coding for hepatitis B surface antigen (HBsAg) in yeast (*Saccharomyces cerevisiae*) or mammalian cells [Chinese hamster ovary (CHO) cells or other suitable cell lines], purification of the resulting HBsAg and the rendering of this antigen into an immunogenic preparation. The suitability and safety of the cells are approved by the competent authority.

The vaccine may contain the product of the S gene (major protein), a combination of the S gene and pre-S2 gene products (middle protein) or a combination of the S gene, the pre-S2 gene and pre-S1 gene products (large protein).

Reference preparation: a part of a batch representative of vaccine batches that have been shown in clinical studies in young healthy adults to produce at least 95 per cent seroconversion (HBsAg antibody titre >10 I.U./litre after a full-course primary immunisation) is used as a reference preparation.

CHARACTERISATION OF THE SUBSTANCE

Development studies are carried out to characterise the antigen. The complete protein, lipid and carbohydrate structure of the antigen is established. The morphological characteristics of the antigen particles are established by electron microscopy. The buoyant density of the antigen particles is determined by a physico-chemical method, for example gradient centrifugation. The antigenic epitopes are characterised. The protein fraction of the antigen is characterised in terms of the primary structure (for example, by determination of the amino-acid composition, by partial amino-acid sequence analysis and by peptide mapping).

CULTURE AND HARVEST

Identity, microbial purity, plasmid retention and consistency of yield are determined at suitable production stages. If mammalian cells are used, tests for extraneous agents and mycoplasmas are performed in accordance with *2.6.16. Tests for extraneous agents in viral vaccines for human use.*

PURIFIED ANTIGEN

Only a purified antigen that complies with the following requirements may be used in the preparation of the final bulk.

Total protein The total protein is determined by a validated method. The content is within the limits approved for the specific product.

Antigen content and identification The quantity and specificity of HBsAg is determined in comparison with the International Standard for HBsAg subtype *ad* or an in-house reference, by a suitable immunochemical method (*2.7.1*) such as radioimmunoassay (RIA), enzyme-linked immunosorbent assay (ELISA), immunoblot (preferably using a monoclonal antibody directed against a protective epitope) or single radial diffusion. The antigen/protein ratio is within the limits approved for the specific product.

The molecular weight of the major band in a sodium dodecyl sulphate polyacrylamide gel electrophoresis (SDS-PAGE) under reduced conditions corresponds to the value expected from the gene sequence and possible glycosylation.

Antigenic purity The purity of the antigen is determined by comparison with a reference preparation using liquid chromatography or other suitable methods such as SDS-PAGE with staining by acid blue 92 and silver. A suitable method is sensitive enough to detect a potential contaminant at a concentration of 1 per cent of total protein. Not less than 95 per cent of the total protein consists of hepatitis B surface antigen.

Composition The content of proteins, lipids, nucleic acids and carbohydrates is determined.

Host-cell- and vector-derived DNA If mammalian cells are used for production, not more than 10 pg of DNA in the quantity of purified antigen equivalent to a single human dose of vaccine.

Caesium If a caesium salt is used during production, a test for residual caesium is carried out on the purified antigen. The content is within the limits approved for the specific product.

Sterility (*2.6.1*). The purified antigen complies with the test for sterility, carried out using 10 ml for each medium.

Additional tests on the purified antigen may be required depending on the production method used: for example, a test for residual animal serum where mammalian cells are used for production or tests for residual chemicals used during extraction and purification.

FINAL BULK VACCINE

An antimicrobial preservative and an adjuvant may be included in the vaccine.

Only a final bulk vaccine that complies with the following requirements may be used in the preparation of the final lot.

Antimicrobial preservative Where applicable, determine the amount of antimicrobial preservative by a suitable chemical or physico-chemical method. The amount is not less than the 85 per cent and not greater than 115 per cent of that stated on the label.

Sterility (*2.6.1*). The final bulk vaccine complies with the test for sterility, using 10 ml for each medium.

FINAL LOT

Only a final lot that complies with each of the requirements given below under Identification, Tests and Assay may be released for use. Provided that the tests for free formaldehyde, antimicrobial preservative content and the assay in animals, where applicable, have been carried out on the final bulk vaccine with satisfactory results, they may be omitted on the final lot.

IDENTIFICATION

The assay or, where applicable, the electrophoretic profile, serves also to identify the vaccine.

TESTS

Aluminium When hydrated aluminium phosphate or aluminium hydroxide is used as the adsorbent, the vaccine complies with the test prescribed in the monograph on *Vaccines for human use (153)*.

Free formaldehyde Where applicable, the vaccine complies with the test prescribed in the monograph on *Vaccines for human use (153)*.

Antimicrobial preservative Where applicable, determine the amount of antimicrobial preservative by a suitable chemical or physico-chemical method. The content is not less than the minimum amount shown to be effective and is not greater than 115 per cent of that stated on the label.

Sterility (*2.6.1*). The vaccine complies with the test for sterility.

Pyrogens (*2.6.8*). The vaccine complies with the test for pyrogens. Inject the equivalent of one human dose into each rabbit.

A validated test for bacterial endotoxins (*2.6.14*) may be used instead of the test for pyrogens.

POTENCY

The potency of the vaccine is determined either in animals by comparing in given conditions its capacity to induce specific anti-HBsAg antibodies in mice or guinea-pigs with the same capacity of the reference preparation or by measuring the antigen content using a validated *in vitro* method (*2.7.1*).

Potency requirement The upper fiducial limit ($P = 0.95$) of the estimated relative potency is not less than 1.0.

Test in animals

Selection and distribution of the test animals Use in the test healthy mice from the same stock, about 5 weeks old. The strain of mice used for this test must give a significant slope for the dose-response curve to the antigen; mice with haplotype H-2^q or H-2^d are suitable. Healthy guinea-pigs, weighing 300 g to 350 g (about 7 weeks old) from the same stock are also suitable. Use animals of the same sex. Distribute the animals in at least seven equal groups of a number appropriate to the requirements of the assay.

Determination of potency of the vaccine to be examined Using a 9 g/l solution of *sodium chloride R* containing the aluminium adjuvant used for the vaccine or another appropriate diluent, prepare at least three dilutions of the vaccine to be examined and matching dilutions of the reference preparation. Allocate the dilutions one to each of the groups of animals and inject intraperitoneally not more than 1.0 ml of each dilution into each animal in the group to which that dilution is allocated. One group of animals remains unvaccinated and is injected intraperitoneally with the same volume of diluent. After an appropriate time interval (for example, 4 to 6 weeks), anaesthetise and bleed all animals, keeping the individual sera separate. Assay the individual sera for specific HBsAg antibody by a suitable immunoassay (*2.7.1*).

Calculations Calculations are carried out by the usual statistical methods for an assay with a quantal response (*5.3. Statistical Analysis of Results of Biological Assays and Tests, section 4*).

From the distribution of reaction levels measured on all the sera in the unvaccinated group, the maximum reaction level that can be expected to occur in an unvaccinated animal for that particular assay is determined. Any response in vaccinated animals that exceeds this level is by definition a seroconversion.

The percentage of animals showing seroconversion in each group is suitably transformed (for example, a probit transformation) and a parallel-line model, using the log dose-response curve, is applied to the data. The potency of the test preparation relative to the reference is established.

Validity conditions The test is not valid unless:

- for both the test and the reference vaccine, the ED_{50} lies between the smallest and the largest doses given to the animals,
- the statistical analysis shows no deviation from linearity or parallelism.
- the fiducial limits of the relative potency fall between 33 and 300 per cent of the estimated potency.

ED_{50}(effective dose 50 per cent): the statistically determined dose of a vaccine that in the conditions of the test induces specific antibodies in 50 per cent of the animals for the relevant vaccine antigens.

In vitro method

An *in vitro* method validated against the test in animals may be used. Enzyme-linked immunosorbent assay (ELISA) and radio-immunoassay (RIA) using monoclonal antibodies specific for protection-inducing epitopes of HBsAg have been shown to be suitable. Suitable numbers of dilutions of the vaccine to be examined and the reference preparation are used and a parallel-line model is used to analyse the data which may be suitably transformed. Kits for measuring HBsAg *in vitro* are commercially available and it is possible to adapt their test procedures for use as an *in vitro* potency assay.

STORAGE

See *Vaccines for human use (153)*.

LABELLING

See *Vaccines for human use (153)*.

The label states:

- the amount of HBsAg per container,
- the type of cells used for production of the vaccine,
- the name and amount of the adjuvant,
- that the vaccine must be shaken before use,
- that the vaccine must not be frozen.

Ph Eur

Inactivated Influenza Vaccine (Whole Virion)

Inactivated Influenza Vaccine (Whole Virion) complies with the requirements of the 3rd edition of the European Pharmacopoeia. [0159]. These requirements are reproduced after the heading 'Definition' below.

The label may state 'Flu/Vac'.

When Inactivated Influenza Vaccine or Influenza Vaccine is prescribed or demanded and the form is not stated, Inactivated Influenza Vaccine (Whole Virion), Inactivated Influenza Vaccine (Split Virion) or Inactivated Influenza Vaccine (Surface Antigen) may be dispensed or supplied.

Ph Eur

DEFINITION

Influenza vaccine (whole virion, inactivated) is a sterile, aqueous suspension of a strain or strains of influenza virus, type A or B, or a mixture of strains of the two types grown individually in fertilised hens' eggs and inactivated in such a manner that their antigenic properties are retained. The stated amount of haemagglutinin antigen for each strain present in the vaccine is 15 µg per dose, unless clinical evidence supports the use of a different amount.

The vaccine is a slightly opalescent liquid.

PRODUCTION

The production method is validated to demonstrate that the product, if tested, would comply with the test for abnormal toxicity for immunosera and vaccines for human use (*2.6.9*).

CHOICE OF VACCINE STRAIN

The World Health Organisation reviews the world epidemiological situation annually and if necessary recommends new strains corresponding to prevailing epidemiological evidence.

Such strains are used in accordance with the regulations in force in the signatory states of the Convention on the Elaboration of a European Pharmacopoeia. It is now common practice to use reassorted strains giving high yields of the appropriate surface antigens. The origin and passage history of virus strains shall be approved by the competent authority.

SUBSTRATE FOR VIRUS PROPAGATION

Influenza virus seed to be used in the production of vaccine is propagated in fertilised eggs from chicken flocks free from specified pathogens *(5.2.2)* or in suitable cell cultures (*5.2.4*), such as chick-embryo fibroblasts or chick kidney cells obtained from chicken flocks free from specified pathogens *(5.2.2)*. For production, the virus of each strain is grown in the allantoic cavity of fertilised hens' eggs from healthy flocks.

VIRUS SEED LOT

The production of vaccine is based on a seed-lot system. Working seed lots represent not more than fifteen passages from the approved reassorted virus or the approved virus isolate. The final vaccine represents one passage from the working seed lot. The haemagglutinin and neuraminidase antigens of each seed lot are identified as originating from the correct strain of influenza virus by suitable methods.

Only a working virus seed lot that complies with the following requirements may be used in the preparation of the monovalent pooled harvest.

Bacterial and fungal contamination Carry out the test for sterility (*2.6.1*), using 10 ml for each medium.

Mycoplasmas (*2.6.7*). Carry out the test for mycoplasmas, using 10 ml.

VIRUS PROPAGATION AND HARVEST

An antimicrobial agent may be added to the inoculum. After incubation at a controlled temperature, the allantoic fluids are harvested and combined to form a monovalent pooled harvest. An antimicrobial agent may be added at the time of harvest. At no stage in the production is penicillin or streptomycin used.

MONOVALENT POOLED HARVEST

To limit the possibility of contamination, inactivation is initiated as soon as possible after preparation. The virus is inactivated by a method that has been demonstrated on three consecutive batches to be consistently effective for the manufacturer. The inactivation process shall have been shown to be capable of inactivating the influenza virus without destroying its antigenicity; the process should cause minimum alteration of the haemagglutinin and neuraminidase antigens. The inactivation process shall also have been shown to be capable of inactivating avian leucosis viruses and mycoplasmas. If the monovalent pooled harvest is stored after inactivation, it is held at a temperature of 5 ± 3°C. If formaldehyde solution is used, the concentration does not exceed 0.2 g/l of CH_2O at any time during inactivation; if betapropiolactone is used, the concentration does not exceed 0.1 per cent *V/V* at any time during inactivation.

Before or after the inactivation process, the monovalent pooled harvest is concentrated and purified by high-speed centrifugation or other suitable method.

Only a monovalent pooled harvest that complies with the following requirements may be used in the preparation of the final bulk vaccine.

Haemagglutinin antigen Determine the content of haemagglutinin antigen by an immunodiffusion test (*2.7.1*), by comparison with a haemagglutinin antigen reference preparation or with an antigen preparation calibrated against it(1). Carry out the test at 20°C to 25°C.

Neuraminidase antigen The presence and type of neuraminidase antigen are confirmed by suitable enzymatic or immunological methods on the first three monovalent pooled harvests from each working seed lot.

Sterility (*2.6.1*). Carry out the test for sterility, using 10 ml for each medium.

Viral inactivation Carry out the test described below under Tests.

FINAL BULK VACCINE

Appropriate quantities of the monovalent pooled harvests are blended to make the final bulk vaccine.

Only a final bulk vaccine that complies with the following requirements may be used in the preparation of the final lot.

Antimicrobial preservative Where applicable, determine the amount of antimicrobial preservative by a suitable chemical method. The content is not less than 85 per cent and not greater than 115 per cent of the intended amount.

Sterility (*2.6.1*). Carry out the test for sterility using 10 ml for each medium.

FINAL LOT

The final bulk vaccine is distributed aseptically into sterile, tamper-proof containers. The containers are closed so as to prevent contamination.

Only a final lot that is satisfactory with respect to each of the requirements given below under Tests and Assay may be released for use. Provided that the test for viral inactivation has been performed with satisfactory results on each monovalent pooled harvest and that the tests for free formaldehyde, ovalbumin and total protein have been performed with satisfactory results on the final bulk vaccine, they may be omitted on the final lot.

IDENTIFICATION

The assay serves to confirm the antigenic specificity of the vaccine.

TESTS

Viral inactivation Inoculate 0.2 ml of the vaccine into the allantoic cavity of each of ten fertilised eggs and incubate at 33°C to 37°C for 3 days. The test is not valid unless at least eight of the ten embryos survive. Harvest 0.5 ml of the allantoic fluid from each surviving embryo and pool the fluids. Inoculate 0.2 ml of the pooled fluid into a further ten fertilised eggs and incubate at 33°C to 37°C for 3 days. The test is not valid unless at least eight of the ten embryos survive. Harvest about 0.1 ml of the allantoic fluid from each surviving embryo and examine each individual harvest for live virus by a haemagglutination test. If haemagglutination is found for any of the fluids, carry out for that fluid a further passage in eggs and test for haemagglutination; no haemagglutination occurs.

Total protein Not more than six times the total haemagglutinin content of the vaccine as determined in the assay, but in any case, not more than 100 µg of protein per virus strain per human dose and not more than a total of 300 µg of protein per human dose.

Free formaldehyde It complies with the test for free formaldehyde prescribed in the monograph on *Vaccines for human use (153)*.

Antimicrobial preservative. Where applicable, determine the amount of antimicrobial preservative by a suitable chemical method. The content is not less than the minimum amount shown to be effective and is not greater than 115 per cent of the quantity stated on the label.

Ovalbumin Not more than 1 µg of ovalbumin per human dose, determined by a suitable technique using a suitable reference preparation of ovalbumin.

Sterility (*2.6.1*). It complies with the test for sterility.

Bacterial endotoxins (*2.6.14*). Not more than 100 I.U. of endotoxin per human dose.

ASSAY

Determine the content of haemagglutinin antigen by an immunodiffusion test (*2.7.1*), by comparison with a haemagglutinin antigen reference preparation or with an antigen preparation calibrated against it(1). Carry out the test at 20°C to 25°C. The confidence interval (P = 0.95) of the assay is not greater than 80 per cent to 125 per cent of the estimated content. The lower confidence limit (P = 0.95) of the estimate of haemagglutinin antigen content is not less than 80 per cent of the amount stated on the label for each strain.

STORAGE

See *Vaccines for human use (153)*.

LABELLING

See *Vaccines for human use (153)*.

The label states:

— that the vaccine has been prepared on eggs,
— the strain or strains of influenza virus used to prepare the vaccine,
— the method of inactivation,
— the haemagglutinin content in micrograms per virus strain per dose,
— the season during which the vaccine is intended to protect.

[1]Reference haemagglutinin antigens are available from the National Institute for Biological Standards and Control, Blanche Lane, South Mimms, Potters Bar, Hertfordshire EN6 3QG, United Kingdom.

Ph Eur

Inactivated Influenza Vaccine (Split Virion)

Inactivated Influenza Vaccine (Split Virion) complies with the requirements of the 3rd edition of the European Pharmacopoeia [0158]. These requirements are reproduced after the heading 'Definition' below.

The label may state 'Flu/Vac/Split'.

When Inactivated Influenza Vaccine or Influenza Vaccine is prescribed or demanded and the form is not stated, Inactivated Influenza Vaccine (Whole Virion), Inactivated Influenza Vaccine (Split Virion) or Inactivated Influenza Vaccine (Surface Antigen) may be dispensed or supplied.

Ph Eur

DEFINITION

Influenza vaccine (split virion, inactivated) is a sterile, aqueous suspension of a strain or strains of influenza virus, type A or B, or a mixture of strains of the two types grown individually in fertilised hens' eggs, inactivated and treated so that the integrity of the virus particles has been disrupted without diminishing the antigenic properties of the haemagglutinin and neuraminidase antigens. The stated amount of haemagglutinin antigen for each strain present in the vaccine is 15 µg per dose, unless clinical evidence supports the use of a different amount.

The vaccine is a slightly opalescent liquid.

PRODUCTION

The production method is validated to demonstrate that the product, if tested, would comply with the test for abnormal toxicity for immunosera and vaccines for human use (*2.6.9*).

CHOICE OF VACCINE STRAIN

The World Health Organisation reviews the world epidemiological situation annually and if necessary recommends new strains corresponding to prevailing epidemiological evidence.

Such strains are used in accordance with the regulations in force in the signatory states of the Convention on the Elaboration of a European Pharmacopoeia. It is now common practice to use reassorted strains giving high yields of the appropriate surface antigens. The origin and passage history of virus strains shall be approved by the competent authority.

SUBSTRATE FOR VIRUS PROPAGATION

Influenza virus seed to be used in the production of vaccine is propagated in fertilised eggs from chicken flocks free from specified pathogens (*5.2.2*) or in suitable cell cultures (*5.2.4*), such as chick-embryo fibroblasts or chick kidney cells obtained from chicken flocks free from specified pathogens (*5.2.2*). For production, the virus of each strain is grown in the allantoic cavity of fertilised hens' eggs from healthy flocks.

VIRUS SEED LOT

The production of vaccine is based on a seed-lot system. Working seed lots represent not more than fifteen passages from the approved reassorted virus or the approved virus isolate. The final vaccine represents one passage from the working seed lot. The haemagglutinin and neuraminidase antigens of each seed lot are identified as originating from the correct strain of influenza virus by suitable methods.

Only a working virus seed lot that complies with the following requirements may be used in the preparation of the monovalent pooled harvest.

Bacterial and fungal contamination Carry out the test for sterility (*2.6.1*), using 10 ml for each medium.

Mycoplasmas (*2.6.7*). Carry out the test for mycoplasmas, using 10 ml.

VIRUS PROPAGATION AND HARVEST

An antimicrobial agent may be added to the inoculum. After incubation at a controlled temperature, the allantoic fluids are harvested and combined to form a monovalent pooled harvest. An antimicrobial agent may be added at the time of harvest. At no stage in the production is penicillin or streptomycin used.

MONOVALENT POOLED HARVEST

To limit the possibility of contamination, inactivation is initiated as soon as possible after preparation. The virus is inactivated by a method that has been demonstrated on three consecutive batches to be consistently effective for the manufacturer. The inactivation process shall have been shown to be capable of inactivating the influenza virus without destroying its antigenicity; the process should cause minimum alteration of the haemagglutinin and neuraminidase antigens. The inactivation process shall also have been shown to be capable of inactivating avian leucosis viruses and mycoplasmas. If the monovalent pooled harvest is stored after inactivation, it is held at a temperature of 5 ± 3°C. If formaldehyde solution is used, the concentration does not exceed 0.2 g/l of CH_2O at any time during inactivation; if betapropiolactone is used, the concentration does not exceed 0.1 per cent *V*/*V* at any time during inactivation.

Before or after the inactivation procedure, the monovalent pooled harvest is concentrated and purified by high-speed centrifugation or other suitable method and the virus particles are disrupted into component subunits by the use of approved procedures. For each new strain, a validation test is carried out to show that the monovalent bulk consists predominantly of disrupted virus particles.

Only a monovalent pooled harvest that complies with the following requirements may be used in the preparation of the final bulk vaccine.

Haemagglutinin antigen Determine the content of haemagglutinin antigen by an immunodiffusion test (*2.7.1*), by comparison with a haemagglutinin antigen reference preparation or with an antigen preparation calibrated against it[(1)]. Carry out the test at 20°C to 25°C.

For some vaccines, the physical form of the haemagglutinin particles prevents quantitative determination by immunodiffusion after inactivation of the virus. For these vaccines, a determination of haemagglutinin antigen is made on the monovalent pooled harvest before inactivation. The production process is validated to demonstrate suitable conservation of haemagglutinin antigen and a suitable tracer is used for formulation, for example, protein content.

Neuraminidase antigen The presence and type of neuraminidase antigen are confirmed by suitable enzymatic or immunological methods on the first three monovalent pooled harvests from each working seed lot.

Sterility (*2.6.1*). Carry out the test for sterility, using 10 ml for each medium.

Viral inactivation Carry out the test described below under Tests.

Chemicals used for disruption Tests are carried out on the monovalent pooled harvest for the chemicals used for disruption, the limits being approved by the competent authority.

FINAL BULK VACCINE

Appropriate quantities of the monovalent pooled harvests are blended to make the final bulk vaccine.

Only a final bulk vaccine that complies with the following requirements may be used in the preparation of the final lot.

Antimicrobial preservative Where applicable, determine the amount of antimicrobial preservative by a suitable chemical method. The content is not less than 85 per cent and not greater than 115 per cent of the intended amount.

Sterility (*2.6.1*). Carry out the test for sterility, using 10 ml for each medium.

FINAL LOT

The final bulk vaccine is distributed aseptically into sterile, tamper-proof containers. The containers are closed so as to prevent contamination.

Only a final lot that is satisfactory with respect to each of the requirements given below under Tests and Assay may be released for use. Provided that the test for viral inactivation has been performed with satisfactory results on each monovalent pooled harvest and that the tests for free formaldehyde, ovalbumin and total protein have been performed with satisfactory results on the final bulk vaccine, they may be omitted on the final lot.

IDENTIFICATION

The assay serves to confirm the antigenic specificity of the vaccine.

TESTS

Viral inactivation Inoculate 0.2 ml of the vaccine into the allantoic cavity of each of ten fertilised eggs and incubate at 33°C to 37°C for 3 days. The test is not valid unless at least eight of the ten embryos survive. Harvest 0.5 ml of the allantoic fluid from each surviving embryo and pool the fluids. Inoculate 0.2 ml of the pooled fluid into a further ten fertilised eggs and incubate at 33°C to 37°C for 3 days. The test is not valid unless at least eight of the ten embryos survive. Harvest about 0.1 ml of the allantoic fluid from each surviving embryo and examine each individual harvest for live virus by a haemagglutination test. If haemagglutination is found for any of the fluids, carry out for that fluid a further passage in eggs and test for haemagglutination; no haemagglutination occurs.

Total protein Not more than six times the total haemagglutinin content of the vaccine as determined in the assay, but in any case, not more than 100 µg of protein per virus strain per human dose and not more than a total of 300 µg of protein per human dose.

Free formaldehyde It complies with the test for free formaldehyde prescribed in the monograph on *Vaccines for human use (153)*.

Antimicrobial preservative Where applicable, determine the amount of antimicrobial preservative by a suitable chemical method. The content is not less than the minimum amount shown to be effective and is not greater than 115 per cent of the quantity stated on the label.

Ovalbumin Not more than 1 µg of ovalbumin per human dose, determined by a suitable technique using a suitable reference preparation of ovalbumin.

Sterility It complies with the test for sterility (*2.6.1*).

Bacterial endotoxins (*2.6.14*). Not more than 100 I.U. of endotoxin per human dose.

ASSAY

Determine the content of haemagglutinin antigen by an immunodiffusion test (*2.7.1*), by comparison with a haemagglutinin antigen reference preparation or with an antigen preparation calibrated against it[(1)]. Carry out the test at 20°C to 25°C. The confidence interval ($P = 0.95$) of the assay is not greater than 80 per cent to 125 per cent of the estimated content. The lower confidence limit ($P = 0.95$) of the estimate of haemagglutinin antigen content is not less than 80 per cent of the amount stated on the label for each strain.

For some vaccines, quantitative determination of haemagglutinin antigen with respect to available reference preparations is not possible. An immunological identification of the haemagglutinin antigen and a semi-quantitative determination are carried out instead by suitable methods.

STORAGE

See *Vaccines for human use (153)*.

LABELLING

See *Vaccines for human use (153)*.

The label states:
— that the vaccine has been prepared on eggs,
— the strain or strains of influenza virus used to prepare the vaccine,
— the method of inactivation,
— the haemagglutinin content in micrograms per virus strain per dose,
— the season during which the vaccine is intended to protect.

---

[1]Reference haemagglutinin antigens are available from the National Institute for Biological Standards and Control, Blanche Lane, South Mimms, Potters Bar, Hertfordshire EN6 3QG, Great Britain.

Ph Eur

Inactivated Influenza Vaccine (Surface Antigen)

Inactivated Influenza Vaccine (Surface Antigen) complies with the requirements of the 3rd edition of the European Pharmacopoeia [0869]. These requirements are reproduced after the heading 'Definition' below.

The label may state 'Flu/Vac/SA'.

When Inactivated Influenza Vaccine or Influenza Vaccine is prescribed or demanded and the form is not stated, Inactivated Influenza Vaccine (Whole Virion), Inactivated Influenza Vaccine (Split Virion) or Inactivated Influenza Vaccine (Surface Antigen) may be dispensed or supplied.

Ph Eur

DEFINITION

Influenza vaccine (surface antigen, inactivated) is a sterile, aqueous suspension of a strain or strains of influenza virus, type A or B, or a mixture of strains of the two types grown individually in fertilised hens' eggs, inactivated and treated so that the preparation consists predominantly of haemagglutinin and neuraminidase antigens, without diminishing the antigenic properties of these antigens. The stated amount of haemagglutinin antigen for each strain present in the vaccine is 15 µg per dose, unless clinical evidence supports the use of a different amount.

The vaccine is a clear liquid.

PRODUCTION

The production method is validated to demonstrate that the product, if tested, would comply with the test for abnormal toxicity for immunosera and vaccines for human use (*2.6.9*).

CHOICE OF VACCINE STRAIN

The World Health Organisation reviews the world epidemiological situation annually and if necessary recommends new strains corresponding to prevailing epidemiological evidence.

Such strains are used in accordance with the regulations in force in the signatory states of the Convention on the Elaboration of a European Pharmacopoeia. It is now common practice to use reassorted strains giving high yields of the appropriate surface antigens. The origin and passage history of virus strains shall be approved by the competent authority.

SUBSTRATE FOR VIRUS PROPAGATION

Influenza virus seed to be used in the production of vaccine is propagated in fertilised eggs from chicken flocks free from specified pathogens (*5.2.2*) or in suitable cell cultures (*5.2.4*), such as chick-embryo fibroblasts or chick kidney cells obtained from chicken flocks free from specified pathogens (*5.2.2*). For production, the virus of each strain is grown in the allantoic cavity of fertilised hens' eggs from healthy flocks.

VIRUS SEED LOT

The production of vaccine is based on a seed-lot system. Working seed lots represent not more than fifteen passages from the approved reassorted virus or the approved virus isolate. The final vaccine represents one passage from the working seed lot. The haemagglutinin and neuraminidase antigens of each seed lot are identified as originating from the correct strain of influenza virus by suitable methods.

Only a working virus seed lot that complies with the following requirements may be used in the preparation of the monovalent pooled harvest.

Bacterial and fungal contamination Carry out the test for sterility (*2.6.1*), using 10 ml for each medium.

Mycoplasmas (*2.6.7*). Carry out the test for mycoplasmas, using 10 ml.

VIRUS PROPAGATION AND HARVEST

An antimicrobial agent may be added to the inoculum. After incubation at a controlled temperature, the allantoic fluids are harvested and combined to form a monovalent pooled harvest. An antimicrobial agent may be added at the time of harvest. At no stage in the production is penicillin or streptomycin used.

MONOVALENT POOLED HARVEST

To limit the possibility of contamination, inactivation is initiated as soon as possible after preparation. The virus is inactivated by a method that has been demonstrated on three consecutive batches to be consistently effective for the manufacturer. The inactivation process shall have been shown to be capable of inactivating the influenza virus without destroying its antigenicity; the process should cause minimum alteration of the haemagglutinin and neuraminidase antigens. The inactivation process shall also have been shown to be capable of inactivating avian leucosis viruses and mycoplasmas. If the monovalent pooled harvest is stored after inactivation, it is held at a temperature of 5 ± 3°C. If formaldehyde solution is used, the concentration does not exceed 0.2 g/l of CH_2O at any time during inactivation; if betapropiolactone is used, the concentration does not exceed 0.1 per cent *V/V* at any time during inactivation.

Before or after the inactivation process, the monovalent pooled harvest is concentrated and purified by high-speed centrifugation or other suitable method. Virus particles are disrupted into component subunits by approved procedures and further purified so that the monovalent bulk consists mainly of haemagglutinin and neuraminidase antigens.

Only a monovalent pooled harvest that complies with the following requirements may be used in the preparation of the final bulk vaccine.

Haemagglutinin antigen Determine the content of haemagglutinin antigen by an immunodiffusion test (*2.7.1*), by comparison with a haemagglutinin antigen reference preparation or with an antigen preparation calibrated against it[(1)]. Carry out the test at 20°C to 25°C.

Neuraminidase antigen The presence and type of neuraminidase antigen are confirmed by suitable enzymatic or immunological methods on the first three monovalent pooled harvests from each working seed lot.

Sterility (*2.6.1*). Carry out the test for sterility, using 10 ml for each medium.

Viral inactivation Carry out the test described below under Tests.

Purity The purity of the monovalent pooled harvest is examined by polyacrylamide gel electrophoresis or by other approved techniques. Mainly haemagglutinin and neuraminidase antigens shall be present.

Chemicals used for disruption and purification Tests are carried out on the monovalent pooled harvest for the chemicals used for disruption and purification, the limits being approved by the competent authority.

FINAL BULK VACCINE

Appropriate quantities of the monovalent pooled harvests are blended to make the final bulk vaccine.

Only a final bulk vaccine that complies with the following requirements may be used in the preparation of the final lot.

Antimicrobial preservative Where applicable, determine the amount of antimicrobial preservative by a suitable chemical method. The content is not less than 85 per cent and not greater than 115 per cent of the intended amount.

Sterility (*2.6.1*). Carry out the test for sterility, using 10 ml for each medium.

FINAL LOT

The final bulk vaccine is distributed aseptically into sterile, tamper-proof containers. The containers are closed so as to prevent contamination.

Only a final lot that is satisfactory with respect to each of the requirements given below under Tests and Assay may be released for use. Provided that the test for viral inactivation has been performed with satisfactory results on each monovalent pooled harvest and that the tests for free formaldehyde, ovalbumin and total protein have been performed with satisfactory results on the final bulk vaccine, they may be omitted on the final lot.

IDENTIFICATION

The assay serves to confirm the antigenic specificity of the vaccine.

TESTS

Viral inactivation Inoculate 0.2 ml of the vaccine into the allantoic cavity of each of ten fertilised eggs and incubate at 33°C to 37°C for 3 days. The test is not valid unless at least eight of the ten embryos survive. Harvest 0.5 ml of the allantoic fluid from each surviving embryo and pool the fluids. Inoculate 0.2 ml of the pooled fluid into a further ten fertilised eggs and incubate at 33°C to 37°C for 3 days. The test is not valid unless at least eight of the ten embryos survive. Harvest about 0.1 ml of the allantoic fluid from each surviving embryo and examine each individual harvest for live virus by a haemagglutination test. If haemagglutination is found for any of the fluids, carry out for that fluid a further passage in eggs and test for haemagglutination; no haemagglutination occurs.

Total protein Not more than 40 µg of protein other than haemagglutinin per virus strain per human dose and not more than a total of 120 µg of protein other than haemagglutinin per human dose.

Free formaldehyde It complies with the test for free formaldehyde prescribed in the monograph on *Vaccines for human use (153)*.

Antimicrobial preservative Where applicable, determine the amount of antimicrobial preservative by a suitable chemical method. The content is not less than the minimum amount shown to be effective and is not greater than 115 per cent of the quantity stated on the label.

Ovalbumin Not more than 1 µg of ovalbumin per human dose, determined by a suitable technique using a suitable reference preparation of ovalbumin.

Sterility It complies with the test for sterility (*2.6.1*).

Bacterial endotoxins (*2.6.14*). Not more than 100 I.U. of endotoxin per human dose.

ASSAY

Determine the content of haemagglutinin antigen by an immunodiffusion test (*2.7.1*), by comparison with a haemagglutinin antigen reference preparation or with an antigen preparation calibrated against it[(1)]. Carry out the test at 20°C to 25°C. The confidence interval (P = 0.95) of the assay is not greater than 80 per cent to 125 per cent of the estimated content. The lower confidence limit (P = 0.95) of the estimate of haemagglutinin antigen content is not less than 80 per cent of the amount stated on the label for each strain.

STORAGE

See *Vaccines for human use (153)*.

LABELLING

See *Vaccines for human use (153)*.

The label states:
- that the vaccine has been prepared on eggs,
- the strain or strains of influenza virus used to prepare the vaccine,
- the method of inactivation,
- the haemagglutinin content in micrograms per virus strain per dose,
- the season during which the vaccine is intended to protect.

[1]Reference haemagglutinin antigens are available from the National Institute for Biological Standards and Control, Blanche Lane, South Mimms, Potters Bar, Hertfordshire EN6 3QG, United Kingdom.

Ph Eur

Measles Vaccine, Live

Measles Vaccine, Live complies with the requirements of the 3rd edition of the European Pharmacopoeia for Measles Vaccine (Live) [0213]. These requirements are reproduced after the heading 'Definition' below.

The label may state 'Meas/Vac (Live)'.

Ph Eur

DEFINITION

Measles vaccine (live) is a freeze-dried preparation of an approved attenuated strain of measles virus. The vaccine is reconstituted immediately before use, as stated on the label, to give a clear liquid that may be coloured owing to the presence of a pH indicator.

PRODUCTION

The production of vaccine is based on a virus seed-lot system and, if the virus is propagated in human diploid cells, a cell-bank system. The production method shall have been shown to yield consistently live measles vaccines of adequate immunogenicity and safety in man. Unless otherwise justified and authorised, the virus in the final vaccine shall have undergone no more passages from the master seed lot than were used to prepare the vaccine shown in clinical studies to be satisfactory with respect to safety and efficacy; even with authorised exceptions, the number of passages beyond the level used for clinical studies shall not exceed five.

The production method is validated to demonstrate that the product, if tested, would comply with the test for abnormal toxicity for immunosera and vaccines for human use (*2.6.9*).

SUBSTRATE FOR VIRUS PROPAGATION

The virus is propagated in human diploid cells (*5.2.3*) or in cultures of chick-embryo cells derived from a chicken flock free from specified pathogens (*5.2.2*).

VIRUS SEED LOT

The strain of measles virus used shall be identified by historical records that include information on the origin of the strain and its subsequent manipulation. To avoid the unnecessary use of monkeys in the test for neurovirulence, virus seed lots are prepared in large quantities and stored at temperatures below –20°C, if freeze-dried, or below –60°C, if not freeze-dried.

Only a virus seed lot that complies with the following requirements may be used for virus propagation.

Identification The master and working seed lots are identified as measles virus by serum neutralisation in cell culture, using specific antibodies.

Virus concentration The virus concentration of the master and working seed lots is determined to monitor consistency of production.

Extraneous agents (*2.6.16*). The working seed lot complies with the requirements for seed lots.

Neurovirulence (*2.6.18*). The working seed lot complies with the test for neurovirulence of live virus vaccines. *Macaca* and *Cercopithecus* monkeys susceptible to measles virus are suitable for the test.

VIRUS PROPAGATION AND HARVEST

All processing of the cell bank and subsequent cell cultures is done under aseptic conditions in an area where no other cells are handled. Approved animal (but not human) serum may be used in the growth medium, but the final medium for maintaining cell growth during virus multiplication does not contain animal serum. Serum and trypsin used in the preparation of cell suspensions and media are shown to be free from extraneous agents. The cell culture medium may contain a pH indicator such as phenol red and approved antibiotics at the lowest effective concentration. It is preferable to have a substrate free from antibiotics during production. Not less than 500 ml of the production cell culture is set aside as uninfected cell cultures (control cells). The viral suspensions are harvested at a time appropriate to the strain of virus being used.

Only a single harvest that complies with the following requirements may be used in the preparation of the final bulk vaccine.

Identification The single harvest contains virus that is identified as measles virus by serum neutralisation in cell culture, using specific antibodies.

Virus concentration The virus concentration in single harvests is determined as prescribed under Assay to monitor consistency of production and to determine the dilution to be used for the final bulk vaccine.

Extraneous agents (*2.6.16*).

Control cells The control cells of the production cell culture comply with a test for identification and with the requirements for extraneous agents (*2.6.16*).

FINAL BULK VACCINE

Virus harvests that comply with the above tests are pooled and clarified to remove cells. A suitable stabiliser may be added and the pooled harvests diluted as appropriate.

Only a final bulk vaccine that complies with the following requirement may be used in the preparation of the final lot.

Bacterial and fungal contamination The final bulk vaccine complies with the test for sterility (*2.6.1*), carried out using 10 ml for each medium.

FINAL LOT

The final bulk vaccine is distributed aseptically into sterile, tamper-proof containers and freeze-dried to a moisture content shown to be favourable to the stability of the vaccine. The containers are then closed so as to prevent contamination and the introduction of moisture.

Only a final lot that complies with the following requirement for thermal stability and with each of the requirements given below under Identification, Tests and Assay may be released for use. Provided that the test for bovine serum albumin has been carried out with satisfactory results on the final bulk vaccine, it may be omitted on the final lot.

Thermal stability An accelerated degradation test is carried out on the freeze-dried vaccine by heating at 37°C for 7 days. The virus concentration after this period is not more than 1 $\log_{10}$ lower than the initial value and, in any case, must not be less than 1×10^3 $CCID_{50}$ per dose.

IDENTIFICATION

When the vaccine reconstituted as stated on the label is mixed with specific measles antibodies, it is no longer able to infect susceptible cell cultures.

TESTS

Bacterial and fungal contamination. The reconstituted vaccine complies with the test for sterility (*2.6.1*).

Bovine serum albumin Not more than 50 ng per single human dose, determined by a suitable immunochemical method (*2.7.1*).

Water (*2.5.12*). Not more than 3.0 per cent, determined by the semi-micro determination of water.

ASSAY

Titrate the vaccine for infective virus at least in triplicate, using at least five cell cultures for each 0.5 $\log_{10}$ dilution step or by a method of equal precision. Use an appropriate virus reference preparation to validate each assay. The estimated virus concentration is not less than that stated on the label; the minimum virus concentration stated on the label is not less than 1×10^3 $CCID_{50}$ per human dose. The assay is not valid if the confidence interval ($P = 0.95$) of the logarithm of the virus concentration is greater than ± 0.3.

STORAGE

See *Vaccines for human use (153)*.

LABELLING

See *Vaccines for human use (153)*.

The label states:

— the strain of virus used for the preparation of the vaccine,
— the type and origin of the cells used for the preparation of the vaccine,
— the minimum virus concentration,
— that contact with disinfectants is to be avoided,
— the time within which the vaccine must be used after reconstitution.

Ph Eur

Measles, Mumps and Rubella Vaccine, Live

Measles, Mumps and Rubella Vaccine, Live complies with the requirements of the 3rd edition of the European Pharmacopoeia for Measles, Mumps and Rubella Vaccine (Live) [1057]. These requirements are reproduced after the heading 'Definition' below.

The label may state 'MMR/Vac(Live)'.

Ph Eur

DEFINITION

Measles, mumps and rubella vaccine (live) is a freeze-dried preparation of suitable attenuated strains of measles virus, mumps virus and rubella virus.

The vaccine is reconstituted immediately before use, as stated on the label, to give a clear liquid that may be coloured owing to the presence of a pH indicator.

PRODUCTION

The three components are prepared as described in the monographs on *Measles vaccine (live) (213), Mumps vaccine (live) (538)* and *Rubella vaccine (live) (162)* and comply with the requirements prescribed therein.

The production method is validated to demonstrate that the product, if tested, would comply with the test for abnormal toxicity for immunosera and vaccines for human use (*2.6.9*).

FINAL BULK VACCINE

Virus harvests for each component are pooled and clarified to remove cells. A suitable stabiliser may be added and the pooled harvests diluted as appropriate. Suitable quantities of the pooled harvest for each component are mixed.

Only a final bulk vaccine that complies with the following requirement may be used in the preparation of the final lot.

Bacterial and fungal contamination. Carry out the test for sterility (*2.6.1*), using 10 ml for each medium.

FINAL LOT

The final bulk vaccine is distributed aseptically into sterile, tamper-proof containers and freeze-dried to a moisture content shown to be favourable to the stability of the vaccine. The containers are then closed so as to prevent contamination and the introduction of moisture.

Only a final lot that complies with the following requirements for thermal stability and each of the requirements given below under Identification, Tests and Assay may be released for use. Provided that the tests for bovine serum albumin and, where applicable, the test for ovalbumin have been carried out with satisfactory results on the final bulk vaccine, they may be omitted on the final lot.

Thermal stability An accelerated degradation test is carried out on the freeze-dried vaccine by heating at 37°C for 7 days. Unless otherwise justified and authorised, at the end of this period:

— the measles virus concentration is not more than 1 $\log_{10}$ lower than the initial value and is not less than 1×10^3 $CCID_{50}$ per single human dose,

— the mumps virus concentration is not more than 1 $\log_{10}$ lower than the initial value and is not less than 5×10^3 $CCID_{50}$ per single human dose,

— the rubella virus concentration is not more than 1 $\log_{10}$ lower than the initial value and is not less than 1×10^3 $CCID_{50}$ per single human dose.

IDENTIFICATION

When the vaccine reconstituted as stated on the label is mixed with antibodies specific for measles virus, mumps virus and rubella virus, it is no longer able to infect cell cultures susceptible to these viruses. When the vaccine reconstituted as stated on the label is mixed with quantities of specific antibodies sufficient to neutralise any two viral components, the third viral component infects susceptible cell cultures.

TESTS

Bacterial and fungal contamination. The reconstituted vaccine complies with the test for sterility (*2.6.1*).

Bovine serum albumin Not more than 50 ng per single human dose, determined by a suitable immunochemical method (*2.7.1*).

Ovalbumin If the mumps component is produced in chick embryos, the vaccine contains not more than 1 µg of ovalbumin per single human dose, determined by a suitable immunochemical method (*2.7.1*).

Water (*2.5.12*). Not more than 3.0 per cent, determined by the semi-micro determination of water.

ASSAY

A. Mix the vaccine with a sufficient quantity of antibodies specific for mumps virus and a sufficient quantity of antibodies specific for rubella virus. Titrate the vaccine for infective measles virus at least in triplicate, using at least five cell cultures for each 0.5 $\log_{10}$ dilution step or by a method of equal precision. Use an appropriate virus reference preparation to validate each assay. The estimated measles virus concentration is not less than that stated on the label; the minimum measles virus concentration stated on the label is not less than 1×10^3 $CCID_{50}$ per single human dose. The assay is not valid if the confidence interval ($P = 0.95$) of the logarithm of the virus concentration is greater than ± 0.3.

B. Mix the vaccine with a sufficient quantity of antibodies specific for measles virus and a sufficient quantity of antibodies specific for rubella virus. Titrate the vaccine for infective mumps virus at least in triplicate, using at least five cell cultures for each 0.5 $\log_{10}$ dilution step or by a method of equal precision. Use an appropriate virus reference preparation to validate each assay. The estimated mumps virus concentration is not less than that stated on the label; the minimum mumps virus concentration stated on the label is not less than 5×10^3 $CCID_{50}$ per single human dose. The assay is not valid if the confidence interval ($P = 0.95$) of the logarithm of the virus concentration is greater than ± 0.3.

C. Mix the vaccine with a sufficient quantity of antibodies specific for measles virus and a sufficient quantity of antibodies specific for mumps virus. Titrate the vaccine for infective rubella virus at least in triplicate, using at least five cell cultures for each 0.5 $\log_{10}$ dilution step or by a method of equal precision. Use an appropriate virus reference preparation to validate each assay. The estimated rubella virus concentration is not less than that stated on the label; the minimum rubella virus concentration stated on the label is not less than 1×10^3 $CCID_{50}$ per single human dose. The assay is not valid if the confidence interval ($P = 0.95$) of the logarithm of the virus concentration is greater than ± 0.3.

STORAGE

See *Vaccines for human use (153)*.

LABELLING

See *Vaccines for human use (153)*.

The label states:

— the strains of virus used in the preparation of the vaccine,

— where applicable, that chick embryos have been used for the preparation of the vaccine,

— the type and origin of the cells used for the preparation of the vaccine,

— the minimum virus concentration for each component of the vaccine,

— that contact with disinfectants is to be avoided,

— the time within which the vaccine must be used after reconstitution,

— that the vaccine must not be given to a pregnant woman and that a woman must not become pregnant within 2 months after having the vaccine.

Ph Eur

Meningococcal Polysaccharide Vaccine

Meningococcal Polysaccharide Vaccine complies with the requirements of the 3rd edition of the European Pharmacopoeia [0250]. These requirements are reproduced after the heading 'Definition' below.

The label may state 'Neimen/Vac'.

Ph Eur

DEFINITION

Meningococcal polysaccharide vaccine is a freeze-dried preparation of one or more purified capsular polysaccharides obtained from one or more suitable strains of *Neisseria meningitidis* group A, group C, group Y and group W135 that are capable of consistently producing polysaccharides.

N. meningitidis group A polysaccharide consists of partly *O*-acetylated repeating units of *N*-acetylmannosamine, linked with 1α→6 phosphodiester bonds.

N. meningitidis group C polysaccharide consists of partly *O*-acetylated repeating units of sialic acid, linked with 2α→9 glycosidic bonds.

N. meningitidis group Y polysaccharide consists of partly *O*-acetylated alternating units of sialic acid and D-glucose, linked with 2α→6 and 1α→4 glycosidic bonds.

N. meningitidis group W135 polysaccharide consists of partly *O*-acetylated alternating units of sialic acid and D-galactose, linked with 2α→6 and 1α→4 glycosidic bonds.

The polysaccharide component or components stated on the label together with calcium ions and residual moisture account for over 90 per cent of the mass of the preparation.

Meningococcal polysaccharide vaccine complies with the monograph on *Vaccines for human use (153)*.

PRODUCTION

Production of the meningococcal polysaccharides is based on a seed-lot system. The method of production shall have been shown to yield consistently meningococcal polysaccharide vaccines of satisfactory immunogenicity and safety for man.

The production method is validated to demonstrate that the product, if tested, would comply with the test for abnormal toxicity for immunosera and vaccines for human use (*2.6.9*).

SEED LOTS

The strains of *N. meningitidis* used for the master seed lots shall be identified by historical records that include information on their origin and by their biochemical and serological characteristics.

Cultures from the working seed lot shall have the same characteristics as the strain that was used to prepare the master seed lot. The strains have the following characteristics:

- colonies obtained from a culture are rounded, uniform in shape and smooth with a mucous, opalescent, greyish appearance,
- Gram staining reveals characteristic Gram-negative diplococci in 'coffee-bean' arrangement,
- the oxidase test is positive,
- the culture utilises glucose and maltose,
- suspensions of the culture agglutinate with suitable specific antisera.

PROPAGATION AND HARVEST

The working seed lots are cultured on solid media that do not contain blood-group substances or ingredients of mammalian origin. The inoculum may undergo one or more subcultures in liquid medium before being used for inoculating the final medium. The liquid media used and the final medium are semisynthetic and free from substances precipitated by cetrimonium bromide (hexadecyltrimethylammonium bromide) and do not contain blood-group substances or high-molecular-mass polysaccharides.

The bacterial purity of the culture is verified by microscopic examination of Gram-stained smears and by inoculation into appropriate media; several fields are observed at high magnification so that at least 10,000 organisms are examined.

The cultures are centrifuged and the polysaccharides precipitated from the supernatant by addition of cetrimonium bromide. The precipitate obtained is harvested and may be stored at −20°C awaiting further purification.

PURIFIED POLYSACCHARIDES

The polysaccharides are purified, after dissociation of the complex of polysaccharide and cetrimonium bromide, using suitable procedures to remove successively nucleic acids, proteins and lipopolysaccharides.

The final purification step consists of ethanol precipitation of the polysaccharides which are then dried and stored at −20°C. The loss on drying is determined by thermogravimetry (*2.2.34*) and the value is used to calculate the results of the other chemical tests with reference to the dried substance.

Only purified polysaccharides that comply with the following requirements may be used in the preparation of the final bulk vaccine.

Protein (*2.5.16*). Not more than 10 mg of protein per gram of purified polysaccharide, calculated with reference to the dried substance.

Nucleic acids (*2.5.17*). Not more than 10 mg of nucleic acids per gram of purified polysaccharide, calculated with reference to the dried substance.

***O*-Acetyl groups** (*2.5.19*). Not less than 2 mmol of *O*-acetyl groups per gram of purified polysaccharide for group A, not less than 1.5 mmol per gram of polysaccharide for group C, not less than 0.3 mmol per gram of polysaccharide for groups Y and W135, all calculated with reference to the dried substance.

Phosphorus (*2.5.18*). Not less than 80 mg of phosphorus per gram of group A purified polysaccharide, calculated with reference to the dried substance.

Sialic acid (*2.5.23*). Not less than 800 mg of sialic acid per gram of group C polysaccharide and not less than 560 mg of sialic acid per gram of purified polysaccharide for groups Y and W135, all calculated with reference to the dried substance. Use the following reference solutions:

Group C polysaccharide: a 150 mg/l solution of N-*acetylneuraminic acid R*.

Group Y polysaccharide: a solution containing 95 mg/l of N-*acetylneuraminic acid R* and 55 mg/l of *glucose R*.

Group W135 polysaccharide: a solution containing 95 mg/l of N-*acetylneuraminic acid R* and 55 mg/l of *galactose R*.

Calcium If a calcium salt is used during purification, a determination of calcium is carried out on the purified polysaccharide; the content is within the limits approved for the product.

Distribution of molecular size Examine by size-exclusion chromatography (*2.2.30)*, using *agarose for chromatography R* or *cross-linked agarose for chromatography R*. Use a column about 0.9 m long and 16 mm in internal diameter equilibrated with a solvent having an ionic strength of 0.2 mol/kg and a pH of 7.0 to 7.5. Apply to the column about 2.5 mg of polysaccharide in a volume of about 1.5 ml and elute at about 20 ml/h. Collect fractions of about 2.5 ml and determine the content of polysaccharide by a suitable method.

At least 65 per cent of group A polysaccharide, 75 per cent of group C polysaccharide, 80 per cent of group Y polysaccharide and 80 per cent of group W135 polysaccharide is eluted before a distribution coefficient (K_D) of 0.50 is reached. In addition, the percentages eluted before this distribution coefficient are within the limits approved for the particular product.

Identification and serological specificity The identity and serological specificity are determined by a suitable immunochemical method (*2.7.1*). Identity and purity of each polysaccharide shall be confirmed; it shall be shown that there is not more than 1 per cent *m/m* of group-heterologous *N. meningitidis* polysaccharide.

Pyrogens (*2.6.8*). The polysaccharide complies with the test for pyrogens. Inject into each rabbit per kilogram of body mass 1 ml of a solution containing 0.025 µg of purified polysaccharide per millilitre.

FINAL BULK VACCINE

One or more purified polysaccharides of one or more *N. meningitidis* groups are dissolved in a suitable solvent that may contain a stabiliser. When dissolution is complete, the solution is filtered through a bacteria-retentive filter.

Only a final bulk vaccine that complies with the following requirement may be used in the preparation of the final lot.

Sterility (*2.6.1*). The final bulk vaccine complies with the test for sterility, carried out using 10 ml for each medium.

FINAL LOT

The final bulk vaccine is distributed aseptically into sterile containers. The containers are then closed so as to avoid contamination.

Only a final lot that is satisfactory with respect to each of the requirements prescribed below under Identification, Tests and Assay may be released for use.

CHARACTERS

A white or cream-coloured powder or pellet, freely soluble in water.

IDENTIFICATION

Carry out an identification test for each polysaccharide present in the vaccine by a suitable immunochemical method (*2.7.1*).

TESTS

Distribution of molecular size Examine by size-exclusion chromatography (*2.2.30*). Use a column about 0.9 m long and 16 mm in internal diameter equilibrated with a solvent having an ionic strength of 0.2 mol/kg and a pH of 7.0 to 7.5. Apply to the column about 2.5 mg of each polysaccharide in a volume of about 1.5 ml and elute at about 20 ml/h. Collect fractions of about 2.5 ml and determine the content of polysaccharide by a suitable method.

For a divalent vaccine (group A + group C), use *cross-linked agarose for chromatography R*. The vaccine complies with the test if:

— 65 per cent of group A polysaccharide is eluted before K_D = 0.50,

— 75 per cent of group C polysaccharide is eluted before K_D = 0.50.

For a tetravalent vaccine (group A+ group C + group Y + group W135), use *cross-linked agarose for chromatography R1* and apply a suitable immunochemical method (*2.7.1*) to establish the elution pattern of the different polysaccharides. The vaccine complies with the test if K_D for the principal peak is:

— not greater than 0.70 for group A and group C polysaccharide,

— not greater than 0.57 for group Y polysaccharide,

— not greater than 0.68 for group W135 polysaccharide.

Water (*2.5.12*). Not more than 3.0 per cent, determined by the semi-micro determination of water.

Sterility (*2.6.1*). It complies with the test for sterility.

Pyrogens (*2.6.8*). It complies with the test for pyrogens. Inject per kilogram of the rabbit's mass 1 ml of a solution containing:

— 0.025 µg of polysaccharide for a monovalent vaccine,

— 0.050 µg of polysaccharide for a divalent vaccine,

— 0.10 µg of polysaccharide for a tetravalent vaccine.

ASSAY

Carry out an assay of each polysaccharide present in the vaccine.

For a divalent vaccine (group A +group C), use measurement of phosphorus (*2.5.18*) to determine the content of polysaccharide A and measurement of sialic acid (*2.5.23*) to determine the content of polysaccharide C. To determine sialic acid, use as reference solution a 150 mg/l solution of N-*acetylneuraminic acid R*.

For a tetravalent vaccine (group A + group C + group Y + group W135) a suitable immunochemical method (*2.7.1*) is used with a reference preparation of purified polysaccharide for each group.

The vaccine contains not less than 70 per cent and not more than 130 per cent of the quantity of each polysaccharide stated on the label.

STORAGE

See *Vaccines for human use (153)*.

LABELLING

See *Vaccines for human use (153)*.

The label states:

— the group or groups of polysaccharides (A, C, Y or W135) present in the vaccine,

— the number of micrograms of polysaccharide per human dose.

Ph Eur

Mumps Vaccine, Live

Mumps Vaccine, Live complies with the requirements of the 3rd edition of the European Pharmacopoeia for Mumps Vaccine (Live) [0213]. These requirements are reproduced after the heading 'Definition' below.

The label may state 'Mump/Vac (Live)'.

Ph Eur

DEFINITION

Mumps vaccine (live) is a freeze-dried preparation of an approved attenuated strain of mumps virus *(Paramyxo-*

virus parotitidis). The vaccine is reconstituted immediately before use, as stated on the label, to give a clear liquid that may be coloured owing to the presence of a pH indicator.

PRODUCTION

The production of vaccine is based on a virus seed-lot system and, if the virus is propagated in human diploid cells, a cell-bank system. The production method shall have been shown to yield consistently live mumps vaccines of adequate immunogenicity and safety in man. Unless otherwise justified and authorised, the virus in the final vaccine shall have undergone no more passages from the master seed lot than were used to prepare the vaccine shown in clinical studies to be satisfactory with respect to safety and efficacy.

The production method is validated to demonstrate that the product, if tested, would comply with the test for abnormal toxicity for immunosera and vaccines for human use (*2.6.9*).

SUBSTRATE FOR VIRUS PROPAGATION

The virus is propagated in human diploid cells (*5.2.3*) or in chick-embryo cells or in the amniotic cavity of chick embryos derived from a chicken flock free from specified pathogens (*5.2.2*).

VIRUS SEED LOT

The strain of mumps virus used shall be identified by historical records that include information on the origin of the strain and its subsequent manipulation. To avoid the unnecessary use of monkeys in the test for neurovirulence, virus seed lots are prepared in large quantities and stored at temperatures below −20°C, if freeze-dried, or below −60°C, if not freeze-dried.

Only a virus seed lot that complies with the following requirements may be used for virus propagation.

Identification The master and working seed lots are identified as mumps virus by serum neutralisation in cell culture, using specific antibodies.

Virus concentration The virus concentration of the master and working seed lots is determined to ensure consistency of production.

Extraneous agents (*2.6.16*). The working seed lot complies with the requirements for virus seed lots.

Neurovirulence (*2.6.18*). The working seed lot complies with the test for neurovirulence of live virus vaccines. *Macaca* and *Cercopithecus* monkeys are suitable for the test.

VIRUS PROPAGATION AND HARVEST

All processing of the cell bank and subsequent cell cultures are done under aseptic conditions in an area where no other cells are handled. Approved animal (but not human) serum may be used in the media. Serum and trypsin used in the preparation of cell suspensions and media are shown to be free from extraneous agents. The cell culture medium may contain a pH indicator such as phenol red and approved antibiotics at the lowest effective concentration. It is preferable to have a substrate free from antibiotics during production. Not less than 500 ml of the production cell cultures is set aside as uninfected cell cultures (control cells). If the virus is propagated in chick embryos, 2 per cent but not less than twenty eggs are set aside as uninfect ed control eggs. The viral suspensions are harvested at a time appropriate to the strain of virus being used.

Only a single harvest that complies with the following requirements may be used in the preparation of the final bulk vaccine.

Identification The single harvest contains virus that is identified as mumps virus by serum neutralisation in cell culture, using specific antibodies.

Virus concentration The virus concentration in single harvests is determined as prescribed under Assay to monitor consistency of production and to determine the dilution to be used for the final bulk.

Extraneous agents (*2.6.16*).

Control cells or eggs The control cells of the production cell culture comply with a test for identity; the control cells and the control eggs comply with the requirements for extraneous agents (*2.6.16*).

FINAL BULK VACCINE

Single harvests that comply with the above tests are pooled and clarified to remove cells. A suitable stabiliser may be added and the pooled harvests diluted as appropriate.

Only a final bulk vaccine that complies with the following requirement may be used in the preparation of the final lot.

Bacterial and fungal contamination The final bulk vaccine complies with the test for sterility (*2.6.1*), carried out using 10 ml for each medium.

FINAL LOT

The final bulk vaccine is distributed aseptically into sterile, tamper-proof containers and freeze-dried to a moisture content shown to be favourable to the stability of the vaccine. The containers are then closed so as to prevent contamination and the introduction of moisture.

Only a final lot that complies with the following requirement for thermal stability and is satisfactory with respect to each of the requirements given below under Identification, Tests and Assay may be released for use. Provided that the tests for bovine serum albumin and, where applicable, ovalbumin have been carried out with satisfactory results on the final bulk vaccine, they may be omitted on the final lot.

Thermal stability An accelerated degradation test is carried out on the freeze-dried vaccine by heating at 37°C for 7 days. The virus concentration after this period is not more than 1 $\log_{10}$ lower than the initial value and, in any case, must not be less than 5×10^3 $CCID_{50\ per}$ dose.

IDENTIFICATION

When the vaccine reconstituted as stated on the label is mixed with specific mumps antibodies, it is no longer able to infect susceptible cell cultures.

TESTS

Bacterial and fungal contamination The reconstituted vaccine complies with the test for sterility (*2.6.1*).

Bovine serum albumin Not more than 50 ng per single human dose, determined by a suitable immunochemical method (*2.7.1*).

Ovalbumin If the vaccine is produced in chick embryos, it contains not more than 1 µg of ovalbumin per single human dose, determined by a suitable immunochemical method (*2.7.1*).

Water (*2.5.12*). Not more than 3.0 per cent, determined by the semi-micro determination of water.

ASSAY

Titrate the vaccine for infective virus at least in triplicate, using at least five cell cultures for each 0.5 $\log_{10}$ dilution step or by a method of equal precision. Use an appropriate virus reference preparation to validate each assay. The estimated virus concentration is not less than that stated on the label; the minimum virus concentration stated on the label is not less than 5×10^3 $CCID_{50}$ per human dose. The assay is not valid if the confidence interval (P = 0.95) of the logarithm of the virus concentration is greater than ± 0.3.

STORAGE

See *Vaccines for human use (153)*.

LABELLING

See *Vaccines for human use (153)*.

The label states:
- the strain of virus used for the preparation of the vaccine,
- that the vaccine has been prepared in chick embryos or the type and origin of cells used for the preparation of the vaccine,
- the minimum virus concentration,
- that contact with disinfectants is to be avoided,
- the time within which the vaccine must be used after reconstitution.

Ph Eur

Pertussis Vaccine

Whooping-cough Vaccine

When Pertussis Vaccine is issued as a plain vaccine, it complies with the requirements of the 3rd edition of the European Pharmacopoeia for Pertussis Vaccine [0160]. These requirements are reproduced after the heading 'Plain Vaccine' below.

When Pertussis Vaccine is issued as an adsorbed vaccine, it complies with the requirements of the 3rd edition of the European Pharmacopoeia for Pertussis Vaccine (Adsorbed) [0161]. These requirements are reproduced after the heading 'Adsorbed Vaccine' below.

The label may state 'Per/Vac' or 'Per/Vac/Ads', as appropriate.

When Pertussis Vaccine is prescribed or demanded and the form is not stated, either the plain or the adsorbed vaccine may be dispensed or supplied.

Ph Eur

PLAIN VACCINE [0160]

DEFINITION

Pertussis vaccine is a sterile saline suspension of inactivated whole cells of one or more strains of *Bordetella pertussis*.

PRODUCTION

Production of the vaccine is based on a seed-lot system. One or more strains of *B. pertussis* with known origin and history are used. Strains, culture medium and cultivation method are chosen in such a way that agglutinogens 1, 2 and 3 are present in the final vaccine. Each strain is grown for 24 h to 72 h in a liquid medium or on a solid medium; the medium used in the final cultivation stage does not contain blood or blood products. Human blood or blood products are not used in any culture media. The bacteria are harvested, washed to remove substances derived from the medium and suspended in a 9 g/l solution of sodium chloride or other suitable isotonic solution. The opacity of the suspension is determined not later than 2 weeks after harvest by comparison with the International Reference Preparation of Opacity and used as the basis of calculation for subsequent stages in vaccine preparation. The equivalence in International Units of the International Reference Preparation is stated by the World Health Organisation.

Single harvests are not used for the final bulk vaccine unless they have been shown to contain *B. pertussis* cells with the same characteristics, with regard to growth and agglutinogens, as the parent strain and to be free from contaminating bacteria and fungi. The bacteria are killed and detoxified in controlled conditions by means of a suitable chemical agent or by heating or by a combination of these two methods. Freedom from live *B. pertussis* is tested using a suitable culture medium. The suspension is maintained at 5 ± 3°C for a suitable period to diminish its toxicity.

FINAL BULK VACCINE

Suitable quantities of the inactivated single harvests are pooled to prepare the final bulk vaccine. Suitable antimicrobial preservatives may be added. The bacterial concentration of the final bulk vaccine does not exceed that corresponding to an opacity of 20 I.U. per single human dose. If two or more strains of *B. pertussis* are used, the composition of consecutive lots of the final bulk vaccine shall be consistent with respect to the proportion of each strain as measured in opacity units.

Only a final bulk vaccine that complies with the following requirements may be used in the preparation of the final lot.

Antimicrobial preservative Where applicable, determine the amount of antimicrobial preservative by a suitable chemical method. The amount is not less than 85 per cent and not greater than 115 per cent of the intended amount.

Sterility (*2.6.1*). Carry out the test for sterility using 10 ml for each medium.

Potency Carry out the test described under Potency.

FINAL LOT

The final bulk vaccine is distributed aseptically into sterile, tamper-proof containers. The containers are closed so as to prevent contamination.

Only a final lot that is satisfactory with respect to each of the requirements given below under Identification, Tests and Potency may be released for use. Provided the tests for specific toxicity, free formaldehyde and antimicrobial preservative and the determination of potency have been carried out with satisfactory results on the final bulk vaccine, they may be omitted on the final lot.

IDENTIFICATION

Identify pertussis vaccine by agglutination of the bacteria in the vaccine by antisera specific to *B. pertussis*.

TESTS

Specific toxicity Use not fewer than ten healthy mice each weighing 14 g to 16 g for the vaccine group and for the saline control. Use mice of the same sex or distribute males and females equally between the groups. Allow the animals access to food and water for at least 2 h before injection and during the test. Inject each mouse of the vaccine group intraperitoneally with 0.5 ml, containing a quantity of the vaccine equivalent to not less than half the single human dose. Inject each mouse of the control group with 0.5 ml of a 9 g/l sterile solution of *sodium chloride R*, preferably containing the same amount of antimicrobial preservative as that injected with the vaccine. Weigh the groups of mice immediately before the injection and 72 h and 7 days after the injection. The vaccine complies with the test if: (a) at the end of 72 h the total mass of the group of vaccinated mice is not less than that preceding the injection; (b) at the end of 7 days the average increase in mass per vaccinated mouse is not less than 60 per cent of that per control mouse; and (c) not more than 5 per cent of the vaccinated mice die during the test.

Free formaldehyde When the bacteria are inactivated with formaldehyde, the vaccine complies with the test prescribed in the monograph on *Vaccines for human use (153)*.

Antimicrobial preservative Where applicable, determine the amount of antimicrobial preservative by a suitable chemical method. The content is not less than the minimum amount shown to be effective and is not greater than 115 per cent of the quantity stated on the label.

Sterility (*2.6.1*). The vaccine complies with the test for sterility.

POTENCY

Carry out the assay of pertussis vaccine (*2.7.7*).

The estimated potency is not less than 4 I.U. per single human dose and the lower confidence limit ($P = 0.95$) of the estimated potency is not less than 2 I.U. per single human dose.

STORAGE

See *Vaccines for human use (153)*.

LABELLING

See *Vaccines for human use (153)*.

The label states:
— the minimum number of International Units per single human dose,
— that the vaccine must be shaken before use,
— that the vaccine is not to be frozen.

ADSORBED VACCINE [0161]

DEFINITION

Pertussis vaccine (adsorbed) is a sterile saline suspension of inactivated whole cells of one or more strains of *Bordetella pertussis*, to which hydrated aluminium phosphate, aluminium hydroxide or calcium phosphate has been added.

PRODUCTION

Production of the vaccine is based on a seed-lot system. One or more strains of *B. pertussis* with known origin and history are used. Strains, culture medium and cultivation method are chosen in such a way that agglutinogens 1, 2 and 3 are present in the final vaccine. Each strain is grown for 24 h to 72 h in a liquid medium or on a solid medium; the medium used in the final cultivation stage does not contain blood or blood products. Human blood or blood products are not used in any culture media. The bacteria are harvested, washed to remove substances derived from the medium and suspended in a 9 g/l solution of sodium chloride or other suitable isotonic solution. The opacity of the suspension is determined not later than 2 weeks after harvest by comparison with the International Reference Preparation of Opacity and used as the basis of calculation for subsequent stages in vaccine preparation. The equivalence in International Units of the International Reference Preparation is stated by the World Health Organisation.

Single harvests are not used for the final bulk vaccine unless they have been shown to contain *B. pertussis* cells with the same characteristics, with regard to growth and agglutinogens, as the parent strain and to be free from contaminating bacteria and fungi. The bacteria are killed and detoxified in controlled conditions by means of a suitable chemical agent or by heating or by a combination of these two methods. Freedom from live *B. pertussis* is tested using a suitable culture medium. The suspension is maintained at 5 ± 3°C for a suitable period to diminish its toxicity.

FINAL BULK VACCINE

Suitable quantities of the inactivated single harvests are pooled to prepare the final bulk vaccine. Hydrated aluminium phosphate, aluminium hydroxide or calcium phosphate is added to the cell suspension. Suitable antimicrobial preservatives may be added. The bacterial concentration of the final bulk vaccine does not exceed that corresponding to an opacity of 20 I.U. per single human dose. If two or more strains of *B. pertussis* are used, the composition of consecutive lots of the final bulk vaccine shall be consistent with respect to the proportion of each strain as measured in opacity units.

Only a final bulk vaccine that complies with the following requirements may be used in the preparation of the final lot.

Antimicrobial preservative Where applicable, determine the amount of antimicrobial preservative by a suitable chemical method. The amount is not less than 85 per cent and not greater than 115 per cent of the intended amount.

Sterility (*2.6.1*). Carry out the test for sterility using 10 ml for each medium.

Potency Carry out the test described under Potency.

FINAL LOT

The final bulk vaccine is distributed aseptically into sterile, tamper-proof containers. The containers are closed so as to prevent contamination.

Only a final lot that is satisfactory with respect to each of the requirements given below under Identification, Tests and Potency may be released for use. Provided the tests for specific toxicity, free formaldehyde and antimicrobial preservative and the determination of potency have been carried out with satisfactory results on the final bulk vaccine, they may be omitted on the final lot.

IDENTIFICATION

Dissolve in the vaccine to be examined sufficient *sodium citrate R* to give a 100 g/l solution. Maintain at 37°C for about 16 h and centrifuge to obtain a bacterial precipitate.

Other suitable methods for separating the bacteria from the adsorbent may also be used. Identify pertussis vaccine by agglutination of the bacteria from the resuspended precipitate by antisera specific to *B. pertussis* or by the assay prescribed under Potency.

TESTS

Specific toxicity Use not fewer than ten healthy mice each weighing 14 g to 16 g for the vaccine group and for the saline control. Use mice of the same sex or distribute males and females equally between the groups. Allow the animals access to food and water for at least 2 h before injection and during the test. Inject each mouse of the vaccine group intraperitoneally with 0.5 ml, containing a quantity of the vaccine equivalent to not less than half the single human dose. Inject each mouse of the control group with 0.5 ml of a 9 g/l sterile solution of *sodium chloride R*, preferably containing the same amount of antimicrobial preservative as that injected with the vaccine. Weigh the groups of mice immediately before the injection and 72 h and 7 days after the injection. The vaccine complies with the test if: (a) at the end of 72 h the total mass of the group of vaccinated mice is not less than that preceding the injection; (b) at the end of 7 days the average increase in mass per vaccinated mouse is not less than 60 per cent of that per control mouse; and (c) not more than 5 per cent of the vaccinated mice die during the test.

Aluminium When hydrated aluminium phosphate or aluminium hydroxide is used as the adsorbent, the vaccine complies with the test prescribed in the monograph on *Vaccines for human use (153)*.

Calcium When calcium phosphate is used as the adsorbent, the vaccine complies with the test prescribed in the monograph on *Vaccines for human use (153)*.

Free formaldehyde When the bacteria are inactivated with formaldehyde, the vaccine complies with the test prescribed in the monograph on *Vaccines for human use (153)*.

Antimicrobial preservative Where applicable, determine the amount of antimicrobial preservative by a suitable chemical method. The content is not less than the minimum amount shown to be effective and is not greater than 115 per cent of the quantity stated on the label.

Sterility (*2.6.1*). The vaccine complies with the test for sterility.

POTENCY

Carry out the assay of pertussis vaccine (*2.7.7*).

The estimated potency is not less than 4 I.U. per single human dose and the lower confidence limit ($P = 0.95$) of the estimated potency is not less than 2 I.U. per single human dose.

STORAGE

See *Vaccines for human use (153)*.

LABELLING

See *Vaccines for human use (153)*.

The label states:

— the minimum number of International Units per single human dose,
— the name and the amount of the adsorbent,
— that the vaccine must be shaken before use,
— that the vaccine is not to be frozen.

Ph Eur

Pneumococcal Polysaccharide Vaccine

Pneumococcal Polysaccharide Vaccine complies with the requirements of the 3rd edition of the European Pharmacopoeia [0966]. These requirements are reproduced after the heading 'Definition' below.

The label may state 'Pneumo/Vac'.

Ph Eur

DEFINITION

Pneumococcal polysaccharide vaccine consists of a mixture of equal parts of purified capsular polysaccharide antigens prepared from suitable pathogenic strains of *Streptococcus pneumoniae* whose capsules have been shown to be made up of polysaccharides that are capable of inducing satisfactory levels of specific antibodies in man. It contains the twenty-three immunochemically different capsular polysaccharides listed in the Table 966-1.

The vaccine is a clear, colourless liquid.

PRODUCTION

Production of the vaccine is based on a seed-lot system for each type. The production method shall have been shown to yield consistently pneumococcal polysaccharide vaccines of adequate safety and immunogenicity in man.

The production method is validated to demonstrate that the product, if tested, would comply with the test for abnormal toxicity for immunosera and vaccines for human use (*2.6.9*) modified as follows for the test in guinea-pigs: inject ten human doses into each guinea-pig and observe for 12 days.

MONOVALENT BULK POLYSACCHARIDES

The bacteria are grown in a suitable liquid medium that does not contain blood-group substances or high-molecular-mass polysaccharides. The bacterial purity of the culture is verified and the culture is inactivated with phenol. Impurities are removed by such techniques as fractional precipitation, enzymatic digestion and ultrafiltration. The polysaccharide is obtained by fractional precipitation, washed, and dried in a vacuum to a residual moisture content shown to be favourable to the stability of the polysaccharide. The residual moisture content is determined by drying under reduced pressure over diphosphorus pentoxide or by thermogravimetric analysis and the value obtained is used to calculate the results of the tests shown below with reference to the dried substance. The monovalent bulk polysaccharide is stored at a suitable temperature in conditions that avoid the uptake of moisture.

Only a monovalent bulk polysaccharide that complies with the following requirements may be used in the preparation of the final bulk vaccine. percentage contents of components, determined by the methods prescribed below, are shown in the Table 966-1.

Protein (*2.5.16*).

Nucleic acids (*2.5.17*).

Total nitrogen (*2.5.9*).

Phosphorus (*2.5.18*).

Molecular size Determine by size-exclusion chromatography (*2.2.30*) using *cross-linked agarose for chromatography R* or *cross-linked agarose for chromatography R1*.

TABLE 966-1 percentage contents of components of monovalent bulk polysaccharaides

Molecular Type*	Proteins	Nucleic acids	Total Nitrogen	Phosphorus	Molecular size (K_D) **	Molecular size (K_D) ***	Uronic acids	Hexos-amines	Methyl-pentoses	O-acetyl Groups
1	≤2	≤2	3.5–6	0–1.5	≤0.15		≤45			≤1.8
2	≤2	≤2	0–1	0–1.0	≤0.15		≤15		≤38	
3	≤5	≤2	0–1	0–1.0	≤0.15		≤40			
4	≤3	≤2	4–6	0–1.5	≤0.15			≤40		
5	≤ 7.5	≤2	2.5–6.0	≤2		≤60	≤12	≤20		
6B	≤2	≤2	0–2	2.5–5.0		≤50			≤15	
7F	≤5	≤2	1.5–4.0	0–1.0	≤0.20				≤13	
8	≤2	≤2	0–1	0–1.0	≤0.15		≤25			
9N	≤2	≤1	2.2–4	0–1.0	≤0.20		≤20	≤28		
9V	≤2	≤2	0.5–3	0–1.0		≤0.45	≤15	≤13		
10A	≤7	≤2	0.5–3.5	1.5–3.5		≤0.65		≤12		
11A	≤3	≤2	0–2.5	2.0–5.0		≤0.40				≤9
12F	≤3	≤2	3–5	0–1.0	≤0.25			≤25		
14	≤5	≤2	1.5–4	0–1.0	≤0.30			≤20		
15B	≤3	≤2	2–5	2.0–4.5		≤0.55		≤15		
17F	≤2	≤2	0–0.5	0–3.5		≤0.45			≤20	
18C	≤3	≤2	0–1	2.4–4.9	≤0.15				≤14	
19A	≤2	≤2	0.6–3.5	3.0–7.0	≤0.45			≤15	≤20	
19F	≤3	≤2	1.4–3.5	3.0–5.5	≤0.20			≤12.5	≤20	
20	≤2	≤2	0.5–2.5	1.5–4.0		≤0.60		≤12		
22F	≤7	≤2	0–2	0–1.0		≤0.55	≤15		≤25	
23F	≤2	≤2	0–1	3.0–4.5	≤0.15				≤37	
33F	≤2.5	≤2	0–1	0–1.0		≤0.50				

Uronic acids (*2.5.22*).

Hexosamines (*2.5.20*).

Methylpentoses (*2.5.21*).

***O*-Acetyl groups** (*2.5.19*).

Identification (*2.7.1*). Confirm the identity of the monovalent bulk polysaccharide by double immunodiffusion or electroimmunodiffusion (except for polysaccharides 7F, 14 and 33F), using specific antisera.

Specificity No reaction occurs when the antigens are tested against all the antisera specific for the other polysaccharides of the vaccine, including factor sera for distinguishing types within groups. The polysaccharides are tested at a concentration of 50 µg/ml using a method capable of detecting 0.5 µg/ml.

FINAL BULK VACCINE

The final bulk vaccine is obtained by aseptically mixing the different polysaccharide powders. The uniform mixture is aseptically dissolved in a suitable isotonic solution so that one human dose of 0.50 ml contains 25 µg of each polysaccharide. An antimicrobial preservative may be added. The solution is sterilised by filtration through a bacteria-retentive filter.

Only a final bulk vaccine that complies with the following requirements may be used in the preparation of the final lot.

Antimicrobial preservative Where applicable, determine the amount of antimicrobial preservative by a suitable chemical method. The content is not less than 85 per cent and not greater than 115 per cent of the intended amount.

Sterility (*2.6.1*). The final bulk vaccine complies with the test for sterility, using 10 ml for each medium.

FINAL LOT

The final bulk vaccine is distributed aseptically into sterile, tamper-proof containers.

Only a final lot that is satisfactory with respect to each of the requirements given below under identification, tests and assay may be released for use. Provided that the tests for phenol and for antimicrobial preservative have been carried out with satisfactory results on the final bulk vaccine, they may be omitted on the final lot. When consistency of production has been established on a suitable number of consecutive batches, the assay may be replaced by a qualitative test that identifies each polysaccharide, provided that an assay has been performed on each monovalent bulk polysaccharide used in the preparation of the final lot.

IDENTIFICATION

The assay serves also to identify the vaccine.

TESTS

pH (*2.2.3*). The pH of the vaccine is 4.5 to 7.4.

Antimicrobial preservative Where applicable, determine the amount of antimicrobial preservative by a suitable chemical method. The content is not less than the minimum amount shown to be effective and is not greater than 115 per cent of the quantity stated on the label.

Phenol (*2.5.15*). Not more than 2.5 g/l.

Sterility (*2.6.1*). It complies with the test for sterility.

Pyrogens (*2.6.8*). It complies with the test for pyrogens. Inject per kilogram of the rabbit's mass 1 ml of a dilution of the vaccine containing 2.5 µg/ml of each polysaccharide.

ASSAY

Determine the content of each polysaccharide by a suitable immunochemical method (*2.7.1*), using antisera specific for each polysaccharide contained in the vaccine, including factor sera for types within groups, and purified polysaccharides of each type as standards.

The vaccine contains not less than 70 per cent and not more than 130 per cent of the quantity stated on the label for each polysaccharide. The confidence interval (P = 0.95) of the assay is not greater than 80 per cent to 120 per cent.

STORAGE

See *Vaccines for human use (153)*.

LABELLING

See *Vaccines for human use (153)*.

The label states:
- the number of micrograms of each polysaccharide per human dose,
- the total amount of polysaccharide in the container.

Ph Eur

Inactivated Poliomyelitis Vaccine

Inactivated Poliomyelitis Vaccine complies with the requirements of the 3rd edition of the European Pharmacopoeia for Poliomyelitis Vaccine (Inactivated) [0214]. These requirements are reproduced after the heading 'Definition' below.

The label may state 'Pol/Vac(Inact)'.

Ph Eur

DEFINITION

Poliomyelitis vaccine (inactivated) is an aqueous suspension of suitable strains of poliomyelitis virus type 1, type 2 and type 3, grown in suitable cell cultures and inactivated by a suitable method. It is a clear liquid.

PRODUCTION

The vaccine is prepared using seed lots and virus used in the final vaccine represents not more than ten subcultures from the seed lots used for the production of the vaccine on which were carried out the laboratory and clinical tests which showed the strains to be suitable.

The production method is validated to demonstrate that the product, if tested, would comply with the test for abnormal toxicity for immunosera and vaccines for human use (*2.6.9*).

Animal serum may be used in the medium for initial cell growth, but the medium for maintaining cell culture during virus multiplication contains no protein. The concentration of serum carried over into the vaccine shall not exceed one part per million. The medium may contain a suitable pH indicator such as phenol red and suitable antibiotics at the smallest effective concentration.

Each virus suspension is tested for identity, bacterial sterility and, after neutralisation with specific antiserum, for freedom from extraneous viruses. The virus suspension is passed through a suitable filter and may then be concentrated and purified. The suspension should contain at least 1×10^7 $CCID_{50}$ per millilitre for each type of virus.

Within a suitable period of time of the last filtration preferably within 24 hours, suitable chemical substances that inactivate the virus filtrate without destroying its antigenicity are added. During inactivation a suitable filtration is made. If necessary, the inactivating substance is later neutralised. Each of the monovalent suspensions is shown by appropriate tests in cell cultures to be free from infective poliomyelitis virus and other human and simian viruses. The trivalent vaccine is prepared by mixing suspensions of each type. Before the addition of any antimicrobial preservative, the trivalent suspension is shown to be free from infective poliomyelitis virus and other human and simian viruses.

IDENTIFICATION

When injected into susceptible animals, it stimulates the production of neutralising antibodies to poliomyelitis virus type 1, type 2 and type 3.

TESTS

Sterility (*2.6.1*). It complies with the test for sterility.

POTENCY

Dilute the vaccine 1 in 20, 1 in 100 and 1 in 500 with a suitable buffered saline solution. Inject 0.5 ml of the dilutions intramuscularly into groups of ten three-week-old chickens or groups of ten guinea-pigs, each weighing 250 g to 350 g, using a separate group for each dilution of vaccine. Bleed the animals on the fifth or sixth day after the injection and separate the sera. Examine the sera for the presence of neutralising antibody, at a dilution of 1 in 4, to each of the poliomyelitis viruses type 1, type 2 and type 3. Mix 100 $CCID_{50}$ of virus with the dilution of serum and incubate at 37°C for 4 h 30 min to 6 h. Keep at 5 ± 3°C for 12 h to 18 h. Inoculate the mixtures into cell cultures for the detection of unneutralised virus and read the results up to 7 days after inoculation. For each group of animals, note the number of sera which have neutralising antibody and calculate the dilution of the vaccine giving an antibody response in 50 per cent of the animals.

The vaccine complies with the test if a dilution of 1 in 100 or more produces an antibody response for each of the three types of virus in 50 per cent of the animals.

STORAGE

See *Vaccines for human use (153)*.

LABELLING

See *Vaccines for human use (153)*.

Ph Eur

Poliomyelitis Vaccine, Live (Oral)

Poliomyelitis Vaccine, Live (Oral) complies with the requirements of the 3rd edition of the European Pharmacopoeia for Poliomyelitis Vaccine (Oral) [0215]. These requirements are reproduced after the heading 'Definition' below.

The label may state 'Pol/Vac(Oral)'.

For vaccine presented in single doses where the individual container is too small to accommodate the abbreviation 'Pol/Vac(Oral)', the code 'OPV' may be stated on the label on the container provided that the code 'OPV' is also stated on the label on the package.

Ph Eur

DEFINITION

Oral poliomyelitis vaccine is a preparation of approved strains of live attenuated poliovirus type 1, 2 or 3 grown in *in vitro* cultures of approved cells, containing any one type or any combination of the three types of Sabin strains, prepared in a form suitable for oral administration.

The vaccine is a clear liquid that may be coloured owing to the presence of a pH indicator.

PRODUCTION

The vaccine strains and the production method shall have been shown to yield consistently vaccines that are both immunogenic and safe in man.

The production of vaccine is based on a virus seed-lot system. Cell lines are used according to a cell-bank system. If primary monkey kidney cells are used, production complies with the requirements indicated below. Unless otherwise justified and authorised, the virus in the final vaccine shall not have undergone more than two passages from the master seed lot.

The production method is validated to demonstrate that the product, if tested, would comply with the test for abnormal toxicity for immunosera and vaccines for human use (*2.6.9*).

SUBSTRATE FOR VIRUS PROPAGATION

The virus is propagated in human diploid cells (*5.2.3*), in continuous cell lines or in monkey kidney cells. Continuous cell lines are approved by the competent authority.

Primary monkey cells *The following special requirements for the substrate for virus propagation apply to primary monkey cells.*

Monkeys used for preparation of kidney cell cultures and for testing of virus. If the vaccine is prepared in monkey kidney cell cultures, animals of a species approved by the competent authority, in good health, and not previously employed for experimental purposes shall be used.

The monkeys shall be kept in well-constructed and adequately ventilated animal rooms in cages spaced as far apart as possible. Adequate precautions shall be taken to prevent cross-infection between cages. Not more than two monkeys shall be housed per cage and cage-mates shall not be interchanged. The monkeys shall be kept in the country of manufacture of the vaccine in quarantine groups for a period of not less than 6 weeks before use. A quarantine group is a colony of selected, healthy monkeys kept in one room, with separate feeding and cleaning facilities, and having no contact with other monkeys during the quarantine period. If at any time during the quarantine period the overall death rate of a shipment consisting of one or more groups reaches 5 per cent (excluding deaths from accidents or where the cause was specifically determined not to be an infectious disease), monkeys from that entire shipment shall continue in quarantine from that time for a minimum of 6 weeks. The groups shall be kept continuously in isolation, as in quarantine, even after completion of the quarantine period, until the monkeys are used. After the last monkey of a group has been taken, the room that housed the group shall be thoroughly cleaned and decontaminated before being used for a fresh group. If kidneys from near-term monkeys are used, the mother is quarantined for the term of pregnancy.

Monkeys from which kidneys are to be removed shall be anaesthetised and thoroughly examined, particularly for evidence of tuberculosis and cercopithecid herpesvirus 1 (B virus) infection.

If a monkey shows any pathological lesion relevant to the use of its kidneys in the preparation of a seed lot or vaccine, it shall not be used, nor shall any of the remaining monkeys of the quarantine group concerned be used unless it is evident that their use will not impair the safety of the product.

All the operations described in this section shall be conducted outside the areas where the vaccine is produced.

The monkeys used shall be shown to be free from antibodies to simian virus 40 (SV40) and simian immunodeficiency virus. If *Macaca* spp. are used for production, the monkeys shall also be shown to be free from antibodies to cercopithecid herpesvirus 1 (B virus). Human herpesvirus has been used as an indicator for freedom from B virus antibodies on account of the danger of handling cercopithecid herpesvirus 1 (B virus).

Monkey kidney cell cultures for vaccine production. Kidneys that show no pathological signs are used for preparing cell cultures. If the monkeys are from a colony maintained for vaccine production, serially passaged monkey kidney cell cultures from primary monkey kidney cells may be used for virus propagation, otherwise the monkey kidney cells are not propagated in series. Virus for the preparation of vaccine is grown by aseptic methods in such cultures. If animal serum is used in the propagation of the cells, the maintenance medium after virus inoculation shall contain no added serum.

Each group of cell cultures derived from a single monkey or from fetuses from no more than ten near-term monkeys is prepared and tested as an individual group.

VIRUS SEED LOTS

The strains of poliovirus used shall be identified by historical records that include information on the origin and subsequent manipulation of the strains.

Working seed lots are prepared by a single passage from a master seed lot and at an approved passage level from the original Sabin virus. Virus seed lots are prepared in large quantities and stored at a temperature below -60°C.

Only a virus seed lot that complies with the following requirements may be used for virus propagation.

Identification Each working seed lot is identified as poliovirus of the given type, using specific antibodies.

Virus concentration Determined by the method described below, the virus concentration is the basis for the quantity of virus used in the neurovirulence test.

Extraneous agents (*2.6.16*). If the working seed lot is produced in human diploid cells (*5.2.3*) or in continuous cell lines, it complies with the requirements for seed lots for virus vaccines. If the working seed lot is produced in primary monkey cells, it complies with the requirements given below under Virus Propagation and Harvest and Monovalent Pooled Harvest and with the tests in adult mice, suckling mice and guinea-pigs given under *2.6.16. Tests for extraneous agents in viral vaccines for human use.*

Neurovirulence (*2.6.19*). Each master and working seed lot complies with the test for neurovirulence of poliomyelitis vaccine (oral). Furthermore, the seed lot shall cease to be used in vaccine production if the frequency of failure of the monovalent pooled harvests produced from it is greater than predicted statistically. Reference preparations of the three types of poliovirus at the Sabin Original +2 passage level are available on application to Biologicals, WHO, Geneva, Switzerland. This statistical prediction is calculated after each test on the basis of all the monovalent pooled harvests tested; it is equal to the probability of false rejection on the occasion of a first test (i.e. 1 per cent), the probability of false rejection on retest being negligible. If the test is carried out only by the manufacturer, the test slides are provided to the control authority for assessment.

Genetic markers Each working seed lot is tested for its replicating properties at temperatures ranging from 36°C to 40°C as described under Monovalent Pooled Harvest.

VIRUS PROPAGATION AND HARVEST

All processing of the cell-banks and subsequent cell-cultures is done under aseptic conditions in an area where no other cells are handled. Approved animal (but not human) serum may be used in the media, but the final medium for maintaining cell growth during virus multiplication does not contain animal serum. Serum and trypsin used in the preparation of cell suspensions and media are shown to be free from live extraneous agents. The cell-culture medium may contain a pH indicator such as phenol red and approved antibiotics at the lowest effective concentration. It is preferable to have a substrate free from antibiotics during production. Not less than 5 per cent and not more than 1000 ml of the cell cultures employed for vaccine production are set aside as uninfected cell cultures (control cells); special requirements, given below, apply to control cells when the vaccine is produced in primary monkey cells The virus suspension is harvested not later than 4 days after virus inoculation. After inoculation of the production cell culture with the virus working seed lot, inoculated cells are maintained at a fixed temperature, shown to be suitable, within the range 33°C to 35°C; the temperature is maintained constant to ± 0.5°C; control cell cultures are maintained at 33°C to 35°C for the relevant incubation periods.

Only a single virus harvest that complies with the following requirements may be used in the preparation of the monovalent pooled harvest.

Virus concentration The virus concentration of virus harvests is determined as prescribed under Assay to monitor consistency of production and to determine the dilution to be used for the final bulk vaccine.

Extraneous agents (*2.6.16*).

Control cells The control cells of the production cell culture from which the virus harvest is derived comply with a test for identity and with the requirements for extraneous agents (*2.6.16*) or, where primary monkey cells are used, as shown below.

Primary monkey cells *The following special requirements apply to virus propagation and harvest in primary monkey cells.*

Cell cultures. On the day of inoculation with virus seed, each cell culture is examined for degeneration caused by an infective agent. If, in this examination, evidence is found of the presence in a cell culture of any extraneous agent, the entire group of cultures concerned shall be rejected.

On the day of inoculation with the virus working seed lot, a sample of at least 30 ml of the pooled fluid removed from the cell cultures of the kidneys of each single monkey or from fetuses from not more than ten near-term monkeys is divided into two equal portions. One portion of the pooled fluid is tested in monkey kidney cell cultures prepared from the same species, but not the same animal, as that used for vaccine production. The other portion of the pooled fluid is, where necessary, tested in monkey kidney cell cultures from another species so that tests on the pooled fluids are done in cell cultures from at least one species known to be sensitive to SV40. The pooled fluid is inoculated into bottles of these cell cultures in such a way that the dilution of the pooled fluid in the nutrient medium does not exceed 1 in 4. The area of the cell sheet is at least 3 cm^2 per millilitre of pooled fluid. At least one bottle of each kind of cell culture remains uninoculated to serve as a control. If the monkey species used for vaccine production is known to be sensitive to SV40, a test in a second species is not required. Animal serum may be used in the propagation of the cells, provided that it does not contain SV40 antibody, but the maintenance medium after inoculation of test material contains no added serum except as described below.

The cultures are incubated at a temperature of 35°C to 37°C and are observed for a total period of at least 4 weeks. During this observation period and after not less than 2 weeks' incubation, at least one subculture of fluid is made from each of these cultures in the same cell culture system. The subcultures are also observed for at least 2 weeks.

Serum may be added to the original culture at the time of subculturing, provided that the serum does not contain SV40 antibody.

Fluorescent-antibody techniques may be useful for detecting SV40 virus and other viruses in the cells.

A further sample of at least 10 ml of the pooled fluid is tested for cercopithecid herpesvirus 1 (B virus) and other viruses in rabbit kidney cell cultures. Serum used in the nutrient medium of these cultures shall have been shown to be free from inhibitors of B virus. Human herpesvirus has been used as an indicator for freedom from B virus inhibitors on account of the danger of handling cercopithecid herpesvirus 1 (B virus). The sample is inoculated into bottles of these cell cultures in such a way that the dilution of the pooled fluid in the nutrient medium does not exceed 1 in 4. The area of the cell sheet is at least 3 cm^2 per millilitre of pooled fluid. At least one bottle of the cell cultures remains uninoculated to serve as a control.

The cultures are incubated at a temperature of 35°C to 37°C and observed for at least 2 weeks.

A further sample of 10 ml of the pooled fluid removed from the cell cultures on the day of inoculation with the seed lot virus is tested for the presence of extraneous agents by inoculation into human cell cultures sensitive to measles virus.

The tests are not valid if more than 20 per cent of the culture vessels have been discarded for non-specific accidental reasons by the end of the respective test periods.

If, in these tests, evidence is found of the presence of an extraneous agent, the single harvest from the whole group of cell cultures concerned is rejected.

If the presence of cercopithecid herpesvirus 1 (B virus) is demonstrated, the manufacture of oral poliomyelitis vaccine shall be discontinued and the competent authority shall be informed. Manufacturing shall not be resumed until a thorough investigation has been completed and precautions have been taken against any reappearance of the infection, and then only with the approval of the competent authority.

If these tests are not done immediately, the samples of pooled cell-culture fluid shall be kept at a temperature of −60°C or below, with the exception of the sample for the test for B virus, which may be held at 4°C, provided that the test is done not more than 7 days after it has been taken.

Control cell cultures. On the day of inoculation with the virus working seed lot 25 per cent (but not more than 2.5 litres) of the cell suspension obtained from the kidneys of each single monkey or from not more than ten near-term monkeys is taken to prepare uninoculated control cell cultures. These control cell cultures are incubated in the same conditions as the inoculated cultures for at least 2 weeks and are examined during this period for evidence of cytopathic changes. The tests are not valid if more than 20 per cent of the control cell cultures have been discarded for non-specific, accidental reasons. At the end of the observation period, the control cell cultures are examined for degeneration caused by an infectious agent. If this examination or any of the tests required in this section shows evidence of the presence in a control culture of any extraneous agent, the poliovirus grown in the corresponding inoculated cultures from the same group shall be rejected.

Tests for haemadsorbing viruses. At the time of harvest or within 4 days of inoculation of the production cultures with the virus working seed lot, a sample of 4 per cent of the control cell cultures is taken and tested for haemadsorbing viruses. At the end of the observation period, the remaining control cell cultures are similarly tested. The tests are made as described in *2.6.16. Tests for extraneous agents in viral vaccines for human use.*

Tests for other extraneous agents. At the time of harvest, or within 7 days of the day of inoculation of the production cultures with the working seed lot, a sample of at least 20 ml of the pooled fluid from each group of control cultures is taken and tested in two kinds of monkey kidney cell culture, as described above.

At the end of the observation period for the original control cell cultures, similar samples of the pooled fluid are taken and the tests referred to in this section in the two kinds of monkey kidney cell culture and in the rabbit cell cultures are repeated, as described above under Cell cultures.

If the presence of cercopithecid herpesvirus 1 (B virus) is demonstrated, the production cell cultures shall not be used and the measures concerning vaccine production described above must be undertaken.

The fluids collected from the control cell cultures at the time of virus harvest and at the end of the observation period may be pooled before testing for extraneous agents. A sample of 2 per cent of the pooled fluid is tested in each of the cell culture systems specified.

Single harvests.

Tests for neutralised single harvests in monkey kidney cell cultures. A sample of at least 10 ml of each single harvest is neutralised by a type-specific poliomyelitis antiserum prepared in animals other than monkeys. In preparing antisera for this purpose, the immunising antigens used shall be prepared in non-simian cells.

Half of the neutralised suspension (corresponding to at least 5 ml of single harvest) is tested in monkey kidney cell cultures prepared from the same species, but not the same animal, as that used for vaccine production. The other half of the neutralised suspension is tested, if necessary, in monkey kidney cell cultures from another species so that the tests on the neutralised suspension are done in cell cultures from at least one species known to be sensitive to SV40.

The neutralised suspensions are inoculated into bottles of these cell cultures in such a way that the dilution of the suspension in the nutrient medium does not exceed 1 in 4. The area of the cell sheet is at least 3 cm^2 per millilitre of neutralised suspension. At least one bottle of each type of cell culture remains uninoculated to serve as a control and is maintained by nutrient medium containing the same concentration of the specific antiserum used for neutralisation.

Animal serum may be used in the propagation of the cells, provided that it does not contain SV40 antibody, but the maintenance medium, after the inoculation of the test material, contains no added serum other than the poliovirus neutralising antiserum, except as described below.

The cultures are incubated at a temperature of 35°C to 37°C and observed for a total period of at least 4 weeks. During this observation period and after not less than 2 weeks' incubation, at least one subculture of fluid is made from each of these cultures in the same cell-culture system. The subcultures are also observed for at least 2 weeks.

Serum may be added to the original cultures at the time of subculturing, provided that the serum does not contain SV40 antibody.

Additional tests are made for extraneous agents on a further sample of the neutralised single harvests by inoculation of 10 ml into human cell cultures sensitive to measles virus.

Fluorescent-antibody techniques may be useful for detecting SV40 virus and other viruses in the cells.

The tests are not valid if more than 20 per cent of the culture vessels have been discarded for non-specific accidental reasons by the end of the respective test periods.

If any cytopathic changes occur in any of the cultures, the causes of these change are investigated. If the cytopathic changes are shown to be due to unneutralised poliovirus, the test is repeated. If there is evidence of the presence of SV40 or other extraneous agents attributable to the single harvest, that single harvest is rejected.

MONOVALENT POOLED HARVEST

Monovalent pooled harvests are prepared by pooling a number of satisfactory single harvests of the same virus type. Monovalent pooled harvests from continuous cell lines may be purified. Each monovalent pooled harvest is filtered through a bacteria-retentive filter.

Only a monovalent pooled harvest that complies with the following requirements may be used in the preparation of the final bulk vaccine.

Identification Each monovalent pooled harvest is identified as poliovirus of the given type, using specific antibodies.

Virus concentration The virus concentration is determined by the method described below and serves as the basis for calculating the dilutions for preparation of the final bulk, for the quantity of virus used in the neurovirulence test and to establish and monitor production consistency.

Neurovirulence (*2.6.19*). Each monovalent pooled harvest complies with the test for neurovirulence of poliomyelitis vaccine (oral). If the test is carried out only by the manufacturer, the test slides are provided to the competent authority for assessment.

Genetic markers A ratio of the replication capacities of the virus in the monovalent pooled harvest is obtained over a temperature range between 36°C and 40°C in comparison with the seed lot or a reference preparation for the marker tests and with appropriate rct/40- and rct/40+ strains of poliovirus of the same type. The incubation temperatures used in this test are controlled to within ± 0.1°C. The monovalent pooled harvest passes the test if, for both the virus in the harvest and the appropriate reference material, the titre determined at 36°C is at least 5.0 log greater than that determined at 40°C. If growth at 40°C is so low that a valid comparison cannot be established, a temperature in the region of 39.0°C to 39.5°C is used, at which temperature the reduction in titre of the reference material must be in the range 3.0 to 5.0 log of its value at 36°C; the acceptable minimum reduction is determined for each virus strain at a given temperature. If the titres obtained for one or more of the reference viruses are not concordant with the expected values, the test must be repeated.

Primary monkey cells *The following special requirements apply to monovalent pooled harvests derived from primary monkey cells.*

Test in rabbits. A sample of the monovalent pooled harvest is tested for cercopithecid herpesvirus 1 (B virus) and other viruses by injection of not less than 100 ml into not fewer than 10 healthy rabbits each weighing 1.5 kg to 2.5 kg. Each rabbit receives not less than 10 ml and not more than 20 ml, of which 1 ml is given intradermally at multiple sites, and the remainder subcutaneously. The rabbits are observed for at least 3 weeks for death or signs of illness.

All rabbits that die after the first 24 h of the test and those showing signs of illness are examined by autopsy, and the brain and organs removed for detailed examination to establish the cause of death.

The test is not valid if more than 20 per cent of the inoculated rabbits show signs of intercurrent infection during the observation period. The monovalent pooled harvest passes the test if none of the rabbits shows evidence of infection with B virus or with other extraneous agents or lesions of any kind attributable to the bulk suspension.

If the presence of B virus is demonstrated, the measures concerning vaccine production described above under Cell cultures are taken.

Test in guinea-pigs. Administer to not fewer than five guinea-pigs, each weighing 350 g to 450 g, 0.1 ml of the monovalent pooled harvest by intracerebral injection and 0.5 ml by intraperitoneal injection. Measure the rectal temperature of each animal on each working day for 6 weeks. At the end of the observation period carry out autopsy on each animal.

In addition, administer to not fewer than five guinea-pigs 0.5 ml by intraperitoneal injection and observe as described above for 2 to 3 weeks. At the end of the observation period, carry out a passage from these animals to not fewer than five guinea-pigs using blood and a suspension of liver or spleen tissue. Measure the rectal temperature of the latter guinea-pigs for 2 to 3 weeks. Examine by autopsy all animals that, after the first day of the test, die or are killed because they show disease or show for three consecutive days a body temperature higher than 39°C; carry out histological examination to detect infection with Marburg virus; in addition, inject a suspension of liver or spleen tissue or of blood intraperitoneally into not fewer than three guinea-pigs. If any signs of infection with Marburg virus are noted, confirmatory serological tests are carried out on the blood of the affected animals. The monovalent pooled harvest complies with the test if not fewer than 80 per cent of the guinea-pigs survive to the end of the observation period and remain in good health and no animal shows signs of infection with Marburg virus.

FINAL BULK VACCINE

The final bulk vaccine is prepared from one or more satisfactory monovalent pooled harvests and may contain more than one virus type. Suitable flavouring substances and stabilisers may be added.

Only a final bulk vaccine that complies with the following requirement may be used in the preparation of the final lot.

Bacterial and fungal contamination Carry out the test for sterility (*2.6.1*), using 10 ml for each medium.

FINAL LOT

Only a final lot that complies with the following requirement for thermal stability and is satisfactory with respect to each of the requirements given below under Identification, Tests and Assay may be released for use.

Thermal stability Maintain samples of the final lot at 37°C for 48 h. Determine the total virus concentration as described under Assay in parallel for the heated vaccine and for unheated vaccine. The estimated difference between the total virus concentration of the unheated and heated vaccines is not greater than 0.5 $\log_{10}$ infectious virus units ($CCID_{50}$) per single human dose.

IDENTIFICATION

The vaccine is shown to contain poliovirus of each type stated on the label, using specific antibodies.

TESTS

Bacterial and fungal contamination The vaccine complies with the test for sterility (*2.6.1*).

ASSAY

Titrate for infectious virus at least in triplicate using the method described below. Use an appropriate virus reference preparation to validate each assay. If the vaccine contains more than one poliovirus type, titrate each type separately, using appropriate type-specific antiserum (or preferably a monoclonal antibody) to neutralise each of the other types present.

For a trivalent vaccine, the estimated mean virus titres must be: not less than $1 \times 10^{6.0}$ infectious virus units ($CCID_{50}$) per single human dose for type 1; not less than $1 \times 10^{5.0}$ infectious virus units ($CCID_{50}$) for type 2; and not less than $1 \times 10^{5.5}$ infectious virus units ($CCID_{50}$) for type 3.

For monovalent or divalent vaccine, the minimum virus titres are decided by the competent authority.

Method. Groups of eight to twelve flat-bottomed wells in a microtitre plate are inoculated with 0.1 ml of each of the selected dilutions of virus followed by a suitable cell suspension of the Hep-2 (Cincinnati) line. The plates are incubated at a suitable temperature. Examine the cultures on days 7 to 9. The assay is not valid if the confidence interval ($P = 0.95$) of the logarithm of the virus concentration is greater than ± 0.3.

STORAGE

See *Vaccines for human use (153)*.

LABELLING

See *Vaccines for human use (153)*.

The label states:
- the types of poliovirus contained in the vaccine,
- the minimum amount of virus of each type contained in one single human dose,
- the cell substrate used for the preparation of the vaccine,
- that the vaccine is not to be injected.

Ph Eur

Rabies Vaccine

Rabies Vaccine complies with the requirements of the 3rd edition of the European Pharmacopoeia for Rabies Vaccine for Human Use Prepared in Cell Cultures [0216]. These requirements are reproduced after the heading 'Definition' below.

The label may state 'Rab/Vac'.

Ph Eur

DEFINITION

Rabies vaccine for human use prepared in cell cultures is a freeze-dried preparation of a suitable strain of fixed rabies virus grown in cell cultures and inactivated by a validated method.

The vaccine is reconstituted immediately before use as stated on the label to give a clear liquid that may be coloured owing to the presence of a pH indicator.

The vaccine complies with the requirements of the monograph on *Vaccines for human use (153)*.

PRODUCTION

The production method shall have been shown to yield consistently vaccines that comply with the requirements for immunogenicity, safety and stability. Unless otherwise justified and authorised, the virus in the final vaccine shall not have undergone more passages from the master seed lot than was used to prepare the vaccine shown in clinical studies to be satisfactory with respect to safety and efficacy; even with authorised exceptions, the number of passages beyond the level used for clinical studies shall not exceed five.

The production method is validated to demonstrate that the product, if tested, would comply with the test for abnormal toxicity for immunosera and vaccines for human use (*2.6.9*).

SUBSTRATE FOR VIRUS PROPAGATION

The virus is propagated in a human diploid cell line (*5.2.3*), in a continuous cell line approved by the competent authority or in cultures of chick-embryo cells derived from a flock free from specified pathogens (*5.2.2*).

SEED LOTS

The strain of rabies virus used shall be identified by historical records that include information on the origin of the strain and its subsequent manipulation.

Working seed lots are prepared by not more than five passages from the master seed lot.

Only a working seed lot that complies with the following tests may be used for virus propagation.

Identification Each working seed lot is identified as rabies virus using specific antibodies.

Virus concentration The virus concentration of each working seed lot is determined by a cell culture method using immunofluorescence, to ensure consistency of production.

Extraneous agents (*2.6.16*). The working seed lot complies with the requirements for virus seed lots. If the virus has been passaged in mouse brain, specific tests for murine viruses are carried out.

VIRUS PROPAGATION AND HARVEST

All processing of the cell bank and subsequent cell cultures are done under aseptic conditions in an area where no other cells are handled. Approved animal (but not human) serum may be used in the media, but the final medium for maintaining cell growth during virus multiplication does not contain animal serum; the media may contain human albumin complying with the monograph *Human albumin solution (255)*. Serum and trypsin used in the preparation of cell suspensions and media are shown to be free from infectious extraneous agents; trypsin complies with the monograph *Trypsin (694)*. The cell culture media may contain a pH indicator such as phenol red and approved antibiotics at the lowest effective concentration. Not less than 500 ml of the cell cultures employed for vaccine production are set aside as uninfected cell cultures (control cells). The virus suspension is harvested on one or more occasions during incubation. Multiple harvests from the same production cell culture may be pooled and considered as a single harvest.

Only a single harvest that complies with the following requirements may be used in the preparation of the inactivated viral harvest.

Identification The single harvest contains virus that is identified as rabies virus using specific antibodies.

Virus concentration Titrate for infective virus in cell cultures; the titre is used to monitor consistency of production.

Control cells The control cells of the production cell culture from which the single harvest is derived comply with a test for identification and with the requirements for extraneous agents (*2.6.16*).

PURIFICATION AND INACTIVATION

The virus harvest may be concentrated and/or purified by suitable methods; the virus harvest is inactivated by a validated method at a fixed, well defined stage of the process which may be before, during or after any concentration or purification. The method shall have been shown to be capable of inactivating rabies virus without destruction of the immunogenic activity. If betapropiolactone is used, the concentration shall at no time exceed 1:3500.

Only an inactivated viral suspension that complies with the following requirements may be used in the preparation of the final bulk vaccine.

Inactivation Carry out an amplification test for residual infectious rabies virus immediately after inactivation or using a sample frozen immediately after inactivation and stored at – 70°C. Inoculate a quantity of inactivated viral suspension equivalent to not less than 25 doses of vaccine into cell cultures of the same type as those used for production of the vaccine. Subculture after 7 days and after 14 days examine the cell cultures for rabies virus using an immunofluorescence test. No rabies virus is detected.

Residual host-cell DNA If a continuous cell line is used for virus propagation, the content of residual host-cell DNA, determined using a suitable method as described in *Products of recombinant DNA technology (784)*, is not greater than 100 pg per single human dose.

FINAL BULK VACCINE

The final bulk vaccine is prepared from one or more inactivated viral suspensions. An approved stabiliser may be added to maintain the activity of the product during and after freeze-drying.

Only a final bulk vaccine that complies with the following requirements may be used in the preparation of the final lot.

Glycoprotein content Determine the glycoprotein content by a suitable immunochemical method (*2.7.1*), for example, single-radial immunodiffusion, enzyme-linked immunosorbent assay or an antibody-binding test. The content is within the limits approved for the particular product.

Sterility (*2.6.1*). The final bulk vaccine complies with the test for sterility, carried out using 10 ml for each medium.

FINAL LOT

The final bulk vaccine is distributed aseptically into sterile containers and freeze-dried to a moisture content shown to be favourable to the stability of the vaccine. The containers are then closed so as to avoid contamination and the introduction of moisture.

Only a final lot that complies with each of the requirements given below under Identification, Tests and Assay may be released for use. Provided that the test for inactivation has been carried out with satisfactory results on the inactivated viral suspension and the test for bovine serum albumin has been carried out with satisfactory results on the final bulk vaccine, these tests may be omitted on the final lot.

IDENTIFICATION

The vaccine is shown to contain rabies virus antigen by a suitable immunochemical method (*2.7.1*) using specific antibodies, preferably monoclonal; alternatively, the assay serves also to identify the vaccine.

TESTS

Inactivation Inoculate a quantity equivalent to not less than 25 human doses of vaccine into cell cultures of the same type as those used for production of the vaccine. Subculture after 7 days and after 14 days examine the cell cultures for rabies virus using an immunofluorescence test. No rabies virus is detected.

Bovine serum albumin Not more than 50 ng per single human dose, determined by a suitable immunochemical method (*2.7.1*).

Sterility (*2.6.1*). The vaccine complies with the test for sterility.

Bacterial endotoxins (*2.6.14*). Not more than 25 I.U. per single human dose.

Pyrogens (*2.6.8*). The vaccine complies with the test for pyrogens. Unless otherwise justified and authorised, inject into each rabbit a single human dose of the vaccine diluted to ten times its volume.

Water (*2.5.12*). Not more than 3.0 per cent, determined by the semi-micro determination of water.

ASSAY

The potency of rabies vaccine is determined by comparing the dose necessary to protect mice against the effects of a lethal dose of rabies virus, administered intracerebrally, with the quantity of a reference preparation of rabies vaccine necessary to provide the same protection. For this comparison a reference preparation of rabies vaccine, calibrated in International Units, and a suitable preparation of rabies virus for use as the challenge preparation are necessary.

The International Unit is the activity contained in a stated quantity of the International Standard. The equivalence in International Units of the International Standard is stated by the World Health Organisation.

The test described below uses a parallel-line model with at least three points for the vaccine to be examined and the reference preparation. Once the analyst has experience with the method for a given vaccine, it is possible to carry out a simplified test using a single dilution of the vaccine to be examined. Such a test enables the analyst to determine that the vaccine has a potency significantly higher than the required minimum but will not give full information on the validity of each individual potency determination. The use of a single dilution allows a considerable reduction in the number of animals required for the test and must be considered by each laboratory in accordance with the provisions of the European Convention for the Protection of Vertebrate Animals used for Scientific and other Experimental Purposes.

Selection and distribution of the test animals. Use in the test healthy female mice about 4 weeks old, each weighing 11 g to 15 g, and from the same stock. Distribute the mice into six groups of a size suitable to meet the requirements for validity of the test and, for titration of the challenge suspension, four groups of five.

Preparation of the challenge suspension. Inoculate mice intracerebrally with the CVS strain of rabies virus and when the mice show signs of rabies, but before they die, sacrifice them, remove the brains and prepare a homogenate of the brain tissue in a suitable diluent. Separate gross particulate matter by centrifugation and use the supernatant liquid as the challenge suspension. Distribute the suspension in small volumes in ampoules, seal and store at a temperature below −60°C. Thaw one ampoule of the suspension and make serial dilutions in a suitable diluent. Allocate each dilution to a group of five mice and inject intracerebrally into each mouse 0.03 ml of the dilution allocated to its group. Observe the mice for 14 days. Calculate the LD_{50} of the undiluted suspension using the number in each group that, between the fifth and fourteenth days, die or develop signs of rabies.

Determination of potency of the vaccine to be examined. Prepare three fivefold serial dilutions of the vaccine to be examined and three fivefold serial dilutions of the reference preparation. Prepare the dilutions such that the most concentrated suspensions may be expected to protect more than 50 per cent of the animals to which they are administered and the least concentrated suspensions may be expected to protect less than 50 per cent of the animals to which they are administered. Allocate the six dilutions one to each of the six groups of sixteen mice and inject intraperitoneally into each mouse 0.5 ml of the dilution allocated to its group. After 7 days, prepare three identical dilutions of the vaccine to be examined and of the reference preparation and repeat the injections. Seven days after the second injection, prepare a suspension of the challenge virus such that, on the basis of the preliminary titration, 0.03 ml contains about 50 LD_{50}. Inject intracerebrally into each vaccinated mouse 0.03 ml of this suspension. Prepare three suitable serial dilutions of the challenge suspension. Allocate the challenge suspension and the three dilutions one to each of the four groups of ten control mice and inject intracerebrally into each mouse 0.03 ml of the suspension or one of the dilutions allocated to its group. Observe the animals in each group for 14 days and record the number in each group that die or show signs of rabies in the period 5 days to 14 days after challenge.

The test is not valid unless: for both the vaccine to be examined and the reference preparation the 50 per cent protective dose lies between the largest and smallest doses given to the mice; the titration of the challenge suspension shows that 0.03 ml of the suspension contained not less than 10 LD_{50}; the statistical analysis shows a significant slope and no significant deviations from linearity or parallelism of the dose-response lines; the fiducial limits of error ($P = 0.95$) are not less than 25 per cent and not more than 400 per cent of the estimated potency.

The vaccine complies with the test if the estimated potency is not less than 2.5 I.U. per human dose.

STORAGE

See *Vaccines for human use (153)*.

LABELLING

See *Vaccines for human use (153)*.

The label states the biological origin of the cells used for the preparation of the vaccine.

Ph Eur

Rubella Vaccine, Live

Rubella Vaccine, Live complies with the requirements of the 3rd edition of the European Pharmacopoeia for Rubella Vaccine (Live) [0162]. These requirements are reproduced after the heading 'Definition' below.

The label may state 'Rub/Vac(Live)'.

Ph Eur

DEFINITION

Rubella vaccine (live) is a freeze-dried preparation of an approved attenuated strain of rubella virus. The vaccine is reconstituted immediately before use, as stated on the label, to give a clear liquid that may be coloured owing to the presence of a pH indicator.

PRODUCTION

The production of vaccine is based on a virus seed-lot system and a cell-bank system. The production method shall have been shown to yield consistently live rubella vaccines of adequate immunogenicity and safety in man. Unless otherwise justified and authorised, the virus in the final vaccine shall have undergone no more passages from the master seed lot than were used to prepare the vaccine shown in clinical studies to be satisfactory with respect to safety and efficacy.

The production method is validated to demonstrate that the product, if tested, would comply with the test for abnormal toxicity for immunosera and vaccines for human use (*2.6.9*).

SUBSTRATE FOR VIRUS PROPAGATION

The virus is propagated in human diploid cells *(5.2.3)*.

VIRUS SEED LOT

The strain of rubella virus used shall be identified by historical records that include information on the origin of the strain and its subsequent manipulation. To avoid the unnecessary use of monkeys in the test for neurovirulence, virus seed lots are prepared in large quantities and stored at temperatures below −20°C, if freeze-dried, or below −60°C, if not freeze-dried.

Only a virus seed lot that complies with the following requirements may be used for virus propagation.

Identification The master and working seed lots are identified as rubella virus by serum neutralisation in cell culture, using specific antibodies.

Virus concentration The virus concentration of the master and working seed lots is determined to ensure consistency of production.

Extraneous agents (*2.6.16*). The working seed lot complies with the requirements for virus seed lots.

Neurovirulence (*2.6.17*). The working seed lot complies with the test for neurovirulence of live virus vaccines. *Macaca* and *Cercopithecus* monkeys are suitable for the test.

VIRUS PROPAGATION AND HARVEST

All processing of the cell bank and subsequent cell cultures are done under aseptic conditions in an area where no other cells are handled. Approved animal (but not human) serum may be used in the growth medium, but the final medium for maintaining cell growth during virus multiplication does not contain animal serum. Serum and trypsin used in the preparation of cell suspensions and media are shown to be free from extraneous agents. The cell culture medium may contain a pH indicator such as phenol red and approved antibiotics at the lowest effective concentration. It is preferable to have a substrate free from antibiotics during production. Not less than 500 ml of the production cell cultures is set aside as uninfected cell cultures (control cells). The temperature of incubation is controlled during the growth of the virus. The virus suspension is harvested, on one or more occasions, within 28 days of inoculation. Multiple harvests from the same production cell culture may be pooled and considered as a single harvest.

Only a single harvest that complies with the following requirements may be used in the preparation of the final bulk vaccine.

Identification The virus harvest contains virus that is identified as rubella virus by serum neutralisation in cell culture, using specific antibodies.

Virus concentration The virus concentration in virus harvests is determined as prescribed under Assay to monitor consistency of production and to determine the dilution to be used for the final bulk vaccine.

Extraneous agents (*2.6.16*).

Control cells The control cells of the production cell culture from which the virus harvest is derived comply with a test for identification and with the requirements for extraneous agents (*2.6.16*).

FINAL BULK VACCINE

Virus harvests that comply with the above tests are pooled and clarified to remove cells. A suitable stabiliser may be added and the pooled harvests diluted as appropriate.

Only a final bulk vaccine that complies with the following requirement may be used in the preparation of the final lot.

Bacterial and fungal contamination The final bulk vaccine complies with the test for sterility (*2.6.1*), carried out using 10 ml for each medium.

FINAL LOT

The final bulk vaccine is distributed aseptically into sterile, tamper-proof containers and freeze-dried to a moisture content shown to be favourable to the stability of the vaccine. The containers are then closed so as to prevent contamination and the introduction of moisture.

Only a final lot that complies with the following requirement for thermal stability and with each of the requirements given below under Identification, Tests and Assay may be released for use. Provided that the tests for bovine serum albumin has been carried out with satisfactory results on the final bulk vaccine, it may be omitted on the final lot.

Thermal stability An accelerated degradation test is carried out on the freeze-dried vaccine by heating at 37°C for 7 days. The virus concentration after this period is not more than 1 $\log_{10}$ lower than the initial value and, in any case, must not be less than 1×10^3 $CCID_{50}$ per dose.

IDENTIFICATION

When the vaccine reconstituted as stated on the label is mixed with specific rubella antibodies, it is no longer able to infect susceptible cell cultures.

TESTS

Bacterial and fungal contamination The reconstituted vaccine complies with the test for sterility (*2.6.1*).

Bovine serum albumin Not more than 50 ng per single human dose, determined by a suitable immunochemical method (*2.7.1*).

Water (*2.5.12*). Not more than 3.0 per cent, determined by the semi-micro determination of water.

ASSAY

Titrate the vaccine for infective virus at least in triplicate, using at least five cell cultures for each 0.5 $\log_{10}$ dilution step or by a method of equal precision. Use an appropriate virus reference preparation to validate each assay. The estimated virus concentration is not less than that stated on the label; the minimum virus concentration stated on the label is not less than 1×10^3 $CCID_{50}$ per human dose. The assay is not valid if the confidence interval ($P = 0.95$) of the logarithm of the virus concentration is greater than ± 0.3.

STORAGE

See *Vaccines for human use (153)*.

LABELLING

See *Vaccines for human use (153)*.

The label states:
— the strain of virus used for the preparation of the vaccine,
— the type and origin of the cells used for the preparation of the vaccine,
— the minimum virus concentration,
— that contact with disinfectants is to be avoided,
— the time within which the vaccine must be used after reconstitution,
— that the vaccine must not be given to a pregnant woman and that a woman must not become pregnant within 2 months after having the vaccine.

Ph Eur

Tetanus Vaccine

Definition Tetanus Vaccine is prepared from tetanus toxin produced by the growth of *Clostridium tetani*. The toxin is converted to tetanus formol toxoid by treatment with Formaldehyde Solution.

The vaccine complies with the requirements stated under Vaccines, with the following modifications.

Identification Flocculates when mixed under appropriate conditions with tetanus antitoxin.

Specific toxicity Inject five times the dose stated on the label subcutaneously or intraperitoneally into each of five guinea-pigs. None of the guinea-pigs shows any symptoms of, or dies from, tetanus within 21 days. If more than one animal dies from non-specific causes within this period repeat the test. None of the second group of animals shows symptoms of tetanus or dies from tetanus or any other cause within 21 days.

Sterility Complies with the *test for sterility*, Appendix XVI A.

Potency Inject into each of no fewer than nine guinea-pigs either a single quantity containing five times the dose stated on the label or two quantities, separated by an interval of not more than 4 weeks, each containing one tenth of the dose stated on the label; some of the guinea-pigs may receive the single dose and the remainder the two doses. Not later than 6 weeks after the single injection or, if two injections have been given, not later than 2 weeks after the second injection, bleed the guinea-pigs and examine the sera of the guinea-pigs for antitoxin using the *biological test for tetanus antitoxin* described below. The serum of each of no fewer than two thirds of the guinea-pigs contains not less than 0.05 Unit of tetanus antitoxin per ml or, alternatively, the serum of each of no fewer than one third of the guinea-pigs contains not less than 0.5 Unit per ml.

Labelling The label states 'Tet/Vac/FT'.

When Tetanus Vaccine is prescribed or demanded and the form is not stated, Adsorbed Tetanus Vaccine may be dispensed or supplied.

BIOLOGICAL TEST FOR TETANUS ANTITOXIN

The potency of tetanus vaccine (or of the tetanus component of a mixed vaccine) is tested by *biological assay*, Appendix XIV, by assessing the ability of the vaccine to stimulate the production of tetanus antitoxin in guinea-pigs to which the vaccine has been administered as prescribed in the test for Potency. The sera of the guinea-pigs are examined for antitoxin by comparing their ability to protect mice from the paralytic effects of a fixed dose of tetanus toxin with the ability of the Standard Preparation of tetanus antitoxin to give the same protection. For this comparison the Standard Preparation of tetanus antitoxin and a suitable preparation of tetanus toxin, for use as a test toxin, are required. The Standard Preparation is used to determine an appropriate dose of the test toxin which is subsequently used in tests of the neutralising properties of the serum or sera being tested.

Standard Preparation

The Standard Preparation is the 3rd British Standard for Tetanus antitoxin, established in 1963, consisting of dried serum, or another suitable preparation the potency of which has been determined in relation to the British Standard.

Suggested method

PREPARATION OF TEST TOXIN Prepare tetanus toxin from a sterile filtrate of an 8 to 10 days culture of *Clostridium tetani*. Test toxin may be prepared by adding this filtrate to *glycerol* in the proportion of 1 volume of the filtrate to 1 or 2 volumes of *glycerol*. This solution of test toxin is stored at or below 0°. Test toxins may also be prepared in stable form by saturating the filtrate with *ammonium sulphate*, collecting the resulting precipitate, drying it over *phosphorus pentoxide* and reducing it to a fine powder. The powder so obtained is preserved in the dry condition at a low temperature, either in sealed ampoules, or over *phosphorus pentoxide* at a pressure of 2 kPa.

DETERMINATION OF THE DOSE OF TEST TOXIN First determine the Limes paralyticum/200 (Lp/200) dose of the test toxin. This is the smallest quantity of the toxin which, when mixed with 0.005 Unit of the Standard Preparation and injected into mice, causes tetanic paralysis within 4 days. The severity of the tetanic paralysis to be regarded as the end point is such that the paralysis is readily recognised but not sufficiently extensive to cause significant suffering.

Prepare a solution of the Standard Preparation by dissolving the contents of one ampoule in 1 ml of *water for injections* and adding sufficient *saline solution* to produce a total volume of 23 ml. Dilute a portion of the solution 200-fold with *saline solution* so that each 0.5 ml contains 0.025 Unit of tetanus antitoxin. Accurately measure or weigh a quantity of the test toxin and dilute with, or dissolve in, *saline solution*. Prepare mixtures such that each contains 0.5 ml of the solution of the Standard Preparation (0.025 Unit), one of a series of graded volumes of the solution of the test toxin and sufficient *saline solution* to give a total volume of 2.5 ml. Allow the mixtures to stand at room temperature, protected from light, for at least 1 hour. After this time inject 0.5 ml of each mixture subcutaneously into mice, four mice being used for each mixture, and observe the mice for 4 days.

The mixture that contains the smallest amount of toxin sufficient to cause tetanic paralysis within the 4-day period after injection contains five times the Lp/200 dose of the test toxin.

NEUTRALISATION TESTS WITH GUINEA-PIG SERA Prepare two dilutions of the serum obtained from each guinea-pig, the first containing 0.5 ml of undiluted serum and 1.0 ml of saline solution and the second 0.5 ml of a 10-fold dilution of guinea-pig serum and 1.0 ml of saline solution. Prepare a fresh 200-fold dilution of the Standard Preparation and use to make a series of further dilutions containing, respectively, 0.3, 0.4, 0.5, 0.6 and 0.7 ml and sufficient saline solution to give a final volume of 1.5 ml. Lastly, prepare a fresh solution of the test toxin such that 1.0 ml contains five times the Lp/200 dose as determined previously and add 1 ml of this solution to each dilution of the guinea-pig sera and of the Standard Preparation. Allow the mixtures so prepared to stand at room temperature and protect from light for at least 1 hour. After this time inject 0.5 ml of each mixture subcutaneously into mice, two or three mice being used for each mixture. Survival of the mice injected with mixtures made with undiluted serum to the fourth day after injection, either without paralysis or with paralysis comparable with that observed in the mice injected with the mixture considered in the determination of the dose of test toxin to contain five Lp/200 doses of toxin, indicates a concentration of antitoxin in the undiluted serum of not less than 0.05 Unit per ml. Survival of the mice injected with mixtures made with serum diluted 10-fold to the fourth day after injection, either without paralysis or with paralysis comparable with that observed in the mice injected with the mixture considered in the determination of the dose of test toxin to contain five Lp/200 doses of the test toxin, indicates a concentration of antitoxin in the undiluted serum of not less than 0.5 Unit per ml.

The test is not valid unless the mice injected with mixtures containing 0.5 ml of the Standard Preparation develop paralysis comparable with that observed in the mice injected with the mixture considered in the determination of the dose of test toxin to contain five Lp/200 doses of toxin, the mice injected with mixtures containing 0.3 ml and 0.4 ml of the Standard Preparation develop paralysis earlier in the observation period and the mice injected with mixtures containing 0.6 ml and 0.7 ml of the

Standard Preparation do not develop paralysis. Record the number of sera containing more than 0.05 Unit per ml and the number containing more than 0.5 Unit per ml.

Adsorbed Tetanus Vaccine

Adsorbed Tetanus Vaccine complies with the requirements of the 3rd edition of the European Pharmacopoeia for Tetanus Vaccine (Adsorbed) [0452]. These requirements are reproduced after the heading 'Definition' below.

The label may state 'Tet/Vac/Ads'.

When Tetanus Vaccine is prescribed or demanded and the form is not stated, Adsorbed Tetanus Vaccine may be dispensed or supplied.

Ph Eur

DEFINITION

Tetanus vaccine (adsorbed) is a preparation of tetanus formol toxoid adsorbed on a mineral carrier. The formol toxoid is prepared from the toxin produced by the growth of *Clostridium tetani*.

PRODUCTION

BULK PURIFIED TOXOID

For the production of tetanus toxin, from which toxoid is prepared, seed cultures are managed in a defined seed-lot system in which toxinogenicity is conserved and, where necessary, restored by deliberate reselection. A highly toxinogenic strain of *Clostridium tetani* with known origin and history is grown in a suitable liquid medium. At the end of cultivation, the purity of each culture is tested and contaminated cultures are discarded. Toxin-containing culture medium is collected aseptically. The toxin content (Lf per millilitre) is checked to monitor consistency of production. Single harvests may be pooled to prepare the bulk purified toxoid. The toxin is purified to remove components likely to cause adverse reactions in humans. The purified toxin is detoxified with formaldehyde by a method that avoids destruction of the immunogenic potency of the toxoid and reversion of toxoid to toxin, particularly on exposure to heat. Alternatively, purification may be carried out after detoxification.

Only bulk purified toxoid that complies with the following requirements may be used in the preparation of the final bulk vaccine.

Sterility (*2.6.1*). Carry out the test for sterility using 10 ml for each medium.

Absence of tetanus toxin Inject subcutaneously at least 500 Lf of purified toxoid in a volume of 1 ml into each of five healthy guinea-pigs, each weighing 250 g to 350 g, that have not previously been treated with any material that will interfere with the test. If within 21 days of the injection any of the animals shows signs of or dies from tetanus, the toxoid does not comply with the test. If more than one animal dies from non-specific causes, repeat the test once; if more than one animal dies in the second test, the toxoid does not comply with the test.

Irreversibility of toxoid Using the buffer for the final vaccine without adsorbent, prepare a dilution of the bulk purified toxoid containing the same toxoid concentration as the final vaccine. Divide the dilution into two equal parts. Keep one of them at 5 ± 3°C and the other at 37°C for 6 weeks. Test both dilutions by a suitable sensitive assay for active tetanus toxin, such as inoculation into mice or guinea-pigs. The toxoid complies with the test if neither sample produces any sign of a toxic reaction attributable to tetanus toxin.

Antigenic purity Not less than 1000 Lf per milligram of protein nitrogen.

FINAL BULK VACCINE

The final bulk vaccine is prepared by adsorption of a suitable quantity of bulk purified toxoid onto hydrated aluminium phosphate, aluminium hydroxide or calcium phosphate; the resulting mixture is approximately isotonic with blood. Suitable antimicrobial preservatives may be added. Certain antimicrobial preservatives, particularly those of the phenolic type, adversely affect the antigenic activity and must not be used.

Only final bulk vaccine that complies with the following requirements may be used in the preparation of the final lot.

Antimicrobial preservative Where applicable, determine the amount of antimicrobial preservative by a suitable chemical method. The amount is not less than 85 per cent and not greater than 115 per cent of the intended amount.

Sterility (*2.6.1*). Carry out the test for sterility using 10 ml for each medium.

Potency Carry out the test described under Potency.

FINAL LOT

The final bulk vaccine is distributed aseptically into sterile, tamper-proof containers. The containers are closed so as to prevent contamination.

Only a final lot that is satisfactory with respect to each of the requirements given below under Identification, Tests and Potency may be released for use. Provided the tests for specific toxicity, free formaldehyde and antimicrobial preservative and the determination of potency have been carried out with satisfactory results on the final bulk vaccine, they may be omitted on the final lot.

IDENTIFICATION

Dissolve in the vaccine to be examined sufficient *sodium citrate R* to give a 100 g/l solution. Maintain at 37°C for about 16 h and centrifuge until a clear supernatant liquid is obtained. The clear supernatant liquid reacts with a suitable tetanus antitoxin, giving a precipitate.

TESTS

Specific toxicity Inject subcutaneously five times the single human dose stated on the label into each of five healthy guinea-pigs, each weighing 250 g to 350 g, that have not previously been treated with any material that will interfere with the test. If within 21 days of the injection any of the animals shows signs of or dies from tetanus, the vaccine does not comply with the test. If more than one animal dies from non-specific causes, repeat the test once; if more than one animal dies in the second test, the vaccine does not comply with the test.

Aluminium When hydrated aluminium phosphate or aluminium hydroxide is used as the adsorbent, the vaccine complies with the test prescribed in the monograph on *Vaccines for human use (153)*.

Calcium When calcium phosphate is used as the adsorbent, the vaccine complies with the test prescribed in the monograph on *Vaccines for human use (153)*.

Free formaldehyde The vaccine complies with the test prescribed in the monograph on *Vaccines for human use (153)*.

Antimicrobial preservative Where applicable, determine the amount of antimicrobial preservative by a suitable chemical method. The content is not less than the minimum amount shown to be effective and is not greater than 115 per cent of the quantity stated on the label.

Sterility (*2.6.1*). The vaccine complies with the test for sterility.

POTENCY

Carry out one of the prescribed methods for the assay of tetanus vaccine (adsorbed) (*2.7.8*).

The lower confidence limit ($P = 0.95$) of the estimated potency is not less than 40 I.U. per single human dose.

STORAGE

See *Vaccines for human use (153)*.

LABELLING

See *Vaccines for human use (153)*.

The label states:
— the minimum number of International Units per single human dose,
— the name and the amount of the adsorbent,
— that the vaccine must be shaken before use,
— that the vaccine is not to be frozen.

Ph Eur

Typhoid Polysaccharide Vaccine

Typhoid Polysaccharide Vaccine complies with the requirements of the 3rd edition of the European Pharmacopoeia [1160]. These requirements are reproduced after the heading 'Definition' below.

The label may state 'Typhoid/Vi/Vac'.

Ph Eur

DEFINITION

Typhoid polysaccharide vaccine is a preparation of purified Vi capsular polysaccharide obtained from *Salmonella typhi* Ty2 strain or some other suitable strain that has the capacity to produce Vi polysaccharide.

Capsular Vi polysaccharide consists of partly 3-*O*-acetylated repeated units of 2-acetylamino-2-deoxy-D-galactopyranuronic acid with α-(1→4) linkages.

PRODUCTION

The production of Vi polysaccharide is based on a seed-lot system. The method of production shall have been shown to yield consistently typhoid polysaccharide vaccines of adequate immunogenicity and safety in man.

The production method is validated to demonstrate that the product, if tested, would comply with the test for abnormal toxicity (*2.6.9*) for immunosera and vaccines for human use.

BACTERIAL SEED LOTS

The strain of *S. typhi* used for the master seed lot shall be identified by historical records that include information on its origin and by its biochemical and serological characteristics. Cultures from the working seed lot shall have the same characteristics as the strain that was used to prepare the master seed lot.

Only a strain that has the following characteristics may be used in the preparation of the vaccine: (a) stained smears from a culture are typical of enterobacteria; (b) the culture utilises glucose without production of gas; (c) colonies on agar are oxidase-negative; (d) a suspension of the culture agglutinates specifically with a suitable Vi antiserum or colonies form haloes on an agar plate containing a suitable Vi antiserum.

CULTURE AND HARVEST

The working seed lot is cultured on a solid medium, which may contain blood-group substances, or a liquid medium; the inoculum obtained is transferred to a liquid medium which is used to inoculate the final medium. The liquid medium used and the final medium are semi-synthetic, free from substances that are precipitated by cetrimonium bromide and do not contain blood-group substances or high-molecular-mass polysaccharides, unless it has been demonstrated that they are removed by the purification process.

The bacterial purity of the culture is verified by microscopic examination of Gram-stained smears and by inoculation into appropriate media; several fields are observed at high magnification so that at least 10,000 organisms are examined. The culture is then inactivated at the beginning of the stationary phase by the addition of formaldehyde. Bacterial cells are eliminated by centrifugation; the polysaccharide is precipitated from the culture medium by addition of hexadecyltrimethylammonium bromide (cetrimonium bromide). The precipitate is harvested and may be stored at −20°C before purification.

PURIFIED VI POLYSACCHARIDE

The polysaccharide is purified, after dissociation of the polysaccharide/cetrimonium bromide complex, using suitable procedures to eliminate successively nucleic acids, proteins and lipopolysaccharides. The polysaccharide is precipitated as the calcium salt in the presence of ethanol and dried at 2°C to 8°C; the powder obtained constitutes the purified Vi polysaccharide. The loss on drying is determined by thermogravimetry (*2.2.34*) and is used to calculate the results of the chemical tests shown below with reference to the dried substance.

Only a purified Vi polysaccharide that complies with the following requirements may be used in the preparation of the final bulk.

Protein (*2.5.16*). Not greater than 10 mg per gram of polysaccharide, calculated with reference to the dried substance.

Nucleic acids (*2.5.17*). Not greater than 20 mg per gram of polysaccharide, calculated with reference to the dried substance.

***O*-Acetyl groups** (*2.5.19*). Not less than 2 mmol per gram of polysaccharide, calculated with reference to the dried substance.

Molecular size Examine by size-exclusion chromatography (*2.2.30*) using *cross-linked agarose for chromato-*

graphy R. Use a column 0.9 m long and 16 mm in internal diameter equilibrated with a solvent having an ionic strength of 0.2 mol/kg and a pH of 7.0 to 7.5. Apply about 5 mg of polysaccharide in a volume of 1 ml to the column and elute at about 20 ml/h. Collect fractions of about 2.5 ml. Determine the point corresponding to K_D = 0.25 and make two pools consisting of fractions eluted before and after this point. Determine *O*-acetyl groups on the two pools *(2.5.19)*. Not less than 50 per cent of the polysaccharide is found in the pool containing fractions eluted before K_D = 0.25.

Identification Carry out an identification test using a suitable immunochemical method *(2.7.1)*.

Bacterial endotoxins *(2.6.14)*. Not more than 150 I.U. per microgram of polysaccharide.

FINAL BULK VACCINE

One or more batches of purified Vi polysaccharide are dissolved in a suitable solvent, which may contain an antimicrobial preservative, so that the volume corresponding to one dose contains 25 µg of polysaccharide and the solution is isotonic with blood (250 mosm/kg to 350 mosm/kg).

Only a final bulk vaccine that complies with the following tests may be used in the preparation of the final lot.

Sterility *(2.6.1)*. The final bulk vaccine complies with the test for sterility, carried out using 10 ml for each medium.

Antimicrobial preservative Where applicable, determine the amount of antimicrobial preservative by a suitable physicochemical method. The amount is not less than 85 per cent and not greater than 115 per cent of the intended amount.

FINAL LOT

The final bulk vaccine is distributed aseptically into sterile tamper-proof containers that are then closed so as to prevent contamination.

Only a final lot that is satisfactory with respect to each of the requirements prescribed below under Identification, Tests and Assay may be released for use. Provided the tests for free formaldehyde and antimicrobial preservative have been carried out on the final bulk vaccine, they may be omitted on the final lot.

CHARACTERS

A clear colourless liquid, free from visible particles.

IDENTIFICATION

Carry out an identification test using a suitable immunochemical method *(2.7.1)*.

TESTS

pH *(2.2.3)*. The pH of the vaccine is 6.5 to 7.5.

***O*-Acetyl groups** 0.085 (± 25 per cent) µmol per dose (25 µg of polysaccharide).

Test solution. Place 3 ml of the vaccine in each of three tubes (two reaction solutions and one correction solution).

Reference solutions. Dissolve 0.150 g of *acetylcholine chloride R* in 10 ml of *water R* (stock solution containing 15 g/l of acetylcholine chloride). Immediately before use, dilute 0.5 ml of the stock solution to 50 ml with *water R* (working dilution containing 150 µg/ml of acetylcholine chloride). In ten tubes, place in duplicate (reaction and correction solutions) 0.1 ml, 0.2 ml, 0.5 ml, 1.0 ml and 1.5 ml of the working dilution.

Prepare a blank using 3 ml of *water R*.

Make up the volume in each tube to 3 ml with *water R*. Add 0.5 ml of a mixture of 1 volume of *water R* and 2 volumes of *dilute hydrochloric acid R* to each of the correction tubes and to the blank. Add 1.0 ml of *alkaline hydroxylamine solution R* to each tube. Allow the reaction to proceed for *exactly* 2 min and add 0.5 ml of a mixture of 1 volume of *water R* and 2 volumes of *dilute hydrochloric acid R* to each of the reaction tubes. Add 0.5 ml of a 200 g/l solution of *ferric chloride R* in *0.2M hydrochloric acid* to each tube, stopper the tubes and shake vigorously to remove bubbles.

Measure the absorbance *(2.2.25)* of each solution at 540 nm using the blank as the compensation liquid. For each reaction solution, subtract the absorbance of the corresponding correction solution. Draw a calibration curve from the corrected absorbances for the five reference solutions and the corresponding content of acetylcholine chloride and read from the curve the content of acetylcholine chloride in the test solution for each volume tested. Calculate the mean of the two values.

1 mol of acetylcholine chloride (181.7 g) is equivalent to 1 mol of *O*-acetyl (43.05 g).

Free formaldehyde It complies with the test for free formaldehyde prescribed in *Vaccines for human use (153)*.

Antimicrobial preservative Where applicable, determine the amount of antimicrobial preservative by a suitable physicochemical method. The content is not less than the minimum amount shown to be effective and not more than 115 per cent of the content stated on the label. If phenol has been used in the preparation, the content *(2.5.15)* is not more than 2.5 g/l.

Sterility *(2.6.1)*. It complies with the test for sterility.

Bacterial endotoxins *(2.6.14)*. Not more than 3750 I.U. per human dose.

ASSAY

Determine Vi polysaccharide by a suitable immunochemical method *(2.7.1)*, using a reference purified polysaccharide. The estimated amount of polysaccharide per dose is 80 per cent to 120 per cent of the content stated on the label. The fiducial limits of error (P = 0.95) of the estimated amount of polysaccharide are not less than 80 per cent and not more than 120 per cent.

STORAGE

See *Vaccines for human use (153)*.

LABELLING

See *Vaccines for human use (153)*.

The label states:

— the number of micrograms of polysaccharide per human dose (25 µg),

— the total quantity of polysaccharide in the container.

Ph Eur

Typhoid Vaccine

When Typhoid Vaccine is issued as a liquid, it complies with the requirements of the 3rd edition of the European Pharmacopoeia for Typhoid Vaccine [0156]. These requirements are reproduced after the heading 'Liquid Vaccine' below.

When Typhoid Vaccine is prepared immediately before use by reconstitution from the dried vaccine, the dried vaccine complies with the requirements of the 3rd edition of the European Pharmacopoeia for Freeze-dried Typhoid Vaccine [0157]. These requirements are reproduced after the heading 'Dried Vaccine' below.

The label may state 'Typhoid/Vac' or 'Dried/Typhoid/Vac', as appropriate.

Ph Eur

LIQUID VACCINE [0156]

DEFINITION

Typhoid vaccine is a sterile suspension of inactivated *Salmonella typhi* containing not less than 5×10^8 and not more than 1×10^9 bacteria (*S. typhi*) per human dose. The human dose does not exceed 1.0 ml.

PRODUCTION

The vaccine is prepared using a seed-lot system from a suitable strain, such as Ty 2[1], of *S. typhi*. The final vaccine represents not more than three subcultures from the strain on which were made the laboratory and clinical tests that showed it to be suitable. The bacteria are inactivated by acetone, by formaldehyde, by phenol or by heating or by a combination of the last two methods.

The production method is validated to demonstrate that the product, if tested, would comply with the test for abnormal toxicity for immunosera and vaccines for human use (*2.6.9*) modified as follows: inject 0.5 ml of the vaccine into each mouse and 1.0 ml into each guinea-pig.

IDENTIFICATION

It is identified by specific agglutination.

TESTS

Phenol (*2.5.15*). If phenol has been used in the preparation, the concentration is not more than 5 g/l.

Antigenic power When injected into susceptible laboratory animals, it elicits anti-O, anti-H and, to a lesser extent, anti-Vi agglutinins.

Sterility (*2.6.1*). It complies with the test for sterility.

STORAGE

See *Vaccines for human use (153)*.

LABELLING

See *Vaccines for human use (153)*.

The label states:
— the method used to inactivate the bacteria,
— the number of bacteria per human dose.

[1]This strain is issued by the World Health Organisation Collaborating Centre for Reference and Research on Bacterial Vaccines, Human Serum and Vaccine Institute, Szallas Utea 5, H-1107, Budapest, Hungary.

DRIED VACCINE [0157]

DEFINITION

Typhoid vaccine, freeze-dried is a freeze-dried preparation of inactivated *Salmonella typhi.* The vaccine is reconstituted as stated on the label to give a uniform suspension containing not less than 5×10^8 and not more than 1×10^9 bacteria (*S. typhi*) per human dose. The human dose does not exceed 1.0 ml of the reconstituted vaccine.

PRODUCTION

The vaccine is prepared using a seed-lot system from a suitable strain, such as Ty 2[1], of *S. typhi.* The final vaccine represents not more than three subcultures from the strain on which were made the laboratory and clinical tests that showed it to be suitable. The bacteria are inactivated either by acetone or by formaldehyde or by heat. Phenol is not used in the preparation. The vaccine is distributed into sterile containers and freeze-dried to a moisture content favourable to the stability of the vaccine. The containers are then closed so as to exclude contamination.

The production method is validated to demonstrate that the product, if tested, would comply with the test for abnormal toxicity for immunosera and vaccines for human use (*2.6.9*) modified as follows: inject 0.5 ml of the vaccine into each mouse and 1.0 ml into each guinea pig.

IDENTIFICATION

The vaccine reconstituted as stated on the label is identified by specific agglutination.

TESTS

The reconstituted vaccine complies with the tests prescribed in the monograph on *Typhoid vaccine (156)*.

STORAGE

See *Vaccines for human use (153)*.

LABELLING

See *Vaccines for human Use (153)*.

The label states:
— the method used to inactivate the bacteria,
— the number of bacteria per human dose,
— that the vaccine should be used within 8 h of reconstitution.

[1]This strain is issued by the World Health Organisation Collaborating Centre for Reference and Research on Bacterial Vaccines, Human Serum and Vaccine Institute, Szallas Utea 5, H-1107, Budapest, Hungary.

Ph Eur

Typhoid (Strain Ty 21a) Vaccine, Live (Oral)

Typhoid (Strain Ty 21a) Vaccine, Live (Oral) complies with the requirements of the 3rd edition of the European Pharmacopoeia for Typhoid Vaccine (Live, Oral, Strain Ty 21a) [1055]. These requirements are reproduced after the heading 'Definition' below.

The label may state 'Typhoid/Vac(Oral)'.

Ph Eur

DEFINITION

Typhoid vaccine (live, oral, strain Ty 21a) is a freeze-dried preparation of live *Salmonella typhi* strain Ty 21a grown in a suitable medium. When presented in capsules, the vaccine complies with the monograph on *Capsules (16)*.

PRODUCTION

CHOICE OF VACCINE STRAIN

The main characteristic of the strain is the defect of the enzyme uridine diphosphate-galactose-4-epimerase. The activities of galactopermease, galactokinase and galactose-1-phosphate uridyl-transferase are reduced by 50 per cent to 90 per cent. Whatever the growth conditions, the strain does not contain Vi antigen. The strain agglutinates to anti-O:9 antiserum only if grown in medium containing galactose. It contains the flagellar H:d antigen and does not produce hydrogen sulphide on Kligler iron agar. The strain is nonvirulent for mice. Cells of strain Ty 21a lyse if grown in the presence of 1 per cent of galactose.

BACTERIAL SEED LOTS

The vaccine is prepared using a seed-lot system. The working seed lots represent not more than one subculture from the master seed lot. The final vaccine represents not more than four subcultures from the original vaccine on which were made the laboratory and clinical tests showing the strain to be suitable.

Only a master seed lot that complies with the following requirements may be used in the preparation of working seed lots.

Galactose metabolism In a spectrophotometric assay, no activity of the enzyme uridine diphosphate-galactose-4-epimerase is found in the cytoplasm of strain Ty 21a compared to strain Ty 2.

Biosynthesis of lipopolysaccharide Lipopolysaccharides are extracted by the hot-phenol method and examined by size-exclusion chromatography. Strain Ty 21a grown in medium free of galactose shows only the rough (R) type of lipopolysaccharide.

Serological characteristics Strain Ty 21a grown in a synthetic medium without galactose does not agglutinate to specific anti-O:9 antiserum. Whatever the growth conditions, strain Ty 21a does not agglutinate to Vi antiserum. Strain Ty 21a agglutinates to H:d flagellar antiserum.

Biochemical markers Strain Ty 21a does not produce hydrogen sulphide on Kligler iron agar. This property serves to distinguish Ty 21a from other galactose-epimerase-negative *S. typhi* strains.

Cell growth Strain Ty 21a cells lyse when grown in the presence of 1 per cent of galactose.

BACTERIAL PROPAGATION AND HARVEST

The bacteria from the working seed lot are multiplied in a preculture, subcultured once and are then grown in a suitable medium containing 0.001 per cent of galactose at 30°C for 13 h to 15 h. The bacteria are harvested. The harvest must be free from contaminating micro-organisms.

Only a single harvest that complies with the following requirements may be used for the preparation of the freeze-dried harvest.

pH The pH of the culture is 6.8 to 7.5.

Optical density The optical density of the culture, measured at 546 nm, is 6.5 to 11.0. Before carrying out the measurement, dilute the culture so that a reading in the range 0.1 to 0.5 is obtained and correct the reading to take account of the dilution.

Identification Culture bacteria on an agar medium containing 1 per cent of galactose and bromothymol blue. Light blue, concave colonies, transparent due to lysis of cells, are formed. No yellow colonies (galactose-fermenting) are found.

FREEZE-DRIED HARVEST

The harvest is mixed with a suitable stabiliser and freeze-dried by a process that ensures the survival of at least 10 per cent of the bacteria and to a water content shown to be favourable to the stability of the vaccine. No anti-microbial preservative is added to the vaccine.

Only a freeze-dried harvest that complies with the following tests may be used for the preparation of the final bulk.

Identification Culture bacteria are examined on an agar medium containing 1 per cent of galactose and bromothymol blue. Light blue, concave colonies, transparent due to lysis of cells, are formed. No yellow colonies (galactose-fermenting) are found.

Number of live bacteria Not fewer than 1×10^{11} live *S. typhi* strain Ty 21a per gram.

Water (*2.5.12*). 1.5 per cent to 4.0 per cent, determined by the semi-micro determination of water.

FINAL BULK VACCINE

The final bulk vaccine is prepared by aseptically mixing one or more freeze-dried harvests with a suitable sterile excipient.

Only a final bulk that complies with the following requirement may be used in the preparation of the final lot.

Number of live bacteria Not fewer than 40×10^9 live *S. typhi* strain Ty 21a per gram.

FINAL LOT

The final bulk vaccine is distributed under aseptic conditions into capsules with a gastro-resistant shell or into suitable containers.

Only a final lot that is satisfactory with respect to each of the requirements given below under Identification, Tests and Number of live bacteria may be released for use, except that in the determination of the number of live bacteria each dosage unit must contain not fewer than 4×10^9 live bacteria.

IDENTIFICATION

Culture bacteria from the vaccine to be examined on an agar medium containing 1 per cent of galactose and bromothymol blue. Light blue, concave colonies, transparent due to lysis of cells, are formed. No yellow colonies (galactose-fermenting) are found.

TESTS

Contaminating micro-organisms (*2.6.12, 2.6.13*). Carry out the test using suitable selective media. Determine the total viable count using the plate-count method. The number of contaminating micro-organisms per dosage unit is not greater than 10^2 bacteria and 20 fungi. No pathogenic bacterium, particularly *Escherichia coli,*

Staphylococcus aureus, Pseudomonas aeruginosa, and no salmonella other than strain Ty 21a are found.

Water (*2.5.12*). 1.5 per cent to 4.0 per cent, determined on the contents of the capsule or of the container by the semi-micro determination of water.

NUMBER OF LIVE BACTERIA

Carry out the test using not fewer than five dosage units. Homogenise the contents of the dosage units in a 9 g/l solution of *sodium chloride R* at 4°C using a mixer in a cold room with sufficient glass beads to emerge from the liquid. Immediately after homogenisation prepare a suitable dilution of the suspension using cooled diluent and inoculate brain heart infusion agar; incubate at 36 ± 1°C for 20 h to 36 h. The vaccine contains not fewer than 2×10^9 live *S. typhi* Ty 21a bacteria per dosage unit.

STORAGE

See *Vaccines for human use (153)*.

LABELLING

See *Vaccines for human use (153)*.

The label states:

— the minimum number of live bacteria per dosage unit,

— that the vaccine is for oral use only.

Ph Eur

Typhoid and Tetanus Vaccine

Definition Typhoid and Tetanus Vaccine is a mixture of a suspension of killed *Salmonella typhi* and tetanus formol toxoid. It contains in 1 ml 1000 million or 2000 million typhoid bacilli (*S. typhi*).

Production The suspension of bacteria is prepared from one or more strains of *S. typhi* that are smooth and have the full complement of O, H and Vi antigens. The bacteria are killed by treatment with formaldehyde or phenol or by heating the suspension.

The vaccine complies with the requirements stated under Vaccines, with the following modifications.

Identification

A. It is agglutinated by specific typhoid antiserum.

B. After removal of the bacteria from the vaccine by centrifugation, the supernatant fluid flocculates when mixed under appropriate conditions with tetanus antitoxin.

Specific toxicity Inject the dose stated on the label subcutaneously or intraperitoneally into each of five guinea-pigs. None of the guinea-pigs shows any symptoms of, or dies from, tetanus within 21 days. If more than one animal dies from non-specific causes within this period repeat the test. None of the second group of animals shows symptoms of tetanus or dies from tetanus or any other cause within 21 days.

Sterility Complies with the *test for sterility*, Appendix XVI A.

Potency Inject into each of no fewer than nine guinea-pigs either a single quantity containing five times the dose stated on the label or two quantities, separated by an interval of not more than 4 weeks, each containing one tenth of the dose stated on the label; some of the guinea-pigs may receive the single dose and the remainder the two doses. Not later than 6 weeks after the single injection or, if two injections have been given, not later than 2 weeks after the second injection, bleed the guinea-pigs and examine the sera of the guinea-pigs for antitoxin using the *biological test for tetanus antitoxin* described under Tetanus Vaccine. The serum of each of no fewer than two thirds of the guinea-pigs contains not less than 0.05 Unit of tetanus antitoxin per ml or, alternatively, the serum of each of no fewer than one-third of the guinea-pigs contains not less than 0.5 Unit per ml.

Labelling The label states (1) 'Typhoid/Tet/Vac'; (2) the number of bacteria in 1 ml.

Typhus Vaccine

Definition Typhus Vaccine is a suspension of killed epidemic typhus rickettsiae.

Production The vaccine may be prepared by the following method. Virulent rickettsiae are injected into the yolk sacs of embryonated eggs that have been incubated for 7 days. After heavy yolk-sac infection has been established (usually within 9 to 13 days), the yolk sacs are collected under aseptic conditions as soon as practicable. Dead or moribund eggs are harvested. The yolk sacs are subjected to suitable treatment to liberate the maximum number of rickettsiae and the material is suspended in a saline or other appropriate solution isotonic with blood to which Formaldehyde Solution has been added so that the concentration of formaldehyde is 0.2 to 0.5% w/v. The suspension so obtained contains from 10 to 15% w/w of yolk-sac tissue. It is purified by treatment with Ether or trichlorotrifluoroethane; the aqueous middle layer of the resultant mixture is collected.

The vaccine may also be prepared from the lungs of small rodents in which rickettsial pneumonias have been caused by inhalation of massive doses of virulent rickettsiae, or from the peritoneal cavities of gerbils that have received intraperitoneal injections of rickettsiae.

The vaccine complies with the requirements stated under Vaccines, with the following modifications.

Characteristics A slightly turbid liquid. On prolonged standing, the rickettsiae settle out as a delicate, powdery, white deposit which is readily redistributed by shaking.

Identification It specifically protects laboratory animals against epidemic typhus.

Sterility Complies with the *test for sterility*, Appendix XVI A.

Potency Carry out the *biological assay of typhus vaccine* described below. The vaccine passes the test if the serum of immunised guinea-pigs, when diluted 32-fold, protects mice against the toxin of epidemic typhus rickettsiae.

Storage When stored under the prescribed conditions, the vaccine may be expected to retain its potency for at least 1 year.

Labelling The label states (1) 'Typhus/Vac'; (2) the nature of the preparation, that is, whether it has been prepared in eggs, rodent's lung or otherwise and whether it has been purified.

BIOLOGICAL ASSAY OF TYPHUS VACCINE

To each of 10 or more guinea-pigs, each weighing between 400 and 500 g, give two subcutaneous injections at an interval of 7 days, each of 0.5 ml of the vaccine being examined. Fourteen days after the second injection bleed the animals and pool aliquots of the sera. Test the pools against a toxic substance that has been prepared from infected yolk sacs of living fertile eggs as described below.

Incubate the eggs for 4 to 10 days after inoculation with epidemic typhus rickettsiae. Harvest the yolk sac in the usual manner and stain a smear by the Macchiavello technique. Use only yolk sacs of living embryos showing 4+ or more rickettsiae. Determine the wet weight of the yolk sac, grind the yolk sac with a suitable grade of aluminium oxide and suspend in sterile milk (pH adjusted to 7.6) or in a mixture of 1 part of fresh egg yolk and 99 parts of *sodium chloride injection* using, for each g of the yolk sac, 10 ml of the vehicle. Centrifuge this suspension for 5 minutes at low speed, decant the supernatant liquid and distribute in ampoules for freezing. Dilute a small amount of this suspension 8-, 16-, 32- and 64-fold with *saline solution.* Inject intravenously doses of 0.5 ml of each dilution into eight white mice, each weighing between 11 and 15 g. Eighteen hours later, estimate the toxicity of the preparation as the LD_{50} per g of yolk sac, calculated from the numbers of mice killed by each dilution. Those toxic suspensions showing 160 or more LD_{50} per g of yolk sac are satisfactory for use in the neutralisation test. The remainder of the suspension may be sealed in ampoules and preserved for 18 months in liquid nitrogen.

Prepare mixtures of the toxic substance and the sera being tested for the neutralisation test in mice and allow to stand for 2 hours before injection. Inject intravenously into mice, each weighing between 11 and 15 g, 0.5 ml containing 2 LD_{50} of the toxic substance together with serial 1 to 2 dilutions of serum. Keep the mice in an incubator at 28° to 30° until the results of the test are recorded. Record the deaths at the end of 24 hours and express the results in terms of the highest dilution giving complete protection.

Varicella Vaccine, Live

Varicella Vaccine, Live complies with the requirements of the 3rd edition of the European Pharmacopoeia for Varicella Vaccine (Live) [0648]. These requirements are reproduced after the heading 'Definition' below.

The label may state 'Var/Vac(Live)'.

Ph Eur

DEFINITION

Varicella vaccine (live) is a freeze-dried preparation of the OKA attenuated strain of *Herpesvirus varicellae.* The vaccine is reconstituted immediately before use, as stated on the label, to give a clear liquid that may be coloured owing to the presence of a pH indicator.

PRODUCTION

The production of vaccine is based on a virus seed-lot system and a cell-bank system. The production method shall have been shown to yield consistently live varicella vaccines of adequate immunogenicity and safety in man. The virus in the final vaccine shall not have been passaged in cell cultures beyond the 38th passage from the original isolated virus.

The production method is validated to demonstrate that the product, if tested, would comply with the test for abnormal toxicity for immunosera and vaccines for human use (*2.6.9*).

SUBSTRATE FOR VIRUS PROPAGATION

The virus is propagated in human diploid cells (*5.2.3*).

VIRUS SEED LOT

The strain of varicella virus shall be identified as OKA by historical records which shall include information on the origin of the strain and its subsequent manipulation. The virus shall at no time have been passaged in continuous cell lines. Seed lots are prepared in the same kind of cells as those used for the production of the final vaccine. To avoid the unnecessary use of monkeys in the test for neurovirulence, virus seed lots are prepared in large quantities and stored at temperatures below −20°C, if freeze-dried, or below −60°C, if not freeze-dried.

Only a virus seed lot that complies with the following requirements may be used for virus propagation.

Identification The master and working seed lots are identified as varicella virus by serum neutralisation in cell culture, using specific antibodies.

Virus concentration The virus concentration of the master and working seed lots is determined as prescribed under assay to monitor consistency of production.

Extraneous agents (*2.6.16*). The working seed lot complies with the requirements for seed lots for live virus vaccines; a sample of 50 ml is taken for the test in cell cultures.

Neurovirulence (*2.6.18*). The working seed lot complies with the test for neurovirulence of live virus vaccines.

VIRUS PROPAGATION AND HARVEST

All processing of the cell bank and subsequent cell cultures is done under aseptic conditions in an area where no other cells are handled. Approved animal (but not human) serum may be used in the media. Serum and trypsin used in the preparation of cell suspensions and media are shown to be free from extraneous agents. The cell culture medium may contain a pH indicator such as phenol red and approved antibiotics at the lowest effective concentration. It is preferable to have a substrate free from antibiotics during production. 5 per cent, but not less than 50 ml, of the cell cultures employed for vaccine production is set aside as uninfected cell cultures (control cells). The infected cells constituting a single harvest are washed, released from the support surface and pooled. The cell suspension is disrupted by sonication.

Only a virus harvest that complies with the following requirements may be used in the preparation of the final bulk vaccine.

Identification The virus harvest contains virus that is identified as varicella virus by serum neutralisation in cell culture, using specific antibodies.

Virus concentration The concentration of infective virus in virus harvests is determined as prescribed under assay to monitor consistency of production and to determine the dilution to be used for the final bulk vaccine.

Extraneous agents (*2.6.16*). Use 50 ml for the test in cell cultures.

Control cells The control cells of the production cell culture from which the single harvest is derived comply with a test for identity and with the requirements for extraneous agents (*2.6.16*).

FINAL BULK VACCINE

Virus harvests that comply with the above tests are pooled and clarified to remove cells. A suitable stabiliser may be added and the pooled harvests diluted as appropriate.

Only a final bulk vaccine that complies with the following requirements may be used in the preparation of the final lot.

Bacterial and fungal contamination Carry out the test for sterility (*2.6.1*) using 10 ml for each medium.

FINAL LOT

The final bulk vaccine is distributed aseptically into sterile, tamper-proof containers and freeze-dried to a moisture content shown to be favourable to the stability of the vaccine. The containers are then closed so as to prevent contamination and the introduction of moisture.

Only a final lot that is satisfactory with respect to each of the requirements given below under identification, tests and assay may be released for use. Provided that the test for bovine serum albumin has been carried out with satisfactory results on the final bulk vaccine, it may be omitted on the final lot.

IDENTIFICATION

When the vaccine reconstituted as stated on the label is mixed with specific *Herpesvirus varicellae* antibodies, it is no longer able to infect susceptible cell cultures.

TESTS

Bacterial and fungal contamination The reconstituted vaccine complies with the test for sterility (*2.6.1*).

Bovine serum albumin Not more than 0.5 µg per human dose, determined by a suitable immunochemical method (*2.7.1*).

Water (*2.5.12*). Not more than 3.0 per cent, determined by the semi-micro determination of water.

ASSAY

Titrate for infective virus, using at least ten cell cultures for each fourfold dilution or by a technique of equal precision. Use a suitable virus reference preparation to validate each assay. The virus concentration is not less than 2.0×10^3 PFU per human dose.

STORAGE

See *Vaccines for human use (153)*.

LABELLING

See *Vaccines for human use (153)*.

The label states:

- the strain of virus used for the preparation of the vaccine,
- the type and origin of the cells used for the preparation of the vaccine,
- that contact with disinfectants is to be avoided,
- the minimum virus concentration,
- that the vaccine is not to be administered to pregnant women,
- the time within which the vaccine must be used after reconstitution.

Ph Eur

Yellow Fever Vaccine, Live

Yellow Fever Vaccine, Live complies with the requirements of the 3rd edition of the European Pharmacopoeia for Yellow Fever Vaccine (Live) [0537]. These requirements are reproduced after the heading 'Definition' below.

The label may state 'Yel/Vac'.

Ph Eur

DEFINITION

Yellow fever vaccine (live) is a freeze-dried preparation of the 17D strain of yellow fever virus *(Flavivirus hominis)* grown in fertilised hen eggs. The vaccine is reconstituted immediately before use, as stated on the label, to give a clear liquid.

PRODUCTION

The production of vaccine is based on a virus seed-lot system. The production method shall have been shown to yield consistently yellow fever vaccine (live) of acceptable immunogenicity and safety for man. The production method is validated to demonstrate that the product, if tested, would comply with the test for abnormal toxicity for immunosera and vaccines for human use (*2.6.9*) modified as follows for the test in guinea-pigs: inject ten human doses into each guinea-pig and observe for 21 days.

SUBSTRATE FOR VIRUS PROPAGATION

Virus for the preparation of master and working seed lots and of all vaccine lots is grown in the tissues of chick embryos from a chicken flock free from specified pathogens (*5.2.2*).

SEED LOTS

The 17D strain shall be identified by historical records that include information on the origin of the strain and its subsequent manipulation. Virus seed lots are prepared in large quantities and stored at a temperature below −60°C. Master and working seed lots shall not contain any human protein or added serum.

Unless otherwise justified and authorised, the virus in the final vaccine shall be between passage levels 204 and 239 from the original isolate of strain 17D. A working seed lot shall be only one passage from a master seed lot. A working seed lot shall be used without intervening passage as the inoculum for infecting the tissues used in the production of a vaccine lot, in order to ensure that no vaccine shall be manufactured that is more than one passage removed from a seed lot that has passed all the safety tests.

Only a virus seed lot that complies with the following requirements may be used for virus propagation.

Identification The master and working seed lots are identified as containing yellow fever virus by serum neutralisation in cell culture, using specific antibodies.

Extraneous agents (*2.6.16*). Each working seed lot complies with the following tests:

Bacterial and fungal sterility
Mycoplasmas
Mycobacteria
Avian viruses
Test in adult mice (intraperitoneal inoculation only)
Test in guinea-pigs

Tests in monkeys Each master and working seed lot complies with the following tests in monkeys for viraemia (viscerotropism), immunogenicity and neurotropism.

The monkeys shall be *Macaca* sp. susceptible to yellow fever virus and shall have been shown to be non-immune to yellow fever at the time of injecting the seed virus. They shall be healthy and shall not have received previously intracerebral or intraspinal inoculation. Furthermore, they shall not have been inoculated by other routes with neurotropic viruses or with antigens related to yellow fever virus. Not fewer than ten monkeys shall be used for each test.

Use a test dose of 0.25 ml containing the equivalent of not less than 5000 mouse LD_{50} and not more than 50,000 mouse LD_{50}, determined by a titration for infectious virus and using the established equivalence between virus concentration and mouse LD_{50} (see under Assay). Inject the test dose into one frontal lobe of each monkey under anaesthesia and observe the monkeys for not less than 30 days.

Viraemia (Viscerotropism). Viscerotropism is indicated by the amount of virus present in serum. Take blood from each of the test monkeys on the second, fourth and sixth days after inoculation and prepare serum from each sample. Prepare 1:10, 1:100 and 1:1000 dilutions from each serum and inoculate each dilution into a group of at least six cell culture vessels used for the determination of the virus concentration. The seed lot complies with the test if none of the sera contains more than the equivalent of 500 mouse LD_{50} in 0.03 ml and at most one serum contains more than the equivalent of 100 mouse LD_{50} in 0.03 ml.

Immunogenicity. Take blood from each monkey 30 days after the injection of the test dose and prepare serum from each sample. The seed lot complies with the test if at least 90 per cent of the test monkeys are shown to be immune, as determined by examining their sera in the test for neutralisation of yellow fever virus described below.

It has been shown that a low dilution of serum (for example, 1:10) may contain non-specific inhibitors that influence this test; such serum shall be treated to remove inhibitors. Mix dilutions of at least 1:10, 1:40 and 1:160 of serum from each monkey with an equal volume of 17D vaccine virus at a dilution that will yield an optimum number of plaques with the titration method used. Incubate the serum-virus mixtures in a water-bath at 37°C for 1 h and then cool in iced water; add 0.2 ml of each serum-virus mixture to each of four cell culture plates and proceed as for the determination of virus concentration. Inoculate similarly ten plates with the same amount of virus plus an equal volume of a 1:10 dilution of monkey serum known to contain no neutralising antibodies to yellow fever virus. At the end of the observation period, compare the mean number of plaques in the plates receiving virus plus non-immune serum with the mean number of plaques in the plates receiving virus plus dilutions of each monkey serum. Not more than 10 per cent of the test monkeys have serum that fails to reduce the number of plaques by 50 per cent at the 1:10 dilution.

Neurotropism. Neurotropism (as indicated by the incidence of clinical manifestations of encephalitis and by the mortality rate) is determined as follows. The monkeys are examined daily by personnel familiar with clinical signs of encephalitis in primates (if necessary the monkeys may be removed from their cages to detect signs of motor weakness or spasticity). Not more than 10 per cent of the test monkeys shall develop severe signs of encephalitis (such as incomplete paralysis, inco-ordination tremors, lethargy, inability to stand spontaneously, motor weakness or spasticity) at a frequency greater than that induced by a laboratory reference vaccine with acceptable properties in man and monkeys. Neither the onset and duration of the febrile reaction nor the nature of the symptoms and pathological findings are such as to indicate a change in the properties of the virus.

VIRUS PROPAGATION AND HARVEST

All processing of the fertilised eggs is done under aseptic conditions in an area where no other infectious agents or cells are handled at the same time. 2 per cent but not less than twenty and not more than fifty eggs are set aside as uninfected control eggs. After inoculation and incubation at a controlled temperature, only living and typical chick embryos are harvested. The age of the embryo at the time of virus harvest is reckoned from the initial introduction of the egg into the incubator and shall be not more than 12 days. After homogenisation and clarification by centrifugation, the extract of embryonic pulp is tested as described below and kept at −70°C or colder until further processing. Virus harvests that comply with the tests may be pooled. No human protein is added to the virus suspension at any stage during production. If stabilisers are added, they shall have been shown to have no antigenic or sensitising properties for man.

Only a single harvest that complies with the following requirements may be used in the preparation of the final bulk vaccine.

Identification The virus harvest contains virus that is identified as yellow fever virus by serum neutralisation in cell culture, using specific antibodies.

Extraneous agents (*2.6.16*). The extract of the embryonic pulp that forms a single harvest complies with the following tests:

Bacterial and fungal sterility
Mycoplasmas
Control eggs (*2.6.16*)

Virus concentration In order to calculate the dilution for formulation of the final bulk, each harvest is tested for virus concentration as described under Assay.

FINAL BULK VACCINE

Virus harvests that comply with the tests prescribed above are pooled and clarified again. A test for protein nitrogen content is carried out. A suitable stabiliser may be added and the pooled harvests diluted as appropriate.

Only a final bulk vaccine that complies with the following requirements may be used in the preparation of the final lot.

Bacterial and fungal contamination Carry out the test for sterility (*2.6.1*), using 10 ml for each medium.

Protein nitrogen content The protein nitrogen content, before the addition of any stabiliser, is not more than 0.25 mg per human dose.

FINAL LOT

The final bulk vaccine is distributed aseptically into sterile, tamper-proof containers and freeze-dried to a moisture content shown to be favourable to the stability of the vaccine. The containers are then closed so as to prevent contamination and the introduction of moisture.

Only a final lot that is satisfactory with respect to thermal stability and each of the requirements given below under Identification, Tests and Assay may be released for use. Provided that the test for ovalbumin has been performed with satisfactory results on the final bulk vaccine, they may be omitted on the final lot.

Thermal stability Maintain samples of the final lot of freeze-dried vaccine in the dry state at 37°C for 14 days. Determine the virus concentration as described under Assay in parallel for the heated vaccine and for unheated vaccine. The difference in the virus concentration between unheated and heated vaccine does not exceed 1.0 $\log_{10}$ and the virus concentration of the heated vaccine is not less than the number of plaque-forming units (PFU) equivalent to 1×10^3 mouse LD_{50} per human dose.

IDENTIFICATION

When the vaccine reconstituted as stated on the label is mixed with specific yellow fever virus antibodies, there is a significant reduction in its ability to infect susceptible cell cultures.

TESTS

Bacterial and fungal contamination The reconstituted vaccine complies with the test for sterility (*2.6.1*).

Ovalbumin Not more than 5 µg of ovalbumin per human dose, determined by a suitable immunochemical method (*2.7.1*).

Bacterial endotoxins (*2.6.14*). Not more than 5 I.U. of bacterial endotoxin per human dose.

Water (*2.5.12*). Not more than 3.0 per cent, determined by the semi-micro determination of water.

ASSAY

Titrate for infective virus in cell cultures. Use an appropriate virus reference preparation to validate each assay.

The virus concentration is not less than the equivalent in PFU of 1×10^3 mouse LD_{50} per human dose. The relationship between mouse LD_{50} and PFU is established by each laboratory and approved by the competent authority.

The method shown below, or another suitable technique, may be used to determine the mouse LD_{50}.

STORAGE

See *Vaccines for human use (153)*.

LABELLING

See *Vaccines for human use (153)*.

The label states:

— the strain of virus used in preparation,
— that the vaccine has been prepared in chick embryos,
— the minimum virus concentration,
— that contact with disinfectants is to be avoided,
— the period of time within which the vaccine is to be used after reconstitution.

Suggested method for determination of the mouse LD_{50}

Mouse LD_{50}. The statistically calculated quantity of virus suspension that is expected to produce fatal specific encephalitis in 50 per cent of mice of a highly susceptible strain, 4 to 6 weeks of age, after intracerebral inoculation.

Appropriate serial dilutions of the reconstituted vaccine are made in diluent for yellow fever virus (a 7.5 g/l solution of *bovine albumin R*, in *phosphate-buffered saline pH 7.4 R*, or any other diluent that has been shown to be equivalent for maintaining the infectivity of the virus).

Mice of a highly susceptible strain, 4 to 6 weeks of age, are injected intracerebrally under anaesthesia with 0.03 ml of the vaccine dilution. Groups of not fewer than six mice are used for each dilution; the series of dilutions is chosen so as to cover the range 0 to 100 per cent mortality of the mice. Injection of the mice is performed immediately after the dilutions have been made. The mice are observed for 21 days and all deaths are recorded. Only survivors and deaths caused by typical yellow fever infections are counted in the computations. Mice paralysed on the twenty-first day of observation are counted as survivors.

Ph Eur

DIAGNOSTIC PREPARATIONS

Schick Test Toxin

Definition Schick Test Toxin is the preparation used in the Schick test to determine susceptibility to diphtheria. It is prepared from a toxigenic strain (a well-characterised PW-8 subculture is satisfactory) of *Corynebacterium diphtheriae*. It contains a suitable antimicrobial preservative.

Production Schick Test Toxin is prepared from a sterile filtrate of a culture in liquid medium of the organism. The toxin may be purified. It is then diluted with a sterile aqueous buffer solution of pH 7.2 to 7.6 that will render the preparation isotonic with blood so that the test dose is contained in 0.1 ml or 0.2 ml.

Schick Test Toxin is distributed in sterile containers which are sealed so as to exclude micro-organisms. When stored at 25° for two months Schick Test Toxin retains its potency.

Characteristics A clear, colourless or very pale straw-coloured liquid.

Identification Causes a local reaction when injected into the skin of a healthy, white guinea-pig or rabbit that has not been previously treated with any material that will interfere with the test but fails to cause this reaction when mixed with a sufficient quantity of Diphtheria Antitoxin.

Alkalinity pH, 7.2 to 7.6, Appendix V L.

Sterility Complies with the *test for sterility*, Appendix XVI A.

Potency

A. *Combining power* Prepare two mixtures of the preparation being examined such that in one mixture one test dose (0.1 ml or 0.2 ml as stated on the label) is mixed with 1/750 of IU of Diphtheria Antitoxin and in the other mixture one test dose is mixed with 1/1250 of 1 IU of Diphtheria Antitoxin. Allow both mixtures to stand at room temperature for 30 to 60 minutes and inject each, on separate flanks, into the depilated skin of a white guinea-pig that weighs not less than 500 g or of a white rabbit that weighs not less than 2.50 kg. Examine the guinea-pig or rabbit 2 days after injection. No reaction occurs at the site injected with the mixture containing 1/750 of 1 IU of Diphtheria Antitoxin. A reaction of the type known as a positive Schick reaction occurs at the site injected with the mixture containing 1/1250 of 1 IU of Diphtheria Antitoxin.

B. *Erythrogenic activity* The estimated potency is 0.5 to 2.0 IU per test dose (0.1 ml or 0.2 ml as stated on the label) when determined in guinea-pigs or rabbits by comparing the effects of intradermal injections of serial dilutions of one test dose of the preparation being examined with those of corresponding dilutions of the Standard Preparation of Diphtheria (Schick) test toxin as follows.

Depilate two healthy, white guinea-pigs or rabbits in such a way that each has an area of denuded skin sufficient for 16 discrete injection sites, two columns of four sites on each flank. Prepare two solutions of the preparation being examined and two solutions of the Standard Preparation such that, for both preparations, one solution contains toxin at one fifth of the concentration of the toxin in the other solution and both evoke erythematous lesions of apposite size when injected intradermally in 0.2-ml volumes into the depilated skin of guinea-pigs or rabbits. Solutions of the preparation being examined prepared by diluting 1 volume of the preparation with 2 volumes of diluent and 1 volume of the preparation with 14 volumes of diluent, respectively, and solutions of the Standard Preparation containing 1/3 and 1/15 of 1 IU in each 0.2 ml are likely to satisfy these requirements. Inject 0.2 ml of each of the four solutions so prepared, in turn, intradermally at each of four sites on each guinea-pig or rabbit. Distribute the four injections of each dilution among the 16 available sites in each animal in a Latin square design.

Measure the longitudinal and transverse axes of the resulting lesions at the injection sites 2 days after the injections have been made. Using for each lesion the geometric mean of the measurements, calculate by regression analysis the erythrogenic activity of one test dose in IU of Schick test toxin.

Standard Preparation The Standard Preparation is the 1st International Standard for Diphtheria (Schick) test toxin, established in 1954, consisting of purified toxin with bovine albumin and phosphate buffer salts, or another suitable preparation, the potency of which has been determined in relation to the International Standard.

Storage Schick Test Toxin should be stored at a temperature of 2° to 8°.

Labelling The label states (1) the total volume in the container; (2) whether the test dose is contained in 0.1 ml or 0.2 ml of the preparation; (3) the name and proportion of the antimicrobial preservative; (4) the date after which the preparation is not intended to be used; (5) the conditions under which the preparation should be stored.

Schick Control

Definition Schick Control is Schick Test Toxin that has been heated at a temperature not lower than 70° and not higher than 85° for not less than five minutes. It may be used in conjunction with Schick Test Toxin in order to exclude reactions due to non-specific substances. It is prepared from the same batch of Schick Test Toxin as that with which it is to be used.

Sterility Complies with the *test for sterility*, Appendix XVI A.

Inactivation Inject 0.2 ml into the depilated skin of a healthy white guinea-pig. Examine the guinea-pig 2 days after injection. No erythematous reaction occurs at the injection site.

Storage Schick Control should be kept with the Schick Test Toxin with which it is to be used and stored at a temperature of 2° to 8°.

Labelling The label states the batch of Schick Test Toxin from which the Schick Control was prepared.

Old Tuberculin

Old Tuberculin complies with the requirements of the 3rd edition of the European Pharmacopoeia for Old Tuberculin for Human Use [0152]. These requirements are reproduced after the heading 'Definition' below.

Ph Eur

DEFINITION

Old tuberculin for human use consists of a filtrate, concentrated by heating, containing the soluble products of the culture and lysis of one or more strains of *Mycobacterium bovis* and/or *Mycobacterium tuberculosis* that is capable of demonstrating a delayed hypersensitivity in an animal sensitised to micro-organisms of the same species.

Old tuberculin for human use in concentrated form is a transparent, viscous, yellow or brown liquid.

PRODUCTION

GENERAL PROVISIONS

The production of old tuberculin is based on a seed-lot system. The production method shall have been shown to yield consistently old tuberculin of adequate potency and safety in man. A batch of old tuberculin, calibrated in International Units by the method described under Assay and for which adequate clinical information is available as to its activity in man, is set aside to serve as a reference preparation.

The International Unit is the activity of a stated quantity of the International Standard. The equivalence in International Units of the International Standard is stated by the World Health Organisation.

SEED LOTS

The strain or strains of mycobacteria used shall be identified by historical records that include information on their origin and subsequent manipulation.

The working seed lots used to inoculate the media for the production of a concentrated harvest shall not have undergone more than four subcultures from the master seed lot.

Only seed lots that comply with the following requirements may be used for propagation.

Identification The species of mycobacterium of the master and working seed lots is identified.

Bacterial and fungal contamination The working seed lot complies with the test for sterility (*2.6.1*), carried out using 10 ml for each medium.

PROPAGATION AND HARVEST

The bacteria are grown in a liquid medium which may be a glycerolated broth or a synthetic medium. Growth must be typical for the strain. The culture is inactivated by a suitable method, such as treatment in an autoclave (121°C for not less than 30 min) or in flowing steam at a temperature not less than 100°C for at least 1 h. The culture liquid, from which the micro-organisms may or may not have been separated by filtration, is concentrated by evaporation, usually to one-tenth of its initial volume. The preparation is free from live mycobacteria. The concentrated harvest is shown to comply with the test for mycobacteria (*2.6.2*) before addition of any antimicrobial preservative or other substance that might interfere with the test. Phenol (5 g/l) or another suitable antimicrobial preservative that does not give rise to false positive reactions may be added.

Only a concentrated harvest that complies with the following requirements may be used in the preparation of the final bulk tuberculin.

pH (*2.2.3*). The pH of the concentrated harvest is 6.5 to 8.

Glycerol Where applicable, determine the glycerol content of the concentrated harvest. The amount is within the limits approved for the particular product.

Antimicrobial preservative Where applicable, determine the amount of antimicrobial preservative by a suitable chemical or physico-chemical method. The content is not less than 85 per cent and not more than 115 per cent of the intended amount. If phenol has been used in the preparation, the concentration is not more than 5 g/l (*2.5.15*).

Sensitisation Carry out the test described under Tests.

Sterility (*2.6.1*). The concentrated harvest complies with the test for sterility, carried out using 10 ml for each medium.

Potency Determine the potency as described under Assay.

FINAL BULK TUBERCULIN

The concentrated harvest is diluted aseptically.

Only a final bulk tuberculin that complies with the following requirement may be used in the preparation of the final lot.

Sterility (*2.6.1*). The final bulk tuberculin complies with the test for sterility, carried out using 10 ml for each medium.

FINAL LOT

The final bulk tuberculin is distributed aseptically into sterile containers which are then closed so as to prevent contamination.

Only a final lot that is satisfactory with respect to each of the requirements given below under Identification, Tests and Assay may be released for use.

The following tests may be omitted on the final lot if they have been carried out at the stages indicated:

live mycobacteria	concentrated harvest
sensitisation	concentrated harvest
toxicity	concentrated harvest or final bulk tuberculin
antimicrobial preservative	final bulk tuberculin.

IDENTIFICATION

Inject increasing doses of the preparation to be examined intradermally into healthy, white or pale-coloured guinea-pigs, specifically sensitised (for example, as described under Assay). A reaction varying from erythema to necrosis is produced at the site of the injection. Similar injections administered to non-sensitised guinea-pigs do not stimulate a reaction. The assay may also serve as identification.

TESTS

Old tuberculin for human use in concentrated form (≥100,000 I.U./ml) complies with each of the tests prescribed below; the diluted product complies with the tests for antimicrobial preservative and sterility.

Toxicity Inject a quantity equivalent to 50,000 I.U. subcutaneously into each of two healthy guinea-pigs weighing 250 g to 350 g and which have not been subjected to any treatment likely to interfere with the test. Observe the animals for 7 days. No adverse effect is produced.

Sensitisation Use three guinea-pigs that have not been subjected to any treatment likely to interfere with the test. On three occasions at intervals of 5 days, inject intradermally into each guinea-pig about 500 I.U. of the preparation to be examined in a volume of 0.1 ml. Two to three weeks after the third injection, administer the same dose intradermally to the same animals and to a control group of three guinea-pigs of the same mass that have not previously received injections of tuberculin. After 24 h to 72 h, the reactions in the two groups of animals are not substantially different.

Antimicrobial preservative Where applicable, determine the amount of antimicrobial preservative by a suitable chemical or physico-chemical method. The content is not less than the minimum amount shown to be effective and not more than 115 per cent of the amount stated on the label. If phenol has been used in the preparation, the concentration is not more than 5 g/l (*2.5.15*).

Live mycobacteria (*2.6.2*). It complies with the test for mycobacteria.

Sterility (*2.6.1*). It complies with the test for sterility.

ASSAY

The potency of old tuberculin is determined by comparing the reactions produced by the intradermal injection of increasing doses of the preparation to be examined into sensitised guinea-pigs with the reactions produced by known concentrations of the reference preparation.

Prepare a suspension containing a suitable amount (0.1 mg to 0.4 mg per millilitre) of heat-inactivated, dried mycobacteria in mineral oil with or without emulsifier; use mycobacteria of a strain of the same species as that used in the preparation to be examined. Sensitise not fewer than six pale-coloured guinea-pigs weighing not less than 300 g by injecting intramuscularly or intradermally a total of about 0.5 ml of the suspension, divided between several sites if necessary. Carry out the test after the period of time required for optimal sensitisation which is usually 4 to 8 weeks after sensitisation. Depilate the flanks of the animals so that it is possible to make at least three injections on each side and not more than a total of twelve injection points per animal. Use at least three different doses of the reference preparation and at least three different doses of the preparation to be examined. For both preparations, use doses such that the highest dose is about ten times the lowest dose. Choose the doses such that when they are injected the lesions produced have a diameter of not less than 8 mm and not more than 25 mm. In any given test, the order of the dilutions injected at each point is chosen at random in a Latin square design. Inject each dose intradermally in a constant volume of 0.1 ml or 0.2 ml. Measure the diameters of the lesions 24 h to 48 h later and calculate the results of the test by the usual statistical methods, assuming that the diameters of the lesions are directly proportional to the logarithm of the concentration of the preparation.

The estimated potency is not less than 80 per cent and not more than 125 per cent of the stated potency. The fiducial limits of error ($P = 0.95$) are not less than 64 per cent and not more than 156 per cent of the stated potency.

STORAGE

Store protected from light.

LABELLING

The label states:
— the number of International Units per millilitre,
— the species of mycobacterium used to prepare the product,
— the name and quantity of any antimicrobial preservative or other substance added to the preparation,
— the expiry date,
— where applicable, that old tuberculin is not to be injected in its concentrated form but diluted so as to administer not more than 100 I.U. per dose.

Ph Eur

Tuberculin Purified Protein Derivative

Tuberculin P.P.D.

Tuberculin Purified Protein Derivative complies with the requirements of the 3rd edition of the European Pharmacopoeia for Tuberculin Purified Derivative for Human Use [0151]. These requirements are reproduced after the heading 'Definition' below.

Ph Eur

DEFINITION

Tuberculin purified protein derivative (tuberculin PPD) for human use is a preparation obtained by precipitation from the heated products of the culture and lysis of *Mycobacterium bovis* and/or *Mycobacterium tuberculosis* and capable of demonstrating a delayed hypersensitivity in an animal sensitised to micro-organisms of the same species.

Tuberculin PPD is a colourless or pale-yellow liquid; the diluted preparation may be a freeze-dried powder which upon dissolution gives a colourless or pale-yellow liquid.

PRODUCTION

GENERAL PROVISIONS

The production of tuberculin PPD is based on a seed-lot system. The production method shall have been shown to yield consistently tuberculin PPD of adequate potency and safety in man. A batch of tuberculin PPD, calibrated in International Units by method A described under Assay and for which adequate clinical information is available as to its activity in man, is set aside to serve as a reference preparation.

The International Unit is the activity of a stated quantity of the International Standard. The equivalence in International Units of the International Standard is stated by the World Health Organisation.

SEED LOTS

The strain or strains of mycobacteria used shall be identified by historical records that include information on their origin and subsequent manipulation.

The working seed lots used to inoculate the media for production of a concentrated harvest shall not have undergone more than four subcultures from the master seed lot.

Only seed lots that comply with the following requirements may be used for propagation.

Identification The species of mycobacterium of the master and working seed lots is identified.

Bacterial and fungal contamination The working seed lot complies with the test for sterility (*2.6.1*), carried out using 10 ml for each medium.

PROPAGATION AND HARVEST

The bacteria are grown in a liquid synthetic medium. Growth must be typical for the strain. The culture is inactivated by a suitable method such as treatment in an autoclave (121°C for not less than 30 min) or in flowing steam at a temperature not less than 100°C for at least 1 h and filtered. The active fraction of the filtrate, consisting mainly of protein, is isolated by precipitation, washed and re-dissolved. The preparation is free from mycobacteria. The concentrated harvest is shown to comply with the test for mycobacteria (*2.6.2*) before addition of any antimicrobial preservative or other substance that might interfere with the test. Phenol (5 g/l) or another suitable antimicrobial preservative that does not give rise to false positive reactions may be added; a suitable stabiliser intended to prevent adsorption on glass or plastic surfaces may be added. The concentrated harvest may be freeze-dried. Phenol is not added to preparations that are to be freeze-dried.

Only a concentrated harvest that complies with the following requirements may be used in the preparation of the final bulk tuberculin.

Antimicrobial preservative Where applicable, determine the amount of antimicrobial preservative by a suitable chemical or physico-chemical method. The content is not less than 85 per cent and not more than 115 per cent of the intended amount. If phenol has been used in the preparation, the concentration is not more than 5 g/l (*2.5.15*).

Sensitisation Carry out the test described under Tests.

Sterility (*2.6.1*). The concentrated harvest, reconstituted if necessary, complies with the test for sterility, carried out using 10 ml for each medium.

Potency Determine the potency as described under Assay.

FINAL BULK TUBERCULIN PPD

The concentrated harvest is diluted aseptically, after reconstitution if necessary.

Only a final bulk that complies with the following requirement may be used in the preparation of the final lot.

Sterility (*2.6.1*). The final bulk tuberculin PPD complies with the test for sterility, carried out using 10 ml for each medium.

FINAL LOT

The final bulk is distributed aseptically into sterile containers which are then closed so as to prevent contamination. It may be freeze-dried.

Only a final lot that is satisfactory with respect to each of the requirements given below under Identification, Tests and Assay may be released for use.

The following tests may be omitted on the final lot if they have been carried out at the stages indicated:

live mycobacteria	concentrated harvest
sensitisation	concentrated harvest
toxicity	concentrated harvest or final bulk tuberculin
antimicrobial preservative	final bulk tuberculin.

IDENTIFICATION

Inject increasing doses of the preparation to be examined intradermally into healthy, white or pale-coloured guinea-pigs, specifically sensitised (for example as described under Assay). A reaction varying from erythema to necrosis is produced at the site of the injection. Similar injections administered to non-sensitised guinea-pigs do not stimulate a reaction. The assay may also serve as identification.

TESTS

Tuberculin purified protein derivative for human use in concentrated form (≥ 100,000 I.U./ml) complies with each of the tests prescribed below; the diluted product complies with the tests for pH, antimicrobial preservative and sterility.

pH (*2.2.3*) The pH of the preparation, reconstituted if necessary as stated on the label, is 6.5 to 7.5.

Toxicity Inject subcutaneously 50,000 I.U. of the preparation to be examined into each of two healthy guinea-pigs weighing 250 g to 350 g and which have not been subjected to any treatment likely to interfere with the test. Observe the animals for 7 days. No adverse effect is produced.

Sensitisation Use three guinea-pigs that have not been subjected to any treatment likely to interfere with the test. On three occasions at intervals of 5 days, inject intradermally into each guinea-pig about 500 I.U. of the preparation to be examined in a volume of 0.1 ml. Two to three weeks after the third injection, administer the same dose intradermally to the same animals and to a control group of three guinea-pigs of the same mass that have not previously received injections of tuberculin. After 24 h to 72 h, the reactions in the two groups of animals are not substantially different.

Antimicrobial preservative Where applicable, determine the amount of antimicrobial preservative by a suitable chemical or physico-chemical method. The content is not less than the minimum amount shown to be effective and not more than 115 per cent of the amount stated on the label. If phenol has been used in the preparation, the concentration is not more than 5 g/l (*2.5.15*).

Live mycobacteria (*2.6.2*). It complies with the test for live mycobacteria.

Sterility (*2.6.1*). It complies with the test for sterility.

ASSAY

Use method A or, where the product contains 1 I.U. to 2 I.U., use method B.

Method A

The potency of tuberculin PPD is determined by comparing the reactions produced by the intradermal injection of increasing doses of the preparation to be examined into sensitised guinea-pigs with the reactions produced by known concentrations of the reference preparation.

Prepare a suspension containing a suitable amount (0.1 mg to 0.4 mg per millilitre) of heat-inactivated, dried mycobacteria in mineral oil with or without emulsifier; use mycobacteria of a strain of the same species as that used in the preparation to be examined. Sensitise not fewer than six pale-coloured guinea-pigs weighing not less than 300 g by injecting intramuscularly or intradermally a total of about 0.5 ml of the suspension, divided between several sites if necessary. Carry out the test after the period of time required for optimal sensitisation which is usually 4 to 8 weeks after sensitisation. Depilate the flanks of the animals so that it is possible to make at least three injections on each side but not more than a total of twelve injection points per animal. Prepare dilutions of the preparation to be examined and of the reference preparation using isotonic phosphate-buffered saline (pH 6.5 to 7.5) containing 50 mg/l of *polysorbate 80 R*. If the preparation to be examined is freeze-dried and does not contain a stabiliser, reconstitute it using the liquid described above. Use at least three different doses of the reference preparation and at least three different doses of the preparation to be examined. For both preparations, use doses such that the highest dose is about ten times the lowest dose. Choose the doses such that when they are injected the lesions produced have a diameter of not less than 8 mm and not more than 25 mm. In any given test, the order of the dilutions injected at each point is chosen at random in a Latin square design. Inject each dose intradermally in a constant volume of 0.1 ml or 0.2 ml. Measure the diameters of the lesions 24 h to 48 h later and calculate the results of the test by the usual statistical methods, assuming that the diameters of the lesions are directly proportional to the logarithm of the concentration of the preparation.

The estimated potency is not less than 80 per cent and not more than 125 per cent of the stated potency. The fiducial limits of error ($P = 0.95$) are not less than 64 per cent and not more than 156 per cent of the stated potency.

Method B

The potency of tuberculin PPD is determined by comparing the reactions produced by the intradermal injection of the preparation to be examined into sensitised guinea-pigs with the reactions produced by known concentrations of the reference preparation.

Prepare a suspension in mineral oil with or without emulsifier and containing a suitable amount (0.1 mg to 0.4 mg per millilitre) of heat-inactivated, dried mycobacteria; use mycobacteria of a strain of the same species as that used in the preparation to be examined. Sensitise not fewer than six pale-coloured guinea-pigs weighing not less than 300 g by injecting intramuscularly or intradermally a total of about 0.5 ml of the suspension, divided between several sites if necessary. Carry out the test after the period of time required for optimal sensitisation which is usually 4 to 8 weeks after sensitisation. Depilate the flanks of the animals so that it is possible to make at least three injections on each side but not more than a total of twelve injection points per animal. Prepare dilutions of the reference preparation using isotonic phosphate-buffered saline (pH 6.5 to 7.5) containing 50 mg/l of *polysorbate 80 R*. Use at least three different doses of the reference preparation such that the highest dose is about ten times the lowest dose and the median dose is the same as that of the preparation to be examined. In any given test, the order of the dilutions injected at each point is chosen at random in a Latin square design. Inject the preparation to be examined and each dilution of the reference preparation intradermally in a constant volume of 0.1 ml or 0.2 ml. Measure the diameters of the lesions 24 h to 48 h later and calculate the results of the test by the usual statistical methods, assuming that the areas of the lesions are directly proportional to the logarithm of the concentration of the preparation to be examined. (This dose relationship applies to this assay and not necessarily to other test systems.)

The estimated potency is not less than 80 per cent and not more than 125 per cent of the stated potency. The fiducial limits of error ($P = 0.95$) are not less than 64 per cent and not more than 156 per cent of the stated potency.

STORAGE

Store protected from light.

LABELLING

The label states:
- the number of International Units per container,
- the species of mycobacteria used to prepare the product,
- the name and quantity of any antimicrobial preservative or other substance added to the preparation,
- the expiry date,
- for freeze-dried products, a statement that the product is to be reconstituted using the liquid provided by the manufacturer,
- where applicable, that tuberculin PPD is not to be injected in its concentrated form but diluted so as to administer not more than 100 I.U. per dose.

If the package does not contain a leaflet warning that the inhalation of concentrated tuberculin PPD may produce toxic effects, this warning must be shown on the label on the container together with a statement that the powder must be handled with care.

Ph Eur

Monographs

Radiopharmaceutical Preparations

RADIOPHARMACEUTICAL PREPARATIONS

A radiopharmaceutical preparation that is the subject of an individual monograph in the European Pharmacopoeia or in the British Pharmacopoeia complies with the requirements of the 3rd edition of the European Pharmacopoeia for Radiopharmaceutical Preparations [0125]. These requirements are reproduced after the heading 'Definition' below.

In the United Kingdom, standardised preparations for the identification and measurement of radiation may be obtained from Amersham International plc, Amersham, HP7 9LL, United Kingdom.

Ph Eur

DEFINITION

The statements in this monograph are intended to be read in conjunction with the monographs on radiopharmaceutical preparations in the Pharmacopoeia. The requirements do not necessarily apply to radiopharmaceutical preparations that are not the subject of such monographs.

Radiopharmaceutical preparations are preparations containing one or more radionuclides.

A nuclide is a species of atom characterised by the number of protons and neutrons in its nucleus (and hence by its atomic number and mass number) and also by its nuclear energy state. Isotopes of an element are nuclides with the same atomic number but different mass numbers. Radionuclides, that is, nuclides which are radioactive, transform spontaneously into other nuclides. The transformation may involve the emission of charged particles, electron capture (EC) or isomeric transition (IT). The charged particles emitted from the nucleus may be alpha particles (helium nucleus of mass number 4) or beta particles (electrons of negative or positive charge, β^- or $\beta+$ respectively, the latter being known as positrons). The emission of charged particles from the nucleus may be accompanied by gamma rays. Gamma rays are also emitted in the process of isomeric transition. These emissions of gamma rays may be partly replaced by the ejection of electrons known as internal-conversion electrons. This phenomenon, like the process of electron capture, causes a secondary emission of X-rays (due to the reorganisation of the electrons in the atom). This secondary emission may itself be partly replaced by the ejection of electrons known as Auger electrons. $\beta+$ particles are annihilated on contact with matter, the process being accompanied by the emission of gamma rays with an energy of 511 keV.

The decay of a radionuclide follows an exponential law. The time in which a given quantity decays to half of its initial value is termed the half-life ($T_{½}$) and is characteristic for each radionuclide.

The penetrating power of each radiation varies considerably according to its nature and its energy. Alpha particles are completely absorbed in a thickness of a few micrometres to some tens of micrometres of solid or liquid. Beta particles are completely absorbed in a thickness of several millimetres to several centimetres. Gamma rays are not completely absorbed but only attenuated and a tenfold reduction may require, for example, several centimetres of lead. The denser the absorbent, the shorter the range of alpha and beta particles and the greater the attenuation of gamma rays.

Each radionuclide is characterised by an invariable half-life, expressed in units of time, and by the nature and energy of its radiation or radiations. The energy is expressed in electronvolts (eV), kilo-electronvolts (keV) or mega-electronvolts (MeV). The radioactivity ("activity") of a preparation is the number of nuclear disintegrations or transformations per unit time.

Quantities of radioactivity were formerly expressed using the curie (Ci), which is 3.7×10^{10} disintegrations per second, the millicurie, the microcurie or the nanocurie.

In the International System (SI), quantities of radioactivity are expressed in the becquerel (Bq) which is 1 nuclear transformation per second. The following factors facilitate conversion between the two systems of units:

1 curie (Ci) = 3.7×10^{10} becquerels
= 37 gigabecquerels (GBq)

1 millicurie (mCi) = 3.7×10^{7} becquerels
= 37 megabecquerels (MBq)

1 microcurie (µCi) = 3.7×10^{4} becquerels
= 37 kilobecquerels (kBq)

1 gigabecquerel (GBq) = 27.027 millicuries (mCi)

1 megabecquerel (MBq) = 27.027 microcuries (µCi)

1 kilobecquerel (kBq) = 27.027 nanocuries (nCi)

The absolute measurement of the quantity of radioactivity in a given sample can be carried out completely and accurately only if the nature and energy of the emitted radiation and the relative contribution of each to the total radiation are known (mode of decay). This measurement requires a specialised laboratory but identification and measurement of radiation can be carried out comparatively and relatively by the use of standardised preparations provided by such laboratories. Standardised preparations are available from laboratories recognised by the relevant competent authority.

DEFINITION

Radioactive source A radioactive material used to provide ionising radiation.

Sealed source A radioactive source intended to be used in such a manner that the radioactive material does not come into immediate contact with its environment. It consists of radioactive material firmly incorporated in inactive solid materials or sealed in a container of sufficient resistance to prevent any dispersion of radioactive material or any possibility of contamination in ordinary conditions of use.

Non-sealed source A radioactive source intended to be used in such a manner that the radioactive material comes into immediate contact with its environment. In a non-sealed source, the radioactive material is directly accessible. It is generally intended that the source will be subjected to physical or chemical manipulation during the course of which it may be transferred from one container to another. Radiopharmaceutical preparations belong to this category.

Radionuclidic purity The ratio, expressed as a percentage, of the radioactivity of the radionuclide concerned to the total radioactivity of the source. The terms "radioactive purity" and "radioisotopic purity" may also be used to describe this ratio.

Radiochemical purity The ratio, expressed as a percentage, of the radioactivity of the radionuclide concerned which is present in the source in the stated chemical form to the total radioactivity of that radionuclide present in the source.

Chemical purity The ratio, expressed as a percentage, of the mass of substance present in the stated chemical form to the total mass contained in the source excluding any excipients or solvents.

Carrier A stable isotope of the radionuclide concerned added to the radioactive preparation in the same chemical form as that in which the radionuclide is present.

Specific radioactivity The radioactivity of a nuclide per unit mass of the element or of the chemical form concerned. For example, the specific radioactivity of sodium [^{32}P]phosphate is expressed as follows: 11.1 MBq (0.3 mCi) of phosphorus-32 per milligram of orthophosphate ion at the date and hour indicated.

Radioactive concentration The radioactivity of a nuclide per unit volume of the solution in which it is present.

IDENTIFICATION

The radionuclide is identified by its half-life or by the nature and energy of its radiation or radiations or by both, as prescribed in the monograph.

Measurement of half-life The half-life is measured with a suitable detection apparatus such as an ionisation chamber, a Geiger-Müller counter or a scintillation counter. The radiopharmaceutical preparation is used as such or diluted or dried in a capsule after appropriate dilution. The quantity of radioactivity chosen, having regard to experimental conditions, must be sufficiently high to allow detection during several presumed half-lives, but should be limited to avoid the phenomenon of "loss of counts". The latter may be due, for example, to the dead time of a Geiger-Müller counter or to random coincidence in a scintillation counter.

The radioactive source is prepared in a manner that will avoid loss of material during handling. If it is a liquid (solution), it is contained in bottles or sealed tubes. If it is a solid (residue from drying in a capsule), it is protected by a cover consisting of a sheet of adhesive cellulose acetate or of some other material whose mass per unit area is sufficiently small not to attenuate a significant amount of the radiation being studied.

The same source is measured in the same geometrical conditions and at intervals usually corresponding to half of the half-life throughout a time equal to about three half-lives. The correct functioning of the apparatus is checked using a source of long half-life and, if necessary, the variations of counting are corrected (see Measurement of Radioactivity).

A graph is drawn with time as the abscissae and the logarithm of the number of impulses counted per unit time (count rate) or the electric current, according to the type of instrument used, as the ordinates. The calculated half-life should not differ by more than 5 per cent from the half-life stated in the Pharmacopoeia.

The curve of exponential decay (decay curve) is described by the equation:

$$A_t = A_0 e^{-\lambda t}$$

A_t = the radioactivity at time t,

A_0 = the radioactivity at time t = 0,

λ = the decay constant characteristic of each radionuclide,

e = the base of Napierian logarithms.

The half-life ($T_{1/2}$) is related to the decay constant (l) by the equation:

$$T_{1/2} = \frac{0.693}{\lambda}$$

The radioactivity of a preparation is measured at a specified time. The radioactivity at other times may be calculated from the exponential equation or from tables, or it may be obtained graphically from a graph drawn for each individual radionuclide.

Determination of the nature and energy of the radiation The nature and energy of the radiation emitted may be determined by several procedures including the construction of an attenuation curve and the use of spectrometry. The attenuation curve is often used for analysis of beta radiation; spectrometry is mostly used for identification of gamma rays.

The attenuation curve is drawn for pure beta emitters when no spectrometer for beta rays is available or for beta/gamma emitters when no spectrometer for gamma rays is available. This method of estimating the maximum energy of beta radiation gives only an approximate value. The source, suitably mounted to give constant geometrical conditions, is placed in front of the thin window of a Geiger-Müller counter or a proportional counter. The source is protected as described above. The count rate of the source is then measured. Between the source and the counter are placed, in succession, at least six aluminium screens of increasing mass per unit area within such limits that, for the screen of highest mass per unit area, a constant count rate is obtained. With a pure beta emitter this count rate is not affected by addition of further screens. The screens are inserted in such a manner that constant geometrical conditions are maintained. A graph is drawn showing, as the abscissae, the mass per unit area of the screen expressed in milligrams per square centimetre and, as the ordinates, the logarithm of the number of impulses counted per unit time for each screen examined. A graph is drawn in the same manner for a standardised preparation. The result is calculated by reference to the median parts of the curves, which are practically rectilinear.

The mass attenuation coefficient μ_m, expressed in square centimetres per milligram, depends on the energy of the beta radiation and on the physical and chemical properties of the screen. It therefore allows beta emitters to be identified. It is calculated from the graphs drawn as described above, using the equation:

$$\mu_m = \frac{2.303}{m_2 - m_1}(\log A_1 - \log A_2)$$

m_1 = mass per unit area of the lightest screen,

m_2 = mass per unit area of the heaviest screen m_1 and m_2 being within the rectilinear part of the curve,

A_1 = count rate for mass per unit area m_1,

A_2 = count rate for mass per unit area m_2.

The mass attenuation coefficient, μ_m, thus calculated must not differ by more than 10 per cent from the coefficient obtained under identical conditions using a standardised preparation of the same radionuclide.

Gamma spectrometry may be based upon the property of certain substances (scintillators) to emit light when struck by a gamma ray. The number of photons produced is proportional to the energy absorbed in the scintillator. The light is transformed into electrical impulses of an amplitude approximately proportional to the energy dissipated by the gamma photons. Examination of the output pulses with a suitable pulse-amplitude analyser gives the energy spectrum of the source. Gamma-ray scintillation spectra show one or more characteristic peaks corresponding to the energies of the gamma radiation of the source. These peaks are accompanied by other peaks of various widths due to secondary effects of radiation on the scintillator or on the material around it. The shape of the spectrum obtained varies with the instrument used and it is necessary to calibrate the apparatus using a reference source of the radionuclide being studied.

The preferred detector for gamma-ray spectrometry is now a lithium-drifted germanium semiconductor detector. Such an instrument can have a resolution (full width of the peak at half maximum height) of 2.0 keV to 2.5 keV at 1.3 MeV, thus making it possible to identify peaks 5 keV apart in the gamma-ray spectrum. A thallium-activated sodium iodide scintillation detector is also used but this has a much lower resolution (about 50 keV). The output from either of these detectors is in the form of electrical pulses whose amplitude is proportional to the energy of the detected gamma ray. After amplification these pulses are analysed in a multichannel analyser which displays the gamma-energy spectrum of the source. The relationship between gamma energy and channel number can easily be established using sources emitting gamma rays of known energy.

The detector system needs to be calibrated because the detection efficiency is a function of the energy of the gamma ray as well as the form of the source and the source-to-detector distance. The detection efficiency may be measured using a calibrated source of the radionuclide to be measured or, for more general work, a graph of efficiency against gamma energy may be constructed from a series of calibrated sources of various radionuclides.

The gamma-ray spectrum of a radionuclide which emits gamma rays is unique to that nuclide and is characterised by the energies and the number of photons of particular energies emitted per transformation. This property can be used to identify which radionuclides are present in a source and the amounts of each. It facilitates the estimation of the degree of radionuclidic impurity by detecting peaks other than those expected.

It is possible to establish the rate of decay of radioactivity in a spectrum since the peaks diminish in amplitude as a function of the half-life. If, in such a source, a radioactive impurity of longer half-life is introduced, it is easy to detect the latter by the isolation and identification of the characteristic peak or peaks whose amplitudes decrease at a different rate from that expected for the particular radionuclide. A determination of the half-life of the interfering peaks by repeated measurements of the sample will help to identify the impurity.

Table 125-1 (see below) summarises the most commonly accepted physical characteristics of radionuclides used in preparations which are the subject of monographs in the Pharmacopoeia. In addition, the Table states the physical characteristics of the main impurities of the radionuclides.

When assessing disintegration patterns, the term "intensity" may be used in two different contexts.

By "intensity of a transition" is meant the probability of the transformation of a nucleus in a given energy state, according to the transition concerned. When used in this way, the word "intensity" is synonymous with "abundance".

By "emission intensity" is meant the probability that a radioactive atom will give rise to the emission of the particle or radiation concerned. This is the meaning attached to the word "intensity" in Table 125-1. Irrespective of whether the one or the other meaning is intended, intensity is usually measured in terms of 100 disintegrations.

MEASUREMENT OF RADIOACTIVITY

The absolute measurement of the radioactivity of a given sample may be carried out only if the decay scheme of the nuclide is known and is usually based on the coincidence method in which counts of, for example, a beta emission and a gamma emission are made separately and in coincidence using special apparatus. The three count rates are sufficient to determine the efficiencies of the counters and the absolute rate of decay. In practice, many corrections are required to obtain accurate results.

It is common to carry out comparisons against a standard source and to use a Geiger-Müller counter, a proportional counter, a scintillation counter or an ionisation chamber. A Geiger-Müller counter is used to measure beta and beta/gamma emitters; scintillation and semiconductor counters are used for measuring gamma rays; low-energy beta emitters require a liquid-scintillation counter.

Whatever apparatus is used, it is essential to work under well-defined geometrical conditions so that the radioactive source is always at the same position in the apparatus and, consequently, its distance from the measuring device is constant and remains the same when the sample being measured is replaced by the standardised preparation. Solutions of radiopharmaceutical preparations may be measured as such using, for example, an ionisation chamber or a well-crystal scintillation detector. However, for certain types of apparatus such as an end-window Geiger-Müller counter or a flat-crystal scintillation counter, it may be preferable to use the residue on evaporation. It is advisable to cover the dry residue with a strip of adhesive cellulose acetate whose mass per unit area should be less than 10 mg/cm^2, so that its absorption of radiation is negligible. The residue on evaporation of the standardised preparation should be as nearly as possible identical with that of the solution to be examined; that is, the two solutions should contain the same substances at the same concentration and the evaporation should be carried out under the same conditions on surfaces of the same material and of identical size. When these precautions are taken, the results obtained are satisfactory, whatever the measuring apparatus used. It is necessary to ensure that the efficiency of the measuring apparatus remains constant during the time of measuring by using a secondary source consisting of a radionuclide of long half-life.

Low-energy beta emitters may be measured by liquid-scintillation counting. The sample is dissolved in a solution containing one or more often two organic fluorescent substances (primary and secondary scintillators), which convert part of the energy of disintegration into photons of light, which are detected by a photomultiplier and converted into electrical impulses. When using a liquid-scintillation counter comparative measurements should be corrected for light-quenching effects.

Direct measurements should be made in conditions which ensure that the geometrical conditions are constant (identical volumes of containers and solutions) for the source to be examined and the standard source. All measurements of radioactivity must be corrected by subtracting the background activity due to radioactivity in the environment and to spurious signals generated in the equipment itself.

With some equipment, when counts are made at high levels of activity, a correction may be required for loss by coincidence due to the finite resolving time of the detector and its associated electronic equipment. For a counting system with a fixed paralysis time t following each count, the correction is:

$$N = \frac{N_o}{1 - N_o\tau}$$

N = the true count rate per second,

N_0 = the observed count rate per second,

τ = the paralysis time in seconds.

It is evident that such a correction will be acceptably small only if the product $N_o\tau$ is very small. With some equipment this correction is made automatically. Corrections for loss by coincidence must be made before the correction for background radiation.

The results of determinations of radioactivity show variations which derive mainly from the random nature of nuclear transformation. A sufficient number of counts must be registered in order to compensate for variations in the number of transformations per unit of time. A count of at least 10,000 is necessary to obtain a standard deviation of not more than 1 per cent.

All statements of radioactive content should be accompanied by a statement of the date and, if necessary, the hour at which the measurement was made. The measurement of radioactivity of a sample in solution is calculated with respect to the original volume of the solution and is expressed per unit volume to give the radioactive concentration or radioactive volume.

RADIONUCLIDIC PURITY

To state the radionuclidic purity of a preparation the radioactivities and hence the identities of every radionuclide present must be known. The most generally useful method of examination for radionuclidic purity is that of gamma spectrometry. It is not a completely reliable method because beta-emitting impurities are not usually detectable and, when sodium iodide detectors are employed, the peaks due to impurities are often obscured by the spectrum of the principal radionuclide.

The individual monographs prescribe the radionuclidic purity required (for example, the gamma-ray spectrum should not be significantly different from that of a standardised preparation) and may set limits for specific radionuclidic impurities (for example, cobalt-60 in cobalt-57). While these requirements are necessary, they are not in themselves sufficient to ensure that the radionuclidic purity of a preparation is sufficient for human use. The manufacturer must examine his products in detail and especially must examine preparations of radionuclides of short half-life for impurities of long half-life after a suitable period of decay. In this way, information on the suitability of his manufacturing processes and the adequacy of his testing procedures may be obtained.

RADIOCHEMICAL PURITY

The determination of radiochemical purity consists in separating the different chemical substances containing the radionuclide and estimating the radioactivity associated with the declared chemical substance. In principle, any method of analytical separation may be used in the determination of radiochemical purity. However, considerations of speed and simplicity have led to the choice of chromatography on flat supports (paper or thin-layer) and, for certain preparations, to electrophoresis (paper or cellulose acetate film). In addition to the technical description of these analytical methods set out in the Pharmacopoeia, certain precautions special to radioactivity must also be taken.

In chromatography, a volume equal to or less than 10 µl should be deposited on the starting-line as prescribed in the general methods for chromatography. It is preferable not to dilute the preparation to be examined but it is important to avoid depositing such a quantity of radioactivity that counting losses by coincidence occur during measurement of the radioactivity. On account of the very small quantities of the radioactive material applied, a carrier may be added when specified in a particular monograph. After development, the support is dried and the positions of the radioactive areas are detected by autoradiography or by measurement of radioactivity over the length of the chromatogram, using suitable collimated counters or by cutting the strips and counting each portion. The positions of the spots or areas permit chemical identification by comparison with solutions of the same chemical substances (non-radioactive) visualised by colour reaction or by examination in ultraviolet light. Visualisation by direct colour reaction of the radioactive substance is not always possible or desirable, since spraying with the visualisation reagents may bring about diffusion of the radioactive substance outside the identified spots or areas.

Measurement of radioactivity may be made by integration using an automatic-plotting instrument or a digital counter. The ratios of the areas under the peaks give the ratios of the radioactive concentration of the chemical substances. When the strips are cut into portions, the ratios of the quantities of radioactivity measured give the ratio of concentrations of the radioactive chemical species.

SPECIFIC RADIOACTIVITY

Specific radioactivity is usually calculated taking into account the radioactive concentration (radioactivity per unit volume) and the concentration of the chemical substance being studied, after verification that the radioactivity is attributable only to the radionuclide (radionuclidic purity) and the chemical species (radiochemical purity) concerned.

STERILITY

Radiopharmaceutical preparations for parenteral administration must be prepared using precautions designed to exclude microbial contamination and to ensure sterility. The test for sterility is carried out as described in (*2.6.1*). Special difficulties arise with radiopharmaceutical preparations because of the small size of batches and the irradiation hazards. Also, it is not always possible to await the results of the test for sterility before authorisation of the release for use of the batch concerned; the test then constitutes a control of the quality of production.

Notwithstanding the requirements concerning the use of antimicrobial preservatives in the monograph on *Parenteral preparations (520)*, their addition to radiopharmaceutical preparations in multidose containers is not obligatory, unless prescribed in the monograph.

PYROGENS

For certain preparations, a test for pyrogens is prescribed but, because of the usually short half-life of the radionuclide present in the preparation and the fairly high radioactivity which these preparations may contain, it is difficult to carry out the test before authorisation of the release for use of the batch. To avoid hyperthermia which might be due not to pyrogens but to the radioactivity of the preparation, it is sometimes necessary to wait until the latter has decayed to the limit prescribed in the monograph and is such that the volume of radioactive solution prescribed in the monograph can be injected. Apart from these details, the test is carried out in accordance with the general method (*2.6.8*), taking the necessary precautions to avoid irradiation of the personnel carrying out the test; the test then constitutes a control of the quality of production. It is advisable for the producer to verify beforehand the absence of pyrogens in the ingredients of radiopharmaceutical preparations.

The official test may be unsuitable for some radiopharmaceutical preparations. For example, it may not be sufficiently sensitive for those intended for administration by any route giving access to the cerebrospinal fluid, or testing after release for use may be unacceptable. In these circumstances, a test for bacterial endotoxins *(2.6.14)* may be useful.

STORAGE

Store in an airtight container in a place that is sufficiently shielded to protect personnel from irradiation by primary or secondary emissions and that complies with national and international regulations concerning the storage of radioactive substances. During storage, containers and solutions may darken due to irradiation. Such darkening does not necessarily involve deterioration of the preparations.

Radiopharmaceutical preparations are intended for use within a short time.

LABELLING

The label states:
- the name of the preparation,
- the name of the manufacturer,
- an identification number,
- for liquid preparations, the total radioactivity in the container, or the radioactive concentration per millilitre, at a stated date and, if necessary, hour, and the volume of liquid in the container,
- for solid preparations such as freeze-dried preparations, the total radioactivity at a stated date and, if necessary, hour,
- for capsules, the radioactivity of each capsule at a stated date and, if necessary, hour and the number of capsules in the container.
- that the preparation is intended for medical use,
- the route of administration,
- the period of validity or the expiry date,
- the name and concentration of any added antimicrobial preservative,
- any special storage conditions.

Ph Eur

Table of physical characteristics of radionuclides mentioned in the Pharmacopoeia:—see following pages

Table of physical characteristics of radionuclides mentioned in the Pharmacopoeia

Radionuclide	Half-life	Electron emission			Photon emission		
		Type	Energy (MeV)	Intensity (per cent)	Type	Energy (MeV)	Intensity (per cent)
Caesium-137 (^{137}Cs) in equilibrium with barium-137m (^{137}Ba)	30.2 years (^{137}Ba: 2.55 min)	e_A	0.004	7.8	X	0.005	1
			0.026	0.8			
		e_c	0.624	8		0.032-0.037	7
			0.656	1.4	γ	0.661	85.4
			0.660	0.4			
		$β^-$	0.511[a]	94.6			
			1.173[a]	5.2			
Chromium-51 (^{51}Cr)	27.7 days	e_A	0.0004	144	X	0.0005	0.33
			0.004	67		0.005	22.3
					γ	0.320	9.83
Cobalt-57 (^{57}Co)	271 days	e_A	0.0007	249	X	0.0007	0.8
		$e_A + e_c$	0.005 - 0.007	175		0.007	56
					γ	0.014	9.5
		e_c	0.014	8.9		0.122	85.6
			0.115	1.9		0.136	10.6
			0.129	1.4		0.692	0.16
Cobalt-58 (^{58}Co)	70.8 days	e_A	0.0007	117	X	0.0007	0.4
			0.006	49.4		0.006	26.2
		$β^+$	0.475[a]	15	γ	0.511	36[b]
						0.811	99.4
						0.864	0.7
						1.675	0.5
Cobalt-60 (^{60}Co)	5.27 years	$β^-$	0.318[a]	99.9	γ	1.173	99.9
						1.332	100
Gallium-66 (^{66}Ga)	9.4 hours	e_A	0.001	56	X	0.001	0.3
			0.008	21		0.008 - 0.010	19
					γ	0.511	113[b]
		$β^+$	0.361[a]	1		0.834	6
			0.720 - 0.820[a]	1.1		1.039	38
			0.924[a]	4.1		1.333	1.3
			1.780[a]	0.4		1.918	2.2
			4.153[a]	50		2.190	5.8
						2.422	2
						2.752	23.5
						4.295	3.5
Gallium-67 (^{67}Ga)	3.26 days	e_A	0.001	169	X	0.001	1
			0.007 - 0.010	60		0.008 - 0.010	55
		e_c	0.081 - 0.084	27	γ	0.091 - 0.093	38.5
			0.090 - 0.093	6		0.185	22
			0.175	0.4		0.209	2.4
						0.300	16.5
						0.394	4.5
						0.494	0.09
						0.888	0.14
Gold-198 (^{198}Au)	2.70 days	e_A	0.005 - 0.015	2.1	X	0.008 - 0.015	1.3
		e_c	0.329	2.9		0.069 - 0.083	2.8
			0.397	1	γ	0.412	95.6
			0.408	0.34		0.676	0.8
		$β^-$	0.290[a]	1		1.088	0.2
			0.966[a]	98.9			

Table of physical characteristics of radionuclides mentioned in the Pharmacopoeia

Radionuclide		Electron emission			Photon emission		
	Half-life	Type	Energy (MeV)	Intensity (per cent)	Type	Energy (MeV)	Intensity (per cent)
Gold-199 (^{199}Au)	3.14 days	e_A	0.005 - 0.015	21	X	0.008 - 0.015	12.9
		$e_A + e_c$	0.035 - 0.054	4.1	γ	0.050	0.33
		e_c	0.075	10.5	X	0.068 - 0.080	15.4
			0.125	5.5			
			0.144	17.1	γ	0.158	36.9
			0.155 - 0.158	5.8		0.208	8.4
			0.193	2			
		β^-	0.245[a]	18.9			
			0.294[a]	66.4			
			0.453[a]	14.7			
Indium-111 (^{111}In)	2.8 days	e_A	0.002 - 0.004	101	X	0.003 - 0.004	6.3
			0.018 - 0.027	16		0.023 - 0.028	82.4
		e_c	0.145	7.9	γ	0.171	90.9
			0.167 - 0.171	1.2		0.245	94.2
			0.219	4.9			
			0.241 - 0.245	0.9			
Indium-114m (^{114m}In)	49.5 days	e_A,e_c	1.99	95	X	0.023 - 0.028	40
Indium-114 (^{114}In)		β^-					
					γ	0.190	17.7
						0.558	4.6
						0.725	4.6
Iodine-123 (^{123}I)	13.2 hours	e_A	0.002 - 0.005	98	X	0.003 - 0.005	8
			0.021 - 0.031	12		0.027 - 0.032	87
			0.127	13.6	γ	0.159	83.4
			0.154	1.8		0.346	0.1
			0.158	0.4		0.440	0.4
						0.505	0.3
						0.529	1.4
						0.538	0.4
Iodine-124 (^{124}I)	4.2 days	e_A	0.003	64	X	0.004	6
		e_c	0.023	8		0.027 - 0.031	59
			0.571	0.3	γ	0.511	46[b]
						0.606	61
		β^+	0.810	0.3		0.723	10
			1.532	11.3		1.325	1.5
			2.135	11.3		1.376	1.7
						1.509	3
						1.691	10.5
Iodine-125 (^{125}I)	60.1 days	$e_A + e_c$	0.002 - 0.005	236	X	0.003 - 0.005	15
			0.021 - 0.035	33		0.027	114
					γ	0.031	25
						0.035	6.7
Iodine-126 (^{126}I)	13.0 days	e_A	0.003	43.5	X	0.004	4.3
		e_c	0.022	5.7		0.027-0.031	40
			0.354	0.5	γ	0.388	34
		β^-	0.634	0.1			
			0.371[a]	3.6		0.491	2.9
		β^+	0.862[a]	32		0.511	6.7[b]
			1.251[a]	8		0.666	33
			1.134[a]	3.3		0.754	4.2
						0.880	0.8
						1.420	0.3

Table of physical characteristics of radionuclides mentioned in the Pharmacopoeia

Radionuclide	Electron emission				Photon emission		
	Half-life	Type	Energy (MeV)	Intensity (per cent)	Type	Energy (MeV)	Intensity (per cent)
Iodine-131 (^{131}I)	8.04 days	e_A	0.003	5.1	X	0.004	0.6
		e_c	0.025	0.6		0.029 - 0.034	5
			0.045	3.5	γ	0.080	2.6
		β^-	0.075 - 0.079	0.6		0.284	6.1
			0.250	0.25		0.365	81.2
			0.330	1.5		0.637	7.3
			1.359	0.25		0.722	1.8
			0.248a	2.1			
			0.304a	0.6			
			0.334a	7.4			
			0.606a	89.4			
			0.807a	0.4			
Krypton-85 (^{85}Kr)	10.7 years	β^-	0.173[a]	0.43	γ	0.514	0.43
			0.687[a]	99.57			
Lead-201 (^{201}Pb)	9.4 hours	e^A,e^c	(*)	(*)	X	0.070 - 0.073	68
						0.083	19
					γ	0.130	1.3
						0.331	79
						0.361	9.9
						0.406	2.0
						0.585	3.5
						0.692	2.7
						0.767	3.3
						0.826	2.3
						0.908	6
						0.946	7.5
Lead-203 (^{203}Pb)	2.17 days	e_A	0.008	54	X	0.010	36
			0.055	3		0.070 - 0.073	68
		e_c	0.194	13	γ	0.083	19
			0.316	0.5		0.279	80
						0.401	3.4
						0.681	0.7
Mercury-197m (^{197m}Hg)	23.8 hours	e_A	0.005 - 0.014	75	X	0.008 - 0.015	44
		e_A + e_c	0.050 - 0.080	36		0.067 - 0.083	40.5
		e_c	0.116 - 0.130	50	γ	0.130	0.23
			0.150	51		0.134	34
			0.161	21		0.164	0.32
			0.198	1.6		0.279	5.1
Mercury-197 (^{197}Hg)	64.1 Hours	e_A	0.005 - 0.014	91	X	0.008 - 0.017	52
		e_A + e_c	0.050 - 0.090	84		0.067 - 0.080	73
					γ	0.077	18.9
						0.191	0.57
						0.269	0.05
Mercury-203 (^{203}Hg)	46.8 days	e_A	0.005 - 0.015	9.3	X	0.009 - 0.015	5.4
			0.055 - 0.085	0.44		0.071 - 0.085	13
		e_c	0.194	13.4	γ	0.270	81.4
			0.264	3.9			
			0.276	1.2			
			0.212	100			

Table of physical characteristics of radionuclides mentioned in the Pharmacopoeia

Radionuclide	Half-life	Electron emission Type	Energy (MeV)	Intensity (per cent)	Photon emission Type	Energy (MeV)	Intensity (per cent)
Molybdenum-99 (^{99}Mo) in equilibrium with technetium-99m (^{99m}Tc)	66.0 hours	$e_A + e_c$	0.002	110	X	0.002	0.7
		e_c	0.015 - 0.020	7	γ	0.018 - 0.021	14
			0.119 - 0.121	9.5		0.140	91
			0.137 - 0.140	1.5		0.181	6
		β^-	0.436[a]	16.6		0.366	1.2
			0.848[a]	1.2		0.740	12.3
			1.214[a]	82		0.778	4.4
						0.823	0.13
Phosphorus-32 (^{32}P)	14.3 days	β^-	1.71[a]	100			
Ruthenium-103 (^{103}Ru) in equilibrium with Rhodium-103m (^{103m}Rh)	39.3 days (^{103m}Rh:56.1 min)	e_A	0.002	77	X	0.003	4
		$e_A + e_c$	0.017	11		0.020 - 0.023	7.7
		e_c	0.036 - 0.039	91	γ	0.053	0.4
						0.295	0.3
						0.444	0.4
						0.497	89.7
						0.557	0.8
		β^-	0.112	6.4		0.610	5.6
			0.225	87			
			0.722	6			
Selenium-75 (^{75}Se)	118.5 days	e_A	0.001	136	X	0.001	1
			0.009	44		0.011	57
		e_c	0.013	4.3		0.066	1
			0.023	1.0	γ	0.097	3.5
			0.054	0.4		0.121	17.7
			0.085	2.7		0.136	61
			0.095	0.4		0.199	1.5
			0.109	0.7		0.265	59.4
			0.124	1.6		0.280	25.2
			0.134	0.2		0.304	1.3
			0.253	0.4		0.401	11.3
			0.268	0.2			
Strontium-89 (^{89}Sr)	50.5 days	β^-	1.492[a]	100			
Strontium-90 (^{90}Sr)	29.1 years	β^-	0.546[a]	100			
Strontium-90 /Yttrium-90 (^{90}Sr/^{90}Y)	29.1 years (^{90}Y : 64.0 h)	β^-	0.546[a]	100			
			2.284[a]	100			
Technetium-99m (^{99m}Tc)	6.02 hours	$e_A + e_c$	0.002	110	X	0.002	0.5
		e_A	0.015 - 0.020	2.1		0.018 - 0.021	7.2
			0.119 - 0.121	9.5			
			0.137 - 0.140	1.5	γ	0.140	89.3
Technetium-99 (^{99}Tc)	2.14×10^5 years	β^-	0.29[a]	100			

Table of physical characteristics of radionuclides mentioned in the Pharmacopoeia

Radionuclide	Half-life	Electron emission Type	Energy (MeV)	Intensity (per cent)	Photon emission Type	Energy (MeV)	Intensity (per cent)
Thallium-200 (^{200}Tl)	1.09 days	e_A	(*)	(*)	X	0.069 - 0.070	66
					γ	0.080 - 0.083	19
						0.368	88.4
						0.579	14
						0.661	2.3
						0.828	11
						0.886	2
						1.206	30.0
						1.226	3.4
						1.274	3.3
						1.363	3.5
						1.515	4.1
Thallium-201 (^{201}Tl)	3.05 days	e_A	0.005 - 0.015	77	X	0.008 - 0.015	45
		e_c	0.015 - 0.020	19	γ	0.031 - 0.032	0.6
		$e_A + e_c$	0.027 - 0.032	6.4	X	0.069 - 0.071	75
			0.052 - 0.085	27.8		0.079 - 0.083	21
		e_c	0.120 - 0.123	1.3	γ	0.135	2.8
			0.132 - 0.135	0.4		0.166 - 0.167	10.7
			0.153 - 0.155	2.8			
			0.164 - 0.167	0.8			
Thallium-202 (^{202}Tl)	12.2 days	e_A	(*)	(*)	X	0.069 - 0.071	65
					γ	0.080 - 0.083	19
						0.440	95
Tritium (^{3}H)	12.3 years	$β^-$	0.019[a]	100			
Xenon-131m (^{131m}Xe)	11.9 days	$e_A e_c$	0.003	26	X	0.004	3
			0.025	6.8			
			0.129	61		0.029 - 0.034	54
			0.158	28.6	γ	0.164	1.92
			0.163	8.2			
Xenon-133 (^{133}Xe)	5.29 days	e_A	0.004	50	X	0.004	6
		e_c	0.025	5			
		$β^-$	0.045	52		0.030 - 0.035	47
			0.075	8.5	γ	0.081	37
			0.266[a]	0.7			
			0.346[a]	99.3			
Xenon-133m (^{133m}Xe)	2.19 days	e_A	0.004	70	X	0.004	8
			0.025	7.1			
		e_c	0.198	64		0.030 - 0.035	57
			0.228	21	γ	0.233	10.3
			0.232	5			
Zinc-65 (^{65}Zn)	243.9 days	e_A	0.001	127	X	0.001	0.8
		$β^-$	0.007 - 0.010	48		0.008 - 0.010	38.7
			0.330[a]	1.46	γ	0.511	2.92[b]
						1.115	50.75

[a] Maximum energy of the beta spectrum
[b] Maximum intensity corresponding to a total annihilation in the source
e_A = Aiger electrons
e_c = Conversion electrons
(*) No precise values are known for the moment.

Iodinated[125I] Albumin Injection

Iodinated[125I] Human Albumin Injection

Definition Iodinated[125I] Albumin Injection is a sterile solution of albumin that has been iodinated with iodine-125 and subsequently freed from iodide[125I] ion, made isotonic with blood by the addition of Sodium Chloride and containing a suitable antimicrobial preservative such as Benzyl Alcohol. It is prepared from Albumin Solution and contains not less than 1% of protein. Before addition of carrier albumin, if this is added, the albumin is uniformly iodinated to an extent that does not exceed the equivalent of one atom of iodine for each molecule of albumin. The content of iodine-125 activity is not less than 85.0% and not more than 115.0% of the content of iodine-125 stated on the label at the date stated on the label.

The injection complies with the requirements stated under Radiopharmaceutical Preparations and with the following requirements.

Characteristics A clear, colourless or faintly yellow solution.

Iodine-125 has a half-life of 60.1 days and emits gamma-radiation and X-rays.

Identification

A. The gamma-ray and X-ray spectrum, measured in a suitable instrument, does not differ significantly from that of a standardised iodine-125 solution other than any differences attributable to the presence of iodine-126. The most prominent gamma-photon of iodine-125 has an energy of 0.027 MeV (corresponding to the K X-ray of tellurium). The presence of iodine-126 is shown by major gamma-photons of 0.388 and 0.666 MeV. Iodine-126 has a half-life of 13.0 days.

B. When examined in an ultracentrifuge, it has the sedimentation coefficient of normal human albumin.

Acidity or alkalinity pH, 6.5 to 8.5, Appendix V L.

Radionuclidic purity Measure the gamma-ray and X-ray spectrum in a suitable instrument by comparison with standardised solutions of iodine-125 and caesium-137. Determine the relative amounts of iodine-125 and iodine-126 present on the assumption that the 0.666 MeV gamma-photon of iodine-126 is emitted in 33% of disintegrations and that the 0.66 MeV gamma-photon of caesium-137 is emitted in 86% of disintegrations. Not more than 1.0% of the total activity is due to iodine-126 at the date stated on the label.

Radiochemical purity Submit a volume containing not less than 0.5 mg of albumin to electrophoresis on a strip of filter paper (30 cm × 5 cm) at 500 volts for 1 hour in a solution containing 5 g of *barbitone sodium*, 3.25 g of *sodium acetate*, 4 g of *sodium octanoate* and 34.2 ml of 0.1M *hydrochloric acid* in sufficient *water* to produce 100 ml. Allow the paper to dry and determine the area of radioactivity using a suitable instrument. Not less than 95% of the activity on the paper occurs in a position corresponding to that which would be occupied by treating normal human albumin at the same time and in the same manner.

Protein

A. To 1 ml in a 75-ml boiling tube add 1 ml of *saline solution* and carry out the method for the *determination of protein in blood products*, Appendix VIII H, Method VI, beginning at the words 'add 2 ml ...' and ending at the words '... as indicator' and taking care to absorb liberated iodine-125. Each ml of 0.02M *hydrochloric acid VS* is equivalent to 1.75 mg of protein.

B. Carry out the test for Radiochemical purity using a volume containing 0.2 to 0.5 mg of albumin but using a strip of cellulose acetate (30 cm × 5 cm) in place of the paper. Dry the strip at about 80° to 100° for 15 minutes and stain for 15 minutes in a solution of 0.2 g of *naphthalene black 12B* in a mixture of 10 ml of *glacial acetic acid* and 90 ml of *methanol*. Wash the strip in a mixture of 12 ml of *glacial acetic acid* and 88 ml of *methanol* until the background is white and then wash for 10 minutes in 1M *acetic acid* and finally in *water*. Dry the strip between blotting paper pressed between glass plates. The distribution of the stained protein does not deviate significantly from that obtained by treating normal human albumin at the same time and in the same manner.

Pyrogens Complies with the *test for pyrogens*, Appendix XIV D. Use per kg of the rabbit's weight either 0.1 ml or a quantity corresponding to 370 kBq at the date stated on the label, whichever is the less.

Assay Determine the activity using suitable counting equipment by comparison with a standardised iodine-125 solution or by measurement in an instrument calibrated with the aid of such a solution. An instrument incorporating a scintillation detector, such as a thin sodium iodide crystal, should be employed and the instrument should be set so that the contribution from iodine-126 is minimal.

Standardised iodine-125 solutions available from Amersham International plc, Amersham, HP7 9LL, England, are suitable.

Storage Iodinated[125I] Albumin Injection should be stored at a temperature of 2° to 8°.

Labelling The label states the concentration of albumin.

Chromium[51Cr] Edetate Injection

Chromium[51Cr] Edetate Injection complies with the requirements of the 3rd edition of the European Pharmacopoeia [0266]. These requirements are reproduced after the heading 'Definition' below.

Ph Eur

DEFINITION

Chromium (51Cr) edetate injection is a sterile solution containing chromium-51 in the form of a complex of chromium(III) with ethylenediaminetetra-acetic acid, the latter being present in excess. It may be made isotonic by the addition of sodium chloride and may contain a suitable antimicrobial preservative such as benzyl alcohol. Chromium-51 is a radioactive isotope of chromium and may be prepared by the neutron irradiation of chromium, either of natural isotopic composition or enriched in chromium-50. The injection contains not less than 90.0 per cent and not more than 110.0 per cent of the declared chromium-51 radioactivity at the date and hour stated on the label. Not less than 95 per cent of the radioactivity corresponds to chromium-51 in the form of chromium edetate. The injection contains a variable quantity of chromium (Cr) not exceeding 1 mg per millilitre.

CHARACTERS

A clear, violet solution.

Chromium-51 has a half-life of 27.7 days and emits gamma radiation.

IDENTIFICATION

A. Record the gamma-ray spectrum using a suitable instrument as described in the monograph on *Radiopharmaceutical preparations (125)*. The spectrum does not differ significantly from that of a standardised chromium-51 solution. Standardised chromium-51 solutions are available from laboratories recognised by the competent authority. The gamma photon has an energy of 0.320 MeV.

B. Examine the electrophoretogram obtained in the test for radiochemical purity. The distribution of radioactivity contributes to the identification of the preparation.

TESTS

pH (*2.2.3*). The pH of the solution is 3.5 to 6.5.

Radionuclidic purity Record the gamma-ray spectrum using a suitable instrument as described in the monograph on *Radiopharmaceutical preparations (125)*. The spectrum does not differ significantly from that of a standardised chromium-51 solution.

Radiochemical purity Examine by zone electrophoresis (*2.2.31*), using a paper strip as the support and a solution containing 0.2 g/l of *barbital sodium R* and 10 g/l of *sodium nitrate R* as the electrolyte solution. A paper with the following characteristics is suitable: mass per unit area 120 g/m^2; thickness 0.22 mm; capillary rise 105 mm to 115 mm per 30 min.

Apply to the paper 10 µl of the injection as a 3 mm band at a position 10 cm from the cathode. Apply an electric field of about 30 V per centimetre for 30 min using a stabilised current. [51Cr]chromium edetate moves about 5 cm towards the anode. [51Cr]Chromate moves about 10 cm towards the anode and [51Cr] chromic ion moves about 7 cm towards the cathode. Determine the distribution of the radioactivity using a suitable detector. Not less than 95 per cent of the total radioactivity is found in the band corresponding to [51Cr]chromium edetate.

Chromium Prepare a reference solution (1 mg per millilitre of Cr) as follows: dissolve 0.96 g of *chromic potassium sulphate R* and 2.87 g of *sodium edetate R* in 50 ml of *water R*, boil for 10 min, cool, adjust to pH 3.5 to 6.5 using *dilute sodium hydroxide solution R* and dilute to 100.0 ml with *water R*. Measure the absorbance (*2.2.25*) of the injection to be examined and the reference solution at the absorption maximum at 560 nm. The absorbance of the injection to be examined is not greater than that of the reference solution.

Sterility It complies with the test for sterility prescribed in the monograph on *Radiopharmaceutical preparations (125)*. The injection may be released for use before completion of the test.

RADIOACTIVITY

Measure the radioactivity as described in the monograph on *Radiopharmaceutical preparations (125)* using suitable equipment by comparison with a standardised chromium-51 solution or by measurement in an instrument calibrated with the aid of such a solution.

STORAGE

See *Radiopharmaceutical preparations (125)*.

LABELLING

See *Radiopharmaceutical preparations (125)*.

Ph Eur

Cyanocobalamin[^{57}Co] Capsules

Cyanocobalamin[^{57}Co] Capsules comply with the requirements of the 3rd edition of the European Pharmacopoeia [0710]. These requirements are reproduced after the heading 'Definition' below.

Ph Eur

DEFINITION

Cyanocobalamin (^{57}Co) capsules contain [^{57}*Co*]-α-(5,6-dimethylbenzimidazol-1-yl)cobamide cyanide and may contain suitable auxiliary substances. Cobalt-57 is a radioactive isotope of cobalt and may be produced by proton irradiation of nickel. Cyanocobalamin (^{57}Co) may be prepared by the growth of suitable micro-organisms on a medium containing (^{57}Co) cobaltous ion. Not less than 90 per cent of the cobalt-57 is in the form of cyanocobalamin. The capsules comply with the requirements for hard capsules in the monograph on *Capsules (16)*, unless otherwise justified and authorised.

CHARACTERS

Hard gelatin capsules.

Cobalt-57 has a half-life of 271 days and emits gamma radiation.

IDENTIFICATION

A. Record the gamma-ray spectrum using a suitable instrument as described in the monograph on *Radiopharmaceutical preparations (125)*. The spectrum does not differ significantly from that of a standardised cobalt-57 solution. Standardised cobalt-57 and cobalt-58 solutions are available from laboratories recognised by the competent authority. The most prominent gamma photon of cobalt-57 has an energy of 0.122 MeV.

B. Examine the chromatograms obtained in the test for radiochemical purity. The principal peak in the radiochromatogram obtained with the test solution has a retention time similar to that of the peak in the chromatogram obtained with the reference solution.

TESTS

Radionuclidic purity Record the gamma-ray spectrum as described in the monograph on *Radiopharmaceutical preparations (125)* using a suitable instrument calibrated with the aid of standardised cobalt-57 and cobalt-58 solutions. The spectrum does not differ significantly from that of the standardised cobalt-57 solution. Determine the relative amounts of cobalt-57, cobalt-56 and cobalt-58 present. Cobalt-56 has a half-life of 78 days and its presence is shown by gamma photons of energy 0.847 MeV. Cobalt-58 has a half-life of 70.8 days and its presence is shown by gamma photons of energy 0.811 MeV. Not more than 0.1 per cent of the total radioactivity is due to cobalt-56, cobalt-58 and other radionuclidic impurities.

Radiochemical purity Examine by liquid chromatography (*2.2.29*).

Test solution. Dissolve the contents of a capsule in 1.0 ml of *water R* and allow to stand for 10 min. Centrifuge at 2000 r/min for 10 min. Use the supernatant.

Reference solution. Dissolve 10 mg of *cyanocobalamin CRS* in the mobile phase and dilute to 100 ml with the mobile phase. Dilute 2 ml of the solution to 100 ml with the mobile phase. Use within 1 h.

The chromatographic procedure may be carried out using:
- a stainless steel column 0.25 m long and 4 mm in internal diameter packed with *octylsilyl silica gel for chromatography R* (5 µm),
- as mobile phase at a flow rate of 1.0 ml per minute a mixture prepared as follows: mix 26.5 volumes of *methanol R* and 73.5 volumes of a 10 g/l solution of *disodium hydrogen phosphate R*, adjust to pH 3.5 using *phosphoric acid R* and use within 2 days,
- a radioactivity detector adjusted for cobalt-57,
- as detector a spectrophotometer set at 361 nm,
- a loop injector.

Inject 100 µl of the test solution and record the chromatogram for three times the retention time of cyanocobalamin. Determine the peak areas and calculate the percentage of cobalt-57 present as cyanocobalamin. Inject 100 µl of the reference solution and record the chromatogram for 30 min.

Disintegration The capsules comply with the test for disintegration of tablets and capsules (*2.9.1*) except that one capsule is used in the test instead of six.

Uniformity of content Determine by measurement in a suitable counting assembly and under identical geometrical conditions the radioactivity of each of not less than ten capsules. Calculate the average radioactivity per capsule. The radioactivity of no capsule differs by more than 10 per cent from the average. The relative standard deviation is less than 3.5 per cent.

RADIOACTIVITY

The average radioactivity determined in the test for uniformity of content is not less than 90.0 per cent and not more than 110.0 per cent of the declared cobalt-57 radioactivity, at the date stated on the label.

STORAGE

Store in an airtight container, protected from light, at a temperature of 2°C to 8°C, in the conditions prescribed in the monograph on *Radiopharmaceutical preparations (125)*.

LABELLING

See *Radiopharmaceutical preparations (125)*.

Ph Eur

Cyanocobalamin[^{57}Co] Solution

Cyanocobalamin[^{57}Co] Solution complies with the requirements of the 3rd edition of the European Pharmacopoeia [0269]. These requirements are reproduced after the heading 'Definition' below.

Ph Eur

DEFINITION

Cyanocobalamin (^{57}Co) solution is a solution of [^{57}*Co*]-α-(5,6-dimethylbenzimidazol-1-yl)cobamide cyanide and may contain a stabiliser and an antimicrobial preservative. Cobalt-57 is a radioactive isotope of cobalt and may be produced by the irradiation of nickel with protons of suitable energy. Cyanocobalamin (^{57}Co) may be prepared by the growth of suitable micro-organisms on a medium containing (^{57}Co) cobaltous ion. The solution contains not less than 90.0 per cent and not more than 110.0 per cent of the declared cobalt-57 radioactivity at the date stated on the label. Not less than 90 per cent of the cobalt-57 is in the form of cyanocobalamin.

CHARACTERS

A clear, colourless or slightly pink solution. Cobalt-57 has a half-life of 271 days and emits gamma radiation.

IDENTIFICATION

A. Record the gamma-ray spectrum using a suitable instrument as described in the monograph on *Radiopharmaceutical preparations (125)*. The spectrum does not differ significantly from that of a standardised cobalt-57 solution. Standardised cobalt-57 and cobalt-58 solutions are available from laboratories recognised by the competent authority. The most prominent gamma photon of cobalt-57 has an energy of 0.122 MeV.

B. Examine the chromatograms obtained in the test for radiochemical purity. The principal peak in the radiochromatogram obtained with the solution to be examined has a retention time similar to that of the peak in the chromatogram obtained with the reference solution.

TESTS

pH (*2.2.3*). The pH of the solution is 4.0 to 6.0.

Radionuclidic purity Record the gamma-ray spectrum as described in the monograph on *Radiopharmaceutical preparations (125)* using a suitable instrument calibrated with the aid of standardised cobalt-57 and cobalt-58 solutions. The spectrum does not differ significantly from that of the standardised cobalt-57 solution. Determine the relative amounts of cobalt-57, cobalt-56 and cobalt-58 present. Cobalt-56 has a half-life of 78 days and its presence is shown by gamma photons of energy 0.847 MeV. Cobalt-58 has a half-life of 70.8 days and its presence is shown by gamma photons of energy 0.811 MeV. Not more than 0.1 per cent of the total radioactivity is due to cobalt-56, cobalt-58 and other radionuclidic impurities.

Radiochemical purity Examine by liquid chromatography (*2.2.29*).

Reference solution. Dissolve 10 mg of *cyanocobalamin CRS* in the mobile phase and dilute to 100 ml with the mobile phase. Dilute 2 ml of the solution to 100 ml with the mobile phase. Use within 1 h.

The chromatographic procedure may be carried out using:
- a stainless steel column 0.25 m long and 4 mm in internal diameter packed with *octylsilyl silica gel for chromatography R* (5 μm),
- as mobile phase at a flow rate of 1.0 ml per minute a mixture prepared as follows: mix 26.5 volumes of *methanol R* and 73.5 volumes of a 10 g/l solution of *disodium hydrogen phosphate R*, adjust to pH 3.5 using *phosphoric acid R* and use within 2 days,
- a radioactivity detector adjusted for cobalt-57,
- as detector a spectrophotometer set at 361 nm,
- a loop injector.

Inject 100 μl of the solution to be examined and record the chromatogram for three times the retention time of cyanocobalamin. Determine the peak areas and calculate the percentage of cobalt-57 present as cyanocobalamin. Inject 100 μl of the reference solution and record the chromatogram for 30 min.

RADIOACTIVITY

Measure the radioactivity as described in the monograph on *Radiopharmaceutical preparations (125)* using suitable counting equipment by comparison with a standardised cobalt-57 solution.

STORAGE

Store protected from light at a temperature of 2°C to 8°C under the conditions prescribed in the monograph on *Radiopharmaceutical preparations (125)*.

LABELLING

See *Radiopharmaceutical preparations (125)*.

Ph Eur

Cyanocobalamin[^{58}Co] Solution

Cyanocobalamin[^{58}Co] Solution complies with the requirements of the 3rd edition of the European Pharmacopoeia [0270]. These requirements are reproduced after the heading 'Definition' below.

Ph Eur

DEFINITION

Cyanocobalamin (^{58}Co) solution is a solution of [^{58}*Co*]-α-(5,6-dimethylbenzimidazol-1-yl)cobamide cyanide and may contain a stabiliser and an antimicrobial preservative. Cobalt-58 is a radioactive isotope of cobalt and may be produced by neutron irradiation of nickel. Cyanocobalamin (^{58}Co) may be prepared by the growth of suitable micro-organisms on a medium containing (^{58}Co) cobaltous ion. The solution contains not less than 90.0 per cent and not more than 110.0 per cent of the declared cobalt-58 radioactivity at the date stated on the label. Not less than 90 per cent of the cobalt-58 is in the form of cyanocobalamin.

CHARACTERS

A clear, colourless or slightly pink solution.

Cobalt-58 has a half-life of 70.8 days and emits beta (β^+) radiation and gamma radiation.

IDENTIFICATION

A. Record the gamma-ray spectrum using a suitable instrument as described in the monograph on *Radiopharmaceutical preparations (125)*. The spectrum does not differ significantly from that of a standardised cobalt-58 solution. Standardised cobalt-58, cobalt-57 and cobalt-60 solutions are available from laboratories recognised by the competent authority. The most prominent gamma photons of cobalt-58 have energies of 0.511 MeV (annihilation radiation) and 0.811 MeV.

B. Examine the chromatograms obtained in the test for radiochemical purity. The principal peak in the radiochromatogram obtained with the solution to be examined has a retention time similar to that of the peak in the chromatogram obtained with the reference solution.

TESTS

pH (*2.2.3*). The pH of the solution is 4.0 to 6.0.

Radionuclidic purity Record the gamma-ray spectrum as described in the monograph on *Radiopharmaceutical preparations (125)* using a suitable instrument having adequate resolution and calibrated with the aid of standardised cobalt-58, cobalt-57 and cobalt-60 solutions. The spectrum does not differ significantly from that of the standardised cobalt-58 solution. Determine the relative amounts of cobalt-58, cobalt-57 and cobalt-60 present. Cobalt-57 has a half-life of 271 days and its presence is shown by gamma photons of energy 0.122 MeV. Cobalt-60 has a half-life of 5.27 years and its presence is shown by gamma photons of energies 1.173 MeV and 1.332 MeV. Not more than 1 per cent of the total radioactivity is due to cobalt-60 and not more than 2 per cent of the total radioactivity is due to cobalt-57, cobalt-60 and other radionuclidic impurities.

Radiochemical purity Examine by liquid chromatography (*2.2.29*).

Reference solution. Dissolve 10 mg of *cyanocobalamin CRS* in the mobile phase and dilute to 100 ml with the mobile phase. Dilute 2 ml of the solution to 100 ml with the mobile phase. Use within 1 h.

The chromatographic procedure may be carried out using:
- a stainless steel column 0.25 m long and 4 mm in internal diameter packed with *octylsilyl silica gel for chromatography R* (5 μm),
- as mobile phase at a flow rate of 1.0 ml per minute a mixture prepared as follows: mix 26.5 volumes of *methanol R* and 73.5 volumes of a 10 g/l solution of *disodium hydrogen phosphate R*, adjust to pH 3.5 using *phosphoric acid R* and use within 2 days,
- a radioactivity detector adjusted for cobalt-58,
- as detector a spectrophotometer set at 361 nm,
- a loop injector.

Inject 100 μl of the solution to be examined and record the chromatogram for three times the retention time of cyanocobalamin. Determine the peak areas and calculate the percentage of cobalt-58 present as cyanocobalamin. Inject 100 μl of the reference solution and record the chromatogram for 30 min.

RADIOACTIVITY

Measure the radioactivity as described in the monograph on *Radiopharmaceutical preparations (125)* using suitable counting equipment by comparison with a standardised cobalt-58 solution or by measurement in an instrument calibrated with the aid of such a solution.

STORAGE

Store protected from light at a temperature of 2°C to 8°C under the conditions prescribed in the monograph on *Radiopharmaceutical preparations (125)*.

LABELLING

See *Radiopharmaceutical preparations (125)*.

Ph Eur

Ferric Citrate[^{59}Fe] Injection

Definition Ferric Citrate[^{59}Fe] Injection is a sterile solution containing iron[^{59}Fe] in the iron(III) state, 1.0% w/v of Sodium Citrate and sufficient Sodium Chloride to make the solution isotonic with blood. Iron-59 is a radioactive isotope of iron and may be prepared by the neutron irradiation of iron-58 sufficiently low in iron-54 to ensure that the final content of iron-55 is not more than 2% of the total activity; cobalt-60 is removed from the irradiated material during preparation. The content of iron-59 activity is not less than 90.0% and not more than 110.0% of the content of iron-59 stated on the label at the date stated on the label. The specific activity is not less than 37 MBq of iron-59 per mg of iron at the date stated on the label.

The injection complies with the requirements stated under Radiopharmaceutical Preparations and with the following requirements.

Characteristics A clear, colourless or faintly orange brown solution.

Iron-59 has a half-life of 44.6 days and emits gamma-radiation.

Identification

A. The gamma-ray spectrum, measured in a suitable instrument, does not differ significantly from that of a standardised iron-59 solution. The most prominent gamma-photons have energies of 1.10 and 1.29 MeV.

B. Boil a suitable quantity with an excess of *mercury(II) sulphate solution*, filter if necessary, boil the filtrate and add 0.15 ml of *dilute potassium permanganate solution*. The colour is discharged and a white precipitate is produced.

Acidity or alkalinity pH, 6.0 to 8.0, Appendix V L.

Radionuclidic purity The gamma-ray spectrum, measured in a suitable instrument, does not differ significantly from that of a standardised iron-59 solution. Iron-55 is not normally detected by an instrument suitable for this measurement.

Total iron Complies with the *limit test for iron*, Appendix VII, using a volume equivalent to 370 kBq of iron-59 at the date stated on the label.

Assay Determine the activity using suitable counting equipment by comparison with a standardised iron-59 solution or by measurement in an instrument calibrated with the aid of such a solution.

Labelling The label states the content of total iron.

Standardised iron-59 solutions available from Amersham International plc, Amersham, HP7 9LL, United Kingdom, are suitable.

Gallium[^{67}Ga] Citrate Injection

Gallium[^{67}Ga] Citrate Injection complies with the requirements of the 3rd edition of the European Pharmacopoeia [0555]. These requirements are reproduced after the heading 'Definition' below.

Ph Eur

DEFINITION

Gallium(^{67}Ga) citrate injection is a sterile solution of gallium-67 in the form of gallium citrate. It may be made isotonic by the addition of sodium chloride and sodium citrate and may contain a suitable antimicrobial preservative such as benzyl alcohol. Gallium-67 is a radioactive isotope of gallium and may be obtained by the irradiation, with protons of suitable energy, of zinc which may be enriched in zinc-68. Gallium-67 may be separated from zinc by solvent extraction or column chromatography. The injection contains not less than 90.0 per cent and not more than 110.0 per cent of the declared gallium-67 radioactivity at the date and hour stated on the label. Not more than 0.2 per cent of the total radioactivity is due to gallium-66.

CHARACTERS

A clear, colourless solution.

Gallium-67 has a half-life of 3.26 days and emits gamma radiation.

IDENTIFICATION

A. Record the gamma-ray spectrum using a suitable instrument as described in the monograph on *Radiopharmaceutical preparations (125)*. The spectrum does not differ significantly from that of a standardised gallium-67 solution when measured either by direct comparison or by use of an instrument calibrated with the aid of such a solution. Standardised gallium-67 solutions are available from laboratories recognised by the competent authority. The most prominent gamma photons have energies of 0.093 MeV, 0.185 MeV and 0.300 MeV.

B. To 0.2 ml of the injection to be examined add 0.2 ml of a solution containing 1 g/l of *ferric chloride R* and 0.1 per cent *V/V* of *hydrochloric acid R* and mix. Compare the colour with that of a solution containing 9 g/l of *benzyl alcohol R* and 7 g/l of *sodium chloride R* treated in the same manner. A yellow colour develops in the test solution only.

TESTS

pH (*2.2.3*). The pH of the injection is 5.0 to 8.0.

Radionuclidic purity Record the gamma-ray spectrum using a suitable instrument as described in the monograph on *Radiopharmaceutical preparations (125)*. The spectrum does not differ significantly from that of a standardised gallium-67 solution, apart from any differences attributable to the presence of gallium-66. Gallium-66 has a half-life of 9.4 h and its most prominent gamma photon has an energy of 1.039 MeV. Not more than 0.2 per cent of the total radioactivity is due to gallium-66.

Zinc To 0.1 ml of the injection to be examined add 0.9 ml of *water R*, 5 ml of *acetate buffer solution pH 4.7 R*, 1 ml of a 250 g/l solution of *sodium thiosulphate R* and 5.0 ml of a dithizone solution prepared as follows: dissolve 10 mg of *dithizone R* in 100 ml of *methyl ethyl ketone R* allow to stand for 5 min, filter and immediately before use dilute the solution to ten times its volume with *methyl ethyl ketone R*. Shake vigorously for 2 min and separate the organic layer. Measure the absorbance (*2.2.25*) of the organic layer at 530 nm, using the organic layer of a blank solution as the compensation liquid. The absorbance is not greater than that of the organic layer obtained with 0.1 ml of *zinc standard solution (5 ppm Zn) R* treated in the same manner.

Sterility It complies with the test for sterility prescribed in the monograph on *Radiopharmaceutical preparations (125)*. The injection may be released for use before completion of the test.

RADIOACTIVITY

Measure the radioactivity as described in the monograph on *Radiopharmaceutical preparations (125)* using suitable counting equipment by comparison with a standardised gallium-67 solution or by measurement in an instrument calibrated with the aid of such a solution.

STORAGE

See *Radiopharmaceutical preparations (125)*.

LABELLING

See *Radiopharmaceutical preparations (125)*.

Ph Eur

Indium[111In] Chloride Solution

Indium[111In] Chloride Solution complies with the requirements of the 3rd edition of the European Pharmacopoeia [1227]. These requirements are reproduced after the heading 'Definition' below.

Ph Eur

DEFINITION

Indium(^{111}In) chloride solution is a sterile solution of indium-111 as the chloride in aqueous hydrochloric acid containing no additives. Indium-111 is a radioactive isotope of indium and may be produced by the irradiation of cadmium with protons of suitable energy. The solution contains not less than 90.0 per cent and not more than 110.0 per cent of the declared indium-111 radioactivity at the date and hour stated on the label. Not more than 0.25 per cent of the total radioactivity is due to radionuclides other than indium-111. Not less than 95 per cent of the radioactivity corresponds to indium-111 in the form of ionic indium(III). The method of preparation is such that no carrier is added and the specific radioactivity is not less than 1.85 GBq of indium-111 per microgram of indium.

CHARACTERS

A clear, colourless solution.

Indium-111 has a half-life of 2.8 days and emits gamma radiation and X-rays.

IDENTIFICATION

A. *Carry out the test after allowing sufficient time for short-lived impurities such as indium-110m to decay.* Record the gamma-ray and X-ray spectrum using a suitable instrument as described in the monograph on *Radiopharmaceutical preparations (125)*. The spectrum does not differ significantly from that of a standardised indium-111 solution apart from any differences due to the presence of indium-114m, when measured either by direct comparison or by using an instrument calibrated with the aid of such a solution. Standardised indium-111 and indium-114m solutions are available from laboratories recognised by the competent authority. The most prominent gamma photons of indium-111 have energies of 0.171 MeV and 0.245 MeV.

B. To 100 ml of *silver nitrate solution R2* add 50 ml of the solution. A white precipitate is formed.

C. It complies with the test for pH (see Tests).

D. Examine the chromatogram obtained in the test for radiochemical purity. The principal peak has an R_f value of 0.5 to 0.8.

TESTS

pH (*2.2.3*). The pH of the solution is 1.0 to 2.0.

Radionuclidic purity Record the gamma-ray and X-ray spectrum using a suitable instrument as described in the monograph on *Radiopharmaceutical preparations (125)*. The spectrum does not differ significantly from that of a standardised solution of indium-111 apart from any differences due to the presence of indium-114m.

Indium-114m *Carry out the test after allowing sufficient time for short-lived impurities such as indium-110m to decay.* Take a volume equivalent to 30 MBq and record the gamma-ray spectrum using a suitable detector with a shield of lead, 6 mm thick, placed between the sample and the detector. The response in the region corresponding to the 0.558 MeV photon and the 0.725 MeV photon of indium-114m does not exceed that obtained using 75 kBq of a standardised solution of indium-114m (0.25 per cent) measured under the same conditions, when all measurements are calculated with reference to the date and hour of administration. Standardised indium-111 and indium-114m solutions are available from laboratories recognised by the competent authority.

Radiochemical purity Examine by thin-layer chromatography (*2.2.27*) as described in the monograph on *Radiopharmaceutical preparations (125)* using silica gel as the coating substance on a glass-fibre sheet.

Apply to the plate 5 µl of the solution to be examined. Develop immediately over a path of 15 cm using a 9.0 g/l solution of *sodium chloride R* adjusted to pH 2.3 ± 0.05 with *dilute hydrochloric acid R*. Allow the plate to dry in a current of cold air. Determine the distribution of radioactivity using a suitable detector. Indium-111 chloride migrates with an R_f value of 0.5 to 0.8. Not less than 95 per cent of the total radioactivity of the chromatogram corresponds to indium-111 chloride.

Cadmium Not more than 0.40 mg/ml, determined by electrothermal atomic absorption spectrometry (*Method I, 2.2.23*).

Test solution. Dilute 0.05 ml of the solution to be examined to a suitable volume with a suitable concentration of *hydrochloric acid R*.

Reference solutions. Prepare the reference solutions using *cadmium standard solution (0.1 per cent Cd) R*, diluted as necessary with the same concentration of *hydrochloric acid R* as in the solution to be examined.

Measure the absorbance at 228.8 nm using a cadmium hollow-cathode lamp as source of radiation.

Copper Not more than 0.15 ml/ml, determined by electrothermal atomic absorption spectrometry (*Method I, 2.2.23*).

Test solution. Dilute 0.1 ml the solution to be examined to a suitable volume with a suitable concentration of *hydrochloric acid R*.

Reference solutions. Prepare the reference solutions using *copper standard solution (0.1 per cent) R* diluted as necessary with the same concentration of *hydrochloric acid R* as the solution to be examined.

Measure the absorbance at 324.8 nm using a copper hollow-cathode lamp as source of radiation.

Iron Not more than 0.60 mg/ml, determined by electrothermal atomic absorption spectrometry (*Method I, 2.2.23*).

Test solution. Dilute 0.1 ml of the solution to be examined to a suitable volume with a suitable concentration of *hydrochloric acid R*.

Reference solutions. Prepare the reference solutions using *iron standard solution (0.1 per cent Fe) R* diluted as necessary with the same concentration of *hydrochloric acid R* as the solution to be examined.

Measure the absorbance at 248.3 nm using an iron hollow-cathode lamp as source of radiation.

Sterility It complies with the test for sterility prescribed in the monograph on *Radiopharmaceutical preparations (125)*. The solution may be released for use before completion of the test.

RADIOACTIVITY

Measure the radioactivity as described in the monograph on *Radiopharmaceutical preparations (125)* using suitable counting equipment by comparison with a standardised indium-111 solution or by measurement in an instrument calibrated with the aid of such a solution.

STORAGE

See *Radiopharmaceutical preparations (125)*.

LABELLING

See *Radiopharmaceutical preparations (125)*.

Ph Eur

Indium[111In] Oxine Solution

$C_{27}H_{18}[^{111}In]N_3O_3$ 547.2

Indium [111In] Oxine Solution complies with the requirements of the 3rd edition of the European Pharmacopoeia [1109]. These requirements are reproduced after the heading 'Definition' below.

Ph Eur

DEFINITION

Indium (^{111}In) oxine solution is a sterile solution of indium-111 in the form of a complex with 8-hydroxyquinoline. It may contain suitable surface active agents and may be made iso- tonic by the addition of sodium chloride and a suitable buffer. Indium-111 is a radioactive isotope of indium and may be produced by the irradiation of cadmium with protons of suitable energy. The solution contains not less than 90.0 per cent and not more than 110.0 per cent of the declared indium-111 radioactivity at the date and hour stated on the label. Not more than 0.25 per cent of the total radioactivity is due to radionuclides other than indium-111. Not less than 90 per cent of the radioactivity corresponds to indium-111 complexed with oxine. The method of preparation is such that no carrier is added and the specific radioactivity is not less than 1.85 GBq of indium-111 per microgram of indium.

CHARACTERS

A clear, colourless solution.

Indium-111 has a half-life of 2.8 days and emits gamma radiation and X-rays.

IDENTIFICATION

A. *Carry out the test after allowing sufficient time for short-lived impurities such as indium-110m to decay.* Record the gamma-ray and X-ray spectrum using a suitable instrument as described in the monograph on *Radiopharmaceutical preparations (125)*. The spectrum does not differ significantly from that of a standardised indium-111 solution apart from any differences due to the presence of indium-114m, when measured either by direct comparison or by using an instrument calibrated with the aid of such a solution. Standardised indium-111 and indium-114m solutions are available from laboratories recognised by the competent authority. The most prominent gamma photons of indium-111 have energies of 0.171 MeV and 0.245 MeV.

B. Place 5 mg to 10 mg of *magnesium oxide R* in a glass container of approximately 20 mm in internal diameter. Add 20 µl of the solution to be examined. Examine in ultraviolet light at 365 nm. Bright yellow fluorescence is produced.

C. The distribution of radioactivity between the organic and aqueous phases in the test for radiochemical purity contributes to the identification of the preparation.

TESTS

pH (*2.2.3*). The pH of the solution is 6.0 to 7.5.

Radionuclidic purity Record the gamma-ray and X-ray spectrum using a suitable instrument as described in the monograph on *Radiopharmaceutical preparations (125)*. The spectrum does not differ significantly from that of a standardised solution of indium-111, apart from any differences due to the presence of indium-114m.

Indium-114m *Carry out the test after allowing sufficient time for short-lived impurities such as indium-110m to decay.* Take a volume equivalent to 30 MBq and record the gamma-ray spectrum using a suitable detector with a shield of lead, 6 mm thick, placed between the sample and the detector. The response in the region corresponding to the 0.558 MeV photon and the 0.725 MeV photon of indium-114m does not exceed that obtained using 75 kBq of a standardised solution of indium-114m (0.25 per cent) measured under the same conditions, when all measurements are calculated with reference to the date and hour of administration. (It should be noted that indium (^{111}In) oxine solution is a precursor used in the *in vitro* labelling of white blood cells or platelets prior to their re-injection into the patient. It is not intended for direct administration.) Standardised indium-111 and indium-114m solutions are available from laboratories recognised by the competent authority.

Radiochemical purity To a silanised separating funnel containing 3 ml of a 9 g/l solution of *sodium chloride R* add 100 µl of the solution to be examined and mix. Add 6 ml of *octanol R* and shake vigorously. Allow the phases to separate and then run the lower layer into a suitable vial for counting. Allow the upper layer to drain completely into a similar vial. Add 1 ml of *octanol R* to the funnel, shake vigorously and drain into the vial containing the organic fraction. Add 5 ml of *dilute hydrochloric acid R* to the funnel, shake vigorously and drain these rinsings into a third vial. Seal each vial and, using a suitable instrument as described in the monograph on *Radiopharmaceutical preparations (125)*, measure the radioactivity in each. Calculate the radiochemical purity by expressing the radioactivity of the indium-111 oxine complex, found in the organic phase, as a percentage of the radioactivity measured in the three solutions. Not less than 90 per cent of the radioactivity corresponds to indium-111 complexed with oxine.

Sterility It complies with the test for sterility prescribed in the monograph on *Radiopharmaceutical preparations (125)*. The solution may be released for use before completion of the test.

RADIOACTIVITY

Measure the radioactivity as described in the monograph on *Radiopharmaceutical preparations* (*125*) using suitable counting equipment by comparison with a standardised indium-111 solution or by measurement in an instrument calibrated with the aid of such a solution.

STORAGE

See *Radiopharmaceutical preparations (125)*.

LABELLING

See *Radiopharmaceutical preparations (125)*.

Ph Eur

Indium[111In] Pentetate Injection

Indium [111In] Pentetate Injection complies with the requirements of the 3rd edition of the European Pharmacopoeia [0670]. These requirements are reproduced after the heading 'Definition' below.

Ph Eur

DEFINITION

Indium (^{111}In) pentetate injection is a sterile and apyrogenic solution containing indium-111 in the form of indium diethylenetriaminepenta-acetate. It may contain calcium and may be made isotonic by the addition of sodium chloride and a suitable buffer. Indium-111 is a radioactive isotope of indium which may be obtained by proton irradiation, of appropriate energy, of cadmium which may be enriched with cadmium-111 or cadmium-112. The injection contains not less than 90 per cent and not more than 110 per cent of the declared indium-111 radioactivity at the date and hour stated on the label. The radioactivity due to indium-114m is not greater than 0.2 per cent of the total radioactivity at the date and hour of administration. Not less than 95 per cent of the radioactivity corresponds to indium-111 complexed with pentetate.

CHARACTERS

A clear, colourless solution.

Indium-111 has a half-life of 2.8 days and emits gamma radiation and X-rays.

IDENTIFICATION

A. Record the gamma-ray and X-ray spectrum using a suitable instrument as described in the monograph on *Radiopharmaceutical preparations (125)*. The spectrum does not differ significantly from that of a standardised indium-111 solution apart from any differences due to the presence of indium-114m, when measured either by direct comparison or by using an instrument calibrated with the aid of such a solution. Standardised indium-111 and indium-114m solutions are available from laboratories recognised by the competent authority. The most prominent gamma photons of indium-111 have energies of 0.171 MeV and 0.245 MeV.

B. Examine the chromatogram obtained in the test for radiochemical purity. The distribution of radioactivity contributes to the identification of the preparation.

TESTS

pH (*2.2.3*). The pH of the injection is 7.0 to 8.0.

Radionuclidic purity Record the gamma-ray and X-ray spectrum using a suitable instrument as described in the monograph on *Radiopharmaceutical preparations (125)*. The spectrum does not differ significantly from that of a standardised solution of indium-111 apart from any differences due to the presence of indium-114m.

Indium-114m Retain a sample of the injection to be examined for a sufficient time to allow the indium-111 radioactivity to decay to a sufficiently low level to permit the detection of radionuclidic impurities. Record the gamma-ray spectrum of the decayed material in a suitable instrument calibrated with the aid of a standardised indium-114m solution. Indium-114m has a half-life of 49.5 days and its most prominent gamma photon has an energy of 0.190 MeV. The radioactivity due to indium-114m is not greater than 0.2 per cent of the total radioactivity at the date and hour of administration.

Radiochemical purity Examine by thin-layer chromatography (*2.2.27*) as described in the monograph on *Radiopharmaceutical preparations (125)*, using silica gel as the coating substance on a glass-fibre sheet. Heat the plate at 110°C for 10 min. Use a plate such that during development the mobile phase migrates over a distance of 10 cm to 15 cm in about 10 min.

Apply to the plate 5 µl to 10 µl of the injection to be examined and allow to dry. Develop over a path of 10 cm to 15 cm using a 9 g/l solution of *sodium chloride R*. Allow the plate to dry in air. Determine the distribution of radioactivity using a suitable detector. Indium pentetate complex migrates near to the solvent front. The radioactivity of the spot corresponding to indium pentetate complex represents not less than 95 per cent of the total radioactivity of the chromatogram.

Cadmium Not more than 5 µg of Cd per millilitre, determined by atomic absorption spectrometry (*Method II, 2.2.23*).

Test solution. Mix 0.1 ml of the injection to be examined with 0.9 ml of a mixture of 1 volume of *hydrochloric acid R* and 99 volumes of *water R.*

Reference solutions. Prepare the reference solutions using *cadmium standard solution (0.1 per cent Cd) R* and diluting with a mixture of 1 volume of *hydrochloric acid R* and 99 volumes of *water R.*

Measure the absorbance at 228.8 nm using a cadmium hollow-cathode lamp as source of radiation and an air-acetylene flame.

Uncomplexed diethylenetriaminepenta-acetic acid In a micro test-tube, mix 100 µl of the injection to be examined with 100 µl of a freshly prepared 1 g/l solution of *hydroxynaphthol blue, sodium salt R* in *1M sodium hydroxide.* Add 50 µl of a 0.15 g/l solution of *calcium chloride R.* The solution remains pinkish-violet or changes from blue to pinkish-violet (0.4 mg per millilitre).

Sterility It complies with the test for sterility prescribed in the monograph on *Radiopharmaceutical preparations (125).* The injection may be released for use before completion of the test.

Bacterial endotoxins (*2.6.14*). Not more than 14/*V* I.U. of endotoxin per millilitre, *V* being the maximum recommended dose in millilitres.

RADIOACTIVITY

Measure the radioactivity as described in the monograph on *Radiopharmaceutical preparations (125)* using suitable counting equipment by comparison with a standardised indium-111 solution or by measurement in an instrument calibrated with the aid of such a solution.

STORAGE

See *Radiopharmaceutical preparations (125).*

LABELLING

See *Radiopharmaceutical preparations (125).*

Ph Eur

Iobenguane[123I] Injection

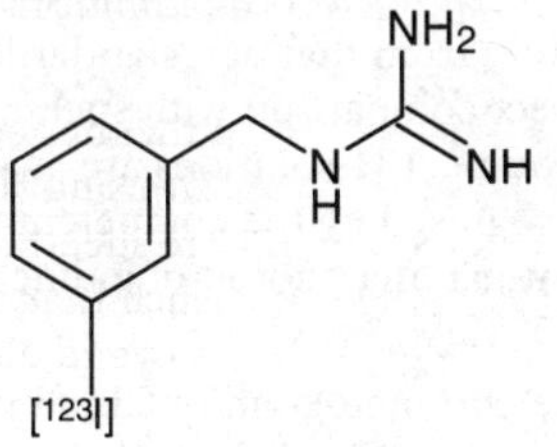

$C_8H_{10}[^{123}I]N_3$

Iobenguane [123I] Injection complies with the requirements of the 3rd edition of the European Pharmacopoeia [1113]. These requirements are reproduced after the heading 'Definition' below.

Ph Eur

DEFINITION

Iobenguane (^{123}I) injection is a sterile, bacterial-endotoxin free solution of (3-[^{123}I]iodobenzyl)guanidine. It may contain a suitable buffer, a suitable labelling catalyst such as ionic copper, a suitable labelling stabiliser such as ascorbic acid and antimicrobial preservatives. Iodine-123 is a radioactive isotope of iodine and may be obtained by proton irradiation of xenon enriched in xenon-124 (not less than 98 per cent) followed by the decay of caesium-123 formed via xenon-123. The injection contains not less than 90.0 per cent and not more than 110.0 per cent of the declared iodine-123 radioactivity at the date and hour stated on the label. Not less than 95 per cent of the radioactivity corresponds to iodine-123 in the form of iobenguane. The specific radioactivity is not less than 10 GBq of iodine-123 per gram of iobenguane base. Not more than 0.35 per cent of the total radioactivity is due to radionuclides other than iodine-123.

CHARACTERS

A clear, colourless or slightly yellow solution.

Iodine-123 has a half-life of 13.2 h and emits gamma radiation and X-rays.

IDENTIFICATION

A. Record the gamma-ray and X-ray spectrum using a suitable instrument as described in the monograph on *Radiopharmaceutical preparations (125).* The spectrum does not differ significantly from that of a standardised iodine-123 solution apart from any differences attributable to the presence of iodine-125, tellurium-121 and other radionuclidic impurities. The most prominent gamma photon of iodine-123 has an energy of 0.159 MeV. Iodine-125 has a half-life of 59.4 days and emits an X-ray of 0.027 MeV and a photon of 0.035 MeV. Tellurium-121 has a half-life of 19.2 days and the most prominent photons have energies of 0.507 MeV and 0.573 MeV. Standardised iodine-123, iodine-125 and tellurium-121 solutions are available from laboratories recognised by the competent authority.

B. Examine the chromatogram obtained in the test for radiochemical purity. The distribution of the radioactivity contributes to the identification of the preparation.

TESTS

pH (*2.2.3*). The pH of the solution is 3.5 to 8.0.

Radionuclidic purity Record the gamma-ray spectrum using a suitable instrument as described in the monograph on *Radiopharmaceutical preparations (125).* Determine the relative amounts of iodine-125, tellurium-121 and other radionuclidic impurities present. No radionuclides with longer half-lives than iodine-125 are detected. For the determination of iodine-125, tellurium-121 and other radionuclidic impurities, retain the solution to be examined for a sufficient time to allow the radioactivity of iodine-123 to decrease to a level which permits the detection of radionuclidic impurities. Record the gamma-ray spectrum and the X-ray spectrum of the decayed material using a suitable instrument as described in the monograph on *Radiopharmaceutical preparations (125).* Not more than 0.35 per cent of the total radioactivity is due to radionuclides other than iodine-123. The injection may be released for use before completion of the test.

Radiochemical purity Examine by liquid chromatography (*2.2.29*).

Test solution. The injection to be examined.

Reference solution (a). Dissolve 0.100 g of *sodium iodide R* in the mobile phase and dilute to 100 ml with the mobile phase.

Reference solution (b). Dissolve 20.0 mg of *iobenguane sulphate CRS* in 50 ml of the mobile phase and dilute to 100.0 ml with the mobile phase.

The chromatographic procedure may be carried out using:
- a stainless steel column 0.25 m long and 4.0 mm in internal diameter packed with *silica gel for chromatography R* (5 µm),
- as mobile phase at a flow rate of 1.0 ml per minute a mixture of 1 volume of an 80 g/l solution of *ammonium nitrate R*, 2 volumes of *dilute ammonia R2* and 27 volumes of *methanol R*,
- a suitable radioactivity detector,
- a spectrophotometer set at 254 nm and provided with a flow-cell,
- a 10 µl loop injector.

Inject the test solution and the reference solutions. Not less than 95 per cent of the radioactivity of the chromatogram is found in the peak corresponding to iobenguane. Not more than 4 per cent of the radioactivity is found in the peak corresponding to iodide and not more than 1 per cent of the radioactivity is found in other peaks.

Specific radioactivity The specific radioactivity is calculated from the results obtained in the test for radiochemical purity. Determine the content of iobenguane sulphate from the areas of the peaks corresponding to iobenguane in the chromatograms obtained with the test solution and reference solution (b). Calculate the concentration as iobenguane base by multiplying the result obtained in the assay by 0.85.

Sterility It complies with the test for sterility prescribed in the monograph on *Radiopharmaceutical preparations (125)*. The injection may be released for use before completion of the test.

Bacterial endotoxins (*2.6.14*). Not more than 175/*V* I.U. of endotoxin per millilitre, *V* being the maximum recommended dose in millilitres.

RADIOACTIVITY

Measure the radioactivity as described in the monograph on *Radiopharmaceutical preparations (125)*, using a suitable counting apparatus by comparison with a standardised iodine-123 solution or by measurement in an instrument calibrated with the aid of such a solution.

STORAGE

Store protected from light in the conditions prescribed in the monograph on *Radiopharmaceutical preparations (125)*.

LABELLING

See *Radiopharmaceutical preparations (125)*.

The label states the specific radioactivity expressed in GBq of iodine-123 per gram of iobenguane base.

Ph Eur

Iobenguane[^{131}I] Injection for Diagnostic Use

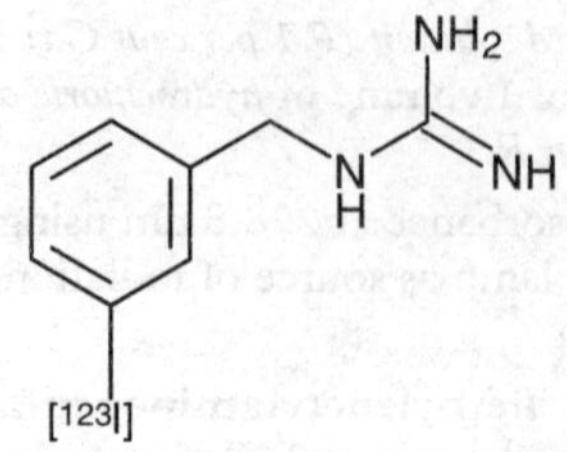

$C_8H_{10}[^{123}I]N_3$

Iobenguane [^{131}I] Injection for Diagnostic Use complies with the requirements of the 3rd edition of the European Pharmacopoeia [1111]. These requirements are reproduced after the heading 'Definition' below.

Ph Eur

DEFINITION

Iobenguane (^{131}I) injection for diagnostic use is a sterile, bacterial endotoxin-free solution of 1-(3-[^{131}I]iodobenzyl)-guanidine. It may contain a suitable buffer. It may also contain a suitable labelling catalyst such as ionic copper and a suitable labelling stabiliser such as ascorbic acid. It may contain antimicrobial preservatives. Iodine-131 is a radioactive isotope of iodine and may be obtained by neutron irradiation of tellurium or by extraction of uranium fission products. The injection contains not less than 90.0 per cent and not more than 110.0 per cent of the declared iodine-131 radioactivity at the date and hour stated on the label. Not less than 94 per cent of the radioactivity corresponds to iodine-131 in the form of iobenguane. The specific radioactivity is not less than 20 GBq of iodine-131 per gram of iobenguane base.

CHARACTERS

A clear, colourless or slightly yellow solution.

Iodine-131 has a half-life of 8.04 days and emits beta and gamma radiation.

IDENTIFICATION

A. Record the gamma-ray spectrum using a suitable instrument as described in the monograph on *Radiopharmaceutical preparations (125)*. The spectrum does not differ significantly from that of a standardised iodine-131 solution by direct comparison with such a solution. Standardised iodine-131 solutions are available from laboratories recognised by the competent authority. The most prominent gamma photon of iodine-131 has an energy of 0.365 MeV.

B. Examine the chromatogram obtained in the test for radiochemical purity. The distribution of the radioactivity contributes to the identification of the preparation.

TESTS

pH (*2.2.3*). The pH of the solution is 3.5 to 8.0.

Radionuclidic purity Record the gamma-ray spectrum using a suitable instrument as described in the monograph on *Radiopharmaceutical preparations (125)*. The spectrum does not differ significantly from that of a standardised iodine-131 solution. Determine the relative amounts of iodine-131, iodine-133, iodine-135 and other radionuclidic impurities present. Iodine-133 has a half-life of 20.8 h and its most prominent gamma photons have energies of 0.530 MeV and 0.875 MeV. Iodine-135 has a half-life of 6.55 h and its most prominent gamma photons have energies of 0.527 MeV, 1.132 MeV and 1.260 MeV. Not less than 99.9 per cent of the total radioactivity is due to iodine-131.

Radiochemical purity Examine by liquid chromatography *(2.2.29)*.

Test solution. The injection to be examined.

Reference solution (a). Dissolve 0.100 g of *sodium iodide R* in the mobile phase and dilute to 100 ml with the mobile phase.

Reference solution (b). Dissolve 20.0 mg of *iobenguane sulphate CRS* in 50 ml of the mobile phase and dilute to 100.0 ml with the mobile phase.

The chromatographic procedure may be carried out using:
— a stainless steel column 0.25 m long and 4.0 mm in internal diameter packed with *silica gel for chromatography R* (5 µm),
— as mobile phase at a flow rate of 1.0 ml per minute a mixture of 1 volume of an 80 g/l solution of *ammonium nitrate R*, 2 volumes of *dilute ammonia R2* and 27 volumes of *methanol R*,
— a suitable radioactivity detector,
— a spectrophotometer set at 254 nm and provided with a flow-cell,
— a 10 µl loop injector.

Inject the test solution and the reference solutions. Not less than 94 per cent of the radioactivity of the chromatogram is found in the peak corresponding to iobenguane. Not more than 5 per cent of the radioactivity is found in the peak corresponding to iodide and not more than 1 per cent of the radioactivity is found in other peaks.

Specific radioactivity The specific radioactivity is calculated from the results obtained in the test for radiochemical purity. Determine the content of iobenguane sulphate from the areas of the peaks corresponding to iobenguane in the chromatograms obtained with the test solution and reference solution (b). Calculate the concentration as iobenguane base by multiplying the result obtained in the assay by 0.85.

Sterility It complies with the test for sterility prescribed in the monograph on *Radiopharmaceutical preparations (125)*. The injection may be released for use before completion of the test.

Bacterial endotoxins *(2.6.14)*. Not more than 175/*V* I.U. of endotoxin per millilitre, *V* being the maximum recommended dose in millilitres.

RADIOACTIVITY

Measure the radioactivity as described in the monograph on *Radiopharmaceutical preparations (125)*, using a suitable counting apparatus by comparison with a standardised iodine-131 solution or by measurement in an instrument calibrated with the aid of such a solution.

STORAGE

Store protected from light in the conditions prescribed in the monograph on *Radiopharmaceutical preparations (125)*.

LABELLING

See *Radiopharmaceutical preparations (125)*.

The label states the specific radioactivity expressed in gigabecquerels of iodine-131 per gram of iobenguane base.

Ph Eur

Iobenguane[^{131}I] Injection for Therapeutic Use

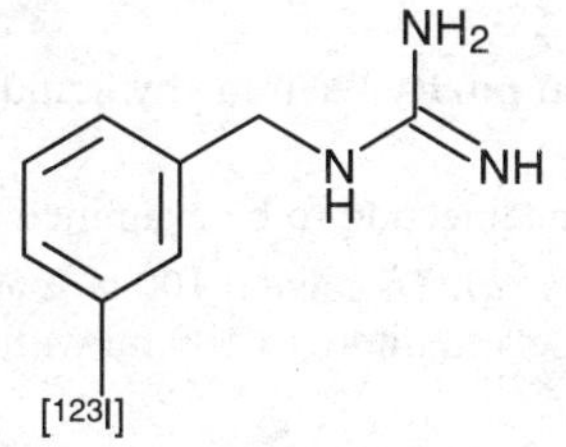

$C_8H_{10}[^{123}I]N_3$

Iobenguane (^{131}I) Injection for Therapeutic Use complies with the requirements of the 3rd edition of the European Pharmacopoeia [1112]. These requirements are reproduced after the heading 'Definition' below.

Ph Eur

DEFINITION

Iobenguane (^{131}I) injection for therapeutic use is a sterile, bacterial endotoxin-free solution of 1-(3-[^{131}I]iodobenzyl)-guanidine. It may contain a suitable buffer, a suitable labelling catalyst such as ionic copper, a suitable labelling stabiliser such as ascorbic acid and antimicrobial preservatives. Iodine-131 is a radioactive isotope of iodine and may be obtained by neutron irradiation of tellurium or by extraction of uranium fission products. The injection contains not less than 90.0 per cent and not more than 110.0 per cent of the declared iodine-131 radioactivity at the date and hour stated on the label. Not less than 92 per cent of the radioactivity corresponds to iodine-131 in the form of iobenguane. The specific radioactivity is not less than 400 GBq of iodine-131 per gram of iobenguane base.

CHARACTERS

A clear, colourless or slightly yellow solution.

Iodine-131 has a half-life of 8.04 days and emits beta and gamma radiation.

IDENTIFICATION

A. Record the gamma-ray spectrum using a suitable instrument as described in the monograph on *Radiopharmaceutical preparations (125)*. The spectrum does not differ significantly from that of a standardised iodine-131 solution by direct comparison with such a solution. Standardised iodine-131 solutions are available from laboratories recognised by the competent authority. The most prominent gamma photon of iodine-131 has an energy of 0.365 MeV.

B. Examine the chromatogram obtained in the test for radiochemical purity. The distribution of the radioactivity contributes to the identification of the preparation.

TESTS

pH *(2.2.3)*. The pH of the solution is 3.5 to 8.0.

Radionuclidic purity Record the gamma-ray spectrum using a suitable instrument as described in the monograph on *Radiopharmaceutical preparations (125)*. The spectrum does not differ significantly from that of a standardised iodine-131 solution. Determine the relative amounts of iodine-131, iodine-133, iodine-135 and other radionuclidic impurities present. Iodine-133 has a half-life of 20.8 h and its most prominent gamma photons have energies of 0.530 MeV and 0.875 MeV. Iodine-135 has a half-life of 6.55 h and its most prominent gamma photons have energies of 0.527 MeV, 1.132 MeV and 1.260 MeV. Not less than 99.9 per cent of the total radioactivity is due to iodine-131.

Radiochemical purity Examine by liquid chromatography *(2.2.29)*.

Test solution. The injection to be examined.

Reference solution (a). Dissolve 0.100 g of *sodium iodide R* in the mobile phase and dilute to 100 ml with the mobile phase.

Reference solution (b). Dissolve 20.0 mg of *iobenguane sulphate CRS* in 50 ml of the mobile phase and dilute to 100.0 ml with the mobile phase.

The chromatographic procedure may be carried out using:
— a stainless steel column 0.25 m long and 4.0 mm in internal diameter packed with *silica gel for chromatography R* (5 µm),
— as mobile phase at a flow rate of 1.0 ml per minute a mixture of 1 volume of an 80 g/l solution of *ammonium nitrate R*, 2 volumes of *dilute ammonia R2* and 27 volumes of *methanol R*,
— a suitable radioactivity detector,
— a spectrophotometer set at 254 nm and provided with a flow-cell,
— a 10 µl loop injector.

Inject the test solution and the reference solutions. Not less than 92 per cent of the radioactivity of the chromatogram is found in the peak corresponding to iobenguane. Not more than 7 per cent of the radioactivity is found in the peak corresponding to iodide and not more than 1 per cent of the radioactivity is found in other peaks.

Specific radioactivity The specific radioactivity is calculated from the results obtained in the test for radiochemical purity. Determine the content of iobenguane sulphate from the areas of the peaks corresponding to iobenguane in the chromatograms obtained with the test solution and reference solution (b). Calculate the concentration as iobenguane base by multiplying the result obtained in the assay by 0.85.

Sterility It complies with the test for sterility prescribed in the monograph on *Radiopharmaceutical preparations (125)*. The injection may be released for use before completion of the test.

Bacterial endotoxins *(2.6.14)*. Not more than 175/*V* I.U. of endotoxin per millilitre, *V* being the maximum recommended dose in millilitres.

RADIOACTIVITY

Measure the radioactivity as described in the monograph on *Radiopharmaceutical preparations (125)*, using a suitable counting apparatus by comparison with a standardised iodine-131 solution or by measurement in an instrument calibrated with the aid of such a solution.

STORAGE

Store protected from light in the conditions prescribed in the monograph on *Radiopharmaceutical preparations (125)*.

LABELLING

See *Radiopharmaceutical preparations (125)*.

The label states the specific radioactivity expressed in gigabecquerels of iodine-131 per gram of iobenguane base.

Ph Eur

Dried Iodinated [^{125}I] Fibrinogen

Dried Iodinated [^{125}I] Fibrinogen complies with the requirements of the 3rd edition of the European Pharmacopoeia for Dried Human Iodinated[^{125}I] Fibrinogen [0604]. These requirements are reproduced after the heading 'Definition' below.

Ph Eur

DEFINITION

Dried iodinated (^{125}I) human fibrinogen is a sterile, apyrogenic preparation of human fibrinogen which has been labelled with iodine-125. The human fibrinogen is prepared from plasma that complies with the monograph on *Human plasma for fractionation (853)*.

The method of preparation is designed to avoid the transmission of or to inactivate known agents of infection and to give a final product with a fibrinogen content not less than 80 per cent of the total protein content. The preparation may contain additives such as sodium citrate and human albumin.

The reconstituted preparation contains not less than 85.0 per cent and not more than 115.0 per cent of the declared iodine-125 radioactivity at the date stated on the label. Not less than 95 per cent of the radioactivity is due to iodine-125 bound to protein and not less than 80 per cent of the total radioactivity is due to substances bound to clottable protein. Not more than 1.0 per cent of the total radioactivity is due to iodine-126.

CHARACTERS

A white or pale yellow powder or friable solid.

Iodine-125 has a half-life of 60.1 days and emits gamma radiation and X-rays.

IDENTIFICATION

A. Record the gamma-ray and X-ray spectrum of the reconstituted preparation using a suitable instrument as described in the monograph on *Radiopharmaceutical preparations (125)*. The spectrum does not differ significantly from that of a standardised iodine-125 solution, apart from any differences attributable to the presence of iodine-126. Standardised iodine-125 and caesium-137 solutions are available from laboratories recognised by the competent authority. The most prominent photon of the preparation has an energy of 0.027 MeV, corresponding to the X-ray of tellurium. Iodine-126 has a half-life of 13.0 days and its most prominent gamma photons have energies of 0.388 MeV and 0.666 MeV.

B. Using a suitable range of species-specific antisera, carry out precipitation tests on the reconstituted preparation. The test is to be carried out using antisera specific for the plasma proteins of each species of domestic animal currently in use for the preparation of materials of biological origin in the country concerned. The preparation is shown to contain proteins of human origin and gives negative results with antisera specific to plasma proteins of other species.

C. The test for clottability also contributes to the identification of the preparation.

TESTS

pH *(2.2.3)*. The pH of the reconstituted preparation is 6.0

to 8.5.

Iodine-126 Record the gamma-ray and X-ray spectrum of the reconstituted preparation using a suitable instrument as described in the monograph on *Radiopharmaceutical preparations (125)* in comparison with standardised solutions of iodine-125 and caesium-137. Determine the relative amounts of iodine-125 and iodine-126 present on the assumption that the 0.666 MeV gamma photon of iodine-126 is emitted in 33 per cent of disintegrations and that the 0.661 MeV gamma photon of caesium-137 is emitted in 85.4 per cent of disintegrations.

Radiochemical purity Examine the reconstituted preparation by zone electrophoresis (*2.2.31*), using a paper strip 200 mm long as the support and *phosphate buffer pH 6.4 R* as the electrolyte solution. Apply to the paper 10 µl of the reconstituted preparation as a band 3 mm wide at a position 100 mm from the anode. Apply an electric potential of about 200 V for 60 min using a stabilised current. Allow the strip to dry. Determine the distribution of radioactivity using a suitable detector. Iodide ion moves about 7 cm towards the anode and iodinated fibrinogen remains almost at the starting point. The radioactivity due to iodine-125 bound to protein represents not less than 95 per cent of the total radioactivity of the electrophoretogram.

Clottability To 0.2 ml of the reconstituted preparation add 5 ml of human plasma, mix and after mixing transfer 1 ml of the mixture to each of two vials each containing 2 ml of *phosphate buffer pH 6.4 R*. Add to one of the vials 0.1 ml of a solution containing 10 units of *bovine thrombin R*. (One unit of thrombin will clot a 2.5 g/l of fibrinogen (>90 per cent clottable) in 15 s at 37°C.) Mix the contents of this vial thoroughly with a glass defibrinating rod and allow to stand for not less than 1 h without removing the rod. Remove the clot from the vial using the glass rod and discard both. Take 1 ml of the remaining solution and 1 ml of the control solution to which no bovine thrombin has been added. Measure the radioactivity of each and determine the percentage of radioactivity removed in the clot.

Not less than 80 per cent of the total radioactivity is present in the clot.

Sterility The reconstituted preparation complies with the test for sterility prescribed in the monograph on *Radiopharmaceutical preparations (125)*. The preparation may be released for use before completion of the test.

Bacterial endotoxins Dissolve the content of one vial in a suitable volume (V ml) of the prescribed solvent. The maximum allowable endotoxin concentration is $175/V$ I.U. of endotoxin per millilitre.

RADIOACTIVITY

Measure the radioactivity of the reconstituted preparation as described in the monograph on *Radiopharmaceutical preparations (125)*, using suitable counting equipment by comparison with a standardised iodine-125 solution or by measurement in an instrument calibrated with the aid of such a solution. Use an instrument incorporating a scintillation detector such as a thin sodium iodide crystal and set the instrument so that the contribution from the radioactivity of iodine-126 is minimised.

STORAGE

See *Radiopharmaceutical preparations (125)*.

LABELLING

See *Radiopharmaceutical preparations (125)*.

The label states:

— the method of reconstitution,

— that the preparation should be used immediately after reconstitution.

Ph Eur

Iodinated[^{131}I] Norcholesterol Injection

Iodinated[^{131}I] Norcholesterol Injection complies with the requirements of the 3rd edition of the European Pharmacopoeia [0939]. These requirements are reproduced after the heading 'Definition' below.

Ph Eur

DEFINITION

Iodinated (^{131}I) norcholesterol injection is a sterile, bacterial endotoxin-free solution of 6β-[^{131}I]iodomethyl-19-norcholest-5(10)-en-3β-ol. It may contain a suitable emulsifier such as polysorbate 80 and a suitable antimicrobial preservative such as benzyl alcohol. Iodine-131 is a radioactive isotope of iodine and may be obtained by neutron irradiation of tellurium or by extraction from uranium fission products. The injection contains not less than 90.0 per cent and not more than 110.0 per cent of the declared iodine-131 radioactivity at the date and hour stated on the label. Not less than 85 per cent of the radioactivity corresponds to iodine-131 in the form of 6β-[^{131}I]iodomethyl-19-norcholest-5(10)-en-3β-ol. Not more than 5 per cent of the radioactivity corresponds to iodine-131 in the form of iodide. The specific radioactivity is 3.7 GBq to 37 GBq per gram of 6β-iodomethylnorcholesterol.

CHARACTERS

A clear or slightly turbid, colourless or pale yellow solution.

Iodine-131 has a half-life of 8.04 days and emits beta and gamma radiation.

IDENTIFICATION

A. Record the gamma-ray spectrum using a suitable instrument as described in the monograph on *Radiopharmaceutical preparations (125)*. The spectrum does not differ significantly from that of a standardised iodine-131 solution by direct comparison with such a solution. The most prominent photon of iodine-131 has an energy of 0.365 MeV. Standardised iodine-131 solutions are available from laboratories recognised by the competent authority.

B. Examine the chromatogram obtained in test (a) for radiochemical purity. The distribution of radioactivity contributes to the identification of the preparation.

TESTS

pH (*2.2.3*). The pH of the solution is between 3.5 and 8.5.

Radionuclidic purity Record the gamma-ray spectrum using a suitable instrument as described in the monograph on *Radiopharmaceutical preparations (125)*. The spectrum does not differ significantly from that of a standardised iodine-131 solution. Determine the relative amounts of iodine-131, iodine-133, iodine-135 and other radionuclidic impurities present. Iodine-133 has a half-life of 20.8 h and its most prominent gamma photons have energies of 0.530 MeV and 0.875 MeV. Iodine-135 has a half-life of 6.55 h and its most prominent gamma photons have energies of 0.527 MeV, 1.132 MeV and 1.260 MeV. Not less than 99.9 per cent of the total radioactivity is due to iodine-131.

Radiochemical purity
(a) Examine by thin-layer chromatography (*2.2.27*) as described in the monograph on *Radiopharmaceutical preparations (125)* using *silica gel* GF_{254} *R* as the coating substance.

Test solution. The injection to be examined.

Carrier solution. Dissolve 10 mg of *potassium iodide R*, 20 mg of *potassium iodate R* and 0.1 g of *sodium hydrogen carbonate R* in *distilled water R* and dilute to 10 ml with the same solvent.

Apply to the plate up to 5 µl of the test solution and 10 µl of the carrier solution on the same spot. Develop over a path of 15 cm (about 60 min) using *chloroform R.* Allow the plate to dry in air and examine in ultraviolet light at 254 nm. Determine the distribution of radioactivity using a suitable detector. In the chromatogram obtained, not less than 85 per cent of the total radioactivity is found in the spot corresponding to 6β-iodomethyl-19-norcholest-5(10)-en-3β-ol at an R_f value of about 0.5. Iodide ion remains near the starting-line.

(b) Examine by thin-layer chromatography (*2.2.27*) as described in the monograph on *Radiopharmaceutical preparations (125)* using *silica gel* GF_{254} *R* as the coating substance.

Test solution. The injection to be examined.

Carrier solution. Dissolve 10 mg *potassium iodide R*, 20 mg of *potassium iodate R* and 0.1 g of *sodium hydrogen carbonate R* in *distilled water R* and dilute to 10 ml with the same solvent.

Apply to the plate 10 µl of the carrier solution and then up to 5 µl of the test solution on the same spot. Develop over a path of 15 cm (about 90 min) using a mixture of equal volumes of *chloroform R* and *ethanol R.* Allow the plate to dry in air. Expose the plate to ultraviolet light at 254 nm for 5 min. A yellow spot corresponding to iodide develops at an R_f value of about 0.5. Determine the distribution of radioactivity using a suitable detector. The main peak of radioactivity is near to the solvent front. Other iodocholesterols migrate near the solvent front. In the chromatogram obtained, not more than 5 per cent of the total radioactivity is found in the spot corresponding to iodide.

Sterility It complies with the test for sterility prescribed in the monograph on *Radiopharmaceutical preparations (125)*. The injection may be released for use before completion of the test.

Bacterial endotoxins (*2.6.14*). Not more than 175/*V* I.U. of endotoxin per millilitre, *V* being the maximum recommended dose in millilitres.

RADIOACTIVITY

Measure the radioactivity as described in the monograph on *Radiopharmaceutical preparations (125)* using suitable counting equipment by comparison with a standardised iodine-131 solution or by measurement in an instrument calibrated with the aid of such a solution.

STORAGE

Store protected from light at a temperature not exceeding −18°C in the conditions prescribed in the monograph on *Radiopharmaceutical preparations (125)*.

LABELLING

See the *Radiopharmaceutical preparations (125)*.

Ph Eur

Sodium Chromate[51Cr] Sterile Solution

Sodium Chromate[51Cr] Sterile Solution complies with the requirements of the 3rd edition of the European Pharmacopoeia [0279]. These requirements are reproduced after the heading 'Definition' below.

Ph Eur

DEFINITION

Sodium chromate (^{51}Cr) sterile solution is a sterile solution of sodium (^{51}Cr) chromate made isotonic by the addition of sodium chloride. Chromium-51 is a radioactive isotope of chromium and may be prepared by neutron irradiation of chromium, either of natural isotopic composition or enriched in chromium-50. The solution contains not less than 90.0 per cent and not more than 110.0 per cent of the declared chromium-51 radioactivity at the date and hour stated on the label. Not less than 90 per cent of the radioactivity corresponds to chromium-51 in the form of chromate. The specific radioactivity is not less than 370 MBq of chromium-51 per milligram of chromate ion.

CHARACTERS

A clear, colourless or slightly yellow solution.

Chromium-51 has a half-life of 27.7 days and emits gamma radiation.

IDENTIFICATION

A. Record the gamma-ray spectrum using a suitable instrument as described in the monograph on *Radiopharmaceutical preparations (125)*. The spectrum does not differ significantly from that of a standardised chromium-51 solution. Standardised chromium-51 solution are available from laboratories recognised by the competent authority. The gamma photon has an energy of 0.320 MeV.

B. Examine the chromatogram obtained in the test for radiochemical purity. The distribution of radioactivity contributes to the identification of the preparation.

TESTS

pH (*2.2.3*). The pH of the solution is 6.0 to 8.5.

Radionuclidic purity Record the gamma-ray spectrum using a suitable instrument as described in the monograph on *Radiopharmaceutical preparations (125)*. The spectrum does not differ significantly from that of a standardised chromium-51 solution.

Radiochemical purity Examine by ascending paper chromatography (*2.2.26*), as described in the monograph on *Radiopharmaceutical preparations (125)*.

Apply to the paper a quantity of the solution sufficient for the detection method. Begin the development immediately and develop for 2.5 h using a mixture of 25 volumes of *ammonia R*, 50 volumes of *alcohol R* and 125 volumes of *water R*. Chromic ions remain on the starting line. Determine the distribution of the radioactivity using a suitable detector. Not less than 90 per cent of the total radioactivity of the chromatogram is found in the spot with an R_f value of about 0.9, corresponding to sodium chromate.

Total chromate Not more than 2.7 µg of chromate ion (CrO_4^{2-}) per megabecquerel. Measure the absorbance of the solution (*2.2.25*) at the absorption maximum at 370 nm. Calculate the content of chromate using the absorbance of a standard consisting of a 1.7 mg/l solution of *potassium chromate R*. If necessary, adjust the solution to be examined and the standard to pH 8.0 by adding *sodium hydrogen carbonate solution R*.

Sterility It complies with the test for sterility prescribed in the monograph on *Radiopharmaceutical preparations (125)*. The solution may be released for use before completion of the test.

RADIOACTIVITY

Measure the radioactivity as described in the monograph on *Radiopharmaceutical preparations (125)* using suitable counting equipment by comparison with a standardised chromium-51 solution or by measurement in an instrument calibrated with the aid of such a solution.

STORAGE

See *Radiopharmaceutical preparations (125)*.

LABELLING

See *Radiopharmaceutical preparations (125)*.

Ph Eur

Sodium Iodide[131I] Capsules for Diagnostic Use

Sodium Iodide[131I] Capsules for Diagnostic Use comply with the requirements of the 3rd edition of the European Pharmacopoeia [0938]. These requirements are reproduced after the heading 'Definition' below.

Ph Eur

DEFINITION

Sodium iodide (^{131}I) capsules for diagnostic use contain iodine-131 in the form of sodium iodide on a suitable solid support. The capsules also contain sodium thiosulphate or other reducing agents and may contain a suitable buffer. Iodine-131 is a radioactive isotope of iodine obtained by neutron irradiation of tellurium or by extraction from uranium fission products. Each capsule contains not less than 90.0 per cent and not more than 110.0 per cent of the declared iodine-131 radioactivity at the date and hour stated on the label. Not more than 0.1 per cent of the total radioactivity is due to radionuclides other than iodine-131. Not less than 95 per cent of the radioactivity corresponds to iodine-131 in the form of iodide. The method of preparation is such that the specific radioactivity is not less than 185 GBq of iodine-131 per milligram of iodine. The capsules comply with the requirements for hard capsules in the monograph on *Capsules (16)*, unless otherwise justified and authorised.

CHARACTERS

Iodine-131 has a half-life of 8.04 days and emits beta and gamma radiation.

IDENTIFICATION

A. Record the gamma-ray spectrum using a suitable instrument as described in the monograph on *Radiopharmaceutical preparations (125)*. The spectrum does not differ significantly from that of a standardised iodine-131 solution. Standardised iodine-131 solutions are available from laboratories recognised by the competent authority. The most prominent gamma photon of iodine-131 has an energy of 0.365 MeV.

B. Examine the chromatograms obtained in the test for radiochemical purity. The distribution of radioactivity contributes to the identification of the preparation.

TESTS

Radionuclidic purity Use a suitable volume of the solution obtained in the test for disintegration. Record the gamma-ray spectrum using a suitable instrument as described in the monograph *Radiopharmaceutical preparations (125)*. The spectrum does not differ significantly from that of a standardised iodine-131 solution.

Determine the relative amounts of iodine-131, iodine-133, iodine-135 and other radionuclidic impurities present. Iodine-133 has a half-life of 20.8 h and its most prominent gamma photons have energies of 0.530 MeV and 0.875 MeV. Iodine-135 has a half-life of 6.55 h and its most prominent gamma photons have energies of 0.527 MeV, 1.132 MeV and 1.260 MeV. Not less than 99.9 per cent of the total radioactivity is due to iodine-131.

Radiochemical purity Examine by ascending paper chromatography (*2.2.26*), as described in the monograph on *Radiopharmaceutical preparations (125)*.

Test solution. Dissolve the contents of one capsule to be examined in 5 ml of *water R*.

On a strip of suitable paper apply 10 µl of the test solution. Add on the same spot, without previously drying, 10 µl of a solution containing 1 g/l of *potassium iodide R*, 2 g/l of *potassium iodate R* and 10 g/l of *sodium hydrogen carbonate R*. Develop without previously drying over a path of 10 cm using a mixture of 30 volumes of *water R* and 70 volumes of *methanol R*. Allow to dry and determine the radioactivity using a suitable detector. In the chromatogram obtained, not less than 95 per cent of the total radioactivity is found in the spot corresponding to iodide. Spray the paper with *palladium chloride solution R* and heat the paper in a current of hot air. Iodide forms a brown spot; iodate forms a yellow spot after heating.

Disintegration In a water-bath at 37°C, warm in a small beaker 10 ml of a 2.0 g/l solution of *potassium iodide R*. Add one of the capsules to be examined. Stir magnetically at a rotation rate of 20 revolutions per minute. The shell and its contents dissolve completely within 15 min.

Uniformity of content Determine by measuring in a suitable counting assembly and under identical geometrical conditions, the radioactivity of each of not less than ten capsules. Calculate the average radioactivity per capsule. The radioactivity of no capsule differs by more than 10 per cent from the average. The relative standard deviation is not greater than 3.5 per cent.

RADIOACTIVITY

The average radioactivity determined in the test for uniformity of content is not less than 90.0 per cent and not more than 110.0 per cent of the declared iodine-131 radioactivity at the date and hour stated on the label.

STORAGE

See *Radiopharmaceutical preparations (125)*.

LABELLING

See *Radiopharmaceutical preparations (125)*.

Ph Eur

Sodium Iodide[^{123}I] Solution

Sodium Iodide[^{123}I] Solution complies with the requirements of the 3rd edition of the European Pharmacopoeia [0563]. These requirements are reproduced after the heading 'Definition' below.

Ph Eur

DEFINITION

Sodium iodide (^{123}I) solution is a solution for oral administration containing iodine-123 in the form of sodium iodide; it also contains sodium thiosulphate or some other suitable reducing agent and may contain a suitable buffer. Iodine-123 is a radioactive isotope of iodine and may be obtained by proton irradiation of xenon enriched in xenon-124 (not less than 98 per cent) followed by the decay of caesium-123 formed via xenon-123. The solution contains not less than 90.0 per cent and not more than 110.0 per cent of the declared iodine-123 radioactivity at the date and hour stated on the label. Not less than 95 per cent of the radioactivity corresponds to iodine-123 in the form of iodide. The specific radioactivity is not less than 185 GBq of iodine-123 per milligram of iodine. Not more than 0.35 per cent of the total radioactivity is due to radionuclides other than iodine-123.

CHARACTERS

A clear, colourless solution.

Iodine-123 has a half-life of 13.2 h and emits gamma radiation and X-rays.

IDENTIFICATION

A. Record the gamma-ray and X-ray spectrum using a suitable instrument as described in the monograph on *Radiopharmaceutical preparations (125)*. The spectrum does not differ significantly from that of a standardised iodine-123 solution apart from any differences attributable to the presence of iodine-125, tellurium-121 and other radionuclidic impurities. Standardised iodine-123, iodine-125 and tellurium-121 solutions are available from laboratories recognised by the competent authority. The most prominent gamma photon of iodine-123 has an energy of 0.159 MeV and is accompanied by an X-ray of 0.027 MeV. Iodine-125 has a half-life of 59.4 days and emits an X-ray of 0.027 MeV and a photon of 0.035 MeV. Tellurium-121 has a half-life of 19.2 days and the most prominent photons have energies of 0.507 MeV and 0.573 MeV.

B. Examine the chromatograms obtained in the test for radiochemical purity. The distribution of radioactivity contributes to the identification of the preparation.

TESTS

pH (*2.2.3*). The pH of the solution is 7.0 to 10.0.

Radionuclidic purity Record the gamma-ray spectrum using a suitable instrument as described in the monograph on *Radiopharmaceutical preparations (125)*. Determine the relative amounts of iodine-125, tellurium-121 and other radionuclidic impurities present. No radionuclides with longer half lives than iodine-125 are detected. For the determination of iodine-125, tellurium-121 and other radionuclidic impurities, retain the solution to be examined for a sufficient time to allow the radioactivity of iodine-123 to decrease to a level which permits the detection of radionuclidic impurities. Record the gamma-ray spectrum and X-ray spectrum of the decayed material using a suitable instrument as described in the monograph on *Radiopharmaceutical preparations (125)*. Not more than 0.35 per cent of the total radioactivity is due to radionuclides other than iodine-123. The solution may be released for use before completion of the test.

Radiochemical purity Examine by ascending paper chromatography (*2.2.26*), as described in the monograph on *Radiopharmaceutical preparations (125)*.

Test solution. Dilute the preparation to be examined with *water R* until the radioactivity is equivalent to about 20,000 counts per minute per 10 μl. Add an equal volume of a solution containing 1 g/l of *potassium iodide R*, 2 g/l of *potassium iodate R* and 10 g/l of *sodium hydrogen carbonate R* and mix.

Reference solution (a). Dissolve 0.1 g of *potassium iodide R* in *water R* and dilute to 10 ml with the same solvent.

Reference solution (b). Dissolve 0.2 g of *potassium iodate R* in *water R* and dilute to 10 ml with the same solvent.

On a strip of suitable paper 250 mm long apply separately 20 μl of the test solution, 10 μl of reference solution (a) and 10 μl of reference solution (b). Develop over a path of 20 cm (about 2 h) using a mixture of 10 volumes of *water R* and 30 volumes of *methanol R*. Allow the paper to dry in air and determine the positions of the inactive potassium iodide and potassium iodate by the application of filter papers impregnated respectively with *acetic acid R* and *potassium iodate R* and *acetic acid R* and *potassium iodide R*. Determine the distribution of radioactivity using a suitable detector. In the chromatogram obtained with the test solution, not less than 95 per cent of the total radioactivity is found in the spot corresponding to iodide and the R_f value of the spot does not differ by more than 5 per cent from the R_f value of the spot corresponding to inactive iodide in the chromatogram obtained with reference solution (a).

RADIOACTIVITY

Measure the radioactivity as described in the monograph on *Radiopharmaceutical preparations (125)* using suitable counting equipment by comparison with a standardised iodine-123 solution or by measurement in an instrument calibrated with the aid of such a solution.

STORAGE

See *Radiopharmaceutical preparations (125)*.

LABELLING

See *Radiopharmaceutical preparations (125)*.

Ph Eur

Sodium Iodide[^{125}I] Solution

Sodium Iodide[^{125}I] Solution complies with the requirements of the 3rd edition of the European Pharmacopoeia [0280]. These requirements are reproduced after the heading 'Definition' below.

Ph Eur

DEFINITION

Sodium iodide (^{125}I) solution is a solution for oral administration containing iodine-125 in the form of sodium iodide; it also contains sodium thiosulphate or some other suitable reducing agent and may contain a suitable buffer. Iodine-125 is a radioactive isotope of iodine and may be prepared by neutron irradiation of xenon. The solution contains not less than 85.0 per cent and not more than 115.0 per cent of the declared iodine-125 radioactivity at the date stated on the label. Not less than 95 per cent of the radioactivity corresponds to iodine-125 in the form of iodide. The method of preparation is such that the specific radioactivity is not less than 74 GBq of iodine-125 per milligram of iodine at the date stated on the label. Not more than 1.0 per cent of the total radioactivity is due to iodine-126.

CHARACTERS

A clear, colourless solution.

Iodine-125 has a half-life of 60.1 days and emits gamma radiation and X-rays.

IDENTIFICATION

A. Record the gamma-ray and X-ray spectrum using a suitable instrument as described in the monograph on *Radiopharmaceutical preparations (125)*. The spectrum does not differ significantly from that of a standardised iodine-125 solution, apart from any differences attributable to the presence of iodine-126. Standardised iodine-125 and caesium-137 solutions are available from laboratories recognised by the competent authority. The most prominent photon of the preparation has an energy of 0.027 MeV, corresponding to the X-ray of tellurium. Iodine-126 has a half-life of 13.0 days and its presence is shown by its most prominent gamma photons with energies of 0.388 MeV and 0.666 MeV.

B. Examine the chromatograms obtained in the test for radiochemical purity. The distribution of radioactivity contributes to the identification of the preparation.

TESTS

pH (*2.2.3*). The pH of the solution is 7.0 to 10.0.

Iodine-126 Record the gamma-ray and X-ray spectrum as described in the monograph on *Radiopharmaceutical preparations (125)* using a suitable instrument in comparison with standardised solutions of iodine-125 and caesium-137. Determine the relative amounts of iodine-125 and iodine-126 present on the assumption that the 0.666 MeV gamma photon of iodine-126 is emitted in 33 per cent of disintegrations, and that the 0.661 MeV gamma photon of caesium-137 is emitted in 85.4 per cent of disintegrations.

Radiochemical purity Examine by ascending paper chromatography (*2.2.26*), as described in the monograph on *Radiopharmaceutical preparations (125)*.

Test solution. Dilute the preparation to be examined with *water R* until the radioactivity is equivalent to about 20,000 counts per minute per 10 µl. Add an equal volume of a solution containing 1 g/l of *potassium iodide R*, 2 g/l of *potassium iodate R* and 10 g/l of *sodium hydrogen carbonate R* and mix.

Reference solution (a). Dissolve 0.1 g of *potassium iodide R* in *water R* and dilute to 10 ml with the same solvent.

Reference solution (b). Dissolve 0.2 g of *potassium iodate R* in *water R* and dilute to 10 ml with the same solvent.

Apply separately to a strip of paper 250 mm long 20 µl of the test solution, 10 µl of reference solution (a) and 10 µl of reference solution (b). Develop over a path of 20 cm using a mixture of 10 volumes of *water R* and 30 volumes of *methanol R* (the development time is about 2 h). Allow the paper to dry in air and determine the positions of the inactive potassium iodide and potassium iodate by the application of filter papers impregnated respectively with *acetic acid R* and *potassium iodate R* and *acetic acid R* and *potassium iodide R*. Determine the distribution of radioactivity using a suitable detector. In the chromatogram obtained with the test solution, not less than 95 per cent of the total radioactivity is found in the spot corresponding to iodide and the R_f value of the spot does not differ by more than 5 per cent from the R_f value of the spot corresponding to inactive potassium iodide in the chromatogram obtained with reference solution (a).

RADIOACTIVITY

Measure the radioactivity as described in the monograph on *Radiopharmaceutical preparations (125)* using suitable counting equipment by comparison with a standardised iodine-125 solution or by measurement in an instrument calibrated with the aid of such a solution. Use an instrument incorporating a scintillation detector such as a thin sodium iodide crystal and set the instrument so that the contribution from the radioactivity of iodine-126 is minimised.

STORAGE

See *Radiopharmaceutical preparations (125)*.

LABELLING

See *Radiopharmaceutical preparations (125)*.

Ph Eur

Sodium Iodide[^{131}I] Solution

Sodium Iodide[^{131}I] Solution complies with the requirements of the 3rd edition of the European Pharmacopoeia [0281]. These requirements are reproduced after the heading 'Definition' below.

Ph Eur

DEFINITION

Sodium iodide (^{131}I) solution is a solution for oral administration containing iodine-131 in the form of sodium iodide; it also contains sodium thiosulphate or some other suitable reducing agent and may contain a suitable buffer. Iodine-131 is a radioactive isotope of iodine and may be obtained by neutron irradiation of tellurium or by extraction from uranium fission products. The solution contains not less than 90.0 per cent and not more than 110.0 per cent of the declared iodine-131 radioactivity at the date and hour stated on the label. Not more than 0.1 per cent of the total radioactivity is due to radionuclides other than iodine-131. Not less than 95 per cent of the radioactivity corresponds to iodine-131 in the form of iodide. The method of preparation is such that the specific radioactivity is not less than 185 GBq of iodine-131 per milligram of iodine at the date and hour stated on the label.

CHARACTERS

A clear, colourless solution.

Iodine-131 has a half-life of 8.04 days and emits beta and gamma radiation.

IDENTIFICATION

A. Record the gamma-ray spectrum using a suitable instrument as described in the monograph on *Radiopharmaceutical preparations (125)*. The spectrum does not differ significantly from that of a standardised iodine-131 solution. Standardised iodine-131 solutions are available from laboratories recognised by the competent authority. The most prominent gamma photon of iodine-131 has an energy of 0.365 MeV.

B. Examine the chromatograms obtained in the test for radiochemical purity. The distribution of radioactivity contributes to the identification of the preparation.

TESTS

pH (*2.2.3*). The pH of the solution is 7.0 to 10.0.

Radionuclidic purity Record the gamma-ray spectrum using a suitable instrument as described in the monograph on *Radiopharmaceutical preparations (125)*. The spectrum does not differ significantly from that of a standardised iodine-131 solution. Determine the relative amounts of iodine-131, iodine-133, iodine-135 and other radionuclidic impurities present. Iodine-133 has a half-life of 20.8 h and its most prominent gamma photons have energies of 0.53 MeV and 0.875 MeV. Iodine-135 has a half-life of 6.55 h and its most prominent gamma photons have energies of 0.527 MeV and 1.260 MeV. Not less than 99.9 per cent of the total radioactivity is due to iodine-131 and not more than 0.1 per cent of the total radioactivity is due to iodine-133, iodine-135 and other radionuclidic impurities.

Radiochemical purity Examine by ascending paper chromatography (*2.2.26*), as described in the monograph on *Radiopharmaceutical preparations (125)*.

Test solution. Dilute the preparation to be examined with *water R* until the radioactivity is equivalent to about 20,000 counts per minute per 10 µl. Add an equal volume of a solution containing 1 g/l of *potassium iodide R*, 2 g/l of *potassium iodate R* and 10 g/l of *sodium hydrogen carbonate R* and mix.

Reference solution (a). Dissolve 0.1 g of *potassium iodide R* in *water R* and dilute to 10 ml with the same solvent.

Reference solution (b). Dissolve 0.2 g of *potassium iodate R* in *water R* and dilute to 10 ml with the same solvent.

Apply separately to a strip of paper 250 mm long 20 µl of the test solution, 10 µl of reference solution (a) and 10 µl of reference solution (b). Develop over a path of 20 cm using a mixture of 10 volumes of *water R* and 30 volumes of *methanol R* (the development time is about 2 h). Allow the paper to dry in air and determine the positions of the inactive potassium iodide and potassium iodate by the application of filter papers impregnated respectively with *acetic acid R* and *potassium iodate R* and *acetic acid R* and *potassium iodide R*. Determine the distribution of radioactivity using a suitable detector. In the chromatogram obtained with the test solution, not less than 95 per cent of the total radioactivity is found in the spot corresponding to iodide and the R_f value of the spot does not differ by more than 5 per cent from that of the spot corresponding to inactive potassium iodide in the chromatogram obtained with reference solution (a).

RADIOACTIVITY

Measure the radioactivity as described in the monograph on *Radiopharmaceutical preparations (125)* using suitable counting equipment by comparison with a standardised iodine-131 solution or by measurement in an instrument calibrated with the aid of such a solution.

STORAGE

See *Radiopharmaceutical preparations (125)*.

LABELLING

See *Radiopharmaceutical preparations (125)*.

Ph Eur

Sodium Iodohippurate[^{123}I] Injection

Sodium Iodohippurate[^{123}I] Injection complies with the requirements of the 3rd edition of the European Pharmacopoeia [0564]. These requirements are reproduced after the heading 'Definition' below.

Ph Eur

DEFINITION

Sodium iodohippurate (^{123}I) injection is a sterile solution of sodium (2-[^{123}I]iodobenzamido)acetate. It may contain a suitable buffer and a suitable antimicrobial preservative such as benzyl alcohol. Iodine-123 is a radioactive isotope of iodine and may be obtained by proton irradiation of xenon enriched in xenon-124 (not less than 98 per cent) followed by the decay of caesium-123 formed via xenon-123. The injection contains not less than 90.0 per cent and not more than 110.0 per cent of the declared iodine-123 radioactivity at the date and hour stated on the label. Not less than 96 per cent of the radioactivity corresponds to iodine-123 in the form of sodium 2-iodohippurate. The specific radioactivity is 0.74 GBq to 10.0 GBq of iodine-123 per gram of sodium 2-iodohippurate. Not more than 0.35 per cent of the total radioactivity is due to radionuclides other than iodine-123.

CHARACTERS

A clear, colourless liquid.

Iodine-123 has a half-life of 13.2 h and emits gamma radiation and X-rays.

IDENTIFICATION

A. Record the gamma-ray and X-ray spectrum using a suitable instrument as described in the monograph on *Radiopharmaceutical preparations (125)*. The spectrum does not differ significantly from that of a standardised iodine-123 solution apart from any differences attributable to the presence of iodine-125, tellurium-121 and other radionuclidic impurities. Standardised iodine-123, iodine-125 and tellurium-121 solutions are available from laboratories recognised by the national authorities. The most prominent gamma photon of iodine-123 has an energy of 0.159 MeV and is accompanied by an X-ray of 0.027 MeV. Iodine-125 has a half-life of 59.4 days and emits an X-ray of 0.027 MeV and a photon of 0.035 MeV. Tellurium-121 has a half-life of 19.2 days and the most prominent photons have energies of 0.507 MeV and 0.573 MeV.

B. Examine the chromatograms obtained in the test for radiochemical purity. The spot corresponding to the main peak of radioactivity in the chromatogram obtained with the test solution is similar in position to the spot corresponding to 2-iodohippuric acid in the chromatogram obtained with the reference solution.

TESTS

pH (*2.2.3*). The pH of the solution is 3.5 to 8.5.

Radionuclidic purity Record the gamma-ray spectrum using a suitable instrument as described in the monograph on *Radiopharmaceutical preparations (125)*. Determine the relative amounts of iodine-125, tellurium-121 and other radionuclidic impurities present. No radionuclides with longer half lives than iodine-125 are detected. For the determination of iodine-125, tellurium-121 and other radionuclidic impurities, retain the solution to be examined for a sufficient time to allow the radioactivity of iodine-123 to decrease to a level which permits the detection of radionuclidic impurities. Record the gamma-ray spectrum and X-ray spectrum of the decayed material using a suitable instrument as described in the monograph on *Radiopharmaceutical preparations (125)*. Not more than 0.35 per cent of the total radioactivity is due to radionuclides other than iodine-123. The injection may be released for use before completion of the test.

Radiochemical purity Examine by thin-layer chromatography (*2.2.27*) as described in the monograph on *Radiopharmaceutical preparations (125)*, using *silica gel GF_{254} R* as the coating substance.

Test solution. Dissolve 1 g of *potassium iodide R* in 10 ml of *water R*, add 1 volume of this solution to 10 volumes of the injection to be examined and use within 10 min of mixing. If necessary, dilute with the reference solution (carrier) to give a radioactive concentration sufficient for the detection method, for example 3.7 MBq per millilitre.

Reference solution (carrier). Dissolve 40 mg of *2-iodohippuric acid R* and 40 mg of *2-iodobenzoic acid R* in 4 ml of *0.1M sodium hydroxide*, add 10 mg of *potassium iodide R* and dilute to 10 ml with *water R*.

Apply separately to the plate 10 µl of each solution. Develop over a path of 12 cm (about 75 min) using a mixture of 1 volume of *water R*, 4 volumes of *glacial acetic acid R*, 20 volumes of *butanol R* and 80 volumes of *toluene R*. Allow the plate to dry in air and examine in ultraviolet light at 254 nm. The chromatogram obtained with the reference solution shows a spot corresponding to 2-iodohippuric acid and nearer to the solvent front a spot corresponding to 2-iodobenzoic acid. Iodide ion remains near the starting-line. Determine the distribution of radioactivity using a suitable detector. In the chromatogram obtained with the test solution, not less than 96 per cent of the total radioactivity is found in the spot corresponding to 2-iodohippuric acid and not more than 2 per cent of the total radioactivity is found in either of the spots corresponding to 2-iodobenzoic acid and to iodide ion.

Sterility It complies with the test for sterility prescribed in the monograph on *Radiopharmaceutical preparations (125)*. The injection may be released for use before completion of the test.

RADIOACTIVITY

Measure the radioactivity as described in the monograph on *Radiopharmaceutical preparations (125)* using suitable counting equipment by comparison with a standardised iodine-123 solution or by measurement in an instrument calibrated with the aid of such a solution.

STORAGE

Store protected from light, in a cool place, in the conditions prescribed in the monograph on *Radiopharmaceutical preparations (125)*.

LABELLING

See *Radiopharmaceutical preparations (125)*.

The label states whether or not the preparation is suitable for renal plasma-flow studies.

Ph Eur

Sodium Iodohippurate[^{131}I] Injection

Sodium Iodohippurate[^{131}I] Injection complies with the requirements of the 3rd edition of the European Pharmacopoeia [0282]. These requirements are reproduced after the heading 'Definition' below.

Ph Eur

DEFINITION

Sodium iodohippurate (^{131}I) injection is a sterile solution of sodium 2-(2-[^{131}I]iodobenzamido)acetate. It may contain a suitable buffer and a suitable antimicrobial preservative such as benzyl alcohol. Iodine-131 is a radioactive isotope of iodine and may be obtained by neutron irradiation of tellurium or by extraction from uranium fission products. The injection contains not less than 90.0 per cent and not more than 110.0 per cent of the declared iodine-131 radioactivity at the date and hour stated on the label. Not less than 96 per cent of the iodine-131 is in the form of sodium 2-iodohippurate. The specific radioactivity is 0.74 GBq to 7.4 GBq of iodine-131 per gram of sodium 2-iodohippurate.

CHARACTERS

A clear, colourless liquid.

Iodine-131 has a half-life of 8.04 days and emits beta and gamma radiation.

IDENTIFICATION

A. Record the gamma-ray spectrum using a suitable instrument as described in the monograph on *Radiopharmaceutical preparations (125)*. The spectrum does not differ significantly from that of a standardised iodine-131 solution. Standardised iodine-131 solutions are available from laboratories recognised by the competent authority. The most prominent gamma photon of iodine-131 has an energy of 0.365 MeV.

B. Examine the chromatograms obtained in the test for radiochemical purity. The main peak of radioactivity in the chromatogram obtained with the test solution is similar in position to the spot corresponding to 2-iodohippuric acid in the chromatogram obtained with the reference solution.

TESTS

pH (*2.2.3*). The pH of the injection is 6.0 to 8.5.

Radionuclidic purity Record the gamma-ray spectrum using a suitable instrument as described in the monograph on *Radiopharmaceutical preparations (125)*. The spectrum does not differ significantly from that of a standardised iodine-131 solution. Determine the relative amounts of iodine-131, iodine-133, iodine-135 and other radionuclidic impurities present. Iodine-133 has a half-life of 20.8 h and its most prominent gamma photons have energies of 0.530 MeV and 0.875 MeV. Iodine-135 has a half-life of 6.55 h and its most prominent gamma photons have energies of 0.527 MeV, 1.132 MeV and 1.260 MeV. Not less than 99.9 per cent of the total radioactivity is due to iodine-131.

Radiochemical purity Examine by thin-layer chromatography (*2.2.27*) as described in the monograph on *Radiopharmaceutical preparations (125)*, using *silica gel* GF_{254} *R* as the coating substance.

Test solution. Dissolve 1 g of *potassium iodide R* in 10 ml of *water R*, add 1 volume of this solution to 10 volumes of the injection to be examined and use within 10 min of mixing. If necessary dilute with the reference solution (carrier) to give a radioactive concentration sufficient for the detection method, for example 3.7 MBq per millilitre.

Reference solution (*carrier*). Dissolve 40 mg of *2-iodohippuric acid R* and 40 mg of *2-iodobenzoic acid R* in 4 ml of *0.1M sodium hydroxide*, add 10 mg of *potassium iodide R* and dilute to 10 ml with *water R*.

Apply separately to the plate 10 µl of each solution. Develop over a path of 12 cm (about 75 min) using a mixture of 1 volume of *water R*, 4 volumes of *glacial acetic acid R*, 20 volumes of *butanol R* and 80 volumes of *toluene R*. Allow the plate to dry in air and examine in ultraviolet light at 254 nm. The chromatogram obtained with the reference solution shows a spot corresponding to 2-iodohippuric acid and nearer to the solvent front a spot corresponding to 2-iodobenzoic acid. Iodide ion remains near the starting-line. Determine the distribution of radioactivity using a suitable detector. In the chromatogram obtained with the test solution, not less than 96 per cent of the total radioactivity is found in the spot corresponding to 2-iodohippuric acid and not more than 2 per cent of the total radioactivity is found in either of the spots corresponding to 2-iodobenzoic acid and to iodide ion.

Sterility It complies with the test for sterility prescribed in the monograph on *Radiopharmaceutical preparations (125)*. The injection may be released for use before completion of the test.

RADIOACTIVITY

Measure the radioactivity as described in the monograph on *Radiopharmaceutical preparations (125)* using suitable counting equipment by comparison with a standardised iodine-131 solution or by measurement in an instrument calibrated with the aid of such a solution.

STORAGE

Store protected from light, in a cool place, in the conditions prescribed in the monograph on *Radiopharmaceutical preparations (125)*.

LABELLING

See *Radiopharmaceutical preparations (125)*.

The label states that the preparation is not necessarily suitable for renal plasma-flow studies.

Ph Eur

Sodium Pertechnetate[^{99m}Tc] Injection (Fission)

Sodium Pertechnetate[^{99m}Tc] Injection (Fission) complies with the requirements of the 3rd edition of the European Pharmacopoeia [0124]. These requirements are reproduced after the heading 'Definition' below.

Ph Eur

This monograph applies to sodium pertechnetate (^{99m}Tc) injection obtained from molybdenum-99 extracted from fission products of uranium. Sodium pertechnetate (^{99m}Tc) injection obtained from molybdenum-99 produced by the neutron irradiation of molybdenum is described in the monograph on Sodium Pertechnetate (^{99m}Tc) Injection (Non-fission) (283).

DEFINITION

Sodium pertechnetate (^{99m}Tc) injection (fission) is a sterile solution containing technetium-99m in the form of pertechnetate ion and made isotonic by the addition of sodium chloride. Technetium-99m is a radionuclide formed by the decay of molybdenum-99. Molybdenum-99 is a radioactive isotope of molybdenum extracted from uranium fission products. The injection contains not less than 90.0 per cent and not more than 110.0 per cent of the declared technetium-99m radioactivity at the date and hour stated on the label. Not less than 95 per cent of the radioactivity corresponds to technetium-99m in the form of pertechnetate ion.

The radioactivity due to radionuclides other than technetium-99m, apart from that due to technetium-99 resulting from the decay of technetium-99m, is not greater than that shown below, expressed as a percentage of the total radioactivity and calculated with reference to the date and hour of administration.

molybdenum-99	0.1 per cent
iodine-131	5×10^{-3} per cent
ruthenium-103	5×10^{-3} per cent
strontium-89	6×10^{-5} per cent
strontium-90	6×10^{-6} per cent
alpha-emitting impurities	1×10^{-7} per cent
other gamma-emitting impurities	0.01 per cent

The injection may be prepared from a sterile preparation of molybdenum-99 under aseptic conditions.

CHARACTERS

A clear, colourless solution.

Technetium-99m has a half-life of 6.02 h and emits gamma radiation.

IDENTIFICATION

Record the gamma-ray spectrum using a suitable instrument as described in the monograph on *Radiopharmaceutical preparations (125)*. The spectrum does not differ significantly from that of a standardised technetium-99m solution either by direct comparison or by measurement in an instrument calibrated with the aid of such a solution. Standardised technetium-99m, molybdenum-99, iodine-131, ruthenium-103, strontium-89 and strontium/yttrium-90 solutions are available from laboratories recognised by the competent authority. The most prominent gamma photon of technetium-99m has an energy of 0.140 MeV.

TESTS

pH (*2.2.3*). The pH of the injection is 4.0 to 8.0.

Radionuclidic purity Operate as described in the monograph on *Radiopharmaceutical preparations (125)*.

Preliminary test. To obtain an approximate estimate before use of the injection, take a volume equivalent to 37 MBq and determine the gamma-ray spectrum using a sodium iodide detector with a shield of lead, of thickness 6 mm, interposed between the sample and the detector. The response in the region corresponding to the 0.740 MeV photon of molybdenum-99 does not exceed that obtained using 37 kBq of a standardised molybdenum-99 solution measured under the same conditions, when all measurements are expressed with reference to the date and hour of administration.

Definitive test. Retain a sample of the injection for a sufficient time to allow the technetium-99m radioactivity to decay to a sufficiently low level to permit the detection of radionuclidic impurities. All measurements of radioactivity are expressed with reference to the date and hour of administration.

Molybdenum-99. Record the gamma-ray spectrum of the decayed material in a suitable instrument calibrated with the aid of a standardised molybdenum-99 solution. The most prominent photons have energies of 0.181 MeV, 0.740 MeV and 0.778 MeV. Molybdenum-99 has a half-life of 66.0 h. Not more than 0.1 per cent of the total radioactivity is due to molybdenum-99.

Iodine-131. Record the gamma-ray spectrum of the decayed material in a suitable instrument calibrated with the aid of a standardised iodine-131 solution. The most prominent photon has an energy of 0.365 MeV. Iodine-131 has a half-life of 8.04 days. Not more than 5×10^{-3} per cent of the total radioactivity is due to iodine-131.

Ruthenium-103. Record the gamma-ray spectrum of the decayed material in a suitable instrument calibrated using a standardised ruthenium-103 solution. The most prominent photon has an energy of 0.497 MeV. Ruthenium-103 has a half-life of 39.3 days. Not more than 5×10^{-3} per cent of the total radioactivity is due to ruthenium-103.

Strontium-89. Determine the presence of strontium-89 in the decayed material with an instrument suitable for the detection of beta rays, by comparison with a standardised strontium-89 solution. It is usually necessary first to carry out chemical separation of the strontium so that the standard and the sample may be compared in the same physical and chemical form. Strontium-89 decays with a beta emission of 1.492 MeV maximum energy and has a half-life of 50.5 days. Not more than 6×10^{-5} per cent of the total radioactivity is due to strontium-89.

Strontium-90. Determine the presence of strontium-90 in the decayed material with an instrument suitable for the detection of beta rays. To distinguish strontium-90 from strontium-89, compare the radioactivity of yttrium-90, the daughter nuclide of strontium-90, with an yttrium-90 standard after the chemical separation of the yttrium. If prior chemical separation of the strontium is necessary, the conditions of radioactive equilibrium must be ensured. The yttrium-90 standard and the sample must be compared in the same physical and chemical form. Strontium-90 and yttrium-90 decay with respective beta emissions of 0.546 MeV and 2.284 MeV maximum energy and half-lives of 29.1 years and 64.0 h. Not more than 6×10^{-6} per cent of the total radioactivity is due to strontium-90.

Other gamma-emitting impurities. Examine the gamma-ray spectrum of the decayed material for the presence of other radionuclidic impurities, which should, where possible, be identified and quantified. The total gamma radioactivity due to these impurities does not exceed 0.01 per cent of the total radioactivity.

Alpha-emitting impurities. Measure the alpha radioactivity of the decayed material to detect any alpha-emitting radionuclidic impurities, which should, where possible, be identified and quantified. The total alpha radio-activity due to these impurities does not exceed 1×10^{-7} per cent of the total radioactivity.

Radiochemical purity Examine by descending paper chromatography (*2.2.26*), as described in the monograph on *Radiopharmaceutical preparations (125)*.

Test solution. Dilute the preparation to be examined with *water R* to a suitable radioactive concentration.

Apply 5 µl of the test solution. Develop for 2 h using a mixture of 20 volumes of *water R* and 80 volumes of *methanol R*. Allow the paper to dry. Determine the distribution of radioactivity using a suitable detector. Not less than 95 per cent of the total radioactivity is in the spot corresponding to pertechnetate ion, which has an R_f value of about 0.6.

Aluminium In a test tube about 12 mm in internal diameter, mix 1 ml of *acetate buffer solution pH 4.6 R* and 2 ml of a 1 in 2.5 dilution of the injection in *water R*. Add 0.05 ml of a 10 g/l solution of *chromazurol S R*. After 3 min, the colour of the solution is not more intense than that of a standard prepared at the same time and in the same manner using 2 ml of *aluminium standard solution (2 ppm Al) R* (5 ppm).

Sterility It complies with the test for sterility prescribed in the monograph on *Radiopharmaceutical preparations (125)*. The injection may be released for use before completion of the test.

RADIOACTIVITY

Measure the radioactivity as described in the monograph on *Radiopharmaceutical preparations (125)* using suitable counting equipment by comparison with a standardised technetium-99m solution or by measurement in an instrument calibrated with the aid of such a solution.

STORAGE

See *Radiopharmaceutical preparations (125)*.

LABELLING

See *Radiopharmaceutical preparations (125)*.

Ph Eur

Sodium Pertechnetate[99mTc] Injection (Non-fission)

Sodium Pertechnetate[99mTc] Injection (Non-fission) complies with the requirements of the 3rd edition of the European Pharmacopoeia [0283]. These requirements are reproduced after the heading 'Definition' below.

Ph Eur

This monograph applies to sodium pertechnetate (^{99m}Tc) injection obtained from molybdenum-99 produced by neutron irradiation of molybdenum. Sodium pertechnetate (^{99m}Tc) injection obtained from molybdenum-99 extracted from fission products of uranium is described in the monograph on Sodium Pertechnetate(^{99m}Tc) Injection (Fission) (124).

DEFINITION

Sodium pertechnetate (^{99m}Tc) injection (non-fission) is a sterile solution containing technetium-99m in the form of pertechnetate ion and made isotonic by the addition of sodium chloride. Technetium-99m is a radionuclide formed by the decay of molybdenum-99. Molybdenum-99 is a radioactive isotope of molybdenum produced by neutron irradiation of molybdenum. The injection contains not less than 90.0 per cent and not more than 110.0 per cent of the declared technetium-99m radioactivity at the date and hour stated on the label. Not less than 95 per cent of the radioactivity corresponds to technetium-99m in the form of pertechnetate ion.

The radioactivity due to radionuclides other than technetium-99m, apart from that due to technetium-99 resulting from the decay of technetium-99m is not greater than that shown below, expressed as a percentage of the total radioactivity and calculated with reference to the date and hour of administration.

Molybdenum-99	0.1 per cent
Other radionuclidic impurities	0.01 per cent

The injection may be prepared from a sterile preparation of molybdenum-99 under aseptic conditions.

CHARACTERS

A clear, colourless solution.

Technetium-99m has a half-life of 6.02 h and emits gamma radiation.

IDENTIFICATION

A. Record the gamma-ray spectrum using a suitable instrument as described in the monograph on *Radiopharmaceutical preparations (125)*. The spectrum does not differ significantly from that of a standardised technetium-99m solution either by direct comparison or by using an instrument calibrated with the aid of such a solution. Standardised technetium-99m and molybdenum-99 solutions are available from laboratories recognised by the competent authority. The most prominent gamma photon of technetium-99m has an energy of 0.140 MeV.

B. Examine the chromatogram obtained in the test for radiochemical purity. The distribution of radioactivity contributes to the identification of the preparation.

TESTS

pH (*2.2.3*). The pH of the injection is 4.0 to 8.0.

Radionuclidic purity Operate as described in the monograph on *Radiopharmaceutical preparations (125)*.

Preliminary test. To obtain an approximate estimate before use of the injection, take a volume equivalent to 37 MBq and record the gamma-ray spectrum using a sodium iodide detector with a shield of lead, of thickness 6 mm, interposed between the sample and the detector. The response in the region corresponding to the 0.740 MeV photon of molybdenum-99 does not exceed that obtained using 37 kBq of a standardised solution of molybdenum-99 measured under the same conditions, when all measurements are expressed with reference to the date and hour of administration.

Definitive test. Retain a sample of the injection for a sufficient time to allow the technetium-99m radioactivity to decay to a sufficiently low level to permit the detection of radionuclidic impurities. All measurements of radioactivity are expressed with reference to the date and hour of administration.

Molybdenum-99. Record the gamma-ray spectrum of the decayed material in a suitable instrument calibrated using a standardised molybdenum-99 solution. The most prominent gamma photons have energies of 0.181 MeV, 0.740 MeV and 0.778 MeV. Molybdenum-99 has a half-life of 66.0 h. Not more than 0.1 per cent of the total radioactivity is due to molybdenum-99.

Other gamma-emitting impurities. Examine the gamma-ray spectrum of the decayed material for the presence of other radionuclidic impurities, which should, where possible, be identified and quantified. The total radioactivity due to other radionuclidic impurities does not exceed 0.01 per cent of the total radioactivity.

Radiochemical purity Examine by descending paper chromatography (*2.2.26*), as described in the monograph on *Radiopharmaceutical preparations (125)*.

Test solution. Dilute the injection with *water R* to a suitable radioactive concentration.

Apply 5 µl of the test solution. Develop for 2 h using a mixture of 20 volumes of *water R* and 80 volumes of *methanol R*. Allow the paper to dry in air. Determine the distribution of radioactivity using a suitable detector. Not less than 95 per cent of the total radioactivity is found in the spot corresponding to pertechnetate ion, which has an R_f value of about 0.6.

Aluminium In a test tube about 12 mm in internal diameter, mix 1 ml of *acetate buffer solution pH 4.6 R* and 2 ml of a 1 in 2.5 dilution of the injection in *water R*. Add 0.05 ml of a 10 g/l solution of *chromazurol S R*. After 3 min, the colour of the solution is not more intense than that of a standard prepared at the same time in the same manner using 2 ml of *aluminium standard solution (2 ppm Al) R* (5 ppm).

Sterility It complies with the test for sterility prescribed in the monograph on *Radiopharmaceutical preparations (125)*. The injection may be released for use before completion of the test.

RADIOACTIVITY

Measure the radioactivity as described in the monograph

on *Radiopharmaceutical preparations (125)* using suitable counting equipment by comparison with a standardised technetium-99m solution or by measurement in an instrument calibrated with the aid of such a solution.

STORAGE

See *Radiopharmaceutical preparations (125)*.

LABELLING

See *Radiopharmaceutical preparations (125)*.

Ph Eur

Sodium Phosphate[^{32}P] Injection

Sodium Phosphate[^{32}P] Injection complies with the requirements of the 3rd edition of the European Pharmacopoeia [0284]. These requirements are reproduced after the heading 'Definition' below.

Ph Eur

DEFINITION

Sodium phosphate (^{32}P) injection is a sterile solution of disodium and monosodium (^{32}P) orthophosphates made isotonic by the addition of sodium chloride. Phosphorus-32 is a radioactive isotope of phosphorus and may be produced by neutron irradiation of sulphur. The injection contains not less than 90.0 per cent and not more than 110.0 per cent of the declared phosphorus-32 radioactivity at the date and hour stated on the label. Not less than 95 per cent of the radioactivity corresponds to phosphorus-32 in the form of orthophosphate ion. The specific radioactivity is not less than 11.1 MBq of phosphorus-32 per milligram of orthophosphate ion.

CHARACTERS

A clear, colourless solution.

Phosphorus-32 has a half-life of 14.3 days and emits beta radiation.

IDENTIFICATION

A. Record the beta-ray spectrum or the beta-ray absorption curve using a suitable method as described in the monograph on *Radiopharmaceutical preparations (125)*. The spectrum or curve does not differ significantly from that of a standardised phosphorus-32 solution obtained under the same conditions. Standardised phosphorus-32 solutions are available from laboratories recognised by the competent authority. The maximum energy of the beta radiation is 1.71 MeV.

B. Examine the chromatogram obtained in the test for radiochemical purity. The distribution of radioactivity contributes to the identification of the preparation.

TESTS

pH (*2.2.3*). The pH of the injection is 6.0 to 8.0.

Radionuclidic purity Record the beta-ray spectrum or the beta-ray absorption curve using a suitable method as described in the monograph on *Radiopharmaceutical preparations (125)*. The spectrum or curve does not differ significantly from that of a standardised phosphorus-32 solution obtained under the same conditions.

Radiochemical purity Examine by ascending paper chromatography (*2.2.26*), as described in the monograph on *Radiopharmaceutical preparations (125)*.

Test solution. Dilute the injection with *water R* until the radioactivity is equivalent to 10,000 to 20,000 counts per minute per 10 μl

Reference solution. Prepare a solution of *phosphoric acid R* containing 2 mg of phosphorus per millilitre.

Using a strip of paper 25 mm wide and about 300 mm long, apply 10 μl of the reference solution. Apply to the same starting-point 10 μl of the test solution. Develop for 16 h using a mixture of 0.3 ml of *ammonia R*, 5 g of *trichloroacetic acid R*, 25 ml of *water R* and 75 ml of *2-propanol R*. Allow the paper to dry in air. Determine the position of the inactive phosphoric acid by spraying with a 50 g/l solution of *perchloric acid R* and then with a 10 g/l solution of *ammonium molybdate R*. Expose the paper to *hydrogen sulphide R*. A blue colour develops. Determine the position of the radioactive spot by autoradiography or by measuring the radioactivity over the whole length of the chromatogram. Not less than 95 per cent of the total radioactivity of the chromatogram is found in the spot corresponding to phosphoric acid.

Phosphates Dilute the injection with *water R* to give a radioactive concentration of 370 kBq of phosphorus-32 per millilitre. Mix in a volumetric flask, with shaking, 1.0 ml of the solution with a mixture of 0.5 ml of a 2.5 g/l solution of *ammonium vanadate R*, 0.5 ml of *ammonium molybdate solution R* and 1 ml of *perchloric acid R* and dilute to 5.0 ml with *water R*. After 30 min, the solution is not more intensely coloured than a standard prepared at the same time in the same manner using 1.0 ml of a solution containing 33 mg of orthophosphate ion per litre.

Sterility It complies with the test for sterility prescribed in the monograph on *Radiopharmaceutical preparations (125)*. The injection may be released for use before completion of the test.

RADIOACTIVITY

Measure the radioactivity as described in the monograph on *Radiopharmaceutical preparations (125)* using suitable counting equipment by comparison with a standardised phosphorus-32 solution or by measurement in an instrument calibrated with the aid of such a solution.

STORAGE

See *Radiopharmaceutical preparations (125)*.

LABELLING

See *Radiopharmaceutical preparations (125)*.

Ph Eur

Technetium[^{99m}Tc] Albumin Injection

Technetium[^{99m}Tc] Albumin Injection complies with the requirements of the 3rd edition of the European Pharmacopoeia for Technetium[^{99m}Tc] Human Albumin Injection [0640]. These requirements are reproduced after the heading 'Definition' below.

Ph Eur

DEFINITION

Technetium (^{99m}Tc) human albumin injection is a sterile, apyrogenic solution of human albumin labelled with technetium-99m. It contains a reducing substance, such as a tin salt in an amount not exceeding 1 mg of Sn per millilitre; it may contain a suitable buffer and an antimicrobial preservative. Although, at present, no definite value for a maximum limit of tin can be fixed, available evidence tends to suggest the importance of keeping the ratio of tin to albumin as low as possible. The human albumin used complies with the requirements of the monograph on *Human albumin solution (255)*. The injection contains not less than 90.0 per cent and not more than 110.0 per cent of the declared technetium-99m radioactivity at the date and hour stated on the label. The injection contains not less than 90.0 per cent and not more than 110.0 per cent of the quantity of albumin stated on the label. Not less than 80 per cent of the radioactivity is associated with the albumin fractions II to V. Not more than 5.0 per cent of the radioactivity due to technetium-99m corresponds to free pertechnetate, as determined by the method described in the test for radiochemical purity.

It is prepared from sodium pertechnetate (^{99m}Tc) injection (fission or non-fission) using suitable sterile and apyrogenic ingredients and calculating the ratio of radionuclidic impurities with reference to the date and hour of administration.

CHARACTERS

A clear, colourless or pale-yellow solution.

Technetium-99m has a half-life of 6.02 h and emits gamma radiation.

IDENTIFICATION

A. Record the gamma-ray spectrum using a suitable instrument as described in the monograph on *Radiopharmaceutical preparations (125)*. The spectrum does not differ significantly from that of a standardised technetium-99m solution either by direct comparison or by using an instrument calibrated with the aid of such a solution. Standardised technetium-99m and molybdenum-99 solutions are available from laboratories recognised by the competent authority. The most prominent gamma photon of technetium-99m has an energy of 0.140 MeV.

B. Using a suitable range of species-specific antisera, carry out precipitation tests on the preparation to be examined. The test is to be carried out using antisera specific to the plasma proteins of each species of domestic animal currently used in the preparation of materials of biological origin in the country concerned. The injection is shown to contain proteins of human origin and gives negative results with antisera specific to plasma proteins of other species.

C. Examine by a suitable immunoelectrophoresis technique. Using antiserum to normal human serum, compare normal human serum and the injection to be examined, both diluted if necessary. The main component of the injection to be examined corresponds to the main component of the normal human serum. The diluted solution may show the presence of small quantities of other plasma proteins.

TESTS

pH (*2.2.3*). The pH of the injection is 2.0 to 6.5.

Radiochemical purity

(a) Examine by thin-layer chromatography (*2.2.27*) as described in the monograph on *Radiopharmaceutical preparations (125)*, using silica gel as the coating substance on a glass-fibre sheet. Heat the plate at 110°C for 10 min. Use a plate such that during development the mobile phase migrates over a distance of 10 cm to 15 cm in about 10 min.

Apply to the plate 5 µl to 10 µl of the injection to be examined and allow to dry. Develop over a path of 10 cm to 15 cm using *methyl ethyl ketone R*. Allow the plate to dry. Determine the distribution of radioactivity using a suitable detector. The technetium-99m human albumin complex remains at the starting-point and pertechnetate ion migrates near to the solvent front. Not more than 5.0 per cent of the technetium-99m radioactivity corresponds to technetium in the form of pertechnetate ion.

(b) Examine by size-exclusion chromatography (*2.2.30*).

Mobile phase (concentrated). Dissolve 1.124 g of *potassium dihydrogen phosphate R*, 4.210 g of *disodium hydrogen phosphate R*, 1.17 g of *sodium chloride R* and 0.10 g of *sodium azide R* in 100 ml of *water R*.

Test solution. Mix 0.25 ml of the injection to be examined with 0.25 ml of the mobile phase (concentrated). Use immediately after dilution.

The chromatographic procedure may be carried out using:
— a stainless steel column 0.6 m long and 7.5 mm in internal diameter, packed with *silica gel for size-exclusion chromatography R*,
— as the mobile phase at a flow rate of 0.6 ml per minute a mixture of equal volumes of mobile phase (concentrated) and *water R*,
— a radioactivity detector set for technetium-99m,
— a loop injector.

Inject 200 µl of the test solution. Continue the chromatography for at least 10 min after background level is reached.

Peaks are eluted with the following retention times:

I	High molecular mass compound	19–20 min
II	Poly III-albumin	23–24 min
III	Poly II-albumin	25–27 min
IV	Poly I-albumin	28–29 min
V	Human serum albumin	32–33 min
VI	Tin colloid	40–47 min
VII	Pertechnetate	48 min

At least 80 per cent of the radioactivity applied to the column is associated with the albumin fractions II to V.

Albumin

Reference solution. Dilute *human albumin solution R* with a 9 g/l solution of *sodium chloride R* to a concentration of 5 mg of albumin per millilitre.

To 1.0 ml of the injection to be examined and to 1.0 ml of the reference solution add 4.0 ml of *biuret reagent R* and mix. After exactly 30 min, measure the absorbance (*2.2.25*) of each solution at 540 nm, using as the compensation liquid a 9 g/l solution of *sodium chloride R* treated in the same manner. From the absorbances measured, calculate the content of albumin in the injection to be examined in milligrams per millilitre.

Tin

Test solution. To 1.0 ml of the injection to be examined add 1.0 ml of *2M hydrochloric acid*. Heat in a water-bath at 100°C for 30 min. Cool and centrifuge at 300 g for 10 min. Dilute 1.0 ml of the supernatant liquid to 10 ml with *1M hydrochloric acid*.

Reference solution. Dissolve 95 mg of *stannous chloride R* in

1M hydrochloric acid and dilute to 1000.0 ml with the same acid.

To 1.0 ml of each solution add 0.4 ml of a 20 g/l solution of *sodium lauryl sulphate R*, 0.05 ml of *thioglycollic acid R*, 0.1 ml of *dithiol reagent R* and 3.0 ml of *0.2M hydrochloric acid*. Mix. Measure the absorbance (*2.2.25*) of each solution at 540 nm, using *0.2M hydrochloric acid* as the compensation liquid. The absorbance of the test solution is not greater than that of the reference solution (1 mg of Sn per millilitre).

Physiological distribution Inject a volume not greater than 0.5 ml and containing not more than 1.0 mg of albumin into a suitable vein such as a caudal vein or a saphenous vein of each of three male rats, each weighing 150 g to 250 g. Measure the radioactivity in the syringe before and after the injection. Kill the rats 30 min after the injection. Take one millilitre of blood by a suitable method and remove the liver and, if a caudal vein has been used for the injection, the tail. Using a suitable instrument as described in the monograph on *Radiopharmaceutical preparations (125)* determine the radioactivity in 1 ml of blood, in the liver and, if a caudal vein has been used for the injection, in the tail. Determine the percentage of radioactivity in the liver and in 1 ml of blood with respect to the total radioactivity calculated as the difference between the measurements made on the syringe minus the activity in the tail (if a caudal vein has been used for the injection). Correct the blood concentration by multiplying by a factor of *m*/200 where m is the body mass of the rat in grams. In not fewer than two of the three rats used, the radioactivity in the liver is not more than 15 per cent and that in blood, after correction, is not less than 3.5 per cent.

Sterility It complies with the test for sterility prescribed in the monograph on *Radiopharmaceutical preparations (125)*. The injection may be released for use before completion of the test.

Bacterial endotoxins (*2.6.14*). Not more than 175/*V* I.U. of endotoxin per millilitre, *V* being the maximum recommended dose in millilitres.

RADIOACTIVITY

Measure the radioactivity as described in the monograph on *Radiopharmaceutical preparations (125)* using suitable counting equipment by comparison with a standardised technetium-99m solution or by measurement in an instrument calibrated with the aid of such a solution.

STORAGE

See *Radiopharmaceutical preparations (125)*.

LABELLING

See *Radiopharmaceutical preparations (125)*.

The label states:

— the amount of albumin,

— the amount of tin, if any.

Ph Eur

Technetium[^{99m}Tc] Colloidal Rhenium Sulphide Injection

Technetium[^{99m}Tc] Colloidal Rhenium Sulphide Injection complies with the requirements of the 3rd edition of the European Pharmacopoeia [0126]. These requirements are reproduced after the heading 'Definition' below.

Ph Eur

DEFINITION

Technetium (^{99m}Tc) colloidal rhenium sulphide injection is a sterile, apyrogenic colloidal dispersion of rhenium sulphide the micelles of which are labelled with technetium-99m. It is stabilised with gelatin. The injection contains not less than 90.0 per cent and not more than 110.0 per cent of the declared technetium-99m radioactivity at the date and hour stated on the label. Not less than 92 per cent of the radioactivity corresponds to technetium-99m in colloidal form. The pH of the injection may be adjusted by the addition of a suitable buffer such as a citrate buffer solution. The injection contains a variable amount of colloidal rhenium sulphide, not exceeding 0.22 mg of rhenium (Re) per millilitre, according to the method of preparation.

It is prepared from sodium pertechnetate (^{99m}Tc) injection (fission or non-fission) using suitable sterile, apyrogenic ingredients and calculating the ratio of radionuclidic impurities with reference to the date and hour of administration.

CHARACTERS

A light-brown liquid.

Technetium-99m has a half-life of 6.02 h and emits gamma radiation.

IDENTIFICATION

A. Record the gamma-ray spectrum using a suitable instrument as described in the monograph on *Radiopharmaceutical preparations (125)*. The spectrum does not differ significantly from that of a standardised technetium-99m solution either by direct comparison or by using an instrument calibrated with the aid of such a solution. Standardised technetium-99m and molybdenum-99 solutions are available from laboratories recognised by the competent authority. The most prominent gamma photon of technetium-99m has an energy of 0.140 MeV.

B. Examine the chromatogram obtained in the test for radiochemical purity. The distribution of radioactivity contributes to the identification of the injection.

C. To 1 ml add 5 ml of *hydrochloric acid R*, 5 ml of a 50 g/l solution of *thiourea R* and 1 ml of a 200 g/l solution of *stannous chloride R* in *hydrochloric acid R*. A yellow colour is produced.

TESTS

pH (*2.2.3*). The pH of the injection is 4.0 to 7.0.

Rhenium

Test solution. Use 1 ml of the injection to be examined.

Reference solutions. Using a solution containing 100 µg of *potassium perrhenate R* (equivalent to 60 ppm of Re) and 240 µg of *sodium thiosulphate R* per millilitre, prepare a suitable range of solutions and dilute to the same final volume with *water R*.

To the test solution and to 1 ml of each of the reference solutions add 5 ml of *hydrochloric acid R*, 5 ml of a 50 g/l solution of *thiourea R* and 1 ml of a 200 g/l solution of *stannous chloride R* in *hydrochloric acid R* and dilute to 25.0 ml with *water R*. Allow to stand for 40 min and measure the absorbance (*2.2.25*) of each solution at 400 nm, using a reagent blank as the compensation liquid. Using the absorbances obtained with the reference solutions, draw a calibration curve and calculate the concentration of rhenium in the injection to be examined.

Radiochemical purity Examine by ascending paper chromatography (*2.2.26*), as described in the monograph on *Radiopharmaceutical preparations (125)*.

Apply to the paper 10 µl of the injection. Develop immediately over a path of 10 cm to 15 cm using a 9 g/l solution of *sodium chloride R*. Allow the paper to dry. Determine the distribution of radioactivity using a suitable detector. Technetium-99m in colloidal form remains at the starting-point and pertechnetate ion migrates with an R_f of about 0.6. There may be other impurities with an R_f of 0.8 to 0.9. The radioactivity corresponding to technetium-99m in colloidal form represents not less than 92 per cent of the total radioactivity of the chromatogram.

Physiological distribution Inject a volume not greater than 0.2 ml into the caudal vein of each of three mice each weighing 20 g to 25 g. Sacrifice the mice 20 min after the injection, remove the liver, spleen and lungs and measure the radioactivity in the organs using a suitable instrument as described in the monograph on *Radiopharmaceutical preparations (125)*. Measure the radioactivity in the rest of the body after having removed the tail. Determine the percentage of radioactivity in the liver, the spleen and the lungs from the expression:

$$\frac{A}{B} \times 100$$

A = radioactivity of the organ concerned,

B = total radioactivity in the liver, the spleen, the lungs and the rest of the body.

In each of the three mice at least 80 per cent of the radioactivity is found in the liver and spleen and not more than 5 per cent in the lungs. If the distribution of radioactivity in one of the three mice does not correspond to the prescribed proportions, repeat the test on a further three mice. The preparation complies with the test if the prescribed distribution of radioactivity is found in five of the six mice used. The injection may be released for use before completion of the test.

Sterility It complies with the test for sterility prescribed in the monograph on *Radiopharmaceutical preparations (125)*. The injection may be released for use before completion of the test.

Pyrogens It complies with the test for pyrogens prescribed in the monograph on *Radiopharmaceutical preparations (125)*. Inject not less than 0.1 ml per kilogram of the rabbit's mass. The injection may be released for use before completion of the test.

RADIOACTIVITY

Measure the radioactivity as described in the monograph on *Radiopharmaceutical preparations (125)* using suitable counting equipment by comparison with a standardised technetium-99m solution or by measurement in an instrument calibrated with the aid of such a solution.

STORAGE

See *Radiopharmaceutical preparations (125)*.

LABELLING

See *Radiopharmaceutical preparations (125)*.

The label states, in particular, the quantity of rhenium per millilitre.

Ph Eur

Technetium[^{99m}Tc] Colloidal Sulphur Injection

Technetium[^{99m}Tc] Colloidal Sulphur Injection complies with the requirements of the 3rd edition of the European Pharmacopoeia [0131]. These requirements are reproduced after the heading 'Definition' below.

Ph Eur

DEFINITION

Technetium (^{99m}Tc) colloidal sulphur injection is a sterile, apyrogenic colloidal dispersion of sulphur, the micelles of which are labelled with technetium-99m. It may be stabilised with a colloid-protecting substance based on gelatin. The injection contains not less than 90.0 per cent and not more than 110.0 per cent of the declared technetium-99m radioactivity at the date and hour stated on the label. Not less than 92 per cent of the radioactivity corresponds to technetium-99m in colloidal form. The pH of the injection may be adjusted by the addition of a suitable buffer, such as an acetate, citrate or phosphate buffer solution. The injection contains a variable amount of colloidal sulphur, according to the method of preparation.

It is prepared from sodium pertechnetate (^{99m}Tc) injection (fission or non-fission) using suitable sterile, apyrogenic ingredients and calculating the ratio of radionuclidic impurities with reference to the date and hour of administration.

CHARACTERS

A clear to opalescent, colourless to yellowish liquid.

Technetium-99m has a half-life of 6.02 h and emits gamma radiation.

IDENTIFICATION

A. Record the gamma-ray spectrum using a suitable instrument as described in the monograph on *Radiopharmaceutical preparations (125)*. The spectrum does not differ significantly from that of a standardised technetium-99m solution either by direct comparison or by using an instrument calibrated with the aid of such a solution. Standardised technetium-99m and molybdenum-99 solutions are available from laboratories recognised by the competent authority. The most prominent gamma photon of technetium-99m has an energy of 0.140 MeV.

B. Examine the chromatogram obtained in the test for radiochemical purity. The distribution of radioactivity contributes to the identification of the injection.

C. In a test-tube 100 mm long and 16 mm in internal diameter, evaporate 0.2 ml of the injection to dryness. Dissolve the sulphur by shaking the residue with 0.2 ml of *pyridine R* and add about 20 mg of *benzoin R*. Cover the open end of the tube with a filter paper moistened with *lead acetate solution R*. Heat the test-tube in a bath containing glycerol at 150°C. The paper slowly becomes brown.

TESTS

pH (*2.2.3*). The pH of the injection is 4.0 to 7.0.

Radiochemical purity Examine by ascending paper chromatography (*2.2.26*), as described in the monograph on *Radiopharmaceutical preparations (125)*.

Apply to the paper 10 µl of the injection. Develop immediately over a path of 10 cm to 15 cm with a 9 g/l solution of *sodium chloride R*. Allow the paper to dry. Determine the distribution of radioactivity using a suitable detector. Technetium-99m in colloidal form remains at the starting-point and pertechnetate ion migrates with an R_f of 0.6. There may be other impurities of R_f 0.8 to 0.9. The radioactivity corresponding to technetium-99m in colloidal form represents not less than 92 per cent of the total radioactivity of the chromatogram.

Physiological distribution Inject a volume not greater than 0.2 ml into the caudal vein of each of three mice, each weighing 20 g to 25 g. Sacrifice the mice 20 min after the injection, remove the liver, spleen and lungs and measure the radioactivity in the organs using a suitable instrument as described in the monograph on *Radiopharmaceutical preparations (125)*. Measure the radioactivity in the rest of the body after having removed the tail. Determine the percentage of radioactivity in the liver, the spleen and the lungs from the expression:

$$\frac{A}{B} \times 100$$

A = radioactivity of the organ concerned,

B = total radioactivity in the liver, the spleen, the lungs and the rest of the body.

In each of the three mice at least 80 per cent of the radioactivity is found in the liver and spleen and not more than 5 per cent in the lungs. If the distribution of radioactivity in one of the three mice does not correspond to the prescribed proportions, repeat the test on a further three mice. The preparation complies with the test if the prescribed distribution of radioactivity is found in five of the six mice used. The injection may be released for use before completion of the test.

Sterility It complies with the test for sterility prescribed in the monograph on *Radiopharmaceutical preparations (125)*. The injection may be released for use before completion of the test.

Pyrogens It complies with the test for pyrogens prescribed in the monograph on *Radiopharmaceutical preparations (125)*. Inject not less than 0.1 ml per kilogram of the rabbit's mass. The injection may be released for use before completion of the test.

RADIOACTIVITY

Measure the radioactivity as described in the monograph on *Radiopharmaceutical preparations (125)* using suitable counting equipment by comparison with a standardised technetium-99m solution or by measurement in an instrument calibrated with the aid of such a solution.

STORAGE

See *Radiopharmaceutical preparations (125)*.

LABELLING

See *Radiopharmaceutical preparations (125)*.

Ph Eur

Technetium[^{99m}Tc] Colloidal Tin Injection

Technetium[^{99m}Tc] Colloidal Tin Injection complies with the requirements of the 3rd edition of the European Pharmacopoeia [0689]. These requirements are reproduced after the heading 'Definition' below.

Ph Eur

DEFINITION

Technetium (^{99m}Tc) colloidal tin injection is a sterile, colloidal dispersion of tin labelled with technetium-99m. The injection contains a variable quantity of tin not exceeding 1 mg of Sn per millilitre; it contains fluoride ions, it may be stabilised with a suitable, apyrogenic colloid-protecting substance and it may contain a suitable buffer. The injection contains not less than 90.0 per cent and not more than 110.0 per cent of the declared technetium-99m radioactivity at the date and hour stated on the label. Not less than 95 per cent of the radioactivity corresponds to technetium-99m in colloidal form.

It is prepared from sodium pertechnetate (^{99m}Tc) injection (fission or non-fission) using suitable sterile ingredients and calculating the ratio of radionuclidic impurities with reference to the date and hour of administration. Syringes for handling the eluate intended for labelling of the final product, or the final product, should not contain rubber parts.

CHARACTERS

A clear or opalescent, colourless liquid.

Technetium-99m has a half life of 6.02 h and emits gamma radiation.

IDENTIFICATION

A. Record the gamma-ray spectrum using a suitable instrument as described in the monograph on *Radiopharmaceutical preparations (125)*. The spectrum does not differ significantly from that of a standardised technetium-99m solution either by direct comparison or by using an instrument calibrated with the aid of such a solution. Standardised technetium-99m and molybdenum-99 solutions are available from laboratories recognised by the competent authority. The most prominent gamma photon of technetium-99m has an energy of 0.140 MeV.

B. Mix 0.05 ml of *zirconyl nitrate solution R* with 0.05 ml of *alizarin S solution R*. Add 0.05 ml of the injection to be examined. A yellow colour is produced.

TESTS

pH (*2.2.3*). The pH of the injection to be examined is 4.0 to 7.0.

Radiochemical purity Examine by thin-layer chromatography (*2.2.27*) as described in the monograph on *Radiopharmaceutical preparations (125)*, using silica gel as the coating substance on a glass-fibre sheet. Heat the plate at 110°C for 10 min. Use a plate such that during development the mobile phase migrates over a distance of 10 cm to 15 cm in about 10 min.

Apply to the plate 5 µl to 10 µl of the injection to be examined. Develop immediately over a path of 10 cm to 15 cm using a 9 g/l solution of *sodium chloride R* purged with *nitrogen R*. Allow the plate to dry. Determine the distribution of radioactivity using a suitable detector. Technetium-99m in colloidal form remains at the starting point and pertechnetate ion migrates near to the solvent front. Not less than 95 per cent of the technetium-99m radioactivity corresponds to technetium in colloidal form.

Tin

Test solution. Dilute 3.0 ml of the injection to be examined to 50.0 ml with *1M hydrochloric acid.*

Reference solution. Dissolve 0.115 g of *stannous chloride R* in *1M hydrochloric acid* and dilute to 1000.0 ml with the same acid.

To 1.0 ml of each solution add 0.4 ml of a 20 g/l solution of *sodium lauryl sulphate R*, 0.05 ml of *thioglycollic acid R*, 0.1 ml of *dithiol reagent R* and 3.0 ml of *0.2M hydrochloric acid.* Mix. Measure the absorbance (*2.2.25*) of each solution at 540 nm, using *0.2M hydrochloric acid* as the compensation liquid. The absorbance of the test solution is not greater than that of the reference solution (1 mg of Sn per millilitre).

Physiological distribution Inject not more than 0.2 ml into a caudal vein of each of three mice, each weighing 20 g to 25 g. Kill the mice 20 min after the injection and remove the liver, spleen and lungs. Measure the radioactivity in the organs using a suitable instrument as described in the monograph on *Radiopharmaceutical preparations (125)*. Measure the radioactivity in the rest of the body, after having removed the tail. Determine the percentage of radioactivity in the liver, the spleen and the lungs with respect to the total radioactivity of all organs and the rest of the body excluding the tail.

In each of the three mice at least 80 per cent of the radioactivity is found in the liver and spleen and not more than 5 per cent in the lungs. If the distribution of radioactivity in one of the three mice does not correspond to the prescribed proportions, repeat the test on a further three mice. The preparation complies with the test if the prescribed distribution of radioactivity is found in five of the six mice used.

Sterility It complies with the test for sterility prescribed in the monograph on *Radiopharmaceutical preparations (125)*. The injection may be released for use before completion of the test.

RADIOACTIVITY

Measure the radioactivity as described in the monograph on *Radiopharmaceutical preparations (125)* using suitable counting equipment by comparison with a standardised technetium-99m solution or by measurement in an instrument calibrated with the aid of such a solution.

STORAGE

See *Radiopharmaceutical preparations (125)*.

LABELLING

See *Radiopharmaceutical preparations (125)*.

Ph Eur

Technetium[^{99m}Tc] Etifenin Injection

Technetium[^{99m}Tc] Etifenin Injection complies with the requirements of the 3rd edition of the European Pharmacopoeia [0585]. These requirements are reproduced after the heading 'Definition' below.

Ph Eur

DEFINITION

Technetium (^{99m}Tc) etifenin injection is a sterile solution which may be prepared by mixing sodium pertechnetate (^{99m}Tc) injection (fission or non-fission) with solutions of etifenin [[(2,6-diethylphenyl)carbamoylmethylimino]diacetic acid; $C_{16}H_{22}N_2O_5$] and stannous chloride. The injection contains a variable quantity of tin (Sn) not exceeding 0.2 mg per millilitre. The injection contains not less than 90.0 per cent and not more than 110.0 per cent of the declared technetium-99m radioactivity at the date and hour stated on the label. Not less than 95.0 per cent of the radioactivity corresponds to technetium-99m complexed with etifenin.

It is prepared from sodium pertechnetate (^{99m}Tc) injection (fission or non-fission) using suitable, sterile ingredients and calculating the ratio of radionuclidic impurities with reference to the date and hour of administration.

CHARACTERS

A clear, colourless solution.

Technetium-99m has a half-life of 6.02 h and emits gamma radiation.

IDENTIFICATION

A. Record the gamma-ray spectrum using a suitable instrument as described in the monograph on *Radiopharmaceutical preparations (125)*. The spectrum does not differ significantly from that of a standardised technetium-99m solution either by direct comparison or by using an instrument calibrated with the aid of such a solution. Standardised technetium-99m and molybdenum-99 solutions are available from laboratories recognised by the competent authority. The most prominent gamma photon of technetium-99m has an energy of 0.140 MeV.

B. Examine by liquid chromatography (*2.2.29*).

Test solution. Dilute the injection to be examined with *methanol R* to obtain a solution containing about 1 mg of etifenin per millilitre.

Reference solution. Dissolve 5.0 mg of *etifenin CRS* in *methanol R* and dilute to 5.0 ml with the same solvent.

The chromatographic procedure may be carried out using:

- a column 0.25 m long and 4.6 mm in internal diameter packed with *octadecylsilyl silica gel for chromatography R* (5 µm to 10 µm),
- as mobile phase at a flow rate of 1 ml per minute a mixture of 20 volumes of *methanol R* and 80 volumes of a 14 g/l solution of *potassium dihydrogen phosphate R* adjusted to pH 2.5 by the addition of *phosphoric acid R*,
- a spectrophotometer set at 230 nm.

Inject 20 µl of each solution. The principal peak in the chromatogram obtained with the test solution has a similar retention time to the principal peak in the chromatogram obtained with the reference solution.

TESTS

pH (*2.2.3*). The pH of the injection is 4.0 to 6.0.

Radiochemical purity Examine by thin-layer chromatography (*2.2.27*), as described in the monograph on *Radiopharmaceutical preparations (125)*, using silicic acid as the coating substance on a glass-fibre sheet. Heat the plate at 110°C for l0 min. The plate used should be such that during development the mobile phase moves over a distance of 10 cm to 15 cm in about 15 min.

Apply to the plate 5 µl to 10 µl of the injection to be examined. Develop immediately over a path of 10 cm to 15 cm using a 9 g/l solution of *sodium chloride R*. Allow the plate to dry. Determine the distribution of radioactivity using a suitable detector. Technetium-99m complexed with etifenin migrates almost to the middle of the chromatogram and pertechnetate ion migrates with the solvent front. Impurities in colloidal form remain at the starting point. The radioactivity corresponding to technetium-99m complexed with etifenin represents not less than 95.0 per cent of the total radioactivity of the chromatogram.

Physiological distribution Inject 0.1 ml (equivalent to about 3.7 MBq) into a caudal vein of each of three mice, each weighing 20 g to 25 g. Kill the mice l h after the injection. Remove the liver, gall-bladder, small intestine, large intestine and kidneys, collecting excreted urine. Measure the radioactivity in the organs using a suitable instrument as described in the monograph on *Radiopharmaceutical preparations (125)*. Measure the radioactivity of the rest of the body, after having removed the tail. Determine the percentage of radioactivity in each organ from the expression:

$$\frac{A}{B} \times 100$$

A = radioactivity of the organ concerned,

B = radioactivity of all organs and the rest of the body, excluding the tail.

In not fewer than two mice the sum of the percentages of radioactivity in the gall-bladder and small and large intestine is not less than 80 per cent. Not more than 3 per cent of the radioactivity is present in the liver, and not more than 2 per cent in the kidneys

Tin

Test solution. Dilute 1.0 ml of the injection to be examined to 5.0 ml with *1M hydrochloric acid.*

Reference solution. Prepare a reference solution containing 0.075 mg of *stannous chloride R* per millilitre in *1M hydrochloric acid.*

To 1.0 ml of each solution add 0.4 ml of a 20 g/l solution of *sodium lauryl sulphate R*, 0.05 ml of *thioglycollic acid R*, 0.l ml of *dithiol reagent R* and 3.0 ml of *0.2M hydrochloric acid.* Mix. Measure the absorbance (*2.2.25*) of each solution at 540 nm, using *0.2M hydrochloric acid* as the compensation liquid. The absorbance of the test solution is not greater than that of the reference solution (0.2 mg of Sn per millilitre).

Sterility It complies with the test for sterility prescribed in the monograph on *Radiopharmaceutical preparations (125)*. The injection may be released for use before completion of the test.

RADIOACTIVITY

Measure the radioactivity as described in the monograph on *Radiopharmaceutical preparations (125)* using suitable counting equipment by comparison with a standardised technetium-99m solution or by measurement in an instrument calibrated with the aid of such a solution.

STORAGE

See *Radiopharmaceutical preparations (125)*.

LABELLING

See *Radiopharmaceutical preparations (125)*.

Ph Eur

Technetium[^{99m}Tc] Gluconate Injection

Technetium[^{99m}Tc] Gluconate Injection complies with the requirements of the 3rd edition of the European Pharmacopoeia [1047]. These requirements are reproduced after the heading 'Definition' below.

Ph Eur

DEFINITION

Technetium (^{99m}Tc) gluconate injection is a sterile solution, which may be prepared by mixing solutions of calcium gluconate and a stannous salt or other suitable reducing agent with sodium pertechnetate (^{99m}Tc) injection (fission or non-fission). The injection contains not less than 90.0 per cent and not more than 110.0 per cent of the declared technetium-99m radioactivity at the date and hour stated on the label. Not less than 90 per cent of the radioactivity corresponds to technetium-99m gluconate complex.

It is prepared from sodium pertechnetate (^{99m}Tc) injection (fission or non-fission) using suitable sterile ingredients and calculating the ratio of radionuclidic impurities with reference to the date and hour of administration.

CHARACTERS

A slightly opalescent solution.

Technetium-99m has a half-life of 6.02 h and emits gamma radiation.

IDENTIFICATION

A. Record the gamma-ray spectrum using a suitable instrument as described in the monograph on *Radiopharmaceutical preparations (125)*. The spectrum does not differ significantly from that of a standardised technetium-99m solution either by direct comparison or by using an instrument calibrated with the aid of such a solution. Standardised technetium-99m and molybdenum-99 solutions are available from laboratories recognised by the competent authority. The most prominent gamma photon of technetium-99m has an energy of 0.140 MeV.

B. 5 µl of the solution complies with identification A prescribed in the monograph on *Calcium gluconate (172)*.

C. Examine the chromatograms obtained in the test for radiochemical purity. The distribution of the radioactivity contributes to the identification of the preparation.

TESTS

pH (*2.2.3*). The pH of the solution is 6.0 to 8.5.

Radiochemical purity Examine by thin-layer chromatography (*2.2.27*) as described in the monograph on *Radiopharmaceutical preparations (125)*, using silica gel as the coating substance on a glass-fibre sheet. Heat the plate at 110°C for 10 min. Use a plate such that during development the mobile phase migrates over a distance of 10 cm to 15 cm in about 10 min.

a) Apply to the plate 5 µl to 10 µl of the solution to be examined. Develop immediately over a path of 10 cm to 15 cm using a 9 g/l solution of *sodium chloride R*. Allow the plate to dry. Determine the distribution of radioactivity using a suitable detector. Impurities in colloidal form remain at the starting point. Technetium gluconate complex and pertechnetate ion migrate near to the solvent front.

b) Apply to the plate 5 µl to 10 µl of the solution to be examined and allow to dry. Develop over a path of 10 cm to 15 cm using *methyl ethyl ketone R*. Dry in a current of warm air. Determine the distribution of radioactivity using a suitable detector. Pertechnetate ion impurity migrates near to the solvent front. Technetium gluconate complex and technetium in colloidal form remain at the starting point.

The sum of the percentages of radioactivity corresponding to impurities in the chromatograms obtained in test (a) and (b) does not exceed 10 per cent.

Physiological distribution Inject a volume not greater than 0.2 ml into the caudal vein of each of three rats weighing 150 g to 250 g. Measure the radioactivity of the syringe before and after injection. Sacrifice the rats 30 min after the injection. Remove at least 1 g of blood by a suitable method and remove the kidneys, the liver, the bladder plus voided urine and the tail. Weigh the sample of blood.

Determine the radioactivity in the organs, the blood sample and the tail using a suitable instrument as described in the monograph on *Radiopharmaceutical preparations (125)*. Calculate the percentage of radioactivity in each organ and in 1 g of blood with respect to the total radioactivity calculated as the difference between the two measurements made on the syringe minus the activity in the tail. Correct the blood concentration by multiplying by a factor of $m/200$ where m is the body mass of the rat in grams.

In not fewer than two of the three rats used, the radioactivity in the kidneys is not less than 15 per cent, that in the bladder plus voided urine is not less than 20 per cent and that in the liver is not more than 5 per cent. The radioactivity in the blood, after correction, is not more than 0.50 per cent.

Sterility It complies with the test for sterility prescribed in the monograph on *Radiopharmaceutical preparations (125)*. The injection may be released for use before completion of the test.

RADIOACTIVITY

Measure the radioactivity as described in the monograph on *Radiopharmaceutical preparations (125)* using suitable counting equipment by comparison with a standardised technetium-99m solution or by measurement in an instrument calibrated with the aid of such a solution.

STORAGE

See *Radiopharmaceutical preparations (125)*.

LABELLING

See *Radiopharmaceutical preparations (125)*.

Ph Eur

Technetium[^{99m}Tc] Macrosalb Injection

Technetium[^{99m}Tc] Macrosalb Injection complies with the requirements of the 3rd edition of the European Pharmacopoeia [0296]. These requirements are reproduced after the heading 'Definition' below.

Ph Eur

DEFINITION

Technetium (^{99m}Tc) macrosalb injection is a sterile, apyrogenic suspension of human albumin in the form of irregular insoluble aggregates obtained by denaturing human albumin in aqueous solution; the particles are labelled with technetium-99m. The injection contains reducing substances, such as tin salts in an amount not exceeding 3 mg of Sn per millilitre; it may contain a suitable buffer such as acetate, citrate or phosphate buffer and also non-denatured human albumin and an antimicrobial preservative such as benzyl alcohol. The human albumin employed complies with the requirements prescribed in the monograph on *Human albumin solution (255)*. The injection contains not less than 90.0 per cent and not more than 110.0 per cent of the declared technetium-99m radioactivity at the date and hour stated on the label. Not less than 90 per cent of the technetium-99m is bound to the particles of the suspension as determined by the test for non-filterable radioactivity. The particles have a typical diameter between 10 µm and 100 µm. The specific radioactivity is not less than 37 MBq of technetium-99m per milligram of aggregated albumin at the date and hour of administration.

It is prepared from sodium pertechnetate (^{99m}Tc) injection (fission or non-fission) using suitable sterile and apyrogenic ingredients and calculating the ratio of radionuclidic impurities with reference to the date and hour of administration.

CHARACTERS

A white suspension which may separate on standing.

Technetium-99m has a half-life of 6.02 h and emits gamma radiation.

IDENTIFICATION

A. Record the gamma-ray spectrum using a suitable instrument as described in the monograph on *Radiopharmaceutical preparations (125)*. The spectrum does not differ significantly from that of a standardised technetium-99m solution either by direct comparison or by using an instrument calibrated with the aid of such a solution. Standardised technetium-99m and molybdenum-99 solutions are available from laboratories recognised by the competent authority. The most prominent gamma photon of technetium-99m has an energy of 0.140 MeV.

B. The tests for non-filterable radioactivity and particle

size contribute to the identification of the preparation.

C. Transfer 1 ml of the injection to a centrifuge tube and centrifuge at 2500 g for 5 min to 10 min. Decant the supernatant liquid. To the residue add 5 ml of *cupri-tartaric solution R2*, mix and allow to stand for 10 min. If necessary, heat to dissolve the particles and allow to cool. Add rapidly 0.5 ml of *dilute phosphomolybdotungstic reagent R*, mixing immediately. A blue colour develops.

TESTS

pH (*2.2.3*). The pH of the injection is 3.8 to 7.5.

Non-filterable radioactivity Use a polycarbonate membrane filter 13 mm to 25 mm in diameter, 10 µm thick and with circular pores 3 µm in diameter. Fit the membrane into a suitable holder. Place 0.2 ml of the injection on the membrane and filter, adding 20 ml of a 9 g/l solution of *sodium chloride R* during the filtration. The radioactivity remaining on the membrane represents not less than 90 per cent of the total radioactivity of the injection.

Particle size Examine using a microscope. Dilute the injection if necessary so that the number of particles is just low enough for individual particles to be distinguished. Using a syringe fitted with a needle having a calibre not less than 0.35 mm, place a suitable volume in a suitable counting chamber such as a haemocytometer cell, taking care not to overfill the chamber. Allow the suspension to settle for 1 min and carefully add a cover slide without squeezing the sample. Scan an area corresponding to at least 5000 particles. Not more than 10 particles have a maximum dimension greater than 100 µm. No particle having a maximum dimension greater than 150 µm is present.

Aggregated albumin

Test solution. Transfer a volume of the injection expected to contain about 1 mg of aggregated albumin to a centrifuge tube and centrifuge at about 2500 g for 5 min to 10 min. Decant the supernatant liquid. Resuspend the sediment in 2.0 ml of a 9 g/l solution of *sodium chloride R*. Centrifuge at 2500 g for 5 min to 10 min. Decant the supernatant liquid. Resuspend the sediment in 5.0 ml of *sodium carbonate solution R1*. Heat in a water-bath at 80°C to 90°C to dissolve the aggregated albumin. Allow to cool, transfer to a volumetric flask and dilute to 10.0 ml with *sodium carbonate solution R1*.

Reference solutions. Prepare a range of reference solutions containing 0.05 mg to 0.2 mg of human albumin per millilitre in *sodium carbonate solution R1*.

Introduce 3.0 ml of each solution separately into 25 ml flasks. To each flask add 15.0 ml of *cupri-tartaric solution R2*, mix and allow to stand for 10 min. Add rapidly 1.5 ml of *dilute phosphomolybdotungstic reagent R* and mix immediately. Allow to stand for 30 min and measure the absorbance (*2.2.25*) at 750 nm using *sodium carbonate solution R1* as the compensation liquid. Using the absorbances obtained with the reference solutions, draw a calibration curve and calculate the content of aggregated albumin in the injection.

Tin

Test solution. To 1.0 ml of the injection add 1.0 ml of *2M hydrochloric acid*. Heat in a water-bath for 30 min. Cool and centrifuge for 10 min at 300 *g*. Dilute 1.0 ml of the supernatant liquid to 25.0 ml with *1M hydrochloric acid*.

Reference solution. Dissolve 0.115 g of *stannous chloride R* in *1M hydrochloric acid* and dilute to 1000.0 ml with the same acid.

To 1.0 ml of each solution add 0.4 ml of a 20 g/l solution of *sodium lauryl sulphate R*, 0.05 ml of *thioglycollic acid R*, 0.1 ml of *dithiol reagent R* and 3.0 ml of *0.2M hydrochloric acid*. Mix. Measure the absorbance (*2.2.25*) of each solution at 540 nm, using *0.2M hydrochloric acid* as the compensation liquid. The absorbance of the test solution is not greater than that of the reference solution (3 mg of Sn per millilitre).

Physiological distribution Inject a volume not greater than 0.2 ml into the caudal vein of each of three rats weighing 150 g to 250 g. Kill the rats 15 min after the injection, remove the liver, the spleen and the lungs and measure the radioactivity in the organs using a suitable instrument as described in the monograph on *Radiopharmaceutical preparations (125)*. Measure the radioactivity in the rest of the body, including the blood, after having removed the tail. Determine the percentage of radioactivity in the lungs, the liver and the spleen from the expression:

$$\frac{A}{B} \times 100$$

A = radioactivity of the organ concerned,

B = total radioactivity in the liver, the spleen, the lungs and the rest of the body.

In not fewer than two of the three rats used, at least 80 per cent of the radioactivity is found in the lungs and not more than a total of 5 per cent in the liver and spleen. The injection may be released for use before completion of the test.

Sterility It complies with the test for sterility prescribed in the monograph on *Radiopharmaceutical preparations (125)*. The injection may be released for use before completion of the test.

Pyrogens It complies with the test for pyrogens prescribed in the monograph on *Radiopharmaceutical preparations (125)*. Inject into the animals not less than 0.1 ml per kilogram of the rabbit's mass. The injection may be released for use before completion of the test.

RADIOACTIVITY

Measure the radioactivity as described in the monograph on *Radiopharmaceutical preparations (125)* using suitable counting equipment by comparison with a standardised technetium-99m solution or by measurement in an instrument calibrated with the aid of such a solution.

STORAGE

See *Radiopharmaceutical preparations (125)*.

LABELLING

See *Radiopharmaceutical preparations (125)*.

The label states:

— that the preparation should be shaken before use,
— the quantity of tin per millilitre, if any,
— that the preparation is not to be used if after shaking, the suspension does not appear homogeneous.

Ph Eur

Technetium[99mTc] Medronate Injection

Technetium[99mTc] Medronate Injection complies with the requirements of the 3rd edition of the European Pharmacopoeia [0641]. These requirements are reproduced after the heading 'Definition' below.

Ph Eur

DEFINITION

Technetium (^{99m}Tc) medronate injection is a sterile solution which may be prepared by mixing solutions of sodium methylenediphosphonate and a stannous salt with sodium pertechnetate (^{99m}Tc) injection (fission or non-fission). The injection contains a variable quantity of tin (Sn) not exceeding 3 mg/ml; it may contain antimicrobial preservatives, antioxidants, stabilisers and buffers. The injection contains not less than 90.0 per cent and not more than 110.0 per cent of the declared technetium-99m radioactivity at the date and hour stated on the label. Radioactivity present as chemical forms other than technetium-99m medronate complex is not greater than 5.0 per cent of the total radioactivity.

It is prepared from sodium pertechnetate (^{99m}Tc) injection (fission or non-fission) using suitable sterile ingredients and calculating the ratio of radionuclidic impurities with reference to the date and hour of administration.

CHARACTERS

A clear, colourless solution.

Technetium-99m has a half life of 6.02 h and emits gamma radiation.

IDENTIFICATION

A. Record the gamma-ray spectrum using a suitable instrument as described in the monograph on *Radiopharmaceutical preparations (125)*. The spectrum does not differ significantly from that of a standardised technetium-99m solution either by direct comparison or by using an instrument calibrated with the aid of such a solution. Standardised technetium-99m and molybdenum-99 solutions are available from laboratories recognised by the competent authority. The most prominent gamma photon of technetium-99m has an energy of 0.140 MeV.

B. Examine the chromatograms obtained in the test for radiochemical purity. The distribution of the radioactivity contributes to the identification of the preparation.

C. Examine by thin-layer chromatography (*2.2.27*) as described in the monograph on *Radiopharmaceutical preparations (125)*, using cellulose as the coating substance.

Test solution. Dilute the injection to be examined with *water R* to obtain a solution containing about 0.1 mg to 0.5 mg of sodium medronate per millilitre.

Reference solution. Dissolve a suitable quantity (1 mg to 5 mg) of *medronic acid CRS* in a mixture of a 9.0 g/l solution of *sodium chloride R* and *water R* and dilute to 10 ml with the same solvent so as to obtain a solution similar to the test solution with regard to medronate and sodium chloride concentrations.

Apply separately to the plate 10 µl of each solution. Develop over a path of 12 cm to 14 cm (development time about 4 h) using a mixture of 20 volumes of *2-propanol R*, 30 volumes of *1M hydrochloric acid* and 60 volumes of *methyl ethyl ketone R*. Allow the plate to dry in air and spray with *ammonium molybdate solution R4*. Expose the plate to ultraviolet light at 254 nm for about 10 min. The principal spot in the chromatogram obtained with the test solution is similar in position and colour to the spot in the chromatogram obtained with the reference solution.

TESTS

pH (*2.2.3*). The pH of the solution is 3.5 to 7.5.

Radiochemical purity. Examine by thin-layer chromatography (*2.2.27*) as described in the monograph on *Radiopharmaceutical preparations (125)*, using silica gel as the coating substance on a glass-fibre sheet. Use plates such that during development, the mobile phase migrates 10 cm to 15 cm in about 10 min. Determine hydrolysed technetium and technetium in colloidal form by test (a) and pertechnetate ion by test (b).

(a) Apply to the plate 5 µl to 10 µl of the injection. Develop immediately over a path of 10 cm to 15 cm using a 136 g/l solution of *sodium acetate R*. Allow the plate to dry in air. Determine the distribution of radioactivity using a suitable detector. Hydrolysed technetium and technetium in colloidal form remain at the starting point. Technetium medronate complex and pertechnetate ion migrate near to the solvent front.

(b) Apply to the plate 5 µl to 10 µl of the injection and dry quickly. Develop over a path of 10 cm to 15 cm using *methyl ethyl ketone R*. Allow the plate to dry. Determine the distribution of radioactivity using a suitable detector. Pertechnetate ion migrates near to the solvent front. Technetium medronate complex and technetium in colloidal form remain at the starting-point.

The percentage of radioactivity corresponding to pertechnetate ion in the chromatogram obtained in test (b) is not greater than 2.0 per cent and the sum of the percentages of radioactivity corresponding to impurities in the chromatograms obtained in test (a) and test (b) (including pertechnetate ion) is not greater than 5.0 per cent.

Tin

Test solution. Dilute 1.0 ml of the solution to 50.0 ml with *1M hydrochloric acid.*

Reference solution. Dissolve 0.115 g of *stannous chloride R* in *1M hydrochloric acid* and dilute to 1000.0 ml with the same acid.

To 1.0 ml of each solution add 0.4 ml of a 20 g/l solution of *sodium lauryl sulphate R*, 0.05 ml of *thioglycollic acid R*, 0.1 ml of *dithiol reagent R* and 3.0 ml of *0.2M hydrochloric acid*. Mix. Measure the absorbance (*2.2.25*) of each solution at 540 nm, using *0.2M hydrochloric acid* as compensation liquid. The absorbance of the test solution is not greater than that of the reference solution (3 mg of Sn per millilitre).

Physiological distribution Inject a volume not greater than 0.2 ml, equivalent to not more than 0.05 mg of sodium medronate into a suitable vein such as a caudal vein or the saphenous vein of each of three rats, each weighing 150 g to 250 g. Measure the radioactivity in the syringe before and after injection. Kill the rats 2 h after the injection. Remove one femur, the liver, and some blood.

Weigh the blood. Remove the tail if a caudal vein has been used for the injection. Using a suitable instrument as described in the monograph on *Radiopharmaceutical preparations (125)* measure the radioactivity in the femurs, liver, and blood, and in the tail if a caudal vein has been used for the injection. Determine the percentage of radioactivity in each sample from the expression:

$$\frac{A}{B}\times 100$$

A = radioactivity of the sample concerned,

B = total radioactivity, which is equal to the difference between the two measurements made on the syringe minus the radioactivity in the tail if a caudal vein has been used for the injection.

Calculate the radioactivity per unit mass in the blood. Correct the blood concentration by multiplying by a factor $m/200$ where m is the body mass of the rat in grams.

In not fewer than two of the three rats: not less than 1.5 per cent of the radioactivity is found in the femurs; not more than 1.0 per cent is found in the liver and not more than 0.05 per cent per gram is found in the blood.

Sterility It complies with the test for sterility prescribed in the monograph on *Radiopharmaceutical preparations (125)*. The injection may be released for use before completion of the test.

RADIOACTIVITY

Measure the radioactivity as described in the monograph on *Radiopharmaceutical preparations (125)* using suitable counting equipment by comparison with a standardised technetium-99m solution or by measurement in an instrument calibrated with the aid of such a solution.

STORAGE

See *Radiopharmaceutical preparations (125)*.

LABELLING

See *Radiopharmaceutical preparations (125)*.

Ph Eur

Technetium[99mTc] Microspheres Injection

Technetium[99mTc] Microspheres Injection complies with the requirements of the 3rd edition of the European Pharmacopoeia [0570]. These requirements are reproduced after the heading 'Definition' below.

Ph Eur

DEFINITION

Technetium (^{99m}Tc) microspheres injection is a sterile, apyrogenic suspension of human albumin which has been denatured to form spherical insoluble particles; the particles are labelled with technetium-99m. The injection contains reducing substances, such as tin salts in an amount not exceeding 3 mg of Sn per millilitre; it may contain a suitable buffer such as acetate, citrate or phosphate and additives such as wetting agents. The human albumin used complies with the requirements of the monograph on *Human albumin solution (255)*. The injection contains not less than 90.0 per cent and not more than 110.0 per cent of the declared technetium-99m radioactivity at the date and hour stated on the label. Not less than 95 per cent of the technetium-99m is bound to the particles of the suspension as determined by the test for non-filterable radioactivity. The particles have a typical diameter between 10 µm and 50 µm. The radioactivity is not less than 185 MBq of technetium-99m per million particles at the date and hour of administration.

Technetium (^{99m}Tc) microspheres injection is prepared from sodium pertechnetate (^{99m}Tc) injection (fission or non-fission) using suitable sterile and apyrogenic ingredients and calculating the ratio of radionuclidic impurities with reference to the date and hour of administration.

CHARACTERS

A suspension of white, yellow or artificially coloured particles which may separate on standing.

Technetium-99m has a half-life of 6.02 h and emits gamma radiation.

IDENTIFICATION

A. Record the gamma-ray spectrum using a suitable instrument as described in the monograph on *Radiopharmaceutical preparations (125)*. The spectrum does not differ significantly from that of a standardised technetium-99m solution either by direct comparison or by using an instrument calibrated with the aid of such a solution. Standardised technetium-99m and molybdenum-99 solutions are available from laboratories recognised by the competent authority. The most prominent gamma photon of technetium-99m has an energy of 0.140 MeV.

B. The tests for non-filterable radioactivity and particle size contribute to the identification of the preparation.

C. Transfer 1 ml of the injection to a centrifuge tube and centrifuge at 2500 g for 5 min to 10 min. Decant the supernatant liquid. To the residue add 5 ml of *cupri-tartaric solution R2*, mix and allow to stand for 10 min. If necessary, heat to dissolve the particles and allow to cool. Add rapidly 0.5 ml of *dilute phosphomolybdotungstic reagent R*, mix immediately and allow to stand. A blue colour develops.

TESTS

pH (*2.2.3*). The pH of the injection is 4.0 to 9.0.

Non-filterable radioactivity Use a polycarbonate membrane filter 13 mm to 25 mm in diameter, 10 µm thick and with circular pores 3 µm in diameter. Fit the membrane into a suitable holder. Place 0.2 ml of the injection on the membrane and filter, adding 20 ml of a 9 g/l solution of *sodium chloride R* during the filtration. The radioactivity remaining on the membrane represents not less than 95 per cent of the total radioactivity of the injection.

Particle size Examine using a microscope. Dilute the injection if necessary so that the number of particles is just low enough for individual particles to be distinguished. Using a syringe fitted with a needle having a calibre not less than 0.35 mm, place a suitable volume in a suitable counting chamber such as a haemocytometer cell, taking care not to overfill the chamber. Allow the suspension to settle for 1 min and carefully add a cover slide without squeezing the sample. Scan an area corresponding to at least 5000 particles. The particles have a uniform spherical appearance. Not more than 10 particles have a maximum dimension greater than 75 µm. No particle having a maximum dimension greater than 100 µm is present.

Number of particles Examine using a microscope. Fill a suitable counting chamber such as a haemocytometer cell with a suitable dilution of the injection taking care that particles do not separate during the transfer. Count the number of particles in the chamber. Repeat this procedure twice and calculate the number of particles per millilitre of the injection.

Tin

Test solution. To 1.0 ml of the injection add 0.5 ml of *sulphuric acid R* and 1.5 ml of *nitric acid R*. Heat and evaporate to approximately 1 ml. Add 2 ml of *water R* and evaporate again to approximately 1 ml. Repeat this procedure twice, cool and dilute to 25.0 ml with *1M hydrochloric acid.*

Reference solution. Dissolve 0.115 g of *stannous chloride R* in *1M hydrochloric acid* and dilute to 1000.0 ml with the same acid.

To 1.0 ml of each solution add 0.4 ml of a 20 g/l solution of *sodium lauryl sulphate R*, 0.05 ml of *thioglycollic acid R*, 0.1 ml of *dithiol reagent R* and 3.0 ml of *0.2M hydrochloric acid.* Mix. Measure the absorbance (*2.2.25*) of each solution at 540 nm, using *0.2M hydrochloric acid* as the compensation liquid. The absorbance of the test solution is not greater than that of the reference solution (3 mg of Sn per millilitre).

Physiological distribution Inject a volume not greater than 0.2 ml into a caudal vein of each of three rats weighing 150 g to 250 g. Sacrifice the rats 15 min after the injection, remove the liver, the spleen and the lungs and measure the radioactivity in the organs using a suitable instrument as described in the monograph on *Radiopharmaceutical preparations (125)*. Measure the radioactivity in the rest of the body, including the blood and voided urine, after having discarded the tail. Determine the percentage of radioactivity in the liver, the spleen and the lungs from the expression:

$$\frac{A}{B} \times 100$$

A = radioactivity of the organ concerned,

B = total radioactivity in the liver, the spleen, the lungs and the rest of the body, including voided urine.

In not fewer than two of the three rats used, not less than 80 per cent of the radioactivity is found in the lungs and not more than a total of 5 per cent in the liver and spleen. The injection may be released for use before completion of the test.

Sterility It complies with the test for sterility prescribed in the monograph on *Radiopharmaceutical preparations (125)*. The injection may be released for use before completion of the test.

Pyrogens It complies with the test for pyrogens prescribed in the monograph on *Radiopharmaceutical preparations (125)*. Inject not less than 0.1 ml per kilogram of the rabbit's mass. The injection may be released for use before completion of the test.

RADIOACTIVITY

Measure the radioactivity as described in the monograph on *Radiopharmaceutical preparations (125)* using suitable counting equipment by comparison with a standardised technetium-99m solution or by measurement in an instrument calibrated with the aid of such a solution.

STORAGE

See *Radiopharmaceutical preparations (125)*.

LABELLING

See *Radiopharmaceutical preparations (125)*.

The label states:

— the quantity of tin per millilitre, if any,

— that the preparation should be shaken before use.

Ph Eur

Technetium[^{99m}Tc] Pentetate Injection

Technetium[^{99m}Tc] Pentetate Injection complies with the requirements of the 3rd edition of the European Pharmacopoeia [0642]. These requirements are reproduced after the heading 'Definition' below.

Ph Eur

DEFINITION

Technetium (^{99m}Tc) pentetate injection is a sterile solution which may be prepared by mixing solutions of sodium diethylenetriaminepenta-acetate or calcium trisodium diethylenetriaminepenta-acetate and a stannous salt with a solution of sodium pertechnetate (^{99m}Tc). It contains a variable quantity of tin (Sn) not exceeding 1 mg per millilitre; it may contain suitable antimicrobial preservatives, antioxidants, stabilisers and buffers. The injection contains not less than 90.0 per cent and not more than 110.0 per cent of the declared technetium-99m radioactivity at the date and hour stated on the label. Not less than 95.0 per cent of the radioactivity corresponds to technetium-99m complexed with sodium pentetate or calcium trisodium pentetate.

It is prepared from sodium pertechnetate (^{99m}Tc) injection (fission or non-fission) using suitable, sterile ingredients and calculating the ratio of radionuclidic impurities with reference to the date and hour of administration.

CHARACTERS

A clear, colourless or slightly yellow solution.

Technetium-99m has a half life of 6.02 h and emits gamma radiation.

IDENTIFICATION

A. Record the gamma-ray spectrum using a suitable instrument as described in the monograph on *Radiopharmaceutical preparations (125)*. The spectrum does not differ significantly from that of a standardised technetium-99m solution either by direct comparison or by using an instrument calibrated with the aid of such a solution. Standardised technetium-99m and molybdenum-99 solutions are available from laboratories recognised by the competent authority. The most prominent gamma photon of technetium-99m has an energy of 0.140 MeV.

B. Examine the chromatograms obtained in the test for radiochemical purity. The distribution of radioactivity contributes to the identification of the preparation.

C. Place in a clean, dry 10 ml glass tube a volume of the injection to be examined containing 2 mg of pentetate. Dilute, if necessary, to 1 ml with *water R*. Place in a second tube 1 ml of *water R* (blank). To each tube add 0.1 ml of a 1 g/l solution of *nickel sulphate R*, 0.5 ml of a 50 per cent *V/V* solution of *glacial acetic acid R* and 0.75 ml of a 50 g/l solution of *sodium hydroxide R*. Mix and verify that the pH is not above 5. To each tube add 0.1 ml of a 10 g/l alcoholic solution of *dimethylglyoxime R*. Mix and allow to stand for 2 min. Adjust the pH in each tube to not less than 12 by adding a 100 g/l solution of *sodium hydroxide R*. Mix and check that the pH is not below 12. Allow to stand for 2 min. Heat the tubes gently on a water-bath for 2 min. The solution in the tube containing the injection to be examined remains clear and colourless throughout. The solution in the blank tube becomes red on addition of dimethylglyoxime solution and a red precipitate is formed when the tube is heated on a water-bath.

TESTS

pH (*2.2.3*). The pH of the injection is 4.0 to 7.5.

Radiochemical purity Examine by thin-layer chromatography (*2.2.27*) as described in the monograph on *Radiopharmaceutical preparations (125)*, using silica gel as the coating substance on a glass-fibre sheet. Heat the plate at 110°C for 10 min. Use a plate such that during development the mobile phase migrates over a distance of 10 cm to 15 cm in about 10 min.

(a) Apply to the plate 5 ml to 10 ml of the injection to be examined. Develop immediately over a path of 10 cm to 15 cm using a 9 g/l solution of *sodium chloride R*. Allow the plate to dry in air. Determine the distribution of radioactivity using a suitable detector. Impurities in colloidal form remain at the starting point. Technetium pentetate complex and pertechnetate ion migrate near to the solvent front.

(b) Apply to the plate 5 ml to 10 ml of the injection to be examined and allow to dry. Develop over a path of 10 cm to 15 cm using *methyl ethyl ketone R*. Allow the plate to dry. Determine the distribution of radioactivity using a suitable detector. Pertechnetate ion migrates near to the solvent front. Technetium pentetate complex and impurities in colloidal form remain at the starting point.

The sum of the percentages of radioactivity corresponding to impurities in the chromatograms obtained in test (a) and (b) does not exceed 5.0 per cent.

Tin

Test solution. Dilute 1.5 ml of the injection to 25.0 ml with *1M hydrochloric acid.*

Reference solution. Dissolve 0.115 g of *stannous chloride R* in *1M hydrochloric acid* and dilute to 1000.0 ml with the same acid.

To 1.0 ml of each solution add 0.4 ml of a 20 g/l solution of *sodium lauryl sulphate R*, 0.05 ml of *thioglycollic acid R*, 0.1 ml of *dithiol reagent R* and 3.0 ml of *0.2M hydrochloric acid*. Mix. Measure the absorbance (*2.2.25*) of each solution at 540 nm, using *0.2M hydrochloric acid* as the compensation liquid. The absorbance of the test solution is not greater than that of the reference solution (1 mg of Sn per millilitre).

Sterility It complies with the test for sterility prescribed in the monograph on *Radiopharmaceutical preparations (125)*.

The injection may be released for use before completion of the test.

RADIOACTIVITY

Measure the radioactivity as described in the monograph on *Radiopharmaceutical preparations (125)* using suitable counting equipment by comparison with a standardised technetium-99m solution or by measurement in an instrument calibrated with the aid of such a solution.

STORAGE

See *Radiopharmaceutical preparations (125)*.

LABELLING

See *Radiopharmaceutical preparations (125)*.

Ph Eur

Technetium[^{99m}Tc] Succimer Injection

Technetium[^{99m}Tc] Succimer Injection complies with the requirements of the 3rd edition of the European Pharmacopoeia [0643]. These requirements are reproduced after the heading 'Definition' below.

Ph Eur

DEFINITION

Technetium (^{99m}Tc) succimer injection is a sterile solution of *meso*-2,3-dimercaptosuccinic acid labelled with technetium-99m. It contains a reducing substance, such as a tin salt in an amount not exceeding 1 mg of Sn per millilitre, and may contain stabilisers, antioxidants such as ascorbic acid, and inert additives. The injection contains not less than 90.0 per cent and not more than 110.0 per cent of the declared technetium-99m radioactivity at the date and hour stated on the label. Not less than 95.0 per cent of the radioactivity corresponds to technetium-99m succimer complex.

It is prepared from sodium pertechnetate (^{99m}Tc) injection (fission or non-fission) using suitable sterile ingredients and calculating the ratio of radionuclidic impurities with reference to the date and hour of administration. Syringes for handling the eluate intended for labelling of the final product, or for handling the final product should not contain rubber parts.

CHARACTERS

A clear, colourless solution.

Technetium-99m has a half life of 6.02 h and emits gamma radiation.

IDENTIFICATION

A. Record the gamma-ray spectrum using a suitable instrument as described in the monograph on *Radiopharmaceutical preparations (125)*. The spectrum does not differ significantly from that of a standardised technetium-99m solution either by direct comparison or by using an instrument calibrated with the aid of such a solution. Standardised technetium-99m and molybdenum-99 solutions are available from laboratories recognised by the competent authority. The most prominent gamma photon of technetium-99m has an energy of 0.140 MeV.

B. Examine the chromatogram obtained in the test for radiochemical purity. The distribution of the radioactivity contributes to the identification of the preparation.

C. Place 1 ml of the injection to be examined in a test-tube and add 1 ml of a 20 g/l solution of *sodium nitroprusside R* and 0.1 ml of *glacial acetic acid R*. Mix. Place carefully at the top of the solution a layer of *concentrated ammonia R*. A violet ring develops between the layers.

TESTS

pH (*2.2.3*). The pH of the injection is 2.3 to 3.5.

Radiochemical purity Examine by thin-layer chromatography (*2.2.27*) as described in the monograph on *Radiopharmaceutical preparations (125)*, using silica gel as the coating substance on a glass-fibre sheet. Heat the plate at 110°C for 10 min. Use a plate such that during development the mobile phase migrates over a distance of 10 cm to 15 cm in about 10 min.

Apply to the plate 5 µl to 10 µl of the injection to be examined. Develop immediately over a path of 10 cm to 15 cm using *methyl ethyl ketone R*. Allow the plate to dry. Determine the distribution of radioactivity using a suitable detector. Technetium succimer complex remains at the starting point. Pertechnetate ion migrates near to the solvent front. Not less than 95.0 per cent of the total radioactivity is found in the spot corresponding to technetium succimer complex. The radioactivity corresponding to pertechnetate ion represents not more than 2.0 per cent of the total radioactivity.

Tin

Test solution. Dilute 1.5 ml of the injection to be examined to 25.0 ml with *1M hydrochloric acid*.

Reference solution. Dissolve 0.115 g of *stannous chloride R* in *1M hydrochloric acid* and dilute to 1000.0 ml with the same acid.

To 1.0 ml of each solution add 0.4 ml of a 20 g/l solution of *sodium lauryl sulphate R*, 0.05 ml of *thioglycollic acid R*, 0.1 ml of *dithiol reagent R* and 3.0 ml of *0.2M hydrochloric acid*. Mix. Allow to stand for 60 min. Measure the absorbance (*2.2.25*) of each solution at 540 nm, using *0.2M hydrochloric acid* as the compensation liquid. The absorbance of the test solution is not greater than that of the reference solution (1 mg of Sn per millilitre).

Physiological distribution Inject a volume not greater than 0.2 ml and containing not more than 0.1 mg of dimercaptosuccinic acid into a suitable vein, such as a caudal vein or a saphenous vein, of each of three rats each weighing 150 g to 250 g. Measure the radioactivity in the syringe before and after the injection. Kill the rats 1 h after the injection. Remove the kidneys, the liver, the stomach, the lungs and, if a caudal vein has been used for the injection, the tail. Using a suitable instrument as described in the monograph on *Radiopharmaceutical preparations (125)*, determine the radioactivity in the organs and, if a caudal vein has been used for injection, in the tail. Determine the percentage of radioactivity in each organ with respect to the total radioactivity calculated as the difference between the two measurements made on the syringe minus the activity in the tail (if a caudal vein has been used for the injection).

In not fewer than two of the three rats used, the radioactivity in the kidneys is not less than 40 per cent, that in the liver is not more than 10.0 per cent, that in the stomach is not more than 2.0 per cent and that in the lungs is not more than 5.0 per cent.

Sterility It complies with the test for sterility prescribed in the monograph on *Radiopharmaceutical preparations (125)*. The injection may be released for use before completion of the test.

RADIOACTIVITY

Measure the radioactivity as described in the monograph on *Radiopharmaceutical preparations (125)* using suitable counting equipment by comparison with a standardised technetium-99m solution or by measurement in an instrument calibrated with the aid of such a solution.

STORAGE

See *Radiopharmaceutical preparations (125)*. Store protected from light.

LABELLING

See *Radiopharmaceutical preparations (125)*.

Ph Eur

Technetium[^{99m}Tc] Tin Pyrophosphate Injection

Technetium[^{99m}Tc] Tin Pyrophosphate Injection complies with the requirements of the 3rd edition of the European Pharmacopoeia [0129]. These requirements are reproduced after the heading 'Definition' below.

Ph Eur

DEFINITION

Technetium (^{99m}Tc) tin pyrophosphate injection is a sterile, apyrogenic solution which may be prepared by mixing solutions of sodium pyrophosphate and stannous chloride with sodium pertechnetate (^{99m}Tc) injection (fission or non-fission). The injection contains not less than 90.0 per cent and not more than 110.0 per cent of the declared technetium-99m radioactivity at the date and hour stated on the label. Not less than 90 per cent of the radioactivity corresponds to technetium-99m complexed with tin pyrophosphate. The injection contains a quantity of sodium pyrophosphate ($Na_4P_2O_7,10H_2O$) that may vary from 1 mg to 50 mg per millilitre and a variable quantity of tin (Sn) not exceeding 3.0 mg per millilitre.

It is prepared from sodium pertechnetate (^{99m}Tc) injection (fission or non-fission) using suitable sterile, apyrogenic ingredients and calculating the ratio of radionuclidic impurities with reference to the date and hour of administration.

CHARACTERS

A clear, colourless solution.

Technetium-99m has a half-life of 6.02 h and emits gamma radiation.

IDENTIFICATION

A. Record the gamma-ray spectrum using a suitable instrument as described in the monograph on *Radiopharmaceutical preparations (125)*. The spectrum does not differ significantly from that of a standardised technetium-99m solution either by direct comparison or by using an instrument calibrated with the aid of such a solution. Standardised technetium-99m and molybdenum-99 solutions are available from laboratories recognised by the competent authority. The most prominent gamma photon of technetium-99m has an energy of 0.140 MeV.

B. Examine the chromatograms obtained in the test for radiochemical purity. The distribution of radioactivity contributes to the identification of the injection.

C. To 1 ml add 1 ml of *acetic acid R*. Heat on a water-bath for 1 h. After cooling, add 10 ml of *nitro-vanadomolybdic reagent R* and allow to stand for 30 min. A yellow colour develops.

D. To 1 ml add 2 ml of a 30 per cent *V/V* solution of *sulphuric acid R*, 1 ml of *hydrochloric acid R*, 0.05 ml of *thioglycollic acid R*, 0.4 ml of a 20 g/l solution of *sodium lauryl sulphate R* and 0.1 ml of *dithiol reagent R* and allow to stand for 30 min. A pink colour develops.

TESTS

pH (*2.2.3*). The pH of the injection is 6.0 to 7.0.

Radiochemical purity

(a) Examine by thin-layer chromatography (*2.2.27*), as described in the monograph on *Radiopharmaceutical preparations (125)* using silica gel as the coating substance on a glass-fibre sheet. Heat the plate at 110°C for 10 min. The plate used should be such that during development the mobile phase migrates over a distance of 10 cm to 15 cm in about 10 min.

Apply to the plate 5 µl to 10 µl of the injection and dry in a stream of nitrogen. Develop over a path of 10 cm to 15 cm using *methyl ethyl ketone R* through which nitrogen has been bubbled in the chromatography tank for 10 min immediately before the chromatography. Allow the plate to dry. Determine the distribution of radioactivity using a suitable detector. The technetium-99m tin pyrophosphate complex remains at the starting-point and pertechnetate ion migrates with an R_f of 0.95 to 1.0.

(b) Examine by thin-layer chromatography (*2.2.27*), as described in the monograph on *Radiopharmaceutical preparations (125)* using silica gel as the coating substance on a glass-fibre sheet. Heat the plate at 110°C for 10 min. The plate used should be such that during development the mobile phase migrates over a distance of 10 cm to 15 cm in about 10 min.

Apply to the plate 5 µl to 10 µl of the injection. Develop immediately over a path of 10 cm to 15 cm using a 136 g/l solution of *sodium acetate R*. Allow the plate to dry and measure the distribution of radioactivity using a suitable detector. Impurities in colloidal form remain at the starting-point and technetium-99m tin pyrophosphate complex and pertechnetate ion migrate with an R_f of 0.9 to 1.0.

Add together the percentages of radioactivity corresponding to impurities in the chromatograms obtained in test (a) and test (b). The sum does not exceed 10 per cent.

Sodium pyrophosphate

Test solution. Use 1 ml of the injection to be examined or a suitable dilution of it.

Reference solutions. Using a solution containing *sodium pyrophosphate R* and *stannous chloride R* in the same proportions as in the injection to be examined, prepare a range of solutions and dilute to the same final volume with *water R*.

To the test solution and to 1 ml of each of the reference solutions add successively 10 ml of a 1 g/l solution of *disodium hydrogen phosphate R*, 10 ml of *iron standard solution (8 ppm Fe) R*, 5 ml of *glacial acetic acid R* and 5 ml of a 1 g/l solution of *hydroxylamine hydrochloride R*. Dilute each solution to 40 ml with *water R* and heat in a water-bath at 40°C for 1 h. To each solution add 4 ml of a 1 g/l solution of *phenanthroline hydrochloride R* and dilute to 50.0 ml with *water R*. Measure the absorbance (*2.2.25*) of each solution at 515 nm using as the compensation liquid a reagent blank containing hydrochloric acid (1.1 g/l HCl) instead of the *iron standard solution (8 ppm Fe) R*. Using the absorbances obtained with the reference solutions, draw a calibration curve and calculate the concentration of sodium pyrophosphate in the injection to be examined.

Tin

Test solution. Use 1 ml of the injection to be examined or a suitable dilution of it.

Reference solutions. Using a solution in hydrochloric acid (6.2 g/l HCl) containing *sodium pyrophosphate R* and *stannous chloride R* in the same proportions as in the injection to be examined, prepare a range of solutions and dilute to the same volume with hydrochloric acid (6.2 g/l HCl).

To the test solution and to 1 ml of each of the reference solutions add 2 ml of a 300 g/l solution of *sulphuric acid R*, 1 ml of *hydrochloric acid R*, 0.05 ml of *thioglycollic acid R*, 0.4 ml of a 20 g/l solution of *sodium lauryl sulphate R* and 0.1 ml of *dithiol reagent R* and dilute to 15 ml with hydrochloric acid (6.2 g/l HCl). Allow the solutions to stand for 30 min and measure the absorbance (*2.2.25*) of each solution at 530 nm, using as the compensation liquid a reagent blank containing the same quantity of *sodium pyrophosphate R* as the injection to be examined. Using the absorbances obtained with the reference solutions, draw a calibration curve and calculate the concentration of tin in the injection to be examined.

Sterility It complies with the test for sterility prescribed in the monograph on *Radiopharmaceutical preparations (125)*. The injection may be released for use before completion of the test.

Pyrogens It complies with the test for pyrogens prescribed in the monograph on *Radiopharmaceutical preparations (125)*. Inject not less than 0.1 ml per kilogram of the rabbit's mass. The injection may be released for use before completion of the test.

RADIOACTIVITY

Measure the radioactivity as described in the monograph on *Radiopharmaceutical preparations (125)* using suitable counting equipment by comparison with a standardised technetium-99m solution or by measurement in an instrument calibrated with the aid of such a solution.

STORAGE

See *Radiopharmaceutical preparations (125)*.

LABELLING

See *Radiopharmaceutical preparations (125)*.

The label states, in particular, the quantity of sodium pyrophosphate per millilitre and the quantity of tin per millilitre.

Ph Eur

Thallous[201Tl] Chloride Injection

Thallous[201Tl] Chloride Injection complies with the requirements of the 3rd edition of the European Pharmacopoeia [0571]. These requirements are reproduced after the heading 'Definition' below.

Ph Eur

DEFINITION

Thallous (^{201}Tl) chloride injection is a sterile solution of thallium-201 in the form of thallous chloride. It may be made isotonic by the addition of sodium chloride and may contain a suitable antimicrobial preservative such as benzyl alcohol. Thallium-201 is a radioactive isotope of thallium formed by the decay of lead-201. Lead-201 is a radioactive isotope of lead and may be obtained by irradiation, with protons of suitable energy, of thallium which may be enriched in thallium-203. Thallium-201 may be separated from lead-201 by passing through a column of an ion-exchange resin. The injection contains not less than 90.0 per cent and not more than 110.0 per cent of the declared thallium-201 radioactivity at the date and hour stated on the label. Not more than 2.0 per cent of the total radioactivity is due to thallium-202 and not less than 97.0 per cent is due to thallium-201. Not less than 95.0 per cent of the radioactivity is due to thallium in the form of thallous ions. The specific radioactivity is not less than 3.7 GBq per milligram of thallium.

CHARACTERS

A clear, colourless solution.

Thallium-201 has a half-life of 3.05 days and emits gamma radiation and X-rays.

IDENTIFICATION

A. Record the gamma-ray and X-ray spectrum using a suitable instrument as described in the monograph on *Radiopharmaceutical preparations (125)*. The spectrum does not differ significantly from that of a standardised thallium-201 solution when measured either by direct comparison or by use of an instrument calibrated with the aid of such a solution. Standardised thallium-201 and thallium-202 solutions are available from laboratories recognised by the competent authority. The most prominent gamma photons have energies of 0.135 MeV, 0.166 MeV and 0.167 MeV. The X-rays have energies of 0.069 MeV to 0.083 MeV.

B. Examine the electrophoretogram obtained in the test for radiochemical purity. The distribution of radioactivity contributes to the identification of the preparation.

TESTS

pH (*2.2.3*). The pH of the injection is 4.0 to 7.0.

Radionuclidic purity Record the gamma-ray and X-ray spectrum as described in the monograph on *Radiopharmaceutical preparations (125)* using a suitable instrument calibrated with the aid of standardised thallium-201 and thallium-202 solutions. The spectrum does not differ significantly from that of the standardised thallium-201 solution. Determine the relative amounts of thallium-201 and thallium-202 and other radionuclidic impurities present. Thallium-202 has a half-life of 12.2 days and its most prominent gamma photon has an energy of 0.440 MeV. Thallium-200 has a half-life of 1.09 days and its most prominent gamma photons have energies of 0.368 MeV, 0.579 MeV, 0.828 MeV and 1.206 MeV. Lead-201 has a half-life of 9.4 h and its most prominent gamma photon has an energy of 0.331 MeV. Lead-203 has a half-life of 2.17 days and its most prominent gamma photon has an energy of 0.279 MeV. Not more than 2.0 per cent of the total radioactivity is due to thallium-202 and not less than 97.0 per cent is due to thallium-201.

Radiochemical purity Examine by zone electrophoresis (*2.2.31*), using a strip of suitable cellulose acetate, 150 mm by 25 mm, as the support and a 18.6 g/l solution of *sodium edetate R* as the electrolyte solution. Soak the strip in the electrolyte solution for 45 min to 60 min. Remove the strip with forceps taking care to handle the outer edges only. Place the strip between two absorbent pads and blot to remove excess solution.

Test solution. Mix equal volumes of the injection to be examined and the electrolyte solution.

Apply not less than 5 µl of the test solution to the centre of the strip and mark the point of application. Apply an electric field of 17 V per centimetre for 30 min. Allow the strip to dry in air. Determine the distribution of radioactivity using suitable equipment. Not less than 95.0 per cent of the radioactivity migrates towards the cathode.

Thallium To 0.5 ml of the injection add 0.5 ml of hydrochloric acid (220 g/l HCl) and 0.05 ml of *bromine water R* and mix. Add 0.1 ml of a 30 g/l solution of *sulphosalicylic acid R*. After decolorisation add 1.0 ml of a 1 g/l solution of *rhodamine* B *R*. Add 4 ml of *toluene R* and shake for 60 s. Separate the toluene layer. The toluene layer is not more intensely coloured than the toluene layer of a standard prepared at the same time in the same manner using 0.5 ml of *thallium standard solution (10 ppm Tl) R*.

Sterility It complies with the test for sterility prescribed in the monograph on *Radiopharmaceutical preparations (125)*. The injection may be released for use before completion of the test.

RADIOACTIVITY

Measure the radioactivity as described in the monograph on *Radiopharmaceutical preparations (125)* using suitable counting equipment by comparison with a standardised thallium-201 solution or by measurement in an instrument calibrated with the aid of such a solution.

STORAGE

See *Radiopharmaceutical preparations (125)*.

LABELLING

See *Radiopharmaceutical preparations (125)*.

Ph Eur

Tritiated[3H] Water Injection

Tritiated[3H] Water Injection complies with the requirements of the 3rd edition of the European Pharmacopoeia [0112]. These requirements are reproduced after the heading 'Definition' below.

Ph Eur

DEFINITION

Tritiated (^3H) water injection is water for injections in which some of the water molecules contain tritium atoms in place of protium atoms. It may be made isotonic by the addition of sodium chloride. Tritium (^3H) may be obtained by the neutron irradiation of lithium. The injection contains not less than 90.0 per cent and not more than 110.0 per cent of the declared tritium activity at the date stated on the label.

CHARACTERS

A clear, colourless liquid.

Tritium has a half-life of 12.3 years and emits beta radiation.

IDENTIFICATION

Record the beta-ray spectrum by the method prescribed in the test for radionuclidic purity. The spectrum does not differ significantly from that of a standardised tritiated (^3H) water. Standardised tritiated (^3H) water is available from laboratories recognised by the competent authority. The maximum energy of the beta radiation is 0.019 MeV.

TESTS

pH (*2.2.3*). The pH of the injection is 4.5 to 7.0.

Radionuclidic purity

(a) Mix 100 µl of a suitable dilution of the injection with 10 ml of a scintillation liquid consisting of 1000 ml of *dioxan R*, 100 g of *naphthalene R*, 7 g of *diphenyloxazole R* and 0.3 g of *methylphenyloxazolylbenzene R*, the reagents being of an analytical grade suitable for liquid scintillation. Measure the radioactivity of the mixture in a liquid scintillation counter fitted with a discriminator. The count should be about 5000 impulses per second at the lowest setting of the discriminator. Record the count at different discriminator settings. For each measurement count at least 10,000 impulses over a period of at least 1 min. Immediately determine in the same conditions the count for a standardised tritiated (3H) water having approximately the same activity.

Plot the counts at each discriminator setting, correcting for background activity, on semi-logarithmic paper, the discriminator settings being in arbitrary units as the abscissae. The vertical distance between the two curves obtained is constant. They obey the mathematical relationship:

$$\frac{\frac{A_1}{B_1}-\frac{A_2}{B_2}}{\frac{A_1}{B_1}}\times 100 < 20$$

A_1 = radioactivity recorded for the standardised preparation at the lowest discriminator setting,

B_1 = radioactivity recorded for the preparation to be examined at the lowest discriminator setting,

A_2 = radioactivity recorded for the standard at the discriminator setting such that $A_2 \approx A_1 \times 10^{-3}$,

B_2 = radioactivity recorded for the preparation to be examined at the latter discriminator setting.

(b) Record the gamma-ray spectrum. The instrument registers only background activity.

Radiochemical purity Place a quantity of the injection equivalent to about 2 µCi (74 kBq), diluted to 50 ml with *water R*, in an all-glass distillation apparatus of the type used for the determination of *Distillation range (2.2.11)*. Determine the radioactive concentration as described in the monograph on *Radiopharmaceutical preparations (125)*. Distil until about 25 ml of distillate has been collected. Precautions must be taken to avoid contamination of the air. If the test is carried out in a fume cupboard, the equipment must be protected from draughts. Determine the radioactive concentration of the distillate and of the liquid remaining in the distillation flask. Neither of the radioactive concentrations determined after distillation differs by more than 5 per cent from the value determined before distillation.

Sterility It complies with the test for sterility prescribed in the monograph on *Radiopharmaceutical preparations (125)*.

RADIOACTIVITY

Determine the radioactivity using a liquid scintillation counter as described in the monograph on *Radiopharmaceutical preparations (125)*.

STORAGE

See *Radiopharmaceutical preparations (125)*.

LABELLING

See *Radiopharmaceutical preparations (125)*.

Ph Eur

Xenon[133Xe] Injection

Xenon[133Xe] Injection complies with the requirements of the 3rd edition of the European Pharmacopoeia [0133]. These requirements are reproduced after the heading 'Definition' below.

Ph Eur

DEFINITION

Xenon (^{133}Xe) injection is a sterile solution of xenon-133 that may be made isotonic by the addition of sodium chloride. Xenon-133 is a radioactive isotope of xenon and is obtained by separation from the other products of uranium fission. The injection contains not less than 80 per cent and not more than 130 per cent of the declared xenon-133 radioactivity at the date and hour stated on the label.

The injection is presented in a container that allows the contents to be removed without introducing air bubbles. The container is filled as completely as possible and any gas bubble present does not occupy more than 1 per cent of the volume of the injection as judged by visual comparison with a suitable standard.

CHARACTERS

A clear, colourless solution.

Xenon-133 has a half-life of 5.29 days and emits beta and gamma radiation and X-rays.

IDENTIFICATION

Record the gamma-ray and X-ray spectrum using a suitable instrument as described in the monograph on

Radiopharmaceutical preparations (125). The spectrum does not differ significantly from that of a standardised xenon-133 solution in a 9 g/l solution of *sodium chloride R*, apart from any differences attributable to the presence of xenon-131m and xenon-133m. If standardised xenon-133 solutions are not readily available, suitable standardised ionisation chambers are obtainable from laboratories recognised by the relevant competent authority. The most prominent gamma photon of xenon-133 has an energy of 0.081 MeV and there is an X-ray (resulting from internal conversion) of 0.030 MeV to 0.035 MeV. Xenon-131m has a half-life of 11.9 days and emits a gamma photon of 0.164 MeV. Xenon-133m has a half-life of 2.19 days and emits a gamma photon of 0.233 MeV.

TESTS

pH (*2.2.3*). The pH of the injection is 5.0 to 8.0.

Radionuclidic purity

(a) Record the gamma-ray and X-ray spectrum using a suitable instrument as described in the monograph on *Radiopharmaceutical preparations (125)*. The spectrum does not differ significantly from that of a standardised xenon-133 solution in a 9 g/l solution of *sodium chloride R*, apart from any differences attributable to the presence of xenon-131 m and xenon-133m.

(b) Transfer 2 ml of the injection to an open flask and pass a current of air through the solution for 30 min, taking suitable precautions concerning the dispersion of radioactivity. Measure the residual beta and gamma activity of the solution. The activity does not differ significantly from the background activity detected by the instrument.

Sterility It complies with the test for sterility prescribed in the monograph on *Radiopharmaceutical preparations (125)*. The injection may be released for use before completion of the test.

RADIOACTIVITY

Weigh the container with its contents. Determine its total radioactivity using suitable counting equipment by comparison with a standardised xenon-133 solution or by measurement in an instrument calibrated with the aid of such a solution, operating in strictly identical conditions. If an ionisation chamber is used its inner wall should be such that the radiation is not seriously attenuated. Remove at least half the contents and re-weigh the container. Measure the radioactivity of the container and the remaining contents as described above. From the measurements, calculate the radioactive concentration of xenon-133 in the injection.

STORAGE

See the monograph on *Radiopharmaceutical preparations (125)*.

LABELLING

See the monograph on *Radiopharmaceutical preparations (125)*.

CAUTION

Significant amounts of xenon-133 may be present in the closures and on the walls of the container. This must be taken into account in applying the rules concerning the transport and storage of radioactive substances and in disposing of used containers.

Ph Eur

Monographs

Surgical Materials

Absorbent Cotton

Absorbent Cotton complies with the requirements of the 3rd edition of the European Pharmacopoeia [0036]. These requirements are reproduced after the heading 'Definition' below.

Ph Eur

DEFINITION

Absorbent cotton consists of hairs or good quality new combers obtained from the seed-coat of various species of the genus *Gossypium L.*, cleaned, purified, bleached and carefully carded. It may not contain any compensatory colouring matter.

CHARACTERS

It is white and is composed of fibres of average length not less than 10 mm and contains not more than traces of leaf residue, pericarp, or seed-coat or of other impurities. It offers appreciable resistance when pulled. It does not shed any appreciable quantity of dust when gently shaken.

IDENTIFICATION

A. Examined under a microscope, each fibre is seen to consist of a single cell, up to about 4 cm long and up to 40 µm wide, in the form of a flattened tube with thick and rounded walls and often twisted.

B. When treated with *iodinated zinc chloride solution R*, the fibres become violet.

C. To 0.1 g add 10 ml of *zinc chloride-formic acid solution R.* Heat to 40°C and allow to stand for 2 h 30 min, shaking occasionally. It does not dissolve.

TESTS

Solution S Place 15.0 g in a suitable vessel, add 150 ml of *water R*, close the vessel and allow to macerate for 2 h. Decant the solution, squeeze the residual liquid carefully from the sample with a glass rod and mix. Reserve 10 ml of the solution for the test for surface-active substances and filter the remainder.

Acidity or alkalinity To 25 ml of solution S add 0.1 ml of *phenolphthalein solution R* and to another 25 ml add 0.05 ml of *methyl orange solution R.* Neither solution is pink.

Foreign fibres Examined under a microscope, it is seen to consist exclusively of typical cotton fibres, except that occasionally a few isolated foreign fibres may be present.

Fluorescence Examine a layer about 5 mm in thickness under ultraviolet light at 365 nm. It displays only a slight brownish-violet fluorescence and a few yellow particles. It shows no intense blue fluorescence, apart from that which may be shown by a few isolated fibres.

Neps Spread about 1 g evenly between two colourless transparent plates each 10 cm square. Examine for neps by transmitted light and compare with the European Pharmacopoeia Standard for Neps. The product to be examined is not more neppy than the standard.

Absorbency *Apparatus.* A dry cylindrical copper wire basket 8.0 cm high and 5.0 cm in diameter. The wire of which the basket is constructed is about 0.4 mm in diameter, the mesh is 1.5 cm to 2.0 cm and the mass of the basket is 2.7 ± 0.3 g.

Sinking time. Not more than 10 s. Weigh the basket to the nearest centigram (m_1). Take 5.00 g in approximately equal quantities from five different places in the product to be examined, place loosely in the basket and weigh the filled basket to the nearest centigram (m_2). Fill a beaker 11 cm to 12 cm in diameter to a depth of 10 cm with *water R* at about 20°C. Hold the basket horizontally and drop it from a height of about 10 mm into the water. Measure with a stopwatch the time taken for the basket to sink below the surface of the water. Calculate the result as the average of three tests.

Water-holding capacity. Not less than 23.0 g of water per gram. After the sinking time has been measured, remove the basket from the water, allow it to drain for exactly 30 s, suspended with its long axis in the horizontal position over the beaker, transfer it to a tared beaker (m_3) and weigh to the nearest centigram (m_4).

$$\text{Water-holding capacity per gram} = \frac{m_4 - (m_2 + m_3)}{m_2 - m_1} \text{ grams}$$

Calculate the result as the average of three tests.

Ether-soluble substances Not more than 0.50 per cent. In an extraction apparatus, extract 5.00 g with *ether R* for 4 h at the rate of at least four extractions per hour. Evaporate the ether extract and dry the residue to constant mass at 100°C to 105°C.

Extractable colouring matter In a narrow percolator, slowly extract 10.0 g with *alcohol R* until 50 ml of extract is obtained. The liquid obtained is not more intensely coloured than reference solution Y_5, GY_6 or blue solution (*Method II, 2.2.2*).

Blue solution. To 3.0 ml of blue primary solution (*2.2.2*) add 7.0 ml of hydrochloric acid (10 g/l HCl). Dilute 0.5 ml of this solution to 10.0 ml with hydrochloric acid (10 g/l HCl).

Surface-active substances Introduce the portion of solution S reserved before filtration into a 25 ml graduated ground-glass-stoppered cylinder with an external diameter of 20 ± 2 mm, previously rinsed with *sulphuric acid R* and then *water R*. Shake vigorously thirty times in 10 s, allow to stand for 1 min and repeat the shaking. After 5 min, the height reached by the froth does not exceed 2 mm above the surface of the liquid.

Water-soluble substances Not more than 0.50 per cent. Boil 5.00 g in 500 ml of *water R* for 30 min, stirring frequently and replacing the water lost by evaporation. Decant the liquid, squeeze the residual liquid carefully from the sample with a glass rod and mix. Filter the liquid whilst hot. Evaporate 400 ml of the extract (corresponding to 4/5th of the mass of the sample taken) and dry the residue to constant mass at 100°C to 105°C.

Loss on drying (*2.2.32*). Not more than 8.0 per cent, determined 5.00 g by drying in an oven at 100°C to 105°C.

Sulphated ash (*2.4.14*). Not more than 0.40 per cent. Introduce 5.00 g into a previously heated and cooled, tared crucible. Heat cautiously over a naked flame and then carefully to dull redness at 600°C. Allow to cool, add a few drops of *dilute sulphuric acid R*, then heat and incinerate until all the black particles have disappeared. Allow to cool. Add a few drops of *ammonium carbonate solution R.* Evaporate and incinerate carefully, allow to cool and weigh again. Repeat the incineration for periods of 5 min to constant mass.

STORAGE

Store in a dust-proof package, in a dry place.

Ph Eur

Sterile Absorbent Cotton

Sterile Absorbent Cotton complies with the requirements of the 3rd edition of the European Pharmacopoeia [0037]. These requirements are reproduced after the heading 'Definition' below.

Ph Eur

DEFINITION

Sterile absorbent cotton complies with the definition, characters, identification and tests prescribed in the monograph on *Cotton, absorbent (36)*. It may, however, become slightly yellowish when sterilised by heat. It also complies with the following test.

Sterility (*2.6.1*). It complies with the test for sterility as applied to surgical dressings.

STORAGE

Store in a package that protects the contents from contamination, in a dry place.

Ph Eur

Absorbent Viscose Wadding

Absorbent Viscose Wadding complies with the requirements of the 3rd edition of the European Pharmacopoeia [0034]. These requirements are reproduced after the heading 'Definition' below.

Ph Eur

DEFINITION

Absorbent viscose wadding consists of bleached, carefully carded, new fibres of regenerated cellulose obtained by the viscose process, with or without the addition of titanium dioxide, of linear density 1.7 dtex to 3.3 dtex (dtex = mass of 10,000 m of fibre, expressed in grams) and cut to a suitable staple length. It does not contain any compensatory colouring matter.

CHARACTERS

It is white or very slightly yellow, has a lustrous or matt appearance, is soft to the touch.

IDENTIFICATION

A. Viscose rayon fibres may be solid or hollow; hollow fibres may have a continuous lumen or be compartmented. The fibres have an average length of 25 mm to 80 mm and when examined under a microscope in the dry state, or when mounted in *alcohol R* and *water R*, the following characters are observed. They are usually of a more or less uniform width, with many longitudinal parallel lines distributed unequally over the width. The ends are cut more or less straight. Matt fibres contain numerous granular particles of approximately 1 µm average diameter.

Solid fibres. In longitudinal view, the surface of the fibres may be uneven or crenated. Fibres having an approximately circular or elliptical cross section have a diameter of about 10 µm to 20 µm and those that are flattened and twisted ribbons appear to vary in width from 15 µm to 20 µm as the twisting of the filament reveals first the major axis and then the minor axis. They are about 4 µm in thickness. Other solid cross sections, such as Y-shaped, have protruding limbs with the major axis 5 µm to 25 µm in length and the minor axis 2 µm to 8 µm wide.

Hollow fibres. Fibres with a continuous, hollow lumen have a diameter up to about 30 µm; they are thin-walled, with a wall thickness of about 5 µm. When mounted in *alcohol R* and *water R*, the lumen is clearly indicated in many fibres by the presence of many entrapped air bubbles.

Compartmented fibres. These fibres may have a diameter of up to 80 µm; they are hollow, having a central lumen which is divided up into several compartments. Individual compartments vary in size but typically may be up to about 60 µm in length and there may be more than one compartment across the width of each fibre. Some compartments show entrapped air bubbles when the fibres are mounted in *alcohol R* and *water R*.

B. When treated with *iodinated zinc chloride solution R*, the fibres become violet.

C. To 0.1 g add 10 ml of *zinc chloride-formic acid solution R*. Heat to 40°C and allow to stand for 2 h 30 min, shaking occasionally. It dissolves completely except for the matt variety where titanium dioxide particles remain.

D. Dissolve the residue obtained in the test for sulphated ash by warming gently with 5 ml of *sulphuric acid R*. Allow to cool and add 0.2 ml of *dilute hydrogen peroxide solution R*. The solution obtained from the lustrous variety undergoes no change in colour; that from the matt variety shows an orange-yellow colour, the intensity of which depends on the quantity of titanium dioxide present.

TESTS

Solution S Place 15.0 g in a suitable vessel, add 150 ml of *water R*, close the vessel and allow to macerate for 2 h. Decant the solution, squeeze the residual liquid carefully from the sample with a glass rod and mix. Reserve 10 ml of the solution for the test for surface-active substances and filter the remainder.

Acidity or alkalinity To 25 ml of solution S add 0.1 ml of *phenolphthalein solution R* and to another 25 ml add 0.05 ml of *methyl orange solution R*. Neither solution is pink.

Foreign fibres Examined under a microscope, it is seen to consist exclusively of viscose fibres, except that occasionally a few isolated foreign fibres may be present.

Fluorescence Examine a layer about 5 mm in thickness under ultraviolet light at 365 nm. It displays only a slight brownish-violet fluorescence but no intense blue fluorescence, apart from that which may be shown by a few isolated fibres.

Absorbency

Apparatus. A dry cylindrical copper-wire basket 8.0 cm high and 5.0 cm in diameter. The wire of which the basket is constructed is about 0.4 mm in diameter, the mesh is 1.5 cm to 2.0 cm, and the mass of the basket is 2.7 ± 0.3 g.

Sinking time. Not more than 10 s. Weigh the basket to the nearest centigram (m_1). Take a total of 5.00 g in approximately equal quantities from five different places in the product to be examined, place loosely in the basket and weigh the filled basket to the nearest centigram (m_2). Fill a beaker 11 cm to 12 cm in diameter to a depth of 10 cm with *water R* at about 20°C. Hold the basket horizontally and drop it from a height of about 10 mm into the water. Measure with a stopwatch the time taken for the basket to sink below the surface of the water. Calculate the result as the average of three tests.

Water-holding capacity. Not less than 18.0 g of *water R* per gram. After the sinking time has been measured, remove the basket from the water, allow it to drain for exactly 30 s suspended with its long axis in the horizontal position over the beaker, transfer it to a tared beaker (m_3) and weigh to the nearest centigram (m_4).

$$\text{Water-holding capacity per gram} = \frac{m_4-(m_2+m_3)}{m_2-m_1} \text{ grams}$$

Calculate the result as the average of three tests.

Ether-soluble substances Not more than 0.30 per cent. In an extraction apparatus extract 5.00 g with *ether R* for 4 h at the rate of at least four extractions per hour. Evaporate the ether extract and dry the residue to constant mass at 100°C to 105°C.

Extractable colouring matter In a narrow percolator, slowly extract 10.0 g with *alcohol R* until 50 ml of extract is obtained. The liquid obtained is not more intensely coloured (*Method II, 2.2.2*) than reference solution Y_5, GY_6 or a reference solution prepared as follows: to 3.0 ml of blue primary solution add 7.0 ml of hydrochloric acid (10 g/l HCl) and dilute 0.5 ml of this solution to 10.0 ml with hydrochloric acid (10 g/l HCl).

Surface-active substances Introduce the 10 ml portion of solution S reserved before filtration into a 25 ml graduated ground-glass-stoppered cylinder with an external diameter of 20 ± 2 mm previously rinsed with *sulphuric acid R* and then with *water R*. Shake vigorously thirty times in 10 s, allow to stand for 1 min and repeat the shaking. After 5 min, the height reached by the froth does not exceed 2 mm above the surface of the liquid.

Water-soluble substances Not more than 0.70 per cent. Boil 5.00 g in 500 ml of *water R* for 30 min, stirring frequently. Replace the water lost by evaporation. Decant the liquid, squeeze the residual liquid carefully from the sample with a glass rod, and mix. Filter the liquid whilst hot. Evaporate 400 ml of the extract (corresponding to 4/5th of the mass of the sample taken) and dry the residue to constant mass at 100°C to 105°C.

Hydrogen sulphide To 10 ml of solution S add 1.9 ml of *water R*, 0.15 ml of *dilute acetic acid R* and 1 ml of *lead acetate solution R*. After 2 min, the solution is not more intensely coloured than a reference solution prepared at the same time using 0.15 ml of *dilute acetic acid R*, 1.2 ml of *thioacetamide reagent R*, 1.7 ml of *lead standard solution (10 ppm Pb) R* and 10 ml of solution S.

Loss on drying (*2.2.32*). Not more than 13.0 per cent, determined on 5.000 g by drying in an oven at 100°C to 105°C.

Sulphated ash (*2.4.14*). Not more than 0.45 per cent for the lustrous variety and not more than 1.7 per cent for the matt variety. Introduce 5.00 g into a previously heated and cooled, tared crucible. Heat cautiously over a naked flame and then carefully to dull redness at 600°C. Allow to cool, add a few drops of *dilute sulphuric acid R*, then heat and incinerate until all the black particles have disappeared. Allow to cool. Add a few drops of *ammonium carbonate solution R*. Evaporate and incinerate carefully, allow to cool and weigh again. Repeat the incineration for periods of 5 min to constant mass.

STORAGE

Store in a dust-proof package in a dry place.

Ph Eur

Sterile Absorbent Viscose Wadding

Sterile Absorbent Viscose Wadding complies with the requirements of the 3rd edition of the European Pharmacopoeia [0035]. These requirements are reproduced after the heading 'Definition' below.

Ph Eur

DEFINITION

Sterile absorbent viscose wadding complies with the definition, characters, identification and tests prescribed in the monograph on *Viscose wadding, absorbent (34)*. It may, however, become slightly yellowish when sterilised by heat. It also complies with the following test.

Sterility (*2.6.1*). It complies with the test for sterility as applied to surgical dressings.

STORAGE

Store in a package that protects the contents from contamination, in a dry place.

Ph Eur

SUTURES

Sutures comply with the requirements of the third edition of the European Pharmacopoeia. The introduction to these requirements is reproduced below.

Ph Eur

INTRODUCTION

The following monographs apply to sutures for human use: Catgut, sterile (317), Sutures, sterile non-absorbable (324), Sutures, sterile synthetic absorbable braided (667) and Sutures, sterile synthetic absorbable monofilament (666). They cover performance characteristics of sutures and may include methods of identification. Sutures are medical devices as defined in Directive 93/42/EEC.

These monographs can be applied to show compliance with essential requirements as defined in Article 3 of Directive 93/42/EEC covering the following:

Physical performance characteristics: diameter, breaking load, needle attachment, packaging, sterility, information supplied by the manufacturer (see Section 13 of Annex 1 of Directive 93/42/EEC), labelling.

To show compliance with other essential requirements, the application of appropriate harmonised standards as defined in Article 5 of Directive 93/42/EEC may be considered.

Ph Eur

Sterile Catgut

Sterile Catgut complies with the requirements of the 3rd edition of the European Pharmacopoeia [0317]. These requirements are reproduced after the heading 'Definition' below.

DEFINITION

Sterile catgut consists of sutures prepared from collagen taken from the intestinal membranes of mammals. After cleaning, the membranes are split longitudinally into strips of varying width, which, when assembled in small numbers, according to the diameter required, are twisted under tension, dried, polished, selected and sterilised. The sutures may be treated with chemical substances such as chromium salts to prolong absorption and glycerol to make them supple, provided such substances do not reduce tissue acceptability.

Appropriate harmonised standards may be considered when assessing compliance with respect to origin and processing of raw materials and with respect to biocompatibility.

Sterile catgut is a surgical wound-closure device. Being an absorbable suture it serves to approximate tissue during the healing period and is subsequently metabolised by proteolytic activity.

PRODUCTION

Appropriate harmonised standards may apply with respect to appropriate validated methods of sterilisation, environmental control during manufacturing, labelling and packaging.

It is essential for the effectiveness and the performance characteristics during use and during the functional lifetime of catgut that the following physical properties are specified: consistent diameter, sufficient initial strength and firm needle attachment.

The requirements outlined below have been established, taking into account stresses which occur during normal conditions of use. These requirements can be used to demonstrate that individual production batches of sterile catgut are suitable for wound closure according to usual surgical techniques.

TESTS

If stored in a preserving liquid, remove the sutures from the sachet and measure promptly and in succession the length, diameter and breaking load. If stored in the dry state, immerse the sutures in alcohol R or a 90 per cent V/V solution of 2-propanol R for 24 h and proceed with the measurements as indicated below.

Length Measure the length without applying to the suture more tension than is necessary to keep it straight. The length of each suture is not less than 90 per cent of the length stated on the label and does not exceed 350 cm.

Diameter Carry out the test on five sutures. Use a suitable instrument capable of measuring with an accuracy of at least 0.002 mm and having a circular pressor foot 10 mm to 15 mm in diameter. The pressor foot and the moving parts attached to it are weighted so as to apply a total load of 100 ± 10 g to the suture being tested. When making the measurement, lower the pressor foot slowly to avoid crushing the suture. Measure the diameter at intervals of 30 cm over the whole length of the suture. For a suture less than 90 cm in length, measure at three points approximately evenly spaced along the suture. The suture is not subjected to more tension than is necessary to keep it straight during measurement. The average of the measurements carried out on the sutures being tested and not less than two-thirds of the measurements taken on

TABLE 317-1.-*Diameters and Breaking Loads*

Gauge number	Diameter (millimetres)				Breaking load (newtons)	
	A		B		C	D
	min.	max.	min.	max.		
0.1	0.010	0.019	0.005	0.025	—	—
0.2	0.020	0.029	0.015	0.035	—	—
0.3	0.030	0.039	0.025	0.045	0.20	0.05
0.4	0.040	0.049	0.035	0.060	0.30	0.10
0.5	0.050	0.069	0.045	0.085	0.40	0.20
0.7	0.070	0.099	0.060	0.125	0.70	0.30
1	0.100	0.149	0.085	0.175	1.8	0.40
1.5	0.150	0.199	0.125	0.225	3.8	0.70
2	0.200	0.249	0.175	0.275	7.5	1.8
2.5	0.250	0.299	0.225	0.325	10	3.8
3	0.300	0.349	0.275	0.375	12.5	7.5
3.5	0.350	0.399	0.325	0.450	20	10
4	0.400	0.499	0.375	0.550	27.5	12.5
5	0.500	0.599	0.450	0.650	38.0	20.0
6	0.600	0.699	0.550	0.750	45.0	27.5
7	0.700	0.799	0.650	0.850	60.0	38.0
8	0.800	0.899	0.750	0.950	70.0	45.0

each suture are within the limits given in the columns under A in Table 317-1 for the gauge number concerned. None of the measurements is outside the limits given in the columns under B in Table 317-1 for the gauge number concerned.

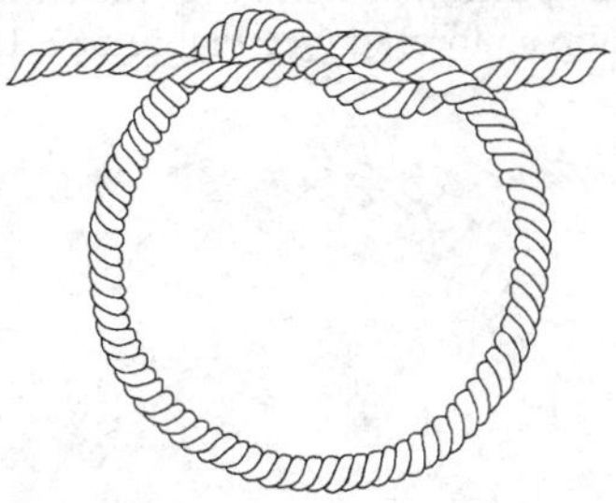

Figure 317-1.-Simple knot

Minimum breaking load The minimum breaking load is determined over a simple knot formed by placing one end of a suture held in the right hand over the other end held in the left hand, passing one end over the suture and through the loop so formed (see Figure 317-1) and pulling the knot tight. Carry out the test on five sutures. Submit sutures of length greater than 75 cm to two measurements and shorter sutures to one measurement. Determine the breaking load using a suitable tensilometer. The apparatus has two clamps for holding the suture, one of which is mobile and is driven at a constant rate of 30 cm per minute. The clamps are designed so that the suture being tested can be attached without any possibility of slipping. At the beginning of the test the length of suture between the clamps is 12.5 cm to 20 cm and the knot is midway between the clamps. Set the mobile clamp in motion and note the force required to break the suture. If the suture breaks in a clamp or within 1 cm of it, the result is discarded and the test repeated on another suture. The average of all the results, excluding those legitimately discarded, is equal to or greater than the value given in column C in Table 317-1 and no individual result is less than that given in column D for the gauge number concerned.

Soluble chromium compounds Place 0.25 g in a conical flask containing 1 ml of *water R per* 10 mg of catgut. Stopper the flask, allow to stand at 37 ± 0.5°C for 24 h, cool and decant the liquid. Transfer 5 ml to a small test tube and add 2 ml of a 10 g/l solution of *diphenylcarbazide R* in *alcohol R* and 2 ml of *dilute sulphuric acid R*. The solution is not more intensely coloured than a standard prepared at the same time using 5 ml of a solution containing 2.83 μg of *potassium dichromate R* per millilitre, 2 ml of *dilute sulphuric acid R* and 2 ml of a 10 g/l solution of *diphenylcarbazide R* in *alcohol R* (1 ppm of Cr).

Needle attachment If the catgut is supplied with an eyeless needle attached that is not stated to be detachable, it complies with the test for needle attachment. Carry out the test on five sutures. Use a suitable tensilometer, such as that described for the determination of the minimum breaking load. Fix the needle and suture (without knot) in the clamps of the apparatus in such a way that the swaged part of the needle is completely free of the clamp and in line with the direction of pull on the suture. Set the mobile clamp in motion and note the force required to break the suture or to detach it from the needle. The average of the five determinations and all individual values are not less than the respective values given in Table 317-2 for the gauge number concerned. If not more than one individual value fails to meet the individual requirement, repeat the test on an additional ten sutures. The catgut complies with the test if none of these ten values is less than the individual value in Table 317-2 for the gauge number concerned.

TABLE 317-2.-*Minimum Strengths of Needle Attachment*

Gauge number	Mean value (newtons)	Individual values (newtons)
0.5	0.50	0.25
0.7	0.80	0.40
1	1.7	0.80
1.5	2.3	1.1
2	4.5	2.3
2.5	5.6	2.8
3	6.8	3.4
3.5	11.0	4.5
4	15.0	4.5
5	18.0	6.0

STORAGE (PACKAGING)

Sterile catgut sutures are presented in individual sachets that maintain sterility and allow the withdrawal and use of the sutures in asetic conditions. Sterile catgut may be stored dry or in a preserving liquid to which an antimicrobial agent but not an antibiotic may be added.

Sutures in their individual sachets (primary packaging) are kept in a protective cover (box) which maintains the physical and mechanical properties until the time of use.

The application of appropriate harmonised standards for packaging of medical devices shall be considered.

LABELLING

Reference may be made to the appropriate harmonised standards for labelling of medical devices.

The details strictly necessary for the user to identify the product properly are indicated on or in each sachet (primary packaging) and on the protective cover (box) and include at least:

— gauge number,
— length in centimetres or metres,
— if appropriate, that the needle is detachable,
— name of the product,
— intended use (surgical suture, absorbable).

Ph Eur

Sterile Synthetic Absorbable Braided Sutures

Sterile Synthetic Absorbable Braided Sutures comply with the requirements of the 3rd edition of the European Pharmacopoeia [0667]. These requirements are reproduced after the heading 'Definition' below.

Ph Eur

DEFINITION

Sterile synthetic absorbable braided sutures consist of sutures prepared from a synthetic polymer, polymers or copolymers which, when introduced into a living organism, are absorbed by that organism and cause no undue tissue irritation. They consist of completely polymerised material. They occur as multifilament sutures consisting of elementary fibres which are assembled by braiding. The sutures may be treated to facilitate handling and they may be coloured.

Appropriate harmonised standards may be considered when assessing compliance with respect to origin and processing of raw materials and with respect to biocompatibility.

Sterile synthetic absorbable braided sutures are wound-closure devices. Being absorbable they serve to approximate tissue during the healing period and subsequently lose tensile strength by hydrolysis.

PRODUCTION

Appropriate harmonised standards may apply with respect to appropriate validated methods of sterilisation, environmental control during manufacturing, labelling and packaging.

It is essential for the effectiveness and the performance characteristics during use and during the functional lifetime of these sutures that the following physical properties are specified: consistent diameter, sufficient initial strength and firm needle attachment.

The requirements below have been established, taking into account stresses which occur during normal conditions of use. These requirements can be used to demonstrate that individual production batches of these sutures are suitable for wound closure according to usual surgical techniques.

TESTS

Carry out the following tests on the sutures in the state in which they are removed from the sachet.

Length Measure the length of the suture without applying more tension than is necessary to keep it straight. The length of each suture is not less than 95 per cent of the length stated on the label and does not exceed 400 cm.

Diameter Unless otherwise prescribed, measure the diameter by the following method, using five sutures in the condition in which they are presented. Use a suitable instrument capable of measuring with an accuracy of at least 0.002 mm and having a circular pressor foot 10 mm to 15 mm in diameter. The pressor foot and the moving parts attached to it are weighted so as to apply a total load of 100 ± 10 g to the suture being tested. When making the measurements, lower the pressor foot slowly to avoid crushing the suture. Measure the diameter at intervals of 30 cm over the whole length of the suture. For a suture less than 90 cm in length, measure at three points approximately evenly spaced along the suture. During the measurement, submit the sutures to a tension not greater than one-fifth of the minimum breaking load shown in column C of Table 667-1 appropriate to the gauge number and type of material or 10 N whichever is the less. For sutures of gauge number above 1.5 make two measurements at each point, the second measurement being made after rotating the suture through 90°. The diameter of that point is the average of the two measurements. The average of the measurements carried out on the sutures being tested and not less than two-thirds of the measurements taken on each suture are within the limits given in the columns under A in Table 667-1 for the gauge number concerned. None of the measurements is outside the limits given in the columns under B in Table 667-1 for the gauge number concerned.

Minimum breaking load The minimum breaking load is determined over a simple knot formed by placing one end of a suture held in the right hand over the other end held in the left hand, passing one end over the suture and through the loop so formed (see Figure 667-1) and pulling the knot tight.

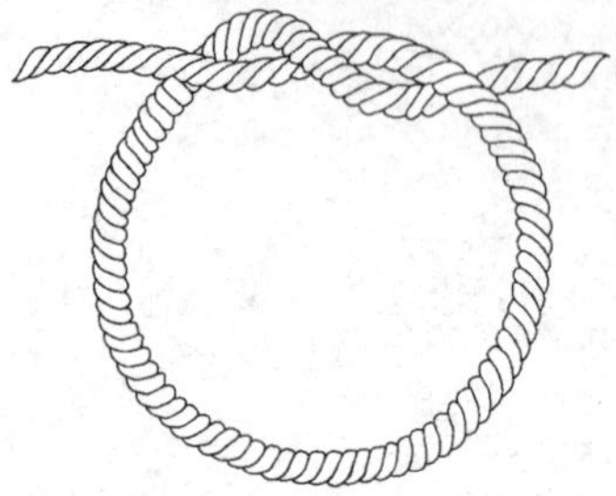

Figure 667-1.-Simple knot

Carry out the test on five sutures. Submit sutures of length greater than 75 cm to two measurements and shorter sutures to one measurement. Determine the breaking load using a suitable tensilometer. The apparatus has two clamps for holding the suture, one of which is mobile and is driven at a constant rate of 25 cm to 30 cm per minute. The clamps are designed so that the suture being tested can be attached without any possibility of slipping. At the beginning of the test the length of suture between the clamps is 12.5 cm to 20 cm and the knot is midway between the clamps. Set the mobile clamp in motion and note the force required to break the suture. If the suture breaks in a clamp or within 1 cm of it, the result is discarded and the test repeated on another suture. The average of all the results excluding those legitimately discarded is equal to or greater than the value given in column C in Table 667-1 and no individual result is less than that given in column D for the gauge number concerned.

Table 667-1.-*Diameters and Breaking Loads*

Gauge number	Diameter (millimetres)				Breaking load (newtons)	
	A		B		C	D
	min.	max.	min.	max.		
0.01	0.001	0.004	0.008	0.005	–	–
0.05	0.005	0.009	0.003	0.012	–	–
0.1	0.010	0.019	0.005	0.025	–	–
0.2	0.020	0.029	0.015	0.035	–	–
0.3	0.030	0.039	0.025	0.045	0.45	0.23
0.4	0.040	0.049	0.035	0.060	0.70	0.35
0.5	0.050	0.069	0.045	0.085	1.4	0.7
0.7	0.070	0.099	0.060	0.125	2.5	1.3
1	0.100	0.149	0.085	0.175	6.8	3.4
1.5	0.150	0.199	0.125	0.225	9.5	4.8
2	0.200	0.249	0.175	0.275	17.7	8.9
2.5	0.250	0.299	0.225	0.325	21.0	10.5
3	0.300	0.349	0.275	0.375	26.8	13.4
3.5	0.350	0.399	0.325	0.450	39.0	18.5
4	0.400	0.499	0.375	0.550	50.8	25.4
5	0.500	0.599	0.450	0.650	63.5	31.8
6	0.600	0.699	0.550	0.750	–	–
7	0.700	0.799	0.650	0.850	–	–

Needle attachment If the suture is supplied with an eyeless needle attached that is not stated to be detachable the attachment, it complies with the test for needle attachment. Carry out the test on five sutures. Use a suitable tensilometer, such as that described for the determination of the minimum breaking load. Fix the needle and suture (without knot) in the clamps of the apparatus in such a way that the swaged part of the needle is completely free of the clamp and in line with the direction of pull on the suture. Set the mobile clamp in motion and note the force required to break the suture or to detach it from the needle. The average of the five determinations and all individual values are not less than the respective values given in Table 667-2 for the gauge number concerned. If not more than one individual value fails to meet the individual requirement, repeat the test on an additional ten sutures. The attachment complies with the test if none of the ten values is less than the individual value in Table 667-2 for the gauge number concerned.

TABLE 667-2.-*Minimum Strengths of Needle Attachment*

Gauge number	Mean value (newtons)	Individual value (newtons)
0.4	0.50	0.25
0.5	0.80	0.40
0.7	1.7	0.80
1	2.3	1.1
1.5	4.5	2.3
2	6.8	3.4
2.5	9.0	4.5
3	11.0	4.5
3.5	15.0	4.5
4	18.0	6.0
5	18.0	7.0

STORAGE (PACKAGING)

Sterile synthetic absorbable braided sutures are presented in a suitable sachet that maintains sterility and allows the withdrawal and use of the sutures in aseptic conditions. The sutures must be stored dry.

They are intended to be used only on the occasion when the sachet is first opened.

Sutures in their individual sachets (primary packaging) are kept in a protective cover (box) which maintains the physical and mechanical properties until the time of use.

The application of appropriate harmonised standards for packaging of medical devices may be considered in addition.

LABELLING

Reference may be made to the appropriate harmonised standards for the labelling of medical devices.

The details strictly necessary for the user to identify the product properly are indicated on or in each sachet (primary packaging) and on the protective cover (box) and include at least:

— gauge number,
— length in centimetres or metres,
— if appropriate, that the needle is detachable,
— name of the product,
— intended use (surgical absorbable suture),
— if appropriate, that the suture is coloured,
— the structure (braided).

Ph Eur

Sterile Synthetic Absorbable Monofilament Sutures

Sterile Synthetic Absorbable Monofilament Sutures comply with the requirements of the 3rd edition of the European Pharmacopoeia [0666]. These requirements are reproduced after the heading 'Definition' below.

Ph Eur

DEFINITION

Sterile synthetic absorbable monofilament sutures consist of sutures prepared from a synthetic polymer, polymers or copolymers which, when introduced into a living organism, are absorbed by that organism and cause no undue tissue irritation. They consist of completely polymerised material. They occur as monofilament sutures. The sutures may be treated to facilitate handling and they may be coloured.

Appropriate harmonised standards may be considered when assessing compliance with respect to origin and processing of raw materials and with respect to biocompatibility.

Sterile synthetic absorbable monofilament sutures are wound-closure devices. Being absorbable they serve to approximate tissue during the healing period and subsequently lose tensile strength by hydrolysis.

PRODUCTION

The appropriate harmonised standards may apply with respect to appropriate validated methods of sterilisation, environmental control during manufacturing, labelling and packaging.

It is essential for the effectiveness and the performance characteristics during use and during the functional lifetime of these sutures that the following physical properties are specified: consistent diameter, sufficient initial strength and firm needle attachment.

The requirements below have been established, taking into account stresses which occur during normal conditions of use. These requirements can be used to demonstrate that individual production batches of these sutures are suitable for wound closure according to usual surgical techniques.

TESTS

Carry out the following tests on the sutures in the state in which they are removed from the sachet.

Length Measure the length of the suture without applying more tension than is necessary to keep it straight. The length of each suture is not less than 95 per cent of the length stated on the label and does not exceed 400 cm.

Diameter Unless otherwise prescribed, measure the diameter by the following method, using five sutures in the condition in which they are presented. Use a suitable instrument capable of measuring with an accuracy of at least 0.002 mm and having a circular pressor foot 10 mm to 15 mm in diameter. The pressor foot and the moving parts attached to it are weighted so as to apply a total load of 100 ± 10 g to the suture being tested. When making the measurements, lower the pressor foot slowly to avoid crushing the suture. Measure the diameter at intervals of 30 cm over the whole length of the suture. For a suture less than 90 cm in length, measure at three points approximately evenly spaced along the suture. During the measurement, submit the sutures to a tension not greater than that required to keep them straight. The average of the measurements carried out on the sutures being tested and not less than two-thirds of the measurements taken on each suture are within the limits given in the columns under A in Table 666-1 for the gauge number concerned. None of the measurements is outside the limits given in the columns under B in Table 666-1 for the gauge number concerned.

Table 666-1.-*Diameters and Breaking Loads*

Gauge number	Diameter (millimetres)				Breaking load (newtons)	
	A		B		C	D
	min.	max.	min.	max.		
0.5	0.050	0.094	0.045	0.125	1.4	0.7
0.7	0.095	0.149	0.075	0.175	2.5	1.3
1	0.150	0.199	0.125	0.225	6.8	3.4
1.5	0.200	0.249	0.175	0.275	9.5	4.7
2	0.250	0.339	0.225	0.375	17.5	8.9
3	0.340	0.399	0.325	0.450	26.8	13.4
3.5	0.400	0.499	0.375	0.550	39.0	18.5
4	0.500	0.570	0.450	0.600	50.8	25.4
5	0.571	0.610	0.500	0.700	63.5	31.8

Minimum breaking load The minimum breaking load is determined over a simple knot formed by placing one end of a suture held in the right hand over the other end held in the left hand, passing one end over the suture and through the loop so formed (see Figure 666-1) and pulling the knot tight.

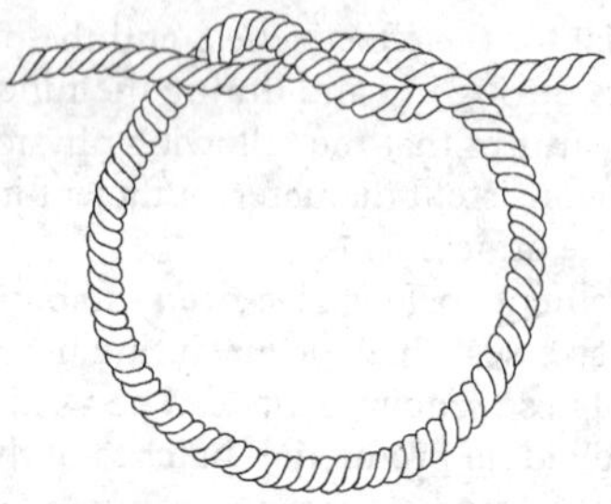

Figure 666-1.-Simple knot

Carry out the test on five sutures. Submit sutures of length greater than 75 cm to two measurements and shorter sutures to one measurement. Determine the breaking load using a suitable tensilometer. The apparatus has two clamps for holding the suture, one of which is mobile and is driven at a constant rate of 25 cm to 30 cm per minute. The clamps are designed so that the suture being tested can be attached without any possibility of slipping. At the beginning of the test the length of suture between the clamps is 12.5 cm to 20 cm and the knot is midway between the clamps. Set the mobile clamp in motion and note the force required to break the suture. If the suture breaks in a clamp or within 1 cm of it, the result is discarded and the test repeated on another suture. The average of all the results excluding those legitimately discarded is equal to or greater than the value given in column C in Table 666-1 and no individual result is less than that given in column D for the gauge number concerned.

Needle attachment If the suture is supplied with an eyeless needle attached that is not stated to be detachable, the attachment complies with the test for needle attachment. Carry out the test on five sutures. Use a suitable tensilometer, such as that described for the determination of the minimum breaking load. Fix the needle and suture (without knot) in the clamps of the apparatus in such a way that the swaged part of the needle is completely free of the clamp and in line with the direction of pull on the suture. Set the mobile clamp in motion and note the force required to break the suture or to detach it from the needle. The average of the five determinations and all individual values are not less than the respective values given in Table 666-2 for the gauge number concerned. If not more than one individual value fails to meet the individual requirement, repeat the test on an additional ten sutures. The attachment complies with the test if none of the ten values is less than the individual value in Table 666-2 for the gauge number concerned.

Table 666-2.-*Minimum Strengths of Needle Attachment*

Gauge number	Mean value (newtons)	Individual value (newtons)
0.5	0.80	0.40
0.7	1.7	0.80
1	2.3	1.1
1.5	4.5	2.3
2	6.8	3.4
2.5	9.0	4.5
3	11.0	4.5
3.5	15.0	4.5
4	18.0	6.0
5	18.0	7.0

STORAGE (PACKAGING)

Sterile synthetic absorbable monofilament sutures are presented in a suitable sachet that maintains sterility and allows the withdrawal and use of the sutures in aseptic conditions. The sutures must be stored dry.

They are intended to be used only on the occasion when the sachet is first opened.

Sutures in their individual sachets (primary packaging) are kept in a protective cover (box) which maintains the physical and mechanical properties until the time of use.

The application of appropriate harmonised standards for packaging of medical devices may be considered in addition.

LABELLING

Reference may be made to appropriate harmonised standards for the labelling of medical devices.

The details strictly necessary for the user to identify the product properly are indicated on or in each sachet (primary packaging) and on the protective cover (box) and include at least:

— gauge number,
— length in centimetres or metres,
— if appropriate, that the needle is detachable,
— name of the product,
— intended use (surgical absorbable suture),
— if appropriate, that the suture is coloured,
— the structure (monofilament).

Ph Eur

Sterile Non-absorbable Sutures

Sterile Non-absorbable Ligatures

Sterile Braided Silk Suture, Sterile Linen Thread (Suture), Sterile Polyethylene Terephthalate (Polyester) Suture, Sterile Polyamide 6 Suture, Sterile Polyamide 6/6 Suture and Sterile Polypropylene Suture comply with the requirements of the 3rd edition of the European Pharmacopoeia for Sterile Synthetic Non-absorbable Sutures [0324]. These requirements are reproduced after the heading 'Definition' below.

NOTE: The name Nylon 6 as a synonym for Polyamide 6 and Nylon 6/6 as a synonym for Polyamide 6/6 may be used freely in many countries, including the United Kingdom, but exclusive proprietary rights in this name are claimed in certain other countries.

Ph Eur

DEFINITION

Sterile non-absorbable sutures are sutures which, when introduced into a living organism, are not metabolised by that organism. Sterile non-absorbable sutures vary in origin, which may be animal, vegetable, metallic or synthetic. They occur as cylindrical monofilaments or as multifilament sutures consisting of elementary fibres which are assembled by twisting, cabling or braiding; they may be sheathed; they may be treated to render them non-capillary, and they may be coloured.

Appropriate harmonised standards may be considered when assessing compliance with respect to origin and processing of raw materials and with respect to biocompatibility.

Sterile non-absorbable surgical sutures serve to approximate tissue during the healing period and provide continuing wound support.

Commonly used materials include the following:

Silk (Filum Bombycis)

Sterile braided silk suture is obtained by braiding a number of threads, according to the diameter required, of degummed silk obtained from the cocoons of the silkworm *Bombyx mori L.*

Linen (Filum Lini)

Sterile linen thread consists of the pericyclic fibres of the stem of *Linum usitatissimum* L. The elementary fibres, 2.5 cm to 5 cm long, are assembled in bundles 30 cm to 80 cm long and spun into continuous lengths of suitable diameter.

Poly(ethylene Terephthalate) (Filum Ethyleni Polyterephthalici)

Sterile poly(ethylene terephthalate) suture is obtained by drawing poly(ethylene terephthalate) through a suitable die. The suture is prepared by braiding very fine filaments in suitable numbers, depending on the gauge required.

Polyamide 6 (Filum Polyamidicum-6)

Sterile polyamide 6 suture is obtained by drawing through a suitable die a synthetic plastic material formed by the polymerisation of ε-caprolactam. It consists of smooth, cylindrical monofilaments or braided filaments, or lightly twisted sutures sheathed with the same material.

Polyamide 6/6 (Filum polyamidicum 6/6)

Sterile polyamide 6/6 suture is obtained by drawing through a suitable die a synthetic plastic material formed by the polycondensation of hexamethylenediamine and adipic acid. It consists of smooth, cylindrical monofilaments or braided filaments, or lightly twisted sutures sheathed with the same material.

TABLE 324-1.-*Diameters and Minimum Breaking Loads*

Gauge number	Diameter (millimetres) A		B		Minimum breaking load (newtons) Linen thread		All other non-absorbable strands	
	min	max	min	max	C	D	C	D
0.05	0.005	0.009	0.003	0.012	–	–	0.01	–
0.1	0.010	0.019	0.005	0.025	–	–	0.03	–
0.15	0.015	0.019	0.012	0.025	–	–	0.06	–
0.2	0.020	0.029	0.015	0.035	–	–	0.1	–
0.3	0.030	0.039	0.025	0.045	–	–	0.35	–
0.4	0.040	0.049	0.035	0.060	–	–	0.60	–
0.5	0.050	0.069	0.045	0.085	–	–	1.0	0.35
0.7	0.070	0.099	0.060	0.125	1.0	0.3	1.5	0.60
1	0.100	0.149	0.085	0.175	2.5	0.6	3.0	1.0
1.5	0.150	0.199	0.125	0.225	5.0	1.0	5.0	1.5
2	0.200	0.249	0.175	0.275	8.0	2.5	9.0	3.0
2.5	0.250	0.299	0.225	0.325	9.0	5.0	13.0	5.0
3	0.300	0.349	0.275	0.375	11.0	8.0	15.0	9.0
3.5	0.350	0.399	0.325	0.450	15.0	9.0	22.0	13.0
4	0.400	0.499	0.375	0.550	18.0	11.0	27.0	15.0
5	0.500	0.599	0.450	0.650	26.0	15.0	35.0	22.0
6	0.600	0.699	0.550	0.750	37.0	18.0	50.0	27.0
7	0.700	0.799	0.650	0.850	50.0	26.0	62.0	35.0
8	0.800	0.899	0.750	0.950	65.0	37.0	73.0	50.0

Polypropylene (Filum polypropylenicum)

Polypropylene suture is obtained by drawing polypropylene through a suitable die. It consists of smooth cylindrical monofilaments.

IDENTIFICATION

Non-absorbable sutures may be identified by chemical tests. Materials from natural origin may also be identified by microscopic examination of the morphology of these fibres. For synthetic materials, identification by infrared spectrophotometry (*2.2.24*) or by differential scanning calorimetry may be applied.

Identification of silk

A. Dissect the end of a suture, using a needle or fine tweezers, to isolate a few individual fibres. The fibres are sometimes marked with very fine longitudinal striations parallel to the axis of the suture. Examined under a microscope, a cross-section is more or less triangular to semicircular, with rounded edges and without a lumen.

B. Impregnate isolated fibres with *iodinated potassium iodide solution R*. The fibres are coloured pale yellow.

Identification of linen

A. Dissect the end of a suture, using a needle or fine tweezers, to isolate a few individual fibres. Examined under a microscope, the fibres are seen to be 12 μm to 31 μm wide and, along the greater part of their length, have thick walls, sometimes marked with fine longitudinal striations, and a narrow lumen. The fibres gradually narrow to a long, fine point. Sometimes there are unilateral swellings with transverse lines.

B. Impregnate isolated fibres with *iodinated zinc chloride solution R*. The fibres are coloured violet-blue.

Identification of poly(ethyleneterephthalate)

It is practically insoluble in most of the usual organic solvents, but is attacked by strong alkaline solutions. It is incompatible with phenols.

A. It dissolves with difficulty when heated in *dimethylformamide R* and in *dichlorobenzene R*.

B. To about 50 mg add 10 ml of *hydrochloric acid R1*. The material remains intact even after immersion for 6 h.

Identification of polyamide 6

It is practically insoluble in the usual organic solvents; it is not attacked by dilute alkaline solutions (for example a 100 g/l solution of *sodium hydroxide R*) but is attacked by dilute mineral acids (for example a 20 g/l solution of *sulphuric acid R*), by hot *glacial acetic acid R* and by a 70 per cent *m/m* solution of *anhydrous formic acid R*.

A. Heat about 50 mg with 0.5 ml of *hydrochloric acid R1* in a sealed glass tube at 110°C for 18 h and allow to stand for 6 h. No crystals appear.

B. It dissolves in a 70 per cent *m/m* solution of *anhydrous formic acid R*.

Identification of polyamide 6/6

It is practically insoluble in the usual organic solvents; it is not attacked by dilute alkaline solutions (for example a 100 g/l solution of *sodium hydroxide R*) but is attacked by dilute mineral acids (for example a 20 g/l solution of *sulphuric acid R*), by hot *glacial acetic acid R* and by an 80 per cent *m/m* solution of *anhydrous formic acid R*.

A. In contact with a flame it melts and burns, forming a hard globule of residue and gives off a characteristic odour resembling that of celery.

B. Place about 50 mg in an ignition tube held vertically and heat gently until thick fumes are evolved. When the fumes fill the tube, withdraw it from the flame and insert a strip of *nitrobenzaldehyde paper R*. A violet-brown colour slowly appears on the paper and fades slowly in air; it disappears almost immediately on washing with *dilute sulphuric acid R*.

C. To about 50 mg add 10 ml of *hydrochloric acid R1*. The material disintegrates in the cold and dissolves within a few minutes.

D. It does not dissolve in a 70 per cent *m/m* solution of *anhydrous formic acid R* but dissolves in an 80 per cent *m/m* solution of *anhydrous formic acid R*.

Identification of polypropylene

Polypropylene is soluble in decahydronaphthalene, 1-chloronaphthalene and trichloroethylene. It is not soluble in alcohol, ether and cyclohexanone.

A. It softens at temperatures between 160°C and 170°C. It burns with a blue flame giving off an odour of burning paraffin wax and of octyl alcohol.

B. To 0.25 g add 10 ml of *toluene R* and boil under a reflux condenser for about 15 min. Place a few drops of the solution on a disc of *sodium chloride R* slide and evaporate the solvent in an oven at 80°C. Examine by infrared absorption spectrophotometry (*2.2.24*), comparing with the spectrum obtained with *polypropylene CRS*.

C. To 2 g add 100 ml of *water R* and boil under a reflux condenser for 2 h. Allow to cool. The relative density (*2.2.5*) of the material is 0.89 g/ml to 0.91 g/ml, determined using a hydrostatic balance.

PRODUCTION

The appropriate harmonised standards may apply with respect to appropriate validated methods of sterilisation, environmental control during manufacturing, labelling and packaging.

It is essential for the effectiveness and the performance characteristics during use and during the functional lifetime of these sutures that the following physical properties are specified: consistent diameter, sufficient initial strength and firm needle attachment.

The requirements below have been established, taking into account stresses which occur during normal conditions of use. These requirements can be used to demonstrate that individual production batches of these sutures are suitable for wound closure in accordance with usual surgical techniques.

TESTS

Remove the sutures from the sachet and measure promptly and in succession the length, diameter and minimum load.

If linen is tested the sutures are conditioned as follows: if stored in the dry state, expose to an atmosphere with a relative humidity of 65 ± 5 per cent at 20 ± 2°C for 4 h immediately before measuring the diameter and for the determination of minimum breaking load immerse in *water R* at room temperature for 30 min immediately before carrying out the test.

Length Measure the length in the condition in which

the sutures are presented and without applying more tension than is necessary to keep them straight. The length of the suture is not less than 95 per cent of the length stated on the label and does not exceed 400 cm.

Diameter Unless otherwise prescribed, measure the diameter by the following method using five sutures in the condition in which they are presented. Use a suitable mechanical instrument capable of measuring with an accuracy of at least 0.002 mm and having a circular pressor foot 10 mm to 15 mm in diameter. The pressor foot and the moving parts attached to it are weighted so as to apply a total load of 100 ± 10 g to the suture being tested. When making the measurements, lower the pressor foot slowly to avoid crushing the suture. Measure the diameter at intervals of 30 cm over the whole length of the suture. For a suture less than 90 cm in length, measure at three points approximately evenly spaced along the suture. During the measurement submit monofilament sutures to a tension not greater than that required to keep them straight. Submit multifilament sutures to a tension not greater than one-fifth of the minimum breaking load shown in column C of Table 324-1 appropriate to the gauge number and type of material concerned or 10 N whichever is the less. For multifilament sutures of gauge number above 1.5 make two measurements at each point, the second measurement being made after rotating the suture through 90°. The diameter of that point is the average of the two measurements. The average of the measurements carried out on the sutures being tested and not less than two-thirds of the measurements taken on each suture are within the limits given in the column under A in Table 324-1 for the gauge number concerned. None of the measurements is outside the limits given in the columns under B in Table 324-1 for the gauge number concerned.

Minimum breaking load Unless otherwise prescribed, determine the minimum breaking load by the following method using sutures in the condition in which they are presented. The minimum breaking load is determined over a simple knot formed by placing one end of a suture held in the right hand over the other end held in the left hand, passing one end over the suture and through the loop so formed (see Figure 324-1) and pulling the knot tight.

Figure 324-1.-Simple knot

Carry out the test on five sutures. Submit sutures of length greater than 75 cm to two measurements and shorter sutures to one measurement. Determine the breaking load using a suitable tensilometer. The apparatus has two clamps for holding the suture, one of which is mobile and is driven at a constant rate of 30 cm per minute. The clamps are designed so that the suture being tested can be attached without any possibility of slipping. At the beginning of the test the length of suture between the clamps is 12.5 cm to 20 cm and the knot is midway between the clamps. Set the mobile clamp in motion and note the force required to break the suture. If the suture breaks in a clamp or within 1 cm of it, the result is discarded and the test repeated on another suture. The average of all the results, excluding those legitimately discarded, is equal to or greater than the value given in column C in Table 324-1 and no value is less than that given in column D for the gauge number and type of material concerned.

Table 324-2.-*Minimum Strengths of Needle Attachment*

Gauge number	Mean value (newtons)	Individual value (newtons)
0.4	0.50	0.25
0.5	0.80	0.40
0.7	1.7	0.80
1	2.3	1.1
1.5	4.5	2.3
2	6.8	3.4
2.5	9.0	4.5
3	11.0	4.5
3.5	15.0	4.5
4	18.0	6.0
5	18.0	7.0

Needle attachment If the sutures are supplied with an eyeless needle attached that is not stated to be detachable, they comply with the test for needle attachment. Carry out the test on five sutures. Use a suitable tensilometer, such as that described for the determination of the minimum breaking load. Fix the needle and suture (without knot) in the clamps of the apparatus in such a way that the swaged part of the needle is completely free of the clamp and in line with the direction of pull on the suture. Set the mobile clamp in motion and note the force required to break the suture or to detach it from the needle. The average of the five determinations and all individual values are not less than the respective values given in Table 324-2 for the gauge number concerned. If not more than one individual value fails to meet the individual requirement, repeat the test on an additional ten sutures. The attachment complies with the test if none of these ten values is less than the individual value in Table 324-2 for the gauge number concerned.

Extractable colour Sutures that are dyed and intended to remain so during use comply with the test for extractable colour. Place 0.25 g of the suture to be examined in a conical flask, add 25.0 ml of *water R* and cover the mouth of the flask with a short-stemmed funnel. Boil for 15 min, cool and adjust to the original volume with *water R*.

Depending on the colour of the suture, prepare the appropriate reference solution as described in Table 324-3 using the primary colour solutions (*2.2.2*).

The test solution is not more intensely coloured than the appropriate reference solution.

Table 324-3.-*Colour Reference Solutions*

Colour of strand	Composition of reference solution (parts by volume)			
	Red primary solution	*Yellow primary solution*	*Blue primary solution*	*Water*
Yellow–brown	0.2	1.2	–	8.6
Pink–red	1.0	–	–	9.0
Green–blue	–	–	2.0	8.0
Violet	1.6	–	8.4	–

Monomer and oligomers Polyamide 6 suture additionally complies with the following test for monomer and oligomers. In a continuous-extraction apparatus, treat 1.00 g with 30 ml of *methanol R* at a rate of at least three extractions per hour for 7 h. Evaporate the extract to dryness, dry the residue at 110°C for 10 min, allow to cool in a desiccator and weigh. The residue weighs not more than 20 mg (2 per cent).

STORAGE (PACKAGING)

Sterile non-absorbable sutures are presented in a suitable sachet that maintains sterility and allows the withdrawal and use of a suture in aseptic conditions. They may be stored dry or in a preserving liquid to which an antimicrobial agent but no antibiotic may be added.

Sterile non-absorbable sutures are intended to be used only on the occasion when the sachet is first opened.

Sutures in their individual sachets (primary packaging) are kept in a protective cover (box) which maintains the physical and mechanical properties until the time of use.

The application of appropriate harmonised standards for packaging of medical devices shall be considered in addition.

LABELLING

Reference may be made to the appropriate harmonised standards for the labelling of medical devices.

The details strictly necessary for the user to identify the product properly are indicated on or in each sachet (primary packaging) and on the protective cover (box) and include at least:

— gauge number,
— length in centimetres or metres,
— if appropriate, that the needle is detachable,
— name of the product,
— intended use (surgical suture, non-absorbable),
— if appropriate, that the suture is coloured,
— if appropriate, the structure (braided, monofilament, sheathed).

Ph Eur

Infrared Reference Spectra

Preparation of Infrared Reference Spectra

All spectra presented in this section were recorded using either a Perkin-Elmer model 682 dispersive infrared spectrophotometer or a Perkin Elmer model 16PC Fourier transform infrared spectrophotometer.

Pressed discs, 13 mm in diameter, were prepared using potassium bromide or potassium chloride. Liquid paraffin mulls and thin films were prepared between potassium bromide plates, and gas and solution spectra were prepared using cells with potassium bromide windows. Solution spectra were prepared against a solvent reference and all other spectra were recorded against air.

For solution spectra the regions of the spectrum within which the solvent shows strong absorption should be disregarded. Solvent 'cut-offs' in the reference spectra are recorded as horizontal straight lines.

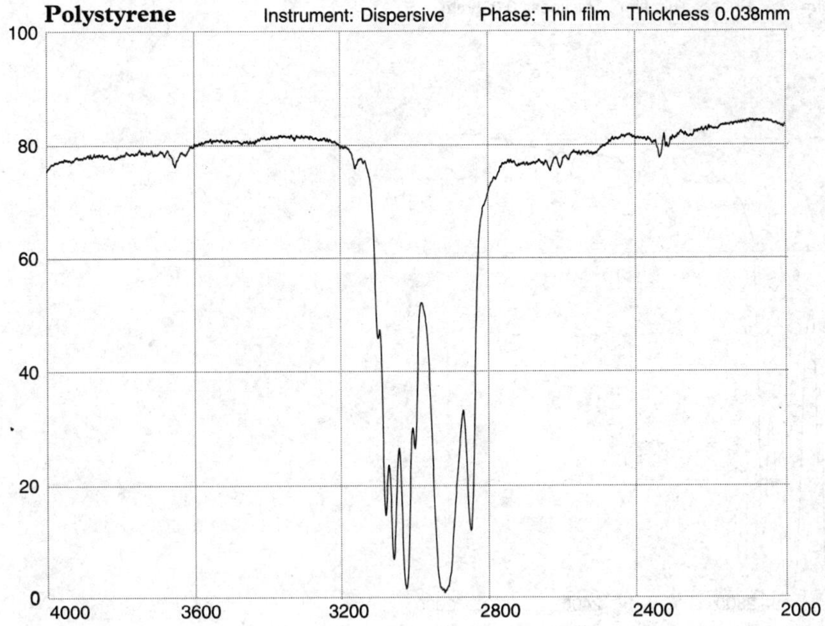
Polystyrene
Instrument: Dispersive
Phase: Thin film
Thickness 0.038mm
100
80
60
40
20
0
4000
3600
3200
2800
2400
2000

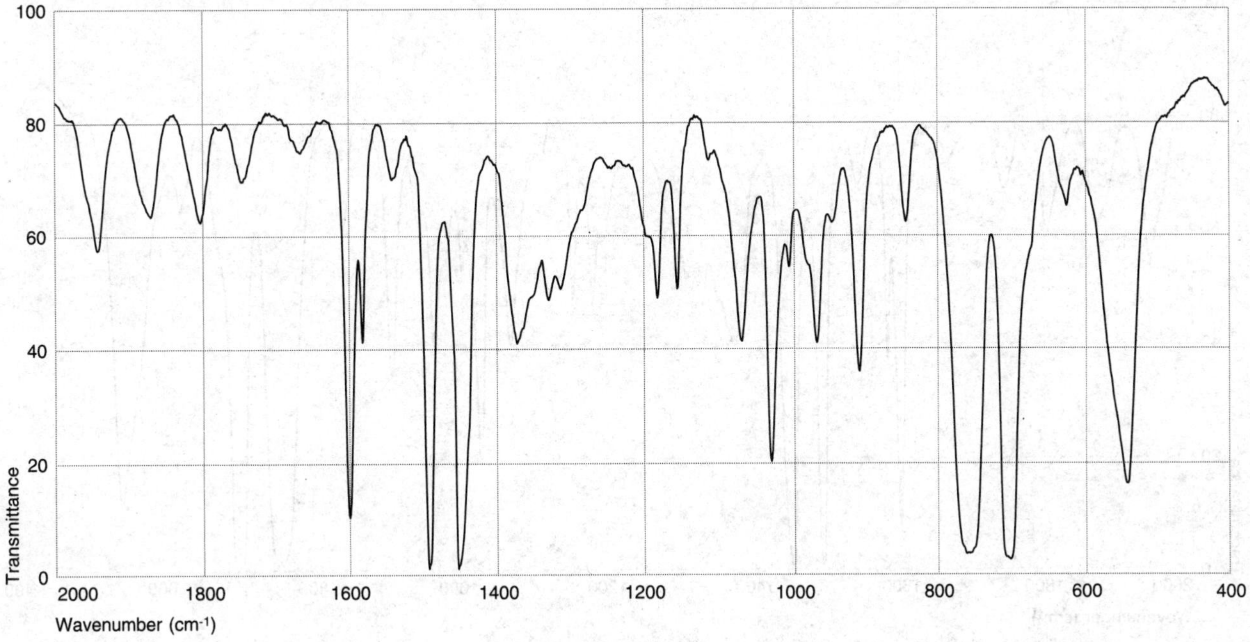
100
80
60
40
20
0
Transmittance
2000
1800
1600
1400
1200
1000
800
600
400
Wavenumber (cm-1)

Polystyrene Instrument: Fourier transform Phase: Thin film Thickness 0.038mm

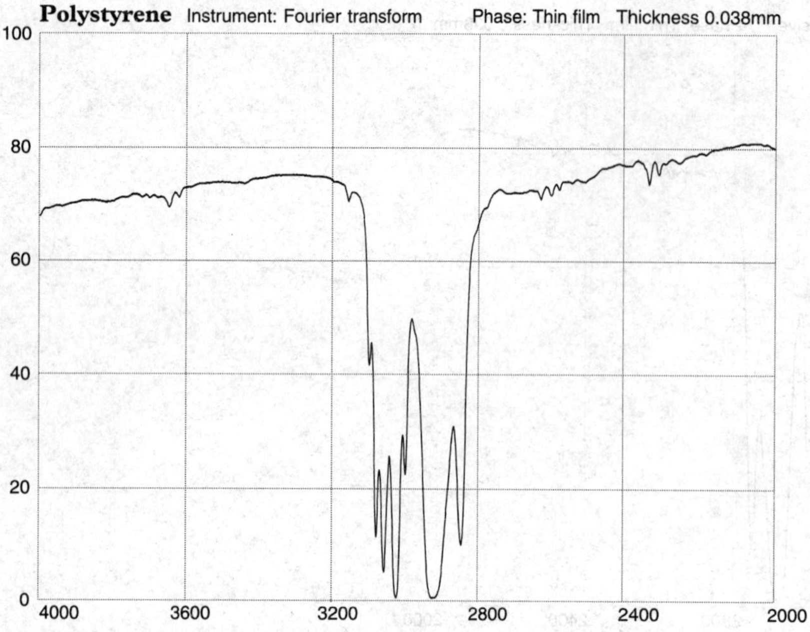

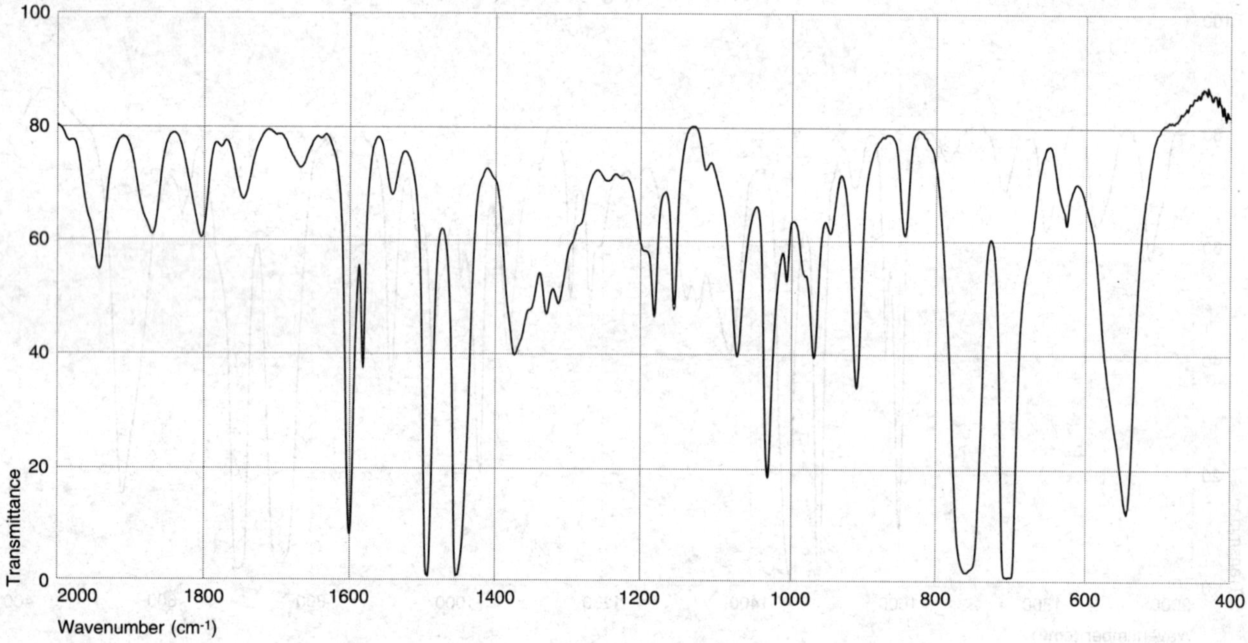

Acenocoumarol

Instrument: Dispersive

Phase: Potassium bromide disc

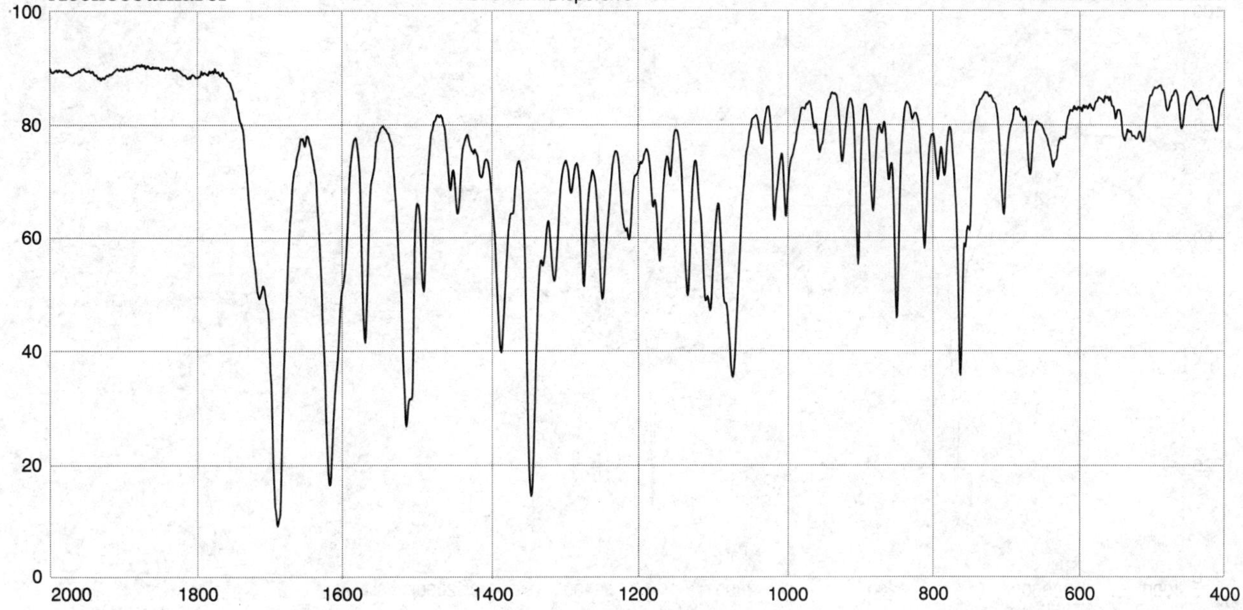

Acetazolamide

Instrument: Dispersive

Phase: Potassium bromide disc

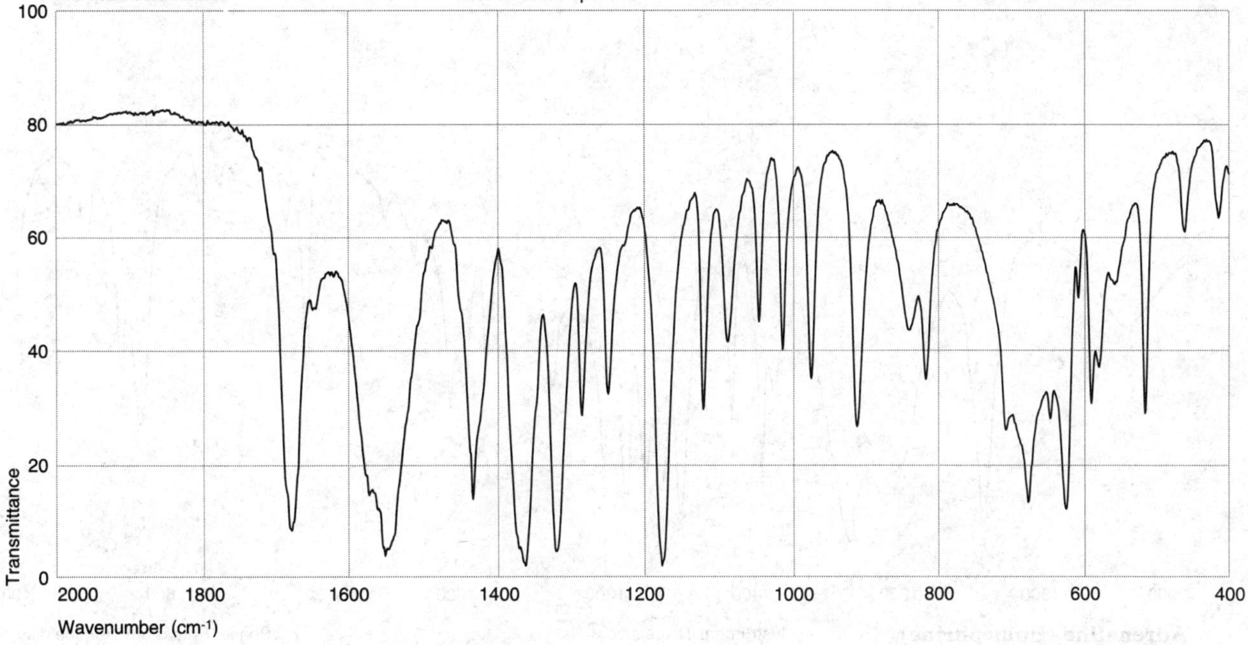

Acetylcysteine Instrument: Dispersive Phase: Potassium bromide disc

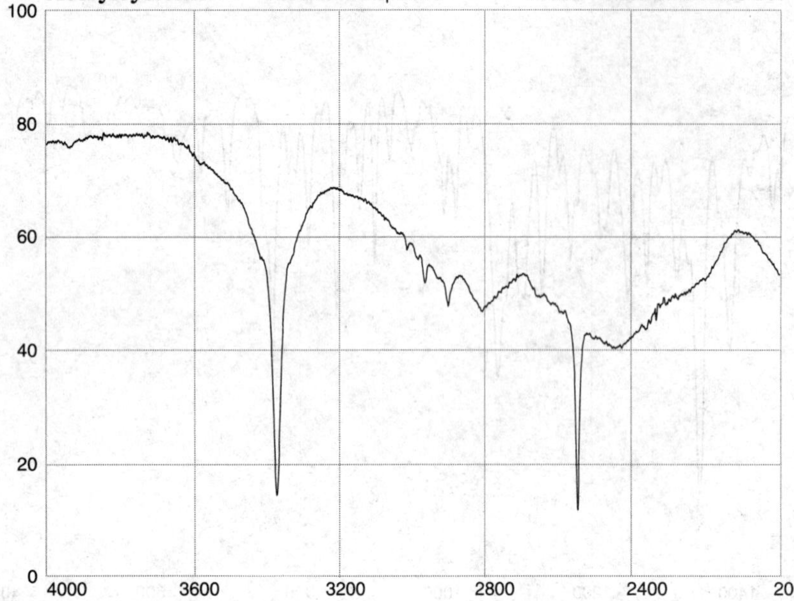

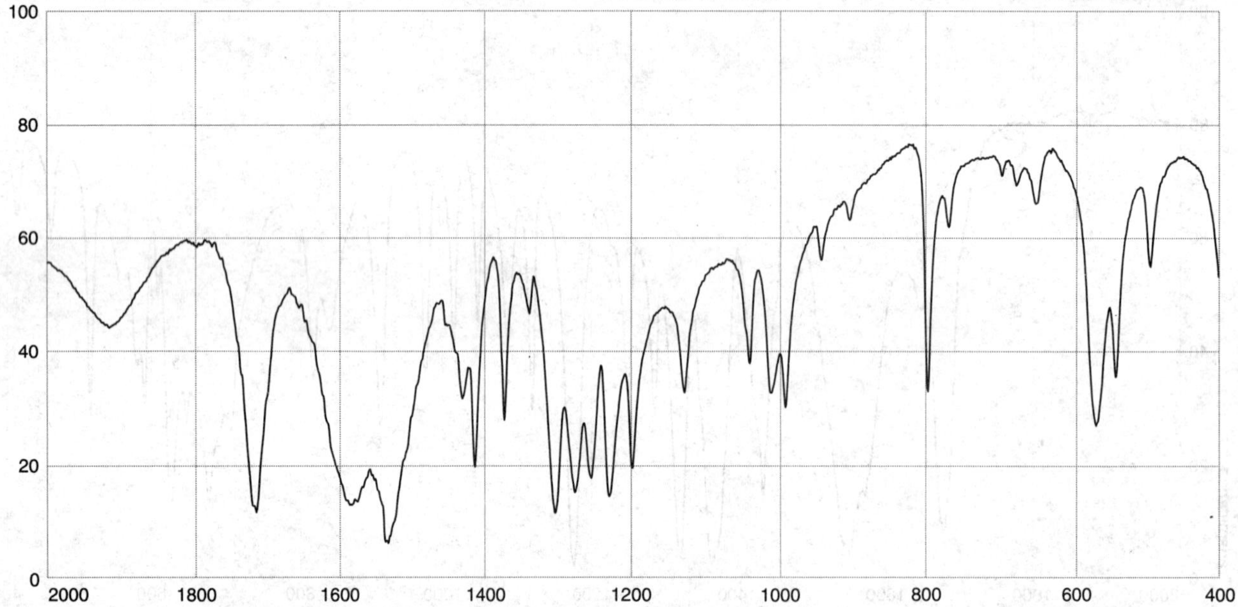

Adrenaline (Epinephrine) Instrument: Dispersive Phase: Potassium bromide disc

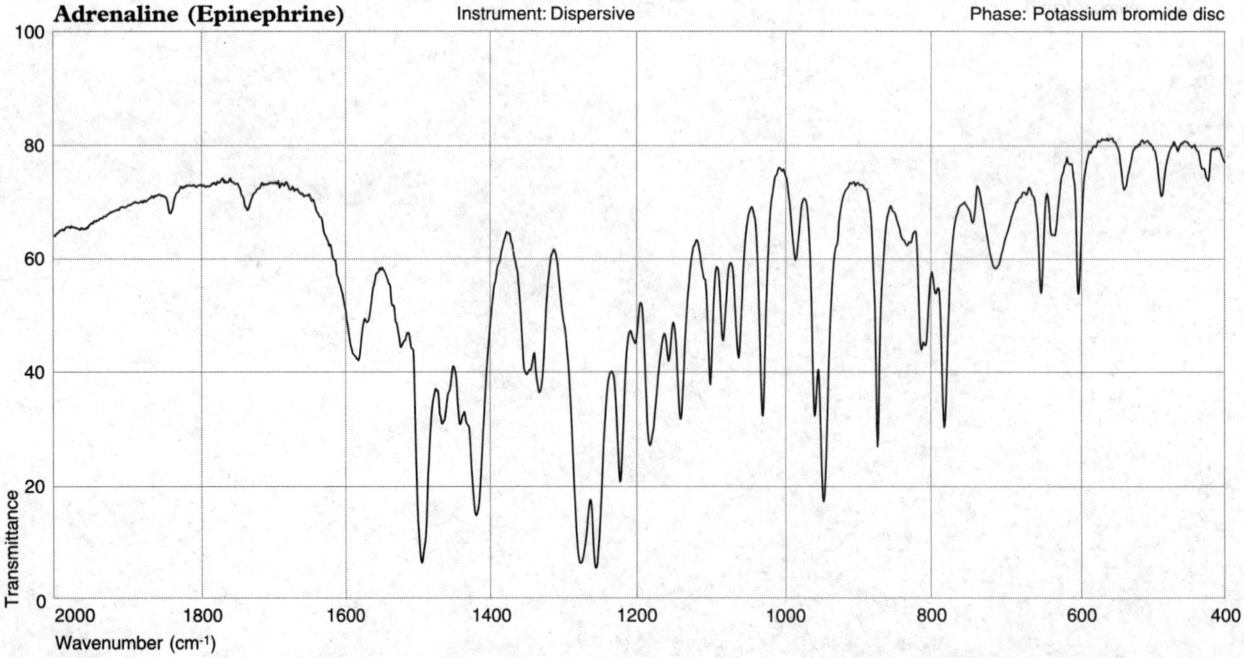

Alimemazine (Trimeprazine) Instrument: Dispersive Phase: 10% w/v solution in chloroform Thickness: 0.1mm

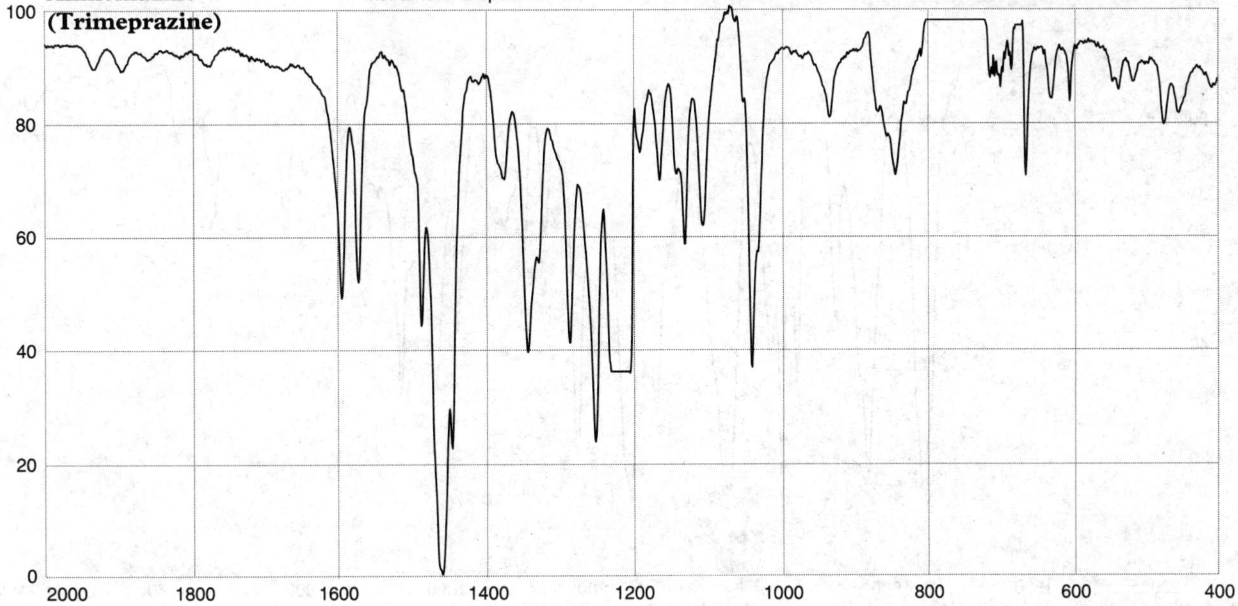

Amantadine Instrument: Dispersive Phase: Potassium bromide disc

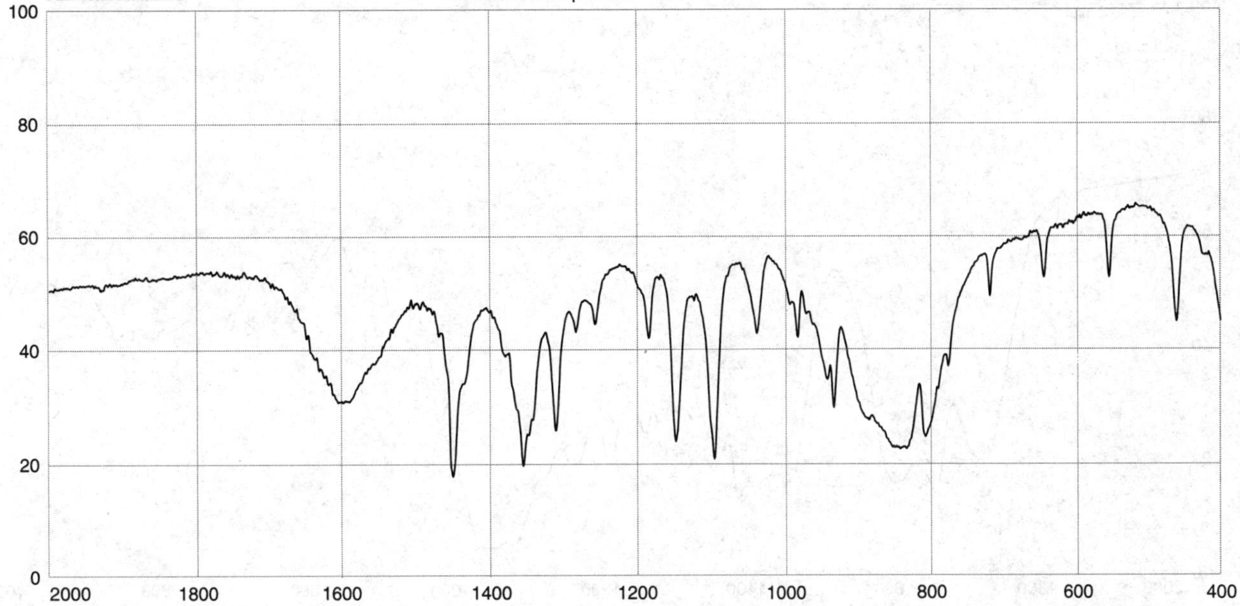

Aminobenzoic Acid Instrument: Dispersive Phase: Potassium bromide disc

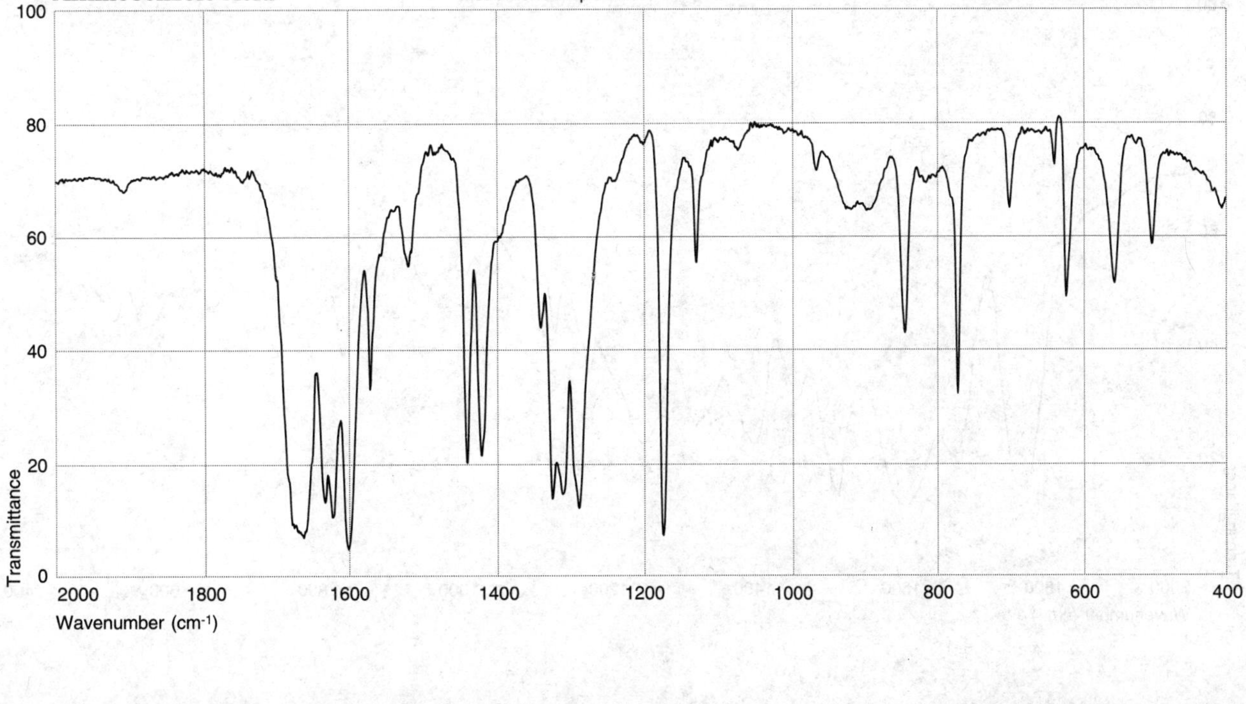

Amiodarone Instrument: Dispersive Phase: 15% w/v solution in dichloromethane Thickness: 0.1mm

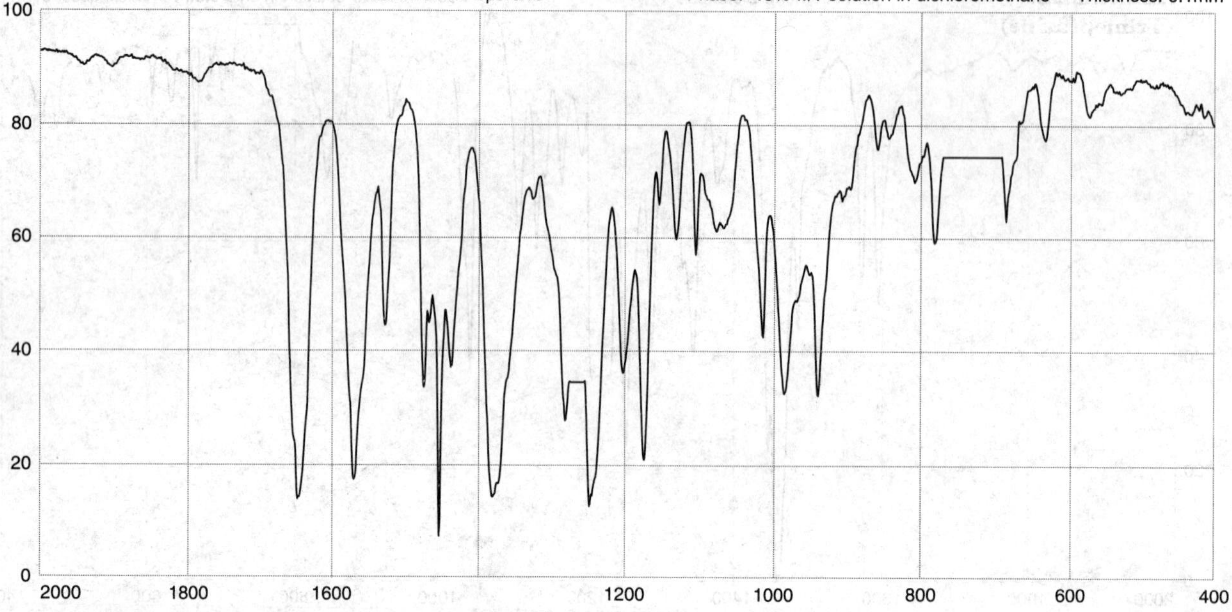

Ammonium Glycyrrhizinate Instrument: Fourier Transform Phase: Potassium bromide disc

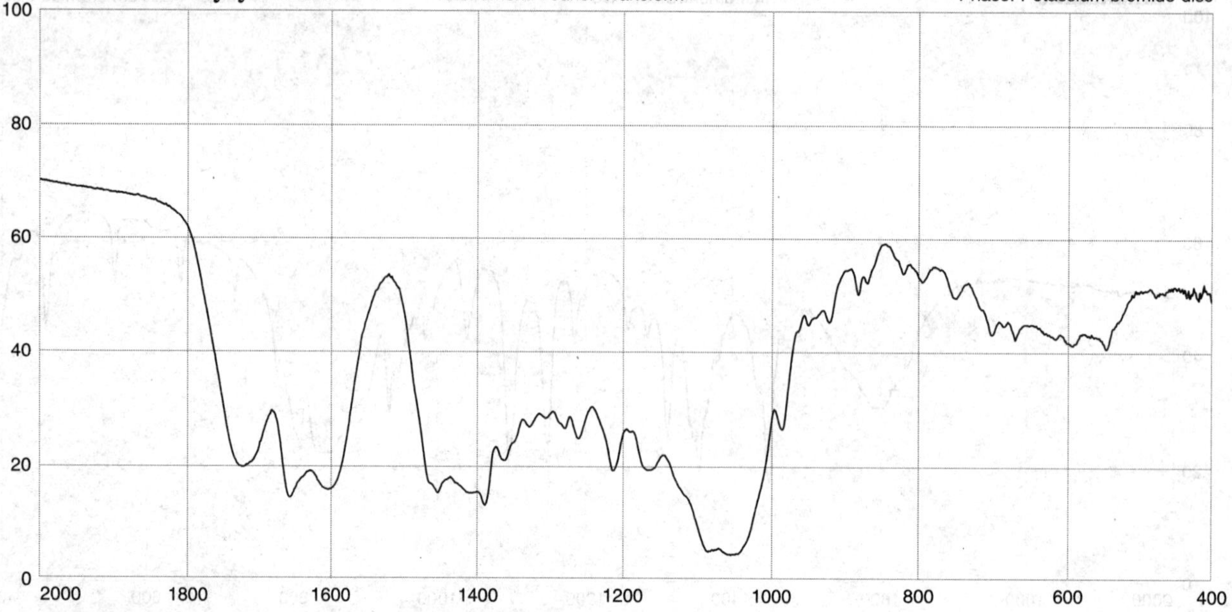

Amoxicillin Sodium Instrument: Dispersive Phase: Potassium bromide disc

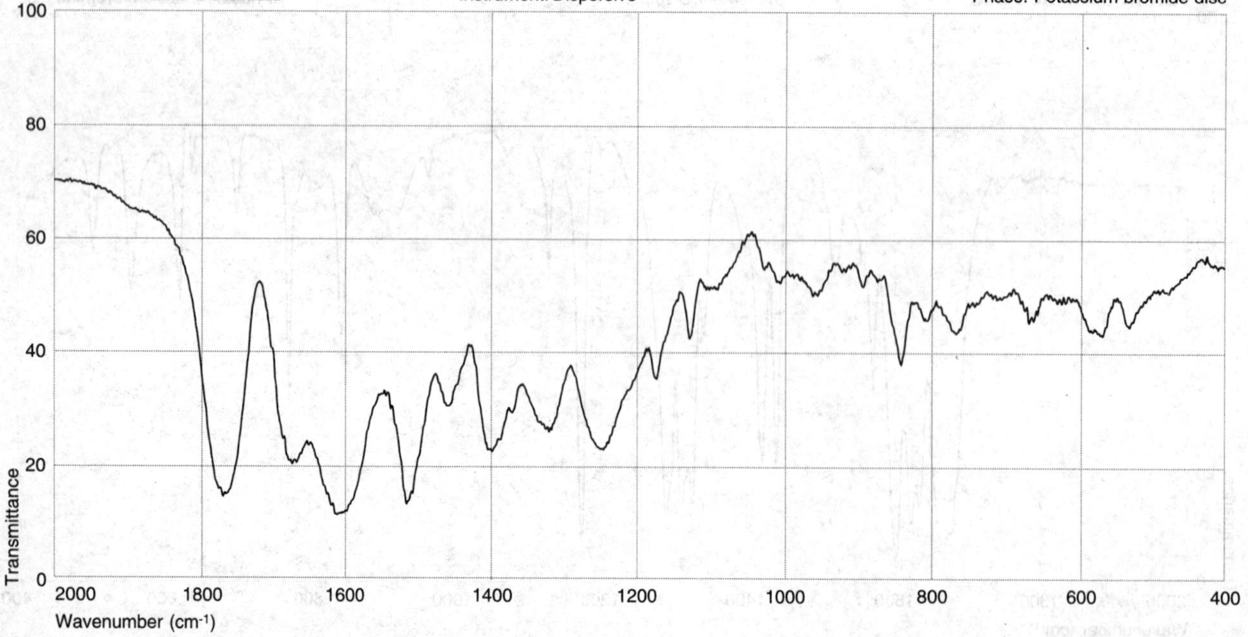

Amoxicillin Trihydrate Instrument: Dispersive Phase: Potassium bromide disc

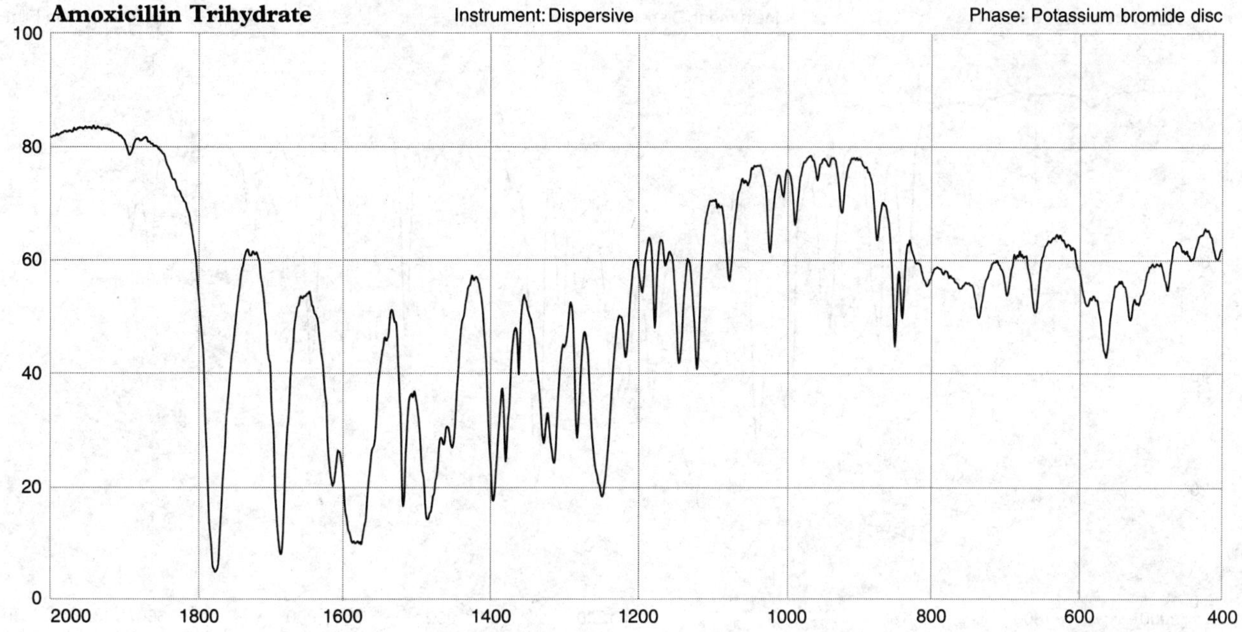

Amphotericin Instrument: Dispersive Phase: Potassium bromide disc

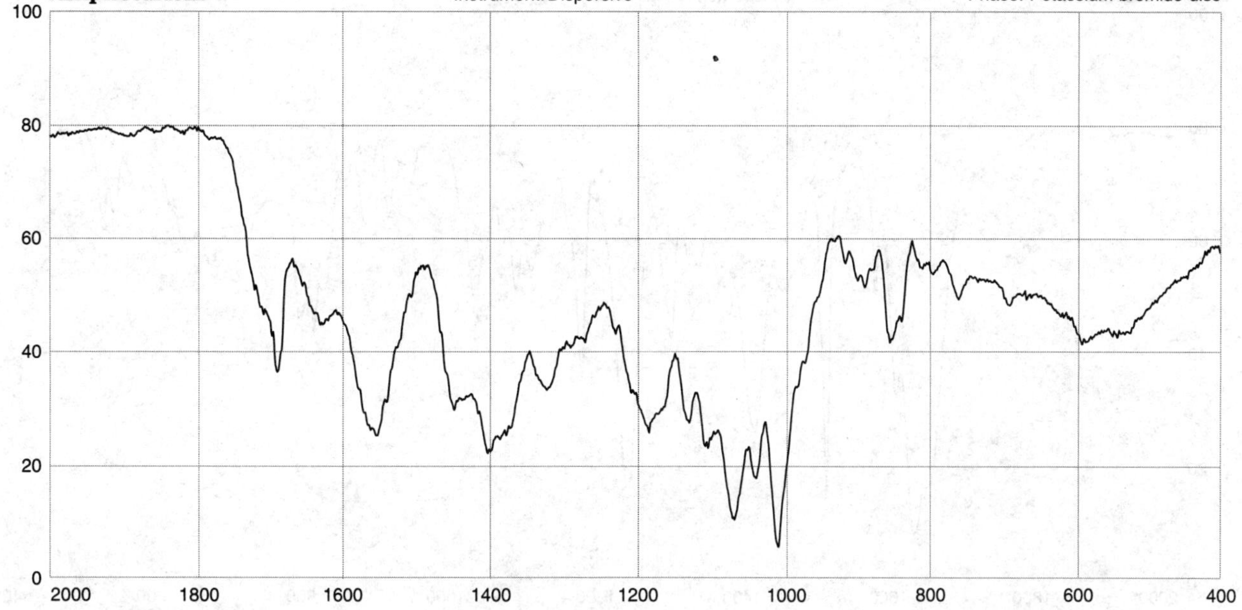

Ampicillin Trihydrate Instrument: Dispersive Phase: Potassium bromide disc

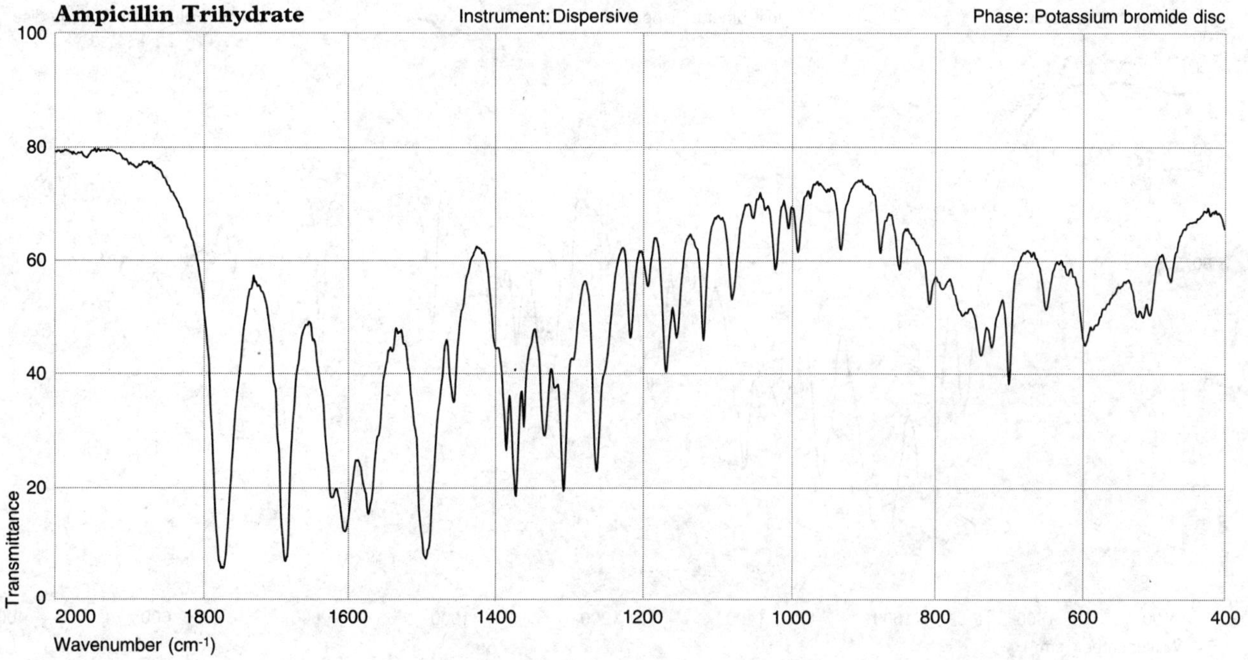

Amylmetacresol

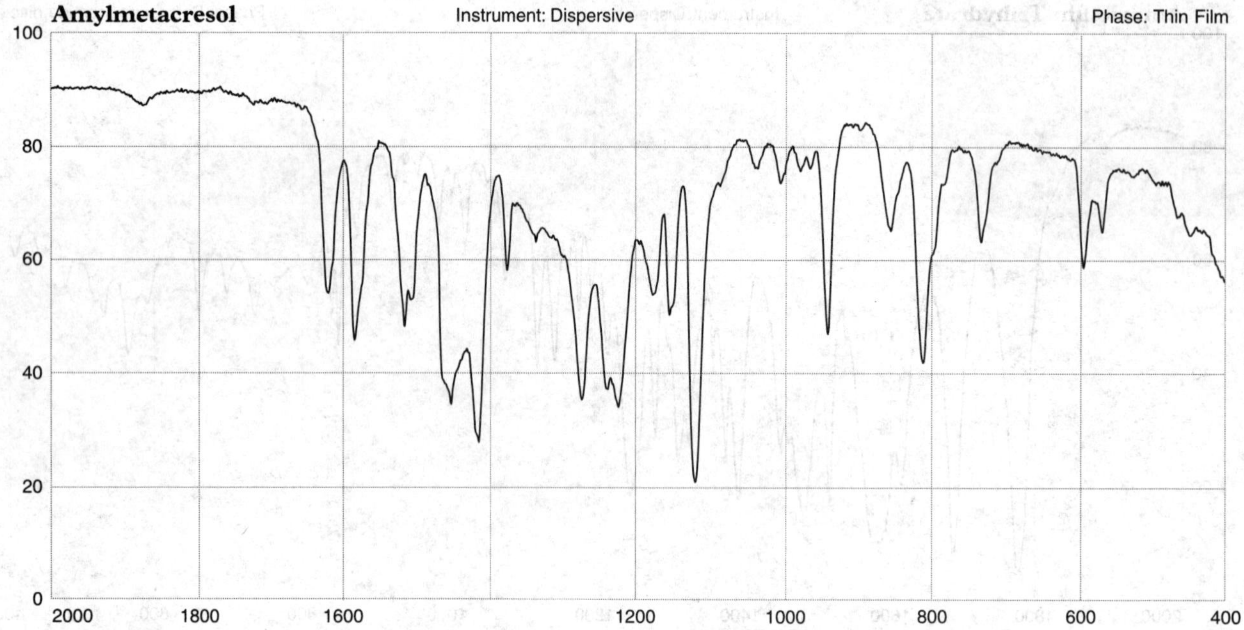

Atenolol

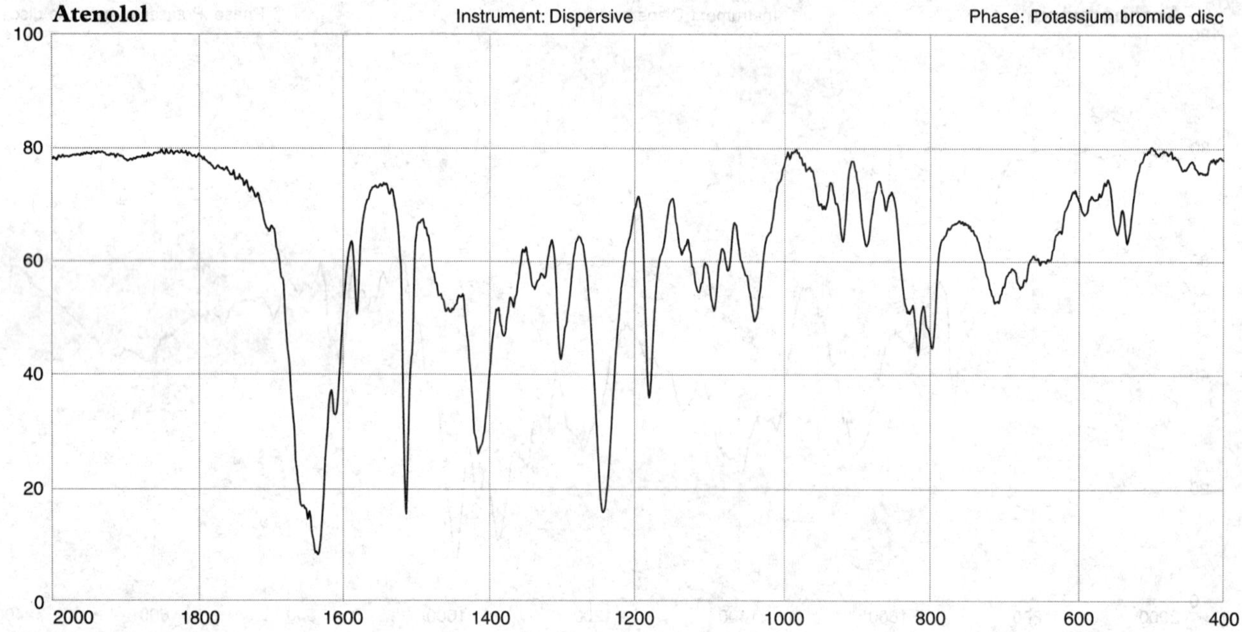

Azapropazone

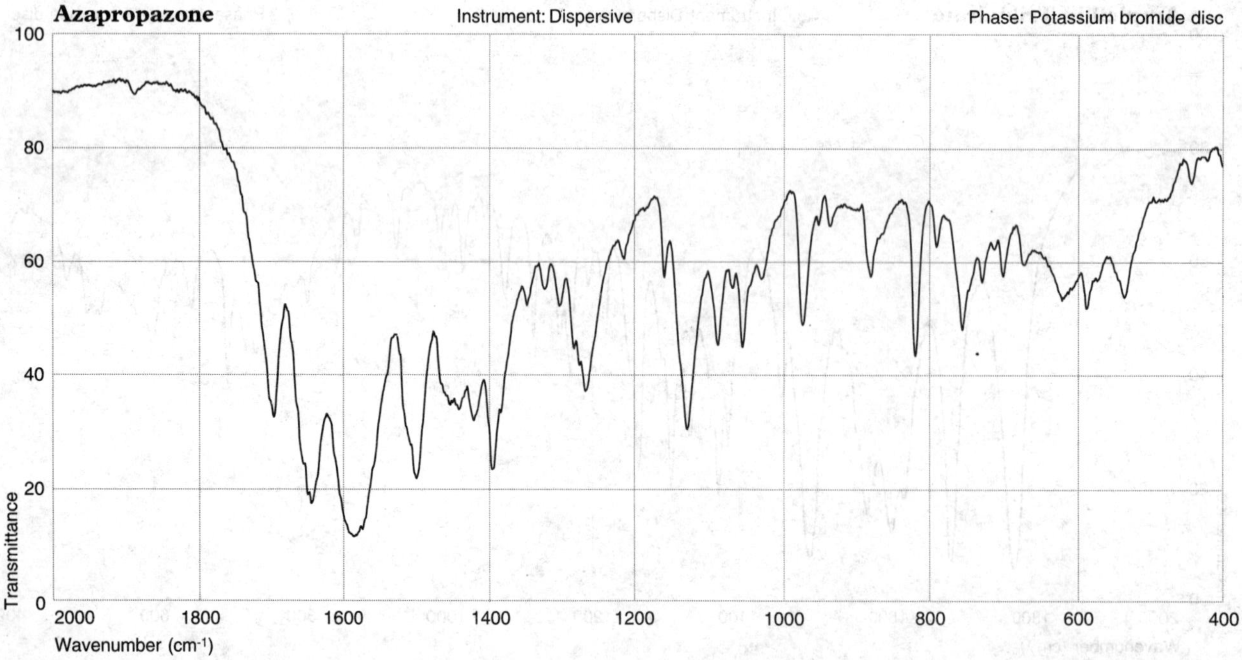

Anhydrous Azapropazone Instrument: Dispersive Phase: Potassium bromide disc

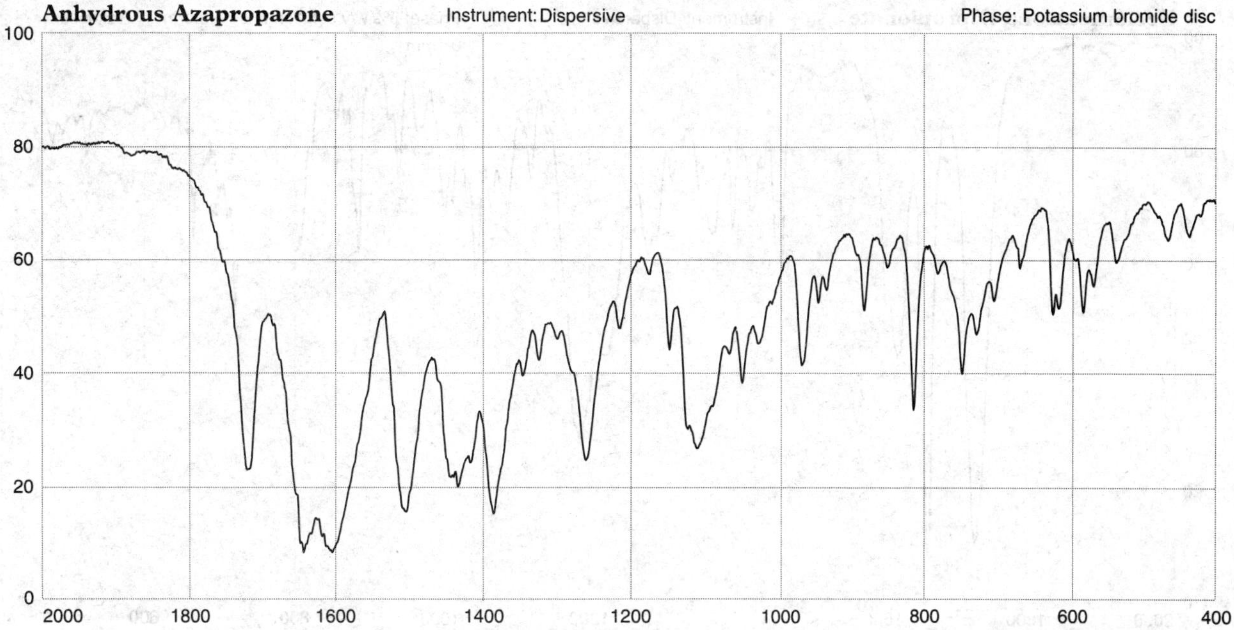

Azelastine Hydrochloride Instrument: Fourier transform Phase: Potassium chloride disc

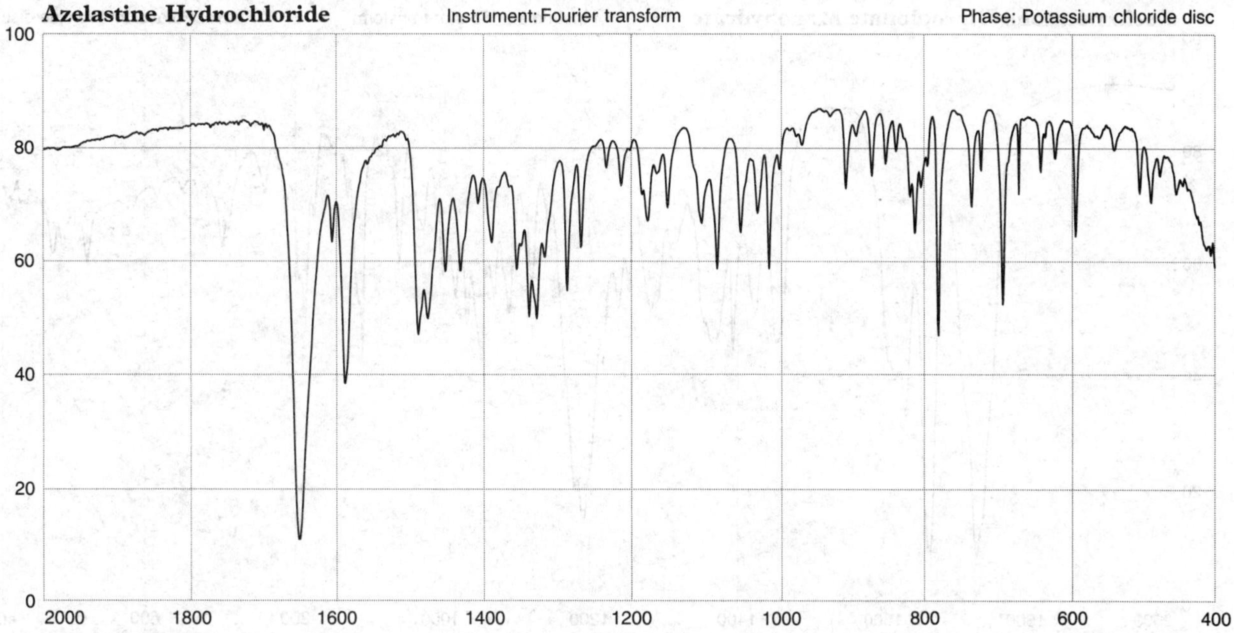

Azlocillin Sodium Instrument: Dispersive Phase: Potassium bromide disc

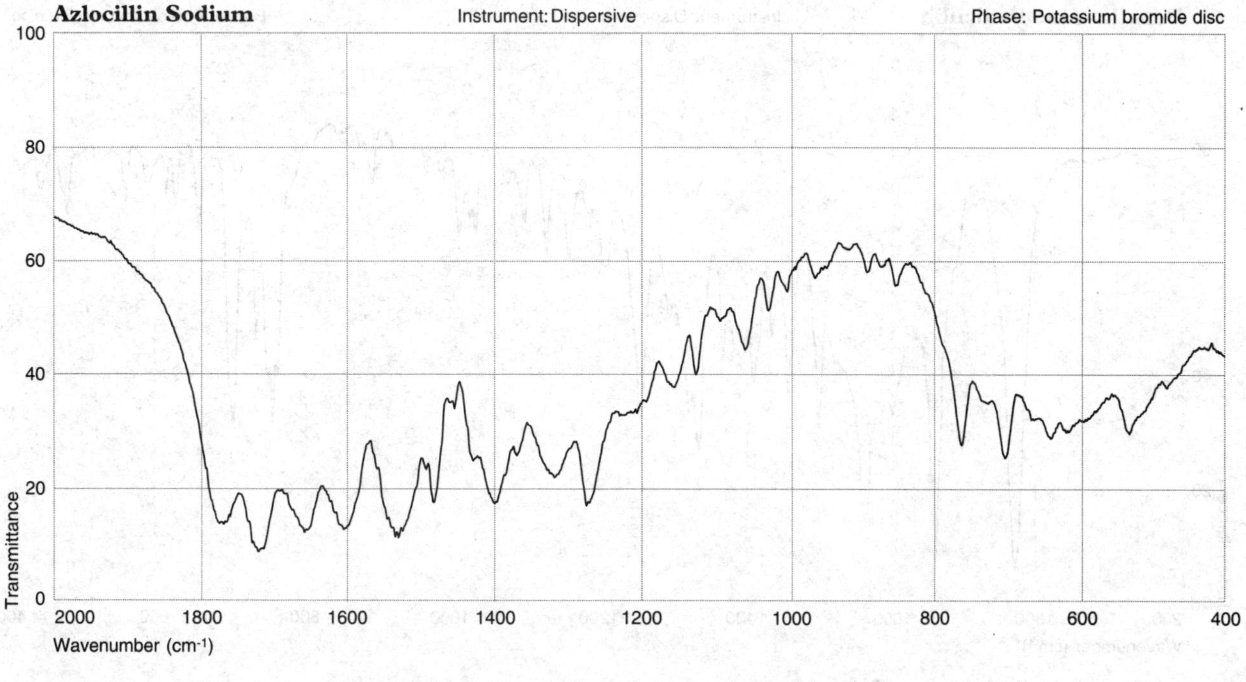

Beclometasone Dipropionate Instrument: Dispersive Phase: 5% w/v solution in chloroform Thickness: 0.1mm

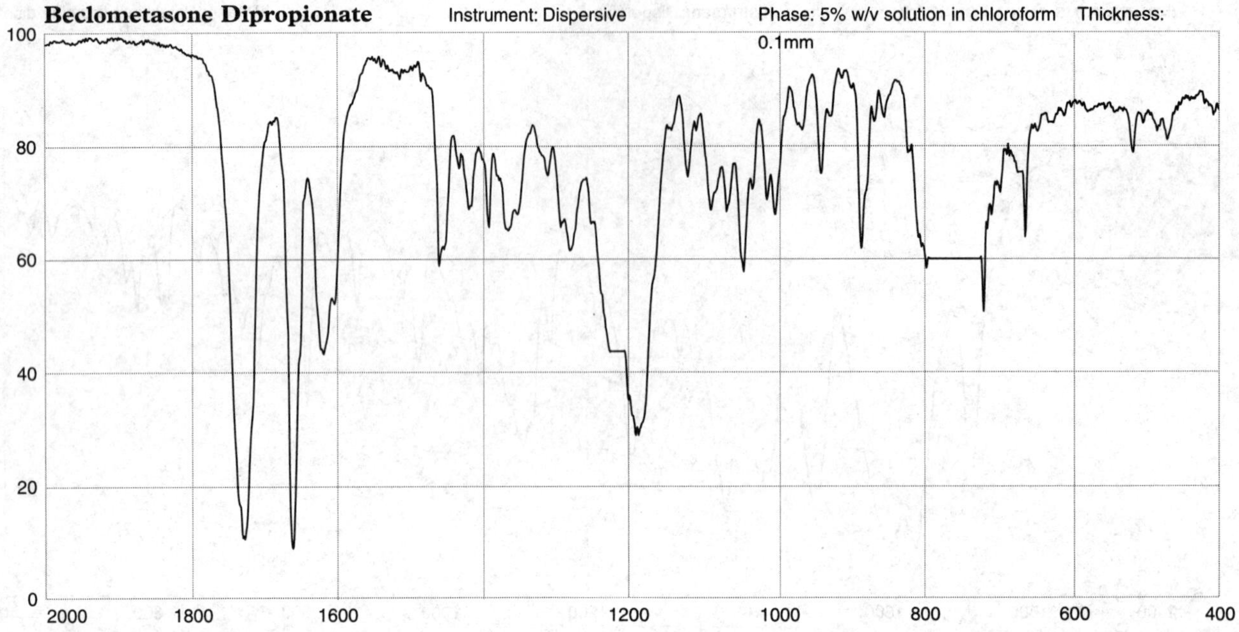

Beclometasone Dipropionate Monohydrate Instrument: Fourier transform Phase: Potassium bromide disc

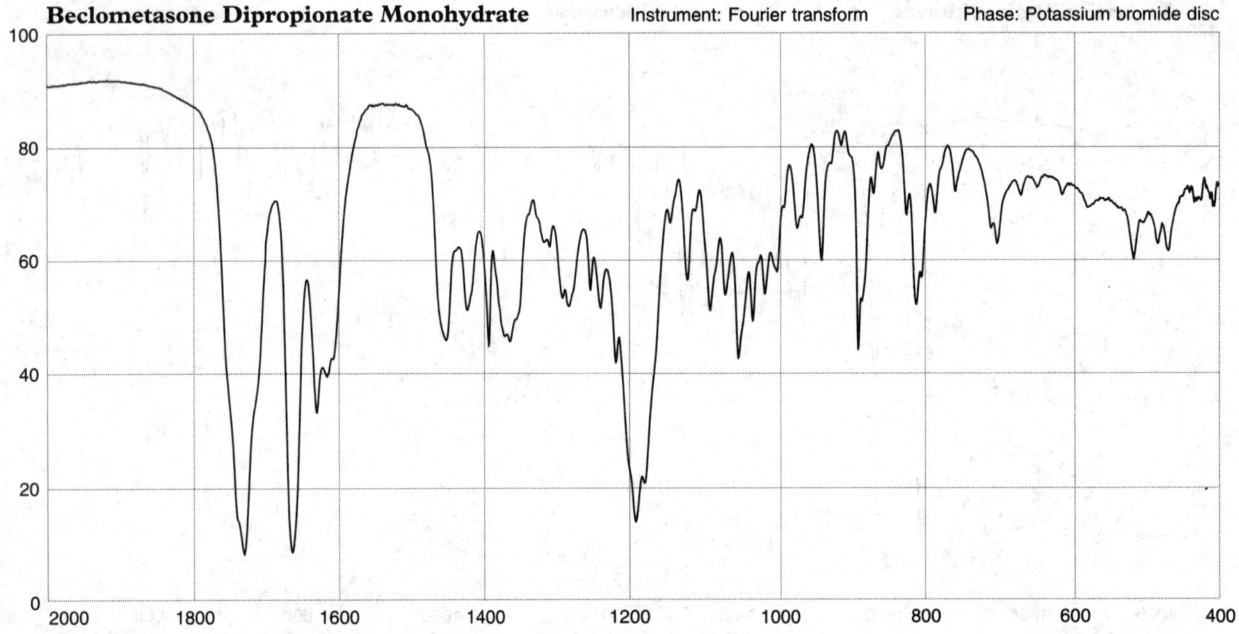

Benethamine Penicillin Instrument: Dispersive Phase: Potassium bromide disc

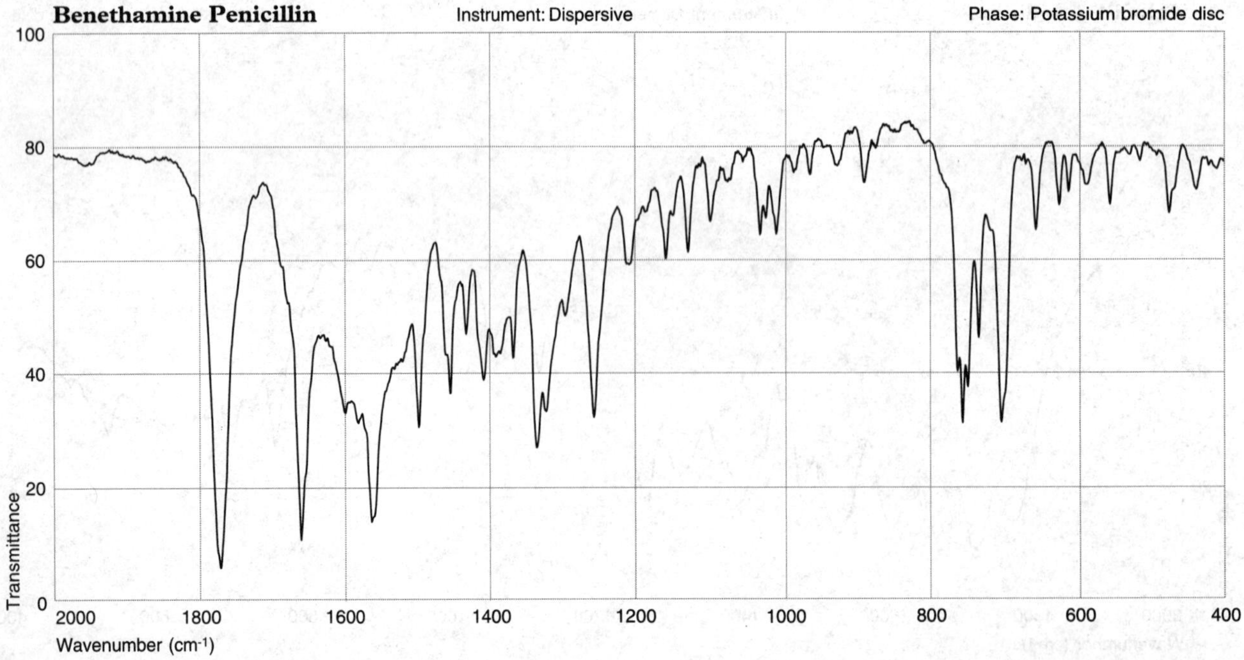

Benorilate Instrument: Dispersive Phase: Potassium bromide disc

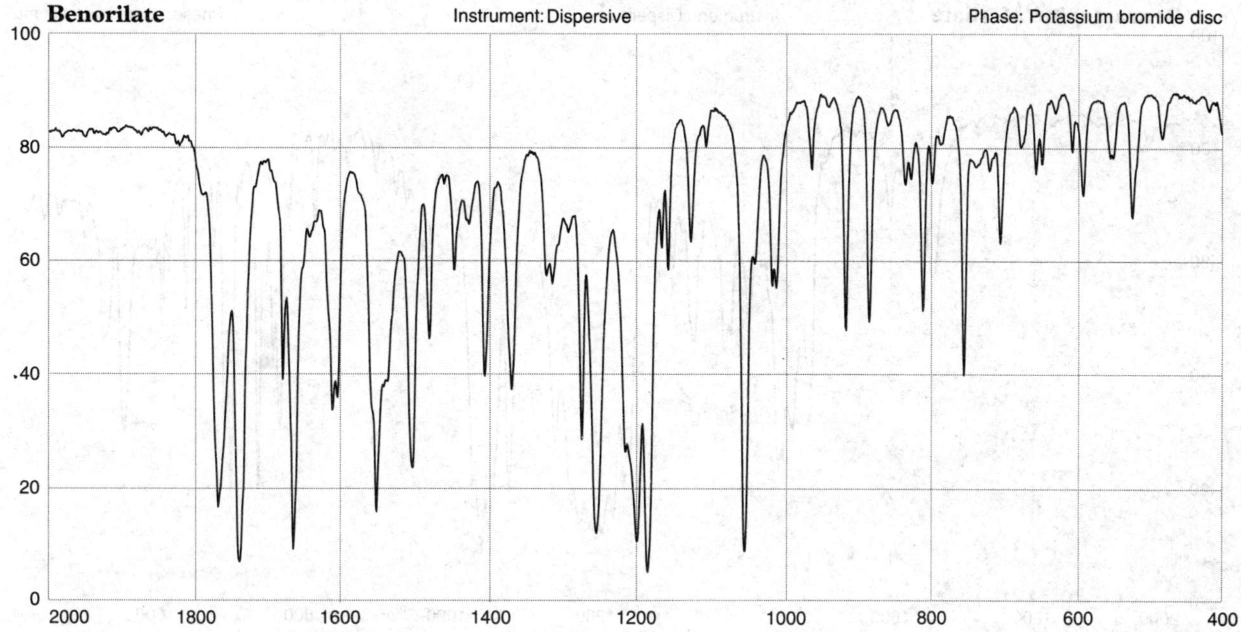

Benzhexol Hydrochloride (Trihexyphenidyl Hydrochloride) Instrument: Dispersive Phase: Potassium chloride disc

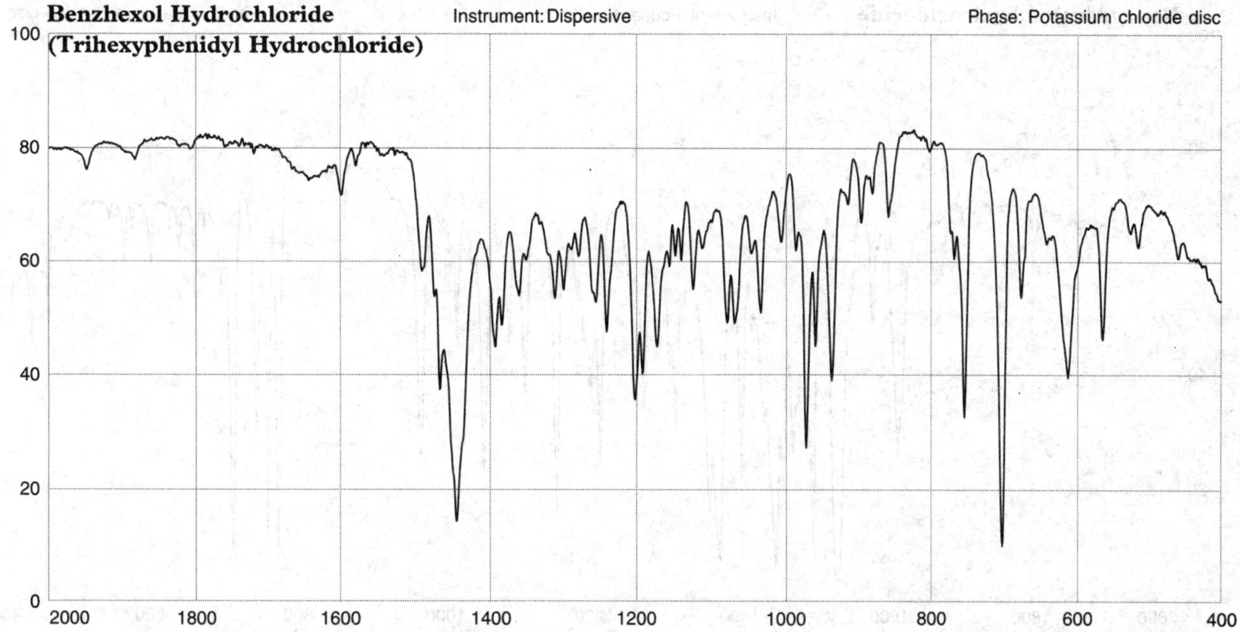

Benzoic Acid Instrument: Dispersive Phase: Potassium bromide disc

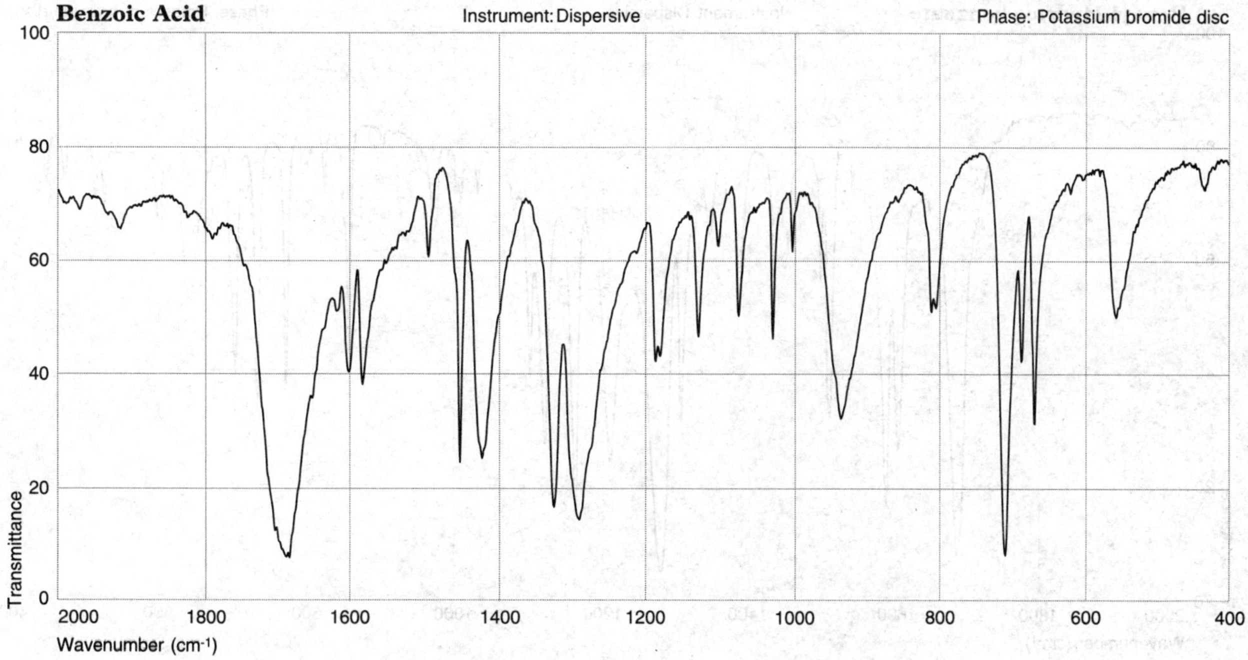

Benzatropine Mesilate Instrument: Dispersive Phase: Liquid paraffin mull

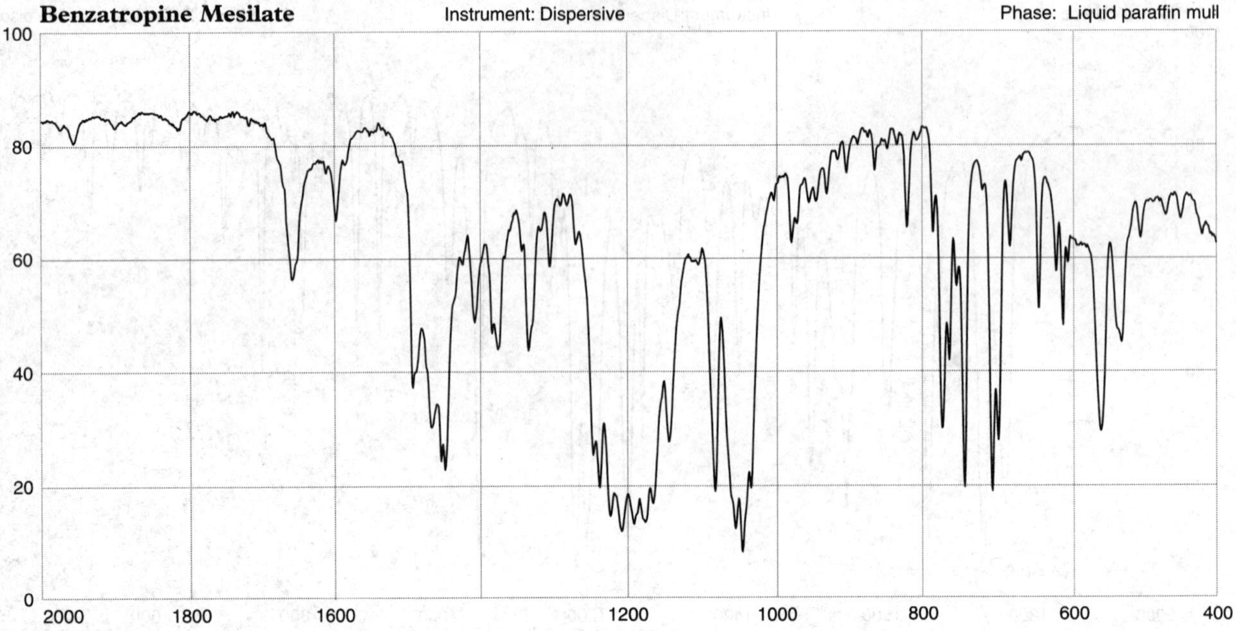

Benzydamine Hydrochloride Instrument: Fourier transform Phase: Potassium chloride disc

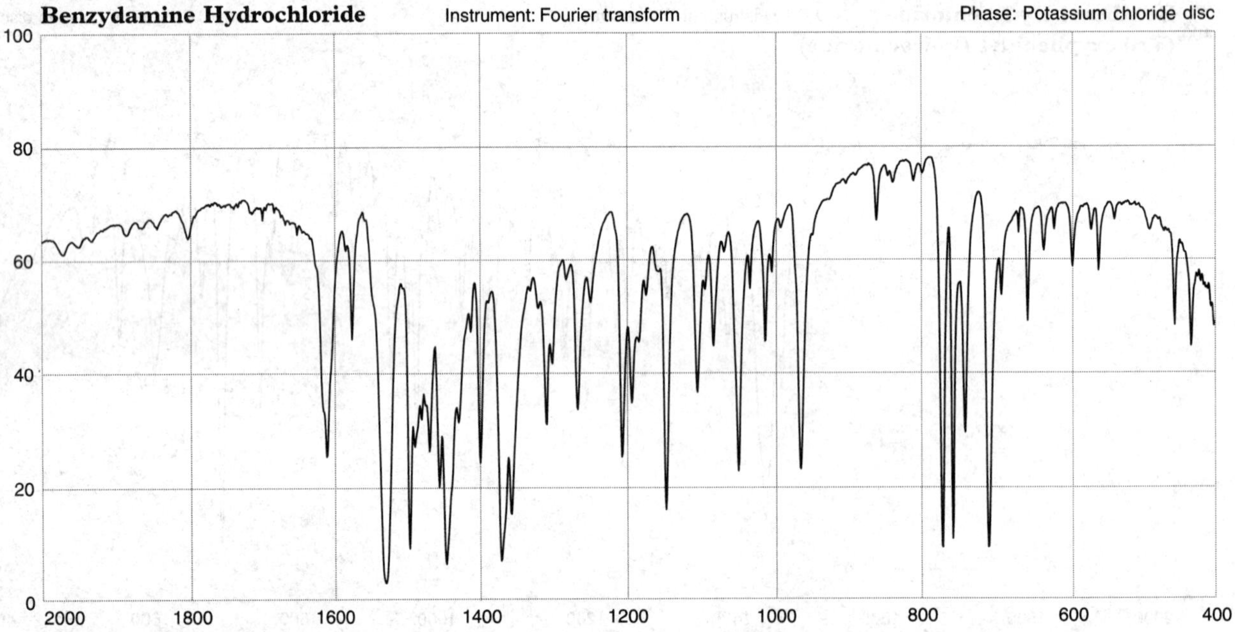

Benzyl Hydroxybenzoate Instrument: Dispersive Phase: Potassium bromide disc

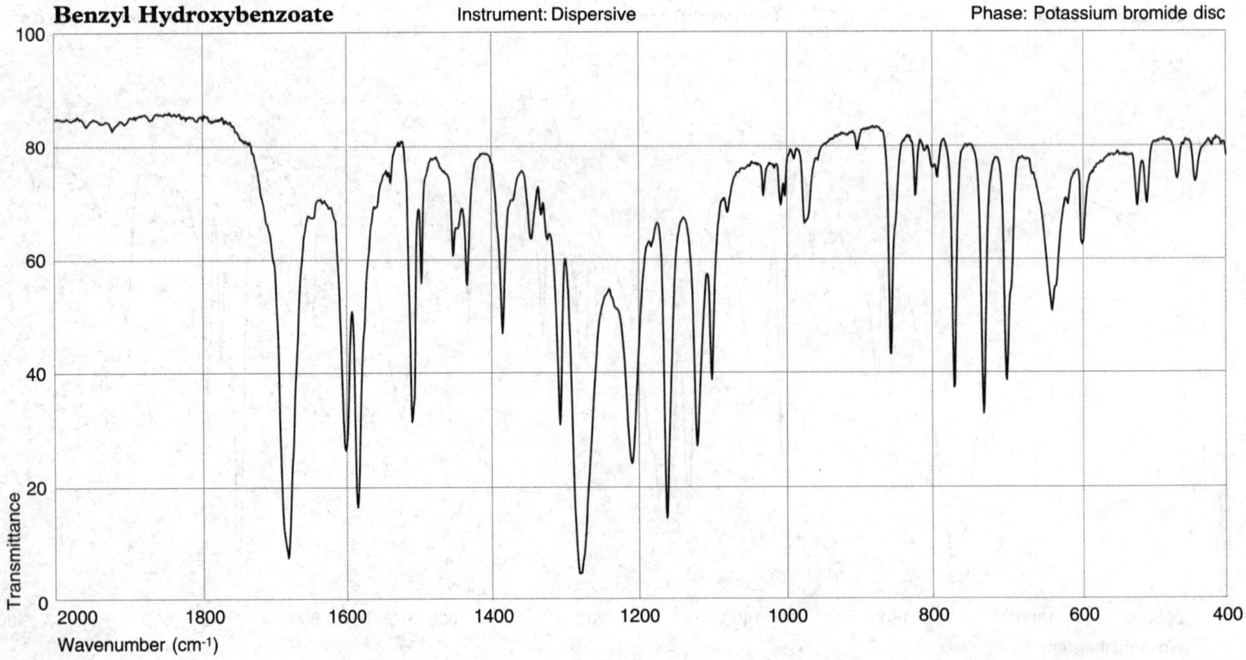

Betamethasone Instrument: Dispersive Phase: Potassium bromide disc

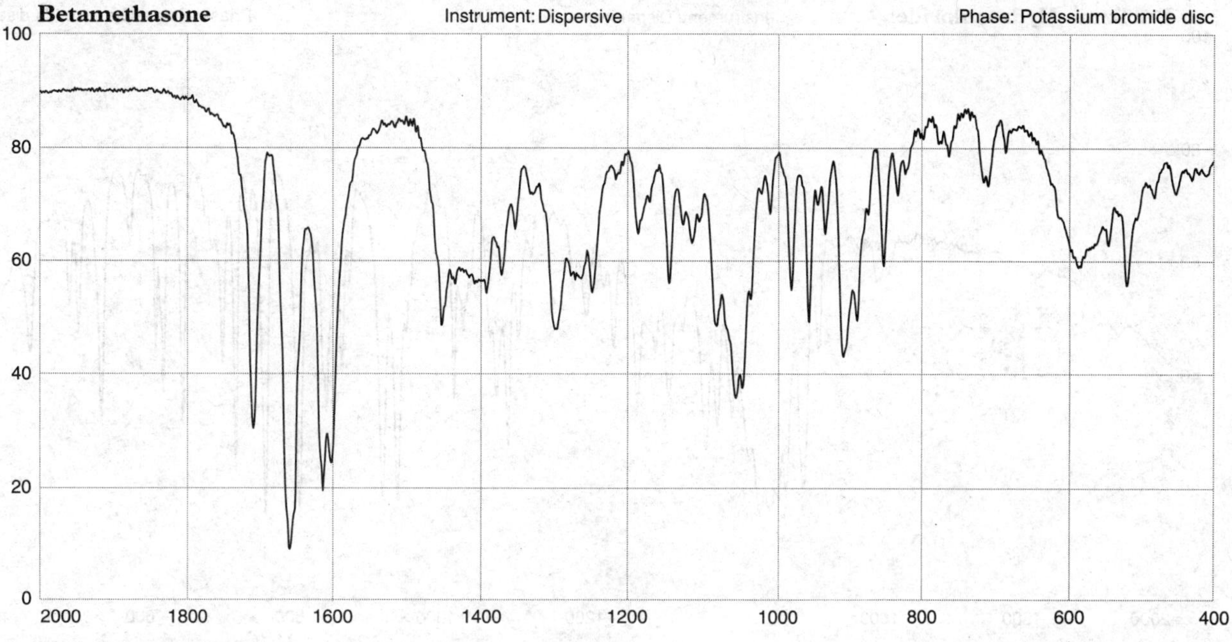

Bretylium Tosilate Instrument: Fourier transform Phase: Potassium bromide disc

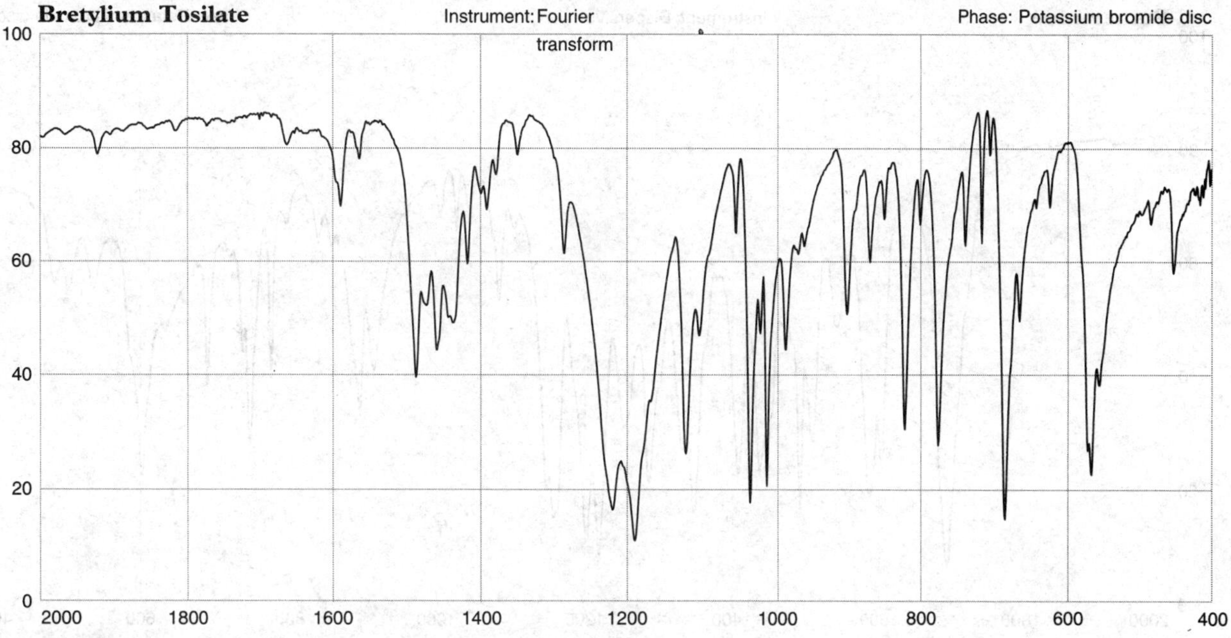

Bronopol Instrument: Dispersive Phase: Potassium bromide disc

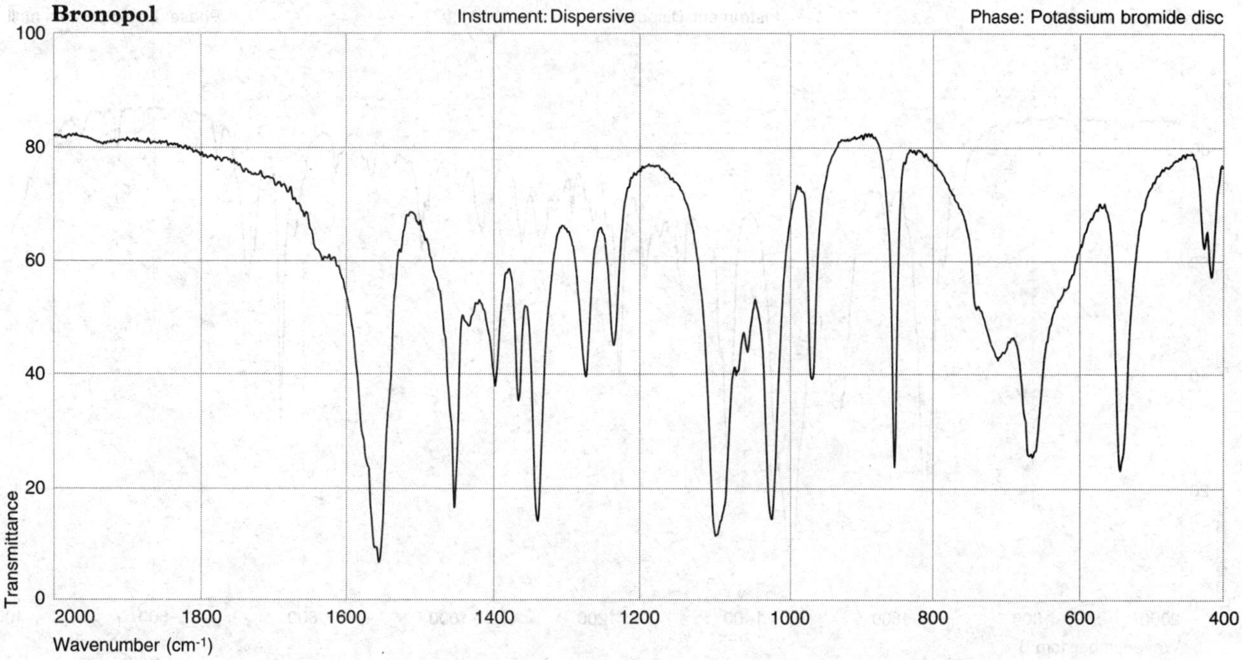

Buclizine Hydrochloride Instrument: Dispersive Phase: Potassium chloride disc

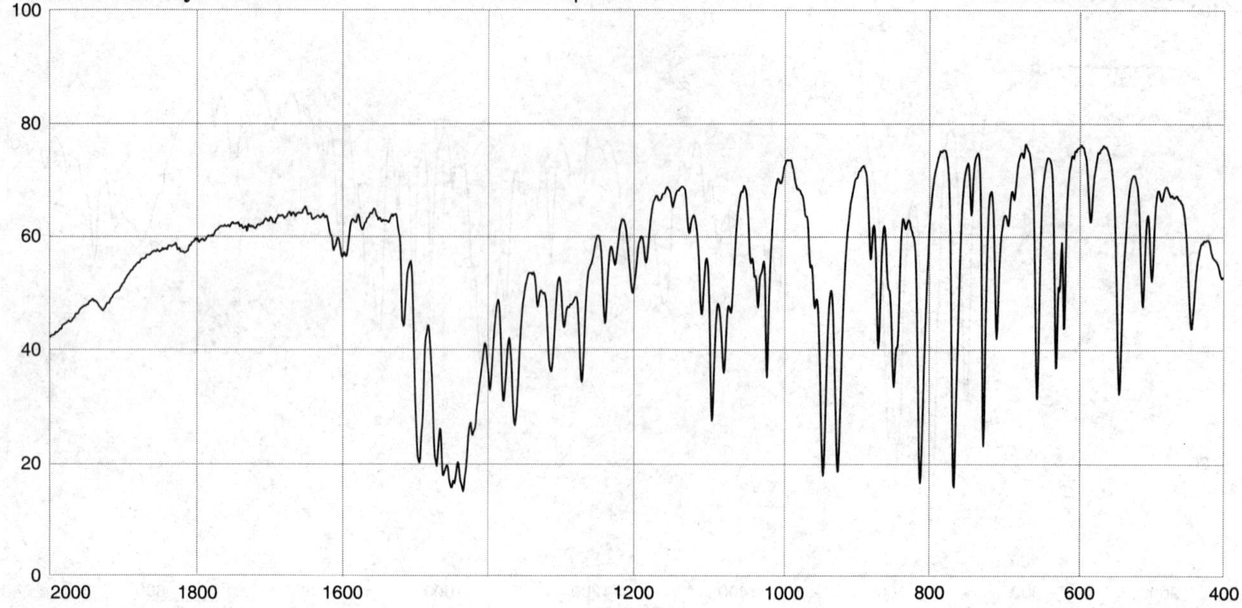

Bumetanide Instrument: Dispersive Phase: Potassium bromide disc

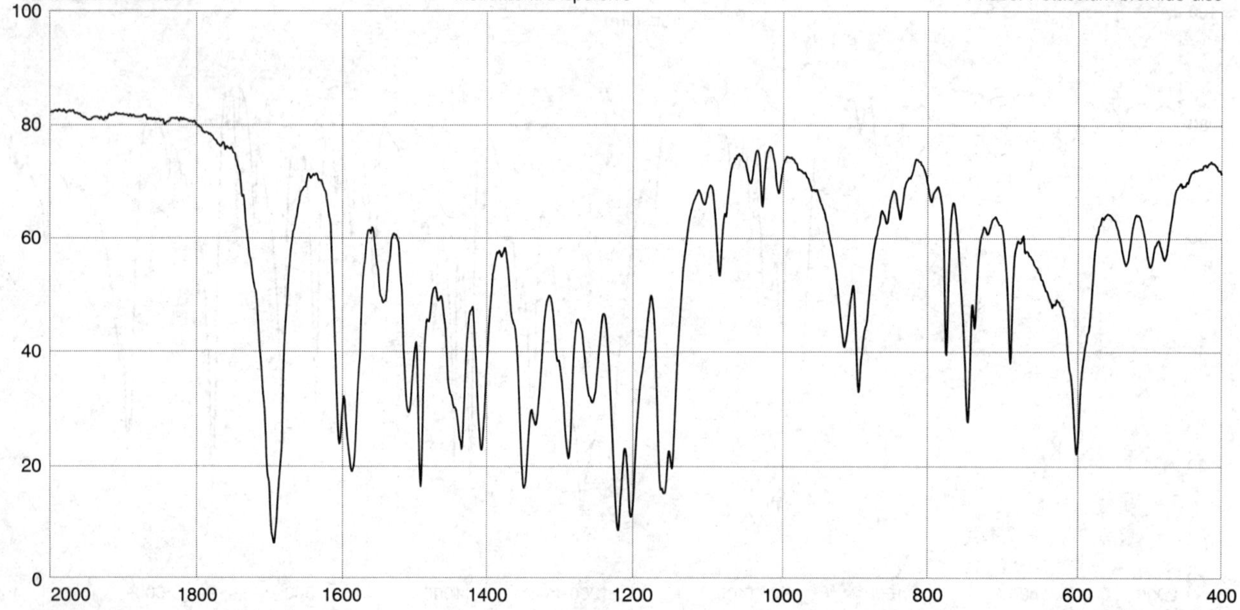

Bupivacaine Instrument: Dispersive Phase: Liquid paraffin mull

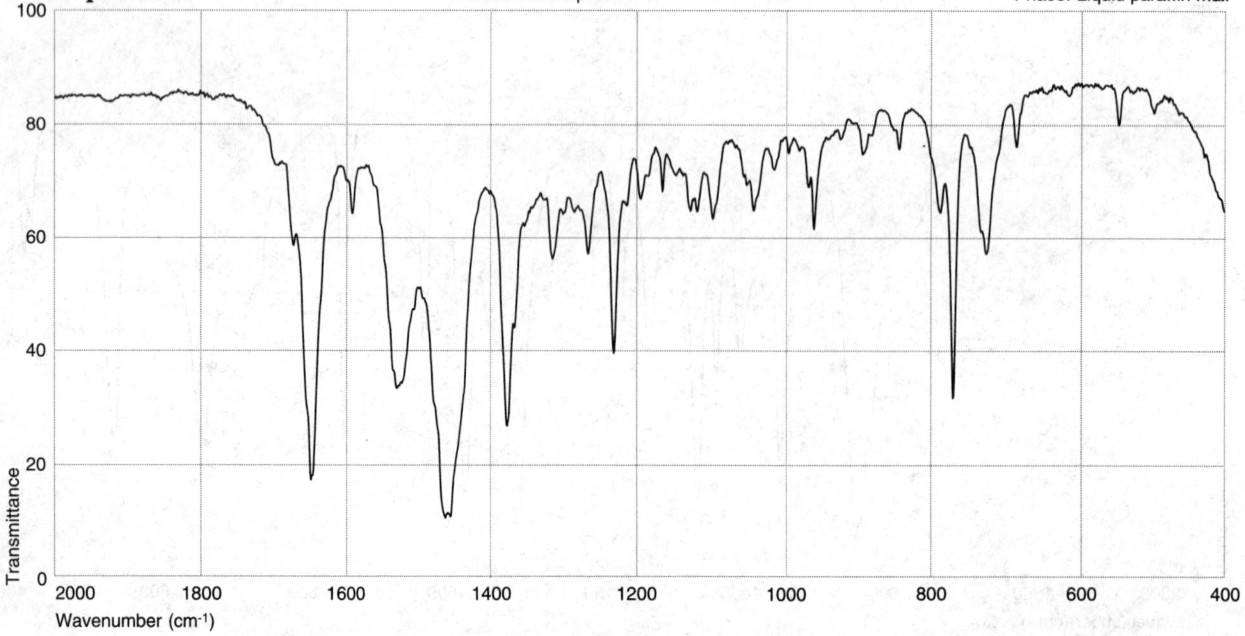

Busulfan Instrument: Dispersive Phase: Potassium bromide disc

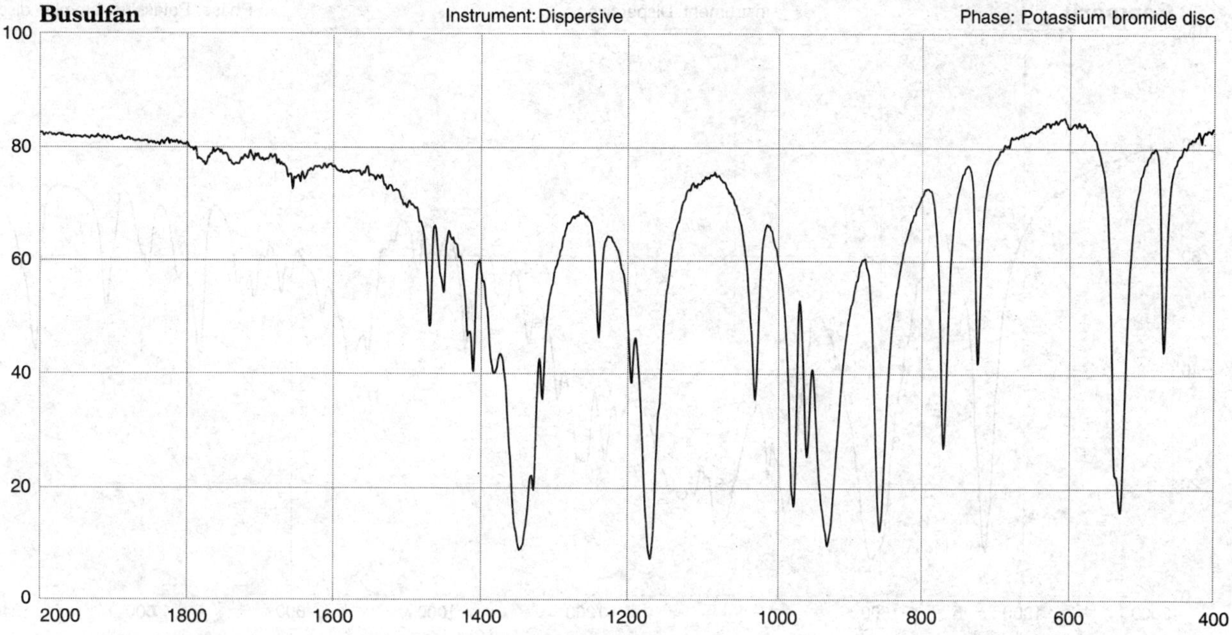

Butyl Hydroxybenzoate Instrument: Dispersive Phase: Potassium bromide disc

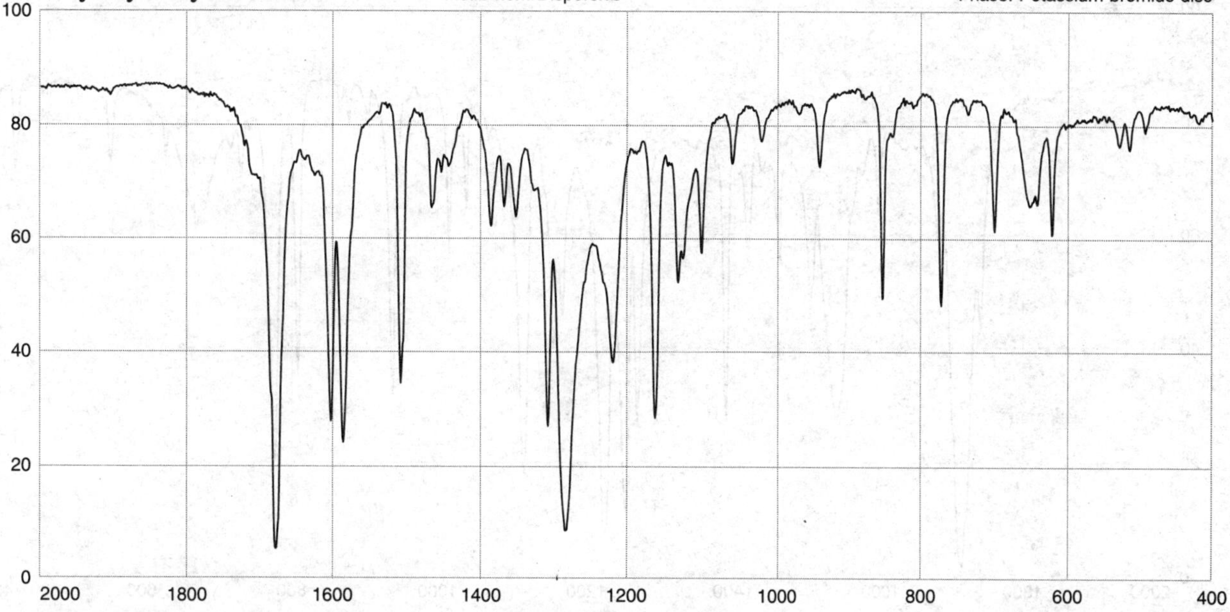

Calcium Polystyrene Sulphonate Instrument: Fourier transform Phase: Potassium bromide disc

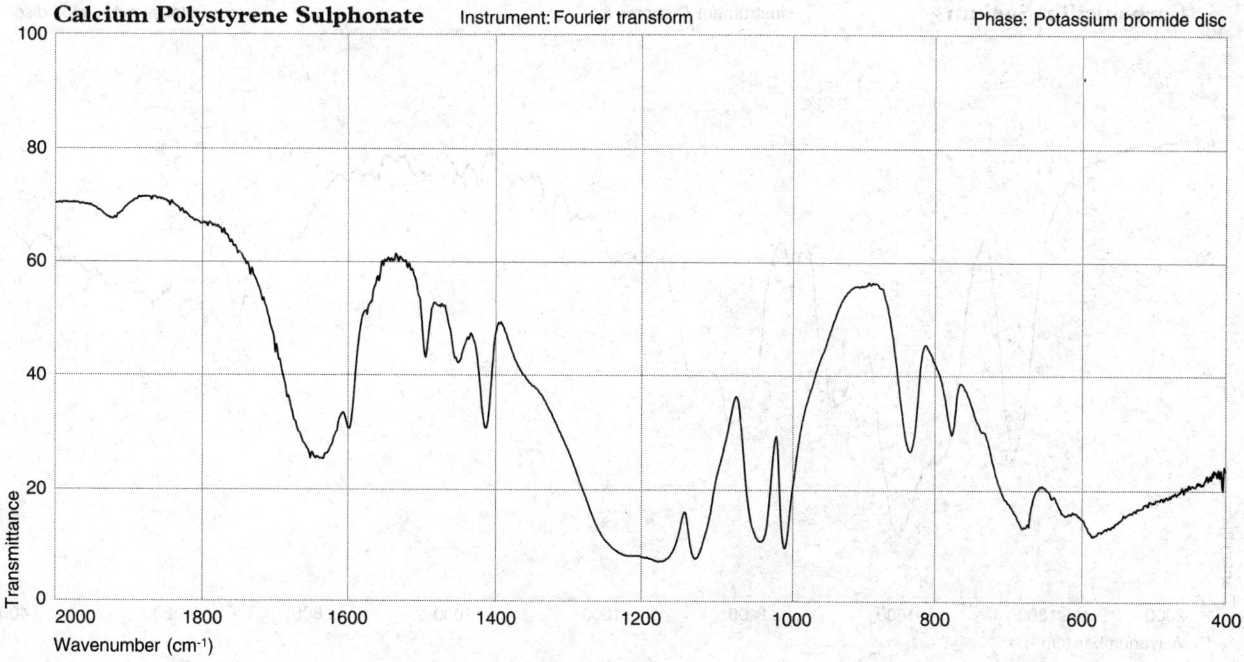

Captopril Instrument: Dispersive Phase: Potassium bromide disc

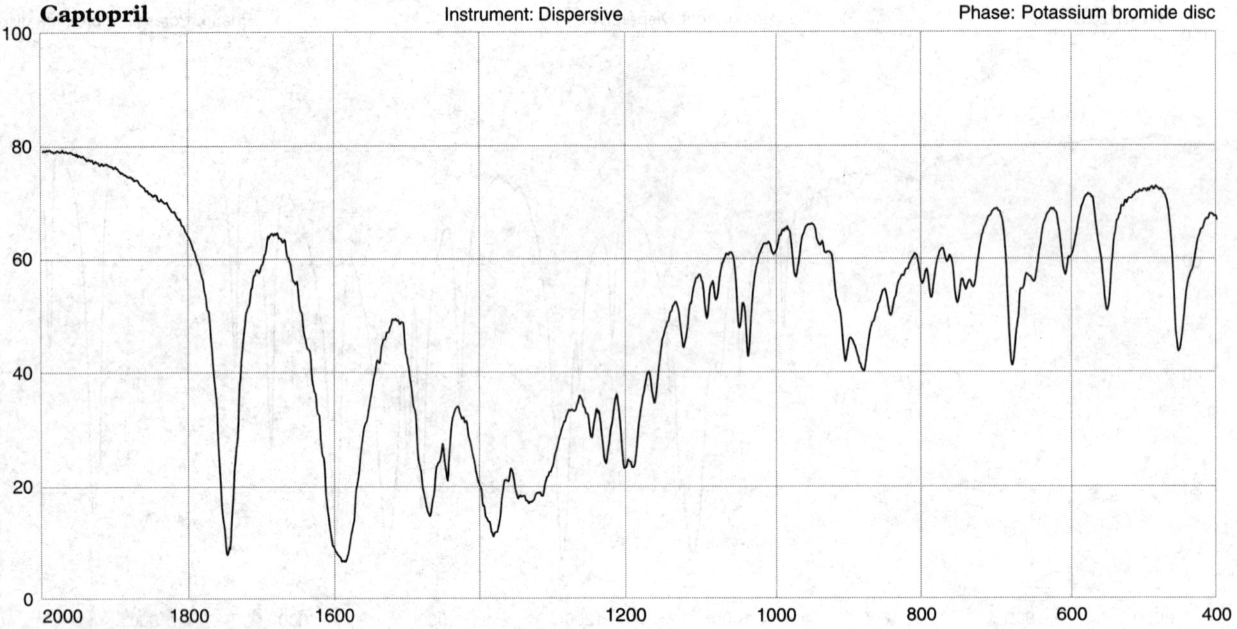

Carbaryl Instrument: Dispersive Phase: Potassium bromide disc

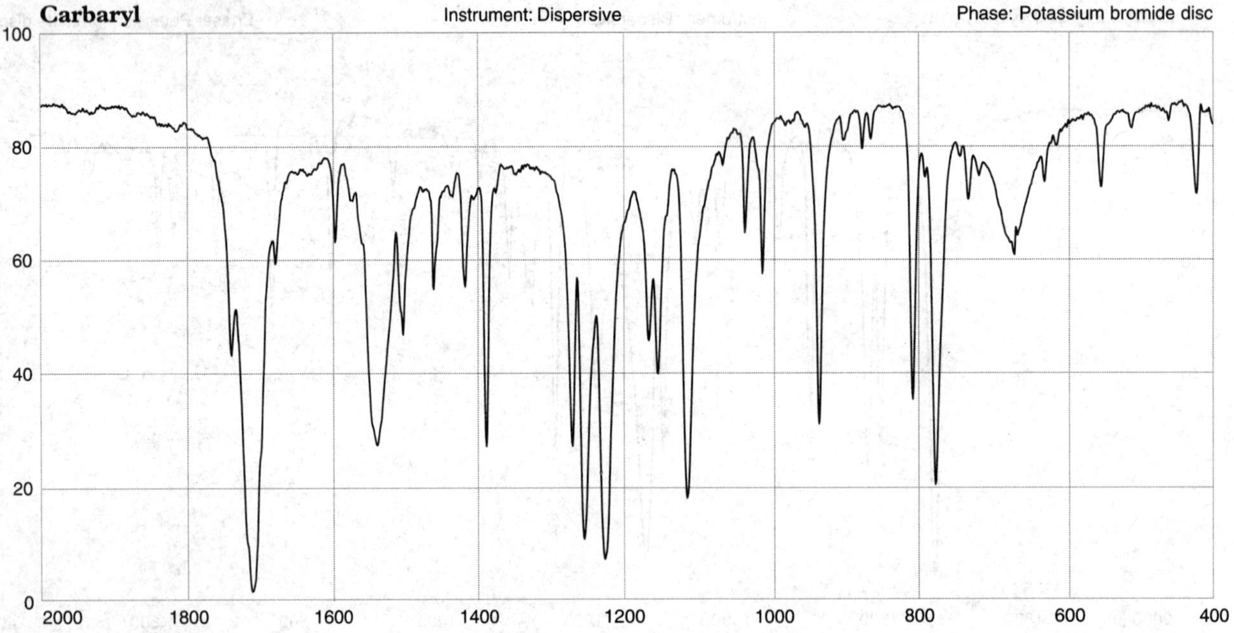

Carbenicillin Sodium Instrument: Dispersive Phase: Potassium bromide disc

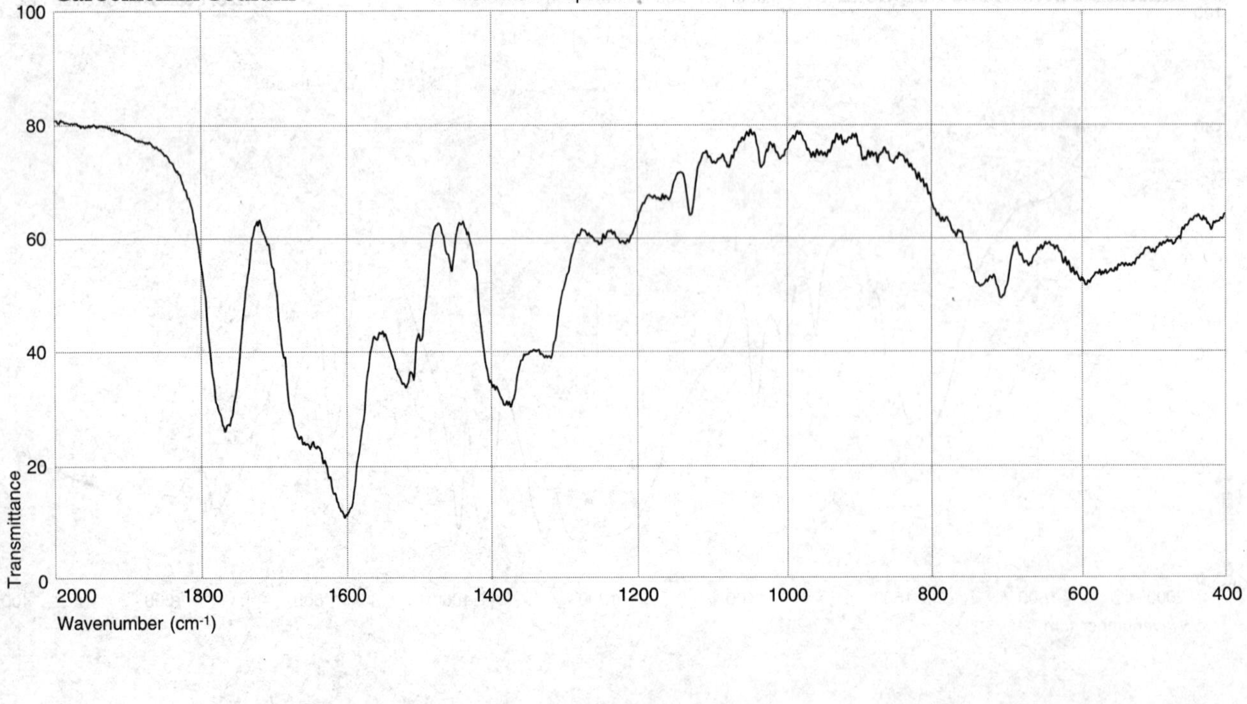

Carbenoxolone Instrument: Dispersive Phase: Potassium bromide disc

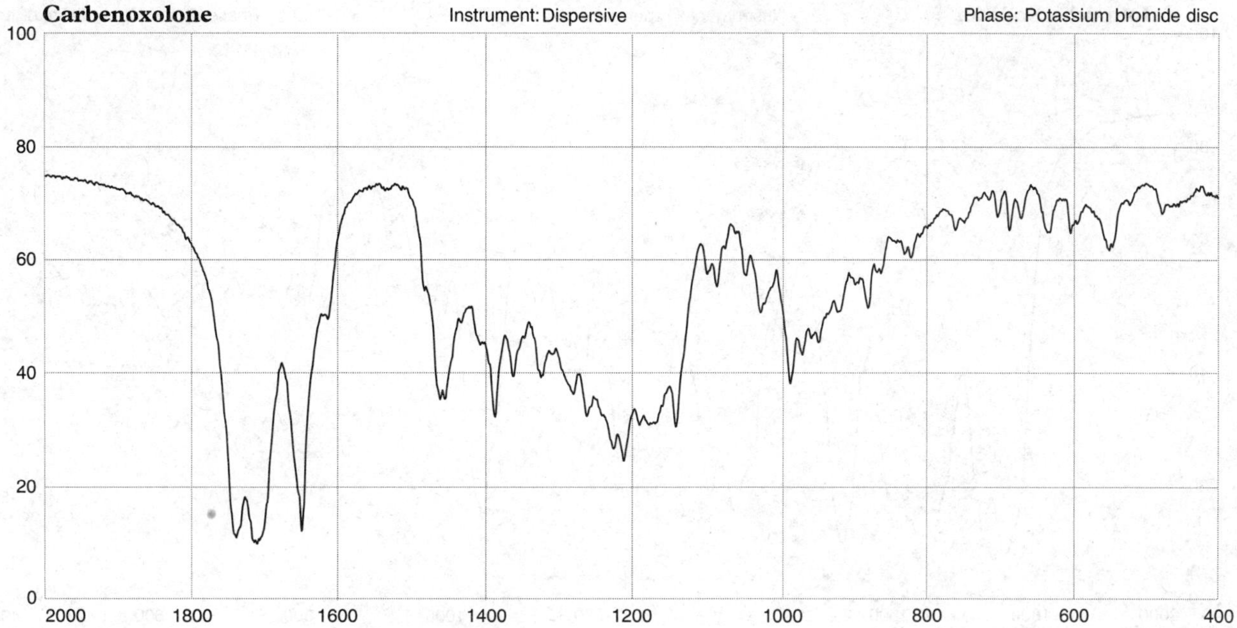

Carbimazole Instrument: Dispersive Phase: Potassium bromide disc

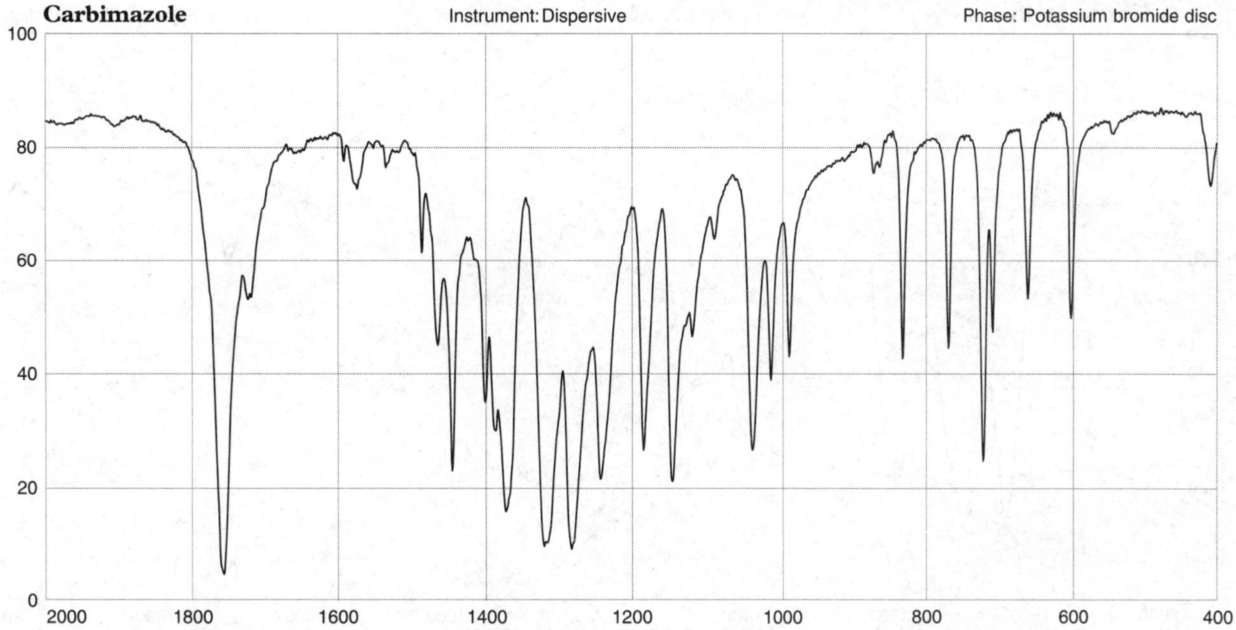

Carteolol Hydrochloride Instrument: Fourier transform Phase: Potassium chloride disc

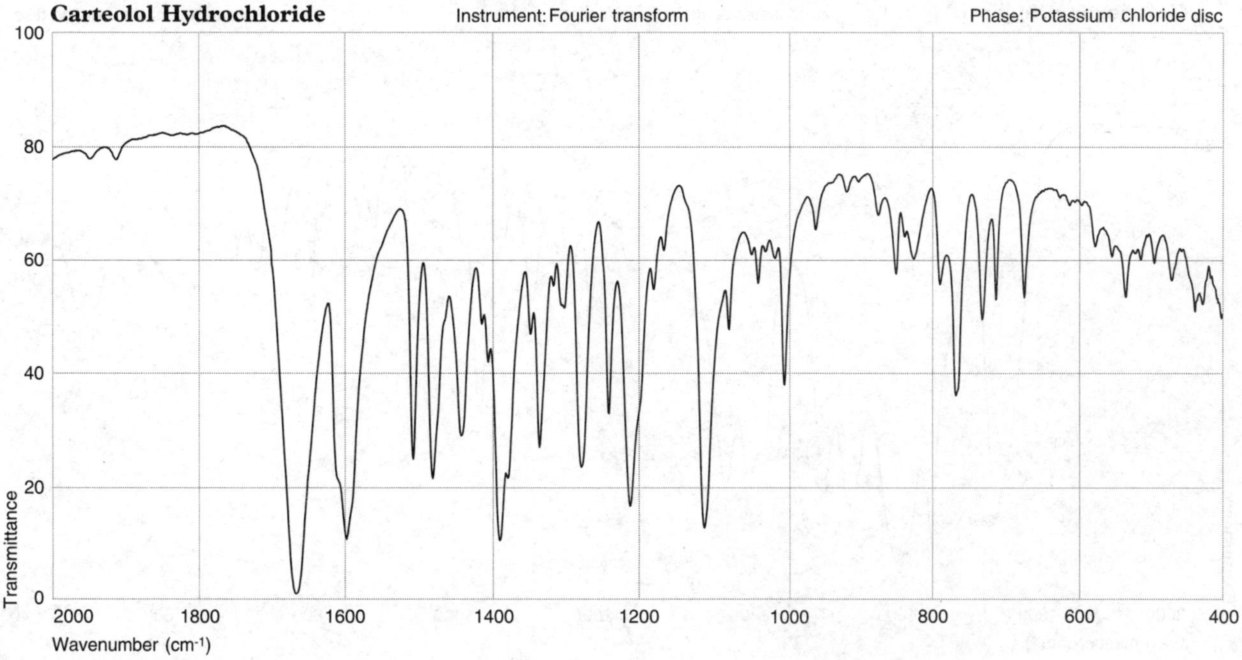

Cefotaxime Sodium Instrument: Dispersive Phase: Potassium bromide disc

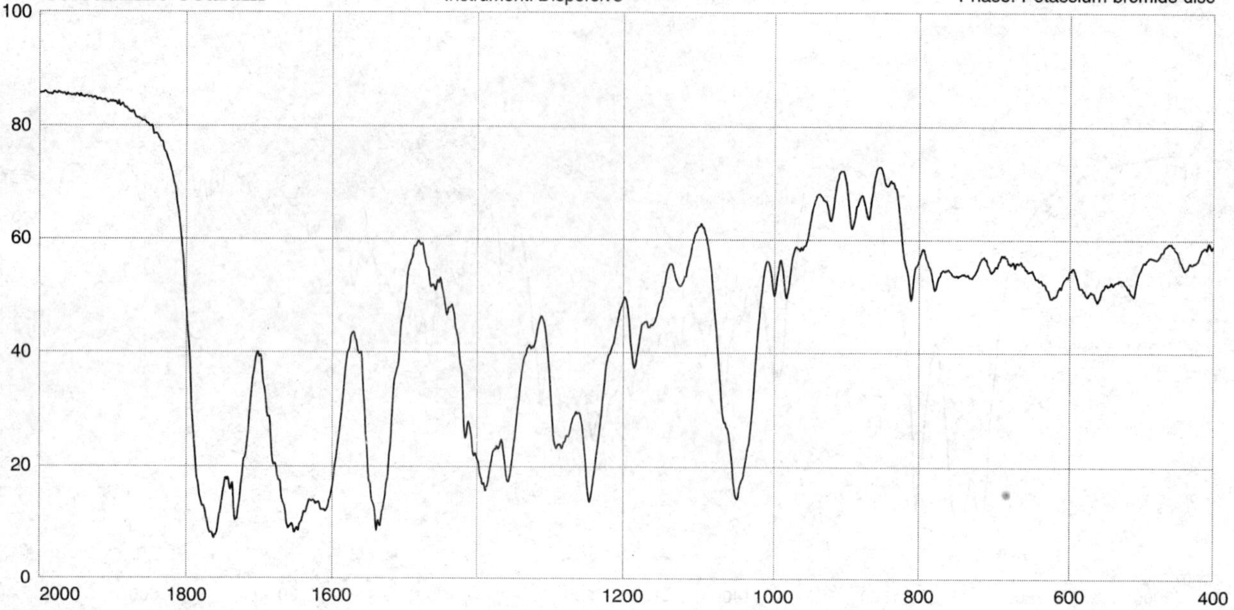

Cefoxitin Sodium Instrument: Fourier transform Phase: Potassium bromide disc

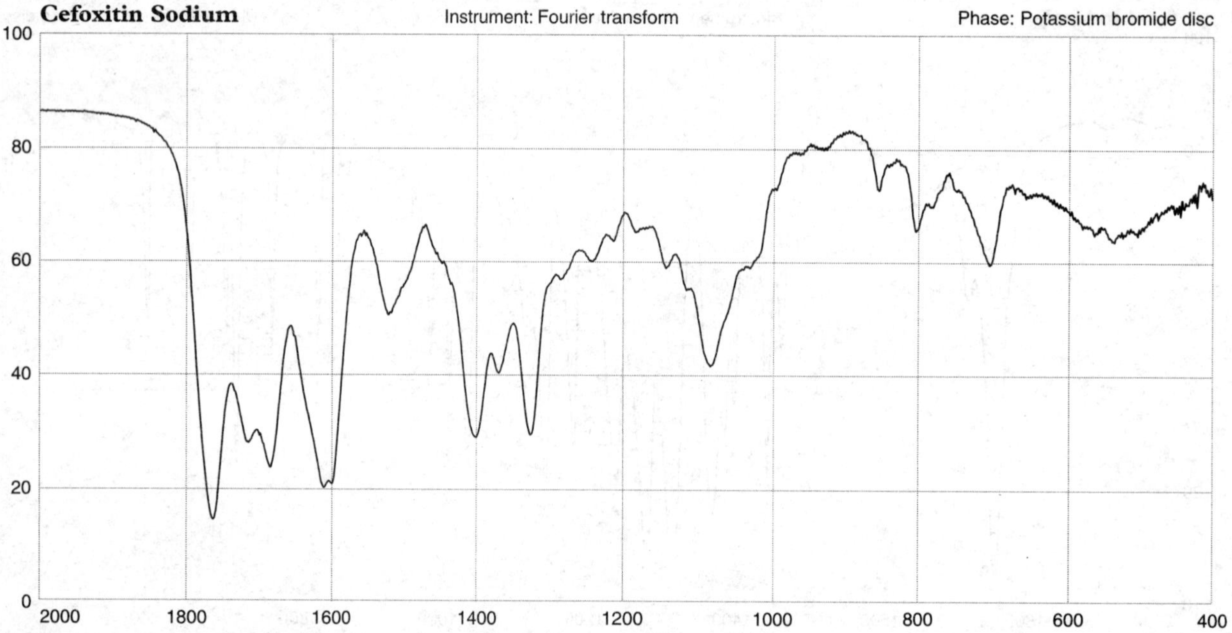

Ceftriaxone Sodium Instrument: Fourier transform Phase: Potassium bromide disc

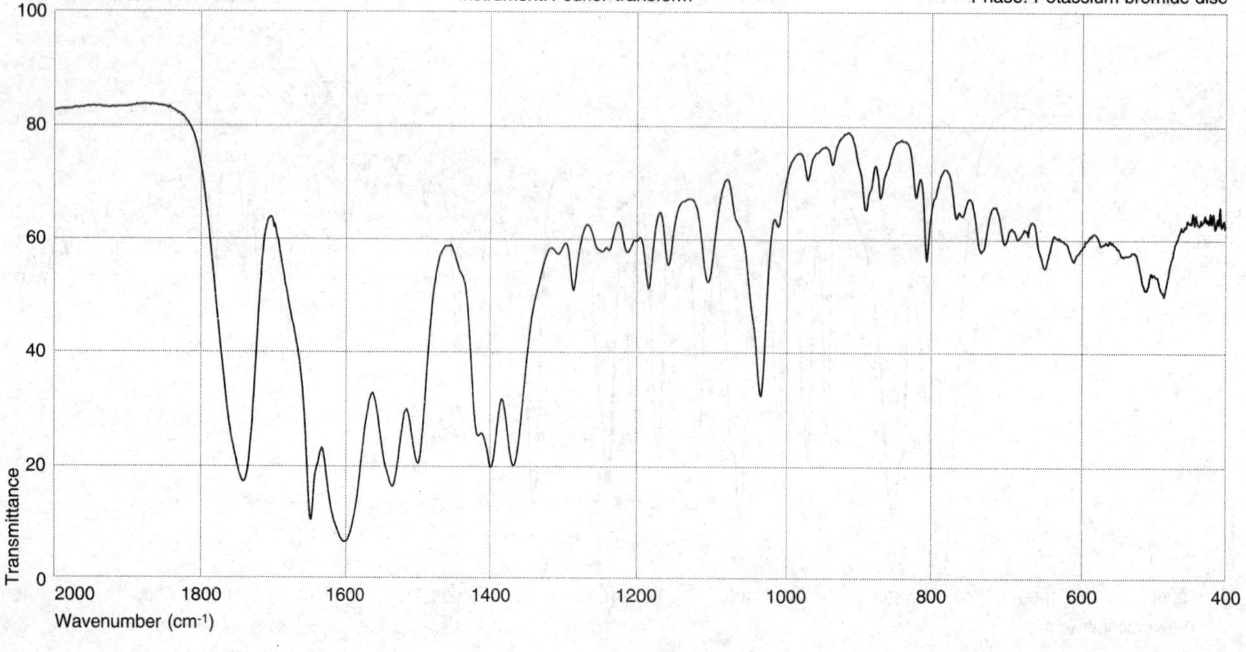

Cefuroxime Axetil Instrument: Dispersive Phase: Potassium bromide disc

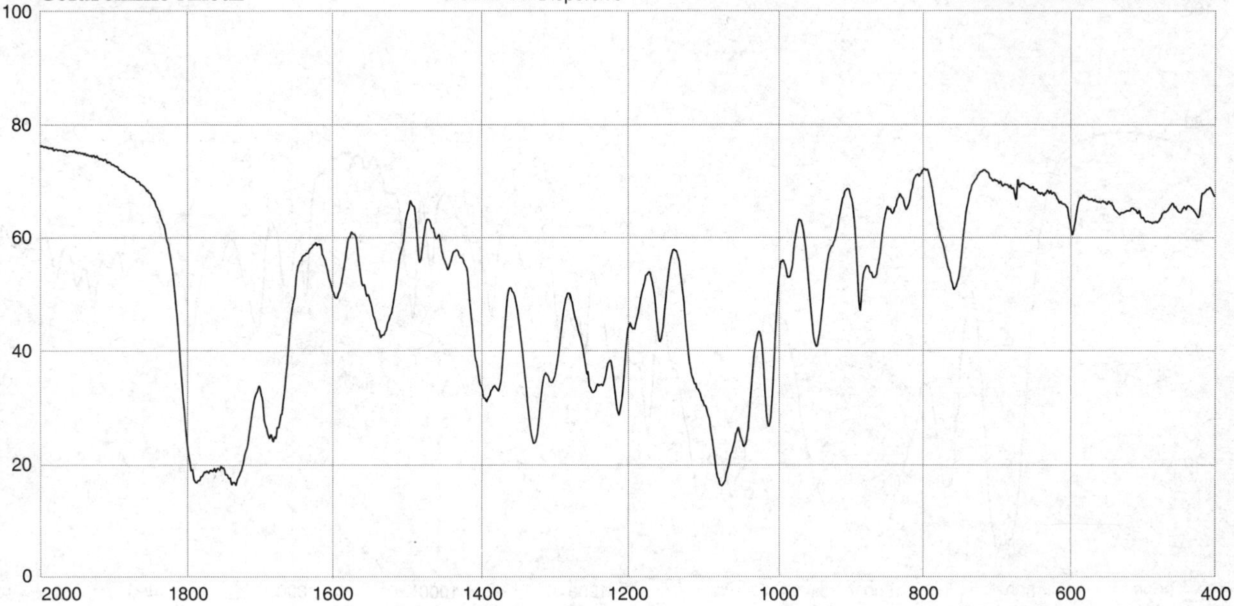

Cefuroxime Sodium Instrument: Fourier transform Phase: Potassium bromide disc

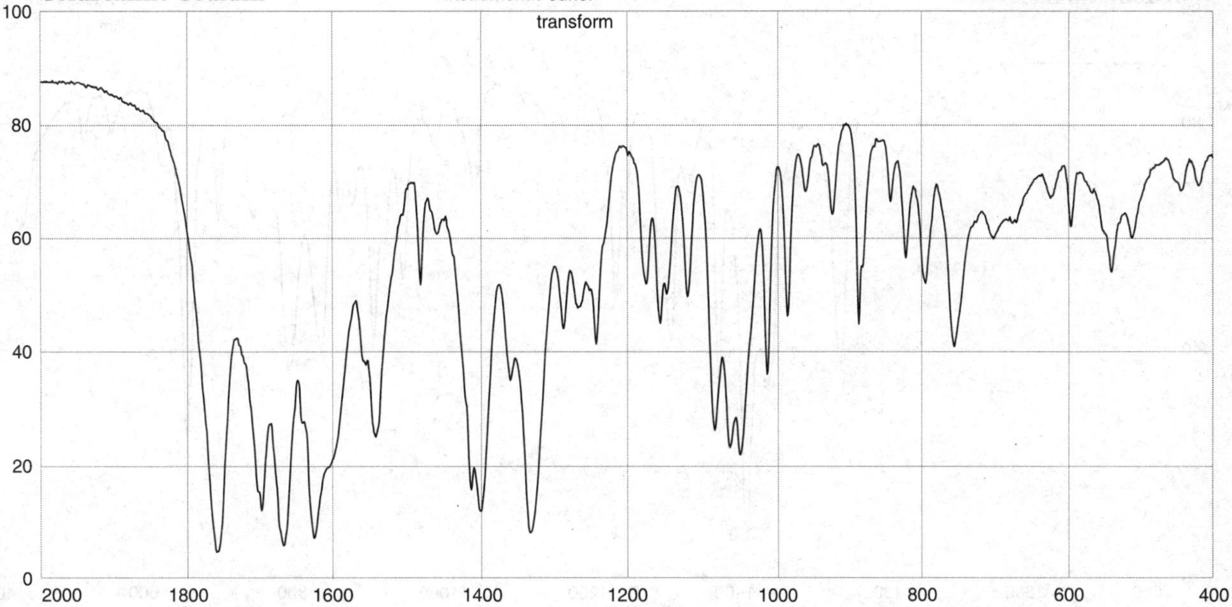

Cefalexin Instrument: Fourier transform Phase: Potassium bromide disc

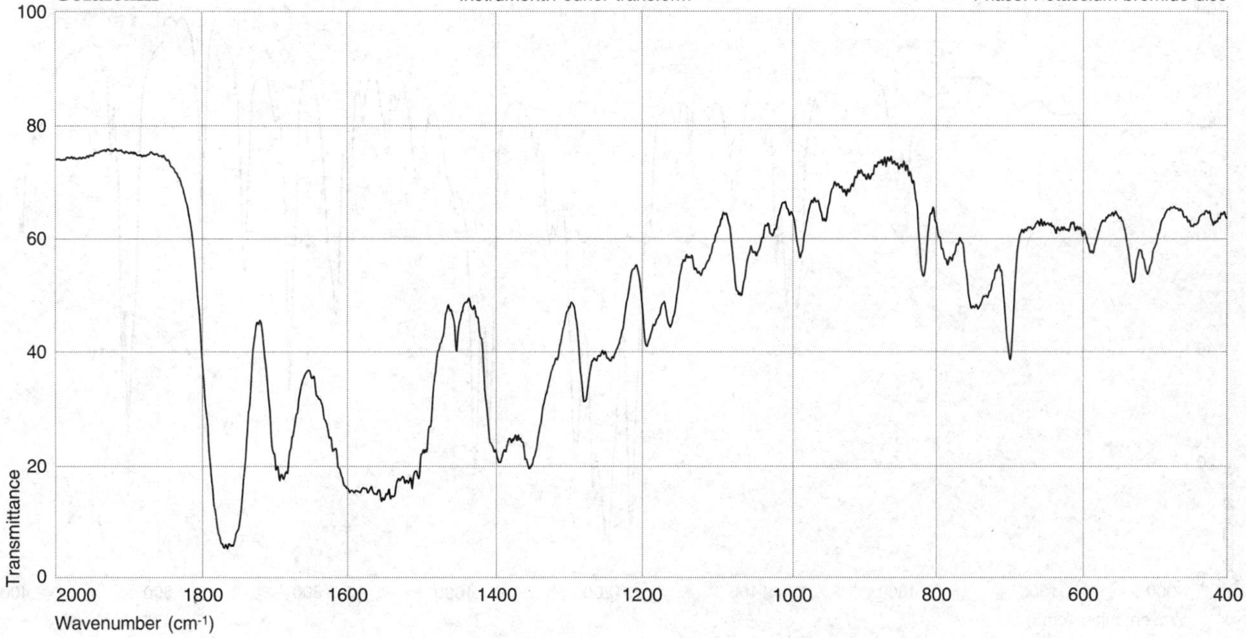

Cefradine

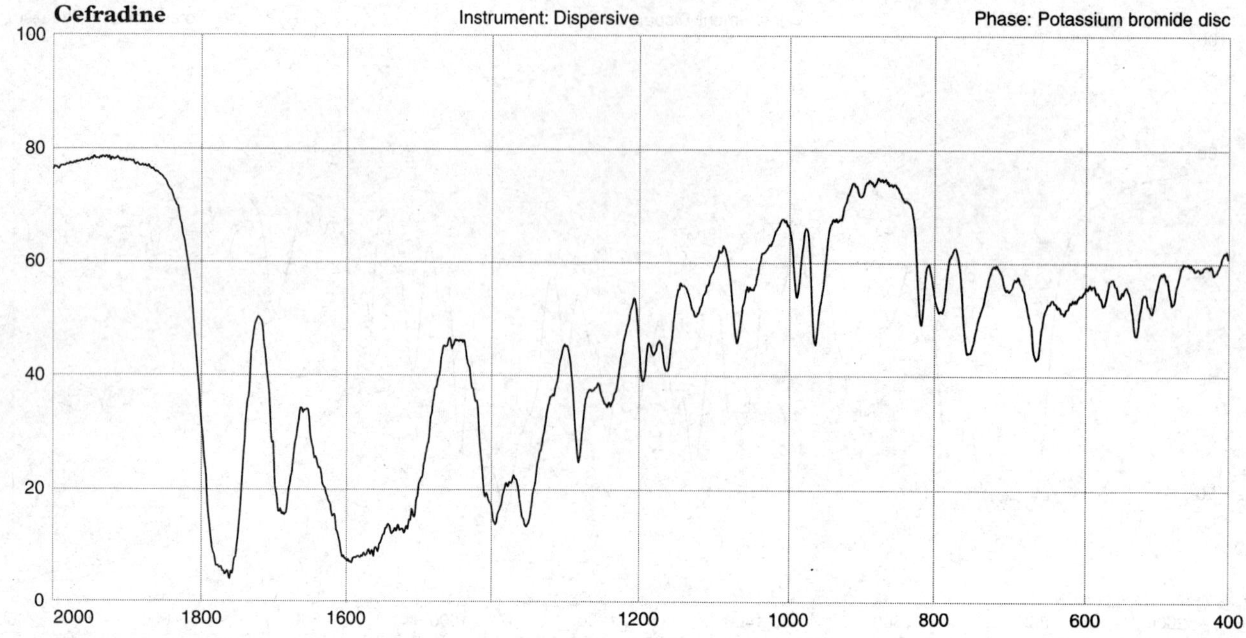

Clomethiazole

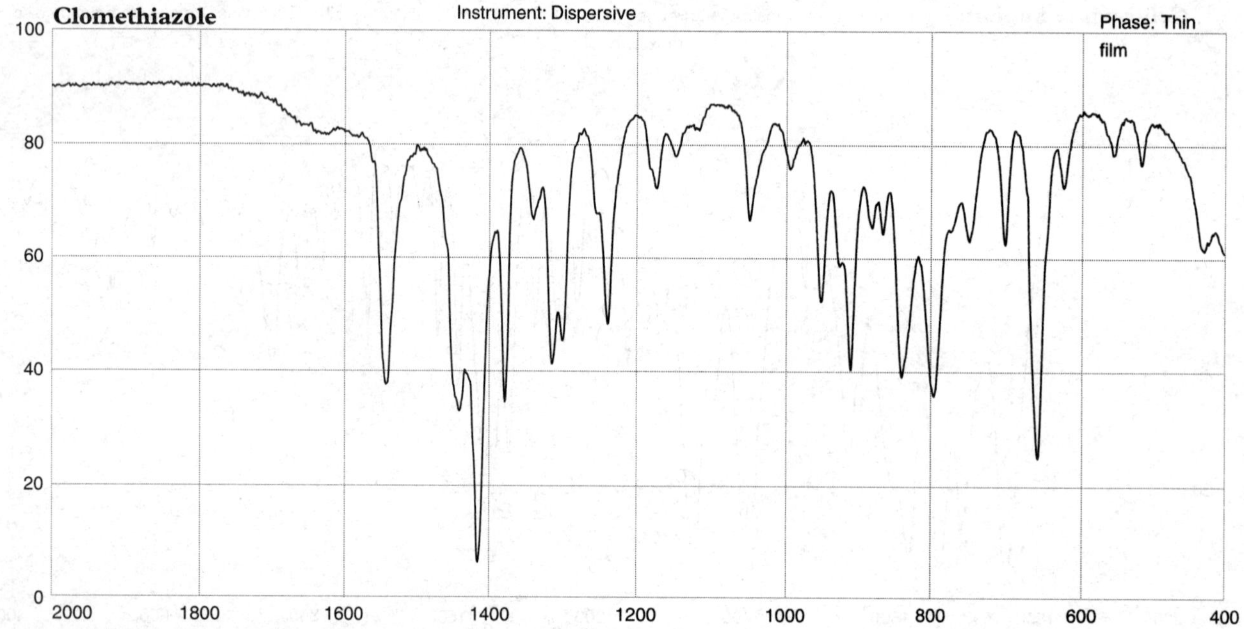

Clomethiazole Edisilate

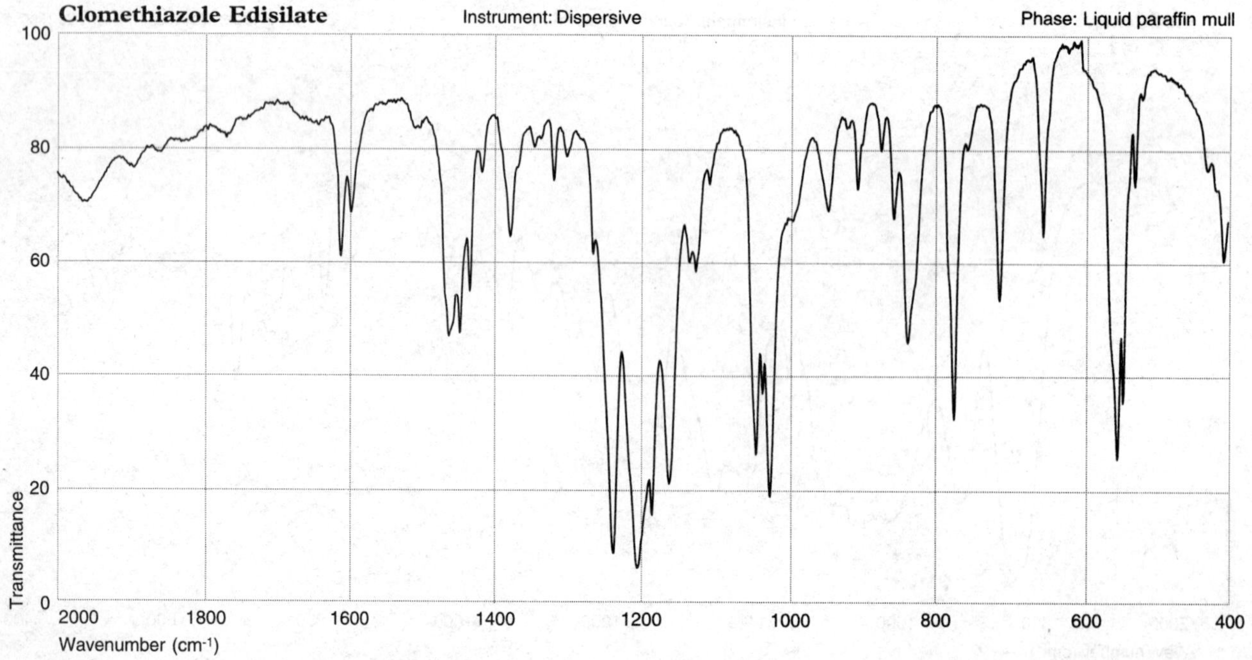

Chloroform Instrument: Dispersive Phase: 0.1mm Layer

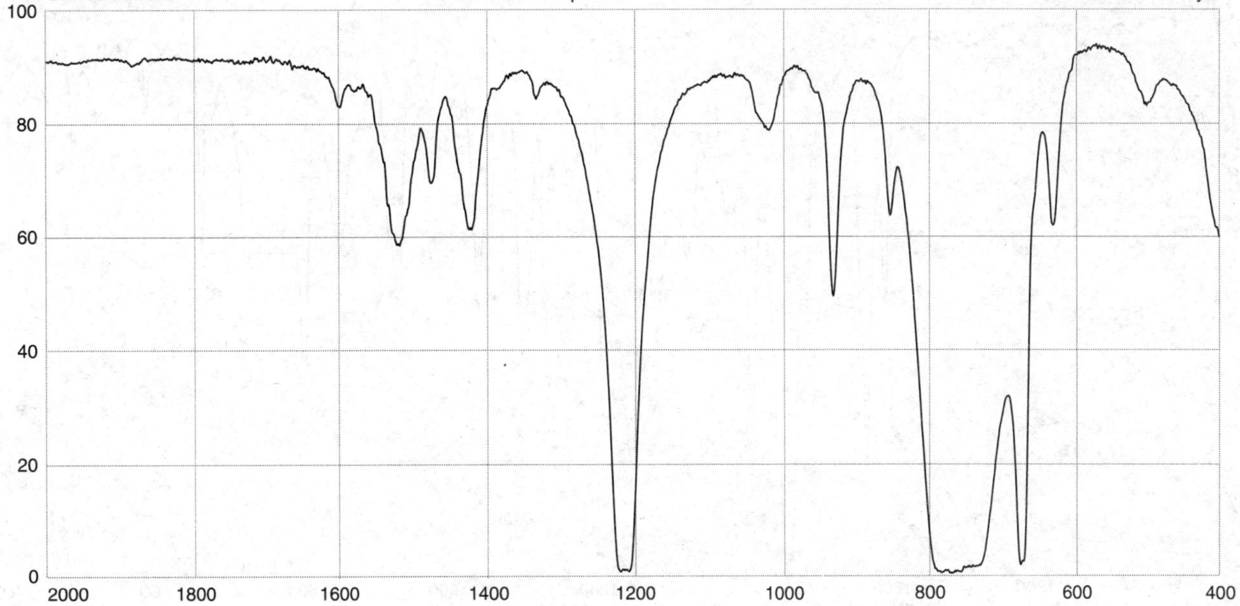

Chloroquine Instrument: Dispersive Phase: 5% w/v solution in chloroform Thickness: 0.1mm

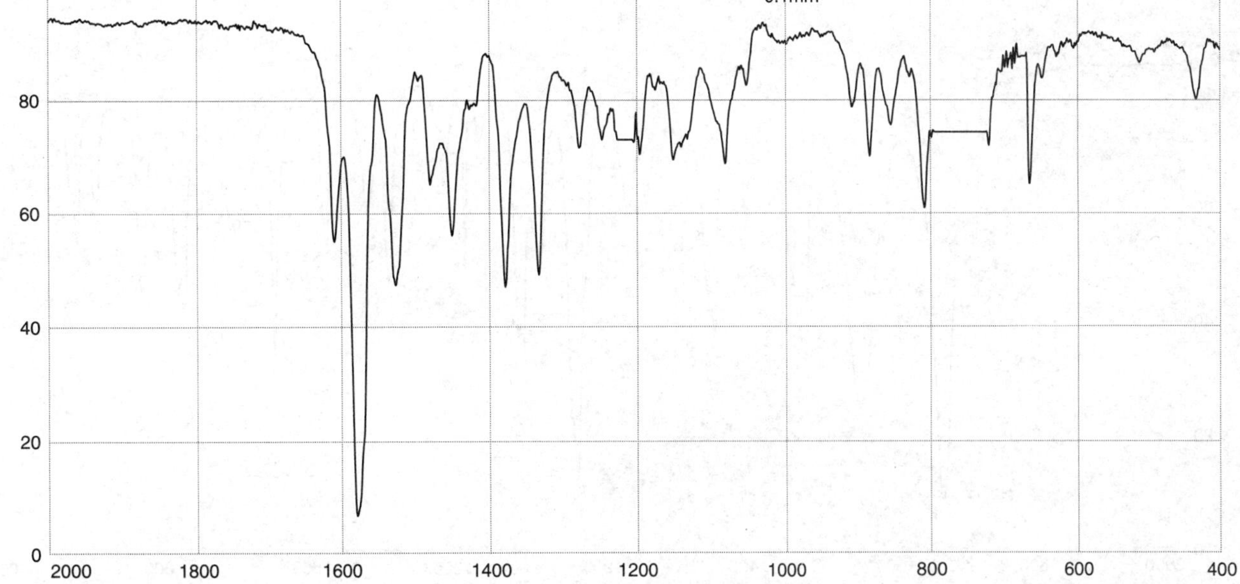

Chloroxylenol Instrument: Dispersive Phase: Potassium bromide disc

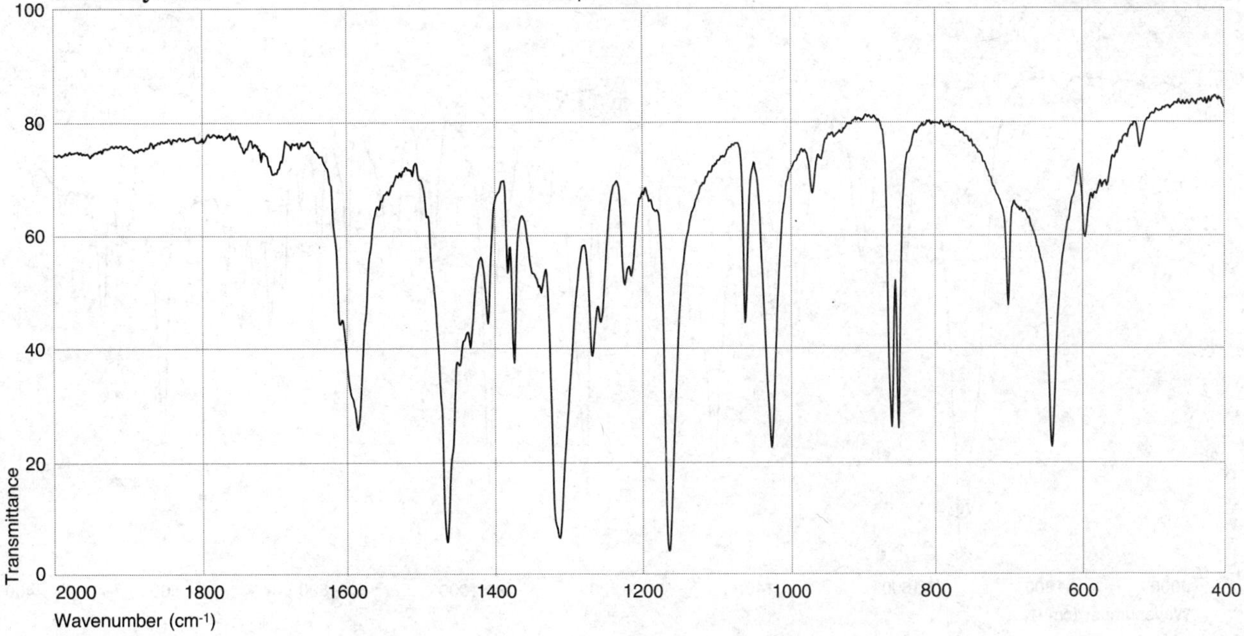

Chlorpromazine Instrument: Dispersive Phase: 5% w/v solution in chloroform Thickness: 0.1mm

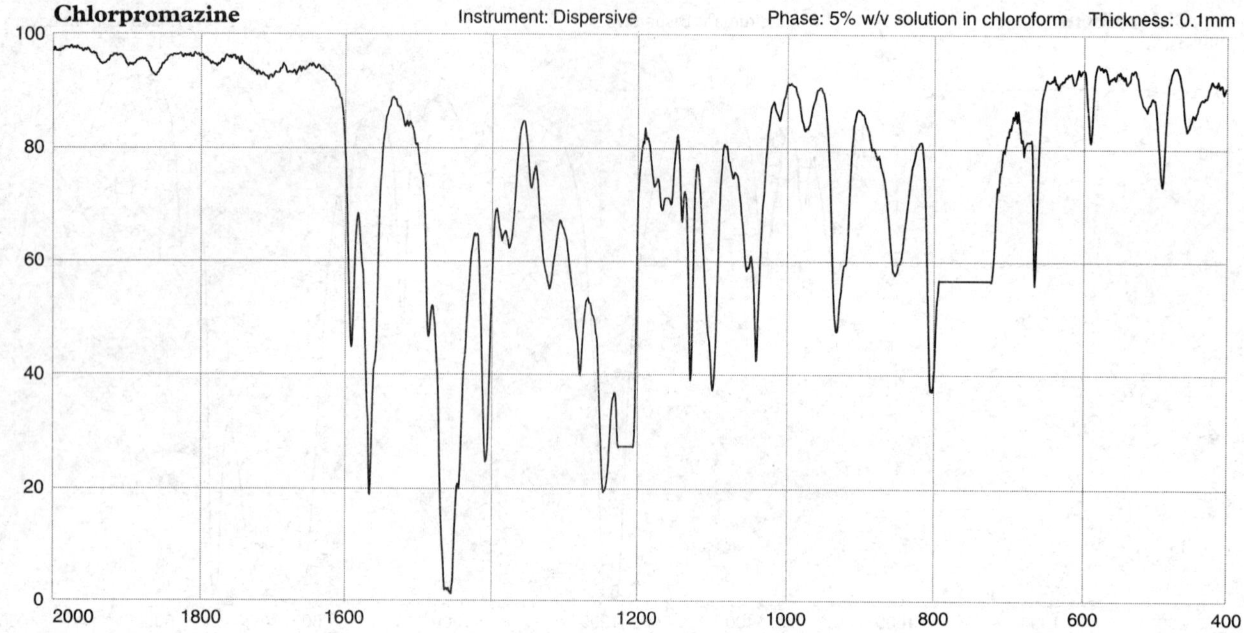

Chlorpropamide Instrument: Dispersive Phase: Potassium bromide disc

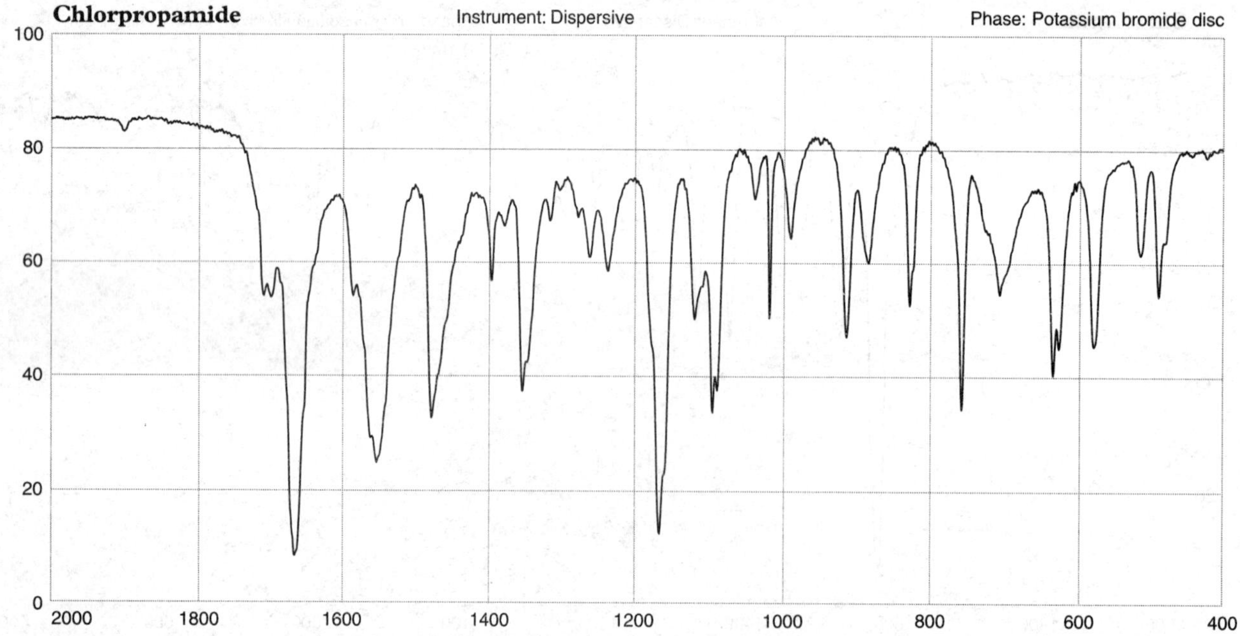

Chlortalidone Instrument: Dispersive Phase: Potassium bromide disc

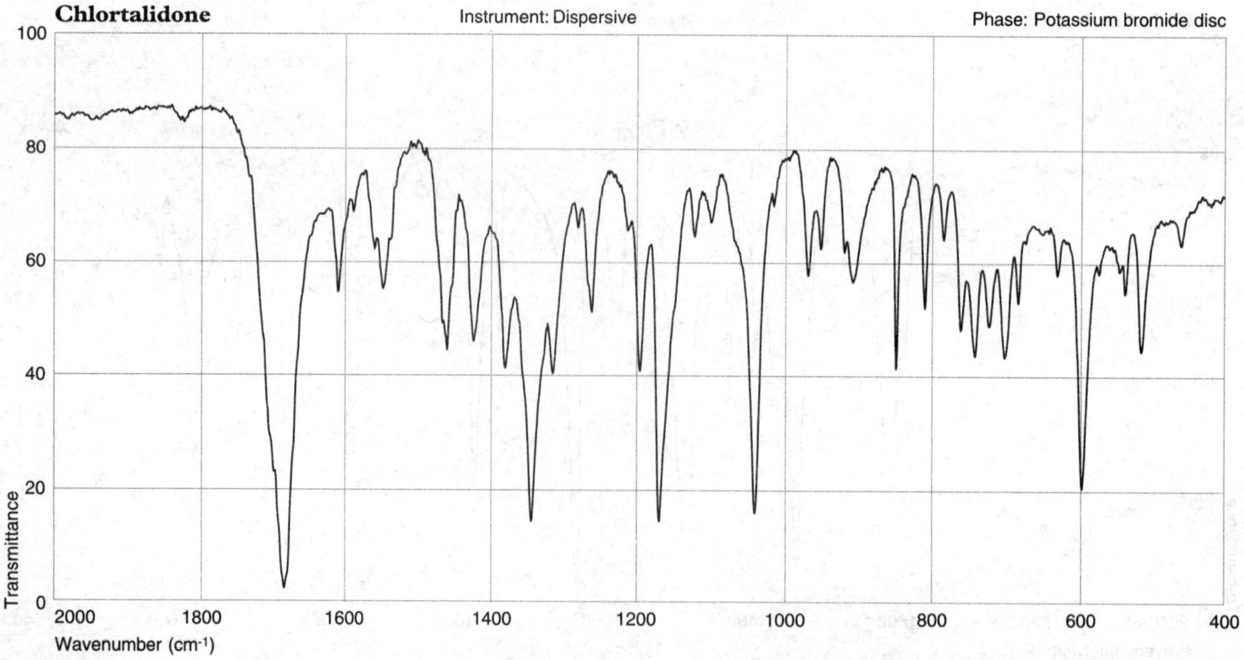

Choline Salicylate Instrument: Dispersive Phase: Thin film

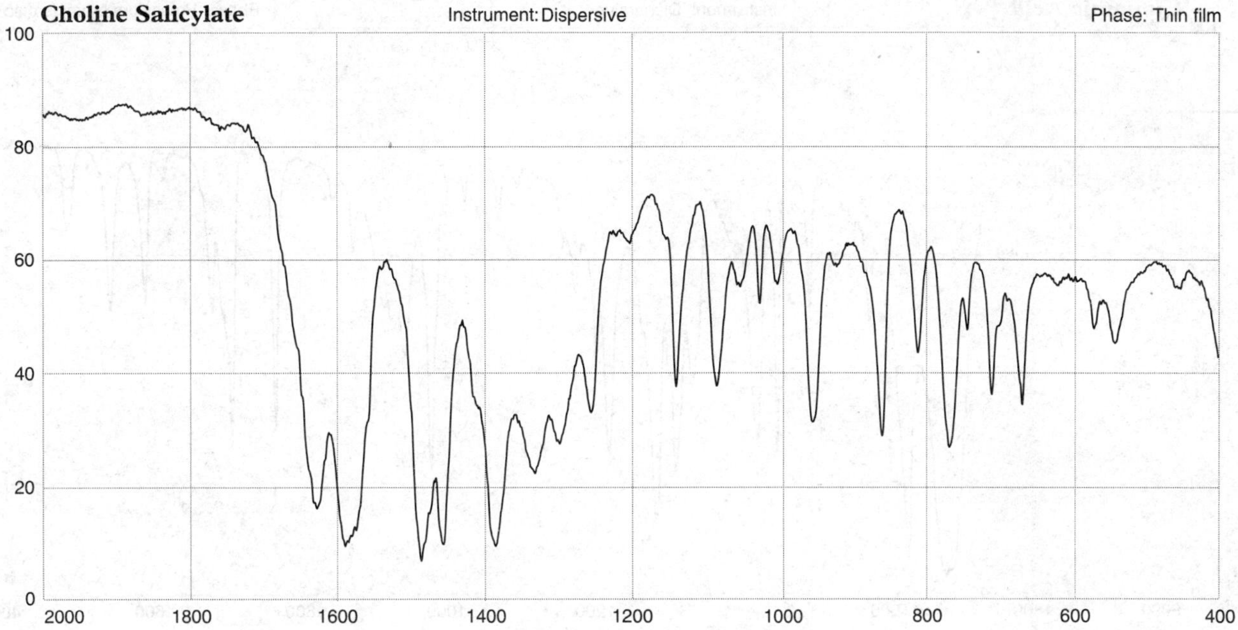

Choline Theophyllinate Instrument: Dispersive Phase: Potassium bromide disc

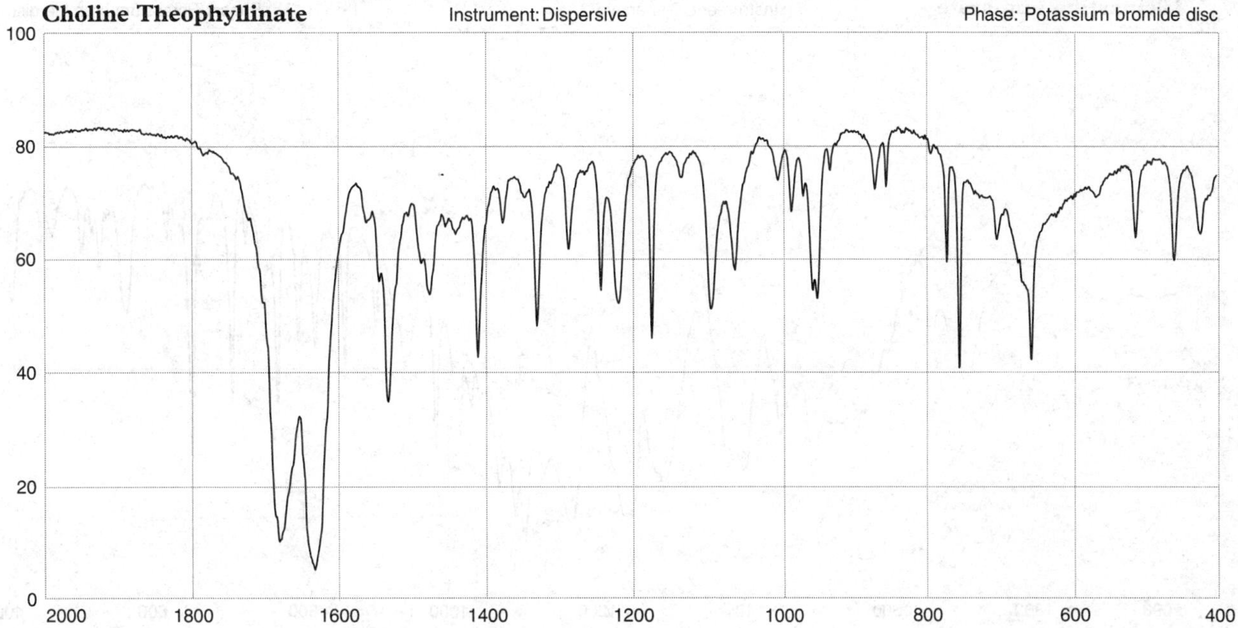

Cimetidine Instrument: Dispersive Phase: Potassium bromide disc

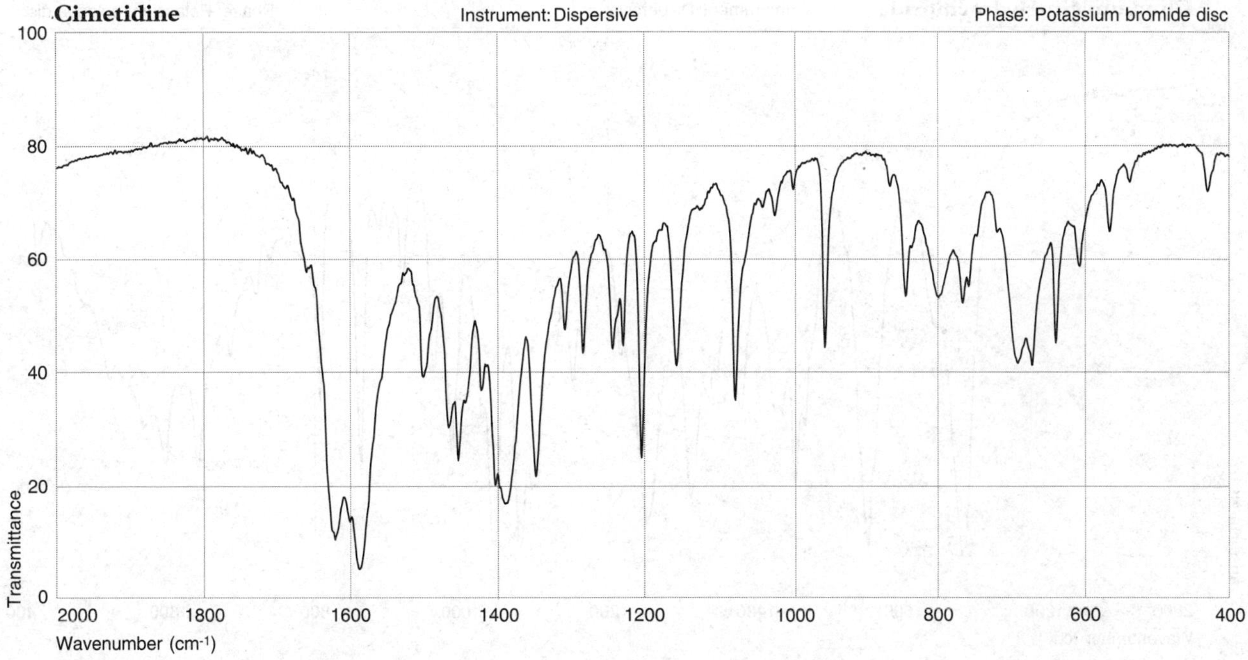

Cinnamic Acid Instrument: Dispersive Phase: Potassium bromide disc

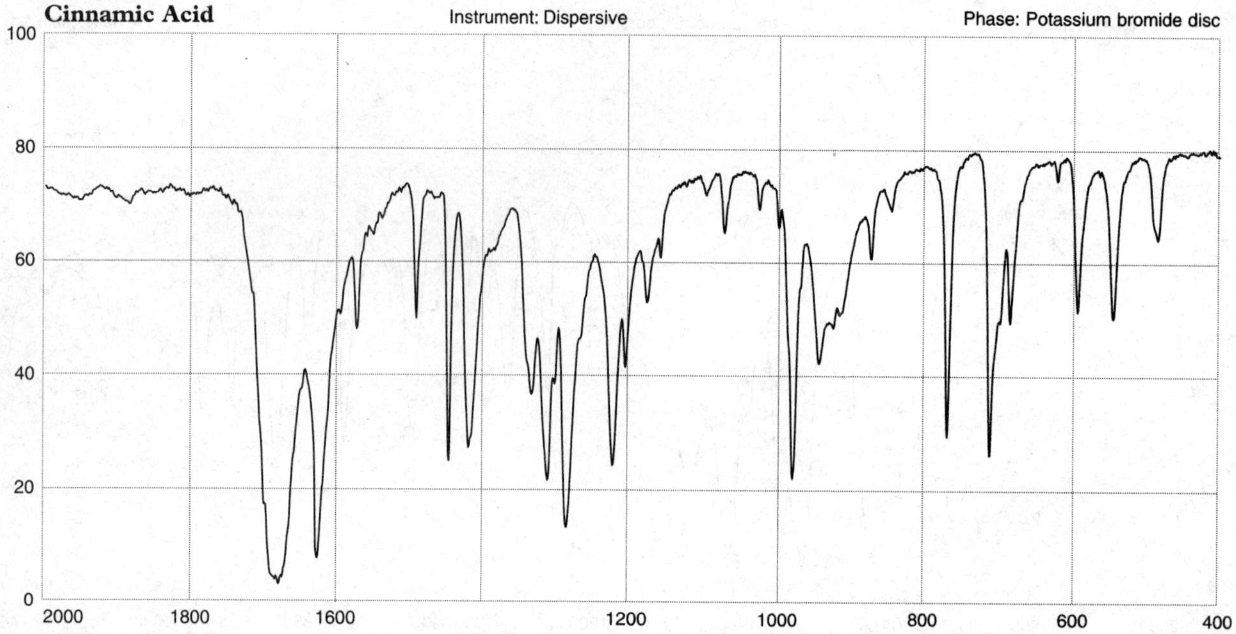

Clemastine Fumarate Instrument: Dispersive Phase: Potassium bromide disc

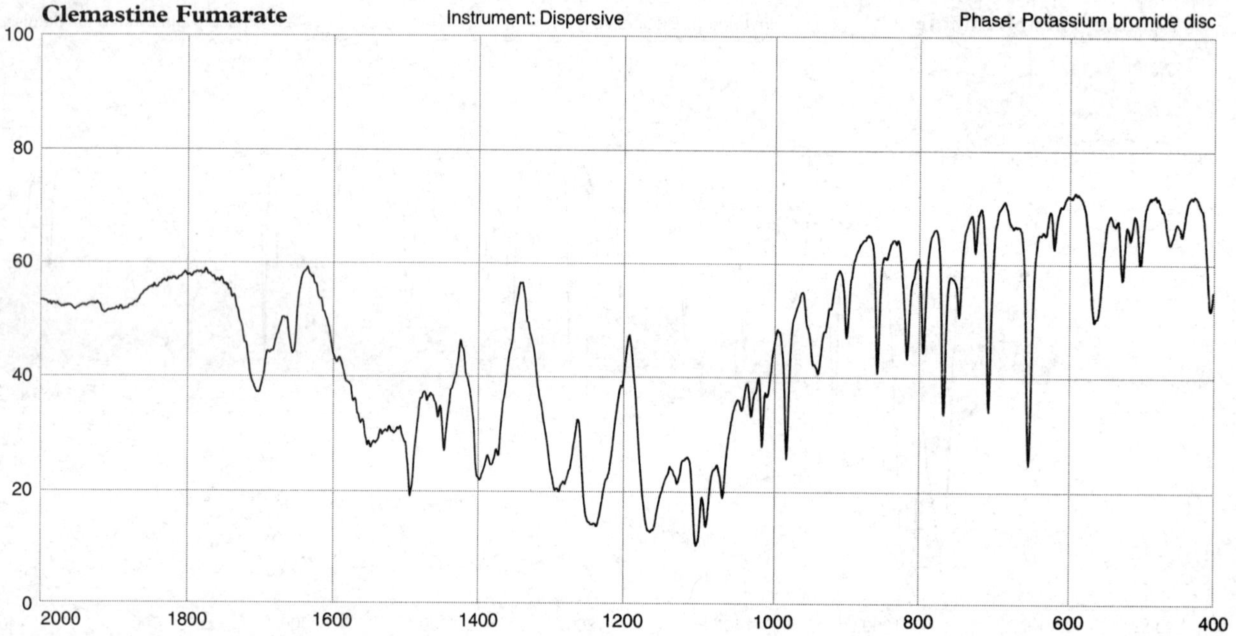

Clindamycin Hydrochloride Instrument: Dispersive Phase: Potassium chloride disc

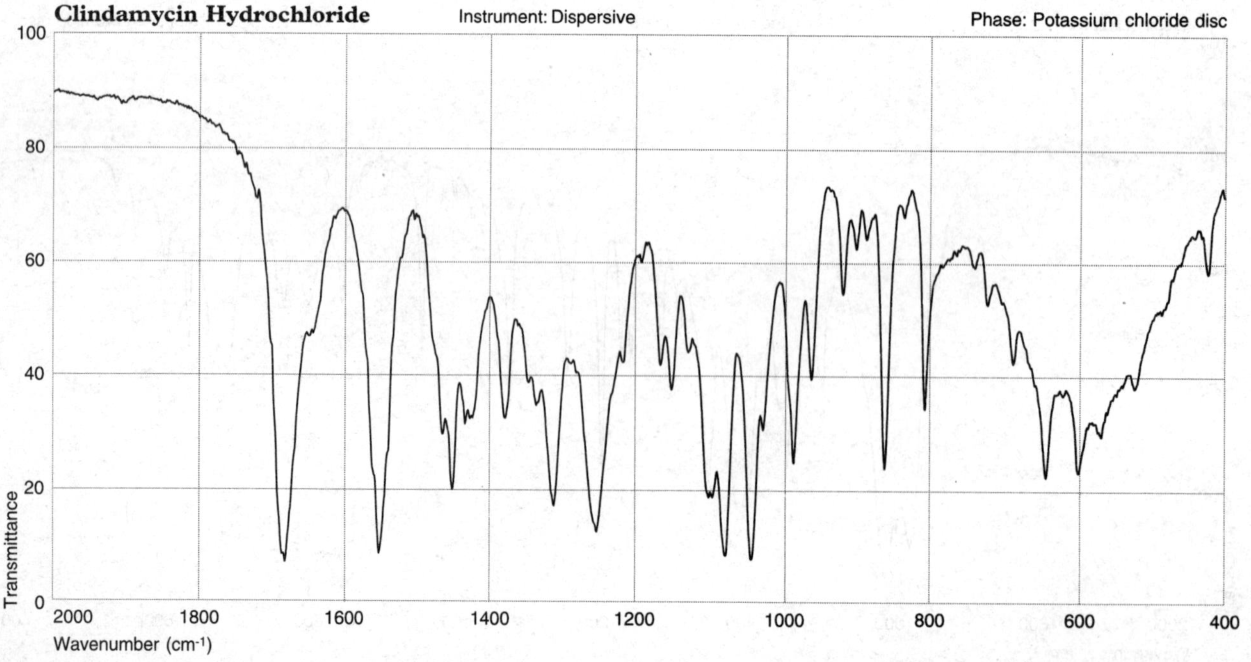

Clioquinol Instrument: Dispersive Phase: Potassium bromide disc

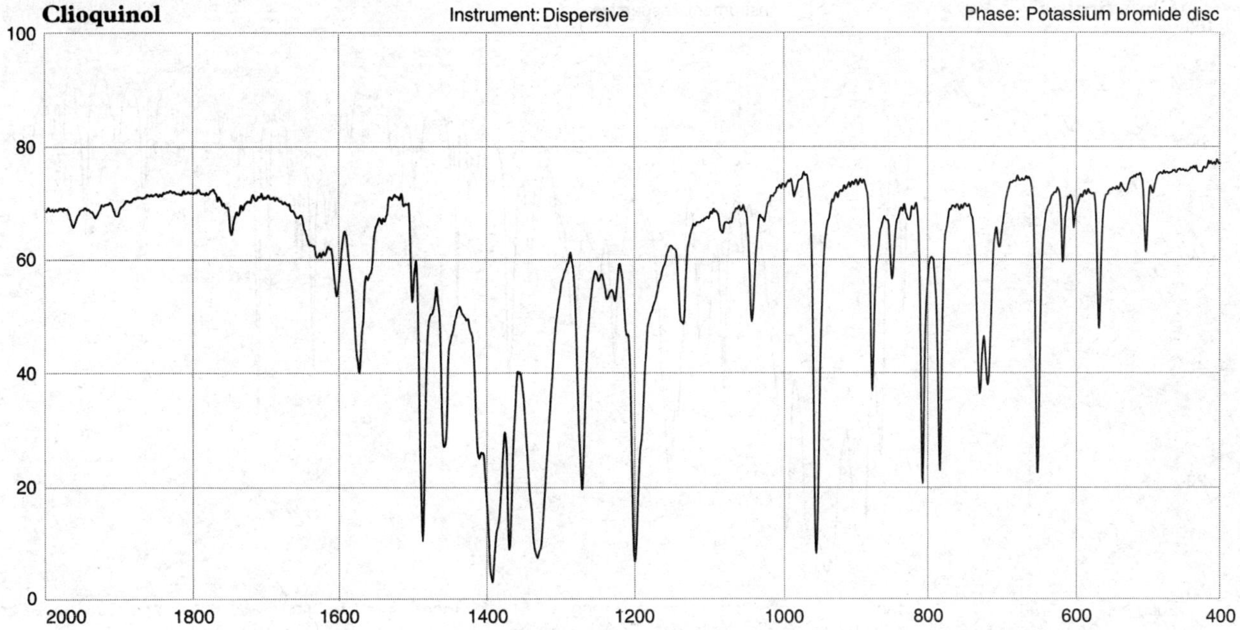

Clobazam Instrument: Dispersive Phase: Potassium bromide disc

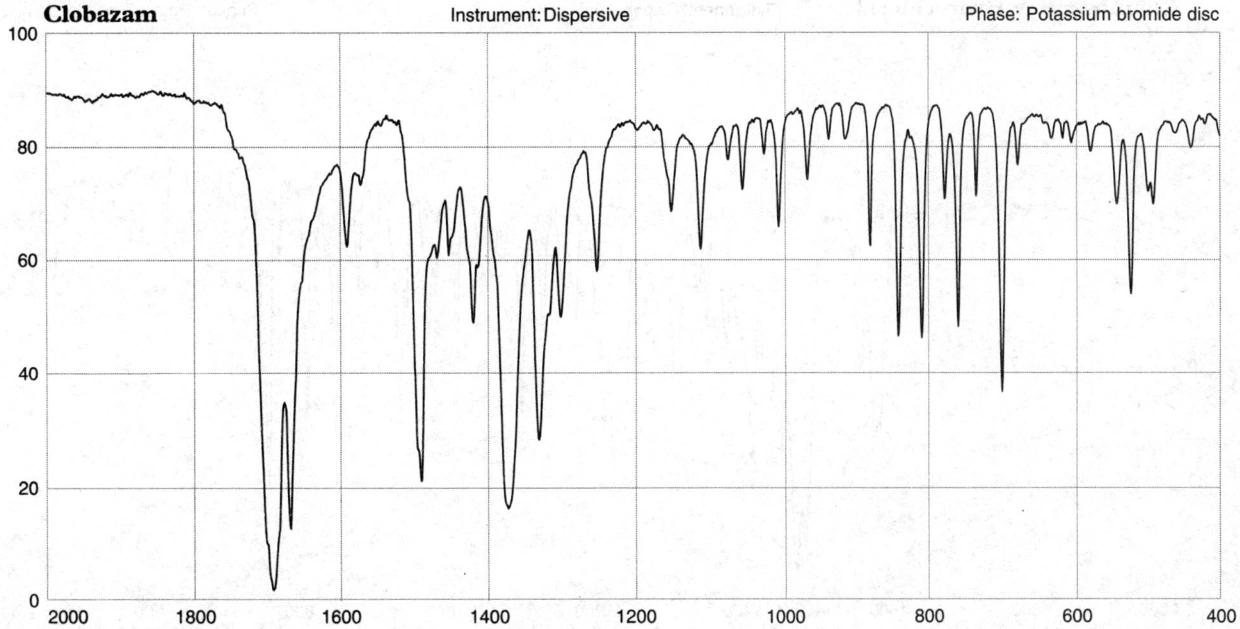

Clobetasol Propionate Instrument: Dispersive Phase: Potassium bromide disc

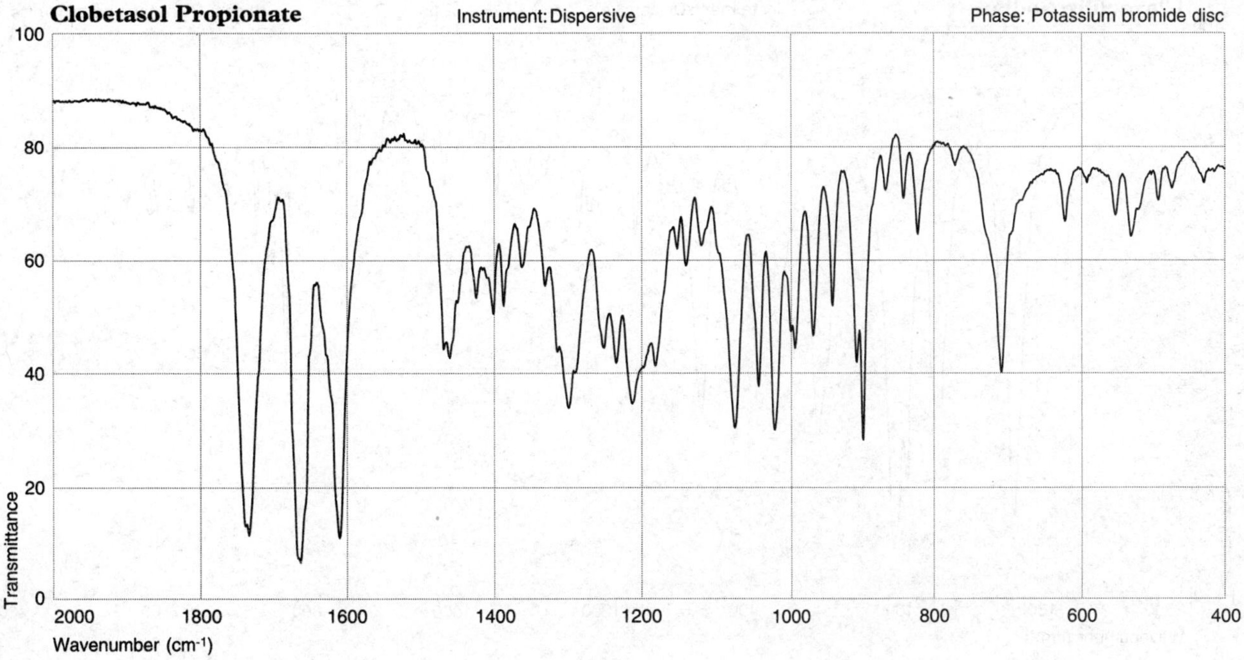

Clofazimine Instrument: Dispersive Phase: Liquid Paraffin mull

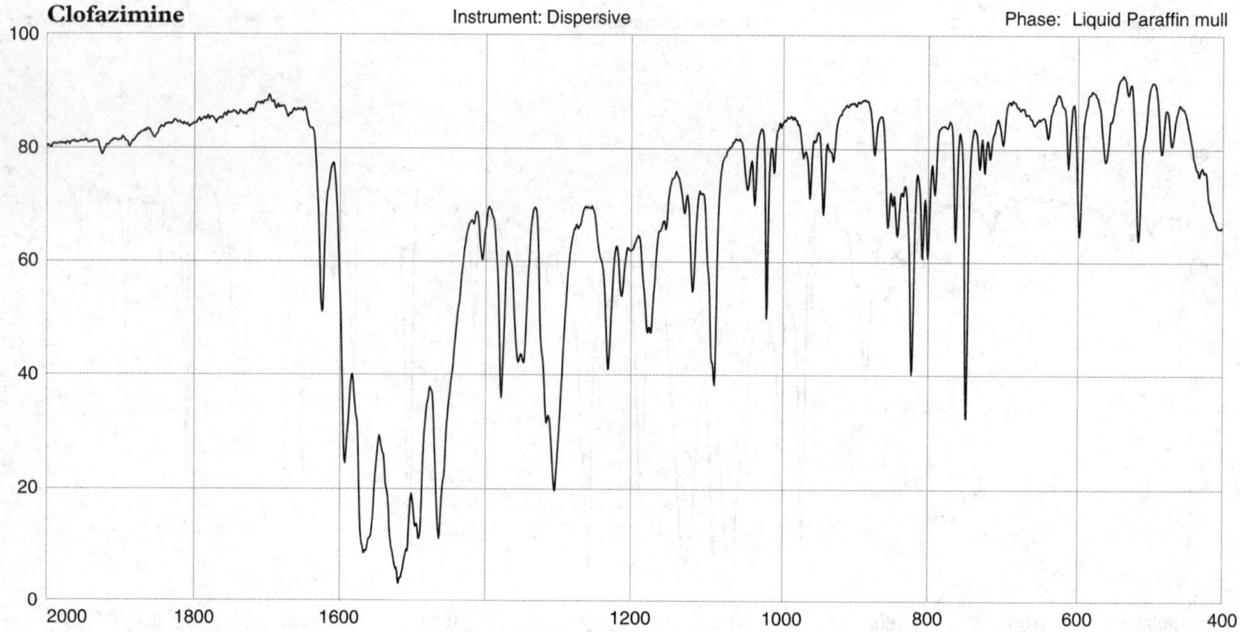

Clomipramine Hydrochloride Instrument: Dispersive Phase: Potassium chloride disc

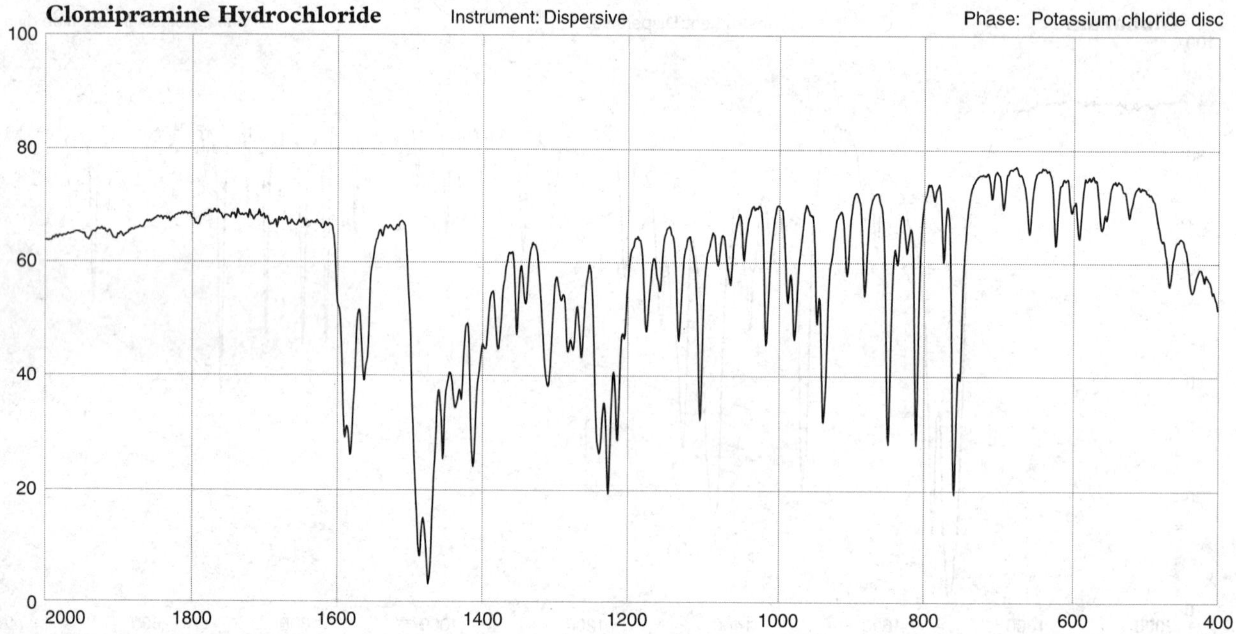

Cloxacillin Sodium Instrument: Dispersive Phase: Potassium bromide disc

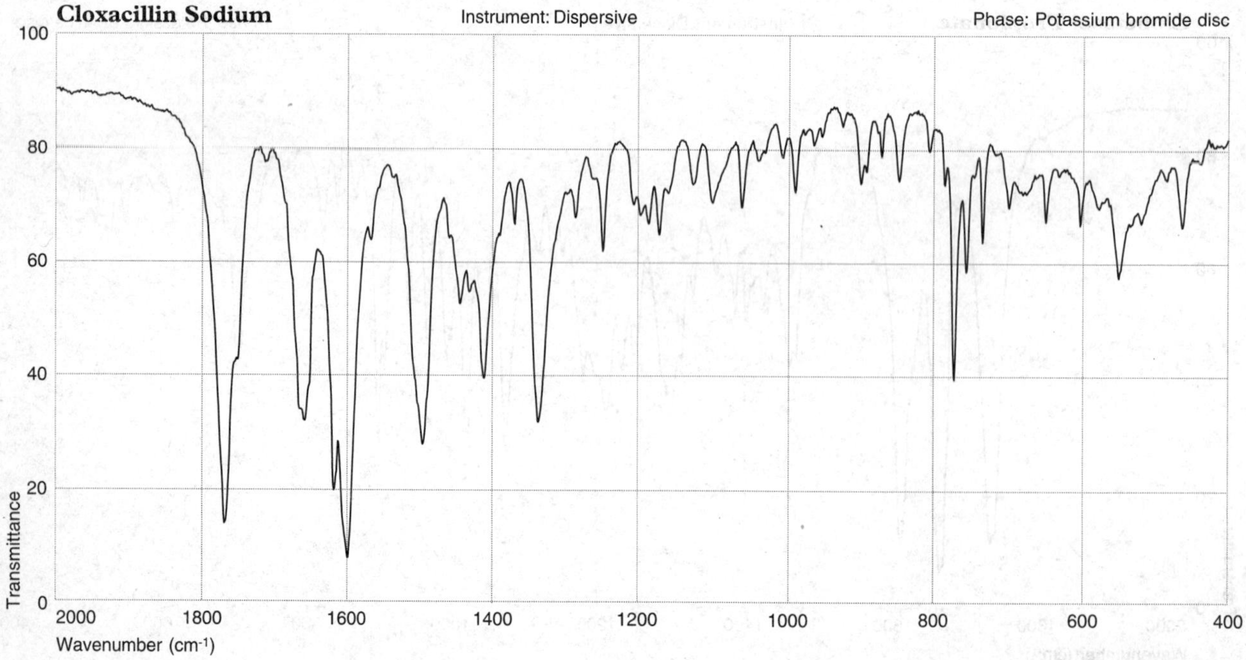

Cocaine

Instrument: Fourier transform

Phase: Potassium bromide disc

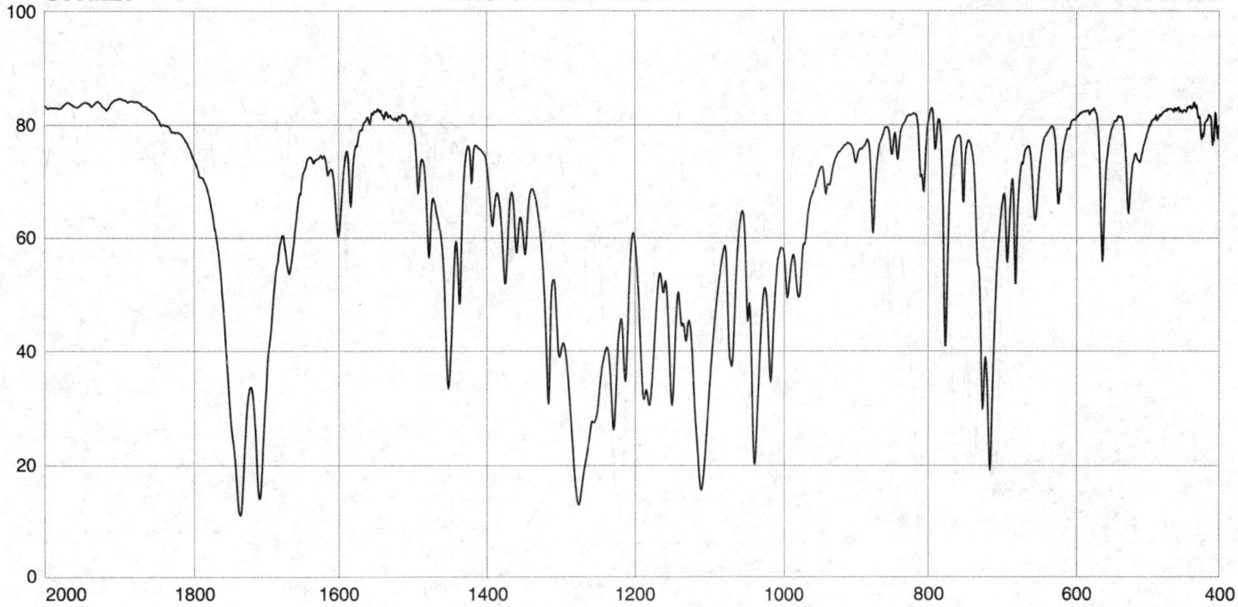

Codeine

Instrument: Dispersive

Phase: Potassium bromide disc

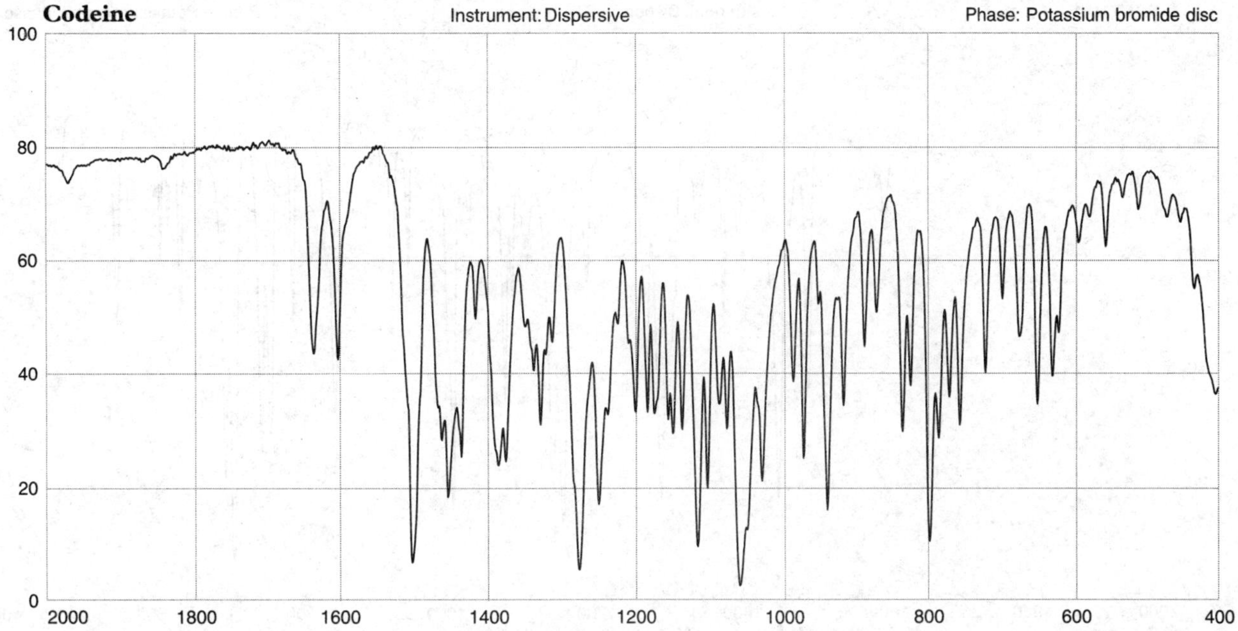

Codeine Hydrochloride

Instrument: Dispersive

Phase: Liquid Paraffin mull

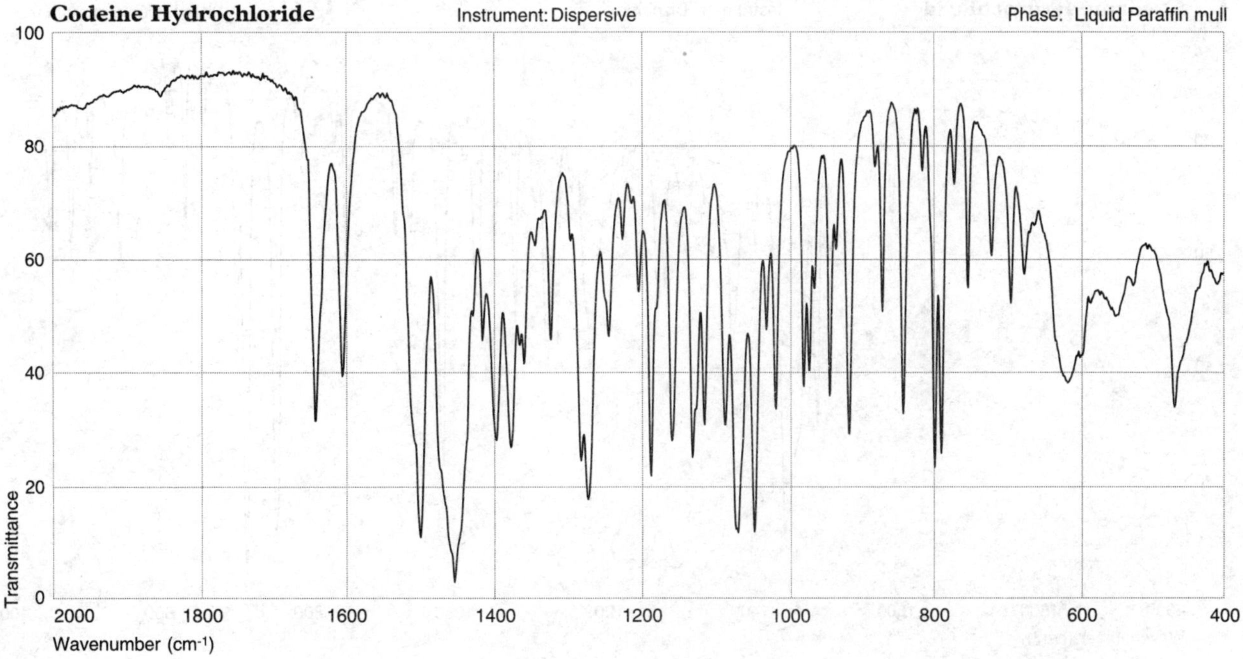

Cortisone Acetate Instrument: Dispersive Phase: Potassium bromide disc

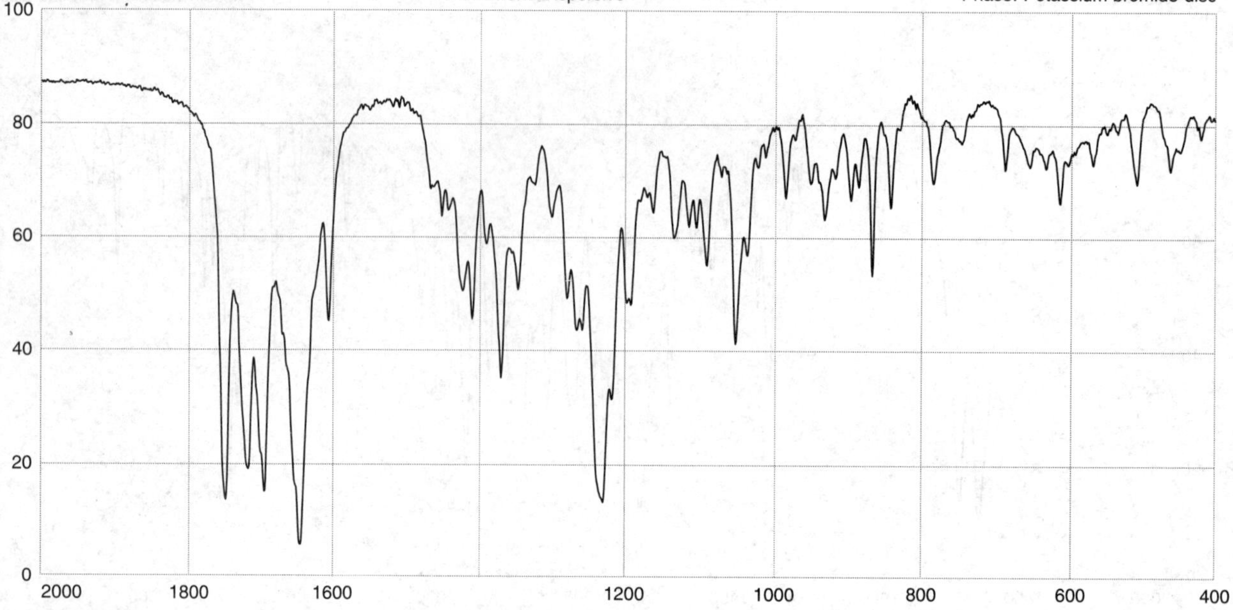

Cyclizine Instrument: Dispersive Phase: Potassium bromide disc

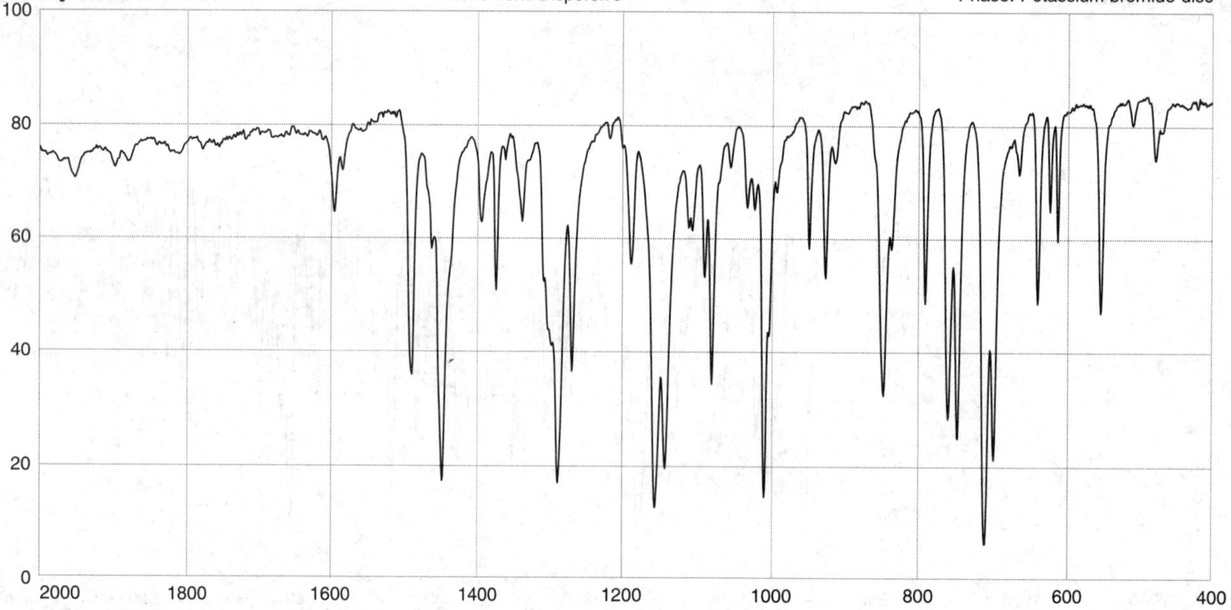

Cyclizine Hydrochloride Instrument: Dispersive Phase: Liquid paraffin mull

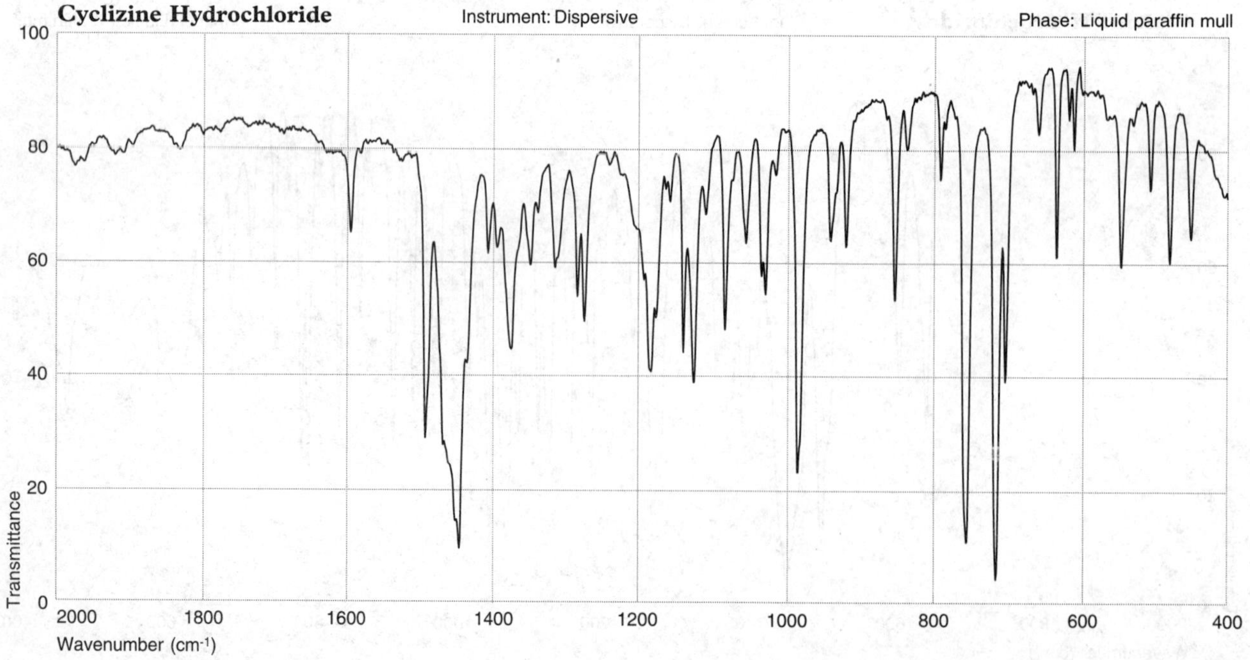

Cyclopenthiazide Instrument: Dispersive Phase: Potassium bromide disc

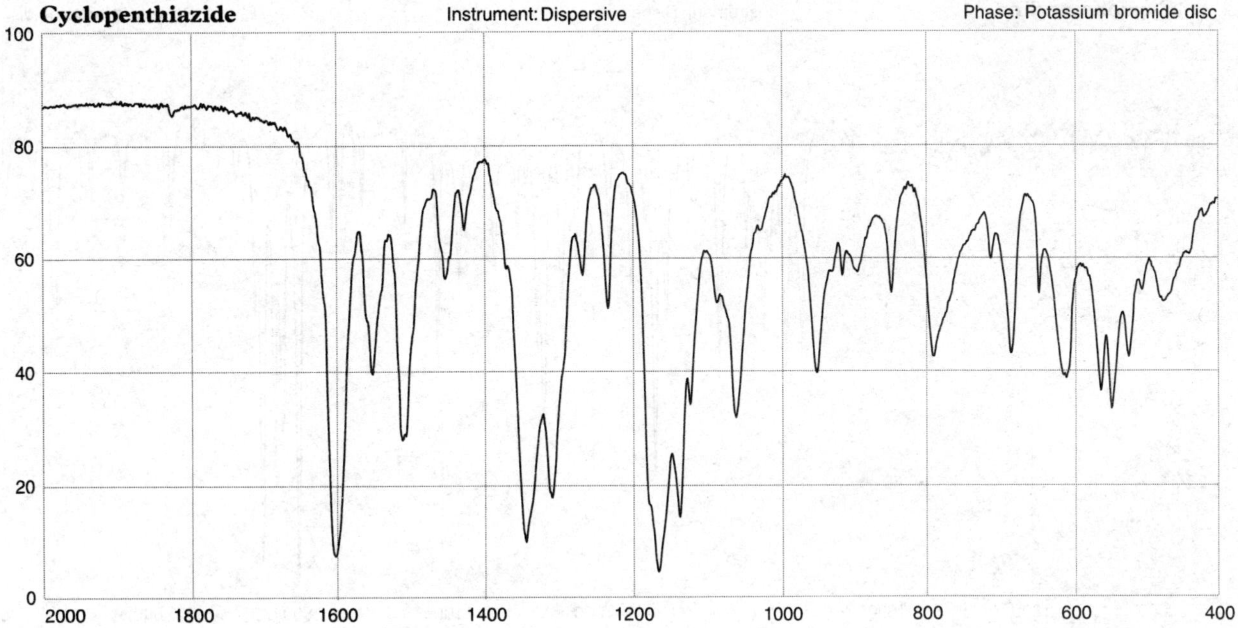

Cyclopentolate Instrument: Dispersive Phase: Thin film

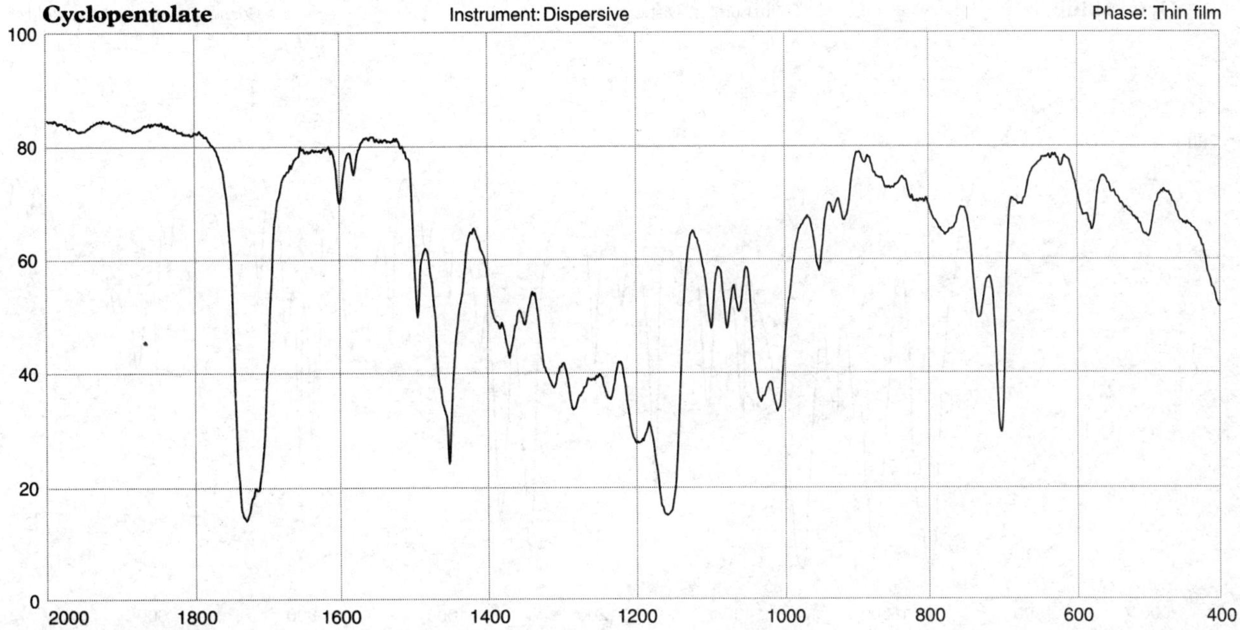

Cyclophosphamide Instrument: Dispersive Phase: 10% w/v solution in chloroform Thickness: 0.1mm

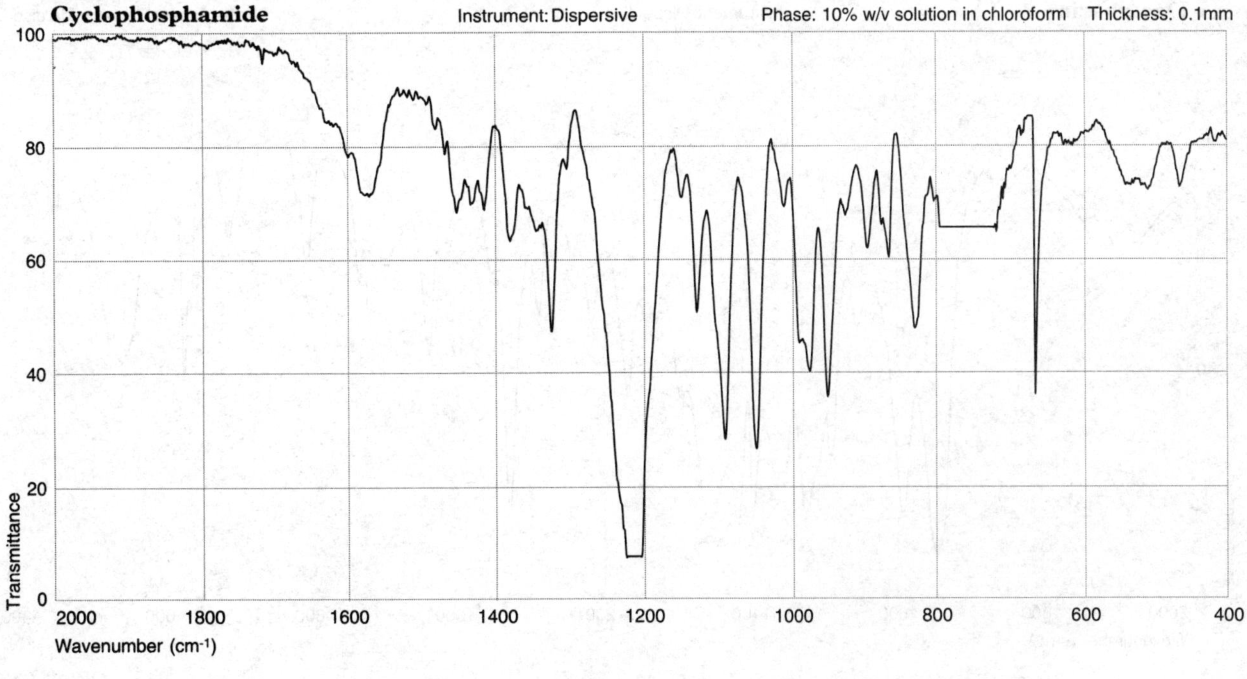

Cyproheptadine Instrument: Dispersive Phase: Potassium bromide disc

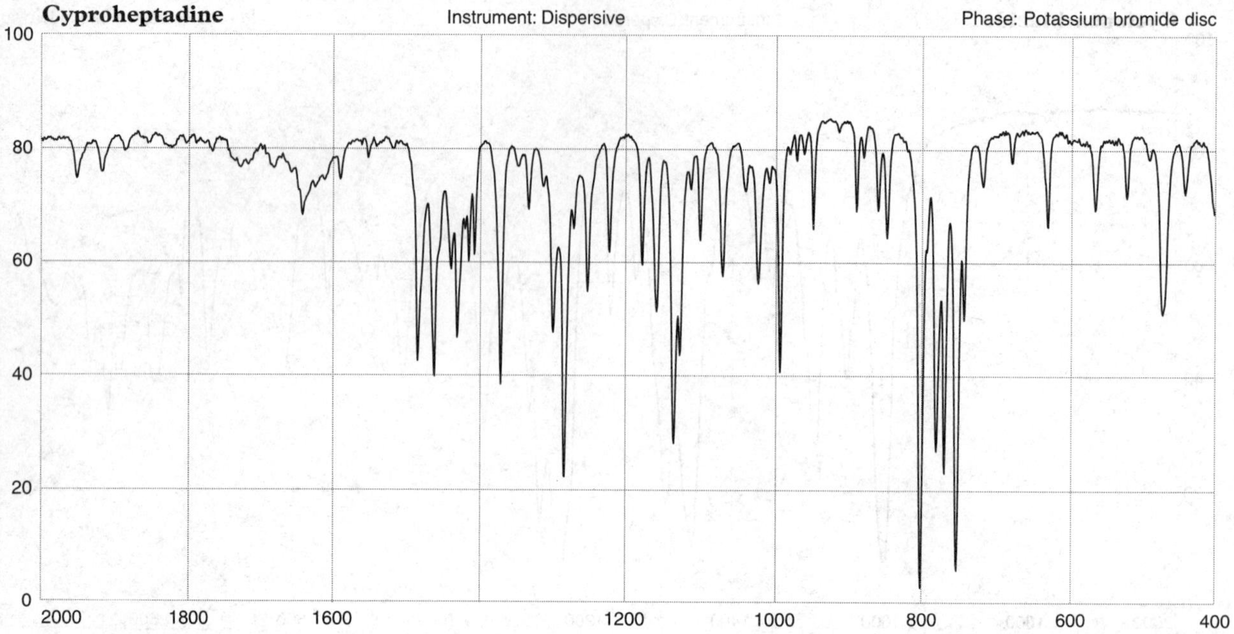

Cytarabine Instrument: Dispersive Phase: Potassium bromide disc

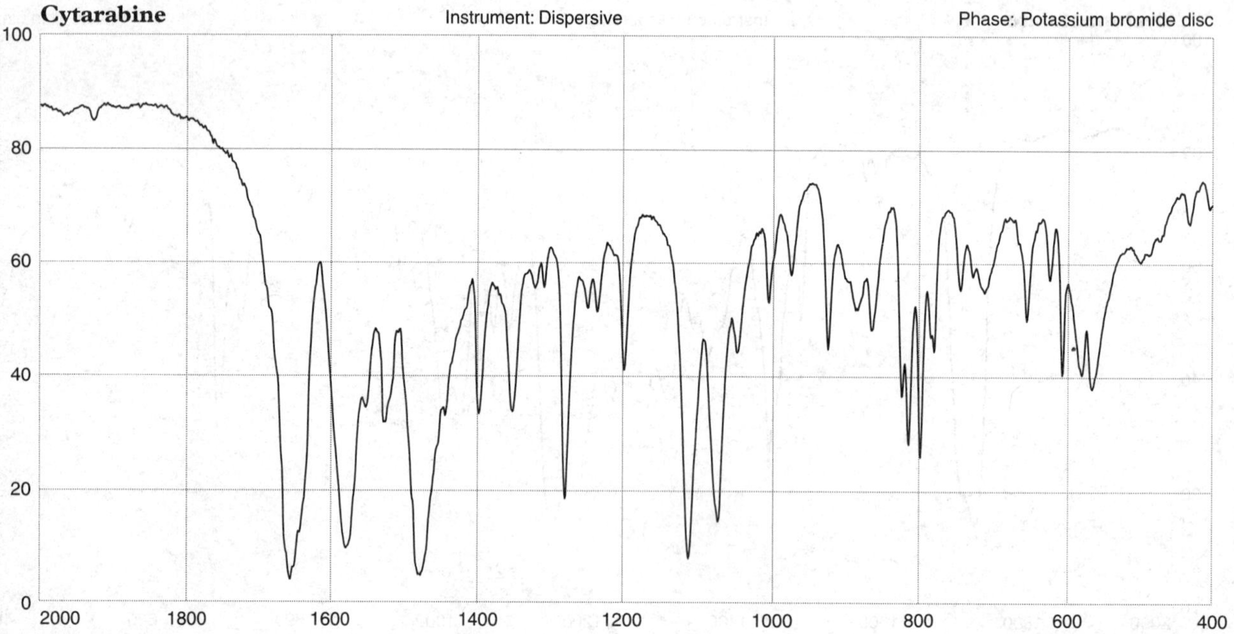

Dacarbazine Instrument: Dispersive Phase: Potassium bromide disc

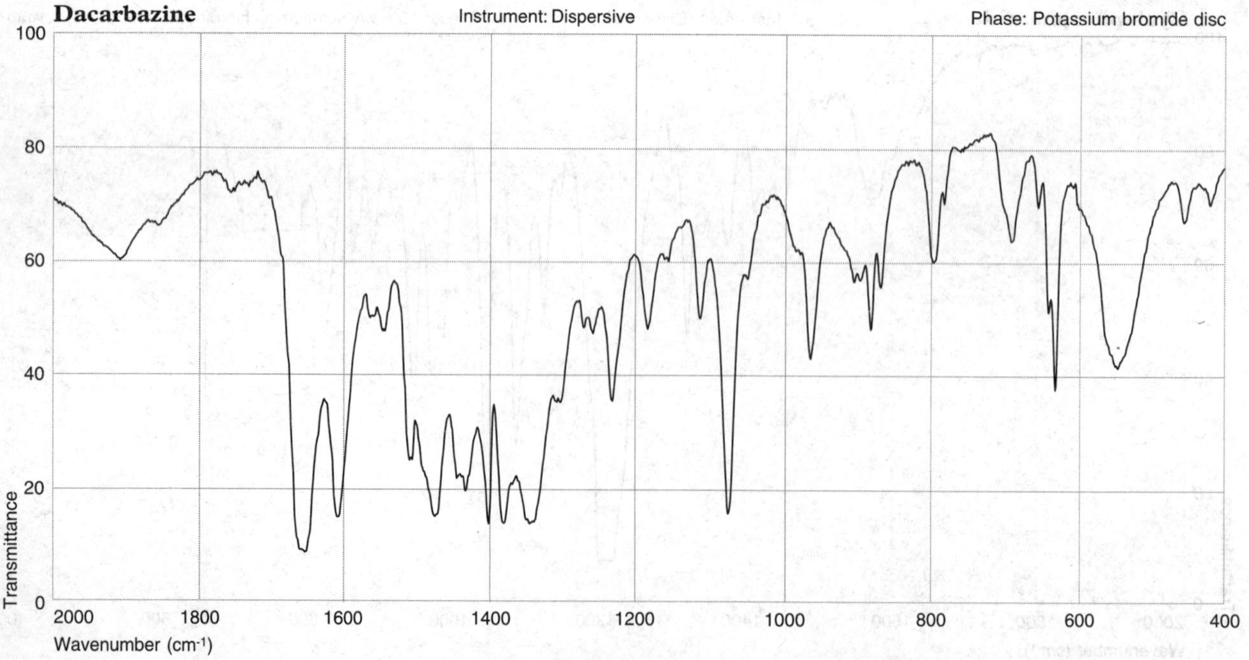

Dantron Instrument: Dispersive Phase: Potassium bromide disc

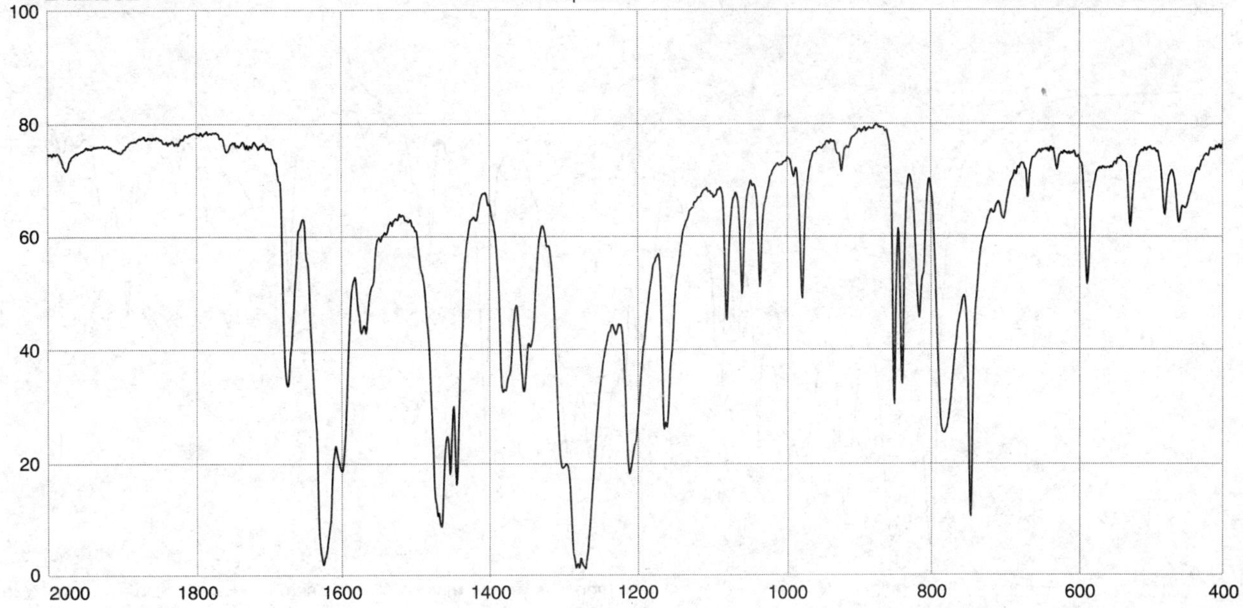

Dapsone Instrument: Dispersive Phase: Potassium bromide disc

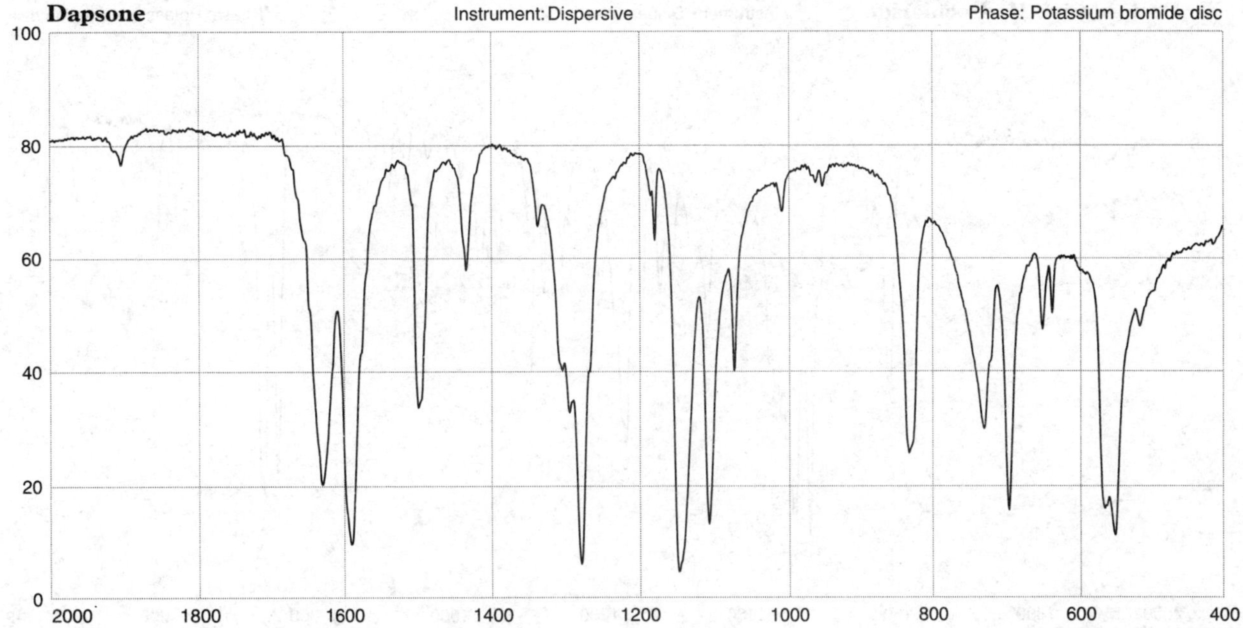

Dequalinium Chloride Instrument: Dispersive Phase: Potassium chloride disc

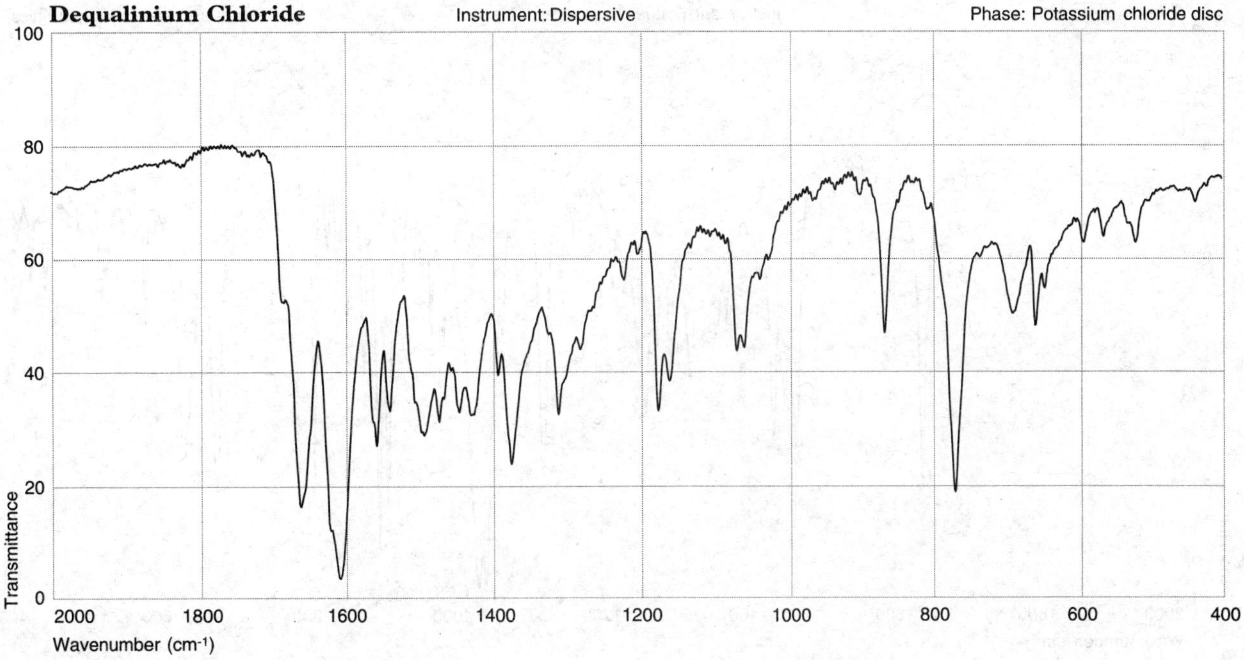

Desferrioxamine Mesilate Instrument: Dispersive Phase: Potassium bromide disc

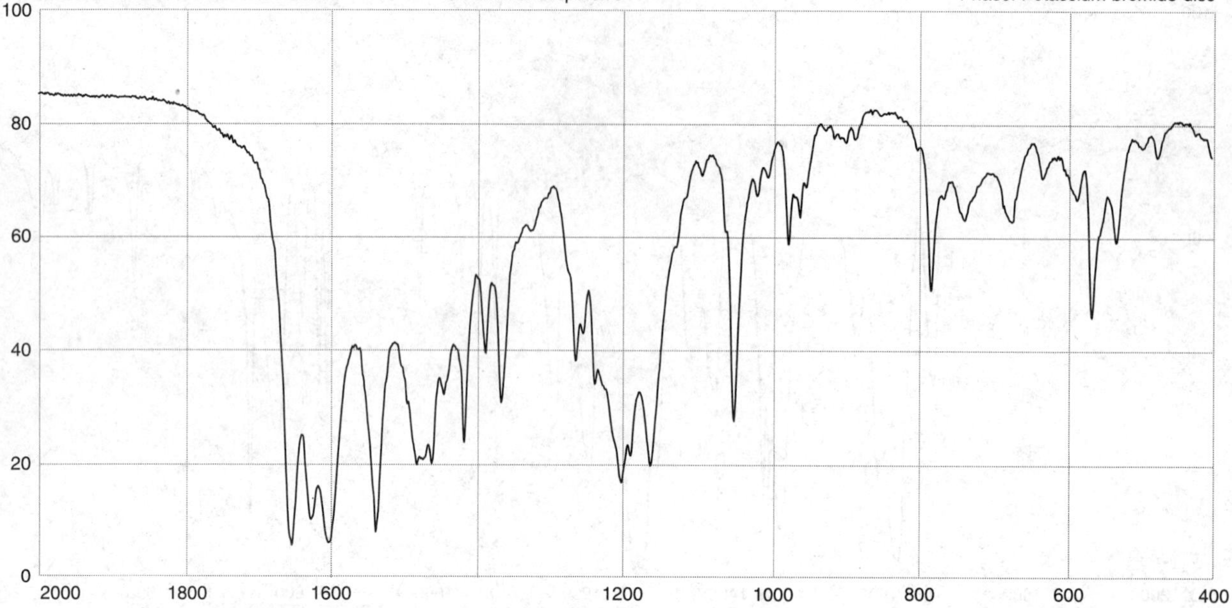

Desipramine Hydrochloride Instrument: Dispersive Phase: Potassium chloride disc

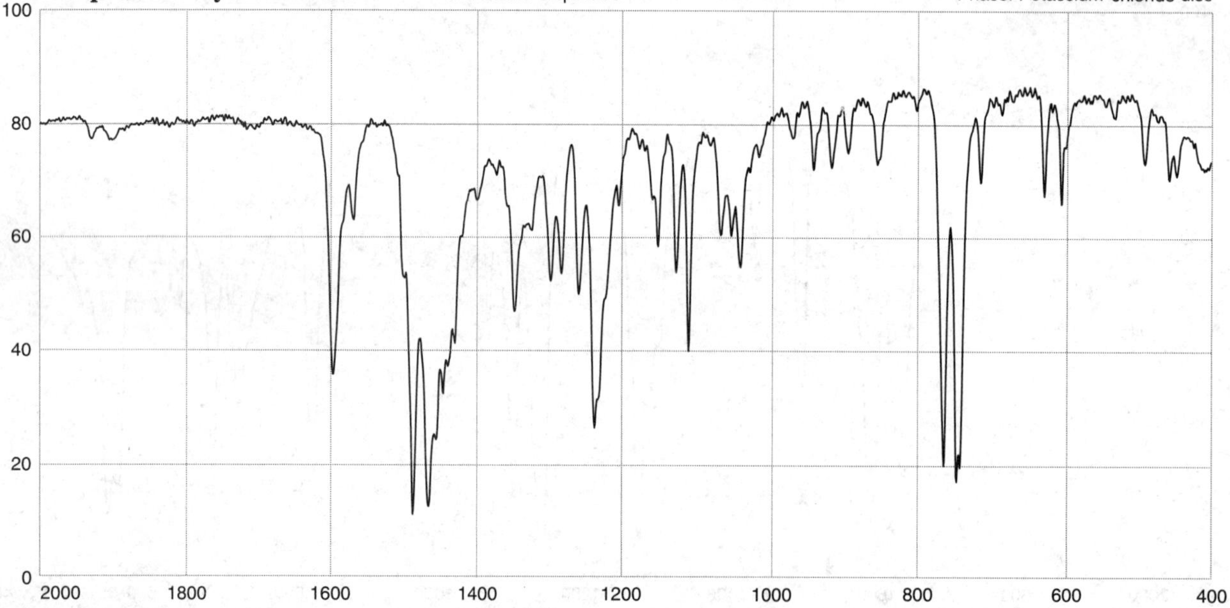

Desogestrel Instrument: Fourier transform Phase: Potassium bromide disc

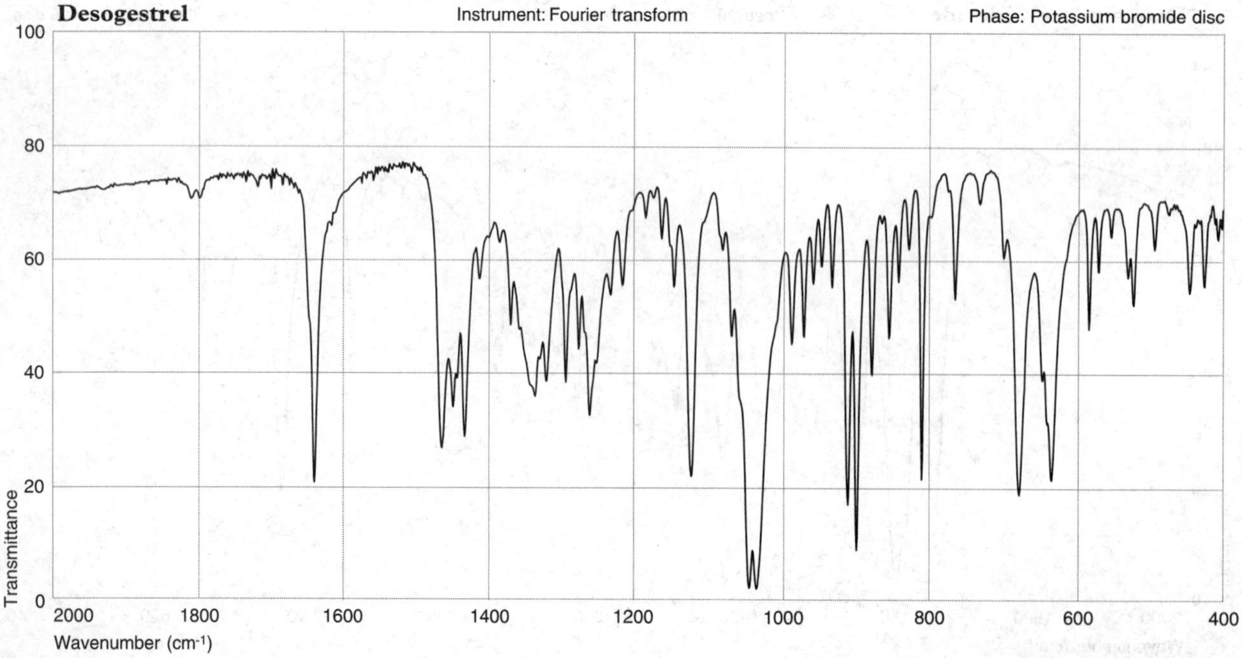

Dexamethasone Instrument: Dispersive Phase: Potassium bromide disc

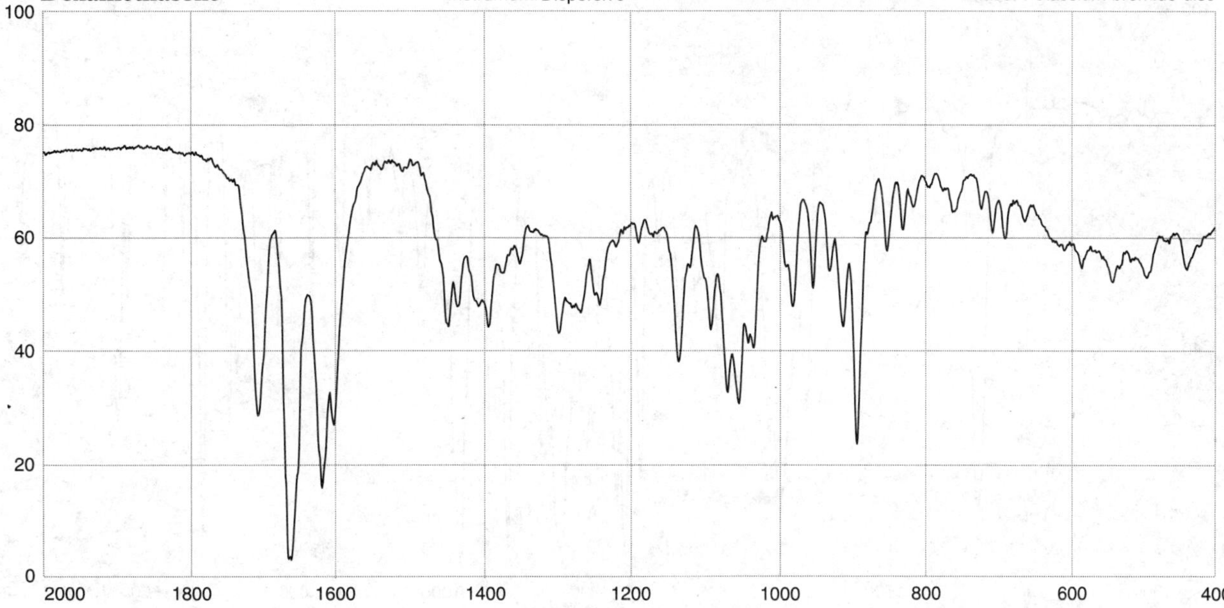

Dextromoramide Instrument: Dispersive Phase: Potassium bromide disc

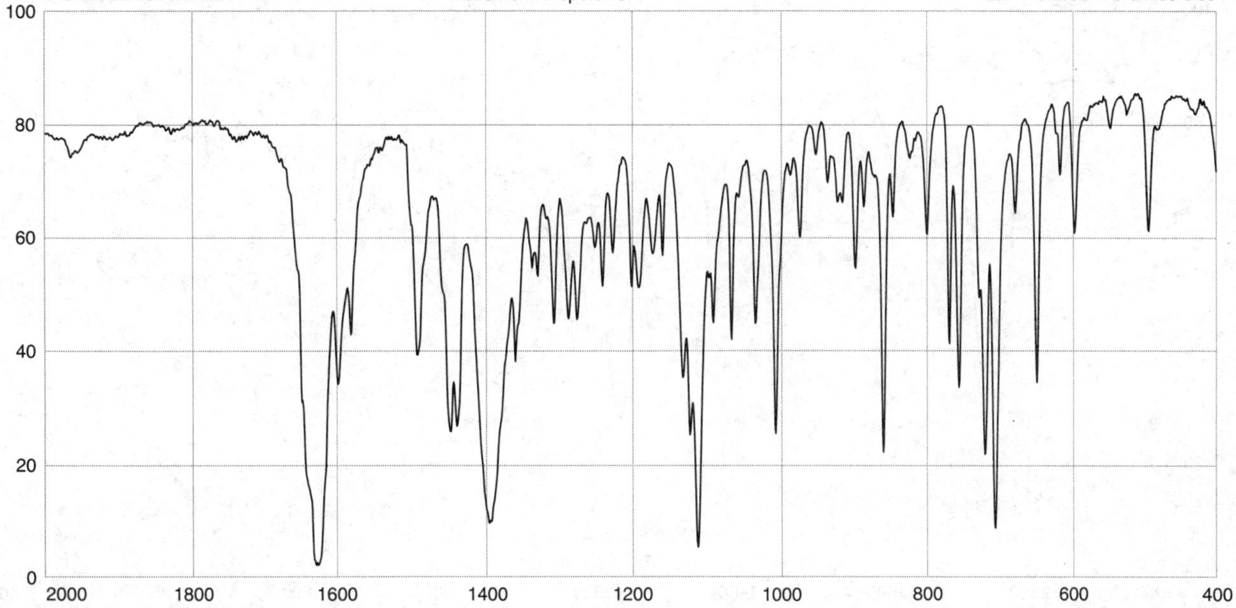

Dextropropoxyphene Instrument: Dispersive Phase: Thin film

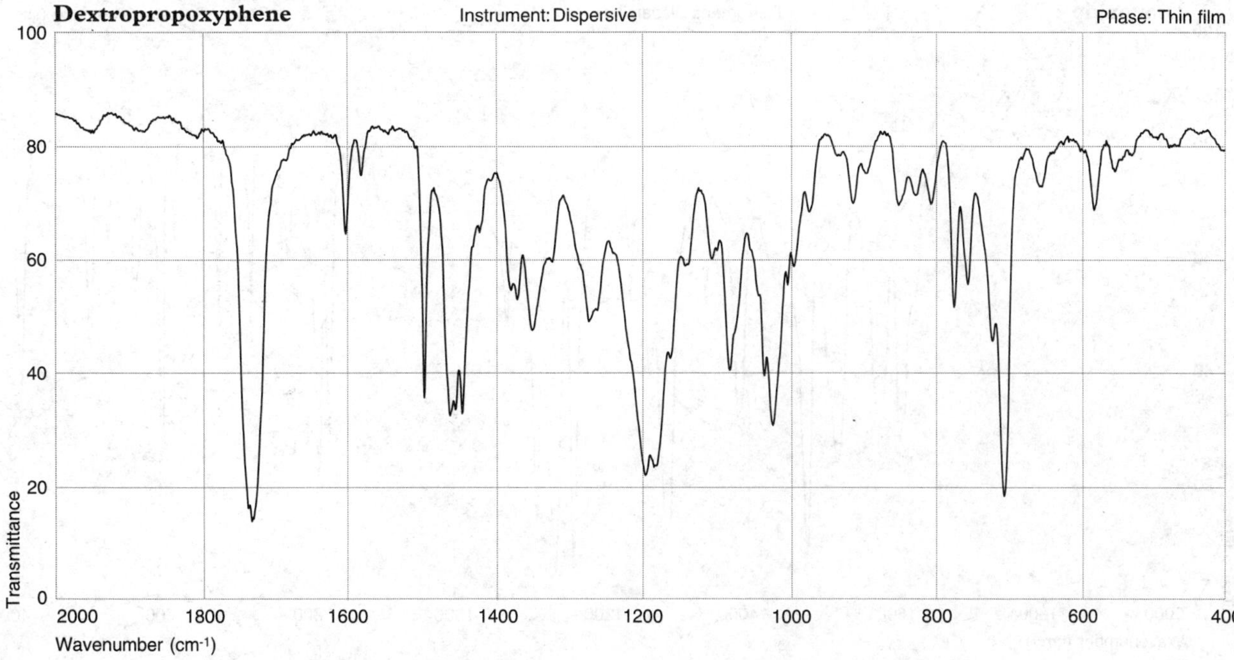

Dextropropoxyphene Napsilate Instrument: Dispersive Phase: Liquid paraffin mull

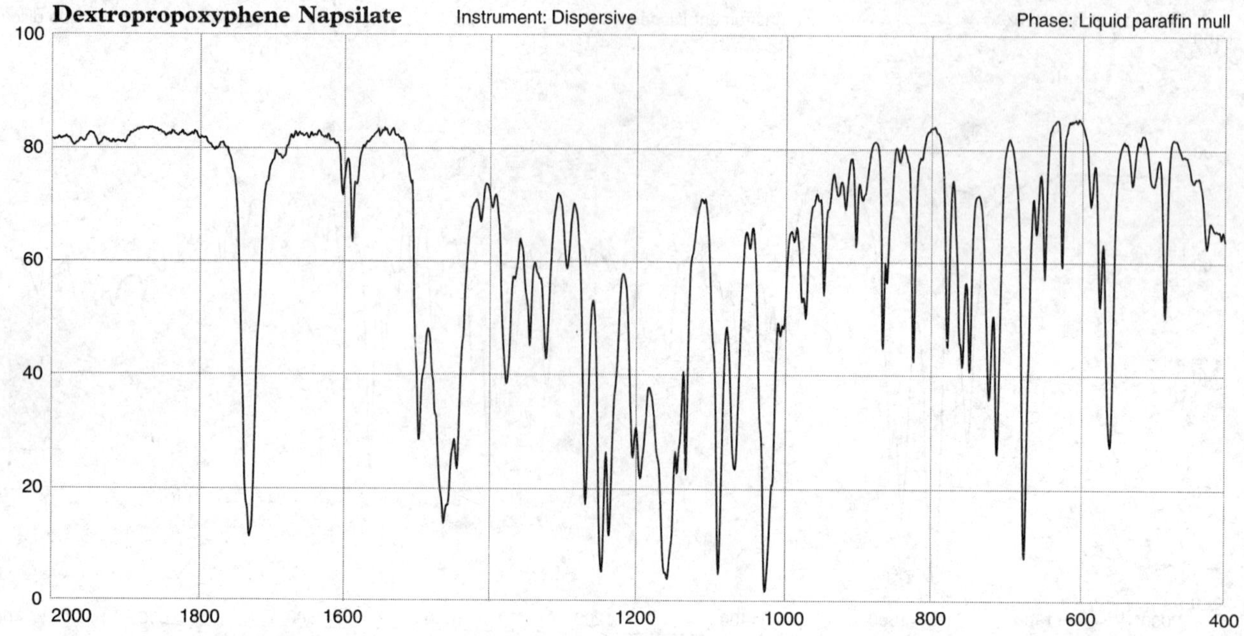

Diamorphine Hydrochloride Instrument: Dispersive Phase: Potassium chloride disc

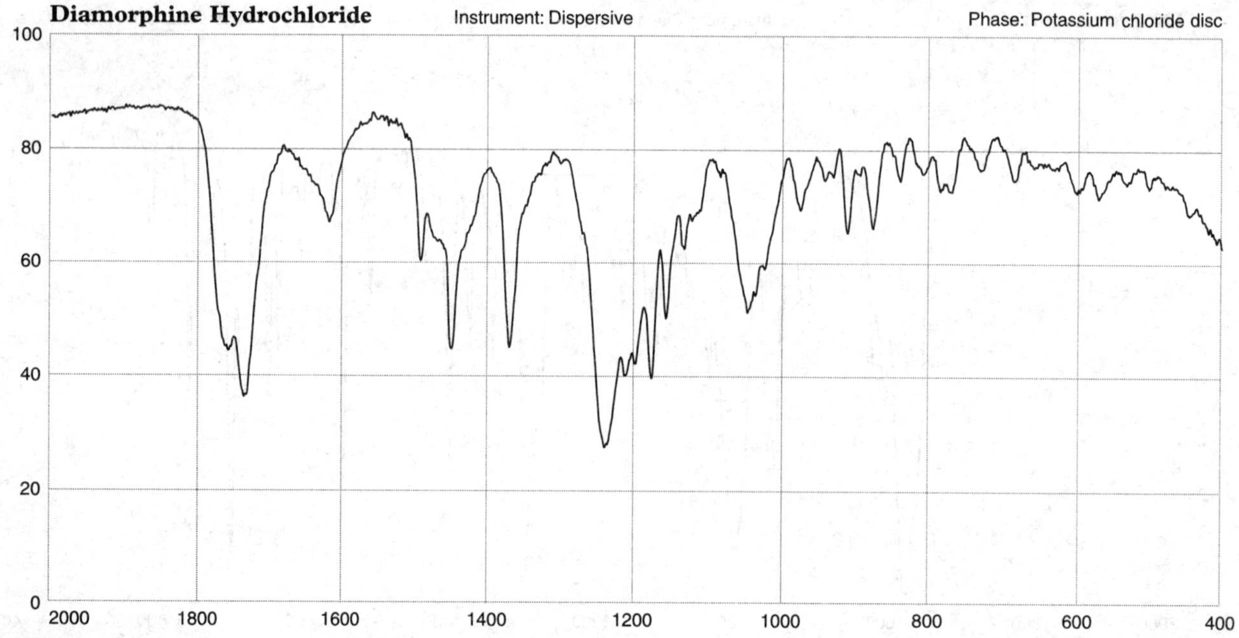

Diazoxide Instrument: Dispersive Phase: Potassium bromide disc

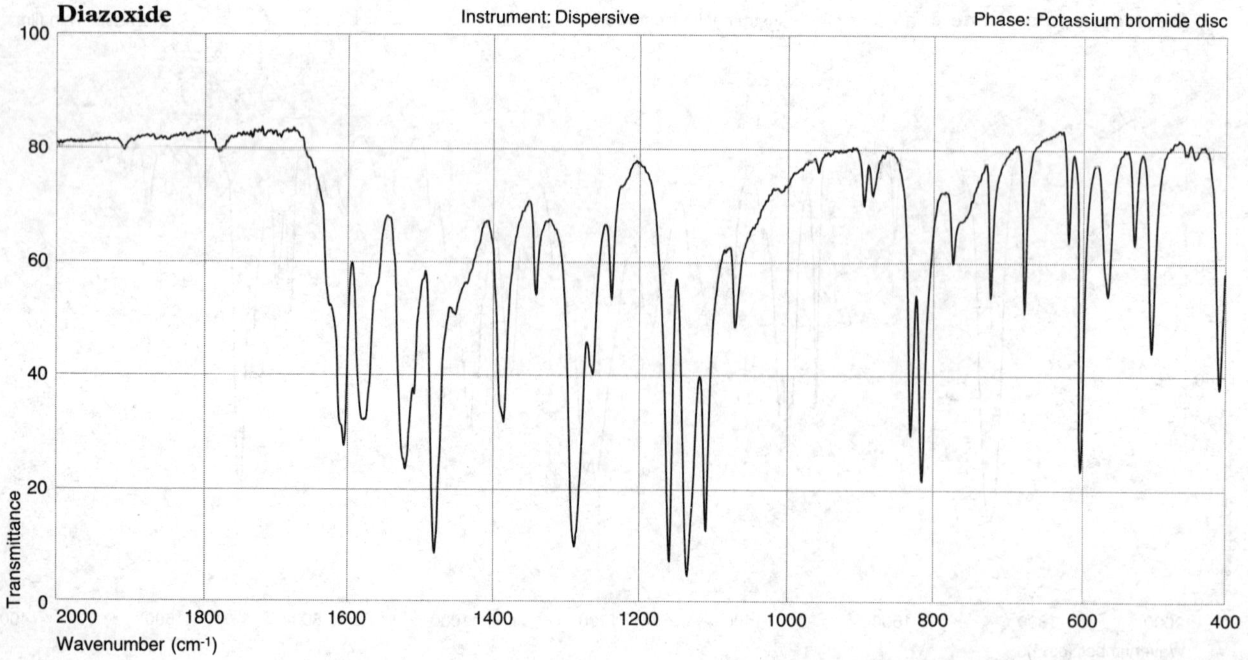

Dibromopropamidine Isetionate Instrument: Dispersive Phase: Potassium bromide disc

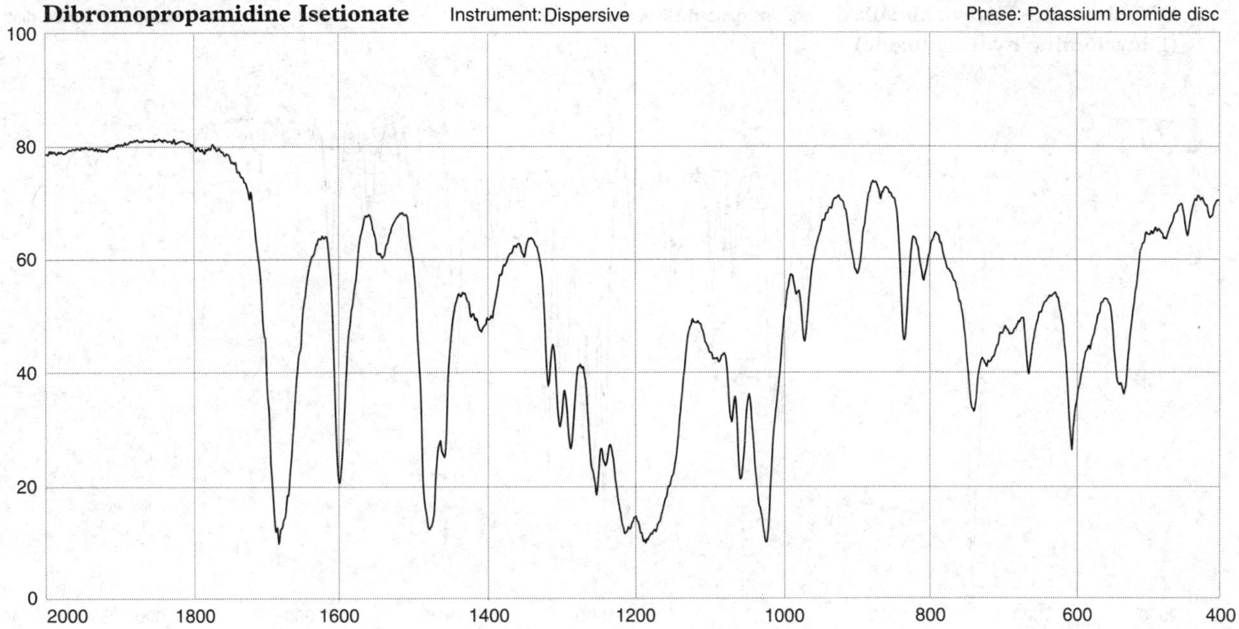

Diclofenac Instrument: Fourier transform Phase: Potassium bromide disc

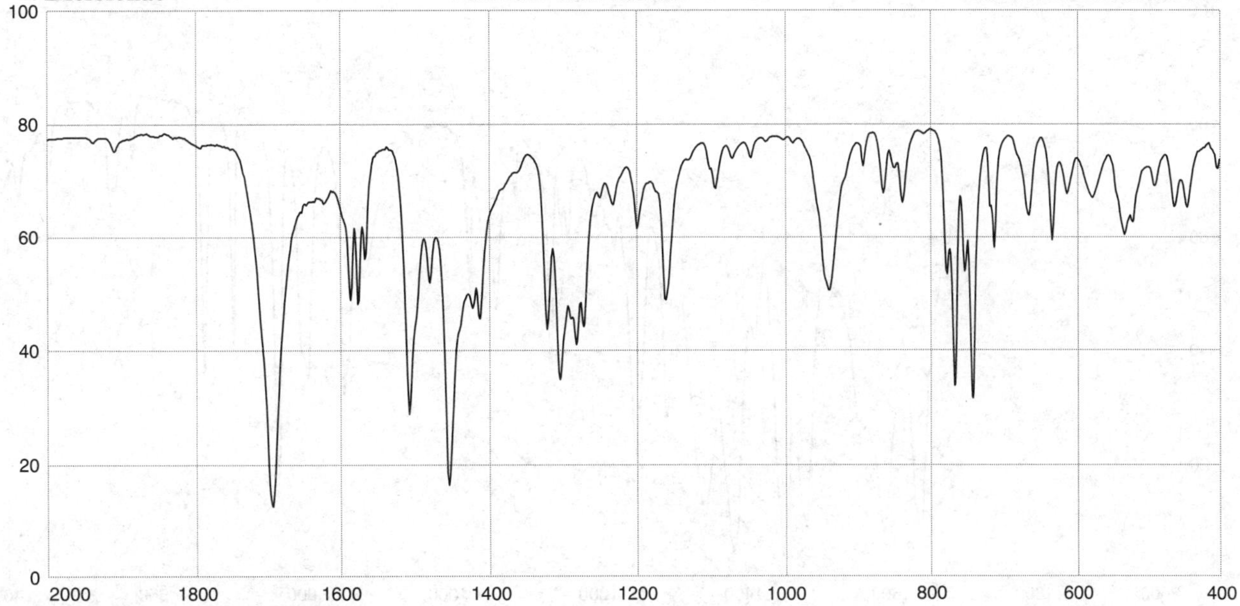

Dicyclomine Hydrochloride (Dicycloverine Hydrochloride) Instrument: Dispersive Phase: Potassium chloride disc

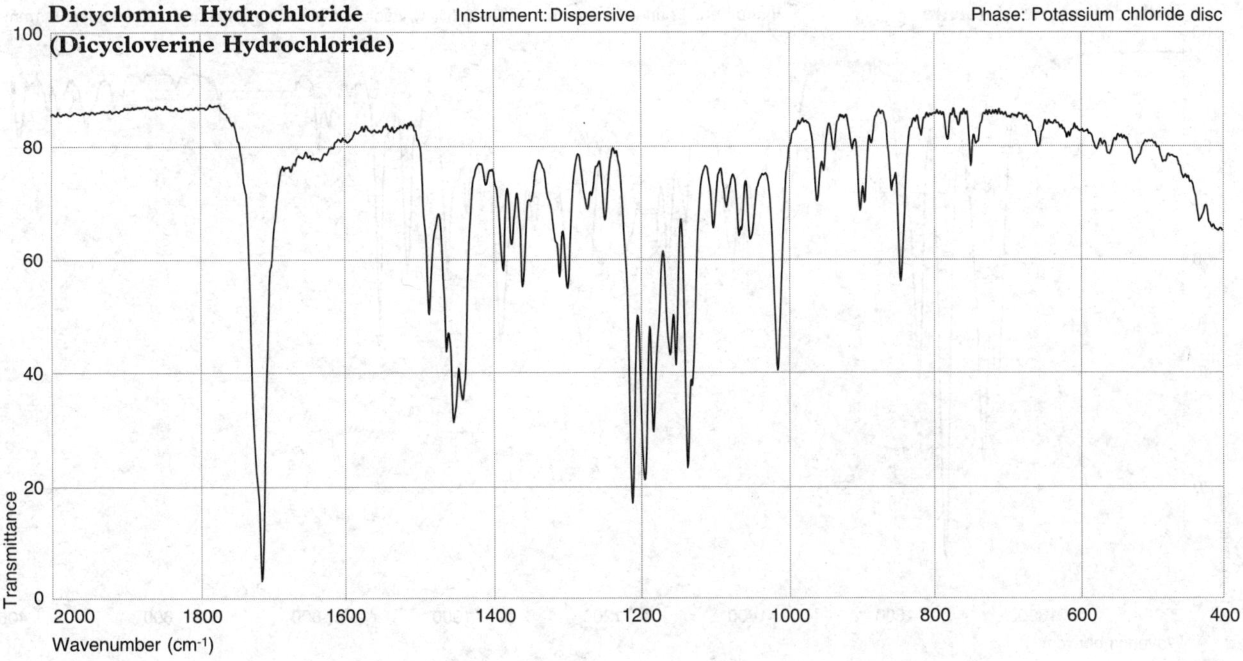

Dicycloverine Hydrochloride (Dicyclomine hydrochloride)

Instrument: Dispersive Phase: Potassium chloride disc

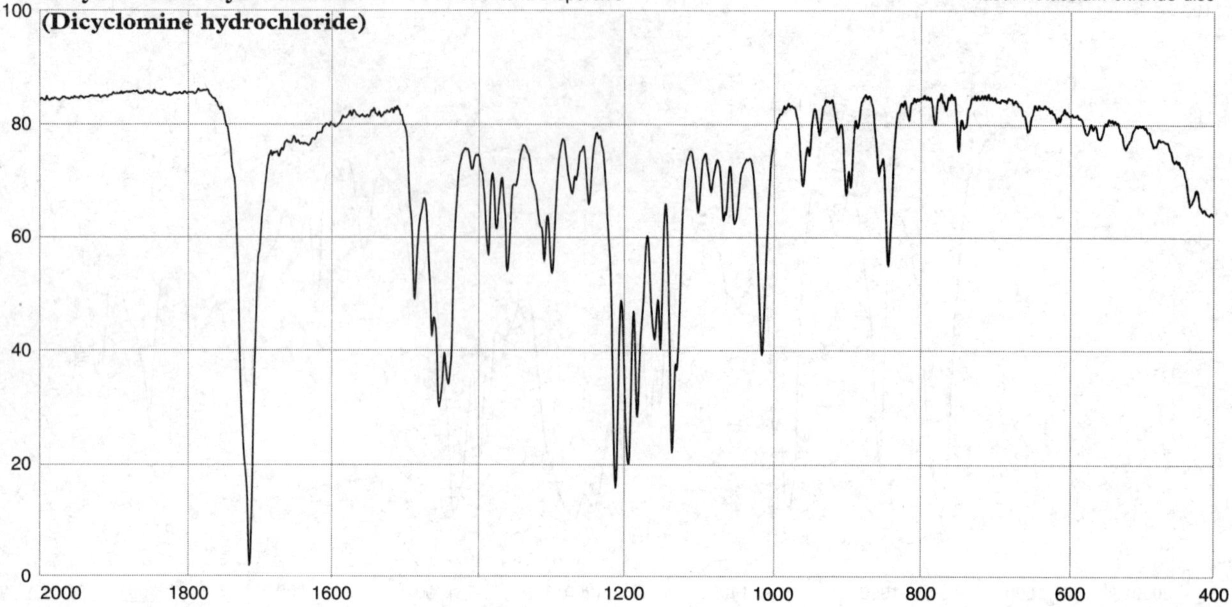

Diethylamine Salicylate

Instrument: Dispersive Phase: Potassium bromide disc

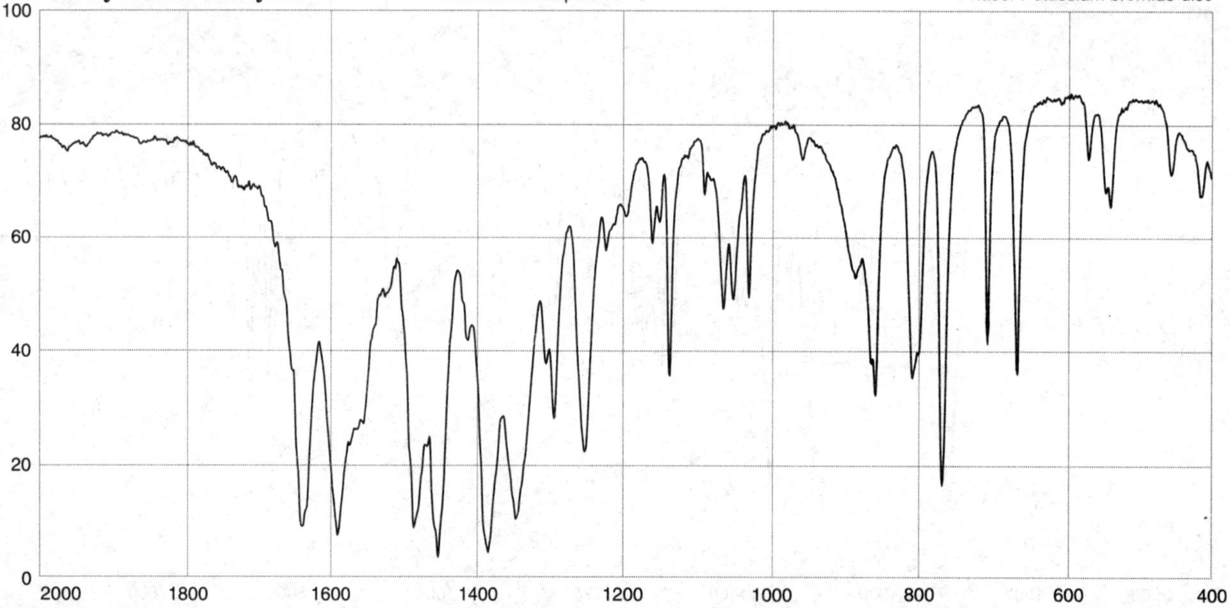

Diflucortolone Valerate

Instrument: Fourier transform Phase: 5% w/v solution in dichloromethane Thickness: 0.1mm

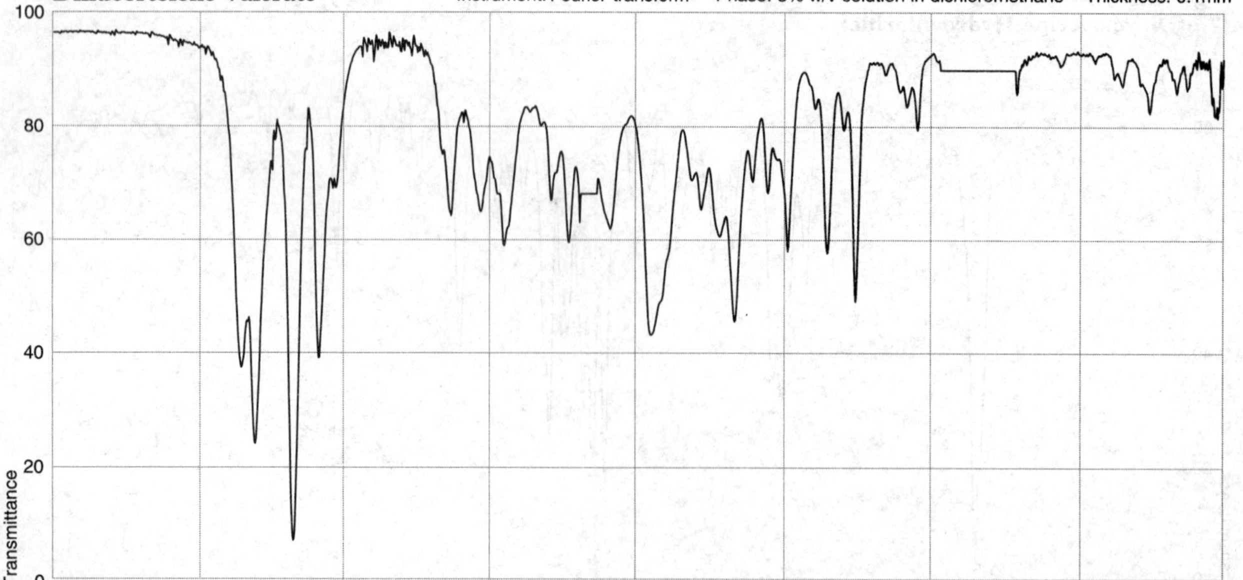

Diflunisal (form B) Instrument: Dispersive Phase: Potassium bromide disc

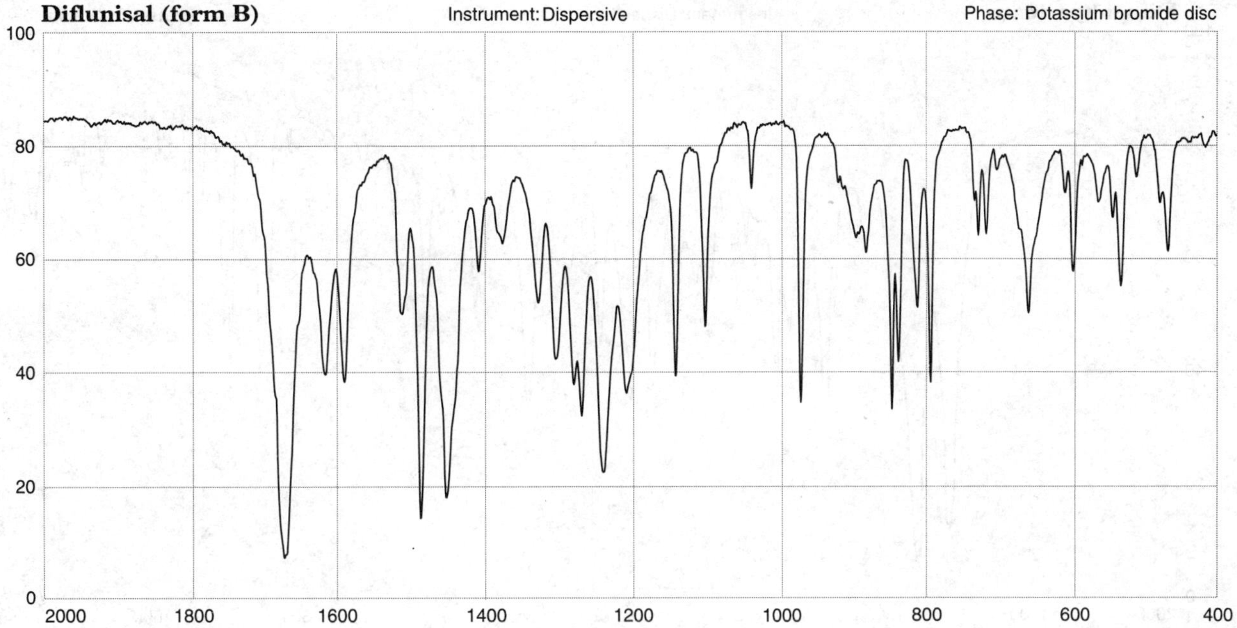

Dihydrocodeine Instrument: Dispersive Phase: Thin film

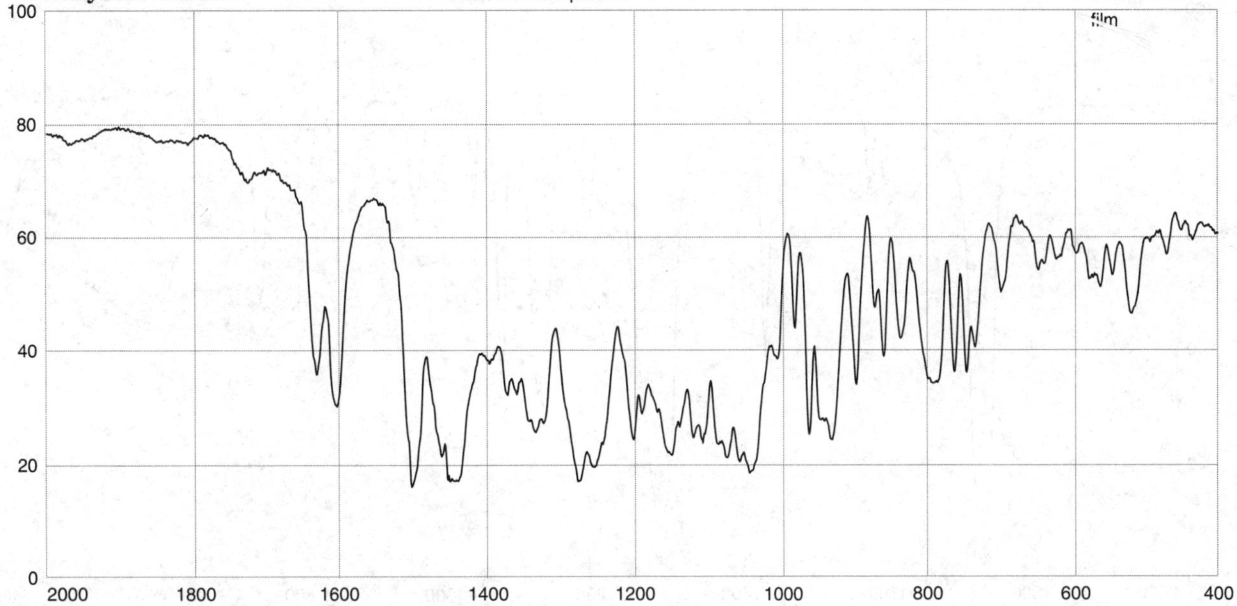

Diloxanide Furoate Instrument: Dispersive Phase: Potassium bromide disc

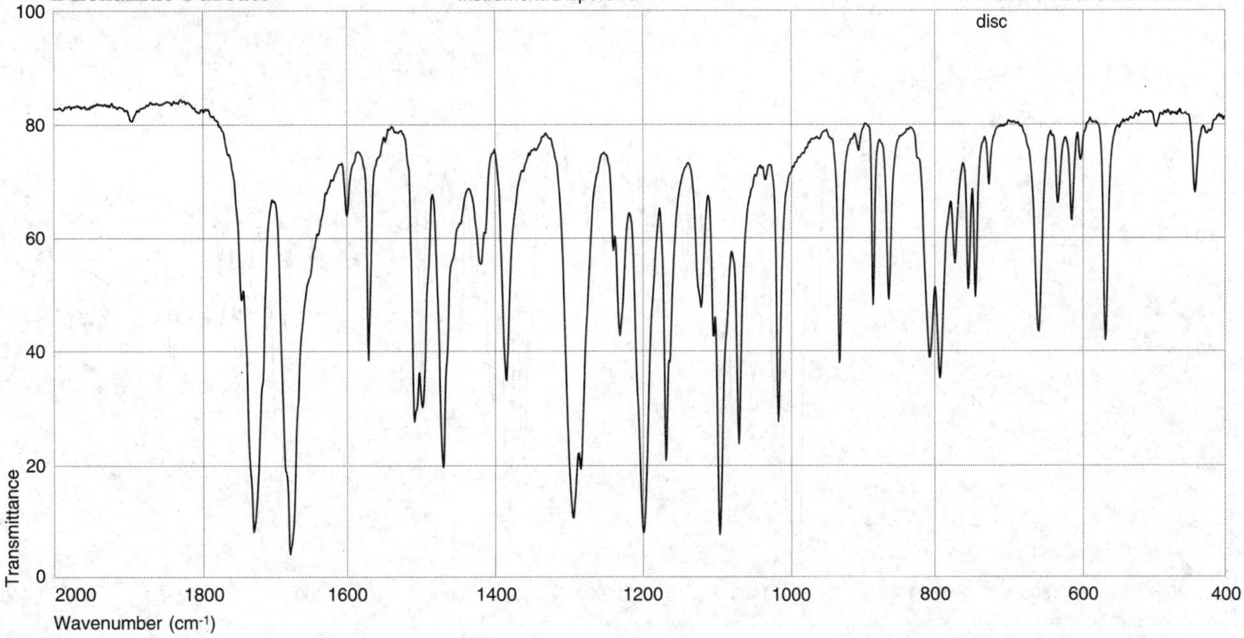

Dimenhydrinate

Instrument: Dispersive

Phase: Potassium bromide disc

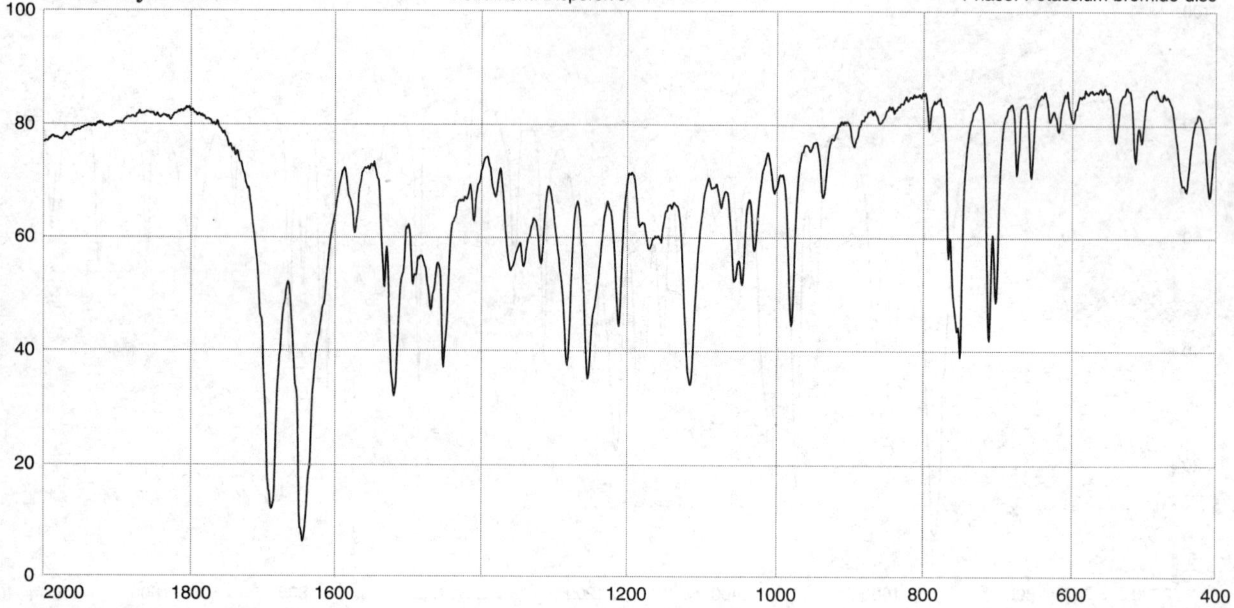

Dimethyl Phthalate

Instrument: Dispersive

Phase: Thin film

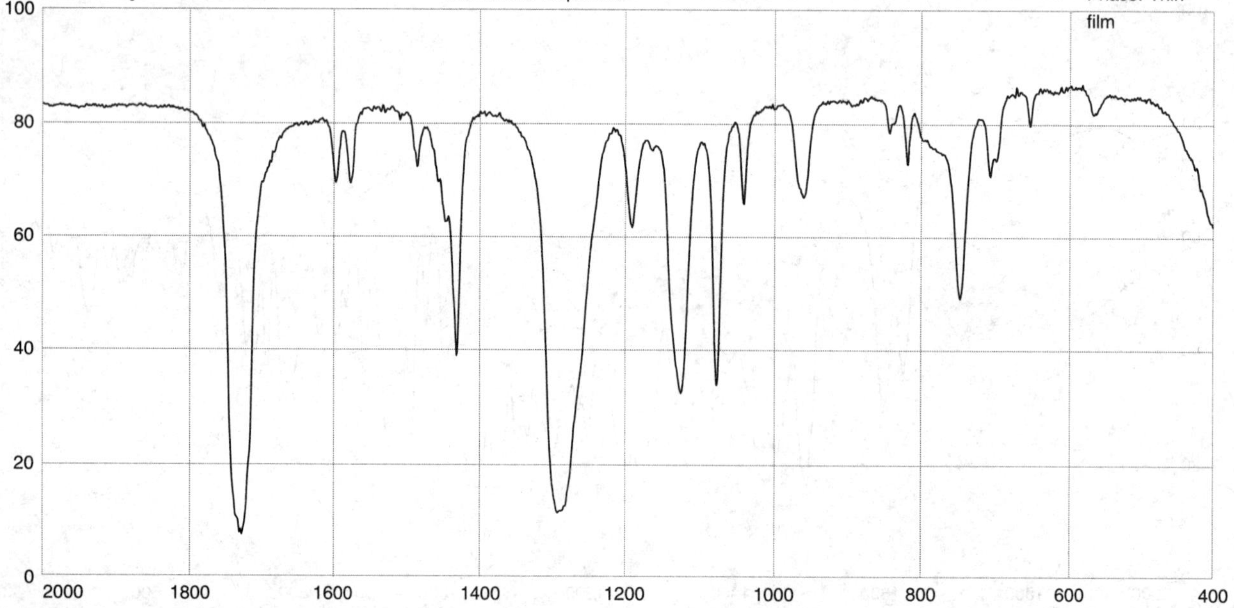

Diphenylpyraline Hydrochloride

Instrument: Dispersive

Phase: Liquid paraffin mull

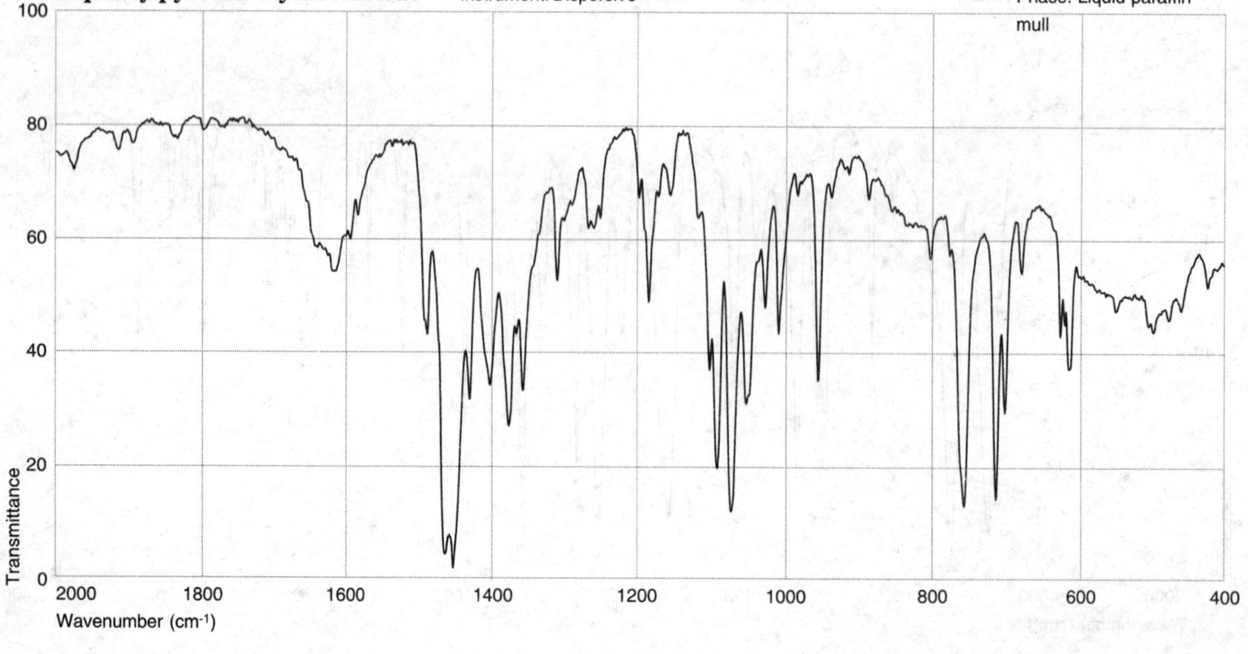

Dipipanone Instrument: Dispersive Phase: Thin film

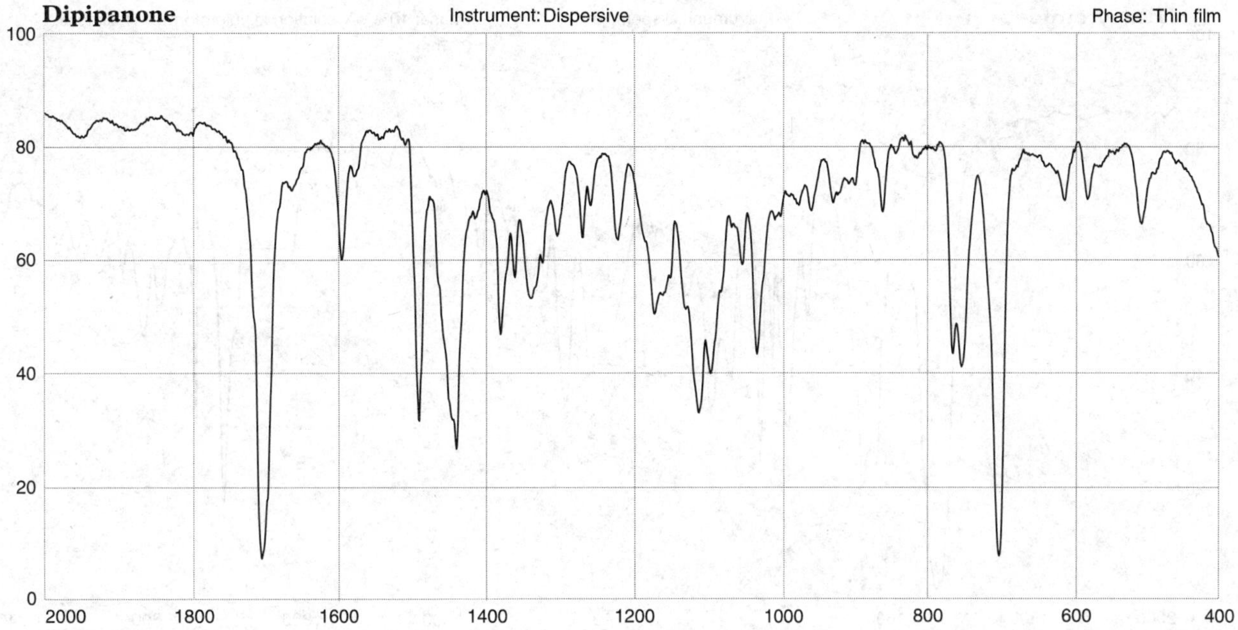

Dipyridamole Instrument: Dispersive Phase: Potassium bromide disc

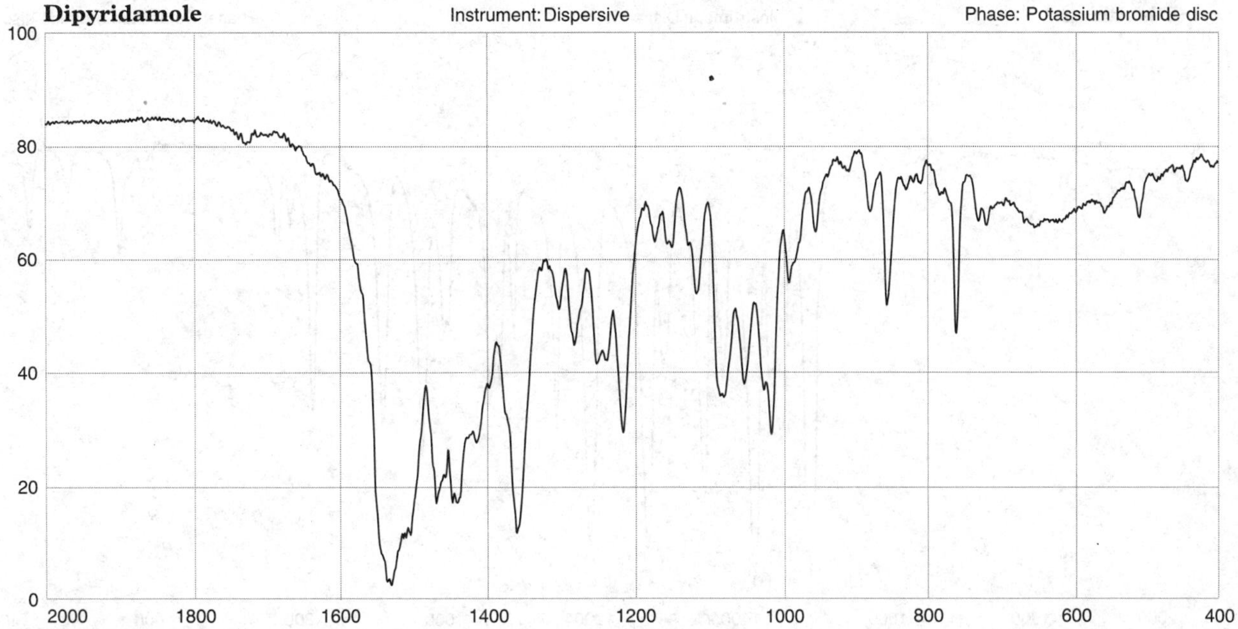

Disodium Pamidronate Instrument: Fourier transform Phase: Potassium bromide disc

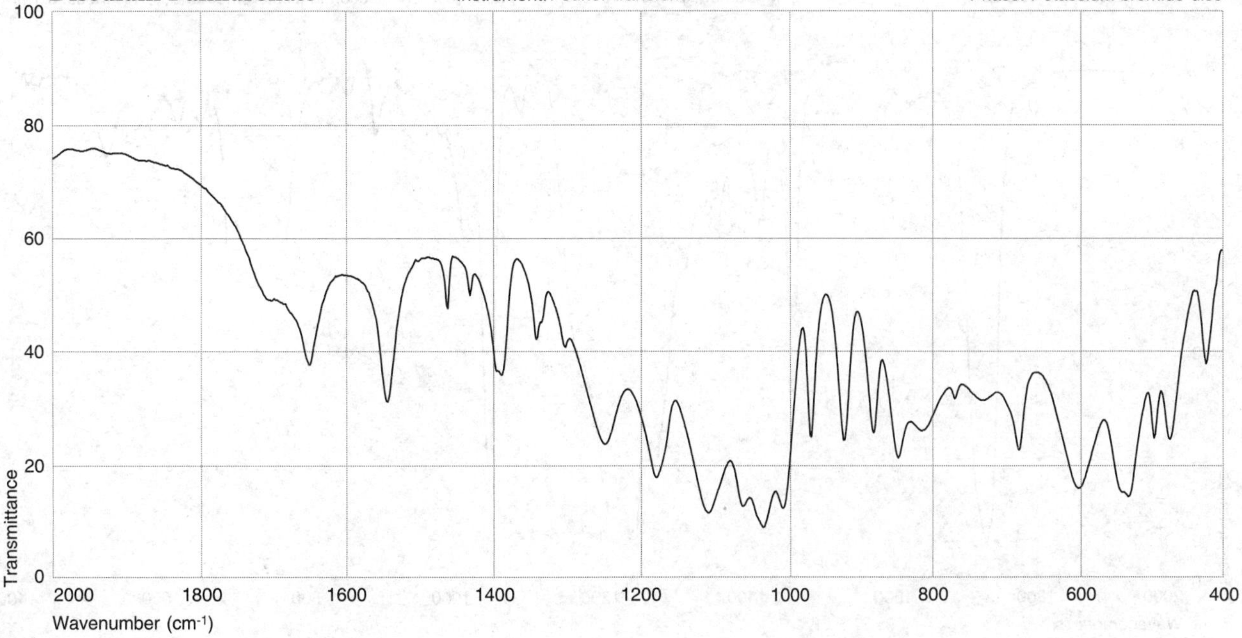

Disopyramide

Instrument: Dispersive Phase: 10% w/v solution in chloroform Thickness: 0.1mm

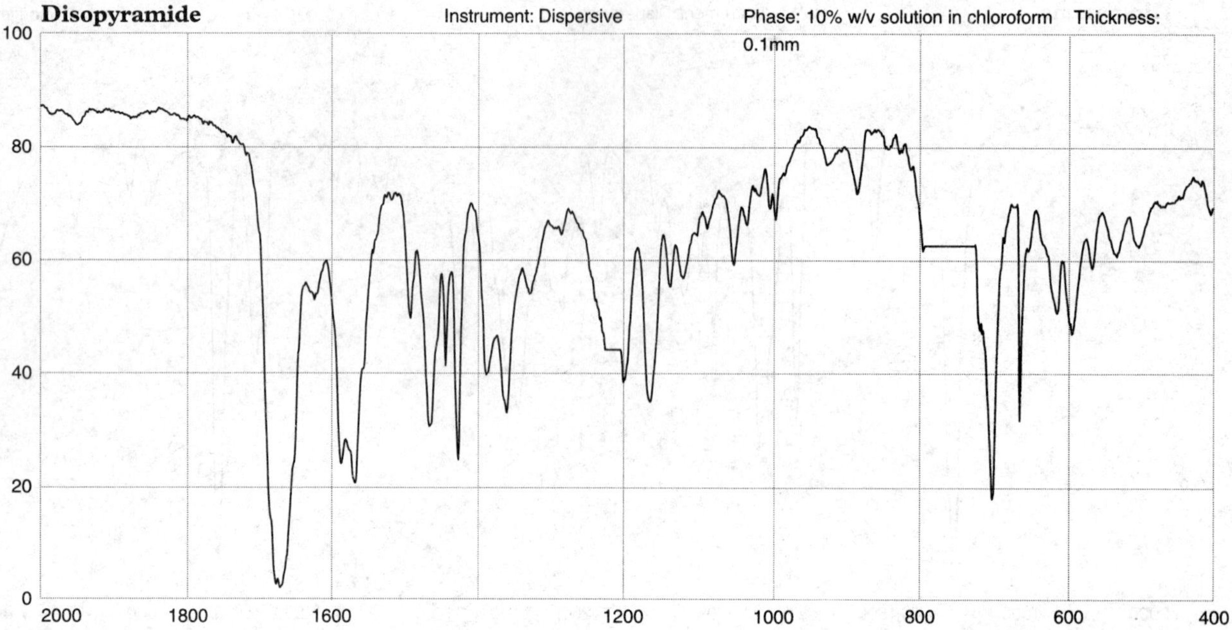

Disulfiram

Instrument: Dispersive Phase: Potassium bromide disc

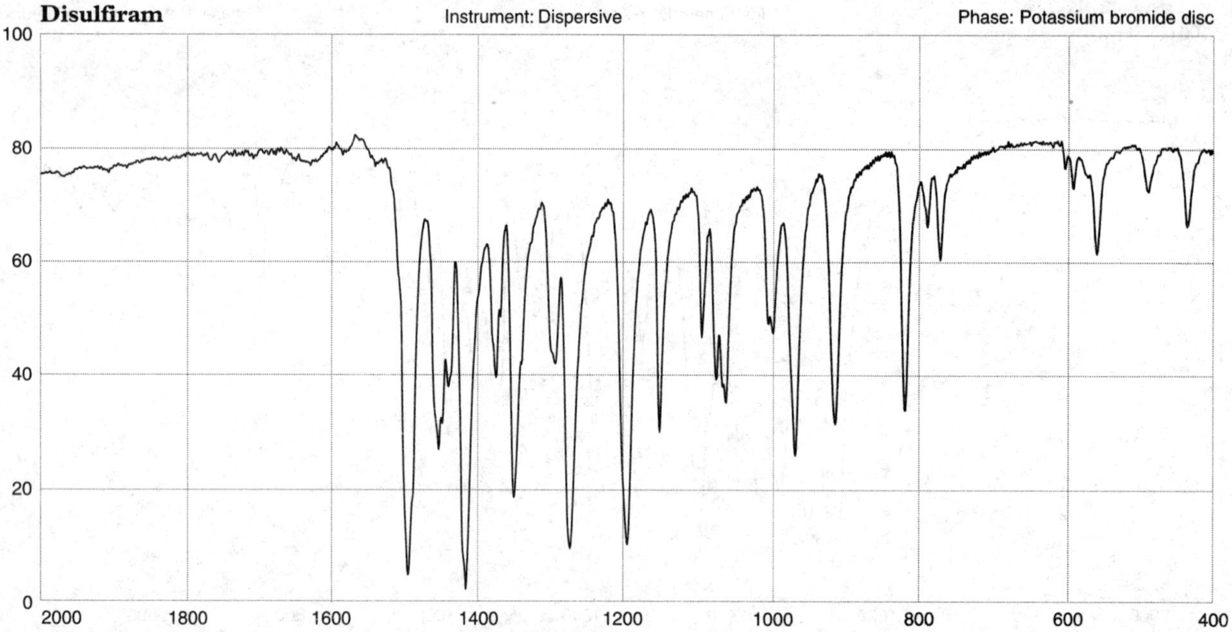

Docusate Sodium

Instrument: Dispersive Phase: 10% w/v solution in dichloromethane Thickness: 0.1mm

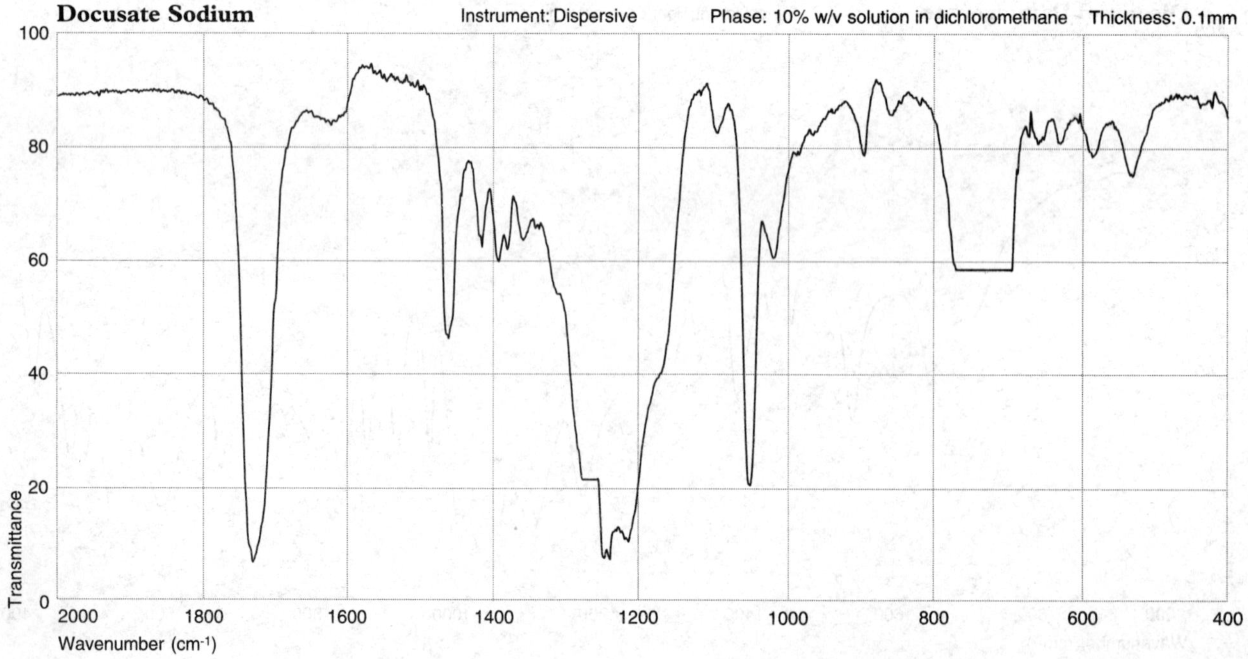

Dopamine Hydrochloride

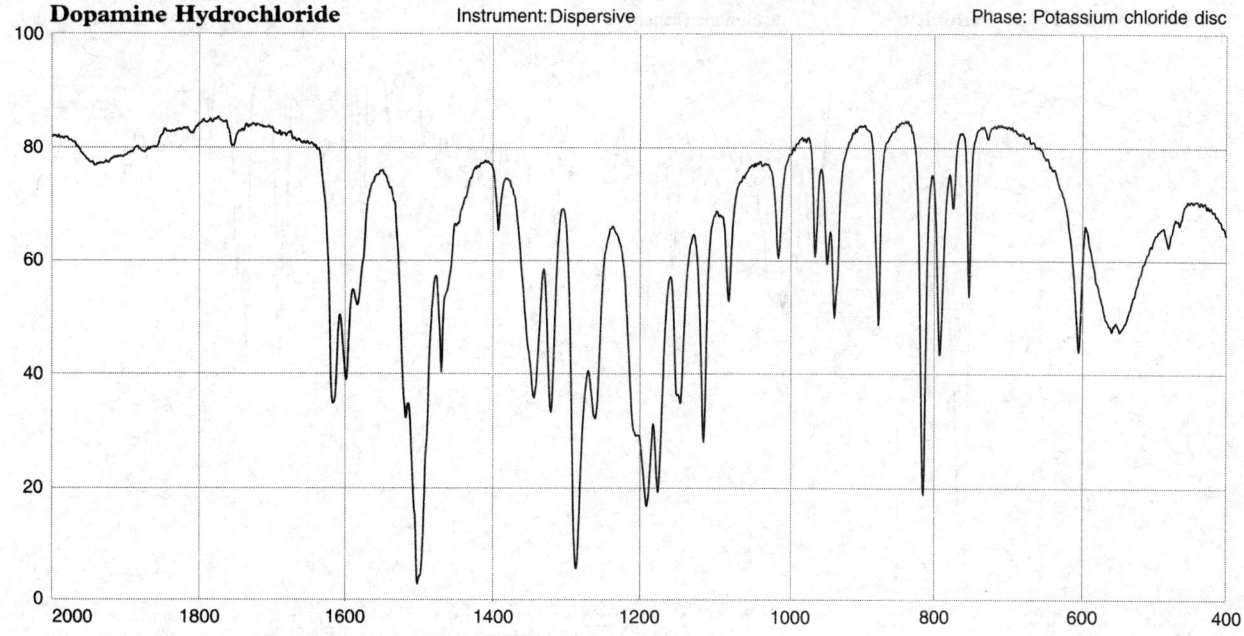

Dosulepin Hydrochloride (Dothiepin Hydrochloride)

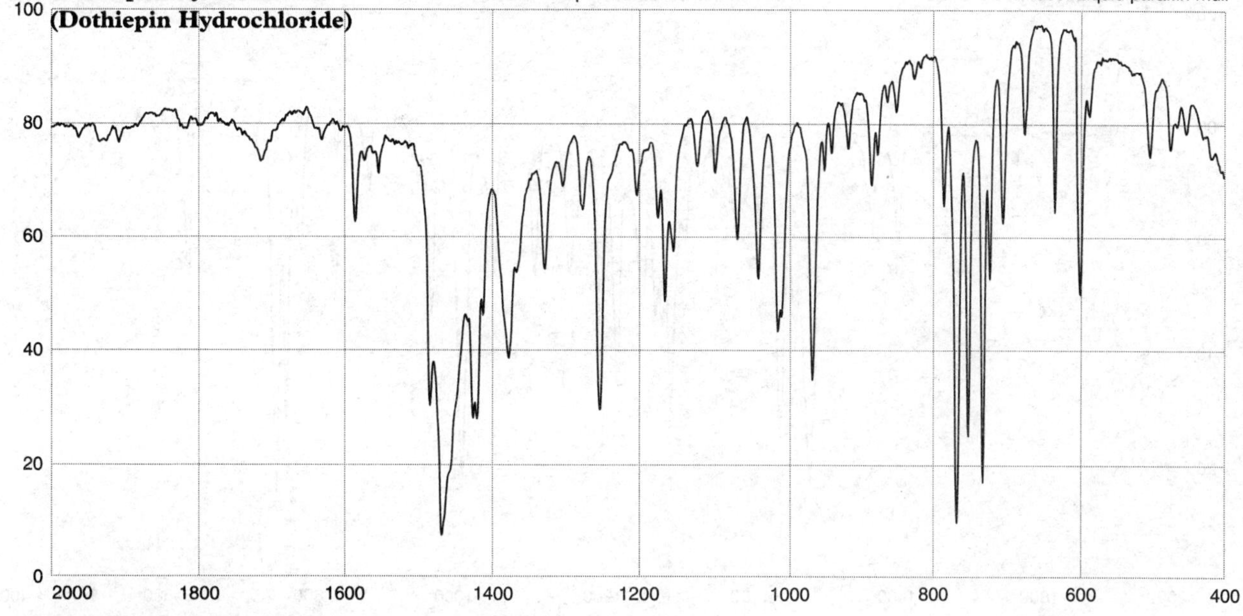

Dothiepin Hydrochloride (Dosulepin Hydrochloride)

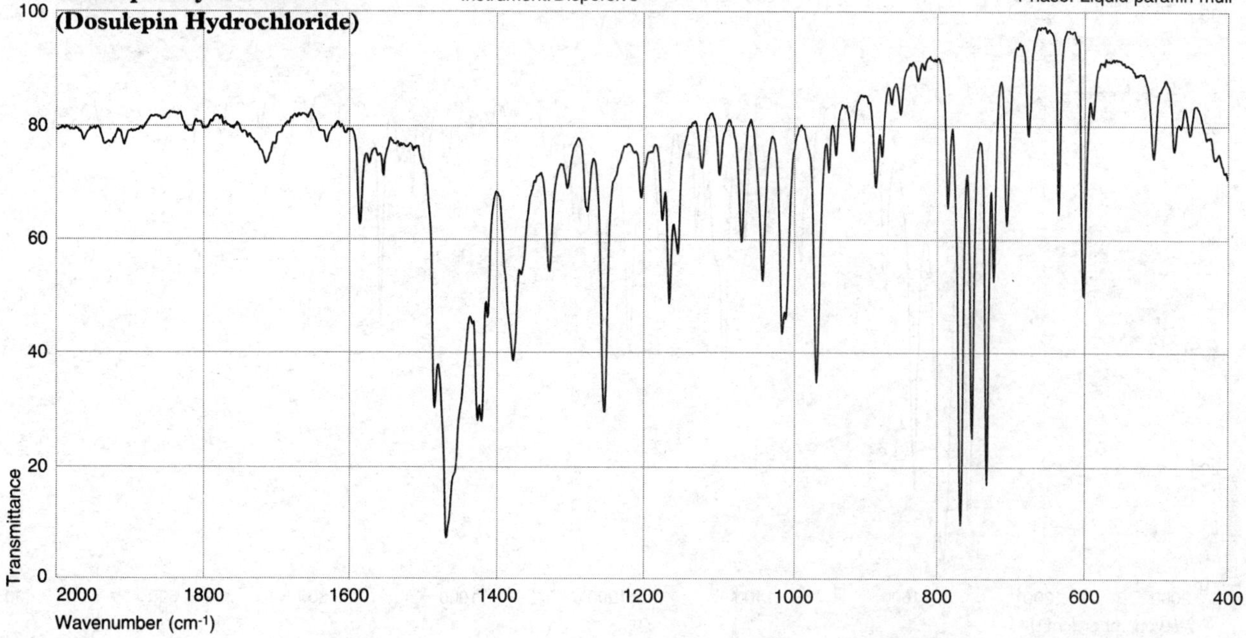

Doxapram Hydrochloride Instrument: Dispersive Phase: Potassium chloride disc

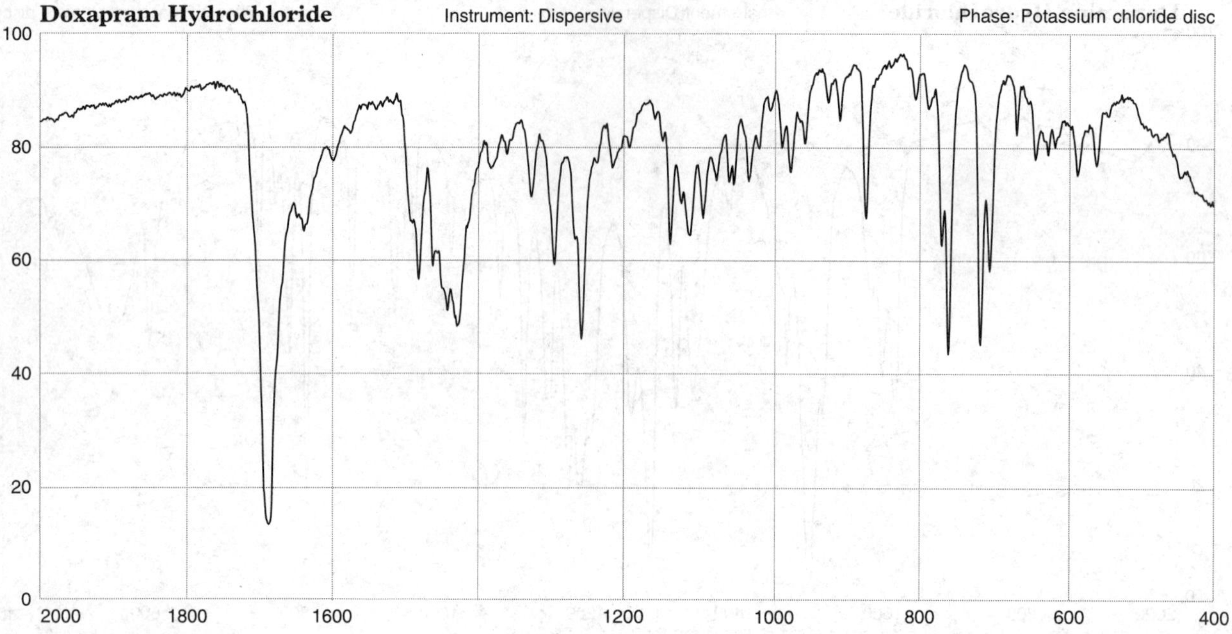

Doxepin Hydrochloride Instrument: Dispersive Phase: Potassium chloride disc

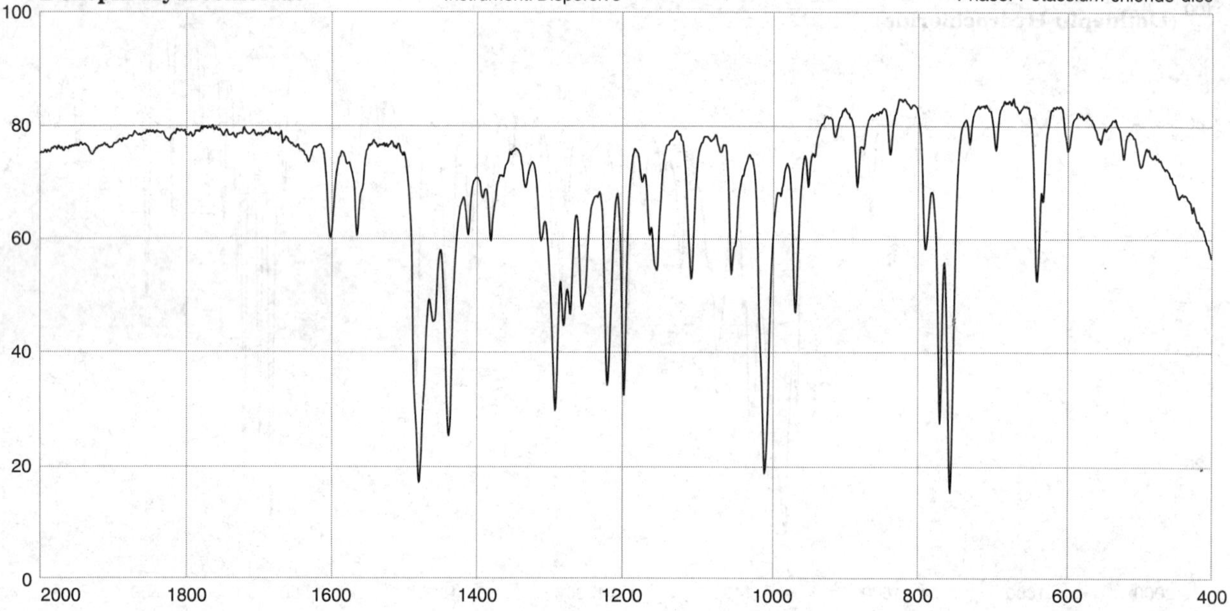

Dydrogesterone Instrument: Dispersive Phase: Potassium bromide disc

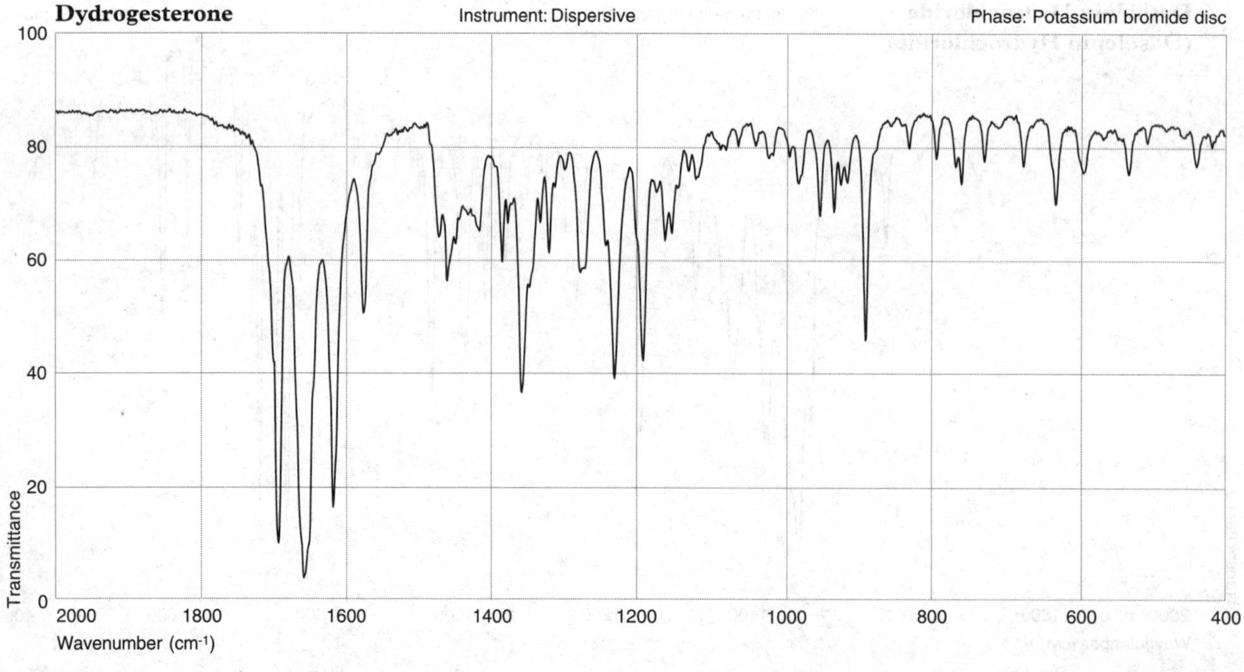

Edetic Acid Instrument: Fourier transform Phase: Potassium bromide disc

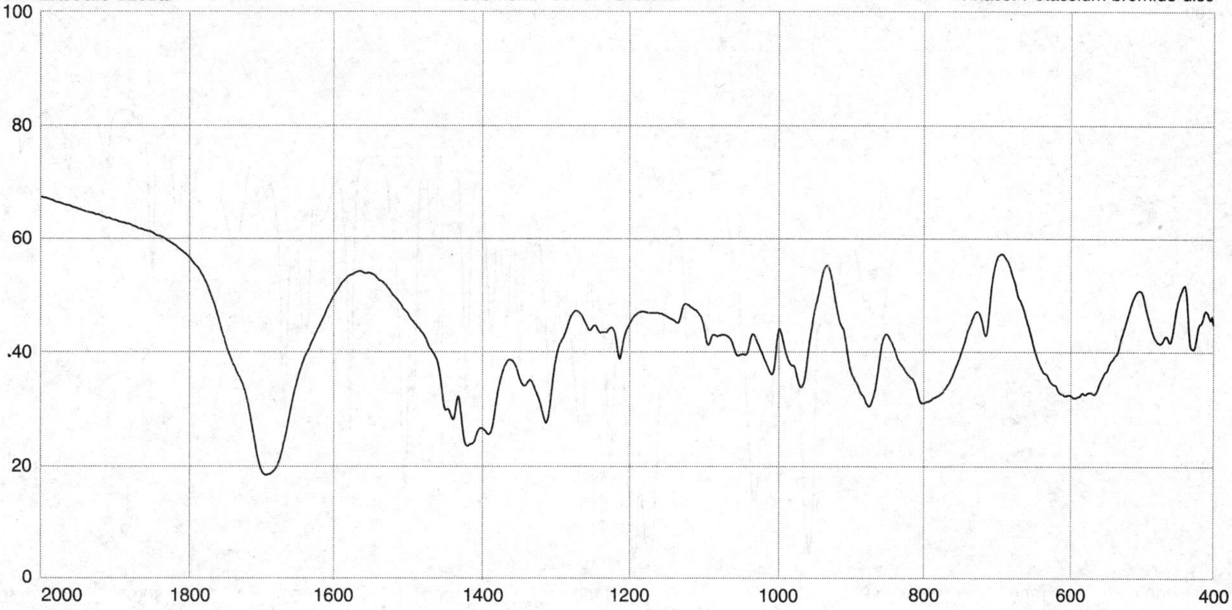

Edrophonium Chloride Instrument: Dispersive Phase: Potassium chloride disc

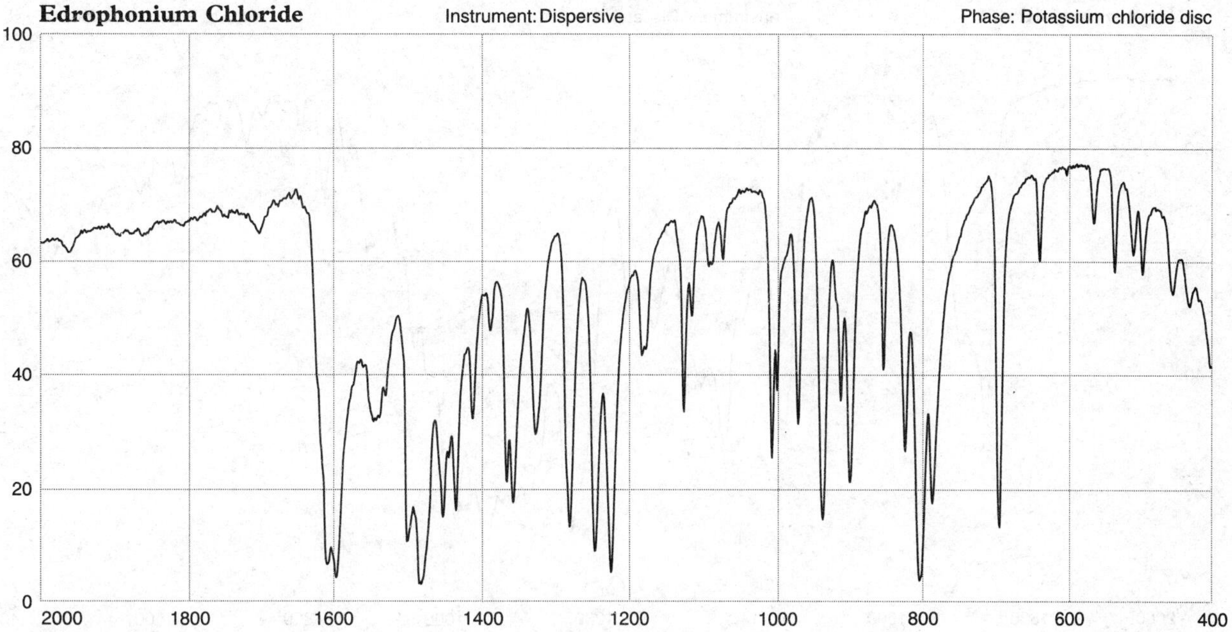

Ephedrine Instrument: Dispersive Phase: Thin film

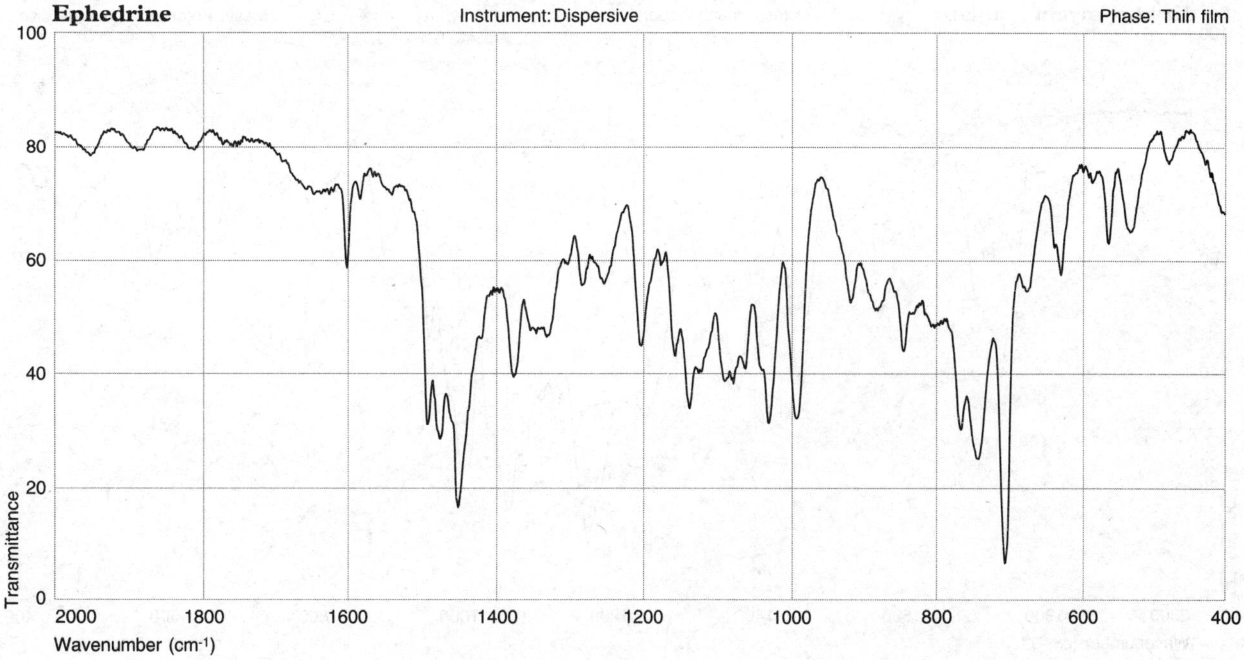

Epinephrine (Adrenaline) Instrument: Dispersive Phase: Potassium bromide disc

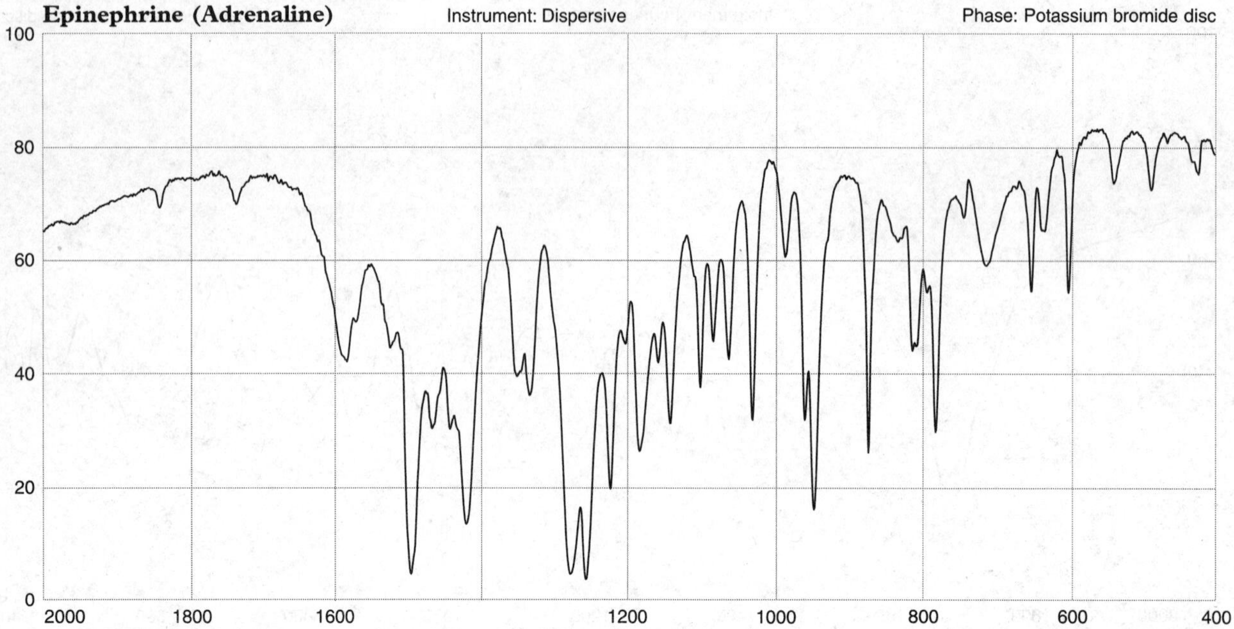

Erythromycin Instrument: Dispersive Phase: Potassium bromide disc

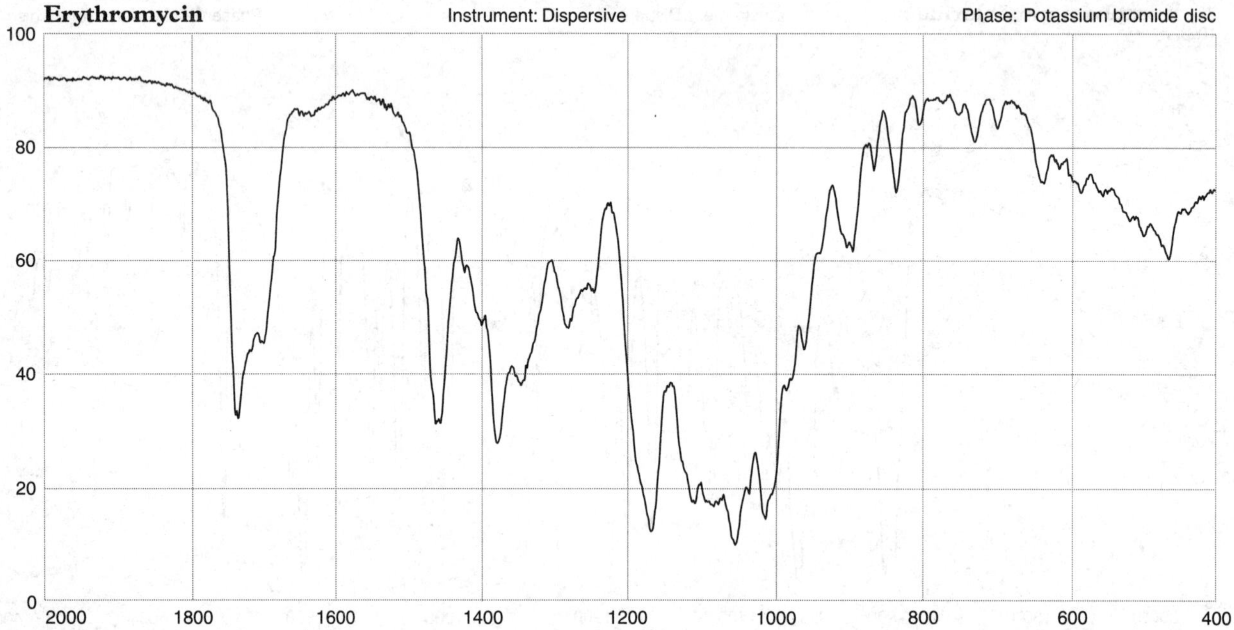

Erythromycin Estolate Instrument: Dispersive Phase: Potassium bromide disc

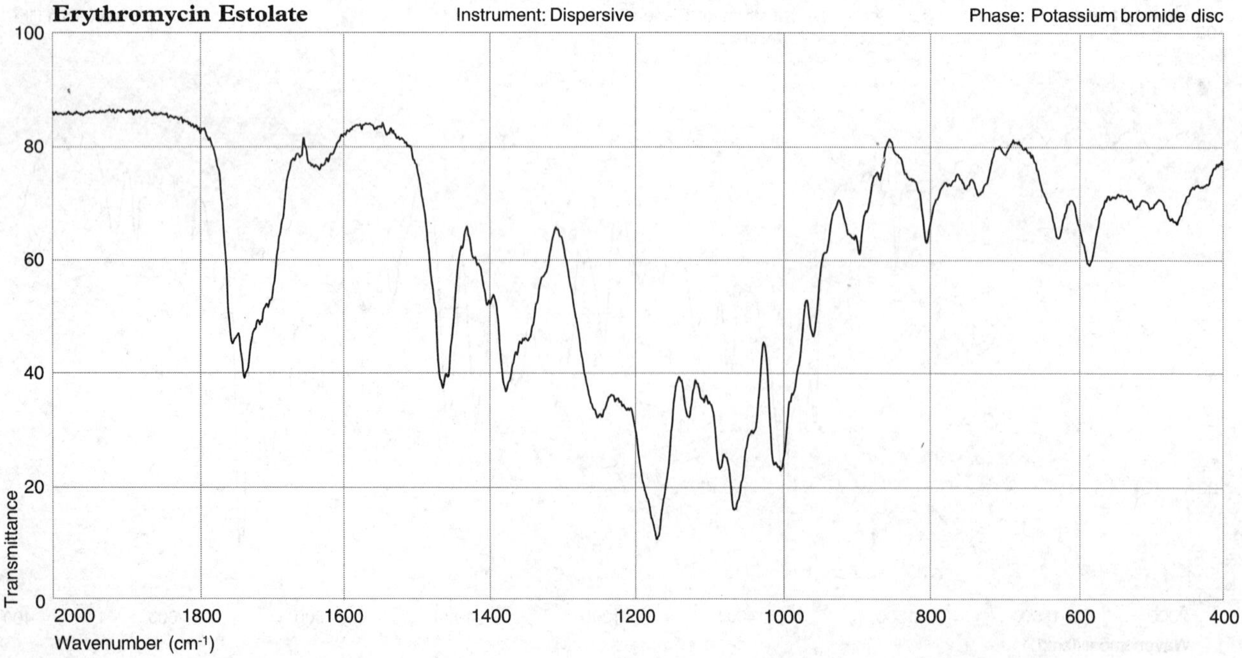

Erythromycin Ethyl Succinate Instrument: Dispersive Phase: Potassium bromide disc

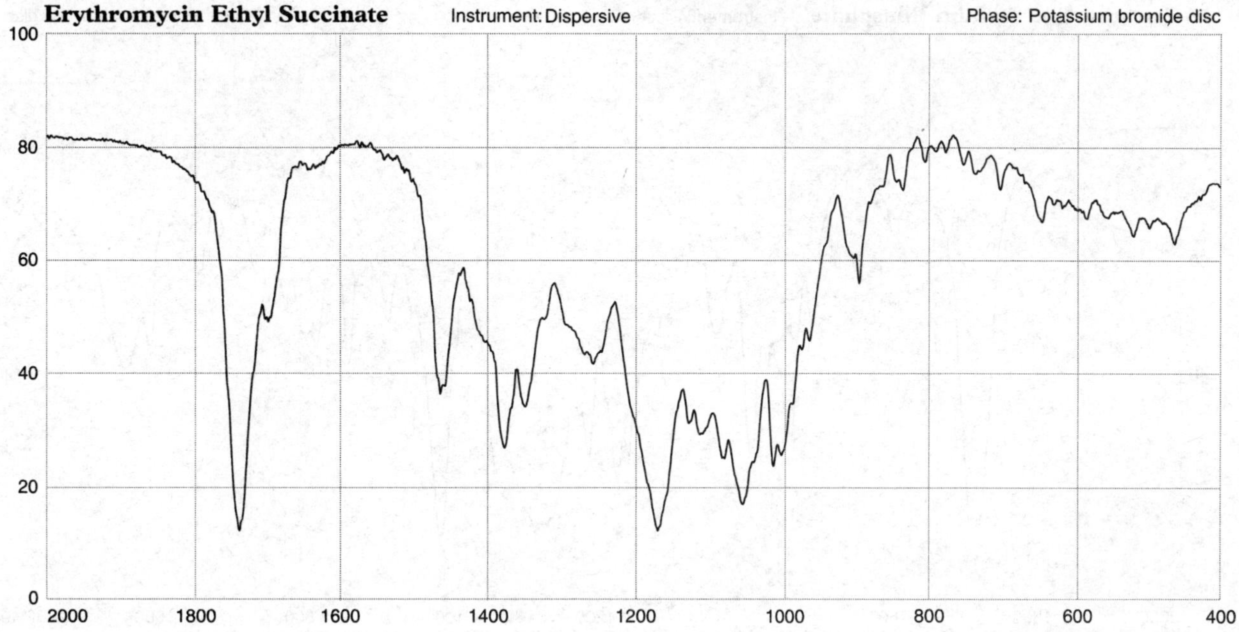

Erythromycin Lactobionate Instrument: Dispersive Phase: Potassium bromide disc

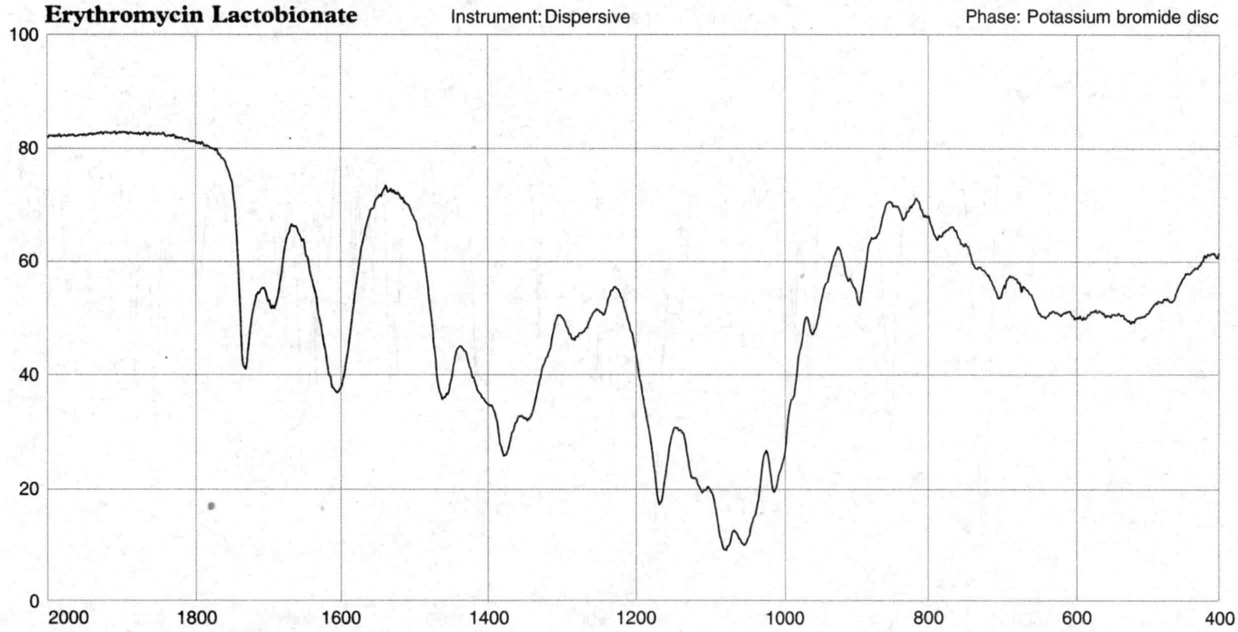

Erythromycin Stearate Instrument: Dispersive Phase: Potassium bromide disc

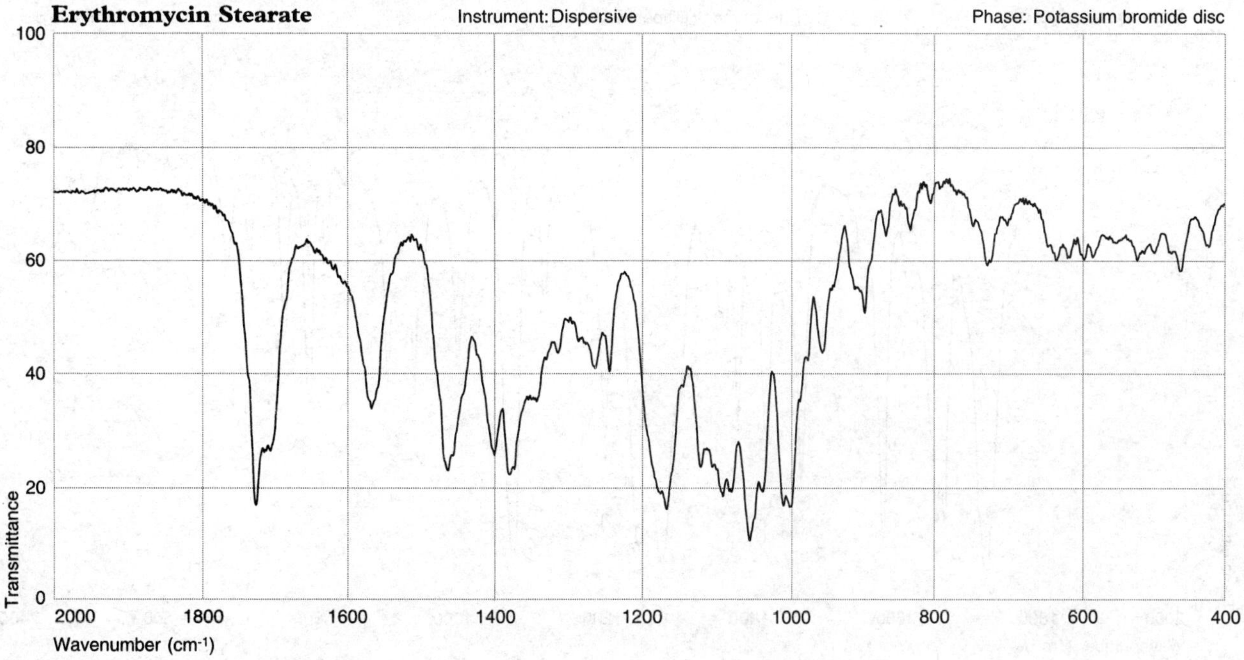

Estramustine Sodium Phosphate Instrument: Dispersive Phase: Potassium bromide disc

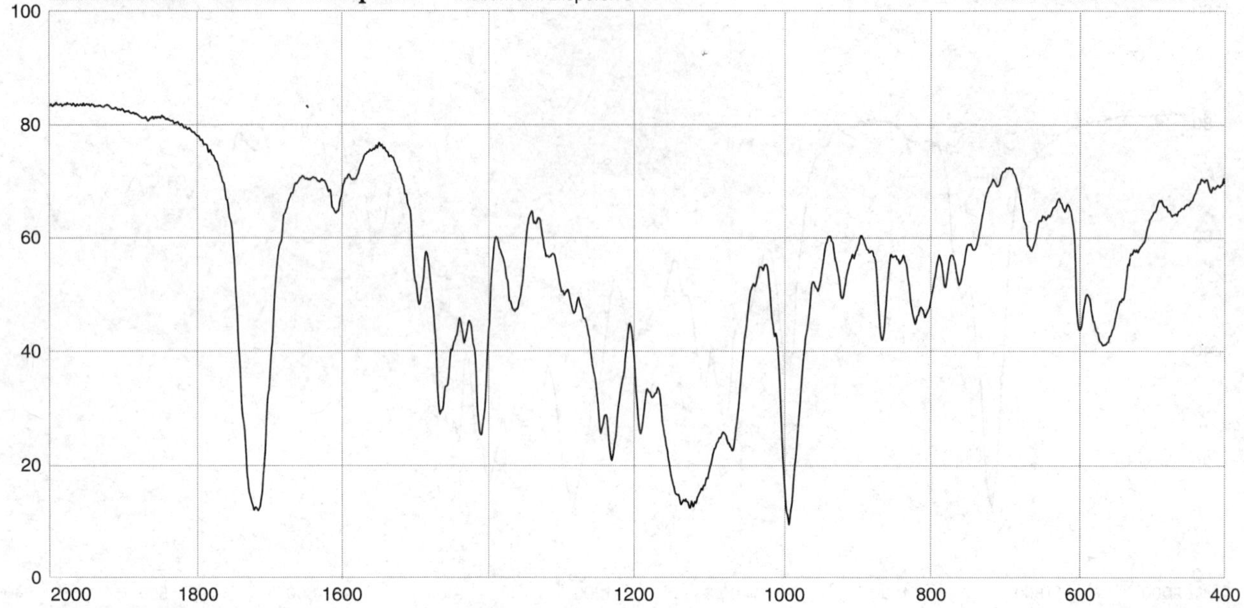

Estropipate Instrument: Fourier transform Phase: Potassium bromide disc

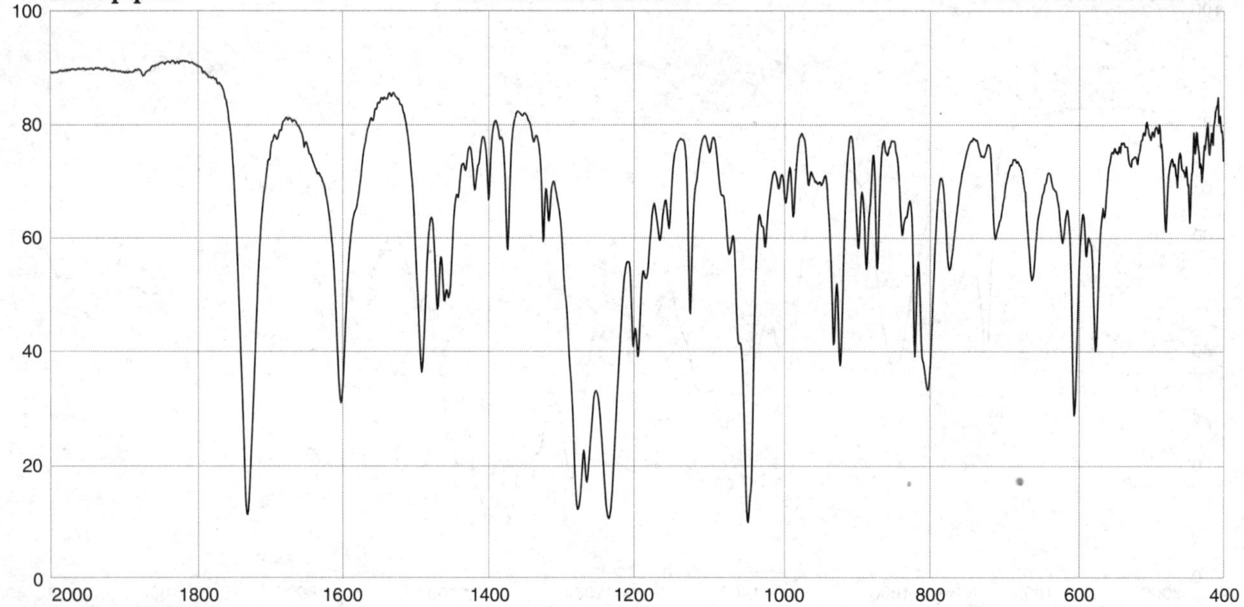

Etacrynic Acid Instrument: Dispersive Phase: Potassium bromide disc

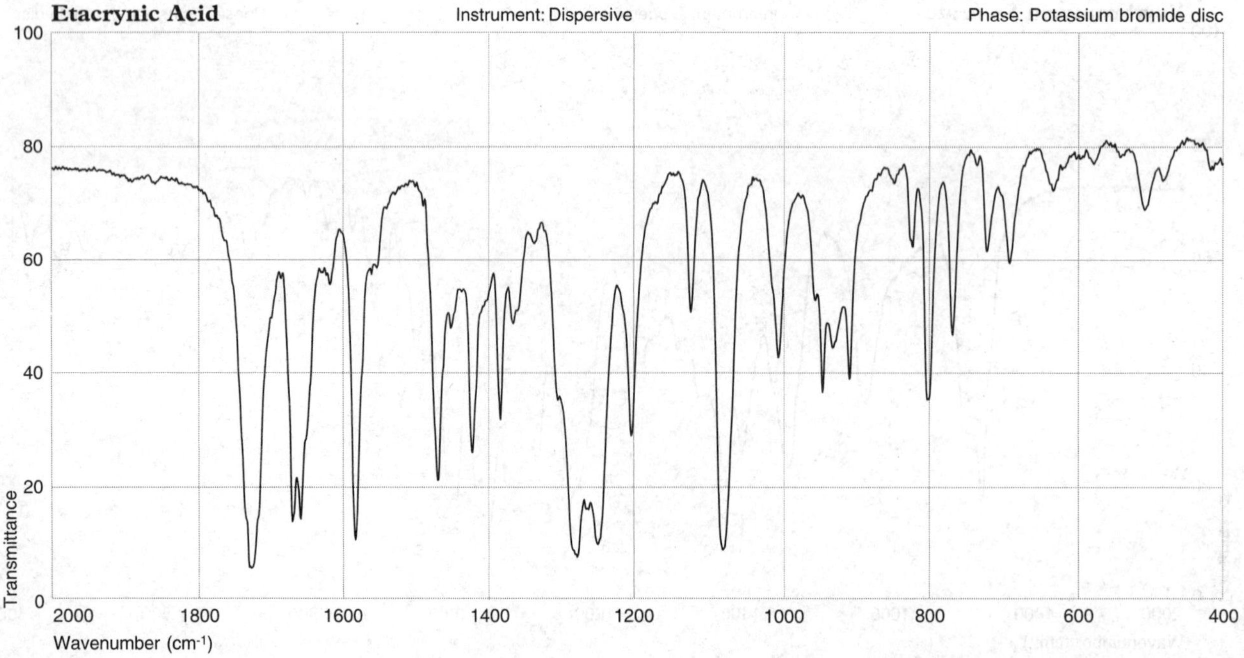

Etamiphylline Instrument: Dispersive Phase: Liquid paraffin mull

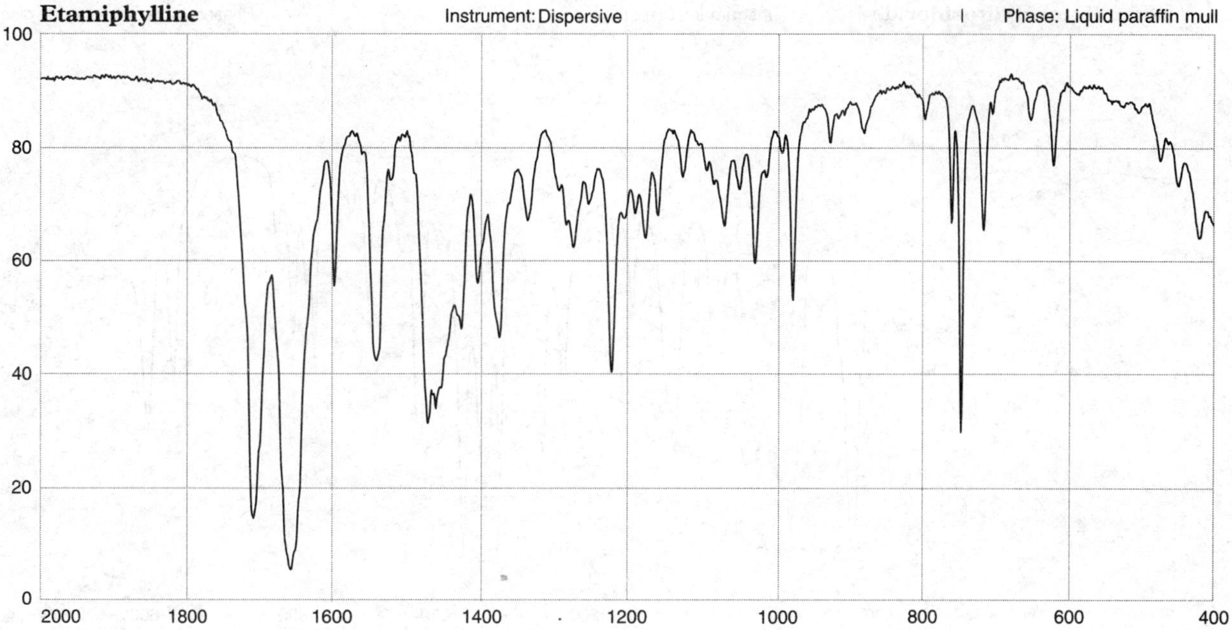

Etamiphylline Camsilate Instrument: Dispersive Phase: Liquid paraffin mull

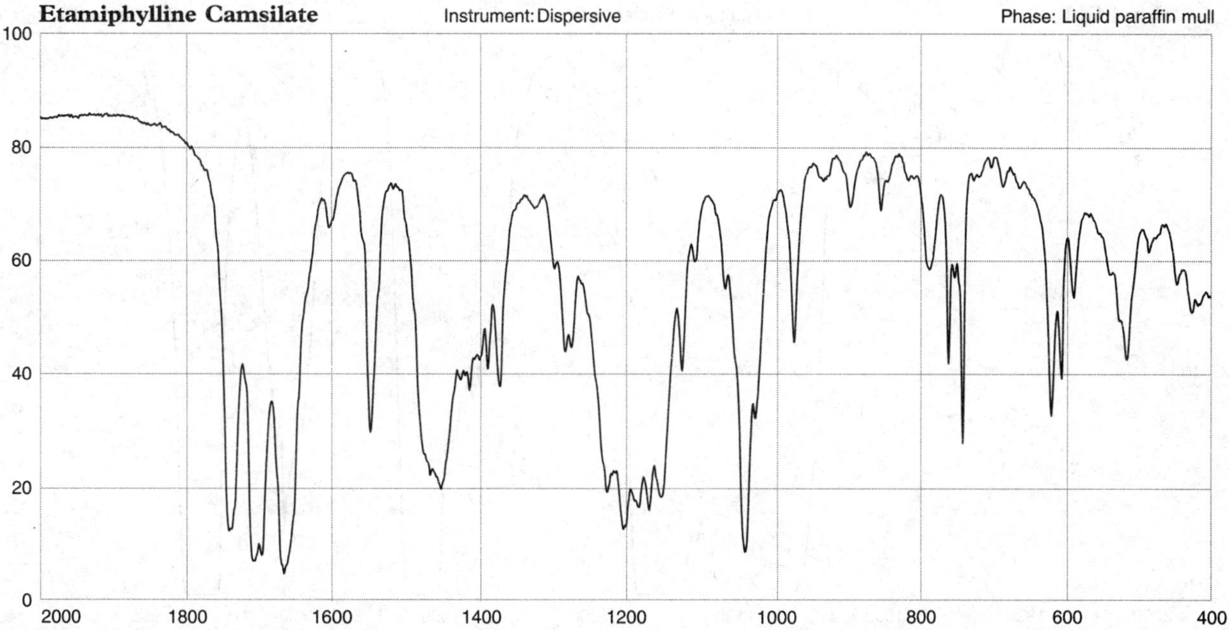

Etamivan Instrument: Dispersive Phase: Potassium chloride disc

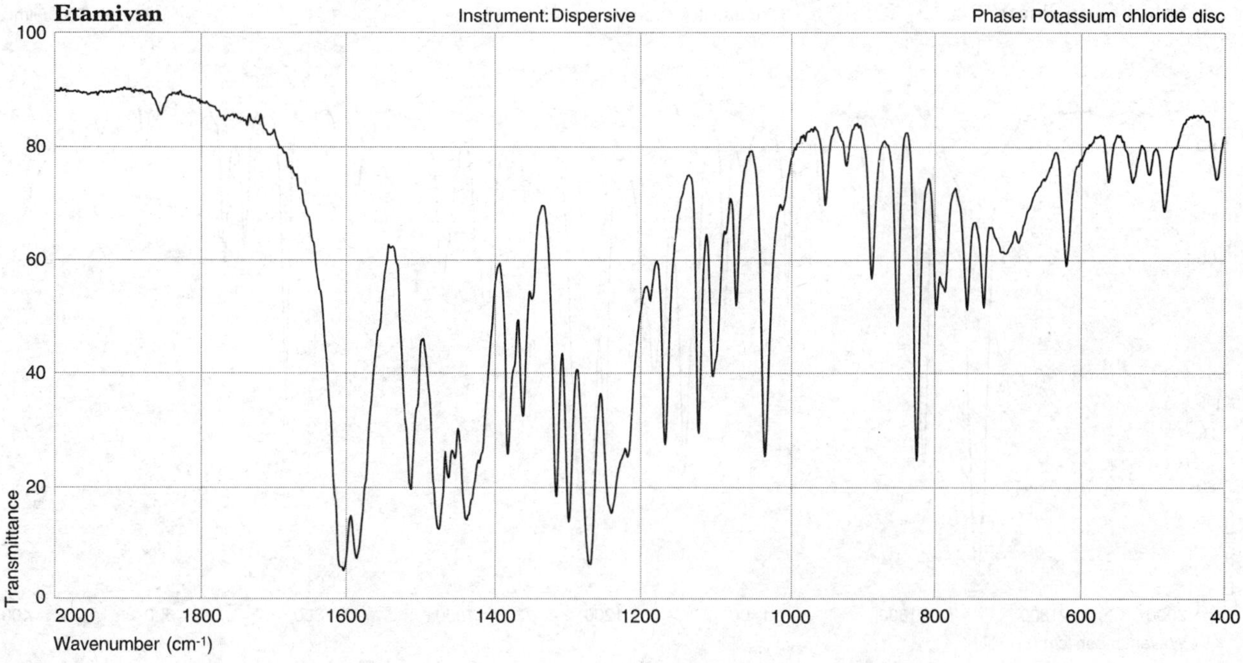

Ethambutol Hydrochloride Instrument: Dispersive Phase: Potassium chloride disc

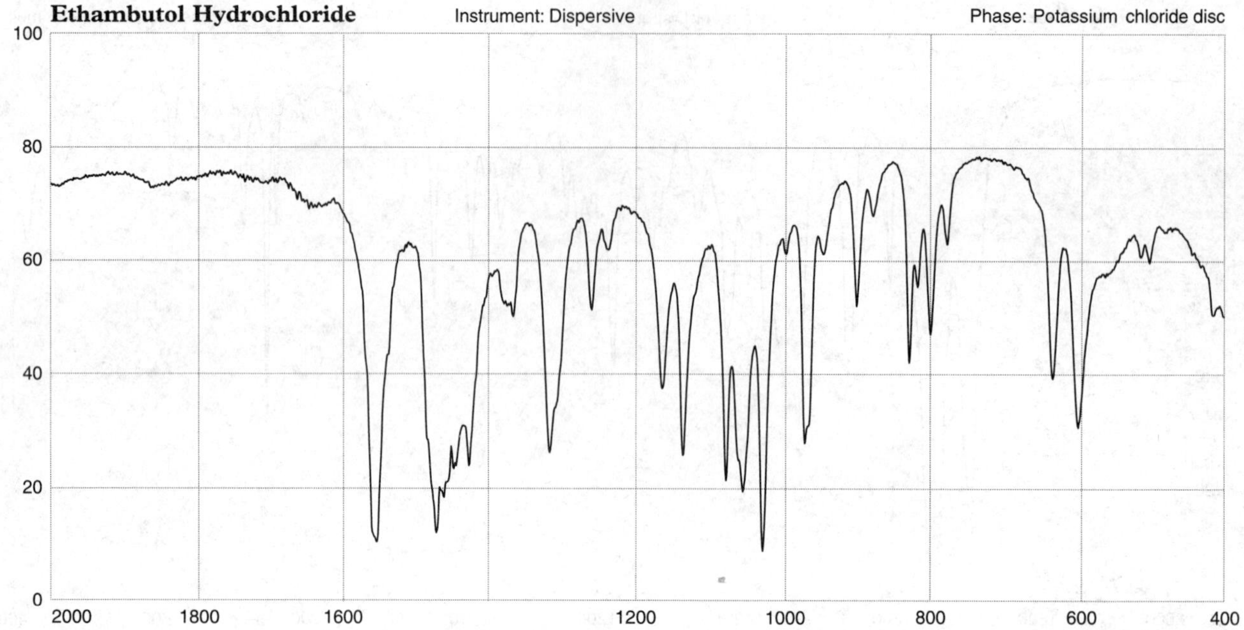

Ethyl Chloride Instrument: Fourier transform Gas Phase: 10 cm cell

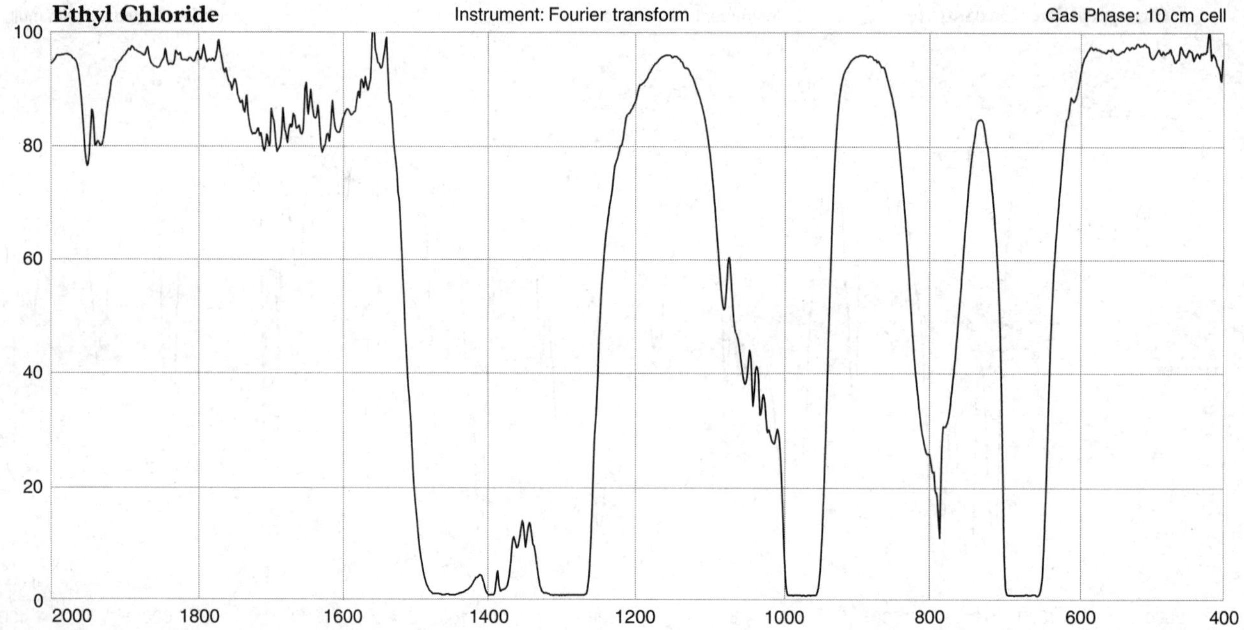

Ethyl Cinnamate Instrument: Dispersive Phase: Thin Film

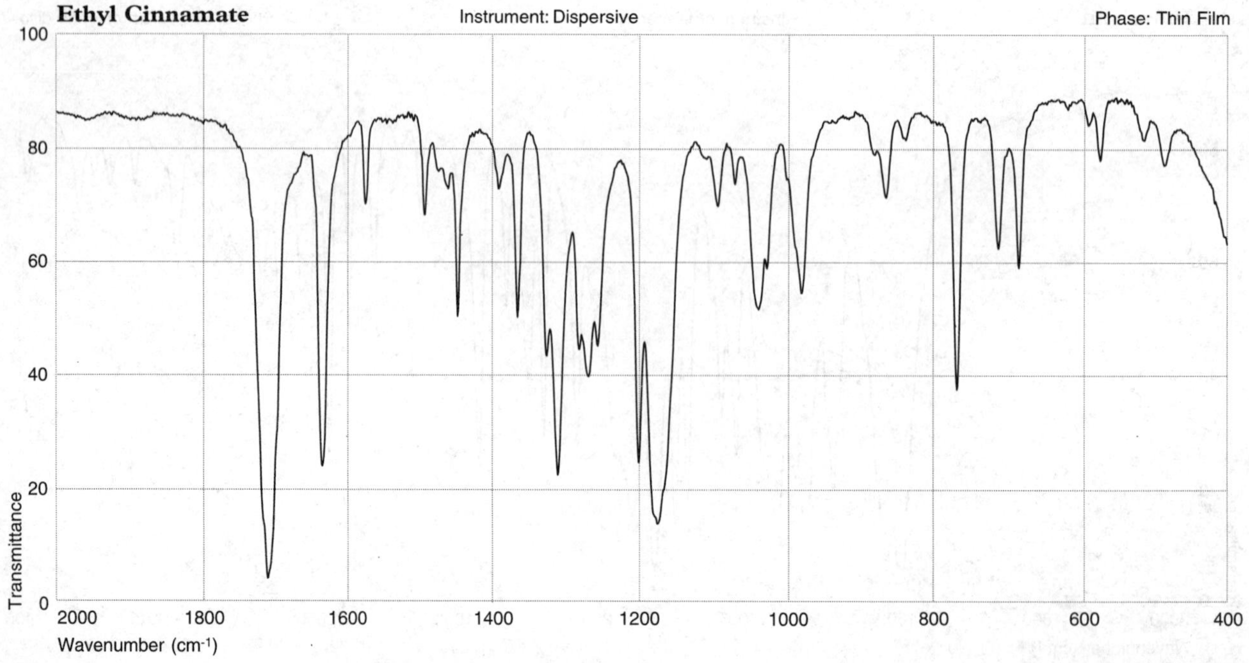

Ethylestrenol

Instrument: Dispersive

Phase: Potassium bromide disc

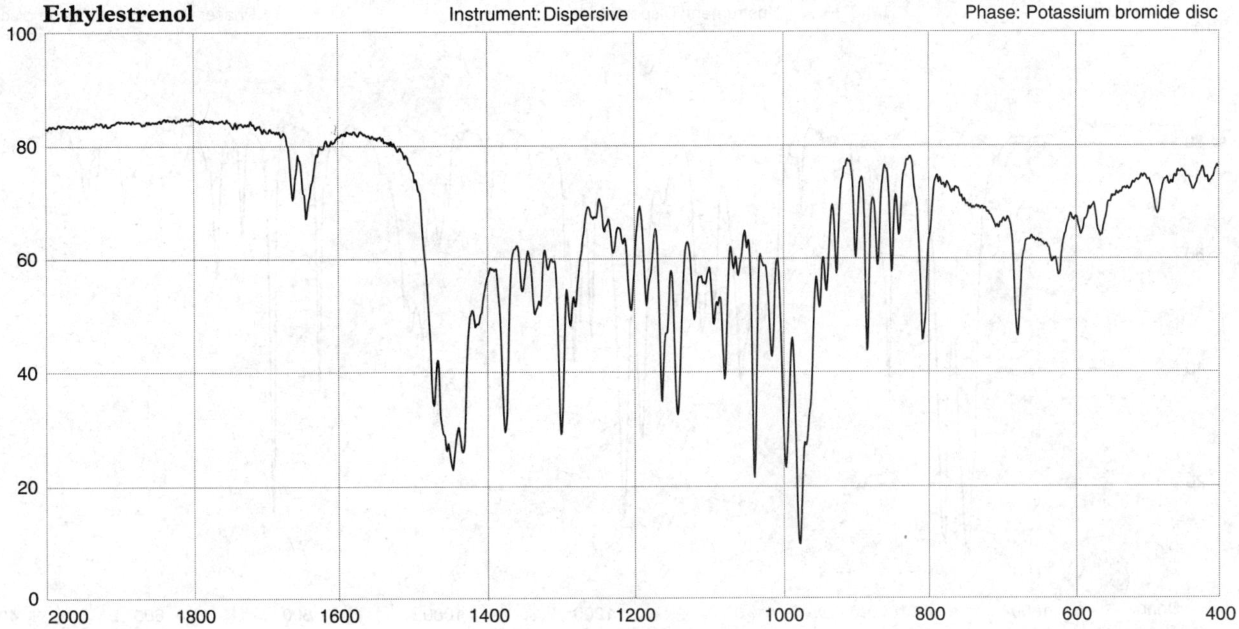

Etynodiol Diacetate

Instrument: Dispersive

Phase: Potassium bromide disc

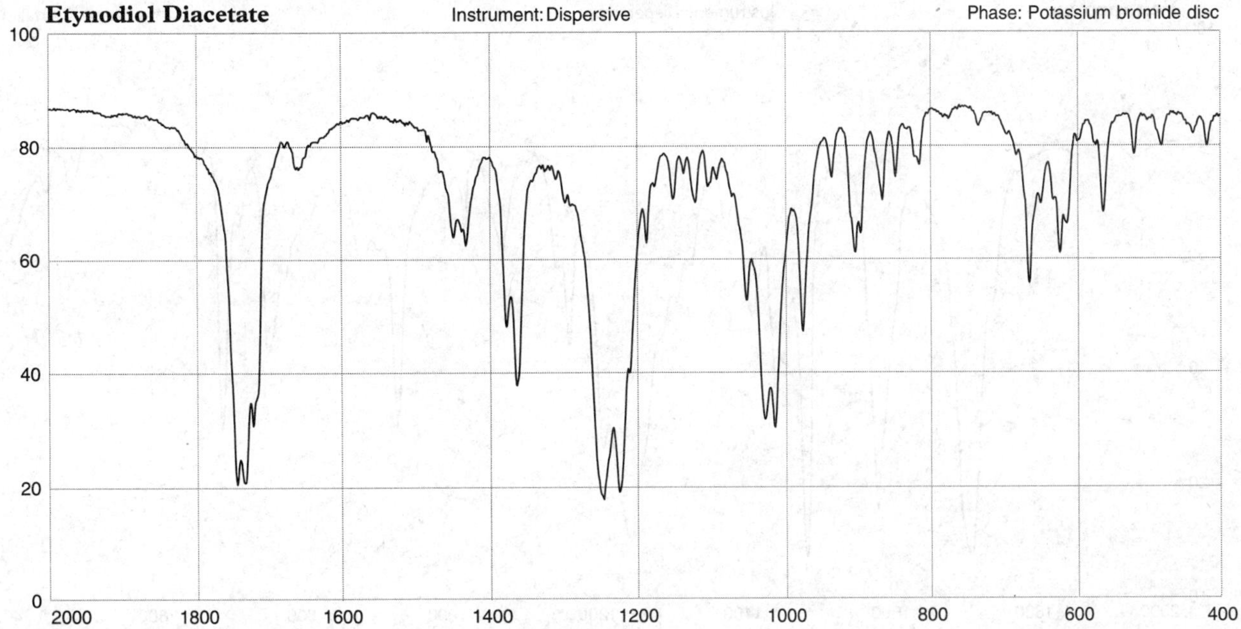

Etodolac

Instrument: Dispersive

Phase: Potassium bromide disc

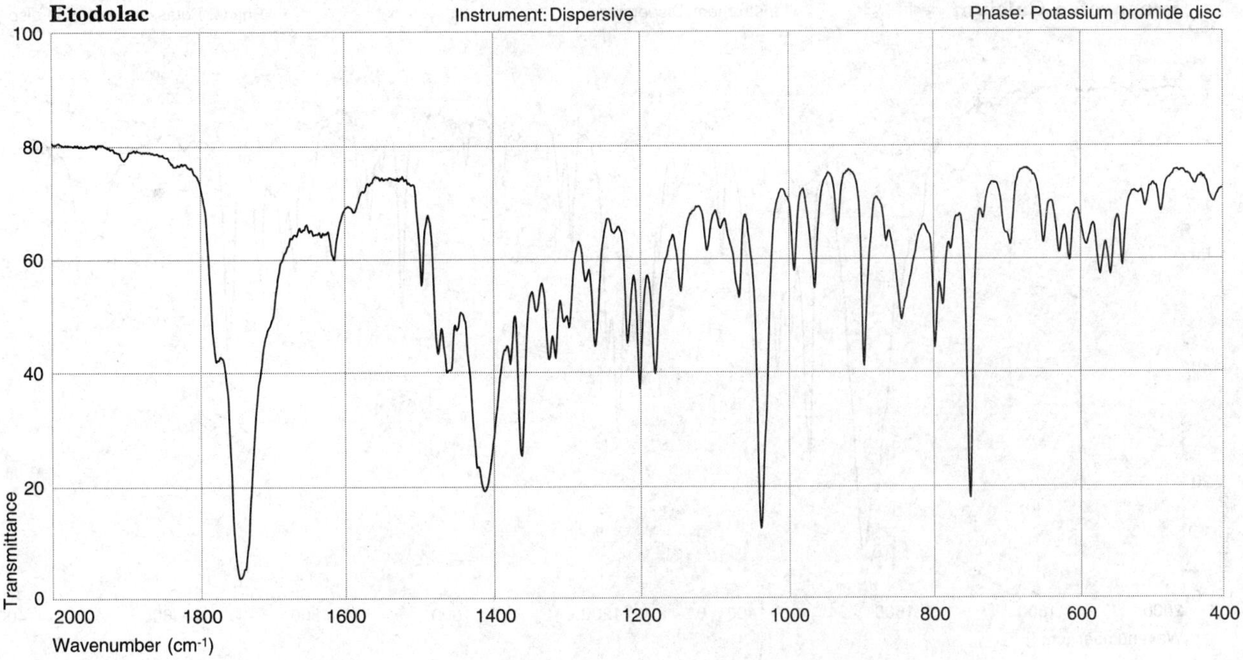

Fenbufen

Instrument: Dispersive

Phase: Potassium bromide disc

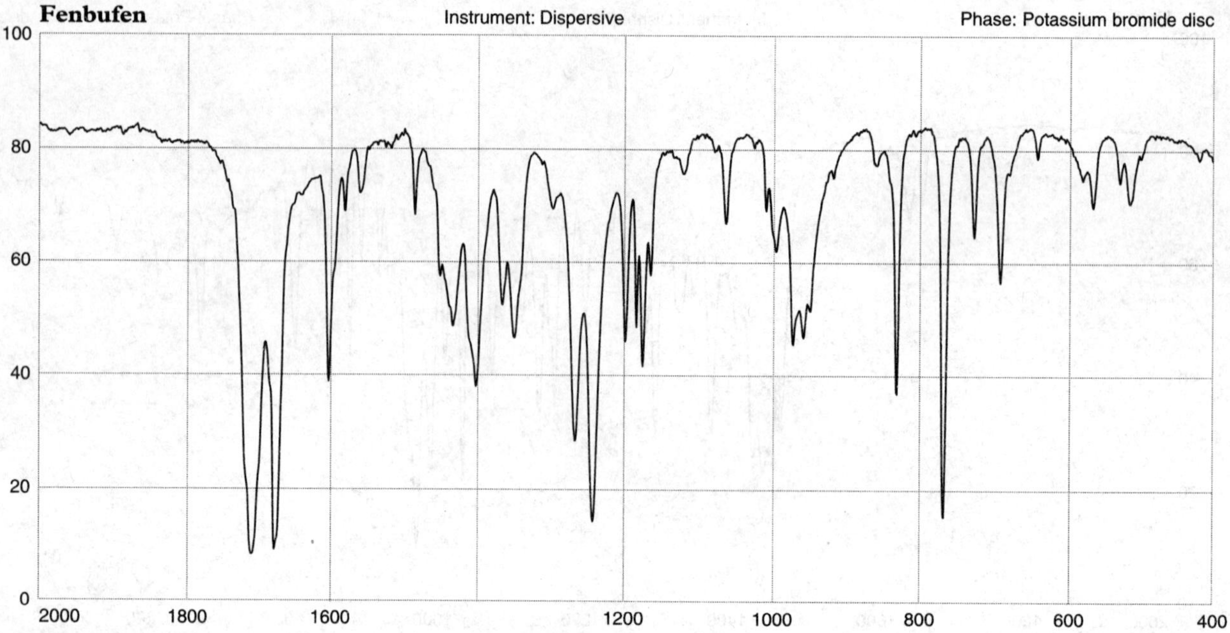

Fenoprofen

Instrument: Dispersive

Phase: Thin film

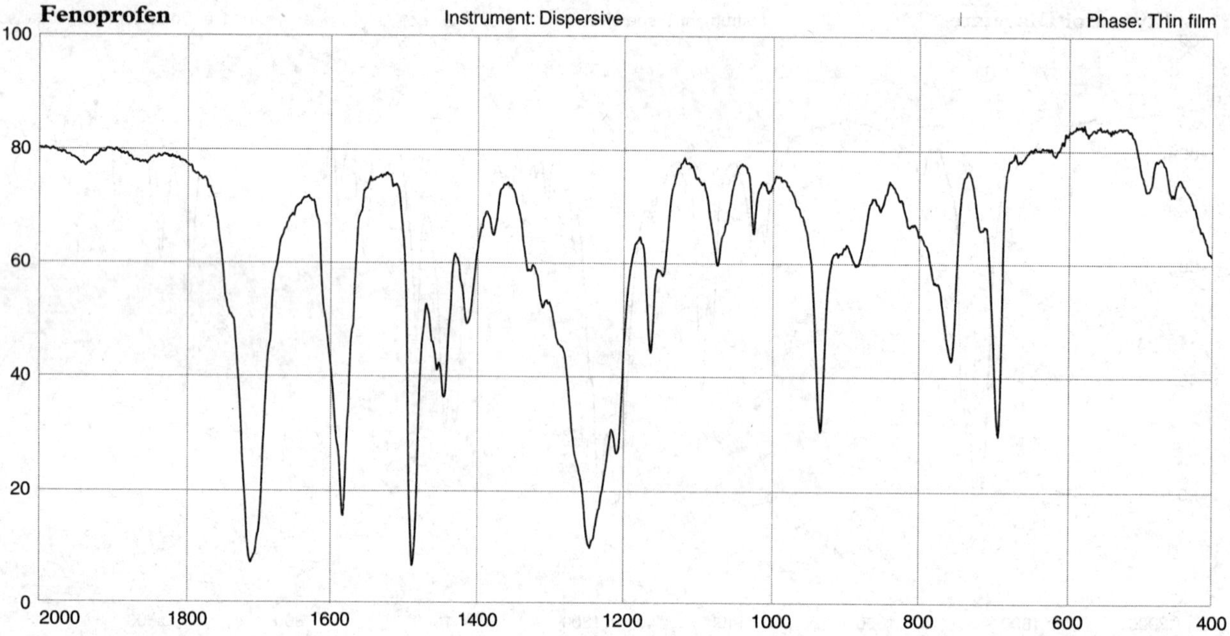

Fenoprofen Calcium

Instrument: Dispersive

Phase: Potassium bromide disc

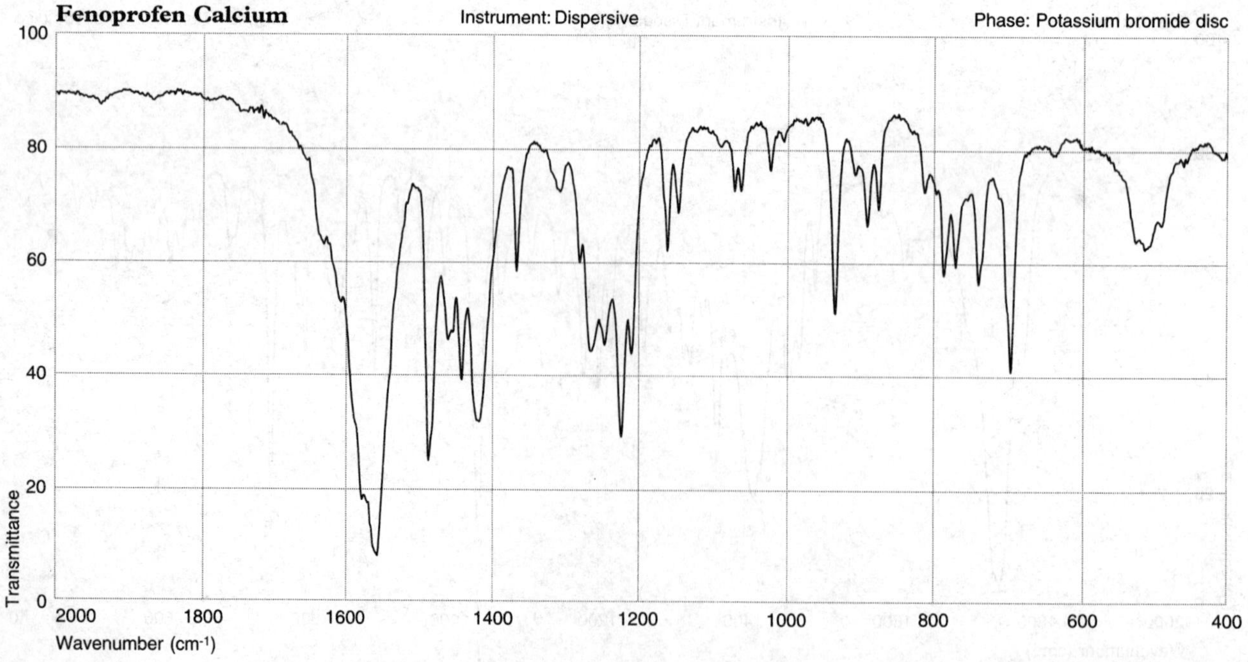

Flavoxate Hydrochloride Instrument: Fourier transform Phase: Potassium chloride disc

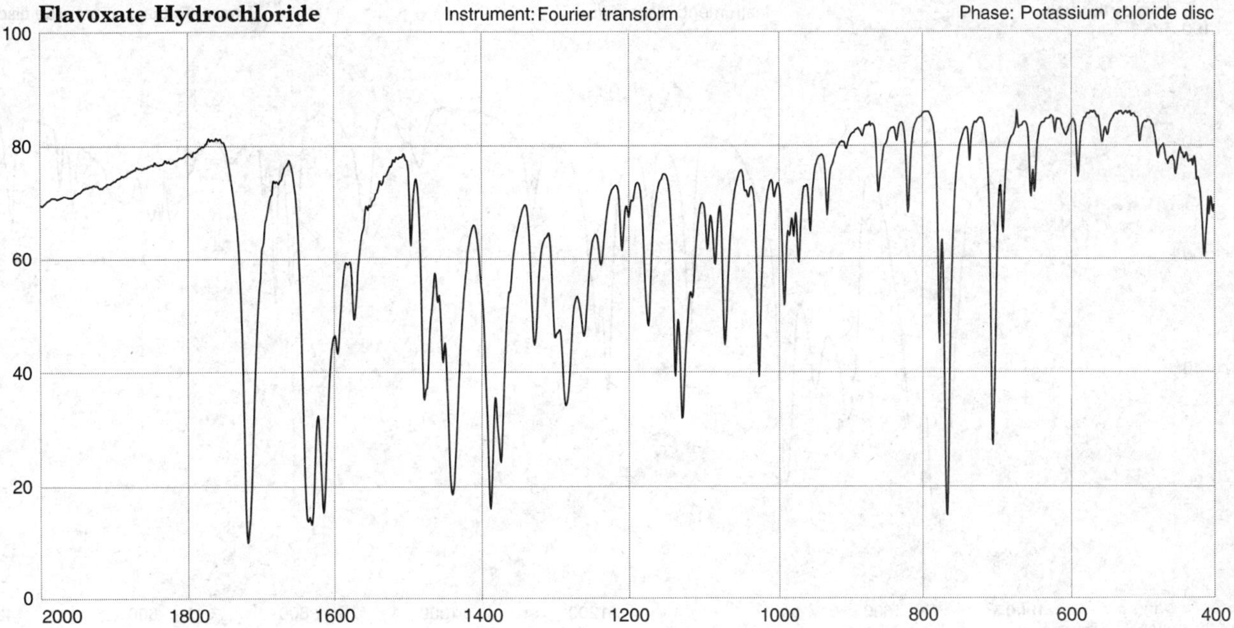

Flucloxacillin Magnesium Instrument: Dispersive Phase: Liquid paraffin mull

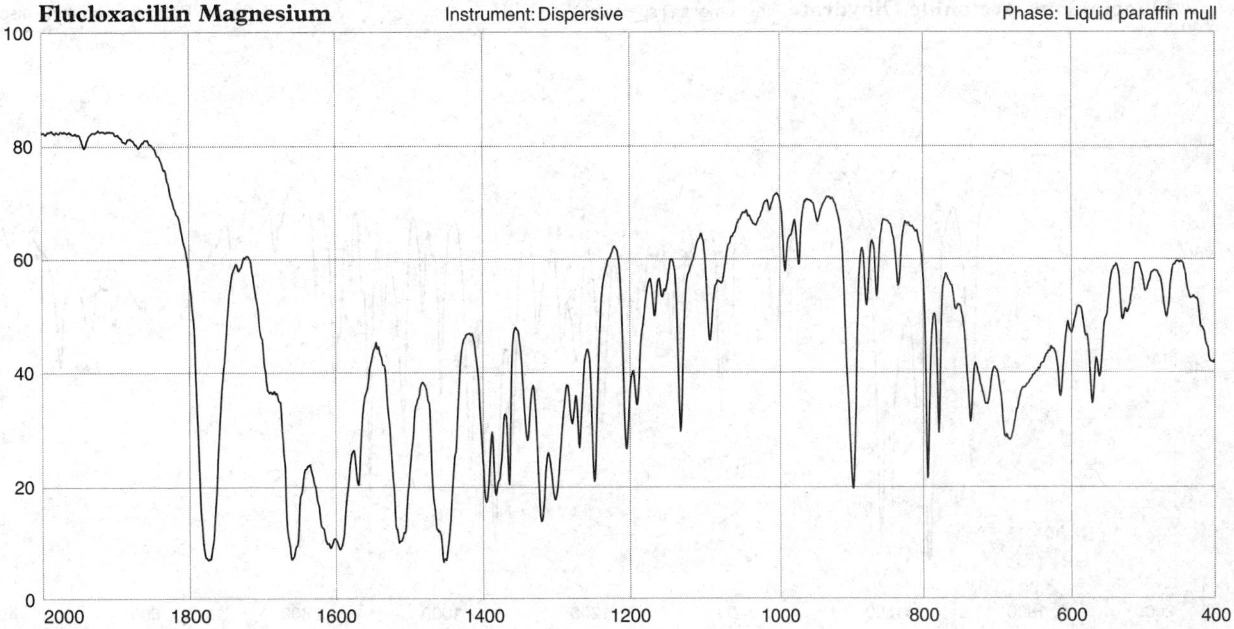

Flucloxacillin Sodium Instrument: Dispersive Phase: Liquid paraffin mull

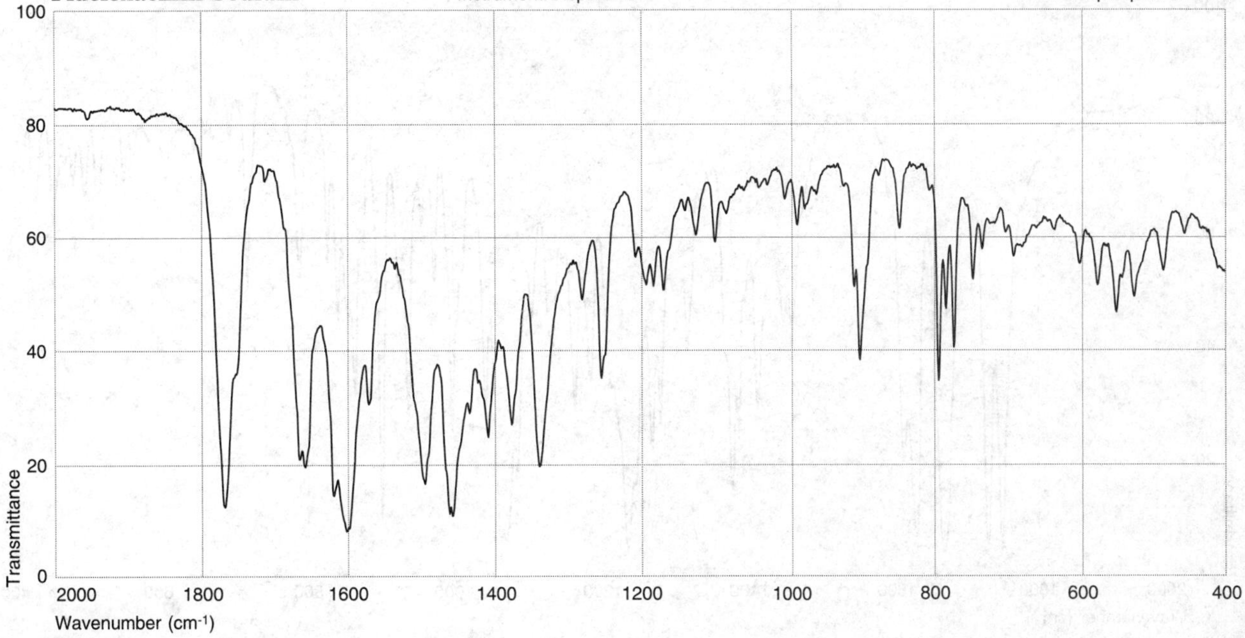

Flucytosine Instrument: Dispersive Phase: Potassium bromide disc

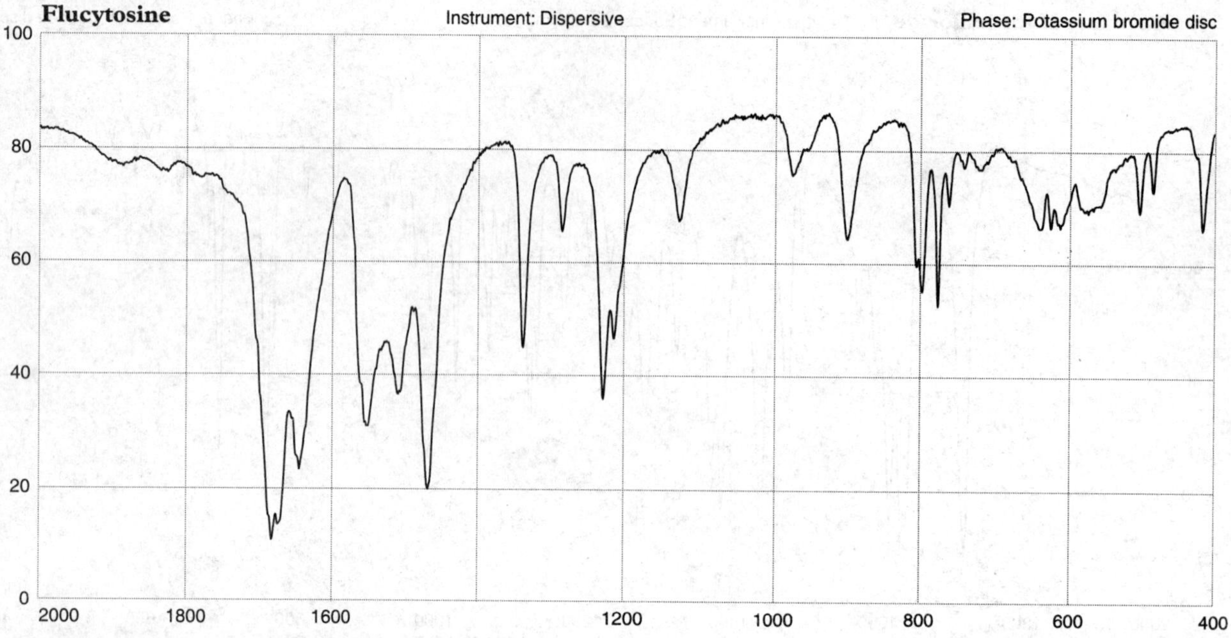

Fluocinolone Acetonide Dihydrate Instrument: Dispersive Phase: Potassium bromide disc

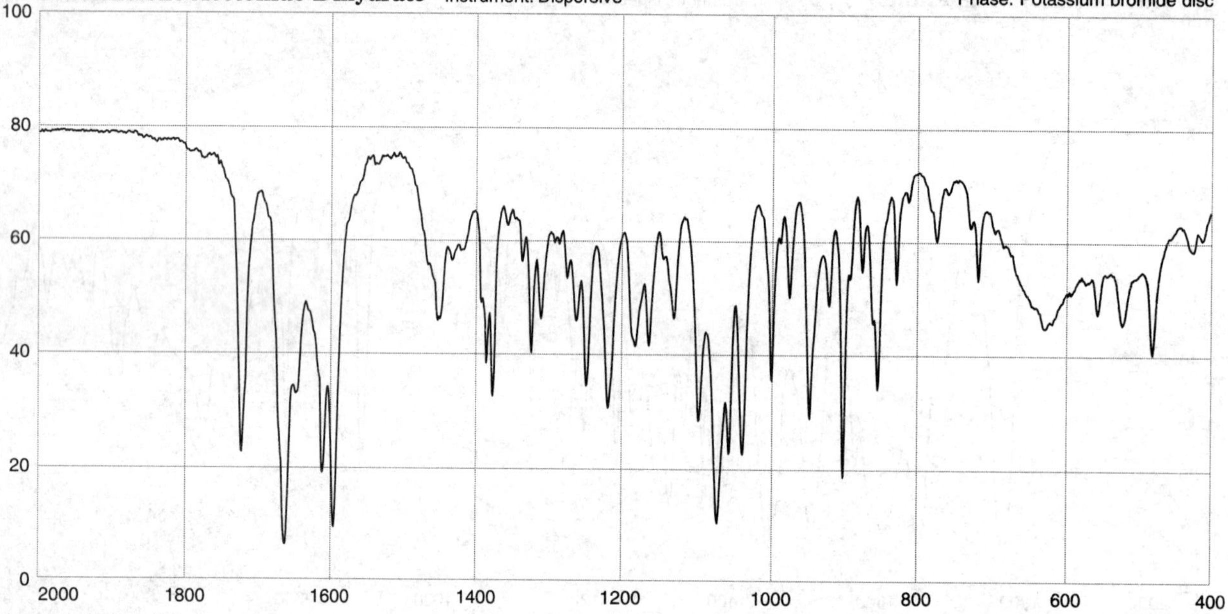

Fluocinonide Instrument: Dispersive Phase: Potassium bromide disc

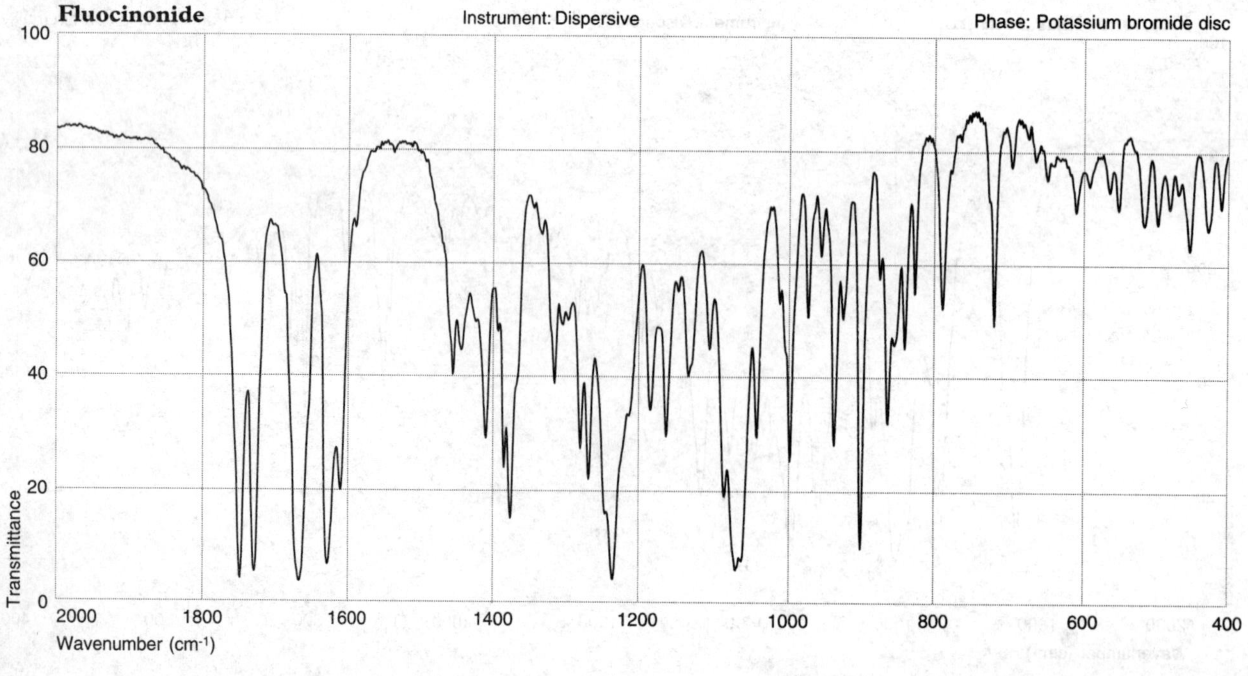

Fluocortolone Hexanoate Instrument: Dispersive Phase: Potassium bromide disc

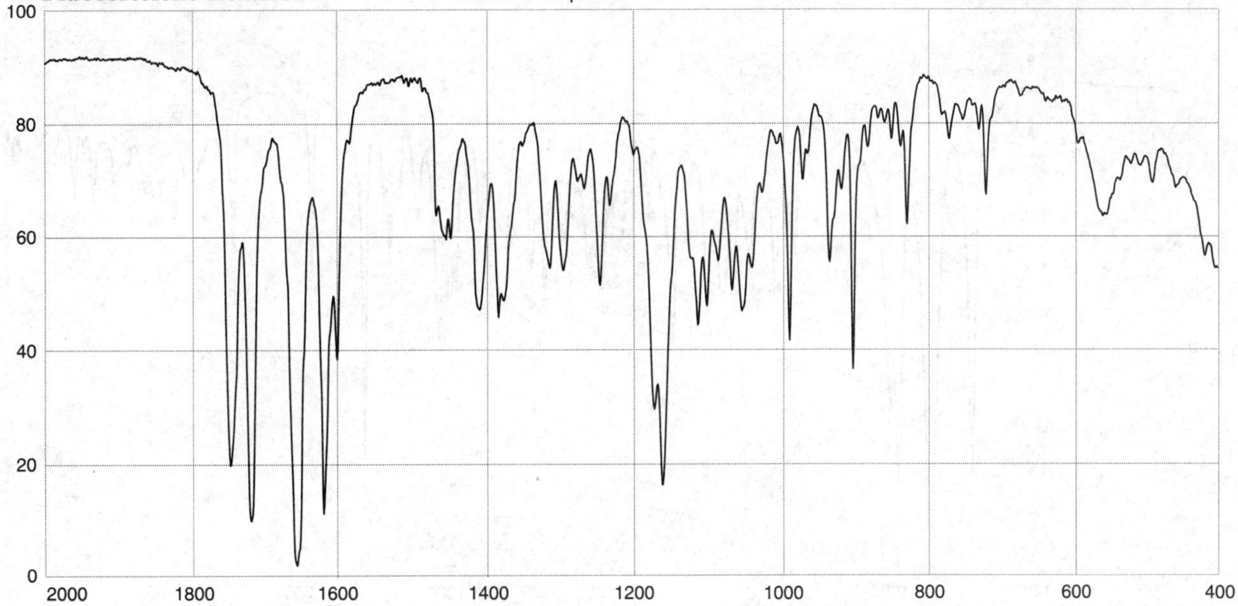

Fluocortolone Pivalate Instrument: Dispersive Phase: 5% w/v solution in chloroform Thickness: 0.1mm

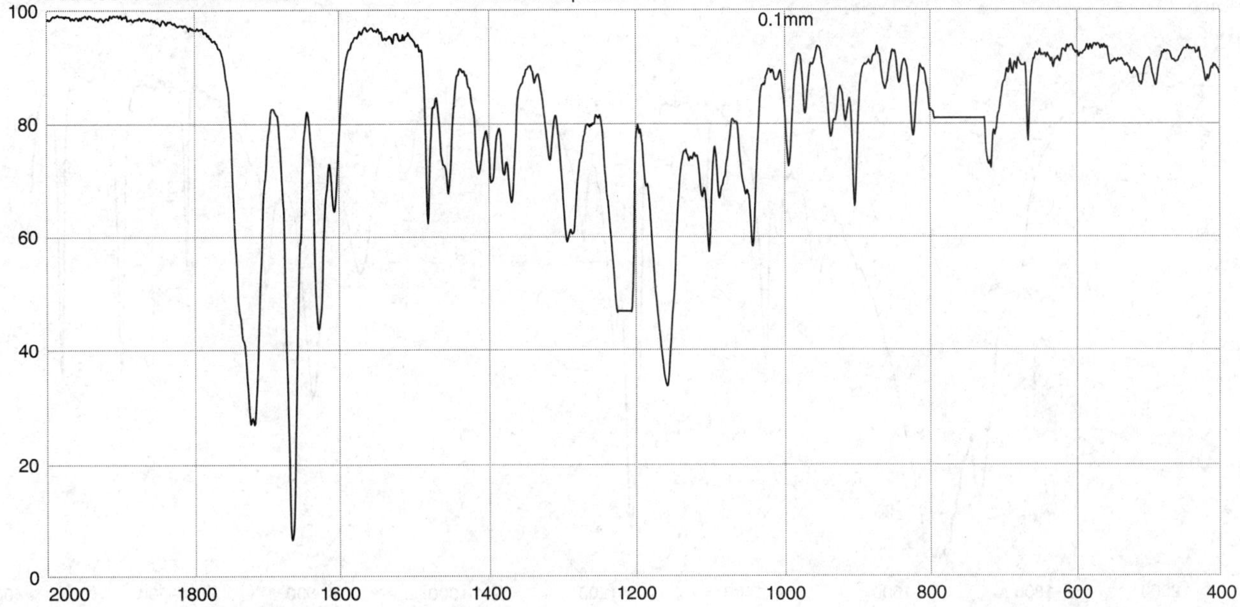

Fluorescein Sodium Instrument: Dispersive Phase: Potassium bromide disc

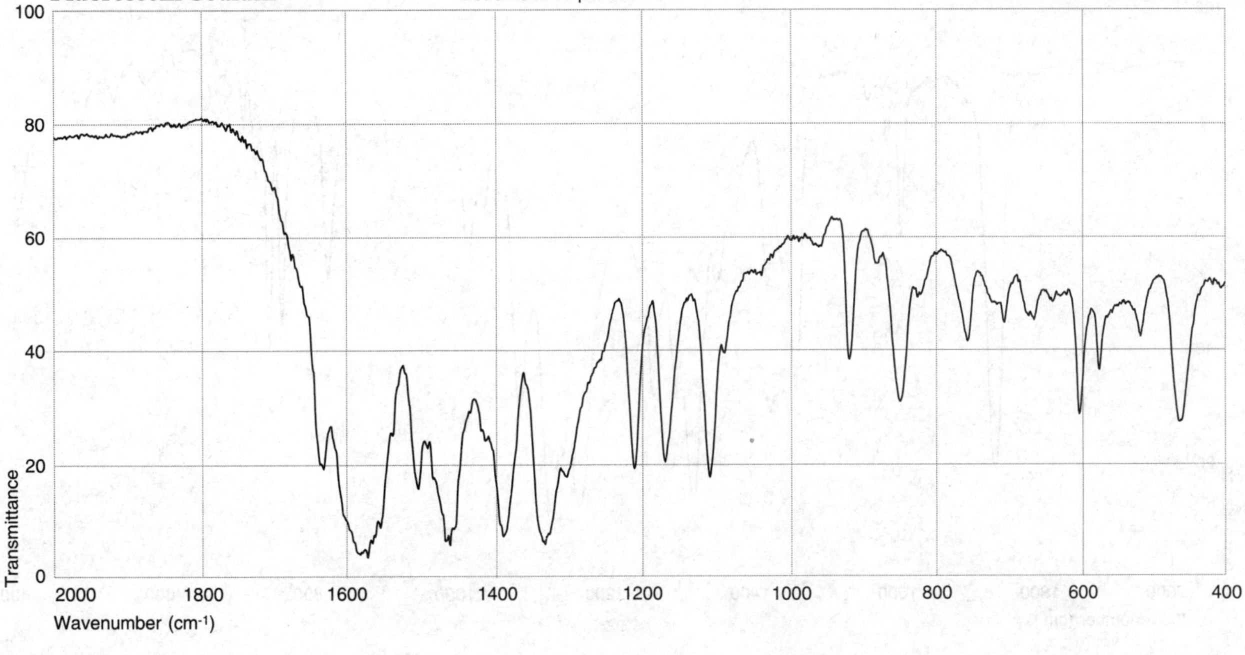

Fluorometholone

Instrument: Fourier transform

Phase: Potassium bromide disc

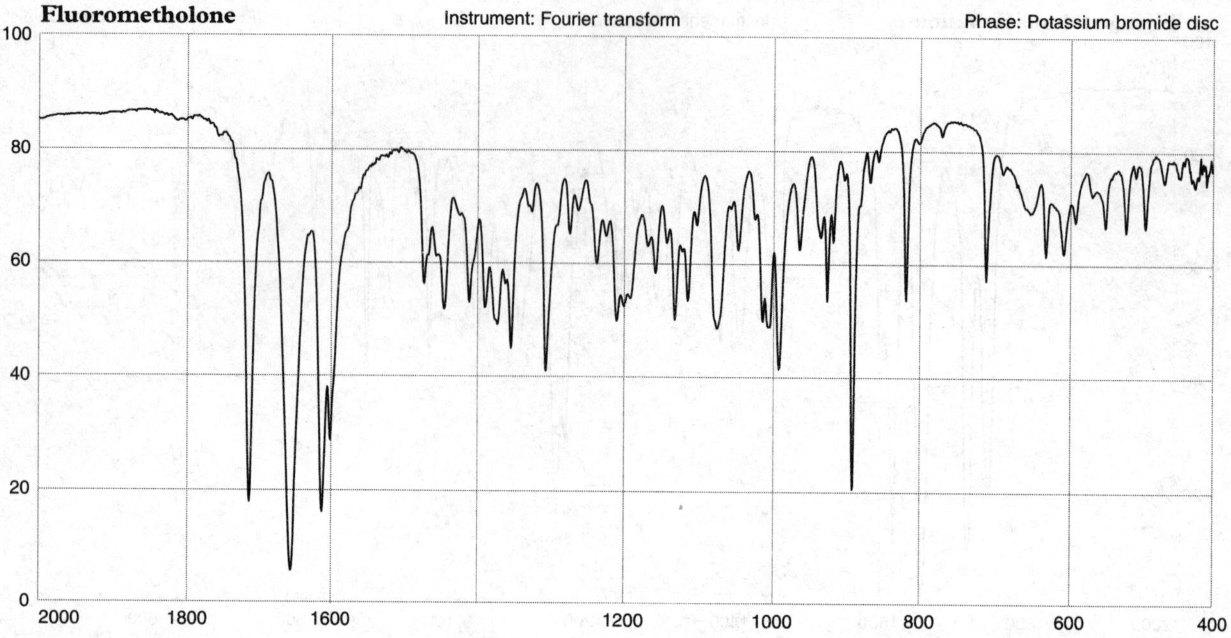

Fluorouracil

Instrument: Dispersive

Phase: Potassium bromide disc

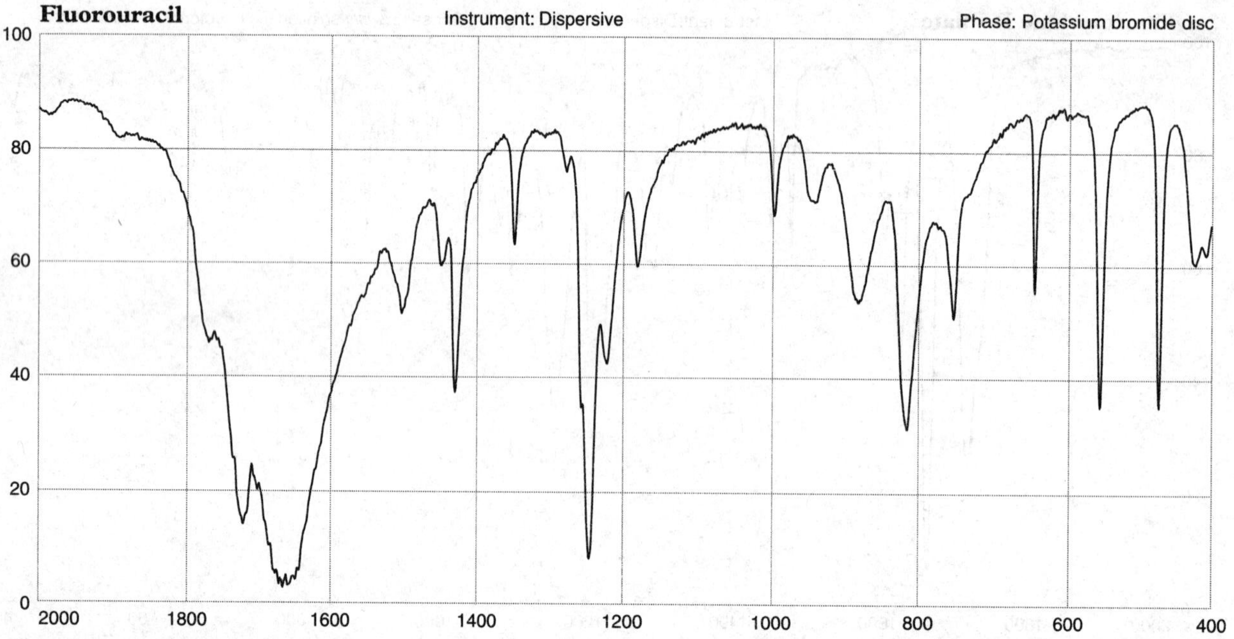

Flupentixol Decanoate

Instrument: Dispersive

Phase: Thin film

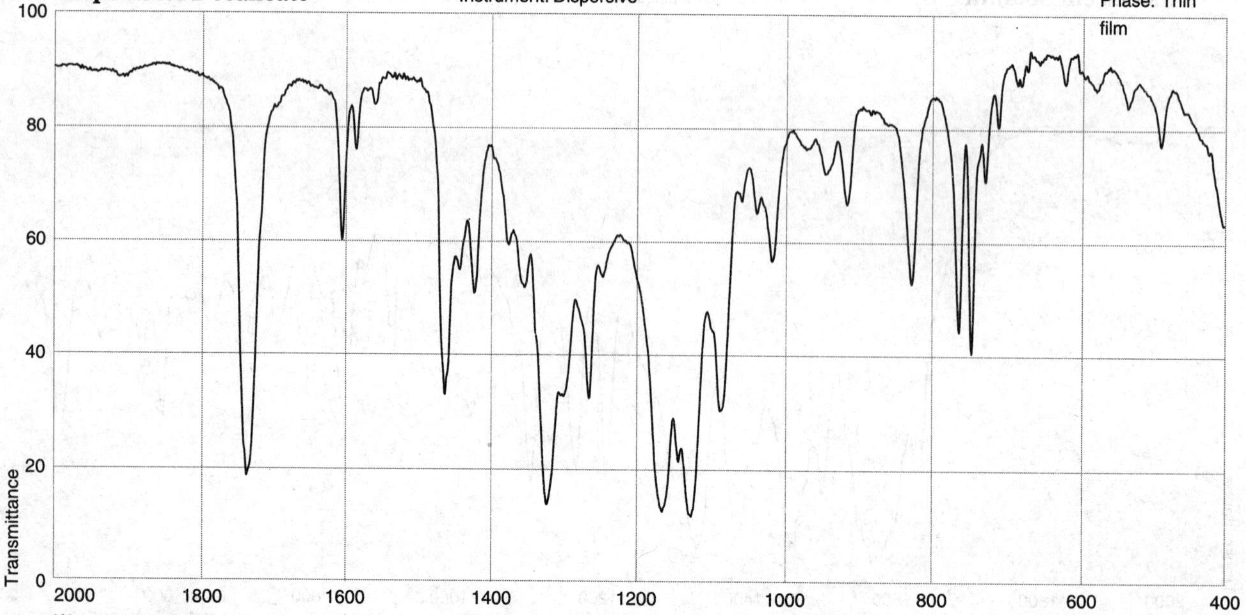

Flurazepam Monohydrochloride Instrument: Dispersive Phase: 5% w/v solution in chloroform Thickness: 0.1mm

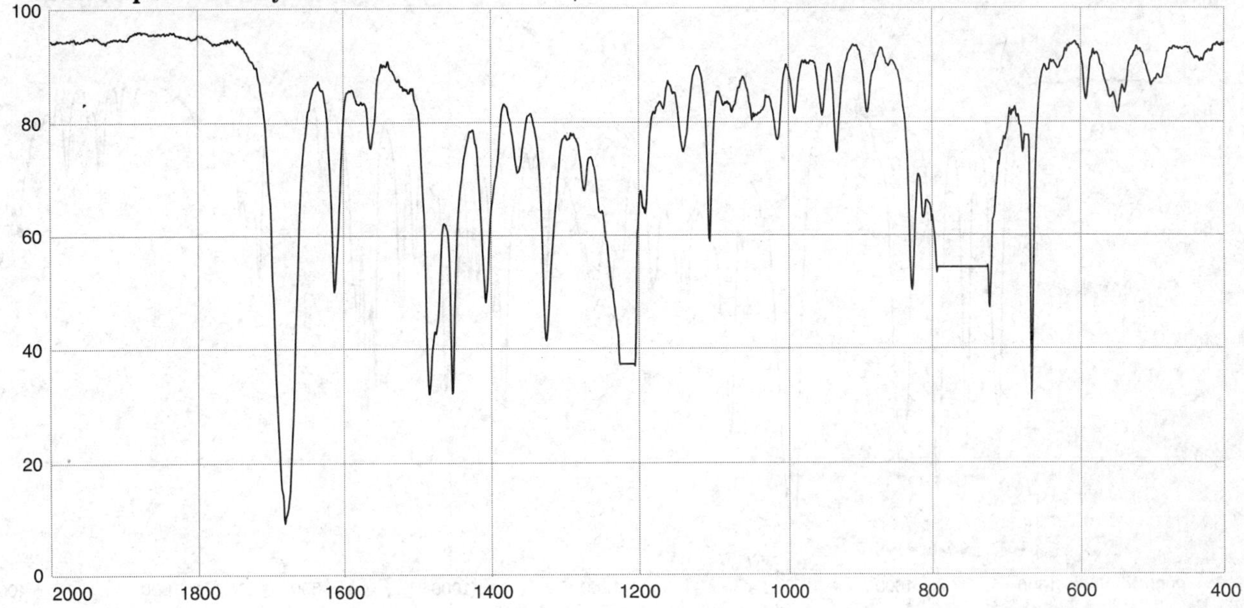

Flurbiprofen Instrument: Dispersive Phase: Potassium bromide disc

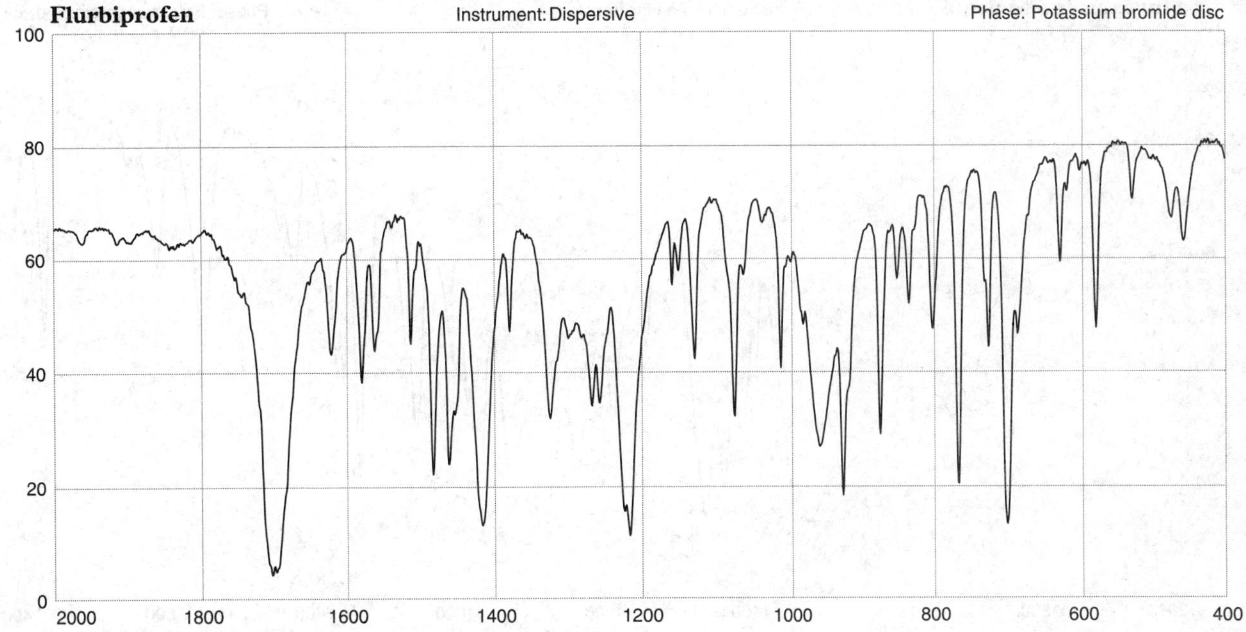

Flurbiprofen Sodium Instrument: Dispersive Phase: Potassium bromide disc

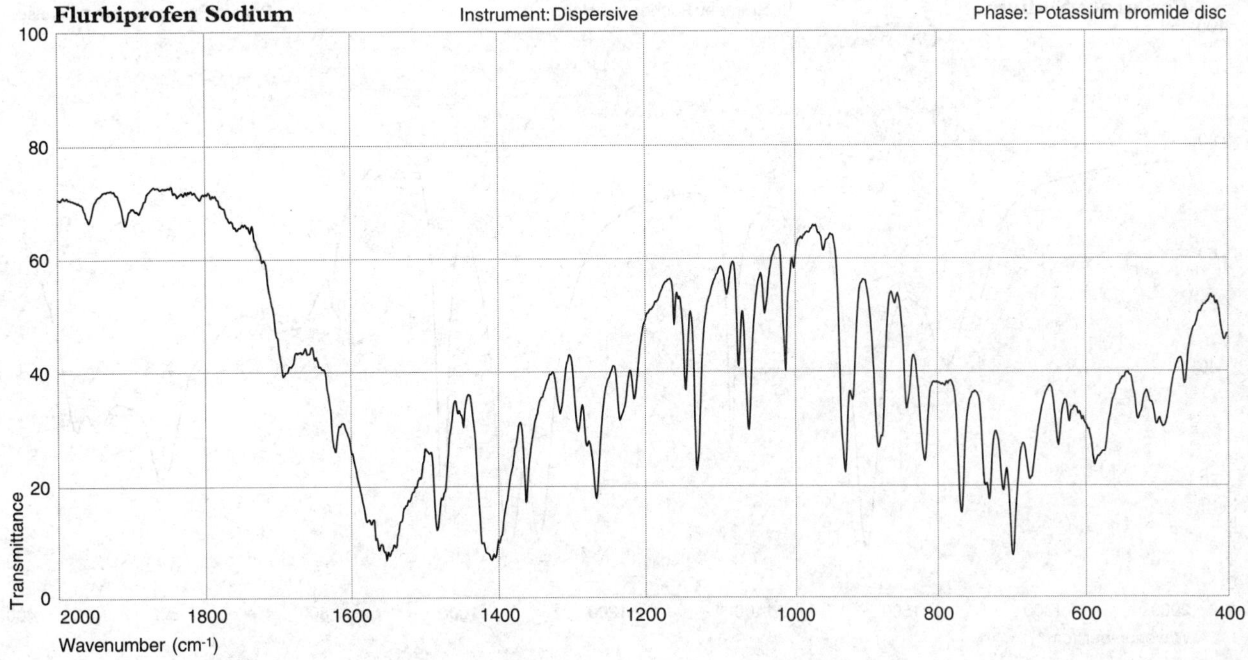

Fluticasone Propionate Instrument: Fourier transform Phase: Liquid paraffin mull

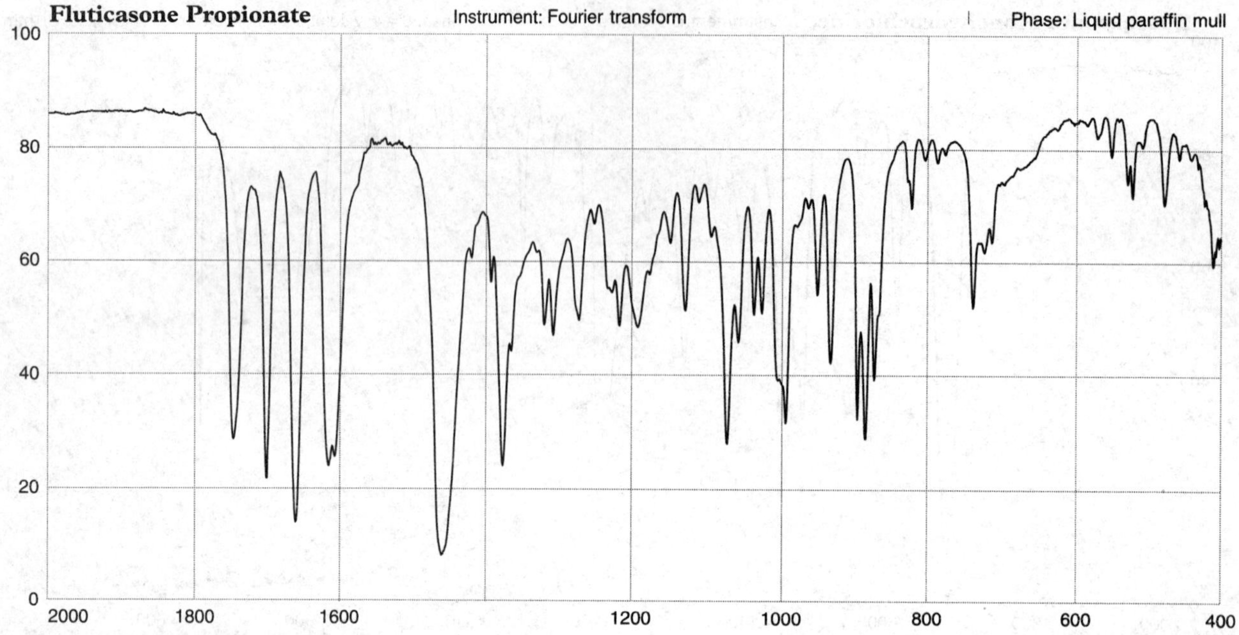

Fluvoxamine Maleate Instrument: Fourier transform Phase: Potassium bromide disc

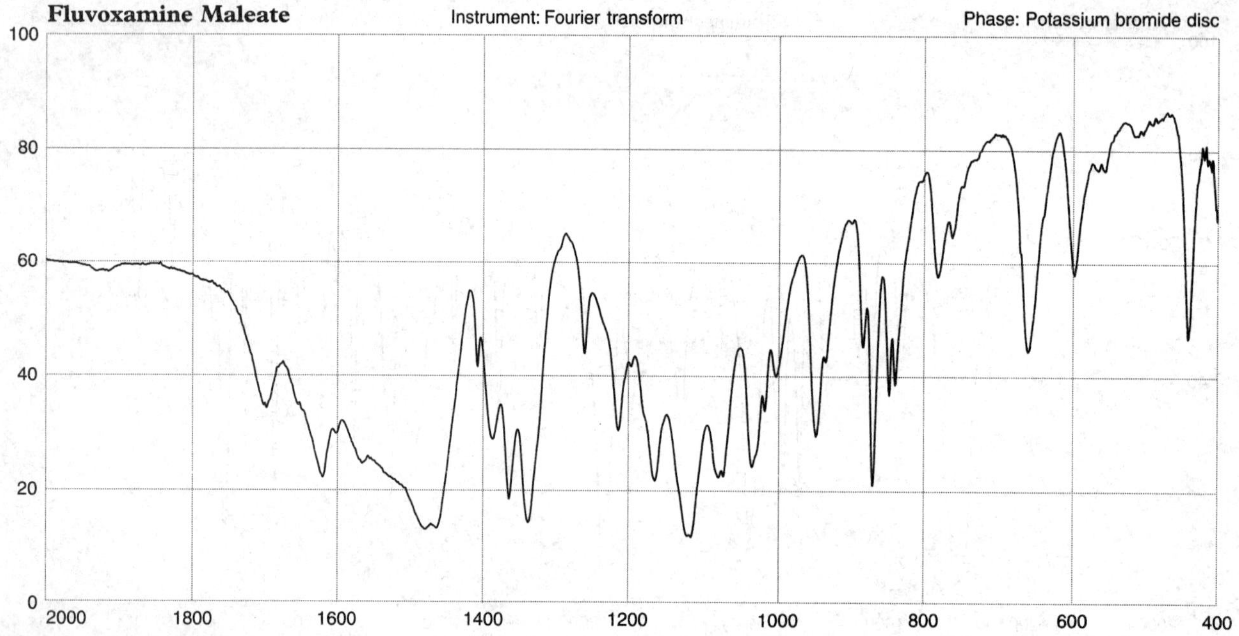

Foscarnet Sodium Instrument: Fourier transform Phase: Potassium bromide disc

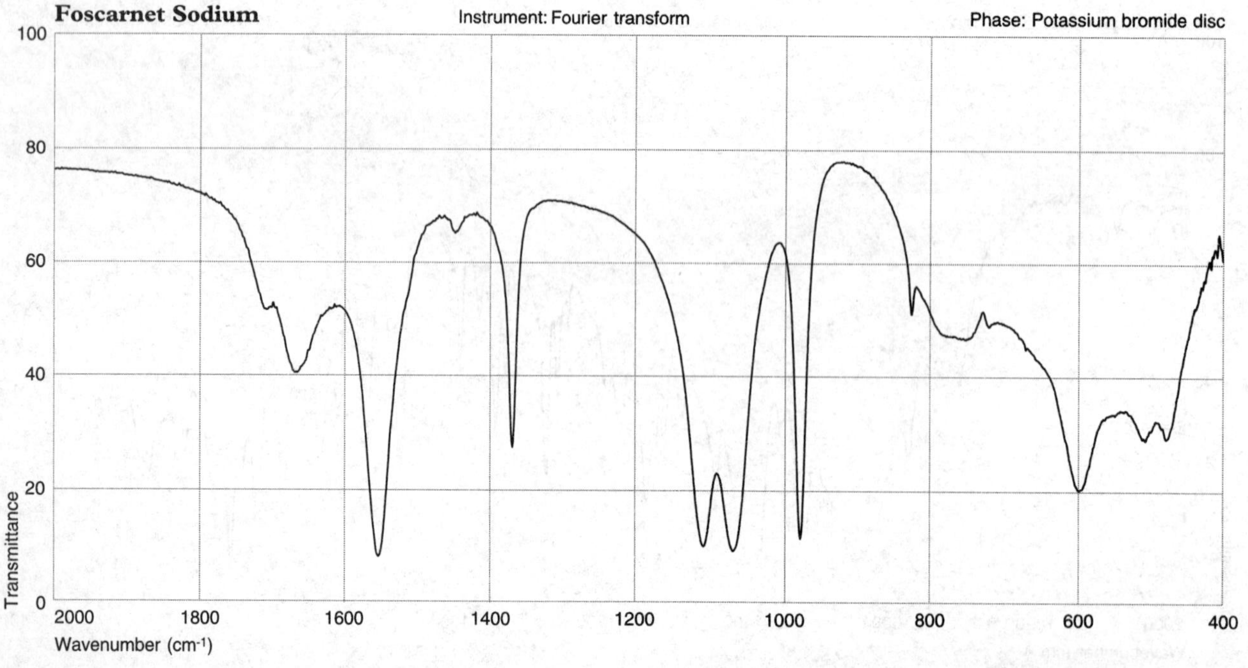

Fosfestrol Sodium Instrument: Dispersive Phase: Liquid paraffin mull

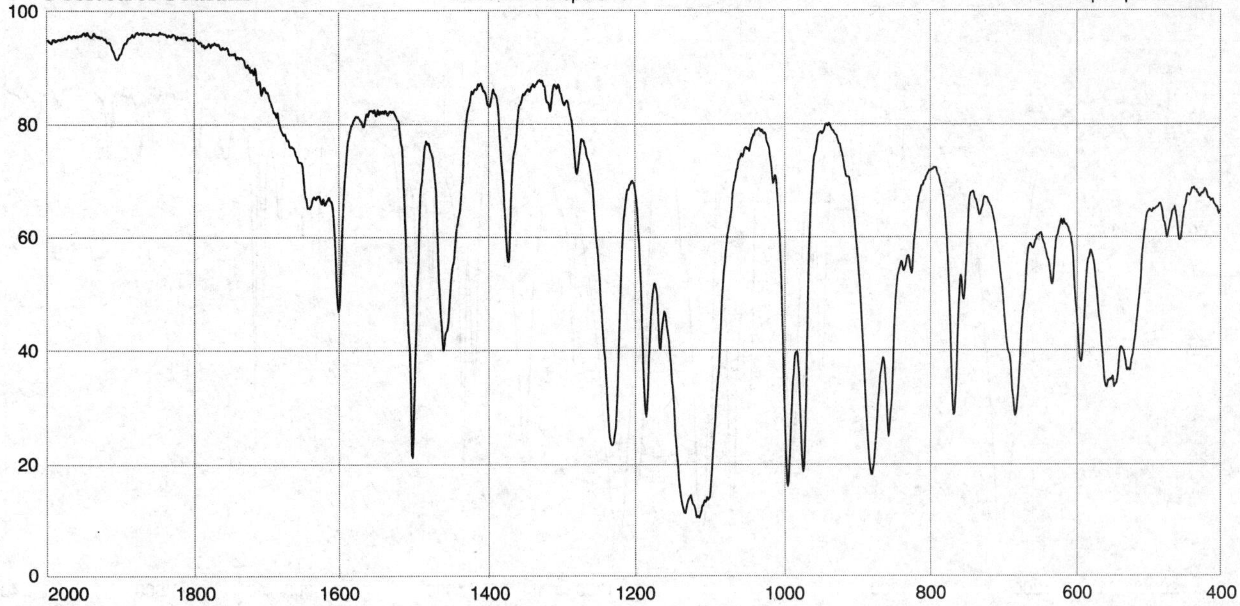

Frusemide (Furosemide) Instrument: Dispersive Phase: Potassium bromide disc

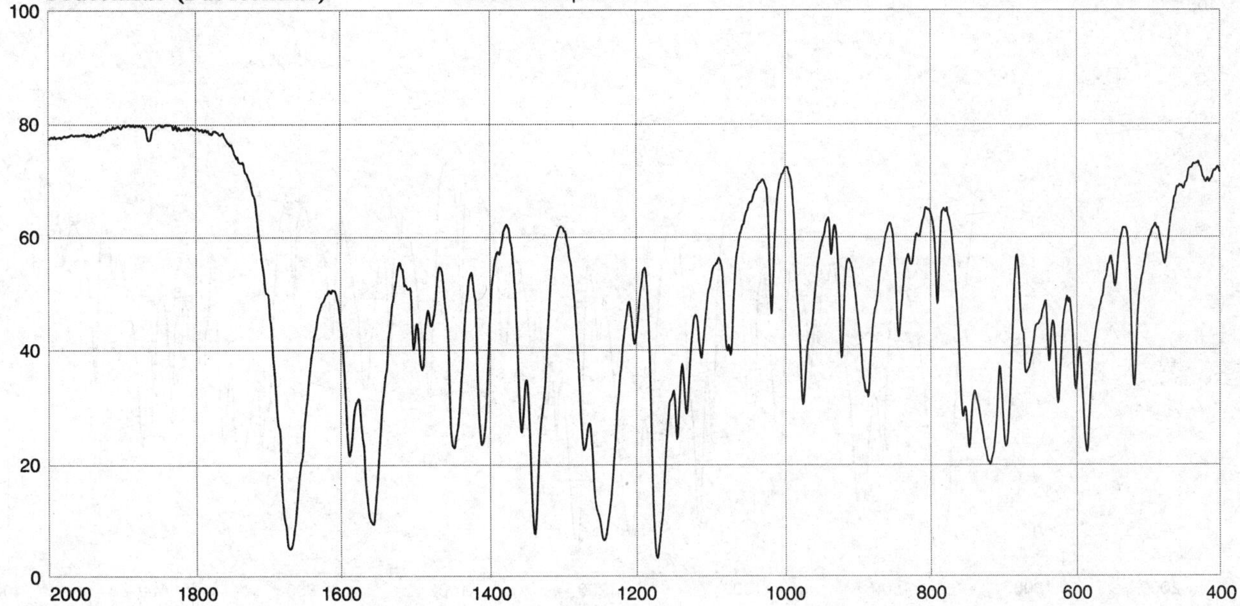

Fumaric Acid Instrument: Dispersive Phase: Potassium bromide disc

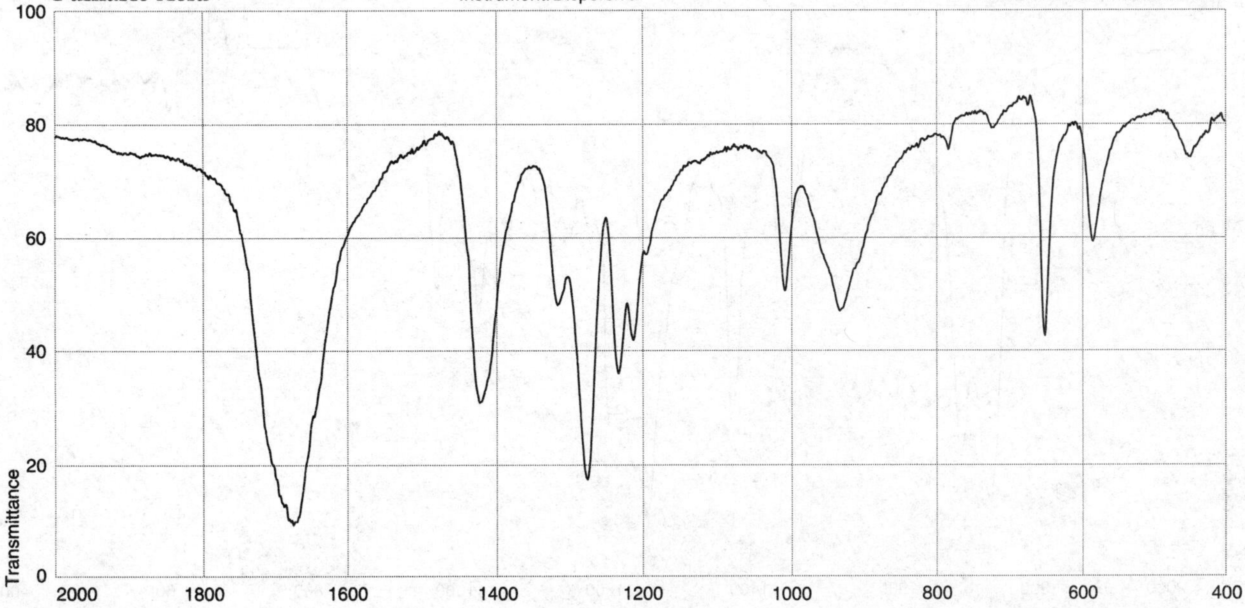

Furazolidone

Instrument: Dispersive | Phase: Potassium bromide disc

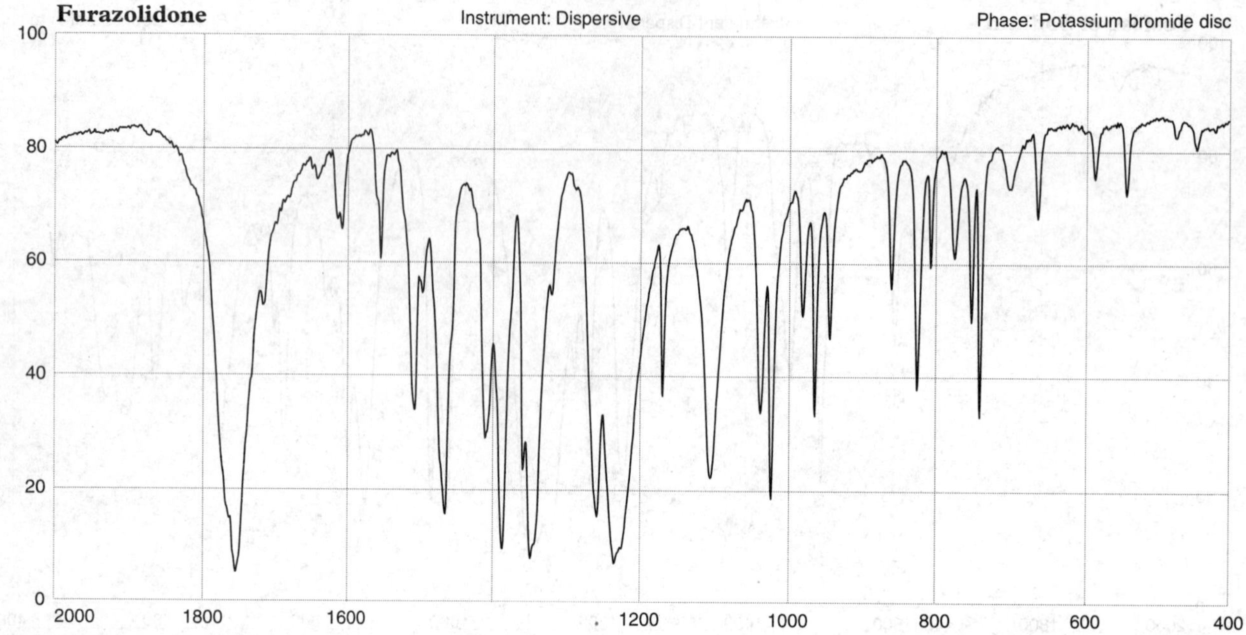

Furosemide (Frusemide)

Instrument: Dispersive | Phase: Potassium bromide disc

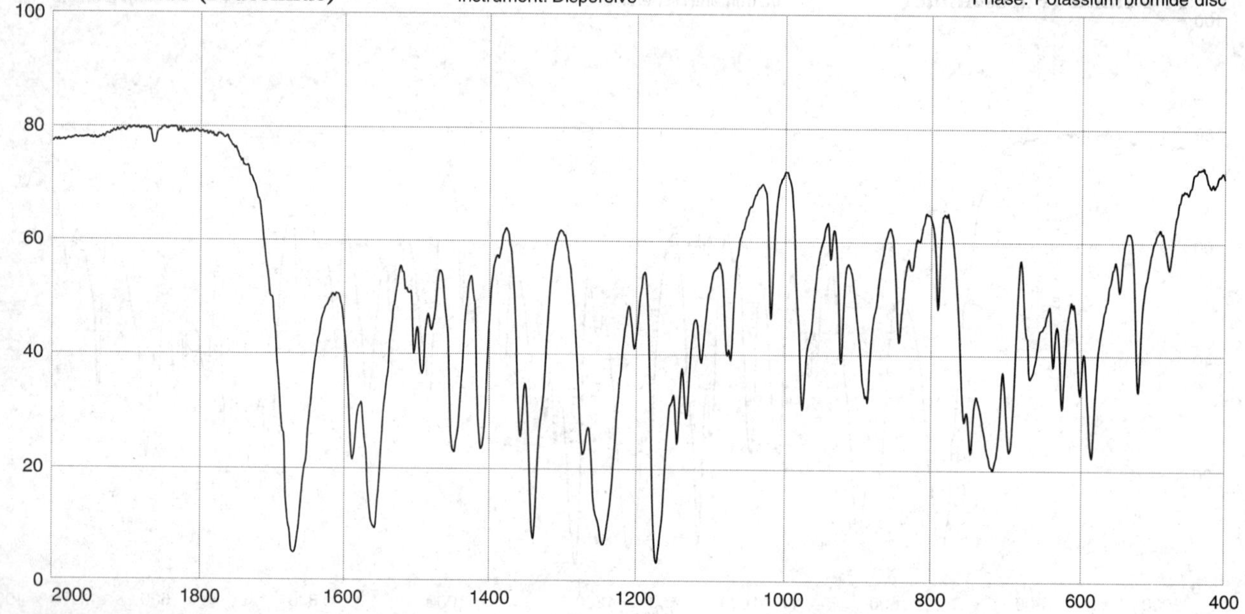

Fusidic Acid

Instrument: Dispersive | Phase: 10% w/v solution in chloroform | Thickness: 0.1mm

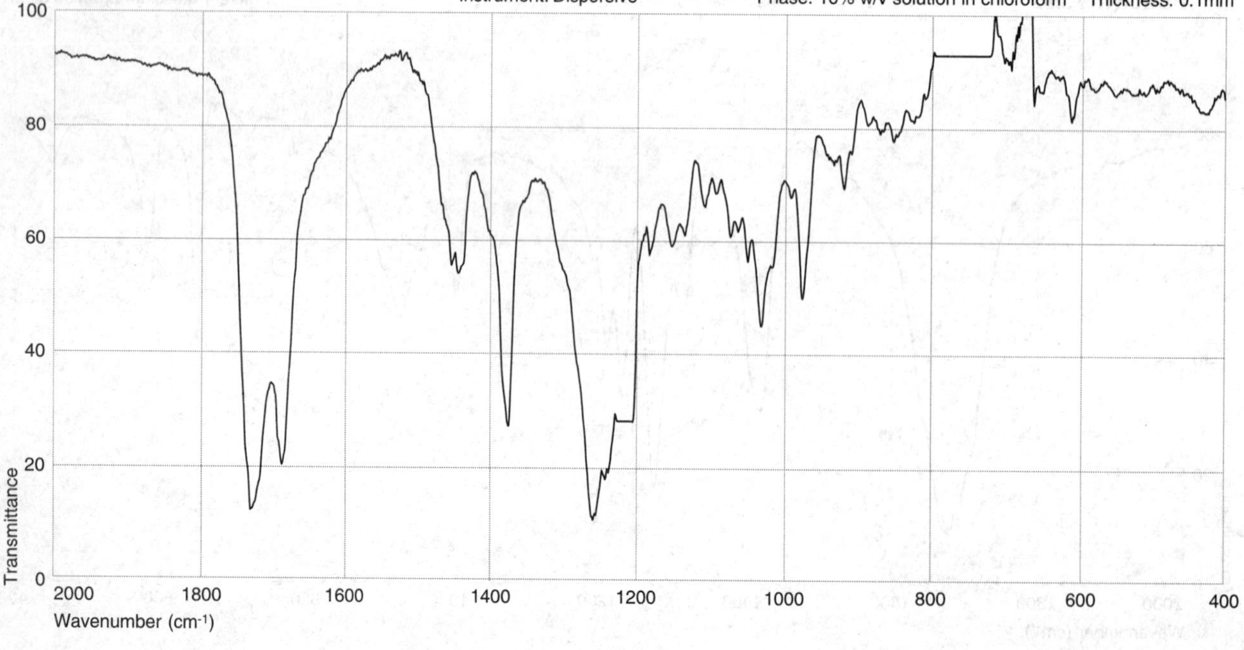

Gemfibrozil Instrument: Dispersive Phase: Potassium bromide disc

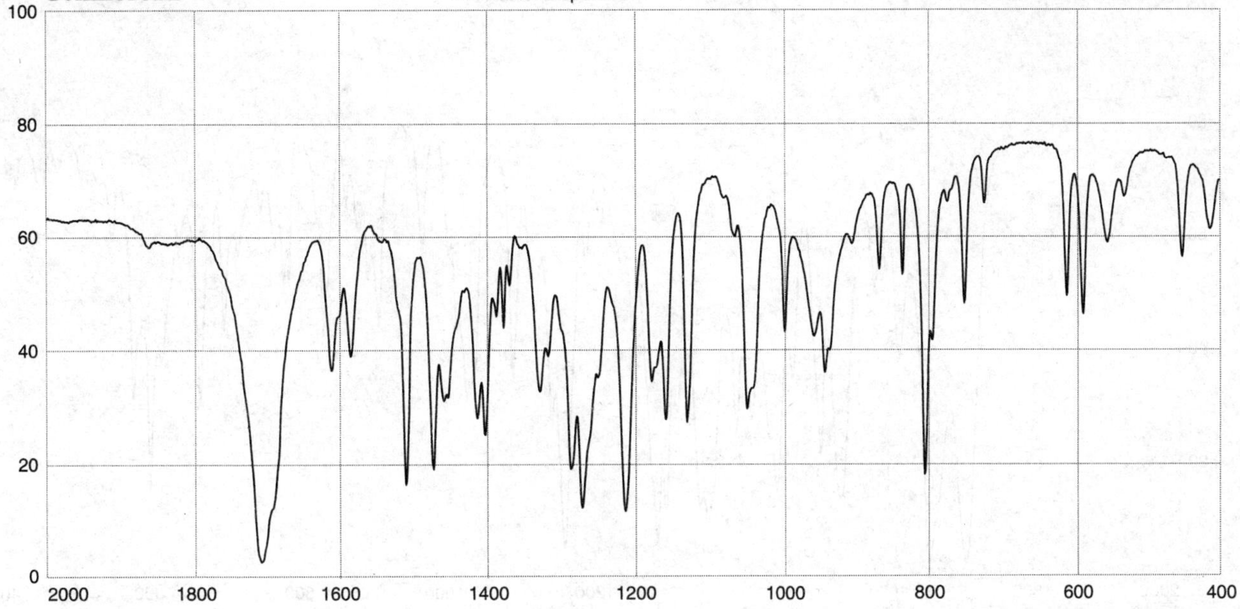

Gliclazide Instrument: Dispersive Phase: Potassium bromide disc

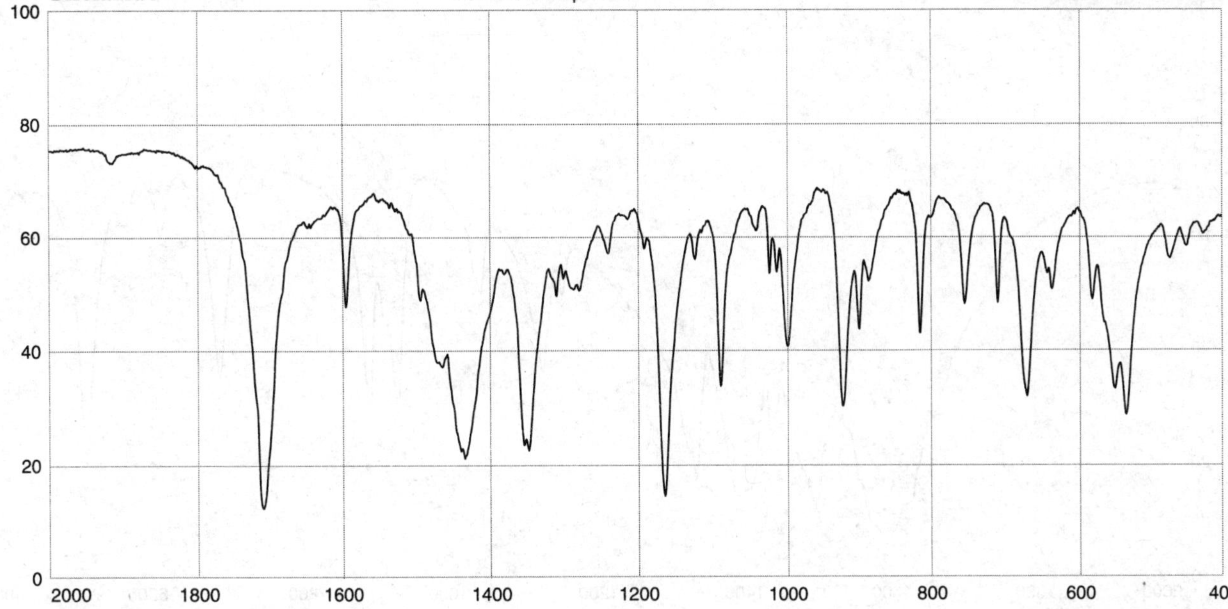

Glipizide Instrument: Dispersive Phase: Potassium bromide disc

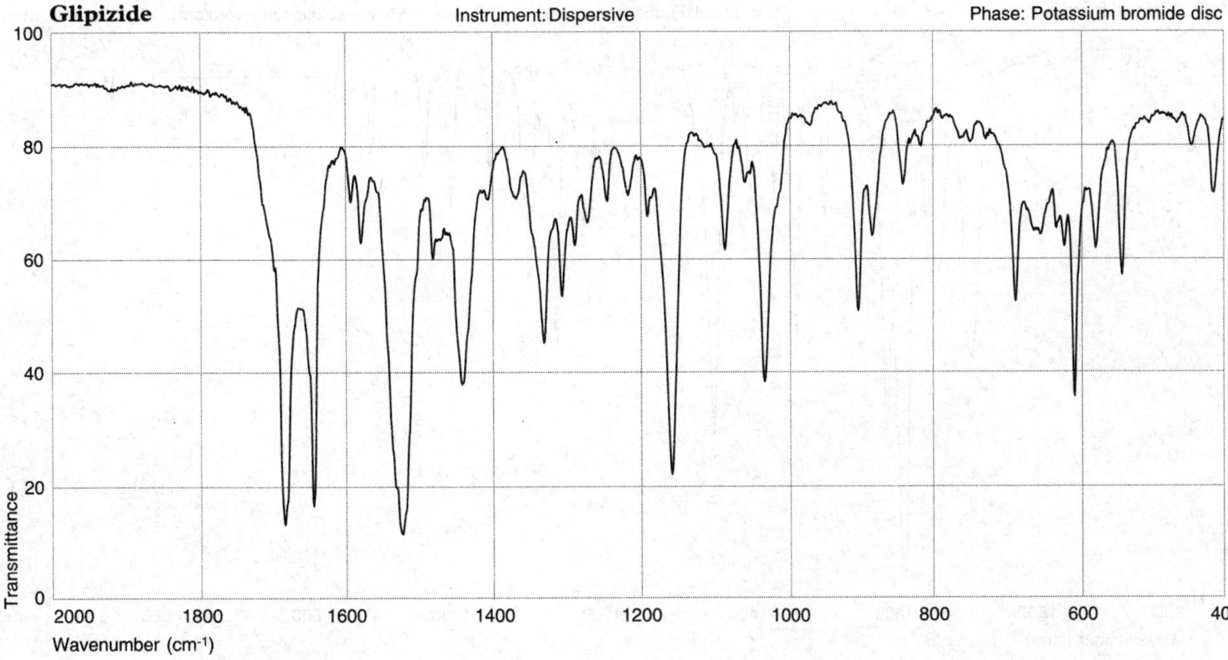

Gliquidone Instrument: Fourier transform Phase: Potassium bromide disc

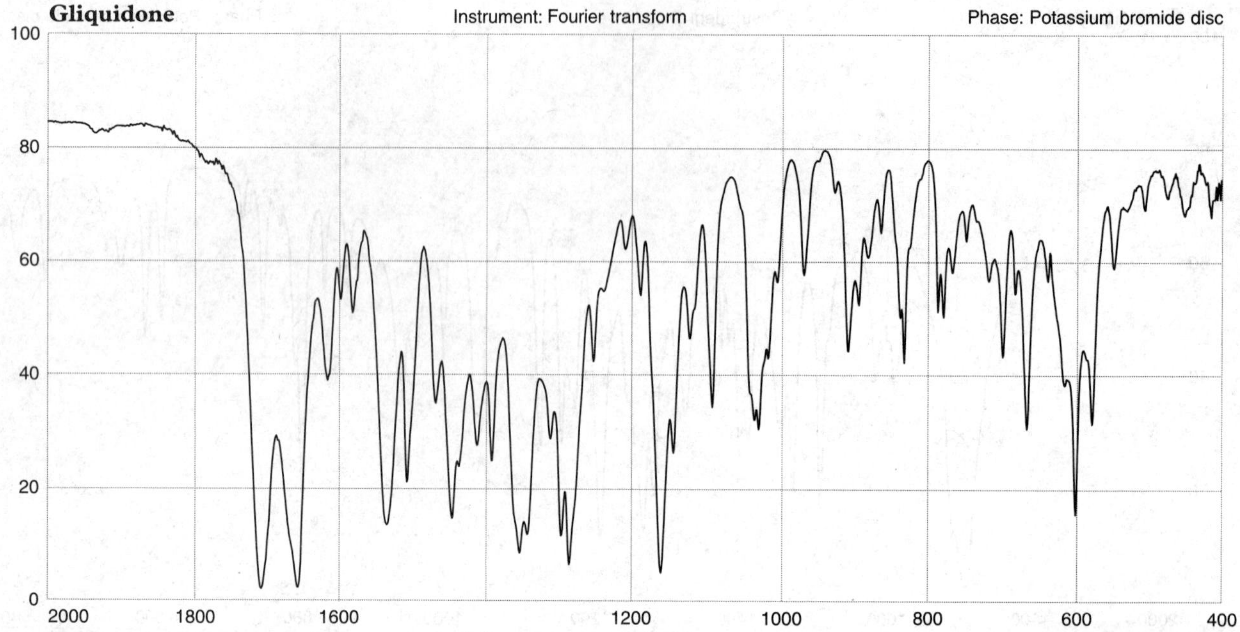

Glycine Instrument: Dispersive Phase: Potassium bromide disc

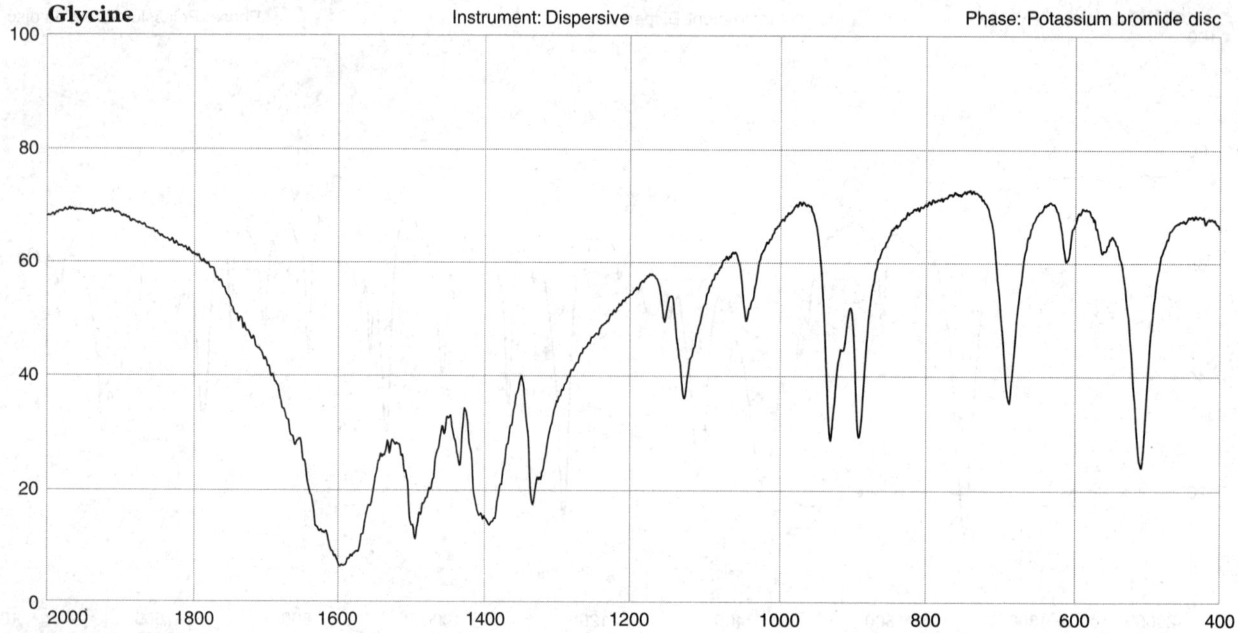

Griseofulvin Instrument: Fourier transform Phase: 1.5% w/v solution in chloroform Thickness: 0.1mm

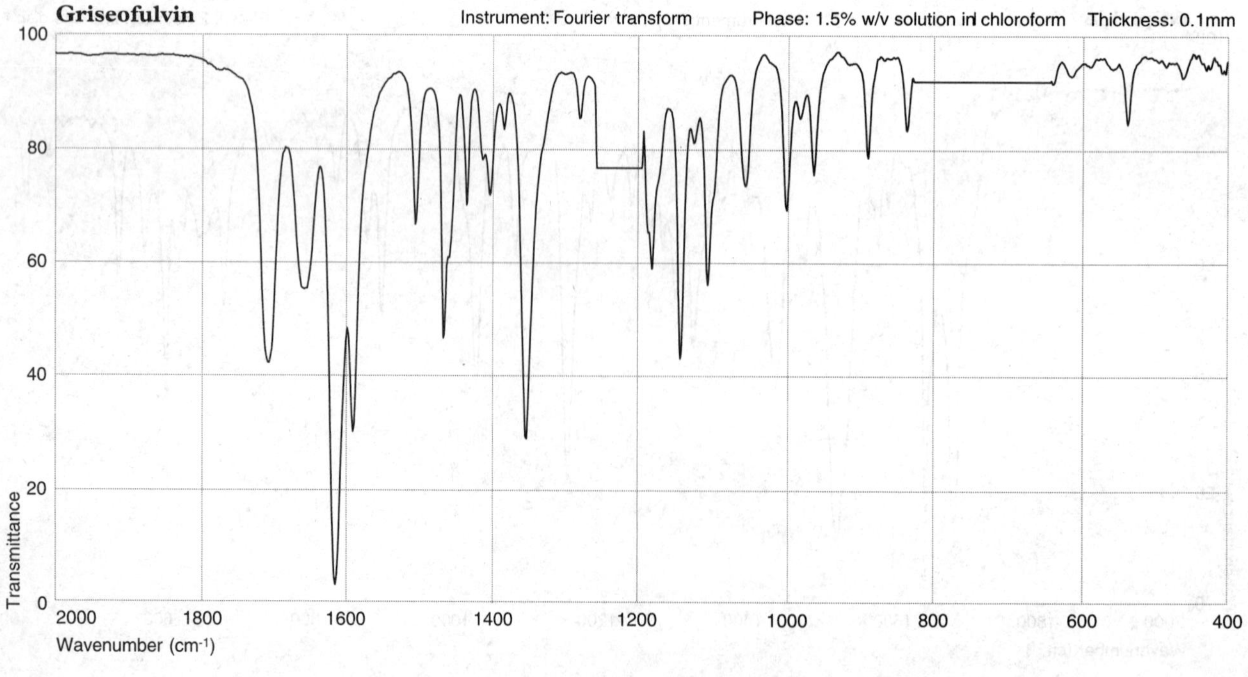

Haloperidol

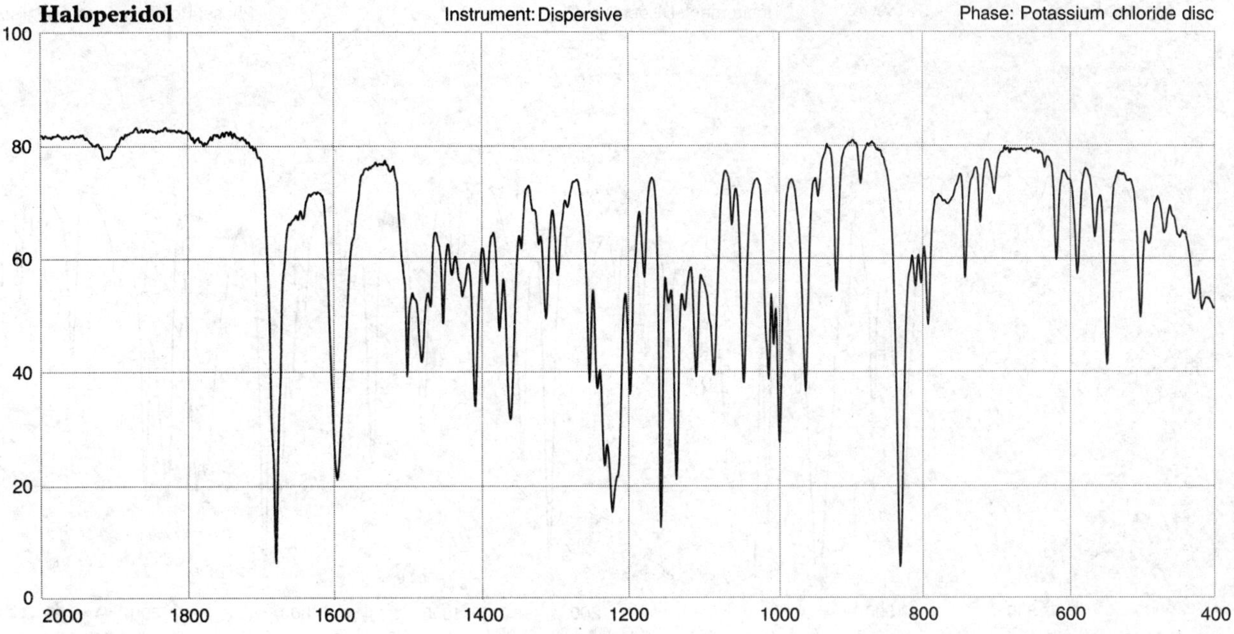

Hexachlorophene

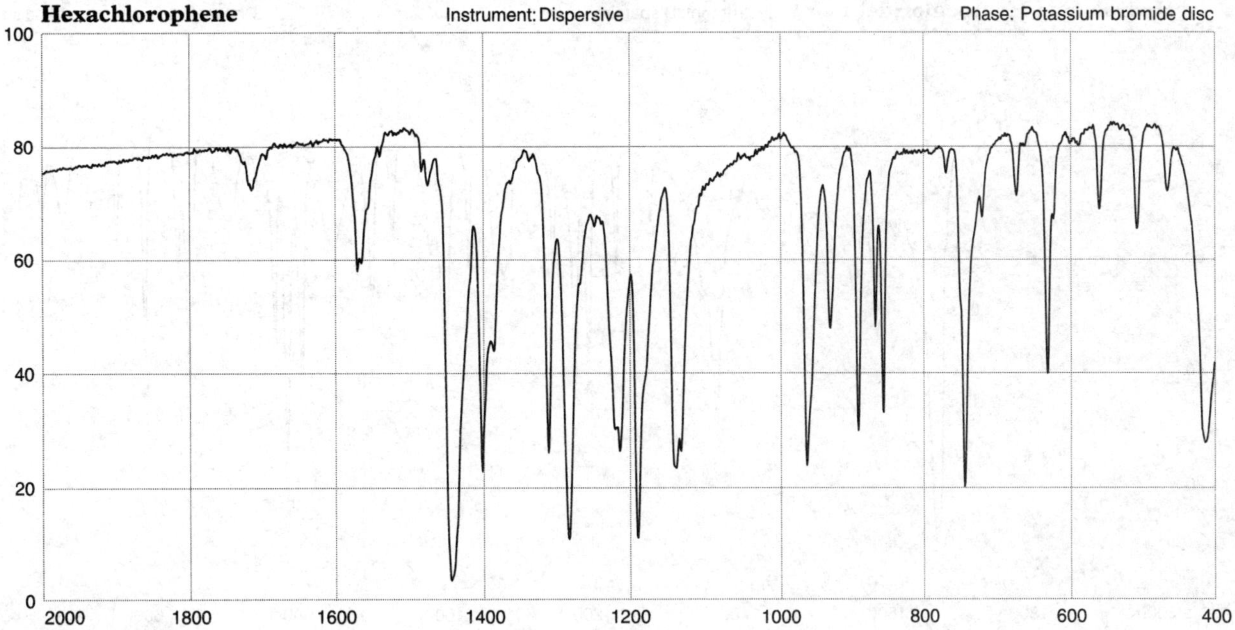

Homatropine

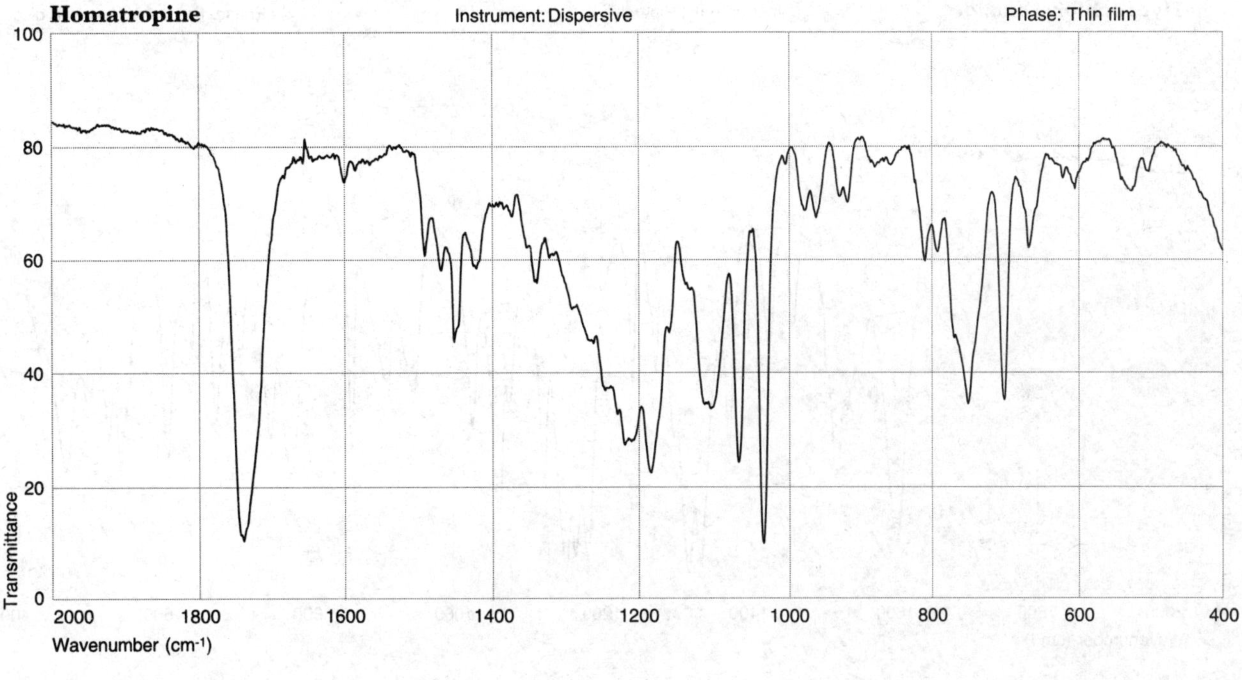

Hydralazine Instrument: Dispersive Phase: Potassium bromide disc

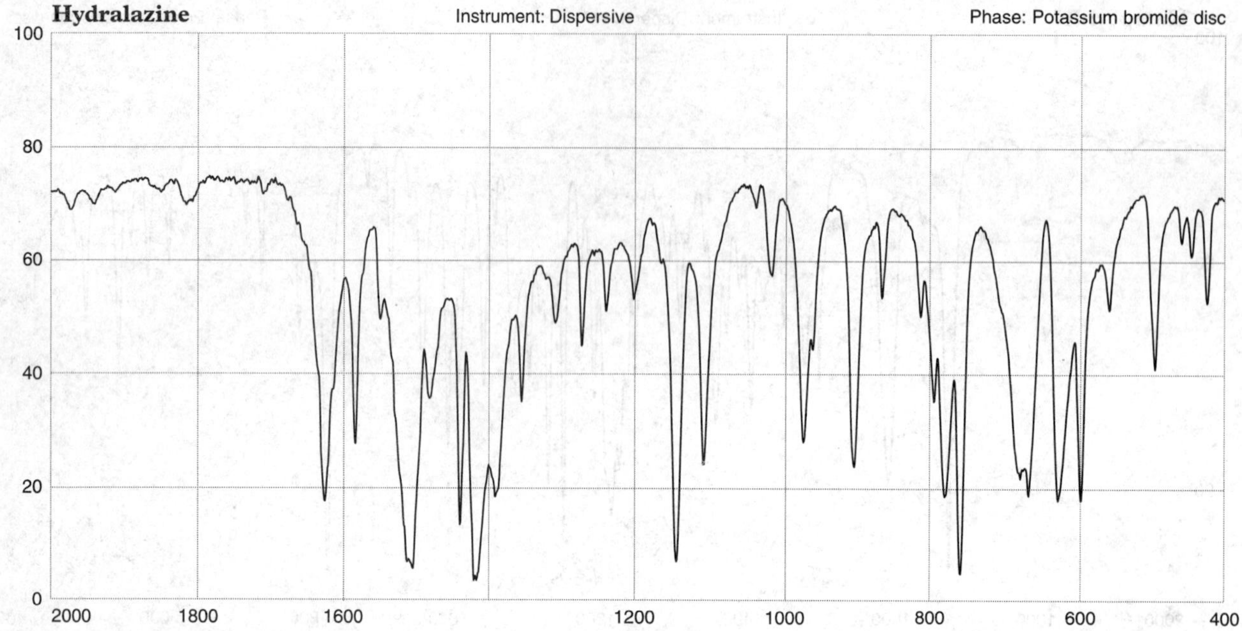

Hydralazine Hydrochloride Instrument: Dispersive Phase: Potassium chloride disc

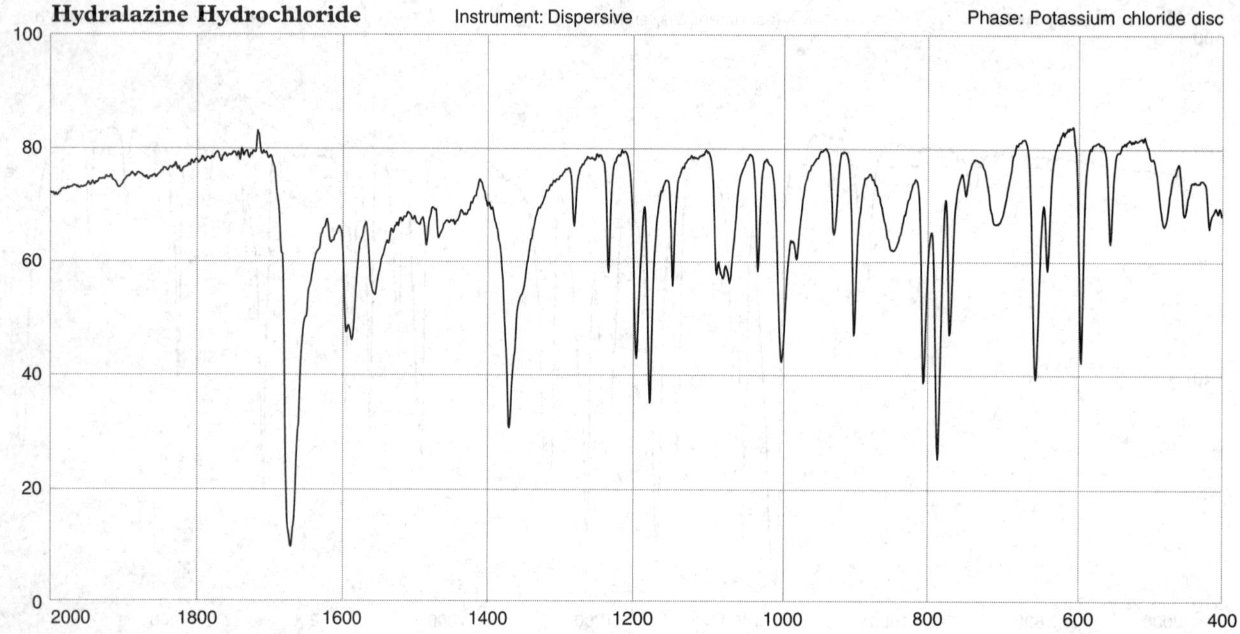

Hydrochlorothiazide Instrument: Dispersive Phase: Potassium bromide disc

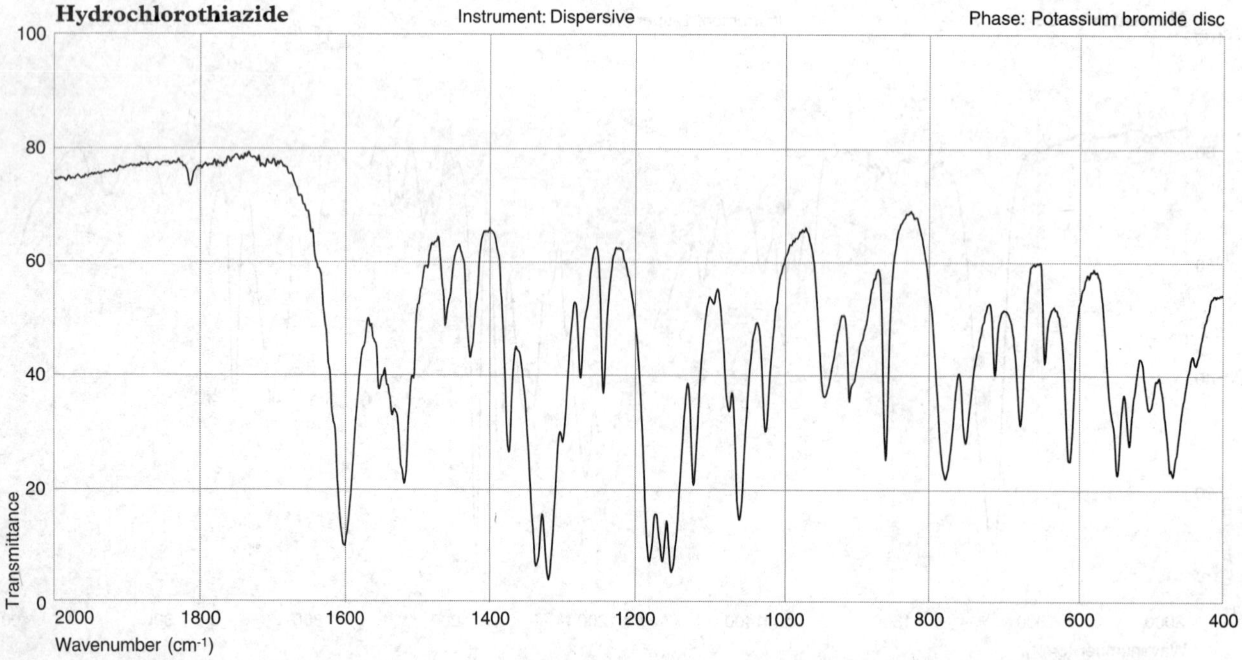

Hydrocortisone Acetate Instrument: Dispersive Phase: Potassium bromide disc

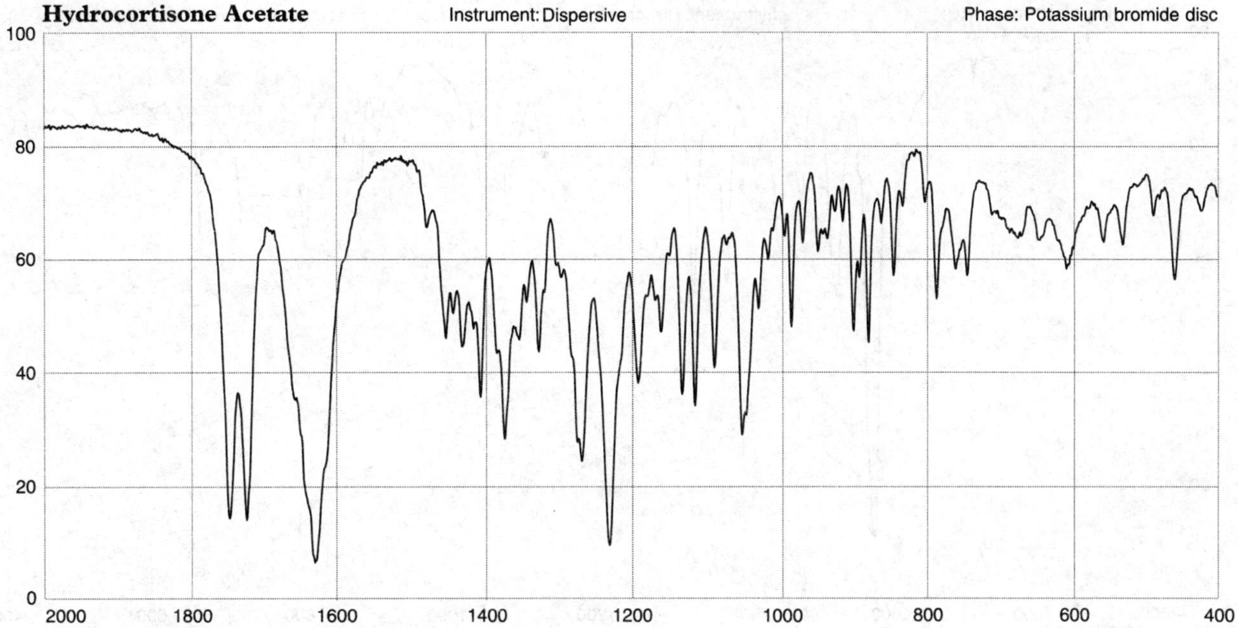

Hydrocortisone Sodium Succinate Instrument: Dispersive Phase: Potassium bromide disc

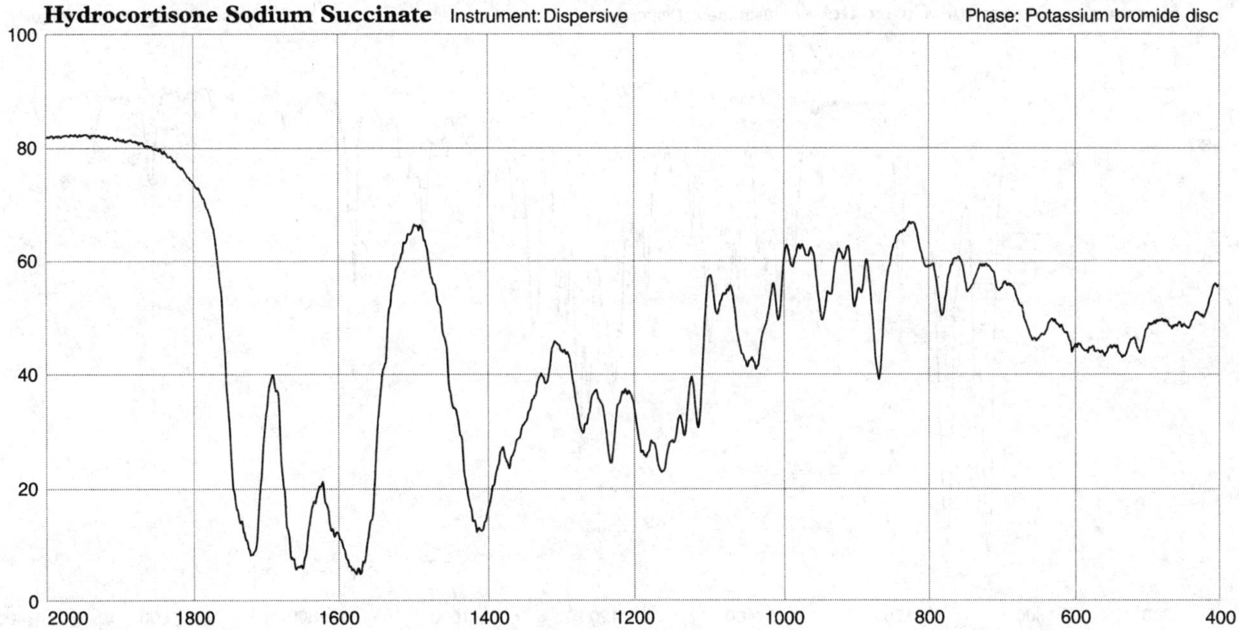

Hydroflumethiazide Instrument: Dispersive Phase: Potassium bromide disc

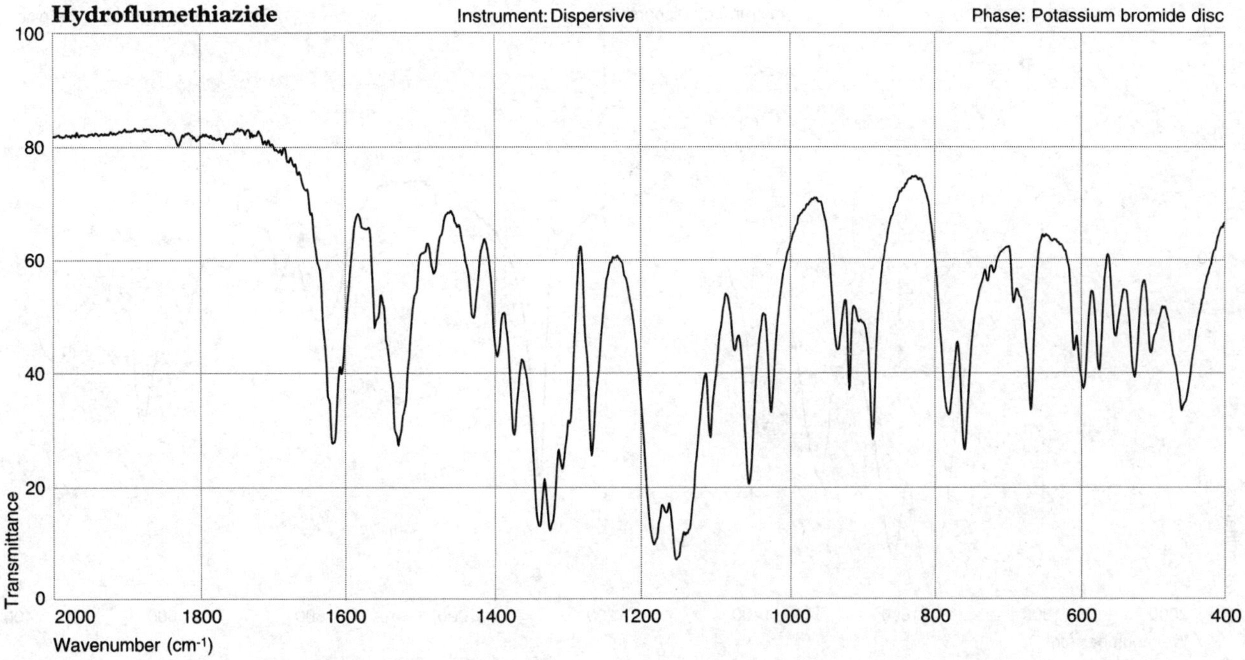

Hydroxychloroquine Instrument: Dispersive Phase: 5% w/v solution in chloroform Thickness: 0.1mm

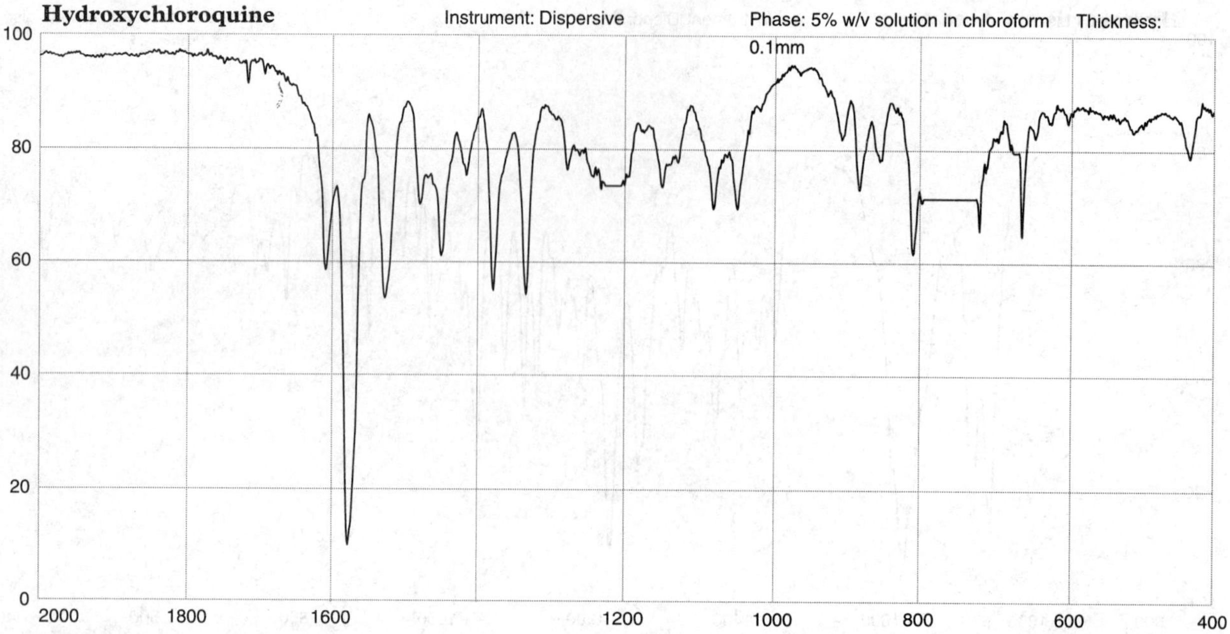

Hydroxyprogesterone Caproate Instrument: Dispersive Phase: Potassium bromide disc

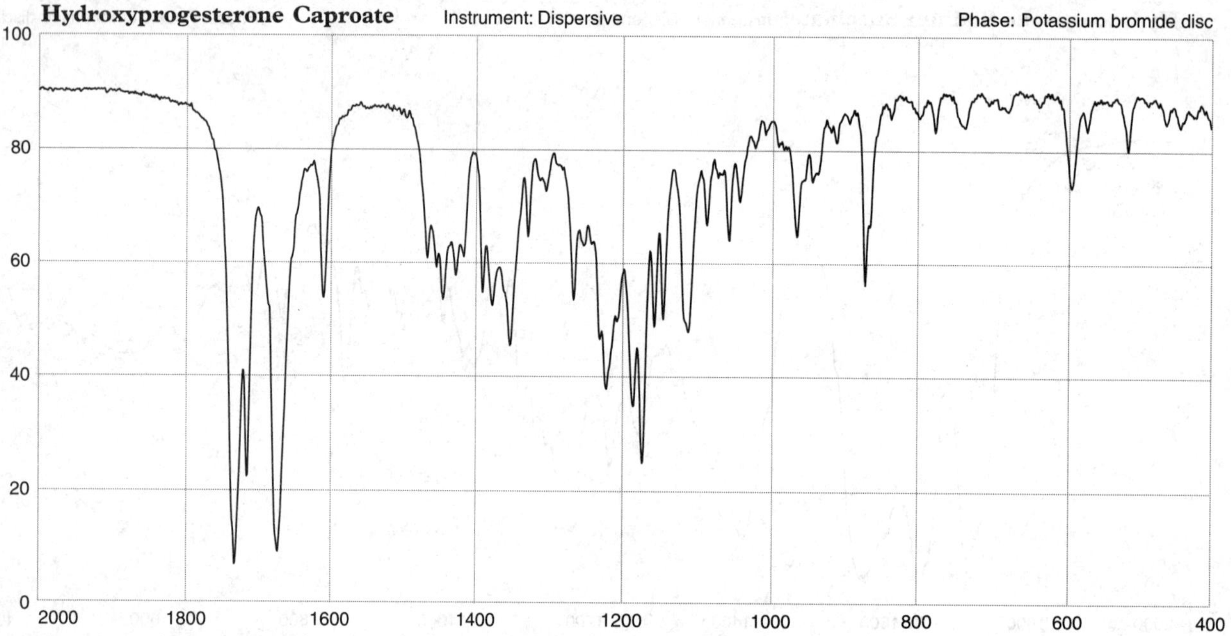

Hydroxycarbamide Instrument: Dispersive Phase: Potassium bromide disc

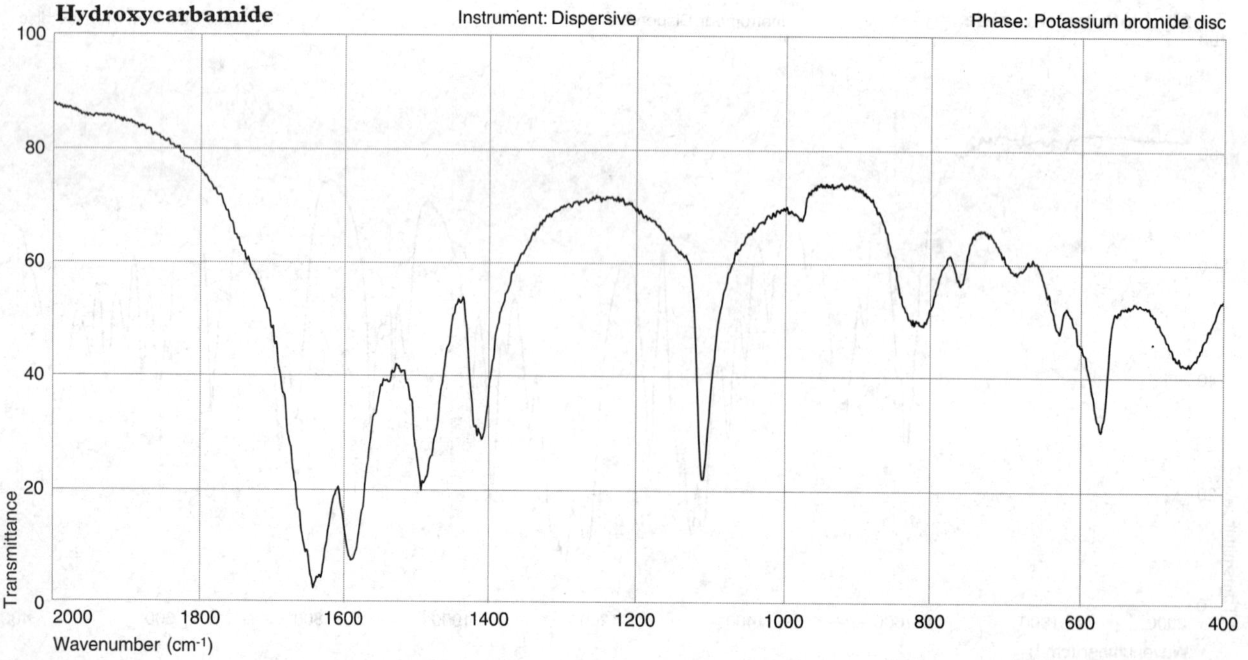

Hyoscine Butylbromide Instrument: Dispersive Phase: Potassium bromide disc

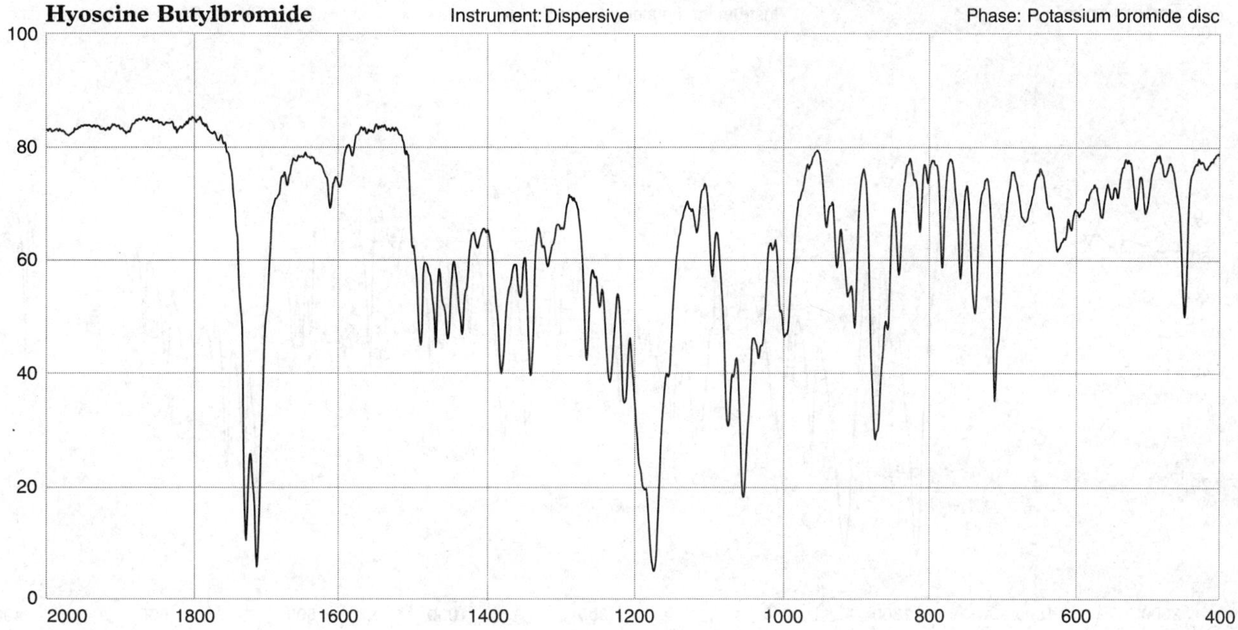

Ibuprofen Instrument: Dispersive Phase: Potassium bromide disc

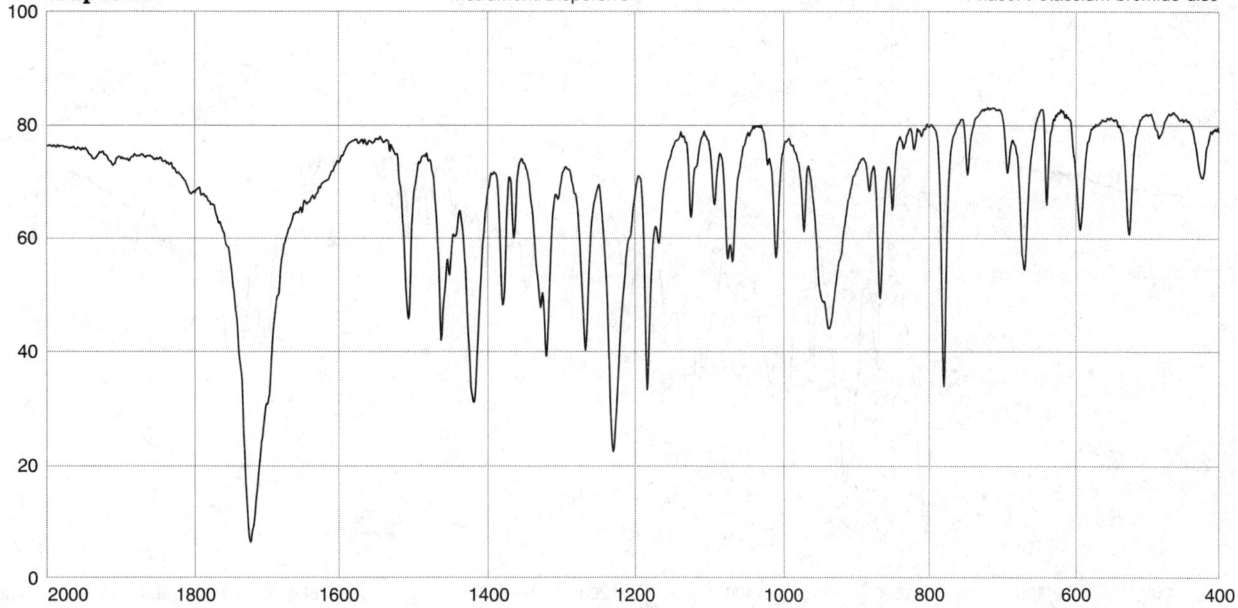

Indometacin Instrument: Dispersive Phase: Liquid paraffin mull

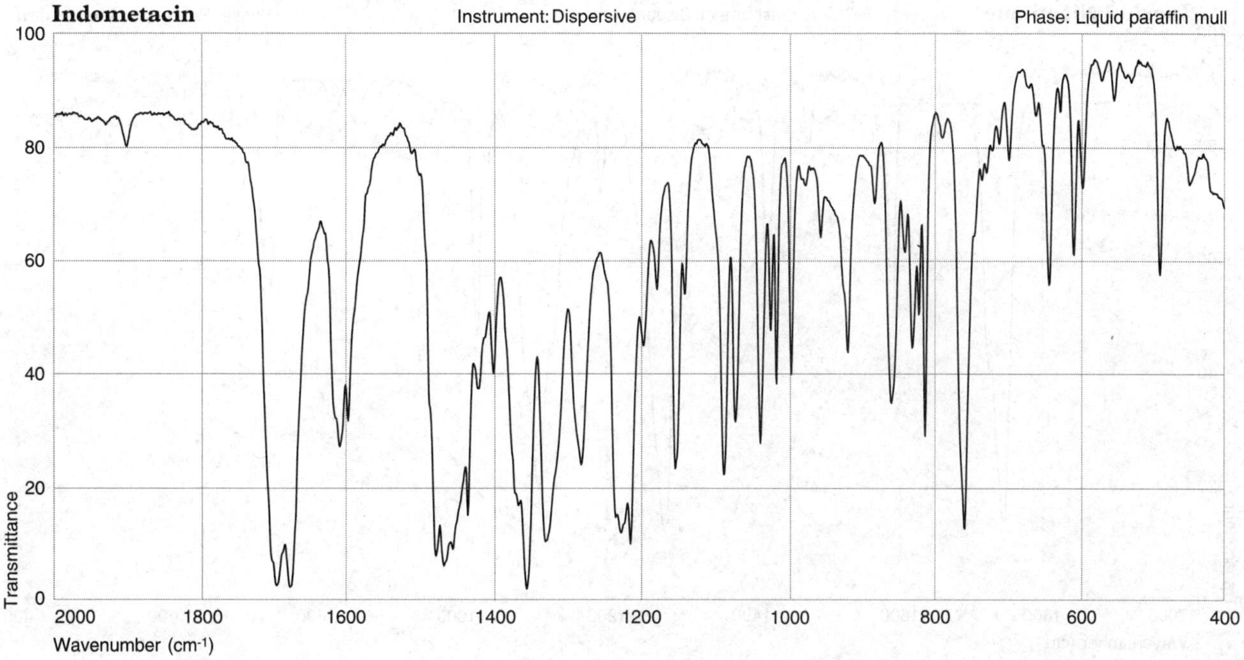

Indoramin Instrument: Fourier transform Phase: Potassium bromide disc

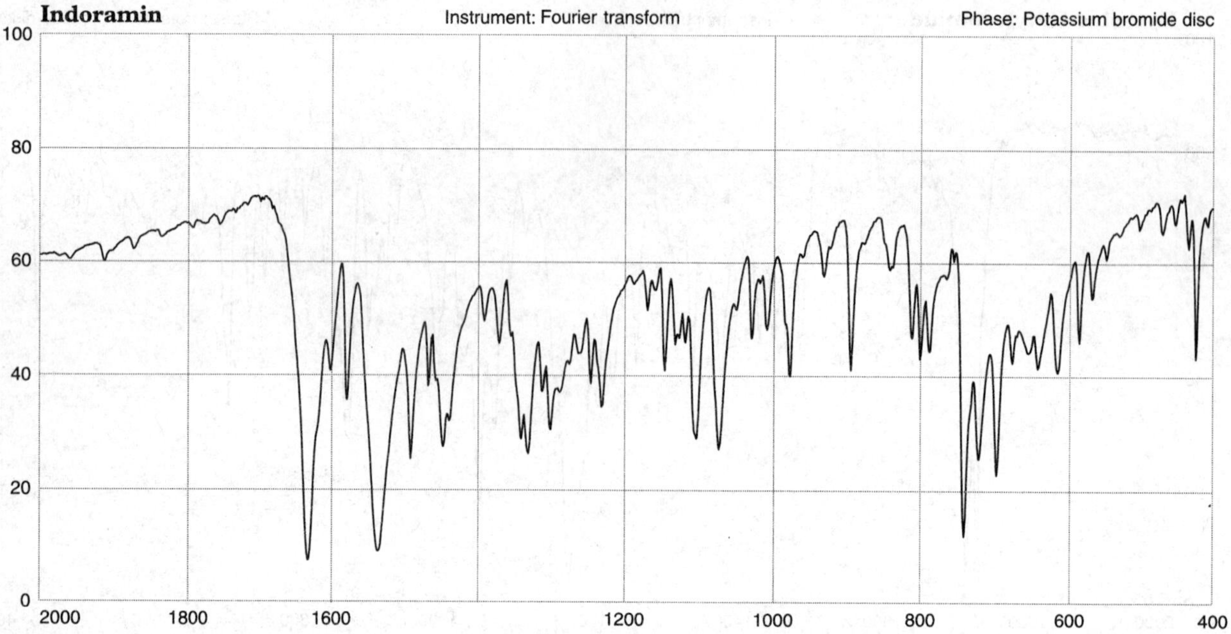

Indoramin Hydrochloride Instrument: Dispersive Phase: Potassium chloride disc

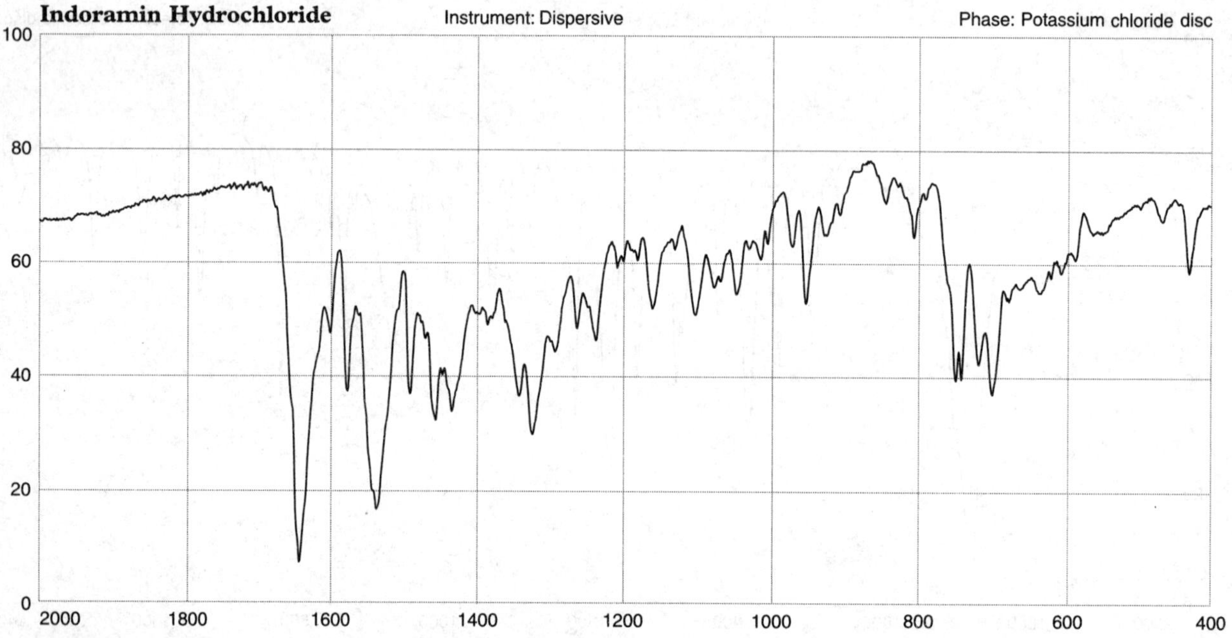

Inositol Nicotinate Instrument: Dispersive Phase: Potassium bromide disc

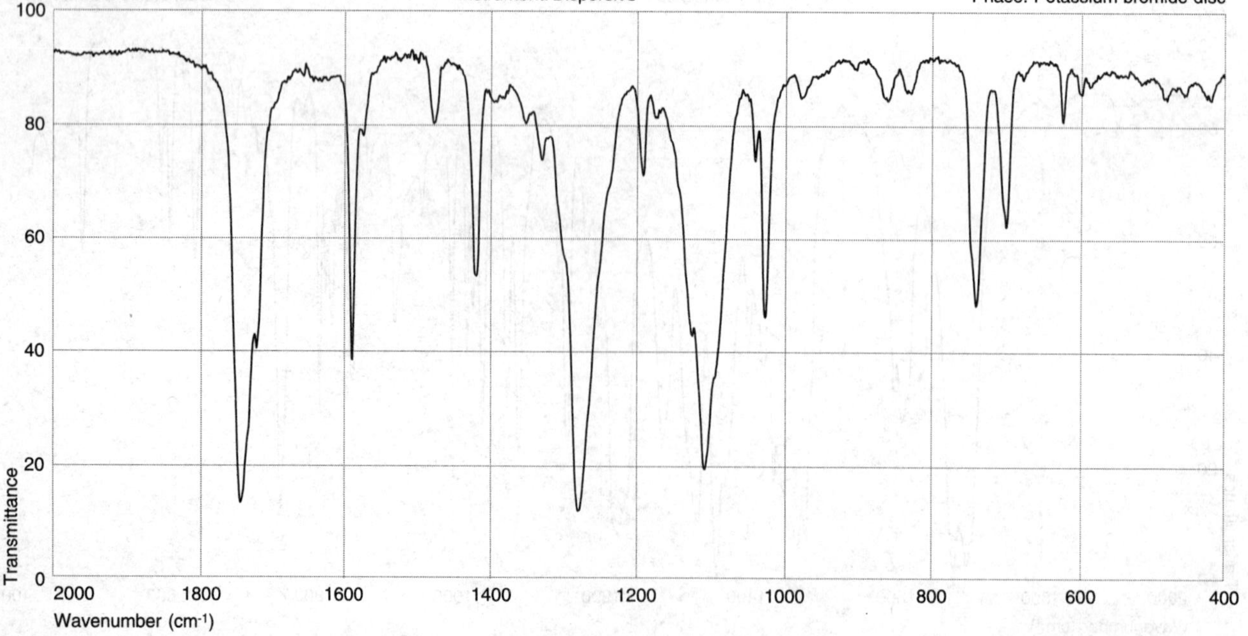

Iodipamide Instrument: Dispersive Phase: Liquid paraffin mull

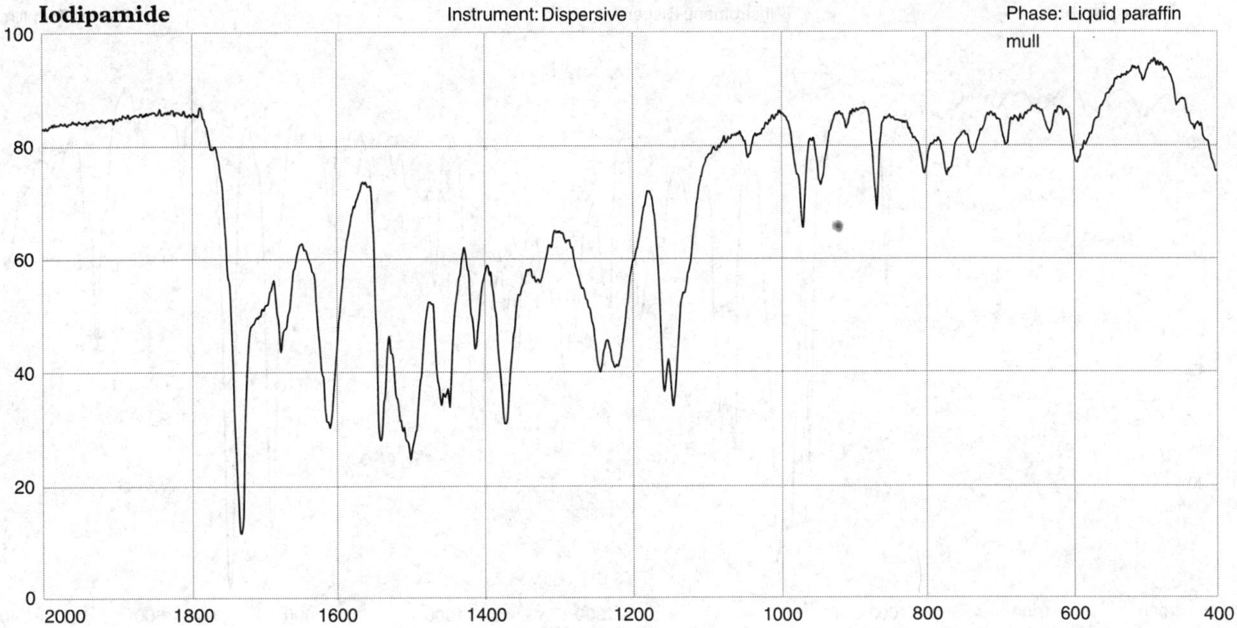

Iopanoic Acid Instrument: Dispersive Phase: Potassium bromide disc

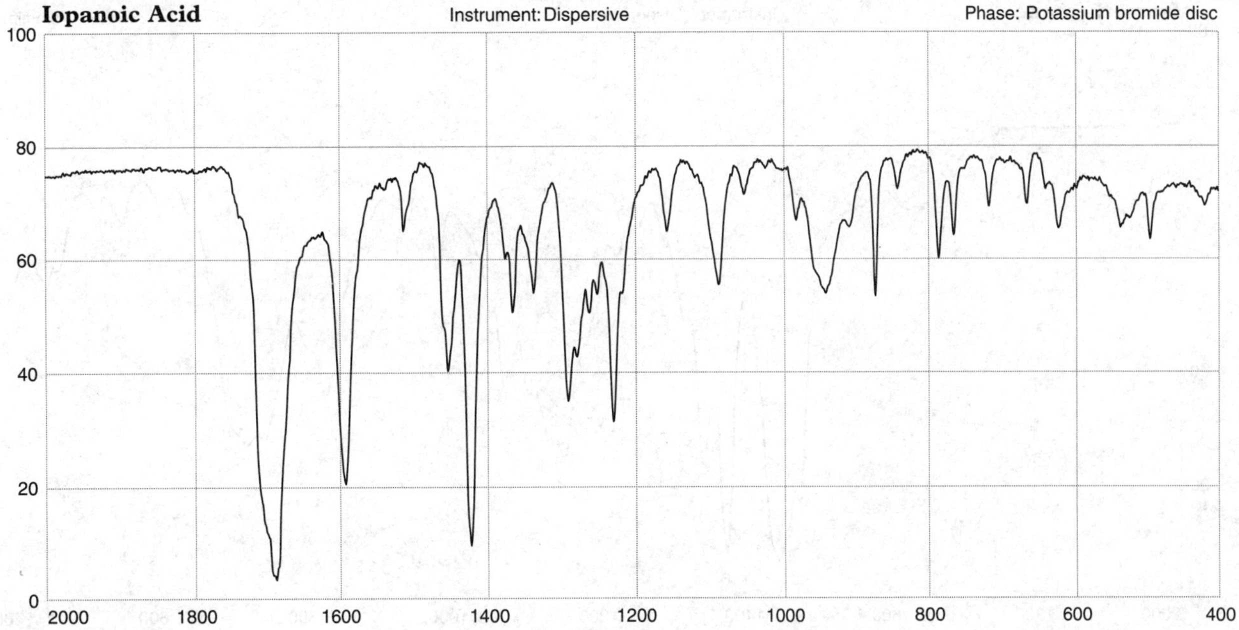

Iotalamic Acid Instrument: Dispersive Phase: Potassium bromide disc

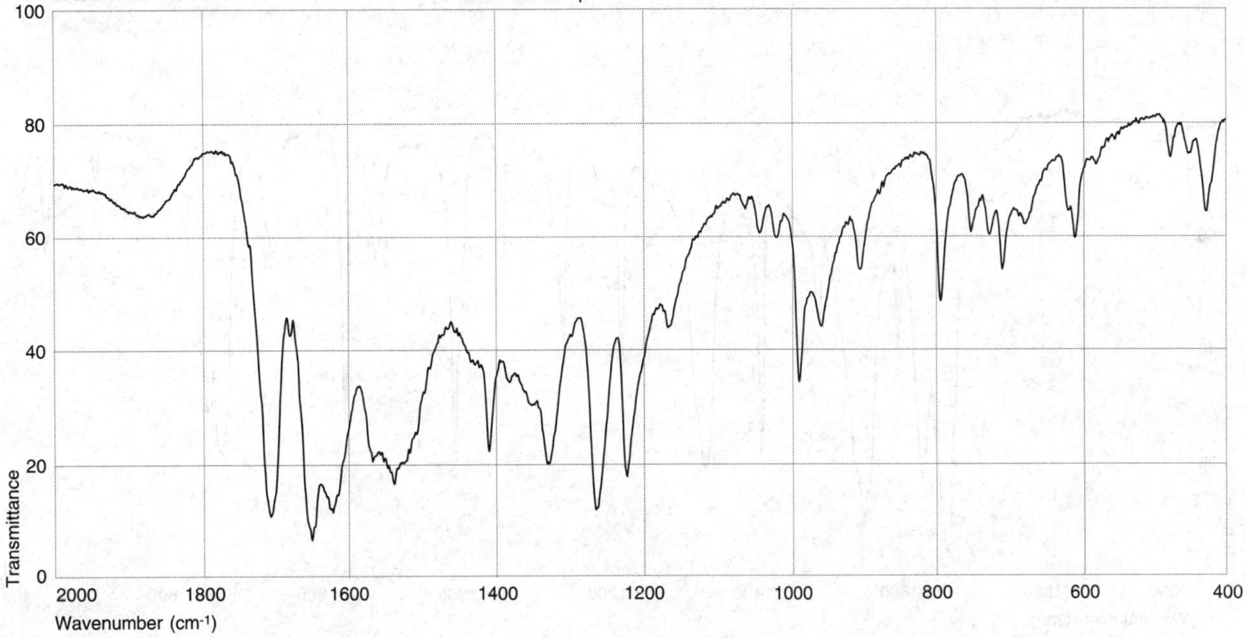

Isoaminile

Instrument: Dispersive | Phase: Thin film

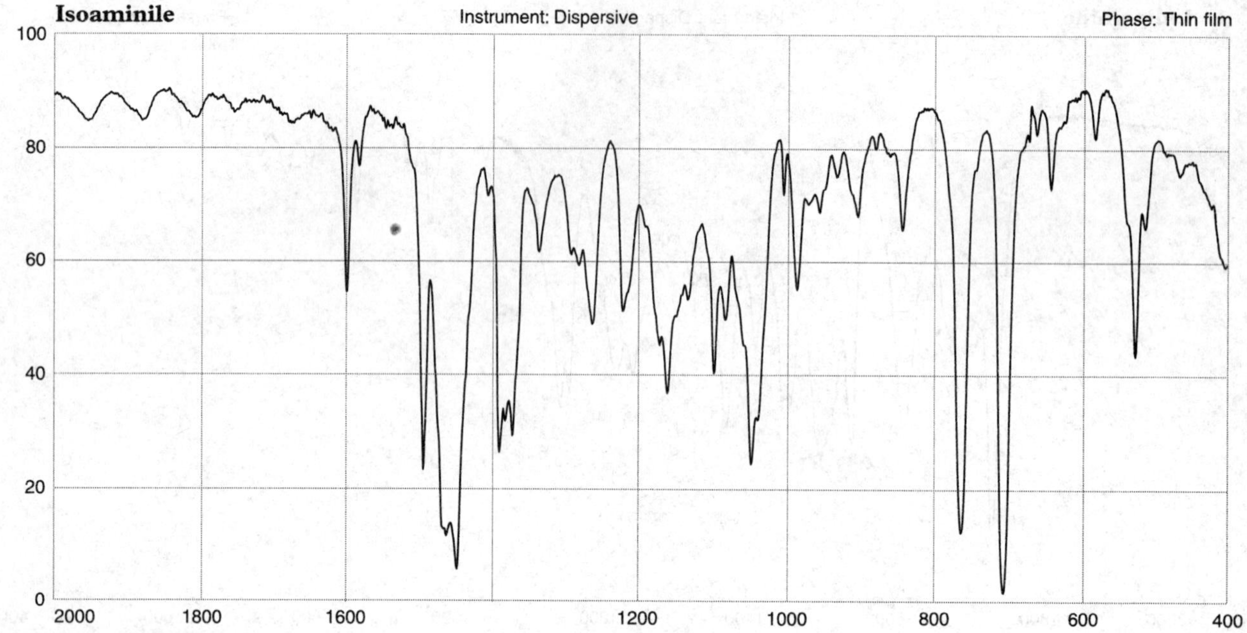

Isometheptene

Instrument: Dispersive | Phase: Thin film

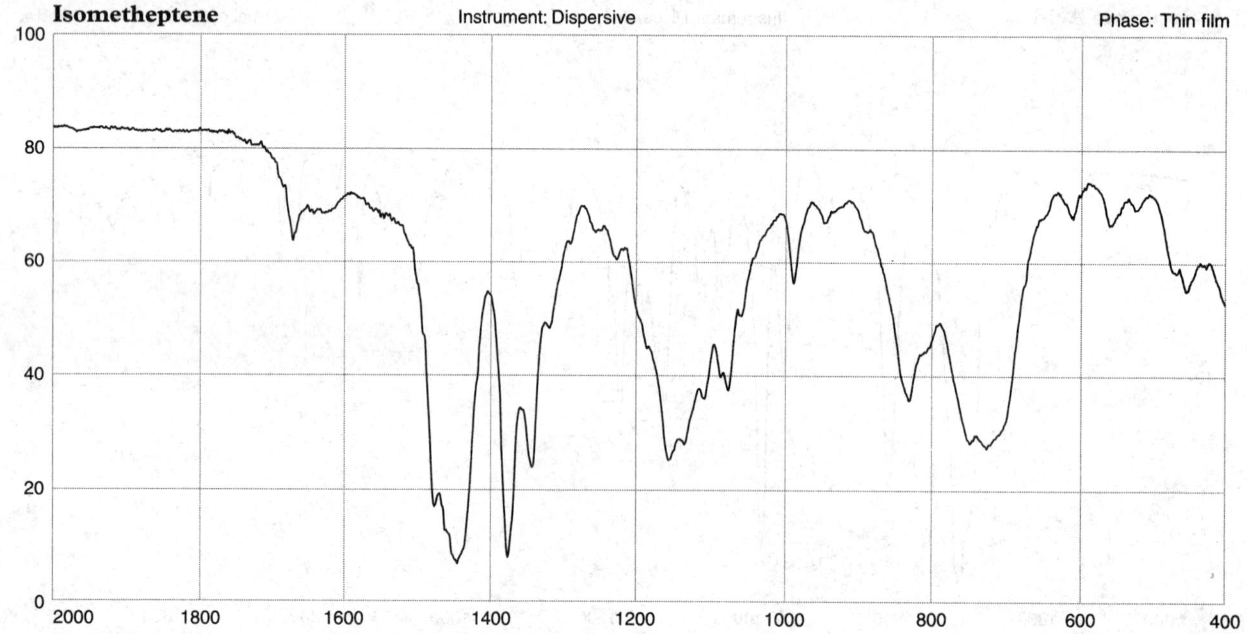

Isoniazid

Instrument: Dispersive | Phase: Potassium bromide disc

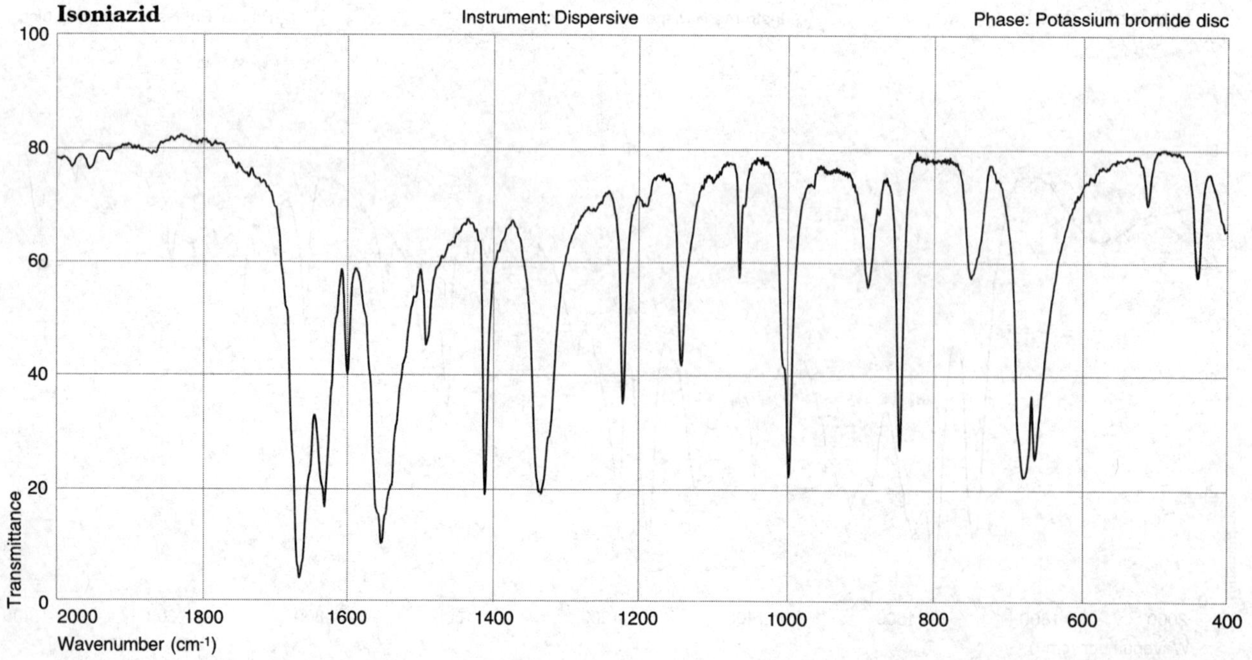

Isoprenaline Hydrochloride Instrument: Dispersive Phase: Potassium chloride disc

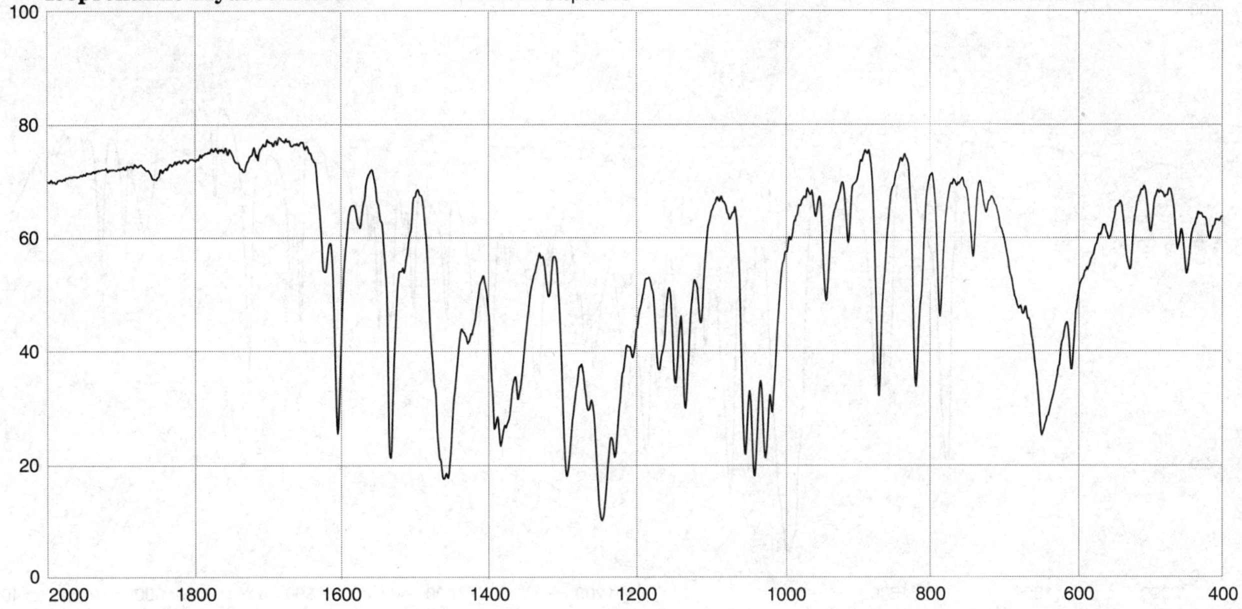

Ketoprofen Instrument: Dispersive Phase: Potassium bromide disc

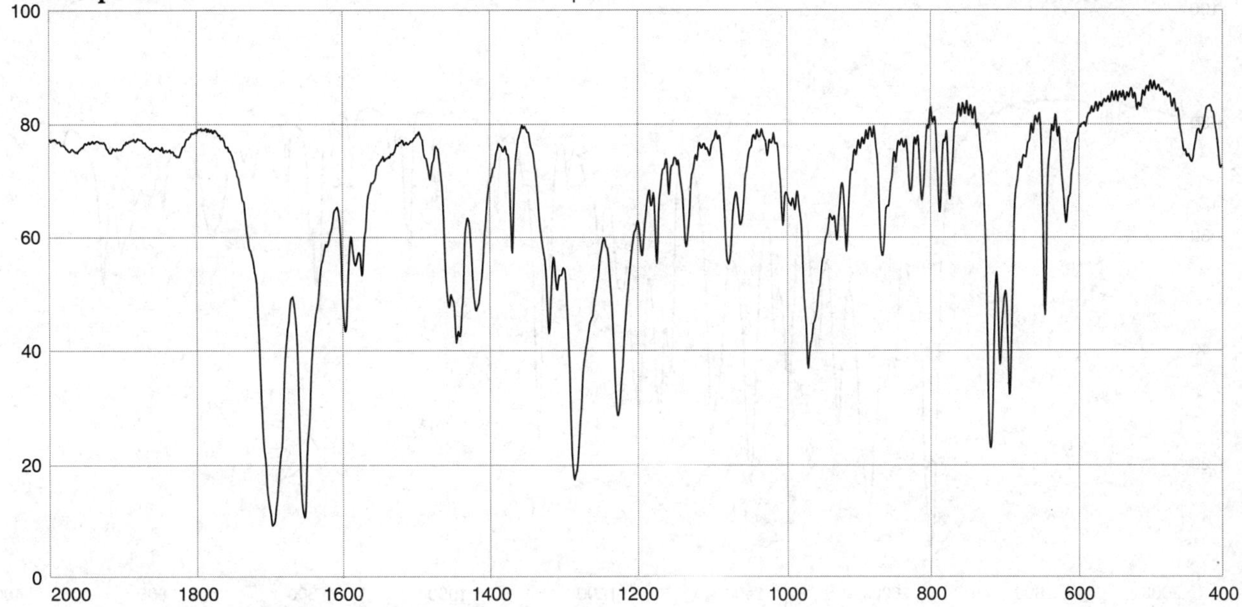

Labetalol Instrument: Dispersive Phase: Potassium bromide disc

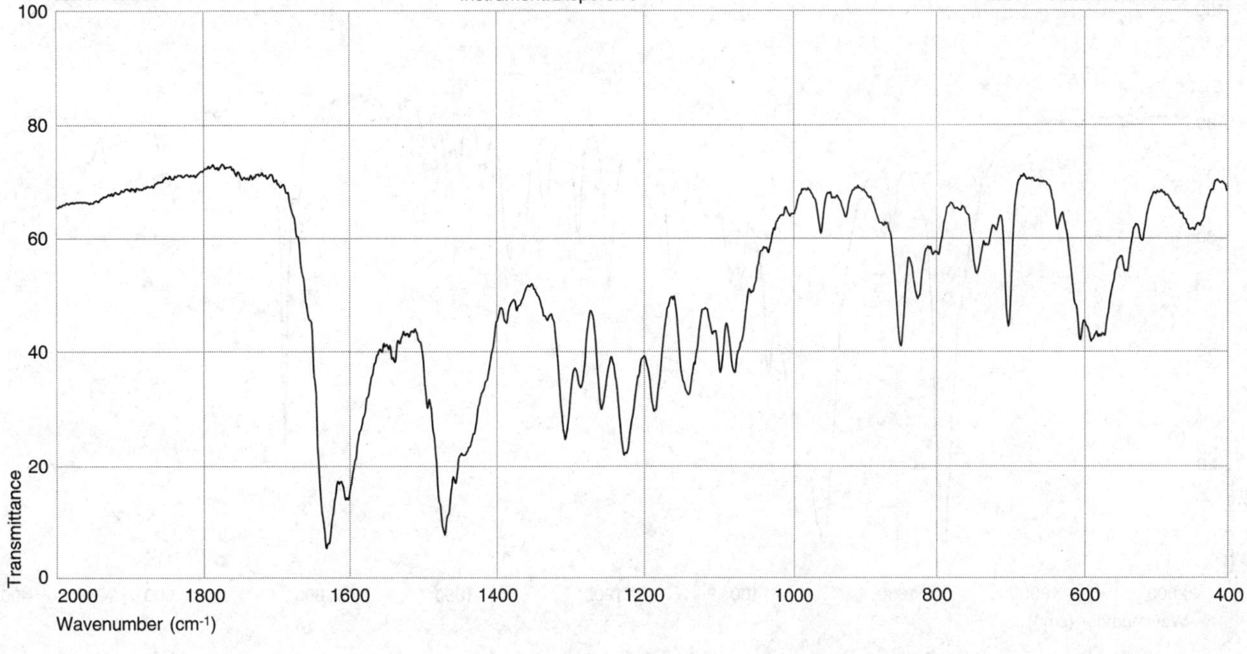

Levobunolol Hydrochloride Instrument: Dispersive Phase: Liquid paraffin mull

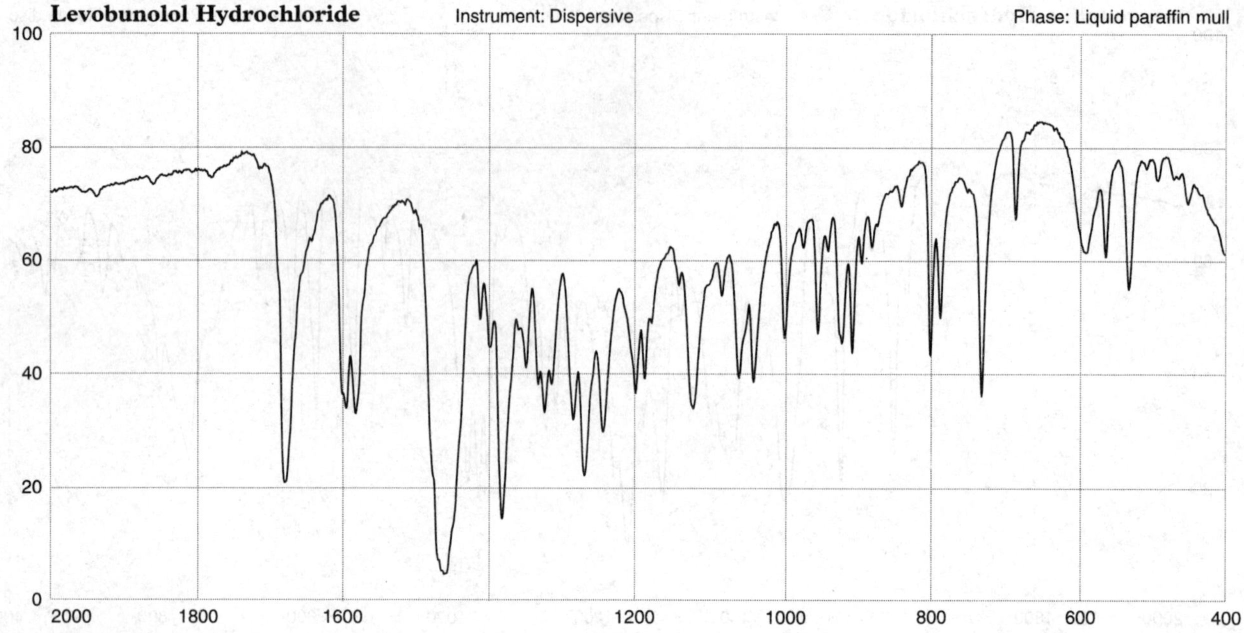

Levodopa Instrument: Dispersive Phase: Potassium bromide disc

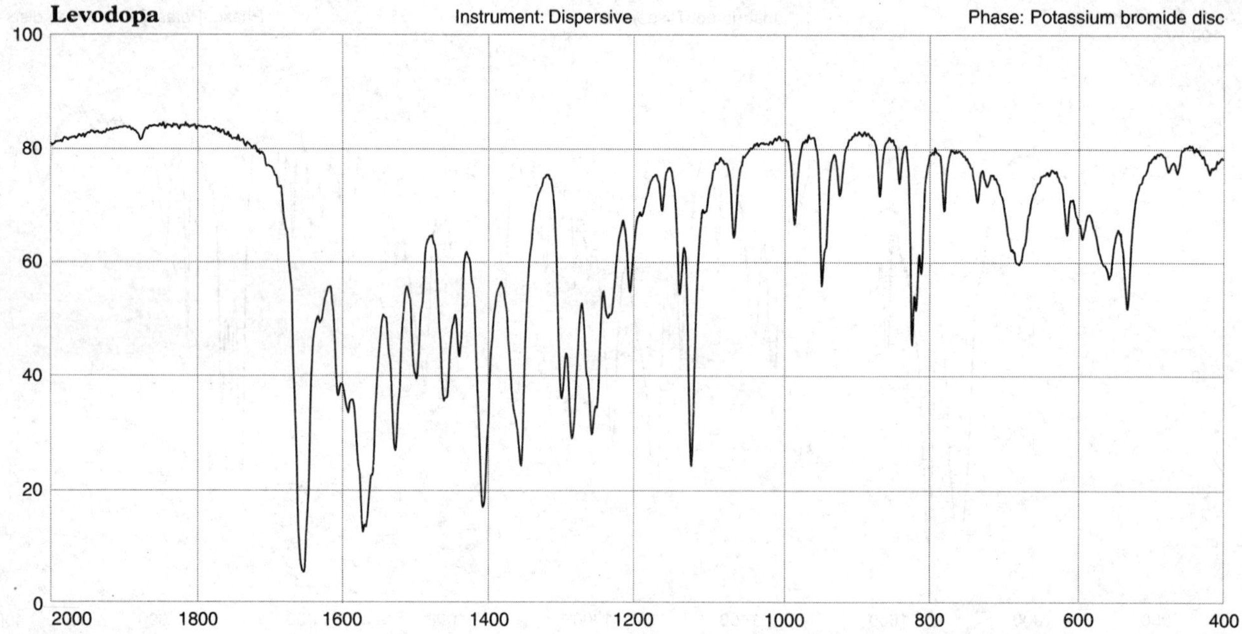

Lidocaine Instrument: Dispersive Phase: Potassium bromide disc

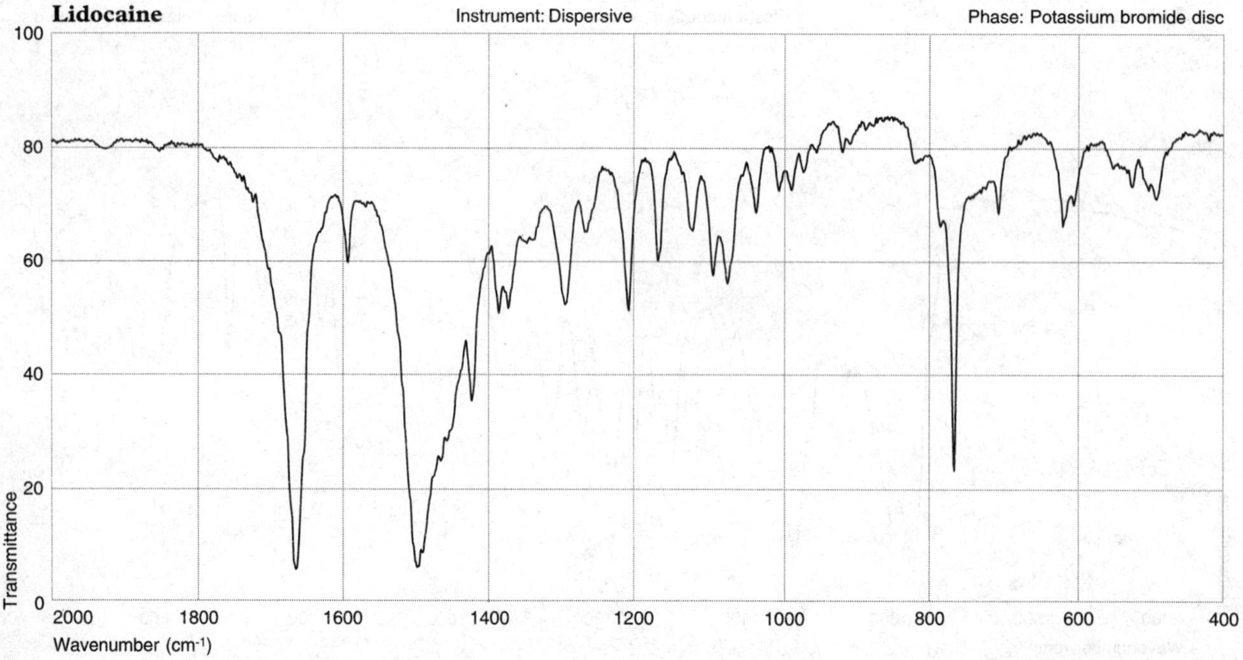

Lincomycin Hydrochloride Instrument: Dispersive Phase: Potassium chloride disc

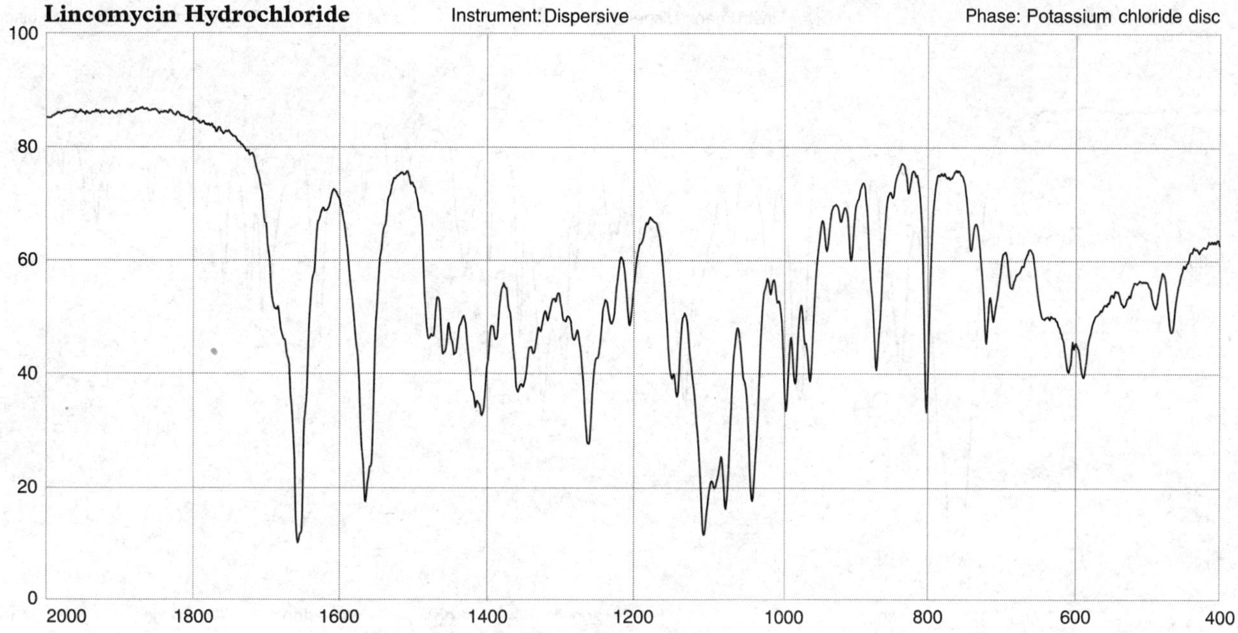

Lomustine Instrument: Dispersive Phase: Potassium bromide disc

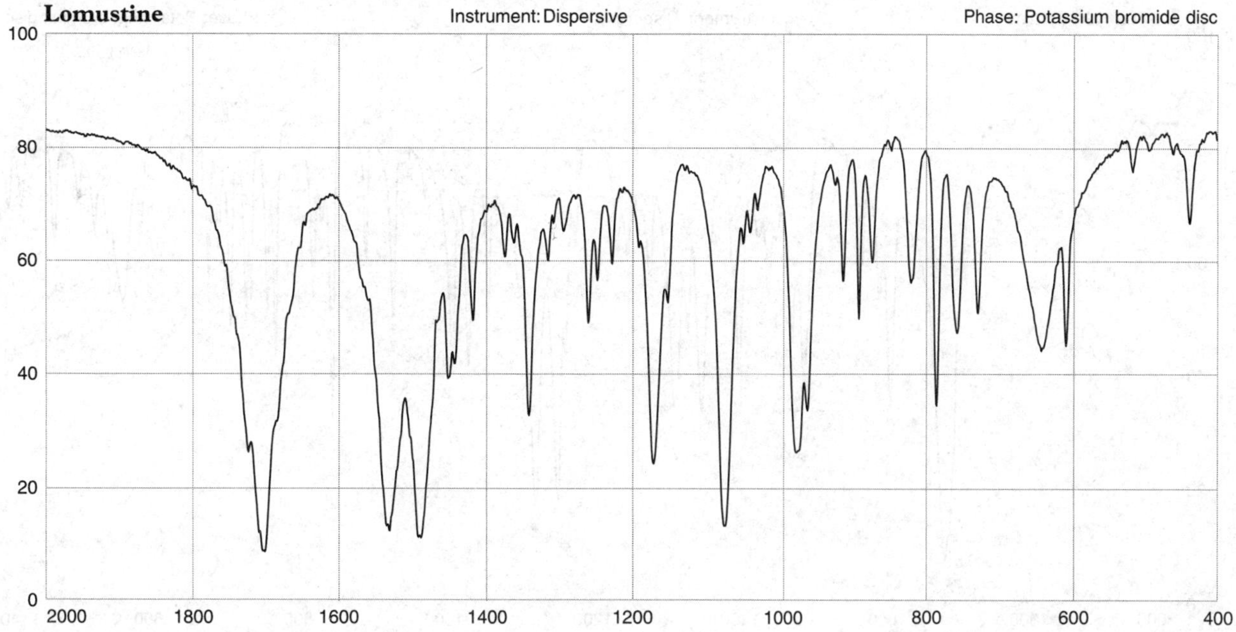

Loprazolam Mesilate Instrument: Dispersive Phase: Potassium bromide disc

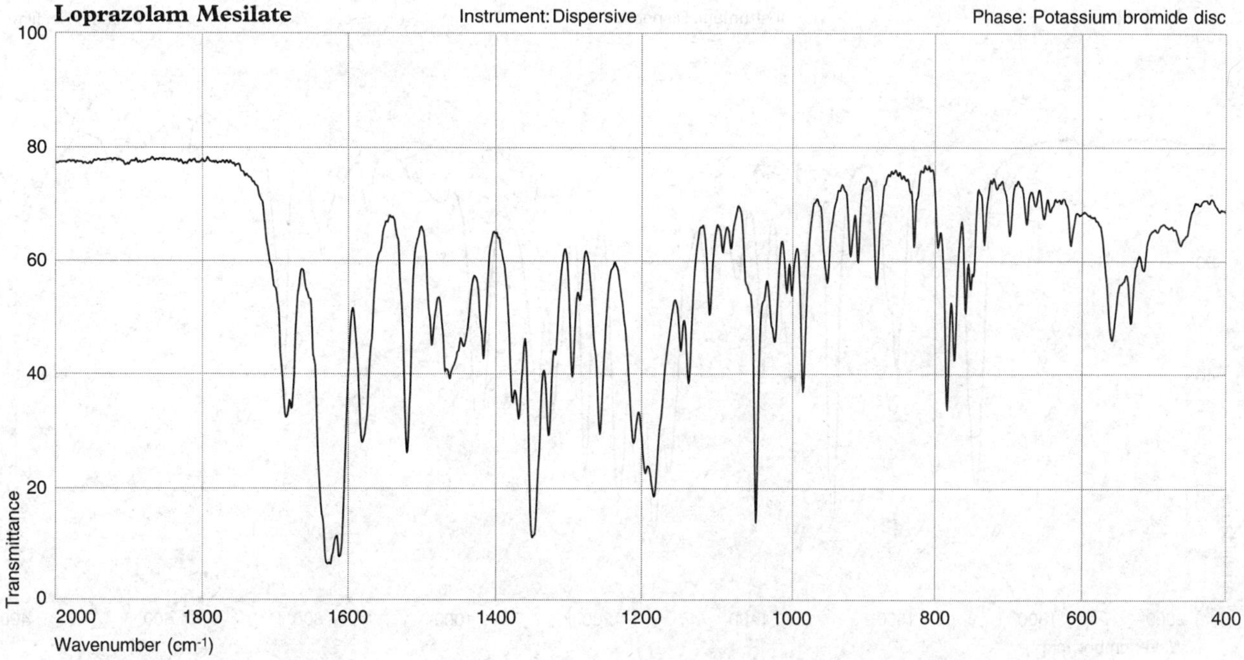

Lorazepam Instrument: Dispersive Phase: Potassium bromide disc

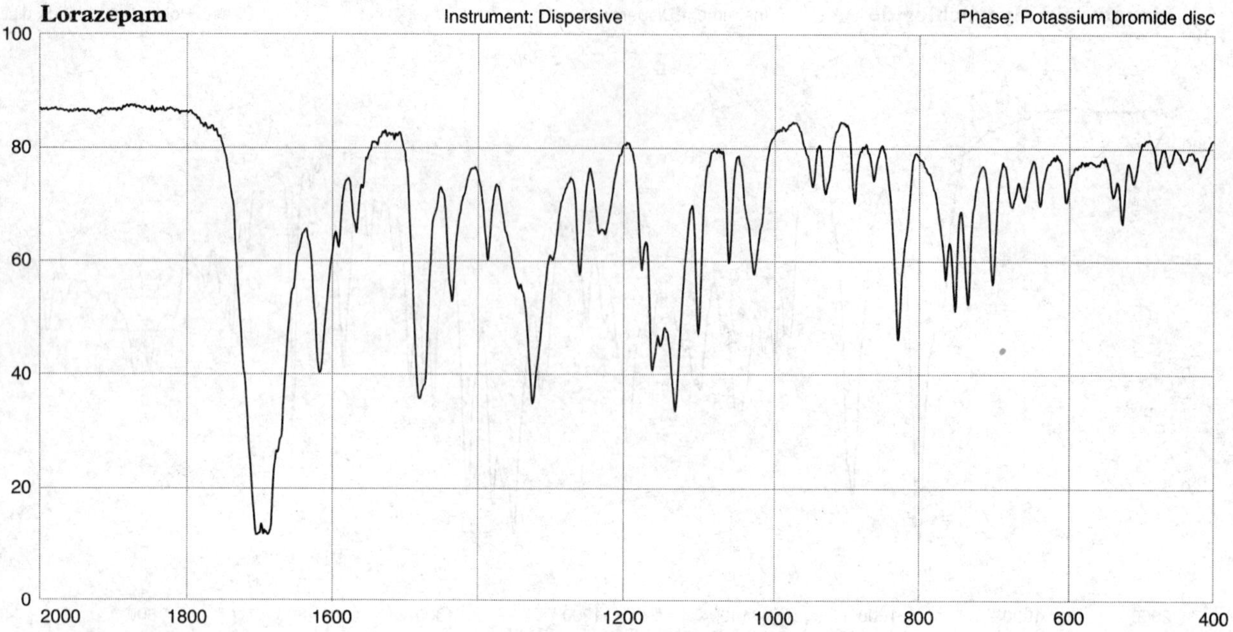

Lormetazepam Instrument: Dispersive Phase: Potassium bromide disc

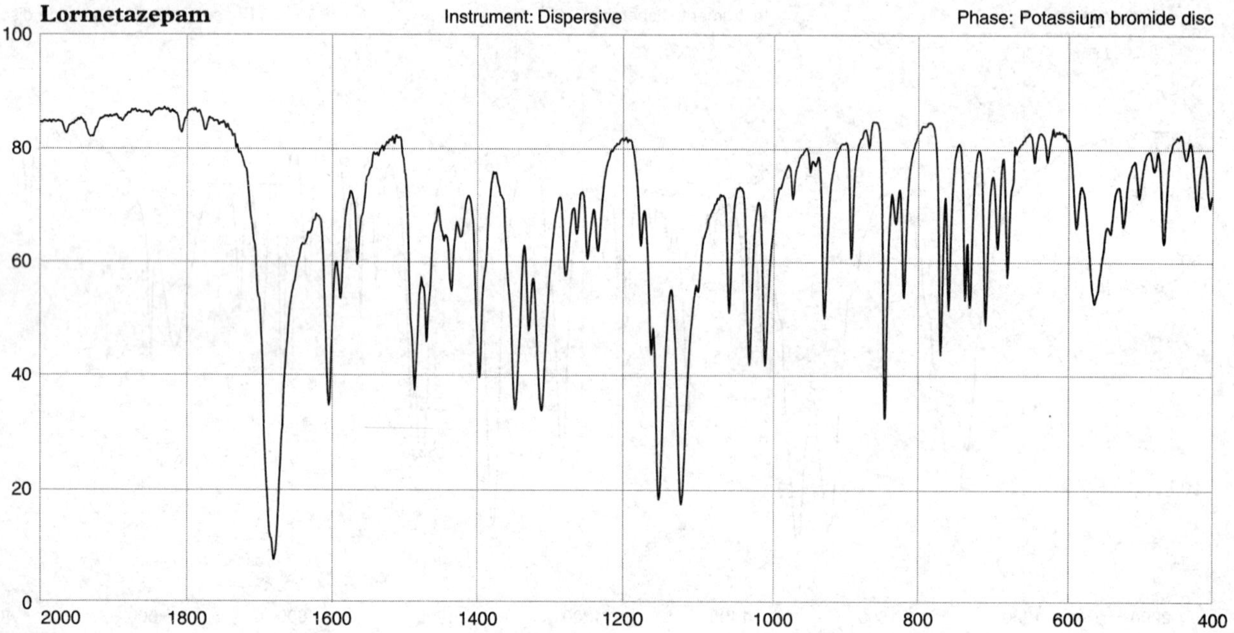

Mebeverine Instrument: Dispersive Phase: Thin film

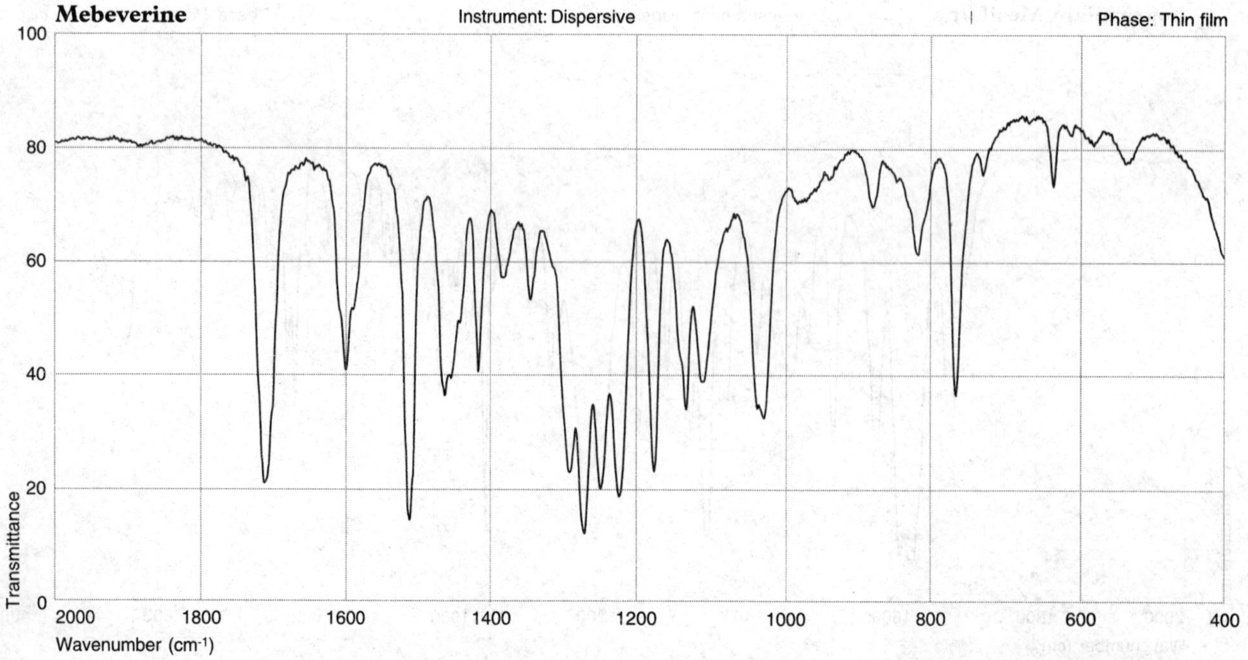

Mebeverine Hydrochloride

Instrument: Dispersive

Phase: Potassium chloride disc

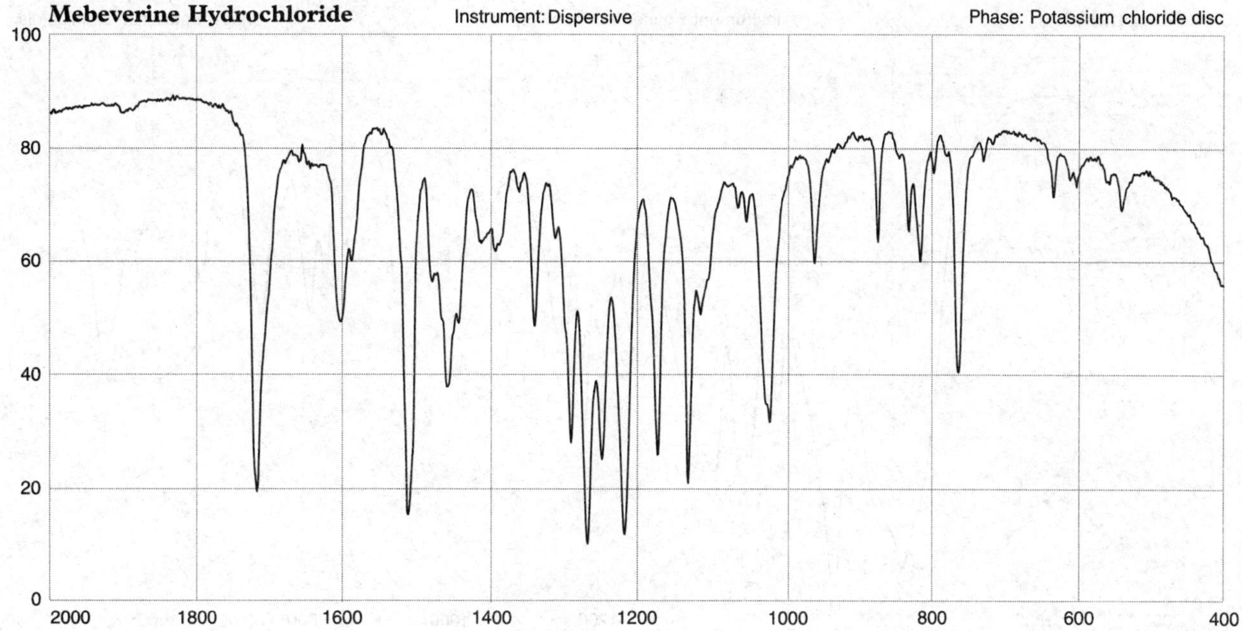

Mefenamic Acid

Instrument: Dispersive

Phase: Liquid paraffin mull

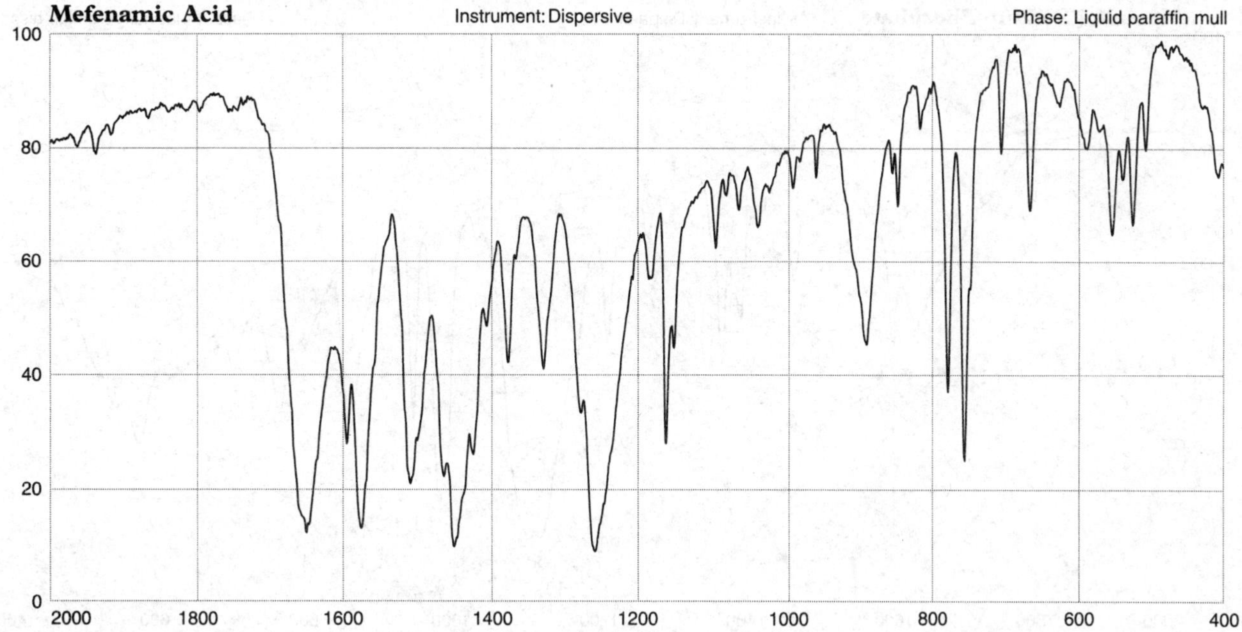

Megestrol Acetate

Instrument: Dispersive

Phase: Potassium bromide disc

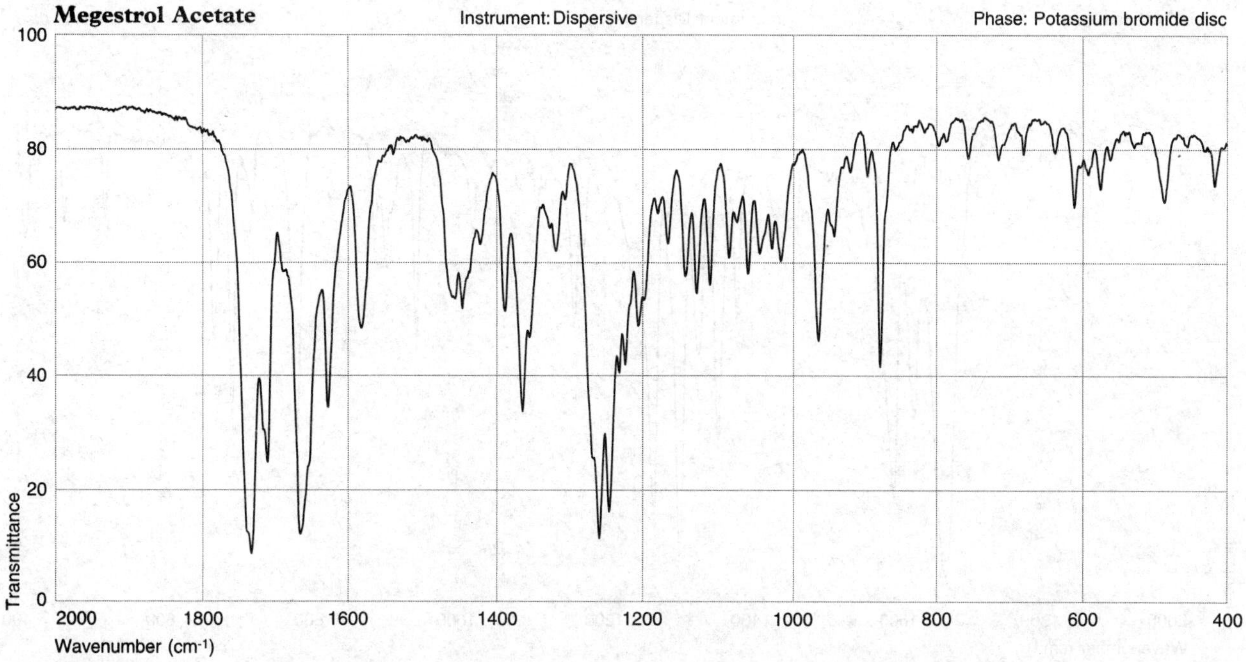

Melphalan Instrument: Fourier transform Phase: Potassium bromide disc

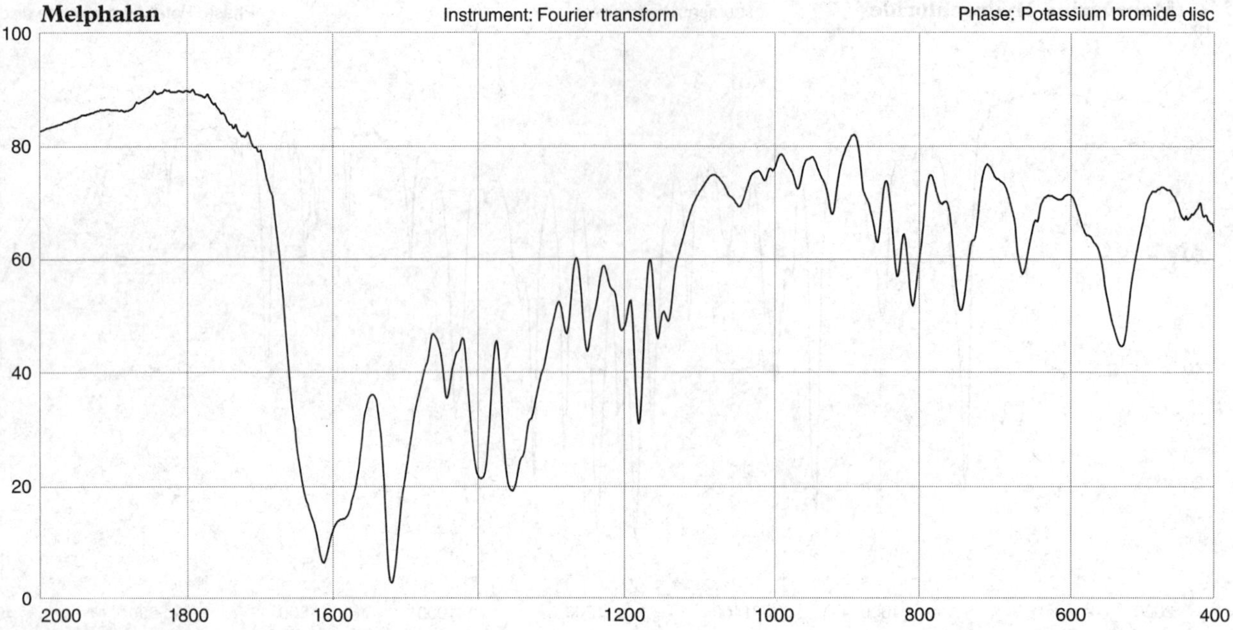

Menadiol Sodium Phosphate Instrument: Dispersive Phase: Potassium bromide disc

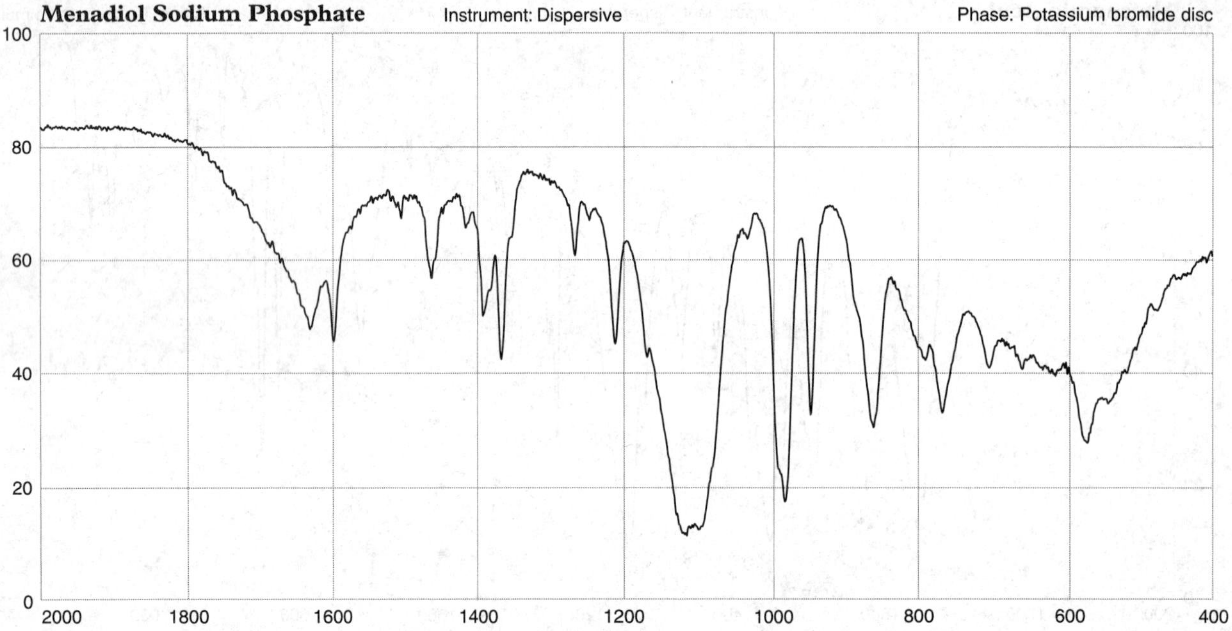

Menadione Instrument: Dispersive Phase: Potassium bromide disc

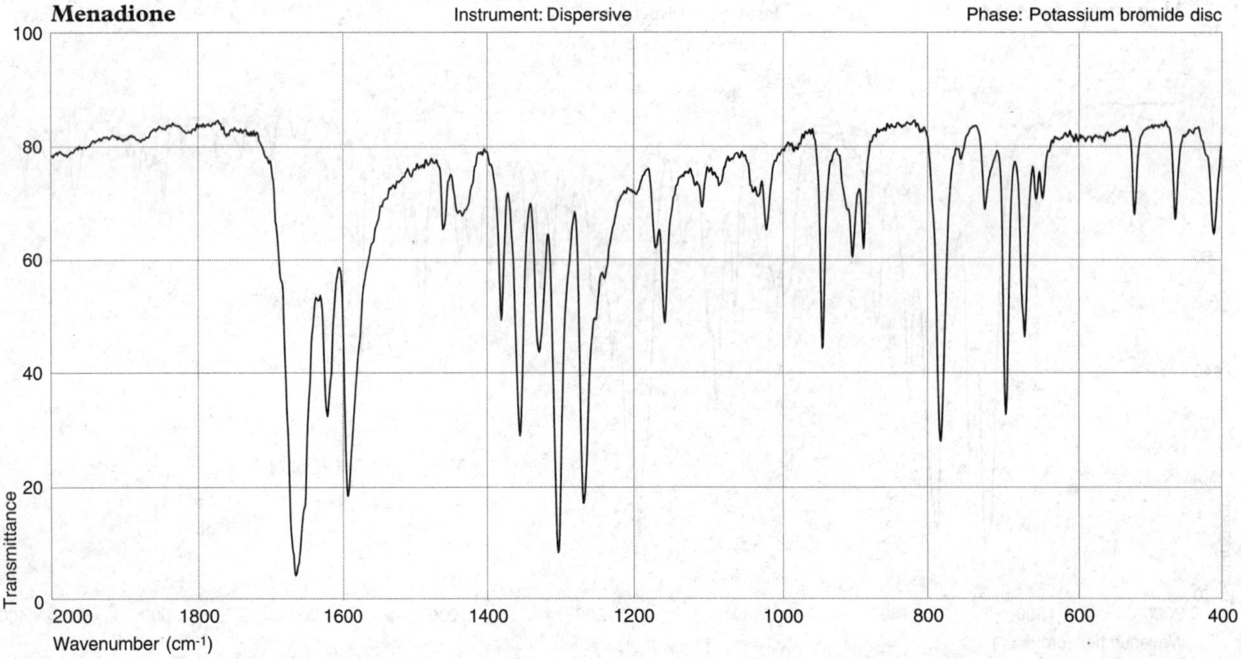

Meptazinol Hydrochloride Instrument: Dispersive Phase: Potassium chloride disc

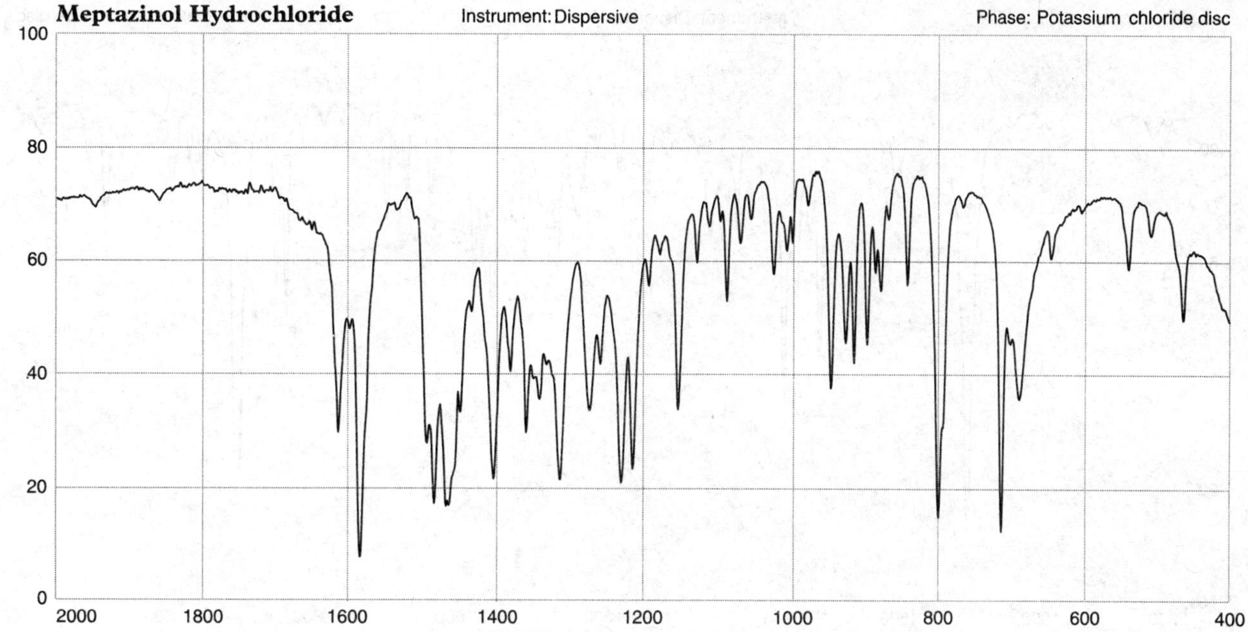

Mepyramine Maleate Instrument: Dispersive Phase: Potassium bromide disc

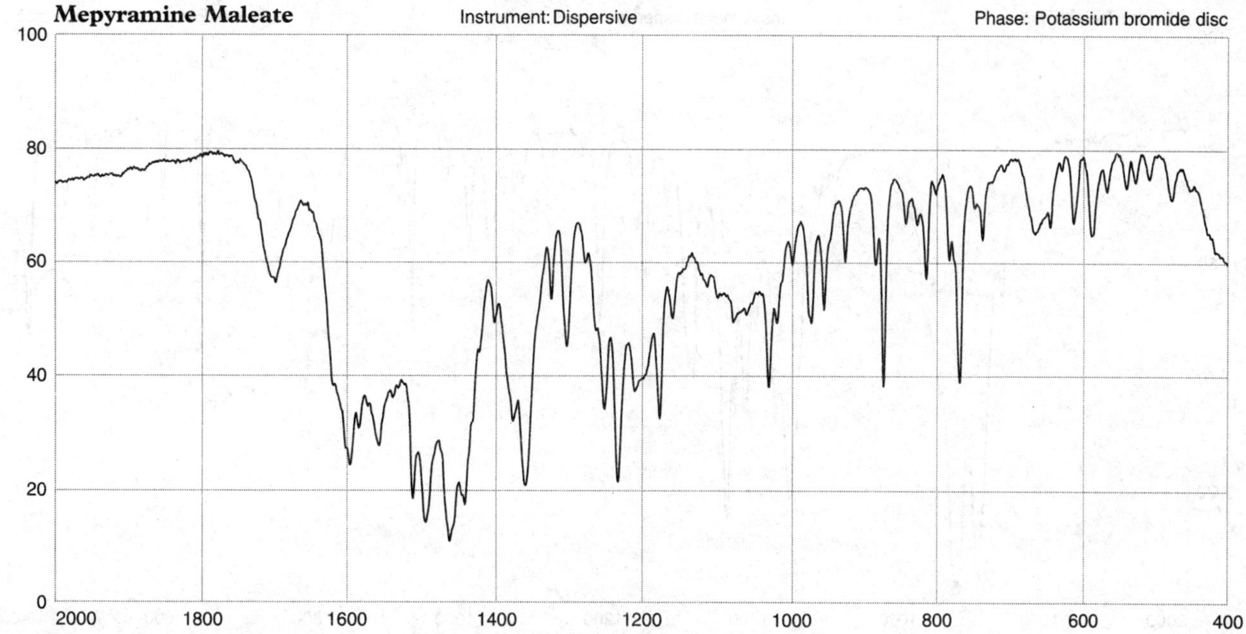

Metformin Hydrochloride Instrument: Dispersive Phase: Potassium chloride disc

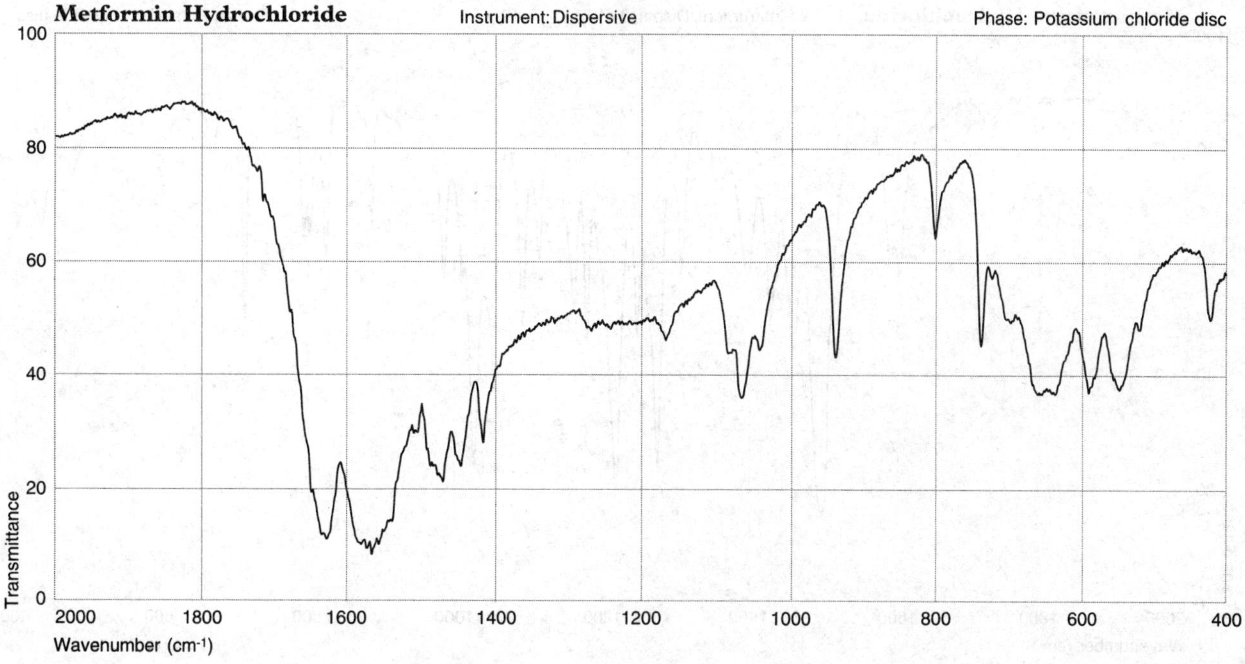

Methadone Instrument: Dispersive Phase: Potassium bromide disc

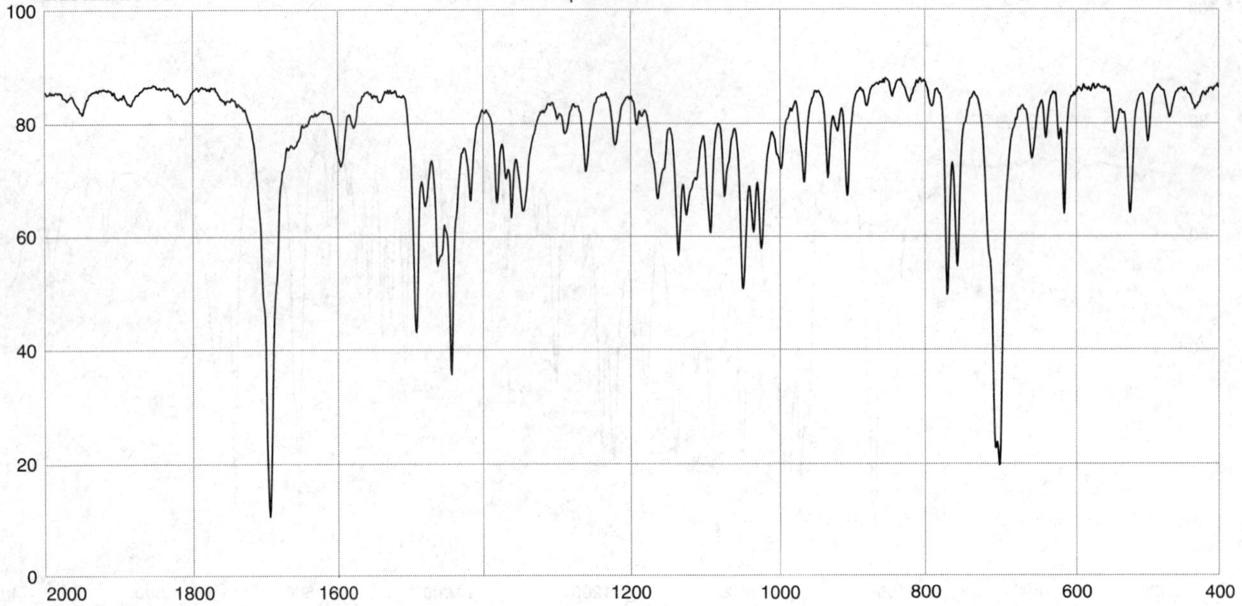

Methohexitone Instrument: Dispersive Phase: Potassium bromide disc

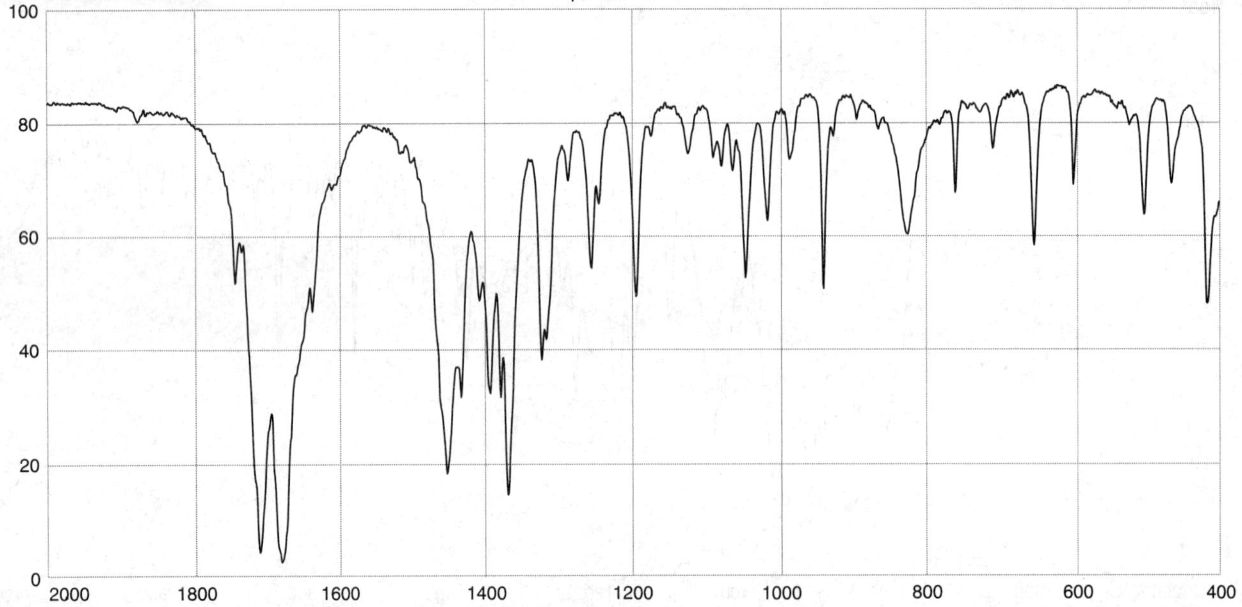

Methoxamine Hydrochloride Instrument: Dispersive Phase: Potassium chloride disc

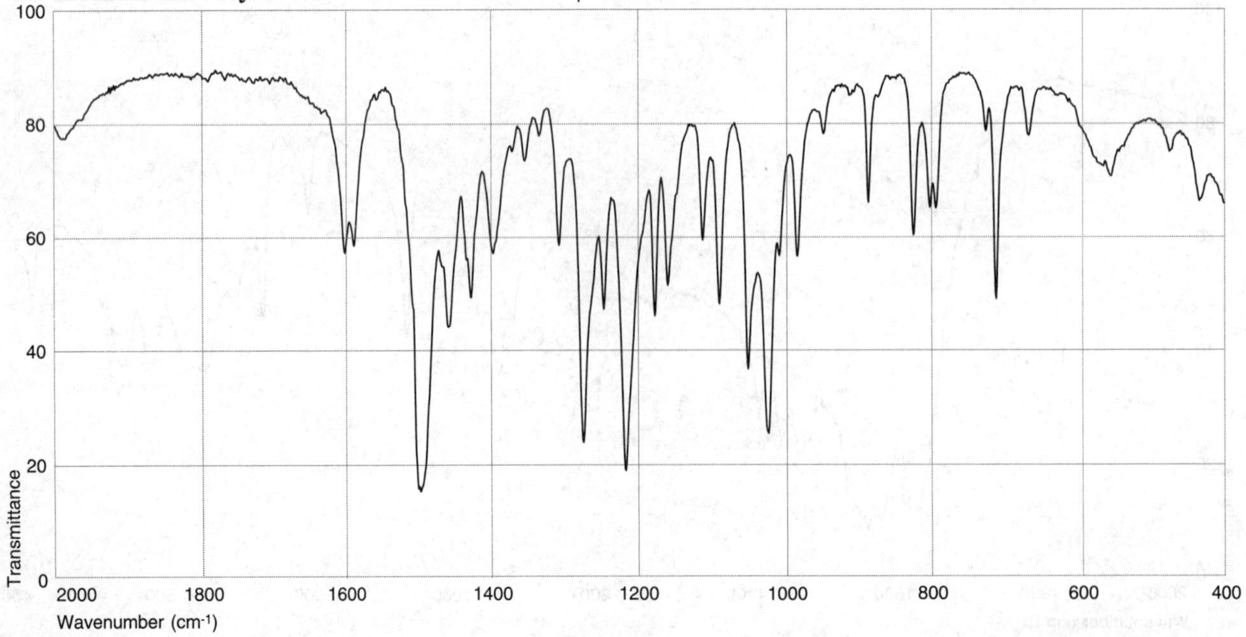

Methyl Hydroxybenzoate Instrument: Dispersive Phase: Potassium bromide disc

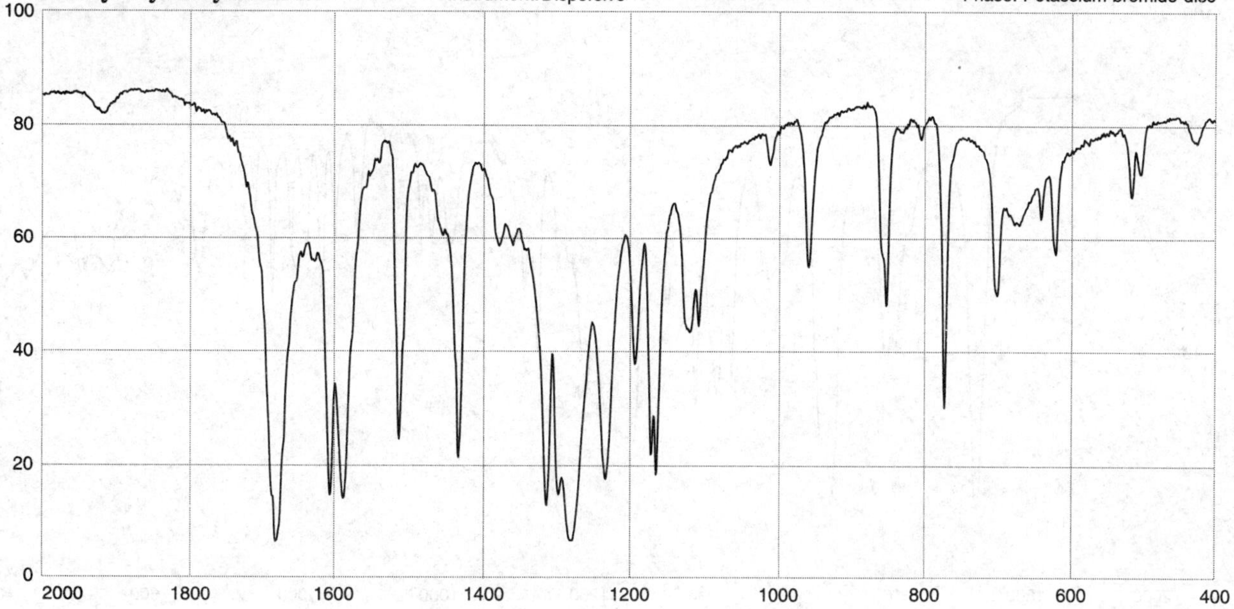

Methyl Nicotinate Instrument: Dispersive Phase: Liquid paraffin mull

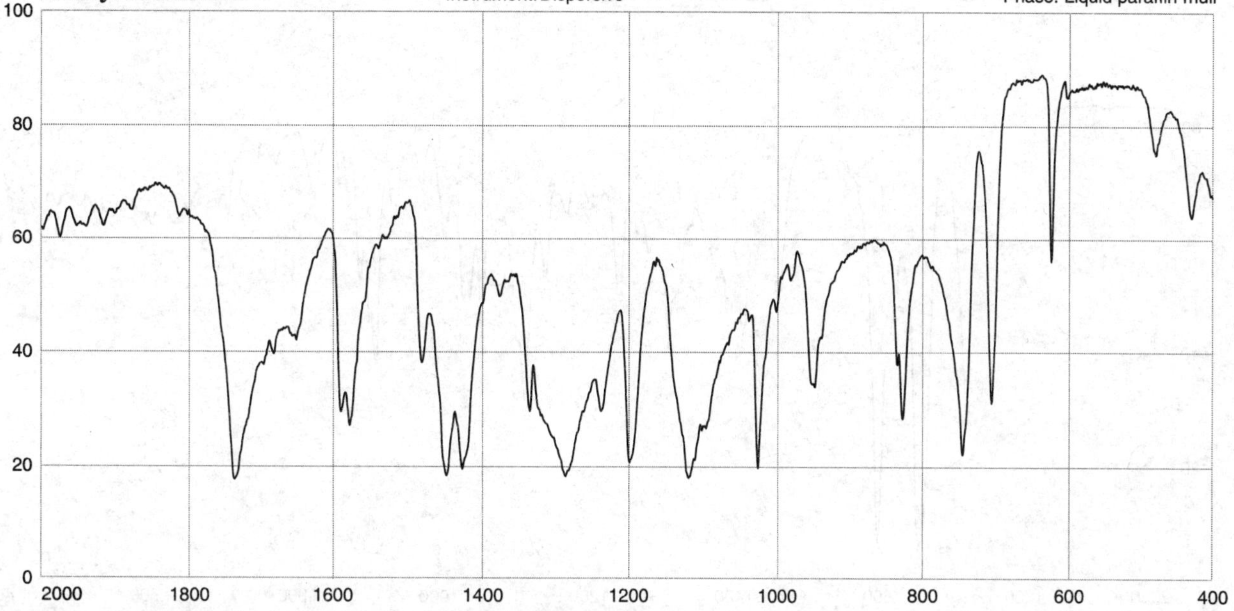

Methyldopa Instrument: Dispersive Phase: Potassium bromide disc

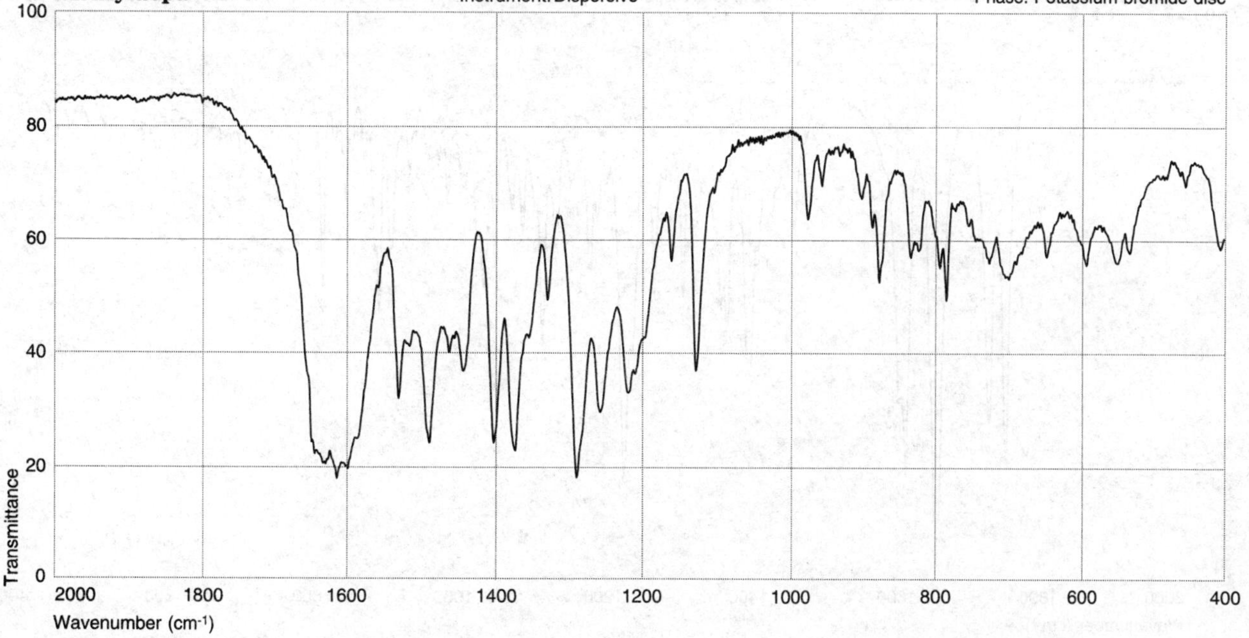

Methyldopate Hydrochloride Instrument: Dispersive Phase: Potassium chloride disc

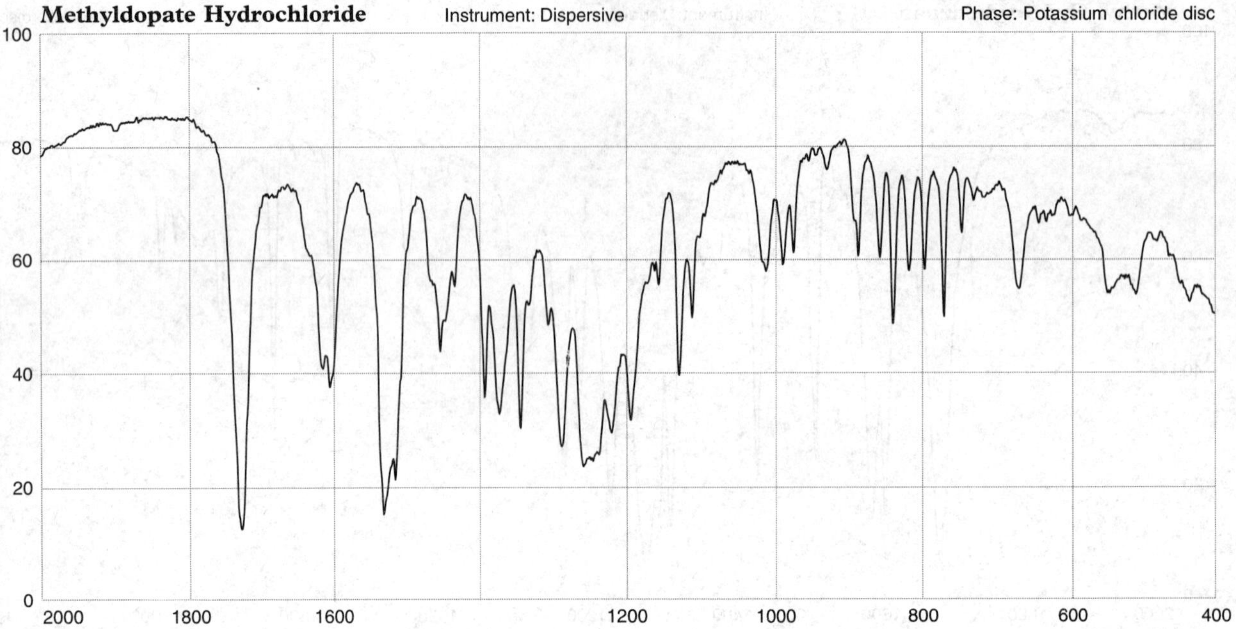

Methylprednisolone Instrument: Dispersive Phase: Potassium bromide disc

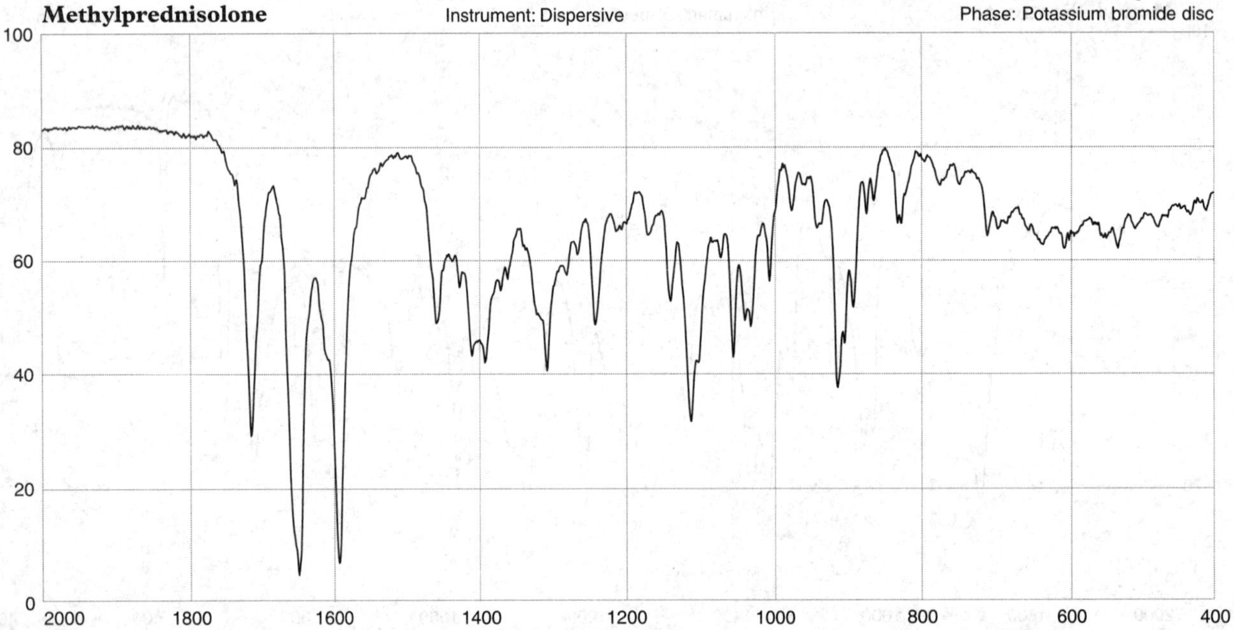

Methylprednisolone Acetate Instrument: Dispersive Phase: Potassium bromide disc

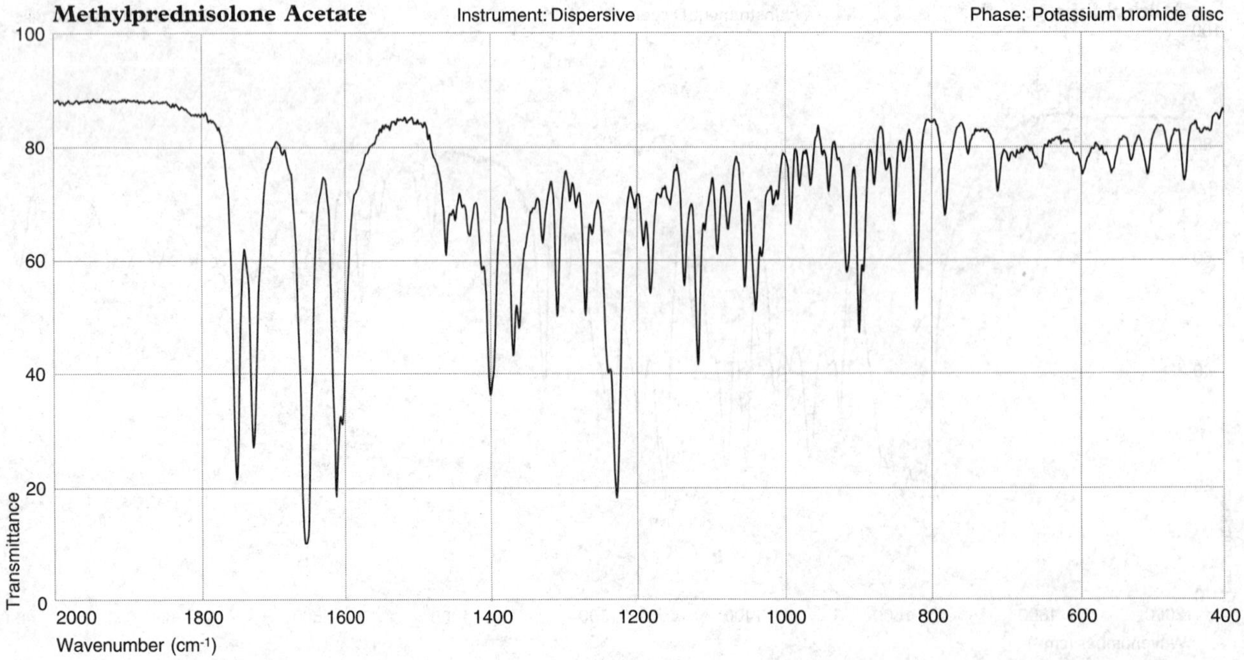

Methysergide Maleate Instrument: Dispersive Phase: Potassium bromide disc

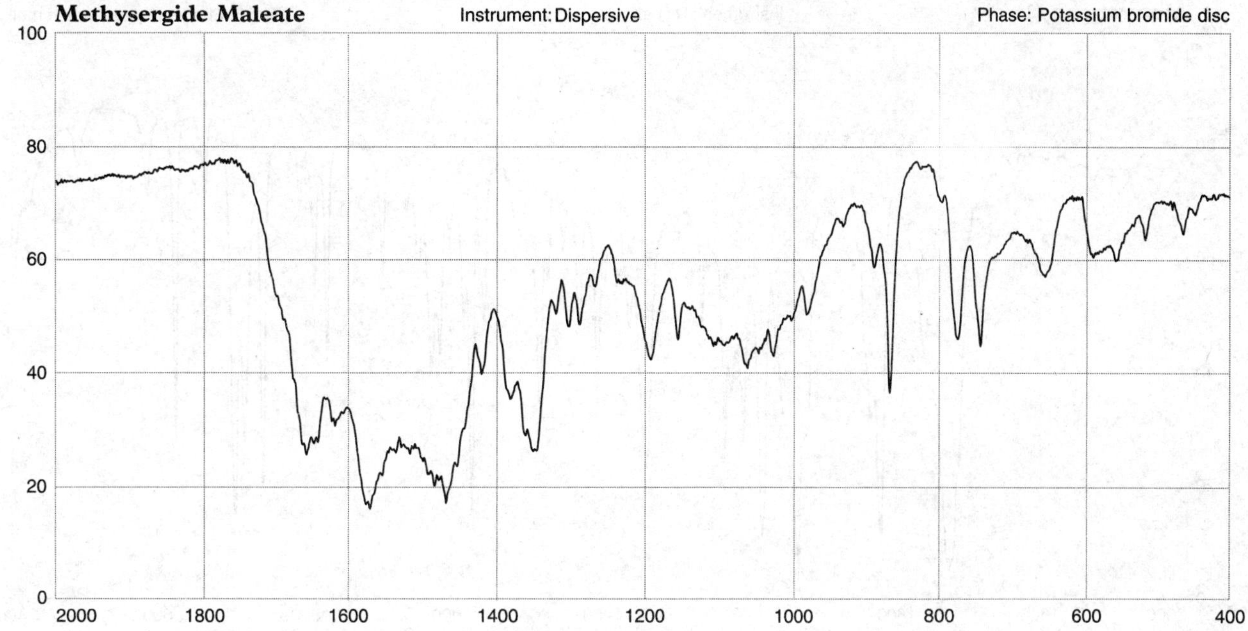

Metoprolol Instrument: Dispersive Phase: Potassium bromide disc

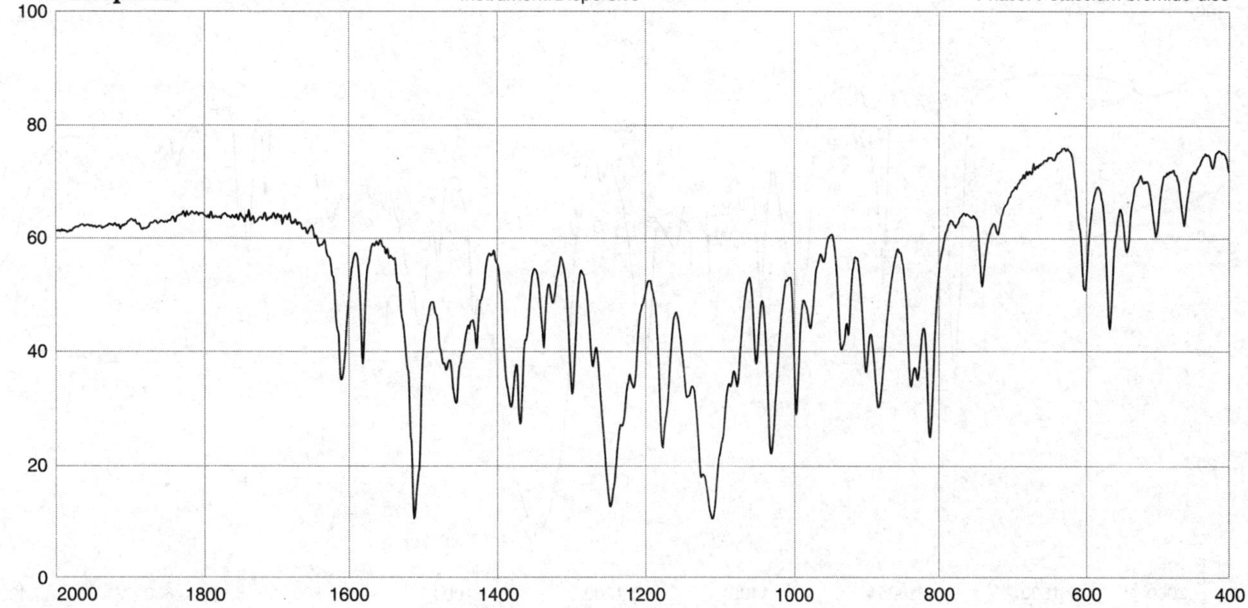

Metronidazole Instrument: Dispersive Phase: Potassium bromide disc

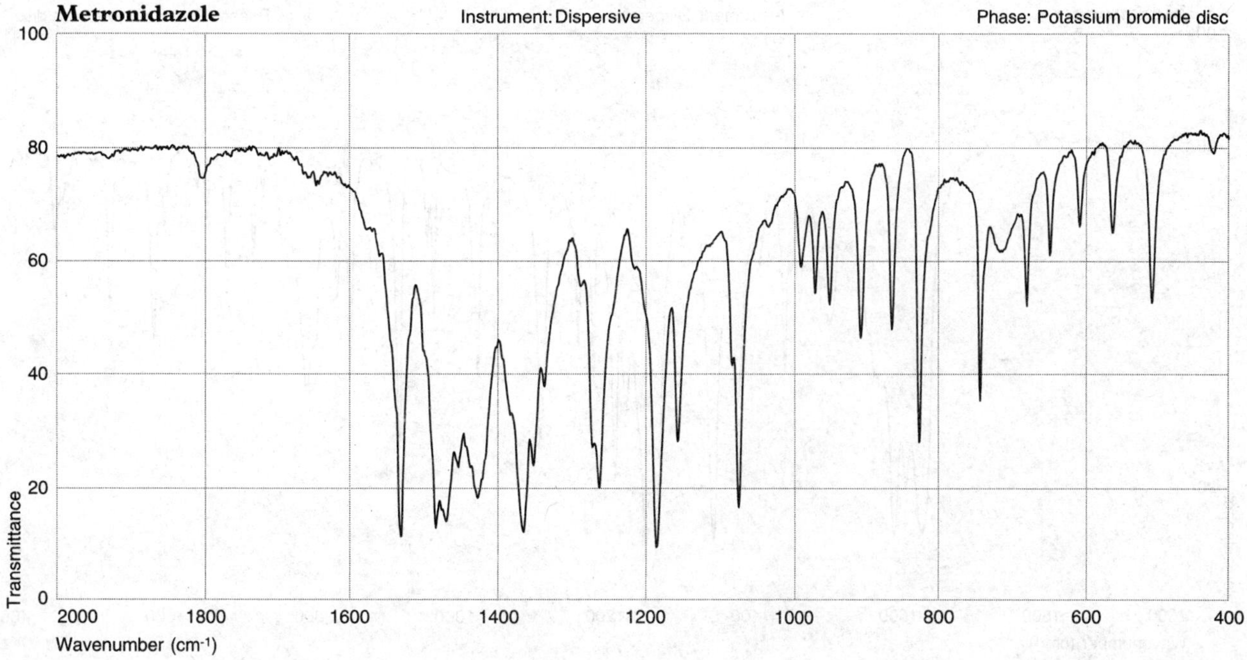

Metyrapone (1)

Instrument: Dispersive

Phase: Liquid paraffin mull

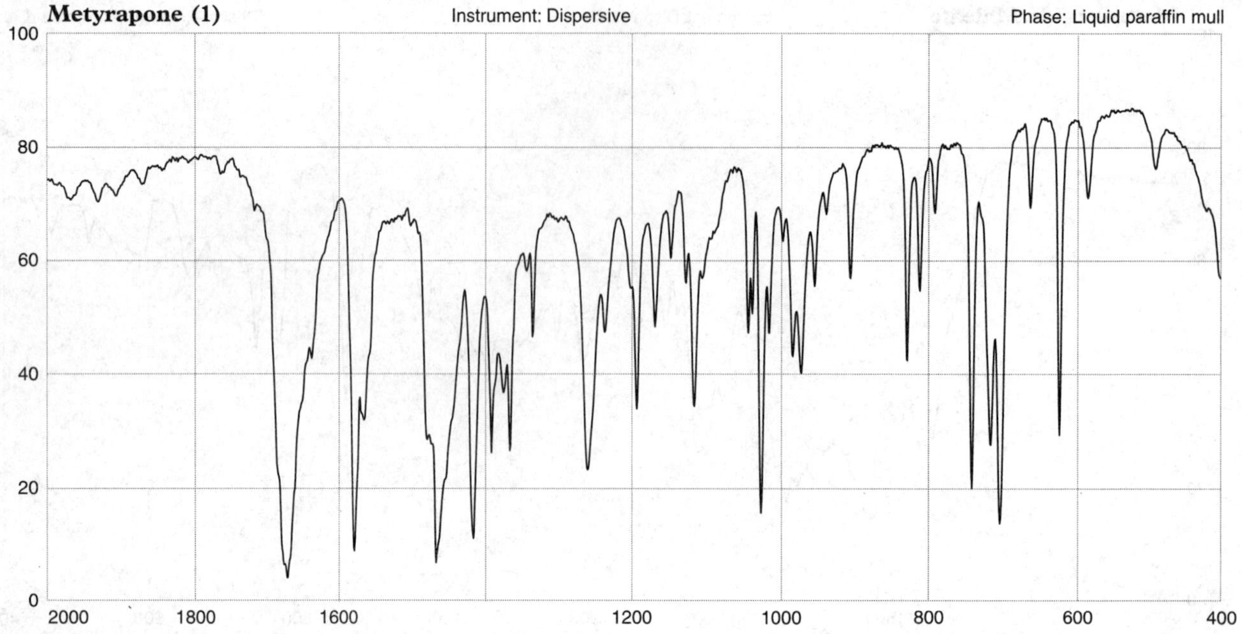

Metyrapone (2)

Instrument: Dispersive

Phase: 50% w/v solution in macrogol 400 Thickness: 0.1mm

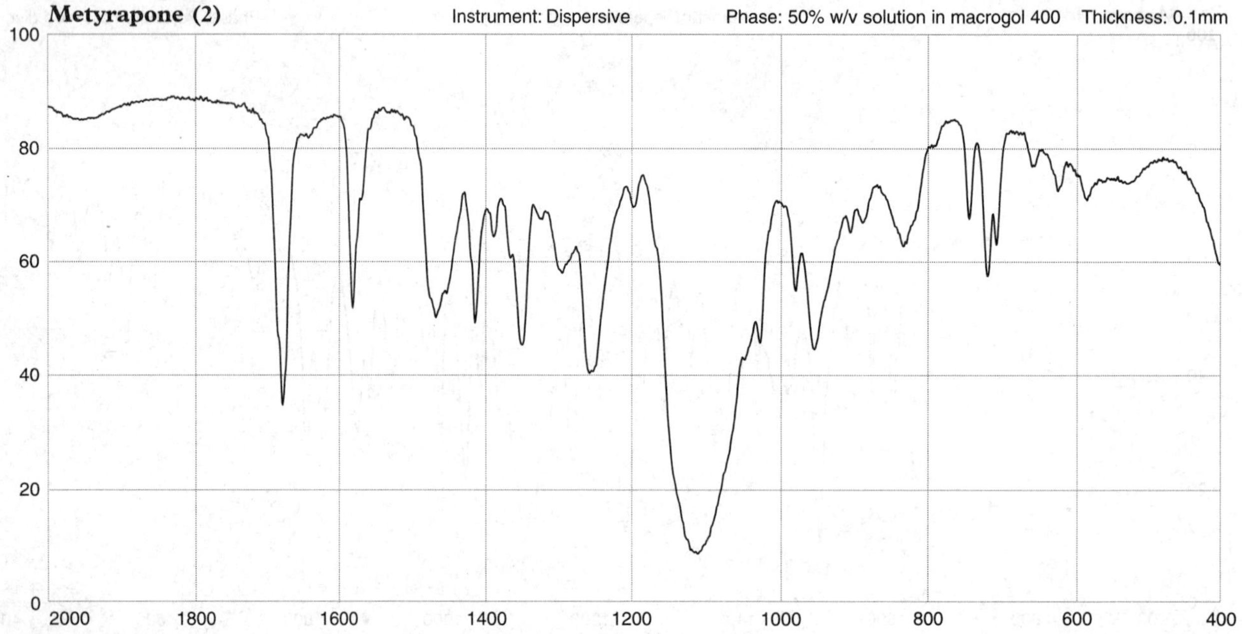

Mexenone

Instrument: Dispersive

Phase: Potassium bromide disc

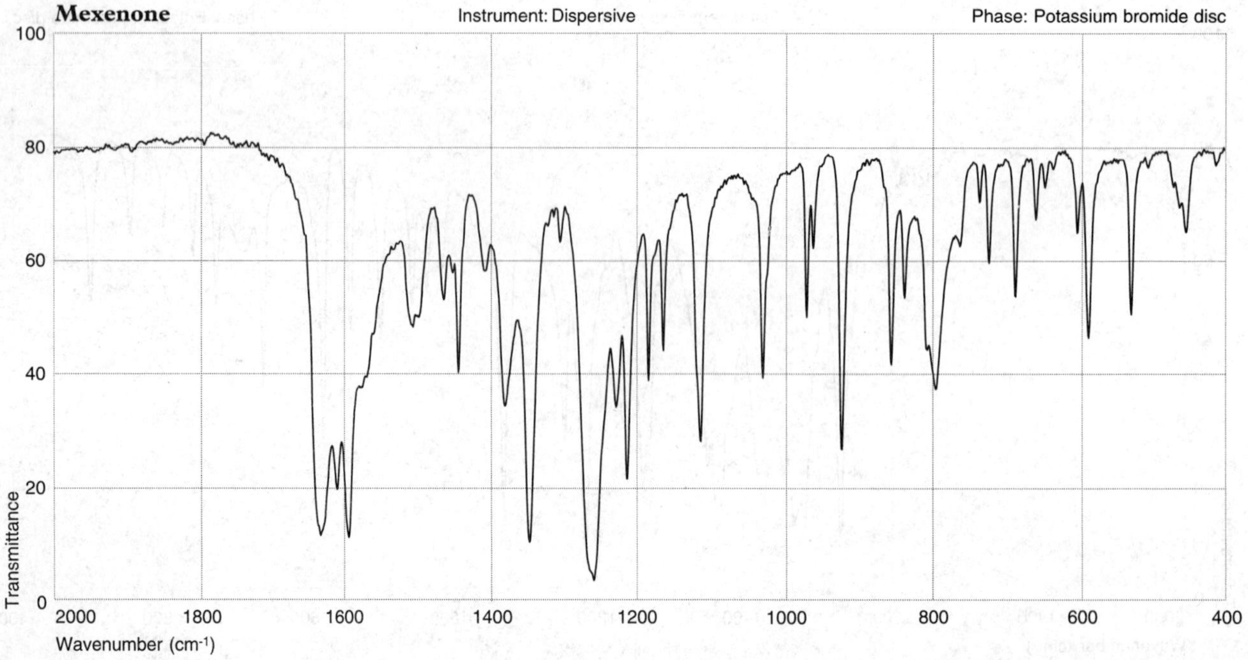

Mexiletine Hydrochloride Instrument: Dispersive Phase: Potassium bromide disc

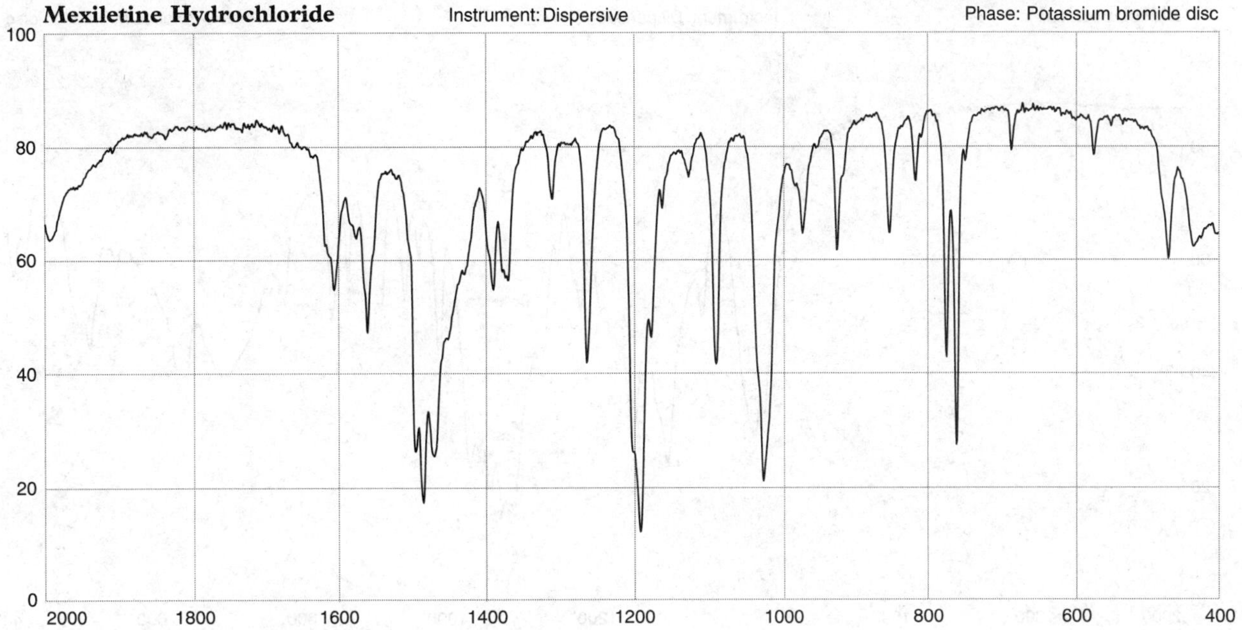

Mianserin Hydrochloride Instrument: Dispersive Phase: Potassium chloride disc

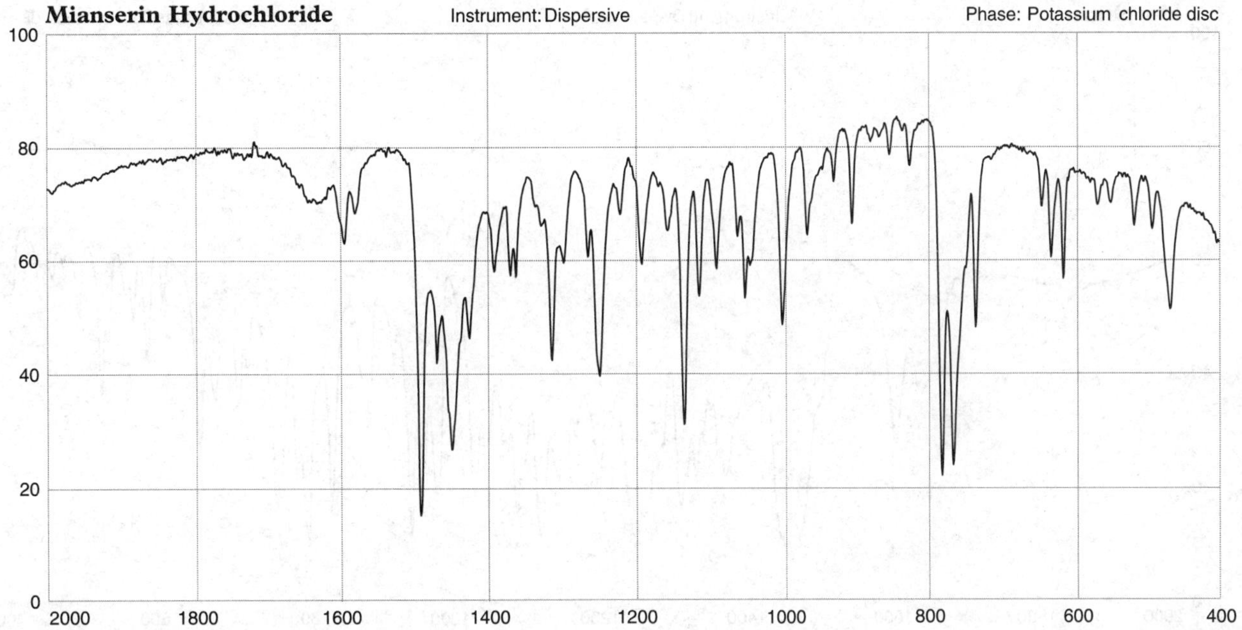

Midazolam Instrument: Dispersive Phase: Potassium bromide disc

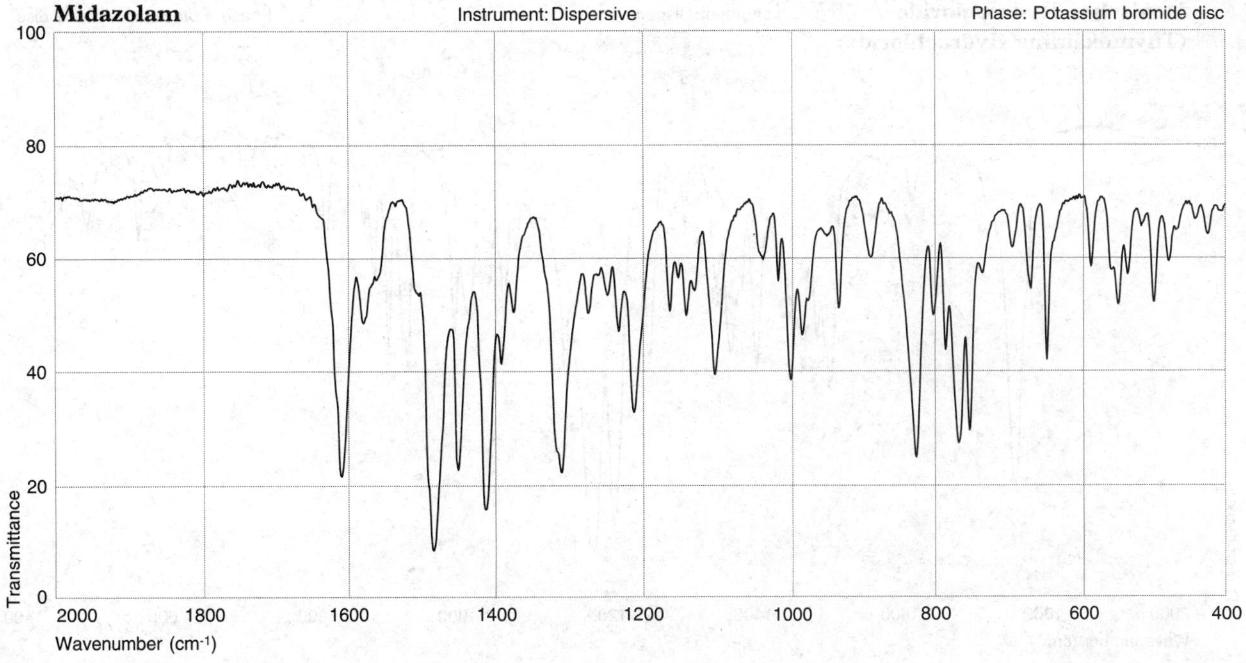

Mitobronitol

Instrument: Dispersive

Phase: Potassium bromide disc

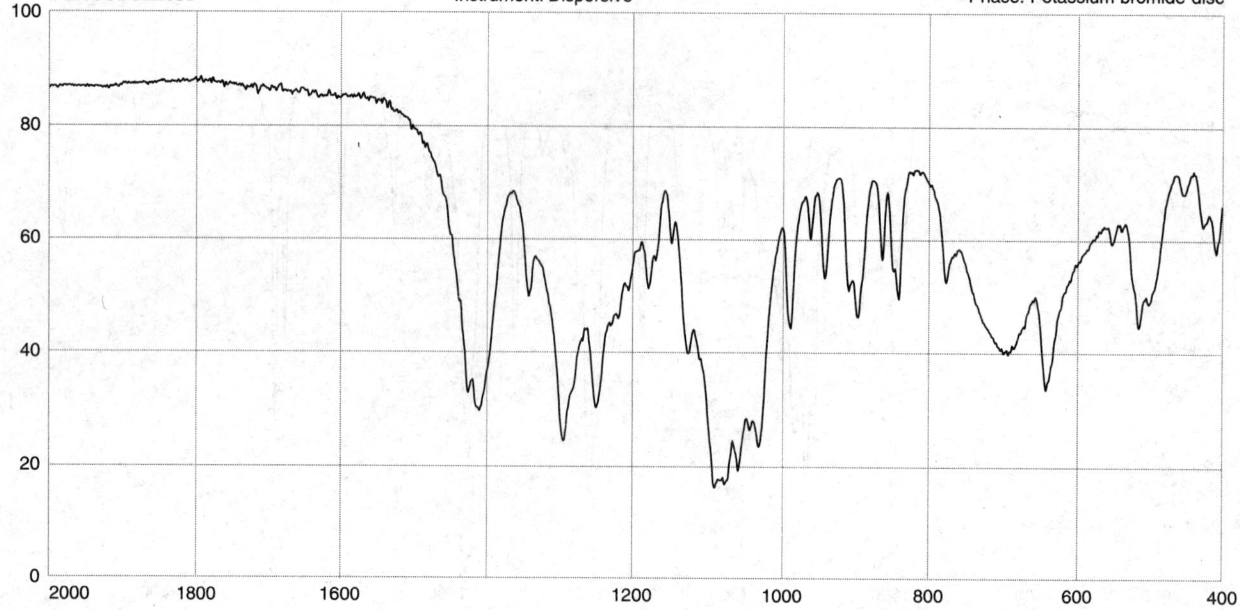

Morphine

Instrument: Dispersive

Phase: Potassium bromide disc

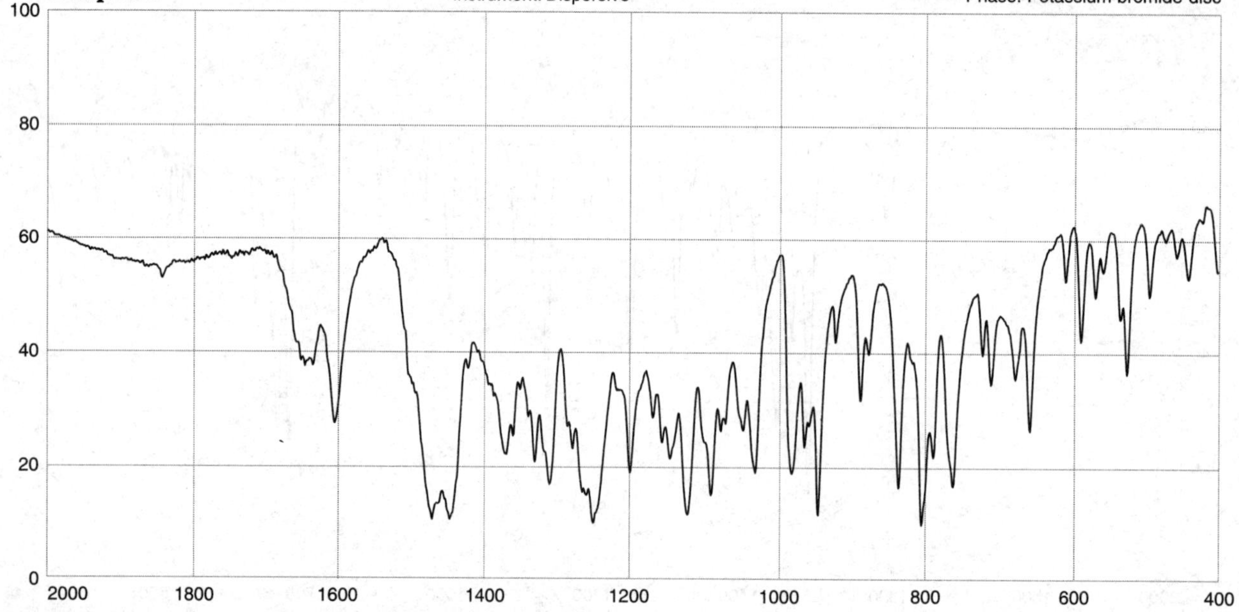

Moxisylyte Hydrochloride (Thymoxamine Hydrochloride)

Instrument: Dispersive

Phase: Potassium chloride disc

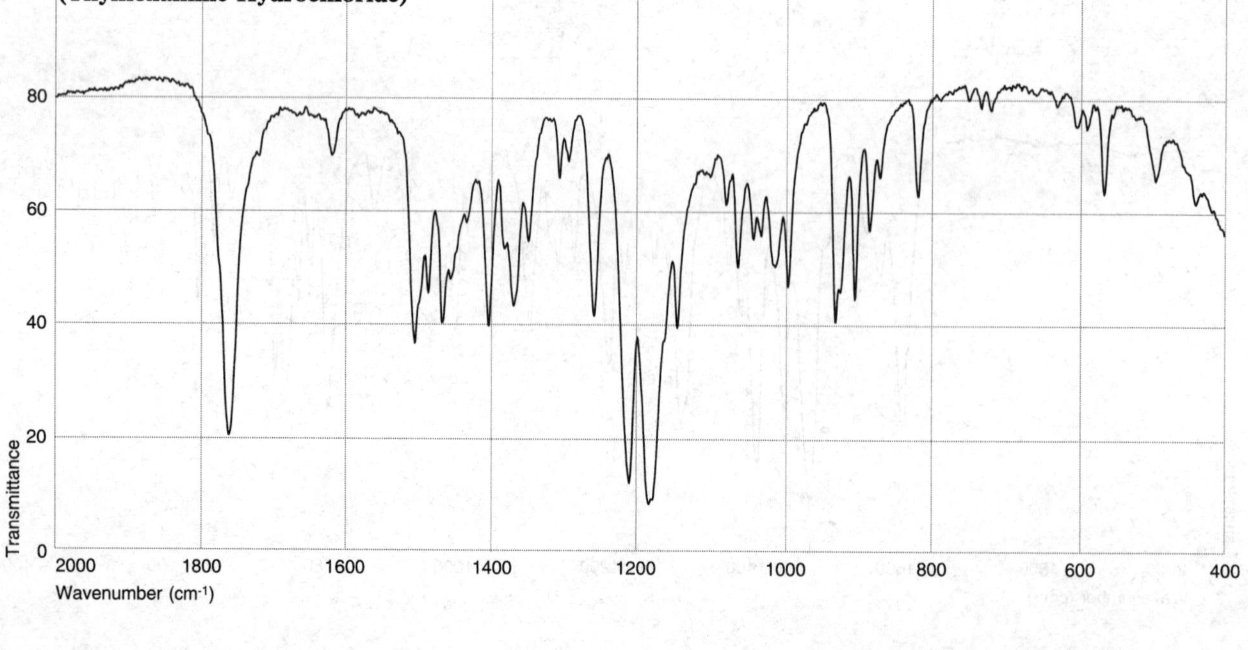

Nabumetone

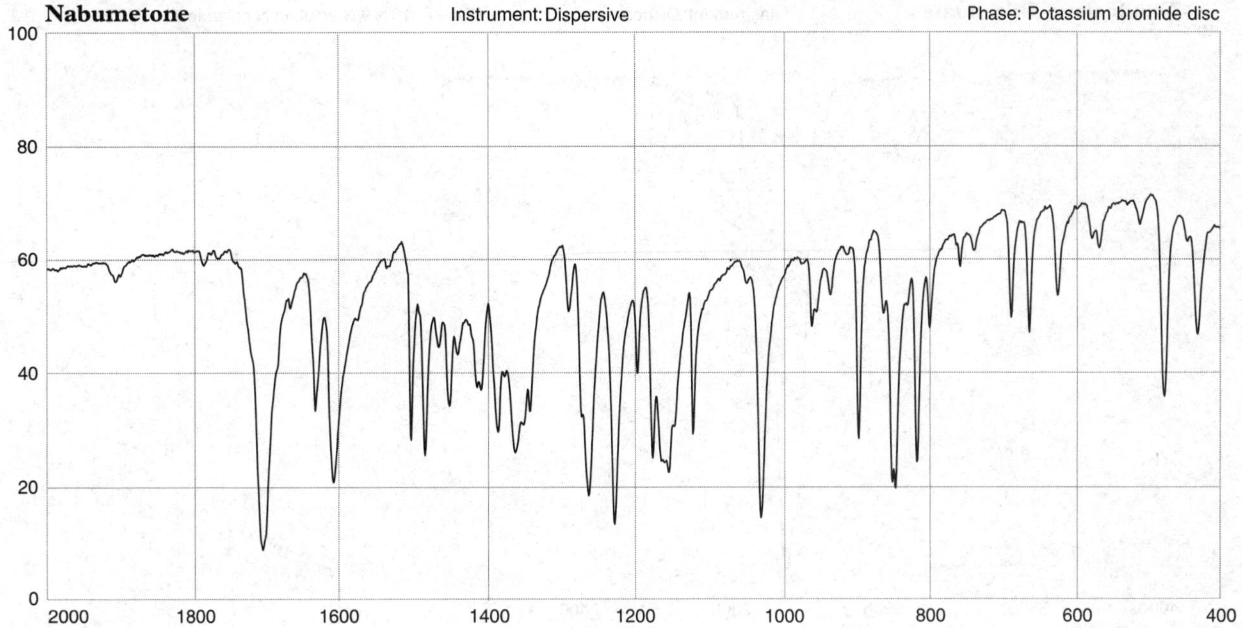

Naftidrofuryl

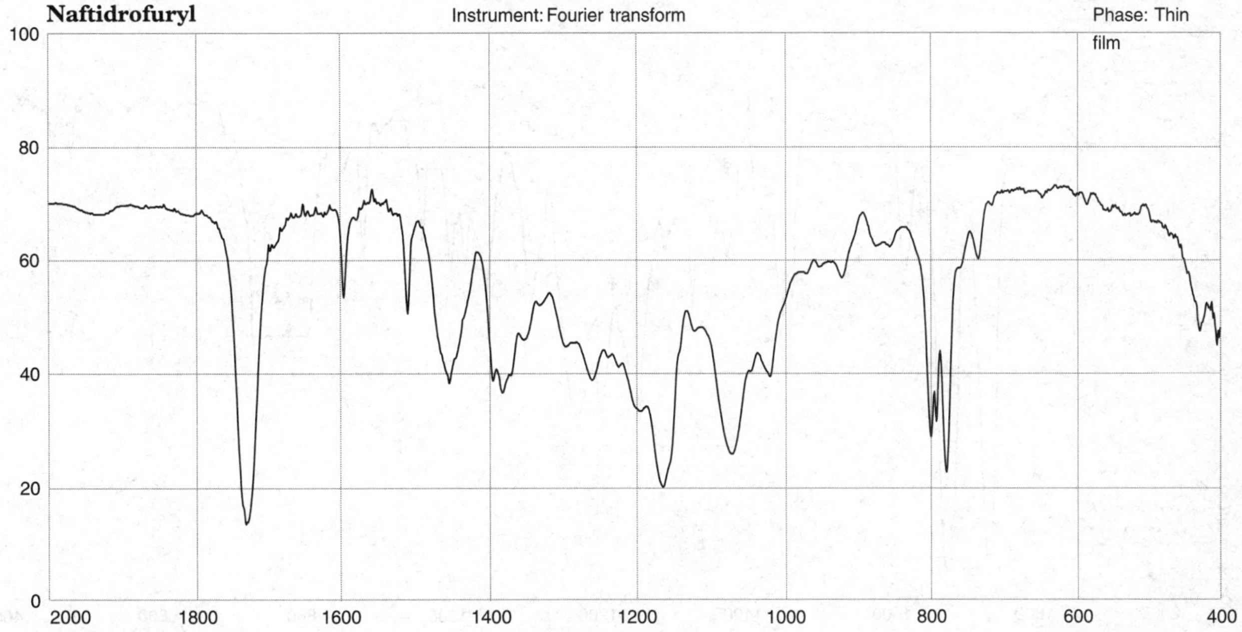

Nalidixic Acid

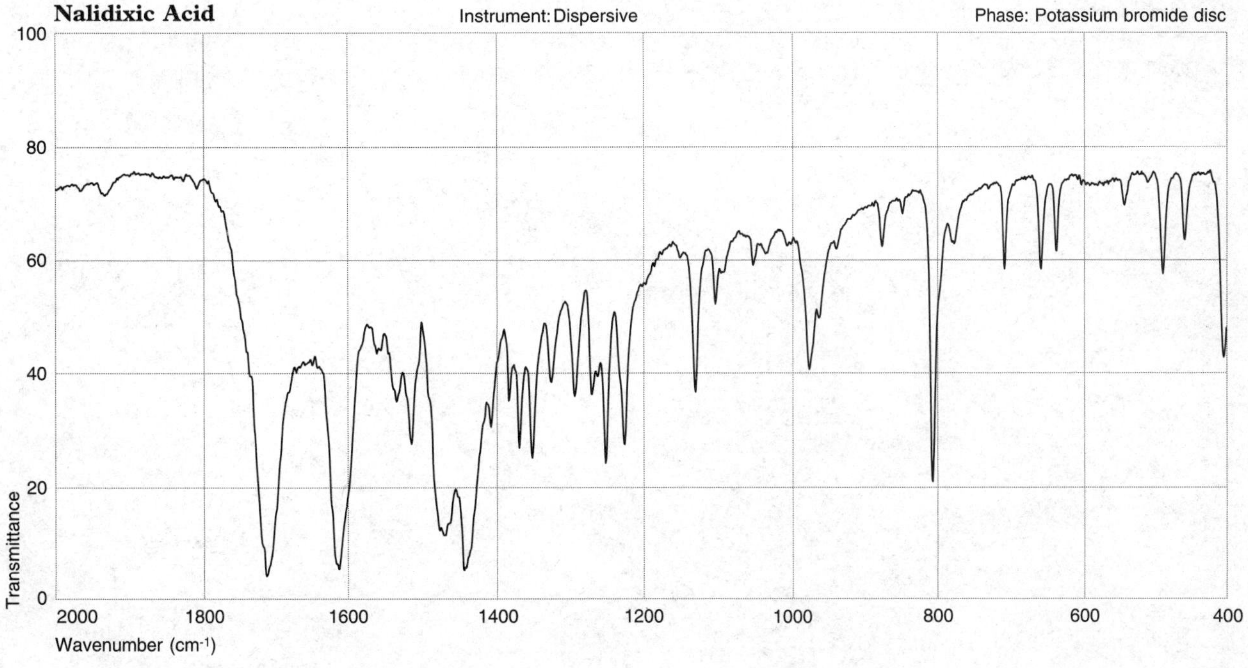

Nandrolone Decanoate

Instrument: Dispersive

Phase: 10% w/v solution in chloroform Thickness: 0.1r

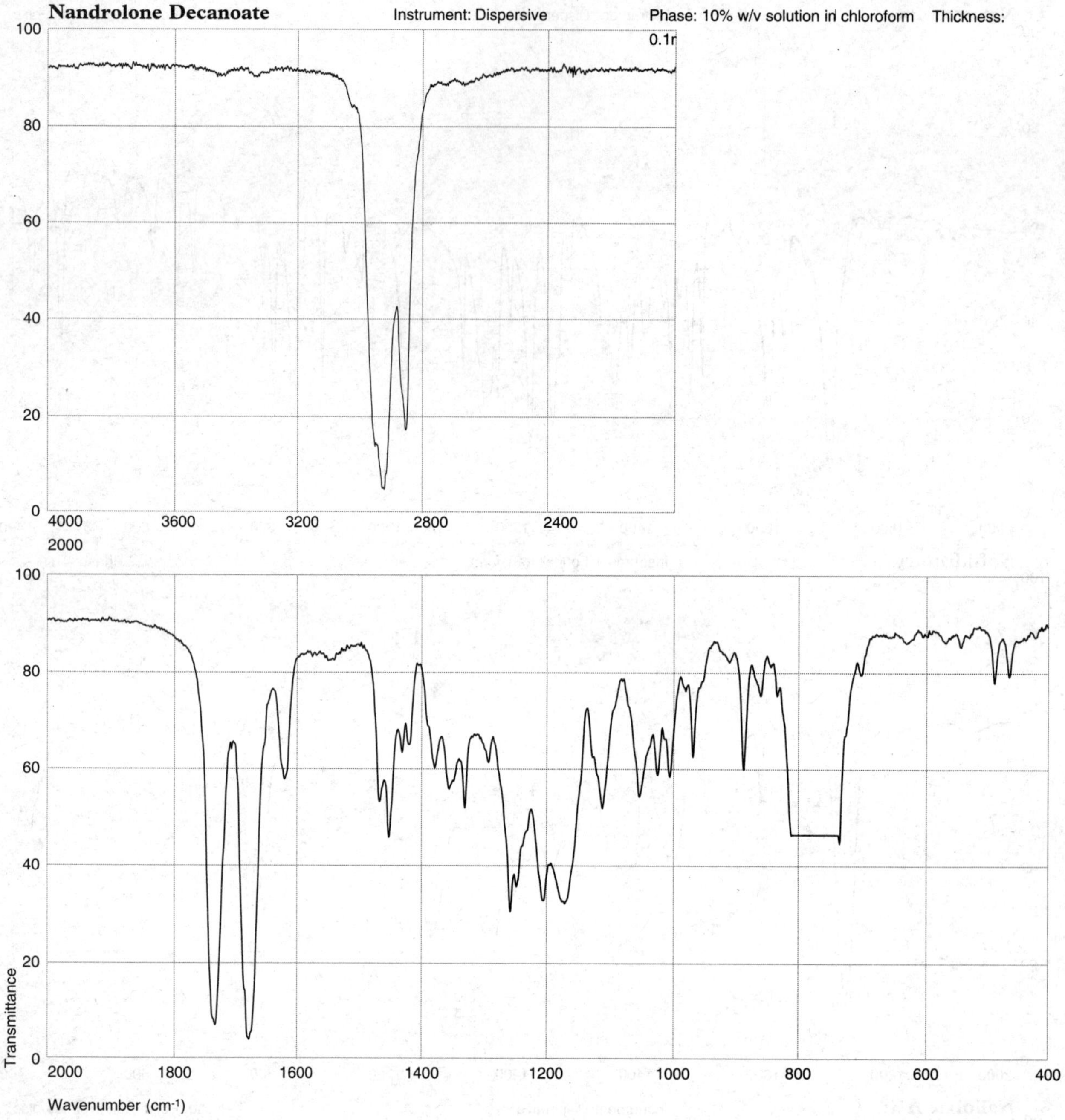

Nandrolone Phenylpropionate

Instrument: Dispersive Phase: 5% w/v solution in chloroform Thickness: 0.1

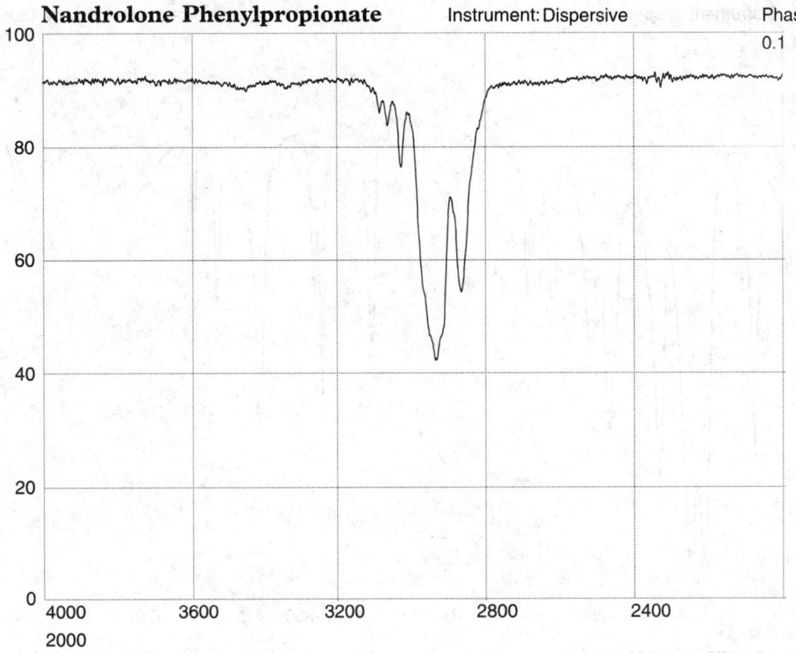

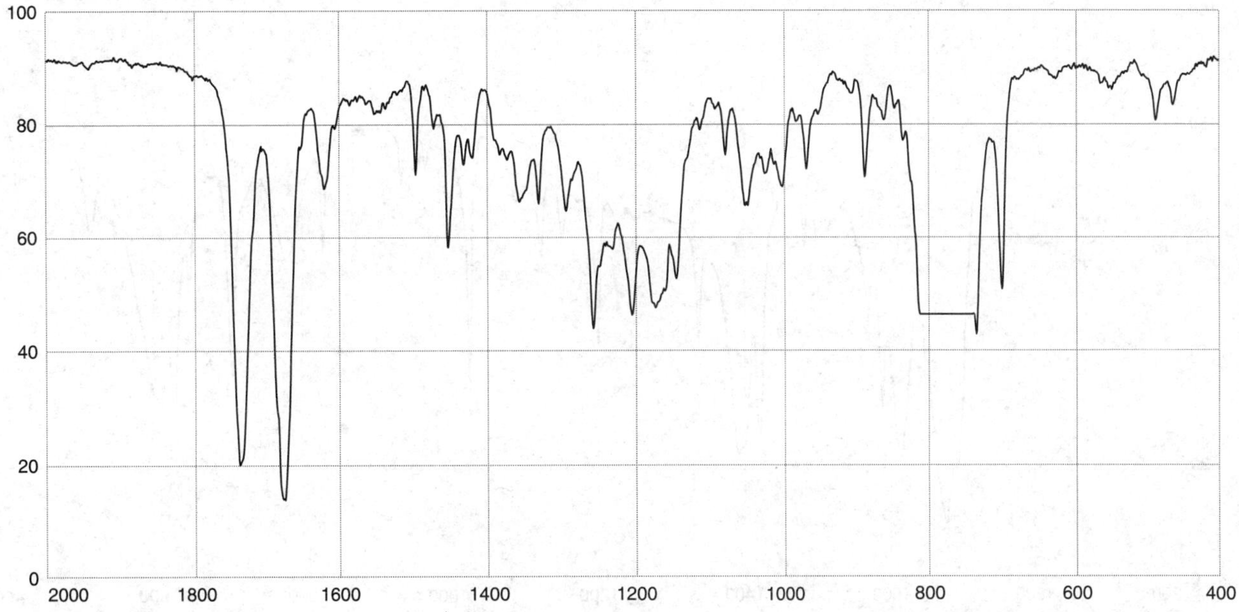

Naproxen

Instrument: Dispersive Phase: Potassium bromide disc

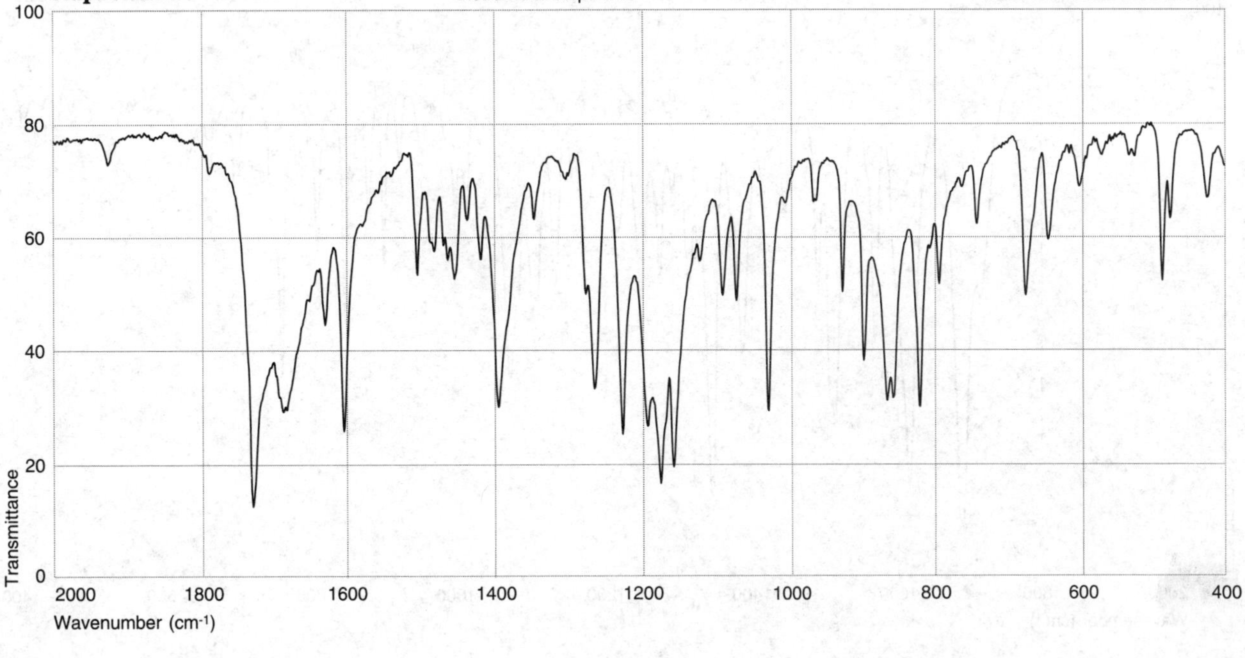

Niclosamide

Instrument: Dispersive

Phase: Potassium bromide disc

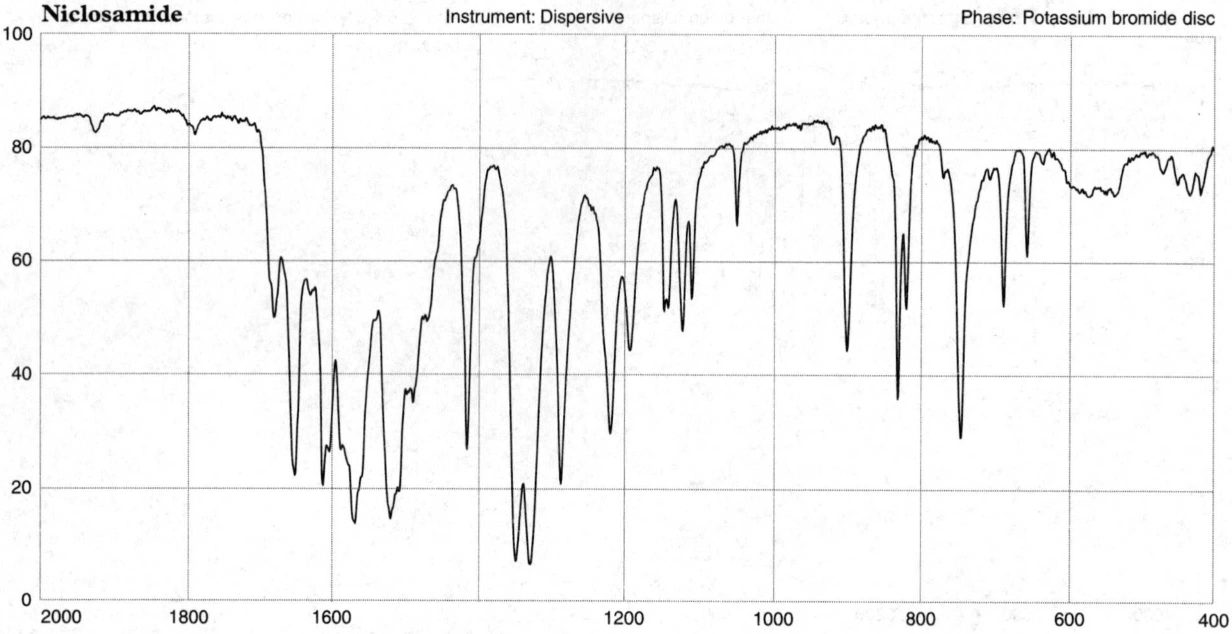

Nicotinamide

Instrument: Dispersive

Phase: Potassium bromide disc

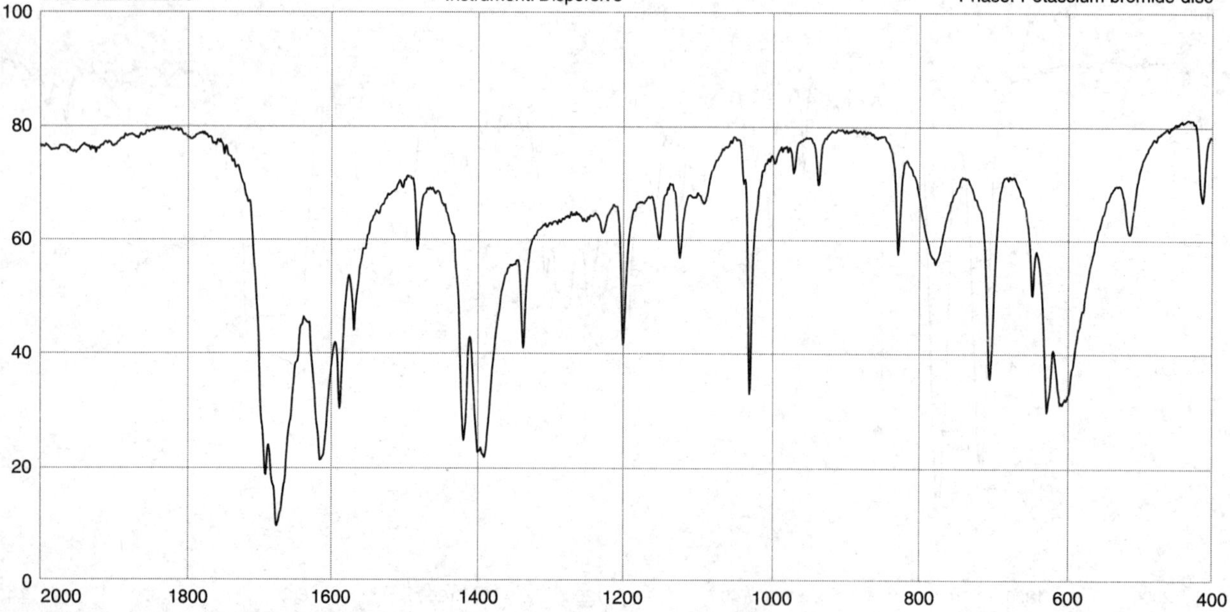

Nicoumalone (Acenocoumarol)

Instrument: Dispersive

Phase: Potassium bromide disc

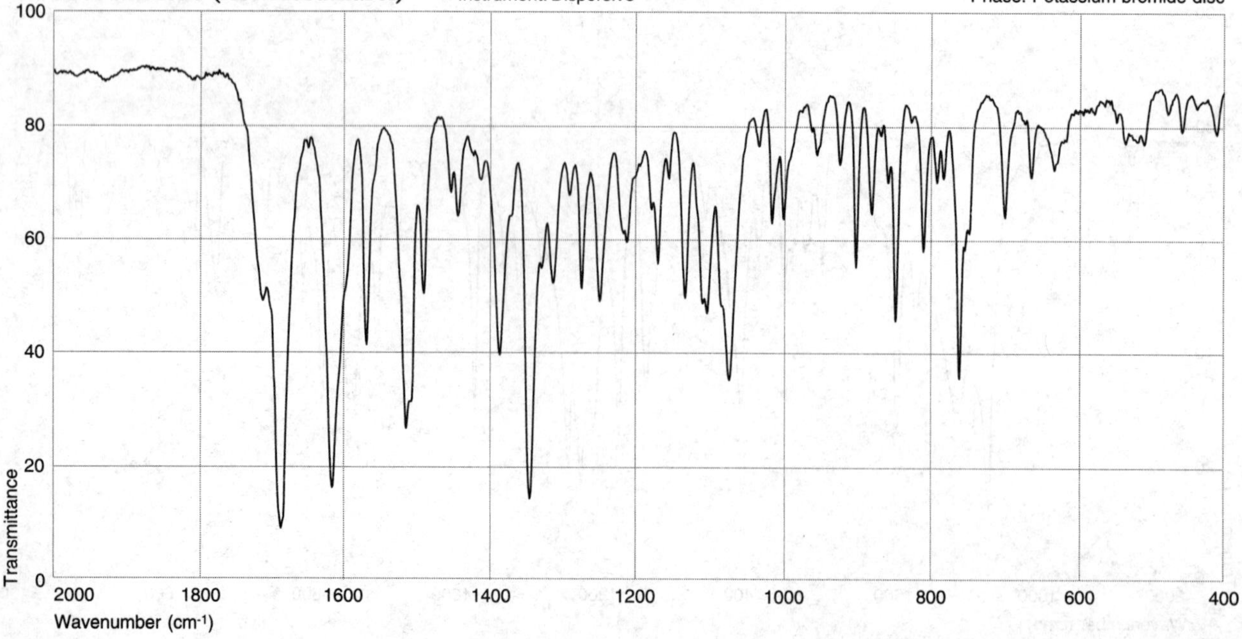

Nifedipine Instrument: Dispersive Phase: Potassium bromide disc

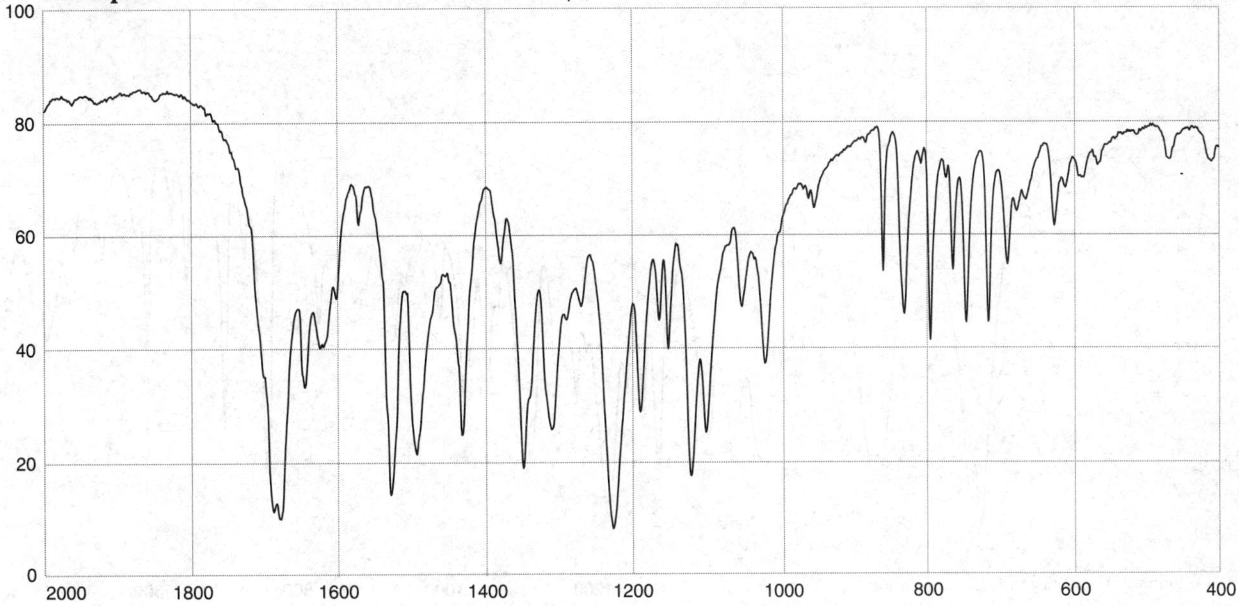

Nikethamide Instrument: Dispersive Phase: Thin film

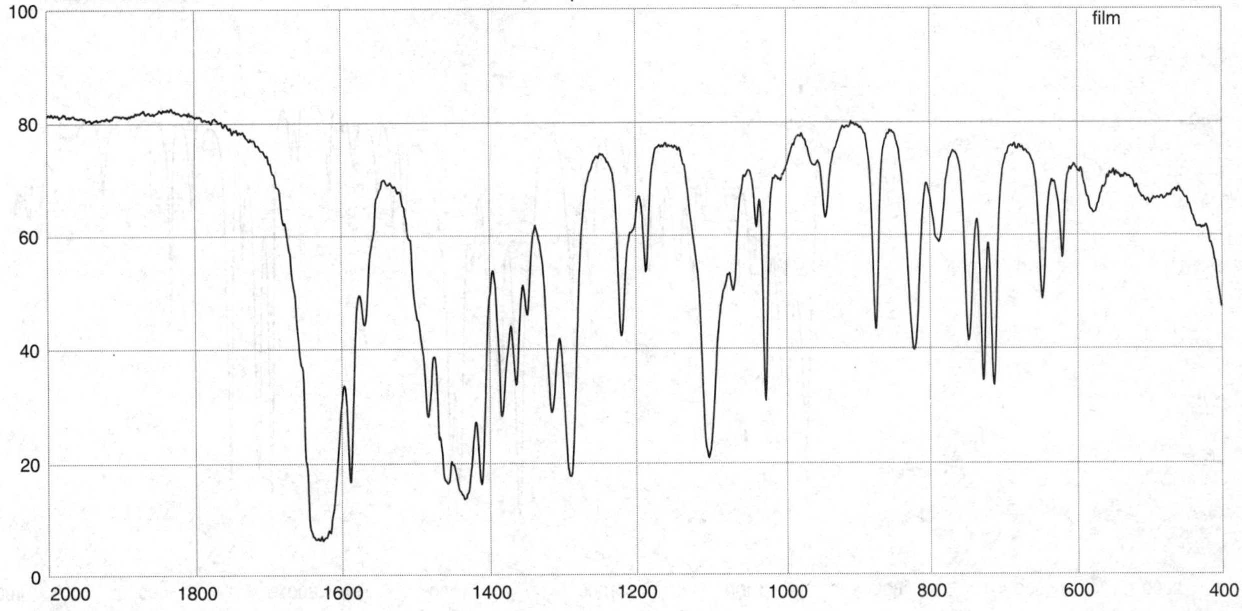

Octanoic Acid Instrument: Dispersive Phase: Thin film

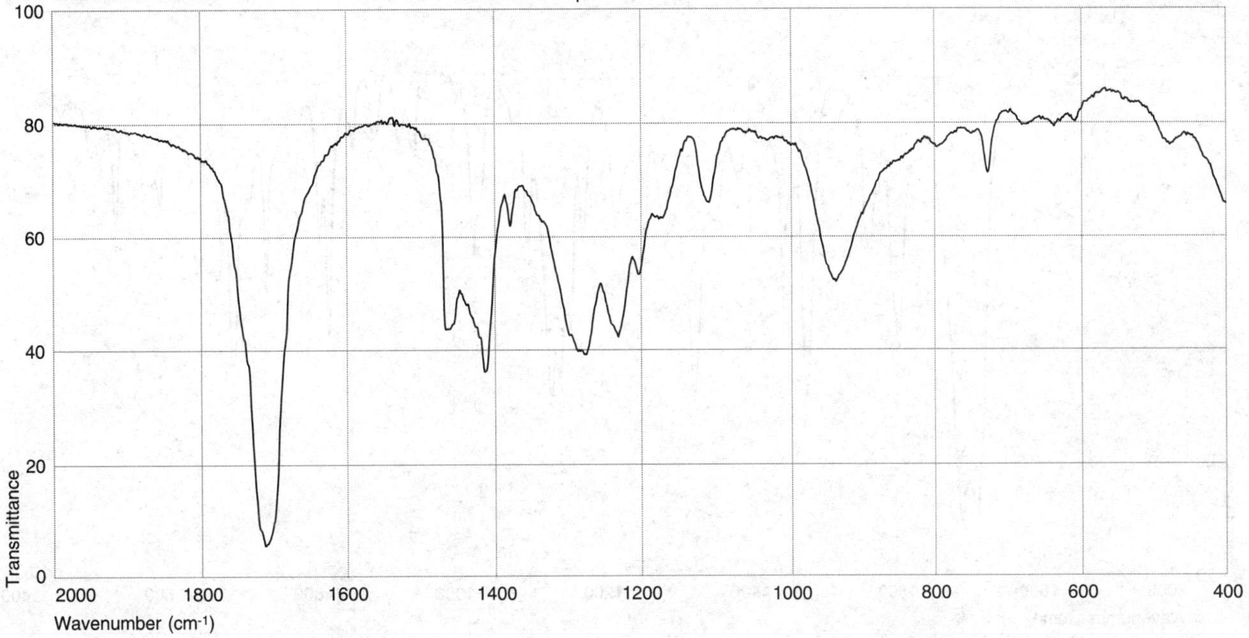

Orphenadrine Citrate Instrument: Fourier transform Phase: Potassium chloride disc

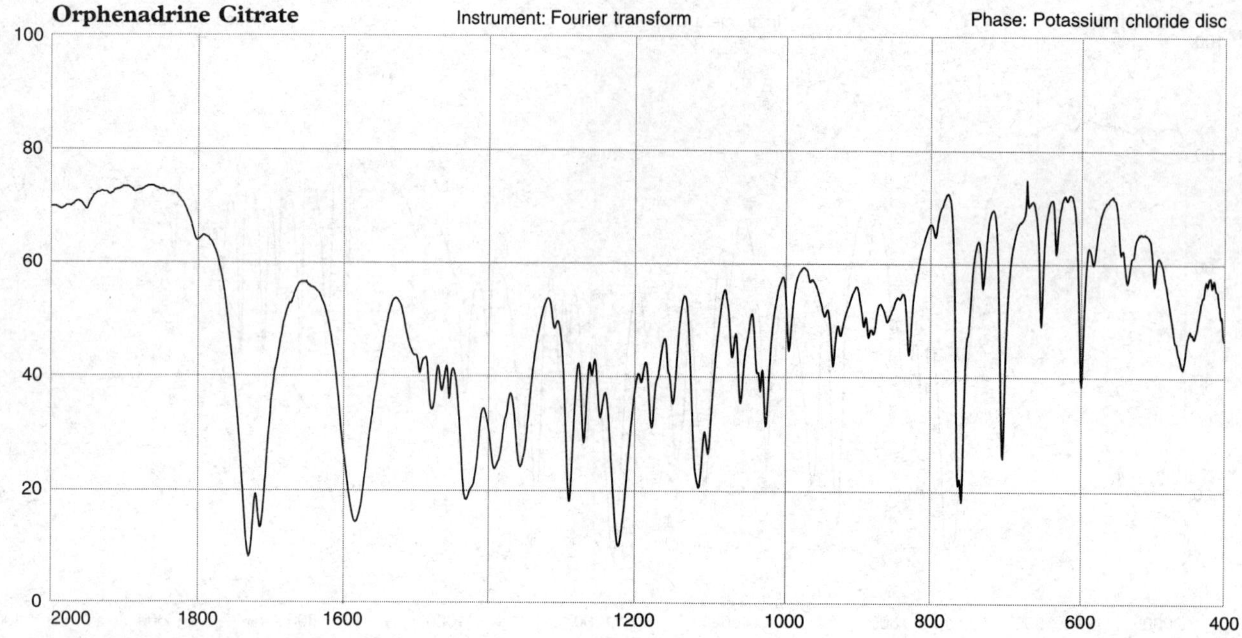

Orphenadrine Hydrochloride Instrument: Fourier transform Phase: Potassium chloride disc

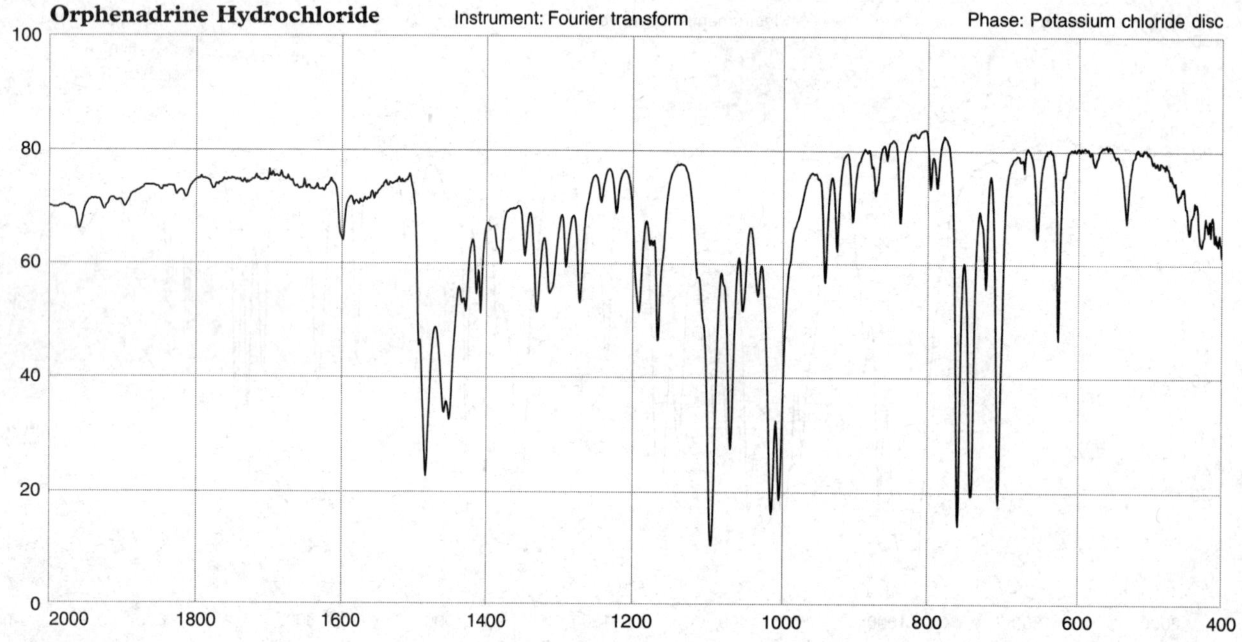

Oxazepam Instrument: Dispersive Phase: Potassium bromide disc

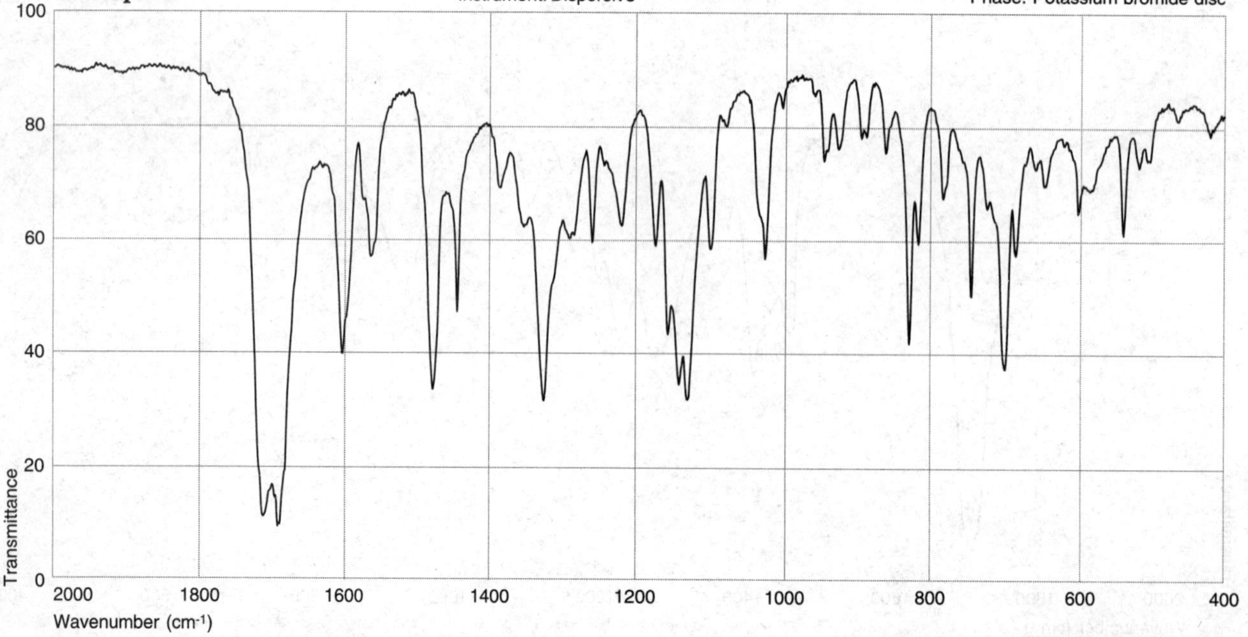

Oxetacaine Instrument: Dispersive Phase: Potassium bromide disc

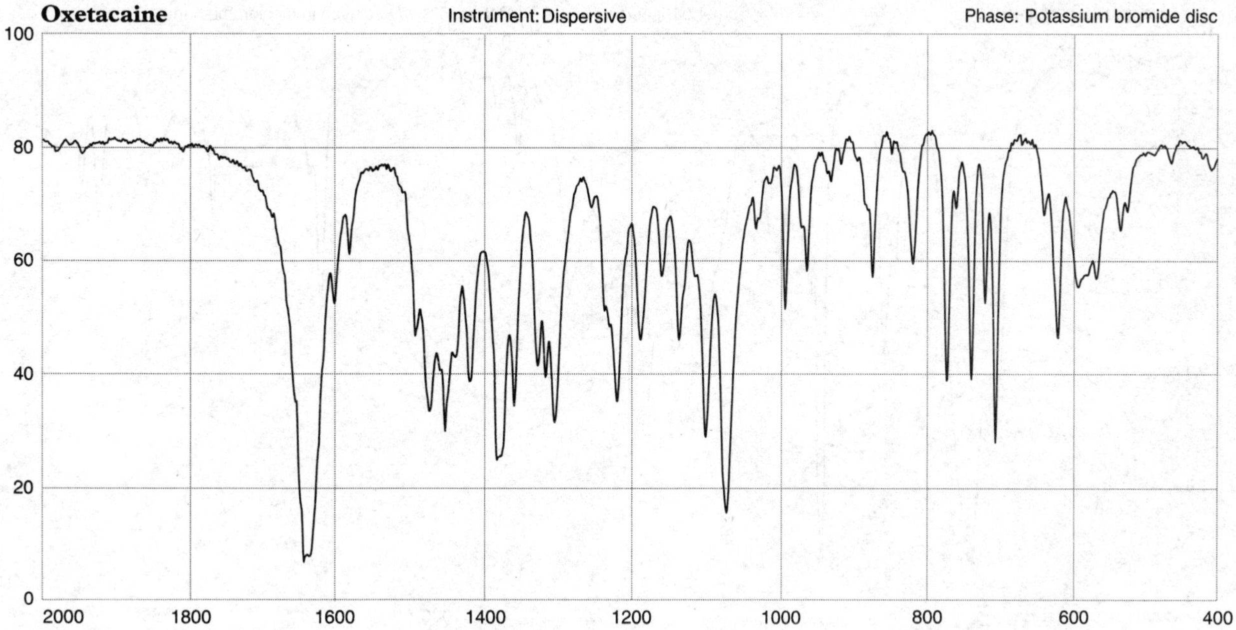

Oxprenolol Instrument: Dispersive Phase: Potassium bromide disc

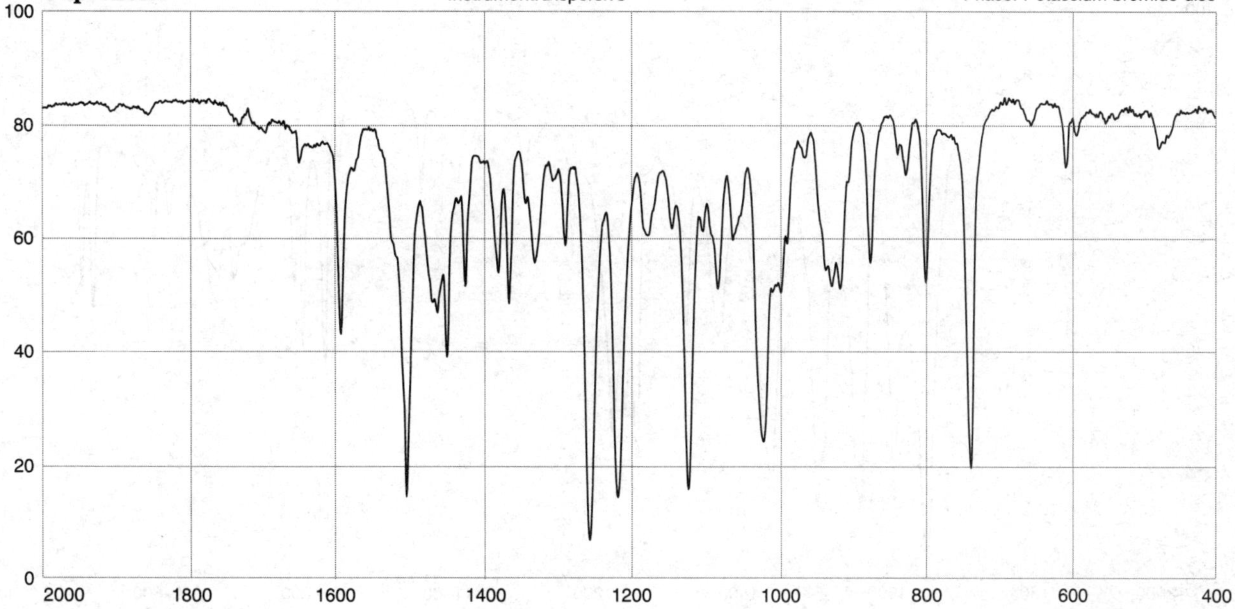

Oxymetholone Instrument: Dispersive Phase: Potassium bromide disc

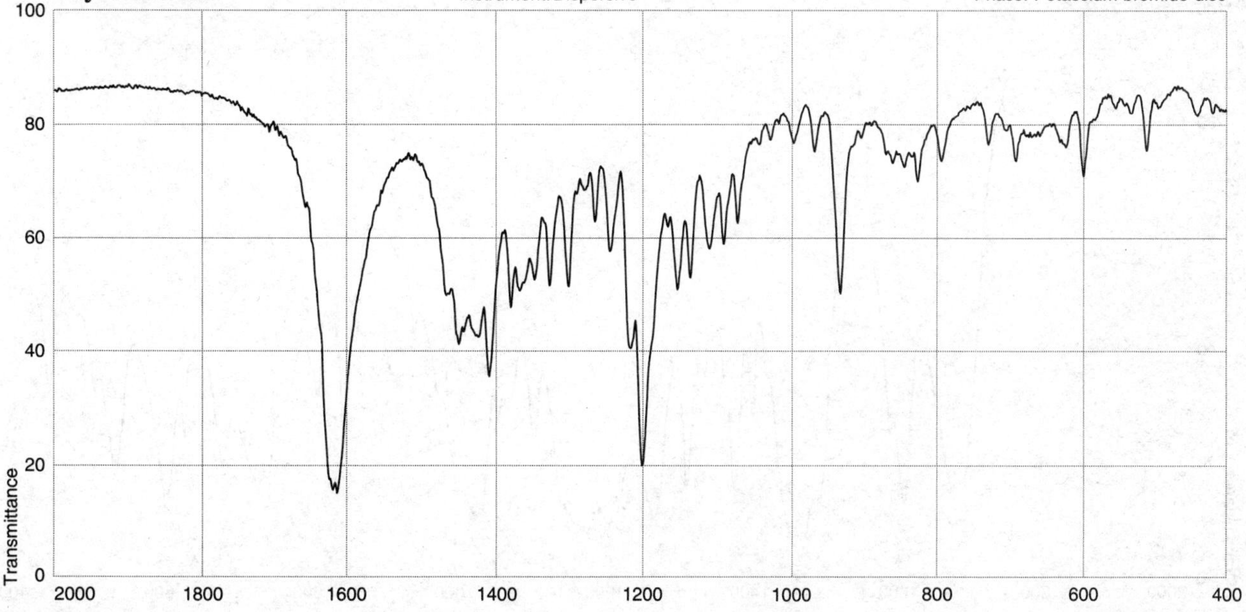

Oxyphenbutazone Instrument: Dispersive Phase: 5% w/v solution in dichloromethane Thickness: 0.1mm

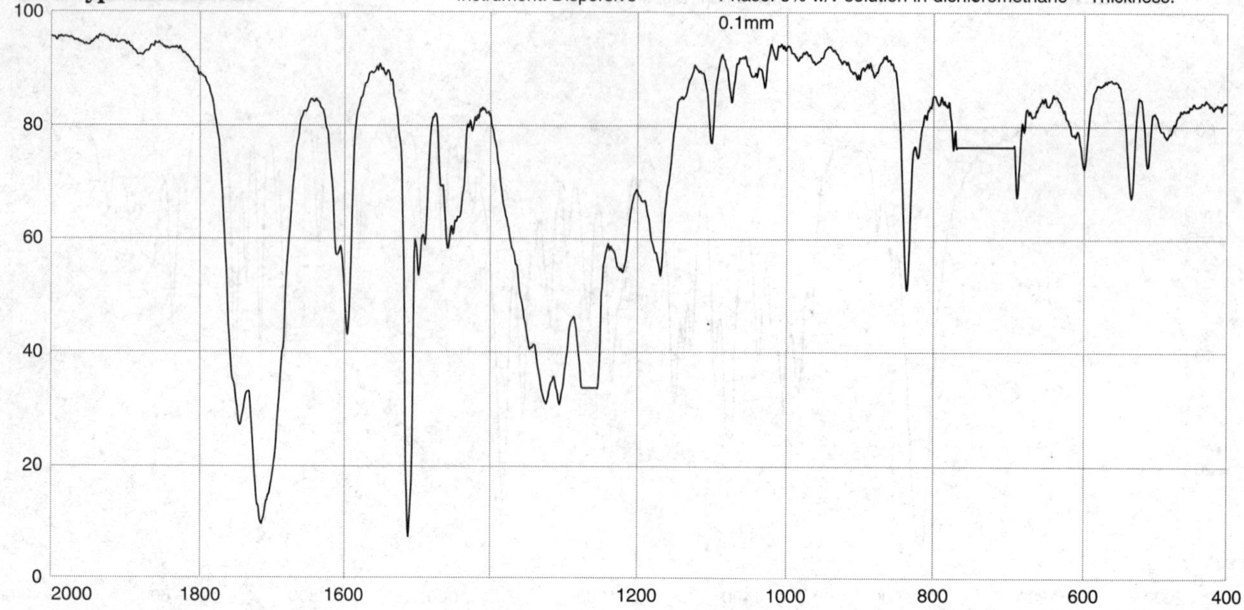

Paracetamol Instrument: Dispersive Phase: Potassium bromide disc

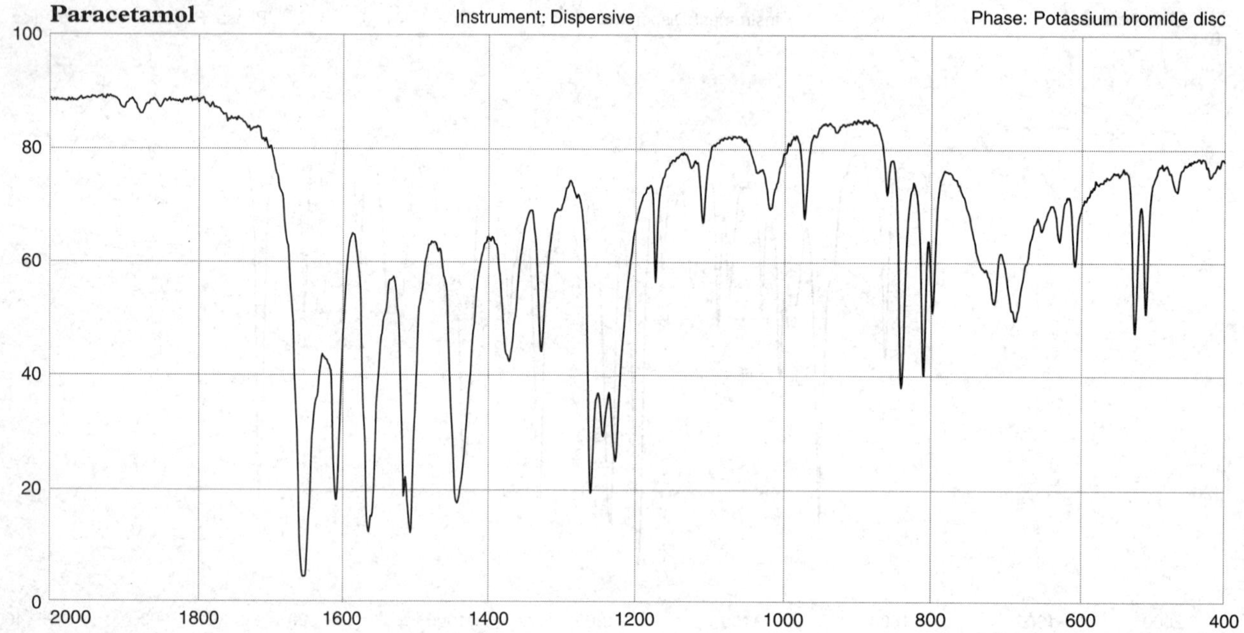

Pentamidine Isetionate Instrument: Dispersive Phase: Liquid paraffin mull

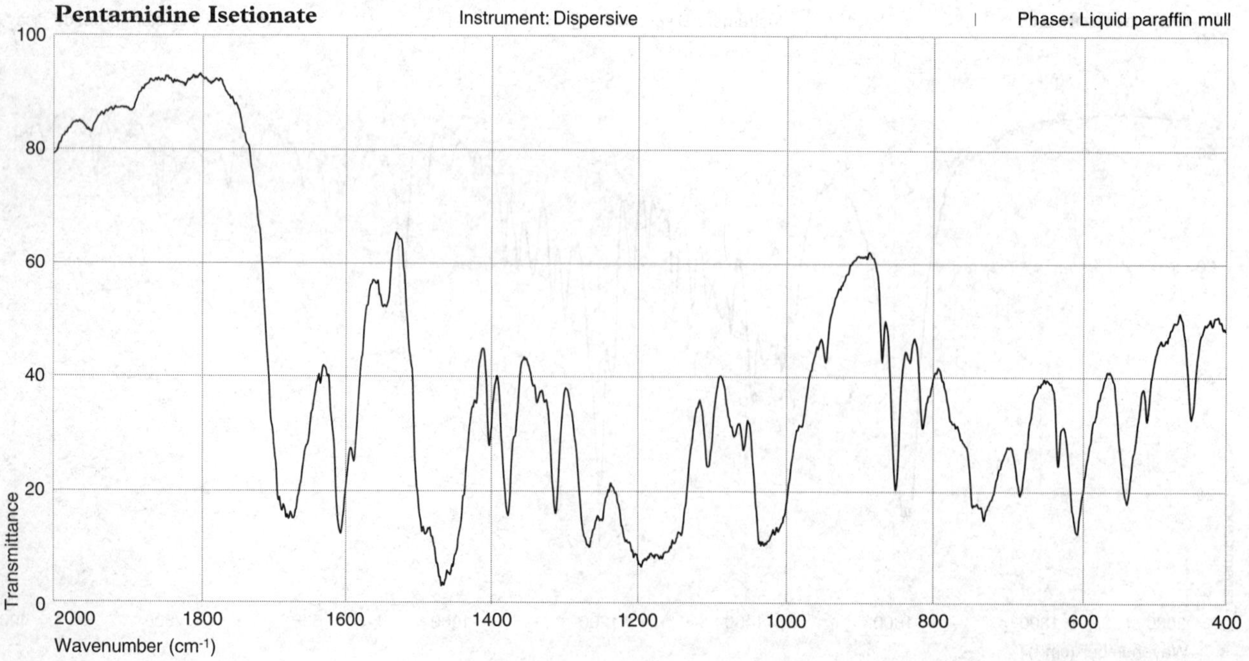

Pentazocine (form A) Instrument: Dispersive Phase: Potassium bromide disc

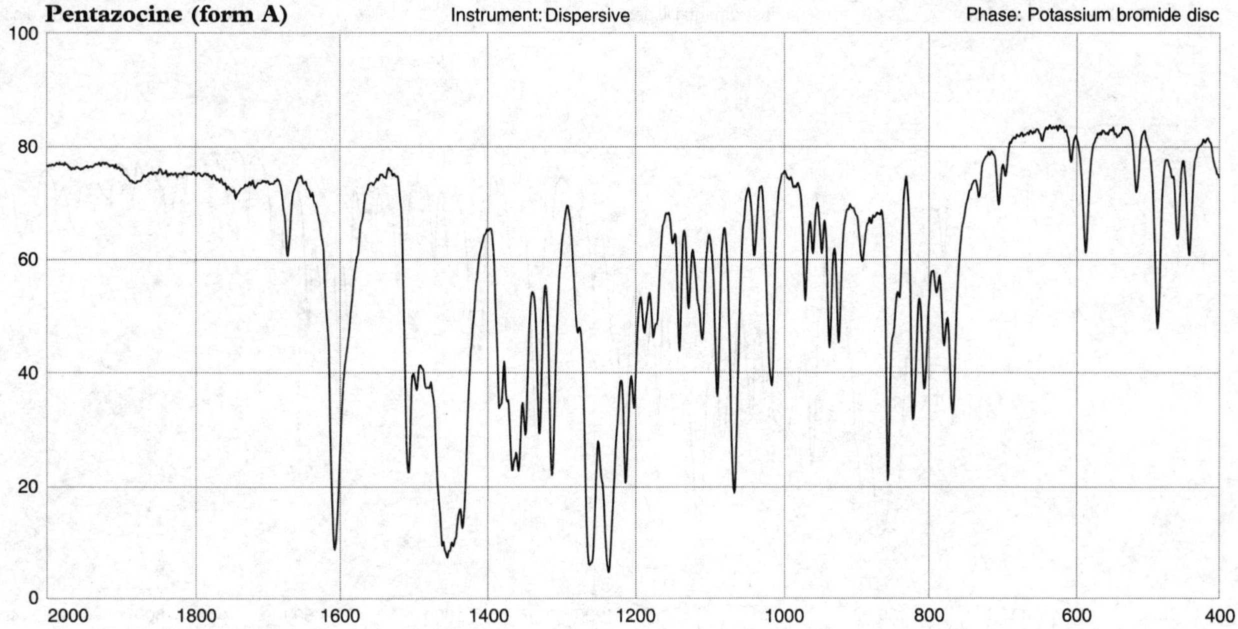

Pentazocine (form B) Instrument: Dispersive Phase: Potassium bromide disc

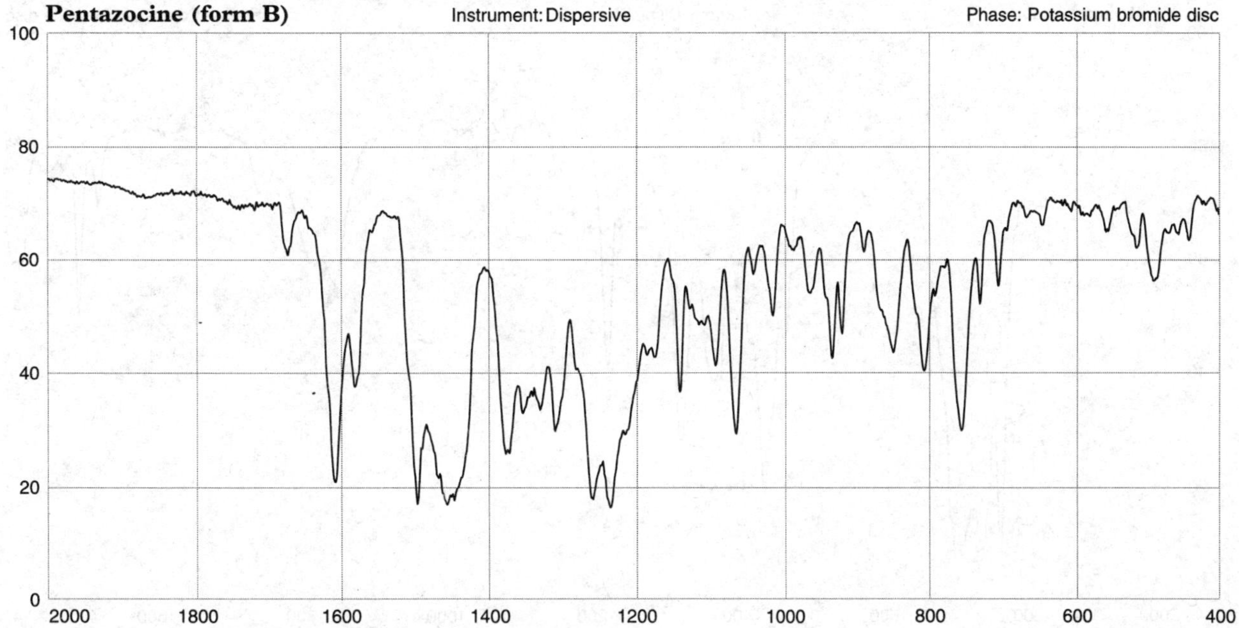

Pentazocine Hydrochloride Instrument: Dispersive Phase: Potassium chloride disc

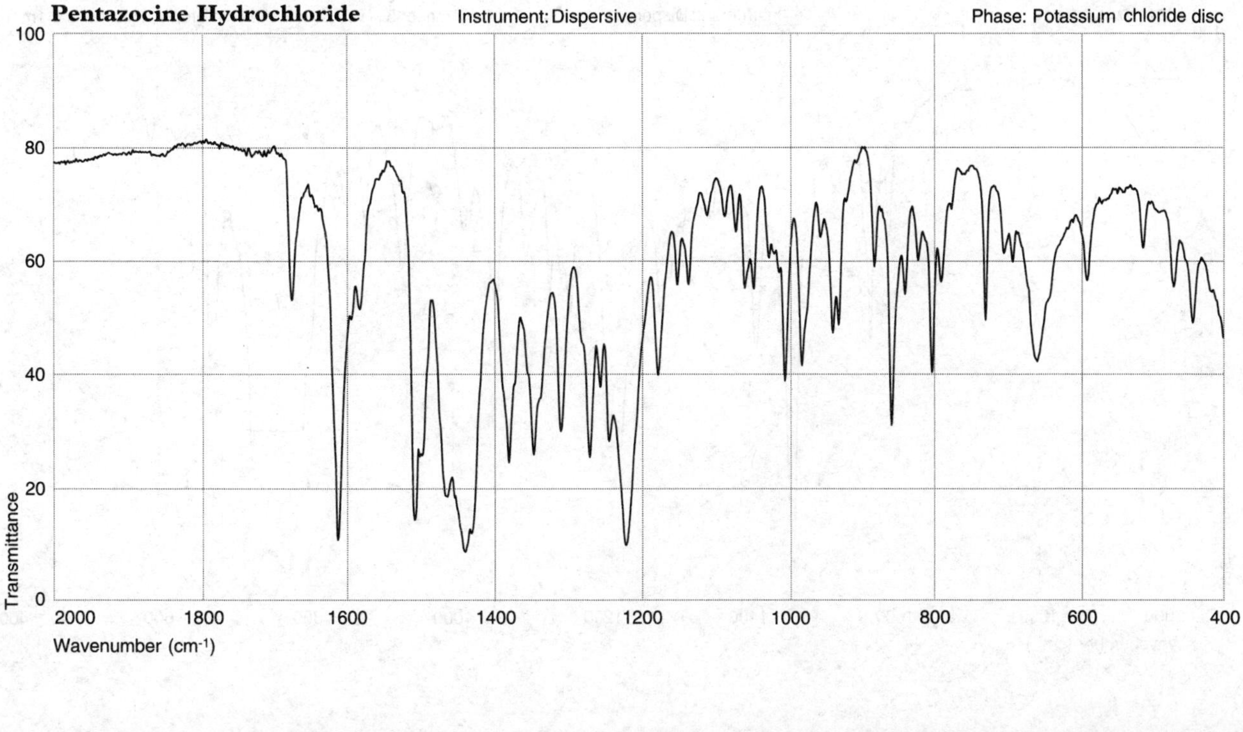

Pentazocine Lactate

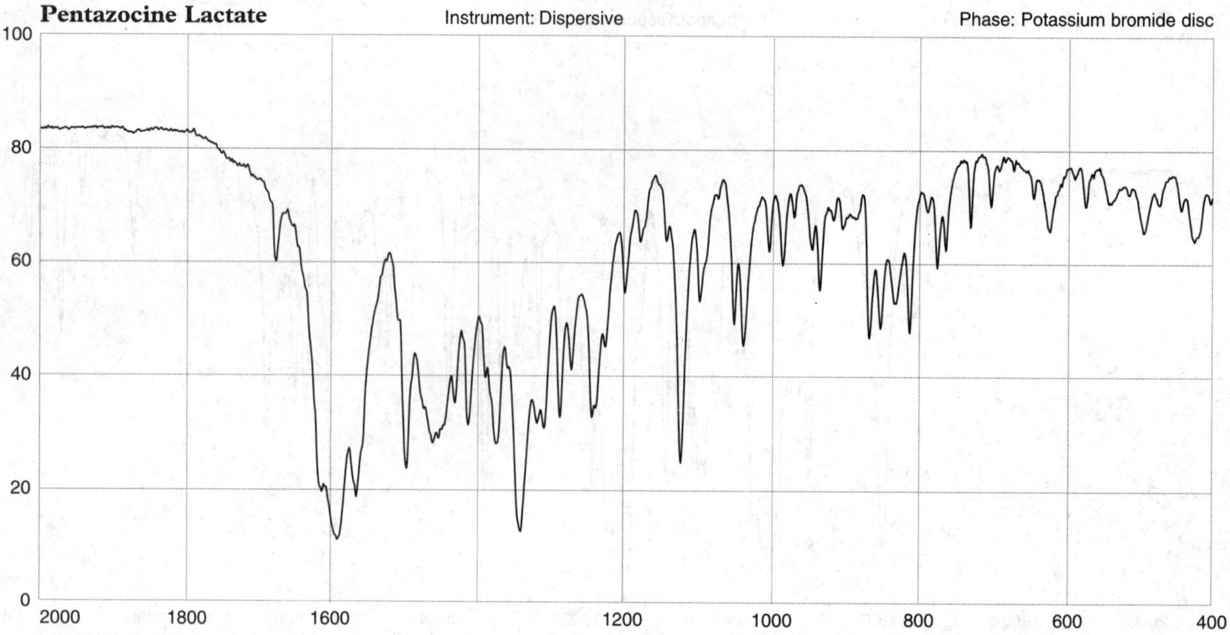

Pentobarbital

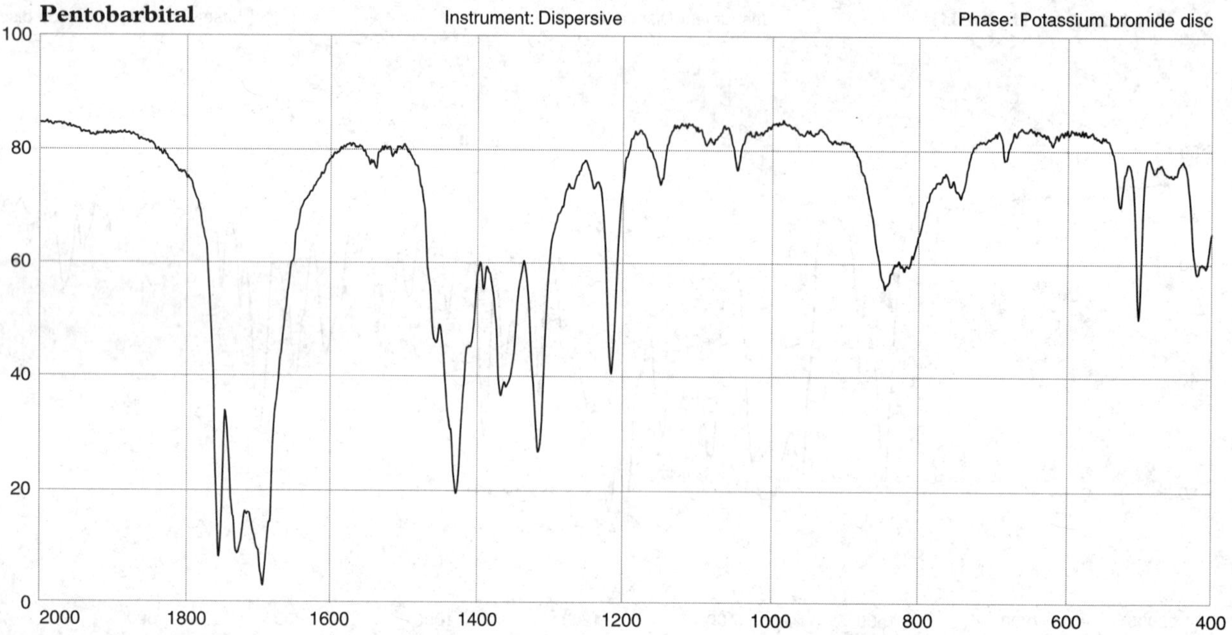

Perphenazine

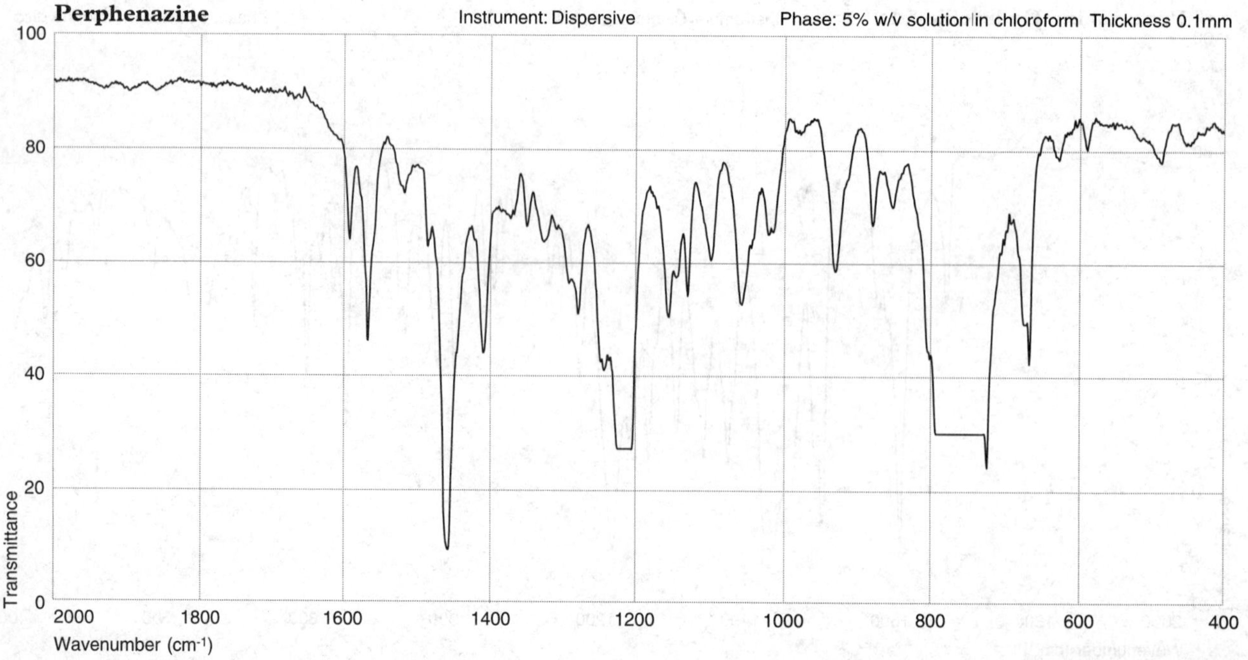

Pethidine

Instrument: Dispersive | Phase: Thin film

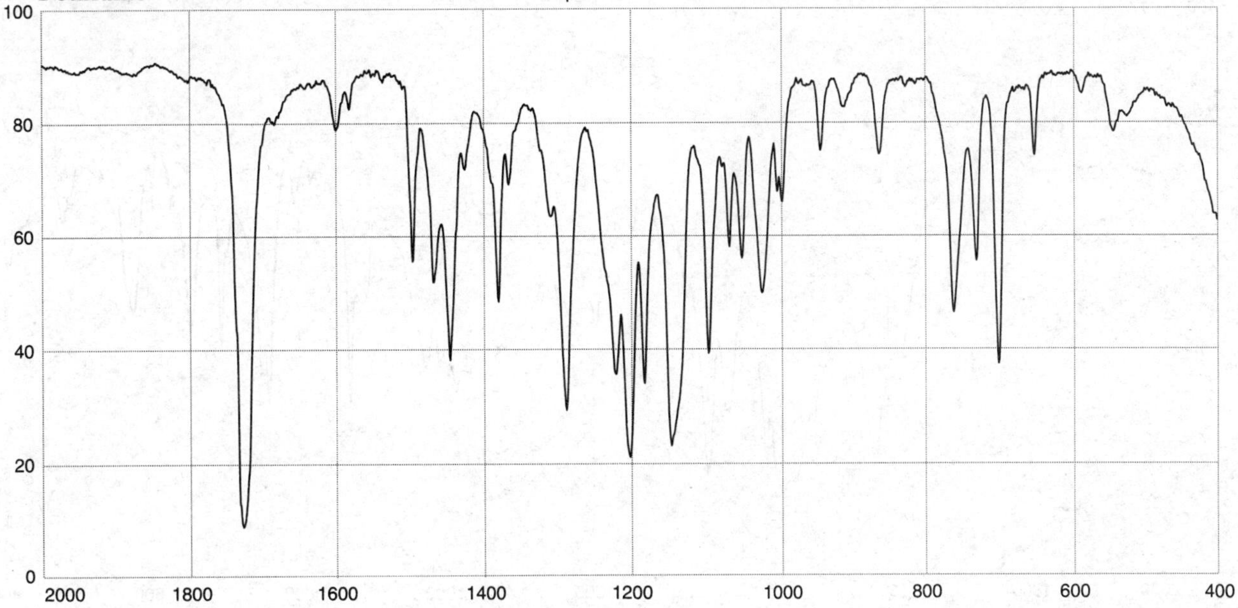

Pethidine Hydrochloride

Instrument: Dispersive | Phase: Potassium chloride disc

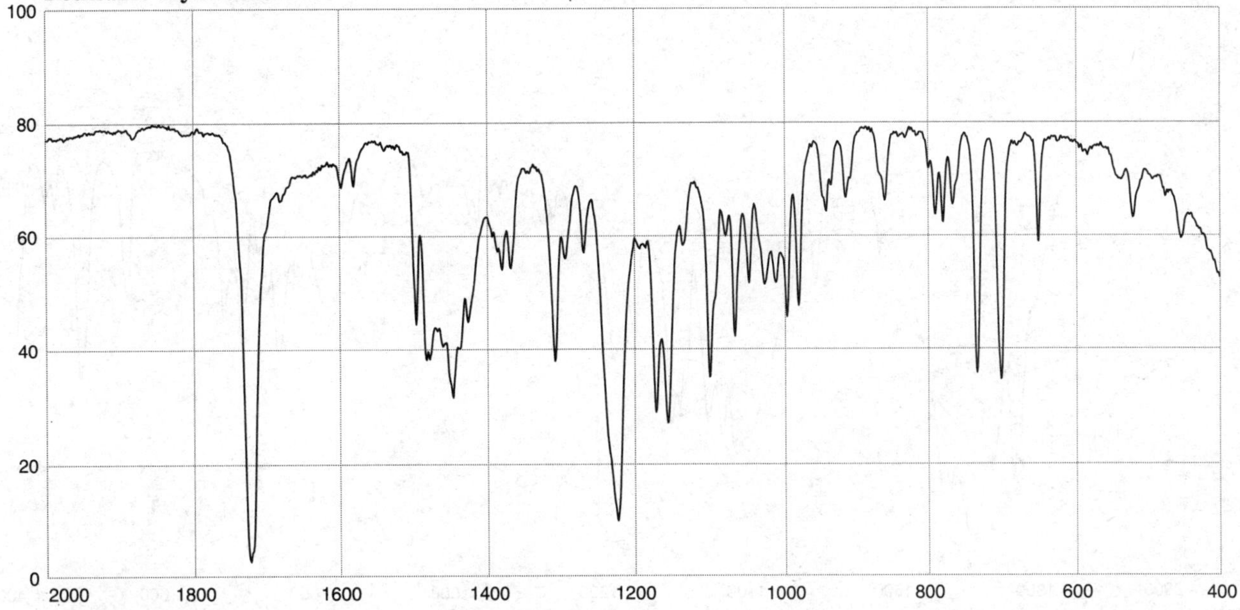

Phenindione

Instrument: Dispersive | Phase: Potassium bromide disc

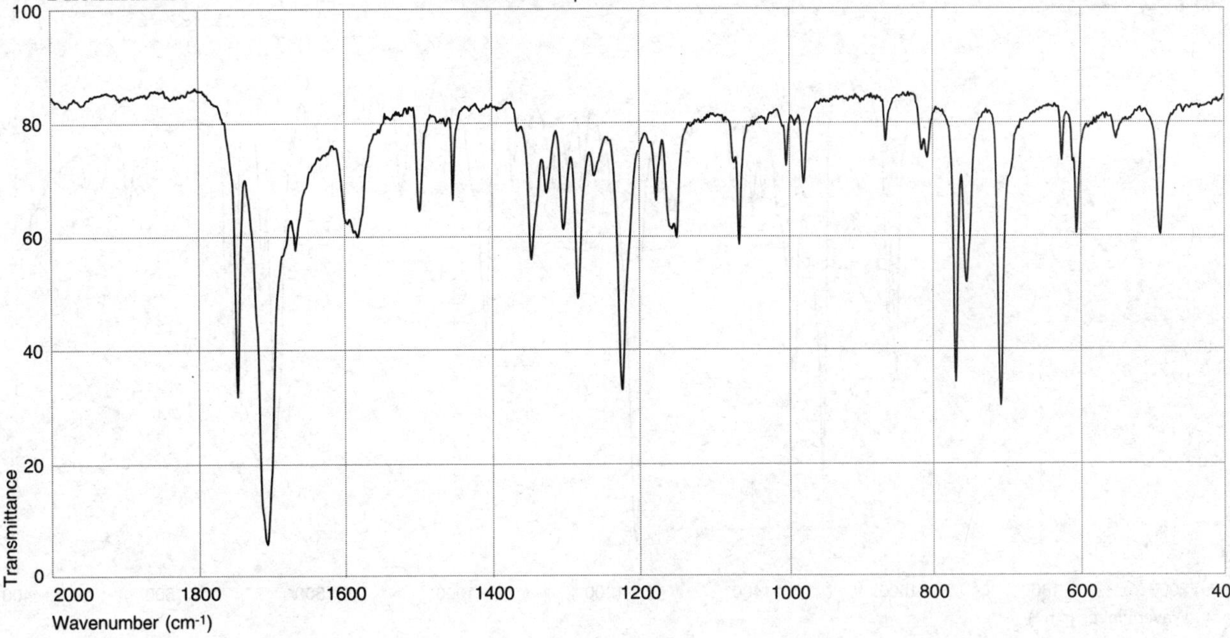

Pheniramine Maleate Instrument: Dispersive Phase: Liquid paraffin mull

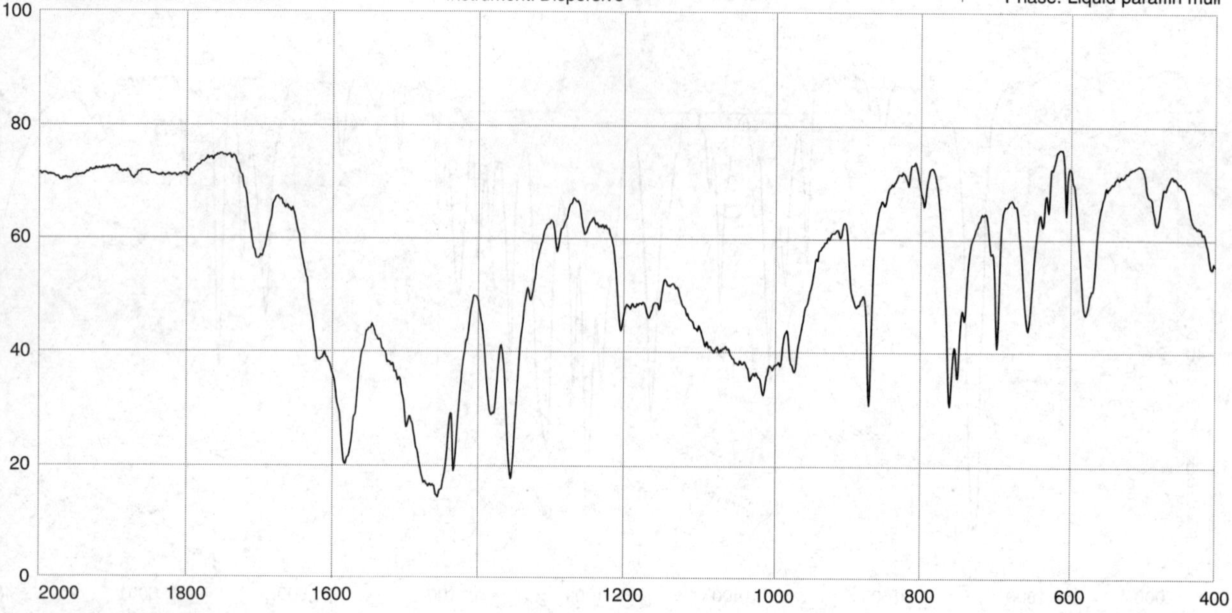

Phenobarbital Instrument: Dispersive Phase: Potassium bromide disc

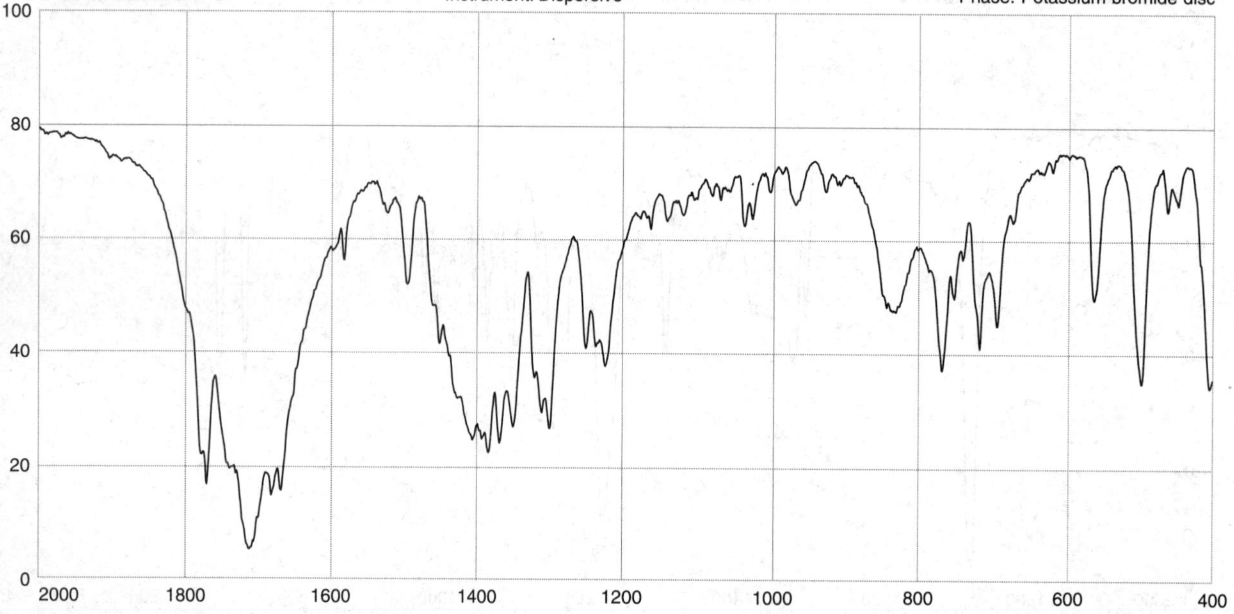

Phenoxybenzamine Hydrochloride Instrument: Dispersive Phase: Potassium chloride disc

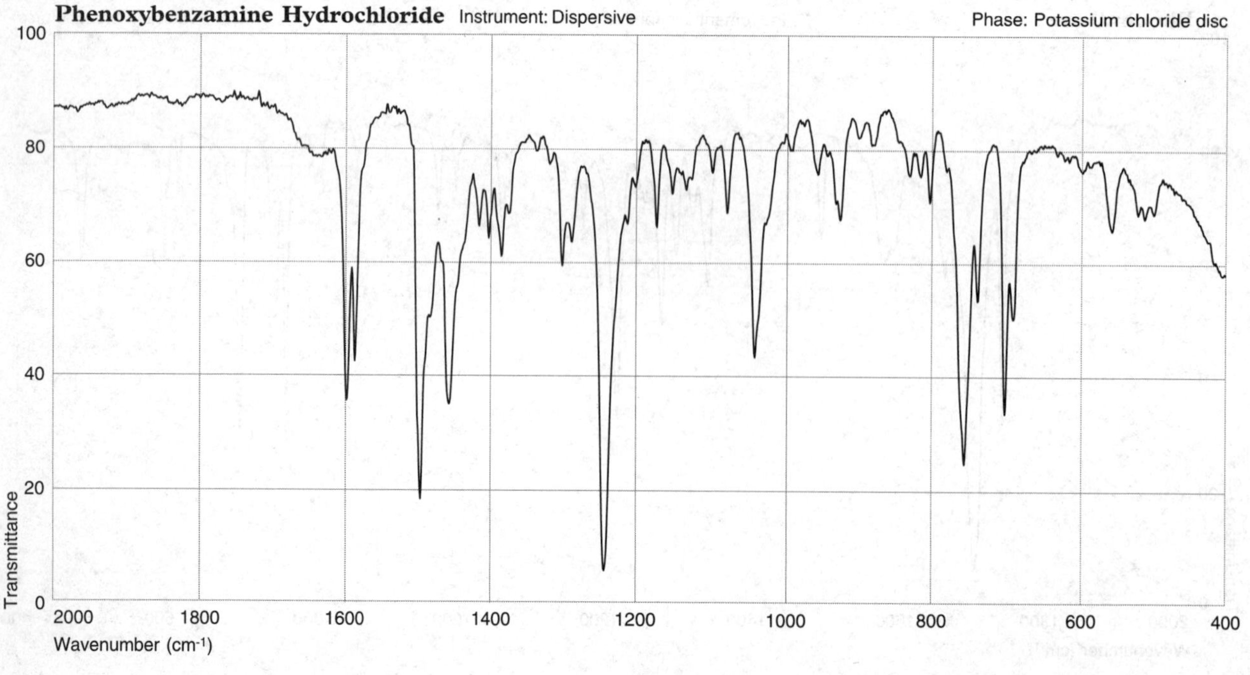

Phenytoin Instrument: Dispersive Phase: Potassium bromide disc

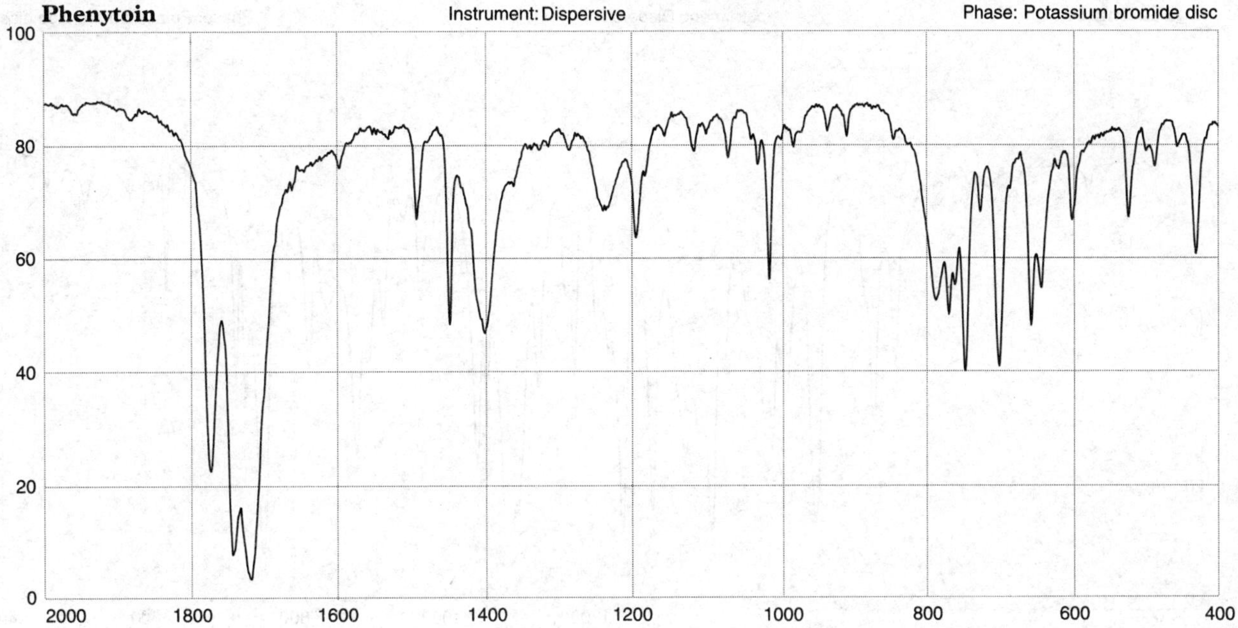

Pholcodine Instrument: Dispersive Phase: Potassium bromide disc

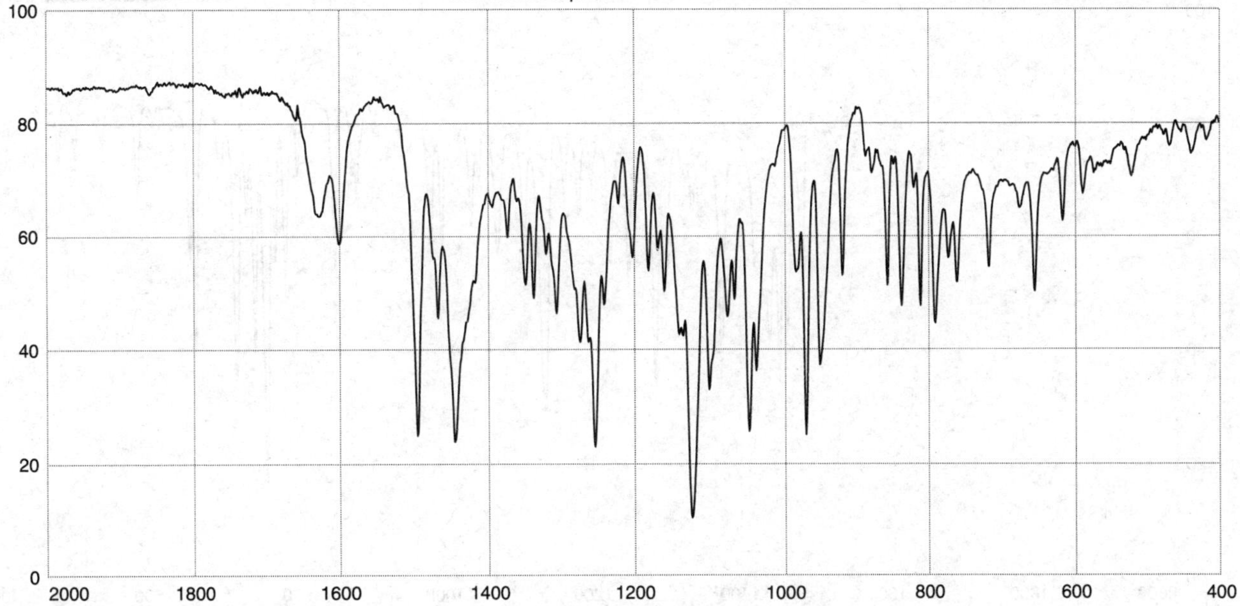

Pilocarpine Nitrate Instrument: Dispersive Phase: Potassium bromide disc

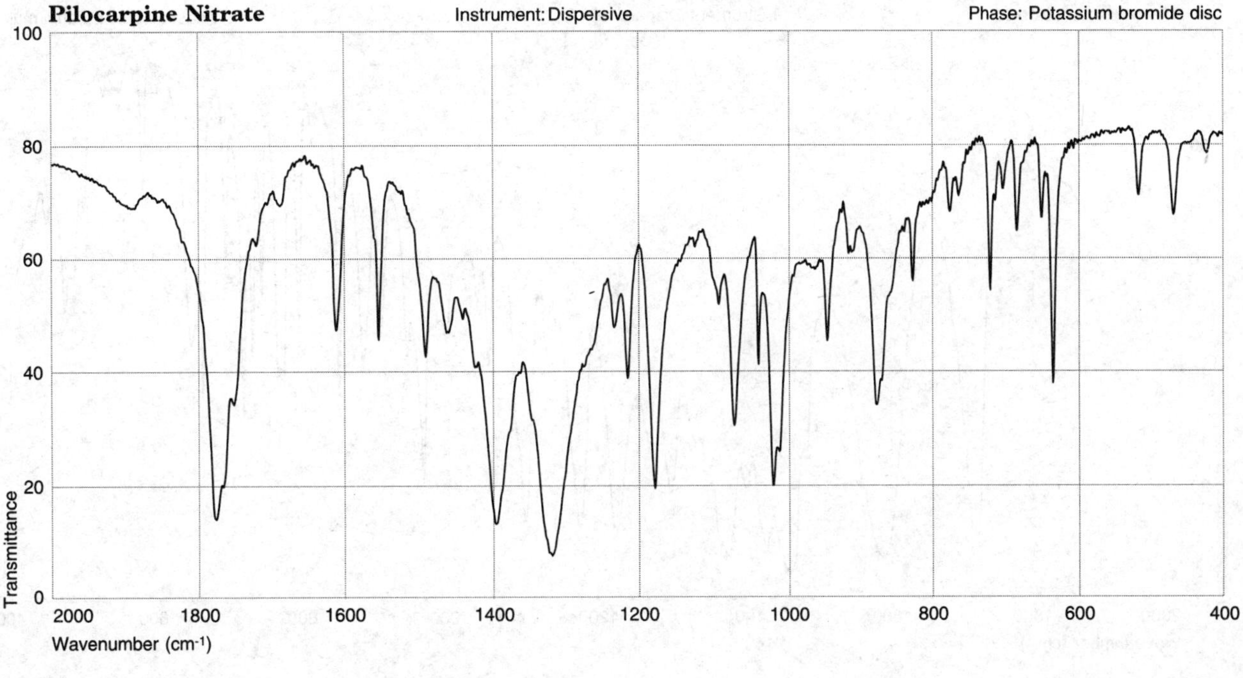

Pindolol Instrument: Dispersive Phase: Potassium bromide disc

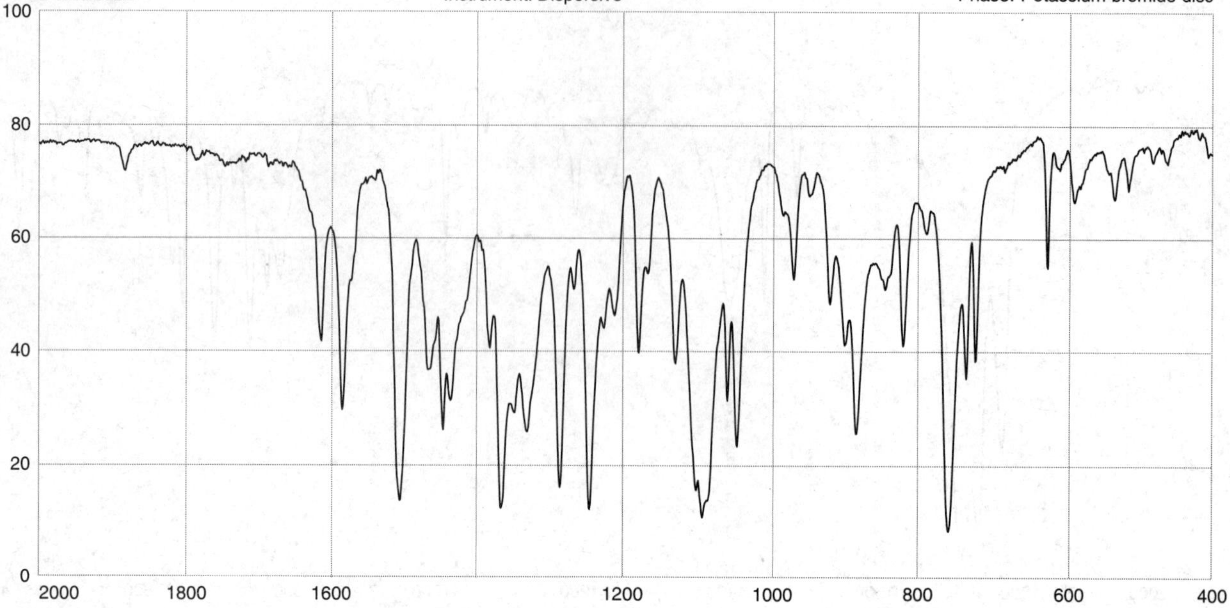

Pizotifen Instrument: Dispersive Phase: Potassium bromide disc

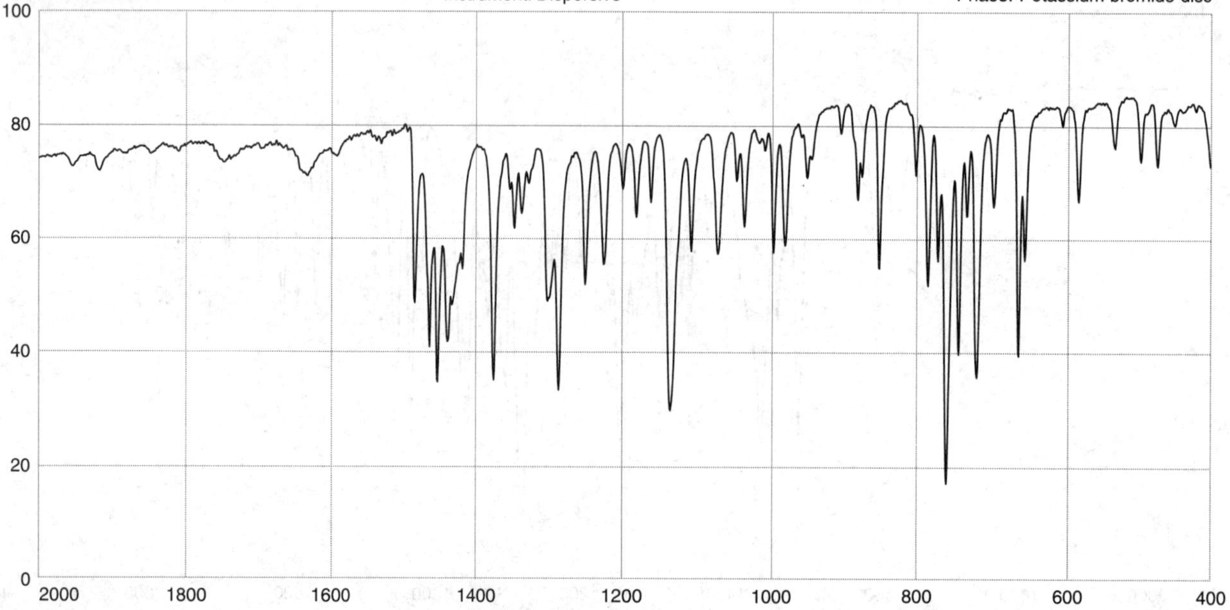

Pizotifen Malate Instrument: Dispersive Phase: Liquid paraffin mull

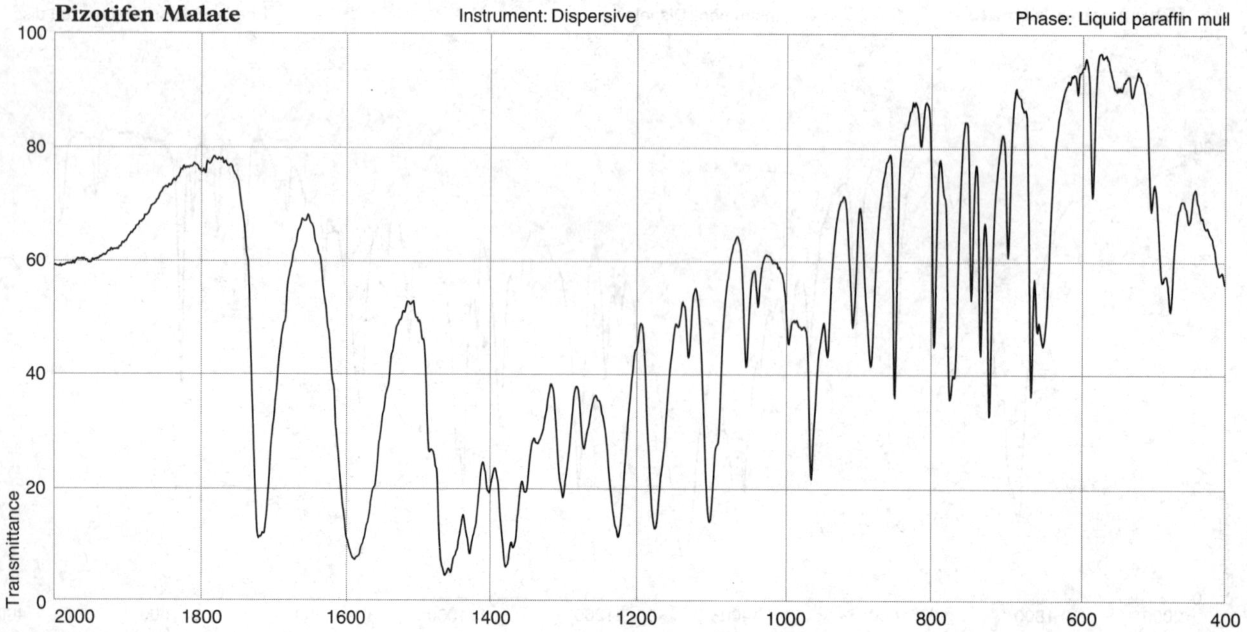

Poldine Metilsulfate Instrument: Dispersive Phase: Liquid paraffin mull

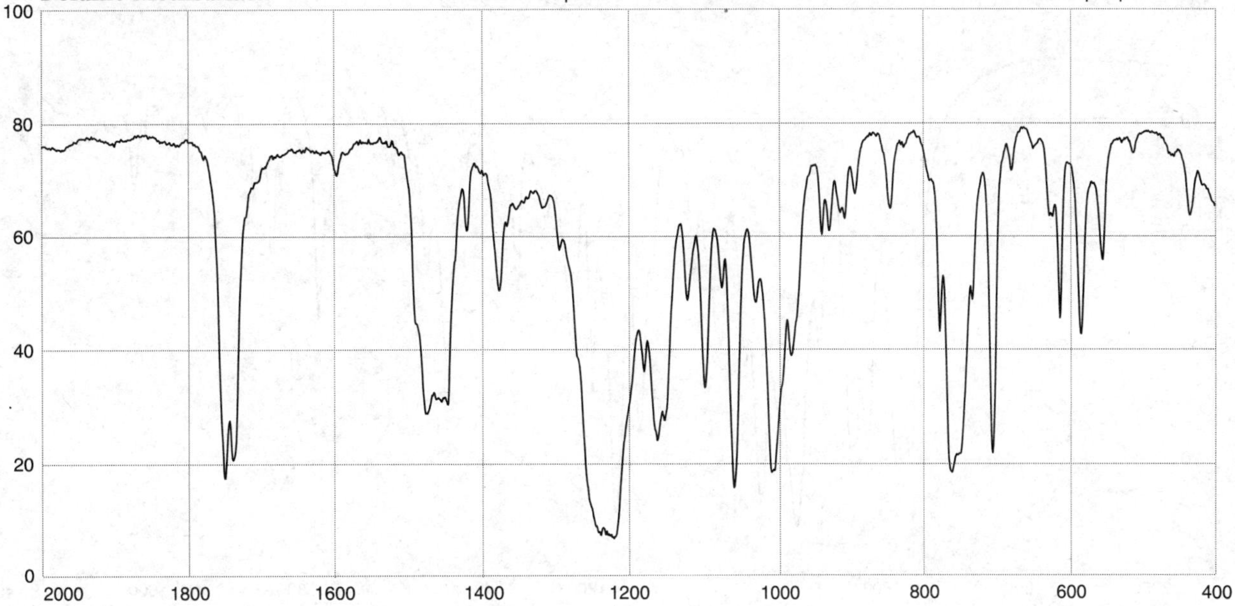

Poloxamer 188 Instrument: Dispersive Phase: Liquid paraffin mull

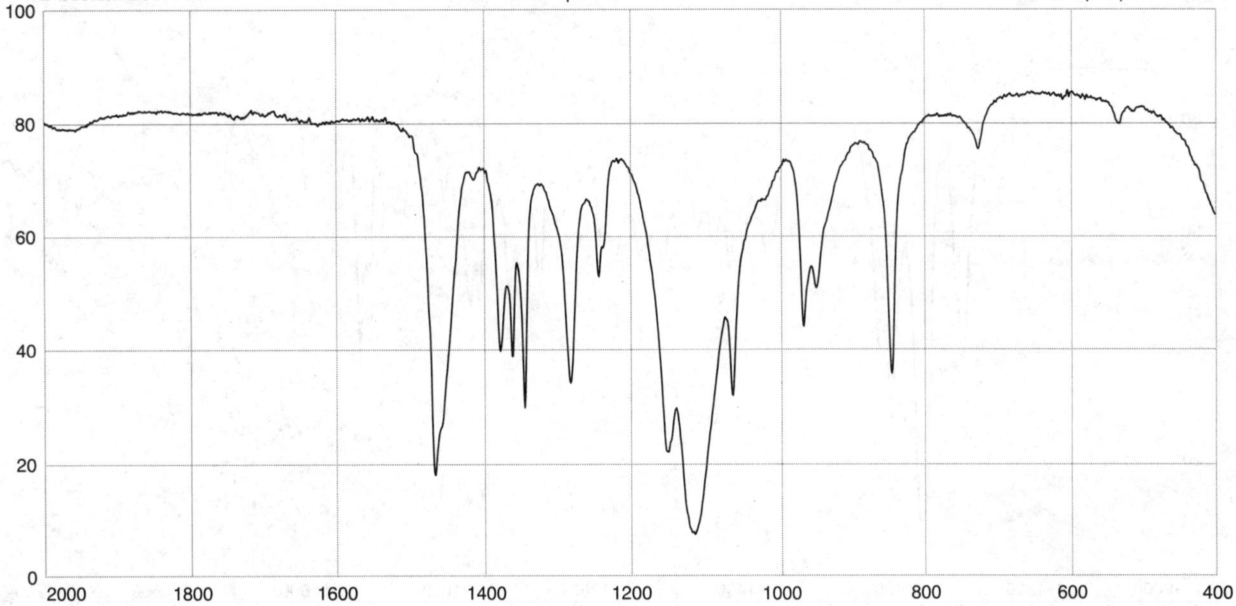

Polythiazide Instrument: Dispersive Phase: Potassium bromide disc

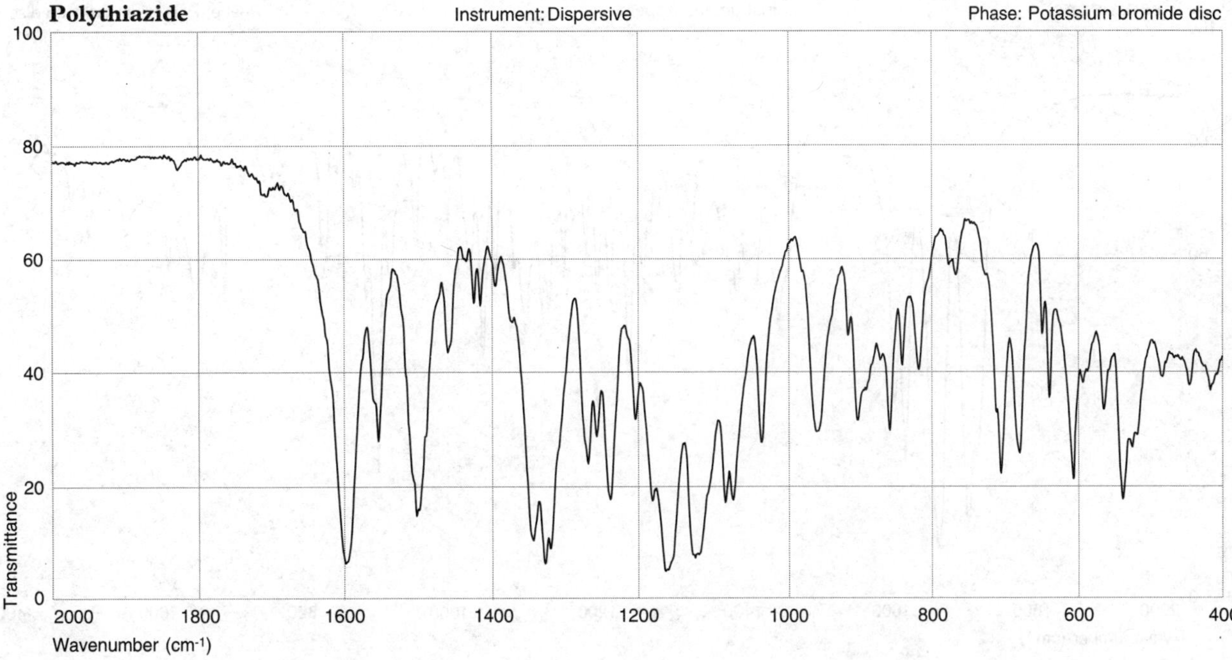

Prazosin

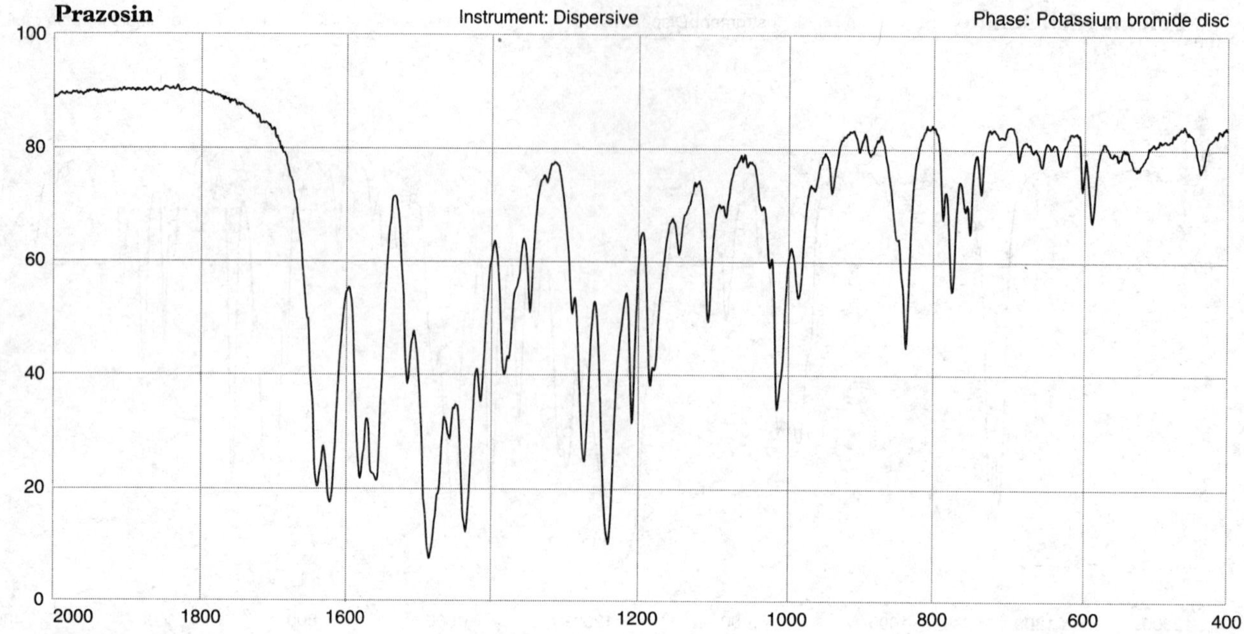

Prednisolone

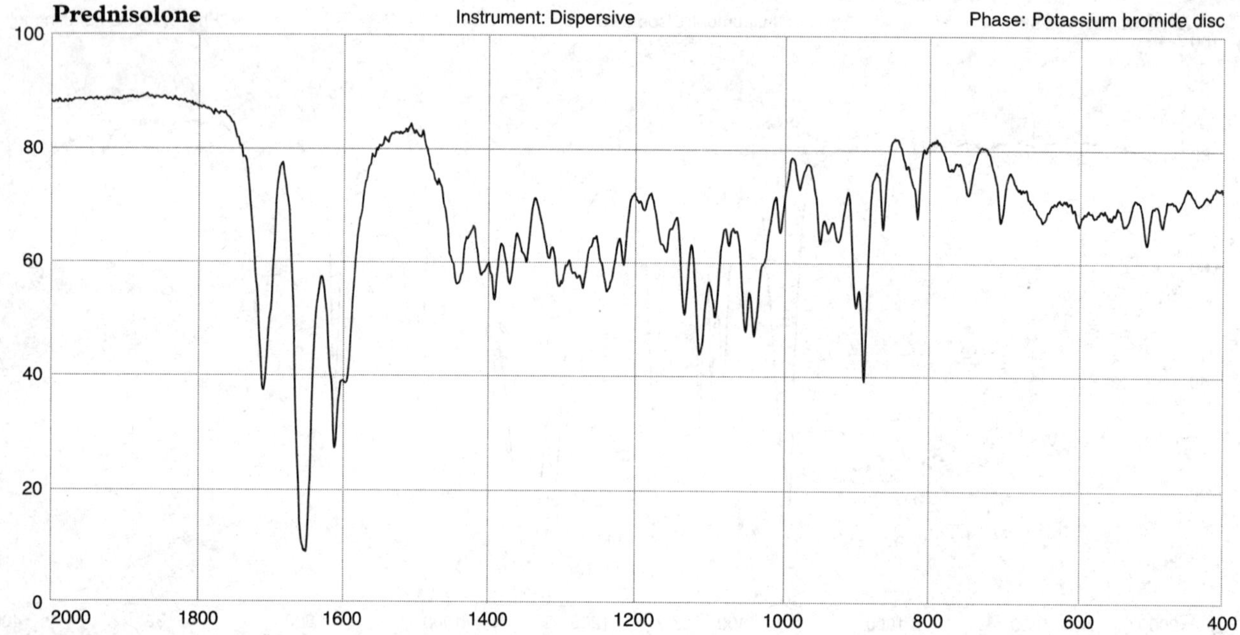

Prednisone

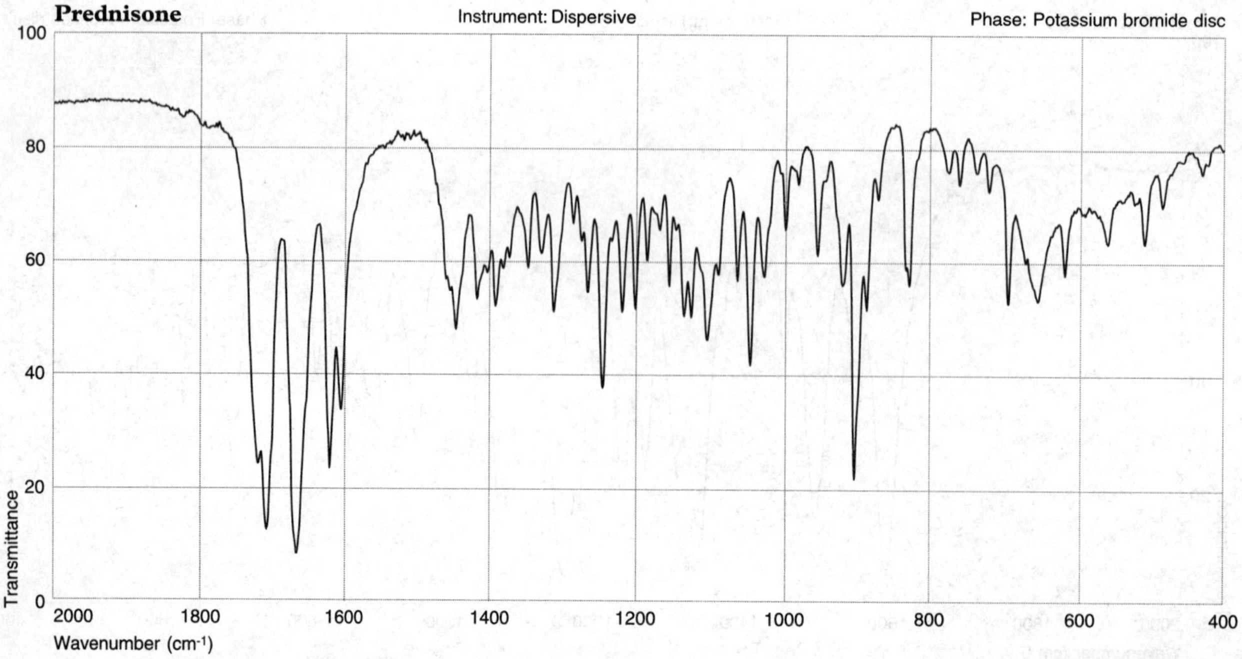

Prilocaine Instrument: Dispersive Phase: Thin film

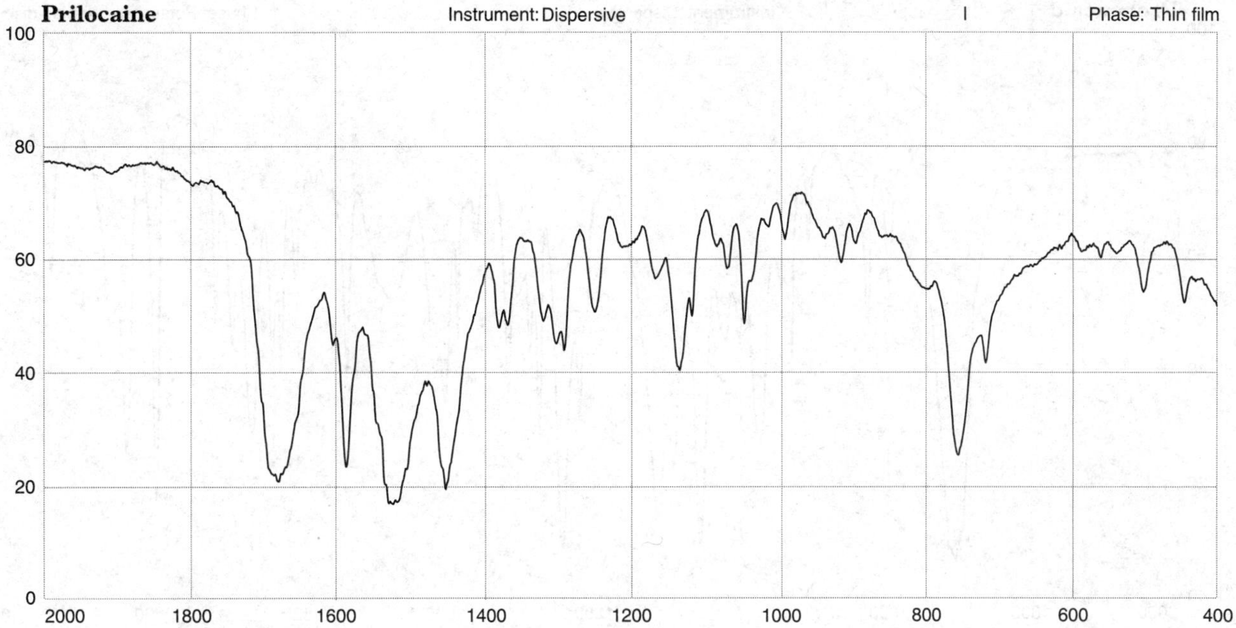

Prilocaine Hydrochloride Instrument: Dispersive Phase: Potassium chloride disc

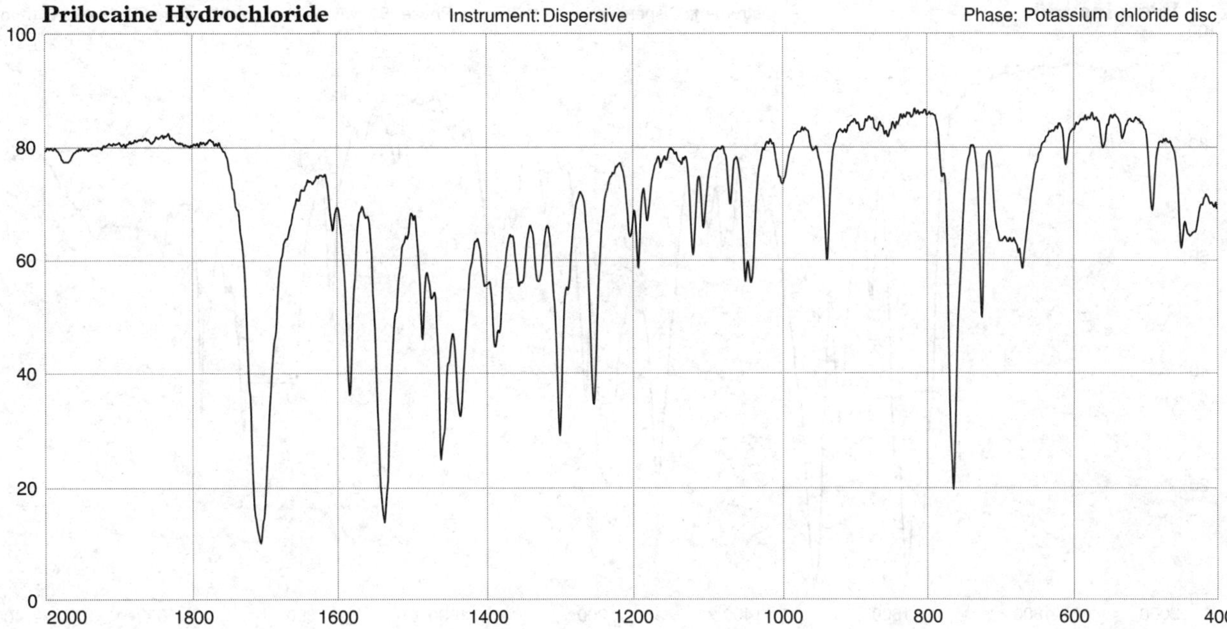

Primidone Instrument: Dispersive Phase: Potassium bromide disc

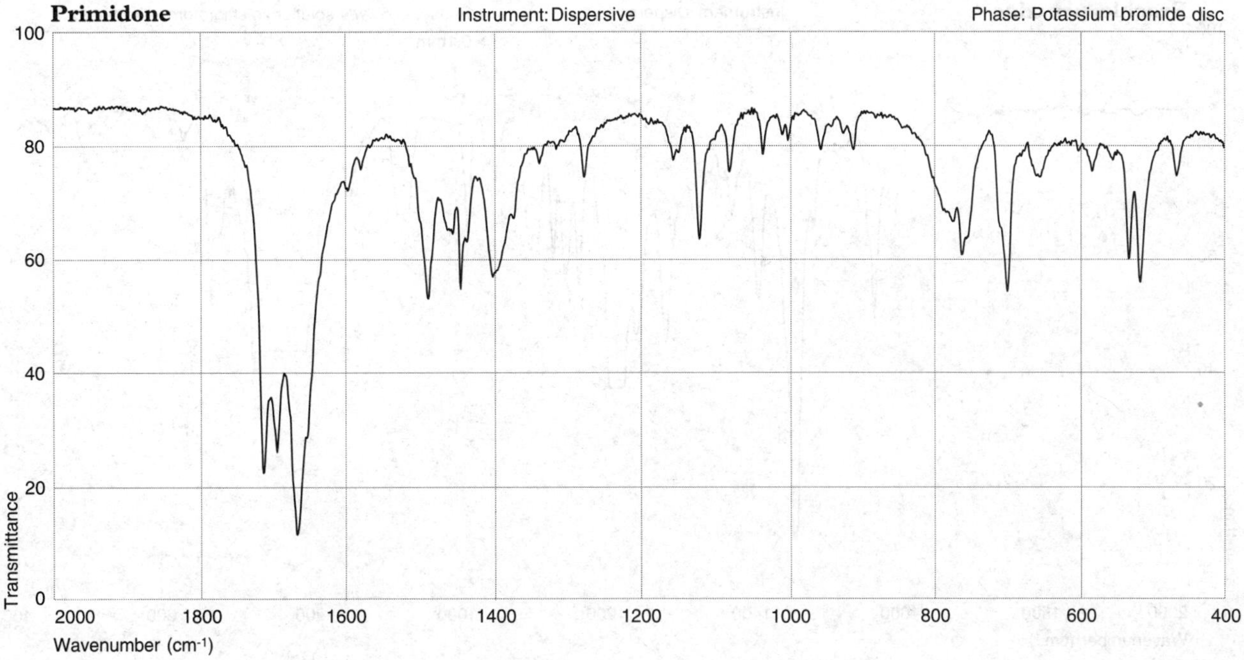

Probenecid

Instrument: Dispersive

Phase: Potassium bromide disc

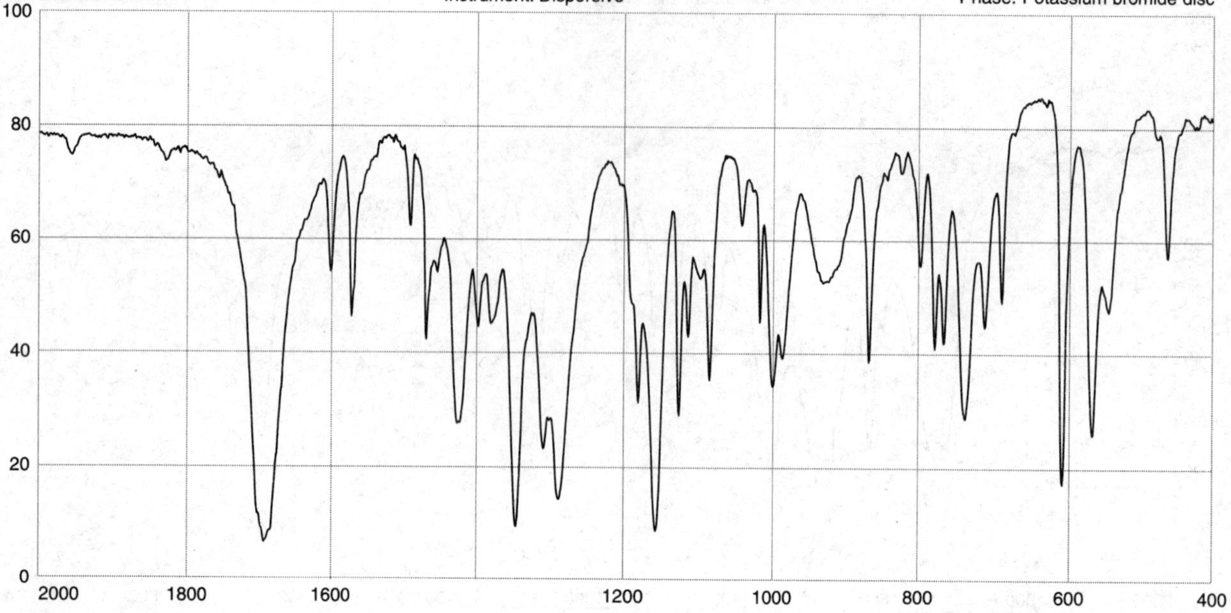

Procainamide

Instrument: Dispersive

Phase: 5% w/v solution in chloroform Thickness 0.1mm

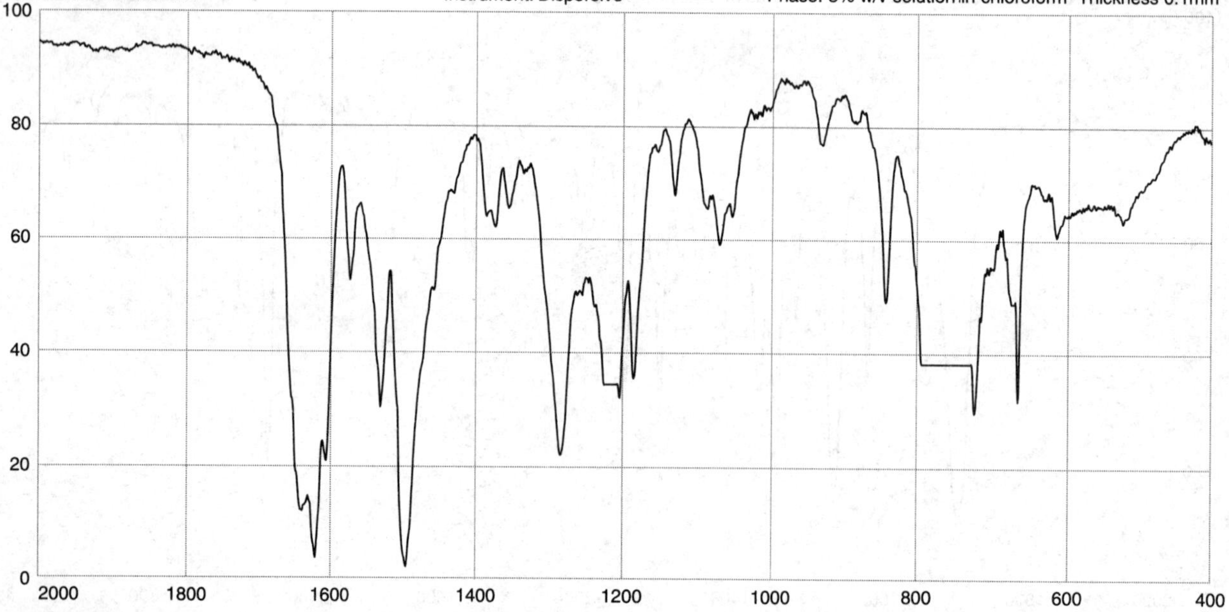

Prochlorperazine

Instrument: Dispersive

Phase: 10% w/v solution in chloroform Thickness 0.1mm

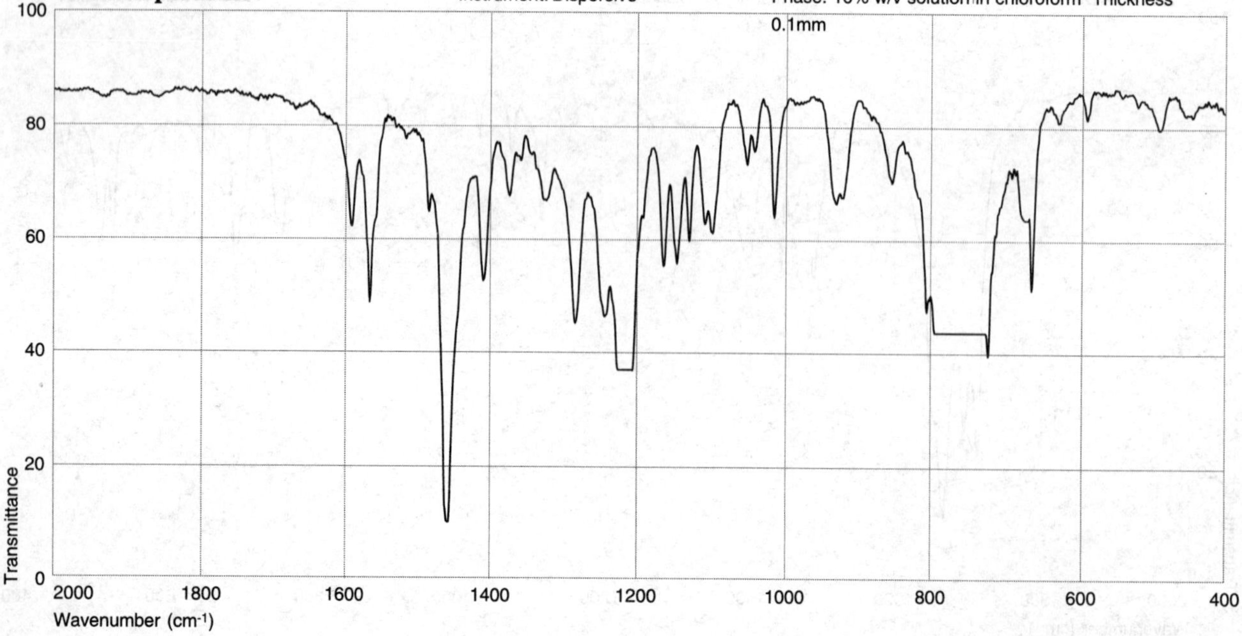

Prochlorperazine Mesilate Instrument: Dispersive Phase: Liquid paraffin mull

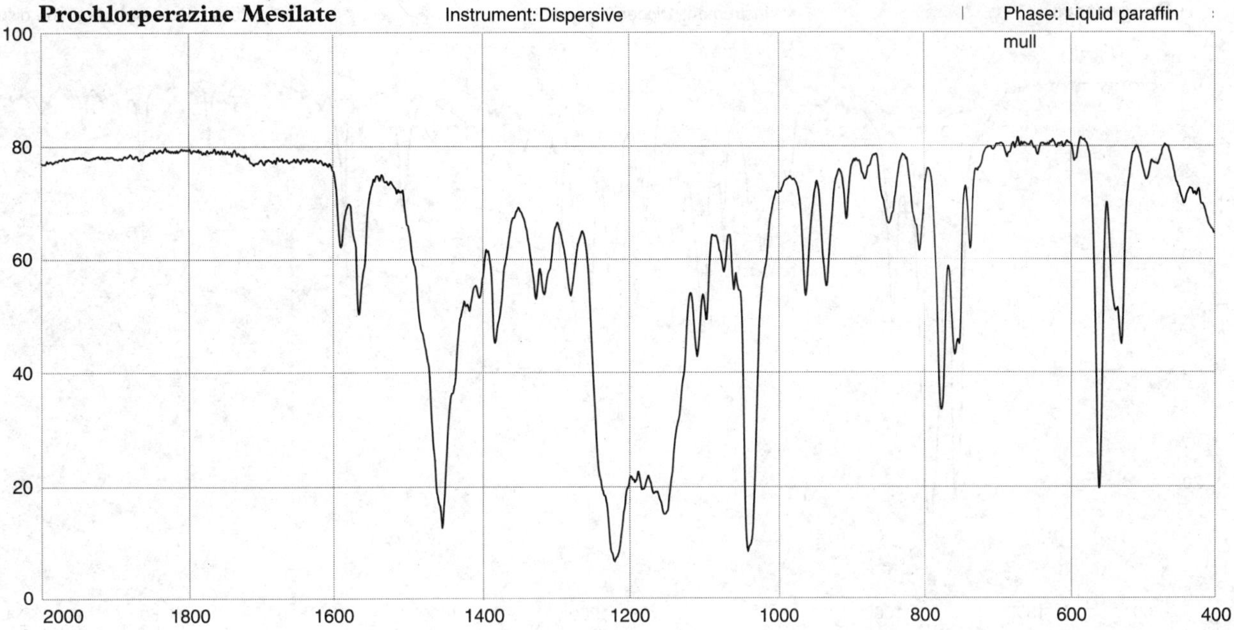

Procyclidine Instrument: Dispersive Phase: Potassium bromide disc

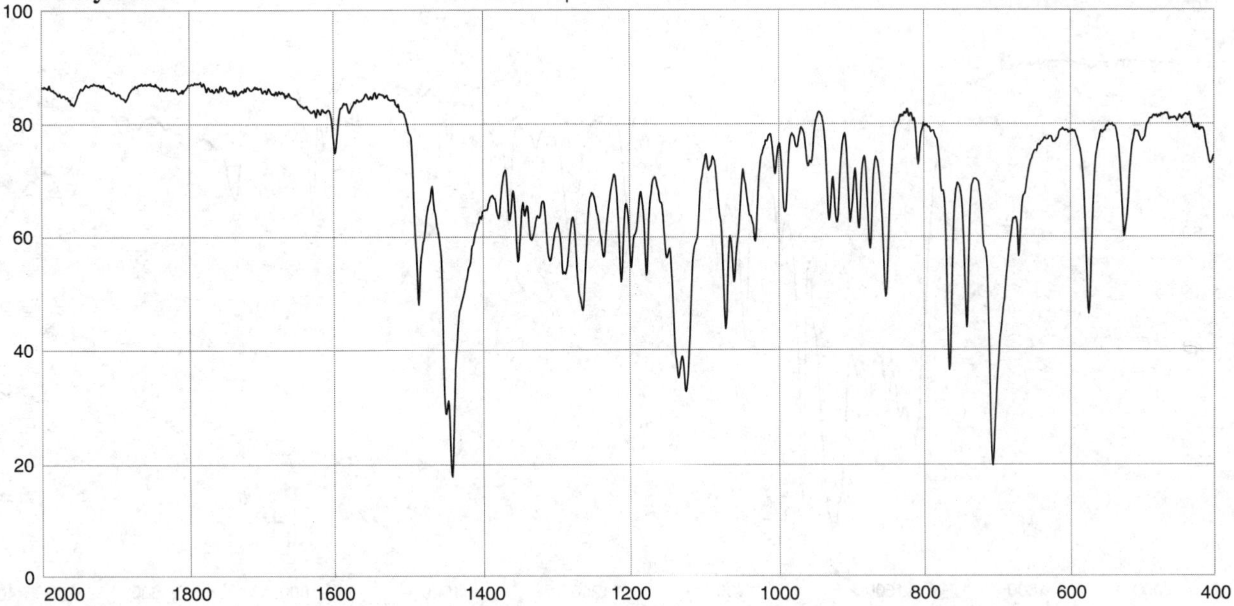

Procyclidine Hydrochloride Instrument: Dispersive Phase: Potassium chloride disc

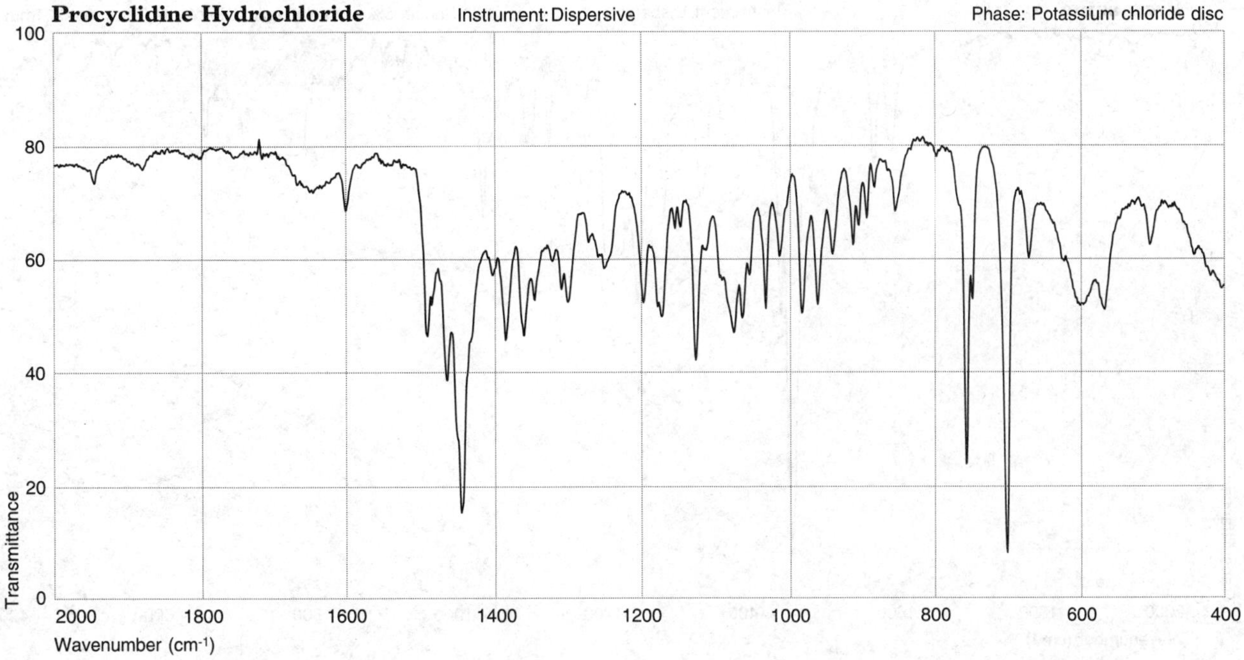

Progesterone Instrument: Dispersive Phase: Potassium bromide disc

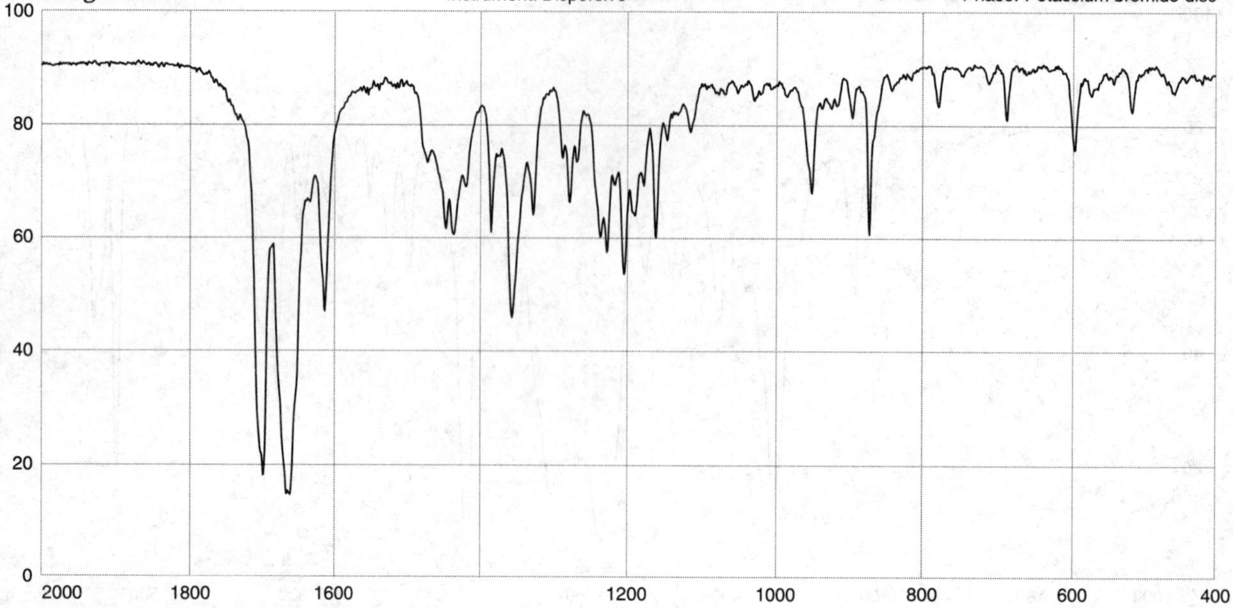

Proguanil Hydrochloride Instrument: Dispersive Phase: Potassium chloride disc

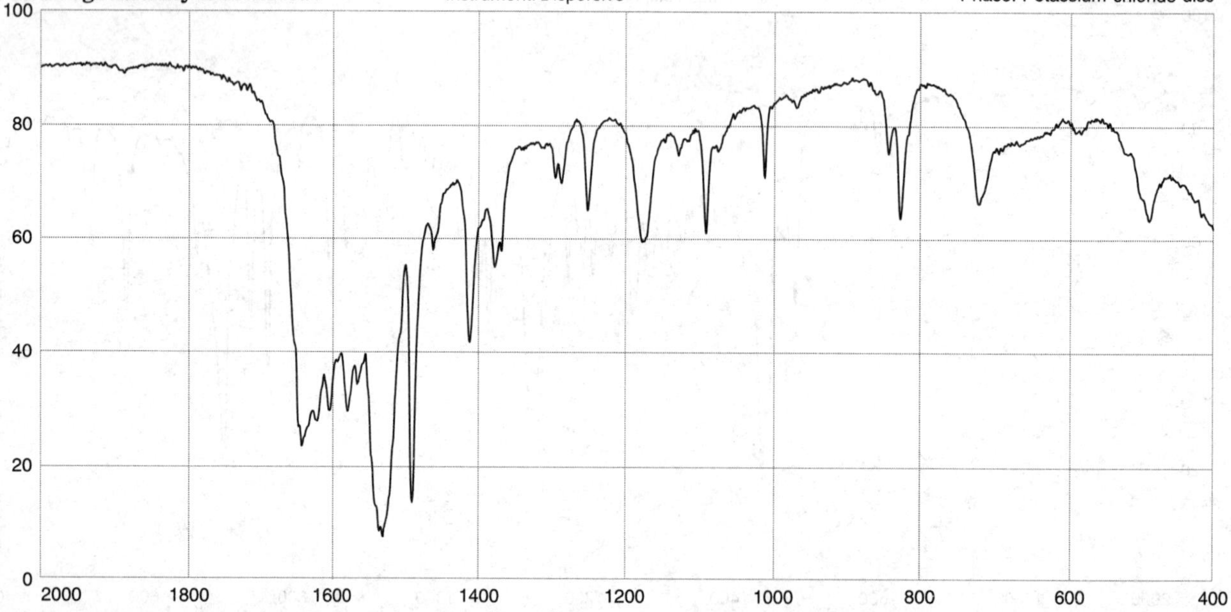

Promazine Instrument: Dispersive Phase: 5% w/v solution in chloroform Thickness 0.1mm

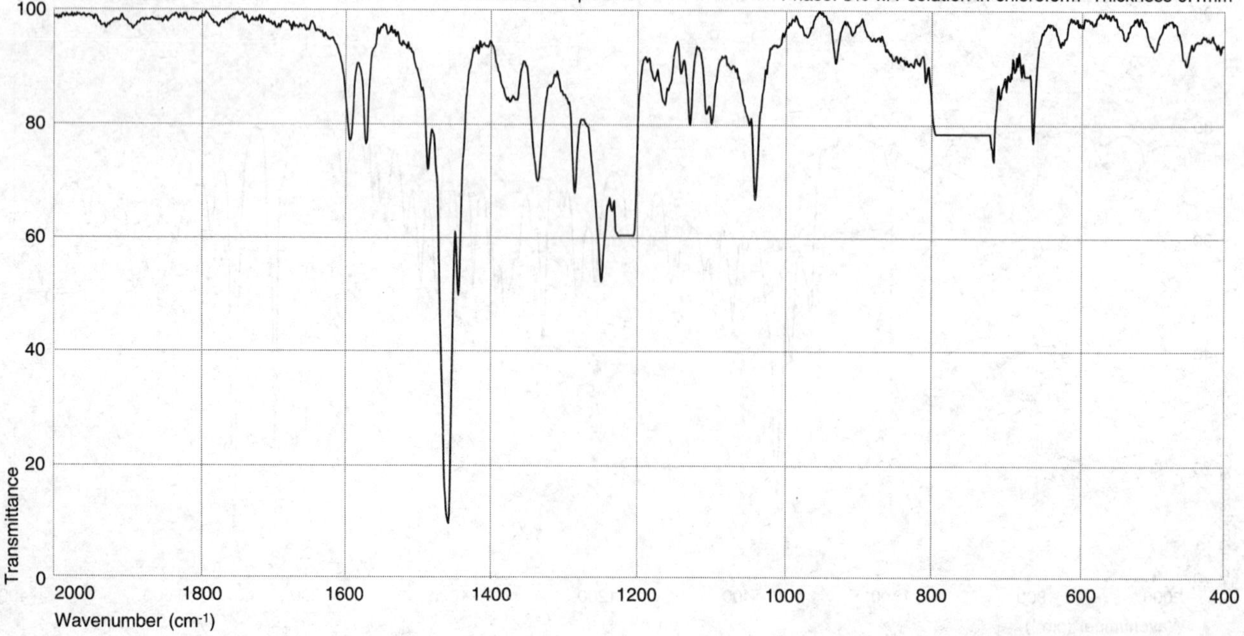

Promazine Hydrochloride Instrument: Dispersive Phase: 5% w/v solution in chloroform Thickness 0.1mm

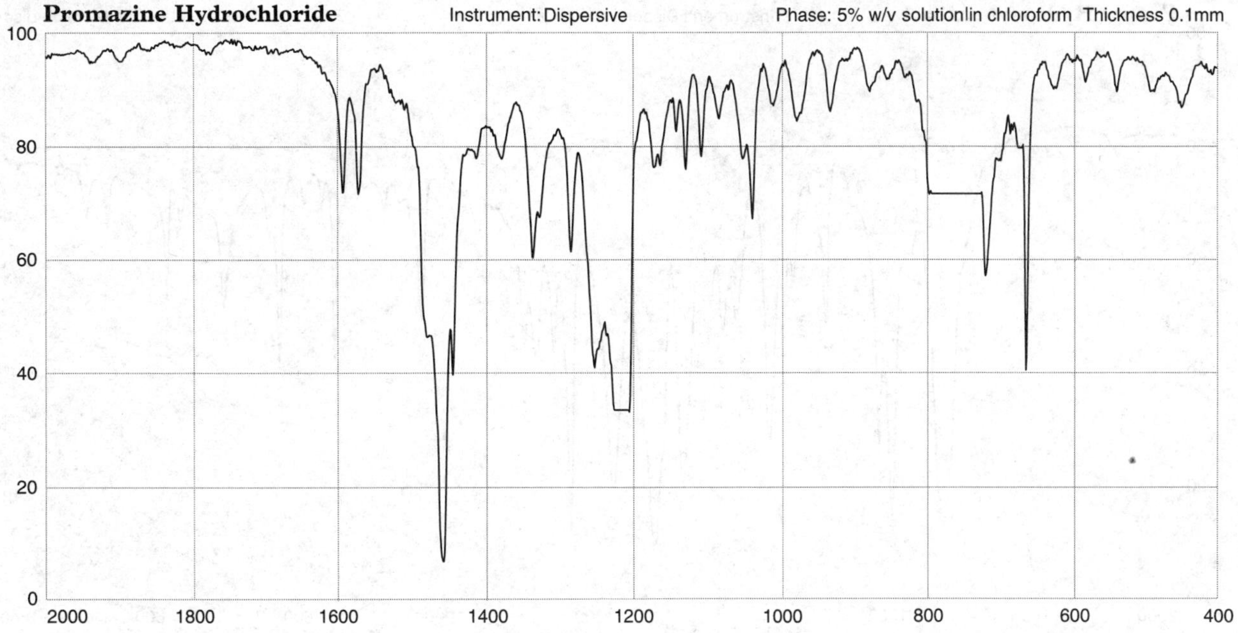

Promethazine Instrument: Dispersive Phase: 5% w/v solution in chloroform Thickness 0.1mm

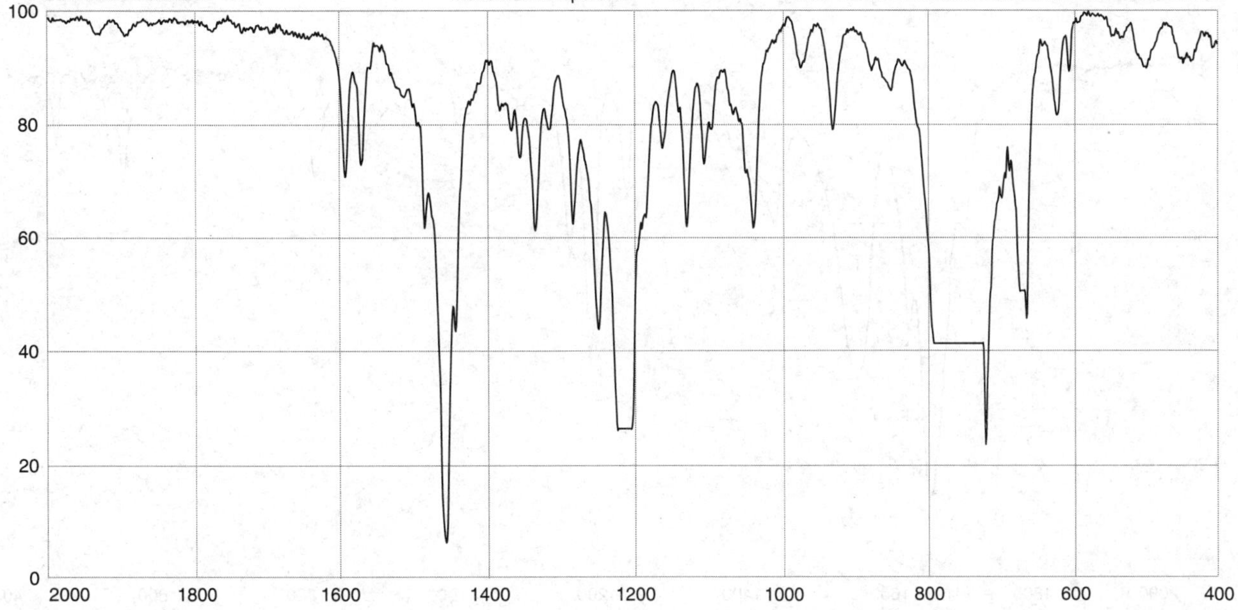

Propranolol Instrument: Dispersive Phase: Potassium bromide disc

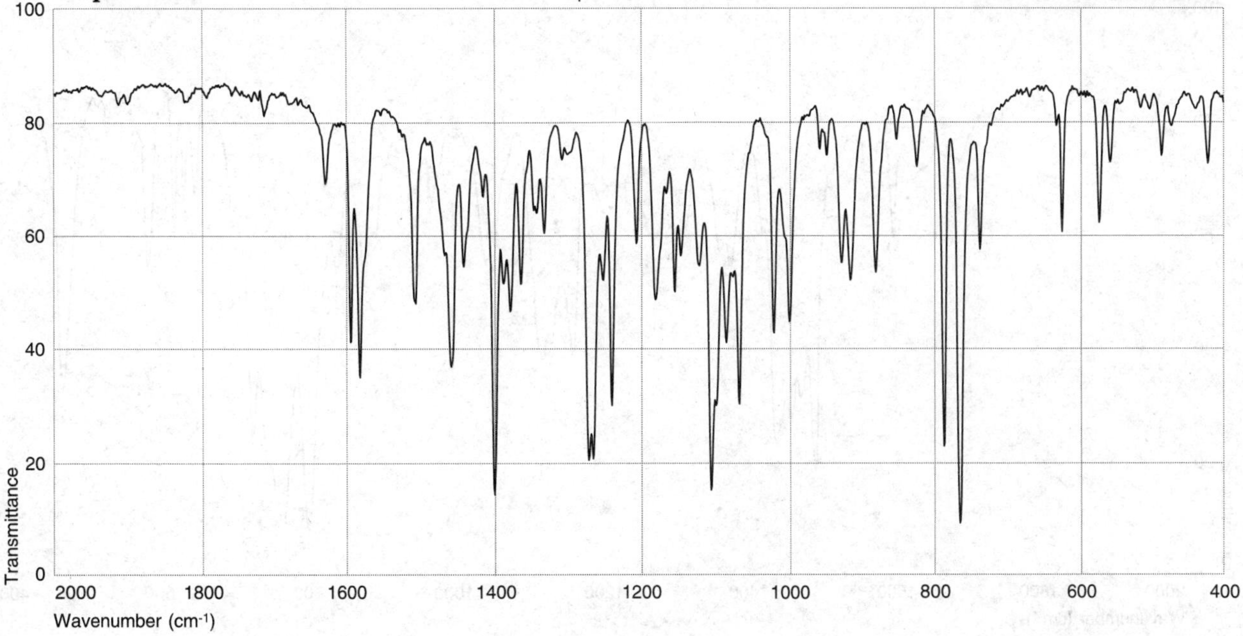

Propyl Hydroxybenzoate Instrument: Dispersive Phase: Potassium bromide disc

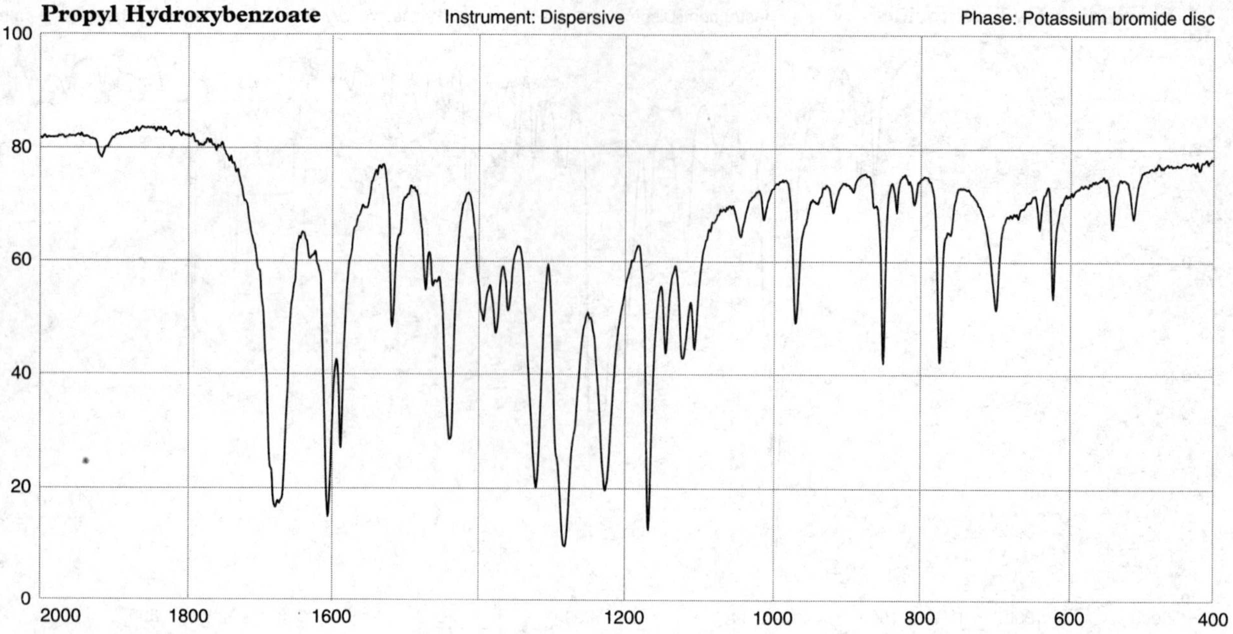

Propylthiouracil Instrument: Dispersive Phase: Potassium bromide disc

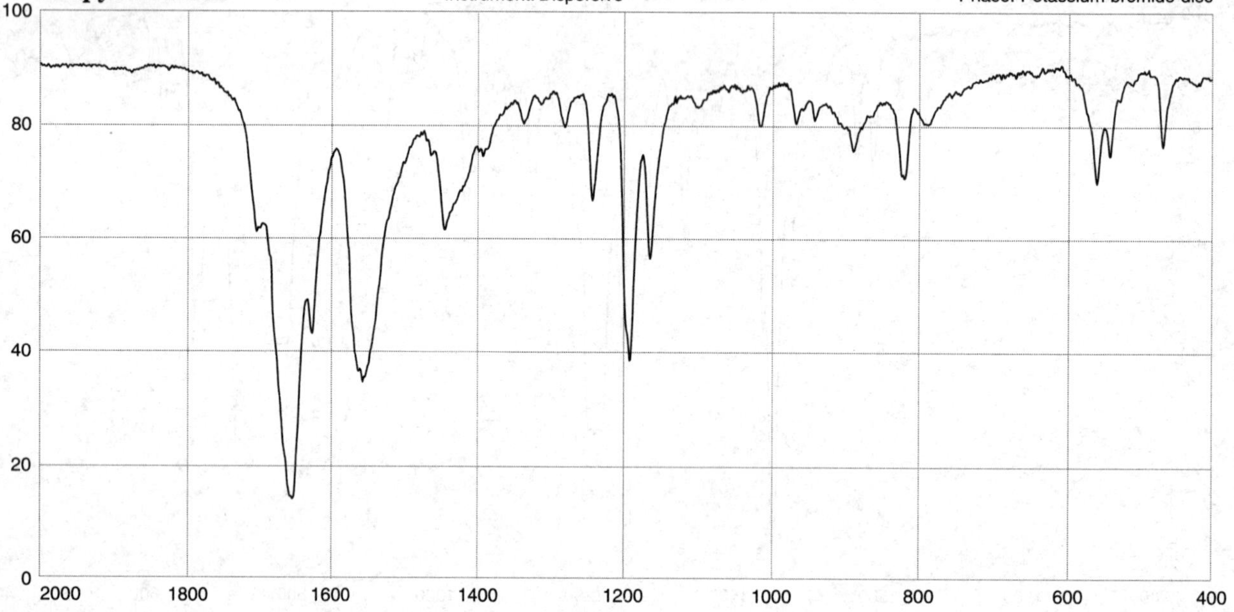

Protriptyline Instrument: Dispersive Phase: Thin film

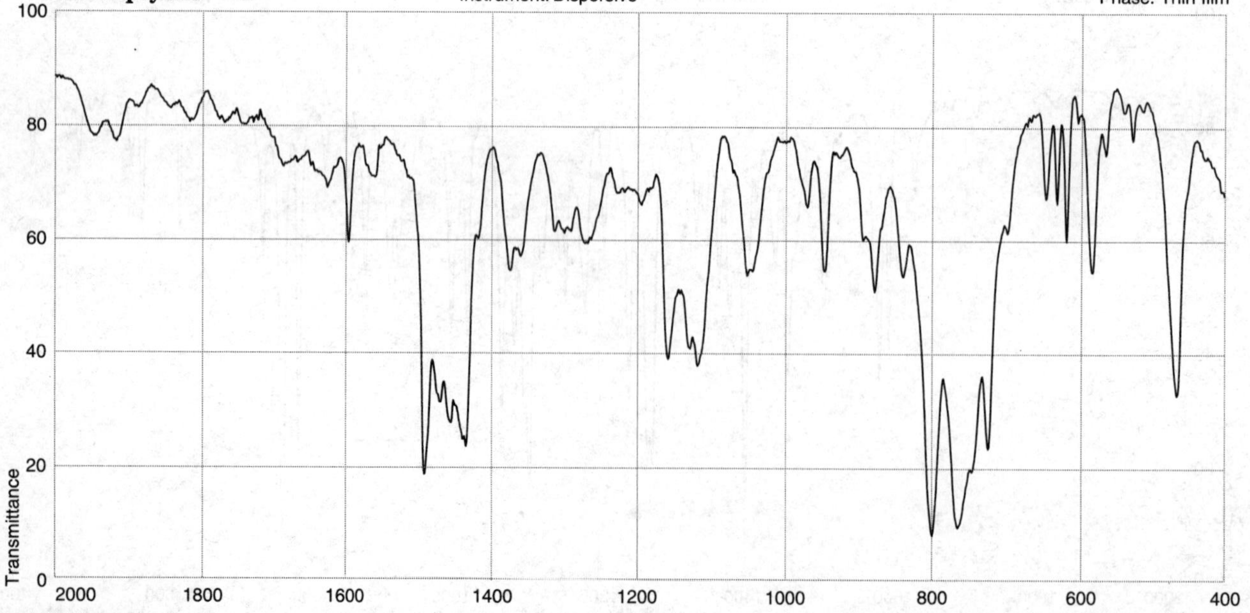

Proxymetacaine Instrument: Dispersive Phase: Thin film

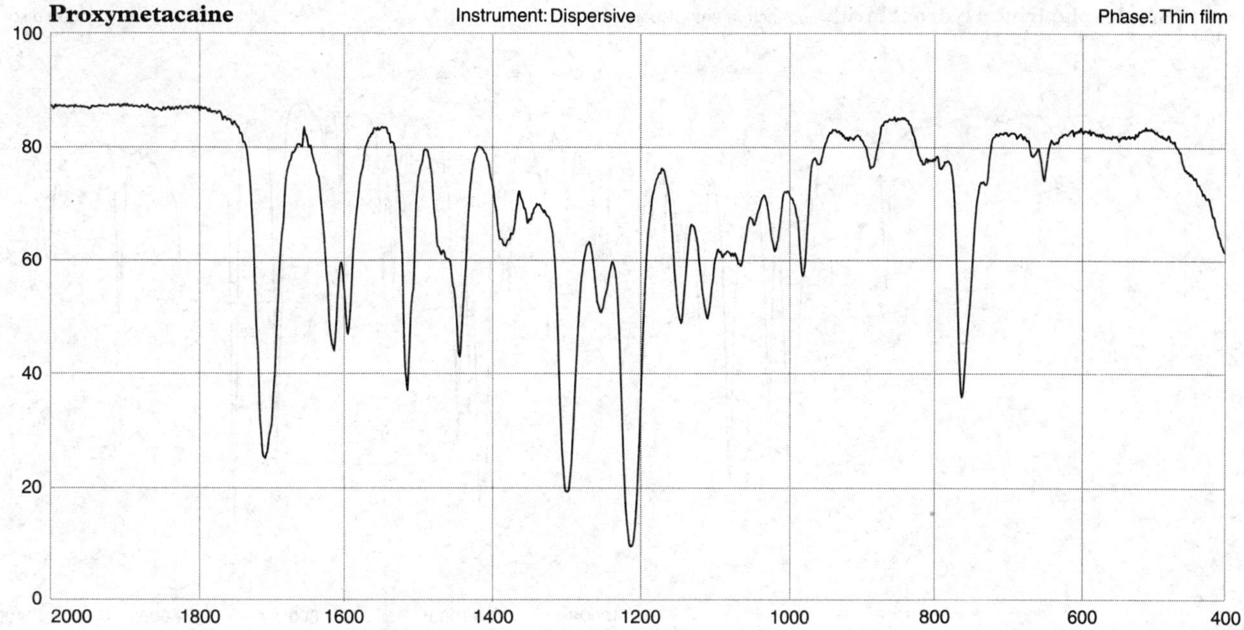

Proxymetacaine Hydrochloride Instrument: Dispersive Phase: Potassium chloride disc

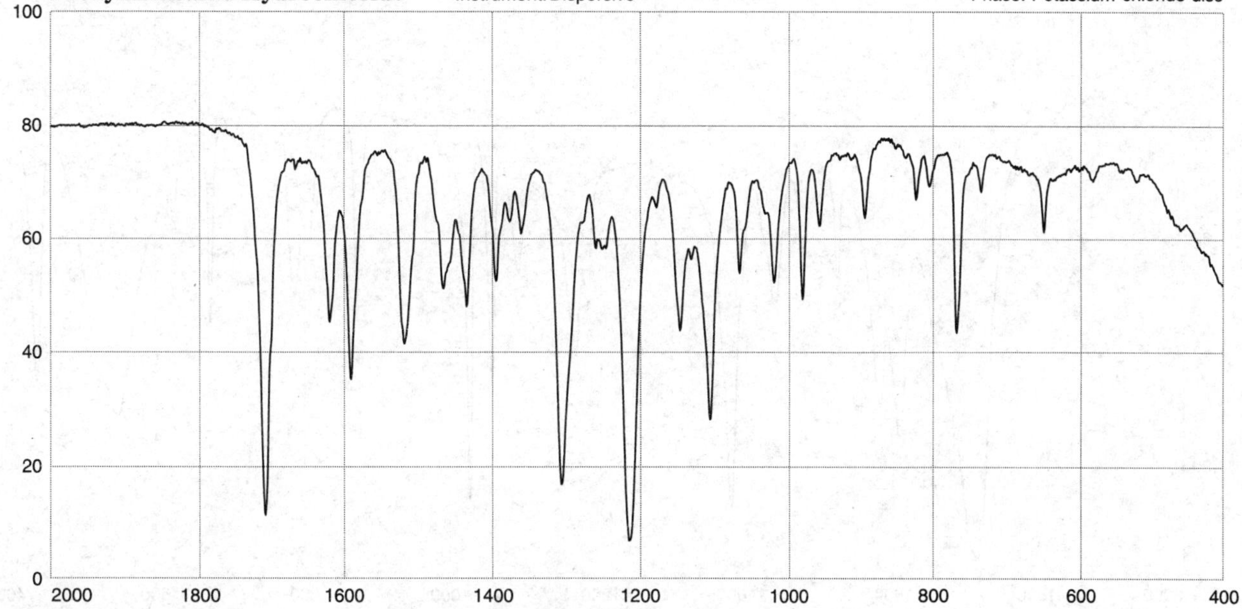

Pseudoephedrine Instrument: Dispersive Phase: Potassium bromide disc

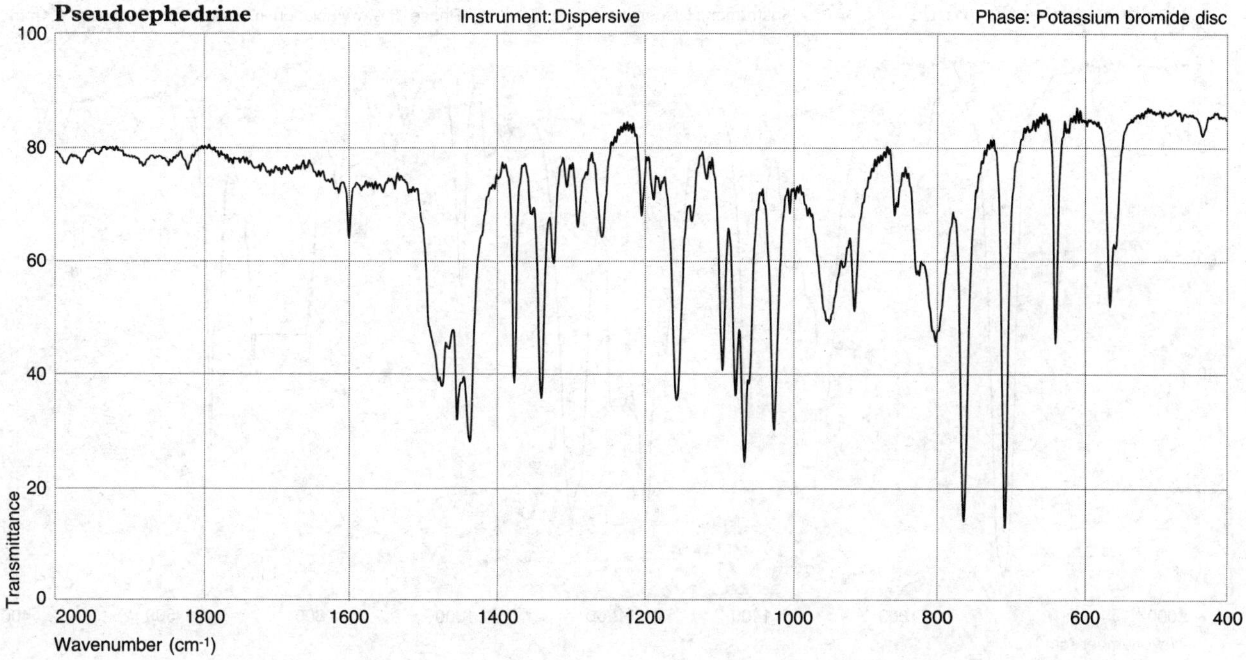

Pseudoephedrine Hydrochloride Instrument: Dispersive Phase: Potassium chloride disc

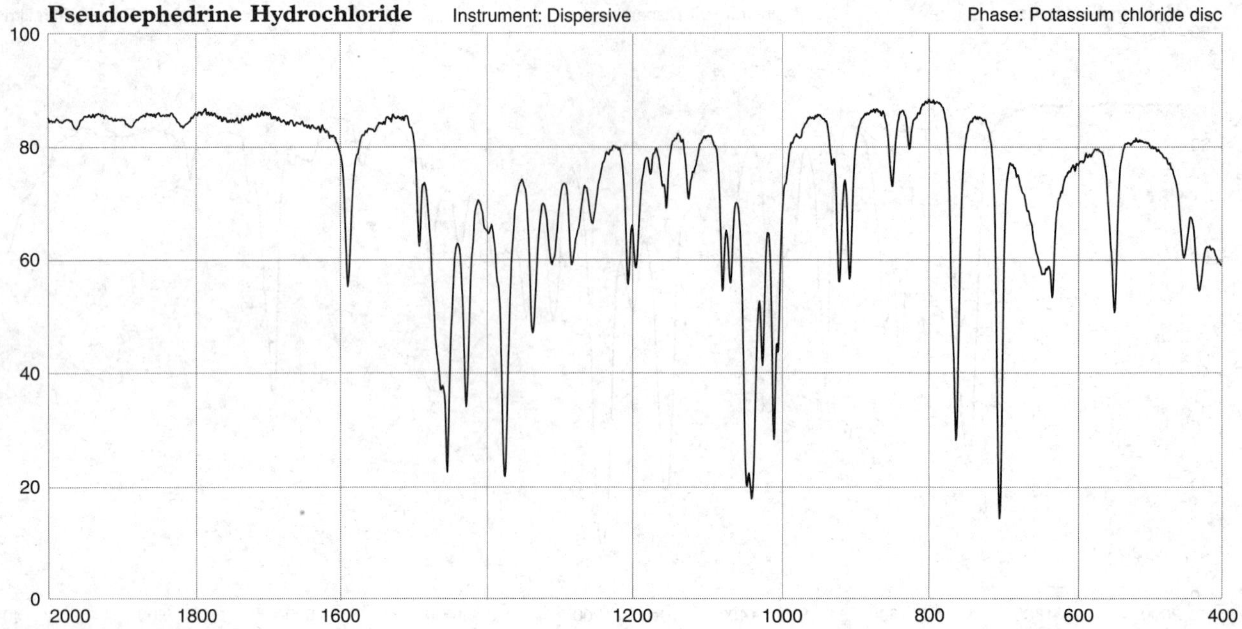

Pyrazinamide Instrument: Dispersive Phase: Potassium bromide disc

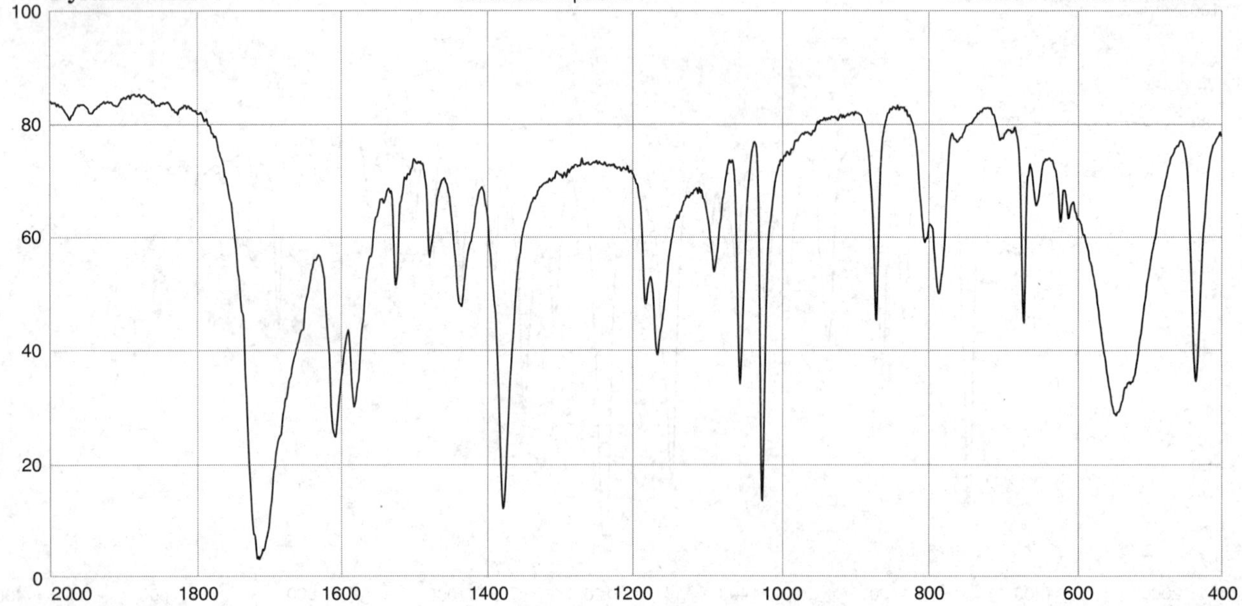

Pyridostigmine Bromide Instrument: Dispersive Phase: 5% w/v solution in chloroform Thickness 0.1mm

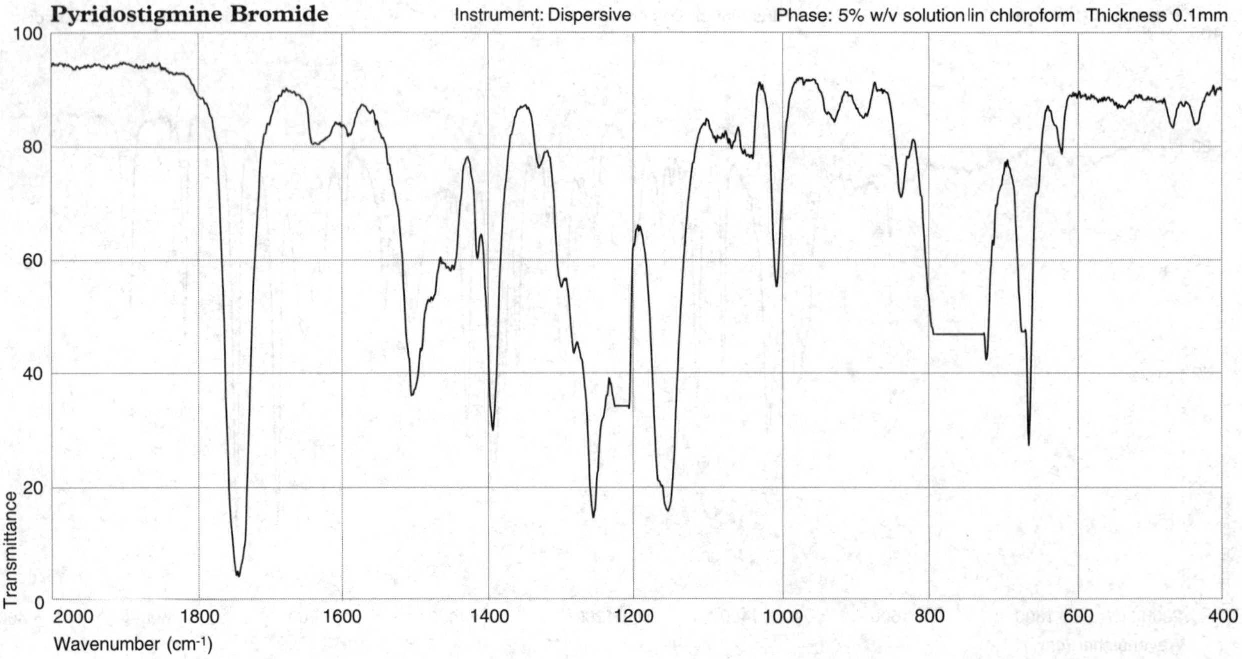

Pyridoxine Hydrochloride Instrument: Dispersive Phase: Potassium chloride disc

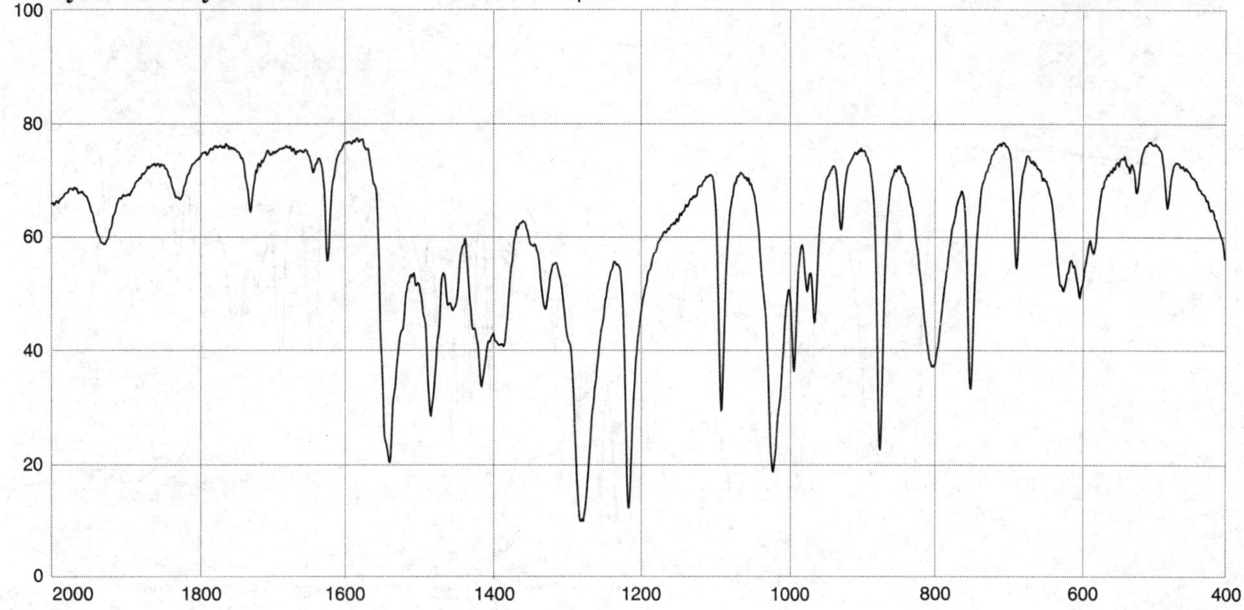

Pyrimethamine Instrument: Dispersive Phase: Potassium bromide disc

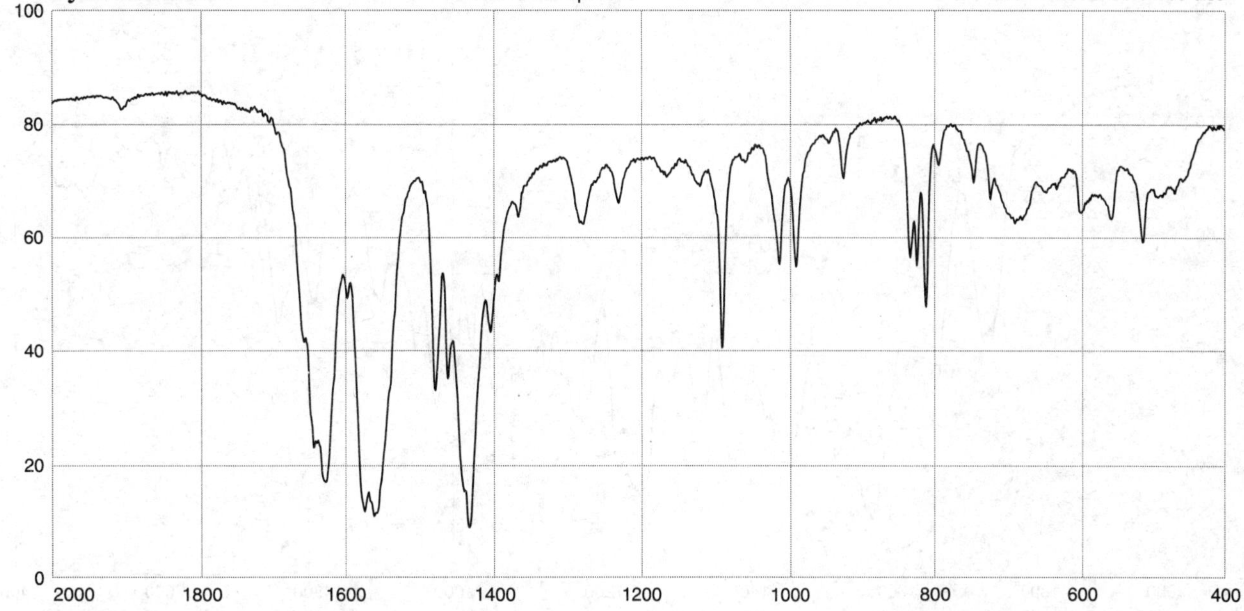

Quinolin-8-ol Instrument: Dispersive Phase: Potassium bromide disc

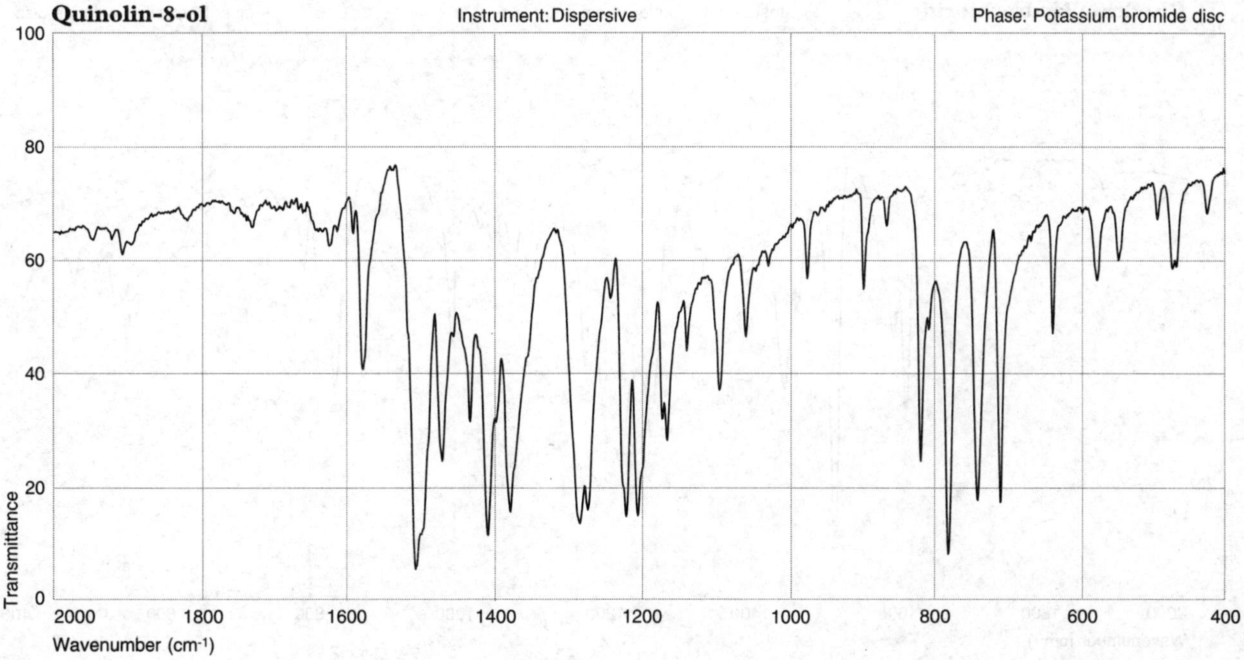

Ranitidine Hydrochloride Instrument: Dispersive Phase: Potassium chloride disc

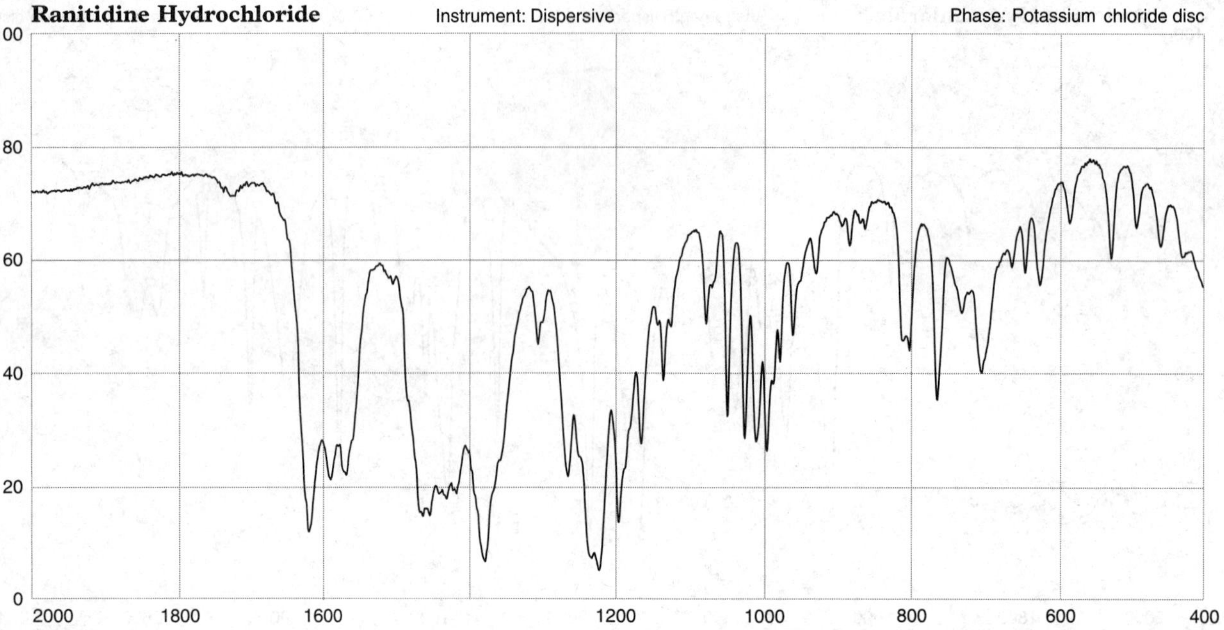

Rifampicin Instrument: Dispersive Phase: Potassium bromide disc

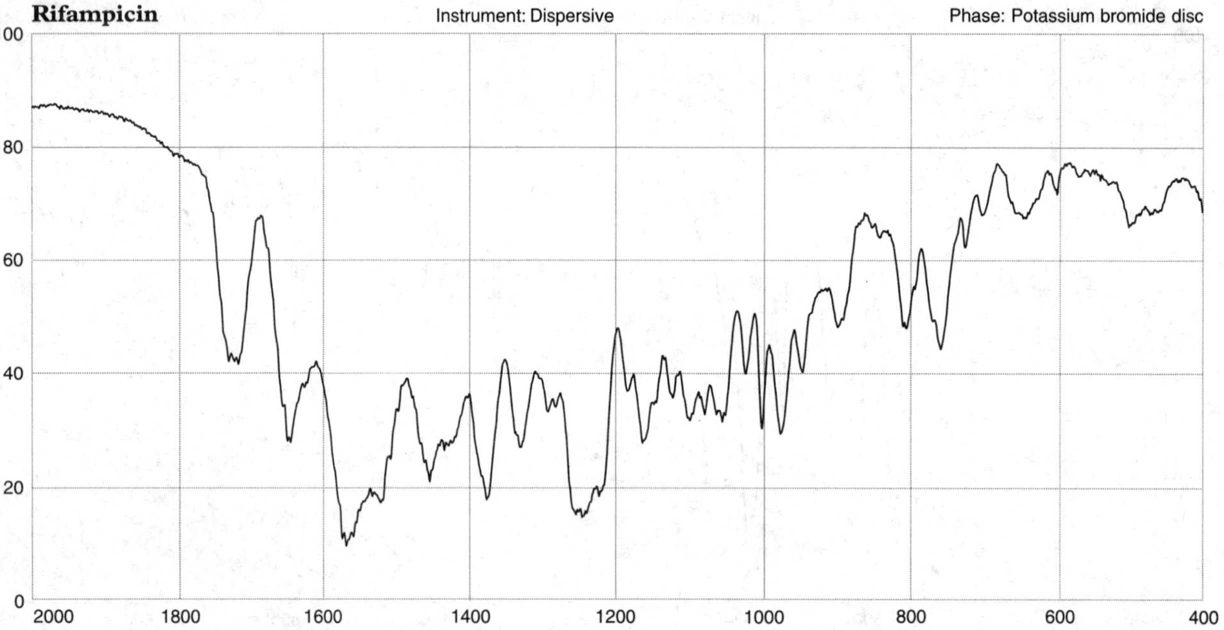

Ritodrine Hydrochloride Instrument: Fourier transform Phase: Potassium chloride disc

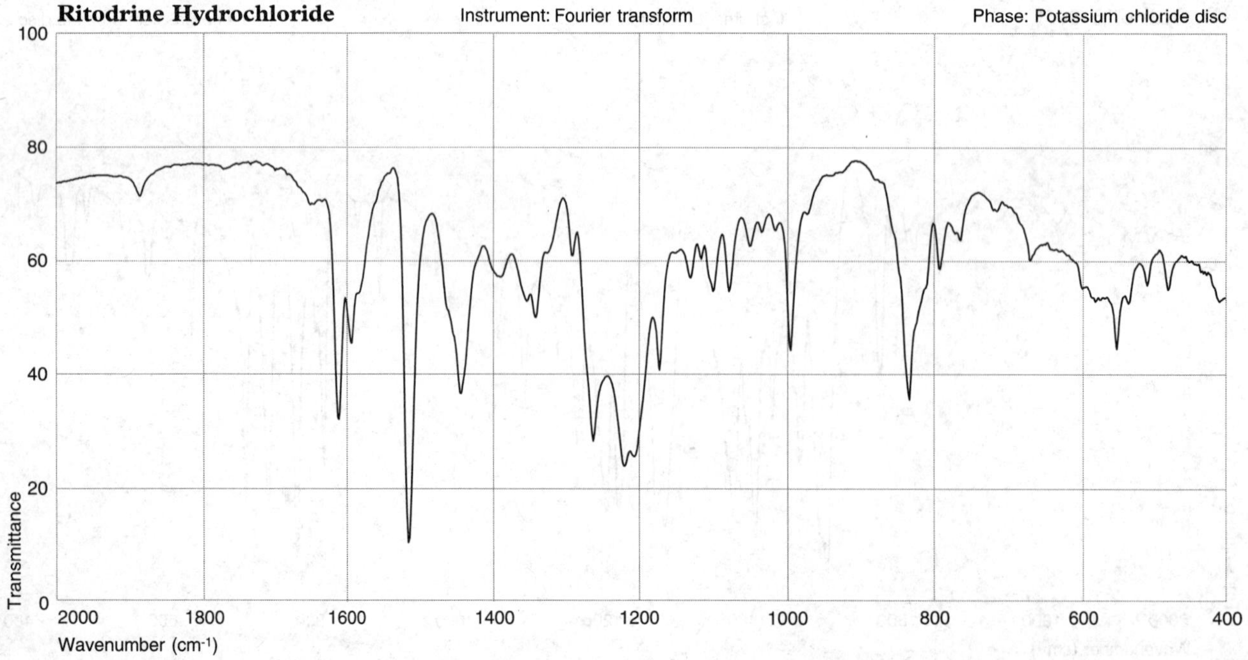

Salbutamol Instrument: Dispersive Phase: Potassium bromide disc

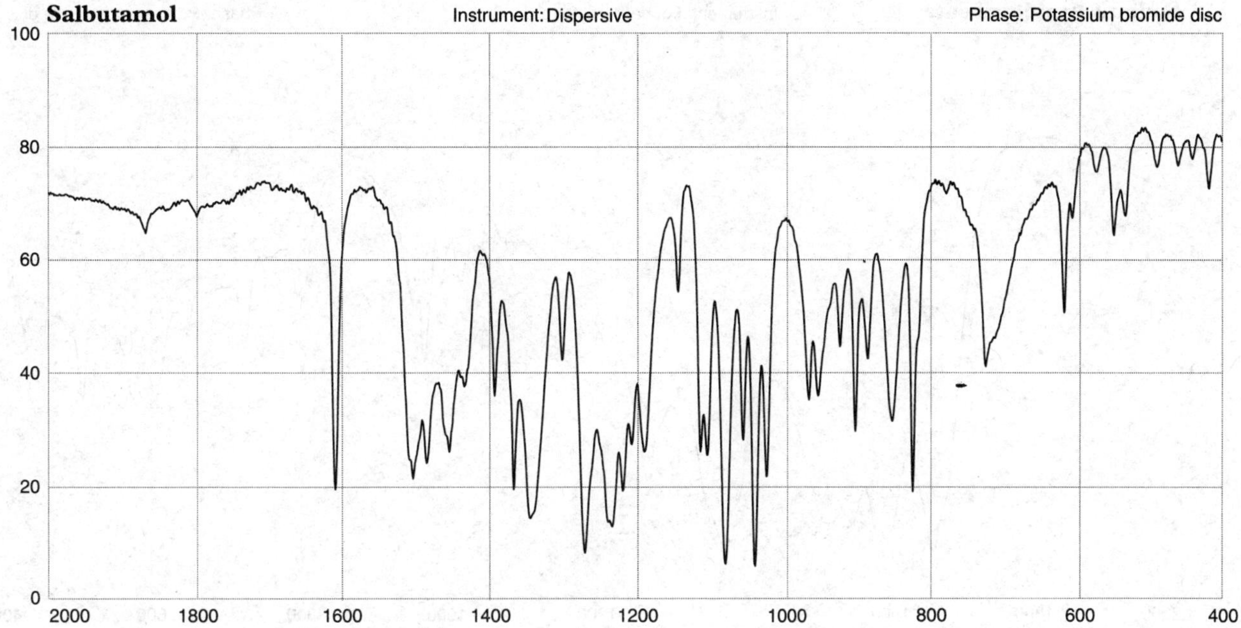

Salbutamol Sulphate Instrument: Dispersive Phase: Potassium bromide disc

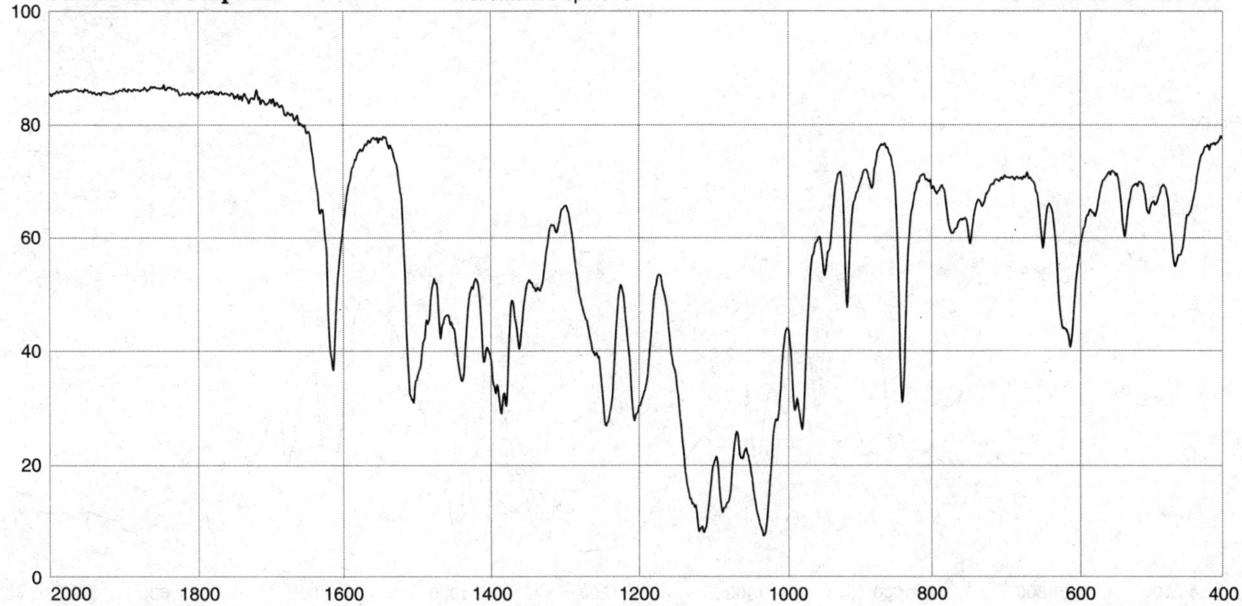

Salicylic Acid Instrument: Dispersive Phase: Potassium bromide disc

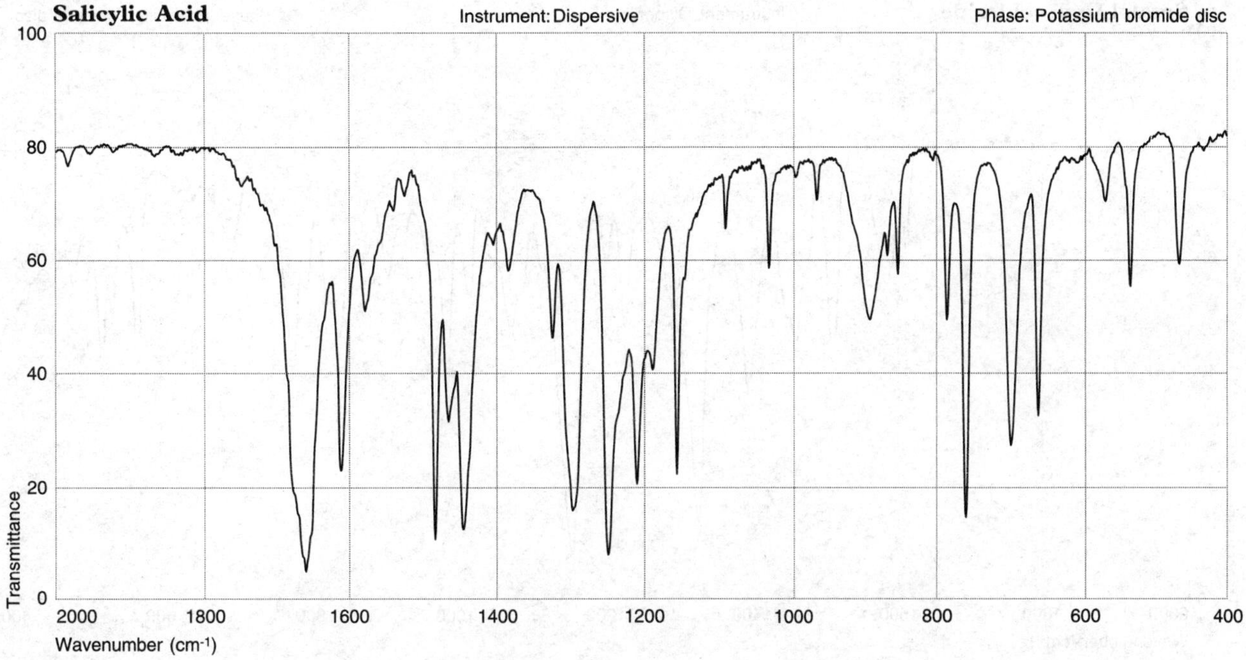

Sodium Amidotrizoate Instrument: Fourier transform Phase: Potassium bromide disc

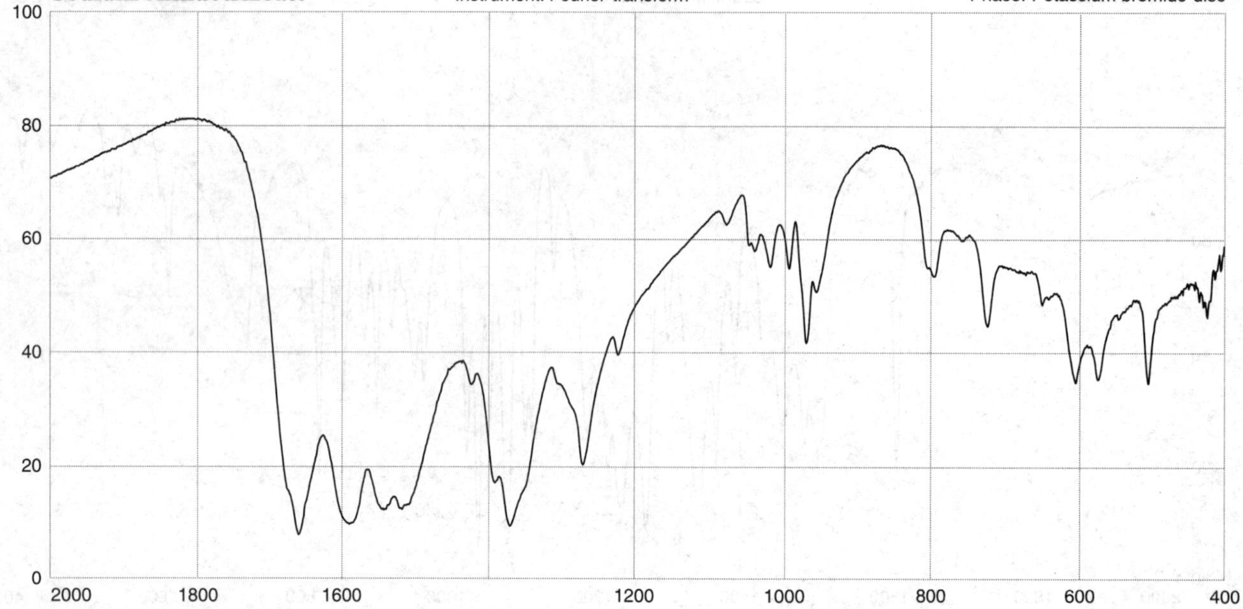

Sodium Polystyrene Sulphonate Instrument: Fourier transform Phase: Potassium bromide disc

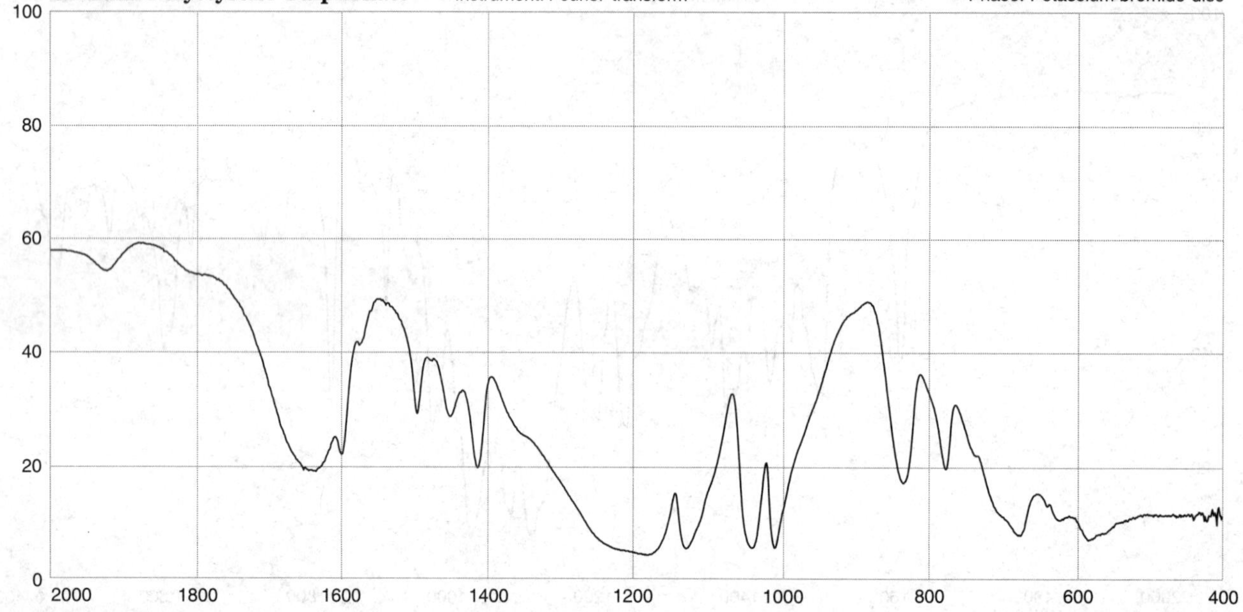

Sotalol Hydrochloride Instrument: Dispersive Phase: Potassium chloride disc

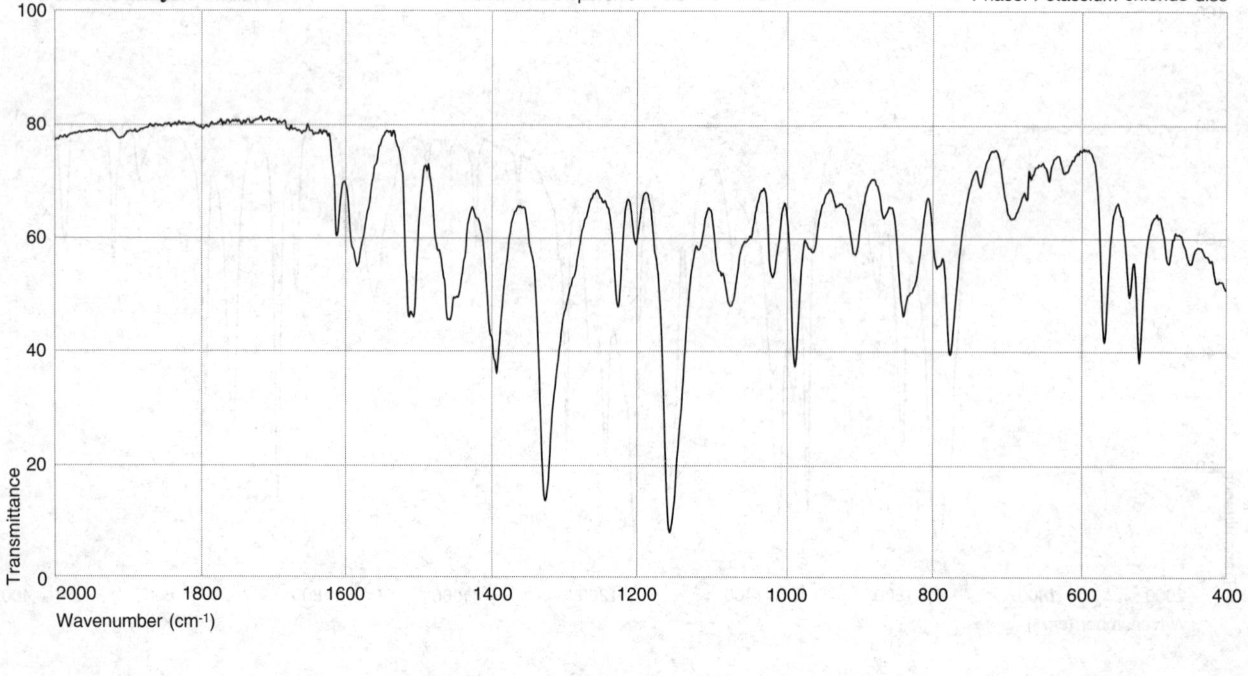

Spectinomycin Hydrochloride Instrument: Dispersive Phase: Potassium chloride disc

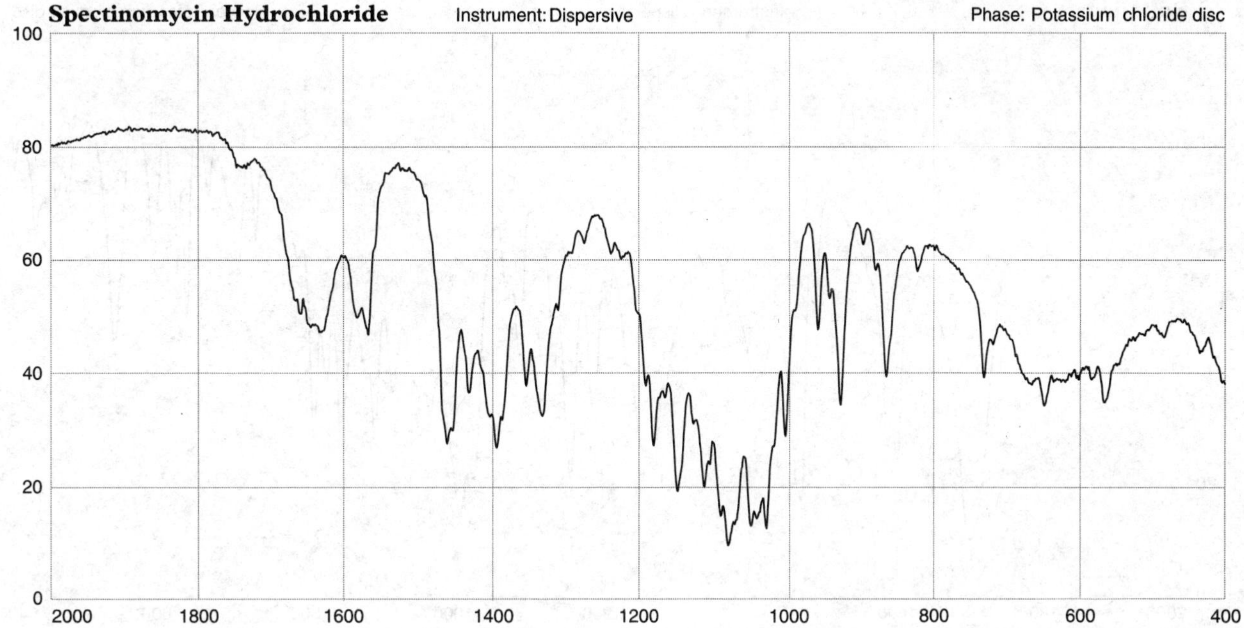

Spironolactone Instrument: Dispersive Phase: 5% w/v solution in chloroform Thickness: 0.1mm

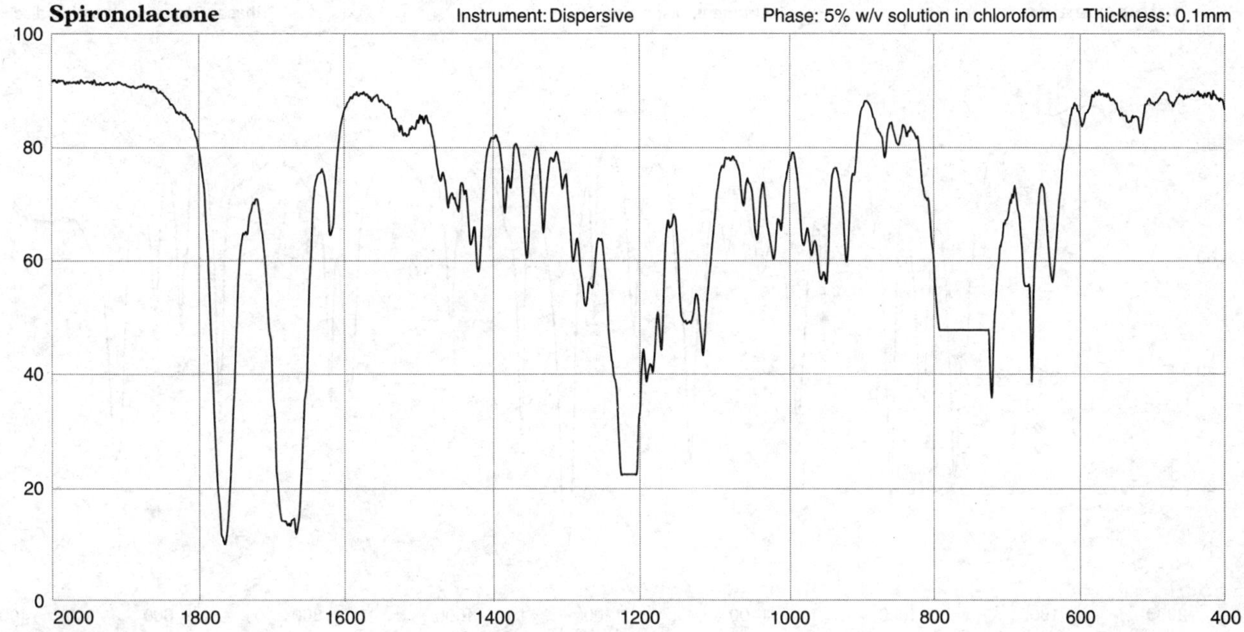

Stanozolol Instrument: Dispersive Phase: Potassium bromide disc

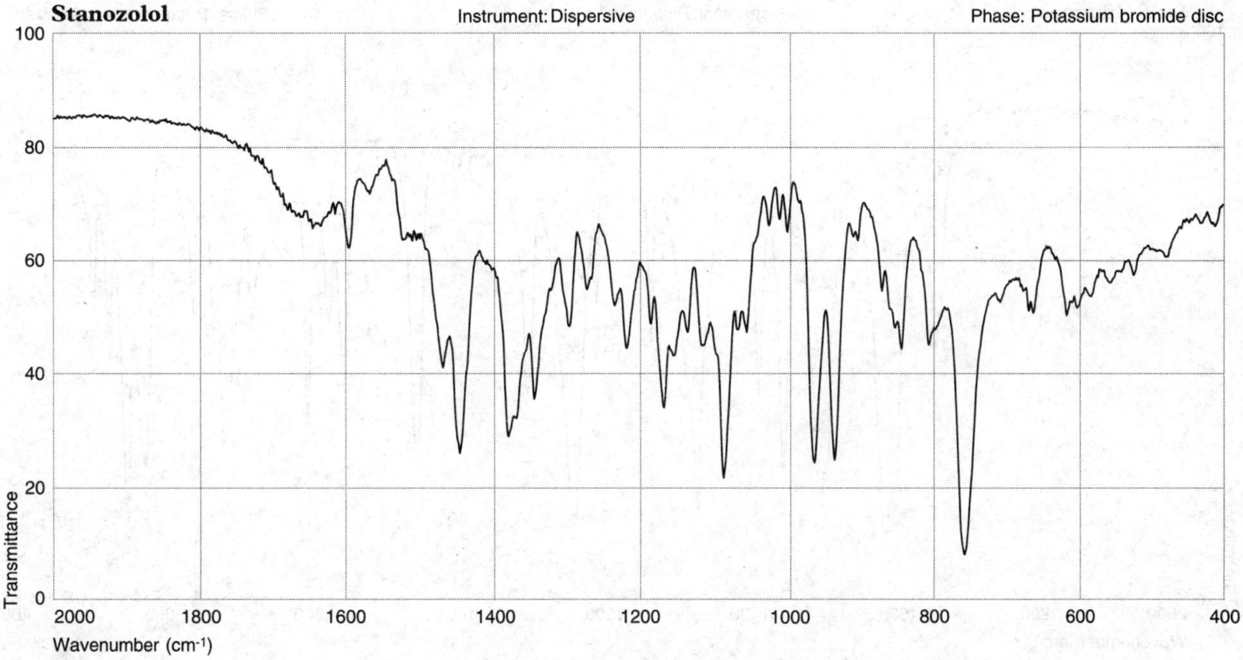

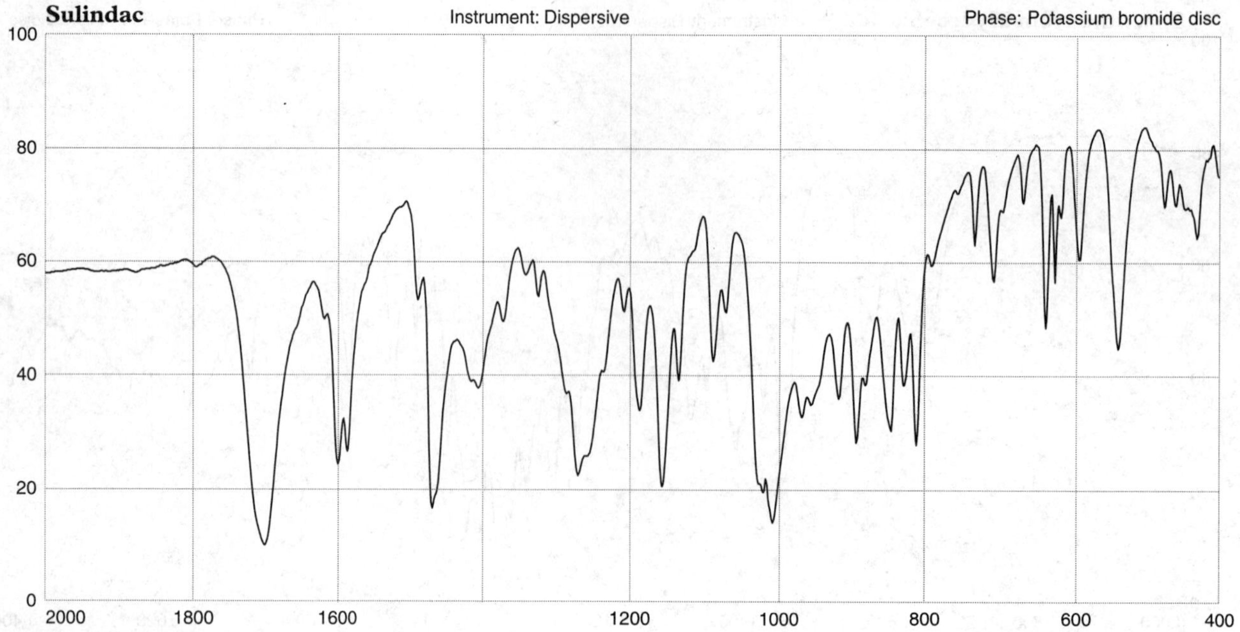
Sulindac
Instrument: Dispersive
Phase: Potassium bromide disc
100
80
60
40
20
0
2000
1800
1600
1200
1000
800
600
400

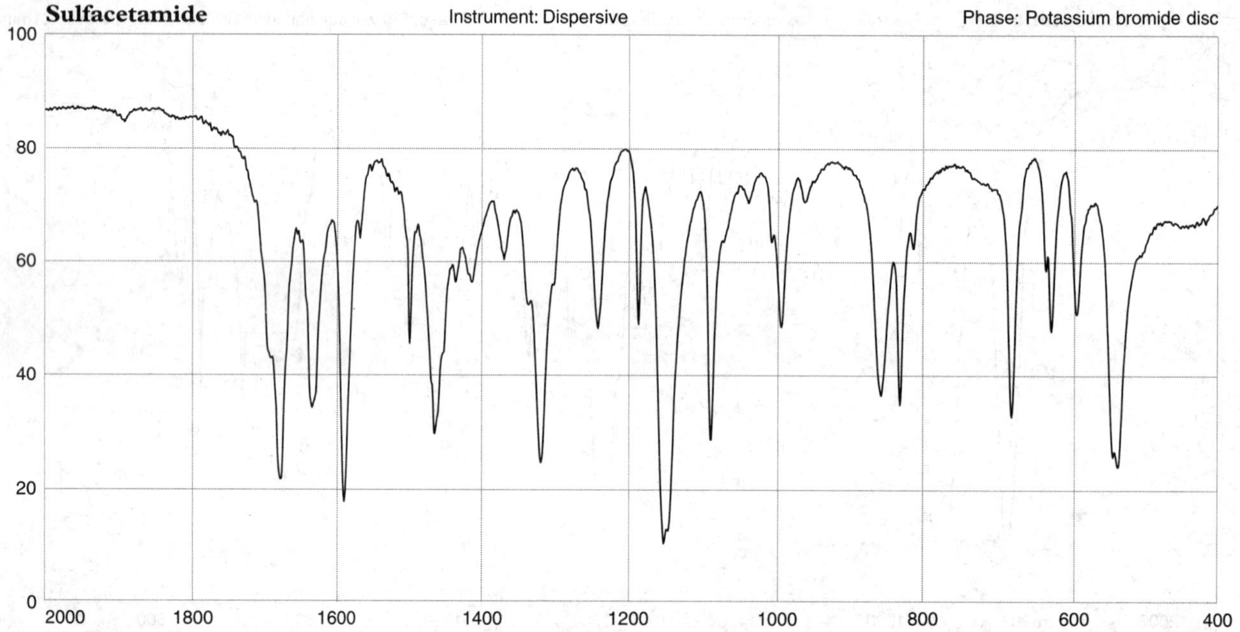
Sulfacetamide
Instrument: Dispersive
Phase: Potassium bromide disc
100
80
60
40
20
0
2000
1800
1600
1400
1200
1000
800
600
400

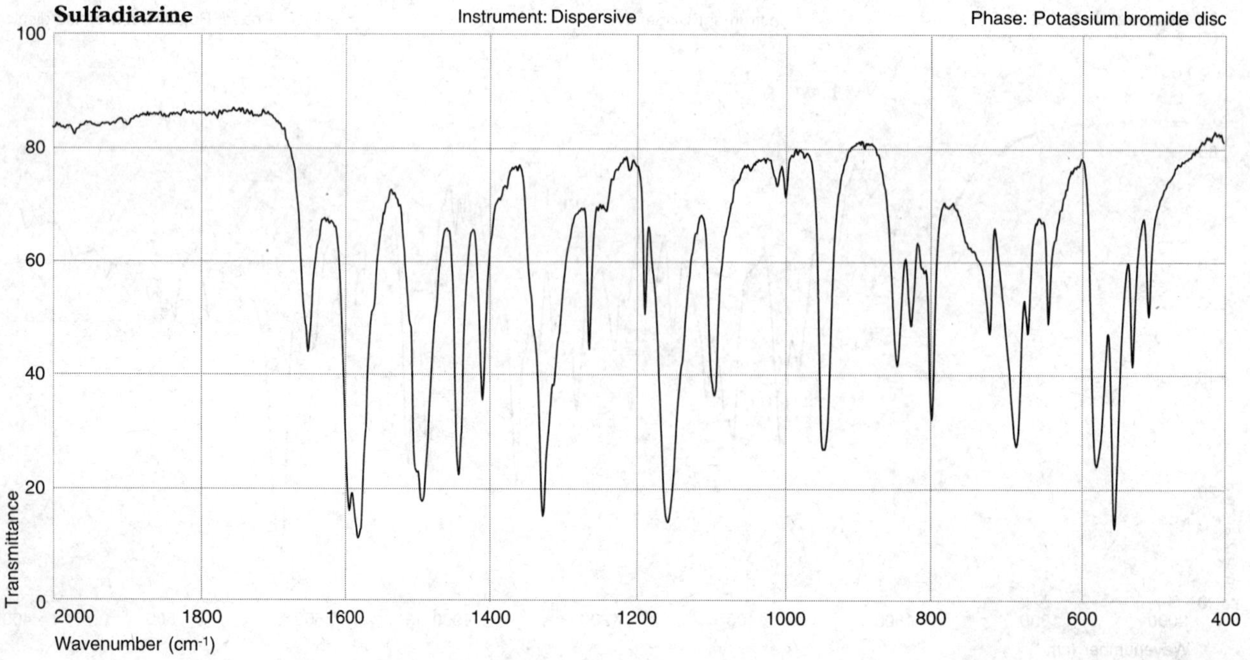
Sulfadiazine
Instrument: Dispersive
Phase: Potassium bromide disc
100
80
60
40
20
0
Transmittance
2000
1800
1600
1400
1200
1000
800
600
400
Wavenumber (cm-1)

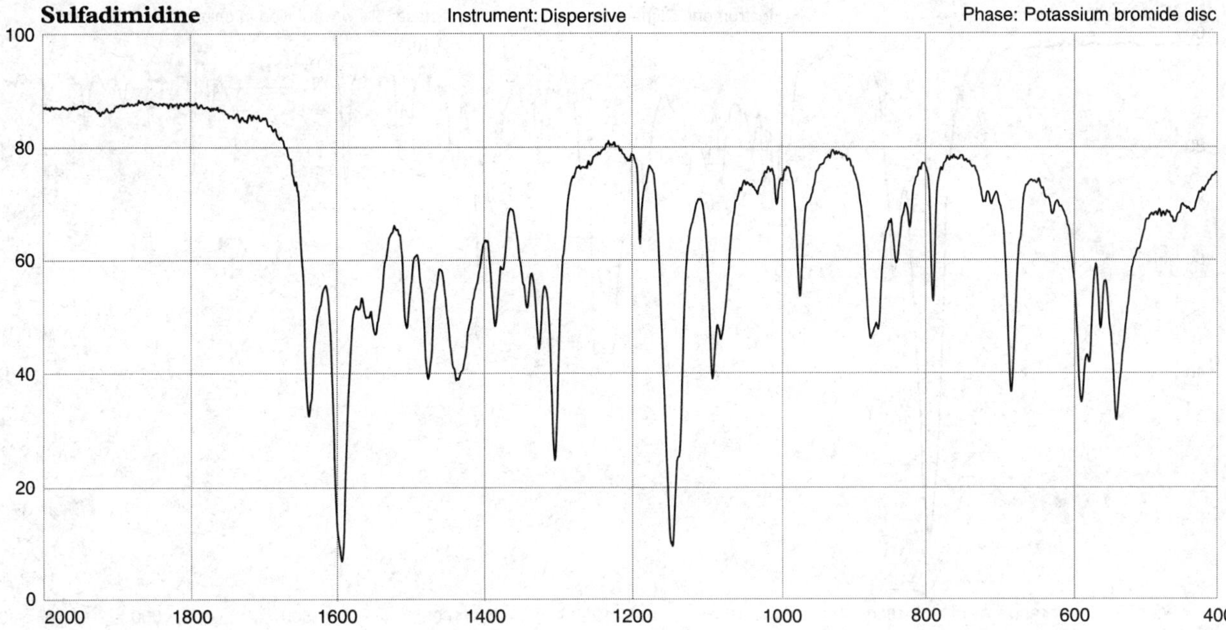
Sulfadimidine
Instrument: Dispersive
Phase: Potassium bromide disc
100
80
60
40
20
0
2000
1800
1600
1400
1200
1000
800
600
400

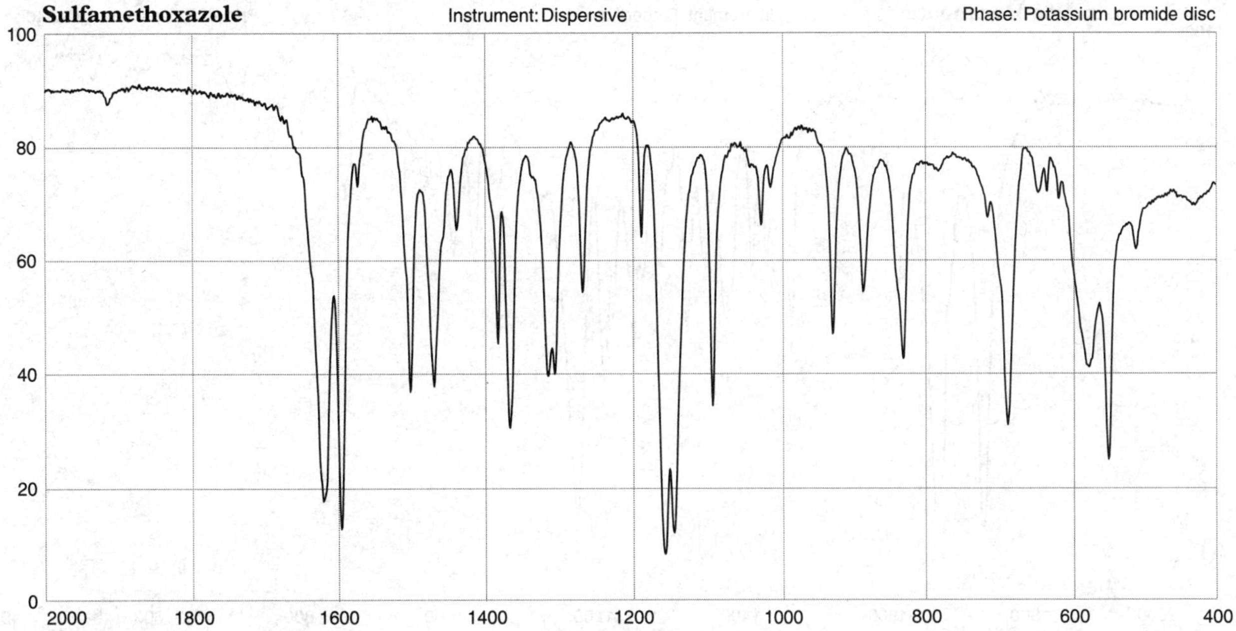
Sulfamethoxazole
Instrument: Dispersive
Phase: Potassium bromide disc
100
80
60
40
20
0
2000
1800
1600
1400
1200
1000
800
600
400

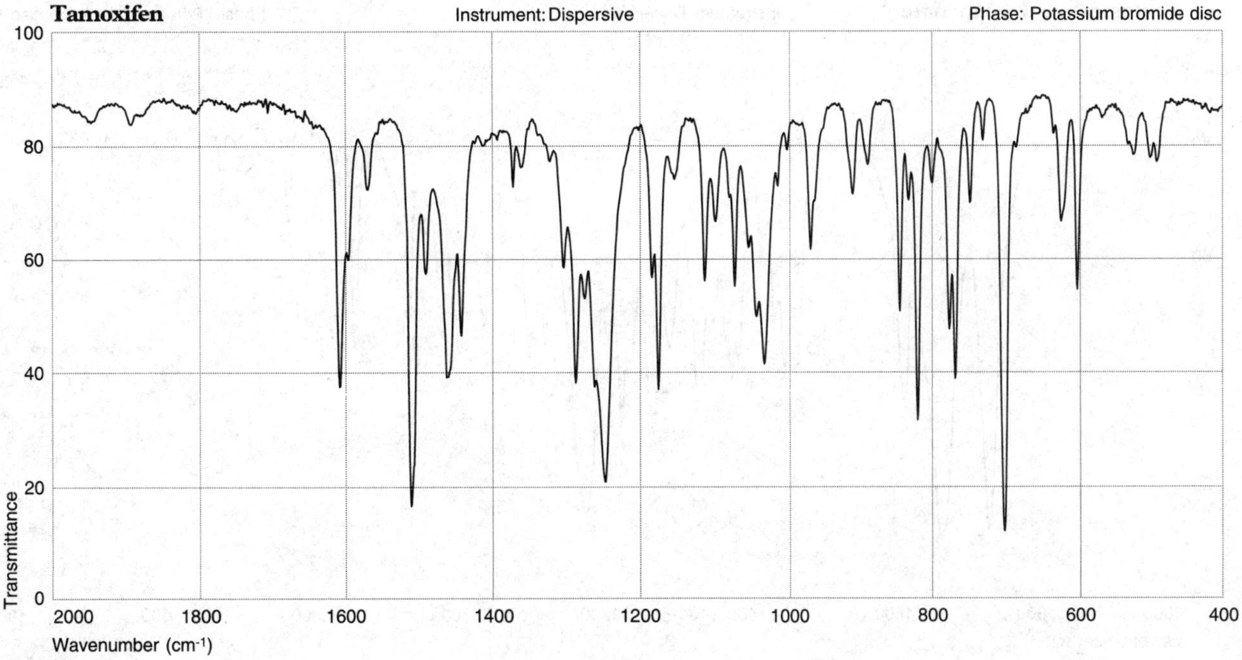
Tamoxifen
Instrument: Dispersive
Phase: Potassium bromide disc
100
80
60
40
20
0
Transmittance
2000
1800
1600
1400
1200
1000
800
600
400
Wavenumber (cm-1)

Testosterone Instrument: Dispersive Phase: 5% w/v solution in chloroform Thickness 0.1mm

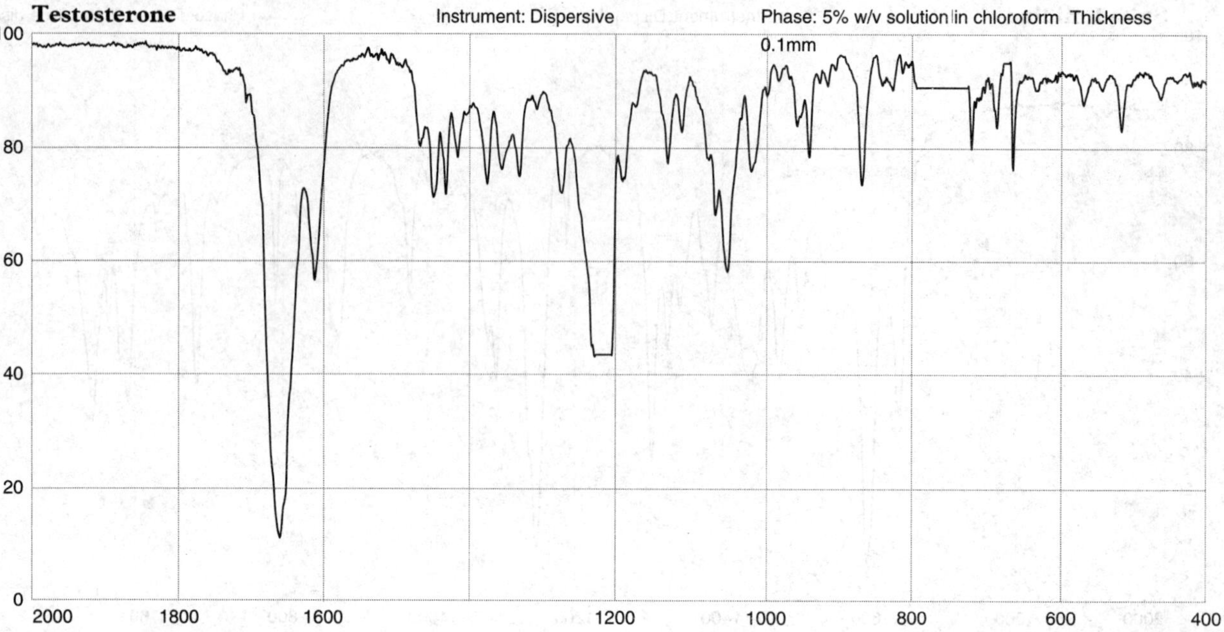

Testosterone Decanoate Instrument: Dispersive Phase: Potassium bromide disc

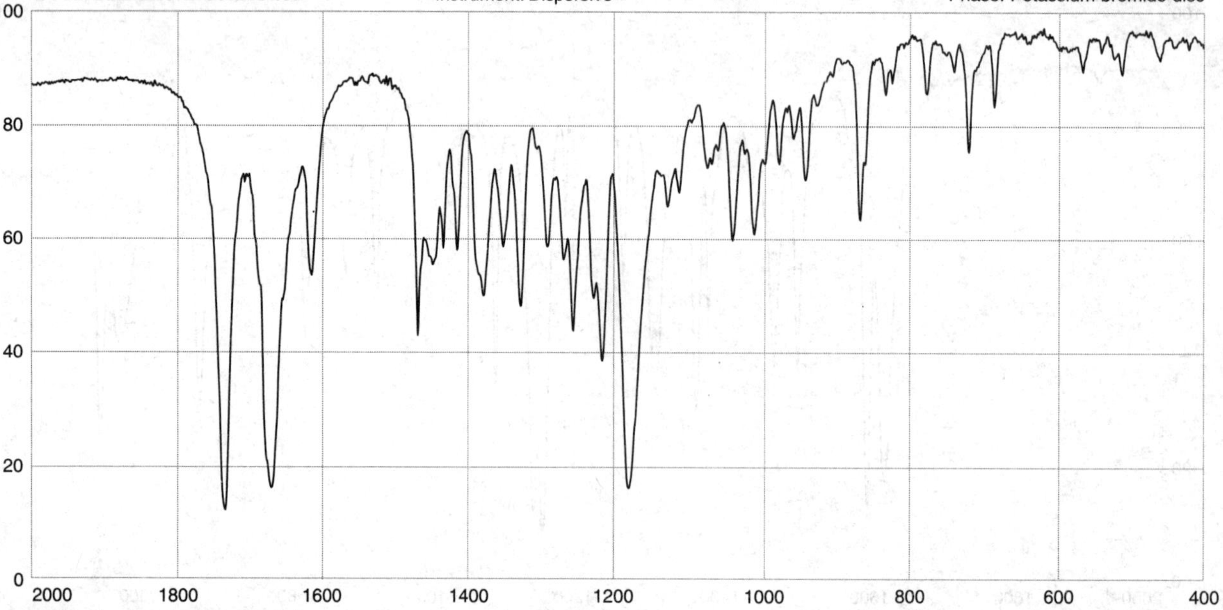

Testosterone Isocaproate Instrument: Dispersive Phase: Potassium bromide disc

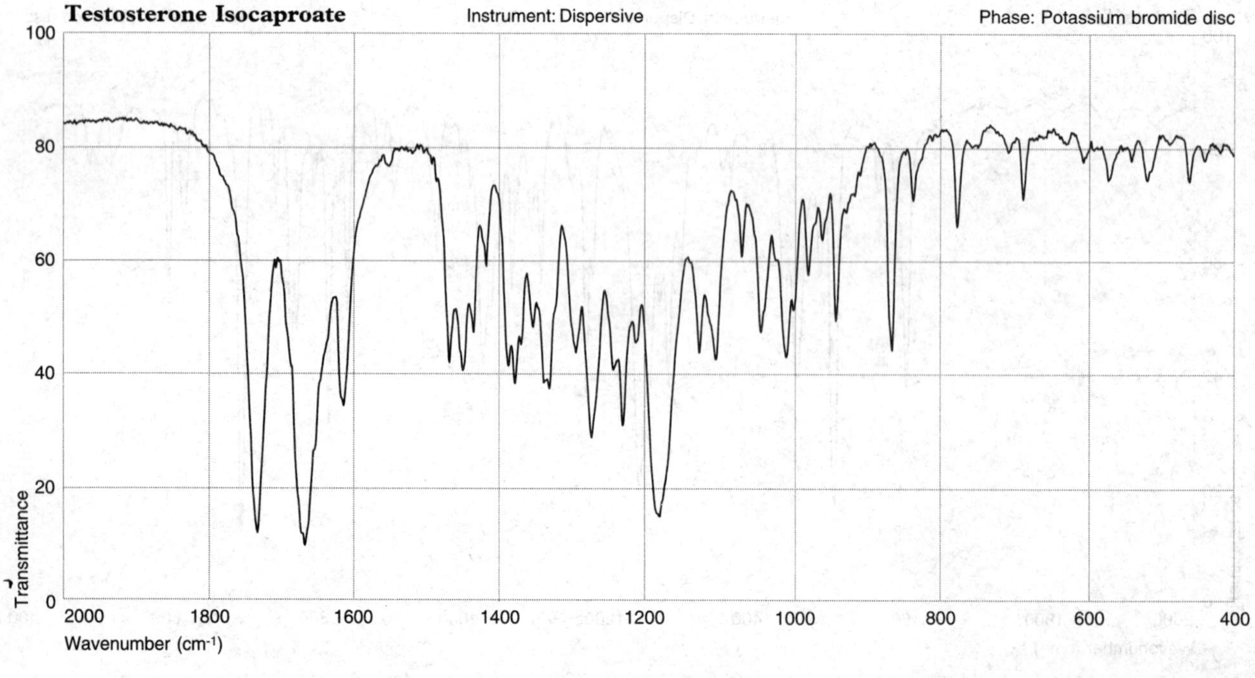

Testosterone Propionate

Instrument: Dispersive

Phase: Potassium bromide disc

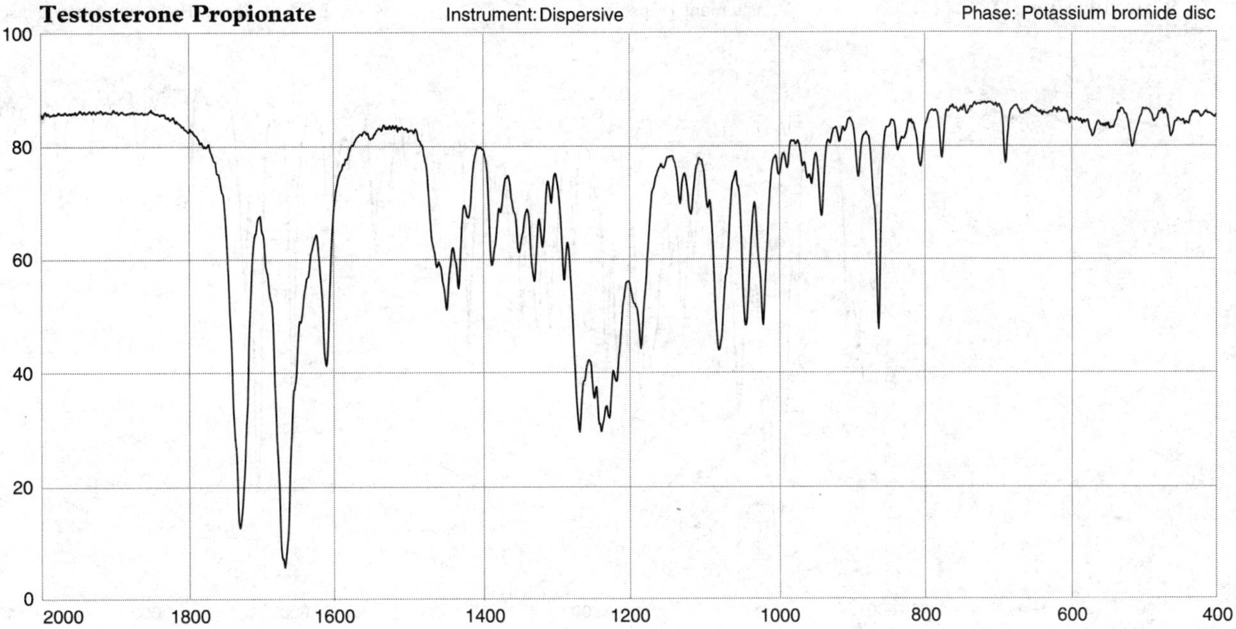

Theophylline

Instrument: Dispersive

Phase: Liquid paraffin mull

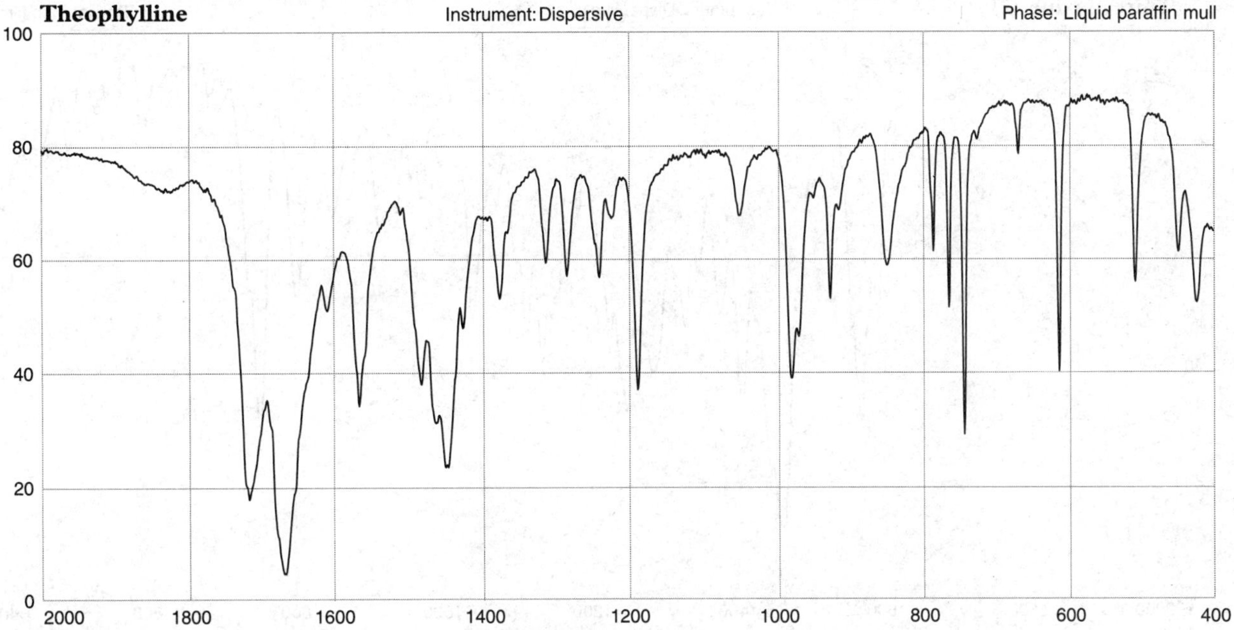

Thiopental

Instrument: Dispersive

Phase: Potassium bromide disc

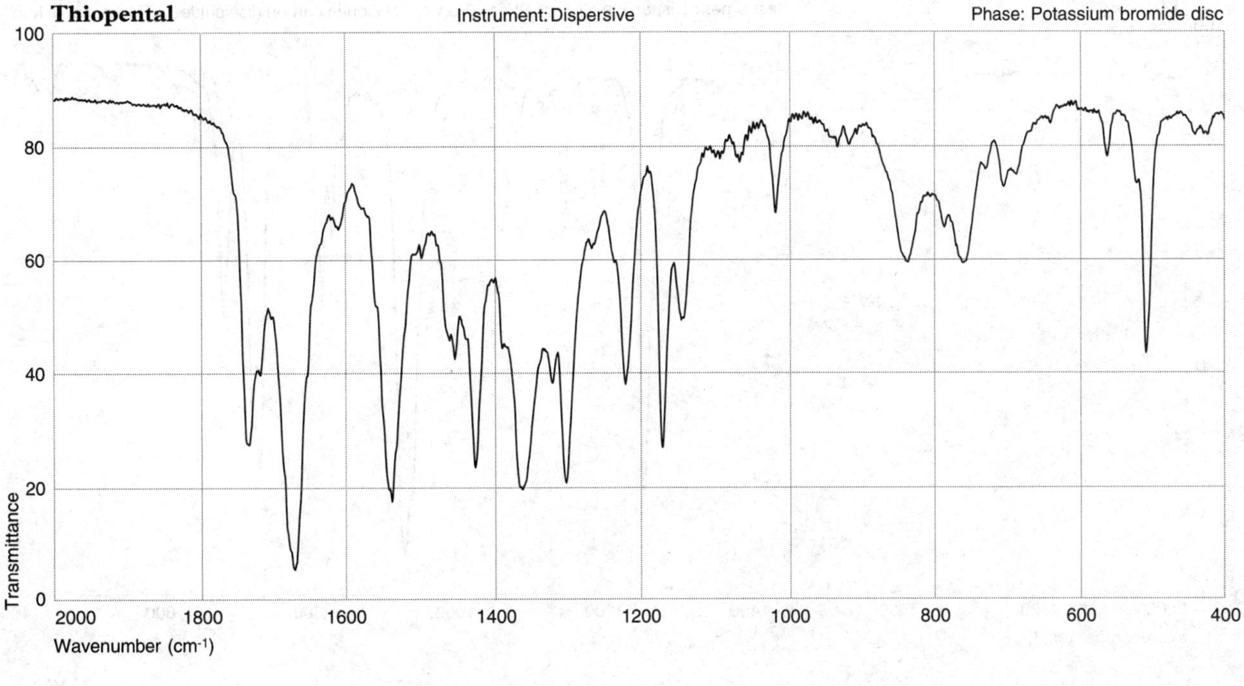

Thioridazine (1) Instrument: Dispersive Phase: Potassium bromide disc

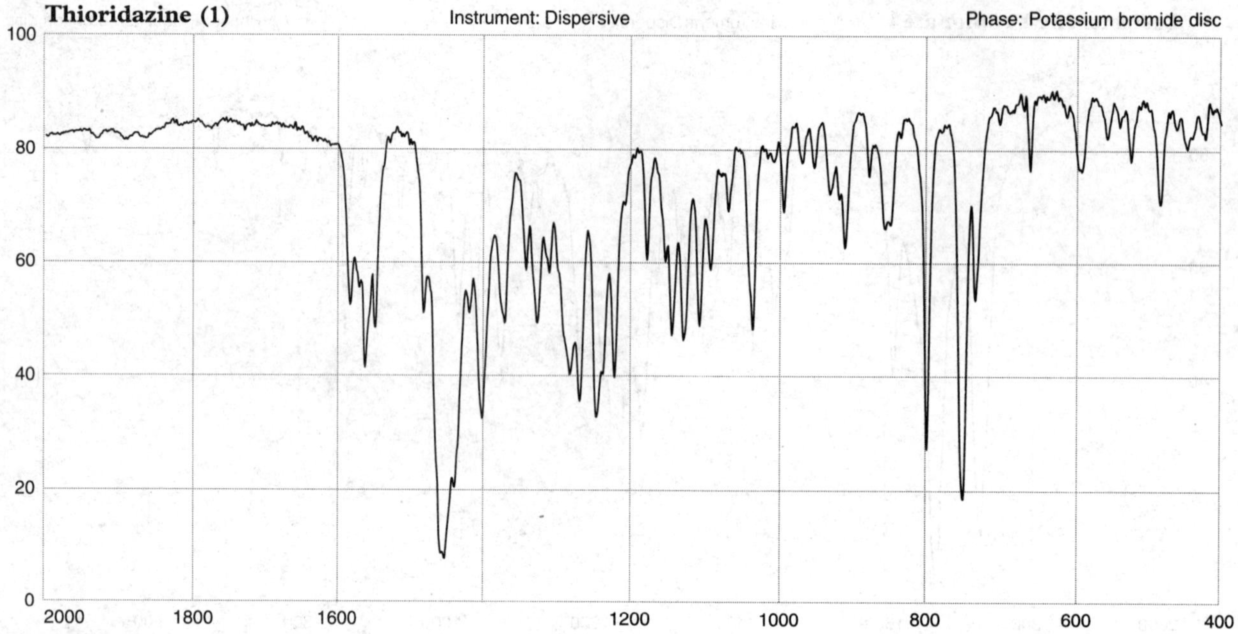

Thioridazine (2) Instrument: Dispersive Phase: Thin film

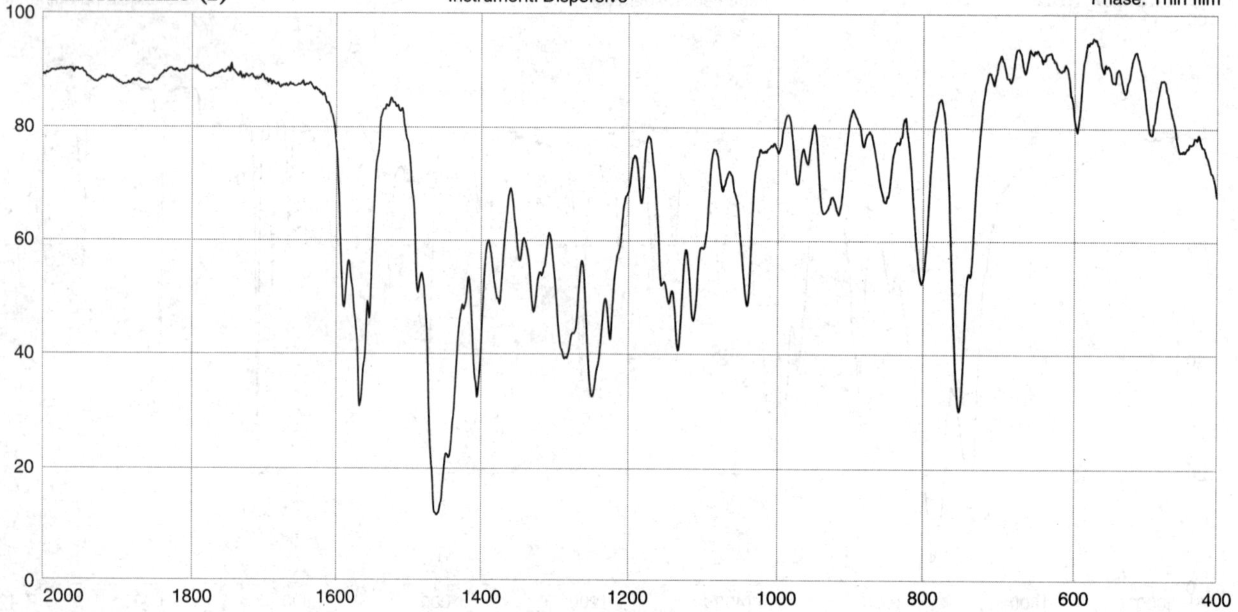

Thiotepa Instrument: Dispersive Phase:2% w/v solution in carbon disulphide Thickness: 0.1mm

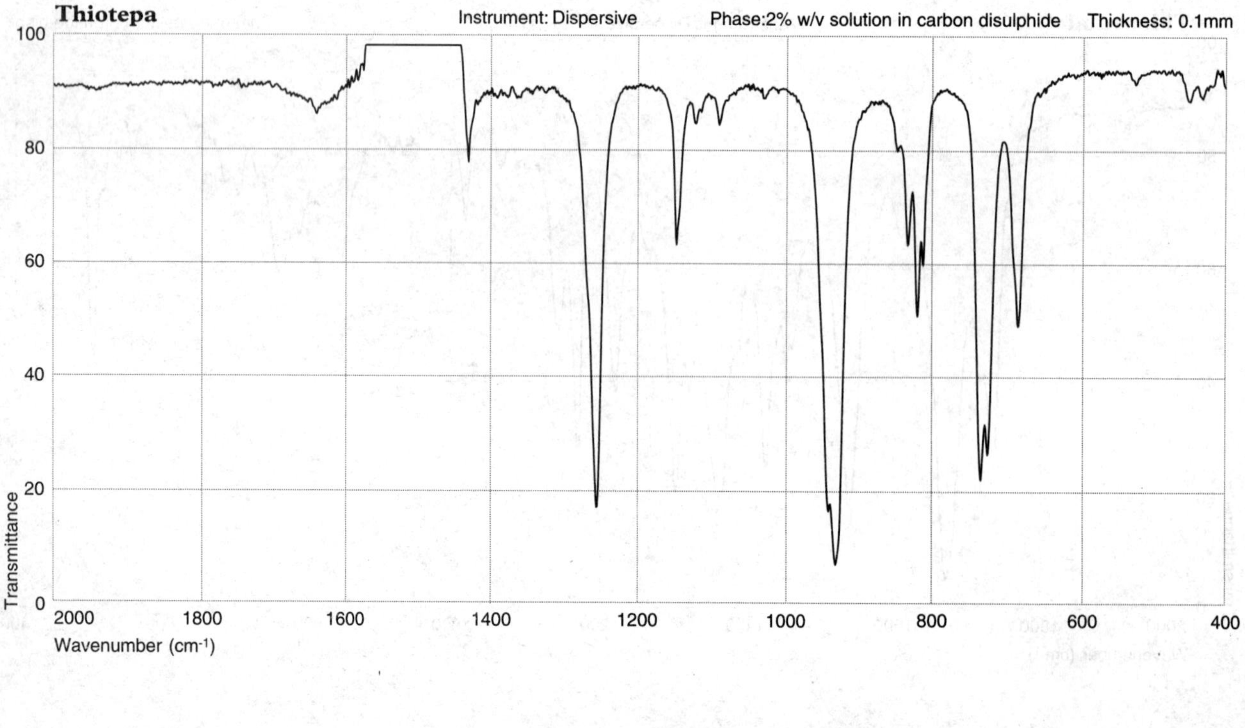

Thymoxamine Hydrochloride (Moxisylyte Hydrochloride)

Instrument: Dispersive

Phase: Potassium chloride disc

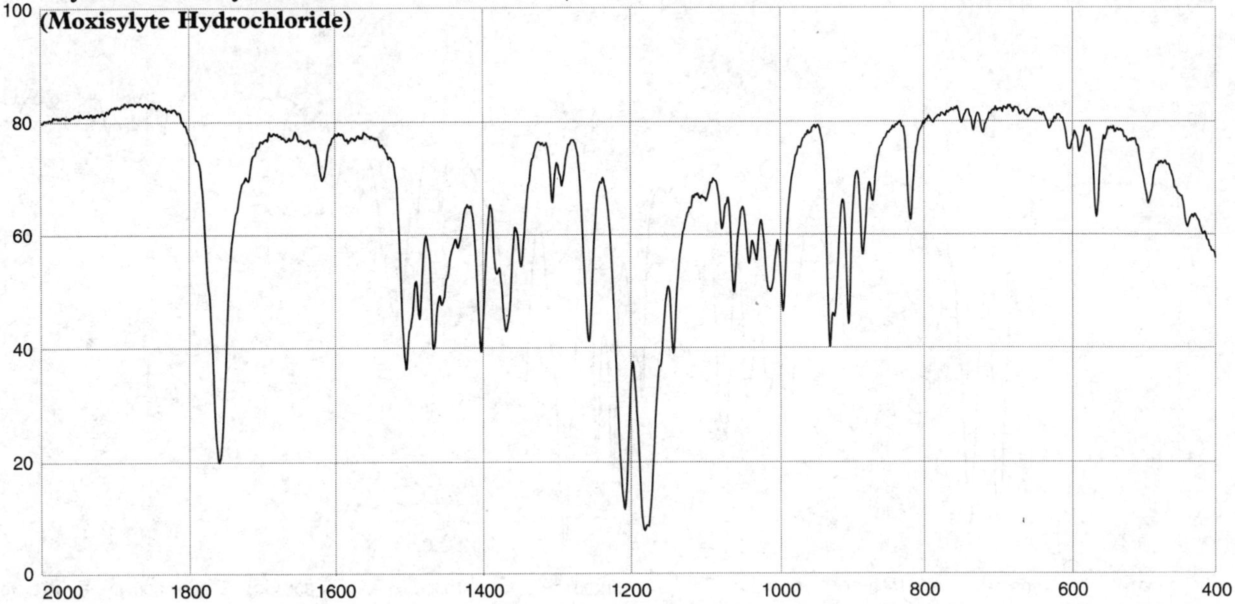

Timolol

Instrument: Dispersive

Phase: 5% w/v solution in carbon tetrachloride Thickness: 0.1mm

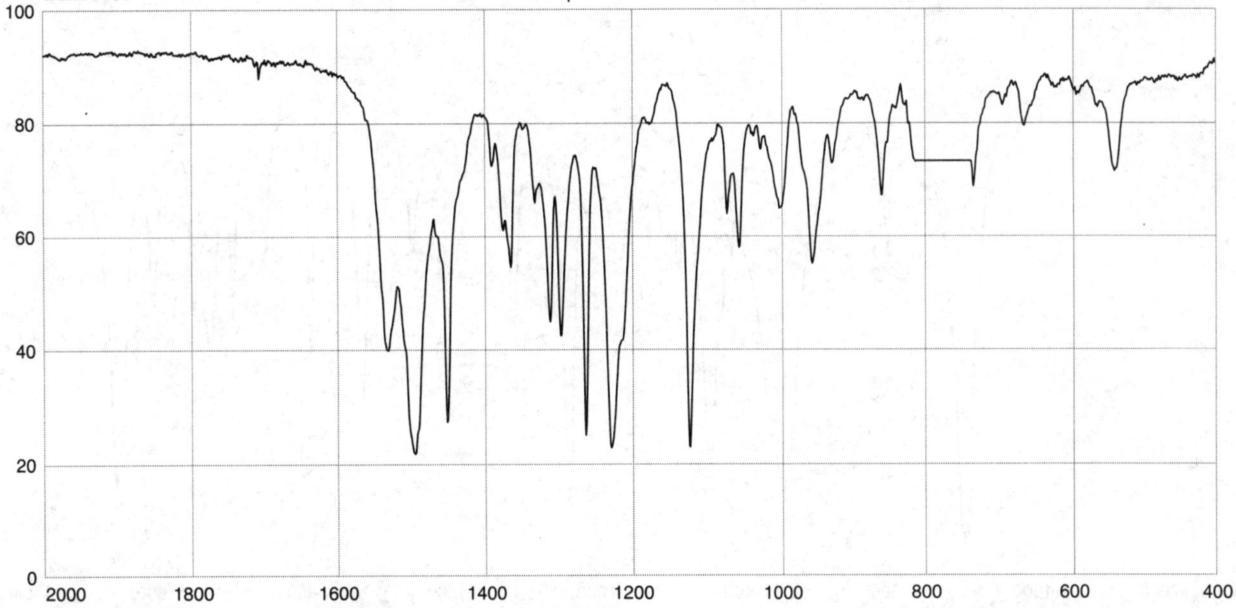

Tioguanine

Instrument: Dispersive

Phase: Potassium bromide disc

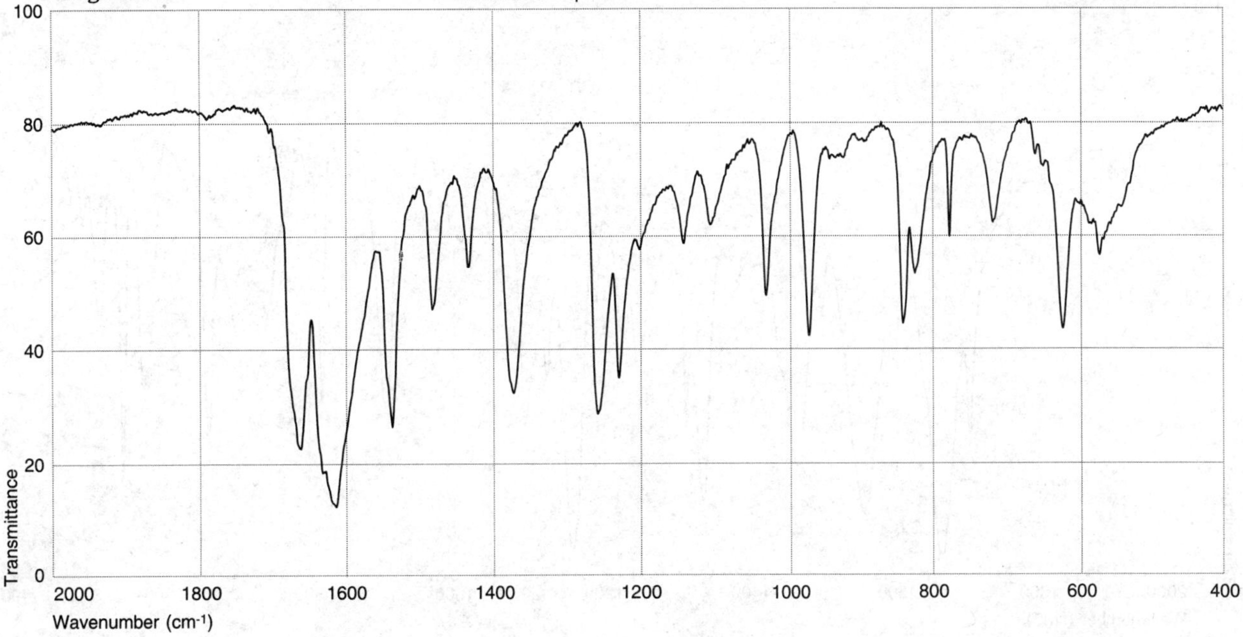

Alpha Tocopheryl Succinate

Instrument: Dispersive

Phase: Potassium bromide disc

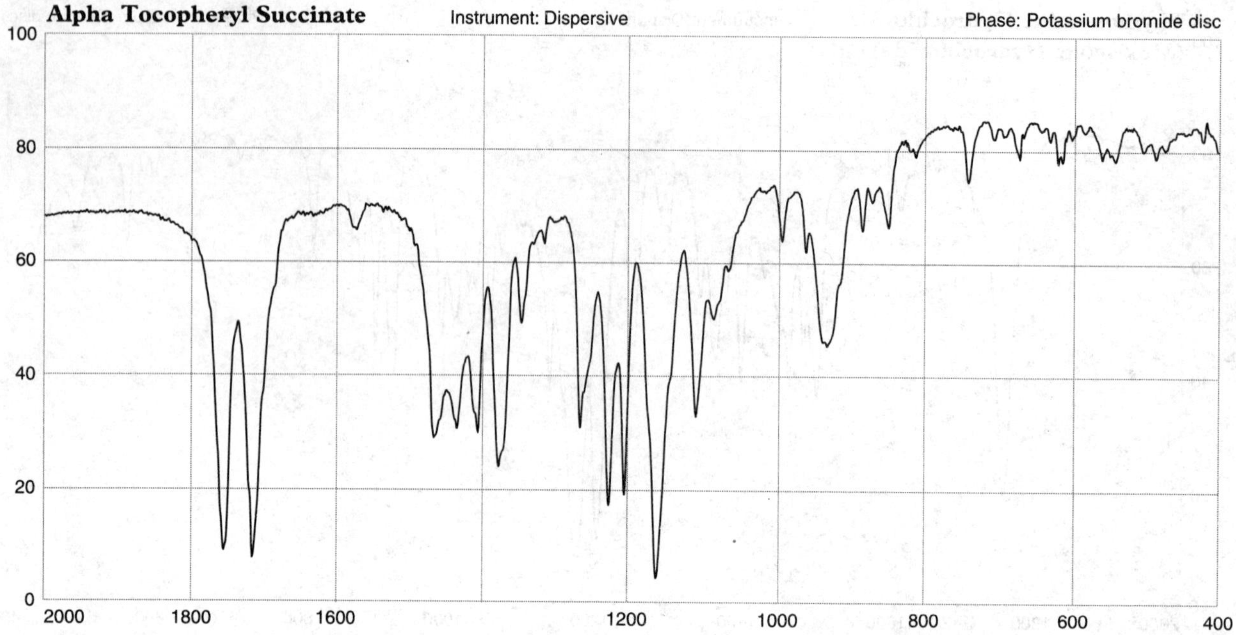

Tolazamide

Instrument: Dispersive

Phase: Potassium bromide disc

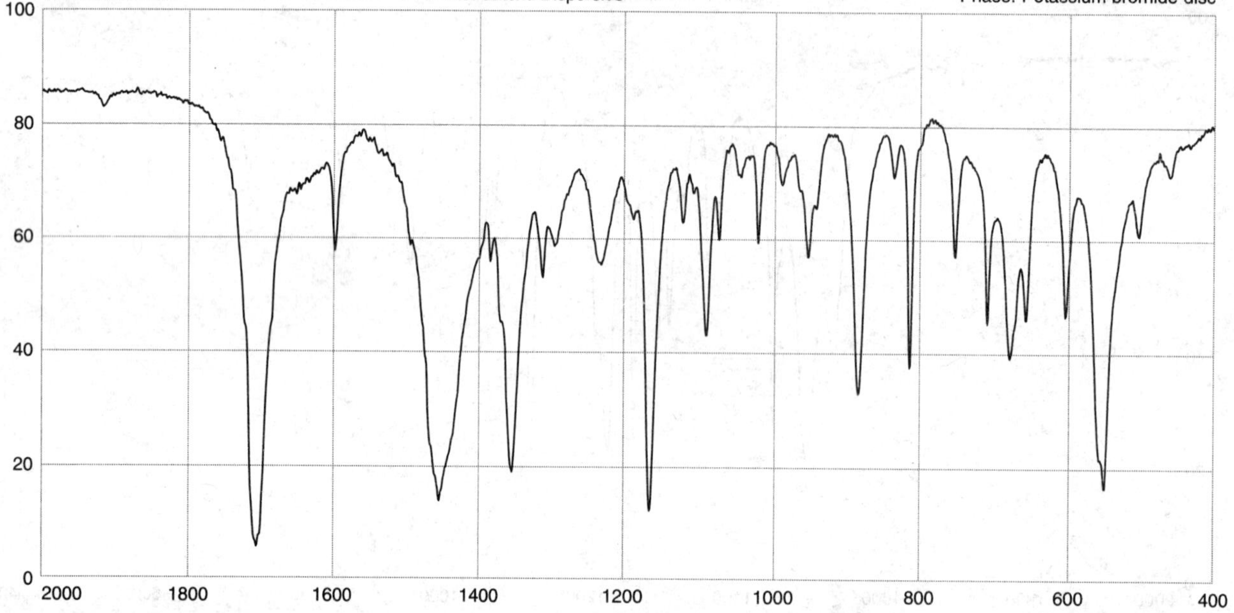

Tolbutamide

Instrument: Dispersive

Phase: Potassium bromide disc

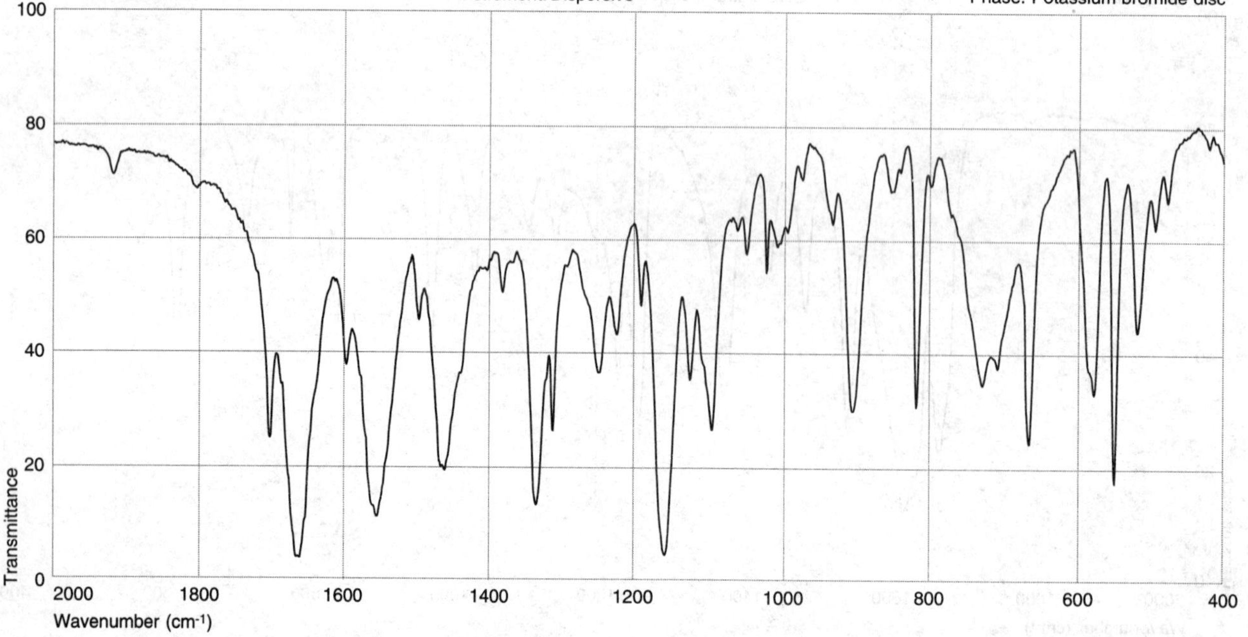

Tranexamic Acid Instrument: Dispersive Phase: Potassium bromide disc

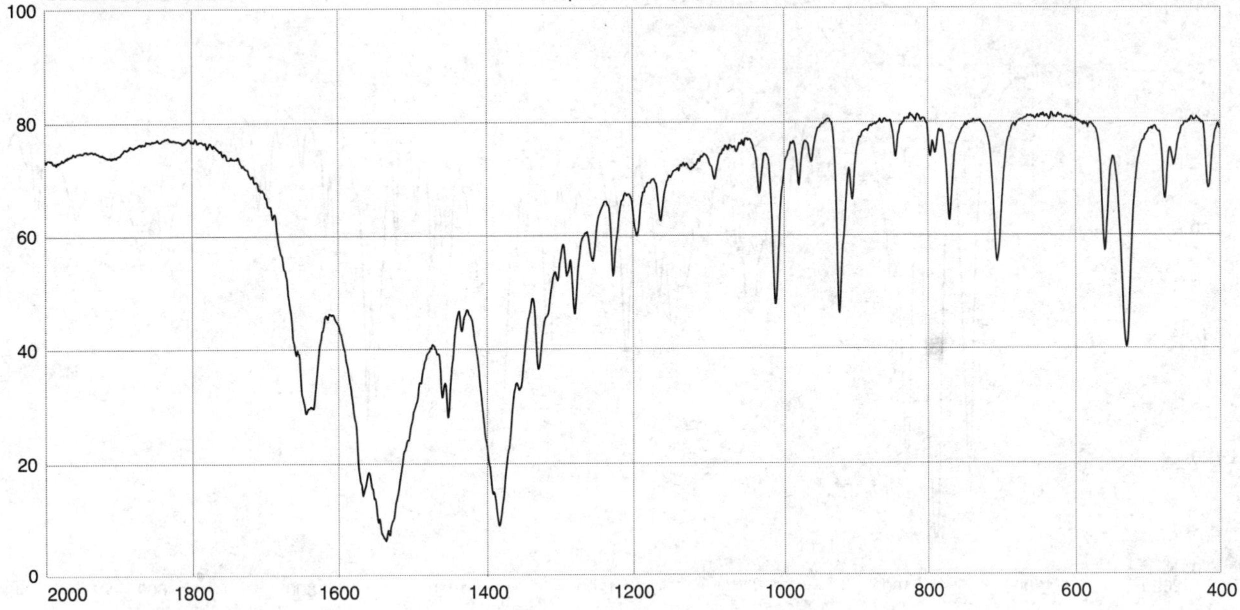

Tranylcypromine Sulphate Instrument: Dispersive Phase: Potassium bromide disc

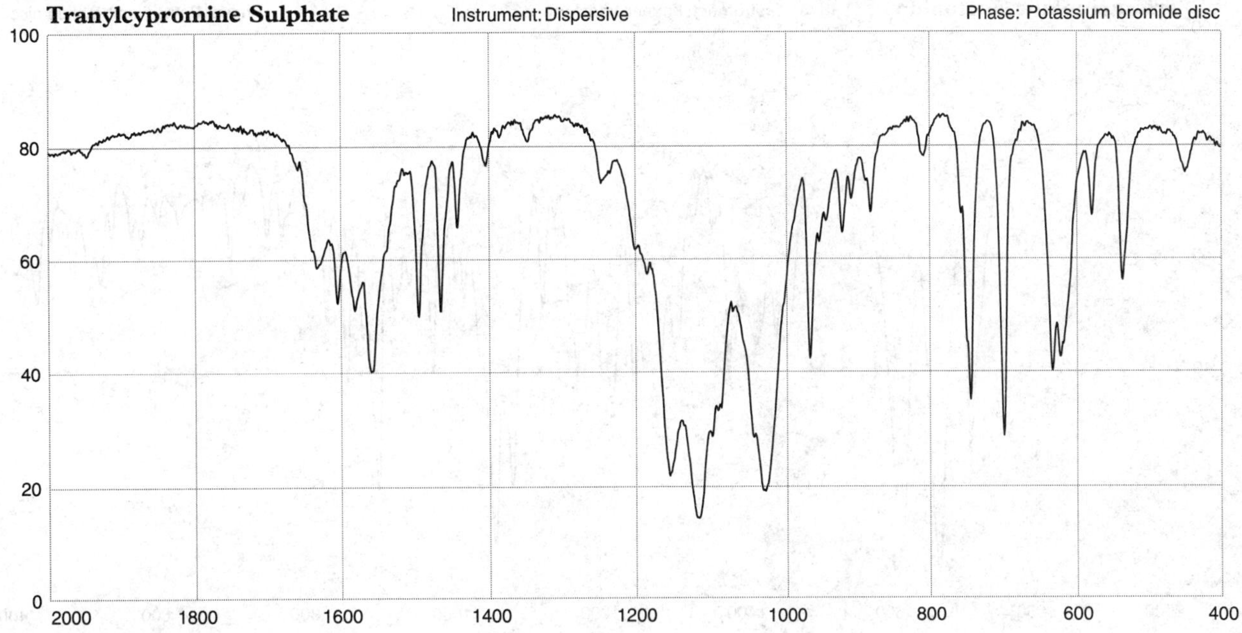

Trazodone Hydrochloride Instrument: Fourier transform Phase: Potassium chloride disc

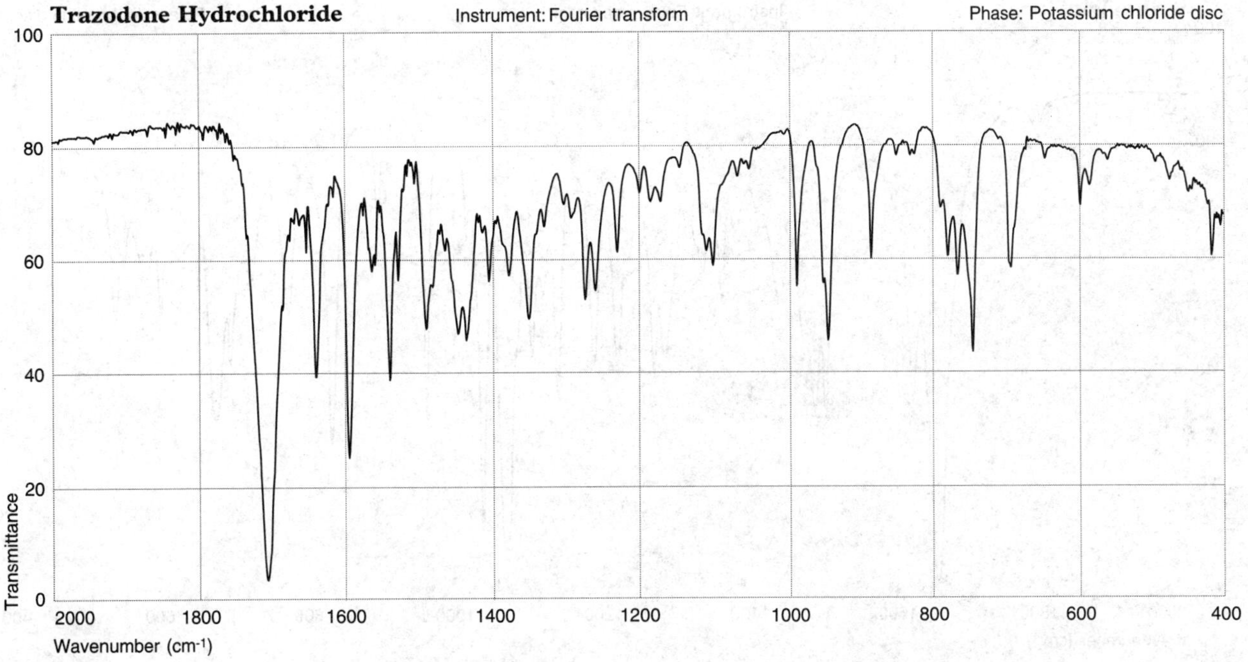

Triamcinolone

Instrument: Dispersive | Phase: Potassium bromide disc

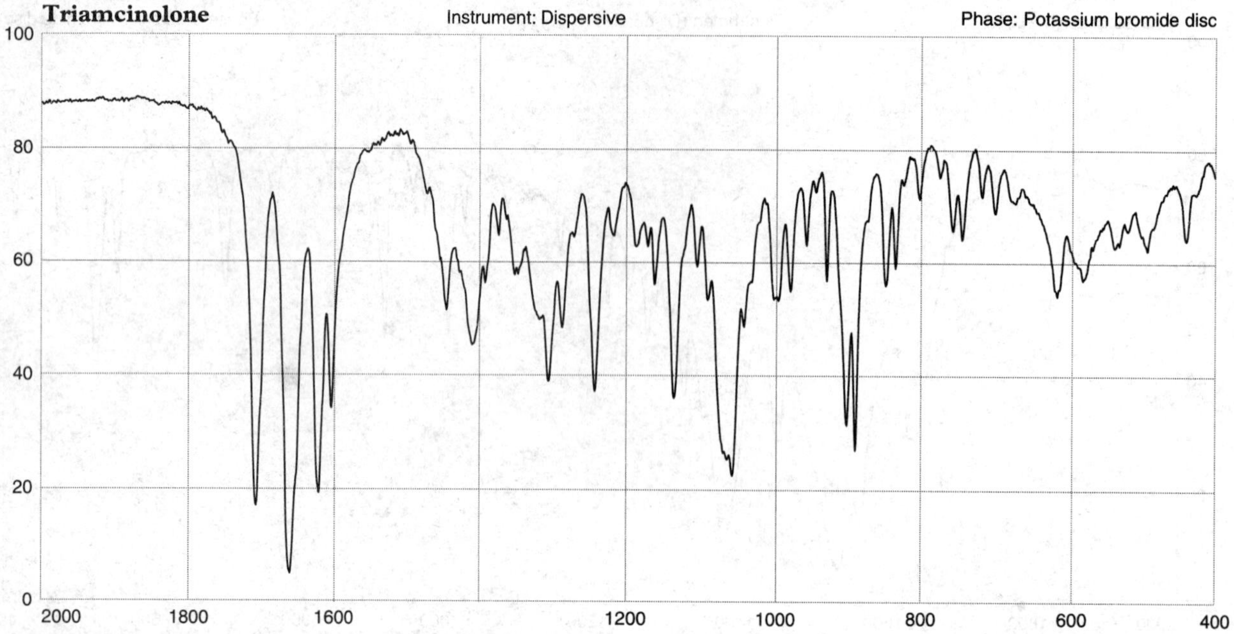

Triamcinolone Acetonide

Instrument: Fourier transform | Phase: Potassium bromide disc

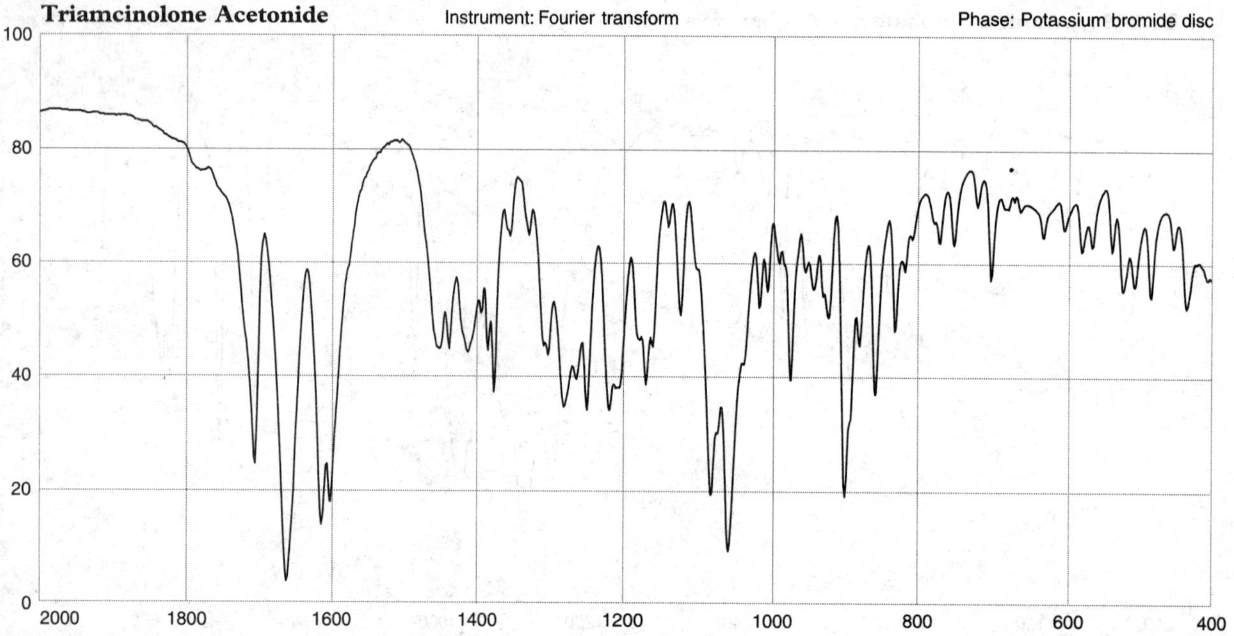

Tribavirin

Instrument: Fourier transform | Phase: Potassium bromide disc

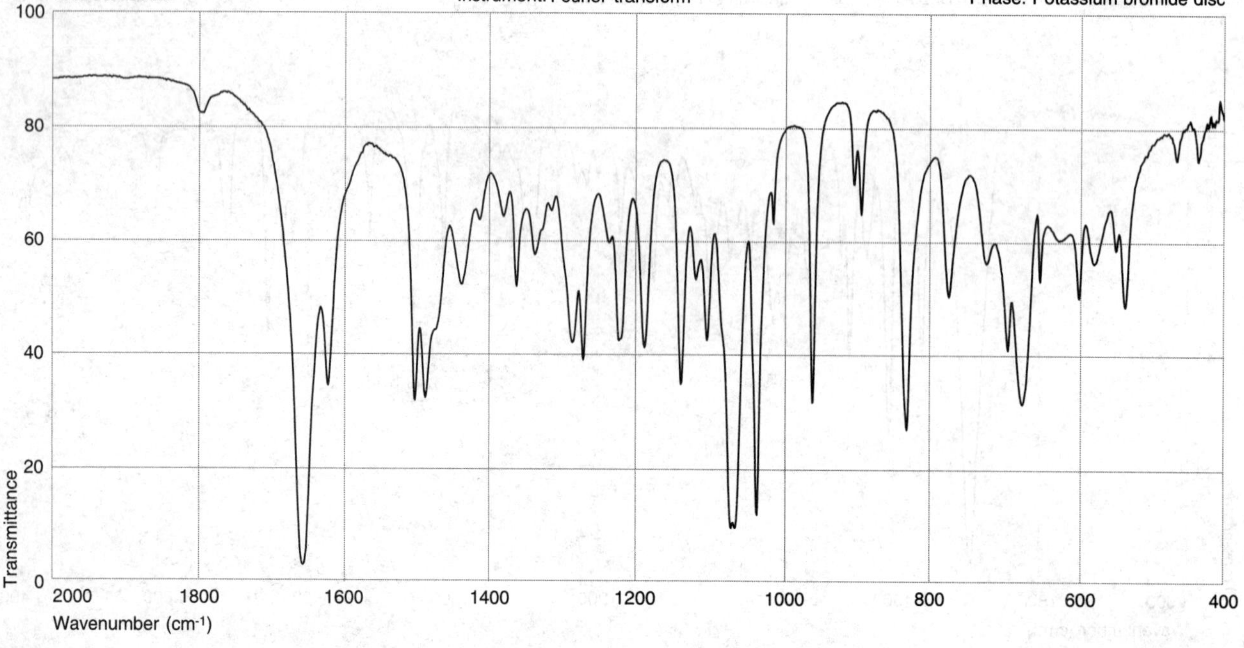

Triclofos Sodium Instrument: Fourier transform Phase: Potassium bromide disc

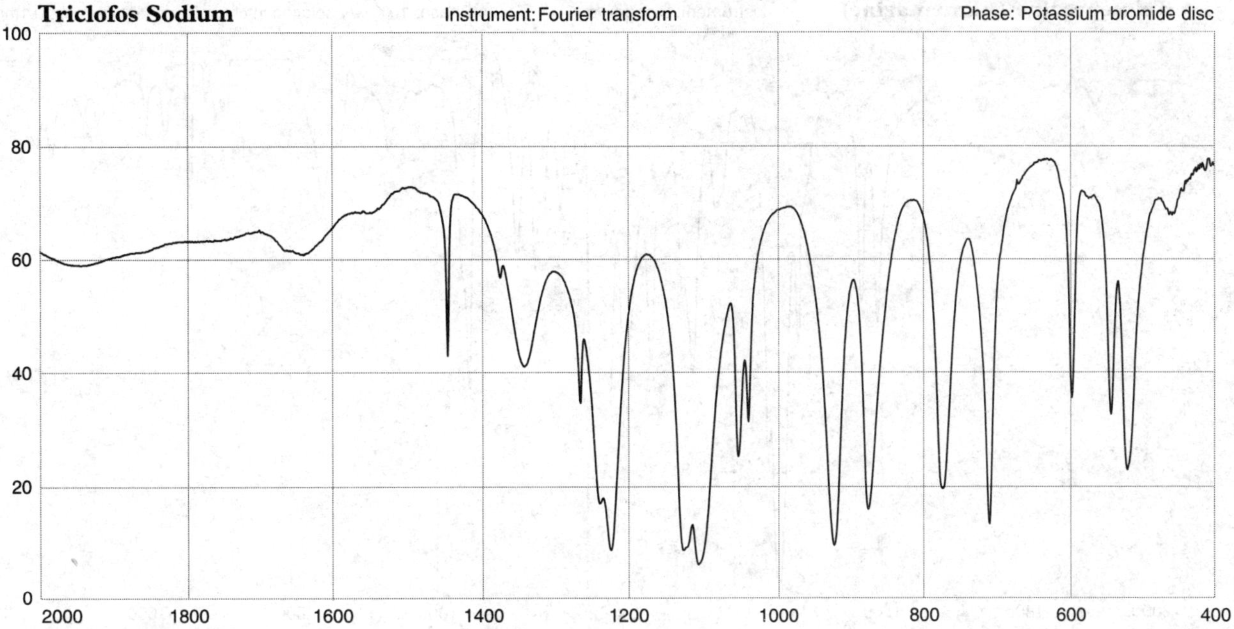

Trifluoperazine Instrument: Dispersive Phase: Thin film

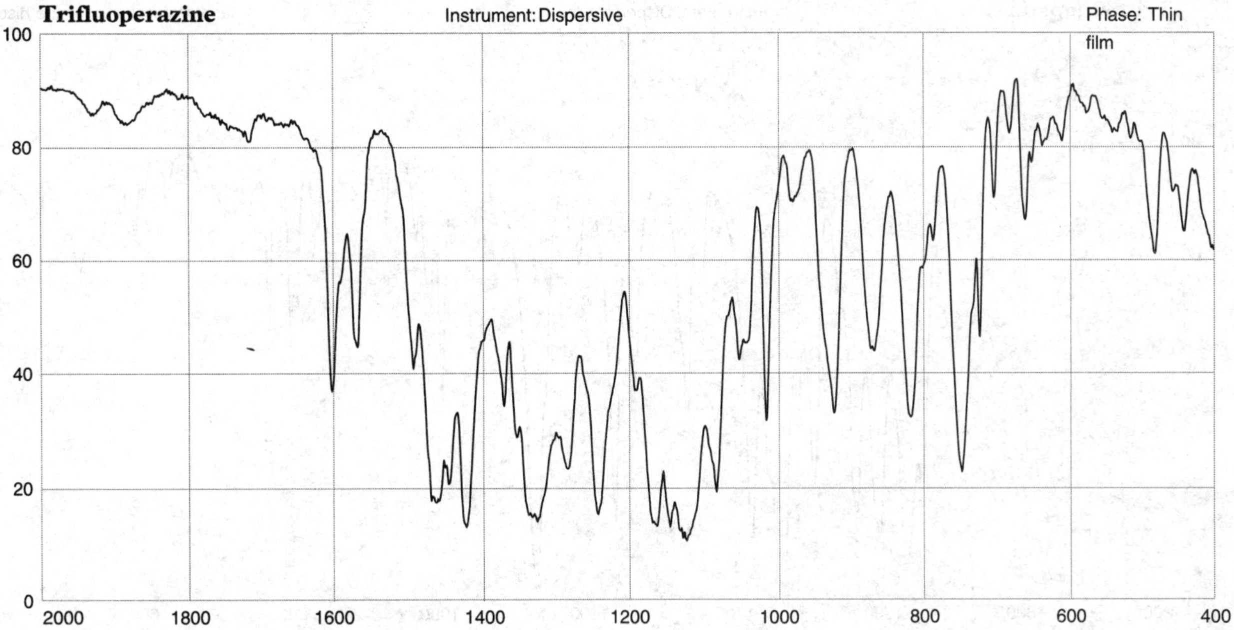

Trihexyphenidyl Hydrochloride (Benzhexol Hydrochloride) Instrument: Dispersive Phase: Potassium chloride disc

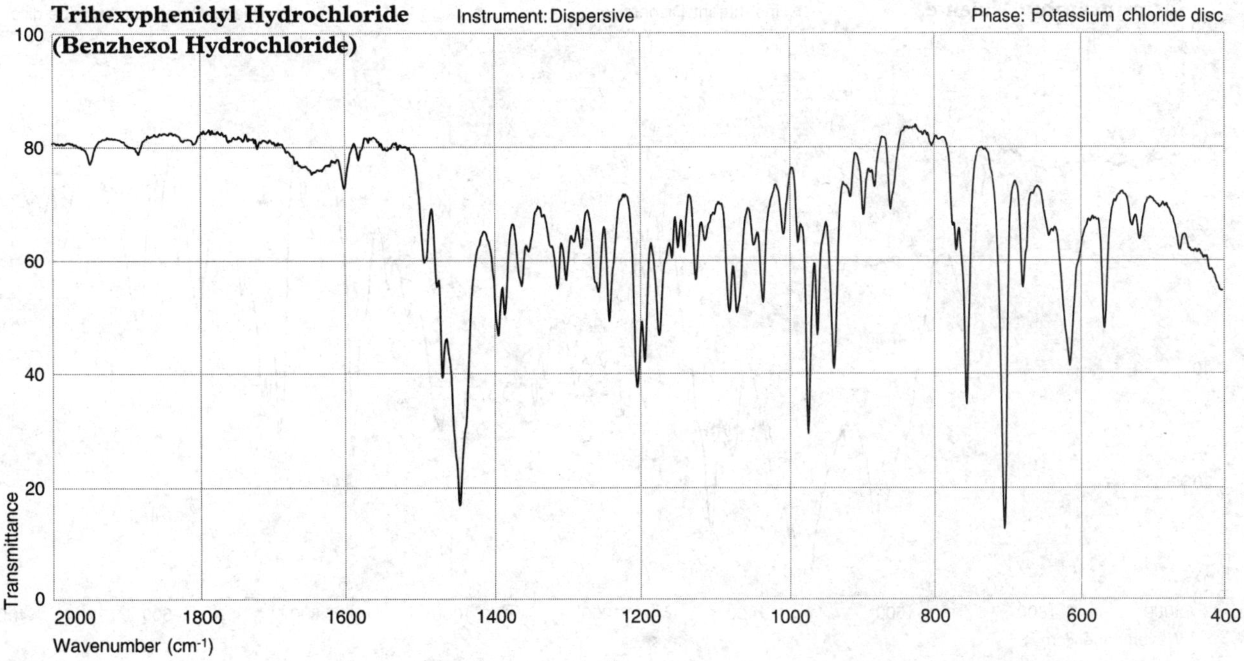

Trimeprazine (Alimemazine) Instrument: Dispersive Phase: 10% w/v solution in chloroform Thickness: 0.1mm

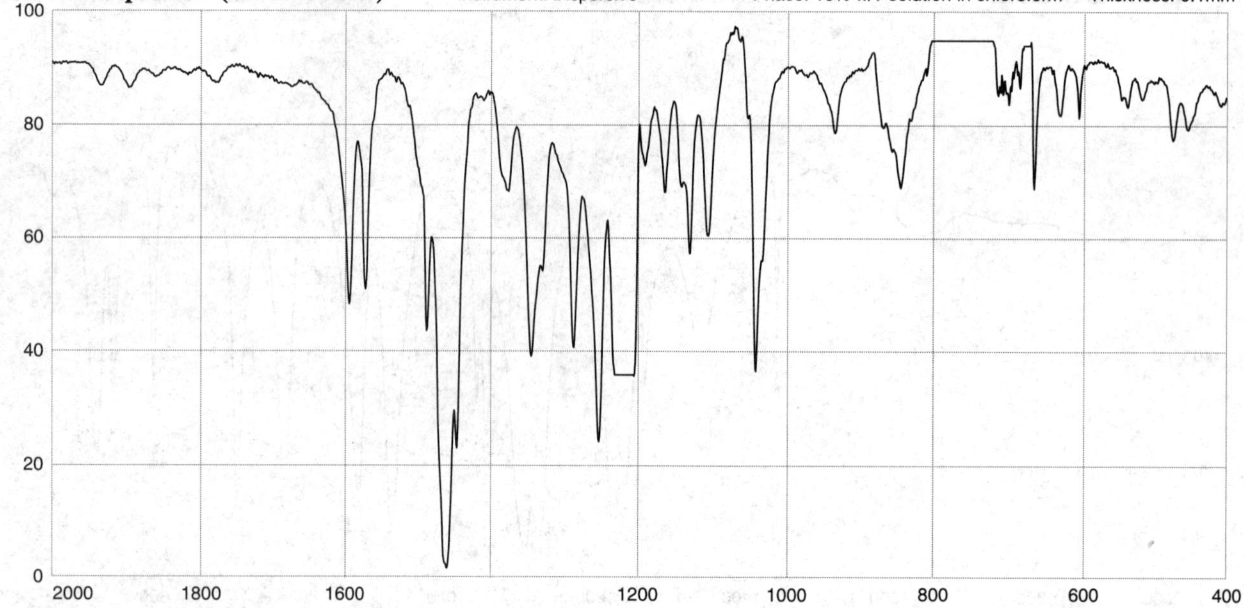

Trimethoprim Instrument: Dispersive Phase: Potassium bromide disc

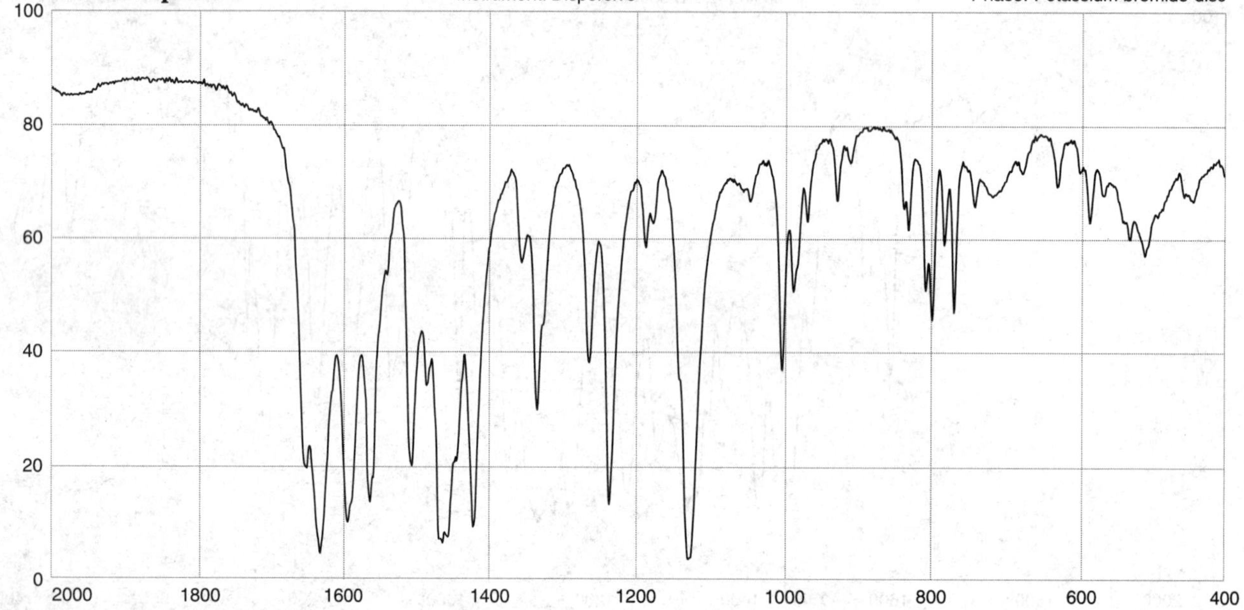

Trimipramine Maleate Instrument: Dispersive Phase: Potassium bromide disc

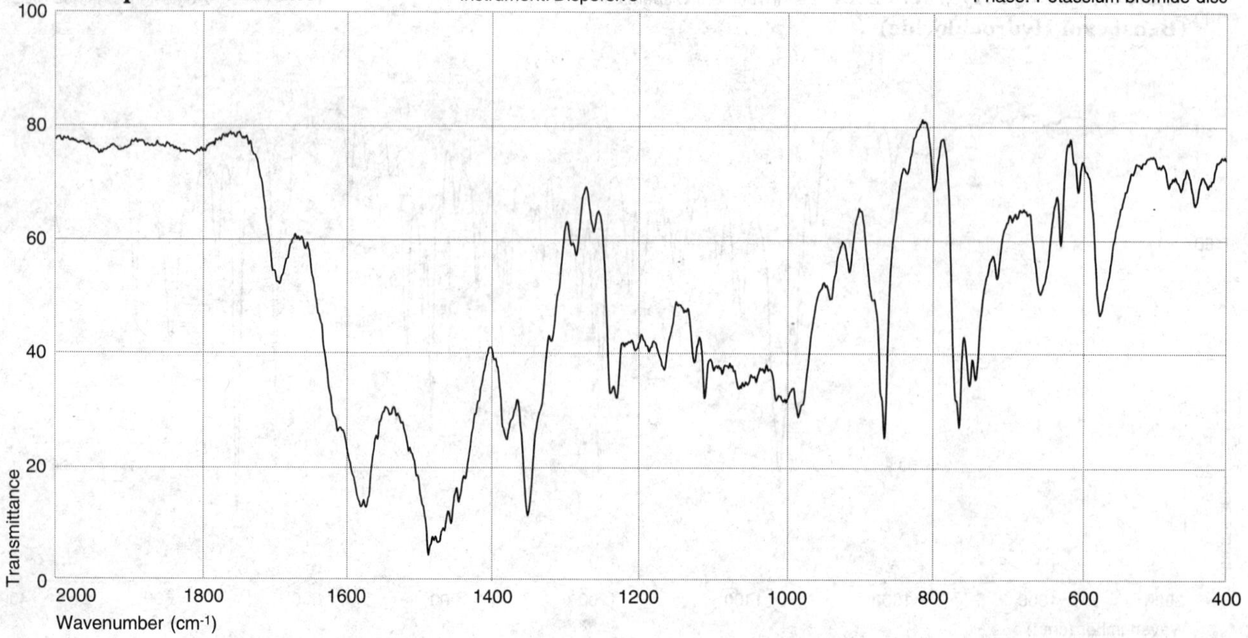

Triprolidine Hydrochloride Instrument: Dispersive Phase: Potassium chloride disc

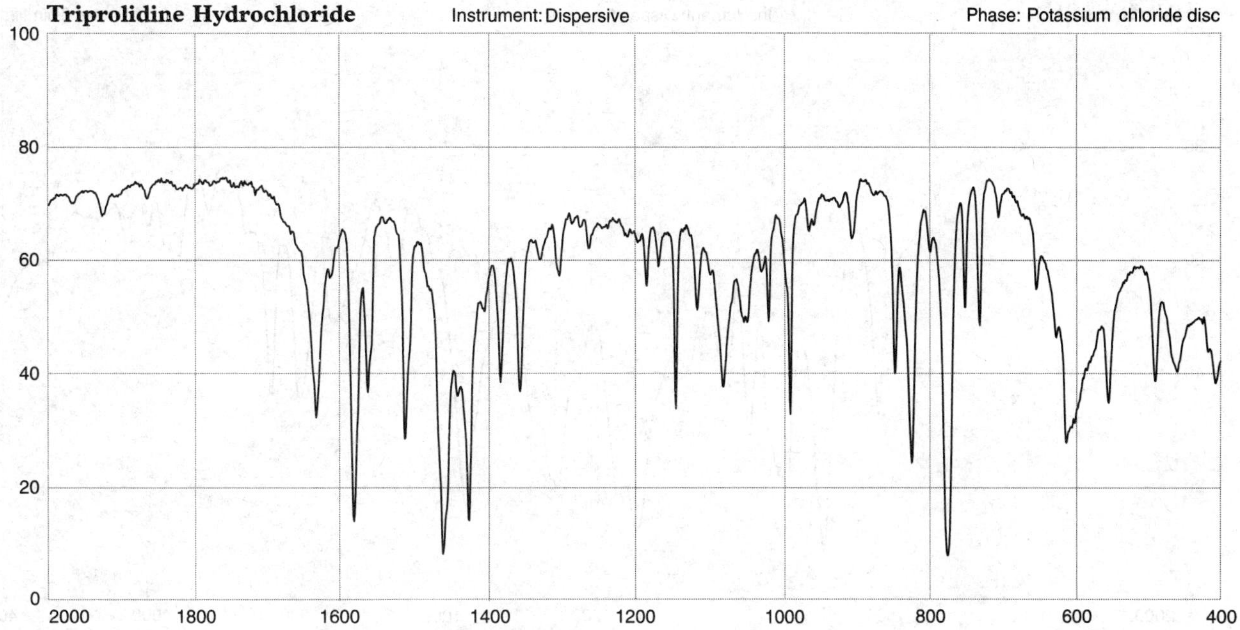

Tropicamide Instrument: Dispersive Phase: Potassium bromide disc

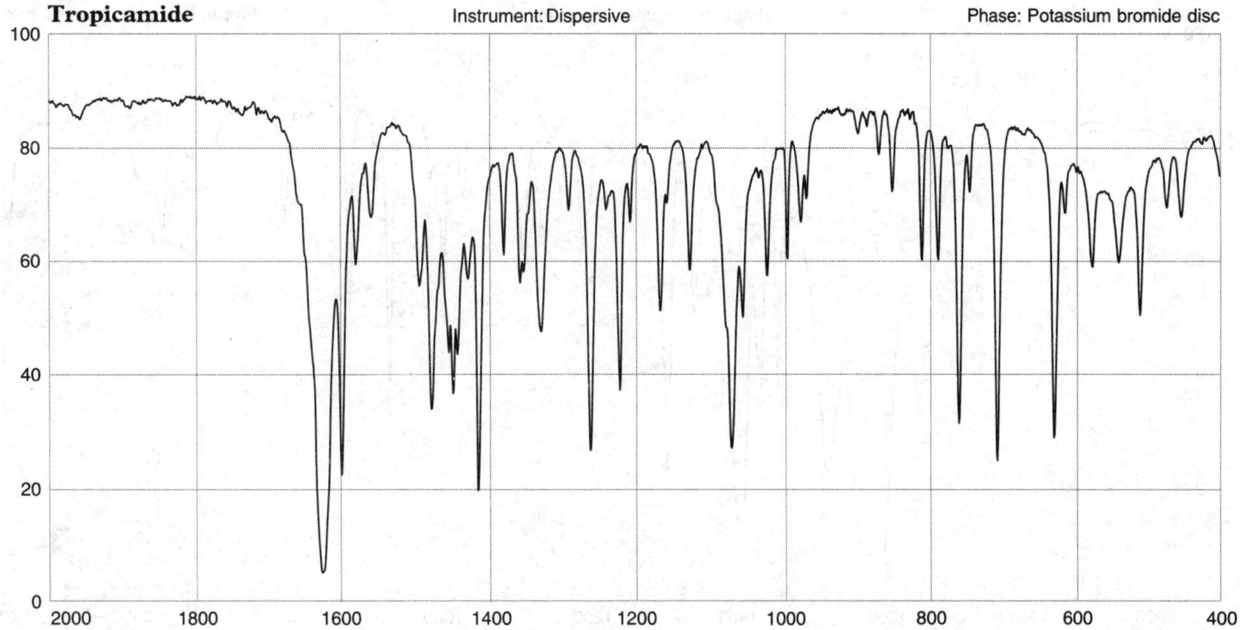

Valproic acid Instrument: Dispersive Phase: Thin film

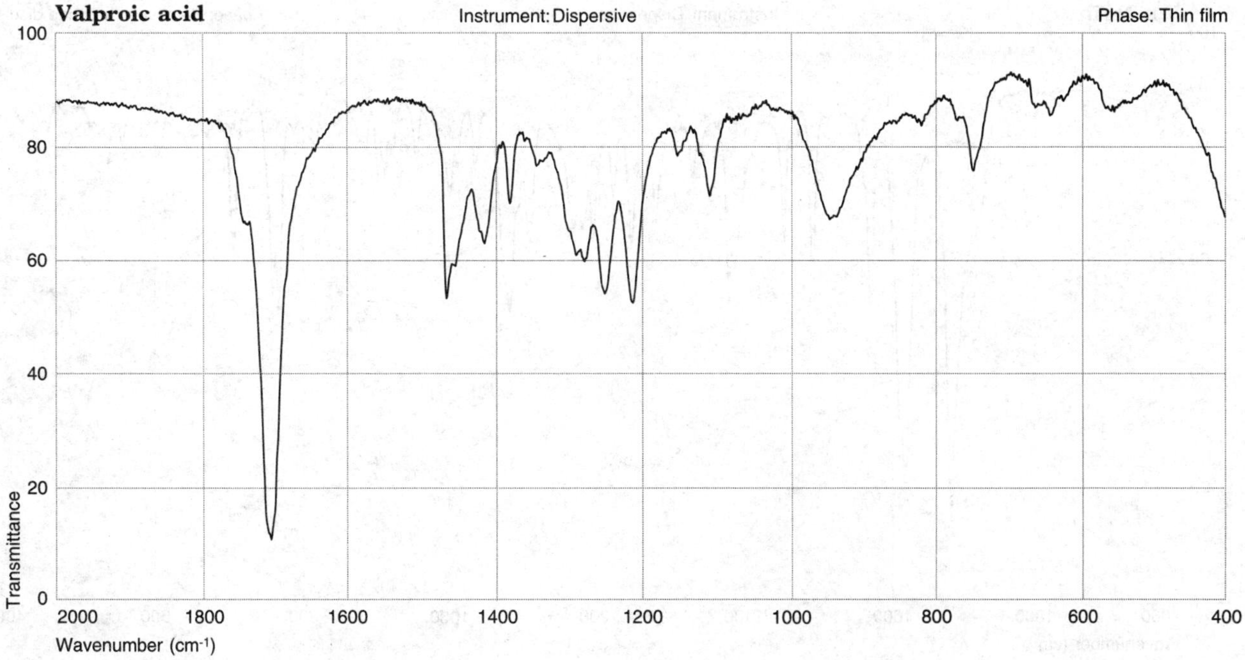

Verapamil

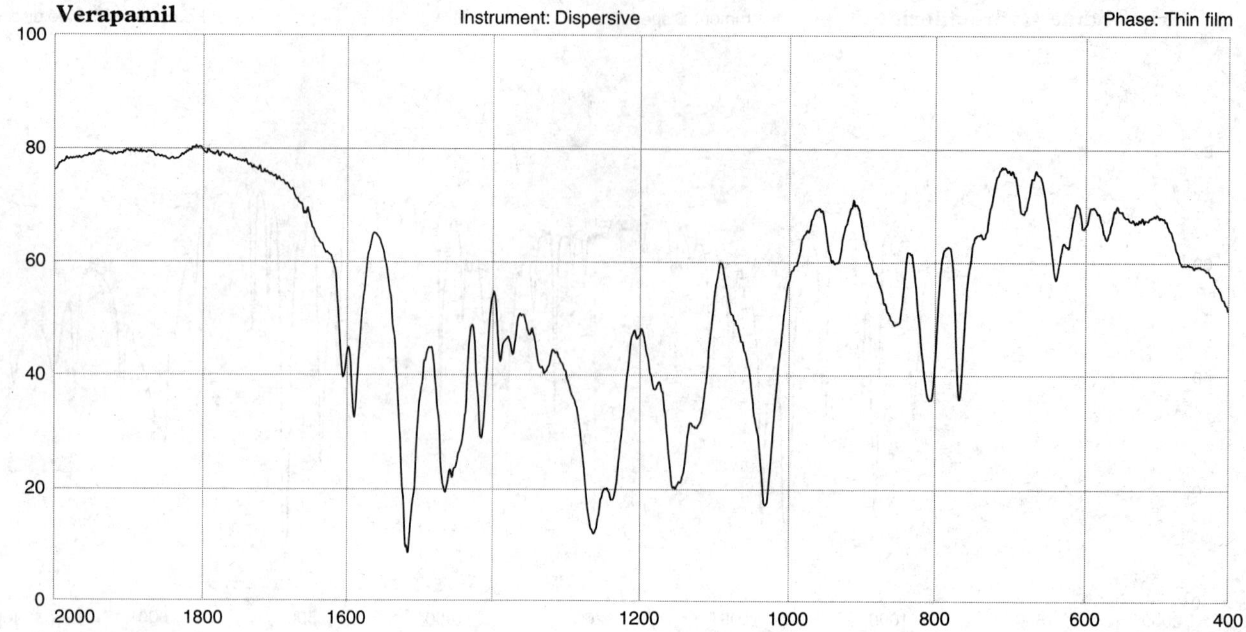

Vigabatrin

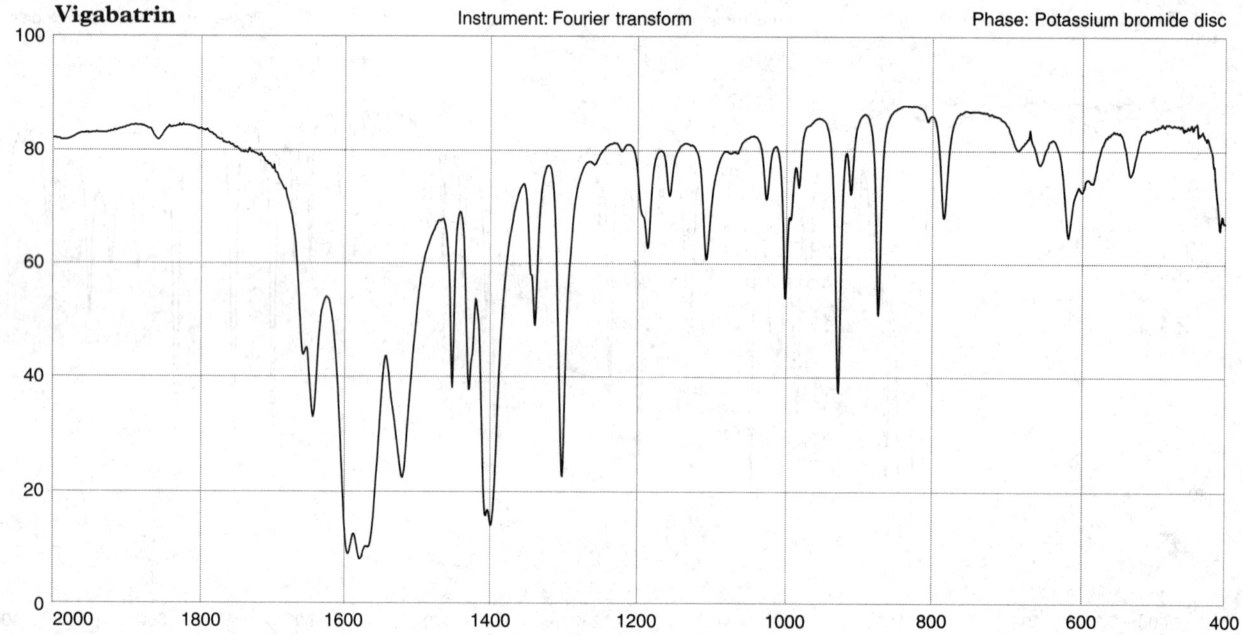

Warfarin

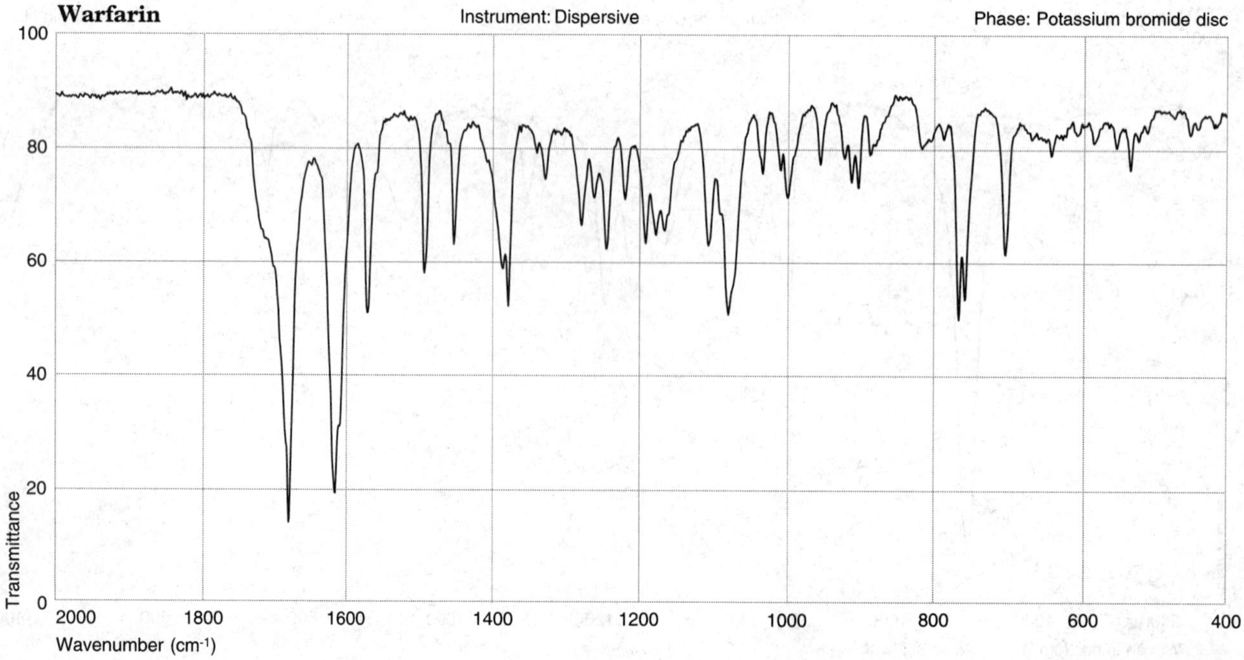

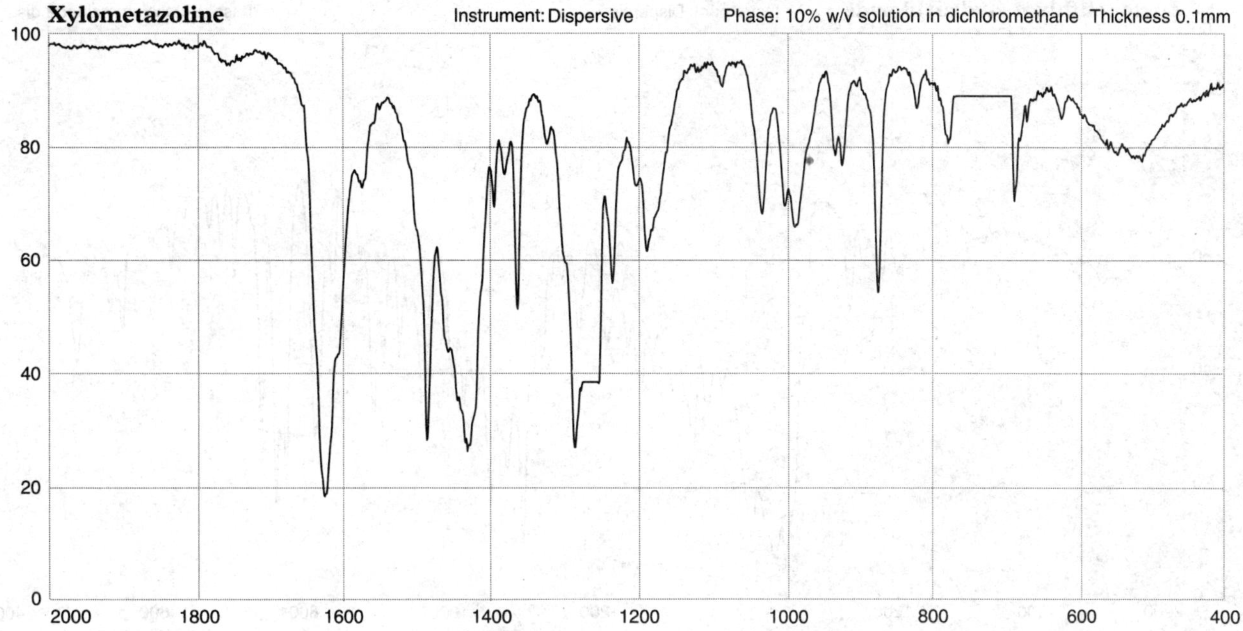
Xylometazoline
Instrument: Dispersive
Phase: 10% w/v solution in dichloromethane Thickness 0.1mm
100
80
60
40
20
0
2000
1800
1600
1400
1200
1000
800
600
400

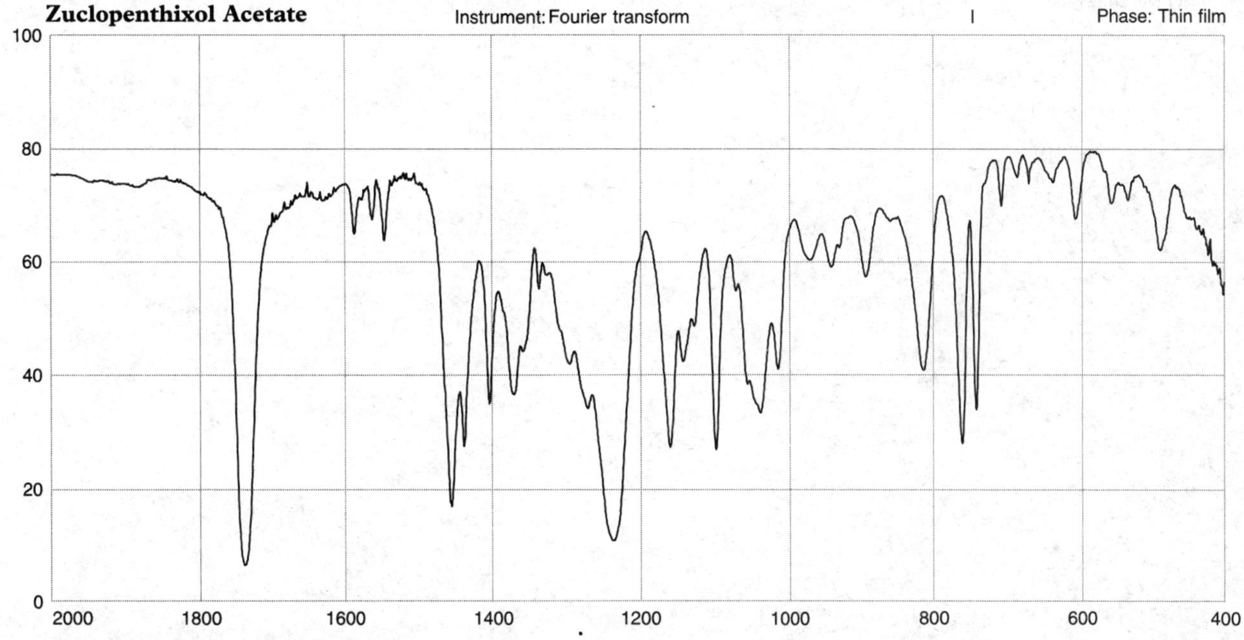
Zuclopenthixol Acetate
Instrument: Fourier transform
Phase: Thin film
100
80
60
40
20
0
2000
1800
1600
1400
1200
1000
800
600
400

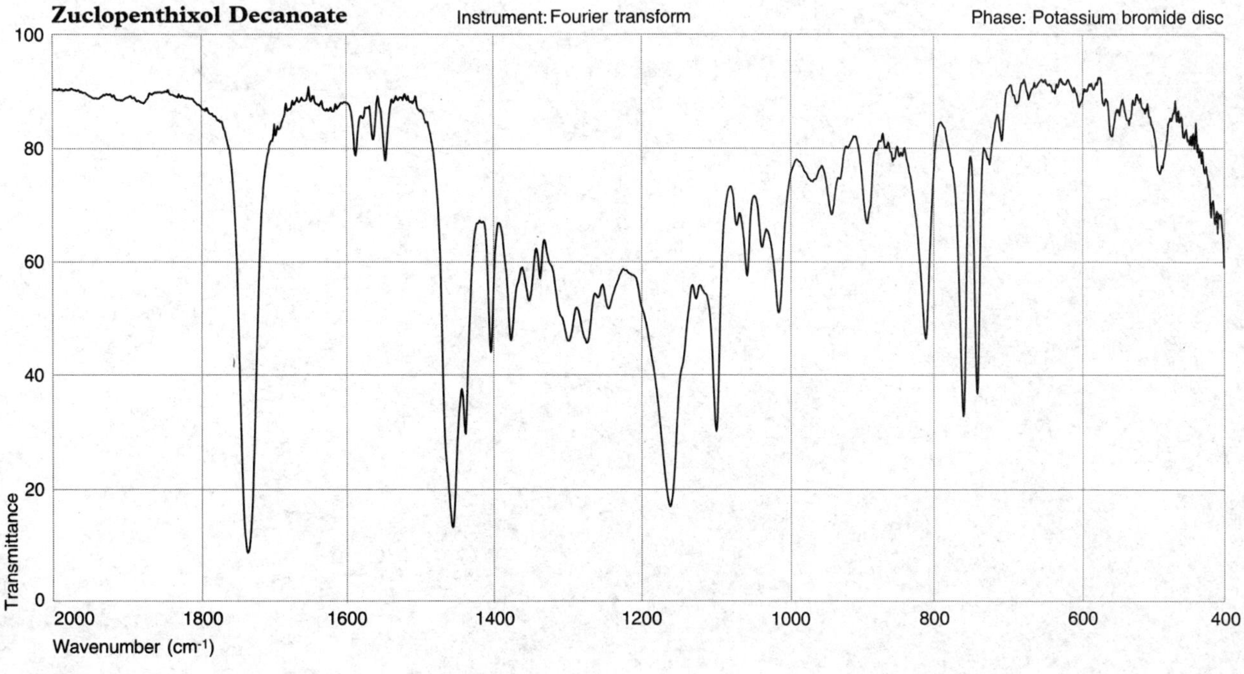
Zuclopenthixol Decanoate
Instrument: Fourier transform
Phase: Potassium bromide disc
100
80
60
40
20
0
Transmittance
2000
1800
1600
1400
1200
1000
800
600
400
Wavenumber (cm-1)

Zuclopenthixol Hydrochloride Instrument: Dispersive Phase: Potassium chloride disc

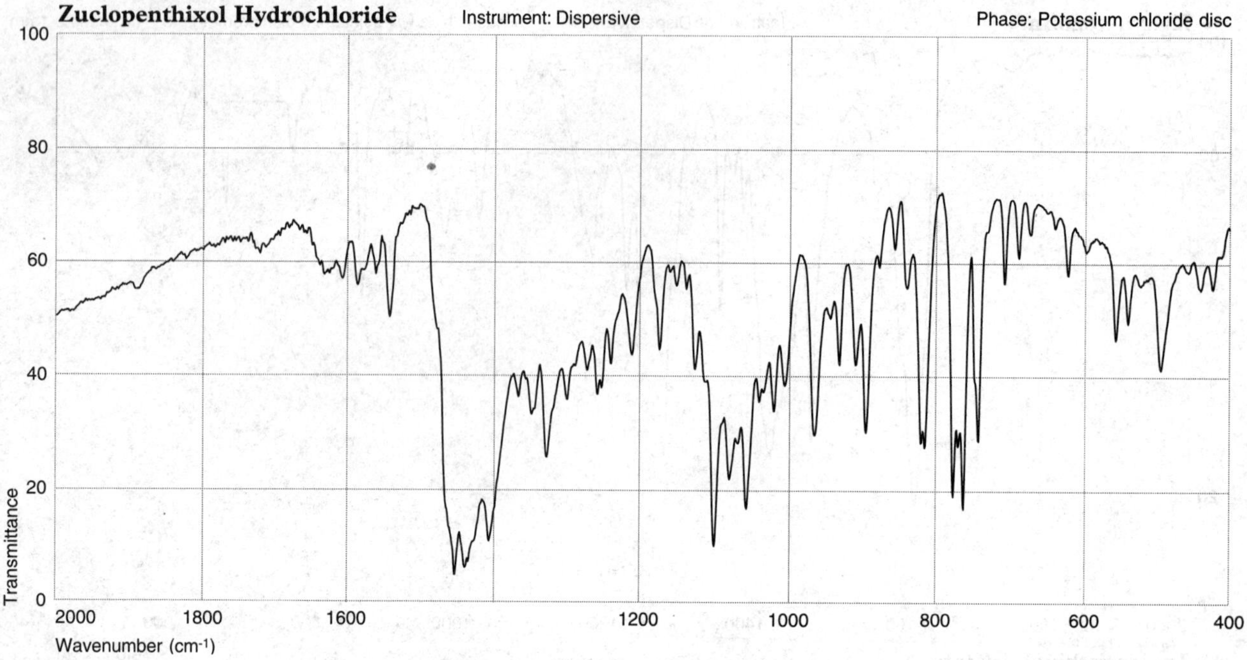

Appendices

When a method, test or other matter described in an appendix is invoked in a monograph reproduced from the European Pharmacopoeia, Part III of the general notices applies. When a method, test or other matter described in an appendix is invoked in any other monograph, Part II of general notices applies.

Contents of the Appendices

APPENDIX I

A. General Reagents A13

B. Volumetric Reagents and Solutions A95

C. Standard Solutions A101

D. Buffer Solutions A104

E. Chemical and Biological Reference Materials A109

APPENDIX II

A. Infrared Spectrophotometry and Near Infrared Spectrophotometry A114

B. Ultraviolet and Visible Spectrophotometry A116

C. Nuclear Magnetic Resonance Spectrometry A118

D. Atomic Spectrophotometry: Emission and Absorption A119

E. Fluorescence Spectrophotometry A121

F. X-Ray Fluorescence Spectrometry A121

APPENDIX III

A. Thin-layer Chromatography A122

B. Gas Chromatography A124

C. Size-exclusion Chromatography A126

D. Liquid Chromatography A129

E. Paper Chromatography A130

F. Electrophoresis A131

APPENDIX IV

A. Clarity of Solution A133

B. Colour of Solution A133

APPENDIX V

Determination of:

A. Melting Point A135

B. Freezing Point A137

C. Distillation Range A137

D. Boiling Point A138

E. Refractive Index A138

F. Optical Rotation and Specific Optical Rotation A139

G. Weight per Millilitre, Density, Relative Density and Apparent Density A139

H. Viscosity A140

J. Circular Dichroism A142

K. Reaction of Indicators A143

L. pH Values A144

M. Thermal Analysis A145

N. Osmolality A145

O. Conductivity A146

APPENDIX VI

Qualitative Reactions and Tests A147

APPENDIX VII

Limit Test for:

Aluminium A151

Ammonium A151

Arsenic A151

Calcium A152

Chlorides A152

Fluorides A152

Heavy Metals A153

Iron A154

Lead in Sugars A154

Magnesium A154

Magnesium and Alkaline-earth Metals A154

Nickel in Polyols A154

Phosphates A155

Potassium A155

Sulphates A155

APPENDIX VIII

A Non-aqueous Titration A155

B. Amperometric and Potentiometric Titrations A155

C. Oxygen-flask Combustion A156

D. Complexometric Titrations A157

E. Ion-selective Potentiometry A157

F. Determination of Ethanol A159

G. Determination of Methanol and Propan-2-ol A160

H. Determination of Nitrogen A161

J. Tetrazolium Assay of Steroids A161

K. Assay of Vitamin A A161

L. Residual Solvents A163

M. Residual Ethylene Oxide and Dioxan A164

APPENDIX IX
Determination of:
A. Sulphated Ash A166
B. Sulphur Dioxide A166
C. Water A167
D. Loss on Drying A168
E. Carbon Monoxide in Medicinal Gases A168
F. Carbon Dioxide in Medicinal Gases A169
G. Nitrogen Monoxide and Nitrogen Dioxide in Medicinal Gases A169
H. Oxygen in Medicinal Gases A169
J. Water in Medicinal Gases A170
K. Impurities in Gases using Gas Detector Tubes A170

APPENDIX X
A. Acetyl Value A171
B. Acid Value A171
C. Ester Value A172
D. Hydroxyl Value A172
E. Iodine Value A172
F. Peroxide Value A173
G. Saponification Value A173
H. Unsaponifiable Matter A173
J. Determination of Cineole A174
K. Determination of Aldehydes A174
L. Oxidising Substances A174
M. Volatile Oils A175
N. Fixed Oils A175

APPENDIX XI
A. Total Solids A180
B. Ethanol-soluble Extractive A180
C. Swelling Index A180
D. Foreign Matter A181
E. Volatile Oil in Drugs A181
F. Continuous Extraction of Drugs A182
G. Complete Extraction of Alkaloids A183
H. Stomata A183
J. Ash A183
K. Acid-insoluble Ash A183
L. Pesticide Residues A184

APPENDIX XII
A. Disintegration Test for Tablets and Capsules A187
B. Disintegration Test for Enteric-coated Tablets A187
C. Disintegration Test for Suppositories and Pessaries A188
D. Dissolution Test for Tablets and Capsules A189
E. Dissolution Test for Transdermal Patches A192
F. Aerodynamic Assessment of Fine Particles A194
G. Uniformity of Weight A201
H. Uniformity of Content A201
J. Extractable Volume A202

APPENDIX XIII
Particulate Contamination
A. Sub-visible Particles A203
B. Visible Particles A203
C. Microscope Method A204

APPENDIX XIV
Biological Assays and Tests
A. Antibiotics A205
B. Immunochemical Methods A211
C. Bacterial Endotoxins A212
D. Pyrogens A216
E. Abnormal Toxicity A217
F. Depressor Substances A218
G. Histamine A218
H. Hormones
1. Corticotropin A219
J. Blood and Related Products
1. Factor VII Fraction A219
2. Factor VIII Fraction A220
3. Factor IX Fraction A222
4. Heparin in Coagulation Factor Concentrates A222
5. Heparin A222
6. Fc Function of Immunoglobulins A223
7. Anti-A and Anti-B Haemagglutinins A224
8. Prekallikrein Activator A224
9. Anticomplementary Activity of Immunoglobulins A225
K. Immunological Products
1. Diphtheria Vaccine (Adsorbed) A226
2. Pertussis Vaccine A228
3. Tetanus Vaccine (Adsorbed) A228

APPENDIX XV
Production and Testing of Vaccines
A. Terminology A230
B. Aluminium A230
C. Calcium A231
D. Free Formaldehyde A231
E. Phenol A231

F. Neurovirulence
- 1. Live Viral Vaccines A231
- 2. Poliomyelitis Vaccine (Oral) A232

G. Composition of Polysaccharide Vaccines A233

H. Specified Pathogen-free Flocks A236

J. Human Diploid Cells for Production of Vaccines A238

APPENDIX XVI

A. Test for Sterility A239

B. Test for Microbial Contamination A243
- 1. Tests for Specified Micro-organisms A243
- 2. Total Viable Aerobic Count A245
- 3. Mycoplasmas A248
- 4. Mycobacteria A250
- 5. Extraneous Agents in Viral Vaccines A250

C. Efficacy of Antimicrobial Preservatives A252

D. Microbial Quality of Pharmaceutical Preparations A253

APPENDIX XVII

A. Particle Size of Powders
- 1. Classification A254
- 2. Limit Test, Microscopy A254

B. Sieves and Filters
- 1. Sieves A255
- 2. Filters A256

C. Specific Surface Area by Air Permeability A257

D. Apparent Volume A258

E. Flowability A259

F. Consistency by Penetrometry A260

G. Friability of Uncoated Tablets A262

H. Resistance to Crushing of Tablets A262

J. Softening Time of Lipophilic Suppositories A263

APPENDIX XVIII

Methods of Sterilisation A264

APPENDIX XIX

Containers

A. Introduction A268

B. Glass Containers for Pharmaceutical Preparations A268

C. Plastic Containers and Closures
- 1. For Aqueous Intravenous Infusions A272

D. Containers for Blood and Blood Components
- 1. Sterile Plastic Containers A273
- 2. Empty Sterile Containers of Plasticised PVC A275
- 3. Empty Sterile Containers of Plasticised PVC with Anticoagulant A276

E. Rubber Closures for Containers for Aqueous Parenteral Preparations A276

F. Sets for the Transfusion of Blood and Blood Components A278

G. Sterile Single-use Plastic Syringes A279

APPENDIX XX

Materials for the Manufacture of Containers

A. Poly(vinyl chloride) Containers
- 1. For Blood, Blood Components and Aqueous Intravenous Infusions A281
- 2. Tubing for Transfusion Sets A283

B. Polyolefines A285

C. Polyethylene
- 1. without Additives A288
- 2. with Additives A289

D. Polypropylene A292

E. Ethylene—Vinyl Acetate Copolymer A296

F. Silicone
- 1. Oil A298
- 2. Elastomer A298

APPENDIX XXI

A. Abbreviated Titles A301

B. Approved Synonyms A302

C. Codes for Eye Drops in Single-dose Containers A310

APPENDIX XXII

Names, Symbols and Atomic Weights of Elements A311

APPENDIX XXIII

Weights and Measures: SI Units A312

APPENDIX XXIV

Abbreviations A313

European Pharmacopoeia Equivalent Texts

In monographs reproduced from the European Pharmacopoeia the analytical methods, tests and other supporting texts are invoked by means of the reference number of the text in the general Chapters of the European Pharmacopoeia.
The table below lists the contents of the General Chapters of the European Pharmacopoeia and gives the British Pharmacopoeia or British Pharmacopoeia (Veterinary) equivalents. It is provided for information but it is emphasised that for texts of the European Pharmacopoeia, in cases of doubt or dispute the text published by the Council of Europe is authoritative. Appendices of the British Pharmacopoeia (Veterinary) are identified by inclusion of '(Vet)' after the Appendix letter, for example, Appendix XV J(Vet) 1.

Ph. Eur. reference	Subject of text	British Pharmacopoeia reference
1	General Notices	†
2.1.1	Droppers	Appendix I A
2.1.2	Sintered-glass filters	Appendix XVII B2
2.1.3	UV lamps	Appendix III A
2.1.4	Sieves	Appendix XVII B
2.1.5	Tubes for comparative tests	Appendix VII
2.1.6	Gas detector tubes	Appendix IX K
2.2.1	Clarity and degree of opalescence of liquids	Appendix IV A
2.2.2	Degree of coloration of liquids	Appendix IV B
2.2.3	Potentiometric determination of pH	Appendix V L
2.2.4	Reaction of solution, pH and indicator colour	Appendix V K
2.2.5	Relative density	Appendix V G
2.2.6	Refractive index	Appendix V E
2.2.7	Optical rotation	Appendix V F
2.2.8	Viscosity	Appendix V H
2.2.9	Capillary viscometer method	Appendix V H, Method II
2.2.10	Rotating viscometer method	Appendix V H, Method III
2.2.11	Distillation range	Appendix V C
2.2.12	Boiling point	Appendix V D
2.2.13	Water by distillation range	Appendix IX C, Method II
2.2.14	Melting point: Capillary method	Appendix V A, Method I
2.2.15	Melting point: Open capillary method	Appendix V A, Method IV
2.2.16	Melting point: Instantaneous method	Appendix V A, Method V
2.2.17	Drop point	Appendix V A, Method III
2.2.18	Freezing point	Appendix V B
2.2.19	Amperometric titrations	Appendix VIII B
2.2.20	Potentiometric titrations	Appendix VIII B

†Reproduced in full as Part III of the General Notices of the British Pharmacopoeia and British Pharmacopoeia (Veterinary)

Ph. Eur. reference	Subject of text	British Pharmacopoeia reference
2.2.21	Fluorimetry	Appendix II E
2.2.22	Atomic emission spectrometry	Appendix II D
2.2.23	Atomic absorption spectrometry	Appendix II D
2.2.24	Infrared spectrophotometry	Appendix II A
2.2.25	Visible and ultraviolet spectrophotometry	Appendix II B
2.2.26	Paper chromatography	Appendix III E
2.2.27	Thin-layer chromatography	Appendix III A
2.2.28	Gas chromatography	Appendix III B
2.2.29	Liquid chromatography	Appendix III D
2.2.30	Size-exclusion chromatography	Appendix III C
2.2.31	Electrophoresis	Appendix III F
2.2.32	Loss on drying	Appendix IX D
2.2.33	Nuclear magnetic resonance spectrometry	Appendix II C
2.2.34	Thermogravimetry	Appendix V M
2.2.35	Osmolality	Appendix V N
2.2.36	Ion-selective potentiometry	Appendix VIII E
2.2.37	X-ray fluorescent spectrophotometry	Appendix II F
2.2.38	Conductivity	Appendix V O
2.2.39	Molecular mass distribution in dextrans	Appendix III C
2.2.40	Near infrared spectrometry	Appendix II A
2.2.41	Circular dichroism	Appendix V J
2.3.1	Identification reactions	Appendix VI
2.3.2	Identification of fatty oils by TLC	Appendix X N
2.3.3	Identification of phenothiazines by TLC	Appendix III A
2.3.4	Odour	Appendix VI
	Limit test for:-	
2.4.1	– ammonium	Appendix VII
2.4.2	– arsenic	Appendix VII
2.4.3	– calcium	Appendix VII
2.4.4	– chloride	Appendix VII
2.4.5	– fluorides	Appendix VII
2.4.6	– magnesium	Appendix VII
2.4.7	– magnesium and alkaline-earth metals	Appendix VII
2.4.8	– heavy metals	Appendix VII
2.4.9	– iron	Appendix VII
2.4.10	– lead in sugars	Appendix VII
2.4.11	– phosphates	Appendix VII
2.4.12	– potassium	Appendix VII
2.4.13	– sulphate	Appendix VII
2.4.14	Sulphated ash	Appendix IX A, Method II
2.4.15	Limit Test for nickel in polyols	Appendix VII
2.4.16	Total ash	Appendix XI J, Method II
2.4.17	Limit test for aluminium	Appendix VII
2.4.18	Free formaldehyde	Appendix XV D
2.4.19	Alkaline impurities in fatty oils	Appendix X N
2.4.20	Antioxidants in fatty oils	Appendix X N
2.4.21	Foreign oils in fatty oils by TLC	Appendix X N
2.4.22	Foreign oils by gas chromatography	Appendix X N
2.4.23	Sterols in fatty oils	Appendix X N

Ph. Eur. reference	Subject of text	British Pharmacopoeia reference
2.4.24	Residual solvents	Appendix VIII L
2.4.25	Residual ethylene oxide and dioxan	Appendix VIII M
2.5.1	Acid value	Appendix X B
2.5.2	Ester value	Appendix X C
2.5.3	Hydroxyl value	Appendix X D
2.5.4	Iodine value	Appendix X E
2.5.5	Peroxide value	Appendix X F
2.5.6	Saponification value	Appendix X G, Method II
2.5.7	Unsaponifiable matter	Appendix X H, Method II
2.5.8	Assay of primary aromatic amino nitrogen	Appendix VIII B
2.5.9	Semi-micro determination of nitrogen by sulphuric acid digestion	Appendix VIII H
2.5.10	Oxygen-flask method	Appendix VIII C
2.5.11	Complexometric titrations	Appendix VIII D
2.5.12	Semi-micro determination of water	Appendix IX C, Method I
2.5.13	Aluminium in adsorbed vaccines	Appendix XV B
2.5.14	Calcium in adsorbed vaccines	Appendix XV C
2.5.15	Phenol in immunosera and vaccines	Appendix XV E
	Polysaccharide vaccines:-	
2.5.16	– protein	Appendix XV G
2.5.17	– nucleic acids	Appendix XV G
2.5.18	– phosphorus	Appendix XV G
2.5.19	– *O*-acetyl	Appendix XV G
2.5.20	– hexosamines	Appendix XV G
2.5.21	– methylpentoses	Appendix XV G
2.5.22	– uronic acids	Appendix XV G
2.5.23	– sialic acid	Appendix XV G
2.5.24	Carbon dioxide in medicinal gases	Appendix IX G
2.5.25	Carbon monoxide in medicinal gases	Appendix IX E
2.5.26	Nitrogen monoxide and nitrogen dioxide in medicinal gases	Appendix IX H
2.5.27	Oxygen in medicinal gases	Appendix IX J
2.5.28	Water in medicinal gases	Appendix IX K
2.5.29	Sulphur dioxide	Appendix IX B
2.5.30	Oxidising substances	Appendix X L
2.5.31	Ribose in polysaccharide vaccines	Appendix XV G
2.6.1	Sterility	Appendix XVI A
2.6.2	Mycobacteria	Appendix XVI B4
2.6.3	Extraneous viruses using fertilised eggs	Appendix XVI B(Vet) 4
2.6.4	Leucosis virus	Appendix XVI B(Vet) 6
2.6.5	Extraneous viruses using cell cultures	Appendix XVI BVet) 7
2.6.6	Extraneous agents using chicks	Appendix XVI B(Vet) 8
2.6.7	Mycoplasmas	Appendix XVI B3 *and* Appendix XVI B(Vet) 3
2.6.8	Pyrogens	Appendix XIV D
2.6.9	Abnormal toxicity	Appendix XIV E
2.6.10	Histamine	Appendix XIV G
2.6.11	Depressor substances	Appendix XIV F
2.6.12	Total viable aerobic count	Appendix XVI B2
2.6.13	Specified micro-organisms	Appendix XVI B1

Ph. Eur. reference	Subject of text	British Pharmacopoeia reference
2.6.14	Bacterial endotoxins	Appendix XIV C
2.6.15	Prekallikrein activator	Appendix XIV J8
2.6.16	Extraneous agents in viral vaccines	Appendix XVI B5
2.6.17	Anticomplementary activity of immunoglobulins	Appendix XIV J9
2.6.18	Neurovirulence of live viral vaccines	Appendix XV F1
2.6.19	Neurovirulence of poliomyelitis vaccine (oral)	Appendix XV F2
2.6.20	Anti-A and anti-B haemagglutinins (indirect method)	Appendix XIV J7
2.7.1	Immunochemical methods	Appendix XIV B
2.7.2	Microbiological assay of antibiotics	Appendix XIV A
2.7.3	Assay of corticotrophin	Appendix XIV H1
2.7.4	Assay of coagulation factor VIII	Appendix XIV J2
2.7.5	Assay of heparin	Appendix XIV J5
2.7.6	Assay of diphtheria vaccine (adsorbed)	Appendix XIV K1
2.7.7	Assay of pertussis vaccine	Appendix XIV K2
2.7.8	Assay of tetanus vaccine (adsorbed)	Appendix XIV K3
2.7.9	Fc function of immunoglobulins	Appendix XIV J6
2.7.10	Assay of coagulation factor VII	Appendix XIV J1
2.7.11	Assay of coagulation factor IX	Appendix XIV J3
2.7.12	Heparin in coagulation factor concentrates	Appendix XIV J4
2.8.1	Ash insoluble in hydrochloric acid	Appendix XI K, Method II
2.8.2	Foreign matter	Appendix XI D, Test B
2.8.3	Stomata and stomatal index	Appendix XI H
2.8.4	Swelling index	Appendix XI C
2.8.5	Water in essential oils	Appendix X M
2.8.6	Foreign esters	Appendix X M
2.8.7	Fatty oils and resinified volatile oils	Appendix X M
2.8.8	Odour and taste of volatile oils	Appendix X M
2.8.9	Residue on evaporation	Appendix X M
2.8.10	Solubility in ethanol (volatile oils)	Appendix X M
2.8.11	Determination of cineole	Appendix X J
2.8.12	Essential oil content of crude drugs	Appendix XI E
2.8.13	Pesticide residues	Appendix XI L
2.9.1	Disintegration: Tablets and capsules	Appendix XII A
2.9.2	Disintegration: Suppositories and pessaries	Appendix XII C
2.9.3	Dissolution: Solid oral dosage forms	Appendix XII D
2.9.4	Dissolution: Transdermal patches	Appendix XII E
2.9.5	Uniformity of mass	Appendix XII G
2.9.6	Uniformity of content	Appendix XII H
2.9.7	Friability of uncoated tablets	Appendix XVII G
2.9.8	Resistance to crushing of tablets	Appendix XVII H
2.9.9	Measurement of consistency by penetrometry	Appendix XVII F
2.9.10	Ethanol content and alcoholimetric tablets	Appendix VIII F, Method III
2.9.11	Methanol and 2-propanol	Appendix VIII G
2.9.12	Sieve test	Appendix XVII A
2.9.13	Particle size by microscopy (limit test)	Appendix XIII
2.9.14	Specific surface area by gas permeability	Appendix XVII C
2.9.15	Apparent volume	Appendix XVII D
2.9.16	Flowability	Appendix XVII E
2.9.17	Extractable volume	Appendix XII J

Ph. Eur. reference	Subject of text	British Pharmacopoeia reference
2.9.18	Aerodynamic assessment of fine particles	Appendix XII F
2.9.19	Particulate contamination: Sub-visible particles	Appendix XIII A
2.9.20	Particulate contamination: Visible particles	Appendix XIII B
2.9.21	Particulate contamination: Microscope method	Appendix XIII C
2.9.22	Softening time of lipophilic suppositories	Appendix XVII J
3.1.1	Materials based on PVC for blood and blood components and for aqueous solutions for IV infusion	Appendix XX A1
3.1.2	Materials based on PVC for tubing used in sets for the transfusion of blood and blood components	Appendix XX A2
3.1.3	Polyolefines	Appendix XX B
3.1.4	Polyethylene - without additives	Appendix XX C1
3.1.5	Polyethylene - with additives	Appendix XX C2
3.1.6	Polypropylene	Appendix XX D
3.1.7	Ethylene—vinyl acetate co-polymer	Appendix XX E
3.1.8	Silicone oil used as a lubricant	Appendix XX F1
3.1.9	Silicone elastomer for closures and tubing	Appendix XX F2
3.2	Containers	Appendix XIX A
3.2.1	Glass containers for pharmaceutical use	Appendix XIX B
3.2.2	Plastic containers and closures	Appendix XIX C
3.2.3	Sterile plastic containers for blood and blood components	Appendix XIX D1
3.2.4	Empty sterile plastic containers for blood and blood components	Appendix XIX D2
3.2.5	Sterile plastic containers with anticoagulant for blood and blood components	Appendix XIX D3
3.2.6	Sets for the transfusion of blood and blood components	Appendix XIX F
3.2.7	Plastic containers for aqueous intravenous infusions	Appendix XIX H
3.2.8	Sterile single-use plastic syringes	Appendix XIX G
3.2.9	Rubber closures for containers for aqueous preparations for parenteral use	Appendix XIX E
4.1.1	Reagents	Appendix I A
4.1.2	Standard solutions	Appendix I C
4.1.3	Buffer solutions	Appendix I D
4.2.1	Reference substances for volumetric solutions	Appendix I B
4.2.2	Volumetric solution	Appendix I B
5.1.1	Methods of preparation of sterile products	Appendix XVIII
5.1.2	Biological indicators (sterilisation)	Appendix XVIII
5.1.3	Efficacy of antimicrobial preservation	Appendix XVI C
5.1.4	Microbial quality of pharmaceutical preparations	Appendix XVI D
5.1.5	F_0 concept (sterilisation)	Appendix XVIII
5.2.1	Terminology: Vaccines	Appendix XV A *and* Appendix XV A(Vet)
5.2.2	SPF Chicken flocks	Appendix XV H *and* Appendix XV H(Vet)
5.2.3	Human diploid cells (vaccine production)	Appendix XV J
5.2.4	Cell cultures (veterinary vaccine production)	Appendix XV J(Vet) 1
5.2.5	Substances of animal origin (veterinary vaccine production)	Appendix XV J(Vet) 2
5.2.6	Safety: Veterinary vaccines	Appendix XV K(Vet) 1
5.2.7	Efficacy: Veterinary vaccines	Appendix XV K(Vet) 2
5.3	Statistical analysis of biological assays and tests	*Not reproduced (see Introduction, Appendices)*

Appendix I

The specifications given below are strictly for the use of the materials as reagents. The inclusion of a material in this Appendix does not imply that it is suitable for use in medicines.

A. General Reagents

In a monograph from the European Pharmacopoeia, the name of a substance or solution followed by the letter R (the whole in italics) indicates a reagent in Appendix I. Where a reagent is described using an expression such as '*hydrochloric acid (10 g/l HCl)*' the solution is prepared by an appropriate dilution with *water* of a more concentrated solution specified in this section.

Where the name of the solvent is not stated, an aqueous solution is intended. Reagents in aqueous solutions are prepared using *water*. Reagent solutions used in the limit tests for barium, calcium and sulphates are prepared using *distilled water*.

The description of a reagent may include a Chemical Abstracts Service Registry number (CAS number) recognisable by its typical format (for example, *9002-93-1*).

Some of the reagents included may be injurious to health unless adequate precautions are taken. They should be handled in accordance with good laboratory practice and any relevant regulations such as those issued in the United Kingdom in accordance with the Health and Safety at Work *etc.* Act (1974). The labelling should comply with relevant national legislation and international agreements. Reagents and reagent solutions should be kept in well-closed containers.

Droppers *(Ph Eur text 2.1.1)*

The term 'drops' means standard drops delivered from a standard dropper as described below.

Standard droppers (Fig. 1.1) are constructed of practically colourless glass. The lower extremity has a circular orifice in a flat surface at right angles to the axis.Other droppers may be used provided they comply with the following test.

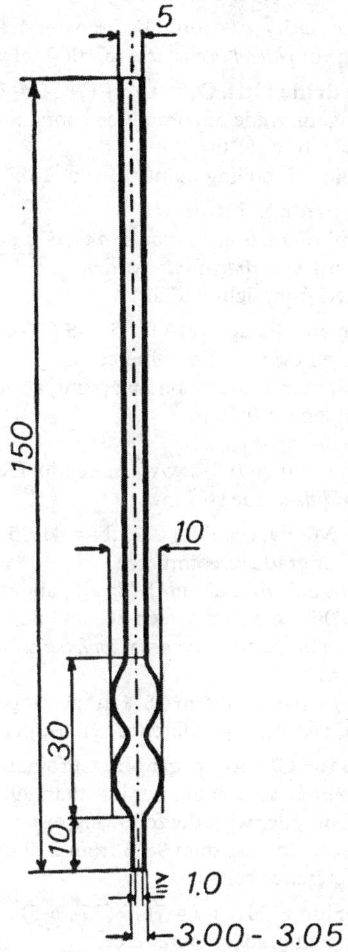

Fig. 1.1 Standard dropper
Dimensions in millimetres

Twenty drops of *water* at 20 ± 1° flowing freely from the dropper held in the vertical position at a constant rate of one drop per second weighs 1000 ± 50 mg. The dropper must be carefully cleaned before use. Carry out three determinations on any given dropper. No result may deviate by more than 5% from the mean of the three determinations

Acacia Of the British Pharmacopoeia.

Acacia Solution Dissolve 100 g of *acacia* in 1000 ml of *water*, stir mechanically for 2 hours, centrifuge at 2000 *g* for 30 minutes to obtain a clear solution.
Store in polyethylene containers of about 250 ml capacity at 0° to –20°.

Acetaldehyde C_2H_4O = 44.1 (*75-07-0*)
General reagent grade of commerce.
A colourless volatile liquid with an acrid, penetrating odour; d^{20}_{20}, about 0.788; n^{20}_{D}, about 1.332; boiling point, about 21°.

Acetamide C_2H_5NO = 59.07 (*60-35-5*)
General reagent grade of commerce.
Melting point, about 78°.

Acetic Acid Dilute 30 g of *glacial acetic acid* to 100 ml with *water*. It contains not less than 29.0% and not more than 31.0% w/v of $C_2H_4O_2$ (5M).

Acetic Acid, Anhydrous Anhydrous glacial acetic acid; $C_2H_4O_2$ = 60.1 (*64-19-7*)
Glacial acetic acid of commerce for use in non-aqueous titrations containing not less than 99.6% w/w of $C_2H_4O_2$. d^{20}_{20}, 1.0152 to 1.053; boiling point, 117° to 119°.
Complies with the following test.
WATER Not more than 0.4% w/w, Appendix IX C. If the water content is greater than 0.4% it may be adjusted by adding the calculated amount of *acetic anhydride*.
Store protected from light.

Acetic Acid, Dilute Dilute 12 g of *glacial acetic acid* to 100 ml with *water*. It contains not less than 11.5% and not more than 12.5% w/v of $C_2H_4O_2$ (2M).

Acetic Acid, Glacial
Analytical reagent grade of commerce.
A colourless liquid with a pungent odour, about 17.5M in strength; freezing point, about 16°; weight per ml, about

1.05 g. It contains not less than 98.0% w/w of $C_2H_4O_2$.
Solutions of molarity *x*M should be prepared by diluting 57*x* ml (60*x* g) of *glacial acetic acid* to 1000 ml with *water.*

Acetic Anhydride $C_4H_6O_3$ = 102.1 (*108-24-7*)
Analytical reagent grade of commerce containing not less than 97.0% w/v of $C_4H_6O_3$.
A colourless liquid; boiling point, 136° to 142°.

Acetic Anhydride Solution R1
Dissolve 25 ml of *acetic anhydride* in *anhydrous pyridine* and dilute to 100 ml with *anhydrous pyridine*.
Store protected from light and air.

Acetone Propan-2-one; C_3H_6O = 58.08 (*67-64-1*)
Analytical reagent grade of commerce.
A volatile, flammable liquid; boiling point, about 56°; weight per ml, about 0.79 g.
Complies with the following test.
WATER Not more than 0.3% w/w, Appendix IX C, using *anhydrous pyridine* as the solvent.

Acetonitrile Methyl cyanide; C_2H_3N = 41.05 (*75-05-8*)
General reagent grade of commerce.
A colourless liquid; d_{20}^{20}, about 0.78; n_D^{20}, about 1.344.
Not less than 95% distils between 80° and 82°.
Acetonitrile used in spectrophotometry complies with the following requirement.
TRANSMITTANCE Not less than 98% in the range 255 to 420 nm using *water* in the reference cell, Appendix II B.

Acetonitrile for Chromatography Chromatographic grade of *acetonitrile* containing not less than 99.8% of C_2H_3N that complies with the following test.
TRANSMITTANCE Not less than 98% from 240 nm using *water* in the reference cell.

Acetyl Chloride C_2H_3ClO = 78.5 (*75-36-5*)
Analytical reagent gradeof commerce.
d_{20}^{20}, about 1.10. Not less than 95% distils between 49° and 53°.

Acetylacetamide 3-Oxobutanamide; $C_4H_7NO_2$ = 101.1 (*5977-14-0*)
General reagent grade of commerce.
Melting point, 53° to 56°.

Acetylacetone Pentane-2,4-dione; $C_5H_8O_2$ = 100.1 (*123-54-6*)
Analytical reagent grade of commerce.
A colourless or slightly yellow, easily flammable liquid.
n_D^{20}, 1.452 to 1.453; boiling point, 138° to 140°.

Acetylacetone Reagent R1
To 100 ml of *ammonium acetate solution* add 0.2 ml of *acetylacetone.*

***N*-Acetyl-ε-caprolactam** $C_8H_{13}NO_2$ = 155.2 (*1888-91-1*)
General reagent grade of commerce.
d_{20}^{20}, about 1.100; n_D^{20}, about 1.489; boiling point, about 135°.

Acetylcholine Chloride $C_7H_{16}ClNO_2$ = 181.7 (*60-31-1*)
General reagent grade of commerce.
Store at –20°.

***N*-Acetyl-L-cysteine** $C_5H_9NO_3S$ = 163.2 (*616-91-1*)
General reagent grade of commerce.
Melting point, about 110°; $[\alpha]_D^{20}$, about +4.6°.

Acetyleugenol $C_{12}H_{14}O_3$ = 206.2 (*93-28-7*)
General reagent grade of commerce.
A yellow, oily liquid; n_D^{20}, about 1.521; boiling point, 281° to 282°.
Acetyleugenol used in gas chromatography complies with the following test.
ASSAY Carry out the test for Chromatographic profile described under Clove Oil using the reagent being examined as the test solution. The area of the principal peak is not less than 98.0% of the total area of the peaks.

***N*-Acetylneuraminic Acid** *O*-Sialic acid; $C_{11}H_{19}NO_9$ = 309.3 (*131-48-6*)
Melting point, about 186°, with decomposition; $[\alpha]_D^{20}$, about –36° (1% w/v in water).

***N*-Acetyltryptophan** $C_{13}H_{14}N_2O_3$ = 246.3 (*1218-34-4*)
General reagent grade of commerce.
Melting point, about 205°.
ASSAY Dissolve 10 mg in sufficient of a mixture of 10 volumes of *acetonitrile* and 90 volumes of *water* to produce 100 ml. Examine as prescribed in the monograph for Tryptophan under 1,1′-Ethylidenebis(tryptophan) and other related substances. The area of the principal peak in the chromatogram obtained is not less than 99.0% of the areas of all the peaks.

Acetyltyrosine Ethyl Ester Ethyl *N*-acetyl-L-tyrosinate; $C_{13}H_{17}NO_4,H_2O$ = 269.3 (*36546-50-6*)
General reagent grade of commerce.
A white, crystalline powder; $[\alpha]_D^{20}$, +21° to +25° (1% w/v in ethanol); A(1%, 1 cm) at 278 nm, 60 to 68 determined in ethanol.

Acetyltyrosine Ethyl Ester, 0.2M 0.2M Ethyl acetyltyrosinate
Dissolve 0.54 g of *acetyltyrosine ethyl ester* in sufficient *ethanol (96%)* to produce 10 ml.

Acid Blue 83 CI 42660; Coomassie brilliant blue R250; brilliant blue R; $C_{45}H_{44}N_3NaO_7S$ = 826 (*6104-59-2*)
General reagent grade of commerce.
A brown powder.

Acid Blue 90 CI 42655; Coomassie brilliant blue G; brilliant blue G; $C_{47}H_{48}N_3NaO_7S_2$ = 854 (*6104-58-1*)
A dark brown powder with a violet sheen; some particles have a metallic lustre.
Complies with the following tests.
LIGHT ABSORPTION A(1%, 1 cm) in a 0.001% w/v solution in *phosphate buffer pH 7.0* at 577 nm, greater than 500, Appendix II B.
LOSS ON DRYING When dried to constant weight at 100° to 105°, loses not more than 5.0% of its weight.

Acid Blue 92 Coomassie blue; CI 13390; trisodium 8-hydroxy-4′-phenylaminoazonaphthalene-3,5′,6-trisulphonate; $C_{26}H_{16}N_3Na_3O_{10}S_3$ = 696 (*3861-73-2*)
General reagent grade of commerce.
Dark blue crystals.

Acid Blue 92 Solution Coomassie blue solution
Dissolve 0.5 g of *acid blue 92* in a mixture of 10 ml of *glacial acetic acid,* 45 ml of *ethanol (96%)* and 45 ml of *water.*

Acrylamide C_3H_5NO = 71.08 (*79-06-1*)
General reagent grade of commerce.
Melting point, about 84°.

Adenosine 6-Amino-9-β-D-ribofuranosyl-9*H*-purine; $C_{10}H_{13}N_5O_4$ = 267.2 (*58-61-7*)
General reagent grade of commerce.
Melting point, about 234°.

Aescin Escin; $C_{54}H_{84}O_{23},2H_2O$ = 1138 (*11072-93-8*)
A mixture of related saponins obtained from the seeds of *Aesculus hippocastum* L.

General reagent grade of commerce complying with the following test.
HOMOGENEITY Carry out the test for Identification described under Senega Root applying 20 µl of solution (2) to the plate. After spraying with *anisaldehyde solution* the chromatogram exhibits a principal spot with an Rf value of about 0.4.

Agar (*9002-18-0*) The dried extract from *Gelidium* sp. and other algae belonging to the class Rhodophyceae.
Microbiological reagent grade of commerce.

Agarose for Chromatography (*9012-36-6*)
Chromatographic reagent grade of commerce.
Swollen beads 60 µm to 140 µm in diameter presented as a 4% suspension in *water*. It is used in size-exclusion chromatography for the separation of proteins with relative molecular masses of 6×10^4 to 20×10^6 and of polysaccharides with relative molecular masses of 3×10^3 to 5×10^6.

Agarose for Chromatography, Cross-linked (*61970-08-9*)
Chromatographic reagent grade of commerce.
Prepared from agarose by reaction with 2,3-dibromopropanol in strongly alkaline conditions.
Swollen beads 60 µm to 140 µm in diameter presented as a 4% suspension in *water*. It is used in size-exclusion chromatography for the separation of proteins with relative molecular masses of 6×10^4 to 20×10^6 and of polysaccharides with relativemolecular masses of 3×10^3 to 5×10^6.

Agarose for Chromatography R1, Cross-linked (*65099-79-8*)
Chromatographic reagent grade of commerce.
Prepared from agarose by reaction with 2,3-dibromopropanol in strongly alkaline conditions.
Swollen beads 60 µm to 140 µm in diameter presented as a 4% suspension in *water*. It is used in size-exclusion chromatography for the separation of proteins with relative molecular masses of 7×10^4 to 40×10^6 and of polysaccharides with relative molecular masses of 1×10^5 to 2×10^7.

Agarose for Electrophoresis (*9012-36-6*)
Electrophoretic reagent grade of commerce.
A neutral, linear polysaccharide, the main component of which is derived from agar.

Agarose-DEAE for Ion Exchange Chromatography
Chromatographic reagent grade of commerce.
Cross-linked agarose substituted with diethylaminoethyl groups, presented as beads.

Agarose/Cross-linked Polyacrylamide
Agarose trapped within a cross-linked polyacrylamide network. It is used for the separation of globular proteins with relative molecular masses of 2×10^4 to 35×10^4.

Alanine L-Alanine; $C_3H_7NO_2$ = 89.1 (*56-41-7*)
General reagent grade of commerce.
Melting point, about 315°, with decomposition.

β-Alanine See *3-aminopropionic acid.*

Albumin, Bovine Bovine serum albumin (*9048-46-8*)
Bovine albumin containing about 96% protein.
A white to light yellowish-brown powder complying with the following test.
WATER Not more than 3.0% w/w, Appendix IX C. Use 0.8 g.
Bovine albumin used in the assay of tetracosactide should be pyrogen-free, free from proteolytic activity when examined by a suitable means, for example using chromogenic substrate, and free from corticosteroid activity by measurement of fluorescence as described in that assay.

Albumin Solution, Human Albumin (*9048-46-8*)
Albumin Solution of the British Pharmacopoeia.

Albumin Solution R1, Human Albumin solution
Dilute *human albumin solution* with sufficient *sodium chloride injection* to produce a protein concentration of 0.1% w/v and adjust the pH to between 3.5 and 4.5 with *glacial acetic acid.*

Alcohol See *Ethanol (96%)*.

Alcohol, Aldehyde-free See *aldehyde-free ethanol (96%)*.
Alcohol (x% v/v) See *ethanol (96%)*.

Aldehyde Dehydrogenase Enzyme obtained from baker's yeast which oxidises acetaldehyde to acetic acid in the presence of nicotinamide-adenine dinucleotide, potassium salts and thiols at pH 8.0.
General reagent grade of commerce.

Aldehyde Dehydrogenase Solution Dissolve in *water* a quantity of *aldehyde dehydrogenase* equivalent to 70 units and dilute to 10 ml with the same solvent. This solution is stable for 8 hours at 4°.

Aleuritic Acid (9*RS*,10*SR*)-9,10,16-Trihydroxyhexadecanoic acid; $C_{16}H_{32}O_5$ = 304.4 (*533-87-9*)
General reagent grade of commerce.
Melting point, about 101°.

Alizarin S CI 58005; alizarin red S; $C_{14}H_7NaO_7S,H_2O$ = 360.3 (*130-22-3*)
General reagent grade of commerce.
A yellowish brown or orange-yellow powder.

Alizarin S Solution A 0.1% w/v solution of *alizarin S*.
Complies with the following test.
SENSITIVITY TO BARIUM To 5 ml of 0.05M *sulphuric acid* add 5 ml of *water*, 50 ml of *acetate buffer pH 3.7* and 0.5 ml of the solution being examined. Add, dropwise, 0.05M *barium perchlorate VS*. The colour changes from yellow to orange-red.
Colour change: pH 3.7 (yellow) to pH 5.2 (violet).

Aluminium Al = 26.98 (*7429-90-5*)
Analytical reagent grade wire of commerce.

Aluminium Chloride Aluminium chloride hexahydrate; $AlCl_3,6H_2O$ = 241.4 (*7784-13-6*)
General reagent grade of commerce containing not less than 98.0% of $AlCl_3,6H_2O$.
Store in an airtight container.

Aluminium Chloride Reagent Dissolve 2.0 g of *aluminium chloride* in 100 ml of a 5% v/v solution of *glacial acetic acid* in *methanol.*

Aluminium Chloride Solution Dissolve 65.0 g of *aluminium chloride* in sufficient *water* to produce 100 ml, add 0.5 g of *activated charcoal*, stir for 10 minutes, filter and add to the filtrate, stirring continuously, sufficient of a 1% w/v solution of *sodium hydroxide* to adjust the pH to about 1.5 (approximately 60 ml is required).

Aluminium Hydroxide Gel $Al(OH)_3$ + aq (*21645-51-2*)
A hydrated grade of aluminium hydroxide of commerce.

Aluminium Nitrate $Al(NO_3)_3,9H_2O$ = 375.1 (*7784-27-2*)
Analytical reagent grade of commerce.
Deliquescent crystals.
Store in an airtight container.

Aluminium Oxide, Anhydrous Al_2O_3 = 102.0 (*1344-28-1*)
Use a grade of commerce consisting of γ-Al_2O_3 dehydrated and activated by heat treatment. The particle size is such that it passes through a 150-µm sieve but is retained on a 75-µm sieve.

Aluminium Oxide, Basic A basic grade of aluminium oxide of commerce suitable for column chromatography.
Complies with the following tests.
ALKALINITY pH of a 10% w/v suspension in *carbon dioxide-free water*, shaken for 5 minutes, 9 to 10, Appendix V L.
ACTIVITY Pack into a chromatographic tube (25 cm × 10 mm) sufficient of the basic aluminium oxide to form a column 50 mm deep. Apply to the column a mixture of 5 ml of *sudan yellow solution* and 5 ml of *sudan red solution* and elute with 20 ml of a mixture of 1 volume of *benzene* and 4 volumes of *petroleum spirit (boiling range, 60° to 80°)*. Sudan red forms a zone about 10 mm in depth on the upper part of the column separated by a colourless zone from a yellow zone of sudan yellow below.

Aluminium Oxide, Deactivated To a suitable basic alumina add 1.5 to 2% of *water*, mix well and allow to stand overnight in a stoppered bottle. The product complies with the following test.

Prepare a column (20 cm × 10 mm) using the alumina and *hexane*. Add a solution of 0.25 g of *calciferol* in 10 ml of *hexane*. When the level of the solution falls just to the top of the column, begin eluting with a 17.5% v/v solution of *ether* in *hexane* adjusting the rate of flow, if necessary, to between 1 and 2 ml per minute. Collect 200 ml of eluate; no calciferol is present. Collect a further 100 ml of eluate; it contains not less than 95% of the calciferol used in the test, when determined by the Assay described under Calciferol Oral Solution.

Aluminium Oxide for Chromatography, Activated Acid Al_2O_3 = 102.1
An almost white, fine, granular powder, very hygroscopic, activated by heating at 200° to 250° for 3 hours.
Mean particle size, 50 to 200 µm.

Aluminium Oxide G A fine, white, homogeneous powder of an average particle size between 10 and 40 µm containing about 10% w/w of calcium sulphate hemihydrate.
CONTENT OF CALCIUM SULPHATE Carry out the test described under *silica gel G*.
ACIDITY OR ALKALINITY pH of a suspension prepared by shaking 1 g with 10 ml of *carbon dioxide-free water*, about 7.5, Appendix V L.

Aluminium Potassium Sulphate Alum; aluminium potassium sulphate dodecahydrate; $AlK(SO_4)_2,12H_2O$ = 474.4 (*7784-24-9*)
Analytical reagent grade of commerce.

Aluminium Sulphate $Al_2(SO_4)_3,16H_2O$ = 630.4 (*10043-01-3*)
Analytical reagent grade of commerce.

Amaranth S CI 16185; acid red 27; $C_{20}H_{11}N_2Na_3O_{10}S_3$ = 604 (*915-67-3*)
General reagent grade of commerce.
A deep brown or deep reddish brown, fine powder.
When used for the titration of iodine and iodides with potassium iodate, the colour changes from orange-red to yellow.

Amaranth Solution A 0.2% w/v solution of *amaranth S*.

Aminoazobenzene α-Aminoazobenzene; 4-Aminoazobenzene; 4-phenylazoaniline; CI 11000; $C_{12}H_{11}N_3$ = 197.2 (*60-09-3*)
General reagent grade of commerce.
Brownish yellow needles with a bluish tinge; melting point, about 128°.

2-Aminobenzoic Acid Anthranilic acid; $C_7H_7NO_2$ = 137.1 (*118-92-3*)
General reagent grade of commerce.
Melting point, about 145°.

4-Aminobenzoic Acid $C_7H_7NO_2$ = 137.1 (*99-05-8*)
General reagent grade of commerce.
Melting point, about 188°.
Complies with the following test.
HOMOGENEITY Carry out the test for Related substances described under Procaine Hydrochloride. The chromatogram obtained shows only one principal spot.
Store protected from light.

4-Aminobenzoic Acid Solution Dissolve 1 g of *4-aminobenzoic acid* in a mixture of 18 ml of *anhydrous acetic acid*, 20 ml of *water* and 1 ml of *orthophosphoric acid*. Immediately before use, mix 2 volumes of the solution with 3 volumes of *acetone*.

(4-Aminobenzoyl)-L-glutamic Acid $C_{12}H_{14}N_2O_5$ = 266.2 (*4271-30-1*)
General reagent grade of commerce.
Melting point, about 173°.

2-Aminobutan-1-ol Aminobutanol; $C_4H_{11}NO$ = 89.14 (*5856-63-3*)
General reagent grade of commerce.
An oily liquid; boiling point, about 180°; d_{20}^{20}, about 0.94; n_D^{20}, about 1.453.

4-Amino-*n*-butyric Acid Gamma amino butyric acid; GABA; $C_4H_9NO_2$ = 103.1 (*2835-81-6*)
General reagent grade of commerce containing not less than 97% of $C_4H_9NO_2$.

2-Amino-5-chlorobenzophenone Aminochlorobenzophenone; $C_{13}H_{10}ClNO$ = 231.7 (*719-59-5*)
General reagent grade of commerce.
A yellow, crystalline powder; melting point, about 97°.
Complies with the following test.
HOMOGENEITY Carry out the test for Related substances described under Chlordiazepoxide Hydrochloride applying to the plate 5 µl of a 0.05% w/v solution in *methanol*. The chromatogram shows only one spot with an Rf value of about 0.9.
Store protected from light.

6-Aminohexanoic Acid 6-Aminocaproic acid; $C_6H_{13}NO_2$ = 131.2 (*60-32-2*)
General reagent grade of commerce.
Melting point, about 205°.

***p*-Aminohippuric Acid** Aminohippuric acid; *N*-(4-Aminobenzoyl)glycine; $C_9H_{10}N_2O_3$ = 194.2 (*61-78-9*)
General reagent grade of commerce.
A white or almost white powder; melting point, about 200°.

Aminohippuric Acid Reagent Dissolve 3 g of *phthalic acid* and 0.3 g of p-*aminohippuric acid* in sufficient *ethanol (96%)* to produce 100 ml.

4-Amino-3-hydroxynaphthalene-1-sulphonic Acid 1-Amino-2-naphthol-4-sulphonic acid; $C_{10}H_9NO_4S$ = 239.3 (*116-63-2*)
General reagent grade of commerce.
A crystalline powder; melting point, about 300°, with decomposition.
Store protected from light.

Aminohydroxynaphthalenesulphonic Acid Solution Dissolve 0.25 g of *4-amino-3-hydroxynaphthalene-1-sulphonic acid* in 75 ml of a 15% w/v solution of *sodium metabisulphite*, warming to assist solution if necessary. Add 2.5 ml of a 20% w/v solution of *sodium sulphite*, mix and add sufficient of the sodium metabisulphite solution to produce 100 ml.

5-Aminoimidazole-4-carboxamide Hydrochloride $C_4H_6N_4O,HCl$ = 162.6 (*72-40-2*)
General reagent grade of commerce.
Melting point, about 251°, with decomposition.

3-Aminomethylalizarin-*N,N*-diacetic Acid Aminomethylalizarindiacetic acid; alizarin complexone; $C_{19}H_{15}NO_8,2H_2O$ = 421.4 (*3952-78-1*)
A fine, ochre to orange-brown powder; melting point, about 185°.
Complies with the following test.
LOSS ON DRYING Not more than 10.0%, determined on 1 g.

Aminomethylalizarindiacetic Acid Reagent
SOLUTION I Dissolve 0.36 g of *cerium(III) nitrate* in sufficient *water* to produce 50 ml.
SOLUTION II Suspend 0.7 g of *3-aminomethylalizarin-*N,N-*diacetic acid* in 50 ml of *water*. Dissolve with the aid of about 0.25 ml of 13.5M *ammonia*, add 0.25 ml of *glacial acetic acid* and dilute to 100 ml with *water*.
SOLUTION III Dissolve 6 g of *sodium acetate* in 50 ml of *water*, add 11.5 ml of *glacial acetic acid* and dilute to 100 ml with *water*.
To 33 ml of *acetone* add 6.8 ml of solution III, 1.0 ml of solution II and 1.0 ml of solution I and dilute to 50 ml with *water*. Use within 5 days.
Complies with the following test.
SENSITIVITY To 1.0 ml of *fluoride standard solution (10 ppm F)* add 19.0 ml of *water* and 5.0 ml of the reagent being examined. After 20 minutes, a distinct blue colour is produced.

Aminomethylalizarindiacetic Acid Solution Dissolve 0.192 g of *3-aminomethylalizarin-*N,N-*diacetic acid* in 6 ml of freshly prepared 1M *sodium hydroxide*. Add 750 ml of *water*, 25 ml of *succinate buffer solution pH 4.6* and, dropwise, 0.5M *hydrochloric acid* until the colour changes from violet-red to yellow (pH 4.5 to 5). Add 100 ml of *acetone* and dilute to 1000 ml with *water*.

3-(Aminomethyl)pyridine (3-Pyridylmethyl)amine; 3-picolylamine; $C_6H_8N_2$ = 108.1 (*3731-52-0*)
General reagent grade of commerce.

8-Aminonaphthalene-2-sulphonic Acid 8-Amino-2-naphthalenesulphonic acid; 1-naphthylamine-7-sulphonic acid; $C_{10}H_9NO_3S$ = 223.2 (*119-28-8*)
General reagent grade of commerce.

Aminonaphthalenesulphonic Acid Solution Mix 0.5 g of *8-aminonaphthalene-2-sulphonic acid*, 30 ml of *glacial acetic acid* and 120 ml of *water* and heat with stirring until dissolved. Allow to cool and filter.
Use the solution within 3 weeks.

Aminonitrobenzophenone See *2-amino-5-nitrobenzophenone*.

2-Amino-5-nitrobenzophenone Aminonitrobenzophenone; $C_{13}H_{10}N_2O_3$ = 242.2 (*1775-95-7*)
General reagent grade of commerce.
A yellow, crystalline powder; melting point, about 160°; A(1%, 1 cm), 690 to 720, determined at 233 nm (0.001% w/v in *methanol*).

4-Aminophenazone Aminopyrazolone; 4-aminoantipyrine; 4-amino-2,3-dimethyl-1-phenyl-5-pyrazolone; $C_{11}H_{13}N_3O$ = 203.3 (*83-07-8*)
General reagent grade of commerce.
Light yellow needles or powder; melting point, about 108°.

Aminophenazone Solution Aminopyrazolone solution
A 0.1% w/v solution of *4-aminophenazone* in *borate buffer pH 9.0*.

4-Aminophenol C_6H_7NO = 109.1 (*123-30-8*)
General reagent grade of commerce.
A white or slightly coloured, crystalline powder; melting point, about 186°, with decomposition.
Store protected from light.

3-Aminopropanol 3-Amino-1-propanol; 3-aminopropan-1-ol; C_3H_9NO = 75.1 (*156-87-6*)
General reagent grade of commerce.
Melting point, about 11°; d_{20}^{20}, about 0.99; n_D^{20}, about 1.461.

3-Aminopropionic Acid β-Alanine; $C_3H_7NO_2$ = 89.1 (*107-95-9*)
General reagent grade of commerce containing not less than 99% of $C_3H_7NO_2$.
Melting point, about 200°, with decomposition.

Aminopyrazolone See *4-aminophenazone*.

Aminopyrazolone Solution See *aminophenazone solution*.

Ammonia NH_3 = 17.03
For 18M and 13.5M *ammonia* use analytical reagent grade solutions of commerce containing 35% and 25% w/w of NH_3 and weighing 0.88 g and 0.91 g per ml, respectively. Solutions of molarity *x*M should be prepared by diluting 75*x* ml of 13.5M *ammonia* or 56*x* ml of 18M *ammonia* to 1000 ml with *water*.

Ammonia, Chloride-free 13.5M *ammonia* that complies with the following test.
CHLORIDE Evaporate 54 ml on a water bath almost to dryness and dilute to 15 ml with *water*. The solution complies with the *limit test for chlorides*, Appendix VII (1 ppm).

Ammonia, Concentrated Strong Ammonia Solution of the British Pharmacopoeia (about 13.5M).

Ammonia, Methanolic Solutions of the requisite molarity may be obtained by diluting 13.5M *ammonia* or 18M *ammonia* with *methanol* as directed under *ammonia*.

Ammonia R1, Concentrated Concentrated ammonia containing not less than 32.0% w/w of NH_3 (about 18M). d_{20}^{20}, 0.883 to 0.889.
Store protected from atmospheric carbon dioxide at a temperature below 20°.

Ammonia R1, Dilute Dilute 41 g of *concentrated ammonia* to 100 ml with *water*. The solution contains not less than 10.0% and not more than 10.4% w/v of NH_3 (about 6M).

Ammonia R2, Dilute Dilute 14 g of *concentrated ammonia* to 100 ml with *water*. The solution contains not less than 3.3% and not more than 3.5% of NH_3 (about 2M).

Ammonium Acetate $C_2H_7NO_2$ = 77.08 (*631-61-8*)
Analytical reagent grade of commerce.
Store in an airtight container.

Ammonium Acetate Solution Dissolve 150 g of *ammonium acetate* in *water*, add 3 ml of *glacial acetic acid* and dilute to 1000 ml with *water*.
Use within 1 week of preparation.

Ammonium and Cerium Nitrate See *ammonium cerium(IV) nitrate.*

Ammonium and Cerium Sulphate See *ammonium cerium(IV) sulphate.*

(1*R*)-(–)-Ammonium 10-Camphorsulphonate 10-Camphorsulphonic acid, ammonium salt; $C_{10}H_{19}O_4S$ = 249.3 (*82509-30-6*)
General reagent grade of commerce containing not less than 97.0% of (1*R*)-(–)-ammonium camphorsulphonate.
$[\alpha]_D^{20}$, –18° ± 2° (5% w/v in *water*).

Ammonium Carbonate (*507-87-6*) Ammonium hydrogen carbonate and ammonium carbamate in approximately equimolecular proportions containing the equivalent of about 30% w/w of NH_3.
Analytical reagent grade of commerce.
Store in a well-closed container at a temperature not exceeding 20°.

Ammonium Carbonate Solution A 15.8% w/v solution of *ammonium carbonate.*

Ammonium Carbonate Solution, Dilute Dissolve 5 g of *ammonium carbonate* in a mixture of 7.5 ml of 5M *ammonia* and 50 ml of *water*, dilute to 100 ml with *water* and filter, if necessary.

Ammonium Cerium(IV) Nitrate Ceric ammonium nitrate; $(NH_4)_2[Ce(NO_3)_6]$ = 548.2 (*16774-21-3*)
Analytical reagent grade of commerce.

Ammonium Cerium(IV) Sulphate Ceric ammonium sulphate; $2(NH_4)_2SO_4,Ce(SO_4)_2,2H_2O$ = 632.6 (*18923-36-9*)
General reagent grade of commerce.

Ammonium Chloride NH_4Cl = 53.49 (*12125-02-9*)
Analytical reagent grade of commerce.

Ammonium Chloride Solution A 10.7% w/v solution of *ammonium chloride.*

Ammonium Citrate Diammonium hydrogen citrate; $C_6H_{14}N_2O_7$ = 226.2 (*3012-65-5*)
General reagent grade of commerce.
ACIDITY pH of 2.26% w/v solution, about 4.3.

Ammonium Citrate Solution Dissolve, with cooling, 500 g of *citric acid* in a mixture of 200 ml of *water* and 200 ml of 13.5M *ammonia*. Filter and dilute to 1000 ml with *water*.

Ammonium Cobaltothiocyanate Solution Dissolve 37.5 g of *cobalt(II) nitrate* and 150 g of *ammonium thiocyanate* in sufficient *water* to produce 1000 ml.
Use within 1 day of preparation.

Ammonium Dihydrogen Orthophosphate Ammonium dihydrogen phosphate; $(NH_4)H_2PO_4$ = 115.0 (*7722-76-1*)
Analytical reagent grade of commerce.
pH of a 2.3% w/v solution, about 4.2, Appendix V L.

Ammonium Hydrogen Carbonate Ammonium bicarbonate; NH_4HCO_3 = 79.06 (*1066-33-7*)
Analytical reagent grade of commerce containing not less than 99% of NH_4HCO_3.

Ammonium Iron(III) Citrate Ferric ammonium citrate (*1185-57-5*)
General reagent grade (brown) of commerce.

Ammonium Iron(II) Sulphate Ferrous ammonium sulphate; $(NH_4)_2Fe(SO_4)_2,6H_2O$ = 392.1 (*7783-85-9*)
Analytical reagent grade of commerce.
Store protected from light.

Ammonium Iron(III) Sulphate Ferric ammonium sulphate; $NH_4Fe(SO_4)_2,12H_2O$ = 482.2 (*7783-83-7*)
Analytical reagent grade of commerce.

Ammonium Iron(III) Sulphate Solution R1 Dissolve 0.2 g of *ammonium iron(III) sulphate* in 50 ml of *water*, add 5 ml of *nitric acid* and dilute to 100 ml with *water.*

Ammonium Iron(III) Sulphate Solution R2 A 10% w/v solution of *ammonium iron(III) sulphate*. If necessary, filter before use.
Produces a deep red colour with ammonium thiocyanate in acid solutions.

Ammonium Iron(III) Sulphate Solution R5 Shake 30.0 g of *ammonium iron(III) sulphate* with 40 ml of *nitric acid* and dilute to 100 ml with *water*. If the solution is turbid, it should be filtered or centrifuged.
Store protected from light.

Ammonium Iron(III) Sulphate Solution R6 Dissolve 20 g of *ammonium iron(III) sulphate* in 75 ml of *water*, add 10 ml of a 2.8% w/v solution of *sulphuric acid (96% w/w)* and dilute to 100 ml with *water.*

Ammonium Mercaptoacetate Solution Add 300 ml of *water* to 50 ml of *mercaptoacetic acid*, neutralise with about 40 ml of 13.5M *ammonia* and dilute to 500 ml with *water.*

Ammonium Mercurithiocyanate Reagent Dissolve 30 g of *ammonium thiocyanate* and 27 g of *mercury(II) chloride* in sufficient *water* to produce 1000 ml.

Ammonium Metavanadate Ammonium vanadate; NH_4VO_3 = 117.0 (*7803-55-6*)
Analytical reagent grade of commerce.

Ammonium Metavanadate Solution Dissolve, with heating, 5 g of *ammonium metavanadate* in a mixture of 10 ml of 5M *sodium hydroxide* and 90 ml of *water*, cool and filter, if necessary, through glass wool.

Ammonium Molybdate $(NH_4)_6Mo_7O_{24},4H_2O$ = 1236 (*12054-85-2*)
Analytical reagent grade of commerce.

Ammonium Molybdate Reagent Mix in the following order 1 volume of a 2.5% w/v solution of *ammonium molybdate*, 1 volume of a 10% w/v solution of *L-ascorbic acid* and 1 volume of 3M *sulphuric acid* and add 2 volumes of *water.*
Use within 1 day of preparation.

Ammonium Molybdate Reagent R1 Mix 10 ml of a 6.0% w/v solution of *disodium arsenate*, 50 ml of *ammonium molybdate solution*, 90 ml of 1M *sulphuric acid* and add sufficient *water* to produce 200 ml.
Condition the mixture at 37° for 24 hours and keep in amber flasks.

Ammonium Molybdate Solution A 10% w/v solution of *ammonium molybdate*.

Ammonium Molybdate Solution R2 Dissolve 5 g of *ammonium molybdate* in 30 ml of *water* with heating, cool, adjust the pH to 7.0 with 2M *ammonia* and dilute to 50 ml with *water*.

Ammonium Molybdate Solution R3
SOLUTION I Dissolve 5 g of *ammonium molybdate* in 20 ml of *water* with the aid of heat.
SOLUTION II Mix 150 ml of *ethanol (96%)* with 150 ml of *water* and add, with cooling, 100 ml of *sulphuric acid*.
Add 80 volumes of solution II to 20 volumes of solution I immediately before use.

Ammonium Molybdate Solution R4 Dissolve 1.0 g of *ammonium molybdate* in sufficient *water* to produce 40 ml, add 3 ml of *hydrochloric acid* and 5 ml of *perchloric acid* and dilute to 100 ml with *acetone*.
Store protected from light and use within 1 month of preparation.

Ammonium Molybdate—Sulphuric Acid Solution Dissolve 10 g of *ammonium molybdate* in sufficient *water* to produce 100 ml and add the solution slowly to 250 ml of cold 10M *sulphuric acid*.
Store in a plastic bottle protected from light.

Ammonium Nitrate NH_4NO_3 = 80.04 (*6484-52-2*)
Analytical reagent grade of commerce.
Store in airtight container.

Ammonium Nitrate R1 *Ammonium nitrate* complying with the following requirements.
ACIDITY A solution is *faintly acid*, Appendix V K.
CHLORIDE 0.5 g complies with the limit test for chlorides, Appendix VII (100 ppm).
SULPHATE 1.0 g complies with the limit test for sulphates, Appendix VII (150 ppm)
SULPHATED ASH Not more than 0.05%, Appendix IX A, Method II. Use 1 g.

Ammonium Oxalate $(CO_2NH_4)_2,H_2O$ = 142.1 (*6009-70-7*)
Analytical reagent grade of commerce.

Ammonium Oxalate Solution A 4% w/v solution of *ammonium oxalate*.

Ammonium Persulphate Ammonium peroxodisulphate; $(NH_4)_2S_2O_8$ = 228.2 (*7727-54-0*)
Analytical reagent grade of commerce.

Ammonium Phosphate See *diammonium hydrogen orthophosphate*.

Ammonium Polysulphide Solution Dissolve a sufficient quantity of *precipitated sulphur* to produce a deep orange solution in a solution prepared in the following manner. Immediately before use saturate 120 ml of 6M *ammonia* with *hydrogen sulphide* and add 80 ml of 6M *ammonia*.

Ammonium Pyrrolidinedithiocarbamate Ammonium tetramethylenedithiocarbamate; $C_5H_{12}N_2S_2$ = 164.3 (*5108-96-3*)
General reagent grade of commerce.
Store in a bottle containing a piece of ammonium carbonate in a muslin bag.

Ammonium Pyrrolidinedithiocarbamate Solution A 1.0% w/v solution of *ammonium pyrrolidinedithiocarbamate* that has been washed immediately before use with three 25-ml quantities of *4-methylpentan-2-one*.

Ammonium Reineckate Ammonium tetrathiocyanatodiamminochromate(III) monohydrate; $NH_4[Cr(NH_3)_2(CNS)_4],H_2O$ = 354.4 (*13573-16-5*)
General reagent grade of commerce.
Red powder or crystals.

Ammonium Reineckate Solution A 1.0% w/v solution of *ammonium reineckate*.
Prepare immediately before use.

Ammonium Sulphamate $NH_2SO_3NH_4$ = 114.1 (*7773-06-0*)
General reagent grade of commerce.
A white, crystalline powder or colourless crystals; melting point, about 130°.
Store in an airtight container.

Ammonium Sulphate $(NH_4)_2SO_4$ = 132.1 (*7783-20-2*)
Analytical reagent grade of commerce.

Ammonium Thiocyanate NH_4SCN = 76.12 (*1762-95-4*)
Analytical reagent grade of commerce.
Store in an airtight container.

Ammonium Thiocyanate Solution A 7.6% w/v solution of *ammonium thiocyanate*.

Ammonium Vanadate See *ammonium metavanadate*

Ammonium Vanadate Solution Dissolve 1.2 g of *ammonium metavanadate* in 95 ml of *water* and dilute to 100 ml with *sulphuric acid*.

Amoxicillin Trihydrate Amoxycillin trihydrate; $C_{16}H_{19}N_3O_5S,3H_2O$ = 419.4 (*61336-70-7*)
General reagent grade of commerce.

Amyl Acetate $C_7H_{14}O_2$ = 130.2
Consists principally of 3-methylbutyl acetate with a small proportion of 2-methylbutyl acetate.
Analytical reagent grade of commerce.
A colourless liquid with a sharp, fruity odour; boiling point, about 140°; weight per ml, about 0.87 g.

Amyl Alcohol Isoamyl alcohol; $C_5H_{12}O$ = 88.15 (*30899-19-5*)
Consists principally of 3-methylbutan-1-ol with a small proportion of 2-methylbutan-1-ol.
Analytical reagent grade of commerce.
A colourless liquid; boiling point, about 130°; weight per ml, about 0.81 g.

α-Amylase 1,4-α-D-glucane-glucanohydrolase
A white to light brown powder.

α-Amylase Solution A solution of *α-amylase* with an activity of 800 FAU per g.

Anethole *p*-Prop-1-enylanisole; $C_{10}H_{12}O$ = 148.2 (*4180-23-8*)
General reagent grade of commerce.
A white crystalline mass at 20° to 21°; liquid above 23°; boiling point, about 230°; n_D^{25}, about 1.56.
Anethole used in gas chromatography complies with the following test.
ASSAY Examine by *gas chromatography*, Appendix III B, under the conditions described in the test for Chromatographic profile in the monograph for Anise Oil using the

reagent being examined as solution (1).

The area of the principal peak, corresponding to *trans*-anethole, with retention time of about 41 minutes, is not less than 99.0% of the total area of the peaks.

***cis*-Anethole** (*Z*)-1-Methoxy-4-prop-1-enylbenzene; $C_{10}H_{12}O$ = 148.2
General reagent grade of commerce.
A white crystalline mass at 20°; liquid above 23°; boiling point, about 230°; n_D^{25}, about 1.56.
Cis-anethole used in gas chromatography complies with the following test.
ASSAY Examine by *gas chromatography*, Appendix III B, under the conditions described in the test for Chromatographic profile in the monograph for Anise Oil using the reagent being examined as solution (1).

The area of the principal peak is not less than 92.0% of the total area of the peaks.

Aniline C_6H_7N = 93.13 (*62-53-3*)
Analytical reagent grade of commerce.
A colourless to pale yellow oily liquid; boiling point, about 183° to 186°; d_{20}^{20}, about 1.02.
Store protected from light.

Aniline Hydrochloride C_6H_7N,HCl = 129.6 (*142-04-1*)
General reagent grade of commerce.

Aniline Hydrochloride Solution Dissolve 2 g of *aniline hydrochloride* in a mixture of 65 ml of *ethanol (96%)* and 35 ml of *water* and add 2 ml of *hydrochloric acid.*
Use within one day of preparation.

Anion Exchange Resin A resin in chlorinated form containing quaternary ammonium groups.
$[CH_2N^+(CH_3)_3]$ attached to a polymer lattice consisting of polystyrene cross-linked with 2% of divinylbenzene. It is available as beads and the particle size is specified in the monograph. Wash the resin with 1M *sodium hydroxide* on a sintered-glass filter until the washings are free from chloride, then wash with *water* until the washings are neutral. Suspend in freshly prepared *ammonia-free water* and protect from atmospheric carbon dioxide.

Anion Exchange Resin, Strongly Basic A gel-type resin in hydroxide form containing quaternary ammonium groups $[-CH_2N^+(CH_3)_3$, type 1] attached to a polymer lattice consisting of polystyrene cross-linked with 8% of divinylbenzene.
Brown, transparent beads containing about 50% of water; particle size, 0.2 mm to 1.0 mm; total exchange capacity, at least 1.2 milliequivalents per ml.

Anisaldehyde 4-Methoxybenzaldehyde; $C_8H_8O_2$ = 136.2 (*123-11-5*)
General reagent grade of commerce.
A colourless to pale yellow, oily liquid with an aromatic odour; boiling point, about 248°; weight per ml, about 1.125 g.
Anisaldehyde used in gas chromatography complies with the following test.
ASSAY Examine by *gas chromatography*, Appendix III B, under the conditions described in the test for Chromatographic profile in the monograph for Anise Oil using the reagent being examined as solution (1).

The area of the principal peak is not less than 99.0% of the total area of the peaks.

Anisaldehyde Solution Mix in the following order 0.5 ml of *anisaldehyde,* 10 ml of *glacial acetic acid,* 85 ml of *methanol* and 5 ml of *sulphuric acid.*

Anisaldehyde Solution R1 To 10 ml of *anisaldehyde* add 90 ml of *ethanol (96%)*, mix, add 10 ml of *sulphuric acid* and mix again.

***p*-Anisidine** C_7H_9NO = 123.2 (*104-94-9*)
General reagent grade of commerce containing not less than 97.0% of C_7H_9NO.
CAUTION *p-Anisidine is a skin irritant and sensitiser.*
Store protected from light at 0° to 4°.
On storage, *p*-anisidine tends to darken as a result of oxidation. A discoloured reagent can be reduced and decolorised in the following manner. Dissolve 20 g of the reagent in 500 ml of *water* at 75°. Add 1 g of *sodium sulphite* and 10 g of *activated charcoal* and stir for 5 minutes. Filer, cool the filtrate to about 0° and allow to stand at this temperature for at least 4 hours. Filter, wash the crystals with a small quantity of water at about 0° and dry the crystals at a pressure of 2 kPa over *phosphorus pentoxide*.

Anthracene $C_{14}H_{10}$ = 178.2 (*120-12-7*)
General reagent grade of commerce.
A white, crystalline powder; melting point, about 218°.

Anthranilic Acid See *2-aminobenzoic acid.*

Anthrone $C_{14}H_{10}O$ = 194.2 (*90-44-8*)
Analytical reagent grade of commerce.
A pale yellow, crystalline powder; melting point, about 155°.
When used in an Assay for glucose or dextrans, complies with the following test.
SENSITIVITY TO GLUCOSE Add, carefully, 6 ml of a 0.2% w/v solution in a mixture of 19 ml of *sulphuric acid* and 1 ml of *water* to 3 ml of a solution containing 5 µg of *D-glucose* per ml and heat in a water bath for 5 minutes. The solution is a darker green than a solution prepared in the same manner but omitting the glucose.

Anthrone Reagent A 0.2% w/v solution of *anthrone* in *nitrogen-free sulphuric acid.* The solution should be allowed to stand for 4 hours before use and should be discarded after 7 days.

Antimony Potassium Tartrate Antimony potassium oxide (+)-tartrate; $KSbO,C_4H_4O_6,½H_2O$ = 333.9 (*28300-74-5*)
Analytical reagent grade of commerce.

Antimony Trichloride $SbCl_3$ = 228.1 (*10025-91-9*)
Analytical reagent grade of commerce.
Colourless crystals or flakes, fuming in moist air.
Store in an airtight container, protected from moisture.

Antimony Trichloride Solution Rapidly wash 30 g of *antimony trichloride* with two 15-ml quantities of *ethanol-free chloroform*. Drain off the washings and dissolve the washed crystals immediately in 100 ml of *ethanol-free chloroform*, warming slightly.
Store over a few grams of *anhydrous sodium sulphate.*

Antimony Trichloride Solution R1 Prepare two stock solutions in the following manner.
SOLUTION A Dissolve 110 g of *antimony trichloride* in 400 ml of *1,2-dichloroethane.* Add 2 g of *anhydrous aluminium oxide,* mix and filter through sintered glass into a 500-ml graduated flask. Dilute to 500 ml with *1,2-dichloroethane* and mix. The *absorbance* of the resulting solution measured in a 2-cm cell at 500 nm, Appendix II B, is not more than 0.07 using *1,2-dichloroethane* in the reference cell.

SOLUTION B In a fume cupboard, mix 100 ml of colourless, distilled *acetyl chloride* and 400 ml of *1,2-dichloroethane* and store in a cool place.
Mix 90 ml of solution A and 10 ml of solution B. Store in an amber, ground-glass-stoppered bottle and use within 7 days. Discard any reagent in which colour develops.

Antithrombin III ATIII (*90170-80-2*)
Reagent grade of commerce.
Antithrombin III is purified from human plasma by heparin agarose chromatography and should have a specific activity of at least 6 IU per mg.

Antithrombin III Solution R1 Reconstitute *antithrombin III* as directed by the manufacturer and dilute with *tris-chloride buffer pH 7.4* to contain 1 IU per ml.

Antithrombin III Solution R2 Reconstitute *antithrombin III* as directed by the manufacturer and dilute with *tris-chloride buffer pH 7.4* to contain 0.5 IU per ml.

Apigenin 4′,5,7-Trihydroxyflavone; $C_{15}H_{10}O$ = 270.2 (*520-36-5*)
General reagent grade of commerce.
Light yellowish powder.
Melting point, about 310°, with decomposition.
Complies with the following test.
CHROMATOGRAPHY Carry out identification test C described under Chamomile Flowers applying 10 µl of a 0.025% w/v solution in *methanol*. The chromatogram shows a principal zone of yellowish-green fluorescence in the upper third.

Apigenin-7-glucoside $C_{21}H_{20}O_{10}$ = 432.6
General reagent grade of commerce.
Light yellowish powder.
Melting point, 198° to 201°.
Complies with the following test.
CHROMATOGRAPHY Carry out identification test C described under Chamomile Flowers applying 10 µl of a 0.025% w/v solution in *methanol*. The chromatogram shows a principal zone of yellowish fluorescence in the middle third.

Aprotinin (*9087-70-1*)
Reagent grade of commerce containing 10 to 20 trypsin inhibitor units per mg.

Arabinose See *L-arabinose.*

L-Arabinose Arabinose; $C_5H_{10}O_5$ = 150.1 (*87-72-9*)
General reagent grade of commerce.
A white, crystalline powder; $[\alpha]_D^{20}$, +103° to +105° (5.0% w/v in *water* containing about 0.05% v/v of NH_3).

Arachidic Alcohol Eicosan-1-ol; Arachidyl alcohol; $C_{20}H_{42}O$ = 298.6 (*629-96-9*)
Purified reagent grade of commerce usually containing not less than 95% of $C_{20}H_{42}O$.
A colourless, waxy or crystalline solid.

Arbutin Arbutoside; 4-hydroxyphenyl-β-D-glucopyranoside; $C_{12}H_{16}O_7$ = 272.3 (*497-76-7*)
General reagent grade of commerce.
Melting point, about 200°; $[\alpha]_D^{20}$, about −64°, determined on a 2.0% w/v solution.
CHROMATOGRAPHY When examined by test C for Identification in the monograph for Bearberry Leaf the chromatogram shows only one principal spot.

Arginine L-Arginine; $C_6H_{14}N_4O_2$ = 174.2 (*74-79-3*)
General reagent grade of commerce.
Melting point, about 235°, with decomposition.

Argon Ar = 39.95 (*7440-37-1*)
Laboratory cylinder grade of commerce containing not less than 99.995% v/v of Ar.
When used in the test for Carbon monoxide in medicinal gases (Appendix IX E), after passage of 10 litres at a flow rate of 4 litres per hour, not more than 0.05 ml of 0.002M *sodium thiosulphate VS* is required for the titration (0.6 ppm).

Arsenious Trioxide Arsenic trioxide; As_2O_3 = 197.8 (*1327-53-3*)
Analytical reagent grade of commerce.

Arsenite Solution Dissolve 0.50 g of *arsenious trioxide* in 5 ml of 2M *sodium hydroxide* solution, add 2.0 g of *sodium hydrogen carbonate* and dilute to 100 ml with *water.*

Ascorbic Acid See *L-ascorbic acid.*

L-Ascorbic Acid $C_6H_8O_6$ = 176.1 (*50-81-7*)
Analytical reagent grade of commerce.
A white, crystalline powder; $[\alpha]_D^{20}$, about +22° (2% w/v in water).

Ascorbic Acid Solution Dissolve 50 mg of *L-ascorbic acid* in 0.5 ml of *water* and dilute to 50 ml with *dimethylformamide.*

L-Aspartyl-L-phenylalanine Aspartame; (*S*)-3-amino-*N*-[(*S*)-1-carboxy-2-phenylethyl]succinamic acid; $C_{13}H_{16}N_2O_5$ = 280.3 (*13433-09-5*)
General reagent grade of commerce.
Melting point, about 210°, with decomposition.

Atenolol $C_{14}H_{22}N_2O_3$ = 266.3 (*56715-13-0*)
General reagent grade of commerce.

Atropine Sulphate $C_{34}H_{46}N_2O_6,H_2SO_4,H_2O$ = 694.8 (*5908-99-6*)
General reagent grade of commerce.
Colourless crystals or a white, crystalline powder; melting point, about 195°.

Azomethine H Azomethine H, monosodium salt hydrate; sodium hydrogen 4-hydroxy-5-(2-hydroxybenzylideneamino)naphthalene-2,7-disulphonate; $C_{17}H_{12}NNaO_8S_2$ = 445.4 (*5941-07-1*)
General reagent grade of commerce; the degree of hydration is variable.

Azomethine H Solution Dissolve 0.45 g of *azomethine H* and 1 g of *ascorbic acid* in *water* with the aid of gentle heat and add sufficient *water* to produce 100 ml.

Barbaloin 1,8-Dihydroxy-3-hydroxymethyl-10-(β-D-glucopyranosyl)anthrone; $C_{21}H_{22}O_9,H_2O$ = 436.4 (*1415-73-2*)
General reagent grade of commerce.
Lemon yellow to dark yellow needles or crystalline powder, darkening on exposure to air and light.
A(1%, 1 cm) determined in *methanol*, about 192 at 269 nm, about 226 at 296.5 nm and about 259 at 354 nm, calculated with reference to the anhydrous substance.
Complies with the following test.
HOMOGENEITY Carry out the test for Other species of *Rhamnus*, anthrones described under Frangula bark applying to the plate a solution containing only the reagent being examined. The chromatogram obtained shows only one major spot.

Barbital See *barbitone.*

Barbital Sodium See *barbitone sodium.*

Barbitone Barbital; 5,5-diethylbarbituric acid; $C_8H_{12}N_2O_3$ = 184.2 (*57-44-3*)
General reagent grade of commerce.
Melting point, about 190°.

Barbitone Sodium Barbital sodium; sodium 5,5-diethylbarbiturate; $C_8H_{11}N_2NaO_3$ = 206.2 (*144-02-5*)
General reagent grade of commerce.

Barbituric Acid 2,4,6-Trihydroxypyrimidine; $C_4H_4N_2O_3$ = 128.1 (*67-52-7*)
General reagent grade of commerce.
A white or almost white powder; melting point, about 253°.

Barium Carbonate $BaCO_3$ = 197.3 (*513-77-9*)
Analytical reagent grade of commerce.

Barium Chloride $BaCl_2,2H_2O$ = 244.3 (*10326-27-9*)
Analytical reagent grade of commerce.

Barium Chloride Solution A 10.0% w/v solution of *barium chloride*.

Barium Chloride Solution R1 A 6.1% w/v solution of *barium chloride*.

Barium Chloride Solution R2 A 3.65% w/v solution of *barium chloride*.

Barium Hydroxide $Ba(OH)_2,8H_2O$ = 315.5 (*12230-71-6*)
Analytical reagent grade of commerce.

Barium Hydroxide Solution A 4.73% w/v solution of *barium hydroxide*.

Barium Sulphate $BaSO_4$ = 233.4 (*7727-43-7*)
Precipitated grade of commerce.

Benzaldehyde C_7H_6O = 106.1 (*100-52-7*)
Analytical reagent grade of commerce.
A colourless to pale yellow, oily liquid with an odour of almonds; d_{20}^{20}, about 1.05; n_D^{20}, about 1.545.
DISTILLATION RANGE Not less than 95% distils between 177° and 180°.
Store protected from light.

Benzalkonium Chloride Of the British Pharmacopoeia.

Benzalkonium Chloride Solution Of the British Pharmacopoeia.

Benzamide C_7H_7NO = 121.1 (*55-21-0*)
General reagent grade of commerce.
Melting point, about 128°.

Benzene C_6H_6 = 78.1 (*71-43-2*)
Analytical reagent grade of commerce.
A flammable, colourless liquid; boiling point, about 80°.

Benzethonium Chloride $C_{27}H_{42}ClNO_2,H_2O$ = 466.1 (*121-54-0*)
General reagent grade of commerce.
A fine, white powder, or colourless crystals; melting point, about 163°.
Store protected from light.

Benzil $C_{14}H_{10}O_2$ = 210.2 (*134-81-6*)
General reagent grade of commerce.
Melting point, about 95°.

Benzilic Acid Diphenylglycollic acid; $C_{14}H_{12}O_3$ = 228.3 (*76-93-7*)
General reagent grade of commerce.
Melting point, about 151°.

Benzoic Acid $C_7H_6O_2$ = 122.1 (*65-85-0*)
Analytical reagent grade of commerce.
Colourless, feathery crystals or a white powder; melting point, about 121°.

Benzoin α-Hydroxy-α-phenylacetophenone; $C_{14}H_{12}O_2$ = 212.3 (*579-44-2*)
General reagent grade of commerce.
Melting point, about 137°.

Benzophenone $C_{13}H_{10}O$ = 182.2 (*119-61-9*)
General reagent grade of commerce.
Melting point, about 48°.

Benzoyl Chloride C_7H_5ClO = 140.6 (*98-88-4*)
Analytical reagent grade of commerce.
A colourless, lachrymatory liquid, fuming in moist air; d_{20}^{20}, about 1.21; boiling point, about 197°.

Benzoyl Peroxide $C_{14}H_{10}O_4$ = 242.2 (*94-36-0*)
General reagent grade of commerce.
White or almost white granules; melting point, after drying, about 104°.
For safety Benzoyl Peroxide should be kept moistened with about 23% w/w of water.

Benzoylarginine Ethyl Ester Hydrochloride $C_{15}H_{23}ClN_4O_3$ = 342.8 (*2645-08-1*)
General reagent grade of commerce.
$[\alpha]_D^{20}$, −15° to −18°, determined in a 1% w/v solution; melting point, about 129°; A(1%, 1 cm), 310 to 340 determined at 227 nm using a 0.001% w/v solution.

***N*-Benzoyl-L-prolyl-L-phenylalanyl-L-arginine 4-nitroanilide acetate** $C_{35}H_{42}N_8O_8$ = 703
General reagent grade of commerce.

Benzyl Alcohol C_7H_8O = 108.1 (*100-51-6*)
General reagent grade of commerce.
A colourless liquid; boiling point, about 204°; weight per ml, about 1.05 g.

Benzyl Benzoate $C_{14}H_{12}O_2$ = 212.3 (*120-51-4*)
General reagent grade of commerce.
Leaflets or an oily liquid; melting point, about 20°; weight per ml, about 1.12 g.
When used in the test for Identification in the monograph for Peru Balsam, complies with the following requirement.
CHROMATOGRAPHY Carry out test B for Identification described in the monograph for Peru Balsam applying to the plate 20 µl of a 0.3% w/v solution of the reagent being examined in *ethyl acetate*. After visualisation, the chromatogram exhibits a principal spot with an Rf value of about 0.8.

Benzyl Cinnamate Benzyl 3-phenylprop-2-enoate; $C_{16}H_{14}O_2$ = 238.3 (*103-41-3*)
General reagent grade of commerce.
Colourless or yellowish crystals; melting point, about 39°.
Complies with the following requirement.
CHROMATOGRAPHY Carry out test B for Identification described in the monograph for Peru Balsam applying to the plate 20 µl of a 0.3% w/v solution of the reagent being examined in *ethyl acetate*. After visualisation, the chromatogram exhibits a principal spot with an Rf value of about 0.6.

Benzylamine C_7H_9N = 107.2
General reagent grade of commerce usually containing not less than 98% of C_7H_9N.
Colourless to pale yellow, oily liquid; boiling point, about 185°; weight per ml, about 0.98 g.

Benzylpenicillin Sodium Of the British Pharmacopoeia.

Bergapten 5-Methoxypsoralen; $C_{12}H_8O_4$ = 216.2 (*484-20-8*)
General reagent grade of commerce.
Melting point, about 188°.

Betamethasone 9α-Fluoro-11β,17α,21-trihydroxy-16β-methylpregna-1,4-diene-3,20-dione; $C_{22}H_{29}FO_5$ = 392.5 *(378-44-9)*
General reagent grade of commerce.
Melting point, about 236°.

Betulin Lup-20(39)-ene-3β,28-diol; $C_{30}H_{50}O_2$ = 442.7 *(473-98-3)*
General reagent grade of commerce.
Melting point, 248° to 251°.

Bibenzyl 1,2-Diphenylethane; $C_{14}H_{14}$ = 182.3 *(103-29-7)*
General reagent grade of commerce.
Colourless or white crystals; melting point, about 50° to 53°.

Biphenyl $C_{12}H_{10}$ = 154.2 *(92-52-4)*
General reagent grade of commerce.
Melting point, about 70°.

Biphenyl-4-ol See *4-hydroxybiphenyl.*

Bisbenzimide 4-{5-[5-(4-Methylpiperazin-1-yl)benzimidazol-2-yl]benzimidazol-2-yl} phenol trihydrochloride pentahydrate; $C_{25}H_{24}N_6O,3HCl,5H_2O$ = 624 *(23491-44-3)*
General reagent grade of commerce.

Bisbenzimide Stock Solution Dissolve 5 mg of *bisbenzimide* in sufficient *water* to produce 100 ml.
Store protected from light.

Bisbenzimide Working Solution Immediately before use, dilute 100 µl of *bisbenzimide stock solution* to 100 ml with *phosphate-buffered saline pH 7.4.*

Bismuth Oxycarbonate Bismuth subcarbonate *(5892-10-4)*
A basic salt corresponding approximately to the formula $(BiO)_2CO_3,½H_2O$, containing the equivalent of about 91% of Bi_2O_3.

Bismuth Oxynitrate Bismuth subnitrate $4[BiNO_3(OH_2),BiO(OH)]$ = 1462 *(1304-85-4)*
A basic salt containing about 80% of Bi_2O_3.

Bismuth Oxynitrate R1 Bismuth subnitrate R1
Bismuth oxynitrate containing not less than 71.5% and not more than 74.0% of bismuth and not less than 14.5% and not more than 16.5% of nitrate, calculated as nitrogen pentoxide, N_2O_5.

Bismuth Oxynitrate Solution Bismuth subnitrate solution
Dissolve 5 g of *bismuth oxynitrate R1* in a mixture of 8.4 ml of *nitric acid* and 50 ml of *water* and dilute to 250 ml with *water*; filter if necessary.
ACIDITY To 10 ml of the reagent add 0.05 ml of *methyl orange solution* and titrate with 1M *sodium hydroxide VS.* Not less than 5.0 ml and not more than 6.25 ml is required to change the colour of the solution.

Bismuth Subcarbonate See *bismuth oxycarbonate.*

Bismuth Subnitrate See *bismuth oxynitrate.*

Bismuth Subnitrate R1 See *bismuth oxynitrate R1.*

Bismuth Subnitrate Solution See *bismuth oxynitrate solution.*

***N,O*-Bis(trimethylsilyl)acetamide** $C_8H_{21}NOSi_2$ = 203.4 *(10416-59-8)*
General reagent grade of commerce.
A colourless liquid; weight per ml, about 0.83 g.

Bis(trimethylsilyl)trifluoroacetamide $C_8H_{18}F_3NOSi_2$ = 257.4 *(25561-30-2)*
General reagent grade of commerce.
Weight per ml, about 0.97 g; n_D^{20}, about 1.384.

Biuret $C_2H_5N_3O_2$ = 103.1 *(108-19-0)*
General reagent grade of commerce.
White, hygroscopic crystals; melting point, 188° to 190°, with decomposition.

Biuret Reagent Dissolve 1.5 g of *copper(II) sulphate* and 6.0 g of *potassium sodium (+)-tartrate* in 500 ml of *water*, add 300 ml of a carbonate-free 10% w/v solution of *sodium hydroxide* and sufficient of the same solution to produce 1000 ml and mix.

Blue Dextran 2000 *(9049-32-5)* Prepared from dextran having an average molecular weight of about 2×10^6 by introduction of a polycyclic chromophore that colours the substance blue. The degree of substitution is 0.017. It is freeze-dried and dissolves rapidly and completely in *water* and aqueous saline solutions.
Complies with the following test.
LIGHT ABSORPTION A 0.1% w/v solution in *phosphate buffer pH 7.0* exhibits a maximum at 280 nm, Appendix II B.

Borate Solution Dissolve 9.55 g of *sodium tetraborate* in *sulphuric acid (96% w/w)*, heating on a water bath, and add sufficient *sulphuric acid (96% w/w)* to produce 1000 ml.

Boric Acid H_3BO_3 = 61.83 *(10043-35-3)*
Analytical reagent grade of commerce.

Boric Acid Solution Dissolve 5 g of *boric acid* in a mixture of 20 ml of *water* and 20 ml of *absolute ethanol* and dilute to 250 ml with *absolute ethanol.*

***d*-Borneol** *endo*-1,7,7-Trimethylbicyclo[2.2.1]heptan-2-ol; $C_{10}H_{18}O$ = 154.3 *(507-70-0)*
General reagent grade of commerce.
Melting point, about 208°.
Complies with the following test.
HOMOGENEITY Carry out the method for *thin-layer chromatography*, Appendix III A, using *silica gel G* as the coating substance and *chloroform* as the mobile phase, but allowing the solvent front to ascend 10 cm above the line of application. Apply to the plate 10 µl of a 0.1% w/v solution of the substance being examined in *toluene*. After removal of the plate, allow it to dry in air and spray with *anisaldehyde solution*, using 10 ml for a plate 200 mm × 200 mm, and heat at 100° to 105° for 10 minutes. The chromatogram obtained shows only one principal spot.

***d*-Bornyl Acetate** $C_{12}H_{20}O_2$ = 196.3 *(5655-61-8)*
General reagent grade of commerce.
Melting point, about 28°; $[\alpha]_D^{20}$, about +44° (10% w/v in ethanol).
Complies with the following test.
HOMOGENEITY Carry out the method for *thin-layer chromatography*, Appendix III A, using *silica gel G* as the coating substance and *chloroform* as the mobile phase, but allowing the solvent front to ascend 10 cm above the line of application. Apply to the plate 10 µl of a 0.2% w/v solution of the reagent being examined in *toluene*. After removal of the plate, allow it to dry in air and spray with *anisaldehyde solution*, using 10 ml for a plate 200 mm × 200 mm, and heat at 100° to 105° for 10 minutes. The chromatogram obtained shows only one principal spot.

Boron Trichloride BCl_3 = 117.2 (*10294-34-5*)
General reagent grade of commerce.
Colourless gas which reacts violently with water. Available as solutions in suitable solvents (2-chloroethanol, dichloromethane, hexane, heptane, methanol).
Boiling point, about 12.6°; n_D^{20}, about 1.420

Boron Trichloride-Methanol Solution A 12% w/v solution of BCl_3 in *methanol.*
Store protected from light at −20°, preferably in sealed tubes.

Boron Trifluoride BF_3 = 67.8 (*7637-07-2*)
General regent grade of commerce.
Colourless gas.

Boron Trifluoride Solution A grade of commerce containing about 14% of BF_3 in *methanol.*

Bovine Coagulation Factor Xa An enzyme which converts prothrombin to thrombin. The semi-purified preparation is obtained from liquid bovine plasma and it may be prepared by activation of the zymogen factor X with a suitable activator such as Russell's viper venom.
Store freeze-dried preparation at −20° and frozen solution at a temperature not higher than −20°.

Bovine Factor Xa Solution Reconstitute *bovine coagulation factor Xa* as directed by the manufacturer and dilute with *tris-chloride buffer pH 7.4*. Any change in the *absorbance* of the solution, Appendix II B, measured at 405 nm using *tris-chloride buffer pH 7.4* in the reference cell, is not more than 0.15 to 0.20 per minute.

Brilliant Blue See *Acid blue 83.*

Brilliant Green CI 42040; basic green 1; $C_{27}H_{34}N_2O_4S$ = 482.6 (*633-03-4*)
Technical grade of commerce.
Small, glistening golden crystals.

Bromelains (*37189-34-7*) A concentrate of proteolytic enzymes derived from *Ananas comosus* Merr.
A dull yellow powder.
Complies with the following test.
ACTIVITY 1 g liberates about 1.2 g of amino nitrogen from a standard *gelatin* solution in 20 minutes at 45° and pH 4.5.

Bromelains Solution A 1.0% w/v solution of *bromelains* in a mixture of 1 volume of *mixed phosphate buffer pH 5.5* and 9 volumes of *saline solution.*

Bromine Br_2 = 159.8 (*7726-95-6*)
Analytical reagent grade of commerce.
A heavy, brownish-red, fuming liquid, highly corrosive to the skin; d_{20}^{20}, about 3.1.

To prepare 0.05M bromine dissolve 3 g of *potassium bromate* and 15 g of *potassium bromide* in sufficient *water* to produce 1000 ml. Weaker solutions should be prepared using proportionately lesser amounts of reagents or by appropriate dilution.

Bromine Solution Dissolve 30 g of *bromine* and 30 g of *potassium bromide* in sufficient *water* to produce 100 ml.

Bromine Solution, Acetic Dissolve 100 g of *potassium acetate* in *glacial acetic acid* and add 4 ml of *bromine* and sufficient *glacial acetic acid* to produce 1000 ml.

Bromine Water A saturated solution obtained by shaking occasionally during 24 hours 3 ml of *bromine* with 100 ml of *water* and allowing to separate.
Store the solution over an excess of *bromine*, protected from light.

Bromine Water R1 Shake 0.5 ml of *bromine* with 100 ml of *water.*
Store protected from light for not longer than 1 week.

α-Bromo-2′-acetonaphthone 2-Bromo-2′-acetonaphthone; $C_{12}H_9BrO$ = 249.1 *(613-54-7)*
General reagent grade of commerce.
Melting point, about 83°.

Bromobenzene C_6H_5Br = 157.0 (*108-86-1*)
General reagent grade of commerce.
A colourless to pale yellow liquid; boiling point, about 156°; n_D^{20}, about 1.56; weight per ml, about 1.50 g.

Bromocresol Green 4,4′-(3*H*-2,1-Benzoxathiol-3-ylidene)bis(2,6-dibromo-*m*-cresol) *S,S*-dioxide; $C_{21}H_{14}Br_4O_5S$ = 698 *(76-60-8)*
Produces a yellow colour in moderately acidic solutions and a blue colour in weakly acidic and alkaline solutions.

Bromocresol Green Solution Dissolve 50 mg of *bromocresol green* in 0.72 ml of 0.1M *sodium hydroxide* and 20 ml of *ethanol (96%)*. After solution is effected add sufficient *water* to produce 100 ml (colour change: pH 3.6 (yellow) to pH 5.2 (blue)).
Complies with the following test.
SENSITIVITY A mixture of 0.2 ml of the solution and 100 ml of *carbon dioxide-free water* is blue. Not more than 0.2 ml of 0.02M *hydrochloric acid VS* is required to change the colour of the solution to yellow.

Bromocresol Green-Methyl Red Solution Dissolve 0.15 g of *bromocresol green* and 0.1 g of *methyl red* in 180 ml of *absolute ethanol* and dilute to 200 ml with *water.*

Bromocresol Purple 4,4′-(3*H*-2,1-Benzoxathiol-3-ylidene)bis(6-bromo-*o*-cresol) *S,S*-dioxide; $C_{21}H_{16}Br_2O_5S$ = 540.2 (*115-40-2*)
Produces a yellow colour in weakly acidic solutions and a bluish violet colour in alkaline, neutral and extremely weakly acidic solutions.

Bromocresol Purple Solution Dissolve 50 mg of *bromocresol purple* in 0.92 ml of 0.1M *sodium hydroxide* and 20 ml of *ethanol (96%)* and add sufficient *water* to produce 100 ml (colour change pH 5.2 (yellow) to pH 6.8 (bluish-violet)).
Complies with the following test.
SENSITIVITY A mixture of 0.2 ml of the solution and 100 ml of *carbon dioxide-free water* to which 0.05 ml of 0.02M *sodium hydroxide VS* has been added is bluish violet. Not more than 0.2 ml of 0.02M *hydrochloric acid VS* is required to change the colour of the solution to yellow.

5-Bromo-2′-deoxyuridine $C_9H_{11}BrN_2O_5$ = 307.1 (*59-14-3*)
General reagent grade of commerce.
Melting point, about 194°.
Complies with the following test.
HOMOGENEITY Examine under the conditions prescribed in the test for Related substances in the monograph for Idoxuridine applying to the plate 5 µl of a 0.025% w/v solution. The chromatogram shows only one principal spot.

Bromophenol Blue 4,4′-(3*H*-2,1-Benzoxathiol-3-ylidene) bis(2,6-dibromophenol) *S,S*-dioxide; $C_{19}H_{10}Br_4O_5S$ = 670 (*115-39-9*)
Produces a yellow colour in moderately acidic solutions and a bluish violet colour in weakly acidic and alkaline solutions.

Bromophenol Blue Solution Dissolve 0.1 g of *bromophenol blue* in 1.5 ml of 0.1M *sodium hydroxide* and 20 ml of *ethanol (96%)* and add sufficient *water* to produce 100 ml (pH range, 2.8 to 4.6).
Complies with the following test.
SENSITIVITY A mixture of 0.05 ml of the solution and 20 ml of *carbon dioxide-free water* to which 0.05 ml of 0.1M *hydrochloric acid VS* has been added is yellow. Not more than 0.1 ml of 0.1M *sodium hydroxide VS* is required to change the colour to bluish violet.

Bromophenol Blue Solution R1 Dissolve 50 mg of *bromophenol blue* with gentle heating in 3.73 ml of 0.02M *sodium hydroxide* and dilute to 100 ml with *water*.

Bromophenol Blue Solution R2 Dissolve with heating 0.2 g of *bromophenol blue* in 3 ml of 0.1M *sodium hydroxide* and 10 ml of *ethanol (96%)*. Allow to cool and dilute to 100 ml with *ethanol (96%)*.

Bromothymol Blue 4,4′-(3*H*-2,1-Benzoxathiol-3-ylidene)bis(2-bromothymol) *S,S*-dioxide; $C_{27}H_{28}Br_2O_5S$ = 624 (*76-59-5*)
Produces a yellow colour in weakly acidic solutions and a blue colour in weakly alkaline solutions. Neutrality is indicated by a green colour.

Bromothymol Blue Solution R1
Dissolve 50 mg of *bromothymol blue* in a mixture of 4 ml of 0.02M *sodium hydroxide* and 20 ml of *ethanol (96%)* and dilute to 100 ml with *water* (pH range, 6.0 to 7.6).
Complies with the following test.
SENSITIVITY A mixture of 0.3 ml of the solution and 100 ml of *carbon dioxide-free water* is yellow. Not more than 0.1 ml of 0.02M *sodium hydroxide VS* is required to change the colour of the solution to blue.

Bromothymol Blue Solution R2 A 1% w/v solution of *bromothymol blue* in *dimethylformamide*.

Bromothymol Blue Solution R3 Warm 0.1 g of *bromothymol blue* with 3.2 ml of 0.05M *sodium hydroxide* and 5 ml of *ethanol (90%)*. After solution is effected, add sufficient *ethanol (90%)* to produce 250 ml.

BRP Indicator Solution Dissolve 0.1 g of *bromothymol blue*, 20 mg of *methyl red* and 0.2 g of *phenolphthalein* in sufficient *ethanol (96%)* to produce 100 ml; filter.

Brucine 10,11-Dimethoxystrychnine; $C_{23}H_{26}N_2O_4,2H_2O$ = 430.5 (*357-57-3*)
General reagent grade of commerce.
Melting point, about 178°.

Butane-1,3-diol $C_4H_{10}O_2$ = 90.1 (*6290-03-5*)
General reagent grade of commerce.
Boiling point, about 203°; n_D^{20}, about 1.440.

Butanol See *butan-1-ol.*

Butan-1-ol *n*-Butyl alcohol; butanol; $C_4H_{10}O$ = 74.12 (*71-36-3*)
Analytical reagent grade of commerce.
A colourless liquid; boiling point, 116° to 119°; d_{20}^{20}, about 0.81.

Butan-1-ol FT
A grade of butan-l-ol specially purified for the determination of 17-ketosteroids.

2-Butanol R1 See *Butan-2-ol R1.*

Butan-2-ol *sec*-Butyl alcohol; 2-butanol; $C_4H_{10}O$ = 74.12 (*78-92-2*)
Analytical reagent grade of commerce.
A colourless liquid; boiling point, about 99°; d_{20}^{20}, about 0.81.

Butan-2-ol R1 *Butan-2-ol* complying with the following requirements.
DISTILLATION RANGE Not less than 95% distils between 99° and 100°, Appendix V C.
ASSAY Contains not less than 99.0% of $C_4H_{10}O$ when examined by the method for Benzene and other related substances in the monograph for Isopropyl Alcohol.

Butan-2-one Methyl ethyl ketone; ethyl methyl ketone; C_4H_8O = 72.11 (*78-93-3*)
Chromatographic reagent grade of commerce.
A colourless, flammable liquid, with a characteristic odour; boiling point, about 79°; d_{20}^{20}, about 0.81.

Butyl Acetate $C_6H_{12}O_2$ = 116.2 (*123-86-4*)
Analytical reagent grade of commerce.
A colourless flammable liquid with a strong, fruity odour; d_{20}^{20}, about 0.88 g; n_D^{20}, about 1.395.

Butyl Acetate R1 A grade of *butyl acetate* specially purified for use in liquid chromatography containing not less than 99.5% of $C_6H_{12}O_2$ and not more than 0.2% of butan-1-ol, 0.1% of *n*-butyl formate, 0.1% of *n*-butyl propionate and 0.1% of water, determined by gas chromatography.

Butyl Chloride See *1-chlorobutane.*

***tert*-Butyl Methyl Ether** *See 1,1-dimethylethyl methyl ether.*

Butyl Parahydroxybenzoate Butyl hydroxybenzoate; $C_{11}H_{14}O_3$ = 194.2 (*94-26-8*)
General reagent grade of commerce.

Butylamine See n-*Butylamine.*

***n*-Butylamine** Butylamine; $C_4H_{11}N$ = 73.1 (*109-73-9*)
General reagent grade of commerce.
A colourless liquid with an ammoniacal odour; boiling point, about 78°; n_D^{20}, about 1.401.
Distil and use within 1 month.

***tert*-Butylamine** See *1,1-dimethylethylamine.*

Butylated Hydroxyanisole 2-*tert*-Butyl-4-methoxyphenol; $C_{11}H_{16}O_2$ = 180.2 (*25013-16-5*)
General reagent grade of commerce.
A white or almost white, crystalline powder; melting point, about 61°.

Butylated Hydroxytoluene 2,6-Di-*tert*-butyl-*p*-cresol; $C_{15}H_{24}O$ = 220.4 (*128-37-0*)
General reagent grade of commerce.
Colourless crystals or a white, crystalline powder; melting point, about 70°.

Butylboronic Acid $C_4H_{11}BO_2$ = 101.9 (*4426-47-5*)
General reagent grade of commerce containing not less than 98% of $C_4H_{11}BO_2$.
Melting point, 90° to 92°.

Butylhydroxytoluene see *butylated hydroxytoluene.*

Butyric Acid *n*-Butyric acid; butanoic acid; $C_4H_8O_2$ = 88.1 (*107-92-6*)
General reagent grade of commerce.
An oily liquid; weight per ml, about 0.96 g.

Butyrolactone Dihydro-2(3*H*)-furanone; γ-butyrolactone; $C_4H_6O_2$ = 86.1
General reagent grade of commerce.
n_D^{25}, about 1.435; boiling point, about 204°.

Cadmium Cd = 112.4 (*10108-64-2*)
A silvery white, lustrous metal; freely soluble in *nitric acid* and hot *hydrochloric acid.*

Cadmium Acetate $C_4H_6O_4Cd,2H_2O$ = 266.5 (*5743-04-4*)
Analytical reagent grade of commerce.

Cadmium and Ninhydrin Solution Dissolve 50 mg of *cadmium acetate* in a mixture of 5 ml of *water* and 1 ml of *glacial acetic acid* and dilute with *butan-2-one* to 50 ml. Immediately before use add and dissolve sufficient *ninhydrin* to produce a solution containing 0.2% w/v.

Cadmium Iodide CdI_2 = 366.2 (*7790-80-9*)
Analytical reagent grade of commerce.

Cadmium Iodide Solution A 5.0% w/v solution of *cadmium iodide.*

Caesium Chloride CsCl = 168.4 (*7647-17-8*)
Analytical reagent grade of commerce.

Caffeic Acid 3,4-Dihydroxycinnamic acid; $C_9H_8O_4$ = 180.2 (*331-39-5*)
General reagent grade of commerce.
White or almost white crystals; melting point, about 225°, with decomposition.
A freshly prepared solution at pH 7.6 shows two absorption maxima, at 293 nm and at 329 nm, Appendix II B.

Caffeine $C_8H_{10}N_4O_2$ = 194.2 (*58-08-2*)
General reagent grade of commerce.
Melting point, about 236°.

Calciferol Ergocalciferol; vitamin D_2; $C_{28}H_{44}O$ = 396.7 (*50-14-6*)
Crystalline reagent grade of commerce.
Colourless crystals or a white, crystalline powder; melting point, about 117°; $[\alpha]_D^{20}$, about +105° (4% w/v in ethanol).

Calcium Acetate, Dried $C_4H_6O_4Ca$ = 158.2 (*62-54-4*)
General reagent grade of commerce.

Calcium Carbonate $CaCO_3$ = 100.1 (*471-34-1*)
Analytical reagent grade of commerce.

Calcium Chloride $CaCl_2,2H_2O$ = 147.0 (*10035-04-8*)
Analytical reagent grade of commerce.

Calcium Chloride, Anhydrous $CaCl_2$ = 111.0 (*10043-52-4*)
Reagent grade of commerce containing not less than 98.0% of $CaCl_2$, calculated with reference to the dried substance.
Deliquescent, white granules.
Complies with the following test.
LOSS ON DRYING When dried to constant weight at 200°, loses not more than 5.0% of its weight.
Store in an airtight container, protected from moisture.

Calcium Chloride R1 Calcium chloride tetrahydrate; $CaCl_2,4H_2O$ = 183.1
General reagent grade of commerce containing not more than 0.05 ppm of Fe.

Calcium Chloride Solution A 7.35% w/v solution of *calcium chloride.*

Calcium Chloride Solution, 0.01M Dissolve 0.147 g of *calcium chloride* in sufficient *water* to produce 100 ml.

Calcium Chloride Solution, 0.02M Dissolve 2.94 g of *calcium chloride* in 900 ml of *water,* adjust to pH 6.0 to 6.2 and dilute to 1000 ml with *water.*
Store at 2° to 8°.

Calcium Hydroxide $Ca(OH)_2$ = 74.09 (*1305-62-0*)
Analytical reagent grade of commerce.

Calcium Hydroxide Solution A freshly prepared saturated solution which may be prepared in the following manner. Shake 10 g of *calcium hydroxide* repeatedly with 1000 ml of *water* and allow to stand until clear.

Calcium Lactate (*41372-22-9*)
Calcium Lactate Pentahydrate of the British Pharmacopoeia.

Calcium Sulphate Calcium sulphate hemihydrate; plaster of Paris; $CaSO_4,\frac{1}{2}H_2O$ = 145.1 (*10101-41-4*)
A white powder which when mixed with half its weight of water rapidly solidifies to a hard and porous mass.

Calcium Sulphate Solution Shake 5 g of *calcium sulphate hemihydrate* for 1 hour with 100 ml of *water* and filter.

Calconcarboxylic Acid Patton and Reeder's reagent; 2-hydroxy-1-(2-hydroxy-4-sulpho-1-naphthylazo)-naphthalene-3-carboxylic acid; $C_{21}H_{14}N_2O_7S,3H_2O$ = 492.5 (*3737-95-9*)
General reagent grade of commerce.
A brownish black powder. Produces a sharp colour change from red to blue in titrations of calcium with disodium edetate.

Calconcarboxylic Acid Triturate A mixture of 1 part of *calconcarboxylic acid* and 99 parts of *sodium chloride.*
Complies with the following test.
SENSITIVITY TO CALCIUM Dissolve 50 mg in a mixture of 100 ml of *water* and 2 ml of 10M *sodium hydroxide*; a blue colour is produced. Add 1 ml of a 1% w/v solution of *magnesium sulphate* and 0.1 ml of a 0.15% w/v solution of *calcium chloride*; a violet colour is produced. Add 0.15 ml of 0.01M *disodium edetate VS*; a pure blue colour is produced.

(1*S*)-(+)-10-Camphorsulphonic Acid $C_{10}H_{16}O_4S$ = 232.3 (*3144-16-9*)
Prismatic crystals; hygroscopic.
General reagent grade of commerce containing not less than 99.0% of $C_{10}H_{16}O_4S$.
Melting point, about 194°, with decomposition; $[\alpha]_D^{20}$, +19° to +21° (4.3% w/v solution in *water*).

ε-Caprolactam Hexane-6-lactam; $C_6H_{11}NO$ = 113.2 (*105-60-2*)
General reagent grade of commerce.
Melting point, about 70°.

Carbazole Dibenzopyrrole; $C_{12}H_9N$ = 167.2 (*86-74-8*)
General reagent grade of commerce.
Melting point, about 245°.

Carbomer (*9007-20-9*) A cross-linked polymer of acrylic acid containing a large proportion (56% to 68%) of carboxylic acid (COOH) groups after drying at 80° for 1 hour.
General reagent grade of commerce.
Average relative molecular weight, about 3×10^6.

Carbon Dioxide CO_2 = 44.01 (*124-38-9*)
Laboratory cylinder grade of commerce.

Carbon Dioxide R1 *Carbon dioxide* containing not less than 99.995% v/v of CO_2.
CARBON MONOXIDE Less than 5 ppm.
OXYGEN Less than 25 ppm.

Carbon Disulphide CS_2 = 76.14 (*75-15-0*)
Analytical reagent grade of commerce.
A colourless, volatile, flammable liquid with an unpleasant odour; boiling point, about 46°; weight per ml, about 1.26 g.

Carbon for Chromatography, Graphitised Carbon chains having a length greater than C_9 with a particle size of 400 to 850 µm.
Chromatographic reagent grade of commerce.
Density, 0.72; surface area, 10 $m^2 g^{-1}$.
Do not use at a temperature higher than 400°.

Carbon Monoxide CO = 28.01 (*630-08-0*)
General reagent grade of commerce containing not less than 99.97% v/v of CO.

Carbon Tetrachloride Tetrachloromethane; CCl_4 = 153.8 (*56-23-5*)
Analytical reagent grade of commerce.
A colourless liquid with a characteristic odour; boiling point, 76° to 77°; d_{20}^{20}, about 1.59.

Carbophenothion *O,O*-Diethyl *S*-{[(4-chlorophenyl)-thio]methyl}phosphorodithioate; $C_{11}H_{16}ClO_2PS_3$ = 342.9 (*786-19-6*)
Chromatographic reagent grade of commerce.
d_4^{25}, about 1.27.

Carob Bean Gum The ground endosperm of the fruit kernels of *Ceratonia siliqua* L. Taub.
A white powder containing 70 to 80% of a water-soluble gum consisting mainly of galactomannoglycone.

Carvacrol 5-Isopropyl-2-methylphenol; $C_{10}H_{14}O$ = 150.2 (*499-75-2*)
General reagent grade of commerce.
d_{20}^{20}, about 0.975; n_D^{20}, about 1.523; boiling point, about 237°.

Carvone *p*-Mentha-6,8-dien-2-one; (+)-2-methyl-5-(1-methylethenyl)cyclohex-2-enone; $C_{10}H_{14}O$ = 150.2 (*2244-16-8*)
General reagent grade of commerce.
d_{20}^{20}, about 0.965; n_D^{20}, about 1.500; $[\alpha]_D^{20}$, about +61°; boiling point, about 230°.
Carvone used in gas chromatography complies with the following test.
ASSAY Examine by gas chromatography, Appendix III B, under the conditions described in the test for Chromatographic profile in the monograph for Peppermint Oil using the reagent being examined.
The area of the principal peak is not less than 98.0% of the total area of the peaks.

β-Caryophyllene (*E*)-(1*R*,9*S*)-4,11,11-Trimethyl-8-methylenebicyclo[7.2.0]undec-4-ene; $C_{15}H_{24}$ = 204.4 (*87-44-5*)
General reagent grade of commerce.
d_4^{17}, about 0.905; n_D^{20}, about 1.492; $[\alpha]_D^{15}$, about −5.2°.
β-Caryophyllene used in gas chromatography complies with the following requirement.
ASSAY Carry out the test for Chromatographic profile in the monograph for Clove Oil using the reagent being examined as the test solution. The area of the principal peak is not less than 98.5% of the total area of the peaks.

Casein (*9000-71-9*) A mixture of related phosphoproteins obtained from milk.
General reagent grade of commerce.
White, amorphous powder or granules.

Casein Substrate, Concentrated Suspend a quantity of *casein EPBRP* equivalent to 2.5 g in 5 ml of *water*, add 18 ml of 0.1M *sodium hydroxide* and stir for 1 minute. Add 60 ml of *water* and stir with a magnetic stirrer until the solution is practically clear. Adjust the pH of the solution to 8.0 with either 0.1M *sodium hydroxide* or 0.1M *hydrochloric acid* and add sufficient *water* to produce 100 ml. Use on the day of preparation.

Catechol Pyrocatechol; benzene-1,2-diol; $C_6H_6O_2$ = 110.1 (*120-80-9*)
General reagent grade of commerce.
A white, crystalline powder; melting point, about 103°.
Store protected from light.

Cation Exchange Resin A resin in protonated form with sulphonic groups attached to a polymer lattice consisting of polystyrene cross-linked with 8% of divinylbenzene. It is available as beads and the particle size is specified after the name of the reagent in tests where it is used.

Cation Exchange Resin (Calcium Form), Strong A resin in calcium form with sulphonic acid groups attached to a polymer lattice consisting of polystyrene cross-linked with 8% of divinylbenzene. The particle size is specified after the name of the reagent in tests where it is used.

Cationic Resin, Weak Polymethacrylic resin
A weak cationic resin, slightly acidic with carboxyl groups present in a protonated form, of particle size 75 to 160 µm. The resin should be used within the pH limits of 5 to 14 and should not be used at temperatures above 120°.

Cedarwood Oil A grade of commerce for microscopy thickened as necessary in temperate or tropical climates.

Cellulose See *cellulose for chromatography*.

Cellulose for Chromatography (*9004-34-6*) A fine, white, homogeneous powder of an average particle size of less than 30 µm.
PREPARATION OF A THIN-LAYER Suspend 15 g in 100 ml of *water* and homogenise in an electric mixer for 60 seconds. Coat carefully cleaned plates with a layer 0.1-mm thick using a spreading device and allow to dry in air.

Cellulose for Chromatography R1 Microcrystalline cellulose
A fine, white, homogeneous powder of an average particle size of less than 30 µm.
PREPARATION OF A THIN-LAYER Suspend 25 g in 90 ml of *water* and homogenise in an electric mixer for 60 seconds. Coat carefully cleaned plates with a layer 0.1-mm thick using a spreading device and allow to dry in air.

Cellulose for Chromatography F_{254} A fine, white, homogeneous powder of an average particle size of less than 30 µm containing a fluorescent indicator with an optimal intensity at 254 nm.
PREPARATION OF A THIN-LAYER Suspend 25 g in 100 ml of *water* and homogenise in an electric mixer for 60 seconds. Coat carefully cleaned plates with a layer 0.1-mm thick using a spreading device and allow to dry in air.

Cellulose F_{254} See *cellulose for chromatography F_{254}*.

Cellulose, Microcrystalline See *cellulose for chromatography R1*.

Cephaeline Dihydrochloride Cephaeline hydrochloride; $C_{28}H_{38}N_2O_4,2HCl,7H_2O$ = 665.6 (*5884-43-5*)
General reagent grade of commerce.
A white to yellowish, crystalline powder; $[\alpha]_D^{20}$, about +25° (2% w/v in water).

Cephalin Reagent Solvents used to prepare this reagent should contain a suitable antioxidant such as *butylated hydroxyanisole* at a concentration of 0.002% w/v.

To 0.5 to 1 g of *acetone-dried ox brain* add 20 ml of *acetone* and leave for 2 hours. Centrifuge for 2 minutes at 500 *g* and decant the supernatant liquid. Dry the residue under reduced pressure and extract the dried material with 20 ml of *chloroform* for 2 hours, shaking the mixture frequently. After removal of the solid material by filtration or centrifugation, evaporate the chloroform from the extract under reduced pressure. Suspend the residue in 5 to 10 ml of *saline solution*. This stock emulsion may be stored frozen or freeze-dried for 3 months.

Cerium(III) Nitrate Cerous nitrate; $Ce(NO_3)_3,6H_2O$ = 434.2 (*10294-41-4*)
General reagent grade of commerce.
A colourless or pale yellow crystalline powder.

Cerium(III) Nitrate Solution Dissolve 0.22 g of *cerium(III) nitrate* in 50 ml of *water*, add 0.1 ml of *nitric acid* and 50 mg of *hydroxylamine hydrochloride* and dilute to 1000 ml with *water*.

Cerium Sulphate See *cerium(IV) sulphate*.

Cerium(IV) Sulphate Ceric sulphate; $Ce(SO_4)_2,4H_2O$ = 404.3 (*123333-60-8*)
General reagent grade of commerce.
Yellow or orange-yellow crystalline powder or crystals.

Cerous Nitrate See *cerium(III) nitrate*.

Cetostearyl Alcohol (*67762-27-0*) Of the British Pharmacopoeia.

Cetrimide (*8044-71-1*) Of the British Pharmacopoeia.

Cetylpyridinium Chloride $C_{21}H_{38}ClN,H_2O$ = 358.0 (*6004-24-6*)
General reagent grade of commerce.
A white powder; melting point, about 81°.

Cetyltrimethylammonium Bromide Cetrimonium bromide; *N*-hexadecyl-*N,N,N*-trimethylammonium bromide; $C_{19}H_{42}BrN$ = 364.5 (*57-09-0*)
General reagent grade of commerce.
A white, crystalline powder; melting point, about 240°.

Charcoal, Activated (*64365-11-3*)
Of the British Pharmacopoeia.

Chloral Hydrate $C_2H_3Cl_3O_2$ = 165.4 (*302-17-0*)
General reagent grade of commerce.
Colourless, hygroscopic crystals with a sharp odour; melting point, about 55°.

Chloral Hydrate Solution Dissolve 80 g of *chloral hydrate* in 20 ml of *water*.

Chloramine See *chloramine T*.

Chloramine Solution A 2% w/v solution of *chloramine T* prepared immediately before use.

Chloramine Solution R1 A 0.01% w/v solution of *chloramine T* prepared immediately before use.

Chloramine Solution R2 A 0.02% w/v solution of *chloramine T* prepared immediately before use.

Chloramine T Chloramine
The sodium salt of *N*-chlorotoluene-*p*-sulphonamide; $C_7H_7ClNNaO_2S,3H_2O$ = 281.7 (*55-86-7*)
General reagent grade of commerce.

Chlorhexidine Acetate Chlorhexidine diacetate; $C_{22}H_{30}Cl_2N_{10},2C_2H_4O_2$ = 625.6 (*56-95-1*)
General reagent grade of commerce.
Melting point, about 154°.

Chlorhexidine Hydrochloride Chlorhexidine dihydrochloride; $C_{22}H_{30}Cl_2N_{10},2HCl$ (*3697-42-5*)
General reagent grade of commerce.

Chloroacetanilide See *4′-chloroacetanilide*.

4′-Chloroacetanilide Chloroacetanilide; C_8H_8ClNO = 169.6 (*539-03-7*)
General reagent grade of commerce.
Colourless, rhombic crystals or plates; melting point, about 178°.

Chloroacetic Acid $C_2H_3ClO_2$ = 94.50 (*79-11-8*)
Analytical reagent grade of commerce.
Colourless, deliquescent crystals; melting point, about 62°.
Store in an airtight container.

Chloroaniline See *4-chloroaniline*.

3-Chloroaniline C_6H_6ClN = 127.6 (*108-42-9*)
General reagent grade of commerce.
n_D^{20}, about 1.594.

4-Chloroaniline Chloroaniline; C_6H_6ClN = 127.6 (*106-47-8*)
General reagent grade of commerce.
White or faintly coloured crystals; melting point, about 71°.

Chloroauric Acid Gold chloride; hydrogen tetrachloroaurate; $HAuCl_4$+aq (*27988-77-8*)
General reagent grade of commerce.
Brown, deliquescent masses.

Chloroauric Acid Solution General reagent grade of commerce containing about 2% w/v of $HAuCl_4,3H_2O$, or a 2.0% w/v solution of *chloroauric acid* in *water*.

Chlorobenzene C_6H_5Cl = 112.6 (*108-90-7*)
Analytical reagent grade of commerce.
A colourless liquid; boiling point, about 131°.

4-Chlorobenzenesulphonamide $C_6H_6ClNO_2S$ = 191.6 (*98-64-6*)
General reagent grade of commerce.
Melting point, about 145°.

4-Chlorobenzoic Acid $C_7H_5ClO_2$ = 156.57 (*74-11-3*)
General reagent grade of commerce.
Melting point, about 240°.

3-(4-Chlorobenzoyl)propionic Acid $C_{10}H_9ClNO_3$ = 212.6 (*3984-34-7*)
General reagent grade of commerce.
Melting point, about 129°.

1-Chlorobutane Butyl chloride; C_4H_9Cl = 92.57 (*109 69-3*)
General reagent grade of commerce.
Boiling point, about 78°; weight per ml, about 0.886 g; n_D^{20}, about 1.402.

Chlorobutanol Anhydrous chlorbutol; 1,1,1-trichloro-2-methylpropan-2-ol; $C_4H_7Cl_3O$ = 177.5 (*57-15-8*)
General reagent grade of commerce.
Melting point, about 95°.

4-Chloro-*o*-cresol 4-Chloro-2-methylphenol; C_7H_7ClO = 142.6 (*1570-64-5*)
General reagent grade of commerce.
Melting point, about 144°.

1-Chloro-2,4-dinitrobenzene $C_6H_3ClN_2O_4$ = 202.6 (*97-00-7*)
Analytical reagent grade of commerce.
Pale yellow crystals or crystalline powder; melting point, about 51°.

2-Chloroethanol Ethylene chlorohydrin; C_2H_5ClO = 80.5 (*107-07-3*)
General reagent grade of commerce.
d_{20}^{20}, about 1.197; n_D^{20}, about 1.442; boiling point, about 130°; melting point, about −89°.

2-Chloroethanol Solution Dissolve 125 mg of *2-chloroethanol* in sufficient *propan-2-ol* to produce 50 ml and dilute 5 ml of the solution to 50 ml with *propan-2-ol.*

(2-Chloroethyl)diethylamine Hydrochloride 2-Diethylaminoethyl chloride hydrochloride; $C_6H_{14}ClN,HCl$ = 172.1 (*869-24-9*)
General reagent grade of commerce.
Melting point, about 211°.

Chloroform Trichloromethane; $CHCl_3$ = 119.4 (*67-66-3*)
Analytical reagent grade of commerce containing 0.4 to 1.0% w/w of ethanol.
A colourless liquid with a sweet, penetrating odour; boiling point, about 60°; d_{20}^{20}, 1.475 to 1.481.

Chloroform, Acidified To 100 ml of *chloroform* add 10 ml of *hydrochloric acid.* Shake, allow to stand and separate the two layers.

Chloroform, Ethanol-free Shake 200 ml of *chloroform* with four 100-ml quantities of *water* and dry over 20 g of *anhydrous sodium sulphate* for 24 hours. Distil the filtrate over 10 g of *anhydrous sodium sulphate* and discard the first 20 ml of distillate.
Prepare immediately before use.

Chloroform IR
Spectroscopic reagent grade of commerce.

Chloroform Stabilised with Amylene $CHCl_3$ = 119.4
Analytical reagent grade of commerce containing not less than 99.8% of $CHCl_3$, determined by gas chromatography.
Complies with the following requirements.
WATER Not more than 0.05%.
RESIDUE ON EVAPORATION Not more than 0.001%.
TRANSMITTANCE Not less than 50% at 255 nm, 80% at 260 nm and 98% at 300 nm using *water* in the reference cell.

Chloroform Water Shake 2.5 ml of *chloroform* with 900 ml of *water* until dissolved and dilute to 1000 ml with *water.*

Chlorogenic Acid $C_{16}H_{18}O_9$ = 354.3 (*327-97-9*)
General reagent grade of commerce.
Melting point, about 208°; $[\alpha]_D^{26}$, about −35.2°.

5-Chloro-8-hydroxyquinoline 5-Chloroquinolin-8-ol; C_9H_6ClNO = 179.6 (*130-16-5*)
General reagent grade of commerce.
Melting point, about 123°.

2-Chloro-4-nitroaniline $C_6H_5ClN_2O_2$ = 172.6 (*121-87-9*)
General reagent grade of commerce.
A yellow to brown, crystalline powder; melting point, about 107°.
Store protected from light.

Chlorophenol See *4-chlorophenol.*

4-Chlorophenol Chlorophenol; C_6H_5ClO= 128.6 (*106-48-9*)
General reagent grade of commerce.
Colourless or slightly coloured crystals; melting point, about 42°.

Chloroplatinic Acid See *chloroplatinic(IV) acid.*

Chloroplatinic(IV) Acid Chloroplatinic acid; platinic chloride; H_2PtCl_6+aq (*18497-13-7*)
General reagent grade of commerce containing not less than 37% w/w of Pt.
Deliquescent, brown, crystalline masses.
ASSAY Ignite 0.2 g to constant weight at 900° and weigh the residue (platinum).
Store protected from light.

Chloroplatinic Acid Solution A solution of *chloroplatinic(IV) acid* in *water,* containing the equivalent of 5.0% w/v of $H_2PtCl_6,6H_2O$.

3-Chloropropane-1,2-diol $C_3H_7ClO_2$ = 110.5 (*96-24-2*)
General reagent grade of commerce.
d_{20}^{20}, about 1.322; n_D^{20}, about 1.480; boiling point, about 213°.

1-Chloropropyl(dimethylamine) Hydrochloride 3-Dimethylaminopropyl chloride hydrochloride; $C_5H_{12}ClN$ = 158.1 (*5407-04-5*)
General reagent grade of commerce.
Melting point, about 142°.

5-Chlorosalicylic Acid $C_7H_5ClO_3$ = 172.6 (*321-14-2*)
General reagent grade of commerce.
A white or almost white, crystalline powder; melting point, about 173°.

Chlorothiazide $C_7H_6ClN_3O_4S_2$ = 295.7 (*58-94-6*)
General reagent grade of commerce.

Chlorotrimethylsilane See *trimethylchlorosilane.*

Chlorotriphenylmethane Triphenylchloromethane; triphenylmethyl chloride; $C_{19}H_{15}Cl$ = 278.8 (*76-83-5*)
General reagent grade of commerce.
A pale yellow or buff, crystalline solid; melting point, about 112°.

Cholesterol $C_{27}H_{46}O$ = 386.7 (*57-88-5*)
General reagent grade of commerce.
A white, waxy powder or leaflets; melting point, about 147°; $[\alpha]_D^{20}$, about −39° (2% w/v in chloroform).

Choline Chloride (2-Hydroxyethyl)trimethylammonium chloride; $C_5H_{14}ClNO$ = 139.6 (*67-48-1*)
General reagent grade of commerce complying with the following test.
HOMOGENEITY Carry out the test for Choline chloride described under Suxamethonium Chloride applying to the plate 5 µl of a 0.02% w/v solution in *methanol.* The chromatogram obtained shows one principal spot.
Store in an airtight container.

Chrome Azurol S CI 43825; Trisodium 5-[(3-carboxylato-5-methyl-4-oxocyclohexa-2,5-dien-1-ylidene)(2,6-dichloro-3-sulphonatophenyl)methyl]-2-hydroxy-3-methylbenzoate; $C_{23}H_{13}Cl_2Na_3O_9S$ = 605 (*1667-99-8*)
Indicator grade of commerce.
A brownish black powder.

Chromic Acid Cleansing Mixture See *chromic—sulphuric acid mixture.*

Chromic Potassium Sulphate See *chromium(III) potassium sulphate.*

Chromic—Sulphuric Acid Mixture A saturated solution of *chromium(VI) oxide* in *sulphuric acid.*

Chromium(VI) Oxide Chromium trioxide; CrO_3 = 99.99 (*1333-82-0*)
Dark brownish-red needles or granules, deliquescent.
Analytical reagent grade of commerce.
Store in an airtight container.

Chromium(III) Potassium Sulphate Chrome alum; chromic potassium sulphate; $CrK(SO_4)_2,12H_2O$ = 499.4 *(7788-99-0)*
Analytical reagent grade of commerce.
Large, violet-red to black crystals.

Chromium(III) Trichloride Hexahydrate $[Cr(H_2O)_4Cl_2]Cl,2H_2O$ = 266.5 *(10060-12-5)*
A dark green, crystalline powder; hygroscopic.
General reagent grade of commerce.
Store protected from humidity and oxidising agents.

Chromium Trioxide *See chromium(VI) oxide.*

Chromophore Substrate R1 Dissolve *N*-α-benzyloxycarbonyl-D-arginyl-L-glycyl-L-arginine *p*-nitroanilide dihydrochloride in *water* to give a 3 millimolar solution. Dilute in *tris—EDTA buffer pH 8.4* to 0.5 millimolar before use.

Chromophore Substrate R2 Dissolve D-phenylalanyl-piperazine-arginine *p*-nitroanilide dihydrochloride in *water* to give a 3 millimolar solution. Dilute in *trisEDTA buffer pH 8.4* to 0.5 millimolar before use.

Chromotrope IIB Chromotrope 2B; CI 16575; $C_{16}H_9N_3Na_2O_{10}S_2$ = 513.4 *(548-80-1)*
General reagent grade of commerce.
A reddish brown powder.

Chromotrope IIB Solution Chromotrope 2B solution
A 0.005% w/v solution of *chromotrope IIB* in *sulphuric acid.*

Chromotropic Acid Sodium Salt Disodium 4,5-dihydroxynaphthalene-2,7-disulphonate; $C_{10}H_6Na_2O_8S_2$, $2H_2O$ = 400.3 *(5808-22-0)*
General reagent grade of commerce.
A pale brown powder.

Chromotropic Acid Solution Dissolve 5 mg of *chromotropic acid sodium salt* in 10 ml of a mixture of 9 ml of *sulphuric acid* and 4 ml of *water.*
Complies with the following test.
SENSITIVITY TO FORMALDEHYDE To 13 ml add 5 ml of a solution containing 1 µg of *formaldehyde* per ml and heat in a water bath for 30 minutes. A violet colour is apparent when compared with a solution prepared in the same manner using *water* in place of the formaldehyde solution.

Cinchonidine $C_{19}H_{22}N_2O$ = 294.4 *(485-71-2)*
General reagent grade of commerce.
A white, crystalline powder; melting point, about 208° with decomposition; $[\alpha]_D^{20}$, −105° to −110° (5% w/v in ethanol).
Store protected from light.

Cinchonine $C_{19}H_{22}N_2O$ = 294.4 *(118-10-5)*
General reagent grade of commerce.
A white, crystalline powder; melting point, about 263°; $[\alpha]_D^{20}$, +225° to +230° (5% w/v in ethanol).
Store protected from light.

Cineole Eucalyptol; 1,8-epoxy-*p*-menthane; $C_{10}H_{18}O$ = 154.3 *(470-82-6)*
Use a grade of commerce specially supplied for *o*-cresol determinations.
A colourless liquid with a camphoraceous odour; boiling point, about 176°; d_{20}^{20}, 0.922 to 0.927; n_D^{20}, 1.465 to 1.459.
Cineole used in gas chromatography complies with the following test.
ASSAY Examine by *gas chromatography*, Appendix III B, under the conditions described in the test for Chromatographic profile in the monograph for Peppermint Oil using the reagent being examined.
The area of the principal peak is not less than 98.0% of the total area of the peaks.

Cinnamaldehyde Cinnamic aldehyde; C_9H_8O = 132.2 *(104-55-2)*
General reagent grade of commerce.
A pale yellow to greenish yellow, oily liquid; d_{20}^{20}, 1.048 to 1.051; n_D^{20}, about 1.620.
Store protected from light in a cool place.

Cinnamic Acid $C_9H_8O_2$ = 148.2 *(140-10-3)*
General reagent grade of commerce.
Melting point, about 133°.

Cinnamic Aldehyde See *cinnamaldehyde.*

Citral 3,7-Dimethylocta-2,6-dienal; $C_{10}H_{16}O$ = 152.2 *(5392-40-5)*
General reagent grade of commerce.
A light yellow liquid; boiling point, about 229°; weight per ml, about 0.89 g; n_D^{20}, about 1.488.
Complies with the following test.
HOMOGENEITY Carry out the method for *thin-layer chromatography*, Appendix III A, using *silica gel GF_{254}* as the coating substance and a mixture of 15 volumes of *ethyl acetate* and 85 volumes of *toluene* as the mobile phase. Apply to the plate 10 µl of a 0.1% w/v solution of the reagent being examined in *toluene.* After removal of the plate, allow it to dry in air and examine under *ultraviolet light (254 nm)*. The chromatogram obtained shows only one principal spot.

Citric Acid $C_6H_8O_7,H_2O$ = 210.1 *(5949-29-1)*
Analytical reagent grade of commerce.
When used in the limit test for iron, *Appendix VII, complies with the following requirement.*
Dissolve 0.5 g in 10 ml of *water*, add 0.1 ml of *mercaptoacetic acid*, mix, make alkaline with 10M *ammonia* and add sufficient *water* to produce 20 ml. No pink colour is produced.

Citric Acid, Anhydrous $C_6H_8O_7$ = 192.1 *(77-92-9)*
General reagent grade of commerce.
Melting point, about 154°.

Citric—Molybdic Acid Solution Mix 54 g of *molybdenum(VI) oxide* with 200 ml of *water*, add 11 g of *sodium hydroxide* and heat, with stirring, until almost complete solution has been obtained. Dissolve 60 g of *citric acid* in 250 ml of *water* and add 140 ml of *hydrochloric acid.* Add the first solution to the second, stirring continuously, cool, filter if necessary, dilute to 1000 ml with *water* and add, dropwise, sufficient of a 1% w/v solution of *potassium bromate* to discharge the green colour.
Store in a well-closed container, protected from light.

Citropten 5,7-Dimethoxycoumarin; $C_{11}H_{10}O_4$ = 206.2 *(487-06-9)*
General reagent grade of commerce.
Melting point, about 145°.
Complies with the following test.
HOMOGENEITY Carry out the method for *thin-layer chromatography*, Appendix III A, using *silica gel GF_{254}* as the coating substance and a mixture of 15 volumes of *ethyl acetate* and 85 volumes of *toluene* as the mobile phase. Apply to the plate 10 µl of a 0.01% w/v solution of the reagent being examined in *toluene.* After removal of the plate, allow it dry in air and examine under *ultraviolet light (254 nm)*. The chromatogram obtained shows only one principal spot.

Clobetasol Propionate 21-Chloro-9-fluoro-11β-hydroxy-16β-methyl-3,20-dioxopregna-1,4-dien-17-yl propionate; $C_{25}H_{32}ClFO_5$ = 467.0 (*25122-46-7*)
General reagent grade of commerce.
Melting point, about 196°; $[\alpha]_D^{20}$, about +104° (in 1,4-dioxan).

Coagulation Factor V Solution Clotting factor V solution
Coagulation Factor V Solution may be prepared by the following method or by any other method that excludes factor VIII. Prepare from fresh oxalated bovine plasma by fractionation at 4° with a saturated solution of *ammonium sulphate* prepared at 4°. Use the fraction precipitating between 38 and 50% saturation (which contains factor V not significantly contaminated with factor VIII), dialysed to remove ammonium sulphate and diluted with *saline solution* to produce a solution containing between 10 and 20% of the amount of factor V present in fresh normal human plasma.

Determine the factor V content of the solution in the following manner. Prepare two dilutions in *imidazole buffer solution pH 7.3* to contain 1 volume of the solution being examined in 10 volumes and 20 volumes, respectively. Test each dilution as follows. Mix 0.1 ml of each of *plasma substrate deficient in factor V*, the dilution being tested, *thromboplastin reagent* and 0.025M *calcium chloride*. Record as the clotting time the interval between the addition of the calcium chloride solution and the first indication of fibrin formation, which may be observed visually or by mechanical means.

Similarly determine the coagulation times, in duplicate, for four dilutions of pooled normal human plasma in *imidazole buffer solution pH 7.3* containing 1 volume in 10 volumes (equivalent to 100% of factor V), in 50 volumes (20%), in 100 volumes (10%) and in 1000 volumes (1%), respectively.

To calculate the result, plot the mean of the coagulation times for each dilution of human plasma on double cycle log/log paper against the equivalent percentage for factor V and read the percentage of factor V for the two dilutions of *coagulation factor V solution* by interpolation from the curve. The mean of the two results is taken as the percentage of factor V in the solution.

Cobalt(II) Acetate Cobaltous acetate; $(CH_3CO_2)_2Co,4H_2O$ = 249.1 (*6147-53-1*)
General reagent grade of commerce.

Cobalt Chloride See *cobalt(II) chloride*.

Cobalt(II) Chloride Cobalt chloride; cobaltous chloride; $CoCl_2,6H_2O$ = 237.9 (*7791-13-1*)
Analytical reagent grade of commerce.
A red, crystalline powder or deep red crystals.

Cobalt Nitrate See *cobalt(II) nitrate*.

Cobalt(II) Nitrate Cobaltous nitrate; $Co(NO_3)_2,6H_2O$ = 291.0 (*10026-22-9*)
Analytical reagent grade of commerce.
Small, garnet red crystals.

Codeine $C_{18}H_{21}NO_3,H_2O$ = 317.4 (*76-57-3*)
General reagent grade of commerce.

Codeine Phosphate $C_{18}H_{21}NO_3,H_3PO_4,½H_2O$ = 406.4 (*41444-62-6*)
General reagent grade of commerce.

2,4,6-Collidine 2,4,6-Trimethylpyridine; $C_8H_{11}N$ = 121.2 (*108-75-8*)
General reagent grade of commerce.
A colourless to pale yellow liquid with a tar-like odour; boiling point, about 170°; weight per ml, about 0.92 g.
It may be stabilised by the addition of aluminium oxide.

Congo Red CI 22120; disodium (4,4′-biphenylbis-2,2′-azo)bis(1-aminonaphthalene-4-sulphonate); $C_{32}H_{22}N_6Na_2O_6S_2$ = 697 (*573-58-0*)
Produces a blue colour in moderately acidic solutions and a red colour in weakly acidic and alkaline solutions.

Congo Red Fibrin Soak washed and shredded fibrin overnight in a 2% w/v solution of *congo red in ethanol (90%)*, strain, wash the product with *water* and store under *ether*.

Congo Red Paper Immerse strips of filter paper for a few minutes in a solution prepared by dissolving 0.1 g of *congo red* in a mixture of 20 ml of *ethanol (96%)* and *water* and adding sufficient *water* to produce 100 ml and allow to dry at room temperature (pH range, 3.0 to 5.0).

Coomassie Blue See *acid blue 92*.

Coomassie Blue Solution See *acid blue 92 solution*.

Copper Cu = 63.54 (*7440-50-8*)
Electrolytic grade of commerce. The physical form to be used is prescribed in the monograph.

Copper Acetate See *copper(II) acetate*.

Copper(II) Acetate Cupric acetate; $C_2H_6CuO_4,H_2O$ = 199.7 (*142-71-2*)
Analytical reagent grade of commerce.

Copper Carbonate Approximately $CuCO_3,Cu(OH)_2,H_2O$ (*12069-69-1*)
General reagent grade of commerce.

Copper(II) Chloride Cupric chloride; $CuCl_2,2H_2O$ = 170.5 (*10125-13-0*)
Analytical reagent grade of commerce.
Store in an airtight container.

Copper Chloride–Pyridine Reagent Dissolve 40 mg of *copper(II) chloride* in *pyridine*, warming until complete dissolution is effected, and cool. Add 1 ml of *carbon disulphide* and sufficient *pyridine* to produce 100 ml.

Copper Edetate Solution To 2 ml of a 2% w/v solution of *copper(II) acetate* add 2 ml of 0.1M *disodium edetate* and dilute to 50 ml with *water*.

Copper Nitrate See *copper(II) nitrate*.

Copper(II) Nitrate Cupric nitrate; copper nitrate; $Cu(NO_3)_2,3H_2O$ = 241.6 (*10031-43-3*)
Analytical reagent grade of commerce.
Store in an airtight container.

Copper Oxide Solution, Ammoniacal Triturate 0.5 g of *copper carbonate* with 10 ml of *water* and gradually add 10 ml of 13.5M *ammonia*.

Copper Sulphate See *copper(II) sulphate*.

Copper(II) Sulphate Cupric sulphate; copper sulphate; $CuSO_4,5H_2O$ = 249.7 (*7758-99-8*)
Analytical reagent grade of commerce.

Copper Sulphate–Pyridine Reagent Dissolve 4 g of *copper(II) sulphate* in 90 ml of *water* and add 30 ml of *pyridine*.
Prepare immediately before use.

Copper Sulphate Solution A 12.5% w/v solution of *copper(II) sulphate*.

Copper Sulphate Solution, Weak A 10% w/v solution of *copper(II) sulphate.*

Copper Tetrammine, Ammoniacal Solution of Dissolve 34.5 g of *copper(II) sulphate* in 100 ml of *water* and whilst stirring, add dropwise 13.5M *ammonia* until the precipitate produced has completely dissolved. Keeping the temperature below 20°, add dropwise 30 ml of 10M *sodium hydroxide,* shaking continuously. Filter the precipitate through a sintered-glass filter (BS porosity No. 3), wash the precipitate with *water* until the filtrate is clear and stir the precipitate with 200 ml of 13.5M *ammonia.* Filter through a sintered-glass filter and repeat the filtration to reduce the residue to a minimum.

Corallin CI 43811; sodium salt of rosolic acid (*603-45-2*)
General reagent grade of commerce.
Hard, dull red masses with a faint phenolic odour.

Corallin Solution, Alkaline Dissolve 5 g of *corallin* in 100 ml of *ethanol (90%).* Immediately before use add 1 ml of the solution to 20 ml of a 20% w/v solution of *sodium carbonate.*

Cortisone Acetate $C_{23}H_{30}O_6$ = 402.5 (*50-04-4*)
General reagent grade of commerce.
Melting point, about 238°; $[\alpha]_D^{20}$, about +211° (1% w/v in dioxan).

Cresol See o-*cresol.*

o-Cresol Cresol; C_7H_8O = 108.1 (*95-48-7*)
General reagent grade of commerce.
A colourless to faintly coloured, crystalline solid or a supercooled liquid with a tarry, phenolic odour; freezing point, not below 30.5°.
d_{20}^{20}, about 1.05; n_D^{20}, 1.540 to 1.550; boiling point, about 190°.
Store protected from light, moisture and oxygen and distil before use.

Cresol Red 4,4′-(3*H*-2,1-Benzoxathiol-3-ylidene)di-*o*-cresol *S,S*-dioxide; $C_{21}H_{18}O_5S$ = 382.4 (*1733-12-6*)
Produces a red colour in very strongly acidic solutions, a yellow colour in less strongly acidic and neutral solutions and a red colour in moderately alkaline solutions.

Cresol Red Solution Dissolve 0.1 g of *cresol red* in a mixture of 2.65 ml of 0.1M *sodium hydroxide* and 20 ml of *ethanol (96%)* and add sufficient *water* to produce 100 ml.
Complies with the following test.
SENSITIVITY A mixture of 0.1 ml of the solution and 100 ml of *carbon dioxide-free water* to which 0.15 ml of 0.02M *sodium hydroxide* has been added is purplish red. Not more than 0.15 ml of 0.02M *hydrochloric acid VS* is required to change the colour of the solution to yellow (pH range, 7.0 (red) to 8.6 (yellow)).

Crystal Violet CI 42555; basic violet 3; $C_{25}H_{30}ClN_3$ = 408.0 (*548-62-9*)
When used for titration in non-aqueous media, it changes from violet (basic) through bluish green (neutral) to yellowish green (acidic).

Crystal Violet Solution A 0.5% w/v solution of *crystal violet* in *anhydrous acetic acid.*
Complies with the following test.
SENSITIVITY A mixture of 0.1 ml of the solution and 50 ml of *anhydrous acetic acid* is bluish purple. Add 0.1 ml of 0.1M *perchloric acid VS.* The colour of the solution changes to bluish green.

Cupric Chloride See *copper(II) chloride.*

Cupri-citric Solution Dissolve 25 g of *copper(II) sulphate,* 50 g of *citric acid* and 144 g of *anhydrous sodium carbonate* in sufficient *water* to produce 1000 ml.

Cupri-citric Solution R1 Dissolve 25 g of *copper(II) sulphate,* 50 g of *citric acid* and 144 g of *anhydrous sodium carbonate* in *water* and dilute to 1000 ml with *water.* Adjust the solution so that it complies with the following tests.
A. To 25 ml add 3 g of *potassium iodide* and then carefully add 25 ml of a 25% w/w solution of *sulphuric acid* in small quantities. Titrate with 0.1M *sodium thiosulphate VS* using 0.5 ml of *starch solution,* added towards the end of the titration, as indicator. 24.5 to 25.5 ml of 0.1M *sodium thiosulphate VS* is required.
B. Dilute 10 ml to 100 ml with *water.* To 10 ml of the resulting solution add 25 ml of 0.1M *hydrochloric acid VS* and heat on a water bath for 1 hour. Cool, restore the original volume with *water* and titrate with 0.1M *sodium hydroxide VS* using *phenolphthalein solution R1* as indicator. 5.7 to 6.3 ml of 0.1M *sodium hydroxide VS* is required.
C. Dilute 10 ml to 100 ml with *water* and titrate 10 ml of the resulting solution with 0.1M *hydrochloric acid VS* using *phenolphthalein solution R1* as indicator. 6.0 to 7.5 ml of 0.1M *hydrochloric acid VS* is required.

Cupri-tartaric Solution
SOLUTION I Dissolve 34.6 g of *copper(II) sulphate* in sufficient *water* to produce 500 ml.
SOLUTION II Dissolve 173 g of *potassium sodium (+)-tartrate* and 50 g of *sodium hydroxide* in 400 ml of *water,* heat to boiling, allow to cool and dilute to 500 ml with freshly boiled and cooled *water.*
Mix equal volumes of solutions I and II immediately before use.

Cupri-tartaric Solution R1 Fehling's solution
SOLUTION A Dissolve 34.6 g of *copper(II) sulphate* in a mixture of 0.5 ml of *sulphuric acid* and sufficient *water* to produce 500 ml.
SOLUTION B Dissolve 176 g of *potassium sodium (+)-tartrate* and 77 g of *sodium hydroxide* in sufficient *water* to produce 500 ml.
Mix equal volumes of solutions A and B immediately before use.

Cupri-tartaric Solution R2 Dilute potassium cupri-tartrate solution
Mix 1 ml of a solution containing 0.5% w/v of *copper(II) sulphate* and 1% w/v of *dipotassium (+)-tartrate* with 50 ml of *sodium carbonate solution R1.*
Prepare immediately before use.

Cupri-tartaric Solution R3 Mix equal volumes of a 1% w/v solution of *copper(II) sulphate* and a 2% w/v solution of *sodium tartrate.* To 1 ml of the mixture add 50 ml of *sodium carbonate solution R1.*
Prepare immediately before use.

Cupri-tartaric Solution R4
SOLUTION A A 15.0% w/v solution of *copper(II) sulphate.*
SOLUTION B Dissolve 2.5 g of *anhydrous sodium carbonate,* 2.5 g of *potassium sodium (+)-tartrate,* 2.0 g of *sodium hydrogen carbonate* and 20.0 g of *anhydrous sodium sulphate* in sufficient *water* to produce 100 ml.
Mix 1 volume of solution A with 25 volumes of solution B immediately before use.

Curcumin 1,7-Bis(4-hydroxy-3-methoxyphenyl)hepta-1,6-diene-3,5-dione; $C_{21}H_{20}O_6$ = 368.4 (*458-37-7*)
General reagent grade of commerce.
An orange-brown, crystalline powder; melting point, about 183°.

Cyanoacetic Acid Malonic acid mononitrile; $C_3H_3NO_2$ = 85.1 *(372-09-8)*
General reagent grade of commerce.
Melting point, about 67°.
Store in an airtight container.

Cyanocobalamin *Coα*-[α-(5,6-Dimethylbenzimidazolyl)]-*Coβ*-cyanocobamide; vitamin B_{12}; $C_{63}H_{88}CoN_{14}O_{14}P$ = 1355 *(68-19-9)*
General reagent grade of commerce.
Hygroscopic, dark red crystals or powder.
Store in an airtight container, protected from light.

Cyanogen Bromide Solution Add, dropwise with cooling, 0.1M *ammonium thiocyanate* to *bromine water* until the colour disappears.
Prepare immediately before use.

Cyanoguanidine See *1-cyanoguanidine*.

1-Cyanoguanidine Dicyandiamide; $C_2H_4N_4$ = 84.1 *(461-58-5)*
General reagent grade of commerce.
Melting point, about 210°.

Cyclohexane C_6H_{12} = 84.16 *(110-82-7)*
Analytical reagent grade of commerce.
A colourless liquid; boiling point, about 81°; d_{20}^{20}, about 0.78.
Cyclohexane used in spectrophotometry complies with the following requirement.
TRANSMITTANCE Not less than 45% at 220 nm, 70% at 235 nm, 90% at 240 nm and 98% at 250 nm, using *water* in the reference cell.

Cyclohexane R1 Spectroscopic reagent grade of commerce complying with the following test.
FLUORESCENCE Under radiation at 365 nm, the *fluorescence* measured at 460 nm in a 1-cm cell is not more intense than that of a solution in 0.05M *sulphuric acid* containing 0.002 µg per ml of *quinine*, Appendix II E.

Cyclohexylamine $C_6H_{13}N$ = 99.18 *(108-91-8)*
General reagent grade of commerce.
Boiling point, about 134°; n_D^{20}, about 1.46.

Cyclohexylenedinitrilotetra-acetic Acid (±)-*trans*-1,2-Diaminocyclohexane-*N,N,N',N'*-tetra-acetic acid; $C_{14}H_{22}N_2O_8,H_2O$ = 364.4 *(13291-61-7)*
General reagent grade of commerce.
A white, crystalline powder; melting point, about 204°.

L-Cysteine $C_3H_7NO_2S$ = 121.2 *(52-90-4)*
General reagent grade of commerce.
$[\alpha]_D^{20}$, about +6.5° (10% w/v in 1M hydrochloric acid).

Cysteine Hydrochloride $C_3H_7NO_2S,HCl,H_2O$ = 175.6 *(7048-04-6)*
General reagent grade of commerce.

L-Cystine $C_6H_{12}N_2O_4S_2$ = 240.3 *(56-89-3)*
General reagent grade of commerce.
$[\alpha]_D^{20}$, −218° to −224°, determined in 1M hydrochloric acid.

Dantron See *1,8-dihydroxyanthraquinone*.

Decane See n-*decane*.

***n*-Decane** $C_{10}H_{22}$ = 142.3 *(124-18-5)*
General reagent grade of commerce.
Boiling point, about 174°; n_D^{20}, about 1.411.

Decanol See *decan-1-ol*.

Decan-1-ol $C_{10}H_{22}O$ = 158.3 *(112-30-1)*
General reagent grade of commerce.
Moderately viscous liquid; boiling point, about 230°; n_D^{20}, about 1.436.

2′-Deoxyuridine $C_9H_{12}N_2O_5$ = 228.2 *(951-78-0)*
General reagent grade of commerce.
A white or almost white, crystalline solid; melting point, about 165°.
Complies with the following test.
HOMOGENEITY Examine under the conditions prescribed in the test for Related substances in the monograph for Idoxuridine applying to the plate 5 µl of a 0.025% w/v solution. The chromatogram shows only one principal spot.

Deuterated Acetic Acid $C_2D_4O_2$ = 64.1 *(1186-52-3)*
General reagent grade of commerce with a minimum isotopic purity of 99.7%.
d_{20}^{20}, about 1.12; n_D^{20}, about 1.368; boiling point, about 115°; melting point, about 16°.

Deuterated Acetone Deuteroacetone; C_3D_6O = 64.1
Spectroscopic grade of commerce with a minimum isotopic purity of 99.5% and containing not more than 0.1% of water and deuterium oxide.
d_{20}^{20}, about 0.87; n_D^{20}, about 1.357; boiling point, about 55°.

Deuterated Chloroform See *deuterochloroform*.

Deuterated Dimethyl Sulphoxide $C_{22}D_6OS$ = 84.2 *(2206-27-1)*
General reagent grade of commerce with a minimum isotopic purity of 99.8% and containing not more than 0.1% of water and deuterium oxide.
A practically colourless, viscous, hygroscopic liquid; d_{20}^{20}, about 1.18; melting point, about 20°.
Store in an airtight container.

Deuterated Methanol CD_4O = 36.1 *(811-98-3)*
General reagent grade of commerce with a minimum isotopic purity of 99.8%.
A colourless liquid; d_{20}^{20}, about 0.888; n_D^{20}, about 1.326; boiling point, 65.4°.

Deuterium Oxide D_2O = 20.03 *(7789-20-0)*
General reagent grade of commerce with a minimum isotopic purity of 99.7%.
A colourless liquid; d_{20}^{20}, about 1.11; n_D^{20}, about 1.328; boiling point, about 101°.

Deuterium Oxide, Isotopically Pure *Deuterium oxide* with a minimum isotopic purity of 99.96%.

Deuterochloroform $CDCl_3$ = 120.4 *(865-49-6)*
Spectroscopic grade of commerce with a minimum isotopic purity of 99.7% and containing not more than 0.05% of water and deuterium oxide.
A colourless liquid; weight per ml, about 1.5 g.
d_{20}^{20}, about 1.51; n_D^{20}, about 1.445; boiling point, about 60°.

Devarda's Alloy *(8049-11-4)* Copper, 50 parts; aluminium, 45 parts; zinc, 5 parts.
General reagent grade of commerce containing not more than 20 ppm of nitrogen as NH_4.

Dexamethasone $C_{22}H_{29}FO_5$ = 392.5 *(50-02-2)*
General reagent grade of commerce.
Melting point, about 263°.

Dextran for Chromatography R2, Cross-linked A bead-form cross-linked dextran with a fraction range suitable for the separation of peptides and proteins with relative molecular weights of 15×10^2 to 30×10^3. When dry, the beads have a diameter of 20 µm to 80 µm.

Dextran for Chromatography R3, Cross-linked A bead-form cross-linked dextran with a fraction range suitable for the separation of peptides and proteins with relative molecular weights of 4×10^3 to 15×10^4. When dry, the beads have a diameter of 40 µm to 120 µm.

Dextrose See *D-glucose.*

3,3′-Diaminobenzidine Tetrahydrochloride
$C_{12}H_{14}N_4,4HCl,2H_2O$ = 396.2 (*7411-49-6*)
General reagent grade of commerce.
An almost white or slightly pink powder.
Melting point, about 280°.

Diammonium Hydrogen Orthophosphate
Ammonium phosphate; $(NH_4)_2HPO_4$ = 132.1 (*7783-28-0*)
Analytical reagent grade of commerce.
Store in an airtight container.

Diatomaceous Earth See *diatomaceous support.*

Diatomaceous Earth for Gas Chromatography See *acid-washed diatomaceous support.*

Diatomaceous Earth for Gas Chromatography R1
Acid-washed diatomaceous support complying with the following requirement.
PARTICLE SIZE Not more than 5% is retained on a *No. 250 sieve* and not more than 10% passes through *No. 180 sieve.*

Diatomaceous Earth for Gas Chromatography R2
Acid-washed diatomaceous support complying with the following requirement.
PARTICLE SIZE Not more than 5% is retained on a *No. 180 sieve* and not more than 10% passes through *No. 125 sieve.*

Diatomaceous Earth for Gas Chromatography R1, Silanised Prepared from crushed pink firebrick and silanised with dimethyldichlorosilane or other suitable silanising agents. The substance is purified by treating with *hydrochloric acid* and washing with *water.*

Diatomaceous Earth for Gas Chromatography, Silanised See *silanised diatomaceous support.*

Diatomaceous Filter-aid, Washed, Flux-calcined To 500 g of flux-calcined, diatomaceous filter-aid (Celite 545 is suitable), add 2000 ml of *hydrochloric acid,* mix, allow to stand with occasional stirring for 12 hours, filter and wash the residue with *water* until the washings are neutral to *litmus paper.* Continue washing the residue on the filter paper, using 500 ml of *methanol* followed by 1000 ml of a mixture of equal volumes of *methanol* and *ether.* Finally dry the washed residue at 100° until the odour of solvent is no longer detectable. It should be stored in an airtight container.

Diatomaceous Support Diatomaceous earth (*91053-39-3*)
A white or almost white, fine granular powder made up of siliceous frustules of fossil diatoms or of debris of fossil diatoms. It may be identified by microscopic examination with a magnification of ×500.

Diatomaceous Support, Acid-washed Diatomaceous earth for gas chromatography
Diatomaceous support that has been purified by treatment with hydrochloric acid and washed with water and that complies with the following requirement.
PARTICLE SIZE Not more than 5% is retained on a *No. 180* sieve and not more than 10% passes through a *No. 125* sieve.

Diatomaceous Support, Alkali-washed
Diatomaceous support that has been treated with potassium hydroxide solution to reduce peak-tailing of basic compounds.

Diatomaceous Support, Silanised Diatomaceous earth for gas chromatography, silanised
Acid-washed diatomaceous support that has been silanised with dimethyldichlorosilane or other suitable silanising agents.

Diazobenzenesulphonic Acid Solution Heat 0.2 g of *sulphanilic acid* with 20 ml of 1M *hydrochloric acid* until dissolved, cool to about 4° and add, dropwise, 2.2 ml of a 4% w/v solution of *sodium nitrite,* swirling continuously. Allow to stand in ice for 10 minutes and add 1 ml of a 5% w/v solution of *sulphamic acid.*

Diazobenzenesulphonic Acid Solution R1 Dissolve 0.9 g of *sulphanilic acid* in a mixture of 30 ml of 2M *hydrochloric acid* and 70 ml of *water.* To 3 ml of the solution add 3 ml of a 5% w/v solution of *sodium nitrite.* Cool in ice for 5 minutes, add 12 ml of the sodium nitrite solution and cool again. Dilute the solution to 100 ml with *water* and keep the reagent in ice. Prepare extemporaneously but allow to stand for 15 minutes before use.

Dibenzosuberone Dibenzo[*a,d*]cyclohepta-1,4-dien-3-one; 10,11-dihydro-5*H*-dibenzo[*a,d*]cyclohepten-5-one; $C_{15}H_{12}O$ = 208.3 (*1210-35-1*)
General reagent grade of commerce.
Melting point, about 34°.

Dibutyl Ether $C_8H_{18}O$ = 130.2 (*142-96-1*)
General reagent grade of commerce.
A colourless, flammable liquid; boiling point, about 140°; d_{20}^{20}, about 0.77; n_D^{20}, about 1.399.
Do not distil unless the dibutyl ether complies with the following test for peroxides.
PEROXIDES Place 8 ml of *potassium iodide and starch solution* in a 12-ml ground-glass-stoppered cylinder about 1.5 cm in diameter. Fill completely with the substance being examined, shake vigorously and allow to stand protected from light for 30 minutes. No colour is produced.

Dibutyl Phthalate Di-*n*-butyl phthalate; $C_{16}H_{22}O_4$ = 278.3 (*84-74-2*)
General reagent grade of commerce.
A colourless or faintly coloured liquid; d_{20}^{20}, 1.043 to 1.048; n_D^{20}, 1.490 to 1.495.

Di-*n*-butylamine $C_8H_{19}N$ = 129.25 (*111-92-2*)
General reagent grade of commerce.
Boiling point, about 159°; n_D^{20}, about 1.417.

Dicarboxidine Hydrochloride 4,4′-[4,4′-Diamino(biphenyl-3,3′-diyl)dioxy]dibutanoic acid dihydrochloride; $C_{20}H_{24}N_2O_6,2HCl$ = 461.3 (*56455-90-4*)
General reagent grade of commerce.

Dichloroacetic Acid $C_2H_3Cl_2O_2$ = 128.9 (*79-43-6*)
General reagent grade of commerce.
Boiling point, about 193°; n_D^{20}, about 1.466; d_{20}^{20}, about 1.566.

Dichloroacetic Acid Solution Dilute 67 ml of *dichloroacetic acid* to 300 ml with *water* and neutralise to *litmus paper* using 10M *ammonia.* Cool, add 33 ml of *dichloroacetic acid* and dilute to 600 ml with *water.*

Dichlorobenzene See *1,2-dichlorobenzene.*

1,2-Dichlorobenzene $C_6H_4Cl_2$ = 147.0 *(95-50-1)*
Analytical reagent grade of commerce.
A clear, oily liquid; n_D^{20}, about 1.551; d_{20}^{20}, about 1.31.

1,2-Dichloroethane Ethylene chloride; $C_2H_4Cl_2$ = 98.96 *(107-06-2)*
Analytical reagent grade of commerce.
A colourless liquid with an odour similar to that of chloroform; boiling point, about 83°; d_{20}^{20}, about 1.25.
Not less than 95% distils between 82° and 84°.

Dichlorofluorescein See *2,7-dichlorofluorescein.*

2,7-Dichlorofluorescein $C_{20}H_{10}Cl_2O_5$ = 401.2 *(76-54-0)*
Adsorption indicator grade of commerce.
A yellowish brown to yellowish orange powder.

5,7-Dichloro-8-hydroxyquinoline 5,7-Dichloroquinolin-8-ol ; $C_9H_5Cl_2NO$ = 214.1 *(773-76-2)*
General reagent grade of commerce.
Melting point, about 181°.

Dichloromethane Methylene chloride; CH_2Cl_2 = 84.93 *(75-09-2)*
Analytical reagent grade of commerce.
A volatile, sweet-smelling liquid; boiling point, about 40°; weight per ml, about 1.32 g.
Dichloromethane used in fluorimetry complies with the following test.
FLUORESCENCE Under radiation at 365 nm, the *fluorescence* measured at 460 nm in a 1-cm cell is not more intense than that of a solution in 0.05M *sulphuric acid* containing 0.002 µg per ml of *quinine*, Appendix II E.

Dichloromethane, Acidified Acidified methylene chloride
To 100 ml of *dichloromethane* add 10 ml of *hydrochloric acid*, shake, allow to stand and separate the two layers. Use the lower layer.

Dichloromethane IR
Spectroscopic reagent grade of commerce.

Dichlorophenolindophenol, Sodium Salt See *2,6-dichlorophenolindophenol sodium salt.*

2,6-Dichlorophenolindophenol Sodium Salt The sodium salt of 2,6-dichloro-*N*-(4-hydroxyphenyl)-1,4-benzoquinone monoimine; Tillman's reagent; $C_{12}H_6Cl_2NNaO_2$ +aq *(620-45-1)*
Analytical reagent grade of commerce.
A dark green powder. Aqueous solutions are dark blue, becoming pink when acidified.

2,6-Dichlorophenolindophenol Solution Warm 0.1 g of *2,6-dichlorophenolindophenol sodium salt* with 100 ml of *water* and filter.
Use within 3 days of preparation.

2,6-Dichlorophenolindophenol Solution, Double-strength Standard Dissolve 0.1 g of *2,6-dichlorophenolindophenol sodium salt* in 100 ml of *water*, filter, standardise by the method described under *standard dichlorophenolindophenol solution* and dilute the solution with *water* so that 1 ml is equivalent to 0.2 mg of ascorbic acid.
Use within 3 days of preparation and standardise immediately before use.

Dichlorophenolindophenol Solution, Standard Dissolve 50 mg of *2,6-dichlorophenolindophenol sodium salt* in 100 ml of *water* and filter. Dissolve 20.0 mg of L-*ascorbic acid* in 10 ml of a freshly prepared 20% w/v solution of *metaphosphoric acid* and dilute to 250 ml with *water*. Titrate 5 ml rapidly with the 2,6-dichlorophenolindophenol sodium salt solution, added from a microburette graduated in units of 0.01 ml, until the pink colour of the dye persists for 10 seconds; the titration should take not more than 2 minutes. Dilute the 2,6-dichlorophenolindophenol sodium salt solution with *water* so that 1 ml of the solution is equivalent to 0.1 mg of ascorbic acid, $C_6H_8O_6$.
Use within 3 days of preparation and standardise immediately before use.

Dichloroquinonechlorimide See *2,6-dichloroquinone-4-chloroimide.*

2,6-Dichloroquinone-4-chloroimide Dichloroquinonechlorimide; $C_6H_2Cl_3NO$ = 210.4 *(101-38-2)*
General reagent grade of commerce.
A yellow or orange, crystalline powder; melting point, about 66°.

Dichlorvos 2,2-Dichlorovinyl dimethyl phosphate; $C_4H_7Cl_2O_4P$ = 221 *(62-73-7)*
Use a grade suitable for the determination of pesticide residues.
n_D^{25}, about 1.452.

Di-2-cyanoethyl Ether (2-Cyanoethyl) ether; $C_6H_8N_2O$ = 124.1 *(1656-48-0)*
Chromatographic grade of commerce.
Boiling point, about 111°; n_D^{20}, 1.4400.

Dicyclohexylamine *N,N*-Dicyclohexylamine; $C_{12}H_{23}N$ = 181.3 *(101-83-7)*
General reagent grade of commerce.
A colourless liquid; n_D^{20}, about 1.484; freezing point, 0° to 1°; boiling point, about 256°.

Dicyclohexylurea See *1,3-dicyclohexylurea.*

1,3-Dicyclohexylurea $C_{13}H_{24}N_2O$ = 224.4 *(2387-23-7)*
General reagent grade of commerce.
Melting point, about 232°.

Didodecyl 3,3′-thiodipropionate $C_{30}H_{58}O_4S$ = 514.8 *(123-28-4)*
General reagent grade of commerce.
Melting point, about 39°.

Diethanolamine $C_4H_{11}NO_2$ = 105.1 *(111-42-2)*
General reagent grade of commerce.
A colourless or slightly yellow, viscous liquid or deliquescent crystals melting at about 28°; d_{20}^{20}, about 1.09.
Complies with the following test.
ALKALINITY pH of a 5% w/v solution, 10.0 to 11.5, Appendix V L.
Diethanolamine used in tests for alkaline phosphatase complies with the following additional test.
ETHANOLAMINE Not more than 1.0% w/w when determined in the following manner. Dissolve 1.00 g of *3-aminopropanol* (internal standard) in sufficient *acetone* to produce 10 ml (solution A). Dissolve 0.5 g of *ethanolamine* in sufficient *acetone* to produce 10 ml (solution B). Carry out the method for *gas chromatography*, Appendix III B, using the following solutions. For solution (1) add 1 ml of solution A to 5 g of the substance being examined and dilute to 10 ml with *acetone*. For solution (2) dissolve 5 g of the substance being examined in sufficient *acetone* to produce 10 ml. For solution (3) add 1 ml of solution A to 0.5 ml of solution B and dilute to 10 ml with *acetone*. Prepare solution (4) in the same manner as solution (3)

but adding 1 ml of solution B in place of 0.5 ml of solution B. Prepare solution (5) in the same manner as solution (3) but adding 2 ml of solution B in place of 0.5 ml of solution B.

The chromatographic procedure may be carried out using a column (1 m × 4 mm) packed with diphenylphenylene oxide porous polymer beads (180 to 250 µm) and using 40 ml per minute as the flow rate of the carrier gas. Maintain the temperature of the column at 125° for 3 minutes and then raise to 300° at a rate of 12° per minute. Maintain the temperature of the injection port at 250° and that of the detector at 280°.
Store in an airtight container.

Diethoxytetrahydrofuran See *2,5-diethoxytetrahydrofuran.*

2,5-Diethoxytetrahydrofuran Diethoxytetrahydrofuran; $C_8H_{16}O_3$ = 160.2 (*3320-90-9*)
General reagent grade of commerce consisting of a mixture of *cis-* and *trans-* isomers.
A colourless or slightly yellow liquid; d_{20}^{20}, about 0.98; n_D^{20}, about 1.418.

Diethylamine $C_4H_{11}N$ = 73.14 (*109-89-7*)
Analytical reagent grade of commerce.
A volatile, colourless liquid; boiling point, about 55°; d_{20}^{20}, about 0.71.

Diethylaminoethyldextran Anion exchange resin presented as the hydrochloride.
A powder forming gels with water.

***N,N*-Diethylaniline** $C_{10}H_{15}N$ = 149.2 (*91-66-7*)
General reagent grade of commerce.
A pale yellow liquid with an ammoniacal odour; boiling point, about 217°; weight per ml, about 0.93 g.

Diethylene Glycol Digol; 2,2′-oxydiethanol; $C_4H_{10}O_3$ = 106.1 (*111-46-6*)
Analytical reagent grade of commerce containing not less than 99.5% w/w of $C_4H_{10}O_3$.
Boiling point, 244° to 246°; d_{20}^{20}, about 1.118; n_D^{20}, about 1.447.

***N,N*-Diethylethylenediamine** *N,N*-Diethyl-1,2-diaminoethane; $C_6H_{16}N_2$ = 116.2 (*100-36-7*)
General reagent grade of commerce.
A colourless or slightly yellow, slightly oily liquid with a strong odour of ammonia; boiling point, about 146°; d_{20}^{20}, 0.827.
Complies with the following test.
WATER Not more than 1.0%, Appendix IX C. Use 0.5 g.

Di(2-ethylhexyl) Phthalate Dioctyl phthalate; $C_{24}H_{38}O_4$ = 390.5 (*117-81-7*)
General reagent grade of commerce.
A colourless, oily liquid; n_D^{20}, about 1.486; d_{20}^{20}, about 0.98; viscosity, about 80 mPa s, Appendix V H, Method II.

Diethylphenylenediamine Sulphate See N,N-*diethyl*-p-*phenylenediamine sulphate.*

***N,N*-Diethyl-*p*-phenylenediamine Sulphate** Diethylphenylenediamine sulphate; $C_{10}H_{16}N_2,H_2SO_4$ = 262.3 (*6283-63-2*)
General reagent grade of commerce.
A white or slightly coloured powder; melting point, about 185° with decomposition.
Store protected from light.

Diethylphenylenediamine Sulphate Solution To 250 ml of *water* add 2 ml of *sulphuric acid* and 25 ml of 0.02M *disodium edetate.* Dissolve in this solution 1.1 g of N,N-*diethyl*-p-*phenylenediamine sulphate* and add sufficient *water* to produce 1000 ml.
Store protected from light and heat use within 1 month; do not use if the solution is not colourless.

Digitonin $C_{56}H_{92}O_{29}$ = 1229 (*11024-24-1*)
General reagent grade of commerce.
A white powder; $[\alpha]_D^{20}$, about −48° (10% w/v in 75% w/w acetic acid).

Digitoxin $C_{41}H_{64}O_{13}$ = 765.0 (*71-63-6*)
General reagent grade of commerce.
Melting point, about 240°, with decomposition.

Digoxin Reagent Add 98 ml of *glacial acetic acid* to 2 ml of *sulphuric acid* and add 0.1 ml of a 5% w/v solution of *anhydrous iron(III) chloride* in *glacial acetic acid.*

10,11-Dihydrocarbamazepine $C_{15}H_{14}N_2O$ = 238.3 (*3564-73-6*)
Analytical reagent grade of commerce.
Melting point, 205° to 210°.

1,8-Dihydroxyanthraquinone Danthron; dantron; $C_{14}H_8O_4$ = 240.2 (*117-10-2*)
General reagent grade of commerce.
An orange, crystalline powder; melting point, about 195°.

1,3-Dihydroxynaphthalene See *naphthalene-1,3-diol.*

2,7-Dihydroxynaphthalene See *naphthalene-2,7-diol.*

2,7-Dihydroxynaphthalene Solution See *naphthalenediol solution.*

5,7-Di-iodo-8-hydroxyquinoline 5,7-Di-iodoquinolin-8-ol; $C_9H_5I_2NO$ = 397.0 (*83-73-8*)
General reagent grade of commerce.
Melting point, about 214°, with decomposition.

1,5-Di-iodopentane $C_5H_{10}I_2$ = 323.9 (*628-77-3*)
General reagent grade of commerce.
A colourless liquid; boiling point, about 101°.

Di-isobutyl Ketone 2,6-Dimethyl-4-heptanone; $C_9H_{18}O$ = 142.2 (*108-83-8*)
General reagent grade of commerce.
n_D^{20}, about 1.414; boiling point, about 168°.

Di-isopropyl Ether Isopropyl ether; $C_6H_{14}O$ = 102.2 (*108-20-3*)
General reagent grade of commerce.
A colourless liquid with a characteristic odour; boiling point, 67° to 69°; d_{20}^{20}, 0.723 to 0.728.
Do not distil unless the di-isopropyl ether complies with the test for peroxides.
PEROXIDES Place 8 ml of *potassium iodide and starch solution* in a 12-ml ground-glass-stoppered cylinder about 1.5 cm in diameter. Fill completely with the reagent being examined, shake vigorously and allow to stand protected from light for 30 minutes. No colour is produced.
Store protected from light. The name and concentration of any added stabiliser are stated on the label.

Di-isopropyl Ether, Stabiliser-free *Di-isopropyl ether* that is free from stabiliser.
Reagent grade of commerce.

Di-isopropylethylamine Ethyldi-isopropylamine; $C_8H_{20}N_2$ = 144.3 (*7087-68-5*)
General reagent grade of commerce.
Boiling point, about 127°; n_D^{20}, about 1.414.

2,5-Dimethoxybenzaldehyde $C_8H_{10}O_3$ = 166.2 *(93-02-7)*
General reagent grade of commerce.
Melting point, about 50°.

4,4′-Dimethoxybenzophenone $C_{15}H_{14}O_3$ = 242.3 *(90-96-0)*
General reagent grade of commerce.
Melting point, about 142°.

3,4-Dimethoxyphenethylamine $C_{10}H_{15}NO_2$ = 181.2 *(120-20-7)*
General reagent grade of commerce.
An oily liquid; n_D^{20}, about 1.546; weight per ml, about 1.07 g.

Dimethoxypropane *See 2,2-dimethoxypropane.*

2,2-Dimethoxypropane Dimethoxypropane; $C_5H_{12}O_2$ = 104.1 *(77-76-9)*
General reagent grade of commerce.
Boiling point, about 83°; n_D^{20}, about 1.378; d_{20}^{20}, about 0.847.

Dimethyl Phthalate $C_{10}H_{10}O_4$ = 194.2 *(131-11-3)*
General reagent grade of commerce.
A colourless or faintly coloured liquid; weight per ml, about 1.19 g.

Dimethyl Sulphone $C_2H_6O_2S$ = 94.13 *(67-71-0)*
General reagent grade of commerce.
Colourless prisms; melting point, 108° to 110°.

Dimethyl Sulphoxide C_2H_6OS = 78.1 *(67-68-5)*
Analytical reagent grade of commerce.
A colourless liquid; odourless or with a slight, but unpleasant, odour; boiling point, about 189°; n_D^{20}, about 1.479; d_{20}^{20}, about 1.10.
Complies with the following test.
WATER Not more than 1.0% w/v, Appendix IX C.
Dimethyl sulphoxide used in spectrophotometry complies with the following requirement and with the modified test for Water given below.
TRANSMITTANCE Not less than 10% at 262 nm, 35% at 270 nm, 70% at 290 nm and 98% at 340 nm and at higher wavelengths using *water* in the reference cell.
WATER Not more than 0.2% w/w.

Dimethyl Yellow CI 11020; 4-dimethylaminoazobenzene; $C_{14}H_{15}N_3$ = 225.3 *(60-11-7)*
Produces a red colour in moderately acidic alcoholic solutions and a yellow colour in weakly acidic and alkaline solutions. (pH range, 2.8 to 4.6).
Complies with the following test.
HOMOGENEITY Carry out the method for *thin-layer chromatography*, Appendix III A, using *silica gel G* as the coating substance and *dichloromethane* as the mobile phase. Apply to the plate 10 µl of a 0.01% w/v solution in *dichloromethane*. The chromatogram shows only one spot.

Dimethyl Yellow Solution A 0.2% w/v solution of *dimethyl yellow* in *ethanol (90%)*.
Complies with the following test.
SENSITIVITY A solution containing 2 g of *ammonium chloride* in 25 ml of *carbon dioxide-free water* to which is added 0.1 ml of the dimethyl yellow solution is yellow. Not more than 0.10 ml of 0.1M *hydrochloric acid VS* is required to change the colour of the solution to red (pH range, 2.8 to 4.6).

Dimethylacetamide C_4H_9NO = 87.12 *(127-19-5)*
General reagent grade of commerce containing not less than 99.5% of C_4H_9NO.
A colourless liquid; boiling point, about 165°; d_{20}^{20}, about 0.94; n_D^{20}, about 1.437.

Dimethylaminobenzaldehyde See *4-dimethylaminobenzaldehyde.*

4-Dimethylaminobenzaldehyde Dimethylaminobenzaldehyde; $C_9H_{11}NO$ = 149.2 *(100-10-7)*
Analytical reagent grade of commerce.
A white or pale yellow, crystalline powder; melting point, about 74°.

Dimethylaminobenzaldehyde Reagent Dissolve 0.5 g of *4-dimethylaminobenzaldehyde* in a cooled mixture of 53 ml of *sulphuric acid* and 50 ml of *water* and add 0.5 ml of *iron(III) chloride solution R1*.
Allow to stand for 2 hours before use.

Dimethylaminobenzaldehyde Solution, Alcoholic Dissolve 1 g of *4-dimethylaminobenzaldehyde* in 30 ml of *ethanol (96%)* and add 180 ml of *butan-1-ol* and 30 ml of *hydrochloric acid.*
Prepare immediately before use and discard if a pink colour develops.

Dimethylaminobenzaldehyde Solution R1 Dissolve 0.2 g of *4-dimethylaminobenzaldehyde* in 20 ml of *ethanol (96%)* and add 0.5 ml of *hydrochloric acid.* Shake the solution with *activated charcoal* and filter. The colour of the solution is less intense than that of freshly prepared 0.0001M *iodine*.
Prepare immediately before use.

Dimethylaminobenzaldehyde Solution R2 Dissolve, without heating, 0.2 g of *4-dimethylaminobenzaldehyde* in a mixture of 4.5 ml of *water* and 5.5 ml of *hydrochloric acid*.
Prepare immediately before use.

Dimethylaminobenzaldehyde Solution R6 Dissolve 0.125 g of *4-dimethylaminobenzaldehyde* in a cooled mixture of 65 ml of *sulphuric acid* and 35 ml of *water* and add 0.1 ml of a 5% w/v solution of *iron(III) chloride hexahydrate*. Allow to stand for 24 hours, protected from light, before use.
When stored at room temperature, it must be used within 1 week; when kept in a refrigerator, it may be stored for several months.

Dimethylaminobenzaldehyde Solution R7 Dissolve 1.0 g of *4-dimethylaminobenzaldehyde* in 50 ml of *hydrochloric acid* and add 50 ml of *ethanol (96%)*.
Store protected from light and use within 4 weeks.

4-Dimethylaminocinnamaldehyde $C_{11}H_{13}NO$ = 175.2 *(6203-18-5)*
General reagent grade of commerce.
Orange or orange-brown crystals or powder; melting point, about 138°.

4-Dimethylaminocinnamaldehyde Solution Dissolve 2 g of *4-dimethylaminocinnamaldehyde* in a mixture of 100 ml of 7M *hydrochloric acid* and 100 ml of *absolute ethanol*. Store in a cool place. Dilute the solution to four times its volume with *absolute ethanol* immediately before use.

Dimethylaminonaphthalenesulphonyl Chloride 5-Dimethylaminonaphthalene-1-sulphonyl chloride; dansyl chloride; $C_{12}H_{12}ClNO_2S$ = 269.8 *(605-65-2)*
General reagent grade of commerce.
Dimethylaminonaphthalenesulphonyl chloride exists in

two crystalline forms; a red form melting at about 70° and a yellow form melting at about 73°.
Store in a cool place.

Dimethylaniline See N,N-*dimethylaniline.*

***N,N*-Dimethylaniline** Dimethylaniline; $C_8H_{11}N$ = 121.2 (*121-69-7*)
Analytical reagent grade of commerce.
A colourless liquid which darkens on storage.
n_D^{20}, about 1.568; not less than 95% distils between 192° and 194°.

2,3-Dimethylaniline 2,3-Xylidine; $C_8H_{11}N$ = 121.2 (*87-59-2*)
General reagent grade of commerce.
Boiling point, about 224°; n_D^{20}, about 1.569; d_{20}^{20}, 0.993 to 0.995.

2,6-Dimethylaniline 2,6-Xylidine; $C_8H_{11}N$ = 121.2 (*87-62-7*)
General reagent grade of commerce.
A colourless liquid; d_{20}^{20}, about 0.98.

1,1-Dimethylethyl Methyl Ether *tert*-Butyl methyl ether ; $C_5H_{12}O$ = 88.1 (*1634-04-4*)
General reagent grade of commerce having a minimum transmittance of 50% at 240 nm, 80% at 255 nm and 98% at 280 nm using *water* in the reference cell.
n_D^{20}, about 1.376.

1,1-Dimethylethylamine 2-Amino-2-methylpropane; *tert*-butylamine; $C_4H_{11}N$ = 73.1 (*75-64-9*)
General reagent grade of commerce.
Boiling point, about 46°; n_D^{20}, about 1.378; d_{20}^{20}, about 0.694.

Dimethylformamide C_3H_7NO = 73.1 (*68-12-2*)
Analytical reagent grade of commerce.
A colourless liquid; boiling point, about 153°; d_{20}^{20}, about 0.95.
Complies with the following test.
WATER Not more than 0.1%, Appendix IX C.

Dimethylglyoxime 2,3-Butanedione dioxime; $C_4H_8N_2O_2$ = 116.1 (*95-45-4*)
Analytical reagent grade of commerce.
A white, crystalline powder or colourless crystals.
Melting point, about 240°, with decomposition; sulphated ash, not more than 0.05%.

***N,N*-Dimethyl-*p*-nitrosoaniline** $C_8H_{10}N_2O$ = 150.2 (*138-89-6*)
General reagent grade of commerce.
Green crystals or a green, crystalline powder; melting point, about 86°.

***N,N*-Dimethyloctylamine** Octyldimethylamine; $C_{10}H_{23}N$ = 157.3 (*7378-99-6*)
General reagent grade of commerce.
Boiling point, about 195°; d_{20}^{20}, about 0.765; n_D^{20}, about 1.424.

2,6-Dimethylphenol $C_8H_{10}O$ = 122.2 (*576-26-1*)
General reagent grade of commerce.
Melting point, 46° to 48°; boiling point, about 203°.

3,4-Dimethylphenol $C_8H_{10}O$ = 122.2 (*95-65-8*)
General reagent grade of commerce.
Melting point, 25° to 27°; boiling point, about 226°.

***N,N'*-Dimethylpiperazine** 1,4-Dimethylpiperazine; $C_6H_{14}N_2$ = 114.2 (*106-58-1*)
General reagent grade of commerce.
A colourless liquid with a characteristic odour; boiling point, about 131°; d_{20}^{20}, about 0.85; n_D^{20}, about 1.446.

Dimethylstearylamide *N,N*-Dimethyloctadecanamide; $C_{20}H_{41}NO$ = 311.5
Chromatographic reagent grade of commerce.
Melting point, about 51°.

***N,N*-Dimethyltetradecylamine** $C_{16}H_{35}N$ = 241.5
General reagent grade of commerce containing 98.0 to 101.0% w/w of $C_{16}H_{35}N$.
A clear or almost clear, colourless or slightly yellow liquid; boiling point, about 260°; d_{20}^{20}, about 0.80.
Complies with the following tests.
WATER Not more than 0.3%, Appendix IX C, Method I A.
ASSAY Dissolve 0.2 g in 10 ml of *ethanol (96%)* and titrate with 0.1M *hydrochloric acid VS* using *methyl red solution* as indicator until a red colour is produced. Each ml of 0.1M *hydrochloric acid VS* is equivalent to 24.15 mg of $C_{16}H_{35}N$.

Dimeticone Dimethicone of the British Pharmacopoeia.

Dimidium Bromide 3,8-Diamino-5-methyl-6-phenylphenanthridinium bromide; $C_{20}H_{18}BrN_3$ = 380.3 (*518-67-2*)
General reagent grade of commerce.
Dark red crystals.

Dimidium Bromide—Sulphan Blue Mixed Solution Dissolve separately 0.5 g of *dimidium bromide* and 0.25 g of *sulphan blue* each in 30 ml of a hot mixture of 1 volume of *absolute ethanol* and 9 volumes of *water*, mix the two solutions and dilute to 250 ml with the same solvent mixture. Mix 20 ml of the resulting solution with a mixture of 20 ml of 2.5M *sulphuric acid* and 250 ml of *water* and dilute to 500 ml with *water*.
Store protected from light.

Dinitrobenzene See *1,3-Dinitrobenzene.*

1,3-Dinitrobenzene Dinitrobenzene; $C_6H_4N_2O_4$ = 168.1 (*528-29-0*)
General reagent grade of commerce.
Pale yellow needles; melting point, about 90°.

Dinitrobenzene Solution A 1% w/v solution of *1,3-dinitrobenzene* in *ethanol (96%)*.

Dinitrobenzoic Acid See *3,5-dinitrobenzoic acid.*

3,5-Dinitrobenzoic Acid Dinitrobenzoic acid; $C_7H_4N_2O_6$ = 212.1 (*99-34-3*)
General reagent grade of commerce.
Almost colourless crystals; melting point, about 206°.

Dinitrobenzoic Acid Solution A 2% w/v solution of *3,5-dinitrobenzoic acid* in *ethanol (96%)*.

Dinitrobenzoyl Chloride See *3,5-dinitrobenzoyl chloride.*

3,5-Dinitrobenzoyl Chloride Dinitrobenzoyl chloride; $C_7H_3ClN_2O_5$ = 230.6 (*99-33-2*)
General reagent grade of commerce.
Yellow needles, decomposing in moist air; melting point, about 68°.

Dinitrophenylhydrazine See *2,4-dinitrophenylhydrazine.*

2,4-Dinitrophenylhydrazine Dinitrophenylhydrazine; $C_6H_6N_4O_4$ = 198.1 (*119-26-6*)
Analytical reagent grade of commerce.
Reddish orange crystals or crystalline powder; melting point, about 203°, Appendix V A, Method V.

Dinitrophenylhydrazine-aceto-hydrochloric Solution Dissolve 0.2 g of *2,4-dinitrophenylhydrazine* in 20 ml of *methanol* and add 80 ml of a mixture of equal volumes of 7M *hydrochloric acid* and 5M *acetic acid*.
Prepare immediately before use.

Dinitrophenylhydrazine-hydrochloric Solution Dissolve 0.5 g of *dinitrophenylhydrazine* in 2M *hydrochloric acid* with the aid of heat and add sufficient 2M *hydrochloric acid* to produce 100 ml. Allow to cool and filter. Prepare immediately before use.

Dinonyl Phthalate $C_{26}H_{24}O_4$ = 418.6 (*28553-12-0*)
Gas chromatographic reagent grade of commerce.
A colourless to pale yellow, viscous liquid; d_{20}^{20}, 0.97 to 0.98; n_D^{20}, about 1.482 to 1.489.
Complies with the following tests.
ACIDITY Shake 5 g with 25 ml of *water* for 1 minute, allow to stand, filter the separated aqueous layer and add 0.1 ml of *phenolphthalein solution*. Not more than 0.3 ml of 0.1M *sodium hydroxide VS* is required to change the colour of the solution (0.05%, calculated as phthalic acid).
WATER Not more than 0.1%, Appendix IX C.

Dioctadecyl Disulphide $C_{36}H_{74}S_2$ = 571.1 (*1844-09-3*)
General reagent grade of commerce.
Melting point, 53° to 58°.

2,2′-Di(octadecyloxy)-5,5′-spirobi(1,3,2-dioxaphosphorinane) $C_{41}H_{82}O_6P_2$ = 733
General reagent grade of commerce.
Melting point, 40° to 70°.

Dioctadecyl 3,3′-Thiodipropionate $C_{42}H_{82}O_4S$ = 683 (*693-36-7*)
General reagent grade of commerce.
Melting point, 58° to 67°.

Dioctyl Sodium Sulphosuccinate $C_{20}H_{37}NaO_7S$ = 444.6 (*577-11-7*)
General reagent grade of commerce.
White, waxy flakes; usually contains about 90% of $C_{20}H_{37}NaO_7S$.

Dioxan See *1,4-dioxan*.

1,4-Dioxan Dioxan; $C_4H_8O_2$ = 88.11 (*123-91-1*)
Analytical reagent grade of commerce containing not more than 0.5% of water.
A colourless liquid with an ethereal odour; freezing point, 9° to 11°; d_{20}^{20}, about 1.03.
Do not distil unless the dioxan complies with the following test for peroxides.
PEROXIDES Place 8 ml of *potassium iodide and starch solution* in a 12-ml ground-glass-stoppered cylinder about 1.5 cm in diameter. Fill completely with the reagent being examined, shake vigorously and allow to stand protected from light for 30 minutes. No colour is produced.

Dioxan Solution Dilute 50 ml of *dioxan stock solution* to 100 ml with *water* (0.5 mg per ml of dioxan).

Dioxan Solution R1 Dilute 10 ml of *dioxan solution* to 50 ml with *water* (0.1 mg per ml of dioxan).

Dioxan Stock Solution Dissolve 1.00 g of *1,4-dioxan* in *water* and dilute to 100 ml with the same solvent. Dilute 5 ml of this solution to 50 ml with *water* (1 mg per ml).

Diphenylamine $C_{12}H_{11}N$ = 169.2 (*122-39-4*)
Analytical reagent grade of commerce.
White crystals with a characteristic odour; melting point, about 55°.
Store protected from light.

Diphenylamine Solution A 0.1% w/v solution of *diphenylamine* in *sulphuric acid*.
Store protected from light.

Diphenylamine Solution R1 A 1% w/v solution of *diphenylamine* in *sulphuric acid*.
The solution is colourless.

Diphenylamine Solution R2 Dissolve 1 g of *diphenylamine* in 100 ml of *glacial acetic acid* and add 2.75 ml of *sulphuric acid*.
Use immediately after preparation.

Diphenylanthracene See *9,10-diphenylanthracene*.

9,10-Diphenylanthracene Diphenylanthracene; $C_{26}H_{18}$ = 330.4 (*1499-10-1*)
General reagent grade of commerce.
Melting point, about 248°.

Diphenylbenzidine See N,N′-*diphenylbenzidine*.

***N,N′*-Diphenylbenzidine** Diphenylbenzidine; $C_{24}H_{20}N_2$ = 336.4 (*531-91-9*)
General reagent grade of commerce.
A white or faintly grey, crystalline powder; melting point, about 248°.
Complies with the following tests.
NITRATE Dissolve 8 mg in a cooled mixture of 45 ml of *nitrogen-free sulphuric acid* and 5 ml of *water*. The solution is colourless or very pale blue.
SULPHATED ASH Not more than 0.1%, Appendix IX A.
Store protected from light.

Diphenylboric Acid Aminoethyl Ester $C_{14}H_{16}BNO$ = 225.1 (*524-95-8*)
General reagent grade of commerce.
A white or pale yellow, crystalline powder; melting point, about 193°.

Diphenylcarbazide See *1,5-diphenylcarbazide*.

1,5-Diphenylcarbazide Diphenylcarbazide; 1,5-diphenylcarbonodihydrazide; $C_{13}H_{14}N_4O$ = 242.3 (*140-22-7*)
Analytical reagent grade of commerce.
A white, crystalline powder gradually turning pink on exposure to air; melting point, about 170°.
Store protected from light.

Diphenylcarbazide Solution Dissolve 0.2 g of *diphenylcarbazide* in 10 ml of *glacial acetic acid* and dilute to 100 ml with *absolute ethanol*.
Prepare immediately before use.

Diphenylcarbazone See *1,5-diphenylcarbazone*.

1,5-Diphenylcarbazone Diphenylcarbazone; $C_{13}H_{12}N_4O$ = 240.3 (*538-62-5*)
General reagent grade of commerce.
An orange, crystalline powder; melting point, about 157°, with decomposition.

Diphenylcarbazone Mercuric Reagent Dissolve 0.1 g of *1,5-diphenylcarbazone* in sufficient *absolute ethanol* to produce 50 ml and, separately, dissolve 1 g of *mercury(II) chloride* in sufficient *absolute ethanol* to produce 50 ml. Mix equal volumes of the two solutions.

Diphenyloxazole 2,5-Diphenyloxazole; $C_{15}H_{11}NO$ = 221.3 (*92-71-7*)
General reagent grade of commerce.
Melting point, about 70°; A(1%, 1 cm), about 1260, determined at 305 nm in *methanol*.
Diphenyloxazole used for liquid scintillation is of a suitable analytical grade.

Diphenylphenylene Oxide Polymer 2,6-Diphenyl-*p*-phenylene oxide polymer
Chromatographic reagent grade of commerce.
White or almost white, porous beads. The size range of the beads is specified after the name of the reagent in tests where it is used.

Diphosphorus Pentoxide See *phosphorus pentoxide.*

Dipotassium Edetate Dipotassium dihydrogen ethylenediaminetetra-acetate; $C_{10}H_{14}N_2K_2O_8,2H_2O$ = 404.5 (*25102-12-9*)
General reagent grade of commerce.

Dipotassium Hydrogen Orthophosphate Dipotassium hydrogen phosphate; K_2HPO_4 = 174.2 (*7758-11-4*)
General reagent grade of commerce.

Dipotassium Hydrogen Phosphate See *dipotassium hydrogen orthophosphate.*

Dipotassium Sulphate See *potassium sulphate.*

Dipotassium (+)-Tartrate Potassium tartrate; $C_4H_4K_2O_6,½H_2O$ = 235.3 (*921-53-9*)
General reagent grade of commerce.

2,2′-Dipyridyl 2,2′-Bipyridine; $C_{10}H_8N_2$ = 156.2 (*366-18-7*)
General reagent grade of commerce.
Melting point, about 72°.

Disodium Arsenate Sodium arsenate heptahydrate; $Na_2HAsO_4,7H_2O$ = 312.0 (*10048-95-0*)
Analytical reagent grade of commerce.
Melting point, about 57°, when rapidly heated.

Disodium Edetate Disodium dihydrogen ethylenediaminetetra-acetate; sodium edetate; $C_{10}H_{14}N_2Na_2O_8,2H_2O$ = 372.2 (*13235-36-4*)
Analytical reagent grade of commerce.

Disodium Ethanedisulphonate 1,2-Ethanedisulphonic acid disodium salt; $C_2H_4Na_2O_6S_2$ = 234.2 (*5325-43-9*)
General reagent grade of commerce.

Disodium Hydrogen Citrate $C_6H_6Na_2O_7,1½H_2O$ = 263.1 (*144-33-2*)
General reagent grade of commerce.

Disodium Hydrogen Orthophosphate Disodium hydrogen phosphate; $Na_2HPO_4,12H_2O$ = 358.1 (*10039-32-4*)
Analytical reagent grade of commerce.

Disodium Hydrogen Orthophosphate, Anhydrous Anhydrous disodium hydrogen phosphate; Na_2HPO_4 = 142.0 (*7558-79-4*)
Analytical reagent grade of commerce.

Disodium Hydrogen Orthophosphate Dihydrate Disodium hydrogen phosphate dihydrate; Na_2HPO_4,H_2O = 178.0 (*10028-24-7*)
Analytical reagent grade of commerce.

Disodium Hydrogen Phosphate See *disodium hydrogen orthophosphate.*

Disodium Hydrogen Phosphate, Anhydrous See *anhydrous disodium hydrogen orthophosphate.*

Disodium Hydrogen Phosphate Dihydrate See *disodium hydrogen orthophosphate dihydrate.*

Disodium Hydrogen Phosphate Solution A 9% w/v solution of *disodium hydrogen orthophosphate.*

Disodium Tetraborate See *sodium tetraborate.*

5,5′-Dithiobis(2-nitrobenzoic) Acid 3-Carboxy-4-nitrophenyldisulphide; $C_{14}H_8N_2O_8S$ = 396.4 (*69-78-3*)
General reagent grade of commerce.
Melting point, about 242°.

Dithiol Toluene-3,4-dithiol; 4-methylbenzene-1,2-dithiol; $C_7H_8S_2$ = 156.3 (*496-74-2*)
General reagent grade of commerce.
Melting point, about 30°.
Store in an airtight container.

Dithiol Reagent Toluenedithiol reagent
To 1 g of *dithiol* add 2 ml of *mercaptoacetic acid* and dilute to 250 ml with a 2% w/v solution of *sodium hydroxide.*
Prepare immediately before use.

Dithiothreitol *threo*-1,4-Dimercapto-2,3-butanediol; $C_4H_{10}O_2S_2$ = 154.2 (*27565-41-9*)
General reagent grade of commerce.
Store in an airtight container.

Dithizone 1,5-Diphenylthiocarbazone; $C_{13}H_{12}N_4S$ = 256.3 (*60-10-6*)
Analytical reagent grade of commerce.
An almost black powder.
Store protected from light.

Dithizone R1 *Dithizone* containing not less than 98.0% of $C_{13}H_{12}N_4S$.

Dithizone Solution A 0.05% w/v solution of *dithizone* in *chloroform.*
Prepare immediately before use.

Dithizone Solution R2 Dissolve 40 mg of *dithizone* in sufficient *chloroform* to produce 1000 ml. Dilute 30 ml of the solution to 100 ml with *chloroform.*

Ascertain its exact concentration in the following manner. Dissolve a quantity of *mercury(II) chloride* equivalent to 0.1354 g of $HgCl_2$ in a mixture of equal volumes of 1M *sulphuric acid* and *water* and dilute to 100 ml with the same solvent. Dilute 2 ml of this solution to 100 ml with a mixture of equal volumes of 1M *sulphuric acid* and *water.* (This solution contains 20 ppm of Hg.) Transfer 1.0 ml of the solution to a separating funnel and add 50 ml of 1M *sulphuric acid,* 140 ml of *water* and 10 ml of a 20% w/v solution of *hydroxylamine hydrochloride.* Titrate with the dithizone solution; after each addition shake the mixture 20 times and towards the end of the titration allow to separate and discard the chloroform layer. Continue the titration until a bluish green colour is obtained. Calculate the equivalent in mg of mercury per ml of the dithizone solution from the expression $20/V$ where V is the volume in ml of the dithizone solution used in the titration.

Divanadium Pentoxide Vanadium(V) oxide; V_2O_5 = 181.9 (*1314-62-1*)
General reagent grade of commerce containing not less than 98.5% of V_2O_5.
Complies with the following test.
SENSITIVITY TO HYDROGEN PEROXIDE Heat 1 g for 30 minutes with 10 ml of *sulphuric acid,* allow to cool and restore the volume to 10 ml with *sulphuric acid.* Dilute cautiously 1 ml of the clear solution to 50 ml with *water.* To 0.5 ml of the resulting solution add 0.1 ml of *hydrogen peroxide solution (20 vol)* diluted to contain 0.01% w/v of H_2O_2; a distinct orange colour is produced in comparison with a blank prepared from 0.5 ml of the solution and 0.1 ml of *water.* Add a further 0.4 ml of the peroxide solution; the colour changes to orange-yellow.

Divanadium Pentoxide Solution in Sulphuric Acid Dissolve 0.2 g of *divanadium pentoxide* in 4 ml of *sulphuric acid* and add sufficient *water* to produce 100 ml.

Docusate Sodium See *dioctyl sodium sulphosuccinate.*

Dodecan-1-ol Lauryl alcohol; $C_{12}H_{26}O$ = 186.3 (*112-53-8*)
Purified general reagent grade of commerce.
Colourless leaflets, or a colourless, oily liquid; freezing point, about 24°.

Domiphen Bromide Dodecyldimethyl-2-phenoxyethyl-ammonium bromide; $C_{22}H_{40}BrNO$ = 414.5 (*538-71-6*)
General reagent grade of commerce.

Dotriacontane $C_{32}H_{66}$ = 450.9 (*544-85-4*)
General reagent grade of commerce.
White plates; melting point, about 69°.
IMPURITIES Not more than 0.1% of impurities with the same retention time as α-tocopherol acetate when determined by the gas chromatographic method described in the monograph for Alpha-Tocopherol Acetate.

***n*-Eicosane** $C_{20}H_{42}$ = 282.6 (*112-95-8*)
General reagent grade of commerce.
Melting point, about 37°.

Emetine Dihydrochloride $C_{29}H_{40}N_2O_4,2HCl,5H_2O$ = 643.6 (*316-42-7 (anhydrous)*)
General reagent grade of commerce.

Emodin 1,3,8-Trihydroxy-6-methylanthraquinone; $C_{15}H_{10}O_5$ = 270.2 (*518-82-1*)
General reagent grade of commerce.
Orange crystals; melting point, about 253°, with decomposition.
Complies with the following test.
HOMOGENEITY Carry out test C for Identification described in the monograph for Rhubarb. The chromatogram obtained with solution (2) shows only one principal spot.

Eosin CI 45380; acid red 87; $C_{20}H_6Br_4Na_2O_5$ = 691.9 (*17372-87-1*)
General reagent grade of commerce.
A red powder.

Erucamide (*Z*)-Docos-13-enoamide; $C_{22}H_{43}NO$ = 337.6 (*112-84-5*)
General reagent grade of commerce.
Melting point, about 70°.

17α-Estradiol $C_{18}H_{24}O$ = 272.4 (*57-91-0*)
General reagent grade of commerce.
Melting point, 178° to 179°.

Estragole 4-Allylanisole; 1-methoxy-4-prop-2-enylbenzene; $C_{10}H_{12}O$ = 148.2 (*140-67-0*)
General reagent grade of commerce.
Boiling point, about 216°; n_D^{20}, about 1.52.
Estragole used in gas chromatography complies with the following test.
ASSAY Examine by *gas chromatography*, Appendix III B, under the conditions described in the test for Chromatographic profile in the monograph for Anise Oil using the reagent being examined as the test solution.

The area of the principal peak is not less than 98.0% of the total area of the peaks.

Ethane-1,2-diol Ethylene glycol; $C_2H_6O_2$ = 62.07 (*107-21-1*)
Analytical reagent grade of commerce.
A colourless, viscous liquid; d_{20}^{20}, 1.113 to 1.115; n_D^{20}, 1.430 to 1.433; boiling point, about 196°.

Ethanol See *absolute ethanol*.

Ethanol, Absolute Ethanol; C_2H_6O = 46.07 (*64-17-5*)
Analytical reagent grade of commerce containing not less than 99.5% v/v of C_2H_6O.
A colourless, hygroscopic liquid with a characteristic odour; boiling point, 78° to 79°; d_{20}^{20}, 0.791 to 0.794.
Store protected from light at a temperature not exceeding 30°.

Ethanol R1 See *absolute ethanol R1*.

Ethanol R1, Absolute Ethanol R1
Absolute ethanol grade of commerce complying with the following test.
METHANOL Not more than 0.005% v/v when determined in the following manner. Carry out the method for *gas chromatography*, Appendix III B, alternately injecting 1 µl of the following solutions three times. For solution (1) use the reagent being examined. For solution (2) dilute 0.5 ml of *anhydrous methanol* to 100 ml with the reagent being examined and further dilute 1 ml to 100 ml.

The chromatographic procedure may be carried out using a glass column (2 m × 2 mm) packed with *ethylvinylbenzene—divinyl benzene copolymer* (75 µm to 100 µm) and using 30 ml per minute as the flow rate of the carrier gas. Maintain the temperature of the column at 130°, that of the injection port at 150° and that of the detector at 200°. After each injection heat the column to 230° for 8 minutes.

Calculate the percentage of methanol using the expression $ab/(c-b)$ where a is the percentage v/v content of methanol in solution (2), b is the area of the methanol peak in the chromatogram obtained with solution (1) and c is the area of the methanol peak in the chromatogram obtained with solution (2).

Ethanol (96%) Alcohol
Analytical reagent grade ethanol of commerce containing not less than 95.1% v/v and not more than 96.9% v/v of C_2H_6O.
A colourless liquid; weight per ml, about 0.81 g.
Diluted ethanols may be prepared by diluting the volumes of *ethanol (96%)* indicated in the following table to 1000 ml with *water*.

Strength % v/v	Volume of *ethanol (96%)* (approx) ml	Weight per ml g
90	934	0.83
85	885	0.85
80	831	0.86
70	727	0.89
65	676	0.90
60	623	0.91
50	519	0.93
45	468	0.94
25	259	0.97
20	207	0.975
10	104	0.986

Ethanol (96%), Aldehyde-free Aldehyde-free alcohol
Mix 1200 ml of *ethanol (96%)* with 5 ml of a 40% w/v solution of *silver nitrate* and 10 ml of a cooled 50% w/v solution of *potassium hydroxide*. Shake, allow to stand for a few days and filter. Distil the filtrate immediately before use.

Ethanolamine 2-Aminoethanol; C_2H_7NO = 61.08 (*141-43-5*)
General reagent grade of commerce.
A colourless, viscous liquid; d_{20}^{20}, about 1.04; n_D^{20}, about 1.454; melting point, about 11°.
Store in an airtight container.

Ether Diethyl ether; $C_4H_{10}O$ = 74.12 (*60-29-7*)
Analytical reagent grade of commerce.
A volatile, highly flammable, colourless liquid; boiling point, 34° to 35°; d_{20}^{20}, 0.713 to 0.715.
Do not distil unless the ether complies with the following test for peroxides.
PEROXIDES Place 8 ml of *potassium iodide and starch solution* in a 12 ml ground-glass-stoppered cylinder about 1.5 cm in diameter. Fill completely with the reagent being examined, shake vigorously and allow to stand in the dark for 30 minutes. No colour is produced.
Store protected from light at a temperature not exceeding 15°. The name and concentration of any added stabiliser are stated on the label.

Ether, Peroxide-free Shake 1000 ml of *ether* with 20 ml of a solution of 30 g of *iron(II) sulphate* in 55 ml of *water* and 3 ml of *sulphuric acid*. Continue shaking until a small sample no longer produces a blue colour when shaken with an equal volume of a 2% w/v solution of *potassium iodide* and 0.1 ml of *starch mucilage*.

Ethoxychrysoidine Hydrochloride 4-*p*-Ethoxyphenylazo-*m*-phenylenediamine hydrochloride; $C_{14}H_{16}N_4O,HCl$ = 292.8
General reagent grade of commerce.
A red powder.

Ethoxychrysoidine Solution A 0.1% w/v solution of *ethoxychrysoidine hydrochloride* in *ethanol (96%)*.
Complies with the following test.
SENSITIVITY TO BROMINE To a mixture of 0.05 ml and 5 ml of 2M *hydrochloric acid* add 0.05 ml of 0.0167M *bromine VS*. The colour changes from red to light yellow within 2 minutes.

2-Ethoxyethanol Ethylene Glycol Monoethyl Ether; $C_4H_{10}O_2$ = 90.1 (*110-80-5*)
General reagent grade of commerce.
Boiling point, about 135°; d_{20}^{20}, about 0.93; n_D^{20}, about 1.406.

Ethyl Acetate $C_4H_8O_2$ = 88.1 (*141-78-6*)
Analytical reagent grade of commerce.
A colourless liquid with a fruity odour; boiling point, about 76° to 78°; d_{20}^{20}, 0.901 to 0.904.

Ethyl Acetate, Treated Disperse 200 g of *sulphamic acid* in sufficient *ethyl acetate* to produce 1000 ml, stir the suspension for 3 days and filter.
Use within 1 month of preparation.

Ethyl Acrylate Ethyl prop-2-enoate; $C_5H_8O_2$ = 100.1 (*140-88-5*)
General reagent grade of commerce.
Melting point, about −71°; boiling point, about 99°; n_D^{20}, about 1.406; d_{20}^{20}, about 1.04.

Ethyl Benzoate $C_9H_{10}O_2$ = 150.2 (*93-89-0*)
General reagent grade of commerce.
A colourless liquid; n_D^{20}, about 1.505; weight per ml, about 1.05 g.

Ethyl Cinnamate $C_{11}H_{12}O_2$ = 176.2 (*103-36-6*)
General reagent grade of commerce.
A colourless or very pale yellow liquid; weight per ml, about 1.05 g.

Ethyl Cyanoacetate $C_5H_7NO_2$ = 113.1 (*105-56-6*)
Analytical reagent grade of commerce.
A colourless or almost colourless liquid; boiling point, 205° to 209°, with decomposition.

Ethyl Formate $C_3H_6O_2$ = 74.1 (*109-94-4*)
General reagent grade of commerce.
d_{20}^{20}, about 0.919; n_D^{20}, about 1.36; boiling point, about 54°.

Ethyl Methyl Ketone See *butan-2-one*.

Ethyl Parahydroxybenzoate Ethyl 4-hydroxybenzoate; $C_9H_{10}O_3$ = 166.2 (*120-47-8*)
General reagent grade of commerce.
Melting point, about 117°.

4-[(Ethylamino)methyl]pyridine $C_8H_{12}N_2$ = 136.2 (*33403-97-3*)
General reagent grade of commerce.
d_{20}^{20}, about 0.98; n_D^{20}, about 1.516; boiling point, about 98°.

Ethylbenzene C_8H_{10} = 106.2 (*100-41-4*)
Reagent grade of commerce containing not less than 99.5% w/w of C_8H_{10} when determined by gas chromatography.
A colourless liquid; d_{20}^{20}, about 0.87; n_D^{20}, about 1.496; boiling point, about 135°.

4-Ethylcatechol 3,4-Dihydroxyethylbenzene; $C_8H_{10}O_2$ = 138.2
General reagent grade of commerce.

Ethylene Bis[3,3-di(3-(1,1-dimethyl)ethyl-4-hydroxyphenyl)butyrate] $C_{50}H_{66}O_8$ = 795 (*32509-66-3*)
General reagent grade of commerce.
Melting point, about 165°.

Ethylene Bis[3,3-di(3-*tert*-butyl-4-hydroxyphenyl)-butyrate] See *ethylene bis[3,3-di(3-(1,1-dimethyl)ethyl-4-hydroxyphenyl)butyrate]*.

Ethylene Chloride See *1,2-dichloroethane*.

Ethylene Glycol See *ethane-1,2-diol*.

Ethylene Glycol Monoethyl Ether See *2-ethoxyethanol*.

Ethylene Glycol Monomethyl Ether See *2-methoxyethanol*.

Ethylene Oxide Oxirane; C_2H_4O = 44.05 (*75-21-8*)
General reagent grade of commerce.
A colourless gas; liquefaction point, about 12°.

Ethylene Oxide Stock Solution *All operations carried out in the preparation of these solutions must be conducted in a fume-hood. The operator must protect both hands and face by wearing polyethylene protective gloves and an appropriate face mask. Store all solutions in airtight containers at 4° to 8°. Cary out all determinations three times.*
Into a dry, clean test tube cooled in a mixture of 1 part of *sodium chloride* and 3 parts of crushed ice introduce a slow current of *ethylene oxide* gas, allowing condensation onto the inner wall of the test tube. Using a glass syringe, previously cooled to −10°, inject about 300 µl (corresponding to about 0.25 g) of liquid *ethylene oxide* into 50 ml of *polyethylene glycol 200 R1*. Determine the absorbed quantity of ethylene oxide by weighing before and after absorption (M_{EO}). Dilute to 100 ml with *polyethylene glycol 200 R1*. Mix well before use. Determine the exact concentration of ethylene oxide in the following manner.
ASSAY To 10 ml of 50% w/v suspension of *magnesium chloride* in *absolute ethanol* add 20 ml of 0.1M *ethanolic hydrochloric acid VS*, shake to obtain a saturated solution and allow to stand overnight to equilibrate. Weigh 5 g of the solution being examined into the flask and allow to stand for 30 minutes. Titrate with 0.1M *ethanolic potassium hydroxide VS*, determining the end point potentio-

metrically, Appendix VIII B. Carry out a blank titration using *polyethylene glycol 200 R1* in place of the substance being examined. The ethylene oxide concentration in mg per g is given by the expression $4.404(V_0 - V_1)/m$, where V_0 and V_1 are the volumes of ethanolic potassium hydroxide used respectively for the blank titration and the assay and *m* is the weight of sample taken, in g.

Ethylene Oxide Solution Weigh a quantity of cool *ethylene oxide stock solution* containing 2.5 mg of ethylene oxide into a cool flask and dilute to 50 g with *polyethylene glycol 200 R1*. Mix well and dilute 2.5 g of this solution to 25 ml with *polyethylene glycol 200 R1* (5 µg of ethylene oxide per g of solution).
Prepare immediately before use.

Ethylene Oxide Solution R1 Dilute 1 ml of cooled *ethylene oxide stock solution* (check the exact volume by weighing) to 50 ml with *ployethylene glycol 200 R1* and mix well. Dilute 2.5 g of this solution to 25 ml with *polyethylene glycol 200 R1* (5 µg of ethylene oxide per g of solution). Calculate the exact amount of ethylene oxide in ppm from the volume determined by weighing and taking the density of polyethylene glycol 200 R1 to be 1.127.
Prepare immediately before use.

Ethylene Oxide Solution R2 *Prepare immediately before use.* Weigh 1 g of cold *ethylene oxide stock solution* (equivalent to 2.5 mg of ethylene oxide) into a cold flask containing 40.0 g of cold *polyethylene glycol 200 R1*. Mix and determine the exact weight and dilute to a calculated weight to obtain a solution containing 50 µg of ethylene oxide per g of solution. Weigh 10 g into a flask containing about 30 ml of *water*, mix and dilute to 50 ml with *water* (10 µg per ml of ethylene oxide).

Ethylene Oxide Solution R3 *Prepare immediately before use.* Dilute 10 ml of *ethylene oxide solution R2* to 50 ml with *water* (2 µg per ml of ethylene oxide).

Ethylenediamine 1,2-Diaminoethane; $C_2H_8N_2$ = 60.10 (*107-15-3*)
General reagent grade of commerce.
Boiling point, about 116°; n_D^{20}, about 1.457; weight per ml, about 0.90 g.

Ethylenediaminetetra-acetic Acid $C_{10}H_{16}N_2O_8$ = 292.2 (*60-00-4*)
General reagent grade of commerce.
Melting point, about 250°.

(Ethylenedinitrilo)tetra-acetic Acid See *ethylenediaminetetra-acetic acid.*

2-Ethylhexane-1,3-diol $C_8H_{18}O_2$ = 146.2 (*94-96-2*)
General reagent grade of commerce.
d_{20}^{20}, about 0.942; n_D^{20}, about 1.451; boiling point, about 244°.

2-Ethylhexanoic Acid 2-Ethylhexoic acid; $C_8H_{16}O_2$ = 144.2 (*149-57-5*)
General reagent grade of commerce.
A colourless liquid; d_{20}^{20}, about 0.91; n_D^{20}, about 1.425.
Complies with the following test.
RELATED SUBSTANCES Carry out the method for *gas chromatography*, Appendix III B, using 1 µl of a solution prepared in the following manner. Suspend 0.2 g of the reagent in 5 ml of *water*, add 3 ml of 2M *hydrochloric acid* and 5 ml of *hexane*, shake for 1 minute, allow the layers to separate and use the upper layer.

The chromatographic procedure described in the test for 2-Ethylhexanoic acid in the monograph for Amoxicillin Sodium may be used.

The sum of the areas of any *secondary peaks* is not greater than 2.5% of the area of the principal peak.

1,1′-Ethylidenebis(tryptophan) $C_{24}H_{26}N_4O_4$ = 434.5 (*132685-02-0*)
General reagent grade of commerce containing not less than 98.0% of $C_{24}H_{26}N_4O_4$.
Melting point, about 223°, with decomposition.
ASSAY Proceed as described in the test for 1,1′-Ethylidenebis(tryptophan) and other related substances in the monograph for Tryptophan. The area of the principal peak in the chromatogram obtained with reference solution (a) is not less than 98.0% of the area of all the peaks.

***N*-Ethylmaleimide** 1-Ethyl-1*H*-pyrrole-2,5-dione; $C_6H_7NO_2$ = 125.1 (*128-53-0*)
General reagent grade of commerce.
Melting point, 41° to 45°.
Store at a temperature between 2° and 8°.

2-Ethyl-2-methylsuccinic Acid 2-Ethyl-2-methylbutanedioic acid; $C_7H_{12}O_4$ = 160.2 (*631-31-2*)
General reagent grade of commerce.
Melting point, 104° to 107°.

Ethylvinylbenzene□Divinylbenzene Copolymer
Porous, rigid, cross-linked polymer beads.
Gas chromatographic grade of commerce.
Several grades are available with different sizes of bead; the size range is specified after the name of the reagent in tests where it is used.

Ethylvinylbenzene—Divinylbenzene Copolymer R1
Porous, rigid, cross-linked polymer beads with a nominal specific surface area of 500m²/g to 600 m²/g and having pores with a mean diameter of 7.5 nm.
Gas chromatographic grade of commerce.
Several grades are available with different sizes of bead; the size range is specified after the name of the reagent in tests where it is used.

Eugenol 4-Allyl-2-methoxyphenol; $C_{10}H_{12}O_2$ = 164.2 (*97-53-0*)
General reagent grade of commerce.
A colourless or pale yellow, oily liquid; d_{20}^{20}, about 1.07.
Eugenol used in gas chromatography complies with the following test.
ASSAY Carry out the test for Chromatographic profile in the monograph for Clove Oil using the reagent being examined as the test solution. The area of the principal peak is not less than 98.0% of the total area of the peaks.
Store protected from light.

Euglobulins, Bovine
For the preparation, use fresh bovine blood collected into an anticoagulant solution (for example sodium citrate solution). Discard any haemolysed blood. Centrifuge at 1500 to 1800 *g* between 15° to 20° to obtain a supernatant plasma poor in platelets.

To 1 litre of the bovine plasma add 75 g of *barium sulphate* and shake for 30 minutes. Centrifuge at not less than 1500 *g* to 1800 *g* between 15° to 20° and draw off the clear supernatant liquid. Add 10 ml of a solution of *aprotinin* containing 0.2 mg per ml and shake to ensure mixing. In a container with a minimum capacity of 30 litres in a chamber at 4° introduce 25 litres of *distilled water* at 4° and add about 500 g of solid carbon dioxide. Immediately add, while stirring, the supernatant liquid obtained from the plasma. A white precipitate is produced. Allow to settle at 4° for 10 to 15 hours. Remove

the clear supernatant solution by siphoning. Collect the precipitate by centrifugation at 4°. Suspend the precipitate by dispersing mechanically in 500 ml of *distilled water* at 4°, shake for 5 minutes and collect the precipitate by centrifugation at 4°. Disperse the precipitate mechanically in 60 ml of a solution containing 0.9% w/v of *sodium chloride* and 0.09% w/v of *sodium citrate* and adjust the pH to 7.2 to 7.4 by adding a 1% w/v solution of *sodium hydroxide*. Filter through a sintered-glass filter; to facilitate the dissolution of the precipitate crush the particles of the precipitate with a suitable implement. Wash the filter and the implement with 40 ml of the chloride—citrate solution described above and dilute to 100 ml with the same solution. Freeze dry the solution. The yields are generally 6 to 8 g of euglobulins per litre of bovine plasma.
SUITABILITY TEST For this test, prepare the solutions using *phosphate buffer pH 7.4* containing 3% w/v of *bovine albumin*. Into a test tube 8 mm in diameter placed in a water bath at 37°, introduce 0.2 ml of a solution of a reference preparation of urokinase containing 100 IU of urokinase activity per ml and 0.1 ml of a solution of *thrombin* containing 20 IU per ml. Add rapidly 0.5 ml of a solution containing 10 mg of the euglobulin fraction per ml. A firm clot is produced in less than 10 seconds. Note the time that elapses between the addition of the solution of the euglobulin fraction and the lysis of the clot. The lysis time does not exceed 15 minutes.
Store protected from moisture at 4° and use within 1 year.

Euglobulins, Human
For the preparation, use fresh human blood collected into an anticoagulant solution (for example sodium citrate solution) or human blood for transfusion collected into plastic blood bags that has just reached its expiry date. Discard any haemolysed blood. Centrifuge at 1500 to 1800 *g* at 15° to obtain a supernatant plasma poor in platelets. Iso-group plasmas may be mixed.

To 1 litre of the human plasma add 75 g of *barium sulphate* and shake for 30 minutes. Centrifuge at not less than 15,000 *g* at 15° and draw off the clear supernatant liquid. Add 10 ml of a 0.02% w/v solution of *aprotinin* and shake to ensure mixing. In a container with a minimum capacity of 30 litres in a chamber at 4° introduce 25 litres of distilled water at 4° and add about 500 g of solid carbon dioxide. Immediately add, while stirring, the supernatant liquid obtained from the plasma. A white precipitate is produced. Allow to settle at 4° for 10 to 15 hours. Remove the clear supernatant solution by siphoning. Collect the precipitate by centrifuging at 4°. Suspend the precipitate by dispersing mechanically in 500 ml of distilled water at 4°, shake for 5 minutes and collect the precipitate by centrifuging at 4°. Disperse the precipitate mechanically in 60 ml of a solution containing 0.9% w/v of *sodium chloride* and 0.09% w/v of *sodium citrate* and adjust the pH to 7.2 to 7.4 by adding a 1% w/v solution of *sodium hydroxide*. Filter through a sintered-glass filter; to facilitate the dissolution of the precipitate crush the particles of the precipitate with a suitable implement. Wash the filter and the implement with 40 ml of the chloride—citrate solution described above and dilute to 100 ml with the same solution. Freeze dry the solution. The yields are generally 6 to 8 g of euglobulins per litre of human plasma.
Complies with the following test.
SUITABILITY TEST Carry out the test described under Bovine Euglobins using *citro-phosphate buffer pH 7.2* containing 3% w/v of *bovine albumin*.
Store in an airtight container at 4° and use within 1 year.

Fast Blue B Salt CI 37235; $C_{14}H_{12}Cl_2N_4O_2$ = 339.2 (*84633-94-3*)
General reagent grade of commerce.
A dark green powder, stabilised by the addition of zinc chloride.
Store in an airtight container at a temperature between 2° and 8°.

Fast Red B Salt CI 37125; 2-methoxy-4-nitrobenzene-diazonium hydrogen naphthalene-1,5-disulphonate; $C_{17}H_{13}N_3O_9S_2$ = 467.4 (*56315-29-8*)
General reagent grade of commerce.
Orange-yellow powder.
Store in an airtight container protected from light at a temperature of 2° to 8°.

Fenbufen $C_{16}H_{14}O_3$ = 254.3 (*36330-85-5*)
General reagent grade of commerce.

Fenchone 1,3,3-Trimethylbicyclo[2.2.1]heptan-2-one; $C_{10}H_{16}O$ = 152.2 (*7787-20-4*)
General reagent grade of commerce.
Boiling point, about 193°; n_D^{20}, about 1.46.
Fenchone used in gas chromatography complies with the following test.
ASSAY Examine by *gas chromatography*, Appendix III B, under the conditions described in the Assay for anethole and fenchone in the monograph for Bitter Fennel using the reagent being examined as solution (1).

The area of the principal peak is not less than 98.0% of the total area of the peaks.

Ferric Ammonium Sulphate See *ammonium iron(III) sulphate*.

Ferric Ammonium Sulphate Solution R2 See *ammonium iron(III) solution R2.*

Ferric Ammonium Sulphate Solution R5 See *ammonium iron(III) solution R5.*

Ferric Ammonium Sulphate Solution R6 See *ammonium iron(III) solution R6.*

Ferric Chloride See *iron(III) chloride.*

Ferric Chloride Solution R1 See *iron(III) chloride solution R1.*

Ferric Chloride Solution R2 See *iron(III) chloride solution R2*

Ferric Chloride-Sulphamic Acid Reagent See *iron(III) chloride—sulphamic acid reagent.*

Ferric Nitrate See *iron(III) nitrate.*

Ferric Sulphate See *iron(III) sulphate.*

Ferrocyphen Dicyanobis(1,10-phenanthroline)iron(II); $C_{26}H_{16}FeN_6$ = 468.3 (*14768-11-7*)
A violet-bronze, crystalline powder.
General reagent grade of commerce.
Store protected from light and moisture.

Ferrocyphen Solution Dissolve, without warming, 0.5 g of *ferrocyphen* in 50 ml of *sulphuric acid.*

Ferrocyphene See *ferrocyphen.*

Ferroin See *ferroin solution.*

Ferroin Solution (*14634-91-4*)
Tris(1,10-phenanthroline)iron(II) sulphate complex prepared in the following manner. Dissolve 0.7 g of *iron(II) sulphate* and 1.76 g of *phenanthroline hydrochloride* in 70 ml of *water* and add sufficient *water* to produce 100 ml.

Complies with the following test.
SENSITIVITY TO CERIUM(IV) Add 0.1 ml of the solution and 0.15 ml of *osmium tetroxide solution* to 50 ml of 1M *sulphuric acid*. Add 0.1 ml of 0.1M *ammonium cerium(IV) nitrate*. The colour changes from red to light blue.

Ferrous Ammonium Sulphate See *ammonium iron(II) sulphate*.

Ferrous Sulphate See *iron(II) sulphate*.

Ferrous Sulphate Solution R2 See *iron(II) sulphate solution R2*.

Fibrin Blue Mix 1.5 g of fibrin with 30 ml of a 0.5% w/v solution of *indigo carmine* in 0.02M *hydrochloric acid*. Heat the mixture to 80° and maintain at this temperature while stirring for about 30 minutes. Allow to cool, filter and wash extensively by resuspension in 0.02M *hydrochloric acid* and mixing for about 30 minutes. Filter and repeat the washing procedure three time. Dry the residue at 50° and grind.

Fibrin Congo Red See *congo red fibrin*.

Fibrinogen *(9001-32-5)*
Complies with the monograph for Dried Fibrinogen.

Flufenamic Acid $C_{14}H_{10}F_3NO_2$ = 281.2 *(530-78-9)*
Pale yellow, crystalline powder or needles.
General reagent grade of commerce.
Melting point, 132° to 135°.

Fluoranthene $C_{16}H_{10}$ = 202.3 *(206-44-0)*
General reagent grade of commerce.
Melting point, 105° to 110°; boiling point, about 384°.

9-Fluorenone $C_{13}H_{18}O$ = 180.2 *(486-25-9)*
General reagent grade of commerce.
Melting point, about 83°.

Fluorenone Solution Dissolve 50 mg of *9-fluorenone* in 10 ml of warm *methanol*, transfer to a 500-ml graduated flask with the aid of 190 ml of *methanol* and add sufficient *water* to produce 500 ml. The solution should be clear. Immediately before use dilute 10 ml of this solution to 100 ml with *methanol*.

(9-Fluorenyl)methyl Chloroformate $C_{15}H_{11}ClO_2$ = 258.7 *(28920-43-6)*
General reagent grade of commerce.
Melting point, about 63°.

Fluorescamine $C_{17}H_{10}O_4$ = 278.3 *(38183-12-9)*
General reagent grade of commerce.
Melting point, about 155°.

Fluorescein $C_{20}H_{12}O_5$ = 332.3 *(2321-07-5)*
An orange-red powder displaying a green fluorescence in solution.
General reagent grade of commerce.
Melting point, about 315°.

Fluorescein Sodium Sodium fluoresceinate; $C_{20}H_{10}Na_2O_5$ = 376.3 *(518-47-8)*
General reagent grade of commerce.

Fluorodinitrobenzene See *1-fluoro-2,4-dinitrobenzene*.

1-Fluoro-2,4-dinitrobenzene 2,4-Dinitrofluorobenzene; $C_6H_3FN_2O_4$ = 186.1 *(70-34-8)*
General reagent grade of commerce.
Pale yellow, vesicatory crystals, lumps or liquid with a lachrymatory vapour.
Melting point, about 29°; weight per ml, about 1.48 g; n_D^{20}, about 1.569.

1-Fluoro-2-nitro-4-trifluoromethylbenzene 4-Fluoro-3-nitrobenzotrifluoride; $C_7H_3F_4NO_2$ = 209.1 *(367-86-2)*
General reagent grade of commerce.
Melting point, about 197°.

Folic Acid $C_{19}H_{19}N_7O_6$ = 441.4 *(75708-92-8)*
General reagent grade of commerce.
A yellow to orange, crystalline powder.
Store in a well-closed container protected from light.

Formaldehyde See *formaldehyde solution*.

Formaldehyde Solution CH_2O = 30.03 *(50-00-0)*
Analytical reagent grade of commerce containing not less than 34.0% w/v and not more than 37.0% w/v of CH_2O.
A colourless, aqueous solution with a lachrymatory vapour; weight per ml, about 1.08 g.
ASSAY Dilute 5 ml to 1000 ml with *water*. To 10 ml of the solution add 25 ml of 0.05M *iodine VS* and 10 ml of 1M *sodium hydroxide*. Allow to stand for 5 minutes, add 11 ml of 1M *hydrochloric acid* and titrate the excess iodine with 0.1M *sodium thiosulphate VS* using 1 ml of *starch solution* added towards the end of the titration as indicator. Each ml of 0.05M *iodine VS* is equivalent to 1.50 mg of CH_2O.
Store at a temperature between 15° and 25°.

Formamide CH_3NO = 45.04 *(75-12-7)*
Analytical reagent grade of commerce.
A colourless, oily liquid; weight per ml, about 1.13 g.
Store in an airtight container.

Formamide, Treated Disperse 1 g of *sulphamic acid* in 20 ml of *formamide* containing 5% v/v of *water*.

Formic Acid CH_2O_2 = 46.03 *(64-18-6)*
Analytical reagent grade of commerce containing about 90% w/w of CH_2O_2 and about 23.6M in strength.
A colourless, corrosive liquid with a pungent odour; weight per ml, about 1.20 g.

Formic Acid, Anhydrous CH_2O_2 = 46.03
Analytical reagent grade formic acid of commerce containing not less than 98.0% w/w of CH_2O_2.
A colourless, corrosive liquid with a pungent odour; d_{20}^{20}, about 1.22.
ASSAY Weigh accurately a conical flask containing 10 ml of *water*, quickly add about 1 ml of the reagent and weigh again. Add 50 ml of *water* and titrate with 1M *sodium hydroxide VS* using 0.5 ml of *phenolphthalein solution* as indicator. Each ml of 1M *sodium hydroxide VS* is equivalent to 46.03 mg of CH_2O_2.

Fructose See *D-fructose*.

D-Fructose Laevulose; $C_6H_{12}O_6$ = 180.2 *(57-48-7)*
General reagent grade of commerce.
A white, crystalline powder; melting point, about 103°, with decomposition; $[\alpha]_D^{20}$, about –92° (10% w/v in water containing 0.05 ml of 5M ammonia).

Fuchsin, Basic Basic violet 14; basic magenta; a mixture of rosaniline hydrochloride, $C_{20}H_{19}N_3$,HCl (337.9) (CI 42510) and pararosaniline hydrochloride, $C_{19}H_{17}N_3$,HCl (323.8) (CI 42500) *(569-61-9)*
A dark red powder or green crystals with a metallic lustre of such a purity that, when used in the preparation of *decolorised fuchsin solution*, an almost colourless solution is obtained. If necessary, purify in the following manner. Dissolve 1 g in 250 ml of 2M *hydrochloric acid*, allow to stand for 2 hours at room temperature, filter and neutralise with 2M *sodium hydroxide* and add 1 ml to 2 ml in excess. Filter the precipitate through a sintered-glass filter

(40) and wash with *water*. Dissolve the precipitate in 70 ml of *methanol*, previously heated to boiling, and add 300 ml of *water* at 80°. Allow to cool to room temperature, filter and dry the crystals at a pressure of 2 kPa. Store protected from light.

Fuchsin Solution, Basic Dissolve 0.1 g of *basic fuchsin* in 3 ml of *methanol*, dilute to 100 ml with *water*, mix and filter.

Fuchsin Solution, Decolorised Dissolve 0.1 g of *basic fuchsin* in 60 ml of *water* and add 1 g of *anhydrous sodium sulphite* dissolved in 10 ml of *water*. Slowly add 2 ml of *hydrochloric acid*, stirring continuously, and dilute to 100 ml with *water*. Allow to stand protected from light for at least 12 hours. Shake with sufficient *activated charcoal* (0.2 to 0.3 g) to remove the colour and then filter immediately. If the solution becomes cloudy, filter before use. If on standing the solution becomes violet, decolorise again by adding *activated charcoal*.
Complies with the following test.
SENSITIVITY TO FORMALDEHYDE To 1.0 ml of the solution add 1.0 ml of *water* and 0.1 ml of *aldehyde-free ethanol (96%)*. Add 0.2 ml of a solution containing 0.01% w/v of formaldehyde. A pale pink colour is produced within 5 minutes.
Store protected from light.

Fuchsin Solution R1, Decolorised To 1 g of *basic fuchsin* add 100 ml of *water*, heat to 50° and allow to cool, shaking occasionally. Allow to stand for 48 hours, shake and filter. To 4 ml of the filtrate add 6 ml of *hydrochloric acid*, mix and dilute to 100 ml with *water*. Allow to stand for at least 1 hour to ensure maximum fading.

Fucose See *L-fucose*.

L-Fucose 6-Deoxy-L-galactose; fucose; $C_6H_{12}O_5$ = 164.2 *(6696-41-9)*
General reagent grade of commerce.
A white powder; melting point, about 140°; $[\alpha]_D^{20}$, about −76° (9% w/v in water measured after 24 hours).

Furfural See *furfuraldehyde*.

Furfuraldehyde Furfural; furan-2-aldehyde; $C_5H_4O_2$ = 96.09 *(98-01-1)*
General reagent grade of commerce.
A colourless or pale brownish yellow, oily liquid; boiling point, about 162°; d_{20}^{20}, 1.155 to 1.161.

Galactose See *D-galactose*.

D-Galactose $C_6H_{12}O_6$ = 180.2 *(59-23-4)*
General reagent grade of commerce.
A white, crystalline powder; melting point, about 164°; $[\alpha]_D^{20}$, about +80° (10% w/v in water containing about 0.05% of NH_3).

Gallic Acid 3,4,5-Trihydroxybenzoic acid monohydrate; $C_7H_6O_5,H_2O$ = 188.1 *(5995-86-8)*
General reagent grade of commerce.
Melting point, about 260°, with decomposition. It loses its water of crystallisation at 120°.
CHROMATOGRAPHY When examined by test C for Identification in the monograph for Bearberry Leaf the chromatogram shows only one spot.

Gastric Juice, Artificial Dissolve 2.0 g of *sodium chloride* and 3.2 g of *pepsin powder* in *water*. Add 80 ml of 1M *hydrochloric acid* and dilute to 1000 ml with *water*.

Gelatin *(9000-70-8)*
General reagent grade of commerce.

Gelatin, Hydrolysed Dissolve 50 g of *gelatin* in 1000 ml of *water*, heat in saturated steam at 121° for 90 minutes and freeze dry.

Geraniol $C_{10}H_{18}O$ = 154.2 *(106-24-1)*
General reagent grade of commerce.
Boiling point, about 230°; n_D^{20}, about 1.476.

Geranyl Acetate (*E*)-3,7-Dimethylocta-2,6-dien-1-yl acetate; $C_{12}H_{20}O_2$ = 196.3 *(105-87-3)*
General reagent grade of commerce.
d_{25}^{25}, 0.896 to 0.913; n_D^{15}, about 1.463.
Geranyl acetate used in gas chromatography complies with the following test.
ASSAY Examine by gas chromatography as prescribed in the monograph for Bitter-orange-flower Oil using the reagent being examined as the test solution. The area of the principal peak is not less than 99.0% of the total area of the peaks.

Gitoxin $C_{41}H_{64}O_{14}$ = 781.0 *(4562-36-1)*
General reagent grade of commerce.
A white, crystalline powder; melting point, about 283°, with decomposition; $[\alpha]_D^{20}$, +20° to +24° (0.5% w/v in a mixture of equal volumes of chloroform and methanol).
Complies with the following test.
HOMOGENEITY Carry out test A for Identification described in the monograph for Digitalis Leaf applying to the plate a solution containing only the reagent being examined. The chromatogram shows only one principal spot.

Glucosamine Hydrochloride $C_6H_{14}ClNO_5$ = 215.6 *(66-84-2)*
General reagent grade of commerce.
$[\alpha]_D^{20}$, +100°, decreasing to +47.5° after 30 minutes, determined on a 10% w/v solution in *water*.

Glucose See *D-glucose*.

D-Glucose Dextrose; $C_6H_{12}O_6$ = 180.2 *(50-99-7)*
Analytical reagent grade of commerce.
A white, crystalline or granular powder; $[\alpha]_D^{20}$, about +52.5° (10% w/v in water containing about 0.2% v/v of ammonia).

D-Glucose Monohydrate $C_6H_{12}O_6,H_2O$ = 198.2 *(5996-10-1)*
General reagent grade of commerce.
Colourless crystals or a white to cream, crystalline powder; $[\alpha]_D^{20}$, about +52.5° (anhydrous) (10% w/v in water containing about 0.2% of NH_3).

Glutamic Acid L-Glutamic acid; $C_5H_9O_4$ = 147.1 *(56-86-0)*
General reagent grade of commerce.
Melting point, about 205°; $[\alpha]_D^{20}$, about +31.5°.

Glutaraldehyde $C_5H_8O_2$ = 100.1 *(111-30-8)*
General reagent grade of commerce.
Boiling point, about 188°; n_D^{25}, about 1.434.

Glycerol Propane-1,2,3-triol; $C_3H_8O_3$ = 92.10 *(56-81-5)*
Analytical reagent grade of commerce.
A colourless viscous liquid; weight per ml, about 1.26 g.

Glycerol (85%) *Glycerol* containing 12.0 to 16.0% w/w of water; weight per ml, 1.22 to 1.24 g.

Glycine Aminoacetic acid; $C_2H_5NO_2$ = 75.1 *(56-40-6)*
Analytical reagent grade of commerce.
Melting point, about 233°, with decomposition.

Glycollic Acid 2-Hydroxyacetic acid; $C_2H_4O_3$ = 76.05 *(79-14-1)*

General reagent grade of commerce.
Melting point, about 80°.

Glycyrrhetic Acid See *glycyrrhetinic acid.*

Glycyrrhetinic Acid Glycyrrhetic acid; a mixture of α- and β-isomers with the β-isomer predominating; $C_{30}H_{46}O_4$ = 470.7 (*471-53-4*)
General reagent grade of commerce.
A white to brownish yellow powder; melting point, about 292°, with decomposition; $[\alpha]_D^{20}$, +145 to 155° (1% w/v in absolute ethanol).
Complies with the following requirement.
HOMOGENEITY Carry out the method for *thin-layer chromatography*, Appendix III A, using a suspension of *silica gel F_{254}*, prepared using a 0.25% v/v solution of *orthophosphoric acid,* to coat the plate and a mixture of 5 volumes of *methanol* and 95 volumes of *chloroform* as the mobile phase but allowing the solvent front to ascend 10 cm above the line of application. Apply to the plate 5 µl of a 0.5% w/v solution of the reagent being examined in the mobile phase. After removal of the plate, examine under *ultraviolet light (254 nm)*. The chromatogram obtained shows a dark spot with an Rf value of about 0.3 (β-glycyrrhetinic acid) and a smaller spot with an Rf value of about 0.5 (α-glycyrrhetinic acid). Spray with *anisaldehyde solution* and heat at 100° to 105° for 10 minutes. Both spots are bluish violet and between them a smaller bluish violet spot may be present.

β-Glycyrrhetinic Acid 3β-Hydroxy-11-oxo-18β,20β-olean-12-enoic acid; $C_{30}H_{46}O_4$ = 470.7 (*471-53-4*)
General reagent grade of commerce.
Melting point, about 293°; $[\alpha]_D^{20}$, about +170° (1% w/v in chloroform).

Glyoxal Bis(2-hydroxyanil) Bis(2-hydroxyphenyl-imino)ethane; glyoxalhydroxyanil; $C_{14}H_{12}N_2O_2$ = 240.3
General reagent grade of commerce.
Melting point, about 200°.

Glyoxal Sodium Bisulphite $C_2H_4Na_2O_8S_2,H_2O$ = 284.2
General reagent grade of commerce.
A white or cream powder.

Glyoxal Solution (*107-22-2*)
General reagent grade of commerce containing about 40% w/w of glyoxal ($C_2H_2O_2$).
ASSAY In a ground-glass stoppered flask place 1 g of the reagent being examined, 20 ml of a 7% w/v solution of *hydroxylamine hydrochloride* and 50 ml of *water.* Allow to stand for 30 minutes and add 1 ml of *methyl red mixed solution* and titrate with 1M *sodium hydroxide VS* until the colour changes from red to green. Carry out a blank titration. Each ml of 1M *sodium hydroxide VS* is equivalent to 29.02 mg of $C_2H_2O_2$.

Glyoxalhydroxyanil See *glyoxal bis(2-hydroxyanil).*

Gonadotrophin, Chorionic (*9002-61-3*)
General reagent grade of commerce.
A white or almost white, amorphous powder.

Gonadotrophin, Serum (*9002-70-4*)
General reagent grade of commerce.
A white or pale grey, amorphous powder.

Guaiacum Resin Gum guaiac
Resin obtained from the heartwood of *Guaiacum officinale* L. and *Guaiacum sanctum* L.
Reddish brown or greenish brown, hard, glassy fragments; fracture, shiny.

Guaiazulene 1,4-Dimethyl-7-isopropylazulene; $C_{15}H_{18}$ = 198.3 (*489-84-9*)
General reagent grade of commerce.
Dark blue crystals or a blue liquid; melting point, about 30°.
Store protected from light and air.

Guanidine Hydrochloride CH_5N_3,HCl = 95.5 (*50-01-1*)
General reagent grade of commerce.

Guanine 2-Aminopurin-6-one; $C_5H_5N_5O$ = 151.1 (*73-40-5*)
General reagent grade of commerce.

Guaiphenesin Guaifenesin; guaiacol glyceryl ether; $C_{10}H_{14}O_4$ = 198.2 (*93-14-1*)
General reagent grade of commerce.
Melting point, about 79°.

Haemoglobin (*9008-02-0*)
General reagent grade of commerce.
Complies with the following requirements.
CONTENT OF IRON 0.2 to 0.3%.
CONTENT OF NITROGEN 15 to 16%.
LOSS ON DRYING Not more than 2%.
SULPHATED ASH Not more than 1.5%.

Haemoglobin Solution Stir 2 g of *haemoglobin* with 75 ml of 0.03M *hydrochloric acid* until dissolution is complete, adjust the pH of the solution to between 1.5 and 1.7 with 1M *hydrochloric acid,* dilute to 100 ml with 0.03M *hydrochloric acid* and add 25 mg of *thiomersal.* Prepare daily, store at a temperature of 2° to 8° and readjust to pH 1.6 before use.

Harpagoside $C_{24}H_{30}O_{11}$ = 494.5
General reagent grade of commerce.
Melting point, 117° to 121°.
Store in an airtight container.

Helium He = 4.003 (*7440-59-7*)
Laboratory cylinder grade of commerce containing not less than 99.995% v/v of He.

Helium for Chromatography See *helium.*

Heparin (*9041-08-1*)
Heparin Sodium of the British Pharmacopoeia.

Heptane See *n-heptane.*

***n*-Heptane** C_7H_{16} = 100.2
General reagent grade of commerce.
A colourless, flammable liquid; d_{20}^{20}, 0.683 to 0.686; n_D^{20}, about 1.387 to 1.388.

2,2′,2″,6,6′,6″-Hexa-(1,1-dimethylethyl)-4,4′,4″-[2,4,6-trimethyl-1,3,5-benzenetriyl)-trismethylene]-triphenol $C_{54}H_{78}O_3$ = 775
General reagent grade of commerce.
Melting point, about 244°.

Hexacosane $C_{26}H_{54}$ = 366.7 (*630-01-3*)
General reagent grade of commerce.
Colourless or white leaflets; melting point, about 57°.

Hexadimethrine Bromide 1,5-Dimethyl-1,5-diazun-decamethylene polymethobromide; poly(1,1,5,5-tetra-methyl-1,5-azoniaundecamethylene dibromide); $(C_{13}H_{30}Br_2N_2)_n$ (*28728-55-4*)
General reagent grade of commerce.
Store in an airtight container.

Hexamethyldisilazane $C_6H_{19}NSi_2$ = 161.4 (*999-97-3*)
General reagent grade of commerce.

A colourless liquid; boiling point, about 125°; d_{20}^{20}, about 0.78; n_D^{20}, about 1.408.
Store in an airtight container.

Hexamethylenetetramine See *hexamine.*

Hexamine Hexamethylenetetramine; $C_6H_{12}N_4$ = 140.2 (*100-97-0*)
Analytical reagent grade of commerce.

Hexane C_6H_{14} = 86.2 (*110-54-3*)
A colourless flammable liquid; d_{20}^{20}, 0.659 to 0.663; n_D^{20}, 1.375 to 1.376. Not less than 95% distils between 67° and 69°.
Hexane used in spectrophotometry has a minimum transmittance of 97% between 260 nm and 420 nm, determined using *water* in the reference cell.

***n*-Hexane** C_6H_{14} = 86.2 (*110-54-3*)
Analytical reagent grade of commerce usually containing not less than 99% of the pure isomer.
A colourless, flammable liquid; boiling point, about 68°; weight per ml, about 0.66 g.

Hexane, Purified A grade of *hexane* containing not more than 0.002% w/v of non-volatile matter.

Hexylamine $C_6H_{15}N$ = 101.2 (*111-26-2*)
General reagent grade of commerce.
A colourless liquid.
Boiling point, 127° to 131°; d_{20}^{20}, about 0.766; n_D^{20}, 1.418.

Histamine Dihydrochloride $C_5H_9N_3,2HCl$ = 184.1 (*56-92-8*)
General reagent grade of commerce.
A white, crystalline powder; melting point, about 250°.

Histamine Phosphate Histamine acid phosphate; $C_5H_9N_3,2H_3PO_4$ = 307.1 (*23297-93-0*)
General reagent grade of commerce.
Colourless crystals.

Histamine Solution A 0.9% w/v solution of *sodium chloride* containing 0.1 µg per ml of histamine, $C_5H_9N_3$ (as the phosphate or the dihydrochloride).

Histidine Monohydrochloride $C_6H_9N_3O_2,HCl,H_2O$ = 191.6 (*123333-71-1*)
General reagent grade of commerce.
Colourless crystals or a white, crystalline powder; melting point, about 250°, with decomposition.
Complies with the following test.
HOMOGENEITY Carry out the method for thin-layer chromatography for Histidine described in the monograph for Histamine Dihydrochloride. The chromatogram obtained shows only one principal spot.

Holmium Oxide Ho_2O_3 = 377.9 (*12055-62-8*)
General reagent grade of commerce.
A yellowish powder.

Holmium Perchlorate Solution
Reagent of commerce for the calibration of spectrophotometers.
Consists of a 4% w/v solution of holmium oxide in 1.4M perchloric acid.

Hyaluronate Solution Dilute *potassium hyaluronate stock solution* with an equal volume of *phosphate-buffered saline pH 6.4*.
Use on the day of preparation.

Hyaluronidase Diluent See *diluent for hyaluronidase solutions.*

Hyaluronidase Solutions, Diluent for Mix 100 ml of *phosphate-buffered saline pH 6.4* with 100 ml of *water* and dissolve 140 mg of *hydrolysed gelatin* in the mixture at 37°. Use the solution within 2 hours.

Hydrazine Hydrate N_2H_4,H_2O = 50.06 (*10217-52-4*)
Analytical reagent grade of commerce.
A colourless liquid with an ammoniacal odour; weight per ml, about 1.03 g.

Hydrazine Sulphate N_2H_4,H_2SO_4 = 130.1 (*10034-93-2*)
Analytical reagent grade of commerce.

Hydrindantin 2,2′-dihydroxy-2,2′-bi-indan-1,1′,3,3′-tetraone dihydrate; $C_{18}H_{10}O_6,2H_2O$ = 358.3 (*5950-69-6*)
General reagent grade of commerce.
Melting point, about 258°.

Hydriodic Acid HI = 127.9 (*10034-85-2*)
Analytical reagent grade of commerce containing about 55% w/w of HI and about 7.5M in strength.
An almost colourless liquid when freshly prepared, rapidly becoming yellow or brown due to the liberation of iodine; weight per ml, about 1.7 g.

Hydrobromic Acid, 30 per cent HBr = 80.92 (*10035-10-6*)
Analytical reagent grade of commerce containing 30% of HBr in *glacial acetic acid.*
Cautiously degas the container before opening.

Hydrobromic Acid, Dilute Place 5 ml of *30 per cent hydrobromic acid* in amber vials equipped with polyethylene stoppers. Seal under *argon* and store in the dark. Add 5 ml of *glacial acetic acid* immediately before use and shake. Store in the dark.

Hydrocarbons (Type L), Low-vapour-pressure
Gas chromatographic reagent grade of commerce (Apiezon L is suitable).
An unctuous mass.

Hydrochloric Acid HCl = 36.46 (*7647-01-0*)
Where no molarity is indicated use analytical reagent grade of commerce with a relative density of about 1.18, containing not less than 35% w/w and not more than 38% w/w of HCl and about 11.5M in strength.
A colourless, fuming liquid.
Solutions of molarity *x*M should be prepared by diluting 85*x* ml of *hydrochloric acid* to 1000 ml with *water.*
Store in a container of polyethylene or other non-reacting material at a temperature not exceeding 30°.

Hydrochloric Acid, Brominated Use brominated hydrochloric acid low in arsenic, of commerce, or prepare by adding 1 ml of *bromine solution* to 100 ml of *hydrochloric acid.*

Hydrochloric Acid, Dilute Dilute 20 g of *hydrochloric acid* to 100 ml with *water.* It contains 7.3% w/v of HCl.

Hydrochloric Acid, Ethanolic Solutions of the requisite molarity may be obtained by diluting *hydrochloric acid* with *ethanol (96%)* in place of water as directed under *hydrochloric acid.* If no molarity is stated, use a solution prepared by diluting 5 ml of 1M *hydrochloric acid* to 500 ml with *ethanol (96%).*

Hydrochloric Acid, Methanolic Solutions of the requisite molarity may be obtained by diluting *hydrochloric acid* with *methanol* in place of water as directed under *hydrochloric acid.*

Hydrochloric Acid R1 Dilute 70 g of *hydrochloric acid* to 100 ml with *water.* It contains 25% w/v of HCl.

Hydrochloric Acid R1, Dilute Dilute 1 ml of *dilute hydrochloric acid* to 200 ml with *water*. It contains 0.037% w/v of HCl.

Hydrochloric Acid R2, Dilute Dilute 30 ml of 1M *hydrochloric acid* to 1000 ml with *water*; adjust to pH 1.5 to 1.7.

Hydrochloric Acid, Stannated
Use stannated hydrochloric acid low in arsenic, of commerce, or prepare by adding 1 ml of *tin(II) chloride solution* to 100 ml of *hydrochloric acid*.

Hydrocortisone $C_{21}H_{30}O_5$ = 362.5 (*50-23-7*)
General reagent grade of commerce.
Melting point, about 214°, with decomposition.

Hydrocortisone Acetate $C_{23}H_{32}O_6$ = 404.5 (*50-03-3*)
General reagent grade of commerce.

Hydrofluoric Acid HF = 20.01 (*7664-39-3*)
Analytical reagent grade of commerce containing not less than 40% w/w of HF.
A colourless, corrosive liquid with a pungent odour; weight per ml, about 1.13 g.
Store in a polyethylene bottle.

Hydrogen H_2 = 2.02 (*1333-74-0*)
Laboratory cylinder grade of commerce containing not less than 99.95% v/v of H_2.

Hydrogen for Chromatography See *hydrogen*.

Hydrogen Peroxide Solution (200 vol) H_2O_2 = 34.02 (*7724-84-1*)
General reagent grade of commerce containing about 60% w/v of H_2O_2.
A colourless liquid; weight per ml, about 1.18 g.

Hydrogen Peroxide Solution (100 vol) Strong hydrogen peroxide solution
Analytical reagent grade of commerce containing about 30% w/v of H_2O_2.
A colourless liquid; weight per ml, about 1.10 g.

Hydrogen Peroxide Solution (20 vol)
Analytical reagent grade of commerce containing about 6% w/v of H_2O_2 or *hydrogen peroxide solution (100 vol)* diluted with 4 volumes of *water*.
A colourless liquid; weight per ml, about 1.02 g.

Hydrogen Peroxide Solution (10 vol) Dilute hydrogen peroxide solution
Dilute *hydrogen peroxide solution (20 vol)* with an equal volume of *water*.

Hydrogen Peroxide Solution, Dilute See *hydrogen peroxide solution (10 vol)*.

Hydrogen Peroxide Solution, Strong See *hydrogen peroxide solution (100 vol)*.

Hydrogen Sulphide H_2S = 34.08 (*7783-06-4*)
Use laboratory cylinder grade of commerce, or prepare the gas by the action of *hydrochloric acid*, diluted with an equal volume of *water*, on iron sulphide; wash the resulting gas by passing it through *water*.
A colourless, poisonous gas, with a characteristic, unpleasant odour.

Hydrogen Sulphide R1 *Hydrogen sulphide* containing not less than 99.7% v/v of H_2S.

Hydrogen Sulphide Solution A freshly prepared, saturated solution of *hydrogen sulphide* in *water*.
It contains about 0.45% w/v of H_2S at 20°.

Hydroquinone Quinol; benzene-1,4-diol; $C_6H_6O_2$ = 110.1 (*123-31-9*)
Analytical reagent grade of commerce.
Colourless or almost colourless crystals or crystalline powder darkening on exposure to air and light; melting point, about 173°.
Store protected from light and air.

4-Hydroxybenzaldehyde $C_7H_6O_2$ = 122.2 (*123-08-0*)
General reagent grade of commerce.
Colourless needles; melting point, about 118°.

4-Hydroxybenzoic Acid Parahydroxybenzoic acid; $C_7H_6O_3$ = 138.1 (*99-96-7*)
General reagent grade of commerce.
Melting point, 214° to 215°.

4-Hydroxybiphenyl 4-Phenylphenol; $C_{12}H_{10}O$ = 170.2 (*90-43-7*)
General reagent grade of commerce.
Colourless crystals or a white, crystalline powder; melting point, about 166°.

4-Hydroxycoumarin $C_9H_6O_3$ = 162.1 (*1076-38-6*)
General reagent grade of commerce.
Melting point, about 214°.

2-[4-(2-Hydroxyethyl)piperazin-1-yl]ethanesulphonic Acid HEPES; $C_8H_{18}N_2SO_4$ = 238.3 (*7365-45-9*)
General reagent grade of commerce.
Melting point, about 236°, with decomposition.

4-Hydroxyisophthalic Acid 4-Hydroxybenzene-1,3-dicarboxylic acid; $C_8H_6O_5$ = 182.1 (*636-46-4*)
General reagent grade of commerce.
Melting point, about 314°, with decomposition.

Hydroxylamine Hydrochloride Hydroxylammonium chloride; NH_2OH,HCl = 69.49 (*5470-11-1*)
Analytical reagent grade of commerce.

Hydroxylamine Hydrochloride Solution R2 Dissolve 2.5 g of *hydroxylamine hydrochloride* in 4.5 ml of hot *water* and add 40 ml of *ethanol (96%)* and 0.4 ml of *bromophenol blue solution R2*. Add 0.5M *ethanolic potassium hydroxide* until a greenish yellow colour is obtained. Dilute to 50 ml with *ethanol (96%)*.

Hydroxylamine Solution, Alcoholic Dissolve 3.5 g of *hydroxylamine hydrochloride* in 95 ml of *ethanol (60%)*, add 0.5 ml of a 0.2% w/v solution of *methyl orange* in *ethanol (60%)* and then add 0.5M *potassium hydroxide* in *ethanol (60%)* until the pure yellow colour of the indicator is produced. Add sufficient *ethanol (60%)* to produce 100 ml.

Hydroxylamine Solution, Alkaline Immediately before use mix equal volumes of a 13.9% w/v solution of *hydroxylamine hydrochloride* and a 15% w/v solution of *sodium hydroxide*.

Hydroxylamine Solution R1, Alkaline
SOLUTION A Dissolve 12.5 g of *hydroxylamine hydrochloride* in *methanol* and dilute to 100 ml with the same solvent.
SOLUTION B Dissolve 12.5 g of *sodium hydroxide* in *methanol* and dilute to 100 ml with the same solvent.
Mix equal volumes of solution A and solution B immediately before use.

5-Hydroxymethylfurfural 5-Hydroxymethylfurfuraldehyde; $C_6H_6O_3$ = 126.1 (*67-47-0*)
General reagent grade of commerce.
Melting point, about 32°.

Hydroxynaphthol Blue Sodium Salt
$C_{20}H_{11}N_2Na_3O_{11}S_3$ = 620 (*63451-35-4*)

General reagent grade of commerce.

Hydroxyquinoline See *8-hydroxyquinoline.*

8-Hydroxyquinoline Quinolin-8-ol; C_9H_7NO = 145.2 (*148-24-3*)
Analytical reagent grade of commerce.
A white to yellowish white, crystalline powder; melting point, about 74°.

12-Hydroxystearic Acid 12-Hydroxyoctadecanoic acid; $C_{18}H_{36}O_3$ = 300.5 (*106-14-9*)
General reagent grade of commerce.
Melting point, 71° to 74°.

5-Hydroxyuracil Isobarbituric acid; pyrimidine-2,4,5-triol; 2,4,5-trihydroxypyrimidine; $C_4H_4N_2O_3$ = 128.1 (*496-76-4*)
General reagent grade of commerce.
Melting point, about 310°, with decomposition.
HOMOGENEITY Carry out the method described under Related substances in the monograph for Fluorouracil. The chromatogram exhibits a principal spot with an Rf value of about 0.3.
Store in an airtight container.

Hyoscine Hydrobromide Scopolamine hydrobromide; $C_{17}H_{21}NO_4,HBr,3H_2O$ = 438.3 (*114-49-8*)
General reagent grade of commerce.
Colourless crystals or a white, crystalline powder; melting point, about 197°; $[\alpha]_D^{20}$, about −25° (5% w/v in water).

Hyoscyamine Sulphate $(C_{17}H_{23}NO_3)_2,H_2SO_4,2H_2O$ = 712.8 (*620-61-1*)
General reagent grade of commerce.
Melting point, about 206°; $[\alpha]_D^{20}$, about −29° (2% w/v in water).

Hyperoside 2-(3,4-Dihydroxyphenyl)-3-β-D-galacto-pyranosyl-5,7-dihydroxy-chromen-4-one; $C_{21}H_{20}O_{12}$ = 464.4
General reagent grade of commerce.
Melting point, about 240°, with decomposition; $[\alpha]_D^{20}$, −8.3°, determined in a 0.2% w/v solution in *pyridine*.

Hypophosphorous Reagent Dissolve, by heating gently, 10 g of *sodium hypophosphite* in 20 ml of *water* and dilute to 100 ml with *hydrochloric acid.* Allow to settle and decant or filter through glass wool.

Hypoxanthine 6-Hydroxypurine; $C_5H_4N_4O$ = 136.1 (*68-94-0*)
General reagent grade of commerce.
Decomposes without melting at about 150°.
Complies with the following test.
HOMOGENEITY Carry out the test for Hypoxanthine described in the monograph for Mercaptopurine applying to the plate a solution containing only the reagent being examined. The chromatogram shows only one principal spot.

Imidazole Glyoxaline; $C_3H_4N_2$ = 68.08 (*288-32-4*)
Purified grade of commerce.
A white, crystalline powder; melting point, about 90°.

Imidazole—Mercury Reagent Dissolve 8.25 g of *recrystallised imidazole* in 60 ml of *water* and add 10 ml of 5M *hydrochloric acid.* Stir the solution magnetically and add, dropwise, 10 ml of a 0.27% w/v solution of *mercury(II) chloride.* If a cloudy solution results, discard and prepare a further solution adding the mercury chloride solution more slowly. Adjust the pH to 6.75 to 6.85 with 5M *hydrochloric acid* (about 4 ml is required) and add sufficient *water* to produce 100 ml.

Imidazole, Recrystallised Twice recrystallise 25 g of *imidazole* from 100 ml of *toluene*, cool in ice with stirring, wash with *ether* and dry at room temperature at a pressure of 2 kPa over *anhydrous silica gel*, or use a purified grade of commerce.
Complies with the following test.
LIGHT ABSORPTION *Absorbance* of an 8% w/v solution at 325 nm, not more than 0.10, Appendix II B.

Imidazole Solution Dissolve 8.25 g of *recrystallised imidazole* in 60 ml of *water*, adjust the pH to 6.75 to 6.85 with 5M *hydrochloric acid* and add sufficient *water* to produce 100 ml.
The hydrochloric acid used in preparing this reagent must be free from stabilising mercury compounds.

Iminodibenzyl 10,11-Dihydro-5*H*-dibenz[*b,f*]azepine; $C_{14}H_{13}N$ = 195.3 (*494-19-9*)
General reagent grade of commerce.
A pale yellow, crystalline powder; melting point, about 106°.

Indigo Carmine CI 73015; acid blue 74; $C_{16}H_8N_2Na_2O_8S_2$ = 466.4 (*860-22-0*)
Analytical reagent grade of commerce.
A deep blue powder or blue granules with a coppery lustre.

Indigo Carmine Solution To a mixture of 10 ml of *hydrochloric acid* and 990 ml of a 20% w/v solution of *nitrogen-free sulphuric acid* in *water*, add sufficient *indigo carmine* (about 0.2 g) to produce a solution that complies with the following test.

Add 10 ml to a solution of 1.0 mg of *potassium nitrate* in 10 ml of *water*, rapidly add 20 ml of *nitrogen-free sulphuric acid* and heat to boiling. The blue colour is discharged within 1 minute.

Indigo Carmine Solution R1 Triturate 4 g of *indigo carmine* with successive portions of *water* (not exceeding 900 ml in total) until dissolved and transfer the solution to a 1000-ml graduated flask. Add 2 ml of *sulphuric acid* and dilute to 1000 ml with *water.*

Ascertain its exact concentration in the following manner. To 10 ml of *nitrate standard solution (100 ppm NO_3)* add 10 ml of *water*, 0.05 ml of the indigo carmine solution and, in a single addition but with caution, 30 ml of *sulphuric acid.* Titrate the solution with the indigo carmine solution until a stable blue colour is produced. The total volume, in ml, of *indigo carmine VS* required is equivalent to 1 mg of NO_3.

Indophenol Blue CI 49700; $C_{18}H_{26}N_2O$ = 276.3 (*132-31-0*)
General reagent grade of commerce.
A dark purple powder complying with the following test.
HOMOGENEITY Carry out the method for *thin-layer chromatography*, Appendix III A, using *silica gel G* as the coating substance and *dichloromethane* as the mobile phase. Apply to the plate 10 µl of a 0.01% w/v solution in *dichloromethane.* After removal of the plate, allow it to dry in air. The chromatogram shows only one spot, but a stain may remain on the line of application.

Iodic Acid HIO_3 = 175.9 (*7782-68-5*)
Analytical reagent grade of commerce.

Iodine I_2 = 253.8 (*7553-56-2*)
Analytical reagent grade of commerce.
To prepare 0.05M iodine dissolve 20 g of *potassium iodide* in the minimum amount of *water*, add 13 g of *iodine*, allow to dissolve and add sufficient *water* to produce 1000 ml.

Weaker solutions should be prepared using proportionately lesser amounts of reagents or by appropriate dilution.

Iodine Bromide IBr = 206.8 *(7789-33-5)*
General reagent grade of commerce.
Bluish black or brownish black crystals with a lachrymatory vapour; melting point, about 40°; boiling point, about 116°.
Store in a cool place protected from light.

Iodine Bromide Solution Dissolve 20 g of *iodine bromide* in sufficient *glacial acetic acid* to produce 1000 ml.
Store protected from light.

Iodine Monochloride Reagent, Strong Dissolve 10 g of *potassium iodide* and 6.4 g of *potassium iodate* in 75 ml of *water*, add 75 ml of *hydrochloric acid* and 5 ml of *chloroform*, shake and, if necessary, add dropwise with vigorous shaking 0.1M *potassium iodide* until a faint iodine colour appears in the chloroform layer. Add in the same manner 0.001M *potassium iodate* until the chloroform is just colourless.
Before use, readjust with either 0.1M *potassium iodide* or 0.001M *potassium iodate* as required.
Store in a cool place protected from light.

Iodine Monochloride Solution Dissolve 8 g of *iodine trichloride* in about 200 ml of *glacial acetic acid* and separately dissolve 9 g of *iodine* in 300 ml of *dichloromethane*. Mix the two solutions and dilute to 1000 ml with *glacial acetic acid*.
Store in a stoppered bottle, protected from light and at a temperature not exceeding 15°.

Iodine Pentoxide, Recrystallised Iodine pentoxide; I_2O_5 = 333.8 *(12029-98-0)*
General reagent grade of commerce recrystallised in the following manner. Boil a saturated solution of commercial iodine pentoxide in *nitric acid* for 1 hour and allow to stand for 24 hours. Decant the supernatant liquid and dry the crystals first in a current of air at room temperature and then over *phosphorus pentoxide* at a pressure not exceeding 0.7 kPa.
A white, crystalline, hygroscopic powder containing not less than 99.5% of I_2O_5.
ASSAY Dissolve 0.1 g in 50 ml of *water* and add 3 g of *potassium iodide* and 10 ml of 2M *hydrochloric acid*. Titrate the liberated iodine with 0.1M *sodium thiosulphate VS* using 1 ml of *starch solution* as indicator. Each ml of 0.1M *sodium thiosulphate VS* is equivalent to 2.782 mg of I_2O_5.
Store in an airtight container protected from light.

Iodine Solution, Alcoholic A 1% w/v solution of *iodine* in *ethanol (96%)*.
Store protected from light.

Iodine Solution, Chloroformic A 0.5% w/v solution of *iodine* in *chloroform*.
Store protected from light.

Iodine Solution R1 To 10 ml of 0.05M *iodine* add 0.6 g of *potassium iodide* and dilute to 100 ml with *water*.
Prepare immediately before use.

Iodine Solution R2 To 10 ml of 0.05M *iodine* add 0.6 g of *potassium iodide* and dilute to 1000 ml with *water*.
Prepare immediately before use.

Iodine Solution R3 Dilute 2 ml of *iodine solution R1* to 100 ml with *water* immediately before use.

Iodine Solution R4 Dissolve 14 g of *iodine* in 100 ml of a 40% w/v solution of *potassium iodide*, add 1 ml of 2M *hydrochloric acid* and dilute to 1000 ml with *water*.
Store protected from light.

Iodine Trichloride ICl_3 = 233.3 *(865-44-1)*
Analytical reagent grade of commerce.
Reddish orange crystals.

Iodoacetic Acid $C_2H_3IO_2$ = 248.0 *(64-69-7)*
General reagent grade of commerce.
Melting point, 82° to 83°.

2-Iodobenzoic Acid $C_7H_5IO_2$ = 248.0 *(88-67-5)*
Microanalytical reagent grade of commerce.
A white or slightly yellow, crystalline powder; melting point, about 160°.
Complies with the following test.
HOMOGENEITY Carry out the method for *thin-layer chromatography*, Appendix III A, using *cellulose* F_{254} as the coating substance and as the mobile phase the upper layer obtained by shaking together 20 volumes of *water*, 40 volumes of *glacial acetic acid* and 40 volumes of *toluene* but allowing the solvent front to ascend 12 cm above the line of application. Apply to the plate 20 µl of a solution prepared by dissolving 40 mg of the reagent being examined in 4 ml of 0.1M *sodium hydroxide* and diluting to 10 ml with *water*. After removal of the plate, allow it to dry in air and examine under *ultraviolet light (254 nm)*. The chromatogram obtained shows only one principal spot.

Iodoethane C_2H_5I = 155.9 *(75-03-6)*
General reagent grade of commerce.
Boiling point, about 72°; d_{20}^{20}, about 1.95; n_D^{20}, about 1.513.
Store in an airtight container.

2-Iodohippuric Acid $C_9H_8INO_3,2H_2O$ = 341.1 *(147-58-0)*
General reagent grade of commerce.
A white, or almost white, crystalline powder; melting point, about 170°.
Complies with the following tests.
HOMOGENEITY Carry out the method for *thin-layer chromatography*, Appendix III A, using *cellulose* F_{254} as the coating substance and as the mobile phase the upper layer obtained by shaking together 20 volumes of *water*, 40 volumes of *glacial acetic acid* and 40 volumes of *toluene*, but allowing the mobile phase to ascend 12 cm above the line of application. Apply to the plate 20 µl of a solution prepared by dissolving 40 mg of the reagent being examined in 4 ml of 0.1M *sodium hydroxide* and diluting to 10 ml with *water*. After removal of the plate, allow it to dry and examine under *ultraviolet light (254 nm)*. The chromatogram shows only one principal spot.
WATER Not less than 9% and not more than 13%, Appendix IX C. Use 1 g.

Iodoplatinate Reagent To 3 ml of a 10% w/v solution of *chloroplatinic(IV) acid* add 97 ml of *water* and 100 ml of a 6% w/v solution of *potassium iodide*.
Store protected from light.

Iodosulphurous Reagent See *Karl Fischer reagent VS*.

5-Iodouracil $C_4H_3IN_2O_2$ = 238.0 *(696-07-1)*
General reagent grade of commerce.
A white or almost white crystalline powder; melting point, about 276°, with decomposition.
Complies with the following test.
HOMOGENEITY Examine under the conditions prescribed in the test for Related substances in the monograph for Idoxuridine applying to the plate 5 µl of a 0.025% w/v solution. The chromatogram shows only one principal spot.

Ion-exchange Resin, Strongly Acidic A strongly acidic resin in bead form (0.3 mm to 1.2 mm).
CAPACITY 4.5 mmol to 5 mmol per gram, with a water content of 50 to 60%.
Preparation of the column Use a glass tube (40 cm × 20 mm) fitted with a sintered-glass disc and with a filling height of about 20 cm. Introduce the resin, mixing it with *water* and pouring the slurry into the tube ensuring that no air bubbles are trapped between the particles. When in use, the liquid must not be allowed to fall below the surface of the resin.

If the resin is in its protonated form, wash with *water* until 50 ml of effluent requires not more than 0.05 ml of 0.1M *sodium hydroxide VS* for neutralisation, using *methyl orange solution* as indicator. If the resin is in its sodium form or if it requires regeneration, pass about 100 ml of a mixture of equal volumes of 7M *hydrochloric acid* and *water* slowly through the column and then wash with *water* as described above.

Iron Fe = 55.85 (*7439-89-6*)
Grey powder or wire, soluble in dilute mineral acids.

Iron(III) Chloride, Anhydrous Iron(III) chloride; anhydrous ferric chloride; $FeCl_3$ = 162.2 (*7705-08-0*)
General reagent grade of commerce.
Greenish black crystals or crystalline powder turning orange on exposure to moist air.

Iron(III) Chloride Hexahydrate Ferric chloride; $FeCl_3,6H_2O$ = 270.3 (*10025-77-1*)
Analytical reagent grade of commerce.
Yellowish orange or brownish, crystalline masses; deliquescent.
Store in an airtight container.

Iron(III) Chloride Solution
Analytical reagent grade of commerce, diluted to contain about 15% w/v of $FeCl_3$.

Iron(III) Chloride Solution, Ethanolic Carefully add 25 ml of *sulphuric acid* dropwise to 75 ml of well-cooled *absolute ethanol,* stirring constantly. Add 2 g of *anhydrous iron(III) chloride,* stir and filter.

Iron(III) Chloride Solution R1 A 10.5% w/v solution of *iron(III) chloride hexahydrate.*

Iron(III) Chloride Solution R2 A 1.3% w/v solution of *iron(III) chloride hexahydrate.*

Iron(III) Chloride—Sulphamic Acid Reagent
A solution containing 1.0% w/v of *iron(III) chloride hexahydrate* and 1.6% w/v of *sulphamic acid.*

Iron(III) Nitrate Ferric nitrate; $Fe(NO_3)_3,9H_2O$ = 404.0 (*7782-61-8*)
Analytical reagent grade of commerce containing not less than 99.0% of $Fe(NO_3)_3,9H_2O$.

Iron(III) Nitrate Solution A 0.1% w/v solution of *iron(III) nitrate* in 0.1% v/v *nitric acid.*

Iron Salicylate Solution Dissolve 0.1 g of *ammonium iron(III) sulphate* in 100 ml of *water* containing 2 ml of 1M *sulphuric acid.* To this solution add 50 ml of a 1.15% w/v solution of *sodium salicylate,* 10 ml of 2M *acetic acid* and 80 ml of a 13.6% w/v solution of *sodium acetate* and dilute to 500 ml with *water.*
The solution should be recently prepared, kept in an airtight container and protected from light.

Iron(II) Sulphate Ferrous sulphate; $FeSO_4,7H_2O$ = 278.0 (*7782-63-0*)
Analytical reagent grade of commerce.

Iron(III) Sulphate Ferric sulphate; $Fe_2(SO_4)_3$+aq (*10028-22-5*)
General reagent grade of commerce.
A very hygroscopic, white to yellow powder which decomposes in air.
Store protected from light.

Iron(II) Sulphate Solution R2 Dissolve 0.45 g of *iron(II) sulphate* in 50 ml of 0.1M *hydrochloric acid* and dilute to 100 ml with *carbon dioxide-free water.* Prepare immediately before use.

Iron(II) Sulphate—Citrate Solution Dissolve 1 g of *sodium metabisulphite* in 200 ml of *water* and add 0.5 ml of 2M *hydrochloric acid,* 1.5 g of *iron(II) sulphate* and 10 g of *sodium citrate.*
Prepare immediately before use.

Isatin $C_8H_5NO_2$ = 147.1 (*91-56-5*)
Analytical reagent grade of commerce.
Orange to red crystals; melting point, about 200°, with partial sublimation.

Isatin Reagent Dissolve 6 mg of *iron(III) sulphate* in 8 ml of *water* and cautiously add 50 ml of *sulphuric acid.* Add 6 mg of *isatin* and stir until dissolved. The reagent should be pale yellow, not orange or red.

Isoamyl Alcohol 3-Methylbutan-1-ol; $C_5H_{12}O$ = 88.1 (*123-51-3*)
General reagent grade of commerce.
Boiling point, about 130°; n_D^{20}, about 1.406; weight per ml, about 0.81 g.

Isoandrosterone Epiandrosterone; 3β-hydroxy-5α-androstan-17-one; $C_{19}H_{30}O_2$ = 290.4 (*481-29-8*)
General reagent grade of commerce.
$[\alpha]_D^{20}$, +88°, determined on a 2% w/v solution in methanol; melting point, 172° to 174°; circular dichroic absorbance, 14.24×10^3, determined at 304 nm on a 0.125% w/v solution.

Isobutyl Acetate $C_6H_{12}O_2$ = 116.2 (*110-19-0*)
General reagent grade of commerce.
A colourless liquid with a fruity odour; boiling point, about 118°; weight per ml, about 0.87 g.

Isomenthol (+)-Isomenthol; (1*S*,2*R*,5*R*)-2-isopropyl-5-methylcyclohexanol; (±)-isomenthol; (1*SR*,2*RS*,5*RS*)-2-isopropyl-5-methylcyclohexanol; $C_{10}H_{20}O$ = 156.3 (*23283-97-8*)
General reagent grade of commerce.
Melting point, about 80° ((+)-isomenthol;), about 53° ((±)-Isomenthol); boiling point, about 218°; $[\alpha]_D^{20}$, about +24° (10% w/v in ethanol (96%) ((+)-isomenthol).

(+)-Isomenthone (1*R*)-*cis*-*p*-Menthan-3-one; (1*R*)-*cis*-2-isopropyl-5-methylcyclohexanone; $C_{10}H_{18}O$ = 154.2
General reagent grade of commerce containing a variable amount of menthone.
d_{20}^{20}, about 0.904; n_D^{20}, about 1.453; $[\alpha]_D^{20}$, +93.2°.
Isomenthone used in gas chromatography complies with the following test.
ASSAY Examine by *gas chromatography,* Appendix III B, under the conditions described in the test for Chromatographic profile in the monograph for Peppermint Oil using the reagent being examined.

The area of the principal peak is not less than 80.0% of the total area of the peaks.

Isoniazid Isonicotinohydrazide; $C_6H_7N_3O$ = 137.1 (*54-85-3*)
General reagent grade of commerce.

Colourless crystals or a white, crystalline powder; melting point, about 171°.

Isoniazid Solution Dissolve 0.1 g of *isoniazid* in 150 ml of *methanol*, add 0.12 ml of *hydrochloric acid* and dilute to 200 ml with *methanol*.

Isonicotinamide $C_6H_6N_2O$ = 122.13 (*1453-82-3*)
General reagent grade of commerce.
Melting point, about 156°.

Isopropyl Myristate Isopropyl tetradecanoate; $C_{17}H_{34}O_2$ = 270.5 (*110-27-0*)
General reagent grade of commerce.

Isopropylamine 2-Propylamine; C_3H_9N = 59.11 (*75-31-0*)
General reagent grade of commerce.
A colourless, volatile liquid with an ammoniacal odour; boiling point, about 33°; weight per ml, about 0.69 g.

4-Isopropylphenol $C_9H_{12}O$ = 136.2 (*99-89-8*)
General reagent grade of commerce contaning not less than 98% of $C_9H_{12}O$.
Melting point, 59° to 61°; boiling point, about 212°.

Kaolin, Light (*1332-58-7*) A purified native hydrated aluminium silicate containing a suitable dispersing agent. A grade of commerce complying with the tests for Coarse particles and Fine particles described in the monograph for Light Kaolin.

Kieselguhr
Acid-purified grade of commerce.

Kieselguhr for Chromatography
Kieselguhr complying with the following requirement.
FILTRATION RATE Use a chromatography column (25 cm × 10 mm) with a sintered-glass (100) plate and two marks at 10 cm and 20 cm above the plate. Place sufficient of the substance being examined in the column to reach the first mark and fill to the second mark with *water*. When the first drops begin to flow from the column, fill to the second mark again with *water* and measure the time required for the first 5 ml to flow from the column. The flow rate is not less than 1 ml per minute. The eluate obtained is colourless.

Kieselguhr G *Kieselguhr* that has been treated with hydrochloric acid and calcined and to which has been added about 15% of calcium sulphate hemihydrate. The average particle size is 10 µm to 40 µm.
Complies with the following test.
CHROMATOGRAPHIC SEPARATION Carry out the method for *thin-layer chromatography*, Appendix III A, using the substance being examined in a 0.27% w/v solution of *sodium acetate* to coat the plate and a mixture of 12 volumes of *water*, 23 volumes of *propan-2-ol* and 65 volumes of *ethyl acetate* as the mobile phase but allowing the solvent front to ascend 14 cm above the line of application; the development time is about 40 minutes. Apply to the plate 5 µl of a solution containing 0.01% w/v of *lactose*, *sucrose*, *D-glucose* and *D-fructose* in *pyridine*. After removal of the plate, allow it to dry in air and spray with about 10 ml of *anisaldehyde solution* and heat for 5 to 10 minutes at 100° to 105°. The chromatogram shows four well-defined spots without tailing and well separated from each other.

Lactic Acid $C_3H_6O_3$ = 90.08 (*50-21-5*)
Analytical reagent grade of commerce.

Lactobionic Acid $C_{12}H_{22}O_{12}$ = 358.3 (*96-82-2*)
General reagent grade of commerce.
Melting point, about 115°.

Lactophenol Dissolve 20 g of *phenol* in a mixture of 20 g of *lactic acid*, 40 g of *glycerol* and 20 ml of *water*, or use microscopic grade of commerce.

Lactose $C_{12}H_{22}O_{11},H_2O$ = 360.3 (*5989-81-1*)
Analytical reagent grade of commerce.
A white, crystalline powder; $[\alpha]_D^{20}$, about +52.4° (10% w/v in water).

Lanthanum Nitrate $La(NO_3)_3,6H_2O$ = 433.0 (*10277-43-7*)
Atomic absorption spectroscopic grade of commerce.
Store in an airtight container.

Lanthanum Nitrate Solution A 5% w/v solution of *lanthanum nitrate*.

Lead Acetate See *lead(II) acetate*.

Lead(II) Acetate $C_4H_6O_4Pb,3H_2O$ = 379.3 (*6080-56-4*)
Analytical reagent grade of commerce.

Lead Acetate Cotton Immerse absorbent cotton in a mixture of 10 volumes of *lead acetate solution* and 1 volume of 2M *acetic acid*. Drain off the excess of liquid by placing it on several layers of filter paper without squeezing the cotton. Allow to dry at room temperature.
Store in an airtight container.

Lead Acetate Paper Immerse white filter paper weighing about 80 g m^{-2} in a mixture of 10 volumes of *lead acetate solution* and 1 volume of 2M *acetic acid*. After drying, cut the paper into strips (40 mm × 15 mm).
Store in an airtight container.

Lead Acetate Solution A 9.5% w/v solution of *lead(II) acetate* in *carbon dioxide-free water*.

Lead Dioxide See *lead(IV) oxide*.

Lead(II) Nitrate $Pb(NO_3)_2$ = 331.2 (*10099-75-8*)
Analytical reagent grade of commerce.

Lead Nitrate Solution A 3.3% w/v solution of *lead(II) nitrate*.

Lead(IV) Oxide Lead dioxide; PbO_2 = 239.2 (*1309-60-0*)
Analytical reagent grade of commerce.

Lead Subacetate Solution Dissolve 40.0 g of *lead(II) acetate* in 90 ml of *carbon dioxide-free water*. Adjust the pH to 7.5 with 10M *sodium hydroxide*, centrifuge and use the clear, supernatant solution. It contains not less than 16.7% w/w and not more than 17.4% w/w of Pb in a form corresponding to the formula $C_8H_{14}O_{10}Pb_3$.
The solution remains clear when stored in a well-closed container.

Lemon Oil Of the British Pharmacopoeia.

Leucine See *L-leucine*.

L-Leucine $C_6H_{13}NO_2$ = 131.2 (*61-90-5*)
General reagent grade of commerce.
A white, crystalline powder; $[\alpha]_D^{20}$, about +14.5° (2% w/v in 6M hydrochloric acid).
Complies with the following test.
HOMOGENEITY Carry out the method for *thin-layer chromatography*, Appendix III A, using *silica gel G* as the coating substance and a mixture of 75 parts of *phenol* and 25 parts of *water* as the mobile phase. Apply to the plate 5 µl of a 0.2% w/v solution of the reagent being examined and expose the plate to the vapour of the mobile phase for 12 hours before development. After removal of the plate, dry it in a current of warm air, spray with a 0.1% w/v solution of *ninhydrin* in *butan-1-ol* saturated with *water* and heat at 100° to 105° for 10 minutes. The chromatogram shows only one spot.

Limonene D-Limonene; (+)-*p*-mentha-1,8-diene; (*R*)-4-isopropenyl-1-methylcyclohex-1-ene; $C_{10}H_{16}$ = 136.2 (*5989-27-5*)
d_{20}^{20}, about 0.84; n_D^{20}, 1.471 to 1.474; $[\alpha]_D^{20}$, +96° to +106°; boiling point, 175° to 177°.
Limonene used in gas chromatography complies with the following test.
ASSAY Examine by *gas chromatography*, Appendix III B, under the conditions described in the test for Chromatographic profile in the monograph for Peppermint Oil using the reagent being examined.
The area of the principal peak is not less than 99.0% of the total area of the peaks.

Linalol See *linalool.*

Linalool (*RS*)-3,7-Dimethylocta-1,6-dien-3-ol; $C_{10}H_{18}O$ = 154.2 (*78-70-6*)
General reagent grade of commerce consisting of a mixture of two stereoisomers, licareol and coriandrol.
d_{20}^{20}, about 0.86; n_D^{20}, about 1.462; boiling point, about 200°.
Linalool used in gas chromatography complies with the following test.
ASSAY Examine by *gas chromatography*, Appendix III B, under the conditions described in the test for Chromatographic profile in the monograph for Anise Oil using the reagent being examined as solution (1).
The area of the principal peak is not less than 98.0% of the total area of the peaks.

Linalyl Acetate (*RS*)-1,5-Dimethyl-1-vinylhex-4-enyl acetate; $C_{12}H_{20}O_2$ = 196.3 *(115-95-7)*
General reagent grade of commerce.
d_{25}^{25}, 0.895 to 0.912; n_D^{20}, 1.448 to 1.451; boiling point, about 215°.
Linalyl acetate used in gas chromatography complies with the following requirement.
ASSAY Examine by gas chromatography as described in the monograph for Bitter-orange-flower Oil using the reagent being examined as the test solution. The area of the principal peak is not less than 95.0% of the total area of the peaks.

Lipase Solvent Dissolve 10 g of *sodium chloride*, 6.06 g of *tris(hydroxymethyl)methylamine* and 4.90 g of *maleic anhydride* in 900 ml of *water*. Adjust to pH 7.0 by the addition of a sufficient quantity (about 13 ml) of 4M *sodium hydroxide*, measuring the pH potentiometrically. Add sufficient *water* to produce 1000 ml.
Store at 2° to 8° and use within 3 days.

Lithium Li = 6.94 (*7439-93-2*)
General reagent grade of commerce.
A soft metal, the freshly cut surface of which is silvery grey. It reacts violently with water. Before use, the paraffin oil in which the metal is supplied should be washed off with toluene.
Store under liquid paraffin or light petroleum.

Lithium and Sodium Molybdotungstophosphate Solution Dissolve 100 g of *sodium tungstate* and 25 g of *sodium molybdate* in 800 ml of *water* in a 1500-ml flask; add 50 ml of *orthophosphoric acid* and 100 ml of *hydrochloric acid* and heat under a reflux condenser for 10 hours. Cool, add 150 g of *lithium sulphate*, 50 ml of *water* and 0.25 ml of *bromine* and allow to stand for 2 hours. Remove the excess of bromine by boiling the mixture for 15 minutes without the condenser. Cool, filter and dilute to 1000 ml with *water.*
Store at a temperature not exceeding 4° and use not later than 4 months after preparation. It has a golden yellow colour and must not be used if any trace of green colour is visible.

Lithium Carbonate Li_2CO_3 = 73.89 (*554-13-2*)
Analytical reagent grade of commerce.

Lithium Chloride LiCl = 42.39 (*7447-41-8*)
Analytical reagent grade of commerce.
Store in an airtight container.

Lithium Hydroxide $LiOH,H_2O$ = 41.96 (*1310-66-3*)
Analytical reagent grade of commerce.
Store in an airtight container.

Lithium Sulphate Li_2SO_4,H_2O = 128.0 (*10102-25-7*)
Analytical reagent grade of commerce.

Litmus (*1393-92-6*) Fragments of indigo blue pigment prepared from various species of *Rocella, Lecanora* or other lichen. The pigment has a faint, characteristic odour. Produces a red colour with acids and a blue colour in alkaline solutions (pH range, 5.0 to 8.0).

Litmus Paper Use *red litmus paper* or *blue litmus paper*, as appropriate.

Litmus Paper, Blue Boil 10 parts of coarsely powdered *litmus* under a reflux condenser for 1 hour with 100 parts of *ethanol (96%)*, decant the ethanol and discard. To the residue add a mixture of 45 parts of *ethanol (96%)* and 55 parts of *water.* After 2 days decant the clear liquid. Impregnate strips of filter paper with the extract and allow to dry.
Complies with the following test.
SENSITIVITY Immerse a strip (60 mm × 10 mm) in 100 ml of 0.002M *hydrochloric acid.* On shaking, the paper turns red within 45 seconds.

Litmus Paper, Red To the extract obtained in the preparation of *blue litmus paper* add 2M *hydrochloric acid* dropwise until the blue solution turns red. Impregnate strips of filter paper with the solution and allow to dry.
Complies with the following test.
SENSITIVITY Immerse a strip, 60 mm × 10 mm, in 100 ml of 0.002M *sodium hydroxide.* On shaking, the paper turns blue within 45 seconds.

Litmus Solution Boil 25 g of coarsely powdered *litmus* with 100 ml of *ethanol (90%)* under a reflux condenser for 1 hour, discard the clear liquid and repeat this operation using two 75-ml quantities of *ethanol (90%)*. Digest the extracted litmus with 250 ml of *water* and filter.

Macrogol 200 See *polyethylene glycol 200.*

Macrogol 200 R1 See *polyethylene glycol 200 R1.*

Macrogol 300 See *polyethylene glycol 300.*

Macrogol 400 See *polyethylene glycol 400.*

Macrogol 1000 See *polyethylene glycol 1000.*

Macrogol 1500 See *polyethylene glycol 1500.*

Macrogol 20,000 See *polyethylene glycol 20,000.*

Macrogol 20,000 2-Nitroterephthalate See *polyethylene glycol 20,000 2-nitroterephthalate.*

Magnesium Mg = 24.31 (*7439-95-4*)
General reagent grade of commerce.
Silver-white ribbon, turnings or wire or a grey powder.

Magnesium Acetate $C_4H_6MgO_4,4H_2O$ = 214.5 (*16674-78--5*)
Analytical reagent grade of commerce.
Store in an airtight container.

Magnesium Chloride $MgCl_2,6H_2O$ = 203.3 (*7791-18-6*)
Analytical reagent grade of commerce.

Magnesium Nitrate $Mg(NO_3)_2,6H_2O$ = 256.4 (*13446-18-9*)
Analytical reagent grade of commerce.
Store in an airtight container.

Magnesium Oxide Light magnesium oxide; MgO = 40.31 (*1309-48-4*)
General reagent grade of commerce.

Magnesium Oxide, Heavy
General reagent grade of commerce.

Magnesium Oxide R1 MgO = 40.31
Use a grade of commerce that complies with the following tests.
ARSENIC Dissolve 0.5 g in a mixture of 5 ml of *water* and 5 ml of 7M *hydrochloric acid*. The resulting solution complies with the *limit test for arsenic*, Appendix VII (2 ppm).
HEAVY METALS Dissolve 0.75 g in a mixture of 3 ml of *water* and 7 ml of 7M *hydrochloric acid*. Add 0.05 ml of *phenolphthalein solution* and sufficient 13.5M *ammonia* to produce a pink colour. Neutralise the excess ammonia by adding *glacial acetic acid*, add 0.5 ml in excess, dilute to 15 ml with *water* and filter if necessary. 12 ml of the solution complies with *limit test A for heavy metals*, Appendix VII (10 ppm). Use a mixture of 5 ml of *lead standard solution (1 ppm Pb)* and 5 ml of *water* to prepare the standard.
IRON Dissolve 0.2 g in 6 ml of 2M *hydrochloric acid* and dilute to 10 ml with *water*. The resulting solution complies with the *limit test for iron*, Appendix VII (50 ppm).

Magnesium Sulphate $MgSO_4,7H_2O$ = 246.8 (*10034-99-8*)
Analytical reagent grade of commerce.

Magneson Azo violet; 4-(4-nitrophenylazo)resorcinol; $C_{12}H_9N_3O_4$ = 259.2 (*74-39-5*)
Indicator grade of commerce.
When used for titration in non-aqueous media, it changes from orange (acidic) through pink (neutral) to blue (basic).

Magneson Reagent A 0.1% w/v solution of *magneson* in a 1% w/v solution of *sodium hydroxide*.

Magneson Solution A 0.2% w/v solution of *magneson* in *toluene*.

Maize Oil
Use oil of commerce that complies with the following requirements.
IDENTIFICATION Carry out the test for *identification of fixed oils by thin-layer chromatography*, Appendix X N. The chromatogram obtained is comparable with that shown for maize oil in Fig. 10N-3.
IODINE VALUE 103 to 128, Appendix X E.
PEROXIDE VALUE Not more than 5, Appendix X F.
SAPONIFICATION VALUE 187 to 195, Appendix X G.

Malachite Green CI 42000; basic green 4; $C_{23}H_{25}ClN_2$ = 364.9 (*123333-61-9*)
General reagent grade of commerce.
Green crystals with a metallic lustre; a 0.001% w/v solution in *ethanol (96%)* shows an absorption maximum at 617 nm.

Malachite Green Solution A 0.5% w/v solution of *malachite green* in *anhydrous acetic acid*.

Maleic Acid (*Z*)-But-2-ene-1,4-dioic acid; $C_4H_4O_4$ = 116.1 (*110-16-7*)
General reagent grade of commerce.
Colourless crystals; melting point, about 135°.

Maleic Anhydride Furan-2,5-dione; $C_4H_2O_3$ = 98.06 (*108-31-6*)
General reagent grade of commerce.
Melting point, about 52°.
Any residue insoluble in toluene does not exceed 5% (maleic acid).

Maleic Anhydride Solution A 5% w/v solution of *maleic anhydride* in *toluene*. Use within 1 month and filter if the solution becomes turbid.

Malic Acid DL-Hydroxysuccinic acid; $C_4H_7O_5$ = 134.1 (*617-48-1*)
General reagent grade of commerce.
Melting point, about 129°.

Manganese Sulphate See *manganese(II) sulphate.*

Manganese(II) Sulphate Manganese sulphate; $MnSO_4,H_2O$ = 169.0 (*10034-96-5*)
Analytical reagent grade of commerce.
Complies with the following test.
LOSS ON IGNITION 10.0 to 12.0%, determined on 1 g at 500°.

Mannitol See *D-mannitol.*

D-Mannitol Mannitol; $C_6H_{14}O_6$ = 182.2 (*69-65-8*)
Analytical reagent grade of commerce.
Melting point, about 167°.

Mannose See *D-mannose.*

D-Mannose Mannose; $C_6H_{12}O_6$ = 180.2 (*3458-28-4*)
General reagent grade of commerce.
Colourless crystals or a white, crystalline powder; melting point, about 132°, with decomposition; $[\alpha]_D^{20}$, +13.7° to +14.2° (20% w/v in water containing about 0.05% w/v of NH_3).

Meclozine Hydrochloride Meclozine dihydrochloride; $C_{25}H_{27}ClN_2,2HCl$ = 463.9 (*1104-22-9*)
General reagent grade of commerce.

Melamine 1,3,5-Triazine-2,4,6-triamine; $C_3H_6N_6$ = 126.1 (*108-78-1*)
General reagent grade of commerce.

Menadione 2-Methyl-1,4-naphthoquinone $C_{11}H_8O_2$ = 172.2 (*58-27-5*)
General reagent grade of commerce.

Menthofuran 3,9-Epoxy-*p*-mentha-3,8-diene; 3,6-dimethyl-4,5,6,7-tetrahydrobenzofuran; $C_{10}H_{14}O$ = 150.2 (*17957-94-7*)
General reagent grade of commerce.
d_{15}^{20}, about 0.965; n_D^{20}, about 1.480; $[\alpha]_D^{20}$, +93°; boiling point, about 196°.
Menthofuran used in gas chromatography complies with the following test.
ASSAY Examine by *gas chromatography*, Appendix III B, under the conditions described in the test for Chromatographic profile in the monograph for Peppermint Oil using the reagent being examined.

The area of the principal peak is not less than 97.0% of the total area of the peaks.

Menthol (−)-*p*-Menthan-3-ol (*2216-51-5*); (±)-*p*-menthan-3-ol (*15356-70-4*); $C_{10}H_{20}O$ = 156.3
General reagent grade of commerce.
A white, crystalline powder with a penetrating odour of peppermint; melting point, about 44° ((−)-menthol);

about 34° (±)-menthol; $[\alpha]_D^{20}$, about −50° (5% w/v in ethanol) ((−)-menthol).

Menthol used in gas chromatography complies with the following test.

ASSAY Examine by *gas chromatography*, Appendix III B, under the conditions described in the test for Chromatographic profile in the monograph for Peppermint Oil using the reagent being examined.

The area of the principal peak is not less than 98.0% of the total area of the peaks.

Menthone (−)-*trans-p*-Menthan-3-one; (2*S*,5*R*)-2-isopropyl-5-methylcyclohexanone; $C_{10}H_{18}O$ = 154.2 (*14073-97-3*)
General reagent grade of commerce containing a variable amount of isomenthone.
d_{20}^{20}, about 0.897; n_D^{20}, about 1.450.
Menthone used in gas chromatography complies with the following test.

ASSAY Examine by *gas chromatography*, Appendix III B, under the conditions described in the test for Chromatographic profile in the monograph for Peppermint Oil using the reagent being examined.

The area of the principal peak is not less than 90.0% of the total area of the peaks.

Menthyl Acetate $C_{12}H_{22}O_2$ = 198.3 (*16409-45-3*)
General reagent grade of commerce.
A colourless liquid with a characteristic odour; d_{20}^{20}, about 0.92; n_D^{20}, about 1.447; boiling point, about 225°.
Menthyl acetate used in gas chromatography complies with the following test.

ASSAY Examine by *gas chromatography*, Appendix III B, under the conditions described in the test for Chromatographic profile in the monograph for Peppermint Oil using the reagent being examined.

The area of the principal peak is not less than 98.0% of the total area of the peaks.

Mercaptoacetic Acid Thioglycollic acid; $C_2H_4O_2S$ = 92.12 (*68-11-1*)
General reagent grade of commerce.
A colourless liquid with an unpleasant odour; weight per ml, about 1.33 g.

2-Mercaptoethanol C_2H_6OS = 78.1 (*60-24-2*)
General reagent grade of commerce.
d_{20}^{20}, about 1.116; boiling point, about 157°.

Mercaptopurine See *6-mercaptopurine.*

6-Mercaptopurine Mercaptopurine; purine-6-thiol; $C_5H_4N_4S,H_2O$ = 170.2 (*6112-76-1*)
General reagent grade of commerce containing not less than 98.5% of $C_5H_4N_4S$.
A yellow, crystalline powder.

Mercuric Acetate See *mercury(II) acetate.*

Mercuric Acetate Solution See *mercury(II) acetate solution.*

Mercuric Bromide See *mercury(II) bromide.*

Mercuric Bromide Paper See *mercury(II) bromide paper.*

Mercuric Chloride See *mercury(II) chloride.*

Mercuric Chloride Solution See *mercury(II) chloride solution.*

Mercuric Iodide See *mercury(II) iodide.*

Mercuric Nitrate See *mercury(II) nitrate.*

Mercuric Oxide See *yellow mercury(II) oxide.*

Mercuric Sulphate Solution See *mercury(II) sulphate solution.*

Mercuric Thiocyanate See *mercury(II) thiocyanate.*

Mercuric Thiocyanate Solution See *mercury(II) thiocyanate solution.*

Mercury Hg = 200.6 (*7439-97-6*)
Analytical reagent grade of commerce.
Weight per ml, about 13.5 g; boiling point, about 357°.

Mercury(II) Acetate Mercuric acetate; $C_4H_6HgO_4$ = 318.7 (*1600-27-7*)
General reagent grade of commerce.

Mercury(II) Acetate Solution Mercuric acetate solution
A 3.19% w/v solution of *mercury(II) acetate* in *anhydrous acetic acid.* Neutralise, if necessary, with 0.1M *perchloric acid VS* using 0.05 ml of *crystal violet solution* as indicator.

Mercury(II) Bromide Mercuric bromide; $HgBr_2$ = 360.4 (*7789-47-1*)
Analytical reagent grade of commerce.

Mercury(II) Bromide Paper Mercuric bromide paper
In a rectangular dish place a 5% w/v solution of *mercury(II) bromide* in *absolute ethanol* and immerse in it pieces of white filter paper weighing 80 g m^{-2} (Whatman No. 1 is suitable), each measuring 20 cm × 15 mm and folded in two. Decant the excess liquid and allow the papers to dry, protected from light, by suspending them over a non-metallic thread. Cut away the folded edges to a width of 1 cm and similarly remove the outer edges. Cut the remaining strips into 15-mm squares or discs of 15 mm diameter.
Store in a glass-stoppered container wrapped with black paper.

Mercury(II) Chloride Mercuric chloride; $HgCl_2$ = 271.5 (*7487-94-7*)
Analytical reagent grade of commerce.

Mercury(II) Chloride Solution Mercuric chloride solution
A 5.4% w/v solution of *mercury(II) chloride.*

Mercury(II) Iodide Mercuric iodide; HgI_2 = 454.4 (*7774-29-0*)
General reagent grade of commerce.
A dense, red, crystalline powder.
Store protected from light.

Mercury(II) Nitrate Mercuric nitrate; $Hg(NO_3)_2,H_2O$ = 342.6 (*7782-86-7*)
Analytical reagent grade of commerce.
Store in an airtight container protected from light.

Mercury, Nitric Acid Solution of
Of commerce, or prepare by dissolving 3 ml of *mercury* in 27 ml of cold *fuming nitric acid* and diluting the solution with an equal volume of *water.*
Store protected from light and use within 2 months.

Mercury(II) Oxide, Yellow Mercuric oxide; HgO = 216.6 (*21908-53-2*)
General reagent grade of commerce.
An orange-yellow, amorphous powder.
Store protected from light.

Mercury(II) Sulphate Solution Mercuric sulphate solution
Dissolve 1 g of *yellow mercury(II) oxide* in a mixture of 20 ml of *water* and 4 ml of *sulphuric acid.*

Mercury(II) Thiocyanate $Hg(SCN)_2$ = 316.8 (*592-85-8*)
General reagent grade of commerce.

Mercury(II) Thiocyanate Solution Mercuric thiocyanate solution
Dissolve 0.3 g of *mercury(II) thiocyanate* in sufficient *absolute ethanol* to produce 100 ml.
Use within 1 week.

Metanil Yellow CI 13065; 4′-anilinoazobenzene-3-sulphonic acid sodium salt; $C_{18}H_{14}N_3NaO_3S$ = 375.4 *(587-98-4)*
When used for titration in non-aqueous media, it changes from yellow (basic) to magenta (acidic).

Metanil Yellow Solution A 0.1% w/v solution of *metanil yellow* in *methanol.*
Complies with the following test.
SENSITIVITY A solution containing 0.1 ml in 50 ml of *anhydrous acetic acid* is pinkish red. Add 0.05 ml of 0.1M *perchloric acid VS*; the colour of the solution changes to violet (pH range, 1.2 to 2.3).

Metaphosphoric Acid $(HPO_3)_x$ *(37267-86-0)*
General reagent grade of commerce.
Hygroscopic, glassy lumps or sticks containing a proportion of sodium metaphosphate.
Complies with the following tests.
NITRATES Boil 1.0 g with 10 ml of *water*, cool, add 1 ml of *indigo carmine solution* and 10 ml of *nitrogen-free sulphuric acid* and heat to boiling. The blue colour is not completely discharged.
REDUCING SUBSTANCES Not more than 0.01%, calculated as H_3PO_3. Dissolve 35 g in 50 ml of *water*, add 5 ml of a 20% w/v solution of *sulphuric acid*, 50 mg of *potassium bromide* and 5 ml 0.02M *potassium bromate VS* and heat on a water bath for 30 minutes. Allow to cool, add 0.5 g of *potassium iodide* and titrate the liberated iodine with 0.1M *sodium thiosulphate VS* using 1 ml of *starch solution* as indicator. Repeat the procedure without the reagent being examined. The difference between the titrations is the amount of potassium bromate required. Each ml of 0.02M *potassium bromate VS* is equivalent to 4.10 mg of H_3PO_3.
Store in an airtight container.

Methacrylic Acid $C_4H_6O_2$ = 86.1 *(79-41-4)*
General reagent grade of commerce.
n_D^{20} , about 1.431; boiling point, about 160°; melting point, about 16°.

Methanesulphonic Acid CH_4O_3S = 96.10 *(75-75-2)*
General reagent grade of commerce.
A colourless, corrosive liquid; d_{20}^{20}, about 1.48; n_D^{20}, about 1.430.

Methanesulphonic Acid, Methanolic Solutions of the requisite molarity may be obtained by dissolving the appropriate quantity of *methanesulphonic acid* in *methanol.*

Methanol Methyl alcohol; CH_4O = 32.04 *(67-56-1)*
Analytical reagent grade of commerce.
A colourless liquid; boiling point, 64° to 65°; d_{20}^{20}, 0.791 to 0.793.
When '*methanol*' is followed by a percentage figure, an instruction to use *methanol* diluted with *water* to produce the specified percentage v/v of methanol is implied.

Methanol, Acidified To 900 ml of *methanol* add 18 ml of *glacial acetic acid* and dilute to 1000 ml with *water.*

Methanol, Aldehyde-free Methanol containing not more than 0.001% of aldehydes and ketones. Dissolve 25 g of *iodine* in 1000 ml of *methanol.* Add this solution, with constant stirring, to 400 ml of 1M *sodium hydroxide* and add 150 ml of *water.* Allow to stand for 16 hours, filter and boil under a reflux condenser until the odour of iodoform is no longer detectable. Distil the resulting solution by fractional distillation.

Methanol, Anhydrous Methanol of commerce specially dried for use in Karl Fischer determinations and other non-aqueous titrations. It may be prepared in the following manner.
Treat 1000 ml of *methanol* with 5 g of *magnesium.* If necessary, initiate the reaction by adding 0.1 ml of *mercury(II) chloride solution.* When the evolution of gas has ceased, distil the liquid and collect the distillate in a dry container protected from moisture.
Complies with the following test.
WATER Not more than 0.03% w/v, Appendix IX C.

Methanol, Hydrochloric Dilute 1 ml of 7M *hydrochloric acid* to 100 ml with *methanol.*

Methanol R1 Spectrophotometric grade of *methanol* having a minimum transmittance of 20% at 210 nm, 50% at 220 nm, 75% at 230 nm, 95% at 250 nm and 98% at 260 nm and above using *water* in the reference cell.

Methimazole Thiamazole; 2-mercapto-1-methylimidazole; $C_4H_6N_2S$ = 114.2 *(60-56-0)*
General reagent grade of commerce.
Melting point, about 145°.

L-Methionine $C_5H_{11}NO_2S$ = 149.2 *(63-68-3)*
General reagent grade of commerce.
A white, crystalline solid; $[\alpha]_D^{20}$, about +23° (5% w/v in 1M hydrochloric acid).

2-Methoxyethanol Ethylene glycol monomethyl ether; $C_3H_8O_2$ = 76.10 *(109-86-4)*
Chromatographic reagent grade of commerce.
A colourless liquid; boiling point, about 125°; d_{20}^{20}, about 0.93; n_D^{20}, about 1.406.

Methoxyphenylacetic Acid $C_9H_{10}O_3$ = 166.2 *(7021-09-2)*
General reagent grade of commerce.
Melting point, about 70°.
Store in a cool place.

Methoxyphenylacetic Acid Reagent Dissolve 2.7 g of *methoxyphenylacetic acid* in 6 ml of *tetramethylammonium hydroxide solution* and add 20 ml of *absolute ethanol.*
Store in a polyethylene container.

Methyl Acetate $C_3H_6O_2$ = 74.1 *(79-20-9)*
General reagent grade of commerce.
d_{20}^{20}, about 0.933; n_D^{20}, about 1.361; boiling point, 56° to 58°.

Methyl Anthranilate Methyl 2-aminobenzoate; $C_8H_9NO_2$ = 151.2 *(134-20-3)*
General reagent grade of commerce.
Melting point, 24° to 25°; boiling point, 134° to 136°.
Methyl anthranilate used in gas chromatography complies with the following test.
ASSAY Examine by gas chromatography as described in the monograph for Bitter-orange-flower Oil using the reagent being examined as the test solution. The area of the principal peak is not less than 95.0% of the total area of the peaks.

Methyl Arachidate Methyl eicosanoate; $C_{21}H_{42}O_2$ = 326.6 *(1120-28-1)*
General reagent grade of commerce containing not less than 98.0% of $C_{21}H_{42}O_2$, determined by gas chromatography.
A white or pale yellow, crystalline mass; melting point, about 46°.

Methyl Behenate See *methyl docosanoate*.

Methyl Cinnamate $C_{10}H_{10}O_2$ = 162.2 (*103-26-4*)
General reagent grade of commerce.
n_D^{20}, about 1.56; melting point, 34° to 36°; boiling point, about 260°.

Methyl Decanoate Methyl caproate; $C_{11}H_{22}O_2$ = 186.3 (*110-42-9*)
General reagent grade of commerce.
A colourless or yellow liquid; n_D^{20},1.425 to 1.426; d_{20}^{20}, 0.871 to 0.876.
Complies with the following test.
RELATED SUBSTANCES Carry out the method for *gas chromatography*, Appendix III B, using solutions of the reagent being examined in *carbon disulphide* containing (1) 0.002% w/v and (2) 0.2% w/v. Solution (3) is *carbon disulphide*.

The chromatographic procedure may be carried out using a glass column (1.5 m × 4 mm) packed with *silanised diatomaceous support* (Diatomite CQ is suitable) (100 to 120 mesh) coated with 10% w/w of silicone gum rubber (methyl) (SE-30 is suitable), maintained at 150° and used in conjunction with a precolumn containing silanised glass wool.

The sum of the areas of any *secondary peaks* in the chromatogram obtained with solution (2) is not greater than the area of the principal peak in the chromatogram obtained with solution (1).

Methyl Docosanoate Methyl behenate; $C_{22}H_{46}O_2$ = 354.6 (*929-77-1*)
General reagent grade of commerce.
Melting point, 54° to 55°.

Methyl Ethyl Ketone See *butan-2-one*.

Methyl Green CI 42585; basic blue 20; $C_{26}H_{33}Cl_2N_3$ = 458.5 (*7114-03-6*)
General reagent grade of commerce.
A green powder.

Methyl Green-Iodomercurate Paper Immerse thin strips of suitable filter paper in a 4% w/v solution of *methyl green* and allow to dry in air. Immerse the strips in a solution containing 14% w/v of *potassium iodide* and 20% w/v of *mercury(II) iodide* for 1 hour. Wash with *distilled water* until the washings are practically colourless and allow to dry in air.
Store protected from light and use within 48 hours.

Methyl 4-Hydroxybenzoate Methyl parahydroxybenzoate; $C_8H_8O_3$ = 152.2 (*99-76-3*)
General reagent grade of commerce.
Melting point, about 127°.

Methyl Isobutyl Ketone See *4-methylpentan-2-one*.

Methyl Isobutyl Ketone R1 See *4-methylpentan-2-one R1*.

Methyl Laurate Methyl dodecanoate; $C_{13}H_{26}O_2$ = 214.4 (*111-82-0*)
Purified reagent grade of commerce containing not less than 98.0% of $C_{13}H_{26}O_2$, determined by gas chromatography.
A colourless or pale yellow liquid; d_{20}^{20}, about 0.87; n_D^{20}, about 1.431; melting point, about 5°.

Methyl Methacrylate Methyl 2-methylprop-2-enoate; $C_5H_8O_2$ = 100.1 (*80-62-6*)
General reagent grade of commerce.
Melting point, about −48°; boiling point, about 100°; n_D^{20}, about 1.414.
It contains a suitable stabilising agent.

Methyl Myristate Methyl tetradecanoate; $C_{15}H_{30}O_2$ = 242.4 (*124-10-7*)
General reagent grade of commerce containing not less than 98.0% of $C_{15}H_{30}O_2$, determined by gas chromatography.
A colourless or slightly yellow liquid; d_{20}^{20}, about 0.87; n_D^{20}, about 1.437; melting point, about 20°.

Methyl Oleate Methyl (*Z*)-octadec-9-enoate; $C_{19}H_{36}O_2$ = 296.5 (*112-62-9*)
Purified reagent grade of commerce containing not less than 98.0% of $C_{19}H_{36}O_2$, determined by gas chromatography.
A colourless or slightly yellow liquid; d_{20}^{20}, about 0.88; n_D^{20}, about 1.452.

Methyl Orange CI 13025; sodium 4′-dimethylaminoazobenzene-4-sulphonate; $C_{14}H_{14}N_3NaO_3S$ = 327.3 (*547-58-0*)
Produces a red colour in moderately acidic solutions and a yellow colour in weakly acidic and alkaline solutions.

Methyl Orange Mixed Solution Dissolve 20 mg of *methyl orange* and 0.1 g of *bromocresol green* in 1 ml of 0.2M *sodium hydroxide* and dilute to 100 ml with *water*.
Colour change: pH 3.0 (orange) to 4.4 (olive-green).

Methyl Orange Solution Dissolve 0.1 g of *methyl orange* in 80 ml of *water* and add sufficient *ethanol (96%)* to produce 100 ml.
Complies with the following test.
SENSITIVITY A mixture of 0.1 ml of the solution and 100 ml of *carbon dioxide-free water* is yellow. Not more than 0.1 ml of 0.1M *hydrochloric acid VS* is required to change the colour of the solution to red.
Colour change: pH 3.0 (red) to 4.4 (yellow).

Methyl Orange—Xylene Cyanol FF Solution Dissolve 0.1 g of *methyl orange* and 0.26 g of *xylene cyanol FF* in 50 ml of *ethanol (96%)* and add sufficient *water* to produce 100 ml.

Methyl Palmitate Methyl hexadecanoate; $C_{17}H_{34}O_2$ = 270.5 (*112-39-0*)
General reagent grade of commerce containing not less than 98.0% of $C_{17}H_{34}O_2$, determined by gas chromatography.
A colourless, waxy solid; freezing point, about 27°; weight per ml at 30°, about 0.86 g.

Methyl Parahydroxybenzoate See *methyl 4-hydroxybenzoate*.

Methyl Red CI 13020; 2-(4-dimethylaminophenylazo)-benzoic acid; $C_{15}H_{15}N_3O_2$ = 269.3 (*493-52-7*)
A dark red powder or violet crystals.

Methyl Red Mixed Solution Dissolve 0.1 g of *methyl red* and 50 mg of *methylene blue* in 100 ml of *ethanol 96%)*.
Colour change: pH 5.2 (reddish violet) to pH 5.6 (green).

Methyl Red Solution Dissolve 50 mg of *methyl red* in a mixture of 1.86 ml of 0.1M *sodium hydroxide* and 50 ml of *ethanol (96%)* and add sufficient *water* to produce 100 ml.
Complies with the following test.
SENSITIVITY A mixture of 0.1 ml of the solution, 100 ml of *carbon dioxide-free water* and 0.05 ml of 0.02M *hydrochloric acid VS* is red. Not more than 0.1 ml of 0.02M *sodium hydroxide VS* is required to change the colour of the solution to yellow.
Colour change: pH 4.4 (red) to pH 6.0 (yellow).

Methyl Salicylate $C_8H_8O_3$ = 152.2 (*119-36-8*)
General reagent grade of commerce.
A colourless or slightly yellow liquid with a strong, persistent, characteristic, aromatic odour; weight per ml, about 1.18 g.

Methyl Stearate $C_{19}H_{38}O_2$ = 298.5 (*112-61-8*)
Use a purified reagent grade of commerce containing not less than 98.0% of $C_{19}H_{38}O_2$, determined by gas chromatography.
A white or pale yellow, crystalline mass; melting point, about 38°.

Methyl Thymol Blue [3*H*-2,1-Benzoxathiol-3-ylidenebis(6-hydroxy-5-isopropyl-2-methyl-*m*-phenylene)-methylenenitrilo]tetra-acetic acid *S,S*-dioxide tetrasodium salt; $C_{37}H_{40}N_2Na_4O_{13}S$ = 845 (*1945-77-3*)
General reagent grade of commerce.
Produces a blue colour with calcium in alkaline solution. When metal ions are absent, for example, in the presence of an excess of disodium edetate, the solution is grey.

Methyl Thymol Blue Mixture A mixture of 1 part of *methyl thymol blue* and 100 parts of *potassium nitrate.*

Methyl Tricosanoate Tricosanoic acid methyl ester; $C_{24}H_{48}O_2$ = 368.6 (*2433-97-8*)
General reagent grade of commerce containing not less than 99.0% of $C_{24}H_{48}O_2$.
Melting point, 55° to 56°.

4-Methylaminophenol Sulphate Metol; $(C_7H_9NO)_2$,H_2SO_4 = 344.4 (*55-55-0*)
General reagent grade of commerce.
Melting point, about 260°.

Methylaminophenol—Sulphite Reagent Dissolve 0.1 g of *4-methylaminophenol sulphate*, 20 g of *sodium metabisulphite* and 0.5 g of *anhydrous sodium sulphite* in sufficient *water* to produce 100 ml.

3-Methylbenzothiazolin-2-one Hydrazone Hydrochloride $C_8H_9N_3S$,HCl,H_2O = 233.7 (*149022-15-1*)
General reagent grade of commerce.
Melting point, about 270°.
When used for the determination of aldehydes, complies with the following test.
SUITABILITY FOR THE DETERMINATION OF ALDEHYDES To 2 ml of *aldehyde-free methanol* add 60 µl of a 0.1% w/v solution of *propionaldehyde* in *aldehyde-free methanol* and 5 ml of a 0.4% w/v solution of the reagent being examined, mix and allow to stand for 30 minutes. Add 25ml of a 0.2% w/v solution of *iron(III) chloride hexahydrate*, dilute to 100 ml with *acetone* and mix. The *absorbance* of the resulting solution at 660 nm is not less than 0.62, Appendix II B. Use in the reference cell a solution prepared at the same time and in the same manner but without the propionaldehyde solution.

Methylbenzothiazolone Hydrazone Hydrochloride See *3-methylbenzothiazolin-2-one hydrazone hydrochloride.*

2-Methylbutane Isopentane; C_5H_{12} = 72.2 (*78-78-4*)
General reagent grade of commerce containing not less than 99.5% of C_5H_{12}.
d_{20}^{20}, about 0.621; n_D^{20}, about 1.354; boiling point, about 29°.
WATER Not more than 0.02%.
TRANSMITTANCE Not more than 50% at 210 nm, 85% at 220 nm and 98% at 240 nm and higher wavelengths using water in the reference cell.

2-Methylbut-2-ene C_5H_{10} = 70.1 (*513-35-9*)
General reagent grade of commerce.
Boiling point, 37.5° to 38.5°; d_4^{15}, about 0.66

Methylcellulose 450 (*9004-67-5*)
General reagent grade of commerce. The nominal viscosity is 450 mPa s.

3-*O*-Methyldopamine Hydrochloride 3-Methoxytyramine hydrochloride; $C_9H_{13}NO_2$,HCl = 203.7 (*1477-68-5*)
General reagent grade of commerce.
Melting point, about 214°.
Complies with the following test.
HOMOGENEITY Examine under the conditions prescribed in the test for Related substances in the monograph for Dopamine Hydrochloride applying to the plate 10 µl of a 0.0075% w/v solution in *methanol.* The chromatogram shows only one principal spot.

4-*O*-Methyldopamine Hydrochloride 3-Hydroxy-4-methoxyphenethylamine hydrochloride; $C_9H_{13}NO_2$,HCl = 203.7 (*645-33-0*)
General reagent grade of commerce.
Melting point, about 208°.
Complies with the following test.
HOMOGENEITY Examine under the conditions prescribed in the test for Related substances in the monograph for Dopamine Hydrochloride applying to the plate 10 µl of a 0.0075% w/v solution in *methanol.* The chromatogram shows only one principal spot.

Methylene Blue CI 52015; basic blue 9; $C_{16}H_{18}ClN_3S$,xH_2O = 319.9 (anhydrous) (*7220-79-3*)
Use a redox indicator grade suitable for biological work.
A hygroscopic, dark green or brown, crystalline powder.

Methylene Chloride See *dichloromethane.*

Methylene Chloride, Acidified See *acidified dichloromethane.*

***N,N'*-Methylenebisacrylamide** $C_7H_{10}N_2O_2$ = 154.2 (*110-26-9*)
General reagent grade of commerce.
A fine, white powder.

4,4'-Methylenebis-*N,N*-dimethylaniline Tetramethyldiaminodiphenylmethane; $C_{17}H_{22}N_2$ = 254.4 (*101-61-1*)
General reagent grade of commerce.
Melting point, about 90°.

4,4'-Methylenebis-*N,N*-dimethylaniline Reagent Tetramethyldiaminodiphenylmethane reagent
SOLUTION A Dissolve 2.5 g of *4,4'-methylenebis-*N,N-*dimethylaniline* in 10 ml of *glacial acetic acid* and add 50 ml of *water.*
SOLUTION B Dissolve 5 g of *potassium iodide* in 100 ml of *water.*
SOLUTION C Dissolve 0.3 g of *ninhydrin* in 10 ml of *glacial acetic acid* and add 90 ml of *water.*
Mix solution A, solution B and 1.5 ml of solution C.

***N*-Methylglucamine** Meglumine; $C_7H_{17}NO_5$ = 195.2 (*6284-40-8*)
General reagent grade of commerce.
Melting point, about 130°.

2-Methyl-1,4-naphthoquinone Menadione; $C_{11}H_8O_2$ = 172.2 (*58-27-5*)
General reagent grade of commerce.
Bright yellow crystals; melting point, about 106°.

2-Methyl-5-nitroimidazole $C_4H_5N_3O_2$ = 127.1 (*88054-22-2*)
General reagent grade of commerce.
Melting point, 252° to 254°.

4-Methylpentan-2-one Methyl isobutyl ketone; $C_6H_{12}O$ = 100.2 (*108-10-1*)
Analytical reagent grade of commerce.
A colourless liquid; boiling point, about 115°; d_{20}^{20}, about 0.80.

4-Methylpentan-2-one R1 Methyl isobutyl ketone R1
Shake 50 ml of freshly distilled *4-methylpentan-2-one* with 0.5 ml of 7M *hydrochloric acid* for 1 minute. Allow the phases to separate and discard the lower phase.
Prepare immediately before use.

Methylpiperazine See N-*methylpiperazine.*

***N*-Methylpiperazine** $C_5H_{12}N_2$ = 100.2 (*74879-18-8*)
General reagent grade of commerce.
A colourless liquid; d_{20}^{20}, about 0.90; n_D^{20}, about 1.466; boiling point, about 138°.

2-Methylpropanol See *2-Methylpropan-1-ol.*

2-Methylpropan-1-ol Isobutyl alcohol; $C_4H_{10}O$ = 74.12 (*78-83-1*)
Analytical reagent grade of commerce.
A colourless liquid with a characteristic odour; d_{20}^{20}, about 0.80; n_D^{15}, 1.397 to 1.399; boiling point, about 107°.

2-Methylpropan-2-ol *tert*-Butyl alcohol; $C_4H_{10}O$ = 74.12 (*75-65-0*)
Analytical reagent grade of commerce.
A colourless, oily liquid or solid with a characteristic odour; freezing point, about 25°; boiling point, about 82°; weight per ml at 26°, about 0.78 g.

Molecular Sieve Molecular sieve composed of sodium aluminosilicate. It is available as beads with a pore size of 0.4 mm and with a diameter of 2 mm.
Reagent grade of commerce.

Molybdenum(VI) Oxide Molybdenum trioxide; MoO_3 = 143.9 (*1313-27-5*)
Analytical reagent grade of commerce.

Molybdovanadic Reagent Suspend 4 g of finely powdered *ammonium molybdate* and 0.1 g of finely powdered *ammonium metavanadate* in 70 ml of *water* and grind until dissolved. Add 20 ml of *nitric acid* and dilute to 100 ml with *water.*

Mordant Black 11 CI 14645; eriochrome black T; solochrome black; $C_{20}H_{12}N_3NaO_7S$ = 461.4 (*1787-61-7*)
General reagent grade of commerce.
A brownish black powder.
Produces a red colour with calcium, magnesium, zinc and certain other metals in alkaline solutions. When metal ions are absent, for example in the presence of an excess of disodium edetate, the solution is blue.
Store in an airtight container protected from light.

Mordant Black 11 Mixed Triturate A mixture of 1 g of *mordant black 11*, 0.4 g of *methyl orange* and 100 g of *sodium chloride.*
Complies with the following test.
SENSITIVITY TO MAGNESIUM Dissolve 50 mg in 100 ml of *water*; a brown colour is produced. Add 0.3 ml of 6M *ammonia*; the colour changes to pale green. Add 0.1 ml of a 1.0% w/v solution of *magnesium sulphate*; the colour changes to red.

Mordant Black 11 Triturate A mixture of 1 part of *mordant black 11* with 99 parts of *sodium chloride.*
Complies with the following test.
SENSITIVITY TO MAGNESIUM Dissolve 50 mg in 100 ml of *water*; a brownish violet colour is produced. Add 0.3 ml of 6M *ammonia*; the colour changes to blue. Add 0.1 ml of a 1% w/v solution of *magnesium sulphate*; the colour changes to violet.
Store in an airtight container protected from light.

Mordant Black 11 Solution A 0.1% w/v solution of *mordant black 11* in *ethanol (96%).*

Mordant Blue 3 CI 43820; chromoxane cyanine R (*3564-18-9*)
General reagent grade of commerce.
A dark red or reddish brown powder.
Produces an intense purple colour with aluminium in weakly acidic solutions. When metal ions are absent, for example, in the presence of an excess of disodium edetate, the solution is pale pink.

Morphine, Anhydrous Add 5M *ammonia*, in slight excess, to a solution of *morphine sulphate* in *water*, wash the precipitated morphine with *water* until free from ammonium salts and dry at 110°.

Morphine Hydrochloride Of the British Pharmacopoeia.

Morpholine Tetrahydro-1,4-oxazine; C_4H_9NO = 87.12 (*110-91-8*)
General reagent grade of commerce.
A colourless liquid; boiling point, about 128°; d_{20}^{20}, about 1.01.

Myristic Acid $C_{14}H_{28}O_2$ = 228.4 (*544-63-8*)
Reagent grade of commerce containing at least 99.5% of $C_{14}H_{28}O_2$.
Melting point, about 55°.

Myristicine 5-Allyl-1-methoxy-2,3-methylenedioxybenzene; $C_{11}H_{12}O_3$ = 192.2 (*607-91-0*)
General reagent grade of commerce.
d_{20}^{20}, about 1.144; n_D^{20}, about 1.540; boiling point, 276° to 277°; melting point, about 173°.
Complies with the following test.
HOMOGENEITY When examined as described in the test for *Ilicium anisatum* in the monograph for Star Anise, the chromatogram obtained shows only one principal spot.

Nalorphine Hydrochloride $C_{19}H_{21}NO_3,HCl$ = 347.8 (*57-29-4*)
General reagent grade of commerce.

Naphthalene $C_{10}H_8$ = 128.2 (*91-20-3*)
Use a grade of commerce suitable for liquid scintillation.
White crystals; melting point, about 81°.

Naphthalene Black 12B CI 20470; amido black 10B; $C_{22}H_{14}N_4Na_2O_9S_2$ = 588.5 (*1064-48-8*)
General reagent grade of commerce.
A dark brown powder.

Naphthalene Black Solution A 1.0% w/v solution of *naphthalene black 12B* in 1M *acetic acid.*

Naphthalene-1,3-diol 1,3-Dihydroxynaphthalene; naphthoresorcinol; $C_{10}H_8O_2$ = 160.2 (*132-86-5*)
General reagent grade of commerce.
Colourless crystals; melting point, about 125°.

Naphthalene-2,7-diol 2,7-Dihydroxynaphthalene; $C_{10}H_8O_2$ = 160.2 (*582-17-2*)
General reagent grade of commerce.
Melting point, about 190°, with decomposition.

Naphthalenediol Solution 2,7-Dihydroxynaphthalene solution
Dissolve 10 mg of *naphthalene-2,7-diol* in 100 ml of *sulphuric acid* and allow to stand until the initial yellow colour has disappeared.
Use within 2 days.

Naphthalenediol Reagent Solution Dissolve 2.5 mg of *naphthalene-2,7-diol* in 90 ml of *methanol* and add 10 mg of *potassium hexacyanoferrate(III)* and 50 mg of *potassium cyanide* dissolved in 10 ml of *water*. Allow to stand for 30 minutes and add 100 ml of 0.05M *sodium hydroxide*.

α-Naphthol See *1-naphthol.*

α-Naphthol Solution See *1-naphthol solution.*

β-Naphthol See *2-naphthol.*

β-Naphthol Solution See *2-naphthol solution.*

1-Naphthol α-Naphthol; $C_{10}H_8O$ = 144.2 *(90-15-3)*
Analytical reagent grade of commerce.
Colourless crystals with a phenolic odour; melting point, about 95°.
Store protected from light.

2-Naphthol β-Naphthol; $C_{10}H_8O$ = 144.2 *(135-19-3)*
Analytical reagent grade of commerce.
A crystalline solid with a faint phenolic odour; melting point, about 122°.
Store protected from light.

1-Naphthol Solution Dissolve 0.1 g of *1-naphthol* in 3 ml of a 15% w/v solution of *sodium hydroxide* and dilute to 100 ml with *water*.
Prepare immediately before use.

1-Naphthol Solution, Strong Dissolve 1 g of *1-naphthol* in a solution of 6 g of *sodium hydroxide* and 16 g of *anhydrous sodium carbonate* in 100 ml of *water*.

2-Naphthol Solution Dissolve 5 g of *2-naphthol*, freshly recrystallised, in 40 ml of 2M *sodium hydroxide* and add sufficient *water* to produce 100 ml.
Prepare immediately before use.

Naphtholbenzein See *1-naphtholbenzein.*

Naphtholbenzein Solution See *1-naphtholbenzein solution.*

1-Naphtholbenzein Phenylbis(4-hydroxynaphthyl)-methanol; $C_{27}H_{20}O_3$ = 392.5 *(6948-88-5)*
A brownish red powder or shiny brownish black crystals.

1-Naphtholbenzein Solution A 0.2% w/v solution of *1-naphtholbenzein* in *anhydrous acetic acid.*
Complies with the following test.
SENSITIVITY Add 0.25 ml of the solution to 50 ml of *glacial acetic acid*. Not more than 0.05 ml of 0.1M *perchloric acid VS* is required to change the colour of the solution from brownish yellow to green.

2-Naphthylacetic Acid 2-Naphthaleneacetic acid; $C_{12}H_{10}O_2$ = 186.2 *(581-96-4)*
General reagent grade of commerce.
Light yellow to light brown crystals; melting point, about 142°.

Naphthylamine See *1-naphthylamine.*

1-Naphthylamine Naphthylamine; $C_{10}H_9N$ = 143.2 *(134-32-7)*
General reagent grade of commerce.
Almost colourless crystals or a white, crystalline powder; melting point, about 51°.
Store protected from light.

Naphthylethylenediamine Dihydrochloride See N-*(1-naphthyl)ethylenediamine dihydrochloride.*

***N*-(1-Naphthyl)ethylenediamine Dihydrochloride** *N*-(1-Naphthyl)ethane-1,2-diammonium dichloride; $C_{12}H_{14}N_2$,2HCl = 259.2 *(1465-25-4)*
General reagent grade of commerce which may contain methanol of crystallisation.
A white or cream powder; melting point, not less than 188°.

***trans*-Nerolidol** 3,7,11-Trimethyldodeca-1,6,10-trien-3-ol; $C_{15}H_{26}O$ = 222.4 *(40716-66-3)*
General reagent grade of commerce.
d_{20}^{20}, about 0.876; n_D^{20}, about 1.479.
trans-*Nerolidol used in gas chromatography complies with the following requirement.*
ASSAY Examine by gas chromatography as described in the monograph for Bitter-orange-flower Oil using the reagent being examined as the test solution. The area of the principal peak is not less than 90.0% of the total area of the peaks.

Neryl Acetate (*Z*)-3,7-Dimethylocta-2,6-dienyl acetate; $C_{12}H_{20}O_2$ = 196.3 *(141-12-8)*
General reagent grade of commerce.
d_{20}^{20}, about 0.907; n_D^{20}, about 1.460.
Neryl acetate used in gas chromatography complies with the following requirement.
ASSAY Examine by gas chromatography as described in the monograph for Bitter-orange-flower Oil using the reagent being examined as the test solution. The area of the principal peak is not less than 93.0% of the total area of the peaks.

Neutral Red CI 50040; basic red 5; $C_{15}H_{17}ClN_4$ = 288.8 *(553-24-2)*
Produces a red colour with acids and an orange colour with alkalis.

Neutral Red Solution A 0.1% w/v solution of *neutral red* in *ethanol (50%)* (pH range, 6.8 to 8.0).

Nickel—Aluminium Alloy Raney nickel catalyst
A powdered alloy containing 48 to 52% of nickel and 48 to 52% of aluminium.
Reduce to *No.180* powder before use.

Nickel Chloride See *nickel(II) chloride.*

Nickel(II) Chloride Anhydrous nickel chloride; $NiCl_2$ = 129.6 *(7718-54-9)*
General reagent grade of commerce.

Nickel(II) Chloride Hexahydrate $NiCl_2,6H_2O$ = 237.7 *(7791-20-0)*
Analytical reagent grade of commerce.

Nickel Chloride Solution, Ammoniacal Dissolve 0.1 g of *nickel(II) chloride hexahydrate* in 10 ml of *water*, add a solution containing 5.4 g of *ammonium chloride*, 8 g of *ammonium hydrogen carbonate* and 1.5 ml of 13.5M *ammonia* and dilute to 100 ml with *water*.

Nickel Sulphate See *nickel(II) sulphate.*

Nickel(II) Sulphate $NiSO_4,7H_2O$ = 280.9 *(10101-98-1)*
Analytical reagent grade of commerce.
A green, crystalline powder or crystals.

Nicotinamide-adenine Dinucleotide NAD^+; $C_{21}H_{27}N_7O_{14}P_2$ = 663 *(7298-93-3)*
General reagent grade of commerce.

Nicotinamide-adenine Dinucleotide Solution Dissolve 40 mg of *nicotinamide-adenine dinucleotide* in *water* and dilute to 10 ml with the same solvent. Prepare immediately before use.

Nicotinic Acid $C_6H_5NO_2$ = 123.1 *(59-67-6)*
General reagent grade of commerce.
A white, crystalline powder; melting point, about 235°.

Nile Blue A CI 51180; 5-amino-9-diethylamino-benzo[*a*]phenoxazinylium hydrogen sulphate; $C_{20}H_{21}N_3O_5S$ = 415.5 *(3625-57-8)*
A green, crystalline powder with a bronze lustre.
Complies with the following test.
LIGHT ABSORPTION A 0.0005% w/v solution in *ethanol (50%)* exhibits a maximum at 640 nm.

Nile Blue A Solution A 1% w/v solution of *nile blue A* in *anhydrous acetic acid.*
Complies with the following test.
SENSITIVITY A solution containing 0.25 ml in 50 ml of *anhydrous acetic acid* is blue. Not more than 0.1 ml of 0.1M *perchloric acid VS* is required to change the colour of the solution to bluish green.
Colour change: pH 9.0 (blue) to 13.0 (red).

Ninhydrin Indane-1,2,3-trione; $C_9H_4O_3,H_2O$ = 178.1 *(485-47-2)*
Analytical reagent grade of commerce.
A very pale yellow, crystalline powder; melting point, about 255°.
Store protected from light.

Ninhydrin and Stannous Chloride Reagent Dissolve 0.2 g of *ninhydrin* in 4 ml of hot *water*, add 5 ml of a 0.16% w/v solution of *tin(II) chloride*, allow to stand for 30 minutes, filter and store at 2° to 8°.
Immediately before use, dilute 2.5 ml of the solution with 5 ml of *water* and 45 ml of *propan-2-ol.*

Ninhydrin and Stannous Chloride Reagent R1 Dissolve 4 g of *ninhydrin* in 100 ml of *2-methoxyethanol*, shake gently with 1 g of a cation exchange resin (hydrogen form) (Dowex 50 is suitable) and filter. Immediately before use, mix equal volumes of this solution and a 0.16% w/v solution of *tin(II) chloride* in *buffer solution pH 5.5.*

Ninhydrin Reagent I Transfer 10 litres of *2-methoxy-ethanol* to a clean, dry 20-litre bottle and purge with *oxygen-free nitrogen* for 2 to 3 minutes. Continue the nitrogen flow and add 10 g of *hydrindantin* and 100 g of *ninhydrin* and allow to dissolve; the solution will be straw coloured when dissolution is complete. Add 2 litres of a solution prepared by dissolving 5.444 kg of *sodium acetate* in 5 litres of *water*, adding 1 litre of *glacial acetic acid*, adjusting the pH to 5.5 with *glacial acetic acid* and adding sufficient *water* to produce 10 litres. Add 6.5 litres of *water* and 20 ml of a 20% w/v solution of *polyoxyethylene 23 lauryl ether.*

The deep red reagent is stable for at least 8 weeks when stored under nitrogen and protected from light; avoid exposure to ammonia.

Ninhydrin Solution A 0.2% w/v solution of *ninhydrin* in a mixture of 95 volumes of *butan-1-ol* and 5 volumes of 2M *acetic acid.*

Ninhydrin Solution R1 Dissolve 1.0 g of *ninhydrin* in 50 ml of *ethanol (96%)* and add 10 ml of *glacial acetic acid.*

Ninhydrin Solution R2 Dissolve 3 g of *ninhydrin* in 100 ml of a 4.55% w/v solution of *sodium metabisulphite.*

Ninhydrin Solution R3 A 0.4% w/v solution of *ninhydrin* in a mixture of 5 volumes of *anhydrous acetic acid* and 95 volumes of *butan-1-ol.*

Nitric Acid HNO_3 = 63.01 *(7697-37-2)*
A corrosive, fuming liquid, about 16M in strength; weight per ml, about 1.42 g.
When no molarity is indicated use analytical reagent grade of commerce containing about 70% w/w of HNO_3.
When solutions of molarity *x*M are required, they should be prepared by diluting 63*x* ml of *nitric acid* to 1000 ml with *water.*
Store protected from light.

Nitric Acid, Cadmium- and Lead-free *Nitric acid* that complies with the following tests.
CADMIUM Not more than 0.1 ppm when determined by *atomic absorption spectrophotometry*, Appendix II D, measuring the absorbance at 228.8 nm using a cadmium hollow-cathode lamp and an air—acetylene or air—propane flame. Use a solution prepared in the following manner. To 100 g add 0.1 g of *anhydrous sodium carbonate* and evaporate to dryness. Dissolve the residue in *water*, heating slightly, and dilute to 50 ml with *water.*
LEAD Not more than 0.1 ppm when determined by *atomic absorption spectrophotometry*, Appendix II D, measuring the absorbance at 283.3 nm or 217 nm using a lead hollow-cathode lamp, an air—acetylene flame and the solution prepared in the test for cadmium.

Nitric Acid, Dilute Dilute 20 g of *nitric acid* to 100 ml with *water.* Contains about 12.5% w/v of HNO_3 (about 2M).

Nitric Acid, Fuming HNO_3 = 63.01
Analytical reagent grade of commerce containing about 95% w/w of HNO_3 and about 22.5M in strength.
A corrosive, fuming, yellow liquid; d_{20}^{20}, about 1.5.

Nitric Acid, Lead-free *Nitric acid* that complies with the following test.
LEAD Not more than 0.1 ppm when determined by *atomic absorption spectrophotometry*, Appendix II D, measuring the absorbance at 283.3 nm or 217 nm using a lead hollow-cathode lamp and an air—acetylene flame. Use a solution prepared in the following manner. To 100 g add 0.1 g of *anhydrous sodium carbonate* and evaporate to dryness. Dissolve the residue in *water*, heating slightly, and dilute to 50 ml with *water.*

Nitrilotriacetic Acid $C_6H_9NO_6$ = 191.1 *(139-13-9)*
General reagent grade of commerce.
Melting point, about 246°, with decomposition.

Nitroaniline See *4-nitroaniline.*

4-Nitroaniline $C_6H_6N_2O_2$ = 138.1 *(100-01-6)*
Microanalytical reagent grade of commerce.
A deep yellow, crystalline powder; melting point, about 148°.

Nitroaniline Solution, Diazotised Dissolve 0.4 g of *4-nitroaniline* in 60 ml of 1M *hydrochloric acid* with the aid of heat, cool to 15° and add a 10% w/v solution of *sodium nitrite* until one drop of the mixture turns *starch iodide paper* blue.
Prepare immediately before use.

Nitrobenzaldehyde See *2-nitrobenzaldehyde.*

2-Nitrobenzaldehyde $C_7H_5NO_3$ = 151.1 *(552-89-6)*
General reagent grade of commerce.
Yellow needles with an almond-like odour; melting point, about 42°.

Nitrobenzaldehyde Paper Dissolve 0.2 g of *2-nitrobenzaldehyde* in 10 ml of 5M *sodium hydroxide*. This solution should be kept for 1 hour only. Immerse the lower half of a hard paper strip (10 cm × 8 to 10 mm) in the solution. Absorb the excess reagent between two sheets of filter paper.
Use within a few minutes of its preparation.

Nitrobenzaldehyde Solution Add 0.12 g of powdered *nitrobenzaldehyde* to 10 ml of 2M *sodium hydroxide*. Allow to stand for 10 minutes, shaking frequently, and filter.
Prepare immediately before use.

Nitrobenzene $C_6H_5NO_2$ = 123.1 (*98-95-3*)
Analytical reagent grade of commerce.
A pale yellow liquid with an almond-like odour; boiling point, about 211°.
Complies with the following test.
DINITROBENZENE To 0.1 ml add 5 ml of *acetone*, 5 ml of *water* and 5 ml of 10M *sodium hydroxide*, shake and allow to stand. The upper layer is almost colourless.

4-Nitrobenzoic Acid $C_7H_5NO_4$ = 167.1 (*62-23-7*)
General reagent grade of commerce.
Yellow crystals; melting point, about 240°.

Nitrobenzoyl Chloride $C_7H_4ClNO_3$ = 185.6 (*122-04-3*)
Analytical reagent grade of commerce.
Yellow crystals; odour, pungent; melting point, about 73°.

4-Nitrobenzyl Bromide $C_7H_6BrNO_2$ = 216.0 (*100-11-8*)
General reagent grade of commerce.
Pale yellow crystals with a lachrymatory vapour; melting point, about 99°.

Nitrobenzyl Chloride See *4-nitrobenzyl chloride*.

4-Nitrobenzyl Chloride Nitrobenzyl chloride; $C_7H_6ClNO_2$ = 171.6 (*100-14-1*)
General reagent grade of commerce.
Pale yellow crystals with a lachrymatory vapour; melting point, about 72°.

4-(4-Nitrobenzyl)pyridine $C_{12}H_{10}N_2O_2$ = 214.2 (*1083-48-3*)
General reagent grade of commerce.
A pale yellow, crystalline powder; melting point, about 70°.

Nitrochromic Reagent Dissolve 0.7 g of *potassium dichromate* in sufficient *nitric acid* to produce 100 ml.

Nitroethane $C_2H_5NO_2$ = 75.07 (*79-24-3*)
General reagent grade of commerce.
Weight per ml, about 1.045 g; boiling point, about 114°.

Nitrofurantoin $C_8H_6N_4O_5$ = 238.2 (*67-20-9*)
General reagent grade of commerce.

(5-Nitro-2-furyl)methylene Diacetate Nitrofurfural diacetate; 5-nitrofurfurylidene diacetate; $C_9H_9NO_7$ = 243.2 (*92-55-7*)
General reagent grade of commerce.
Yellow crystals; melting point, about 90°.

Nitrogen N_2 = 28.01 (*7727-37-9*)
Laboratory cylinder grade of commerce, washed with *water* and dried.

Nitrogen R1 *Nitrogen* containing not less than 99.999% v/v of N_2.
CARBON MONOXIDE Less than 1 ppm.
OXYGEN Less than 5 ppm.

Nitrogen for Chromatography *Nitrogen* containing not less than 99.95% v/v of N_2.

Nitrogen Monoxide Nitric oxide; NO = 30.01 (*10102-43-9*)
General reagent grade of commerce containing not less than 98.0% of NO.

Nitrogen, Oxygen-free *Nitrogen* that has been freed from oxygen by passage through *alkaline pyrogallol solution*.

Nitromethane CH_3NO_2 = 61.04 (*75-52-5*)
General reagent grade of commerce.
A colourless liquid; d_{20}^{20}, 1.132 to 1.134; n_D^{20}, 1.381 to 1.383; boiling point, about 102°.

Nitrosodipropylamine Dipropylnitrosamine; $C_6H_{14}N_2O$ = 130.2 (*621-64-7*)
General reagent grade of commerce suitable for chemiluminescence determination.
d_{20}^{20}, about 0.915; boiling point, about 78°.

Nitrosodipropylamine Solution Inject 78.62 g of *absolute ethanol* through the septum of the vial containing *nitrosodipropylamine*. Dilute 1 volume to 100 volumes with *absolute ethanol* and place 0.5-ml aliquots in crimp-sealed vials.
Store in the dark at 5°.

Nitrotetrazolium Blue Nitro blue tetrazolium; 3,3′-(3,3′-dimethoxybiphenyl-4,4′-diyl)bis[2-(4-nitrophenyl)-5-phenyl-2*H*-tetrazolium] dichloride; $C_{40}H_{30}Cl_2N_{10}O_6$ = 818 (*298-83-9*)
General reagent grade of commerce.
Melting point, about 189°, with decomposition.

Nitrous Oxide N_2O = 44.01 (*10024-97-2*)
General reagent grade of commerce containing not less than 99.99% v/v of N_2O and less than 1 ppm of each of nitrogen monoxide and carbon monoxide.

Nitro-vanado-molybdic Reagent
SOLUTION A Dissolve 10 g of *ammonium molybdate* in *water*, add 1 ml of 10M *ammonia* and dilute to 100 ml with *water*.
SOLUTION B Dissolve 2.5 g of *ammonium metavanadate* in hot *water*, add 14 ml of *nitric acid* and dilute to 500 ml with *water*.
To 96 ml of *nitric acid* add 100 ml of solution A and 100 ml of solution B and dilute to 500 ml with *water*.

Nonadecanoic Acid $C_{19}H_{38}O_2$ = 298.5 (*646-30-0*)
General reagent grade of commerce.
Melting point, about 69°.

Nonan-5-one Di-*n*-butyl ketone; $C_9H_{18}O$ = 142.2 (*502-56-7*)
General reagent grade of commerce.
Weight per ml, about 0.83 g; boiling point, about 188°.

Noradrenaline Acid Tartrate Noradrenaline bitartrate; $C_8H_{11}NO_3,C_4H_6O_6$ = 319.3 (*69815-49-2*)
General reagent grade of commerce.
A white, crystalline powder, melting point, about 102°.

Nordazepam 7-Chloro-2,3-dihydro-5-phenyl-1*H*-1,4-benzodiazepin-2-one; desmethyldiazepam; $C_{15}H_{11}ClN_2O$ = 270.7 (*340-57-8*)
General reagent grade of commerce.
Melting point, about 216°.

DL-Norleucine (*RS*)-2-Aminohexanoic acid; $C_6H_{13}NO_2$ = 131.2 (*616-06-8*)
General reagent grade of commerce.
Shiny crystals.

Noroxymorphone $C_{16}H_{17}NO_4$ = 287.3 (*33522-95-1*)
General reagent grade of commerce.

Norpseudoephedrine Hydrochloride $C_9H_{13}NO,HCl$ = 187.7 (*53643-20-2*)
General reagent grade of commerce.
A crystalline powder; melting point, 180° to 181°.

Noscapine Hydrochloride $C_{22}H_{23}NO_7,HCl,H_2O$ = 467.9 (*912-60-7*)
General reagent grade of commerce.

Octadecan-1-ol Stearyl alcohol; $C_{18}H_{38}O$ = 270.5 (*112-92-5*)
Purified general reagent grade of commerce.
White flakes or granules; melting point, about 58°.

Octadecyl 3-(3,5-Di-(1,1-dimethylethyl)-4-hydroxyphenyl)propionate $C_{35}H_{62}O_3$ = 530.9 (*2082-79-3*)
General reagent grade of commerce.
Melting point, 49° to 55°.

Octanoic Acid Caprylic acid; $C_8H_{16}O_2$ = 144.2 (*124-07-2*)
General reagent grade of commerce.
A colourless, oily liquid; boiling point, about 237°; weight per ml, about 0.92 g.

Octanol See *octan-1-ol*.

Octan-1-ol *n*-Octyl alcohol; Octanol; $C_8H_{18}O$ = 130.2
Purified general reagent grade of commerce.
A colourless liquid with a penetrating aromatic odour; d_{20}^{20}, about 0.828; boiling point, about 195°.

Octan-2-ol *sec*-Octyl alcohol; $C_8H_{18}O$ = 130.2 (*6169-06-8*)
General reagent grade of commerce.
An oily liquid; boiling point, about 178°; weight per ml, about 0.82 g.

Octoxinol 10 α-[4-(1,1,3,3-Tetramethylbutyl)phenyl]-ω-hydroxypoly(oxyethylene); $C_{34}H_{62}O_{11}$ (average) = 647 (*9002-93-1*)
General reagent grade of commerce (Triton X-100 is suitable).
A clear, pale yellow, viscous liquid.
Store in an airtight container.

Octylamine *n*-Octylamine; 1-amino-octane; $C_8H_{19}N$ =129.3 (*111-86-4*)
General reagent grade of commerce.

Oleamide (*Z*)-Octadec-9-enoamide; $C_{18}H_{35}NO$ = 281.5
General reagent grade of commerce.
Melting point, about 80°.

Olive Oil (*8001-25-0*) Of the British Pharmacopoeia.

Olive Oil Substrate Emulsion Homogenise 40 ml of *olive oil*, 330 ml of *acacia solution* and 30 ml of *water* in an 800-ml beaker placed in a vessel containing a mixture of ice and ethanol as cooling mixture. Emulsify using a mixer at an average speed of 1000 to 2000 revolutions per minute. Cool to 5° to 10°. Increase the mixing speed to 8000 revolutions per minute. Mix for 30 minutes keeping the temperature below 25° by the continuous addition of crushed ice into the cooling mixture (a mixture of calcium chloride and crushed ice is also suitable). Store this preparation (the stock emulsion) in a refrigerator and use within 14 days. The emulsion must not separate into two distinct layers. Check the diameter of the globules of the emulsion under a microscope. At least 90% have a diameter below 3 μm and none has a diameter greater than 10 μm. Shake the emulsion thoroughly before preparing the substrate emulsion.

For 10 determinations mix the following solutions in the order indicated: 100 ml of the stock emulsion, 80 ml of *tris— chloride buffer solution*, 20 ml of a freshly prepared 8% w/v solution of *sodium taurocholate EPBRP* and 95 ml of *water*. Use on the day of preparation.

Oracet Blue B Solvent blue 19
A mixture of 1-methylamino-4-anilinoanthraquinone ($C_{21}H_{16}N_2O_2$) and 1-amino-4-anilinoanthraquinone ($C_{20}H_{14}N_2O_2$). When used for titration in non-aqueous media, it changes from blue (basic) through purple (neutral) to pink (acidic).

Oracet Blue B Solution A 0.5% w/v solution of *oracet blue B* in *anhydrous acetic acid*.

Oracet Blue 2R 1-Amino-4-(phenylamino)anthracene-9,10-dione; CI 61110; $C_{20}H_{14}N_2O_2$ = 314.3 (*4395-65-7*)
General reagent grade of commerce.
Melting point, about 174°.

Orcinol 5-Methylbenzene-1,3-diol monohydrate; $C_7H_8O_2,H_2O$ = 142.2 (*6153-39-5*)
General reagent grade of commerce.
Melting point, 58° to 61°; boiling point, about 290°.
Orcinol is sensitive to light.

Orthophosphorous Acid Phosphorous acid; H_3PO_3 = 82.0 (*13598-36-2*)
General reagent grade of commerce.

Orthophosphoric Acid Phosphoric acid; H_3PO_4 = 98.00 (*7664-38-2*)
Analytical reagent grade of commerce containing not less than 84% w/w of H_3PO_4 and about 15.7M in strength.
A corrosive liquid; weight per ml, about 1.75 g.

Osmium Tetroxide Osmic acid; OsO_4 = 254.2 (*20816-12-0*)
General reagent grade of commerce.
Light yellow needles or a yellow, crystalline mass; melting point, about 40°.
Store in an airtight container.

Osmium Tetroxide Solution A 0.25% w/v solution of *osmium tetroxide* in 0.05M *sulphuric acid*.

Ox Brain, Acetone-dried Cut into small pieces a fresh ox brain previously freed from vascular and connective tissue. Place in *acetone* for preliminary dehydration. Complete the dehydration by pounding in a mortar 30 g of this material with successive 75-ml quantities of *acetone* until a dry powder remains after filtration. Finally dry at 37° for 2 hours until all traces of acetone are removed.

Oxalic Acid Ethanedioic acid dihydrate; $C_2H_2O_4,2H_2O$ = 126.1 (*6153-56-6*)
General reagent grade of commerce.

Oxalic Acid and Sulphuric Acid Solution A 5% w/v solution of *oxalic acid* in a cooled mixture of equal volumes of *sulphuric acid* and *water*.

Oxygen O_2 = 32.00 (*7782-44-7*)
General reagent grade of commerce containing not less than 99.99% v/v of oxygen.
NITROGEN AND ARGON Less than 100 ppm.
CARBON DIOXIDE Less than 10 ppm.
CARBON MONOXIDE Less than 5 ppm.

Palladium Chloride See *palladium(II) chloride*.

Palladium(II) Chloride Palladous chloride; $PdCl_2$ = 177.3 (*7647-10-1*)
General reagent grade of commerce containing not less

than 59% of Pd.
A hygroscopic, brownish red powder or red crystals; melting point, 678° to 680°.

Palladium Chloride Solution Dissolve 1 g of *palladium(II) chloride* in 10 ml of warm *hydrochloric acid*. Dilute the solution to 250 ml with a mixture of equal volumes of 2M *hydrochloric acid* and *water*. Dilute this solution immediately before use with 2 volumes of *water*.

Palmitic Acid Hexadecanoic acid; $C_{16}H_{32}O_2$ = 256.4 (*57-10-3*)
General reagent grade of commerce.
White, crystalline scales; melting point, about 63°.
Complies with the following test.
HOMOGENEITY Carry out test A for Identification described in the monograph for Chloramphenicol Palmitate applying to the plate 4 µl of a 0.2% w/v solution in *acetone*. The chromatogram shows only one principal spot.

Pancreas Powder Of the British Pharmacopoeia.

Papaverine Hydrochloride $C_{20}H_{21}NO_4,HCl$ = 375.9 (*61-25-6*)
General reagent grade of commerce.

Paracetamol 4′-Hydroxyacetanilide; 4-acetamidophenol; $C_8H_9NO_2$ = 151.2 (*103-90-2*)
General reagent grade of commerce.
Melting point, about 171°.

Paracetamol, 4-Aminophenol-free Paracetamol of the British Pharmacopoeia or *paracetamol* that has been recrystallised from *water* and dried at a pressure of 2 kPa at 70°. Repeat the procedure until it complies with the following test.
Dissolve 5 g of the dried material in sufficient *methanol (50%)* to produce 100 ml, add 1 ml of a freshly prepared solution containing 1% w/v of each of *sodium nitroprusside* and *anhydrous sodium carbonate,* mix and allow to stand for 30 minutes protected from light. No blue or green colour is produced.

Paraffin, Liquid (*8042-47-5*)
Use a spectroscopic grade of commerce, except for solubility tests for which a colourless grade weighing 0.83 to 0.89 g per ml may be used.

Paraffin, White Soft A semi-liquid mixture of hydrocarbons obtained from petroleum and bleached.

Pararosaniline Hydrochloride CI 42500; pararosaniline chloride; basic red 9; $C_{19}H_{18}ClN_3$ = 323.8 (*569-61-9*)
General reagent grade of commerce.
A bluish red, crystalline powder; melting point, about 270°, with decomposition.

Pararosaniline Solution, Decolorised To 0.1 g of *pararosaniline hydrochloride* add 60 ml of *water* and a solution of 1.0 g of *anhydrous sodium sulphite* or 2.0 g of *sodium sulphite* or 0.75 g of *sodium metabisulphite* in 10 ml of *water*. Add slowly, with stirring, 6 ml of 2M *hydrochloric acid*, stopper the flask and continue stirring until completely dissolved. Dilute to 100 ml with *water*. Allow to stand for 12 hours before use.
Store protected from light.

Penicillinase Solution Dissolve 10 g of casein hydrolysate, 2.72 g of *potassium dihydrogen orthophosphate* and 5.88 g of *sodium citrate* in 200 ml of *water*, adjust the pH to 7.2 with 5M *sodium hydroxide* and dilute to 1000 ml with *water*. Dissolve 0.41 g of *magnesium sulphate* in 5 ml of *water* and add 1 ml of a 0.16% w/v solution of *ammonium iron(II) sulphate* and sufficient *water* to produce 10 ml. Sterilise both solutions by *heating in an autoclave*, cool, mix, distribute in shallow layers in conical flasks and inoculate with *Bacillus cereus* (NCTC 9946). Incubate the flasks at 18° to 37° until growth is observed and then maintain at 35° to 37° for 16 hours, agitating constantly to ensure maximum aeration. Centrifuge and sterilise the supernatant fluid by filtration through a suitable membrane filter.

1.0 ml of Penicillinase Solution should hydrolyse benzylpenicillin to benzylpenicilloic acid at the rate of at least 500 mg per hour at 30° and pH 7, provided that the concentration of benzylpenicillin does not fall below the level necessary for enzyme saturation. The Michaelis constant for benzylpenicillin of the penicillinase in *penicillinase solution* is approximately 12 µg per ml.
STERILITY Complies with the *test for sterility*, Appendix XVI A.
Store at 0° to 2° and use within 2 or 3 days. When freeze dried and kept in sealed ampoules it may be stored for several months.

Pentaerythrityl Tetrakis[3-(3,5-di-*tert*-butyl-4-hydroxyphenyl)propionate] $C_{73}H_{108}O_{12}$ = 1178 (*6683-19-8*)
General reagent grade of commerce.
A white to slightly yellowish, crystalline powder; melting point, 110° to 125°; α-form, 120° to 125°; β-form, 110° to 115°.

Pentane See *n*-pentane.

***n*-Pentane** Pentane; C_5H_{10} = 72.15 (*109-66-0*)
General reagent grade of commerce.
A colourless, volatile liquid; boiling point, about 36°; d_{20}^{20}, about 0.63; n_D^{20}, about 1.359.
Pentane used in spectrophotometry complies with the following requirement.
TRANSMITTANCE Not less than 20% at 200 nm, 50% at 210 nm, 85% at 220 nm, 93% at 230 nm and 98% at 240 nm, Appendix II B, determined using *water* in the reference cell.

Pentanol See *pentan-1-ol.*

Pentan-1-ol *n*-Pentyl alcohol; Pentanol; $C_5H_{12}O$ = 88.15 (*71-41-0*)
General reagent grade of commerce.
A colourless liquid; boiling point, about 137°; n_D^{20}, about 1.410.

***tert*-Pentyl Alcohol** 2-Methylbutan-2-ol; *tert*-amyl alcohol; $C_5H_{12}O$ = 88.1 (*75-85-4*)
General reagent grade of commerce.
Not less than 95% distils between 100° and 104°; d_{20}^{20}, about 0.81.
Store protected from light.

Pepsin A substance containing a proteolytic enzyme of the gastric secretion of animals, diluted, if necessary, by admixture with Lactose or Sucrose. Use a grade of commerce capable of digesting 2500 times its own weight of coagulated egg albumen.

Pepsin Powder (*9001-75-6*) Of the British Pharmacopoeia.

Perchloric Acid $HClO_4$ = 100.5 (*7601-90-3*)
When no molarity is indicated, use analytical reagent grade of commerce containing not less than 70.0% and not more than 73.0% w/w of $HClO_4$ and about 12M in strength; a corrosive liquid; weight per ml, about 1.7 g.

For 9M perchloric acid use analytical reagent grade solution of commerce containing about 60% w/w of $HClO_4$; weight per ml, about 1.54 g.
Solutions of any other molarity *x*M should be prepared by diluting 82*x* ml of *perchloric acid* with *water* to 1000 ml.

Perchloric Acid Solution Dilute 8.5 ml of *perchloric acid* to 100 ml with *water* (about 0.1M).

Periodic Acetic Acid Solution Dissolve 0.446 g of *sodium periodate* in 2.5 ml of *sulphuric acid (25%)* and dilute to 100 ml with *glacial acetic acid.*

Periodic Acid H_5IO_6 = 227.9 *(10450-60-9)*
General reagent grade of commerce.
Melting point, about 122°.

Periodic Acid Reagent Dissolve 0.5 g of *sodium periodate* in 5 ml of *water*, add 1 ml of 2M *sulphuric acid* and dilute to 10 ml with *water*.
Prepare immediately before use.

Periodic Acid Solution General reagent grade of commerce containing about 50% w/v of $HIO_4,2H_2O$.

Peroxyacetic Acid Solution Dilute 1 ml of *hydrogen peroxide (100 volumes)* to 100 ml with *glacial acetic acid.* Mix and allow to stand for 12 hours before use.
Discard 24 hours after preparation.

Petroleum, Light See *petroleum spirit (boiling range, 50° to 70°).*

Petroleum R1, Light See *petroleum spirit (boiling range, 40° to 60°).*

Petroleum R2, Light See *petroleum spirit (boiling range, 30° to 40°).*

Petroleum R3, Light *Petroleum spirit* distilling between 40° and 80° .
d_{20}^{20}, 0.659 to 0.671.

Petroleum Spirit Petroleum ether; light petroleum
Analytical reagent grades of commerce.
Colourless, volatile, highly flammable liquids obtained from petroleum, consisting of a mixture of the lower members of the paraffin series of hydrocarbons supplied in the following fractions:
boiling range, 30° to 40°; weight per ml, about 0.63 g
boiling range, 40° to 60°; weight per ml, about 0.64 g
boiling range, 50° to 70°; weight per ml, about 0.66 g
boiling range, 60° to 80°; weight per ml, about 0.67 g
boiling range, 80° to 100°; weight per ml, about 0.70 g
boiling range, 100° to 120°; weight per ml, about 0.72 g
boiling range, 120° to 160°; weight per ml, about 0.75 g.

Petroleum Spirit (boiling range, 40° to 60°), Aromatic-free *Petroleum spirit (boiling range, 40° to 60°)* complying with the following additional test.
LIGHT ABSORPTION *Absorbance* against air at 235 nm, not more than 0.7, Appendix II B.

Phenacetin *p*-Ethoxyacetanilide; $C_{10}H_{13}NO_2$ = 179.2 *(62-44-2)*
General reagent grade of commerce.
Melting point, about 135°.

Phenanthrene $C_{14}H_{10}$ = 178.1 *(85-01-8)*
General reagent grade of commerce.
Melting point, about 100°.

Phenanthroline Hydrochloride $C_{12}H_8N_2,HCl,H_2O$ = 234.7 *(3829-86-5)*
General reagent grade of commerce.
A white or almost white powder; melting point, about 215°, with decomposition.

Phenazone 2,3-Dimethyl-1-phenyl-3-pyrazolin-5-one; $C_{11}H_{12}N_2O$ = 188.2 *(60-80-0)*
General reagent grade of commerce.
A colourless, crystalline powder; melting point, about 112°.

Phenol C_6H_6O = 94.11 *(108-95-2)*
Analytical reagent grade of commerce.
Caustic, deliquescent crystals with a characteristic odour; freezing point, not less than 40°; boiling point, about 180°.
Store protected from light in a cool place.

Phenol, Liquefied
General reagent grade of commerce.
A solution of phenol in water containing about 80% w/w of C_6H_6O.

Phenol Red 4,4′-(3*H*-2,1-Benzoxathiol-3-ylidene)-diphenol *S,S*-dioxide; phenolsulphonphthalein; $C_{19}H_{14}O_5S$ = 354.4 *(143-74-8)*
General reagent grade of commerce.
Produces a yellow colour in neutral and very faintly acidic solutions and a red colour in weakly alkaline solutions.

Phenol Red Solution Dissolve 0.1 g of *phenol red* in 2.82 ml of 0.1M *sodium hydroxide* and 20 ml of *ethanol (96%)* and add sufficient *water* to produce 100 ml.
Complies with the following test.
SENSITIVITY A mixture of 0.1 ml and 100 ml of *carbon dioxide-free water* is yellow. Not more than 0.1 ml of 0.02M *sodium hydroxide VS* is required to change the colour of the solution to reddish violet.
Colour change: pH 6.8 (yellow) to pH 8.4 (reddish violet).

Phenol Red Solution R1 Buffered phenol red solution
Dissolve 33 mg of *phenol red* in 1.5 ml of 2M *sodium hydroxide* and dilute to 100 ml with *water* (solution A). To 250 ml of 2M *sodium hydroxide* add 325 ml of 2M *acetic acid* and 575 ml of *water* (solution B). Mix 25 ml of solution A with 475 ml of solution B.

Phenol Red Solution R2
SOLUTION I Dissolve 33 mg of *phenol red* in 1.5 ml of 2M *sodium hydroxide* and dilute to 100 ml with *water*.
SOLUTION II Dissolve 25 mg of *ammonium sulphate* in 235 ml of *water*, add 105 ml of 2M *sodium hydroxide* and 135 ml of 2M *acetic acid.*
Add 25 ml of solution I to solution II. If necessary, adjust the pH of the mixture to 4.7.

Phenol Red Solution R3
SOLUTION I Dissolve 33 mg of *phenol red* in 1.5 ml of 2M *sodium hydroxide* and dilute to 50 ml with *water*.
SOLUTION II Dissolve 50 mg of *ammonium sulphate* in 235 ml of *water*; add 105 ml of 2M *sodium hydroxide* and 135 ml of 2M *acetic acid.*
Add 25 ml of solution I to solution II and adjust the pH of the mixture to 4.7, if necessary.

Phenoldisulphonic Acid Solution A clear liquid which may develop a pale brown colour on storage, prepared either by heating 3 g of *phenol* with 20 ml of *sulphuric acid* on a water bath for 6 hours and transferring the resulting liquid to a stoppered vessel, or by diluting a 25% w/v solution of commerce with *sulphuric acid* to contain 15% w/v of phenol. The solution complies with the following test.
SENSITIVITY TO NITRATE Evaporate a solution containing

0.1 mg of *potassium nitrate* to dryness in a porcelain dish on a water bath. To the cooled residue add 1 ml of the reagent and allow to stand for 10 minutes. Add 10 ml of *water*, cool, add 10 ml of 5M *ammonia* and dilute to 25 ml with *water*. A distinct yellow colour is produced when compared with a solution prepared in the same manner but omitting the potassium nitrate.

Phenolphthalein 3,3-Bis(4-hydroxyphenyl)phthalide; $C_{20}H_{14}O_4$ = 318.3 (*77-09-8*)
General reagent grade of commerce.

Phenolphthalein Solution Dissolve 0.1 g of *phenolphthalein* in 80 ml of *ethanol (96%)* and add sufficient *water* to produce 100 ml.
Complies with the following test.
SENSITIVITY A mixture of 0.1 ml of the reagent and 100 ml of *carbon dioxide-free water* is colourless. Not more than 0.2 ml of 0.02M *sodium hydroxide VS* is required to change the colour of the solution to pink.
Colour change: pH 8.2 (colourless) to pH 10.0 (red).

Phenolphthalein Solution R1 A 1.0% w/v solution of *phenolphthalein* in *ethanol (96%)*.

Phenolphthalein—Thymol Blue Solution Dissolve 0.1 g of *thymol blue* in a mixture of 2.2 ml of 0.1M *sodium hydroxide* and 50 ml of *ethanol (96%)* and dilute to 100 ml with *water*. Mix 3 volumes of this solution with 2 volumes of *phenolphthalein solution*.

Phenoxyacetic Acid 2-Phenoxyethanoic acid; $C_8H_8O_3$ = 152.1 (*122-59-8*)
General reagent grade of commerce.
White or almost white crystals; melting point, about 98°.
Complies with the following test.
HOMOGENEITY Examine under the conditions and at the concentration prescribed in the test for Phenoxyacetic acid described in the monograph for Phenoxymethylpenicillin applying to the plate 10 µl of a 0.010% w/v solution in *methanol (50%)*. The chromatogram shows only one principal spot.

Phenoxybenzamine Hydrochloride *N*-(2-Chloroethyl)-*N*-(1-methyl-2-phenoxyethyl)benzylamine hydrochloride; $C_{18}H_{23}Cl_2NO$ = 340.3 (*63-92-3*)
General reagent grade of commerce.
Melting point, about 138°.

Phenoxyethanol See *2-phenoxyethanol*.

2-Phenoxyethanol Phenoxyethanol; $C_8H_{10}O_2$ = 138.2 (*122-99-6*)
General reagent grade of commerce.
A colourless, oily liquid; d_{20}^{20}, about 1.11; n_D^{20}, about 1.537; freezing point, not less than 12°.

Phenyl Benzoate $C_{13}H_{10}O_2$ = 198.2 (*93-99-2*)
General reagent grade of commerce.
Melting point, about 70°.

Phenylalanine See *L-phenylalanine*.

L-Phenylalanine $C_9H_{11}NO_2$ = 165.2 (*63-91-2*)
General reagent grade of commerce.
A white, crystalline powder; melting point, about 272°, with decomposition; $[\alpha]_D^{20}$, about −34° (2% w/v in water).
Complies with the following test.
HOMOGENEITY Carry out the method for *thin-layer chromatography*, Appendix III A, protected from light, using *silica gel G* as the coating substance and a mixture of 25 parts of *water* and 75 parts of *phenol* as the mobile phase, but allowing the solvent front to ascend 12 cm above the line of application. Apply to the plate 5 µl of a 0.2% w/v solution and keep the plate in the vapour of the mobile phase for 12 hours before development. After removal of the plate, dry it, spray with a 0.1% w/v solution of *ninhydrin* in *butan-1-ol* saturated with *water* and heat at 100° to 105° for 10 minutes. The chromatogram shows only one principal spot.

(*E*)-4-Phenylbut-3-en-2-one Benzalacetone; $C_{10}H_{10}O$ = 146.2 (*1896-62-4*)
General reagent grade of commerce.
Melting point, about 41°.

***N*-Phenylcarbazole** $C_{18}H_{13}N$ = 243.3 (*1150-62-5*)
General reagent grade of commerce.
A white to pale tan, crystalline powder; melting point, about 96°.

***p*-Phenylenediamine Dihydrochloride** 1,4-Diaminobenzene dihydrochloride; $C_6H_8N_2$,2HCl = 181.1 (*615-28-1*)
General reagent grade of commerce.
A white to pale tan, crystalline powder, turning pink on exposure to air.

α-Phenylglycine See *DL-phenylglycine*.

DL-Phenylglycine 2-Amino-2-phenylacetic acid; $C_8H_9NO_2$ = 151.2 (*2835-06-5*)
General reagent grade of commerce.
A white, crystalline solid; melting point, about 290°, with sublimation.

Phenylhydrazine $C_6H_8N_2$ = 108.1 (*100-63-0*)
General reagent grade of commerce.
A colourless or yellowish liquid turning yellow or dark red on exposure to light and air; freezing point, not less than 18°.
Store protected from light and distil under reduced pressure before use.

Phenylhydrazine Hydrochloride Phenylhydrazinium chloride; $C_6H_8N_2$,HCl = 144.6 (*59-88-1*)
Analytical reagent grade of commerce.
A white or almost white, crystalline powder, becoming brown on exposure to air; melting point, about 245°, with decomposition.
Store protected from light.

Phenylhydrazine Hydrochloride Solution Strong phenylhydrazine hydrochloride solution
Dissolve 0.9 g of *phenylhydrazine hydrochloride* in 50 ml of *water*. Decolorise with *activated charcoal* and filter. To the filtrate add 30 ml of *hydrochloric acid* and dilute to 250 ml with *water*.

Phenylhydrazine—Sulphuric Acid Solution
Dissolve 65 mg of *phenylhydrazine hydrochloride*, previously recrystallised from *ethanol (85%)*, in sufficient of a mixture of 170 volumes of *sulphuric acid* and 80 volumes of *water* to produce 100 ml.
Prepare immediately before use.

Phloroglucinol Benzene-1,3,5-triol; $C_6H_6O_3,2H_2O$ = 162.1 (*6099-90-7*)
Analytical reagent grade of commerce.
White or pale cream crystals; melting point, about 223°, Appendix V A, Method V.

Phloroglucinol Solution To 1 ml of a 10% w/v solution of *phloroglucinol* in *ethanol (96%)* add 9 ml of *hydrochloric acid*.
Store protected from light.

Phospholipid Wash a quantity of human or bovine brain freed from meninges and blood vessels and macerate in a suitable blender. Weigh 1000 to 1300 g of the macerate and measure its volume (V ml). Extract with three quantities, each of $4V$ ml, of *acetone*, filter by suction and dry the precipitate at 37° for 18 hours. Extract the dried precipitate with two quantities, each of $2V$ ml, of a mixture of 2 volumes of *petroleum spirit (boiling range, 30° to 40°)* and 3 volumes of *petroleum spirit (boiling range, 40° to 60°)*, filtering each extract through a filter paper previously washed with the petroleum spirit mixture. Combine the extracts and evaporate to dryness at 45° at a pressure not exceeding 0.7 kPa. Dissolve the residue in $0.2V$ ml of *ether* and allow to stand at 4° until a deposit is produced. Centrifuge and evaporate the clear supernatant liquid under reduced pressure until the volume is about 100 ml per kg of the original macerate. Allow to stand at 4° until a precipitate is produced (12 to 24 hours) and centrifuge. To the clear supernatant liquid add 5 volumes of *acetone*, centrifuge, discard the supernatant liquid, dry the precipitate and store protected from light in a vacuum desiccator.

Phosphomolybdic Acid Dodecamolybdophosphoric acid; approximately $H_3PO_4,12MoO_3,24H_2O$ = 2258 *(51429-74-4)*
Analytical reagent grade of commerce.
Fine, orange-yellow crystals.

Phosphomolybdic Acid Solution To 40 ml of a 10% w/v solution of *phosphomolybdic acid* add, cautiously and with cooling, 60 ml of *sulphuric acid*.
Prepare immediately before use.

Phosphomolybdotungstic Reagent Folin Ciocalteau phenol reagent of commerce.
Dissolve 100 g of *sodium tungstate* and 25 g of *sodium molybdate* in 700 ml of *water*, add 100 ml of *hydrochloric acid* and 50 ml of *orthophosphoric acid* and heat the mixture under a reflux condenser for 10 hours. Add 150 g of *lithium sulphate*, 50 ml of *water* and 0.2 ml of *bromine* and boil to remove excess bromine (about 15 minutes), cool, dilute to 1000 ml with *water* and filter. The reagent should be yellow in colour. If it acquires a greenish tint, it is unsatisfactory for use but may be regenerated by boiling with 0.2 ml of *bromine*. Care must be taken to remove excess bromine by boiling.
Store at 2° to 8°.

Phosphomolybdotungstic Reagent, Dilute Dilute 1 volume of *phosphomolybdotungstic reagent* with 2 volumes of *water*.

Phosphoric Acid See *orthophosphoric acid*.

Phosphoric Acid, Dilute Use 2M *orthophosphoric acid*.

Phosphorus Pentoxide Diphosphorus pentoxide; P_2O_5 = 142.0 *(1314-56-3)*
Use a grade specially supplied for use in desiccators.
A white, amorphous, deliquescent powder hydrated by water with the evolution of heat.
Store in an airtight container.

Phosphotungstic Acid Solution Dissolve 10 g of *sodium tungstate* in 75 ml of *water* and add 8 ml of *orthophosphoric acid*. Heat under a reflux condenser for 3 hours, allow to cool, filter and add sufficient *water* to produce 100 ml.

Phthalaldehyde $C_8H_6O_2$ = 134.1 *(643-79-8)*
General reagent grade of commerce.
Melting point, about 55°.
Store protected from light and air.

Phthalaldehyde Reagent Dissolve 2.47 g of *boric acid* in 75 ml of *water*, adjust the pH to 10.4 with a 45% w/v solution of *potassium hydroxide* and add sufficient *water* to produce 100 ml. Dissolve 1.0 g of *phthalaldehyde* in 5 ml of *methanol*, add 95 ml of the boric acid solution and 2 ml of *mercaptoacetic acid* and adjust the pH to 10.4 with the potassium hydroxide solution.
Store protected from light and use within 3 days of preparation.

Phthalazine $C_8H_6N_2$ = 130.1 *(253-52-1)*
General reagent grade of commerce.
Melting point, 89° to 92°.

Phthalein Purple Metalphthalein; $C_{32}H_{32}N_2O_{12}$ +aq *(2411-89-4)*
Indicator grade of commerce.
A creamy white to brown powder complying with the following test.
SENSITIVITY Dissolve 10 mg in 1 ml of 13.5M *ammonia* and dilute to 100 ml with *water*. To 5 ml of the solution add 95 ml of *water*, 4 ml of 13.5M *ammonia*, 50 ml of *ethanol (96%)* and 0.1 ml of 0.1M *barium chloride VS*; the solution is bluish violet. Add 0.15 ml of 0.1M *disodium edetate VS*; the solution becomes colourless.

Phthalic Acid Benzene-1,2-dicarboxylic acid; $C_8H_6O_4$ = 166.1 *(88-99-3)*
General reagent grade of commerce.
A white, crystalline powder.

Phthalic Anhydride Isobenzofuran-1,3-dione; $C_8H_4O_3$ = 148.1 *(85-44-9)*
General reagent grade of commerce containing not less than 99.0% of $C_8H_4O_3$.
Melting point, 130° to 132°.

Phthalic Anhydride Solution Dissolve 42 g of *phthalic anhydride* in 300 ml of *anhydrous pyridine*. Allow to stand for 16 hours.
Store protected from light and use within 1 week.

Picric Acid 2,4,6-Trinitrophenol; $C_6H_3N_3O_7$ = 229.1 *(88-89-1)*
Analytical reagent grade of commerce.
Yellow prisms or plates moistened with an equal weight of water for safety; explodes when heated rapidly or subjected to percussion.
Store moistened with *water*.

Picric Acid Solution A 1% w/v solution of *picric acid*.

Picric Acid Solution R1 Add 0.25 ml of 10M *sodium hydroxide* to 100 ml of a saturated solution of *picric acid* in *water*.

Picrolonic Acid 3-Methyl-4-nitro-1-(4-nitrophenyl)-5-pyrazolone; $C_{10}H_8N_4O_5$ = 264.2 *(550-74-3)*
General reagent grade of commerce.
A yellow or brownish yellow, crystalline powder; melting point, about 116°.
Complies with the following test.
SENSITIVITY Dissolve 25 mg in 10 ml of warm *water* containing 0.1 ml of *glacial acetic acid*; to 1 ml of this solution add 1 ml of a 0.05% w/v solution of *calcium chloride* previously heated to 60°. A bulky precipitate is produced within 5 minutes.

β-Pinene 6,6-Dimethyl-2-methylenebicyclo[3.1.1]-heptane; $C_{10}H_{16}$ = 136.2 *(19902-08-0)*
General reagent grade of commerce.
d_{20}^{20}, about 0.867; n_D^{20}, about 1.474; boiling point, 155° to 156°.
β-Pinene used in gas chromatography complies with the following requirement.

ASSAY Examine by gas chromatography as described in the monograph for Bitter-orange-flower Oil using the reagent being examined as the test solution. The area of the principal peak is not less than 99.0% of the total area of the peaks.

Piperazine Dipicrate Solution Dissolve 0.2 g of *piperazine hydrate* in 3.5 ml of 0.5M *sulphuric acid* and 10 ml of *water*. Add 100 ml of *picric acid solution R1*, heat on a water bath for 15 minutes, cool and filter. Wash the precipitate with *water* until the washings are free from sulphate. Shake the precipitate with *water* to produce a saturated solution and filter.

Piperazine Hydrate $C_4H_{10}N_2,6H_2O$ = 194.2 (*142-63-2*)
General reagent grade of commerce.
Colourless, glossy, deliquescent crystals; melting point, about 44°.

Piperidine Hexahydropyridine; $C_5H_{11}N$ = 85.2 (*110-89-4*)
General reagent grade of commerce.
Boiling point, about 106°.

Plasma, Citrated Rabbit Collect blood by intracardiac puncture from a rabbit that has been fasted for 12 hours prior to the collection, using a plastic syringe with a No. 1 needle containing a suitable volume of a 3.8% w/v solution of *sodium citrate* so that the final volume ratio of citrate solution to blood is 1:9. Separate the plasma by centrifugation at 1500 to 1800 *g* at 15° to 20° for 30 minutes.
Store at 0° to 6° and use within 4 hours of collection.

Plasma, Platelet-poor Withdraw 45 ml of human blood into a 50 ml plastic syringe containing 5 ml of a sterile 3.8% w/v solution of *sodium citrate*. Immediately centrifuge the citrated whole blood at 1150 *g* for 30 minutes at 4°. Remove the upper two thirds of the supernatant plasma using a plastic syringe and immediately centrifuge at 3500 *g* for 30 minutes at 4°. Remove the upper two thirds of the liquid and freeze it rapidly in suitable quantities in plastic tubes at a temperature of –40° or below. Use plastic or siliconised equipment throughout.

Plasma Substrate Substrate plasma
Separate the plasma from 9 volumes of human or bovine blood collected in 1 volume of a 3.8% w/v solution of *sodium citrate* or from 3.5 volumes of human or bovine blood collected in 1 volume of a solution containing 2% w/v of *disodium hydrogen citrate* and 2.5% w/v of *D-glucose*. In the former case, prepare the substrate plasma on the day of collection of the blood. In the latter case, the substrate plasma may be prepared up to 2 days after collection of the blood.
Store at –20°.

Plasma Substrate Deficient in Factor V Preferably use congenitally deficient plasma or, alternatively, prepare in the following manner. Separate the plasma from human blood collected in 0.1 of its volume of a 1.34% w/v solution of *sodium oxalate* and incubate at 37° for 24 to 36 hours. This plasma should have a clotting time, when tested by the assay method given under *coagulation factor V solution*, of 70 to 100 seconds; if the clotting time is less than 70 seconds, incubate the plasma for a further 12 to 24 hours.
Store, in small amounts, at –20° or below.

Plasma Substrate R1 Substrate plasma R1
Use water-repellent equipment (made from materials such as suitable plastics or suitably siliconised glass) for taking and handling the blood. Collect a suitable volume of blood from each of an appropriate number of sheep. (A volume of 285 ml of blood added to 15 ml of anticoagulant solution is considered suitable; smaller volumes may be collected. Whatever volume is collected it is considered advisable to use at least 5 sheep.) Take the blood, either from a live animal or immediately after slaughter, using a needle attached to a suitable cannula which is long enough to reach the bottom of the collecting vessel. Discarding the first few millilitres and collecting only free-flowing blood, collect the blood into sufficient of an anticoagulant solution containing 8.7 g of *sodium citrate* and 4 mg of *aprotinin* in 100 ml of *water* to give a final ratio of blood to anticoagulant solution of 19:1. During and immediately after collection swirl the flask gently to ensure mixing, but do not allow frothing to occur. When collection is complete, close the flask, cool to 10° to 15° and then pool the contents of all the flasks with the exception of any that show obvious haemolysis or clots and keep the pooled blood at 10° to 15°.

As soon as possible and, in any case, within 4 hours of collection, centrifuge the pooled blood at 1000 to 2000 *g* at 10° to 15° for 30 minutes. Separate the resulting supernatant liquid and centifuge it at 5000 *g* for 30 minutes. (More powerful centrifugation, for example at 20,000 *g* for 30 minutes, may be used if necessary to clarify the plasma at this stage but filtration procedures should not be used.) Separate the resulting supernatant liquid and, without delay, mix thoroughly and distribute the resulting substrate plasma into small stoppered containers in portions sufficient for a complete heparin assay (for example, 10 to 30 ml). Without delay, freeze rapidly at a temperature below –70° (for example, by plunging the containers into liquid nitrogen) and store at a temperature below –30°.

The prepared plasma is considered suitable for use as substrate plasma in the assay for heparin if, under the conditions of the assay, it gives a clotting time appropriate to the method of detection used and if it provides reproducible, steep log dose—response curves. When required, thaw a portion of substrate plasma in a water bath at 37°, gently swirling until thawing is complete; once thawed it should be kept at 10° to 20° and used without delay. The thawed substrate plasma may be lightly centrifuged if necessary; filtration procedures should not be used.

Plasma Substrate R2 Prepare from human blood containing less than 1% of the normal amount of factor IX. Collect 9 volumes of the blood into 1 volume of a 3.8% w/v solution of *sodium citrate*. Store in small amounts in plastic tubes at a temperature of –30° or below.

Plasminogen, Human *(9001-91-6)*
A substance present in blood which may be activated to plasmin, an enzyme that lyses fibrin in blood clots.

Platelet Substitute To 0.5 to 1 g of *phospholipid* add 20 ml of *acetone* and allow to stand for 2 hours with frequent shaking. Centrifuge for 2 minutes and discard the supernatant liquid. Dry the residue using a water pump, mix with 20 ml of *chloroform* and shake for 2 hours. Filter under vacuum and suspend the residue obtained in 5 to 10 ml of *saline solution*.

Prepare a dilution in *saline solution* so that it will give clotting time differences between consecutive dilutions of the reference preparation used in the Assay of factor IX fraction of about 10 seconds.

Store the dilute suspensions at –30° and use within 6 weeks.

Poloxamer 124
General reagent grade of commerce.

Poly[(cyanopropyl)methylphenylmethylsiloxane]
Gas chromatographic reagent grade of commerce with an average molecular weight of 8000 containing 25% of cyanopropyl groups, 25% of phenyl groups and 50% of methyl groups.

Poly(cyanopropyl)(phenylmethyl)siloxane
Gas chromatographic reagent grade of commerce containing 90% cyanopropyl and 10% phenylmethyl groups.

Poly(cyanopropyl)(7)(phenyl)(7)methyl)(86)siloxane
Gas chromatographic reagent grade of commerce.
Polysiloxane substituted with 7% of cyanopropyl groups, 7% of phenyl groups and 86% of dimethyl groups.

Poly(cyanopropyl)siloxane Polysiloxane substituted with 100% of cyanopropyl groups.
Gas chromatographic grade of commerce.

Poly(dimethyl)(diphenyl)(divinyl)siloxane
Chromatographic reagent grade of commerce containing 94% of methyl groups, 5% of phenyl groups and 1% of vinyl groups.

Poly(dimethyl)(diphenyl)siloxane
Chromatographic reagent grade of commerce containing 95% of methyl groups and 5% of phenyl groups.

Poly(dimethyl)siloxane Silicone gum rubber (methyl)
Gas chromatographic reagent grade of commerce.
Organosilicon polymer with the appearance of a semi-liquid, colourless gum. The *infrared absorption spectrum*, Appendix II A, obtained by applying the reagent, if necessary dispersed in a few drops of *carbon tetrachloride*, to a sodium chloride plate does not show absorption at 3053 cm^{-1}, corresponding to vinyl groups.

Polyether Hydroxylated Gel for Chromatography
Chromatographic reagent grade of commerce.
Gel with a small particle size having a hydrophilic surface with hydroxyl groups. It has an exclusion limit for dextran of molecular weight 2×10^5 to 2.5×10^6.

Polyethylene Glycol 200 Macrogol 200 *(25322-68-3)*
General reagent grade of commerce.
A viscous liquid; d_{20}^{20}, about 1.127; n_D^{20}, about 1.450.

Polyethylene Glycol 200 R1 Macrogol 200 R1
Place 500 ml of *polyethylene glycol 200* in a 1000-ml round-bottomed flask. Using a rotary evaporator remove any volatile components by applying a temperature of 60° and a pressure of 1.5 to 2.5 kPa for 6 hours.

Polyethylene Glycol 300 Macrogol 300 *(25322-68-3)*
General reagent grade of commerce.
A viscous liquid; weight per ml, about 1.13 g; n_D^{20}, about 1.465; viscosity at 25°, about 80 mPa s, Appendix V H, Method II.

Polyethylene Glycol 400 Macrogol 400 *(25322-68-3)*
General reagent grade of commerce.
A viscous liquid; weight per ml, about 1.13 g; freezing point, about 6°; viscosity, about 130 mPa s, Appendix V H, Method II.

Polyethylene Glycol 1000 Macrogol 1000 *(25322-68-3)*
General reagent grade of commerce.
A white, waxy mass; freezing point, about 35°; viscosity, about 25 mPa s for a 50% w/w solution, Appendix V H, Method II.

Polyethylene Glycol 1500 Macrogol 1500 *(25322-68-3)*
General reagent grade of commerce.
A white, waxy mass; freezing point, 43° to 48°; viscosity, about 70 mPa s for a 50% w/w solution, Appendix V H, Method II.

Polyethylene Glycol 20,000 Macrogol 20,000
Chromatographic reagent grade of commerce.
A hard, white, waxy solid; soluble in water with gel formation.

Polyethylene Glycol 20,000 2-Nitroterephthalate
General reagent grade of commerce.
A white or almost white, hard, waxy solid.

Polyethylene Glycol Adipate Macrogol adipate
Gas chromatographic reagent grade of commerce.
A white, waxy mass; melting point, about 43°.

Polyethylene Glycol Succinate Macrogol succinate
Gas chromatographic reagent grade of commerce.
A white, crystalline powder; melting point, about 102°.

Polymethylphenylsiloxane Average molecular weight, 4000.
Chromatographic grade of commerce containing about 50% of methyl groups and 50% of phenyl groups.
A very viscous liquid (about 1300 mPa s); weight per ml, about 1.09 g.

Poly[methyl(95)phenyl(5)]siloxane Polysiloxane containing 95% of methyl groups and 5% of phenyl groups.
Chromatographic reagent grade of commerce.

Poly[methyl(94)phenyl(5)vinyl(1)]siloxane Polysiloxane containing 94% of methyl groups, 5% of phenyl groups and 1% of vinyl groups.
Chromatographic reagent grade of commerce.

Polyoxyethylated Castor Oil
General reagent grade of commerce.
A light yellow liquid which becomes clear above 26°.

Polyoxyethylene 23 Lauryl Ether Brij 35; $C_{58}H_{120}O_{24}$ = 1199.6 *(9002-92-0)*
General reagent grade of commerce.
Melting point, about 43°; boiling point, about 100°.

Polysorbate 20 Polyoxyethylene(20) sorbitan monolaurate *(9005-64-5)*
General reagent grade of commerce (Tween 20 is suitable).
A yellow or brownish yellow, oily liquid; weight per ml, about 1.073 to 1.078 g.

Polysorbate 80 Polyoxyethylene(20) sorbitan monooleate *(9005-65-6)*
General reagent grade of commerce (Tween 80 is suitable).
A yellow to amber coloured, oily liquid; weight per ml, about 1.10 g.

Polystyrene 900-1000 *(9003-53-6)*
Organic standard used for calibration in gas chromatography.
Molecular weight, about 950.

Potassium Acetate $C_2H_3O_2K$ = 98.14 *(127-08-2)*
General reagent grade of commerce.

Potassium Antimonate(v) Potassium pyroantimonate; $KSbO_3,3H_2O$ = 262.9 *(12208-13-8)*
Analytical reagent grade of commerce.

Potassium Antimonate(v) Solution Potassium pyro-

antimonate solution
Dissolve 2 g of *potassium antimonate(v)* in 95 ml of hot *water*, cool rapidly and add a solution containing 2.5 g of *potassium hydroxide* in 50 ml of *water* and 1 ml of 2M *sodium hydroxide*. Allow to stand for 24 hours, filter and dilute to 150 ml with *water*.

Potassium Bicarbonate See *potassium hydrogen carbonate*.

Potassium Bicarbonate Solution, Saturated Methanolic See *saturated methanolic potassium hydrogen carbonate solution*.

Potassium Borohydride Potassium tetrahydroborate; KBH_4 = 53.94 (*13762-51-1*)
General reagent grade of commerce.

Potassium Bromate $KBrO_3$ = 167.0 (*7758-01-2*)
Analytical reagent grade of commerce.
White, granular powder or crystals.

Potassium Bromide KBr = 119.0 (*7758-02-3*)
Analytical reagent grade of commerce.
Potassium bromide used for infrared absorption spectrophotometry complies with the following requirement.
The *infrared absorption spectrum*, Appendix II A, of a disc 2 mm thick prepared from material previously dried at 250° for 1 hour has a substantially flat baseline over the range 4000 to 620 cm^{-1}; it exhibits no maxima with an absorbance greater than 0.02 above the baseline with the exception of maxima due to water at 3440 and 1630 cm^{-1}.

Potassium Carbonate Anhydrous potassium carbonate; K_2CO_3 = 138.2 (*584-08-7*)
Analytical reagent grade of commerce.
A white, granular, hygroscopic powder.
Store in an airtight container.

Potassium Carbonate Sesquihydrate $K_2CO_3,1\frac{1}{2}H_2O$ = 165.2 (*6381-79-9*)
General reagent grade of commerce.

Potassium Chlorate $KClO_3$ = 122.6 (*3811-04-9*)
Analytical reagent grade of commerce.
A white powder, granules or crystals.

Potassium Chloride KCl = 74.55 (*7447-40-7*)
Analytical reagent grade of commerce.
Potassium chloride used for infrared absorption spectrophotometry complies with the following requirement.
The *infrared absorption spectrum*, Appendix II A, of a disc 2 mm thick prepared from material previously dried at 250° for 1 hour has a substantially flat baseline over the range 4000 to 620 cm^{-1}; it exhibits no maxima with an absorbance greater than 0.02 above the baseline with the exception of maxima due to water at 3440 and 1630 cm^{-1}.

Potassium Chloride, 0.1M A solution of *potassium chloride* containing 7.46 g of KCl in 1000 ml.

Potassium Chromate K_2CrO_4 = 194.2 (*7789-00-6*)
Analytical reagent grade of commerce.
Yellow crystals.

Potassium Chromate Solution A 5% w/v solution of *potassium chromate*.
Produces a red precipitate with silver nitrate in neutral solutions.

Potassium Citrate Tripotassium citrate; $C_6H_5K_3O_7,H_2O$ = 324.4 (*6100-05-6*)
General reagent grade of commerce.

Potassium Cyanide KCN = 65.12 (*151-50-8*)
Analytical reagent grade of commerce.
A white, crystalline powder or white mass or crystals.

Potassium Cyanide Solution A 10% w/v solution of *potassium cyanide*.

Potassium Cyanide Solution PbT Dissolve 10 g of *potassium cyanide* in 90 ml of *water*, add 2 ml of *hydrogen peroxide solution (20 vol)*, allow to stand for 24 hours, dilute to 100 ml with *water* and filter.

Potassium Dichromate Dipotassium dichromate $K_2Cr_2O_7$ = 294.2 (*7778-50-9*)
Analytical reagent grade of commerce.
Potassium dichromate used for the calibration of spectrophotometers contains not less than 99.9% of $K_2Cr_2O_7$, calculated with reference to the substance dried at 130°.
ASSAY Dissolve 1 g in sufficient *water* to produce 250 ml. Add 50 ml of this solution to a freshly prepared solution of 4 g of *potassium iodide*, 2 g of *sodium hydrogen carbonate* and 6 ml of *hydrochloric acid* in 100 ml of *water* in a 500-ml flask. Stopper the flask and allow to stand protected from light for 5 minutes. Titrate with 0.1M *sodium thiosulphate VS* using 1 ml of *iodide-free starch solution* as indicator. Each ml of 0.1M *sodium thiosulphate VS* is equivalent to 4.903 mg of $K_2Cr_2O_7$.

Potassium Dichromate Solution A 10.6% w/v solution of *potassium dichromate*.

Potassium Dichromate Solution, Dilute A 7.0% w/v solution of *potassium dichromate*.

Potassium Dichromate Solution R1 A 0.5% w/v solution of *potassium dichromate*.

Potassium Dihydrogen Citrate $C_6H_7KO_7$ = 230.2
General reagent grade of commerce.

Potassium Dihydrogen Orthophosphate Potassium dihydrogen phosphate; KH_2PO_4 = 136.1 (*7778-77-0*)
Analytical reagent grade of commerce.
Colourless crystals.

Potassium Dihydrogen Phosphate See *potassium dihydrogen orthophosphate*.

Potassium Dihydrogen Phosphate, 0.2M A solution of *potassium dihydrogen orthophosphate* containing 27.22 g per litre of KH_2PO_4.

Potassium Ferricyanide See *potassium hexacyanoferrate(III)*.

Potassium Ferricyanide Solution See *potassium hexacyanoferrate(III) solution*.

Potassium Ferriperiodate Solution Dissolve 1 g of *potassium periodate* in 5 ml of a freshly prepared 12% w/v solution of *potassium hydroxide*, add 20 ml of *water* and 1.5 ml of *iron(III) chloride solution R1* and add sufficient of a freshly prepared 12% w/v solution of *potassium hydroxide* to produce 50 ml.

Potassium Ferrocyanide See *potassium hexacyanoferrate(II)*.

Potassium Ferrocyanide Solution See *potassium hexacyanoferrate(II) solution*.

Potassium Hexacyanoferrate(II) Potassium ferrocyanide; $K_4Fe(CN)_6,3H_2O$ = 422.4 (*14459-95-1*)
Analytical reagent grade of commerce.
Transparent, yellow crystals.

Potassium Hexacyanoferrate(III) Potassium ferricyanide; $K_3Fe(CN)_6$ = 329.3 (*13746-66-2*)
Analytical reagent grade of commerce.
Red crystals.

Potassium Hexacyanoferrate(II) Solution A 5.3% w/v solution of *potassium hexacyanoferrate(II)*.

Potassium Hexacyanoferrate(III) Solution Wash 5 g of *potassium hexacyanoferrate(III)* crystals with a little *water* and dissolve in sufficient *water* to produce 100 ml.
Prepare immediately before use.

Potassium Hexacyanoferrate(III) Solution, Dilute Wash about 1 g of *potassium hexacyanoferrate(III)* crystals with a little *water* and dissolve the washed crystals in 100 ml of *water*.
Produces a blue colour with solutions of iron(II) salts.
Prepare immediately before use.

Potassium Hyaluronate (*31799-91-4*)
General reagent grade of commerce obtained from human umbilical cords and freeze-dried.
Protein, not more than 2%; chondroitin sulphate, not more than 3%.

Potassium Hyaluronate Stock Solution A 0.05% w/v solution of *potassium hyaluronate*.
Store below 0° and use within 30 days.

Potassium Hydrogen Carbonate Potassium bicarbonate; $KHCO_3$ = 100.1 (*298-14-6*)
Analytical reagent grade of commerce.

Potassium Hydrogen Carbonate Solution, Saturated Methanolic Dissolve 0.1 g of *potassium hydrogen carbonate* in 0.4 ml of *water* by heating on a water bath. Add 25 ml of *methanol* and swirl, keeping the solution on the water bath until dissolution is complete.
Use a freshly prepared solution.

Potassium Hydrogen Phthalate $C_8H_5KO_4$ = 204.2 (*877-24-7*)
Analytical reagent grade of commerce.

Potassium Hydrogen Phthalate, 0.2M A solution of *potassium hydrogen phthalate* containing 40.84 g of $C_8H_5KO_4$ in 1000 ml.

Potassium Hydrogen Sulphate Potassium bisulphate; $KHSO_4$ = 136.2 (*7646-93-7*)
Analytical reagent grade of commerce.
Colourless, transparent, hygroscopic crystals.
Store in an airtight container.

Potassium Hydrogen Tartrate See *potassium hydrogen (+)-tartrate*.

Potassium Hydrogen (+)-Tartrate $C_4H_5KO_6$ = 188.2 (*868-14-4*)
Analytical reagent grade of commerce.
A white, crystalline powder or colourless, slightly opaque crystals.

Potassium Hydroxide KOH = 56.11 (*1310-58-3*)
Analytical reagent grade of commerce containing not less than 85.0% of total alkali calculated as KOH and not more than 2.0% of K_2CO_3.
Deliquescent pellets, sticks or slabs.
Store in an airtight container.

Potassium Hydroxide, 2M Alcoholic Dissolve 12 g of *potassium hydroxide* in 10 ml of *water* and add sufficient *ethanol (96%)* to produce 100 ml.

Potassium Hydroxide, Ethanolic Solutions of the requisite molarity may be obtained by dissolving the appropriate amount of *potassium hydroxide* in sufficient *ethanol (96%)* to produce 1000 ml.

Potassium Hydroxide in Alcohol (10% v/v), 0.5M Dissolve 28 g of *potassium hydroxide* in 100 ml of *ethanol (96%)* and add sufficient *water* to produce 1000 ml.

Potassium Hydroxide, Methanolic Solutions of the requisite molarity may be obtained by dissolving the appropriate amount of *potassium hydroxide* in sufficient *methanol* to produce 1000 ml.

Potassium Hydroxide Solution, Alcoholic Dissolve 3 g of *potassium hydroxide* in 5 ml of *water* and dilute to 100 ml with *aldehyde-free ethanol (96%)* and decant the clear solution. The solution should be almost colourless.

Potassium Hydroxide Solution R1, Alcoholic Dissolve 6.6 g of *potassium hydroxide* in 50 ml of *water* and dilute to 1000 ml with *absolute ethanol*.

Potassium Iodate KIO_3 = 214.0 (*7758-05-6*)
Analytical reagent grade of commerce.
A white, crystalline powder.

Potassium Iodide KI = 166.0 (*7681-11-0*)
Analytical reagent grade of commerce.
A white, crystalline powder.

Potassium Iodide and Starch Solution Dissolve 0.75 g of *potassium iodide* in 100 ml of *water*, heat to boiling and add, whilst stirring, a solution of 0.5 g of *soluble starch* in 35 ml of *water*. Boil for 2 minutes and allow to cool.
Complies with the following test.
SENSITIVITY TO IODINE To 15 ml of the reagent add 0.05 ml of *glacial acetic acid* and 0.3 ml of 0.0005M *iodine VS*. A blue colour is produced.

Potassium Iodide Solution A 16.6% w/v solution of *potassium iodide*.

Potassium Iodide Solution, Dilute A 10% w/v solution of *potassium iodide*.

Potassium Iodide Solution, Iodinated Dissolve 2 g of *iodine* and 4 g of *potassium iodide* in 10 ml of *water*. When solution is complete, add sufficient *water* to produce 100 ml.

Potassium Iodide Solution, Saturated A saturated solution of *potassium iodide* in *carbon dioxide-free water*; it contains some undissolved crystals.
Store protected from light and discard if it fails to comply with the following test.
Add 0.1 ml of *starch solution* to 0.5 ml of the reagent in 30 ml of a mixture of 3 volumes of 6M *acetic acid* and 2 volumes of *chloroform*. If a blue colour is produced it is discharged on the addition of not more than 0.05 ml of 0.1M *sodium thiosulphate VS*.

Potassium Iodobismuthate Solution Dissolve 8 g of *potassium iodide* in sufficient *water* to produce 20 ml and add the solution to a mixture of 0.85 g of *bismuth oxynitrate*, 40 ml of *water* and 10 ml of *glacial acetic acid*.

Potassium Iodobismuthate Solution, Acid Dissolve 1.7 g of *bismuth oxynitrate* in a mixture of 80 ml of *water* and 20 ml of *glacial acetic acid*, warming if necessary, cool, add 100 ml of a 50% w/v solution of *potassium iodide* and mix. Dilute 10 ml to 100 ml with *water*, add 10 ml of *glacial acetic acid*, mix, add 0.12 g of *iodine* and shake until the iodine has completely dissolved.
Store at a temperature of 2° to 8° and use within 2 weeks.

Potassium Iodobismuthate Solution, Dilute Dissolve 100 g of *(+)-tartaric acid* in 500 ml of *water* and add 50 ml of *potassium iodobismuthate solution R1*.

Potassium Iodobismuthate Solution R1 Dissolve 100 g of *(+)-tartaric acid* in 400 ml of *water* and add 8.5 g of *bismuth oxynitrate*. Shake for 1 hour, add 200 ml of a

40% w/v solution of *potassium iodide* and shake well. Allow to stand for 24 hours and filter.
Store protected from light.

Potassium Iodobismuthate Solution R2 Suspend 1.7 g of *bismuth oxynitrate* and 20 g of *(+)-tartaric acid* in 40 ml of *water*. To the suspension add 40 ml of a 40% w/v solution of *potassium iodide*, stir for 1 hour and filter. This stock solution may be kept for several days protected from light.
Immediately before use, mix 5 ml of the stock solution with 15 ml of *water*.

Potassium Iodoplatinate Solution Add 5 ml of a 5% w/v solution of *chloroplatinic(IV) acid* to 45 ml of *dilute potassium iodide solution* and dilute to 100 ml with *water*. Store in an amber glass container.

Potassium Mercuri-iodide Solution, Alkaline To 3.5 g of *potassium iodide* add 1.25 g of *mercury(II) chloride* dissolved in 80 ml of *water* and a cold, saturated solution of *mercury(II) chloride* in *water*, stirring continuously, until a slight red precipitate remains. Dissolve 12 g of *sodium hydroxide* in the resulting solution and add a little more of the saturated solution of mercury(II) chloride and sufficient *water* to produce 100 ml. Allow to stand and decant the clear, supernatant liquid.

Potassium Nitrate KNO_3 = 101.1 (*7757-79-1*)
Analytical reagent grade of commerce.
Colourless crystals.

Potassium Periodate Potassium metaperiodate; KIO_4 = 230.0 (*7790-21-8*)
Analytical reagent grade of commerce.
A white, crystalline powder or colourless crystals.

Potassium Permanganate $KMnO_4$ = 158.0 (*7722-64-7*)
Analytical reagent grade of commerce.

Potassium Permanganate and Phosphoric Acid Solution Dissolve 3 g of *potassium permanganate* in a mixture of 15 ml of *orthophosphoric acid* and 70 ml of *water* and add sufficient *water* to produce 100 ml.

Potassium Permanganate Solution A 3% w/v solution of *potassium permanganate*.

Potassium Permanganate Solution, Dilute A 1.0% w/v solution of *potassium permanganate*.

Potassium Perrhenate $KReO_4$ = 289.3 (*10466-65-6*)
General reagent grade of commerce.

Potassium Persulphate Dipotassium peroxodisulphate; $K_2S_2O_8$ = 270.3 (*7727-21-1*)
General reagent grade of commerce.
Aqueous solutions decompose at room temperature and more rapidly on warming.
Store in a cool place.

Potassium Plumbite Solution Dissolve 1.7 g of *lead acetate*, 3.4 g of *potassium citrate* and 50 g of *potassium hydroxide* in sufficient *water* to produce 100 ml.

Potassium Pyroantimonate See *potassium antimonate(V)*.

Potassium Pyroantimonate Solution See *potassium antimonate(V) solution*.

Potassium Sodium (+)-Tartrate Sodium potassium (+)-tartrate; $C_4H_4KNaO_6,4H_2O$ = 282.2 (*6381-59-5*)
Analytical reagent grade of commerce.

Potassium Sulphate Dipotassium sulphate; K_2SO_4 = 174.3 (*7778-80-5*)
Analytical reagent grade of commerce.

Potassium Tartrate See *dipotassium (+)-tartrate*.

Potassium Tetraiodomercurate Solution Dissolve 1.35 g of *mercury(II) chloride* in 50 ml of *water*, add 5 g of *potassium iodide*, mix and add sufficient *water* to produce 100 ml.

Potassium Tetraiodomercurate Solution, Alkaline Dissolve 11 g of *potassium iodide* and 15 g of *mercury(II) iodide* in *water* and dilute to 100 ml with *water*. Immediately before use, mix the solution with an equal volume of a 25% w/v solution of *sodium hydroxide*.

Potassium Tetraoxalate Potassium trihydrogen dioxalate; $C_4H_3KO_8,2H_2O$ = 254.2 (*6100-20-5*)
Analytical reagent grade of commerce.
A white, crystalline powder.

Potassium Thiocyanate KCNS = 97.18 (*333-20-0*)
Analytical reagent grade of commerce.
Colourless crystals; deliquescent.
Store in an airtight container.

Potassium Thiocyanate Solution A 9.7% w/v solution of *potassium thiocyanate*.

Povidone Polyvidone; PVP (*9003-39-8*)
A mixture of linear polymers of 1-vinylpyrrolidin-2-one with an average relative molecular weight of about 10,000 to 700,000, containing 12 to 13% of N, calculated with reference to the dried substance.
A fine, white or almost white powder.
Complies with the following tests.
LOSS ON DRYING When dried at 100° to 105°, loses not more than 5.0% of its weight. Use 1 g.
ASSAY Carry out the *determination of nitrogen*, Appendix VIII H, Method I, using 16 mg. Continue the heating for 1 hour.

Prednisolone $C_{21}H_{28}O_5$ = 360.5 (*50-24-8*)
General reagent grade of commerce.
Hygroscopic crystalline powder; melting point, about 230°, with decomposition; $[\alpha]_D^{20}$, about +97° (1% w/v in 1,4-dioxan).

Prednisolone 21-Acetate $C_{23}H_{30}O_6$ = 402.5 (*52-21-1*)
General reagent grade of commerce.

Procaine Hydrochloride $C_{13}H_{20}N_2O_2,HCl$ = 272.8 (*51-05-8*)
General reagent grade of commerce.
Melting point, about 156°.

D-Prolyl-L-phenylalanyl-L-arginine 4-Nitroanilide Hydrochloride $C_{26}H_{36}Cl_2N_8O_5$ = 612 (*62354-56-7*)
General reagent grade of commerce.

Propane-1,2-diol Propylene glycol; $C_3H_8O_2$ = 76.10 (*57-55-6*)
General reagent grade of commerce.
A colourless, viscous, hygroscopic liquid; boiling point, about 187°; weight per ml, about 1.04 g.

Propanol See *propan-1-ol*.

2-Propanol See *propan-2-ol*.

2-Propanol R1 See *propan-2-ol R1*.

Propan-1-ol Propanol; *n*-Propyl alcohol; C_3H_8O = 60.10 (*71-23-8*)
Analytical reagent grade of commerce.
A colourless liquid; boiling point, about 97°; d_{20}^{20}, 0.802 to 0.806. Not less than 95% distils between 96° and 99°.

Propan-2-ol Isopropyl alcohol; 2-propanol; C_3H_8O = 60.10 (*67-63-0*)

Analytical reagent grade of commerce.
A colourless liquid with a characteristic odour; boiling point, 81° to 83°; d_{20}^{20}, about 0.785.

Propan-2-ol R1 *Propan-2-ol* complying with the following requirements.
REFRACTIVE INDEX About 1.378.
TRANSMITTANCE Not less than 25% at 210 nm, 55% at 220 nm, 75% at 230 nm, 95% at 250 nm and 98% at 260 nm, determined using *water* in the reference cell.
WATER Not more than 0.05% w/w, Appendix IX C. Use 10 g.

Propanolamine See *3-Aminopropanol.*

Propionaldehyde Propanal; C_3H_6O = 58.1 (*123-38-6*)
General reagent grade of commerce.
Melting point, about –81°; boiling point, about 49°; n_D^{20}, about 1.365; d_{20}^{20}, about 0.81.

Propionic Acid $C_3H_6O_2$ = 74.1 (*79-09-4*)
General reagent grade of commerce.
d_{20}^{20}, about 0.993; n_D^{20}, about 1.387; boiling point, about 141°.

Propionic Anhydride $C_6H_{10}O_3$ = 130.1 (*123-62-6*)
General reagent grade of commerce.
A colourless liquid with a pungent odour; weight per ml, about 1.01 g; boiling point, about 167°.
A clear, colourless liquid.

Propionic Anhydride Reagent Dissolve 1 g of *toluene-p-sulphonic acid* in 30 ml of *glacial acetic acid,* add 5 ml of *propionic anhydride* and allow to stand for at least 15 minutes.
Use within 24 hours of preparation.

Propyl Acetate $C_5H_{10}O_2$ = 102.1 (*109-60-4*)
General reagent grade of commerce.
Boiling point, about 102°; d_{20}^{20}, about 0.888.

Propyl 4-Hydroxybenzoate Propyl parahydroxybenzoate; $C_{10}H_{12}O_3$ = 180.2 (*94-13-3*)
General reagent grade of commerce.
Melting point, about 97°.

Propyl Parahydroxybenzoate See *propyl 4-hydroxybenzoate.*

Propylene Glycol See *propane-1,3-diol.*

Protamine Sulphate (*53597-25-4* (salmine); *9007-31-2* (clupeine))
A mixture of the sulphates of basic peptides extracted from the sperm or roe of fish, usually species of Salmonidae or Clupeidae. It binds with heparin, inhibiting its anticoagulant activity.

Pulegone (+)-*p*-Menth-4-en-3-one; (*R*)-2-isopropylidene-5-methylcyclohexanone; $C_{10}H_{16}O$ = 152.2 (*89-82-7*)
General reagent grade of commerce.
d_{15}^{20}, about 0.937; n_D^{20}, about 1.485 to 1.489; $[\alpha]_D^{20}$, +19.5° to +22.5°; boiling point, 222° to 224°.
Pulegone used in gas chromatography complies with the following test.
ASSAY Examine by gas chromatography under the conditions described in the test for Chromatographic profile in the monograph for Peppermint Oil using the reagent being examined.
The area of the principal peak is not less than 98.0% of the total area of the peaks.

Pumice Powder
Pumice of commerce, powdered and sifted, which passes through a 710 µm sieve, but is retained on a 250 µm sieve.

Pyridine C_5H_5N = 79.10 (*110-86-1*)
Analytical reagent grade of commerce.
A colourless liquid with an unpleasant odour; boiling point, about 115°.
Store in an airtight container.

Pyridine, Anhydrous
Dry *pyridine* over *anhydrous sodium carbonate,* filter and distil.
Complies with the following test.
WATER Not more than 0.01% w/w, Appendix IX C.

Pyridine Bromide Solution Dissolve 8 g of *pyridine* and 5.4 ml of *sulphuric acid* in 20 ml of *glacial acetic acid,* keeping the mixture cool. Add 2.6 ml of *bromine* dissolved in 20 ml of *glacial acetic acid* and dilute to 1000 ml with *glacial acetic acid.*
Prepare immediately before use.

Pyridine-3-carboxaldehyde Nicotinaldehyde; C_6H_5NO = 107.1 (*500-22-1*)
General reagent grade of commerce.
Weight per ml, 1.14 g.

Pyrid-2-ylamine See *2-pyridylamine.*

2-Pyridylamine 2-Aminopyridine; pyrid-2-ylamine; $C_5H_6N_2$ = 94.1 (*504-29-0*)
General reagent grade of commerce.
Melting point, about 58°; boiling point, about 210°.

Pyridylazonaphthol PAN; 1-(2-pyridylazo)-2-naphthol; $C_{15}H_{11}N_3O$ = 249.3 (*85-85-8*)
General reagent grade of commerce.
A brick red powder; melting point, about 138°.

Pyridylazonaphthol Solution A 0.1% w/v solution in *absolute ethanol.*
Complies with the following test.
SENSITIVITY TO COPPER To 50 ml of *water* add 10 ml of *acetate buffer pH 4.4,* 0.1 ml of 0.02M *disodium edetate VS* and 0.25 ml of the reagent being examined; a yellow colour is produced. Add 0.15 ml of a 0.5% w/v solution of *copper(II) sulphate*; the colour changes to violet.

Pyrocatechol See *catechol.*

Pyrogallol Benzene-1,2,3-triol; $C_6H_6O_3$ = 126.1
Analytical reagent grade of commerce.
White crystals becoming brownish on exposure to air and light; melting point, about 131°.
Store protected from light.

Pyrogallol Solution, Alkaline Dissolve 0.5 g of *pyrogallol* in 2 ml of *carbon dioxide-free water*; dissolve 12 g of *potassium hydroxide* in 8 ml of *carbon dioxide-free water.* Mix the two solutions immediately before use.

Pyruvic Acid 2-Oxopropanoic acid; $C_3H_4O_3$ = 88.1 (*127-17-3*)
General reagent grade of commerce.
d_{20}^{20}, about 1.267; n_D^{20}, about 1.413; boiling point, about 165°.

Quinaldine Red 2-(4-Dimethylaminostyryl)quinoline ethiodide; $C_{21}H_{23}IN_2$ = 430.3 (*117-92-0*)
When used for titration in glacial acetic acid, it changes from magenta (basic) to almost colourless (acidic).

Quinaldine Red Solution A 0.1% w/v solution of *quinaldine red* in *methanol* (pH range, 1.4 to 3.2).

Quinalizarin CI 58500; 1,2,5,8-tetrahydroxyanthraquinone; $C_{14}H_8O_6$ = 272.2 (*81-61-8*)

General reagent grade of commerce.
A reddish brown powder.

Quinhydrone Cyclohexa-2,5-diene-1,4-dione compound with benzene-1,4-diol; $C_{12}H_{10}O_4$ = 218.2 (*106-34-3*)
Analytical reagent grade of commerce.
Dark green, lustrous crystals or crystalline powder; melting point, about 170°.

Quinidine $C_{20}H_{24}N_2O_2$ = 324.4 (*56-54-2*)
General reagent grade of commerce.
White crystals; melting point, about 172°; $[\alpha]_D^{20}$, about +260° (1% w/v in absolute ethanol).
Store protected from light.

Quinidine Sulphate $C_{40}H_{48}N_4O_4,H_2SO_4,2H_2O$ = 783.0 (*6591-63-5*)
General reagent grade of commerce.
White, fine crystals; melting point, about 213°, with decomposition; $[\alpha]_D^{20}$, about +220° (1% w/v in ethanol).
Store protected from light.

Quinine $C_{20}H_{24}N_2O_2$ = 324.4 (*130-95-0*)
General reagent grade of commerce.
A microcrystalline powder; melting point, about 175°; $[\alpha]_D^{20}$, about −167° (1% in absolute ethanol).
Store protected from light.

Quinine Hydrochloride $C_{20}H_{24}N_2O_2,HCl,2H_2O$ = 396.9 (*6119-47-7*)
General reagent grade of commerce.
Melting point, about 115°, with decomposition.
Store protected from light.

Quinine Sulphate $C_{40}H_{48}N_4O_4,H_2SO_4,2H_2O$ = 783.0 (*6119-70-6*)
General reagent grade of commerce.
A white or off-white, efflorescent, crystalline solid; melting point, about 234°, with decomposition; $[\alpha]_D^{20}$, about −220° (0.5% w/v in 0.5M hydrochloric acid).
Store protected from light.

Quinoline C_9H_7N = 129.2 (*91-22-5*)
General reagent grade of commerce, suitable for phosphate assay.
A pale yellow liquid with an unpleasant odour; n_D^{20}, 1.624 to 1.627.
Complies with the following requirement.
TARRY IMPURITIES Dissolve 1.0 g in a mixture of 2.5 ml of *water* and 2.5 ml of *hydrochloric acid.* Add 3 ml of *water* and 1 ml of *potassium chromate solution* and heat to boiling. The solution shows no darkening and no black deposit.
Store protected from light.

Quinoline Solution Dissolve 50 ml of *quinoline* in a mixture of 60 ml of *hydrochloric acid* and 300 ml of *water* previously heated to 70°, cool and filter.

Rabbit Erythrocyte Suspension Prepare a 1.6% w/v suspension of rabbit erythrocytes in the following manner. Defibrinate 15 ml of freshly drawn rabbit blood by shaking with glass beads, centrifuge at 2000 *g* for 10 minutes and wash the erythrocytes with three 30-ml quantities of a 0.9% w/v solution of *sodium chloride.* Dilute 1.6 ml of the suspension of erythrocytes to 100 ml with a mixture of 1 volume of *phosphate buffer pH 7.2* and 9 volumes of a 0.9% w/v solution of *sodium chloride.*

Rabies Antiserum, Fluorescein-conjugated Immunoglobulin fraction with a high rabies antibody titre, prepared from the sera of suitable animals that have been immunised with inactivated rabies virus. The immunoglobulin is conjugated with fluorescein isothiocyanate.

Rapeseed Oil Rape seed oil
The fatty oil obtained by expression from the seeds of different varieties of *Brassica napus* L. The fatty-acid fraction contains 40 to 55% of erucic acid.
A clear, yellow to dark yellow, oily liquid.
Complies with the following tests.
IODINE VALUE 94 to 120 *(iodine bromide method)*, Appendix X E.
PEROXIDE VALUE Not more than 5, Appendix X F.
SAPONIFICATION VALUE 168 to 181, Appendix X G, Method II.
CONTENT OF ERUCIC ACID Carry out the *test for foreign oils by thin-layer chromatography*, Appendix X N, applying separately to the plate 3 µl of each of the following solutions. Solution (1) contains 0.5% w/v of the mixture of fatty acids in *chloroform.* For solution (2) dilute 2 ml of solution (1) with *chloroform* to 50 ml.

The chromatogram obtained with solution (1) shows five distinct spots. The spot with the lowest Rf value (about 0.25) is the most intense or one of the most intense and corresponds to erucic acid. The spot corresponding to erucic acid is also clearly visible on the chromatogram obtained with solution (2).

Reducing Mixture Hydrazine reducing mixture
Grind 20 mg of *potassium bromide*, 0.5 g of *hydrazine sulphate* and 5 g of *sodium chloride* in the order listed to obtain a homogeneous mixture.

Resorcinol Benzene-1,3-diol; $C_6H_6O_2$ = 110.1 (*108-46-3*)
Analytical reagent grade of commerce.
Colourless crystals or crystalline powder; melting point, about 111°.

Resorcinol Reagent To 80 ml of *hydrochloric acid* add 10 ml of a 2% w/v solution of *resorcinol* and 0.25 ml of a 2.5% w/v solution of *copper(II) sulphate* and dilute to 100 ml with *water.* Prepare the solution at least 4 hours before use.
Store at 2° to 8° and use within 1 week.

Rhamnose See *L-rhamnose.*

L-Rhamnose $C_6H_{12}O_5,H_2O$ = 182.2 (*6155-35-7*)
General reagent grade of commerce.
A white, crystalline powder; melting point, about 96°; $[\alpha]_D^{20}$, +7.8° to +8.3° (5% w/v in water containing about 0.05% of NH_3).

Rhaponticin Rhapontin; 4′-methoxystilbene-3,3′,5-triol 3-glucoside; $C_{21}H_{24}O_9$ = 420.4 (*155-58-8*)
General reagent grade of commerce.
Yellowish grey crystalline powder.
Complies with the following test.
HOMOGENEITY Carry out the test for *Rheum rhaponticum* described in the monograph for Rhubarb. The chromatogram obtained with the reference solution shows only one principal spot.

Rhodamine B CI 45170; basic violet 10; $C_{28}H_{31}ClN_2O_3$ = 479.0 (*81-88-9*)
General reagent grade of commerce.
Green crystals or a reddish violet powder.

Ribose D-Ribose; $C_5H_{10}O_5$ = 150.1 (*50-69-1*)
General reagent grade of commerce.
Melting point, 88° to 92°.

Ricinoleic Acid 12-Hydroxyoleic acid; $C_{18}H_{34}O_3$ = 298.5 (*141-22-0*)
General reagent grade of commerce.

d_{20}^{20}, about 0.942; n_D^{20}, about 1.472; melting point, about 285°, with decomposition.

Ruthenium Red Ammoniated ruthenium oxychloride; $H_{42}Cl_6N_{14}O_2Ru_3,4H_2O$ = 858 (*11103-72-3*)
Microscopical staining grade of commerce.
A brownish red powder.

Ruthenium Red Solution A 0.08% w/v solution of *ruthenium red* in *lead acetate solution*.

Rutin Vitamin P; rutoside; 3,3′,4′,5,7-pentahydroxyflavone 3-rutinoside; $C_{27}H_{30}O_{16},3H_2O$ = 664.6 (*153-18-4*)
General reagent grade of commerce.
A yellow, crystalline powder, darkening on exposure to light.
Melting point, about 210°, with decomposition; a solution in *ethanol (96%)* exhibits absorption maxima at 259 nm and 362 nm, Appendix II B.
Store protected from light.

Sabinene 4-Methylene-1-isopropylbicyclo[3.1.0]hexane; $C_{10}H_{16}$ = 136.2 (*2009-00-9*)
General reagent grade of commerce.
d_{25}^{25}, about 0.843; n_D^{20}, about 1.468; boiling point, 163° to 165°.

Saccharin $C_7H_5NO_3S$ = 183.2 (*81-07-2*)
General reagent grade of commerce.
Melting point, about 230°.

Salicylaldehyde 2-Hydroxybenzaldehyde; $C_7H_6O_2$ = 122.1 (*90-02-8*)
General reagent grade of commerce.
A colourless, oily liquid with a characteristic odour; d_{20}^{20}, about 1.167; n_D^{20}, about 1.574; melting point, about −7°; boiling point, about 196°.

Salicylaldehyde Azine $C_{14}H_{12}N_2O_2$ = 240.3
Dissolve 0.30 g of *hydrazine sulphate* in 5 ml of *water*, add 1 ml of *glacial acetic acid* and 2 ml of a freshly prepared 20% v/v solution of *salicylaldehyde* in *propan-2-ol*. Mix and allow to stand until a yellow precipitate is produced. Shake with two 15-ml quantities of *dichloromethane*, allow to separate, dry the combined dichloromethane layers over *anhydrous sodium sulphate* and evaporate to dryness. Recrystallise the residue from a mixture of 60 volumes of *toluene* and 40 volumes of *methanol* with cooling. The melting point of the resulting crystals, after drying over *phosphorus pentoxide* at a pressure of 1.5 to 2.5 kPa, is about 213°.
Complies with the following test.
HOMOGENEITY Examine under the conditions prescribed in the test for Hydrazine in the monograph for Povidone. The chromatogram shows only one spot.

Salicylic Acid $C_7H_6O_3$ = 138.1 (*69-72-7*)
Analytical reagent grade of commerce.
Colourless crystals; melting point, about 160°.

Saline Solution A 0.9% w/v solution of *sodium chloride* in freshly prepared *water*, sterilised by *heating in an autoclave*.

Sand White or slightly greyish grains of silica with a particle size between 150 µm and 300 µm.

Selenious Acid Selenous acid; selenic(IV) acid; H_2SeO_3 = 129.0 (*7783-00-8*)
General reagent grade of commerce.
Store in an airtight container.

Selenium Se = 78.96 (*7782-49-2*)
Analytical reagent grade of commerce.
Very dark red to black powder; melting point, about 220°.

Selenium Dioxide SeO_2 = 111.0 (*7446-08-4*)
General reagent grade of commerce.

Semicarbazide Acetate Solution Triturate 2.5 g of *semicarbazide hydrochloride* with 3.3 g of *sodium acetate*, add 10 ml of *methanol*, mix, transfer to a flask with the aid of 20 ml of *methanol* and allow to stand at a temperature of about 4° for 30 minutes; filter and add sufficient *methanol* to produce 100 ml.

Semicarbazide Hydrochloride CH_5N_3O,HCl = 111.5 (*563-41-7*)
Analytical reagent grade of commerce.
A white, crystalline powder; melting point, about 175°, with decomposition.

Serine See *L-serine*.

L-Serine $C_3H_7NO_3$ = 105.1 (*56-45-1*)
General reagent grade of commerce
A white, crystalline solid; melting point, about 222°, with decomposition; $[\alpha]_D^{20}$, about +14° (10% in 1M hydrochloric acid).
Complies with the following test.
HOMOGENEITY Carry out the method for *thin-layer chromatography*, Appendix III A, using *silica gel G* as the coating substance and a mixture of 25 parts of *water* and 75 parts of *phenol* as the mobile phase but allowing the mobile phase to ascend 12 cm above the line of application. Apply 5 µl of a 0.2% w/v solution to the plate and keep the plate in the vapour of the mobile phase for 12 hours before development. After removal of the plate, dry it in air, spray with a 0.1% w/v solution of *ninhydrin* in *butan-1-ol* saturated with *water* and heat at 100° to 105° for 10 minutes. The chromatogram shows only one principal spot.

Serum Solution Dilute 1 volume of *serum stock solution* with 3 volumes of solution prepared by dissolving 14 g of *potassium acetate* in *water*, adding 20.5 ml of *glacial acetic acid* and diluting to 1000 ml with *water* and adjust to room temperature.
Use on the day of preparation.

Serum Stock Solution Dilute 1 volume of cattle or horse serum (native or reconstituted with *water* to its original volume) with 9 volumes of a solution prepared by dissolving 14 g of *potassium acetate* in *water*, adding 20.5 ml of *glacial acetic acid* and diluting to 1000 ml with *water*. Adjust the pH to 3.1 with 4M *hydrochloric acid* and allow to stand for 18 to 24 hours.
Store at 0° to 4° and use within 30 days.

Silica Gel, Anhydrous Partially dehydrated, polymerised, colloidal silicic acid containing cobalt(II) chloride as an indicator.
Of commerce.
Blue granules, becoming pink when the moisture adsorption capacity is exhausted. Anhydrous silica gel adsorbs about 30% of its weight of water at 20°. Its adsorptive capacity may be regenerated by heating at 150° for 2 hours.

Silica Gel, Butylsilyl
Chromatographic reagent grade of commerce.
A very finely divided silica gel (3 to 10 µm) chemically modified at the surface by the introduction of butylsilyl groups. The particle size is indicated after the name of the reagent in tests where it is used.
Spheroidal silica 30 nm; pore volume, 0.6 cm³ g⁻¹; specific surface area, 80 m² g⁻¹.

Silica Gel for Chromatography Silica gel
Use a grade of commerce suitable for column chromatography.
The particle size may be indicated after the name of the reagent in tests where it is used.

Silica Gel for Chromatography, Aminopropylmethylsilyl
Liquid chromatographic reagent grade of commerce.
A silica gel with a fine particle size (3 to 10 µm) the surface of which has been modified by chemically bonding aminopropylmethylsilyl groups. The particle size is indicated after the name of the reagent in tests where it is used.

Silica Gel for Chromatography, Aminopropylsilyl
Liquid chromatographic reagent grade of commerce.
A silica gel with a fine particle size (3 to 10 µm) the surface of which has been modified by chemically bonding aminopropylsilyl groups. The particle size is indicated after the name of the reagent in tests where it is used.

Silica gel for Chromatography, Amylose-derivative
Chromatographic reagent grade of commerce.
A very finely divided (10 µm) silica gel, chemically modified at the surface by the introduction of an amylose derivative. The particle size is indicated after the name of the reagent in tests where it is used.

Silica Gel for Chromatography, Base-deactivated, End-capped Octadecylsilyl
A very finely divided (3 to 10 µm) silica gel, treated before the introduction of octadecylsilyl groups by washing and hydrolysing most of the superficial siloxane bridges. To minimise any interaction with basic compounds further it is carefully end-capped to cover most the remaining silanol groups. The particle size is stated after the name of the reagent in tests where it is used.

Silica Gel for Chromatography, Base-deactivated Octadecylsilyl
Chromatographic reagent grade of commerce.
A very finely divided (3 to 10 µm) silica gel chemically modified at the surface by the introduction of octadecylsilyl groups and deactivated for the separation of basic components by careful washing and hydrolysing most of the superficial siloxane bridges. The particle size is stated after the name of the reagent in tests where it is used.

Silica gel for Chromatography, Cyanosilyl
Chromatographic reagent grade of commerce.
A very finely divided silica gel, chemically modified at the surface by the introduction of cyanosilyl groups. The particle size is indicated after the name of the reagent in tests where it is used.

Silica gel for Chromatography, Diol
Chromatographic reagent grade of commerce.
Spherical particles of silica to which dihydroxypropyl groups are bonded. Pore size, 10 nm.

Silica Gel for Chromatography, End-capped Octylsilyl
Chromatographic reagent grade of commerce.
Silanol deactivated octylsilyl silica gel.

Silica Gel for Chromatography, Hexylsilyl
Chromatographic reagent grade of commerce.
A very finely divided (3 to 10 µm) silica gel chemically modified at the surface by the introduction of hexylsilyl groups. The particle size is indicated after the name of the reagent in tests where it is used.

Silica Gel for Chromatography, Hydrophilic
A very finely divided (3 to 10 µm) silica gel, the surface of which has been modified to provide hydrophilic characteristics. The particle size is stated after the name of the reagent in tests where it is used.

Silica Gel for Chromatography, Nitrile
Liquid chromatographic grade of commerce.
A very finely divided silica gel the surface of which has been modified by the introduction of cyanopropylsilyl groups. The particle size is indicated after the name of the reagent in tests where it is used.

Silica Gel for Chromatography, Octadecylsilyl
Liquid chromatographic reagent grade of commerce.
A very finely divided silica gel (3 to 10 µm) chemically modified at the surface by the introduction of octadecylsilyl groups.
The particle size is specified after the name of the reagent in tests where it is used.

Silica Gel for Chromatography, Octylsilyl
Chromatographic reagent grade of commerce.
A very finely divided (3 to 10 µm) silica gel chemically modified at the surface by the introduction of octylsilyl groups. The particle size is indicated after the name of the reagent in tests where it is used.

Silica Gel for Chromatography R1, Octadecylsilyl
Liquid chromatographic reagent grade of commerce.
Ultrapure silica (10 nm pore size) chemically modified at the surface by bonding C18 groups (19% carbon load). Less than 20 ppm of metals.

Silica Gel for Chromatography R1, Nitrile
Chromatographic reagent grade of commerce.
A very finely divided silica gel consisting of porous, spherical particles with chemically bonded nitrile groups. The particle size is indicated after the name of the reagent in tests where it is used.

Silica Gel for Chromatography, Phenyl
Liquid chromatographic reagent grade of commerce.
A very finely divided (5 to 10 µm) silica gel chemically modified at the surface by the introduction of phenyl groups.

Silica Gel for Chromatography, Strong-anion-exchange
Chromatographic reagent grade of commerce.
A very finely divided (3 to 10 µm) silica gel, chemically modified at the surface by the introduction of quaternary ammonium groups. The particle size is indicated after the name of the reagent in tests where it is used.

Silica Gel for Size-exclusion Chromatography
Chromatographic reagent grade of commerce.
A very finely divided (10 µm) silica gel with a very hydrophilic surface. The average diameter of the pores is about 30 nm. It is compatible with aqueous solutions between pH 2 and 8 and with organic solvents. It is suitable for the separation of proteins with relative molecular weights of 1×10^3 to $3 \times$ to 10^5.

Silica Gel OD for Chiral Separations
Chromatographic reagent grade of commerce.
A very finely divided silica gel for chromatography (5 µm) coated with the following derivative.

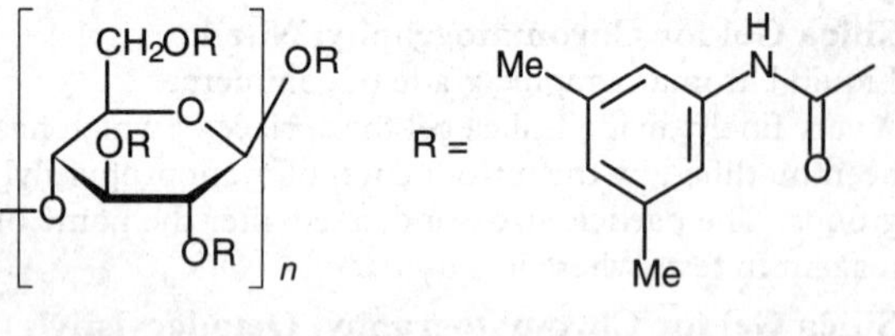

Silica Gel G (*112926-00-8*)
A fine, white, homogeneous powder of an average particle size of about 15 µm containing about 13% of calcium sulphate hemihydrate and complying with the following requirements.
CONTENT OF CALCIUM SULPHATE To 0.25 g add 3 ml of 2M *hydrochloric acid* and 100 ml of *water* and shake vigorously for 30 minutes. Filter, wash the residue with *water* and carry out the *complexometric titration of calcium*, Appendix VIII D, on the combined filtrate and washings. Each ml of 0.1M *disodium edetate VS* is equivalent to 14.51 mg of $CaSO_4,\frac{1}{2}H_2O$.
ACIDITY OR ALKALINITY pH of a suspension prepared by shaking 1 g with 10 ml of *carbon dioxide-free water* for 5 minutes, about 7, Appendix V L.

Silica Gel GF_{254} A fine, white, homogeneous powder of an average particle size of about 15 µm containing about 13% of calcium sulphate hemihydrate and about 1.5% of a fluorescent indicator having a maximum intensity at 254 nm. It complies with the tests for Content of calcium sulphate and Acidity or alkalinity described under silica gel G and with the following requirement.
FLUORESCENCE Carry out the method for *thin-layer chromatography* using a mixture of 10 volumes of *anhydrous formic acid* and 90 volumes of *propan-2-ol* as the mobile phase, but allowing the solvent front to ascend 10 cm above the line of application. Apply separately to the plate 10 quantities from 1 to 10 µl of a 0.1% w/v solution of *benzoic acid* in the mobile phase. After removal of the plate, dry it in a current of warm air and examine under *ultraviolet light (254 nm)*. The benzoic acid appears as dark spots on a fluorescent background in the upper third of the chromatogram at levels of 2 µg and greater.

Silica Gel H A fine, white, homogeneous powder of an average particle size of about 15 µm. It complies with the test for Acidity or alkalinity described under *silica gel G*.

Silica Gel H, Silanised A fine, white homogeneous powder which, after shaking with water, floats on the surface because of its water-repellent properties. It complies with the test for Acidity or alkalinity described under *silica gel G*.

Use a suspension prepared by vigorously shaking 30 g of the silica gel for 2 minutes with 60 ml of *methanol (33%)* and spreading it to form a uniform layer about 0.25 mm thick on a series of carefully cleaned glass plates (200 mm × 50 mm). Allow the coated plates to dry in air and heat in an oven at 105° to 110° for 30 minutes.

Complies with the test for Separating power prescribed under *silanised silica gel HF_{254}*.

Silica Gel HF_{254} A fine, white homogeneous powder of an average particle size of about 15 µm containing about 1.5% of a fluorescent indicator having a maximum intensity at 254 nm. It complies with the test for Acidity or alkalinity described under *silica gel G* and with the test for Fluorescence described under *silica gel GF_{254}*.

Silica Gel HF_{254}, Silanised A fine, white, homogeneous powder which, after shaking with water, floats on the surface because of its water-repellent properties. It contains about 1.5% of a fluorescent indicator having a maximum intensity at 254 nm.

Use a suspension prepared by vigorously shaking 30 g of the silica gel for 2 minutes with 60 ml of *methanol (33%)* and spreading it to form a uniform layer about 0.25 mm thick on a series of carefully cleaned glass plates (200 mm × 50 mm). Allow the coated plates to dry in air and heat in an oven at 105° to 110° for 30 minutes.
Complies with the following test.
SEPARATING POWER Carry out the method for *thin-layer chromatography* using a plate prepared as described above and a mixture of 10 volumes of *glacial acetic acid*, 25 volumes of *water* and 65 volumes of *1,4-dioxan* as the mobile phase. Apply separately to the plate three 10-µl quantities of a solution prepared in the following manner. To a mixture of 0.1 g each of *methyl laurate*, *methyl myristate*, *methyl palmitate* and *methyl stearate* add 40 ml of *alcoholic potassium hydroxide solution* and heat under a reflux condenser on a water bath for 1 hour. Allow to cool, add 100 ml of *water*, acidify the mixture with 2M *hydrochloric acid* and extract with three 10-ml quantities of *chloroform*. Dry the combined chloroform extracts over *anhydrous sodium sulphate*, filter and evaporate to dryness on a water bath. Dissolve the residue in 50 ml of *chloroform*. After removal of the plate, heat it at 120° for 30 minutes. Allow to cool, spray with a 3.5% w/v solution of *phosphomolybdic acid* in *propan-2-ol* and heat at 150° until spots become visible. Expose the plate to ammonia vapour until the background turns white. Each chromatogram shows four clearly separated, well-defined spots.

Silica Gel, Phenyl A very finely divided silica gel (5 µm) chemically modified at the surface by the bonding of phenyl groups. The particle size is indicated after the name of the reagent in tests where it is used.
Spheroidal silica, 8 nm; specific surface area, 180 $m^2 g^{-1}$; carbon loading, 5.5%.

Silicotungstic Acid Dodecatungstosilicic acid; $H_4SiW_{12}O_{40}$,+aq (*11130-20-4*)
General reagent grade of commerce.
White or yellowish white crystals; deliquescent.
Store in an airtight container.

Silver Diethyldithiocarbamate Diethyldithiocarbamic acid silver salt; $C_5H_{10}AgNS_2$ = 256.1 (*1470-61-7*)
General reagent grade of commerce.
Protect from light; do not use if a strong odour develops or the colour is other than pale yellow or greyish yellow.

Silver Manganese Paper Immerse strips of slow filter paper in a solution containing 0.85% w/v of *manganese(II) sulphate* and 0.85% w/v of *silver nitrate* and leave for a few minutes. Allow the paper to dry over *phosphorus pentoxide* protected from acidic or alkaline vapours.

Silver Nitrate $AgNO_3$ = 169.9 (*7761-88-8*)
Analytical reagent grade of commerce.

Silver Nitrate Solution A freshly prepared 5.0% w/v solution of *silver nitrate*.
Store protected from light.

Silver Nitrate Solution, Ammoniacal Dissolve 2.5 g of *silver nitrate* in 80 ml of *water*, add 6M *ammonia* dropwise until the precipitate just dissolves and dilute to 100 ml with *water*.
Prepare immediately before use.

Silver Nitrate Solution in Pyridine An 8.5% w/v solution of *silver nitrate* in *pyridine*.
Store protected from light.

Silver Nitrate Solution R1 A 4.25% w/v solution of *silver nitrate*.
Store protected from light.

Silver Nitrate Solution R2 A 1.7% w/v solution of *silver nitrate*.
Store protected from light.

Silver Oxide Ag_2O = 231.7 (*20667-12-3*)
General reagent grade of commerce.
A brownish black powder.
Store protected from light.

Sinensetine 3′,4′,5,6,7-Pentamethoxyflavone; $C_{20}H_{20}O_7$ = 372 (*2306-27-6*)
General reagent grade of commerce.

Sodium Na = 22.99 (*7440-23-5*)
General reagent grade of commerce.
A soft silvery grey metal.
Sodium should be kept under light petroleum or liquid paraffin.

Sodium Acetate $C_2H_3O_2Na,3H_2O$ = 136.1 (*6131-90-4*)
Analytical reagent grade of commerce.

Sodium Acetate, Anhydrous $C_2H_3O_2Na$ = 82.03 (*127-09-3*)
Analytical reagent grade of commerce.
Complies with the following requirement.
LOSS ON DRYING When dried at 100° to 105°, loses not more than 2.0% of its weight.

Sodium Ascorbate Solution Dissolve 3.5 g of *L-ascorbic acid* in 20 ml of 1M *sodium hydroxide*.
Prepare immediately before use.

Sodium Azide NaN_3 = 65.0 (*26628-22-8*)
Analytical reagent grade of commerce.

Sodium Bicarbonate See *sodium hydrogen carbonate*.

Sodium Bismuthate $NaBiO_3$ = 280.0 (*12232-99-4*)
Analytical reagent grade of commerce containing not less than 85.0% of $NaBiO_3$.
A yellow to yellowish brown powder, slowly decomposing when moist or at a high temperature.
ASSAY Suspend 0.2 g in 10 ml of a 20% w/v solution of *potassium iodide* and add 20 ml of 1M *sulphuric acid*. Titrate with 0.1M *sodium thiosulphate VS* using 1 ml of *starch solution* as indicator until an orange solution is produced. Each ml of 0.1M *sodium thiosulphate VS* is equivalent to 14.00 mg of $NaBiO_3$.

Sodium Butanesulphonate 1-Butanesulphonic acid sodium salt; $C_4H_9NaO_3S$ = 160.2 (*2386-54-1*)
Chromatographic reagent grade of commerce.

Sodium Carbonate $Na_2CO_3,10H_2O$ = 286.2 (*5968-11-6*)
Analytical reagent grade of commerce.

Sodium Carbonate, Anhydrous Na_2CO_3 = 106.0 (*497-19-8*)
Analytical reagent grade of commerce.
A white, hygroscopic powder which loses not more than 1% of its weight on heating to about 300°.
Store in an airtight container.

Sodium Carbonate Solution A 10.6% w/v solution of *anhydrous sodium carbonate*.

Sodium Carbonate Solution, Dilute A 10% w/v solution of *sodium carbonate*.

Sodium Carbonate Solution R1 A 2% w/v solution of *anhydrous sodium carbonate* in 0.1M *sodium hydroxide*.

Sodium Cetostearyl Sulphate
Of the British Pharmacopoeia.

Sodium Chloride NaCl = 58.44 (*7647-14-5*)
Analytical reagent grade of commerce.

Sodium Chloride Injection Sodium Chloride Intravenous Infusion of the British Pharmacopoeia containing 0.9% w/v of Sodium Chloride.

Sodium Chloride Solution A 20% w/v solution of *sodium chloride*.

Sodium Cholate Cholic acid sodium salt hydrate; $C_{24}H_{39}NaO_5$ = 430.5 (*73163-53-8*)
General reagent grade of commerce.
$[\alpha]_D^{20}$, +31.3° (0.5% w/v in water).

Sodium Citrate Trisodium citrate; $C_6H_5Na_3O_7,2H_2O$ = 294.1 (*6132-04-3*)
Analytical reagent grade of commerce.

Sodium Cobaltinitrite Sodium hexanitritocobaltate(III); $Na_3Co(NO_2)_6$ = 403.9 (*13600-98-1*)
Analytical reagent grade of commerce.
Orange-yellow powder.

Sodium Cobaltinitrite Solution A 10% w/v solution of *sodium cobaltinitrite*. Prepare immediately before use.

Sodium Decanesulphonate $C_{10}H_{22}NaO_3S$ = 245.3 (*13419-61-9*)
Chromatographic reagent grade of commerce.

Sodium Deoxyribonucleate (*73049-39-5*)
Reagent grade of commerce containing not less than 86% of material with a molecular weight of 2×10^7 or greater.
A 0.1% w/v solution in *imidazole buffer solution pH 6.5* (solution A) complies with the following tests. All spectrophotometric measurements are made at 260 nm, Appendix II B.
A. Dilute 1 ml of solution A to 25 ml with the buffer solution. The *absorbance* is 0.4 to 0.8.
B. Mix 0.5 ml of solution A with 0.5 ml of the buffer solution, add 3.0 ml of *perchloric acid* (2.5% w/v $HClO_4$) and centrifuge. The *absorbance* of the supernatant liquid is not more than 0.3, using in the reference cell a mixture of 1 ml of the buffer solution and 3 ml of the perchloric acid.
C. To each of two tubes add 0.5 ml of solution A and 0.5 ml of a reference preparation containing 10 IU per ml of streptodornase in *imidazole buffer solution pH 6.5*. Add 3 ml of *perchloric acid* (2.5% w/v ($HClO_4$) to one tube, incubate the other at 37° for 15 minutes and then add 3 ml of the perchloric acid and centrifuge. The *absorbance* of the incubated supernatant liquid is not less than 0.15, using in the reference cell the untreated supernatant liquid.

Sodium Diethyldithiocarbamate $C_5H_{10}NNaS_2,3H_2O$ = 225.3 (*20624-25-3*)
Analytical reagent grade of commerce.

Sodium Diethyldithiocarbamate Solution A 0.1% w/v solution of *sodium diethyldithiocarbamate* in *water*.
Prepare immediately before use.

Sodium Dihydrogen Orthophosphate Sodium dihydrogen phosphate; $NaH_2PO_4,2H_2O$ = 156.0 (*10028-24-7*)
Analytical reagent grade of commerce.

Sodium Dihydrogen Orthophosphate, Anhydrous Anhydrous sodium dihydrogen phosphate; NaH_2PO_4 = 120.0 (*7558-80-7*)
Analytical reagent grade of commerce.
Store in an airtight container.

Sodium Dihydrogen Orthophosphate Monohydrate Sodium dihydrogen phosphate monohydrate; NaH_2PO_4,H_2O = 138.0 (*10049-21-5*)
Analytical reagent grade of commerce.
Store in an airtight container.

Sodium Dihydrogen Phosphate See *sodium dihydrogen orthophosphate.*

Sodium Dihydrogen Phosphate, Anhydrous See *anhydrous sodium dihydrogen orthophosphate.*

Sodium Dihydrogen Phosphate Monohydrate See *sodium dihydrogen orthophosphate monohydrate.*

Sodium Dithionite $Na_2S_2O_4$ = 174 (*7775-14-6*)
General reagent grade of commerce.
A white or greyish white, crystalline powder.
Store in an airtight container.

Sodium Dodecyl Sulphate Sodium lauryl sulphate; $C_{12}H_{25}NaO_4S$ = 288.4 (*151-21-3*)
Purified grade of commerce containing not less than 99.0% of $C_{12}H_{25}NaO_4S$.
White, crystalline flakes.

Sodium Edetate See *disodium edetate.*

Sodium Fluoresceinate See *fluorescein sodium.*

Sodium Fluoride NaF = 41.99 (*7681-49-4*)
Analytical reagent grade of commerce.

Sodium Formate HCO_2Na = 68.01 (*3996-15-4*)
General reagent grade of commerce.

Sodium Glucuronate D-Glucuronic acid, sodium salt; $C_6H_9NaO_7,H_2O$ = 234.1
General reagent grade of commerce.
$[\alpha]_D^{20}$, about +21.5°, determined in a 2% w/v solution.

Sodium Heptanesulphonate 1-Heptanesulphonic acid sodium salt; $C_7H_{15}NaO_3S$ = 202.3 (*22767-50-6*)
Chromatographic reagent grade of commerce containing not less than 96.0% of $C_7H_{15}NaO_3S$

Sodium Heptanesulphonate Monohydrate 1-Heptanesulphonic acid sodium salt monohydrate; $C_7H_{15}NaO_3S,H_2O$ = 220.3
Chromatographic reagent grade of commerce containing not less than 96.0% of $C_7H_{15}NaO_3S$, calculated with reference to the anhydrous substance.
Complies with the following tests.
WATER Not more than 8%, Appendix IX C. Use 0.3 g.
ASSAY Dissolve 0.15 g in 50 ml of *anhydrous acetic acid* and carry out Method I for *non-aqueous titration,* Appendix VIII A, determining the end point potentiometrically. Each ml of 0.01M *perchloric acid VS* is equivalent to 20.22 mg of $C_7H_{15}NaO_3S$.

Sodium Hexanesulphonate Hexanesulphonic acid sodium salt; $C_6H_{13}NaO_3S$ = 188.2 (*2832-45-3*)
Chromatographic reagent grade of commerce.

Sodium Hydrogen Carbonate Sodium bicarbonate; $NaHCO_3$ = 84.01 (*144-55-8*)
Analytical reagent grade of commerce.

Sodium Hydrogen Carbonate Solution A 4.2% w/v solution of *sodium hydrogen carbonate.*

Sodium Hydroxide NaOH = 40.00 (*1310-73-2*)
Analytical reagent grade of commerce containing not less than 97% of total alkali calculated as NaOH and not more than 2.0% of Na_2CO_3.
White, deliquescent pellets, sticks or slabs.
ASSAY Dissolve 2 g in 25 ml of *water* and add 25 ml of *barium chloride solution R1* and 0.3 ml of *phenolphthalein solution.* Titrate with 1M *hydrochloric acid VS,* add 0.3 ml of *bromophenol blue solution* and continue the titration with 1M *hydrochloric acid VS.* Each ml of 1M *hydrochloric acid* used in the second part of the titration is equivalent to 52.99 mg of Na_2CO_3. Each ml of 1M *hydrochloric acid VS* used in the combined titrations is equivalent to 40.00 mg of total alkali, calculated as NaOH.
Store in an airtight container.

Sodium Hydroxide, Ethanolic Solutions of the requisite molarity may be obtained by dissolving the appropriate amount of *sodium hydroxide* in sufficient *ethanol (96%)* to produce 1000 ml.

Sodium Hydroxide, Methanolic Solutions of the requisite molarity may be obtained by dissolving the appropriate amount of *sodium hydroxide* in sufficient *methanol* to produce 1000 ml.

Sodium Hydroxide Solution A 20% w/v solution of *sodium hydroxide.* Verify the concentration by titration with 1M *hydrochloric acid VS* using *methyl orange solution* as indicator and adjust, if necessary (5M).

Sodium Hydroxide Solution, Dilute An 8.5% w/v solution of *sodium hydroxide* (about 2M).

Sodium Hydroxide Solution, Methanolic Dissolve 40 mg of *sodium hydroxide* in 50 ml of *water,* cool and add 50 ml of *methanol.*

Sodium Hydroxide Solution, Strong A 42% w/v solution of *sodium hydroxide* (about 10M).

Sodium Hypobromite Solution Mix 20 ml of 10M *sodium hydroxide* and 500 ml of *water* in an ice bath, add 5 ml of *bromine solution* and stir gently until solution is complete.
Prepare immediately before use.

Sodium Hypochlorite Solution
General reagent grade of commerce containing 10 to 14% w/v of available chlorine.

Sodium Hypochlorite Solution (3% Cl) Strong sodium hypochlorite solution
General reagent grade sodium hypochlorite solution of commerce diluted to contain not less than 2.5% and not more than 3.0% w/v of available chlorine.
ASSAY Add to a flask, successively, 50 ml of *water,* 1 g of *potassium iodide* and 12.5 ml of 2M *acetic acid.* Dilute 10 ml of the reagent being examined to 100 ml with *water,* add 10 ml of this solution to the flask and titrate with 0.1M *sodium thiosulphate VS* using 1 ml of *starch solution* as indicator. Each ml of 0.1M *sodium thiosulphate VS* is equivalent to 3.546 mg of active chlorine.
Store protected from light.

Sodium Hypochlorite Solution, Dilute Dilute 35 ml of *sodium hypochlorite solution* to 100 ml with *water* immediately before use.
The solution contains approximately 3.5% w/v of available chlorine.

Sodium Hypochlorite Solution, Strong See *sodium hypochlorite solution (3% Cl)*.

Sodium Hypophosphite Sodium phosphinate monohydrate; NaH_2PO_2,H_2O = 106.0 (*10039-56-2*)
General reagent grade of commerce.
Store in an airtight container.

Sodium Iodide NaI = 149.9 (*7681-82-5*)
Analytical reagent grade of commerce.

Sodium Iodobismuthate Solution Boil for a few minutes a mixture of 2.6 g of *bismuth oxycarbonate*, 7.0 g of *sodium iodide* and 25 ml of *glacial acetic acid*. Allow to stand for 12 hours and filter, if necessary, through sintered glass. To 20 ml of the filtrate add 80 ml of *ethyl acetate* (solution A). Immediately before use, mix 2 ml of solution A, 20 ml of *glacial acetic acid* and 40 ml of *ethyl acetate*.

For use in connection with thin-layer chromatography the sensitivity may be increased by spraying first with this solution and then with *sulphuric acid (0.2%)*.
Solution A should be kept in a well-closed container.

Sodium Lauryl Sulphate See *sodium dodecyl sulphate*.

Sodium Metabisulphite Sodium pyrosulphite; $Na_2S_2O_5$ = 190.1 (*7681-57-4*)
Analytical reagent grade of commerce containing not less than 95.0% of $Na_2S_2O_5$.

Sodium Methanesulphonate Methanesulphonic acid, sodium salt; CH_3SO_3Na = 118.1 (*2386-57-4*)
General reagent grade of commerce.
Hygroscopic; store in an airtight container.

Sodium Molybdate $Na_2MoO_4,2H_2O$ = 242.0 (*10102-40-6*)
Analytical reagent grade of commerce.

Sodium Molybdotungstophosphate Solution Boil under a reflux condenser 350 ml of *water*, 50 g of *sodium tungstate*, 12 g of *phosphomolybdic acid* and 25 ml of *orthophosphoric acid* for 2 hours. Cool and add sufficient *water* to produce 500 ml.

Sodium Naphthoquinonesulphonate See *sodium 1,2-naphthoquinone-4-sulphonate*.

Sodium 1,2-Naphthoquinone-4-sulphonate Sodium naphthoquinonesulphonate; $C_{10}H_5NaO_5S$ = 260.2 (*521-24-4*)
General reagent grade of commerce.
A yellow or orange-yellow, crystalline powder.

Sodium Nitrate $NaNO_3$ = 85.0 (*7631-99-4*)
Analytical reagent grade of commerce.
A white powder or colourless, transparent crystals; deliquescent in moist air.
Store in an airtight container.

Sodium Nitrite $NaNO_2$ = 69.00 (*7632-00-0*)
Analytical reagent grade of commerce containing not less than 97.0% of $NaNO_2$.

Sodium Nitrite Solution A 10% w/v solution of *sodium nitrite*.
Prepare immediately before use.

Sodium Nitroprusside Sodium pentacyanonitrosylferrate(III) dihydrate; $Na_2[Fe(CN)_5(NO)],2H_2O$ = 298.0 (*13755-38-9*)
Analytical reagent grade of commerce.
Reddish brown powder or crystals.

Sodium Nitroprusside—Carbonate Solution Dissolve 1 g of *sodium nitroprusside* and 1 g of *anhydrous sodium carbonate* in sufficient *water* to produce 100 ml.

Sodium Octanesulphonate Octanesulphonic acid sodium salt; $C_8H_{17}NaO_3S$ = 216.3 (*5324-84-5*)
General reagent grade of commerce containing not less than 98% of $C_8H_{17}NaO_3S$.

Sodium Octanoate Sodium caprylate; octanoic acid sodium salt; $C_8H_{15}NaO_2$ = 166.2 (*1984-06-1*)
General reagent grade of commerce.

Sodium Octyl Sulphate 4-Octyl sulphate sodium salt; $C_8H_{17}NaO_4S$ = 232.3 (*142-31-4*)
Chromatographic reagent grade of commerce.

Sodium Oxalate $C_2Na_2O_4$ = 134.0 (*62-76-0*)
Analytical reagent grade of commerce.
A white crystalline powder.

Sodium Pentanesulphonate 1-Pentanesulphonic acid sodium salt; $C_5H_{11}NaO_3S$ = 174.2 (*22767-49-3*)
Chromatographic reagent grade of commerce.

Sodium Perchlorate $NaClO_4,H_2O$ = 140.5 (*7791-07-3*)
Analytical reagent grade of commerce containing not less than 99.0% of $NaClO_4,H_2O$; deliquescent.
Store in a well-closed container.

Sodium Periodate Sodium metaperiodate; $NaIO_4$ = 213.9 (*7790-28-5*)
Analytical reagent grade of commerce containing not less than 99.0% of $NaIO_4$.

Sodium Periodate Solution Dissolve 1.07 g of *sodium periodate* in *water*, and add 5 ml of 1M *sulphuric acid* and sufficient *water* to produce 100 ml.
It should be freshly prepared.

Sodium Phosphite Disodium phosphite; sodium phosphonate; $Na_2HPO_3,5H_2O$ = 216 (*13517-23-2*)
General reagent grade of commerce.

Sodium Picrate Solution, Alkaline Mix 20 ml of *picric acid solution* with 10 ml of a 5% w/v solution of *sodium hydroxide* and dilute to 100 ml with *water*.
Use within 2 days of preparation.

Sodium Potassium Tartrate See *potassium sodium (+)-tartrate*.

Sodium Pyrophosphate $Na_4P_2O_7,10H_2O$ = 446.1 (*13472-36-1*)
Analytical reagent grade of commerce.
Colourless, slightly efflorescent crystals.

Sodium Salicylate $C_7H_5NaO_3$ = 160.1 (*54-21-7*)
General reagent grade of commerce.

Sodium Starch Glycollate
General reagent grade of commerce complying with the following test.
SENSITIVITY TO IODINE Dissolve 10 mg in 7 ml of *water* and add 0.2 ml of 0.005M *iodine VS*. A distinct blue colour is produced.

Sodium Sulphate $Na_2SO_4,10H_2O$ = 322.2 (*7727-73-3*)
Analytical reagent grade of commerce.

Sodium Sulphate, Anhydrous Na_2SO_4 = 142.0 (*7757-82-6*)
Analytical reagent grade of commerce complying with the following test.
LOSS ON DRYING When dried at 130°, loses not more than 0.5% of its weight.

Sodium Sulphide Na_2S +aq (*1313-84-4*)
Analytical reagent grade of commerce.
Deliquescent, crystalline masses which turn yellow on storage.

Store in an airtight container.

Sodium Sulphide Solution Dissolve, with heating, 12 g of *sodium sulphide* in 45 ml of a mixture of 10 volumes of *water* and 29 volumes of *glycerol (85%)*, allow to cool and dilute to 100 ml with the same mixture.
It should be colourless.

Sodium Sulphite $Na_2SO_3,7H_2O$ = 252.2 (*27610-45-3*)
General reagent grade of commerce containing not less than 95.0% of $Na_2SO_3,7H_2O$.

Sodium Sulphite, Anhydrous Na_2SO_3 = 126.0 (*7757-83-7*)
Analytical reagent grade of commerce containing not less than 95.0% of Na_2SO_3.

Sodium Tartrate See *sodium (+)-tartrate*.

Sodium (+)-Tartrate Sodium tartrate; $C_4H_4O_6Na_2,2H_2O$ = 230.1 (*6106-24-7*)
Analytical reagent grade of commerce.

Sodium Tetraborate Borax; disodium tetraborate; $Na_2B_4O_7,10H_2O$ = 381.4 (*1330-43-4*)
Analytical reagent grade of commerce.

Sodium Tetradeuteriodimethylsilapentanoate
Sodium (2,2,3,3-D_4)-4,4-dimethyl-4-silapentanoate; $C_6H_9D_4NaO_2Si$ = 172.3
General reagent grade of commerce with an isotopic purity of not less than 99% and containing not more than 0.5% of water and deuterium oxide.

Sodium Tetraphenylborate $(C_6H_5)_4BNa$ = 342.2 (*143-66-8*)
General reagent grade of commerce.
A white or slightly yellowish, bulky powder.

Sodium Tetraphenylborate Solution A 1% w/v solution of *sodium tetraphenylborate*.
Use within 1 week and filter before use, if necessary.

Sodium Thioglycollate Sodium mercaptoacetate; $C_2H_3NaO_2S$ = 114.1 (*367-51-1*)
General reagent grade of commerce.
Store in an airtight container.

Sodium Thiosulphate $Na_2S_2O_3,5H_2O$ = 248.2 (*10102-17-7*)
Analytical reagent grade of commerce.

Sodium 3-Trimethylsilylpropanesulphonate
$C_6H_{15}NaO_3SSi$ = 236.3 (*2039-96-5*)
Use a grade of commerce suitable for NMR spectroscopy.
A white, hygroscopic, crystalline powder; melting point, about 125°, with decomposition.

Sodium Tungstate $Na_2WO_4,2H_2O$ = 329.9 (*10213-10-2*)
Analytical reagent grade of commerce.

Solochrome Dark Blue CI 15705; calcon; mordant black 17; $C_{20}H_{13}N_2NaO_5S$ = 416.4 (*2538-85-4*)
General reagent grade of commerce.
A brownish black powder with a violet sheen. Produces a purplish red colour with calcium ions in alkaline solutions. When metal ions are absent, for example, in the presence of an excess of disodium edetate, the solution is blue.

Solochrome Dark Blue Mixture A mixture of 1 part of *solochrome dark blue* with 99 parts of freshly ignited *anhydrous sodium sulphate*.
Complies with the following test.
SENSITIVITY TO CALCIUM Dissolve 0.2 g in 5 ml of *water*. To 1 ml of the solution add 50 ml of *water*, 10 ml of 1M *sodium hydroxide* and 1 ml of a 1% w/v solution of *magnesium sulphate*; a blue colour is produced. Add 0.1 ml of a 0.15% w/v solution of *calcium chloride*; a violet colour is produced. Add 0.1 ml of 0.01M *disodium edetate VS*; a pure blue colour is produced.

Sorbic Acid Hexa-2,4-dienoic acid; $C_6H_8O_2$ = 112.1 (*110-44-1*)
General reagent grade of commerce.
Melting point, about 136°.

Sorbitol See *D-sorbitol*.

D-Sorbitol Sorbitol; $C_6H_{14}O_6$ = 182.2 (*50-70-4*)
General reagent grade of commerce.
A white, microcrystalline powder; melting point, about 95°; $[\alpha]_D^{20}$, about +15° (5% w/v in 1M sodium hydroxide containing 15% w/v of sodium tetraborate).

Squalane 2,6,10,15,19,23-Hexamethyltetracosane; $C_{30}H_{62}$ = 422.8 (*111-01-3*)
Gas chromatographic reagent grade of commerce.
A colourless, oily liquid; d_{20}^{20}, 0.811 to 0.813; n_D^{20}, 1.451 to 1.453.

Stannous Chloride See *tin(II) chloride*.

Stannous Chloride Solution See *tin(II) chloride solution*.

Stannous Chloride Solution R1 See *tin(II) chloride solution R1*.

Stannous Chloride Solution R2 See *tin(II) chloride solution R2*.

Starch
Potato starch of commerce.

Starch, Hydrolysed
Electrophoretic grade of commerce.

Starch Iodate Paper Immerse strips of filter paper in 100 ml of *iodide-free starch solution* containing 0.1 g of *potassium iodate*. Drain and allow to dry protected from light.

Starch Iodide Paper Immerse strips of filter paper in 100 ml of *starch solution* containing 0.5 g of *potassium iodide*. Drain and allow to dry protected from light.
Complies with the following test.
SENSITIVITY Mix 0.05 ml of 0.1M *sodium nitrite* with 4 ml of *hydrochloric acid* and dilute to 100 ml with *water*. Deposit 0.05 ml of the solution on the paper. A blue spot appears.

Starch Iodide Solution Dissolve 0.5 g of *soluble starch* in 100 ml of *water* containing 0.5 g of *potassium iodide*.

Starch Mucilage Triturate 0.5 g of *starch* or *soluble starch* with 5 ml of *water* and add, stirring continuously, to sufficient *water* to produce about 100 ml. Boil for a few minutes, cool and filter.
Produces a blue colour with free iodine in the presence of a soluble iodide.
It must be recently prepared.

Starch, Soluble (*9005-84-9*)
Analytical reagent grade of commerce.
A 2% w/v solution in hot *water* is at most slightly opalescent and remains fluid on cooling.

Starch Solution Triturate 1.0 g of *soluble starch* with 5 ml of *water* and add, stirring continuously, to 100 ml of boiling *water* containing 10 mg of *mercury(II) iodide*.
Complies with the following test, which should be carried out each time the reagent is used.
SENSITIVITY TO IODINE A mixture of 1 ml with 20 ml of *water*, about 50 mg of *potassium iodide* and 0.05 ml of 0.005M *iodine VS* is blue.

Starch Solution, Iodide-free Triturate 1.0 g of *soluble starch* with 5 ml of *water* and add, stirring continuously, to 100 ml of boiling *water*.
Prepare immediately before use.

Starch Substrate Determine the water content of *starch EPBRP* by heating at 120° for 4 hours. Stir a quantity of *starch EPBRP* equivalent to 2.0 g of the dried substance with 10 ml of *water* and add, stirring continuously, to 160 ml of boiling *water*. Rinse the container with several 10-ml quantities of *water*, add the washings to the hot starch solution and heat to boiling, stirring continuously. Cool to 20° and add sufficient *water* to produce 200 ml. Use on the day of preparation.

Stearic Acid Octadecanoic acid; $C_{18}H_{36}O_2$ = 284.5 (*57-11-4*)
General reagent grade of commerce.
Melting point, about 70°.

Stearic Anhydride $C_{36}H_{70}O_3$ = 551.0 (*638-08-4*)
General reagent grade of commerce.
White, waxy flakes; melting point, about 70°.

Streptomycin Sulphate $(C_{21}H_{39}N_7O_{12})_2,3H_2SO_4$ = 1457 (*3810-74-0*)
General reagent grade of commerce.

Strontium Chloride $SrCl_2,6H_2O$ = 266.6 (*10025-70-4*)
Analytical reagent grade of commerce.

Styrene C_8H_8 = 104.2 (*100-42-5*)
General reagent grade of commerce containing not less than 99% of C_8H_8.
Boiling point, about 145°; n_D^{20}, about 1.547.

Styrene—Divinylbenzene Copolymer
Gas chromatographic reagent grade of commerce.
Porous, rigid, cross-linked polymer beads. Several grades are available with different sizes of beads. The size range of the beads is specified after the name of the reagent in the tests where it is used.

Succinic Acid Butanedioic acid; $C_4H_6O_4$ = 118 (*110-15-6*)
General reagent grade of commerce.
Melting point, 184° to 187°.

Sucrose $C_{12}H_{22}O_{11}$ = 342.3 (*57-50-1*)
Analytical reagent grade of commerce.
When sucrose is used for polarimetry, it must be kept dry in a sealed ampoule.

Sudan Orange See *Sudan yellow*.

Sudan Red CI 26100; sudan III; solvent red 23; 1-(4-phenylazophenylazo)-2-naphthol; $C_{22}H_{16}N_4O$ = 352.4 (*85-86-9*)
Technical reagent grade of commerce.
A reddish brown powder.

Sudan Red G CI 12150; sudan red I; 1-(2′-methoxyphenylazo)-2-naphthol; $C_{17}H_{14}N_2O_2$ = 278.3
HOMOGENEITY Carry out the method for *thin-layer chromatography*, Appendix III A, using *silica gel G* as the coating substance and *dichloromethane* as the mobile phase, but allowing the solvent front to ascend 10 cm above the line of application. Apply to the plate 10 µl of a 0.1% w/v solution in *dichloromethane*. The chromatogram shows only one principal spot.

Sudan Red Solution A 0.5% w/v solution of *sudan red* in *anhydrous acetic acid*.

Sudan Yellow CI 12055; Sudan orange; Sudan I; solvent yellow 14; 1-phenylazo-2-napththol; $C_{16}H_{14}N_4O$ = 278.3 (*842-07-9*)
Technical reagent grade of commerce.
A yellow, crystalline powder; melting point, about 160°.
Complies with the following test.
HOMOGENEITY Carry out the method for *thin-layer chromatography*, Appendix III A, using *silica gel G* as the coating substance and *dichloromethane* as the mobile phase. Apply to the plate 10 µl of a 0.01% w/v solution in *chloroform*. The chromatogram shows only one principal spot.

Sudan Yellow Solution A 0.2% w/v solution of *sudan yellow* in a mixture of 1 volume of *benzene* and 4 volumes of *petroleum spirit (boiling range, 60° to 80°)*.

Sulfathiazole See *sulphathiazole*.

Sulphamic Acid H_3NO_3S = 97.1 (*5329-14-6*)
General reagent grade of commerce.
White crystals or crystalline powder; melting point, about 205°, with decomposition.

Sulphan Blue CI 42045; patent blue VF, acid blue 1; $C_{27}H_{31}N_2NaO_6S_2$ = 566.7 (*129-17-9*)
General reagent grade of commerce.
A violet powder.

Sulphanilamide $C_6H_8N_2O_2S$ = 172.2 (*63-74-1*)
General reagent grade of commerce.
A white or almost white, crystalline powder; melting point, about 165°.

Sulphanilic Acid $C_6H_7NO_3S$ = 173.2 (*121-57-3*)
Analytical reagent grade of commerce.

Sulphanilic Acid, Diazotised Dissolve, with warming, 0.2 g of *sulphanilic acid* in 20 ml of 1M *hydrochloric acid*, cool in ice, add dropwise, stirring continuously, 2.2 ml of a 4% w/v solution of *sodium nitrite*, allow to stand in ice for 10 minutes and then add 1 ml of a 5% w/v solution of *sulphamic acid*.

Sulphanilic Acid Solution Mix 0.5 g of *sulphanilic acid*, 30 ml of *glacial acetic acid* and 120 ml of *water* and heat with stirring until dissolved. Allow to cool and filter.
Use the solution within 3 weeks.

Sulphathiazole N^1-Thiazol-2-ylsulphanilamide; $C_9H_9N_3O_2S$ = 255.3 (*72-14-0*)
General reagent grade of commerce.
A white or yellowish white powder or crystals; melting point about 200°.

Sulphomolybdic Reagent R2 Dissolve about 50 mg of *ammonium molybdate* in 10 ml of *sulphuric acid*.

Sulphomolybdic Reagent R3 Dissolve, with heating, 2.5 g of *ammonium molybdate* in 20 ml of *water*. Separately, with care, add 28 ml of *sulphuric acid* to 50 ml of *water* and cool. Mix the two solutions and dilute to 100 ml with *water*.
Store in a polyethylene container.

Sulphosalicylic Acid 5-Sulpho-2-hydroxybenzoic acid; 3-sulpho-6-hydroxybenzoic acid; $C_7H_6O_6S,2H_2O$ = 254.2 (*5965-83-3*)
Analytical reagent grade of commerce.
A white, crystalline powder or crystals; melting point, about 109°.

Sulphur See *precipitated sulphur*.

Sulphur Dioxide SO_2 = 64.05 (*7446-09-5*)
Laboratory cylinder grade of commerce.
A colourless gas with an acrid, penetrating odour.

Sulphur Dioxide R1 *Sulphur dioxide* containing not less than 99.9% v/v of SO_2.

Sulphur Dioxide Solution Sulphurous acid; H_2SO_3 = 82.08
Use a solution of commerce containing about 5% w/v of SO_2; weight per ml, about 1.03 g.

Sulphur, Precipitated S = 32.1 *(7704-34-9)*
Precipitated grade of commerce.
A pale, greyish yellow or greenish yellow, soft powder.

Sulphuric Acid H_2SO_4 = 98.08 *(7664-93-9)*
When no molarity is indicated use analytical reagent grade of commerce containing about 96% w/w of sulphuric acid and about 18M in strength; an oily, corrosive liquid; weight per ml, about 1.84 g.

When solutions of molarity *x*M are required, they should be prepared by carefully adding 54*x* ml of *sulphuric acid* to an equal volume of *water* and diluting to 1000 ml with *water*.

When '*sulphuric acid*' is followed by a percentage figure, an instruction to add, carefully, *sulphuric acid* to *water* to produce the specified percentage v/v (or, if required, w/w) proportion of sulphuric acid is implied.

Sulphuric Acid, 2.5M Alcoholic Carefully and with constant cooling stir 14 ml of *sulphuric acid* into 60 ml of *absolute ethanol*, allow to cool and add sufficient *absolute ethanol* to produce 100 ml. Prepare immediately before use.

Sulphuric Acid, 0.25M Alcoholic Dilute 10 ml of 2.5M *alcoholic sulphuric acid* to 100 ml with *absolute ethanol*. Prepare immediately before use.

Sulphuric Acid, Dilute Add 5.5 ml of *sulphuric acid* to 60 ml of *water*, allow to cool and add sufficient *water* to produce 100 ml. Contains 9.8% w/v of H_2SO_4 (about 1M)

Sulphuric Acid, Ethanolic Solutions of the requisite molarity may be obtained by mixing *sulphuric acid* with *ethanol (96%)* as directed under *sulphuric acid*.

When '*ethanolic sulphuric acid*' is followed by a percentage figure, an instruction to use *sulphuric acid* diluted with *ethanol (96%)* to produce the specified percentage v/v proportion of sulphuric acid is implied.

Sulphuric Acid-Formaldehyde Reagent Mix 2 ml of *formaldehyde solution* with 100 ml of *sulphuric acid (96% w/w)*.

Sulphuric Acid, Methanolic Solutions of the requisite molarity may be obtained by mixing *sulphuric acid* with *methanol* as directed under *sulphuric acid*.

When '*methanolic sulphuric acid*' is followed by a percentage figure, an instruction to use *sulphuric acid* diluted with *methanol* to produce the specified percentage v/v proportion of sulphuric acid is implied.

Sulphuric Acid, Nitrogen-free
Nitrogen-free sulphuric acid of commerce containing about 96% w/w of H_2SO_4.
Complies with the following test.
NITRATES To 5 ml of *water* add carefully 45 ml of the reagent being examined, allow to cool to 40° and add 8 mg of N,N′-*diphenylbenzidine*. The solution is faint pink or very pale blue.

Sunflower Oil
The fixed oil obtained by expression from the seeds of *Helianthus annuus* L.
A clear, pale yellow liquid complying with the following tests.
HYDROXYL VALUE 14 to 16, Appendix X D.
IODINE VALUE 125 to 136 *(iodine bromide method)*, Appendix X E.
SAPONIFICATION VALUE 188 to 194, Appendix X G, Method II.

Tagatose D-*lyxo*-Hexulose; $C_6H_{12}O_6$ = 180.16 *(87-81-0)*
General reagent grade of commerce.
Melting point, 134° to 135°; $[\alpha]_D^{20}$, −2.3° (2.19% w/v solution in water).

Talc *(14807-96-6)*
Purified grade of commerce.
A very fine, white powder.

Tannic Acid *(1401-55-4)*
General reagent grade of commerce.
Yellowish to light brown, glistening scales or amorphous powder.
Store protected from light.

Tannic Acid Reagent Dissolve 25 mg of *tannic acid* in 20 ml of *glacial acetic acid* and add 80 ml of *orthophosphoric acid*.
Prepare immediately before use.

Tartaric Acid See *(+)-tartaric acid.*

(+)-Tartaric Acid $C_4H_6O_6$ = 150.1 *(87-69-4)*
Analytical reagent grade of commerce.

α-Terpineol (*RS*)-2-(4-Methylcyclohex-3-enyl)propan-2-ol; $C_{10}H_{18}O$ = 154.2 *(98-55-5)*
General reagent grade of commerce.
It may contain 1% to 3% of β-terpineol.
Melting point, about 35°; d_{20}^{20}, about 0.935; n_D^{20}, about 1.483; $[\alpha]_D^{20}$, about 92.5°.
α-Terpineol used in gas chromatography complies with the following test.
ASSAY Examine by *gas chromatography*, Appendix III B, under the conditions described in the test for Chromatographic profile in the monograph for Anise Oil using as solution (1) a 10% w/v solution of the reagent being examined in *hexane*.

The area of the principal peak is not less than 97.0% of the total area of the peaks. Disregard the peak due to hexane.

Testosterone $C_{19}H_{28}O_2$ = 288.4 *(58-22-0)*
General reagent grade of commerce.
Melting point, about 154°.

Testosterone Propionate $C_{22}H_{32}O_3$ = 344.5 *(57-85-2)*
General reagent grade of commerce.
Melting point, about 121°.

Tetrabutylammonium Bromide $C_{16}H_{36}BrN$ = 322.4 *(1643-19-2)*
General reagent grade of commerce.
Melting point, 102° to 104°.

Tetrabutylammonium Dihydrogen Orthophosphate
Tetrabutylammonium dihydrogen phosphate; $C_{16}H_{38}NO_4P$ = 339.5 *(5574-97-0)*
General reagent grade of commerce.
Melting point, about 153°.
Store in an airtight container.

Tetrabutylammonium Dihydrogen Phosphate See *tetrabutylammonium dihydrogen orthophosphate.*

Tetrabutylammonium Hydrogen Sulphate
$C_{16}H_{37}NO_4S$ = 339.5 *(32503-27-8)*
Analytical reagent grade of commerce.
A white, crystalline powder; melting point, 169° to 173°.
Complies with the following tests.

ABSORBANCE *Absorbance* of a 5.0% w/v solution in the range 240 nm to 300 nm, Appendix II B, not greater than 0.05.
pH A 1.7% w/v solution has a pH of about 1.5, Appendix V L.

Tetrabutylammonium Hydroxide $C_{16}H_{37}NO$ = 259.5 (*2052-49-5*)
General reagent grade of commerce containing about 40% w/v of $C_{16}H_{37}NO$.
Weight per ml, about 0.990 g.

Tetrabutylammonium Hydroxide Solution
General reagent grade of commerce containing 40.0% w/v of $C_{16}H_{37}NO$.

Tetrabutylammonium Hydroxide Solution (104 g/l)
Dilute *tetrabutylammonium hydroxide* to contain 10.4% w/v of $C_{16}H_{37}NO$.

Tetrabutylammonium Iodide $C_{16}H_{36}IN$ = 369.4 (*311-28-4*)
General reagent grade of commerce containing not less than 98.0% of $C_{16}H_{36}IN$.
Complies with the following requirements.
SULPHATED ASH Not more than 0.02%.
ASSAY Dissolve 1.2 g in 30 ml of *water* and add 50 ml of 0.1M *silver nitrate VS* and 5 ml of 2M *nitric acid*. Titrate the excess of silver nitrate with 0.1M *ammonium thiocyanate VS* using 2 ml of *ammonium iron(III) sulphate solution R2* as indicator. Each ml of 0.1M *silver nitrate VS* is equivalent to 36.94 mg of $C_{16}H_{36}IN$.

Tetrachloroethane 1,1,2,2-Tetrachloroethane; $C_2H_2Cl_4$ = 167.9 (*79-34-5*)
General reagent grade of commerce.
d_{20}^{20}, about 1.59; n_D^{20}, about 1.495. Not less than 95% distils between 145° and 147°.

Tetracycline $C_{22}H_{24}N_2O_8$ = 444.4 (*60-54-8*)
General reagent grade of commerce.
Melting point, about 176°.
Store protected from light.

***n*-Tetradecane** $C_{14}H_{30}$ = 198.4 (*629-59-4*)
General reagent grade of commerce containing not less than 99.5% of $C_{14}H_{30}$.
A colourless liquid; d_{20}^{20}, about 0.76; n_D^{20}, about 1.429; melting point, about –5°; boiling point, about 253°.

Tetradecylammonium Bromide $C_{40}H_{84}BrN$ = 659.0 (*14937-42-9*)
Chromatographic reagent grade of commerce.
Melting point, 88° to 89°.

Tetraethylammonium Hydroxide Solution $C_8H_{21}NO$ = 147.3 (*77-98-5*)
Chromatographic reagent grade of commerce containing 20% w/v of $C_8H_{21}NO$.
d_{20}^{20}, about 1.01; n_D^{20}, about 1.372.

Tetraethylene Pentamine 3,6,9-Triazaundecan-1,11-diamine; $C_8H_{21}N_5$ = 189.3 (*112-57-2*)
General reagent grade of commerce.
n_D^{20}, about 1.506.
Store protected from humidity and heat.

Tetraheptylammonium Bromide $C_{28}H_{60}BrN$ = 490.7 (*4368-51-8*)
Chromatographic reagent grade of commerce.
Melting point, 89° to 91°.

Tetrahexylammonium Hydrogen Sulphate
$C_{24}H_{52}N,HSO_4$ = 451.8 (*32503-34-7*)
Chromatographic reagent grade of commerce.

Tetrahydrofuran Tetramethylene oxide; C_4H_8O = 72.11 (*109-99-9*)
Analytical reagent grade of commerce.
A clear, colourless, flammable liquid; boiling point, about 66°; d_{20}^{20}, about 0.89.
Do not distil unless it complies with the following test.
PEROXIDES Place 8 ml of *potassium iodide and starch solution* in a ground-glass-stoppered cylinder with a capacity of 12 ml and about 1.5 cm in diameter and add sufficient of the substance being examined to fill the cylinder completely, shake vigorously and allow to stand for 30 minutes protected from light. No colour is produced.
Tetrahydrofuran used in spectrophotometry complies with the following additional requirement.
TRANSMITTANCE Not less than 20% at 255 nm, 80% at 270 nm and 98% at 310 nm determined using *water* in the reference cell.

Tetrahydrofuran, Stabiliser-free *Tetrahydrofuran* that is free from stabilisers and inhibitors.
Reagent grade of commerce.

Tetramethylammonium Chloride $C_4H_{12}ClN$ = 109.6 (*75-57-0*)
General reagent grade of commerce.
Melting point, about 300°, with decomposition.

Tetramethylammonium Hydrogen Sulphate
$C_4H_{13}NO_4S$ = 171.2 (*80526-82-5*)
Chromatographic grade of commerce.
Tetramethylammonium hydrogen sulphate used in liquid chromatography complies with the following requirement.
TRANSMITTANCE Not less than 50% at 200 nm and 90% at 220 nm determined using a 0.005M solution.

Tetramethylammonium Hydroxide Pentahydrate
$C_4H_{13}NO,5H_2O$ = 181.2 (*10424-65-4*)
General reagent grade of commerce.
Melting point, about 66°.

Tetramethylammonium Hydroxide Solution
General reagent grade of commerce containing not less than 10.0% w/w of $C_4H_{13}NO$.
A clear, colourless or very pale liquid.
ASSAY To 1 g add 50 ml of *water* and titrate with 0.05M *sulphuric acid VS* using *methyl red solution* as indicator. Each ml of 0.05M *sulphuric acid VS* is equivalent to 9.115 mg of $C_4H_{13}NO$.

Tetramethylammonium Hydroxide Solution, Dilute
Dilute 10 ml of *tetramethylammonium hydroxide solution* to 100 ml with *aldehyde-free ethanol (96%)*. It contains about 1% w/v of $C_4H_{13}NO$.
Prepare immediately before use.

Tetramethyldiaminodiphenylmethane See *4,4′-methylenebis-(*N,N*-dimethylaniline)*.

Tetramethyldiaminodiphenylmethane Reagent See *4,4′-methylenebis-(*N,N*-dimethylaniline) reagent*.

Tetramethylethylenediamine Tetramethylethane-1,2-diamine; *N,N,N′,N′*-Tetramethylethylenediamine; $C_6H_{16}N_2$ = 116.2 (*110-18-9*)
General reagent grade of commerce.
A colourless liquid; boiling point, about 121°; d_{20}^{20}, about 0.78.

***N,N,N′,N′*-Tetramethyl-*p*-phenylenediamine Dihydrochloride** $C_{10}H_{16}N_2,2HCl$ = 237.2 (*637-01-4*)
General reagent grade of commerce.
Whitish grey crystals.

Tetramethylsilane $(CH_3)_4Si$ = 88.23 *(75-76-3)*
Spectroscopic reagent grade of commerce.
A colourless liquid; d_{20}^{20}, about 0.64; n_D^{20}, about 1.358; boiling point, about 26°.
When used in nuclear magnetic spectrometry, complies with the following test.
NUCLEAR MAGNETIC RESONANCE In the NMR spectrum of a 10% v/v solution of the reagent being examined in *deuterochloroform*, the intensity of any foreign signal, excluding those due to spinning side bands and to chloroform, is not greater than the intensity of the ^{13}C-satellite signals located at a distance of 59.1 Hz on each side of the principal signal of tetramethylsilane.

1,2,3,4-Tetraphenylcyclopenta-1,3-diene $C_{29}H_{22}$ = 370.5 *(15570-45-3)*
General reagent grade of commerce.
Melting point, about 178°.

1,2,3,4-Tetraphenylcyclopenta-1,3-dienone Tetraphenylcyclopentadienone; $C_{29}H_{20}O$ = 384.5 *(479-33-4)*
General reagent grade of commerce.
Melting point, about 218°.

Tetraphenylethylene $C_{26}H_{20}$ = 332.5 *(632-51-9)*
General reagent grade of commerce.
Melting point, about 223°.

Tetrazolium Blue Blue tetrazolium salt; 3,3′-(3,3′-dimethoxy-4,4′-biphenylylene)bis(2,5-diphenyl-2*H*-tetrazolium chloride); $C_{40}H_{32}Cl_2N_8O_2$ = 727.7 *(1871-22-3)*
General reagent grade of commerce.
Yellow crystals; melting point, about 245°, with decomposition.

Tetrazolium Blue Solution, Alkaline Immediately before use mix 1 volume of a 0.2% w/v solution of *tetrazolium blue* in *methanol* with 3 volumes of a 12% w/v solution of *sodium hydroxide* in *methanol*.

Thallium(I) Nitrate Thallous nitrate; $TlNO_3$ = 266.4 *(10102-45-1)*
General reagent grade of commerce.

Thallium(I) Sulphate Thallous sulphate; Tl_2SO_4 = 504.8 *(7446-18-6)*
White, rhomboid prisms.

Thallous Sulphate See *thallium(I) sulphate.*

Thebaine (5*R*,9*R*,13*S*)-4,5-Epoxy-3,6-dimethoxy-9a-methylmorphina-6,8-diene; $C_{19}H_{21}N)_3$ = 311.4 *(115-37-7)*
General reagent grade of commerce.
A white or pale yellow powder; melting point, about 193°.
Complies with the following test.
CHROMATOGRAPHY Carry out Identification test B in the monograph for Opium applying to the plate as a band (20 mm × 3 mm) 20 µl of a 0.05% w/v solution. The chromatogram obtained shows an orange-red or red principal spot with a Rf value of about 0.5.

Theophylline $C_7H_8N_4O_2$ = 180.2 *(58-55-9)*
General reagent grade of commerce.
Melting point, about 272°.

Thiamazole See *methimazole.*

2-(2-Thienyl)acetic Acid 2-Thiopheneacetic acid; $C_6H_6O_2S$ = 142.1 *(1918-77-0)*
General reagent grade of commerce.
Melting point, about 65°.

Thioacetamide C_2H_5NS = 75.13 *(62-55-5)*
General reagent grade of commerce.
White crystals or crystalline powder; melting point, about 113°.

Thioacetamide Reagent Add 1 ml of a mixture of 15 ml of 1M *sodium hydroxide*, 5 ml of *water* and 20 ml of *glycerol (85%)* to 0.2 ml of *thioacetamide solution*, heat in a water bath for 20 seconds, cool and use immediately.

Thioacetamide Solution A 4% w/v solution of *thioacetamide.*

Thiobarbituric Acid 4,6-Dihydroxy-2-mercaptopyrimidine; $C_4H_4N_2O_2S$ = 144.2 *(504-17-6)*
General reagent grade of commerce.

Thiodiglycol Thiodiethanol; $C_4H_{10}O_2S$ = 122.2 *(111-48-8)*
General reagent grade of commerce.
n_D^{20}, about 1.522.

Thioglycollic Acid See *mercaptoacetic acid.*

Thiomersal $C_9H_9HgNaO_2S$ = 404.8 *(54-64-8)*
General reagent grade of commerce.
A light, yellowish white, crystalline powder; melting point, about 233°, with decomposition.

Thiourea CH_4N_2S = 76.12 *(62-56-6)*
Analytical reagent grade of commerce.
Melting point, about 178°.

Threonine See *L-threonine.*

L-Threonine $C_4H_9NO_3$ = 119.1 *(72-19-5)*
Chromatographic reagent grade of commerce.
A white, crystalline powder; $[\alpha]_D^{20}$, about −28° (2% w/v in water).
Complies with the following test.
HOMOGENEITY Carry out the method for *thin-layer chromatography*, Appendix III A, protected from light, using *silica gel G* as the coating substance and a mixture of 25 parts of *water* and 75 parts of *phenol* as the mobile phase but allowing the solvent front to ascend 12 cm from the line of application. Apply to the plate 5 µl of a 0.2% w/v solution of the reagent being examined and keep the plate in the vapour of the mobile phase for 12 hours before development. After removal of the plate, dry it, spray with a 0.1% w/v solution of *ninhydrin* in *butan-1-ol* saturated with *water* and heat at 100° to 105° for 10 minutes. The chromatogram shows only one spot.

Thrombin Human thrombin
Dried human thrombin obtained from liquid plasma. It may be prepared by precipitation with suitable salts and organic solvents under controlled conditions of pH, ionic strength and temperature.
General reagent grade of commerce.
A yellowish white powder.
Store in a sealed, sterile container under nitrogen, protected from light and at a temperature below 25°.

Thrombin, Bovine A preparation of the enzyme that converts fibrinogen into fibrin.
General reagent grade of commerce.

Thrombin, Human See *thrombin.*

Thrombin Solution Human thrombin solution
Reconstitute *thrombin* as directed by the manufacturer and dilute with *tris–chloride buffer pH 7.4* to contain 5 IU per ml.
Store below 0°.

Thrombin Solution, Human See *thrombin solution.*

Thromboplastin Reagent Thrombokinase extract
Extract 1.5 g of *acetone-dried ox brain* with 60 ml of *water* for 10 to 15 minutes at 50°, centifuge for 2 minutes at 1500 revolutions per minute and decant the supernatant liquid. This extract will retain its activity for several days when stored in a refrigerator. It may contain 0.3% w/v of o-*cresol* as an antimicrobial preservative.

Thymine 5-Methylpyrimidine-2,4(1*H*,3*H*)-dione; $C_5H_6N_2O_2$ = 126.1 *(65-71-4)*
General reagent grade of commerce.

Thymol 2-Isopropyl-5-methylphenol; $C_{10}H_{14}O$ = 150.2 *(89-83-8)*
General reagent grade of commerce.
Colourless crystals with an aromatic odour; melting point, about 50°.

Thymol Blue Thymolsulphonphthalein; 4,4′-(3*H*)-2,1-Benzoxathiol-3-ylidene)dithymol *S,S*-dioxide; $C_{27}H_{30}O_5S$ = 466.6 *(76-61-9)*
A brownish green to greenish blue crystalline powder.

Thymol Blue Solution Dissolve 0.1 g of *thymol blue* in 2.15 ml of 0.1M *sodium hydroxide* and 20 ml of *ethanol (96%)* and add sufficient *water* to produce 100 ml.
Complies with the following test.
SENSITIVITY A mixture of 0.1 ml and 100 ml of *carbon dioxide-free water* to which 0.2 ml of 0.02M *sodium hydroxide VS* has been added is blue. Not more than 0.1 ml of 0.02M *hydrochloric acid VS* is required to change the colour of the solution to yellow.
Colour change pH 1.2 (red) to pH 2.8 (yellow); pH 8.0 (olive green) to pH 9.6 (blue).

Thymolphthalein 3,3-Bis(4-hydroxy-5-isopropyl-2-methylphenyl)phthalide; $C_{28}H_{30}O_4$ = 430.5 *(125-20-2)*
Produces a colourless solution in acidic and weakly alkaline solutions and a blue colour in more strongly alkaline solutions.

Thymolphthalein Solution A 0.1% w/v solution of *thymolphthalein* in *ethanol (96%).*
Complies with the following test.
SENSITIVITY A mixture of 0.2 ml and 100 ml of *carbon dioxide-free water* is colourless. Not more than 0.05 ml of 0.1M *sodium hydroxide VS* is required to change the colour of the solution to blue.
Colour change: pH 9.3 (colourless) to pH 10.5 (blue).

Tin Granulated tin; Sn = 118.7 *(7440-31-5)*
Analytical granulated grade of commerce complying with the following test.
ARSENIC 0.1 g complies with *limit test A for arsenic,* Appendix VII (10 ppm).

Tin(II) Chloride Stannous chloride; $SnCl_2,2H_2O$ = 225.6 *(10025-69-1)*
Analytical reagent grade of commerce containing not less than 97.0% of $SnCl_2,2H_2O$.
ASSAY Dissolve 0.5 g in 15 ml of *hydrochloric acid* in a ground-glass-stoppered flask and add 10 ml of *water* and 5 ml of *chloroform.* Titrate rapidly with 0.05M *potassium iodate VS* until the chloroform layer is colourless. Each ml of 0.05M *potassium iodate VS* is equivalent to 22.56 mg of $SnCl_2,2H_2O$.

Tin(II) Chloride Solution Stannous chloride solution
Heat 20 g of *tin* with 85 ml of *hydrochloric acid* until no more hydrogen is evolved.
Store over an excess of tin and protected from air.

Tin(II) Chloride Solution AsT
Stannous chloride solution, low in arsenic, of commerce, or prepare from *tin(II) chloride solution* by adding an equal volume of *hydrochloric acid,* reducing the original volume by boiling and filtering through a fine-grain filter paper.
Complies with the following test.
To 10 ml add 6 ml of *water* and 10 ml of *hydrochloric acid,* distil and collect 16 ml. To the distillate add 50 ml of *water,* 0.1 ml of the solution, 5 ml of 0.1M *potassium iodide* and 5 g of *activated zinc.* Using the apparatus and procedure described for the *limit test for arsenic,* Appendix VII, the stain produced on *mercuric bromide paper* is not more intense than that produced when the test is repeated with the addition of 1 ml of *arsenic standard solution (1 ppm As).*

Tin(II) Chloride Solution R1 Stannous chloride solution R1
Immediately before use, dilute 1 volume of *tin(II) chloride solution* with 10 volumes of 2M *hydrochloric acid.*

Tin(II) Chloride Solution R2 Stannous chloride solution R2
To 8 g of *tin(II) chloride* add 100 ml of a 20% v/v solution of *hydrochloric acid.* Shake until dissolved, heating, if necessary, on a water bath at 50°. Pass a current of *nitrogen* through the solution for 15 minutes.
Prepare immediately before use.

Titan Yellow CI 19540; thiazol yellow; $C_{28}H_{19}N_5Na_2O_6S_4$ = 696 *(1829-00-1)*
A yellowish brown powder.

Titan Yellow Paper Impregnate filter paper with *titan yellow solution.* Allow to dry at room temperature.

Titan Yellow Solution A 0.05% w/v solution of *titan yellow.*
Complies with the following test.
SENSITIVITY To 0.1 ml add 10 ml of *water,* 0.2 ml of *magnesium standard solution (10 ppm mg)* and 1.0 ml of 1M *sodium hydroxide.* A distinct pink colour is visible by comparison with a reference solution prepared in the same manner but omitting the magnesium solution.

Titanium Ti = 47.9 *(7440-32-6)*
Metal powder, fine wire (diameter not more than 0.5 mm) or sponge containing not less than 99% of Ti.
Melting point, about 1668°; density, 4.507 g cm^{-3}.

Titanium(III) Chloride Titanium trichloride; $TiCl_3$ = 154.3 *(7705-07-9)*
General reagent grade of commerce.
Reddish violet crystals; melting point, about 440°.
Store in an airtight container.

Titanium(III) Chloride Solution Titanium trichloride solution
General reagent grade of commerce containing about 15% w/v of $TiCl_3$ in *hydrochloric acid* (10% w/v HCl).
Weight per ml, about 1.2 g.

Titanium(III) Chloride-Sulphuric Acid Reagent
Titanium trichloride-sulphuric acid reagent
Carefully mix 20 ml of *titanium(III) chloride solution* with 13 ml of *sulphuric acid,* add sufficient *hydrogen peroxide solution (100 vol)* to produce a yellow colour, heat until white fumes are evolved and allow to cool. Dilute with *water* and repeat the evaporation and addition of water until a colourless solution is obtained. Dilute this solution to 100 ml with *water.*

Titanium Dioxide Titanium(IV) oxide; TiO_2 = 79.90 *(1317-80-2)*
General reagent grade of commerce.

Titanium Trichloride See *titanium(III) chloride.*

Titanium Trichloride Solution See *titanium(III) chloride solution.*

Titanium Trichloride-Sulphuric Acid Reagent See *titanium(III) chloride-sulphuric acid reagent.*

Toluene Methylbenzene; C_7H_8 = 92.14 (*108-88-3*)
Analytical reagent grade of commerce.
A colourless liquid with a characteristic odour; weight per ml, 0.865 to 0.870 g; boiling point, about 110°.

Toluene, Sulphur-free *Toluene* that complies with the following tests.
SULPHUR COMPOUNDS To 10 ml add 1 ml of *absolute ethanol* and 3 ml of *potassium plumbite solution* and boil under a reflux condenser for 15 minutes. Allow to stand for 15 minutes; no darkening is produced in the aqueous layer.
THIOPHENE-RELATED SUBSTANCES Shake 2 ml with 5 ml of *isatin reagent* for 5 minutes and allow to stand for 15 minutes. No blue colour is produced in the lower layer.

Toluenesulphonamide See *toluene-p-sulphonamide.*

***o*-Toluenesulphonamide** See *toluene-o-sulphonamide.*

***p*-Toluenesulphonamide** See *toluene-p-sulphonamide.*

Toluene-*o*-sulphonamide *o*-Toluenesulphonamide; 2-methylbenzenesulphonamide; $C_7H_9NO_2S$ = 171.2 (*88-19-7*)
General reagent grade of commerce.
Melting point, about 156°.

Toluene-*p*-sulphonamide *p*-Toluenesulphonamide; toluene sulphonamide; 4-methylbenzenesulphonamide; $C_7H_9NO_2S$ = 171.2 (*70-55-3*)
General reagent grade of commerce.
Melting point, about 136°.
Complies with the following test.
HOMOGENEITY Carry out the test for Related substances described in the monograph for Tolbutamide applying to the plate 5 µl of a 0.015% w/v solution in *acetone*. The chromatogram shows only one principal spot.

Toluenesulphonic Acid See *toluene-p-sulphonic acid.*

Toluene-*p*-sulphonic Acid Toluenesulphonic acid; 4-methylbenzenesulphonic acid; $C_7H_8O_3S,H_2O$ = 190.2 (*6192-52-5*)
General reagent grade of commerce containing not less than 87.0% of $C_7H_8O_3S$.
A white, crystalline powder or crystals.

***o*-Toluic Acid** $C_8H_8O_2$ = 136.2 (*118-90-1*)
General reagent grade of commerce.
A white, crystalline powder; melting point, about 104°.

***o*-Toluidine** 2-Methylaniline; C_7H_9N = 107.2 (*95-53-4*)
General reagent grade of commerce.
A pale yellow liquid becoming reddish-brown on exposure to air and light; d_{20}^{20}, about 1.01; n_D^{20}, about 1.569; boiling point, about 200°.
Store in an airtight container protected from light.

***p*-Toluidine** 4-Methylaniline; C_7H_9N = 107.2 (*106-49-0*)
General reagent grade of commerce.
Lustrous plates or flakes; melting point, about 44°.

Toluidine Blue Toluidine blue O; CI 52040; 3-amino-7-dimethylamino-2-methylphenothiazin-5-ium chloride; $C_{15}H_{16}ClN_3S$ = 305.8 (*92-31-9*)
General reagent grade of commerce.
A dark green powder.

***o*-Toluidine Hydrochloride** 2-Methylaniline hydrochloride; C_7H_9N,HCl = 143.6 (*636-21-5*)
General reagent grade of commerce.
Melting point, about 216°.

Tosylarginine Methyl Ester Hydrochloride Methyl *N*-tosyl-L-argininate hydrochloride; $C_{14}H_{22}N_4O_4S,HCl$ = 378.9 (*1784-03-8*)
Use a grade of commerce suitable for the assay of trypsin.
A white, crystalline powder; melting point, about 145°; $[\alpha]_D^{20}$, −12° to −16° (4% w/v in water).

Tosylarginine Methyl Ester Hydrochloride Solution Dissolve 98.5 mg of *tosylarginine methyl ester hydrochloride* in 5 ml of *tris—chloride buffer, pH 8.1*, shaking to effect dissolution, add 2.5 ml of *methyl red mixed solution* and dilute to 25 ml with *water*.

Tosyl-lysyl-chloromethane Hydrochloride (3*S*)-7-Amino-1-chloro-3-tosylamido-2-heptanone hydrochloride; *N*-tosyl-L-lysylchloromethane hydrochloride; $C_{14}H_{21}ClN_2O_3S,HCl$ = 369.3 (*4238-41-9*)
General reagent grade of commerce.
Melting point, about 155°, with decomposition; $[\alpha]_D^{20}$, −7° to −9° (2% w/v); A(1%, 1 cm) at 230 nm, 310 to 340 (water).

Tosylphenylalanylchloromethane *N*-Tosyl-L-phenylalanylchloromethane; L-Tosylaminophenethyl chloromethyl ketone; $C_{17}H_{18}ClNO_3S$ = 351.9 (*402-71-1*)
General reagent grade of commerce.
A white, crystalline solid, melting point, about 105°; $[\alpha]_D^{20}$, −85° to −89° [1% w/v in ethanol (96%)]; A(1%, 1 cm), 290 to 320 determined at 228.5 nm in *ethanol (96%)*.

Tragacanth (*9000-65-1*)
Of the British Pharmacopoeia.

Triacetin Propane-1,2,3-triyl triacetate; $C_9H_{14}O_6$ = 218.2 (*102-76-1*)
General reagent grade of commerce.
d_{20}^{20}, about 1.16; n_D^{20}, about 1.43; boiling point, about 260°

Triamcinolone $C_{21}H_{27}FO_6$ = 394.4 (*124-94-7*)
General reagent grade of commerce.
Melting point, 262° to 263°.

Tributyl Orthophosphate Tributyl phosphate; $C_{12}H_{27}O_4P$ = 266.3 (*126-73-8*)
General reagent grade of commerce washed before use with three quantities, each of one-sixth of its volume, of a solution containing 10% w/v of *sodium chloride* and 1.0% w/v of *disodium hydrogen orthophosphate*.
A colourless liquid; weight per ml, about 0.98 g.

Trichloroacetic Acid $C_2HCl_3O_2$ = 163.4 (*76-03-9*)
Analytical reagent grade of commerce.
Colourless, deliquescent crystals with a pungent odour.
Store in an airtight container.

Trichloroacetic Acid Solution Dissolve 40 g of *trichloroacetic acid* in sufficient *water* to produce 1000 ml. Verify the concentration by titration with 0.1M *sodium hydroxide VS* and adjust, if necessary, to 40 ± 1 g/l.

1,1,1-Trichloroethane Methylchloroform; $C_2H_3Cl_3$ = 133.4 (*71-55-6*)
General reagent grade of commerce.
d_{20}^{20}, about 1.34; n_D^{20}, about 1.438; boiling point, about 74°.

Trichloroethylene C_2HCl_3 = 131.4 *(79-01-6)*
Technical grade of commerce.
A colourless liquid with a chloroform-like odour; d_{20}^{20}, about 1.46; n_D^{20}, about 1.477.

Trichlorotrifluoroethane 1,1,2-Trichlorotrifluoroethane; $C_2Cl_3F_3$ = 187.4 *(76-13-1)*
General reagent grade of commerce.
A colourless, volatile liquid; boiling point, about 47°; d_{20}^{20}, about 1.58.
Complies with the following requirement.
DISTILLATION RANGE Not less than 98% distils between 47° and 48°, Appendix V C.

Tricosane $C_{23}H_{48}$ = 324.6 *(638-67-5)*
General reagent grade of commerce.
White crystals; melting point, about 48°; n_D^{20}, about 1.447.

Triethanolamine $C_6H_{15}NO_3$ = 149.2 *(102-71-6)*
General reagent grade of commerce.
A viscous, very hygroscopic, colourless liquid with a slight ammoniacal odour, which becomes brown on exposure to air and light; d_{20}^{20}, about 1.13.
Store in an airtight container protected from light.

Triethylamine $C_6H_{15}N$ = 101.2 *(121-44-8)*
General reagent grade of commerce.
A colourless liquid with an ammoniacal odour; d_{20}^{20}, about 0.727; n_D^{20}, about 1.401; boiling point, about 90°.

Triethylamine Hydrogen Carbonate Solution Pass a gentle current of *carbon dioxide* through a 5% w/v solution of *triethylamine* for 16 hours.

Triethylenediamine 1,4-Diazobicyclo[2.2.2]octane; $C_6H_{12}N_2$ = 112.2 *(280-57-9)*
General reagent grade of commerce.
Hygroscopic crystals which sublime readily at room temperature; melting point, about 158°; boiling point, about 174°.
Store in an airtight container.

Trifluoroacetic Acid $C_2HF_3O_2$ = 114.0 *(76-05-1)*
Reagent grade of commerce suitable for protein sequencing containing not less than 99% of $C_2HO_2F_3$.
Boiling point, about 72°; d_{20}^{20}, about 1.53.
Store in an airtight container.

Trifluoroacetic Anhydride $C_4F_6O_3$ = 210.0 *(407-25-0)*
General reagent grade of commerce.
A colourless liquid with an acrid, penetrating odour; d_{20}^{20}, about 1.5.

Trimethylchlorosilane Chlorotrimethylsilane; C_3H_9ClSi = 108.7 *(75-77-4)*
General reagent grade of commerce.
A colourless liquid; d_{20}^{20}, about 0.86; n_D^{20}, about 1.388; boiling point, about 57°.

Trimethylpentane See *2,2,4-trimethylpentane.*

2,2,4-Trimethylpentane Iso-octane; trimethylpentane; C_8H_{18} = 114.2 *(540-84-1)*
General reagent grade of commerce.
A colourless, flammable liquid; d_{20}^{20}, 0.691 to 0.696; n_D^{20}, 1.391 to 1.393.
Complies with the following requirement.
DISTILLATION RANGE Not less than 95% distils between 98° and 100°.
2,2,4-Trimethylpentane used in spectrophotometry complies with the following additional requirement.
TRANSMITTANCE Not less than 98% between 250 and 420 nm, Appendix II B, using *water* in the reference cell.

Trimethylpentane R1 *2,2,4-Trimethylpentane* complying with the following test.
ABSORBANCE Not more than 0.07 from 220 nm to 360 nm determined using *water* in the reference cell.

***N*-Trimethylsilylimidazole** $C_6H_{12}N_2Si$ = 140.3 *(18156-74-6)*
Analytical reagent grade of commerce.
A colourless, hygroscopic liquid; d_{20}^{20}, about 0.96; n_D^{20}, about 1.48.
Store in an airtight container.

Triphenylamine $C_{18}H_{15}N$ = 245.3 *(603-34-9)*
General reagent grade of commerce.
A white, crystalline solid; melting point, about 126°.

Triphenylethylene $C_{20}H_{16}$ = 256.4 *(58-72-0)*
General reagent grade of commerce.
Melting point, about 70°.

Triphenylmethanol Triphenylcarbinol; $C_{19}H_{16}O$ = 260.3 *(76-84-6)*
General reagent grade of commerce.

2,3,5-Triphenyltetrazolium Chloride Tetrazolium salt; $C_{19}H_{15}ClN_4$ = 334.8 *(298-96-4)*
Analytical reagent grade of commerce containing not less than 98.0% of $C_{19}H_{15}ClN_4$.
A pale yellow or cream powder; melting point, about 240°, with decomposition.
ASSAY Dissolve 1 g in a mixture of 5 ml of 2M *nitric acid* and 45 ml of *water*, add 50 ml of 0.1M *silver nitrate VS* and heat to boiling. Allow to cool, add 3 ml of *dibutyl phthalate*, shake vigorously and titrate with 0.1M *ammonium thiocyanate VS* using 2 ml of *ammonium iron(III) sulphate solution R2* as indicator. Each ml of 0.1M *silver nitrate VS* is equivalent to 33.48 mg of $C_{19}H_{15}ClN_4$.
Store protected from light.

Triphenyltetrazolium Chloride Solution A 0.5% w/v solution of *2,3,5-triphenyltetrazolium chloride* in *aldehyde-free ethanol (96%).*
Store protected from light.

Triscyanoethoxypropane 1,2,3-Tris(cyanoethoxy)-propane; $C_{12}H_{17}N_3O_3$ = 251.3
Chromatographic reagent grade of commerce.
A viscous, brownish yellow liquid; d_{20}^{20}, about 1.11; viscosity, about 172 mPa s, Appendix V H, Method II.

1,3,5-Tris(3,5-di-(1,1-dimethylethyl)-4-hydroxybenzyl)-1*H*,3*H*,5*H*-1,3,5-triazine-2,4,6-trione
Tris(3,5-di-*tert*-butyl-4-hydroxybenzyl isocyanurate; $C_{48}H_{69}N_3O_6$ = 784.1 *(27676-62-6)*
General reagent grade of commerce.
Melting point, 218° to 222°.

Tris(2,4-di-(1,1-dimethylethyl)phenyl) Phosphite $C_{42}H_{63}O_3P$ = 647 *(31570-04-4)*
General reagent grade of commerce.
Melting point, 182° to 186°.

Tris(hydroxymethylaminoethane) See *tris(hydroxymethyl)methylamine.*

Tris(hydroxymethylaminoethane) Solution See *tris(hydroxymethyl)methylamine solution.*

Tris(hydroxymethyl)methylamine Tris(hydroxymethyl)aminomethane; trometamol; $C_4H_{11}NO_3$ = 121.1 *(77-86-1)*
Analytical reagent grade of commerce.
Melting point, about 170°.

Tris(hydroxymethyl)methylamine Solution

Tris(hydroxymethyl)aminoethane solution
A 2.422% w/v solution of *tris(hydroxymethyl)methylamine* (0.1M).

Tris(hydroxymethyl)methylamine Solution, Methanolic Dissolve 6.07 g of *tris(hydroxymethyl)methylamine* in 900 ml of *methanol*, add 50 ml of 0.5M *hydrochloric acid* and dilute to 1000 ml with *water*.

Trisodium Orthophosphate Trisodium phosphate dodecahydrate; $Na_3PO_4,12H_2O$ = 380.1 (*10101-89-0*)
General reagent grade of commerce.

Trisodium Phosphate Dodecahydrate See *trisodium orthophosphate*.

Tropine (*1R*,3*r*,5*S*)-Tropan-3-ol; $C_8H_{15}NO$ = 141.2 (*120-29-6*)
General reagent grade of commerce.
Colourless crystals; melting point, about 54°.

Trypsin (*9002-07-7*) A proteolytic enzyme obtained by activation of trypsinogen extracted from the pancreas of cattle (*Bos taurus* L.).
A white, crystalline or amorphous powder.

Trypsin for Peptide Mapping
Trypsin of high purity treated to eliminate chymotryptic activity.

Tryptophan $C_{11}H_{12}N_2O_2$ = 204.2 (*73-22-3*)
General reagent grade of commerce.

$[\alpha]_D^{20}$, about –30°, determined in a 1% w/v solution.

Tyrosine See *L-tyrosine*.

L-Tyrosine 2-Amino-3-(4-hydroxyphenyl)propionic acid; tyrosine; $C_9H_{11}NO_3$ = 181.2 (*60-18-4*)
General reagent grade of commerce complying with the following test.
HOMOGENEITY Carry out the test for Related substances in the monograph for Levodopa. The chromatogram shows only one spot.

Undecanoic Acid $C_{11}H_{22}O_2$ = 186.3 (*112-37-8*)
General reagent grade of commerce.
Melting point, about 28.5°.

Urea CH_4N_2O = 60.06 (*57-13-6*)
Analytical reagent grade of commerce.
White crystals or crystalline powder; melting point, about 133°.

Urease-active Meal (*9002-13-5*)
General reagent grade of commerce.
ACTIVITY Each mg of urease-active meal hydrolyses 3 mg of urea in 30 minutes at 37°.

Uridine 1-β-D-Ribofuranosyluracil; $C_9H_{12}N_2O_6$ = 244.2 (*58-96-8*)
Chromatographic reeagent grade of commerce.
Melting point, about 165°.

Valeric Acid *n*-Valeric acid; pentanoic acid; $C_5H_{10}O_2$ = 102.1 (*109-52-4*)
General reagent grade of commerce.
Boiling point, about 186°; d_{20}^{20}, about 0.94; n_D^{20}, about 1.409.

Vanillic Acid 4-Hydroxy-3-methoxybenzoic acid; $C_8H_8O_4$ = 168.2 (*121-34-6*)
General reagent grade of commerce.
A white, crystalline solid; melting point, about 212°.

Vanillin 4-Hydroxy-3-methoxybenzaldehyde; $C_8H_8O_3$ = 152.2 (*121-33-5*)
Analytical reagent grade of commerce.
White to yellowish white, needles or crystalline powder, with an odour of vanilla.
Melting point, about 81°, determined without previous drying.

Vanillin Reagent Carefully add, dropwise, 2 ml of *sulphuric acid* to 100 ml of a 1% w/v solution of *vanillin* in *ethanol (96%)*.
Use within 48 hours.

Vanillin Solution, Phosphoric Dissolve 1 g of *vanillin* in 25 ml of *ethanol (96%)* and add 25 ml of *water* and 35 ml of *orthophosphoric acid*.

Veratric Acid 3,4-Dimethoxybenzoic acid; $C_9H_{10}O_4$ = 182.2 (*93-07-2*)
General reagent grade of commerce.
Melting point, about 180°.

Vinyl Acetate $C_4H_6O_2$ = 86.1 (*108-05-4*)
General reagent grade of commerce.
d_{20}^{20}, about 0.930; melting point, about –93°; boiling point, about 72°.

Vinyl Chloride C_2H_3Cl = 62.5 (*75-01-4*)
General reagent grade of commerce.

2-Vinylpyridine C_7H_7N = 105.1 (*100-69-6*)
General reagent grade of commerce.
A yellow liquid; d_{20}^{20}, about 0.97; n_D^{20}, about 1.549.

1-Vinylpyrrolidin-2-one C_6H_9NO = 111.1 (*88-12-0*)
General reagent grade of commerce.
When used in the test for Vinylpyrrolidone in the monograph for Povidone, complies with the following requirements.
WATER Not more than 0.1% determined on 2.5 g, Appendix IX C. Use as the solvent a mixture of 50 ml of *anhydrous methanol* and 10 ml of *butyrolactone*.
ASSAY Not less than 99.0% of C_6H_9NO, determined by the following method. Examine by *gas chromatography*, Appendix III B.

The chromatographic procedure may be carried out using:

(a) a fused silica column (30 m × 0.5 mm) the inner wall of which is coated with a 1.0-µm layer of *polyethylene glycol 20,000*,
(b) *helium* as the carrier gas,
(c) a flame ionisation detector

maintaining the temperature of the injection port at 190° and programming the temperature of the column as follows: maintain the temperature at 80° for 1 minute and then increase it to 190° at a rate of 10° per minute. Maintain at 190° for 15 minutes. Inject 0.3 µl of the reagent being examined and adjust the flow rate of the carrier gas so that the retention time of the peak corresponding to 1-vinylpyrrolidin-2-one is about 17 minutes. Determine the content of C_6H_9NO by *normalisation*.

Water (*7732-18-5*) Purified Water of the British Pharmacopoeia.

Water, Ammonia-free Ammonium-free water
To 100 ml of *water* add 0.1 ml of *sulphuric acid (96% w/w)* and distil using the apparatus described in Appendix V C. Discard the first 10 ml and collect the following 50 ml.

Water, Ammonium-free See *ammonia-free water*.

Water, Carbon Dioxide-free *Water* that has been boiled vigorously for a few minutes and protected from the atmosphere during cooling and storage.

Water, Distilled Purified Water of the British Pharmacopoeia that has been prepared by distillation.

Water for Chromatography Deionised *water* with a resistivity of not less than 0.18 Mohm m.

Water for Injections Of the British Pharmacopoeia.

Water, Nitrate-free To 100 ml of *water* add about 5 mg each of *potassium permanganate* and *barium hydroxide* and distil using the apparatus described under *determination of distillation range*, Appendix V C. Discard the first 10 ml and collect the following 50 ml.

Water, Particle-free
Filter *water* through a membrane with a pore size of 0.22 µm.

Weak Cationic Resin Polymethacrylic resin, slightly acidic, with carboxyl groups present in a protonated form. Particle size, 75 µm to 160 µm; pH limits of use, 5 to 14; maximum temperature of use, 120°.

Xanthydrol 9-Hydroxyxanthene; xanthen-9-ol; $C_{13}H_{10}O_2$ = 198.2 (*90-46-0*)
General reagent grade of commerce containing not less than 90.0% of $C_{13}H_{10}O_2$.
A white to pale yellow powder; melting point, about 123°.
Xanthydrol is also available as a solution in methanol containing 9.0 to 11.0% w/v of $C_{13}H_{10}O_2$.
ASSAY In a 250-ml flask dissolve 0.3 g in 3 ml of *methanol* or use 3 ml of the solution. Add 50 ml of *glacial acetic acid* and add, dropwise with shaking, 25 ml of a 2% w/v solution of *urea*. Allow to stand for 12 hours, collect the precipitate on a sintered-glass filter (16 mm), wash with 20 ml of *ethanol (96%)*, dry the precipitate at 100° to 105° and weigh. Each g of precipitate is equivalent to 0.9429 g of xanthydrol.
Store protected from light. If a methanolic solution is used, store in small, sealed ampoules and filter before use, if necessary.

Xanthydrol R1
Xanthydrol containing not less than 98.0% of $C_{13}H_{10}O_2$.

Xanthydrol Reagent Dissolve about 0.125 g of *xanthydrol* in 100 ml of *anhydrous acetic acid*. Add 1 ml of *hydrochloric acid* immediately before use.

Xanthydrol Solution To 0.1 ml of a 10% w/v solution of *xanthydrol* in *methanol* add 100 ml of *anhydrous acetic acid* and 1 ml of *hydrochloric acid*; allow to stand for 24 hours.

Xylene A mixture of *o*-, *m*- and *p*- isomers; C_8H_{10} = 106.2 (*1330-20-7*)
Analytical reagent grade of commerce.
A colourless, clear, flammable liquid; d_{20}^{20}, about 0.867; n_D^{20}, about 1.497; boiling point, about 138°.

***o*-Xylene** 1,2-Dimethylbenzene; C_8H_{10} = 106.2 (*95-47-6*)
General reagent grade of commerce.
d_{20}^{20}, about 0.881; n_D^{20}, about 1.505; boiling point, about 144°; melting point, about –25°.

Xylene Cyanol FF CI 42135 (*2650-17-1*)
A blue, alcohol-soluble dye used as a screening agent in *methyl orange—xylene cyanol FF solution*.

Xylenol Orange [3*H*-2,1-Benzoxathiol-3-ylidenebis(6-hydroxy-5-methyl-*m*-phenylene)methylenenitrilo]tetra-acetic acid *S,S*-dioxide tetrasodium salt; $C_{31}H_{28}N_2Na_4O_{13}S$ = 761 (*3618-43-7*)
General reagent grade of commerce.
A reddish brown, crystalline powder.
Produces a violet colour with mercury, lead, zinc and certain other metal ions, in alkaline solutions. When metal ions are absent, for example in the presence of an excess of disodium edetate, the solution is yellow.

Xylenol Orange Triturate Triturate 1 part of *xylenol orange* with 99 parts of *potassium nitrate*.
Complies with the following test.
SENSITIVITY Add 50 mg to a mixture of 50 ml of *water*, 1 ml of 2M *acetic acid* and 0.05 ml of *lead nitrate solution*. Add sufficient *hexamine* to change the colour from yellow to violet-red, and add 0.1 ml of 0.1M *disodium edetate VS*. The colour changes to yellow.

Xylenol Orange Solution Shake 0.1 g of *xylenol orange* with 100 ml of *water* and filter if necessary.

Xylose See *D-xylose*.

D-Xylose Xylose; $C_5H_{10}O_5$ = 150.1 (*58-86-6*)
Analytical reagent grade of commerce.
A white, crystalline powder; $[\alpha]_D^{20}$, about +20° (10% w/v solution in water measured after 10 hours).

Zinc Zn = 65.38 (*7440-66-6*)
Analytical reagent grade of commerce containing not less than 99.5% of Zn.
Silver-white cylinders, granules, pellets or filings with a blue sheen.
Complies with the following test.
ARSENIC 5.0 g complies with *limit test A for arsenic*, Appendix VI (0.2 ppm). Use 15 ml of *hydrochloric acid AsT* and 25 ml of *water* as the solvent.

Zinc, Activated Cover a quantity of *zinc*, in granules, pellets or cylinders, with a solution containing 50 µg of *chloroplatinic(IV) acid* per ml. Allow to stand for 10 minutes, wash, drain and dry immediately.
Complies with the following tests.
ARSENIC To 5 g add 15 ml of *hydrochloric acid* and 25 ml of *water*. Add 0.1 ml of *tin(II) chloride solution AsT* and 5 ml of 0.1M *potassium iodide*. Using the apparatus and procedure described for the *limit test for arsenic*, Appendix VII, no stain is produced on the *mercury(II) bromide paper*.
ACTIVITY Repeat the test for arsenic using the same reagents and adding 1 ml of *arsenic standard solution (1 ppm As)*. An appreciable stain appears on the *mercury(II) bromide paper*.

Zinc Acetate $(C_2H_3O_2)_2Zn,2H_2O$ = 219.5 (*5970-45-6*)
General reagent grade of commerce.
Melting point, about 237°.

Zinc Acetate Solution Mix 600 ml of *water* with 150 ml of *glacial acetic acid*, add 54.9 g of *zinc acetate* and stir to dissolve. Continue stirring while adding 150 ml of 13.5M *ammonia*, cool to room temperature, adjust to pH 6.4 with *ammonium hydroxide* and add sufficient *water* to produce 1000 ml.

Zinc Chloride $ZnCl_2$ = 136.3 (*7646-85-7*)
Purified granular grade of commerce.
A white or almost white, granular powder.

Zinc Chloride-Formic Acid Solution Dissolve 20 g of *zinc chloride* in 80 g of an 85% w/v solution of *anhydrous formic acid*.

Zinc Chloride Solution, Iodinated Dissolve 20 g of *zinc chloride* and 6.5 g of *potassium iodide* in 10.5 ml of *water*. Add 0.5 g of *iodine* and shake for 15 minutes, filtering if necessary.
Store protected from light.

Zinc Iodide ZnI_2 = 319.2 (*10139-47-6*)
General reagent grade of commerce.

Zinc Oxide ZnO = 81.4 (*1341-13-2*)
General reagent grade of commerce.

Zinc Powder Zn = 65.38 (*7440-66-6*)
Analytical reagent grade of commerce containing not less than 90.0% of Zn.

Zinc Shot Zn = 65.38
Analytical reagent grade of commerce.
Shot, 0.5 to 2.0 mm (about 8 to 30 mesh).

Zinc Sulphate $ZnSO_4,7H_2O$ = 287.5 (*7446-20-0*)
Analytical reagent grade of commerce.

Zirconyl Chloride $ZrOCl_2,8H_2O$ = 322.3 (*15461-27-5*)
Use a grade of commerce supplied especially for fluoride determinations containing not less than 96.0% of $ZrOCl_2, 8H_2O$.
ASSAY Dissolve 0.6 g in a mixture of 5 ml of *nitric acid* and 50 ml of *water*, add 50 ml of 0.1M *silver nitrate VS* and 3 ml of *dibutyl phthalate* and shake. Titrate with 0.1M *ammonium thiocyanate VS* using 2 ml of *ammonium iron(III) sulphate solution R2* as indicator until a reddish yellow colour is obtained. Each ml of 0.1M *silver nitrate VS* is equivalent to 16.11 mg of $ZrOCl_2,8H_2O$.

Zirconyl Nitrate Approximately $ZrO(NO_3)_2$+aq (*14985-18-3*)
General reagent grade of commerce.
Usually contains about 44.5% of ZrO_2.
Store in an airtight container.

Zirconyl Nitrate Solution Dissolve 0.1 g of *zirconyl nitrate* in a mixture of 60 ml of *hydrochloric acid* and 40 ml of *water*.

B. Volumetric Reagents and Solutions

Terminology Volumetric solutions are prepared according to the usual chemical analytical methods. The accuracy of the apparatus used is verified to ensure that it is appropriate for the intended use.

The concentration of volumetric solutions is indicated in terms of *molarity* (M). The molarity of a solution is the number of moles of substance contained in 1000 ml of the solution. A solution that contains *x* moles of substance per litre is said to be *x*M.

Volumetric reagents do not differ from the prescribed strength by more than 10% and the molarity is determined with a precision of 0.2%.

In monographs other than those of the European Pharmacopoeia, solutions to be standardised before use in assays and other quantitative tests are designated by appending the letters *VS* to the name of the reagent.

Primary standards

The following materials, after drying under the specified conditions, are recommended for use as primary standards in the standardisation of volumetric solutions. Analytical reagent grade materials of commerce must be used.

Arsenic Trioxide Arsenious trioxide
Sublime in a suitable apparatus and store over *anhydrous silica gel*.

Benzoic Acid Sublime in a suitable apparatus.

Potassium Bromate Recrystallise from boiling *water*, collect the crystals and dry to constant weight at 180°.

Potassium Dichromate Dry to constant weight at 150°.

Potassium Hydrogen Phthalate Recrystallise from boiling *water*, collect the crystals at a temperature above 35° and dry to constant weight at 110°.

Potassium Iodate Dry to constant weight at 130°.

Sodium Carbonate, Anhydrous Filter a saturated solution of *sodium carbonate* at room temperature and introduce slowly into the filtrate a current of *carbon dioxide* with constant stirring and cooling. After about 2 hours collect the precipitate on a sintered-glass filter. Wash the filter with iced *water* containing carbon dioxide. After drying at 100° to 105°, heat to constant weight at 270° to 300°, stirring occasionally.

Sodium Chloride To 1 volume of a saturated solution of *sodium chloride* add 2 volumes of *hydrochloric acid*, collect the crystals produced and wash with 7M *hydrochloric acid*. Remove the hydrochloric acid by heating on a water bath and dry the crystals to constant weight at 300°.

Sulphanilic Acid Recrystallise from boiling *water*, filter and dry to constant weight at 100° to 105°.

Zinc Use a granulated form containing not less than 99.9% w/w of Zn.

Preparation and standardisation

For each solution the preparation and standardisation of the most commonly used strengths are described. Solutions more concentrated than those described are prepared and standardised using proportionate amounts of the reagents. Aqueous solutions less concentrated than those described are prepared by making an exact dilution of a more concentrated solution with *carbon dioxide-free water*. The correction factors of these solutions are the same as those from which the dilutions were prepared. Aqueous solutions of molarity below 0.1M are freshly prepared using *carbon dioxide-free water*.

The water used in preparing volumetric solutions complies with the requirements of the monograph for Purified Water. When used for the preparation of unstable solutions such as potassium permanganate and sodium thiosulphate, it should be freshly boiled and cooled. When a solution is to be used in an assay in which the end point is determined by an electrochemical process, the exact concentration of the solution must be determined in the same way. The composition of the medium in which a volumetric solution is standardised should be the same as that in which it is to be used.

All volumetric solutions should, if practicable, be prepared, standardised and used at 20°; if a titration is carried out at a markedly different temperature from that at which the standardisation took place, a suitable temperature correction should be made.

Volumetric solutions

Acetic Acid VS $C_2H_4O_2$ = 60.1
For a 0.1M solution Dilute 6.0 g of *glacial acetic acid* to 1000 ml with *water*.

Ascertain its exact concentration in the following manner. To 25 ml of the solution add 0.5 ml of *phenolphthalein solution* and titrate with 0.1M *sodium hydroxide VS*. Each ml of 0.1M *sodium hydroxide VS* is equivalent to 6.01 mg of $C_2H_4O_2$.

Ammonium Cerium(IV) Nitrate VS Ammonium and cerium nitrate; $(NH_4)_2Ce(NO_3)_6$ = 548.2
For a 0.1M solution Shake a solution containing 56 ml of *sulphuric acid* and 54.82 g of *ammonium cerium(IV) nitrate*

for 2 minutes and carefully add five successive 100-ml quantities of *water*, shaking after each addition. Dilute the clear solution to 1000 ml with *water*.

After 10 days, ascertain its exact concentration as described for 0.1M *ammonium cerium(IV) sulphate VS*. Each ml of 0.1M *ammonium cerium(IV) nitrate VS* is equivalent to 4.946 mg of As_2O_3.
Store protected from light.
For a 0.01M solution To 100 ml of 0.1M *ammonium cerium(IV) nitrate VS* add, while cooling, 30 ml of *sulphuric acid* and sufficient *water* to produce 1000 ml.

Ammonium Cerium(IV) Sulphate VS Ammonium and cerium sulphate; $2(NH_4)_2SO_4,Ce(SO_4)_2,2H_2O$ = 632.6
For a 0.1M solution Dissolve 65 g of *ammonium cerium(IV) sulphate* in a mixture of 30 ml of *sulphuric acid* and 500 ml of *water*. Allow to cool and dilute to 1000 ml with *water*.

Ascertain its exact concentration in the following manner. Dissolve 80 mg of *arsenic trioxide*, by heating gently in 15 ml of 0.2M *sodium hydroxide*, add to the clear solution 50 ml of 1M *sulphuric acid*, 0.15 ml of a 0.25% w/v solution of *osmium tetroxide* in 1M *sulphuric acid* and 0.1 ml of *ferroin solution*. Titrate this solution with the ammonium cerium(IV) sulphate solution until the red colour is discharged, titrating slowly towards the end point. Each ml of 0.1M *ammonium cerium(IV) sulphate VS* is equivalent to 4.946 mg of As_2O_3.
For a 0.01M solution To 100 ml of 0.1M *ammonium cerium(IV) sulphate VS* add, while cooling, 30 ml of *sulphuric acid* and sufficient *water* to produce 1000 ml.

Ammonium Iron(II) Sulphate VS $(NH_4)_2Fe(SO_4)_2,6H_2O$ = 392.1
For a 0.1M solution Dissolve 40 g of *ammonium iron(II) sulphate* in 100 ml of 2M *sulphuric acid* and dilute with sufficient freshly boiled and cooled *water* to produce 1000 ml.

Ascertain its exact concentration in the following manner. To 25 ml add 10 ml of 1M *sulphuric acid* and 1 ml of *orthophosphoric acid* and titrate with 0.02M *potassium permanganate VS*. Each ml of 0.02M *potassium permanganate VS* is equivalent to 39.21 mg of $(NH_4)_2Fe(SO_4)_2,6H_2O$.

Ammonium Iron(III) Sulphate VS Ferric ammonium sulphate; $NH_4Fe(SO_4)_2,12H_2O$ = 482.2
For a 0.1M solution Dissolve 50 g of *ammonium iron(III) sulphate* in a mixture of 300 ml of *water* and 6 ml of *sulphuric acid* and dilute to 1000 ml with *water*.

Ascertain its exact concentration in the following manner. To 25 ml add 3 ml of *hydrochloric acid* and 2 g of *potassium iodide*, allow to stand for 10 minutes and titrate the liberated iodine with 0.1M *sodium thiosulphate VS* using *starch mucilage* as indicator. Each ml of 0.1M *sodium thiosulphate VS* is equivalent to 48.22 mg of $NH_4Fe(SO_4)_2,12H_2O$.

Ammonium Thiocyanate VS NH_4SCN = 76.12
For a 0.1M solution Dissolve 7.612 g in sufficient *water* to produce 1000 ml.

Ascertain its exact concentration in the following manner. To 20 ml of 0.1M *silver nitrate VS* add 25 ml of *water*, 2 ml of 2M *nitric acid* and 2 ml of *ammonium iron(III) sulphate solution R2* and titrate with the ammonium thiocyanate solution until a reddish yellow colour is obtained. Each ml of 0.1M *silver nitrate VS* is equivalent to 7.612 mg of NH_4SCN.

Barium Chloride VS $BaCl_2,2H_2O$ = 244.3
For a 0.1M solution Dissolve 24.4 g of *barium chloride* in sufficient *water* to produce 1000 ml.

Ascertain its exact concentration in the following manner. To 10 ml of the solution add 60 ml of *water*, 3 ml of 13.5M *ammonia* and 0.5 to 1 mg of *phthalein purple* as indicator and titrate with 0.1M *disodium edetate VS*. As the solution begins to decolorise, add 50 ml of *ethanol (96%)* and titrate until the bluish violet colour is discharged. Each ml of 0.1M *disodium edetate VS* is equivalent to 24.43 mg of $BaCl_2,2H_2O$.

Barium Perchlorate VS $Ba(ClO_4)_2$ = 336.2
For a 0.05M solution Dissolve 15.8 g of *barium hydroxide* in a mixture of 75 ml of *water* and 7.5 ml of *perchloric acid*, adjust to pH 3 with *perchloric acid* and filter if necessary. To the solution add 150 ml of *ethanol (96%)*, dilute to 250 ml with *water* and add sufficient *buffer solution pH 3.7* to produce 1000 ml.

Ascertain its exact concentration immediately before use in the following manner. To 5 ml of 0.05M *sulphuric acid VS* add 5 ml of *water*, 50 ml of *acetate buffer pH 3.7* and 0.5 ml of *alizarin S solution* and titrate with the barium perchlorate solution until an orange-red colour appears. Each ml of 0.05M *sulphuric acid VS* is equivalent to 16.81 mg of $Ba(ClO_4)_2$.

Benzethonium Chloride VS, 0.004M Dissolve 1.792 g of *benzethonium chloride*, previously dried to constant weight at 100° to 105°, in sufficient *water* to produce 1000 ml.

Calculate the molarity of the solution from the content of $C_{27}H_{42}ClNO_2$ in the dried benzethonium chloride determined in the following manner. Dissolve 0.35 g of the dried substance in 30 ml of *anhydrous acetic acid*, add 6 ml of *mercury(II) acetate solution* and carry out Method I for *non-aqueous titration*, Appendix VIII A, using 0.05 ml of *crystal violet solution* as indicator. Carry out a blank titration. Each ml of 0.1M *perchloric acid VS* is equivalent to 44.81 mg of $C_{27}H_{42}ClNO_2$.

Bromine VS Bromide-bromate; Br_2 = 159.8
For a 0.05M solution Dissolve 2.7835 g of *potassium bromate* and 13 g of *potassium bromide* in sufficient *water* to produce 1000 ml. (This solution is equivalent to *0.0167M bromide-bromate* of the European Pharmacopoeia).
Store in a dark amber-coloured bottle.

Cerium(IV) Sulphate VS Cerium sulphate; $Ce(SO_4)_2,4H_2O$ = 404.3
For a 0.1M solution Dissolve 40.4 g of *cerium(IV) sulphate* in a mixture of 500 ml of *water* and 50 ml of *sulphuric acid (96% w/w)*. Allow to cool and dilute to 1000 ml with *water*.

Ascertain its exact concentration immediately before use in the following manner. To 25 ml of the solution add 2 g of *potassium iodide*, 150 ml of *water* and 1 ml of *starch solution* and titrate immediately with 0.1M *sodium thiosulphate VS*. Each ml of 0.1M *sodium thiosulphate VS* is equivalent to 40.43 mg of $Ce(SO_4)_2,4H_2O$.

Cetylpyridinium Chloride VS $C_{21}H_{38}ClN,H_2O$ = 358.0
For a 0.005M solution Dissolve 1.8 g of *cetylpyridinium chloride* in 10 ml of *ethanol (96%)* and dilute to 1000 ml with *water*.

Ascertain its exact concentration in the following manner. Transfer 25 ml to a separating funnel, add 25 ml of *chloroform*, 10 ml of 0.01M *sodium hydroxide* and 10 ml of a freshly prepared 0.5% w/v solution of *potassium iodide*. Shake well, allow to separate and discard the chloroform layer. Shake the aqueous layer with three further 10-ml quantities of *chloroform* and discard the chloroform solutions. Add 40 ml of *hydrochloric acid*, cool and titrate with 0.005M *potassium iodate VS* until the solution becomes pale brown in colour. Add 2 ml of *chloroform* and continue the titration, shaking vigorously and allowing the layers to separate after each addition, until the chloroform becomes colourless. Titrate a mixture of 20 ml of *water*, 10 ml of the potassium iodide solution and 40 ml of *hydrochloric acid* with 0.005M *potassium iodate VS* in the same manner. The difference between the titrations represents the amount of potassium iodate required. Each ml of 0.005M *potassium iodate VS* is equivalent to 3.580 mg of $C_{21}H_{38}ClN,H_2O$.

Copper Sulphate VS $CuSO_4,5H_2O$ = 249.7

For a 0.02M solution Dissolve 5.0 g of *copper(II) sulphate* in *water* and dilute to 1000 ml with *water*.

Ascertain its exact concentration in the following manner. To 20 ml add 2 g of *sodium acetate* and titrate with 0.02M *disodium edetate VS*, using 0.1 ml of *pyridylazonaphthol solution* as indicator, until the colour changes from violet-blue to bright green. Titrate slowly towards the end point. Each ml of 0.02M *disodium edetate VS* is equivalent to 4.994 mg of $CuSO_4,5H_2O$.

Cupriethylenediamine Hydroxide Solution Use a 1M solution in which the molar ratio of ethylenediamine to copper is 2.00 ± 0.04.

Dioctyl Sodium Sulphosuccinate VS $C_{20}H_{37}NaO_7S$ = 444.6

For a 0.01M solution Dissolve 4.5 g of *dioctyl sodium sulphosuccinate* in warm *water*, cool and dilute to 1000 ml with *water*.

Ascertain its exact concentration in the following manner. To 25 ml add 25 ml of a solution containing 20% w/v of *anhydrous sodium sulphate* and 2% w/v of *sodium carbonate*, 50 ml of *chloroform* and 1.5 ml of *bromophenol blue solution* and mix. Titrate with 0.01M *tetrabutylammonium iodide VS* until about 1 ml from the end point. Stopper the flask, shake vigorously for 2 minutes and continue the titration, in 0.05-ml increments, shaking vigorously and allowing the flask to stand for about 10 seconds after each addition. Continue the titration until a blue colour just appears in the chloroform layer. Each ml of 0.01M *tetrabutylammonium iodide VS* is equivalent to 4.446 mg of $C_{20}H_{37}NaO_7S$.

Disodium Edetate VS Sodium edetate; $C_{10}H_{14}N_2Na_2O_8,2H_2O$ = 372.2

For a 0.1M solution Dissolve 37.5 g of *disodium edetate* in sufficient *water* to produce 500 ml, add 100 ml of 1M *sodium hydroxide* and dilute to 1000 ml with *water*.

Ascertain its exact concentration in the following manner. Dissolve 0.120 g of *zinc*, in granules, in 4 ml of 7M *hydrochloric acid* and add 0.1 ml of *bromine water*. Boil to remove excess bromine, cool, add 2M *sodium hydroxide* until the solution is weakly acidic or neutral and carry out the method for the *complexometric titration of zinc*, Appendix VIII D. Each ml of 0.1M *disodium edetate VS* is equivalent to 6.54 mg of Zn.

Store in a polyethylene container.

For a 0.02M solution Dissolve 7.444 g of *disodium edetate* in sufficient *water* to produce 1000 ml.

Ascertain its exact concentration in the following manner. Dissolve 0.100 g of *zinc*, in granules, in 4 ml of 7M *hydrochloric acid* and add 0.1 ml of *bromine water*. Boil to remove excess bromine, cool and dilute to 100 ml with *water*. Dilute 25 ml of this solution to 200 ml with *water*, add about 50 mg of *xylenol orange triturate* and *hexamine* until the solution becomes violet-pink and add 2 g of *hexamine* in excess. Titrate with the disodium edetate solution until the violet-pink colour changes to yellow. Each ml of 0.02M *disodium edetate VS* is equivalent to 1.308 mg of Zn.

Hydrochloric Acid VS HCl = 36.46

For a 0.1M solution Dilute 8.5 ml of *hydrochloric acid* with sufficient *water* to produce 1000 ml.

Ascertain its exact concentration in the following manner. Dissolve 0.1 g of *anhydrous sodium carbonate* in 20 ml of *water*, add 0.1 ml of *methyl orange solution* and titrate with the hydrochloric acid until the solution becomes reddish yellow. Boil for 2 minutes and continue the titration until the reddish yellow colour is restored. Each ml of 0.1M *hydrochloric acid VS* is equivalent to 5.30 mg of Na_2CO_3.

For a 1M solution Dilute 103.0 g of *hydrochloric acid* to 1000 ml with *water*.

Ascertain its exact concentration as described for the 0.1M solution using 1.000 g of *anhydrous sodium carbonate* dissolved in 50 ml of *water*. Each ml of 1M *hydrochloric acid VS* is equivalent to 53.00 mg of Na_2CO_3.

For a 2M solution Dilute 206.0 g of *hydrochloric acid* to 1000 ml with *water*.

For a 3M solution Dilute 309.0 g of *hydrochloric acid* to 1000 ml with *water*.

For a 6M solution Dilute 618.0 g of *hydrochloric acid* to 1000 ml with *water*.

Iodine VS I_2 = 253.8

For a 0.05M solution Dissolve 20 g of *potassium iodide* in the minimum amount of *water*, add 12.7 g of *iodine*, allow to dissolve and dilute to 1000 ml with *water*.

Ascertain its exact concentration in the following manner. Dissolve 80 mg of *arsenic trioxide* in 20 ml of 1M *sodium hydroxide*, add 10 ml of 2M *hydrochloric acid* and 3 g of *sodium hydrogen carbonate* and titrate with the iodine solution using 1 ml of *starch solution* as indicator. Each ml of 0.05M *iodine VS* is equivalent to 4.946 mg of As_2O_3. Store protected from light.

For a 0.01M solution Add 0.3 g of *potassium iodide* to 20 ml of 0.05M *iodine VS* and add sufficient *water* to produce 100 ml.

Iron(II) Sulphate VS Ferrous sulphate; $FeSO_4,7H_2O$ = 278.0

For a 0.1M solution Dissolve 27.80 g of *iron(II) sulphate* in 500 ml of 1M *sulphuric acid* and add sufficient *water* to produce 1000 ml.

Ascertain its exact concentration immediately before use in the following manner. To 25 ml of the solution add 3 ml of *orthophosphoric acid* and titrate immediately with 0.02M *potassium permanganate VS*. Each ml of 0.02M *potassium permanganate VS* is equivalent to 27.80 mg of $FeSO_4,7H_2O$.

Karl Fischer Reagent VS Iodosulphurous reagent

The apparatus, which must be kept closed and dry during the preparation, consists of a 3000- to 4000-ml round-bottomed flask with inlets for a thermometer and a stirrer and fitted with a drying tube. To 700 ml of *anhydrous pyridine* and 700 ml of *2-methoxyethanol* add, stirring constantly, 220 g of finely powdered *iodine*, previously dried over *phosphorus pentoxide*. Continue stirring until the iodine has completely dissolved (about 30 minutes), cool to −10° and add quickly, while stirring, 190 g of *sulphur dioxide*. Do not allow the temperature to exceed 30°; cool.

Determine the water-equivalent of the reagent immediately before use in the following manner. Transfer 20 ml of *anhydrous methanol* to the titration vessel and titrate to the electrometric end point with the reagent, Appendix IX C. Add in an appropriate form a suitable amount of water, accurately weighed, and titrate to the end point. Calculate the water-equivalent of the reagent in mg per ml. The minimum water equivalent is 3.5 mg of water per ml of reagent. Work protected from humidity.

The composition of commercially available Karl Fischer reagents often differs from that above by the replacement of pyridine with other basic compounds. The use of these reagents must be validated in order to verify in each individual case the stoichiometry and the absence of incompatibility between the substance under test and the reagent.

Lead Nitrate VS $Pb(NO_3)_2$ = 331.2

For a 0.05M solution Dissolve 16.5 g of *lead(II) nitrate* in sufficient *water* to produce 1000 ml.

Ascertain its exact concentration in the following manner. To 50 ml of the solution add 300 ml of *water* and carry out the method for the *complexometric titration of lead*, Appendix VIII D. Each ml of 0.1M *disodium edetate VS* is equivalent to 33.12 mg of $Pb(NO_3)_2$.

For a 0.1M solution Dissolve 33.0 g of *lead(II) nitrate* in sufficient *water* to produce 1000 ml.

Ascertain its exact concentration in the following manner. To 20 ml of the solution add 300 ml of *water* and carry out the method for the *complexometric titration of lead*, Appendix VIII D. Each ml of *disodium edetate VS* is equivalent to 33.12 mg of $Pb(NO_3)_2$.

Lithium Methoxide VS $LiOCH_3$ = 37.97

For a 0.1M solution Dissolve in small portions 0.694 g of *lithium* in 150 ml of *anhydrous methanol* and add sufficient *toluene* to produce 1000 ml.

Ascertain its exact concentration immediately before use in the following manner. To 10 ml of *dimethylformamide* add 0.05 ml of a 0.3% w/v solution of *thymol blue* in *methanol* and titrate with the lithium methoxide solution until a pure blue colour is produced. Immediately add 0.2 g of *benzoic acid*, stir to effect solution and titrate with the lithium methoxide solution until the pure blue colour is restored. Protect the solution from atmospheric carbon dioxide throughout the titration. The volume of titrant used in the second titration represents the amount of lithium methoxide required. Each ml of 0.1M *lithium methoxide VS* is equivalent to 12.21 mg of $C_7H_6O_2$.

Magnesium Chloride VS $MgCl_2,6H_2O$ = 203.3

For a 0.1M solution Dissolve 20.33 g of *magnesium chloride* in sufficient *water* to produce 1000 ml.

Ascertain its exact concentration by carrying out the method for the *complexometric titration of magnesium*, Appendix VIII D, using 25 ml of the magnesium chloride solution. Each ml of 0.1M *disodium edetate VS* is equivalent to 20.33 g of $MgCl_2,6H_2O$.

Magnesium Sulphate VS $MgSO_4,7H_2O$ = 246.5

For a 0.05M solution Dissolve 12.5 g of *magnesium sulphate* in sufficient *water* to produce 1000 ml.

Ascertain its exact concentration by carrying out the method for the *complexometric titration of magnesium*, Appendix VIII D, using 40 ml of the magnesium sulphate solution. Each ml of 0.1M *disodium edetate VS* is equivalent to 24.65 mg of $MgSO_4,7H_2O$.

Mercury(II) Nitrate VS Mercuric nitrate; $Hg(NO_3)_2$ + aq

For a 0.02M solution Dissolve 6.85 g of *mercury(II) nitrate* in 20 ml of 1M *nitric acid* and add sufficient *water* to produce 1000 ml.

Ascertain its exact concentration in the following manner. Dissolve 15 mg of *sodium chloride* in 50 ml of *water* and titrate with the mercury nitrate solution determining the end point potentiometrically, using a platinum or mercury indicator electrode and a mercury—mercury(I) sulphate reference electrode. Each ml of 0.02M *mercury(II) nitrate VS* is equivalent to 2.338 mg of NaCl.

Nitric Acid VS HNO_3 = 63.01

For a 1M solution Dilute 96.6 g of *nitric acid* with sufficient *water* to produce 1000 ml.

Ascertain its exact concentration in the following manner. Dissolve 2 g of *anhydrous sodium carbonate* in 50 ml of *water* and titrate with the nitric acid solution using 0.1 ml of *methyl orange solution* as indicator until the solution becomes reddish yellow. Boil for 2 minutes, cool and continue the titration until the reddish yellow colour is restored. Each ml of 1M *nitric acid VS* is equivalent to 53.00 mg of Na_2CO_3.

Perchloric Acid VS $HClO_4$ = 100.5

For a 0.1M solution To 900 ml of *glacial acetic acid* add 8.5 ml of *perchloric acid*, mix, add 30 ml of *acetic anhydride*, dilute to 1000 ml with *glacial acetic acid*, mix and allow to stand for 24 hours. Determine the water content, Appendix IX A, without addition of methanol and if necessary adjust the water content to between 0.1 and 0.2% by adding either *acetic anhydride* or *water*; allow to stand for 24 hours.

Ascertain its exact concentration in the following manner. Dissolve 0.35 g of *potassium hydrogen phthalate* in 50 ml of *anhydrous acetic acid*, warming gently if necessary. Allow to cool protected from the air and titrate with the perchloric acid solution using 0.05 ml of *crystal violet solution* as indicator. Each ml of 0.1M *perchloric acid VS* is equivalent to 20.42 mg of $C_8H_5KO_4$. Record the temperature at which the standardisation was carried out. If the temperature at which an assay is carried out is different from that at which the perchloric acid has been standardised the volume used in the assay becomes

$$V_c = V[1 + 0.0011(t_1 - t_2)$$

where t_1 is the temperature during standardisation, t_2 is the temperature during the assay, V is the observed volume and V_c is the corrected volume.

Other strengths of perchloric acid should be prepared by diluting 0.1M *perchloric acid VS* appropriately with *anhydrous acetic acid*.

Potassium Bromate VS $KBrO_3$ = 167.0

For a 0.0167M solution Dissolve 2.783 g of *potassium bromate* in sufficient *water* to produce 1000 ml.

For a 0.02M solution Dissolve 3.340 g of *potassium bromate* in sufficient *water* to produce 1000 ml.

For a 0.033M solution Dissolve 5.567 g of *potassium bromate* in sufficient *water* to produce 1000 ml.

Potassium Dichromate VS $K_2Cr_2O_7$ = 294.2

For a 0.0167M solution Dissolve 4.9 g of *potassium dichromate* in sufficient *water* to produce 1000 ml.

Ascertain its exact concentration in the following manner. To 20 ml of the solution add 1 g of *potassium iodide* and 7 ml of 2M *hydrochloric acid.* Add 250 ml of *water* and titrate with 0.1M *sodium thiosulphate VS*, using 3 ml of *starch solution* as indicator, until the colour changes from blue to light green. Each ml of 0.1M *sodium thiosulphate VS* is equivalent to 4.9 mg of $K_2Cr_2O_7$.

Potassium Hydrogen Phthalate VS $C_8H_5O_4K$ = 204.2
For a 0.1M solution Dissolve 20.42 g of *potassium hydrogen phthalate* in about 800 ml of *anhydrous acetic acid,* heat on a water bath until completely dissolved, protected from humidity, cool to 20° and add sufficient *anhydrous acetic acid* to produce 1000 ml.

Potassium Hydroxide VS KOH = 56.11
For a 0.1M solution Dissolve 6 g of *potassium hydroxide* in sufficient *carbon dioxide-free water* to produce 1000 ml.
Ascertain its exact concentration in the following manner. Titrate 20 ml of the solution with 0.1M *hydrochloric acid VS* using 0.5 ml of *phenolphthalein solution* as indicator. Each ml of 0.1M *hydrochloric acid VS* is equivalent to 5.611 mg of KOH.
For a 1M solution Dissolve 60 g of *potassium hydroxide* in sufficient *carbon dioxide-free water* to produce 1000 ml.
Ascertain its exact concentration in the following manner. Titrate 20 ml of the solution with 1M *hydrochloric acid VS* using 0.5 ml of *phenolphthalein solution* as indicator. Each ml of 1M *hydrochloric acid VS* is equivalent to 56.11 mg of KOH.

Potassium Hydroxide VS, Ethanolic Alcoholic potassium hydroxide
For a 0.1M solution Dissolve 6 g of *potassium hydroxide* in 50 ml of *water* and dilute to 1000 ml with *aldehyde-free ethanol (96%).*
Ascertain its exact concentration immediately before use in the following manner. Titrate 20 ml of the solution with 0.1M *hydrochloric acid VS* using 0.5 ml of *phenolphthalein solution* as indicator. Each ml of 0.1M *hydrochloric acid VS* is equivalent to 5.611 mg of KOH.
For a 0.5M solution Dissolve 3 g of *potassium hydroxide* in 5 ml of *water* and add sufficient *aldehyde-free ethanol (96%)* to produce 100 ml. Allow the solution to stand for 24 hours and decant the clear solution.
Ascertain its exact concentration in the following manner. Titrate 20 ml of the solution with 0.5M *hydrochloric acid VS* using 0.5 ml of *phenolphthalein solution* as indicator. Each ml of 0.5M *hydrochloric acid VS* is equivalent to 28.06 mg of KOH.
Store in a well-closed container protected from light.

Potassium Hydroxide in Ethanol (60%) VS Potassium hydroxide in alcohol (60% v/v)
For a 0.5M solution Prepare and standardise as directed for 0.5M *ethanolic potassium hydroxide VS* but using *aldehyde-free ethanol (60%)* in place of the aldehyde-free ethanol (96%).

Potassium Hydroxide in Ethanol (90%) VS
For a 1M solution Dissolve 60 g of *potassium hydroxide* in sufficient *aldehyde-free ethanol (90%)* to produce 1000 ml, allow the solution to stand for 24 hours, decant the clear solution and ascertain its exact concentration by the method described under 0.5M *ethanolic potassium hydroxide VS.*

Potassium Iodate VS KIO_3 = 214.0
For a 0.05M solution Dissolve 10.7 g of *potassium iodate* in sufficient *water* to produce 1000 ml.
Ascertain its exact concentration in the following manner. Dilute 25 ml of the solution to 100 ml with *water* and to 20 ml of this solution add 2 g of *potassium iodide* and 10 ml of 1M *sulphuric acid VS.* Titrate with 0.1M *sodium thiosulphate VS* using 1 ml of *starch solution*, added towards the end of the titration, as indicator. Each ml of 0.1M *sodium thiosulphate VS* is equivalent to 3.566 mg of KIO_3.

Potassium Iodide VS KI = 166.0
For a 0.001M solution Dilute 10.0 ml of *potassium iodide solution* to 100.0 ml with *water.* Dilute 5 ml of this solution to 500.0 ml with *water.*

Potassium Permanganate VS $KMnO_4$ = 158.0
For a 0.02M solution Dissolve 3.2 g of *potassium permanganate* in 1000 ml of *water*, heat on a water bath for 1 hour, cool and filter through a sintered-glass filter.
Ascertain its exact concentration immediately before use in the following manner. To 20 ml of the solution add 2 g of *potassium iodide* and 10 ml of 1M *sulphuric acid* and titrate with 0.1M *sodium thiosulphate VS* using 1 ml of *starch solution,* added towards the end of the titration, as indicator. Each ml of 0.1M *sodium thiosulphate VS* is equivalent to 3.161 mg of $KMnO_4$.
Store protected from light.

Silver Nitrate VS $AgNO_3$ = 169.9
For a 0.1M solution Dissolve 17.0 g of *silver nitrate* in sufficient *water* to produce 1000 ml.
Ascertain its exact concentration in the following manner. Dissolve 0.1 g of *sodium chloride* in 30 ml of *water* and titrate with the silver nitrate solution determining the end point potentiometrically, Appendix VIII B. Each ml of 0.1M *silver nitrate VS* is equivalent to 5.844 mg of NaCl.
Store protected from light.
For a 0.001M solution Dilute 5 ml of 0.1M *silver nitrate VS* to 500 ml with *water.*

Sodium Arsenite VS
For a 0.1M solution Dissolve 4.946 g of *arsenic trioxide* in a mixture of 20 ml of 10M *sodium hydroxide* and 20 ml of *water*, dilute to 400 ml with *water* and add 2M *hydrochloric acid* until the solution is neutral to *litmus paper.* Dissolve 2 g of *sodium hydrogen carbonate* in the solution and dilute to 500 ml with *water.*

Sodium Dodecyl Sulphate VS $C_{12}H_{25}NaO_4S$ = 288.4
For a 0.001M solution Dissolve 0.2884 g of *sodium dodecyl sulphate*, calculated with reference to the substance dried at 105° for 2 hours, in sufficient *water* to produce 1000 ml.
Ascertain its exact concentration in the following manner. To 50 ml add 15 ml of *chloroform*, 10 ml of 1M *sulphuric acid* and 1 ml of a solution containing 0.003% w/v of each of *dimethyl yellow* and *oracet blue B* in *chloroform* and titrate with *0.004M benzethonium chloride VS*, shaking vigorously and allowing the layers to separate after each addition, until the chloroform layer acquires a permanent clear green colour. Each ml of *0.004M benzethonium chloride VS* is equivalent to 1.154 mg of $C_{12}H_{25}NaO_4S$.

Sodium Hydroxide VS NaOH = 40.00
For a 0.1M solution Dissolve 4.2 g of *sodium hydroxide* in sufficient *carbon dioxide-free water* to produce 1000 ml.
Ascertain its exact concentration immediately before use in the following manner. Titrate 20 ml of the solution with 0.1M *hydrochloric acid VS* using the indicator prescribed in the assay in which the solution is to be used. Each ml of 0.1M *hydrochloric acid VS* is equivalent to 4.00 mg of NaOH.

When a carbonate-free solution is specified it is prepared using the following method. Dissolve *sodium hydroxide* in an equal weight of *water* and allow to stand overnight. Taking precautions to avoid absorption of carbon dioxide, siphon off or decant the clear supernatant liquid and dilute with *carbon dioxide-free water* to the desired molarity. The solution complies with the following test.

Titrate 20 ml of *hydrochloric acid VS* of the same molarity as the solution being examined with the sodium hydroxide solution using 0.5 ml of *phenolphthalein solution* as indicator. At the end point add just sufficient of the acid to discharge the pink colour and boil to reduce the volume to 20 ml. Add, whilst boiling, sufficient of the acid again to discharge the pink colour which does not re-appear after prolonged boiling. Not more than 0.1 ml of the acid is required.

For a 1M solution Dissolve 42 g of sodium hydroxide in sufficient carbon dioxide-free water to produce 1000 ml.

Ascertain its exact concentration immediately before use in the following manner. Titrate 20 ml of the solution with 1M *hydrochloric acid VS* using the indicator prescribed in the assay in which the solution is to be used. Each ml of 1M *hydrochloric acid VS* is equivalent to 4.00 mg of NaOH.

Sodium Hydroxide VS, Ethanolic

For a 0.1M solution Add 3.3 g of 10M *sodium hydroxide solution* to 250 ml of *absolute ethanol*.

Ascertain its exact concentration immediately before use in the following manner. Dissolve 0.2 g of *benzoic acid* in a mixture of 10 ml of *ethanol (96%)* and 2 ml of *water* and titrate with the ethanolic sodium hydroxide solution using 0.2 ml of *thymolphthalein solution* as indicator. Each ml of 0.1M *ethanolic sodium hydroxide VS* is equivalent to 12.21 mg of $C_7H_6O_2$.

Sodium Methoxide VS

For a 0.1M solution Cool 175 ml of *anhydrous methanol* in ice and add, in small portions, about 2.5 g of freshly cut *sodium*. When the metal has dissolved add sufficient *toluene* to produce 1000 ml.

Ascertain its exact concentration immediately before use in the following manner. To 10 ml of *dimethylformamide* add 0.05 ml of a 0.3% w/v solution of *thymol blue* in *methanol* and titrate with the sodium methoxide solution until a pure blue colour is produced. Immediately add 0.2 g of *benzoic acid*, stir to effect solution and titrate with the sodium methoxide solution until the pure blue colour is restored. Protect the solution from atmospheric carbon dioxide throughout the titration. The volume of titrant used in the second titration represents the amount of sodium methoxide required. Each ml of 0.1M *sodium methoxide VS* is equivalent to 12.21 mg of $C_7H_6O_2$.

Sodium Nitrite VS $NaNO_2$ = 69.00

For a 0.1M solution Dissolve 7.5 g of *sodium nitrite* in sufficient *water* to produce 1000 ml.

Ascertain its exact concentration immediately before use in the following manner. Dissolve 0.3 g of *sulphanilic acid* in 50 ml of 2M *hydrochloric acid*, add 3 g of *potassium bromide*, cool in ice and titrate with 0.1M *sodium nitrite VS* determining the end point electrometrically. Each ml of 0.1M *sodium nitrite VS* is equivalent to 17.32 mg of $C_6H_7NO_3S$.

Sodium Tetraphenylborate VS $B(C_6H_5)_4Na$ = 342.2

For a 0.01M solution Dissolve 3.5 g of *sodium tetraphenylborate* in 50 ml of *water*, shake for 20 minutes with 0.5 g of *aluminium hydroxide gel*, add 250 ml of *water* and 16.6 g of *sodium chloride* and allow to stand for 30 minutes. Filter, add 600 ml of *water*, adjust the pH to 8.0 to 9.0 with 0.1M *sodium hydroxide* and dilute to 1000 ml with *water*.

Ascertain its exact concentration in the following manner. Dissolve 7 mg of *potassium chloride*, previously dried at 150° for 1 hour, in 5 ml of *acetate buffer pH 3.7* and 5 ml of *water*, add 15 ml of the sodium tetraphenylborate solution, allow to stand for 5 minutes and filter through a dry, sintered-glass filter. To 20 ml of the filtrate add 0.5 ml of *bromophenol blue solution* and titrate the excess of sodium tetraphenylborate with 0.005M *cetylpyridinium chloride VS* to the blue colour of the indicator. Repeat the procedure without the potassium chloride. The molarity of the solution is given by the expression:

$$aw/[15(a-b)0.07455]$$

where *a* is the volume of 0.005M *cetylpyridinium chloride VS* required when the potassium chloride is omitted, *b* is the volume of 0.005M *cetylpyridinium chloride VS* required when the potassium chloride is present and *w* is the weight, in g, of potassium chloride taken.

Sodium Thiosulphate VS $Na_2S_2O_3,5H_2O$ = 248.2

For a 0.1M solution Dissolve 25 g of *sodium thiosulphate* and 0.2 g of *sodium carbonate* in sufficient *carbon dioxide-free water* to produce 1000 ml.

Ascertain its exact concentration in the following manner. To 20 ml of 0.0167M *potassium bromate VS* add 40 ml of *water*, 10 ml of *potassium iodide solution* and 5 ml of 7M *hydrochloric acid*. Titrate with the sodium thiosulphate solution using 1 ml of *starch solution*, added towards the end of the titration, as indicator. Each ml of 0.1M *sodium thiosulphate VS* is equivalent to 2.784 mg of $KBrO_3$.

Sulphuric Acid VS H_2SO_4 = 98.08

For a 0.5M solution Carefully add 28 ml of *sulphuric acid* to 50 ml of *water* and dilute to 1000 ml with the same solvent.

Ascertain its exact concentration in the following manner. Dissolve 1.0 g of *anhydrous sodium carbonate* in 50 ml of *water*, add 0.1 ml of *methyl orange solution* and titrate with the sulphuric acid solution until the solution begins to turn reddish yellow. Boil the solution for 2 minutes, cool and titrate again until the reddish yellow colour is restored. Each ml of 0.5M *sulphuric acid VS* is equivalent to 53.00 mg of Na_2CO_3.

For a 0.05M solution Dilute 100 ml of 0.5M *sulphuric acid VS* to 1000 ml with *water*.

Ascertain its exact concentration as described above using 0.10 g of *anhydrous sodium carbonate* dissolved in 20 ml of *water*.

Tetrabutylammonium Hydroxide VS $C_{16}H_{37}NO$ = 259.5

For a 0.1M solution Dissolve 40 g of *tetrabutylammonium iodide* in 90 ml of *anhydrous methanol*, add 20 g of finely powdered *silver oxide* and shake vigorously for 1 hour. Centrifuge a few ml of the mixture and test the supernatant liquid for iodides. If a positive reaction is obtained, add a further 2 g of *silver oxide* and shake for 30 minutes. Repeat this procedure until the mixture is free from iodides, filter through a fine sintered-glass filter and wash the reaction vessel and filter with three 50-ml quantities of *toluene*. Add the washings to the filtrate and add sufficient *toluene* to produce 1000 ml. Pass dry carbon dioxide-free nitrogen through the solution for 5 minutes.

Ascertain its exact concentration immediately before use in the following manner. To 10 ml of *dimethylformamide* add 0.05 ml of a 0.3% w/v solution of *thymol blue* in *methanol* and titrate with the tetrabutylammonium hydroxide solution until a pure blue colour is produced. Immediately add 0.2 g of *benzoic acid*, stir to effect solution and titrate with the tetrabutylammonium hydroxide solution until the pure blue colour is restored. Protect the solution from atmospheric carbon dioxide throughout the titration. The volume of titrant used in the second titration represents the amount of tetrabutylammonium hydroxide required. Each ml of 0.1M *tetrabutylammonium hydroxide VS* is equivalent to 12.21 mg of $C_7H_6O_2$.

Tetrabutylammonium Hydroxide in Propan-2-ol VS Tetrabutylammonium hydroxide in 2-propanol
For a 0.1M solution Prepare as described for 0.1M *tetrabutylammonium hydroxide VS* using *propan-2-ol* in place of *toluene* and ascertain its exact concentration immediately before use as described above.

Tetrabutylammonium Iodide VS $C_{16}H_{36}IN$ = 369.4
For a 0.01M solution Dissolve 4 g of *tetrabutylammonium iodide* in sufficient *water* to produce 1000 ml.

Ascertain its exact concentration in the following manner. To 25 ml add 50 ml of 0.01M *silver nitrate VS* and 0.5 ml of 2M *nitric acid* and titrate the excess of silver nitrate with 0.01M *ammonium thiocyanate VS* using *ammonium iron(III) sulphate solution R1* as indicator. Each ml of 0.01M *silver nitrate VS* is equivalent to 3.694 mg of $C_{16}H_{36}IN$.

Titanium(III) Chloride VS $TiCl_3$ = 154.3
For a 0.1M solution Dilute 100 ml of *titanium(III) chloride solution* with 200 ml of *hydrochloric acid* and add sufficient freshly boiled and cooled *water* to produce 1000 ml.

Ascertain its exact concentration immediately before use by titrating with it, in an atmosphere of carbon dioxide, 25 ml of 0.1M *ammonium iron(III) sulphate VS* acidified with *sulphuric acid*, using *ammonium thiocyanate solution*, added just before the end point, as indicator. Each ml of 0.1M *ammonium iron(III) sulphate VS* is equivalent to 15.43 mg of $TiCl_3$.

Zinc Chloride VS $ZnCl_2$ = 136.3
For a 0.05M solution Dissolve 6.82 g of *zinc chloride*, weighed with appropriate precautions, in *water*. If necessary, add 2M *hydrochloric acid* dropwise until the opalescence disappears and add sufficient *water* to produce 1000 ml.

Ascertain its exact concentration in the following manner. To 20 ml add 5 ml of 2M *acetic acid* and carry out the method for the *complexometric titration of zinc*, Appendix VIII D. Each ml of 0.1M *disodium edetate VS* is equivalent to 13.63 mg of $ZnCl_2$.

Zinc Sulphate VS $ZnSO_4,7H_2O$ = 287.5
For a 0.1M solution Dissolve 29 g of *zinc sulphate* in sufficient *water* to produce 1000 ml.

Ascertain its exact concentration in the following manner. To 20 ml add 5 ml of 2M *acetic acid* and carry out the method for the *complexometric titration of zinc*, Appendix VIII D. Each ml of 0.1M *disodium edetate VS* is equivalent to 28.75 mg of $ZnSO_4,7H_2O$.

C. Standard Solutions

The following solutions are used as reference standards in limit tests and should, unless experience has shown it to be unnecessary, be prepared immediately before use.

In monographs of the European Pharmacopoeia, the symbol '%' may be replaced by the words 'per cent'. In such cases the reagent described below is to be used.

Acetaldehyde Standard Solution (100 ppm C_2H_4O) Dissolve 1.0 g of *acetaldehyde* in sufficient *propan-2-ol* to produce 100 ml and dilute 5.0 ml of the solution to 500.0 ml with *propan-2-ol*. Prepare immediately before use.

Acetaldehyde Standard Solution (100 ppm C_2H_4O) R1 Dissolve 1 g of *acetaldehyde* in *water* and dilute to 100 ml with the same solvent. Dilute 5 ml of the solution to 500 ml with *water*. Prepare immediately before use.

Aluminium Standard Solution (200 ppm Al) Dissolve in *water* a quantity of *aluminium potassium sulphate* containing 0.352 g of $AlK(SO_4)_2,12H_2O$. Add 10 ml of 1M *sulphuric acid* and dilute to 100 ml with *water*.

Aluminium Standard Solution (10 ppm Al) Dilute 1 volume of a 1.39% w/v solution of *aluminium nitrate* to 100 volumes with *water* immediately before use.

Aluminium Standard Solution (2 ppm Al) Dilute 1 volume of a 0.352% w/v solution of *aluminium potassium sulphate* in 0.1M *sulphuric acid* to 100 volumes with *water* immediately before use.

Ammonium Standard Solution (100 ppm NH_4) Dilute 10.0 ml of a 0.0741% w/v solution of *ammonium chloride* to 25.0 ml with *water*.

Ammonium Standard Solution (2.5 ppm NH_4) Dilute 1 volume of a 0.0741% w/v solution of *ammonium chloride* to 100 volumes with *water*.

Ammonium Standard Solution (1 ppm NH_4) Dilute 1 volume of *ammonium standard solution (2.5 ppm NH_4)* to 2.5 volumes with *water* immediately before use.

Antimony Standard Solution (1 ppm Sb) Dissolve 0.274 g of *antimony potassium tartrate* in 20 ml of 7M *hydrochloric acid* and dilute the clear solution to 100.0 ml with *water*. To 10.0 ml of this solution add 200 ml of 7M *hydrochloric acid* and dilute with *water* to 1000.0 ml. To 100.0 ml of this solution add 300 ml of 7M *hydrochloric acid* and dilute to 1000.0 ml with *water*. Prepare the dilute solutions immediately before use.

Arsenic Standard Solution (10 ppm As) Dissolve 0.330 g of *arsenic trioxide* in 5 ml of 2M *sodium hydroxide* and dilute to 250.0 ml with *water*. Dilute 1 volume of this solution to 100 volumes with *water* immediately before use.

Arsenic Standard Solution (1 ppm As) Dilute 1 volume of *arsenic standard solution (10 ppm As)* to 10 volumes with *water* immediately before use.

Arsenic Standard Solution (0.1 ppm As) Dilute 1 volume of *arsenic standard solution (1 ppm As)* to 10 volumes with *water* immediately before use.

Barium Standard Solution (0.1% Ba) Dissolve 1.778 g of *barium chloride* in sufficient *water* to produce 1000 ml.

Barium Standard Solution (50 ppm Ba) Dilute 1 volume of a 0.178% w/v solution of *barium chloride* in *distilled water* to 20 volumes with *distilled water* immediately before use.

Cadmium Standard Solution (0.1% Cd) Dissolve a quantity of *cadmium* containing 0.100 g of Cd in the minimum quantity of a mixture of equal volumes of *hydrochloric acid* and *water* and dilute to 100.0 ml with a 1% v/v solution of *hydrochloric acid*.

Cadmium Standard Solution (10 ppm Cd) Dilute 1 volume of *cadmium standard solution (0.1% Cd)* to 100 volumes with a 1% v/v solution of *hydrochloric acid* immediately before use.

Calcium Standard Solution (400 ppm Ca) Dissolve 1.0 g of *calcium carbonate* in 23 ml of 1M *hydrochloric acid* and add sufficient *distilled water* to produce 100 ml. Dilute 1 volume of this solution to 10 volumes with *distilled water* immediately before use.

Calcium Standard Solution (100 ppm Ca) Dissolve 0.624 g of dried *calcium carbonate* in *distilled water* containing 3 ml of 5M *acetic acid* and add sufficient *distilled water* to produce 250 ml. Immediately before use dilute 1 volume of this solution to 10 volumes with *distilled water*.

Calcium Standard Solution (100 ppm Ca), Alcoholic Dissolve 2.50 g of dried *calcium carbonate* in 12 ml of 5M *acetic acid* and dilute to 1000.0 ml with *distilled water*. Dilute 1 volume of this solution to 10 volumes with *ethanol (96%)* immediately before use.

Calcium Standard Solution (10 ppm Ca) Dissolve 0.624 g of dried *calcium carbonate* in *distilled water* containing 3 ml of 5M *acetic acid* and dilute to 250 ml with *distilled water*. Dilute 1 volume of this solution to 100 volumes with *distilled water* immediately before use.

Chloride Standard Solution (8 ppm Cl) Dilute 1 volume of a 0.132% w/v solution of *sodium chloride* to 100 volumes with *water* immediately before use.

Chloride Standard Solution (5 ppm Cl) Dilute 1 volume of a 0.0824% w/v solution of *sodium chloride* to 100 volumes with *water* immediately before use.

Chromium Standard Solution (100 ppm Cr) Dissolve 0.283 g of dried *potassium dichromate* in sufficient *water* to produce 1000 ml.

Chromium Standard Solution (0.1 ppm Cr) Dilute 1 volume of *chromium standard solution (100 ppm Cr)* to 1000 volumes with *water* immediately before use.

Copper Standard Solution (0.1% Cu) Dissolve 0.393 g of *copper sulphate* in sufficient *water* to produce 100 ml.

Copper Standard Solution (10 ppm Cu) Dilute 1 volume of a 0.393% w/v solution of *copper(II) sulphate* to 100 volumes with *water* immediately before use.

Copper Standard Solution (0.1 ppm Cu) Dilute 1 volume of *copper standard solution (10 ppm Cu)* to 100 volumes with *water* immediately before use.

Digitoxin Standard Solution Dissolve 0.1250 g of *digitoxin EPCRS* in sufficient *glacial acetic acid* to produce 100.0 ml. Dilute 4.0 ml of the solution to 100.0 ml with *glacial acetic acid*. To 25.0 ml of the resulting solution add 3.0 ml of *water* and mix well.

Digoxin Standard Solution Dissolve 0.1250 g of *digoxin EPCRS* in sufficient *glacial acetic acid* to produce 100 ml. Dilute 4.0 ml of the solution to 100 ml with *glacial acetic acid*. To 25.0 ml of the resulting solution add 3.0 ml of *water* and mix well.

Ferricyanide Standard Solution (50 ppm $Fe(CN)_6$) Dilute 1 volume of a 0.78% w/v solution of *potassium hexacyanoferrate(III)* to 100 volumes with *water* immediately before use.

Ferrocyanide Standard Solution (100 ppm $Fe(CN)_6$) Dilute 1 volume of a 0.20% w/v solution of *potassium hexacyanoferrate(II)* to 100 volumes with *water*.

Fluoride Standard Solution (10 ppm F) Immediately before use, dilute 1 volume of a 0.0442% w/v solution of *sodium fluoride*, previously dried at 300° for 12 hours, to 20 volumes with *water*. Keep the concentrated solution in a polyethylene container.

Fluoride Standard Solution (1 ppm F) Dilute *fluoride standard solution (10 ppm F)* to 10 times its volume with *water* immediately before use.

Formaldehyde Standard Solution (5 ppm CH_2O) Dilute 1 volume of a solution containing 3.0 g of *formaldehyde solution* in 1000.0 ml to 200 volumes with *water* immediately before use.

Glucose Standard Solution Dissolve 0.10 g of *glucose* in a saturated solution of *benzoic acid in water*, dilute to 100 ml with the saturated benzoic acid solution and dilute 2 ml of this solution to 100 ml with *water*.
Glucose Standard Solution contains 20 µg of glucose per ml.

Glyoxal Standard Solution (20 ppm $C_2H_2O_2$) Dilute a quantity of *glyoxal solution* containing 0.200 g of $C_2H_2O_2$ to 100 ml with *absolute ethanol*. Dilute 1 volume to 100 volumes with *absolute ethanol* immediately before use.

Iodide Standard Solution (20 ppm I) Dilute 10.0 ml of a 0.026% w/v solution of *potassium iodide* to 100.0 ml with *water*.

Iodide Standard Solution (10 ppm I) Dilute 1 volume of a 0.131% w/v solution of *potassium iodide* to 100 volumes immediately before use.

Iron Standard Solution (0.1% Fe) Dissolve 0.10 g of *iron* in the smallest amount necessary of a mixture of equal volumes of *hydrochloric acid* and *water* and add sufficient *water* to produce 100 ml.

Iron Standard Solution (20 ppm Fe) Dissolve 0.863 g of *ammonium iron(III) sulphate* in *water* containing 25 ml of 1M *sulphuric acid* and add sufficient *water* to produce 500 ml. Dilute 1 volume to 10 volumes with *water* immediately before use.

Iron Standard Solution (10 ppm Fe) Dissolve 7.022 g of *ammonium iron(II) sulphate* in *water* containing 25 ml of 1M *sulphuric acid* and add sufficient *water* to produce 1000.0 ml. Dilute 1 volume to 100 volumes with *water*.

Iron Standard Solution (8 ppm Fe) Dilute 1 volume of a solution containing 80 mg of *iron* and 50 ml of *hydrochloric acid (220 g/l HCl)* in 1000 ml to 10 volumes with *water* immediately before use.

Iron Standard Solution (2 ppm Fe) Dilute 1 volume of *iron standard solution (20 ppm Fe)* to 10 volumes with *water* immediately before use.

Iron Standard Solution (1 ppm Fe) Dilute 1 volume of *iron standard solution (20 ppm Fe)* to 20 volumes with *water* immediately before use.

Lead Standard Solution (0.1% Pb) Dissolve 0.400 g of *lead(II) nitrate* in sufficient *water* to produce 250.0 ml.

Lead Standard Solution (100 ppm Pb) Dilute 1 volume of *lead standard solution (0.1% Pb)* to 10 volumes with *water* immediately before use.

Lead Standard Solution (20 ppm Pb) Dissolve 0.80 g of *lead(II) nitrate* in *water* containing 2 ml of *nitric acid* and add sufficient *water* to produce 250 ml. Dilute 1 volume to 100 volumes with *water* immediately before use.

Lead Standard Solution (10 ppm Pb) Dilute 1 volume of *lead standard solution (100 ppm Pb)* to 10 volumes with *water* immediately before use.

Lead Standard Solution (2 ppm Pb) Dilute 1 volume of *lead standard solution (10 ppm Pb)* to 5 volumes with *water* immediately before use.

Lead Standard Solution (1 ppm Pb) Dilute 1 volume of *lead standard solution (10 ppm Pb)* to 10 volumes with *water* immediately before use.

Lead Standard Solution (0.1 ppm Pb) Dilute 1 volume of *lead standard solution (1 ppm Pb)* to 10 volumes with *water* immediately before use.

Magnesium Standard Solution (0.1% Mg) Dissolve 9 g of *magnesium chloride* in sufficient *water* to produce 500 ml. Ascertain its exact strength in the following manner. To 25 ml of the solution add 25 ml of *water* and 10 ml of *ammonia buffer pH 10.9* and titrate with 0.1M *disodium edetate VS* using 0.1 g of *mordant black 11 triturate* as indicator. Each ml of 0.1M *disodium edetate VS* is equivalent to 1.215 mg of Mg. Dilute the remainder of the prepared solution with *water* so that 1 ml contains 1 mg of Mg.

Magnesium Standard Solution (100 ppm Mg) Dilute 1 volume of a solution containing 1.010% w/v of *magnesium sulphate* to 10 volumes with *water* immediately before use.

Magnesium Standard Solution (10 ppm Mg) Dilute 1 volume of a 1.01% w/v solution of *magnesium sulphate* to 100 volumes with *water.*

Mercury Standard Solution (1000 ppm Hg) Dissolve 1.354 g of *mercury(II) chloride* in 50 ml of 2M *nitric acid* and dilute to 1000.0 ml with *water.*

Mercury Standard Solution (100 ppm Hg) Dissolve 1.080 g of *yellow mercury(II) oxide* in the minimum volume of 2M *hydrochloric acid* and add sufficient *water* to produce 1000 ml.

Mercury Standard Solution (5 ppm Hg) Dilute 1.0 ml of a 0.0675% w/v solution of *mercury(II) chloride* to 100.0 ml with *water.*

Nickel Standard Solution (10 ppm Ni) Dilute 1 volume of a 0.478% w/v solution of *nickel(II) sulphate* to 100 volumes with *water* immediately before use.

Nickel Standard Solution (0.1 ppm Ni) Dilute 1 volume of *nickel standard solution (10 ppm Ni)* to 100 volumes with *water* immediately before use.

Nitrate Standard Solution (100 ppm NO_3) Dilute 1 volume of a 0.163% w/v solution of *potassium nitrate* to 10 volumes with *water* immediately before use.

Nitrate Standard Solution (10 ppm NO_3) Dilute 1 volume of *nitrate standard solution (100 ppm NO_3)* to 10 volumes with *water* immediately before use.

Nitrate Standard Solution (2 ppm NO_3) Dilute 1 volume of *nitrate standard solution (10 ppm NO_3)* to 5 volumes with *water* immediately before use.

Nitrite Standard Solution (20 ppm NO_2) Dissolve 0.6 g of *sodium nitrite* in sufficient *water* to produce 100 ml and dilute 1 ml of this solution to 200 ml with *water.*

Phosphate Standard Solution (100 ppm PO_4) Dilute 10.0 ml of a 0.143% w/v solution of *potassium dihydrogen orthophosphate* to 100.0 ml with *water* immediately before use.

Phosphate Standard Solution (5 ppm PO_4) Dilute 1 volume of a 0.0716% w/v solution of *potassium dihydrogen orthophosphate* to 100 volumes with *water* immediately before use.

Platinum Standard Solution (30 ppm Pt) Dilute 1 volume of a 0.080% w/v solution of *chloroplatinic(IV) acid* in 1M *hydrochloric acid* to 10 volumes with the same solvent immediately before use.

Potassium Standard Solution (600 ppm K) Dissolve 1.144 g of *potassium chloride,* previously dried at 100° to 105° for 3 hours, in sufficient *water* to produce 1000 ml.

Potassium Standard Solution (100 ppm K) Dilute 1 volume of a 0.446% w/v solution of *potassium sulphate* to 20 volumes with *water* immediately before use.

Potassium Standard Solution (20 ppm K) Dilute 1 volume of *potassium standard solution (100 ppm K)* to 5 volumes with *water* immediately before use.

Selenium Standard Solution (100 ppm Se) Dissolve 0.100 g of *selenium* in 2 ml of *nitric acid,* evaporate to dryness, dissolve the residue in 2 ml of *water* and evaporate to dryness; carry out three times. Dissolve the residue in sufficient 2M *hydrochloric acid* to produce 1000.0 ml.

Selenium Standard Solution (1 ppm Se) Dilute 25.0 ml of a 0.00654% w/v solution of *selenious acid* to 1000 ml with *water* immediately before use.

Silver Standard Solution (5 ppm Ag) Dilute 1 volume of a 0.079% w/v solution of *silver nitrate* to 100 volumes with *water.*

Sodium Standard Solution (200 ppm Na) Dilute a solution containing 0.509 g of *sodium chloride* in 100 ml to 10 times its volume with *water* immediately before use.

Sodium Standard Solution (50 ppm Na) Dilute 1 volume of *sodium standard solution (200 ppm Na)* to 4 volumes with *water.*

Sulphate Standard Solution (10 ppm SO_4) Dilute 1 volume of a 0.181% w/v solution of *potassium sulphate* in *distilled water* to 100 volumes with the same solvent immediately before use.

Sulphate Standard Solution (10 ppm SO_4) R1 Dilute 1 volume of a 0.181% w/v solution of *potassium sulphate* in *ethanol (30%)* to 100 volumes with *ethanol (30%).*

Sulphite Standard Solution (1.5 ppm SO_2) Dilute 5.0 ml of a 0.152% w/v solution of *sodium metabisulphite* to 100.0 ml with *water.* To 3.0 ml of this solution add 4.0 ml of 0.1M *sodium hydroxide VS* and dilute to 100.0 ml with *water.*

Thallium Standard Solution (10 ppm Tl) Dilute 10.0 ml of a 0.01235% w/v solution of *thallium(I) sulphate* in a 0.9% w/v solution of *sodium chloride* to 100.0 ml with the same solution.

Tin Standard Solution (5 ppm Sn) Dissolve 0.500 g of *tin* in a mixture of 5 ml of *water* and 25 ml of *hydrochloric acid* and add sufficient *water* to produce 1000 ml. Dilute 1 volume of this solution to 100 volumes with a 2.5% v/v solution of *hydrochloric acid* immediately before use.

Tin Standard Solution (0.1 ppm Sn) Dilute 1 volume of *tin standard solution (5 ppm Sn)* to 50 volumes with *water.*

Titanium Standard Solution (100 ppm Ti) Dissolve 0.10 g of *titanium* in 100 ml of *hydrochloric acid* diluted to 150 ml with *water*, heating if necessary. Allow to cool and dilute to 1000 ml with *water*.

Vanadium Standard Solution (0.1% V) Dissolve 0.230 g of *ammonium metavanadate* in sufficient *water* to produce 100 ml.

Zinc Standard Solution (5 mg/ml Zn) Dissolve 3.15 g of *zinc oxide* in 15 ml of *hydrochloric acid* and dilute to 500 ml with *water*.

Zinc Standard Solution (100 ppm Zn) Dissolve 0.440 g of *zinc sulphate* in *water* containing 1 ml of 5M *acetic acid* and add sufficient *water* to produce 100.0 ml. Immediately before use dilute 1 volume of this solution to 10 volumes with *water*.

Zinc Standard Solution (25 ppm Zn) Dilute 25.0 ml of *zinc standard solution (100 ppm Zn)* to 100.0 ml with *water* immediately before use.

Zinc Standard Solution (10 ppm Zn) Dilute 1 volume of *zinc standard solution (100 ppm Zn)* to 10 volumes with *water* immediately before use.

Zinc Standard Solution (5 ppm Zn) Dilute 1 volume of *zinc standard solution (100 ppm Zn)* to 20 volumes with *water* immediately before use.

Zirconium Standard Solution (0.1% Zr) Dissolve 0.293 g of *zirconyl nitrate* in sufficient of a mixture of 2 volumes of *hydrochloric acid* and 8 volumes of *water* to produce 100 ml.

D. Buffer Solutions

Buffer solutions should be prepared using *carbon dioxide-free water*.

Acetate Buffer pH 2.45 Mix 200 ml of 1M *hydrochloric acid* with 200 ml of 1M *sodium acetate* and dilute to 1000 ml with *water*. Immediately before use adjust the pH to 2.45 by the addition of 1M *hydrochloric acid* or 1M *sodium acetate*, as required.

Acetate Buffer pH 2.8 Dissolve 4 g of *anhydrous sodium acetate* in about 840 ml of *water*, add sufficient *glacial acetic acid* to adjust the pH to 2.8 (about 155 ml) and dilute to 1000 ml with *water*.

Acetate Buffer pH 3.4 Mix 5 volumes of 0.1M *sodium acetate* with 95 volumes of 0.1M *acetic acid*.

Acetate Buffer pH 3.5 Buffer solution pH 3.5
Dissolve 25 g of *ammonium acetate* in 25 ml of *water* and add 38 ml of 7M *hydrochloric acid*. Adjust the pH to 3.5 with either 2M *hydrochloric acid* or 6M *ammonia* and dilute to 100 ml with *water*.

Acetate Buffer pH 3.7 Dissolve 10 g of *anhydrous sodium acetate* in 300 ml of *water*, adjust to pH 3.7 with *glacial acetic acid* and dilute to 1000 ml with *water*. If necessary, readjust to pH 3.7 with *glacial acetic acid* or *anhydrous sodium acetate* as required, before use.

Acetate Buffer pH 4.4 Acetate buffer solution pH 4.4
Dissolve 136 g of *sodium acetate* and 77 g of *ammonium acetate* in *water* and dilute to 1000 ml with *water*. Add 250 ml of *glacial acetic acid* and mix.

Acetate Buffer pH 4.6 Acetate buffer solution pH 4.6
Dissolve 5.4 g of *sodium acetate* in 50 ml of *water*, add 2.4 g of *glacial acetic acid* and dilute to 100 ml with *water*. Adjust the pH if necessary.

Acetate Buffer Solution pH 4.7 Dissolve 136.1 g of *sodium acetate* in 500 ml of *water*. Mix 250 ml of this solution with 250 ml of 2M *acetic acid*. Shake twice with a freshly prepared, filtered 0.01% w/v solution of *dithizone* in *chloroform*. Shake with *carbon tetrachloride* until the extract is colourless and filter the aqueous layer to remove traces of carbon tetrachloride.

Acetate Buffer pH 5.0 Dissolve 13.6 g of *sodium acetate* and 6 ml of *glacial acetic acid* in sufficient *water* to produce 1000 ml.

Acetate Buffer pH 6.0 Acetate buffer solution pH 6.0
Dissolve 100 g of *ammonium acetate* in 300 ml of *water*, add 4.1 ml of *glacial acetic acid*, adjust the pH, if necessary, using 10M *ammonia* or 5M *acetic acid* and dilute to 500 ml with *water*.

Acetone Solution, Buffered Dissolve 8.15 g of *sodium acetate* and 42 g of *sodium chloride* in *water*, add 68 ml of 0.1M *hydrochloric acid* and 150 ml of *acetone* and dilute to 500 ml with *water*.

Acetate-edetate Buffer Solution pH 5.5 Dissolve 250 g of *ammonium acetate* and 15 g of *disodium edetate* in 400 ml of *water* and add 125 ml of *glacial acetic acid*.

Ammonia Buffer pH 10.0 Ammonium chloride buffer solution pH 10.0
Dissolve 5.4 g of *ammonium chloride* in 20 ml of *water*, add 35 ml of 10M *ammonia* and dilute to 100 ml with *water*.

Ammonia Buffer pH 10.9 Buffer solution pH 10.9
Dissolve 67.5 g of *ammonium chloride* in sufficient 10M *ammonia* to produce 1000 ml.

Ammonia Buffer pH 10.9, Dilute Dilute 2 ml of *ammonia buffer pH 10.9* to 1000 ml with *water*.

Ammonium Chloride Buffer Solution pH 9.5
Ammonia buffer pH 9.5
Dissolve 33.5 g of *ammonium chloride* in 150 ml of *water*, add 42 ml of 13.5M *ammonia* and dilute to 250 ml with *water*.
Store in a polyethylene container.

Barbitone Buffer pH 7.4 Barbital buffer solution pH 7.4
Mix 50 ml of a solution containing 1.944% w/v of *sodium acetate* and 2.946% w/v of *barbitone sodium* with 50.5 ml of 0.1M *hydrochloric acid*, add 20 ml of an 8.5% w/v solution of *sodium chloride* and dilute to 250 ml with *water*.

Barbitone Buffer pH 8.4 Barbital buffer solution pH 8.4
Dissolve 8.25 g of *barbitone sodium* in sufficient *water* to produce 1000 ml.

Barbitone Buffer pH 8.6 R1 Barbital buffer solution pH 8.6 R1
Dissolve 1.38 g of *barbitone*, 8.76 g of *barbitone sodium* and 0.38 g of *calcium lactate* in sufficient *water* to produce 1000 ml.

Borate Buffer pH 7.5 Borate buffer solution pH 7.5
Dissolve 2.5 g of *sodium chloride*, 2.85 g of *sodium tetraborate* and 10.5 g of *boric acid* in sufficient *water* to produce 1000 ml. Adjust the pH if necessary.
Store at 2° to 8°.

Borate Buffer pH 8.0 To 50 ml of a solution containing 0.6189 g of *boric acid* and 0.7456 g of *potassium chloride* add 3.97 ml of 0.2M *sodium hydroxide VS* and dilute to 200 ml with *water*.
At 20°, the solution may be used as a solution of standard pH.

Borate Buffer pH 9.0 Buffer solution pH 9.0
SOLUTION A Dissolve 6.18 g of *boric acid* in sufficient 0.1M *potassium chloride* to produce 1000 ml.
SOLUTION B 0.1M *sodium hydroxide*.
Mix 1000 ml of solution A with 420 ml of solution B.
At 20°, the solution may be used as a solution of standard pH.

Borate Buffer pH 9.6 To 50 ml of a solution containing 0.6189 g of *boric acid* and 0.7456 g of *potassium chloride* add 36.85 ml of 0.2M *sodium hydroxide VS* and dilute with *water* to 200 ml.
At 20°, the solution may be used as a solution of standard pH.

Borate Buffer Solution pH 8.0, 0.0015M Dissolve 0.572 g of *sodium tetraborate* and 2.94 g of *calcium chloride* in 800 ml of *water*, adjust to pH 8.0 with 1M *hydrochloric acid* and dilute to 1000 ml with *water*.

Boric Buffer pH 9.0 Buffer solution pH 9.0 R1
Dissolve 6.20 g of *boric acid* in 500 ml of *water*, adjust to pH 9.0 with 1M *sodium hydroxide* (about 41.5 ml) and dilute to 1000 ml with *water*.

Buffer (Phosphate) Solution pH 9.0 Dissolve 1.74 g of *potassium dihydrogen orthophosphate* in 80 ml of *water*, adjust the pH, if necessary, with 1M *potassium hydroxide* and dilute to 100 ml with *water*.

Buffer Solution pH 2.5 Phosphate buffer pH 2.5
Dissolve 100 g of *potassium dihydrogen orthophosphate* in 800 ml of *water*, adjust to pH 2.5 with *hydrochloric acid* and add sufficient *water* to produce 1000 ml.

Buffer Solution pH 2.5 R1 Phosphate buffer pH 2.5 R1
To 4.9 g of 2M *orthophosphoric acid* add 250 ml of *water*. Adjust the pH with 2M *sodium hydroxide* and dilute to 500 ml with *water*.

Buffer Solution pH 3.7 Ethanolic aceticammonia buffer pH 3.7
To 15 ml of 5M *acetic acid* add 60 ml of *ethanol (96%)* and 20 ml of *water*. Adjust the pH of the solution to 3.7 with 10M *ammonia* and dilute to 100 ml with *water*.

Buffer Solution pH 5.2 Dissolve 1.02 g of *potassium hydrogen phthalate* in 30.0 ml of 0.1M *sodium hydroxide VS* and dilute with *water* to 100 ml.
At 20°, the solution may be used as a solution of standard pH.

Buffer Solution pH 5.5 Dissolve 54.4 g of *sodium acetate* in 50 ml of *water*, heating to 35° if necessary. After cooling, slowly add 10 ml of *anhydrous acetic acid*, shake and add sufficient *water* to produce 100 ml.

Buffer Solution pH 6.5 Dissolve 60.5 g of *disodium hydrogen orthophosphate* and 46 g of *potassium dihydrogen orthophosphate* in *water*, add 100 ml of 0.02M *disodium edetate* and 20 mg of *mercury(II) chloride* and dilute to 1000 ml with *water*.

Buffer Solution pH 6.6 Use *phosphate buffer pH 6.6* described under phosphate buffers below.

Buffer Solution pH 7.0 To 1000 ml of a solution containing 1.8% w/v of *disodium hydrogen orthophosphate* and 2.3% w/v of *sodium chloride* add sufficient (about 280 ml) of a solution containing 0.78% w/v of *sodium dihydrogen orthophosphate* and 2.3 % w/v of *sodium chloride* to adjust the pH. Dissolve in the solution sufficient *sodium azide* to give a 0.02% w/v solution.

Buffer Solution pH 7.2 Use *phosphate buffer pH 7.2* described under phosphate buffers below.

Buffer Solution pH 7.4 Dissolve 0.6 g of *potassium dihydrogen orthophosphate*, 6.4 g of *disodium hydrogen orthophosphate* and 5.85 g of *sodium chloride* in sufficient *water* to produce 1000 ml and adjust the pH if necessary.

Buffer Solution pH 8.0 Use *phosphate buffer pH 8.0* described under phosphate buffers below.

Buffered Salt Solution pH 7.2 Dissolve in *water* 8.0 g of *sodium chloride*, 0.2 g of *potassium chloride*, 0.1 g of *anhydrous calcium chloride*, 0.1 g of *magnesium chloride*, 3.18 g of *disodium hydrogen orthophosphate* and 0.2 g of *potassium dihydrogen orthophosphate* and dilute to 1000 ml with *water*.

Carbonate Buffer pH 9.7 Dissolve 8.4 g of *sodium hydrogen carbonate* and 10.6 g of *sodium carbonate* in sufficient *water* to produce 500 ml.

Chloride Buffer pH 2.0, 0.1M Buffer solution pH 2.0
Dissolve 6.57 g of *potassium chloride* in *water*, add 119.0 ml of 0.1M *hydrochloric acid VS* and dilute to 1000 ml with *water*.

Citro-phosphate Buffer pH 4.5 To 30 volumes of 0.2M *disodium hydrogen orthophosphate* add sufficient 0.1M *citric acid* to give a pH of 4.5 (about 36 volumes).

Citro-phosphate Buffer pH 5.0 Mix 48.5 ml of 0.1M *citric acid* with sufficient 0.2M *disodium hydrogen orthophosphate* to produce 100 ml.

Citro-phosphate Buffer pH 6.0 Phosphate buffer solution pH 6.0
Mix 36.8 ml of a 2.1% w/v solution of *citric acid* with 63.2 ml of a 7.15% w/v solution of *disodium hydrogen orthophosphate*.

Citro-phosphate Buffer pH 6.5 Mix 29.0 ml of 0.1M *citric acid* with sufficient 0.2M *disodium hydrogen orthophosphate* to produce 100 ml.

Citro-phosphate Buffer pH 6.8 Phosphate buffer solution pH 6.8
Mix 77.3 ml of a 7.15% w/v solution of *disodium hydrogen orthophosphate* with 22.7 ml of a 2.1% w/v solution of *citric acid*.

Citro-phosphate Buffer pH 7.0 Phosphate buffer solution pH 7.0
Mix 82.4 ml of a 7.15% w/v solution of *disodium hydrogen orthophosphate* with 17.6 ml of a 2.1% w/v solution of *citric acid*.

Citro-phosphate Buffer pH 7.2 Phosphate buffer solution pH 7.2
Mix 87.0 ml of a 7.15% w/v solution of *disodium hydrogen orthophosphate* with 13.0 ml of a 2.1% w/v solution of *citric acid*.

Citro-phosphate Buffer pH 7.6 Dissolve 67.1 g of *disodium hydrogen orthophosphate* and 1.33 g of *citric acid* in sufficient *water* to produce 1000 ml.

Copper Sulphate Solution pH 4.0, Buffered Dissolve 0.25 g of *copper(II) sulphate* and 4.5 g of *ammonium acetate* in sufficient 2M *acetic acid* to produce 100 ml.

Copper Sulphate Solution pH 5.2, Buffered Dissolve 15.22 g of *anhydrous disodium hydrogen orthophosphate* in sufficient *water* to produce 536 ml and add a 2.1% w/v solution of *citric acid* until the pH of the solution is between 5.15 and 5.25 (about 464 ml). Mix 985 ml of the resulting solution with 15 ml of a 0.393% w/v solution of *copper(II) sulphate*.

Diethanolamine Buffer Solution pH 10.0 Dissolve 96.4 g of *diethanolamine* in sufficient *water* to produce 400 ml. Add 0.5 ml of an 18.6% w/v solution of *magnesium chloride*, adjust to pH 10.0 with 1M *hydrochloric acid* and dilute to 500 ml with *water*.

Diethylammonium Phosphate Buffer Solution pH 6.0 Dilute 68 ml of *orthophosphoric acid* to 500 ml with *water*. To 25 ml of this solution add 450 ml of *water* and 6 ml of *diethylamine*, adjust to pH 5.95 to 6.05, if necessary, using *diethylamine* or *orthophosphoric acid* and dilute to 500 ml with *water*.

Glycine Buffer pH 2.9 Dissolve 6.0 g of *glycine* and 4.68 g of *sodium chloride* in 10 litres of *water*. Adjust the pH with 1M *hydrochloric acid* (about 30 ml).

Glycine Buffer pH 11.3 Mix a solution containing 0.75% w/v of *glycine* and 0.58% w/v of *sodium chloride* with an equal volume of 0.1M *sodium hydroxide* and adjust the pH if necessary.

Glycine Buffer Solution Mix 42 g of *sodium hydrogen carbonate* and 50 g of *potassium hydrogen carbonate* with 180 ml of *water* and add a solution containing 37.5 g of *glycine* and 15 ml of 13.5M *ammonia* in 180 ml of *water*. Dilute to 500 ml with *water* and stir until solution is complete.

Imidazole Buffer Solution pH 6.5 Dissolve 6.81 g of *imidazole* and 1.23 g of *magnesium sulphate* in 752 ml of 0.1M *hydrochloric acid VS*, adjust the pH if necessary and dilute to 1000 ml with *water*.

Imidazole Buffer Solution pH 7.3 Dissolve 3.4 g of *imidazole* and 5.8 g of *sodium chloride* in *water*, add 18.6 ml of 1M *hydrochloric acid* and dilute to 1000 ml with *water*. Adjust the pH if necessary.

Maleate Buffer Solution pH 7.0 Dissolve 10 g of *sodium chloride*, 6.06 g of *tris(hydroxymethyl)methylamine* and 4.90 mg of *maleic anhydride* in 900 ml of *water*. Adjust the pH using a 17.0% w/v solution of *sodium hydroxide* and dilute to 1000 ml with *water*.
Store at 2° to 8° and use within 3 days.

Octylamine Phosphate Buffer pH 3.0 Dilute 3.32 ml of *octylamine* to 1000 ml, adjust the pH to 3.0 using *orthophosphoric acid* and filter through a membrane filter with a nominal pore size not greater than 0.5 µm.

Phosphate Buffers Solutions from pH 5.8 to pH 8.0 may be prepared by mixing 50 ml of 0.2M *potassium dihydrogen orthophosphate* with the quantities of 0.2M *sodium hydroxide VS* specified in the following table and diluting to 200 ml with *water*.
At 20° the solutions may be used as solutions of standard pH.

pH	5.8	6.0	6.2	6.4	6.6
ml of 0.2M *sodium hydroxide VS*	3.72	5.70	8.60	12.60	17.80
pH	7.0	7.2	7.4	7.6	7.8
ml of 0.2M *sodium hydroxide VS*	29.63	35.00	39.50	42.80	45.20

Phosphate Buffer pH 3.0 Dissolve 34 g of *potassium dihydrogen orthophosphate* in 250 ml of *water* and adjust the pH of the solution to 3.0 with *orthophosphoric acid*.

Phosphate Buffer pH 3.5 Phosphate buffer solution pH 3.5
Dissolve 68 g of *potassium dihydrogen orthophosphate* in 1000 ml of *water* and adjust the pH of the solution to 3.5 with *orthophosphoric acid*.

Phosphate Buffer pH 4.0 Dissolve 6.8 g of *potassium dihydrogen orthophosphate* in 700 ml of *water*, adjust the pH, if necessary, with a 10% v/v solution of *orthophosphoric acid* and add sufficient *water* to produce 1000 ml.

Phosphate Buffer pH 4.0, Mixed Dissolve 5.04 g of *disodium hydrogen orthophosphate* and 3.01 g of *potassium dihydrogen orthophosphate* in sufficient *water* to produce 1000 ml and adjust the pH with *glacial acetic acid*.

Phosphate Buffer pH 4.75 Dilute 100 ml of 0.5M *potassium dihydrogen orthophosphate* to 800 ml with *water*, adjust to pH 4.75 with 0.1M *sodium hydroxide* and dilute to 1000 ml with *water*.

Phosphate Buffer pH 4.9 Dissolve 40 g of *sodium dihydrogen orthophosphate* and 1.2 g of *sodium hydroxide* in sufficient *water* to produce 100 ml. If necessary, adjust the pH with 1M *sulphuric acid* or 1M *sodium hydroxide* as required.

Phosphate Buffer pH 5.4, Mixed Dissolve 1.76 g of *disodium hydrogen orthophosphate* and 13.61 g of *potassium dihydrogen orthophosphate* in sufficient *water* to produce 1000 ml. Adjust the pH with 0.05M *orthophosphoric acid*, if necessary.

Phosphate Buffer pH 6.8, Mixed Dissolve 28.80 g of *disodium hydrogen orthophosphate* and 11.45 g of *potassium dihydrogen orthophosphate* in sufficient *water* to produce 1000 ml.

Phosphate Buffer pH 6.8, 0.2M Mixed Phosphate buffer solution pH 6.8 R1
Mix 51 ml of a 2.72% w/v solution of *potassium dihydrogen orthophosphate* with 49 ml of a 7.16% w/v solution of *disodium hydrogen orthophosphate* and adjust the pH if necessary.
Store at 2° to 8°.

Phosphate Buffer pH 7.0, Mixed Dissolve 0.50 g of *anhydrous disodium hydrogen orthophosphate* and 0.301 g of *potassium dihydrogen orthophosphate* in sufficient *water* to produce 1000 ml.

Phosphate Buffer pH 7.0, 0.067M Mixed 0.067M Mixed phosphate buffer solution pH 7.0
SOLUTION A Dissolve 0.908 g of *potassium dihydrogen orthophosphate* in sufficient *water* to produce 100 ml.
SOLUTION B Dissolve 2.38 g of *disodium hydrogen orthophosphate* in sufficient *water* to produce 100 ml.
Mix 38.9 ml of solution A with 61.1 ml of solution B.

Phosphate Buffer pH 7.0, 0.1M Mixed 0.1M Phosphate buffer solution pH 7.0
Dissolve 1.361 g of *potassium dihydrogen orthophosphate* in sufficient *water* to produce 100 ml and adjust the pH using a 3.5% w/v solution of *disodium hydrogen orthophosphate*.

Phosphate Buffer pH 7.5, 0.2M 0.2M Phosphate buffer solution pH 7.5
Dissolve 27.22 g of *potassium dihydrogen orthophosphate* in 930 ml of *water*, adjust the pH of the solution to 7.5 with a 30% w/v solution of *potassium hydroxide* and add sufficient *water* to produce 1000 ml.

Phosphate Buffer pH 10, Mixed To 100 ml of 0.2M *disodium hydrogen orthophosphate* add 6.0 ml of 0.25M *trisodium orthophosphate*.

Phosphate Buffer, 0.025M Standard Dissolve 3.40 g of *potassium dihydrogen orthophosphate* and 3.55 g of *anhydrous disodium hydrogen orthophosphate,* both previously dried at 110° to 130° for 2 hours, in sufficient *water* to produce 1000 ml.

Phosphate Buffer Solution pH 2.0 Dissolve 8.95 g of *disodium hydrogen orthophosphate* and 3.40 g of *potassium dihydrogen orthophosphate* in sufficient *water* to produce 1000 ml. If necessary, adjust the pH with *orthophosphoric acid.*

Phosphate Buffer Solution pH 3.0 R1 Mix 0.7 ml of *orthophosphoric acid* with 100 ml of *water* and dilute to 900 ml with *water.* Adjust to pH 3.0 with 10M *sodium hydroxide* and add sufficient *water* to produce 1000 ml.

Phosphate Buffer Solution pH 3.2 To 900 ml of a 0.4% w/v solution of *sodium dihydrogen orthophosphate* add 100 ml of a 0.25% w/v solution of *orthophosphoric acid* and adjust the pH if necessary.

Phosphate Buffer Solution pH 3.2 R1 Adjust a 3.58% w/v solution of *disodium hydrogen orthophosphate* to pH 3.2 with 2M *orthophosphoric acid.* Dilute 100 ml of the solution to 2000 ml with *water.*

Phosphate Buffer Solution pH 5.5
SOLUTION A Dissolve 13.61 g of *potassium dihydrogen orthophosphate* in sufficient *water* to produce 1000 ml.
SOLUTION B Dissolve 35.81 g of *disodium hydrogen orthophosphate* in sufficient *water* to produce 1000 ml.
Mix 96.4 ml of solution A with 3.6 ml of solution B.

Phosphate Buffer Solution pH 5.8 Dissolve 1.19 g of *disodium hydrogen orthophosphate dihydrate* and 8.25 g of *potassium dihydrogen orthophosphate* in sufficient *water* to produce 1000 ml.

Phosphate Buffer Solution pH 6.0 R1 Dissolve 6.8 g of *sodium dihydrogen orthophosphate* in sufficient *water* to produce 1000 ml and adjust the pH with 10M *sodium hydroxide.*

Phosphate Buffer Solution pH 6.0 R2 To 250 ml of 0.2M *potassium dihydrogen orthophosphate* add 28.5 ml of 0.2M *sodium hydroxide* and sufficient *water* to produce 1000 ml.

Phosphate Buffer Solution pH 7.0 R1 Use *phosphate buffer pH 7.0* described under phosphate buffers above.

Phosphate Buffer Solution pH 7.0 R2 Mix 50 ml of a 13.6% w/v solution of *potassium dihydrogen orthophosphate* with 29.5 ml of 1M *sodium hydroxide* and dilute to 100 ml with *water.* Adjust the pH to 6.9 to 7.1, Appendix V L.

Phosphate Buffer Solution pH 7.0 R3 Dissolve 5 g of *potassium dihydrogen orthophosphate* and 11 g of *dipotassium hydrogen orthophosphate* in 900 ml of *water.* Adjust to pH 7.0 with 2M *orthophosphoric acid* or 2M *sodium hydroxide,* dilute to 1000 ml with *water* and mix.

Phosphate Buffer Solution pH 7.4 Add 250 ml of 0.2M *potassium dihydrogen orthophosphate* to 393.4 ml of 0.1M *sodium hydroxide.*

Phosphate Buffer Solution pH 7.5, 0.33M
SOLUTION A Dissolve 119.31 g of *disodium hydrogen orthophosphate* in sufficient *water* to produce 1000 ml.
SOLUTION B Dissolve 45.36 g of *potassium dihydrogen orthophosphate* in sufficient *water* to produce 1000 ml.
Mix 85 ml of solution A and 15 ml of solution B and adjust the pH if necessary.

Phosphate Buffer Solution pH 8.0, 0.02M Mix 50 ml of 0.2M *potassium dihydrogen orthophosphate* with 46.8 ml of 0.2M *sodium hydroxide* and add sufficient *water* to produce 500 ml.

Phosphate Buffer Solution pH 8.0, 0.1M Dissolve 0.523 g of *potassium dihydrogen orthophosphate* and 16.73 g of *dipotassium hydrogen orthophosphate* in sufficient *water* to produce 1000 ml.

Phosphate Buffer Solution pH 8.0, 1M Dissolve 136.1 g of *potassium dihydrogen orthophosphate* in *water,* adjust the pH with 1M *sodium hydroxide* and add sufficient *water* to produce 1000 ml.

Phosphate-citrate Buffer Solution pH 5.5 Mix 56.85 ml of a 2.84% w/v solution of *anhydrous disodium hydrogen orthophosphate* and 43.15 ml of a 2.1% w/v solution of *citric acid.*

Phthalate Buffer pH 3.6 Buffer solution pH 3.6
To 250 ml of 0.2M *potassium hydrogen phthalate* add 11.94 ml of 0.2M *hydrochloric acid VS* and dilute to 1000 ml with *water.*
At 20°, the solution may be used as a solution of standard pH.

Phthalate Buffer Solution pH 4.4 Dissolve 2.042 g of *potassium hydrogen phthalate* in 50 ml of *water,* add 7.5 ml of 0.2M *sodium hydroxide VS* and dilute to 200 ml with *water.*
At 20°, the solution may be used as a solution of standard pH.

Saline pH 6.4, Phosphate-buffered Phosphate buffer solution pH 6.4 R1
Dissolve 1.79 g of *disodium hydrogen orthophosphate,* 1.36 g of *potassium dihydrogen orthophosphate* and 7.02 g of *sodium chloride* in sufficient *water* to produce 1000 ml.

Saline pH 6.8, Phosphate-buffered Dissolve 1.0 g of *potassium dihydrogen orthophosphate,* 2.0 g of *dipotassium hydrogen orthophosphate* and 8.5 g of *sodium chloride* in 900 ml of *water,* adjust the pH if necessary and sufficient *water* to produce 1000 ml.

Saline pH 7.2, Phosphate-albumin Buffered Dissolve 10.75 g of *disodium hydrogen orthophosphate,* 7.6 g of *sodium chloride* and 10 g of *bovine albumin* in sufficient *water* to produce 1000 ml. Immediately before use adjust to pH 7.2 with either 2M *sodium hydroxide* or a 10% w/w solution of *orthophosphoric acid,* as required.

Saline pH 7.4, Phosphate-buffered Dissolve 2.38 g of *disodium hydrogen orthophosphate,* 0.19 g of *potassium dihydrogen orthophosphate* and 8.0 g of *sodium chloride* in sufficient *water* to produce 1000 ml and adjust the pH if necessary.

Sodium Acetate Solution pH 6.0, Buffered Dissolve 4.1 g of *anhydrous sodium acetate* in 1000 ml of *water* and adjust the pH to 6.0 with *glacial acetic acid.*

Succinate Buffer Solution pH 4.6 Dissolve 11.8 g of *succinic acid* in a mixture of 600 ml of *water* and 82 ml of 1M *sodium hydroxide* and dilute to 1000 ml with *water.*

Thiobarbituric Acid–Citrate Buffer Dissolve 5.0 g of *thiobarbituric acid* in 5 ml of 4M *sodium hydroxide* and dilute to 500 ml with *water.* Dissolve separately 37 g of *sodium citrate* in 32 ml of *hydrochloric acid* and dilute to 250 ml with *water.* Mix the two solutions and adjust the pH of the resulting solution to 2.0.

Total-ionic-strength-adjustment Buffer Dissolve 58.5 g of *sodium chloride*, 57 ml of *glacial acetic acid*, 61.5 g of *sodium acetate* and 5.0 g of *cyclohexylenedinitrilotetra-acetic acid* in sufficient *water* to produce 500 ml. Adjust to a pH between 5.0 and 5.5 with a 33.5% w/v solution of *sodium hydroxide* and dilute to 1000 ml with *distilled water*.

Total Ionic Strength Adjustment Buffer R1
SOLUTION A Dissolve 210 g of *citric acid* in 400 ml of *distilled water*, adjust to pH 7.0 with *concentrated ammonia* and add sufficient *distilled water* to produce 1000 ml.
SOLUTION B Dissolve 132 g of *ammonium phosphate* in sufficient *distilled water* to produce 1000 ml.
SOLUTION C To a suspension of 292 g of *(ethylene-dinitrilo) tetra-acetic acid* in about 500 ml of *distilled water* add about 200 ml of *concentrated ammonia* to dissolve. Adjust the pH to 6 to 7 with *concentrated ammonia* and add sufficient *water* to produce 1000 ml.
Mix equal volumes of solutions A, B and C and adjust to pH 7.5 with *concentrated ammonia*.

Tris Acetate Buffer Solution pH 8.5 Dissolve 0.294 g of *calcium chloride* and 12.11 g of *tris(hydroxymethyl)-methylamine* in *water*. Adjust the pH with 5M *acetic acid* and add sufficient *water* to produce 1000 ml.

Tris-chloride Buffer pH 7.4 Tris(hydroxymethyl)-aminomethane sodium chloride buffer solution pH 7.4 Dissolve 6.08 g of *tris(hydroxymethyl)methylamine* and 8.77 g of *sodium chloride* in 500 ml of *distilled water*. Add 10 g of *bovine albumin*. Adjust the pH to 7.4 using *hydrochloric acid* and add sufficient *distilled water* to produce 1000 ml.

Tris-chloride Buffer pH 7.5 Tris(hydroxymethyl)-aminomethane sodium chloride buffer solution pH 7.5 Dissolve 7.27 g of *tris(hydroxymethyl)methylamine* and 5.27 g of *sodium chloride* in *water*, adjust the pH if necessary and dilute to 1000 ml with *water*.

Tris-chloride Buffer pH 7.5 R1 Tris(hydroxymethyl)-aminomethane sodium chloride buffer solution pH 7.5 R1 Dissolve 6.057 g of *tris(hydroxymethyl)methylamine* in *water* and adjust the pH with *hydrochloric acid*, if necessary. Dilute to 1000 ml with *water*.

Tris-chloride Buffer pH 8.1 Tris(hydroxymethyl)-aminomethane sodium chloride buffer solution pH 8.1 Dissolve 0.294 g of *calcium chloride* and 0.969 g of *tris(hydroxymethyl)methylamine* in *water*, adjust the pH to 8.1 with 1M *hydrochloric acid* and add sufficient *water* to produce 100 ml.

Tris-chloride Buffer pH 8.6 Dissolve 2.0 g of *tris-(hydroxymethyl)methylamine* and 2.4 g of *sodium chloride* in about 100 ml of *water*, adjust the pH to 8.6 with 1M *sodium hydroxide* or 1M *hydrochloric acid* and dilute with *water* to 200 ml.

TrisEDTA Buffer pH 8.4 Tris(hydroxymethyl)-aminomethane EDTA buffer solution pH 8.4 Dissolve 5.12 g of *sodium chloride*, 3.03 g of *tris(hydroxy-methyl)methylamine* and 1.4 g of *disodium edetate* in 250 ml of *distilled water*. Adjust to pH 8.4 using *hydrochloric acid* and add sufficient *distilled water* to produce 500 ml.

Tris-EDTA BSA Buffer Solution pH 8.4 Dissolve 6.1 g of *tris(hydroxymethyl)methylamine*, 2.8 g of *disodium edetate*, 10.2 g of *sodium chloride* and 10 g of *bovine albumin* in *water*, adjust to pH 8.4 using 1M *hydrochloric acid* and dilute to 1000 ml with *water*.

Tris-glycine Buffer Solution pH 8.3 Dissolve 6 g of *tris(hydroxymethyl)methylamine* and 28.8 g of *glycine* in sufficient *water* to produce 1000 ml. Dilute 1 volume of the solution to 10 volumes with *water* immediately before use.

E. Chemical and Biological Reference Materials

Where the letters *BPCRS* appear after the name of a substance in a test or assay, the British Pharmacopoeia Chemical Reference Substance is to be used. A list of the British Pharmacopoeia Chemical Reference Substances and the quantity supplied in each pack is given below. The substances are available from the Medicines Control Agency Laboratory, Government Buildings (Block 2), Honeypot Lane, Stanmore HA7 1AY, England, from which the conditions of supply may be obtained (telephone 0171-972 3608; facsimile 0181-951 3069. Telephone orders cannot be accepted).

Where the letters *CRS* or *EPCRS* appear, the Chemical Reference Substance issued by the European Pharmacopoeia Commission is to be used, and where the letters *BRP* or *EPBRP* appear, the Biological Reference Preparation issued by the European Pharmacopoeia Commission is to be used. These materials are obtainable from the European Pharmacopoeia Commission Secretariat, Council of Europe, BP 907, 67029 Strasbourg Cedex 1, France.

Other sources of specific substances are shown below.

Alpha Benzene Hexachloride CRS [BHC (alpha)] Certified reference preparation of the Office of Reference Materials, Laboratory of the Government Chemist, Teddington, TW11 0LW, England.

Gamma Benzene Hexachloride CRS [BHC (gamma)] Certified reference preparation of the Office of Reference Materials, Laboratory of the Government Chemist, Teddington TW11 0LY, England.

Opacity, Standard Preparation of The Standard Preparation is the 5th International Reference Preparation, established in 1975, and consists of a rod of plastic simulating the optical properties of a bacterial suspension (10 Units of opacity). It may be obtained from the National Institute for Biological Standards and Control, South Mimms, Potters Bar, Hertfordshire, EN6 3QG, England.

Piperonyl Butoxide CRS Certified reference preparation of the Office of Reference Materials, Laboratory of the Government Chemist, Teddington TW11 0LY, England.

Sodium Taurocholate CRS The *Fédération Internationale Pharmaceutique* (FIP) standard preparation of sodium taurocholate. It may be obtained from the International Commission on Pharmaceutical Enzymes, Centre for Standards, Wolterslaan 12, B–9000 Ghent, Belgium.

^{12}C-2,3,7,8-Tetrachloro-*p*-dioxin CRS; **^{13}C-2,3,7,8-Tetrachloro-*p*-dioxin CRS** May be obtained from the National Institute for Standards and Technology, Office of Standard Reference Materials, Room B311, Chemistry Building, Gathersburg, MD 20899, United States of America, or from Promochem Ltd, PO Box 255, St Albans, Hertfordshire AL1 4LN, England

Catalogue No.	Pack size	British Pharmacopoeia Chemical Reference Substance
001	50 mg	acepromazine maleate
402	25 mg	3-acetylbenzophenone
438	50 mg	aciclovir
003	100 mg	adrenaline acid tartrate (*epinephrine acid tartrate*)
560	25 mg	9-allyl-2-chlorothioxanthen-9-ol
006	100 mg	alfadolone acetate (*alphadolone acetate*)
007	100 mg	alfaxalone (*alphaxalone*)
415	100 mg	alimemazine tartrate (*trimeprazine tartrate*)
530	200 mg	amantadine hydrochloride
008	100 mg	amiloride hydrochloride
624	25 mg	2-amino-4-chloro-5-sulphamoylbenzoic acid
010	50 mg	4-amino-6-chlorobenzene-1,3-disulphonamide
374	50 mg	3-amino-6-chloro-1-methyl-4-phenylquinolin-2-ol
485	25 mg	3-amino-4-(2-chlorophenyl)-6-nitroquinolin-2-one
012	50 mg	2-amino-4,6-dichlorophenol
013	50 mg	*N*-(2-aminoethyl)-4-*tert*-butyl-2,6-xylylacetamide
486	25 mg	2-amino-2′-chloro-5-nitrobenzophenone
602	25 mg	4-amino-2-ethylidenebutyric acid
417	50 mg	2-amino-1-(4-nitrophenyl)propane-1,3-diol
601	25 mg	3-aminopent-4-ene-1,1-dicarboxylic acid
536	25 mg	3-amino-4-phenoxy-5-sulphamoylbenzoic acid
014	50 mg	3-amino-4-propoxybenzoic acid
532	200 mg	amiodarone hydrochloride
015	200 mg	amitraz
016	150 mg	amitriptyline hydrochloride
017	100 mg	ammonium dihydrogen glycyrrhizinate
019	500 mg	amoxicillin trihydrate (*amoxycillin trihydrate*)
020	100 mg	amphotericin B
021	500 mg	ampicillin trihydrate
022	100 mg	amprolium hydrochloride
546	250 mg	apramycin
461	50 mg	ascorbic acid
617	100 mg	aspirin
492	200 mg	atenolol
370	50 mg	atenolol impurity standard
023	200 mg	atropine sulphate
366	30 mg	1-(3-azabicyclo[3.3.0]oct-3-yl)-3-*o*-tolylsulphonylurea
024	50 mg	2-azahypoxanthine
025	100 mg	azaperone
534	100 mg	azapropazone
515	10 mg	azapropazone impurity A
516	10 mg	azapropazone impurity B
517	10 mg	azapropazone impurity C
527	50 mg	azapropazone impurity standard
519	100 mg	azlocillin sodium
028	150 mg	baclofen
535	25 mg	baclofen lactam
030	150 mg	beclometasone dipropionate (*beclomethasone dipropionate*)
031	50 mg	beclometasone 17-propionate (*beclomethasone 17-propionate*)
432	50 mg	benethamine penicillin
036	100 mg	benzatropine mesilate (*benztropine mesylate*)
037	50 mg	(1*S*,2*R*)-1-benzyl-3-dimethylamino-2-methyl-1-phenylpropyl acetate
610	200 mg	benzydamine hydrochloride
426	100 mg	benzyl benzoate
611	50 mg	1-benzyl-3-(3-diethylaminopropoxy)-1*H*-indazole
609	50 mg	1-benzyl-1*H*-indazol-3-ol
575	100 mg	betamethasone
041	100 mg	betamethasone sodium phosphate
042	100 mg	betamethasone valerate
043	50 mg	betamethasone 21-valerate
046	25 mg	2-(biphenyl-4-yl) propionic acid
441	25 mg	1,4-bis(4-chlorobenzhydryl)piperazine
049	25 mg	17β,17′β-bis{3-[bis-(2-chloroethyl)carbamoyloxy]estra-1,3,5,(10)-trienyl} pyrophosphate
612	200 mg	bretylium tosilate
613	50 mg	2-bromobenzyldimethylamine hydrochloride
050	100 mg	bromocriptine mesilate (*bromocriptine mesilate*)
440	100 mg	buclizine hydrochloride impurity standard
537	100 mg	bumetanide
479	100 mg	bupivacaine hydrochloride
403	25 mg	busulfan (*busulphan*)
055	200 mg	butyl aminobenzoate
531	25 mg	2-butyl 3-(4-hydroxy-3,5-di-iodobenzoyl)benzofuran
192	25 mg	2-*tert*-butylamino-1-(4-hydroxy-3-methylphenyl)ethanol sulphate

Catalogue No.	Pack size	British Pharmacopoeia Chemical Reference Substance
355	100 mg	calcitonin (salmon) (*salcatonin*)
059	50 mg	capreomycin sulphate
538	100 mg	captopril
500	25 mg	captopril disulphide
477	25 mg	2-carbamoyl-1-methyl-3-[2-(5-methylimidazol-4-ylmethylthio)ethyl]guanidine hydrochloride
523	100 mg	carbaryl
060	100 mg	carbidopa
506	25 mg	2-(3-carboxyphenyl)propionic acid
567	100 mg	carteolol hydrochloride
062	500 mg	cefalotin sodium (*cephalothin sodium*)
063	200 mg	cefradine (*cephradine*)
502	100 mg	cefuroxime axetil
562	100 mg	cephalonium
064	100 mg	chlorambucil
065	100 mg	chloramphenicol palmitate
066	100 mg	chloramphenicol palmitate (polymorph A)
067	100 mg	chlorcyclizine hydrochloride
068	100 mg	chlorhexidine acetate
069	100 mg	chlorhexidine hydrochloride
604	25 mg	4-chlorobenzylphthalazinone
524	0.25 ml	4-chloro-1,1-diphenylethanol
376	50 mg	6-chloro-4-(2-chlorophenyl)quinazoline-2-carboxaldehyde
442	25 mg	6-chloro-1,4-dihydro-1-methyl-4-phenylquinazolin-4-ol
470	25 mg	7-chloro-1,5-dihydro-5-phenyl-1,5-benzodiazepine-2,4(3*H*)-dione
070	25 mg	4-(2-chloroethyl)-1-ethyl-3,3-diphenyl-2-pyrrolidone
446	25 mg	5-(2-chloroethyl)-4-methyl-3-[2-(4-methylthiazol-5-yl)ethyl]thiazolium chloride
071	50 mg	4-[2-(5-chloro-2-methoxybenzamido)ethyl]benzenesulphonamide
378	50 mg	5-chloro-2-methylaminobenzophenone
072	50 mg	3-chloro-4-methylumbelliferone
443	25 mg	6-(2-chlorophenyl)-2,4-dihydro-2-[(dimethylamino)methylene]8-nitroimidazo[1,2-a][1,4]benzodiazepin-1-one
074	25 mg	4-chloro-5-sulphamoylanthranilic acid
559	25 mg	2-chlorothioxanthone
077	25 mg	2-(6-chlorothymoxy)ethyldimethylamine hydrochloride
079	25 mg	2-chlorotritanol
080	500 mg	chloroxylenol
081	100 mg	chlorphenamine maleate (*chlorpheniramine maleate*)
467	50 mg	chlorpromazine sulphoxide
491	100 mg	chlortalidone (*chlorthalidone*)
618	100 mg	cholic acid
475	100 mg	cimetidine
597	100 mg	*cis*-flupentixol propionate dihydrochloride (cis-*flupenthixol propionate dihydrochloride*)
525	200 mg	clemastine fumarate
083	200 mg	clindamycin hydrochloride
419	100 mg	clindamycin phosphate
084	200 mg	clioquinol
507	100 mg	clobazam
522	25 mg	clobetasol impurity A
521	100 mg	clobetasol propionate
482	100 mg	clobetasone butyrate
406	100 mg	clocortolone hexanoate
543	100 mg	clomethiazole edisilate (*chlormethiazole edisylate*)
484	100 mg	clonazepam
085	100 mg	clonidine hydrochloride
565	50	*trans*-clopenthixol acetate dihydrochloride
565	25	*trans*-clopenthixol decanoate dihydrochloride
561	25 mg	*trans*-clopenthixol hydrochloride
628	20 mg	cloprostenol sodium
086	2 ml	cloprostenol sodium injection
087	5 ml	cloprostenol sodium solution
379	50 mg	clotrimazole
088	250 mg	cloxacillin benzathine
089	300 mg	cloxacillin sodium
514	100 mg	codeine hydrochloride *(controlled drug—permit required)*
090	200 mg	codeine phosphate *(controlled drug—permit required)*
091	50 mg	co-dergocrine mesilate (*co-dergocrine mesylate*)
614	50 mg	colestipol hydrochloride
094	100 mg	crotamiton
585	100 mg	cortisone acetate
466	100 mg	cyanocobalamin
478	25 mg	2-cyano-1-methyl-3-[2-(5-methylimidazol-4-ylmethylsulphinyl)ethyl]guanidine
096	100 mg	cyclizine hydrochloride
098	100 mg	cyclopenthiazide
380	100 mg	cyclopentolate hydrochloride
383	100 mg	cytarabine

Catalogue No.	Pack size	British Pharmacopoeia Chemical Reference Substance
100	25 mg	dacarbazine
428	50 mg	dantron (*danthron*)
429	150 mg	dantron impurity standard (danthron impurity standard)
102	100 mg	dapsone
103	100 mg	debrisoquine sulphate
104	50 mg	decoquinate
572	25 mg	deltamedrane
568	100 mg	desogestrel
594	25 mg	desogestrel Δ^3-isomer
578	100 mg	dexamethasone
108	50 mg	dexamethasone sodium phosphate
465	100 mg	dextropropoxyphene hydrochloride *(controlled drug—permit required)*
111	100 mg	diazepam
112	100 mg	diazoxide
113	50 mg	dibenzocycloheptatriene
114	25 mg	6*H*-dibenzo[*b,e*]thiepin-11-one
608	25 mg	3-(1,5-dibenzyl-1*H*-indazole-3-yl)oxypropyldimethylamine hydrochloride
430	50 mg	3,5-dichloro-4-hydroxybenzenesulphonamide
116	100 mg	dichlorophen
420	100 mg	dichlorophen impurity standard
619	100 mg	diclofenac sodium
404	100 mg	diclofenamide (*dichlorphenamide*)
117	50 mg	dicloxacillin sodium
118	100 mg	diethanolamine fusidate
361	25 mg	2-diethylaminoethyl 3-(1-naphthyl)-2-(1-naphthylmethyl)propionate oxalate
119	50 mg	diethyl 4-decyloxy-3-ethoxyanilinomethylene malonate
401	100 mg	diflucortolone valerate
397	25 mg	diflucortolone valerate impurity standard
431	100 mg	dihydrocodeine tartrate *(controlled drug—permit required)*
120	25 mg	dihydroergocristine mesilate (*dihydroergocristine mesylate*)
122	50 mg	2,3-dihydro-6-phenylimidazo[2,1,*b*]thiazole
582	25 mg	6,6′-dimethoxy-2,2′-binaphthyl
195	50 mg	4-dimethylamino-3-methyl-1,2-diphenylbutan-2-ol hydrochloride
607	25 mg	3-dimethylaminopropyl-2-benzylaminobenzoate hydrochloride
124	25 mg	11-(3-dimethylaminopropylidene)-6*H*-dibenzo[*b,e*]thiepin-5-oxide
456	50 mg	1,5-dimethylhexyl(methyl)amine
511	25 mg	dimethyl{5-[2-(1-methylamino-2-nitrovinylamino)ethylsulphinylmethyl]furfuryl}amine
364	25 mg	2,2-dimethyl-5-(2,4-xylyloxy)valeric acid
487	20 mg	dinoprost trometamol
128	100 mg	dipipanone hydrochloride *(controlled drug—permit required)*
589	100 mg	diprenorphine
130	100 mg	1,3-dipropylurea
131	100 mg	dipyridamole
384	25 mg	N^1,N^2-diquinoxalin-2-ylsulphanilamide
577	25 mg	disodium ethoxyphosphinatoformate
615	200 mg	disodium pamidronate
132	50 mg	disulfiram
385	100 mg	dithranol
386	50 mg	dithranol dimer
133	200 mg	docusate sodium
468	100 mg	dopamine hydrochloride
134	100 mg	dosulepin hydrochloride (*dothiepin hydrochloride*)
135	100 mg	doxapram hydrochloride
136	100 mg	doxepin hydrochloride
139	100 mg	econazole nitrate
387	100 mg	ephedrine hydrochloride
405	100 mg	ergometrine maleate
141	50 mg	ergotamine tartrate
488	100 mg	erythromycin stearate
396	50 mg	estradiol benzoate (*oestradiol benzoate*)
142	25 mg	estramustine
279	50 mg	estrone (*oestrone*)
616	100 mg	estropipate
143	100 mg	etacrynic acid (*ethacrynic acid*)
421	100 mg	ethinylestradiol (*ethinyloestradiol*)
145	50 mg	ethopabate
146	200 mg	ethosuximide
150	25 mg	ethyldimethyl[2-(2-methylbenzhydryloxy)ethyl]ammonium chloride
437	500 mg	*N*-ethylglucamine hydrochloride
148	25 mg	1-ethyl-4-[2-(2-hydroxyethyl)aminoethyl]-3,3-diphenyl-2-pyrrolidone
149	25 mg	ethyl meclofenamate
152	25 mg	17α-ethylestran-17β-ol (*17α-ethyloestran-17β-ol*)
153	100 mg	ethylestrenol (*ethyloestrenol*)
529	100 mg	etodolac

Catalogue No.	Pack size	British Pharmacopoeia Chemical Reference Substance
533	25 mg	etodolac acid dimer
541	50 mg	etodolac 1-methyl analogue
542	50 mg	etodolac 8-methyl analogue
354	100 mg	fenbufen
154	100 mg	fenfluramine hydrochloride
156	0.25 ml	fenthion
571	100 mg	flavoxate hydrochloride
157	100 mg	fluclorolone acetonide
158	250 mg	flucloxacillin sodium
159	50 mg	fludrocortisone acetate
160	50 mg	fluocinolone acetonide
489	100 mg	fluocinonide
161	50 mg	fluocortolone hexanoate
162	50 mg	fluocortolone pivalate
163	25 mg	4′-fluoro-4-chlorobutyrophenone
573	100 mg	fluorometholone
164	50 mg	fluoxymesterone
554	100 mg	flupentixol decanoate dihydrochloride (*flupenthixol decanoate hydrochloride*)
556	25 mg	*trans*-flupentixol decanoate dihydrochloride (trans-*flupenthixol decanoate dihydrochloride*)
165	150 mg	fluphenazine decanoate
167	100 mg	fluphenazine hydrochloride
574	100 mg	flurbiprofen sodium
587	100 mg	fluticasone propionate
588	25 mg	fluticasone *S*-methyl impurity
600	100 mg	fluvoxamine maleate
627	25 mg	3-formylrifamycin SV
623	100 mg	foscarnet sodium
170	50 mg	framycetin sulphate
171	50 mg	fumaric acid
172	50 mg	furazolidone
547	100 mg	furosemide (*frusemide*)
363	300 mg	gemfibrozil
303	25 mg	gemfibrozil impurity A
365	0.2 ml	gemfibrozil methyl ester
175	100 mg	glibenclamide
368	200 mg	gliclazide
580	150 mg	gliquidone
581	25 mg	gliquidone sulphonamide
177		glyceryl trinitrate tablets (20 × 0.5-mg tablets)
180	100 mg	griseofulvin
181	100 mg	guanethidine monosulphate
407	150 mg	haloperidol
182	300 mg	haloxon
185	200 mg	homatropine hydrobromide
186	200 mg	hydrochlorothiazide
576	100 mg	hydrocortisone
584	100 mg	hydrocortisone acetate
188	100 mg	hydrocortisone sodium phosphate
189	50 mg	hydrocortisone sodium succinate
190	100 mg	hydroflumethiazide
481	25 mg	1-hydroxy-9-anthrone
197	200 mg	hydroxycarbamide (*hydroxyurea*)
526	0.25 ml	2-(2-hydroxyethyl)-1-methylpyrrolidine
196	50 mg	5-[1-hydroxy-2-(1-methyl-3-phenylpropylamino)ethyl]salicylic acid hydrochloride
193	50 mg	hydroxyprogesterone caproate (*hydroxyprogesterone hexanoate*)
194	25 mg	2-(6-hydroxythymoxy)ethyldimethylamine hydrochloride
198	100 mg	hyoscine butylbromide
199	200 mg	hyoscine hydrobromide
539	200 mg	ibuprofen
202	100 mg	idoxuridine
625	100 mg	ipratropium bromide
557	0.25 ml	4′-isobutylacetophenone
205	100 mg	isoprenaline hydrochloride
499	25 mg	4′-(2-isopropylaminoethyl)methylsulphonanilide hydrochloride
626	25 mg	8*s*-isopropyl-3β-hydroxytropanium bromide
206	100 mg	isosorbide dinitrate, diluted
209	25 mg	3-ketofusidic acid
212	100 mg	levamisole hydrochloride
356	100 mg	levobunolol hydrochloride
501	100 mg	levonorgestrel
214	50 mg	lidocaine hydrochloride (*lignocaine hydrochloride*)
215	200 mg	lincomycin hydrochloride
216	100 mg	liquiritigenin
508	200 mg	lithium clavulanate
433	100 mg	lithium lactate
447	50 mg	loprazolam mesilate (*loprazolam mesylate*)

Catalogue No.	Pack size	British Pharmacopoeia Chemical Reference Substance
434	50 mg	lorazepam
528	100 mg	lormetazepam
218	100 mg	lymecycline
222	25 mg	megestrol
223	100 mg	megestrol acetate
391	100 mg	melphalan
583	100 mg	meptazinol hydrochloride
496	50 mg	mesoridazine besilate (*mesoridazine besylate*)
226	100 mg	metaraminol tartrate
359	25 mg	5-(6-methoxy-2-naphthyl)-3-methylcyclohexan-1-one
232	25 mg	1-(2-methoxyphenyl)piperazine
606	25 mg	1-methylazepan-4-one hydrochloride
605	25 mg	1-methyl-4-(2-benzoylhydrazino)azepan hydrochloride
234	0.5 ml	*N*-(3-methylbenzyl)piperazine
237	25 mg	methyl *N*-4[2-(5-chloro-2-methoxybenzamido)ethyl]benzenesulphonylcarbamate
238	50 mg	methyl 3,5-diamino-6-chloropyrazine-2-carboxylate
239	50 mg	3-methyl-2,2-diphenyl-4-piperidinobutyronitrile
240	100 mg	methyldopa
241	100 mg	methyldopate hydrochloride
569	25 mg	3-methylflavone-8-carboxylic acid
570	25 mg	3-methylflavone-8-carboxylic acid ethyl ester
444	25 mg	4-methyl-5-(2-hydroxyethyl)thiazole
457	50 mg	2-methyl-6-methylaminoheptan-2-ol
233	50 mg	methyl[2-(2-methylbenzhydryloxy)ethyl]amine hydrochloride
243	25 mg	3-*O*-methylmethyldopa
476	25 mg	1-methyl-3-[2-(5-methylimidazol-4-ylmethylthio)ethyl]guanidine dihydrochloride
244	50 mg	2-methyl-5-nitroimidazole
245	25 mg	(1-methyl-5-nitroimidazol-2-yl)methanol
246	25 mg	methyl-5-phenylthio-1*H*-benzamidazol-2-yl carbamate
248	50 mg	methylprednisolone
249	200 mg	methylprednisolone acetate
392	50 mg	4-[2-(5-methylpyrazine-2-carboxamido)ethyl]benzenesulphonamide
445	25 mg	4-methyl-5-vinylthiazole edisilate (*4-methyl-5-vinylthiazole edisylate*)
409	50 mg	methysergide maleate
357	100 mg	metoclopramide hydrochloride
540	100 mg	metoprolol tartrate
603	150 mg	metronidazole
251	100 mg	mexenone
393	50 mg	mexiletine hydrochloride
252	100 mg	mianserin hydrochloride
253	100 mg	miconazole nitrate
254	100 mg	monosulfiram
255	100 mg	morphine hydrochloride *(controlled drug—permit required)*
358	200 mg	nabumetone
362	100 mg	naftidrofuryl oxalate
548	100 mg	naloxone hydrochloride
257	100 mg	nandrolone
425	50 mg	nandrolone decanoate
259	50 mg	nandrolone laurate
260	100 mg	nandrolone phenylpropionate
360	25 mg	3-(1-naphthyl)-2-tetrahydrofurfurylpropionic acid
435	100 mg	naproxen
261	25 mg	neostigmine metilsulfate (*neostigmine methylsulphate*)
460	100 mg	nicotinamide
395	50 mg	nicotinyl alcohol tartrate
462	100 mg	nifedipine
262	100 mg	nitrazepam
263	50 mg	nitrofurfural diacetate
264	25 mg	5-nitrofurfurylidene azine
367	0.20 ml	3-nitroso-3-azabicyclo[3.3.0]octane
512	100 mg	noradrenaline acid tartrate (*norepinephrine acid tartrate*)
266	50 mg	norethisterone
269	200 mg	nortriptyline hydrochloride
270	50 mg	noscapine hydrochloride
271	100 mg	nystatin
272	100 mg	orciprenaline sulphate
273	200 mg	oxyclozanide
416	250 mg	oxyphenbutazone
275	100 mg	oxytetracycline hydrochloride
448	200 mg	palmitic acid
276	25 mg	pancuronium bromide
277	100 mg	papaverine hydrochloride
371	100 mg	paracetamol

Catalogue No.	Pack size	British Pharmacopoeia Chemical Reference Substance
278	0.1 mg	pentagastrin
422	100 mg	perphenazine
280	250 mg	phenethicillin potassium
282	500 mg	phenoxymethylpenicillin potassium
520	50 mg	phentolamine mesilate (*phentolamine mesylate*)
284	100 mg	phenylephrine hydrochloride
035	50 mg	1-phenyl-3-pyrrolidinopropan-1-one hydrochloride
423	100 mg	phytomenadione
503	200 mg	pilocarpine nitrate
450	50 mg	3-piperidylpropiophenone hydrochloride
463	100 mg	piroxicam
411	50 mg	pizotifen malate
288	100 mg	poldine metilsulfate (*poldine methylsulphate*)
289	100 mg	polythiazide
399	100 mg	prazosin hydrochloride
464	100 mg	prednisolone
292	100 mg	prednisolone sodium phosphate
553	250 mg	prednisone
497	100 mg	prilocaine hydrochloride
293	100 mg	primidone
295	100 mg	procaine benzylpenicillin (*procaine penicillin*)
294	100 mg	procaine hydrochloride
493	100 mg	prochlorperazine mesilate (*prochlorperazine mesylate*)
494	25 mg	prochlorperazine sulphoxide
296	100 mg	procyclidine hydrochloride
449	50 mg	progesterone
297	100 mg	proguanil hydrochloride
412	100 mg	promethazine hydrochloride
505	25 mg	promethazine sulphoxide
413	100 mg	pseudoephedrine hydrochloride
458	100 mg	pyridoxine hydrochloride
299	100 mg	pyrimethamine
300	200 mg	rafoxanide
471	100 mg	ranitidine hydrochloride
473	25 mg	ranitidine impurity B
459	50 mg	riboflavin sodium phosphate (*riboflavine sodium phosphate*)
400	25 mg	rifampicin *N*-oxide
586	200 mg	ritodrine hydrochloride
451	100 mg	salbutamol
302	100 mg	salbutamol sulphate
436	1 g	senna powder
304	100 mg	silica in dimeticone suspension (*silica in dimethicone suspension*)
453	200 mg	sodium nitroprusside
490	100 mg	sodium picosulfate (*sodium picosulphate*)
452	500 mg	sodium valproate
498	200 mg	sotalol hydrochloride
454	200 mg	stearic acid
312	100 mg	sulfadiazine (*sulphadiazine*)
310	100 mg	sulfadoxine
314	100 mg	sulfamethoxazole (*sulphamethoxazole*)
315	50 mg	tamoxifen citrate
316	100 mg	tamoxifen citrate impurity standard
455	100 mg	temazepam *(controlled drug—permit required)*
318	100 mg	terbutaline sulphate
319	100 mg	testosterone decanoate
320	100 mg	testosterone enantate (*testosterone enanthate*)
321	100 mg	testosterone isocaproate
322	100 mg	testosterone phenylpropionate
480	100 mg	tetracycline hydrochloride
325	100 mg	tetramisole hydrochloride
327	100 mg	theophylline
414	100 mg	thiamine mononitrate
495	100 mg	thioridazine
331	100 mg	thiotepa
332	25 mg	2-thymoxyethyldimethylamine hydrochloride
328	300 mg	tiabendazole (*thiabendazole*)
513	500 mg	α-tocopheryl succinate
334	100 mg	tolnaftate
544	25 mg	transplatin
591	50 mg	trazodone hydrochloride impurity standard
338	100 mg	triamcinolone
339	50 mg	triamcinolone acetonide
340	200 mg	triamterene

Catalogue No.	Pack size	British Pharmacopoeia Chemical Reference Substance
593	100 mg	tribavirin
592	25 mg	tribavirin impurity standard
341	50 mg	3,5,6-trichloro-2-hydroxybenzoic acid
579	25 mg	triethyl phosphonoformate
555	25 mg	2-trifluoromethylthioxanthone
034	200 mg	trihexyphenidyl hydrochloride (*benzhexol hydrochloride*)
344	100 mg	trimethoprim
346	50 mg	*Z*-triprolidine
347	100 mg	triprolidine hydrochloride
349	50 mg	tylosin
350	1 g	urea
563	150 mg	vigabatrin
564	25 mg	5-vinyl-2-pyrrolidone
518	100 mg	warfarin sodium
353	100 mg	xylometazoline hydrochloride
599	100 mg	zuclopenthixol acetate dihydrochloride
596	25 mg	zuclopenthixol decanaote dihydrochloride
558	100 mg	zuclopenthixol hydrochloride

Appendix II

A. Infrared Spectrophotometry

(Ph. Eur. method 2.2.24)

Spectrophotometers

Spectrophotometers for recording spectra in the infrared region consist of an optical system capable of providing monochromatic light in the region of 4000 to 670 cm^{-1} (about 2.5 to 15 µm) or in some cases down to 200 cm^{-1} (50 µm) and a means of measuring the quotient of the intensities of the transmitted radiation and the incident radiation.

Preparation of the substance being examined

Substances are examined in one of the following forms.

Liquids Examine a liquid as a thin film held between two plates or in a cell of suitable path length constructed of material transparent to infrared radiation in the region being examined.

Liquids or solids prepared as solutions Prepare a solution in a suitable solvent and use a concentration and pathlength to give a satisfactory spectrum over a sufficiently wide wavelength range. Compensation for absorption due to the solvent should be made by placing in the reference beam a similar cell containing the solvent used. Suitable concentrations of the solute will vary with the substance being examined but typical concentrations are 1% to 10% w/v for a pathlength of 0.5 to 0.1 mm.

Solids Examine a solid after dispersion in a suitable liquid (mull) or solid (halide disc), as appropriate. If prescribed in the monograph, make a film of a molten mass between two plates transparent to infrared radiation.

Mulls Triturate a small quantity of the substance with the minimum amount of *liquid paraffin* or other suitable liquid; 5 to 10 mg of the substance is usually sufficient to make an adequate mull. Compress a portion of the mull between two plates transparent to infrared radiation.

Discs Unless otherwise specified, triturate 1 to 2 mg of the substance with 0.3 to 0.4 g of dried, finely powdered *potassium bromide* or *potassium chloride*. These quantities are usually suitable for a disc 13 mm in diameter and a spectrum of suitable intensity. Grind the mixture carefully, spread it uniformly in a suitable die and compress under vacuum at a pressure of about 800 MPa. Commercial dies are available and the manufacturer's instructions should be followed. Several factors, such as inadequate or excessive grinding, moisture or other impurities in the dispersion medium and an insufficient reduction of the particle size may give rise to unsatisfactory discs. A disc should be discarded if visual inspection shows lack of uniformity or if the transmittance at about 2000 cm^{-1} (5 µm) in the absence of a specific absorption band is less than 75% without compensation. If the other ingredients of tablets, injections or other dosage forms are not completely removed from the substance being examined, they may contribute to the spectrum.

Gases Examine a gas in a cell transparent to infrared radiation and having an optical path length of about 100 mm. Evacuate the cell and fill to the desired pressure through a stopcock or needle valve using a suitable gas transfer line between the cell and the container of the substance being examined. If necessary adjust the pressure using a gas transparent to infrared radiation, for example, *nitrogen* or *argon*. To avoid absorption interferences due to water vapour, carbon dioxide or other atmospheric gases place in the reference beam an identical cell that is either evacuated or filled with a gas transparent to infrared radiation.

For recording by multiple reflection

When prescribed in the monograph, prepare the substance by one of the following methods.

Solutions Dissolve the substance in the appropriate solvent under the conditions described in the monograph. Evaporate the solution on a thallium bromo-iodide plate or on another suitable plate.

Solids Place the substance on a thallium bromo-iodide plate or on another suitable plate in a manner giving uniform contact.

Identification

Identification by chemical reference substances
Unless otherwise directed in the monograph, prepare the substance being examined and the reference substance by the same procedure and record the spectra between 4000 cm^{-1} and 670 cm^{-1} (2.5 µm to 15 µm) under the same operational conditions. The absorption maxima in the spectrum obtained with the substance being examined correspond in position and relative intensity to those in the spectrum obtained with the reference substance (CRS or EPCRS). When the spectra recorded in the solid state show differences in the positions of the absorption maxima, treat the substance being examined and the reference substance in the same manner so that they crystallise or are produced in the same form, or otherwise proceed as directed in the monograph, then record the spectra.

Identification by European Pharmacopoeia reference spectra

Resolution performance of the apparatus Record the spectrum of a polystyrene film 0.05 mm thick. The difference x between the percentage transmittance at the absorption minimum A at 2870 cm^{-1} (3.48 µm) and that at the absorption maximum B at 2851 cm^{-1} (3.51 µm) should be greater than 18. The difference y between the percentage transmittance at the absorption minimum C at 1589 cm^{-1} (6.29 µm) and that at the absorption maximum D at 1583 cm^{-1} (6.32 µm) should be greater than

Verification of the wave-number scale The wave-number scale may be verified using a polystyrene film which has maxima at the wave-numbers (in cm^{-1}) shown. The numbers in parentheses indicate the accuracy with which these values have been established.

3027.1	(±0.3)	1583.1	(±0.3)
2924	(±2)	1181.4	(±0.3)
2850.7	(±0.3)	1154.3	(±0.3)
1944	(±1)	1069.1	(±0.3)
1871.0	(±0.3)	1028.0	(±0.3)
1801.6	(±0.3)	906.7	(±0.3)
1601.4	(±0.3)	698.9	(±0.5)

Method Prepare the substance being examined according to the instructions accompanying the reference spectrum. Using the operating conditions that were used when verifying the resolution performance, record the spectrum of the substance being examined and superimpose on it the polystyrene absorption bands at 2851 cm^{-1} (3.51 μm), 1601 cm^{-1} (6.25 μm) and 1028 cm^{-1} (9.73 μm). Compare the two spectra and the maxima of polystyrene indicated above. Using the positions of the maxima of polystyrene as references, the positions of the significant maxima in the spectrum of the substance being examined and the reference spectrum should correspond to within 0.5% of the wave-number scale. The relative intensities of the maxima should be concordant in the two spectra.

Reference spectra of the European Pharmacopoeia are obtainable from the Secretariat of the European Pharmacopoeia Commission, BP 907, F67029, Strasbourg Cedex 1, France.

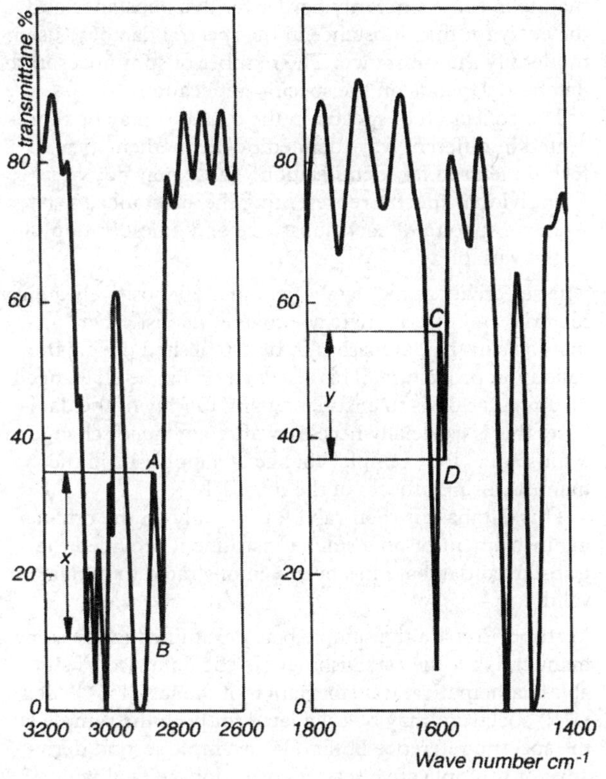

Fig. 2A-1 Typical spectrum of polystyrene used to verify the resolution performance

Identification by British Pharmacopoeia reference spectra

Resolution performance of the apparatus The instrument used for recording infrared spectra should comply with the following test for resolution.

Record the spectrum of a polystyrene film 0.038 mm thick. The difference *x* between the depth of the trough from the maximum absorption at 2851 cm^{-1} (3.51 μm) to the minimum at 2870 cm^{-1} (3.48 μm) should be greater than 18% transmittance and that from the maximum at 1583 cm^{-1} (6.32 μm) to the minimum at 1589 cm^{-1} (6.29 μm) should be greater than 12% transmittance.

Verification of the wave-number scale The wave-number scale may be verified as described under identification by European Pharmacopoeia reference spectrum.

Method Unless otherwise directed in the monograph or on the reference spectrum prepare the substance as a disc in a dispersion of *potassium bromide* and record the spectrum from 2000 to 625 cm^{-1} (5 to 16 μm); in some cases the spectrum should be scanned from 4000 cm^{-1} (2.5 μm) (where required, the 4000 to 2000 cm^{-1} region of the reference spectrum is printed separately). The spectrum should be scanned using the same instrumental conditions as were used to demonstrate compliance with the requirement for resolution.

When the spectrum of the substance being examined is compared with a reference spectrum of the British Pharmacopoeia, the positions and relative intensities of the absorption bands of the spectrum of the substance being examined should conform to those of the reference spectrum. When comparing the two spectra, care should be taken to allow for the possibility of differences in resolving power between the instrument on which the *reference spectrum* was prepared and the instrument being used to examine the substance. A *reference spectrum* of a polystyrene film recorded on the same instrument as the *reference spectrum* of the substance is included for assessing these differences. It should be noted that the greatest variations due to differences in resolving power are likely to occur in the region between 4000 and 2000 cm^{-1} (2.5 to 5 μm).

The reference spectra are provided on pages S1 and following.

Impurities in gases

For the analysis of impurities use a cell transparent to infrared radiation and of suitable optical path length (for example, 1 to 20 m). Fill the cell as prescribed under Gases. For detection and quantification of the impurities proceed as prescribed in the monograph.

NEAR-INFRARED SPECTROPHOTOMETRY

(Ph. Eur. method 2.2.40)

Near infrared spectrophotometry is a technique particularly useful for identifying organic substances. Although the spectra are restricted to C—H, N—H, O—H and S—H resonances they usually have a high informative content. However, the spectra depend on a number of parameters such as particle size, polymorphism, residual solvents, humidity... which cannot always be controlled. For this reason, direct comparison of the spectrum obtained with the substance being examined with the reference spectrum is usually impossible and some suitable validated mathematical treatment of the data is required.

Apparatus Spectrophotometers for recording spectra in the near-infrared region consist of:

— a filter, grating or interferometer system capable of providing the whole range of electromagnetic radiation in the region of about 780 nm to about 2500 nm (12821 cm^{-1} to 4000 cm^{-1}),

— a means of collecting and measuring the intensity of the transmitted or reflected radiation (transmission or reflection), such as an integration sphere, a fibre optic probe, etc, coupled to an appropriate detector,

— a means of mathematical treatment of the spectral data obtained.

Preparation of the substance being examined

For measurement by transmission This method generally applies to liquids, diluted or undiluted, and to solids in solution.

Examine the samples in a cell of suitable path length (generally 0.5 mm to 4 mm), transparent to near-infrared radiation, or by immersion of a fibre optic probe of a suitable configuration, which yields a spectrum situated in a zone of transmittance compatible with the specifications of the apparatus and appropriate for the intended purpose. When recording the near-infrared spectrum of a liquid sample, the hazards of temperature dependent perturbations or any other effects of spectral disturbances must be taken into consideration.

In all cases, compensation for background interferences must be made in a manner appropriate to the optical configuration of the apparatus, for example, a reference scan of air (for liquids) or solvent (for solutions) may be subtracted from the sample spectrum.

For measurement by diffuse reflection This method generally applies to solids.

Examine the samples in a suitable device. When immersing a fibre optic probe in the sample, care must be taken in the positioning of the probe to ensure that it remains stationary during the acquisition of the spectra and that the measuring conditions are as reproducible as possible from one sample to another.

In all cases, compensation for background interferences must be made in a manner appropriate to the optical configuration of the instrument, for example, a reference scan of an internal or external reflection standard must be subtracted from the sample spectrum. The particle size and the state of hydration or of solvation must also be taken into consideration.

For measurement by transflection This method generally applies to liquids, diluted or undiluted, and to solids in solution or in suspension.

Examine the sample in a cell with a suitable diffuse reflector, made of either metal or of an inert substance (for example titanium oxide), not exhibiting a spectrum in the near-infrared region and introduced at a suitable concentration into the sample. The samples are examined as described above under For measurement by transmission or For measurement by diffuse reflection.

Control of instrument performance

Use the apparatus according to the manufacturer's instructions and carry out the prescribed verifications at regular intervals, according to the use of the apparatus and the substances to be tested.

Verification of the wavelength scale (except for filter apparatus) Verify the wavelength scale employed, generally in the region between 780 nm and 2500 nm using (a) suitable wavelength standard(s) which has characteristic maxima at the wavelengths under investigation, for example polystyrene or rare-earth oxides.

Verification of the wavelength repeatability (except for filter apparatus) Verify the wavelength repeatability using (a) suitable standard(s), for example polystyrene or rare-earth oxides. The standard deviation of the wavelengths is consistent with the spectrophotometer specification.

Verification of response repeatability Verify the response repeatability using (a) suitable standard(s), for example reflective thermoplastic resins doped with carbon black. The standard deviation of the maxima response is consistent with the spectrophotometer specification.

Verification of photometric noise Determine the photometric noise using a suitable reflectance standard, for example white reflective ceramic tiles or reflective thermoplastic resins. Scan the reflection standard in accordance with the spectrophotometer manufacturer's recommendation and calculate the photometric noise, either peak to peak, or for a given wavelength. In the latter case, the photometric noise is represented by the standard deviation of the responses. The photometric noise is consistent with the spectrophotometer specification.

Establishment of a spectral reference library

Record the spectra of a suitable number of batches of the substance which have been fully tested as prescribed in the monograph and which exhibit the variation typical (e.g. manufacturer, particle size...) of the substance being analysed. The set of spectra represents the information that defines the similarity border for that substance and is the entry for that substance in the spectral database used to identify the substance. The number of substances in the database depends on the specific application.

The collection of spectra in the database may be represented in different ways defined by the mathematical technique used for identification. These may be:

— individual spectra representing the substance,
— mean spectra of each substance and a description of the variability.

The selectivity of the database to identify positively a given material and discriminate adequately against other materials in the database is to be established during the validation procedure. This selectivity must be challenged on a regular basis to ensure ongoing validity of the database; this is especially necessary after any major change in a substance, for example: change of supplier or in the manufacturing process of the material.

This database is then valid for use only on the originating instrument or on a similar instrument provided the transferred database has been demonstrated to remain valid.

Method Prepare the sample being examined in the same manner as for the establishment of the database. A suitable mathematical transformation of the log $(1/T)$ or log $(1/R)$ spectrum may be calculated for both the sample and the spectral reference library, for example second derivative or multiplicative scatter correction, to facilitate spectral comparison.

Comparison of the transforms of the sample and the spectral reference library involves the use of a suitable chemometric classification technique.

B. Ultraviolet and Visible Absorption Spectrophotometry

(Ph. Eur. method 2.2.25)

The *absorbance*, *A*, of a solution is defined as the logarithm to base 10 of the reciprocal of the transmittance, *T*, for monochromatic light, and is expressed by the equation:

$$A = \log_{10}(1/T) = \log_{10}(I_o/I)$$

where I = the intensity of transmitted monochromatic light,

I_o = the intensity of incident monochromatic light and

$T = I/I_o$.

In the absence of other physico-chemical factors, the

measured absorbance (A) is proportional to the path length (d) through which the light passes and to the concentration (c) of the substance in accordance with the expression:

$$A = \varepsilon cd$$

where ε is the molar absorptivity when d is expressed in cm and c in moles per litre.

The expression A(1%, 1 cm) representing the *specific absorbance* of a dissolved substance refers to the absorbance of a 1.0% w/v solution in a 1 cm cell and measured at a defined wavelength so that

$$A(1\%, 1\ cm) = 10\varepsilon/M$$

where M is the molecular weight of the substance being examined.

The *specific absorbance* is therefore the notional absorbance of a 1-cm layer of a 1% w/v solution of the absorbing solute, its value at a particular wavelength in a given solvent being a property of the solute.

Unless otherwise prescribed, measure the *absorbance* at the prescribed wavelength using a path-length of 1 cm at 19° to 21°. Unless otherwise prescribed, carry out the measurements with reference to the solvent or mixture of solvents used to prepare the solution being examined. In measuring the absorbance of a solution at a given wavelength, the absorbance of the reference cell and its contents should not exceed 0.4 and is preferably less than 0.2 when measured with reference to air at the same wavelength. Plot the absorption spectrum with absorbance or function of absorbance as ordinate against wavelength or function of wavelength as abscissa.

A statement in an assay or test of the wavelength at which maximum absorption occurs implies the maximum occurring either precisely at or within ±2 nm of the given wavelength.

Apparatus Spectrophotometers suitable for measuring in the ultraviolet and visible range of the spectrum consist of an optical system capable of producing monochromatic light in the range 200 to 800 nm and a device suitable for determining the absorbance.

Control of wavelengths Verify the wavelength scale using the absorption maxima of *holmium perchlorate solution,* the line of a hydrogen or deuterium discharge lamp or the lines of a mercury vapour arc shown below. The permitted tolerance is ±1 nm for the ultraviolet range and ±3 nm for the visible range.

241.15 nm	(Ho)	404.66 nm	(Hg)
253.7 nm	(Hg)	435.83 nm	(Hg)
287.15 nm	(Ho)	486.0 nm	(Dβ)
302.25 nm	(Hg)	486.1 nm	(Hβ)
313.16 nm	(Hg)	536.3 nm	(Ho)
334.15 nm	(Hg)	546.07 nm	(Hg)
361.5 nm	(Ho)	576.96 nm	(Hg)
365.48 nm	(Hg)	579.07 nm	(Hg)

Control of absorbances Check the absorbance using a solution of *potassium dichromate* at the wavelengths indicated in the following Table, which gives for each wavelength the exact value of the specific absorbance [A(1%, 1 cm)] and the permitted limits. The tolerance for the absorbance is ±0.01.

Wavelength nm	A(1%, 1 cm)	Maximum tolerance
235	124.5	122.9 to 126.2
257	144.0	142.4 to 145.7
313	48.6	47.0 to 50.3
350	106.6	104.9 to 109.2

Use a solution of potassium dichromate prepared in the following manner. Dissolve 57.0 to 63.0 mg of *potassium dichromate,* previously dried to constant weight at 130°, in sufficient 0.005M *sulphuric acid* to produce 1000 ml.

The absorbances of a potassium dichromate solution containing exactly 60.06 mg of K2Cr2O7 in 1000 ml of 0.005M *sulphuric acid* were used as the basis for the Table above. Measured at a path length of 1 cm, the absorbances are as shown in the Table below.

Wavelength (nm)	Absorbance
235	0.748
257	0.865
313	0.292
350	0.640

Limit of stray light Stray light may be detected at a given wavelength with suitable filters or solutions. For example, the absorbance of a 1.2% w/v solution of *potassium chloride* with a path-length of 1 cm should be more than 2 at 200 nm when compared with *water* as reference liquid.

Resolution When prescribed in a monograph, record the spectrum of a 0.02% v/v solution of *toluene* in *hexane.* The ratio of the absorbance at the maximum at 269 nm to that at the minimum at 266 nm is stated in the monograph.

Spectral slit width When measuring the absorbance at an absorption maximum and when using an instrument the slit-width of which is variable at the selected wavelength, the slit-width should be small compared with the half-width of the absorption band. However, it should be as large as possible to obtain a high value of I and should be such that further reduction does not result in an increased absorbance reading.

Cells The absorbances of the cells intended to contain the solution being examined and the solvent liquid, when filled with the same solvent, should be the same. If this is not the case, an appropriate correction must be applied. The tolerance on the path length of the cells used is ±0.005 cm. The cells should be cleaned and handled with care.

Determination of absorbance for monographs other than those from the European Pharmacopoeia

Unless otherwise prescribed, measure the *absorbance* at the prescribed wavelength using a path-length of 1 cm at 19° to 21°. If this is not appropriate for a particular instrument, the path-length should be varied, or, alternatively, the concentration may be varied provided that compliance with Beer's Law has been shown over the range in question. Unless otherwise prescribed, carry out the measurements with reference to the solvent or mixture of solvents used to prepare the solution being examined. The solvent in the reference cell should be of the same batch as that used to prepare the solution. In certain cases measurements are carried out with reference to a mixture of reagents, details of which are prescribed in the monograph.

When an assay or test prescribes the use of a reference substance, make the spectrophotometric measurements with the solution prepared from the reference substance by the official directions and then with the corresponding solution prepared from the substance being examined. Carry out the second measurement as quickly as possible after the first, using the same cell and the same experimental conditions.

SECOND DERIVATIVE SPECTROPHOTOMETRY

(no Ph. Eur. equivalent method)

Derivative spectrophotometry involves the transformation of absorption spectra into first, second or higher order derivative spectra. A first derivative spectrum is a plot of the gradient of the absorption curve (rate of change of the absorbance with wavelength, $dA/d\lambda$) against wavelength. A second-derivative spectrum is a plot of the curvature of the absorption spectrum ($d^2A/d\lambda^2$) against wavelength. If the absorbance follows the Beer-Lambert relationship, the second derivative at any wavelength, λ, is related to concentration by the following equation.

$$\frac{d^2A}{d\lambda^2} = \frac{d^2A(1\%,\ 1\ \text{cm})}{d\lambda^2} \times cd$$

where A = the absorbance at wavelength l,

A(1%, 1 cm) = the specific absorbance at wavelength l,

c = the concentration of the absorbing solute expressed as a percentage w/v,

d = the thickness of the absorbing layer in cm.

Apparatus A spectrophotometer complying with the requirements for Control of wavelengths and Control of absorbances above and equipped with an analogue resistance—capacitance differentiation module or a digital differentiator or another means of producing second-derivative spectra should be used in accordance with the manufacturer's instructions. Some methods of producing second-derivative spectra lead to a wavelength shift relative to the zero order spectrum and this should be taken into account when necessary. Unless otherwise stated in the monograph, the spectral slit width of the spectrophotometer, where variable, should be set as described under Spectral slit width above. The cells used should comply with the statements given under the heading Cells.

Reagents The temperatures of all solutions used in the test should not differ by more than 0.5°.

Resolution When prescribed in a monograph, record the second-derivative spectrum in the range 255 to 275 nm of a 0.020% v/v solution of *toluene* in *methanol* using *methanol* in the reference cell. A small negative extremum (or trough) located between two large negative extrema (or troughs) at about 261 nm and 268 nm should be clearly visible.

C. Nuclear Magnetic Resonance Spectrometry

(Ph. Eur. method 2.2.33)

Nuclear magnetic resonance (NMR) spectrometry is based on the fact that nuclei such as ^{1}H, ^{13}C, ^{19}F and ^{31}P possess a permanent nuclear magnetic moment. When placed in an external magnetic field (main field) they take certain well-defined orientations with respect to the direction of this field which correspond to distinct energy levels. For a given field value, transitions between neighbouring energy levels take place due to absorption of electromagnetic radiation of characteristic wavelengths at radio frequencies.

The determination of these frequencies may be made either by sequential search of the resonance conditions (continuous-wave spectrometry) or by simultaneous excitation of all transitions with a multi-frequency pulse followed by computer analysis of the free-induction decay of the irradiation emitted as the system returns to the initial state (pulsed spectrometry).

A proton magnetic resonance spectrum appears as a set of signals which correspond to protons and are characteristic of their nuclear and electronic environment within the molecule. The separation between a given signal and that of a reference compound is called a chemical shift (δ) and is expressed in part per million (ppm); it characterises the kind of proton in terms of electronic environment. Signals are frequently split into groups of related peaks, called doublets, triplets, ... multiplets; this splitting is due to the presence of permanent magnetic fields emanating from adjacent nuclei, particularly from other protons within two to five valence bonds. The intensity of each signal, determined from the area under the signal, is proportional to the number of equivalent protons.

Apparatus

A nuclear magnetic resonance spectrometer for continuous-wave spectrometry consists of a magnet, a low-frequency sweep generator, a sample holder, a radio-frequency transmitter and a computer for the acquisition, storage and mathematical transformation of the data into a conventional spectrum.

Unless otherwise directed in the monograph, use a nuclear magnetic resonance spectrometer operating at not less than 60 MHz in accordance with the manufacturer's instructions and the following operating conditions.

Before recording the spectrum, verify the following.

(1) The resolution is equal to 0.5 Hz or less by measuring the peak width at half-height using an adequate scale expansion of either

(i) the band at δ7.33 ppm or at δ7.51 ppm of the symmetrical multiplet of a 20% v/v solution of *1,2-dichlorobenzene* in *deuterated acetone* or

(ii) the band at δ0.00 ppm of a 5% v/v solution of *tetramethylsilane* in *deuterochloroform*.

(2) The signal-to-noise ratio (S/N), measured over the range from δ2 to 5 ppm on the spectrum obtained with a 1% v/v solution of *ethylbenzene* in *carbon tetrachloride*, is at least 25:1. This ratio is calculated as the mean of five successive determinations from the expression

$$S/N = 2.5A/H$$

where A is the amplitude, measured in millimetres, of the

largest peak of the methylene quartet of ethylbenzene centred at δ2.65 ppm and *H* is the peak-to-peak amplitude of the base line noise measured in millimetres obtained between δ4 and δ5 ppm. The amplitude is measured from a base line constructed from the centre of the noise on either side of this quartet and at a distance of at least 1 ppm from its centre.

(3) The amplitude of spinning side bands is not greater than 2% of the sample peak height in a tube rotating at a speed appropriate for the spectrometer used.

(4) For quantitative measurements verify the repeatability of the integrator responses using a 5% v/v solution of *ethylbenzene* in *carbon tetrachloride*. Carry out five successive scans of the protons of the phenyl and ethyl groups and determine the mean of the values obtained. None of the individual values differs by more than 2.5% from the mean.

Method

Dissolve the substance being examined as prescribed in the monograph and filter; the solution must be clear. Unless otherwise specified in the monograph, an internal chemical shift standard should be used; for solutions in deuterated organic solvents, 0.5 to 1.0% v/v of *tetramethylsilane* may be added; for solutions in *deuterium oxide*, 0.5 to 1.0% w/v of *sodium tetradeuterodimethylsilapentanoate* may be added. Take the necessary quantity and record the spectrum.

Continuous wave spectrometry Adjust the spectrometer so that it is operating as closely as possible in the pure absorption mode and use a radio frequency setting that avoids saturation of the signals. Adjust the spectrometer controls so that the height of the strongest peak of the spectrum of the substance being examined reaches almost to full-scale deflection and the peak associated with the internal reference standard registers on the chart at δ0.00 ppm. Record the spectrum over the prescribed spectral width, using a scan speed of not more than 2 Hz per second unless otherwise specified. It is advisable to record an integral spectrum over the same spectral range, using a suitable scan speed.

Directions for quantitative measurements are given in individual monographs.

Pulsed spectrometry Set the spectrometer controls, for example pulse flip angle, pulse amplitude, pulse interval, spectral width, number of data points (resolution) and data acquisition rate, as indicated in the manufacturer's instructions and collect the necessary number of free induction decays. After mathematical transformation of the data by the computer, adjust the phase control in order to obtain as far as possible a pure absorption spectrum and calibrate the spectrum relative to the resonance frequency of the chemical shift internal reference compound. Display the spectrum stored in the computer on a suitable output device and, for quantitative measurements, process the integral according to the facility of the instrument.

D. Atomic Spectrophotometry: Emission and Absorption

These techniques are used to determine the concentration of certain metallic ions by measuring the intensity of emission or absorption of light at a particular wavelength by the atomic vapour of the element generated from the substance, for example, by introducing a solution of the substance into a flame.

ATOMIC EMISSION SPECTROMETRY

(*Ph. Eur. method 2.2.22*)

Atomic emission spectrometry is a method for determining the concentration of an element in a substance by measuring the intensity of one of the emission lines of the atomic vapour of the element generated from the substance. The determination is carried out at the wavelength corresponding to this emission line.

Apparatus

This consists essentially of an atomic generator of the element being determined (flame, plasma, arc, etc), a monochromator and a detector. If the generator is a flame, water is the solvent of choice for preparing test and reference [standard] solutions, although organic solvents may also be used if precautions are taken to ensure that the solvent does not interfere with the stability of the flame.

Method

Operate an atomic emission spectrometer in accordance with the manufacturer's instructions at the prescribed wavelength setting. Introduce a blank solution into the atomic generator and adjust the instrument reading to zero. Introduce the most concentrated reference [standard] solution and adjust the sensitivity to give a suitable reading.

Determinations are made by comparison with reference [standard] solutions with known concentrations of the element to be determined either by the method of direct calibration (Method I) or the method of standard additions (Method II).

Use Method I unless otherwise directed.

Method I: Method of direct calibration

Prepare the solution of the substance to be examined (test solution) as prescribed. Prepare not fewer than three reference [standard] solutions of the element being determined the concentrations of which span the expected value in the test solution. Any reagents used in the preparation of the test solution are added to the reference [standard] solutions in the same concentration. Introduce the test solution and each reference [standard] solution into the instrument at least three times and record the steady reading. Rinse the apparatus with blank solution each time and ascertain that the reading returns to its initial blank value. Prepare a calibration curve from the mean of the readings obtained with the reference [standard] solutions and determine the concentration of the element in the test solution from the curve so obtained.

Method II: Method of standard addition

Add to at least three similar volumetric flasks equal volumes of the solution of the substance being examined (test solution) prepared as prescribed. Add to all but one of the flasks progressively larger volumes of a reference [standard] solution containing a known concentration of the element to be determined to produce a series of solutions containing increasing concentrations of that element known to give responses in the linear part of the curve. Dilute the contents of each flask to volume with solvent.

Introduce each of the solutions into the instrument at least three times and record the steady reading. Rinse the apparatus with solvent each time and ascertain that the reading returns to its initial blank value. Calculate the linear equation of the graph using a least-squares fit and derive from it the concentration of the element being determined in the test solution. Alternatively, plot on a graph the mean of readings against the added quantity of the element being determined. Extrapolate the line joining the points on the graph until it meets the concentration axis. The distance between this point and the intersection of the axes represents the concentration of the element to be determined in the test solution.

If a solid sampling technique is required, full details of the procedure to be followed are provided in the monograph.

ATOMIC ABSORPTION SPECTROMETRY

(*Ph. Eur. method 2.2.23*)

Atomic absorption spectrometry is a method for determining the concentration of an element in a substance by measuring the absorption of radiation by atomic vapour of the element generated from the substance. The determination is carried out at the wavelength of one of the absorption lines of the element concerned.

Apparatus

This consists essentially of a source of radiation, an atomic generator of the element to be determined (flame, furnace etc), a monochromator and a detector.

The method of introducing the substance to be analysed depends on the type of atomic generator used. If it is a flame, substances are nebulised and *water* is the solvent of choice for preparing test and reference [standard] solutions although organic solvents may also be used if precautions are taken to ensure that the solvent does not interfere with the stability of the flame. When a furnace is used, substances may be introduced dissolved in *water* or an organic solvent, but with this technique solid sampling is also possible.

The atomic vapour may also be generated outside the spectrometer, for example, the cold vapour method for mercury or certain hydrides. For mercury, atoms are generated by chemical reduction and the atomic vapour is swept by a stream of an inert gas into an absorption cell mounted in the optical path of the instrument. Hydrides are either mixed with the gas feeding the burner or swept by an inert gas into a heated cell in which they are dissociated into atoms.

Method

Operate an atomic absorption spectrometer in accordance with the manufacturer's instructions at the prescribed wavelength setting. Introduce a blank solution into the atomic generator and adjust the instrument reading so that it indicates maximum transmission. Introduce the most concentrated reference [standard] solution and adjust the sensitivity to obtain a suitable absorbance reading.

Determinations are made by comparison with reference solutions with known concentrations of the element being determined either by the method of direct calibration (Method I) or the method of standard additions (Method II).

Use Method I unless otherwise directed.

Method I: Method of direct calibration

Prepare the solution of the substance being examined (test solution) as prescribed. Prepare not fewer than three reference [standard] solutions of the element to be determined the concentrations of which span the expected value in the test solution. Any reagents used in the preparation of the test solution are added to the reference [standard] and blank solutions at the same concentration. Introduce the test solution and each reference [standard] solution into the instrument at least three times and record the steady reading. Rinse the apparatus with blank solution each time and ascertain that the reading returns to its initial blank value. If a furnace is being used, it is fired between readings.

Prepare a calibration curve from the mean of the readings obtained with the reference [standard] solutions and determine the concentration of the element in the test solution from the curve so obtained.

If a solid sampling technique is required, full details of the procedure to be followed are provided in the monograph.

Method II: Method of standard addition

Add to at least three similar volumetric flasks equal volumes of the solution of the substance being examined (test solution) prepared as prescribed. Add to all but one of the flasks progressively larger volumes of a reference [standard] solution containing a known concentration of the element being determined to produce a series of solutions containing increasing concentrations of that element known to give responses in the linear part of the curve. Dilute the contents of each flask to volume with solvent.

Introduce each of the solutions into the instrument at least three times and record the steady reading. Rinse the apparatus with solvent each time and ascertain that the reading returns to its initial blank value. If a furnace is being used, it is fired between readings.

Calculate the linear equation of the graph using a least-squares fit and derive from it the concentration of the element to be determined in the test solution. Alternatively, plot on a graph the mean of readings against the added quantity of the element to be determined. Extrapolate the line joining the points on the graph until it meets the concentration axis. The distance between this point and the intersection of the axes represents the concentration of the element being determined in the test solution.

If a solid sampling technique is required, full details of the procedure to be followed are provided in the monograph.

E. Fluorescence Spectrophotometry [Fluorimetry]

(Ph. Eur. method 2.2.21)

Fluorescence spectrophotometry [fluorimetry] is a procedure that uses the measurement of the intensity of the fluorescent light emitted by the substance being examined in relation to that emitted by a given standard.

Apparatus

Operate a spectrophotofluorimeter in accordance with the manufacturer's instructions.

Method

Prepare a solution as prescribed in the monograph, transfer the solution to the cell of the spectrophotofluorimeter and illuminate it with an excitant light beam of the nominal wavelength prescribed in the monograph and as nearly monochromatic as possible. Measure the intensity of the emitted light at an angle of 90° to the excitant beam, after passing it through a filter which transmits predominantly light of the wavelength of the fluorescence. Other types of apparatus may be used provided that the results obtained are identical.

For quantitative determinations, introduce into the apparatus the solvent or mixture of solvents used to dissolve the substance being examined and set the instrument to zero. Introduce the prescribed standard solution and adjust the sensitivity of the instrument so that the reading is greater than 50. If the second adjustment is made by altering the width of the slits, a new zero setting must be made and the intensity of the standard must be measured again. Finally introduce the solution of unknown concentration and read the result on the instrument. Calculate the concentration c_x of the substance in the solution being examined using the formula:

$$c_x = (I_x c_s)/I_s$$

where c_x = concentration of the solution being examined,

c_s = concentration of the standard solution,

I_x = intensity of the light emitted by the solution being examined and

I_s = intensity of the light emitted by the standard solution.

If the intensity of the fluorescence is not strictly proportional to the concentration, the determination may be effected using a calibration graph. In some cases, measurement can be made with reference to a fixed standard (for example, a fluorescent glass or a solution of another fluorescent substance). In such cases, the concentration of the substance being examined must be determined using a calibration graph previously prepared under the same conditions.

F. X-Ray Fluorescence Spectrometry

(Ph. Eur. method 2.2.37)

Wavelength dispersive X-ray fluorescence spectrometry is a procedure that uses the measurement of the intensity of the fluorescent radiation emitted by an element having an atomic weight between 11 and 92 excited by a continuous primary X-ray radiation. The intensity of the fluorescence produced by a given element depends on the concentration of this element in the sample but also on the absorption by the matrix of the incident and fluorescent radiation. At trace levels, where the calibration curve is linear, the intensity of the fluorescent radiation emitted by an element in a given matrix, at a given wavelength, is proportional to the concentration of this element and inversely proportional to the mass absorption coefficient of the matrix at this wavelength.

Method Set and use the instrument in accordance with the instructions given by the manufacturer. Liquid samples are placed directly in the instrument; solid samples are first compressed into pellets, sometimes after mixing with a suitable binder.

To determine the concentration of an element in a sample, it is necessary to measure the net impulse rate produced by one or several standard preparations containing known amounts of this element in given matrices and to calculate or measure the weight absorption coefficient of the matrix of the sample being analysed.

Calibration From a calibration solution or a series of dilutions of the element to be analysed in various matrices, determine the slope of the calibration curve, b_0, from the following equation:

$$b_0 \frac{1}{\mu_M} = \frac{I_C^N}{C}$$

where μ_M = absorption coefficient of the matrix, calculated or measured,

I_C^N = net impulse rate,

C = concentration of the element being assayed in the standard preparation.

Weight absorption coefficient of the matrix of the sample If the empirical formula of the sample being analysed is known, calculate its weight absorption coefficient from the known elemental composition and the tabulated elemental weight absorption coefficients. If the elemental composition is unknown, determine the weight absorption coefficient of the sample matrix by measuring the intensity of the scattered X-radiation I_U (Compton scattering) from the following equation:

$$\frac{1}{\mu_{MP}} = a + bI_U$$

where μ_{MP} = weight absorption coefficient of the sample and

I_U = scattered X-radiation.

Determination of the net impulse rate of the element to be determined in the sample Calculate the net impulse rate I_{EP}^N of the element being determined from the measured intensity of the fluorescence line and the intensity of the background line(s), allowing for any tube contaminants present.

Calculation of the trace content If the concentration of the element is in the linear part of the calibration curve, it can be calculated using the following equation:

$$C = \frac{I_{EP}^N}{b_0 \frac{1}{\mu_{MP}}} \times f$$

where f = dilution factor.

Appendix III

A. Thin-layer Chromatography

(*Ph. Eur. method 2.2.27*)

Thin-layer chromatography is a separation technique in which a stationary phase consisting of an appropriate material is spread in a uniform thin layer and fixed on a support (plate or sheet) of glass, metal or plastic. The separation is carried out by migration (development) through the thin layer of solutes in a solvent or suitable mixture of solvents (mobile phase).

Unless otherwise prescribed, use the following apparatus, plates and method.

Apparatus

The apparatus consists of:

(a) plates or sheets, precoated or prepared as described below, of appropriate size (generally 100 mm × 100 mm or 200 mm × 200 mm) for the application of the solutions to be chromatographed and the migration path prescribed. The thickness of the active layer is generally 0.1 mm to 0.3 mm.

(b) a chromatographic tank with a flat bottom or a twin trough of inert, transparent material, of a size suitable for the plates or sheets used and provided with a tightly fitting lid.

(c) micropipettes, microsyringes, calibrated disposable capillary tubes or other applicator devices suitable for the proper application of the solutions.

Preparation of plates The chromatography is carried out using precoated plates or plates prepared as described below. Both types of plate comply with the verification of the detecting power and, if prescribed, with the verification of the separating power. These tests are carried out at the same time as the chromatography of the substance being examined by applying the prescribed reference solutions. At the time of use, plates may be activated, if necessary, by heating at 100° to 105° for 1 hour.

Unless otherwise specified in the monograph, prepare the plates in the following manner. Prepare a homogeneous suspension of the coating substance in accordance with the instructions of the supplier and, using a spreading device designed for the purpose, spread the suspension to form a uniform layer 0.1 to 0.3 mm thick on the carefully cleaned plates. Allow the coated plates to dry in air, heat at 100° to 105° for 1 hour and allow to cool protected from moisture. At the time of use, remove a narrow band of the coating substance from the two sides of the plate that will be vertical during development.

Method

Unless otherwise prescribed, prepare the tank by lining the walls with sheets of filter paper; pour the mobile phase into the tank, saturating the filter paper in the process, to a depth of 5 to 10 mm, close the tank and allow to stand at 20° to 25° for 1 hour (saturated conditions).

Apply the prescribed volumes of the solutions being examined in the form of circular spots about 2 to 6 mm in diameter, or, if prescribed, in the form of bands (10 to 20 mm × 2 to 6 mm unless otherwise specified) on a line parallel with, and 15 to 20 mm from, one end of the plate and not nearer than 10 mm to the sides; the spots should be at least 10 mm apart. If necessary, the solutions may be applied in portions, drying between applications. Allow the solvent to evaporate and place the plate in the tank, ensuring that it is as nearly vertical as possible and that the spots or bands are above the level of the mobile phase. Close the tank and allow to stand at 20° to 25°, unless otherwise stated in the monograph, until the mobile phase has ascended over the distance indicated in the monograph. Remove the plate and dry and visualise as directed in the monograph. For two-dimensional chromatography dry the plate after the first development and carry out the second development in a direction perpendicular to the first.

Verification of separating power

The requirements for the verification of the separating power are prescribed in the monograph.

Verification of detecting power

The detecting power is satisfactory if a spot or band is clearly visible in the chromatogram obtained with the most dilute reference solution.

Additional points for monographs other than those from the European Pharmacopoeia

When the method prescribed in a monograph carries the instructions ‘protected from light’ or ‘in subdued light’ it is intended that the entire procedure is carried out under these conditions.

Unless otherwise indicated in the monograph, the mobile phase should be allowed to ascend 15 cm above the line of application.

The phrase *ultraviolet light (254 nm)* indicates that the plate should be examined under an ultraviolet lamp having a maximum output at 254 nm (see below); other wavelength maxima may be specified.

The term *secondary spot* means any spot other than the principal spot. Similarly, a *secondary band* is any band other than the principal band.

Where a spraying technique is prescribed it is essential that the reagent is evenly applied as a fine spray. The following method of visualisation is used when directed in the monograph.

Method I Spray the dried plate with *ethanolic sulphuric acid (20%)*, heat at 105° for 30 minutes and immediately expose to nitrous fumes in a closed glass tank for 15 minutes (the nitrous fumes may be generated by adding 7M *sulphuric acid* dropwise to a solution containing 10% w/v of *sodium nitrite* and 3% w/v of *potassium iodide*). Place the plate in a current of warm air for 15 minutes and spray with a 0.5% w/v solution of N-*(1-naphthyl)ethylenediamine dihydrochloride* in *ethanol (96%)*. If necessary, allow to dry and repeat the spraying.

Materials The coating substances are described in Appendix I A: General Reagents. They are used to prepare thin-layer plates in accordance with the procedure described under Method. Prepare suspensions of the coating substances as recommended by the manufacturer unless otherwise prescribed. Commercial pre-coated plates may be used for Pharmacopoeial tests provided that they comply with the test for chromatographic separation described for the corresponding coating substance and with any additional test for verification of separating power required in the monograph test.

ULTRAVIOLET RAY LAMPS FOR ANALYTICAL PURPOSES

(Ph. Eur. text 2.1.3)

Mercury vapour in quartz lamps is used as the source of ultraviolet light. A suitable filter may be fitted to eliminate the visible part of the spectrum emitted by the lamp. When the Pharmacopoeia prescribes in a test the use of ultraviolet light of wavelength 254 nm or 365 nm, an instrument consisting of a mercury vapour lamp and a filter which gives an emission band with maximum intensity at about 254 nm or 365 nm is used. The lamp used should be capable of revealing without doubt a standard spot of sodium salicylate with a diameter of about 5 mm on a support of *silica gel G R*, the spot being examined while in a position normal to the radiation.

For this purpose apply 5 µl of a 0.4 g/l solution of *sodium salicylate R* in *alcohol R*[1] for lamps of maximum output at 254 nm and 5 µl of a 2 g/l solution in *alcohol R*[1] for lamps of maximum output at 365 nm. The distance between the lamp and the chromatographic plate under examination used in a pharmacopoeial test should never exceed the distance used to carry out the above test.

---

[1]The *alcohol R* used must be free from fluorescence

IDENTIFICATION OF PHENOTHIAZINES

(*Ph. Eur. method 2.3.3*)

Carry out the method for *thin-layer chromatography* protected from light using *kieselguhr G* as the coating substance. Impregnate the dry plate by placing it in a tank containing a shallow layer of a solution containing 1.0% w/v of *2-phenoxyethanol* and 5.0% w/v of *polyethylene glycol 300* in *acetone* so that the plate dips about 5 mm beneath the surface of the liquid and allowing the impregnating solvent to ascend at least 17 cm above the line of application. Remove the plate from the tank and use it immediately. Carry out the chromatography in the same direction as the impregnation. For the mobile phase shake a mixture of 100 volumes of *petroleum spirit (boiling range, 50° to 70°)* and 2 volumes of *diethylamine* with 6 to 8 volumes of *2-phenoxyethanol* until a persistent cloudiness is obtained, decant and use the supernatant layer even if cloudy. Apply separately to the plate 2 µl of each of two solutions in *chloroform* containing (1) 0.2% w/v of the substance being examined and (2) 0.2% w/v of the corresponding European Pharmacopoeia Chemical Reference Substance. After removal of the plate, examine under *ultraviolet light (365 nm)* and observe the fluorescence produced after a few minutes. The spot in the chromatogram obtained with solution (1) is similar in position, colour, fluorescence and size to that in the chromatogram obtained with solution (2). Spray the plate with *ethanolic sulphuric acid (10%)* and observe the colour produced. The colour of the spot in the chromatogram obtained with solution (1) is the same as that in the chromatogram obtained with solution (2) and has a similar stability over a period of at least 20 minutes after spraying.

IDENTIFICATION OF STEROIDS

Carry out the method for *thin-layer chromatography* using *kieselguhr G* as the coating substance. Impregnate the dry plate by placing it in a tank containing a shallow layer of the specified impregnating solvent, allowing the solvent to ascend to the top, removing the plate from the tank and allowing the solvent to evaporate; use within 2 hours, with the flow of the mobile phase in the direction in which impregnation was carried out. Unless otherwise specified, apply separately to the plate 2 µl of each of the following three solutions in a mixture of 9 volumes of *chloroform* and 1 volume of *methanol*. Solution (1) contains 0.25% w/v of the substance being examined. Solution (2) contains 0.25% w/v of the corresponding British Pharmacopoeia Chemical Reference Substance or European Pharmacopoeia Chemical Reference Substance. Solution (3) is a mixture of equal volumes of solutions (1) and (2). Use the specified mobile phase. After removal of the plate, allow the solvent to evaporate, heat at 120° for 15 minutes and spray the hot plate with *ethanolic sulphuric acid (20%)*. Heat at 120° for a further 10 minutes, allow to cool and examine in daylight and under *ultraviolet light (365 nm)*. The principal spot in the chromatogram obtained with solution (1) is similar in position, colour in daylight, fluorescence in ultraviolet light (365 nm) and size to that in the chromatogram obtained with solution (2). The principal spot in the chromatogram obtained with solution (3) appears as a single, compact spot.

Impregnating Solvents

I. A mixture of 1 volume of *formamide* and 9 volumes of *acetone*.

II. A mixture of 1 volume of *propane-1,2-diol* and 9 volumes of *acetone*.

III. A mixture of 1 volume of *liquid paraffin* and 9 volumes of *petroleum spirit (boiling range, 40° to 60°* or *50° to 70°)*.

Mobile phases

A. *Chloroform*.

B. A mixture of 25 volumes of *chloroform* and 75 volumes of *toluene*.

C. *Toluene*.

D. A mixture of 20 volumes of *toluene* and 80 volumes of *cyclohexane*.

E. A mixture of equal volumes of *cyclohexane* and *petroleum spirit (boiling range, 40° to 60°* or *50° to 70°)*.

F. A mixture of 40 volumes of *glacial acetic acid* and 60 volumes of *water*.

G. A mixture of 20 volumes of *1,4-dioxan* and 80 volumes of *hexane*.

H. A mixture of 29 volumes of *toluene*, 56 volumes of *chloroform* and 115 volumes of *cyclohexane*.

RELATED SUBSTANCES IN PHENOTHIAZINES

Carry out the method for *thin-layer chromatography* protected from light using *silica gel* GF_{254} as the coating substance and the mobile phase prescribed in the monograph, but allowing the solvent front to ascend 12 cm above the line of application. Unless otherwise specified, apply separately to the plate 10 µl of each of two solutions of the substance being examined prepared immediately before use in a mixture of 95 volumes of *methanol* and 5 volumes of *diethylamine* containing (1) 2.0% w/v and (2) 0.010% w/v. After removal of the plate, allow it to dry in air and examine under *ultraviolet light (254 nm)*. Disregard any spot remaining on the line of application. Unless otherwise specified any *secondary spot* in the chromatogram obtained with solution (1) is not more intense than the spot in the chromatogram obtained with solution (2) (0.5%).

Mobile phases

A. A mixture of 10 volumes of *acetone*, 10 volumes of *diethylamine* and 80 volumes of *cyclohexane*.

B. A mixture of 5 volumes of *diethylamine*, 10 volumes of *acetone* and 85 volumes of *hexane*.

C. A mixture of 18 volumes of 1M *ammonia* and 90 volumes of *butan-1-ol*.

B. Gas Chromatography

(Ph. Eur. method 2.2.28)

Gas chromatography is a method of separation in which the mobile phase is a gas (the carrier gas) and the stationary phase, contained in a column, is either a solid or a liquid coated on a solid inert support or a liquid film evenly coated on the walls of the column. Gas chromatography is based on mechanisms of adsorption and partition.

Apparatus

The apparatus consists of a gas supply, a sample injection port, a chromatographic column and a detection and recording system.

The column is usually made of glass or of stainless steel and contains the stationary phase. Its dimensions are stated in the monograph as (length × internal diameter) where this is not explicit. The carrier gas flows through the column at a constant rate or pressure and then through a detector. The temperature of the column is either maintained at a constant value or varied according to a predetermined programme, as specified in the monograph. Where necessary, the temperatures of the injection and detection ports are stated in the monograph. The detector used must enable the amounts of the substances of interest present in the column eluate to be determined. It is usually based on flame ionisation, thermal conductivity, thermionic or electron capture phenomena.

Performance

When a *column efficiency* is stated in a monograph, it is defined in terms of the number of *theoretical plates* (n) either as theoretical plates per metre or per column. Theoretical plates per metre may be calculated from data obtained under isothermal conditions from the expression

$$n = \frac{5.54 V_R{}^2}{L W_h{}^2}$$

where V_R = the distance along the baseline between the point of injection and a perpendicular dropped from the maximum of the peak of interest,

L = the length of the column in metres,

W_h = the width of the peak of interest at half peak height, expressed in the same units as V_R.

Theoretical plates per column (referred to as 'theoretical plates') may be calculated from data obtained under isothermal conditions from the expression:

$$n = \frac{5.54 V_R^2}{W_h^2}$$

When a *capacity factor, k¢, (also* known as mass distribution ratio, D_m) is stated in a monograph, it is defined by the expression

$$D_m = k' = K\frac{V_S}{V_m}$$

where K = the equilibrium distribution coefficient,

V_s = the volume of the stationary phase and

V_m = the volume of the mobile phase.

The capacity factor (mass distribution ratio) of a component may be determined from the chromatogram using the formula

$$k' = \frac{V_R - V_0}{V_0}$$

where V_R = the distance along the baseline between the point of injection and a perpendicular dropped from the maximum of the peak of interest,

V_0 = the distance along the baseline between the point of injection and a perpendicular dropped from the maximum of the peak of an unretained component.

The values of V_R and V_0 must be expressed in the same unit of measurement.

Unless otherwise stated in the monograph, the *resolution factor* (R_s) or resolution between measured peaks on the chromatogram must be greater than 1.0. It is defined by the expression

$$R_s = \frac{1.18(V_{Rb} - V_{Ra})}{W_{ha} + W_{hb}}$$

where V_{Rb} and V_{Ra}

= the distances along the baseline between the point of injection and perpendiculars dropped from the maxima of two adjacent peaks,

and W_{hb} and W_{ha}

= the respective peak widths measured at half peak height.

The values of W_{ha}, W_{hb}, V_{Ra} and V_{Rb} must be expressed in the same unit of measurement.

The *symmetry factor* of a peak is calculated from the expression $W_x/2A$, where W_x is the width of the peak at one-twentieth of the peak height and A is the distance between the perpendicular dropped from the peak maximum and the leading edge of the peak at one-twentieth of the peak height.

In some cases reference is made to a signal-to-noise ratio (S/N). The *signal-to-noise* ratio is determined using the expression $2H/h_n$, where H is the height of the peak corresponding to the component concerned in the chromatogram obtained with the prescribed solution and h_n is the absolute value of the largest noise fluctuation from the baseline in a chromatogram obtained after injection of a blank solution and observed over a distance equal to 20 times the width at half-height of the peak in the chromatogram obtained with the prescribed solution and situated equally around the place where this peak would be found.

Method

Equilibrate the column, injection port and detector at the prescribed temperatures. Prepare the solutions as described in the monograph. Using the reference solutions determine experimentally suitable instrument settings and volumes of the solutions to be injected to produce an adequate response. Carry out replicate injections to verify the repeatability of response and check, if required, the number of theoretical plates.

Inject the solutions and record the resulting chromatograms. Carry out replicate injections to verify the repeatability of response. Determine the peak areas or, alternatively, when the symmetry factor is between 0.80 and 1.20, determine the peak heights corresponding to the components of interest. From the values obtained calculate the content of the component or components being determined. In applications where an internal standard is used, determine whether any peak is present that will interfere with that of the internal standard. If an interfering peak is present, a suitable correction should be made. In applications requiring temperature programmes, peak-area determinations are to be used.

From the values obtained, calculate the content of the component or components being determined.

Normalisation

In certain cases, reference is made to *normalisation* for the assessment of one or more components or related substances. In these cases the total area of the peak or peaks due to the components or related substances is expressed as a percentage of the sum of the areas of all the peaks derived from the substance being examined. In such determinations, the use of an automatic integrator and a wide-range amplifier is desirable.

Additional points for monographs other than those from the European Pharmacopoeia

Apparatus The design of a particular chromatograph may require modification of the conditions detailed in the monograph. In such a case, the analyst should be satisfied that the modified conditions produce comparable results. If necessary, adjust the flow rate of the carrier gas to improve the quality of the chromatogram or to modify the retention times of the peaks of interest.

Method Unless otherwise stated in the monograph, use nitrogen as the carrier gas and a flame ionisation detector. Occasionally reference is made to on-column injection, in which case the sample is injected directly on to the packing material without the use of an inlet heater. When non-volatile material is to be injected on to the column, a suitable interchangeable pre-column may be used.

Reagents Solvents and reagents used in the preparation of solutions for examination should be of a quality suitable for use in gas chromatography. A wide range of chemical substances is used as stationary phases, including polyethylene glycols, high-molecular weight esters and amides, hydrocarbons, silicone gums and fluids (polysiloxanes often substituted with methyl, phenyl, nitrilo, vinyl or fluoroalkyl groups or mixtures of these) and microporous cross-linked polyaromatic beads. A suitable stationary phase, its concentration and the nature and grade of a suitable solid support are stated in the monograph. The column should be conditioned in accordance with the manufacturer's instructions. In most cases reference is made to a particular commercial brand that has been found to be suitable for the purpose, but such statements do not imply that a different but equivalent commercial brand may not be used.

Internal standards Reagents used as internal standards should not contain any impurity that would produce a peak likely to interfere in the determination described in the monograph.

Secondary peaks Reference may be made to a secondary peak. A *secondary peak* is a peak in the chromatogram other than the principal peak and any peaks due to internal standard, solvent and derivatising agents.

HEAD-SPACE GAS CHROMATOGRAPHY

(*Ph. Eur. method 2.2.28*)

Head-space gas chromatography is a method particularly suitable for separating and determining volatile compounds present in solid or liquid samples. The method is based on the analysis of the vapour phase in equilibrium with the solid or liquid phase.

Apparatus

The apparatus consists of a gas chromatograph provided with a device for introducing the test sample. The device may be connected to a module that automatically controls the pressure and the temperature. If necessary, a device for eliminating solvents can be added. The sample is introduced into a container fitted with a suitable stopper and a valve system which permits the passage of the carrier gas. The container is placed in a thermostatically controlled chamber at a temperature set according to the nature of the sample and held at this temperature long enough to allow equilibrium between the solid or liquid phase and the vapour phase to be established. The carrier gas is introduced into the container and, after the prescribed time, a suitable valve is opened so that the gas expands towards the chromatographic column, taking the volatilised compounds with it.

Instead of using a chromatograph specifically equipped for the introduction of samples, it is also possible to use airtight syringes and a conventional chromatograph. Equilibration is then carried out in a separate chamber and the vapour phase is carried onto the column taking the precautions necessary to avoid any changes in the equilibrium.

Method

Using the reference preparations, determine suitable instrument settings to produce an adequate response.

Direct calibration Separately introduce into identical containers the substance being examined and each of the reference preparations, as prescribed in the monograph, avoiding contact between the sampling device and the samples. Close the containers hermetically and place in the thermostatically controlled chamber. Equilibrate and carry out the chromatography under the conditions prescribed in the monograph.

Standard addition Add to a set of identical suitable containers equal volumes of the preparation being examined. Add to all but one of the containers suitable quantities of a reference preparation containing a known concentration of the substance being determined so as to produce a series of standards containing steadily increasing concentrations of the substance. Close the containers hermetically and place in the thermostatically controlled chamber. Equilibrate and carry out the chromatography under the conditions described in the monograph.

Plot the mean concentrations determined against the quantity of the reference preparation added. Calculate the linear equation of the graph using a least-squares fit, and derive from it the concentration of the substance being determined in the preparation. Alternatively, extrapolate the line joining the points on the graph until it meets the concentration axis. The distance between this point and the intersection of the axes represents the concentration of the substance being determined in the preparation.

Successive withdrawal If prescribed, the successive withdrawal method is fully described in the monograph.

C. Size-exclusion Chromatography

(*Ph. Eur. method 2.2.30*)

Size-exclusion chromatography is a method of separation which separates molecules in solution according to their size. With organic mobile phases, the technique is known as gel-permeation chromatography and with aqueous mobile phases, the term gel-filtration chromatography has been used. The sample is introduced onto a column, which is filled with a gel or a porous packing material, and is carried by the mobile phase through the column. The size separation takes place by repeated exchange of the solute molecules between the solvent of the mobile phase and the same solvent in the stagnant liquid phase (stationary phase) within the pores of the column-packing material. The pore size range of the packing material determines the molecular size range within which separation can occur.

Molecules small enough to penetrate all the pore spaces elute at the total permeation volume, V_t. Molecules apparently larger than the maximum pore size of the packing material migrate along the column only through the spaces between the particles of the packing material without being retained and elute at the exclusion volume (void volume), V_o. Separation according to molecular size occurs between the exclusion volume and the total permeation volume, useful separation usually occurring in the first two thirds of this range.

Apparatus

The apparatus consists of a chromatographic column of appropriate dimension, if necessary temperature-controlled, packed with a separation material that is capable of fractionation in the appropriate range of molecular sizes. The dimensions of the column are stated in the monograph as (length × internal diameter) where this is not explicit. The mobile phase is passed through the column at a constant rate either by gravity or by means of a suitable pump. One end of the column is usually fitted with a suitable device for applying the sample such as a flow adaptor, a syringe through a septum or an injection valve and may also be connected to a suitable pump for controlling the flow of eluent. Alternatively, the sample may be applied directly to the drained bed surface or, where the sample is denser than the eluent, it may be layered beneath the eluent.

The outlet from the column is connected to a detector fitted with an automatic recorder that allows the monitoring of the relative concentrations of the separated components of the sample. Detectors are usually based on photometric, refractometric or luminescent properties. An automatic fraction collector may be attached if necessary. The packing material may be a soft support such as a swollen gel or a rigid support composed of a material such as glass, silica or a solvent-compatible, cross-linked organic polymer. Rigid supports usually require pressurised systems giving faster separations. The mobile phase is chosen according to sample type, separation medium and method of detection.

The packing material should be treated, and the column packed, as described in the monograph or in accordance with the manufacturer's instructions.

Performance

When a *column efficiency* is stated in a monograph, it is defined in terms of the number of *theoretical plates* (n) either as theoretical plates per metre or per column. Theoretical plates per metre may be calculated from the expression

$$n = \frac{5.54 V_R^2}{L W_h^2}$$

where V_R = the distance along the baseline between the point of injection and a perpendicular dropped from the maximum of the peak of interest,

L = the length of the column in metres,

W_h = the width of the peak of interest at half peak height, expressed in the same units as V_R.

Theoretical plates per column (referred to as 'theoretical plates') may be calculated from the expression:

$$n = \frac{5.54 V_R^2}{W_h^2}$$

The elution characteristics of a compound in a particular column may be given by the *distribution coefficient*. When a distribution coefficient (K_D) is stated in a monograph it is defined by the expression

$$K_D = \frac{V_R - V_0}{V_T - V_0}$$

where V_R, V_0 and V_T are the *retention volumes* for the component of interest, a non-retained component (*exclusion volume*) and a component that has full access to all the pores in the support (*total permeation volume*) respectively. The retention volume is measured from the application point to that of the peak maximum.

V_R, V_0 and V_T must be expressed in the same unit of measurement.

Determination of relative component composition

Carry out the method using the conditions stated in the monograph. If possible, monitor the elution of the components continuously and measure the corresponding peak areas. If the sample is monitored by a physico-chemical property to which all of the components of the sample exhibit equivalent responses (for example, they have the same specific absorbance), then the relative amount of each component can be determined by dividing each peak area by the sum of the peak areas of the components of interest. If the responses are not equivalent, calculate the relative component composition either from calibration curves obtained with the calibration standards specified in the monograph or by any other means stated in the monograph.

Determination of molecular weight [mass]

Carry out the method on the sample and calibration standards using the procedure specified in the monograph. Plot a graph of the retention volume of the calibration standards as a function of the logarithm of the molecular weight. The curve usually approximates to a straight line within the exclusion and total permeation limits. The molecular weight of the component of interest may be estimated from the calibration curve. The calibration is valid only for the particular system used under the specified experimental conditions.

Determination of molecular size distribution of polymers

Size-exclusion chromatography may be used to determine the distribution of the molecular size of polymers. However, sample comparison may be valid only for results obtained under the same experimental conditions. The material used for the calibration and the methods for the determination of the distribution of the molecular sizes of polymers are specified in the monograph.

MOLECULAR WEIGHT [MASS] DISTRIBUTION IN DEXTRANS

(*Ph. Eur. method 2.2.39*)

Examine by *size-exclusion chromatography*.

Solution (1) Dissolve 0.20 g of the substance being examined in the mobile phase and dilute to 10 ml with the mobile phase.

Marker solution Dissolve 5 mg of *dextrose* and 2 mg of *dextran V_0 EPCRS* in 1 ml of the mobile phase.

Calibration solutions Dissolve separately in 1 ml of the mobile phase 15 mg of *dextran 4 for calibration EPCRS*, 15 mg of *dextran 10 for calibration EPCRS*, 20 mg of *dextran 40 for calibration EPCRS*, 20 mg of *dextran 70 for calibration EPCRS* and 20 mg of *dextran 250 for calibration EPCRS*.

System suitability solution Dissolve either 20 mg of *dextran 40 for performance test EPCRS* (for dextran 40) or 20 mg of *dextran 60/70 for performance test EPCRS* (for dextran 60 and dextran 70) in 1 ml of the mobile phase.

The chromatographic procedure may be carried out using:

(a) a column (0.3 m × 10 mm) packed with *cross-linked agarose for chromatography* or a series of columns, (0.3 m × 10 mm) packed with *polyether hydroxylated gel for chromatography*,

(b) a solution containing 7 g of *anhydrous sodium sulphate* and 1 g of *anhydrous chlorbutol* in 1 litre of *water* as the mobile phase, at a flow rate of 0.5 ml to 1 ml per minute, kept constant to ±1% per hour,

(c) as detector a differential refractometer,

(d) a 100-µl to 200-µl loop injector,

maintaining the system at a constant temperature (± 0.1°).

Calibration of the chromatographic system Carry out replicate injections of the chosen volume of the marker solution. The chromatogram shows two peaks the first of which is dextran V_0 EPCRS and the second of which is dextrose. From the elution volume of the peak corresponding to dextran V_0, calculate the void volume V_0 and from the peak corresponding to dextrose, calculate the total volume V_t.

Inject the chosen volume of each of the calibration solutions. Draw carefully the baseline of each of the chromatograms. Divide each chromatogram into p (at least 60) equal vertical sections (corresponding to equal elution volumes).

In each section, i, corresponding to an elution volume V_i, measure the height (y_i) of the chromatogram line above the baseline and calculate the coefficient of distribution K_i, using the expression:

$$\frac{(V_i - V_0)}{(V_t - V_0)} \qquad (1)$$

where V_0 = void volume of the column, determined using the peak corresponding to *dextran V_0 EPCRS* in the chromatogram obtained with the marker solution,

V_t = total volume of the column, determined using the peak corresponding to *dextrose* in the chromatogram obtained with the marker solution and

V_i = elution volume of section i in the chromatogram obtained with each of the calibration solutions.

Carry out the calibration using either of the following methods.

Calibration by plotting of the curve For each of the dextrans for calibration EPCRS calculate the coefficient of distribution, K_{max}, corresponding to the maximum height of the chromatographic line, using expression (1). Plot on semi-logarithmic paper, the values of K_{max} (on the x-axis) against the declared molecular weight [mass] at the maximum height of the chromatographic line (M_{max}) of each of the dextrans for calibration EPCRS and *dextrose*. Draw a first calibration curve through the points obtained, extrapolating it from the point K_{max} obtained with *dextran 250 for calibration EPCRS* to the lowest K value obtained for this EPCRS (see Fig. 3C-1). Using this first calibration curve, transform, for each chromatogram, all K_i values into the corresponding molecular weight [mass] M_i thus obtaining the molecular weight [mass] distribution. Calculate for each dextran for calibration EPCRS the average molecular weight M_w using equation (3) below. If the calculated values for M_w do not differ by more than 5% from those declared for each of the dextrans for calibration EPCRS and the mean difference is within 3%, the calibration curve is approved. If not, move the calibration curve along the y-axis and repeat the procedure above until the calculated and the declared values for M_w do not differ by more than 5%.

Calibration by calculation of the curve Calculate from equations (2) and (3) below, using a suitable method[1], values for b_1, b_2, b_3, b_4 and b_5 that give values of M_w within 5% of the declared values of each of the dextrans for calibration EPCRS and 180±2 for dextrose.

$$M_i = b_5 + e^{(b_4 + b_1 K_i + b_2 K_i^2 + b_3 K_i^3)} \qquad (2)$$

$$\overline{M_w} = \frac{\sum_{i=1}^{p} (y_i M_i)}{\sum_{i=1}^{p} y_i} \qquad (3)$$

where p = number of sections dividing the chromatograms,

y = height of the chromatographic line above the baseline in section i and

M_i= molecular weight [mass] in section i.

System suitability Inject the chosen volume of the appropriate system suitability solution.

Average molecular mass of dextran for performance test EPCRS Calculate the average molecular weight M_w as indicated under Calibration of the chromatographic system, using either the plotted calibration curve or the values obtained above for b_1, b_2, b_3, b_4 and b_5. The test is not valid unless M_w is:

41,000 to 47,000 (dextran 40 for performance test EPCRS),
67,000 to 75,000 (dextran 60/70 for performance test EPCRS).

Average molecular weight [mass] of the 10% high-fraction dextran Calculate M_w for the 10% high-fraction dextran eluted through section n using the equation:

$$M_w = \frac{\sum_{i=1}^{n}(y_i M_i)}{\sum_{i=1}^{n} y_i} \tag{4}$$

in which n is defined by the expressions:

$$\sum_{i=1}^{n} y_i \le 0.1\left(\sum_{i=1}^{p} y_i\right) \tag{5}$$

$$\sum_{i=1}^{n+1} y_1 > 0.1\left(\sum_{i=1}^{p} y_1\right) \tag{6}$$

where p = number of sections dividing the chromatograms,
y_i = height of the chromatographic line above the baseline in section i and
M_i = molecular weight [mass] in section i.

The test is not valid unless M_w of the high fraction dextran is:

110,000 to 130,000 (dextran 40 for performance test EPCRS),
190,000 to 230,000 (dextran 60/70 for performance test EPCRS).

Average molecular weight [mass] of the 10% low-fraction dextran Calculate M_w for the 10% low-fraction dextran eluted in and after section m using the expression:

$$M_w = \frac{\sum_{i=m}^{p}(y_i M_i)}{\sum_{i=m}^{p} y_i} \tag{7}$$

in which m is defined by the expressions:

$$\sum_{i=m}^{p} y_1 \le 0.1\left(\sum_{i=1}^{p} y_1\right) \tag{8}$$

$$\sum_{i=m}^{p} y_1 > 0.1\left(\sum_{i=1}^{p} y_1\right) \tag{9}$$

where p = number of sections dividing the chromatograms
y_i = height of the chromatographic line above the baseline in section i and
M_i = molecular weight [mass] in section i.

The test is not valid unless M_w of the low-fraction dextran is:

6,000 to 8,500 (dextran 40 for performance test EPCRS),
7,000 to 11,000 (dextran 60/70 for performance test EPCRS).

Molecular weight [mass] distribution of the dextran being analysed Inject the chosen volume of solution (1) and calculate M_w of the total molecular weight distribution, M_w of the 10% high-fraction dextran and M_w of the 10% low-fraction dextran as indicated under System suitability.

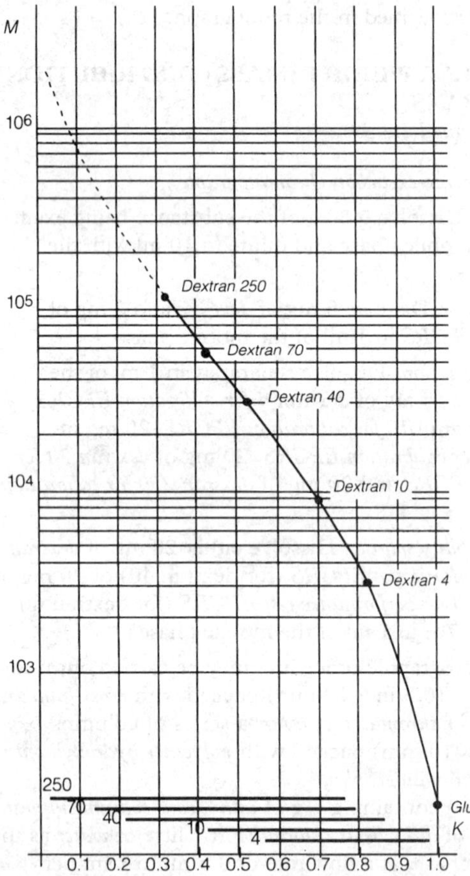

Fig. 3C-1

Example of a calibration curve. The dotted line corresponds to the part of the curve that is extrapolated. Horizontal lines at the bottom of the figure represent the width and the position of the chromatographic line obtained with each of the *dextrans for calibration EPCRS.*

(1) An iterative method such as the Gauss-Newton method modified by Hartley is suitable (see O Hartley, *Tecnometrics*, 3 (1961) and G Nilsson and K Nilsson, *J. Chromat.* **101**, 137 (1974)). A curve-fitting program for micro-computers, capable of non-linear regression, may be used.

D. Liquid Chromatography

(*Ph. Eur. method 2.2.29*)

Liquid chromatography is a method of separation in which the mobile phase is a liquid and the stationary phase, contained in a column, is either a finely divided solid or a liquid coated on a solid support or a solid support which has been chemically modified by the introduction of organic groups. Liquid chromatography is based on mechanisms of absorption, partition, ion exchange or size exclusion.

Apparatus

The apparatus usually consists of a pumping system, an injector (syringe or injection valve), a chromatographic column, a detector and a recorder.

The mobile phase is usually supplied under pressure from one or several reservoirs and flows through the column at a constant rate and then through the detector. The temperature of the chromatographic column is kept constant. The composition of the prescribed mobile phase may either be constant throughout the whole chromatographic procedure (isocratic elution) or may vary according to a defined programme (gradient elution).

The detector used must enable the amount of the substances of interest present in the column eluate to be determined. It is usually based on absorption spectrophotometry; differential refractometry, fluorimetry, combustion and electro-chemical methods are also used.

Method

Equilibrate the column with the prescribed mobile phase. Prepare the solutions as prescribed in the monograph. The solutions must be free from solid particles. Using the reference solutions determine suitable instrument settings and the quantities to be injected to produce an adequate response. Carry out replicate injections to verify the repeatability of response and check, if required, the number of theoretical plates.

Inject the solutions and record the resulting chromatograms. Carry out replicate injections to verify the repeatability of response. Determine the peak areas of the components of interest unless otherwise directed or, alternatively, when the symmetry factor is between 0.80 and 1.20 determine the peak heights corresponding to the components of interest. In applications requiring gradient elution, peak area determinations are to be used. Where an internal standard is used, check that no peak of the substance being examined is masked by that of the internal standard. From the values obtained calculate the content of the component or components being determined.

Normalisation

In certain cases, reference is made to *normalisation* for the assessment of one or more substances. In these cases the total area of the peak or peaks due to the components or related substances is expressed as a percentage of the sum of the areas of all the peaks derived from the substance being examined. In such determinations, the use of a wide range amplifier and an automatic integrator is desirable.

Performance

When a *column efficiency* is stated in a monograph, it is defined in terms of the number of *theoretical plates* (n) either as theoretical plates per metre or per column.

Theoretical plates per metre may be calculated from data obtained under isothermal conditions from the expression

$$n = \frac{5.54 V_R^2}{L W_h^2}$$

where V_R = the distance along the baseline between the point of injection and a perpendicular dropped from the maximum of the peak of interest,

L = the length of the column in metres,

W_h = the width of the peak of interest at half peak height, expressed in the same units as V_R.

Theoretical plates per column (referred to as 'theoretical plates') may be calculated from data obtained under isothermal conditions from the expression:

$$n = \frac{5.54 V_R^2}{W_h^2}$$

Unless otherwise stated in the monograph, the *resolution* or *resolution factor* (R_s) between measured peaks on the chromatogram must be greater than 1.0. It is defined by the expression

$$R_s = \frac{1.18(V_{Rb} - V_{Ra})}{W_{ha} + W_{hb}}$$

where V_{Rb} and V_{Ra}

= distances along the baseline between the point of injection and perpendiculars dropped from the maxima of two adjacent peaks,

and W_{hb} and W_{ha}

= the respective peak widths measured at half peak height.

The values of W_{ha}, W_{hb}, V_{Ra} and V_{Rb} must be expressed in the same unit of measurement.

The *symmetry factor* of a peak is calculated from the expression $W_x/2A$ where W_x is the width of the peak at one twentieth of the peak height and A is the distance between the perpendicular dropped from the peak maximum and the leading edge of the peak at one twentieth of the peak height.

When a *capacity factor*, k',(also known as mass distribution ratio, D_m) is stated in a monograph, it is defined by the expression

$$D_m = k' = K \frac{V_S}{V_m}$$

where K = the equilibrium distribution coefficient,

V_s = the volume of the stationary phase and

V_m = the volume of the mobile phase.

The capacity factor (mass distribution ratio) of a component may be determined from the chromatogram using the formula

$$k' = \frac{V_R - V_0}{V_0}$$

where V_R = the distance along the baseline between the point of injection and a perpendicular dropped from the maximum of the peak of interest,

V_0 = the distance along the baseline between the point of injection and a perpendicular dropped from the maximum of the peak of an unretained component.

The values of V_R and V_0 must be expressed in the same unit of measurement.

In some cases reference is made to a signal-to-noise ratio. The *signal-to-noise* ratio is determined using the expression $2H/h_n$ where H is the height of the peak corresponding to the component concerned in the chromatogram obtained with the prescribed solution and h_n is the absolute value of the largest noise fluctuation from the baseline in a chromatogram obtained after injection of a blank solution and observed over a distance equal to 20 times the width at half-height of the peak in the chromatogram obtained with the prescribed solution and situated equally around the place where this peak would be found.

Additional points for monographs other than those from the European Pharmacopoeia

The composition and flow rate of the mobile phase are stated in the monograph. It is advisable to use as the mobile phase solvent mixtures that have been de-aerated using a vacuum pump or other suitable means of de-aeration that has no effect on the composition of the mixture.

In quantitative work, particularly where the use of an internal standard is not specified in the monograph, the use of a fixed-volume loop injector is recommended. In certain exceptional cases the use of peak heights alone is prescribed in the monograph; where this is the case peak heights should be used irrespective of the symmetry factor.

The column is usually made of stainless steel and its dimensions are stated in the monograph. The dimensions are stated as (length × internal diameter). When the monograph prescribes the use of a stationary phase designated by a letter, the relevant stationary phase defined below is intended. The nominal diameter of the particles of the stationary phase is stated in parentheses immediately following the designating letter. In most cases reference is made to a particular commercial brand that has been found to be suitable for the purpose, but such statements do not imply that a different but equivalent commercial brand may not be used. The separation should be carried out at a constant ambient temperature unless otherwise specified in the monograph.

Unless otherwise specified in the monograph the detector consists of a photometric detector fitted with a low-volume flow cell (about 10 µl is suitable); the wavelength setting is specified in the monograph.

The design of a particular chromatograph may require modification of the conditions detailed in the monograph. In such a case the analyst should be satisfied that the modified conditions produce comparable results.

Secondary peaks Reference may be made to a secondary peak. A *secondary peak* is a peak in the chromatogram other than the principal peak and any peaks due to internal standard, solvent or derivatising agents.

Materials Solvents and reagents used in the preparation of solutions for examination should be of a quality suitable for use in liquid chromatography.

When the monograph prescribes the use of a stationary phase designated by a letter, the following stationary phases are intended.

Stationary Phase A Particles of silica.

Stationary Phase B Particles of silica the surface of which has been modified by chemically-bonded octylsilyl groups.

Stationary Phase C Particles of silica the surface of which has been modified by chemically-bonded octadecylsilyl groups.

E. Paper Chromatography

(Ph. Eur. method 2.2.26)

Apparatus

The apparatus consists of a glass tank of suitable dimensions to accommodate the chromatographic paper used, ground at the top to take a closely-fitting glass lid and adapted as necessary for ascending or descending chromatography.

The chromatographic paper consists of suitable absorbent paper, cut into strips of convenient length and not less than 25 mm wide; the paper is cut so that the mobile phase runs in the direction of the grain of the paper. A fine pencil line is drawn horizontally across the paper, either 30 mm from one end for ascending paper chromatography or, for descending paper chromatography, at such a distance from one end that when this end is secured in the solvent trough with the remainder of the paper hanging freely over the guide rod, the line is parallel to and a few centimetres below the rod. The volume of the solution specified in the monograph is applied to a point on the pencil line. If the total volume to be applied would produce a spot more than 10 mm in diameter, the solution is applied in portions, each being allowed to dry before the next application. When more than one chromatogram is to be run on the same strip of paper, the solutions are spaced along the pencil line at points not less than 30 mm apart.

Descending paper chromatography

The glass lid is supplied with a central hole about 15 mm in diameter, closed by a heavy glass plate or a stopper. Suspended in the upper part of the tank is a solvent trough with a device such as a heavy glass rod for holding the chromatographic paper. On each side of the trough, parallel to and slightly above its upper edges, are two glass guide rods to support the paper in such a way that no part of it is in contact with the walls of the tank.

Use sufficient of the solvent (saturating solvent) prescribed in the monograph to form a 25-mm layer in the bottom of the tank. Close the tank, allow to stand for 24 hours at 20° to 25° and maintain at this temperature throughout the subsequent procedure. Insert the prepared paper into the tank, close the lid and allow to stand for 90 minutes. Through the hole in the lid, introduce into the solvent trough a sufficient quantity of the prescribed mobile phase, close the tank and allow development to proceed for the distance or the time prescribed in the monograph. The paper should be protected from bright light during the development. Remove the paper from the tank and allow it to dry in air. The method of visualisation is described in the monograph.

Ascending paper chromatography

The top of the tank contains a device from which the chromatographic paper is suspended and which is capable of being lowered without opening the chamber. In the bottom of the tank is a dish to contain the mobile phase, into which the paper may be lowered.

Use sufficient of the prescribed mobile phase to form a 25-mm layer in the dish, and, if prescribed, pour the saturating solvent between the dish and the walls of the tank. Close the tank and allow to stand for 24 hours at 20° to 25° and maintain the tank at this temperature throughout the subsequent procedure. Insert the prepared paper into the tank, close the lid and allow to stand for 90 minutes. Lower the paper into the mobile phase and allow development to proceed for the distance or the time prescribed in the monograph. The paper should be protected from bright light during the development. Remove the paper from the tank and allow it to dry in air. The method of visualisation is described in the monograph.

F. Electrophoresis

(Ph. Eur. method 2.2.31)

Electrophoresis is a physical method of analysis based on the migration of charged particles dissolved or dispersed in an electrolyte solution under the action of an electric field.

The electrophoretic mobility is the rate of movement in metres per second of the charged particles under the action of an electric field of 1 volt per metre and is expressed in square metres per volt second. For practical reasons it is given in square centimetres per volt second. The mobility can be defined only for a given electrolyte under precisely determined operational conditions. It is influenced by many factors such as:

— the characteristics of charged particles: nature, size, form, electrical charge, friction coefficient,

— the liquid in which the charged particles are in motion: solvent, nature and concentration of the conducting electrolyte, ionic strength, pH, viscosity of the solution.

The direction of movement depends on the nature of the electrical charge; the charged particles travel towards the electrode that bears the charge opposite to their own.

Free or moving boundary electrophoresis

This method is mainly used for the determination of mobility, the experimental characteristics being directly measurable and reproducible. It is chiefly employed with substances of high relative molecular mass and low diffusibility. The boundaries are initially located by a physical process such as refractometry or conductimetry. After applying a given electric field for an accurately measured time, the new boundaries and their respective positions are observed. The operating conditions must be such as to make it possible to determine as many boundaries as there are components.

Zone electrophoresis using a supporting medium

This method requires the use of small samples only.

The nature of the support, such as paper, agar gel, cellulose acetate, starch, agarose, methacrylamide, mixed gel, introduces a number of additional factors modifying the mobility:

(a) owing to channelling in the supporting medium, the apparent distance covered is less than the real distance,

(b) some supporting media are not electrically neutral. As the medium is a stationary phase it may sometimes give rise to a considerable electroendosmotic flow,

(c) any heating due to the joule effect may cause some evaporation of the liquid from the supporting medium which, by capillarity, causes the solution to move from the ends towards the centre. The ionic strength therefore tends to increase gradually.

The rate of migration then depends on four main factors, namely, the mobility of the charged particle, the electroendosmotic flow, the evaporation flow, and the field strength. Hence it is necessary to operate under clearly defined experimental conditions and to use, wherever possible, reference substances.

Apparatus The apparatus for electrophoresis consists of the following components.

(1) A generator supplying direct current the voltage of which can be controlled and, preferably, stabilised.

(2) An electrophoresis chamber which is usually rectangular and made of glass or rigid plastic, with two separate compartments, the anodic and the cathodic, containing the electrolyte solution. In each compartment is immersed an electrode, for example of platinum or graphite. These are connected by means of an appropriately isolated circuit to the corresponding terminal of the power supply to form the anode and the cathode. The level of the liquid in the two compartments is kept equal to prevent siphoning. The electrophoresis chamber is fitted with an airtight lid which maintains a moisture-saturated atmosphere during operation and reduces evaporation of the solvent. A safety device may be used to cut off the power when the lid is removed. If the electrical power measured across the strip exceeds 10 W, it is preferable to cool the support.

(3) A support carrying device.

Strip electrophoresis The supporting strip, previously wetted with the same conducting solution and dipping at each end into an electrode compartment, is appropriately tightened and fixed on to a suitable carrier designed to prevent diffusion of the conducting electrolyte, such as a horizontal frame, inverted-V stand or a uniform surface with contact points at suitable intervals.

Gel electrophoresis The device consists essentially of a glass plate (for example, a microscope slide) over the whole surface of which is deposited a firmly adhering layer of gel of uniform thickness. The connection between the gel and the conducting solution is effected in various ways according to the type of apparatus used. Precautions must be taken to avoid condensation of moisture or drying of the solid layer.

(4) A measuring device or means of detection.

Method Introduce the electrolyte solution into the electrode compartments. Place the support suitably impregnated with electrolyte in the chamber under the conditions prescribed for the type of apparatus used. Locate the starting line and apply the sample. Apply the electric current for the prescribed time. After the current has been switched off, remove the support from the chamber, dry and visualise.

Polyacrylamide gel electrophoresis

In polyacrylamide gel electrophoresis, the stationary phase is a gel which is prepared from a mixture of acrylamide and *N,N′*-methylenebisacrylamide. Gels may be prepared in tubes 7.5 cm long and 0.5 cm in internal diameter (rod gels), one solution being applied to each rod. Gels may also be prepared between glass plates giving slab gels to each of which several solutions may be applied.

Apparatus This consists of two buffer reservoirs made of suitable material such as poly(methyl methacrylate) and mounted vertically one above the other. Each reservoir is fitted with a platinum electrode. The electrodes are connected to a power supply allowing operation either at constant current or at constant voltage. For rod gels the apparatus has in the base of the upper reservoir a number of holders equidistant from the electrode. For slab gels, developing chambers are available which allow either vertical development or horizontal development.

Method The solutions should usually be degassed before polymerisation and the gels used immediately after preparation.

(a) *Rod gels* Prepare the gel mixture as prescribed and pour into suitable glass tubes, stoppered at the bottom, to an equal height in each tube and to about 1 cm from the top, taking care to ensure that no air bubbles are trapped in the tubes. Cover the gel mixture with a layer of *water* to exclude air and allow to set. Gel formation usually takes about 30 minutes and is complete when a sharp interface appears between the gel and the water layer. Remove the water layer. Fill the lower reservoir with the prescribed buffer solution and remove the stoppers from the tubes. Fit the tubes into the holders of the upper reservoir and adjust so that the bottom of the tubes are immersed in the buffer solution in the lower reservoir. Carefully fill the tubes with the prescribed buffer solution. Prepare the test and reference solutions containing the prescribed marker dye and make them dense, for example by dissolving *sucrose* in them. Apply the solutions to the surface of a gel using a different tube for each solution. Add the same buffer to the upper reservoir. Connect the electrodes to the power supply and allow electrophoresis to proceed at the prescribed temperature and using the prescribed constant voltage or current. Switch off the power supply when the marker dye has migrated almost into the lower reservoir. Immediately remove each tube from the apparatus and extrude the gel. Locate the position of the bands in the electrophoretogram as prescribed.

(b) *Slab gels* Prepare the gel mixture as prescribed and introduce into a suitable mould either by pumping or pouring, taking care to ensure that no air bubbles are trapped in the gel. Sample wells may be cast directly in the gels using suitable plastic well formers. When gel formation is complete, remove the slab with the supporting plates, trim free of excess polyacrylamide and remove the well formers. Mount in a suitable tank and fill the lower reservoir with the prescribed buffer solution. Carefully fill the wells with the prescribed buffer solution. Prepare the test and reference solutions containing the prescribed marker dye and make them dense for example, by dissolving *sucrose* in them. Introduce the solutions into the wells using a different well for each solution. Add the prescribed buffer to the upper reservoir. Connect the electrodes to the power supply and allow electrophoresis to proceed at the prescribed temperature and using the prescribed constant voltage or current. Switch off the power supply when the marker dye has migrated almost to the bottom of the gel. Immediately remove the plates from the apparatus and extrude the gel. Locate the position of the bands in the electrophoretogram as prescribed.

Stacking gel When the use of a separate stacking gel is prescribed in the monograph, proceed as described above with the following modifications. Fill approximately three-quarters of the total gel length with the separation gel mixture and allow to set. Remove the water layer and fill the remaining gel length with the stacking gel mixture prepared as described in the monograph. If necessary, introduce the appropriate well formers and allow to set. When gel formation is complete, the distance between the sample wells and the surface of the separation gel should be at least 1 cm to 2 cm.

Appendix IV

A. Clarity of Solution

(Ph. Eur. method 2.2.1)

Into separate matched, flat-bottomed test tubes, 15 to 25 mm in internal diameter and of colourless, transparent, neutral glass, place sufficient of the solution being examined and of the appropriate reference suspension, freshly prepared as specified below, such that the test tubes are filled to a depth of 40 mm. Five minutes after preparation of the reference suspension, compare the contents of the test tubes against a black background by viewing in diffused daylight down the vertical axes of the tubes. The diffusion of the light must be such that *reference suspension I* can be readily distinguished from *water* and from *reference suspension II*.

Standard of opalescence Dissolve 1.0 g of *hydrazine sulphate* in sufficient *water* to produce 100.0 ml and allow to stand for 4 to 6 hours. Add 25.0 ml of this solution to a solution containing 2.5 g of *hexamine* in 25.0 ml of *water*, mix well and allow to stand for 24 hours. This suspension is stable for 2 months provided that it is stored in a glass container free from surface defects. The suspension must not adhere to the glass and must be well mixed before use.

To prepare the *standard of opalescence*, dilute 15.0 ml of the suspension to 1000.0 ml with *water*. This suspension must be used within 24 hours of preparation.

Reference suspensions Reference suspensions I to IV are prepared as indicated in Table I. Each suspension is to be mixed and shaken before use.

	I	II	III	IV
standard of opalescence (ml)	5.0	10.0	30.0	50.0
water (ml)	95.0	90.0	70.0	50.0

Expression of clarity and degree of opalescence

A liquid is considered *clear* if its clarity is the same as that of *water* or of the solvent used when examined under the conditions described above or if its opalescence is not more pronounced than that of *reference suspension I*.

Requirements for degree of opalescence are expressed in terms of *reference suspensions I, II, III* and *IV*.

B. Colour of Solution

(Ph. Eur. method 2.2.2)

The examination of the colour of solution in the range brown—yellow—red is carried out by one of the two following methods, as prescribed in the monograph. A solution is considered *colourless* if it has the appearance of *water* or the solvent or is not more intensely coloured than *reference solution* B_9.

Method I

Using identical tubes of colourless, transparent, neutral glass 12 mm in external diameter compare 2.0 ml of the liquid being examined with 2.0 ml of *water* or of the solvent or of the reference solution (Tables II A to II E) prescribed in the monograph. Compare the colours in diffused daylight, viewing horizontally against a white background.

Method II

Using identical tubes of colourless, transparent, neutral glass with a flat base and an internal diameter of 15 to 25 mm compare a 40-mm layer of the liquid being examined with a 40-mm layer of *water* or of the solvent or of the reference solution (Tables II A to II E) prescribed in the monograph. Examine the columns of liquid in diffused daylight by viewing down the vertical axes of the tubes against a white background.

Reagents

Yellow Primary Solution Dissolve 46 g of *iron(III) chloride* in about 900 ml of a mixture of 25 ml of *hydrochloric acid* and 975 ml of *water* and dilute to 1000 ml with the same mixture. Assay the solution and dilute it with the dilute hydrochloric acid mixture to contain 45 mg of $FeCl_3,6H_2O$ per ml. The solution should be protected from light.

ASSAY To 10 ml of the solution add 15 ml of *water*, 5 ml of *hydrochloric acid* and 4 g of *potassium iodide*, close the flask, allow to stand in the dark for 15 minutes and add 100 ml of *water*. Titrate the liberated iodine with 0.1M *sodium thiosulphate VS* using 0.5 ml of *starch solution*, added towards the end of the titration, as indicator. Each ml of 0.1M *sodium thiosulphate VS* is equivalent to 27.03 mg of $FeCl_3,6H_2O$.

Red Primary Solution Dissolve 60 g of *cobalt(II) chloride* in about 900 ml of a mixture of 25 ml of *hydrochloric acid* and 975 ml of *water* and dilute to 1000 ml with the same mixture. Assay the solution and dilute it with the dilute hydrochloric acid to contain 59.5 mg of $CoCl_2,6H_2O$ per ml.

ASSAY To 5 ml of the solution add 5 ml of *hydrogen peroxide solution (10 vol)* and 10 ml of a 30% w/v solution of *sodium hydroxide*. Boil gently for 10 minutes, allow to cool and add 60 ml of 1M *sulphuric acid* and 2 g of *potassium iodide*. Close the flask and dissolve the precipitate by shaking gently. Titrate the liberated iodine with 0.1M *sodium thiosulphate VS* using 0.5 ml of *starch solution*, added towards the end of the titration, as indicator. The end point is reached when the solution turns pink. Each ml of 0.1M *sodium thiosulphate VS* is equivalent to 23.79 mg of $CoCl_2,6H_2O$.

Blue Primary Solution Dissolve 63 g of *copper(II) sulphate* in about 900 ml of a mixture of 25 ml of *hydrochloric acid* and 975 ml of *water* and dilute to 1000 ml with the same mixture. Assay the solution and dilute it with the dilute hydrochloric acid to contain 62.4 mg of $CuSO_4,5H_2O$ per ml.

ASSAY To 10 ml of the solution add 50 ml of *water*, 12 ml of 2M *acetic acid* and 3 g of *potassium iodide*. Titrate the liberated iodine with 0.1M *sodium thiosulphate VS* using 0.5 ml of *starch solution*, added towards the end of the titration, as indicator. The end point is reached when the solution exhibits a slight pale brown colour. Each ml of 0.1M *sodium thiosulphate VS* is equivalent to 24.97 mg of $CuSO_4,5H_2O$.

Standard solutions

Using the three *primary solutions* prepare five *standard solutions* as indicated in Table 4B-1.

TABLE 4B-1

Standard solution	*Yellow primary solution* ml	*Red primary solution* ml	*Blue primary solution* ml	hydrochloric acid (1% w/v of HCl) ml
B (brown)	30	30	24	16
BY (brownish yellow)	24	10	4	62
Y (yellow)	24	6	0	70
GY (greenish yellow)	96	2	2	0
R (red)	10	20	0	70

Reference Solutions for Methods I and II

Using the five *standard solutions*, prepare the following *reference solutions.*

TABLE 4B-2 Reference solutions B

Reference solution	Standard solution B ml	Hydrochloric acid (1% w/v of HCl) ml
B_1	75.0	25.0
B_2	50.0	50.0
B_3	37.5	62.5
B_4	25.0	75.0
B_5	12.5	87.5
B_6	5.0	95.0
B_7	2.5	97.5
B_8	1.5	98.5
B_9	1.0	99.0

TABLE 4B-3Reference solutions BY

Reference solution	Standard solution BY ml	Hydrochloric acid (1% w/v of HCl) ml
BY_1	100.0	0.0
BY_2	75.0	25.0
BY_3	50.0	50.0
BY_4	25.0	75.0
BY_5	12.5	87.5
BY_6	5.0	95.0
BY_7	2.5	97.5

TABLE 4B-4 Reference solutions Y

Reference solution	Standard solution Y ml	Hydrochloric acid (1% w/v of HCl) ml
Y_1	100.0	0.0
Y_2	75.0	25.0
Y_3	50.0	50.0
Y_4	25.0	75.0
Y_5	12.5	87.5
Y_6	5.0	95.0
Y_7	2.5	97.5

TABLE 4B-5 Reference solutions GY

Reference solution	Standard solution GY ml	Hydrochloric acid (1% w/v of HCl) ml
GY_1	25.0	75.0
GY_2	15.0	85.0
GY_3	8.5	91.5
GY_4	5.0	95.0
GY_5	3.0	97.0
GY_6	1.5	98.5
GY_7	0.75	99.25

TABLE 4B-6 Reference solutions R

Reference solution	Standard solution R ml	Hydrochloric acid (1% w/v of HCl) ml
R_1	100.0	0.0
R_2	75.0	25.0
R_3	50.0	50.0
R_4	37.5	62.5
R_5	25.0	75.0
R_6	12.5	87.5
R_7	5.0	95.0

Storage

For Method I, the reference solutions may be stored in sealed tubes of colourless, transparent, neutral glass of 12 mm external diameter and protected from light.

For Method II, prepare the reference solutions immediately before use from the standard solutions.

Appendix V

A. Determination of Melting Point

For monographs from the European Pharmacopoeia, use the method indicated in the monograph. For other monographs, use Method II unless otherwise directed.

Method I *(Ph. Eur. method 2.2.14)*

The melting point determined by the capillary method is the temperature at which the last solid particle of a compact column of a substance in a tube passes into the liquid phase. When prescribed in the monograph, the same apparatus and method are used for the determination of other factors, such as meniscus formation or melting range, that characterise the melting behaviour of a substance.

Apparatus

(*a*) A suitable glass vessel containing a suitable liquid, for example water, liquid paraffin or silicone oil, and fitted with an appropriate means of heating.
(*b*) A suitable stirring device capable of maintaining the uniformity of temperature of the liquid.
(*c*) A thermometer suitable for the substance under examination, graduated at not more than 0.5° intervals and provided with an immersion mark. The range of the thermometer is not more than 100°.
(*d*) Capillary tubes of alkali-free hard glass, closed at one end, with a wall thickness of 0.10 to 0.15 mm and of internal diameter 0.9 to 1.1 mm.

The apparatus may be calibrated using certified reference substances of declared melting point, such as those of the World Health Organization or other suitable substances[1].

Method Unless otherwise specified, dry a small quantity of the finely powdered substance at a pressure of 1.5 to 2.5 kPa over *anhydrous silica gel* for 24 hours. Transfer a sufficient portion to a dry capillary tube to form a compact column 4 to 6 mm in height. Raise the temperature of the bath to about 10° below the presumed melting point and then adjust the rate of heating to about 1° per minute. When the temperature is 5° below the presumed melting point, adjust the height of the thermometer so that the immersion mark is level with the surface of the liquid and insert the capillary tube so that its lower end is near the middle of the thermometer bulb. The temperature at which the last solid particle passes into the liquid phase is the melting point of the substance.

Method II *(No Ph. Eur. equivalent method)*

Apparatus

(*a*) A glass heating vessel of suitable construction and capacity containing one of the following, or another suitable liquid, to a height of not less than 14 cm.
(i) A liquid paraffin of sufficiently high boiling point.
(ii) A silicone fluid of sufficiently high boiling point.
(iii) Water.
(*b*) A suitable stirring device capable of rapidly mixing the liquid.
(*c*) An accurately standardised thermometer suitable for the substance being examined complying with the requirements of British Standard 1365:1990 (Specification for short-range short-stem thermometers) for thermometers designated by one of the following Schedule Marks.

Schedule mark	Range °C	Graduated at each	Diameter of stem mm	Overall length mm
SA 55C/80	−10 to 55	0.5	5.5 to 8	200 max
SA 105C/80	45 to 105			
SA 155C/80	95 to 155			
SA 205C/80	145 to 205			
SA 225C/80	195 to 255			
SA 305C/80	245 to 305			
SA 360C/80	295 to 360			

(*d*) Thin-walled capillary glass tubes of hard glass, closed at one end, with a wall thickness of 0.10 to 0.15 mm, at least 12 cm in length and of internal diameter 0.9 to 1.1 mm. The tubes should preferably be kept sealed at both ends and cut as required.

Method Dry a small quantity of the finely powdered substance at a temperature considerably below its melting point or at a pressure of 2 kPa over a suitable desiccant, unless otherwise directed. Transfer a portion to a dry capillary tube and pack the powder by tapping on a hard surface so as to form a tightly packed column 4 to 6 mm in height. Heat a suitable liquid in the heating vessel and regulate the rate of rise of temperature, prior to the introduction of the capillary tube, to 3° per minute, unless otherwise directed, stirring constantly. When the temperature reaches 10° below the lowest figure of the range for the substance being tested, adjust the height of the thermometer so that the immersion mark is at the level of the surface of the liquid and insert the capillary tube so that the closed end is near the middle of the bulb of the thermometer. Note the temperature at which the liquefaction of the substance occurs, which is indicated by the formation of a definite meniscus or, for substances that decompose, the temperature at which frothing begins. Correct the observed temperature for any error in the calibration of the thermometer and for the difference, if any, between the temperature of the emergent stem of the thermometer and the temperature of the emergent stem under the conditions of standardisation of the thermometer. The temperature of the emergent stem is determined by placing the bulb of a second thermometer in contact with the emergent stem at a point approximately midway along the mercury thread in the emergent stem.

The correction to be applied is given by the following equation

$$t_c = 0.00016n(t_s - t_d)$$

where t_c = correction to be added to the observed temperature of the melting point,

t_s = mean temperature of the emergent column when standardised,

t_d = mean temperature of the emergent column at the observed melting point,

n = number of °C over which the exposed column extends.

The corrected temperature is regarded as the melting point of the substance. When the melting point in the monograph is expressed as a range, the melting point of the substance being tested must fall within that range.

Method III *(Ph. Eur. method 2.2.17)*

The drop point is the temperature at which the first drop of the melting substance falls from a cup under defined conditions.

Apparatus The apparatus (Fig. 5A-1) consists of the following parts.

A metal sheath (A) fixed to a mercury thermometer and screwed to another metal sheath (B). A metal cup (F) is loosely fixed to the lower part of sheath (B) by two tightening bands (E). The exact position of the cup is determined by two fixed supports (D), 2 mm long, which are also used to centre the thermometer. A hole (C) pierced in the wall of sheath (B) is used to balance the pressure. The draining surface of the cup must be flat and the edges of the outflow orifice at right angles to it. The mercury thermometer is of the form shown in Fig. xx with a mercury reservoir 3.3 to 3.7 mm in diameter and 5.7 to 6.3 mm long; it is calibrated from 0° to 110° and on its scale a distance of 1 mm represents a difference of 1°. The apparatus is placed in the axis of a tube (about 20 cm × 4 cm) and fixed by means of a stopper through which the thermometer passes and which is provided with a side groove. The opening of the cup should be about 15 mm from the bottom of the tube. The tube is immersed in a 1-litre beaker filled with water so that the bottom of the tube is about 25 mm above the bottom of the beaker and the water level reaches the upper part of sheath (A). A stirrer is used to ensure that the temperature of the water remains uniform.

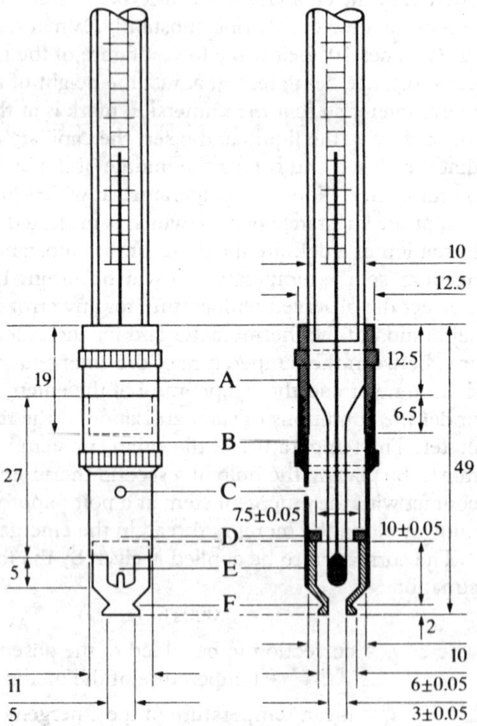

Fig. 5A-1

Apparatus for the determination of melting point (Method III)

Dimensions in mm

Method Unless otherwise specified, fill the cup to the brim with the substance being examined without melting it and remove excess at the top and bottom with a spatula. Press the cup into its housing in sheath (B) until it touches the supports and remove with a spatula material displaced by the thermometer. Heat the water bath. When the temperature is about 10° below the presumed melting or drop point adjust the heating rate to about 1° per minute and record the temperature at the fall of the first drop. Carry out at least three determinations, each time with a fresh sample of the substance being examined. The difference between the readings must not exceed 3°. The mean of the three determinations is taken as the melting or drop point.

Method IV *(Ph. Eur. method 2.2.15)*

For certain substances, the point of liquefaction, commonly called the melting point, is determined by the following method.

Apparatus Use the apparatus described under Method I using glass capillary tubes open at both ends and of internal diameter 1.0 to 1.2 mm, of external diameter 1.4 to 1.5 mm and about 8 cm long.

Method Introduce into each of five capillary tubes a sufficient amount of the substance treated as described in the monograph to form a column about 1 cm high. Allow the tubes to stand at the specified temperature for the appropriate time. Attach the tube to the thermometer, graduated in 0.2° increments, so that the column of the substance is level with the mercury bulb. Suspend the thermometer in the heating vessel containing water to a depth of 5 cm and at a temperature at least 5° below the expected melting point, so that the lower end of the capillary tube is 1 cm above the bottom of the beaker. Heat the water so that the temperature rises at the rate of 1° per minute, stirring continuously. The temperature at which the substance begins to rise in the tube is regarded as the melting point. Repeat the operation with the other four capillary tubes and determine the mean of the five readings.

Method V *(Ph. Eur method 2.2.16)*

The instantaneous melting point is calculated using the expression $(t_1 + t_2)/2$, in which t_1 is the first temperature and t_2 the second temperature read under the conditions stated below.

Apparatus A block of suitable metal (such as brass) not susceptible to corrosion by the substance being examined and of good heat-conducting capacity with a carefully polished plane upper surface. The block is heated uniformly throughout its mass by means of an adjustable gas microburner or an electric heating device with fine adjustment. The block has a cylindrical cavity parallel to and about 3 mm below its upper polished surface, of suitable dimensions to accommodate the thermometer, such that the mercury column is in the same position during calibration of the apparatus and the determination. The apparatus is calibrated using suitable substances of declared melting point as described in Method I.

Method Heat the block at a suitably rapid rate to a temperature about 10° below the presumed melting point and then adjust the rate of rise of temperature to about 1° per minute. At regular intervals, drop a few particles of the powdered substance, previously dried at a pressure of 1.5 to 2.5 kPa over *anhydrous silica gel* for 24 hours if appropriate, on to the block in the vicinity of the thermometer bulb, cleaning the surface after each test. Record the temperature (t_1) at which the substance melts instantaneously for the first time as soon as it touches the metal and stop the heating at that moment. During cooling drop a few particles of the substance at regular intervals on to the block, cleaning the surface after each test. Record the temperature (t_2) at which the substance ceases to melt instantaneously on contact with the block.

[1]In the United Kingdom certified melting point reference materials may be obtained from the National Physical Laboratory, Teddington TW11 0LW.

B. Determination of Freezing Point

(Ph. Eur. method 2.2.18)

The freezing point is the maximum temperature occurring during the solidification of a supercooled liquid.

Apparatus A test tube about 150 mm × 25 mm placed inside a test tube about 160 mm × 40 mm; the inner tube is closed by a stopper which carries a stirrer and a thermometer (about 175 mm long and with 0.2° graduations) fixed so that the bulb is about 15 mm above the bottom of the tube (Fig. 5B-1). The stirrer is made from a glass rod or other suitable material formed at one end into a loop of about 18 mm overall diameter at right angles to the rod. The inner tube with its jacket is supported centrally in a litre beaker containing a suitable cooling liquid to within 20 mm of the top. A thermometer is supported in the cooling bath.

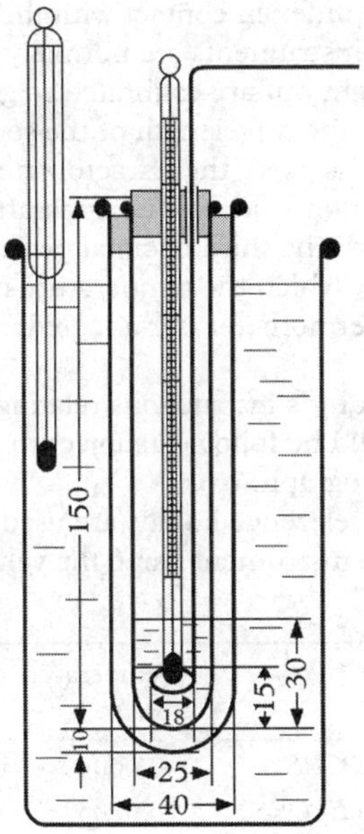

Fig. 5B-1

Apparatus for Determination of Freezing Point

Dimensions in mm

Method Place a quantity of the substance, previously melted if necessary, in the inner tube such that the thermometer bulb is well-covered and determine the approximate freezing point by cooling rapidly. Place the inner tube in a bath about 5° above the approximate freezing point until all but the last traces of crystals are melted.

Fill the beaker with water or a saturated solution of sodium chloride at a temperature about 5° lower than the approximate freezing point, insert the inner tube into the outer tube, ensuring that some seed crystals are present, and stir thoroughly until solidification takes place. The highest temperature observed during solidification of the substance is regarded as the freezing point of the substance.

C. Determination of Distillation Range

(Ph. Eur. method 2.2.11)

The distillation range of a liquid is the temperature interval, corrected to a pressure of 101.3 kPa, within which the liquid, or a specified fraction of the liquid, distils under the following conditions.

Apparatus A distillation flask with a straight tube condenser fitted to its side arm and an adaptor attached to the end of the condenser, the dimensions of which are shown in Fig. 5C-1. Alternatively the lower end of the condenser may be bent to provide a corresponding end piece. During the determination the flask, including its neck, is protected from draught by a suitable screen. A thermometer, which has a scale covering about 50° graduated in 0.2° increments, is inserted in the neck of the flask so that the upper end of the mercury reservoir is 5 mm below the lower wall of the side arm. The distillate is collected in a 50-ml cylinder graduated in 1-ml increments. For liquids distilling below 150° the condenser must be cooled by water circulation.

Method Place in the flask 50 ml of the liquid being examined, add a few pieces of porous material and heat rapidly to boiling. Record the temperature at which the first drop of distillate falls into the cylinder and adjust the rate of heating to obtain a regular distillation rate of 2 to 3 ml per minute. Record the temperature at which the prescribed fraction of the liquid, measured at 20° has distilled. Correct the temperature reading for barometric pressure using the following expression

$$t_1 = t_2 + K(101.3 - b)$$

where t_1 = the corrected temperature,

t_2 = the measured temperature,

b = the barometric pressure in kPa at the time of the determination,

K = the correction factor indicated in Table 5C-1, unless otherwise specified in the monograph.

TABLE 5C-1 Variation of correction factor with temperature

Boiling point °C	K
<100	0.30
100 to 140	0.34
140 to 190	0.38
190 to 240	0.41
>240	0.45

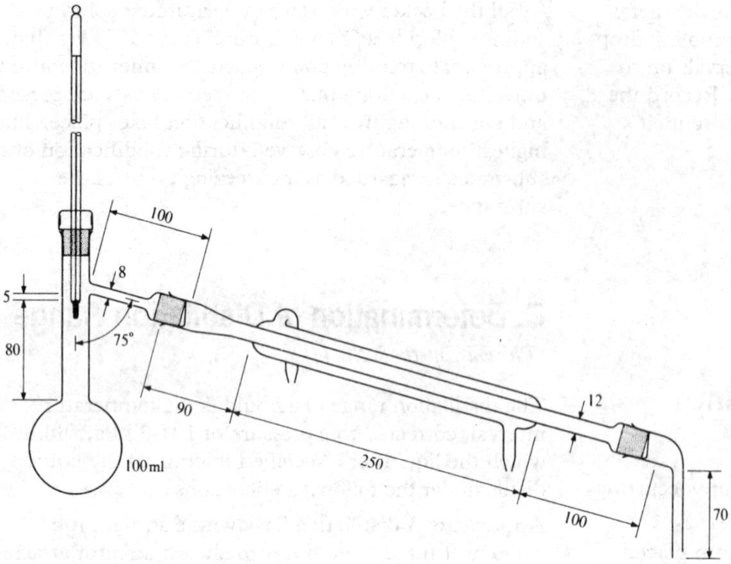

Fig. 5C-1
Apparatus for Determination of Distillation Range
Dimensions in mm

D. Determination of Boiling Point

(Ph. Eur. method 2.2.12)

The boiling point of a liquid is the corrected temperature at which the vapour pressure of the liquid reaches 101.3 kPa.

Apparatus The apparatus and its dimensions are shown in Fig. 5C-1 in Appendix V C, except that the thermometer is inserted in the neck of the flask so that the lower end of the mercury reservoir is level with the lower end of the neck of the flask and the flask is placed on a sheet of insulating material pierced by a hole 35 mm in diameter.

Method Place in the flask 20 ml of the liquid being examined, add a few pieces of porous material and heat rapidly to boiling. Record the temperature at which liquid begins to run from the side arm into the condenser.

Correct the temperature reading for the effect of barometric pressure using the following expression:

$$t_1 = t_2 + K(101.3 - b)$$

where t_1 = the corrected temperature,
t_2 = the measured temperature,
b = the barometric pressure in kPa at the time of the determination,
K = the correction factor, indicated in Table I under Determination of Distillation Range, Appendix V C.

E. Determination of Refractive Index

(Ph. Eur. method 2.2.6)

The *refractive index* (n) of a substance with reference to air is the ratio of the sine of the angle of incidence to the sine of the angle of refraction of a beam of light passing from air into the substance. It varies with the wavelength of the light used in its measurement.

Refractive indices, n_D^{20}, are stated in terms of the wavelength of the sodium D-line (589.3 nm) at a temperature of 19.5° to 20.5° unless otherwise specified.

Apparatus

Commercial refractometers normally determine the critical angle. In such apparatus the essential part is a prism of known refractive index in contact with the liquid being examined. Such instruments are normally constructed for use with white light but are calibrated to give the refractive index in terms of the wavelength of the sodium D-line. When white light is used, the refractometer is provided with a compensation system. The apparatus gives readings accurate to at least the third decimal place and is provided with a method by which the temperature may be varied, if required. The thermometer is graduated in increments of 0.5° or less.

The manufacturer's instructions relating to a suitable light source should be followed subject to the directions given in the monograph.

The following reference liquids are used to verify the calibration of the instrument using the value of n_D^{20} stated on the label.

Reference liquid	Temperature coefficient $\Delta n/\Delta t$
Trimethylpentane EPCRS	–0.00049
Carbon tetrachloride EPCRS	–0.00057
Toluene EPCRS	–0.00056
Methylnaphthalene EPCRS	–0.00048

F. Determination of Optical Rotation and Specific Optical Rotation

(Ph. Eur. method 2.2.7)

The *optical rotation* of a substance is the angle through which the plane of polarisation is rotated when polarised light passes through the substance, if liquid, or a solution of the substance, if solid. Substances are described as dextrorotatory or laevorotatory according to whether the plane of polarisation is rotated clockwise or anticlockwise, respectively, as determined by viewing towards the light source. Dextrorotation is designated (+) and laevorotation is designated (–).

The *optical rotation*, α, unless otherwise specified, is measured at the wavelength of the sodium D-line (589.3 nm) at a temperature of 20° in a layer 1 dm thick.

The *specific optical rotation*, $[\alpha]_D^{20}$, of a liquid is determined by measuring the angle of rotation at the wavelength of the sodium D-line at a temperature of 20°, unless otherwise specified, calculating the optical rotation with reference to a layer 1 dm thick and dividing by the *relative density* at 20°, Appendix V G.

The *specific optical rotation* of a solid substance is determined, using the solution specified in the monograph, by measuring the angle of rotation at the wavelength of the sodium D-line at a temperature of 20°, unless otherwise specified, and calculating the result with reference to a layer 1 dm thick of a solution containing 1 g of the substance per ml. The *specific optical rotation* of a solid is always expressed with reference to a given solvent and concentration.

In the conventional system adopted by the Pharmacopoeia the specific optical rotation is expressed in degree millilitres per decimetre gram.

Polarimeters

Commercial instruments are normally constructed for use with a sodium or mercury vapour lamp. For certain applications the use of a photoelectric polarimeter capable of making measurements at specified wavelengths may be necessary. The polarimeter must be capable of giving readings to the nearest 0.01°. The scale is usually checked by means of certified quartz plates. The linearity of the scale may be checked using solutions of sucrose.

Method

Determine the angle of rotation of the substance being examined at 19.5° to 20.5°, unless otherwise specified, using the D-line of polarised sodium light. Measurements may be carried out at other temperatures only where the monograph indicates the temperature correction to be made to the measured optical rotation. Carry out at least five measurements and determine the mean value. Determine the zero point of the polarimeter with the tube empty and closed for liquid substances and filled with the specified solvent for solutions of solid substances.

Calculate the *specific optical rotation* using the expression

$$\text{For liquids, } [\alpha]_D^{20} = \alpha/ld,$$

$$\text{For solids, } [\alpha]_D^{20} = 100\alpha/lc,$$

Calculate the content in g/l or in % w/w of a dissolved substance using the following formulae:

$$\text{concentration (g/l)} = 1000\alpha/l[\alpha]_D^{20}$$

$$\text{concentration (\% w/w)} = 100\alpha/ld[\alpha]_D^{20}$$

where l = the length in dm of the polarimeter tube,

d = the relative density of the substance,

c = the concentration of the substance expressed as a percentage w/w.

G. Determination of Weight per Millilitre, Density, Relative Density and Apparent Density

Weight per Millilitre

(No Ph. Eur. equivalent method)

The *weight per millilitre* of a liquid is the weight in g of 1 ml of a liquid when weighed in air at 20°, unless otherwise specified in the monograph.

The *weight per millilitre* is determined by dividing the weight in air, expressed in g, of the quantity of liquid that fills a pycnometer at the specified temperature by the capacity, expressed in ml, of the pycnometer at the same temperature. The capacity of the pycnometer is ascertained from the weight in air, expressed in g, of the quantity of *water* required to fill the pycnometer at that temperature. The weight of a litre of *water* at specified temperatures when weighed against brass weights in air of density 0.0012 g per ml is given in the following table. Ordinary deviations in the density of air from the above value, here taken as the mean, do not affect the result of a determination in the significant figures prescribed for Pharmacopoeial substances.

Temperature °C	Weight of a litre of water g
20	997.18
25	996.02
30	994.62

Density

(No Ph. Eur. equivalent method)

The *density*, ρ_{20}, of a substance is the ratio of its mass to its volume at 20°. It is expressed in kg m^{-3}.

The *density* is determined by dividing the weight in air of the quantity of the liquid being examined that fills a pycnometer at 20° by the weight in air of *water* required to fill the pycnometer after making allowance for the thrust of the air.

The *density* is calculated from the expression

$$\rho_{20} = \frac{998.2(M_1 + A)}{M_2 + A}$$

where M_1 = weight in air (apparent mass) in grams of the substance being examined,

M_2 = weight in air (apparent mass) in grams of *water*,

A = the correction factor for the thrust of the air, $0.0012M_2$,

998.2 = the density of water at 20° in kg m^{-3}.

In most cases, the correction for the thrust of the air may be disregarded.

Relative Density

(Ph. Eur. method 2.2.5)

The *relative density*, d_{20}^{20}, of a substance is the ratio of the mass of a given volume of the substance to the mass of an equal volume of *water*, both weighed at 20°.

The *relative density* is determined, with the precision indicated in the monograph, using a pycnometer, a density bottle, a hydrostatic balance or a hydrometer, as appropriate. The thrust of air is disregarded during the weighing; this may introduce an error of one unit in the third decimal place.

One other definition is commonly used.

The *relative density*, d_{4}^{20}, of a substance is the ratio of the mass of a given volume of the substance at 20° to the mass of an equal volume of *water*, weighed at 4°.

The numerical relationships between the relative density and the density expressed in kg m^{-3} are:

$$\rho_{20} = 998.202 d_{20}^{20} \text{ or } d_{20}^{20} = 1.00180 \times 10^{-3} \rho_{20}$$

$$\rho_{20} = 999.972 d_{4}^{20} \text{ or } d_{4}^{20} = 1.00003 \times 10^{-3} \rho_{20}$$

$$d_{4}^{20} = 0.998230 d_{20}^{20}$$

Apparent Density

(No Ph. Eur. equivalent method)

The term 'Apparent density' is used in the monographs for Ethanol, Ethanol (96 per cent), Dilute Ethanols, Industrial Methylated Spirit and Industrial Methylated Spirit (Ketone-free). It is defined as weight in air per unit volume and expressed in kg m^{-3}. It is named 'density' in the *Laboratory Alcohol Table for Laboratory Use* (HM Customs and Excise 1979).

The *apparent density* is calculated from the following expression

$$\textit{apparent density} = 997.2 \times d_{20}^{20}$$

where d_{20}^{20} is the *relative density* of the substance being examined and 997.2 is the weight in air in kg of a cubic metre of water.

H. Determination of Viscosity

(Ph. Eur. general text 2.2.8)

The dynamic viscosity or viscosity coefficient, η, is the tangential force per unit surface, known as shearing stress, τ, and expressed in pascals, necessary to move, parallel to the sliding plane, a layer of liquid of 1 square metre at a rate (v) of 1 metre per second relative to a parallel layer at a distance (x) of 1 metre.

The ratio dv/dx is a speed gradient giving the rate of shear D expressed in reciprocal seconds (s^{-1}), so that $\eta = \tau/D$. The unit of dynamic viscosity is the pascal second (Pa s). The most commonly used submultiple is the millipascal second (mPa s).

The kinematic viscosity, v, expressed in square metres per second, is obtained by dividing the dynamic viscosity, η, by the density, ρ, expressed in kilograms per cubic metre, of the liquid measured at the same temperature, that is, $v = \eta/\rho$. The kinematic viscosity is usually expressed in square millimetres per second.

A capillary viscometer may be used for determining the viscosity of Newtonian liquids and a rotating viscometer for determining the viscosity of Newtonian and non-Newtonian liquids. Other viscometers may be used provided that the accuracy and precision is not less than that obtained with the viscometers described below.

The apparatus and methods described in Methods I and II are in agreement in all essentials with International Standards ISO 3104-1976 and 3105-1976 (Methods for the determination of the viscosity of liquids).

Method I *(No Ph. Eur equivalent method)*

Apparatus The apparatus consists of a glass U-tube viscometer (Fig.5H-1) made of clear borosilicate glass and constructed in accordance with the dimensions shown in the figure and in Table I. The monograph states the size of viscometer to be used.

Method Fill the viscometer with the liquid being examined through tube L to slightly above the mark G, using a long pipette to minimise wetting the tube above the mark. Place the tube vertically in a water bath and when it has attained the specified temperature, adjust the volume of the liquid so that the bottom of the meniscus settles at the mark G. Suck or blow the liquid to a point about 5 mm above the mark E. After releasing pressure or suction, measure the time taken for the bottom of the meniscus to fall from the top edge of mark E to the top edge of mark F.

Calculate, as required, either the *kinematic viscosity* (v) in square millimetres per second (mm^2 s^{-1}) from the expression

$$v = Kt,$$

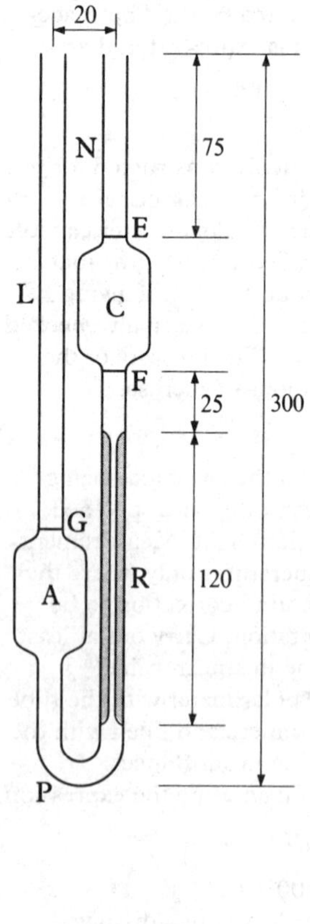

Fig. 5H-1
U-Tube Viscometer

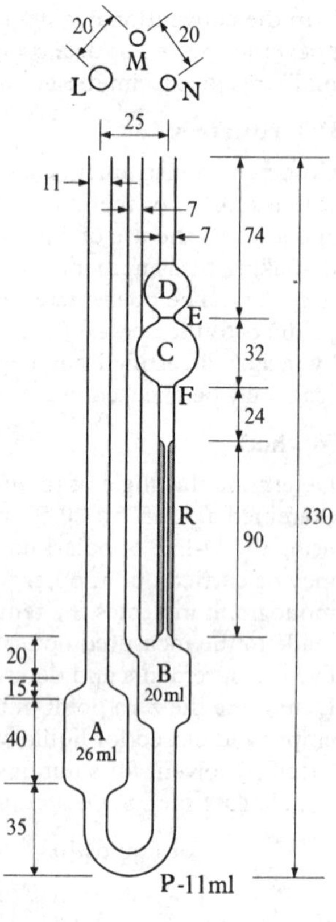

Fig. 5H-2
Suspended-level Viscometer

Dimensions in mm unless otherwise stated; tolerances are ±10% or ±10 mm, whichever is the less.

or the *dynamic viscosity* (η) in millipascal seconds (mPa s) from the expression

$$\eta = K\rho t,$$

where t = time in seconds for the meniscus to fall from E to F,

ρ = mass/volume (g cm^{-3}) obtained by multiplying the *relative density*, Appendix V G, of the fluid being examined by 0.9982.

The constant (K) of the instrument is determined using the appropriate European Pharmacopoeia reference liquid for viscometers.

Method II *(Ph. Eur. method 2.2.9)*

Apparatus The apparatus consists of a glass suspended-level viscometer (Fig. 5H-2) made of clear borosilicate glass and constructed in accordance with the dimensions shown in Table 5H-2.

Method Fill the viscometer through tube L with a sufficient quantity of the liquid being examined at 20° to fill bulb A but ensuring that the level of liquid in bulb B is below the exit to ventilation tube M. After the tube has been placed vertically in a water bath at 19.9° to 20.1° unless otherwise specified, allow it to stand for not less than 30 minutes. Close tube M and apply suction to tube N until the liquid reaches a level about 8 mm above mark E. Hold the liquid at this level by closing tube N and open tube M. When the liquid is clear of the capillary end of tube N and the lower end of tube M, open tube N. Measure the time taken, to the nearest 0.2 of a second, for the bottom of the meniscus to fall from the top edge of mark E to the top edge of mark F.

The result is not valid unless two consecutive readings do not differ by more than 1%. The average of not fewer than three readings gives the flow time of the liquid being examined.

Calculate the *kinematic viscosity* (ν) in square millimetres per second ($mm^2\ s^{-1}$) from the expression

$$\nu = Kt,$$

where t = time in seconds for the meniscus to fall from E to F.

Calculate the *dynamic viscosity* (η) in millipascal seconds (mPa s) from the expression

$$\eta = K\rho t,$$

where t = time in seconds for the meniscus to fall from E to F,

ρ = mass/volume (g cm^{-3}) obtained by multiplying the relative density, d_{20}^{20}, of the fluid being examined by 0.9982.

The constant (K) of the instrument is determined using the appropriate European Pharmacopoeia reference liquid for viscometers.

Method III *(Ph. Eur. method 2.2.10)*

Commonly used types of rotating viscometers are based on the measurement of shearing forces in a liquid medium placed between two coaxial cylinders, one of which is driven by a motor and the other is made to revolve by the rotation of the first. Under these conditions, the viscosity (or apparent viscosity) becomes a measurement (*M*) of the angle of deflection of the cylinder made to revolve, which corresponds to a moment of force expressed in Newton metres. For laminar flow, the *dynamic viscosity*, h, expressed in pascal seconds is given by the formula:

$$\eta = \frac{1}{\omega}\left(\frac{M}{4\pi h}\right)\left(\frac{1}{R_A^2} - \frac{1}{R_B^2}\right)$$

where h = the height of immersion in metres of the cylinder made to revolve in the liquid medium,

R_A and R_B = the radii in metres of the cylinders, R_A being smaller than R_B, and

ω = the angular velocity in radians per second.

The constant k of the apparatus may be determined at various speeds of rotation using a Pharmacopoeia viscometer calibration liquid. Commercially available apparatus is supplied with tables giving the constants of the apparatus in relation to the surface area of the cylinders used and their speed of rotation. The viscosity then corresponds to the formula:

$$\eta = k(M/\omega)$$

TABLE 5H-1U-Tube Viscometer – Dimensions

Size	Nominal viscometer constant	Kinematic viscosity range	Inside diameter of tube R	Outside diameter of tubes		Volume of bulb C	Vertical distance F to G	Outside diameter of bulbs A and C
				L and P	N			
	mm^2s^{-2}	mm^2s^{-1}	mm(±2%)	mm	mm	mm(±5%)	mm	mm
A	0.003	0.9 to 3	0.50	8 to 9	6 to 7	5.0	91±4	21 to 23
B	0.01	2.0 to 10	0.71	8 to 9	6 to 7	5.0	87±4	21 to 23
C	0.03	6 to 30	0.88	8 to 9	6 to 7	5.0	83±4	21 to 23
D	0.1	20 to 100	1.40	9 to 10	7 to 8	10.0	78±4	25 to 27
E	0.3	60 to 300	2.00	9 to 10	7 to 8	10.0	73±4	25 to 27
F	1.0	200 to 1000	2.50	9 to 10	7 to 8	10.0	70±4	25 to 27
G	3.0	600 to 3000	4.00	10 to 11	9 to 10	20.0	60±3	32 to 35
H	10.0	2000 to 10,000	6.10	10 to 11	9 to 10	20.0	50±3	32 to 35

[1]Use 1 to 1.25 mm wall tubing for L, N and P.

[2]300 s minimum flow time; 200 s minimum flow time for all other sizes.

TABLE 5H-2 Suspended-level Viscometer – Dimensions

Size No.	Nominal viscometer constant	Kinematic viscometer range	Inside diameter of tube R	Volume of bulb C	Inside diameter of tube N
	mm^2s^{-2}	mm^2s^{-1}	mm(±2%)	ml (±5%)	mm
1[1]	0.01	3.5 to 10	0.64	5.6	2.8 to 3.2
1A	0.03	6 to 30	0.84	5.6	2.8 to 3.2
2	0.1	20 to 100	1.15	5.6	2.8 to 3.2
2A	0.3	60 to 300	1.51	5.6	2.8 to 3.2
3	1.0	200 to 1100	2.06	5.6	3.7 to 4.3
3A	3.0	600 to 3000	2.74	5.6	4.6 to 5.4
4	10	2000 to 10,000	3.70	5.6	4.6 to 5.4
4A	30	6000 to 30,000	4.97	5.6	5.6 to 6.4
5	100	20,000 to 100,000	6.76	5.6	6.8 to 7.5

[1]Use 1 to 1.25 mm-wall tubing for L, N and P

[2]300 s minimum flow time; 200 s minimum for all other sizes

Method

Measure the viscosity according to the instructions for the operation of the rotating viscometer. The temperature for measuring the viscosity is indicated in the monograph. For pseudoplastic and other non-Newtonian systems, the monograph indicates the type of viscometer to be used and the angular velocity or the shear rate at which the measurement is made. If it is impossible to obtain the indicated shear rate exactly, use a shear rate slightly higher and a shear rate slightly lower and interpolate.

J. Circular Dichroism

(Ph. Eur. method 2.2.41)

The difference in absorbance of optically active substances within an absorption band for left and right circularly polarised light is referred to as circular dichroism.

Direct measurement gives a mean algebraic value:

$$\Delta A = A_L - A_R$$

where ΔA = circular dichroic absorbance,

A_L = absorbance of left circularly polarised light,

A_R = absorbance of right circularly polarised light.

Circular dichroism is calculated using the equation:

$$\Delta\varepsilon = \varepsilon_L - \varepsilon_R = \frac{\Delta A}{c \times l}$$

where $\Delta\varepsilon$=molar circular dichroism or molar differential dichroic absorptivity expressed in litre.mole^{-1}cm^{-1},

ε_L=molar absorptivity (*2.2.25*) of left circularly polarised light,

ε_R=molar absorptivity of right circularly polarised light,

c=concentration of the test solution in mole.litre^{-1},

l=optical path of the cell in centimetres.

The following units may also be used to characterise circular dichroism:

Dissymmetry factor:

$$g = \frac{\Delta\varepsilon}{\varepsilon}$$

where ε =molar absorptivity (*2.2.25*).

Molar ellipticity:

Certain types of instruments display directly the value of ellipticity Θ, expressed in degrees. When such instruments are used, the molar ellipticity $[\Theta]$ may be calculated using the following equation:

$$[\Theta] = \frac{\Theta \times M}{c \times l \times 10}$$

where $[\Theta]$ = molar ellipticity, expressed in degrees.cm^2.decimole^{-1},

Θ = value of ellipticity given by the instrument,

M = relative molecular weight [mass] of the substance to be examined,

c = concentration of the solution to be examined in g/ml,

l = optical path of the cell in centimetres.

Molar ellipticity is also related to molar circular dichroism by the following equation:

$$[\Theta] = 2.303\Delta\varepsilon\frac{4500}{\pi} \approx 3300\Delta\varepsilon$$

Molar ellipticity is often used in the analysis of proteins and nucleic acids. In this case, molar concentration is expressed in terms of monomeric residue, calculated using the expression:

$$\frac{\text{molecular mass}}{\text{number of amino acids}}$$

The mean relative molecular weight [mass]of the monomeric residue is 100 to 120 (generally 115) for proteins and about 330 for nucleic acids (as the sodium salt).

Apparatus. The light source (S) is a xenon lamp; the light passes through a double monochromator (M) equipped with quartz prisms (P_1, P_2). The linear beam from the first

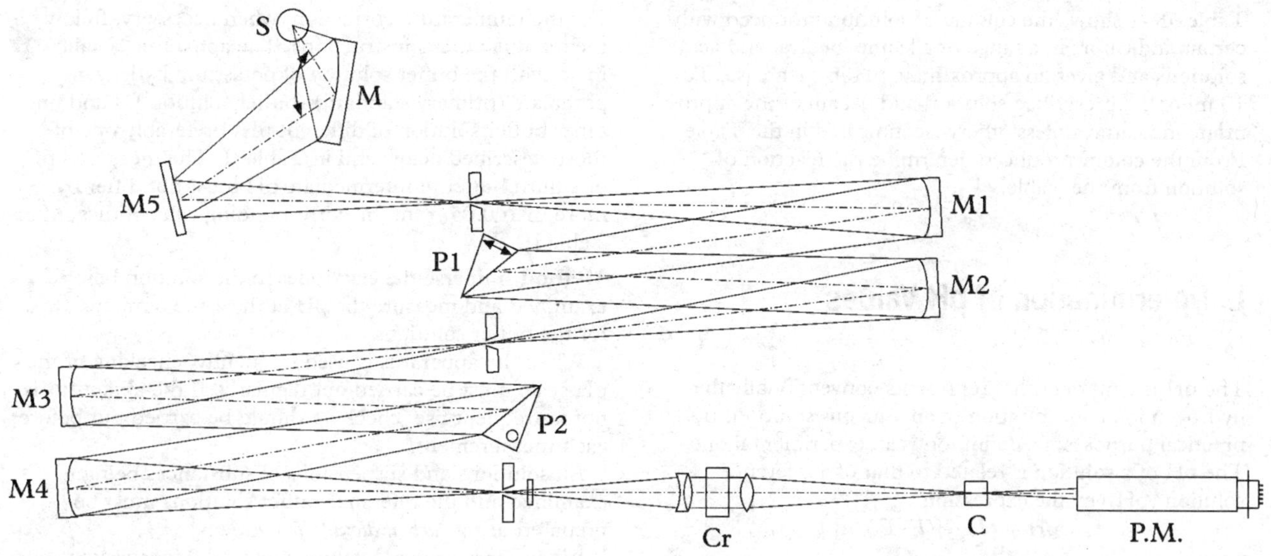

Fig. 5J-1 Optical scheme of a dichrograph

monochromator is split into two components polarised at right angles in the second monochromator. The exit slit of the monochromator eliminates the extraordinary beam. The polarised and monochromatic light passes through a birefringent modulator (Cr): the result is alternating circularly polarised light. The beam then passes through the sample to be examined (C) and reaches a photomultiplier (PM) followed by an amplifier circuit which produces two electrical signals: one is a direct current V_c and the other is an alternating current at the modulation frequency V_{ac} characteristic of the sample to be examined. The phase gives the sign of the circular dichroism. The ratio V_{ac}/V_c is proportional to the differential absorption ΔA which created the signal. The region of wavelengths normally covered by a dichrograph is 170 nm to 800 nm.

Calibration of the apparatus.

Accuracy of absorbance scale. Dissolve 10.0 mg of *isoandrosterone R* in *dioxan R* and dilute to 10.0 ml with the same solvent. Record the circular dichroism spectrum of the solution between 280 nm and 360 nm. Measured at the maximum at 304 nm, Δε is +3.3.

The solution of *(1S)-(+)-camphorsulphonic acid R* may also be used.

Linearity of modulation. Dissolve 10.0 mg of *(1S)-(+)-10-camphorsulphonic acid R* in *water R* and dilute to 10.0 ml with the same solvent. Determine the exact concentration of camphorsulphonic acid in the solution by ultraviolet spectrophotometry (*2.2.25*), taking the specific absorbance to be 1.49 at 285 nm. Record the circular dichroism spectrum between 185 nm and 340 nm. Measured at the maximum at 290.5 nm, Δε is +2.2 to +2.5. Measured at the maximum at 192.5 nm, Δε is −4.3 to −5.

(1S)-(+)- or antipodal *(1R)-(−)-ammonium 10-camphorsulphonate R* can also be used.

K. Relationship between reaction of solution and colour of certain indicators

(Ph. Eur. method 2.2.4)

TABLE 5K-1 Relationship between reaction of solution and colour of certain indicators

Reaction	Indicator	Colour	pH
Alkaline	Litmus paper Thymol blue	Blue Grey or violet-blue	>8
Slightly alkaline	Phenolphthalein[1] Thymol Blue	Colourless to pink Grey	8.0 to 10.0
Strongly alkaline	Phenolphthalein paper Thymol blue	Red Violet-blue	>10
Neutral	Methyl red Phenol red[1]	Yellow Yellow or pink	6.0 to 8.0
Neutral to tropaeolin OO	Tropaeolin OO	Yellow	>3.0
Neutral to dimethyl yellow	Dimethyl yellow[1]	Yellow; red after adding 0.1 ml of 0.1M acid	>4.0
Neutral to methyl red	Methyl red	Orange-red	4.5 to 6.0
Neutral to phenolphthalein	Phenolphthalein[1]	Colourless; pink or red after adding 0.05 ml of 0.1M alkali	<8.0
Acid	Methyl red Bromothymol blue[2]	Orange or red Yellow	<6.0
Faintly acid	Methyl red Bromocresol green	Orange Green or blue	4.0 to 6.0
Strongly acid	Congo red Dimethyl yellow[1]	Green or blue Orange or red	<4.0

[1]Use 0.05 ml

[2]Use bromothymol blue solution R1

Table 5K-1 shows the colours of solution produced with certain indicators in a range of alkaline, neutral and acid solutions and gives an approximate pH in each case. To 10 ml of the prescribed solution add 0.1 ml of the appropriate indicator, unless otherwise indicated in the Table. From the colour produced determine the reaction of solution from the Table.

L. Determination of pH Values

(Ph. Eur. method 2.2.3)

The pH is a number that represents conventionally the hydrogen ion concentration of an aqueous solution. For practical purposes, its definition is an experimental one. The pH of a solution is related to that of a reference solution (pH_s) by the expression

$$pH = pH_s - [(E - E_s)/k]$$

where E is the potential, in volts, of the cell containing the solution being examined, E_s is the potential, in volts, of the cell containing the solution of known pH and k varies with the temperature as shown in Table 5L-1.

TABLE 5L-1 Values of k at different temperatures

Temperature	k
15°	0.0572
20°	0.0582
25°	0.0592
30°	0.0601
35°	0.0611

Apparatus The pH value of a solution is determined potentiometrically by measuring the potential difference between an indicator electrode sensitive to hydrogen ions (usually a glass electrode) and a reference electrode, for example, a saturated calomel electrode. The measuring apparatus is a voltmeter with an input resistance at least 100 times that of the electrodes used. It is usually graduated in pH units and is sufficiently sensitive to detect changes of 0.05 pH unit or at least 0.003 V. [Suitable glass electrodes and pH meters of both the analogue and digital type are described in British Standards 2586:1979 and 3145:1978.]

Operate the pH meter and electrode system according to the manufacturer's instructions. All measurements should be made at the same temperature of 20° to 25° unless otherwise specified in the monograph. Table 2 shows the variation of pH with respect to temperature of a number of reference buffer solutions used for calibration.

For the temperature correction, when necessary, follow the manufacturer's instructions. The apparatus is calibrated with the buffer solution of potassium hydrogen phthalate (primary standard) (buffer solution D) and one other buffer solution of different pH, preferably one of those described below and in Table II. The measured pH of a third buffer of intermediate pH must not differ by more than 0.05 from the corresponding value indicated in Table II.

Method Immerse the electrodes in the solution being examined and measure the pH at the same temperature as for the buffer solutions.

When the apparatus is used frequently, checking of the pH scale must be carried out regularly. If the apparatus is not in frequent use, checking should be carried out before each measurement.

All solutions and suspensions of substances being examined and the reference buffer solutions must be prepared using *carbon dioxide-free water.*

When measuring pH values above 10.0, ensure that the glass electrode is suitable for use under alkaline conditions and apply any correction that is necessary.

For monographs other than those from the European Pharmacopoeia , record the pH of the solution used to standardise the meter and electrodes at the end of a set of measurements. If the difference between this reading and the original value is greater than 0.05, the set of measurements must be repeated.

Reference buffer solutions

Buffer Solution A Dissolve 12.61 g of *potassium tetraoxalate* in sufficient *water* to produce 1000 ml (0.05M).

Buffer Solution B Shake an excess of *potassium hydrogen (+)-tartrate* vigorously with *water* at 25° and filter or decant. Prepare immediately before use.

Buffer solution C Dissolve 11.41 g of *potassium dihydrogen citrate* in sufficient *water* to produce 1000 ml (0.05M). Prepare immediately before use.

Buffer solution D Dissolve 10.13 g of *potassium hydrogen phthalate*, previously dried at 110° to 135°, in sufficient *water* to produce 1000 ml (0.05M).

Buffer solution E Dissolve 3.39 g of *potassium dihydrogen orthophosphate* and 3.53 g of *anhydrous disodium hydrogen orthophosphate*, both previously dried at 110° to 130° for 2 hours, in sufficient *water* to produce 1000 ml (0.025M in each salt).

Buffer solution F Dissolve 1.18 g of *potassium dihydrogen orthophosphate* and 4.30 g of *anhydrous disodium hydrogen orthophosphate*, both previously dried at 110° to 130° for 2 hours, in sufficient *water* to produce 1000 ml (0.0087M and 0.0303M respectively).

TABLE 5L-2 pH of Reference Buffer Solutions at various temperatures

Temperature	Buffer Solutions							
t°	A	B	C	D	E	F	G	H
15	1.67	-	3.80	4.00	6.90	7.45	9.28	10.12
20	1.68	-	3.79	4.00	6.88	7.43	9.23	10.06
25	1.68	3.56	3.78	4.01	6.87	7.41	9.18	10.01
30	1.68	3.55	3.77	4.02	6.85	7.40	9.14	9.97
35	1.69	3.55	3.76	4.02	6.84	7.39	9.10	9.93
ΔpH/Δt	+0.001	−0.0014	−0.0022	+0.0012	−0.0028	−0.0028	−0.0082	−0.0096

ΔpH/Δt = pH variation per degree Celsius.

Buffer solution G Dissolve 3.80 g of *sodium tetraborate* in sufficient *water* to produce 1000 ml (0.01M).
Store protected from atmospheric carbon dioxide.

Buffer solution H Dissolve 2.64 g of *anhydrous sodium carbonate* and 2.09 g of *sodium hydrogen carbonate* in sufficient *water* to produce 1000 ml (0.025M in each salt).

M. Thermal Analysis

(Ph. Eur. method 2.2.34)

Thermal analysis is a group of techniques in which the variation of a physical property of a substance is measured as a function of temperature. The most commonly used techniques are those that measure changes of energy or changes in weight of the substance being examined.

Thermogravimetry

Definition Thermogravimetry is a technique in which the weight of a sample is recorded as a function of temperature according to a controlled temperature programme.

Apparatus A thermobalance consisting of a device for heating or cooling the substance being examined according to a given temperature programme, a sample holder in a controlled atmosphere, an electrobalance and a recorder. The instrument may be coupled to a device permitting the analysis of volatile products.

Temperature verification Check the temperature scale using nickel or other suitable material according to the manufacturer's instructions.

Calibration of the electrobalance Place a suitable quantity of *calcium oxalate monohydrate EPCRS* in the sample holder and record the weight. Set the heating rate according to the manufacturer's instructions and start the temperature programme. Record the thermogravimetric curve as a graph with temperature on the abscissa, increasing from left to right, and weight on the ordinate, increasing upwards. Stop the temperature increase at about 230°. Measure the distance on the graph between the initial and final weight—temperature plateaux that correspond to the loss of weight. The declared loss of weight for *calcium oxalate monohydrate EPCRS* is stated on the label.

Method Apply the same procedure to the substance being examined, using the conditions prescribed in the monograph. Calculate the loss of weight of the substance being examined from the distance measured on the graph obtained and express as a percentage w/w of the substance taken.

If the apparatus is in frequent use, carry out temperature verification and calibration regularly. Otherwise, carry out such checks before each measurement.

N. Osmolality

(Ph. Eur. method 2.2.35)

Osmolality is a practical means of giving an overall measure of the contribution of the various solutes present in a solution to the osmotic pressure of the solution.

An acceptable approximation for the osmolality ξ_m of a given aqueous solution is given by:

$$\xi_m = \nu m \Phi$$

where m = molality of the solution, that is the number of moles of solute per kilogram of solvent,

Φ = molal osmotic coefficient which takes account of the interactions between ions of opposite charge in the solution. It is dependent on the value of m. As the complexity of solutions increases, Φ becomes difficult to measure.

If the solute is not ionised ν is 1, otherwise ν is the total number of ions already present or formed by solvolysis from one molecule of solute.

The unit of osmolality is osmole per kilogram (osmol kg^{-1}), but the submultiple milliosmole per kilogram (mosmol kg^{-1}) is usually used.

Unless otherwise prescribed, osmolality is determined by measurement of the depression of freezing point. The following relationship exists between the osmolality and the depression of freezing point ΔT:

$$\xi_m = \frac{\Delta T}{1.86} \times 1000 \text{mosmol / kg}$$

Apparatus
The apparatus (osmometer) consists of:
(a) a means of cooling the container used for the measurement,
(b) a system for measuring temperature consisting of a resistor sensitive to a temperature (thermistor), with an appropriate current or potential difference measurement device that may be graduated in temperature depression or directly in osmolality,
(c) a means of mixing the sample is usually included.

Method
Prepare reference solutions as described in Table 5N-1, as required. Determine the zero of the apparatus using *distilled water*. Calibrate the apparatus using the reference solutions: introduce 50 to 250 µl of sample into the measurement cell and start the cooling system. Usually, the mixing device is programmed to operate at a temperature below that expected through cryoscopic depression to

TABLE 5N-1 Reference solution for osmometer calibration

Weight of *sodium chloride* per kg of water g	Real osmolality mosmol /kg	Ideal osmolality mosmol /kg	Molal osmotic coefficient Φ	Cryoscopic depression °C
3.087	100	105.67	0.9463	0.186
6.260	200	214.20	0.9337	0.372
9.463	300	323.83	0.9264	0.558
12.684	400	434.07	0.9215	0.744
19.147	600	655.24	0.9157	1.116
22.380	700	765.86	0.9140	1.302

prevent supercooling. A suitable device indicates attainment of equilibrium. Before each measurement, rinse the measurement cell with the solution being examined.

Carry out the same operations with the test sample. Read directly the osmolality or calculate it from the measured depression of freezing point. The test is not valid unless the value is within two values of the calibration scale.

O. Conductivity

(Ph. Eur. method 2.2.38)

The conductivity of a solution (κ) is, by definition, the reciprocal of resistivity (ρ). Resistivity is defined as the quotient of the electric field and the density of the current. The resistance R (Ω) of a conductor of cross-section S (cm^2) and length L (cm) is given by the expression:

$$R = \rho \frac{L}{S}$$

$$\text{thus: } R = \frac{1}{\kappa} \times \frac{L}{S} \text{ or } \kappa = \frac{1}{R} \times \frac{L}{S}$$

The unit of conductivity in the International System is the siemens per metre ($S\ m^{-1}$). In practice, the electrical conductivity of a solution is expressed in siemens per centimetre ($S\ cm^{-1}$) or in microsiemens per centimetre ($\mu S\ cm^{-1}$). The unit of resistivity in the International System is the ohm-metre (Ω m). The resistivity of a solution is generally expressed in ohm-centimetres (Ω cm). Unless otherwise prescribed, the reference temperature for the expression of conductivity or resistivity is 20°.

Apparatus The apparatus used (conductivity meter or resistivity meter) measures the resistance of the column of liquid between the electrodes of the immersed measuring device (conductivity cell). The apparatus is supplied with alternating current to avoid the effects of electrode polarisation. It is equipped with a temperature compensation device or a precision thermometer. The conductivity cell contains two parallel platinum electrodes coated with platinum black, each with a surface area S, and separated from the other by a distance L. Both are generally protected by a glass tube that allows good exchange between the solution and the electrodes.

The cell constant C of the conductivity cell is given in cm^{-1} according to the equation:

$$C = \alpha \frac{L}{S}$$

where α = a dimensionless numerical coefficient, which is characteristic of the cell design.

Reagents Prepare three standard solutions of *potassium chloride* containing 0.7455 g, 0.0746 g and 0.0149 g, respectively, of *potassium chloride* per 1000 g of solution, using *carbon dioxide-free water*, prepared from *distilled water* the conductivity of which does not exceed 2 $\mu S\ cm^{-1}$.

The conductivity and resistivity of these three solutions at 20° are given in the Table.

If the determination cannot be made at the temperature of 20°, use the following equation to correct the conductivity of the potassium chloride solutions indicated in the Table. This equation is valid only for temperatures in the range 15° to 25°.

$$C_T = C_{20^\circ}[1 + 0.021(T - 20)]$$

where T = measurement temperature prescribed in the monograph,

C_T = conductivity of KCl at T° and

C_{20° = conductivity of KCl at 20°.

Table 5O-1 Conductivity and resistivity of potassium chloride solutions

Concentration in g per 1000.0 g	Conductivity $\mu S\ cm^{-1}$	Resistivity Ω cm
0.7455	1330	752
0.0746	133.0	7519
0.0149	26.6	37594

Operating procedure

Determination of the cell constant Choose a conductivity cell that is appropriate for the conductivity of the solution being examined. The higher the expected conductivity, the higher the cell constant that should be chosen (low ρ) so that the value R measured is as large as possible for the apparatus used. Commonly used conductivity cells have cell constants of the order of 0.1 cm^{-1}, 1 cm^{-1} and 10 cm^{-1}. Use a standard solution of *potassium chloride* that is appropriate for the measurement. Rinse the cell several times with *carbon dioxide-free water* prepared from *distilled water* and at least twice with the potassium chloride solution used for the determination of the cell constant of the conductivity cell. Measure the resistance of the conductivity cell using the potassium chloride solution at 20° ± 0.1° or at the temperature prescribed in the monograph. The constant C (in cm^{-1}) of the conductivity cell is given by the expression:

$$C = R_{KCl} \times \kappa_{KCl}$$

where R_{KCl} = measured resistance, expressed in megaohms and

κ_{KCl} = conductivity of the standard solution of *potassium chloride* used, expressed in $\mu s\ cm^{-1}$.

The measured constant C of the conductivity cell must be within 5% of the given value.

Determination of the conductivity of the solution being examined After calibrating the apparatus with one of the standard solutions, rinse the conductivity cell several times with *carbon dioxide-free water* prepared from *distilled water* and at least twice with the aqueous solution being examined at 20° ± 0.1° or at the temperature prescribed in the monograph. Carry out successive measurements as described in the monograph.

Appendix VI

Qualitative Reactions and Tests

(*Ph. Eur. method 2.3.1*)

Acetates

A. Heat the substance being examined with an equal quantity of *oxalic acid*. Acidic vapours with the characteristic odour of acetic acid are evolved.

B. To about 30 mg of the substance being examined dissolved in 3 ml of *water* or to 3 ml of the prescribed solution add successively 0.25 ml of *lanthanum nitrate solution*, 0.1 ml of 0.05M *iodine* and 0.05 ml of 2M *ammonia* and heat the mixture carefully to boiling. After a few minutes a blue precipitate or a dark blue colour is produced.

Acetyl Groups

In a test tube (about 180 mm × 18 mm) place about 15 mg of the substance being examined or the prescribed quantity and 0.15 ml of *orthophosphoric acid*. Close the tube with a stopper through which passes a small test tube (about 100 mm × 10 mm) containing water to act as a condenser. Hang a drop of *lanthanum nitrate solution* on the outside of the smaller tube.

Except for substances hydrolysable only with difficulty, place the apparatus in a water bath for 5 minutes and remove the smaller tube. Mix the drop with 0.05 ml of 0.01M *iodine* on a tile and add, at the edge, 0.05 ml of 2M *ammonia*. After 1 or 2 minutes a blue colour is produced at the junction of the two drops which intensifies and persists for a short time.

For substances hydrolysable only with difficulty, proceed as described above but heat the mixture slowly to boiling point over an open flame instead of using a water bath.

Alkaloids

Dissolve a few mg or the prescribed quantity of the substance being examined in 5 ml of *water*, acidify with 2M *hydrochloric acid* and add 1 ml of *potassium iodobismuthate solution*. An orange or orange-red precipitate is produced immediately.

Aluminium Salts

For monographs from the European Pharmacopoeia, use test A only.

A. To about 15 mg of the substance being examined dissolved in 2 ml of *water* or to 2 ml of the prescribed solution add about 0.5 ml of 2M *hydrochloric acid* and about 0.5 ml of *thioacetamide reagent*; no precipitate is produced. Add 2M *sodium hydroxide* dropwise; a gelatinous white precipitate is produced which dissolves on further addition of 2M *sodium hydroxide*. Gradually add *ammonium chloride solution;* the gelatinous white precipitate reappears.

B. To a solution of the substance being examined add 5M *ammonia* until a faint precipitate is produced and then add 0.25 ml of a freshly prepared 0.05% w/v solution of *quinalizarin* in a 1.0% w/v solution of *sodium hydroxide*. Heat to boiling, cool and acidify with an excess of 5M *acetic acid*. A reddish violet colour is produced.

Amines, Primary Aromatic

Acidify the prescribed solution with 2M *hydrochloric acid* or dissolve 0.1 g in 2 ml of 2M *hydrochloric acid* and add 0.2 ml of *sodium nitrite solution*. After 1 to 2 minutes add the solution to 1 ml of *2-naphthol solution*. An intense orange or red colour and, usually, a precipitate of the same colour are produced.

Ammonium Salts

To the prescribed solution add 0.2 g of *magnesium oxide*. Pass a current of air through the mixture and direct the gas that escapes just beneath the surface of a mixture of 1 ml of 0.1M *hydrochloric acid* and 0.05 ml of *methyl red solution;* the colour of the solution changes to yellow. Add 1 ml of a freshly prepared 10% w/v solution of *sodium cobaltinitrite*; a yellow precipitate is produced.

Ammonium Salts and Salts of Volatile Bases

To about 20 mg of the substance being examined dissolved in 2 ml of *water* or to 2 ml of the prescribed solution add 2 ml of 2M *sodium hydroxide* and heat. A vapour is evolved which can be identified by its odour and which is *alkaline*, Appendix V K.

Antimony Compounds

Dissolve with gentle heating about 10 mg of the substance being examined in a solution of 0.5 g of *potassium sodium (+)-tartrate* in 10 ml of *water* and allow to cool. To 2 ml of this solution or to 2 ml of the prescribed solution add *sodium sulphide solution* dropwise. An orange-red precipitate is produced which dissolves on addition of 2M *sodium hydroxide*.

Arsenic Compounds

Heat 5 ml of the prescribed solution on a water bath with 5 ml of *hypophosphorous reagent*. A brown precipitate is produced.

Barbiturates, Non-nitrogen Substituted

Dissolve about 5 mg of the substance being examined in 3 ml of *methanol*, add 0.1 ml of a solution containing 10% w/v of *cobalt(II) nitrate* and 10% w/v of *calcium chloride*, mix and add, with shaking, 0.1 ml of 2M *sodium hydroxide*. A violet blue colour and precipitate are produced.

Benzoates

A. To 1 ml of a 10% w/v neutral solution of the substance being examined or to 1 ml of the prescribed solution add 0.5 ml of *iron(III) chloride solution R1*. A dull yellow precipitate is produced which is soluble in *ether*.

B. Moisten 0.2 g of the substance being examined, treated as prescribed if necessary, with 0.2 to 0.3 ml of *sulphuric acid* and gently warm the bottom of the tube. A white sublimate is deposited on the inner wall of the tube.

C. To 0.5 g of the substance being examined dissolved in 10 ml of *water* or to 10 ml of the prescribed solution add 0.5 ml of *hydrochloric acid*. The *melting point* of the precipitate, after recrystallisation from *water* and drying at a pressure of 2 kPa, is 120° to 124°, Appendix V A, Method I.

Bicarbonates

A. Introduce into a test tube 0.1 g of the substance being examined suspended in 2 ml of *water* or use 2 ml of the prescribed solution. Add 3 ml of 2M *acetic acid*, close the tube immediately using a stopper fitted with a glass tube bent at two right angles. The solution or suspension effervesces. Heat gently and collect the gas in 5 ml of a 4.73% w/v solution of *barium hydroxide*. A white precipitate is produced which dissolves on addition of an excess of 7M *hydrochloric acid*.

B. Treat a solution of the substance being examined with a solution of *magnesium sulphate*; no precipitate is produced (distinction from carbonates). Boil; a white precipitate is produced.

C. A solution liberates carbon dioxide when boiled.

Bismuth and Bismuth Compounds

A. To 0.5 g of the substance being examined add 10 ml of 2M *hydrochloric acid* or use 10 ml of the prescribed solution. Boil for 1 minute, cool, filter if necessary and to 1 ml of the resulting solution add 20 ml of *water*. A white or slightly yellow precipitate is produced which turns brown on addition of 0.05 to 0.1 ml of *sodium sulphide solution*.

B. To about 45 mg of the substance being examined add 10 ml of 2M *nitric acid* or use 10 ml of the prescribed solution. Boil for 1 minute, allow to cool, filter if necessary and to 5 ml of the resulting solution add 2 ml of a 10% w/v solution of *thiourea*; a yellowish orange colour or an orange precipitate is produced. Add 4 ml of a 2.5% w/v solution of *sodium fluoride*; the solution is not decolorised within 30 minutes.

Bromides

A. Dissolve a quantity of the substance being examined containing about 3 mg of bromide ion in 2 ml of *water* or use 2 ml of the prescribed solution. Acidify with 2M *nitric acid*, add 0.4 ml of *silver nitrate solution R1*, shake and allow to stand; a curdy, pale yellow precipitate is produced. Centrifuge and wash the precipitate with three 1-ml quantities of *water*. Carry out this operation rapidly in subdued light disregarding the fact that the supernatant solution may not become perfectly clear. Suspend the precipitate obtained in 2 ml of *water* and add 1.5 ml of 10M *ammonia*; the precipitate dissolves with difficulty.

B. Introduce into a small test tube a quantity of the substance being examined containing about 5 mg of bromide ion or the prescribed quantity, add 0.25 ml of *water*, about 75 mg of *lead(IV) oxide* and 0.25 ml of 5M *acetic acid* and shake gently. Dry the inside of the upper part of the test tube with filter paper and allow to stand for 5 minutes. Moisten a strip of suitable filter paper of appropriate size by dipping the tip in a drop of *decolorised fuchsin solution* and introduce the moistened part immediately into the tube. Starting from the tip, a violet colour is produced within 10 seconds which is clearly distinguishable from the red colour of fuchsin, which may be visible on a small area at the top of the moistened part of the paper strip.

Calcium and Calcium Salts

For monographs from the European Pharmacopoeia, use tests A and B only.

A. To 0.2 ml of a neutral solution containing about 0.2 mg of calcium ion per ml or to 0.2 ml of the prescribed solution add 0.5 ml of a 0.2% w/v solution of *glyoxal bis(2-hydroxyanil)* in *ethanol (96%)*, 0.2 ml of 2M *sodium hydroxide* and 0.2 ml of *sodium carbonate solution*. Extract with 1 to 2 ml of *chloroform* and add 1 to 2 ml of *water*. The chloroform layer is red.

B. Dissolve about 20 mg of the substance being examined or the prescribed quantity in 5 ml of 5M *acetic acid* and add 0.5 ml of *potassium hexacyanoferrate(II) solution*; the solution remains clear. Add about 50 mg of *ammonium chloride*; a white, crystalline precipitate is produced.

C. To 5 ml of 0.4% w/v solution of the substance being examined add 0.2 ml of a 2% w/v solution of *ammonium oxalate*. A white precipitate is produced which is only sparingly soluble in 6M *acetic acid* but is soluble in *hydrochloric acid*.

Carbonates

A. Introduce into a test tube 0.1 g of the substance being examined suspended in 2 ml of *water* or use 2 ml of the prescribed solution. Add 3 ml of 2M *acetic acid*, close the tube immediately using a stopper fitted with a glass tube bent at two right angles. The solution or suspension effervesces evolving a colourless and odourless gas. Heat gently and collect the gas in 5 ml of 0.1M *barium hydroxide*. A white precipitate is produced which dissolves on addition of an excess of 7M *hydrochloric acid*.

B. Treat a solution of the substance being examined with a solution of *magnesium sulphate*. A white precipitate is produced (distinction from bicarbonates).

Carbonates and Bicarbonates

Introduce into a test tube 0.1 g of the substance being examined suspended in 2 ml of *water* or use 2 ml of the prescribed solution. Add 3 ml of 2M *acetic acid*, close the tube immediately using a stopper fitted with a glass tube bent at two right angles. The solution or suspension effervesces evolving a colourless and odourless gas. Heat gently and collect the gas in 5 ml of 0.1M *barium hydroxide*. A white precipitate is produced which dissolves on addition of an excess of 7M *hydrochloric acid*.

Chlorides

A. Dissolve a quantity of the substance being examined containing about 2 mg of chloride ion in 2 ml of *water* or use 2 ml of the prescribed solution. Acidify with 2M *nitric acid*, add 0.4 ml of *silver nitrate solution R1*, shake and allow to stand; a curdy, white precipitate is produced. Centrifuge and wash the precipitate with three 1-ml quantities of *water*. Carry out this operation rapidly in subdued light, disregarding the fact that the supernatant solution may not become perfectly clear. Suspend the precipitate in 2 ml of *water* and add 1.5 ml of 10M *ammonia*; the precipitate dissolves easily with the possible exception of a few large particles which dissolve slowly.

B. Introduce into a test tube a quantity of the substance being examined containing about 15 mg of chloride ion or the prescribed quantity, add 0.2 g of *potassium dichromate* and 1 ml of *sulphuric acid* and place a filter paper strip moistened with 0.1 ml of *diphenylcarbazide solution* over the opening of the test tube. The paper turns violet-red. The moistened paper must not come into contact with the potassium dichromate solution.

Citrates

For monographs of the European Pharmacopoeia, use test A only.

A. To a quantity of the substance being examined corresponding to about 50 mg of citric acid dissolved in 5 ml of *water* or to 5 ml of the prescribed solution add 0.5 ml of *sulphuric acid* and 1 ml of *potassium permanganate solution* and warm until the colour of the permanganate is discharged. Add 0.5 ml of a 10% w/v solution of *sodium nitroprusside* in 1M *sulphuric acid* and 4 g of *sulphamic acid* and add 13.5M *ammonia* dropwise until all the sulphamic acid has dissolved. On addition of an excess of 13.5M *ammonia* a violet colour is produced which changes to violet-blue.

B. To a neutral solution of the substance being examined add a solution of *calcium chloride*; no precipitate is produced. Boil the solution; a white precipitate is produced which is soluble in 6M *acetic acid.*

Esters

To about 30 mg of the substance being examined or to the prescribed quantity add 0.5 ml of a 7% w/v solution of *hydroxylamine hydrochloride* in *methanol* and 0.5 ml of a 10% w/v solution of *potassium hydroxide* in *ethanol (96%)*. Heat to boiling, cool, acidify with 2M *hydrochloric acid* and add 0.2 ml of a 1% w/v solution of *iron(III) chloride hexahydrate.* A bluish red or red colour is produced.

Iodides

A. Dissolve a quantity of the substance being examined containing about 4 mg of iodide ion in 2 ml of *water* or use 2 ml of the prescribed solution. Acidify with 2M *nitric acid,* add 0.4 ml of *silver nitrate solution R1,* shake and allow to stand; a curdy, pale yellow precipitate is produced. Centrifuge and wash with three 1-ml quantities of *water.* Carry out these operations rapidly in subdued light disregarding the fact that the supernatant solution may not become perfectly clear. Suspend the precipitate in 2 ml of *water* and add 1.5 ml of 10M *ammonia*; the precipitate does not dissolve.

B. To 0.2 ml of a solution of the substance being examined containing about 5 mg of iodide ion per ml or to 0.2 ml of the prescribed solution add 0.5 ml of 1M *sulphuric acid,* 0.1 ml of *potassium dichromate solution,* 2 ml of *water* and 2 ml of *chloroform.* Shake for a few seconds and allow to stand. The chloroform layer is violet or violet-red.

Iron and Iron Salts

A. To a quantity of the substance being examined containing about 10 mg of iron(II) dissolved in 1 ml of *water* or to 1 ml of the prescribed solution add 1 ml of *potassium hexacyanoferrate(III) solution.* A blue precipitate is produced which is insoluble in 2M *hydrochloric acid* (iron(II) salts).

B. To 3 ml of a solution containing about 0.1 mg of iron(III) or to 3 ml of the prescribed solution add 1 ml of 2M *hydrochloric acid* and 1 ml of *potassium thiocyanate solution;* the solution is red. To 1 ml of the solution add 5 ml of *amyl alcohol* or *ether,* shake and allow to stand; the organic layer is pink. To a further 1 ml of the solution add 2 ml of *mercury(II) chloride solution;* the red colour is discharged (iron(III) salts).

C. To 1 ml of a solution containing not less than 1 mg of iron(III) or to 1 ml of the prescribed solution add 1 ml of *potassium hexacyanoferrate(II) solution.* A blue precipitate is produced which is insoluble in 5 ml of 2M *hydrochloric acid* (iron(III) salts).

Lactates

To 5 ml of a solution of the substance being examined corresponding to about 5 mg of lactic acid or to 5 ml of the prescribed solution add 1 ml of *bromine water* and 0.5 ml of 1M *sulphuric acid* and heat on a water bath until the colour is discharged, stirring occasionally with a glass rod. Add 4 g of *ammonium sulphate,* mix and add dropwise, without mixing, 0.2 ml of a 10% w/v solution of *sodium nitroprusside* in 1M *sulphuric acid.* Still without mixing add 1 ml of 13.5M *ammonia* and allow to stand for 30 minutes. A dark green ring is produced at the interface of the two liquids.

Lead and Lead Compounds

A. To 0.1 g of the substance being examined dissolved in 1 ml of 5M *acetic acid* or to 1 ml of the prescribed solution add 2 ml of *potassium chromate solution.* A yellow precipitate is produced which is soluble in 2 ml of 10M *sodium hydroxide.*

B. To 50 mg of the substance being examined dissolved in 1 ml of 5M *acetic acid* or to 1 ml of the prescribed solution add 10 ml of *water* and 0.2 ml of *potassium iodide solution;* a yellow precipitate is produced. Heat to boiling for 1 to 2 minutes and allow to cool; the precipitate reappears as glistening, yellow plates.

Lignin

A. Lignin cell walls are coloured bright red by soaking them in a 1% w/v solution of *phloroglucinol* in *ethanol (90%)* and adding 0.1 to 0.2 ml of *hydrochloric acid.*

B. Lignified tissues are coloured yellow by *aniline hydrochloride solution.*

Magnesium and Magnesium Salts

For European Pharmacopoeia monographs, use test A only.

A. To about 15 mg of the substance being examined dissolved in 2 ml of *water* or to 2 ml of the prescribed solution add 1 ml of 6M *ammonia*; a white precipitate is produced which is dissolved by adding 1 ml of *ammonium chloride solution.* Add 1 ml of *disodium hydrogen phosphate solution;* a white crystalline precipitate is produced.

B. To 0.5 ml of a neutral or slightly acidic solution of the substance being examined add 0.2 ml of a 0.1% w/v solution of *titan yellow* and 0.5 ml of 0.1M *sodium hydroxide.* A bright red turbidity is produced which gradually settles to give a bright red precipitate.

Mercury and Mercury Compounds

A. Place about 0.1 ml of a solution of the substance being examined on well-scraped copper foil; a dark grey stain is produced which becomes shiny on rubbing. Heat the dried copper foil in a test tube; the spot disappears.

B. To the prescribed solution add 2M *sodium hydroxide* until *strongly alkaline,* Appendix V K. A dense, yellow precipitate is produced (mercury(II) compounds).

Nitrates

To a mixture of 0.1 ml of *nitrobenzene* and 0.2 ml of *sulphuric acid* add a quantity of the powdered substance containing about 1 mg of nitrate ion or the prescribed quantity and allow to stand for 5 minutes. Cool in ice, add slowly with stirring 5 ml of *water,* then 5 ml of 10M *sodium hydroxide* and 5 ml of *acetone,* shake and allow to stand. The upper layer is deep violet.

Odour

(Ph. Eur. method 2.3.4)

Spread 0.5 to 2.0 g of the substance being examined in a thin layer on a watch glass 6 to 8 cm in diameter. After 15 minutes determine the odour or verify the absence of odour.

Phosphates (orthophosphates)

A. To 5 ml of the prescribed solution, neutralised if necessary, add 5 ml of *silver nitrate solution R1*. A yellow precipitate is produced the colour of which is not changed on boiling and which is soluble in 10M *ammonia*.

B. Mix 1 ml of the prescribed solution with 2 ml of *molybdovanadic reagent*. A yellow colour develops.

Potassium and Potassium Salts

A. To 0.1 g of the substance being examined dissolved in 2 ml of *water* or to 2 ml of the prescribed solution add 1 ml of *sodium carbonate solution* and heat; no precipitate is produced. Add while hot 0.05 ml of *sodium sulphide solution;* no precipitate is produced. Cool in ice and add 2 ml of a 15% w/v solution of *(+)-tartaric acid* and allow to stand; a white, crystalline precipitate is produced.

B. To about 40 mg of the substance being examined dissolved in 1 ml of *water* or to 1 ml of the prescribed solution add 1 ml of 2M *acetic acid* and 1 ml of a freshly prepared 10% w/v solution of *sodium cobaltinitrate*. A yellow or orange-yellow precipitate is produced immediately.

Salicylates

A. To 1 ml of a 10% w/v neutral solution of the substance being examined or to 1 ml of the prescribed solution add 0.5 ml of *iron(III) chloride solution R1*. A violet colour is produced which is not discharged on the addition of 0.1 ml of 5M *acetic acid*.

B. To 0.5 g of the substance being examined dissolved in 10 ml of *water* or to 10 ml of the prescribed solution add 0.5 ml of *hydrochloric acid*. The *melting point* of the precipitate, after recrystallisation from hot *water* and drying at a pressure of 2 kPa, is 156° to 161°, Appendix V A, Method I.

Silicates

In a lead or platinum crucible mix to a thin slurry using a copper wire the prescribed quantity of the substance being examined with 10 mg of *sodium fluoride* and 0.2 ml of *sulphuric acid*. Cover the crucible with a thin, transparent plate of plastic from which a drop of *water* is suspended and warm gently. A white ring is rapidly produced around the drop of water.

Silver and Silver Compounds

To 10 mg of the substance being examined dissolved in 10 ml of *water* or to 10 ml of the prescribed solution add 0.3 ml of 7M *hydrochloric acid*; a curdy, white precipitate is produced which is soluble in 3 ml of 6M *ammonia*.

Sodium and Sodium Salts

A. To 0.1 g of the substance being examined dissolved in 2 ml of *water* or to 2 ml of the prescribed solution add 2 ml of a 15% w/v solution of *potassium carbonate* and heat to boiling; no precipitate is produced. Add 4 ml of freshly prepared *potassium antimonate(V) solution* and heat to boiling. Allow to cool in ice and if necessary scratch the inside of the tube with a glass rod; a dense, white precipitate is produced.

B. To 0.5 ml of a solution containing about 2 mg of sodium ion or to 0.5 ml of the prescribed solution add 1.5 ml of *methoxyphenylacetic acid reagent* and cool in ice for 30 minutes; a voluminous, white, crystalline precipitate is produced. Warm in water at 20° and stir for 5 minutes; the precipitate does not dissolve. Add 1 ml of 6M *ammonia*; the precipitate dissolves completely. Add 1 ml of a 16% w/v solution of *ammonium carbonate*; no precipitate is produced.

Sulphates

A. To about 45 mg of the substance being examined dissolved in 5 ml of *water* or to 5 ml of the prescribed solution add 1 ml of 2M *hydrochloric acid* and 1 ml of *barium chloride solution R1*. A white precipitate is produced.

B. Add 0.1 ml of 0.05M *iodine* to the suspension obtained in reaction A; the suspension remains yellow (distinction from sulphites and dithionites) but is decolorised by adding, dropwise, *tin(II) chloride solution* (distinction from iodates). Boil the mixture; no coloured precipitate is produced (distinction from selenates and tungstates).

Tartrates

A. To about 15 mg of the substance being examined dissolved in 5 ml of *water* or to 5 ml of the prescribed solution add 0.05 ml of a 1% w/v solution of *iron(II) sulphate* and 0.05 ml of *hydrogen peroxide solution (10 vol)*; a transient yellow colour is produced. After the colour has disappeared add 2M *sodium hydroxide* dropwise; an intense blue colour is produced.

B. To 0.1 ml of a solution containing the equivalent of about 15 mg of tartaric acid per ml or to 0.1 ml of the prescribed solution add 0.1 ml of a 10% w/v solution of *potassium bromide*, 0.1 ml of a 2% w/v solution of *resorcinol* and 3 ml of *sulphuric acid* and heat on a water bath for 5 to 10 minutes. A dark blue colour is produced which changes to red when the solution is allowed to cool and poured into *water*.

Xanthines

Mix a few mg of the substance being examined or the prescribed quantity with 0.1 ml of *hydrogen peroxide solution (100 vol)* and 0.3 ml of 2M *hydrochloric acid*, heat to dryness on a water bath until a yellowish red residue is produced and add 0.1 ml of 2M *ammonia*. The colour of the residue changes to violet-red.

Zinc and Zinc Salts

To 0.1 g of the substance being examined dissolved in 5 ml of *water* or to 5 ml of the prescribed solution add 0.2 ml of 10M *sodium hydroxide*; a white precipitate is produced. Add a further 2 ml of 10M *sodium hydroxide*; the precipitate dissolves. Add 10 ml of *ammonium chloride solution;* the solution remains clear. Add 0.1 ml of *sodium sulphide solution;* a flocculent, white precipitate is produced.

Appendix VII

Limit Tests

Nessler cylinders

Where the use of *Nessler cylinders* is prescribed in a test of the Pharmacopoeia, Nessler cylinders complying with the following requirements should be used.

Nessler cylinders comply with British Standard 612:1966 (Specification for Nessler cylinders). They are of clear glass with a nominal capacity of 50 ml; the overall height is about 15 cm, the external height to the 50-ml mark 11.0 to 12.4 cm, the thickness of the wall 1.0 to 1.5 mm and the thickness of the base 1.0 to 3.0 mm. The external heights to the 50-ml mark of cylinders used for a test must not differ by more than 1 mm.

Tubes used for comparative tests

(Ph. Eur. text 2.1.5)

Unless otherwise prescribed, tubes used for comparative tests are matched tubes of colourless glass with a uniform internal diameter of 16 mm. The base is transparent and flat. A column of the liquid is examined down the vertical axis of the tube against a white background or, if necessary, against a black background. The examination is carried out in diffused light.

Limit Test for Aluminium

(Ph. Eur. method 2.4.17)

Extract the prescribed solution with successive quantities of 20, 20 and 10 ml of a 0.5% w/v solution of *8-hydroxyquinoline* in *chloroform* and dilute the combined extracts to 50 ml with *chloroform*. Unless otherwise stated in the monograph use as the blank solution a mixture of 10 ml of *acetate buffer pH 6.0* and 100 ml of *water* treated in the same manner and as the standard solution a mixture of 2 ml of *aluminium standard solution (2 ppm Al)*, 10 ml of *acetate buffer pH 6.0* and 98 ml of *water* treated in the same manner. Measure the *fluorescence* of the test solution (I_1), of the standard solution (I_2) and of the blank (I_3), Appendix II E, using an excitation wavelength of 392 nm and a secondary filter with a transmission band centred at 518 nm, or a monochromator set to transmit at this wavelength. The fluorescence of the test solution ($I_1 - I_3$) is not greater than that of the standard solution ($I_2 - I_3$).

Limit Tests for Ammonium

(Ph. Eur. method 2.4.1)

Use method A unless otherwise prescribed in the monograph.

Method A Dissolve the prescribed quantity of the substance being examined in 14 ml of *water* in a test tube, if necessary make alkaline with 2M *sodium hydroxide* and dilute to 15 ml with *water*. Add 0.3 ml of *alkaline potassium tetraiodomercurate solution,* stopper the tube, mix and allow to stand for 5 minutes. Any yellow colour produced is not more intense than that obtained by treating a mixture of 10 ml of *ammonium standard solution (1 ppm NH_4)* and 5 ml of *water* in the same manner.

Method B In a 25-ml jar fitted with a polyethylene cap place the prescribed quantity of the finely powdered substance being examined and dissolve or suspend in 1 ml of *water*. Add 0.3 g of *heavy magnesium oxide*. Close immediately after placing a piece of *silver manganese paper* 5 mm square, wetted with a few drops of *water*, under the polyethylene cap. Swirl, avoiding projection s of liquid, and allow to stand at 40° for 30 minutes. If the silver manganese paper shows a grey colour, it is not more intense than that of a standard prepared at the same time and in the same manner using the prescribed quantity of ammonium standard solution, 1 ml of *water* and 0.3 g of *heavy magnesium oxide*.

Limit Tests for Arsenic

(Ph. Eur. method 2.4.2)

Use Test [Method] A unless otherwise directed in the monograph.

Test A The apparatus (Fig. 7-1) consists of a 100-ml conical flask closed with a ground-glass stopper through which passes a glass tube about 200 mm long and 5 mm in internal diameter. The lower part of the tube is drawn to an internal diameter of 1.0 mm and 15 mm from its tip is a lateral orifice 2 to 3 mm in diameter. When the tube is in position in the stopper the lateral orifice should be at least 3 mm below the lower surface of the stopper. The upper end of the tube has a perfectly flat, ground surface

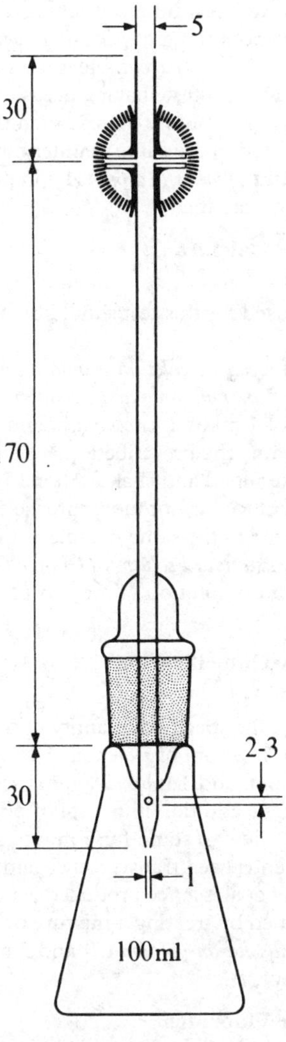

Fig. 7-1
Apparatus for Limit Test for Arsenic
Dimensions in mm

at right angles to the axis of the tube. A second glass tube of the same internal diameter and 30 mm long, with a similar flat ground surface, is placed in contact with the first and is held in position by two spiral springs. Into the lower tube insert 50 to 60 mg of *lead acetate cotton*, loosely packed, or a small plug of cotton and a rolled piece of *lead acetate paper* weighing 50 to 60 mg. Between the flat surfaces of the tubes place a disc or a small square of *mercury(II) bromide paper* large enough to cover the orifice of the tube (15 mm × 15 mm).

In the conical flask dissolve the prescribed quantity of the substance being examined in 25 ml of *water* or, in the case of a solution, dilute the prescribed volume to 25 ml with *water*. Add 15 ml of *hydrochloric acid*, 0.1 ml of *tin(II) chloride solution AsT* and 5 ml of *potassium iodide solution*, allow to stand for 15 minutes and add 5 g of *activated zinc*. Immediately assemble the two parts of the apparatus and immerse the flask in a water bath at a temperature such that a uniform evolution of gas is maintained. After not less than 2 hours any stain produced on the mercury(II) bromide paper is not more intense than that obtained by treating 1 ml of *arsenic standard solution (1 ppm As)* diluted to 25 ml with *water* in the same manner.

Test B Add the prescribed quantity of the substance being examined to a test tube containing 4 ml of *hydrochloric acid* and about 5 mg of *potassium iodide* and add 3 ml of *hypophosphorous reagent*. Heat the mixture on a water bath for 15 minutes, shaking occasionally. Any colour produced is not more intense than that obtained in a solution prepared in the same manner but using 0.5 ml of *arsenic standard solution (10 ppm As)* in place of the substance being examined.

Limit Test for Calcium

(Ph. Eur. method 2.4.3)

The solutions used for this test should be prepared with *distilled water*.

To 0.2 ml of *alcoholic calcium standard solution (100 ppm Ca)* add 1 ml of *ammonium oxalate solution*. After 1 minute add a mixture of 1 ml of 2M *acetic acid* and 15 ml of a solution containing the prescribed quantity of the substance being examined and shake. After 15 minutes any opalescence produced is not more intense than that of a standard prepared in the same manner using a mixture of 10 ml of *calcium standard solution (10 ppm Ca)* and 5 ml of *water* in place of the solution of the substance being examined.

Limit Test for Chlorides

(Ph. Eur. method 2.4.4)

To a solution of the specified quantity of the substance being examined in 15 ml of *water* or to 15 ml of the prescribed solution add 1 ml of 2M *nitric acid*, pour the mixture as a single addition into 1 ml of *silver nitrate solution R2* and allow to stand for 5 minutes protected from light. When viewed transversely against a black background any opalescence produced is not more intense than that obtained by treating a mixture of 10 ml of *chloride standard solution (5 ppm Cl)* and 5 ml of *water* in the same manner.

Limit Test for Fluorides

(Ph. Eur. method 2.4.5)

Introduce into the inner tube of the apparatus (Fig. 7.2) the specified quantity of the substance being examined, 0.1 g of acid-washed *sand* and 20 ml of *sulphuric acid (50% v/v)*. Place tetrachloroethane in the outer jacket and heat to maintain at its boiling point (146°). Attach a steam generator and distil, collecting the distillate in a 100-ml graduated flask containing 0.3 ml of 0.1M *sodium hydroxide* and 0.1 ml of *phenolphthalein solution*. Maintain a constant volume (20 ml) in the tube during distillation and ensure that the distillate remains alkaline, adding 0.1M *sodium hydroxide* if necessary. Dilute the distillate to 100 ml with *water*. Prepare a standard by distillation in the same manner, using 5 ml of *fluoride standard solution (10 ppm F)* in place of the substance being examined. Into two glass-stoppered cylinders separately place 20 ml of the test solution and 20 ml of the standard and add 5 ml of *aminomethylalizarindiacetic acid reagent* to each solution. After 20 minutes any blue colour in the test solution (originally red) is not more intense than that in the standard solution.

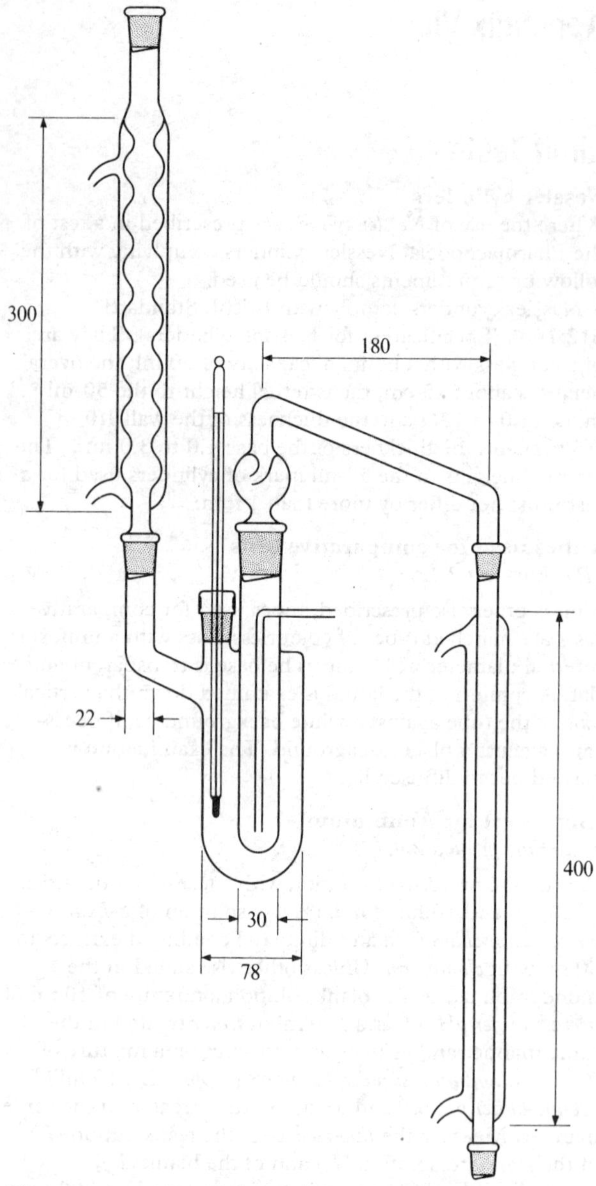

Fig. 7-2
Apparatus for Limit Test for Fluorides
Dimensions in mm

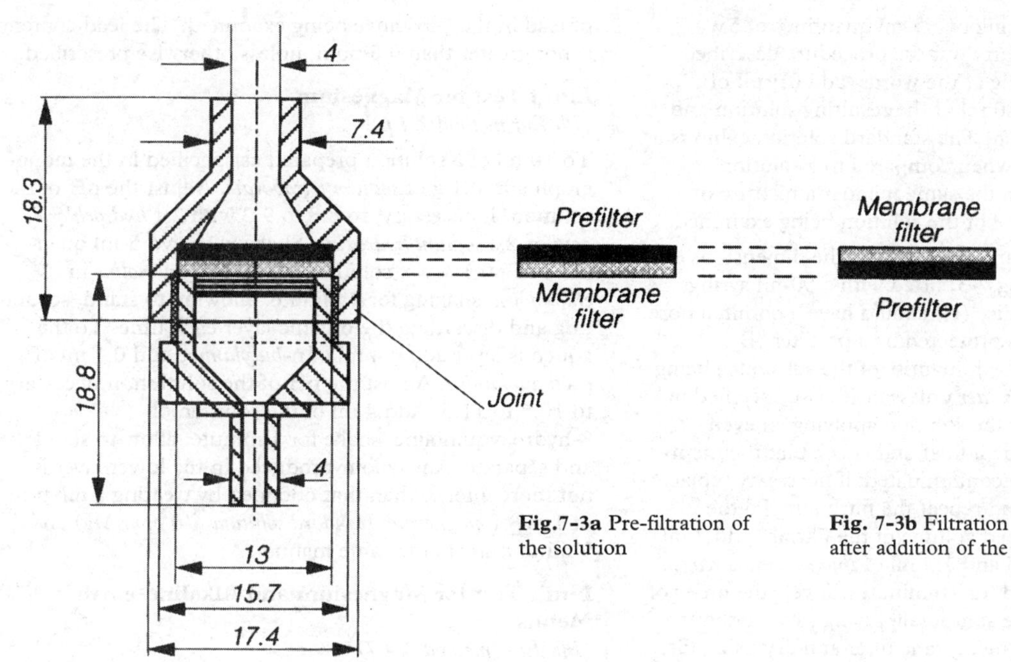

Fig.7-3a Pre-filtration of the solution

Fig. 7-3b Filtration of the solution after addition of the reagents

Fig. 7-3
Apparatus for Limit Test E for Heavy Metals
Dimensions in mm

Limit Tests for Heavy Metals
(Ph. Eur. method 2.4.8)

Test A To 12 ml of the prescribed aqueous solution add 2 ml of *acetate buffer pH 3.5*, mix, add 1.2 ml of *thioacetamide reagent*, mix immediately and allow to stand for 2 minutes. Any brown colour produced is not more intense than that obtained by treating in the same manner a mixture of 10 ml of either *lead standard solution (1 ppm Pb)* or *lead standard solution (2 ppm Pb)*, as prescribed, and 2 ml of the solution being examined. The standard solution exhibits a slightly brown colour when compared to a solution prepared by treating in the same manner a mixture of 10 ml of *water* and 2 ml of the solution being examined.

Test B Dissolve the specified quantity of the substance being examined in an organic solvent containing a minimum percentage of water, such as *1,4-dioxan* or *acetone* containing 15% v/v of *water*, and carry out Test A but prepare the standard by diluting *lead standard solution (100 ppm Pb)* with the solvent used to prepare the test solution to contain 1 or 2 ppm of Pb, as specified. The standard solution exhibits a slightly brown colour when compared to a solution prepared by treating in the same manner a mixture of 10 ml of the solvent used to prepare the test solution and 2 ml of the solution being examined.

Test C Place the prescribed quantity (usually not more than 2 g) of the substance being examined in a silica crucible with 4 ml of a 25% w/v solution of *magnesium sulphate* in 1M *sulphuric acid*. Mix using a fine glass rod and heat cautiously. If the mixture is liquid, evaporate gently to dryness on a water bath. Progressively heat to ignition, not allowing the temperature to exceed 800°, and continue heating until a white or at most greyish residue is produced. Allow to cool, moisten the residue with 0.2 ml of 1M *sulphuric acid*, evaporate, ignite again and allow to cool. The total period of ignition must not exceed 2 hours. Dissolve the residue using two 5-ml quantities of 2M *hydrochloric acid*. Add 0.1 ml of *phenolphthalein solution* and 13.5M *ammonia* dropwise until a pink colour is produced. Cool, add *glacial acetic acid* until the solution is decolorised and add a further 0.5 ml. Filter if necessary and dilute the solution to 20 ml with *water*.

To 12 ml of the resulting solution add 2 ml of *acetate buffer pH 3.5*, mix, add 1.2 ml of *thioacetamide reagent*, mix immediately and allow to stand for 2 minutes. Any brown colour produced is not more intense than that obtained by treating in the same manner a mixture of 2 ml of the test solution obtained above and 10 ml of the 20 ml of solution obtained by repeating the procedure using the prescribed volume of *lead standard solution (10 ppm Pb)* in place of the substance being examined, adding 4 ml of a 25% w/v solution of *magnesium sulphate* in 1M *sulphuric acid* and beginning at the words 'Mix with a fine glass rod...'. The standard solution exhibits a slightly brown colour when compared to a solution prepared by treating in the same manner a mixture of 10 ml of *water* and 2 ml of the solution being examined.

Test D Mix the prescribed quantity of the substance being examined with 0.5 g of *magnesium oxide R1* in a silica crucible. Ignite to dull red heat until a homogeneous white or greyish white mass is produced. If after 30 minutes of ignition the mixture remains coloured, allow to cool, mix with a fine glass rod and repeat the ignition. If necessary, repeat the operation. Finally heat at 800° for about 1 hour, dissolve the residue using two 5-ml quantities of 5M *hydrochloric acid* and carry out the procedure described under Test C beginning at the words 'Add 0.1 ml of...'.

To prepare the standard add the prescribed volume of *lead standard solution (10 ppm Pb)* to 0.5 g of *magnesium oxide R1* contained in a silica crucible, dry the mixture in an oven at 100° to 105°, ignite as described above, dissolve the residue using two 5-ml quantities of 5M *hydrochloric acid* and carry out the procedure described under Test C beginning at the words 'add 0.1 ml of...', and use a mixture of 10 ml of the resulting solution and 2 ml of the test solution. The standard solution exhibits a slightly brown colour when compared to a solution prepared by treating in the same manner a mixture of 10 ml of *water* and 2 ml of the solution being examined.

Test E Use a membrane filter holder, the dimensions of which are shown in Fig.7-3, fitted with a 50-ml syringe. The membrane filter disc (C) should have a nominal pore diameter of 3 μm. It is protected by a prefilter (B).

Dissolve the prescribed quantity of the substance being examined in 30 ml of *water* unless otherwise specified in the monograph. Filter the solution applying an even pressure. Dismantle the holder and check that the membrane filter remains uncontaminated; if necessary replace the membrane filter and repeat the filtration. To the filtrate, or the prescribed volume of the filtrate, add 2 ml of *acetate buffer pH 3.5* and 1.2 ml of *thioacetamide reagent*, mix and allow to stand for 10 minutes. Invert the order of the filters and filter the solution applying slow and even pressure. Remove the membrane filter and dry using filter paper. The intensity of any stain produced on the membrane filter is not more intense than that obtained by treating the prescribed volume of *lead standard solution (1 ppm Pb)* in the same manner.

Limit Test for Iron

(Ph. Eur. method 2.4.9)

Dissolve the specified quantity of the substance being examined in sufficient *water* to produce 10 ml or use 10 ml of the solution prescribed in the monograph and transfer to a *Nessler cylinder*. Add 2 ml of a 20% w/v solution of *citric acid* and 0.1 ml of *mercaptoacetic acid*, mix, make alkaline with 10M *ammonia*, dilute to 20 ml with *water* and allow to stand for 5 minutes. Any pink colour produced is not more intense than that obtained by treating 10 ml of *iron standard solution (1 ppm Fe)* in the same manner.

Limit Test for Lead in Sugars

(Ph. Eur. method 2.4.10)

Carry out Method II for *atomic absorption spectrophotometry*, Appendix II D, using an air—acetylene flame, a lead hollow-cathode lamp and the following solutions.

TEST SOLUTION Dissolve 20.0 g of the substance being examined in sufficient 1M *acetic acid* to produce 100.0 ml. Add 2.0 ml of a saturated solution of *ammonium pyrrolidinedithiocarbamate* (about 1% w/v) and 10.0 ml of *4-methylpentan-2-one* and shake for 30 seconds protected from bright light. Allow the two layers to separate and use the methylpentanone layer.

REFERENCE SOLUTIONS Prepare three reference solutions in the same manner as the test solution using 0.5 ml, 1.0 ml and 1.5 ml respectively of *lead standard solution (10 ppm Pb)* in addition to 20.0 g of the substance being examined. Prepare a blank solution in the same manner as the test solution but without the substance being examined.

Examine the test solution, the three reference solutions and the blank solution at the maximum at 283.3 nm using the blank solution to set the zero of the instrument. Construct a calibration curve and determine the content of lead in the substance being examined. The lead content is not greater than 0.5 ppm, unless otherwise prescribed.

Limit Test for Magnesium

(Ph Eur method 2.4.6)

To 10 ml of a solution prepared as specified in the monograph add 0.1 g of *sodium tetraborate*. Adjust the pH of the solution, if necessary, to 8.8 to 9.2 with 2M *hydrochloric acid* or 2M *sodium hydroxide*. Shake with two 5-ml quantities of a 0.1% w/v solution of *8-hydroxyquinoline* in *chloroform*, shaking for 1 minute, allowing to stand, separating and discarding the organic layer each time. To the aqueous layer add 0.4 ml of *n-butylamine* and 0.1 ml of *triethanolamine*. Adjust the pH of the solution, if necessary, to 10.5 to 11.5. Add 4 ml of the solution of 8-hydroxyquinoline, shake for 1 minute, allow to stand and separate. Any colour produced in the lower layer is not more intense than that obtained by treating a mixture of 1 ml of *magnesium standard solution (10 ppm Mg)* and 9 ml of *water* in the same manner.

Limit Test for Magnesium and Alkaline-earth Metals

(Ph. Eur. method 2.4.7)

To 200 ml of *water* add 0.1 g of *hydroxylamine hydrochloride*, 10 ml of *ammonia buffer pH 10.0*, 1 ml of 0.1M *zinc sulphate* and about 15 mg of *mordant black 11 triturate*. Heat to about 40° and titrate with 0.01M *disodium edetate VS* until the violet colour changes to a full blue. To the solution add the specified quantity of the substance being examined dissolved in 100 ml of *water* or use the prescribed solution. If the colour of the solution changes to violet, titrate with 0.01M *disodium edetate VS* until the full blue colour is again produced. The volume of 0.01M *disodium edetate VS* used in the second titration does not exceed the prescribed quantity.

Limit Test for Nickel in Polyols

(Ph. Eur. method 2.4.15)

Carry out Method II for *atomic absorption spectrophotometry*, Appendix II D, using an air—acetylene flame, a nickel hollow-cathode lamp and the following solution s.

TEST SOLUTION Dissolve 20.0 g of the substance being examined in 1M *acetic acid* and dilute to 100.0 ml with the same solvent. Add 2.0 ml of a saturated solution of *ammonium pyrrolidinedithiocarbamate* (about 1% w/v) and 10.0 ml of *4-methylpentan-2-one* and shake for 30 seconds protected from bright light. Allow the two layers to separate and use the methylpentanone layer.

REFERENCE SOLUTIONS Prepare three reference solutions as described for the test solution using 0.5 ml, 1.0 ml and 1.5 ml respectively of *nickel standard solution (10 ppm Ni)* in addition to 20.0 g of the substance being examined. Prepare a blank solution in the same manner as for the test solution but without the substance being examined and use this solution to set the zero of the instrument.

Examine the test solution, the three reference solutions and the blank solution at the maximum at 232.0 nm. Construct a calibration curve and determine the content of nickel in the substance being examined. The nickel content is not greater than 1 ppm unless otherwise prescribed.

Limit Test for Phosphates

(Ph. Eur. method 2.4.11)

To 100 ml of the solution prepared and, if necessary, neutralised as prescribed add 4 ml of *sulphomolybdic reagent R3*, shake, add 0.1 ml of *tin(II) chloride solution R1*, allow to stand for 10 minutes and examine 20 ml of the resulting solution. Any colour produced is not more intense than that produced in 20 ml of a solution obtained by treating a mixture of 2 ml of *phosphate standard solution (5 ppm PO_4)* and 98 ml of *water* in the same manner.

Limit Test for Potassium

(Ph. Eur. method 2.4.12)

To 10 ml of the prescribed solution add 2 ml of a freshly prepared 1% w/v solution of *sodium tetraphenylborate* and allow to stand for 5 minutes. Any opalescence produced is not more intense than that obtained by treating a mixture of 5 ml of *potassium standard solution (20 ppm K)* and 5 ml of *water* in the same manner.

Limit Test for Sulphates

(Ph. Eur. method 2.4.13)

The solutions used for this test should be prepared with *distilled water.*

Add 1 ml of a 25% w/v solution of *barium chloride* to 1.5 ml of *sulphate standard solution (10 ppm SO_4) R1*, shake and allow to stand for 1 minute. Add 15 ml of the prescribed solution or a solution of the specified quantity of the substance being examined in 15 ml of *water* and 0.5 ml of 5M *acetic acid* and allow to stand for 5 minutes. Any opalescence produced is not more intense than that of a standard prepared in the same manner but using 15 ml of *sulphate standard solution (10 ppm SO_4)* in place of the solution being examined.

Appendix VIII

A. Non-aqueous Titration

(No Ph. Eur. method)

Method I

Dissolve the prescribed quantity of the substance being examined in a suitable volume of *anhydrous acetic acid* previously neutralised using the indicator specified in the monograph, warming and cooling if necessary, or prepare a solution as directed. When the substance is a salt of hydrochloric or hydrobromic acid, add 15 ml of *mercury(II) acetate solution* before neutralising the solvent, unless otherwise directed in the monograph. Titrate with 0.1M *perchloric acid VS* to the colour change of the indicator that corresponds to the maximum absolute value of dE/dV (where E is the electromotive force and V is the volume of titrant) in a *potentiometric titration,* Appendix VIII B, of the substance being examined. The indicator specified in the monograph is also used for the neutralisation of the *mercury(II) acetate solution* and the standardisation of the titrant.

When the temperature (t_2) of the titrant at the time of the assay differs from the temperature (t_1) of the titrant when it was standardised, multiply the volume of the titrant required by $[1+0.0011(t_1-t_2)]$ and calculate the result of the assay from the corrected volume.

Carry out a blank titration when necessary.

Method II

The titrant, solvent and, where necessary, the indicator to be used are stated in the monograph.

Protect the solution and titrant from atmospheric carbon dioxide and moisture throughout the determination.

Dissolve the substance being examined in a suitable volume of the solvent previously neutralised to the indicator, warming and cooling if necessary, or prepare a solution as directed. Titrate to the colour change of the indicator that corresponds to the maximum absolute value of dE/dV (where E is the electromotive force and V is the volume of titrant) in a *potentiometric titration,* Appendix VIII B, of the substance under examination. The titrant is standardised using the same solvent and indicator as specified for the substance.

Carry out a blank titration when necessary.

B. Amperometric and Potentiometric Titrations

Amperometric titration

(Ph. Eur. method 2.2.19)

In amperometric titration the end point is determined by following, as a function of the quantity of titrant added, the variation of the current measured between two electrodes, either one indicator electrode and one reference electrode or two indicator electrodes, immersed in the solution being examined and maintained at a constant potential difference.

The potential of the measuring electrode is sufficient to ensure a diffusion current for the electroactive substance.

Apparatus The apparatus comprises an adjustable voltage source and a sensitive microammeter; the detection system generally consists of an indicator electrode (for example, a platinum electrode, a dropping-mercury electrode, a rotating-disc electrode or a carbon electrode) and a reference electrode (for example, a calomel electrode or a silversilver chloride electrode). A three-electrode apparatus is sometimes used, consisting of an indicator electrode, a reference electrode and a polarised auxiliary electrode.

Method Set the potential of the indicator electrode as prescribed and plot a graph of the initial current and the values obtained during the titration as function s of the quantity of titrant added. Add the titrant in not fewer than three successive quantities equal to a total of about 80% of the theoretical volume corresponding to the presumed equivalence point. The three values must fall on a straight line. Continue adding the titrant beyond the presumed equivalence point in not fewer than three successive quantities. The values obtained must fall on a straight line. The point of intersection of the two lines represents the end point of the titration.

For amperometric titration with two indicator electrodes, the whole titration curve is recorded and used to determine the end point.

Potentiometric titration

(Ph. Eur. method 2.2.20)

In a potentiometric titration the end point of the titration is determined by following, as a function of the quantity of titrant added, the variation of the potential difference between two electrodes, either one indicator electrode and one reference electrode or two indicator electrodes, immersed in the solution being examined.

The potential is usually measured at zero or practically zero current.

Apparatus The apparatus used (a simple potentiometer or electronic device) comprises a voltmeter allowing readings to the nearest millivolt. The choice of indicator electrode depends on the substance being examined and may be a glass or metal electrode (for example, platinum, gold, silver or mercury). The reference electrode is generally a calomel or a silver—silver chloride electrode. For acid–base titration s and unless otherwise prescribed, a glass-calomel or glass–silver—silver chloride electrode combination is used.

Method Plot a graph of the variation of potential difference as a function of the quantity of the titrant added, continuing the addition of the titrant beyond the presumed equivalence point. The end point corresponds to a sharp variation of potential difference.

Determination of primary aromatic amino nitrogen

(Ph. Eur. method 2.5.8)

Dissolve the prescribed quantity of the substance being examined in 50 ml of 2M *hydrochloric acid* or in another prescribed solvent and add 3 g of *potassium bromide*. Cool in iced water and titrate by slowly adding 0.1M *sodium nitrite VS* with constant stirring. Determine the end-point electrometrically or by the use of the prescribed indicator.

C. Oxygen-flask Combustion

(Ph. Eur. method 2.5.10)

Apparatus

Unless otherwise prescribed in the monograph the combustion flask is a borosilicate-glass conical flask of at least 500-ml capacity with a ground-glass stopper fitted with a suitable carrier for the sample, for example made of platinum or platinumiridium.

Method

Finely grind the substance being examined, place the prescribed quantity in the centre of a piece of filter paper (40 mm × 30 mm), secure the package in the sample carrier and insert one end of a narrow strip (10 mm × 30 mm) of filter paper in the roll. If paper impregnated with *lithium carbonate* is prescribed, moisten the centre of the paper with a saturated solution of *lithium carbonate* and dry at 100° to 105° before use. Envelop the substance in the paper and place it in the sample carrier. Place the specified absorbing liquid in the flask, flush the flask with *oxygen* using a tube with its end just above the level of liquid, moisten the neck with *water*, fill it with *oxygen*, ignite the free end of the narrow strip of filter paper by suitable means with the usual precaution s and immediately insert the stopper. Hold the stopper firmly in place. When vigorous burning has begun, invert the flask so as to provide a liquid seal but taking care to prevent incompletely burned material falling into the liquid. Immediately combustion is complete, shake the flask vigorously to dissolve the combustion products completely, cool and after about 5 minutes, unless otherwise prescribed, carefully withdraw the stopper and rinse the stopper, platinum wire, platinum gauze and sides of the flask with *water* and proceed as described below or in the monograph.

For liquids place the specified quantity on about 15 mg of ashless filter-paper flock contained in one part of a methylcellulose capsule of a suitable size, close the capsule, inserting one end of a narrow strip of filter paper between the two parts, and secure the capsule in the platinum gauze.

Ointments should be enclosed in grease-proof paper before wrapping in filter paper.

FOR IODINE

Burn the specified quantity of the substance being examined in the prescribed manner using a mixture of 10 ml of *water* and 2 ml of 1M *sodium hydroxide* as the absorbing liquid. When the process is complete, add to the flask an excess of *acetic bromine solution* (between 5 and 10 ml) and allow to stand for 2 minutes. Remove the excess of bromine by the addition of *formic acid* (about 0.5 to 1 ml), rinse the sides of the flask with *water* and displace any bromine vapour above the liquid with a current of air. Add 1 g of *potassium iodide* and titrate with 0.02M *sodium thiosulphate VS* using *starch mucilage*, added towards the end of the titration, as indicator. Each ml of 0.02M *sodium thiosulphate VS* is equivalent to 0.4230 mg of I.

D. Complexometric Titrations

(Ph. Eur. method 2.5.11)

Aluminium

To 20 ml of the prescribed solution in a 500 ml conical flask add 25 ml of 0.1M *disodium edetate VS* and 10 ml of a mixture of equal volumes of a 15.5% w/v solution of *ammonium acetate* and 2M *acetic acid*. Heat to boiling for 2 minutes, cool and add 50 ml of *absolute ethanol* and 3 ml of a freshly prepared 0.025% w/v solution of *dithizone* in *absolute ethanol*. Titrate the excess of disodium edetate with 0.1M *zinc sulphate VS* until the colour changes from greenish blue to reddish violet. Each ml of 0.1M *disodium edetate VS* is equivalent to 2.698 mg of Al.

Bismuth

Dilute the prescribed solution in *nitric acid* to 250 ml with *water* and unless otherwise directed add, with shaking, 13.5M *ammonia* dropwise until cloudiness is first observed. Add 0.5 ml of *nitric acid* and heat to 70°, maintaining the solution at this temperature until the solution becomes completely clear. Add about 50 mg of *xylenol orange triturate* and titrate with 0.1M *disodium edetate VS* until the colour changes from pinkish violet to yellow. Each ml of 0.1M *disodium edetate VS* is equivalent to 20.90 mg of Bi.

Calcium

In a 500 ml conical flask dilute the prescribed solution with *water* to 300 ml, add 6 ml of 10M *sodium hydroxide* and about 15 mg of *calconcarboxylic acid triturate* and titrate with 0.1M *disodium edetate VS* until the colour changes from violet to full blue. Each ml of 0.1M *disodium edetate VS* is equivalent to 4.008 mg of Ca.

Lead

In a 500 ml conical flask dilute the prescribed solution to 200 ml with *water* and add about 50 mg of *xylenol orange triturate* and sufficient *hexamine* to produce a violet-pink colour. Titrate with 0.1M *disodium edetate VS* until the colour changes to yellow. Each ml of 0.1M *disodium edetate VS* is equivalent to 20.72 mg of Pb.

Magnesium

In a 500 ml conical flask dilute the prescribed solution to 300 ml with *water* or dissolve the prescribed quantity of the substance being examined in 5 to 10 ml of *water* or in the minimum volume of 2M *hydrochloric acid* and dilute to 50 ml with *water*. To the resulting solution add 10 ml of *ammonia buffer pH 10.0* and about 50 mg of *mordant black 11 triturate*. Heat to 40° and titrate at this temperature with 0.1M *disodium edetate VS* until the colour changes from violet to full blue. Each ml of 0.1M *disodium edetate VS* is equivalent to 2.431 mg of Mg.

Zinc

In a 500 ml conical flask dilute the prescribed solution to 200 ml with *water* and add about 50 mg of *xylenol orange triturate* and sufficient *hexamine* to produce a violet-pink colour. Add a further 2 g of *hexamine* and titrate with 0.1M *disodium edetate VS* until the colour changes to yellow. Each ml of 0.1M *disodium edetate VS* is equivalent to 6.54 mg of Zn.

E. Potentiometric Determination of Ionic Concentration Using Ion-selective Electrodes

(Ph. Eur. method 2.2.36)

Ideally, the potential, E, of an ion-selective electrode varies linearly with the logarithm of the activity, a_i, of a given ion, as expressed by the Nernst equation :

$$E = E_0 + 2.303\frac{RT}{z_i F}\log a_i$$

where E_0 = part of the constant potential due to the apparatus used,

R = gas constant,

T = absolute temperature,

F = Faraday's number and

z_i = charge number of the ion including its sign.

At a constant ionic strength, the following holds:

$$E = E_0 + \frac{k}{z_i}\log fC_i$$

where C_i = molar concentration of the ion,

f = the activity coefficient ($a_i = fC_i$) and

$k = RT/F$

$$\text{If: } E_0 + \frac{k}{z_i}\log f = E_0^{\star} \text{ and } S = \frac{k}{z_i}$$

where S = slope of the calibration curve of the electrode,

the following holds: $E = E_0^{\star} + S\log C_i$

and for $-\log C_i = pC_i$ $E = E_0^{\star} - SpC_i$

The potentiometric determination of the ion concentration is carried out by measuring the potential difference between two suitable electrodes immersed in the solution being examined; the indicator electrode is selective for the ion being determined and the other is a reference electrode.

Apparatus

Use a voltmeter allowing measurements to the nearest 0.1 millivolt and the input impedance of which is at least 100 times greater than that of the electrodes used. Ion-selective electrodes may be primary electrodes with a crystal or non-crystal membrane or with a rigid matrix (for example, glass electrodes), or electrodes with charged (positive or negative) or uncharged mobile carriers, or sensitised electrodes (enzymatic-substrate electrodes, gas-indicator electrodes). The reference electrode is generally a silver—silver chloride electrode or a calomel electrode, with suitable junction liquids, producing no interference.

Procedure

Carry out each measurement at a temperature constant to ±0.5°, taking into account the variation of the slope of the electrode with temperature (see Table). Adjust the ionic strength and possibly the pH of the solution being analysed using the buffer reagent described in the monograph and equilibrate the electrode by immersing it in the solution to be analysed, under slow and uniform stirring, until a constant reading is obtained. If the electrode system is used frequently, check regularly the repeatability and the stability of responses, and the linearity of the calibration curve or the calculation algorithm in the range of concentration s of the test solution; if not, carry out the test before each set of measurements. The response of the electrode may be regarded as linear if the slope S of the calibration curve is approximately equal to k/z_i, per unit of pC_i.

Temperature (°C)	k
20	0.0582
25	0.0592
30	0.0602

Method I *(direct calibration)* Measure at least three times in succession the potential of at least three reference solutions spanning the expected concentration of the test solution. Calculate the calibration curve or plot on a chart the mean potential E obtained against the concentration of the ion being determined expressed as $-\log C_i$ or pC_i. Prepare the test solution as prescribed in the monograph; measure the potential three times and, from the mean potential, calculate the concentration of the ion being determined using the calibration curve.

Method II *(multiple standard addition s)* Prepare the test solution as prescribed in the monograph. Measure the potential at equilibrium E_T of a volume V_T of this solution of unknown concentration C_T of the ion being determined. Make at least three consecutive addition s of a volume V_S negligible compared to V_T ($V_S \le 0.01 V_T$) of a reference solution of a concentration C_S known to be within the linear part of the calibration curve. After each addition, measure the potential and calculate the difference of potential ΔE between the measured potential and E_T. ΔE is related to the concentration of the ion being determined by the equation :

$$\Delta E = S \log\left(1 + \frac{C_S V_S}{C_T V_T}\right)$$

or

$$10^{\frac{\Delta E}{S}} = 1 + \frac{C_S V_S}{C_T V_T}$$

where V_T = volume of the test solution,
C_T = concentration of the ion being determined in the test solution,
V_S = added volume of the reference solution,
C_S = concentration of the ion being determined in the reference solution,
S = slope of the electrode determined experimentally, at constant temperature, by measuring the difference between the potentials obtained with two reference solutions the concentration s of which differ by a factor of 10 and are situated within the range where the calibration curve is linear.

Plot on a graph $10^{\frac{\Delta E}{S}}$ (y-axis) against V_S (x-axis) and extrapolate the line obtained until it intersects the x-axis. At the intersection, the concentration C_T of the ion being determined in the test solution is given by the equation :

$$C_T = \frac{C_T V_S}{V_T}$$

Method III (*single standard addition*) To a volume V_T of the test solution prepared as described in the monograph, add a volume V_S of a reference solution containing an amount of the ion being determined known to give a response situated in the linear part of the calibration curve. Prepare a blank solution in the same condition s. Measure at least three times the potentials of the test solution and the blank solution, before and after adding the reference solution. Calculate the concentration C_T of the ion being analysed using the following equation and making the necessary correction s for the blank:

$$C_T = \frac{C_S V_S}{10^{\frac{\Delta E}{S}}(V_T + V_S) - V_T}$$

where V_T = volume of the test solution or the blank,
C_T = concentration of the ion being determined in the test solution,
V_S = added volume of the reference solution,
C_S = concentration of the ion being determined in the reference solution,
ΔE = difference between the average potentials measured before and after adding V_S and
S = slope of the electrode determined experimentally, at constant temperature, by measuring the difference between the potentials obtained from two reference solutions the concentration s of which differ by a factor of 10 and are situated within the range where the calibration curve is linear.

F. Determination of Ethanol

Use Method I or, where appropriate, Method II unless otherwise prescribed in the monograph.

Method I *(No Ph. Eur. method)*

Carry out the method for *gas chromatography*, Appendix III B, using the following solution s. Solution (1) contains 5.0% v/v of *absolute ethanol* and 5.0% v/v of *propan-1-ol* (internal standard). For solution (2) dilute a volume of the preparation being examined with *water* to contain between 4.0 and 6.0% v/v of ethanol. Prepare solution (3) in the same manner as solution (2) but adding sufficient of the internal standard to produce a final concentration of 5.0% v/v.

The chromatographic procedure may be carried out using a column (1.5 m × 4 mm) packed with porous polymer beads (100 to 120 mesh) (Porapak Q and Chromosorb 101 are suitable) and maintained at 150° with both the inlet port and the detector at 170°.

Calculate the percentage content of ethanol from the areas of the peaks due to ethanol in the chromatograms obtained with solutions (1) and (3).

Method II *(No Ph. Eur. method)*

For preparation s in which, in accordance with the authority given in the monographs, Industrial Methylated Spirit has been used, determine the content of ethanol as described in Method I but using as solution (2) a volume of the preparation being examined diluted with *water* to contain between 4.0 and 6.0% v/v of total ethanol and methanol.

Determine the concentration of methanol in the following manner. Carry out the chromatographic procedure described under Method I but using the following solutions. Solution (1) contains 0.25% v/v of *methanol* and 0.25% v/v of *propan-1-ol* (internal standard). For solution (2) dilute a volume of the preparation being examined with *water* to contain between 0.2% and 0.3% v/v of methanol. Prepare solution (3) in the same manner as solution (2) but adding sufficient of the internal standard to produce a final concentration of 0.25% v/v.

The sum of the contents of ethanol and methanol is within the range specified in the monograph and the ratio of the content of methanol to that of ethanol is commensurate with Industrial Methylated Spirit having been used.

Table 8F-1 Relationship between density, relative density and ethanol content

ρ_{20} (kg m^{-3})	Relative density of the distillate measured in air d^{20}_{20}	Ethanol content %v/v at 20°	ρ_{20} (kg m^{-3})	Relative density of the distillate measured in air d^{20}_{20}	Ethanol content %v/v at 20°
968.0	0.9697	25.09	983.5	0.9853	11.02
968.5	0.9702	24.64	984.0	0.9858	10.60
969.0	0.9707	24.19	984.5	0.9863	10.18
969.5	0.9712	23.74	985.0	0.9868	9.76
970.0	0.9717	23.29	985.5	0.9873	9.35
970.5	0.9722	22.83	986.0	0.9878	8.94
971.0	0.9727	22.37	986.5	0.9883	8.53
971.5	0.9733	21.91	987.0	0.9888	8.13
972.0	0.9738	21.45	987.5	0.9893	7.73
972.5	0.9743	20.98	988.0	0.9898	7.34
973.0	9.9748	20.52	988.5	0.9903	6.95
973.5	0.9753	20.05	989.0	0.9908	6.56
974.0	0.9758	19.59	989.5	0.9913	6.17
974.5	0.9763	19.12	990.0	09918	5.79
975.0	0.9768	18.66	990.5	0.9923	5.42
975.5	0.9773	18.19	991.0	0.9928	5.04
976.0	0.9778	17.73	991.5	0.9933	4.67
976.5	0.9883	17.25	992.0	0.9938	4.30
977.0	0.9788	16.80	992.5	0.9943	3.94
977.5	0.9793	16.34	993.0	0.9948	3.58
978.0	0.9798	15.88	993.5	0.9953	3.22
978.5	0.9803	15.43	994.0	0.9958	2.86
979.0	0.9808	14.97	994.5	0.9963	2.51
979.5	0.9813	14.52	995.0	0.9968	2.16
980.0	0.9818	14.07	995.5	0.9973	1.82
980.5	0.8923	13.63	996.0	0.9978	1.47
981.0	0.9828	13.18	996.5	0.9983	1.13
981.5	0.9833	12.74	997.0	0.9988	0.80
982.0	0.9838	12.31	997.5	0.9993	0.46
982.5	0.9843	11.87	998.0	0.9998	0.13
983.0	0.9848	11.44			

Method III *(Ph. Eur. method 2.9.10)*

This method is intended only for the examination of certain liquid pharmaceutical preparation s containing ethanol together with dissolved substances that must be separated from the ethanol to be determined by distillation. When distillation would distil volatile substances other than ethanol and water the appropriate precaution s are stated in the monograph.

The ethanol content of a liquid is expressed as the number of volumes of ethanol contained in 100 volumes of the liquid, the volumes being measured at 19.9° to 20.1°. This is known as the 'percentage of ethanol by volume'. The content may also be expressed in grams of ethanol per 100 g of the liquid. This is known as the 'percentage of ethanol by weight'.

The relation between the density at 19.9° to 20.1°, the relative density (corrected to vacuum) and the ethanol content of a mixture of water and ethanol is given in the tables of the International Organisation for Legal Metrology (1972), International Recommendation No. 22.

Apparatus The apparatus (see Fig. 8F-1) consists of a round-bottomed flask fitted with a distillation head with a steam trap and attached to a vertical condenser. A tube is fitted to the lower part of the condenser and carries the distillate into the lower part of a 100-ml or 250-ml graduated flask. The graduated flask is immersed in a mixture of ice and water during the distillation. A disc with a circular aperture 6 cm in diameter is placed under the distillation flask to reduce the risk of charring of any dissolved substances.

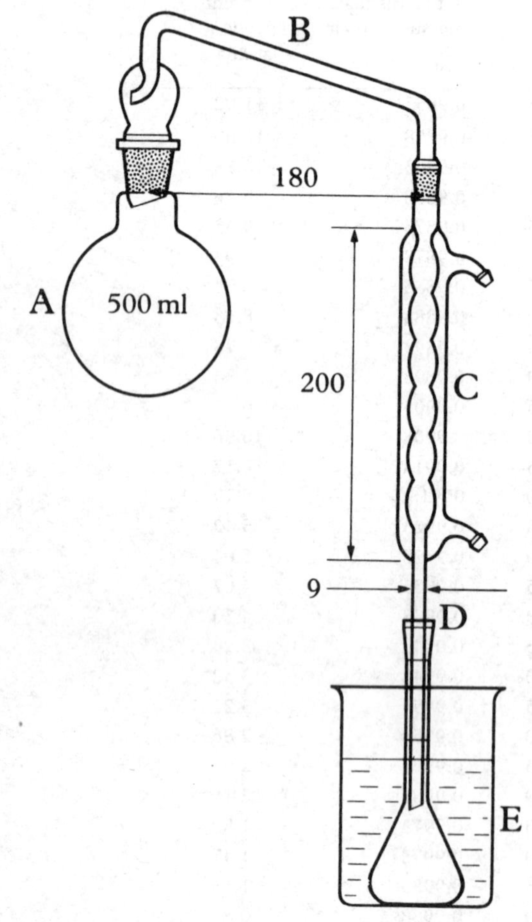

Fig. 8F-1
Apparatus for the Determination of Ethanol Content
Dimensions in millimetres

Pycnometer method Transfer 25 ml of the preparation, measured at 19.9° to 20.1°, to the distillation flask. Dilute with 100 to 150 ml of *distilled water* and add a few pieces of pumice. Attach the distillation head and condenser. Distil and collect not less than 90 ml of distillate in a 100-ml graduated flask. Adjust the temperature to 19.9° to 20.1° and dilute to 100 ml with *distilled water* at 19.9° to 20.1°. Determine the relative density at 19.9° to 20.1° using a pycnometer.

The values indicated in column 3 of Table 8F-1 are multiplied by 4 in order to obtain the percentage of ethanol by volume contained in the preparation. After calculation of the ethanol content using the Table, report the result to one decimal place.

Hydrometer method Transfer 50 ml of the preparation, measured at 19.9° to 20.1°, to the distillation flask, add 200 to 300 ml of *distilled water* and distil, as described above, into a graduated flask until at least 180 ml has been collected. Adjust the temperature to 19.9° to 20.1° and dilute to 250 ml with *distilled water* at 19.9° to 20.1°.

Transfer the distillate to a cylinder the diameter of which is at least 6 mm wider than the bulb of the hydrometer. If the volume is insufficient, double the quantity of the sample and dilute the distillate to 500 ml with *distilled water* at 19.9° to 20.1°. Multiply the strength by 5 to allow for the dilution during the determination. After calculation of the ethanol content using the Table, report the result to one decimal place.

G. Determination of Methanol and Propan-2-ol

(Ph. Eur. method 2.9.11)

Method

Carry out the method for *gas chromatography*, Appendix III B, using the following solutions.

Test solution To the distillate obtained by Method III for the *determination of ethanol*, Appendix VIII F, add 2.0 ml of the internal standard, adjust the ethanol content to 10.0% v/v by dilution to 50 ml with *water* or addition of *ethanol R1* diluted to contain 90% v/v of ethanol.

Reference solution Prepare 50 ml of a solution containing 2.0 ml of the internal standard, 10% v/v of *ethanol R1*, 0.05% v/v of *propan-2-ol* and sufficient *anhydrous methanol* to give a total of 0.05% v/v of methanol taking into account the methanol content of *ethanol R1*.

Internal standard solution Prepare a solution containing 2.5% v/v of *propan-1-ol*.

The chromatographic procedure may be carried out using a glass column (2 m × 2 mm) packed with ethylvinylbenzene divinylbenzene copolymer (125 to 150 µm) and maintained at 130°, with the inlet port at 200° and the detector at 220°.

Inject 1 µl of each solution and calculate the content of methanol and propan-2-ol in the original sample.

The sensitivity of the method is such that less than 0.025% v/v of methanol and propan-2-ol can be detected.

H. Determination of Nitrogen

Use Method I unless otherwise specified in the monograph.

Method I *(Ph. Eur. method 2.5.9)*

Place the specified quantity, containing about 2 mg of nitrogen, in a 200-ml Kjeldahl flask and add three glass beads and 4 g of a powdered mixture containing 100 g of *potassium sulphate*, 5 g of *copper(II) sulphate* and 2.5 g of *selenium*. Add 5 ml of *sulphuric acid*, allowing it to run down the sides of the flask, mix by rotation and loosely stopper the flask, for example by means of a glass bulb with a short stem, to avoid excessive loss of sulphuric acid. Heat gradually to boiling and, unless otherwise directed, boil vigorously for a further 30 minutes so that sulphuric acid condenses in the neck of the flask, taking precaution s to prevent any part of the flask above the surface of the liquid from becoming overheated. Cool, dissolve the residue by cautiously adding 25 ml of *water*, cool again and connect the flask to a steam-distillation apparatus. Add 30 ml of 10M *sodium hydroxide* and distil immediately by passing steam through the mixture. Collect about 40 ml of the distillate in a mixture of 20 ml of 0.01M *hydrochloric acid VS* and sufficient *water* to cover the tip of the condenser, taking precaution s to prevent water from the outer surface of the condenser from reaching the receiver. Towards the end of the distillation lower the receiver so that the top of the condenser is above the surface of the acid. Titrate the excess of acid with 0.01M *sodium hydroxide VS* using *methyl red mixed solution* as indicator. Repeat the operation using 50 mg of *D-glucose* in place of the substance being examined. The difference between the titration s represents the ammonia liberated by the substance being examined. Each ml of 0.01M *hydrochloric acid VS* is equivalent to 0.1401 mg of N.

Method II (Determination of protein in blood products)

For dried blood products prepare a solution of the preparation as directed in the monograph.

To a volume expected to contain about 0.1 g of protein add sufficient *saline solution* to produce 20 ml. To 2 ml of the resulting solution, in a 75-ml boiling tube, add 2 ml of a solution containing 75% v/v of *nitrogen-free sulphuric acid*, 4.5% w/v of *potassium sulphate* and 0.5% w/v of *copper(II) sulphate*, mix and loosely stopper the tube. Heat gradually to boiling, boil vigorously for 1.5 hours and cool. If the solution is not clear add 0.25 ml of *hydrogen peroxide solution (20 vol)*, continue heating until a clear solution is produced and cool. During heating, take precaution s to ensure that the upper part of the tube is not overheated.

Transfer the solution to a distillation apparatus using three 3-ml quantities of *water*, add 10 ml of 10M *sodium hydroxide* and distil rapidly for 4 minutes, collecting the distillate in a mixture of 5 ml of a saturated solution of *boric acid* and 5 ml of *water* and keeping the tip of the condenser below the level of the acid. Lower the collection flask so that the condenser can drain freely and continue the distillation for a further 1 minute. Titrate with 0.02M *hydrochloric acid VS* using *methyl red mixed solution* as indicator (V_1 ml).

To a further volume of the preparation being examined, or of the solution prepared from it, expected to contain about 0.1 g of protein, add 12 ml of *saline solution*, 2 ml of a 7.5% w/v solution of *sodium molybdate* and 2 ml of a mixture of 1 volume of *nitrogen-free sulphuric acid* and 30 volumes of *water*. Shake, allow to stand for 15 minutes, add sufficient *water* to produce 20 ml, shake again and centrifuge. Using 2 ml of the resulting clear supernatant liquid repeat the procedure described above beginning at the words 'in a 75-ml boiling tube...' (V_2 ml). Calculate the protein content in mg per ml of the preparation being examined, using the expression $6.25 \times 0.280(V_1 - V_2)$ and taking into account the initial dilution.

J. Tetrazolium Assay of Steroids

(No Ph. Eur. method)

The coloured reaction products tend to adsorb onto the surface of the glassware. To avoid low results, the glassware should be treated with the coloured reaction products before use. The treated glassware should be reserved for this assay and should be washed only with water *between assays.*

Carry out the following procedure protected from light. Dissolve a quantity of the substance being examined in sufficient *aldehyde-free absolute ethanol* to produce a solution containing 300 to 350 µg in 10 ml unless otherwise specified in the monograph. Transfer 10 ml to a 25-ml graduated flask, add 2 ml of *triphenyltetrazolium chloride solution*, displace the air in the flask with *oxygen-free nitrogen*, immediately add 2 ml of *dilute tetramethylammonium hydroxide solution* and again displace the air with *oxygen-free nitrogen*. Stopper the flask, mix the contents by gently swirling and allow to stand in a water bath at 30° for 1 hour unless otherwise specified in the monograph. Cool rapidly, add sufficient *aldehyde-free absolute ethanol* to produce 25 ml, mix and immediately determine the *absorbance* of the resulting solution in a stoppered cell at the maximum at 485 nm, Appendix II B, using in the reference cell a solution prepared at the same time and in the same manner using 10 ml of *aldehyde-free absolute ethanol*. Repeat the operation using the specified BPCRS or EPCRS in place of the substance being examined ensuring that the period of time that elapses between the addition of the tetramethylammonium hydroxide solution and the measurement of the absorbance is the same as for the test solution.

K. Assay of Vitamin A

(No Ph. Eur. method)

The potency of vitamin A is calculated from measurements of its ultraviolet absorption spectrum and expressed in terms of the Unit, which is 0.344 µg of *all-trans*-vitamin A acetate, equivalent to 0.3 µg of *all-trans*-vitamin A alcohol.

Since a measured absorbance may be the sum of that due to vitamin A and that contributed by other substances, a simple measurement of the absorption maximum may be misleading. In certain conditions defined below, the irrelevant absorption of non-vitamin A substances can be allowed for by applying correcting equations. In other cases, when these conditions are not satisfied, preliminary treatment by chemical or a combination of chemical and physical methods and the use of correcting equations must be employed before the spectrophotometric method can yield a valid assay.

Method

All procedures should be carried out as rapidly as possible and care must be taken to avoid exposure to actinic light and to oxidising agents.

Since the position of the absorption maximum is an important criterion and since the correcting equations require measurements at exact wavelengths, it is essential that the wavelength scale of the spectrophotometer should be checked immediately before the assay, Appendix II B. The mercury lines at 313.16 and 334.15 nm provide suitable points and for convenience the setting of the instrument on these lines may be related to its setting on the hydrogen lines at 379.7 and 486.1 nm. The precision of a corrected absorbance is appreciably less than that of the three directly determined absorbances from which it is calculated and the absorbance measurements therefore require special care and at least two assays should be performed.

Vitamin A in Ester Form A preparation not directly soluble in cyclohexane may be fraction ated by extraction or other means not involving saponification. If this is not possible the preparation is dealt with as described below under 'Other Vitamin A'.

Dissolve a quantity of the preparation being examined in sufficient *cyclohexane* to give a solution containing 9 to 15 IU per ml. Determine the wavelength of maximum absorption. Measure the *absorbances*, Appendix II B, at the wavelengths given in Table 8K-1 and calculate them as fractions relative to that at 328 nm. Calculate also the absorbance at 328 nm in terms of the A(1%, 1 cm) for the preparation.

TABLE 8K-1

Wavelength nm	Relative absorbance
300	0.555
316	0.907
340	0.811
360	0,299

If the wavelength of maximum absorption lies between 326 and 329 nm and the observed relative absorbances are within 0.02 of those in Table II calculate the potency of the preparation in IU per g from the expression

$$A_{328}(1\%, 1\text{ cm}) \times 1900.$$

If the wavelength of maximum absorption lies between 326 and 329 nm but the relative absorbances are not within 0.02 of those in Table 8K-1, calculate a corrected absorbance at 328 nm by applying the observed values to the equation

$$A_{328}(\text{corr.}) = 3.52(2A_{328} - A_{316} - A_{340}).$$

If the corrected absorbance lies within ±3.0% of the uncorrected absorbance, disregard the corrected absorbance and calculate the potency from the uncorrected absorbance.

If the corrected absorbance lies within −15% and −3% of the uncorrected absorbance, calculate the potency from the corrected absorbance.

If the corrected absorbance lies outside −15% to +3% of the uncorrected absorbance or if the wavelength of maximum absorption does not lie between 326 and 329 nm, the preparation must be dealt with as described under 'Other Vitamin A'.

Other Vitamin A Mix a quantity of the preparation being examined containing not less than 500 Units of vitamin A and not more than 1 g of fat with 30 ml of *absolute ethanol* and 3 ml of a 50% w/w solution of *potassium hydroxide*. Boil gently under a reflux condenser in a current of *oxygen-free nitrogen* for 30 minutes, cool rapidly and add 30 ml of *water*. Transfer the hydrolysate to a separating funnel using three 50-ml quantities of *ether* and extract the vitamin A by shaking for 1 minute. After complete separation discard the aqueous layer and wash the extract with four 50-ml quantities of *water*, mixing very cautiously during the first two washes to avoid the formation of emulsions. Evaporate the separated extract to about 5 ml and remove the remaining solvent in a current of *oxygen-free nitrogen* without the application of heat. Dissolve the residue in sufficient *propan-2-ol R1* to produce a solution containing 9 to 15 Units per ml and measure the *absorbance* at 300, 310, 325 and 334 nm. Determine the wavelength of maximum absorption.

If the wavelength of maximum absorption lies between 323 and 327 nm and the absorbance at 300 nm relative to that at 325 nm does not exceed 0.73, a corrected absorbance is derived from the equation

$$A_{325}(\text{corr.}) = 6.815\,A_{325} - 2.555A_{310} - 4.260A_{334}.$$

Calculate the potency of the preparation in Units per g from the expression

$$A_{325}(1\%, 1\text{ cm}) \times 1830$$

but if the corrected absorbance lies within ±3.0% of the uncorrected absorbance, calculate the potency from the uncorrected absorbance.

If the wavelength of maximum absorption lies outside the range 323 to 327 nm, or if the relative absorbance at 300 nm exceeds 0.73, the unsaponifiable fraction of the preparation must be further purified by chromatography.

***all-trans*-Vitamin A Acetate**

CHARACTERISTICS White to very pale yellow, free-flowing crystals.

Practically insoluble in *water*; very soluble in *chloroform*, in *ethanol (96%)*, in *ether*, in petroleum spirit, in fats and in fixed oils.

LIGHT ABSORPTION *Absorbance* of a 0.0003% w/v solution in *propan-2-ol R1* at 325 nm, not less than 0.4575, in *cyclohexane* at 327.5 nm, not less than 0.4545, and in *absolute ethanol* at 326 nm, not less than 0.4635, Appendix II B.

MELTING POINT 57.0° to 60.0°, Appendix V A.

RELATIVE ABSORBANCES Measure the *absorbance*, Appendix II B, of a 0.0003% w/v solution in *cyclohexane* at 327.5 nm and at the following wavelengths. The relative absorbances, calculated with reference to the absorbance at 327.5 nm, are within the limits stated in Table 8K-2.

TABLE 8K-2

Wavelength nm	Relative absorbance
300	0.545 to 0.565
312.5	0.845 to 0.865
337.5	0.845 to 0.865
345	0.685 to 0.705
360	0.290 to 0.310

L. Residual Solvents

(Ph. Eur. method 2.4.24)

The test is intended for the control of residual solvents in substances that are soluble in water. For substances insoluble or insufficiently soluble in water, the diluent used for the preparation of the sample solution and the static head-space conditions to be employed are given in the individual monograph.

Method

Examine by *gas chromatography* with static head-space injection, Appendix III B.

Sample solution Unless otherwise prescribed, dissolve 0.20 g of the substance being examined in *water* and dilute to 20 ml with the same solvent.

Solvent solution (a) Dissolve 0.50 g each of *acetonitrile* and *chloroform* and 1.0 g each of *benzene, 1,4-dioxan, dichloromethane, pyridine* and *trichloroethylene* in *dimethyl sulphoxide* and dilute to 100 ml with the same solvent. Dilute 1 ml to 100 ml with *water*. Dilute 1 ml of this solution to 50 ml with *water*.

Solvent solution (b) Prepare as for solvent solution (a) but use only the solvent or solvents present in the substance being examined and dilute to give a concentration of 1/20 the limit(s) stated in the monograph.

Blank solution Prepare as described for solvent solution (b) but without the addition of solvent or solvents (used to verify the absence of interfering peaks).

Test solution Introduce 5 ml of the sample solution and 1 ml of the blank solution into an injection vial.

Reference solution Introduce 5 ml of the sample solution and 1 ml of solvent solution (b) into an injection vial.

Close the vials with a tight rubber membrane stopper coated with polytetrafluoroethylene and secure with an aluminium crimped cap. Shake to obtain a homogeneous solution.

The following static head-space injection conditions may be used:

equilibration temperature: 80°,
equilibration time: 60 minutes,
transfer-line temperature: 85°,
carrier gas: *nitrogen for chromatography* or *helium* at an appropriate pressure,
pressurisation time: 30 seconds,
injection volume: 1 ml.

The chromatographic procedure may be carried out using:

System A

(a) a fused-silica capillary or wide-bore column (30 m × 0.32 mm or 0.53 mm) coated on the inner wall with cross-linked 6% polycyanopropylphenylsiloxane and 94% polydimethylsiloxane (film thickness 1.8 µm or 3 µm),
(b) *helium* as the carrier gas, split ratio 1:5 with a linear velocity of about 35 cm per second,
(c) a flame-ionisation detector (or an electron-capture detector may be used, if necessary, for chlorinated solvents),

maintaining the temperature of the column at 40° for 20 minutes, then raising the temperature at a rate of 10° per minute to 240° and maintaining it at 240° for 20 minutes and maintaining the temperature of the injection port at 140° and that of the detector at 250°.

Where there is interference from the matrix, use:

System B

(a) a fused-silica capillary or wide-bore column (30 m × 0.32 mm or 0.53 mm) coated on the inner wall with *polyethyleneglycol 20,000* (film thickness 0.25 µm),
(b) *helium* as the carrier gas, split ratio 1:5 with a linear velocity of about 35 cm per second,
(c) a flame-ionisation detector (or an electron-capture detector may be used, if necessary, for chlorinated solvents),

maintaining the temperature of the column at 50° for 20 minutes, then raising the temperature at a rate of 6° per minute to 165° and maintaining it at 165° for 20 minutes and maintaining the temperature of the injection port at 140° and that of the detector at 250°.

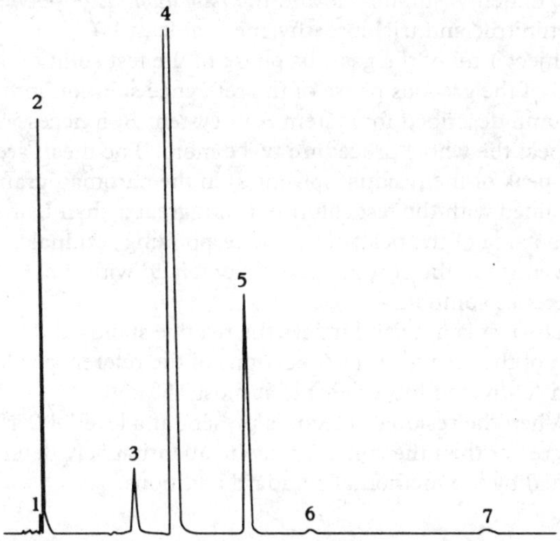

Fig. 8M-2
Chromatogram of solvent solution (a) using System A

1. methylene chloride
2. benzene
3. trichloroethylene
5. chloroform
6. dioxan
7. pyridine
8. acetonitrile

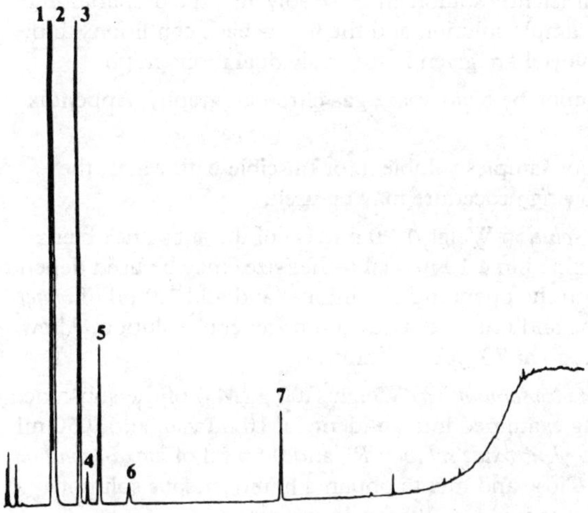

Fig. 8M-1
Chromatogram of solvent solution (a) using System B

1. acetonitrile
2. methylene chloride
3. chloroform
5. trichloroethylene
6. dioxan
7. pyridine
8.benzene

Inject 1 ml of the gaseous phase of solvent solution (a) on to the column described in system A or in system B and record the chromatogram under such conditions that the *signal-to-noise ratio* for chloroform can be measured; the signal-to-noise ratio must be at least 3. The system is not suitable unless in the chromatogram obtained using system A (see Fig. 8M-1) the solvents are eluted in the following order: acetonitrile, methylene chloride (dichloromethane), chloroform, benzene, trichloroethylene, 1,4-dioxan, pyridine and dimethyl sulphoxide and the *resolution factor* between acetonitrile and methylene chloride (dichloromethane) is at least 1.0, or, using system B (see Fig. **xx**b) the solvents elute in the following order: methylene chloride (dichloromethane), benzene, trichloroethylene, acetonitrile, chloroform, 1,4-dioxan, pyridine and dimethyl sulphoxide and the *resolution factor* between acetonitrile and trichloroethylene is at least 1.0.

Inject 1 ml of the gaseous phase of the test solution and 1 ml of the gaseous phase of the reference solution into the column described for system A or system B, if necessary. Repeat the whole procedure twice more. The mean area of the peak of the residual solvent(s) in the chromatograms obtained with the test solution is not greater than half the mean area of the peak of the corresponding residual solvent(s) in the chromatograms obtained with the reference solution.

The test is not valid unless the relative standard deviation of the area for three injections of the reference solution (corrected for weight) is at most 15%.

When the residual solvent is present at a level of 0.1% or greater then the content may be quantitatively determined by the method of standard additions.

M. Residual Ethylene Oxide and Dioxan

(Ph. Eur. method 2.4.25)

The test is intended for the determination of residual ethylene oxide and dioxan in samples soluble in water or dimethylacetamide. For substances that are insoluble or insufficiently soluble in these solvents, the preparation of the sample solution and the head-space conditions to be employed are given in the individual monograph.

Examine by head-space gas chromatography, Appendix III B.

A. For samples soluble in or miscible with water, the following procedure may be used.

Test solution Weigh 1.00 g (M_T) of the substance being examined in a 10 ml vial (other sizes may be used depending on the operating conditions) and add 1.0 ml of *water*. Close and mix to obtain a homogeneous solution. Allow to stand at 70° for 45 minutes.

Reference solution (a) Weigh 1.00 g (M_R) of the substance being examined into an identical 10 ml vial, add 0.50 ml of *ethylene oxide solution R3* and 0.50 ml of *dioxan solution R1*. Close and mix to obtain a homogeneous solution. Allow to stand at 70° for 45 minutes.

Reference solution (b) To 0.50 ml of *ethylene oxide solution R3* in a 10 ml vial add 0.1 ml of a freshly prepared 0.001% w/v solution of *acetaldehyde* and 0.1 ml of *dioxan solution R1*. Close and mix to obtain a homogeneous solution. Allow to stand at 70° for 45 minutes.

B. For samples soluble in or miscible with dimethylacetamide, the following procedure may be used.

Test solution Weigh 1.00 g (M_T) of the substance being examined in a 10 ml vial (other sizes may be used depending on the operating conditions) and add 1.0 ml of *dimethylacetamide R* and 0.20 ml of *water*. Close and mix to obtain a homogeneous solution. Allow to stand at 90° for 45 minutes.

Reference solution (a) Weigh 1.00 g (M_R) of the substance being examined into a 10 ml vial, add 1.0 ml of *dimethylacetamide*, 0.10 ml of *dioxan solution* and 0.10 ml of *ethylene oxide solution R2*. Close and mix to obtain a homogeneous solution. Allow to stand at 90° for 45 minutes.

Reference solution (b) To 0.10 ml of *ethylene oxide solution R2* in a 10 ml vial, add 0.1 ml of a freshly prepared 0.001% w/v solution of *acetaldehyde* and 0.10 ml of *dioxan solution.* Close and mix to obtain a homogeneous solution

The following static head-space injection conditions may be used:

- equilibration temperature: 70° (90° for solutions in dimethylacetamide),
- equilibration time: 45 minutes,
- transfer-line temperature: 75° (150° for solutions in dimethylacetamide),
- carrier gas: *helium for chromatography,*
- pressurisation time: 1 minute,
- injection time: 12 seconds.

The chromatographic procedure may be carried out using:

- a capillary glass or quartz column 30 m long and 0.32 mm in internal diameter the inner surface of which is coated with a 1.0 µm thick layer of *polydimethylsiloxane,*
- *helium for chromatography* or *nitrogen for chromatography* as the carrier gas with a linear velocity of about 20 cm per second and a split ratio 1:20,
- a flame-ionisation detector,

maintaining the temperature of the column at 50° for 5 minutes, then raising the temperature at a rate of 5° per minute to 180° and then raising the temperature at a rate of 30° per minute to 230° and maintaining at 230° for 5 minutes; maintaining the temperature of the injection port at 150° and that of the detector at 250°.

Inject a suitable volume, for example 1.0 ml, of the gaseous phase of reference solution (b). Adjust the sensitivity of the system so that the heights of the peaks due to ethylene oxide and acetaldehyde in the chromatogram obtained are at least 15% of the full scale of the recorder. The test is not valid unless the *resolution factor* between the peaks corresponding to acetaldehyde and ethylene oxide is at least 2.0 and the peak of ethylene oxide is detected with a *signal-to-noise ratio* of at least five.

Inject separately suitable volumes, for example 1.0 ml (or the same volume used for reference solution (b)), of the gaseous phases of the test solution and reference solution (a). Repeat the procedure twice more. The mean areas of the ethylene oxide and dioxan peaks in the chromatogram obtained with the test solution are not greater than half the mean area of the corresponding peak in the chromatogram obtained with reference solution (a) (1 ppm of ethylene oxide and 50 ppm of dioxan).

Verification of precision

For each pair of injections, calculate for ethylene oxide and for dioxan the difference in area between the peaks obtained with the test solution and reference solution (a). The test is not valid unless the relative standard deviation of the three values obtained for ethylene oxide is not greater than 15% and the relative standard deviation of the three values obtained for dioxan is not greater than 10%. If the weighings used for the test solution and reference solution differ from 1.00 g by more than 0.5%, the appropriate corrections must be made.

The content of ethylene oxide in parts per million is calculated from the expression:

$$\frac{A_T \times C}{(A_R \times M_T) - (A_T \times M_R)}$$

where A_T = area of the peak corresponding to ethylene oxide in the chromatogram obtained with the test solution,

A_R = area of the peak corresponding to ethylene oxide in the chromatogram obtained with reference solution (a),

M_T = mass of the substance to be examined in the test solution in grams,

M_R = mass of the substance to be examined in the reference solution in grams,

C = the amount of ethylene oxide added to reference solution (a) in micrograms.

The content of dioxan in parts per million is calculated from the expression:

$$\frac{D_T \times C}{(D_R \times M_T) - (D_T \times M_R)}$$

where D_T = area of the peak corresponding to dioxan in the chromatogram obtained with the test solution,

D_R = area of the peak corresponding to dioxan in the chromatogram obtained with reference solution (a),

C = the amount of dioxan added to reference solution (a) in micrograms.

Appendix IX

A. Determination of Sulphated Ash

Use Method I unless otherwise directed.

Method I *(No Ph. Eur. method)*

Heat a platinum dish to redness for 10 minutes, allow to cool in a desiccator and weigh. Unless otherwise specified in the monograph, place 1 g of the substance being examined in the dish, moisten with *sulphuric acid*, ignite gently, again moisten with *sulphuric acid* and ignite at about 800°. Cool, weigh again, ignite for 15 minutes and repeat this procedure until two successive weighings do not differ by more than 0.5 mg.

Method II *(Ph. Eur. method 2.4.14)*

Heat a silica or platinum crucible to redness for 30 minutes, allow to cool in a desiccator and weigh. Place a suitable quantity of the substance being examined, in the crucible, add 2 ml of 1M *sulphuric acid* and heat, first on a water bath, then cautiously over a flame and then progressively to about 600°. Continue incineration until all black particles have disappeared and then allow to cool. Add a few drops of 1M *sulphuric acid*, incinerate as before and allow to cool. Add a few drops of a 15.8% w/v solution of *ammonium carbonate*, evaporate to dryness and incinerate carefully. Allow to cool, weigh, incinerate for 15 minutes and repeat this procedure to constant weight.

B. Determination of Sulphur Dioxide

Use Method II for monographs of the European Pharmacopoeia and Method I for all other monographs.

Method I *(No Ph. Eur. method)*

Apparatus A round-bottomed flask of 1000- to 1500-ml capacity is fitted with a water-cooled reflux condenser the upper end of which is connected to two absorption tubes in series. The flask is fitted with a gas inlet tube which reaches nearly to the bottom of the flask. Each absorption tube contains 10 ml of *hydrogen peroxide solution (20 vol)* previously neutralised with 0.1M *sodium hydroxide VS* using *bromophenol blue solution* as indicator.

Method Place in the flask 500 ml of *water* and 20 ml of *hydrochloric acid.* Pass through the flask a steady current of *nitrogen* or *carbon dioxide* that has been bubbled through *dilute sodium carbonate solution* and gradually heat the liquid until it boils. Maintain the current of *nitrogen* or *carbon dioxide,* allow the solution to boil for about 10 minutes and cool the flask by gradual immersion in water. Introduce, while momentarily removing the stopper of the flask, a weighed quantity of 50 to 100 g of the substance being examined, heat gently and boil for 45 minutes. Disconnect the absorption tubes before turning off the current of *nitrogen* or *carbon dioxide* and titrate the combined contents with 0.1M *sodium hydroxide VS.* Each ml of 0.1M *sodium hydroxide VS* is equivalent to 3.203 mg of sulphur dioxide.

Repeat the operation without the substance being examined. The solution in the absorption tubes remains neutral.

Method II *(Ph. Eur. method 2.5.29)*

Introduce 150 ml of *water* into the flask (*A*) (see Fig.9B-1) and pass *carbon dioxide* through the whole system for 15 minutes at a rate of 100 ml per minute. Place 10 ml of *dilute hydrogen peroxide solution* neutralised with a 0.1% w/v solution of *bromophenol blue* in *ethanol (20% v/v)* in the test-tube (*D*). Without interrupting the stream of carbon dioxide, remove the funnel (*B*) and introduce through the opening into the flask (*A*) 25.0 g of the substance being examined with the aid of 100 ml of *water.* Add through the funnel 80 ml of *dilute hydrochloric acid* and boil for 1 hour. Open the tap of the funnel and stop the flow of carbon dioxide and also the heating and the cooling water. Transfer the contents of the test-tube with the aid of a little *water* to a 200 ml wide-necked, conical flask. Heat on a water-bath for 15 minutes and allow to cool. Add 0.1 ml of 0.1 w/v solution of *bromophenol blue* in *alcohol (20% v/v)* and titrate with 0.1M *sodium hydroxide VS* until the colour changes from yellow to violet-blue. Calculate the content of sulphur dioxide in parts per million from the expression 128*a* where *a* is the volume of 0.1M *sodium hydroxide VS* used.

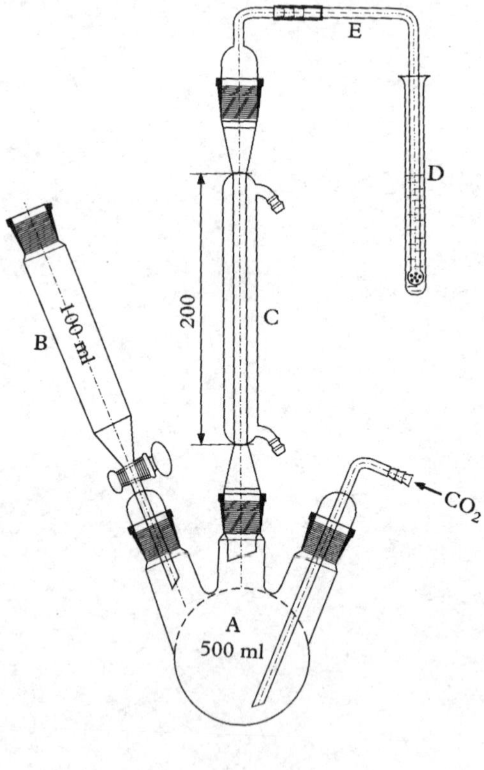

Fig.9B-1

Apparatus for the Determination of Sulphur Dioxide
Dimensions in millimetres

C. Determination of Water

Use Method IA unless otherwise directed.

Method I *(Ph. Eur. method 2.5.12)*

Apparatus The apparatus consists of a titration vessel of about 60-ml capacity fitted with two platinum electrodes, a nitrogen inlet tube, a stopper which accommodates the burette tip and a vent tube protected by a suitable desiccant. The substance being examined is introduced through an inlet tube or side arm which can be closed by a ground-glass stopper. Stirring is effected magnetically or by means of a stream of dried nitrogen passed through the solution during the titration. The end point is determined by amperometry. A suitable circuit consists of a potentiometer of about 2000 ohms resistance connected across a 1.5 volt battery to supply a variable potential. The potential is adjusted so that a low initial current passes through the platinum electrodes connected in series with a microammeter. After addition of the reagent the microammeter shows a deflection but returns immediately to its original position. At the end of the reaction a deflection is obtained which persists for not less than 30 seconds.

The reagents and solutions used must be kept anhydrous and precautions must be taken throughout to prevent exposure to atmospheric moisture. *Karl Fischer reagent VS* (*iodosulphurous reagent R*) should be protected from light and preferably stored in a bottle fitted with an automatic burette. Its water-equivalent is determined before use.

The composition of commercially available reagents may differ from that of *Karl Fischer reagent VS* by the replacement of pyridine with various other basic compounds. The use of these reagents must be validated in order to verify in each case the stoichiometry and the absence of incompatibility between the substance being examined and the reagent.

Method IA Unless otherwise prescribed, add about 20 ml of *anhydrous methanol* or the solvent prescribed in the monograph to the titration vessel and titrate to the amperometric end point with *Karl Fischer reagent VS*. Quickly add the prescribed amount of the substance being examined, stir for 1 minute and again titrate to the amperometric end point with *Karl Fischer reagent VS*.

Method IB Unless otherwise prescribed, add about 10 ml of *anhydrous methanol* or the solvent prescribed in the monograph to the titration vessel and titrate to the amperometric end point with *Karl Fischer reagent VS*. Quickly add the prescribed amount of the substance being examined in a suitable state of division followed by sufficient *Karl Fischer reagent VS*, accurately measured, to give an excess of about 1 ml, or the volume prescribed in the monograph. Unless otherwise prescribed, allow the closed vessel to stand for 1 minute, protected from light, stirring occasionally. Unless otherwise directed, titrate the excess of *Karl Fischer reagent VS* with *anhydrous methanol* to which has been added an accurately measured amount of *water* equivalent to about 0.25% w/v, until the low initial current is attained.

Method II *(Ph. Eur. method 2.2.13)*

Apparatus The apparatus (Fig. 9C-1) consists of a glass flask (A) connected by a tube (D) to a cylindrical tube (B) fitted with a graduated receiving tube (E) and reflux condenser (C). The receiving tube (E) is graduated in 0.1-ml increments. The source of heat is preferably an electric heater with rheostat control or an oil bath. The upper portion of the flask and the connecting tube may be insulated.

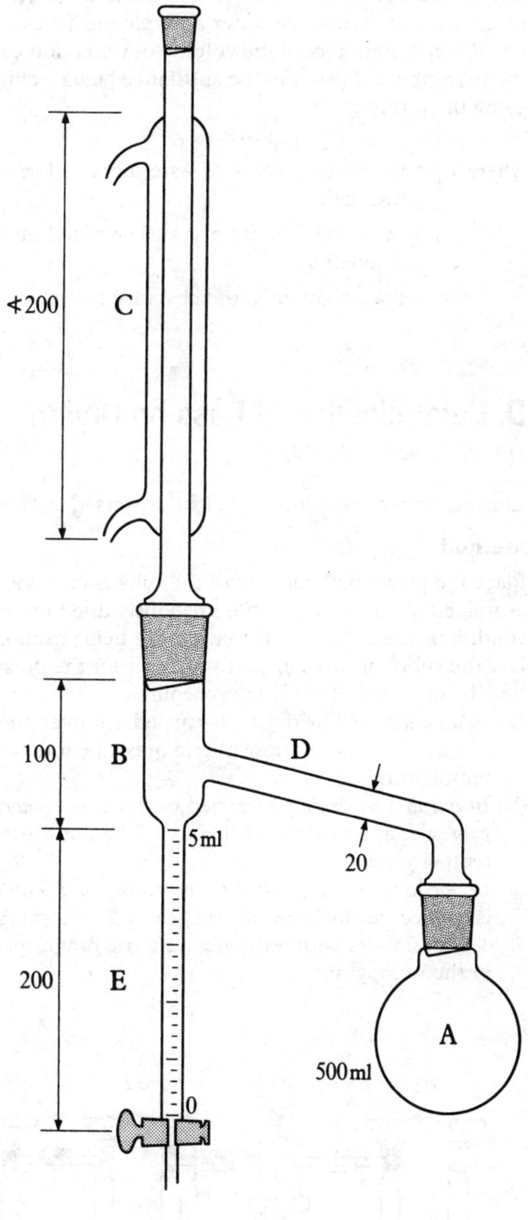

Fig. 9C-1
Apparatus for the Determination of Water (Method II)
Dimensions in mm unless otherwise stated

Method Clean the receiving tube and the condenser of the apparatus, thoroughly rinse with *water* and dry. Add 200 ml of *toluene* and about 2 ml of *water* to the dry flask. Distil for 2 hours, allow to cool for about 30 minutes and read the water volume to an accuracy of 0.05 ml. Add to the flask a quantity of the substance being examined, weighed with an accuracy of 1%, expected to give about 2 to 3 ml of water. If the substance is of a pasty consistence, weigh it in a boat of metal foil. Add a few pieces of porous material and heat the flask gently for 15 minutes. When the toluene begins to boil, distil at a rate of 2 drops per second until most of the water has distilled over and then increase the rate of distillation to about 4 drops per second. When the water has completely distilled, rinse the inside of the condenser tube with *toluene*. Continue the distillation for 5 minutes, remove from the heat, allow the receiving tube to cool to room temperature and dislodge any droplets of water that adhere to the walls of the receiving tube. When the water and toluene have completely separated, record the volume of water and calculate the percentage of water in the substance being examined using the formula

$$100(n_2-n_1)/w$$

where n_1 = the number of ml of water obtained in the first distillation,

n_2 = the number of ml of water obtained in the two distillations,

w = the weight, in g, of substance taken.

D. Determination of Loss on Drying

(Ph. Eur. method 2.2.32)

Loss on drying is the loss of weight expressed as % w/w.

Method

Place the prescribed quantity of the substance being examined in a weighing bottle previously dried under the conditions prescribed for the substance being examined. Dry the substance to constant weight or for the prescribed time by one of the following procedures.

(a) *In a desiccator* The drying is carried out over *phosphorus pentoxide* at atmospheric pressure and at room temperature.

(b) *In vacuo* The drying is carried out over *phosphorus pentoxide* at a pressure of 1.5 to 2.5 kPa at room temperature.

(c) *In vacuo within a specified temperature range* The drying is carried out over *phosphorus pentoxide* at a pressure of 1.5 to 2.5 kPa within the temperature range specified in the monograph.

(d) *In an oven within a specified temperature range* The drying is carried out in an oven within the temperature range specified in the monograph.

(e) *Under high vacuum* The drying is carried out over *phosphorus pentoxide* at a pressure not exceeding 0.1 kPa at the temperature prescribed in the monograph.

If other conditions are prescribed, the procedure to be used is described in full in the individual monograph.

E. Limit Test for Carbon Monoxide in Medicinal Gases

(Ph. Eur. method 2.5.25)

Method I

Apparatus The apparatus consists of the following parts connected in series (see Fig. 9E-1):

(*a*) a U-tube containing *anhydrous silica gel* impregnated with *chromium(VI) oxide*,

(*b*) a wash bottle containing 100 ml of a 40% w/v solution of *potassium hydroxide*,

(*c*) a U-tube containing pellets of *potassium hydroxide*,

(*d*) a U-tube containing *phosphorus pentoxide* dispersed on previously granulated fused pumice,

(*e*) a U-tube containing 30 g of *recrystallised iodine pentoxide* in granules, previously dried at 200° and maintained at a temperature of 120° throughout the test. The iodine pentoxide is packed in the tube in 1-cm columns separated by 1-cm columns of glass wool to give an effective length of 5 cm,

(*f*) a reaction tube containing 2.0 ml of *potassium iodide solution* and 0.15 ml of *starch solution*.

Method Flush the apparatus with 5.0 litres of *argon* and, if necessary, discharge any blue colour in the iodide solution by adding the smallest necessary quantity of freshly prepared 0.002M *sodium thiosulphate VS*. Continue flushing until not more than 0.045 ml of 0.002M *sodium thiosulphate VS* is required after passing 5.0 litres of *argon*.

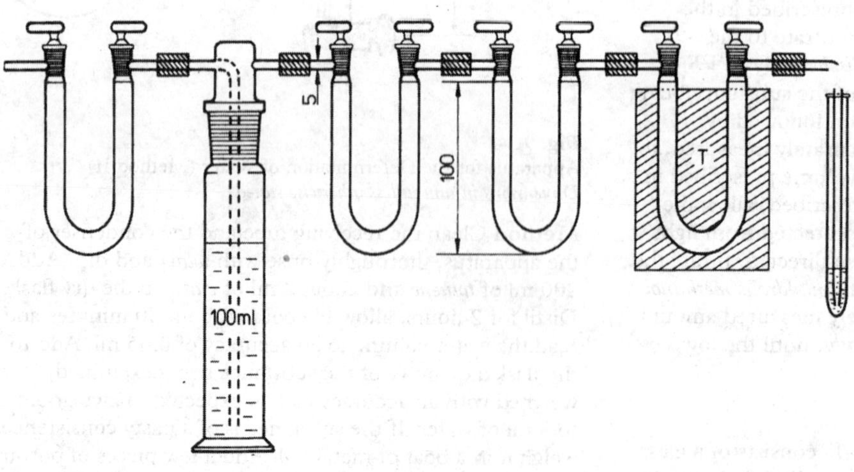

Fig. 9E-1
Apparatus for the determination of carbon monoxide in medicinal gases
Dimensions in mm

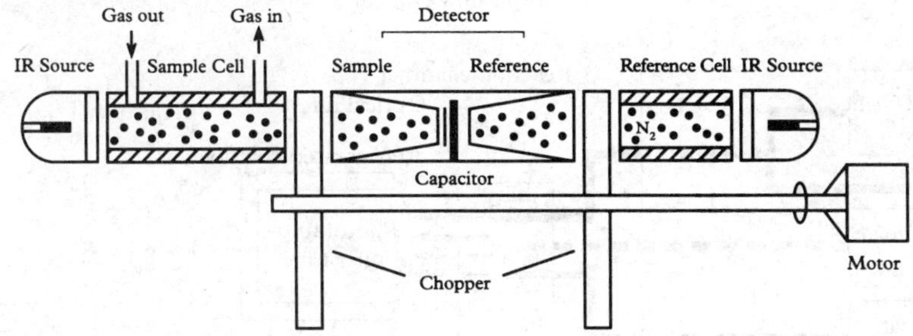

Fig. 9E-2
Infrared analyser
Dimensions in mm

Pass the gas being examined from the cylinder through the apparatus, using the volume and the rate of flow prescribed in the monograph. Flush the last traces of liberated iodine into the reaction tube by passing through the apparatus 1.0 litre of *argon*. Titrate the liberated iodine with 0.002M *sodium thiosulphate VS*.

Carry out a blank determination under the same conditions using the volume of argon prescribed in the monograph. The difference between the volumes of 0.002M *sodium thiosulphate VS* used in the two titrations is not greater than the limit prescribed in the monograph.

Method II

Carbon monoxide in medicinal gases may be determined using an infrared analyser (see Fig. 9E-2). The analyser includes a system generating two identical infrared beams consisting of coils electrically heated to low red heat and equipped with reflectors. One beam crosses a sample cell and the other beam crosses a reference cell. The sample cell receives a stream of the gas being analysed and the reference cell contains *nitrogen R1*. The two chambers of the detector are filled with *carbon monoxide* and the radiation is automatically received selectively. The absorption of this radiation produces heat and differential expansion of the gas in the two chambers, owing to the absorption of some of the emitted radiation by the carbon monoxide in the gas being examined. The pressure difference between the two chambers of the detector causes distension of the metal diaphragm that separates them. This diaphragm is part of a capacitor, the capacitance of which varies with the pressure difference, which itself depends on the carbon monoxide content in the gas being examined. Since the infrared beams are periodically blocked by a rotating chopper, the electric signal is frequency modulated.

F. Determination of Carbon Dioxide in Medicinal Gases

(Ph. Eur. method 2.5.24)

Carbon dioxide in medicinal gases may be determined using an infrared analyser (see Fig. 9E-2). The analyser includes a system generating two identical infrared beams consisting of coils electrically heated to low red heat and equipped with reflectors. One beam crosses a sample cell and the other beam crosses a reference cell. The sample cell receives a stream of the gas being analysed and the reference cell contains *nitrogen R1*. The two chambers of the detector are filled with *carbon dioxide R1* and the radiation is automatically received selectively. The absorption of this radiation produces heat and differential expansion of the gas in the two chambers, owing to the absorption of some of the emitted radiation by the carbon dioxide in the gas being examined. The pressure difference between the two chambers of the detector causes distension of the metal diaphragm that separates them. This diaphragm is part of a capacitor, the capacitance of which varies with the pressure difference, which itself depends on the carbon dioxide content in the gas being examined. Since the infrared beams are periodically blocked by a rotating chopper, the electric signal is frequency modulated.

G. Determination of Nitrogen Monoxide and Nitrogen Dioxide in Medicinal Gases

(Ph. Eur. method 2.5.26)

Nitrogen monoxide and nitrogen dioxide in medicinal gases may be determined using a chemiluminescence analyser (see Fig. 9G-1). The apparatus consists of the following parts:

(*a*) a device for filtering, checking and controlling the flow of the gas being examined,

(*b*) a converter that reduces nitrogen dioxide to nitrogen monoxide, to determine the combined content of nitrogen monoxide and nitrogen dioxide; it consists of a stainless steel, glass or quartz oven maintained at a temperature not exceeding 550°,

(*c*) a controlled flow-rate ozone generator; the ozone is produced by high-voltage electric discharges across two electrodes; the ozone generator is supplied with pure oxygen or with dehydrated ambient air and the concentration of ozone obtained must greatly exceed the maximum content of any detectable nitrogen oxides,

(*d*) a chamber in which nitrogen monoxide and ozone can react,

(*e*) a system for detecting light radiation emitted at a wavelength of 1.2 µm, consisting of a selective optical filter and a photomultiplier tube.

H. Determination of Oxygen in Medicinal Gases

(Ph. Eur. method 2.2.27)

Oxygen in medicinal gases may be determined using a paramagnetic analyser. The principle of the method is based on the high paramagnetic sensitivity of the oxygen molecule. Oxygen exerts a strong interaction on magnetic fields, which is measured electronically, amplified and

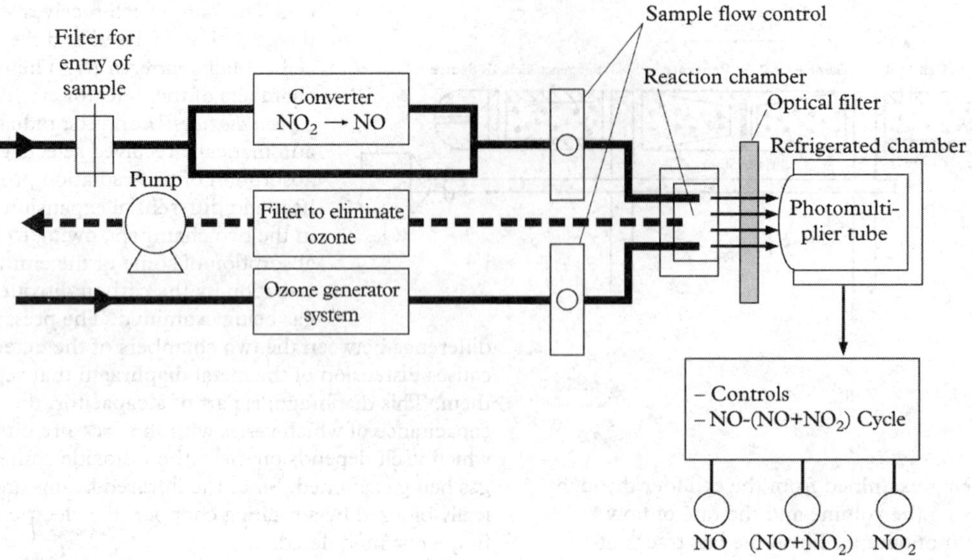

Fig.9G-
Chemiluminescence analyser

converted to a reading of oxygen concentration. The measurement of oxygen concentration is dependent upon the pressure and temperature and, if the analyser is not automatically compensated for variations in temperature and pressure, it must be calibrated immediately before use. As the paramagnetic effect of oxygen is linear, the instrument must have a suitable range with a readability of 0.1% or better.

Calibration of the instrument Make the setting in the following manner. Set the zero by passing *nitrogen R1* through the instrument at a suitable flow rate until a constant reading is obtained. It should be set to zero according to the manufacturer's instructions. Set the appropriate limit by passing air (20.9% v/v O_2) through the instrument until a constant reading is obtained. The limit should be set to 20.9% v/v in accordance with the manufacturer's instructions.

Assay Pass the gas through the instrument at a suitable flow rate until a suitable reading is obtained.

J. Determination of Water in Medicinal Gases

(Ph. Eur. method 2.5.28)

Water in medicinal gases may be determined using an electrolytic hygrometer, described below.

The measuring cell consists of a thin film of phosphorus pentoxide between two coiled platinum wires which act as electrodes. The water vapour in the gas being examined is absorbed by the phosphorus pentoxide, which is transformed to phosphoric acid, an electrical conductor. A continuous voltage applied across the electrodes produces electrolysis of the water and the regeneration of the phosphorus pentoxide. The resulting electric current, which is proportional to the water content in the gas being examined, is measured. This system is self-calibrating since it obeys Faraday's law.

Take a sample of the gas being examined. Allow the gas to stabilise at room temperature. Purge the cell continuously until a stable reading is obtained. Measure the water content in the gas being examined, making sure that the temperature is constant throughout the device used to introduce the gas into the apparatus.

K. Gas Detector Tubes

(Ph. Eur. text 2.1.6)

Gas detector tubes are cylindrical, sealed tubes consisting of an inert transparent material and constructed to allow the passage of gas. They contain reagents adsorbed onto inert substrates that are suitable for the visualisation of the substance to be detected and, if necessary, they also contain preliminary layers and/or adsorbent filters to eliminate substances that interfere with the substance to be detected. The layer of indicator contains either a single reagent for the detection of a given impurity or several reagents for the detection of several substances (monolayer tube or multilayer tube).

The test is carried out by passing the required volume of the gas to be examined through the indicator tube. The length of the coloured layer or the intensity of a colour change on a graduated scale gives an indication of the impurities present.

The calibration of the detector tubes is verified according to the instructions of the manufacturer.

Operating conditions. Examine according to the instructions of the manufacturer or proceed as follows:

The gas supply is connected to a suitable pressure regulator and needle valve. Connect the flexible tubing fitted with a Y piece to the valve and adjust the flow of gas to be examined to purge the tubing to an appropriate flow (see Fig. 9K-1). Prepare the indicator tube and fit to the metering pump following the manufacturer's instructions. Connect the open end of the indicator tube to the short leg of the tubing and operate the pump by the appropriate number of strokes to pass a suitable volume of gas to be examined through the tube. Read the value corresponding to the length of the coloured layer or the intensity of the colour on the graduated scale. If a negative result is achieved, indicator tubes can be verified with a calibration gas containing the appropriate impurity. For the verification of the oil tube, use another tube from the same batch.

Carbon dioxide detector tube Sealed glass tube containing adsorbent filters and suitable supports for hydrazine and crystal violet indicators. The minimum value indicated is 100 ppm with a relative standard deviation of at most ± 15 per cent.

Sulphur dioxide detector tube Sealed glass tube containing adsorbent filters and suitable supports for the iodine and starch indicator. The minimum value indicated is 0.5 ppm with a relative standard deviation of at most ±15 per cent.

Oil detector tube Sealed glass tube containing adsorbent filters and a suitable support for the sulphuric acid indicator. The minimum value indicated is 0.1 mg/m^3 with a relative standard deviation of at most ± 30 per cent.

Nitrogen monoxide and nitrogen dioxide detector tube Sealed glass tube containing adsorbent filters and suitable supports for an oxidising layer Cr(VI) salt and the diphenylbenzidine indicator. The minimum value indicated is 0.5 ppm with a relative standard deviation of at most ±15 per cent.

Carbon monoxide detector tube Sealed glass tube containing adsorbent filters and suitable supports for di-iodine pentoxide, selenium dioxide and fuming sulphuric acid indicators. The minimum value indicated is 5 ppm or less, with a relative standard deviation of at most ±15 per cent.

Hydrogen sulphide detector tube Sealed glass tube containing adsorbent filters and suitable supports for an appropriate lead salt indicator. The minimum value indicated is 1 ppm or less, with a relative standard deviation of at most ±10 per cent.

Water vapour detector tube Sealed glass tube containing adsorbent filters and suitable supports for the magnesium perchlorate indicator. The minimum value indicated is 60 ppm or less, with a relative standard deviation of at most ±20 per cent.

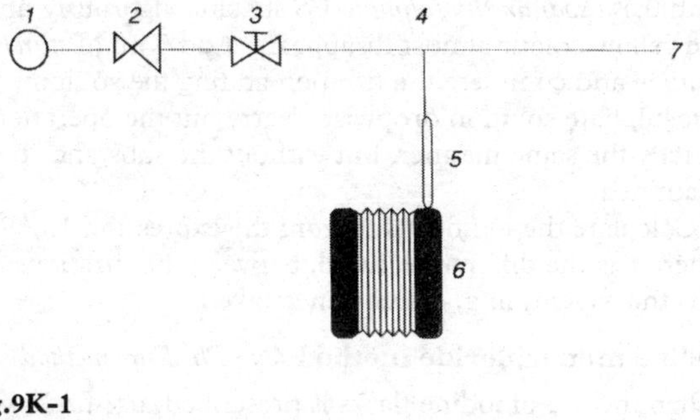

Fig.9K-1
Apparatus for gas detector tubes

1. gas supply
2. pressure regulator
3. needle valve
4. "Y" piece
5. indicator tube
6. indicator tube pump
7. end open to atmosphere

Appendix X

A. Acetyl Value

(No Ph. Eur. method)

The acetyl value of a substance is the number of mg of potassium hydroxide required to neutralise the acetic acid liberated by the hydrolysis of 1 g of the acetylated substance.

Determine the *saponification value*, Appendix X G.

Acetylate by the following method. To 10 g in a 200-ml Kjeldahl flask add 20 ml of *acetic anhydride*. Support the flask on a sheet of heat resistant material in which a hole about 4 cm in diameter has been cut and heat with a small, naked flame, not more than 25 mm in height and which does not impinge on the bottom of the flask. Boil gently under a reflux air condenser for 2 hours, allow to cool, pour into 600 ml of *water* contained in a large beaker, add 0.2 g of *pumice powder* and boil for 30 minutes. Cool, transfer to a separating funnel and discard the lower layer. Wash the acetylated product with three or more 50-ml quantities of a warm, saturated solution of *sodium chloride* until the washings are no longer acidic to *litmus paper*. Finally shake with 20 ml of warm *water* and remove the aqueous layer as completely as possible. Pour the acetylated substance into a small dish, add 1 g of powdered *anhydrous sodium sulphate*, stir thoroughly and filter through a dry, pleated filter paper. Determine the *saponification value* of the acetylated substance.

Calculate the acetyl value from the expression $1335(b-a)/(1335-a)$ where a is the saponification value of the substance and b is the saponification value of the acetylated substance.

B. Acid Value

(Ph. Eur. method 2.5.1)

The acid value is the number of mg of potassium hydroxide required to neutralise the free acid in 1 g of the substance when determined by the following method, unless otherwise specified in the monograph.

Unless otherwise specified in the monograph weigh 10 g of the substance being examined and add 50 ml of a mixture of equal volumes of *ethanol (96%)* and *ether* that has been neutralised with 0.1M *potassium hydroxide VS* using 0.5 ml of *phenolphthalein solution R1* as indicator. When the substance has completely dissolved, titrate with 0.1M *potassium hydroxide VS*, shaking constantly until a pink colour that persists for at least 15 seconds is produced.

Calculate the acid value from the expression $5.610v/w$, where v is the volume, in ml, of potassium hydroxide solution required and w is the weight, in g, of substance taken.

C. Ester Value

(Ph. Eur. method 2.5.2)

The ester value is the number of mg of potassium hydroxide required to saponify the esters present in 1 g of the substance.

Determine the *acid value*, Appendix X B, of the substance being examined and the *saponification value*, Appendix X G, using Method II.

Calculate the ester value by subtracting the acid value from the saponification value.

D. Hydroxyl Value

(Ph. Eur. method 2.5.3)

The hydroxyl value of a substance is the number of mg of potassium hydroxide required to neutralise the acid combined by acylation in 1 g of the substance.

Use Method A unless otherwise specified in the monograph.

Method A

Unless otherwise specified in the monograph place the quantity of the substance being examined prescribed in the Table in a 150-ml acetylation flask fitted with an air condenser and add the corresponding volume of *acetic anhydride solution R1*. Heat for 1 hour in a water bath, maintaining the level of the water about 2.5 cm above the level of the liquid in the flask throughout. Remove the flask and condenser, allow to cool and add 5 ml of *water* through the top of the condenser; if this causes cloudiness, add sufficient *pyridine* to produce a clear liquid, recording the volume added. Shake the flask, replace in the water bath for 10 minutes, remove and allow to cool. Rinse the condenser and the walls of the flask with 5 ml of *ethanol (96%)*, previously neutralised to *phenolphthalein solution R1*. Titrate with 0.5M *ethanolic potassium hydroxide VS* using 0.2 ml of *phenolphthalein solution R1* as indicator. Repeat the operation without the substance being examined.

Calculate the hydroxyl value from the expression $a + 28.05v/w$ where v is the difference, in ml, between the titrations, a is the acid value and w is the weight, in g, of the substance taken.

Presumed hydroxyl value	Quantity of substance g	Volume of *acetic anhydride solution R1* ml
10 to 100	2.0	5.0
100 to 150	1.5	5.0
150 to 200	1.0	5.0
200 to 250	0.75	5.0
250 to 300	0.60 or 1.20	5.0 or 10.0
300 to 350	1.0	10.0
350 to 700	0.75	15.0
700 to 950	0.5	15.0

Method B

To the specified quantity of the substance being examined in a perfectly dry 5-ml conical flask add 2 ml of *propionic anhydride reagent*, close the flask with a ground-glass or suitable plastic stopper and shake gently to dissolve the substance. Allow to stand for 2 hours, unless otherwise prescribed, remove the stopper and transfer the flask and its contents to a 500-ml wide-necked conical flask containing 25.0 ml of a 0.9% w/v solution of *aniline* in *cyclohexane* and 30 ml of *glacial acetic acid*, swirl, allow to stand for 5 minutes and titrate with 0.1M *perchloric acid VS*, using 0.05 ml of *crystal violet solution* as indicator, until the solution is emerald green. Repeat the operation without the substance being examined.

Calculate the hydroxyl value from the expression $5.610v/w$ where v is the difference, in ml, between the titrations and w is the weight, in g, of substance taken.

Determine the water content (A%) of the substance, Appendix IX C. Calculate the corrected hydroxyl value from the expression (hydroxyl value $-$ $31.1A$).

E. Iodine Value

The iodine value of a substance is the weight of iodine absorbed by 100 parts by weight of the substance when determined by one of the following methods.

Methods

Iodine bromide method *(Ph. Eur. method 2.5.4)*

Unless otherwise specified in the individual monograph, use the following quantity of the substance being examined:

presumed iodine value less than 20	1.0 g
presumed iodine value 20 to 60	0.25 to 0.5 g
presumed iodine value 60 to 100	0.15 to 0.25 g
presumed iodine value more than 100	0.10 to 0.15 g.

Dissolve the specified quantity in 15 ml of *chloroform* in an iodine flask fitted with a ground-glass stopper which is dry or has been rinsed with *glacial acetic acid*, unless otherwise specified in the monograph. Add slowly 25 ml of *iodine bromide solution*, insert the stopper and allow to stand in the dark for 30 minutes, unless otherwise specified in the monograph, shaking frequently. Add 10 ml of a 10% w/v solution of *potassium iodide* and 100 ml of *water* and titrate with 0.1M *sodium thiosulphate VS* shaking vigorously until the yellow colour almost disappears. Add 5 ml of *starch solution* and complete the titration adding the sodium thiosulphate solution dropwise. Carry out the operation in exactly the same manner, but without the substance being examined.

Calculate the iodine value from the expression $1.269v/w$ where v is the difference, in ml, between the titrations and w is the weight, in g, of substance taken.

Iodine monochloride method *(No Ph. Eur. method)*

When the use of iodine flasks is prescribed, use flasks with a nominal capacity of 250 ml and complying with British Standard 2735:1956 (Specification for iodine flasks), unless otherwise specified.

Dissolve the specified quantity of the substance being examined in 10 ml of *dichloromethane* in a dry iodine flask. Add 20 ml of *iodine monochloride solution*, insert the stopper, previously moistened with *dilute potassium iodide solution*, and allow to stand in the dark at 15° to 25° for 30 minutes. Place 15 ml of *dilute potassium iodide solution* in the top cup, carefully remove the stopper, rinse the stopper and the sides of the flask with 100 ml of *water*, shake and titrate with 0.1M *sodium thiosulphate VS* using *starch mucilage*, added towards the end of the titration, as indicator. At the same time carry out the operation in exactly the same manner, but without the substance being examined. Calculate the iodine value from the expression $1.269v/w$ where v is the difference, in ml, between the titrations and w is the weight, in g, of the substance taken. The approximate weight, in g, of the substance to be taken may be calculated by dividing 20 by the highest expected iodine value. If more than half of the available halogen is absorbed, the test must be repeated, using a smaller quantity of the substance.

F. Peroxide Value

(Ph. Eur. method 2.5.5)

The peroxide value is the number of milli-equivalents of active oxygen that expresses the amount of peroxide contained in 1000 g of the substance when determined by the following method.

To 5 g in a 250-ml glass-stoppered conical flask add 30 ml of a mixture of 30 volumes of *glacial acetic acid* and 20 volumes of *chloroform*, shake until dissolved and add 0.5 ml of *saturated potassium iodide solution*. Shake for exactly 1 minute, add 30 ml of *water* and titrate slowly, shaking continuously, with 0.01M *sodium thiosulphate VS* until the yellow colour almost disappears. Add 5 ml of *starch solution* and continue the titration, shaking vigorously, until the blue colour disappears. Repeat the operation without the substance being examined.

Calculate the peroxide value from the expression $10v/w$ where v is the difference, in ml, between the titrations and w is the weight, in g, of substance taken.

The volume of 0.01M *sodium thiosulphate VS* used in the blank determination must be not greater than 0.1 ml.

G. Saponification Value

The saponification value is the number of mg of potassium hydroxide required to neutralise the free acids and to saponify the esters in 1 g of the substance.

Use Method I unless otherwise specified in the monograph.

Method I *(No Ph. Eur. method)*

Dissolve 35 to 40 g of *potassium hydroxide* in 20 ml of *water* and add sufficient *ethanol (96%)* to produce 1000 ml. Allow to stand overnight and pour off the clear liquid.

Weigh 2 g of the substance into a 200-ml flask, add 25 ml of the ethanolic solution of potassium hydroxide and boil under a reflux condenser for 1 hour, rotating the contents frequently. While the solution is still hot, titrate the excess of alkali with 0.5M *hydrochloric acid VS* using 1 ml of *phenolphthalein solution R1* as indicator. Repeat the operation without the substance being examined.

Calculate the saponification value from the expression $28.05v/w$ where v is the difference, in ml, between the titrations and w is the weight, in g, of substance taken.

Method II *(Ph. Eur. method 2.5.6)*

Unless otherwise specified in the monograph weigh 2 g of the substance into a 250-ml borosilicate-glass flask, add 25 ml of 0.5M *ethanolic potassium hydroxide VS* and a few glass beads and heat under a reflux condenser for 30 minutes, unless otherwise specified. Titrate immediately with 0.5M *hydrochloric acid VS* using 1 ml of *phenolphthalein solution R1* as indicator. Repeat the operation without the substance being examined.

Calculate the saponification value from the expression $28.05v/w$ where v is the difference, in ml, between the titrations and w is the weight, in g, of substance taken.

H. Unsaponifiable Matter

The unsaponifiable matter is the percentage content, w/w, of material not volatile at 100° to 105° that is obtained by extraction with an organic solvent from the saponified substance being examined.

Use Method I unless otherwise specified in the monograph.

Method I *(No Ph. Eur. method)*

To 2.0 to 2.5 g of the substance being examined in a 250-ml flask add 25 ml of 0.5M *ethanolic potassium hydroxide* and boil under a reflux condenser in a water bath for 1 hour, swirling the contents frequently. Wash the contents of the flask into a separating funnel with the aid of 50 ml of *water* and, while the liquid is still slightly warm, extract by shaking vigorously with three 50-ml quantities of *peroxide-free ether*, rinsing the flask with the first quantity of ether. Mix the ether solutions in a separating funnel containing 20 ml of *water*. (If the ether solutions contain solid suspended matter, filter them into the separating funnel through a fat-free filter paper and wash the filter paper with *peroxide-free ether*.) Gently rotate the separating funnel for a few minutes without violent shaking, allow the liquids to separate and discard the aqueous layer. Wash the ether solution by shaking vigorously with two 20-ml quantities of *water* and then treat with three 20-ml quantities of 0.5M *potassium hydroxide*, shaking vigorously on each occasion, each treatment being followed by washing with 20 ml of *water*. Finally wash with successive 20-ml quantities of *water* until the aqueous layer is no longer alkaline to *phenolphthalein solution R1*. Transfer the ether extract to a weighed flask, rinsing the separating funnel with *peroxide-free ether*, distil the ether and add 3 ml of *acetone* to the flask. With the aid of a gentle current of air, remove the solvent completely from the flask, which is almost entirely immersed in boiling water and preferably held obliquely and rotated. Dry to constant weight at a temperature not exceeding 80° and dissolve the contents of the flask in 10 ml of freshly boiled *ethanol (96%)*, previously neutralised to *phenolphthalein solution R1*. Titrate with 0.1M *ethanolic sodium hydroxide VS* using *phenolphthalein solution R1* as indicator.

If the volume of 0.1M *ethanolic sodium hydroxide VS* required does not exceed 0.1 ml, the amount of residue weighed is to be taken as the unsaponifiable matter. Calculate the unsaponifiable matter as a percentage of the substance being examined.

If the volume of 0.1M *ethanolic sodium hydroxide VS* required exceeds 0.1 ml, the amount of residue weighed cannot be taken as the unsaponifiable matter and the test must be repeated.

Method II *(Ph. Eur. method 2.5.7)*

Add 50 ml of 2M *ethanolic potassium hydroxide* to the prescribed quantity of the substance being examined (*w* g) in a 250-ml flask and heat under a reflux condenser on a water bath for 1 hour, swirling frequently. Cool to below 25°, wash the contents of the flask into a separating funnel with the aid of 100 ml of *water* and extract carefully with three 100-ml quantities of *peroxide-free ether*. Mix the ether solutions in a separating funnel containing 40 ml of *water*, shake gently for a few minutes, allow to separate and discard the aqueous layer. Wash the ether solution with two 40-ml quantities of *water* and then with three 40-ml quantities of a 3% w/v solution of *potassium hydroxide*, each treatment being followed by washing with 40 ml of *water*. Finally wash the ether solution with successive 40-ml quantities of *water* until the aqueous layer is no longer alkaline to phenolphthalein. Transfer the ether solution to a weighed flask, washing out the separating funnel with *peroxide-free ether*. Distil off the ether with suitable precautions and add 6 ml of *acetone* to the residue. Remove the solvent in a current of air and dry to constant weight at 100° to 105°. Allow to cool in a desiccator and weigh (*a* g). The percentage content of the unsaponifiable matter is given by the expression $100a/w$.

Dissolve the residue in 20 ml of *ethanol (96%)*, previously neutralised to *phenolphthalein solution*, and titrate with 0.1M *ethanolic sodium hydroxide VS*. If the volume of 0.1M *ethanolic sodium hydroxide VS* exceeds 0.2 ml, the separation of the layers has been incomplete; the amount of residue weighed cannot be taken as the unsaponifiable matter and the test must be repeated.

J. Determination of Cineole

(Ph. Eur. method 2.8.11)

Weigh 3.00 g of the oil, recently dried with *anhydrous sodium sulphate*, into a dry test tube and add 2.10 g of melted o-*cresol*. Place the tube in the apparatus for the *determination of freezing point*, Appendix V B, and allow to cool, stirring continuously. When crystallisation takes place there is a small rise in temperature; note the highest temperature reached (t_1).

Remelt the mixture on a water bath ensuring that the temperature does not exceed t_1 by more than 5° and place the tube in the apparatus maintained at a temperature 5° below t_1. When recrystallisation takes place, or when the temperature of the mixture has fallen 3° below t_1, stir continuously; note the highest temperature at which the mixture freezes (t_2). Repeat the operation until the two highest values obtained for t_2 do not differ by more than 0.2°. If supercooling occurs, induce crystallisation by the addition of a small crystal of a complex consisting of 3.00 g of *cineole* and 2.10 g of melted o-*cresol*. If t_2 is below 27.4°, repeat the determination after the addition of 5.10 g of the complex.

Determine the percentage w/w of cineole corresponding to the freezing point (t_2) from the Table, obtaining intermediate values by interpolation. If 5.10 g of the cineole—*o*-cresol complex was added, calculate the percentage w/w of cineole from the expression $2(A-50)$, where A is the value corresponding to a freezing point of t_2 taken from the Table.

t_2°	cineole % w/w	t_2°	cineole % w/w
24	45.5	40	67.0
25	47.0	41	68.5
26	48.5	42	70.0
27	49.5	43	72.5
28	50.5	44	74.0
29	52.0	45	76.0
30	53.5	46	78.0
31	54.5	47	80.0
32	56.0	48	82.0
33	57.0	49	84.0
34	58.5	50	86.0
35	60.0	51	88.5
36	61.0	52	91.0
37	62.5	53	93.5
38	63.5	54	96.0
39	65.0	55	99.0

K. Determination of Aldehydes

(No Ph. Eur. method)

To 1 g of the oil in a glass-stoppered tube (approximately 150 mm × 25 mm) add 5 ml of *toluene* and 15 ml of *alcoholic hydroxylamine solution*, shake vigorously and titrate immediately with 0.5M *potassium hydroxide in ethanol (60%) VS* until the red colour changes to yellow. Continue shaking and neutralising until the full yellow colour of the indicator is permanent in the lower layer after shaking vigorously for 2 minutes and allowing to separate; the reaction is complete in about 15 minutes. This procedure gives an approximate value for the aldehyde content of the oil.

Repeat this procedure, using as the colour standard for the end point of the titration the titrated liquid of the first determination with the addition of 0.5 ml of 0.5M *potassium hydroxide in ethanol (60%) VS*. Calculate the content of aldehydes from the second determination, using the equivalent given in the monograph.

L. Oxidising Substances

(Ph. Eur. method 2.5.30)

Transfer 4.0 g to a glass-stoppered, 125 ml conical flask and add 50.0 ml of *water*. Insert the stopper and swirl for 5 minutes. Transfer to a glass-stoppered 50 ml centrifuge tube and centrifuge. Transfer 30.0 ml of the clear supernatant liquid to a glass-stoppered 125 ml conical flask. Add 1 ml of *glacial acetic acid* and 0.5 g to 1.0 g of *potassium iodide*. Insert the stopper, swirl, and allow to stand for 25 minutes to 30 minutes in the dark. Add 1 ml of *starch solution* and titrate with 0.002M *sodium thiosulphate VS* until the starch—iodine colour disappears. Carry out a blank determination. Not more than 1.4 ml of 0.002M *sodium thiosulphate VS* is required (0.002%, calculated as H_2O_2). Each ml of 0.002M *sodium thiosulphate VS* is equivalent to 34 µg of oxidising substances, calculated as hydrogen peroxide.

M. Volatile Oils

Fixed oils and resinified volatile oils *(Ph. Eur. method 2.8.7)*

Allow 0.05 ml of the substance being examined to fall onto a filter paper. The substance evaporates completely within 24 hours without leaving a translucent or greasy mark.

Foreign esters *(Ph. Eur. method 2.8.6)*

Heat 1 ml with 3.0 ml of a freshly prepared 10% w/v solution of *potassium hydroxide* in *ethanol (96%)* on a water bath for 2 minutes. No crystals form within 30 minutes, even after cooling.

Odour and taste *(Ph. Eur. method 2.8.8)*

Mix 0.15 ml with 5 ml of *ethanol (90%)* and stir in 10 g of *sucrose*, in powder. The odour and taste are similar to those of the plant or the parts of the plant from which the volatile oil was obtained.

Residue on evaporation *(Ph. Eur. method 2.8.9)*

The residue on evaporation is the percentage by weight of the oil that remains after evaporation when determined by the following method. Unless otherwise specified in the monograph place 5 g of the oil in a heat-resistant glass evaporating dish, which has been weighed after heating on a water bath for 1 hour and cooling in a desiccator; place the evaporating dish over a water bath on a cover with holes 70 mm in diameter and maintain the water level in the water bath so that it is about 50 mm below the cover throughout the test (Fig. 10M-1). Vigorously boil the water in the water bath in a draught-free atmosphere for the time specified in the monograph. Allow the evaporating dish to cool in a desiccator and weigh.

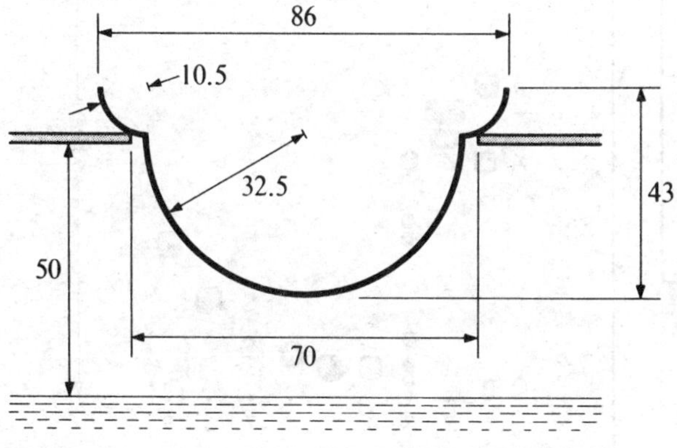

Fig. 10M-1
Apparatus for Determination of Residue on Evaporation of Volatile Oils
Dimensions in mm

Solubility in ethanol *(Ph. Eur. method 2.8.10)*

Weigh 1 ml of the oil with an accuracy of 5 mg into a 25- or 30-ml glass-stoppered cylinder and place in a constant-temperature device maintained at 19.8° to 20.2°. Using a burette with a capacity of not less than 20 ml, add ethanol of the strength specified in the monograph by 0.1-ml increments until solution is complete and then by 0.5-ml increments to 20 ml, shaking frequently and vigorously. Record the volume of the ethanol required to produce a clear solution. Continue to add more of the ethanol in the same manner. If the solution becomes cloudy or opalescent before 20 ml of the ethanol has been added, record the volume at the point at which the cloudiness or opalescence appears and, if appropriate, the volume at which it disappears. If a clear solution is not obtained when 20 ml of the ethanol has been added, repeat the test using the next highest concentration of ethanol.

The following definitions are applied.

Soluble in n *volumes or more of ethanol (*a*%)*: when the clear solution in *n* volumes remains clear when compared with the undiluted oil after further addition of ethanol of the same strength up to a total of 20 volumes of the ethanol.

Soluble in n *volumes of ethanol (*a*%), becoming cloudy when diluted*: when the clear solution in *n* volumes becomes cloudy in n_1 volumes (where n_1 is less than 20) and remains so after further gradual addition of ethanol of the same strength up to a total of 20 volumes of the ethanol.

Soluble in n *volumes of ethanol (*a*%), with cloudiness between* n_1 *and* n_2 *volumes*: when the clear solution in *n* volumes becomes cloudy in n_1 volumes (where n_1 is less than 20) and remains so after further gradual addition of ethanol of the same strength up to a total of n_2 volumes (where n_2 is less than 20) and then becomes clear.

Soluble with opalescence: when the ethanolic solution shows a bluish tinge similar to that produced by mixing 0.5 ml of *silver nitrate solution R2* with 0.05 ml of *nitric acid*, adding 50 ml of a 0.0012% w/v solution of *sodium chloride*, mixing and allowing to stand protected from light for 5 minutes.

Water *(Ph. Eur. method 2.8.5)*

Mix 0.5 ml with 1 ml of *carbon disulphide*. The solution remains clear on standing.

N. Fixed Oils

Alkaline impurities *(Ph. Eur. method 2.4.19)*

Mix 10 ml of recently distilled *acetone* and 0.3 ml of *water* in a test tube, add 0.05 ml of a 0.04% w/v solution of *bromophenol blue* in *ethanol (96%)* and neutralise the solution, if necessary, with 0.01M *hydrochloric acid* or 0.01M *sodium hydroxide*. Add 10 ml of the oil, shake and allow to stand. Not more than 0.1 ml of 0.01M *hydrochloric acid VS* is required to change the colour of the upper layer to yellow.

Antioxidants *(Ph. Eur. method 2.4.20)*

Carry out the method for *thin-layer chromatography*, Appendix III A, using *silica gel G* as the coating substance and drying the plate at 130° for 2 hours before use. Prepare three solutions in the following manner. For solution (1) dilute 20 g of the substance being examined, taken from the centre of the sample, or 20 g of the oil with 50 ml of *petroleum spirit (boiling range, 50° to 70°)*, shake vigorously with two 30-ml quantities of *methanol (75%)*, remove and reserve the upper layer after clear separation is obtained. Evaporate the combined methanolic solutions (lower layers) at as low a temperature as possible at a pressure of 2 kPa and in an atmosphere of nitrogen. Dissolve the residue in 5 ml of *ethanol-free chloroform* and keep the resulting solution in a well-closed container. For solution (2) evaporate carefully to dryness the combined petroleum spirit layers (upper layers) reserved from the preparation of solution (1), add 0.5 g of *pyrogallol* dissolved in 100 ml of *ethanol (96%)* and boil under a reflux condenser for 30 minutes with 15 ml of a freshly prepared 33% w/v solution of *potassium hydroxide.* Allow to cool, dilute with 250 ml of *water* and extract the unsaponifiable matter with three 100-ml quantities of *petroleum spirit (boiling range, 50° to 70°)*. Wash the combined extracts with *water* until free from alkali, evaporate to dryness and dissolve the residue in 5 ml of *ethanol-free chloroform.* Keep the resulting solution in a well-closed container. Solution (3) contains 0.01% w/v each of *dimethyl yellow, sudan red G* and *indophenol blue* in *benzene.*

For non-polyhydroxy antioxidants Using *ethanol-free chloroform* as the mobile phase, allow the solvent front to ascend 12 cm, remove the plate and allow it to dry in air for 20 minutes and then in a desiccator at a pressure of 2 kPa for a further 20 minutes. Apply at point (a) (see Fig. 10N-1) as a spot not more than 5 mm in diameter a suitable volume, usually between 2 and 10 µl, of solution (1). Apply 2 µl of solution (3) at each of points (b) and (c). Using *ethanol-free chloroform* as the mobile phase allow the solvent front to ascend 10 cm above the line of application, remove the plate and allow it to dry in air for 10 minutes. Turn the plate through 90° and, using *benzene* as the mobile phase, allow the solvent front to ascend 10 cm. After removal of the plate, allow it to dry in air for 5 minutes and spray with a 20% w/v solution of *phosphomolybdic acid* in *ethanol (96%)* until a permanent yellow colour is obtained. Blue spots begin to appear within 2 minutes. After a further 5 to 10 minutes, expose the plate to ammonia vapour until the background is clear white. Antioxidants appear as blue, slightly violet or greenish spots; if a blue spot remains at point (a), carry out the method for *polyhydroxy antioxidants* described below.

Evaluate the chromatogram by reference to Fig. 10N-1.

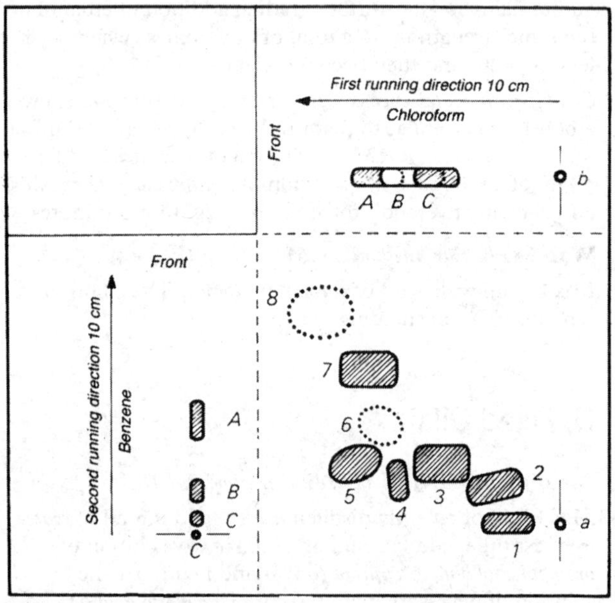

Fig. 10N-1
Typical Chromatograms of Non-polyhydroxy and Methanol-insoluble Antioxidants

a = application point for solution (1); position of polyhydroxy antioxidants and nordihydroguaiaretic acid after development

b, c = application positions for colour reference solutions. A = yellow; B = red; C = blue.

For the method *for non-polyhydroxy antioxidants*

1 = guaiacum resin
2 = 3-*tert*-butyl-4-methoxyphenol
3 = 2-*tert*-butyl-4-methoxyphenol
4 = 2,2,5,7,8-pentamethyl-6-chromanol
5 = tetraethylthiuram disulphide
8 = butylated hydroxytoluene

For the method *for antioxidants not extractable with methanol*

3 = beta- and gamma-tocopherol
6 = alpha-tocopherol
7 = dibutylhydroxyanisole

For polyhydroxy antioxidants Apply separately to the plate 1, 2, 4 and 6 µl of solution (1) and 1 to 2 µl of solution (3).

Using a mixture of 30 volumes of *glacial acetic acid,* 60 volumes of *benzene* and 60 volumes of *petroleum spirit (boiling range, 50° to 70°)* as the mobile phase, allow the solvent front to ascend 13 cm above the line of application. After removal of the plate, dry it in air and spray with a 20% w/v solution of *phosphomolybdic acid* in *ethanol (96%)* until a permanent yellow colour is obtained. Blue spots begin to appear within 2 minutes. After a further 5 to 10 minutes expose the plate to ammonia vapour until the background is clear white. Antioxidants appear as blue, slightly violet or greenish spots.

Evaluate the chromatogram by reference to Fig. 10N-2.

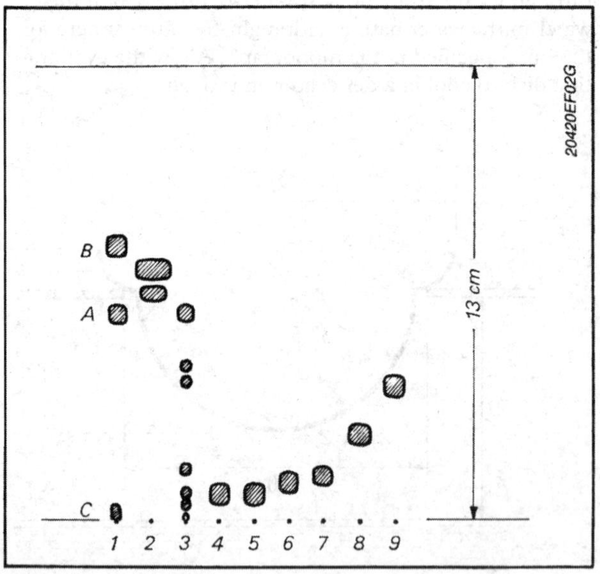

Fig. 10N-2
Typical Chromatograms of Polyhydroxy Antioxidants
A = yellow; B = red; C = blue.

1 = solution (3)
2 = butylated hydroxyanisole
3 = guaiacum resin
4 = nordihydroguaiaretic acid
5 = methyl gallate
6 = ethyl gallate
7 = propyl gallate
8 = octyl gallate
9 = dodecyl gallate

For antioxidants not extractable with methanol Using a separate plate, carry out the method *for non-polyhydroxy antioxidants* but using solution (2) in place of solution (1). After removal of the plate, allow it to dry in air and spray with a 1% w/v solution of *2,6-dichloroquinone-4-chloroimide* in *ethanol (96%)*. The spots become clearly visible within 15 minutes.

Evaluate the chromatogram by reference to Fig. 10N-1.

Identification of fixed oils by thin-layer chromatography *(Ph. Eur. method 2.3.2)*

Examine by *thin-layer chromatography*, Appendix III A, using as the coating substance a suitable octadecylsilyl silica gel for high performance thin-layer chromatography (Merck HPTLC silica gel RP-18 is suitable).

Solution (1) Unless otherwise prescribed, dissolve about 20 mg (1 drop) of the oil in 3 ml of *dichloromethane*.

Solution (2) Dissolve about 20 mg (1 drop) of *maize oil* in 3 ml of *dichloromethane*.

Apply separately to the plate 1 µl of each solution. Develop twice over a path of 0.5 cm using *ether*. Develop twice over a path of 8 cm using a mixture of 20 volumes of *dichloromethane*, 40 volumes of *glacial acetic acid* and 50 volumes of *acetone*. Allow the plate to dry in air and spray with a 10% w/v solution of *phosphomolybdic acid* in *ethanol (96%)*. Heat the plate at 120° for about 3 minutes and examine in daylight. The chromatogram obtained typically shows spots comparable to those in Figure 10N-3.

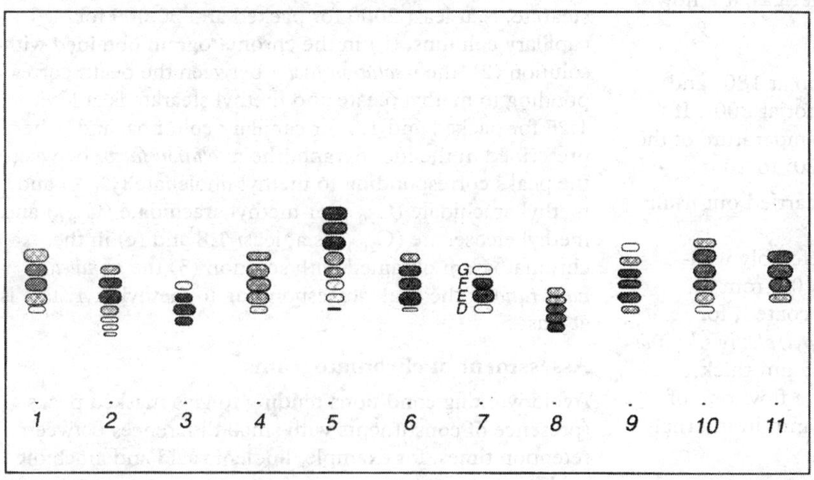

Fig. 10N-3

Typical chromatograms for the identification of fatty oils

1. Maize oil
2. Arachis oil
3. Theobroma oil
4. Sesame oil
5. Linseed oil
6. Almond oil
7. Olive oil
8. Rapeseed oil
9. Rapeseed oil (erucic acid-free)
10. Soya-bean oil
11. Sunflower oil

Test for foreign oils by thin-layer chromatography *(Ph. Eur. method 2.4.21)*

Carry out the method for *thin-layer chromatography*, Appendix III A, using *kieselguhr G* as the coating substance. Impregnate the dry plate by placing it to a depth of about 5 mm in a tank containing a shallow layer of a mixture of 10 volumes of *liquid paraffin* and 90 volumes of *petroleum spirit (boiling range, 50° to 70°)*, allowing the impregnating solvent to ascend at least 12 cm, removing the plate and allowing it to dry in air for 5 minutes; use with the flow of the mobile phase in the direction in which impregnation was carried out. Use a mixture of 10 volumes of *water* and 90 volumes of *glacial acetic acid* as the mobile phase and allow the solvent front to ascend 8 cm above the line of application. Apply separately to the plate 3 µl of each of the following solutions. For solution (1) heat 2 g of the oil with 30 ml of 0.5M *ethanolic potassium hydroxide* under a reflux condenser for 45 minutes, dilute with 50 ml of *water*, allow to cool, transfer to a separating funnel, shake with three 50-ml quantities of *ether* and discard the ether extracts. Acidify the aqueous layer with *hydrochloric acid* and extract with three 50-ml quantities of *ether*; combine the ether extracts, wash with three 10-ml quantities of *water*, dry the ether over *anhydrous sodium sulphate* and filter. Evaporate the ether on a water bath and dissolve 40 mg of the residue in 4 ml of *chloroform*. The fatty acids may also be obtained from the soap solution prepared during the determination of the unsaponifiable matter. Prepare solution (2) in the same manner as solution (1) but using 2 g of a mixture of 19 volumes of *maize oil* and 1 volume of *rapeseed oil* in place of the oil being examined. After removal of the plate, dry it at 110° for 10 minutes and, unless otherwise prescribed, expose it to iodine vapour in a saturated chamber; after some time, brown or yellowish brown spots become visible. Remove the plate and allow it to stand for a few minutes until the brown background colour has disappeared. Spray the plate with *starch solution*. Blue spots appear which may become brown on drying and again become blue after spraying with *water*. In the chromatogram obtained with solution (1) spots are always obtained with Rf values of about 0.5 (oleic acid) and about 0.65 (linoleic acid), corresponding to spots in the chromatogram obtained with solution (2). In the chromatogram obtained with solution (1) a spot with an Rf value of about 0.75 (linolenic acid) may be present but no spot is present with an Rf value of about 0.25 (erucic acid) corresponding to a spot in the chromatogram obtained with solution (2).

Test for foreign oils by gas chromatography

(Ph. Eur. method 2.4.22)

The test for foreign oils is carried out on the methyl esters of the fatty acids contained in the oil being examined.

This method is not applicable to oils that contain glycerides of fatty acids with an epoxy-, hydro-epoxy-, cyclopropanic or cyclopropenic group, or those that contain a large proportion of fatty acids of chain length less than 8 carbon atoms or to oils with an acid value greater than 2.

Method

Examine by *gas chromatography*, Appendix III B (packed column or capillary column).

Solution (1) When prescribed in the monograph, dry the oil being examined before the methylation. Weigh 4.0 g of the oil into a 100-ml round-bottomed flask with a ground-glass neck fitted with a reflux condenser and a means of passing gas into the flask. Add 40 ml of *anhydrous methanol* and 0.5 ml of a 6% w/v solution of *potassium hydroxide in methanol*. Attach the reflux condenser, pass *nitrogen* through the mixture at the rate of about 100 ml per minute, shake and heat to boiling. When the solution is clear (usually about 10 minutes), continue heating for a further 5 minutes. Cool under running water and transfer to a separating funnel. Rinse the flask with 20 ml of n-*heptane* and transfer the rinsings to the separating funnel. Add about 40 ml of *water* and shake gently. If an emulsion forms, add n-*heptane* or *water* dropwise from a pipette. Allow to separate, remove the aqueous layer and shake it with a further 20 ml of n-*heptane*. Allow to separate and combine the upper layers. Wash with two quantities, each of 20 ml, of *water*, dry over *anhydrous sodium sulphate* and filter. If necessary, the solution may be concentrated by evaporating on a water bath in a current of *nitrogen*. For capillary gas chromatography dilute the solution with n-*heptane* in order to obtain a 0.5 to 1% w/v solution of the fatty acid methyl ester mixture.

Solution (2) Prepare 0.50 g of the mixture of calibrating substances with the composition described in Table 10N-1; dissolve in n-*heptane* and dilute to 50 ml with the same solvent.

Solution (3) Dilute 1 ml of solution (2) to 10 ml with n-*heptane*.

The chromatographic procedure may be carried out using:
— a glass or stainless steel column (2 m to 3 m × 2 mm to 4 mm) packed with *acid-washed diatomaceous support* (125 µm to 200 µm), impregnated with 5% to 15% of *polyethylene glycol succinate* or *polyethylene glycol adipate*,
— *nitrogen for chromatography* as the carrier gas at a flow rate of 25 ml per minute,
— a flame ionisation detector,

maintaining the temperature of the column at 180° and that of the injection port and of the detector at 200°. If necessary or where prescribed, raise the temperature of the column at a rate of 5° per minute from 120° to 200°.

The chromatographic procedure may be carried out using alternatively:
— a capillary glass or quartz column (preferably wall-coated open tubular) (10 m to 25 m × 0.2 mm to 0.8 mm) the inner surface of which is coated, for instance, with a layer of *poly(cyanopropyl)phenylsiloxane* or of *polyethylene glycol 20,000* (0.1 to 5 µm thick),
— *helium* or *hydrogen* as the carrier gas at a flow rate of 1.3 ml per minute (for a column 0.32 mm in internal diameter),
— a flame-ionisation detector,
— a split ratio of 1:100 or less according to the internal diameter of the column used (1:50 for a 0.32 mm column),

maintaining the temperature of the column at 160° to 200°, according to the length and type of column used (for a column 30 m long coated with polyethylene glycol 20,000, 200°), and that of the injection port and of the detector at 250°. If necessary or where prescribed, raise the temperature of the column at a rate of 3° per minute from 170° to 230° (for a polyethylene glycol 20,000 column).

Inject 0.5 µl of solution (2). Adjust the sensitivity of the detector so that the height of the principal peak in the chromatogram obtained is 50% to 70% of the full scale of the recorder. Determine the retention times of the various constituent fatty acids. Inject 1 µl of solution (3) and check the *signal-to-noise ratio* of the peak corresponding to methyl myristate. Inject from 0.5 µl to 1 µl of solution (1) and adjust the sensitivity of the detector appropriately. Record the chromatograms for 2.5 times the retention time of methyl oleate. Assess the chromatogram as indicated below.

TABLE 10N-1 Calibrating Substances[1]

A mixture of the following reagents	Equivalent chain length[2]	Composition (% w/w) Isothermal	Composition (% w/w) Linear temperature programme
Methyl laurate	12.0	5	10
Methyl myristate	14.0	5	15
Methyl palmitate	16.0	10	15
Methyl stearate	18.0	20	20
Methyl arachidate	20.0	40	20
Methyl oleate	18.6	20	20

[1]For GC with capillary column and split inlet system, it is recommended that the component with the longest chain length of the mixture being examined is added to the calibration mixture.

[2]This value, which is calculated using calibration curves, is given as an example for a column of polyethylene glycol succinate.

The test is not valid unless: (a) in the chromatogram obtained with solution (2), the number of *theoretical plates (n)*, calculated for the peak corresponding to methyl stearate, is at least 2000 for packed and 30,000 for capillary columns, (b) in the chromatogram obtained with solution (2), the *resolution factor* between the peaks corresponding to methyl oleate and methyl stearate is at least 1.25 for packed and 1.8 for capillary columns, and, where prescribed in the monograph, the *resolution factor* between the peaks corresponding to methyl linolenate ($C_{18.3}$) and methyl arachidate ($C_{20.0}$) or methyl arachidate ($C_{20.0}$) and methyl eicosenate ($C_{20.1}$) is at least 1.8 and (c) in the chromatogram obtained with solution (3) the *signal-to-noise ratio* of the peak corresponding to methyl myristate is at least 5.

Assessment of chromatograms

Avoid working conditions tending to give masked peaks (presence of constituents with small differences between retention times, for example, linolenic acid and arachidic acids).

Qualitative analysis Draw calibration curves using the chromatogram obtained with the calibration solution and the information in the Table:
(a) using isothermal operating conditions giving the logarithms of reduced retention time as a function of the number of carbon atoms of the fatty acid; identify the peaks by means of the straight line thus obtained and of the 'equivalent chain lengths' of the different peaks. The calibration curve of the saturated acids is a straight line. The logarithms of reduced retention times of non-saturated acids are situated on this line at points corresponding to non-integral numbers known as 'equivalent chain length'.
(b) using linear temperature programming giving the retention time according to the number of carbon atoms of the fatty acid; identify by reference to the calibration curve.

Quantitative analysis The method of *normalisation* is used in which the sum of the areas of the peaks in the chromatogram, except that of the solvent, is set at 100%. The use of an electronic integrator is recommended. The content of a constituent is calculated by determining the area of the corresponding peak as a percentage of the sum of the area of all the peaks. Disregard any peak with an area less than 0.05% of the total area.

Sterols in fatty oils *(Ph. Eur. method 2.4.23)*

Separation of the sterol fraction Prepare the unsaponifiable matter and then isolate the sterol fraction of the fatty oil by *thin-layer chromatography*, Appendix III A, using *silica gel G* in a 0.3 mm to 0.5 mm layer as the coating substance.

Solution (1) In a 150-ml flask fitted with a reflux condenser place a volume of a 0.2% w/v solution of *betulin* in *dichloromethane* containing betulin corresponding to about 10% of the sterol content of the sample used for the determination (e.g. in the case of olive oil add 500 µl, in the case of other vegetable oils add 1500 µl of the betulin solution). If the monograph requires the content of the individual sterols as a percentage of the sterol fraction, the addition of betulin may be omitted. Evaporate to dryness under a current of *nitrogen*. Add 5 g (*m* g) of the substance being examined. Add 50 ml of 2M *ethanolic potassium hydroxide* and heat on a water bath for 1 hour, swirling frequently. Cool to a temperature below 25° and transfer the contents of the flask to a separating funnel with 100 ml of *water*. Shake the liquid carefully with three quantities, each of 100 ml, of *peroxide-free ether*. Combine the ether layers in another separating funnel containing 40 ml of *water*, shake gently for a few minutes, allow to separate and discard the aqueous phase. Wash the ethereal phase with several quantities, each of 40 ml, of *water* until the aqueous phase is no longer alkaline to phenolphthalein. Transfer the ethereal phase to a tared flask, washing the separating funnel with *peroxide-free ether*. Distil off the ether with suitable precautions and add 6 ml of *acetone*. Carefully remove the solvent in a current of air. Dry to a constant weight at 100° to 105°. Allow to cool in a desiccator and weigh. Dissolve the residue in a minimal volume of *dichloromethane*.

Solution (2) Treat 5 g of *rapeseed oil* as prescribed for the substance being examined, beginning at the words 'Add 50 ml of 2M *ethanolic potassium hydroxide*...'.

Solution (3) Treat 5 g of *sunflower oil* as prescribed for the substance being examined, beginning at the words 'Add 50 ml of 2M *ethanolic potassium hydroxide*...'.

Solution (4) Dissolve 50 mg of *cholesterol* and 50 mg of *betulin* in 1 ml of *dichloromethane*.

Use a separate plate for each of solutions (1) to (3). Apply separately as a band of 10 mm by 3 mm 5 µl of solution (4) and as a band of 40 mm by 3 mm 0.2 ml of either solution (1), solution (2) or solution (3). Develop over a path of 18 cm using a mixture of 35 volumes of *ether* and 65 volumes of *hexane*. Dry the plates in a current of *nitrogen*. Spray the plates with a 0.2% w/v solution of *2,7-dichlorofluorescein* in *absolute ethanol* and examine in *ultraviolet light (254 nm)*. The chromatogram obtained with solution (4) shows bands corresponding to cholesterol and betulin. The chromatograms obtained with solutions (1) to (3) show bands with similar Rf values due to sterols. From each of the chromatograms, remove an area of coating corresponding to the area occupied by the sterol bands and additionally the area of the zones 2 to 3 mm above and below the visible zones corresponding to solution (4). Place separately in three 50-ml flasks. To each flask add 15 ml of hot *dichloromethane* and shake. Filter each solution through a sintered-glass filter (40) and wash each filter with three quantities, each of 15 ml, of *dichloromethane*. Place the combined filtrate and washings from each filter separately in three tared flasks, evaporate to dryness under a stream of *nitrogen* and weigh.

Determination of the sterols Examine by *gas chromatography*, Appendix III B. Carry out the operations protected from humidity and prepare the solutions immediately before use.

Solution (1) To the sterols separated from the substance being examined by thin-layer chromatography add, per milligram of residue, 0.02 ml of a freshly prepared mixture of 1 volume of *trimethylchlorosilane*, 3 volumes of *hexamethyldisilazane* and 9 volumes of *anhydrous pyridine*. Shake carefully until the sterols are completely dissolved. Allow to stand in a desiccator over *phosphorus pentoxide* for 30 minutes. Centrifuge if necessary and use the supernatant liquid.

Solution (2) To 9 parts of the sterols separated from rapeseed oil by thin-layer chromatography add 1 part of *cholesterol*. To the mixture add, per milligram of residue, 0.02 ml of a freshly prepared mixture of 1 volume of *trimethylchlorosilane*, 3 volumes of *hexamethyldisilazane* and 9 volumes of *anhydrous pyridine*. Shake carefully until the sterols are completely dissolved. Allow to stand in a desiccator over *phosphorus pentoxide* for 30 minutes. Centrifuge if necessary and use the supernatant liquid.

Solution (3) To the sterols separated from sunflower oil by thin-layer chromatography add, per milligram of residue, 0.02 ml of a freshly prepared mixture of 1 volume of *trimethylchlorosilane*, 3 volumes of *hexamethyldisilazane* and 9 volumes of *anhydrous pyridine*. Shake carefully until the sterols are completely dissolved. Allow to stand in a desiccator over *phosphorus pentoxide* for 30 minutes, centrifuge if necessary and use the supernatant liquid.

The chromatographic procedure may be carried out using:

— a fused-silica column (20 m to 30 m × 0.25 mm to 0.32 mm) coated with *poly[methyl(95)phenyl(5)]-siloxane* or with *poly[methyl(94)phenyl(5)vinyl(1)]-siloxane* (film thickness, 0.25 mm),

— *hydrogen* at a linear flow rate of 30 cm to 50 cm per minute or *helium* at a linear flow rate of 20 cm to 35 cm per minute, as the carrier gas. Measure the linear flow rate as follows: maintaining the indicated operating conditions for the determination of the sterols, inject 1 ml to 3 ml of methane or propane. Measure the time in seconds required by the gas to pass through the column from the moment of the injection to the appearance of the peak (tm). The linear flow rate is given by L/t_m, where L is the length of the column in centimetres,

— a flame-ionisation detector,

— a split injector (1/50 or 1/100),

maintaining the temperature of the column at 260°, that of the injection port at 280° and that of the detector at 290°.

Inject 1 µl of each solution. The chromatogram obtained with solution (2) shows four major peaks corresponding respectively to cholesterol, brassicasterol, campesterol and β-sitosterol and the chromatogram obtained with solution (3) shows four major peaks corresponding respectively to campesterol, stigmasterol, β-sitosterol and Δ^7-stigmastenol. The retention times of the sterols relative to that for β-sitosterol are given in Table 10N-2. The peak of the internal standard (betulin) must be clearly separated from the peaks of the sterols being determined.

	Poly[methyl-(95)phenyl(5)]-siloxane	Poly[methyl(94)-phenyl(5)vinyl-(1)]siloxane
Cholesterol	0.63	0.67
Brassicasterol	0.71	0.73
24-Methylenecholesterol	0.80	0.82
Campesterol	0.81	0.83
Campestanol	0.82	0.85
Stigmasterol	0.87	0.88
Δ^7-Campesterol	0.92	0.93
$\Delta^{5,23}$-Stigmastadienol	0.95	0.95
Clerosterol	0.96	0.96
β-Sitosterol	1	1
Sitostanol	1.02	1.02
Δ^5-Avenasterol	1.03	1.03
$\Delta^{5,24}$-Stigmastadienol	1.08	1.08
Δ^7-Stigmastenol	1.12	1.12
Δ^7-Avenasterol	1.16	1.16
Betulin	1.4	1.6

For the chromatogram obtained with solution (1), identify the peaks and calculate the percentage content of each sterol in the sterol fraction of the substance being examined using the expression $100(A/S)$ where A is the area of the peak corresponding to the component being determined and S is the sum of the areas of the peaks corresponding to the components indicated in the Table. If required in the monograph, calculate the content of each sterol in mg per 100 g of the substance being examined using the following expression:

$$\frac{A \times m_S \times 100}{A_S \times m}$$

where A = area of the peak corresponding to the component being determined,
A_S = area of the peak corresponding to betulin,
m = weight of the sample of the substance being examined in g,
m_S = weight of betulin added in mg.

Appendix XI

A. Total Solids

(No Ph. Eur. method)

The term 'total solids' is applied to the residue obtained when the prescribed amount of the preparation is dried to constant weight under the conditions specified below.

Apparatus

A shallow, flat-bottomed, flanged dish, about 75 mm in diameter and about 25 mm deep, made of nickel or other suitable metal of high heat conductivity and low specific heat and which is not affected by boiling water. Suitable dishes are described in British Standard 1742:1951 (Methods for the chemical analysis of condensed milk).

Method

Place the quantity stated in the monograph in a tared dish, evaporate at as low a temperature as possible until the ethanol is removed and heat on a water bath until the residue is apparently dry. Transfer to an oven operating without a fan and dry to constant weight at 105° unless otherwise stated in the monograph. It may be necessary, for residues of a hygroscopic nature, to use a dish provided with a well-fitting cover and to cool in a desiccator.

B. Ethanol-soluble Extractive

(No Ph. Eur. method)

Macerate 5 g of the air-dried drug, coarsely powdered, with 100 ml of ethanol of the specified strength in a closed flask for 24 hours, shaking frequently during the first 6 hours and then allowing to stand for 18 hours. Filter rapidly, taking precautions against loss of ethanol, evaporate 20 ml of the filtrate to dryness in a tared, flat-bottomed, shallow dish and dry at 105° to constant weight. Calculate the percentage of ethanol-soluble extractive with reference to the air-dried drug.

C. Swelling Index

(Ph. Eur. method 2.8.4)

The swelling index is the volume in ml occupied by 1 g of a drug, including any adhering mucilage, after it has swollen in an aqueous liquid for 4 hours.

Place 1 g of the drug, whole or of the degree of comminution specified in the monograph, in a 25-ml ground-glass-stoppered cylinder graduated over a height of about 120 to 130 mm in 0.5 ml divisions. Unless otherwise specified, moisten the drug with 1.0 ml of *ethanol (96%)*, add 25 ml of *water* and close the cylinder. Shake vigorously every 10 minutes for 1 hour and then allow to stand for 3 hours. At 1.5 hours after the beginning of the test, release any large volumes of liquid retained in the layer of the drug and any particles of the drug floating at the surface of the liquid by rotating the cylinder about a vertical axis. Measure the volume occupied by the drug, including any adhering mucilage. Carry out three tests at the same time. Calculate the swelling index from the mean of the three tests.

D. Foreign Matter

Use Test A unless otherwise specified.

Test A *(No Ph. Eur. method)*

Vegetable drugs are as free as possible from moulds, insects and other animal contamination and are not visibly spoilt. The amount of foreign matter is not more than the percentage prescribed in the monograph.

Foreign matter is material consisting of any or all of the following:

(i) parts of the organ or organs from which the drug is derived other than the parts named in the monograph under Definition or under Characteristics or for which a limit is prescribed in the monograph;

(ii) any organs other than those named in the monograph under Definition or under Characteristics.

Method Weigh 100 to 500 g of the substance being examined or the quantity specified in the monograph and spread it in a thin layer. Detect the foreign matter by inspecting with the unaided eye or with the use of a ×6 lens, separate, weigh and calculate the percentage present.

Test B *(Ph. Eur. method 2.8.2)*

Vegetable drugs should be free from moulds, insects and other animal contamination. Unless otherwise prescribed in the monograph, the amount of foreign matter is not greater than 2% w/w.

Foreign matter is material consisting of any or all of the following:

(i) *Foreign organs*: matter coming from the source plant but not defined as the drug.

(ii) *Foreign elements*: matter not coming from the source plant and of either vegetable or mineral origin.

Method Weigh 100 to 500 g of the substance being examined or the quantity specified in the monograph and spread it in a thin layer. Detect the foreign matter by inspecting with the unaided eye or with the use of a ×6 lens, separate, weigh and calculate the percentage present.

E. Volatile Oil in Drugs

(Ph. Eur. method 2.8.12)

The determination of volatile oil in drugs is carried out by steam distillation in the apparatus described below. The distillate is collected in a graduated tube and the aqueous phase is automatically recirculated into the distillation flask. The volume of volatile oil may be measured directly or *xylene* may be used to take up the volatile oil.

The content of volatile oil is expressed as a percentage v/w.

Apparatus

The apparatus is constructed of glass of low coefficient of expansion and consists of the following parts:

(a) a suitable round-bottomed flask with a short, ground-glass neck having an internal diameter of about 29 mm at the wide end,

(b) a condenser assembly (see Figure 11E-1) that closely fits the flask, the different parts being fused into one piece; the glass used has a low coefficient of expansion; the stopper K′ is vented and the tube K has an orifice of diameter about 1 mm that coincides with the vent; the wide end of the tube K is of ground-glass and has an internal diameter of 10 mm; a pear-shaped swelling, J, of 3 ml capacity; the tube JL is graduated in 0.01 ml; the bulb-shaped swelling L has a capacity of about 2 ml; M is a three-way tap; the junction B is at a level 20 mm higher than the uppermost graduation,

(c) a suitable heating device, allowing a fine control,

(d) a vertical support with a horizontal ring covered with insulating material.

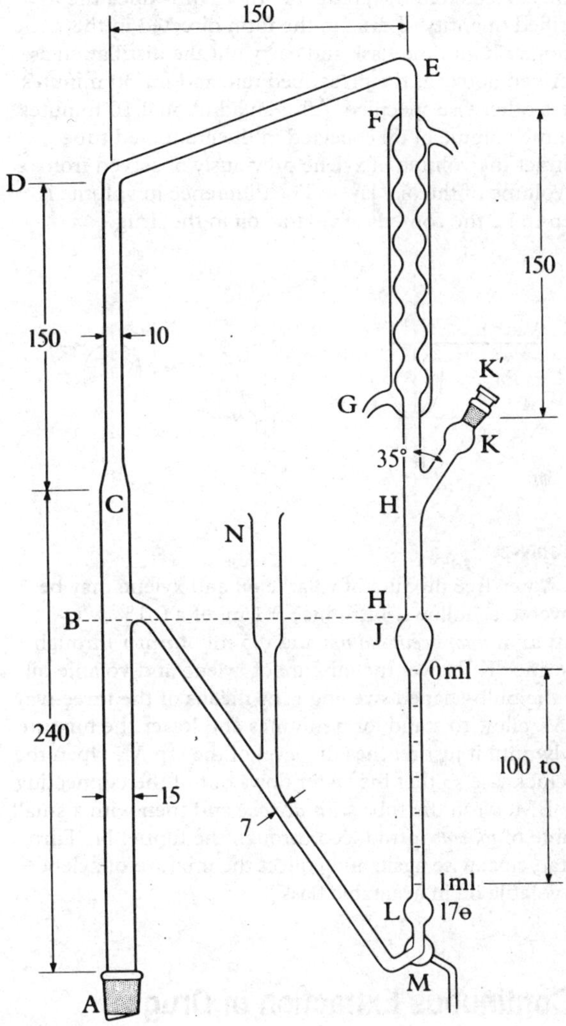

Fig. 10N-1
Apparatus for the Determination of Volatile Oils in Drugs
Dimensions in mm

Method

Clean the glass apparatus thoroughly before each distillation.

Carry out the assay according to the nature of the material being examined. Connect the distillation flask of the apparatus, containing the prescribed volume of distillation liquid and a few small pieces of porous earthenware, to the still head (Fig. 10N-1). Add *water* through the funnel N until it is at the level B. Introduce the prescribed volume of *xylene* at K by means of a pipette, the tip of which is inserted into the lower part of orifice K. Heat the flask until ebullition begins and adjust the distillation rate to 2 to 3 ml per minute unless otherwise prescribed. Determine the rate of distillation by lowering the level of the distillation liquid by means of the three-way tap M until the meniscus is level with the lower mark (a) (see Fig. 10N-2), closing the tap and simultaneously starting a stop watch. When the level reaches the upper mark (b) stop the watch and note the time. Open the tap and continue the distillation, modifying the heat to regulate the distillation rate. After 30 minutes discontinue heating and after at least a further 10 minutes read the volume of xylene collected in the graduated tube. Introduce the specified quantity of drug in the form directed in the monograph into the flask and carry out the distillation as described above at the prescribed rate and for 30 minutes, unless otherwise specified. After an additional 10 minutes, read the volume of oil collected in the graduated tube. Subtract the volume of xylene previously observed from the volume of the oily layer. The difference in volume is taken to be the content of volatile oil in the drug.

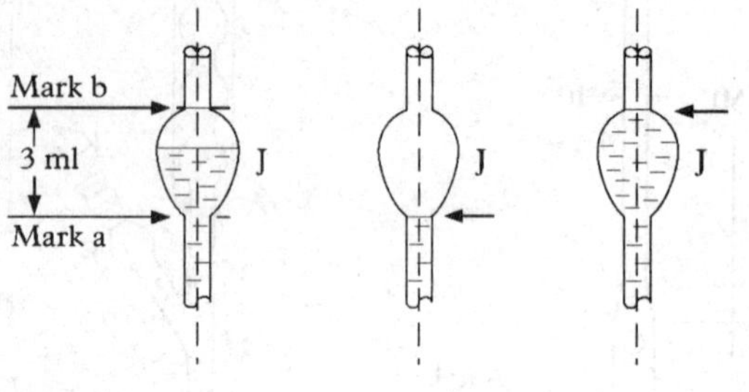

Fig. 10N-2

The water-free mixture of volatile oil and xylene may be recovered as follows. Introduce 0.1 ml of a 0.1% w/v solution of *fluorescein sodium* and 0.5 ml of *water* through the orifice K. Lower the mixture of xylene and volatile oil into the bulb-shaped swelling L by means of the three-way tap M, allow to stand for 5 minutes and lower the mixture slowly until it just reaches the level of the tap M. Open the tap clockwise so that the water flows out of the connecting tube BM, wash the tube with *acetone* and then with a small volume of *toluene* introduced through the funnel N. Turn the tap clockwise again and collect the mixture of xylene and volatile oil in a suitable flask.

F. Continuous Extraction of Drugs

(No Ph. Eur. method)

Where the process of *maceration* or *percolation* is specified in a monograph, carry out the following procedures with any modification indicated in the monograph.

Maceration Place the solid materials with the whole of the menstruum in a closed vessel and allow to stand for 7 days, shaking occasionally. Strain, press the marc and mix the liquids obtained. Clarify by subsidence or filtration.

Percolation Moisten the solid materials with a sufficient quantity of the menstruum, allow to stand for 4 hours in a well-closed vessel, pack in a percolator and add sufficient of the menstruum to saturate the materials. When the liquid begins to drop from the percolator, close the outlet, add sufficient of the menstruum to leave a layer above the drug and allow to macerate for 24 hours. Allow percolation to proceed slowly until the percolate measures about three-quarters of the required volume. Press the marc, mix the expressed liquid with the percolate and add sufficient of the menstruum to produce the required volume. Clarify by subsidence or filtration.

Continuous extraction of a drug for the purpose of an assay consists of percolating the drug with the solvent stated in the monograph at a temperature approximately that of the boiling point of the solvent.

The apparatus described below, or any similar apparatus, may be used, provided that it permits the uniform percolation of the drug and the regular flow of the vapour of the solvent around the percolator.

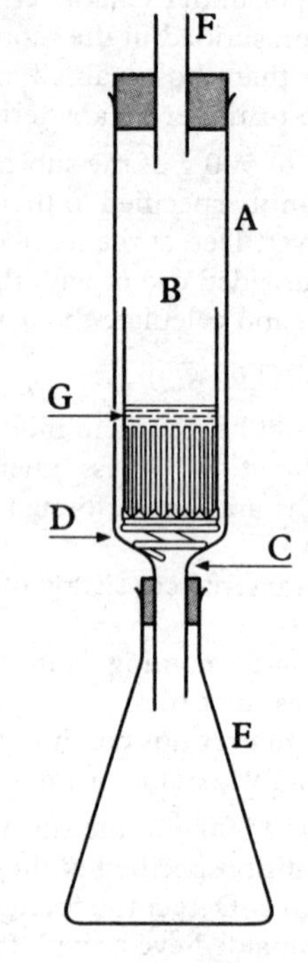

Fig. 11F-1
Apparatus for the Continuous Extraction of Drugs

The apparatus is shown in Fig. 11F-1. A is an outer tube of stout glass; the wider part is about 18 cm long and has an internal diameter of 4.8 to 5 cm; the lower end C is about 5 cm long and has an external diameter of about 1.6 cm. B is a straight glass tube open at both ends, about 9 cm long and with an external diameter of about 3.8 cm; over its lower, flanged end is tied firmly a piece of calico or other suitable material. D is a glass coil which supports the margin of the tube B and prevents it from resting in contact with the outer tube A. The lower end C of the outer tube A is fitted by a cork or ground-glass joint to the distillation flask E, in which a suitable quantity of the solvent has been placed. The drug to be extracted, previously moistened with the solvent or subjected to any preliminary treatment required, is introduced into the inner tube B, which is supported so that the percolate drops into the outer tube. A pad of absorbent cotton G is placed on the top of the drug, the inner tube is lowered into position and the outer tube connected by means of a suitable cork or ground-glass joint with the tube of a reflux condenser F. The flask is heated and the extraction continued as directed.

G. Complete Extraction of Alkaloids

(No Ph. Eur. method)

Complete extraction is indicated by the following tests.

Extraction with an aqueous or alcoholic liquid

After extracting at least three times with the liquid, add to 0.1 to 0.2 ml of the next portion, after acidifying with 2M *hydrochloric acid* if necessary, 0.05 ml of *potassium tetraiodomercurate solution* or, for solanaceous alkaloids, 0.05 ml of *potassium iodobismuthate solution R1*. No precipitate or turbidity is produced.

Extraction with an immiscible solvent

After extracting at least three times with the solvent, add to 1 to 2 ml of the next portion 1 to 2 ml of 0.1M *hydrochloric acid*, remove the organic solvent by evaporation, transfer the aqueous residue to a test tube and add 0.05 ml of *potassium tetraiodomercurate solution* or, for solanaceous alkaloids, 0.05 ml of *potassium iodobismuthate solution R1* or, for emetine, 0.05 ml of *iodinated potassium iodide solution*. Not more than a very faint opalescence is produced.

Continuous extraction

After percolating for at least 2 hours, collect 1 to 2 ml of the effluent and carry out the procedure described under 'Extraction with an aqueous or alcoholic liquid' or 'Extraction with an immiscible solvent', as appropriate.

H. Stomata

(Ph. Eur. method 2.8.3)

There are several types of stomata (Fig.11H-1), distinguished by the form and arrangement of the surrounding cells. The following descriptions apply to mature stomata. In describing an epidermis where certain stomata differ from the predominant type, the term applying to the majority of stomata is used.

(1) *Anisocytic* (unequal-celled) The stoma is usually surrounded by three subsidiary cells, of which one is markedly smaller than the others.

1 2 3 4

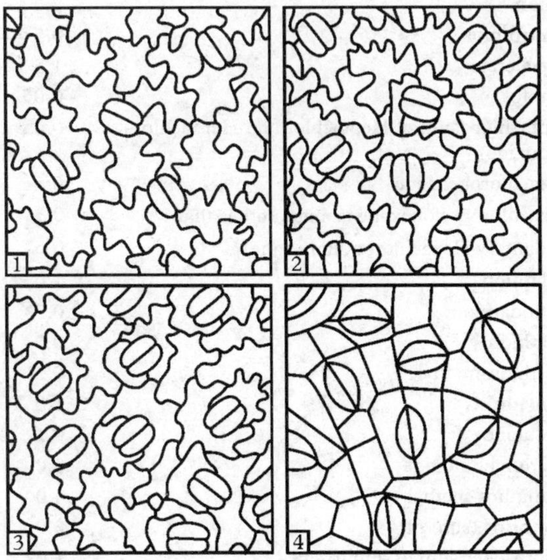

Fig.11H-1

(2) *Anomocytic* (irregular-celled) The stoma is surrounded by a varying number of cells in no way differing from those of the epidermis generally.

(3) *Diacytic* (cross-celled) The stoma is accompanied by two subsidiary cells the common wall of which is at right angles to the guard cells.

(4) *Paracytic* (parallel-celled) The stoma has on each side one or more subsidiary cells parallel to the long axis of the pore and guard cells.

Stomatal index

For each sample of leaf make not fewer than 10 determinations of the numbers of stomata and epidermal cells (including trichomes) in the same area of leaf and calculate the mean. Calculate the stomatal index from the following expression:

$$\text{stomatal index} = \frac{100 \times \text{number of stomata}}{\text{number of epidermal cells} + \text{number of stomata}}$$

J. Ash

Use Method I unless otherwise directed in the monograph.

Method I *(No Ph. Eur. method)*

For vegetable drugs Incinerate 2 to 3 g of the ground drug in a tared platinum or silica dish at a temperature not exceeding 450° until free from carbon, cool and weigh. If a carbon-free ash cannot be obtained in this way, exhaust the charred mass with hot *water*, collect the residue on an ashless filter paper, incinerate the residue and filter paper, add the filtrate, evaporate to dryness and ignite at a temperature not exceeding 450°. Calculate the percentage of ash with reference to the air-dried drug.

For other substances Carry out the above method using 1 g, unless otherwise stated. Calculate the percentage of ash.

Method II *(Ph. Eur. method 2.4.16)*

Heat a silica or platinum crucible to red heat for 30 minutes, allow to cool in a desiccator and weigh. Unless otherwise specified in the monograph, evenly distribute 1 g of the substance being examined in the crucible, dry at 100° to 105° for 1 hour and ignite to constant weight in a muffle furnace at 575° to 625°. Allow the crucible to cool in a desiccator after each ignition. Flames should not be produced at any time during the procedure. If after prolonged ignition a carbon-free ash cannot be obtained, take up with hot *water*, filter through an ashless filter paper and ignite the residue and the filter paper. Combine the filtrate with the ash, carefully evaporate to dryness and ignite to constant weight.

K. Acid-insoluble Ash

Use Method I unless otherwise directed in the monograph.

Method I *(No Ph. Eur. method)*

Boil the *ash* for 5 minutes with 25 ml of 2M *hydrochloric acid*, collect the insoluble matter in a sintered-glass crucible or on an ashless filter paper, wash with hot *water* and ignite. Calculate the percentage of acid-insoluble ash with reference to the air-dried drug.

Method II *(Ph. Eur. method 2.8.1)*

Ash insoluble in hydrochloric acid is the residue obtained after extracting the sulphated ash or total ash with *hydrochloric acid*, calculated with reference to 100 g of drug.

Place the *ash* or the *sulphated ash*, as specified in the monograph, in a crucible, add 15 ml of *water* and 10 ml of *hydrochloric acid*, cover with a watch glass, boil gently for 10 minutes and allow to cool. Collect the insoluble matter on an ashless filter paper, wash with hot *water* until the filtrate is neutral, dry, ignite to dull redness, allow to cool in a desiccator and weigh. Reheat until the difference between two successive weighings is not more than 1 mg. Calculate the percentage of acid-insoluble ash.

L. Pesticide Residues

(Ph. Eur. method 2.8.13)

Definition For the purposes of the Pharmacopoeia, a pesticide is any substance or mixture of substances intended for preventing, destroying or controlling any pest, unwanted species of plants or animals causing harm during or otherwise interfering with the production, processing, storage, transport or marketing of vegetable drugs. The item includes substances intended for use as growth-regulators, defoliants or desiccants and any substance applied to crops either before or after harvest to protect the commodity from deterioration during storage and transport.

Limits Unless otherwise indicated in the monograph, the drug being examined at least complies with the limits indicated in Table I. The limits applying to pesticides that are not listed in Table I and the presence of which is suspected for any reason comply with the limits set by European Community Directives EEC/76/895 and EEC/90/642, including their annexes and successive updates. Limits for pesticides that are not listed in Table 11L-1nor in EC directives are calculated using the following expression:

$$\frac{ADI \times M}{MDD \times 100}$$

where ADI = acceptable daily intake, as published by FAO-WHO in milligrams per kilogram of body weight,

M = body weight in kilograms (60 kg)

MDD = daily dose of the drug in kilograms.

If the drug is intended for the preparation of extracts, tinctures or other pharmaceutical forms the preparation method of which modifies the content of pesticides in the finished product, the limits are calculated using the following expression:

$$\frac{ADI \times M \times E}{MDD \times 100}$$

where E = extraction factor of the method of preparation, determined experimentally.

Higher limits can also be authorised, in exceptional cases, especially when a plant requires a particular cultivation method or has a metabolism or a structure that gives rise to a higher than normal content of pesticides.

The competent authority may grant total or partial exemption of the test when the complete history (nature and quantity of the pesticides used, date of each treatment during cultivation and after the harvest) of the treatment of the batch is known and can be checked precisely.

Sampling

Method For containers up to 1 kg, take one sample from the total content, thoroughly mixed, sufficient for the tests. For containers between 1 kg and 5 kg, take three samples, equal in volume, from the upper, middle and lower parts of the container, each being sufficient to carry out the tests. Thoroughly mix the samples and take from the mixture an amount sufficient to carry out the tests. For containers of more than 5 kg, take three samples, each of at least 250 g from the upper, middle and lower parts of the container. Thoroughly mix the samples and take from the mixture an amount sufficient to carry out the tests.

TABLE 11L-1

Substance	Limit (mg/kg)
Alachlor	0.02
Aldrin and Dieldrin (sum of)	0.05
Azinphos-methyl	1.0
Bromopropylate	3.0
Chlordane (sum of *cis*, *trans*- and Oxychlordane)	0.05
Chlorfenvinphos	0.5
Chlorpyrifos	0.2
Chlorpyrifos-methyl	0.1
Cypermethrin (and isomers)	1.0
DDT (sum of *p,p'*-DDT, *o,p'*-DDT, *p,p'*-DDE and *p,p'*-TDE)	1.0
Deltamethrin	0.5
Diazinon	0.5
Dichlorvos	1.0
Dithiocarbamates (as CS_2)	2.0
Endosulfan (sum of isomers and Endosulfan sulphate)	3.0
Endrin	0.05
Ethion	2.0
Fenitrothion	0.5
Fenvalerate	1.5
Fonofos	0.05
Heptachlor (sum of Heptachlor and Heptachlor-epoxide)	0.05
Hexachlorobenzene	0.1
Hexachlorocyclohexane isomers (other than γ)	0.3
Lindane (γ-Hexachlorocyclohexane)	0.6
Malathion	1.0
Methidathion	0.2
Parathion	0.5
Parathion-methyl	0.2
Permethrin	1.0
Phosalone	0.1
Piperonyl butoxide	3.0
Pirimiphos-methyl	4.0
Pyrethrins (sum of)	3.0
Quintozene (sum of quintozene, pentachloroanaline and methyl pentachlorophenyl sulphide)	1.0

Size of sampling If the number (n) of containers is three or fewer, take samples from each container as indicated above under Method. If the number of containers is more than three, take samples as indicated under Method, from $\sqrt{n}+1$ containers, rounding up to the nearest unit if necessary.

The samples are to be analysed immediately to avoid possible degradation of the residues. If this is not possible, the samples are stored in airtight containers suitable for food contact, at a temperature below 0°, protected from light.

Reagents All reagents and solvents are free from any contaminants, especially pesticides, which might interfere with the analysis. It is often necessary to use special quality solvents or if this is not possible, solvents that have recently been re-distilled in an apparatus made entirely of glass. In any case, suitable blank tests must be carried out.

Apparatus Clean the apparatus and especially glassware to ensure that they are free from pesticides, for example, soak for at least 16 hours in a solution of phosphate-free detergent, rinse with large quantities of distilled water, and wash with acetone and hexane or heptane.

Qualitative and quantitative analysis of pesticide residues The analytical procedures used are validated according to the regulations in force. In particular, they satisfy the following criteria:

(a) the chosen method, especially the purification steps, is suitable for the substance being analysed, and not susceptible to interference from co-extractives; the limits of detection and quantification are measured for each pesticide-matrix combination being analysed,
(b) between 70% and 110% of each pesticide is recovered,
(c) the repeatability of the method is not less than the values indicated in Table 11L-2,
(d) the reproducibility of the method is not less than the values indicated in Table 11L-2,
(e) the concentration of test and reference solutions and the setting of the apparatus are such that a linear response is obtained from the analytical detector.

Table 11L-2

Concentration of the analyte (mg/kg)	Repeatability (difference ±mg/kg)	Reproducibility (difference ±mg/kg)
0.010	0.005	0.01
0.100	0.025	0.05
1.000	0.125	0.25

ANNEX

This section is given for information and guidance; it does not form a mandatory part of the general method.

Organochlorine, organophosphorus and pyrethroid insecticides

The following methods may be used, in connection with the general method above. Depending on the substance being examined, it may be necessary to modify, sometimes extensively, the procedure described hereafter. In any case, it may be necessary to use, in addition, another column with a different polarity or another detection method (for example, mass spectrometry) or a different method (for example, immunochemical methods) to confirm the results obtained.

This procedure is valid only for the analysis of samples of vegetable drugs containing less than 15% of water. Samples with a higher content of water may be dried, provided it has been shown that the drying procedure does not affect significantly the pesticide content.

1. Extraction

To 10 g of the substance being examined, coarsely powdered, add 100 ml of *acetone* and allow to stand for 20 minutes. Add 1 ml of a solution containing 1.8 µg per millilitre of *carbophenothion* in *toluene*. Homogenise using a high-speed blender for 3 minutes. Filter and wash the filter cake with two quantities, each of 25 ml, of *acetone*. Combine the filtrate and the washings and heat using a rotary evaporator at a temperature not exceeding 40° until the solvent has almost completely evaporated. To the residue add a few millilitres of *toluene* and heat again until the acetone is completely removed. Dissolve the residue in 8 ml of *toluene*. Filter through a membrane filter (45 µm), rinse the flask and the filter with *toluene* and dilute to 10 ml with the same solvent (solution A).

2. Purification

2.1. ORGANOCHLORINE, ORGANOPHOSPHORUS AND PYRETHROID INSECTICIDES Examine by *size-exclusion chromatography*, Appendix III C.

The chromatographic procedure may be carried out using:

— a stainless steel column (0.30 m × 7.8 mm) packed with *styrene—divinylbenzene copolymer* (5 µm),
— *toluene* as mobile phase at a flow rate of 1 ml per minute.

Performance of the column Inject 100 µl of a solution containing 0.05% w/v of *methyl red* and 0.05% w/v of *oracet blue 2R* in *toluene* and proceed with the chromatography. The column is not suitable unless the colour of the eluate changes from orange to blue at an elution volume of about 10.3 ml. If necessary calibrate the column, using a solution containing, in *toluene*, at a suitable concentration, the insecticide being analysed with the lowest molecular weight (for example, dichlorvos) and that with the highest molecular weight (for example, deltamethrin). Determine which fraction of the eluate contains both pesticides.

Purification of the test solution Inject a suitable volume of solution A (100 µl to 500 µl) and proceed with the chromatography. Collect the fraction as determined above (solution B). Organophosphorus insecticides are usually eluted between 8.8 ml and 10.9 ml. Organochlorine and pyrethroid insecticides are usually eluted between 8.5 ml and 10.3 ml.

2.2. ORGANOCHLORINE AND PYRETHROID INSECTICIDES In a chromatography column (0.10 m × 5 mm) introduce a piece of defatted cotton and 0.5 g of silica gel treated as follows: heat *silica gel for chromatography* in an oven at 150° for 4 hours. Allow to cool and add dropwise a quantity of *water* corresponding to 1.5% of the weight of silica gel used; shake vigorously until agglomerates have disappeared and continue shaking for 2 hours using a mechanical shaker. Condition the column using 1.5 ml of *hexane*. Prepacked columns containing about 500 mg of a suitable silica gel may also be used provided they are previously validated.

Concentrate solution B in a current of *helium* or *oxygen-free nitrogen* almost to dryness and dilute to a suitable volume with *toluene* (200 µl to 1 ml according to the volume injected in the preparation of solution B). Transfer quantitatively onto the column and proceed to the chromatography using 1.8 ml of *toluene* as the mobile phase. Collect the eluate (solution C).

3. Quantitative analysis

3.1. ORGANOPHOSPHORUS INSECTICIDES Examine by *gas chromatography*, Appendix III B, using *carbophenothion* as the internal standard. It may be necessary to use a second internal standard to identify possible interferences with the peak due to carbophenothion.

Solution (1) Concentrate solution B in a current of *helium* almost to dryness and dilute to 100 µl with *toluene*.

Solution (2) Prepare at least three solutions in *toluene* containing the insecticides being determined and *carbophenothion* at concentrations suitable for plotting a calibration curve.

The chromatographic procedure may be carried out using:

— a fused-silica column (30 m × 0.32 mm) the internal wall of which is covered with a layer 0.25 mm thick of *poly(dimethyl) siloxane*,

— *hydrogen* as the carrier gas; other gases such as *helium* or *nitrogen for chromatography* may also be used provided the chromatography is suitably validated,

— a phosphorus—nitrogen flame-ionisation detector or a flame-photometry detector,

maintaining the temperature of the column at 80° for 1 minute, then raising it at a rate of 30° per minute to 150°, maintaining at 150° for 3 minutes, then raising the temperature at a rate of 4° per minute to 280° and maintaining at this temperature for 1 minute, and maintaining the temperature of the injector port at 250° and that of the detector at 275°. Inject the chosen volume of each solution. When the chromatograms are recorded in the prescribed conditions, the relative retention times are approximately those listed in Table III. Calculate the content of each insecticide from the peak areas and the concentrations of the solutions.

Table 11L-3

Substance	Relative retention times
Dichlorvos	0.20
Fonofos	0.50
Diazinon	0.52
Parathion-methyl	0.59
Chlorpyrifos-methyl	0.60
Pirimiphos-methyl	0.66
Malathion	0.67
Parathion	0.69
Chlorpyrifos	0.70
Methidathion	0.78
Ethion	0.96
Carbophenothion	1.00
Azinphos-methyl	1.17
Phosalone	1.18

3.2. ORGANOCHLORINE AND PYRETHROID INSECTICIDES Examine by *gas chromatography*, Appendix III B, using *carbophenothion* as internal standard. It may be necessary to use a second internal standard to identify possible interferences with the peak due to carbophenothion.

Solution (1) Concentrate solution C in a current of *helium* or *oxygen-free nitrogen* almost to dryness and dilute to 500 µl with *toluene*.

Solution (2) Prepare at least three solutions in *toluene* containing the insecticides being determined and *carbophenothion* at concentrations suitable for plotting a calibration curve.

The chromatographic procedure may be carried out using:

— a fused silica column (30 m × 0.32 mm) the internal wall of which is covered with a layer 0.25 µm thick of *poly(dimethyl) (diphenyl) siloxane*,

— *hydrogen* as the carrier gas; other gases such as *helium* or *nitrogen for chromatography* may also be used provided the chromatography is suitably validated,

— an electron-capture detector,

— a device allowing direct cold on-column injection,

maintaining the temperature of the column at 80° for 1 minute, then raising it at a rate of 30° per minute to 150°, maintaining at 150° for 3 minutes, then raising the temperature at a rate of 4° per minute to 280° and maintaining at this temperature for 1 minute, and maintaining the temperature of the injector port at 250° and that of the detector at 275°. Inject the chosen volume of each solution. When the chromatograms are recorded in the prescribed conditions, the relative retention times are approximately those listed in Table11L-4. Calculate the content of each insecticide from the peak areas and the concentrations of the solutions.

Table 11L-4

Substance	Relative retention times
α-Hexachlorocyclohexane	0.44
Hexachlorobenzene	0.45
β-Hexachlorocyclohexane	0.49
Lindane	0.49
δ-Hexachlorocyclohexane	0.54
ε-Hexachlorocyclohexane	0.56
Heptachlor	0.61
Aldrin	0.68
cis-Heptachlor-epoxide	0.76
o,p' -DDE	0.81
α-Endosulfan	0.82
Dieldrin	0.87
p,p' -DDE	0. 87
o,p' -DDD	0.89
Endrin	0.91
β-Endosulfan	0.92
o,p' -DDT	0.95
Carbophenothion	1.00
p,p' -DDT	1.02
cis-Permethrin	1.29
trans-Permethrin	1.31
Cypermethrin	1.40
Fenvalerate*	1.47, 1.49
Deltamethrin	1.54

*The substance shows several peaks

Appendix XII

A. Disintegration Test for Tablets and Capsules

(Ph. Eur. method 2.9.1)

The disintegration test determines whether tablets or capsules disintegrate within a prescribed time when placed in a liquid medium under the prescribed experimental conditions.

Disintegration is considered to be achieved when no residue, except fragments of undissolved tablet coating or of capsule shell, remains on the screen of the test apparatus or adheres to the lower surface of the disc if a disc has been used; if any other residue remains, it consists of a soft mass having no palpably firm, unmoistened core.

Apparatus

(*a*) A rigid basket-rack assembly supporting six cylindrical glass tubes 75.0 to 80.0 mm long, 21.5 mm in internal diameter and with a wall thickness of about 2 mm (see Fig. 12A-1).

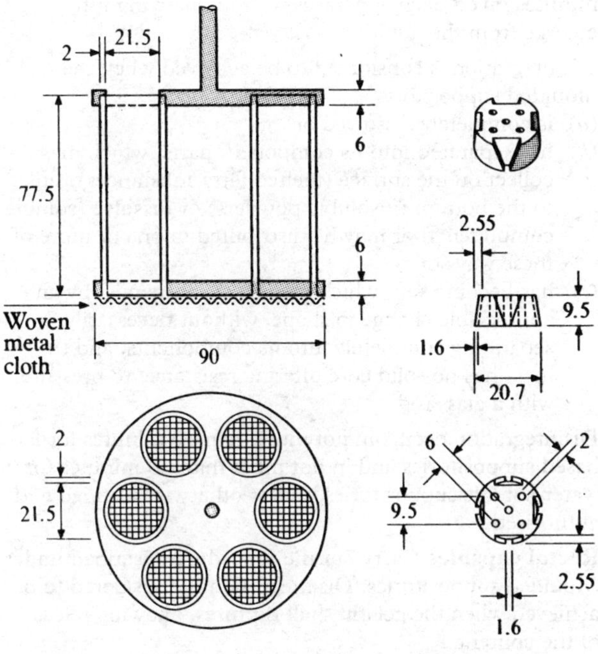

Fig. 12A-1
Apparatus for the Disintegration of Tablets and Capsules
Dimensions in mm

(*b*) A cylindrical disc for each tube, each 20.55 to 20.85 mm in diameter and 9.35 to 9.65 mm thick, made of transparent plastic with a relative density of 1.18 to 1.20, pierced with five holes, each 2 mm in diameter, one in the centre and the other four spaced equally on a circle of radius 6 mm from the centre of the disc. Four equally-spaced grooves are cut in the lateral surface of the disc in such a way that at the upper surface of the disc they are 9.5 mm wide and 2.55 mm deep and at the lower surface 1.6 mm square.

(*c*) The tubes are held vertically by two superimposed transparent plastic plates 90 mm in diameter and 6 mm thick, perforated by six holes. The holes are equidistant from the centre of the plate and are equally spaced from one another. Attached to the under side of the lower plate is a piece of woven gauze made from stainless steel wire 0.635 mm in diameter and having nominal mesh apertures of 2.00 mm.

(*d*) The plates are held rigidly in position and 77.5 mm apart by vertical metal rods at the periphery and a metal rod is also fixed to the centre of the upper plate to enable the assembly to be attached to a mechanical device capable of raising and lowering it smoothly through a distance of 50 to 60 mm at a constant frequency of between 28 and 32 cycles per minute.

(*e*) The assembly is suspended in the specified liquid medium in a suitable vessel, preferably a 1000-ml beaker. The volume of liquid is such that when the assembly is in the highest position the wire mesh is at least 15 mm below the surface of the liquid and when the assembly is in the lowest position the wire mesh is at least 25 mm above the bottom of the beaker and the upper open ends of the tubes remain above the surface of the liquid.

(*f*) A suitable device maintains the temperature of the liquid at 36° to 38°.

The design of the basket-rack assembly may be varied provided that the specifications for the glass tubes and wire mesh are maintained.

Method

Unless otherwise stated in the individual monograph, introduce one tablet or capsule into each tube and, if prescribed in the appropriate general monograph, add a disc to each tube. Suspend the assembly in the beaker containing the specified liquid and operate the apparatus for the specified time. Remove the assembly from the liquid. The tablets or capsules pass the test if all six have disintegrated.

B. Disintegration Test for Enteric-coated Tablets

(Included in Ph. Eur. general monograph for Tablets)

Use the apparatus described under *disintegration test for tablets and capsules*, Appendix XII A.

Method

Introduce one tablet into each tube, suspend the assembly in the beaker containing 0.1M *hydrochloric acid* and operate without the discs for 120 minutes, unless otherwise stated in the individual monograph. Remove the assembly from the liquid. No tablet shows signs of cracks that would allow the escape of the contents or disintegration, apart from fragments of coating.

Replace the liquid in the beaker with *mixed phosphate buffer pH 6.8*, add a disc to each tube and operate the apparatus for a further 60 minutes. Remove the assembly from the liquid. The tablets pass the test if all six have disintegrated.

C. Disintegration Test for Suppositories and Pessaries

(Ph. Eur. method 2.9.2)

The test for disintegration of suppositories and pessaries determines whether suppositories and pessaries disintegrate or soften within a prescribed time when placed in a liquid medium under the prescribed experimental conditions.

Apparatus

(*a*) A transparent sleeve of glass or suitable plastic, of height 60 mm with an internal diameter of 52 mm and an appropriate wall thickness (see Fig. 2.9.2-1).

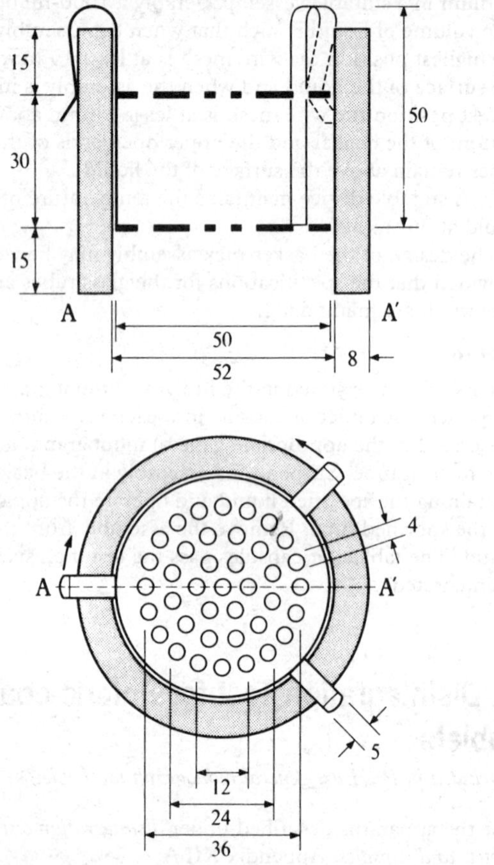

Fig. 12C-1
Apparatus for the Disintegration of Suppositories and Pessaries
Dimension in mm

(*b*) A metal device consisting of two stainless metal discs, each of which contains 39 holes, each 4 mm in diameter, being distributed as indicated in Fig. 12C-1. The diameter of the discs is closely similar to the internal diameter of the sleeve. The discs are separated by a distance of about 30 mm. The metal device is attached to the outer sleeve by means of three equally-spaced hooks.

For vaginal tablets use with the hook-end downwards as in Fig. 12C-2.

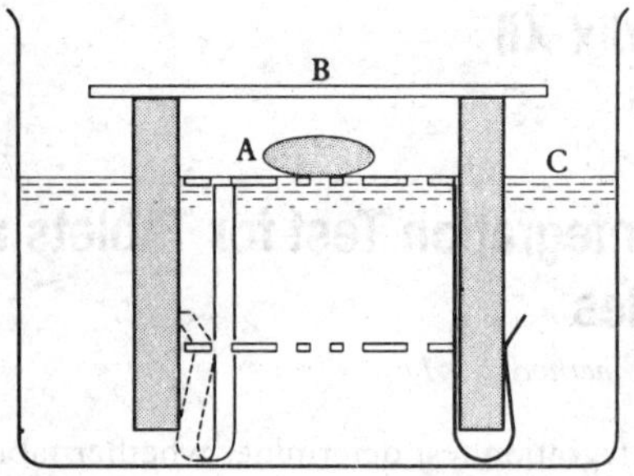

Fig. 12C-2
Apparatus for the Disintegration of Vaginal Tablets
A – Vaginal tablet
B – Glass plate
C – Water surface

Method

Moulded suppositories Place a suppository on the lower perforated disc of the metal device and then insert the device into the cylinder and attach this to the sleeve. Repeat the operation with a further two suppositories and metal devices and sleeves. Unless otherwise specified, place each piece of apparatus in a vessel containing at least 4 litres[1] of *water* at 36° to 37° and fitted with a slow stirrer and a means of holding the apparatus vertically 90 mm below the surface of the water. After each 10 minutes invert each apparatus without allowing it to emerge from the liquid.

Disintegration is considered to be achieved when the moulded suppository

(*a*) is completely dissolved or

(*b*) has separated into its component parts, which may collect on the surface (melted fatty substances), sink to the bottom (insoluble powders) or dissolve (soluble components) or may be distributed in one or more of these ways or

(*c*) has become soft, which may be accompanied by an appreciable change in shape, without necessarily separating completely into its components, and the mass has no solid core offering resistance to pressure with a glass rod.

Disintegration occurs in not more than 30 minutes for fat-based suppositories and in not more than 60 minutes for water-soluble suppositories, unless otherwise justified and authorised.

Rectal capsules Carry out the procedure described under Moulded suppositories. Disintegration is considered to be achieved when the gelatin shell ruptures, allowing release of the contents.

Disintegration occurs in not more than 30 minutes.

Moulded pessaries Carry out the procedure and use the criteria for disintegration described under Moulded suppositories.

Disintegration occurs in not more than 60 minutes unless otherwise justified and authorised.

Vaginal capsules Carry out the procedure described under Moulded suppositories and use the criterion for disintegration described under Rectal capsules.

Disintegration occurs in not more than 30 minutes.

Vaginal Tablets Place the apparatus in a vessel of suitable diameter containing *water* at 36° to 37°. Adjust the level of the liquid by the gradual addition of *water* at 36°

to 37° until the perforations in the metal disc are just covered by a uniform layer of *water*. Place one vaginal tablet on the upper perforated disc and cover the apparatus with a glass plate to maintain appropriate conditions of humidity. Repeat the operation with a further two vaginal tablets.

Disintegration is considered to be achieved when

(*a*) there is no residue on the perforated plate or

(*b*) if a residue remains, it consists only of a soft or frothy mass having no solid core offering resistance to pressure with a glass rod.

Disintegration occurs in not more than 30 minutes, unless otherwise justified and authorised.

---

[1]All three pieces of apparatus may alternatively be placed together in a vessel containing at least 12 litres.

D. Dissolution Test for Tablets and Capsules (Dissolution Test for Solid Dosage Forms)

(Ph. Eur. method 2.9.3)

The test is used to determine the dissolution rate of the active ingredients of solid dosage forms (for example, tablets, capsules and suppositories).

The choice of the apparatus to be used depends on the physico-chemical characteristics of the dosage form. When this Appendix is invoked in an individual tablet or capsule monograph of the British Pharmacopoeia, use Apparatus I unless otherwise directed. All parts of the apparatus that may come into contact with the preparation being examined or with the dissolution medium are chemically inert and do not adsorb, react with or interfere with the preparation being examined. All metal parts of the apparatus that may come into contact with the preparation or the dissolution medium must be made from a suitable stainless steel or coated with a suitable material to ensure that such parts do not react or interfere with the preparation being examined or the dissolution medium.

No part of the assembly, including the environment in which the assembly is placed, contributes significant motion, agitation or vibration beyond that due to the smoothly rotating element or from the flow-through system.

An apparatus that permits observation of the preparation being examined and the stirrer during the test is preferable.

The dissolution medium is that specified in the individual monograph. If the dissolution medium is a buffered solution, adjust the solution so that its pH is within 0.05 units of the pH specified in the monograph. The dissolution medium is de-aerated prior to testing.

The dimensions and tolerances of the apparatus are specified in Figs. 12D1 to 12D6.

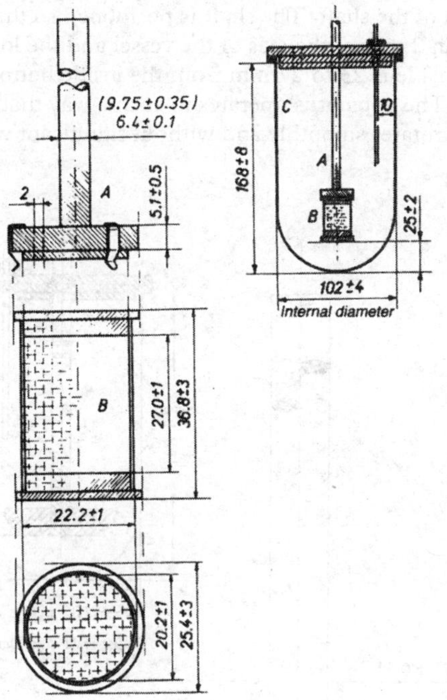

Fig. 12D-1
Basket apparatus
Dimensions in mm

Apparatus I (Basket apparatus)

(a) A cylindrical vessel, C, made of borosilicate glass or other suitable transparent material, with a hemispherical bottom and with a nominal capacity of 1000 ml (Fig. 12D-1). The vessel has a flanged upper rim and is fitted with a lid that has a number of openings, one of which is central.

(b) A motor with a speed regulator capable of maintaining the speed of rotation of the basket within ±4% of that specified in the individual monograph. The motor is fitted with a stirring element which consists of a drive shaft, A, and a cylindrical basket, B (Fig. 12D-1). The metallic shaft rotates smoothly and without significant wobble. The basket consists of two components. The top part, with a vent, is attached to the shaft. It is fitted with three spring clips, or other suitable means, that allow removal of the lower part for introduction of the preparation being examined and that firmly hold the lower part of the basket concentric with the axis of the vessel during rotation. The lower detachable part of the basket is made of welded-seam cloth, with a wire thickness of 0.254 mm diameter and with 0.381 mm square openings, formed into a cylinder with a narrow rim of sheet metal around the top and the bottom. For use with acidic media the basket may be plated with a 2.5-µm layer of gold. The distance between the inside bottom of the vessel and the basket is maintained at 23 to 27 mm during the test.

(c) A water bath that will maintain the dissolution medium at 36.5° to 37.5°.

Apparatus II (Paddle apparatus)

Use Apparatus I described above, except that in the stirring element the basket is replaced by a paddle, D (Fig. 12D-2). The blade passes through the diameter of the shaft so that the bottom of the blade is flush with the bottom of the shaft. The shaft is positioned so that its axis is within 2 mm of the axis of the vessel and the lower edge of the blade is 23 to 27 mm from the inside bottom of the vessel. The apparatus operates in such a way that the paddle rotates smoothly and without significant wobble.

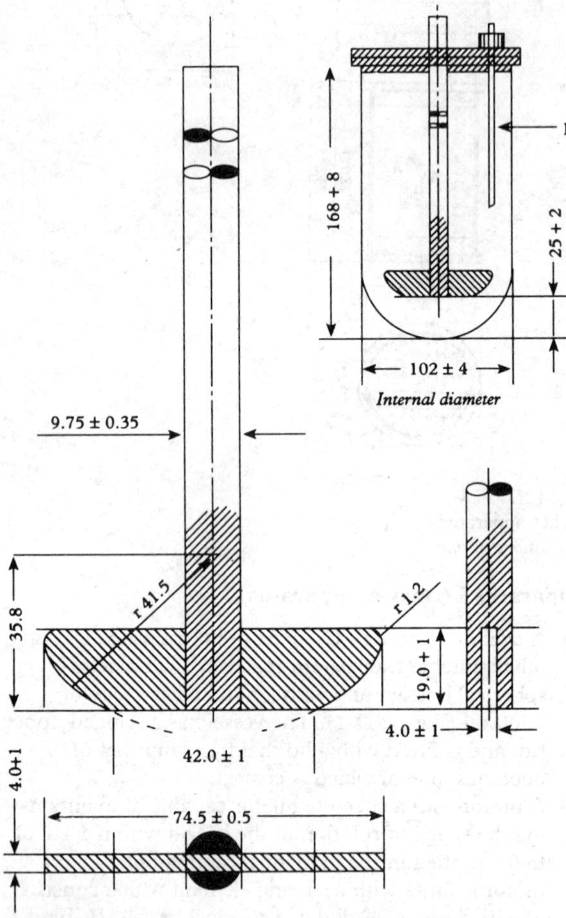

Fig. 12D-2
Paddle apparatus
Dimensions in mm

Apparatus III (Flow-through cell apparatus)

(a) A reservoir for the dissolution medium (Fig. 12D-3).
(b) A pump that forces the dissolution medium upwards through the flow-through cell (Fig. 12D-3).
(c) A flow-through cell of transparent material mounted vertically with a filter system preventing escape of undissolved particles (Fig. 12D-4/5/6).
(d) A water bath that will maintain the dissolution medium at 36.5° to 37.5°.

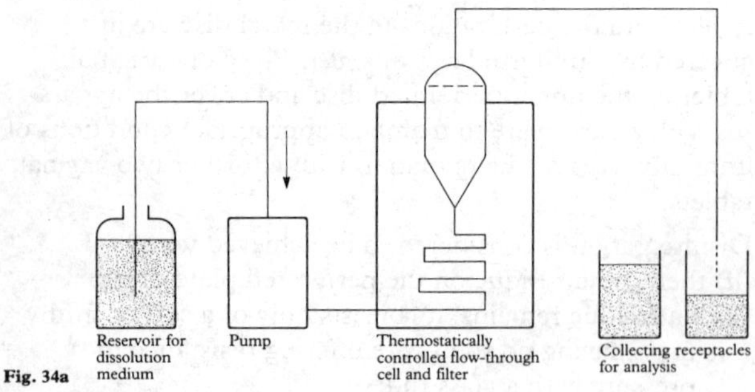

Fig. 12D-3
Apparatus for the Dissolution of Tablets and Capsules (flow-through cell).
Dimensions in mm

Method

Introduce the stated volume of the dissolution medium, free from dissolved air, into the vessel of the apparatus. Warm the dissolution medium to between 36.5° and 37.5°. Unless otherwise stated use one tablet or capsule.

When Apparatus I is used, place the tablet or capsule in a dry basket at the beginning of each test. Lower the basket into position before rotation. When Apparatus II is used, allow the tablet or capsule to sink to the bottom of the vessel prior to the rotation of the paddle. A suitable device such as a wire or glass helix is used to keep tablets

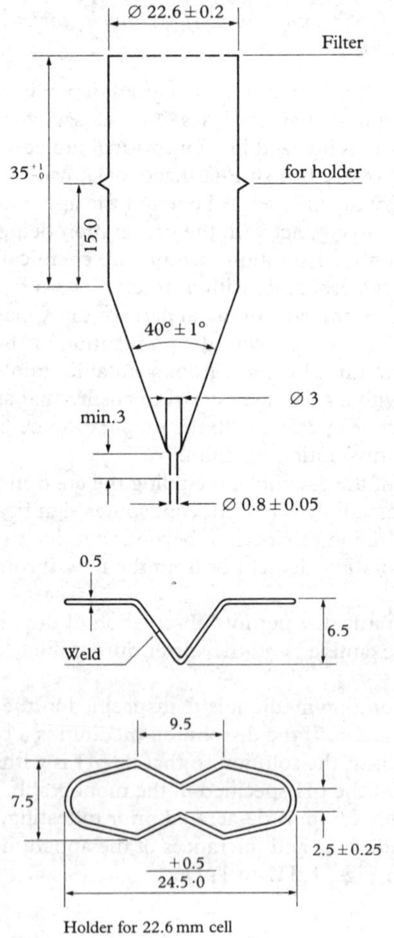

Fig. 12D-4
Flow-through cell
Dimensions in mm

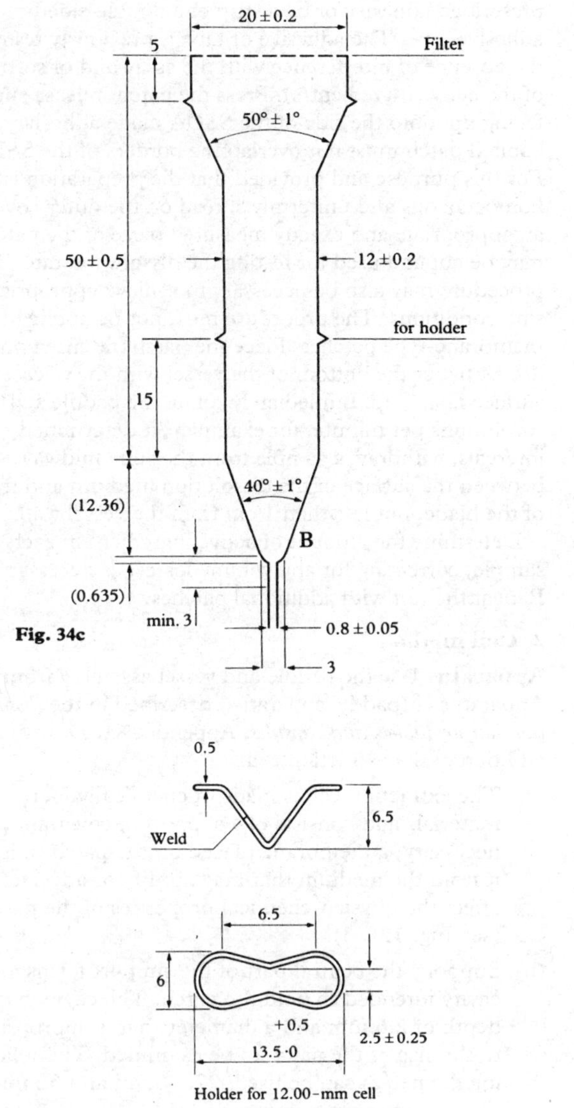

Fig. 12D-5
Flow-through cell
Dimensions in mm

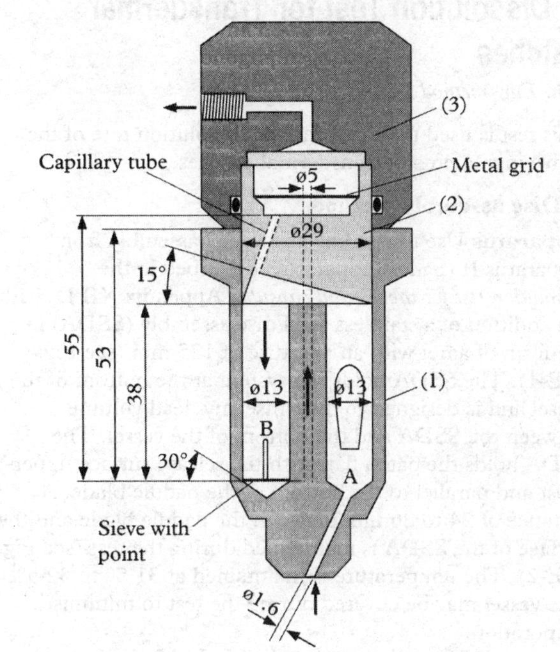

Fig
Flow-through cell
Dimensions in mm

or capsules that would otherwise float horizontal at the bottom of the vessel. Care should be taken to ensure that air bubbles are excluded from the surface of the tablet or capsule. Operate the apparatus immediately at the speed of rotation specified in the individual monograph. When Apparatus III is used, place glass beads of a suitable size, preferably 0.9 to 1.1 mm in diameter, with one bead of 4.5 to 5.5 mm in diameter at the bottom of the cone to protect the fluid entry of the tube and introduce the tablet or capsule in the cell on or within the layer of glass beads or by means of a holder. Assemble the filter head and fix the parts together by means of a suitable clamping device. Warm the dissolution medium to between 36.5° and 37.5° and introduce it through the bottom of the cell using a suitable pump to obtain a suitable continuous flow at the specified rate (± 5%).

Take samples at 45 minutes or at the prescribed intervals or continuously. Withdraw the samples from a point half-way between the surface of the dissolution medium and the top of the rotating basket or blade, not less than 10 mm from the wall of the vessel, or from the continuously flowing medium of the flow-through cell. Except in the cases of continuous flow with the paddle or basket method, where the liquid removed is returned to the dissolution vessel, and single sampling, add a volume of dissolution medium equal to the volume of the samples withdrawn or compensate by calculation. Filter the samples at 36.5° to 37.5° and determine the amount of active ingredient present by the method prescribed in the individual monograph. The filter used is inert, causes no significant absorption of the active ingredient from the solution, contains no materials extractable by the dissolution medium that would interfere with the prescribed analytical procedures and has an appropriate pore size.

Repeat the complete operation five times. Where one tablet or capsule is directed to be placed in the apparatus, for each of the six tablets or capsules tested the amount of active ingredient in solution is not less than 70% of the prescribed or stated amount, unless otherwise specified in the monograph, except that if one fails this requirement a further six may be tested individually and all must comply. Where two or more tablets or capsules are directed to be placed together in the apparatus, a total of six replicate tests are carried out. In each test the amount of active ingredient in solution per tablet or capsule is not less than 70% of the prescribed or stated amount, unless otherwise specified in the monograph No retesting is permitted.

Where capsule shells interfere with the analysis, remove the contents of no fewer than six capsules as completely as possible and dissolve the empty capsule shells in the specified volume of dissolution medium. Carry out the test as directed in the individual monograph and make any necessary correction. Correction factors should not be greater than 25% of the labelled content.

E. Dissolution Test for Transdermal Patches

(Ph. Eur. method 2.9.4)

This test is used to determine the dissolution rate of the active ingredients of transdermal patches.

1. Disc assembly method

Apparatus Use the paddle and vessel assembly from Apparatus II (paddle apparatus) described in the *dissolution test for tablets and capsules*, Appendix XII D, with the addition of a stainless steel disc assembly (SSDA) in the form of a net with an aperture of 125 mm (see Fig. 12E-1). The SSDA holds the system at the bottom of the vessel and is designed to minimise any dead volume between the SSDA and the bottom of the vessel. The SSDA holds the patch flat, with the release surface uppermost and parallel to the bottom of the paddle blade. A distance of 24 to 26 mm between the paddle blade and the surface of the SSDA is maintained during the test (see Fig. 12E-2). The temperature is maintained at 31.5° to 32.5°. The vessel may be covered during the test to minimise evaporation.

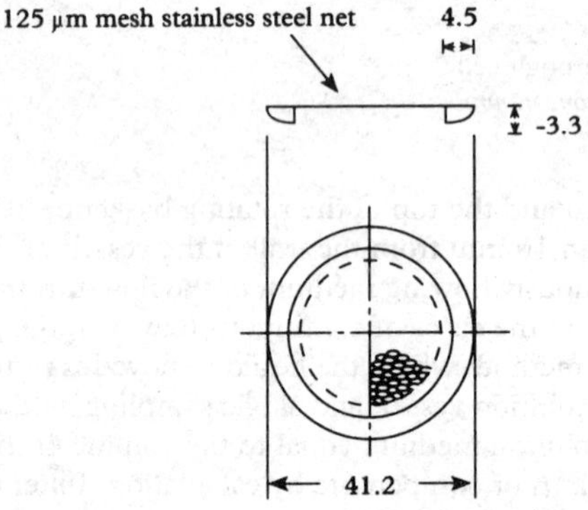

Fig. 12E-1
Paddle Apparatus
Dimensions in mm

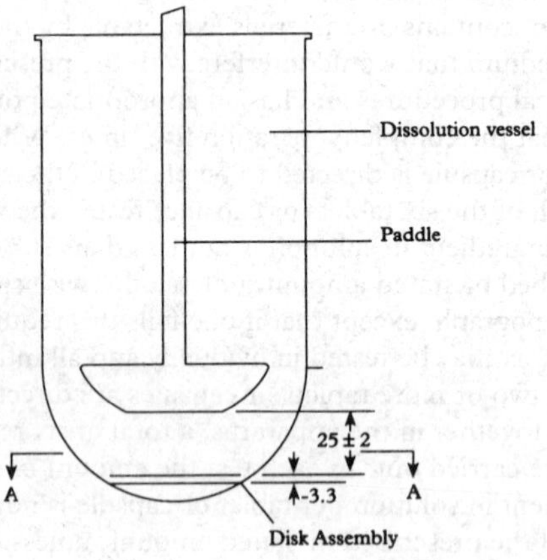

Fig 12E-2
Paddle and disc
Dimensions in mm

Method Place the prescribed volume of the dissolution medium in the vessel and equilibrate the medium to the prescribed temperature. Apply the patch to the SSDA, ensuring that the release surface of the patch is as flat as possible. The patch may be attached to the SSDA by a prescribed adhesive or by a strip of a double-sided adhesive tape. The adhesive or tape is previously tested for the absence of interference with the assay and of sorption of the active ingredient(s). Press the patch, release surface facing up, onto the side of the SSDA made adhesive. The applied patch must not overlap the borders of the SSDA. For this purpose and provided that the preparation is homogeneous and uniformly spread on the outer covering, an appropriate and exactly measured piece of the patch may be cut and used for testing the dissolution rate. This procedure may also be necessary to achieve appropriate sink conditions. The procedure must not be applied to membrane-type patches. Place the patch mounted on the SSDA flat at the bottom of the vessel with the release surface facing up. Immediately rotate the paddle at 100 revolutions per minute, for example. At determined intervals, withdraw a sample from the zone midway between the surface of the dissolution medium and the top of the blade, not less than 1 cm from the vessel wall.

Determine the amount of active ingredient in each sample, correcting for any volume losses, as necessary. Repeat the test with additional patches.

2. Cell method

Apparatus Use the paddle and vessel assembly from Apparatus II (paddle apparatus) described in the *dissolution test for tablets and capsules,* Appendix XII D, with the addition of the extraction cell.

(a) The extraction cell is made of chemically inert materials and consists of a support, a cover and, if necessary, a membrane placed on the patch to isolate it from the medium that may modify or adversely affect the physico-chemical properties of the patch (see Fig. 12E-3).

(b) Support: the central part of the support forms a cavity intended to hold the patch. The cavity has a depth of 2.6 mm and a diameter that is appropriate to the size of the patch to be examined. The following diameters can be used: 27, 38, 45 and 52 mm, corresponding to volumes of 1.48, 2.49, 4.13 and 5.52 ml, respectively.

(c) Cover: the cover has a central opening with a diameter selected according to the size of the patch to be examined. The patch can thus be precisely centred, and its releasing surface limited. The following diameters may be used: 20, 32, 40 and 50 mm corresponding to areas of 3.14, 8.03, 12.56 and 19.63 cm^2, respectively. The cover is held onto the reservoir by nuts screwed onto bolts projecting from the support. The cover is sealed to the support by a rubber ring set on the reservoir.

The extraction cell holds the patch flat, with the release surface uppermost and parallel to the bottom of the paddle blade. A distance of 24 to 26 mm is maintained between the paddle blade and the surface of the patch (see Fig.12E-4). The temperature is maintained at 31.5° to 32.5°. The vessel may be covered during the test to minimise evaporation.

Method Place the prescribed volume of the dissolution medium in the vessel and equilibrate the medium to the prescribed temperature. Precisely centre the patch in the cell with the releasing surface uppermost. Close the cell, if necessary applying a hydrophobic substance (for example, soft paraffin) to the flat surfaces to ensure the seal, and ensure that the patch stays in place. Introduce the cell flat into the bottom of the vessel with the cover facing up. Immediately rotate the paddle, at 100 revolutions per minute for example. At determined intervals, withdraw a sample from the zone midway between the surface of the dissolution medium and the top of the blade, not less than 1 cm from the vessel wall.

Perform the assay on each sample, correcting for any volume losses, as necessary. Repeat the test with additional patches.

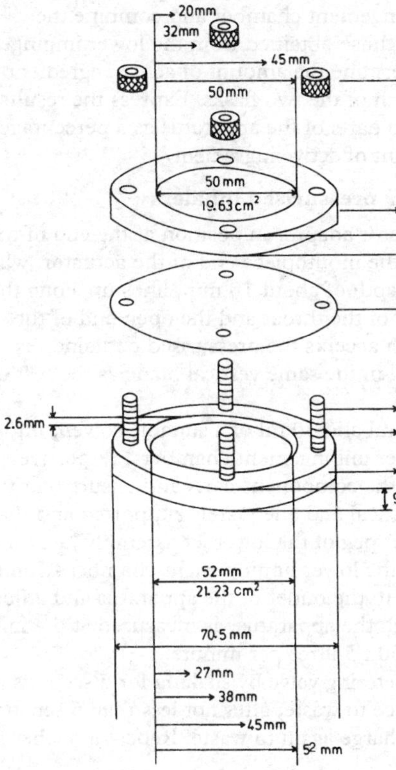

Fig 12E-3
Extraction cell
Dimensions in mm

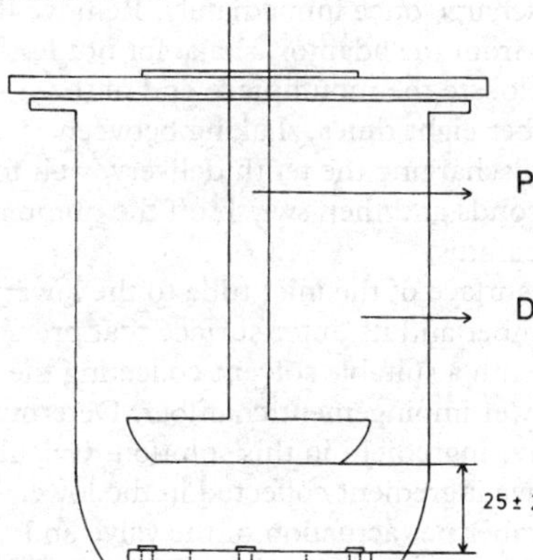

Fig 12E-4
Paddle over extraction cell
Dimensions in mm

3. Rotating cylinder method

Apparatus Use the assembly of Apparatus II (paddle apparatus) described in the *dissolution test for tablets and capsules*, Appendix XII D. Replace the paddle and shaft with a stainless steel cylinder stirring element (cylinder; see Fig. 12E-5). The patch is placed on the cylinder at the beginning of each test. The distance between the inside bottom of the vessel and the cylinder is maintained at 31.5° to 32.5°. The vessel is covered during the test to minimise evaporation.

Method Place the prescribed volume of the dissolution medium in the vessel and equilibrate the medium to the prescribed temperature. Remove the protective liner from the patch and place the adhesive side on a piece of suitable inert porous membrane that is at least 1 cm larger on all sides than the patch. Place the patch on a clean surface with the membrane in contact with this surface. Two systems for adhesion to the cylinder may be used:

(a) apply a suitable adhesive to the exposed membrane borders and, if necessary, to the back of the patch,

(b) apply a double-sided adhesive tape to the external wall of the cylinder.

Using gentle pressure, carefully apply the patch to the adhesive tape by the side of the outer covering, so that the release surface is in contact with the dissolution medium and the long axis of the patch fits around the circumference of the cylinder.

The system for adhesion used is previously tested for absence of interference with the assay and of adsorption of the active ingredient(s).

Place the cylinder in the apparatus, and immediately rotate the cylinder at 100 revolutions per minute for example. At determined intervals, withdraw a sample of dissolution medium from a zone midway between the surface of the dissolution medium and the top of the rotating cylinder, and not less than 1 cm from the vessel wall.

Perform the assay on each sample as directed in the individual monograph, correcting for any volume withdrawn, as necessary. Repeat the test with additional patches.

Interpretation

The requirements are met if the quantity of active ingredient(s) released from the patch, expressed as the amount per surface area per time unit is within the prescribed limits at the defined sampling times.

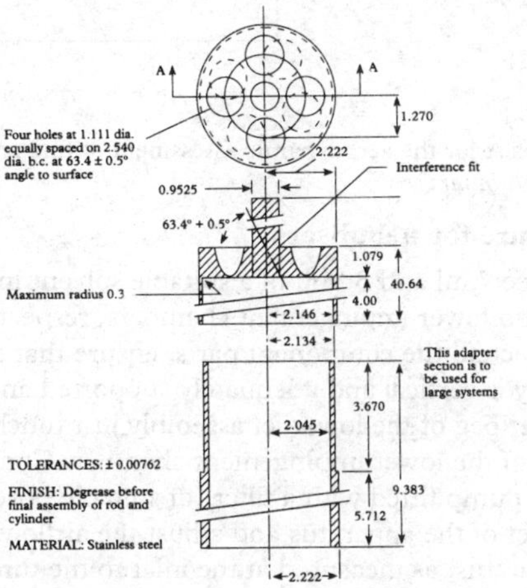

Fig 12E-5
Cylinder stirring element
Dimensions in cm

F. Aerodynamic Assessment of Fine Particles

(Ph. Eur. method 2.9.18)

This test is used to determine the fine particles fraction in the aerosols generated by preparations for inhalation.

Unless otherwise justified and authorised, one of the following apparatus and test procedures is used.

Apparatus A (Glass Impinger)

The apparatus is shown in Fig. 12-1 (see also Table 12F-1).

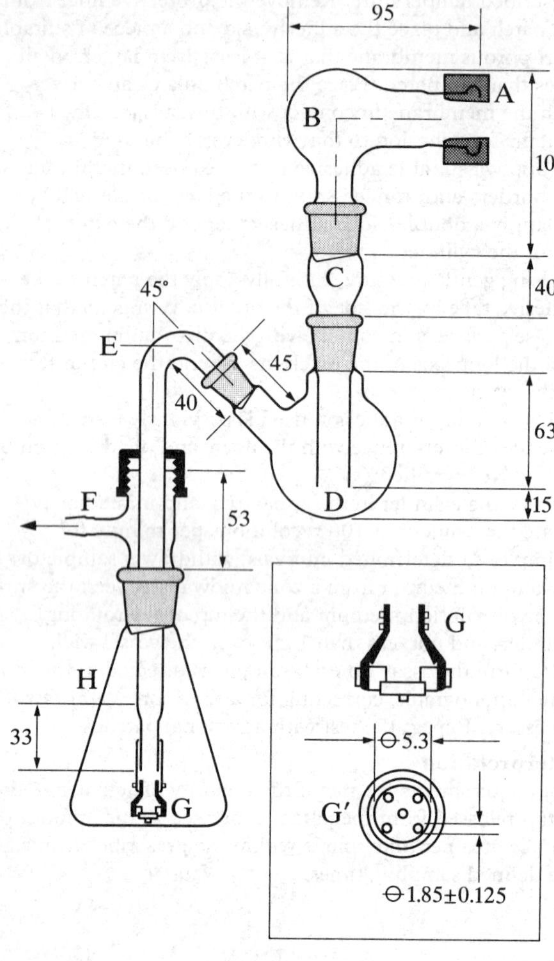

Fig. 12F-1
Apparatus A for the aerodynamic assessment of fine particles
Dimensions in mm

Procedure for nebulisers

Introduce 7 ml and 30 ml of a suitable solvent into the upper and lower impingement chambers, respectively.

Connect all the component parts, ensure that the assembly is vertical and adequately supported and that the jet spacer peg of the lower jet assembly just touches the bottom of the lower impingement chamber. Connect a suitable pump fitted with a filter (of suitable pore size) to the outlet of the apparatus and adjust the airflow through the apparatus, as measured at the inlet to the throat, to 60±5 litres per minute.

Introduce the liquid preparation for inhalation into the reservoir of the nebuliser. Fit the mouthpiece and connect it by means of an adaptor to the device.

Switch on the pump of the apparatus and after 10 seconds switch on the nebuliser.

After 60 seconds, unless otherwise justified, switch off the nebuliser, wait for about 5 seconds and then switch off the pump of the apparatus. Dismantle the apparatus and wash the inner surface of the upper impingement chamber collecting the washings in a volumetric flask. Wash the inner surface of the lower impingement chamber collecting the washings in a second volumetric flask. Finally, wash the filter preceding the pump and its connections to the lower impingement chamber and combine the washings with those obtained from the lower impingement chamber. Determine the amount of active ingredient collected in each of the two flasks. Express the results for each of the two parts of the apparatus as a percentage of the total amount of active ingredient.

Procedure for pressurised inhalers

Place the actuator adaptor in position at the end of the throat so that the mouthpiece end of the actuator, when inserted to a depth of about 10 mm, lines up along the horizontal axis of the throat and the open end of the actuator, which accepts the pressurised container, is uppermost and in the same vertical plane as the rest of the apparatus.

Introduce 7 ml and 30 ml of a suitable solvent into the upper and lower impingement chambers, respectively.

Connect all the component parts and ensure that the assembly is vertical and adequately supported and that the lower jet-spacer peg of the lower jet assembly just touches the bottom of the lower impingement chamber. Connect a suitable pump to the outlet of the apparatus and adjust the air flow through the apparatus, as measured at the inlet to the throat, to 60±5 litres per minute.

Prime the metering valve by shaking for 5 seconds and discharging once to waste; after not less than 5 seconds, shake and discharge again to waste. Repeat a further three times.

Shake for about 5 seconds, switch on the pump to the apparatus and locate the mouthpiece end of the actuator in the adaptor, discharge once immediately. Remove the assembled inhaler from the adaptor, shake for not less than 5 seconds, relocate the mouthpiece end of the actuator for a further eight times, shaking between actuations. After discharging the tenth delivery, wait for not less than 5 seconds and then switch off the pump. Dismantle the apparatus.

Wash the inner surface of the inlet tube to the lower impingement chamber and its outer surface that projects into the chamber with a suitable solvent collecting the washings in the lower impingement chamber. Determine the content of active ingredient in this solution. Calculate the amount of active ingredient collected in the lower impingement chamber per actuation of the valve and express the results as a percentage of the dose stated on the label.

Procedure for powder inhalers

Introduce 7 ml and 30 ml of a suitable solvent into the upper and lower impingement chambers, respectively.

Connect all the component parts and ensure that the assembly is vertical and adequately supported and that the jet spacer peg of the lower jet assembly just touches the bottom of the lower impingement chamber. Without the inhaler in place, connect a suitable pump to the outlet of the apparatus and adjust the air flow through the appara-

TABLE I Details of Apparatus A

Item	Description	Identifying Code[1]	Dimensions[2] mm
Mouthpiece adapter	Moulded rubber adapter for actuator mouthpiece	A	
Throat	Modified round-bottomed flask	B	50 ml
	ground-glass inlet socket		29/32
	ground-glass outlet cone		24/29
Neck	Modified glass adaptor	C	
	ground-glass inlet socket		24/29
	ground-glass outlet cone		24/29
	Lower outlet section of precision-bore glass tubing		
	bore diameter		14
	Selected-bore light-wall glass tubing		
	external diameter		17
Upper impingement chamber	Modified round-bottomed flask	D	100 ml
	ground-glass inlet socket		24/29
	ground-glass outlet cone		24/29
Coupling tube	Medium wall glass tubing	E	
	ground-glass cone		14/23
	Bent section and upper vertical section		
	external diameter		13
	Lower vertical section		
	external diameter		8
Screwthread, side-arm adapter	Plastic screw cap	F	28/13
	Silicone rubber ring		28/11
	PTFE washer		28/11
	Glass screwhead, *threadsize*		28
	Side-arm outlet to vacuum pump,		
	minimum bore diameter		5
Lower jet assembly	Modified polypropylene[3] filter holder connected to lower vertical section of coupling tube by PTFE tubing	G	See Fig. 60
	Acetal circular disc with the centres of four jets arranged on a projected circle of diameter 5.3 mm with an integral jet spacer peg	G′	10
	peg diameter		2
	peg protrusion		2
Lower impingement chamber	Conical flask	H	250 ml
	ground-glass inlet socket		24/29

[1]On Fig. 12F-1

[2]Dimensions of ground-glass sockets and cones are specified in terms of the ISO designation in accordance with British Standard 572:1960. Quickfit apparatus is suitable.

[3]A modified Millipore Swinnex 13 polypropylene filter holder is suitable.

tus, as measured at the inlet to the throat, to 60±5 litres per minute.

Prepare the inhaler for use and locate the mouthpiece in the apparatus by means of a suitable adaptor. Switch on the pump for 5 seconds. Switch off the pump and remove the inhaler. Repeat for a further nine discharges. Dismantle the apparatus.

Wash the inner surface of the inlet tube to the lower impingement chamber and its outer surface that projects into the chamber with a suitable solvent, collecting the washings in the lower impingement chamber. Determine the content of active ingredient in this solution. Calculate the amount of active ingredient collected in the lower impingement chamber per discharge and express the results as a percentage of the dose stated on the label.

Apparatus B (Metal Impinger)

The apparatus is shown in Figs. 12F-1and 12F-2.

Procedure for nebulisers

The deposition of emitted droplets is tested using the impingement apparatus, which is connected to the filled nebuliser by means of a suitable adaptor. The outlet of the apparatus to the pump is fitted with a suitable filter (for example pores of 0.25 µm).

In this procedure, the impingement chamber is used dry. Connect all the component parts and ensure that the base of the impinger is placed on a flat, horizontal and adequately supported surface. Connect a suitable pump to the outlet of the apparatus and adjust the air flow through the apparatus, as measured at the inlet to the throat, to 60±5 litres per minute.

Introduce the liquid preparation for inhalation into the reservoir of a suitable nebuliser. Fit the mouthpiece and connect it to the adaptor of the device.

Switch on the pump of the apparatus and after 10 seconds, switch on the nebuliser.

After 60 seconds, unless otherwise justified, switch off the nebuliser, wait for about 5 seconds and then switch off the pump of the apparatus. Dismantle the apparatus. Wash the inner surface of the throat, the top and bottom portions of the chamber, collecting the washings in a volumetric flask. Wash the filter assembly by passing a suitable solvent through the filter and collecting in a suitable graduated flask. Determine the content of active ingredient in these solutions. Express the results for each of the two parts of the apparatus as a percentage of the total amount of active ingredient.

Procedure for pressurised inhalers

Place the actuator adaptor in position at the end of the throat so that the mouthpiece end of the actuator, when inserted, lines up along the horizontal axis of the throat and the open end of the actuator, which accepts the pressurised container, is uppermost and in the same vertical plane as the rest of the apparatus.

In this procedure, the impingement chamber is used dry. Connect all the component parts and ensure that the base of the impinger is placed on a flat, horizontal and adequately supported surface so that the open end of the actuator, which accepts the pressurised container, is in a vertical position. Connect a suitable pump to the outlet of the apparatus and adjust the air flow through the apparatus, as measured at the inlet to the throat, to 60±5 litres per minute.

Prime the metering valve by shaking for 5 seconds and discharging once to waste; after not less than 5 seconds, shake and discharge again to waste. Repeat a further three times.

Shake for about 5 seconds, switch on the pump to the apparatus and locate the mouthpiece end of the actuator in the adaptor and discharge once immediately. Remove the assembled inhaler from the adaptor, shake for about 5 seconds, relocate the mouthpiece end of the actuator in the adaptor and discharge again. Repeat the discharge sequence for a further eight times shaking between actuations. After discharging the tenth delivery, wait for about 5 seconds and then switch off the pump. Dismantle the apparatus.

Wash the filter assembly by passing a suitable solvent through the filter. Determine the content of active ingredient in this solution. Calculate the amount of active ingredient collected on the filter assembly per actuation of the valve and express the results as a percentage of the dose stated on the label.

Procedure for powder inhalers

Introduce 25-ml amounts of a suitable solvent into the impingement chamber so as to cover the sintered-glass disk.

Connect all the component parts and ensure that the base of the impinger is placed on a flat, horizontal and adequately supported surface. Without the inhaler in place, connect a suitable pump to the outlet of the apparatus and adjust the air flow through the apparatus, as measured at the inlet to the throat, to 60±5 litres per minute.

Prepare the inhaler for use and locate the mouthpiece in the apparatus by means of a suitable adaptor. Switch on the pump for 5 seconds. Switch off the pump and remove the inhaler. Repeat the discharge for a further nine discharges. Dismantle the apparatus.

Wash the filter assembly by passing a suitable solvent through the filter. Determine the content of active ingredient in this solution. Calculate the amount of active ingredient collected on the filter assembly per discharge and express the results as a percentage of the dose stated on the label.

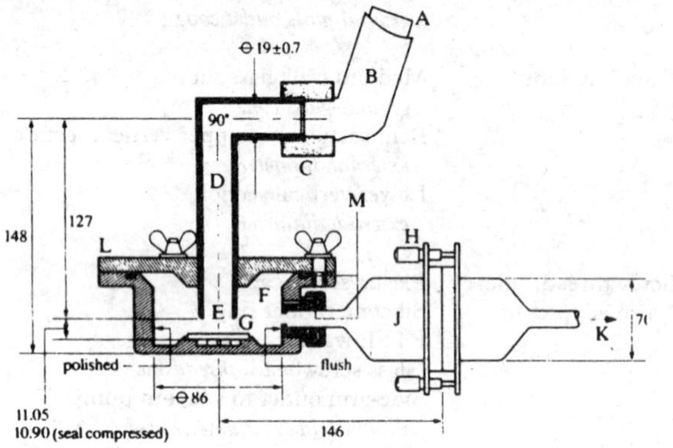

Fig. 12F-2
Apparatus B for the aerodynamic assessment of fine particles
Dimensions in mm

A – Pressurised inhalation container	G – Sintered-glass disc (BS porosity No. 1)
B – Actuator	H – Stainless steel filter clamp
C – Adaptor	J – Glass filter assembly
D – Throat	K – Vacuum Pump
E – Jet	L – Aluminium impingement chamber pump
F – Impingement chamber	M – Rubber O-rings

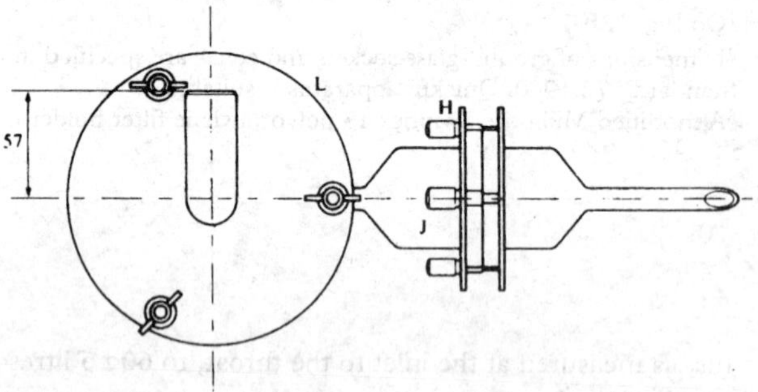

Fig. 12F-3
Apparatus B for the aerodynamic assessment of fine particles (top elevation)

Apparatus C (Multistage Liquid Impinger)

The apparatus is shown in Figures 62a, 62b and 62c.

The apparatus consists of a glass inlet throat (A), impaction stages 1, 2 and 3 and an integral filter stage (stage 4). An impaction stage comprises an upper horizontal metal partition wall (B) through which a metal inlet jet tube (C) with its impaction plate (D) protrudes, a glass

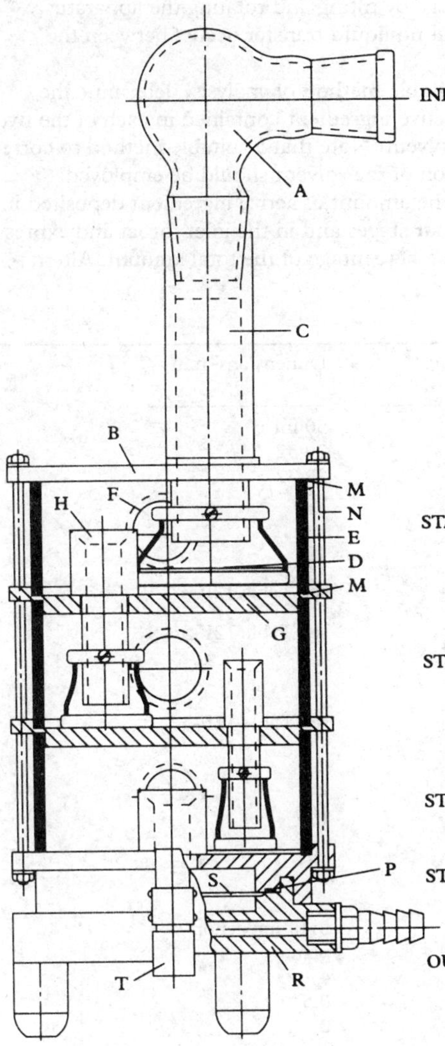

Fig. 12F-4
Apparatus C for the aerodynamic assessment of fine particles
Dimensions in mm

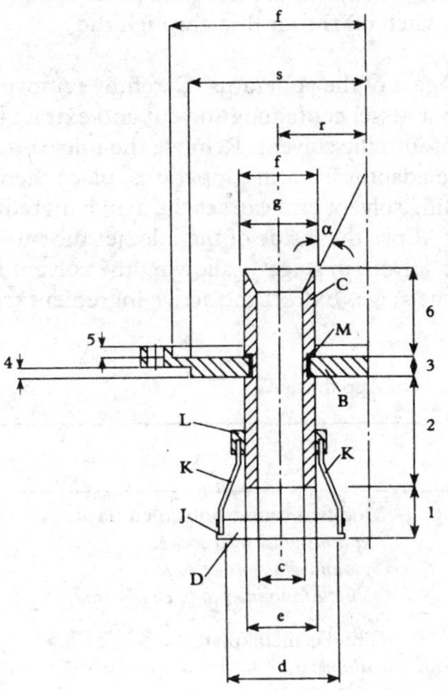

Fig. 12F-5
Details of Apparatus C
Dimensions in mm

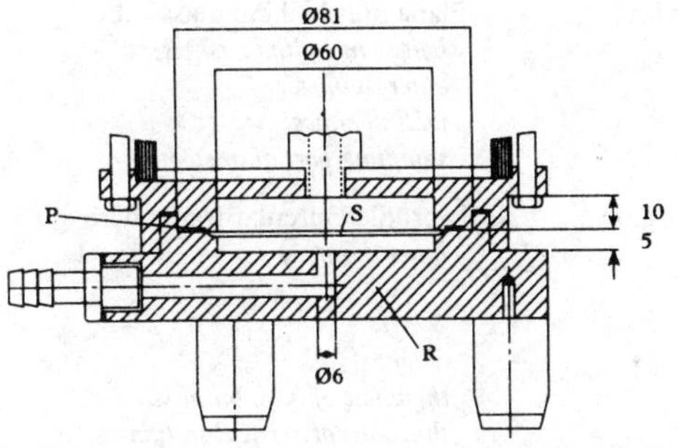

Fig. 12F-6
Details of filter stage for Apparatus C (stage 4)
Dimensions in mm

cylinder (E) with a sampling port (F) forming the vertical wall of the stage, and a lower horizontal metal partition wall (G) through which a jet tube (H) connects to the next lower stage. The impaction plate (D) is secured in a metal frame (J) which is fastened by two wires (K) to a sleeve (L) secured on the jet tube (C). The horizontal plane of the collection plate is perpendicular to the axis of the jet tube and centrally aligned. The upper surface of the impaction plate is slightly raised above the edge of the metal frame. A recess around the perimeter of the horizontal partition wall guides the position of the glass cylinder. The glass cylinders are sealed against the horizontal partition walls with gaskets (M) and clamped together by six bolts (N). The sampling ports are closed by stoppers. The bottom-side of the lower partition wall of stage 3 has a concentrical protrusion fitted with a rubber O-ring (P) which seals against the edge of a filter placed in the filter holder. The filter holder (R) is constructed as a basin with a concentric recess in which a perforated filter support (S) is flush-fitted. The assembly of impaction stages is clamped onto the filter holder by two snap-locks (T). The filter holder is dimensioned for 76-mm diameter filters. Details and dimensions of the apparatus are given in Tables 12F-1 and 12F-2.

Procedure for nebulisers

Dispense 20 ml of a suitable solvent into each of the three upper stages of the apparatus. Place a suitable filter in stage 4 and assemble the apparatus. Place a suitable adaptor in position at the end of the throat so that the mouthpiece end of the nebuliser, when inserted, lines up along the horizontal axis of the throat and the nebuliser unit is positioned in the same orientation as the intended use. Connect a suitable pump to the outlet of the apparatus and adjust the air flow through the apparatus, as measured at the inlet to the throat, to 60±5 litres per minute. Switch off the air flow.

Introduce the liquid preparation for inhalation into the reservoir of a suitable nebuliser and prepare the nebuliser for operation. Connect the mouthpiece of the nebuliser to the adaptor of the apparatus.

Switch on the pump of the apparatus and after 10 seconds switch on the nebuliser. After 60 seconds, unless otherwise justified, switch off the nebuliser, wait for about 5 seconds and switch off the air flow through the apparatus.

Dismantle stage 4 of the apparatus. Carefully remove the filter, place it in a vessel containing solvent and extract the active ingredient into the solvent. Remove the inlet throat and mouthpiece adaptor from the apparatus, place them in a vessel containing solvent and extract the active ingredient into the solvent. Rinse the inside of the inlet jet tube to stage 1 with the solvent in stage 1, allowing the solvent to flow back into the stage. Extract the active ingredient from the inner walls and the collection plate of each of the three upper stages of the apparatus into the solution in the respective stage by tilting and rotating the apparatus, observing that no liquid transfer occurs between the stages.

Using a suitable method of analysis, determine the quantity of active ingredient contained in each of the five volumes of solvent. Note that a suitable method to correct for evaporation of the solvent should be employed.

Calculate the amount of active ingredient deposited in each of the four stages and in the inlet throat and express the results as a percentage of the total amount. Alterna-

Table 12F-2 Details of Apparatus C

Item	Description	Identifying code[1]	Dimensions[2] mm
Throat	Modified round-bottomed flask	A	50 ml
	ground-glass inlet socket		29/32
	ground-glass outlet cone		29/32
	length from inlet to back of throat		95
Partition wall	Circular metal plate	B, G	
	diameter		120
	thickness		see Table 12F-3
Jet tube	Metal tube screwed onto partition wall sealed by *gasket, polished inner surface*	C, H	see Table 12F-3
Impaction plate	Porosity 0 sintered-glass disk	D	
	diameter		see Table 12F-3
Glass cylinder	Plane polished cut glass tube	E	
	height including gaskets		46
	outer diameter		100
	wall thickness		3.5
	sampling port diameter	F	18
Metal Frame	L-profiled circular frame with slit	J	
	inner diameter		to fit impaction plate
	height		4
	thickness of horizontal section		0.5
	thickness of vertical section		2
Wire	Steel wire interconnecting metal frame and sleeve (two for each frame)	K	
	diameter		1
Sleeve	Metal sleeve secured on jet tube by screw	L	
	inner diameter		to fit jet tube
	height		6
	thickness		5
Bolt	Metal bolt with nut (six pairs), *length*	N	157
	diameter		4
O-ring	Rubber O-ring	P	
	diameter		66.34
	thickness		2.62
Filter holder	Metal housing with stand and outlet	R	see Fig. 62c
Filter support	Perforated metal sheet	S	
	diameter		65
	hole diameter		3
	distance between centre points of holes		4

[1]Refer to Figs. 12F-4 and 12F-6

[2]Dimensions of ground-glass sockets and cones are specified in terms of the ISO designation in accordance with British Standard 572:1960. Quickfit apparatus is suitable.

tively, combine the results from stage 3 with stage 4 and the results from the inlet throat with stage 1 and stage 2.

Procedure for pressurised inhalers

Dispense 20 ml of a suitable solvent into each of the three upper stages of the apparatus. Place a suitable filter in stage 4 and assemble the apparatus. Place a suitable mouthpiece adaptor in position at the end of the throat so that the mouthpiece end of the actuator, when inserted lines up along the horizontal axis of the throat and the inhaler unit is positioned in the same orientation as the intended use. Connect a suitable pump to the outlet of the apparatus and adjust the air flow through the apparatus, as measured at the inlet to the throat, to 60±5 litres per minute. Switch off the air flow.

Prime the metering valve by shaking for 5 seconds and discharge once to waste; after not less than 5 seconds, shake and discharge again to waste. Repeat a further three times.

Shake for about 5 seconds, switch on the pump to the apparatus and locate the mouthpiece end of the actuator in the adaptor and discharge once immediately. Remove the assembled inhaler from the adaptor, shake for about 5 seconds, relocate the mouthpiece end of the actuator in the adaptor and discharge again. Repeat the discharge sequence for a further eight times shaking between actuations. After discharging the tenth delivery, wait for about 5 seconds and then switch off the pump.

Dismantle stage 4 of the apparatus. Carefully remove the filter, place it in a vessel containing solvent and extract the active ingredient into the solvent. Remove the inlet throat and mouthpiece adaptor from the apparatus, place them in a vessel containing solvent and extract the active ingredient into the solvent. Rinse the inside of the inlet jet tube to stage 1 with the solvent in stage 1, allowing the solvent to flow back into the stage. Extract the active ingredient from the inner walls and the collection plate of each of the three upper stages of the apparatus into the solution in the respective stage by tilting and rotating the apparatus, observing that no liquid transfer occurs between the stages.

Using a suitable method of analysis, determine the quantity of active ingredient contained in each of the five volumes of solvent. Note that a suitable method to correct for evaporation of the solvent should be employed.

Calculate the accumulated mass of active ingredient per discharge deposited in stage 4, in stage 3 + 4, in stage 2 + 3 + 4, in stage 1 + 2 + 3 + 4 and in stage 1 + 2 + 3 + 4 + inlet throat + mouthpiece adaptor (the total dose delivered per discharge to the apparatus).

Alternatively, only the two volumes of solvent from stage 3 and stage 4 may be analysed, and the amount of active ingredient per discharge deposited in stage 3 + 4 is expressed as a percentage of the dose stated on the label.

Procedure for powder inhalers

Dispense 20 ml of a suitable solvent into each of the three upper stages of the apparatus. Place a suitable filter in stage 4 and assemble the apparatus. Place a suitable adaptor in position at the end of the throat so that the mouthpiece of the inhaler, when inserted, lines up along the horizontal axis of the throat and the inhaler unit is positioned in the same orientation as the intended use. Without the device in place, connect a suitable pump to the outlet of the apparatus and adjust the air flow through the apparatus, as measured at the inlet to the throat to 60±5 litres per minute. Switch off the air flow.

Prepare the inhaler for use and locate the mouthpiece in the apparatus by means of a suitable adaptor. Switch on the pump for 5 seconds, switch off the pump and remove the inhaler. Repeat for a further nine discharges.

Dismantle stage 4 of the apparatus. Carefully remove the filter, place it in a vessel containing solvent and extract the active ingredient into the solvent. Remove the inlet throat and mouthpiece adaptor from the apparatus, place them in a vessel containing solvent and extract the active ingredient into the solvent. Rinse the inside of the inlet jet tube to stage 1 with the solvent in stage 1, allowing the solvent to flow back into the stage. Extract the active ingredient from the inner walls and the collection plate of each of the three upper stages of the apparatus into the solution in the respective stage by tilting and rotating the apparatus, observing that no liquid transfer occurs between the stages.

Using a suitable method of analysis, determine the quantity of active ingredient contained in each of the five volumes of solvent. Note that a suitable method to correct for evaporation of the solvent should be employed. This may involve the use of an internal standard or the use of quantitative transfer followed by dilution to a fixed volume.

Calculate the accumulated mass of active ingredient per discharge deposited in stage 4, in stage 3 + 4, in stage 2 + 3 + 4, in stage 1 + 2 + 3 + 4 and in stage 1 + 2 + 3 + 4 + inlet throat + mouthpiece adapator (the total dose delivered per discharge to the apparatus).

Alternatively, only the two volumes of solvent from stage 3 and stage 4 may be analysed, and the amount of active ingredient per discharge deposited in stage 3 + 4 is expressed as a percentage of the dose stated on the label.

Table 12F-3 Dimensions[1] of jet tube with impaction plate of Apparatus C

Type	Code[2]	Stage 1	Stage 2	Stage 3	Filter 4 (Stage 4)
Distance	1	9.5	5.5	4.0	–
Distance	2	26	31	33	0
Distance	3	8	5	5	5
Distance	4	3	3	3	–
Distance	5	0	3	3	3
Distance	6[3]	90	25	25	25
Diameter	c	25	14	8	14
Diameter	d	50	30	20	–
Diameter	e	27.9	16.5	10.5	–
Diameter	f	32	22	14	22
Diameter	g	27.5	21	13	21
Radius[4]	r	16	22	27	0
Radius[4]	s	46	46	46	–
Radius[4]	t	–	50	50	50
Angle	α	2.86°	26.5°	26.5°	26.5°
cone		1/10	1/2	1/2	1/2

[1]Dimensions in mm unless otherwise stated
[2]Refer to Fig. 12F-6
[3]Including gasket
[4]Relative centre point of stage compartment

Apparatus D (Multistage Cascade Impactor)

Suitable configurations of a multistage cascade impactor, for which the following text applies, are given in Figure 12F-7 (see also Table 12F-4). Other suitable induction ports may also be used.

Procedure for pressurised inhalers

Assemble the multistage cascade impactor and ensure that the system is airtight. Connect a pump to the apparatus and adjust the air flow through the apparatus, as measured at the inlet to the throat, for that prescribed for the apparatus. Switch off the pump.

Place a moulded adaptor in position on the ground glass socket at the end of the throat piece such that the inhaler actuator mouthpiece, when inserted into the adaptor, will be lined up along the horizontal axis of the throat piece and the open end of the actuator which accepts the canister will be uppermost and in the same vertical plane as the rest of the apparatus.

Prime the metering valve by shaking for 5 seconds and discharge once to waste; after about 5 seconds, shake and discharge again to waste. Repeat a further three times.

Shake for about 5 seconds, switch on the pump to the apparatus and locate the mouthpiece end of the actuator in the adaptor, discharge once immediately. Remove the assembled inhaler from the adaptor, shake for about 5 seconds, relocate the mouthpiece end of the actuator in the adaptor and discharge again. Repeat the discharge sequence for a further eight times, shaking between actuations. After discharging the tenth delivery, wait for not less than 5 seconds and then switch off the pump. Dismantle the apparatus.

Wash the rubber adaptor and the inside of the throat with a suitable solvent and collect the washings.

Rinse the residues of each impaction stage with a suitable solvent. Determine the content of active ingredient on each stage and in the throat.

Procedure for powder inhalers

If necessary, coat each plate with a suitable liquid, for example, silicone oil. Assemble the multistage cascade impactor with a suitable pre-separator and ensure that the system is airtight. Connect a pump to the apparatus and, without the inhaler in place, adjust the air flow through the apparatus, as measured at the inlet to the throat, to that prescribed for the apparatus. Switch off the pump.

Prepare the inhaler for use and locate the mouthpiece in the apparatus by means of a suitable adaptor. Switch on the pump for 5 seconds. Switch off the pump and remove the inhaler. Repeat for a further nine discharges. Dismantle the apparatus.

TABLE 12F-3 Component units of Apparatus D

Item	Description	Identifying code[1]	Dimensions
Mouthpiece adaptor	Moulded rubber adaptor for actuator mouthpiece	A	
Throat[2]	Modified round-bottom flask *ground-glass inlet socket*	B	50 ml 29/32
Adaptor	Plastic tube	C	
Multistage cascade impactor	Manufacturer's description	D	

[1]Refer to Fig. 63

[2]A suitable induction port design is given in Fig. 63. Different configurations may also be employed.

Rinse the residues of each impaction stage with a suitable solvent. Determine the content of active ingredient on each stage and in the throat.

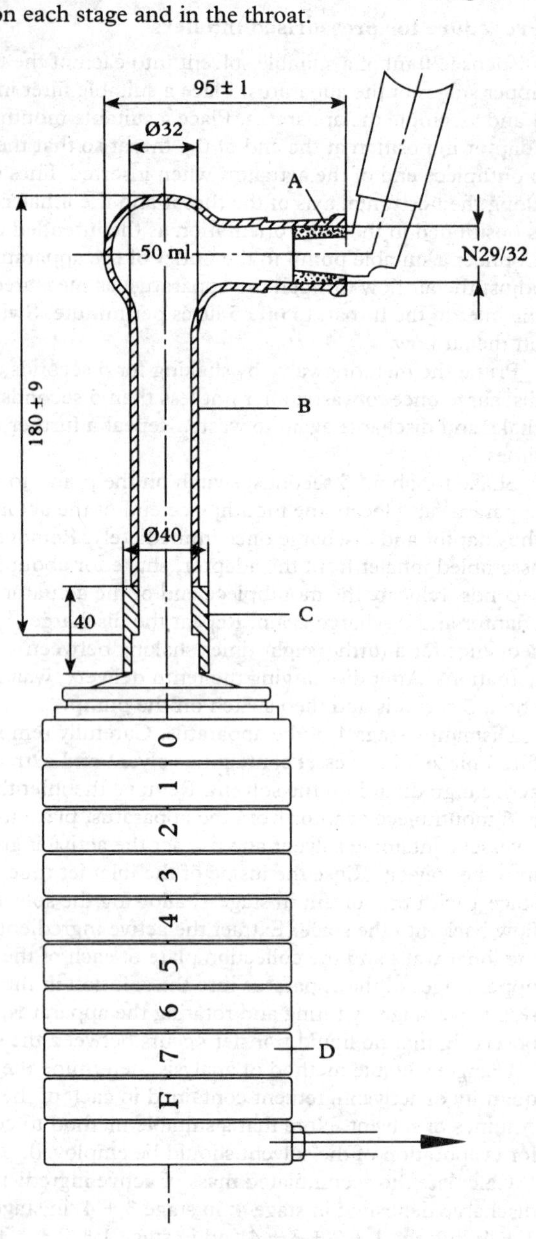

Fig. 12F-7
Apparatus D for the aerodynamic assessment of fine particles
Dimensions in mm

G. Uniformity of Weight (Mass)

(Ph. Eur. method 2.9.5)

Weigh individually twenty units taken at random or, for single-dose preparations presented in individual containers, contents of twenty units, and determine the average weight (mass). Not more than two of the individual weights (masses) deviate from the average weight (mass) by more than the percentage deviation shown in Table 12G-1 and none deviates by more than twice that percentage.

Table 12G-1

Pharmaceutical form	Average weight (mass)	Percentage deviation
Tablets (uncoated and film-coated	80 mg or less	10
	More than 80 mg and less than 250 mg	7.5
	250 mg or more	5
Capsules, Granules (uncoated, single-dose) and Powders (single-dose)	Less than 300 mg	10
	300 mg or more	7.5
Powders for Parenteral Use(*) (single-dose)	More than 40 mg	10
Suppositories and Pessaries	All weights (masses)	5

When the average weight (mass) is equal to or below 40 mg, the preparation is not submitted to the test for uniformity of weight (mass) but to the test for uniformity of content, Appendix XII H. For capsules and powders for parenteral use, proceed as described below.

Capsules

Weigh an intact capsule. Open the capsule without losing any part of the shell and remove the contents as completely as possible. For soft shell capsules, wash the shell with ether or other suitable solvent and allow to stand until the odour of the solvent is no longer perceptible. Weigh the shell. The weight (mass) of the contents is the difference between the weighings. Repeat the procedure with another nineteen capsules.

Powders for parenteral use

Remove any paper labels from a container and wash and dry the outside. Open the container and without delay weigh the container and its contents. Empty the container as completely as possible by gentle tapping, rinse it if necessary with *water* and *ethanol (96%)* and dry at 100° to 105° for 1 hour, or, if the nature of the container precludes heating at this temperature, dry at a lower temperature to constant weight (mass). Allow to cool in a desiccator and weigh. The weight (mass) of the contents is the difference between the weighings. Repeat the procedure with another nineteen containers.

H. Uniformity of Content

(Ph. Eur. method 2.9.6)

The test for uniformity of content is based on the assay of the individual contents of active ingredient of a number of single-dose units to determine whether the individual contents are within limits set with reference to the average content of the sample.

The test is not required for multivitamin and trace-element preparations and in other justified and authorised circumstances.

Method

Using a suitable analytical method, determine the individual contents of active ingredient of ten dosage units taken at random.

Apply the criteria of test A, test B or test C as specified in the monograph for the dosage form in question.

Test A

Tablets, powders for parenteral use and suspensions for injection The preparation complies with the test if each individual content is between 85% and 115% of the average content. The preparation fails to comply with the test if more than one individual content is outside these limits or if one individual content is outside the limits of 75% to 125% of the average content.

If one individual content is outside the limits of 85% to 115% but within the limits of 75% to 125%, determine the individual contents of another twenty dosage units taken at random. The preparation complies with the test if not more than one of the individual contents of the thirty units is outside 85%to 115% of the average content and none is outside the limits of 75% to 125% of the average content.

Test B

Capsules, powders other than for parenteral use, granules, suppositories and pessaries The preparation complies with the test if not more than one individual content is outside the limits of 85% to 115% of the average content and none is outside the limits of 75% to 125% of the average content. The preparation fails to comply with the test if more than three individual contents are outside the limits 85% to 115% of the average content or if one or more individual contents are outside the limits of 75% to 125% of the average content.

If two or three individual contents are outside the limits of 85% to 115% but within the limits of 75% to 125%, determine the individual contents of another twenty dosage units taken at random. The preparation complies with the test if not more than three individual contents of the thirty units are outside the limits of 85% to 115% of the average content and none is outside the limits of 75% to 125% of the average content.

Test C

Transdermal patches The preparation complies with the test if the average content of the ten dosage units is between 90% and 110% of the labelled content and if the individual content of each dosage unit is between 75% and 125% of the average content.

J. Extractable Volume

(Ph. Eur. method 2.9.17)

The determination of extractable volume applies to preparations for parenteral use: injections and parenteral infusions.

INJECTIONS

Single-dose preparations may be supplied in single-dose containers, cartridges or prefilled syringes.

Single-dose containers

The volume of the injection in a single-dose container is sufficient to permit withdrawal of the nominal dose. The single-dose container does not hold a quantity relative to the declared volume that would present a risk should the whole contents be administered.

Compliance with the requirement for extractable volume is assured by making the filling volume greater than the nominal volume to a degree determined by the characteristics of the product.

Suspensions and emulsions must be shaken before withdrawal of the contents and before the determination of the density.

Oily or viscous preparations may be heated, if necessary, and thoroughly shaken immediately before removing the contents. The contents are then cooled before the determination.

CONTAINERS WITH A NOMINAL VOLUME LESS THAN 5 ML Take six containers, five for the test and one to rinse the syringe and the needle used.

Choose a syringe with a capacity not greater than twice the volume to be measured and fitted with a suitable needle. Take into the syringe a small quantity of the injection being examined from the container intended for rinsing and discharge the liquid from the syringe held vertically with the needle pointed upwards to expel any air. Withdraw as much as possible of the contents from one of the five containers to be used in the test, expel any bubbles and transfer this quantity, without emptying the needle, into a dry tared container. Weigh the whole and determine the weight of the contents. Repeat the procedure with the four other containers. Determine the density of the preparation at the temperature at which the test is carried out. From the weight of the contents of each container, calculate the corresponding volume by dividing by the density.

The preparation complies with the test for extractable volume if the volume measured for each of the five containers is not less than the nominal volume.

CONTAINERS WITH A NOMINAL VOLUME OF 5 ML OR MORE Take six containers, five for the test and one to rinse the syringe and the needle used.

Choose a syringe with a capacity not greater than twice the volume to be measured and fitted with an appropriate needle. Fill the syringe with a small quantity of the injection being examined from the container intended for rinsing and discharge the liquid from the syringe held vertically with the needle pointed upwards to expel any air. Withdraw as much as possible of the contents from one of the five containers to be used in the test, expel any bubbles and transfer this quantity, without emptying the needle, into a dry measuring cylinder of such a capacity that the volume to be measured occupies not less than 40% of the nominal volume of the cylinder. Measure the volume transferred. Repeat the procedure with the four other containers.

The preparation complies with the test for extractable volume if the volume measured for each of the five containers is not less than the nominal volume.

Cartridges and prefilled syringes

The volume of the injection contained in a cartridge or a prefilled syringe is sufficient to permit the discharge of the nominal dose.

Suspensions and emulsions must be shaken before withdrawal of the contents and before determination of the density. Oily or viscous preparations may be heated, if necessary, and thoroughly shaken immediately before removing the contents. The contents are then cooled before the determination.

Take five containers. If necessary, fit the first container with the accessories required for its use (needle, piston, syringe) and transfer the entire contents (without emptying the needle) into a dry tared container by slowly and constantly depressing the piston. Weigh the whole and determine the weight of the contents. Repeat the procedure with the four other containers. Determine the density of the preparation at the temperature at which the test is carried out. From the weight of the contents of each container, calculate the corresponding volume by dividing by the density.

The preparation complies with the test for extractable volume if the volume measured for each of the five containers is not less than the nominal volume.

PARENTERAL INFUSIONS

Take one container. Transfer its content into a dry measuring cylinder of such a capacity that the volume to be determined fills at least 40% of the nominal volume of the cylinder. Measure the volume transferred.

The volume measured is not less than the nominal volume stated on the container.

Appendix XIII

Particulate Contamination

A. Sub-visible Particles

(Ph. Eur. method 2.9.19)

Particulate contamination of injections and parenteral infusions consists of extraneous, mobile undissolved particles, other than gas bubbles, unintentionally present in the solutions.

The types of preparation for which this test is required and the requirements to be applied are stated in the relevant monograph.

Apparatus

Use a suitable apparatus based on the principle of light blockage which allows an automatic determination of the size of particles and the number of particles according to size.

Calibration The apparatus is calibrated using dispersions of *spherical particles EPCRS* of known size between 5 µm and 25 µm. These standard particles are dispersed in *particle-free water*. Care must be taken to avoid aggregation of particles during dispersion.

General precautions

The test is carried out under conditions limiting particulate contamination, preferably in a laminar-flow cabinet.

Clean, particle-free glassware may be obtained by very carefully washing the glassware and filtration equipment used, except for the membrane filters, with a warm detergent solution and rinsing with abundant amounts of *water* to remove all traces of detergent. Immediately before use, rinse the equipment from top to bottom, outside and then inside, with *particle-free water*.

Take care not to introduce air bubbles into the preparation being examined, especially when fractions of the preparation are being transferred to the container in which the determination is to be carried out.

In order to check that the environment is suitable for the test and that the glassware is properly cleaned and to verify that the water to be used is particle-free, the following test is carried out. Determine the particle contamination of five samples of *particle-free water*, each of 5 ml, according to the method described below. If the number of particles of 10 µm or greater size exceeds 25 for the combined 25 ml, the precautions taken for the test are not sufficient. The preparatory steps must be repeated until environment, glassware and water are suitable for the test.

Method

Mix the contents of the sample by slowly inverting the container five times successively. If necessary, cautiously remove the sealing closure. Clean the outer surfaces of the container opening using a jet of *particle-free water* and remove the closure, avoiding any contamination of the contents. Eliminate gas bubbles by allowing to stand for 2 minutes.

Remove four portions, each of not less than 5 ml, and count the number of particles with sizes equal to or greater than the limits specified below or in the individual monograph, as appropriate. Disregard the result obtained for the first portion, and calculate the mean number of particles for the preparation being examined.

For preparations that are required to comply with this test, the mean number of particles does not exceed 100 per ml greater than 5 µm and does not exceed 50 per ml greater than 10 µm, unless otherwise stated in the monograph.

B. Visible Particles

(Ph. Eur. method 2.9.20)

Particulate contamination of injections and parenteral infusions consists of extraneous, mobile undissolved particles, other than gas bubbles, unintentionally present in the solutions.

The test provides a simple method for the detection of visible particles. It is performed in accordance with the provisions of good manufacturing practice.

Apparatus

The apparatus (see Fig. 13-1) consists of a viewing station comprising:

(a) a matt black panel of appropriate size held in a vertical position,

(b) a non-glare white panel of appropriate size held in a vertical position next to the black panel,

(c) an adjustable lampholder fitted with a suitable shaded, white-light source and with a suitable light diffuser (a viewing illuminator containing two 13-watt fluorescent tubes, each 525 mm in length is suitable). The intensity of illumination at the viewing point is maintained between 2000 lux and 3750 lux, although higher values are preferable for coloured glass and plastic containers.

Method

Gently swirl or invert each individual container, ensuring that air bubbles are not introduced, and observe for about 5 seconds in front of the white panel. Repeat the procedure in front of the black panel.

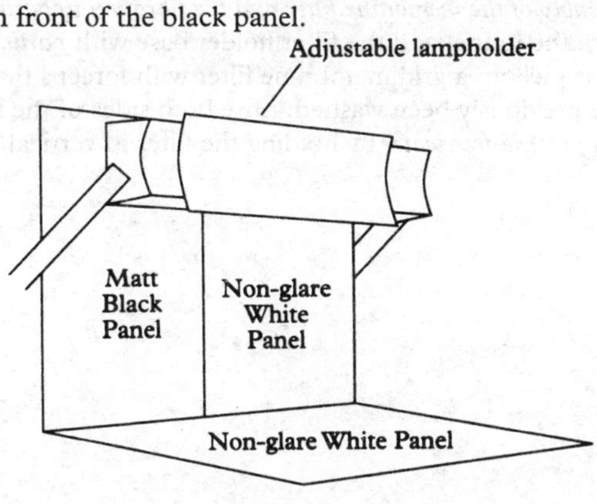

Fig. 13-1
Apparatus for visible particles

C. Microscope Method

(Ph. Eur. method 2.9.21)

Particulate contamination of injections and parenteral infusions consists of extraneous, mobile undissolved particles, other than gas bubbles, unintentionally present in the solutions.

The test is intended to provide a qualitative method for identifying any particles that may be present in a solution and for determining their characteristics. This may provide an indication of the possible origin of the contamination. From such information it may be possible for a manufacturer to develop means to avoid the contamination.

General precautions

Carry out manipulative procedures in a laminar-flow cabinet.

Preparation of materials: very carefully wash the glassware and filtration equipment used, except for the membrane filters, with a warm detergent solution and rinse with abundant amounts of water to remove all traces of detergent. Immediately before use, rinse the equipment from top to bottom, outside and then inside with *particle-free water*.

Apparatus

Use a stainless-steel or glass vacuum-filtration system equipped with a grid membrane filter having a suitable porosity and colour.

A binocular microscope equipped as follows may be used:

(a) an achromatic objective with a magnifying power of 10,

(b) eyepieces with a magnifying power of 10, of which at least one is equipped with a reticle allowing the accurate measurement of particles 10 µm or larger in size,

(c) an illumination system for observation with incident or reflected light,

(d) an object micrometer to calibrate the eyepiece reticle.

Method

Assembly of the membrane filter and the filtration apparatus Rinse the funnel and the filter holder base with *particle-free water*; pick up a grid membrane filter with forceps that have previously been washed; rinse both sides of the filter with *particle-free water* by holding the filter in vertical position and sweeping the stream slowly back and forth from top to bottom to eliminate all particles. Place the rinsed filter, grid upwards, on the filter holder base of the vacuum-filtration apparatus, making sure that the filter is well centred on the holder base. Install the filtering funnel on the base without sliding the funnel over the grid side of the filter. Invert the assembled unit and rinse the inside of the funnel and the filter surface with a jet of *particle-free water* for about 15 seconds. Place the unit on the filter flask.

Filtration of the sample Transfer 25 ml of the homogenised preparation being examined to the filtration apparatus. Allow to stand for about 1 minute. Apply the vacuum and filter. Release the vacuum gently and rinse the inner walls of the funnel with a jet of *particle-free water*. Avoid directing the jet onto the filter surface. After turbulence has dissipated, vacuum-filter the rinsing. Maintain the vacuum for a moment to dry the filter. Release the vacuum. Carefully remove the funnel; pick up the filter with steel forceps previously washed with a jet of *particle-free water* and place the filter in a clean Petri dish. Position the clean cover of the dish so that is slightly ajar. Put the dish in the laminar flow cabinet to dry the filter slightly, avoiding the formation of folds, and then place the Petri dish on the microscope stage and count the particles present on the filter as described below.

Preparation of the blank Prepare a blank under the same conditions as the sample. The blank consists of 25 ml of *particle-free water* passed directly through the funnel of the vacuum filtration apparatus.

Calibration under the microscope Calibrate the reticle of the microscope eyepiece using an object micrometer.

Determination Either visual examination or an electronic recording device can be used. Examine the entire surface of the filter at a magnification of 100 and illuminated with incident light or reflected light. Count and classify the particles according to the sizes previously chosen, ≥10 µm. For each class, subtract the blank count from that of the sample. If the blank contains more than five particles 25 µm in size or larger, the operational conditions are unsatisfactory and the test must be repeated.

Interpretation Where possible, identify the type of particles detected and determine their characteristics. Where relevant, the number of particles detected can also be recorded.

Appendix XIV

Biological Assays and Tests

General guidance concerning biological assays and tests is provided in Supplementary Chapter I H.

A. Biological Assay of Antibiotics

The potency of an antibiotic is estimated by comparing the inhibition of growth of sensitive micro-organisms produced by known concentrations of the antibiotic being examined and a reference substance.

The reference substances used in the assays are substances whose activity has been precisely determined with reference to the corresponding International Standard or International Reference Preparation.

The assay must be designed in a way that will permit examination of the validity of the mathematical model on which the potency equation is based. If a parallel-line model is chosen, the two log dose-response (or transformed response) lines of the preparation being examined and the reference preparation must be parallel; they must be linear over the range of doses used in the calculation. These conditions must be verified by validity tests for a given probability, usually (P = 0.05). Other mathematical models, such as the slope ratio model, may be used provided that proof of validity is demonstrated.

Unless otherwise stated in the monograph, the fiducial limits of error (P = *0.95*) of the assay for potency are not less than 95% and not more than 105% of the estimated potency.

Carry out the assay by Method A or Method B unless otherwise specified in the monograph.

A. Diffusion Method

Liquefy a medium suitable for the conditions of the assay and inoculate it at a suitable temperature, for example 48° to 50° for vegetative forms, with a known quantity of a suspension of micro-organisms sensitive to the antibiotic being examined, such that clearly defined zones of inhibition of suitable diameter are produced with the concentrations of the antibiotic used for the assay. Immediately pour into Petri dishes or large rectangular dishes a quantity of the inoculated medium to form a uniform layer 2 mm to 5 mm thick. Alternatively, the medium may consist of two layers, only the upper layer being inoculated. Store the dishes so that no appreciable growth or death of the micro-organisms occurs before the dishes are used and so that the surface of the medium is dry at the time of use.

Using the solvent and the buffer solution indicated in the Table 14A-1, prepare solutions of the reference substance and of the antibiotic being examined having known concentrations and presumed to be of equal activity. Apply the solutions to the surface of the medium, for example, in sterile cylinders of porcelain, stainless steel or other suitable material, or in cavities prepared in the agar. The same volume of solution must be added to each cylinder or cavity. Alternatively, use sterile absorbent paper discs of suitable quality; impregnate the discs with the solutions of the reference substance or the solutions of the antibiotic being examined and place on the surface of the agar.

In order to assess the validity of the assay, use not fewer than three doses of the reference substance and three doses of the antibiotic being examined having the same presumed activity as the doses of the reference substance. It is preferable to use a series of doses in geometric progression. In routine assays when the linearity of the system has been demonstrated over an adequate number of experiments using a three-point assay, a two-point assay may be sufficient, subject to agreement by the competent authority. However, in all cases of dispute, a three-point assay as described above must be applied.

Arrange the solutions on each Petri dish or on each rectangular dish according to a statistically suitable design, except for small Petri dishes that cannot accomodate more than six solutions, arrange the solutions of the antibiotic being examined and the solutions of the reference substance in an alternate manner to avoid interaction of the more concentrated solutions.

Incubate at a suitable temperature for about 18 hours. A period of diffusion prior to incubation, usually 1 to 4 hours, at room temperature or at about 4°, as appropriate, may be used to minimise the effects of the variation in time between the application of the solutions and to improve the regression slope.

Measure the diameters with a precision of at least 0.1 mm or the areas of the circular inhibition zones with a corresponding precision and calculate the potency using appropriate statistical methods.

Use in each assay the number of replications per dose sufficient to ensure the required precision. The assay may be repeated and the results combined statistically to obtain the required precision and to ascertain whether the potency of the antibiotic being examined is not less than the minimum required.

B. Turbidimetric Method

Inoculate a suitable medium with a suspension of the chosen micro-organism having a sensitivity to the antibiotic being examined such that a sufficiently large inhibition of microbial growth occurs in the conditions of the test. Use a known quantity of the suspension chosen so as to obtain a readily measurable opacity after an incubation period of about 4 hours.

Use the inoculated medium immediately after its preparation.

Using the solvent and the buffer solution indicated in the Table 14A-2 prepare solutions of the reference substance and of the antibiotic being examined having known concentrations presumed to be of equal activity. In order that the validity of the assay may be assessed, use not fewer than three doses of the reference substance and three doses of the antibiotic being examined having the same presumed activity as the doses of the reference substance. It is preferable to use a series of doses in geometric progression. In order to obtain the required linearity, it may be necessary to select from a large number three consecutive doses, using corresponding doses for the reference substance and the antibiotic being examined.

Distribute an equal volume of each of the solutions into identical test-tubes and add to each tube an equal volume of inoculated medium (for example, 1 ml of the solution and 9 ml of the medium).

Table 14A-1 Diffusion Assay

Antibiotic	Reference substance	Solvent to be used in preparing the stock solution	Buffer solution (pH)	Micro-organism	Medium and final pH (± 0.1 pH unit)	Incubation temperature
Bacitracin zinc	*Bacitracin zinc CRS*	*0.01M hydrochloric acid*	pH 7.0 (0.05M)	*Micrococcus flavus* NCTC 7743 CIP 53.160 ATCC 10240	A; 7.0	35-39°
Bleomycin sulphate	*Bleomycin sulphate CRS*	*Water*	pH 6.8 (0.1M)	*Mycobacterium smegmatis* ATCC 607	G; 7.0	35-37°
Colistin sulphate Colistimethate sodium	*Colistin sulphate CRS* *Colistimethate sodium CRS*	*Water*	pH 6.0 (0.05M)	*Bordetella bronchiseptica* NCTC 8344 CIP 53.157 ATCC 4617	B; 7.3	35-39°
				Escherichia coli NCIMB 8879 CIP 54.127 ATCC 10536	B; 7.3	35-39°
Dihydrostreptomycin sulphate	*Dihydrostreptomycin sulphate CRS*	*Water*	pH 8.0 (0.05M)	*Bacillus subtilis* NCTC 8236 CIP 1.83	A; 7.9	30-37°
				Bacillus subtilis NCTC 10400 CIP 52.62 ATCC 6633	A; 7.9	30-37°
Erythromycin estolate Erythromycin ethylsuccinate	*Erythromycin CRS*	*Methanol* (see the monographs)	pH 8.0 (0.05M)	*Bacillus pumilus* NCTC 8241 CIP 76.18	A; 7.9	30-37°
Erythromycin stearate		*Methanol*		*Bacillus subtilis* NCTC 10400 CIP 52.62 ATCC 6633	A; 7.9	30-37°
Framycetin sulphate	*Framycetin sulphate CRS*	*Water*	pH 8.0 (0.05M)	*Bacillus subtilis* NCTC 10400 CIP 52.62 ATCC 6633	E; 7.9	30-37°
				Bacillus pumilus NCTC 8241 CIP 76.18	E; 7.9	30-37°
Gentamicin sulphate	*Gentamicin sulphate CRS*	*Water*	pH 8.0 (0.05M)	*Bacillus pumilus* NCTC 8241 CIP 76.18	A; 7.9	35-39°
				Staphylococcus epidermidis NCIMB 8853 CIP 68.21 ATCC 12228	A; 7.9	35-39°
Kanamycin Sulphate Kanamycin acid sulphate	*Kanamycin monosulphate CRS*	*Water*	pH 8.0 (0.05M)	*Bacillus subtilis* NCTC 10400 CIP 52.62 ATCC 6633	A; 7.9	30-37°
				Staphylococcus aureus NCTC 7447 CIP 53.156 ATCC 6538 P	A; 7.9	35-39°
Neomycin sulphate	*Neomycin sulphate CRS*	*Water*	pH 8.0 (0.05M)	*Bacillus pumilus* NCTC 8241 CIP 76.18	E; 7.9	30-37°
				Bacillus subtilis NCTC 10400 CIP 52.62 ATCC 6633	E; 7.9	30-37°

cont....

Table 14A-1 Diffusion Assay *(continued)*

Antibiotic	Reference substance	Solvent to be used in preparing the stock solution	Buffer solution (pH)	Micro-organism	Medium and final pH (± 0.1 pH unit)	Incubation temperature
Nystatin	*Nystatin CRS*	*Dimethylformamide*	*	*Saccharomyces cerevisiae* NCYC 87 CIP 1432-83 ATCC 9763	F; 6.0	30-32°
Polymyxin B sulphate	*Polymyxin B sulphate CRS*	*Water*	pH 6.0 (0.05M)	*Bordetella bronchiseptica* NCTC 8344 CIP 53.157 ATCC 4617	B; 7.3	35-39°
Rifamycin sodium	*Rifamycin sodium CRS*	*Methanol*	pH 7.0 (0.05M)	*Micrococcus flavus* NCTC 8340 CIP 53.45 ATCC 9341	A; 6.6	35-39°
Spiramycin	*Spiramycin CRS*	*Methanol*	pH 8.0 (0.05M)	*Bacillus subtilis* NCTC 10400 CIP 52.62 ATCC 6633	A; 7.9	30-32°
Streptomycin sulphate	*Streptomycin sulphate CRS*	*Water*	pH 8.0 (0.05M)	*Bacillus subtilis* NCTC 8236 CIP 1.83	A; 7.9	30-37°
				Bacillus subtilis NCTC 10400 CIP 52.62 ATCC 6633	A; 7.9	30-37°
Tobramycin	*Tobramycin CRS*	*Water*	pH 8.0 (0.05M)	*Bacillus subtilis* NCTC 10400 CIP 52.62 ATCC 6633	A; 7.9	30-37°
Tylosin Tylosin tartrate	*Tylosin CRS*	†	‡	*Micrococcus flavus* NCTC 8340 ATCC 9341 CIP 53.45	A; 8.0	32-35°
Vancomycin hydrochloride	*Vancomycin hydrochloride CRS*	*Water*	pH 8.0	*Bacillus subtilis* NCTC 8236 ATCC 6633 CIP 52.62	A; 8.0	37-39°

* pH 6.0 (0.05M) containing 5 %V/V of *dimethylformamide*

†2.5 per cent V/V solution of *methanol* in 0.1M *phosphate buffer solution pH 7.0*

‡ A mixture of 40 volumes of *methanol* and 60 volumes of 0.1M *phosphate buffer solution pH 8.0*

Additional section for monographs other than those from the European Pharmacopoeia.

Antibiotic	Reference substance	Solvent to be used in preparing the stock solution	Buffer solution (pH)	Micro-organism	Medium and final pH (± 0.1 pH unit)	Incubation temperature
Amphotericin	Amphotericin B 1st Int. Stand., 1963		§	*Saccharomyces cerevisiae* (NCYC 87)	F; 6.1	35 - 37°
Capreomycin Sulphate	Capreomycin 1st Int. Ref., 1967		pH 8.0	*Bacillus subtilis* (NCTC 10,400)	A; 7.8	35 - 37°
Lymecycline	Lymecycline 2nd Int. Ref., 1971		pH 5.8	*Bacillus pumilus* (NCTC 8241)	A; 6.6	37 - 39°
Oxytetracycline Hydrochloride	Oxytetracycline 2nd Int. Ref., 1966		pH 5.8	*Bacillus pumilus* (NCTC 8241)	A; 6.6	30 - 37°

§Solution prepared by dissolving 35 g of *dipotassium hydrogen orthophosphate* in *water* and adding 20 ml of 1M *sodium hydroxide* and sufficient *water* to produce 1000 ml. The dilutions of the reference and test solutions are prepared taking precautions to exclude light and adjusted to contain 8% v/v of *dimethylformamide*. They are prepared immediately before use and the time between the preparation of a dilution and its application to the inoculated plate is the same for the reference and test solutions.

Table 14A-2 Turbidimetric Assay

Antibiotic	Reference substance	Solvent to be used in preparing the stock solution	Buffer solution (pH)	Micro-organism	Medium and final pH (± 0.1 pH unit)	Incubation temperature
Colistin sulphate Colistimethate sodium	*Colistinsulphate CRS* *Colistimethate sodium CRS*	*Water*	pH 7.0	*Escherichia coli* NCIMB 8666 CIP 2.83 ATCC 9637	C ; 7.0	35-37°
Dihydrostreptomycin sulphate	*Dihydrostreptomycin CRS*	*Water*	pH 8.0	*Klebsiella pneumoniae* NCTC 7427 CIP 53.153 ATCC 10031	C ; 7.0	35-37°
Erythromycin estolate Erythromycin ethylsuccinate Erythromycinstearate	*Erythromycin CRS*	*Methanol R (see the monographs)* *Methanol*	pH 8.0	*Klebsiella pneumoniae* NCTC 7427 CIP 53.153 ATCC 10031 *Staphylococcus aureus* NCTC 7447 CIP 53.156 ATCC 6538 P	D; 7.0 C ; pH 7.0	35-37° 35-37°
Framycetin sulphate	*Framycetin sulphate CRS*	*Water*	pH 8.0	*Staphylococcus aureus* NCTC 7447 CIP 53.156 ATCC 6538 P	C ; 7.0	35-37°
Gentamicin sulphate	*Gentamicin sulphate CRS*	*Water*	pH 7.0	*Staphylococcus aureus* NCTC 7447 CIP 53.156 ATCC 6538 P	C; 7.0	35-37°
Gramicidin	*Gramicidin CRS*	*Methanol*	*	*Streptococcus faecalis* ATCC 10541 *Staphylococcus aureus* ATCC 6538P	C; 7.0	35-37°
Kanamycin sulphate Kanamycin acid sulphate	*Kanamycin monosulphate CRS*	*Water*	pH 8.0	*Staphylococcus aureus* NCTC 7447 CIP 53.156 ATCC 6538 P	C; 7.0	35-37°
Neomycin sulphate	*Neomycin sulphate CRS*	*Water*	pH 8.0	*Staphylococcus aureus* NCTC 7447 CIP 53.156 ATCC 6538P	C; 7.0	35-37°
Rifamycin sodium	*Rifamycin sodium CRS*	*Methanol*	pH 7.0	*Escherichia coli* NCIMB 8879 CIP 54.127 ATCC 10536	C; 7.0	35-37°
Spiramycin	*Spiramycin CRS*	*Methanol*	pH 7.0	*Staphylococcus aureus* NCTC 7447 CIP 53.156 ATCC 6538 P	C; 7.0	35-37°
Streptomycin sulphate	*Streptomycin sulphate CRS*	*Water*	pH 8.0	*Klebsiella pneumoniae* NCTC 7427 CIP 53.153 ATCC 10031	C; 7.0	35-37°
Tobramycin	*Tobramycin CRS*	*Water*	pH 7.0	*Staphylococcus aureus* NCTC 7447 ATCC 6538 P CIP 53.136 ATCC 9144	C; 7.0	35-37°
Tylosin Tylosin tartrate	*Tylosin CRS*	†	pH 7.0	*Staphylococcus aureus* NCTC 6571 ATCC 9144 CIP 53.154	C; 7.0	37°

cont....

Table 14A-2 Turbidimetric Assay *(continued)*

Antibiotic	Reference substance	Solvent to be used in preparing the stock solution	Buffer solution (pH)	Micro-organism	Medium and final pH (± 0.1 pH unit)	Incubation temperature
Vancomycin hydrochloride	*Vancomycin hydrochloride CRS*	*Water*	pH 8.0	*Staphylococcus aureus* ATCC 6538 P CIP 53.156	C; 8.0	37-39°

*pH 7.0 Addition of a detergent may be necessary to avoid adsorption on the material during the dilutions, forexample mg/ml of polysorbate 80.

†2.5 per cent *V/V* solution of *methanol* in 0.1M *phosphate buffer solution pH 7.0*

Additional section for monographs other than those from the European Pharmacopoeia.

Antibiotic	Reference substance	Solvent to be used in preparing the stock solution	Buffer solution (pH)	Micro-organism	Medium and final pH (± 0.1 pH unit)	Incubation temperature
Apramycin	*Apramycin BPCRS*		*	*Salmonella cholerasuis*	H; 8.0	37°
Oxytetracycline Hydrochloride	Oxytetracycline 2nd Int., 1966		†	*Staphylococcus aureus* (NCTC 6571)	C; 6.6	35 - 37°

*Solution prepared by dissolving 16.73 g of *dipotassium hydrogen orthophosphate* and 0.523 g of *potassium dihydrogen orthophosphate* in about 750 ml of *water*, if necessary adjusting to pH 8.0 with 0.1M *sodium hydroxide* or 0.1M *orthophosphoric acid*, and diluting to 1000 ml with *water*.

†Solution prepared by dissolving 13.61 g of *potassium dihydrogen orthophosphate* in about 750 ml of *water*, adjusting the pH to 4.5 with 0.1M *sodium hydroxide* and diluting to 1000 ml with *water*.

Prepare at the same time two control tubes without antibiotic, both containing the inoculated medium and to one of which is added immediately 0.5 ml of *formaldehyde*. These tubes are used to set the optical apparatus used to measure the growth.

Place all the tubes, randomly distributed or in a Latin square or randomised block arrangement, in a water-bath or other suitable apparatus fitted with a means of bringing all the tubes rapidly to the appropriate incubation temperature and maintain them at that temperature for 3 to 4 hours, taking precautions to ensure uniformity of temperature and identical incubation time.

After incubation, stop the growth of the micro-organisms by adding 0.5 ml of *formaldehyde* to each tube or by heat treatment and measure the opacity to three significant figures using suitable optical apparatus. Alternatively use a method which allows the opacity of each tube to be measured after exactly the same period of incubation.

Calculate the potency using appropriate statistical methods.

Linearity of the dose-response relationship, transformed or untransformed, is often obtained only over a very limited range. It is this range which must be used in calculating the activity and it must include at least three consecutive doses in order to permit linearity to be verified. In routine assays when the linearity of the system has been demonstrated over an adequate number of experiments using a three-point assay, a two-point assay may be sufficient, subject to agreement by the competent authority. However, in all cases of dispute, a three-point assay must be applied.

Use in each assay the number of replications per dose sufficient to ensure the required precision. The assay may be repeated and the results combined statistically to obtain the required precision and to ascertain whether the potency of the antibiotic being examined is not less than the minimum required.

ANNEX

The following section is given for information and guidance; it does not form a mandatory part of the general method.

RECOMMENDED MICRO-ORGANISMS

The following text shows the recommended micro-organisms and the conditions of use. Other micro-organisms may be used provided that they are shown to be sensitive to the antibiotic being examined and are used in appropriate media and appropriate conditions of temperature and pH. The concentrations of the solutions used should be chosen so as to ensure that a linear relationship exists between the logarithm of the dose and the response in the conditions of the test.

Preparation of inocula *Bacillus cereus* var. *mycoides*; *Bacillus subtilis*; *Bacillus pumilus*. Spore suspensions of the organisms to be used as inocula are prepared as follows.

Grow the organism at 35° to 37° for 7 days on the surface of a suitable medium to which has been added 0.001 g/l of *manganese(II) sulphate*. Using sterile *water*, wash off the growth, which consists mainly of spores. Heat the suspension at 70° for 30 minutes and dilute to give an appropriate concentration of spores, usually 10×10^6 to 100×10^6 per ml. The spore suspensions may be stored for long periods at a temperature not exceeding 4°.

Alternatively, spore suspensions may be prepared by cultivating the organisms in medium C at 26° for 4 days to 6 days, then adding, aseptically, sufficient *manganese(II) sulphate* to give a concentration of 0.001 g/l and incubating for a further 48 hours. Examine the suspension microscopically to ensure that adequate spore formation has taken place (about 80%) and centrifuge. Re-suspend the sediment in sterile *water* to give a concentration of 10×10^6 to 100×10^6 spores per millilitre, and then heat to 70° for 30 minutes. Store the suspension at a temperature not exceeding 4°.

Bordetella bronchiseptica. Grow the test organism on medium B at 35° to 37° for 16 to18 hours. Wash off the bacterial growth with sterile *water* and dilute to a suitable opacity.

Staphylococcus aureus; Klebsiella pneumoniae; Escherichia coli; Micrococcus flavus; Staphylococcus epidermidis. Prepare as described above for *B. bronchiseptica* but using medium A and adjusting the opacity to one which has been shown to produce a satisfactory dose-response relationship in the turbidimetric assay, or to produce clearly defined zones of inhibition of convenient diameter in the diffusion assay, as appropriate.

Saccharomyces cerevisiae; Candida tropicalis. Grow the test organism on medium F at 30° to 37° for 24 hours. Wash off the growth with a sterile 9 g/l solution of *sodium chloride*. Dilute to a suitable opacity with the same solution.

Buffer solutions. Buffer solutions having a pH between 5.8 and 8.0 are prepared by mixing 50.0 ml of *0.2M potassium dihydrogen phosphate* with the quantity of *0.2M sodium hydroxide* indicated in Table 14A-3. Dilute with freshly prepared distilled *water* to produce 200.0 ml.

TABLE 14A-3

pH	0.2M *sodium hydroxide* ml	pH	0.2M *sodium hydroxide* ml
5.8	3.72	7.0	29.63
6.0	5.70	7.2	35.00
6.2	8.60	7.4	39.50
6.4	12.60	7.6	42.80
6.6	17.80	7.8	45.20
6.8	23.65	9.0	46.80

These buffer solutions are used for all microbiological assays shown in Table 14A.-1 with the exception of bleomycin sulphate. The buffer solution (pH 6.8) for bleomycin sulphate is prepared by dissolving 6.4 g of *potassium dihydrogen* and 18.9 g of *disodium hydrogen phosphate* in *water* and diluting to 1000 ml.

Culture media. The following media or equivalent media may be used.

Medium A

Peptone	6 g
Pancreatic digest of casein	4 g
Beef extract	1.5 g
Yeast extract	3 g
Glucose monohydrate	1 g
Agar	15 g
Water to produce	1000 ml

Medium B

Pancreatic digest of casein	17 g
Papaic digest of soya bean	3 g
Sodium chloride	5 g
Dipotassium hydrogen phosphate	2.5 g
Glucose monohydrate	2.5 g
Agar	15 g
Polysorbate 80	10 g
Water to produce	1000 ml

The polysorbate 80 is added to the hot solution of the other ingredient after boiling, and immediately before adjusting to volume.

Medium C

Peptone	6 g
Beef extract	1.5 g
Yeast extrac	t3 g
Sodium chloride	3.5 g
Glucose monohydrate	1 g
Dipotassium hydrogen phosphate	3.68 g
Potassium dihydrogen phosphate	1.32 g
Water to produce	1000 ml

Medium D

Heart extract	1.5 g
Yeast extract	1.5 g
Peptone-casein	5 g
Glucose monohydrate	1 g
Sodium chloride	3.5 g
Dipotassium hydrogen phosphate	3.68 g
Potassium dihydrogen phosphate	1.32 g
Potassium nitrate	2 g
Water to produce	1000 ml

Medium E

Peptone	5 g
Meat extract	3 g
Disodium hydrogen phosphate,$12H_2O$	26.9 g
Agar	10 g
Water to produce	1000 ml

The disodium hydrogen phosphate is added as a sterile solution after sterilisation of the medium.

Medium F

Peptone	9.4 g
Yeast extract	4.7 g
Beef extract	2.4 g
Sodium chloride	30.0 g
Glucose monohydrate	10.0 g
Agar	23.5 g
Water to produce	1000 ml

Medium G

Glycerol	10 g
Peptone	10 g
Meat extract	10 g
Sodium chloride	3 g
Agar	15 g
Water to produce	1000 ml

pH 7±0.1 after sterilisation.

Medium H

D-Glucose	10 g
Tryptone	6 g
Yeast extract	2 g

(Ardamine yeats extract supplied by Champlain Industries Inc., Clifton, NJ 07012, USA is suitable)

Water	sufficient to produce 1000 ml

Adjust to pH 8.0 with 1M *sodium hydroxide* or 0.1M *orthophosphoric acid*.

Additional information and guidance for monographs other than those from the European Pharmacopoeia

The required minimum precision for an acceptable assay of any particular antibiotic or preparation is defined in the appropriate monograph in the paragraph on the Assay. This degree of precision is the minimum acceptable for determining that the final product complies with the official requirements. It may be inadequate for a decision about the potency that should be stated on the label or used as the basis for calculating the quantity of an antibiotic to be incorporated in a preparation. In such circumstances, assays of greater precision may be desirable with, for instance, fiducial limits of error of the order of 98 to 102%. With this degree of precision, the lower fiducial limit lies close to the estimated potency. By using this limit, instead of the estimated potency, to assign a potency to the antibiotic either for labelling or for calculating the quantity to be included in a preparation, there is less likelihood of the final preparation subsequently failing to comply with the official requirements for potency.

B. Immunochemical Methods

(Ph. Eur. method 2.7.1)

Immunochemical methods are based on the selective, reversible and non-covalent binding of antigens by antibodies. These methods are employed to detect or quantify either antigens or antibodies. The formation of an antigen—antibody complex may be detected, and the amount of complex formed may be measured, by a variety of techniques. The provisions of this general method apply to immunochemical methods using labelled or unlabelled reagents, as appropriate.

The results of immunochemical methods depend on the experimental conditions and the nature and quality of the reagents used. It is essential to standardise the components of an immunoassay and to use, wherever available, international reference preparations for immunoassays.

The reagents necessary for many immunochemical methods are available as commercial assay kits, that is a set including reagents (particularly the antigen or the antibody) and materials intended for the *in vitro* estimation of a specified substance as well as instructions for their proper use. The kits are used in accordance with the manufacturers' instructions; it is important to ascertain that the kits are suitable for the analysis of the substance being examined, with particular reference to selectivity and sensitivity. Guidance concerning immunoassay kits is provided by the World Health Organization, *Technical Report Series* **658** (1981).

Methods in which a labelled antigen or a labelled antibody is used

Methods using labelled substances may employ suitable labels such as enzymes, fluorophores, luminophores and radioisotopes. Where the label is a radioisotope, the method is described as a 'radio-immunoassay'. The recommendations for the measurement of radioactivity given under Radiopharmaceutical Preparations are applicable to immunoassays involving radioisotopes. All work with radioactive materials must be carried out in conformity with national legislation and internationally accepted codes of practice for protection against radiation hazards.

Methods in which an unlabelled antigen or antibody is used

Immunoprecipitation methods Immunoprecipitation methods include flocculation and precipitation reactions. When a solution of an antigen is mixed with its corresponding antibody under suitable conditions, the reactants form flocculating or precipitating aggregates. The ratio of the reactants that gives the shortest flocculation time or the most marked precipitation is called the optimal ratio, and is usually produced by equivalent amounts of antigen and antibody. Immunoprecipitation can be assessed visually or by light-scattering techniques (nephelometric or turbidimetric assay). An increase in sensitivity can be obtained by using antigen- or antibody-coated particles (such as latex) as reactants.

In flocculation methods, stepwise dilutions of one of the reactants are usually used whereas in immunodiffusion (ID) methods the dilution is obtained by diffusion in a gel medium. Concentration gradients of one or both of the reactants are obtained, thus creating zones in the gel medium where the ratio of the reactants favours precipitation. Whereas flocculation methods are performed in tubes, immunodiffusion methods may be performed using different supports such as tubes, plates, slides, cells or chambers.

Where the immunoprecipitating system consists of one antigen combining with its corresponding antibody, the system is referred to as *simple*; when it involves related but not serologically identical reactants, the system is *complex* and where several serologically unrelated reactants are involved, the system is *multiple*.

In *simple diffusion methods*, a concentration gradient is established for only one of the reactants diffusing from an external source into the gel medium containing the corresponding reactant at a comparatively low concentration.

Single radial immunodiffusion (SRID) is a *simple* quantitative immunodiffusion technique. When the equilibrium between the external and the internal reactant has been established, the circular precipitation area, originating from the site of the external reactant, is directly proportional to the amount of the antigen applied and inversely proportional to the concentration of the antibody in the gel.

In *double diffusion methods*, concentration gradients are established in a neutral (inert) gel by allowing both reactants to diffuse into the gel from separate sites.

Comparative double diffusion methods are used for qualitatively comparing various antigens versus a suitable antibody or *vice versa*. The comparison is based on the presence or absence of interaction between the precipitation patterns. Reactions of identity, non-identity or partial identity of antigens/antibodies can be distinguished.

Immunoelectrophoretic methods *Immunoelectrophoresis* (IE) is a qualitative technique combining two methods: gel electrophoresis followed by immunodiffusion.

Crossed immunoelectrophoresis is a modification of the IE method. It is suitable for both qualitative and quantitative analysis. The first part of the procedure is an ordinary gel electrophoresis, after which a longitudinal gel strip, containing the separated fractions to be determined, is cut out and transferred to another plate. The electrophoresis in the second direction is carried out at an angle of 90° to the previous electrophoretic run in a gel containing a comparatively low concentration of antibodies corresponding to the antigens. For a given antibody concentration and gel thickness, the relationship between the area of the respective precipitation peaks and the amount of the corresponding antigen is linear.

Electroimmunoassay, often referred to as *rocket immunoelectrophoresis*, is a rapid quantitative method for determining antigens with a charge differing from that of the antibodies or *vice versa*. The electrophoresis of the antigen being determined is carried out in a gel containing a comparatively lower concentration of the corresponding antibody. The test material and dilutions of a standard antigen used for calibration are introduced into different wells in the gel. During electrophoresis, migrating peak-shaped precipitation zones originating from the wells are developed. The edge of the precipitate becomes stationary when the antigen is no longer in excess. For a given antibody concentration, the relationship between the distance travelled by the precipitate and the amount of antigen applied is linear.

Counter-immunoelectrophoresis is a rapid quantitative method allowing concentration gradients of external antigen and external antibody to be established in an electric field depending on the different charges. Dilutions of a standard for calibration and dilutions of the test material are introduced into a row of wells in a gel and a fixed amount of the corresponding reactant is introduced into an opposite row of wells. The titre of the test material may be determined as the highest dilution showing a precipitation line.

A number of modifications of crossed immunoelectrophoresis and electroimmunoassay methods exist. Other techniques combine separation of antigens by molecular size and serological properties.

Visualisation and characterisation of immunoprecipitation lines These may be performed by selective or non-selective stains, by fluorescence, by enzyme or isotope labelling or other relevant techniques. Selective staining methods are usually performed for characterisation of non-protein substances in the precipitates. In translucent gels such as agar or agarose, the precipitation line becomes clearly visible in the gel, provided that the concentration of each of the reactants is appropriate.

Validation of the method

Validation criteria A quantitative immunochemical method is not valid:

(1) if the antibody or antigen significantly discriminates between the test and standard, or if, for a labelled reactant, the corresponding reactant significantly discriminates between labelled and unlabelled compound;

(2) unless the method is unaffected by the assay matrix, that is, any component of the test sample or its excipients, that can vary between samples. These may include high concentrations of other proteins, salts, preservatives or contaminating proteolytic activity;

(3) unless the limit of quantitation is below the acceptance criteria stated in the individual monograph;

(4) unless the precision of the assay is such that the variance of the results meets the requirements stated in the individual monographs;

(5) if the order in which the assay is performed gives rise to systematic errors.

Validation methods In order to verify the validation criteria, the validation design includes the following:

(1) the assay is performed at least in triplicate;

(2) the assay includes at least three different dilutions of the standard preparation and three dilutions of sample preparations of presumed activity similar to that of the standard preparation;

(3) the assay layout is randomised;

(4) if the test sample is presented in serum or formulated with other components, the standard is likewise prepared;

(5) the test includes measurements of non-specific binding of the labelled reactant;

(6) for displacement immunoassay: (a) maximum binding (zero displacement) is determined; (b) dilutions cover the complete response range from values close to non-specific binding to maximum binding, preferably for both standard and test preparations.

Statistical calculation

To analyse the results, response curves for test and standard may be analysed by the methods described in the European Pharmacopoeia general text 5.3 *Statistical Analysis of Biological Assays and Tests*. Significant non-parallelism indicates that the antibody or antigen discriminates between test and standard and the results are not valid.

In displacement immunoassays, the values for non-specific binding and maximum displacement at high test or standard concentration must not be significantly different. Differences may indicate effects due to the matrix, either inhibition of binding or degradation of tracer.

C. Test for Bacterial Endotoxins

(Ph. Eur. method 2.6.14)

The five methods described in this monograph have been designed to determine whether the endotoxin concentration in a product, subject to a monograph in the Pharmacopoeia containing a limit for bacterial endotoxins, complies with this limit. Manufacturers wishing to ascertain, for example, whether their production methods reduce the endotoxin concentration in their product in the course of production are not limited to the procedures described in this monograph. Guidelines concerning the use of this test are provided in Supplementary Chapet I C.

The test for bacterial endotoxins uses a lysate of amoebocytes from the horseshoe crab, *Limulus polyphemus* (LAL test). The addition of a solution containing endotoxins to a solution of the lysate produces turbidity, precipitation or gelation of the mixture. The rate of reaction depends on the concentration of endotoxin, the pH and the temperature. The reaction requires the presence of certain divalent cations, a proclotting enzyme system and clottable protein, which are provided by the lysate. The lysis of a chromogenic peptide in a solution of the lysate after activation by endotoxins in the solution may also be used to determine the concentration of endotoxins from the concentration of dye liberated.

The five following methods are described in the present chapter:

Method A. Gelation method: limit test
Method B. Semiquantitative gelation method
Method C. Turbidimetric kinetic method
Method D. Chromogenic peptide kinetic method
Method E. Chromogenic peptide endpoint method

When a monograph contains a test for endotoxins without mentioning a method, the test is carried out by the gelation method A, which has been validated for the product. Otherwise, the test is carried out by the method validated for the product and specified in the monograph.

Monographs state requirements for bacterial endotoxins in terms of the endotoxin limit concentration (ELC); a product complies if it has *not more than* the endotoxin limit concentration. However, compliance with this requirement can only be demonstrated by showing that the endotoxin concentration of the product is *less* than the endotoxin limit concentration.

The test is carried out in a manner that avoids microbial contamination.

Before carrying out the test for endotoxins on the preparation being examined, it is necessary to verify:

— that the equipment used does not adsorb endotoxins;
— the value of lambda (λ) of the lysate used. Lambda is defined as the labelled lysate sensitivity (gelation methods) or the lowest endotoxin concentration used

to generate the standard curve (quantitative methods);
— the absence of interfering factors.

If necessary, equipment is treated to eliminate endotoxins.

Unless stated otherwise in the monograph on the product being examined the same criteria are applied in the five methods described in Method A to Method E.

In this appendix the term tube includes any other receptacle such as the well of a micro-titre plate.

The following reagents and reference preparation are used in the test.

Endotoxin standard BRP Endotoxin standard BRP is calibrated in International Units (IU) of endotoxin by comparison with the International Standard.

Limulus amoebocyte lysate This must be manufactured in accordance with the regulations of the competent authority of the country of manufacture. Reconstitute the lysate as stated on the label. For each batch, confirm the stated sensitivity (λ); it is expressed in IU of endotoxin per ml.

Water BET (Water LAL) Water is suitable if it gives a negative result in the conditions prescribed in the test for endotoxins in the preparation being examined. It may be prepared by distilling water three times in an apparatus fitted with an effective device to prevent the entrainment of droplets or by other means which give water of the requisite quality.

0.1M Hydrochloric acid BET and **0.1M Sodium Hydroxide BET (0.1M Hydrochloric acid LAL** and **0.1M Sodium Hydroxide LAL)** Prepare from *hydrochloric acid* and *sodium hydroxide*, respectively, using *water BET*. Each reagent is suitable if, after adjustment to pH 6.0–8.0 it gives a negative result in the conditions of the test.

Unless otherwise prescribed, the solutions and dilutions used in the test are prepared using water BET.

Gelation methods

Methods A and B both use the formation of a firm gel in a solution containing bacterial endotoxins incubated after mixing with lysate. Both these methods require that the sensitivity of the lysate specified by the manufacturer be confirmed as described under Sensitivity of the lysate and that the presence of interfering factors is examined as described under Interfering factors.

Methods A and B differ in that method A tests whether both the replicate solutions of the preparation being examined contain less endotoxin than the endotoxin limit concentration specified in the relevant monograph whereas in method B the endotoxin concentration of the preparation being examined is determined semiquantitatively, and the geometric mean endotoxin concentration must be less than the endotoxin limit concentration specified in the monograph.

The following paragraphs Procedure, Sensitivity of the lysate and Interfering factors apply to both methods A and B.

Procedure Add a volume of the lysate appropriate to the chosen receptacle (for example a slide or a tube) to each of the requisite number of such receptacles maintained at 37° ± 1°. At intervals that will permit the reading of each result, add to each receptacle an equal volume of the solution being examined and immediately mix gently with the lysate. Incubate the reaction mixture, without vibration and minimising loss of water by evaporation, for a constant period that has been found suitable in the experimental conditions (usually 20 to 60 minutes), and read the results. A positive result is indicated by the formation of a firm gel that does not disintegrate when the receptacle is gently inverted. A result is negative if such a gel is not formed.

Sensitivity of the lysate Prepare not fewer than four replicate series of two-fold dilutions of *endotoxin standard BRP* to give concentrations of 2λ, l, 1/2λ, and 1/4λ, where λ is the stated sensitivity of the lysate used. At least the final dilution in each series must give a negative result. Examine the dilutions and a negative control solution consisting of *water BET* as described under Procedure. Calculate the average of the logarithms of the lowest concentration of endotoxin in each series of dilutions for which a positive result is found. The antilogarithm of this average gives the estimated lysate sensitivity. If the latter does not differ by more than a factor of two from the stated sensitivity, the stated sensitivity is confirmed and is used in all tests performed using this lysate.

Interfering factors The pH of the solutions must be in the range specified by the manufacturer of the lysate. This is usually achieved by a product with a pH in the range of 6.0 to 8.0. If necessary add 0.1M *hydrochloric acid BET,* 0.1M *sodium hydroxide BET* or a suitable buffer to the solution before addition of the lysate to correct it.

Operate as prescribed under Sensitivity of the lysate but to prepare the dilutions of *endotoxin standard BRP* use untreated specimens of the preparation being examined in which no endotoxins are detectable. Use these specimens at a dilution not exceeding the maximum valid dilution (MVD) calculated from the expression:

$$\text{maximum valid dilution} = \frac{\text{endotoxin limit concentration}}{\text{sensitivity of the lysate}}$$

both values being expressed in IU of endotoxin per ml.

When the endotoxin limit is specified in the individual monograph in terms of IU of endotoxin per milligram of product or in the case of a biologically assayed product per IU of product, multiply the endotoxin limit by the concentration of the product in the solution tested (in mg per ml or in IU of the product tested per ml) to obtain the endotoxin limit concentration in IU of endotoxin per ml of solution tested. Where relevant the multiplication described above applies to a solution of the product constituted as prescribed on the label.

In monographs other than those of the European Pharmacopoeia, the limit for a given material or preparation is usually expressed as the endotoxin limit concentration in IU per ml for a *defined solution* of that material or preparation. In such cases the above calculations are unnecessary.

If the sensitivity of the lysate determined in the presence of the preparation being examined does not differ by more than a factor of two from that determined in the absence of the preparation being examined, the latter does not contain factors which interfere in the experimental conditions and may be examined without further treatment. Otherwise the preparation being examined acts as an inhibitor or an activator and the interfering factors are eliminated by suitable treatment such as dilution, filtration, neutralisation, dialysis or addition of substances which displace adsorbed endotoxins. The use of a more sensitive lysate permits a greater dilution of the preparation being examined and this may contribute to the elimination of interference.

If the preparation being examined does not comply with the test in a dilution less than the MVD, repeat the test using the MVD.

Ultrafiltration may be used when the interfering factor passes through a filter with a nominal separation limit corresponding to a relative molecular mass of 10,000 to 20,000. Asymmetric membrane filters of cellulose triacetate may be used. They must be checked for the presence of components causing false positive results. The material retained on the filter, which contains the endotoxins, is rinsed with *water BET* or a suitable buffer and the endotoxins are recovered in *water BET* or a suitable buffer. The test volume and the final volume used to recover the endotoxins are determined for each preparation being examined.

To establish that the treatment chosen effectively eliminated interference without removing endotoxins, repeat the test for interfering factors using the preparation being examined to which *endotoxin standard BRP* has been added and which has then been submitted to the chosen treatment.

Method A: Gelation method (limit test)

Endotoxins in the preparation being examined Perform the test in duplicate as described under Procedure using a dilution not exceeding the maximum valid dilution of the preparation being examined which has been treated if necessary to eliminate interfering factors.

Examine at the same time a negative control consisting of *water BET* and two positive controls both of which contain *endotoxin standard BRP* at a concentration corresponding to twice the stated sensitivity of the lysate and one of which contains the preparation being examined (treated if necessary to eliminate interfering factors after the addition of the endotoxin standard) at the concentration being used in the test. The test is valid if the negative and both positive controls give the appropriate result.

The preparation being examined complies with the test if a negative result is found for both test mixtures. The preparation being examined does not comply with the test if a positive result is found for both test mixtures. If a positive result is found for one test mixture and a negative one for the other, repeat the test; the preparation being examined then complies with the test if a negative result is found for both test mixtures.

Method B: Semiquantitative gelation method

Endotoxins in the preparation being examined Treat the preparation being examined if necessary to eliminate interfering factors. Prepare the following solutions:

(a) two independent replicate solutions of the preparation being examined at the dilution with which the test for interfering factors was completed. Use *water BET* to make two independent dilution series of four tubes containing the preparation being examined at concentrations of 1, 1/2, 1/4 and 1/8 relative to the dilution with which the test for interfering factors was completed;

(b) two series of four tubes of *water BET* containing *endotoxin standard BRP* at a concentration of 2λ, λ, 1/2λ and 1/4λ respectively;

(c) two independent replicate solutions of the preparation being examined at the dilution with which the test for interfering factors was completed and *endotoxin standard BRP* at a concentration of 2λ;

(d) *water BET* (as a negative control).

Carry out the assay as described under Sensitivity of the lysate. The test is valid if the following three conditions are met:

— the result obtained with solution (d) is negative;
— the results obtained with the solutions (c) are positive;
— the geometric mean of the endotoxin concentration obtained with the solutions (b) is in the range of 1/2λ to 2λ.

Determine for each of the series (a) the lowest concentration of the preparation giving a positive result, hence containing λ IU of endotoxin per ml. If the original solution of the preparation was diluted by a factor d_1 to complete the test for interfering factors, and this solution, further diluted by a factor d_2 resulted in the lowest concentration yielding a positive result, the product ($\lambda \times d_1 \times d_2$) estimates the number of IU of endotoxin per ml of the original solution of the preparation being examined. Calculate the geometric mean of the two estimates for the two series (a). The preparation being examined passes the test if the geometric mean endotoxin concentration is less than the endotoxin limit concentration specified in the relevant monograph.

Kinetic methods

Both the turbidimetric kinetic method (Method C) and the chromogenic peptide kinetic method (Method D) make use of the linear regression of the logarithm of the response on the logarithm of the endotoxin concentration. The techniques of the method are described under Procedure respectively for each method separately; the sections on Assurance of the criteria for the standard curve, Interfering factors and the determination of Endotoxins in the preparation being examined apply both to the turbidimetric kinetic method and the chromogenic peptide kinetic method.

Method C. Turbidimetric kinetic method

Procedure Measure the reaction time needed for the development of a predetermined degree of turbidity of a solution to which lysate has been added, using a suitable instrument. The endotoxin concentration of the solution may be derived from the logarithm of the reaction time with the aid of a calibration line prepared as described under Assurance of the criteria for the standard curve.

The rate of change of turbidity in the linear part of the regression curve may also be used to measure the endotoxin concentration.

Method D. Chromogenic peptide kinetic method

Procedure Measure the reaction time needed for the development of a predetermined intensity of colour after the liberation of dye from a suitable chromogenic peptide by the endotoxin-lysate complex, using a spectrophotometer set at a suitable wavelength. The endotoxin concentration of the solution may be derived from the logarithm of the reaction time with the aid of a calibration line prepared as described under Assurance of the criteria for the standard curve.

Method C and Method D

Assurance of the criteria for the standard curve This is required when a new batch of lysate is used or when any other condition changes which is likely to influence the result of the test.

Prepare at least two independent series of at least four concentrations of *endotoxin standard BRP* extending over the range required. Limits beyond the ones given by the manufacturer are not recommended. Use at least one concentration per unit under logarithmic scale and a negative control of *water BET*. To each tube add an equal volume of lysate, and, in method D, the appropriate volume of chromogenic peptide. Measure the reaction time as defined above.

For each tube plot the logarithm of the reaction time as a function of the logarithm of the concentration of endotoxin and analyse the regression of the log reaction time on the log concentration of endotoxin, using standard methods of analysis (the method of least squares).

The regression line must have a significant slope and significant linearity, both at the 95% level of significance, for the range of endotoxin concentrations indicated by the manufacturer of the lysate.

Determine the number of logarithmically equidistant concentrations for which the regression curve is linear. If this number is three (λ_1, λ_2 and λ_3), use the second concentration (λ_2) as λ_m in the test for interfering factors and in the test for endotoxins in the preparation being examined. If this number equals 4 or 5, use the third concentration (λ_3) as the λ_m for these purposes.

In addition to these requirements any other test or requirement specified by the manufacturer of the lysate must also be met.

Interfering factors Prepare four independent replicate solutions containing *endotoxin standard BRP* at a concentration of λ_m and the preparation being examined with the dilution factor calculated from the expression:

$$\frac{\text{endotoxin limit concentration}}{\lambda_m}$$

The pH of the solutions must be in the range specified by the manufacturer of the lysate. This is usually achieved by a product with a pH in the range of 6.0 to 8.0. If necessary, to correct the pH add *0.1M hydrochloric acid BET*, 0.1M *sodium hydroxide BET* or a suitable buffer to the solution before addition of the lysate.

Perform the assay with these four replicate solutions, and calculate the mean endotoxin concentration as the anti-logarithm of the mean logarithmic endotoxin concentration.

When the mean endotoxin concentration is at least 50% of λ_m the preparation being examined does not contain factors which interfere with the activity of the lysate under the conditions of the test; samples of this preparation may be examined without further treatment for removal of interfering factors.

When the mean endotoxin concentration is less than 50% of λ_m the interfering factors must be removed as described in method A.

When the mean endotoxin concentration exceeds the highest concentration in the linear part of the regression curve, repeat the test with a higher dilution factor for the preparation being examined, calculated from the expression:

$$\frac{\text{endotoxin limit concentration}}{\lambda_{m'}}$$

in which $\lambda_1 < \lambda_{m'} < \lambda_m$

Endotoxins in the preparation being examined Treat the preparation being examined if necessary to eliminate interfering factors. The pH of the solutions must be in the range specified by the manufacturer of the lysate. This is usually achieved by a product with a pH in the range of 6.0 to 8.0. If necessary add 0.1M *hydrochloric acid BET*, 0.1M *sodium hydroxide BET* or a suitable buffer to the solution before addition of the lysate to correct it.

Prepare the following solutions:

(a) two independent replicate solutions of the preparation being examined at the dilution with which the test for interfering factors was completed;

(b) two independent replicate solutions containing *endotoxin standard BRP* at a concentration of λ_m or $\lambda_{m'}$ whichever is applicable, and the preparation being examined at the dilution described under (a);

(c) three logarithmically equidistant concentrations of *endotoxin standard BRP*, covering the linear part of the regression curve. Test each solution in duplicate;

(d) *water BET* as a negative control.

Carry out the assay as described under Assurance of the criteria for the standard curve. Calculate the endotoxin concentration of each of the replicate solutions (a) and (b), using the regression line generated by the control series (c).

The test is valid if the following three conditions are met:

— the result of the negative control (d) does not exceed the limit for the blank value obtained in the validation of the sensitivity of the lysate.

— the results of the control series (c) comply with the requirements for validation defined under Assurance of the criteria for the standard curve.

— the recovery of endotoxin, calculated from the geometric mean endotoxin concentration of solutions (b) after subtracting the geometric mean endotoxin concentration of solutions (a) is more than 50% and less than 200%. Calculate the percentage recovery by dividing the result of the subtraction by λ_m or $\lambda_{m'}$, whichever is applicable, and multiplying the result by 100.

The preparation being examined passes the test when the endotoxin concentration of each of the two solutions (a) is less than $_m$ or $\lambda_{m'}$ IU of endotoxin per ml, whichever is applicable. If the endotoxin concentration of one of the two solutions is lower and the other one is higher than this limit, repeat the test. The preparation being examined then passes the test if both the solutions (a) comply with the limit.

Method E: Chromogenic peptide endpoint method

Procedure Measure the concentration of dye liberated from a suitable chromogenic peptide by a solution containing endotoxin, incubated with lysate and chromogenic peptide, using a spectrophotometer set at a suitable wavelength. The endotoxin concentration of the solution may be derived from the absorbance at the wavelength chosen with the aid of a calibration line prepared as described under Assurance of the criteria for the standard curve.

Assurance of the criteria for the standard curve This is required when a new batch of lysate is used or when any other condition changes which is likely to influence the result of the test.

Prepare four independent series of dilutions of the *endotoxin standard BRP* in *water BET* which extend over the range indicated by the manufacturer of the lysate; the range must include the limit (λ) indicated by the manufacturer. Use a reagent blank prepared according to the instructions of the manufacturer of the lysate.

Add the prescribed volume of lysate and chromogenic peptide to each tube and incubate for the time specified by the manufacturer. Stop the reaction and measure the absorbance at a suitable wavelength.

For each tube, plot the absorbance at each concentration of the four replicate series as a function of the endotoxin concentration and analyse the regression of the absorbance on the concentration, using standard methods of analysis (the method of least squares).

The regression line must have a significant slope and significant linearity, both at the 95% level of significance, for the range of endotoxin concentrations indicated by the manufacturer of the lysate.

Determine the endotoxin concentration λ_m which is the arithmetic mean of the highest (λ_h)and the lowest (λ_l) endotoxin concentrations for which the regression curve is linear, all values being expressed in IU of endotoxin per ml.

In addition to these requirements any other test or requirement specified by the manufacturer of the lysate must also be met.

Interfering factors Prepare four independent replicate solutions containing *endotoxin standard BRP* at a concentration of λ_m and the preparation being examined with the dilution factor calculated from the expression:

$$\frac{\text{endotoxin limit concentration}}{\lambda_m}$$

The pH of the solutions must be in the range specified by the manufacturer of the lysate. This is usually achieved by a product with a pH in the range of 6.0 to 8.0. If necessary add 0.1M *hydrochloric acid BET,* 0.1M *sodium hydroxide BET* or a suitable buffer to the solution before addition of the lysate to correct it.

Perform the assay with these four replicate solutions, and calculate the mean endotoxin concentration.

When the mean endotoxin concentration is at least 50% and not more than 200%of λ_m, the preparation being examined does not contain factors which interfere with the activity of the lysate under the conditions of the test; samples of this preparation may be examined without further treatment for removal of interfering factors.

When the mean endotoxin concentration is less than 50% or more than 200% of λ_m, the interfering factors must be removed as described in method A.

When the mean endotoxin concentration exceeds the highest concentration in the linear part of the regression curve, repeat the test with a higher dilution factor for the preparation being examined, calculated from the expression:

$$\frac{\text{endotoxin limit concentration}}{\lambda_{m'}}$$

in which $\lambda_l < \lambda_{m'} < \lambda_m$.

Endotoxins in the preparation being examined Treat the preparation being examined if necessary to eliminate interfering factors. The pH of the solutions must be in the range specified by the manufacturer of the lysate. This is usually achieved by a product with a pH in the range of 6.0 to 8.0. If necessary add 0.1M *hydrochloric acid BET,* 0.1M *sodium hydroxide BET* or a suitable buffer to the solution before addition of the lysate to correct the pH.

Prepare the following solutions:

(a) two independent replicate solutions of the preparation being examined at the dilution with which the test for interfering factors was completed;

(b) two independent replicate solutions containing *endotoxin standard BRP* at a concentration of λ_m or $\lambda_{m'}$, whichever is applicable, and the preparation being examined at the dilution described under (a);

(c) two replicate solutions of *endotoxin standard BRP* at a concentration of λ_h and two replicate solutions of *endotoxin standard BRP* at a concentration of λ_l;

(d) *water BET* as a negative control.

Carry out the assay as described under Assurance of the criteria for the standard curve. Determine the absorbance after the incubation for each of the solutions (a), (b), (c) and (d). Use the absorbance of the solutions (c) and (d) to calculate the regression line and calculate the endotoxin concentrations of the solutions (a) and (b).

The test is valid if the following three conditions are met:

— the result of the negative control (d) does not exceed the limit for the blank value obtained in the validation of the sensitivity of the lysate;

— the results of the control solutions (c) comply with the calibration line used to check the sensitivity of the lysate;

— the recovery of endotoxin, calculated from the arithmetic mean endotoxin concentration of solutions (b) after subtracting the arithmetic mean endotoxin concentration of solutions (a) is more than 50% and less than 200%. Calculate the percentage recovery by dividing the result of the subtraction by $_m$ or $\lambda_{m'}$, whichever is applicable, and multiplying the result by 100.

The preparation being examined passes the test if the endotoxin concentration of each of the two solutions (a) is less than λ_m or $\lambda_{m'}$ IU of endotoxin per ml, whichever is applicable. If the endotoxin concentration of one of the two solutions is lower and the other one is higher than this limit, repeat the test. The preparation being examined then passes the test if both the solutions (a) comply with the limit.

D. Test for Pyrogens

(Ph. Eur. method 2.6.8)

The test consists of measuring the rise in body temperature evoked in rabbits by the intravenous injection of a sterile solution of the substance being examined.

Where under the heading Pyrogens in an individual monograph it states that the substance being examined is to be dissolved in *albumin solution*, this reagent may be replaced by a solution in *water for injections* containing an appropriate amount of a suitable protein that has been shown to be pyrogen-free and also shown, by a suitable method, to be free from proteolytic activity; the solution is adjusted to an appropriate pH.

Selection of animals

Use healthy, adult rabbits of either sex, weighing not less than 1.5 kg, fed a complete and balanced diet not containing antibiotics and showing no loss of body weight during the week preceding the test. The rabbits must not have been used in a similar test (*a*) during the preceding 3 days or (*b*) during the preceding 3 weeks unless the material being examined passed the test. Rabbits used in a test for pyrogens where the mean rise in the rabbits' temperature has exceeded 1.2° are permanently excluded.

Animals' quarters

Keep the rabbits individually in a quiet area with an appropriate uniform temperature. Carry out the test in a quiet room where there is no risk of disturbance exciting the animals and in which the room temperature is within 3° of that of the rabbits' living quarters or in which the rabbits have been kept for at least 18 hours before the test. Withhold food from the rabbits overnight and until the test is completed; withhold water during the test.

Equipment

Thermometers The thermometer or electrical device used indicates the temperature with a precision of 0.1° and is inserted in the rectum of the rabbit to a depth of about 5 cm. The depth of insertion is constant for any one rabbit in any one test. When an electrical device is used it should be inserted in the rectum of the rabbit 90 minutes before the injection of the solution being examined and left in position throughout the test.

Glassware, syringes and needles All glassware, syringes and needles must be thoroughly washed with *water for injections* and heated in a hot air oven at 250° for 30 minutes or at 200° for 1 hour.

Retaining boxes The retaining boxes for rabbits in which the temperature is being measured by an electrical device are made in such a way that the animals are retained only by loosely-fitting neck-stocks; the rest of the body remains relatively free so that the rabbits may sit in a normal position. The rabbits are not restrained by the use of straps or other similar methods that may harm the animal. The animals must be put into the boxes not less than 1 hour before the test and remain in them throughout the test.

Preliminary test

One to three days before testing the product, inject intravenously into animals, selected as prescribed above but that have not been used during the 2 previous weeks, 10 ml per kg of body weight of a pyrogen-free, 0.9% w/v solution of sodium chloride warmed to about 38.5°.

Record the temperatures of the animals, beginning at least 90 minutes before injection and continuing for 3 hours after injection of the solution being examined. Any animal showing a temperature variation greater than 0.6° must not be used in the main test.

Main test

Carry out the test using a group of three rabbits.

Preparation and injection of the sample The preparation being examined may be dissolved in, or diluted with, a pyrogen-free, 0.9% w/v solution of sodium chloride or other solution prescribed in the monograph. Warm the liquid being examined to approximately 38.5° before injection. Inject the solution slowly into the marginal vein of the ear of each rabbit over a period not exceeding 4 minutes, unless otherwise prescribed in the monograph. The amount of the sample to be injected varies according to the preparation being examined and is prescribed in the monograph. The volume of the injection is 0.5 to 10 ml per kg of body weight.

Determination of the initial and maximum temperatures The 'initial temperature' of each rabbit is the mean of two temperature readings recorded for that rabbit at an interval of 30 minutes in the 40 minutes immediately preceding the injection of the material being examined. The 'maximum temperature' of each rabbit is the highest temperature recorded for that rabbit in the 3 hours after the injection. Record the temperature of each animal at intervals of not more than 30 minutes, beginning at least 90 minutes before the injection of the solution being examined and continuing for 3 hours after the injection. The difference between the initial temperature and the maximum temperature of each rabbit is taken to be its response. When this difference is negative, the result is counted as a zero response. Rabbits showing a temperature difference greater than 0.2° between any two successive readings taken during the 90 minutes before the injection are withdrawn from the test. In any one test, only rabbits having initial temperatures that do not differ from one another by more than 1° may be used. All rabbits having an initial temperature higher than 39.8° or lower than 38.0° are excluded from the test.

Interpretation of results Having carried out the test first on a group of three rabbits, repeat if necessary on further groups of three rabbits to a total of four groups, depending on the results obtained. If the summed response of the first group does not exceed the figure given in the second column of the following table, the preparation being examined passes the test. If the summed response exceeds the figure in the second column but does not exceed the figure in the third column of the table repeat the test as indicated above. If the summed response is greater than the figure given in the third column of the table, the preparation being examined fails the test.

Number of rabbits	Material passes if summed response does not exceed	Material fails if summed response exceeds
3	1.15°	2.65°
6	2.80°	4.30°
9	4.45°	5.95°
12	6.60°	6.60°

E. Test for Abnormal Toxicity

(Ph. Eur. method 2.6.9)

General Test

Inject intravenously into each of five healthy mice, weighing 17 g to 22 g, the quantity of the substance being examined prescribed in the monograph, dissolved in 0.5 ml of *water for injections* R or of a 9 g/l sterile solution of sodium chloride. Inject the solution over a period of 15 to 30 seconds, unless otherwise prescribed.

The substance passes the test if none of the mice dies within 24 hours or within such time as is specified in the individual monograph. If more than one animal dies the preparation fails the test. If one of the animals dies, repeat the test. The substance passes the test if none of the animals in the second group dies within the time interval specified.

Antisera and Vaccines (Immunosera)

Unless otherwise prescribed, inject intraperitoneally one human dose but not more than 1.0 ml into each of five healthy mice, weighing 17 g to 22 g. The human dose is that stated on the label of the preparation being examined or on the accompanying leaflet. Observe the animals for 7 days. The preparation passes the test if none of the animals shows signs of ill health. If more than one animal dies, the preparation fails the test. If one of the animals dies or shows signs of ill health, repeat the test. The preparation passes the test if none of the animals in the second group dies or shows signs of ill health in the time interval specified.

The test must also be carried out on two healthy guinea-pigs weighing 250 g to 350 g. Inject intraperitoneally into each animal one human dose but not more than 5.0 ml. The human dose is that stated on the label of the preparation being examined or on the accompanying leaflet. Observe the animals for 7 days. The preparation passes the test if none of the animals shows signs of ill health. If more than one animal dies the preparation fails the test. If one of the animals dies or shows signs of ill health, repeat the test. The preparation passes the test if none of the animals in the second group dies or shows signs of ill health in the time interval specified.

F. Test for Depressor Substances

(Ph. Eur. method 2.6.11)

Carry out the test on a cat weighing not less than 2 kg and anaesthetised with chloralose or with a barbiturate that allows the maintenance of uniform blood pressure. Protect the animal from loss of body heat and maintain it so that the rectal temperature remains within physiological limits. Introduce a cannula into the trachea. Insert a cannula filled with heparinised *saline solution* into the common carotid artery and connect it to a device capable of giving a continuous record of the blood pressure. Insert into the femoral vein another cannula filled with heparinised *saline solution* through which can be injected solutions of histamine and of the substance being examined.

Determine the sensitivity of the animal to histamine by injecting intravenously, at regular intervals, doses of *histamine solution* corresponding to 0.1 and 0.15 µg of histamine base per kg of the cat's weight. Repeat the lower dose at least a further three times. Administer the second and subsequent injections not less than 1 minute after the blood pressure has returned to a constant level. The animal is used for the test only if a readily discernible decrease in blood pressure that is constant for the lower dose is obtained and if the higher dose causes greater responses.

Dissolve the substance being examined in sufficient *saline solution*, or other solvent prescribed in the monograph, to give the concentration specified in the monograph. Inject intravenously per kg of the cat's weight, 1.0 ml of *histamine solution*, followed by two successive injections of the specified volume of the solution being examined and, finally, 1.0 ml of *histamine solution*. The second, third and fourth injections are given not less than 1 minute after the blood pressure has returned to a constant level. Repeat this series of injections twice and conclude the test by giving 1.5 ml of *histamine solution* per kg of the cat's weight.

The test is not valid unless the response to 1.5 ml of *histamine solution* per kg of the cat's weight is greater than that to 1.0 ml. The substance fails the test if the mean of the series of responses to the substance is greater than the mean of the responses to 1.0 ml of *histamine solution* per kg of body weight or if any one dose of the substance causes a greater depressor response than the concluding dose of the histamine solution. The test animal must not be used in another test for depressor substances if the second criterion applies or if the response to the high dose of histamine given after the administration of the substance being examined is less than the mean response to the low doses of histamine previously injected.

G. Test for Histamine

(Ph. Eur. method 2.6.10)

Kill a guinea-pig weighing 250 to 350 g that has been deprived of food for the preceding 24 hours. Remove a portion of the distal small intestine 2 cm in length and empty the isolated part by rinsing carefully with *solution B* using a syringe. Attach a fine thread to each end and make a small transverse incision in the middle of the piece of intestine. Place it in an organ bath with a capacity of 10 to 20 ml containing *solution B* maintained at a constant temperature (34° to 36°) and pass through the solution a current of a mixture of 95 volumes of oxygen and 5 volumes of carbon dioxide. Attach one of the threads near to the bottom of the organ bath. Attach the other thread to an isotonic myograph and record the contraction of the organ on a kymograph or other suitable means of giving a permanent record. If a lever is used, its length is such that the movements of the organ are amplified about 20 times. The tension on the intestine should be about 9.8 mN and it should be adjusted to the sensitivity of the organ. Flush out the organ bath with *solution B*. Allow it to stand for 10 minutes. Flush two or three times more with *solution B*. Add measured volumes of 0.2 to 0.5 ml of a solution of *histamine dihydrochloride* having a strength that produces reproducible submaximal responses. This dose is termed the 'high' dose. Flush the organ bath (preferably by overflow without emptying the bath) three times with *solution B* before each addition of histamine. The successive additions should be made at regular intervals allowing a complete relaxation between additions (about 2 minutes). Add equal volumes of a weaker solution of *histamine dihydrochloride* that produces reproducible responses approximately half as great as the 'high' dose. This dose is termed the 'low' dose. Continue the regular additions of 'high' and 'low' doses of the histamine solution as indicated above and alternate each addition with an equal volume of a dilution of the solution being examined, adjusting the dilution so that the contraction of the intestine, if any, is smaller than that due to the 'high' dose of histamine. Determine whether the contraction, if any, is reproducible and whether the responses to the 'high' and 'low' doses of histamine given subsequently are unchanged. Calculate the activity of the substance being examined in terms of its equivalent in micrograms of histamine base from the dilution determined as above. The quantity so determined does not exceed the quantity prescribed in the monograph.

If the substance being examined does not produce a

contraction, prepare a fresh solution adding a quantity of histamine corresponding to the maximum tolerated in the monograph and note whether the contractions produced by the preparation with the added histamine correspond to the amount of histamine added. If this is not the case, or if the contractions caused by the substance being examined are not reproducible or if subsequent responses to the 'high' and 'low' doses of histamine are diminished, the results of the test are invalid and the *test for depressor substances*, Appendix XIV F, must be carried out.

Solution A

Sodium chloride	160 g
Potassium chloride	4.0 g
Anhydrous calcium chloride	2.0 g
Anhydrous magnesium chloride	1.0 g
Disodium hydrogen orthophosphate	50 mg
Water for injections	sufficient to produce 1000 ml

Solution B

Solution A	50 ml
Atropine sulphate	0.5 mg
Sodium hydrogen carbonate	1.0 g
D-Glucose	0.5 g
Water for injections	sufficient to produce 1000 ml

Solution B should be freshly prepared and used within 24 hours.

H . Hormones

1. ASSAY OF CORTICOTROPIN
(Ph. Eur. method 2.7.3)

The potency of corticotropin is determined by comparing one or more of its biological effects with the same effect of the International Standard, or of a reference preparation calibrated in International Units, under the same conditions.

The International Unit is the activity contained in a stated amount of the International Standard, which consists of freeze-dried, purified pig corticotropin with lactose. The equivalence in International Units of the International Standard is stated by the World Health Organization.

Corticotropin BRP is calibrated in International Units in comparison with the International Standard.

Use rats of either sex weighing between 100 g and 200 g, the difference in weight between the heaviest and the lightest animal being not greater than 15 g. Maintain the rats under uniform conditions for at least 7 days before the test. On the day before the test, weigh the rats and carry out a hypophysectomy. After the operation, allow access to a 50 g/l solution of *glucose* in a 1.8 g/l solution of *sodium chloride* in addition to rat diet and water and keep the animals in a room at a constant temperature between 24° and 27°. Carry out the test between 18 and 36 hours after hypophysectomy.

On the day of the test reweigh the animals and assign them at random to six groups of eight to ten animals. Choose three doses of the reference preparation and three doses of the substance being examined, such that the smallest dose produces some depletion, and the largest dose does not produce maximal depletion of the adrenal ascorbic acid content. Administer doses adjusted to the body weight of the animals in random order by subcutaneous injection. Doses of the order of 1.0 IU, 0.5 IU and 0.25 IU per 100 g of body weight are usually suitable. Unless otherwise prescribed, dissolve the reference preparation and the substance being examined in 0.01 M *hydrochloric acid* and make subsequent dilutions with *water* containing 150 g/l of *gelatin*. Inject the solutions within 4 hours of preparation.

Three hours after injection, remove both adrenal glands from the anaesthetised rat, free them from extraneous tissue and weigh as quickly as possible to avoid losses of weight. Kill the rat and examine for completeness of hypophysectomy.

Crush and homogenise the pair of adrenal glands in a freshly prepared 25 g/l solution of *metaphosphoric acid* and dilute to 10 ml with the same solution. Allow the homogenate to stand for 30 minutes and centrifuge. Add 7 ml of the clear supernatant liquid to a freshly prepared mixture consisting of 7 ml of a 45.3 g/l solution of *sodium acetate* adjusted to pH 7 by the addition of *acetic acid*, 3 ml of *water* and 2 ml *of standard 2,6-dichlorophenolindophenol solution*. Thirty seconds after mixing, measure the light absorption in a colorimeter, using a filter with maximum transmission at 470 nm and a transmission range of 450 nm to 520 nm. Calculate the ascorbic acid content from a standard curve prepared by treating suitable volumes of a freshly prepared solution of L-*ascorbic acid* in the 25 g/l solution of *metaphosphoric acid* in the same manner. Express the result in milligrams per 100 g of adrenal gland. Calculate the result of the assay by the usual statistical methods.

J. Blood and Related Products

1. ASSAY OF FACTOR VII FRACTION (COAGULATION FACTOR VII)
(Ph Eur. method 2.7.10)

Factor VII Fraction (coagulation factor VII) is assayed by its biological activity as a factor VIIa-tissue factor complex in the activation of factor X in the presence of calcium ions and phospholipids. The potency of a factor VII preparation is estimated by comparing the quantity necessary to achieve a certain rate of factor Xa formation in a test mixture containing the substances that take part in the activation of factor X, and the quantity of the International Standard, or of a reference preparation calibrated in International Units, required to produce the same rate of factor Xa formation.

The International Unit is the factor VII activity of a stated amount of the International Standard which consists of freeze-dried plasma. The equivalence in International Units of the International Standard is stated by the World Health Organization.

The chromogenic assay method consists of two consecutive steps: the factor VII-dependent activation of factor X reagent mixture containing tissue factor, phospholipids and calcium ion, followed by enzymatic cleavage of a chromogenic factor Xa substrate into a chromophore that can be quantified spectrophotometrically. Under appropriate assay conditions, there is a linear relation between the rate of factor Xa formation and the factor VII concentration. The assay is summarised in Figure 2.7.10.–1.

Step 1 a) Factor VII —(Tissue factor + Ca^{++})→ Factor VIIa

b) Factor X —(Factor VII a + Ca^{++} + Tissue factor/Phospholipid)→ Factor Xa

Step 2 Chromogenic substrate —(Factor Xa)→ Peptide + chromophore

Fig. 16J-1 Schematic representation of the assay of human coagulation Factor VII

Both steps employ reagents that may be obtained commercially from a variety of sources. Although the composition of individual reagents may be subject to some variation, their essential features are described in the following specification.

Reagents

The coagulation factor reagent comprises purified proteins derived from human or bovine sources. These include factor X and thromboplastin tissue factor/phospholipid as factor VII activator. These proteins are partly purified and do not contain impurities that interfere with the activation of factor VII or factor X. Factor X is present in amounts giving a final concentration during the first step of the assay of 10 to 350 nmol per litre, preferably 14 to 70 nmol per litre. Thromboplastin from natural sources (bovine or rabbit brain) or synthetic preparations may be used as the tissue factor/phospholipid component. Thromboplastin suitable for use in prothrombin time determination is diluted 1:5 to 1:50 in buffer such that the final concentration of Ca^{++} is 15 to 25 mmol per litre. The final factor Xa generation is performed in a solution containing human or bovine albumin at a concentration such that adsorption losses do not occur and which is appropriately buffered at pH 7.3 to 8.0. In the final incubation mixture, factor VII must be the only rate-limiting component and each reagent component must lack the ability to generate factor Xa on its own.

The second step comprises the quantification of the formed factor Xa employing a chromogenic substrate that is specific for factor Xa. Generally this consists of a short peptide of between three and five amino acids, bound to a chromophore group. On cleavage of this group from the peptide substrate, its absorption maximum shifts to a wavelength allowing its spectrophotometric quantification. The substrate is usually dissolved in *water* and used at a final concentration of 0.2 to 2 mmol per litre. The substrate may also contain appropriate inhibitors to stop further factor Xa generation (addition of edetate).

Assay procedure

Reconstitute the entire contents of one ampoule of the reference preparation and the preparation being examined by adding the appropriate quantity of *water*; use within 1 hour. Add sufficient prediluent to the reconstituted preparations to produce solutions containing between 0.5 and 2.0 IU of factor VII per ml.

Prepare further dilutions of reference and test preparations using an isotonic non-chelating buffer containing 1% of bovine or human albumin, buffered preferably between pH 7.3 and 8.0. Prepare at least three separate, independent dilutions for each material, preferably in duplicate. Prepare the dilutions such that the final factor VII concentration is below 0.005 IU per ml.

Prepare a control solution that includes all components except factor VII.

Prepare all dilutions in plastic tubes and use within 1 hour.

Step 1 Mix dilutions of the factor VII reference preparation and the preparation being examined with an appropriate volume of the prewarmed coagulation factor reagent or a combination of its separate constituents, and incubate the mixture in plastic tubes or microplate wells at 37°. The concentrations of the various components during the factor Xa generation must be as specified above under the description of the reagents.

Allow the activation of factor X to proceed for a suitable time, usually terminating the reaction before the factor Xa concentration has reached its maximal level in order to obtain a satisfactory linear dose-response relationship. The activation time is also chosen to achieve linear production of factor Xa in time. Appropriate activation times are usually between 2 minutes and 5 minutes, but deviations are permissible if acceptable linearity of the dose-response relationship is thus obtained.

Step 2 Terminate the activation by the addition of a prewarmed reagent containing a chromogenic substrate. Quantify the rate of substrate cleavage, which must be linear with the concentration of factor Xa formed, by measuring the absorbance change at an appropriate wavelength using a spectrophotometer, either monitoring the absorbance continuously, thus allowing the initial rate of substrate cleavage to be calculated, or terminating the hydrolysis reaction after a suitable interval by lowering the pH by the addition of a suitable reagent, such as acetic acid (500 g/l $C_2H_4O_2$) or a citrate solution (1 mol per litre) at pH 3. Adjust the hydrolysis time to achieve a linear development of chromophore with time. Appropriate hydrolysis times are usually between 3 minutes and 15 minutes, but deviations are permissible if better linearity of the dose-response relationship is thus obtained.

Check the validity of the assay and calculate the potency of the test preparation by the usual statistical methods (for example, *Ph Eur general text 5.3. Statistical Analysis of Results of Biological Assays and Tests*).

2. ASSAY OF FACTOR VIII FRACTION (BLOOD COAGULATION FACTOR VIII)

(Ph. Eur. method 2.7.4)

Factor VIII fraction (coagulation factor VIII) is assayed by its biological activity as a cofactor in the activation of factor X by activated factor IX (factor IXa) in the presence of calcium ions and phospholipids. The potency of a factor VIII preparation is estimated by comparing the quantity necessary to achieve a certain rate of factor Xa formation in a test mixture containing the substances that take part in the activation of factor X, and the quantity of the International Standard, or of a reference preparation calibrated in International Units, required to produce the same rate of factor Xa formation.

The International Unit is the factor VIII activity of a stated amount of the International Standard which consists of a freeze-dried human blood coagulation factor VIII concentrate. The equivalence in International Units of the International Standard is stated by the World Health Organization.

Human coagulation factor VIII BRP is calibrated in International Units by comparison with the International Standard.

The chromogenic assay method consists of two consecutive steps: the factor VIII-dependent activation of factor X in a coagulation-factor reagent composed of purified components, and the enzymatic cleavage of a chromogenic factor Xa substrate to yield a chromophore that can be quantified spectrophotometrically. Under appropriate assay conditions, there is a linear relation between the rate of factor Xa formation and the factor VIII concentration. The assay is summarised by the following scheme:

Step 1 a) $\text{Factor X} \xrightarrow[\text{factor IXa, phospholipid } Ca^{2+}]{\text{activated factor VIII}} \text{factor Xa}$

Step 2 $\text{chromogenic substrate} \xrightarrow{\text{factor Xa}} \text{peptide + chromophore}$

Both steps employ reagents that may be obtained commercially from a variety of sources. Although the composition of individual reagents may be subject to some variation, their essential features are described in the following specification. Deviations from this description may be permissible provided that it has been shown, using the International Standard for Human Blood Coagulation Factor VIII concentrate as the standard, that the results obtained do not differ significantly.

Commercial assay kits are to be used in accordance with the manufacturers' instructions; it is important to ascertain the suitability for the assay of the kit used.

Reagents

The coagulation factor reagent comprises purified proteins derived from human or bovine sources. These include factor X, factor IXa, and a factor VIII activator, usually thrombin. These proteins are partly purified, preferably to at least 50%, and do not contain impurities that interfere with the activation of factor VIII or factor X. Factor X is present in amounts giving a final concentration during the first step of the assay of 10 to 350 nmol per litre, preferably 15 to 30 nmol per litre. Factor IXa is prepared by activating purified factor IX to factor IXaβ using factor XIa, and by subsequent purification of factor IXaβ from the reaction mixture. Its final concentration during factor Xa generation is less than 30% of the factor X concentration, usually 1 to 100 nmol per litre, preferably 1 to 10 nmol per litre. Thrombin may be present in its precursor form prothrombin, provided that its activation in the reagent is sufficiently rapid to give almost instantaneous, complete activation of factor VIII in the assay. Phospholipids may be obtained from natural sources such as bovine brain or spinal cord or soya-bean extract, or synthetically prepared, and must consist to a substantial extent, usually 15 to 35%, of the species phosphatidylserine. The final phospholipid concentration during factor Xa generation is 1 to 50 nmol per litre, preferably 10 to 35 nmol per litre. The reagent contains calcium ions to give a final concentration of 5 to 15 nmol per litre. The final factor Xa generation is performed in a solution containing at least 1 mg per ml of human or bovine albumin which is appropriately buffered, at a pH of 7.3 to 8.0.

The components of the complete reagent are usually divided into at least two separate reagents each lacking the ability to generate factor Xa on its own. After reconstitution, these may be combined provided that no substantial amounts of factor Xa are generated in the absence of factor VIII. In the final incubation mixture, factor VIII must be the only rate-limiting component.

The second step comprises the quantification of the formed factor Xa employing a chromogenic substrate that is specific for factor Xa. Generally this consists of a derivatised short peptide of between three and five amino acids, joined to a chromophore group. On cleavage of this group from the peptide substrate, its chromophoric properties shift to a wavelength allowing its spectrophotometric quantification. The substrate is usually dissolved in water and used at a final concentration of 0.2 to 2 mmol per litre. The substrate may further contain appropriate inhibitors to stop further factor Xa generation and to suppress thrombin activity, thereby improving selectivity for factor Xa.

Assay procedure

Reconstitute the entire contents of one ampoule of the reference preparation and the preparation being examined by adding the appropriate quantity of *water*; use immediately. Add sufficient prediluent to the reconstituted preparations to produce solutions containing between 0.5 and 2.0 IU per ml.

The prediluent consists of plasma from a patient with severe haemophilia A, or of an artificially prepared reagent that gives results that do not differ significantly from those obtained employing haemophilic plasma and the same reference and test preparations. The prediluted materials must be stable beyond the time required for the assay, for at least 30 minutes at 20° and must be used within 15 minutes.

Prepare further dilutions of reference and test preparations using an isotonic non-chelating buffer containing 1% of human or bovine albumin and for example, tris(hydroxymethyl)aminomethane or imidazole, buffered preferably between pH 7.3 and 8.0. Prepare at least three separate, independent dilutions for each material, preferably with each one prepared in duplicate. Prepare the dilutions such that the final factor VIII concentration is below 0.03 IU per ml, and preferably below 0.01 IU per ml, during the step of factor Xa generation. Prepare a control solution that includes all components except factor VIII. Prepare all dilutions in plastic tubes and use without delay.

Step 1 Mix prewarmed dilutions of the factor VIII reference preparation and the preparation being examined with an appropriate volume of the prewarmed coagulation factor reagent or a combination of its separate constituents, and incubate the mixture in plastic tubes or microplate wells at 37°. The concentrations of the various components during the factor Xa generation must be as specified above under the description of the reagents. Allow the activation of factor X to proceed for a suitable time, preferably terminating the reaction before the factor Xa concentration has reached its maximal level in order to obtain a satisfactory linear dose-response relationship. The activation time is also chosen to achieve linear production of factor Xa in time. Appropriate activation times are usually between 2 min and 5 min, but deviations are permissible if better linearity of the dose-response relationship is thus obtained.

Step 2 Terminate the activation by addition of a prewarmed reagent containing a chromogenic substrate. Quantify the rate of substrate cleavage, which must be linear with the concentration of factor Xa formed, by measuring the absorbance change at an appropriate wavelength using a spectrophotometer, either monitoring the absorbance continuously, thus allowing the initial rate of substrate cleavage to be calculated, or terminating the hydrolysis reaction after a suitable interval by lowering the pH by addition of a suitable reagent, such as acetic acid (50% v/v $C_2H_4O_2$) or a citrate solution (1 mol per litre) at pH 3. Adjust the hydrolysis time to achieve a linear development of chromophore in time. Appropriate hydrolysis times usually are between 3 and 15 minutes, but deviations are permissible if better linearity of the dose–response relationship is thus obtained. Check the validity of the assay and calculate the potency of the test preparation by the usual statistical methods for a slope-ratio assay (for example, *Ph. Eur general text 5.3. Statistical Analysis of Results of Biological Assays and Tests*).

3. ASSAY OF FACTOR IX FRACTION (HUMAN COAGULATION FACTOR IX)

(Ph. Eur. method 2.7.11)

The potency is determined by comparing the quantity of the preparation being examined necessary to reduce the coagulation time of a test mixture containing the substances, other than factor IX, that take part in the coagulation of blood and the quantity of a reference preparation, calibrated in International Units, required to produce the same effect.

The International Unit is the activity of a stated amount of the International Standard, which consists of a freeze-dried concentrate of human blood coagulation factor IX. The equivalence in International Units of the international standard is stated by the World Health Organization.

Reconstitute separately the preparation being examined and the reference preparation as stated on the label and use immediately. Where applicable, determine the amount of heparin present, Appendix XIV J4 (*Ph Eur method 2.7.12*) and neutralise the heparin by addition of *protamine sulphate* (10 µg of protamine sulphate neutralises 1 IU of heparin). Dilute the preparation being examined and the reference preparation with a sufficient quantity of *imidazole buffer solution pH 7.3* to produce solutions containing 0.5 to 2.0 IU per ml. Prepare twofold dilutions in the range 1:10 to 1:80 using a mixture of 1 volume of a 38 g/1 solution of *sodium citrate* and 5 volumes of *imidazole buffer solution pH 7.3*. Make these dilutions accurately and use immediately.

Use, for example, incubation tubes maintained in a waterbath at 37°. Place in each tube 0.1 ml of *plasma substrate R2* and 0.1 ml of one of the dilutions of the reference preparation or of the preparation being examined. Add to each tube 0.1 ml of a suitable dilution of *cephalin* or *platelet substitute* and 0.1 ml of a suspension of 0.5 g of *light kaolin* in 100 ml of a 9 g/1 solution of *sodium chloride* and allow to stand for about 10 minutes, tilting the tubes regularly. To each tube, add 0.1 ml of a 7.4 g/1 solution of *calcium chloride*. Using a timer, measure the coagulation time, i.e. the interval between the moment of the addition of the calcium chloride and the first indication of the formation of fibrin, which may be observed visually or by the use of a suitable apparatus. Calculate the potency using the usual statistical methods (for example, *Ph Eur general text 5.3. Statistical analysis of results of biological assays and tests*).

To ensure that there is no appreciable contamination of *plasma substrate R2* by factor IX, carry out a blank test using, instead of the preparation being examined, a corresponding volume of a mixture of 1 volume of a 38 g/1 solution of *sodium citrate* and 5 volumes of *imidazole buffer solution pH 7.3*. The test is not valid unless the coagulation time measured in the blank test is 100 to 200 seconds.

4. ASSAY OF HEPARIN IN COAGULATION FACTOR CONCENTRATES

(Ph. Eur. method 2.7.12)

The test sample is incubated with a defined excess of thrombin and a thrombin-specific chromogenic substrate and the rate of increase of absorbance (related to the amount of *p*-nitroaniline released) is measured at 405 nm. The rate of increase is inversely proportional to the heparin content of the sample.

Test solutions Reconstitute the preparation as stated on the label and dilute with a suitable buffer solution (for example, 7 g/1 of *sodium chloride*, 6 g/1 of *sodium citrate*, pH 7.3) to approximately 0.25 IU of heparin per ml. Prepare serial dilutions, using the dilution buffer (see under reference solutions), up to 1:32. Allow the dilutions to stand for 30 minutes.

Reference solutions Dilute a heparin reference preparation with a suitable dilution buffer (for example, 6 g/1 of *tris(hydroxymethyl)aminomethane*, 2.2 g/l of *(ethylene-dinitrilotetra-acetic acid*, 11.3 g/1 of *sodium chloride*, pH 8.4) to approximately 0.25 IU of heparin per ml. Prepare serial dilutions up to 1:32.

Pipette 200 µl of the test solution, reference solution or blank (dilution buffer) and 200 µl of a solution of *anti-thrombin III* (3 IU/ml) into a series of plastic tubes. Allow the mixture to stand for 30 minutes and add 200 µl of a solution of *bovine thrombin* (20 IU/ml). Mix thoroughly using a vortex mixer and maintain at 37° for 90 seconds.

Prepare a solution of a thrombin-specific chromogenic substrate at a concentration equivalent to at least twice the K_m (Michaelis constant) value.

Preheat the substrate solution to 37° and add 200 µl to each tube containing the test sample, the reference preparation or the blank. Mix thoroughly using a vortex mixer. Incubate at 37° for 90 seconds, stop the reaction by adding 200 µl of a solution of *acetic acid* (500 g/l $C_2H_4O_2$) and measure the absorbance at 405 nm.

Calculate the heparin content of the test preparation by the usual statistical methods (for example, *Ph Eur general text 5.3. Statistical analysis of results of biological assays and tests*).

5. ASSAY OF HEPARIN

(Ph. Eur. method 2.7.5)

The anticoagulant activity of heparin is determined *in vitro* by comparing its ability in given conditions to delay the clotting of recalcified citrated sheep plasma with the same ability of a reference preparation of heparin calibrated in International Units.

The International Unit is the activity contained in a stated amount of the International Standard, which consists of a quantity of freeze-dried heparin sodium from pork intestinal mucosa. The equivalence in International

Units of the International Standard is stated by the World Health Organization.

Heparin sodium BRP is calibrated in International Units by comparison with the International Standard by means of the assay given below.

Carry out the assay using one of the following methods for determining the onset of clotting and using tubes and other equipment appropriate to the chosen method:
a) direct visual inspection, preferably using indirect illumination and viewing against a matt black background;
b) spectrophotometric recording of the change in optical density at a wavelength of approximately 600 nm;
c) visual detection of the change in fluidity on manual tilting of the tubes;
d) mechanical recording of the change in fluidity on stirring, care being taken to cause the minimum disturbance of the solution during the earliest phase of clotting.

Assay procedure

The volumes in the text are given as examples and may be adapted to the apparatus used provided that the ratios between the different volumes are respected.

Dilute *heparin sodium BRP* with a 9 g/l solution of *sodium chloride* to contain a precisely known number of IU per ml and prepare a similar solution of the preparation being examined which is expected to have the same activity. Using a 9 g/l solution of *sodium chloride*, prepare from each solution a series of dilutions in geometric progression such that the clotting time obtained with the lowest concentration is not less than 1.5 times the blank recalcification time, and that obtained with the highest concentration is such as to give a satisfactory log dose-response curve, as determined in a preliminary test.

Place twelve tubes in a bath of iced water, labelling them in duplicate: T1, T2 and T3 for the dilutions of the preparation being examined and S1, S2 and S3 for the dilutions of the reference preparation. To each tube add 1.0 ml of thawed *plasma substrate R1* and 1.0 ml of the appropriate dilution of the preparation being examined or the reference preparation. After each addition, mix but do not allow bubbles to form. Treating the tubes in the order S1, S2, S3, T1, T2, T3, transfer each tube to a water-bath at 37°, allow to equilibrate at 37° for about 15 minutes and add to each tube 1 ml of a dilution of *cephalin reagent* to which has been added an appropriate activator such as kaolin so that a suitable blank recalcification time not exceeding 60 seconds is obtained. When kaolin is used, prepare just before use, a mixture of equal volumes of *cephalin reagent* and a 4 g/l suspension of *light kaolin* in a 9 g/l solution of *sodium chloride*. After exactly 2 min add 1 ml of a 3.7 g/l solution of *calcium chloride* and record as the clotting time the interval in seconds between this last addition and the onset of clotting determined by the chosen technique. Determine the blank recalcification time at the beginning and at the end of the procedure in a similar manner, using 1 ml of a 9 g/l solution of *sodium chloride* R in place of one of the heparin dilutions; the two blank values obtained should not differ significantly. Transform the clotting times to logarithms, using the mean value for the duplicate tubes. Repeat the procedure using fresh dilutions and carrying out the incubation in the order T1, T2, T3, S1, S2, S3. Calculate the results by the usual statistical methods.

Carry out not fewer than three independent assays. For each such assay prepare fresh solutions of the reference preparation and the preparation being examined and use another, freshly thawed portion of plasma substrate.

Calculate the potency of the preparation being examined by combining the results of these assays by the usual statistical methods. When the variance due to differences between assays is significant at $P = 0.01$ a combined estimate of potency may be obtained by calculating the non-weighted mean of potency estimates.

6. TEST FOR FC FUNCTION OF IMMUNOGLOBULIN

(Ph. Eur. method 2.7.9)

Stabilised human blood Collect group O human red blood into ACD anticoagulant solution. Store the stabilised blood at 4° for not more than 3 weeks.

Phosphate buffered saline pH 7.2 Dissolve 1.022 g of *anhydrous disodium hydrogen orthophosphate*, 0.336 g of *anhydrous sodium dihydrogen orthophosphate* and 8.766 g of *sodium chloride* in 800 ml of *water* and dilute to 1000 ml with the same solvent.

Magnesium and calcium stock solution Dissolve 1.103 g of *calcium chloride* and 5.083 g of *magnesium chloride* in *water* and dilute to 25 ml with the same solvent.

Barbital buffer stock solution Dissolve 207.5 g of *sodium chloride* and 25.48 g of *barbitone sodium* in 4000 ml of *water* and adjust to pH 7.3 using 1M *hydrochloric acid.* Add 12.5 ml of *magnesium and calcium stock solution* and dilute to 5000 ml with water. Filter through a membrane filter (pore size 0.22 µm). Store at 4° in glass containers.

Albumin barbital buffer solution Dissolve 0.150 g *of bovine albumin* in 20 ml of *barbital buffer stock solution* and dilute to 100 ml with *water.*

Tannic acid solution Dissolve 10 mg of tannic acid in 100 ml of *phosphate-buffered saline pH 7.2.* Prepare immediately before use.

Guinea-pig complement Prepare a pool of serum from the blood of not fewer than 10 guinea-pigs. Separate the serum from the clotted blood by centrifugation at about 4°. Store the serum in small amounts below –70 °C. Immediately before starting complement-initiated haemolysis, dilute to 125 to 200 CH_{50} per millilitre with *albumin barbital buffer solution* and store in an ice-bath during the test.

Rubella antigen Suitable rubella antigen for haemagglutination-inhibition titre (HIT). Titre >256 HA units.

PREPARATION OF TANNED HUMAN RED BLOOD CELLS Separate human red blood cells by centrifuging an appropriate volume of stabilised human blood and wash the cells at least three times with *phosphate-buffered saline pH 7.2* and suspend at 2 per cent v/v in *phosphate-buffered saline pH 7.2.* Dilute 0.1 ml of *tannic acid solution* to 7.5 ml with *phosphate-buffered saline pH 7.2* (final concentration 1.3 mg/l). Mix 1 volume of the freshly prepared dilution with 1 volume of human red blood cell suspension and incubate at 37° for 10 minutes. Collect the cells by centrifugation (400 to 800*g* for 10 minutes), discard the supernatant and wash the cells once *with phosphate-buffered saline pH 7.2.* Resuspend the tanned cells at 1 per cent v/v in *phosphate-buffered saline pH 7.2.*

ANTIGEN COATING OF TANNED HUMAN RED BLOOD CELLS Take a suitable volume (V_s) of tanned cells, add 0.2 ml of *rubella antigen* per 1.0 ml of tanned cells and incubate at

37° for 30 minutes. Collect the cells by centrifugation (400 to 800*g* for 10 minutes) and discard the supernatant, leaving a volume of 200 µl. Add a volume of *albumin barbital buffer solution* equivalent to the discarded supernatant, resuspend and collect the cells as described and repeat the washing procedure. Make up the remaining 200 µl to three-quarters of V_s, thereby obtaining the initial volume (V_i). Mix 900 µl of *albumin barbital buffer solution* with 100 µl of V_i, which is thereby reduced to the residual volume (V_r), and determine the initial absorbance at 541 nm (A). Dilute V_r by a factor equal to A using *albumin barbital buffer solution*, thereby obtaining the final adjusted volume $V_f = V_r \times A$ of sensitised human red blood cells and adjusting A to 1.0 ± 0.1 for a tenfold dilution.

ANTIBODY BINDING OF ANTIGEN-COATED TANNED HUMAN RED BLOOD CELLS Prepare the following solutions in succession and in duplicate, using for each solution a separate half-micro cuvette (for example, disposable type) or test-tube:

(1) *Test solutions* If necessary, adjust the immunoglobulin being examined to pH 7, for example by addition of 1 M *sodium hydroxide.* Dilute volumes of the preparation being examined containing 30 mg and 40 mg of immunoglobulin with albumin barbital buffer solution and adjust the volume to 900 ml.

(2) *Reference solutions* Prepare as for the test solutions using *human immunoglobulin BRP.*

(3) *Complement control* 900 ml of *albumin barbital buffer solution.*

Add to each cuvette/test-tube 100 ml of sensitised human red blood cells and mix well.

Incubate at room temperature for 15 minutes, add 1000 µl of *albumin barbital buffer solution,* collect the cells by centrifugation (1000 *g* for 10 minutes) of the cuvette/test-tube and remove 1900 µl of the supernatant. Replace the 1900 µl with *albumin barbital buffer solution* and repeat the whole of the washing procedure, finally leaving a volume of 200 µl. Test samples may be stored in sealed cuvette/test-tubes at 4° for 24 hours.

COMPLEMENT-INITIATED HAEMOLYSIS. To measure haemolysis, add 600 µl of albumin barbital buffer solution warmed to 37° to the test sample, resuspend the cells carefully by repeated pipetting (not fewer than five times) and place the cuvette in the thermostatted cuvette holder of a spectrophotometer. After 2 minutes, add 200 µl of diluted guinea-pig complement (125 to 200 CH_{50}/ml), mix thoroughly by pipetting twice and start immediately after the second pipetting the time-dependent recording of absorbance at 541 nm, using *albumin barbital buffer solution* as the compensation liquid. Stop the measurement if absorbance as a function of time has clearly passed the inflexion point.

EVALUATION Determine the slope (S) of the haemolysis curve at the approximate inflexion point by segmenting the steepest section in suitable time intervals Δt (for example, Δt = 1 minute) and calculate S between adjacent intersection points, expressed as ΔA per minute. The largest value for S serves as (S_{exp}). In addition, determine the absorbance at the start of measurement (A_s) by extrapolating the curve, which is almost linear and parallel to the time axis within the first few minutes. Correct (S_{exp}) using the expression $S' = S_{exp}/A_s$

Calculate the arithmetic mean of the values of S' for each preparation. Calculate the index of Fc function (I_{Fc}) from the expression:

$$I_{Fc} = \frac{100 \times (\overline{S'} - \overline{S'_c})}{\overline{S'_S} - \overline{S'_c}}$$

where $\overline{S'}$ = arithmetic mean of the corrected slope for the preparation being examined,

$\overline{S'_s}$ = arithmetic mean of the corrected slope for the reference preparation,

$\overline{S'_c}$ = arithmetic mean of the corrected slope for the complement control.

Calculate the index of Fc function for the preparation being examined: the value is not less than that stated in the leaflet accompanying the reference preparation.

7. ANTI-A AND ANTI-B HAEMAGGLUTININS

(Ph. Eur. method 2.6.20)

Prepare in duplicate serial dilutions of the preparation being examined in a 9 g/l solution of *sodium chloride.* To each dilution of one series add an equal volume of a 5% v/v suspension of group A1 red blood cells previously washed three times with the sodium chloride solution. To each dilution of the other series add an equal volume of a 5% v/v suspension of group B red blood cells previously washed three times with the sodium chloride solution. Incubate the suspensions at 37° for 30 minutes then wash the cells three times with the sodium chloride solution. Leave the cells in contact with a polyvalent anti-human globulin reagent for 30 minutes. Without centrifuging, examine each suspension for agglutination under a microscope.

8. TEST FOR PREKALLIKREIN ACTIVATOR

Prekallikrein activator (PKA) activates prekallikrein to kallikrein and may be assayed by its ability to cleave a chromophore from a synthetic peptide substrate so that the rate of cleavage can be measured spectrophotometrically and the concentration of PKA calculated by comparison with a standard preparation calibrated in Units.

Standard Preparation

The Standard Preparation is the 1st International Standard for Prekallikrein activator, established in 1984 consisting of prekallikrein activator in human serum albumin (supplied in ampoules containing 85 Units) or another suitable preparation the potency of which has been determined in relation to the International Standard.

Method

PREPARATION OF PREKALLIKREIN SUBSTRATE *To avoid coagulation activation, blood or plasma used for the preparation of prekallikrein must come into contact only with plastics or silicone-treated glass surfaces.*

Draw 9 volumes of human blood into 1 volume of anticoagulant solution (ACD, CPD or 3.8% w/v *sodium citrate*) to which 1 mg per ml of *hexadimethrine bromide* has been added. Centrifuge the mixture at 3600 *g* for 5 minutes. Separate the plasma and centrifuge again at 6000 *g* for 20 minutes to sediment platelets. Separate the platelet-poor plasma and dialyse against 10 volumes of buffer A for 20 hours. Apply the dialysed plasma to a chromatography column containing *agarose-DEAE for ion exchange chromatography* which has been equilibrated in *buffer A* and is equal to twice the volume of the plasma. Elute from the column with *buffer A* at about 20 ml per cm^2 per hour. Collect the eluate in fractions and record the *absorbance* at 280 nm, Appendix II B. Pool the fractions containing the first protein peak so that the volume of the pool is about 1.2 times the volume of the platelet-poor plasma.

Test the substrate pool for absence of kallikrein activity by mixing 1 part with 20 parts of the pre-warmed chromogenic substrate solution to be used in the assay and incubate at 37° for 2 minutes. The substrate is suitable if the increase in absorption is less than 0.001 per minute. Add to the pooled solution 7 g per litre of *sodium chloride* and filter using a membrane filter (porosity 0.45 µm). Freeze the filtrate in portions and store at –25°; the substrate may be freeze-dried.

Carry out all procedures from the beginning of the chromatography to freezing in portions during a single working day.

DETERMINATION OF ACTIVATOR

The determination is preferably carried out using an automated enzyme analyser at 37°, with volumes, concentration of substrates and incubation times adjusted so that the reaction rate is linear at least up to 35 Units per ml. Standards, samples and prekallikrein substrate may be diluted as necessary using *buffer B*.

Incubate diluted standards or samples with prekallikrein substrate for 10 minutes such that the volume of the undiluted simple does not exceed 1/10 of the total volume of the incubation mixture to avoid errors caused by variation in ionic strength and pH in the incubation mixture. Incubate the mixture or a part thereof with at least an equal volume of a solution of a suitable synthetic chromogenic substrate, known to be specific for kallikrein (for example, *N-benzoyl-L-prolyl-L-phenylalanyl-L-arginine-4-nitroanilide acetate* or *D-prolyl-L-phenylalanyl-L-arginine 4-nitroanilide dihydrochloride*), dissolved in *buffer B*. Record the rate of change in absorbance per minute for 2 minutes to 10 minutes at the wavelength specific for the substrate used. Prepare a blank for each mixture of sample or standard using buffer B instead of prekallikrein substrate.

Correct ΔA per minute by subtracting the value obtained for the corresponding blank. Plot a calibration curve using the values thus obtained for the reference preparation and the respective concentrations. Use the curve to determine the PKA activity of the preparation being examined.

Buffer A

Tris(hydroxymethyl)methylamine	6.055 g
Sodium chloride	1.17 g
Hexadimethrine bromide	50 mg
Sodium azide	0.100 g

Dissolve the ingredients in *water*, adjust to pH 8.0 with 2M *hydrochloric acid* and dilute to 1000 ml with *water*.

Buffer B

Tris(hydroxymethyl)methylamine	6.055 g
Sodium chloride	8.77 g

Dissolve the ingredients in *water*, adjust to pH 8.0 with 2M *hydrochloric acid* and dilute to 1000 ml with *water*.

9. TEST FOR ANTICOMPLEMENTARY ACTIVITY OF IMMUNOGLOBULIN

(Ph. Eur. method 2.6.17)

For the measurement of anticomplementary activity (ACA) of immunoglobulin. a defined amount of test material (10 mg of immunoglobulin) is incubated with a defined amount of guinea pig complement (20 CH_{50}) and the remaining complement is titrated; the anticomplementary activity is expressed as the percentage consumption of complement relative to the complement control as 100%.

The haemolytic unit of complement activity (CH_{50}) is the amount of complement that, in the given reaction conditions, will produce the lysis of 2.5×10^8 out of a total of 5×10^8 optimally sensitised red blood cells.

Magnesium and calcium stock solution Dissolve 1.103 g of *calcium chloride* and 5.083 g of *magnesium chloride* in *distilled water* and dilute to 25 ml with the same solvent.

TABLE 14J-3

Required dilution of haemolysin	Prepared using		
	Gelatin barbital buffer solution	*Haemolysin*	
	volume ml	Dilution (1:...)	volume ml
7.5	0.65	undiluted	0.1
10	0.90	undiluted	0.1
75	1.80	7.5	0.2
100	1.80	10	0.2
150	1.0	75	1.
200	1.00	100	1.0
300	1.00	150	1.0
400	1.00	200	1.0
600	1.00	300	1.0
800	1.00	400	1.0
1200	1.00	600	1.0
1600	1.00	800	1.0
2400	1.00	1200	1.0
3200	1.00	1600	1.0*
4800	1.00	2400	1.0*

Barbitone buffer stock solution Dissolve 207.5 g of *sodium chloride* and 25.48 g of *barbitone sodium* in 4000 ml of *water* and adjust to pH 7.3 using 1M *hydrochloric acid.* Add 12.5 ml of *magnesium and calcium stock solution* and dilute to 5000 ml with *water*. Filter through a membrane filter (pore size 0.22 µm). Store at 4° in glass containers.

Gelatin solution Dissolve 12.5 g of *gelatin* in about 800 ml of *water* and heat to boiling in a water bath. Cool to 20° and dilute to 10 litres with *water*. Filter through a membrane filter (pore size 0.22 µm). Store at 4°. Use clear solutions only.

Citrate solution Dissolve 8.0 g of *sodium citrate*, 4.2 g of *sodium chloride* and 20.5 g of *glucose* in 750 ml of *water*. Adjust to pH 6.1 using a 10% w/v solution of *citric acid* and dilute to 1000 ml with *water*.

Gelatin barbitone buffer solution Add 4 volumes of *gelatin solution* to 1 volume of *barbitone buffer stock solution* and mix. Adjust to pH 7.3, if necessary, using 1M *sodium hydroxide* or 1M hydro*chloric acid.* Maintain at 4°. Prepare fresh solution daily.

Stabilised sheep blood Collect one volume of sheep blood into one volume of *citrate solution* and mix. Store at 4° for not less than 7 days and not more than 28 days. (Stabilised sheep blood or sheep red blood cells are available from a number of commercial sources.)

Haemolysin Antiserum against sheep red blood cells prepared in rabbits. (Such antisera are available from a number of commercial sources.)

Guinea-pig complement Prepare a pool of serum from the blood of not fewer than 10 guinea pigs. Separate the serum from the clotted blood by centrifugation at about 4°. Store the serum in small amounts below –70°. It may also be stored after freeze drying. Suitable guinea pig complement has an activity of not less than 200 CH_{50} per ml. (Freeze dried guinea pig complement is available from a number of commercial sources.)

Method

PREPARATION OF STANDARDISED 5% SHEEP RED BLOOD CELL SUSPENSION Separate sheep red blood cells by centrifuging an appropriate volume of *stabilised sheep blood* and wash the cells at least three times with *gelatin barbitone buffer solution* and prepare as a 5% v/v suspension in the same solution. Measure the cell density of the suspension as follows. Add 0.2 ml to 2.8 ml of *water* and centrifuge the lysed solution for 5 minutes at 1000 *g*; the cell density is suitable if the *absorbance*, Appendix II B, of the supernatant liquid at 541 nm is 0.62±0.01. Correct the cell density by adding *gelatin barbitone buffer solution* according to the formula:

$$V_f = \frac{V_i \times A}{0.62}$$

where V_f = final adjusted volume,
V_i = the initial volume,
A = absorbance of the original suspension at 541 nm.

The adjusted suspension contains about 1×10^9 cells per ml.

HAEMOLYSIN TITRATION Prepare haemolysin dilutions as shown in Table 14J-3.

Add 1.0 ml of the standardised 5% sheep red blood cell suspension to each tube of the haemolysin dilution series, starting at the 1:75 dilution, and mix. Incubate at 37° for 30 minutes.

Transfer 0.2 ml of each of these incubated mixtures to new tubes and add 1.10 ml of *gelatin barbitone buffer solution* and 0.2 ml of diluted *guinea-pig complement* (for example, 1:150). Perform this in duplicate.

As the unhaemolysed cell control, prepare three tubes with 1.4 ml of *gelatin barbitone buffer solution* and 0.1 ml of the standardised 5% sheep red blood cell suspension.

As the fully haemolysed control, prepare three tubes with 1.4 ml of *water* and 0.1 ml of the standardised 5% sheep red blood cell suspension.

Incubate all tubes at 37° for 60 minutes and centrifuge at 1000 *g* for 5 minutes. Measure the *absorbance*, Appendix II B, of the supernatants at 541 nm and calculate the percentage degree of haemolysis in each tube using the expression:

$$\frac{A_a - A_1}{A_b - A_1} \times 100$$

where A_a = absorbance of tubes with haemolysin dilution.
A_b = mean absorbance of the three tubes with full haemolysis,
A_1 = mean absorbance of the three tubes with no haemolysis

TABLE 14J-4

Tube No.	Volume of diluted complement (for example 1: 250) ml	Volume of *gelatin barbital buffer solution* ml
1	0.1	1.2
2	0.2	1.1
3	0.3	1.0
4	0.4	0.9
5	0.5	0.8
6	0.6	0.7
7	0.7	0.6
8	0.8	0.5
9	0.9	0.4
10	1.0	0.3
11	1.1	0.2
12	1.2	0.1
Three tubes as cell control at 0% haemolysis	—	1.3
Three tubes at 100% haemolysis	—	1.3 (*water*)

Plot the percentage degree of haemolysis (Y) as the ordinate against the corresponding reciprocal value of the haemolysin dilution as the abscissa on linear graph paper. Determine the optimal dilution of the haemolysin from the graph by inspection. Select a dilution such that further increase in the amount of haemolysin does not cause appreciable change in the degree of haemolysis. This dilution is defined as one minimal haemolytic unit (1 MHU) in 1.0 ml. The optimal haemolytic haemolysin dilution for preparation of sensitised sheep red blood cells contains 2 MHU per ml.

The haemolysin titration is not valid unless the maximum degree of haemolysis is 50 to 70%. If the maximum degree of haemolysis is not in this range, repeat the titration with more or less diluted complement solution.

PREPARATION OF OPTIMISED SENSITISED SHEEP RED BLOOD CELLS (HAEMOLYTIC SYSTEM) Prepare an appropriate volume of diluted haemolysin containing 2 MHU per ml and an equal volume of the standardised 5% sheep red blood cell suspension. Add the haemolysin dilution to the standardised cell suspension and mix. Incubate at 37° for 15 minutes, store at 2° to 8° and use within 6 hours.

TITRATION OF COMPLEMENT Prepare an appropriate dilution of complement (for example, 1:250) with *gelatin barbitone buffer solution* and perform the titration in duplicate as shown in Table 14J-4.

Add 0.2 ml of the optimised sensitised sheep red blood cells to each tube, mix well and incubate at 37° for 60 minutes. Cool the tubes in an ice bath and centrifuge at 1000 *g* for 5 minutes. Measure the absorbance of the supernatant liquid at 541 nm and calculate the degree of haemolysis using the expression:

$$\frac{A_c - A_1}{A_b - A_1}$$

where A_c = absorbance of tubes 1 to 12,

A_b = mean absorbance of tubes with 100% haemolysis,

A_l = mean absorbance of cell controls with 0% haemolysis.

Plot $Y/(1 - Y)$ as the ordinate against the amount of complement in ml on log—log graph paper. Fit the best line to the points and read the 50% haemolytic complement dose at the intersection of this line with the ordinate, *ie* where $Y/(1 - Y) = 1.0$. Calculate the activity in haemolytic units (CH_{50} per ml) from the expression $C_d/(C_a \times 5)$ where C_d is the reciprocal value of the complement dilution, C_a is the volume of complement in millilitres resulting in 50% haemolysis, and 5 is the scaling factor.

The test is not valid unless the plot is a straight line between 15% and 85% haemolysis and the slope is 0.18 to 0.30.

TEST FOR ANTICOMPLEMENTARY ACTIVITY Prepare a complement dilution having 100 CH_{50} per ml by diluting titrated *guinea-pig complement* with *gelatin barbitone buffer solution.* If necessary, adjust the immunoglobulin being examined to pH 7. Prepare incubation mixtures as shown in Table 14J-5 for an immunoglobulin containing 50 mg per ml:

TABLE 14J-5

	Immunoglobulin to be examined ml	Complement control (in duplicate) ml
Immunoglobulin (50 mg/ml)	0.2	—
Gelatin barbitone buffer solution	0.6	0.8
Complement	0.2	0.2

Carry out the test in parallel on the immunoglobulin being examined and on *immunoglobulin (ACA negative control) EPBRP* and *immunoglobulin (ACA positive control) EPBRP.* Higher or lower volumes of sample and of *gelatin barbitone buffer solution* are added if the immunoglobulin concentration varies from 50 mg per ml; for example, 0.47 ml of *gelatin barbitone buffer solution* is added to 0.33 ml of immunoglobulin containing 30 mg per ml to give 0.8 ml. Close the tubes and incubate at 37° for 60 minutes. Add 0.2 ml of each incubation mixture to 9.8 ml of *gelatin barbitone buffer solution* to dilute the complement. Perform complement titrations as described above on each tube to determine the remaining complement activity (see Table II). Calculate the anticomplementary activity of the preparation being examined relative to the complement control considered as 100%, from the expression $a - b/100a$ where a is the mean complement activity (CH_{50} per ml) of complement control and b is the complement activity (CH_{50} per ml) of tested sample.

The test is not valid unless the anticomplementary activities found for *immunoglobulin (ACA negative control) EPBRP* and *immunoglobulin (ACA positive control) EPBRP* are within the limits stated in the leaflet accompanying the reference preparation and the complement activity of the complement control (a) is in the range 80 to 120 CH_{50} per ml.

K. Immunological Products

1. ASSAY OF ADSORBED DIPHTHERIA VACCINE

(Ph. Eur. method 2.7.6 An alternative method in which the potency is determined by comparing the dose necessary to protect guinea-pigs against the lethal effect of a subcutaneous injection of diphtheria toxin with the dose of a reference preparation calibrated in International Units necessary to give the same protection is also described in the European Pharmacopoeia.)

The potency of adsorbed diphtheria vaccine is determined by comparing the dose of the vaccine required to protect guinea-pigs from the effects of an erythrogenic dose of diphtheria toxin administered intradermally with the dose of a reference preparation, calibrated in International Units, needed to give the same protection.

The International Unit is the activity contained in a stated amount of the International Standard which consists of a quantity of diphtheria toxoid adsorbed on aluminium hydroxide. The equivalence in International Units of the International Standard is stated by the World Health Organization.

Method of intradermal challenge

SELECTION AND DISTRIBUTION OF THE TEST ANIMALS Use in the test, healthy, white guinea-pigs from the same stock and of a size suitable for the prescribed number of challenge sites, the difference in body mass between the heaviest and the lightest animal being not greater than 100 g. Distribute the guinea-pigs in not fewer than six equal groups; use groups containing a number of animals sufficient to obtain results that fulfil the requirements for a valid assay prescribed below. If the challenge toxin to be used has not been shown to be stable or has not been adequately standardised, include five guinea-pigs as unvaccinated controls. Use guinea-pigs of the same sex or with males and females equally distributed between the groups.

SELECTION OF THE CHALLENGE TOXIN Select a preparation of diphtheria toxin containing 67 to 133 lr/100 in 1 Lf and 25,000 to 50,000 minimal reacting doses for guinea-pig skin in 1 Lf. If the challenge toxin preparation has been shown to be stable, it is not necessary to verify the activity for every assay.

PREPARATION OF THE CHALLENGE TOXIN SOLUTION Immediately before use, dilute the challenge toxin with a suitable diluent to obtain a challenge toxin solution containing about 0.0512 Lf in 0.2 ml. Prepare from this a further series of five four-fold dilutions containing about 0.0128, 0.0032, 0.0008, 0.0002 and 0.00005 Lf in 0.2 ml.

DETERMINATION OF POTENCY OF THE VACCINE Using a 9 g/l solution of *sodium chloride*, prepare dilutions of the vaccine being examined and of the reference preparation, such that for each, the dilutions form a series differing by not more than 2.5-fold steps and in which the intermediate dilutions, when injected subcutaneously at a dose of 1.0 ml per guinea-pig, will result in an intradermal score of approximately three when the animals are challenged. Allocate the dilutions one to each of the groups of guinea-pigs and inject subcutaneously 1.0 ml of each dilution into each guinea-pig in the group to which that dilution is allocated. After 28 days, shave both flanks of each guinea-pig and inject 0.2 ml of each of the six toxin dilutions intradermally into six separate sites on each of the vaccinated guinea-pigs in such a way as to minimise interference between adjacent sites.

DETERMINATION OF THE ACTIVITY OF THE CHALLENGE TOXIN If necessary, inject the unvaccinated control animals with dilutions containing 8×10^{-5}, 4×10^{-5}, 2×10^{-5}, 1×10^{-5} and 5×10^{-6} Lf of the challenge toxin.

READING AND INTERPRETATION OF RESULTS Examine all injection sites 48 hours after injection of the challenge toxin and record the incidence of specific diphtheria erythema. Record also the number of sites free from such reactions as the intra-dermal challenge score. Tabulate together the intradermal challenge scores for all the animals receiving the same dilution of vaccine and use those data with a suitable transformation, such as $(\text{score})^2$ or $\arcsin[(\text{score}/6)^2]$, to obtain an estimate of the relative potency for each of the test preparations by parallel-line quantitative analysis.

REQUIREMENTS FOR A VALID ASSAY The test is not valid unless:

- for both the vaccine being examined and the reference preparation, the mean score obtained at the lowest dose level is less than three and the mean score at the highest dose level is more than three,
- if applicable, the toxin dilution that contains 4×10^{-5} Lf gives a positive erythema in at least 80% of the control guinea-pigs and the dilution containing 2×10^{-5} Lf gives no reaction in at least 80% of the guinea-pigs (if these criteria are not met a different toxin has to be selected),
- the fiducial limits of the assay (P = 0.95) fall between 50 per cent and 200 per cent of the estimated potency,
- the statistical analysis shows no deviation from linearity and parallelism.

The test may be repeated but when more than one test is performed the results of all valid tests must be combined in the estimate of potency.

2. ASSAY OF PERTUSSIS VACCINE

(Ph. Eur. method 2.7.7)

The potency of pertussis vaccine is determined by comparing the dose necessary to protect mice against the effects of a lethal dose of *Bordetella pertussis*, administered intracerebrally, with the quantity of a reference preparation, calibrated in International Units, needed to give the same protection.

The International Unit is the activity contained in a stated amount of the International Standard which consists of a quantity of dried pertussis vaccine. The equivalence in International Units of the International Standard is stated by the World Health Organization.

SELECTION AND DISTRIBUTION OF THE TEST ANIMALS Use in the test, healthy mice less than 5 weeks old of a suitable strain from the same stock, the difference in weight between the heaviest and the lightest being not greater than 5 g. Distribute the mice in six groups of not fewer than 16 and four groups of 10. The mice must all be of the same sex or the males and females should be distributed equally between the groups.

SELECTION OF THE CHALLENGE STRAIN AND PREPARATION OF THE CHALLENGE SUSPENSION Select a suitable strain of *B. pertussis* capable of causing the death of mice within 14 days of intracerebral injection. If more than 20% of the mice die within 48 hours of the injection the strain is not suitable. Make one subculture from the strain and suspend the *harvested B. pertussis* in a solution containing 10 g/l of *casein hydrolysate* and 6 g/l of *sodium chloride* and having a pH of 7.0 to 7.2 or in another suitable solution. Determine the opacity of the suspension. Prepare a series of dilutions in the same solution and allocate each dilution to a group of 10 mice. Inject intracerebrally into each mouse a dose (0.02 ml or 0.03 ml) of the dilution allocated to its group. After 14 days, count the number of mice surviving in each group. From the results, calculate the expected opacity of a suspension containing 100 LD_{50} in each challenge dose. For the test of the vaccine being examined make a fresh subculture from the same strain of *B. pertussis* and prepare a suspension of the harvested organisms with an opacity corresponding to about 100 LD_{50} in each challenge dose. Prepare three dilutions of the challenge suspension.

DETERMINATION OF POTENCY Prepare three serial dilutions of the vaccine being examined and three similar dilutions of the reference preparation such that in each the intermediate dilution may be expected to protect about 50% of the mice from the lethal effects of the challenge dose of *B. pertussis*. Suggested doses are 1/8, 1/40 and 1/200 of the human dose of the vaccine being examined and 0.5 IU, 0.1 IU and 0.02 IU of the reference preparation, each dose being contained in a volume not exceeding 0.5 ml. Allocate six dilutions one to each of the groups of not fewer than 16 mice and inject intraperitoneally into each mouse one dose of the dilution allocated to its group. After 14 to 17 days inject intracerebrally into each animal in the groups of not fewer than 16, one dose of the challenge suspension. Allocate the challenge suspension and the three dilutions made from it one to each of the groups of ten mice and inject intracerebrally one dose of each suspension into each mouse in the group to which that suspension is allocated. Exclude from consideration any mice that die within 48 hours of challenge. Count the number of mice surviving in each of the groups after 14 days. Calculate the potency of the vaccine being examined relative to the potency of the reference preparation on the basis of the numbers of animals surviving in each of the groups of not fewer than 16.

The test is not valid unless:

- for both the vaccine being examined and the reference preparation, the 50% protective dose lies between the largest and the smallest doses given to the mice;
- the number of animals which die in the four groups of 10 injected with the challenge suspension and its dilutions indicates that the challenge dose is approximately 100 LD_{50};
- and the statistical analysis shows no deviation from linearity or parallelism.

The test may be repeated but when more than one test is performed the results of all valid tests must be combined.

3. ASSAY OF ADSORBED TETANUS VACCINE

(Ph. Eur method 2.7.8. The European Pharmacopoeia text states 'In countries where the paralysis method is not obligatory the LD_{50} method may be used. For the LD_{50} method, the number of animals and the procedure are identical with those described for the paralysis method but the end-point is the death of the animal rather than paralysis.')

The potency of adsorbed tetanus vaccine is determined by comparing the dose of the vaccine required to protect guinea-pigs or mice from the effects of a subcutaneous injection of a paralytic dose of tetanus toxin with the dose of a reference preparation, calibrated in International Units, needed to give the same protection.

The International Unit is the activity contained in a stated amount of the International Standard which consists of a quantity of tetanus toxoid adsorbed on aluminium hydroxide.. The equivalence in International Units of the International Standard is stated by the World Health Organization

Test in guinea-pigs

SELECTION AND DISTRIBUTION OF THE TEST ANIMALS Use in the test healthy guinea-pigs from the same stock, each weighing 250 g to 350 g. Distribute the guinea-pigs in not fewer than six equal groups; use groups containing a number of animals sufficient to obtain results that fulfil the requirements for a valid assay prescribed below. If the challenge toxin to be used has not been shown to be stable or has not been adequately standardised, include four further groups of five guinea-pigs as unvaccinated controls. Use guinea-pigs of the same sex or with the males and females equally distributed between the groups.

SELECTION OF THE CHALLENGE TOXIN Select a preparation of tetanus toxin containing not less than fifty times the 50% paralytic dose per ml. If the challenge toxin preparation has been shown to be stable, it is not necessary to verify the paralytic dose for every assay.

PREPARATION OF THE CHALLENGE TOXIN SOLUTION Immediately before use, dilute the challenge toxin with a suitable diluent to obtain a challenge toxin solution containing approximately fifty times the 50% paralytic dose per ml. If necessary, dilute portions of the challenge toxin solution 1 in 16, 1 in 50 and 1 in 160 with the same diluent.

DETERMINATION OF POTENCY OF THE VACCINE Using a 9 g/l solution of *sodium chloride*, prepare dilutions of the vaccine being examined and of the reference preparation, such that for each, the dilutions form a series differing by not more than 2.5-fold steps and in which the intermediate dilutions, when injected subcutaneously at a dose of 1.0 ml per guinea-pig, protect approximately 50% of the animals from the paralytic effects of the subcutaneous injection of the quantity of tetanus toxin prescribed for this test. Allocate the dilutions one to each of the groups of guinea-pigs and inject subcutaneously 1.0 ml of each dilution into each guinea-pig in the group to which that dilution is allocated. After 28 days, inject subcutaneously into each animal 1.0 ml of the challenge toxin solution (containing fifty times the 50% paralytic dose).

DETERMINATION OF THE ACTIVITY OF THE CHALLENGE TOXIN If necessary, allocate the challenge toxin solution and the three dilutions made from it, one to each of the four groups of five guinea-pigs, and inject subcutaneously 1.0 ml of each solution into each guinea-pig in the group to which that solution is allocated.

READING AND INTERPRETATION OF RESULTS Examine the guinea-pigs twice daily, remove and humanely kill all animals showing definite signs of tetanus paralysis. Count the number of guinea-pigs without paralysis five days after injection of the challenge toxin. Calculate the potency of the vaccine being examined relative to the potency of the reference preparation on the basis of the proportion of challenged animals without paralysis in each of the groups of vaccinated guinea-pigs, using the usual statistical methods.

REQUIREMENTS FOR A VALID ASSAY. The test is not valid unless:

— for both the vaccine being examined and the reference preparation the 50% protective dose lies between the largest and smallest doses of the preparations given to the guinea-pigs,
— if applicable, the number of paralysed animals in the four groups of five injected with the challenge toxin solution and its dilutions indicates that the challenge was approximately fifty times the 50% paralytic dose,
— the fiducial limits of the assay (P = 0.95) fall between 50% and 200% of the estimated potency,
— the statistical analysis shows no deviation from linearity and parallelism.

The test may be repeated but when more than one test is performed the results of all valid tests must be combined in the estimate of potency.

Test in mice

SELECTION AND DISTRIBUTION OF THE TEST ANIMALS Use in the test healthy mice from the same stock, each weighing 14 g to 20 g. Distribute the mice in not fewer than six equal groups; use groups containing a number of animals sufficient to obtain results that fulfil the requirements for a valid assay prescribed below. If the challenge toxin to be used has not been shown to be stable or has not been adequately standardised, include four groups of six mice to serve as unvaccinated controls. Use mice of the same sex or with males and females equally distributed between the groups.

SELECTION OF THE CHALLENGE TOXIN Select a preparation of tetanus toxin containing not less than one hundred times the 50% paralytic dose per ml. If the challenge toxin preparation has been shown to be stable, it is not necessary to verify the paralytic dose for every assay.

PREPARATION OF THE CHALLENGE TOXIN SOLUTION Immediately before use, dilute the challenge toxin with a suitable diluent to obtain a challenge toxin solution containing approximately fifty times the 50% paralytic dose in 0.5 ml. If necessary, dilute portions of the challenge toxin solution 1 in 16, 1 in 50 and 1 in 160 with the same diluent.

Appendix XV

Production and Testing of Vaccines

A. Terminology Used in Monographs on Vaccines and Certain Other Products

(Ph. Eur. general text 5.2.1)

For some items, alternative terms commonly used in connection with vaccines for veterinary use are shown in parenthesis.

Seed-lot system A seed-lot system is a system according to which successive batches of a product are derived from the same master seed lot. For routine production, a working seed lot may be prepared from the master seed lot. The origin and the passage history of the master seed lot and the working seed lot are recorded.

Master seed lot A culture of a micro-organism distributed from a single bulk into containers and processed together in a single operation in such a manner as to ensure uniformity and stability and to prevent contamination. A master seed lot in liquid form is usually stored at or below −70°. A freeze-dried master seed lot is stored at a temperature known to ensure stability.

Working seed lot A culture of a micro-organism derived from the master seed lot and intended for use in production. Working seed lots are distributed into containers and stored as described above for master seed lots.

Cell-bank system (Cell-seed system) A system whereby successive final lots (batches) of a product are manufactured by culture in cells derived from the same master cell bank (master cell seed). A number of containers from the master cell bank (master cell seed) are used to prepare a working cell bank (working cell seed). The cell-bank system (cell-seed system) is validated for the highest passage level achieved during routine production.

Master cell bank (Master cell seed) A culture of cells distributed into containers in a single operation, processed together and stored in such a manner as to ensure uniformity and stability and to prevent contamination. A master cell bank (master cell seed) is usually stored at −70° or lower.

Working cell bank (Working cell seed) A culture of cells derived from the master cell bank (master cell seed) and intended for use in the preparation of production cell cultures. The working cell bank (working cell seed) is distributed into containers, processed and stored as described for the master cell bank (master cell seed).

Primary cell cultures Cultures of cells obtained by trypsination of a suitable tissue or organ. The cells are essentially identical to those of the tissue of origin and are no more than five *in vitro* passages from the initial preparation from the animal tissue.

Cell lines Cultures of cells that have a high capacity for multiplication in *vitro*. In diploid cell lines, the cells have essentially the same characteristics as those of the tissue of origin. In continuous cell lines, the cells are able to multiply indefinitely in culture and may be obtained from healthy or tumoral tissue. Some continuous cell lines have oncogenic potential under certain conditions.

Production cell culture A culture of cells intended for use in production; it may be derived from one or more containers of the working cell bank (working cell seed) or it may be a primary cell culture.

Control cells A quantity of cells set aside, at the time of virus inoculation, as uninfected cell cultures. The uninfected cells are incubated under similar conditions to those used for the production cell cultures.

Single harvest Material derived on one or more occasions from a single production cell culture inoculated with the same working seed lot or a suspension derived from the working seed lot, incubated, and harvested in a single production run.

Monovalent pooled harvest Pooled material containing a single strain or type of micro-organism or antigen and derived from a number of eggs, cell culture containers etc. that are processed at the same time.

Final bulk vaccine Material that has undergone all the steps of production except for the final filling. It consists of one or more monovalent pooled harvests, from cultures of one or more species or types of micro-organism, after clarification, dilution or addition of any adjuvant or other auxiliary substance. It is treated to ensure its homogeneity and is used for filling the containers of one or more final lots (batches).

Final Lot (Batch) A collection of closed, final containers or other final dosage units that are expected to be homogeneous and equivalent with respect to risk of contamination during filling or preparation of the final product. The dosage units are filled, or otherwise prepared, from the same final bulk vaccine, freeze dried together (if applicable) and closed in one continuous working session. They bear a distinctive number or code identifying the final lot (batch). Where a final bulk vaccine is filled and/or freeze dried in several separate sessions, there results a related set of final lots (batches) that are usually identified by the use of a common part in the distinctive number or code; these related final lots (batches) are sometimes referred to as sub-lots, filling lots ot sub-batches.

Combined vaccine A multicomponent preparation formulated so that different antigens are administered simultaneously. The different antigenic components are intended to protect against different strains or types of the same organism and/or different organisms. A combined vaccine may be supplied by the manufacturer either as a single liquid or freeze-dried preparation or as several constituents with directions for admixture before use.

B. Aluminium in Adsorbed Vaccines

(Ph. Eur. method 2.5.13)

Homogenise the preparation being examined and transfer a suitable quantity, presumed to contain 5 to 6 mg of aluminium, to a 50-ml combustion flask. Add 1 ml of *sulphuric acid*, 0.1 ml of *nitric acid* and some glass beads. Heat the solution until thick, white fumes are evolved. If there is charring at this stage add a few more drops of *nitric acid* and continue boiling until the colour disappears. Allow to cool for a few minutes, carefully add 10 ml of *water* and boil until a clear solution is obtained. Allow to cool, add 0.05 ml of *methyl orange solution* and neutralise with *strong sodium hydroxide solution* (6.5 to 7 ml). If a precipitate forms dissolve it by adding, dropwise, sufficient dilute *sulphuric acid*. Transfer the solution to a 250-ml conical flask, rinsing the combustion flask with 25 ml of *water*. Add 25.0 ml of 0.02 M *disodium edetate VS*, 10 ml of *acetate buffer solution pH 4.4* and a few glass beads and boil gently for 3 minutes. Add 0.1 ml of *pyridylazonaphthol solution* and titrate the hot solution with 0.02 M *copper sulphate VS* until the colour changes to purplish-brown. Carry out a blank titration omitting the vaccine.

1 ml of 0.02 M *disodium edetate VS* is equivalent to 0.5396 mg of Al.

C. Calcium in Adsorbed Vaccines

(Ph. Eur. method 2.5.14)

All solutions used for this test must be prepared using *water*.

Determine the calcium by *atomic emission spectrometry*, Method I, Appendix II D. Homogenise the preparation being examined. To 1.0 ml add 0.2 ml of *dilute hydrochloric acid* and dilute to 3.0 ml with *water*. Measure the absorbance at 620 nm.

D. Free Formaldehyde

(Ph. Eur. method 2.4.18)

For vaccines containing formaldehyde, not more than 0.02% w/v of free formaldehyde. Use test A unless otherwise prescribed.

Test B is suitable for vaccines where sodium metabisulphite has been used to neutralise excess formaldehyde.

Test A.

To 1 ml of a 10-fold dilution of the vaccine in *water* add 4 ml of *water* and 5 ml of *acetylacetone reagent R1*. Warm in a water bath at 40° and allow to stand for 40 minutes. The solution is not more intensely coloured than a reference solution prepared at the same time and in the same manner using 1 ml of a solution containing 0.002% w/v of formaldehyde, CH_2O, in place of the dilution of the vaccine. The comparison should be made examining the tubes down their vertical axes.

Test B.

To 0.5 ml of a 100-fold dilution of the preparation being examined add 5 ml of a 0.05% w/v solution of *3-methylbenzothiazolin-2-one hydrazone hydrochloride* and 0.05 ml of *polysorbate 80*, close the tube, shake and allow to stand for 60 minutes. Add 1 ml of *iron(III) chloride—sulphamic acid solution* and allow to stand for 15 minutes (solution A). Prepare solution B in the same manner as for solution A but using 0.5 ml of *water* in place of the dilution of the preparation being examined. Measure the *absorbance* of solution A at 628 nm, Appendix II B, using solution B in the reference cell. The absorbance is not greater than that of a reference solution prepared at the same time and in the same manner using 0.5 ml of a solution containing 0.0005% w/v of formaldehyde, CH_2O, in place of the dilution of the preparation being examined.

If the preparation being examined is an emulsion, separate the aqueous phase by the following method. Add an equal volume of *isopropyl myristate* to the vaccine and mix. To 3 volumes of the mixture add 2 volumes of 1M *hydrochloric acid*, 3 volumes of *chloroform* and 4 volumes of a 0.9% w/v solution of *sodium chloride* and mix thoroughly. Centrifuge at 15,000 *g* for 60 minutes. Remove the aqueous phase and measure its volume. Use 0.5 ml of 100-fold dilution of the aqueous phase and carry out the procedure described above, adjusting the concentration of formaldehyde in the reference solution to allow for the dilution of the vaccine during the separation of the phases. If the procedure described fails to separate the aqueous phase, add 10% w/v of *polysorbate 20* to the sodium chloride solution and repeat the procedure but centrifuging at 22,500 *g*.

E. Phenol in Antisera (Immunosera) and Vaccines

(Ph. Eur. method 2.5.15)

Homogenise the preparation being examined. Dilute an appropriate volume with *water* so as to obtain a solution presumed to contain 15 µg of phenol per ml. Prepare a series of reference solutions with *phenol* containing 5 µg, 10 µg, 15 µg, 20 µg and 30 µg of phenol per millilitre respectively. To 5 ml of the solution being examined and to 5 ml of each of the reference solutions respectively, add 5 ml of *borate buffer pH 9.0*, 5 ml of *aminophenazone solution* and 5 ml of *potassium hexacyanoferrate (III) solution*. Allow to stand for 10 minutes and measure the intensity of colour at 546 nm.

Plot the calibration curve and calculate the phenol content of the preparation being examined.

F. Neurovirulence

1. TEST FOR NEUROVIRULENCE OF LIVE VIRAL VACCINES
(Ph. Eur. method 2.4.18)

For each test, use no fewer than 10 monkeys that are seronegative for the virus to be tested. For each monkey, inject not more than 0.5 ml of the material being examined into the thalamic region of each hemisphere, unless otherwise prescribed. The total amount of virus inoculated in each monkey must be not less than the amount contained in the recommended single dose of the vaccine. As a check against the introduction of wild neurovirulent virus, keep a group of no fewer than four control monkeys as cage-mates or in the immediate vicinity of the inoculated monkeys. Observe the inoculated monkeys for 17 to 21 days for symptoms of paralysis and other evidence of neurological involvement; observe the control monkeys for the same period plus 10 days. Animals that die within 48 hours of injection are considered to have died from non-specific causes and may be replaced. The test is not valid if: more than 20% of the inoculated monkeys die from nonspecific causes; serum samples taken from the control monkeys at the time of inoculation of the test animals and 10 days after the latter are killed show evidence of infection by wild virus of the type being tested or by measles virus. At the end of the observation period, carry out autopsy and histopathological examinations of appropriate areas of the brain for evidence of central nervous system involvement. The material complies with the test if there is no unexpected clinical or histopathological evidence of involvement of the central nervous system attributable to the inoculated virus.

2. TEST FOR NEUROVIRULENCE OF POLIOMYELITIS VACCINE (ORAL)

(Ph. Eur. method 2.4.19)

Monkeys used in the neurovirulence test comply with the requirements given under Poliomyelitis Vaccine, Live (Oral) and weigh not less than 1.5 kg. The pathogenicity for *Macaca* or *Cercopithecus* monkeys is tested in comparison with that of a reference virus preparation for neurovirulence testing by inoculation into the lumbar region of the central nervous system after sedation with a suitable substance, for example, ketamine hydrochloride. A sample of serum taken before the injection shall be shown not to contain neutralising antibody at a dilution of 1:4 when tested against not more than 1000 $CCID_{50}$ of each of the three types of poliovirus.

Number of monkeys The vaccine and the appropriate homotypic reference virus are tested concurrently in the same group of monkeys. Equal numbers of animals are inoculated with the vaccine being examined and the reference preparation. The animals are allocated randomly to treatment groups and cages and their identity is coded so that the treatment received by each animal is concealed from the observers and the evaluators of the sections. The number of monkeys inoculated is such that in the evaluation of both the vaccine and the reference preparation no fewer than 11 positive monkeys are included for type 1 and type 2 virus and no fewer than 18 positive monkeys for type 3 virus (positive monkeys are those that show specific neuronal lesions of poliovirus in the central nervous system). More than one batch of vaccine may be tested with the same homotypic reference. Monkeys from the same quarantine group are used wherever possible, otherwise monkeys from two groups are used and equal numbers from each group are treated with the vaccine and the reference preparation. If the test is carried out on two working days, an equal number of monkeys from each group are inoculated on each day with the vaccine and the homotypic reference preparation.

Virus content The virus contents of the vaccine and the homotypic reference preparation are adjusted so as to be as near as possible equal and between $10^{5.5}$ and $10^{6.5}$ $CCID_{50}$ per 0.1 ml.

Observation All monkeys are observed for 17 to 22 days for signs of poliomyelitis or other virus infection. Monkeys that survive the first 24 hours but die before the 11th day after inoculation are autopsied to determine whether poliomyelitis was the cause of death. Animals that die from causes other than poliomyelitis are excluded from the evaluation. Animals that become moribund or are severely paralysed are killed and autopsied. All animals that survive until the end of the observation period are autopsied. The test is not valid if more than 20% of the animals show intercurrent infection during the observation period.

Number of sections examined The lumbar cord, the cervical cord, the lower and upper medulla oblongata, the midbrain, the thalamus and the motor cortex of each monkey, as a minimum, are subjected to histological examination. Sections are cut with a thickness of 15 µm and stained with gallocyanin. The minimum number of sections examined is as follows:

(a) 12 sections representative of the whole of the lumbar enlargement,
(b) 10 sections representative of the whole of the cervical enlargement,
(c) 2 sections from the medulla oblongata,
(d) 1 section from the pons and cerebellum,
(e) 1 section from the midbrain,
(f) 1 section from the left and the right of the thalamus,
(g) 1 section from the left and the right motor cerebral cortex.

Scoring of virus activity For the evaluation of virus activity in the hemisections of the spinal cord and brain-stem, a score system for the severity of lesions is used, differentiating cellular infiltration and destruction of neurons as follows:

1. Cellular infiltration only (the monkey is not counted as positive),
2. Cellular infiltration with minimal neuronal damage,
3. Cellular infiltration with extensive neuronal damage,
4. Massive neuronal damage with or without cellular infiltration.

The scores are recorded on a standard form[2]. A monkey with neuronal lesions in the sections but that shows no needle tract is counted as positive. A monkey showing a needle tract in the sections, but no neuronal lesions is not regarded as positive. A section that shows damage from trauma but no specific virus lesions is not included in the score.

Severity scores are based on hemisection readings of the lumbar (L), cervical (C) and brain (B) histological sections. The lesion score (LS) for each positive monkey is calculated as follows:

$$LS = \left[\frac{\text{Sum of L score}}{\text{Number of hemisections}}\right] + \left[\frac{\text{Sum of C score}}{\text{Number of hemisections}}\right] + \left[\frac{\text{Sum of B score}}{\text{Number of hemisections}}\right] \div 3$$

A mean lesion score is calculated for each group of positive monkeys.

Evaluation The comparison of the virus activity in the vaccine and the reference preparation is based on the activity in the lumbar enlargement of the cord and the degree of spread of activity from this region to the cervical enlargement and the brain. Acceptance or rejection is based on the total score of all the test animals. Individual animals showing evidence of unusually high activity, either in the lumbar region or as the result of spread from this region, are also taken into consideration in the final evaluation. The monovalent bulk passes the test if the required number of animals is positive and if none of the clinical and histopathological examinations shows a significant difference in pathogenicity between the vaccine virus and the reference material. Criteria for acceptance are given below.

Criteria A suitable number of neurovirulence qualifying tests (for example, four tests) is carried out on each reference vaccine (types 1, 2 and 3) to provide data on the activity of such vaccines that will serve as the basis of the criteria for vaccines to be tested. The overall mean lesion score (M) for the replicate tests on each reference virus is calculated together with the pooled estimate of the within-test variance (s^2) and the within-test deviation (s).

Validity criteria for the results of a test on a reference preparation are established on the basis of the cumulative data from the qualifying tests. No generally applicable criteria can be given; for laboratories with limited experience, the following empirical method for setting acceptable limits for the mean lesion score for the reference preparation (X_{ref}) may be helpful:

	Lower limit	Upper limit
Types 1 and 2	$M - s$	$M + s$
Type 3	$M - s/2$	$M + s$

If the mean lesion score for the vaccine to be tested is X_{test} and C_1, C_2 and C_3 are constants determined as described below, then:

the vaccine is not acceptable if:

$$X_{test} - X_{ref} > C_1$$

the vaccine may be retested once if:

$$C_1 < X_{test} - X_{ref} < C_2$$

If the vaccine is retested, the means of the lesion scores for the vaccine to be tested and the reference vaccine are recalculated. The vaccine is not acceptable if:

$$\frac{X(test\,1 + test\,2) - X(ref\,1 + ref\,2)}{2} > C_3$$

The constants C_1, C_2 and C_3 are calculated from the expressions:

$$C_1 = 2.3\sqrt{\frac{2s^2}{N_1}}$$

$$C_2 = 2.6\sqrt{\frac{2s^2}{N_1}}$$

$$C_3 = 1.6\sqrt{\frac{2s^2}{N_2}}$$

where N_1 = number of positive monkeys per vaccine test,
N_2 = number of positive monkeys in the two tests,
2.3 = normal deviate at the 1% level,
2.6 = normal deviate at the 0.5% level,
1.6 = normal deviate at the 5% level.

A neurovirulence test in which the mean lesion score for the reference (X_{ref}) is not compatible with previous experience is not used for assessing a test vaccine. If the test is valid, the mean lesion score for the vaccine to be tested (X_{test}) is calculated and compared with that of the homotypic reference vaccine.

G. Composition of Polysaccharide Vaccines

(Ph. Eur. methods 2.5.16 to 2.5.23 and 2.5.31)

Protein *(Ph. Eur. method 2.5.16)*

Test solution Use a graduated flask with a suitable volume for preparation of a solution containing about 5 mg per ml of dry polysaccharide. Transfer the contents of a container quantitatively to the flask and dilute to volume with *water*. Place 1 ml of the solution in a glass tube and add 0.15 ml of a 40% w/v solution of *trichloroacetic acid*. Shake, allow to stand for 15 minutes, centrifuge for 10 minutes at 5000 revolutions per minute and discard the supernatant liquid. Add 0.4 ml of 0.1M *sodium hydroxide* to the centrifugation residue.

Standard solutions Dissolve 0.100 g of *bovine albumin* in 100 ml of 0.1M *sodium hydroxide* (stock solution containing 1 g of protein per litre). Dilute 1 ml of the stock solution to 20 ml with 0.1M *sodium hydroxide* (working dilution 1:50 mg of protein per litre). Dilute 1 ml of the stock solution to 4 ml with 0.1M *sodium hydroxide* (working dilution 2: 0.25 g of protein per litre). Place in six glass tubes 0.1 ml, 0.2 ml and 0.4 ml of working dilution 1 and 0.15 ml, 0.2 ml and 0.25 ml of working dilution 2. Make up the volume in each tube to 0.4 ml using 0.1M *sodium hydroxide*. Prepare a blank using 0.4 ml of 0.1M *sodium hydroxide*.

Method Add 2 ml of *cupri-tartaric solution R3* to each tube, shake and allow to stand for 10 minutes. Add to each tube 0.2 ml of a mixture of equal volumes of *phosphomolybdotungstic reagent* and *water*, prepared immediately before use. Stopper the tubes, mix by inverting and allow to stand in the dark for 30 minutes. The blue colour is stable for 60 minutes. If necessary, centrifuge to obtain clear solutions.

Measure the *absorbance*, Appendix II B, of each solution at 760 nm using the blank as compensation liquid. Draw a calibration curve from the absorbances of the six standard solutions and the corresponding protein contents and read from the curve the content of protein in the test solution.

Nucleic Acids *(Ph. Eur. method 2.5.17)*

Test solution Use a graduated flask with a suitable volume for preparation of a solution containing about 5 mg per ml of dry polysaccharide. Transfer the contents of a container quantitatively to the flask and dilute to volume with water.

Method Dilute the test solution if necessary to obtain an absorbance value suitable for the instrument used. Measure the *absorbance*, Appendix II B at 260 nm using *water* as compensation liquid. The *absorbance* of a 0.1% w/v solution of nucleic acid at 260 nm is 20.

Phosphorus *(Ph. Eur. method 2.5.18)*

Test solution Use a graduated flask with a suitable volume for preparation of a solution containing about 5 mg per ml of dry polysaccharide. Transfer the contents of a container quantitatively to the flask and dilute to volume with *water*. Dilute the solution so that the volume used in the test solution (1 ml) contains about 6 mg of phosphorus. Transfer 1 ml of the solution to a 10 ml ignition tube.

Standard solutions Dissolve 0.2194 g of *potassium dihydrogen orthophosphate* in 500 ml of *water* to give a solution containing the equivalent of 0.1 mg of phosphorus per ml.

Dilute 5 ml of the solution to 100 ml with *water*. Transfer respectively 0.5 ml, 1 ml and 2 ml of the dilute solution to three ignition tubes. Prepare a blank solution using 2 ml of *water* in an ignition tube.

Method To all the tubes add 0.2 ml of *sulphuric acid (96% w/w)* and heat in an oil bath at 120° for 1 hour then at 160° until white fumes appear (about 1 hour). Add 0.1 ml of *perchloric acid* and heat at 160° until the solution is decolorised (about 90 minutes). Cool and add to the tubes 4 ml of *water* and 4 ml of *ammonium molybdate reagent*. Heat in a water bath at 37° for 90 minutes and cool. Adjust the volume to 10 ml with *water*. The blue colour is stable for several hours.

Measure the *absorbance*, Appendix II B, of each solution at 820 nm using the blank solution as compensation liquid. Draw a calibration curve with the absorbances of the three reference solutions as a function of the quantity of phosphorus in the solutions and read from the curve the quantity of phosphorus in the test solution.

O-Acetyl Groups *(Ph. Eur. method 2.5.19)*

Test solution Use a graduated flask with a suitable volume for preparation of a solution containing about 5 mg per ml of dry polysaccharide. Transfer the contents of a container quantitatively to the flask and dilute to volume with *water*. Dilute the solution so that the volumes used in solution (1) contain 30 to 600 µg of acetylcholine (*O*-acetyl). Introduce 0.3 ml, 0.5 ml and 1 ml in duplicate into six tubes (three reaction solutions and three correction solutions).

Standard solutions Dissolve 0.150 g of *acetylcholine chloride* in 10 ml of *water* (stock solution containing 15 g of *acetylcholine chloride* per litre). Immediately before use, dilute 1 ml of the stock solution to 50 ml with *water* (working dilution 1:300 µg of *acetylcholine chloride* per ml). Immediately before use, dilute 1 ml of the stock solution to 25 ml with *water* (working dilution 2:600 µg of *acetylcholine chloride* per ml). Introduce 0.1 ml and 0.4 ml of working dilution 1 in duplicate (reaction and correction solutions) in four tubes and 0.6 ml and 1 ml of working dilution 2 in duplicate (reaction and correction solutions) in another four tubes. Prepare a blank using 1 ml of water.

Method Make up the volume in each tube to 1 ml with *water*. Add 1 ml of 4M *hydrochloric acid* to each of the correction tubes and to the blank. Add 2 ml of *alkaline hydroxylamine solution* to each tube. Allow the reaction to proceed for exactly 2 minutes and add 1 ml of 4M *hydrochloric acid* to each of the reaction tubes. Add 1 ml of a 10% w/v solution of *iron(III) chloride hexahydrate* in 0.1M *hydrochloric acid* to each tube, stopper the tubes and shake vigorously to remove bubbles.

Measure the *absorbance*, Appendix II B of each solution at 540 nm using the blank as compensation liquid. For each reaction solution, subtract the absorbance of the corresponding correction solution. Draw a calibration curve from the corrected absorbances for the four reference solutions and the corresponding content of acetylcholine chloride and read from the curve the content of acetylcholine chloride in the test solution for each volume tested. Calculate the mean of the three values. 1 mole of acetylcholine chloride (181.7 g) is equivalent to 1 mole of *O*-acetyl (43.05 g).

Hexosamines *(Ph. Eur. method 2.5.20)*

Test solution Use a graduated flask with a suitable volume for preparation of a solution containing about 5 mg per ml of dry polysaccharide. Transfer the contents of a container quantitatively to the flask and dilute to volume with *water*. Dilute the solution so that the volumes used in the test contain 0.125 to 0.500 mg of glucosamine (hexosamine). Introduce 1 ml of the diluted solution into a graduated tube.

Standard solutions Dissolve 60 mg of *D-glucosamine hydrochloride* in 100 ml of *water* (stock solution containing 0.500 g of glucosamine per litre). Introduce 0.25 ml, 0.5 ml, 0.75 ml, and 1 ml of the working dilution into four graduated tubes. Prepare a blank using 1 ml of *water*.

Method Make up the volume in each tube to 1 ml with *water*. Add 1 ml of 8M *hydrochloric acid* to each tube. Stopper the tubes and place in a water bath for 1 hour. Cool to room temperature. Add to each tube 0.05 ml of a 0.5% w/v solution of *thymolphthalein* in *ethanol (96%)*; add 5M *sodium hydroxide* until a blue colour is obtained and then 1M *hydrochloric acid* until the solution is colourless. Dilute the volume in each tube to 10 ml with *water* (neutralised hydrolysates).

In a second series of 10-ml graduated tubes, place 1 ml of each neutralised hydrolysate. Add 1 ml of acetylacetone reagent (a mixture, prepared immediately before use, of 1 volume of *acetylacetone* and 50 volumes of a 5.3% w/v solution of *anhydrous sodium carbonate*) to each tube. Stopper the tubes and place in a water bath at 90° for 45 minutes. Cool to room temperature. Add to each tube 2.5 ml of *ethanol (96%)* and 1 ml of dimethylaminobenzaldehyde solution (prepared immediately before use by dissolving 0.8 g of *dimethylaminobenzaldehyde* in 15 ml of *ethanol (96%)* and adding 15 ml of *hydrochloric acid*) and dilute the volume in each tube to 10 ml with *ethanol (96%)*. Stopper the tubes, mix by inverting and allow to stand in the dark for 90 minutes. Measure the *absorbance*, Appendix II B, of each solution at 530 nm using the blank as compensation liquid.

Draw a calibration curve from the absorbances for the four reference solutions and the corresponding content of hexosamine and read from the curve the quantity of hexosamine in the test solution.

Methylpentoses *(Ph. Eur. method 2.5.21)*

Test solution Use a graduated flask with a suitable volume for the preparation of a solution containing about 5 mg per ml of dry polysaccharide. Transfer the contents of a container quantitatively to the flask and dilute to volume with *water*. Dilute the solution so that the volumes used in the test contain 2 to 20 µg of rhamnose (methylpentoses). Introduce 0.25 ml, 0.5 ml and 1 ml of the diluted solution into three tubes.

Standard solutions Dissolve 0.100 g of *L-rhamnose* in 100 ml of *water* (stock solution containing 1 g of methylpentose per litre). Immediately before use, dilute 1 ml of th stock solution to 50 ml with *water* (working dilution: 20 mg of methylpentose per litre). Introduce 0.1 ml, 0.25 ml, 0.5ml, 0.75 ml and 1 ml of the working dilution into five tubes. Prepare a blank using 1 ml of *water*.

Method Make up the volume in each tube to 1 ml with *water*. Place the tubes in iced water and add dropwise and with continuous stirring to each tube 4.5 ml of a cooled mixture of 1 volume of *water* and 6 volumes of *sulphuric acid (96% w/w)*.Warm the tubes to room temperature and place in a water bath. Cool to room temperature. Add to each tube 0.1 ml of a 3% w/v solution of *cysteine hydrochloride*, prepared immediately before use. Shake and allow to stand for 2 hours.

Measure the *absorbance*, Appendix II B, of each solution at 396 nm and at 430 nm using the blank as compensation liquid. For each solution, calculate the difference between the absorbance measured at 396 nm and that measured at 430 nm. Draw a calibration curve from the absorbance differences for the five standard solutions and the corresponding content of methylpentose and read from the curve the quantity of methylpentose in the test solution for each volume tested. Calculate the mean of the three values.

Uronic Acids *(Ph. Eur. method 2.5.22)*

Test solution Use a graduated flask with a suitable volume for preparation of a solution containing about 5 mg per ml of dry polysaccharide. Transfer the contents of a container quantitatively to the flask and dilute to volume with water. Dilute the solution so that the volumes used in the test contain 4 to 40 µg of glucuronic acid (uronic acids). Introduce 0.25 ml, 0.5 ml and 1 ml of the diluted solution into three tubes.

Standard solutions Dissolve 50 mg of *sodium glucuronate* in 100 ml of *water* (stock solution containing 0.4 g of *glucuronic acid* per litre). Immediately before use, dilute 5 ml of the stock solution to 50 ml with *water* (working dilution: 40 mg of *glucuronic acid* per litre). Introduce 0.1 ml, 0.25 ml, 0.5 ml, 0.75 ml and 1 ml of the working dilution into five tubes. Prepare a blank using 1 ml of *water*.

Method Make up the volume in each tube to 1 ml with *water*. Place the tubes in iced water and add dropwise and with continuous stirring to each tube 5 ml of *borate solution*. Stopper the tubes and place in a water bath for 15 minutes. Cool to room temperature. Add 0.2 ml of a 0.125% w/v solution of *carbazole* in *absolute ethanol* to each tube. Stopper the tubes and place in a water bath for 15 minutes. Cool to room temperature. Measure the *absorbance,* Appendix II B, of each solution at 530 nm using the blank as compensation liquid.

Draw a calibration curve from the absorbances for the five standard solutions and the corresponding content of glucuronic acid and read from the curve the quantity of glucuronic acid in the test solution for each volume tested. Calculate the mean of the three values.

Sialic acid *(Ph. Eur. method 2.5.23)*

Test solution Transfer quantitatively the contents of one or several containers to a volumetric flask of a suitable volume that will give a solution with a known concentration of about 250 µg per ml of polysaccharide and dilute to volume with *water*. Using a syringe, transfer 4.0 ml of this solution to a 10 ml ultrafiltration cell suitable for the passage of molecules of relative molecular mass less than 50,000. Rinse the syringe twice with *water* and transfer the rinsings to the ultrafiltration cell. Carry out the ultrafiltration, with constant stirring, under *nitrogen* at a pressure of about 150 kPa. Refill the cell with *water* each time the volume of liquid in it has decreased to 1 ml and continue until 200 ml has been filtered and the remaining volume in the cell is about 2 ml. Using a syringe, transfer this residual liquid to a 10 ml volumetric flask. Wash the cell with three quantities, each of 2 ml, of *water*, transfer the washings to the flask and dilute to 10.0 ml with *water* (test solution). In each of two test-tubes place 2.0 ml of the test solution.

Reference solutions Use the reference solutions prescribed in the monograph.

Prepare two series of three test-tubes, place in the tubes of each series 0.5 ml, 1.0 ml and 1.5 ml respectively, of the reference solution corresponding to the type of vaccine being examined and adjust the volume in each tube to 2.0 ml with *water*. Prepare blank solutions using 2.0 ml of *water* in each of two test-tubes. To all the tubes add 5.0 ml of *resorcinol reagent*. Heat at 105° for 15 minutes, cool in cold water and transfer the tubes to a bath of iced water. To each tube add 5 ml of *isoamyl alcohol* and mix thoroughly. Place in the bath of iced water for 15 minutes. Centrifuge the tubes and keep them in the bath of iced water until the examination by absorption spectrophotometry. Measure the *absorbance*, Appendix II B, of each supernatant solution at 580 nm and 450 nm using *isoamyl alcohol* as the compensation liquid. For each wavelength, calculate the absorbance as the mean of the values obtained with two identical solutions. Subtract the mean value for the blank solution from the mean values obtained for the other solutions. Draw a graph showing the difference between the absorbances at 580 nm and 450 nm of the reference solution as a function of the content of *N*-acetylneuraminic acid and read from the graph the quantity of N-acetylneuraminic acid (sialic acid) in the test solution.

Ribose *(Ph. Eur. method 2.5.31)*

Test solution Use a volumetric flask with a suitable volume for preparation of a solution containing about 5 mg per millilitre of dry polysaccharide. Transfer the contents of a container quantitatively to the flask and dilute to volume with *water*. Dilute the solution so that the volumes used in the test contain 2.5 mg to 25 mg of ribose. Introduce 0.20 ml and 0.40 ml of the diluted solution into tubes in triplicate.

Reference solutions Dissolve 25 mg of *ribose* in *water* and dilute to 100.0 ml with the same solvent (stock solution containing 0.25 g/l of ribose). Immediately before use, dilute 1 ml of the stock solution to 10.0 ml with *water* (working dilution: 25 mg/l of ribose). Introduce 0.10 ml, 0.20 ml, 0.40 ml, 0.60 ml, 0.80 ml and 1.0 ml of the working dilution into six tubes.

Prepare a blank using 2 ml of *water*.

Make up the volume in each tube to 2 ml with *water*. Shake. Add 2 ml of a 0.5 g/l solution of *ferric chloride* in *hydrochloric acid* to each tube. Shake. Add 0.2 ml of a 100 g/l solution of *orcinol* in *absolute ethanol*. Place the tubes in a water-bath for 20 minutes. Cool in iced water. Measure the *absorbance*, Appendix II B, of each solution at 670 nm using the blank as the compensation liquid. Draw a calibration curve from the absorbance readings for the six reference solutions and the corresponding content of ribose and read from the curve the quantity of ribose in the test solution for each volume tested. Calculate the mean of the three values.

H. Chicken Flocks Free from Specified Pathogens for the Production and Quality Control of Vaccines

(Ph. Eur. general text 5.2.2)

Where specified in a monograph, chickens, embryos or cell cultures used for the production or quality control of vaccines are derived from eggs produced by chicken flocks free from specified pathogens (SPF). The SPF status of a flock is ensured by means of the system described below. The list of micro-organisms given is based on current knowledge and will be updated as necessary.

General principles and procedures

A flock is defined as a group of birds sharing a common environment and having their own caretakers who have no contact with non-SPF flocks. Once a flock is defined, no non-SPF birds are added to it.

For SPF flocks established on a rolling basis, all replacements are hatched and reared in the controlled environment house. Subject to the agreement of the competent authorities, SPF embryos derived from a tested SPF flock from another house on the same site may be introduced. From 8 weeks of age, these replacement birds are regarded as a flock and monitored monthly in accordance with the Subsequent testing requirements. At point of lay, all these replacement birds are tested in accordance with the Initial testing requirements.

The flock is housed so as to minimise the chance of contamination. It is not sited near to non-SPF flocks of birds and is housed in an isolator or on wire in a building with filtered air under positive pressure. Appropriate measures are taken to prevent access of rodents, wild birds, insects and unauthorised people.

Personnel authorised to enter must have no contact with other birds or with agents likely to infect the flock. It is advisable for personnel to shower and change clothing or to wear protective clothing before entering the chicken house.

Items taken into the flock are sterilised. The feed is suitably treated to avoid the introduction of undesirable micro-organisms and water is obtained from a chlorinated supply. No medication is given that could interfere with detection of disease in the flock.

A permanent record is kept of the general health of the flock and any abnormality is investigated. Factors to be monitored include morbidity, mortality, general physical condition, feed consumption, daily egg production and egg quality, fertility and hatchability. Dirty eggs are discarded; clean eggs may be surface-disinfected whilst warm.

The flock originates from chickens shown to be free from vertically-transmitted agents. In particular, each chicken from which the flock is derived is tested repeatedly to ensure freedom from leucosis viruses and their antibodies. In order to establish the SPF status of a flock, it is kept under SPF conditions for a test period of not less than 4 months. Each bird in the entire flock is shown to be free from evidence of infection with the agents listed below under Initial testing after 6 weeks and at the end of the test period.

TABLE 15H-1 INITIAL TESTING *Subject to agreement by the competent authority, other types of test may be used provided they are as least as sensitive as those indicated and are of appropriate specificity.*

Micro-organism	Type of test
Avian adenoviruses	Enzyme-linked immunosorbent assay
Avian encephalomyelitis virus	Enzyme-linked immunosorbent assay
Avian infectious bronchitis virus	Enzyme-linked immunosorbent assay
Avian infectious laryngo-tracheitis virus	Serum neutralisation
Avian leucosis viruses	Enzyme-linked immunosorbent assay for virus and serum neutralisation for antibody
Avian nephritis virus	Fluorescent antibody
Avian reoviruses	Enzyme-linked immunosorbent assay
Avian reticuloendotheliosis virus	Fluorescent antibody
Haemagglutinating avian adenovirus (Egg drop syndrome 76 adenovirus; EDS 76 virus)	Haemagglutination inhibition
Infectious bursal disease virus	Serum neutralisation against each serotype present in the country of origin
Influenza A virus	Enzyme-linked immunosorbent assay
Marek's disease virus	Enzyme-linked immunosorbent assay
Newcastle disease virus	Haemagglutination inhibition
Turkey rhinotracheitis virus	Enzyme-linked immunosorbent assay
Mycoplasma gallisepticum	Agglutination and, to confirm a positive test, haemagglutination inhibition
Mycoplasma synoviae	Agglutination and, to confirm a positive test, haemagglutination inhibition
Salmonella pullorum	Agglutination

For each new generation in an established flock, all of the birds in the flock are tested at not later than 20 weeks of age, using the tests prescribed below under Initial testing. After the initial test, monthly tests are carried out on a representative 5% sample (but not less than ten and not more than two hundred birds), using the tests prescribed below under Subsequent testing, with a final test at 4 weeks after the last collection of eggs.

For all tests, blood samples are collected from an appropriate number of birds at the specified time. The resultant serum samples are examined for antibodies against the relevant agents. Serum-neutralisation tests are done on pools of not more than five sera. All other tests are done on each individual serum. Positive and negative controls are used in all tests. The reagents used in the tests are standardised against international or European standard reagents where these are available. For avian leucosis virus, in addition to tests for antibodies carried out on serum samples, appropriate samples are taken for testing for the virus.

In addition to serological tests, clinical examination is carried out at least once per week to verify that the birds are free from fowl-pox and signs of other infections. Necropsy and, where necessary to confirm diagnosis, histopathological examination are carried out on any bird that dies to verify that there is no sign of infection. The absence of *Salmonella* species is determined by cultural examination of faecal samples at least once every 4 weeks; a pool of up to ten samples may be used for the tests.

If a positive result is obtained in any test carried out to establish the SPF status of a flock, the flock may not be designated as an SPF flock. If a positive result is obtained in any test carried out on an established flock, the flock loses its SPF status. Special provisions apply to chick anaemia agent (CAA) as described below. Any chickens, embryos or cell cultures collected since the previous negative test are not suitable for use: any product made from them must be discarded and any quality control tests done with them are invalid and must be repeated.

In order to regain SPF status, the flock is maintained under SPF conditions and routine 5% monthly testing shall continue except that every bird in the entire flock is tested every month for infection with the particular agent that gave the positive result. Infected birds and their progeny are removed from the flock. SPF status is regained after two such consecutive tests have yielded completely negative results.

A positive result for CAA does not necessarily exclude use of material derived from the flock, but live vaccines for use in birds less than 7 days old must be produced using material from CAA-negative flocks. Inactivated vaccines for use in birds less than 7 days old may be produced using material from flocks that have not been shown to be free from CAA, provided it has been demonstrated that the inactivation process inactivates CAA.

Permanent records of mortality and of results of flock testing are kept for a minimum of five years. Details of any deterioration in egg production or hatchability, except for accidental cases identified as being of non-infectious origin, and of any test results indicating infection with a specified agent, are immediately submitted to the user of the eggs.

TABLE 15H-2 SUBSEQUENT TESTING *Subject to agreement by the competent authority, other types of test may be used provided they are as least as sensitive as those indicated and are of appropriate specificity.*

Micro-organism	Type of test
Avian adenoviruses	Enzyme-linked immunosorbent assay
Avian encephalomyelitis virus	Enzyme-linked immunosorbent assay
Avian infectious bronchitis virus	Enzyme-linked immunosorbent assay
Avian infectious laryngo-tracheitis virus	Serum neutralisation
Avian leucosis viruses	Enzyme-linked immunosorbent assay for the antibody
Avian nephritis virus	Fluorescent antibody
Avian reoviruses	Fluorescent antibody
Avian reticuloendotheliosis virus	Fluorescent antibody
Chick anaemia agent	Fluorescent antibody
Haemagglutinating avian adenovirus	Haemagglutination inhibition
Infectious bursal disease virus	Serum neutralisation against each serotype present in the country of origin
Influenza A virus	Enzyme-linked immunosorbent assay
Marek's disease virus	Enzyme-linked immunosorbent assay
Newcastle disease virus	Haemagglutination inhibition
Turkey rhinotracheitis virus	Enzyme-linked immunosorbent assay
Mycoplasma gallisepticum	Agglutination and, to confirm a positive test, haemagglutination inhibition
Mycoplasma synoviae	Agglutination and, to confirm a positive test, haemagglutination inhibition
Salmonella pullorum	Agglutination

J. Human Diploid Cells for the Production of Vaccines

(Ph. Eur. general text 5.2.3)

Production of vaccines on human diploid cells is based on a cell-bank system. An early population doubling level of a diploid cell culture (the cell seed) is subcultured to a level convenient for the establishment of a working cell bank.

Cell seed The cell seed from which the working cell bank is to be derived is characterised with respect to genealogy, identity (isoenzymes, serology, nucleic acid fingerprinting), genetic markers (HLA), karyotype (as described below under Chromosomal characterisation), growth characteristics, virus susceptibility, viability during storage and finite life-span.

A late passage (at or beyond production level) of the cell strain is tested for freedom from tumorigenicity, for identity and normal karyotype.

Working cell bank The working cell bank is characterised with respect to identity and karyotype (as described below under Chromosomal monitoring). Using the tests shown below, it is shown to be free from bacterial, fungal and mycoplasmal contamination and, by the tests in animals, eggs and cell cultures, to be free from extraneous agents. Other suitable tests may also be necessary in particular cases.

Production cell culture Each production cell culture consists of a passage at a level up to two-thirds of the life-span of the accepted cell strain and is tested for identity using markers such as isoenzymes, HLA or karyotype of at least one metaphase spread of chromosomes. The production cell culture is also tested as prescribed below under Extraneous agents in viral vaccines.

Methods

Tests in animals and eggs Inject intramuscularly (or, for suckling mice, by deep subcutaneous route) into each of the following groups of animals at least 10^7 viable cells divided equally between the animals in each group:

(a) two litters of suckling mice less than 24 hours old, comprising no fewer than 10 animals,

(b) 10 adult mice,

(c) five guinea-pigs,

(d) five rabbits.

Observe the animals for at least 4 weeks. Investigate animals that become sick or show any abnormality to establish the cause of illness. No evidence of any extraneous agent is found. The test is not valid unless at least 80% of the animals in each group remain healthy and survive to the end of the observation period.

Inject at least 10^6 viable cells into the allantoic cavity of each of 10 fertilised hen eggs, 9 to 11 days old. Incubate for 3 days and test the allantoic fluids for the presence of haemagglutinins using guinea-pig, chick or other avian red blood cells. No evidence of any extraneous agent is found. The test is not valid unless at least 80% of the embryos remain healthy and survive to the end of the observation period.

Tumorigenicity Cells at or beyond the production level are shown to be free from tumorigenicity by suitable tests. Cells of the MRC-5 strain and of the WI-38 strain are recognised as being non-tumorigenic and further testing is not necessary.

Chromosomal characterisation Examine at least four samples, each consisting of 1000 metaphase cells, at approximately equal intervals over the life-span of the cell line during serial cultivation. Examine for frequency of polyploidy, for exact counts of chromosomes, for frequency of breaks, structural abnormalities and other abnormalities, such as despiralisation or marked attenuations of the primary and secondary constrictions. All cells showing abnormalities are subjected to detailed examination and records are maintained according to the detailed criteria applied to particular abnormalities evaluated in the karyotype analysis. Permanent stained slide preparations or photographs of the slides, are kept as part of the record for each batch of vaccine.

The World Health Organization has recommended the following criteria applicable to MRC-5 and Wl-38 cells.

For cells examined in the metaphase the upper limits [higher confidence limit (P = 0.95) (Poisson)] for abnormalities are as follows:

Abnormality	1000 cells	500 cells
Chromatid and chromosome breaks	47/1000	26/500
Structural abnormalities	17/1000	10/500
Hyperploidy	8/1000	5/500
Hypoploidy	180/1000	90/500
Polyploidy	30/1000	17/500

Chromosomal monitoring Examine at least 500 cells in metaphase at the production level or at any passage thereafter. Carry out examination for the same features and in the same manner as described above. Only cell banks that have normal karyotype are used for vaccine production.

Bacterial and fungal sterility A 10-ml sample complies with the *test for sterility*, Appendix XVI A.

Mycoplasmas A 10-ml sample complies with the *test for absence of mycoplasmas*, Appendix XVI B3.

Mycobacteria A 5-ml sample is tested for the presence of Mycobacterium spp. by culture methods known to be sensitive for the detection of these organisms. Use the method described in Appendix XVI B4.

Test for extraneous agents in cell cultures The material complies with the test for Haemadsorbing viruses and with the tests in cell cultures for Other extraneous agents given in the section on Production cell culture: control cells described under *extraneous agents in viral vaccines*, Appendix XVI B5.

Appendix XVI

A. Test for Sterility

(Ph. Eur. method 2.6.1)

The test is applied to substances, preparations or articles which, according to the Pharmacopoeia, are required to be sterile. However, a satisfactory result only indicates that no contaminating micro-organism has been found in the sample examined in the conditions of the test. Guidance on the further requirements for demonstrating the sterility of the batch is given at the end of this text.

Precautions against microbial contamination

The test for sterility is carried out under conditions equivalent to those required for aseptic manufacture of pharmaceutical products, using, for example, a class A laminar-air-flow cabinet located within a class B clean-room, or an isolator located within a class D clean-room environment. The precautions taken to avoid contamination are such that they do not affect any micro-organisms which should be revealed in the test. The working conditions in which the tests are performed are monitored regularly by appropriate sampling of the working area and by carrying out appropriate controls such as those indicated in the appropriate European Community Directives and associated Notes for guidance on GMP.

Culture media

The following culture media have been found to be suitable for the test for sterility. Fluid thioglycollate medium is primarily intended for the culture of anaerobic bacteria; however, it will also detect aerobic bacteria. Soya-bean casein digest medium is primarily intended for the culture of aerobic bacteria but is also suitable for fungi. Other media may be used provided that they have been shown to sustain the growth of a wide range of micro-organisms.

Fluid thioglycollate medium

L-Cystine	0.5 g
Agar, granulated (moisture content not in excess of 15%)	0.75 g
Sodium chloride	2.5 g
Glucose monohydrate	5.5 g
Yeast extract (water-soluble)	5.0 g
Pancreatic digest of casein	15.0 g
Sodium thioglycollate or	0.5 g
Thioglycollic acid	0.3 ml
Resazurin sodium solution (1 in 1000), freshly prepared	1.0 ml
Water	1000 ml

pH after sterilisation 7.1 ± 0.2

Mix the L-cystine, agar, sodium chloride, glucose, water-soluble yeast extract and pancreatic digest of casein with the *water*, and heat until solution is effected. Dissolve the sodium thioglycollate or thioglycollic acid in the solution and, if necessary, add 1M *sodium hydroxide* so that, after sterilisation, the solution will have a pH of 7.1 ± 0.2. If filtration is necessary, heat the solution again without boiling and filter while hot through moistened filter paper. Add the resazurin sodium solution, mix and place the medium in suitable vessels which provide a ratio of surface to depth of medium such that not more than the upper third of the medium has undergone a colour change indicative of oxygen uptake at the end of the incubation period. Sterilise using a validated process. Store at a temperature between 2° and 25° in a sterile, sealed container, unless it is intended for immediate use. If necessary, regenerate the medium just before use, for example by heating in a water-bath for 20 minutes and cooling quickly, taking care to prevent the introduction of non-sterile air into the container.

Soya-bean casein digest medium

Pancreatic digest of casein	17.0 g
Papaic digest of bean meal	3.0 g
Sodium chloride	5.0 g
Dipotassium hydrogen phosphate	2.5 g
Glucose monohydrate	2.5 g
Water	1000 ml

pH after sterilisation 7.3 ± 0.2

Dissolve the solids in the water, warming slightly to effect solution. Cool the solution to room temperature. Add 1M *sodium hydroxide*, if necessary, so that after sterilisation the solution will have a pH of 7.3 ± 0.2. Filter, if necessary, to clarify, distribute into suitable vessels and sterilise using a validated process. Store at a temperature between 2° and 25° in a sterile, sealed container, unless it is intended for immediate use.

The media used, whether they are those described above or others, comply with the following tests, carried out before or in parallel with the test on the product being examined.

Sterility Incubate portions of the media at the temperatures indicated in Table 16A-1 for 14 days. No growth of micro-organisms occurs.

Growth promotion test of aerobes, anaerobes and fungi Inoculate portions of the chosen media respectively with a small number of one of the types of micro-organisms (10-100 CFU is suitable) indicated in Table 16A-1 and incubate them under the conditions indicated in Table 16A-1 for not more than 3 days in the case of bacteria and not more than 5 days in the case of fungi. The list of suitable species and strains in the table is not exclusive; other micro-organisms may also be suitable.

Seed lot culture maintenance techniques (seed-lot systems) are used so that the viable micro-organisms used for inoculation are not more than five passages removed from the original master seed-lot.

The media are suitable if a clearly visible early growth of the micro-organisms occurs.

Validation test

For each type of micro-organism specified in Table 16A-1 carry out a test as described below under Test for sterility of the product being examined using exactly the same method except for the following modifications.

Membrane filtration After transferring the contents of the container or containers being tested to the membrane add an inoculum of a small number of viable micro-organisms (10-100 CFU is suitable) to the final portion of the sterile diluent used to rinse the filter.

Direct inoculation After transferring the contents of the container or containers being tested to the culture medium add an inoculum of a small number of viable micro-organisms (10-100 CFU is suitable) to the medium.

In both cases perform a growth promotion test as a positive control. Incubate all the containers containing medium at the temperatures indicated in Table 16A-2 for not more than 3 days for bacteria and 5 days for fungi. If clearly visible early growth of micro-organisms is obtained after the inoculation, visually comparable to that in the control vessel without product, either the product possesses no antimicrobial activity under the conditions of the test or such activity has been satisfactorily eliminated. The test for sterility may then be carried out without further modification. If clearly visible early growth is not obtained in the presence of the product to be tested, visually comparable to that in the control vessels without product, the product possesses antimicrobial activity that has not been satisfactorily eliminated under the conditions of the test. Modify the conditions in order to eliminate the antimicrobial activity and repeat the validation test.

This validation is performed:

a) when the test for sterility has to be carried out on a new product;
b) whenever there is a change in the experimental conditions of the test.

The validation may be performed simultaneously with the Test for sterility of the product being examined, but before the results of this test are interpreted.

Test for sterility of the product being examined

The test may be carried out using the technique of membrane filtration or by direct inoculation of the culture media with the product being examined. Appropriate negative controls are included in either case. The technique of membrane filtration is used whenever the nature of the product permits, that is, for filterable aqueous preparations, for alcoholic or oily preparations and for preparations miscible with or soluble in aqueous or oily solvents which do not have an antimicrobial effect in the conditions of the test.

Membrane filtration Use membrane filters having a nominal pore size not greater than 0.45 µm whose effectiveness to retain micro-organisms has been established. Cellulose nitrate filters, for example, are used for aqueous, oily and weakly alcoholic solutions and cellulose acetate filters, for example, for strongly alcoholic solutions. Specially adapted filters may be needed for certain products, e.g. for antibiotics. The technique described below assumes that membranes about 50 mm in diameter will be used. If filters of a different diameter are used the volumes of the dilutions and the washings should be adjusted accordingly. The filtration apparatus and membrane are sterilised by appropriate means. The apparatus is so designed that the solution being examined can be introduced and filtered under aseptic conditions; it permits the aseptic removal of the membrane for transfer to the medium or it is suitable for carrying out the incubation after adding the medium to the apparatus itself.

Aqueous solutions If appropriate, transfer a small quantity of a suitable, sterile diluent such as a 1 g/l neutral solution of meat or casein peptone pH 7.1 ± 0.2 onto the membrane in the apparatus and filter. The diluent may contain suitable neutralising substances and/or appropriate inactivating substances for example in the case of antibiotics. Transfer the contents of the container or containers being tested to the membrane or membranes, if necessary after diluting to about 100 ml with the chosen sterile diluent but in any case using not less than the quantities of the product being examined prescribed in Table 16A-2. Filter immediately. Wash the membrane at least three times by filtering through it each time, the volume of the chosen sterile diluent used in the validation test. Transfer the whole membrane to the culture medium or cut it aseptically into two equal parts and transfer one half to each of two suitable media. Use the same volume of each medium as in the validation test. Alternatively, transfer the medium onto the membrane in the apparatus. Unless otherwise prescribed, incubate the media for not less than 14 days, at 32.5 ± 2.5° in the test intended mainly to detect bacteria and at 22.5 ± 2.5° in the test intended mainly to detect fungi.

Table 16A-1 Test micro-organisms suitable for use in the growth promotion Test and the Validation Test.

Medium	Micro-organism		Incubation	
	Species	Suitable Strain	Temperature °C	Maximum Duration
	Type: aerobic bacteria		For all aerobes	
Fluid thioglycollate	*Staphylococcus aureus*	ATCC 6538P CIP 53.156 NCTC 7447		
	Bacillus subtilis	ATCC 6633 CIP 52.62 NCIB 8054	32.5±2.5	3 days
	Pseudomonas aeruginosa	ATCC 9027 NCIMB 8626 CIP 82.118		
	Type: Anaerobes		For all anaerobes	
	Clostridium sporogenes	ATCC 19404 CIP 79.3	32.5±2.5	3 days
	Type: Fungi*		For all fungi	
Soya-bean casein digest	*Candida albicans*	ATCC 10231 IP 4872 ATCC 2091 IP 1180.79	22.5±2.5	5 days
	Aspergillus niger	ATCC 16404		

**Bacillus subtilis* (ATCC 6633 or CIP 52.62) also grows in this medium.

TABLE 16A-2 Quantities of the product being examined in the test for sterility

Type of preparation	Quantity per container	Minimum quantity to be used for each container, unless otherwise justified and authorised
Parenteral preparations	*Liquids*	
	Less than 1 ml	The whole contents of a container
	1 ml or more	Half the contents of a container but not more than 20 ml
	Solids	
	Less than 50 mg	The whole contents of a container
	50 mg or more but less than 300 mg	Half the contents of a container
	300 mg or more	150 mg
Eye preparations and other non-injectable preparations	Aqueous solutions	The whole contents of one or more containers to provide not less than 2.5 ml
	Other preparations soluble in water or isopropyl myristate	The whole contents of one or more containers to provide not less than 0.25 g
	Insoluble preparations, creams and ointments to be suspended or emulsified	The whole contents or one or more containers to provide not less than 0.25 g

Soluble solids Use for each medium not less than the quantity prescribed in Table 16A-2 of the product dissolved in a suitable solvent such as a 1 g/l neutral solution of meat or casein peptone and proceed with the test as described above for aqueous solutions using a membrane appropriate to the chosen solvent.

Oils and oily solutions Use for each medium not less than the quantity of the product prescribed in Table 16A-2. Oils and oily solutions of sufficiently low viscosity may be filtered without dilution through a dry membrane. Viscous oils may be diluted as necessary with a suitable sterile diluent such as isopropyl myristate shown not to have antimicrobial activity in the conditions of the test. Allow the oil to penetrate the membrane by its own weight then filter, applying the pressure or suction gradually. Wash the membrane not fewer than three times by filtering through it each time about 100 ml of a suitable sterile solution such as 1 g/l neutral meat or casein peptone containing 1 g/l of (*p-tert*-octylphenoxy)polyoxyethanol or 10 g/l of polysorbate 80. Transfer the membrane or membranes to the culture medium or media or vice versa as described above for aqueous solutions and incubate at the same temperatures and for the same times.

Ointments and creams Use for each medium not less than the quantities of the product prescribed in Table 16A-2. Ointments in a fatty base and emulsions of the water-in-oil type may be diluted to 1% in isopropyl myristate as described above, by heating, if necessary, to not more than 40°. In exceptional cases it may be necessary to heat to not more than 44°. Filter as rapidly as possible and proceed as described above for oils and oily solutions.

Direct inoculation of the culture medium Transfer the quantity of the preparation being examined prescribed in Table 16A-2 directly into the culture medium so that the volume of the product is not more than 10% of the volume of the medium, unless otherwise prescribed.

Oily liquids Use media to which have been added 10 g/l of polysorbate 80 or 1 g/l of (*p-tert*-octylphenoxy)polyoxyethanol or other emulsifying agents in appropriate concentration shown not to have any antimicrobial action in the conditions of the test.

Ointments and creams Prepare by diluting to about 1 in 10 by emulsifying with the chosen emulsifying agent in a suitable sterile diluent such as a 1 g/l neutral solution of meat or casein peptone. Transfer the diluted product to a medium not containing an emulsifying agent.

If the product being examined has antimicrobial activity, carry out the test after neutralising this with a suitable neutralising substance or by dilution in a sufficient quantity of culture medium. When it is necessary to use a large volume of the product it may be preferable to use a concentrated culture medium prepared in such a way that it takes account of the subsequent dilution. Where appropriate the concentrated medium may be added directly to the product in its container.

Incubate the inoculated media for at least 14 days unless otherwise prescribed at the temperatures indicated in Table 16A-1. Observe the cultures several times during the incubation period. Shake cultures containing oily products gently each day. However when thioglycollate medium or other similar medium is used for the detection of anaerobic micro-organisms keep shaking or mixing to a minimum in order to maintain anaerobic conditions.

Observation and interpretation of results

At intervals during the incubation period and at its conclusion examine the media for macroscopic evidence of microbial growth. When the material being tested renders the medium turbid, so that the presence or absence of microbial growth cannot be determined readily by visual examination 14 days after the incubation started, transfer suitable portions of the medium to fresh vessels of the same medium. Continue incubation of the original and of the transfer vessels for a total of not less than 14 + 7 days from the original inoculation.

If no evidence of microbial growth is found, the product being examined complies with the test for sterility. If evidence of microbial growth is found the product being examined does not comply with the test for sterility, unless it can be clearly demonstrated that the test was invalid for causes unrelated to the product being examined. The test may be considered invalid only when one or more of the following conditions are fulfilled:

a) the data of the microbiological monitoring of the sterility testing facility show a fault;
b) a review of the testing procedure used during the test in question reveals a fault;

c) microbial growth is found in the negative controls;
d) after determination of the identity of the micro-organisms isolated from the test the growth of this species or these species may be ascribed unequivocally to faults with respect to the material and/or the technique used in conducting the sterility test procedure.

If the test is declared to be invalid it is repeated with the same number of units as in the original test. If no evidence of microbial growth is found in the repeat test the product examined complies with the test for sterility. If microbial growth is found in the repeat test the product examined does not comply with the test for sterility.

Application of the test to parenteral preparations and to eye preparations and other non-injectable preparations required to comply with the test for sterility

When using the technique of membrane filtration, use, whenever possible, the whole contents of the container, but not less than the quantities indicated in Table 16A-2, diluting where necessary to about 100 ml with a suitable sterile solution, such as 1 g/l neutral meat or casein peptone. The total volume washed through one single membrane does not exceed 1000 ml, unless otherwise justified and authorised.

When using the technique of direct inoculation of media, use the quantities shown in Table 16A-2. The tests for bacterial and fungal sterility are carried out on the same sample of the product being examined. When the volume or the quantity in a single container is insufficient to carry out the tests, the contents of two or more containers are used to inoculate the different media. When the volume of liquid in a container is greater than 100 ml the membrane filtration method is used, unless otherwise justified and authorised.

ANNEX

Guidelines for using the test for sterility

The purpose of the test for sterility, as that of all pharmacopoeial tests, is to provide an independent control analyst with the means of verifying that a particular material meets the requirement of the Pharmacopoeia. Manufacturers are neither obliged to carry out such tests nor precluded from using modifications of or alternatives to the stated method provided they are satisfied that, if tested by the official method, the material in question would comply with the requirements of the Pharmacopoeia.

Guidance to manufacturers The level of assurance provided by a satisfactory result of a test for sterility (the absence of contaminated units in the sample) as applied to the quality of the batch is a function of the homogeneity of the conditions of manufacture and of the efficiency of the adopted sampling plan. Hence for the purpose of this text a batch is defined as a homogeneous collection of sealed containers prepared in such a manner that the risk of contamination is the same for each of the units contained therein.

In the case of terminally sterilised products, physical proofs, biologically based and automatically documented, showing correct treatment throughout the batch during sterilisation are of greater assurance than the sterility test. The circumstances in which parametric release may be considered appropriate are described under *5.1.1. Methods of preparation of sterile products* (Appendix XVIII). The method of media-fill runs may be used to evaluate the process of aseptic production. Apart from that the sterility test is the only analytical method available for products prepared under aseptic conditions and furthermore it is, in all cases, the only analytical method available to the authorities who have to examine a specimen of a product for sterility.

The probability of detecting micro-organisms by the test for sterility increases with their number present in the sample tested and varies according to the readiness of growth of micro-organism present. The probability of detecting very low levels of contamination even when it is homogeneous throughout the batch is very low. The interpretation of the results of the test for sterility rests on the assumption that the contents of the every container in the batch, had they been tested, would have given the same result. Since it is manifest that every container cannot be tested, an appropriate sampling plan should be adopted. Guidance on the minimum number of items recommended being tested in relation to the size of the batch is given in Table 16A-3, assuming that the preparation has been manufactured under conditions designed to exclude contamination. The application of the recommendations must have regard to the volume of preparation per container, to the validation of the sterilisation method and to any other special considerations concerning the intended sterility of the product.

TABLE 16A-3 Minimum number of items recommended to be tested

Number of items in the batch	Minimum number of items to be tested for each medium*
Parenteral preparations	
Not more than 100 containers	10% or 4 containers, whichever is the greater
More than 100 but not more than 500 containers	10 containers
More than 500 containers	2% or 30 containers, whichever is the lesser
Eye preparations and other non-injectable preparations	
Not more than 200 containers	5% or 2 containers whichever is the greater
More than 200 containers	10 containers
If the product is presented in the form of single-dose containers, apply the scheme shown above for parenteral preparations	
Bulk solid products	
Up to 4 containers	Each container
More than 4 containers but not more than 50 containers	20% of 4 containers, whichever is the greater
More than 50 containers	2% or 10 containers, whichever is the greater

*If the contents of one container are enough to inoculate the two media, this column gives the number of containers needed for both the media together.

B. Tests for Microbial Contamination

(Ph. Eur. method2 2.6.13 and 2.6.12)

Tests for microbial contamination are carried out under conditions designed to avoid accidental contamination of the preparation during the test. The precautions taken to avoid contamination must be such that they do not adversely affect any micro-organisms that should be revealed in the test.

To obtain the required quantity for any of the tests described below mix several portions selected at random from the bulk material or from the contents of a sufficient number of containers. Depending on the nature of the preparation being examined, dilute, dissolve, suspend or emulsify it using a suitable liquid. Eliminate any antimicrobial properties of the preparation being examined by dilution, neutralisation or filtration.

1. TESTS FOR SPECIFIED MICRO-ORGANISMS

(Ph. Eur. method 2.6.13)

Pretreatment of the preparation being examined

WATER-SOLUBLE PRODUCTS Dissolve or dilute 10 g or 10 ml of the preparation being examined, unless otherwise prescribed, in *lactose broth* or another suitable medium shown not to have antimicrobial activity under the conditions of the test and adjust the volume to 100 ml[1] with the same medium. If necessary, adjust the pH to about 7.

NON-FATTY PRODUCTS INSOLUBLE IN WATER Suspend 10 g or 10 ml of the preparation being examined, unless otherwise prescribed, in *lactose broth* or another suitable medium shown not to have antimicrobial activity under the conditions of the test and dilute to 100 ml[2] with the same medium. If necessary divide the preparation being examined and homogenise the suspension mechanically.

A suitable surface-active agent such as 0.1% w/v of *polysorbate 80* may be added to assist the suspension of poorly wettable substances. If necessary, adjust the pH of the suspension to about 7.

FATTY PRODUCTS Homogenise 10 g or 10 ml of the preparation being examined, unless otherwise prescribed, with 5 g of *polysorbate 20* or *polysorbate 80*. If necessary, heat[3] to not more than 40°. Mix carefully while maintaining the temperature in a water bath or in an oven. Add 85 ml of *lactose broth* or another suitable medium shown not to have antimicrobial activity in the conditions of the test, heated to not more than 40° if necessary. Maintain this temperature for the shortest time necessary for formation of an emulsion and in any case for not more than 30 minutes. If necessary, adjust the pH of the emulsion to about 7.

Clostridia

The tests described below are intended for distinct purposes. The first method is intended for products where exclusion of pathogenic clostridia is essential and it is necessary to test for their absence. These products generally have a low total count. The second method is a semi-quantitative test for *Clostridium perfringens* and is intended for products where the level of this species is a criterion of quality.

DETECTION OF CLOSTRIDIA Homogenise the preparation being examined as described above. Take two equal portions corresponding to 1 g or 1 ml of the preparation being examined. Heat one portion to 80° for 10 minutes and cool rapidly. Do not heat the other portion. Transfer 10 ml of each of the homogenised portions to two tubes (38 mm × 200 mm) or other suitable containers containing 100 ml of *reinforced medium for clostridia*. Incubate under anaerobic conditions at 35° to 37° for 48 hours.

After incubation, make subcultures from each tube on *Columbia agar* to which gentamicin has been added and incubate under anaerobic conditions at 35° to 37° for 48 hours. The preparation being examined passes the test if no growth of micro-organisms is detected.

Where growth occurs, subculture each distinct colony form on *Columbia agar*, without gentamicin, and incubate in both aerobic and anaerobic conditions. The occurence of only anaerobic growth of Gram-positive bacilli (with or without endospores) giving a negative catalase reaction indicates the presence of Clostridium species. Compare, if necessary, the colonial growth on the two plates and apply the catalase test to eliminate aerobic and facultatively anaerobic Bacillus species that give a positive catalase reaction. This test may be applied to discrete, uniform colonies on agar, or indirectly following transfer to a glass slide, by application of a drop of *hydrogen peroxide solution (10 vol)*. The formation of gas bubbles indicates a positive catalase reaction.

SEMI-QUANTITATIVE EVALUATION OF CLOSTRIDIUM PERFRINGENS Using the preparation being examined prepared as described above, prepare appropriate dilutions containing 10 mg and 1 mg or 10 µl and 1 µl of the product.

Determine the most probable number of micro-organisms as described under Total viable aerobic count, Appendix XVI B2, transferring each time 1 ml of homogenate into a tube (16 mm × 160 mm) or other suitable container containing 9 ml of culture Lactose Sulphite Medium and a small Durham tube. Mix with minimum shaking and incubate at 45.5° to 46.5° for 24 hours to 48 hours.

The tubes showing a blackening due to iron sulphide and abundant formation of gas in the Durham tube (at least one tenth the volume) indicate the presence of *C. perfringens*. Determine from Table 16B-1 the most probable number of *C. perfringens*.

Enterobacteriaceae and certain other Gram-negative bacteria

DETECTION OF BACTERIA Homogenise the preparation being examined appropriately pretreated as described above and incubate at 35° to 37° for a time sufficient to revivify the bacteria but not sufficient to encourage multiplication of the organisms (usually 2 to 5 hours). Shake the container, transfer a quantity of the homogenate containing 1 g or 1 ml of the product to 100 ml of *Enterobacteriaceae enrichment broth—Mossel* and incubate at 35° to 37° for 18 to 48 hours. Subculture on a plate of *violet-red bile agar with glucose and lactose*. Incubate at 35° to 37° for 18 to 24 hours. The preparation being examined passes the test if there is no growth of colonies of Gram-negative bacteria on the plate.

QUANTITATIVE EVALUATION Inoculate suitable quantities of *Enterobacteriaceae enrichment broth—Mossel* with quantities of a homogenate prepared as described under Detection of bacteria, appropriately diluted as necessary, containing 1.0 g, 0.1 g and 10 mg or 1.0 ml, 0.1 ml and 10 µl of the preparation being examined. Incubate at 35° to 37° for 24 to 48 hours. Subculture each of the cultures on a plate of *violet-red bile agar with glucose and lactose* to obtain selective isolation. Incubate at 35° to 37° for 18 to 24 hours. Growth of well-developed colonies, generally red or reddish, of Gram-negative bacteria constitutes a positive result. Note the smallest quantity of the preparation that gives a positive result and the largest quantity that gives a negative result. Determine from Table 16B-1 the probable number of bacteria.

TABLE 16B-1

Results of each quantity of products			Probable number of bacteria per gram of product
1.0 g or 1.0 ml	0.1 g or 0.1 ml	0.1 g or 0.1 ml	
+	+	+	more than 10^2
+	+	–	fewer than 10^2 but more than 10
+	–	–	fewer than 10 but more than 1
–	–	–	fewer than 1

Escherichia coli

Transfer a quantity of the homogenate in *lactose broth* containing 1 g or 1 ml of the preparation being examined, prepared and incubated as for the test for Enterobacteriaceae and certain other Gram-negative bacteria, to 100 ml of *MacConkey broth* and incubate at 43° to 45° for 18 to 24 hours. Subculture on a plate of *MacConkey agar* and incubate at 43° to 45° for 18 to 24 hours. Growth of red, generally non-mucoid colonies of Gram-negative rods, sometimes surrounded by a reddish precipitation zone, indicates the possible presence of *E. coli*. This may be confirmed by the formation of indole at 43.5° to 44.5° and by other biochemical reactions. The preparation being examined passes the test if such colonies are not seen or if the confirmatory biochemical reactions are negative.

Salmonella

Incubate the solution, suspension or emulsion obtained by appropriately pretreating the preparation being examined as described above at 35° to 37° for 5 to 24 hours, as appropriate for enrichment.

Primary test Transfer 10 ml of the enrichment culture to 100 ml of *tetrathionate bile brilliant green broth* and incubate at 42° to 43° for 18 to 24 hours. Subculture on at least two of the following three agar media: *deoxycholate citrate agar*, *xylose, lysine, deoxycholate agar* and *brilliant green agar*. Incubate at 35° to 37° for 24 to 48 hours. If any colonies conforming to the description in Table 16B-2 are produced, carry out the secondary test.

Secondary test Subculture any colonies showing characteristics given in Table 16B-2 on *triple sugar iron agar* using surface and deep inoculation. (This can be done by first inoculating the surface of the slope and then making a stab culture with the same inoculating needle and incubating at 35° to 37° for 18 to 24 hours.) The presence of salmonellae is provisionally confirmed if, in the deep culture but not in the surface culture, there is a change of colour from red to yellow and usually a formation of gas, with or without production of hydrogen sulphide in the agar. Precise confirmation may be carried out by appropriate biochemical and serological tests.

The preparation being examined passes the test if, in the primary test, cultures of the type described do not appear or if, in the secondary test, the confirmatory biochemical and serological tests are negative.

TABLE 116B-2

Medium	Description of colony
Brilliant green agar	Small, transparent and colourless, or opaque, pink or white (frequently surrounded by a pink to red zone)
Deoxycholate citrate agar	Well-developed, colourless
Xylose, lysine, deoxycholate agar	Well-developed, red with or without black centres

Pseudomonas aeruginosa

Pretreat the preparation being examined as described above but using *buffered sodium chloride—peptone solution pH 7.0*, or another suitable medium shown not to have antimicrobial activity under the conditions of the test, in place of *lactose broth*. Inoculate 100 ml of *casein soya bean digest broth* with a quantity of the solution, suspension or emulsion thus obtained containing 1 g or 1 ml of the preparation being examined. Mix and incubate at 35° to 37° for 24 to 48 hours. Subculture on a plate of *cetrimide agar* and incubate at 35° to 37° for 24 to 48 hours. If no growth of micro-organisms is detected, the preparation being examined passes the test. If growth of colonies of Gram-negative rods, usually with a greenish fluorescence, occurs, apply an oxidase test and test the growth in *casein soya bean digest broth* at 42°.

The preparation being examined passes the test if cultures of the type described do not appear or if the confirmatory biochemical test is negative.

Staphylococcus aureus

Prepare an enrichment culture as described for *Ps. aeruginosa*. Subculture on a suitable medium such as *Baird-Parker agar*. Incubate at 35° to 37° for 24 to 48 hours. If no growth of micro-organisms is detected, the preparation being examined passes the test. Black colonies of Gram-positive cocci often surrounded by clear zones may indicate the presence of *S. aureus*. For catalase-positive cocci, confirmation may be obtained, for example, by coagulase and deoxyribonuclease tests.

The preparation being examined passes the test if cultures of the type described do not appear or if the confirmatory biochemical tests are negative.

Nutritive and selective properties of the media and validity of the test for specified micro-organisms

When necessary, grow separately the test strains listed in Table 16B-3 in the media indicated at 30° to 35° for 18 to 24 hours.

Dilute portions of each of the cultures using *buffered sodium chloride—peptone solution pH 7.0* to make test suspensions containing about 10^3 viable micro-organisms per ml. Mix equal volumes of each suspension and use 0.4 ml (approximately 10^2 micro-organisms of each strain) as an inoculum in tests for *E. coli*, salmonellae, *Ps. aeruginosa* and *S. aureus*, in the presence and absence of the preparation being examined if necessary. When testing the method, a positive result for the respective strain of micro-organism should be obtained.

2. TOTAL VIABLE AEROBIC COUNT
(Ph. Eur. method 2.6.12)

Pretreatment of the preparation being examined

Pretreat the preparation being examined as described under Tests for specified micro-organisms, but using *buffered sodium chloride—peptone solution pH 7.0*, or another suitable medium shown not to have antimicrobial activity under the conditions of the test, in place of *lactose broth*.

Examination of the preparation being examined

Determine the total viable aerobic count of the preparation being examined by the membrane filtration method, the plate count method or the serial dilution method as prescribed. Suitable degrees of dilution should be used so that the number of colony-forming units is within the limits suggested for the method to be used. Unless otherwise prescribed, use 10 g or 10 ml of the preparation being examined.

Membrane filtration Use membrane filters having a nominal pore size not greater than 0.45 µm the effectiveness of which in retaining bacteria has been established. For example, cellulose nitrate filters are used for aqueous, oily and weakly alcoholic solutions and cellulose acetate filters for strongly alcoholic solutions.

The technique described below assumes that filter discs about 50 mm in diameter will be used. If filters of a different diameter are used the volumes of the dilutions and the washings should be adjusted accordingly. The filtration apparatus and membrane are sterilised by appropriate means and are designed so that the solution being examined can be introduced and filtered under aseptic conditions and so as to permit the removal of the membrane for transfer to the culture medium.

Transfer 10 ml or a quantity of each dilution containing 1 g of the preparation being examined to each of two membrane filters and filter immediately. If necessary, dilute the pretreated preparation so that a colony count of 10 to 100 may be expected. Wash each membrane by filtering through it three or more successive quantities, each of approximately 100 ml, of a suitable liquid such as *buffered sodium chloride—peptone solution pH 7.0*. For fatty substances, this liquid may contain a suitable surface-active agent such as *polysorbate 20* or *polysorbate 80*. Transfer one of the membrane filters, intended primarily for the enumeration of bacteria, to the surface of a plate of *casein soya bean digest agar* and the other, intended primarily for the enumeration of fungi, to the surface of a plate of *Sabouraud glucose agar with antibiotics*.

Incubate the plates for 5 days, unless a more reliable count is obtained in a shorter time, at 30° to 35° in the test intended to detect bacteria and at 20° to 25° in the test intended to detect fungi. Count the number of colonies that are formed. Calculate the number of micro-organisms per gram or per millilitre of the preparation being examined, if necessary counting bacteria and fungi separately.

Plate count

For bacteria Using Petri dishes 9 to 10 cm in diameter, add to each dish a mixture of 1 ml of the pretreated preparation and about 15 ml of liquefied *casein soya bean digest agar* at not more than 45°. Alternatively, spread the pretreated preparation on the surface of the solidified medium in a Petri dish of the same diameter. If necessary, dilute the pretreated preparation as described above so that a colony count of not more than 300 may be expected. Prepare at least two such Petri dishes using the same dilution and incubate at 30° to 35° for 5 days, unless a more reliable count is obtained in a shorter time. Count the number of colonies that are formed. Calculate the results using plates with the greatest number of colonies but taking 300 colonies per plate as the maximum consistent with good evaluation.

For fungi Using Petri dishes 9 to 10 cm in diameter, add to each dish a mixture of 1 ml of the pretreated preparation and about 15 ml of liquefied *Sabouraud glucose agar with antibiotics* at not more than 45°. Alternatively, spread the pretreated preparation on the surface of the solidified medium in a Petri dish of the same diameter. If necessary, dilute the pretreated preparation as described above so that a colony count of not more than 100 may be expected. Prepare at least two such plates using the same dilution and incubate at 20° to 25° for 5 days, unless a more reliable count is obtained in a shorter time. Count the colonies that are formed. Calculate the results using plates with not more than 100 colonies.

Serial dilution Prepare a series of 12 tubes each containing 9 to 10 ml of *casein soya bean digest broth*. To each of the first three tubes add 1 ml of the preparation diluted, dissolved or homogenised in the proportion 1 in 10, as described above. To the next three tubes add 1 ml of a 1 in 100 dilution of the preparation and to the next three tubes add 1 ml of a 1 in 1000 dilution of the preparation.

TABLE 16B-3

Micro-organism	Strain number	Medium
Staphylococcus aureus	such as NCIMB 8625 (ATCC 6538 P, CIP 53.156) or NCIMB 9518(ATCC 6538, CIP 4.83)	Casein soya bean digest broth
Pseudomonas aeruginosa	such as NCIMB 8626 (ATCC 9027, CIP 82.118)	Casein soya bean digest broth
Escherichia coli	such as NCIMB 8545 (ATCC 8739, CIP 53.126)	Lactose broth
Salmonella typhimurium	[1]	Lactose broth
Clostridium sporogenes (for detection of Clostridia)	such as NCTC 532 (ATCC 19404, CIP 79.03)	
Clostridium perfringens (for semi-quantitive evaluation)[2]	such as NCIMB 6125 (ATCC 13124. CIP 103 409)	

[1]No strain number is recommended. A salmonella not pathogenic for man, such as *Salmonella abony* (NCTC 6017, CIP 80.39), may be used.

[2]If necessary, combine with *C. sporogenes* to check selectivity and anaerobic conditions.

To the last three tubes add 1 ml of the diluent. Incubate the tubes at 30° to 35° for at least 5 days. The last three tubes should show no microbial growth. If the reading of the results is difficult or uncertain owing to the nature of the preparation being examined, subculture on a liquid or solid medium and read the results after a further period of incubation. Determine the most probable number of micro-organisms per gram or per millilitre of the preparation being examined from Table 16B-4.

Effectiveness of culture media and validity of the counting methods

When necessary, operate as follows. Grow the following test strains separately in tubes containing *casein soya bean digest broth* at 30° to 35° for 18 to 24 hours or, for *Candida albicans*, at 20° to 25° for 48 hours.

Staphylococcus aureus such as NCIMB 8625 (ATCC 6538P, CIP 53.156) or NCIMB 9518 (ATCC 6538, CIP 4.83)

Bacillus subtilis, such as NCIMB 8054 (ATCC 6633, CIP 52.62)

Escherichia coli, such as NCIMB 8545 (ATCC 8739, CIP 53.126)

Candida albicans, such as ATCC 2091 (CIP 1180.79) or ATCC 10 231 (NCPF 3179, CIP 48.72)

Dilute portions of each of the cultures using *buffered sodium chloride—peptone solution pH 7.0* to make test suspensions containing about 100 viable micro-organisms per millilitre. Use the suspension of each of the micro-organisms separately as a control of the counting methods in the presence and absence of the preparation being examined if necessary.

When testing the method, a count for any of the test organisms differing by not more than a factor of 10 from the calculated value for the inoculum should be obtained. To test the sterility of the medium and of the diluent and the aseptic performance of the test, carry out the total viable aerobic count method using sterile *buffered sodium chloride—peptone solution pH 7.0* as the test preparation. There should be no growth of micro-organisms.

Table 16B-4

Number of tubes in microbial growth is seen for each quantity of the preparation being examined			Most probable number of micro-organisms per gram or per millilitre
100 mg or 0.1 ml per tube	10 mg or 0.01 ml per tube	1 mg or 0.001 ml per tube	
3	3	3	>1100
3	3	2	1100
3	3	1	500
3	3	0	200
3	2	3	290
3	2	2	210
3	2	1	150
3	2	0	9
3	1	3	160
3	1	2	120
3	1	1	70
3	1	0	40
3	0	3	95
3	0	2	60
3	0	1	40
3	0	0	23

Interpretation of results

If a limit is prescribed, it is to be interpreted as follows:

10^2 micro-organisms,
maximum limit of acceptance: 5×10^2;

10^3 micro-organisms,
maximum limit of acceptance: 5×10^3; *etc.*

ANNEX

Media

The following media have been found satisfactory for the purposes for which they are prescribed in the test for microbial contamination. Other media may be used if they have similar nutritive and selective properties for the micro-organisms to be tested.

Baird-Parker Agar

Pancreatic digest of casein	10.0 g
Beef extract	5.0 g
Yeast extract	1.0 g
Lithium chloride	5.0 g
Agar	20.0 g
Glycine	12.0 g
Sodium pyruvate	10.0 g
Water	950 ml

Heat to boiling for 1 minute, shaking frequently. Adjust the pH so that after sterilisation it is 6.6 to 7.0. Sterilise by heating in an autoclave at 121° for 15 minutes, cool to 45° to 50° and add 10 ml of a sterile 1% w/v solution of *potassium tellurite* and 50 ml of egg-yolk emulsion.

Violet-Red Bile Agar with Glucose and Lactose

Yeast extract	3.0 g
Pancreatic digest of gelatin	7.0 g
Bile salts	1.5 g
Lactose	10.0 g
Sodium chloride	5.0 g
D-Glucose monohydrate	10.0 g
Agar	15.0 g
Neutral red	30 mg
Crystal violet	2 mg
Water	1000 ml

Adjust the pH so that after heating it is 7.2 to 7.6. Heat to boiling but do not heat in an autoclave.

Brilliant Green Agar

Peptones (meat and casein)	10.0 g
Yeast extract	3.0 g
Sodium chloride	5.0 g
Lactose	10.0 g
Sucrose	10.0 g
Agar	20.0 g
Phenol red	80 mg
Brilliant green	12.5 mg
Water	1000 ml

Heat to boiling for 1 minute. Adjust the pH so that after sterilisation it is 6.7 to 7.1. Immediately before use, sterilise by heating in an autoclave at 121° for 15 minutes, cool to 50° and pour into Petri dishes.

Buffered Sodium Chloride—Peptone Solution pH 7.0

Potassium dihydrogen orthophosphate	3.56 g
Disodium hydrogen orthophosphate	7.23 g
Sodium chloride	4.30 g
Peptone (meat or casein)	1.0 g
Water	1000 ml

0.1 to 1.0% w/v of polysorbate 20 or polysorbate 80 may be added. Sterilise by heating in an autoclave at 121° for 15 minutes.

Casein Soya Bean Digest Agar

Pancreatic digest of casein	15.0 g
Papaic digest of soya bean	5.0 g
Sodium chloride	5.0 g
Agar	15.0 g
Water	1000 ml

Adjust the pH so that after sterilisation it is 7.1 to 7.5. Sterilise by heating in an autoclave at 121° for 15 minutes.

Casein Soya Bean Digest Broth

Pancreatic digest of casein	17.0 g
Papaic digest of soya bean	3.0 g
Sodium chloride	5.0 g
Dipotassium hydrogen orthophosphate	2.5 g
D-Glucose monohydrate	2.5 g
Water	1000 ml

Adjust the pH so that after sterilisation it is 7.1 to 7.5. Sterilise by heating in an autoclave at 121° for 15 minutes.

Cetrimide Agar

Pancreatic digest of gelatin	20.0 g
Magnesium chloride	1.4 g
Potassium sulphate	10.0 g
Cetrimide	0.3 g
Agar	13.6 g
Glycerol	10.0 ml
Water	1000 ml

Heat to boiling for 1 minute with shaking. Adjust the pH so that after sterilisation it is 7.0 to 7.4. Sterilise by heating in an autoclave at 121° for 15 minutes.

Reinforced Medium for Clostridia

Beef extract	10.0 g
Peptone	10.0 g
Yeast extract	3.0 g
Soluble starch	1.0 g
D-Glucose monohydrate	5.0 g
Cysteine hydrochloride	0.5 g
Sodium chloride	5.0 g
Sodium acetate	3.0 g
Agar	0.5 g
Water	1000 ml

Hydrate the agar, dissolve by heating to boiling with continuous stirring. If necessary, adjust the pH so that after sterilisation it is about 6.8. Sterilise by heating in an autoclave at 121° for 15 minutes.

Columbia Agar

Pancreatic digest of casein	10.0 g
Meat peptic digest	5.0 g
Heart pancreatic digest	3.0 g
Yeast extract	5.0 g
Maize starch	1.0 g
Sodium chloride	5.0 g
Agar according to gelling power	10.0 to 15.0 g
Water	1000 ml

Hydrate the agar, dissolve by heating to boiling with continous stirring. If necessary, adjust the pH so that after sterilisation it is 7.1 to 7.5. Sterilise by heating in an autoclave at 121° for 15 minutes. Allow to cool to 45° to 50°, add, where necessary, gentamicin sulphate corresponding to 20 mg of gentamicin base and pour into Petri dishes.

Deoxycholate Citrate Agar

Beef extract	10.0 g
Meat peptone	10.0 g
Lactose	10.0 g
Sodium citrate	20.0 g
Iron(III) citrate	1.0 g
Sodium deoxycholate	5.0 g
Agar	13.5 g
Neutral red	20 mg
Water	1000 ml

Adjust the pH so that after heating it is 7.1 to 7.5. Heat gently to boiling and boil for 1 minute, cool to 50° and pour into Petri dishes; do not heat in an autoclave.

Enterobacteriaceae Enrichment Broth—Mossel

Pancreatic digest of gelatin	10.0 g
D-Glucose monohydrate	5.0 g
Dehydrated ox bile	20.0 g
Potassium dihydrogen orthophosphate	2.0 g
Disodium hydrogen orthophosphate	8.0 g
Brilliant green	15 mg
Water	1000 ml

Adjust the pH so that after heating it is 7.0 to 7.4. Heat at 100° for 30 minutes and cool immediately.

Lactose Broth

Beef extract	3.0 g
Pancreatic digest of gelatin	5.0 g
Lactose	5.0 g
Water	1000 ml

Adjust the pH so that after sterilisation it is 6.7 to 7.1. Sterilise by heating in an autoclave at 121° for 15 minutes and cool immediately.

Lactose Sulphite Medium

Pancreatic digest of casein	5.0 g
Yeast extract	2.5 g
Sodium chloride	2.5 g
Lactose	10.0 g
Cysteine hydrochloride	0.3 g
Purified water	1000 ml

Dissolve, adjust to pH 7.0 to 7.2 and fill to 8 ml in 16 mm × 160 mm tubes containing a small Durham tube. Sterilise by heating in an autoclave at 121° for 15 minutes and store at 4°.

Before use, heat the medium for 5 minutes in a water bath and cool. Add to each tube 0.5 ml of a 1.2% w/v solution of sodium metabisulphite and 0.5 ml of a 1.0% w/v solution of ammonium iron(III) citrate both solutions being freshly prepared and filtered through membranes (pore size: 0.45 µm).

MacConkey Agar

Pancreatic digest of gelatin	17.0 g
Peptones (meat and casein)	3.0 g
Lactose	10.0 g
Sodium chloride	5.0 g
Bile salts	1.5 g
Agar	13.5 g

Neutral red	30 mg
Crystal violet	1 mg
Water	1000 ml

Adjust the pH so that after sterilisation it is 6.9 to 7.3. Boil for 1 minute with constant shaking then sterilise by heating in an autoclave at 121° for 15 minutes.

3.TEST FOR ABSENCE OF MYCOPLASMAS

(Ph. Eur. method 2.6.7 as applied to vaccines for human use)

Where the test for mycoplasmas is prescribed for a master cell bank, for a working cell bank, for a virus seed lot or for control cells, both the culture method and the indicator cell culture method are used. Where the test for mycoplasmas is prescribed for a virus harvest, for a bulk vaccine or for the final lot (batch), the culture method is used. The indicator cell culture method may also be used, where necessary, for screening of media.

Culture method

Choice of culture media The test is carried out using a sufficient number of both solid and liquid media to ensure growth in the chosen incubation conditions of small numbers of mycoplasmas that may be present in the product being examined. Liquid media must contain phenol red. The range of media chosen is shown to have satisfactory nutritive properties for at least the organisms shown below. The nutritive properties of each new batch of medium are verified for the appropriate organisms in the list.

Acholeplasma laidlawii (vaccines where an antibiotic has been used during production)
Mycoplasma gallisepticum (where avian material has been used during production)
Mycoplasma orale
Mycoplasma pneumoniae or other suitable species of D-glucose fermenter
Mycoplasma synoviae (where avian material has been used during production).

The test strains are field isolates having undergone not more than fifteen subcultures and are stored frozen or freeze-dried. After cloning the strains are identified as being of the required species by a suitable method, by comparison with type cultures, for example:

A. laidlawii	NCTC 10116	CIP 75.27	ATCC 23206
M. gallisepticum	NCTC 10115	CIP 104967	ATCC 19610
M. orale	NCTC 10112	CIP 104969	ATCC 23714
M. pneumoniae	NCTC 10119	CIP 103766	ATCC 15531
M. synoviae	NCTC 10124	CIP 104970	ATCC 25204

Incubation conditions Divide inoculated media into two equal parts and incubate one in aerobic conditions and the other in microaerophilic conditions; for solid media maintain an atmosphere of adequate humidity to prevent desiccation of the surface. For aerobic conditions, incubate in an atmosphere of air containing, for solid media, 5 to 10% of carbon dioxide. For microaerophilic conditions, incubate in an atmosphere of nitrogen containing, for solid media, 5 to 10% of carbon dioxide.

Nutritive properties *Carry out the test for nutritive properties for each new batch of medium.* Inoculate the chosen media with the appropriate test organisms; use not more than 100 colony-forming units per 60 mm plate containing 9 ml of solid medium and not more than 40 colony-forming units per 100 ml container of the corresponding liquid medium; use a separate plate and container for each species of organism. Incubate the media in the conditions that will be used for the test of the product being examined (aerobically, microaerophilically or both, depending on the requirements of the test organism). The media comply with the test for nutritive properties if there is adequate growth of the test organisms accompanied by an appropriate colour change in liquid media.

Inhibitory substances Carry out the test for nutritive properties in the presence of the product being examined. If growth of the test organisms is notably less than that found in the absence of the product being examined, the latter contains inhibitory substances that must be neutralised (or their effect otherwise countered, for example, by dilution) before the test for mycoplasmas is carried out. The effectiveness of the neutralisation or other process is checked by repeating the test for inhibitory substances after neutralisation.

Test for mycoplasmas in the product being examined For solid media, use plates 60 mm in diameter and containing 9 ml of medium. Inoculate each of not fewer than two plates of each solid medium with 0.2 ml of the product being examined and inoculate 10 ml per 100 ml of each liquid medium. Incubate at 35° to 38°, aerobically and microaerophilically, for 21 days and at the same time incubate an uninoculated 100 ml portion of each liquid medium for use as a control. If any significant pH change occurs on addition of the product being examined, restore the liquid medium to its original pH value by the addition of a solution of either sodium hydroxide or hydrochloric acid. On the first, second or third day after inoculation subculture each liquid culture by inoculating each of two plates of each solid medium with 0.2 ml and incubating at 35° to 38° aerobically and microaerophilically for not less than 21 days. Repeat the procedure on the sixth, seventh or eighth day and again on the thirteenth or fourteenth day of the test. Observe the liquid media every 2 or 3 days and if any colour change occurs subculture immediately. Observe solid media once per week.

If the liquid media show bacterial or fungal contamination, repeat the test. If, not earlier than 7 days after inoculation, not more than one plate at each stage of the test is accidentally contaminated with bacteria or fungi, or broken, that plate may be ignored provided that on immediate examination it shows no evidence of mycoplasmal growth. If, at any stage of the test, more than one plate is accidentally contaminated with bacteria or fungi, or broken, the test is invalid and must be repeated.

Include in the test positive controls prepared by inoculating not more than 100 colony-forming units of suitable species such as *M. orale* and *M. pneumoniae.*

At the end of the incubation periods, examine all the inoculated solid media microscopically for the presence of mycoplasmas. The product passes the test if growth of mycoplasmas has not occurred in any of the inoculated media. If growth of mycoplasmas has occurred, the test may be repeated once using twice the amount of inoculum, media and plates; if growth of mycoplasmas does not occur, the product complies with the test. The test is invalid if the positive controls do not show growth of the relevant test organism.

Indicator cell culture method

Cell cultures are stained with a fluorescent dye that binds to DNA. Mycoplasmas are detected by their characteristic particulate or filamentous pattern of fluorescence on the cell surface and, if contamination is heavy, in surrounding areas.

Verification of the substrate Using a Vero cell culture substrate, pre-test the procedure using an inoculum of not more than 100 CFU (colony-forming units) of a strain growing readily in liquid or solid medium and demonstrate its ability to detect potential mycoplasma contaminants such as suitable strains of *Mycoplasma orale*. A different cell substrate may be used, for example the production cell line, if it has been demonstrated that it will provide at least equal sensitivity for the detection of potential mycoplasma contaminants.

Test method Take not less than 1 ml of the product being examined and use it to inoculate in duplicate, as described under Procedure, indicator cell cultures representing not less than 25 cm^2 of cell culture area at confluence.

Include in the test a negative (non-infected) control and two positive mycoplasma controls, such as *M. orale* and another suitable species. Use an inoculum of not more than 100 CFU for the positive controls.

If for viral suspensions the interpretation of results is affected by marked cytopathic effects, the virus may be neutralised using a specific antiserum that has no inhibitory effects on mycoplasmas or a cell culture substrate that does not allow growth of the virus may be used. To demonstrate the absence of inhibitory effects of serum, carry out the positive control tests in the presence and absence of the antiserum.

Procedure

1. Seed culture at a regular density (2×10^4 to 2×10^5 cells/ml, 4×10^3 to 2.5×10^4 cells/cm^2) and incubate at 36°±1° for at least 2 days. Inoculate the product being examined and incubate for at least 2 days; make not fewer than one subculture. Grow the last subculture on coverslips in suitable containers or on some other surface suitable for the test procedure. Do not allow the last subculture to reach confluence since this would inhibit staining and impair visualisation of mycoplasmas.
2. Remove and discard the medium.
3. Rinse the monolayer with *phosphate buffered saline pH 7.4*, then with a mixture of equal volumes of *phosphate buffered saline pH 7.4* and a suitable fixing solution and finally with the fixing solution; when *bisbenzimide* is used for staining, a freshly prepared mixture of 1 volume of *glacial acetic acid* and 3 volumes of *methanol* is a suitable fixing solution.
4. Add the fixing solution and allow to stand for 10 min.
5. Remove the fixing solution and discard.
6. If the monolayer is to be stained later, dry it completely. (Particular care is needed for staining of the slides after drying because of artefacts that may be produced.)
7. If the monolayer is to be stained directly, wash off the fixing solution twice with sterile water and discard the wash.
8. Add *bisbenzimide working solution* or some other suitable DNA staining agent and allow to stand for 10 minutes.
9. Remove the stain and rinse the monolayer with water.
10. Mount each coverslip, where applicable, with a drop of a mixture of equal volumes of *glycerol* and *phosphate-citrate buffer solution pH 5.5*; blot off surplus mountant from the edge of the coverslip.
11. Examine by epifluorescence (330 nm/380 nm excitation filter, LP 440 nm barrier filter) at 100–400 × magnification or greater.
12. Compare the microscopic appearance of the test cultures with that of the negative and positive controls, examining for extranuclear fluorescence. Mycoplasmas give pinpoints or filaments over the cytoplasm and sometimes in intercellular spaces.

The product being examined complies with the test if there is no evidence of the presence of mycoplasmas in the test cultures inoculated with it. The test is invalid if the positive controls do not show the presence of the appropriate test organisms.

The following section is given for information and guidance; it does not form a mandatory part of the general method.

Recommended media for the culture method

The following media are recommended. Other media may be used providing their ability to sustain the growth of mycoplasmas has been demonstrated on each batch in the presence and absence of the product being examined.

I. Recommended media for the detection of *Mycoplasma gallisepticum*

(a) *Liquid medium*

Beef heart infusion broth (1)	90.0 ml
Horse serum (unheated)	20.0 ml
Yeast extract (250 g/l)	10.0 ml
Thallium acetate (10 g/l solution)	1.0 ml
Phenol red (0.6 g/l solution)	5.0 ml
Penicillin (20 000 I.U. per millilitre)	0.25 ml
Deoxyribonucleic acid (2 g/l solution)	1.2 ml

Adjust to pH 7.8.

(b) *Solid medium*

Prepare as described above replacing beef heart infusion broth by beef heart infusion agar containing 15 g/l of agar.

II. Recommended media for the detection of *Mycoplasma synoviae*

(a) *Liquid medium*

Beef heart infusion broth (1)	90.0 ml
Essential vitamins (2)	0.025 ml
Glucose monohydrate (500 g/l solution)	2.0 ml
Swine serum (inactivated at 56° for 30 minutes)	12.0 ml
β-Nicotinamide adenine dinucleotide (10 g/l solution)	1.0 ml
Cysteine hydrochloride (10 g/l solution)	1.0 ml
Phenol red (0.6 g/l solution)	5.0 ml
Penicillin (20,000 I.U. per millilitre)	0.25 ml

Mix the solutions of β-nicotinamide adenine dinucleotide and cysteine hydrochloride and after 10 minutes add to the other ingredients. Adjust to pH 7.8.

(b) *Solid medium*

Beef heart infusion broth (1)	90.0 ml
Ionagar (3)	1.4 g

Adjust to pH 7.8, sterilise by autoclaving then add:

Essential vitamins (2)	0.025 ml
Glucose monohydrate (500 g/l solution)	2.0 ml
Swine serum (unheated)	12.0 ml
β-Nicotinamide adenine dinucleotide (10 g/l solution)	1.0 ml
Cysteine hydrochloride (10 g/l solution)	1.0 ml
Phenol red (0.6 g/l solution)	5.0 ml
Penicillin (20,000 I.U. per millilitre)	0.25 ml

III. Recommended media for the detection of non-avian mycoplasmas

(a) *Liquid medium*

Hanks' balanced salt solution (modified) (4)	800 ml
Distilled water	67 ml
Brain heart infusion (5)	135 ml
PPLO Broth (6)	248 ml
Yeast extract (170 g/l)	60 ml
Bacitracin	250 mg
Meticillin	250 mg
Phenol red (5 g/l)	4.5 ml
Thallium acetate (56 g/l)	3 ml
Horse serum	165 ml
Swine serum	165 ml

Adjust to pH 7.4–7.45.

(b) *Solid medium*

Hanks' balanced salt solution (modified) (4)	200 ml
DEAE-dextran	200 mg
Ionagar (3)	15.65 g

Mix well and sterilise by autoclaving. Cool to 100°. Add to 1740 ml of liquid medium as described above.

(1) *Beef heart infusion broth*

Beef heart (for preparation of the infusion)	500 g
Peptone	10 g
Sodium chloride	5 g
Distilled water	to 1000 ml

Sterilise by autoclaving.

(2) *Essential vitamins*

Biotin	100 mg
Calcium pantothenate	100 mg
Choline chloride	100 mg
Folic acid	100 mg
i-Inositol	200 mg
Nicotinamide	100 mg
Pyridoxal hydrochloride	100 mg
Riboflavine	10 mg
Thiamine hydrochloride	100 mg
Distilled water	to 1000 mg

(3) *Ionagar*

A highly refined agar for use in microbiology and immunology prepared by an ion-exchange procedure which results in a product having superior purity, clarity and gel strength. It contains about:

Water	12.2%
Ash	1.5%
Acid-insoluble ash	0.2%
Phosphate (calculated as P_2O_5)	0.3%
Total nitrogen	0.3%
Copper	8 ppm
Iron	170 ppm
Calcium	0.28%
Magnesium	0.32%

(4) *Hanks' balanced salt solution (modified)*

Sodium chloride	6.4 g
Potassium chloride	0.32 g
Magnesium sulphate heptahydrate	0.08 g
Magnesium chloride hexahydrate	0.08 g
Calcium chloride, anhydrous	0.112 g
Disodium hydrogen phosphate dihydrate	0.0596 g
Potassium dihydrogen phosphate, anhydrous	0.048 g
Distilled water	to 800 ml

(5) *Brain heart infusion*

Calf-brain infusion	200 g
Beef-heart infusion	250 g
Proteose peptone	10 g
Glucose	2 g
Sodium chloride	5 g
Disodium hydrogen phosphate, anhydrous	2.5 g
Distilled water	to 1000 ml

(6) *PPLO broth*

Beef-heart infusion	50 g
Peptone	10 g
Sodium chloride	5 g
Distilled water	to 1000 ml

4. MYCOBACTERIA

(*Ph. Eur. Method 2.6.2*)

If the sample being examined may be contaminated by micro-organisms other than mycobacteria, treat it with a suitable decontamination solution, such as acetylcysteine-NaOH solution or sodium lauryl sulphate solution.

Inoculate 0.2 ml of the sample in triplicate onto each of two suitable solid media (Löwenstein-Jensen medium and Middlebrook 7H10 medium are considered suitable). Inoculate 0.5 ml in triplicate into a suitable liquid medium. Incubate all media at 37° for 56 days.

Establish the fertility of the media in the presence of the preparation being examined by inoculation of a suitable strain of *Mycobacterium tuberculosis* such as BCG and if necessary use a suitable neutralising substance.

If contaminating micro-organisms develop during the first 8 days of incubation, repeat the test and carry out at the same time a bacteriological sterility test.

If at the end of the incubation time no growth of mycobacteria occurs in any of the test media, the preparation complies with the test.

5. EXTRANEOUS AGENTS IN VIRAL VACCINES

(*Ph. Eur. method 2.6.16*)

In those tests that require prior neutralisation of the virus, use specific antibodies of non-human, non-simian origin; if the virus has been propagated in avian tissues, the antibodies must also be of non-avian origin. To prepare antiserum, use an immunising antigen produced in cell culture from a species different from that used for the production of the vaccine and free from extraneous agents. Where the use of SPF eggs is prescribed, the eggs comply with the requirements prescribed above under Chicken flocks free from specified pathogens for the production and quality control of vaccines, Appendix XV H.

Virus seed lot

Take samples of the virus seed lot at the time of harvesting and, if not tested immediately, keep them at a temperature below –40°.

Adult mice Inoculate each of at least 10 adult mice, each weighing 15 g to 20 g, intracerebrally with 0.03 ml and intraperitoneally with 0.5 ml of the virus seed lot. Observe the mice for at least 21 days. Carry out autopsy of all mice that die after the first 24 hours of the test or that show signs of illness and examine for evidence of viral infection, both by direct macroscopical observation and by subinoculation of appropriate tissue suspensions by the intracerebral and intraperitoneal routes into at least five additional mice which are observed for 21 days. The virus seed lot complies with the test if no mouse shows evidence of infection attributable to the seed lot. The test is not valid unless at least 80% of the original inoculated mice survive the observation period.

Suckling mice Inoculate each of at least 20 mice, less than 24 hours old, intracerebrally with 0.01 ml and intraperitoneally with at least 0.1 ml of the virus seed lot. Observe the mice daily for at least 14 days. Carry out autopsy of all mice that die after the first 24 hours of the test or that show signs of illness and examine for evidence of viral infection, both by direct macroscopical observation and by subinoculation of appropriate tissue suspensions by the intracerebral and intraperitoneal routes into at least five additional suckling mice which are observed daily for 14 days. The virus seed lot passes the test if no mouse shows evidence of infection attributable to the seed lot. The test is not valid unless at least 80% of the original inoculated mice survive the observation period.

Guinea-pigs Inoculate intraperitoneally into each of at least five guinea pigs, each weighing 350 g to 450 g, 5 ml of the virus seed lot. Observe the animals for at least 42 days for signs of disease. Carry out autopsy of all guinea-pigs that die after the first 24 hours of the test, or that show signs of illness and examine macroscopically; examine the tissues both microscopically and culturally for evidence of infection. Kill animals that survive the observation period and examine in a similar manner. The virus seed lot passes the test if no guinea-pig shows evidence of infection attributable to the seed lot. The test is not valid unless at least 80% of the guinea-pigs survive the observation period.

Virus seed lot and virus harvest

Take samples at the time of harvesting and, if not tested immediately, keep them at a temperature below –40°.

Bacterial and fungal sterility A 10-ml sample complies with the test for sterility, Appendix XVI A.

Mycoplasmas A 10-ml sample complies with the test for mycoplasmas, Appendix XVI B3; use only the method for non-avian mycoplasmas and ureaplasmas unless avian material has been used in production.

Mycobacteria A 5-ml sample is tested for the presence of *Mycobacterium* spp. by culture methods known to be sensitive for the detection of these organisms. Use the method described in Appendix XVI B4.

Other extraneous agents *(test in cell culture)* Samples equivalent, unless otherwise prescribed, to 500 doses of vaccine or 50 ml, whichever is the greater, are tested for the presence of extraneous agents by inoculation into continuous simian kidney and human cell cultures. If the virus is grown in human diploid cells, the neutralised virus harvest is also tested on a separate culture of the diploid cells. If the vaccine virus is grown in a cell system other than simian or human, cells of that species, from a separate culture, are also inoculated. The cells are incubated at 35° to 37° and observed for a period of 14 days. The virus seed lot or harvest passes the tests if none of the cell cultures show evidence of the presence of any extraneous agents not attributable to accidental contamination. The test is not valid unless at least 80% of the cell cultures remain viable.

Avian viruses *(required only for virus propagated in avian tissues)* Neutralise a sample equivalent to 100 doses or 10 ml, whichever is the greater. Using 0.5 ml per egg, inoculate a group of fertilised SPF eggs, 9 to 11 days old, by the allantoic route and a second group, 5 to 7 days old, into the yolk sac. Incubate for 7 days. The virus seed lot or harvest complies with the test if the allantoic and yolk sac fluids show no sign of the presence of any haemagglutinating agent and if all embryos and chorio-allantoic membranes, examined for gross pathology, are normal. The test is not valid unless at least 80% of the inoculated eggs survive for 7 days.

Production cell culture: control cells

Examine the control cells microscopically for freedom from any virus causing cytopathic degeneration throughout the time of incubation of the inoculated production cell cultures or for not less than 14 days beyond the time of inoculation of the production vessels, whichever is the longer. The test is not valid unless at least 80% of the control cell cultures survive to the end of the observation period.

At 14 days or at the time of the last virus harvest, whichever is the longer, carry out the tests described below.

Haemadsorbing viruses Examine not fewer than 25% of the control cultures for the presence of haemadsorbing viruses by the addition of guinea pig red blood cells. If the guinea pig red blood cells have been stored, they shall have been stored at 2° to 8° for not more than 7 days. Read half of the cultures after incubation at 2° to 8° for 30 minutes and the other half after incubation at 20° to 25° for 30 minutes. No evidence of haemadsorbing agents is found.

Other extraneous agents *(tests in cell cultures)* Pool the supernatant fluids from the control cells and examine for the presence of extraneous agents by inoculation of simian kidney and human cell cultures. If the vaccine virus is grown in a cell system other than simian or human, cells of that species, but from a separate culture, are also inoculated. In each cell system, at least 5 ml is tested. Incubate the inoculated cultures at a temperature of 35° to 37° and observe for a period of 14 days. No evidence of extraneous agents is found.

Avian leucosis viruses (required only if the virus is propagated in avian tissues) Carry out a test for avian leucosis viruses using 5 ml of the supernatant fluid from the control cells.

Control eggs

Haemagglutinating agents Examine 0.25 ml of the allantoic fluid from each egg for haemagglutinating agents by mixing directly with chicken red blood cells and after a passage in SPF eggs carried out as follows: inoculate a 5-ml sample of the pooled amniotic fluids from the control eggs in 0.5 ml volumes into the allantoic cavity and into the amniotic cavity of SPF eggs. The control eggs comply with the test if no evidence of the presence of haemagglutinating agents is found in either test.

Avian leucosis viruses Use a 10-ml sample of the pooled amniotic fluids from the control eggs. Carry out amplification by five passages in leucosis-free, chick-embryo cell cultures; carry out a test for avian leucosis using cells from the fifth passage. The control eggs comply with the test if no evidence of the presence of avian leucosis viruses is found.

Other extraneous agents Inoculate 5-ml samples of the pooled amniotic fluids from the control eggs into human and simian cell cultures. Observe the cell cultures for 14 days. The control eggs comply with the test if no evidence of the presence of extraneous agents is found. The test is not valid unless 80% of the inoculated cultures survive to the end of the observation period.

C. Efficacy of Antimicrobial Preservation

(Ph. Eur. general text 5.1.3)

Guidelines concerning the use of this test are reproduced in Supplementary Chapter I J.

If a pharmaceutical preparation does not itself have adequate antimicrobial activity, antimicrobial preservatives may be added, particularly to aqueous preparations, to prevent proliferation or to limit microbial contamination which, during normal conditions of storage and use, particularly for multidose containers, could occur in a product and present a hazard to the patient from infection and spoilage of the preparation. Antimicrobial preservatives must not be used as a substitute for good manufacturing practice.

The efficacy of an antimicrobial preservative may be enhanced or diminished by the active constituent of the preparation or by the formulation in which it is incorporated or by the container and closure used. The antimicrobial activity of the preparation in its final container is investigated over the claimed shelf-life (period of validity) to ensure that such activity has not been impaired by storage. Such investigations may be carried out on samples removed from the container immediately prior to testing.

During development of a pharmaceutical preparation, it shall be demonstrated that the antimicrobial activity of the preparation as such or, if necessary, with the addition of a suitable preservative or preservatives, provides adequate protection from adverse effects that may arise from microbial contamination or proliferation during storage and use of the preparation.

The efficacy of the antimicrobial activity may be demonstrated by the test described below. The test is not intended to be used for routine control purposes.

The test consists of challenging the preparation, wherever possible in its final container, with a prescribed inoculum of suitable micro-organisms, storing the inoculated preparation at a prescribed temperature, withdrawing samples from the container at specified intervals of time and counting the organisms in the samples so removed.

The preservative properties of the preparation are adequate if, in the conditions of the test, there is a significant fall or no increase, as appropriate, in the number of micro-organisms in the inoculated preparation after the times and at the temperatures prescribed. The criteria of acceptance, in terms of decrease in the number of micro-organisms with time, vary for different types of preparation according to the degree of protection intended as shown in the appropriate Table below.

Test organisms

Aspergillus niger IMI 149 007 (ATCC 16404, IP 1431.83)
Candida albicans NCPF 3179 (ATCC 10231, IP 48.72)
Pseudomonas aeruginosa NCIMB 8626 (ATCC 9027, CIP 82.118)
Staphylococcus aureus NCTC 10788 (NCIMB 9518, ATCC 6538, CIP 4.83)

Single-strain challenges are used and the designated micro-organisms are supplemented by other strains or species that may represent likely contaminants to the preparation. For example, *Escherichia coli* [NCIMB 8545 (ATCC 8739, CIP 53.126)] is used for all oral preparations and *Zygosaccharomyces rouxii* [NCYC 381 (IP 2021.92)] for oral preparations containing a high concentration of sugar.

Preparation of inoculum

Preparatory to the test, inoculate the surface of a *tryptone soya agar* plate for bacteria or *Sabouraud agar* plate for fungi, with the recently grown stock culture of each of the specified micro-organisms. Incubate the bacterial cultures at 30° to 35° for 18 to 24 hours, the culture of *Candida albicans* at 20° to 25° for 48 hours, and the culture of *Aspergillus niger* at 20° to 25° for 7 days or until good sporulation is obtained. Subcultures may be needed after revival before the organism is in its optimal state, but it is recommended that the number of subcultures be kept to a minimum.

To harvest the bacterial and *Candida albicans* cultures, use a sterile suspending fluid containing 0.9% w/v of *sodium chloride* and 0.1% w/v of *peptone* for dispersal and transfer of the surface growth into a suitable vessel. Add sufficient suspending fluid to reduce the microbial count to about 10^8 micro-organisms per ml. To harvest the *Aspergillus niger* culture, use a sterile suspending fluid containing 0.9% w/v of *sodium chloride* and 0.05% w/v of *polysorbate 80* and adjust the spore count to about 10^8 per ml by adding the same solution.

Remove immediately a suitable sample from each suspension and determine the number of colony-forming units per ml in each suspension by plate count or by membrane filtration, Appendix XVI B2. This value serves to determine the inoculum and the baseline to use in the test. The suspensions shall be used immediately.

Test procedure

To count the viable micro-organisms in the inoculated products, use the agar medium used for the initial cultivation of the respective micro-organisms.

Inoculate a series of containers of the product to be examined, each with a suspension of one of the test organisms to give an inoculum of 10^5 to 10^6 micro-organisms per g or per ml of the preparation. The volume of the suspension of inoculum does not exceed 1% of the volume of the product. Mix thoroughly to ensure homogeneous distribution.

Maintain the inoculated product at 20° to 25°, protected from light. Remove a suitable sample from each container, typically 1-ml or 1-g quantities, at zero hour and at appropriate intervals according to the type of the product and determine the number of viable micro-organisms by plate count or membrane filtration,

Appendix XVI B2. Ensure that any residual antimicrobial activity of the product is eliminated by dilution, by filtration or by the use of a specific inactivator. When dilution procedures are used, due allowance is made for the reduced sensitivity in the recovery of small numbers of viable micro-organisms. When a specific inactivator is used, the ability of the system to support the growth of the test organisms is confirmed by the use of appropriate controls.

The procedure is validated to verify its ability to demonstrate the required reduction in count of viable micro-organisms.

Criteria of acceptance

The criteria for evaluation of antimicrobial activity are given in the appropriate table below in terms of the log reduction in the number of viable micro-organisms using as baseline the value obtained for the inoculum.

TABLE 16C-1 Parenteral and Ophthalmic Preparations

		Log reduction				
		6 h	24 h	7 d	14 d	28 d
Bacteria	A	2	3	–	–	NR
	B	–	1	3	–	NI
Fungi	A	–	–	2	–	NI
	B	–	–	–	2	NI

The A criteria express the recommended efficacy to be achieved. In justified cases where the A criteria cannot be attained, for example, for reasons of an increased risk of adverse reactions, the B criteria must be satisfied.

NI: no increase
NR: no recovery

TABLE 16C-2 Oral Preparations

	Log reduction	
	14 d	28 d
Bacteria	3	NI
Fungi	1	NI

The above criteria express the recommended efficacy to be achieved.

NI: no increase
NR: no recovery

TABLE 16C-3 Topical Preparations

	Log reduction			
	48 h	7 d	14 d	28 d
Bacteria	3	NR	NR	NR
Fungi	–	–	2	NR

The A criteria express the recommended efficacy to be achieved. In justified cases where the A criteria cannot be attained, for example, for reasons of an increased risk of adverse reactions, the B criteria must be satisfied.

NI: No increase

TABLE 16C-4 Ear Preparations

	Log reduction				
	6 h	24 h	7 d	14 d	28 d
Bacteria	2	3	–	–	NR
Fungi	–	–	2	–	NI

In the absence of any criteria for ear preparations in the European Pharmacopoeia, the above criteria express the recommended efficacy to be achieved.

NI: no increase
NR: no recovery

ANNEX

Media

Tryptone soya agar (casein soya bean digest agar)

Pancreatic digest of casein	15.0 g
Papaic digest of soya bean	5.0 g
Sodium chloride	5.0 g
Agar	15.0 g
Water	1000 ml

Dissolve the ingredients in the water, filter, adjust to give an expected pH after sterilisation of 7.1 to 7.5 and sterilise by heating in an autoclave at 121° for 15 minutes.

Sabouraud agar (Sabouraud glucose agar)

D-Glucose monohydrate	40.0 g
Peptones (meat and casein)	10.0 g
Agar	15.0 g
Water	1000 ml

Dissolve the ingredients in the water, adjust to give an expected pH after sterilisation of 5.4 to 5.8 and sterilise by heating in an autoclave at 121° for 15 minutes.

D. Microbial Quality of Pharmaceutical Preparations

(Ph. Eur. general text 5.1.4)

This text is published for information and does not form a mandatory part of the Pharmacopoeia.

In the manufacture, packaging, storage and distribution of pharmaceutical preparations, suitable means must be taken to ensure their microbial quality. The pharmaceutical preparations should comply with the criteria given below.

CATEGORY 1: Preparations required to be sterile by the relevant monograph on the dosage form and other preparations labelled sterile

Sterility Comply with the *test for sterility*, Appendix XVI A.

CATEGORY 2: Preparations for topical use and for use in the respiratory tract except where required to be sterile

(a) Total viable aerobic count. Not more than a total of 10^2 aerobic bacteria and fungi per gram or per millilitre, Appendix XVI B2.

(b) Not more than 10^1 enterobacteriaceae and certain other Gram-negative bacteria per gram or per millilitre, Appendix XVI B1.

(c) Absence of *Pseudomonas aeruginosa* (1.0 g or 1.0 ml), Appendix XVI B1.
(d) Absence of *Staphylococcus aureus* (1.0 g or 1.0 ml), Appendix XVI B1.

CATEGORY 3

A. Preparations for oral and rectal administration

(a) Total viable aerobic count. Not more than 10^3 aerobic bacteria and not more than 10^2 fungi per gram or per millilitre, Appendix XVI B2.
(b) Absence of *Escherichia coli* (1.0 g or 1.0 ml), Appendix XVI B1.

B. Preparations for oral administration containing raw materials of natural origin (animal, vegetable or mineral) for which antimicrobial pretreatment is not feasible and for which the competent authority accepts a microbial contamination of the raw material exceeding 10^3 viable micro-organisms per gram or per millilitre. Herbal remedies described in category 4 are excluded.

(a) Total viable aerobic count. Not more than 10^4 aerobic bacteria and not more than 10^2 fungi per gram or per millilitre, Appendix XVI B2.
(b) Not more than 10^2 enterobacteriaceae and certain other Gram-negative bacteria per gram or per millilitre, Appendix XVI B1.
(c) Absence of *Salmonella* (10.0 g or 10.0 ml), Appendix XVI B1.
(d) Absence of *Escherichia coli* (1.0 g or 1.0 ml), Appendix XVI B1.
(e) Absence of *Staphylococcus aureus* (1.0 g or 1.0 ml), Appendix XVI B1.

CATEGORY 4: Herbal remedies consisting solely of one or more vegetable drugs (whole, reduced or powdered)

A. Herbal remedies to which boiling water is added before use

(a) Total viable aerobic count. Not more than 10^7 aerobic bacteria and not more than 10^5 fungi per gram or per millilitre, Appendix XVI B2.
(b) Not more than 10^2 *Escherichia coli* per gram or per millilitre, Appendix XVI B1, using suitable dilutions.

B. Herbal remedies to which boiling water is not added before use

(a) Total viable aerobic count. Not more than 10^5 aerobic bacteria and not more than 10^4 fungi per gram or per millilitre, Appendix XVI B2.
(b) Not more than 10^3 enterobacteriaceae and certain other Gram-negative bacteria per gram or per millilitre, Appendix XVI B1.
(c) Absence of *Escherichia coli* (1.0 g or 1.0 ml), Appendix XVI B1.
(d) Absence of *Salmonella* (10.0 g or 10.0 ml), Appendix XVI B1.

Appendix XVII

A. Particle Size of Powders

1. PARTICLE SIZE CLASSIFICATION OF POWDERS

(Ph. Eur. method 2.9.12)

The degree of fineness of a powder may be expressed by reference to sieves which comply with the specifications for non-analytical sieves (Appendix XVII B1).

Where the degree of fineness of powders is determined by sieving, it is defined in relation to the sieve number(s) used either by means of the following terms or, where such terms cannot be used, by expressing the fineness of the powder as a percentage w/w passing the sieve(s) used.

If a single sieve number is given, not less than 97% of the powder passes through the sieve of that number, unless otherwise prescribed.

Assemble the sieves and operate in a suitable manner until sifting is practically complete. Weigh the separated fractions of the powder.

The following terms are used in the description of powders:

Coarse powder Not less than 95% by weight passes through a number 1400 sieve and not more than 40% by weight passes through a number 355 sieve.

Moderately fine powder Not less than 95% by weight passes through a number 355 sieve and not more than 40% by weight passes through a number 180 sieve.

Fine powder Not less than 95% by weight passes through a number 180 sieve and not more than 40% by weight passes through a number 125 sieve.

Very fine powder Not less than 95% by weight passes through a number 125 sieve and not more than 40% by weight passes through a number 90 sieve.

Additional points for monographs other than those of the European Pharmacopoeia

Within the monographs of the British Pharmacopoeia, the above terms may be used to specify the degree of coarseness or fineness of a medicinal or pharmaceutical substance in powder form that is to be incorporated into a formulated preparation. The following terms may also be used for such purposes.

When the use of sieves is inappropriate, the definition is expressed in terms of the particle size as determined by suitable microscopical examination.

Moderately coarse powder Not less than 95% by weight passes through a number 710 sieve and not more than 40% by weight passes through a number 250 sieve.

Microfine powder Not less than 90% by weight of the particles passes through a number 45 sieve.

Superfine powder Not less than 90% by number of the particles are less than 10 µm in size.

2. LIMIT TEST OF PARTICLE SIZE BY MICROSCOPY

(Ph. Eur. method 2.9.13)

Weigh a suitable quantity of the powder being examined (for example 10 mg to 100 mg) and suspend it in 10.0 ml of a suitable medium in which the powder does not dissolve, adding, if necessary, a wetting agent. Introduce a portion of the homogeneous suspension into a suitable counting cell and scan under a microscope an area corresponding to not less than 10 μg of the powder to be examined. Count all the particles having a maximum dimension greater than the prescribed size limit. The size limit and the permitted number of particles exceeding the limit are stated in the monograph.

B. Sieves and Filters

(Ph. Eur. text 2.1.4)

1. SIEVES

Wire mesh sieves used in sifting powdered drugs are identified by numbers indicating the nominal mesh aperture in micrometres.

The sieves are made of suitable materials with square meshes. For purposes other than analytical procedures, sieves with circular meshes may be used, the internal diameters of which are 1.25 times the aperture of the square mesh of the corresponding sieve size. There must be no reaction between the material of the sieve and the substance being sifted.

Maximum tolerance[1] *for an aperture* (+X): no aperture size shall exceed the nominal size by more than X, where

$$X = (2/3)w^{0.75} + 4w^{0.25}$$

where w is the width of aperture.

Tolerance for mean aperture (±Y): the average aperture size shall not depart from the nominal size by more than ±Y, where

$$Y = (1/27)w^{0.98} + 1.6$$

Intermediary tolerance (+Z): not more than 6% of the total number of apertures shall have sizes between "nominal + X" and "nominal + Y", where

$$Z = \frac{X+Y}{2}$$

Wire diameter d: the wire diameters given in Table 17B-1 apply to woven metal cloth mounted in a frame. The nominal sizes of the wire diameters may depart from these values within the limits d_{max} and d_{min}. The limits define a permissible range of choice ±0.15 per cent of the recommended nominal dimensions. The wires in a test sieve shall be of a similar diameter in warp and weft directions.

[1]see the International Standard ISO 3310/1 (1975)

TABLE 17B-1

Sieve numbers (Nominal dimensions of aperture)	Tolerances for apertures			Wire diameters			Approximate percentage sieving area
	Maximum tolerance for an aperture	Tolerance for mean aperture	Intermediary tolerance	Recommended nominal dimensions	Admissible limits		
	+X	±Y	+Z	d	d_{max}	d_{min}	
11200	770	350	560	2500	2900	2100	-
8000	600	250	430	2000	2300	1700	-
5600	470	180	320	1600	1900	1300	-
4000	370	130	250	1400	1700	1200	55
2800	290	90	190	1120	1300	950	51
2000	230	70	150	900	1040	770	48
1700	-	60	-	800	-	-	46
1400	180	50	110	710	820	600	44
1000	140	30	90	560	640	480	41
710	112	25	69	450	520	380	37
500	89	18	54	315	360	270	38
355	72	13	43	224	260	190	38
250	58	9.9	34	160	190	130	37
180	47	7.6	27	125	150	106	35
125	38	5.8	22	90	104	77	34
90	32	4.6	18	63	72	54	35
63	26	3.7	15	45	52	38	34
45	22	3.1	13	32	37	27	34
38	-	-	-	30	35	24	-

Dimensions in μm.

2. FILTERS

(Ph. Eur. text 2.1.2)

COMPARATIVE TABLE OF POROSITY OF SINTERED-GLASS FILTERS[1]

TABLE 917B-2

Porosity number (Ph. Eur.)[2]	Maximum diameter of pores in micrometres	Germany	France	United Kingdom
1.6	Less than 1.6	5f	–	–
–	1–2.5	5		5
4	1.6–4	–	–	–
–	4–6	–	5	–
10	4–10	4f	–	4
16	10–16	4	4	–
40	16–40	3	3	3
–	40–50	–	–	2
100	40–100	2	2	–
–	100–120	–	–	1
160	100–160	1	1	–
–	150–200	0	0	–
250	160–250	200-250		00

Diameters in micrometres

Special Uses

<2.5	Bacteriological filtration
4–10	Ultra-fine filtration, separation of micro-organisms of large diameter
10–40	Analytical filtration, very fine filtration of mercury, very fine dispersion of gases
40–100	Fine filtration, filtration of mercury, fine dispersion of gases
100–160	Filtration of coarse materials, dispersion and washing of gases, support for other filter materials
160–500	Filtration of very coarse materials, dispersion and washing of gases.

[1]The given limits are only approximate.

[2]The European Pharmacopoeia has adopted the system proposed by the International Organisation for Standardisation (ISO).

C. Specific Surface Area by Air Permeability

(Ph. Eur. method 2.9.14)

The test is intended for the determination of the specific surface area of dry powders expressed in square metres per gram in the sub-sieve region. The effect of molecular flow ('slip flow') which may be important when testing powders consisting of particles less than a few micrometers is not taken into account in the equation used to calculate the specific surface area.

Apparatus

The apparatus consists of the following parts:

(a) a permeability cell (see Fig. 17C-1), which consists of a cylinder with an inner diameter of 12.5 to 12.7 mm (A), constructed of glass or non-corroding metal. The bottom of the cell forms an airtight connection (for example, via an adaptor) with the manometer (see Fig. 50). A ledge 0.5 to 1 mm in width is located 35 to 65 mm from the top of the cell. It is an integral part of the cell or firmly fixed so as to be air-tight. It supports a perforated metal disc (B), constructed of non-corroding metal. The disc has a thickness of 0.8 to 1.0 mm and is perforated with 30 to 40 holes 1 mm in diameter evenly distributed over this area. The plunger (C) is made of non-corroding metal and fits into the cell with a clearance of not more than 0.1 mm. The bottom of the plunger has sharp square edges at right angles to the principal axis. There is an air vent 3 mm long and 0.3 mm deep on one side of the plunger. The top of the plunger has a collar such that when the plunger is placed in the cell and the collar is brought into contact with the top of the cell, the distance between the bottom of the plunger and the top of the perforated disc (B) is 14 to 16 mm. The filter paper discs (D) have smooth edges and the same diameter as the inside of the cell.

(b) a U-tube manometer (E) (see Fig. 17C-2) is made of nominal 9 mm outer diameter and 7 mm inner diameter glass tubing with standard walls. The top of one arm of the manometer forms an airtight connection with the permeability cell (F). The manometer arm connected to the permeability cell has a line etched around the tube at 125 to 145 mm below the top of the side outlet and three other lines at distances of 15, 70 and 110 mm above that line (G). The side outlet 250 to 305 mm above the bottom of the manometer is used to evacuate the manometer arm connected to the permeability cell. A tap is provided on the side outlet not more than 50 mm from the manometer arm.

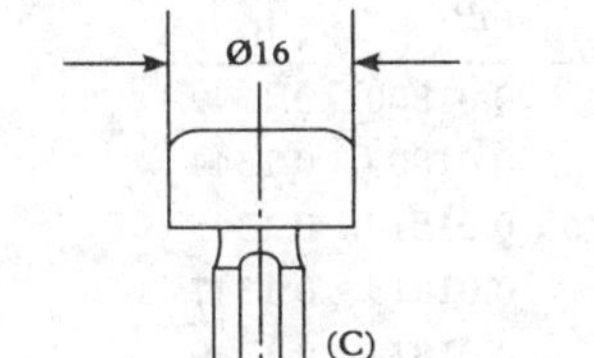

Fig. 17C-1
Permeability cell
Dimensions in mm

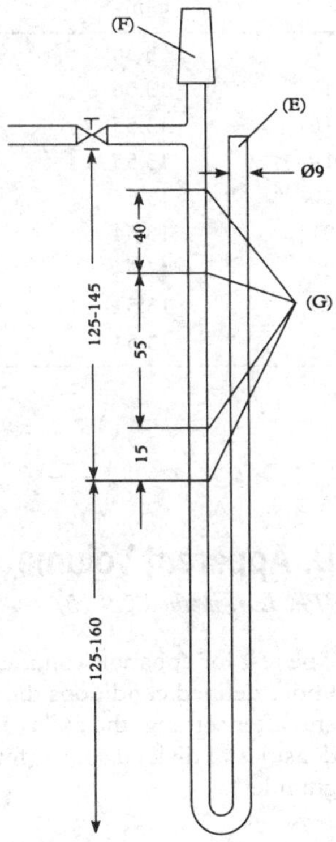

Fig. 17C-2
Manometer

The manometer is mounted firmly in such a manner that the arms are vertical. It is filled to the lowest mark with *dibutyl phthalate* containing a lipophilic dye.

Method

If prescribed, dry the powder to be examined and sift through a suitable sieve (for example No. 125) to disperse agglomerates. Calculate the weight (W) of the powder to be used from the following expression:

$$W = V \times \rho \times (1 - \varepsilon) \quad (1)$$

where V = bulk volume of the compacted bed of powder,

ρ = density of the substance to be examined in g ml^{-1} and

ε = porosity of the compacted bed of powder.

Assume first a porosity of 0.5 and introduce this value in equation 1 to calculate the weight W of the powder to be examined.

Place a filter paper disc on top of the perforated metal disk (B). Weigh the calculated weight W of the powder to be examined to the nearest 1 mg. Carefully transfer the powder into the cleaned, tared permeability cell and carefully tap the cell so that the surface of the powder bed is level and cover it with a second filter paper disc. Slowly compact the powder by means of the plunger, avoiding rotary movement. Maintain the pressure until the plunger is completely inserted into the permeability cell. If this is not possible, decrease the quantity of the powder used. If, on the contrary, there is not enough resistance, increase the quantity of the powder. In this case calculate the porosity again. After at least 10 seconds, remove the plunger.

Attach the permeability cell to the tube of the manometer by means of an airtight connection. Evacuate the air from the manometer by means of a rubber bulb until the level of the coloured liquid is at the highest mark. Close the tap and check that the apparatus is airtight by closing the upper end of the cell, for example with a rubber stopper. Remove the stopper and, using a timer, measure the time taken for the liquid to fall from the second to the third mark.

Apparatus

Use a drum with an internal diameter of about 286 mm and about 39 mm in depth, made of transparent synthetic polymer with polished internal surfaces and not subject to static build-up (see Figure 65). One side of the drum is removable. The tablets are tumbled at each turn of the drum by a curved projection that extends from the middle

Apparatus

Use a drum with an internal diameter of about 286 mm and about 39 mm in depth, made of transparent synthetic polymer with polished internal surfaces and not subject to static build-up (see Figure 65). One side of the drum is removable. The tablets are tumbled at each turn of the drum by a curved projection that extends from the middle

Using the measured flow time, calculate the specific surface area (S), expressed in square metres per gram, from the following expression.

$$S = \frac{K \times \sqrt{\varepsilon^3} \times \sqrt{t}}{\rho \times (1-\varepsilon) \times \sqrt{\eta}} \qquad (2)$$

where t = flow time in seconds,

η = dynamic viscosity of the air in mPa s (see Table),

K = apparatus constant determined according to equation 4,

ρ = density of the substance to be examined in g ml^{-1} and

ε = porosity of the compacted bed of powder.

Calibration of the apparatus

(a) The bulk volume of the compacted bed of powder is determined by the mercury displacement method as follows:

Place two filter paper discs in the permeability cell, pressing down the edges with a rod slightly smaller than the cell diameter until the filter discs lie flat on the perforated metal disc; fill the cell with mercury, removing any air bubbles adhering to the wall of the cell and wipe away the excess to create a plane surface of mercury at the top of the cell. If the cell is made of material that will amalgamate, grease the cell and the metal disc first with a thin layer of liquid paraffin. Pour out the mercury into a tared beaker and determine the weight (W_A) and the temperature of the mercury.

Make a compacted bed using the reference powder and again fill the cell with mercury with a planar surface at the top of the cell. Pour out the mercury in a tared beaker and again determine the weight of the mercury (W_B). Calculate the bulk volume (V) of the compacted bed of powder from the following expression:

$$V = \frac{W_A - W_B}{\rho_{Hg}} \qquad (3)$$

where $W_A - W_B$ = difference between the determined weights of mercury in grams and

ρ_{Hg} = density of mercury at the determined temperature in g ml^{-1}.

Repeat the procedure twice, changing the powder each time; the range of values for the calculated volume (V) is not greater than 0.01 ml. Use the mean value of the three determined volumes for the calculations.

(b) The apparatus constant K is determined by using a reference powder with known specific surface area and density as follows:

Calculate the required quantity of the reference powder to be used (equation 1) using the stated density and the determined volume of the compacted powder bed (equation 3).

Homogenise and loosen up the powder by shaking it for 2 minutes in a 100-ml bottle. Prepare a compacted powder bed and measure the flow time of air as previously described. Calculate the apparatus constant (K) from the following expression:

$$K = \frac{S_{sp} \times \rho \times (1-\varepsilon) \times \sqrt{\eta}}{\sqrt{\varepsilon^3} \times \sqrt{t}} \qquad (4)$$

where S_{sp} = stated specific surface area of the reference powder,

ρ = density of the substance to be examined in g ml^{-1},

ε = porosity of the compacted bed of powder,

t = flow time in seconds and

η = dynamic viscosity of the air in mPa s (see Table),

The density of mercury and the viscosity of air over a range of temperatures are shown in the Table.

Temperature	Density of mercury	Viscosity of air (η)	
°C	g ml^{-1}	mPa s	$\sqrt{\eta}$
16	13.56	0.01800	0.1342
17	13.56	0.01805	0.1344
18	13.55	0.01810	0.1345
19	13.55	0.01815	0.1347
20	13.55	0.01819	0.1349
21	13.54	0.01824	0.1351
22	13.54	0.01829	0.1353
23	13.54	0.01834	0.1354
24	13.54	0.01839	0.1356

D. Apparent Volume

(Ph. Eur. method 2.9.15)

The test for apparent volume is intended to determine under defined conditions the apparent volumes, before and after settling, the ability to settle and the apparent densities of divided solids (for example, powders, granules).

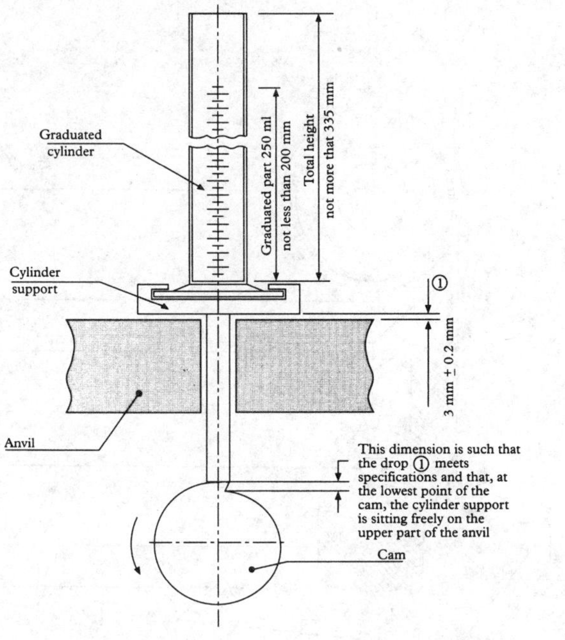

Fig. 17D-1

Apparatus

The apparatus is specified in Fig. 17D-1 and consists of the following components:

(a) A settling apparatus, A, capable of producing in 1 minute 250±15 taps from a height of 3±0.2 mm. The support, B, for the graduated cylinder, with its holder, has a mass of 450±5 g.

(b) A 250-ml graduated cylinder (2-ml intervals), C, with a mass of 220±40 g.

Method

Into the dry cylinder, introduce without compacting 100.0 g (m) of the substance being examined. If this is not possible, select a test sample with an apparent volume between 50 ml and 250 ml and specify the weight in the expression of results. Secure the cylinder in its holder. Read the unsettled apparent volume, V_0, to the nearest millilitre. Carry out 10, 500 and 1250 taps and read the corresponding volumes V_{10}, V_{500} and V_{1250}, to the nearest millilitre. If the difference between V_{500} and V_{1250} is greater than 2 ml, carry out another 1250 taps.

Expression of the results

(a) *Apparent volumes*
apparent volume before settling or bulk volume:
V_0 ml;
apparent volume after settling or settled volume:
V_{1250} or V_{2500} ml.

(b) *Ability to settle*
difference:
$V_{10} - V_{500}$ ml.

(c) *Apparent densities*
apparent density before settling or density of bulk product:
m/V_0, in g per ml (poured density);
apparent density after settling or density of settled product:
m/V_{1250} or m/V_{2500}, in g per ml (tapped density).

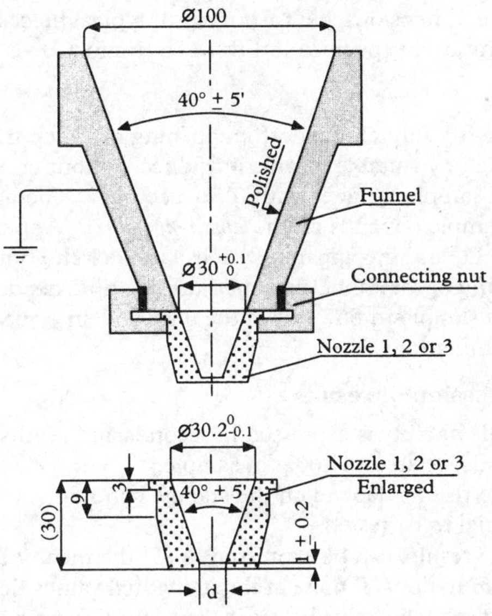

Fig. 17E-1
Dimensions in mm

Nozzle	Diameter (d) of the outflow opening *mm*
1	10 ± 0.01
2	15 ± 0.01
3	25 ± 0.01

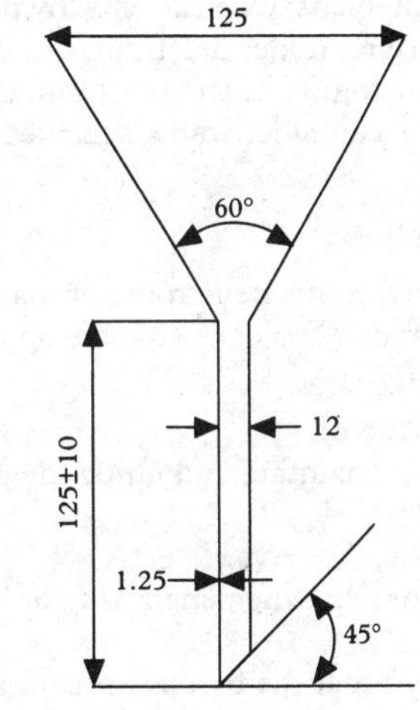

Fig. 17E-2
Dimensions in mm

E. Flowability

(Ph. Eur. method 2.9.16)

The test for flowability is intended to determine the ability of divided solids (for example, powders and granules) to flow vertically under defined conditions.

Apparatus

According to the flow properties of the material to be tested, funnels with or without stem, with different angles and orifice diameters are used. The funnel is maintained upright by a suitable device. The assembly must be protected from vibrations.

The dimensions and tolerances of typical pieces of apparatus are specified in Figs. 17E-1 and 17E-2.

Method

Into a dry funnel, the bottom opening of which has been blocked by suitable means, introduce without compacting a test sample weighed with 0.5% accuracy. The amount of the sample depends on the *apparent volume*, Appendix XVII D, and the apparatus used. Unblock the bottom opening of the funnel and measure the time needed for the entire sample to flow out of the funnel. Carry out three determinations.

Expression of results

The flowability is expressed in seconds and tenths of seconds, related to 100 g of sample.

The results depend on the storage conditions of the material to be tested.

The results can be expressed as (1) the mean of the determinations, if none of the individual values deviates from the mean value by more than 10%; (2) as a range, if the individual values deviate from the mean value by more than 10%; (3) as a plot of the mass against the flow time; (4) as an infinite time, if the entire sample fails to flow through.

F. Measurement of Consistency by Penetrometry

(Ph. Eur. method 2.9.9)

The test for measurement of consistency by penetrometry is intended to measure, under determined and validated conditions, the penetration of an object into the product to be examined in a container with a specified shape and size.

Apparatus

The apparatus consists of a penetrometer made up of a stand and a penetrating object. A suitable apparatus is shown in Fig 17F-1.

The stand is made up of:

(a)a vertical shaft to maintain and guide the penetrating object,
(b)a horizontal base,
(c)a device to ensure that the penetrating object is vertical,
(d)a device to check that the base is horizontal,
(e)a device to retain and release the penetrating object,
(f) a scale showing the depth of penetration (0.1 mm intervals).

The penetrating object, made of a suitable material, has a smooth surface and is characterised by its shape, size and weight. Suitable penetrating objects are shown in Figs. 45a and 45b.

Method

Prepare the test samples by one of the following procedures.

A. Carefully and completely fill three containers, without forming air bubbles. Level if necessary to obtain a flat surface. Store the samples at 24.5° to 25.5° for 24 hours, unless otherwise prescribed.

B. Store three samples at 24.5° to 25.5° for 24 hours. Apply a suitable shear to the samples for 5 minutes.

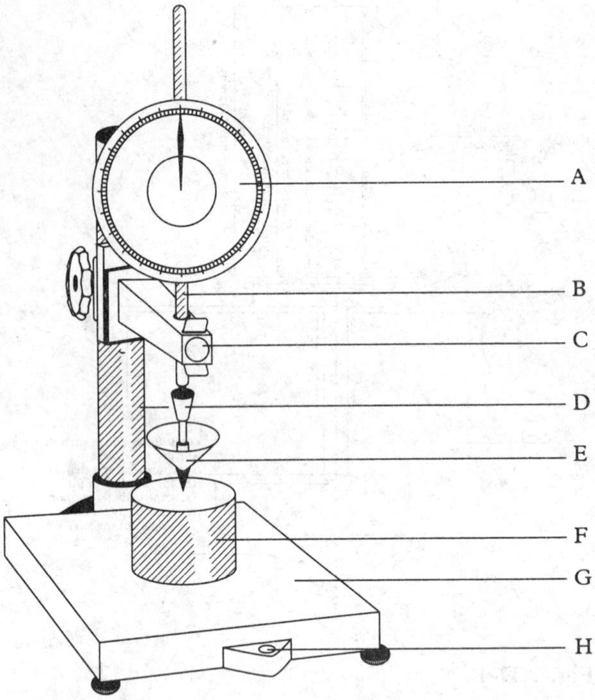

Fig. 17F-1 Penetrometer

A - scale showing the depth of penetration, graduated in tenths of millimetres

B - vertical shaft to maintain and guide the penetrating object

C - device to retain and to release the penetrating object automatically and for a constant time

D - device to ensure thet the penetrating object is vertival and that the base is horizontal

E - penetrating object (see Figs. 17F-2 and 17F-3)

F - container

G - horizontal base

H - control for the horizontal base

Carefully and completely fill three containers, without forming air bubbles, and level if necessary to obtain a flat surface.

C. Melt three samples and carefully and completely fill three containers, without forming air bubbles. Store the samples at 24.5° to 25.5° for 24 hours, unless otherwise prescribed.

Determination of penetration

Place the test sample on the base of the penetrometer. Verify that its surface is perpendicular to the vertical axis of the penetrating object. Bring the temperature of the penetrating object to 24.5° to 25.5° and then adjust its position such that its tip just touches the surface of the sample. Release the penetrating object and hold it free for 5 seconds. Clamp the penetrating object and measure the depth of penetration. Repeat the test with the two remaining containers.

Expression of the results

The penetration is expressed in tenths of millimetres as the arithmetic mean of the three measurements. If any of the individual results deviate from the mean value by more than 3%, repeat the test and express the results of the six measurements as the mean and the relative standard deviation.

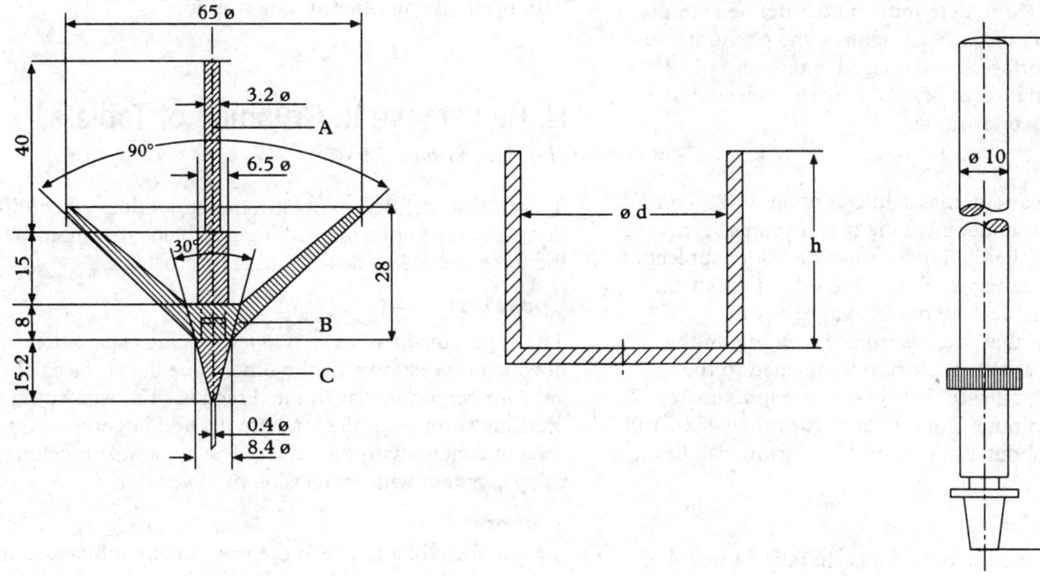

Fig. 17F-2

Cone (w = 102.5 g), suitable container (d = 102 mm or 75 mm, h = 62 mm) and shaft (l = 162 mm, w = 47.5 g)

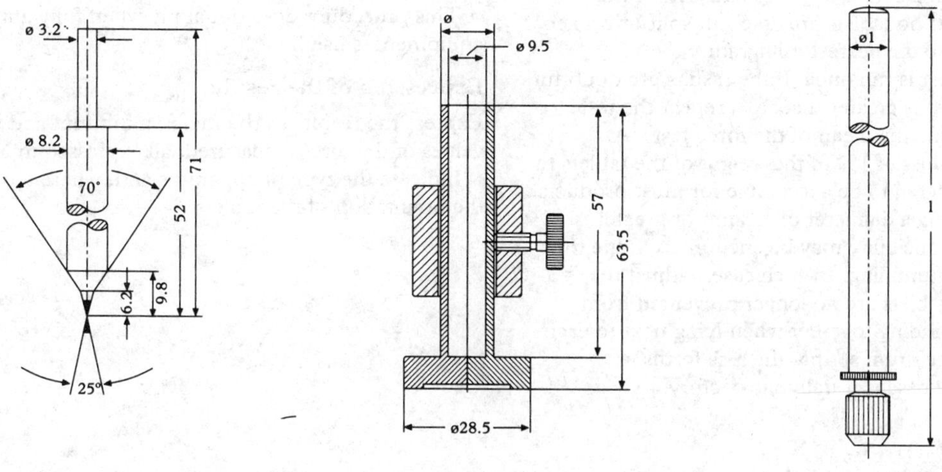

Fig. 17F-3

Cone (w = 102.5 g), suitable container (d = 102 mm or 75 mm, h = 62 mm) and shaft (l = 162 mm, w = 47.5 g)

G. Friability of Uncoated Tablets

(Ph. Eur. method 2.9.7)

The test is intended to determine, under defined conditions, the friability of uncoated tablets, the phenomenon whereby tablet surfaces are damaged and/or show evidence of lamination or breakage when subjected to mechanical shock or attrition.

Apparatus

Use a drum with an internal diameter of about 286 mm and about 39 mm in depth, made of transparent synthetic polymer with polished internal surfaces and not subject to static build-up.(see Fig. 17G-1). One side of the drum is removable. The tablets are tumbled at each turn by a curved projection that extends from the middle of the drum to the outer wall. The drum is attached to the horizontal axis of a device that rotates at approximately 25 revolutions per minute. Thus, at each turn the tablets roll or slide and fall about 130 mm onto the drum wall or onto each other.

Method

For tablets weighing up to 0.65 g each, take a sample of 20 tablets; for tablets weighing more than 0.65 g each, take 10 tablets. Place the tablets on a sieve no. 1000 and remove any loose dust with the aid of air pressure or a soft brush. Accurately weigh the tablet sample and place the tablets in the drum. Rotate the drum 100 times and remove the tablets. Remove any loose dust from the tablets as before. If no tablets are cracked, split or broken, weigh the tablets to the nearest milligram.

Generally the test is run once. If the results are doubtful or if the weight loss is greater than 1%, repeat the test twice and determine the mean of the three tests. A maximum weight loss of 1% of the weight of the tablets to be tested is considered to be acceptable for most products.

For tablets having a diameter of 13 mm or greater, problems of reproducibility may be encountered due to frequent irregular tumbling. In such cases, adjust the drum so that the tablets are no longer prevented from falling freely, by binding together when lying next to each other; adjusting the drum so that the axis forms a 10°-angle with the base is usually satisfactory.

Expression of the results

The friability is expressed as the loss of weight and it is calculated as a percentage of the initial weight.

Indicate the number of tablets used.

H. Resistance to Crushing of Tablets

(Ph. Eur. method 2.9.8)

This test is intended to determine, under defined conditions, the resistance to crushing of tablets, measured by the force needed to disrupt them by crushing.

Apparatus

The apparatus consists of two jaws facing each other, one of which moves towards the other. The flat surfaces of the jaws are perpendicular to the direction of movement. The crushing surfaces of the jaws are flat and larger than the zone of contact with the tablet. The apparatus is calibrated using a system with a precision of 1 Newton.

Method

Place the tablet between the jaws, taking into account, where applicable, the shape, the break-mark and the inscription; for each measurement orient the tablet in the same way with respect to the direction of application of the force. Carry out the measurement on 10 tablets, taking care that all fragments of the tablets have been removed before each determination.

This procedure does not apply when fully automated equipment is used.

Expression of the results

Express the results as the mean, minimum and maximum values of the forces measured, all expressed in Newtons.

Indicate the type of apparatus and, where applicable, the orientation of the tablets.

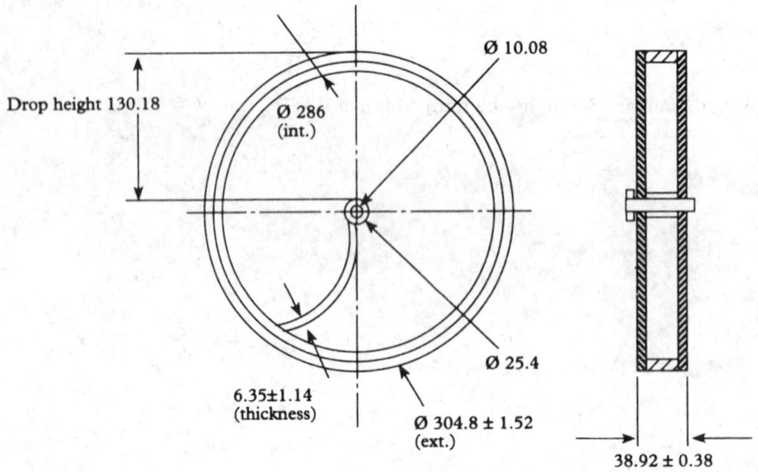

Fig. 17G-1
Dimensions in mm

J. Softening Time Determination of Lipophilic Suppositories

(Ph. Eur. method 2.9.22)

The test is intended to determine, under defined conditions, the time which elapses until a suppository maintained in water softens to the extent that it no longer offers resistance when a defined weight is applied.

Apparatus

The apparatus (see Figure 17J–1) consists of a glass tube 15.5 mm in internal diameter with a flat bottom and a length of about 140 mm. The tube is closed by a removable plastic cover having an opening 5.2 mm in diameter. The apparatus comprises a rod 5.0 mm in diameter which becomes wider towards the lower end, reaching a diameter of 12 mm. A metal needle 2 mm in length and 1 mm in diameter is fixed on the flat underside.

The rod consists of two parts, a lower part made of plastic material and an upper part made of plastic material or metal with a weight disk. The upper and lower parts are either fitted together (manual version) or separate (automated version). The weight of the entire rod is 30 ± 0.1 g. The upper part of the rod carries a sliding mark ring. When the rod is introduced into the glass tube so that it touches the bottom, the mark ring is adjusted to coincide with the upper level of the plastic cover.

Method

Place the glass tube containing 10 ml of water in the water-bath and equilibrate at 36.5 ± 0.5°. Fix the glass tubes vertically and immerse to a depth of at least 7 cm below the surface but without touching the bottom of the water-bath. Introduce a suppository, tip first, into the tube followed by the rod with the free gliding plastic cover into the glass tube until the metal needle touches the flat end of the suppository. Put the cover on the tube. Note the time which elapses until the rod sinks down to the bottom of the glass tube and the mark ring reaches the upper level of the plastic cover.

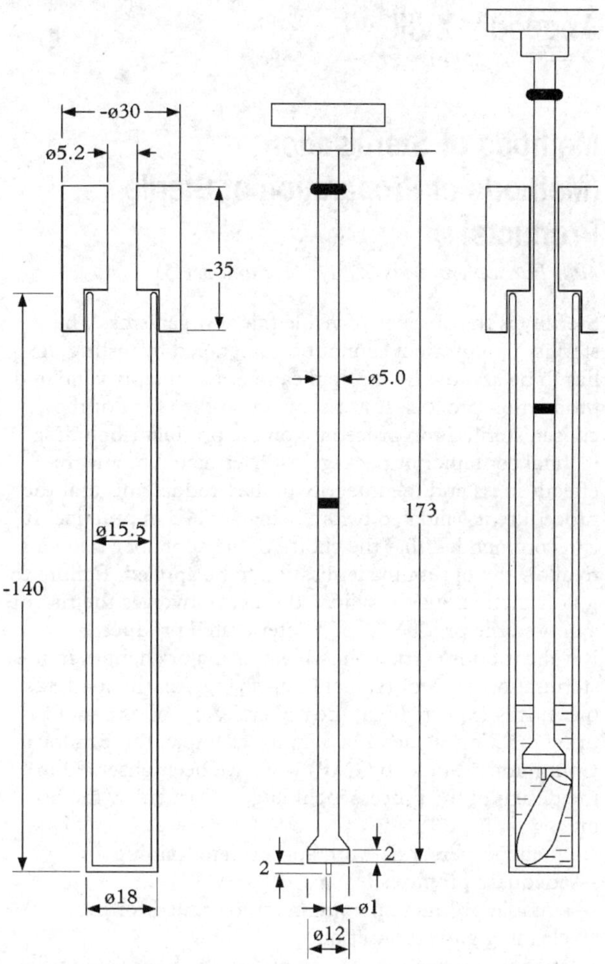

Fig. 17J-1

Dimensions in millimetres

Appendix XVIII

Methods of Sterilisation (Methods of Preparation of Sterile Products)

(Ph. Eur. general texts 5.1.1, 5.1.2 and 5.1.5)

Sterility is the absence of viable micro-organisms. The sterility of a product cannot be guaranteed by testing; it has to be assured by the application of a suitably validated production process. It is essential that the effect of the chosen sterilisation procedure on the product (including its final container or package) is investigated to ensure effectiveness and the integrity of the product and that the procedure is validated before being applied in practice. It is recommended that the choice of the container is such as to allow the optimum sterilisation to be applied. Failure to follow meticulously a validated process involves the risk of a non-sterile product or of a deteriorated product. Revalidation is carried out whenever major changes in the sterilisation procedure, including changes in the load, take place. It is expected that the principles of good manufacturing practice (as described in, for example, the European Community Guide to GMP) will have been observed in the design of the process including, in particular, the use of:

— qualified personnel with appropriate training,
— adequate premises,
— suitable production equipment, designed for easy cleaning and sterilisation,
— adequate precautions to minimise the bioburden prior to sterilisation,
— validated procedures for all critical production steps,
— environmental monitoring and in-process testing procedures.

The precautions necessary to minimise the pre-sterilisation bioburden include the use of components with an acceptable low degree of microbial contamination. Microbiological monitoring and setting of suitable action limits may be advisable for ingredients which are liable to be contaminated because of their origin, nature or method of preparation.

The methods described here apply mainly to the inactivation or removal of bacteria, yeasts and moulds. For biological products of animal or human origin or in cases where such material has been used in the production process, it is necessary during validation to demonstrate that the process is capable of the removal or inactivation of relevant viral contamination. Guidance on this aspect is provided in, for example, the appropriate European Community Notes for Guidance.

Wherever possible, a process in which the product is sterilised in its final container (terminal sterilisation) is chosen. When a fully validated terminal sterilisation method by steam, dry heat or ionising radiation is used, parametric release, that is the release of a batch of sterilised items based on process data rather than on the basis of submitting a sample of the items to sterility testing, may be carried out, subject to the approval of the competent authority.

If terminal sterilisation is not possible, filtration through a bacteria-retentive filter or aseptic processing is used; wherever possible, appropriate additional treatment of the product (for example, heating of the product) in its final container is applied. In all cases, the container and closure are required to maintain the sterility of the product throughout its shelf-life.

Sterility Assurance Level (SAL) Where appropriate reference is made within the methods described below, to a 'sterility assurance level' or 'SAL'. The achievement of sterility within any one item in a population of items submitted to a sterilisation process cannot be guaranteed nor can it be demonstrated. The inactivation of micro-organisms by physical or chemical means follows an exponential law; thus there is always a finite statistical probability that a micro-organism may survive the sterilising process. For a given process, the probability of survival is determined by the number, types and resistance of the micro-organisms present and by the environment in which the organisms exist during treatment. The SAL of a sterilising process is the degree of assurance with which the process in question renders a population of items sterile. The SAL for a given process is expressed as the probability of a non-sterile item in that population. An SAL of 10^{-6}, for example, denotes a probability of not more than one viable micro-organism in 1×10^6 sterilised items of the final product. The SAL of a process for a given product is established by appropriate validation studies.

METHODS AND CONDITIONS OF STERILISATION

Sterilisation may be carried out by one of the methods described below. Modifications to, or combinations of, these methods may be used provided that the chosen procedure is validated both with respect to its effectiveness and the integrity of the product including its container or package. For all methods of sterilisation the critical conditions of the operation are monitored in order to confirm that the previously determined required conditions are achieved throughout the batch during the whole sterilisation process This applies in all cases including those where the reference conditions are used.

Terminal Sterilisation

For terminal sterilisation it is essential to take into account the non-uniformity of the physical and, where relevant, chemical conditions within the sterilising chamber. The location within the sterilising chamber that is least accessible to the sterilising agent is determined for each loading configuration of each type and size of container or package (for example, the coolest location in an autoclave). The minimum lethality delivered by the sterilising cycle and the reproducibility of the cycle are also determined in order to ensure that all loads will consistently receive the specified treatment.

Having established a terminal sterilisation process, knowledge of its performance in routine use is gained wherever possible, by monitoring and suitably recording the physical and, where relevant, chemical conditions achieved within the load in the chamber throughout each sterilising cycle.

Steam sterilisation (Heating in an autoclave) Sterilisation by saturated steam under pressure is preferred, wherever applicable, especially for aqueous preparations. For this method of terminal sterilisation the reference conditions for aqueous preparations are heating at a minimum of 121° for 15 minutes. Other combinations of time and temperature may be used provided that it has been satisfactorily demonstrated that the process chosen delivers an adequate and reproducible level of lethality when operating routinely within the established tolerances. The procedures and precautions employed are such, as to give an SAL of 10^{-6} or better. Guidance concerning validation by means of the F_0 concept is provided below [Annex 2 (*Ph. Eur general text 5.1.5*)].

Knowledge of the physical conditions (temperature and pressure) within the autoclave chamber during the sterilisation procedure is obtained. The temperature is usually measured by means of temperature-sensing elements inserted into representative containers together with additional elements at the previously established coolest part of the loaded chamber. The conditions throughout each cycle are suitably recorded, for example, as a temperature-time chart, or by any other suitable means.

Where a biological assessment is carried out, this is obtained using a suitable biological indicator [Annex 1 (*Ph. Eur. general text 5.1.2*)].

Dry heat sterilisation For this method of terminal sterilisation the reference conditions are a minimum of 160° for at least 2 hours. Other combinations of time and temperature may be used provided that it has been satisfactorily demonstrated that the process chosen delivers an adequate and reproducible level of lethality when operated routinely within the established tolerances. The procedures and precautions employed are such as to given an SAL of 10^{-6} or better.

Dry heat sterilisation is carried out in an oven equipped with forced air circulation or other equipment specially designed for the purpose. The steriliser is loaded in such a way that a uniform temperature is achieved throughout the load. Knowledge of the temperature within the steriliser during the sterilisation procedure is usually obtained by means of temperature-sensing elements inserted into representative containers together with additional elements at the previously established coolest part of the loaded steriliser. The temperature throughout each cycle is suitably recorded.

Where a biological assessment is carried out, this is obtained using a suitable biological indicator [Annex 1 (*Ph. Eur. general text 5.1.2*)].

Dry heat at temperatures greater than 220° is frequently used for sterilisation and depyrogenation of glassware. In this case demonstration of a 3-log reduction in heat resistant endotoxin can be used as a replacement for biological indicators [Annex 1 (*Ph. Eur. general text 5.1.2*)].

Ionising radiation sterilisation Sterilisation by this method is achieved by exposure of the product to ionising radiation in the form of gamma radiation from a suitable radioisotopic source (such as cobalt 60) or of a beam of electrons energised by a suitable electron accelerator.

In some countries there are regulations that lay down rules for the use of ionising radiation for sterilisation purposes, for example, in the appropriate European Community Notes for Guidance.

For this method of terminal sterilisation the reference absorbed dose is 25 kGy. Other doses may be used provided that it has satisfactorily been demonstrated that the dose chosen delivers an adequate and reproducible level of lethality when the process is operated routinely within the established tolerances. The procedures and precautions employed are such as to give an SAL of 10^{-6} or better.

During the sterilisation procedure the radiation absorbed by the product is monitored regularly by means of established dosimetry procedures that are independent of dose rate. Dosimeters are calibrated against a standard source at a reference radiation plant on receipt from the supplier and at suitable intervals of not longer than one year thereafter.

Where a biological assessment is carried out, this is obtained using a suitable biological indicator [Annex 1 (*Ph. Eur. general text 5.1.2*)].

Gas sterilisation This method of sterilisation is only to be used where there is no suitable alternative. It is essential that penetration by gas and moisture into the material to be sterilised is ensured and that it is followed by a process of elimination of the gas under conditions that have been previously established to ensure that any residue of gas or its transformation products in the sterilised product is below the concentration that could give rise to toxic effects during use of the product. Guidance on this aspect with respect to the use of ethylene oxide is provided, for example, in the appropriate European Community Notes for Guidance.

Wherever possible, the gas concentration, relative humidity, temperature and duration of the process are measured and recorded. Measurements are made where sterilisation conditions are least likely to be achieved, as determined at validation.

The effectiveness of the process applied to each sterilisation load is checked using a suitable biological indicator [Annex 1 (*Ph. Eur. general text 5.1.2*)].

A suitable sample of each batch is tested for sterility, Appendix XVI A (*Ph. Eur method 2.6.1*), before the batch is released.

Filtration

Certain active ingredients and products that cannot be terminally sterilised may be subjected to a filtration procedure using a filter of a type that has been demonstrated to be satisfactory by means of a microbial challenge test using a suitable test micro-organism. A suspension of Pseudomonas diminuta (ATCC 19146, NCIMB 11091 or CIP 103020) may be suitable. It is recommended that a challenge of at least 10^7 cfu per cm^2 of active filter surface is used and that the suspension is prepared in tryptone soya broth which, after passage through the filter, is collected aseptically and incubated aerobically at 32°. Such products need special precautions. The production process and environment are designed to minimise microbial contamination and are regularly subjected to appropriate monitoring procedures. The equipment, containers and closures and, wherever possible, the ingredients are subjected to an appropriate sterilisation process. It is recommended that the filtration process is carried out as close as possible to the filling point. The operations following filtration are carried out under aseptic conditions.

Solutions are passed through a bacteria-retentive membrane with a nominal pore size of 0.22 µm or less or any other type of filter known to have equivalent properties of bacteria retention. Appropriate measures are taken to avoid loss of solute by adsorption on to the filter and to avoid the release of contaminants from the filter. Attention is given to the bioburden prior to filtration, filter capacity, batch size and duration of filtration. The filter is not used for a longer period than has been approved by validation of the combination of the filter and the product in question.

The integrity of an assembled sterilising filter is verified before use and confirmed after use by carrying out tests appropriate to the type of filter used and the stage of testing, for example bubble-point, pressure hold or diffusion rate tests.

Due to the potential additional risks of the filtration method as compared with other sterilisation processes, a prefiltration through a bacteria-retentive filter may be advisable in cases where a low bioburden cannot be ensured by other means.

ASEPTIC PREPARATION

The objective of aseptic processing is to maintain the sterility of a product that is assembled from components, each of which has been sterilised by one of the above methods. This is achieved by using conditions and facilities designed to prevent microbial contamination. Aseptic processing may include aseptic filling of products into container/closure systems, aseptic blending of formulations followed by aseptic filling and aseptic packaging.

In order to maintain the sterility of the components and the product during processing, careful attention needs to be given to:

— environment,
— personnel,
— critical surfaces,
— container/closure sterilisation and transfer procedures,
— maximum holding period of the product before filling into the final container.

Process validation includes appropriate checks on all the above and checks on the process are regularly carried out by means of process simulation tests using microbial growth media which are then incubated and examined for microbial contamination (media fill tests). In addition, a suitable sample of each batch of any product that is sterilised by filtration and/or aseptically processed is tested for sterility, Appendix XVI A (*Ph. Eur. method 2.6.1*), before the batch is released.

ANNEX 1

Biological indicators of sterilisation

(Ph. Eur. general text 5.1.2)

Biological indicators are standardised preparations of selected micro-organisms used to assess the effectiveness of a sterilisation procedure. They usually consist of a population of bacterial spores placed on an inert carrier, for example a strip of filter paper, a glass slide or a plastic tube. The inoculated carrier is covered in such a way that it is protected from any deterioration or contamination, while allowing the sterilising agent to enter into contact with the micro-organisms. Spore suspensions may be presented in sealed ampoules. Biological indicators are prepared in such a way that they can be stored under defined conditions; an expiry date is set.

Micro-organisms of the same bacterial species as the bacteria used to manufacture the biological indicators may be inoculated directly into a liquid product to be sterilised or into a liquid product similar to that to be sterilised. In this case, it must be demonstrated that the liquid product has no inhibiting effect on the spores used, especially as regards their germination.

A biological indicator is characterised by the name of the species of bacterium used as the reference micro-organism, the number of the strain in the original collection, the number of viable spores per carrier and the D-value. The D-value is the value of a parameter of sterilisation (duration or absorbed dose) required to reduce the number of viable organisms to 10 per cent of the original number. It is of significance only under precisely defined experimental conditions. Only the stated micro-organisms are present. Biological indicators consisting of more than one species of bacteria on the same carrier may be used. Information on the culture medium and the incubation conditions is supplied.

It is recommended that the indicator organisms are placed at the locations presumed, or wherever possible, found by previous physical measurement to be least accessible to the sterilising agent. After exposure to the sterilising agent, aseptic technique is used to transfer carriers of spores to the culture media, so that no contamination is present at the time of examination. Biological indicators that include an ampoule of culture medium placed directly in the packaging protecting the inoculated carrier may be used.

A choice of indicator organisms is made such that:

(a) the resistance of the test strain to the particular sterilisation method is great compared to the resistance of all pathogenic micro-organisms and to that of micro-organisms potentially contaminating the product,
(b) the test strain is non-pathogenic,
(c) the test strain is easy to culture.

After incubation, growth of the reference micro-organisms subjected to the sterilisation procedure demonstrates that this procedure is unsatisfactory.

1. Steam sterilisation

The use of biological indicators intended for steam sterilisation is recommended for the validation of sterilisation cycles. Spores of *Bacillus stearothermophilus* (for example, ATCC 7953, NCTC 10007, NCIMB 8157 or CIP 52.81) are recommended. The number of viable spores exceeds 5×10^5 per carrier. The D value at 121° exceeds 1.5 minutes. It is verified that exposing the biological indicators to steam at 121 ± 1° for 6 minutes leaves revivable spores, and that there is no growth of the reference micro-organisms after the biological indicators have been exposed to steam at 121 ± 1° for 15 minutes.

2. Dry-heat sterilisation

Spores of Bacillus subtilis (for example, var. niger ATCC 9372, NCIMB 8058 or CIP 77.18) are recommended for the preparation of biological indicators. The number of viable spores exceeds 1×10^5 per carrier and the D-value at 160° is approximately 5 to 10 minutes. Dry heat at temperatures greater than 220° is frequently used for sterilisation and depyrogenation of glassware. In this case, demonstration of a 3 log reduction in heat resistant bacterial endotoxin can be used as a replacement for biological indicators.

3. Ionising radiation sterilisation

Biological indicators may be used to monitor routine operations, as an additional possibility to assess the effectiveness of the set dose of radiation energy, especially in the case of accelerated electron sterilisation. The spores of Bacillus pumilus (for example, ATCC 27.142, NCTC

10327, NCIMB 10692 or CIP 77.25) are recommended. The number of viable spores exceeds 1×10^7 per carrier. The D-value exceeds 1.9 kGy. It is verified that there is no growth of the reference micro-organisms after the biological indicators have been exposed to 25 kGy (minimum absorbed dose).

4. Gas sterilisation

The use of biological indicators is necessary for all gas sterilisation procedures, both for the validation of the cycles and for routine operations. The number of viable spores exceeds 5×10^5 per carrier. For hydrogen peroxide and peracetic acid spores of *Bacillus stearothermophilus* (for example ATCC 7953, NCTC 10007, NCIMB 8157 or CIP 52.81), for ethylene oxide and formaldehyde spores of Bacillus subtilis (for example, var. niger ATCC 9372, NCIMB 8058 or CIP 77.18) are recommended. The parameters of resistance are known for the procedure used: for example, for ethylene oxide, the D-value exceeds 2.5 minutes for a test cycle involving 600 mg/l of ethylene oxide, at 54° and at 60 per cent relative humidity. It is verified that there is no growth of the reference micro-organisms after the biological indicators have been exposed to the test cycle described above for 60 minutes and that exposing the indicators to a reduced temperature cycle (600 mg/l, 30° and 60% relative humidity) for 15 min leaves revivable spores. It is essential that the biological indicator is able to reveal insufficient humidification in the steriliser and the product to ensure dehydrated micro-organisms are inactivated. Exposing the indicators to 600 mg/l of ethylene oxide at 54° for 60 minutes without humidification must leave revivable spores.

Annex 2

Application of the F_0 concept to steam sterilisation of aqueous preparations

(Ph. Eur. general text 5.1.5)

This section is published for information and guidance and does not form a mandatory part of the Pharmacopoeia.

The F_0 value of a saturated steam sterilisation process is the lethality expressed in terms of the equivalent time in minutes at a temperature of 121° delivered by the process to the product in its final container with reference to micro-organisms possessing a Z-value of 10.

The total F_0 of a process takes account of the heating up and cooling down phases of the cycle and can be calculated by integration of lethal rates with respect to time at discrete temperature intervals.

When a steam sterilisation cycle is chosen on the basis of the F_0 concept, great care must be taken to ensure that an adequate assurance of sterility is consistently achieved. In addition to validating the process, it may also be necessary to perform continuous, rigorous microbiological monitoring during routine production to demonstrate that the microbiological parameters are within the established tolerances so as to given an SAL of 10^{-6} or better.

In connection with sterilisation by steam, the Z-value relates the heat resistance of a micro-organism to changes in temperature. The Z-value is the change in temperature required to alter the D-value by a factor of 10.

The D-value (or decimal reduction value) is the value of a parameter of sterilisation (duration or absorbed dose) required to reduce the number of viable organisms to 10% of the original number. It is only of significance under precisely defined experimental conditions.

The following mathematical relationships apply:

$$F_0 = D_{121}(\log N_0 - \log N) = D_{121}\log IF$$

where D_{121} = D-value of the reference spores (Annex 1) at 121°,
N_0 = initial number of viable micro-organisms
N = final number of viable micro-organisms
IF = inactivation factor

$$Z = (T_2 - T_1)/\log D_1 - \log D_2)$$

where D_1 = D-value of the micro-organism at temperature T_1
D_2 = D-value of the micro-organism at temperature T_2

$$IF = N_0 - N = 10^{t/D}$$

where t = exposure time
D = D-value of micro-organism in the exposure conditions

Appendix XIX

Containers

A. Introduction

(Ph. Eur. text 3.2)

This Appendix provides requirements, guidance and information on containers for pharmaceutical use. Additional guidance is provided in a number of British Standards. Attention is drawn in particular, to British Standards 795:1983 and 1679.

A container for pharmaceutical use is an article that contains or is intended to contain a medicinal substance or preparation and is, or may be, in direct contact with it. The closure is a part of the container.

The container is designed so that the contents may be removed in a manner appropriate to the intended use of the preparation. It provides a varying degree of protection depending on the nature of the product and the hazards of the environment. It minimises the loss of constituents. The container should not interact physically or chemically with the contents in a way that will alter their quality beyond the limits tolerated by official requirements.

The selection of containers for products containing a volatile ingredient should be made with particular attention to the properties of that ingredient. In particular, it is advised that such products should not be stored or dispensed in plastic containers unless these have been shown to be satisfactory for that purpose.

Single-dose container A single-dose container holds a quantity of the preparation intended for total or partial use as a single administration.

Multidose container A multidose container holds a quantity of the preparation suitable for two or more doses.

Well closed container A well closed container protects the contents from contamination with extraneous solids and liquids and from loss of contents under ordinary conditions of handling, storage and transport.

Airtight container An airtight container is impermeable to solids, liquids and gases under ordinary conditions of handling, storage and transport. If the container is intended to be opened on more than one occasion, it must be so designed that it remains airtight after reclosure.

Sealed container A sealed container is a container closed by fusion of the material of the container. This definition does not necessarily apply when the term 'sealed container' is used with reference to a Powder for Injections in an individual monograph of the British Pharmacopoeia. In this latter context, the container may be sealed by appropriate means other than by fusion of the material.

Tamper-proof container A tamper-proof container is a closed container fitted with a device that reveals irreversibly whether the container has been opened.

B. Glass Containers for Pharmaceutical Use

(Ph. Eur. text 3.2.1)

Glass containers for pharmaceutical use are glass articles intended to come into direct contact with pharmaceutical preparations.

Several types of glass container exist, such as the following.

Ampoules These are thin-walled glass containers which, after filling, are sealed by fusion of the glass. The contents are withdrawn after rupture of the glass, on a single occasion only.

Bottles, vials, syringes and carpules These are more or less thick-walled containers with closures of glass or of material other than glass such as plastic materials or elastomers. The contents may be removed in several portions on one or more occasions.

Containers for blood and blood components These are cylindrical more or less thick-walled containers of various capacities and of colourless and transparent neutral glass.

Quality of glass

Colourless glass is highly transparent in the visible spectrum.

Coloured glass is obtained by the addition of small amounts of metal oxides, chosen according to the desired spectral absorbance.

Neutral glass is a borosilicate glass containing significant amounts of boric oxide, aluminium and/or alkaline earth oxides. Due to its composition neutral glass has a high thermal shock resistance and a very high hydrolytic resistance.

Soda-lime—silica glass is a silica glass containing alkali metal oxides, mainly sodium oxide, and alkaline earth oxides, mainly calcium oxide. Due to its composition soda-lime—silica glass has only a moderate hydrolytic resistance.

The chemical stability of glass containers for pharmaceutical use is expressed by the hydrolytic resistance, that is, the resistance to release of soluble mineral substances into water under the prescribed conditions of contact between the interior surface of the container or powdered glass and water. The hydrolytic resistance is evaluated by titrating released alkalinity.

According to their hydrolytic resistance glass containers are classified as follows.

Type I glass containers They are of neutral glass and have a high hydrolytic resistance due to the chemical composition of the glass itself.

Type I glass containers are in general suitable for all preparations whether or not for parenteral use and for human blood and blood components.

Type II glass containers They are usually of soda-lime—silica glass and have high hydrolytic resistance resulting from suitable treatment of the surface.

Type II glass containers are in general suitable for aqueous preparations for parenteral use with a pH lower than 7. It is necessary to check the stability of each preparation in these containers.

Type III glass containers They are usually of soda-lime–silica glass and have only moderate hydrolytic resistance.

Type III glass containers are suitable for non-aqueous preparations for parenteral use, for Powders for Parenteral Use and for preparations not for parenteral use. Ampoules up to 20 ml in capacity for liquids for oral use may be made from glass with a hydrolytic resistance superior to that of Type III glass containers.

Type IV glass containers They are usually of soda-lime–silica glass and have a low hydrolytic resistance.

Type IV glass containers are in general suitable for solid preparations that are not for parenteral use and for some liquid or semi-solid preparations that are not for parenteral use.

Glass containers with a hydrolytic resistance higher than that prescribed for the preparations to be contained may always be used.

For preparations that are not for parenteral use, colourless or coloured glass may be used. Preparations for parenteral use are normally presented in colourless glass, but coloured glass may be used for substances known to be light-sensitive. All glass containers for liquid preparations and for Powders for Parenteral Use should permit the visual inspection of the contents.

The inner surface of glass containers may be specially treated to improve hydrolytic resistance, to confer water-repellancy, etc. The external surface may also be treated, for example to reduce friction and to improve resistance to abrasion. The external treatment is such that it does not contaminate the internal surface of the container.

Except for Type I glass containers, glass containers for pharmaceutical preparations must not be re-used. Containers for blood and blood products must not be re-used.

Glass containers for pharmaceutical use comply with the relevant test or tests for hydrolytic resistance. When glass containers have non-glass components the tests apply only to the glass part of the container.

To define the quality of glass containers according to the intended use, one or more of the following tests are necessary.

Hydrolytic resistance

Apparatus

(a) A mortar, pestle (see Fig. 19B-1) and hammer in tempered, magnetic steel.

(b) A nest of three square-mesh sieves of stainless steel, mounted on frames of the same material and having nominal mesh apertures of 710, 425 and 250 µm.

(c) A permanent magnet.

(d) 'Aged' neutral-glass flasks and covers, that is, flasks and covers already used for the test or flasks that have been filled with water and kept in an autoclave at 121° for at least 1 hour.

(e) Foils of inert metal such as aluminium.

(f) An autoclave capable of maintaining a temperature of 120° to 122° equipped with a thermometer, a pressure gauge, a vent cock and a tray, and of sufficient capacity to accommodate above the water level the number of containers needed to carry out the test.

(g) A hot-air oven, capable of maintaining a temperature of 105° to 115°.

(h) A balance, capable of weighing up to 500 g with an accuracy of 5 mg.

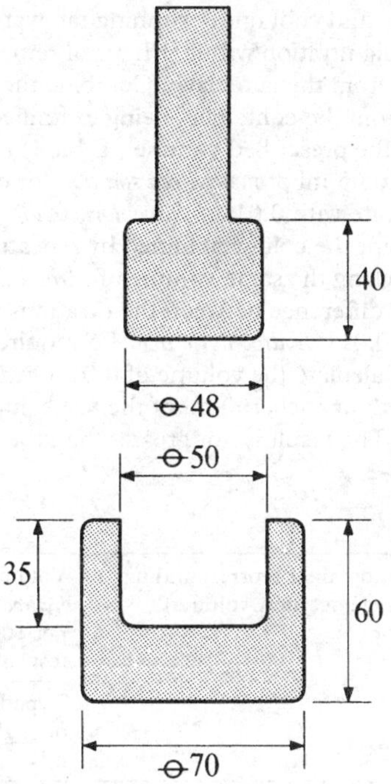

Fig. 19B-1
Apparatus for powdered glass method
Dimensions in millimetres

Filling volume The filling volume is the volume of water to be filled in the container for the purpose of the test. For vials and bottles the filling volume is 90% of the brimful capacity. For ampoules it is the volume up to the height of the shoulder.

A. Test for surface hydrolytic resistance The determination is carried out on the unused containers. The number of containers to be examined and the volumes of the test liquid necessary for the final determination are indicated in Table19B-1.

TABLE 19B-1

Nominal capacity of container ml	Number of containers to be used	Volume of test solution to be used for titration ml
3 or less	at least 10	25.0
3 to 30	at least 5	50.0
more than 30	at least 3	100.0

Shortly before the test, rinse each container carefully at least three times with *carbon dioxide-free water*, allow to drain and fill the containers with *carbon dioxide-free water* to their filling volume. Cover vials and bottles with neutral glass dishes or aluminium foil previously rinsed with *carbon dioxide-free water*. Seal the ampoules by fusion of the glass. Place the containers on the tray of the autoclave. Place the tray in the autoclave containing a quantity of water such that the tray remains clear of the water. Close the autoclave and carry out the following operations. (1) Heat to 100° and allow the steam to issue from the vent cock for 10 minutes; (2) raise the temperature from 100° to 121° over 20 minutes; (3) maintain the temperature at 120° to 122° for 60 minutes; (4) lower the temperature from 121° to 100° over 40 minutes, venting to prevent vacuum.

Remove the containers from the autoclave using normal precautions and cool under running tap water. Carry out the following titration within 1 hour of removing the containers from the autoclave. Combine the liquids obtained from the containers being examined and mix. Introduce the prescribed volume (Table I) into a conical flask. Add 0.05 ml of *methyl red solution* for each 25 ml of liquid. Titrate with 0.01M *hydrochloric acid VS* taking as the end point the colour obtained by repeating the operation using the same volume of *carbon dioxide-free water*. The difference between the titrations represents the volume of 0.01M *hydrochloric acid VS* required by the test solution. Calculate the volume of 0.01M *hydrochloric acid VS* required for each 100 ml of the test solution, if necessary. The result is not greater than the value stated in Table 19B-2.

TABLE 19B-2

Capacity of container (corresponding to 90% average overflow volume) ml	Volume of 0.01M *hydrochloric acid* VS per 100 ml of test solution: Type I or II glass ml	Type III glass ml
Not more than 1	2.0	20.0
More than 1 but not more than 2	1.8	17.6
More than 2 but not more than 5	1.3	13.2
More than 5 but not more than 10	1.0	10.2
More than 10 but not more than 20	0.80	8.1
More than 20 but not more than 50	0.60	6.1
More than 50 but not more than 100	0.50	4.8
More than 100 but not more than 200	0.40	3.8
More than 200 but not more than 500	0.30	2.9
More than 500	0.20	2.2

B. Test for hydrolytic resistance of powdered glass Rinse the containers to be tested with *water* and dry in the hot-air oven. Coarsely break about 100 g of the glass from at least three containers with the hammer into coarse fragments so that the largest fragments are not greater than 25 mm. Transfer a part of the sample to the mortar. Insert the pestle and strike heavily once with the hammer. Transfer the contents of the mortar to the coarsest sieve of the nest. Repeat the operation a sufficient number of times until all the fragments have been transferred to the sieve. Rapidly sift the glass and remove the portion retained by the 710-µm and 425-µm sieves. Submit these fractions to further fracture, repeating the operation until about 20 g of glass is retained by the 710-µm sieve. Reject this portion and the portion that passes through the 250-µm sieve. Shake the nest of sieves manually or mechanically for 5 minutes. Reserve the portion of glass grains that passes through the 425-µm sieve but that is retained on the 250-µm sieve. Remove any metal particle from the glass grains by passing a magnet over them. Transfer about 22 g to a conical flask and wash with 60 ml of *acetone*. Shake to suspend the grains and decant the supernatant liquid. Carry out the operation five times. Spread the glass grains in an evaporating dish. Allow the acetone to evaporate, dry in an oven at 110° for 20 minutes and allow to cool.

Introduce 20.00 g of the glass grains so treated into a 250-ml conical flask. Add 100 ml of *carbon dioxide-free water* and weigh. In a second identical flask place 100 ml of *carbon dioxide-free water* to serve as the blank and weigh. Close the two flasks with neutral glass dishes or aluminium foil rinsed with *carbon dioxide-free water*. Ensure that the glass grains are uniformly spread over the bottom of the flask. Place the flasks in the autoclave and maintain at 121° for 30 minutes, carrying out operations similar to those described in Test A for surface hydrolytic resistance. After cooling, remove the closures, wipe the flasks carefully and adjust to the original weight by the addition of *carbon dioxide-free water*.

Transfer 50.0 ml (corresponding to 10.0 g of glass grains) of the clear supernatant liquid to a conical flask. Prepare the blank in a similar flask using 50 ml of water. To each flask add 0.1 ml of *methyl red solution* and titrate with 0.01M *hydrochloric acid VS*. Titrate the test liquid with the same acid to the same colour as that obtained in the blank titration. Subtract the value found for the blank titration from that found for the test liquid, and express the results in millilitres of 0.01M *hydrochloric acid VS* per 10.0 g of glass. Glass from Type I glass containers requires not more than 2.0 ml, glass from containers of Type II or Type III requires not more than 17.0 ml and glass from containers of Type IV requires not more than 30.0 ml of 0.01M *hydrochloric acid VS*.

C. Test for hydrolytic resistance of the etched surface of the container The number of containers to be tested and the volume of test liquid required are shown in Table I.

Rinse the containers twice with *carbon dioxide-free water*, fill completely with a mixture of 1 volume of *hydrofluoric acid* and 9 volumes of *hydrochloric acid* and allow to stand for 10 minutes. Empty the containers and rinse carefully five times with *carbon dioxide-free water*. Immediately before the test, rinse once again with *carbon dioxide-free water*. Submit the containers thus prepared to the same autoclaving and titrating procedure as that described in Test A for surface hydrolytic resistance.

Distinction between Type I and Type II glass containers Compare the results obtained in Test C to those obtained in Test A. The meaning is shown in Table 19B-3.

TABLE 19B-3 Distinction between Types I and II glass containers

Type I	Type II
The values are closely similar to those found in the test for surface hydrolytic resistance for Type I glass containers	The values greatly exceed those found in the test for surface hydrolytic resistance and are similar but not larger than those for Type III glass containers

Chlorides The release of chlorides from glass containers for parenteral use filled with *water* and heated at 121° for 30 minutes is not greater than 0.5 ppm, Appendix VII.

Arsenic *The test applies to glass containers for aqueous parenteral preparations.*

Apparatus The apparatus (see Fig. 19B-2) consists of an arsine generator (A) fitted with a scrubber unit (C) and an absorber tube (E) with standard-taper or ground glass ball-and-socket joints (B and D) between the units. Any other suitable apparatus embodying the principle of the described assembly may be used.

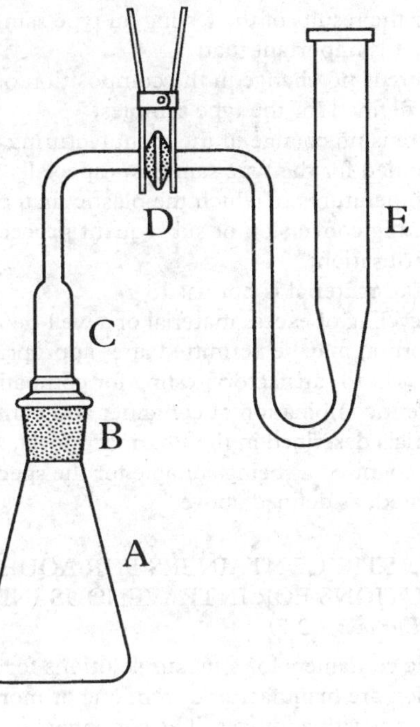

Fig. 19B-2
Apparatus for arsenic determination

Method Prepare a reference solution by diluting 3.5 ml of *arsenic standard solution (1 ppm As)* to 35 ml with *water* and introduce into the generator flask. Prepare a test solution by transferring to the generator flask 35 ml of the liquid prepared as directed under Test A for surface hydrolytic resistance, from the glass container for aqueous parenteral preparations. For smaller containers, transfer 35 ml of the combined contents of several glass containers so prepared. Treat the reference solution and the test solution under the same conditions as follows. Mix 20 ml of a 35% w/v solution of *sulphuric acid*, 2 ml of *potassium iodide solution*, 0.5 ml of *tin(II)* chloride solution and 1 ml of *propan-2-ol* and allow to stand for 30 minutes. Pack the scrubber tube (C) with two pledgets of *lead acetate cotton* in such a manner that there is a 2-mm space between the two pledgets. Lubricate the joints (B and D) with an appropriate stopcock grease and connect the scrubber unit to the absorber tube (E). Transfer 3.0 ml of a 0.5% w/v solution of *silver diethyldithiocarbamate* in *anhydrous pyridine* to the absorber tube. Add 3.0 g of *zinc* in granules (710 µm) to the mixture in the flask, immediately connect the assembled scrubber unit, place the generator flask (A) in a water bath maintained at a temperature of 22° to 28° and allow the evolution of hydrogen and the colour development to proceed for 45 minutes, swirling the flask gently at 10-minute intervals. Disconnect the absorber tube from the generator and scrubber units and transfer the solution to a tube for comparative tests. Any red colour in the test solution is not more intense than that in the reference solution. The evaluation may also be carried out using a spectrophotometer or a colorimeter using the silver diethyldithiocarbamate solution as blank. Measure between 535 nm and 540 nm using a 1-cm layer. The test solution does not contain more than 0.1 ppm of arsenic (As).

Light transmission for coloured light-protecting glass containers Break the glass container or cut it with a circular saw fitted with a wet abrasive wheel, such as a carborundum or a bonded-diamond wheel. Select sections representative of the wall thickness and trim them as suitable for mounting in a spectrophotometer. If the specimen is too small to cover the opening in the specimen holder, mask the uncovered portion with opaque paper or tape, provided that the length of the specimen is greater than that of the slit. Before placing in the holder, wash, dry and wipe the specimen with lens tissue. Mount the specimen with the aid of wax, or by other convenient means, taking care to avoid leaving fingerprints or other marks.

Place the specimen in the spectrophotometer with its cylindrical axis parallel to the slit and in such a way that the light beam is perpendicular to the surface of the section and that the losses due to reflection are at a minimum. Measure the transmission of the specimen with reference to air in the spectral region of 290 to 450 nm, continuously or at intervals of 20 nm.

The observed light transmission for coloured glass containers for preparations that are not for parenteral use does not exceed 10% at any wavelength in the range from 290 to 450 nm, irrespective of the Type and the capacity of the glass container. The observed light transmission in coloured glass containers for parenteral preparations does not exceed the limits given in Table19B-4.

TABLE19B-4 Limits of light transmission for coloured glass containers of Types I, II and III

	Maximum percentage of light transmission at any wavelength between 290 nm and 450 nm	
	Flame-sealed containers	Containers with closures
Up to 1	50	25
Above 1 and up to 2	45	20
Above 2 and up to 5	40	15
Above 5 and up to 10	35	13
Above 10 and up to 20	30	12
Above 20	15	10

Containers for blood and blood components

Resistance to thermal shock The containers do not break, crack or split when they are (a) placed empty in an autoclave and the temperature is raised in about 30 minutes to 140° and kept at this temperature for 30 minutes; (b) placed empty in an oven the temperature of which is raised in about 30 minutes to 250° and kept at this temperature for 1 hour; (c) filled to 70% of the maximum marked volume with a 0.9% w/v solution of *sodium chloride* and gradually cooled to −20° in air and kept at this temperature for 24 hours (after restoring to room temperature, the containers comply with the test for resistance to centrifugation); (d) submitted to a rapid drop of temperature by placing the containers filled with tap water successively in two water baths with a difference of temperature of at least 40°.

Resistance to centrifugation Fill the container with water to the maximum marked volume and place in a suitable centrifuge. Balance the centrifuge and accelerate to 2000 *g* over a period of at least 1 minute. The container resists these conditions for at least 30 minutes.

Labelling Containers for blood and blood components are labelled according to the relevant national legislation and international agreements.

C. Plastic Containers and Closures

(Ph. Eur. text 3.2.2)

Introduction

A plastic container for pharmaceutical use is a plastic article which contains or is intended to contain a pharmaceutical product and is, or may be, in direct contact with it. The closure is a part of the container.

The materials of which the containers for pharmaceutical use are made consist of one or more polymers with which may be included certain additives. These materials do not include in their composition any substance that can be extracted by the contents in such quantities as to alter the efficacy or the stability of the product or increase its toxicity.

The most commonly used polymers are polyethylene (low and high density), polypropylene, poly(vinyl chloride), poly(ethylene terephthalate) and ethylene-vinyl acetate copolymers.

The nature and amount of the additives are determined by the type of the polymer, the process used to convert the plastic into the article and the intended purpose. Additives may consist of antioxidants, stabilisers, plasticisers, lubricants, colouring matter and impact modifiers. Antistatic agents and mould-release agents may be used only for containers for preparations for oral use or for external use for which they are authorised. Acceptable additives are indicated in the type specification for each material described in the Pharmacopoeia, Appendix XX. Other additives may be used provided they are approved in each case by the competent authority responsible for the licensing for sale of the preparation.

For selection of a suitable plastic container, it is necessary to know the full manufacturing formula of the plastic, including all materials added during formation of the container so that the potential hazards can be assessed. The plastic container chosen for any particular preparation should be such that:

— the ingredients of the product in contact with the plastic material are not significantly adsorbed on its surface and do not significantly migrate into or through the plastic,

— the plastic material does not yield to the contents substances in quantities sufficient to affect the stability of the preparation or to present a risk of toxicity.

Using the material or materials selected to satisfy these criteria, a number of identical type samples of the container are made by a well-defined procedure and submitted to practical testing in conditions that reproduce those of the intended use, including, where appropriate, sterilisation. In order to confirm the compatibility of the container and the contents and to ensure that there are no changes detrimental to the quality of the preparation, various tests are carried out such as verification of the absence of changes in physical characteristics; assessment of any loss or gain through permeation; detection of pH changes; assessment of changes caused by light; chemical tests; and, where appropriate, biological tests.

The method of manufacture is such as to ensure reproduc-ibility for subsequent bulk manufacture and the conditions of manufacture are chosen so as to preclude the possibility of contamination with other plastic materials or their ingredients. The manufacturer of the product must ensure that containers made in production are similar in every respect to the type samples.

For the results of the testing on type samples to remain valid, it is important that:

— there is no change in the composition of the material as defined for the type samples;

— here is no change in the manufacturing process as defined for the type samples, especially as regards the temperatures to which the plastic material is exposed during conversion or subsequent procedures such as sterilisation;

— scrap material is not used.

Recycling of excess material of a well-defined nature and proportion may be permitted after appropriate validation.

Subject to satisfactory testing for compatibility of each different combination of container and contents, the materials described in the Pharmacopoeia, Appendix XX, are recognised as being suitable for the specific purposes indicated, as defined above.

1. PLASTIC CONTAINERS FOR AQUEOUS SOLUTIONS FOR INTRAVENOUS INFUSION

(Ph. Eur text 3.2.7)

Plastic containers for aqueous solutions for intravenous infusion are manufactured from one or more polymers, if necessary with additives. The containers described in this section are not necessarily suitable for emulsions. The polymers most commonly used are polyethylene, polypropylene and poly(vinyl chloride).

The containers may be bags or bottles. They have a site suitable for the attachment of an infusion set designed to ensure a secure connection. They may have a site that allows an injection to be made at the time of use. They usually have a part that allows them to be suspended and which will withstand the tension occurring during use. The containers must withstand the sterilisation conditions to which they will be submitted. The design of the container and the method of sterilisation chosen are such that all parts of the containers that may be in contact with the infusion are sterilised. The containers are impermeable to micro-organisms after closure. The containers are such that after filling they are resistant to damage from accidental freezing which may occur during transport of the final preparation. The containers are and remain sufficiently transparent to allow the appearance of the contents to be examined at any time, unless otherwise justified and authorised.

The empty containers display no defects that may lead to leakage and the filled and closed container shows no leakage.

For satisfactory storage of some preparations, the container has to be enclosed in a protective envelope. The initial evaluation of storage has then to be carried out using the container enclosed in the envelope.

TESTS

Solution S Fill a container to its nominal capacity with *water R* and close it, if possible using the usual means of closure; otherwise close using a sheet of pure aluminium. Heat in an autoclave so that a temperature of 121 ± 2° is reached within 20 to 30 minutes and maintain at this temperature for 30 minutes. If heating at 121° leads to deterioration of the container, heat at 100° for 2 hours. Use solution S within 4 hours of preparation.

Blank Prepare a blank by heating *water R* in a borosilicate-glass flask closed by a sheet of pure aluminium at the temperature and for the time used for the preparation of solution S.

Appearance of solution S Solution S is clear (2.2.1) and colourless (Method II, 2.2.2).

Acidity or alkalinity To a volume of solution S corresponding to 4 per cent of the nominal capacity of the container add 0.1 ml of *phenolphthalein solution R*. The solution is colourless. Add 0.4 ml of 0.01M sodium hydroxide. The solution is pink. Add 0.8 ml of 0.01M hydrochloric acid and 0.1 ml of *methyl red solution R*. The solution is orange-red or red.

Absorbance (2.2.25). Measure the absorbance of solution S from 230 nm to 360 nm, using the blank (see solution S) as the compensation liquid. At these wavelengths, the absorbance is not greater than 0.20.

Oxidisable substances To 20.0 ml of solution S add 1 ml of *dilute sulphuric acid R* and 20.0 ml of 0.002M *potassium permanganate*. Boil for 3 min. Cool immediately. Add 1 g of *potassium iodide R* and titrate immediately with 0.01M sodium thiosulphate, using 0.25 ml of *starch solution R* as indicator. Carry out a titration using 20.0 ml of the blank. The difference between the titration volumes is not greater than 1.5 ml.

Transparency Fill a container previously used for the preparation of solution S with a volume equal to the nominal capacity of the primary opalescent suspension (2.2.1) diluted 1 in 200 for a container made from polyethylene or polypropylene and 1 in 400 for other containers. The cloudiness of the suspension is perceptible when viewed through the container and compared with a similar container filled with *water R*.

LABELLING

The label accompanying a batch of empty containers includes a statement of:
-the name and address of the manufacturer,
— a batch number which enables the history of the container and of the plastic material of which it is manufactured to be traced

D. Containers for Blood and Blood Components

This section is to be read in conjunction with the Introduction to Appendix XIX C (*Ph. Eur. section 3.2.2 Plastic Containers and Closures*).

1. STERILE PLASTIC CONTAINERS FOR BLOOD AND BLOOD COMPONENTS
(Ph. Eur. text 3.2.3)

Plastic containers for the collection, storage, processing and administration of blood and its components are supplied sterile. In normal conditions of use, the materials of the different parts of the containers do not release monomers or other substances in amounts likely to be harmful and do not lead to any abnormal modifications of the blood. The containers may contain anticoagulant solutions depending on their intended use.

Each container is fitted with attachments suitable for its intended use. The container may be in the form of a single unit or the collecting container may be connected by one or more tubes to one or more secondary containers to allow separation of the blood components to be effected within a closed system. The outlets are of a shape and size allowing for adequate connection of the container with the blood transfusion equipment. The protective coverings on the blood-taking needle and on the appendages are designed to ensure that sterility is maintained. They are easily removable but are tamper-evident. The containers are fitted with a suitable device for suspending or fixing which does not hinder the collection, storage, processing or administration of blood.

The capacity of the containers is related to the nominal capacity, that is, to the volume of blood to be collected in the container and to the appropriate volume of anticoagulant solution. The containers are shaped in such a manner that when filled they may be centrifuged. They are enclosed in sealed, protective envelopes.

Characteristics The container is sufficiently transparent to allow adequate visual examination of its contents before and after taking the blood. It is also sufficiently flexible to offer minimal resistance during filling and emptying under normal conditions of use. The container contains not more than 5 ml of air.

Resistance to centrifugation Introduce into the container a sufficient volume of *water*, previously acidified with 1 ml of 2M *hydrochloric acid*, to fill it to its nominal capacity. Envelop the container with absorbent paper that has been impregnated with a 5-fold dilution of *bromophenol blue solution R1* or other suitable indicator and then dried. Centrifuge at 5000 *g* for 10 minutes. No leakage is detectable on the indicator paper and no permanent distortion occurs.

Resistance to stretch Introduce into the container a sufficient volume of *water* previously acidified with 1 ml of 2M *hydrochloric acid* to fill it to its nominal capacity. Suspend the container by the suspending device at the opposite end from the blood-taking tube, apply an immediate force of 20 N along the axis of the tube and maintain the traction for 5 seconds. Repeat the test with the force applied to each of the parts for filling and emptying. No break and no deterioration occur.

Leakage Place the container that has been used in the test for Resistance to stretch between two plates covered with absorbent paper that has been impregnated with a 5-fold dilution of *bromophenol blue solution R1* or other suitable indicator and then dried. Apply a force progressively to the plates to press the container so that its internal pressure (that is, the difference between the applied and atmospheric pressure) reaches 67 kPa within 1 minute. Maintain the pressure for 10 minutes. No signs of leakage are detectable on the indicator paper or at any point of attachment (seals, joints, etc).

Vapour permeability For a container containing an anticoagulant solution, fill with a volume of a 0.9% w/v solution of *sodium chloride* equal to the nominal capacity. For an empty container, fill with the same mixture of anticoagulant solution and sodium chloride solution. Close the container, weigh and store at 4° to 6° in an atmosphere with a relative humidity of 45 to 55% for 21 days. At the end of this period, the loss in weight is not more than 1%.

Emptying under pressure Fill the container with a volume of *water*, at 4° to 6°, equal to the nominal capacity. Attach a transfusion set without an intravenous cannula to one of the connectors. Compress the container so as to maintain an internal pressure of 40 kPa throughout the emptying. The container empties in less than 2 minutes.

Speed of filling Attach the container by means of the blood-taking tube fitted with the needle to a reservoir containing a suitable solution having a viscosity equal to that of blood (a 33.5% w/v solution of *sucrose* at 37° is suitable). Maintain the internal pressure of the reservoir at 9.3 kPa with the base of the reservoir and the upper part of the container at the same level. The volume of liquid that flows into the container in 8 minutes is not less than the nominal capacity of the container.

Resistance to temperature variations Place the container in a suitable chamber having an initial temperature of 20° to 23°. Cool rapidly to −80° and maintain at this temperature for 24 hours. Raise the temperature to 50° and maintain for 12 hours. Allow to cool to room temperature. The container complies with the tests for Resistance to centrifugation, Resistance to stretch, Leakage, Vapour permeability, Emptying under pressure and Speed of filling.

Transparency Prepare an approximately 16-fold dilution of the suspension prepared for the *standard of opalescence*, Appendix IV A, Method I, so as to give an *absorbance* at 640 nm of 0.37 to 0.43, Appendix II B. Fill the empty container to its nominal capacity with the diluted suspension. The cloudiness of the diluted suspension is detectable when viewed through the container, as compared with a similar container filled with *water*.

Extractable matter Carry out suitable tests by methods designed to simulate as far as possible the conditions of contact between the container and its contents that occur in conditions of use.

Haemolytic effects in buffered systems Introduce into the container a volume of *water for injections* corresponding to the intended volume of anticoagulant solution. Close the container and heat in an autoclave so that the contents are maintained at 110° for 30 minutes. Cool and add sufficient *water for injections* to fill the container to its nominal capacity (solution A). If the container being examined contains an anticoagulant solution, empty it and then rinse with 250 ml of *water for injections* at 19° to 21° and discard the rinsings.

Prepare a stock buffer solution by dissolving 90.0 g of *sodium chloride*, 34.6 g of *disodium hydrogen orthophosphate* and 2.43 g of *sodium dihydrogen orthophosphate* in *water* and diluting to 1000 ml with the same solvent. Prepare three buffer solutions as follows. For solution (1) add 10 ml of *water* to 30 ml of stock buffer solution. For solution (2) add 20 ml of *water* to 30 ml of stock buffer solution. For solution (3) add 85 ml of *water* to 15 ml of stock buffer solution.

Introduce 1.4 ml of solution A into each of three centrifuge tubes. To the first tube add 0.1 ml of solution (1), to the second tube add 0.1 ml of solution (2) and to the third tube add 0.1 ml of solution (3). To each tube add 0.02 ml of fresh, heparinised human blood[1], mix well and warm on a water bath at 29° to 31° for 40 minutes.

Prepare a further three solutions as follows. For solution (4) add 12 ml of *water* to 3 ml of solution (1). For solution(5) add 11 ml of *water* to 4 ml of solution (2). For solution (6) add 10.25 ml of *water* to 4.75 ml of solution (2).

To the three tubes add, respectively, 1.5 ml of solution (4), 1.5 ml of solution (5) and 1.5 ml of solution (6). At the same time and in the same manner prepare three other tubes but using *water* in place of solution A. Centrifuge simultaneously all six tubes at exactly 2500 *g* in the same horizontal centrifuge for 5 minutes. After centrifuging, measure the *absorbances* of the liquids at 540 nm, Appendix II B, using the stock buffer solution in the reference cell. Calculate the *haemolytic value* as a percentage from the expression $100(A/A_3)$ where A_3 is the absorbance of the third tube and A is the absorbance of the first or second tube or of the corresponding control tube.

The solution in the first tube gives a *haemolytic value* of not more than 10% and the *haemolytic value* of the solution in the second tube does not differ by more than 10% from that of the corresponding control tube.

Sterility Comply with the *test for sterility*, Appendix XVI A, with the following modifications. Introduce aseptically into the container 100 ml of *saline solution* and shake the container to ensure that the internal surfaces have been entirely wetted. Filter the contents through a membrane filter and place the membrane in the appropriate culture medium.

Pyrogens If the container being examined contains an anticoagulant solution, empty it, rinse the container with 250 ml of *water for injections* at 19° to 21° and discard the rinsings. Fill the container with 100 ml of *sodium chloride injection*. Close the container and heat it in an autoclave so that the contents are maintained at 110° for 30 minutes (solution B). Solution B complies with the *test for pyrogens*, Appendix XIV D. Use 10 ml of the solution per kg of the rabbit's weight.

Abnormal toxicity Solution B complies with the *test for abnormal toxicity*, Appendix XIV E, using 0.5 ml of the solution.

Packaging Sterile plastic containers for human blood and blood components are packed in protective tamper-evident envelopes. The protective envelopes are sufficiently robust to withstand normal handling.

On removal from its protective envelope the container shows no signs of leakage and no growth of micro-organisms.

Labelling The label states (1) the date after which the container is not intended to be used; (2) that, once withdrawn from its protective envelope, the container must be used within 10 days.

A part of the label is reserved for the information required concerning the blood or blood component for which the container is intended to be used.

The ink or other substance used to print the labels or the writing does not diffuse into the plastic material of the container and it remains legible up to the time of use.

2. EMPTY STERILE CONTAINERS OF PLASTICISED POLY(VINYL CHLORIDE) FOR BLOOD AND BLOOD COMPONENTS

(Ph. Eur. text 3.2.4)

Unless otherwise authorised as described in the Introduction to Appendix XIX C, the nature and composition of the material from which the containers are made should meet the type specification for materials based on plasticised poly(vinyl chloride) for containers for human blood and blood components, Appendix XX A1.

Empty sterile containers of plasticised poly(vinyl chloride) for blood and blood components comply with the tests stated under Sterile plastic containers for blood and blood components, Appendix XIX D1, and with the following tests.

Acidity or alkalinity Introduce into the container a volume of *water for injections* corresponding to the intended volume of anticoagulant solution. Close the container and heat in an autoclave so that the contents are maintained at 110° for 30 minutes. Cool and add sufficient *water for injections* to fill the container to its nominal capacity (solution A). To a volume of solution A corresponding to 4% of the nominal capacity of the container add 0.1 ml of *phenolphthalein solution*; the solution remains colourless. Add 0.4 ml of 0.01M *sodium hydroxide VS*; the solution is pink. Add 0.8 ml of 0.01M *hydrochloric acid VS* and 0.1 ml of *methyl red solution*; the solution is orange-red or red.

Light absorption Heat *water for injections* in a borosilicate-glass flask in an autoclave at 110° for 30 minutes (solution B). Measure the *light absorption* of solution A, Appendix II B, in the range 230 to 360 nm using solution B in the reference cell. The *absorbance* is not more than 0.30 at any wavelength from 230 to 250 nm and not more than 0.10 at any wavelength from 251 to 360 nm.

Ammonium Dilute 5 ml of solution A to 14 ml with *water*. The resulting solution complies with the *limit test for ammonium*, Appendix VII (2 ppm).

Chloride 15 ml of solution A complies with the *limit test for chlorides*, Appendix VII. Use a mixture of 1.2 ml of *chloride standard solution (5 ppm Cl)* and 13.8 ml of *water* to prepare the standard (0.4 ppm).

Extractable di(2-ethylhexyl) phthalate *Extraction solvent* Ethanol having a *relative density* of 0.9389 to 0.9395, Appendix V G, verified with a pycnometer.

Stock solution Dissolve 0.1 g of *di(2-ethylhexyl) phthalate* in the extraction solvent and dilute to 100 ml with the same solvent.

Standard solutions

(a) Dilute 20 ml of stock solution to 100 ml with extraction solvent.

(b) Dilute 10 ml of stock solution to 100 ml with extraction solvent.

(c) Dilute 5 ml of stock solution to 100 ml with extraction solvent.

(d) Dilute 2 ml of stock solution to 100 ml with extraction solvent.

(e) Dilute 1 ml of stock solution to 100 ml with extraction solvent.

Measure the *absorbances*, Appendix II B, of the standard solutions at the maximum at 272 nm, using the extraction solvent as compensation liquid and plot a curve of absorbance against the concentration of di(2-ethylhexyl) phthalate.

Extraction procedure Using the donor tubing and the needle or adaptor, fill the empty container with a volume equal to half the nominal volume with the extraction solvent, previously heated to 37° in a well-stoppered flask. Expel the air completely from the container and seal the donor tube. Immerse the filled container in a horizontal position in a water bath maintained at 37°±1° for 60±1 minutes without shaking. Remove the container from the water bath, invert it gently ten times and transfer the contents to a glass flask. Immediately measure the *absorbance*, Appendix II B, at the maximum at 272 nm, using the extraction solvent as compensation liquid.

Determine the concentration of di(2-ethylhexyl) phthalate in milligrams per 100 ml of extract from the calibration curve. The concentration does not exceed:
10 mg per 100 ml for containers of nominal volume greater than 300 ml but not greater than 500 ml;
13 mg per 100 ml for containers of nominal volume greater than 150 ml but not greater than 300 ml;
14 mg per 100 ml for containers of nominal volume up to 150 ml.

Oxidisable substances Immediately after the preparation of solution A transfer a quantity corresponding to 8% of the nominal capacity of the container to a borosilicate-glass flask. At the same time prepare a blank solution using an equal volume of freshly prepared solution B in another borosilicate-glass flask. To each solution add 20 ml of 0.002M *potassium permanganate VS* and 1 ml of 1M *sulphuric acid*. Allow to stand at room temperature, protected from light, for 15 minutes. To each solution add 0.1 g of *potassium iodide*, allow to stand protected from light for 5 minutes and titrate immediately with 0.01M *sodium thiosulphate VS* using 0.25 ml of *starch solution*, added towards the end of the titration, as indicator. The difference between the two titrations is not more than 2.0 ml.

Residue on evaporation Evaporate to dryness 100 ml of solution A in a borosilicate-glass beaker previously heated to 105°. At the same time and in the same manner evaporate 100 ml of solution B. Dry to constant weight at 100° to 105°. The difference between the weights of the residues is not more than 3 mg.

3. STERILE CONTAINERS OF PLASTICISED POLY(VINYL CHLORIDE) FOR BLOOD CONTAINING AN ANTICOAGULANT SOLUTION

(Ph. Eur text 3.2.5)

Unless otherwise authorised as described in the Introduction to Appendix XIX C, the nature and composition of the material from which the containers are made should meet the type specification for materials based on plasticised poly(vinyl chloride) for containers for human blood and blood components, Appendix XX A1.

Sterile plastic containers containing an anticoagulant solution that complies with the monograph for Anticoagulant and Preservative Solutions for Blood are used for the collection, storage and administration of blood. Before filling they comply with the description and characteristics stated under Empty sterile containers of plasticised poly(vinyl chloride) for blood and blood components, Appendix XIX D2.

After addition of the anticoagulant solution the containers comply with the tests stated under Sterile plastic containers for blood and blood components, Appendix XIX D1, and with the following tests.

Light absorption Measure the *light absorption*, Appendix II B, of the anticoagulant solution from the container in the range 250 to 350 nm using in the reference cell an anticoagulant solution of the same composition that has not been in contact with a plastic material. The *absorbance* at the maximum at 280 nm is not more than 0.5.

Extractable di(2-ethylhexyl) phthalate Carefully remove the anticoagulant solution by means of the flexible transfer tube. Using a funnel fitted to the tube, completely fill the container with *water*, leave in contact for 1 minute squeezing the container gently and empty completely. Repeat the rinsing. The container then complies with the test described under Empty sterile containers of plasticised poly(vinyl chloride) for human blood and blood components.

Volume of anticoagulant solution The volume does not differ by more than ± 10% from the stated volume when determined by emptying the container and collecting the anticoagulant solution in a graduated cylinder.

[1]Use blood collected less than 3 hours previously or blood collected into anticoagulant Citrate Phosphate Dextrose Solution (CPD) less than 24 hours previously.

E. Rubber Closures for Containers for Aqueous Parenteral Preparations

(Ph. Eur. text 3.2.9)

Rubber closures for containers for aqueous parenteral preparations[1] are made of materials obtained by vulcanisation (cross-linking) of macromolecular organic substances (elastomers), with appropriate additives. The elastomers are produced from natural or synthetic substances by polymerisation, polyaddition or polycondensation. The nature of the principal components and of the various additives, for example, vulcanisers, accelerators, stabilising agents and pigments, depends on the properties required for the finished article.

Rubber closures may be classified into two types. Type I closures are those that meet the strictest requirements and are to be preferred. Type II closures are those that have mechanical properties suitable for special uses, for example, multiple piercing, and cannot meet requirements as severe as those for Type I closures because of their chemical composition.

The closures chosen for use with a particular preparation are such that the components of the preparation in contact with the closure are not adsorbed onto the surface of the closure and do not migrate into or through the closure to an extent sufficient to affect the preparation adversely. The closure does not yield to the preparation substances in quantities sufficient to affect its stability or to present a risk of toxicity. The closures are compatible with the preparation for which they are used throughout its period of validity.

The manufacturer of the preparation must obtain an assurance from the supplier that the composition of the closure does not vary and that it is identical to that of the closure used during compatibility testing. When the manufacturer of the preparation is informed of changes in the composition, compatibility testing must be repeated, totally or partly, depending on the nature of the changes.

The closures are washed and may be sterilised before use.

Characteristics Rubber closures are elastic and either translucent or opaque; the colour depends on the additives used. They are homogeneous and practically free from flash and adventitious materials, for example, fibres, foreign particles and waste rubber.

Rubber closures are practically insoluble in *tetrahydrofuran* in which, however, a considerable reversible swelling may occur.

Identification of the type of rubber used for the closures is not within the scope of this specification. The identification test given below distinguishes elastomer and non-elastomer closures but does not differentiate the various types of rubber. Other identity tests may be carried out with the aim of detecting differences in a batch compared to the closures used for compatibility testing. One or more of the following analytical methods may be applied for this purpose: determination of relative density, determination of sulphated ash, determination of sulphur content, thin-layer chromatography carried out on an extract, ultraviolet absorption spectrophotometry of an extract, infrared absorption spectrophotometry of a pyrolysate.

For the tests for Fragmentation, Penetrability and Self-sealing, treat the closures in the same manner as that for the preparation of solution A described under the test for Acidity or alkalinity and allow to dry.

Identification The elasticity is such that a strip of material with a cross-section of 1 to 5 mm^2 can be stretched by hand to at least twice its original length. Once stretched to twice its length for 1 minute, it contracts to less than 1.2 times its original length within 30 seconds.

Acidity or alkalinity Place a number of uncut closures, corresponding to a surface area of about 100 cm^2, in a suitable glass container, cover with *water*, boil for 5 minutes and rinse 5 times with cold *water*. Place the washed closures in a wide-necked flask of Type I glass (Appendix XIX B), add 200 ml of *water* per 100 cm^2 surface area of the closures and weigh. Cover the mouth of the flask with aluminium foil or a borosilicate-glass beaker. Heat in an autoclave so that a temperature of 119° to 123°

is reached within 20 to 30 minutes and maintain at that temperature for 30 minutes. Cool to room temperature over about 30 minutes and make up to the original weight with *water*. Shake and immediately separate the solution from the closures by decantation (solution A). Shake solution A before use in this or any other test.

To 20 ml of solution A add 0.1 ml of *bromothymol blue solution R1*. Not more than 0.3 ml of 0.01M *sodium hydroxide VS* or 0.8 ml of 0.01M *hydrochloric acid VS* is required to change the colour of the solution to blue or yellow respectively.

Clarity and colour of solution Solution A is not more opalescent than *reference suspension II*, Appendix IV A, for Type I closures and is not more opalescent than *reference suspension III* for Type II closures. Solution A is not more intensely coloured than *reference solution* GY_5, Appendix IV B, Method II.

Fragmentation For closures intended to be pierced by a hypodermic needle, carry out the following test. For closures that are intended to be used for aqueous preparations, place a volume of *water* corresponding to the nominal volume minus 4 ml in each of 12 clean vials, close the vials with the closures being examined, secure with a cap and allow to stand for 16 hours. For closures that are intended to be used for dry preparations, close 12 clean vials with the closures being examined. Using a lubricated, long-bevel[2] (bevel angle of 10° to 14°) hypodermic needle with an external diameter of 0.8 mm fitted to a clean syringe, inject 1 ml of *water* into the vial and remove 1 ml of air; carry out this operation 4 times for each closure, piercing each time at a different site. Use a new needle for each closure and check that the needle is not blunted during the test. Pass the liquid in the vials through a filter with a nominal pore size of 0.5 µm. Count the fragments of rubber visible to the naked eye. The total number of fragments is not more than five. This limit is based on the assumption that fragments with a diameter equal to or greater than 50 µm are visible to the naked eye. In cases of doubt or dispute, examine the fragments with a microscope to verify their nature and size.

Light absorption Carry out the test within 4 hours of preparing solution A. Filter solution A on a membrane filter with a nominal pore size of 0.5 µm and reject the first few ml of filtrate. Measure the *light absorption* of the filtrate, Appendix II B, in the range 220 to 360 nm using in the reference cell a solution prepared in the same manner as solution A but using 200 ml of *water* without the closures. The *absorbance* is not more than 0.2 for Type I closures and not more than 4.0 for Type II closures. If necessary, dilute the filtrate before measurement and correct the result for the dilution.

Penetrability For closures intended to be pierced by a hypodermic needle, carry out the following test. Fill 10 suitable vials with *water* to the nominal volume, close the vials with the closures being examined and secure with a cap. For each closure, use a new, lubricated, long-bevel[3] (bevel angle of 10° to 14°) hypodermic needle with an external diameter of 0.8 mm and pierce the closures with the needle perpendicular to the surface. The force required for piercing, determined with an accuracy of ±0.25 N, is not greater than 10 N for each closure.

Self-sealing test For closures intended to be used with multidose containers, carry out the following test. Fill 10 suitable vials with *water* to the nominal volume, close the vials with the closures being examined and secure with a cap. For each closure, use a new hypodermic needle with an external diameter of 0.8 mm and pierce the closure 10 times, piercing each time at a different site. Immerse the vials upright in a 0.1% w/v solution of *methylene blue* and reduce the external pressure by 27 kPa for 10 minutes. Restore atmospheric pressure and leave the vials immersed for 30 minutes. Rinse the outside of the vials. None of the vials contains any trace of coloured solution.

Ammonium Make 5 ml of solution A alkaline, if necessary, by adding 2M *sodium hydroxide* and dilute to 15 ml with *water*. To the resulting solution add 0.3 ml of *alkaline potassium tetraiodomercurate solution*. After 30 seconds, any yellow colour is not more intense than that of a solution prepared in the same manner and at the same time but using 10 ml of *ammonium standard solution (1 ppm* NH_4*)* and adding the same volume of 2M *sodium hydroxide* as in the preparation of the test solution (2 ppm in solution A).

Heavy metals Solution A complies with *limit test A for heavy metals*, Appendix VII. Use *lead standard solution (2 ppm Pb)* to prepare the standard (2 ppm in solution A).

Soluble zinc Not more than 5 µg of Zn per ml of solution A when determined by the following method. To 10 ml of solution A, add 0.5 ml of 0.1M *hydrochloric acid* and dilute to 100 ml with *water*. Carry out the method for *atomic absorption spectrophotometry*, Appendix II D, measuring at 214 nm but using a single standard solution prepared in the following manner. To 10 ml of a 0.1% v/v solution of *zinc solution ASp* add 0.5 ml of 0.1M *hydrochloric acid* and dilute to 100 ml with *water*.

Volatile sulphides Place closures, cut if necessary, with a total surface area of 19 to 21 cm^2 in a 100-ml conical flask and add 50 ml of a 2% w/v solution of *citric acid*. Place a piece of *lead acetate paper* over the mouth of the flask and maintain the paper in position by placing an inverted weighing bottle over it. Heat in an autoclave at 119° to 123° for 30 minutes. Any black stain on the paper is not more intense than that of a standard prepared at the same time and in the same manner using 0.154 mg of *sodium sulphide* and 50 ml of a 2% w/v solution of *citric acid*.

Reducing substances Carry out the test within 4 hours of preparing solution A. To 20 ml of solution A, add 1 ml of 1M *sulphuric acid* and 20 ml of 0.002M *potassium permanganate VS* and boil for 3 minutes. Cool, add 1 g of *potassium iodide* and titrate immediately with 0.01M *sodium thiosulphate VS*, using 0.25 ml of *starch solution* as indicator. Repeat the operation using 20 ml of the blank solution prepared in the test for Light absorption. The difference between the titration volumes is not more than 3.0 ml for Type I closures and 7.0 ml for Type II closures.

Residue on evaporation Evaporate 50 ml of solution A to dryness on a water bath and dry at 100° to 105°. The residue weighs not more than 2.0 mg for Type I closures and not more than 4.0 mg for Type II closures. [1]This text also applies to closures for containers for powders and freeze-dried products to be dissolved in water immediately before use. It does not apply to closures made from silicone elastomer (see European Pharmacopoeia, section VI.1.3.2 Silicone elastomer for closures and tubing), to laminated closures or to lacquered closures.

[1]This text also applies to closures for containers for powders and freeze-dried products to be

dissolved in water immediately before use. It does not apply to closures made from silicone elastomer (see European Pharmacopoeia, section VI.1.3.2 Silicone elastomer for closures and tubing), to laminated closures or to lacquered closures.

[2]See ISO 7864: Sterile hypodermic needles for single use.

[3]See ISO 7864: Sterile hypodermic needles for single use.

F. Sets for the Transfusion of Blood and Blood Components

(Ph. Eur. text 3.2.6)

Sets for the transfusion of blood and blood components consist principally of plastic tubing to which are fitted the parts necessary to enable the set to be used for transfusion in the appropriate manner. The sets include a closure-piercing device, a blood filter, a drip chamber, a flow regulator and a Luer connector. Provision to allow an injection to be made into the transfusion line during use is also usually included. When the sets are to be used with containers requiring an air filter, this may be incorporated in the closure-piercing device or a separate air-inlet device may be used. The chamber enclosing the blood filter, the drip chamber and the main tubing are transparent.

All parts of the set that may be in contact with blood and blood components are sterile and pyrogen-free. The sets are not to be resterilised or reused. Each set is presented in an individual package that maintains the sterility of the contents.

Sets for the transfusion of blood and blood components are manufactured in accordance with the requirements of good manufacturing practice for medical devices. The materials chosen and the design of the set are such as to ensure the absence of haemolytic effects.

For use in the United Kingdom it is recommended that the sets comply with British Standard BS 2463:Part 2:1989 (Specifications for administration sets) with regard to dimensions and performance.

Carry out the following tests on sterilised sets.

Acidity or alkalinity Make a closed circulation system from three sets and a 300-ml borosilicate-glass vessel. Fit a thermostat device to the vessel so that the temperature of the liquid in the vessel is maintained at 36° to 38°. Circulate 250 ml of *water for injections* through the system in the direction used for transfusion for 2 hours at a rate of 1 litre per hour using for example a peristaltic pump applied to a piece of suitable silicone tubing as short as possible. Collect the whole of the solution and allow to cool (solution A).

To 25 ml of solution A add 0.15 ml of a solution containing 0.1% w/v of *bromothymol blue*, 0.02% w/v of *methyl red* and 0.2% w/v of *phenolphthalein* in *ethanol (96%)*. Not more than 0.5 ml of 0.01M *sodium hydroxide VS* is required to change the colour of the solution to blue.

To a further 25 ml of solution A add 0.2 ml of *methyl orange solution*. Not more than 0.5 ml of 0.01M *hydrochloric acid VS* is required to begin the change in colour of the indicator.

Clarity and colour of solution Solution A is *clear*, Appendix IV A, and *colourless*, Appendix IV B, Method II.

Flow rate Using a complete set with the flow regulator fully open, pass 50 ml of a solution having a viscosity of 3 mPa s (a 3.3% w/v solution of polyethylene glycol 4000 at 20° is suitable) under a static head of 1 m. The time taken for the passage of the solution is not more than 90 seconds.

Light absorption Measure the *light absorption* of solution A, Appendix II B, in the range 230 to 250 nm and in the range 251 to 360 nm. The *absorbance* is not more than 0.30 at any wavelength in the range 230 to 250 nm and not more than 0.15 at any wavelength in the range 251 to 360 nm.

Resistance to pressure Make tight the extremities of the set and any air-inlet device. Connect the set to a compressed air outlet fitted with a pressure regulator. Immerse the set in a tank of water at 20° to 23°. Apply progressively an excess pressure of 100 kPa and maintain for 1 minute. No air bubble escapes from the set.

Transparency Prepare an 8-fold dilution of the suspension prepared for the *standard of opalescence*, Appendix IV A, Method I, for sets having tubing with an external diameter of less than 5 mm and a 16-fold dilution of the suspension for sets having tubing with an external diameter equal to or greater than 5 mm. The opalescence of and presence of bubbles in the diluted suspension are discernible when it is circulated through the set, as compared with a set from the same batch filled with *water*.

Ethylene oxide Not more than 10 ppm if the label states that ethylene oxide has been used for sterilisation. Use the following method. Carry out the method for *gas chromatography*, Appendix III B, using the following gaseous solutions. For solution (1) remove the set from the packaging and weigh. Cut the set into pieces with a maximum dimension of 1 cm and place the pieces in a 250- to 500-ml vial containing 150 ml of *dimethylacetamide*. Close the vial with a suitable stopper and secure the stopper. Place the vial in an oven at 69° to 71° for 16 hours. Remove 1 ml of the hot gas from the vial and inject it onto the column. Prepare solution (2) under a ventilated hood as follows. Place 50 ml of *dimethylacetamide* in a 50-ml vial, stopper, secure the stopper and weigh to the nearest 0.1 mg. Fill a 50-ml polyethylene or polypropylene syringe with gaseous *ethylene oxide*, allow the gas to remain in contact with the syringe for about 3 minutes, empty the syringe and fill again with 50 ml of gaseous *ethylene oxide*. Fit a hypodermic needle to the syringe and reduce the volume of gas in the syringe from 50 ml to 25 ml. Inject the remaining 25 ml of gas slowly into the vial, shaking gently and avoiding contact between the needle and the dimethylacetamide. Weigh the vial again. The increase in weight is 45 to 60 mg. Using this increase in weight calculate the exact concentration of the solution (about 1 g per litre).

Prepare a calibration curve using a series of seven vials of the same type as that used in the preparation of solution (1), each containing 150 ml of *dimethylacetamide*. Introduce respectively 0, 0.05, 0.10, 0.20, 0.50, 1.00 and 2.00 ml of solution (2), that is, about 0, 50, 100, 200, 500, 1000 and 2000 µg of ethylene oxide. Stopper the vials, secure the stoppers and place the vials in an oven at 69° to 71° for 16 hours. Inject 1 ml of the hot gas from each vial onto the column and prepare a calibration curve from the heights of the peaks and the weight of ethylene oxide in each flask.

The chromatographic procedure may be carried out using a stainless steel column (1.5 m × 6.4 mm) packed with *acid-washed silanised diatomaceous support* coated with 30% w/w of *polyethylene glycol 1500* and maintained at 40° with the inlet port at 100°, the detector at 150° and using *helium* as the carrier gas with a flow rate of 20 ml per minute. Verify the absence of peaks interfering with the ethylene oxide peak by carrying out the test using an unsterilised set or using the chromatographic procedure prescribed above but using a column such as a stainless steel column (3 m × 3.2 mm) packed with *acid-washed silanised diatomaceous support* coated with 20% w/w of triscyanoethoxypropane and maintained at 60°.

Calculate the weight of ethylene oxide in the vial used in the preparation of solution (1) from the calibration curve prepared as described above and from the height of the peak obtained in the chromatogram obtained with solution (1).

Extraneous particles Using the normal inlet, fill the set with a 0.01% w/v solution of *sodium dodecyl sulphate* previously filtered through a sintered-glass filter (pore size 10 to 16 µm) and heated to 37°. Collect the liquid through the normal outlet. When examined under suitable conditions of visibility, the liquid is clear and practically free from visible particles and filaments. (It is assumed that particles and filaments with a diameter equal to or greater than 50 µm are visible to the naked eye.)

Reducing substances Carry out the test within 4 hours of preparing solution A. To 20 ml of solution A, add 1 ml of 1M *sulphuric acid* and 20 ml of 0.002M *potassium permanganate VS* and boil for 3 minutes. Cool immediately, add 1 g of *potassium iodide* and titrate with 0.01M *sodium thiosulphate VS* using 0.25 ml of *starch solution* as indicator. Repeat the operation using 20 ml of *water for injections*. The difference between the titration volumes is not more than 2.0 ml.

Residue on evaporation Evaporate 50 ml of solution A to dryness on a water bath and dry to constant weight at 100° to 105°. Repeat the operation using 50 ml of *water for injections*. The difference between the weights of the residues is not more than 1.5 mg.

Sterility Comply with the *test for sterility*, Appendix XVI A, with the following modifications.

If the sets are stated to be sterile internally only, pass 50 ml of *sodium chloride—peptone solution pH 7.0* through the set and use to carry out the test by Method I: Membrane filtration.

If the sets are stated to be sterile both internally and externally, open the packaging using aseptic precautions. When carrying out the test by Method I: Membrane filtration, place the set or its components in a suitable container containing a sufficient quantity of *buffered sodium chloride—peptone solution pH 7.0* to allow total rins-ing for 10 minutes. When carrying out the test by Method II: Direct inoculation, place the set or its components in a suitable container containing a sufficient quantity of the culture medium to ensure complete immersion.

Pyrogens Connect together five sets and pass through the assembly 250 ml of *sodium chloride injection* with a flow rate not exceeding 10 ml per minute. Collect the solution aseptically in a pyrogen-free container. The solution complies with the *test for pyrogens*, Appendix XIV D. Use 10 ml of the solution per kg of the rabbit's weight.

Labelling The label states, where applicable, that the set has been sterilised using ethylene oxide.

G. Sterile Single-use Plastic Syringes

(Ph. Eur. text 3.2.8)

Sterile single-use plastic syringes are medical devices intended for immediate use for the administration of injectable preparations. They consist of a syringe barrel and a piston that may have an elastomer sealing ring and may be fitted with a needle that may be non-detachable. The barrel of the syringe is sufficiently transparent to permit dosages to be read without difficulty and to allow air bubbles and foreign particles to be discerned. Silicone oil may be applied to the internal wall of the barrel to assist in the smooth operation of the syringe but no excess remains that is capable of contaminating the contents at the time of use.

The plastics and elastomer materials from which the barrel and piston are made are commonly polypropylene and polyethylene, type specifications for which are provided in the European Pharmacopoeia in the section on Plastic Materials (VI.1.2).

Sterile single-use plastic syringes are supplied sterile and pyrogen-free and are not to be resterilised or reused. Each syringe is presented in an individual package that maintains its sterility.

The inks, glues and adhesives for the marking on the syringe or on the package and, where necessary, the assembly of the syringe and its package, do not migrate across the walls.

For use in the United Kingdom it is recommended that the syringes comply with British Standard BS 5081: Parts 1 and 2:1987 (Sterile Hypodermic Syringes and Needles).

Acidity or alkalinity Using a sufficient number of syringes to produce 50 ml of solution, fill the syringes to their nominal capacity with *water for injections* and maintain at 37° for 24 hours. Combine the contents of the syringes in a suitable borosilicate-glass vessel (solution A). Prepare solution A in a manner that avoids contamination by foreign particles. To 20 ml of solution A add 0.1 ml of *bromothymol blue solution R1*. Not more than 0.3 ml of 0.01M *sodium hydroxide VS* or 0.01M *hydrochloric acid VS* is required to change the colour of the solution.

Clarity and colour of solution Solution A is *clear*, Appendix IV A, and *colourless*, Appendix IV B, Method II, and is practically free from foreign solid particles.

Light absorption *Absorbance* of solution A in the range 220 to 360 nm, not more than 0.40, Appendix II B.

Transparency Prepare a 10-fold dilution of the suspension prepared for the *standard of opalescence*, Appendix IV A, Method I, previously allowing the suspension to stand at 18° to 22° for 24 hours. Fill a syringe with *water* (reference) and another with the diluted suspension. Compare with the naked eye in diffuse light against a dark background. The opalescence of the diluted suspension is detectable when compared with the reference.

Ethylene oxide Not more than 10 ppm if the label states that ethylene oxide has been used for sterilisation. Use the following method. Carry out the method for *gas chromatography*, Appendix III B, using the following gaseous solutions. For solution (1) remove the syringe from the packaging and weigh. Cut the syringe into pieces with a maximum dimension of 1 cm and place the pieces in a 250- to 500-ml vial containing 150 ml of *dimethylacetamide*. Close the vial with a suitable stopper and secure the stopper. Place the vial in an oven at 69° to 71° for 16 hours. Remove 1 ml of the hot gas from the vial and inject it onto the column. Prepare solution (2) under a ventilated hood as follows. Place 50 ml of *dimethylacetamide* in a 50-ml vial, stopper, secure the stopper and weigh to the nearest 0.1 mg. Fill a 50-ml polyethylene or polypropylene syringe with gaseous *ethylene oxide,* allow the gas to remain in contact with the syringe for about 3 minutes, empty the syringe and fill again with 50 ml of gaseous *ethylene oxide.* Fit a hypodermic needle to the syringe and reduce the volume of gas in the syringe from 50 ml to 25 ml. Inject the remaining 25 ml of gas slowly into the vial, shaking gently and avoiding contact between the needle and the dimethylacetamide. Weigh the vial again. The increase in weight is 45 to 60 mg. Using this increase in weight calculate the exact concentration of the solution (about 1 g per litre).

Prepare a calibration curve using a series of seven vials of the same type as that used in the preparation of solution (1), each containing 150 ml of *dimethylacetamide.* Introduce respectively 0, 0.05, 0.10, 0.20, 0.50, 1.00 and 2.00 ml of solution (2), that is, about 0, 50, 100, 200, 500, 1000 and 2000 µg of ethylene oxide. Stopper the vials, secure the stoppers and place the vials in an oven at 69° to 71° for 16 hours. Inject 1 ml of the hot gas from each vial onto the column and prepare a calibration curve from the heights of the peaks and the weight of ethylene oxide in each flask.

The chromatographic procedure may be carried out using a stainless steel column (1.5 m × 6.4 mm) packed with *acid-washed silanised diatomaceous support* coated with 30% w/w of *polyethylene glycol 1500* and maintained at 40° with the inlet port at 100°, the detector at 150° and using *helium* as the carrier gas with a flow rate of 20 ml per minute. Verify the absence of peaks interfering with the ethylene oxide peak by carrying out the test using an unsterilised syringe or using the chromatographic procedure prescribed above but using a column such as a stainless steel column (3 m × 3.2 mm) packed with *acid-washed silanised diatomaceous support* coated with 20% w/w of triscyanoethoxypropane and maintained at 60°.

Calculate the weight of ethylene oxide in the vial used in the preparation of solution (1) from the calibration curve prepared as described above and from the height of the peak obtained in the chromatogram obtained with solution (1).

Silicone oil Calculate the internal surface area of a syringe in cm² using the expression $2(\pi hv)^{1/2}$ where h is the height of the graduation in cm and v is the nominal volume of the syringe in cm³. Use a sufficient number of syringes to give an internal surface area of 100 to 200 cm². Aspirate into each syringe a volume of *dichloromethane* equal to half the nominal volume and make up to the nominal volume with air. Rinse the internal surface corresponding to the nominal volume with the solvent by inverting the syringe 10 times in succession with the needle fitting closed by a finger covered by a plastic film inert to dichloromethane. Expel the extracts into a tared dish and repeat the operation. Evaporate the combined extracts to dryness on a water bath and dry at 100° to 105° for 1 hour. The residue weighs not more than 0.25 mg per square centimetre of internal surface area.

The *infrared absorption spectrum* of the residue, Appendix II A, shows absorption bands typical of silicone oil at 805, 1020, 1095, 1260 and 2960 cm^{-1}.

Reducing substances To 20 ml of solution A add 2 ml of *sulphuric acid* and 20 ml of 0.002M *potassium permanganate* and boil for 3 minutes. Cool immediately, add 1 g of *potassium iodide* and titrate immediately with 0.01M *sodium thiosulphate VS* using 0.25 ml of *starch solution* as indicator. Repeat the operation using 20 ml of *water for injections* in place of solution A. The difference between the titration volumes is not more than 3.0 ml.

Sterility Comply with the *test for sterility,* Appendix XVI A, with the following modifications.

For syringes stated to be sterile, using aseptic technique, open the package, withdraw the syringe, separate the components and place each in a suitable container containing sufficient culture medium to cover the part completely. Use both the recommended media.

For syringes stated to be sterile only internally, use 50 ml of inoculation medium for each test syringe. Using aseptic technique, remove the needle protector and submerge the needle in the culture medium. Flush the syringe five times by withdrawing the plunger to its fullest extent.

Pyrogens Syringes with a nominal capacity equal to or greater than 15 ml comply with the *test for pyrogens,* Appendix XIV D. Fill a minimum of three syringes to their nominal volume with a pyrogen-free 0.9% w/v solution of *sodium chloride* and maintain at 37° for 2 hours. Combine the solutions aseptically in a pyrogen-free container and carry out the test immediately using 10 ml of the solution per kg of the rabbit's weight.

Labelling The label states (1) the batch number; (2) the identity of the manufacturer; (3) a description of the syringe; (4) that the syringe is for single-use only; (5) the method of sterilisation; (6) that the syringe is sterile or that it is sterile only internally; (7) that the syringe is not to be used if the packaging is damaged or the sterility protector is loose.

Appendix XX

Materials Used for the Manufacture of Containers

(Ph. Eur. text 3.1)

The materials described below are used for the manufacture of containers for pharmaceutical use. Materials other than those described in the Pharmacopoeia may be used subject to approval in each case by the national authority responsible for the licensing for sale of the preparation in the container.

A. Material Based on Plasticised Poly(Vinyl Chloride)

1. FOR CONTAINERS FOR BLOOD AND BLOOD COMPONENTS AND FOR CONTAINERS FOR AQUEOUS SOLUTIONS FOR INTRAVENOUS INFUSION

(Ph. Eur. text 3.1.1)

Materials based on plasticised poly(vinyl chloride) contain various additives, in addition to the high-molecular-mass polymer obtained by polymerisation of vinyl chloride.

Materials based on plasticised poly(vinyl chloride) for containers for human blood and blood components and for containers for aqueous solutions for intravenous infusion are defined by the nature and the proportions of the substances used in their manufacture.

They contain not less than 55 per cent of poly(vinyl chloride) and may contain the following additives:

- — not more than 40 per cent of di(2-ethylhexyl) phthalate,
- — not more than 1 per cent of zinc octanoate (zinc 2-ethylhexanoate),
- — not more than 1 per cent of calcium stearate or zinc stearate or 1 per cent of a mixture of the two,
- — not more than 1 per cent of *N,N'*-diacylethylenediamines (in this context acyl means in particular palmitoyl and stearoyl),
- — not more than 10 per cent of one of the following epoxidised oils or 10 per cent of a mixture of the two:
- - epoxidised soya oil of which the oxiran oxygen content is 6 per cent to 8 per cent and the iodine value is not greater than 6,
- - epoxidised linseed oil of which the oxiran oxygen content is not greater than 10 per cent and iodine value is not greater than 7.

No antioxidant additive may be added to the polymer.

When colouring matter is added, only ultramarine blue is to be added. No colouring material is added to poly(vinyl chloride) for the manufacture of containers for blood and blood products.

CHARACTERS

Powder, beads, granules or translucent sheets of varying thicknesses, colourless to pale yellow.

IDENTIFICATION

If necessary, cut the material to be examined into pieces with a maximum dimension of 1 cm.

To 2.0 g of the material to be examined add 200 ml of *peroxide-free ether R* and heat under a reflux condenser for 12 h. Separate the residue (*B*) and the solution (*A*) by filtration.

Evaporate solution *A* to dryness under reduced pressure on a water-bath at 30°C. Dissolve the residue in 10 ml of *toluene R* (solution A_1). Dissolve the residue *B* in 60 ml of *ethylene chloride R*, heating on a water-bath under a reflux condenser. Filter. Add the solution dropwise and with vigorous shaking to 600 ml of *heptane R* heated almost to boiling. Filter the hot mixture through a hot filter to separate the coagulum (B_1) and the organic solution. Allow the latter to cool; separate the precipitate (B_2) that forms and filter through a tared sintered-glass filter (40).

A. Dissolve the coagulum B_1 in 30 ml of *tetrahydrofuran R* and add, in small quantities with shaking, 40 ml of *ethanol R*. Separate the precipitate (B_3) by filtration and dry *in vacuo* at a temperature not exceeding 50°C over *diphosphorus pentoxide R* or *anhydrous calcium chloride R*. Dissolve a few milligrams of precipitate B_3 in 1 ml of *tetrahydrofuran R*, place a few drops of the solution obtained on a sodium chloride plate and evaporate to dryness in an oven at 100°C to 105°C. Examine by infrared absorption spectrophotometry (*2.2.24*), comparing with the spectrum obtained with *poly(vinyl chloride) CRS*.

B. Examine by thin-layer chromatography (*2.2.27*), using *silica gel G R* as the coating substance.

Test solution. Use solution A_1.

Reference solution. Dissolve 0.8 g of *di(2-ethyl-hexyl)-phthalate CRS* in *toluene R* and dilute to 10 ml with the same solvent.

Apply separately to the plate 5 µl of each solution. Develop over a path of 15 cm using *toluene R*. Dry the plate carefully and examine in ultraviolet light at 254 nm. The spot in the chromatogram obtained with the test solution is similar in position and fluorescence to the spot in the chromatogram obtained with the reference solution.

C. Examine the residue obtained in the test for di(2-ethylhexyl) phthalate by infrared absorption spectrophotometry (*2.2.24*), comparing with the spectrum obtained with *di(2-ethylhexyl) phthalate CRS*.

TESTS

Solution S_1 Place 5.0 g in a combustion flask. Add 30 ml of *sulphuric acid R* and heat until a black, syrupy mass is obtained. Cool and add carefully 10 ml of *strong hydrogen peroxide solution R*. Heat gently. Allow to cool and add 1 ml of *strong hydrogen peroxide solution R*; repeat by alternating evaporation and addition of hydrogen peroxide solution until a colourless liquid is obtained. Reduce the volume to about 10 ml. Cool and dilute to 50.0 ml with *water R*.

Solution S_2 Place 25 g in a borosilicate-glass flask. Add 500 ml of *water R* and cover the neck of the flask with aluminium foil or a borosilicate-glass beaker. Heat in an autoclave at 121 ± 2° for 20 min. Allow to cool and decant the solution.

Appearance of solution S_2 Solution S_2 is clear (*2.2.1*) and colourless (*Method II, 2.2.2*).

Acidity or alkalinity To 100 ml of solution S_2, add 0.15 ml of *BRP indicator solution R*. Not more than 1.5 ml of *0.01M sodium hydroxide* is required to change the colour of the indicator to blue. To 100 ml of solution S_2 add

0.2 ml of *methyl orange solution R*. Not more than 1.0 ml of *0.01M hydrochloric acid* is required to initiate the colour change of the indicator.

Absorbance (*2.2.25*). Evaporate 100 ml of solution S_2 to dryness. Dissolve the residue in 5 ml of *hexane R*. At no wavelength in the range 250 nm to 310 nm is the absorbance greater than 0.25.

Reducing substances *Carry out the test within 4 h of preparation of solution* S_2. To 20.0 ml of solution S_2 add 1 ml of *dilute sulphuric acid R* and 20.0 ml of *0.002M potassium permanganate*. Boil under a reflux condenser for 3 min and cool immediately. Add 1 g of *potassium iodide R* and titrate immediately with *0.01M sodium thiosulphate*, using 0.25 ml of *starch solution R* as indicator. Carry out a blank titration using 20 ml of *water for injections R*. The difference between the titration volumes is not more than 2.0 ml.

Primary aromatic amines To 2.5 ml of solution A_1 obtained during the identification, add 6 ml of *water R* and 4 ml of *0.1M hydrochloric acid*. Shake vigorously and discard the organic layer. To the aqueous layer add 0.4 ml of a freshly prepared 10 g/l solution of *sodium nitrite R*. Mix and allow to stand for 1 min. Add 0.8 ml of a 25 g/l solution of *ammonium sulphamate R*, allow to stand for 1 min and add 2 ml of a 5 g/l solution of *naphthylethylenediamine dihydrochloride R*. After 30 min, any colour in the solution is not more intense than that in a standard prepared at the same time in the same manner using a mixture of 1 ml of a 0.01 g/l solution of *naphthylamine R* in *0.1M hydrochloric acid*, 5 ml of *water R* and 4 ml of *0.1M hydrochloric acid* instead of the aqueous layer (20 ppm).

Di(2-ethylhexyl) phthalate Examine the chromatogram obtained in the test for epoxidised oils in ultraviolet light at 254 nm and locate the zone corresponding to di(2-ethylhexyl) phthalate. Remove the area of silica gel corresponding to this zone and shake with 40 ml of *ether R*. Filter without loss and evaporate to dryness. The residue weighs not more than 40 mg.

***N,N′*-diacylethylenediamines** Wash precipitate B_2 obtained during the identification and contained in the tared sintered-glass filter (40) with *ethanol R*. Dry to constant mass over *diphosphorus pentoxide R* and weigh the filter. The precipitate weighs not more than 20 mg. Examine the residue by infrared absorption spectrophotometry (*2.2.24*). The absorption maxima in the spectrum obtained with the residue correspond in position and relative intensity to those in the spectrum obtained with *N,N′-diacylethylenediamines CRS*.

Epoxidised oils Examine by thin-layer chromatography (*2.2.27*), using *silica gel G R* in a 1 mm layer as the coating substance.

Apply separately to the plate as a band 30 mm by 3 mm 0.5 ml of solution A_1 obtained during the identification. Develop over a path of 15 cm using *toluene R*. Dry the plate carefully. Expose the plate to iodine vapour for 5 min. Examine the chromatogram and locate the band with an R_f of 0 and possibly the secondary band with an R_f of about 0.7, both corresponding to epoxidised oils. Remove the area of silica gel corresponding to the band or bands. Similarly remove a corresponding area of silica gel as blank reference. Separately shake both samples for 15 min with 40 ml of *methanol R*. Filter and evaporate to dryness. Weigh the two residues. The difference between the masses is not more than 10 mg.

Examine each of the residues by infrared absorption spectrophotometry (*2.2.24*). The absorption maxima in the spectrum obtained with the test residue correspond in position and relative intensity to those in the spectrum obtained with *epoxidised soya oil CRS* or *epoxidised linseed oil CRS* or with a mixture of the two, taking into consideration the absorption maxima of the blank reference if necessary.

Vinyl chloride Not more than 1 ppm, determined by head-space gas chromatography (*2.2.28*), using *ether R* as the internal standard.

Internal standard solution. Using a microsyringe, inject 10 µl of *ether R* into 20.0 ml of *dimethylacetamide R*, immersing the tip of the needle in the solvent. Immediately before use, dilute the solution to 1000 times its volume with *dimethylacetamide R*.

Test solution. Place 1.000 g of the material to be examined in a 50 ml vial and add 10.0 ml of the internal standard solution. Close the vial and secure the stopper. Shake, avoiding contact between the stopper and the liquid. Place the vial in a water-bath at 60 ±1° for 2 h.

Vinyl chloride primary solution. Prepare under a ventilated hood. Place 50.0 ml of *dimethylacetamide R* in a 50 ml vial, stopper the vial, secure the stopper and weigh to the nearest 0.1 mg. Fill a 50 ml polyethylene or polypropylene syringe with gaseous *vinyl chloride R*, allow the gas to remain in contact with the syringe for about 3 min, empty the syringe and fill again with 50 ml of gaseous *vinyl chloride R*. Fit a hypodermic needle to the syringe and reduce the volume of gas in the syringe from 50 ml to 25 ml. Inject these 25 ml of vinyl chloride slowly into the vial shaking gently and avoiding contact between the liquid and the needle. Weigh the vial again; the increase in mass is about 60 mg (1 µl of the solution thus obtained contains about 1.2 µg of vinyl chloride).

Vinyl chloride standard solution. To 1 volume of the vinyl chloride primary solution add 3 volumes of *dimethylacetamide R*.

Reference solutions. Place 10.0 ml of the internal standard solution in each of six 50 ml vials. Close the vials and secure the stoppers. Inject 1 µl, 2 µl, 3 µl, 5 µl and 10 µl, respectively, of the vinyl chloride standard solution into five of the vials. The six solutions thus obtained contain respectively, 0 µg, about 0.3 µg, 0.6 µg, 0.9 µg, 1.5 µg and 3 µg of vinyl chloride. Shake, avoiding contact between the stopper and the liquid. Place the vials in a water-bath at 60 ±1° for 2 h.

The chromatographic procedure may be carried out using:

— a stainless steel column 3 m long and 3 mm in internal diameter packed with *silanised diatomaceous earth for gas chromatography R* impregnated with 5 per cent *m/m* of *dimethylstearylamide R* and 5 per cent *m/m* of *macrogol 400 R*,

— *nitrogen for chromatography R* as the carrier gas at a flow rate of 30 ml per minute,

— a flame-ionisation detector,

maintaining the temperature of the column at 45°, that of the injection port at 100° and that of the detector at 150°. Inject 1 ml of the head-space of each vial. Calculate the content of vinyl chloride.

Total phosphorus Ignite 0.25 g in a platinum crucible with 0.2 g of *anhydrous sodium carbonate R* and 50 mg of *potassium nitrate R*. After cooling, take up the residue with *water R* and transfer to a 50 ml volumetric flask. Rinse the crucible with *water R*, add the washings to the flask, acidify with a 60 per cent *m/m* solution of *sulphuric acid R* until effervescence ceases, add 25 ml of *molybdovanadic reagent R* and dilute to 50.0 ml with *water R*. Any yellow colour in the solution is not more intense than that in a standard prepared at the same time by mixing 0.5 ml of a solution containing 0.219 g of *potassium dihydrogen phosphate R* in 1000.0 ml, 10 ml of *water R* and 25 ml of *molybdovanadic reagent R* and diluting to 50.0 ml with *water R* (100 ppm).

Barium Ignite 2.0 g in a silica crucible. Take up the residue in 10 ml of *hydrochloric acid R* and evaporate to dryness on a water-bath. Take up this residue with two quantities, each of 1 ml, of *distilled water R*. Filter and add 3 ml of *calcium sulphate solution R*. Any opalescence in the solution is not more intense than that in a standard prepared using 1.2 ml of *barium standard solution (50 ppm Ba) R*, 0.8 ml of *distilled water R* and 3 ml of *calcium sulphate solution R* (30 ppm).

Cadmium Not more than 0.6 ppm of Cd, determined by atomic absorption spectrometry (*Method I, 2.2.23*).

Test solution. Evaporate 10 ml of solution S_1 to dryness. Take up the residue using 5 ml of a 1 per cent *V/V* solution of *hydrochloric acid R*, filter and dilute the filtrate to 10.0 ml with the same acid.

Reference solutions. Prepare the reference solutions using *cadmium standard solution (0.1 per cent Cd) R*, diluted with a 1 per cent *V/V* solution of *hydrochloric acid R*.

Measure the absorbance at 228.8 nm using a cadmium hollow-cathode lamp as the source of radiation and an air-acetylene flame.

Calcium Not more than 0.07 per cent of Ca, determined by atomic absorption spectrometry (*Method I, 2.2.23*).

Test solution. Ignite 2.0 g of the material to be examined in a silica crucible. Take up the residue using 10 ml of *hydrochloric acid R* and evaporate to dryness on a water-bath. Take up this residue using 5 ml of *water R*, filter and dilute to 25.0 ml with the same solvent.

Reference solutions. Prepare the reference solutions using *calcium standard solution (400 ppm Ca) R*, diluted with *water R*.

Measure the absorbance at 422.7 nm using a calcium hollow-cathode lamp as the source of radiation and an air-acetylene flame.

Heavy metals (*2.4.8*). To 10 ml of solution S_1 add 0.5 ml of *phenolphthalein solution R* and then *strong sodium hydroxide solution R* until a pale pink colour is obtained. Dilute to 25 ml with *water R*. 12 ml of the solution complies with limit test A for heavy metals (50 ppm). Prepare the standard using *lead standard solution (2 ppm Pb) R*.

Tin To 10 ml of solution S_1 add 0.3 ml of *thioglycollic acid R* and 30 ml of *water R*. Mix, add 2 ml of a 10 g/l solution of *sodium lauryl sulphate R* and 1 ml of a freshly prepared 5 g/l solution of *dithiol R* in *ethanol R* and dilute to 50 ml with *water R*. After 15 min, any colour in the solution is not more intense than that in a standard prepared at the same time in the same manner using 10 ml of a 20 per cent *V/V* solution of *sulphuric acid R* and 6 ml of *tin standard solution (5 ppm Sn) R* (30 ppm).

Zinc Dilute 1 ml of solution S_1 to 100 ml with *water R*. To 10 ml of the solution add 5 ml of *acetate buffer solution pH 4.4 R*, 1 ml of *0.1M sodium thiosulphate* and 5.0 ml of a 0.01 g/l solution of *dithizone R* in *chloroform R* and shake. After 2 min, if the lower layer of the solution is slightly violet in colour, it is not more intense than that in the lower layer of a standard prepared at the same time and in the same manner using a mixture of 2 ml of *zinc standard solution (10 ppm Zn) R* and 8 ml of *water R* (0.2 per cent). Prepare a blank using 10 ml of *water R*. The test is not valid unless the lower layer obtained with the blank is green.

Residue on evaporation Evaporate 50 ml of solution S_2 to dryness on a water-bath and dry at 100° to 105°. The residue weighs not more than 7.5 mg (0.3 per cent).

ASSAY

Carry out the oxygen-flask method (*2.5.10*), using 50.0 mg. Absorb the combustion products in 20 ml of *1M sodium hydroxide*. To the solution obtained add 2.5 ml of *nitric acid R*, 10.0 ml of *0.1M silver nitrate*, 5 ml of *ferric ammonium sulphate solution R2* and 1 ml of *dibutyl phthalate R*. Titrate with *0.05M ammonium thiocyanate* until a reddish-yellow colour is obtained. Carry out a blank test.

1 ml of *0.1M silver nitrate* is equivalent to 6.25 mg of poly(vinyl chloride).

2. FOR TUBING USED IN SETS FOR THE TRANSFUSION OF BLOOD AND BLOOD COMPONENTS

(Ph. Eur. text 3.1.2)

Materials based on plasticised poly(vinyl chloride) for tubing used in sets for transfusion of blood and blood components contain not less than 55 per cent of poly(vinyl chloride) with di(2-ethylhexyl) phthalate as plasticiser.

CHARACTERS

Almost colourless or pale-yellow material with a slight odour. On combustion it gives off dense, black smoke with a pungent odour.

IDENTIFICATION

A. To 0.5 g add 30 ml of *tetrahydrofuran R*. Heat with stirring on a water-bath under a hood for 10 min. The material dissolves completely. Add *methanol R* dropwise with stirring. A granular precipitate is formed. Filter the precipitate and dry at 60°. Examine the precipitate by infrared absorption spectrophotometry (*2.2.24*). Dissolve 50 mg in 2 ml of *tetrahydrofuran R* and pour on a glass slide. Dry in an oven at 80°, remove the film and fix on a suitable mount. The absorption maxima in the spectrum obtained with the precipitate correspond in position and relative intensity to those in the spectrum obtained with *poly(vinyl chloride) CRS*.

B. Examine by thin-layer chromatography (*2.2.27*), using *silica gel G R* as the coating substance.

Test solution. To 2.0 g of the material to be examined add 200 ml of *peroxide-free ether R* and heat under a reflux condenser for 12 h. Filter. Evaporate the filtrate to dryness under reduced pressure on a water-bath at 30°. Dissolve the residue in 10 ml of *toluene R*.

Reference solution. Dissolve 0.8 g of *di(2-ethylhexyl) phthalate CRS* in *toluene R* and dilute to 10 ml with the same solvent.

Apply separately to the plate 5 µl of each solution. Develop over a path of 15 cm using *toluene R*. Dry the plate carefully and examine in ultraviolet light at 254 nm.

The spot in the chromatogram obtained with the test solution is similar in position and fluorescence to the spot in the chromatogram obtained with the reference solution. Spray the plate with a 0.5 g/l solution of *sodium fluorescein-ate R* and examine in ultraviolet light at 254 nm. The chromatogram obtained with the test solution shows a single spot, at the starting-point.

TESTS

Solution S_1 Place 5.0 g of the material to be examined in a combustion flask. Add 30 ml of *sulphuric acid R* and heat until a black, syrupy mass is obtained. Cool and add carefully 10 ml of *strong hydrogen peroxide solution R*. Heat gently. Allow to cool and add 1 ml of *strong hydrogen peroxide solution R*; repeat by alternating evaporation and addition of hydrogen peroxide solution until a colourless liquid is obtained. Reduce the volume to about 10 ml. Cool and dilute to 50.0 ml with *water R*.

Solution S_2 Place 25 g of the material to be examined in a borosilicate-glass flask. Add 500 ml of *water R* and cover the neck of the flask with aluminium foil or a borosilicate-glass beaker. Heat in an autoclave at 121 ±2° for 20 min. Allow to cool and decant the solution.

Appearance of solution S_2 Solution S_2 is clear (*2.2.1*) and colourless (*Method II, 2.2.2*). It is practically odourless.

Vinyl chloride Not more than 1 ppm. Examine by gas chromatography (*2.2.28*), using *ether R* as the internal standard.

Internal standard solution. Using a microsyringe, inject 10 µl of *ether R* into 20.0 ml of *dimethylacetamide R*, immersing the tip of the needle in the solvent. Immediately before use, dilute the solution to 1000 times its volume with *dimethyl-acetamide R*.

Test solution. Place 1.000 g of the material to be examined in a 50 ml vial and add 10.0 ml of the internal standard solution. Close the vial and secure the stopper. Shake, avoiding contact between the stopper and the liquid. Place the vial in a water-bath at 60 ±1° for 2 h.

Vinyl chloride primary solution. Prepare under a ventilated hood. Place 50.0 ml of *dimethylacetamide R* in a 50 ml vial, stopper the vial, secure the stopper and weigh to the nearest 0.1 mg. Fill a 50 ml polyethylene or polypropylene syringe with gaseous *vinyl chloride R*, allow the gas to remain in contact with the syringe for 3 min, empty the syringe and fill again with 50 ml of gaseous *vinyl chloride R*. Fit a hypodermic needle to the syringe and reduce the volume of gas in the syringe from 50 ml to 25 ml. Inject these 25 ml of vinyl chloride slowly into the vial shaking gently and avoiding contact between the liquid and the needle. Weigh the vial again: the increase in mass is about 60 mg (1 µl of the solution thus obtained contains about 1.2 µg of vinyl chloride).

Vinyl chloride standard solution. To 1 volume of the vinyl chloride primary solution add 3 volumes of *dimethyl-acetamide R*.

Reference solutions. Place 10.0 ml of the internal standard solution in each of six 50 ml vials. Close the vials and secure the stoppers. Inject 0 µl, 1 µl, 2 µl, 3 µl, 5 µl and 10 µl of the vinyl chloride standard solution, respectively, into the vials. The six solutions thus obtained contain respectively, 0 µg, about 0.3 µg, 0.6 µg, 0.9 µg, 1.5 µg and 3 µg of vinyl chloride. Shake, avoiding contact between the stopper and the liquid. Place the vials in a water-bath at 60 ±1° for 2 h.

The chromatographic procedure may be carried out using:

— a stainless steel column 3 m long and 3 mm in internal diameter packed with *silanised diatomaceous earth for gas chromatography R* impregnated with 5 per cent *m/m* of *dimethylstearylamide R* and 5 per cent *m/m* of *macrogol 400 R*,

— *nitrogen for chromatography R* as the carrier gas at a flow rate of 30 ml per minute,

— a flame-ionisation detector,

maintaining the temperature of the column at 45°, that of the injection port at 100° and that of the detector at 150°

Inject 1 ml of the gaseous phase above the test solution and above each of the reference solutions.

Barium Ignite 2.0 g in a silica crucible. Take up the residue in 10 ml of *hydrochloric acid R* and evaporate to dryness on a water-bath. Take up this residue with two quantities, each of 1 ml, of distilled *water R*. Filter and add 3 ml of *calcium sulphate solution R*. Any opalescence in the solution is not more intense than that in a standard prepared using 1.2 ml of *barium standard solution (50 ppm Ba) R*, 0.8 ml of *distilled water R* and 3 ml of *calcium sulphate solution R* (30 ppm).

Cadmium Not more than 0.6 ppm of Cd, determined by atomic absorption spectrophotometry (*Method I, 2.2.23*).

Test solution. Evaporate 10.0 ml of solution S_1 to dryness. Take up the residue using 5 ml of a 1 per cent *V/V* solution of *hydrochloric acid R*, filter and dilute the filtrate to 10.0 ml with the same acid.

Reference solutions. Prepare the reference solutions using *cadmium standard solution (0.1 per cent Cd) R*, diluted with a 1 per cent *V/V* solution of *hydrochloric acid R*.

Measure the absorbance at 228.8 nm using a cadmium hollow-cathode lamp as source of radiation and an air-acetylene flame.

Heavy metals (*2.4.8*). To 10 ml of solution S_1 add 0.5 ml of *phenolphthalein solution R* and then *strong sodium hydroxide solution R* until a pale pink colour is obtained. Dilute to 25 ml with *water R*. 12 ml of the solution complies with limit test A for heavy metals (50 ppm). Prepare the standard using *lead standard solution (2 ppm Pb) R*.

Tin To 10 ml of solution S_1 add 0.3 ml of *thioglycollic acid R* and 30 ml of *water R*. Mix, add 2 ml of a 10 g/l solution of *sodium lauryl sulphate R* and 1 ml of a freshly prepared 5 g/l solution of *dithiol R* in *ethanol R* and dilute to 50 ml with *water R*. After 15 min, any colour in the solution is not more intense than that in a standard prepared at the same time in the same manner using 10 ml of a 20 per cent *V/V* solution of *sulphuric acid R* and 6 ml of *tin standard solution (5 ppm Sn) R* (30 ppm).

ASSAY

To 0.500 g add 30 ml of *tetrahydrofuran R* and heat with stirring on a water-bath under a hood for 10 min. The material dissolves completely. Add 60 ml of *methanol R* dropwise with stirring. A granular precipitate of poly(vinyl chloride) is formed. Allow to stand for a few minutes. Continue addition of *methanol R* until no further precipitation is observed. Transfer to a sintered-glass filter (40), using three small quantities of *methanol R* to aid transfer and to wash the precipitate. Dry the filter and the precipitate to constant mass at 60° and weigh.

B. Polyolefines

(Ph. Eur. text 3.1.3)

Polyolefines are obtained by polymerisation of ethylene or propylene or by copolymerisation of these substances with not more than 20 per cent of higher homologues (C_4 to C_{10}) or of carboxylic acids or of esters. Certain materials may be mixtures of polyolefines.

They may contain at most three stabilisers, one or several lubricants or antiblocking agents as well as titanium dioxide as opacifying agent when the material must provide protection from light.

All these additives are chosen from the appended list which specifies for each product the maximum allowable content and the appropriate method by which it may be controlled. The list of additives included in the material will be communicated by the manufacturer to the user.

This text is applicable to all polyolefines used for medico-pharmaceutical purposes with the exception of those materials whose uses are already described in texts of the Pharmacopoeia.

CHARACTERS

Powder, beads, granules or sheets of varying thickness. They are practically insoluble in water, soluble in hot aromatic hydrocarbons, practically insoluble in ethanol, in hexane and in methanol. They soften at temperatures between 90° and 150°. They burn with a blue flame giving off an odour of burning paraffin wax.

IDENTIFICATION

A. To 0.25 g add 10 ml of *toluene R* and boil under a reflux condenser for about 15 min. Place a few drops of the solution obtained on a sodium chloride slide and evaporate the solvent in an oven at 80°. Examine by infrared absorption spectrophotometry (*2.2.24*). The spectrum of the material to be examined shows maxima in particular at 2920 cm^{-1}, 2850 cm^{-1}, 1475 cm^{-1}, 1465 cm^{-1}, 1380 cm^{-1}, 1170 cm^{-1}, 737 cm^{-1}, 722 cm^{-1}; the spectrum obtained is identical to the spectrum obtained with the material selected for the type sample. If the material to be examined is in the form of sheets, the spectrum may be determined directly on a cut piece of suitable size.

B. It complies with the supplementary tests corresponding to the additives present.

C. In a platinum crucible, mix about 20 mg with 1 g of *potassium hydrogen sulphate R* and heat until completely melted. Allow to cool and add 20 ml of *dilute sulphuric acid R*. Heat gently. Filter the resulting solution. To the filtrate add 1 ml of *phosphoric acid R* and 1 ml of *strong hydrogen peroxide solution R*. If the substance is opacified with titanium dioxide, an orange-yellow colour develops.

TESTS

If necessary, cut samples of the material to be examined into pieces of maximum dimension not greater than l cm.

Solution S_1 Place 25 g in a borosilicate-glass flask with a ground-glass neck. Add 500 ml of *water R* and boil under a reflux condenser for 5 h. Allow to cool and decant. Reserve a portion of the solution for the test for appearance of solution S_1 and filter the rest through a sintered-glass filter (16). *Use solution S_1 within 4 h of preparation.*

Solution S_2 Place 2.0 g in a conical borosilicate-glass flask with a ground-glass neck. Add 80 ml of *toluene R* and boil under a reflux condenser with constant stirring for 90 min. Allow to cool to 60°C and add with continued stirring 120 ml of *methanol R*. Filter the solution through a sintered-glass filter (16). Rinse the flask and the filter with 25 ml of a mixture of 40 ml of *toluene R* and 60 ml of *methanol R*, add the rinsings to the filtrate and dilute to 250 ml with the same solvent. Prepare a blank solution.

Solution S_3 Place 100 g in a conical borosilicate-glass flask with a ground-glass neck. Add 250 ml of *0.1M hydrochloric acid* and boil under a reflux condenser with constant stirring for 1 h. Allow to cool and decant the solution.

GENERAL TESTS

Appearance of solution S_1 Solution S_1 is clear (*2.2.1*) and colourless (*Method II, 2.2.2*).

Acidity or alkalinity To 100 ml of solution S_1, add 0.15 ml of *BRP indicator solution R*. Not more than 1.5 ml of *0.01M sodium hydroxide* is required to change the colour of the indicator to blue. To 100 ml of solution S_1 add 0.2 ml of *methyl orange solution R*. Not more than 1 ml of *0.01M hydrochloric acid* is required to initiate the colour change of the indicator from yellow to orange.

Absorbance (*2.2.25*). At wavelengths from 220 nm to 340 nm, the absorbance of solution S_1 is not greater than 0.2.

Reducing substances To 20 ml of solution S_1 add 1 ml of *dilute sulphuric acid R* and 20 ml of *0.002M potassium permanganate*. Boil under a reflux condenser for 3 min and cool immediately. Add 1 g of *potassium iodide R* and titrate immediately with *0.01M sodium thiosulphate*, using 0.25 ml of *starch solution R* as indicator. Carry out a blank titration. The difference between the titration volumes is not more than 3.0 ml.

Extractable heavy metals (*2.4.8*). 12 ml of solution S_3 complies with limit test A for heavy metals (2.5 ppm). Prepare the standard using 10 ml of *lead standard solution (1 ppm Pb) R*.

Sulphated ash (*2.4.14*). Not more than 1.0 per cent, determined on 5.0 g. This limit does not apply to material that has been opacified with titanium dioxide.

SUPPLEMENTARY TESTS

These tests are to be carried out, in whole or in part, only if required by the stated composition or the use of the material.

Phenolic antioxidants Examine by liquid chromatography (*2.2.29*).

The chromatographic procedure may be carried out using:

— a stainless steel column 0.25 m long and 4.6 mm in internal diameter packed with *octadecylsilyl silica gel for chromatography R* (5 µm),

— as mobile phase one of the three following mixtures:

Mobile phase 1 at a flow rate of 2 ml per minute:

30 volumes of *water R*,

70 volumes of *acetonitrile R*,

Mobile phase 2 at a flow rate of 1.5 ml per minute:

10 volumes of *water R*,

30 volumes of *tetrahydrofuran R*,

60 volumes of *acetonitrile R*,

Mobile phase 3 at a flow rate of 1.5 ml per minute:
5 volumes of *water R*,
45 volumes of *2-propanol R*,
50 volumes of *methanol R*,
— as detector a spectrophotometer set at 280 nm.

The chromatographic system must ensure the following:
— a resolution of not less than 8 between the peaks corresponding to butylhydroxytoluene and ethylene bis[3,3-di(3-1,1-dimethylethyl-4-hydroxyphenyl)-butyrate] with mobile phase 1;
— a resolution of not less than 2 between the peaks corresponding to pentaerythrityl tetrakis[3-(3,5-di-1,1-dimethylethyl-4-hydroxyphenyl)propionate] and 2,2′,2″,6,6′,6″-hexa-1,1-dimethylethyl-4,4′,4″-[(2,4,6-trimethyl-1,3,5-benzenetriyl)tris-methylene]triphenol, with mobile phase 2;
— a resolution of not less than 2 between the peaks corresponding to octadecyl 3-(3,5-di-1,1-dimethylethyl-4-hydroxy-phenyl)propionate and tris(2,4-di-1,1-dimethylethylphenyl) phosphite with mobile phase 3.

Test solution S_{21}. Evaporate 50 ml of solution S_2 to dryness *in vacuo* at 45°C. Dissolve the residue in 5 ml of a mixture of equal volumes of *acetonitrile R* and *tetrahydrofuran R*. Prepare a blank solution from the blank solution corresponding to solution S_2.

Test solution S_{22}. Evaporate 50 ml of solution S_2 to dryness *in vacuo* at 45°. Dissolve the residue with 5 ml of *methylene chloride R*. Prepare a blank solution from the blank solution corresponding to solution S_2.

Of the following reference solutions, prepare only those that are necessary for the analysis of the phenolic antioxidants stated in the composition of the substance to be examined.

Reference solution (a). Dissolve 25 mg of *butylhydroxytoluene R* and 60 mg of *ethylene bis[3,3-di(3-1,1-dimethylethyl-4-hydroxyphenyl)butyrate] R* in 10 ml of a mixture of equal volumes of *acetonitrile R* and *tetrahydrofuran R*. Dilute 2 ml to 50 ml with the same solvent.

Reference solution (b). Dissolve 60 mg of *pentaerythrityl tetrakis[3-(3,5-di-1,1-dimethylethyl-4-hydroxyphenyl)-propionate] R* and 60 mg of *2,2′,2″,6,6′,6″-hexa-1,1-dimethylethyl-4,4′,4″-[(2,4,6-trimethyl-1,3,5-benzenetriyl)-trismethylene]-triphenol R* in 10 ml of a mixture of equal volumes of *acetonitrile R* and *tetrahydrofuran R*. Dilute 2 ml to 50 ml with the same solvent.

Reference solution (c). Dissolve 60 mg of *octadecyl 3-(3,5-di-1,1-dimethylethyl-4-hydroxyphenyl)propionate R* and 60 mg of *tris(2,4-di-1,1-dimethylethylphenyl) phosphite R* in 10 ml of *methylene chloride R*. Dilute 2 ml to 50 ml with the same solvent.

Reference solution (d). Dissolve 25 mg of *butylhydroxytoluene R* in 10 ml of a mixture of equal volumes of *acetonitrile R* and *tetrahydrofuran R*. Dilute 2 ml to 50 ml with the same solvent.

Reference solution (e). Dissolve 60 mg of *ethylene bis[3,3-di(3-1,1-dimethylethyl-4-hydroxyphenyl)butyrate] R* in 10 ml of a mixture of equal volumes of *acetonitrile R* and *tetrahydrofuran R*. Dilute 2 ml to 50 ml with the same solvent.

Reference solution (f). Dissolve 60 mg of *1,3,5-tris(3,5-di-1,1-dimethylethyl-4-hydroxybenzyl)-1H,3H,5H-1,3,5-triazine-2,4,6-trione R* in 10 ml of a mixture of equal volumes of *acetonitrile R* and *tetrahydrofuran R*. Dilute 2 ml to 50 ml with the same solvent.

Reference solution (g). Dissolve 60 mg of *pentaerythrityl tetrakis[3-(3,5-di-1,1-dimethylethyl-4-hydroxyphenyl)-propionate] R* in 10 ml of a mixture of equal volumes of *acetonitrile R* and *tetrahydrofuran R*. Dilute 2 ml to 50 ml with the same solvent.

Reference solution (h). Dissolve 60 mg of *2,2′,2″,6,6′,6″-hexa-1,1-dimethylethyl-4,4′,4″-[(2,4,6-trimethyl-1,3,5-benzene-triyl)trismethylene]triphenol R* in 10 ml of a mixture of equal volumes of *acetonitrile R* and *tetrahydrofuran R*. Dilute 2 ml to 50 ml with the same solvent.

Reference solution (i). Dissolve 60 mg of *octadecyl 3-(3,5-di-1,1-dimethylethyl-4-hydroxyphenyl)propionate R* in 10 ml of *methylene chloride R*. Dilute 2 ml to 50 ml with the same solvent.

Reference solution (j). Dissolve 60 mg of *tris(2,4-di-1,1-dimethylethylphenyl) phosphite R* in 10 ml of *methylene chloride R*. Dilute 2 ml to 50 ml with the same solvent.

If the substance to be examined contains butylhydroxytoluene and/or ethylene bis[3,3-di(3-1,1-dimethylethyl-4-hydroxyphenyl)-butyrate], use mobile phase 1 and inject 20 µl of solution S_{21}, 20 µl of the corresponding blank solution, 20 µl of reference solution (a), and either 20 µl of solutions (d) or (e) or 20 µl of solutions (d) and (e).

If the substance to be examined contains one or more of the following antioxidants:
— 1,3,5-tris(3,5-di-1,1-dimethylethyl-4-hydroxybenzyl)-1*H*,3*H*,5*H*-1,3,5-triazine-2,4,6-trione,
— pentaerythrityl tetrakis[3-(3,5-di-1,1-dimethylethyl-4-hydroxyphenyl) propionate],
— 2,2′,2″,6,6′,6″-hexa-1,1-dimethylethyl-4,4′,4″-[(2,4,6-trimethyl-1,3,5-benzene-triyl)trismethylene]triphenol,
— octadcyl 3-(3,5-di-1,1-dimethylethyl-4-hydroxyphenyl)propionate,
— tris(2,4-di-1,1-dimethylethylphenyl) phosphite,

use mobile phase 2 and inject 20 µl of solution S_{21}, 20 µl of the corresponding blank solution, 20 µl of reference solution (b) and 20 µl of each of the reference solutions of the antioxidants on the list above that are stated in the composition.

If the substance to be examined contains octadecyl 3-(3,5-di-1,1-dimethylethyl-4-hydroxyphenyl)propionate and/or tris(2,4-di-1,1-dimethylethylphenyl) phosphite, use mobile phase 3 and inject 20 µl of solution S_{22}, 20 µl of the corresponding blank solution, 20 µl of reference solution (c), and either 20 µl of reference solution (i) or (j) or 20 µl of solutions (i) and (j).

In all cases, record the chromatogram for 30 min; the chromatograms corresponding to solutions S_{21} and S_{22} only show peaks due to antioxidants stated in the composition and minor peaks that also appear in the chromatograms corresponding to the blank solutions. The areas of the peaks of solutions S_{21} and S_{22} are less than the corresponding areas of the peaks in the chromatograms obtained with reference solutions (d) to (j).

Non-phenolic antioxidants Examine by thin-layer chromatography (*2.2.27*), using *silica gel GF$_{254}$ R* as the coating substance.

Test solution S_{23}. Evaporate 100 ml of solution S_2 to dryness *in vacuo* at 45°. Dissolve the residue in 2 ml of *acidified methylene chloride R*.

Reference solution (k). Dissolve 60 mg of *2,2′-di(octadecyloxy)-5,5¢-spirobi(1,3,2-dioxaphosphorinane) R* in 10 ml of *methylene chloride R*. Dilute 2 ml of the solution to 10 ml with *acidified methylene chloride R*.

Reference solution (l). Dissolve 60 mg of *dioctadecyl disulphide R* in 10 ml of *methylene chloride R.* Dilute 2 ml of the solution to 10 ml with *acidified methylene chloride R.*

Reference solution (m). Dissolve 60 mg of *didodecyl 3,3′-thiodipropionate R* in 10 ml of *methylene chloride R.* Dilute 2 ml of the solution to 10 ml with *acidified methylene chloride R.*

Reference solution (n). Dissolve 60 mg of *dioctadecyl 3,3′-thiodipropionate R* in 10 ml of *methylene chloride R.* Dilute 2 ml of the solution to 10 ml with *acidified methylene chloride R.*

Reference solution (o). Dissolve 60 mg of *didodecyl 3,3′-thiodipropionate R* and 60 mg of *dioctadecyl 3,3′-thiodipropionate R* in 10 ml of *methylene chloride R.* Dilute 2 ml of the solution to 10 ml with *acidified methylene chloride R.*

Apply separately to the plate 20 µl of test solution S_{23}, 20 µl of reference solution (o) and 20 µl of each of the reference solutions corresponding to all the phenolic and non-phenolic antioxidants mentioned in the type composition of the material to be examined.

Develop over a path of 18 cm using *hexane R.* Allow the plate to dry. Develop a second time over a path of 17 cm using *methylene chloride R.* Allow the plate to dry and examine in ultraviolet light at 254 nm. Spray with *alcoholic iodine solution R* and examine in ultraviolet light at 254 nm after 10 min to 15 min. Any spots in the chromatogram obtained with test solution S_{23} are not more intense than the spots in the corresponding locations in the chromatograms obtained with the reference solutions. The test is not valid unless the chromatogram obtained with reference solution (o) shows two clearly separated spots.

Amides and stearates Examine by thin-layer chromatography (*2.2.27*), using two plates with *silica gel GF_{254} R* as the coating substance.

Test solution. Solution S_{23}.

Reference solution (p). Dissolve 20 mg of *stearic acid R* in 10 ml of *methylene chloride R.*

Reference solution (q). Dissolve 40 mg of *oleamide R* in 20 ml of *methylene chloride R.*

Reference solution (r). Dissolve 40 mg of *erucamide R* in 20 ml of *methylene chloride R.*

Apply to two plates 10 µl of solution S_{23}. Apply 10 µl of reference solution (p) to the first plate and 10 µl of each of reference solutions (q) and (r) to the second plate.

Develop the first plate over a path of 10 cm using a mixture of 25 volumes of *ethanol R* and 75 volumes of *trimethyl-pentane R.* Allow the plate to dry in air. Spray with a 2 g/l solution of *dichlorophenolindophenol sodium R* in *ethanol R* and heat in an oven at 120°C for a few minutes to intensify the spots. Any spot corresponding to stearic acid in the chromatogram obtained with test solution S_{23} is identical in position to (R_f about 0.5) but not more intense than the spot in the chromatogram obtained with reference solution (p).

Develop the second plate over a path of 13 cm using *hexane R.* Allow the plate to dry in air. Develop a second time over a path of 10 cm using a mixture of 5 volumes of *methanol R* and 95 volumes of *methylene chloride R.* Allow the plate to dry. Spray with a 40 g/l solution of *phosphomolybdic acid R* in *ethanol R.* Heat in an oven at 120° until spots appear. Any spots corresponding to erucamide or oleamide in the chromatogram obtained with test solution S_{23} are identical in position to (R_f about 0.2) but not more intense than the corresponding spots in the chromatograms obtained with reference solutions (q) and (r).

Substances soluble in hexane Place 1.00 g in a 250 ml conical borosilicate-glass flask with a ground-glass neck. Add 100 ml of *hexane R* and boil under a reflux condenser for 4 h, stirring constantly. Cool in iced water and filter rapidly (*the filtration time must be less than 5 min; if necessary the filtration may be accelerated by applying pressure to the solution*) through a sintered-glass filter (16) maintaining the solution at about 0°. Evaporate 20 ml of the filtrate in a tared glass dish in a water-bath. Dry the residue in an oven at 100° to 105° for 1 h. The mass of the residue obtained must be within 10 per cent of that of the residue obtained with the type sample and does not exceed 5 per cent.

Extractable aluminium Not more than 1 ppm of extractable Al, determined by atomic absorption spectrometry (*Method I, 2.2.23*).

Test solution. Evaporate to dryness 100 ml of solution S_3 on a water-bath. Dissolve the residue in 2 ml of *hydrochloric acid R* and dilute to 10.0 ml with *0.1M hydrochloric acid.*

Reference solutions. Prepare the reference solutions using *aluminium standard solution (200 ppm Al) R,* diluted with *0.1M hydrochloric acid.*

Measure the absorbance at 309.3 nm using an aluminium hollow-cathode lamp as a source of radiation and a nitrous oxide-acetylene flame.

Extractable titanium Not more than 1 ppm of extractable Ti, determined by atomic absorption spectrometry (*Method I, 2.2.23*).

Test solution. Evaporate to dryness 100 ml of solution S_3 on a water-bath. Dissolve the residue in 2 ml of *hydrochloric acid R* and dilute to 10.0 ml with *0.1M hydrochloric acid.*

Reference solutions. Prepare the reference solutions using *titanium standard solution (100 ppm Ti) R,* diluted with *0.1M hydrochloric acid.*

Measure the absorbance at 364.3 nm using a titanium hollow-cathode lamp as a source of radiation and a nitrous oxide-acetylene flame.

Extractable zinc Not more than 1 ppm of extractable Zn, determined by atomic absorption spectrometry (*Method I, 2.2.23*).

Test solution. Solution S_3.

Reference solutions. Prepare the reference solutions using *zinc standard solution (10 ppm Zn) R,* diluted with *0.1M hydrochloric acid.*

Measure the absorbance at 213.9 nm using a zinc hollow-cathode lamp as a source of radiation and an air-acetylene flame.

LIST OF ADDITIVES

— butylhydroxytoluene, not more than 0.125 per cent;

— pentaerythrityl tetrakis[3-(3,5-di-1,1-dimethylethyl-4-hydroxyphenyl)-]propionate, not more than 0.3 per cent;

— 1,3,5-tris(3,5-di-1,1-dimethylethyl-4-hydroxybenzyl)-1*H*,3*H*,5*H*-1,3,5-triazine-2,4,6-trione, not more than 0.3 per cent;

— octadecyl 3-(3,5-di-1,1-dimethylethyl-4-hydroxyphenyl)propionate, not more than 0.3 per cent;

— ethylene bis[3,3-di-(3-1,1-dimethylethyl-4-hydroxyphenyl)butyrate], not more than 0.3 per cent;
— dioctadecyl disulphide, not more than 0.3 per cent;
— 2,2′,2″,6,6′,6″-hexa-1,1-dimethylethyl-4,4′,4″-[(2,4,6-trimethyl-1,3,5-benzene-triyl)trismethylene]triphenol, not more than 0.3 per cent;
— 2,2′-di(octadecyloxy)-5,5′-spirobi(1,3,2-dioxaphosphane), not more than 0.3 per cent;
— didodecyl 3,3′-thiodipropionate, not more than 0.3 per cent;
— dioctadecyl 3,3′-thiodipropionate, not more than 0.3 per cent;
— tris(2,4-di-1,1-dimethylethylphenyl) phosphite, not more than 0.3 per cent;

The total of antioxidant additives listed above does not exceed 0.3 per cent.
— hydrotalcite, not more than 0.5 per cent;
— alkanamides, not more than 0.5 per cent;
— alkenamides, not more than 0.5 per cent;
— sodium silico-aluminate, not more than 0.5 per cent;
— silica, not more than 0.5 per cent;
— sodium benzoate, not more than 0.5 per cent;
— fatty acid esters or salts, not more than 0.5 per cent;
— trisodium phosphate, not more than 0.5 per cent;
— paraffin oil, not more than 0.5 per cent;
— zinc oxide, not more than 0.5 per cent;
— talc, not more than 0.5 per cent;
— calcium or zinc stearate or a mixture of both, not more than 0.5 per cent;
— titanium dioxide not more than 4 per cent.

C. Polyethylene

1. WITHOUT ADDITIVES FOR CONTAINERS FOR PARENTERAL AND OPHTHALMIC PREPARATIONS

(Ph. Eur. Text 3.1.4)

DEFINITION

Polyethylene without additives is obtained by the polymerisation of ethylene under high pressure in the presence of oxygen or free-radical-forming initiators as catalyst.

CHARACTERS

Beads, granules, powder or translucent sheets of varying thickness, practically insoluble in water, soluble in hot aromatic hydrocarbons, practically insoluble in ethanol, in hexane and in methanol. It softens as temperatures above 65°.

The relative density (*2.2.5*) of the material is 0.910 to 0.937.

IDENTIFICATION

A. To 0.25 g add 10 ml of *toluene R* and boil under a reflux condenser for about 15 min. Place a few drops of the solution on a sodium chloride disc and evaporate the solvent in an oven at 80°. Examine by infrared absorption spectrophotometry (*2.2.24*). The spectrum of the substance to be examined shows maxima in particular at 2920 cm^{-1}- 2850 cm^{-1}, 1465 cm^{-1}, 730 cm^{-1}, 720 cm^{-1}; the spectrum obtained is identical to that obtained with the material selected for the type sample. If the material to be examined is in the form of sheets, the identification may be performed directly on a cut piece of suitable size.

B. The substance to be examined complies with the test for additives specified under Tests.

TESTS

If necessary, cut the material into pieces of maximum dimension on a side not greater than 1 cm.

Solution S1 Place 25 g in a borosilicate-glass flask with a ground-glass neck. Add 500 ml of *water R* and heat under a reflux condenser for 5 h. Allow to cool and decant. Keep part of the solution for the test for appearance of solution. Filter the rest through a sintered-glass filter (16). Use solution S1 within 4 h of preparation.

Solution S2 Place 2.0 g in a conical borosilicate-glass flask with a ground-glass neck. Add 80 ml of *toluene R* and boil under a reflux condenser with constant stirring for 1 h 30 min. Allow to cool to 60°C and add with continued stirring 120 ml of *methanol R*. Filter the solution through a sintered-glass filter (16). Rinse the flask and the filter with 25 ml of a mixture of 40 ml of *toluene R* and 60 ml of *methanol R*, add the rinsings to the filtrate and dilute to 250 ml with the same mixture of solvents. Prepare a blank solution.

Solution S3 Place 100 g in a conical borosilicate-glass flask with a ground-glass neck. Add 250 ml of *0.1M hydrochloric acid* and boil under a reflux condenser with constant stirring for 1 h. Allow to cool and decant the solution.

Appearance of solution Solution S1 is clear (*2.2.1*) and colourless (*Method II, 2.2.2*).

Acidity or alkalinity To 100 ml of solution S1 add 0.15 ml of *BRP indicator solution R*. Not more than 1.5 ml of *0.01M sodium hydroxide* is required to change the colour of the indicator to blue. To 100 ml of solution S1 add 0.2 ml of *methyl orange solution R*. Not more than 1.0 ml of *0.01M hydrochloric acid* is required to reach the beginning of the colour change of the indicator from yellow to orange.

Absorbance (*2.2.25*). At wavelengths from 220 nm to 340 nm, the absorbance of solution S1 is not greater than 0.2.

Reducing substances To 20 ml of solution S1 add 1 ml of *dilute sulphuric acid R* and 20 ml of *0.002M potassium permanganate*. Boil under a reflux condenser for 3 min and cool immediately. Add 1 g of *potassium iodide R* and titrate immediately with *0.01M sodium thiosulphate*, using 0.25 ml of *starch solution R* as indicator. Carry out a blank titration. The difference between the titration volumes is not more than 0.5 ml.

Substances soluble in hexane Place 1.00 g in a 250 ml conical borosilicate-glass flask with a ground-glass neck. Add 100 ml of *hexane R* and boil under a reflux condenser for 4 h, stirring constantly. Cool in iced water and filter rapidly through a sintered-glass filter (16) maintaining the solution at 0° (*the filtration time must be less than 5 min; if necessary the filtration may be accelerated by applying pressure to the solution*). Evaporate 20 ml of the filtrate in a tared glass dish on a water-bath. Dry the residue in an oven at 100° to 105° for 1 h. The mass of the residue obtained must be within 10 per cent of the residue obtained with the type sample and does not exceed 5 per cent.

Additives Examine by thin-layer chromatography (*2.2.27*), using *silica gel G R* as the coating substance.

Test solution. Evaporate 50 ml of solution S2 to dryness *in vacuo* at 45°. Dissolve the evaporation residue with 5 ml of *methylene chloride R*. Prepare a blank solution from the blank solution corresponding to solution S2.
Reference solution. Dissolve 20 mg of *dioctadecyl disulphide R* and 20 mg of *ethylene bis[3,3-di[3-(1,1-dimethylethyl)-4-hydroxyphenyl]butyrate] R* in *methylene chloride R* and dilute to 10 ml with the same solvent.

Apply separately to the plate 10 µl of each solution. Develop over a path of 13 cm using *hexane R*. Allow the plate to dry in air. Carry out a second development over a path of 10 cm using a mixture of 5 volumes of *methanol R* and 95 volumes of *methylene chloride R*. Allow the plate to dry in air, spray with a 40 g/l solution of *phosphomolybdic acid R* in *alcohol R* and heat at 120° until the spots appear in the chromatogram obtained with the reference solution. No spot appears in the chromatogram obtained with the test solution, except for a spot which may be at the solvent front from the first development and which corresponds to oligomers. Disregard any spots corresponding to those obtained in the chromatogram with the blank solution. The chromatogram obtained with the reference solution shows two distinct spots.

Extractable heavy metals (*2.4.8*). 12 ml of solution S3 complies with limit test A for heavy metals (2.5 ppm). Prepare the standard using 10 ml of *lead standard solution (1 ppm Pb) R*.

Sulphated ash (*2.4.14*). Not more than 0.2 per cent, determined on 5.0 g.

2. WITH ADDITIVES FOR CONTAINERS FOR PARENTERAL AND OPHTHALMIC PREPARATIONS

(Ph. Eur. method 3.1.5)

DEFINITION

Polyethylene with additives is obtained by the polymerisation of ethylene under pressure in the presence of a catalyst or by copolymerisation of ethylene with up to 20 per cent of higher alkene homologues (C_3 to C_{10}).

CHARACTERS

Powder, beads, granules or translucent sheets of varying thickness. It is practically insoluble in water, soluble in hot aromatic hydrocarbons, practically insoluble in ethanol, in hexane and in methanol. It softens at temperatures between 70°C and 140°C.

The relative density (*2.2.5*) of the material is 0.890 to 0.965.

IDENTIFICATION

A. To 0.25 g add 10 ml of *toluene R* and boil under a reflux condenser for about 15 min. Place a few drops of the solution on a sodium chloride slide and evaporate the solvent in an oven at 80°C. Examine by infrared absorption spectrophotometry (*2.2.24*). The spectrum of the material being examined shows maxima in particular at 2920 cm^{-1} - 2850 cm^{-1}, 1465 cm^{-1}, 1375 cm^{-1}, 1170 cm^{-1}, 730 cm^{-1}, 720 cm^{-1}; the spectrum obtained is identical to the spectrum obtained with the material selected for the type sample. If the material being examined is in the form of sheets, the identification may be performed directly on a cut piece of suitable size.

B. It complies with the supplementary tests corresponding to the additives present (see Tests).

TESTS

If necessary, cut the material into pieces of maximum dimension on a side of not greater than 1 cm.

Solution S1 Place 25 g in a borosilicate-glass flask with a ground-glass neck. Add 500 ml of *water R* and boil under a reflux condenser for 5 h. Allow to cool and decant. Reserve a portion of the solution for the test for appearance of solution and filter the rest through a sintered-glass filter (16). *Use solution S1 within 4 h of preparation.*

Solution S2 Place 2.0 g in a conical borosilicate-glass flask with a ground-glass neck. Add 80 ml of *toluene R* and boil under a reflux condenser with constant stirring for 1 h 30 min. Allow to cool to 60°C and add with continued stirring 120 ml of *methanol R*. Filter the solution through a sintered-glass filter (16). Rinse the flask and the filter with 25 ml of a mixture of 40 ml of *toluene R* and 60 ml of *methanol R*, add the rinsings to the filtrate and dilute to 250.0 ml with the same mixture of solvents. Prepare a blank solution.

Solution S3 Place 100 g in a conical borosilicate-glass flask with a ground-glass neck. Add 250 ml of *0.1M hydrochloric acid* and boil under a reflux condenser with constant stirring for 1 h. Allow to cool and decant the solution.

Appearance of solution Solution S1 is clear (*2.2.1*) and colourless (*Method II, 2.2.2*).

Acidity or alkalinity To 100 ml of solution S1 add 0.15 ml of *BRP indicator solution R*. Not more than 1.5 ml of *0.01M sodium hydroxide* is required to change the colour of the indicator to blue. To 100 ml of solution S1 add 0.2 ml of *methyl orange solution R*. Not more than 1.0 ml of *0.01M hydrochloric acid* is required to reach the beginning of the colour change of the indicator from yellow to orange.

Absorbance (*2.2.25*). At wavelengths from 220 nm to 340 nm, the absorbance of solution S1 is not greater than 0.2.

Reducing substances To 20 ml of solution S1 add 1 ml of *dilute sulphuric acid R* and 20 ml of *0.002M potassium permanganate*. Boil under a reflux condenser for 3 min and cool immediately. Add 1 g of *potassium iodide R* and titrate immediately with *0.01M sodium thiosulphate*, using 0.25 ml of *starch solution R* as indicator. Carry out a blank titration. The difference between the titration volumes is not more than 0.5 ml.

Substances soluble in hexane Place 1.00 g in a 250 ml conical borosilicate-glass flask with a ground-glass neck. Add 100 ml of *hexane R* and boil under a reflux condenser for 4 h, stirring constantly. Cool in iced water and filter rapidly through a sintered-glass filter (16) maintaining the solution at 0°C (*the filtration time must be less than 5 min; if necessary the filtration may be accelerated by applying pressure to the solution*). Evaporate 20 ml of the filtrate in a tared glass dish on a water-bath. Dry the residue in an oven at 100°C to 105°C for 1 h. The mass of the residue obtained must be within 10 per cent of the residue obtained with the type sample and does not exceed 5 per cent.

Extractable aluminium Not more than 1 ppm of extractable Al, determined by atomic emission spectrometry in an argon plasma (*Method I, 2.2.22*).

Test solution. Use solution S3.

Reference solutions. Prepare the reference solutions using *aluminium standard solution (200 ppm Al) R*, diluted with *0.1M hydrochloric acid.*

Carry out the determination using the emission of aluminium at 396.15 nm, the spectral background being taken as 396.25 nm.

Verify the absence of aluminium in the hydrochloric acid used.

Extractable chromium Not more than 0.05 ppm of extractable Cr, determined by atomic emission spectrometry in an argon plasma (*Method I, 2.2.22*).

Test solution. Use solution S3.

Reference solutions. Prepare the reference solutions using *chromium standard solution (100 ppm Cr) R*, diluting with a mixture of 2 volumes of *hydrochloric acid R* and 8 volumes of *water R*.

Carry out the determination using the emission of chromium at 205.55 nm, the spectral background being taken as 205.50 nm.

Verify the absence of chromium in the hydrochloric acid used.

Extractable heavy metals (*2.4.8*). 12 ml of solution S3 complies with limit test A for heavy metals (2.5 ppm). Prepare the standard using 10 ml of *lead standard solution (1 ppm Pb) R*.

Extractable titanium Not more than 1 ppm of extractable Ti, determined by atomic emission spectrometry in an argon plasma (*Method I, 2.2.22*).

Test solution. Use solution S3.

Reference solutions. Prepare the reference solutions using *titanium standard solution (100 ppm Ti) R*, diluted with *0.1M hydrochloric acid.*

Carry out the determination using the emission of titanium at 336.12 nm, the spectral background being taken as 336.16 nm.

Verify the absence of titanium in the hydrochloric acid used.

Extractable vanadium Not more than 10 ppm of extractable V, determined by atomic emission spectrometry in an argon plasma (*Method I, 2.2.22*).

Test solution. Use solution S3.

Reference solutions. Prepare the reference solutions using *vanadium standard solution (1 g/l V) R*, diluting with a mixture of 2 volumes of *hydrochloric acid R* and 8 volumes of *water R*.

Carry out the determination using the emission of vanadium at 292.40 nm, the spectral background being taken as 292.35 nm.

Verify the absence of vanadium in the hydrochloric acid used.

Extractable zinc Not more than 1 ppm of extractable Zn, determined by atomic absorption spectrometry (*Method I, 2.2.23*).

Test solution. Use solution S3.

Reference solutions. Prepare the reference solutions using *zinc standard solution (10 ppm Zn) R*, diluted with *0.1M hydrochloric acid.*

Measure the absorbance at 213.9 nm using a zinc hollow-cathode lamp as a source of radiation and an air-acetylene flame.

Extractable zirconium Not more than 100 ppm of extractable, determined by atomic emission spectrometry in an argon plasma (*Method I, 2.2.22*).

Test solution. Use solution S3.

Reference solutions. Prepare the reference solutions using *zirconium standard solution (1 g/l Zr) R*, diluting with a mixture of 2 volumes of *hydrochloric acid R* and 8 volumes of *water R*.

Carry out the determination using the emission of zirconium at 343.82 nm, the spectral background being taken as 343.92 nm.

Verify the absence of zirconium in the hydrochloric acid used.

Sulphated ash (*2.4.14*). Not more than 1.0 per cent, determined on 5.0 g. This limit does not apply to material opacified with titanium dioxide.

SUPPLEMENTARY TESTS

These tests are to be carried out, in whole or in part, only if required by the stated composition of the material.

Phenolic antioxidants Examine by liquid chromatography (*2.2.29*).

The chromatographic procedure may be carried out using:

— a stainless steel column 0.25 m long and 4.6 mm in internal diameter packed with *octadecylsilyl silica gel for chromatography R* (5 mm),

— as mobile phase one of the following mixtures:

— Mobile phase 1 at a flow rate of 2 ml per minute;
30 volumes of *water R*,
70 volumes of *acetonitrile R*,

— Mobile phase 2 at a flow rate of 1.5 ml per minute;
10 volumes of *water R*,
30 volumes of *tetrahydrofuran R*,
60 volumes of *acetonitrile R*,

— Mobile phase 3 at a flow rate of 1.5 ml per minute;
5 volumes of *water R*,
45 volumes of *2-propanol R*,
50 volumes of *methanol R*,

— as detector a spectrophotometer set at 280 nm.

The chromatographic system must ensure the following:

— a resolution of not less than 8 between the peaks corresponding to butylhydroxytoluene and ethylene bis[3,3-di[3-(1,1-dimethylethyl)-4-hydroxyphenyl]-butyrate], with mobile phase 1;

— a resolution of not less than 2 between the peaks corresponding to pentaerythrityl tetrakis[3-[3,5-di(1,1-dimethylethyl)-4-hydroxyphenyl]propionate] and 2,2′,2″,6,6′,6″-hexa(1,1-dimethylethyl)-4,4′,4″-[(2,4,6-trimethyl-1,3,5-benzenetriyl)trismethylene]-triphenol, with mobile phase 2;

— a resolution of not less than 2 between the peaks corresponding to octadecyl 3-[3,5-di-(1,1-dimethyl-ethyl)-4-hydroxyphenyl]propionate and tris[2,4-di(1,1-dimethyl-ethyl)phenyl] phosphite, with mobile phase 3.

Test solution S21. Evaporate 50.0 ml of solution S2 to dryness *in vacuo* at 45°C. Dissolve the residue with 5.0 ml of a mixture of equal volumes of *acetonitrile R* and *tetrahydrofuran R*. Prepare a blank solution from the blank solution corresponding to solution S2.

Test solution S22. Evaporate 50.0 ml of solution S2 to dryness *in vacuo* at 45°C. Dissolve the residue with 5.0 ml of *methylene chloride R*. Prepare a blank solution from the blank solution corresponding to solution S2.

Of the following reference solutions, prepare only those that are necessary for the analysis of the phenolic anti-oxidants stated in the composition of the substance being examined.

Reference solution (a). Dissolve 25.0 mg of *butylhydroxytoluene R* and 60.0 mg of *ethylene bis[3,3-di[3-(1,1 dimethyl-ethyl)-4-hydroxyphenyl]butyrate] R* in 10 ml of a mixture of equal volumes of *acetonitrile R* and *tetrahydrofuran R.* Dilute 2.0 ml of the solution to 50.0 ml with the same mixture of solvents.

Reference solution (b). Dissolve 60.0 mg of *pentaerythrityl tetrakis[3-[3,5-di(1,1-dimethylethyl)-4-hydroxyphenyl]-propionate] R* and 60.0 mg of *2,2′,2″,6,6′,6″-hexa(1,1-dimethylethyl)-4,4′,4″-[(2,4,6-trimethyl-1,3,5-benzenetriyl)-trismethylene]triphenol R* in 10.0 ml of a mixture of equal volumes of *acetonitrile R* and *tetrahydrofuran R.* Dilute 2.0 ml of the solution to 50.0 ml with the same mixture of solvents.

Reference solution (c). Dissolve 60.0 mg of *octadecyl 3-[3,5-di(1,1-dimethylethyl)-4-hydroxyphenyl]propionate R* and 60.0 mg of *tris[2,4-di(1,1-dimethylethyl)phenyl] phosphite R* in 10 ml of *methylene chloride R.* Dilute 2.0 ml of the solution to 50.0 ml with the same solvent.

Reference solution (d). Dissolve 25.0 mg of *butylhydroxy-toluene R* in 10.0 ml of a mixture of equal volumes of *acetonitrile R* and *tetrahydrofuran R.* Dilute 2.0 ml of the solution to 50.0 ml with the same mixture of solvents.

Reference solution (e). Dissolve 60.0 mg of *ethylene bis[3,3-di[3-(1,1-dimethylethyl)-4-hydroxyphenyl]butyrate] R* in 10.0 ml of a mixture of equal volumes of *acetonitrile R* and *tetrahydrofuran R.* Dilute 2.0 ml of the solution to 50.0 ml with the same mixture of solvents.

Reference solution (f). Dissolve 60.0 mg of *1,3,5-tris[3,5-di(1,1-dimethylethyl)-4-hydroxybenzyl]-1H,3H,5H-1,3,5-triazine-2,4,6-trione R* in 10.0 ml of a mixture of equal volumes of *acetonitrile R* and *tetrahydrofuran R.* Dilute 2.0 ml of the solution to 50.0 ml with the same mixture of solvents.

Reference solution (g). Dissolve 60.0 mg of *pentaerythrityl tetrakis[3-[3,5-di-(1,1-dimethylethyl)-4-hydroxyphenyl]-propionate] R* in 10.0 ml of a mixture of equal volumes of *acetonitrile R* and *tetrahydrofuran R.* Dilute 2.0 ml of the solution to 50.0 ml with the same mixture of solvents.

Reference solution (h). Dissolve 60.0 mg of *2,2′,2″,6,6′,6″-hexa(1,1-dimethylethyl)-4,4′,4″-[(2,4,6-trimethyl-1,3,5-benzenetriyl)trismethylene]triphenol R* in 10.0 ml of a mixture of equal volumes of *acetonitrile R* and *tetrahydro-furan R.* Dilute 2.0 ml of the solution to 50.0 ml with the same mixture of solvents.

Reference solution (i). Dissolve 60.0 mg of *octadecyl 3-[3,5-di(1,1-dimethylethyl)-4-hydroxyphenyl]propionate R* in 10.0 ml of *methylene chloride R.* Dilute 2.0 ml of the solution to 50.0 ml with the same solvent.

Reference solution (j). Dissolve 60.0 mg of *tris[2,4-di(1,1-dimethylethyl)phenyl] phosphite R* in 10.0 ml of *methylene chloride R.* Dilute 2.0 ml of the solution to 50.0 ml with the same solvent.

If the substance being examined contains butylhydroxy-toluene and/or ethylene bis[3,3-di[3-(1,1-dimethylethyl)-4-hydroxy-phenyl[butyrate], use mobile phase 1 and inject 20 ml of solution S21, 20 ml of the corresponding blank solution and 20 ml of reference solutions (a), (d) or (e) or (d) and (e).

If the substance being examined contains one or more of the following antioxidants:

— 1,3,5-tris[3,5-di(1,1-dimethylethyl)-4-hydroxybenzyl]-1*H*,3*H*, 5*H*-1,3,5-triazine-2,4,6-trione,
— pentaerythrityl tetrakis[3-[3,5-di(1,1-dimethylethyl)-4-hydroxyphenyl]propionate],
— 2,2′,2″,6,6′,6″-hexa(1,1-dimethylethyl)-4,4′,4″- [(2,4,6-trimethyl-1,3,5-benzenetriyl)trismethylene]triphenol,
— octadecyl 3-[3,5-di(1,1-dimethylethyl)-4-hydroxy-phenyl]-propionate,
— tris[2,4-di(1,1-dimethylethyl)phenyl] phosphite,

use mobile phase 2 and inject 20 ml of solution S21, 20 ml of the corresponding blank solution, 20 ml of reference solution (b) and 20 ml of the reference solutions of the antioxidants on the list above that are stated in the composition.

If the substance being examined contains octadecyl 3-[3,5-di (1,1-dimethylethyl)-4-hydroxyphenyl]propionate and/or tris[2,4-di(1,1-dimethylethyl)phenyl] phosphite, use mobile phase 3 and inject 20 ml of solution S22, 20 ml of the corresponding blank solution, 20 ml of reference solutions (c), (i) or (j) or (i) and (j).

In all cases record the chromatogram for 30 min; the chromatograms corresponding to solutions S21 and S22 only show peaks due to antioxidants stated in the composi-tion and minor peaks that also appear in the chromatograms corresponding to the blank solutions. The areas of the peaks of solutions S21 and S22 are less than the areas of the corresponding peaks in the chromatograms obtained with reference solutions (d) to (j).

Non-phenolic antioxidants. Examine by thin-layer chromatography (*2.2.27*), using *silica gel* GF_{254} as the coating substance.

Test solution S23. Evaporate 100 ml of solution S2 to dryness *in vacuo* at 45°C. Dissolve the residue in 2 ml of *acidified methylene chloride R.*

Reference solution (k). Dissolve 60 mg of *2, 2′-di(octa-decyloxy)-5,5′-spirobi(1,3,2-dioxaphosphorinane) R* in *methylene chloride R* and dilute to 10 ml with the same solvent. Dilute 2 ml of the solution to 10 ml with *acidified methylene chloride R.*

Reference solution (l). Dissolve 60 mg of *dioctodecyl disulphide R* in *methylene chloride R* and dilute to 10 ml with the same solvent. Dilute 2 ml of the solution to 10 ml with *acidified methylene chloride R.*

Reference solution (m). Dissolve 60 mg of *didodecyl 3,3′-thiodipropionate R* in *methylene chloride R* and dilute to 10ml with the same solvent. Dilute 2 ml of the solution to 10 ml with *acidified methylene chloride R.*

Reference solution (n). Dissolve 60 mg of *dioctadecyl 3,3′-thiodipropionate R* in *methylene chloride R* and dilute to 10 ml with the same solvent. Dilute 2 ml of the solution to 10 ml with *acidified methylene chloride R.*

Reference solution (o). Dissolve 60 mg of *didodecyl 3,3′-thiodipropionate R* and 60 mg of *dioctadecyl 3,3′-thiodipro-pionate R* in *methylene chloride R* and dilute to 10 ml with the same solvent. Dilute 2 ml of the solution to 10 ml with *acidified methylene chloride R.*

Apply separately to the plate 20 ml of test solution S23, reference solution (o) and the reference solutions corresp-onding to all the phenolic and non-phenolic antioxidants mentioned in the type composition of the material being examined.

Develop over a path of 18 cm using *hexane R*. Allow the plate to dry. Develop a second time over a path of 17 cm using *methylene chloride R*. Allow the plate to dry and examine in ultraviolet light at 254 nm. Spray with *alcoholic iodine solution R* and examine in ultraviolet light at 254 nm after 10 min to 15 min. Any spots in the chromatogram obtained with test solution S23 are not more intense than the spots in the same locations in the chromatograms obtained with the reference solutions. The test is not valid unless the chromatogram obtained with reference solution (o) shows two clearly separated spots.

Amides and stearates Examine by thin-layer chromatography (*2.2.27*), using two plates with *silica gel* GF_{254} as the coating substance.

Test solution. Use solution S23.

Reference solution (p). Dissolve 20 mg of *stearic acid R* in *methylene chloride R* and dilute to 10 ml with the same solvent.

Reference solution (q). Dissolve 40 mg of *oleamide R* in *methylene chloride R* and dilute to 20 ml with the same solvent.

Reference solution (r). Dissolve 40 mg of *erucamide R* in *methylene chloride R* and dilute to 20 ml with the same solvent.

Apply to each of the two plates 10 ml of solution S23. Apply 10 ml of reference solution (p) to the first and 10 ml of reference solutions (q) and (r) to the second. Develop the first plate over a path of 10 cm using a mixture of 25 volumes of *ethanol R* and 75 volumes of *trimethylpentane R*. Allow the plate to dry in air. Spray with a 2 g/l solution of *sodium dichlorophenolindophenol R* in *ethanol R* and heat in an oven at 120°C for a few minutes to intensify the spots. Any spot corresponding to stearic acid in the chromatogram obtained with test solution S23 is identical in position (R_f about 0.5) but not more intense than the spot in the same location in the chromatogram obtained with reference solution (p).

Develop the second plate over a path of 13 cm using *hexane R*. Allow the plate to dry in air. Develop a second time over a path of 10 cm using a mixture of 5 volumes of *methanol R* and 95 volumes of *methylene chloride R*. Allow the plate to dry. Spray with a 40 g/l solution of *phosphomolybdic acid R* in *ethanol R*. Heat in an oven at 120°C until spots appear. Any spots corresponding to erucamide or oleamide in the chromatogram obtained with test solution S23 are identical in position (R_f about 0.2) but not more intense than the corresponding spots in the chromatograms obtained with reference solutions (q) and (r).

LIST OF ADDITIVES

It may contain not more than three of the following antioxidants:

- butylhydroxytoluene, not more than 0.125 per cent;
- pentaerythrityl tetrakis[3-[3,5-di(1,1-dimethylethyl)-4-hydroxyphenyl]]propionate, not more than 0.3 per cent;
- 1,3,5-tris[3,5-di(1,1-dimethylethyl)-4-hydroxybenzyl]-1*H*,3*H*,5*H*-1,3,5-triazine-2,4,6-trione, not more than 0.3 per cent;
- octadecyl 3-[3,5-di(1,1-dimethylethyl)-4-hydroxyphenyl]-propionate, not more than 0.3 per cent;
- ethylene bis[3,3-di-[3-(1,1-dimethylethyl)-4-hydroxyphenyl]-butyratel], not more than 0.3 per cent;
- dioctadecyl disulphide, not more than 0.3 per cent;
- 2,2′,2″,6,6′,6″-hexa(1,1-dimethylethyl)-4,4′,4″-[(2,4,6-trimethyl-1,3,5-benzenetriyl)trismethylene]-triphenol, not more than 0.3 per cent;
- 2,2′-di(octadecyloxy)-5,5′-spirobi(1,3,2-dioxaphosphorinane), not more than 0.3 per cent;
- didodecyl 3,3′-thiodipropionate, not more than 0.3 per cent;
- dioctadecyl 3,3′-thiodipropionate, not more than 0.3 per cent;
- tris[2,4-di(1,1-dimethylethyl)phenyl] phosphite, not more than 0.3 per cent.

The total amount of the antioxidant additives listed above does not exceed 0.3 per cent.

- hydrotalcite, not more than 0.5 per cent;
- alkane amides, not more than 0.5 per cent;
- alkene amides, not more than 0.5 per cent;
- sodium silico-aluminate, not more than 0.5 per cent;
- silica, not more than 0.5 per cent;
- sodium benzoate, not more than 0.5 per cent;
- fatty acid esters or salts, not more than 0.5 per cent;
- sodium triphosphate, not more than 0.5 per cent;
- liquid paraffin, not more than 0.5 per cent;
- zinc oxide, not more than 0.5 per cent;
- calcium or zinc stearate or a mixture of the two, not more than 0.5 per cent;
- titanium oxide, not more than 4 per cent.

D. Polypropylene for Containers and Closures for Parenteral and Ophthalmic Preparations

(Ph. Eur. text 3.1.6)

DEFINITION

Polypropylene consists of the homopolymer of propylene or of a copolymer of propylene with up to 20 per cent of ethylene or of a mixture (alloy) of polypropylene with up to 20 per cent of polyethylene. It may contain additives.

CHARACTERS

Powder, beads, granules or translucent sheets of varying thickness. It is practically insoluble in water, soluble in hot aromatic hydrocarbons, practically insoluble in ethanol, in hexane and in methanol. It softens at temperatures above about 120°.

IDENTIFICATION

A. To 0.25 g add 10 ml of *toluene R* and boil under a reflux condenser for about 15 min. Place a few drops of the hot solution on a sodium chloride disc and evaporate the solvent in an oven at 80°. Examine by infrared absorption spectrophotometry (*2.2.24*). The spectrum obtained with the material to be examined presents a certain number of maxima, in particular at 1375 cm^{-1}, 1170 cm^{-1}, 995 cm^{-1} and 970 cm^{-1}. The spectrum obtained is identical to the spectrum obtained with the material selected for the type sample. If the material to be examined is in the form of sheets, the identification may be performed directly on a cut piece of suitable size.

B. It complies with the supplementary tests corresponding to the additives present (see Tests).

TESTS

If necessary, cut the material into pieces of maximum dimension on a side of not greater than 1 cm.

Solution S1 Place 25 g in a borosilicate-glass flask with a ground-glass neck. Add 500 ml of *water R* and boil under a reflux condenser for 5 h. Allow to cool and decant. Reserve a portion of the solution for the test for appearance of solution and filter the rest through a sintered-glass filter (16). *Use solution S1 within 4 h of preparation.*

Solution S2 Place 2.0 g in a conical borosilicate-glass flask with a ground-glass neck. Add 80 ml of *toluene R* and boil under a reflux condenser with constant stirring for 1 h 30 min. Allow to cool to 60° and add with continued stirring 120 ml of *methanol R*. Filter the solution through a sintered-glass filter (16). Rinse the flask and the filter with 25 ml of a mixture of 40 ml of *toluene R* and 60 ml of *methanol R*, add the rinsings to the filtrate and dilute to 250.0 ml with the same mixture of solvents. Prepare a blank solution.

Solution S3 Place 100 g in a conical borosilicate-glass flask with a ground-glass neck. Add 250 ml of *0.1M hydrochloric acid* and boil under a reflux condenser with constant stirring for 1 h. Allow to cool and decant the solution.

Appearance of solution Solution S1 is not more opalescent than reference suspension II (*2.2.1*) and is colourless (*Method II, 2.2.2*).

Acidity or alkalinity To 100 ml of solution S1 add 0.15 ml of *BRP indicator solution R*. Not more than 1.5 ml of *0.01M sodium hydroxide* is required to change the colour of the indicator to blue. To 100 ml of solution S1 add 0.2 ml of *methyl orange solution R*. Not more than 1.0 ml of *0.01M hydrochloric acid* is required to reach the beginning of the colour change of the indicator from yellow to orange.

Absorbance (*2.2.25*). At wavelengths from 220 nm to 340 nm, the absorbance of solution S1 is not greater than 0.2.

Reducing substances To 20 ml of solution S1 add 1 ml of *dilute sulphuric acid R* and 20 ml of *0.002M potassium permanganate*. Boil under a reflux condenser for 3 min and cool immediately. Add 1 g of *potassium iodide R* and titrate immediately with *0.01M sodium thiosulphate*, using 0.25 ml of *starch solution R* as indicator. Carry out a blank titration. The difference between the titration volumes is not more than 0.5 ml.

Substances soluble in hexane Place 1.00 g in a 250 ml conical borosilicate-glass flask with a ground-glass neck. Add 100 ml of *hexane R* and boil under a reflux condenser for 4 h, stirring constantly. Cool in iced water and filter rapidly through a sintered-glass filter (16) maintaining the solution at 0°C (*the filtration time must be less than 5 min; if necessary the filtration may be accelerated by applying pressure to the solution*). Evaporate 20 ml of the filtrate in a tared glass dish on a water-bath. Dry the residue in an oven at 100°C to 105°C for 1 h. The mass of the residue obtained must be within 10 per cent of the residue obtained with the type sample and does not exceed 5 per cent.

Extractable aluminium Not more than 1 ppm of extractable Al, determined by atomic emission spectrometry in an argon plasma (*Method I, 2.2.22*).

Test solution. Use solution S3.

Reference solutions. Prepare the reference solutions using *aluminium standard solution (200 ppm Al) R*, diluted with *0.1M hydrochloric acid.*

Carry out the determination using the emission of aluminium at 396.15 nm, the spectral background being taken as 396.25 nm.

Verify the absence of aluminium in the hydrochloric acid used.

Extractable chromium Not more than 0.05 ppm of extractable Cr, determined by atomic emission spectrometry in an argon plasma (*Method I, 2.2.22*).

Test solution. Use solution S3.

Reference solutions. Prepare the reference solutions using *chromium standard solution (100 ppm Cr) R*, diluting with a mixture of 2 volumes of *hydrochloric acid R* and 8 volumes of *water R*.

Carry out the determination using the emission of chromium at 205.55 nm, the spectral background being taken as 205.50 nm.

Verify the absence of chromium in the hydrochloric acid used.

Extractable heavy metals (*2.4.8*). 12 ml of solution S3 complies with limit test A for heavy metals (2.5 ppm). Prepare the standard using 10 ml of *lead standard solution (1 ppm Pb) R*.

Extractable titanium Not more than 1 ppm of extractable Ti, determined by atomic emission spectrometry in an argon plasma (*Method I, 2.2.22*).

Test solution. Use solution S3.

Reference solutions. Prepare the reference solutions using *titanium standard solution (100 ppm Ti) R*, diluted with *0.1M hydrochloric acid.*

Carry out the determination using the emission of titanium at 336.12 nm, the spectral background being taken as 336.16 nm.

Verify the absence of titanium in the hydrochloric acid used.

Extractable vanadium Not more than 10 ppm of extractable V, determined by atomic emission spectrometry in an argon plasma (*Method 1, 2.2.22*).

Test solution. Use solution S3.

Reference solutions. Prepare the reference solutions using *vanadium standard solution (1 g/l V) R*, diluting with a mixture of 2 volumes of *hydrochloric acid R* and 8 volumes of *water R*.

Carry out the determination using the emission of vanadium at 292.40 nm, the spectral background being taken as 292.35 nm.

Verify the absence of vanadium in the hydrochloric acid used.

Extractable zinc Not more than 1 ppm of extractable Zn, determined by atomic absorption spectrometry (*Method 1, 2.2.23*).

Test solution. Use solution S3.

Reference solutions. Prepare the reference solutions using *zinc standard solution (10 ppm Zn) R*, diluted with *0.1M hydrochloric acid.*

Measure the absorbance at 213.9 nm using a zinc hollow-cathode lamp as a source of radiation and an air-acetylene flame.

Sulphated ash (*2.4.14*). Not more than 1.0 per cent, determined on 5.0 g. This limit does not apply to material that has been opacified with titanium dioxide.

SUPPLEMENTARY TESTS

These tests are to be carried out, in whole or in part, only if required by the stated composition of the material.

Phenolic antioxidants. Examine by liquid chromatography (*2.2.29*).

The chromatographic procedure may be carried out using:

— a stainless steel column 0.25 m long and 4.6 mm in internal diameter packed with *octadecylsilyl silica gel for chromatography R* (5 µm),

— as mobile phase one of the following mixtures:
Mobile phase 1 at a flow rate of 2 ml per minute;
30 volumes of *water R*,
70 volumes of *acetonitrile R*,
Mobile phase 2 at a flow rate of 1.5 ml per minute;
10 volumes of *water R*,
30 volumes of *tetrahydrofuran R*,
60 volumes of *acetonitrile R*,
Mobile phase 3 at a flow rate of 1.5 ml per minute;
5 volumes of *water R*,
45 volumes of *2-propanol R*,
50 volumes of *methanol R*,

— as detector a spectrophotometer set at 280 nm.

The chromatographic system must ensure the following:

— resolution of not less than 8 between the peaks corresponding to butylhydroxytoluene and ethylene bis[3,3-di[3-(1,1-dimethylethyl)-4-hydroxyphenyl]-butyrate], with mobile phase 1;

— a resolution of not less than 2 between the peaks corresponding to pentaerythrityl tetrakis[3-[3,5-di(1,1-dimethylethyl)-4-hydroxyphenyl]propionate] and 2,2′,2″6,6′,6″-hexa(1,1-dimethylethyl)-4,4′,4″-[(2,4,6-trimethyl-1,3,5-benzenetriyl)trismethylene]-triphenol, with mobile phase 2;

— a resolution of not less than 2 between the peaks corresponding to octadecyl 3-[3,5-di-(1,1-dimethyl-ethyl)-4-hydroxyphenyl]propionate and tris[2,4-di(1,1-dimethyl-ethyl)phenyl] phosphite, with mobile phase 3.

Test solution S21. Evaporate 50.0 ml of solution S2 to dryness *in vacuo* at 45°. Dissolve the residue with 5.0 ml of a mixture of equal volumes of *acetonitrile R* and *tetrahydrofuran R*. Prepare a blank solution from the blank solution corresponding to solution S2.

Test solution S22. Evaporate 50.0 ml of solution S2 to dryness *in vacuo* at 45°. Dissolve the residue with 5.0 ml of *methylene chloride R*. Prepare a blank solution from the blank solution corresponding to solution S2.

Of the following reference solutions, prepare only those that are necessary for the analysis of the phenolic antioxidants stated in the composition of the substance to be examined.

Reference solution (a). Dissolve 25.0 mg of *butylhydroxytoluene R* and 60.0 mg of *ethylene bis[3,3-di[3-(1,1 dimethyl-ethyl)-4-hydroxyphenyl]butyrate] R* in 10 ml of a mixture of equal volumes of *acetonitrile R* and *tetrahydrofuran R*. Dilute 2.0 ml of the solution to 50.0 ml with the same mixture of solvents.

Reference solution (b). Dissolve 60.0 mg of *pentaerythrityl tetrakis[3-[3,5-di(1,1-dimethylethyl)-4-hydroxyphenyl]-propionate] R* and 60.0 mg of *2,2′,2″,6,6′,6″-hexa(1,1-dimethylethyl)-4,4′,4″-[(2,4,6-trimethyl-1,3,5-benzenetriyl)-trismethylene]triphenol R* in 10.0 ml of a mixture of equal volumes of *acetonitrile R* and *tetrahydrofuran R*. Dilute 2.0 ml of the solution to 50.0 ml with the same mixture of solvents.

Reference solution (c). Dissolve 60.0 mg of *octadecyl 3-[3,5-di(1,1-dimethylethyl)-4-hydroxyphenyl]propionate R* and 60.0 mg of *tris[2,4-di(1,1-dimethylethyl)phenyl] phosphite R* in 10 ml of *methylene chloride R*. Dilute 2.0 ml of the solution to 50.0 ml with the same solvent.

Reference solution (d). Dissolve 25.0 mg of *butylhydroxytoluene R* in 10.0 ml of a mixture of equal volumes of *acetonitrile R* and *tetrahydrofuran R*. Dilute 2.0 ml of the solution to 50.0 ml with the same mixture of solvents.

Reference solution (e). Dissolve 60.0 mg of *ethylene bis[3,3-di[3-(1,1-dimethylethyl)-4-hydroxyphenyl]butyrate] R* in 10.0 ml of a mixture of equal volumes of *acetonitrile R* and *tetrahydrofuran R*. Dilute 2.0 ml of the solution to 50.0 ml with the same mixture of solvents.

Reference solution (f). Dissolve 60.0 mg of *1,3,5-tris[3,5-di(1,1-dimethylethyl)-4-hydroxybenzyl]-1H,3H,5H-1,3,5-triazine-2,4,6-trione R* in 10.0 ml of a mixture of equal volumes of *acetonitrile R* and *tetrahydrofuran R*. Dilute 2.0 ml of the solution to 50.0 ml with the same mixture of solvents.

Reference solution (g). Dissolve 60.0 mg of *pentaerythrityl tetrakis[3-[3,5-di-(1,1-dimethylethyl)-4-hydroxyphenyl]-propionate] R* in 10.0 ml of a mixture of equal volumes of *acetonitrile R* and *tetrahydrofuran R*. Dilute 2.0 ml of the solution to 50.0 ml with the same mixture of solvents.

Reference solution (h). Dissolve 60.0 mg of *2,2′,2″,6,6′,6″-hexa(1,1-dimethylethyl)-4,4′,4″-[(2,4,6-trimethyl-1,3,5-benzenetriyl)trismethylene]triphenol R* in 10.0 ml of a mixture of equal volumes of *acetonitrile R* and *tetrahydrofuran R*. Dilute 2.0 ml of the solution to 50.0 ml with the same mixture of solvents.

Reference solution (i). Dissolve 60.0 mg of *octadecyl 3-[3,5-di(1,1-dimethylethyl)-4-hydroxyphenyl]propionate R* in 10.0 ml of *methylene chloride R*. Dilute 2.0 ml of the solution to 50.0 ml with the same solvent.

Reference solution (j). Dissolve 60.0 mg of *tris[2,4-di(1,1-dimethylethyl)phenyl] phosphite R* in 10.0 ml of *methylene chloride R*. Dilute 2.0 ml of the solution to 50.0 ml with the same solvent.

If the substance to be examined contains butylhydroxytoluene and/or ethylene bis[3,3-di[3-(1,1-dimethylethyl)-4-hydroxy-phenyl[butyrate], use mobile phase 1 and inject 20 ml of solution S21, 20 ml of the corresponding blank solution and 20 ml of reference solutions (a), (d) or (e) or (d) and (e).

If the substance to be examined contains one or more of the following antioxidants:

— 1,3,5-tris[3,5-di(1,1-dimethylethyl)-4-hydroxybenzyl]-1*H*,3*H*, 5*H*-1,3,5-triazine-2,4,6-trione,

— pentaerythrityl tetrakis[3-[3,5-di(1,1-dimethylethyl)-4-hydroxyphenyl]propionate],

— 2,2′,2″,6,6′,6″-hexa(1,1-dimethylethyl)-4,4′,4″-[(2,4,6-trimethyl-1,3,5-benzenetriyl)trismethylene]-triphenol,

— octadecyl 3-[3,5-di(1,1-dimethylethyl)-4-hydroxy-phenyl]-propionate,

— tris[2,4-di(1,1-dimethylethyl)phenyl] phosphite,

use mobile phase 2 and inject 20 µl of solution S21, 20 µl of the corresponding blank solution, 20 µl of reference solution (b) and 20 µl of the reference solutions of the antioxidants on the list above that are stated in the composition.

If the substance to be examined contains octadecyl 3-[3,5-di (1,1-dimethylethyl)-4-hydroxyphenyl]propionate and/or tris[2,4-di(1,1-dimethylethyl)phenyl] phosphite, use mobile phase 3 and inject 20 µl of solution S22, 20 µl of the corresponding blank solution, 20 µl of reference solutions (c), (i) or (j) or (i) and (j).

In all cases record the chromatogram for 30 min; the chromatograms corresponding to solutions S21 and S22 only show peaks due to antioxidants stated in the composition and minor peaks that also appear in the chromatograms corresponding to the blank solutions. The areas of the peaks of solutions S21 and S22 are less than the areas of the corresponding peaks in the chromatograms obtained with reference solutions (d) to (j).

Non-phenolic antioxidants. Examine by thin-layer chromatography (*2.2.27*), using *silica gel* GF_{254} as the coating substance.

Test solution S23. Evaporate 100 ml of solution S2 to dryness *in vacuo* at 45°. Dissolve the residue in 2 ml of *acidified methylene chloride R*.

Reference solution (k). Dissolve 60 mg of *2,2′-di(octadecyloxy)-5,5′-spirobi(1,3,2-dioxaphosphorinane) R* in *methylene chloride R* and dilute to 10 ml with the same solvent. Dilute 2 ml of the solution to 10 ml with *acidified methylene chloride R*.

Reference solution (l). Dissolve 60 mg of *dioctodecyl disulphide R* in *methylene chloride R* and dilute to 10 ml with the same solvent. Dilute 2 ml of the solution to 10 ml with *acidified methylene chloride R*.

Reference solution (m). Dissolve 60 mg of *didodecyl 3,3′-thiodipropionate R* in *methylene chloride R* and dilute to 10 ml with the same solvent. Dilute 2 ml of the solution to 10 ml with *acidified methylene chloride R*.

Reference solution (n) Dissolve 60 mg of *dioctadecyl 3,3′-thiodipropionate R* in *methylene chloride R* and dilute to 10 ml with the same solvent. Dilute 2 ml of the solution to 10 ml with *acidified methylene chloride R*.

Reference solution (o). Dissolve 60 mg of *didodecyl 3,3′-thiodipropionate R* and 60 mg of *dioctadecyl 3,3′-thiodipropionate R* in *methylene chloride R* and dilute to 10 ml with the same solvent. Dilute 2 ml of the solution to 10 ml with *acidified methylene chloride R*.

Apply separately to the plate 20 µl of test solution S23, reference solution (o) and the reference solutions corresponding to all the phenolic and non-phenolic antioxidants mentioned in the type composition of the material to be examined.

Develop over a path of 18 cm using *hexane R*. Allow the plate to dry. Develop a second time over a path of 17 cm using *methylene chloride R*. Allow the plate to dry and examine in ultraviolet light at 254 nm. Spray with *alcoholic iodine solution R* and examine in ultraviolet light at 254 nm after 10 min to 15 min. Any spots in the chromatogram obtained with test solution S23 are not more intense than the spots in the same locations in the chromatograms obtained with the reference solutions. The test is not valid unless the chromatogram obtained with reference solution (o) shows two clearly separated spots.

Amides and stearates Examine by thin-layer chromatography (*2.2.27*), using two plates with *silica gel* GF_{254} as the coating substance.

Test solution. Use solution S23.

Reference solution (p). Dissolve 20 mg of *stearic acid R* in *methylene chloride R* and dilute to 10 ml with the same solvent.

Reference solution (q). Dissolve 40 mg of *oleamide R* in *methylene chloride R* and dilute to 20 ml with the same solvent.

Reference solution (r). Dissolve 40 mg of *erucamide R* in *methylene chloride R* and dilute to 20 ml with the same solvent.

Apply to each of the two plates 10 µl of solution S23. Apply 10 µl of reference solution (p) to the first and 10 µl of reference solutions (q) and (r) to the second. Develop the first plate over a path of 10 cm using a mixture of 25 volumes of *ethanol R* and 75 volumes of *trimethylpentane R*. Allow the plate to dry in air. Spray with a 2 g/l solution of *sodium dichlorophenolindophenol R* in *ethanol R* and heat in an oven at 120° for a few minutes to intensify the spots. Any spot corresponding to stearic acid in the chromatogram obtained with test solution S23 is identical in position (R_f about 0.5) but not more intense than the spot in the same location in the chromatogram obtained with reference solution (p).

Develop the second plate over a path of 13 cm using *hexane R*. Allow the plate to dry in air. Develop a second time over a path of 10 cm using a mixture of 5 volumes of *methanol R* and 95 volumes of *methylene chloride R*. Allow the plate to dry. Spray with a 40 g/l solution of *phosphomolybdic acid R* in *ethanol R*. Heat in an oven at 120° until spots appear. Any spots corresponding to erucamide or oleamide in the chromatogram obtained with test solution S23 are identical in position (R_f about 0.2) but not more than the corresponding spots in the chromatograms obtained with reference solutions (q) and (r).

LIST OF ADDITIVES

It may contain not more than three of the following antioxidants:

— butylhydroxytoluene, not more than 0.125 per cent;
— pentaerythrityl tetrakis[3-[3,5-di(1,1-dimethylethyl)-4-hydroxyphenyl]]propionate, not more than 0.3 per cent;
— 1,3,5-tris[3,5-di(1,1-dimethylethyl)-4-hydroxybenzyl]-1*H*,3*H*,5*H*-1,3,5-triazine-2,4,6-trione, not more than 0.3 per cent;
— octadecyl 3-[3,5-di(1,1-dimethylethyl)-4-hydroxyphenyl]-propionate, not more than 0.3 per cent;
— ethylene bis[3,3-di-[3-(1,1-dimethylethyl)-4-hydroxyphenyl]-butyratel], not more than 0.3 per cent;
— dioctadecyl disulphide, not more than 0.3 per cent;
— 2,2′,2″,6,6′,6″-hexa(1,1-dimethylethyl)-4,4′,4″-[(2,4,6-trimethyl-1,3,5-benzenetriyl)trismethylene]-triphenol, not more than 0.3 per cent;
— 2,2′-di(octadecyloxy)-5,5′-spirobi(1,3,2-dioxaphosphorinane), not more than 0.3 per cent;
— didodecyl 3,3′-thiodipropionate, not more than 0.3 per cent;
— dioctadecyl 3,3′-thiodipropionate, not more than 0.3 per cent;
– tris[2,4-di(1,1-dimethylethyl)phenyl] phosphite, not more than 0.3 per cent.

The total amount of the antioxidant additives listed above does not exceed 0.3 per cent
— hydrotalcite, not more than 0.5 per cent;
— alkane amides, not more than 0.5 per cent;
— alkene amides, not more than 0.5 per cent;
— sodium silico-aluminate, not more than 0.5 per cent;
— silica, not more than 0.5 per cent;
— sodium benzoate, not more than 0.5 per cent;
— fatty acid esters or salts, not more than 0.5 per cent;
— sodium triphosphate, not more than 0.5 per cent;
— liquid paraffin, not more than 0.5 per cent;
— zinc oxide, not more than 0.5 per cent;
— calcium or zinc stearate or a mixture of the two, not more than 0.5 per cent;
— titanium oxide, not more than 4 per cent.

E. Ethylene—Vinyl Acetate Copolymer For Containers And Tubing For Total Parenteral Nutrition Preparations

(Ph Eur text 3.1.7)

Ethylene—vinyl acetate copolymer complying with the following requirements is suitable for the manufacture of containers and tubing for total parenteral nutrition preparations.

Ethylene-vinyl acetate copolymer is obtained by copolymerisation of mixtures of ethylene and vinyl acetate. This copolymer contains a defined quantity of up to 25 per cent of vinyl acetate for material to be used for containers and up to 30 per cent for material to be used for tubing.

Ethylene-vinyl acetate copolymer may contain not more than three of the following stabilisers:
— not more than 0.125 per cent of butylhydroxytoluene,
— not more than 0.2 per cent of each of:
— pentaerythrityl tetrakis[3-(3,5-di-1,1-dimethylethyl-4-hydroxyphenyl)propionate],
— octadecyl 3-(3,5-di-1,1-dimethylethyl-4-hydroxyphenyl)propionate,
—tris(2,4-di-1,1-dimethylethylphenyl) phosphite,
— 2,2′,2″,6,6′,6″-hexa-1,1-dimethylethyl-4,4′,4″-[(2,4,6-trimethyl-1,3,5-benzenetriyl)trismethylene]triphenol.

It may also contain:
— not more than 0.2 per cent of oleamide or not more than 0.2 per cent of erucamide,
— not more than 0.5 per cent of calcium stearate or zinc stearate or 0.5 per cent of a mixture of the two,
— not more than 0.5 per cent of calcium carbonate or not more than 0.5 per cent of potassium hydroxide,
— not more than 0.2 per cent of silicon dioxide.

CHARACTERS

Pellets, granules or translucent sheets or tubing of varying thickness. It is practically insoluble in water, soluble in hot aromatic hydrocarbons, practically insoluble in ethanol, in methanol and in hexane which dissolves, however, low molecular mass polymers. It burns with a blue flame giving off an odour of burning paraffin wax and a faint odour of acetic acid. The temperature at which the substance softens changes with the vinyl acetate content; it decreases from about 100° for contents of a few per cent to about 70° for contents of 30 per cent.

IDENTIFICATION

To 0.25 g add 10 ml of *toluene R* and boil under a reflux condenser for about 15 min. Place a few drops of the solution on a disc of *sodium chloride R* and evaporate the solvent in an oven at 80°. Examine by infrared absorption spectrophotometry (*2.2.24*). The spectrum obtained shows absorption maxima corresponding to vinyl acetate at the following positions: 1740 cm^{-1}; 1374 cm^{-1}; 1240 cm^{-1}; 1020 cm^{-1}; 610 cm^{-1}; and maxima corresponding to ethylene at the following positions: 2920 cm^{-1} to 2850 cm^{-1}; 1470 cm^{-1}; 1460 cm^{-1}; 1374 cm^{-1}; 730 cm^{-1}; 720 cm^{-1}. The spectrum obtained is, in addition, identical to the spectrum obtained with the reference substance provided by the manufacturer. If the material to be examined is in the form of sheets, the spectrum may be determined directly on a cut piece of suitable size.

TESTS

If necessary, cut the material into pieces of maximum dimension not greater than 1 cm.

Solution S_1 Place 2.0 g in a borosilicate-glass flask with a ground-glass neck. Add 80 ml of *toluene R* and heat under a reflux condenser with constant agitation for 90 min. Allow to cool to 60° and add 120 ml of *methanol R* to the flask with constant stirring. Filter the solution through a sintered-glass filter (16). Rinse the flask and the filter with 25 ml of a mixture of 40 ml of *toluene R* and 60 ml of *methanol R*, add the rinsing mixture to the filtrate and dilute to 250 ml with the same mixture of solvents.

Solution S_2 Place 25 g in a borosilicate-glass flask with a ground-glass neck. Add 500 ml of *water R* and boil under a reflux condenser for 5 h. Allow to cool and decant. Reserve a portion of the solution for the test for appearance of solution S_2 and filter the rest through a sintered-glass filter (16). Use within 4 h of preparation.

Appearance of solution S_2 Solution S_2 is clear (*2.2.1*) and colourless (*Method II, 2.2.2*).

Acidity or alkalinity To 100 ml of solution S_2 add 0.15 ml of *BRP indicator solution R*. Not more than 1.0 ml of *0.01M sodium hydroxide* is required to change the colour of the indicator to blue. To 100 ml of solution S_2 add 0.2 ml of *methyl orange solution R*. Not more than 1.5 ml of *0.01M hydrochloric acid* is required to reach the beginning of the colour change of the indicator from yellow to orange.

Absorbance (*2.2.25*). At wavelengths from 220 nm to 340 nm, the absorbance of solution S_2 is not greater than 0.20.

Reducing substances To 20 ml of solution S_2 add 1 ml of *dilute sulphuric acid R* and 20 ml of *0.002M potassium permanganate*. Boil under a reflux condenser for 3 min and cool immediately. Add 1 g of *potassium iodide R* and titrate immediately with *0.01M sodium thiosulphate*, using 0.25 ml of *starch solution R* as indicator. Carry out a blank titration. The difference between the titration volumes is not more than 0.5 ml.

Amides and stearic acid Examine by thin-layer chromatography (*2.2.27*), using *silica gel GF_{254} R* as the coating substance.

Test solution. Evaporate 100 ml of solution S_1 to dryness *in vacuo* at 45°. Dissolve the residue in 2 ml of *acidified methylene chloride R.*

Reference solution (a). Dissolve 20 mg of *stearic acid R* in 10 ml of *methylene chloride R.*

Reference solution (b). Dissolve 40 mg of *oleamide R* in 10 ml of *methylene chloride R.* Dilute 1 ml of the solution to 5 ml with *methylene chloride R.*

Reference solution (c). Dissolve 40 mg of *erucamide R* in 10 ml of *methylene chloride R.* Dilute 1 ml of the solution to 5 ml with *methylene chloride R.*

Apply separately 10 µl of each solution to two plates.

Develop the first plate over a path of 10 cm using a mixture of 25 volumes of *ethanol R* and 75 volumes of *trimethyl-pentane R.* Allow the plate to dry. Spray with a 2 g/l solution of *dichlorophenolindophenol sodium salt R* in *ethanol R* and heat in an oven at 120°C for a few minutes to intensify the spots. Any spot corresponding to stearic acid in the chromatogram obtained with the test solution is not more intense than the spot in the chromatogram obtained with reference solution (a).

Develop the second plate over a path of 13 cm using *hexane R.* Allow the plate to dry. Develop a second time over a path of 10 cm using a mixture of 5 volumes of *methanol R* and 95 volumes of *methylene chloride R.* Allow the plate to dry. Spray with a 40 g/l solution of *phosphomolybdic acid R* in *ethanol R.* Heat in an oven at 120° until spots appear. Any spots corresponding to erucamide or oleamide in the chromatogram obtained with the test solution are not more intense than the spots in the chromatograms obtained with reference solutions (b) and (c) respectively.

Phenolic antioxidants Examine by liquid chromatography (*2.2.29*).

Test solution (a). Evaporate 50 ml of solution S_1 to dryness *in vacuo* at 45°. Dissolve the residue in 5 ml of a mixture of 50 volumes of *acetonitrile R* and 50 volumes of *tetrahydrofuran R.*

Test solution (b). Evaporate 50 ml of solution S_1 to dryness *in vacuo* at 45°. Dissolve the residue in 5 ml of *methylene chloride R.*

Reference solution (a). Dissolve 25 mg of *butylhydroxytoluene R,* 40 mg of *2,2′,2″,6,6′,6″-hexa-1,1-dimethylethyl-4,4′,4″-[(2,4,6-trimethyl-1,3,5-benzenetriyl)trismethylene]-triphenol R,* 40 mg of *pentaerythrityl tetrakis[3-(3,5-di-1,1-dimethylethyl-4-hydroxyphenyl)propionate] R* and 40 mg of *octadecyl 3-(3,5-di-1,1-dimethylethyl-4-hydroxyphenyl)-propionate R* in 10 ml of a mixture of 50 volumes of *acetonitrile R* and 50 volumes of *tetrahydrofuran R.* Dilute 2 ml to 50 ml with a mixture of 50 volumes of *acetonitrile R* and 50 volumes of *tetrahydrofuran R.*

Reference solution (b). Dissolve 40 mg of *octadecyl 3-(3,5-di-1,1-dimethylethyl-4-hydroxyphenyl)propionate R* and 40 mg of *tris(2,4-di-1,1-dimethylethylphenyl) phosphite R* in 10 ml of *methylene chloride R.* Dilute 2 ml to 50 ml with *methylene chloride R.*

The chromatographic procedure may be carried out using:

- a stainless steel column 0.25 m long and 4.6 mm in internal diameter packed with *octadecylsilyl silica gel for chromatography R* (5 µm),
- as mobile phase at a flow rate of 1.5 ml per minute one of the following mixtures:

  Mobile phase 1;

  10 volumes of *water R,*

  30 volumes of *tetrahydrofuran R,*

  60 volumes of *acetonitrile R,*

  Mobile phase 2;

  5 volumes of *water R,*

  45 volumes of *2-propanol R,*

  50 volumes of *methanol R,*
- as detector a spectrophotometer set at 280 nm.

Using mobile phase 1, inject 20 µl of test solution (a) and 20 µl of reference solution (a).

The chromatogram obtained with test solution (a) shows only principal peaks corresponding to the peaks in the chromatogram obtained with reference solution (a) with a retention time greater than 2 min.

The areas of the peaks in the chromatogram obtained with test solution (a) are not greater than those of the corresponding peaks in the chromatogram obtained with reference solution (a), except for the last peak eluted in the chromatogram obtained with reference solution (a).

The test is not valid unless, with mobile phase 1, the number of theoretical plates calculated for the peak corresponding to butylhydroxytoluene is at least 2500 and the resolution between the peaks corresponding to pentaerythrityl tetrakis[3-(3,5-di-1,1,-dimethylethyl-4-hydroxyphenyl)propionate] and 2,2′,2″,6,6′,6″-hexa-1,1,-dimethylethyl-4,4′,4″-[(2,4,6-trimethyl-1,3,5-benzenetriyl)trismethylene]triphenol is not less than 2.0.

If the chromatogram obtained with test solution (a) shows a peak with the same retention time as the last antioxidant eluted from reference solution (a), use mobile phase 2 as follows:

Inject 20 µl of test solution (b) and 20 µl of reference solution (b).

The chromatogram obtained with test solution (b) shows only principal peaks corresponding to the peaks in the chromatogram obtained with reference solution (b) with a retention time greater than 3 min.

The areas of the peaks in the chromatogram obtained with test solution (b) are not greater than those of the corresponding peaks in the chromatogram obtained with reference solution (b).

The test is not valid unless the resolution between the peaks corresponding to octadecyl 3-(3,5-di-(1,1-dimethylethyl)-l-4-hydroxy-phenyl)propionate and tris(2,4-di-(1,1-dimethylethyl)phenyl) phosphite is at least 2.0.

Substances soluble in hexane Place 5 g in a borosilicate-glass flask with a ground-glass neck. Add 50 ml of *hexane R,* fit a condenser and boil under reflux with constant stirring for 4 h. Cool in iced water; a gel may form. Adapt a cooling jacket filled with iced water to a sintered-glass filter (16) fitted with a device allowing pressure to be applied during filtration. Allow the filter to cool for 15 min. Filter the hexane solution applying a gauge pressure of 27 kPa and without washing the residue; the filtration time must not exceed 5 min. Evaporate 20 ml of the solution to dryness on a water-bath. Dry at 100° for 1 h. The mass of the residue is not greater than 40 mg (2 per cent) for copolymer to be used for containers and not greater than 0.1 g (5 per cent) for copolymer to be used for tubing.

Sulphated ash (*2.4.14*). Not more than 1.2 per cent, determined on 5.0 g.

ASSAY

Introduce 0.250 g to 1.000 g of the substance to be examined, according to the vinyl acetate content of the copolymer to be examined, into a 300 ml conical flask with a ground-glass neck containing a magnetic stirrer.

Add 40 ml of *xylene R*. Boil under a reflux condenser with stirring for 4 h. Stirring continously, allow to cool until precipitation begins before slowly adding 25.0 ml of *alcoholic potassium hydroxide solution R1*. Boil again under a reflux condenser with stirring for 3 h. Allow to cool with continued stirring, rinse the condenser with 50 ml of *water R* and add 30.0 ml of *0.05M sulphuric acid* to the flask. Transfer the contents of the flask into a 400 ml beaker; rinse the flask with two quantities, each of 50 ml, of a 200 g/l solution of *anhydrous sodium sulphate R* and three quantities, each of 20 ml, of *water R* and add all the rinsings to the beaker containing the initial solution. Titrate the excess sulphuric acid with *0.1M sodium hydroxide*, determining the end-point potentiometrically (*2.2.20*). Carry out a blank titration.

1 ml of *0.05M sulphuric acid* is equivalent to 8.609 mg of vinyl acetate.

F. Silicone

1. SILICONE OIL USED AS A LUBRICANT
(Ph. Eur. Text 3.1.8)

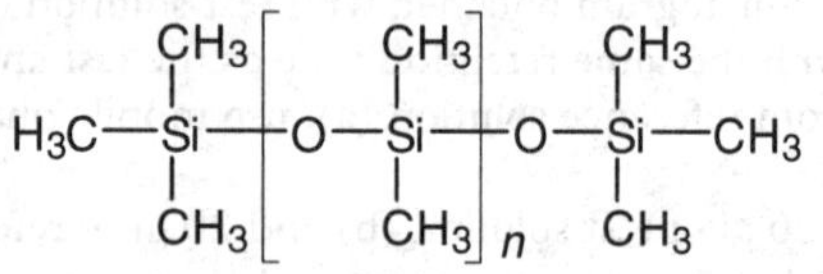

Silicone oil used as a lubricant is a poly(dimethylsiloxane) obtained by hydrolysis and polycondensation of dichlorodimethylsilane and chlorotrimethylsilane. Different grades exist which are characterised by a number indicating the nominal viscosity placed after the name.

Their degree of polymerisation (n = 400 to 1200) is such that their kinematic viscosities are nominally between 1000 $mm^2.s^{-1}$ and 30,000 $mm^2.s^{-1}$.

CHARACTERS

Clear, colourless liquids of various viscosities, practically insoluble in water and in methanol, miscible with carbon tetrachloride, with chloroform, with ether, with ethyl acetate, with methyl ethyl ketone and with toluene, very slightly soluble in ethanol.

IDENTIFICATION

A. It is identified by its kinematic viscosity at 25° (see Tests).

B. Examine by infrared absorption spectrophotometry (*2.2.24*). The absorption maxima in the spectrum obtained with the substance to be examined correspond in position and relative intensity to those in the spectrum obtained with *silicone oil CRS*. The region of the spectrum from 850 cm^{-1} to 750 cm^{-1} is not taken into account since it may show slight differences depending on the degree of polymerisation.

C. Heat 0.5 g in a test-tube over a small flame until white fumes begin to appear. Invert the tube over a second tube containing 1 ml of a 1 g/l solution of chromotropic acid, *sodium salt R* in *sulphuric acid R* so that the fumes reach the solution. Shake the second tube for about 10 s and heat on a water-bath for 5 min. The solution is violet.

D. In a platinum crucible, prepare the sulphated ash (*2.4.14*) using 50 mg. The residue is a white powder that gives the reaction of silicates (*2.3.1*).

TESTS

Acidity To 2.0 g add 25 ml of a mixture of equal volumes of *ethanol R* and *ether R*. Add 0.2 ml of *bromothymol blue solution R1* and shake. Not more than 0.15 ml of *0.01M sodium hydroxide* is required to change the colour of the indicator to blue.

Viscosity (*2.2.10*). Determine the dynamic viscosity at 25°. Calculate the kinematic viscosity taking the relative density to be 0.97. The kinematic viscosity is not less than 95 per cent and not more than 105 per cent of the nominal viscosity stated on the label.

Mineral oils Place 2 ml in a test-tube and examine in ultraviolet light at 365 nm. The fluorescence is not more intense than that of a solution containing 0.1 ppm of *quinine sulphate R* in *0.005M sulphuric acid* examined in the same conditions.

Phenylated compounds The refractive index (*2.2.6*) is not greater than 1.410.

Volatile matter Not more than 2.0 per cent, determined on 2.00 g by heating in an oven at 150° for 24 h. Carry out the test using a dish 60 mm in diameter and 10 mm deep.

Heavy metals Mix 1.0 g with *chloroform R* and dilute to 20 ml with the same solvent. Add 1.0 ml of a freshly prepared 0.02 g/l solution of *dithizone R* in *chloroform R*, 0.5 ml of *water R* and 0.5 ml of a mixture of 1 volume of *dilute ammonia R2* and 9 volumes of a 2 g/l solution of *hydroxylamine hydrochloride R*. At the same time, prepare a standard as follows: to 20 ml of *chloroform R* add 1.0 ml of a freshly prepared 0.02 g/l solution of *dithizone R* in *chloroform R*, 0.5 ml of *lead standard solution (10 ppm Pb) R* and 0.5 ml of a mixture of 1 volume of *dilute ammonia R2* and 9 volumes of a 2 g/l solution of *hydroxylamine hydrochloride R*. Immediately shake each solution vigorously for 1 min. Any red colour in the test solution is not more intense than that in the standard (5 ppm).

LABELLING

The label indicates the nominal viscosity by a number placed after the name of the product. The label also states that the contents are to be used as a lubricant.

2. SILICONE ELASTOMER FOR CLOSURES AND TUBING
(Ph. Eur. Text 3.1.9)

Silicone elastomer complying with the following requirements is suitable for the manufacture of closures and tubing.

Silicone elastomer is obtained by cross-linking a linear polysiloxane constructed mainly of dimethylsiloxy units with small quantities of methylvinylsiloxy groups; the chain ends are blocked by trimethylsiloxy or dimethylvinylsiloxy groups. The general formula of the polysiloxane is:

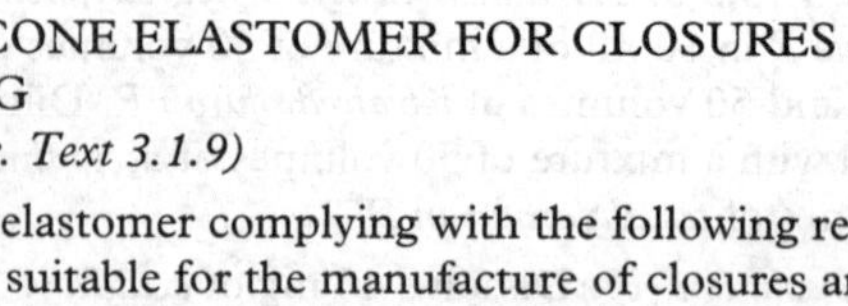

M and M' = 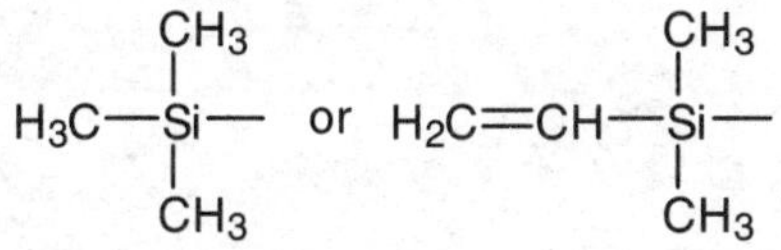

The cross-linking is carried out in the hot state either with:
- — 2,4-dichlorobenzoyl peroxide for extruded products,
- — 2,4-dichlorobenzoyl peroxide or dicumyl peroxide or *OO*-(1,1-dimethylethyl) *O*-isopropyl monoperoxycarbonate or 2,5-bis(*t*(1,1-dimethylethyl)dioxy)-2,5-dimethylhexane for moulded products,
- — or by hydrosilylation by means of polysiloxane with -SiH groups using platinum as a catalyst.

In all cases, appropriate additives are used such as silica and sometimes small quantities of organosilicon additives (α,ω-dihydroxypolydimethylsiloxane).

CHARACTERS

A transparent or translucent, odourless material, practically insoluble in organic solvents, some of which, for example, cyclohexane, hexane and chlorinated hydrocarbons, cause a reversible swelling of the material.

IDENTIFICATION

A. Examine by infrared absorption spectrophotometry recording the spectrum by the multiple reflection method for solids (*2.2.24*). The absorption maxima in the spectrum obtained with the substance to be examined correspond in position and relative intensity to those in the spectrum obtained with *silicone elastomer CRS*.

B. Heat 1.0 g in a test-tube over a small flame until white fumes begin to appear. Invert the tube over a second tube containing 1 ml of a 1 g/l solution of *chromotropic acid, sodium salt R* in *sulphuric acid R* so that the fumes reach the solution. Shake the second tube for about 10 s and heat on a water-bath for 5 min. The solution is violet.

C. 50 mg of the residue of combustion gives the reaction of silicates (*2.3.1*).

TESTS

If necessary, cut the material into pieces of maximum dimension not greater than 1 cm.

Solution S Place 25 g in a borosilicate-glass flask with a ground-glass neck. Add 500 ml of *water R* and boil under a reflux condenser for 5 h. Allow to cool and decant the solution.

Appearance of solution Solution S is clear (*2.2.1*).

Acidity or alkalinity To 100 ml of solution S add 0.15 ml of *bromothymol blue solution R1*. Not more than 2.5 ml of *0.01M sodium hydroxide* is required to change the colour of the indicator to blue. To a further 100 ml of solution S, add 0.2 ml of *methyl orange solution R*. Not more than 1.0 ml of *0.01M hydrochloric acid* is required to reach the beginning of the colour change of the indicator from yellow to orange.

Relative density (*2.2.5*). 1.05 to 1.25, determined using a density bottle with *ethanol R* as the immersion liquid.

Reducing substances To 20 ml of solution S add 1 ml of *dilute sulphuric acid R* and 20 ml of *0.002M potassium permanganate*. Allow to stand for 15 min. Add 1 g of *potassium iodide R* and titrate immediately with *0.01M sodium thiosulphate* using 0.25 ml of *starch solution R* as indicator. Carry out a blank titration using 20 ml of *water R* instead of solution S. The difference between the titration volumes is not more than 1.0 ml.

Substances soluble in hexane Evaporate 25 ml of the solution obtained in the test for phenylated compounds in a glass evaporating dish on a water-bath and dry in an oven at 100° to 105° for 1 h. The residue weighs not more than 15 mg (3 per cent).

Volatile matter Weigh 10.0 g of the substance previously stored for 48 h in a desiccator over *anhydrous calcium chloride R*. Heat in an oven at 200° for 4 h, allow to cool in a desiccator and weigh again. For silicone elastomer prepared using peroxides, the volatile matter is not greater than 0.5 per cent. For silicone elastomer prepared using platinum, the volatile matter is not greater than 2.0 per cent.

Mineral oils Place 2 g in a 100 ml conical flask containing 30 ml of a mixture of 5 volumes of *ammonia R* and 95 volumes of *pyridine R*. Allow to stand for 2 h, shaking frequently. Decant the pyridine solution and examine in ultraviolet light at 365 nm. The fluorescence is not greater than that of a solution containing 1 ppm of *quinine sulphate R* in *0.005M sulphuric acid* examined in the same conditions.

Phenylated compounds Place 2.0 g in a borosilicate-glass flask with a ground-glass neck and add 100 ml of *hexane R*. Boil under a reflux condenser for 4 h. Cool, then filter rapidly through a sintered-glass filter (16). Collect the filtrate and close the container immediately to avoid evaporation. At wavelengths from 250 nm to 340 nm (*2.2.25*), the absorbance is not greater than 0.4.

Silicone elastomer prepared using peroxides complies with the following additional test:

Residual peroxides Place 5 g in a borosilicate-glass flask, add 150 ml of *methylene chloride R* and close the flask. Stir with a mechanical stirrer for 16 h. Filter rapidly, collecting the filtrate in a container with a ground-glass neck. Replace the air in the container with *oxygen-free nitrogen R*, introduce 1 ml of a 200 g/l solution of *sodium iodide R* in *anhydrous acetic acid R*, close the flask, shake thoroughly and allow to stand protected from light for 30 min. Add 50 ml of *water R* and titrate immediately with *0.01M sodium thiosulphate*, using 0.25 ml of *starch solution R* as indicator. Carry out a blank titration. The difference between the titration volumes is not greater than 2.0 ml (0.08 per cent calculated as dichlorobenzoyl peroxide).

Silicone elastomer prepared using platinum complies with the following additional test:

Platinum In a quartz crucible, ignite 1.0 g of the material to be examined, raising the temperature very gradually until a white residue is obtained. Transfer the residue to a graphite crucible. To the quartz crucible add 10 ml of a freshly prepared mixture of 1 volume of *nitric acid R* and 3 volumes of *hydrochloric acid R*, heat on a water-bath for 1 min to 2 min and transfer to the graphite crucible. Add 5 mg of *potassium chloride R* and 5 ml of *hydrofluoric acid R* and evaporate to dryness on a water-bath. Add 5 ml of *hydrofluoric acid R* and evaporate to dryness again; repeat this operation twice. Dissolve the residue in 5 ml of *1M hydrochloric acid*, warming on a water-bath. Allow to cool and add the solution to 1 ml of a 250 g/l solution of *stannous chloride R* in *1M hydrochloric acid*, rinse the graphite crucible with a few millilitres of *1M hydrochloric* *acid* and dilute to 10.0 ml with the same acid. Prepare simultaneously a standard as follows: to 1 ml of a 250 g/l solution of *stannous chloride R* in *1 M hydrochloric acid* add 1.0 ml of *platinum standard solution (30 ppm Pt) R* and dilute to 10.0 ml with *1M hydrochloric acid.* The colour of the test solution is not more intense than that of the standard (30 ppm).

LABELLING

The label states whether the material was prepared using peroxides or platinum.

Appendix XXI

A. Abbreviated Titles

In accordance with the General Notices the main title of each monograph may be abbreviated using the following abbreviations. An abbreviated title has the same significance as the main title.

Cations

Alum.	Aluminium
Ammon.	Ammonium
Bism.	Bismuth
Calc.	Calcium
Ferr.	Ferrous
Mag.	Magnesium
Pot.	Potassium
Sod.	Sodium

Anions

Acet.	Acetate
Benz.	Benzoate
Brom.	Bromide
Chlor.	Chloride
Cit.	Citrate
Dihydrochlor.	Dihydrochloride
Fumar.	Fumarate
Hydrobrom.	Hydrobromide
Hydrochlor.	Hydrochloride
Hydrox.	Hydroxide
Iod.	Iodide
Lact.	Lactate
Mal.	Maleate
Methonit.	Methonitrate
Methyllsulph.	Methylsulphate
Metilsulf.	Metilsulfate
Nit.	Nitrate
Ox.	Oxide
Phenylprop.	Phenylpropionate
Phos.	Phosphate
Prop.	Propionate
Succin.	Succinate
Sulph.	Sulphate
Tart.	Tartrate

Adjectives

Ammon.	Ammoniated
Arom.	Aromatic
Camph.	Camphorated
Co.	Compound
Conc.	Concentrated
Cryst.	Crystalline
Efferv.	Effervescent
Emulsif.	Emulsifying
Liq.	Liquefied; Liquid
Prep.	Prepared
Simp.	Simple

Preparations

Applic.	Application
Caps.	Capsules
Ext.	Extract
Inf.	Infusion
Inj.	Injection
Lin.	Liniment
Lot.	Lotion
Mixt.	Mixture
Oint.	Ointment
Pess.	Pessaries
Soln.	Solution
Suppos.	Suppositories
Tabs.	Tablets
Tinct.	Tincture

B. Approved Synoyms

In accordance with the General Notice on Titles, the name or names given in the right-hand column of the list below are Approved Synonyms for the names at the head of the monograph of the European Pharmacopoeia given in the left-hand column.

Names made by changing the order of the words in an Approved Synonym, with the addition of a preposition when necessary, are also Approved Synonyms.

Where square brackets are used in a title these may be replaced by round brackets, and *vice versa.* The words 'per cent' may be replaced by the symbol '%'.

Where the word 'Injection' appears in the title or synonym of a monograph in the European Pharmacopoeia, the abbreviation 'Inj.' is declared to be an approved synonym for that part of the title.

Monographs included in the British Pharmacopoeia (Veterinary) 1998 are identified by means of a superscript number:[1].

Medicinal Substances and Formulated Preparations	
Acetylsalicylic Acid	Aspirin
Activated Charcoal	Decolorising Charcoal
Adrenaline Tartrate	Adrenaline Acid Tartrate/ Epinephrine Acid Tartrate
Alexandrian Senna Pods	Alexandrian Senna Fruit
Alum	Aluminium Potassium Sulphate Potash Alum
Anhydrous Ampicillin	Ampicillin
Anhydrous Citric Acid	Citric Acid
Anhydrous Niclosamide	Niclosamide
Anise Oil	Aniseed Oil
Aniseed	Anise
Anticoagulant and Preservative Solutions for Human Blood	Anticoagulant and Preservative Solutions for Blood
Arachis Oil	Ground-nut Oil Peanut Oil
Barbados Aloes	Curaçao Aloes
Belladonna Leaf	Belladonna Herb
Bendroflumethiazide	Bendroflumethiazide/ Bendrofluazide
Betacyclodextrin	Betadex
Biphasic Insulin Injection	Biphasic Insulin
Biphasic Isophane Insulin Injection	Biphasic Isophane Insulin
Bismuth Subcarbonate	Bismuth Carbonate
Borax	Sodium Borate Sodium Tetraborate
Butyl Parahydroxybenzoate	Butyl Hydroxybenzoate Butylparaben
Butylhydroxyanisole	Butylated Hydroxyanisole
Butylhydroxytoluene	Butylated Hydroxytoluene
Caffeine	Anhydrous Caffeine
Caffeine Monohydrate	Caffeine Hydrate
Calcitonin (Salmon)	Calcitonin (Salmon)/ Salcatonin
Calcium Chloride	Calcium Chloride Dihydrate
Calcium Hydrogen Phosphate Dihydrate	Calcium Hydrogen Phosphate Dibasic Calcium Phosphate
Calcium Lactate Pentahydrate	Calcium Lactate

Calcium Phosphate	Tribasic Calcium Phosphate
Caraway Fruit	Caraway
Cellulose Acetate Phthalate	Cellacefate
Cellulose Powder	Powdered Cellulose
Cetirizine Dihydrochloride	Cetirizine Hydrochloride
Chloramine	Chloramine T
Chlorhexidine Diacetate	Chlorhexidine Acetate
Chlorhexidine Digluconate Solution	Chlorhexidine Gluconate Solution
Chlorhexidine Dihydrochloride	Chlorhexidine Hydrochloride
Chlorobutanol Hemihydrate	Chlorobutanol
Chlorphenamine Maleate	Chlorphenamine Maleate/ Chlorpheniramine Maleate
Cholecalciferol	Colecalciferol
Cholecalciferol Concentrate (Oily Form)	Colecalciferol Concentrate (Oily Form)
Cholecalciferol Concentrate (Powder Form)	Colecalciferol Concentrate (Powder Form)
Cholecalciferol Concentrate (Water-dispersible Form)	Colecalciferol Concentrate (Water-dispersible Form)
Ciclosporin	Cyclosporin
Cinchona Bark	Cinchona Red Cinchona Bark
Cinnamon	Cinnamon Bark Ceylon Cinnamon
Clemastine Fumarate	Clemastine Hydrogen Fumarate
Codeine Phosphate Hemihydrate	Codeine Phosphate
Concentrated Ammonia Solution	Strong Ammonia Solution
Concentrated Hydrochloric Acid	Hydrochloric Acid
Concentrated Phosphoric Acid	Phosphoric Acid
Copper Sulphate Pentahydrate	Copper Sulphate
Cysteine Hydrochloride Monohydrate	Cysteine Hydrochloride
Deferoxamine Mesilate	Desferrioxamine Mesilate
Devil's Claw Root	Devil's Claw Harpagophytum
Digitalis Leaf	Digitalis
Dipotassium Phosphate	Dipotassium Hydrogen Phosphate
Disodium Phosphate Dihydrate	Disodium Hydrogen Phosphate Dihydrate Sodium Phosphate Dihydrate
Disodium Phosphate Dodecahydrate	Disodium Hydrogen Phosphate Dodecahydrate Disodium Hydrogen Phosphate Sodium Phosphate
Dried Iodinated (^{125}I) Human Fibrinogen	Dried Iodinated[^{125}I] Fibrinogen
Emetine Hydrochloride Heptahydrate	Emetine Hydrochloride
Ephedrine Hemihydrate	Ephedrine
Equine Serum Gonadotrophin for Veterinary Use	Serum Gonadotrophin[1]
Erythromycin Ethylsuccinate	Erythromycin Ethyl Succinate
Ethyl Parahydroxybenzoate	Ethyl Hydroxybenzoate Ethylparaben
Fluorescein Sodium	Soluble Fluorescein

Formaldehyde Solution (35 per cent)	Formaldehyde Solution Formalin
Furosemide	Furosemide/ Frusemide
Gentian Root	Gentian
Glucose Monohydrate	Glucose
Glycerol	Glycerin
Glycerol Triacetate	Triacetin
Human Albumin Solution	Albumin Solution Albumin Human Albumin
Human Anti-D (Rh_0) Immunoglobulin	Anti-D (Rh_0) Immunoglobulin
Human Antithrombin III Concentrate, Freeze-dried	Antithrombin III Concentrate
Human Coagulation Factor VII, Freeze-dried	Dried Factor VII Fraction
Human Coagulation Factor VIII, Freeze-dried	Dried Factor VIII Fraction Dried Human Antihaemophilic Fraction
Human Coagulation Factor IX, Freeze-dried	Dried Factor IX Fraction
Human Fibrinogen, Freeze-dried	Dried Fibrinogen
Human Hepatitis A Immunoglobulin	Hepatitis A Immunoglobulin
Human Hepatitis B Immunoglobulin	Hepatitis B Immunoglobulin
Human Hepatitis B Immunoglobulin for Intravenous Use	Hepatitis B Immunoglobulin for Intravenous Use
Human Measles Immunoglobulin	Measles Immunoglobulin
Human Normal Immunoglobulin	Normal Immunoglobulin Normal Immunoglobulin Injection
Human Normal Immunoglobulin for Intravenous Administration	Normal Immunoglobulin for Intravenous Use
Human Plasma for Fractionation	Plasma for Fractionation
Human Prothrombin Complex, Freeze-dried	Dried Prothrombin Complex
Human Rabies Immunoglobulin	Rabies Immunoglobulin
Human Rubella Immunoglobulin	Rubella Immunoglobulin
Human Tetanus Immunoglobulin	Tetanus Immunoglobulin
Human Varicella Immunoglobulin	Varicella Immunoglobulin
Hydrated Aluminium Oxide	Dried Aluminium Hydroxide
Hydrogen Peroxide Solution (3 per cent)	Dilute Hydrogen Peroxide Solution
Hydrous Wool Fat	Lanolin
Ichthammol	Ammonium Ichthosulphonate
Injectable Insulin Preparations	Insulin Preparations
Insulin Zinc Injectable Suspension	Insulin Zinc Suspension Insulin Zinc Suspension (Mixed) I.Z.S. I.Z.S. (Mixed)
Insulin Zinc Injectable Suspension (Amorphous)	Insulin Zinc Suspension (Amorphous) Amorph. I.Z.S.
Insulin Zinc Injectable Suspension (Crystalline)	Insulin Zinc Suspension (Crystalline) Cryst. I.Z.S.
Ipecacuanha Root	Ipecacuanha
Isophane Insulin Injection	Isophane Insulin Isophane Insulin (NPH)
Kanamycin Monosulphate	Kanamycin Sulphate

Lactose Monohydrate	Lactose
Light Magnesium Oxide	Light Magnesia
Liquid Lactulose	Lactulose Solution
Liquorice Root	Liquorice
Low-molecular-mass Heparins	Low-molecular-weight Heparins
Magnesium Chloride Hexahydrate	Magnesium Chloride
Magnesium Sulphate	Epsom Salts
Matricaria Flower	Matricaria Flowers
Medium-chain Triglycerides	Fractionated Coconut Oil (when prepared from the endosperm of *Cocos nucifera* L.)
Methyl Parahydroxybenzoate	Methyl Hydroxybenzoate Methylparaben
Methylatropine Bromide	Atropine Methobromide
Methylatropine Nitrate	Atropine Methonitrate
Methylene Chloride	Dichloromethane
Methylhydroxyethylcellulose	Hydroxyethylmethylcellulose
Nitrofural	Nitrofurazone
Noradrenaline Tartrate	Noradrenaline Acid Tartrate/ Norepinephrine Acid Tartrate
Oxytetracycline	Oxytetracycline Dihydrate
Pancreas Powder	Pancreatic Extract
Pentamidine Diisetionate	Pentamidine Isetionate
Pepsin Powder	Pepsin
Polysorbate 20	Polyoxyethylene 20 Sorbitan Monolaurate
Polysorbate 60	Polyoxyethylene 20 Sorbitan Monostearate
Polysorbate 80	Polyoxyethylene 20 Sorbitan Mono-oleate
Potassium Hydrogen Carbonate	Potassium Bicarbonate
Potassium Hydroxide	Caustic Potash
Prepared Belladonna	Prepared Belladonna Herb
Primaquine Diphosphate	Primaquine Phosphate
Procaine Benzylpenicillin	Procaine Benzylpenicillin/ Procaine Penicillin
Propyl Parahydroxybenzoate	Propyl Hydroxybenzoate Propylparaben
Racemic Ephedrine Hydrochloride	Racephedrine Hydrochloride
Racemic Menthol	Racementhol
Raw Opium	Opium
Rhatany Root	Krameria
Riboflavine	Riboflavin
Riboflavine Sodium Phosphate	Riboflavin Sodium Phosphate
Roman Chamomile Flower	Chamomile Flowers
Saccharin Sodium	Soluble Saccharin
Selenium Disulphide	Selenium Sulphide
Senega Root	Senega
Sodium Citrate	Trisodium Citrate
Sodium Diclofenac	Diclofenac Sodium
Sodium Dihydrogen Phosphate Dihydrate	Sodium Acid Phosphate

Sodium Hydrogen Carbonate	Sodium Bicarbonate
Sodium Hydroxide	Caustic Soda
Sodium Laurilsulfate	Sodium Lauryl Sulphate
Sodium Metabisulphite	Sodium Pyrosulphite
Sodium Methyl Parahydroxybenzoate	Sodium Methyl Hydroxybenzoate
Sodium Propyl Parahydroxybenzoate	Sodium Propyl Hydroxybenzoate
Sodium Sulphate Decahydrate	Sodium Sulphate Glauber's Salt
Sodium Sulphite Heptahydrate	Sodium Sulphite
Soluble Insulin Injection	Insulin Injection Neutral Insulin Neutral Insulin Injection Soluble Insulin
Sorbitol 70 per cent (Crystallising)	Sorbitol Solution (70 per cent) (Crystallising) Sorbitol Solution (70 per cent)
Sorbitol 70 per cent (Non-crystallising)	Sorbitol Solution (70 per cent) (Non-crystallising)
Soya-bean Oil	Soya Oil Soyabean Oil
Soya-bean Oil, Hydrogenated	Hydrogenated Soya Oil Hydrogenated Soyabean Oil
Starch, Pregelatinised	Pregelatinised Maize Starch (when prepared from *Zea mays* L.)
Sterile Non-absorbable Sutures	Sterile Non-absorbable Ligatures
Sucrose	Refined Sugar
Sulfacetamide Sodium	Soluble Sulfacetamide
Synthetic Vitamin A Concentrate (Oily Form)	Synthetic Retinol Concentrate (Oily Form)
Synthetic Vitamin A Concentrate (Powder Form)	Synthetic Retinol Concentrate (Powder Form)
Synthetic Vitamin A Concentrate (Water-dispersible Form)	Synthetic Retinol Concentrate (Water-dispersible Form)
Talc	Purified Talc
Technetium (^{99m}Tc) Human Albumin Injection	Technetium[^{99m}Tc] Albumin Injection
Tetracaine Hydrochloride	Tetracaine Hydrochloride/ Amethocaine Hydrochloride
Theophylline—Ethylenediamine	Aminophylline
Theophylline—Ethylenediamine Hydrate	Aminophylline Hydrate
Theophylline Monohydrate	Theophylline Hydrate
Thiopental Sodium and Sodium Carbonate	Thiopental Sodium
Tinnevelly Senna Pods	Tinnevelly Senna Fruit
α-Tocopherol	Alpha Tocopherol
α-Tocopherol Acetate	Alpha Tocopherol Acetate
α-Tocopherol Acetate Concentrate (Powder Form)	Alpha Tocopheryl Acetate Concentrate (Powder Form)
DL-α-Tocopheryl Hydrogen Succinate	Alpha Tocopheryl Hydrogen Succinate
RRR-α-Tocopherol	*RRR*-Alpha Tocopherol
RRR-α-Tocopheryl Acetate	*RRR*-Alpha Tocopheryl Acetate
RRR-α-Tocopheryl Hydrogen Succinate	*RRR*-Alpha Tocopheryl Hydrogen Succinate
Tylosin For Veterinary Use	Tylosin[1]

Tylosin Tartrate For Veterinary Use	Tylosin Tartrate[1]
Undecylenic Acid	Undecenoic Acid
Valerian Root	Valerian
Wool Alcohols	Wool Wax Alcohols
Wool Fat	Anhydrous Lanolin
Zinc Undecylenate	Zinc Undecenoate

Immunological Products (Human)	
BCG Vaccine, Freeze-dried	Bacillus Calmette-Guérin Vaccine BCG Vaccine
Cholera Vaccine, Freeze-dried	Cholera Vaccine
Diphtheria and Tetanus Vaccine (Adsorbed)	Adsorbed Diphtheria and Tetanus Vaccine Adsorbed Diphtheria—Tetanus Prophylactic
Diphtheria and Tetanus Vaccine (Adsorbed) for Adults and Adolescents	Adsorbed Diphtheria and Tetanus Vaccine for Adults and Adolescents
Diphtheria Vaccine (Adsorbed)	Adsorbed Diphtheria Vaccine Adsorbed Diphtheria Prophylactic
Diphtheria Vaccine (Adsorbed) for Adults and Adolescents	Adsorbed Diphtheria Vaccine for Adults and Adolescents
Diphtheria, Tetanus and Pertussis Vaccine (Adsorbed)	Adsorbed Diphtheria, Tetanus and Pertussis Vaccine Adsorbed Diphtheria—Tetanus—Whooping-cough Prophylactic
Gas-gangrene Antitoxin (Novyi)	Gas-gangrene Antitoxin (Oedematiens)
Hepatitis A Vaccine (Inactivated, Adsorbed)	Inactivated Hepatitis A Vaccine
Influenza Vaccine (Split Virion, Inactivated)	Inactivated Influenza Vaccine (Split Virion)
Influenza Vaccine (Surface Antigen, Inactivated)	Inactivated Influenza Vaccine (Surface Antigen)
Influenza Vaccine (Whole Virion, Inactivated)	Inactivated Influenza Vaccine (Whole Virion)
Measles Vaccine (Live)	Measles Vaccine, Live
Measles, Mumps and Rubella Vaccine (Live)	Measles, Mumps and Rubella Vaccine, Live
Mumps Vaccine (Live)	Mumps Vaccine, Live
Old Tuberculin for Human Use	Old Tuberculin
Pertussis Vaccine	Whooping-cough Vaccine
Pertussis Vaccine (Adsorbed)	Pertussis Vaccine Whooping-cough Vaccine
Poliomyelitis Vaccine (Inactivated)	Inactivated Poliomyelitis Vaccine
Poliomyelitis Vaccine (Oral)	Poliomyelitis Vaccine, Live (Oral)
Rabies Vaccine for Human Use Prepared in Cell Cultures	Rabies Vaccine
Rubella Vaccine (Live)	Rubella Vaccine, Live
Tetanus Antitoxin for Human Use	Tetanus Antitoxin
Tetanus Vaccine (Adsorbed)	Adsorbed Tetanus Vaccine
Tuberculin Purified Protein Derivative for Human Use	Tuberculin Purified Protein Derivative Tuberculin P.P.D.
Typhoid Vaccine, Freeze-dried	Typhoid Vaccine
Typhoid Vaccine (Live, Oral, Strain Ty 21a)	Typhoid (Strain Ty 21a) Vaccine, Live (Oral)
Varicella Vaccine (Live)	Varicella Vaccine, Live
Yellow Fever Vaccine (Live)	Yellow Fever Vaccine, Live

Immunological Products (Veterinary)	
Monographs included in the British Pharmacopoeia (Veterinary) 1998	
Anthrax Spore Vaccine (Live) for Veterinary Use	Anthrax Vaccine, Living
Aujeszky's Disease Vaccine (Inactivated) for Pigs	Aujeszky's Disease Vaccine, Inactivated
Aujeszky's Disease Vaccine (Live) for Pigs for Parenteral Administration, Freeze-dried	Aujeszky's Disease Vaccine, Living
Avian Infectious Bronchitis Vaccine (Live), Freeze-dried	Avian Infectious Bronchitis Vaccine, Living
Avian Infectious Bursal Disease Vaccine (Inactivated)	Infectious Bursal Disease Vaccine, Inactivated Gumboro Disease Vaccine, Inactivated
Avian Infectious Bursal Disease (Gumboro Disease) Vaccine (Live), Freeze-dried	Infectious Bursal Disease Vaccine, Living Gumboro Disease Vaccine, Living
Avian Infectious Encephalomyelitis Vaccine (Live)	Infectious Avian Encephalomyelitis Vaccine, Living Epidemic Tremor Vaccine, Living
Avian Infectious Laryngotracheitis Vaccine (Live) for Chickens	Laryngotracheitis Vaccine, Living
Bovine Parainfluenza Virus Vaccine (Live), Freeze-dried	Bovine Parainfluenza Virus Vaccine, Living
Bovine Respiratory Syncytial Virus Vaccine (Live), Freeze-dried	Bovine Respiratory Syncytial Virus Vaccine, Living
Brucellosis Vaccine (Live) (Brucella Melitensis Rev. 1 Strain) Freeze-dried, for Veterinary Use	Brucella Melitensis (Strain Rev. 1) Vaccine, Living
Canine Contagious Hepatitis Vaccine (Live), Freeze-dried	Canine Contagious Hepatitis Vaccine, Living
Canine Distemper Vaccine (Live), Freeze-dried	Canine Distemper Vaccine, Living
Canine Parvovirosis Vaccine (Inactivated)	Inactivated Canine Parvovirus Vaccine
Canine Parvovirosis Vaccine (Live)	Canine Parvovirus Vaccine, Living
Clostridium Botulinum Vaccine for Veterinary Use	Clostridium Botulinum Vaccine Botulinum Vaccine
Clostridium Chauvoei Vaccine for Veterinary Use	Clostridium Chauvoei Vaccine Blackleg Vaccine
Clostridium Novyi (Type B) Vaccine for Veterinary Use	Clostridium Novyi Type B Vaccine Clostridium Oedematiens Type B Vaccine Black Disease Vaccine
Clostridium Novyi Alpha Antitoxin for Veterinary Use	Clostridium Novyi Alpha Antitoxin Clostridium Oedematiens Alpha Antitoxin Black Disease Antiserum
Clostridium Perfringens Epsilon Antitoxin for Veterinary Use	Clostridium Perfringens Type D Antitoxin Enterotoxaemia Antiserum Pulpy Kidney Antiserum

cont...

Clostridium Perfringens Vaccine for Veterinary Use	Clostridium Perfringens Vaccines Clostridium Perfringens Type B Vaccine
Type B	Lamb Dysentery Vaccine
Type C	Clostridium Perfringens Type C Vaccine Struck Vaccine
Type D	Clostridium Perfringens Type D Vaccine Enterotoxaemia Vaccine Pulpy Kidney Vaccine
Clostridium Septicum Vaccine for Veterinary Use	Clostridium Septicum Vaccine Braxy Vaccine Malignant Oedema Vaccine
Distemper Vaccine (Live) for Mustelids, Freeze-dried	Ferret and Mink Distemper Vaccine, Living
Egg Drop Syndrome '76 Vaccine (Inactivated)	Egg Drop Syndrome '76 (Adenovirus) Vaccine
Equine Influenza Vaccine (Inactivated)	Equine Influenza Vaccine Equine Influenza Vaccine, Inactivated
Feline Calicivirosis Vaccine (Inactivated)	Feline Calicivirus Vaccine, Inactivated
Feline Calicivirosis Vaccine (Live), Freeze-dried	Feline Calicivirus Vaccine, Living
Feline Infectious Enteritis (Feline Panleucopenia) Vaccine (Inactivated)	Feline Infectious Enteritis Vaccine, Inactivated Feline Panleucopenia Vaccine, Inactivated
Feline Infectious Enteritis (Feline Panleucopenia) Vaccine (Live)	Feline Infectious Enteritis Vaccine, Living Feline Panleucopenia Vaccine, Living
Feline Viral Rhinotracheitis Vaccine (Inactivated), Freeze-dried	Feline Viral Rhinotracheitis Vaccine, Inactivated
Feline Viral Rhinotracheitis Vaccine (Live), Freeze-dried	Feline Viral Rhinotracheitis Vaccine, Living
Foot-and-mouth Disease (Ruminants) Vaccine (Inactivated)	Foot and Mouth Disease (Ruminants) Vaccine Foot and Mouth Disease Vaccine Foot and Mouth Disease Vaccine, Inactivated
Fowl-pox Live Vaccine, Freeze-dried	Fowl Pox Vaccine, Living
Infectious Bovine Rhinotracheitis Vaccine (Live), Freeze-dried	Infectious Bovine Rhinotracheitis Vaccine, Living
Leptospira Vaccine for Veterinary Use	Leptospira Veterinary Vaccine
Marek's Disease Vaccine (Live)	Marek's Disease Vaccine, Living
Neonatal Piglet Colibacillosis Vaccine (Inactivated)	Porcine E. Coli Vaccine, Inactivated Porcine Escherichia Coli Vaccine, Inactivated
Neonatal Ruminant Colibacillosis Vaccine (Inactivated)	Ruminant E. Coli Vaccine, Inactivated Ruminant Escherichia Coli Vaccine, Inactivated
Newcastle Disease Vaccine (Inactivated),	Newcastle Disease Vaccine, Inactivated
Newcastle Disease Vaccine (Live), Freeze-dried	Newcastle Disease Vaccine, Living
Porcine Influenza Vaccine (Inactivated)	Swine Influenza Vaccine, Inactivated
Porcine Parvovirosis Vaccine (Inactivated)	Porcine Parvovirus Vaccine, Inactivated
Rabies Vaccine (Inactivated) for Veterinary Use	Rabies Veterinary Vaccine, Inactivated
Rabies Vaccine (Live, Oral) for Foxes	Rabies Vaccine for Foxes, Living

Swine Erysipelas Vaccine (Inactivated)	Swine Erysipelas Vaccine, Inactivated Erysipelothrix Rhusiopathiae Vaccine, Inactivated
Swine-fever Vaccine (Live), Classical, Freeze-dried	Swine Fever Vaccine, Living
Tetanus Antitoxin for Veterinary Use	Clostridium Tetani Antitoxin Tetanus Antitoxin (Veterinary)
Tetanus Vaccine for Veterinary Use	Clostridium Tetani Vaccines Clostridium Tetani Vaccine for Equidae *(for vaccines with an appropriate potency)* Tetanus Toxoids (Veterinary) *(for vaccines with an appropriate potency)* Tetanus Toxoid for Equidae
Tuberculin Purified Protein Derivative, Avian	Avian Tuberculin Purified Protein Derivative Avian Tuberculin P.P.D.
Tuberculin Purified Protein Derivative, Bovine	Bovine Tuberculin Purified Protein Derivative Bovine Tuberculin P.P.D.

C. Eye Drops

Codes for eye drops in single-dose containers

The following codes are approved for use on single unit doses of eye drops where the individual container may be too small to bear all of the appropriate labelling information (see the general monograph for Eye Drops).

The inclusion of a preparation in this list does not necessarily mean that a monograph is or will be included in the British Pharmacopoeia.

Eye Drops	Code	Eye Drops	Code
Adrenaline/Epinephrine	ADN/EPN	Lachesine	LAC
Apraclonidine	APR	Lidocaine and Fluorescein	LIDFLN
Atropine Sulphate	ATR	Metipranolol	MPR
Betamethasone	BET	Neomycin	NEO
Carbachol	CAR	Oxybuprocaine[1]	BNX
Castor Oil	CASOIL	Phenylephrine	PHNL
Chloramphenicol	CPL	Phenylephrine and Cyclopentolate	PHNCYC
Cocaine	CCN	Pilocarpine	PIL
Cyclopentolate	CYC	Prednisolone	PRED
Diclofenac	DICL	Proxymetacaine	PROX
Fluorescein	FLN	Proxymetacaine and Fluorescein	PROXFLN
Dexamethasone Sodium Phosphate	DSP	Rose Bengal	ROS
Gentamicin	GNT	Sodium Chloride	SALINE[2]
Homatropine	HOM	Sulfacetamide	SULF
Hydrocortisone	HCOR	Tetracaine/Amethocaine	TET/AME
Hydroxyethylcellulose and Sodium Chloride	HECL	Thymoxamine	THY
		Timolol	TIM
Hyoscine	HYO	Tropicamide	TRO
Hypromellose	HPRM	Zinc Sulphate	ZSU

[1]The United States Adopted Name is *benoxinate*

[2]The term 'Saline' indicates that the contents of the container are a 0.9% w/v solution of Sodium Chloride.

Appendix XXII

Names, Symbols and Atomic Weights of Elements

The following atomic weights are those published in 1989 by the International Union of Pure and Applied Chemistry (*Pure App. Chem.* 1991, **63**, 978).

Element*	Symbol	Atomic Weight	Element*	Symbol	Atomic Weight
Aluminium	Al	26.9815	Molybdenum	Mo	95.94
Antimony	Sb	121.757	Neodymium	Nd	144.24
Argon	Ar	39.948	Neon	Ne	20.1797
Arsenic	As	74.9216	Nickel	Ni	58.6934
Barium	Ba	137.327	Niobium	Nb	92.9064
Beryllium	Be	9.0122	Nitrogen	N	14.0067
Bismuth	Bi	208.9804	Osmium	Os	190.2
Boron	B	10.811	Oxygen	O	15.9994
Bromine	Br	79.904	Palladium	Pd	106.42
Cadmium	Cd	112.411	Phosphorus	P	30.9738
Caesium	Cs	132.9054	Platinum	Pt	195.08
Calcium	Ca	40.078	Potassium	K	39.0983
Carbon	C	12.011	Praseodymium	Pr	140.9077
Cerium	Ce	140.115	Rhenium	Re	186.207
Chlorine	Cl	35.4527	Rhodium	Rh	102.9055
Chromium	Cr	51.9961	Rubidium	Rb	85.4678
Cobalt	Co	58.9332	Ruthenium	Ru	101.07
Copper	Cu	63.546	Samarium	Sm	150.36
Dysprosium	Dy	162.50	Scandium	Sc	44.9559
Erbium	Er	167.26	Selenium	Se	78.96
Europium	Eu	151.965	Silicon	Si	28.0855
Fluorine	F	18.9984	Silver	Ag	107.8682
Gadolinium	Gd	157.25	Sodium	Na	22.9898
Gallium	Ga	69.723	Strontium	Sr	87.62
Germanium	Ge	72.61	Sulphur	S	32.066
Gold	Au	196.9665	Tantalum	Ta	180.9479
Hafnium	Hf	178.49	Technetium	Tc	(97)
Helium	He	4.0026	Tellurium	Te	127.60
Holmium	Ho	163.9303	Terbium	Tb	158.9253
Hydrogen	H	1.0079	Thallium	Tl	204.3833
Indium	In	114.82	Thorium	Th	232.0381
Iodine	I	126.9045	Thulium	Tm	168.9342
Iridium	Ir	192.22	Tin	Sn	118.70
Iron	Fe	55.847	Titanium	Ti	47.88
Krypton	Kr	83.80	Tungsten	W	183.85
Lanthanum	La	138.9055	Uranium	U	238.0289
Lead	Pb	207.2	Vanadium	V	50.9415
Lithium	Li	6.941	Xenon	Xe	131.29
Lutetium	Lu	174.967	Ytterbium	Yb	173.04
Magnesium	Mg	24.3050	Yttrium	Y	88.9059
Manganese	Mn	54.9381	Zinc	Zn	65.39
Mercury	Hg	200.59	Zirconium	Zr	91.224

*Elements that lack a characteristic terrestrial isotopic composition have not been included in this table.

Appendix XXIII

Weights and Measures: SI Units

The International System of Units (SI) comprises three categories of units, namely basic units, derived units and supplementary units. The basic units are set out in Table I.

The derived units may be formed by combining the basic units according to certain algebraic relationships between the corresponding quantities. Some of these derived units have special names and symbols which are shown in Table II.

Certain units of the SI have not yet been classified as basic or derived; they are known as supplementary units and are shown in Table III.

Some important and widely used units outside the international system are shown in Table IV.

The prefixes shown in Table V are used to form the names and symbols of the decimal multiples and sub-multiples of SI units.

Further information relating to the use of SI units and their interconversion with CGS metric units can be found in the following publications:

BS 5555:1981 *Specification for SI Units and recommendations for the use of their multiples and of certain other units* (ISO 1000).

SI— International System of Units, 6th edition, HMSO, 1993, ISBN 0 11 887 5388.

TABLE 23-1 Basic Units

Quantity	Name of basic SI Unit	Symbol
Length	metre	m
Mass	kilogram	kg
Time	second	s
Electric current	ampere	A
Thermodynamic temperature	kelvin	K
Amount of substance	mole	mol
Luminous intensity	candela	cd

TABLE 23-2 Derived SI Units used in the *British Pharmacopoeia 1998* and their equivalence with other units

Quantity	Name of derived SI unit	Symbol	Expressions in basic SI units	Equivalence with other units
Absorbed dose of ionising radiation	gray	Gy	$m^2\ s^{-2}$	1 Gy = 1 joule per kg
Energy, work, quantity of heat	joule	J	$kg\ m^2\ s^{-2}$	1 J = 10^7 ergs
Electrical potential, potential	volt	V	$kg\ m^2\ A^{-1}\ s^{-3}$	
Electric resistance	ohm	Ω	$kg\ m^2\ A^{-2}\ s^{-3}$	
Force	newton	N	$kg\ m\ s^{-2}$	1 N = 10^5 dynes
Frequency	hertz	Hz	s^{-1}	1 Hz = 1 cycle per second
Power	watt	W	$kg\ m^2\ s^{-3}$	
Pressure	pascal	Pa	$kg\ m^{-1}\ s^{-2}$	1 kPa = 7.5 mm Hg = 7.5 torr
Radioactivity	becquerel	Bq	s^{-1}	1 Bq = 2.703 x 10^{-11} curies

TABLE 23-3 Supplementary Units

Quantity	Name of derived SI unit	Symbol
Plane angle	radian	rad
Solid angle	steradian	sr

TABLE 23-4 Units used with the International System

Quantity	Unit Name	Unit Symbol	Value in SI units
Time	minute	min	1 min = 60 s
	hour	h	1 h = 60 min = 3600 s
	day	d	1 d = 24 h = 86,400 s
Plane angle	degree	°	1° = (π/180) rad
	minute	'	1' = (1/60)° = (π/10,800)
	second	"	1" = (1/60)' = (π/648,000)
Volume	litre	l	1 l = 1 dm^3 = $10^{-3}\ m^3$
Light	lux	lx	1 lx = 1 lumen m^2
	lumen	lm	1 lm = luminous flux emitted per unit solid angle from a uniform source of 1 candela
Mass	tonne	t	1 t = 10^3 kg

TABLE 23-5 Decimal multiples and sub-multiples

Factor	Prefix	Symbol
10^{18}	exa	E
10^{15}	peta	P
10^{12}	tera	T
10^{9}	giga	G
10^{6}	mega	M
10^{3}	kilo	k
10^{2}	hecto	h
10^{1}	deca	da
10^{-1}	deci	d
10^{-2}	centi	c
10^{-3}	milli	m
10^{-6}	micro	µ
10^{-9}	nano	n
10^{-12}	pico	p
10^{-15}	femto	f
10^{-16}	atto	A

Appendix XXIV

Abbreviations

ATCC	*American Type Culture Collection.
BPCRS	British Pharmacopoeia Chemical Reference Substance (see Appendix I E).
BRP	Biological reference preparation (see Appendix I E).
BS	British Standard.
$CCID_{50}$	Cell culture infective dose (the dose of the micro-organism that infects 50% of the cell cultures inoculated).
CIP	*Collection de Bactéries de l'Institut Pasteur.
CRS	Chemical reference substance (see Appendix I E).
DNA	Deoxyribonucleic Acid.
EID_{50}	Egg embryos infective dose (the dose of the micro-organism that infects 50% of the embryonated eggs inoculated).
EPBRP	European Pharmacopoeia Biological Reference Preparation (see Appendix I E).
EPCRS	European Pharmacopoeia Chemical Reference Substance (see Appendix I E).
HIV	Human immunodeficiency virus
FIP	International Pharmaceutical Federation.
g	Acceleration due to gravity.
ID_{50}	Infective dose 50 (the dose of the micro-organism that infects 50% of the animals inoculated).
IMI	*Commonwealth Mycological Institute.
IP	*Collection Nationale de Cultures de Microorganismes (CNCM)
ISO	International Organization for Standardization.
IU	International Unit
IUPAC	International Union of Pure and Applied Chemistry.
LD_{50}	Lethal dose 50 (the dose of the preparation or organism that kills 50% of the animals inoculated).
MID	Minimum infective dose.
MLD	Minimum lethal dose.
NCIMB	*National Collection of Industrial and Marine Bacteria.
NCPF	*National Collection of Pathogenic Fungi.
NCTC	*National Collection of Type Cultures.
NCYC	*National Collection of Yeast Cultures.
PD_{50}	Protective dose 50 (the dose of the preparation that protects 50% of the animals inoculated).
ppm	Parts per million by weight.
SN_{50}	Serum neutralising dose 50 (the amount of serum that will protect 50% of the cultures against the specified amount of virus).
SSI	Statens Serum Institute (Copenhagen).
VS	Volumetric solution (see Appendix I B).
μkat	Microkatal: the enzyme activity that, under defined conditions, produces 1 micromole of the reaction product per second or consumes one micromole of the reaction substrate per second.

---

*Strains of the micro-organisms referred to in the Pharmacopoeia may be obtained from:

ATCC	American Type Culture Collection, 12301 Parklawn Drive, Rockville, MD 20852, USA.
CIP	Collection de Bactéries de l'Institut Pasteur, BP 52, 25 Rue du Dr-Roux, F-75724, Paris Cedex 15, France.
IMI	Commonwealth Mycological Institute, Ferry Lane, Kew TW9 3AF, England.
IP	Service de la Collection Nationale de Culture de Microorganismes (CNCM), Institut Pasteur, 25 Rue de Dr Roux, F-75724, Paris Cedex 15, France
NCIMB	National Collection of Industrial and Marine Bacteria Ltd, 23, St Machar Drive, Aberdeen , AB2 1RY, Scotland.
NCPF	National Collection of Pathogenic Fungi, London School of Hygiene and Tropical Medicine, Keppel Street, London WC1E 7HT, England.
NCTC	National Collection of Type Cultures, Central Public Health Laboratory, Colindale Avenue, London NW9 5HT, England.
NCYC	National Collection of Yeast Cultures, AFRC Food Research Institute, Colney Lane, Norwich NR4 7UA, England.

Supplementary Chapters

Supplementary Chapters contain no standards, tests or assays nor any other mandatory specifications with respect to any Pharmacopoeial article. They comprise explanatory and other ancillary texts and are provided for the assistance and information of users of the Pharmacopoeia.

Contents of the Supplementary Chapters

SUPPLEMENTARY CHAPTER I
Basis of Pharmacopoeial Requirements A319
- A. Control of Impurities A320
- B. Polymorphism A323
- C. Bacterial Endotoxin Testing A324
- D. Excipients A329
- E. Dissolution Testing of Solid Oral Dosage Forms A329
- F. Declaration of Content A333
- G. Labelling A333
- H. Biological Assays and Tests A334
- J. Efficacy of Antimicrobial Preservation A335
- K. Stereochemistry A335

SUPPLEMENTARY CHAPTER II
Names of Medicinal Substances and Preparations A336

SUPPLEMENTARY CHAPTER III
Pharmacopoeial Organisation
- A. Contact Points A339
- B. Monograph Development: Mechanism A340
- C. Monograph development: Guidance to Manufacturers A341
- D. Monograph development: Methods of Analysis A342
- E. British Pharmacopoeia Chemical Reference Substances (BPCRS) A344

SUPPLEMENTARY CHAPTER IV
European Pharmacopoeia
- A. European Pharmacopoeia Commission and Groups of Experts A345
- B. Dates of Implementation A347
- C. Certification Scheme A347

Supplementary Chapter I

Basis of Pharmacopoeial Requirements

Introduction

This chapter provides explanatory text and guidance on the pharmacopoeial approach to a range of subjects.

Separate, lettered sections of this chapter explain the current approach to a particular aspect of pharmacopoeial control and, where appropriate, give an indication of future developments. The British Pharmacopoeia Commission's policies continue to evolve and these sections will be updated as and when necessary to reflect further developments.

While these texts outline general policies that are adopted in the Pharmacopoeia, each monograph is considered individually. Departures from the general rule are accepted where justified and are accommodated by appropriate statements in the individual monographs.

In providing these texts to users of the Pharmacopoeia it is emphasised that the specifications of the Pharmacopoeia are one facet of the overall control of the quality of medicinal products and their constituents. Those concerned with the manufacture of medicinal substances and those responsible for their incorporation into pharmaceutical dosage forms must also pay due attention to the requirements and recommendations of other competent authorities. Within the European Community the information required for marketing authorization is laid down in the relevant Directives, Notice to Applicants and associated Notes for Guidance available from the Commission of the European Communities as the series 'The Rules Governing Medicinal Products in the European Community'.

Dialogue with users is an essential element of pharmacopoeial development and the British Pharmacopoeia Commission hopes that this chapter will provide insight into certain features of pharmacopoeial requirements. The Commission places great value on the assistance it receives from manufacturers and others with the necessary knowledge to assist it in its work. It welcomes suggestions for improvement of published texts and constructive comment on any issues of interest and concern to users.

General considerations

1. A proper understanding of the basis on which the requirements of the Pharmacopoeia are established is essential to the correct interpretation of the requirements.

2. The Pharmacopoeia contributes significantly to the overall control of the quality of medicinal products and provides a publicly available statement concerning the quality that a product or a component of a product is expected to meet at any time during its period of use. Pharmacopoeial specifications are used within licensing systems and by manufacturers, suppliers, purchasers and those acting on behalf of consumers of medicinal products.

3. A manufacturer must recognise that a product or material may be challenged at any time during its claimed period of use by the methods of the Pharmacopoeia and that it must then comply with the pharmacopoeial requirements. These requirements allow for acceptable levels of change that may occur during storage and distribution and reject articles showing unacceptable levels of change. Frequently a manufacturer will need to apply more stringent test limits at the time of release of a batch of the product or material in order to ensure compliance. As stated in the General Notices, a manufacturer may assure himself that the requirements of the Pharmacopoeia will be met by means other than routinely performing all of the tests prescribed in the Pharmacopoeia. It is emphasised that the circumstances under which, and the frequency with which, tests of the Pharmacopoeia should be performed by a manufacturer as part of his overall quality assurance are ultimately matters for agreement between the manufacturer and the competent authority.

4. The requirements included in a monograph, other than any instructions given under the side-heading Production, are designed to provide the means by which an independent judgement can be made as to the overall quality of a particular article. A manufacturer in possession of detailed knowledge of the manufacturing process may have no need to carry out certain tests. The example of some impurity tests in monographs for formulated preparations is discussed in more detail in section A of this chapter. The methods described in the Pharmacopoeia must be robust because they are intended to be used by analysts in a wide range of laboratories, sometimes on an infrequent basis. Understandably, a manufacturer may wish to use other methods that may be more suitable for frequent use or automation and is entitled to do so. However in the event of any doubt or dispute as to whether or not a material is of pharmacopoeial quality, as the General Notice on Assays and Tests makes clear, the methods of the Pharmacopoeia alone are authoritative.

5. This view of pharmacopoeial requirements is also significant when considering the size of sample to be taken for test. In an overall programme designed to give assurance of quality of a manufactured product, the statistical validity of any sampling programme must be beyond doubt. The standards of the Pharmacopoeia, on the other hand, are intended to apply to the sample available, perhaps the container of dispensed tablets provided to a patient in accordance with a prescription. The Pharmacopoeia requires that twenty of those tablets should meet the test for Uniformity of weight. A manufacturer establishing a sampling and testing protocol designed to ensure ultimate compliance with the pharmacopoeial requirements will need to operate at a level designed to show with an acceptable degree of confidence that any twenty tablets, taken at random from a given batch, will meet the requirements.

6. Pharmacopoeial methods and limits are set with the intention that they should be used as compliance requirements and not as requirements to guarantee total quality assurance. An article is not of pharmacopoeial quality if any sample of the size stipulated in the monograph taken at any time during storage, distribution and use within the accepted shelf-life fails to meet all of the requirements.

7. Arising from this it may be useful to underline that compliance of a product with pharmacopoeial requirements demands that the product meets *all* mandatory aspects of the appropriate monograph and that those requirements shall be interpreted in the light of any relevant General Notices. In certain cases individual requirements of particular tests may seem to be incom-

patible with those of other tests; where this is apparently the case such requirements have been framed intentionally. For example, the requirement for the overall content of active ingredient in a tablet preparation, as determined on a powdered sample of twenty tablets, might be 95.0 to 105.0% of the prescribed or stated amount. Thus an assay result of 96.0% would indicate compliance. For the Uniformity of content test a further ten tablets might be individually examined, each tablet being required to contain between 85 and 115% of the mean value, with the possibility of a single exception between 75 and 125%. Thus if nine out of ten tablets fall within the range (assuming the mean to be 96.0%) 81.6 and 110.4% and the tenth falls within the range 72.0 to 120.0% then the tablets examined comply with that requirement. For the Dissolution test each tablet examined might be required to yield at least 70% of the labelled claim into solution within 45 minutes. It has been suggested that since a single outlier tablet might contain as little as 72.0% of the labelled claim and yet still fall within the acceptance limits for content, the requirements for dissolution should be relaxed to take this into account. In framing requirements, however, the view is taken that it is neither realistic nor profitable to attempt to compound the results of various tests in this way. Each test in a Pharmacopoeial monograph and the acceptance limit is therefore framed as an individual entity with requirements based on values encountered in practice; compliance with the monograph requires compliance with each and every test.

8. The philosophy outlined above has an important bearing on the construction of a monograph for the Pharmacopoeia. To achieve maximum benefit from the examination of a product the recommended approach is that, wherever possible, a variety of different analytical techniques should be employed. The monographs of the British Pharmacopoeia are, therefore, usually constructed to use fundamentally different procedures for assay and for the examination for impurities. For a medicinal substance the general approach has been to employ spectrophotometric or other appropriate techniques for identification, spectrophotometric techniques for the control of impurities and a precise, albeit non-specific method for assay. It has been held that this approach confers greater confidence in the verification of the identity and quality of the substance and in the detection of unexpected impurities than would be the case in using, for example, a single stability-indicating liquid chromatographic method for all three purposes. The British Pharmacopoeia Commission recognises, however, that as chromatographic methods become more precise it will become increasingly possible to use them for assay purposes thereby combining precision with specificity and economising upon analytical effort and time. For dosage forms this concept has already been adopted and more specific assay methods, such as those employing liquid chromatography, are being employed increasingly.

9. A discussion of the basis of pharmacopoeial requirements would be incomplete without reminding users that any article described by a name at the head of a monograph in the current edition of the Pharmacopoeia, *whether or not it is referred to as 'BP'*, must comply with that monograph. The name at the head of a monograph is to be interpreted in accordance with the General Notice on Titles. In particular, a formulated preparation that is labelled with a title that includes the full nonproprietary name of the active ingredient, where this is not included in the title of the monograph, must also comply with the monograph. Thus, for example, a preparation labelled Labetalol Hydrochloride Tablets must comply with the monograph for Labetalol Tablets.

A. Control of Impurities

This section provides a guide to the pharmacopoeial approach to the control of impurities in medicinal substances and formulated preparations.

1. This section relates primarily to totally synthetic organic medicinal substances and those substances obtained by synthetic modification of a naturally-produced precursor. It is not necessarily applicable to other organic substances (*eg*, those of plant or animal origin), inorganic substances and excipients.

Certain additional information of specific relevance to impurity control in the formulated preparation monographs of the British Pharmacopoeia is also provided.

2.The control provided by chemical tests limiting the levels of particular impurities or classes of impurities is often augmented by physical tests such as absorbance, specific optical rotation, melting point and clarity and colour of solution and, for a liquid, refractive index, boiling point range and weight per ml.

3. Tests such as sulphated ash, heavy metals and loss on drying are non-specific but they contribute to an assurance of the general quality of the material, the use of good pharmaceutical manufacturing practice in its production, the avoidance of contamination especially by inorganic substances and the removal of volatile solvents. Typical limits are 0.1% for sulphated ash, 10 or 20 ppm for heavy metals and 0.5% for loss on drying.

4.Tests for purity are intended to provide appropriate limitation of known potential or actual impurities rather than to provide against all possible impurities. The tests are not necessarily designed to detect any adventitious contaminants or adulteration. Material found to contain an impurity not detectable by means of the prescribed tests is not of pharmacopoeial quality if the nature or amount of the impurity found is incompatible with good pharmaceutical practice.

5. Some medicinal substances are mixtures of closely related compounds. Where these components have similar activity they are not usually regarded as impurities and may indeed contribute to the result obtained in the assay. Examples include Erythromycin, Gentamicin Sulphate and Sodium Lauryl Sulphate. It may however be appropriate to control the relative amounts of such components, *eg*, gentamicins C_1, C_{1a}, C_2 and C_{2a} in Gentamicin Sulphate in order to ensure batch to batch consistency for material from one manufacturer and uniformity between supplies of the same substance from different manufacturers.

6. Many medicinal substances already on the market have been made available as racemic mixtures with little or nothing known about the biological activities of the separate isomers. This has been reflected in the monograph in the Pharmacopoeia and a test to show that the substance is the racemic mixture has not usually been included unless it was known that at least one of the separate enantiomers was also available commercially.

Nevertheless, with increasing concern by regulatory authorities for substances to be made available as single isomers, tests for enantiomeric composition will become more common. When a medicinal substance is a racemate, an indication is given by means of the graphic formula [see also Supplementary Chapter I K; Stereochemistry].

Related Substances

7. It is usual to include a test for related substances in a monograph for a medicinal substance. These may be manufacturing impurities (intermediates or by-products) or degradation products or both. When preparation of a monograph is initiated the manufacturer is asked to provide information concerning the nature of such impurities, the reason for their presence, the amounts that may be encountered in material prepared under conditions of good pharmaceutical manufacturing practice and the manner in which proportions may vary on storage, together with an indication of the toxicity of any impurities in relation to that of the substance itself. Where there is only one manufacturer of a substance, pharmacopoeial limits are set in the knowledge that the level of impurities in production batches of the substance will have been accepted by the registration authority after a full consideration of the toxicity studies and clinical trials carried out before the granting of a licence. Such studies and trials will have been carried out on material with an impurity profile that is qualitatively and quantitatively similar to that of subsequent production batches. Any subsequent changes to the manufacturing process by the original manufacturer or the introduction of material from another manufacturer utilising a different route of synthesis will be subject to the need to demonstrate essential similarity or to provide equivalent data to the relevant registration authority. In some cases a change in production or source may give rise to impurities that are not adequately controlled by the published pharmacopoeial monograph. Appropriate revision of the monograph will be carried out provided that the pharmacopoeial authority is notified of the need and that it is supplied with the relevant information [see paragraph below].

8. Tests for related substances may be specific or general.

9. **Specific tests for named impurities** A specific test is included where a particular impurity arising from the manufacturing process or from degradation needs to be limited on grounds of toxicity or for another special reason. Where an impurity is known to be particularly toxic, this is taken into account in setting the limit; for example a limit of 0.5% is specified for 4-epianhydrotetracycline in the monograph for Tetracycline and a limit of 1 ppm is specified for hydrazine in the monograph for Povidone.

9.1 Such specific tests usually employ a chromatographic or colorimetric comparison with a sample of the named substance, for example, 4-chloroaniline in Chlorhexidine Acetate and 4-aminophenol in Paracetamol.

9.2 Where a specimen of the impurity is required in the test, this will be made available as a Chemical Reference Substance unless it is known that specimens of the requisite quality can readily be obtained through the usual suppliers of chemical reagents.

9.3 Specific control may be included within a more general test controlling other impurities; an example is 4-epianhydrotetracycline in the monograph for Tetracycline.

9.4 In other cases, an absolute method is more appropriate. Such a test may be for a group of potentially toxic impurities, *eg*, polycyclic aromatic hydrocarbons in Liquid Paraffin.

9.5 Sometimes an impurity may be named in the Pharmacopoeia because it is necessary to use a named substance in its control for analytical reasons, such as different response factors in the specified test method. Examples are iminodibenzyl in Imipramine Hydrochloride, hypoxanthine in Mercaptopurine and dibenzosuberone in Amitriptyline Hydrochloride. Typical wording is as follows:

> *Any spot corresponding to [x] in the chromatogram obtained with solution (1) is not more intense than the principal spot in the chromatogram obtained with solution (2). [Solution (1) contains the substance being examined and solution (2) contains a named impurity [x].]*

10. **General tests for unnamed impurities** It is unusual for the Pharmacopoeia to require the absence of a visible spot in a thin-layer chromatogram or the absence of a peak in a liquid chromatogram. Reasons for this include the difficulty of interpreting and defining absence that is a consequence of variations in the sensitivity of a method when performed in different laboratories by different analysts. It is more usual to limit the levels of impurities. This may be done in a simple test by comparison with a spot or peak obtained with a dilute solution of the substance being examined. An example is Amethocaine Hydrochloride:

> *Any secondary spot in the chromatogram obtained with solution (1) is not more intense than the spot in the chromatogram obtained with solution (2). [Solutions (1) and (2) contain the substance being examined at high and low concentrations respectively.]*

10.1 In the absence of evidence that the limit for a particular impurity needs to be set on the basis of its toxicity, control is often provided by a two-level test requiring, say, not more than one related substance at a nominal concentration of up to 0.5% and any others at nominal concentrations of up to 0.1%. The actual limits may be chosen on the basis of batch data for material manufactured in accordance with good pharmaceutical manufacturing practice and will take account of a number of factors, including the dose regimen of the substance and the number of impurities commonly present. An example is Oxetacaine:

> *Any secondary spot in the chromatogram obtained with solution (1) is not more intense than the spot in the chromatogram obtained with solution (2) (0.5%) and not more than one such spot is more intense than the spot in the chromatogram obtained with solution (3) (0.1%).*

Another example, with different limits, is Chlorambucil:

> *Any secondary spot in the chromatogram obtained with solution (1) is not more intense than the spot in the chromatogram obtained with solution (2) (2%) and not more than one such spot is more intense than the spot in the chromatogram obtained with solution (3) (0.5%).*

10.2 Where it is known that several impurities are likely to be present at significant concentrations, a three-level test may be appropriate. An example is Pentazocine:

In the chromatogram obtained with solution (1) any secondary spot is not more intense than the spot in the chromatogram obtained with solution (2) (1%), not more than one such spot is more intense than the spot in the chromatogram obtained with solution (3) (0.5%) and not more than four such spots are more intense than the spot in the chromatogram obtained with solution (4) (0.25%).

10.3 General tests with an 'open' design such as those described above have the great advantage that they provide a means of limiting the levels of related substances that may arise from modified or alternative synthetic routes not in use at the time the test was elaborated. In this context, thin-layer chromatography has the advantage over liquid chromatography and gas chromatography that it allows detection of impurities completely retained or those not retained at all by the stationary phase.

11. **Total impurity limits** In gas chromatographic and liquid chromatographic tests, it is increasingly common to limit the total areas of peaks due to related substances. In monographs currently in force the limit for the sum is commonly in the range 1 to 2% but these values are applicable at the end of the shelf-life. This procedure is rarely adopted in thin-layer chromatographic tests, because of the semi-quantitative nature of estimating individual spots and resulting imprecision in expression of results for the totals. This apparent drawback to the use of thin-layer chromatography is largely overcome by means of two- and three-level tests as described in paragraphs 10.1 and 10.2, above.

12. In response to requests from users of the Pharmacopoeia statements of the approximate real or nominal levels of impurities controlled by tests for impurities are being introduced, where appropriate, for information [see paragraphs 14 and 15 below].Conformity with the requirements will still be determined on the basis of compliance or otherwise with the stated test.

Test design and expression of limits

13. For **known impurities**, several aspects are taken into account in designing the test. These include the nature of the impurity, its toxicity and the levels likely to be found in routine production. Analytical considerations such as the response factor (defined in paragraph 16) for the impurity and practical issues such as availability of the impurity as a reference material or reagent also influence the test design.

14. If a major and/or toxic impurity in a material is known to have a significantly different response (more than ±20%) from that of the substance being examined in the conditions of the test, the preferred manner of limiting this impurity is to use a reference substance of the impurity. If this is not possible, a reference solution of the substance being examined containing a known amount of the impurity may be used. Using either of these approaches, the concentration limit indicated in the monograph for information in parentheses expresses the approximate limit as a real percentage of the impurity in question. When neither of these approaches is possible, a dilution of the solution of the substance being examined may be used as a reference solution. This approach is also commonly used in tests where an impurity that is known (but not named within the test) has a response within ±20% of that of the substance being examined.

15. Unless explicitly stated otherwise, an indication of the approximate concentration limit provided in *any* test where a dilution of the substance being examined is used as the reference solution should be interpreted as an expression in terms of a nominal percentage of the substance being examined (in accordance with the General Notices) rather than as a real percentage of the impurity.

16. No reference is made in a test to a **response factor** for a named impurity unless unavoidable. When used, the term is defined as follows:

The response factor (k) is a relative term, being the response of equal weights of one substance relative to that of another in the conditions described in the test.

In the context of a Related substances test where a response factor is quoted for an impurity, unless otherwise stated, this is the expected response for that impurity in relation to a response of unity for the substance being examined. The way in which a response factor is to be used in any subsequent calculation is stated in the monograph.

17. Response factors of less than 0.2 or more than 5 are not used. If the difference between the response of an impurity and that of the substance being examined is outside these limits, a different method of determination, such as a different detection wavelength (*l) or a different method of visualisation, is used.

18. For a response factor quoted in a pharmacopoeial test, the following points are observed:

(a) the peak to which the factor applies is identified unambiguously, recognising the difficulties associated with such identification in chromatograms showing peaks of similar retention times (see paragraph 8) [the use of a sample containing an unquantified amount of the relevant impurity can sometimes be used to assist such identification],

(b) the response factor quoted is a confirmed value and preferably is based on relative peak areas of equal weights of the impurity and the sample under the conditions of the test [alternatively an absolute figure based on the A(1%, 1 cm) for the detection wavelength used (or similar for other methods of detection) of the impurity and the sample may be used],

(c) the response factor is stated in a way that does not imply an unrealistic or misleading degree of precision [declaration to several significant figures is not meaningful when placed in context of the nature of the test and the amount of the impurity likely to be present (typically, less than 0.5%); factors quoted to 1 significant figure (*eg*, 1.4, 2.5, 3, 0.5) or 1 decimal place (*eg*, 1.4, 7.5) are generally appropriate],

(d) the formula for the calculation is included within the test [the correction factor to be applied in such calculations is the reciprocal of the response factor (defined in paragraph 5) (1/k)].

19. Identification of peaks is not based on absolute retention times since these may be too 'system dependent'; however, advice such as 'the principal peak

has a retention time of about *x* minutes' may be given. In some cases, for example, where a simple chromatogram is expected to show a limited number of impurities, an expected *relative* retention time may be given to designate impurities. In other cases where potential impurities have similar retention times, a sample containing the components of interest and a sample chromatogram may be provided.

20. **Unknown impurities** may be limited by reference to a dilution of the solution of the substance being examined used as a reference solution together with an open design of statement limiting 'any' or 'any other' *secondary peak* or *spot*. Such a reference solution may be used in addition to those containing named impurities (any other secondary peak/spot) or, in some simple tests, control of unknown and known (but unnamed) impurities may be exerted by means of a comparison between the sample solution and a dilution of this solution (any secondary peak/spot).

21. An indication of the approximate limit concentration for an unknown impurity would only be given in terms of a nominal percentage of the substance being examined (see paragraph 16) since no assumption can be made about the response of an unknown impurity. While such nominal limits are not quantitatively fully transparent and caution is needed in attempting to use them to set a total impurity limit, their use is less misleading than quoting an arbitrary/assumed response factor of 1 for an unknown impurity.

Formulated Preparations

22. Many monographs for formulated preparations in the British Pharmacopoeia also include tests for impurities. In general, wherever possible a test for impurities based on that in the monograph for the active ingredient is included with any necessary modification.

23. Wider limits and/ or additional controls may be required for impurities arising on manufacture or storage of the dosage form.

24. Tests for impurities in monographs for formulated preparation are used to control not only degradation products but also by-products of the synthetic route used for manufacture of the active ingredient. It has been argued that by-products of synthesis have been controlled already during examination of the substance before formulation and that further testing for these impurities is unnecessary. Clearly it would be repetitious and wasteful of resources for tests, often complex in nature, to be repeated simply to demonstrate acceptably low levels of impurities that could arise only during synthesis (as opposed to degradation) of the active ingredient. However, this information is available only to those who know the detailed attributes of the active raw material that has been used. For an analyst who has access only to the dosage form, the profile of synthesis-related impurities offers one means of establishing whether or not the dosage form has been prepared from an active ingredient of pharmacopoeial quality. It is for this reason that such tests are included in British Pharmacopoeia monographs for formulated preparations.

Current and future developments

25. **Transparency** Following requests by a number of users of the Pharmacopoeia, a statement giving the identities of impurities that are known to be limited by the specifications is being added to appropriate monographs for medicinal substances and formulated preparations. For example the monograph for Azelastine Hydrochloride contains the following information at the end of the monograph:

IMPURITIES 4-chlorobenzylphthalazinone,
1-methyl-4-(2-benzoylhydrazino)azepan,
1-methlyazepan-4-one.

This increase in the transparency of pharmacopoeial specifications is of assistance to licensing authorities and others when considering whether the standards in the monograph are appropriate to a new source of supply. It is emphasised that other, unnamed impurities may also be limited. The Commission is actively seeking information that will allow the statements to be extended in future.

26. **Systems suitability** In chromatographic tests increasing use is being made of system suitability tests to enable the analyst to confirm that performance of the chosen column or plate is satisfactory under the chosen conditions. In liquid chromatographic and gas chromatographic tests, peak separation between impurities and the substance being examined is generally considered to offer the best indication of performance of the system.

27. **Residual solvents** A general test for residual solvents has been included in the European Pharmacopoeia (Appendix VIII L). Its sphere of application is currently under consideration. At present, a test for solvent residues is included only where variation in levels of known solvents requires control, eg, methanol in Gentamicin Sulphate.

28. The Commission welcomes suggestions for improving the monographs. In particular, where it is found that significant impurities are not controlled by the monograph, the Commission would be glad to receive details of validated methods that can be considered for adoption.

B. Polymorphism

1. Polymorphism (the occurrence of more than one morphic form) is a function of the internal structure of crystalline solids. Its occurrence cannot be predicted and, as it can be induced in many materials in appropriate conditions, its absence is difficult to demonstrate using a single, specific test. Different polymorphs may exhibit different physicochemical properties such as melting point, dissolution rate and infrared absorption spectrum. In some cases these may affect the handling characteristics of the material, the stability of formulated preparations and bioavailability. Control of morphic form by a manufacturer is necessary during processing of active ingredients and excipients and during production of a formulated product to ensure the correct physical characteristics of the product. Its main importance to the control of medicinal products is in the areas of bioavailability and stability.

2. The morphic form of a readily soluble starting material that is incorporated into a solution, for example, an injection, an oral solution or eye drops, is not usually important. (An exception to this statement might be if the concentration of the solution is such that it is close to the limit of solubility of one of the possible polymorphs.) The morphic form may be important when the material is included in a solid dosage form or as a suspension in a liquid dosage form when the characteristics of the different polymorphs are such as to affect the bioavailability of the material.

3. For most pharmaceutical and medicinal substances it will not usually be appropriate or necessary for the monograph to control the morphic form. In the British Pharmacopoeia the subject usually has not been addressed directly, although the monographs for Spironolactone and Cimetidine, for example, state under Characteristics that the substance exhibits polymorphism. The existence of polymorphism in some cases can be deduced from the tests of the monograph. There are currently around 50 instances of infrared identification tests in pharmaceutical and medicinal substances where the analyst is instructed to prepare a solution spectrum or recrystallise the sample if the spectrum obtained is not concordant with the reference spectrum or spectrum of a reference substance, for example, Prednisolone Sodium Phosphate. This procedure recognises but does not limit polymorphism. In some cases where polymorphism is recognised no deviation from the spectrum/form of the reference substance prescribed is permitted, for example, Tamoxifen Citrate. This effectively restricts the substance to a single polymorph. In some cases the morphic form is controlled by a melting point range. An example is Carbamazepine where the range permitted excludes the polymorph of lower melting point.

4. In future the British Pharmacopoeia will include a specific statement that the material exhibits polymorphism, where it is known that this readily occurs under normal laboratory and manufacturing conditions. In the rare cases where it is considered necessary, there will be a specific statement that the pharmacopoeial material is limited to one polymorph. This approach will provide for amendment of the monograph if it becomes apparent that the material is unjustifiably restricted to one polymorph.

5. Polymorphism is a potential problem in solid dosage forms, such as tablets, or in liquid or semi-solid preparations where the active ingredient is present as a solid, for example, in oral suspensions. In most cases it is difficult to demonstrate that the material contains the desired polymorph as the process of extracting a sufficient sample of the material in question for analysis may itself change the form of the material. For a solid dosage form where the active ingredient is known to exist in forms with significant differences in solubility, a dissolution test may be the method of choice. The side heading 'Production' will be used to draw attention to control of morphic form in future editions the British Pharmacopoeia as attention is drawn to cases where control of morphic form is known to be important.

6. The General Monographs of the European Pharmacopoeia are applicable to all dosage forms of the type described. The European Pharmacopoeia Commission has been asked to consider amending the general monographs for solid dosage forms, or those where the active ingredient may be a solid, to state that where the active ingredient is known to exist in more than one morphic form and the choice of polymorph is critical with regard to bioavailability and/or stability, the method of manufacture should ensure the presence of the correct amount of the desired polymorph in the preparation. Such Production statements might also include reference to the need during product development to examine drug sensitivity to polymorphic change due to granulation conditions or compressional forces and to make appropriate processing adjustments to control potential variation.

7. The Commission would find it helpful to be advised of instances where control of morphic form is important so that a suitable Production statement may be added. In such cases it would also appreciate receiving details of any validated test methods that will appropriately limit the undesirable form.

C. Bacterial Endotoxin Testing

This section provides an exposition of the Commission's policy and information on its implementation. The guidelines of the European Pharmacopoeia are included as an Annex.

The test for bacterial endotoxins of the European Pharmacopoeia (Ph Eur) is included as Appendix XIV C of the British Pharmacopoeia 1998.

1. This *in vitro* test is being progressively applied in appropriate monographs of both the British and European Pharmacopoeia in place of the *in vivo* test for pyrogens.

2. Methods for the detection of Gram-negative bacterial endotoxins are based on the use of a lysate of amoebocytes from the horseshoe crab, *Limulus polyphemus*. Addition of endotoxin to this lysate may result in gelation, precipitation or turbidity. The method used in the monographs of the European and British Pharmacopoeias is, unless otherwise stated, that using a gelation end-point.

3. A European Pharmacopoeia Biological Reference Preparation (BRP) of Endotoxin calibrated in International Units (IU) has been established for use in this test. The current BRP (batch 3) was established following an international collaborative study. It consists of endotoxin from the same bulk as the Second International Standard established by the World Health Organization and the current standard established by the Food and Drug Administration and the United States Pharmacopeia for use in the United States of America (EC6). Following adoption of the recommendations in the report of the collaborative study[1] global harmonisation of endotoxin unitage has been achieved, that is, the FDA/USP Endoxin Unit (EU) is equivalent to the International Unit (IU).

General policy

4. In any individual monograph only one test is required, either that for pyrogens or that for bacterial endotoxins.

5. In the absence of evidence to the contrary, the test for bacterial endotoxins is preferred, since it is considered usually to provide equal or better protection to the patient.

6. Before including a test for bacterial endotoxins in a monograph, evidence is required that a test, as described in Appendix XIV C, can be applied satisfactorily to the item in question.

7. The necessary information is sought from manufacturers. Companies are invited to provide any validation data that they have concerning the applicability of the test for bacterial endotoxins to the substances and formulations of interest.

Poole, S., Dawson, P., Gaines Das, R.E. (1997). Second international standard for endotoxin: calibration in an international collaborative study. *Journal of Endotoxin Research 4 (3), 221-231.*

7.1 Such data should include details of sample preparation and of any procedures necessary to eliminate interfering factors.7.2 In addition, any available parallel data for rabbit pyrogen testing that would contribute to an assurance that the replacement of a rabbit pyrogen test by the test for bacterial endotoxin is appropriate, should be provided.

7.3 For formulated preparations, a distinction should be made between any sample treatment necessitated by excipients included in a particular product and any required due to the nature of the active constituent. Attention should also be drawn to any manipulation normally required for the active constituent that is rendered redundant by the composition of the formulation for example, pH adjustment.

8. In order to set an appropriate limit for bacterial endotoxins it is necessary to know the intended route of parenteral administration (in particular, if the substance may be administered intrathecally) together with the maximum dose as recommended in relevant product data sheets. The limit for a given material or preparation is expressed as the endotoxin limit concentration (ELC). The ELC may be expressed in IU of endotoxin per millilitre *for a defined solution* of the material or preparation, or, for some medicinal substances, in IU of endotoxin in relation to a defined quantity of the material (that is, per milligram or, for biologically assayed materials, per IU) of material. The limit, which is stated in the monograph, is usually established on the following basis:

$$ELC = K/M$$

8.1 *K*, sometimes referred to as the minimum pyrogenic dose, is the maximum number of IU of endotoxin which the patient may receive without suffering toxic reactions. The appropriate value for *K* will be taken from the table below.

8.2 *M* is the maximum dose of the drug substance per person (or per kg) per hour. This is interpreted as the maximum amount that might be administered within one hour. For subcutaneous (SC), intramuscular (IM) or bolus intravenous (IV) injections this will be an entire single dose. For intravenous infusions given over a prolonged period it is the proportion of the dose that would be infused during one hour and depends upon the rate of infusion. The value used is the maximum dose recommended by the manufacturer and stated in the relevant product data sheet. It is accepted that in exceptional circumstances this dose may be exceeded at the discretion of the physician; such use is outside the scope of the Pharmacopoeia.

Implementation

9. The British Pharmacopoeia Commission is seeking to replace the test for pyrogens by that for bacterial endotoxins wherever possible in the Pharmacopoeia. The European Pharmacopoeia Commission has a similar policy and has indicated that, for monographs already published, the change will be carried out, where appropriate, whenever the monograph in question is revised.

9.1 The test for bacterial endotoxins is now specified in the European Pharmacopoeia monograph for Water for Injections and in many other monographs including a range of antibiotics (for example, Doxorubicin Hydrochloride and Oxytetracycline Hydrochloride), biological materials (for example, Somatropin and Heparin) and radiopharmaceutical preparations.

9.2 Revision of the European Pharmacopoeia monograph for Parenteral Preparations to permit the use of the test for bacterial endotoxins in defined circumstances opened the way for the test for pyrogens to be replaced by that for bacterial endotoxins in individual monographs for parenteral preparations in the British Pharmacopoeia. The necessary change has already been made in a wide range of monographs including those for certain biological formulations such as Calcitonin (Pork) Injection and in the monographs for a number of widely used intravenous infusions such as Sodium Chloride Intravenous Infusion. Appropriate data are being sought from manufacturers for the remaining monographs for which a test for pyrogens is specified.

ANNEX

Guidelines concerning the test for Bacterial endotoxins have been published as an Annex to the method text 2.6.14 in the European Pharmacopoeia and are reproduced here.

The following section is given for information and guidance, it does not form a mandatory part of the Pharmacopoeia.

1. Introduction

Endotoxins stemming from Gram-negative microorganisms are the most common cause of the toxic reactions attributed to contamination of pharmaceutical products with pyrogens; their pyrogenic activity is much higher than that of most other pyrogenic substances. These endotoxins are lipopolysaccharides. Although there are a small number of pyrogens which possess a different structure, the conclusion is generally justified that absence

Type of product	Route of administration	K per person	K per kg
All parenteral preparations	Intrathecal[1]	14	0.2
Radiopharmaceuticals	Intravenous	175	2.5
All parenteral preparations except radiopharmaceuticals	All parenteral routes except intrathecal	350	5.0

[1]Where a product can be administered both intrathecally and by another parenteral route, the more stringent value of *K* for the intrathecal route will be taken as the basis of establishing the ELC.

of bacterial endotoxins in a product implies absence of pyrogenic components, provided the presence of non-endotoxin pyrogenic substances can be ruled out.

The presence of endotoxins in a product may be masked by factors interfering with the reaction between the endotoxins and the amoebocyte lysate. Hence the analyst who wishes to replace the rabbit pyrogen test required in a pharmacopoeial monograph by a test for bacterial endotoxins has to demonstrate that a valid test can be carried out on the product concerned; this may entail a procedure for removing interfering factors.

As indicated in the test for bacterial endotoxins, information must be available on the following aspects before a test on a sample can be regarded as valid.

1.1. The suitability of the material to be used for the test has to be established. The absence of endotoxins in the LAL water and in the other reagents must be assured and the sensitivity of the amoebocyte lysate must be checked to confirm the sensitivity declared by the manufacturer.

1.2. As the product to be examined may interfere with the test, the sensitivity of the amoebocyte lysate is determined in the presence and in the absence of the product under examination. There should be no significant difference between the two sensitivity values.

The test for bacterial endotoxins indicates methods for removing the interference (see under Gelation methods); in the case of interference another test must be carried out after such a method has been applied to check whether the interference has indeed been neutralised or removed.

When the product under examination appears to fail the test (positive result) a repeat test is permitted. Apparent failure of the product to meet the requirements may be due to faults in the preparation or dilution or to another adventitious contamination by the analyst.

This section explains the reasons for the requirements in the test for bacterial endotoxins, and then deals with the reading and interpretation of the results.

Substitution of the rabbit pyrogen test required in a pharmacopoeial monograph by an amoebocyte lysate test constitutes the use of an alternative method of analysis and hence requires validation; some guidance on how to proceed is given in this section.

The reference method for bacterial endotoxins is stated in the monograph on a given product; where no method is stated, method A is the reference method. If a method other than the reference method is to be used, the analyst must demonstrate that the method is appropriate for this product and gives a result consistent with that obtained with the reference method (see also paragraph 11).

Although the test for bacterial endotoxins specifies the species *Limulus polyphemus* as the source of the lysate, an active lysate may also be obtained from closely related species, such as those belonging to the genus *Tachypleus*. The term 'amoebocyte lysate' is used in this text to indicate a validated amoebocyte lysate irrespective of its biological origin.

2. Method

The addition of endotoxins to amoebocyte lysate may result in turbidity, precipitation or gelation; only gelation was used as an endpoint in the first type of test for bacterial endotoxins. The advantage was the simplicity of basing the decision to pass or fail the product under examination on the absence or presence of gelation, visible with the naked eye. The quantitative methods described as methods C, D, E were developed later: they require more instrumentation, but they are easier to automate for the regular testing of large numbers of samples of the same product.

Endotoxins may be adsorbed onto the surface of tubes or pipettes made from certain plastics or types of glass. Interference may appear due to the release of substances from plastic materials. Hence the materials used should be checked; subsequent batches of tubes or pipettes may have a slightly different composition, and hence the analyst is advised to repeat such tests on starting with new batches of materials.

Whereas the result of the rabbit pyrogen test depends on the *dose* of pyrogen, the result of the test for bacterial endotoxins depends on the *concentration* of endotoxin in the reaction mixture. The decision to use the test for bacterial endotoxins as a limit test implies first of all that a threshold endotoxin concentration must be defined for the products to be tested and secondly, that the analyst performing the test needs to know whether the endotoxin concentration in the product under examination is below or above this threshold. The quantitative methods C, D, E make it possible to determine the endotoxin concentration in the sample under examination, but in routine quality control the final question is whether this concentration does or does not exceed a defined limit.

In setting a threshold concentration of endotoxin for the product to be tested, due attention should be paid to the human dose of the product: the aim should be to ensure that as long as the endotoxin concentration in the product remains below this threshold even the maximal dose administered by the intended route per hour does not contain sufficient endotoxin to cause a toxic reaction.

When the endotoxin concentration in the product exactly equals the threshold value, gelation will occur, as is the case when the endotoxin concentration is much higher, and the product will fail the test, because the all-or-none character of the test makes it impossible to differentiate between a concentration exactly equal to the threshold concentration and one that is higher. It is only when no gelation occurs that the analyst may conclude that the endotoxin concentration does not exceed the threshold concentration.

For products in the solid state, this threshold concentration of endotoxin per mass unit or per International Unit of product has to be translated into a concentration of endotoxin per millilitre of solution to be tested, as the test can be carried out only on a solution. The case of products that already exist in the liquid state (such as infusion fluids) is discussed below.

Determination of the threshold concentration of endotoxin in International Units of endotoxin per unit of product (mass unit or International Unit) requires the definition of:

M = the maximum adult dose of the product in units of mass (or International Units) per kilogram body mass per hour when given by the intended route of administration. When the maximum dose is stated for an adult, 70 kg should be used as the mass of an adult person. The paediatric dose per kilogram body mass per hour should be used when this is higher than the corresponding maximum dose for an adult.

K = the maximum dose of endotoxin in International Units of endotoxin per kilogram body mass per hour that a patient may receive by the intended route without any untoward effect (see Table below).

Suppose a solution containing c mg (or International Units) of the product per millilitre is available for the test. Then a volume of M/c ml is the volume containing the maximum dose M. When this volume contains K International Units of endotoxin, it should give a positive test.

Hence the Endotoxin Limit Concentration (ELC) in International Units of endotoxin per millilitre which is equivalent with the threshold concentration of endotoxin per milligram or per International Unit of product in the solid state is equal to:

$$ELC = (K \times c)/M$$

where K = maximum acceptable dose of endotoxin in International Units per kilogram per hour,

c = concentration of the solution in milligrams or International Units of product per millilitre,

M = maximum dose in milligrams or International Units of product per kilogram per hour.

For products that already exist in the liquid state, the maximum adult dose per kilogram body mass per hour is expressed in millilitres. The above expression for the endotoxin limit concentration is also applicable to these products, provided the value for the maximum dose in millilitres per kilogram body mass per hour is substituted for M and c is given the value of one.

The threshold concentration of endotoxin was defined in the past as the 'Maximum Allowable Endotoxin Concentration' or MAEC. However, in practice a product containing exactly this MAEC of endotoxin would fail the test, just as a product containing more endotoxin. The only way of assuring that the MAEC is not exceeded in the product consists of demonstrating that the endotoxin concentration in the product is less than the MAEC; hence it is more logical to use the term 'endotoxin limit concentration' (or ELC) as the concentration of endotoxin that must not be attained.

The Endotoxin Limit Concentration depends on the product and its use and is stated in the individual monographs which are to be consulted. Values for K are suggested in the following Table.

Intended route of administration	K in IU of endotoxin per kg of body mass per hour
Intravenous	5.0
Intravenous, for radiopharmaceuticals	2.5
Intrathecal	0.2

The value of the ELC in the eluate of disposable or implantable medical devices depends not only on the values of K and M but also on the preparation of the eluate. The specific monograph is to be consulted for the relevant information.

Which dilution of the product should be used in the test to obtain maximal assurance that a negative test means that the endotoxin concentration of the product is less than the ELC and that a positive test means that the lysate detected at least the ELC? This dilution depends on the ELC and on the sensitivity of the lysate: it is called the Maximum Valid Dilution (MVD) and its value may be calculated as follows:

$$MVD = ELC/\lambda = (K \times c)/(M \times \lambda)$$

where λ = the stated sensitivity of the lysate in International Units of endotoxin per millilitre.

When the value of the maximum valid dilution is not a whole number, a convenient whole number smaller than the MVD may be used for routine purposes (which means diluting the solution of the product less than the MVD indicates). In this case a negative test indicates that the endotoxin concentration of the product lies below the limit value. However, when the endotoxin concentration of the product in such a test is less than the ELC but high enough to make the reaction with the lysate result in a clot, the test may be positive under these conditions. Hence, when a test with this 'convenient' dilution factor is positive, the product should be diluted to the MVD and the test should be repeated. In any case of doubt or dispute the MVD must be used.

This stresses the importance of the confirmation of the sensitivity of the lysate.

Example

A solution of phenytoin sodium containing 50 mg/ml (intended for intravenous injection) has to be tested. Determine the MVD, given the following variables:

M = maximum human dose

= 15 mg per kilogram body mass per hour.

c = 50 mg/ml.

K = 5 I.U. of endotoxin per kilogram per hour.

λ = 0.4 I.U. of endotoxin per millilitre.

Solution:

$$ELC = (K \times c)/M = (5 \times 50)/15$$

$$\text{MVD} = ELC/\lambda = (5 \times 50)/15 \times (1/0.4) = 41.67$$

For routine tests on this product, it may be expedient to dilute 1 ml of the solution under test to 20 ml (MVD/2 rounded to the next lower whole number). However, if this test is positive the analyst will have to dilute 1 ml to 41.67 ml and repeat the test. A dilution to 41.67 ml is also necessary when the test is performed to settle a dispute.

3. Reference Material

Endotoxin standard BRP is intended for use as the reference preparation. It has been assayed against the WHO International Standard for Endotoxin and its potency is expressed in International Units of endotoxin per millilitre. The International Unit of endotoxin is defined as the specific activity of a defined mass of the International Standard.

For routine purposes, another preparation of endotoxin may be used, provided it has been assayed against the International Standard for Endotoxin or the BRP and its potency is expressed in International Units of endotoxin.

The ampoule of the reference preparation usually contains more material than the quantity needed for one test and the analyst may wonder how long the contents of an opened ampoule may be used. No loss of activity has been found in ampoules which have been closed with a suitable material after opening in a laminar flow cabinet and stored at 4° for periods up to 2 weeks. Of course the analyst is advised to check the activity of such ampoules when a routine laboratory regime is devised for prolonged use of opened ampoules.

4. Water LAL [Water BET]

Testing the absence of endotoxin in this reagent by a technique derived from the rabbit pyrogen test was rejected for practical and theoretical reasons:

- the rabbit is not sensitive enough to detect endotoxin in water LAL intended for tests on products with a very low endotoxin limit concentration;
- the relatively low precision of the temperature response in rabbits would call for many replications in rabbits;
- the terms 'pyrogens' and 'endotoxins' denote groups of entities that do not coincide completely.

The text of the test for bacterial endotoxins indicates that methods other than triple distillation may be used to prepare water LAL. Reverse osmosis has been used with good results; some analysts may prefer to distil the water more than three times. Whatever method is used, the resultant product must be free of detectable endotoxins.

5. pH of the mixture

Optimum gelation in the test for bacterial endotoxins occurs for a mixture at pH 6.0 to 7.5. However, the addition of the lysate to the sample may result in a lowering of the pH. To be sure that the pH of the mixture is not lower than 6.0, the analyst should make certain that the pH of the sample to be examined is not less than 6.5.

6. Validation of the lysate

It is important to follow the instructions of the manufacturer for preparing the solutions of the lysate.

The positive end-point dilution factors in the gelation methods A and B are converted to logarithms. The reason is that if the frequency distribution of these logarithmic values is plotted, it usually approaches a normal distribution curve much more closely than the frequency distribution of the dilution factors themselves; in fact it is so similar that it is acceptable to use the normal frequency distribution as a mathematical model and calculate fiducial limits with Student's *t*-test.

The kinetic methods C and D use the logarithm of the endotoxin concentration because the model of linear regression of the log reaction time on the log endotoxin concentration may be used. The chromogenic endpoint method E uses a different model. In this case the effect (the absorbance due to liberated dye) may be regarded as a linear function of the concentration of endotoxin in the concentration range used.

7. Preliminary test for interfering factors

Some products cannot be tested directly for the presence of endotoxins because they are not miscible with the reagents, cannot be adjusted to pH 6.5 to 7.5 or inhibit or activate gel formation. Therefore a preliminary test is required to check for the presence of interfering factors; when these are found the analyst must demonstrate that the procedure to remove them has been effective.

The object of the preliminary test is to test the null hypothesis, that the sensitivity of the lysate in the presence of the product under examination does not differ significantly from the sensitivity of the lysate in the absence of the product. A simple criterion is used in the methods A and B: the null hypothesis is accepted when the sensitivity of the lysate in the presence of the product is at least 0.5 times and not more than twice the sensitivity of the lysate by itself.

A classical approach would have been to calculate the means of the log dilution factor for the sensitivity with and without the product and to test the difference between the two means with Student's *t*-test.

The test for interfering factors in the gelation methods A and B requires the use of a sample of the product in which no endotoxins are detectable. This presents a theoretical problem when an entirely new product has to be tested. Hence a different approach was designed for the quantitative methods C, D and E.

8. Removal of interfering factors

The procedures to remove interference must not increase or decrease the amount of endotoxin in the product under examination (for example, decrease by adsorption). The correct way of checking this is to apply the procedures to a spiked sample of the product, that is, a sample to which a known amount of endotoxin has been added, and then to measure the recovery of the endotoxin.

Methods C and D. If the nature of the product to be analysed presents interference which cannot be removed by classical methods, it may be possible to carry out the CSE curve in the same type of product freed from endotoxins by appropriate treatment or by dilution of the product. The endotoxins test is then carried out by comparison with this standard curve.

Ultrafiltration with asymmetric membrane filters of cellulose triacetate described in the test for bacterial endotoxins has been found to be adequate in most cases. The filters should be adequately validated, because under some circumstances cellulose derivatives (β-D-glycans) can cause false positive results.

The polysulphone filters mentioned in the previous text have been found to be unsuitable because false positive results were obtained by some users.

9. The purpose of the controls

The purpose of the positive control made up with water LAL and the reference preparation of endotoxin at twice the concentration of the labelled lysate sensitivity is to verify the activity of the lysate at the time and under the conditions of the test. The purpose of the negative control is to verify the absence of a detectable concentration of endotoxin in water LAL.

The second positive control, which contains the product to be examined at the concentration used in the test, is intended to show the absence of inhibiting factors at the time and under the conditions of the test.

10. Reading and interpretation of the results

As stated in the introductory paragraphs of the text, the amoebocyte lysate test is used as a limit test and the choice of the limit depends on the factors described. Minute amounts of endotoxin in the water LAL or in any other reagent or material to which the lysate is exposed during the test may escape detection as long as they do not reach the sensitivity limit of the lysate. However, they may raise the amount of endotoxin in the solution containing the product under examination to just above the sensitivity limit and cause a positive reaction.

The risk of this happening may be reduced by testing the water LAL and the other reagents and materials with the most sensitive lysate available, or at least one that is more sensitive than the one used in the test on the product. Even then, the risk of such a 'false positive test' cannot be ruled out completely. It should be realised, however, that in this respect the test design is 'fail-safe' in contrast to a test design permitting a false negative test, which could lead to the release of an unsatisfactory product endangering the patient's health.

11. Replacement of the rabbit pyrogen test or a test for endotoxin prescribed in a Ph Eur monograph

Monographs on pharmaceutical products intended for parenteral use that may contain toxic amounts of bacterial endotoxins require either a rabbit pyrogen test or a test for bacterial endotoxins. When a test for bacterial endotoxins is prescribed and none of the five methods (A to E) described in 2.6.14 is specified, then method A, the gelation method limit test, has been validated for this product. If one of the other methods (B to E) is specified, this is the one which has been validated for this product. Replacement of a rabbit pyrogen test by a bacterial endotoxin test or replacement of a stated or implied method for bacterial endotoxins by another method is to be regarded as the use of an alternative method in replacement of a pharmacopoeial test, as described in 1. General Notices:

The test and assays described are the official methods upon which the standards of the Pharmacopoeia are based. With the agreement of the competent authority, alternative methods of analysis may be used for control purposes, provided that the methods used enable an unequivocal decision to be made as to whether compliance with the standards of the monographs would be achieved if the official methods were used. In the event of doubt or dispute, the methods of analysis of the Pharmacopoeia are alone authoritative.

The following procedures are suggested as a guideline for validating another method for bacterial endotoxins other than the one implied or indicated in the monograph:

11.1. The procedure and the materials and reagents used in the method should be validated as described for the test concerned;

11.2. The presence of interfering factors (and, if needed, the procedure for removing them) should be tested on samples of at least three production batches. It should be borne in mind that methods D and E using a chromogenic peptide require reagents that are absent in methods A, B and C, and hence compliance of methods A, B or C with the requirements for interfering factors cannot be extrapolated to method D or method E without further testing.

11.3. If samples of production batches that gave a positive result in the method implied or indicated in the monograph are available, they should be tested also with the method intended to be used as an alternative method. If such samples are not available, then a comparison of the alternative method with the one in the monograph on the same samples is useless.

12. Validation of the test for new products

The procedures described under 11.1 and 11.2 should be applied to all new products intended for parenteral use that have to be tested for the presence of bacterial endotoxins according to the requirements of the Pharmacopoeia.

13. New products that affect body temperature

Where a new product has shown during the developmental stage that it may affect body temperature, one of the methods (A to E) may be used to demonstrate the absence of bacterial endotoxins; especially a quantitative method (B, C, D or E) may give useful information. In such a case, the analyst should proceed as indicated under 11.1 and 11.2. However, if there are indications of contamination of the product with non-endotoxin pyrogenic substances, it may be necessary to collect information from more extensive tests.

D. Excipients

1. The General Notice on Excipients states that 'any substances added in preparing an official preparation shall... not interfere with the assays and tests of the Pharmacopoeia'.

2. The British Pharmacopoeia Commission wishes to stress that any preparation described by a name at the head of a monograph in the current edition of the Pharmacopoeia, *whether or not it is referred to as BP*, is not of pharmacopoeial quality unless it meets all of the requirements of the monograph when tested by the methods set down.

3. It is recognised that new formulations of existing preparations may from time to time be developed and that the excipients and other ingredients used might result in interference with the official assays and tests. In such cases the Commission is prepared to consider modification of methods to overcome the difficulties thus caused.

4. When seeking modification manufacturers are invited to submit details of the nature of the interference together with proposals for change that will allow the valid testing, by an independent analyst, not only of the proposed new formulation *but also of all similar preparations already on the market.* Practical evaluation in the Laboratory will usually be necessary before any amendments to a British Pharmacopoeia monograph can be considered. It is therefore in the interests of a manufacturer to submit any proposals at the earliest possible date.

E. Dissolution Testing of Solid Oral Dosage Forms

This section provides information on the pharmacopoeial dissolution test and guidance on its function and application in individual monographs of the British Pharmacopoeia for tablets and capsules.

1. Apparatus

Three types of apparatus are now described in the British and European Pharmacopoeias; the basket, the paddle and the flow-through cell. The descriptions are concordant with those published in the United States Pharmacopeia (USP). Of the two established apparatus (basket and paddle) the paddle is now the apparatus of choice for many preparations. However, where a published test uses the basket, work to validate a change to the paddle method is not contemplated. The flow-through cell may be more appropriate for preparations of poorly soluble active ingredients (see section 5).

2. Test conditions and acceptance criteria

2.1 **Test conditions** Pharmacopoeial tests using either the basket or the paddle are based on the principle of operating under 'sink conditions', that is, in a manner such that material already in solution does not exert a modifying effect on the rate of dissolution of the remainder. 'Sink conditions' normally occur in a volume of dissolution medium that is at least 5 to10 times the saturation volume. The standardised conditions have been chosen to provide a gentle hydrodynamic regimen. 'Physiological' media are preferred to water/organic solvent mixtures or solutions incorporating surfactants.

2.2 In the interests of international harmonisation the British Pharmacopoeia Commission reviewed the testing conditions specified in the British Pharmacopoeia 1993 and adopted a dissolution medium volume of 900 ml instead of 1000 ml as the norm and now requires the analyst to test 6 individual tablets or capsules instead of 5. The latter change was made by means of an amendment to Appendix XII D included in the Addendum 1995 to the British Pharmacopoeia 1993. Following consultation of manufacturers, the published tests, wherever appropriate, were also amended by means of this Addendum to conform to the revised standardised conditions. However, changes to the volume of the dissolution medium were not made in cases such as Digoxin Tablets, where there was an indication of correlation between the results of *in-vivo* bioavailability and the established pharmacopoeial test and in other justified cases.

2.3 The revised standardised BP conditions for published tests using either the basket or the paddle are:

rotation speed:100 rpm (basket), 50 rpm (paddle)
dissolution medium volume: 900 ml
dissolution medium composition: aqueous, commonly 0.1M HCl or phosphate buffers of pH 6.8 to 7.6
number of units tested: 6 (plus 6, if retest).

The number of units tested is specified in Appendix XII D; other conditions are specified in the relevant individual monographs.

2.4 **Acceptance criteria** The standardised BP criteria for published tests using either the basket or the paddle are that, for each unit tested, not less than 70% of the active ingredient or ingredients dissolves within 45 minutes. If one unit fails to meet this requirement, a retest may be carried out using the same number of units; all units in the retest must comply. These criteria are specified in Appendix XII D and apply unless otherwise stated in the individual monograph. It is intended to maintain these standardised criteria as the norm in published monographs.

2.5 It should be noted that the 70% dissolution requirement must be met by *each* of the tablets or capsules tested (or by all but one of the total number of units if a retest is performed) and that the percentage is in terms of the prescribed or *stated* amount (that is, the labelled claim). Taking account of permissible assay ranges and content uniformity, this pharmacopoeial (that is, shelf-life) dissolution requirement is considered to offer an acceptable degree of assurance of 'total dissolution'. The choice of a time is, of necessity, somewhat arbitrary but 45 minutes is considered satisfactory for the majority of conventional-release (non-modified-release) products.

2.6 Compliance with the standard BP requirement provides an assurance that *most* of the active ingredient will be dissolved in a *reasonable* time when the preparation is subjected to mild agitation in an aqueous environment. While such an assurance does not, of course, guarantee bioavailability, it significantly reduces the likelihood of unsatisfactory bioavailability due to inadequate dissolution.

2.7 Standardised conditions and limits are considered appropriate for a pharmacopoeial test that is intended for application to monographs covering products from different manufacturers. It might be argued that non-standardised conditions and limits would be more discriminatory but 'tailor-made' test conditions and limits may introduce product bias and may discriminate unnecessarily between products that are equally acceptable from a clinical view-point. Similarly with sufficient manipulation of the test conditions dissolution of almost any product can be achieved. Ideally the test should reflect clinically significant differences in bioavailability arising from differences in dissolution in such a way that clinically acceptable formulations will pass whereas clinically unacceptable formulations will fail.

2.8 Another issue that has been considered in relation to test conditions and criteria is that of multiple-point dissolution profiles as opposed to single-point dissolution tests. It has been concluded that for conventional-release preparations such an extension of testing is not generally necessary or appropriate for pharmacopoeial purposes.

3. Function

3.1 The BP policy of selective application of dissolution testing is based on an assumption that such testing is relevant to the clinical situation and that, *in general,* a conventional-release preparation of already proven bioavailability, which consistently complies with the requirement, is unlikely to give rise to major problems of bioavailability. While the ultimate objective of dissolution testing might be described as ensuring adequate and reproducible bioavailability without recourse to routine *in-vivo* testing, this ideal goal is considered unrealistic in relation to the majority of pharmacopoeial applications. It may be achieved sometimes by a manufacturer's in-house dissolution testing of a particular product for which *in vitro/in vivo* correlation has been demonstrated.

3.2 The published standards of the British Pharmacopoeia are applied to products that have received a product licence in accordance with the relevant regulations. Such products will have met any necessary requirements for bioavailability and bioequivalence and dissolution testing will have been carried out as part of the development studies. Once a product is licensed, a dissolution test may be required routinely as part of quality assurance to demonstrate consistency of process before the release of each batch of the finished product or, when necessary, to provide evidence to support changes in manufacture such as minor changes in formulation or process, changes in site or changes in immediate packaging materials.

3.3 Compliance with a pharmacopoeial dissolution test does not by itself guarantee bioavailability and is not necessarily an adequate basis for judging bioequivalence between preparations. However, such a pharmacopoeial test contributes to an overall assurance of the consistency of the quality of a preparation with respect to its drug release properties.

4. Application

4.1 In reviewing the future application of dissolution testing in the British Pharmacopoeia, the British Pharmacopoeia Commission decided that dissolution testing would be applied to a wider range of capsules and tablets than before. It did not, however, adopt a policy of universal application and a dissolution requirement will not be included automatically in every capsule and tablet monograph.

4.2 As a *general guideline*, it is expected that all new monographs for conventional-release capsules and tablets will contain a dissolution requirement except (i) where the solubility of the active ingredient is 10% or better in water or in dilute hydrochloric acid, at approximately 20°; (ii) where the nature or intended use of the preparation renders a dissolution test inappropriate (for example, liquid-containing capsules, dispersible, effervescent or soluble tablets) or (iii) in other justified circumstances.

4.3 The same guideline is being applied to a review of those capsule and tablet monographs that were published in the British Pharmacopoeia 1993. Each case is being judged on its merits and departures from the norm accepted where appropriate. A provisional list of published monographs for which it is *not* intended to develop a pharmacopoeial dissolution test is provided at the end of this text. Addition of tests to the remaining monographs is being carried out under the Commission's revision programme in accordance with defined priorities and available resources.

4.4 Tests were added to a considerable number of monographs by means of the Addendum 1997 to the British Pharmacopoeia 1993 and more have been added in this new edition. It is emphasised that, while the objective is to include a 'standard' pharmacopoeial test wherever appropriate, the circumstances for each preparation are considered individually in consultation with the manufacturers. It should be appreciated, however, that the retrospective addition of dissolution tests is not without its difficulties. The problems are most acute for those well-established preparations that are manufactured by a wide range of companies, each with its own dissolution specification. A pragmatic approach is being taken to developing compromise test procedures in these circumstances. It has sometimes been possible to harmonise with the test conditions specified in the corresponding monograph in the USP.

4.5 Development of a test for preparations containing active substances of low aqueous solubility, for which application of the paddle method using standard aqueous media may not be technically feasible, has been deferred pending the outcome of further collaborative work (see section 5).

5. Low-solubility preparations

5.1 Certain BP monographs for tablets or capsules containing active substances of low solubility in aqueous media were originally identified as requiring a dissolution specification. Progress in developing suitable specifications for these preparations has been difficult.

5.2 One way of resolving the problem is use of media modified by the addition of an organic solvent, such as ethanol, or a surfactant. This approach has been adopted by the USP and as an *interim* measure in certain BP monographs. Dissolution tests based on those in the USP using modified media were published in the Addendum 1992 to the British Pharmacopoeia 1988 for Cortisone Tablets (30% propanol), Griseofulvin Tablets (1.5% sodium dodecyl sulphate) and Spironolactone Tablets (0.1% sodium dodecyl sulphate), following laboratory work to demonstrate applicability to products on the UK market and in the knowledge that, in the absence of a published BP test, that in the USP was usually cited.

5.3 While such an approach may be validated by *in vivo* correlation on a product-specific basis, doubt has continued to be expressed as to its validity for pharmacopoeial purposes. Departure from the gentle hydrodynamic regimen represented by the aqueous media normally used in BP tests calls into question the relevance of the specification especially as an indicator of bioavailability and in relation to product comparisons. With respect to the two types of modifier, some have argued that the use of surfactants is more likely to give problems of product bias while others have suggested that water/organic solvent mixtures can adversely affect the initial disintegration of the tablet. A consensus has emerged, however, that in circumstances where use of a modified medium is unavoidable, a low concentration of sodium dodecyl sulphate is the modifier of choice.

5.4 Another approach to dealing with low-solubility preparations is to use a flow-through cell apparatus. This is described in the European Pharmacopoeia (Ph Eur, 2.9.3; BP, Appendix XII D) and it was proposed that this method should now be investigated as a possible method of choice for low-solubility preparations since it would overcome the objections to the use of 'non-physiological' media. In view of the lack of wide experience of the use of this method in the United Kingdom, it was recognised that collaborative practical work would be necessary to standardise the technique and explore its potential for pharmacopoeial applications. A working party was established under the auspices of BP Committee F: Pharmacy to carry out this work with participation from industry, control laboratories and licensing assessors. The study would focus on preparations of two or three poorly soluble active substances. In addition to investigating the use of the flow-through apparatus, the study would look at the use of sodium dodecyl sulphate in conjunction with the paddle apparatus. Based on the preliminary findings from the first phase of the trial, it has been recommended that this latter approach should be adopted for Cortisone Tablets and suggested that it might usefully be explored for other formulations. Further work will be carried out when resources permit.

6. Modified-release preparations

6.1 Any consideration of the quality of modified-release preparations in relation to their safety and efficacy must include attention to the release characteristics of these products. A manufacturer must be able to provide the licensing authority with an assurance that the dissolution profile reflects *in vivo* performance, which in turn is compatible with the recommended dosage schedule for the specific product.

6.2 The general monographs for Capsules and Tablets include a Production requirement that a suitable test is carried out to demonstrate the appropriate release of the active ingredient or ingredients. With respect to providing tests in individual monographs, however, it has been concluded reluctantly, following detailed discussion and practical investigation, that it is not possible to provide satisfactory pharmacopoeial control of the dissolution profile of the majority of modified-release preparations. Data obtained in a study of theophylline formulations, for example, indicated that it was not possible even to devise simplified dissolution criteria for such preparations to ensure that dose-dumping did not occur and that an acceptable amount of the active ingredient was eventually released. Between-product differences are such as to preclude the setting of meaningful pharmacopoeial limits even for these more limited objectives.

Solid oral-dosage form monographs for which it is not intended to develop a dissolution test

Capsules

Amantadine Capsules
Ampicillin Capsules
Chlormethiazole Capsules
Clofibrate Capsules
Clomipramine Capsules
Cloxacillin Capsules
Co-danthrusate Capsules
Cyanocobalamin[^{57}Co] Capsules
Dothiepin Capsules
Doxepin Capsules
Estramustine Phosphate Capsules
Ethosuximide Capsules
Flucloxacillin Capsules
Flurazepam Capsules
Halibut-liver Oil Capsules
Hydroxyurea Capsules
Lincomycin Capsules
Lymecycline Capsules
Mexiletine Capsules

Tablets

Aluminium Hydroxide Tablets
Amitriptyline Tablets
Ascorbic Acid Tablets
Aspirin Tablets, Dispersible
Aspirin Tablets, Effervescent Soluble
Atenolol Tablets
Atropine Tablets
Benztropine Tablets
Betamethasone Sodium Phosphate Tablets
Brompheniramine Tablets
Busulphan Tablets
Calcium Gluconate Tablets, Effervescent
Calcium Lactate Tablets
Cascara Tablets
Chlordiazepoxide Hydrochloride Tablets
Chlorpheniramine Tablets
Choline Theophyllinate Tablets
Clonidine Tablets
Co-codaprin Tablets, Dispersible
Codeine Phosphate Tablets
Colchicine Tablets
Colistin Tablets
Co-magaldrox Tablets
Co-trimoxazole Tablets, Dispersible
Desipramine Tablets
Dexamphetamine Tablets
Dextromoramide Tablets
Dicyclomine Tablets
Digitoxin Tablets
Dihydrocodeine Tablets
Docusate Tablets
Dothiepin Tablets
Ephedrine Hydrochloride Tablets
Etamiphylline Tablets[1]
Ethambutol Tablets
Ferrous Gluconate Tablets
Ferrous Sulphate Tablets
Fluphenazine Tablets
Glyceryl Trinitrate Tablets
Guanethidine Tablets
Hydrotalcite Tablets
Hydroxychloroquine Tablets
Hyoscine Butylbromide Tablets
Hyoscine Tablets
Imipramine Tablets
Labetalol Tablets
Lincomycin Tablets[1]
Lithium Carbonate Tablets
Magnesium Trisilicate Tablets, Compound
Mebeverine Tablets
Menadiol Phosphate Tablets
Mepyramine Tablets
Methadone Tablets
Metoclopramide Tablets
Metoprolol Tablets
Neomycin Tablets
Neostigmine Tablets
Nicotinamide Tablets
Nicotinyl Alcohol Tablets
Nitrofurantoin Tablets
Orciprenaline Tablets
Orphenadrine Hydrochloride Tablets
Oxprenolol Tablets
Pancreatin Tablets
Penicillamine Tablets

Pentaerythritol Tetranitrate Tablets
Pentobarbitone Tablets
Pethidine Tablets
Phenelzine Tablets
Pindolol Tablets
Piperazine Citrate Tablets[1]
Poldine Tablets
Potassium Chloride Tablets, Effervescent
Promazine Tablets
Promethazine Hydrochloride Tablets
Propantheline Tablets
Propranolol Tablets
Protriptyline Tablets
Pseudoephedrine Tablets
Pyridostigmine Tablets
Pyridoxine Tablets
Ranitidine Tablets
Salbutamol Tablets
Senna Tablets
Sodium Bicarbonate Tablets, Compound
Sodium Chloride Tablets
Sodium Citrate Tablets
Sotalol Tablets
Stilboestrol Tablets
Terbutaline Tablets
Thiamine Tablets
Thioridazine Tablets
Thymoxamine Tablets
Timolol Tablets
Tranexamic Acid Tablets
Trifluoperazine Tablets
Trimeprazine Tablets
Triprolidine Tablets

1. Monograph of the British Pharmacopoeia (Veterinary)

F. Declaration of Content

This section describes the way in which the content of active substance in a preparation is declared and the method adopted to express the content of the medicinal substances themselves. A proper understanding of such statements is essential to their correct interpretation.

Medicinal substances

1. The purpose of the assay in monographs for medicinal substances, taken in conjunction with the tests for impurities, is to determine the purity of the medicinal substance and the limits are therefore usually stated in terms of the molecular entity (salt, ester, etc) and calculated with reference to the anhydrous or dried substance as appropriate (depending on whether the monograph includes a test for water or for loss on drying).

2. One advantage of this form of expression in 'parent' monographs is that it gives an indication 'at a glance' of the purity of the substance. For example (albeit an extreme example) the purity of Amitriptyline Embonate is stated as not less than 98.5% of $(C_{20}H_{23}N)_2$, $C_{23}H_{16}O_6$ calculated with reference to the anhydrous substance rather than as not less than 57.9% of $C_{20}H_{23}N$ calculated with reference to the anhydrous substance.

3. The mode of expression chosen for the 'parent' monograph in no way circumscribes that which may be used in the monograph for a preparation. There is no reason why the two should be the same and there is frequently good reason why they should be different. In the example of Amitriptyline Embonate, the assay limits for the preparation Amitriptyline Oral Suspension are stated in terms of amitriptyline, $C_{20}H_{23}N$.

Formulated preparations

4. The purpose of the assay in monographs for formulated preparations is to determine whether the content of the active ingredient is within acceptable limits of the labelled claim and the limits are therefore of necessity stated in terms of the moiety declared on the label as established by the manufacturer.

5. Every effort is made in the British Pharmacopoeia to achieve internal consistency within monographs, that is, to use the same terms for content statement, assay and label. The British Pharmacopoeia Commission, however, has no means of achieving external (inter-monograph) consistency since, unless it perceives there to be a potentially serious risk, it would not seek to obtain a change in a manufacturer's established practice. Problems arise when a manufacturer is not consistent or does not state clearly to what the strength refers and, in particular, when different manufacturers of the same preparation express the content in different terms.

6. Ideally in many cases where several salts or hydrated forms of the same drug substance are available, the label and dose (and therefore all monograph statements) should be in terms of the anhydrous free base or acid, that is, the active moiety, in order to facilitate comparison and equivalent dosage.

7. Implementation of such a policy would clearly require that each case should be judged on its merits since there would be instances when, for example, a different salt is considered as a different active moiety or where it would be misleading to suggest that two different forms are therapeutically equivalent. Nevertheless it is strongly recommended that as a general rule *for new drug substances*, doses and strengths of preparations should be expressed in terms of the active moiety.

8. Meanwhile, for established materials the Pharmacopoeia will continue to reflect current practice. In this respect it should be noted that the labelling requirements of the Pharmacopoeia are not comprehensive. Thus a monograph requirement to state the content of active ingredient in terms of the entire drug substance molecule does not preclude an additional indication of the content expressed in terms of the active moiety where such an indication is considered desirable.

G. Labelling

This section provides guidance on the status and interpretation of pharmacopoeial labelling sections.

1. The General Notice on Labelling distinguishes between the mandatory status of those Pharmacopoeial labelling statements that are necessary to demonstrate compliance with the monograph and the advisory status of other labelling statements included in the Pharmacopoeia.

2. This distinction, which is consistent with the approach adopted in the European Pharmacopoeia, is made in recognition of the complexity of the statutory and advisory framework within which the labelling of medicines is determined. It is hoped that by thus restricting mandatory

pharmacopoeial labelling statements to those that are essential for pharmacopoeial purposes, the potential for conflict between pharmacopoeial and other statutory provisions will be minimised.

3. Within the context of any particular monograph, it should be apparent which of the labelling statements are necessary to demonstrate compliance with the monograph and are thus mandatory. As guidance, a labelling statement is considered essential for a medicinal substance
(i) where a test or assay requirement is expressed in relation to a declared value, the 'labelled claim' (for example, the apparent viscosity of Carmellose Sodium or the potency of Capreomycin Sulphate and of Salcatonin);
(ii) where different test requirements or limits apply to materials derived from different sources (for example, the requirements for matter insoluble in 5M ammonia depend on the botanical source of Podophyllum Resin), or intended for different purposes (for example, the sterility of Benzylpenicillin Sodium when intended for use in the manufacture of a parenteral dosage form without a further sterilisation process);
(iii) in other special circumstances.

4. Likewise a labelling statement is considered essential for a formulated preparation
(i) where a test requirement is expressed in relation to a declared value, the 'labelled claim';
(ii) where the content of active ingredient is required to be expressed in terms other than the weight of the official medicinal substance used in making the formulation (for example, Primaquine Tablets contain Primaquine Phosphate but the content is expressed in terms of the equivalent amount of primaquine base);
(iii) where different test requirements or limits apply to the formulated preparation manufactured from different bulk drug substances (for example, Heparin Injection manufactured from Heparin Calcium or Heparin Sodium) or intended for different purposes (for example, Isosorbide Dinitrate Tablets intended to be chewed before swallowing or allowed to dissolve in the mouth);
(iv) in other special circumstances.

5. Advisory labelling statements for formulated preparations may be included either in the general monograph or in the monograph for the individual preparation, as appropriate. Such statements commonly relate to features such as the expiry date, the storage conditions, the name and amount of any excipients and the directions for making the final preparations. Additional advisory labelling statements may relate to the directions for using the preparation or the precautions relating to the handling and use of the preparation.

H. Biological Assay and Tests

This section provides information and guidance concerning the biological assays and test of the Pharmacopoeia and the standard preparations required for them.

Biological, including biochemical or immunochemical, methods are described for the determination of potency or other specific properties of certain substances and preparations where these properties cannot be adequately determined by chemical or physical means. The principle applied wherever possible throughout these methods is that of comparison with a standard preparation so as to determine how much of a sample being examined produces the same effect as a given quantity, the Unit, defined by the standard preparation. It is an essential condition of such methods that the tests on the standard preparation and on the sample, the potency or other property of which is being determined, shall be carried out at the same time and, in all other respects, under strictly comparable conditions.

Standard Preparations, as defined in the biological assays and tests of the Pharmacopoeia, are of two kinds: primary standards which are established, held and distributed by the appropriate international or national organisation and secondary (working) standards which are preparations the potencies of which have been determined by an adequate number of comparative tests in relation to the relevant primary standard.

A primary standard is a selected representative sample of the substance for which it is to serve as a basis of measurement. It is essential that primary standards shall be of uniform quality and as stable as possible. These conditions are usually ensured by providing the preparations in the dry state, dispensing them in sealed containers free from moisture and oxygen and storing them continuously at a low temperature and in the absence of light.

For the majority of biological assays of the Pharmacopoeia, the primary standards are the International Standards and Reference Preparations, established by the World Health Organization. Laboratories in the United Kingdom may obtain these for the purposes of the biological assays described in the Pharmacopoeia from the National Institute for Biological Standards and Control, Blanche Lane, South Mimms, Potters Bar, Hertfordshire EN6 3QG, England.

For the assay of certain enzymes in the Pharmacopoeia the Standard Preparations, as defined in the appropriate method, are the primary standards established by the International Commission on Pharmaceutical Enzymes of the International Pharmaceutical Federation (FIP). These standards may be obtained from the Centre for Standards, Wolterslaan 12, B–9000, Ghent, Belgium or, where these standards have been established in co-operation with, and adopted as official preparations by, the European Pharmacopoeia Commission, they may be obtained from the European Pharmacopoeia Commission Secretariat, Council of Europe, BP 907, F–67029 Strasbourg Cedex 1, France.

As a measure of economy in the use of the primary standards it is recommended that working standards should be prepared and used in those biological methods of the Pharmacopoeia where the definition of the Standard Preparation is so worded as to permit this. However, in some instances the complexity or lack of precision of the method or difficulties associated with the preparation of a secondary standard render such a practice inadvisable and in any country in which a particular assay is controlled by law it may be necessary to obtain the approval of the appropriate authority for the use of working standards. The biological properties of the samples selected as working standards should conform as closely as possible to those of the primary standard and an assurance that these conditions have been fulfilled is usually obtained by comparing the behaviour of the two samples under varying conditions of comparative testing. In such tests a detailed study of the dose—response curves may indicate whether the sample selected to serve as a working standard is a suitable preparation. For the assay of certain biological materials in the Pharmacopoeia, for example oxytocin, European Pharmacopoeia Biological Reference

Preparations have been established and are recommended for use as the working standards. Such preparations may be obtained from the European Pharmacopoeia Commission (address as above).

Wherever possible the primary standard is the International Standard, and the biological activity is expressed in International Units.

In other cases, where Units are referred to in the official assays and tests, the Unit for a particular substance is, for the United Kingdom, the specific biological activity contained in such an amount of the respective primary standard as the appropriate international or national organisation indicates. The necessary information is provided with the samples of the primary standard.

For enzymes in the Pharmacopoeia, where the assay is such that the stoichiometry of the reaction is known, for example, where the substrate is a synthetic ester, the activity is measured in microkatals or nanokatals. A microkatal is defined as the enzyme activity that under defined conditions, produces one micromole of the reaction product per second or alternatively consumes one micromole of the reaction substrate per second. For other enzymes in the Pharmacopoeia, where the reaction involved in the assay is more complex, for example, where the substrate is a naturally occurring macromolecule such as a protein, the activity is measured in Units as previously defined.

The methods of biological assay described in the Pharmacopoeia have been found satisfactory but will not necessarily be the best methods for use in all circumstances. In most instances they may be replaced by other methods if it can be shown that such methods are at least equally accurate and precise and provide a measurement of the same active principles.

Any estimate of potency derived from a biological assay is subject to random error due to the inherent variability of biological responses and calculations of error should be made, if possible, from the results of each assay and recorded with the potency estimate even when the official method of assay is used. Guidance on the design of assays, the statistical analysis of results and the calculation of potency is provided in general text 5.3 of the European Pharmacopoeia. The methods described therein take account of the inherent random error but assume that systematic errors, for example, errors in weighing or dilution, will not represent a major source of variation in the potency estimates. Alternative assay designs and methods of calculation may be used provided that they are not less reliable.

Where an immunoassay, that is an assay procedure based on the reversible and non-covalent binding of an antigen by antibody, is described in the Pharmacopoeia for detecting or quantifying either an antigen or an antibody, the considerations described in Appendix XIV B apply in addition to the general points referred to above.

J.Efficacy of Antimicrobial Preservation

This section of Supplementary Chapter I provides background information on the purpose and scope of the test for effficacy of antimicrobial preservation.

1. The test for efficacy of antimicrobial preservation, included in Appendix XVI C, has been accorded non-mandatory status in the Pharmacopoeia. This status is reflected in the test's inclusion as a general text in the section 5 of the European Pharmacopoeia and in the form of reference to the test within Production sections of relevant general monographs of the European Pharmacopoeia.

2. It is intended to serve as a model offering a manufacturer guidance concerning this aspect of quality and a foundation on which he can build to meet his own particular needs. The testing procedure is intended to serve as a means whereby, during product development, a manufacturer can assess the efficacy of any antimicrobial preservative included in the product.

3. If during development a fully quantitative, comparative evaluation of different preservative systems would be useful, the procedure described in the appendix could be extended to incorporate an estimation of initial microbial death rates.

4. The present European Pharmacopoeia text provides criteria for parenteral, ophthalmic, topical and oral preparation. The British Pharmacopoeia continues also to provide criteria for ear preparations in Appendix XVI C. The criteria for ear preparations are equivalent to the A criteria now specified for ophthalmic preparations thus maintaining parity between these two types of product.

5. An unusual feature of the European Pharmacopoeia text is the inclusion of two sets of criteria (A and B) for parenteral and ophthalmic preparations. The A criteria express the recommended efficacy to be achieved, that is, they represent generally applicable 'target' criteria.

6. It is recognised that for a number of products these target criteria are unlikely to be achieved except at the expense of some other property of equal or greater importance. The alternative criteria to be met in these circumstances are a matter for agreement between the manufacturer and the competent authority and should take account of any special considerations relevant to the specific product. The B criteria for parenteral and ophthalmic products were adopted by the European Pharmacopoeia Commission in deference to those member states that wanted published guidance on the minimum values below which any alternative criteria should not fall.

K. Stereochemistry

This section describes the way in which the stereochemistry of a substance is indicated in the chemical definitions and graphic formulae of the British Pharmacopoeia and the way it may be identified and/or controlled within the tests in a monograph.

1. Many medicinal substances that contain one or more chiral centres and that are already on the market have been made available for pharmaceutical use as racemic mixtures with little known about the biological activities of the separate isomers. This has been reflected in the monograph in the Pharmacopoeia and a test to show that the substance is the racemic mixture has not usually been included unless it was known that at least one of the separate enantiomers was also available commercially. Nevertheless, with increasing concern by regulatory authorities for substances to be made available as single isomers, tests for enantiomeric composition will become more common (see section on tests below).

Chemical definition (monographs other than those of the European Pharmacopoeia)

2. In the case of substances containing a single chiral centre, the descriptor '(*RS*)-' is included at the appropriate position in the chemical definition of the substance to indicate a racemic mixture.

3. For substances containing multiple chiral centres and comprising a mixture of all possible stereoisomers the term '*all-rac-*' has been used, for example Isoaminile. In those few substances existing as diastereoisomeric mixtures, that is where in one or more centres the stereochemistry is explicit but in other centres it is not, each centre is defined either as the specific (*R*)- or (*S*)- configuration, or as racemic (*RS*)-, respectively.

Graphic formulae

4.When a medicinal substance is a racemate, an indication is given by means of the graphic formula.

5. Because in graphic formulae there is no generally accepted convention for depicting a racemate, each racemic substance with one chiral centre is shown in the (*R*)- form with the appended text 'and enantiomer' for example, Carteolol Hydrochloride. For the *all-rac-* mixtures, such as Docusate Sodium and Alpha Tocopheryl Acetate, non-stereospecific graphic formulae are drawn and the legend 'mixture of *n* stereoisomers' added beneath (where *n* is the number of possible stereoisomers); the stereogenic carbon atoms concerned are identified by means of asterisks

6. In diastereoisomeric mixtures, the unique configuration centres are drawn as such, while each racemic centre (with equal amounts of the (*R*) and (*S*) configuration) are indictated by an asterisk and the legend 'racemic at C*' appended. For example, Carbenicillin Sodium is drawn in this way; the chiral atoms in the penicillanic acid ring each in their single specific configuration and the phenylmalonyl side-chain chiral atom marked with an asterisk.

Tests

7. In future, when a monograph describes an enantiomer, it will include both a test for specific optical rotation under Identification and a test, using methods such as chiral chromatography, to control enantiomeric purity.

8. When both the racemic mixture and the enantiomer are available, the monograph for the racemic mixture will specify a test for angle of rotation together with a cross reference under Identification. The test for angle of rotation will normally specify limits of + 0.10° to - 0.10° in order to limit the presence of optically active impurities and demonstrate equal proportions of the enantiomers.

9. When only the racemic mixture is available, the monograph for the racemic mixture will simply specify a test for angle of rotation.

SUPPLEMENTARY CHAPTER II

Names of Medicinal Substances and Preparations

The following section is included as Appendix A to British Approved Names 1997; it is reproduced here for the convenience of the user of the British Pharmacopoeia.

Structures and Nomenclature of Substances of Natural or Semi-synthetic Origin

These notes provide a guide to the semi-systematic chemical nomenclature of certain groups of natural and semi-synthetic products. The following literature should be consulted for further information.

1. The definitive rules of the International Union of Pure and Applied Chemistry (IUPAC) for organic substances are contained in *Nomenclature of Organic Chemistry*, Section A to F and H, Pergamon Press, Oxford, 1979.
2. The IUPAC rules for inorganic substances are given in *Nomenclature of Inorganic Chemistry*, Blackwells, Oxford, 1990.
3. *Biochemical Nomenclature and Related Documents*, The Biochemical Society for the International Union of Biochemistry (IUB), 2nd. edn. London, 1992. The following topics are included.

   Stereochemistry (Nomenclature of Organic chemistry, Section E)
   Natural products are related compounds (Nomenclaure of Organic Chemistry, Section F)
   Abbreviations and Symbols
   Amino-acids, peptides, peptide hormones and immunoglobulins
   Steroids
   Carotenoids and tocopherols
   Carbohydrates and cyclitols
   Vitamins

A. Aminoglycoside Antibiotics

A.1 The aminoglycoside antibiotics are conveniently named by reference to 2-D-deoxystreptamine, **1**, in which name the configuration and numbering shown are implicit.

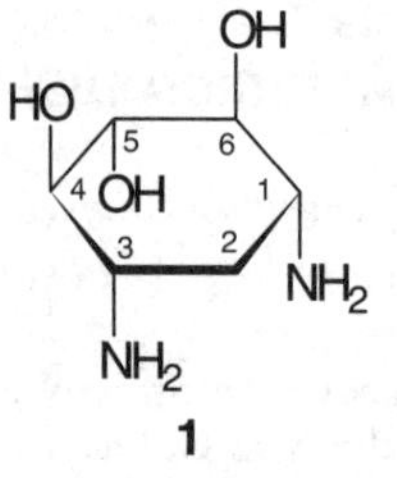

1

A.2 The aminoglycoside antibiotics commonly carry glycosyl radicals on the oxygen atoms attached to C-4 and C-6. The configuration and numbering shown in 1 should be strictly observed if confusion is to be avoided.

A.3 When one glycosyl radical is linked to another the names are separated by two locants which indicate the respective positions involved in this glycosidic union; these locants are enclosed in parentheses and separated by an arrow (pointing from the locant corresponding to the glycosyl carbon atom to the locant corresponding to the hydroxylic carbon atom involved).

B Cephalosporin Antibiotics

B.1 The cephalosporin antibiotics are conveniently named by reference to either cephalosporanic acid (**2**, *R* = CH_2OAc, X = H) or cephem-4-carboxylic acid (**2**, R = X = H).

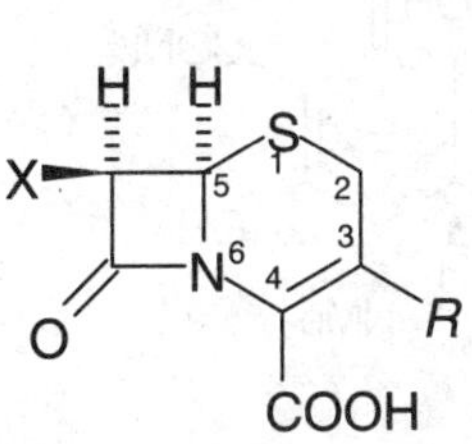

2

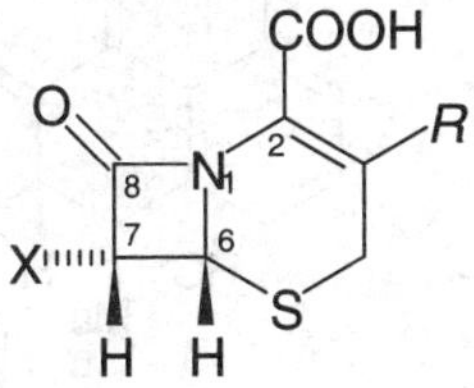

3

B.2 When names are based on cephalosporanic acid or cephem-carboxylic acid the traditional numbering shown in **2** is used.

B.3 Cephalosporanic acid is systematically named as (6*R*)-3-acetoxymethyl-8-oxo-5-thia-1-azabicyclo-[4.2.0]oct-2-ene-2-carboxylic acid. Compounds that are named systematically use the numbering and orientation shown in **3**.

B.4 The cephalosporin antibiotics bear an acylamino group (X) at position 7 (under both numbering systems)

.

C Ergot Alkaloids

C.1 Members of the ergoline group of substances are conveniently named by reference to either ergoline itself, **4**, or to D-lysergamide, **5**. When names are so based the traditional numbering shown in **4** is used. In 9,10-dihydro compounds the configuration at position-10 needs to be specified.

C.2 Members of the ergotamine group of substances are conveniently named by reference to ergotaman, **6**. Ergotamine itself is (5¢*R*)-5¢-benzyl-12¢-hydroxy-2¢-methyl-18-oxoergotaman-3¢,6¢-dione.

D Morphines

D.1 Members of the morphine and codeine group of substances have traditionally been named with reference to morphine itself, **7**, using the numbering shown. However, names may be based more conveniently on either morphinan, **8**, or *ent*-morphinan, **9**.

D.2 Morphine, **7**, is (5*R*, 6*S*)-4,5-epoxy-9a-methyl-7,8-didehydromorphinan-3,6-diol.

D.3 In certain morphine derivatives, an etheno or ethano bridge is present joining positions 6 and 14 and a hydroxyalkyl side chain is present at position 7.

E Penicillin Antibiotics

E.1 The penicillin antibiotics are conveniently named by reference to penicillanic acid (**10**, X = H) when the classical numbering shown is used.

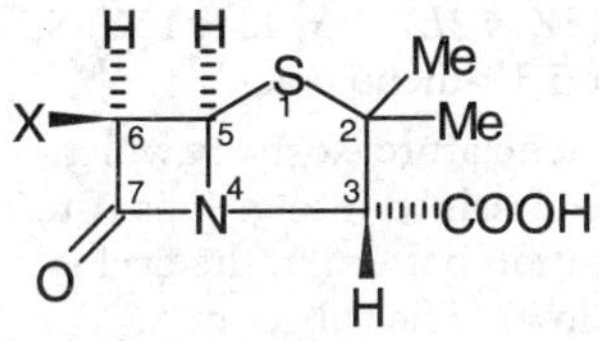

10

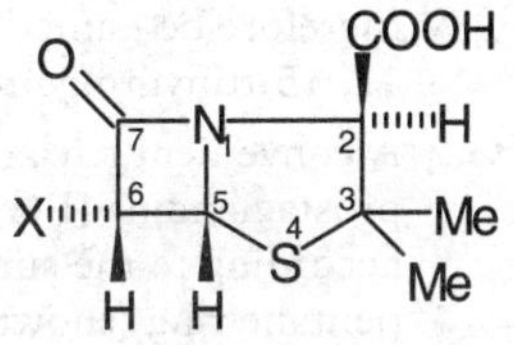

11

E.2 Penicillanic acid is systematically named as (2*S*, 5*R*)-3,3-dimethyl-7-oxo-4-thia-1-azabicyclo[3.2.0]heptane-2-carboxylic acid. Compounds that are named systematically use the orientation and numbering shown in **11**.

E.3 The penicillin antibiotics are usually 6-acylamino penicillanic acid derivatives in which the configuration at position 6 is *R*.

F Polypeptides

F.1 The following 3-letter and 1-letter symbols for amino-acids, authorised by the IUPAC-IUB Joint Commission on Biochemical Nomenclature, are used for representing the sequences of polypeptides:

Alanine	Ala	A	*Leucine*	Leu	L
Arginine	Arg	R	*Lysine*	Lys	K
Asparagine	Asn	N	*Methionine*	Met	M
Aspartic Acid	Asp	D	*Phenylalanine*	Phe	F
Cysteine	Cys	C	*Proline*	Pro	P
Glutamine	Gln	Q	*Serine*	Ser	S
Glutamic acid	Glu	E	*Threonine*	Thr	T
Glycine	Gly	G	*Tryptophan*	Trp	W
Histidine	His	H	*Tyrosine*	Try	Y
Isoleucine	Ile	I	*Valine*	Val	V

F.2 The following symbols recommended by the Joint Commission are also used:

2-Aminohexanoic acid	Ahx
Sarcosine	Sar
Pyroglutamic acid	<Glu
tert-*Butoxycarbonyl*	Boc

F.3 When interpreting sequences of amino-acid residues, the hyphen should be considered as part of the symbol. Its use to separate the individual residues or radicals may be illustrated by the following example:

$$\text{Gly} = NH_2CH_2COOH$$
$$\text{Gly-} = NH_2CH_2CO\text{-}$$
$$\text{-Gly} = \text{-}NHCH_2COOH$$
$$\text{-Gly-} = \text{-}NHCH_2CO\text{-}$$

and thus,

$$\text{Gly-Gly-Gly} = NH_2CH_2CONHCH_2CONHCH_2\,COOH$$

The residues are conventionally written with the amino group to the left and the carboxyl group to the right. This is implicit in the symbolism.

F.4 Where peptide sequences are shown using 3-letter symbols all amino-acids except glycine have the 'L-' configuration unless otherwise indicated.

G Prostaglandins

G.1 Members of the prostaglandin group of substances are conveniently named by reference to prostanoic acid, **12**, using the numbering shown. Prostanoic acid may be systematically named as 7-[(1*S*, 2*S*)-2-octylcyclopentyl]heptanoic acid. *Dinoprost*, **13**, may therefore be named as (5Z, 12*E*)-(9*S*, 11*R* 15*S*)-9, 11, 15-trihydroxyprosta-5,13-dienoic acid.

G.2 A convenient trivial nomenclature exists by which prostaglandins (PG) are classified into groups A to F according to the substitution pattern in the cyclopentane ring (shown below). The subscript numerals 1, 2 and 3 refer to the number of double bonds found in the side-chains and subscript a refers to the configuration of the C-9 hydroxy group. Thus, **13** is referred to as PGF_{2a} .

H Steroids

H.1 Steroids are drawn and numbered, and the rings lettered, as shown in **14**.

H.2 Steroids are named with reference to certain basic carbocycles some of which are defined in Table 1. When so drawn, dotted bonds are regarded as lying below the plane of the paper and are designated a, thickened bonds are regarded as lying above the plane of the paper and are designated b and bonds of unknown configuration are shown by a wavy line and are designated x.

TABLE I

	R_1	R_2	R_3
Gonane	H	H	H
Estrane	H	Me	H
Androstane	Me	Me	H
Pregnane	Me	Me	Et

H.3 When the hydrogen atom at C-5 is present, its configuration is always specified, eg 5a-pregnane, 5b-androstane. The configuration at centres, 8,9,10,13,14 and 17 is assumed to be as shown in 15 unless otherwise specified.

H.4 When inversion of the normal configuration occurs, the positions concerned are specified; and thus 16 is named 5b, 17a-pregnane.

H.5 When inversion occurs at all of the defined asymmetric centres, the original name is preceded by the italicised prefix *ent-*. Racemates are indicated by use of the italicised prefix *rac-*.

H.6 Further fundamental carbocycles are defined thus:

TABLE II

Side-chain	carbon positions present
Cholane	20 - 24
Cholestane	20 - 27
Ergostane	20 - 27, 24^1

In addition to retaining the configuration shown in 15, C-20 has an R-configuration in each carbocycle and C-24 in ergostane has an S-configuration. However, additional substituents at positions C-17, C-20, C-21 may alter the *R* and *S* propriety descriptions without any change at C-20.

H.7 A large number of therapeutically active steroids bear a carbonyl group at position 3 and unsaturation across positions 4 and 5. Ring A is often aromatic in estrogens.

J Tetracyclines

J.1 The tetracycline antibiotics are conveniently named by reference to tetracycline itself, **17**, (*R* = H), which may be defined as (4*S*,4a*S*,5a*S*,6*S*,12a*S*)4-dimethylamino-1,4,4a,5a,6,11,12a-octahydro-3,6,10,12, 12a-pentahydroxy-6-methyl-1,11-dioxonaphthacene-2-carboxamide.

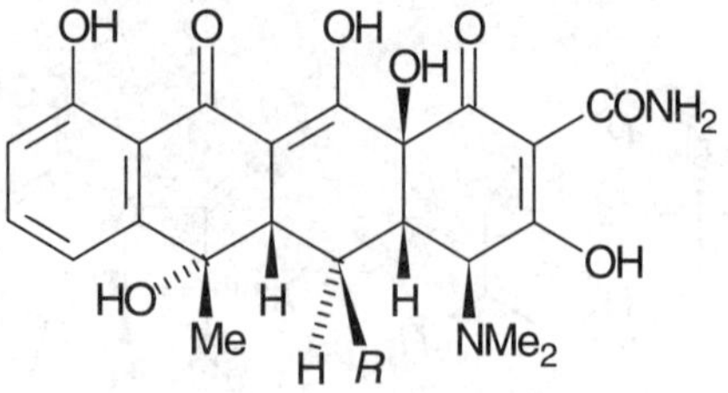

17

J.2 When analogues of tetracycline are named the stereodescriptors *R* and *S* may be subject to change even though the steric configuration usually remains unchanged. For example, in oxytetracycline, the hydroxyl group at position 5 imposes assignment inversions at positions 4a and 5a from *S* to *R* although the steric configuration at these positions remains unchanged.

TABLE III

	Position					
	4	**4a**	**5**	**5a**	**6**	**12a**
Chlortetracycline	*S*	*S*	¾	*S*	*S*	*S*
Clomocycline	*S*	*S*	¾	*S*	*S*	*S*
Demeclocycline	*S*	*S*	¾	*S*	*S*	*S*
Doxycycline	*S*	*R*	*S*	*R*	*R*	*S*
Meclocycline	*S*	*R*	*S*	*R*	¾	*S*
Methacycline	*S*	*R*	*S*	*R*	¾	*S*
Minocycline	*S*	*S*	¾	*R*	¾	*S*
Oxytetracycline	*S*	*R*	*S*	*R*	*S*	*S*
Tetracycline	*S*	*S*	¾	*S*	*S*	*S*

J.3 When fully systematic names based on naphthacene-2-carboxamide are used, the stereodescriptors given in Table III should be used.

K Tropanes

K.1 Members of the tropane group of substances are conveniently named by references to tropane itself, **18**, when the numbering and orientation shown are used. Tropane is defined as (8*r*)-*N*-methyl-8-azabicyclo[3.2.1]octane.

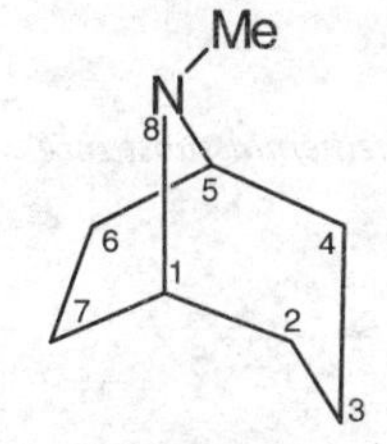

18

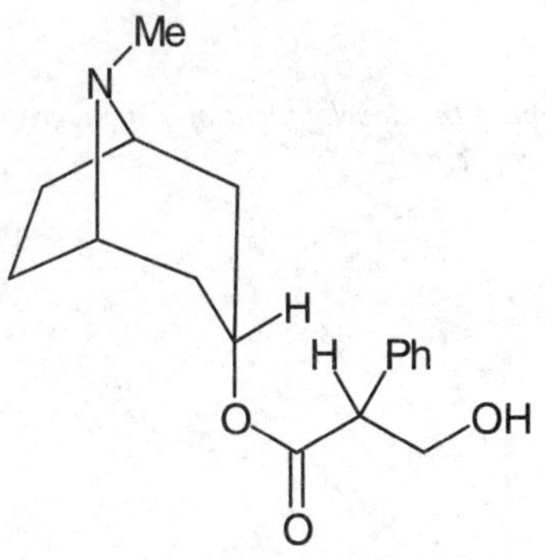

19

K.2 Atropine, **19**, is (1*R*,3*r*,5*S*,8*r*,)-tropan-3-yl (*RS*)-tropate where the term *tropate* represents 3-hydroxy-2-phenylpropionate.

K.3 In the (-) -series the tropoyl side-chain has the (*S*) configuration, **20**.

K.4 In y-tropane compounds, **21**, the configuration at position-3 is designated as '3s'.

K.5 In hyoscine and other atropine derivatives bearing a 6,7-epoxy bridge, the configuration is as shown in **22**.

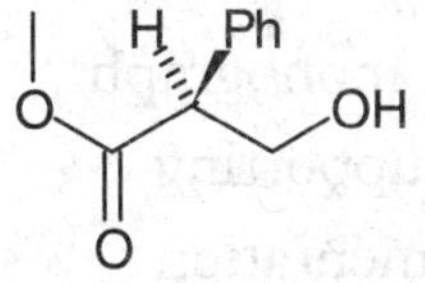

20

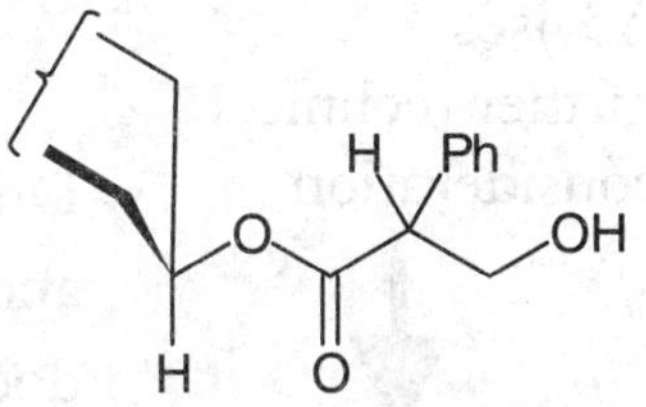

21

L Xanthines

Members of the xanthine group of substances are conveniently named by references to purine, **24**, when the non-systematic numbering shown is used.

Supplementary Chapter III

Pharmacopoeial Organisation

This Supplementary Chapter provides information that may be helpful to those wishing to communicate with the British Pharmacopoeia Commission.

A. Contact points

The following list gives an indication of which member of the British Pharmacopoeia Secretariat is responsible for particular areas of the Commission's work.

For matters concerning British Pharmacopoeia Chemical Reference Substances (BPCRS) please contact Mr C Woollam at the Laboratory (telephone: +44 (0)171 972 3608; facsimile: +44 (0)181 951 3069).

Facsimile number: +44 (0)171 272 0566

Telephone: direct lines +44 (0) 171 273-

Antibiotics	Mr R B Trigg	0557
Analytical methods (general)	Mrs H J Judd	0558
Biological materials	Miss M L Rabouhans	0560
European Pharmacopoeia (general matters)[1]	Mrs M Vallender	0562
General monographs	Miss M L Rabouhans	0560
Immunological products	Miss M L Rabouhans	0560
Information technology	Mr R B Trigg	0557
Inorganic chemicals	Mrs H J Judd	0558
Labelling	Miss M L Rabouhans	0560
Microbiological aspects	Miss M L Rabouhans	0560
Nomenclature	Mr R B Trigg	0557
Organic Chemicals	Mrs H J Judd *or*	0558
	Mr R B Trigg	0557
Pharmaceutical aspects	Miss M L Rabouhans	0560
Radioactive materials	Mrs H J Judd	0558
Reagents	Mrs H J Judd	0558
Surgical materials	Mrs M Vallender	0562
Vegetable drugs	Mrs H J Judd	0558

[1]For specific matters see under relevant subject entry

B. Monograph Development: Mechanism

The following diagram provides a simplified, schematic representation of the development of a monograph for a medicinal substance or an associated formulated preparation for inclusion in the Pharmacopoeia.

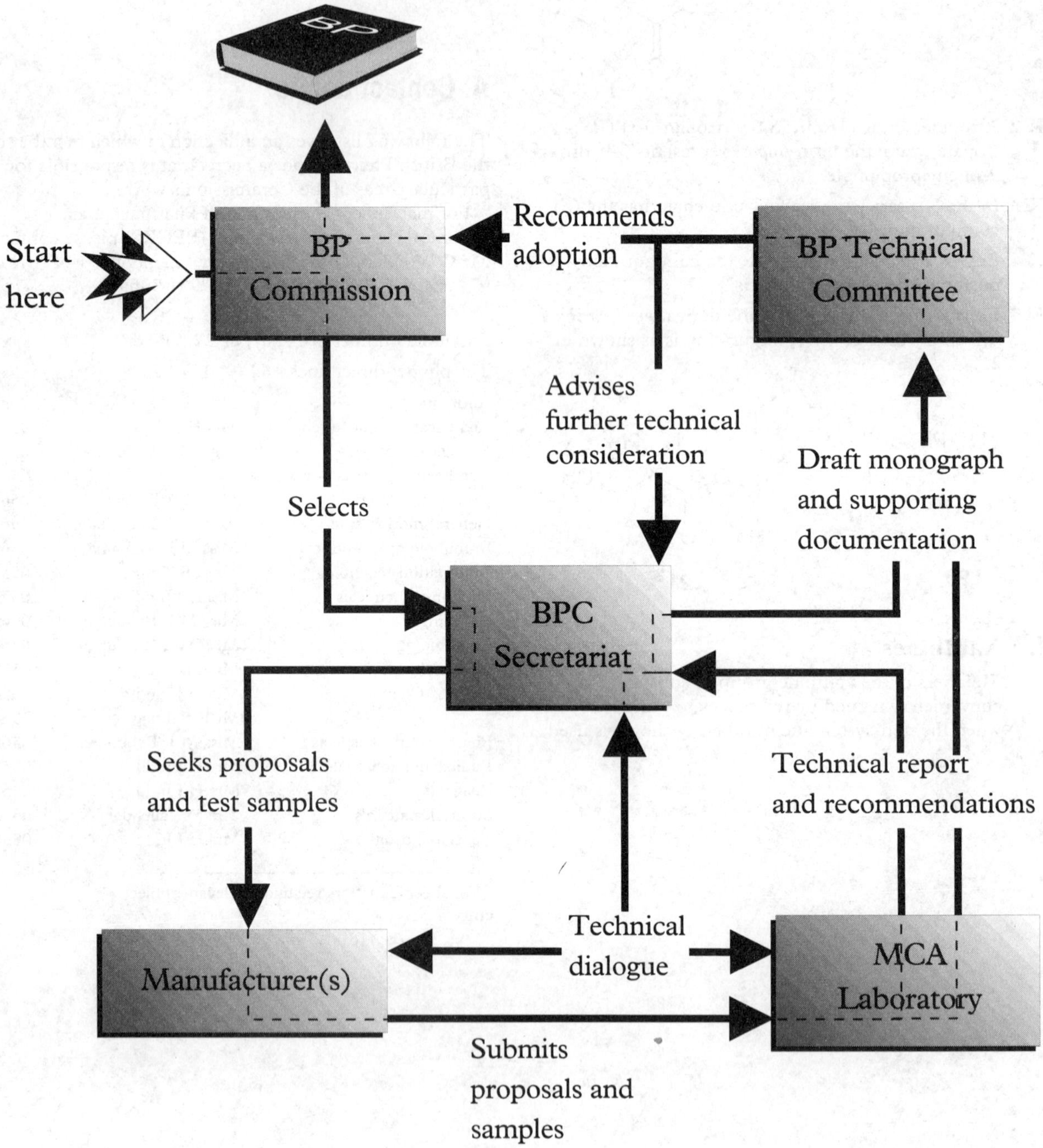

C. Monograph Development: Guidance to Manufacturers

BULK DRUG SUBSTANCES

Each monograph, taken as a whole, should provide a reliable basis for making an independent judgement as to the quality of the substance in the interests of the protection of the public. General guidance as to the types of test required and the level of control considered appropriate can be obtained by reference to current BP monographs for similar chemical entities where such are available. In general any monograph for a bulk drug substance should include the features listed below.

Attention is drawn to the General Notices of the Pharmacopoeia, to the general methods described in the Appendices, to the basis of pharmacopoeial requirements as described in the Introduction and to other information provided in the Supplementary Chapters of the Pharmacopoeia.

1. **Definition/ Description** Brief description of physical form of material, whether hygroscopic, odour if readily apparent. It would be helpful if information concerning polymorphism could be provided (see Supplementary Chapter I B).

2. **Solubility** Solubility in a number of common solvents, expressed quantitatively or using defined BP terms.

3. **Identification** 2 or 3 identification tests including infrared spectrometry where possible/appropriate.

4. **Impurities** (see also Supplementary Chapter I A) Both related substances and any other impurities that may be present in the substance as a result of the method of manufacture or from degradation on storage. It would be helpful to know the nature of such impurities, the reason for their presence, the amounts that may be encountered in material prepared under conditions of good manufacturing practice and the manner in which the proportions may vary on storage. An indication of the toxicity of any impurities in relation to that of the substance itself and methods for their detection and control would enable the Committee preparing the monograph to decide whether control tests are necessary and, if so, the methods and limits to be applied.

Impurities other than related substances that might require control include inorganic impurities, heavy metals (especially for chronically administered or high-dosage materials) and residues of solvents and reagents used during synthesis and purification. Non-specific purity tests such as light absorption, specific optical rotation and sulphated ash should also be considered.

5. **Transparency** In keeping with BP policy on monograph transparency a suitable statement will be added to appropriate new monographs for medicinal substances giving the identities of impurities known to be limited by the specifications. It is to be emphasised that such statements are not intended to be exclusive and other, unnamed impurities may also be limited. Manufacturers are requested to provide information for such statements (see paragraph 4 above).

6. **Assay** Method and proposed limits calculated with reference to the anhydrous, dried or solvent-free material as appropriate. For bulk drug substances, it has been BP policy *generally* to use a robust and precise method of assay (such as titration) rather than a specific, but sometimes less precise, stability-indicating method (such as liquid chromatography). Wherever possible, control of potential impurities is provided separately by means of specific impurity tests (see paragraph 4 above). It is appreciated, however, that a manufacturer may use, and therefore propose, a chromatographic method for both related substances and assay. In such circumstances, each case is judged on its merits on the basis of the data provided, which must relate to validated methods. Adequate means of demonstrating system suitability will need to be included in the monograph so that the analyst has an assurance that the results are accurate. As stated above, each monograph, taken as a whole, should provide a reliable basis for making an independent judgement as to the quality of the substance.

7. **Other tests** A test for water or for loss on drying is usually required.

8. **Storage** Any special storage conditions such as protection from light.

9. **Labelling** Any special labelling statements (see Supplementary Chapter I G).

10. **Preparations** Pharmaceutical dosage forms normally available and information on dose.

11. **Samples** A quantity of the material sufficient to carry out in duplicate all the tests and the assay in the proposed specification should be supplied (10 g is usually suitable). This sample should be taken from a typical production batch, that is it should not be specially purified. In addition appropriate amounts of possible impurities should be supplied. Many monographs require the use of one or more reference substances (BPCRS); these are established by the Laboratory before publication of the monograph (see Supplementary Chapter III E).

When sending samples, material safety data sheets that comply with COSHH Regulations should be supplied for all materials including impurities, so that Pharmacopoeia staff are aware of possible hazards when handling these materials.

12. **Validation data** Appropriate and relevant validation data relating to the proposed analytical procedures and methodology should be provided (see Supplementary Chapter III D). This information will be kept confidential to the BP Secretariat and Laboratory. However, manufacturers will be requested to allow wider consideration of such data by the relevant Committee(s) of the British Pharmacopoeia Commission should this become necessary during the monograph elaboration process.

FORMULATED PREPARATIONS

Each monograph, taken as a whole, should provide a reliable basis for making an independent judgement as to the quality of the preparation in the interests of the protection of the public. General guidance as to the types of test required and the level of control considered appropriate can be obtained by reference to current BP monographs for the same dosage form of similar chemical entities where such are available. Reference should also be made to any general monograph for the dosage form in question for general requirements and any exceptions to, or modifications of, those requirements noted. In general any monograph for a formulated preparation should include the features listed below.

Attention is drawn to the General Notices of the Pharmacopoeia, to the general methods described in the Appendices, to the basis of pharmacopoeial requirements as described in the Introduction and to other information provided in the Supplementary Chapters of the Pharmacopoeia.

1. **Definition/Description** A definition of the preparation in terms of the active ingredient(s) together with information on its presentation.

For sterile preparations (parenteral, ophthalmic and others) this should include information on the nature of the vehicle; the nature of any additives (eg antimicrobial preservatives, buffers) present; the method of sterilisation. In addition, for parenteral preparations information should be provided on whether it is a solution, a suspension, a dry powder or a concentrate for dilution.

For topical semi-solid preparations this should include information on the type of basis (water-in-oil, oil-in-water, etc) and the particle size of the active ingredient, if significant.

For tablets this should include whether or not they are coated and, if so, the type of coating and whether or not coating is considered essential (with reason).

Information concerning polymorphism should be included where relevant (see Supplementary Chapter I B).

2. **Content statement** Proposed limits as a percentage of the stated content of the active ingredient (see Supplementary Chapter I F).

The purpose of the assay in preparation monographs is to determine whether the content of the active ingredient is within acceptable limits of the labelled claim and the limits are therefore of necessity stated in terms of *the moiety declared on the label*. That is, the same method of expression is used in the content statement as under the headings Assay and Labelling. The preferred means of expression is in terms of the therapeutically active part of the molecule. It should be noted that the mode of expressions chosen for the assay limits in the monograph for the bulk drug substance in no way circumscribes that which may be used in the monograph for the formulation.

3. **Identification** 2 or 3 identification tests – based on those for the parent drug substance, where applicable, with details of any necessary preliminary treatment such as extraction.

4. **Impurities** [As under Bulk drug substances] Additional information on any impurities arising on manufacture or storage of the dosage form.

The tests applied to the bulk drug substance, including those for impurities arising in manufacture of the bulk drug substance, should be applied, wherever possible – with any necessary modification – in order to demonstrate that material of pharmacopoeial quality has been used in making the formulation.

5. **Transparency** In keeping with BP policy on monograph transparency a suitable statement will be added to appropriate new monographs for formulated preparations giving the identities of impurities known to be limited by the specifications. It is to be emphasised that such statements are not intended to be exclusive and other, unnamed impurities may also be limited. Manufacturers are requested to provide information for such statements (see paragraph 4 above).

6. **Assay** The method of assay will not necessarily be that used for the bulk drug substance. For formulations a specific, stability-indicating method is preferred.

7. **Other tests** Tests such as pH and clarity and colour of solution may be necessary depending on the type of dosage form. In addition, for single-dose preparations a test for uniformity of content and, in the case of solid dosage forms, a dissolution test may be required (see Supplementary Chapter I E).

8. **Storage** Any special storage conditions/containers.

9. **Labelling** Any special labelling statements (see Supplementary Chapter I G).

Please provide sample labels, outer packages, leaflets and a copy of the relevant summary of product characteristics (SPC) or data sheet.

10. **Strengths available/Dose** While no longer included in the published monograph, this information is of assistance during monograph development.

11. **Samples** A quantity of the formulation sufficient to carry out in duplicate all the tests (including those under 6) and the assay in the proposed specification should be supplied. Samples should be taken from a typical production batch.

The following suggested quantities are provided as a rough guide of the order of sample size for each strength of different dosage forms:

Solid single-dose formulations (Tablets, Capsules, etc) 100 units

Liquid formulations

i)	Topical and Oral formulations	100 ml
ii)	Parenteral formulations	50 ml
	Semi-solid topical formulations	50 to 100 g

In addition appropriate amounts of possible impurities (arising from synthesis or degradation) should be supplied. Many monographs require the use of one or more reference substances (BPCRS); these are established by the Laboratory before publication of the monograph (see Supplementary Chapter III E).

When sending samples, material safety data sheets that comply with COSHH Regulations should be supplied for all materials including impurities, so that Pharmacopoeia staff are aware of possible hazards when handling these materials.

12. **Validation data** Appropriate and relevant validation data relating to the proposed analytical procedures and methodology should be provided routinely (see Supplementary Chapter III D). This information will be kept confidential to the BP Secretariat and Laboratory. However, manufacturers will be requested to allow wider consideration of such data by the relevant Committee(s) of the British Pharmacopoeia Commission should this become necessary during the monograph elaboration process.

D. Monograph Development: Methods of Analysis

1. This supplementary chapter concerns the methods described in the Pharmacopoeia for the analysis of medicinal and pharmaceutical substances, pharmaceutical dosage forms and other articles. It provides information on

the development, validation and use of pharmacopoeial methods so that users of the Pharmacopoeia may understand the purpose and limitations of a monograph and to guide manufacturers and other users when participating in the development of new monographs and the revision of existing monographs.

2. The chapter does not set out the nature and extent of validation required in particular instances. Guidelines on such matters with respect to product registration are available from other sources such as the International Conference on Harmonisation (ICH) (Commission of the European Communities, III/5626/93 Final) and the World Health Organization (World Health Organization Technical Report Series 823, Annex 5, 1992). The terms used throughout the chapter are as defined in the ICH Guidelines and a glossary taken from these guidelines is provided as an Annex.

Method origin

3. Proposals for new or revised methods for inclusion are often provided by manufacturers and other users of the Pharmacopoeia either in response to a request from the Secretariat or Laboratory or, for revised methods, when a published method has been found to be unsuitable for any reason. A method may become unsuitable when, for example, a reagent or piece of apparatus is no longer readily available, knowledge of the material has increased, regulatory requirements have altered or a more specific or sensitive test has been developed.

4. Any method that is to be considered for inclusion in a monograph has to be suitable for pharmacopoeial purposes and, wherever possible, accompanied by appropriate validation data. A pharmacopoeial monograph applies throughout the shelf-life of a formulated preparation or throughout the period of use of a medicinal or pharmaceutical substance. A pharmacopoeial method therefore, should be able to be carried out by a competent analyst using readily available apparatus and reagents.

4.1 Guidance on the suitability of any method for inclusion in the Pharmacopoeia may be obtained by reference to the General Notices (in particular, those dealing with official standards, excipients, identification and assays and tests) and Supplementary Chapter I concerning the basis of pharmacopoeial requirements. Each monograph, taken as a whole, should provide a reliable basis for making an independent judgement as to the quality of an article in the interests of the protection of the public.

4.2 Other than in exceptional circumstances, methods should not specify the use of apparatus that is not widely available in reasonably equipped laboratories nor should they require extensive additional training of laboratory staff. An example of a case where a specialised method is specified is in the GC-MS test for traces of the toxic impurity 2,3,7,8-tetrachlorodibenzo-*p*-dioxin in Hexachlorophane. Reagents and reference materials required for a proposed pharmacopoeial method should be generally available from the common sources of supply in the United Kingdom or a manufacturer should be able to supply sufficient quantity for use as a British Pharmacopoeia Chemical Reference Substance (BPCRS). The method should be described in sufficient detail that a competent analyst is able to repeat it.

4.3 Methods proposed by manufacturers should have been adequately validated in accordance with appropriate guidelines (paragraph 2 refers). Exceptionally, full validation data may not be available in some circumstances. For example, not all contributors to the Pharmacopoeia are able to demonstrate the *specificity* of a test method for application to a monograph for a formulated preparation since the nature of the excipients may be unknown; in this case a note of the extent of any validation carried out, with its limitations, is helpful.

4.4 It is of particular importance that a pharmacopoeial method is *robust* and *reproducible*. Data that demonstrate the transferability of a method are, therefore, especially helpful.

Method elaboration

5. All proposals for new and revised methods for publication are carefully examined. The nature and extent of the evaluation is determined by a number of factors including the following:

whether the proposal is for a new monograph or for revision of an existing monograph,

extent of validation and batch data available,

how many specifications and/or samples are available for examination,

complexity of the proposed method.

6. The evaluation of methods is carried out by the Commission's advisory Committees and Consultative Groups, the Secretariat and the Laboratory; practical evaluation is included in many cases. If necessary, more extensive practical work is carried out in consultation with the proposer of the method. Such practical work may be necessary, for example, where a proposed method is not directly applicable to other sources of the material or preparation or is shown to be insufficiently *robust* for pharmacopoeial use.

7. After initial evaluation, the method is drafted in the style of the Pharmacopoeia and those known to have an interest in the material or preparation are invited to comment. If necessary, further modifications may be made to the method and the consultation process repeated before the method is published. A diagrammatic representation of the process of monograph elaboration is provided as Supplementary Chapter III B.

Published methods

8. The user can expect that published methods:

are suitable for the purpose for which they are described in the Pharmacopoeia,have been evaluated and, where necessary, modified as described in the preceding section, have been shown to be adequately validated, as appropriate to the type of test, and include tests to demonstrate the continuing suitability of the method, where necessary, are described in sufficient detail that a competent analyst can perform the test using readily available apparatus and reagents and that any necessary reference materials are available,will be reviewed and revised when experience shows this to be necessary.

9. The user cannot, however, assume that a method forming part of a pharmacopoeial monograph will have been applied to all sources of a raw material or to all formulations of a dosage form currently available. The user is responsible for confirming that the method is applicable to the particular material being examined. It is essential that a manufacturer carries out sufficient checks to demonstrate that, for example, impurities arising from a new route of synthesis are controlled by the methods described in the monograph or that the excipients in a

formulated preparation do not interfere with any of the tests in a monograph. It should be noted that an article cannot claim to be of pharmacopoeial quality unless it can be shown to comply with all of the tests specified in a monograph (see General Notice on Official Standards). The British Pharmacopoeia Commission welcomes constructive comments from users on the tests of the Pharmacopoeia and it is through such feedback that revision of the tests is initiated.

ANNEX

Glossary of terms used for Analytical Validation

The definitions are taken from the ICH Guidelines referred to in paragraph 2.

Specificity is the ability to assess unequivocally the analyte in the presence of components which may be expected to be present.

Accuracy expresses the closeness of agreement between the value which is accepted either as a conventional true value or an accepted reference value and the value found.

Precision expresses the closeness of agreement (degree of scatter) between a series of measurements obtained from multiple sampling of the same homogeneous sample under the prescribed conditions.

Repeatability expresses the precision under the same operating conditions over a short interval of time.

Reproducibility expresses the precision between laboratories.

Detection limit is the lowest amount of analyte in a sample which can be detected, but not necessarily quantitated, as an exact value.

Quantitation limit is the lowest amount of analyte in a sample which can be quantitatively determined with suitable precision and accuracy.

Linearity of an analytical procedure is its ability, within a given range, to obtain test results which are directly proportional to the concentration of analyte in the sample.

Range of an analytical procedure is the interval between the upper and lower concentration of analyte in the sample (including these concentrations) for which it has been demonstrated that the analytical procedure has a suitable level of precision, accuracy and linearity.

Robustness of an analytical procedure is a measure of its capacity to remain unaffected by small, but deliberate, variations in method parameters and provides an indication of its reliability during normal use.

E. British Pharmacopoeia Chemical Reference Substances (BPCRS)

1. The current list of BPCRS may be found in Appendix I E. The quantity of material supplied is sufficent to carry out twice each of the tests in which it is used.

Establishment

2. The establishment of a new British Pharmacopoeia Chemical Reference Substance is based on scientific necessity following advice from the British Pharmacopoeia Commission's analytical committees. The following criteria are taken into account when determining whether a new BPCRS is required.

Availability of the material A commercially available reagent is specified wherever it is found to be suitable and justified.

Existence of a European Pharmacopoeia Chemical Reference Substance (EPCRS) A new BPCRS is established only when an existing EPCRS is not suitable for the purpose. (For example, if a reference substance with a declared content is required for the assay of a BP dosage form monograph where the EPCRS is used only for identification in the bulk drug substance monograph.)

Analytical convenience Wherever possible, either the same EPCRS or the same BPCRS is specified throughout any one monograph.

Monitoring and Replacement

3. All substances used for quantitative analyses are re-tested every three years and materials used for qualitative analysis every five years unless experience has shown that more frequent testing is necessary.

4. When a BPCRS is due for replacement (because of a fall in quality or exhaustion), a review of the use of the material and the number of units supplied is carried out. If an EPCRS that is suitable for the BP application has been established since the last review, the BPCRS is normally replaced by the EPCRS with publication of the necessary amendments in the affected monographs.

Continued Availability

5. When a monograph is omitted from the Pharmacopoeia the last published monograph remains the legal standard. As the usual reason for omission is low and declining use or withdrawal of the material from the market, demand for any associated reference substances from within the United Kingdom is normally low.

6. It is not possible to maintain reference substances for omitted materials indefinitely and, for materials no longer marketed in the United Kingdom, it is difficult to obtain replacement stocks. As a service to analysts, reference substances for monographs omitted from the current edition of the Pharmacopoeia are normally retained for about five years from the date of publication of the current edition unless the material becomes unsatisfactory or the supply is exhausted before that date.

7. Demand is monitored and any significant increase in demand for a reference substance for an omitted monograph is noted. If such increased demand appears to stem from a renewed interest in the medicinal or pharmaceutical product, consideration may be given to reinstating the monograph in the Pharmacopoeia.

Supplementary Chapter IV

European Pharmacopoeia

This Supplementary Chapter provides information concerning the European Pharmacopoeia.

A. Membership of the European Pharmacopoeia Commission

The membership of the European Pharmacopoeia Commission on 1 September 1997 was as follows:

Chairman:	D Schnädelbach
Austria *(A)*:	K Liszka, E Luszczak, E Schlederer, H Halbich-Zankl*, K Pfleger*, J Trenker*
Belgium *(B)*:	L Angenot, J Hoogmartens, P Jacqmain, J De Beer*, L Delattre*, A Vlietinck*
Croatia *(CR)*:	L Stefanini Oresic
Cyprus *(CY)*:	E Kkolos
Denmark *(DK)*:	P Frandsen, P Helboe, H G Kristensen, K Brønnum-Hansen*, S Grell*, A Sørensen*
Finland *(SF)*:	P Paronen, K Sinivuo, L Turakka, A Huikari*
France *(F)*:	J P Fournier, M H Loulergue, A Nicolas, H J De Jong*, M Gachon*, C Nicolas*
Germany *(D)*:	D Krüger, U Kullmann, J Mohr, A Baeckmann*, S Ebel*, R Kurth*
Greece *(GR)*:	M Koupparis, S Philianos, A Tsoka
Iceland *(ISL)*:	E Magnusson, V G Skulason
Ireland *(IRL)*:	T McGuinn, M Morris, J O'Riordan
Italy *(I)*:	A Cassonne, M Cignitti, A Farina, E Ciranni*, A Macri* G Orefici*
Luxembourg *(L)*:	J Genoux-Hames, M Backes-Lies*, J L Robert*
The Netherlands *(NL)*:	J W Dorpema, J Nienhuis, P H Vree, D de Kaste*, H H M Tummers*, H L Vos*
Norway *(N)*:	G Brugaard, V Holten, R Winsnes,
Portugal *(P)*:	J M Correia Neves Sousa Lobo, R M R Morgado, L V Nogueira Prista*
Slovakia *(SLK)*:	M Chalabala, R Martincova, J Slany, D Grancai*, J Lucansky*, L Sovik*
Slovenia *(SLO)*:	M Cvelbar, D Hrobat, S Primozic
Spain *(E)*:	A Vardulaki
Sweden *(S)*:	M Ek, I Sjöholm, J Vessman, L Sjödin*
Switzerland *(CH)*:	U Salzmann, E Wachberger, S Weber Brunner, V Eckert*, I Kapetanidis*, H Partenheimer*
Turkey *(T)*:	K Akalin, E Izgü
United Kingdom *(UK)*:	D H Calam, D Ganderton, R C Hutton, J A Goldsmith*, J M Midgley*, M L Rabouhans*
Former Yugoslav Republic of Macedonia *(MAC)*:	N Poposki, A Simov
European Union *(EU)*:	B Hughes, S Fairchild, M F Lutz
	*alternate member
Observers:	
Australia:	E Walker
Bulgaria:	L Ljubomirova Kostova
Canada:	G L Mattok
China:	Chen Yin-Qing
Czech Republic:	J Portych
Estonia:	M Jaagola
Hungary:	J J Liptak
Lithuania:	A Gendrolis
Poland:	W Wieniawski
Roumania:	D Enach
Syrian Arab Republic:	H Abboud
World Health Organization (WHO):	S Kopp-Kubel

MEMBERSHIP OF GROUPS OF EXPERTS OF THE EUROPEAN PHARMACOPOEIA COMMISSION

The membership of the Groups of Experts on 1 September 1997 was as follows:

Group No 1CM: Microbial Contamination — D Krüger *(Chairman)*, J Dony *(B)*, H P Riniker *(CH)*, H Seyfarth *(D)*, L V Frederiksen,*(DK)*, J C Darbord*(F)*, J Lavdiotis *(GR)*, G Orefici *(I)*, H van Doorne *(NL)*, L Hamilton *(S)*, A L Davison *(UK)*

Group No 1L: Limulus Amoebocyte Lysate Test *(LAL)* — C Borensztejn, *(B)*, D Witthauer *(CH)*, D Krüger *(D)*, V Montejo *(E)*, J Giroux *(F)*, L Bellentani *(I)*, A M Gommer *(NL)*, L Sjödin*(S)*, S Poole *(UK)*

Group No 3: P Jacqmain *(Chairman)*

Group No 6: Biological Substances — J W Dorpema *(Chairman)*, A Lauwers *(B)*, H Windemann *(CH)*, T Doll *(D)*, S Grell *(DK)*, J C Diez-Masa *(E)*, A Bayol *(F)*, M Vannini *(I)*, R W Skare *(N)*, P M J M Jongen *(NL)*, L Sjödin *(S)*, J J Himberg *(SF)*, F Izgü *(T)*, A F Bristow *(UK)*

Group No 6B: Human Blood and Blood Products — I Sjöholm *(Chairman)*, H Igel *(A)*, D Van Gysegem *(B)*, N Chariatte *(CH)*, R Seitz *(D)*, E Sandberg *(DK)*, C Alonso Verduras *(E)*, L Mouillot *(F)*, M Orlando *(I)*, J O'Riordan *(IRL)*, M K Fagerhol *(N)*, F G Korse *(NL)*, B Karlen *(S)*, R Soininen *(SF)*, T J Snape *(UK)*, A M Padilla Marroquin *(WHO)*

Group No 6I: Insulin Preparations — G Seipke *(D)*, M Møller Christensen *(DK)*, M V Griffoul *(F)*, P M J M Jongen *(NL)*, J Olivie *(NL)*, L Sjödin *(S)*, A F Bristow *(UK)*

Group No 7: Antibiotics — D H Calam *(Chairman)*, P Inama *(A)*, J Hoogmartens *(B)*, E Wachberger *(CH)*, C P Christiansen *(D)*, L Thomsen *(DK)*, E Porqueras *(E)*, S Guyomard *(F)*, S Tedeschi *(I)*, C van der Vlies *(NL)*, K Gröningsson *(S)*, F Aktan *(T)*, R C Hutton *(UK)*

Group No 8: Sutures — D Ganderton *(Chairman)*, B Hinsch *(D)*, P R Montenoise *(F)*, G S Groot *(NL)*, P Newlands *(UK)*

Group No 9: Inorganic Chemistry — S Ebel *(Chairman)*, J M Kauffman *(B)*, H Altorfer *(CH)*, M Türck *(D)*, M Mazza *(F)*, G Zanni *(I)*, A D Förch *(NL)*, S Holmqvist *(S)*, N Noyanalpan *(T)*, A Rixon *(UK)*

Sub-group No 9G: Medicinal Gases — H Tschiersky-Schöneburg *(Chairman)*, H Müller *(D)*, P Andre *(F)*, M B Marie *(F)*, V Zurletti *(I)*, J den Hartigh *(NL)*, E Sundström *(S)*, P Henrys *(UK)*

Group No 10A: Organic Chemistry—Synthetic Products — J P Fournier *(Chairman)*, J Bonnard *(B)*, E Schläfli *(CH)*, J Iwan *(D)*, K Brønnum-Hansen *(DK)*, A Martin-Gonzalez Hernan *(E)*, G Gernez *(F)*, F La Torre *(I)*, L Borka *(N)*, O M van Berkel-Geldof *(NL)*, K G Svensson *(S)*, B M Everett *(UK)*

Group No 10B: Organic Chemistry—Synthetic Products — S Weber Brunner *(Chairman)*, J Trenker *(A)*, J F H Van Rompay *(B)*, E Keller *(CH)*, V Schulze *(D)*, A Sørensen *(DK)*, J M de Ciurana Gay *(E)*, H J de Jong *(F)*, E Souli *(GR)*, L Valvo *(I)*, J L Robert *(L)*, E A Hagen *(N)*, A van den Hoek *(NL)*, M Ek *(S)*, K Sinivuo *(SF)*, A Holbrook *(UK)*

Group No 10C: Organic Chemistry—Synthetic Products — J Vessman *(Chairman)*, J de Beer *(B)*, H Ludwig *(CH)*, W Arz *(D)*, M Handlos*(DK)*, D Mauleon *(E)*, T Bourquin *(F)*, G Colli *(I)*, F J van der Vaart *(NL)*, K J Leiper *(UK)*

Group No 11: Organic Chemistry—Natural Products — H Partenheimer *(Chairman)*, J Crommen *(B)*, M Richter *(CH)*, A Müller *(D)*, J Ruiz Combalia *(E)*, M Gachon *(F)*, V Hartofylax *(GR)*, C Galeffi *(I)*, K Øydvin *(N)*, D de Kaste*(NL)*, E Ehrin *(S)*, H Can Baser *(T)*, A G Davidson *(UK)*

Sub-group No 11A: Vitamins A and D — B Borsje *(Chairman)*, E Wachberger *(CH)*, E Ohst *(D)*, Y Roché *(F)*, G G L M Feenstra-Bielders *(NL)*, G F Phillips *(UK)*

Sub-group No 11C: Cellulose Ethers — G Rotzler *(Chairman)*, E Doelker *(CH)*, W Schmidt *(D)*, J Rabiant *(F)*, M Pedrani *(I)*, E Izeboud *(NL)*, L J Blackwell *(UK)*

Group No 12: Galenical Products — H G Kristensen *(Chairman)*, L Delattre *(B)*, J Schrank *(CH)*, W Pohler *(D)*, A Velazquez Carvajal *(E)*, M Veillard *(F)*, A Gazzaniga *(I)*, A Simov *(MAC)*, J Karlsen *(N)*, H Burger *(NL)*, S Wahlgren *(S)*, L Turakka *(SF)*, K Canefe *(T)*, M C R Johnson *(UK)*

Group No 13: Phytochemistry — M H Loulergue *(Chairman)*, T Kartnig *(A)*, A Vlietinck *(B)*, O Sticher *(CH)*, G Harnischfeger *(D)*, I Fouraste *(F)*, S Philianos *(GR)*, A de Pasquale *(I)*, J H Zwaving *(NL)*, L Bohlin *(S)*, E Sezik *(T)*, K Helliwell *(UK)*

Group No 13H: Fatty Oils and Derivatives	A Vlietinck *(Chairman)*, M Thevenin *(CH)*, V Bühler *(D)*, G Nain *(F)*, S Philianos *(GR)*, M Pedrani *(I)*, J H Zwaving *(NL)*, L Svensson *(S)*, M R Harrison *(UK)*
Group No 14: Radioactive Compounds	C J Fallais *(Chairman)*, A Verbruggen *(B)*, C Wastiel *(CH)*, R Suchi *(D)*, B Pedersen*(DK)*, M Roca *(E)*, L Merlin *(F)*, P Salvadori *(I)*, P O Bremer *(N)*, M Kroon *(NL)*, G Antoni *(S)*, R D Pickett *(UK)*
Group No 15: Sera and Vaccines	R Winsnes *(Chairman)*, W Maurer *(A)*, R Dobbelaer *(B)*, F Reigel *(CH)*, M Schwanig *(D)*, A Bjerregaard *(DK)*, F Fuchs *(F)*, L Nicoletti *(I)*, H H M Tummers *(NL)*, T Kuronen *(SF)*, I G S Furminger *(UK)*, E Griffiths *(WHO)*
Group No 15V: Veterinary Sera and Vaccines	J M Person *(Chairman)*, J P Binder *(A)*, M Pensaert *(B)*, L Bruckner *(CH)*, M Moos *(D)*, R Hoff-Jørgensen *(DK)*, P van Houwelingen *(EEC)*, C Guittré *(F)*, M Tollis *(I)*, P J O'Connor *(IRL)*, A Lillehaug (*N*), H H Lensing *(NL)*, A M T Lee *(UK)*
Group No 16: Plastic Containers for Pharmaceutical Use	G Gernez *(Chairman)*, P Hoet *(B)*, U Schönhausen *(CH)*, M E Spingler *(CH)*, R Rößler *(D)*, D Baylocq-Ferrier *(F)*, L Gramiccioni Valsecchi *(I)*, L R Berkenbosch *(NL)*, A Arbin *(S)*, N Hasirci *(T)*, I D Newton *(UK)*,

B. Dates of Implementation

Under the 1964 Convention[1] on the Elaboration of a European Pharmacopoeia the standards of the European Pharmacopoeia are required to take precedence over the standards of the national pharmacopoeia of the contracting parties, thus ensuring a common standard. In the United Kingdom this has been achieved by means of section 65(7) of the Medicines Act 1968. In addition to the United Kingdom the countries party to the Convention are Austria, Belgium, Bosnia-Herzegovina, Croatia, Cyprus, Denmark, Finland, France, Germany, Greece, Iceland, Ireland, Italy, Luxembourg, The Netherlands, Norway, Portugal, Slovakia, Slovenia, Spain, Sweden, Switzerland, Turkey and the Former Yugoslav Republic of Macedonia. The European Community is also party to the Convention.

The current edition of the European Pharmacopoeia is the Third Edition the main volume of which was published in 1996 and the first supplement to which was published in 1997. The date of entry into force of each publication is agreed by the member states of the Convention. For new texts and monographs the agreed date is the latest date by which all member states must have implemented the standard but for replacement texts and monographs the standard enters into force on the same day in all states party to the Convention. In the United Kingdom implementation is by means of a notice published in the London, Belfast and Edinburgh Gazettes. For convenience, dates of implementation are also publicised through other channels.

The date of entry into force of the monographs of the main volume of the Third Edition of the European Pharmacopoeia is 1 January 1997 and of those in the first supplement is 1 January 1998.

To provide the user of the British Pharmacopoeia with a comprehensive collection of pharmacopoeial standards applicable in the United Kingdom the monographs of the European Pharmacopoeia are included in the British Pharmacopoeia (see the General Notice on the European Pharmacopoeia).

Monographs of the European Pharmacopoeia relevant only to veterinary medicine are published in the British Pharmacopoeia (Veterinary) 1993.

Where the title of the monograph entry included in the British Pharmacopoeia is different from the English title of the European Pharmacopoeia monograph (see Appendix XXI B), the latter is also given in the italicised introduction to the entry.

The Convention on the Elaboration of a European Pharmacopoeia (European Treaty Series No. 50; UK Treaty Series No.32 (1974) CMND 5763) as amended by the Protocol (European Treaty Series No. 134; UK Treaty Series No. MISC16 (1990) CMND 1133)

C. Certification Scheme

The scheme is operated in accordance with the procedures described in Council of Europe Resolution AP-CSP(93)5 which is available from the European Pharmacopoeia Secretariat, BP 907, F 67029, Strasbourg, Cedex 1, France. Additional information, including a list of certificates granted, is published from time to time in Pharmeuropa (for example, Pharmeuropa 9.2, June 1997).

The certificate is a '*Certificate of Suitability of a Monograph of the European Pharmacopoeia*'. It certifies that the relevant Ph. Eur. monograph adequately controls the drug substance as manufactured by the company concerned at the time that the certificate is granted (mainly that the impurity tests are adequate to control the impurity profile associated with the particular source/route of synthesis). It is *not a certificate of compliance.* It does not certify that the drug substance as manufactured by the company concerned at the time that the certificate is granted complies with the requirements of the relevant Ph. Eur. monograph.

The certificate is intended to facilitate the licensing process. It can be used to simplify the data required within the Control of starting materials section of an application as stated in the amended Annex to European Community Directive 75/318/EEC and the associated EC Guideline on Requirements in relation to active substances (*Rules Governing Medicinal Products in the European Community*, Volume I, page 45 and Volume III, Addendum No. 2, May 1992, page 321). The Certification Scheme is intended to operate in an analogous fashion to that for Drug Master Files (DMFs) for which it is an alternative.

Index

A

Abbreviated Titles, A301
Abbreviated Titles, Status of, 7, 1397
Abbreviations, A313
Abbreviations and Symbols, 24, 1414
Abdominal Pad, X-Ray Detectable, xxvi
Abnormal Toxicity, Test for, A219
Absolute Alcohol, **548**
Absolute Ethanol, A41
Absolute Ethanol R1, A41
Absorbable Braided Sutures, Sterile Synthetic, 2159
Absorbable Dusting Powder, *see Sterilisable Maize Starch*
Absorbable Gelatin Sponge, xxvi
Absorbable Monofilament Sutures, Sterile Synthetic, **2161**
Absorbance, Definition of, A116
Absorbance, Specific, Definition of, A116
Absorbent Cotton, **2155**
Absorbent Cotton, Sterile, **2156**
Absorbent Dressing, Perforated Film, xxvi
Absorbent Viscose Wadding, **2156**
Absorbent Viscose Wadding, Sterile, **2157**
Absorption Spectrophotometry, Atomic, A119
Absorption Spectrophotometry, Ultraviolet and Visible, A116
Acacia, **31**, A13
Acacia, Powdered, xxv, *see also Acacia*
Acacia Solution, A13
Acacia, Spray-dried, **32**
Acebutolol Hydrochloride, **32**
Aceclofenac, **33**
Acenocoumarol, **35**, S5, S88
Acenocoumarol Tablets, **1465**
Acesulfame Potassium, **35**
Acetaldehyde, A13
Acetaldehyde Standard Solution (100 ppm C_2H_4O), A98
Acetaldehyde Standard Solution (100 ppm C_2H_4O) R1, A98
Acetamide, A13
Acetate Buffer pH 2.45, A101
Acetate Buffer pH 2.8, A101
Acetate Buffer pH 3.4, A101
Acetate Buffer pH 3.5, A101
Acetate Buffer pH 3.7, A101
Acetate Buffer pH 4.4, A101
Acetate Buffer pH 4.6, A101
Acetate Buffer pH 5.0, A101
Acetate Buffer pH 6.0, A101
Acetate Buffer Solution pH 4.4, *see acetate buffer pH 4.4*
Acetate Buffer Solution pH 4.6, *see acetate buffer pH 4.6*
Acetate Buffer Solution pH 4.7, A101
Acetate Buffer Solution pH 6.0, *see acetate buffer pH 6.0*
Acetate-edetate Buffer Solution pH 5.5, A101
Acetates, Reactions of, A147
Acetazolamide, **37**, S5
Acetazolamide Tablets, **1465**
Acetic Acid, **38**, A13, *see also acetic acid VS*
Acetic Acid (6 per cent), **39**
Acetic Acid (33 per cent), **38**
Acetic Acid, Anhydrous, A13
Acetic Acid, Deuterated, A33
Acetic Acid, Dilute, **39**, A13
Acetic Acid, Glacial, **38**, A13
Acetic Acid VS, A92
Acetic–Ammonia Buffer pH 3.7, Ethanolic, *see buffer solution pH 3.7*
Acetic Anhydride, A14
Acetic Anhydride Solution R1, A14
Acetic Bromine Solution, A24
Acetohexamide, xxv
Acetohexamide Tablets, xxv
Acetone, **39**, A14
Acetone, Deuterated, A33
Acetone Solution, Buffered, A101
Acetone-dried Ox Brain, A64
Acetonitrile, A14
Acetonitrile for Chromatography A14
Acetyl Chloride, A14
O-Acetyl Groups in Polysaccharide Vaccines, Test for, A234
Acetyl Groups, Reactions of, A147
Acetyl Value, Determination of, A171
Acetylacetamide, A14
Acetylacetone, A14
Acetylacetone Reagent R1, A14
N-Acetyl-ε-caprolactam, A14
Acetylcholine Chloride, A14
Acetylcysteine, **40**, S6
N-Acetyl-L-cysteine, A14
Acetylcysteine Injection, **1466**
Acetyleugenol A14
N-Acetylneuraminic Acid, A14
Acetylsalicylic Acid, *see Aspirin*
Acetylsalicylic Acid Tablets, **1492**
N-Acetyltryptophan, A14
Acetyltyrosine Ethyl Ester, A14
Acetyltyrosine Ethyl Ester, 0.2M, A14
Aciclovir, **42**
Aciclovir Cream, **1466**
Aciclovir Eye Ointment, **1467**
Aciclovir Intravenous Infusion, **1467**
Aciclovir Oral Suspension, **1468**
Aciclovir Sodium for Intravenous Infusion, **1467**
Aciclovir Tablets, **1469**
Acid Aluminium Oxide for Chromatography, Activated, A16
Acid Blue 83, A14
Acid Blue 90, A14
Acid Blue 92, A14
Acid Blue 92 Solution, A14
Acid Gentian Mixture, **1707**
Acid Gentian Oral Solution, **1707**
Acid Potassium Iodobismuthate Solution, A72
Acid Value, Determination of, A171
Acid-insoluble Ash, Determination of, A184
Acid-washed Diatomaceous Support, A34
Acidified Chloroform, A29
Acidified Dichloromethane, A35
Acidified Methanol, A57
Acidified Methylene Chloride, *see acidified dichloromethane*
Acknowledgements, xxiii
Acrylamide, A14
Action and Use Statements, Status of, 15, 1405
Activated Acid Aluminium Oxide for Chromatography A16
Activated Attapulgite, **127**
Activated Charcoal, **302**, A28
Activated Zinc, A91
Active Moiety, A331
Additions to the British Pharmacopoeia, xv, xxiii
Adenine, **43**
Adenosine, A14
Adhesive Bandage, Elastic, xxvi
Adhesive Bandage, Titanium Dioxide Elastic, xxvi
Adhesive Bandage, Ventilated Elastic, xxvi
Adhesive Dressing, Elastic, xxvi
Adhesive Film Dressing, Vapour-permeable, xxvi
Adrenaline, S6, S46
Adrenaline Acid Tartrate, **45**
Adrenaline Acid Tartrate/Epinephrine Acid Tartrate, **45**
Adrenaline Eye Drops, Neutral/ Epinephrine Eye Drops, Neutral, **1469**
Adrenaline Eye Drops/Epinephrine Eye Drops, **1469**
Adrenaline Injection 1 in 10,000, Dilute/ Epinephrine Injection 1 in 10,000, Dilute, **1470**
Adrenaline Injection, Bupivacaine and/ Epinephrine Injection, Bupivacaine and, **1528**
Adrenaline Injection/Epinephrine Injection, **1470**
Adrenaline Injection, Lidocaine and/ Epinephrine Injection, Lidocaine and, **1778**
Adrenaline Solution/Epinephrine Solution, **1471**
Adrenaline Tartrate, *see Adrenaline Acid Tartrate/Epinephrine Acid Tartrate*
Adrenaline Tartrate Injection/ Epinephrine Tartrate Injection **1470**
Adrenaline Tartrate Solution/ Epinephrine Tartrate Solution, **1471**
Adrenaline/Epinephrine, **44**
Adsorbed Diphtheria and Tetanus Vaccine, **2046**
Adsorbed Diphtheria and Tetanus Vaccine for Adults and Adolescents, **2048**
Adsorbed Diphtheria Prophylactic, **2043**
Adsorbed Diphtheria–Tetanus Prophylactic, **2046**
Adsorbed Diphtheria, Tetanus and Pertussis Vaccine, **2050**
Adsorbed Diphtheria Vaccine, **2043**
Adsorbed Diphtheria Vaccine, Assay of, A229
Adsorbed Diphtheria Vaccine for Adults and Adolescents, **2045**
Adsorbed Diphtheria–Tetanus–Whooping Cough Prophylactic, **2050**

Adsorbed Pertussis Vaccine, *see Pertussis Vaccine*
Adsorbed Tetanus Vaccine, **2085**
Adsorbed Tetanus Vaccine, Assay of, A231
Aerodynamic Assessment of Fine Particles, A194
Aescin, A14
Agar, **46**, A15
Agar, Powdered, xxv
Agarose for Chromatography, A15
Agarose for Chromatography, Cross-linked, A15
Agarose for Chromatography R1, Cross-linked, A15
Agarose for Electrophoresis, A15
Agarose-DEAE for Ion Exchange Chromatography, A15
Agarose/Cross-linked Polyacrylamide, A15
Air, Medical, **47**
Air Permeability, Specific Surface Area by, A257
Airtight Container, A268
β-Alanine, *see 3-aminopropionic acid*
Alanine, **50**, A15
Albumin, *see human albumin solution*
Albumin, **2005**
Albumin, Bovine, A15
Albumin, Human, **2005**
Albumin Injection, Iodinated[^{125}I], **2113**
Albumin Solution, *see human albumin solution R1*
Albumin Solution, **2005**
Albumin Solution, Human, A15
Albumin Solution R1, Human, A15
Alcohol, *see ethanol (96%)*
Alcohol (20 per cent), **550**
Alcohol (25 per cent), **550**
Alcohol (45 per cent), **550**
Alcohol (50 per cent), **550**
Alcohol (60 per cent), **550**
Alcohol (70 per cent), **550**
Alcohol (80 per cent), **549**
Alcohol (90 per cent), **549**
Alcohol (96 per cent), **549**
Alcohol, Absolute, **548**
Alcohol, Aldehyde-free, *see aldehyde-free ethanol;*
Alcohol, Dehydrated, **548**
Alcoholic Calcium Standard Solution (100 ppm Ca), A99
Alcoholic Dimethylaminobenzaldehyde Solution, A37
Alcoholic Hydroxylamine Solution, A49
Alcoholic Iodine Solution, **1758**, A51
Alcoholic Potassium Hydroxide, *see ethanolic potassium hydroxide VS*
Alcoholic Potassium Hydroxide, 2M, A72
Alcoholic Potassium Hydroxide Solution, A72
Alcoholic Potassium Hydroxide Solution R1, A72
Alcoholic Sulphuric Acid, 0.25M, A84
Alcoholic Sulphuric Acid, 2.5M, A84
Aldehyde Dehydrogenase, A15
Aldehyde Dehydrogenase Solution, A15
Aldehyde-free Alcohol, *see aldehyde-free ethanol;*
Aldehyde-free Ethanol (96%), A41
Aldehyde-free Methanol, A57
Aldehydes, Determination of, A174
Aleuritic Acid, A15
Alexandrian Senna, *see Senna Leaf*
Alexandrian Senna Fruit, **1156**
Alexandrian Senna Fruit, Powdered, xxv, *see also Alexandrian Senna Fruit*
Alexandrian Senna Pods, *see Alexandrian Senna Fruit*
Alfentanil Hydrochloride, **51**
Alginate Dressing, xxvi
Alginate Fibre, xxvi
Alginate Packing, xxvi
Alginic Acid, **52**
Alimemazine, S7, S124
Alimemazine Oral Solution, Paediatric,/Trimeprazine Oral Solution, Paediatric, **1472**
Alimemazine Oral Solution, Strong Paediatric,/Trimeprazine Oral Solution, Strong Paediatric, **1472**
Alimemazine Tablets/Trimeprazine Tablets, **1473**
Alimemazine Tartrate/Trimeprazine Tartrate, **53**
Alizarin S, A15
Alizarin S Solution, A15
Alkali-washed Diatomaceous Support, A34
Alkaline Corallin Solution, A32
Alkaline Eye Drops, **1744**
Alkaline Gentian Mixture, **1707**
Alkaline Gentian Oral Solution, **1707**
Alkaline Hydroxylamine Solution, A49
Alkaline Hydroxylamine Solution R1, A49
Alkaline Impurities in Fixed Oils, Test for, A175
Alkaline Potassium Mercuri-iodide Solution, A73
Alkaline Potassium Tetraiodomercurate Solution, A73
Alkaline Pyrogallol Solution, A74
Alkaline Sodium Picrate Solution, A81
Alkaline Tetrazolium Blue Solution, A86
Alkaline-earth Metals, Magnesium and, Limit Test for, A154
Alkaloids, Complete Extraction of, Tests for, A183
Alkaloids, Reactions of, A147
Allergen Products, **54**
Allopurinol, **56**
Allopurinol Tablets, **1473**
Almond Oil, **57**
Almond Oil Ear Drops, **1474**
Almond Oil, Refined, **57**
Aloes, Barbados, **58**
Aloes, Cape, **59**
Aloes, Curaçao, **58**
Aloes Dry Extract, Standardised, **1474**
Aloxiprin, **60**
Aloxiprin Tablets, **1475**
Alpha Benzene Hexachloride CRS, A106
Alpha Tocopherol and Esters, *see under tocopherols*
Alpha Tocopheryl Succinate, S120
Alpha Tocopheryl Succinate Tablets, **1972**
Alprazolam, **61**
Alprenolol Benzoate, **63**
Alprenolol Hydrochloride, **64**
Alteplase for Injection, **66**
Alum, *see aluminium potassium sulphate*
Alum, **70**
Aluminium, A15
Aluminium Acetate Ear Drops, **1476**
Aluminium Acetate Solution, *see Aluminium Acetate Ear Drops*
Aluminium Chloride, A15
Aluminium Chloride Hexahydrate, **70**
Aluminium Chloride Reagent, A15
Aluminium Chloride Solution, **1476**, A15
Aluminium, Complexometric Titration of, A157
Aluminium Glycinate, **71**
Aluminium Hydroxide and Magnesium Trisilicate Tablets, **1791**
Aluminium Hydroxide, Dried, **72**
Aluminium Hydroxide Gel, A15
Aluminium Hydroxide Oral Suspension, **1477**
Aluminium Hydroxide Oral Suspension, Magnesium Hydroxide and, **1605**
Aluminium Hydroxide Tablets, **1478**
Aluminium Hydroxide Tablets, Magnesium Hydroxide and, **1606**
Aluminium in Adsorbed Vaccines, A230
Aluminium, Limit Test for, A151
Aluminium Magnesium Silicate, **72**
Aluminium Nitrate, A16
Aluminium Oxide, Anhydrous, A16
Aluminium Oxide, Basic, A16
Aluminium Oxide, Deactivated, A16
Aluminium Oxide for Chromatography, Activated Acid, A16
Aluminium Oxide G, A16
Aluminium Oxide, Hydrated, *see Dried Aluminium Hydroxide*
Aluminium Paste, Compound, **1476**
Aluminium Phosphate, Dried, **73**
Aluminium Potassium Sulphate, **70**, A16
Aluminium Powder, **73**
Aluminium Salts, Reactions of, A147
Aluminium Standard Solution (2 ppm Al), A98
Aluminium Standard Solution (10 ppm Al), A98
Aluminium Standard Solution (200 ppm Al), A98
Aluminium Sulphate, **74**, A16
Amantadine, S7
Amantadine Capsules, **1478**
Amantadine Hydrochloride, **75**
Amantadine Oral Solution, **1479**
Amaranth S, A16
Amaranth Solution, A16
Amethocaine Hydrochloride and Preparations, *see under Tetracaine*
Amfetamine Sulphate, **76**
Amidotrizoic Acid Dihydrate, **76**
Amiloride and Furosemide Tablets/Amiloride and Frusemide Tablets, **1590**
Amiloride and Hydrochlorothiazide Oral Solution, **1590**

Amiloride and Hydrochlorothiazide Tablets, **1591**
Amiloride Hydrochloride, **78**
Amiloride Tablets, **1479**
Amines, Reactions of Primary Aromatic, A147
Amino Acids, Use of Codes for, 8, 1398
α-Aminoazobenzene, *see aminoazobenzene*
Aminoazobenzene, A16
Aminobenzoic Acid, **79**, S7
Aminobenzoic Acid Lotion, xxv
2-Aminobenzoic Acid, A16
4-Aminobenzoic Acid, A16
4-Aminobenzoic Acid Solution, A16
(4-Aminobenzoyl)-L-glutamic Acid, A16
2-Aminobutan-1-ol, A16
Aminobutanol, *see 2-aminobutan-1-ol*
4-Amino-*n*-butyric Acid, A16
Aminocaproic Acid, **80**
2-Amino-5-chlorobenzophenone, A16
Aminochlorobenzophenone, *see 2-amino-5-chlorobenzophenone*
6-Aminohexanoic Acid, A16
Aminohippuric Acid, *see* p-*aminohippuric acid*
p-Aminohippuric Acid, A16
Aminohippuric Acid Reagent, A17
4-Amino-3-hydroxynaphthalene-1-sulphonic Acid, A17
Aminohydroxynaphthalenesulphonic Acid Solution, A17
5-Aminoimidazole-4-carboxamide Hydrochloride, A17
3-Aminomethylalizarin-*N*,*N*-diacetic Acid, A17
Aminomethylalizarindiacetic Acid, *see 3-aminomethylalizarin-*N,N*-diacetic acid*
Aminomethylalizarindiacetic Acid Reagent, A17
Aminomethylalizarindiacetic Acid Solution, A17
3-(Aminomethyl)pyridine, A17
8-Aminonaphthalene-2-sulphonic Acid, A17
Aminonaphthalenesulphonic Acid Solution, A17
2-Amino-5-nitrobenzophenone, A17
Aminonitrobenzophenone, *see 2-amino-5-nitrobenzophenone*
4-Aminophenazone, A17
Aminophenazone Solution, A17
4-Aminophenol, A17
4-Aminophenol-free Paracetamol, A65
Aminophylline, **81**
Aminophylline Hydrate, **82**
Aminophylline Injection, **1480**
Aminophylline Tablets, **1480**
3-Aminopropanol, A17
3-Aminopropionic Acid, A17
Aminopropylmethylsilyl Silica Gel for Chromatography, A77
Aminopropylsilyl Silica Gel for Chromatography, A77
Aminopyrazolone, *see 4-aminophenazone*
Aminopyrazolone Solution, *see aminophenazone solution*
Amiodarone, S8
Amiodarone Concentrate, Sterile, **1481**
Amiodarone Hydrochloride, **82**
Amiodarone Intravenous Infusion, **1481**
Amiodarone Tablets, **1482**
Amitriptyline Embonate, **83**
Amitriptyline Hydrochloride, **84**
Amitriptyline Oral Suspension, **1482**
Amitriptyline Tablets, **1483**
Ammonia, A17
Ammonia and Ipecacuanha Mixture, **1484**
Ammonia and Ipecacuanha Oral Solution, **1484**
Ammonia Buffer pH 9.5, *see ammonium chloride buffer solution pH 9.5*
Ammonia Buffer pH 10.0, A101
Ammonia Buffer pH 10.9, A101
Ammonia Buffer pH 10.9, Dilute, A101
Ammonia, Chloride-free, A17
Ammonia, Concentrated, A17
Ammonia, Methanolic, A17
Ammonia R1, Concentrated, A17
Ammonia R1, Dilute, A18
Ammonia R2, Dilute, A18
Ammonia Solution, *see Dilute Ammonia Solution,*
Ammonia Solution, Aromatic, **1484**
Ammonia Solution, Concentrated, *see Strong Ammonia Solution*
Ammonia Solution, Dilute, **1484**
Ammonia Solution, Strong, **85**
Ammonia Spirit, Aromatic, **1485**
Ammonia-free Water, A90
Ammoniacal Copper Oxide Solution, A31
Ammoniacal Nickel Chloride Solution, A61
Ammoniacal Silver Nitrate Solution, A79
Ammoniacal Solution of Copper Tetrammine, A32
Ammonium Acetate, A18
Ammonium Acetate Solution, *see Strong Ammonium Acetate Solution*
Ammonium Acetate Solution, A18
Ammonium Acetate Solution, Dilute, *see Strong Ammonium Acetate Solution*
Ammonium Acetate Solution, Strong, **1485**
Ammonium and Cerium Nitrate, *see ammonium cerium(IV) nitrate and ammonium cerium(IV) nitrate VS*
Ammonium and Cerium Sulphate, *see ammonium cerium(IV) sulphate and ammonium cerium(IV) sulphate VS*
Ammonium Bicarbonate, **86**
(1*R*)-(−)-Ammonium 10-Camphorsulphonate, A18
Ammonium Carbonate, *see Ammonium Bicarbonate*
Ammonium Carbonate, A18
Ammonium Carbonate Solution, A18
Ammonium Carbonate Solution, Dilute, A18
Ammonium Cerium(IV) Nitrate, A18
Ammonium Cerium(IV) Nitrate VS, A92
Ammonium Cerium(IV) Sulphate, A18
Ammonium Cerium(IV) Sulphate VS, A93
Ammonium Chloride, **87**, A18
Ammonium Chloride and Morphine Mixture, xxv
Ammonium Chloride Buffer Solution pH 9.5, A101
Ammonium Chloride Buffer Solution pH 10.0, *see ammonia buffer pH 10.0*
Ammonium Chloride Mixture, **1485**
Ammonium Chloride Oral Solution, **1485**
Ammonium Chloride Solution, A18
Ammonium Citrate, A18
Ammonium Citrate Solution, A18
Ammonium Cobaltothiocyanate Solution, A18
Ammonium Dihydrogen Orthophosphate, A18
Ammonium Dihydrogen Phosphate, *see ammonium dihydrogen orthophosphate*
Ammonium Glycyrrhizinate, **87**, S8
Ammonium Hydrogen Carbonate, A18
Ammonium Ichthosulphonate, **715**
Ammonium Iron(II) Sulphate, A18
Ammonium Iron(II) Sulphate VS, A93
Ammonium Iron(III) Citrate, A18
Ammonium Iron(III) Sulphate, A18
Ammonium Iron(III) Sulphate Solution R1, A18
Ammonium Iron(III) Sulphate Solution R2, A18
Ammonium Iron(III) Sulphate Solution R5, A18
Ammonium Iron(III) Sulphate Solution R6, A18
Ammonium Iron(III) Sulphate VS, A93
Ammonium, Limit Tests for, A151
Ammonium Mercaptoacetate Solution, A18
Ammonium Mercurithiocyanate Reagent, A18
Ammonium Metavanadate, A18
Ammonium Metavanadate Solution, A18
Ammonium Molybdate, A18
Ammonium Molybdate Reagent, A18
Ammonium Molybdate Reagent R1, A19
Ammonium Molybdate Solution, A19
Ammonium Molybdate Solution R2, A19
Ammonium Molybdate Solution R3, A19
Ammonium Molybdate Solution R4, A19
Ammonium Molybdate–Sulphuric Acid Solution, A19
Ammonium Nitrate, A19
Ammonium Nitrate R1, A19
Ammonium Oxalate, A19
Ammonium Oxalate Solution, A19
Ammonium Persulphate, A19
Ammonium Phosphate, *see diammonium hydrogen orthophosphate*
Ammonium Polysulphide Solution, A19
Ammonium Pyrrolidinedithiocarbamate, A19
Ammonium Pyrrolidinedithiocarbamate Solution, A19
Ammonium Reineckate, A19
Ammonium Reineckate Solution, A19

Ammonium Salts and Salts of Volatile Bases, Reactions of, A147
Ammonium Salts, Reactions of, A147
Ammonium Standard Solution (1 ppm NH_4), A98
Ammonium Standard Solution (2.5 ppm NH_4), A98
Ammonium Standard Solution (100 ppm NH_4), A98
Ammonium Sulphamate, A19
Ammonium Sulphate, A19
Ammonium Thiocyanate, A19
Ammonium Thiocyanate Solution, A19
Ammonium Thiocyanate VS, A93
Ammonium Vanadate, *see ammonium metavanadate*
Ammonium Vanadate Solution, A19
Ammonium-free Water, *see ammonia-free water*
Amobarbital, **88**
Amobarbital Sodium, **89**
Amorph. I.Z.S., **1755**
Amoxicillin and Potassium Clavulanate Tablets, **1592**
Amoxicillin Capsules, **1486**
Amoxicillin Injection, **1486**
Amoxicillin Oral Suspension, **1487**
Amoxicillin Sodium, **90**, S8
Amoxicillin Sodium for Injection, **1486**
Amoxicillin Trihydrate, **93**, S9, A19
Amoxycillin and Preparations, *see under Amoxicillin*
Amperometric Titration, A155
Amphetamine Sulphate, *see Amfetamine Sulphate*
Amphotericin, **94**, S9
Amphotericin Lozenges, **1488**
Ampicillin, **95**
Ampicillin, Anhydrous, *see Ampicillin*
Ampicillin Capsules, **1488**
Ampicillin Capsules, Flucloxacillin and, **1601**
Ampicillin Injection, **1488**
Ampicillin Oral Suspension, **1490**
Ampicillin Oral Suspension, Flucloxacillin and, **1602**
Ampicillin Sodium, **98**
Ampicillin Sodium for Injection, **1489**
Ampicillin Trihydrate, **100**, S9
Ampoules, A268
Amyl Acetate, A19
Amyl Alcohol, A19
α-Amylase, A19
α-Amylase Solution, A19
Amylmetacresol, **102**, S10
Amylobarbitone, *see Amobarbital*
Amylobarbitone Sodium, *see Amobarbital Sodium*
Amylose-derivative Silica Gel for Chromatography, A77
Anaesthetic Ether, **551**
Analysis, Methods of, A340
Analytical Validation, A341
Analytical Validation, Glossary of Terms, A342
Anethole, A19
cis-Anethole, A20
Anhydrous Acetic Acid, A13
Anhydrous Aluminium Oxide, A16
Anhydrous Ampicillin, *see Ampicillin*
Anhydrous Azapropazone, S11
Anhydrous Caffeine, **210**
Anhydrous Calcium Chloride, A26
Anhydrous Calcium Hydrogen Phosphate, **228**
Anhydrous Chlorbutol, *see Anhydrous Chlorobutanol*
Anhydrous Chlorobutanol, **311**
Anhydrous Citric Acid, **350**
Anhydrous Citric Acid, A30
Anhydrous Copper Sulphate, **403**
Anhydrous Disodium Hydrogen Orthophosphate, A40
Anhydrous Disodium Hydrogen Phosphate, *see anhydrous disodium hydrogen orthophosphate*
Anhydrous Ephedrine, **527**
Anhydrous Formic Acid, A45
Anhydrous Glacial Acetic Acid, *see anhydrous acetic acid*
Anhydrous Glucose, **642**
Anhydrous Iron(II) Chloride, A52
Anhydrous Lactose, **771**
Anhydrous Lanolin, **1370**
Anhydrous Methanol, A57
Anhydrous Morphine, A60
Anhydrous Niclosamide, **925**
Anhydrous Potassium Carbonate, *see potassium carbonate*
Anhydrous Pyridine, A74
Anhydrous Silica, Colloidal, **1164**
Anhydrous Silica Gel, A76
Anhydrous Sodium Acetate, A79
Anhydrous Sodium Carbonate, **1175**, A79, A92
Anhydrous Sodium Dihydrogen Orthophosphate, A80
Anhydrous Sodium Dihydrogen Phosphate, **1183**
Anhydrous Sodium Dihydrogen Phosphate, *see anhydrous sodium dihydrogen orthophosphate*
Anhydrous Sodium Sulphate, **1199**, A81
Anhydrous Sodium Sulphite, **1200**
Aniline, A20
Aniline Hydrochloride, A20
Aniline Hydrochloride Solution, A20
Animals, Use of, 14, 1404
Anion Exchange Resin, A20
Anion Exchange Resin, Strongly Basic, A20
Anionic Emulsifying Wax, **1658**
Anisaldehyde, A20
Anisaldehyde Solution, A20
Anisaldehyde Solution R1, A20
Anise, **105**
Anise Oil, **102**
Anise, Star, **104**
Anise Water, Concentrated, **1490**
Aniseed, **105**
Aniseed Oil, **102**
Aniseed, Powdered, xxv, *see also Aniseed*
p-Anisidine, A20
Anisocytic Stomata, A183
Anomocytic Stomata, A183
Antazoline Hydrochloride, **106**
Anthracene, A20
Anthranilic Acid, *see 2-aminobenzoic acid*
Anthrone, A20
Anthrone Reagent, A20
Anti-A and Anti-B Haemagglutinins, Test for, A226
Anti-D (Rh_0) Immunoglobulin, **2020**
Antibiotics, Biological Assay of, A207
Antibiotics, Potency of, 13, 1403
Anticoagulant and Preservative Solutions for Blood, **2001**
Anticomplementary Activity of Immunoglobulin, Tests for, A227
Antihaemophilic Fraction, Dried Human, **2010**
Antimicrobial Preservation, Efficacy of, A252, A333
Antimicrobial Preservatives, Definition of Suitability of, 10, 1400
Antimony Compounds, Reactions of, A147
Antimony Potassium Oxide (+)-Tartrate, *see antimony potassium tartrate*
Antimony Potassium Tartrate, A20
Antimony Standard Solution (1 ppm Sb), A98
Antimony Trichloride, A20
Antimony Trichloride Solution, A20
Antimony Trichloride Solution R1, A20
Antioxidants in Fixed Oils, Test for, A175
Antisera, **2029**, *see also under name of antiserum*
Antisera, Test for Phenol in, A231
Antithrombin III, A21
Antithrombin III Concentrate, **2006**
Antithrombin III Solution R1, A21
Antithrombin III Solution R2, A21
Apigenin, A21
Apigenin-7-glucoside, A21
Apomorphine Hydrochloride, **107**
Apparent Density, Determination of, A140
Apparent Volume, Determination of, A258
Appendices, xxii
Appendices, Contents of the, A3
Applications, 1424, *see also under name of substance*
Applications of the BP, List of, 1425
Approved Synonyms, xix, A289
Approved Synonyms, Status of, 7, 1397
Aprotinin, **108**, A21
Aprotinin Concentrated Solution, **109**
Aprotinin Injection, **1490**
Aqueous Calamine Cream, **1530**
Aqueous Cream, **1491**
Aqueous Iodine Oral Solution, **1758**
Aqueous Solutions for Intravenous Infusion, Containers for, A281
L-Arabinose, A21
Arabinose, *see L-arabinose*
Arachidic Alcohol, A21
Arachis Oil, **111**
Arachis Oil Enema, **1491**
Arachis Oil, Hydrogenated, **112**
Arbutin, A21
Arginine, **113**, A21

Arginine Hydrochloride, **114**
Argon, A21
Aromatic Amino Nitrogen, Determination of Primary, A156
Aromatic Ammonia Solution, **1484**
Aromatic Ammonia Spirit, **1485**
Aromatic Cardamom Tincture, **1540**
Aromatic Magnesium Carbonate Mixture, **1788**
Aromatic Magnesium Carbonate Oral Suspension, **1788**
Aromatic Waters, 1462, *see also under name of substance*
Aromatic Waters of the BP, List of, 1462
Aromatic-free Petroleum Spirit, (boiling range, 40° to 60°), A66
Arsenic Compounds, Reactions of, A147
Arsenic, Limit Tests for, A151
Arsenic Standard Solution (0.1 ppm As), A98
Arsenic Standard Solution (1 ppm As), A98
Arsenic Standard Solution (10 ppm As), A98
Arsenic Trioxide, A92, *see also arsenious trioxide*
Arsenious Trioxide, A21, *see also arsenic trioxide,*
Arsenite Solution, A21
Artificial Gastric Juice, A46
Artificial Tears, **1744**
Ascending Paper Chromatography, A131
L-Ascorbic Acid, A21
Ascorbic Acid, *see L-ascorbic acid*
Ascorbic Acid, **115**
Ascorbic Acid Injection, **1492**
Ascorbic Acid Solution, A21
Ascorbic Acid Tablets, **1492**
Ascorbyl Palmitate, **116**
Aseptic Preparation, A266
Ash, Acid-insoluble, Determination of, A184
Ash, Determination of, A183
Ash, Sulphated, Determination of, A166
Aspartame, **116**
Aspartic Acid, **118**
L-Aspartyl-L-phenylalanine, A21
Aspirin, **119**
Aspirin and Caffeine Tablets, **1494**
Aspirin and Codeine Tablets, **1595**
Aspirin and Codeine Tablets, Dispersible, **1596**
Aspirin Tablets, **1492**
Aspirin Tablets, Dispersible, **1493**
Aspirin Tablets, Effervescent, **1493**
Aspirin Tablets, Effervescent Soluble, **1493**
Aspirin Tablets, Soluble, *see Dispersible Aspirin Tablets,*
Assays and Tests, 11, 21, 1401, 1411
Assays and Tests, Biological, 13, 1403, A332
Astemizole, **120**
ATCC, A313
Atenolol, **122**, S10, A21
Atenolol and Chlortalidone Tablets, **1608**
Atenolol Injection, **1494**
Atenolol Oral Solution, **1495**
Atenolol Tablets, **1495**
Atomic Absorption Spectrometry, A120
Atomic Emission Spectrometry, A119
Atomic Spectrophotometry: Emission and Absorption A119
Atomic Weights of Elements, A311
Atomic Weights, 5, 1395
Atropine Eye Drops, **1496**
Atropine Eye Ointment, **1496**
Atropine Injection, **1497**
Atropine Injection, Morphine and, **1820**
Atropine Methobromide, **123**
Atropine Methonitrate, **124**
Atropine Sulphate, **125**, A21
Atropine Tablets, **1497**
Attapulgite, **126**
Attapulgite, Activated, **127**
Azapropazone, **127**, S10
Azapropazone, Anhydrous, S11
Azapropazone Capsules, **1498**
Azapropazone Tablets, **1498**
Azathioprine, **128**
Azathioprine Tablets, **1499**
Azelastine Hydrochloride, **129**, S11
Azlocillin Injection, **1499**
Azlocillin Sodium, **130**, S11
Azlocillin Sodium for Injection, **1499**
Azomethine H, A21
Azomethine H Solution, A21

B

B.A.L., *see Dimercaprol*
Bacampicillin Hydrochloride, **131**
Bacillus Calmette-Guérin Vaccine, **2040**
Bacillus Calmette-Guérin Vaccine, Percutaneous, **2042**
Bacitracin, **133**
Bacitracin Eye Ointment, Polymyxin and, **1880**
Bacitracin Zinc, **134**
Baclofen, **135**
Baclofen Oral Solution, **1500**
Baclofen Tablets, **1501**
Bacterial Endotoxin Test, Guidelines, A323
Bacterial Endotoxin Testing, A322
Bacterial Endotoxins, Test for, A214
Bacterial Endotoxins in Formulated Preparations, *see appropriate general monograph*
Balsam, Peru, **1012**
Baltimore Paste, **1476**
Barbados Aloes, **58**
Barbaloin, A21
Barbital, **136**, *see also barbitone*
Barbital Buffer Solution pH 7.4, *see barbitone buffer pH 7.4*
Barbital Buffer Solution pH 8.4, *see barbitone buffer pH 8.4*
Barbital Buffer Solution pH 8.6 R1, *see barbitone buffer pH 8.6 R1*
Barbital Sodium, *see barbitone sodium*
Barbitone, A22, *see also Barbital*
Barbitone Buffer pH 7.4, A101
Barbitone Buffer pH 8.4, A101
Barbitone Buffer pH 8.6 R1, A101
Barbitone Sodium, A22
Barbiturates, Non-nitrogen Substituted, Reactions of, A147
Barbituric Acid, A22
Barium Carbonate, A22
Barium Chloride, A22
Barium Chloride Solution, A22
Barium Chloride Solution R1, A22
Barium Chloride Solution R2, A22
Barium Chloride VS, A93
Barium Hydroxide, A22
Barium Hydroxide Solution, A22
Barium Perchlorate VS, A93
Barium Standard Solution (50 ppm Ba), A98
Barium Standard Solution (0.1% Ba), A98
Barium Sulphate, **137**, A22
Barium Sulphate for Suspension, **138**
Barium Sulphate Oral Suspension, **1501**
Base-deactivated End-capped Octadecylsilyl Silica Gel for Chromatography, A77
Base-deactivated Octadecylsilyl Silica Gel for Chromatography, A77
Basic Aluminium Oxide, A16
Basic Anion Exchange Resin, Strongly, A20
Basic Fuchsin, A45
Basic Fuchsin Solution, A46
Basic Magenta, *see basic fuchsin*
Basis of Pharmacopoeial Requirements, xix, A317
Batch Release, 8, 1398
BCG Vaccine, **2040**
BCG Vaccine. Percut., **2042**
Bearberry Leaf, **138**
Beclometasone Cream, **1502**
Beclometasone Dipropionate, **139**, S12
Beclometasone Dipropionate Monohydrate, **141**, S12
Beclometasone Nasal Spray, **1503**
Beclometasone Ointment, **1503**
Beclometasone Pressurised Inhalation, **1503**
Beclomethasone Dipropionate and Preparations, *see under Beclometasone*
Beeswax, White, **142**
Beeswax, Yellow, **143**
Belladonna Dry Extract, **1504**
Belladonna Herb, **143**
Belladonna Herb, Powdered, xxv, *see also Belladonna Herb*
Belladonna Herb, Prepared, **145**
Belladonna Leaf, *see Belladonna Herb*
Belladonna, Prepared, *see Prepared Belladonna Herb*
Belladonna Tincture, **1505**
Bendrofluazide and Preparations, *see under Bendroflumethiazide*
Bendroflumethazide Tablets/Bendrofluazide Tablets, **1506**
Bendroflumethiazide/Bendrofluazide, **145**
Benethamine Penicillin, **146**, S12
Benethamine Penicillin Injection, Fortified, xxv
Benorilate, **147**, S13

Benorilate Oral Suspension, **1506**
Benorilate Tablets, **1507**
Benorylate and Preparations, *see under Benorilate*
Benperidol, **148**
Benserazide Hydrochloride, **150**
Bentonite, **151**
Benzaldehyde, **152**, A22
Benzaldehyde Spirit, **1507**
Benzalkonium Chloride, **152**, A22
Benzalkonium Chloride Solution, **153**, A22
Benzamide, A22
Benzathine Benzylpenicillin, **154**
Benzathine Penicillin, *see Benzathine Benzylpenicillin*
Benzatropine Injection, **1507**
Benzatropine Mesilate, **155**, S14
Benzatropine Tablets, **1508**
Benzene, A22
Benzene Hexachloride CRS, Alpha, A106
Benzene Hexachloride CRS, Gamma, A106
Benzethonium Chloride, **156**, A22
Benzethonium Chloride VS, 0.004M, A93
Benzhexol Hydrochloride, S13, S123
Benzhexol Hydrochloride and Preparations, *see under Trihexyphenidyl*
Benzil, A22
Benzilic Acid, A22
Benzoates, Reactions of, A147
Benzocaine, **156**
Benzoic Acid, **157**, S13, A22, A92
Benzoic Acid Ointment, Compound, **1509**
Benzoic Acid Solution, **1509**
Benzoin, **158**, A22
Benzoin Inhalation, **1509**
Benzoin Inhalation, Menthol and, **1799**
Benzoin, Sumatra, **158**
Benzoin Tincture, Compound, **1510**
Benzophenone, A22
Benzoyl Chloride, A22
Benzoyl Peroxide, A22
Benzoyl Peroxide Cream, **1510**
Benzoyl Peroxide Cream, Potassium Hydroxyquinoline Sulphate and, **1885**
Benzoyl Peroxide Gel, **1510**
Benzoyl Peroxide, Hydrous, **159**
Benzoyl Peroxide Lotion, **1511**
Benzoylarginine Ethyl Ester Hydrochloride, A22
N-Benzoyl-L-prolyl-L-phenylalanyl-L-arginine, *A22*
Benztropine Mesylate and Preparations, *see under Benzatropine*
Benzydamine Cream, **1511**
Benzydamine Hydrochloride, **160**, S14
Benzydamine Mouthwash, **1511**
Benzydamine Oromucosal Spray, **1512**
Benzyl Alcohol, **161**, A22
Benzyl Benzoate, **162**, A22
Benzyl Benzoate Application, **1512**
Benzyl Cinnamate, A22
Benzyl Hydroxybenzoate, **163**, S14
Benzylamine, A22
Benzylparaben, **163**
Benzylpenicillin for Injection, **1513**
Benzylpenicillin Injection, **1513**
Benzylpenicillin Potassium, **164**
Benzylpenicillin Sodium, **166**, A22
Bephenium Granules, xxv
Bephenium Hydroxynaphthoate, xxv
Bergapten, A22
Betacarotene, **168**
Betacyclodextrin, *see Betadex*
Betadex, **168**
Betahistine Mesilate, **170**
Betahistine Mesylate, *see Betahistine Mesilate*
Betamethasone, **171**, S15, A23
Betamethasone Acetate, **173**
Betamethasone and Clioquinol Cream, **1514**
Betamethasone and Clioquinol Ointment, **1518**
Betamethasone Dipropionate, **175**
Betamethasone Eye Drops, **1515**
Betamethasone Injection, **1516**
Betamethasone Sodium Phosphate, **176**
Betamethasone Sodium Phosphate Tablets, **1519**
Betamethasone Tablets, **1519**
Betamethasone Valerate, **178**
Betamethasone Valerate Cream, **1514**
Betamethasone Valerate Lotion, **1517**
Betamethasone Valerate Ointment, **1517**
Betamethasone Valerate Scalp Application, **1514**
Betanidine Sulphate, **180**
Betaxolol Hydrochloride, **181**
Bethanidine Sulphate, *see Betanidine Sulphate*
Betulin, A23
Bibenzyl, A23
Bicarbonates, Carbonates and, Reactions of, A148
Bicarbonates, Reactions of, A147
Biological Assay of Antibiotics, A207
Biological Assays, A207
Biological Assays and Tests, 13, 1403, A332
Biological Indicators of Sterilisation, A266
Biological Reference Materials, A106
Biological Reference Preparations, European Pharmacopoeia, A106
Biological Tests, A207
Biotin, **182**
Biperiden Hydrochloride, **183**
Biphasic Insulin, **1753**
Biphasic Insulin Injection, **1753**
Biphasic Isophane Insulin, **1753**
Biphasic Isophane Insulin Injection, **1753**
Biphenyl, A23
Biphenyl-4-ol, *see 4-hydroxybiphenyl*
Birch Leaf, **184**
Bisacodyl, **185**
Bisacodyl Suppositories, **1520**
Bisacodyl Tablets, **1520**
Bisbenzimide, A23
Bisbenzimide Stock Solution, A23
Bisbenzimide Working Solution, A23
Bismuth Carbonate, **186**
Bismuth, Complexometric Titration of, A157
Bismuth Compounds, Reactions of, A148
Bismuth Oxycarbonate, A23
Bismuth Oxynitrate, A23
Bismuth Oxynitrate R1, A23
Bismuth Oxynitrate Solution, A23
Bismuth, Reactions of, A148
Bismuth Subcarbonate, *see bismuth oxycarbonate*
Bismuth Subcarbonate, **186**
Bismuth Subnitrate, *see bismuth oxynitrate*
Bismuth Subnitrate R1, *see bismuth oxynitrate R1*
Bismuth Subnitrate Solution, *see bismuth oxynitrate solution*
N,O-Bis(trimethylsilyl)acetamide, A23
Bis(trimethylsilyl)trifluoroacetamide, A23
Bitter Fennel, **576**
Bitter-Orange Flower Oil, **963**
Bitter-Orange Peel, Dried, **965**
Biuret, A23
Biuret Reagent, A23
Black Currant, **187**
Black Currant Syrup, **1521**
Bleomycin Sulphate, **187**
Blood and Blood Components, Containers for, A268, A271, A273, A281
Blood and Blood Components, Sets for the Transfusion of, A278
Blood and Blood Components, Sterile Plastic Containers for, A273
Blood, Anticoagulant and Preservative Solutions for, **2001**
Blue Dextran 2000, A23
Blue Primary Solution, A133
Boiling Point, Determination of, A138
Borate Buffer pH 7.5, A101
Borate Buffer pH 8.0, A101
Borate Buffer pH 9.0, A102
Borate Buffer pH 9.6, A102
Borate Buffer Solution pH 7.5, *see borate buffer pH 7.5*
Borate Buffer Solution pH 8.0, 0.0015M, A102
Borate Solution, A23
Borax, **188**
Boric Acid, **189**, A23
Boric Acid Solution, A23
Boric Acid Solution, Chlorinated Lime and, xxv
Boric Buffer pH 9.0, A102
D-Borneol, A23
D-Bornyl Acetate, A23
Boron Trichloride, A24
Boron Trichloride–Methanol Solution, A24
Boron Trifluoride, A24
Boron Trifluoride Solution, A24
Bot/Ser, *see Botulinum Antitoxin*
Bottles, Glass, A268
Botulinum Antitoxin, **2030**
Bovine Albumin, A15
Bovine Coagulation Factor Xa, A24
Bovine Euglobulins, A43
Bovine Factor Xa Solution, A24
Bovine Serum Albumin, *see bovine albumin*

Bovine Thrombin, A86
BP, 3, 1393
BPCRS, A106, A313, A342
Braided Silk Suture, Sterile, *see Non-absorbable Sutures, Sterile*
Braided Sutures, Sterile Synthetic Absorbable, 2159
Bretylium Injection, **1521**
Bretylium Tosilate, **190**, S15
Bretylium Tosylate, *see Bretylium Tosilate*
Brilliant Blue, *see acid blue 83*
Brilliant Green, A24
British Pharmacopoeia Chemical Reference Substance, A106, A342
British Pharmacopoeia Commission, ix
British Pharmacopoeia Commission, Membership of the, x
Bromazepam, **191**
Bromelains, A24
Bromelains Solution, A24
Bromhexine Hydrochloride, **192**
Bromide–Bromate, *see bromine VS*
Bromides, Reactions of, A148
Brominated Hydrochloric Acid, A48
Bromine, A24
Bromine Solution, A24
Bromine Solution, Acetic, A24
Bromine VS, A93
Bromine Water, A24
Bromine Water R1, A24
α-Bromo-2′-acetonaphthone, A24
Bromobenzene, A24
Bromocresol Green, A24
Bromocresol Green Solution, A24
Bromocresol Green–Methyl Red Solution, A24
Bromocresol Purple, A24
Bromocresol Purple Solution, A24
Bromocriptine Capsules, **1522**
Bromocriptine Mesilate, **193**
Bromocriptine Mesylate, *see Bromocriptine Mesilate*
Bromocriptine Tablets, **1523**
5-Bromo-2′-deoxyuridine, A24
Bromophenol Blue, A24
Bromophenol Blue Solution, A25
Bromophenol Blue Solution R1, A25
Bromophenol Blue Solution R2, A25
Bromothymol Blue, A25
Bromothymol Blue Solution R1, A25
Bromothymol Blue Solution R2, A25
Bromothymol Blue Solution R3, A25
Bromperidol, **194**
Brompheniramine Maleate, **196**
Brompheniramine Tablets, **1523**
Bronopol, **197**, S15
BRP, A106, A313
BRP Indicator Solution, A25
Brucine, A25
BS, A313
Buclizine Hydrochloride, **198**, S16
Budesonide, **198**
Bufexamac, **200**
Buffer (Phosphate) Solution pH 9.0, A102
Buffer Solution for Determination of pH, Reference, A144
Buffer Solution pH 2.0, *see 0.1M chloride buffer pH 2.0*
Buffer Solution pH 2.5, A102
Buffer Solution pH 2.5 R1, A102
Buffer Solution pH 3.5, *see acetate buffer pH 3.5*
Buffer Solution pH 3.6, *see phthalate buffer pH 3.6*
Buffer Solution pH 3.7, A102
Buffer Solution pH 5.2, A102
Buffer Solution pH 5.5, A102
Buffer Solution pH 6.5, A102
Buffer Solution pH 6.6, A102
Buffer Solution pH 7.0, A102
Buffer Solution pH 7.2, A102
Buffer Solution pH 7.4, A102
Buffer Solution pH 8.0, A102
Buffer Solution pH 9.0, *see borate buffer pH 9.0*
Buffer Solution pH 9.0 R1, *see boric buffer pH 9.0*
Buffer Solution pH 10.9, *see ammonia buffer pH 10.9*
Buffer Solutions, A101
Buffer Solutions, Water for, A101
Buffered Acetone Solution, A101
Buffered Copper Sulphate Solution pH 4.0, A102
Buffered Copper Sulphate Solution pH 5.2, A102
Buffered Cream, **1524**
Buffered Phenol Red Solution, *see phenol red solution R1*
Buffered Salt Solution pH 7.2, A102
Buffered Sodium Acetate Solution pH 6.0, A104
Bumetanide, **201**, S16
Bumetanide and Slow Potassium Tablets, **1526**
Bumetanide Injection, **1524**
Bumetanide Oral Solution, **1525**
Bumetanide Tablets, **1525**
Bupivacaine, S16
Bupivacaine and Adrenaline Injection/Bupivacaine and Epinephrine Injection, **1528**
Bupivacaine Hydrochloride, **202**
Bupivacaine Injection, **1527**
Buprenorphine, **204**
Buprenorphine Hydrochloride, **205**
Burow's Solution, *see Aluminium Acetate Ear Drops*
Buserelin, **206**
Busulfan, **207**, S17
Busulfan Tablets, **1529**
Busulphan and Preparations, *see under Busulfan*
Butane-1,3-diol, A25
Butanol, *see butan-1-ol*
Butan-1-ol, A25
Butan-1-ol FT, A25
Butan-2-ol, A25
Butan-2-ol R1, A25
2-Butanol R1, *see butan-2-ol R1*
Butan-2-one, A25
Butyl Acetate, A25
Butyl Acetate R1, A25
n-Butyl Alcohol, *see butan-1-ol*
sec-Butyl Alcohol, *see butan-2-ol*
Butyl Chloride, *see 1-chlorobutane*
Butyl Hydroxybenzoate, **208**, S17
tert-Butyl Methyl Ether, *see 1,1-dimethylethyl methyl ether*
Butyl Parahydroxybenzoate, A25, *see Butyl Hydroxybenzoate*
Butylamine, *see n-butylamine*
n-Butylamine, A25
tert-Butylamine, *see 1,1-dimethylethylamine*
Butylated Hydroxyanisole, **209**, A25
Butylated Hydroxytoluene, **210**, A25
Butylboronic Acid, A25
Butylhydroxyanisole, *see Butylated Hydroxyanisole*
Butylhydroxytoluene, *see Butylated Hydroxytoluene; butylated hydroxytoluene*
Butylparaben, **208**
Butylsilyl Silica Gel, A76
Butyric Acid, A25
n-Butyric Acid, *see butyric acid*
Butyrolactone, A25

C

Cadmium, A26
Cadmium Acetate, A26
Cadmium and Ninhydrin Solution, A26
Cadmium Iodide, A26
Cadmium Iodide Solution, A26
Cadmium Standard Solution (10 ppm Cd), A99
Cadmium Standard Solution (0.1% Cd), A99
Cadmium- and Lead-free Nitric Acid, A62
Caesium Chloride, A26
Caffeic Acid, A26
Caffeine, **210**, A26
Caffeine, Anhydrous, **210**
Caffeine Hydrate, **211**
Caffeine Monohydrate, *see Caffeine Hydrate*
Caffeine Tablets, Aspirin and, **1494**
Calamine, **212**
Calamine and Clioquinol Bandage, Zinc Paste, xxvi
Calamine and Coal Tar Ointment, **1530**
Calamine Cream, Aqueous, **1530**
Calamine Lotion, **1530**
Calamine Ointment, **1530**
Calamine Ointment, Compound, **1530**
Calamine, Prepared, **212**
Calciferol, A26, *see also Ergocalciferol*
Calciferol Injection, **1531**
Calciferol Oral Drops, **1531**
Calciferol Oral Solution, **1531**
Calciferol Tablets, **1532**
Calcitonin (Pork), **212**
Calcitonin (Pork) for Injection, **1533**
Calcitonin (Pork) Injection, **1533**
Calcitonin (Salmon) Injection/Salcatonin Injection, **1533**
Calcitonin (Salmon)/Salcatonin, **214**
Calcitriol, **217**
Calcitriol Capsules, **1534**
Calcium Acetate, **218**
Calcium Acetate, Dried, A26
Calcium Ascorbate, **219**
Calcium Carbonate, **220**, A26

Calcium Chloride, **220**, A26
Calcium Chloride, Anhydrous, A26
Calcium Chloride Dihydrate, **220**
Calcium Chloride Hexahydrate, **221**
Calcium Chloride Injection, **1534**
Calcium Chloride Intravenous Infusion, **1534**
Calcium Chloride R1, A26
Calcium Chloride Solution, A26
Calcium Chloride Solution, 0.02M, A26
Calcium Chloride Solution, 0.1M, A26
Calcium, Complexometric Titration of, A157
Calcium Dobesilate Monohydrate, **222**
Calcium Folinate, **222**
Calcium Gluconate, **225**
Calcium Gluconate for Injection, **225**
Calcium Gluconate Injection, **1534**
Calcium Gluconate Tablets, **1535**
Calcium Gluconate Tablets, Effervescent, **1535**
Calcium Glycerophosphate, **227**
Calcium Hydrogen Phosphate, **228**
Calcium Hydrogen Phosphate, Anhydrous, **228**
Calcium Hydrogen Phosphate Dihydrate, *see Calcium Hydrogen Phosphate*
Calcium Hydroxide, **229**, A26
Calcium Hydroxide Solution, **1535**, A26
Calcium in Adsorbed Vaccines, A231
Calcium Lactate, **230**, A26
Calcium Lactate Pentahydrate, **230**
Calcium Lactate Tablets, **1536**
Calcium Lactate Trihydrate, **231**
Calcium, Limit Test for, A152
Calcium Pantothenate, **231**
Calcium Phosphate, **232**
Calcium Phosphate, Dibasic, **228**
Calcium Phosphate, Tribasic, **232**
Calcium Polystyrene Sulphonate, **233**, S17
Calcium, Reactions of, A148
Calcium Salts, Reactions of, A148
Calcium Sodium Lactate, **234**
Calcium Standard Solution (10 ppm Ca), A99
Calcium Standard Solution (100 ppm Ca), A99
Calcium Standard Solution (100 ppm Ca), Alcoholic, A99
Calcium Standard Solution (400 ppm Ca), A99
Calcium Stearate, **234**
Calcium Sulphate, A26
Calcium Sulphate Dihydrate, **236**
Calcium Sulphate, Dried, **236**
Calcium Sulphate, Exsiccated, **236**
Calcium Sulphate Hemihydrate, *see calcium sulphate*
Calcium Sulphate Solution, A26
Calconcarboxylic Acid, A26
Calconcarboxylic Acid Triturate, A26
Camphor, Racemic, **236**
Camphor Water, Concentrated, **1536**
Camphorated Opium Tincture, **1843**
Camphorated Opium Tincture, Concentrated, **1843**
(1*S*)-(+)-10-Camphorsulphonic Acid, A26
Capacity Factor, Definition of, A124, A130
Cape Aloes, **59**
Capital Initial Letters, Significance of, 7, 1397
Capreomycin Injection **1536**
Capreomycin Sulphate, **237**
Capreomycin Sulphate for Injection **1536**
ε-Caprolactam, A26
Caprylic Acid, **950**
Caprylocaproyl Macrogolglycerides, **238**
Capsules, 1421, *see also under name of substance*
Gastro-resistant, 1422
Hard, 1421
Modified-release, 1422
Rectal, 1449
Soft, 1421
Vaginal, 1462
Capsules, Disintegration Test for, A187
Capsules, Dissolution Test for, A189
Capsules of the BP, Additional Requirements for, 1422
Capsules of the BP, List of, 1422
Captopril, **239**, S18
Captopril Tablets, **1537**
Caraway, **240**
Caraway Fruit, *see Caraway*
Caraway Oil, **241**
Caraway, Powdered, xxv, *see also Caraway*
Carbamazepine, **242**
Carbamazepine Tablets, **1537**
Carbaryl, **243**, S18
Carbaryl Lotion, **1538**
Carbasalate Calcium, **244**
Carbazole, A26
Carbenicillin Injection, **1539**
Carbenicillin Sodium, **245**, S18
Carbenicillin Sodium for Injection, **1539**
Carbenoxolone, S19
Carbenoxolone Sodium, **246**
Carbenoxolone Tablets, xxv
Carbidopa, **247**
Carbidopa Tablets, Levodopa and, **1593**
Carbimazole, **248**, S19
Carbimazole Tablets, **1540**
Carbocisteine, **249**
Carbomer, A26
Carbomers, **250**
Carbon Dioxide, **251**, A26
Carbon Dioxide in Medicinal Gases, Determination of, A169
Carbon Dioxide R1, A26
Carbon Dioxide-free Water, A90
Carbon Disulphide, A27
Carbon for Chromatography, Graphitised, A27
Carbon Monoxide, A27
Carbon Monoxide in Medicinal Gases, Limit Test for, A168
Carbon Tetrachloride, A27
Carbonate Buffer pH 9.7, A102
Carbonates and Bicarbonates, Reactions of, A148
Carbonates, Reactions of, A148
Carbophenothion, A27
Carboplatin, **252**
Cardamom Fruit, **253**
Cardamom Oil, **254**
Cardamom Tincture, Aromatic, **1540**
Cardamom Tincture, Compound, **1540**
Carmellose Calcium, **254**
Carmellose Sodium, **255**
Carmellose Sodium, Low-substituted, **256**
Carmustine, **257**
Carnauba Wax, **258**
Carob Bean Gum, A27
Carpules, Glass, A268
Carteolol Eye Drops, **1541**
Carteolol Hydrochloride, **258**, S19
Carvacrol, A27
Carvone, A27
β-Caryophyllene, A27
Cascara, **259**
Cascara Dry Extract, **1541**
Cascara, Powdered, xxv, *see also Cascara*
Cascara Tablets, **1542**
Casein, A27
Casein Substrate, Concentrated, A27
Cassava Starch, **1257**
Castor Oil, **261**
Castor Oil Cream, Zinc and, **1994**
Castor Oil, Hydrogenated Polyoxyl, **263**
Castor Oil Ointment, Zinc and, **1994**
Castor Oil, Polyoxyethylated, A70
Castor Oil, Polyoxyl, **262**
Catechol, A27
Catgut, Sterile, **2158**
Cation Exchange Resin, A27
Cation Exchange Resin (Calcium Form), Strong, A27
Cationic Resin, Weak, A27, A91
Caustic Potash, **1068**
Caustic Soda, **1186**
Caution Statements, 6, 1396, *see also Warnings*
$CCID_{50}$, A313
Cedarwood Oil, A27
Cefaclor, **265**
Cefadroxil, **266**
Cefalexin, **268**, S21
Cefalexin Capsules, **1542**
Cefalexin Oral Suspension, **1543**
Cefalexin Tablets, **1544**
Cefalotin Sodium, **270**
Cefazolin Injection, **1544**
Cefazolin Sodium, **272**
Cefazolin Sodium for Injection, **1544**
Cefixime, **274**
Cefotaxime Injection, **1545**
Cefotaxime Sodium, **275**, S20
Cefotaxime Sodium for Injection, **1545**
Cefoxitin Injection, **1546**
Cefoxitin Sodium, **277**, S20
Cefoxitin Sodium for Injection, **1546**
Cefradine, **279**, S22
Cefradine Capsules, **1547**
Ceftriaxone Injection, **1548**
Ceftriaxone Sodium, **281**, S20
Ceftriaxone Sodium for Injection, **1548**
Cefuroxime Axetil, **283**, S21
Cefuroxime Axetil Tablets, **1550**
Cefuroxime Injection, **1549**
Cefuroxime Sodium, **284**, S21

Cefuroxime Sodium for Injection, **1549**
Cellacefate, **286**
Cells for Use in Ultraviolet and Visible Spectrophotometers, A117
Cells, Red, xxvi
Cellulose, *see cellulose for chromatography*
Cellulose Acetate, **291**
Cellulose Acetate Phthalate, *see Cellacefate*
Cellulose, Dispersible, **287**
Cellulose F_{254}, *see cellulose for chromatography*
Cellulose for Chromatography, A27
Cellulose for Chromatography F_{254}, A27
Cellulose for Chromatography R1, A27
Cellulose, Microcrystalline, *see cellulose for chromatography R1*
Cellulose, Microcrystalline, **287**
Cellulose Nitrate, **1122**
Cellulose, Oxidised, xxvi
Cellulose, Powdered, **288**
Cephaeline Dihydrochloride, A27
Cephalexin and Preparations, *see under Cefalexin*
Cephalin Regent, A28
Cephaloridine Injection, xxv
Cephalothin Injection, xxv
Cephalothin Sodium and Preparations, *see under Cefalotin Sodium*
Cephazolin, Salts and Preparations, *see under Cefazolin*
Cephazolin Sodium and Preparations, *see under Cefazolin Sodium*
Cephradine, Salts and Preparations, *see under Cefradine*
Ceric Ammonium Nitrate, *see ammonium cerium(IV) nitrate*
Ceric Ammonium Sulphate, *see ammonium cerium(IV) sulphate*
Cerium Sulphate, *see cerium(IV) sulphate and cerium(IV) sulphate VS*
Cerium(III) Nitrate, A28
Cerium(III) Nitrate Solution, A28
Cerium(IV) Ammonium Nitrate, *see ammonium cerium(IV) nitrate*
Cerium(IV) Ammonium Sulphate, *see ammonium cerium(IV) sulphate*
Cerium(IV) Sulphate, A28
Cerium(IV) Sulphate VS, A93
Cerous Nitrate, *see cerium(III) nitrate*
Certification, European Pharmacopoeia, A345
Cetirizine Dihydrochloride, *see Cetirizine Hydrochloride*
Cetirizine Hydrochloride, **292**
Cetomacrogol 1000, **293**
Cetomacrogol Emulsifying Ointment, **1551**
Cetomacrogol Emulsifying Wax, **1551**
Cetostearyl Alcohol, **294**, A28
Cetostearyl Alcohol (Type A), Emulsifying, **294**
Cetostearyl Alcohol (Type B), Emulsifying, **296**
Cetostearyl Isononanoate, **297**
Cetrimide, **298**, A28
Cetrimide Cream, **1551**
Cetrimide Emulsifying Ointment, **1552**
Cetrimide Solution, **1552**
Cetrimide Solution, Sterile, **1552**
Cetrimide Solution, Strong, **299**
Cetyl Alcohol, **300**
Cetylpyridinium Chloride, **300**, A28
Cetylpyridinium Chloride VS, A93
Cetyltrimethylammonium Bromide, A28
Ceylon Cinnamon, **341**
Chalk, **301**
Chalk, Prepared, **301**
Chamomile Flower, Roman, *see Chamomile Flowers*
Chamomile Flowers, **301**
Changes in Title, Introduction, xvii, xxviii
Characteristics, Status of, 11, 1401
Characters, Status of, 21, 1411
Charcoal, Activated, **302**, A28
Charcoal, Decolorising, **302**
Chemical Abstracts Service Registry Number, Status of, 4, 1394
Chemical Formulae, 7, 1397
Chemical Reference Materials, A106
Chemical Reference Substances, British Pharmacopoeia, A106
Chemical Reference Substances, European Pharmacopoeia, A106
Chenodeoxycholic Acid, **303**
Chewing Gums, Medicated, 1423
Chloral Elixir, Paediatric, **1552**
Chloral Hydrate, **305**, A28
Chloral Hydrate Mixture, **1553**
Chloral Hydrate Solution, A28
Chloral Mixture, **1553**
Chloral Oral Solution, **1553**
Chloral Oral Solution, Paediatric, **1552**
Chlorambucil, **305**
Chlorambucil Tablets, **1553**
Chloramine, **306**, *see also chloramine T*
Chloramine Solution, A28
Chloramine Solution R1, A28
Chloramine Solution R2, A28
Chloramine T, **306**, A28
Chloramphenicol, **307**
Chloramphenicol Capsules, **1553**
Chloramphenicol Ear Drops, **1554**
Chloramphenicol Eye Drops, **1554**
Chloramphenicol Eye Ointment, **1555**
Chloramphenicol Oral Suspension, xxv
Chloramphenicol Palmitate, **308**
Chloramphenicol Sodium Succinate, **309**
Chloramphenicol Sodium Succinate for Injection, **1555**
Chloramphenicol Sodium Succinate Injection, **1555**
Chlorbutol, *see Chlorobutanol*
Chlorbutol, Anhydrous, *see Anhydrous Chlorobutanol*
Chlorcyclizine Hydrochloride, **311**
Chlordiazepoxide, **312**
Chlordiazepoxide Capsules, **1556**
Chlordiazepoxide Hydrochloride, **313**
Chlordiazepoxide Hydrochloride Tablets, **1557**
Chlordiazepoxide Tablets, xxv
Chlorhexidine Acetate, **315**, A28
Chlorhexidine Diacetate, *see Chlorhexidine Acetate*
Chlorhexidine Digluconate Solution, *see Chlorhexidine Gluconate Solution*
Chlorhexidine Dihydrochloride, *see Chlorhexidine Hydrochloride*
Chlorhexidine Gauze Dressing, xxvi
Chlorhexidine Gel, Lidocaine and, **1777**
Chlorhexidine Gluconate Solution, **316**
Chlorhexidine Hydrochloride, **317**, A28
Chlorhexidine Irrigation Solution, **1557**
Chloride Buffer pH 2.0, 0.1M, A102
Chloride Standard Solution (5 ppm Cl), A99
Chloride Standard Solution (8 ppm Cl), A99
Chloride-free Ammonia, A17
Chlorides, Limit Test for, A152
Chlorides, Reactions of, A148
Chlorinated Lime, **319**
Chlorinated Lime and Boric Acid Solution, xxv
Chlormethiazole, Esters and Preparations, *see under Clomethiazole*
Chlormethine Hydrochloride for Injection/Mustine Hydrochloride for Injection, **1558**
Chlormethine Hydrochloride/Mustine Hydrochloride, **319**
Chlormethine Injection/Mustine Injection, **1558**
4′-Chloroacetanilide, A28
Chloroacetanilide, *see 4′-chloroacetanilide*
Chloroacetic Acid, A28
3-Chloroaniline, A28
4-Chloroaniline, A28
Chloroaniline, *see 4-chloroaniline*
Chloroauric Acid, A28
Chloroauric Acid Solution, A28
Chlorobenzene, A28
4-Chlorobenzenesulphonamide, A28
4-Chlorobenzoic Acid, A28
3-(4-Chlorobenzoyl)propionic Acid, A28
1-Chlorobutane, A28
Chlorobutanol A28
Chlorobutanol, **310**
Chlorobutanol, Anhydrous, **311**
Chlorobutanol Hemihydrate, *see Chlorobutanol*
4-Chloro-*o*-cresol, A28
Chlorocresol, **319**
1-Chloro-2,4-dinitrobenzene, A28
Chlorodyne, **1559**
2-Chloroethanol, A29
2-Chloroethanol Solution, A29
(2-Chloroethyl)diethylamine Hydrochloride, A29
Chloroform, **320**, S23, A29
Chloroform, Acidified, A29
Chloroform and Morphine Tincture, **1559**
Chloroform, Deuterated, *see deuterochloroform*
Chloroform, Ethanol-free, A29
Chloroform IR, A29
Chloroform Spirit, **1559**
Chloroform Stabilised with Amylene, A29
Chloroform Water, **1560**, A29
Chloroform Water, Double-strength, **1560**
Chloroformic Iodine Solution, A51
Chlorogenic Acid, A29

5-Chloro-8-hydroxyquinoline, A29
2-Chloro-4-nitroaniline, A29
4-Chlorophenol, A29
Chlorophenol, *see 4-chlorophenol*
Chloroplatinic Acid, *see chloroplatinic(IV) acid*
Chloroplatinic Acid Solution, A29
Chloroplatinic(IV) Acid, A29
3-Chloropropane-1,3-diol, A29
1-Chloropropyl(dimethyl)amine Hydrochloride, A29
Chloroquine, S23
Chloroquine Phosphate, **321**
Chloroquine Phosphate Injection, xxv
Chloroquine Phosphate Tablets, **1560**
Chloroquine Sulphate, **322**
Chloroquine Sulphate Injection, **1560**
Chloroquine Sulphate Tablets, **1561**
5-Chlorosalicylic Acid, A29
Chlorothiazide, **323**, A29
Chlorothiazide Tablets, **1561**
Chlorotrimethylsilane, *see trichloromethylsilane*
Chlorotriphenylmethane, A29
Chloroxylenol, **324**, S23
Chloroxylenol Solution, **1562**
Chlorphenamine Injection/ Chlorpheniramine Injection, **1562**
Chlorphenamine Maleate/ Chlorpheniramine Maleate, **325**
Chlorphenamine Oral Solution/ Chlorpheniramine Oral Solution, **1563**
Chlorphenamine Tablets/ Chlorpheniramine Tablets, **1563**
Chlorpheniramine Maleate and Preparations, *see under Chlorphenamine*
Chlorpromazine, **326**, S24
Chlorpromazine Elixir, **1564**
Chlorpromazine Hydrochloride, **326**
Chlorpromazine Injection, **1564**
Chlorpromazine Oral Solution, **1564**
Chlorpromazine Suppositories, **1565**
Chlorpromazine Tablets, **1565**
Chlorpropamide, **327**, S24
Chlorpropamide Tablets, **1566**
Chlorprothixene Hydrochloride, **328**
Chlortalidone, **329**, S24
Chlortalidone Tablets, **1566**
Chlortalidone Tablets, Atenolol and, **1608**
Chlortetracycline Capsules, xxv
Chlortetracycline Eye Ointment, **1567**
Chlortetracycline Hydrochloride, **331**
Chlortetracycline Ointment, **1567**
Chlorthalidone and Preparations, *see under Chlortalidone*
Chocolate Basis for Tablets, 1453
Cholecalciferol and Preparations, *see under Colecalciferol*
Cholecalciferol Injection, *see Calciferol Injection*
Cholecalciferol Oral Solution, *see Calciferol Oral Solution*
Cholecalciferol Tablets, *see Calciferol Tablets*
Cholera Vaccine, **2042**
Cholesterol, **332**, A29
Choline Chloride, A29
Choline Salicylate, S25
Choline Salicylate Dental Gel, **1568**
Choline Salicylate Ear Drops, **1568**
Choline Salicylate Solution, **334**
Choline Theophyllinate, **334**, S25
Choline Theophyllinate Tablets, **1568**
Chorionic Gonadotrophin, **335**, A47
Chorionic Gonadotrophin for Injection, **1569**
Chorionic Gonadotrophin Injection, **1569**
Cho/Vac, *see Cholera Vaccine*
Chromatography, *see under type of chromatography*
Chrome Alum, *see chromium(III) potassium sulphate*
Chrome Azurol S, A29
Chromic Acid Cleansing Mixture, *see chromic–sulphuric acid mixture*
Chromic Potassium Sulphate, *see chromium(III) potassium sulphate*
Chromic–Sulphuric Acid Mixture, A29
Chromium Standard Solution (0.1 ppm Cr), A99
Chromium Standard Solution (100 ppm Cr), A99
Chromium Trioxide, *see chromium(VI) oxide*
Chromium(III) Potassium Sulphate, A30
Chromium(VI) Oxide, A29
Chromium(III) Trichloride Hexahydrate, *A30*
Chromium[^{51}Cr] Edetate Injection, **2113**
Chromophore Substrate R1, A30
Chromophore Substrate R2, A30
Chromotrope 2B, *see chromotrope IIB*
Chromotrope 2B solution, *see chromotrope IIB solution*
Chromotrope IIB, A30
Chromotrope IIB Solution, A30
Chromotropic Acid Sodium Salt, A30
Chromotropic Acid Solution, A30
Chymotrypsin, **336**
Ciclosporin, *see Cyclosporin*
Cimetidine, **337**, S25
Cimetidine Injection, **1569**
Cimetidine Oral Solution, **1570**
Cimetidine Oral Suspension, **1571**
Cimetidine Tablets, **1571**
Cinchocaine Hydrochloride, **338**
Cinchona, **339**
Cinchona Bark, **339**
Cinchona Bark, Powdered, xxv, *see also Cinchona Bark*
Cinchona Bark, Red, **339**
Cinchonidine, A30
Cinchonine, A30
Cineole, A30
Cineole, Determination of, A174
Cinnamaldehyde, A30
Cinnamic Acid, **340**, S26, A30
Cinnamic Aldehyde, *see cinnamaldehyde*
Cinnamon, **341**
Cinnamon Bark, **341**
Cinnamon, Ceylon, **341**
Cinnamon Oil, **342**
Cinnamon, Powdered, xxv, *see also Cinnamon*
Cinnamon Water, Concentrated, **1572**
Cinnarizine, **342**
CIP, A313
Ciprofloxacin, **344**
Ciprofloxacin Hydrochloride, **345**
Ciprofloxacin Intravenous Infusion, **1572**
Ciprofloxacin Tablets, **1573**
Circular Dichroism, Determination of, A142
Cisapride, **347**
Cisplatin, **348**
Cisplatin for Injection, **1574**
Cisplatin Injection, **1574**
Citral, A30
Citrated Rabbit Plasma, A69
Citrates, Reactions of, A148
Citric Acid, **350**, A30
Citric Acid, Anhydrous, **350**, A30
Citric Acid Monohydrate, **351**
Citric—Molybdic Acid Solution, A30
Citro-phosphate Buffer pH 4.5, A102
Citro-phosphate Buffer pH 5.0, A102
Citro-phosphate Buffer pH 6.0, A102
Citro-phosphate Buffer pH 6.5, A102
Citro-phosphate Buffer pH 6.8, A102
Citro-phosphate Buffer pH 7.0, A102
Citro-phosphate Buffer pH 7.2, A102
Citro-phosphate Buffer pH 7.6, A102
Citropten, A30
Clarity of Solution, Determination of, A133
Classification of Particle Size of Powders, A254
Clemastine Fumarate, **352**, S26
Clemastine Oral Solution, **1574**
Clemastine Tablets, **1575**
Clindamycin Capsules, **1576**
Clindamycin Hydrochloride, **353**, S26
Clindamycin Injection, **1577**
Clindamycin Phosphate, **355**
Clioquinol, **356**, S27
Clioquinol Bandage, Zinc Paste, Calamine and, xxvi
Clioquinol Cream, **1577**
Clioquinol Cream, Betamethasone and, **1514**
Clioquinol Cream, Hydrocortisone and, **1729**
Clioquinol Ointment, Betamethasone and, **1518**
Clioquinol Ointment, Hydrocortisone and, **1736**
Clobazam, **357**, S27
Clobazam Capsules, **1578**
Clobetasol Cream, **1578**
Clobetasol Ointment, **1579**
Clobetasol Propionate, **358**, S27, A31
Clobetasone Butyrate, **359**
Clobetasone Cream, **1580**
Clobetasone Ointment, **1580**
Clofazimine, **360**, S28
Clofazimine Capsules, **1581**
Clofibrate, **361**
Clofibrate Capsules, **1581**
Clomethiazole, **362**, S22
Clomethiazole Capsules, **1582**
Clomethiazole Edisilate, **363**, S22
Clomethiazole Intravenous Infusion, **1583**

Clomethiazole Oral Solution, **1583**
Clomifene Citrate, **364**
Clomifene Tablets, **1584**
Clomiphene Citrate and Preparations, *see under Clomifene*
Clomipramine Capsules, **1584**
Clomipramine Hydrochloride, **366**, S28
Clonazepam, **367**
Clonazepam Concentrate, Sterile, **1585**
Clonazepam Injection, **1585**
Clonidine Hydrochloride, **368**
Clonidine Injection, **1585**
Clonidine Tablets, **1586**
Clostridia, Test for, A243
Clotrimazole, **369**
Clotrimazole Cream, **1586**
Clotrimazole Pessaries, **1587**
Clotting Factor V Solution, *see coagulation factor V solution*
Clove, **370**
Clove Oil, **371**
Clove, Powdered, xxv, *see also Clove*
Cloxacillin Capsules, **1588**
Cloxacillin Injection, **1588**
Cloxacillin Oral Solution **1589**
Cloxacillin Sodium, **372**, S28
Cloxacillin Sodium for Injection, **1588**
Clozapine, **374**
Coagulation Factor VII, Assay of Human, A221
Coagulation Factor VIII, Assay of Human A222
Coagulation Factor IX, Assay of Human, A224
Coagulation Factor V Solution, A31
Coagulation Factors, *see under name of factor*
Coal Tar, **1258**
Coal Tar and Salicylic Acid Ointment, **1957**
Coal Tar and Zinc Ointment, **1957**
Coal Tar Bandage, Zinc Paste and, xxvi
Coal Tar Ointment, Calamine and, **1530**
Coal Tar Paste, **1958**
Coal Tar Paste, Zinc and, **1994**
Coal Tar Solution, **1958**
Coal Tar Solution, Strong, **1958**
Co-amilofruse Tablets, **1590**
Co-amilozide Oral Solution, **1590**
Co-amilozide Tablets, **1591**
Co-amoxiclav Tablets, **1592**
Coarse Powder, Definition of, A254
Coated Granules, 1432
Coated Tablets, 1452
Cobalt Chloride, *see cobalt(II) chloride*
Cobalt Nitrate, *see cobalt(II) nitrate*
Cobalt(II) Acetate, A31
Cobalt(II) Chloride, A31
Cobalt(II) Nitrate, A31
Cocaine, **375**, S29
Cocaine Hydrochloride, **375**
Co-careldopa Tablets, **1593**
Cochineal, **376**
Cocillana, **376**
Cocillana, Powdered, xxv, *see also Cocillana*
Cocoa Butter, **1277**
Co-codamol Tablets, **1593**
Co-codaprin Tablets, **1595**
Co-codaprin Tablets, Dispersible, **1596**
Coconut Oil, **377**
Coconut Oil, Fractionated, *see Medium-chain Triglycerides*
Co-danthrusate Capsules, **1596**
Codeine, **377**, S29, A31
Codeine Hydrochloride, **378**, S29
Codeine Linctus, **1597**
Codeine Linctus, Diabetic, *see Codeine Linctus*
Codeine Linctus, Paediatric, **1598**
Codeine Phosphate, **379**, A31
Codeine Phosphate and Paracetamol Tablets, **1593**
Codeine Phosphate Hemihydrate, *see Codeine Phosphate*
Codeine Phosphate Oral Solution, **1598**
Codeine Phosphate Sesquihydrate, **380**
Codeine Phosphate Tablets, **1598**
Codeine Tablets, Aspirin and, **1595**
Codeine Tablets, Dispersible Aspirin and, **1596**
Co-dergocrine Mesilate, **380**
Co-dergocrine Mesylate, *see Co-dergocrine Mesilate*
Co-dergocrine Tablets, **1599**
Codes for Eye Drops in Single-dose Containers, A310
Cod-liver Oil (Type A), **381**
Cod-liver Oil (Type B), **385**
Co-dydramol Tablets, **1600**
Co-fluampicil Capsules, **1601**
Co-fluampicil Oral Suspension, **1602**
Colchicine, **389**
Colchicine Tablets **1603**
Colecalciferol, **391**
Colecalciferol Concentrate (Oily Form), **392**
Colecalciferol Concentrate (Powder Form), **394**
Colecalciferol Concentrate (Water-dispersible Form), **396**
Colecalciferol Oral Drops, *see Calciferol Oral Drops*
Colestipol Granules, **1603**
Colestipol Hydrochloride, **398**
Colistimethate Sodium for Injection, **1604**
Colistimethate Injection, **1604**
Colistimethate Sodium, **399**
Colistin Sulphate, **400**
Colistin Sulphomethate Sodium and Preparations, *see under Colistimethate Sodium*
Colistin Tablets, **1604**
2,4,6-Collidine, A31
Collodion, Flexible, **1680**
Collodion for the Preparation of Flexible Collodion, **1681**
Collodions, 1424, *see also under name of substance,*
Collodions of the BP List of, 1425
Colloidal Anhydrous Silica, **1164**
Colloidal Hydrated Silica, **1164**
Colophony, **401**
Colour of Certain Indicators, Relationship with Reaction of Solution, A143
Colour of Solution, Determination of, A133
Coloured Glass, A268
Colouring Agents, Permitted Alternatives, 10, 1400
Colourless Glass, A268
Column Efficiency, Definition of, A124, A126, A129
Columns
for Gas Chromatography, A125
for Liquid Chromatography, A130
for Size-exclusion Chromatography, A126
Co-magaldrox Oral Suspension, **1605**
Co-magaldrox Tablets, **1606**
Competent Authority, Definition of, 4, 17, 1394, 1407
Complete Extraction of Alkaloids, Tests for, A183
Complexometric Titrations, A157
Composition of Polysaccharide Vaccines, A233
Compound Aluminium Paste, **1476**
Compound Benzoic Acid Ointment, **1509**
Compound Benzoin Tincture, **1510**
Compound Calamine Ointment, **1530**
Compound Cardamom Tincture, **1540**
Compound Fig Elixir, xxv
Compound Gentian Infusion, **1707**
Compound Gentian Infusion, Concentrated, **1707**
Compound Magnesium Trisilicate Mixture, **1790**
Compound Magnesium Trisilicate Oral Powder, **1791**
Compound Magnesium Trisilicate Tablets, **1791**
Compound Orange Spirit, **1844**
Compound Podophyllin Paint, **1880**
Compound Rhubarb Tincture, **1916**
Compound Sodium Bicarbonate Tablets, **1928**
Compound Sodium Chloride Mouthwash, **1930**
Compound Sodium Lactate Injection, **1936**
Compound Sodium Lactate Intravenous Infusion, **1936**
Compound Squill Linctus, **1947**
Compound Tolu Linctus, Paediatric, **1973**
Compound Zinc Paste, **1994**
Concentrated Ammonia, A17
Concentrated Ammonia R1, A17
Concentrated Ammonia Solution, *see Strong Ammonia Solution*
Concentrated Anise Water, **1490**
Concentrated Camphor Water, **1536**
Concentrated Camphorated Opium Tincture, **1843**
Concentrated Casein Substrate, A27
Concentrated Cinnamon Water, **1572**
Concentrated Compound Gentian Infusion, **1707**
Concentrated Glyceryl Trinitrate Solution, **650**
Concentrated Haemodialysis Solutions, Water for Diluting, **1718**

Concentrated Hydrochloric Acid, *see Hydrochloric Acid*
Concentrated Interferon Alfa-2 Solution, **728**
Concentrated Orange Peel Infusion, **1844**
Concentrated Peppermint Emulsion, **1862**
Concentrated Phosphoric Acid, *see Phosphoric Acid*
Concentrated Red Blood Cells, xxvi
Concentrated Solutions for Haemodialysis, **1716**
Concentrated Solutions for Injections, 1445
Concentrates for Injections, 1444
Concentrates for Intravenous Infusions, 1444
Concentrations, Expression of, 6, 1396
Conductivity, Determination of, A146
Congo Red, A31
Congo Red Fibrin, A31
Congo Red Paper, A31
Consistency by Penetrometry, Measurement of, A260
Constant Mass, Definition of, 18, 1408
Constant Weight, Definition of, 5, 1395
Contact Points, A337
Containers, 19, 1409, A268
Containers for Pharmaceutical Use, Glass, A268
Containers, Materials Used for the Manufacture of, A281
Content, Declaration of, A331
Content, Limits of, 20, 1410
Content of Active Ingredient of
- Capsules, 1422
- Tablets, 1453

Content, Standards for, 5, 1395
Content, Test for Uniformity of, A203
Contents of the
- Appendices, A3
- British Pharmacopoeia, v, xxxix
- General Notices, 2, 1392
- Supplementary Chapters, A316

Continuous Extraction of Drugs, A182
Continuous Wave Spectrometry, A119
Control of Impurities, A318
Conventional Terms, 17, 1407
Coomassie Blue, *see acid blue 92*
Coomassie Blue Solution, *see acid blue 92 solution*
Copovidone, **401**
Copper, A31
Copper Acetate, *see copper(II) acetate*
Copper Carbonate, A31
Copper Chloride–Pyridine Reagent, A31
Copper Edetate Solution, A31
Copper Nitrate, *see copper(II) nitrate*
Copper Oxide Solution, Ammoniacal, A31
Copper Standard Solution (0.1 ppm Cu), A99
Copper Standard Solution (10 ppm Cu), A99
Copper Standard Solution (0.1% Cu), A99
Copper Sulphate, *see copper(II) sulphate*
Copper Sulphate, **402**
Copper Sulphate, Anhydrous, **403**
Copper Sulphate Pentahydrate, **402**
Copper Sulphate–Pyridine Reagent, A31
Copper Sulphate Solution, A31
Copper Sulphate Solution pH 4.0, Buffered, A102
Copper Sulphate Solution pH 5.2, Buffered, A102
Copper Sulphate Solution, Weak, A32
Copper Sulphate VS, A94
Copper Tetrammine, Ammoniacal Solution of, A32
Copper(II) Acetate, A31
Copper(II) Chloride, A31
Copper(II) Nitrate, A31
Copper(II) Sulphate, A31
Co-proxamol Tablets, **1606**
Corallin, A32
Corallin Solution, Alkaline, A32
Coriander, **404**
Coriander Oil, **404**
Coriander, Powdered, xxv, *see also Coriander*
Corticotrophin, *see Corticotropin*
Corticotropin, **404**
Corticotropin, Assay of, A221
Cortisone Acetate, S30, A32
Cortisone Tablets, **1607**
Co-tenidone Tablets, **1608**
Co-triamterzide Tablets, **1609**
Co-trimoxazole Concentrate, Sterile, **1610**
Co-trimoxazole Intravenous Infusion, **1610**
Co-trimoxazole Oral Suspension, **1610**
Co-trimoxazole Oral Suspension, Paediatric, **1611**
Co-trimoxazole Tablets, **1611**
Co-trimoxazole Tablets, Dispersible, **1612**
Co-trimoxazole Tablets, Paediatric, **1613**
Cotton, Absorbent, **2155**
Cotton and Rubber Elastic Bandage, xxvi
Cotton and Rubber Elastic Bandage, Heavy, xxvi
Cotton and Viscose Gauze, X-Ray-Detectable, xxvi
Cotton and Viscose Ribbon Gauze, X-Ray-Detectable, xxvi
Cotton Gauze, X-Ray-Detectable, xxvi
Cotton Ribbon Gauze, X-Ray-Detectable xxvi
Cotton, Sterile Absorbent, **2156**
Cream, Aqueous, **1491**
Cream, Buffered, **1524**
Cream of Tartar, **1067**
Cream, Oily, **1738**
Creams, 1459, *see also under name of substance*
Creams of the BP, List of, 1460
Cresol, **409**, *see also* o-*cresol*
o-Cresol, A32
Cresol Red, A32
Cresol Red Solution, A32
Critical Physical Properties, 17, 23, 1407, 1413
Croscarmellose Sodium, **410**
Crospovidone, **411**
Cross-linked Agarose for Chromatography, A15
Cross-linked Agarose for Chromatography R1, A15
Cross-linked Dextran for Chromatography R2, A34
Cross-linked Dextran for Chromatography R3, A34
Crotamiton, **412**
Crotamiton Cream, **1613**
Crotamiton Lotion, **1614**
CRS, A106, A313
Crude Drugs, 15, 1405
Cryst. I.Z.S., **1755**
Crystal Violet, A32
Crystal Violet Solution, A32
Cupric Chloride, *see copper(II) chloride*
Cupri-citric Solution, A32
Cupri-citric Solution R1, A32
Cupriethylenediamine Hydroxide Solution, A94
Cupri-tartaric Solution, A32
Cupri-tartaric Solution R1, A32
Cupri-tartaric Solution R2, A32
Cupri-tartaric Solution R3, A32
Cupri-tartaric Solution R4, A32
Curaçao Aloes, **58**
Curcumin, A32
Cutaneous Application, Liquids for, 1424
Cutaneous Application, Liquids for, of the BP, Additional Requirements for, 1424
Cutaneous Foams, 1424
Cyanoacetic Acid, A33
Cyanocobalamin, **413**, A33
Cyanocobalamin Injection, **1614**
Cyanocobalamin[^{57}Co] Capsules, **2114**
Cyanocobalamin[^{57}Co] Solution, **2115**
Cyanocobalamin[^{58}Co] Solution, **2116**
Cyanogen Bromide Solution, A33
1-Cyanoguanidine, A33
Cyanoguanidine, *see 1-cyanoguanidine*
Cyanosilyl Silica Gel for Chromatography, A77
Cyclizine, **414**, S30
Cyclizine Hydrochloride, **415**, S30
Cyclizine Injection, **1615**
Cyclizine Tablets, **1615**
Cyclizine Tablets, Dipipanone and, **1644**
Cyclohexane, A33
Cyclohexane R1, A33
Cyclohexylamine, A33
Cyclohexylenedinitrilotetra-acetic Acid, A33
Cyclopenthiazide, **416**, S31
Cyclopenthiazide Tablets, **1616**
Cyclopentolate, S31
Cyclopentolate Eye Drops, **1616**
Cyclopentolate Hydrochloride, **416**
Cyclophosphamide, **417**, S31
Cyclophosphamide for Injection, **1617**
Cyclophosphamide Injection, **1617**
Cyclophosphamide Tablets, **1617**
Cyclosporin, **418**
Cyproheptadine, S32
Cyproheptadine Hydrochloride, **419**
Cyproheptadine Tablets **1618**

Cyproterone Acetate, **420**
L-Cysteine, A33
Cysteine Hydrochloride, **421**, A33
L-Cystine, A33
Cystine, **423**
Cytarabine, **424**, S32
Cytarabine for Injection, **1619**
Cytarabine Injection, **1618**

D

Dacarbazine, **424**, S32
Dacarbazine for Injection, **1619**
Dacarbazine Injection, **1619**
Dalteparin Sodium, **425**
Dansyl Chloride, *see dimethylaminonaphthalenesulphonyl chloride*
Danthron and Preparations, *see under Dantron*
Dantron, **427**, S33 *see also 1,8-dihydroxyanthraquinone*
Dantron and Docusate Sodium Capsules, **1596**
Dapsone, **427**, S33
Dapsone Tablets, **1620**
Dates of Implementation, European Pharmacopoeia, A345
Daunorubicin Hydrochloride, **428**
Deactivated Aluminium Oxide, A16
Debrisoquine Sulphate, **430**
Debrisoquine Tablets, **1620**
Decane, *see n-decane*
n-Decane, A33
Decan-1-ol, A33
Decanol, *see decan-1-ol*
Declaration of Content, A331
Decolorised Fuchsin Solution, A46
Decolorised Fuchsin Solution R1, A46
Decolorised Pararosaniline Solution, A65
Decolorising Charcoal, **302**
Deferoxamine Mesilate, *see Desferrioxamine Mesilate*
Definition, Status of, 8, 20, 1398, 1410
Deglycyrrhizinised Liquorice Extract, xxv
Dehydrated Alcohol, **548**
Demeclocycline Capsules, **1621**
Demeclocycline Hydrochloride, **430**
Dementholised Mint Oil, **906**
Density, Apparent, Determination of, A140
Density, Determination of, A139
Density, Relative, Determination of, A140
Dental Gel, Choline Salicylate, **1568**
Dental Paste, Triamcinolone, **1978**
Deoxycortone Acetate, *see Desoxycortone Acetate*
2′-Deoxyuridine, A33
Depressor Substances, Test for, A220
Dequalinium Chloride, **432**, S33
Descending Paper Chromatography, A130
Desferrioxamine Injection, **1622**
Desferrioxamine Mesilate, **432**, S34
Desferrioxamine Mesilate for Injection, **1622**
Desferrioxamine Mesylate, *see Desferrioxamine Mesilate*
Design of Biological Assays, A333
Desipramine Hydrochloride, **434**, S34
Desipramine Tablets, **1623**
Deslanoside, **435**
Desmopressin, **436**
Desmopressin Injection, **1623**
Desmopressin Intranasal Solution, **1623**
Desogestrel, **438**, S34
Desoxycortone Acetate, **439**
Deuterated Acetic Acid, A33
Deuterated Acetone, A33
Deuterated Chloroform, *see deuterochloroform*
Deuterated Dimethyl Sulphoxide, A33
Deuterated Methanol, A33
Deuterium Oxide, A33
Deuterium Oxide, Isotopically Pure, A33
Deuteroacetone, *see deuterated acetone*
Deuterochloroform, A33
Devarda's Alloy, A33
Devil's Claw, **440**
Devil's Claw Root, *see Devil's Claw*
Dexamethasone, **441**, S35, A33
Dexamethasone Acetate, **443**
Dexamethasone Sodium Phosphate, **444**
Dexamethasone Tablets, **1624**
Dexamfetamine Sulphate, **446**
Dexamfetamine Tablets, **1624**
Dexamphetamine Sulphate and Preparations, *see under Dexamfetamine*
Dexchlorpheniramine Maleate, **446**
Dexpanthenol, **448**
Dextran 40 for Injection, **449**
Dextran 40 Injection, **1625**
Dextran 40 Intravenous Infusion, **1625**
Dextran 60 for Injection, **450**
Dextran 70 for Injection, **450**
Dextran 70 Injection, **1625**
Dextran 70 Intravenous Infusion, **1625**
Dextran 110 Injection, **1626**
Dextran 110 Intravenous Infusion, **1626**
Dextran 2000, Blue, A23
Dextran for Chromatography R2, Cross-linked, A34
Dextran for Chromatography R3, Cross-linked, A34
Dextrans, Molecular Weight [Mass] Distribution in, A127
Dextrin, **451**
Dextromethorphan Hydrobromide, **452**
Dextromoramide, S35
Dextromoramide Injection, **1627**
Dextromoramide Tablets, **1627**
Dextromoramide Tartrate, **453**
Dextropropoxyphene, S35
Dextropropoxyphene Capsules, **1628**
Dextropropoxyphene Hydrochloride, **454**
Dextropropoxyphene Hydrochloride and Paracetamol Tablets, **1606**
Dextropropoxyphene Napsilate, **455**, S36
Dextropropoxyphene Napsylate, *see Dextropropoxyphene Napsilate*
Dextrose and Preparations, *see D-glucose and under Glucose*
Diabetic Codeine Linctus, *see Codeine Linctus*
Diacytic Stomata, A183
Diagnostic Preparations, 2095
3,3′-Diaminobenzidine Tetrahydrochloride, A34
Diammonium Hydrogen Orthophosphate, A34
Diamorphine Hydrochloride, **455**, S36
Diamorphine Hydrochloride for Injection, **1628**
Diamorphine Injection, **1628**
Diatomaceous Earth, *see diatomaceous support*
Diatomaceous Earth for Gas Chromatography, Silanised, *see silanised diatomaceous earth for gas chromatography*
Diatomaceous Earth for Gas Chromatography R1, A34
Diatomaceous Earth for Gas Chromatography R1, Silanised, *see silanised diatomaceous support*
Diatomaceous Earth for Gas Chromatography R2, A34
Diatomaceous Earth for Gas Chromatography, Silanised, *see silanised diatomaceous support*
Diatomaceous Filter-aid, Washed, Flux-calcined, A34
Diatomaceous Support, A34
Diatomaceous Support, Acid-washed, A34
Diatomaceous Support, Alkali-washed, A34
Diatomaceous Support, Silanised, A34
Diatrizoic Acid Dihydrate, *see Amidotrizoic Acid Dihydrate*
Diazepam, **456**
Diazepam Capsules, **1629**
Diazepam Injection, **1629**
Diazepam Oral Solution, **1630**
Diazepam Rectal Solution, **1630**
Diazepam Tablets, **1631**
Diazobenzenesulphonic Acid Solution, A34
Diazobenzenesulphonic Acid Solution R1, A34
Diazotised Nitroaniline Solution, A62
Diazotised Sulphanilic Acid, A83
Diazoxide, **457**, S36
Diazoxide Injection, **1631**
Diazoxide Tablets, **1632**
Dibasic Calcium Phosphate, **228**
Dibenzosuberone, A34
Dibromopropamidine Isethionate, *see Dibromopropamidine Isetionate*
Dibromopropamidine Isetionate, **458**, S37
Dibutyl Ether, A34
Dibutyl Phthalate, **459**, A34
Di-*n*-butylamine, A34
Dicarboxidine Hydrochloride, A34
Dichloroacetic Acid, A34
Dichloroacetic Acid Solution, A34
1,2-Dichlorobenzene, A35
Dichlorobenzene, *see 1,2-dichlorobenzene*
1,2-Dichloroethane, A35
Dichlorofluorescein, *see 2,7-dichlorofluorescein*
2,7-Dichlorofluorescein, A35
5,7-Dichloro-8-hydroxyquinoline, A35

Dichloromethane, **460**, A35
Dichloromethane, Acidified, A35
Dichloromethane IR, A35
Dichlorophen, **461**
Dichlorophen Tablets, **1632**
2,6-Dichlorophenolindophenol Sodium Salt, A35
Dichlorophenolindophenol, Sodium Salt, *see 2,6-dichlorophenolindophenol sodium salt*
2,6-Dichlorophenolindophenol Solution, A35
2,6-Dichloroindophenol Solution, Double-strength Standard, A35
Dichlorophenolindophenol Solution, Standard, A35
Dichloroquinonechlorimide, *see 2,6-dichloroquinone-4-chlorimide*
2,6-Dichloroquinone-4-chloroimide, A35
Dichlorphenamide, xxv
Dichlorphenamide Tablets, xxv
Dichlorvos, A35
Diclofenac, S37
Diclofenac Sodium, **462**
Diclofenac Tablets, **1632**
Diclofenac Tablets, Slow, **1633**
Dicloxacillin Sodium, **463**
Di-2-cyanoethyl Ether, A35
Dicyclohexylamine, A35
1,3-Dicyclohexylurea, A35
Dicyclohexylurea, *see 1,3-dicyclohexylurea*
Dicyclomine Hydrochloride, S37
Dicyclomine Hydrochloride and Preparations, *see under Dicyloverine*
Dicycloverine Hydrochloride, S37, S38
Dicycloverine Hydrochloride/ Dicyclomine Hydrochloride, **465**
Dicycloverine Oral Solution/Dicyclomine Oral Solution, **1634**
Dicycloverine Tablets/Dicyclomine Tablets, **1634**
Didodecyl 3,3′-thiodipropionate, A35
Dienestrol, **466**
Dienoestrol, *see Dienestrol*
Diethanolamine, A35
Diethanolamine Buffer Solution pH 10.0, A103
2,5-Diethoxytetrahydrofuran, A36
Diethoxytetrahydrofuran, *see 2,5-diethoxytetrahydrofuran*
Diethyl Phthalate, **467**
Diethylamine, A36
Diethylamine Salicylate, **468**, S38
Diethylamine Salicylate Cream, **1635**
Diethylaminoethyldextran, A36
Diethylammonium Phosphate Buffer Solution pH 6.0, A103
N,N-Diethylaniline, A36
Diethylcarbamazine Citrate, **468**
Diethylene Glycol, A36
Diethylene Glycol Monoethyl Ether, **469**
N,N-Diethylethylenediamine, A36
Di(2-ethylhexyl) Phthalate, A36
Diethylphenylenediamine Sulphate, *see* N,N-*diethyl*-p-*phenylenediamine sulphate*
Diethylphenylenediamine Sulphate Solution, A36
N,N-Diethyl-*p*-phenylenediamine Sulphate, A36
Diethylpropion Hydrochloride, xxv
Diethylstilbestrol, **470**
Diethylstilbestrol Pessaries, **1635**
Diethylstilbestrol Tablets, **1635**
Diflucortolone Cream, **1636**
Diflucortolone Oily Cream, **1636**
Diflucortolone Ointment, **1637**
Diflucortolone Valerate, **472**, S38
Diflunisal, **471**
Diflunisal (form B), S39
Diflunisal Tablets, **1637**
Digitalis, **473**
Digitalis Leaf, **473**
Digitalis Leaf, Powdered, xxv, *see also under Digitalis Leaf*
Digitonin, A36
Digitoxin, **475**, A36
Digitoxin Standard Solution, A99
Digitoxin Tablets, **1638**
Digoxin, **476**
Digoxin Injection, **1638**
Digoxin Injection, Paediatric, **1639**
Digoxin Oral Solution, Paediatric, **1639**
Digoxin Reagent, A36
Digoxin Standard Solution, A99
Digoxin Tablets, **1639**
10,11-Dihydrocarbamazepine, A36
Dihydrocodeine, S39
Dihydrocodeine and Paracetamol Tablets, **1600**
Dihydrocodeine Injection, **1640**
Dihydrocodeine Oral Solution, **1640**
Dihydrocodeine Tablets, **1641**
Dihydrocodeine Tartrate, **477**
Dihydroergotamine Injection, xxv
Dihydroergotamine Mesilate, **478**
Dihydroergotamine Mesylate, *see Dihydroerogotamine Mesilate*
Dihydroergotamine Oral Solution, xxv
Dihydroergotamine Tablets, xxv
Dihydroergotamine Tartrate, **479**
Dihydrotachysterol, **480**
1,8-Dihydroxyanthraquinone, A36
1,3-Dihydroxynaphthalene, *see naphthalene-1,3-diol*
2,7-Dihydroxynaphthalene, *see naphthalene-2,7-diol*
2,7-Dihydroxynaphthalene Solution, *see naphthalenediol solution*
5,7-Di-iodo-8-hydroxyquinoline, A36
1,5-Di-iodopentane, A36
Di-isopropylethylamine, A36
Di-isobutyl Ketone, A36
Di-isopropyl Ether, A36
Di-isopropyl Ether, Stabiliser-free, A36
Dill Oil, **481**
Diloxanide Furoate, **481**, S39
Diloxanide Tablets, **1641**
Diltiazem Hydrochloride, **482**
Diluent for Hyaluronidase Solutions, A48
Dilute Acetic Acid, **39**, A13
Dilute Adrenaline Injection 1 in 10,000/ Dilute Epinephrine Injection 1 in 10,000, **1470**
Dilute Ammonia Buffer pH 10.9, A101
Dilute Ammonia R1, A18
Dilute Ammonia R2, A18
Dilute Ammonia Solution, **1484**
Dilute Ammonium Acetate Solution, *see Strong Ammonium Acetate Solution*
Dilute Ammonium Carbonate Solution, A18
Dilute Ethanols, **549**
Dilute Hydrobromic Acid, A48
Dilute Hydrochloric Acid, **684**, A48
Dilute Hydrochloric Acid R1, A49
Dilute Hydrochloric Acid R2, A49
Dilute Hydrogen Peroxide Solution, *see hydrogen peroxide solution (10 vol) and Hydrogen Peroxide Solution (3 per cent)*
Dilute Nitric Acid, A62
Dilute Orthophosphoric Acid, A68
Dilute Phosphomolybdotungstic Reagent, A68
Dilute Phosphoric Acid, **1037**
Dilute Potassium Cupri-tartrate Solution, *see cupri-tartaric solution R2*
Dilute Potassium Dichromate Solution, A71
Dilute Potassium Hexacyanoferrate(III) Solution, A72
Dilute Potassium Iodide Solution, A72
Dilute Potassium Iodobismuthate Solution, A72
Dilute Potassium Permanganate Solution, A73
Dilute Sodium Carbonate Solution, A79
Dilute Sodium Hydroxide Solution, A80
Dilute Sodium Hypochlorite Solution, **1935**, A80
Dilute Sulphuric Acid, **1252**, A84
Dilute Tetramethylammonium Hydroxide Solution, A85
Diluted Isosorbide Dinitrate, **752**
Diluted Isosorbide Mononitrate, **753**
Diluted Sorbide Nitrate, *see Diluted Isosorbide Dinitrate*
Dilution of Creams, 1459
Dilution of Ointments, 1459
Dimenhydrinate, **483**, S40
Dimenhydrinate Tablets, **1642**
Dimercaprol, **484**
Dimercaprol Injection, **1642**
Dimethicone, *see Dimeticone*
2,5-Dimethoxybenzaldehyde, A37
4,4′-Dimethoxybenzophenone, A37
5,7-Dimethoxycoumarin, *see citropten*
3,4-Dimethoxyphenethylamine, A37
Dimethoxypropane, *see 2,2-dimethoxypropane*
2,2-Dimethoxypropane, A37
Dimethyl Phthalate, **485**, S40, A37
Dimethyl Sulfoxide, **486**
Dimethyl Sulphone, A37
Dimethyl Sulphoxide, A37, *see also Dimethyl Sulfoxide*
Dimethyl Sulphoxide, Deuterated, A33
Dimethyl Yellow, A37
Dimethyl Yellow Solution, A37
Dimethylacetamide, A37
4-Dimethylaminobenzaldehyde, A37
Dimethylaminobenzaldehyde, *see 4-dimethylbenzaldehyde*

Dimethylaminobenzaldehyde Reagent, A37
Dimethylaminobenzaldehyde Solution, Alcoholic, A37
Dimethylaminobenzaldehyde Solution R1, A37
Dimethylaminobenzaldehyde Solution R2, A37
Dimethylaminobenzaldehyde Solution R6, A37
Dimethylaminobenzaldehyde Solution R7, A37
4-Dimethylaminocinnamaldehyde, A37
4-Dimethylaminocinnamaldehyde Solution, A37
Dimethylaminonaphthalenesulphonyl Chloride, A37
2,3-Dimethylaniline, A38
2,6-Dimethylaniline, A38
Dimethylaniline, *see* N,N-*dimethylaniline*
N,N-Dimethylaniline, A38
1,1-Dimethylethyl Methyl Ether, A38
1,1-Dimethylethylamine, A38
Dimethylformamide, A38
Dimethylglyoxime, A38
N,N-Dimethyl-*p*-nitrosoaniline A38
N,N-Dimethyloctylamine, A38
2,6-Dimethylphenol, A38
3,4-Dimethylphenol, A38
N,N-Dimethylpiperazine, A38
Dimethylstearylamide, A38
N,N-Dimethyltetradecylamine, A38
Dimeticone, **486**, A38
Dimidium Bromide, A38
Dimidium Bromide—Sulphan Blue Mixed Solution, A38
1,3-Dinitrobenzene, A38
Dinitrobenzene, *see 1,3-dinitrobenzene*
Dinitrobenzene Solution, A38
3,5-Dinitrobenzoic Acid, A38
Dinitrobenzoic Acid, *see 3,5-dinitrobenzoic acid*
Dinitrobenzoic Acid Solution, A38
3,5-Dinitrobenzoyl Chloride, A38
Dinitrobenzoyl Chloride, *see 3,5-Dinitrobenzoyl Chloride*
2,4-Dinitrophenylhydrazine, A38
Dinitrophenylhydrazine, *see 2,4-dinitrophenylhydrazine*
Dinitrophenylhydrazine–aceto-hydrochloric Solution A38
Dinitrophenylhydrazine–hydrochloric Solution, A39
Dinonyl Phthalate, A39
Dinoprost Injection, **1643**
Dinoprost Trometamol, **487**
Dioctadecyl Disulphide, A39
Dioctadecyl 3,3′-Thiodipropionate, A39
2,2′-Di(octadecyloxy)-5,5′-spirobi(1,3,2-dioxaphosphorinane), A39
Dioctyl Sodium Sulphosuccinate, **504**, A39
Dioctyl Sodium Sulphosuccinate Tablets, **1650**
Dioctyl Sodium Sulphosuccinate VS, A94
Diol Silica Gel for Chromatography, A77
1,4-Dioxan, A39
Dioxan, *see 1,4-dioxan*
Dioxan, Determination of Residual Ethylene Oxide and, A164
Dioxan Solution, A39
Dioxan Solution R1, A39
Dioxan Stock Solution, A39
Diphenhydramine Hydrochloride, **488**
Diphenhydramine Oral Solution, **1643**
Diphenoxylate Hydrochloride, **489**
Diphenylamine, A39
Diphenylamine Solution, A39
Diphenylamine Solution R1, A39
Diphenylamine Solution R2, A39
9,10-Diphenylanthracene, A39
Diphenylanthracene, *see 9,10-diphenylanthracene*
Diphenylbenzidine, *see* N,N-*diphenylbenzidine*
N,N-Diphenylbenzidine, A39
Diphenylboric Acid Aminoethyl Ester, A39
1,5-Diphenylcarbazide, A39
Diphenylcarbazide, *see 1,5-diphenylcarbazide*
Diphenylcarbazide Solution, A39
1,5-Diphenylcarbazone, A39
Diphenylcarbazone, *see 1,5-diphenylcarbazone*
Diphenylcarbazone Mercuric Reagent, A39
Diphenyloxazole, A39
Diphenylphenylene Oxide Polymer, A39
Diphenylpyraline Hydrochloride, **490**, S40
Diphosphorus Pentoxide, *see phosphorus pentoxide*
Diphtheria and Tetanus Vaccine, Adsorbed, **2046**
Diphtheria and Tetanus Vaccine for Adults and Adolescents, Adsorbed, **2048**
Diphtheria Antitoxin, **2031**
Diphtheria Prophylactic, Adsorbed, **2043**
Diphtheria, Tetanus and Pertussis Vaccine, Adsorbed **2050**
Diphtheria–Tetanus Prophylactic, Adsorbed, **2046**
Diphtheria Vaccine, Adsorbed, **2043**
Diphtheria Vaccine, Adsorbed, Assay of, A229
Diphtheria Vaccine for Adults and Adolescents, Adsorbed, **2045**
Diphtheria–Tetanus–Whooping-cough Prophylactic, **2050**
Dipipanone, S41
Dipipanone and Cyclizine Tablets, **1644**
Dipipanone Hydrochloride, **490**
Diploid Cells for the Production of Vaccines, A238
Dipotassium Clorazepate, **491**
Dipotassium Edetate, A40
Dipotassium Hydrogen Orthophosphate, A40
Dipotassium Hydrogen Phosphate, *see dipotassium hydrogen orthophosphate*
Dipotassium Hydrogen Phosphate, **492**
Dipotassium Phosphate, *see Dipotassium Hydrogen Phosphate*
Dipotassium Sulphate, *see potassium sulphate*
Dipotassium (+)-Tartrate, A40
Diprophylline, **493**
Dip/Ser, *see Diphtheria Antitoxin*
Dip/Vac/Ads(Adult), *see Adsorbed Diphtheria Vaccine for Adults and Adolescents*
Dip/Vac/Ads(Child), *see Adsorbed Diphtheria Vaccine*
Dipyridamole, **494**, S41
Dipyridamole Tablets, **1644**
2,2′-Dipyridyl, A40
Disintegration of Formulated Preparations, *see appropriate general monograph*
Disintegration Test for Enteric-coated Tablets, A187
Disintegration Test for Suppositories and Pessaries, A187
Disintegration Test for Tablets and Capsules, A187
Disodium Arsenate, A40
Disodium Edetate, **495**, A40
Disodium Edetate VS, A94
Disodium Ethanedisulphonate, A40
Disodium Hydrogen Citrate, **1168**, A40
Disodium Hydrogen Orthophosphate, A40
Disodium Hydrogen Orthophosphate, Anhydrous, A40
Disodium Hydrogen Orthophosphate Dihydrate, A40
Disodium Hydrogen Phosphate, **496**, *see also disodium hydrogen orthophosphate*
Disodium Hydrogen Phosphate, Anhydrous, *see anhydrous disodium hydrogen orthophosphate*
Disodium Hydrogen Phosphate Dihydrate, **495**, *see disodium hydrogen orthophosphate dihydrate*
Disodium Hydrogen Phosphate Dodecahydrate, **496**
Disodium Hydrogen Phosphate Solution, A40
Disodium Pamidronate, **497**, S41
Disodium Pamidronate for Intravenous Infusion, **1645**
Disodium Pamidronate Intravenous Infusion, **1645**
Disodium Phosphate Dihydrate, *see Disodium Hydrogen Phosphate Dihydrate*
Disodium Phosphate Dodecahydrate, *see Disodium Hydrogen Phosphate Dodecahydrate*
Disodium Tetraborate, *see sodium tetraborate*
Disopyramide, **498**, S42
Disopyramide Capsules, **1646**
Disopyramide Phosphate, **499**
Disopyramide Phosphate Capsules, **1646**
Dispersible Aspirin and Codeine Tablets, **1596**
Dispersible Aspirin Tablets, **1493**
Dispersible Cellulose, **287**
Dispersible Co-codaprin Tablets, **1596**
Dispersible Co-trimoxazole Tablets, **1612**
Dispersible Paracetamol Tablets, **1855**
Dispersible Tablets, 1452

Dispersible Trimethoprim and Sulphamethoxazole Tablets, **1612**
Dissolution of Formulated Preparations, *see appropriate general monograph*
Dissolution Test for Tablets and Capsules, A189
Dissolution Test for Transdermal Patches, A192
Dissolution Testing of Solid Oral Dosage Forms, A327
Distillation Range, Determination of, A137
Distilled Water, A90
Distribution Coefficient, Definition of, A126
Disulfiram, **500**, S42
Disulfiram Tablets, **1647**
5,5′-Dithiobis(2-nitrobenzoic) Acid, A40
Dithiol, A40
Dithiol Reagent, A40
Dithiothreitol, A40
Dithizone, A40
Dithizone R1, A40
Dithizone Solution, A40
Dithizone Solution R2, A40
Dithranol, **501**
Dithranol Cream, **1647**
Dithranol Ointment, **1648**
Dithranol Paste, **1649**
Divanadium Pentoxide, A40
Divanadium Pentoxide Solution in Sulphuric Acid, A40
DNA, A313
Dobutamine Hydrochloride, **502**
Docusate Sodium, *see dioctyl sodium sulphosuccinate*
Docusate Sodium, **504**, S42
Docusate Sodium Capsules, Dantron and, **1596**
Docusate Tablets, **1650**
Dodecan-1-ol, A40
Dodecyl Gallate, **504**
Domiphen Bromide, **505**, A41
Domperidone, **506**
Domperidone Maleate, **507**
L-Dopa and Preparations, *see under Levodopa*
Dopamine Concentrate, Sterile, **1651**
Dopamine Hydrochloride, **509**, S43
Dopamine Hydrochloride for Injection, **1652**
Dopamine Intravenous Infusion, **1651**
Dosulepin Capsules/Dothiepin Capsules, **1652**
Dosulepin Hydrochloride, S43
Dosulepin Hydrochloride/Dothiepin Hydrochloride, **510**
Dosulepin Tablets/Dothiepin Tablets, **1653**
Dothiepin Hydrochloride, S43
Dothiepin Hydrochloride and Preparations, *see under Dosulepin*
Dotriacontane, A41
Double-strength Chloroform Water, **1560**
Double-strength Standard 2,6-Dichlorophenolindophenolindophenol Solution, A35
Doxapram Hydrochloride, **511**, S44
Doxapram Injection, **1653**
Doxepin Capsules, **1654**
Doxepin Hydrochloride, **512**, S44
Doxorubicin Hydrochloride, **513**
Doxorubicin Hydrochloride for Injection, **1655**
Doxorubicin Injection, **1654**
Doxycycline, **515**
Doxycycline Capsules, **1656**
Doxycycline Hyclate, **516**
Doxycycline Hydrochloride, *see Doxycycline Hyclate*
Dried Aluminium Hydroxide, **72**
Dried Aluminium Phosphate, **73**
Dried Bitter-Orange Peel, **965**
Dried Calcium Acetate, A26
Dried Calcium Sulphate, **236**
Dried Coagulation Factors, *see under name of factor*
Dried Epsom Salts, **835**
Dried Ferrous Sulphate, **587**
Dried Iodinated[^{125}I] Fibrinogen, **2124**
Dried Lemon Peel, **780**
Dried Magnesium Sulphate, **835**
Dried/Cho/Vac, *see Cholera Vaccine*
Dried/Tub/Vac/BCG, *see Bacillus Calmette-Guérin Vaccine*
Dried/Typhoid/Vac, *see Typhoid Vaccine*
Droperidol, **518**
Droppers, A13
Drops, Ear, 1426, *see also under under name of substance*
Drops, Eye, 1428, *see also under name of substance*
Drops, Nasal, 1438, *see also under name of substance*
Drops, Oral, 1441, *see also under name of substance*
Dry Extracts, 1428
Dry Heat Sterilisation, A265
Dry Residue of
Liquid Extracts, 1427
Soft Extracts 1427
Tinctures, 1456
Drying, Determination of Loss on, A168
DT/Vac/Ads(Adult), *see Adsorbed Diphtheria and Tetanus Vaccine for Adults and Adolescents*
DT/Vac/Ads(Child), *see Adsorbed Diphtheria–Tetanus Prophylactic*
DT/Per/Vac/Ads, *see Adsorbed Diphtheria, Tetanus and Pertussis Vaccine*
Dusting Powder, Absorbable, *see Sterilisable Maize Starch*
Dusting Powders, 1458, *see also under name of substance*
Dusting Powders of the BP, List of, 1458
Dydrogesterone, **520**, S44
Dydrogesterone Tablets, **165**

E

Ear Drops, 1426, *see also under name of substance*
Ear Drops of the BP, List of, 1426
Ear Powders, 1426
Ear Preparations, 1425
Ear Preparations of the BP, Additional Requirements for, 1426
Ear Sprays, 1426
Ear Tampons, Medicated, 1426
Ear Washes, 1426
Econazole Cream, **1657**
Econazole Nitrate, **520**
Econazole Pessaries, **1657**
Edetic Acid, **521**, S45
Edrophonium Chloride, **522**, S45
Edrophonium Injection, **1658**
Effervescent Aspirin Tablets, **1493**
Effervescent Calcium Gluconate Tablets, **1535**
Effervescent Granules, 1432
Effervescent Potassium Chloride Tablets, **1883**
Effervescent Powders, 1442
Effervescent Soluble Aspirin Tablets, **1493**
Effervescent Tablets, 1452
Efficacy of Antimicrobial Preservation, A252, A333
n-Eicosane, A41
EID_{50}, A313
Elastic Adhesive Bandage, xxvi
Elastic Adhesive Bandage, Titanium Dioxide, xxvi
Elastic Adhesive Bandage, Ventilated, xxvi
Elastic Adhesive Dressing, xxvi
Elastic Bandage, Cotton and Rubber, xxvi
Elastic Bandage, Heavy Cotton and Rubber, xxvi
Elastic Web Bandage, xxvi
Elasticated Tubular Bandage, xxvi
Elder Flower, **522**
Electrophoresis, A131
Elements, Names, Symbols and Atomic Weights of, A311
Elixirs, 1440, *see also under name of substance,*
Elixirs of the BP, List of, 1441
Embrocation, White, **1992**
Emetine Dihydrochloride, A41
Emetine Hydrochloride, **524**
Emetine Hydrochloride Heptahydate, *see Emetine Hydrochloride*
Emetine Hydrochloride Pentahydrate, **525**
Emission Spectrophotometry, Atomic, A119
Emodin, A41
Emulsifying Cetostearyl Alcohol (Type A), **294**
Emulsifying Cetostearyl Alcohol (Type B), **296**
Emulsifying Ointment, **1658**
Emulsifying Wax, **1658**
Emulsifying Wax, Anionic, **1658**
Emulsifying Wax, Cetomacrogol, **1551**
Emulsifying Wax, Non-ionic, **1551**
Emulsions, *see under name of substance*
Emulsions, Oral, 1441, *see also under name of substance*
Endotoxin Standard, A325
Endotoxin Standard BRP, A215

Endotoxin Testing, Bacterial, A322
Endotoxins, Bacterial, Test for, A214
Enemas, 1450, *see also under name of substance*
Enemas of the BP, List of, 1450
Enoxaparin Sodium, **525**
Enteric-coated Prednisolone Tablets, **1890**
Enteric-coated Tablets, Disintegration Test for, A187
Enterobacteriaceae, Test for, A243
Eosin, A41
EPBRP, A106, A313
EPCRS, A106, A313, A342
Ephedrine, **526**, S45
Ephedrine, Anhydrous, **527**
Ephedrine Elixir, **1659**
Ephedrine Hemihydrate, *see Ephedrine*
Ephedrine Hydrochloride, **528**
Ephedrine Hydrochloride, Racemic, **1132**
Ephedrine Hydrochloride Tablets, **1660**
Ephedrine Nasal Drops, **1659**
Ephedrine Oral Solution, **1659**
Epinephrine, S6, S46
Epinephrine, Salts and Preparations, *see under Adrenaline*
Epsom Salts, **835**
Epsom Salts, Dried, **835**
Ergocalciferol, **529**, *see also calciferol*
Ergocalciferol Injection, *see Calciferol Injection*
Ergocalciferol Oral Drops, *see Calciferol Oral Drops*
Ergocalciferol Oral Solution, *see Calciferol Oral Solution*
Ergocalciferol Tablets, *see Calciferol Tablets*
Ergometrine and Oxytocin Injection, **1661**
Ergometrine Injection, **1661**
Ergometrine Maleate, **530**
Ergometrine Tablets, **1662**
Ergotamine Injection, **1663**
Ergotamine Tablets, xxv
Ergotamine Tartrate, **531**
Error, Fiducial Limits of, 13, 1403
Erucamide, A41
Erythromycin, **533**, S46
Erythromycin Estolate, **535**, S46
Erythromycin Estolate Capsules, **1663**
Erythromycin Ethyl Succinate, **536**, S47
Erythromycin Ethyl Succinate Oral Suspension, **1665**
Erythromycin Ethyl Succinate Tablets, **1667**
Erythromycin Ethylsuccinate, *see Erythromycin Ethyl Succinate*
Erythromycin Lactobionate, **537**, S47
Erythromycin Lactobionate Intravenous Infusion, **1664**
Erythromycin Stearate, **538**, S47
Erythromycin Stearate Tablets, **1667**
Erythromycin Tablets, **1666**
Escherichia coli, Test for, A244
Ester Value, Determination of, A172
Esters in Volatile Oils, Test for Foreign, A175
Esters, Reactions of, A149
Estimated Potency, 13, 1403
17α-Estradiol, A41
Estradiol Benzoate, **539**
Estradiol Hemihydrate, **540**
Estradiol Injection, **1668**
Estragole, A41
Estramustine Phosphate Capsules, **1668**
Estramustine Sodium Phosphate, **542**, S48
Estriol, **543**
Estropipate, **544**, S48
Estropipate Tablets, **1669**
Etacrynic Acid, **545**, S48
Etacrynic Acid Tablets, **1669**
Etamiphylline, S49
Etamiphylline Camsilate, **546**, S49
Etamiphylline Camsylate, *see Etamiphylline Camsilate*
Etamiphylline Injection, **1670**
Etamiphylline Suppositories, **1670**
Etamivan, **546**, S49
Etamivan Oral Solution, **1671**
Etamsylate, **547**
Ethacrynic Acid and Preparations, *see under Etacrynic Acid*
Ethambutol Hydrochloride, **548**, S50
Ethambutol Tablets, **1671**
Ethamivan and Preparations, *see under Etamivan*
Ethane-1,2-diol, A41
Ethanol, *see absolute ethanol*
Ethanol, **548**
Ethanol (20 per cent), **550**
Ethanol (25 per cent), **550**
Ethanol (45 per cent), **550**
Ethanol (50 per cent), **550**
Ethanol (60 per cent), **550**
Ethanol (70 per cent), **550**
Ethanol (80 per cent), **549**
Ethanol (90 per cent), **549**
Ethanol (96 per cent), **549**
Ethanol (96%), A41
Ethanol (96%), Aldehyde-free, A41
Ethanol, Absolute, A41
Ethanol Content of
Liquid Extracts, 1427
Tinctures, 1456
Ethanol, Determination of, A159
Ethanol R1, *see Absolute Ethanol R1*
Ethanol R1, Absolute, A41
Ethanol-free Chloroform, A29
Ethanol-soluble Extractive, Determination of, A180
Ethanolamine, **550**, A41
Ethanolamine Oleate Injection, **1671**
Ethanolic Acetic–Ammonia Buffer pH 3.7, *see buffer solution pH 3.7*
Ethanolic Hydrochloric Acid, A48
Ethanolic Iron(III) Chloride Solution, A52
Ethanolic Potassium Hydroxide, A72
Ethanolic Potassium Hydroxide VS, A96
Ethanolic Sodium Hydroxide, A80
Ethanolic Sodium Hydroxide VS, A97
Ethanolic Sulphuric Acid, A84
Ethanols, Dilute, **549**
Ether, **550**, A42
Ether, Anaesthetic, **551**
Ether, Peroxide-free A42
Ether, Solvent, **552**
Ethinylestradiol, **552**
Ethinylestradiol Tablets, **1672**
Ethinylestradiol Tablets, Levonorgestrel and, **1775**
Ethinyloestradiol and Preparations, *see under Ethinylestradiol*
Ethionamide, **553**
Ethisterone, **554**
Ethosuximide, **555**
Ethosuximide Capsules, **1672**
Ethosuximide Oral Solution, **1672**
Ethoxychrysoidine Hydrochloride, A42
Ethoxychrysoidine Solution, A42
2-Ethoxyethanol, A42
Ethyl Acetate, **556**, A42
Ethyl Acetate, Treated, A42
Ethyl *N*-Acetyl-L-tyrosinate, *see acetyltyrosine ethyl ester*
Ethyl Acetyltyrosinate, 0.2M, *see 0.2M acetyltyrosine ethyl ester*
Ethyl Acrylate, A42
Ethyl Benzoate, A42
Ethyl Chloride, **557**, S50
Ethyl Cinnamate, **557**, S50, A42
Ethyl Cyanoacetate, A42
Ethyl Formate, A42
Ethyl Gallate, **558**
Ethyl Hydroxybenzoate, **558**
Ethyl Methyl Ketone, *see butan-2-one*
Ethyl Oleate, **559**
Ethyl Parahydroxybenzoate, A42
4-[(Ethylamino)methyl]pyridine, A42
Ethylbenzene, A42
4-Ethylcatechol, A42
Ethylcellulose, **560**
Ethyldi-isopropylamine, *see di-isopropylethylamine*
Ethylene Bis[3,3-di(3-(1,1-dimethyl)-ethyl-4-hydroxyphenyl)butyrate], A42
Ethylene Bis[3,3-di(3-*tert*-butyl-4-hydroxyphenyl)butyrate], *see ethylene bis[3,3-di(3-(1,1-dimethyl)ethyl-4-hydroxyphenyl)butyrate]*
Ethylene Chloride, *see 1,2-dichloroethane,*
Ethylene Glycol, *see ethane-1,2-diol,*
Ethylene Glycol Monoethyl Ether, *see 2-ethoxyethanol*
Ethylene Glycol Monomethyl Ether, *see 2-methoxyethanol*
Ethylene Glycol Monostearate, **561**
Ethylene Oxide, A42
Ethylene Oxide and Dioxan, Determination of Residual, A164
Ethylene Oxide Solution, A43
Ethylene Oxide Solution R1, A43
Ethylene Oxide Solution R2, A43
Ethylene Oxide Solution R3, A43
Ethylene Oxide Stock Solution, A42
Ethylene–Vinyl Acetate Copolymer, Containers of, A296
Ethylenediamine, **562**, A43
Ethylenediaminetetra-acetic Acid, A43
(Ethylenedinitrilo)tetra-acetic Acid, *see ethylenediaminetetra-acetic acid*

Ethylestrenol, **563**, S51
Ethylestrenol Tablets, **1673**
2-Ethylhexane-1,3-diol, A43
2-Ethylhexanoic Acid, A43
1,1′-Ethylidenebis(tryptophan), A43
N-Ethylmaleimide, A43
2-Ethyl-2-methylsuccinic Acid, A43
Ethylmorphine Hydrochloride, **564**
Ethyloestrenol and Preparations, *see under Ethylestrenol*
Ethylparaben, **558**
Ethylvinylbenzene–Divinylbenzene Copolymer, A43
Ethylvinylbenzene–Divinyl Benzene Copolymer R1, A43
Ethynodiol Diacetate, *see Etynodiol Diacetate*
Etilefrine Hydrochloride, **564**
Etodolac, **566**, S51
Etodolac Capsules, **1673**
Etodolac Tablets, **1674**
Etofylline, **567**
Etoposide, **568**
Etynodiol Diacetate, **569**, S51
Eucalyptus Oil, **570**
Eugenol, **571**, A43
Euglobulins, Bovine, A43
Euglobulins, Human, A44
European Pharmacopoeia, 3, 1393, A343
European Pharmacopoeia Biological Reference Preparation, A106
European Pharmacopoeia Chemical Reference Substances, A106, A342
European Pharmacopoeia Commission, Membership of the, A343
European Pharmacopoeia General Methods, A7
European Pharmacopoeia, Introduction, xvi
European Pharmacopoeia Reference Spectra, A115
European Viper Venom Antiserum, **2032**
Excipients, A327
Excipients in Parenteral Preparations, 1443
Excipients, Use of 10, 1400
Exclusion Volume, Definition of, A126
Expression of Content, 19, 1409
Expression of Standards, 5, 1395
Exsiccated Calcium Sulphate, **236**
Extemporaneous Preparation, Status of, 9, 1399
Extension Strapping, xxvi
Extractable Volume, A204
Extraction of Alkaloids, Complete, Tests for, A183
Extraction of Drugs, Continuous, A182
Extractive, Ethanol-soluble, Determination of, A180
Extracts, 1427, *see also under name of substance*
 Dry, 1428
 Liquid, 1427
 Soft, 1427
Extracts of the BP, List of, 1428
Extraneous Agents in Viral Vaccines, A250
Eye Drops, 1428, 1430, *see also under name of substance*
Eye Drops, Alkaline, **1744**
Eye Drops in Single-dose Containers, Codes for, A310
Eye Drops of the BP, List of, 1430
Eye Lotions, 1429, *see also under name of substance*
Eye Lotions of the BP, List of 1431
Eye Ointment Basis, **1925**
Eye Ointment, Simple, **1925**
Eye Ointments 1430, *see also under name of substance,*
Eye Preparations, 1428
Eye Preparations of the BP, Additional Requirements for, 1430

F

F_0 Concept in Steam Sterilisation, A267
Factor VII Fraction, Assay of, A221
Factor VII Fraction, Dried, **2008**
Factor VIII Fraction, Assay of, A222
Factor VIII Fraction, Dried, **2010**
Factor IX Fraction, Assay of, A224
Factor IX Fraction, Dried, **2011**
Factor Xa Solution, Bovine, A24
Famotidine, **572**
Fast Blue B Salt, A44
Fast Red B Salt, A44
Fat, Hard, **573**
Fc Function of Immunoglobulin, Test for, A225
Felodipine, **574**
Fenbufen, **575**, S52, A44
Fenbufen Capsules, **1675**
Fenbufen Tablets, **1676**
Fenchone, A44
Fenfluramine Hydrochloride, xxv
Fenfluramine Tablets, xxv
Fennel, Bitter, **576**
Fennel, Sweet, **577**
Fenoprofen, S52
Fenoprofen Calcium, **578**, S52
Fenoprofen Tablets, **1676**
Fenoterol Hydrobromide, **579**
Fentanyl, **580**
Fentanyl Citrate, **581**
Fenticonazole Nitrate, **583**
Ferric Ammonium Citrate, *see ammonium iron(III) citrate*
Ferric Ammonium Sulphate, *see ammonium iron(III) sulphate and ammonium iron(III) sulphate VS*
Ferric Ammonium Sulphate Solution R2, *see ammonium iron(III) sulphate solution R2,*
Ferric Ammonium Sulphate Solution R5, *see ammonium iron(III) sulphate solution R5*
Ferric Ammonium Sulphate Solution R6, *see ammonium iron(III) sulphate solution R6*
Ferric Chloride, *see iron(III) chloride*
Ferric Chloride Solution R1, *see iron(III) chloride solution R1*
Ferric Chloride Solution R2, *see iron(III) chloride solution R2*
Ferric Chloride–Sulphamic Acid Reagent, *see iron(III) chloride–sulphamic acid reagent*
Ferric[59Fe] Citrate Injection, **2117**
Ferric Nitrate, *see iron(III) nitrate*
Ferric Sulphate, *see iron(III) sulphate*
Ferricyanide Standard Solution (50 ppm $Fe(CN)_6$), A99
Ferrocyanide Standard Solution (100 ppm $Fe(CN)_6$), A99
Ferrocyphen, A44
Ferrocyphen Solution, A44
Ferrocyphene, *see ferrocyphen*
Ferroin, *see ferroin solution*
Ferroin Solution, A44
Ferrous Ammonium Sulphate, *see ammonium iron(II) sulphate and ammonium iron(II) sulphate VS*
Ferrous Fumarate, **584**
Ferrous Fumarate and Folic Acid Tablets, **1678**
Ferrous Fumarate Oral Suspension, **1677**
Ferrous Fumarate Tablets, **1678**
Ferrous Gluconate, **585**
Ferrous Gluconate Tablets, **1679**
Ferrous Succinate, xxv
Ferrous Succinate Capsules, xxv
Ferrous Succinate Tablets, xxv
Ferrous Sulphate, *see iron(II) sulphate and iron(II) sulphate VS*
Ferrous Sulphate, **586**
Ferrous Sulphate, Dried, **587**
Ferrous Sulphate Oral Solution, Paediatric, **1679**
Ferrous Sulphate Solution R2, *see iron(II) sulphate solution R2*
Ferrous Sulphate Tablets, **1679**
Fibrin Blue, A45
Fibrin Congo Red, *see Congo red fibrin*
Fibrin Sealant Kit, **2015**
Fibrinogen, A45
Fibrinogen, Dried, **2014**
Fibrinogen, Dried Iodinated[125I], **2124**
Fibrinogen, Freeze-dried Human, *see Fibrinogen, Dried*
Fiducial Limits of Error, 13, 1403
Fig, **588**
Fig Elixir, Compound, xxv
Filtration, Sterilisation by, A265
Fine Particles, Aerodynamic Assessment of, A194
Fine Powder, Definition of, A254
Fineness of
 Dispersion of Dispersible Tablets, 1452
 Oral Powders, 1442
 Topical Powders, 1457
FIP, A313
Fixed Oils in Volatile Oils, Test for, A175
Fixed Oils, Methods for, A175
Flavoxate Hydrochloride, **588**, S53
Flavoxate Tablets, **1680**
Flexible Collodion, **1680**
Flowability, Determination of, A259
Flucloronlone Acetonide, xxv
Fluclorolone Ointment, xxv

Flucloxacillin and Ampicillin Capsules, **1601**
Flucloxacillin and Ampicillin Oral Suspension, **1602**
Flucloxacillin Capsules, **1681**
Flucloxacillin Injection, **1681**
Flucloxacillin Magnesium, **589**, S53
Flucloxacillin Oral Solution, **1682**
Flucloxacillin Oral Suspension, **1683**
Flucloxacillin Sodium, **590**, S53
Flucloxacillin Sodium for Injection, **1681**
Flucytosine, **592**, S54
Flucytosine Tablets, **1683**
Fludrocortisone Acetate, **593**
Fludrocortisone Tablets, **1684**
Flufenamic Acid, A45
Flunitrazepam, **595**
Fluocinolone Acetonide, **596**
Fluocinolone Acetonide Dihydrate, **597**, S54
Fluocinolone Cream, **1684**
Fluocinolone Ointment, **1685**
Fluocinonide, **598**, S54
Fluocinonide Cream, **1686**
Fluocinonide Ointment, **1686**
Fluocortolone Cream, **1687**
Fluocortolone Hexanoate, **599**, S55
Fluocortolone Ointment, **1687**
Fluocortolone Pivalate, **599**, S55
Fluoranthene, A45
9-Fluorenone, A45
Fluorenone Solution, A45
9-Fluorenylmethyl Chloroformate, A45
Fluorescamine, A45
Fluorescein, A45
Fluorescein Eye Drops, **1688**
Fluorescein Injection, **1689**
Fluorescein Sodium, **601**, S55, A45
Fluorescein, Soluble, **601**
Fluorescein-conjugated Rabies Antiserum, A75
Fluorescence Spectrometry, X-Ray, A121
Fluorescence Spectrophotometry, A121
Fluoride Standard Solution (1 ppm F), A99
Fluoride Standard Solution (10 ppm F), A99
Fluorides, Limit Test for, A152
Fluorimetry, A121
1-Fluoro-2,4-dinitrobenzene, A45
Fluorodinitrobenzene, *see 1-fluoro-2,4-dinitrobenzene,*
Fluorometholone, **602**, S56
Fluorometholone Eye Drops, **1689**
1-Fluoro-2-nitro-4-trifluoromethylbenzene, A45
Fluorouracil, **603**, S56
Fluorouracil Cream, **1690**
Fluorouracil Injection, **1690**
Fluoxetine Hydrochloride, **604**
Flupenthixol Esters and Preparations, *see under Flupentixol*
Flupentixol Injection, **1691**
Flupentixol Decanoate, **606**, S56
Fluphenazine Decanoate, **607**
Fluphenazine Decanoate Injection, **1692**
Fluphenazine Enantate, **608**
Fluphenazine Enanthate, *see Fluphenazine Enantate*
Fluphenazine Enanthate Injection, xxv
Fluphenazine Hydrochloride, **609**
Fluphenazine Tablets, **1692**
Flurazepam Capsules, **1693**
Flurazepam Monohydrochloride, **610**, S57
Flurbiprofen, **612**, S57
Flurbiprofen Eye Drops, **1694**
Flurbiprofen Sodium, **612**, S57
Flurbiprofen Tablets, **1694**
Fluticasone Cream, **1695**
Fluticasone Ointment, **1696**
Fluticasone Propionate, **613**, S58
Flu/Vac, *see Inactivated Influenza Vaccine (Whole Virion)*
Flu/Vac/SA, *see Inactivated Influenza Vaccine (Surface Antigen)*
Flu/Vac/Split, *see Inactivated Influenza Vaccine (Split Virion)*
Fluvoxamine Maleate, **615**, S58
Fluvoxamine Tablets, **1696**
Flux-calcined Diatomaceous Filter-aid, Washed, A34
Foams, Cutaneous, 1424
Foams, Medicated, 1431
Foams, Rectal, 1449
Foams, Vaginal, 1462
Folic Acid, **616**, A45
Folic Acid Tablets, **1697**
Folic Acid Tablets, Ferrous Fumarate and, **1678**
Foreign Esters in Volatile Oils, Test for, A175
Foreign Matter in Vegetable Drugs, Determination of, A181
Foreign Oils by Gas Chromatography, Test for, A177
Formaldehyde, *see formaldehyde solution*
Formaldehyde Solution, **617**, A45
Formaldehyde Standard Solution (5 ppm CH_2O), A99
Formaldehyde, Test for Free, A231
Formalin, **617**
Formamide, A45
Formamide, Treated, A45
Formic Acid, A45
Formic Acid, Anhydrous, A45
Formulated Preparations, xx
Formulated Preparations, General Monographs for, 3, 5, 1393, 1395
Formulated Preparations, Manufacture of, 9, 1399
Fortified Benethamine Penicillin Injection, xxv
Fortified Procaine Benzylpenicillin Injection/Fortified Procaine Penicillin Injection, **1895**
Foscarnet Intravenous Infusion, **1698**
Foscarnet Sodium, **618**, S58
Fosfestrol Sodium, **619**, S59
Fractionated Coconut Oil, *see Medium-chain Triglycerides*
Fractionated Palm Kernel Oil, **986**
Framycetin Gauze Dressing, xxvi
Framycetin Sulphate, **620**
Frangula Bark, **621**
Frangula Bark Dry Extract, Standardised, **1699**
Frangula Bark, Powdered, xxv, *see also Frangula Bark*
Free Formaldehyde, Test for, A231
Freeze-dried Blood Products, *see under name of blood product*
Freeze-dried Vaccines, *see under name of vaccine*
Freezing Point, Determination of, A137
Fresh Frozen Plasma, xxvi
Freshly Prepared, Definition of, 10, 1400
Friability of Uncoated Tablets, A262
Friars' Balsam, **1510**
D-Fructose, A45
Fructose, *see D-fructose*
Fructose, **623**
Fructose Intravenous Infusion, **1700**
Frusemide, S59, S60
Frusemide and Preparations, *see under Furosemide*
Fuchsin, Basic, A45
Fuchsin Solution, Basic, A46
Fuchsin Solution, Decolorised, A46
Fuchsin Solution R1, Decolorised, A46
L-Fucose, A46
Fucose, *see L-fucose*
Fumaric Acid, S59
Fuming Nitric Acid, A62
Furazolidone, **624**, S60
Furfural, *see furfuraldehyde*
Furfuraldehyde, A46
Furosemide, S59, S60
Furosemide Injection/Frusemide Injection, **1700**
Furosemide Tablets, Amiloride and/Frusemide Tablets, Amiloride and, **1590**
Furosemide Tablets/Frusemide Tablets, **1701**
Furosemide/Frusemide, **624**
Fusidic Acid, **625**, S60
Fusidic Acid Oral Suspension, **1702**

G

g, A313
D-Galactose A46
Galactose, **626**, *see also D-galactose*
Gallamine Injection, **1702**
Gallamine Triethiodide, **627**
Gallic Acid, A46
Gallium[^{67}Ga] Citrate Injection, **2117**
Gamma Benzene Hexachloride, *see Lindane*
Gamma Benzene Hexachloride CRS, A106
Garlic Powder, **629**
Gas Chromatography, A125
Gas Chromatography, Head-space, A125
Gas Detector Tubes, A170
Gas Sterilisation, A265
Gas-gangrene Antitoxin (Novyi), **2033**
Gas-gangrene Antitoxin (Oedematiens), **2033**
Gas-gangrene Antitoxin (Perfringens), **2034**

Gas-gangrene Antitoxin (Septicum), **2035**
Gas-gangrene Antitoxin, Mixed, **2036**
Gas/Ser, *see Mixed Gas-gangrene Antitoxin*
Gastric Juice, Artificial, A46
Gastro-resistant Capsules, 1422
Gastro-resistant Granules, 1432
Gastro-resistant Prednisolone Tablets, **1890**
Gastro-resistant Tablets, 1452
Gauze Pledget, X-Ray-Detectable, xxvi
Gauze Swab, X-Ray-Detectable, xxvi
Gee's Linctus, **1947**
Gel Electrophoresis, A131
Gelatin, **629**, A46
Gelatin, Hydrolysed, A46
Gelatin Sponge, Absorbable, xxvi
Gels, 1459, *see also under name of substance*
Gels of the BP, List of, 1460
Gemfibrozil, **631**, S61
Gemfibrozil Capsules, **1703**
Gemfibrozil Tablets, **1704**
General Methods of the European Pharmacopoeia, A7
General Monographs for Formulated Preparations, 3, 5, 1393, 1395
General Notices, xvii, xx, 1, 1391
General Notices, Contents of, 2, 1392
General Reagents, A13
Gentamicin Cream, **1704**
Gentamicin Eye Drops, **1705**
Gentamicin Injection, **1705**
Gentamicin Ointment, **1706**
Gentamicin Sulphate, **633**
Gentian, **634**
Gentian Infusion, Compound, **1707**
Gentian Infusion, Concentrated Compound, **1707**
Gentian Mixture, Acid, **1707**
Gentian Mixture, Alkaline, **1707**
Gentian Oral Solution, Acid, **1707**
Gentian Oral Solution, Alkaline, **1707**
Gentian, Powdered, xxv
Gentian Root, *see Gentian*
Geraniol, A46
Geranyl Acetate, A46
Ginger, **635**
Ginger Essence, **1707**
Ginger, Powdered, *see Ginger*
Ginger, Powdered, xxv
Ginger Tincture, Strong, **1707**
Ginger Tincture, Weak, **1707**
Ginger, Unbleached, *see Ginger*
Gitoxin, A46
Glacial Acetic Acid, **38**, A13
Glacial Acetic Acid, Anhydrous, *see anhydrous acetic acid*
Glass Containers for Pharmaceutical Use, A268
Glassware, Requirements for, 5, 18, 1395, 1408
Glauber's Salt, **1200**
Glibenclamide, **636**
Glibenclamide Tablets, **1708**
Gliclazide, **637**, S61
Gliclazide Tablets, **1708**
Glipizide, **638**, S61
Glipizide Tablets, **1709**
Gliquidone, **640**, S62
Gliquidone Tablets, **1709**
Glucagon, **640**
Glucagon for Injection, **1710**
Glucagon Injection, **1710**
Glucosamine Hydrochloride, A46
D-Glucose, A46
Glucose, **643**, *see also D-glucose*
Glucose, Anhydrous, **642**
Glucose Injection, Potassium Chloride and, **1882**
Glucose Injection, Potassium Chloride, Sodium Chloride and, **1883**
Glucose Injection, Sodium Chloride and, **1930**
Glucose Intravenous Infusion, **1711**
Glucose Intravenous Infusion, Potassium Chloride and, **1882**
Glucose Intravenous Infusion, Potassium Chloride, Sodium Chloride and, **1883**
Glucose Intravenous Infusion, Sodium Chloride and, **1930**
Glucose Irrigation Solution, **1711**
D-Glucose Monohydrate, A46
Glucose Monohydrate, *see Glucose*
Glucose Standard Solution, A99
Glutamic Acid, **644**, A46
Glutaraldehyde, A46
Glutaraldehyde Solution, **1712**
Glutaraldehyde Solution, Strong, **645**
Glutethimide, **645**
Glycerin, **646**
Glycerin Suppositories, **1712**
Glycerol, **646**, A46
Glycerol (85 per cent), **647**
Glycerol (85%), A46
Glycerol Injection, Phenol and, **1868**
Glycerol Suppositories, **1712**
Glycerol Triacetate, *see Triacetin*
Glyceryl Monostearate 40-50, **648**
Glyceryl Monostearate, Self-emulsifying, **649**
Glyceryl Trinitrate Solution, Concentrated, **650**
Glyceryl Trinitrate Tablets, **1712**
Glycine, **650**, S62, A46
Glycine Buffer pH 2.9, A103
Glycine Buffer pH 11.3, A103
Glycine Buffer Solution, A103
Glycine Irrigation Solution, **1713**
Glycollic Acid, A46
Glycyrrhetic Acid, *see glycyrrhetinic acid*
Glycyrrhetinic Acid, A47
β-Glycyrrhetinic Acid, A47
Glyoxal Bis(2-hydroxyanil), A47
Glyoxal Sodium Bisulphite, A47
Glyoxal Solution, A47
Glyoxal Standard Solution (20 ppm $C_2H_2O_2$), A99
Glyoxalhydroxyanil, *see glyoxal bis(2-hydroxyanil)*
Gonadorelin Acetate, **651**
Gonadorelin for Injection, **1714**
Gonadorelin Hydrochloride, **653**
Gonadorelin Injection, **1714**
Gonadotrophin, Chorionic, **335**, A47
Gonadotrophin Injection, Chorionic, **1569**
Gonadotrophin, Serum, A47
Graduated Glassware, Requirements for, 5, 1395
Gramicidin, **654**
Granulated Tin, *see tin*
Granules, 1432, *see also under name of substance*
Coated, 1432
Effervescent, 1432
for Oral Solutions and Suspension, 1440
Gastro-resistant, 1432
Modified-release, 1433
Granules of the BP, Additional Requirements for, 1433
Granules of the BP, List of, 1433
Graphic Formula, Status of, 4, 1394
Graphitised Carbon for Chromatography, A27
Griseofulvin, **655**, S62
Griseofulvin Tablets, **1715**
Ground-nut Oil, **111**
Guaiacum Resin, A47
Guaiazulene, A47
Guaifenesin, **656**
Guaiphenesin, A47, *see also Guaifenesin*
Guanethidine Monosulphate, **657**
Guanethidine Tablets, **1715**
Guanidine Hydrochloride, A47
Guanine, A47
Guar, **658**
Guar Galactomannan, **658**
Guidance to Manufacturers, Monograph Development, A339
Guidelines for Bacterial Endotoxin Testing, A323
Guidelines on the Test for Sterility, A242
Guinea-pigs, 14, 1404

H

Haemagglutinins, Anti-A and Anti-B, A226
Haemodialysis Solutions, **1716**
Haemodialysis Solutions, Water for Diluting Concentrated, **1718**
Haemofiltration Solutions, **1720**
Haemoglobin, A47
Haemoglobin Solution, A47
Haemolytic Value, A274
Haemophilus Type B Conjugate Vaccine, **2052**
Half-life, Measurement of, 2104
Halibut-liver Oil, **659**
Halibut-liver Oil Capsules, **1722**
Haloperidol, **660**, S63
Haloperidol Capsules, **1722**
Haloperidol Injection, **1722**
Haloperidol Oral Drops, **1723**
Haloperidol Oral Drops, Strong, **1723**
Haloperidol Oral Solution, **1723**
Haloperidol Oral Solution, Strong, **1723**
Haloperidol Tablets, **1724**
Halothane, **661**
Hamamelis Leaf, **663**
Hard Capsules, 1421
Hard Fat, **573**
Hard Paraffin, **995**

Harpagophytum, **440**
Harpagoside, A47
Hartmann's Solution for Injection, **1936**
Hawthorn Berries, **664**
Head-space Gas Chromatography, A125
Heating in an Autoclave, A264
Heavy Cotton and Rubber Elastic Bandage, xxvi
Heavy Kaolin, **761**
Heavy Magnesium Carbonate, **830**
Heavy Magnesium Oxide, **833**, A55
Heavy Metals, Limit Tests for, A153
Helium, A47
Helium for Chromatography, *see helium*
Hep A/Vac, *see Inactivated Hepatitis A Vaccine*
Hep B/Vac, *see Hepatitis B Vaccine (rDNA)*
Heparin, A47
Heparin, Assay of, A225
Heparin Calcium, **665**
Heparin in Coagulation Factor Concentrates, Assay of, A224
Heparin Injection, **1724**
Heparin Sodium, **666**
Heparins, Low-molecular-mass, *see Low-molecular weight Heparins,*
Heparins, Low-molecular-weight, **667**
Hepatitis A Immunoglobulin, **2021**
Hepatitis A Vaccine Inactivated, **2055**
Hepatitis B Immunoglobulin, **2021**
Hepatitis B Immunoglobulin for Intravenous Use, **2022**
Hepatitis B Vaccine (rDNA), **2058**
Heptane, *see n-heptane*
n-Heptane, A47
Hexachlorophane and Preparations, *see under Hexachlorophene*
Hexachlorophene, **670**, S63
Hexachlorophene Dusting Powder, **1725**
Hexachlorophene Dusting Powder, Zinc and, **1725**
Hexacosane, A47
Hexadimethrine Bromide, A47
2,2′,2″,6,6′,6″-Hexa-(1,1-dimethylethyl)-4,4′,4″-[2,4,6-trimethyl-1,3,5-benzenetriyl)-trismethylene]triphenol, A47
Hexamethyldisilazane, A47
Hexamethylenentetramine, *see hexamine*
Hexamine, A48
Hexane, A48
n-Hexane, A48
Hexane, Purified, A48
Hexetidine, **671**
Hexobarbital, **672**
Hexobarbitone, *see Hexobarbital*
Hexosamines in Polysaccharide Vaccines, Test for, A234
Hexylamine, A48
Hexylresorcinol, **673**
Hexylsilyl Silica Gel for Chromatography, A77
Hib/Vac, *see Haemophilus Type B Conjugate Vaccine*
Histamine Dihydrochloride, **674**
Histamine Dihydrochloride, A48
Histamine Phosphate, **674**, A48
Histamine Solution, A48
Histamine, Test for, A220
Histidine, **675**
Histidine Hydrochloride Monohydrate, **676**
Histidine Monohydrochloride, A48
HIV, A313
Holmium Oxide, A48
Holmium Perchlorate Solution, A48
Homatropine, S63
Homatropine Eye Drops, **1725**
Homatropine Hydrobromide, **678**
Homatropine Methylbromide, **678**
Homoeopathic Preparations, **679**
Hop Strobile, **680**
Human Albumin, **2005**
Human Albumin Solution, A15
Human Albumin Solution R1, A15
Human Blood Products, *see under name of blood product*
Human Diploid Cells for the Production of Vaccine, A238
Human Euglobulins, A44
Human Immunoglobulins, *see under name of immunoglobulin*
Human Insulin, **727**
Human Plasminogen, A69
Human Thrombin, *see thrombin*
Human Thrombin Solution, *see thrombin solution*
Hyaluronate Solution, A48
Hyaluronidase, **681**
Hyaluronidase Diluent, *see diluent for hyaluronidase solutions*
Hyaluronidase for Injection, **1726**
Hyaluronidase Injection, **1726**
Hyaluronidase Solutions, Diluent for, A48
Hydralazine, S64
Hydralazine Hydrochloride, **682**, S64
Hydralazine Hydrochloride for Injection, **1726**
Hydralazine Injection, **1726**
Hydralazine Tablets, **1727**
Hydrated Aluminium Oxide, *see Dried Aluminium Hydroxide*
Hydrated Silica, Colloidal, **1164**
Hydrazine Reducing Mixture, *see reducing mixture*
Hydrazine Sulphate, A48
Hydrindantin, A48
Hydriodic Acid, A48
Hydrobromic Acid, A48
Hydrobromic Acid, 30 per cent, A48
Hydrobromic Acid, Dilute, A48
Hydrocarbons (Type L), Low-vapour-pressure, A48
Hydrochloric Acid, **683**, A48
Hydrochloric Acid BET, A215
Hydrochloric Acid, Brominated, A48
Hydrochloric Acid, Concentrated, *see Hydrochloric Acid*
Hydrochloric Acid, Dilute, **684**, A48
Hydrochloric Acid, Ethanolic, A48
Hydrochloric Acid LAL, A215
Hydrochloric Acid, Methanolic, A48
Hydrochloric Acid R1, A48
Hydrochloric Acid R1, Dilute, A49
Hydrochloric Acid R2, Dilute, A49
Hydrochloric Acid, Stannated A49
Hydrochloric Acid VS, A94
Hydrochloric Methanol, A57
Hydrochlorothiazide, **684**, S64
Hydrochlorothiazide Oral Solution, Amiloride and, **1590**
Hydrochlorothiazide Tablets, **1727**
Hydrochlorothiazide Tablets, Amiloride and, **1591**
Hydrochlorothiazide Tablets, Triamterene and, **1609**
Hydrocolloid Dressing, Semipermeable, xxvi
Hydrocortisone, **686**, A49
Hydrocortisone Acetate, **688**, S65, A49
Hydrocortisone Acetate and Neomycin Ear Drops, **1731**
Hydrocortisone Acetate and Neomycin Eye Drops, **1732**
Hydrocortisone Acetate and Neomycin Eye Ointment, **1732**
Hydrocortisone Acetate Cream, **1728**
Hydrocortisone Acetate Injection, **1733**
Hydrocortisone Acetate Ointment, **1736**
Hydrocortisone and Clioquinol Cream, **1729**
Hydrocortisone and Clioquinol Ointment, **1736**
Hydrocortisone and Neomycin Cream, **1730**
Hydrocortisone and Neomycin Ear Drops, **1731**
Hydrocortisone and Neomycin Eye Drops, **1732**
Hydrocortisone Cream, **1728**
Hydrocortisone Hydrogen Succinate, **689**
Hydrocortisone Ointment, **1735**
Hydrocortisone Sodium Phosphate, **691**
Hydrocortisone Sodium Phosphate Injection, **1734**
Hydrocortisone Sodium Succinate, S65
Hydrocortisone Sodium Succinate for Injection, **1734**
Hydrocortisone Sodium Succinate Injection, **1734**
Hydroflumethiazide, **692**, S65
Hydroflumethiazide Tablets, **1737**
Hydrofluoric Acid, A49
Hydrogen, A49
Hydrogen for Chromatography, *see hydrogen*
Hydrogen Peroxide Mouthwash, **1737**
Hydrogen Peroxide Solution, **693**
Hydrogen Peroxide Solution (3 per cent), **694**
Hydrogen Peroxide Solution (6 per cent), **693**
Hydrogen Peroxide Solution (27 per cent), xxv
Hydrogen Peroxide Solution (30 per cent), **692**
Hydrogen Peroxide Solution (10 vol), A49
Hydrogen Peroxide Solution (20 vol), A49
Hydrogen Peroxide Solution (100 vol), A49
Hydrogen Peroxide Solution (200 vol), A49

Hydrogen Peroxide Solution, Dilute, *see hydrogen peroxide solution (10 vol) and Hydrogen Peroxide Solution (3 per cent)*
Hydrogen Peroxide Solution, Strong, *see hydrogen peroxide solution (100 vol)*
Hydrogen Sulphide, A49
Hydrogen Sulphide R1, A49
Hydrogen Sulphide Solution, A49
Hydrogenated Arachis Oil, **112**
Hydrogenated Polyoxyl Castor Oil, **263**
Hydrogenated Soya Oil, **1219**
Hydrogenated Soya-bean Oil, **1219**
Hydrogenated Soyabean Oil, **1219**
Hydrogenated Vegetable Oil, **1353**
Hydrogenated Wool Fat, **1371**
Hydrolysed Gelatin, A46
Hydrolysed Starch, A82
Hydrolytic Resistance of Glass Containers, A268
Hydrophilic Silica Gel for Chromatography, A77
Hydroquinone, A49
Hydrotalcite, **694**
Hydrotalcite Tablets, **1738**
Hydrous Benzoyl Peroxide, **159**
Hydrous Ointment, **1738**
Hydrous Wool Fat, **1372**
Hydroxocobalamin Acetate, **695**
Hydroxocobalamin Chloride, **696**
Hydroxocobalamin Injection, **1738**
Hydroxocobalamin Sulphate, **697**
4′-Hydroxyacetanilide, *see paracetamol*
4-Hydroxybenzaldehyde, A49
4-Hydroxybenzoic Acid, A49
4-Hydroxybiphenyl, A49
Hydroxycarbamide, **698**, S66
Hydroxycarbamide Capsules, **1739**
Hydroxychloroquine, S66
Hydroxychloroquine Sulphate, **699**
Hydroxychloroquine Tablets, **1739**
4-Hydroxycoumarin, A49
Hydroxyethyl Salicylate, **700**
Hydroxyethylcellulose, **701**
Hydroxyethylmethylcellulose, **703**
2-[4-(2-Hydroxyethyl)piperazin-1-yl]-ethanesulphonic Acid, A49
4-Hydroxyisophthalic Acid, A49
Hydroxyl Value, Determination of, A172
Hydroxylamine Hydrochloride, A49
Hydroxylamine Hydrochloride Solution R2, A49
Hydroxylamine Solution, Alcoholic, A49
Hydroxylamine Solution, Alkaline, A49
Hydroxylamine Solution R1, Alkaline, A49
5-Hydroxymethylfurfural, A49
Hydroxynaphthol Blue Sodium Salt, A49
Hydroxyprogesterone Caproate, **704**, S66
Hydroxyprogesterone Hexanoate, *see Hydroxyprogesterone Caproate*
Hydroxyprogesterone Injection, **1740**
Hydroxypropylcellulose, **704**
8-Hydroxyquinoline, A50
Hydroxyquinoline, *see 8-hydroxyquinoline*
12-Hydroxystearic Acid, A50
5-Hydroxyuracil, A50
Hydroxyurea and Preparations, *see under Hydroxycarbamide*
Hydroxyzine Hydrochloride, **705**
Hyoscine Butylbromide, **707**, S67
Hyoscine Butylbromide Injection, **1740**
Hyoscine Butylbromide Tablets, **1741**
Hyoscine Eye Drops, **1742**
Hyoscine Hydrobromide, **708**, A50
Hyoscine Injection, **1742**
Hyoscine Tablets, **1743**
Hyoscyamine Sulphate, **709**, A50
Hyoscyamus Dry Extract, **1744**
Hyoscyamus Leaf, **709**
Hyoscyamus Leaf, Powdered, xxv, *see also Hyoscyamus Leaf*
Hyoscyamus, Prepared, **711**
Hyperoside, A50
Hypophosphorous Reagent, A50
Hypoxanthine, A50
Hypromellose, **711**
Hypromellose Eye Drops, **1744**
Hypromellose Phthalate, **712**

I

Ibuprofen, **713**, S67
Ibuprofen Cream, **1745**
Ibuprofen Gel, **1745**
Ibuprofen Oral Suspension, **1746**
Ibuprofen Tablets, **1747**
Ichthammol, **715**
Ichthammol Bandage, Zinc Paste and, xxvi
Ichthammol Cream, Zinc and, **1993**
ID_{50}, A313
Identification, 11, 21, 1401, 1411
Identification by Infrared Reference Spectra, A114
Identification of Fixed Oils by Thin-layer Chromatography, A177
Idoxuridine, **716**
Idoxuridine Eye Drops, **1748**
IMI, A313
Imidazole, A50
Imidazole Buffer Solution pH 6.5, A103
Imidazole Buffer Solution pH 7.3, A103
Imidazole–Mercury Reagent, A50
Imidazole, Recrystallised, A50
Imidazole Solution, A50
Iminodibenzyl, A50
Imipenem, **717**
Imipramine Hydrochloride, **718**
Imipramine Tablets, **1748**
Immunoassays, A333
Immunochemical Methods, A207, A213
Immunoglobulin for Intravenous Use, Normal, **2018**
Immunoglobulin Injection, Normal, **2016**
Immunoglobulin, Normal, **2016**
Immunoglobulins, *see under name of immunoglobulin*
Immunosera, Test for Phenol in, A231
Impermeable Plastic Wound Dressing, xxvi
Implants, 1444, *see also under name of substance*
Implants of the BP, List of, 1445
Implementation, Dates of, European Pharmacopoeia, A345
Impurities, Control of, A318
Impurities, Expression of Limits for, A320
Impurities, Limitation of Potential, 4, 1394
Impurities, Statements of, A321
Impurity Limits, Status of, 12, 22, 1402, 1412
Impurity Statements, Status of, 4, 23, 1394, 1413
IMS, **875**
Inactivated Hepatitis A Vaccine, **2055**
Inactivated Influenza Vaccine (Split Virion), **2061**
Inactivated Influenza Vaccine (Surface Antigen), **2063**
Inactivated Influenza Vaccine (Whole Virion), **2060**
Inactivated Poliomyelitis Vaccine, **2075**
Indapamide, **719**
Index, xxiii
Indian Squill, **1224**
Indian Squill, Powdered, *see Squill*
Indian Squill, Powdered, xxv
Indicators of Sterilisation, Biological, A266
Indicators, Use of Chemical, 6, 18, 1396, 1408
Indigo Carmine, A50
Indigo Carmine Solution, A50
Indigo Carmine Solution R1, A50
Indium[111In] Chloride Solution, **2118**
Indium[111In] Oxine Solution, **2119**
Indium[111In] Pentetate Injection, **2120**
Indometacin, **721**, S67
Indometacin Capsules, **1749**
Indometacin Suppositories, **1749**
Indomethacin and Preparations, *see under Indometacin*
Indophenol Blue, A50
Indoramin, S68
Indoramin Hydrochloride, **722**, S68
Indoramin Tablets, **1750**
Industrial Methylated Spirit, **875**
Industrial Methylated Spirit (Ketone-free), **875**
Industrial Methylated Spirits, **875**
Influenza Vaccine (Split Virion), Inactivated, **2061**
Influenza Vaccine (Surface Antigen), Inactivated, **2063**
Influenza Vaccine (Whole Virion), Inactivated, **2060**
Infrared Reference Spectra, Identification by, A114
Infrared Reference Spectra, Preparation of, S2
Infrared Spectrophotometry, A114
Infrared Spectrophotometry, Spectrophotometers for, A114
Infusions, 1433, *see also under name of substance*
Infusions, Intravenous, 1444, 1445, *see also under name of substance*
Infusions of the BP, List of, 1433

Inhalation,
Liquid Preparations for, 1434
Powders for, 1435
Preparations for, 1433
Pressurised Metered-dose Preparations for, 1434
Inhalations, *see under name of substance*
Inhalations, Aerodynamic Assessment of Fine Particles A194
Inhalations of the BP, List of, 1436
Inhalations, Preparation for, of the BP, Additional Requirements for, 1435
Inhalations, Pressurised, *see under Pressurised Inhalations and name of substance*
Injectable Insulin Preparations, *see Insulin Preparations*
Injections, 1443, *see also under name of substance*
Injections of the BP List of, 1445
Inositol Nicotinate, 722, S68
Inositol Nicotinate Tablets, **1750**
Insulin, **723**
Insulin, Human, **725**
Insulin Injection, **1754**
Insulin Injection, Biphasic, **1753**
Insulin Injection, Biphasic Isophane, **1753**
Insulin Injection, Isophane, **1756**
Insulin Injection, Neutral, **1754**
Insulin Injection, Soluble, *see Soluble Insulin*
Insulin, Neutral, **1754**
Insulin Preparations, **1751**
Insulin, Soluble, **1754**
Insulin Zinc Suspension, **1754**
Insulin Zinc Suspension (Amorphous), **1755**
Insulin Zinc Suspension (Crystalline), **1755**
Insulin Zinc Suspension (Mixed), **1754**
Interferon Alfa-2 Solution, Concentrated, **728**
International Reference Preparation, 14, 1404
International Standard, 18, 1408
International Unit, Definition of, 13, 1403
International Units, xx
Intranasal Solutions, 1439, *see also under name of substance*
Intranasal Solutions of the BP, List of, 1439
Intranasal Suspensions, 1439
Intravenous Infusions, 1444, **1445**, *see also under name of substance*
Intravenous Infusions of the BP, List of, 1447
Introduction, xv
Inulin, **731**
Inulin Injection, **1756**
Invert Syrup, **1757**
Iobenguane[^{123}I] Injection, **2121**
Iobenguane[^{131}I] Injection for Diagnostic Use, **2122**
Iobenguane[^{131}I] Injection for Therapeutic Use, **2123**
Iodic Acid, A50
Iodide Standard Solution (10 ppm I), A99
Iodide Standard Solution (20 ppm I), A99
Iodide-free Starch Solution, A83
Iodides, Reactions of, A149
Iodinated Potassium Iodide Solution, A72
Iodinated Povidone **1074**
Iodinated Zinc Chloride Solution, A91
Iodinated[^{125}I] Albumin Injection, **2113**
Iodinated[^{125}I] Fibrinogen, Dried, **2124**
Iodinated[^{125}I] Human Albumin Injection, **2113**
Iodinated[^{131}I] Norcholesterol Injection, **2125**
Iodine, **732**, A50
Iodine Bromide, A51
Iodine Bromide Method, A172
Iodine Bromide Solution, A51
Iodine Monochloride Method, A172
Iodine Monochloride Reagent, Strong, A51
Iodine Monochloride Solution, A51
Iodine Oral Solution, Aqueous, **1758**
Iodine, Oxygen-flask Combustion Method for, A156
Iodine Pentoxide, *see recrystallised iodine pentoxide*
Iodine Pentoxide, Recrystallised, A51
Iodine Solution, Alcoholic, **1758**, A51
Iodine Solution, Chloroformic, A51
Iodine Solution, Povidone–, **1886**
Iodine Solution R1, A51
Iodine Solution R2, A51
Iodine Solution R3, A51
Iodine Solution R4, A51
Iodine Tincture, *see Alcoholic Iodine Solution*
Iodine Trichloride, A51
Iodine Value, Determination of, A172
Iodine VS, A94
Iodipamide, S69
Iodised Oil Fluid Injection, **1759**
Iodoacetic Acid, A51
2-Iodobenzoic Acid, A51
Iodoethane, A51
2-Iodohippuric Acid, A51
Iodoplatinate Reagent, A51
Iodosulphurous Reagent, *see Karl Fischer reagent VS*
5-Iodouracil, A51
Iofendylate Injection, **1759**
Iohexol, **732**
Ion-exchange Resin, Strongly Acidic, A52
Ion-selective Potentiometry, A157
Ionic Concentration, Determination of, A157
Ionising Radiation Sterilisation, A265
Iopamidol, **735**
Iopanoic Acid, **737**, S69
Iopanoic Acid Tablets, **1759**
Iophendylate Injection, *see Iofendylate Injection*
Iotalamic Acid, **738**, S69
Iothalamic Acid and Preparations, *see under Iotalamic Acid*
IP, A313
Ipecacuanha, **739**
Ipecacuanha Emetic Mixture, Paediatric, **1760**
Ipecacuanha Emetic, Paediatric, **1760**
Ipecacuanha Liquid Extract, **1760**
Ipecacuanha Mixture, Ammonia and, **1484**
Ipecacuanha Oral Solution, Ammonia and, **1484**
Ipecacuanha Oral Solution, Paediatric, **1760**
Ipecacuanha, Powdered, xxv, *see also Ipecacuanha*
Ipecacuanha, Prepared, **740**
Ipecacuanha Root, *see Ipecacuanha*
Ipecacuanha Tincture, **1761**
Ipecacuanha Wine, *see Ipecacuanha Tincture*
Ipratropium Bromide, **740**
Ipratropium Pressurised Inhalation, **1761**
Iron, A52
Iron Dextran Injection, **1763**
Iron, Limit Test for, A154
Iron, Reactions of, A149
Iron Salicylate Solution, A52
Iron Salts, Reactions of, A149
Iron Sorbitol Injection, **1764**
Iron Standard Solution (1 ppm Fe), A99
Iron Standard Solution (2 ppm Fe), A99
Iron Standard Solution (8 ppm Fe), A99
Iron Standard Solution (10 ppm Fe), A99
Iron Standard Solution (20 ppm Fe), A99
Iron Standard Solution (0.1% Fe), A99
Iron(II) Sulphate, A52
Iron(II) Sulphate–Citrate Solution, A52
Iron(II) Sulphate Solution R2, A52
Iron(II) Sulphate VS, A94
Iron(III) Chloride, Anhydrous, A52
Iron(III) Chloride Hexahydrate, A52
Iron(III) Chloride Solution, A52
Iron(III) Chloride Solution, Ethanolic, A52
Iron(III) Chloride Solution R1, A52
Iron(III) Chloride Solution R2, A52
Iron(III) Chloride–Sulphamic Acid Reagent, A52
Iron(III) Nitrate, A52
Iron(III) Nitrate Solution, A52
Iron(III) Sulphate, A52
Irrigation, Preparations for, 1436
Irrigation, Preparations for, of the BP, Additional Requirements for, 1437
Irrigation Solutions, 1437, *see also under name of substance*
Irrigation Solutions of the BP, List of, 1437
Irrigation, Water for, **1991**
Isatin, A52
Isatin Reagent, A52
ISO, A313
Isoaminile, **742**, S70
Isoamyl Alcohol, *see amyl alcohol*
Isoamyl Alcohol, A52
Isoandrosterone, A52
Isobutyl Acetate, A52
Isoconazole, **742**
Isoconazole Nitrate, **744**
Isoleucine, **745**

Isomenthol, A52
(+)-Isomenthone, A52
Isometheptene, S70
Isometheptene Mucate, **746**
Isoniazid, **747**, S70, A52
Isoniazid Injection, **1765**
Isoniazid Solution, A53
Isoniazid Tablets, **1766**
Isonicotinamide, A53
Isophane Insulin, **1756**
Isophane Insulin (NPH), **1756**
Isophane Insulin Injection, **1756**
Isophane Insulin Injection, Biphasic, **1753**
Isoprenaline Hydrochloride, **748**, S71
Isoprenaline Injection, **1766**
Isoprenaline Sulphate, **749**
Isopropyl Alcohol, **749**
Isopropyl Ether, *see di-isopropyl ether*
Isopropyl Myristate, **750**, A53
Isopropyl Palmitate, **751**
Isopropylamine, A53
4-Isopropylphenol, A53
Isosorbide Dinitrate, Diluted, **752**
Isosorbide Dinitrate Tablets, **1767**
Isosorbide Mononitrate, Diluted, **753**
Isotopically Pure Deuterium Oxide, A33
Isotretinoin, **755**
Isoxsuprine Hydrochloride, **756**
Isoxsuprine Injection, xxv
Isoxsuprine Tablets, xxv
Ispaghula Husk, **758**
Italic Type, Significance of, 7, 16, 1397, 1406
IU, Definition of, 13, 1403
IUPAC, A313
I.Z.S., **1754**
I.Z.S. (Mixed), **1754**

J

Java Tea, **758**
Justified and Authorised, Definition of, 4, 17, 1394, 1407

K

Kanamycin Acid Sulphate, **759**
Kanamycin Acid Sulphate for Injection, **1768**
Kanamycin Injection, **1767**
Kanamycin Sulphate, **760**
Kaolin, *see Light Kaolin*
Kaolin and Morphine Mixture, **1769**
Kaolin and Morphine Oral Suspension, **1769**
Kaolin, Heavy, **761**
Kaolin, Light, **762**, A53
Kaolin, Light (Natural), **763**
Kaolin Mixture, **1768**
Kaolin Oral Suspension, **1768**
Kaolin Poultice, **1770**
Karaya Gum, **1228**
Karl Fischer Reagent VS, A94
Ketamine Hydrochloride, **763**
Ketamine Injection, **1770**
Ketoconazole, **764**
Ketoprofen, **766**, S71
Ketoprofen Capsules, **1771**
Khartoum Senna, *see Senna Leaf*
Kieselguhr, A53
Kieselguhr for Chromatography, A53
Kieselguhr G, A53
Knitted Viscose Primary Dressing, xxvi
Krameria, **1136**

L

Labelling, A331
Labelling of Formulated Preparations, *see appropriate general monograph*
Labelling of Radiopharmaceutical Preparations, 2107
Labelling of Vaccines, 2040
Labelling, Requirements for, 15, 22, 1405, 1412
Labetalol, S71
Labetalol Hydrochloride, **768**
Labetalol Injection, **1771**
Labetalol Tablets, **1772**
Lactates, Reactions of, A149
Lactic Acid, **769**, A53
Lactic Acid Pessaries, **1772**
Lactobionic Acid, A53
Lactophenol, A53
Lactose, **770**, A53
Lactose, Anhydrous, **771**
Lactose Monohydrate, *see Lactose*
Lactulose, **772**
Lactulose, Liquid, *see Lactulose Solution*
Lactulose Solution, **774**
LAL Test, A214
Lanatoside C, **776**
Lanolin, **1372**
Lanolin, Anhydrous, **1370**
Lanthanum Nitrate, A53
Lanthanum Nitrate Solution, A53
Lassar's Paste, **1995**
Lauroyl Macrogolglycerides, **778**
LD_{50}, A313
Lead Acetate, *see lead(II) acetate*
Lead Acetate Cotton, A53
Lead Acetate Paper, A53
Lead Acetate Solution, A53
Lead, Complexometric Titration of, A157
Lead Compounds, Reactions of, A149
Lead Dioxide, *see lead(IV) oxide*
Lead in Sugars, Limit Test for, A154
Lead Nitrate Solution, A53
Lead Nitrate VS, A95
Lead, Reactions of, A149
Lead Standard Solution (0.1 ppm Pb), A100
Lead Standard Solution (1 ppm Pb), A100
Lead Standard Solution (2 ppm Pb), A100
Lead Standard Solution (10 ppm Pb), A100
Lead Standard Solution (20 ppm Pb), A100
Lead Standard Solution (100 ppm Pb), A99
Lead Standard Solution (0.1% Pb), A99
Lead Subacetate Solution, A53
Lead(II) Acetate, A53
Lead(II) Nitrate, A53
Lead(IV) Oxide, A53
Lead-free Nitric Acid, A62
Lemon Oil, **779**, A53
Lemon Oil, Terpeneless, **780**
Lemon Peel, Dried, **780**
Lemon Spirit, **1773**
Lemon Syrup, **1773**
Leucine, **781**, *see L-leucine*
L-Leucine, A53
Levamisole Hydrochloride, **782**
Levobunolol Eye Drops, **1773**
Levobunolol Hydrochloride, **783**, S72
Levodopa, **783**, S72
Levodopa and Carbidopa Tablets, **1593**
Levodopa Capsules, **1774**
Levodopa Tablets, **1774**
Levomenthol, **785**
Levomepromazine Hydrochloride, **786**
Levomepromazine Maleate, **787**
Levonorgestrel, **788**
Levonorgestrel and Ethinylestradiol Tablets, **1775**
Levothyroxine Sodium, **788**
Levothyroxine Tablets, **1776**
Lidocaine, **790**, S72
Lidocaine and Adrenaline Injection/ Lidocaine and Epinephrine Injection, **1778**
Lidocaine and Chlorhexidine Gel, **1777**
Lidocaine Gel, **1776**
Lidocaine Hydrochloride, **790**
Lidocaine Injection, **1778**
Lidocaine Solution, Sterile, **1779**
Light Kaolin, **762**, A53
Light Kaolin (Natural), **763**
Light Liquid Paraffin, **996**
Light Magnesia, **833**
Light Magnesium Carbonate, **831**
Light Magnesium Oxide, *see magnesium oxide*
Light Magnesium Oxide, **833**
Light Petroleum, *see petroleum spirit (boiling range 50° to 70°)*
Light Petroleum R1, *see petroleum spirit (boiling range, 40° to 60°)*,
Light Petroleum R2, *see petroleum spirit (boiling range, 30° to 40°)*,
Light Petroleum R3, A66
Light, Protected from, Definition of, 12, 22, 1402, 1412
Light, Protected from, Storage Statements, 14, 1404
Light, Subdued, Definition of, 12, 1402
Lignin, Reactions of, A149
Lignocaine, Salts and Preparations, *see under Lidocaine*
Lime and Boric Acid Solution, Chlorinated, xxv
Lime, Chlorinated, **319**
Lime Flower, **791**
Lime Water, **1535**
Limit Tests, A151
Limitation of Impurities, Expression of, A320
Limits, Application of, 12, 21, 1402, 1411
Limonene, A54
Limulus Amoebocyte Lysate, A215
Linalol, *see linalool*

Linalool, A54
Linalyl Acetate, A54
Lincomycin Capsules, **1779**
Lincomycin Hydrochloride, **792**, S73
Lincomycin Injection, **1780**
Linctus, Paediatric Simple, **1925**
Linctus, Simple, **1925**
Linctuses, 1440, *see also under name of substance*
Linctuses of the BP, List of, 1441
Lindane, **794**
Lindane Application, xxv
Lindane Cream, xxv
Lindane Lotion, xxv
Lindane Shampoo, xxv
Linen Thread, Sterile, *see Non-absorbable Sutures, Sterile*
Liniment, White, **1992**
Liniments, 1424, *see also under name of substance*
Liniments of the BP, List of, 1425
Linoleoyl Macrogolglycerides, **794**
Linseed, **795**
Linseed Oil, **796**
Linseed, Powdered, xxv, *see also Linseed*
Liothyronine Sodium, **796**
Liothyronine Tablets, **1780**
Lipase Solvent, A54
Lipophilic Suppositories, Softening Time Determination of, A263
Liquefied Phenol, **1020**, A66
Liquid Chromatography, A129
Liquid Chromatography, Stationary Phases for, A130
Liquid Extracts, 1427
Liquid Lactulose, *see Lactulose Solution*
Liquid Maltitol, **839**
Liquid Nasal Sprays, 1438
Liquid Paraffin, **996**, A65
Liquid Paraffin and Magnesium Hydroxide Oral Emulsion, **1857**
Liquid Paraffin Emulsion, **1856**
Liquid Paraffin, Light, **996**
Liquid Paraffin Oral Emulsion, **1856**
Liquid Preparations for Inhalation, 1434
Liquids for Cutaneous Application, 1424
Liquids for Cutaneous Application of the BP, Additional Requirements for, 1424
Liquids for Nebulisation, 1434
Liquids, Oral, 1439
Liquorice, **797**
Liquorice Extract, Deglycyrrhizinised, xxv
Liquorice Liquid Extract, **1781**
Liquorice, Powdered, xxv, *see Liquorice*
Liquorice Root, *see Liquorice*
Lisinopril Dihydrate, **799**
Lithium, A54
Lithium and Sodium Molybdotungstophosphate Solution, A54
Lithium Carbonate, **800**, A54
Lithium Carbonate Tablets, **1781**
Lithium Carbonate Tablets, Slow, **1782**
Lithium Chloride, A54
Lithium Citrate, **801**
Lithium Hydroxide, A54
Lithium Methoxide VS, A95
Lithium Sulphate, A54
Litmus, A54
Litmus Paper, A54
Litmus Paper, Blue, A54
Litmus Paper, Red, A54
Litmus Solution, A54
Live Measles, Mumps and Rubella Vaccine, **2066**
Live Measles Vaccine, **2065**
Live Mumps Vaccine, **2069**
Live Poliomyelitis Vaccine (Oral), **2076**
Live Rubella Vaccine, **2082**
Live Typhoid (Strain Ty 21a) Vaccine (Oral), **2088**
Live Varicella Vaccine, **2091**
Live Yellow Fever Vaccine, **2092**
Lomustine, **802**, S73
Lomustine Capsules, **1782**
Loperamide Hydrochloride, **803**
Loprazolam Mesilate, **805**, S73
Loprazolam Mesylate, *see Loprazolam Mesilate*
Loprazolam Tablets, **1783**
Lorazepam, **806**, S74
Lorazepam Injection, **1783**
Lorazepam Tablets **1784**
Lormetazepam, **807**, S74
Lormetazepam Tablets, **1785**
Loss on Drying, Definition of Temperature Range, 12, 1402
Loss on Drying, Determination of, A168
Loss on Drying of Soft Extracts, 1428
Lotions, 1425, *see also under name of substance*
Lotions, Eye, 1429, *see also under name of substance*
Lotions of the BP, List of, 1425
Lovage Root, **807**
Low-molecular-weight Heparins, **667**
Low-substituted Carmellose Sodium, **256**
Low-vapour-pressure Hydrocarbons (Type L), A48
Lozenges, *see under Tablets for Use in the Mouth and name of substance*
Lozenges of the BP, List of, 1456
Lymecycline, **808**
Lymecycline Capsules, **1785**
Lynestrenol, **809**
Lynoestrenol, *see Lynestrenol*
Lypressin Injection, **1786**
Lysine Hydrochloride, **810**

M

M, Definition of, 6, 1396
Maceration, Definition of, A182
Maceration, Production of Extracts by, 1427
Maceration, Production of Tinctures by, 1456
Macrogol, *see polyethylene glycols for reagent grades*
Macrogol 300, **811**, *see also polyethylene glycol 300*
Macrogol 400, **812**, *see also polyethylene glycol 400*
Macrogol 1000, **814**, *see also polyethylene glycol 1000*
Macrogol 1500, **815**, *see also polyethylene glycol 1500*
Macrogol 1540, xxv
Macrogol 3000, **816**
Macrogol 4000, **817**
Macrogol 6000, **818**
Macrogol 20,000, **819**, *see polyethylene glycol 20,000*
Macrogol 20,000 2-Nitroterephthalate, *see polyethylene glycol 20,000 2-nitroterephthalate*
Macrogol 35,000, **820**
Macrogol Cetostearyl Ether, **821**
Macrogol 7 Glycerol Cocoate, **823**
Macrogol Lauryl Ether, **824**
Macrogol Ointment, **1787**
Macrogol Oleyl Ether, **826**
Macrogol Stearate, **827**
Macroscopical Characteristics of Crude Drugs, 15, 1405
Magaldrate, **828**
Magaldrate Oral Suspension, **1788**
Magenta, Basic, *see basic fuchsin,*
Magnesia, Light, **833**
Magnesium, A54
Magnesium Acetate, **829**, A54
Magnesium and Alkaline-earth Metals, Limit Test for, A154
Magnesium Carbonate, Heavy, **830**
Magnesium Carbonate, Light, **831**
Magnesium Carbonate Mixture, Aromatic, **1788**
Magnesium Carbonate Oral Suspension, Aromatic, **1788**
Magnesium Chloride, **831**, A55
Magnesium Chloride Hexahydrate, *see Magnesium Chloride*
Magnesium Chloride VS, A95
Magnesium, Complexometric Titration of, A157
Magnesium Hydroxide, **832**
Magnesium Hydroxide and Aluminium Hydroxide Tablets **1606**
Magnesium Hydroxide Mixture, **1789**
Magnesium Hydroxide Oral Emulsion, Liquid Paraffin and, **1857**
Magnesium Hydroxide Oral Suspension, **1789**
Magnesium Hydroxide Oral Suspension, Aluminium Hydroxide and, **1605**
Magnesium, Limit Test for, A154
Magnesium Nitrate, A55
Magnesium Oxide, A55
Magnesium Oxide, Heavy, **833**, A55
Magnesium Oxide, Light, **833**, *see also magnesium oxide*
Magnesium Oxide R1, A55
Magnesium, Reactions of, A149
Magnesium Salts, Reactions of, A149
Magnesium Standard Solution (10 ppm Mg), A100
Magnesium Standard Solution (100 ppm Mg), A100
Magnesium Standard Solution (0.1% Mg), A100
Magnesium Stearate, **834**
Magnesium Sulphate, **835**, A55
Magnesium Sulphate, Dried, **835**
Magnesium Sulphate Injection, **1789**

Magnesium Sulphate Mixture, **1789**
Magnesium Sulphate Oral Suspension, **1789**
Magnesium Sulphate Paste, **1790**
Magnesium Sulphate VS, A95
Magnesium Trisilicate, **836**
Magnesium Trisilicate Mixture, **1790**
Magnesium Trisilicate Mixture, Compound, **1790**
Magnesium Trisilicate Oral Powder, Compound, **1791**
Magnesium Trisilicate Oral Suspension, **1790**
Magnesium Trisilicate Tablets, Aluminium Hydroxide and, **1791**
Magnesium Trisilicate Tablets, Compound, **1791**
Magneson, A55
Magneson Reagent, A55
Magneson Solution, A55
Maize Oil, A55
Maize Starch, **836**
Maize Starch, Pregelatinised, *see Pregelatinised Starch*
Maize Starch, Sterilisable, **837**
Malachite Green, A55
Malachite Green Solution, A55
Maleate Buffer Solution pH 7.0, A103
Maleic Acid, **838**, A55
Maleic Anhydride, A55
Maleic Anhydride Solution, A55
Malic Acid, A55
Maltitol, **838**
Maltitol, Liquid, **839**
Manganese Sulphate, **840**, *see also manganese(II) sulphate*
Manganese Sulphate Monohydrate, **841**
Manganese(II) Sulphate, A55
Mannitol, **842**, *see D-mannitol*
D-Mannitol, A55
Mannitol Intravenous Infusion, **1792**
Mannose, *see D-mannose*
D-Mannose, A55
Manufacture of Formulated Preparations, 9, 1399
Manufacturers, Guidance to, A339
Maprotiline Hydrochloride, **843**
Marshmallow Root, **844**
Mass Distribution Ratio, Definition of, A124, A130
Mass, Test for Uniformity of, A203
Materials Used for the Manufacture of Containers, A281
Matricaria Flowers, **845**
Measles Immunoglobulin, **2022**
Measles, Mumps and Rubella Vaccine, Live, **2066**
Measles Vaccine, Live, **2065**
Meas/Vac(Live), *see Measles Vaccine, Live*
Measures, Expression of Weights and, 5, 1395
Measures, Weights and, A312
Mebendazole, **846**
Mebeverine, S74
Mebeverine Hydrochloride, **847**, S75
Mebeverine Tablets, **1792**
Mechanism of Monograph Development, A338
Meclozine Hydrochloride, **847**
Meclozine Hydrochloride, A55
Medazepam, xxv
Medazepam Capsules, xxv
Medical Air, **47**
Medicated Chewing Gums, 1423
Medicated Ear Tampons, 1426
Medicated Foams, 1431
Medicated Tampons, 1456
Medicinal Preparations, Names of, A334
Medicinal Substances, Names of, A334
Medium-chain Triglycerides, **1329**
Medroxyprogesterone Acetate, **848**
Mefenamic Acid, **849**, S75
Mefenamic Acid Capsules, **1793**
Mefloquine Hydrochloride, **851**
Megestrol Acetate, **852**, S75
Megestrol Tablets, **1793**
Meglumine, **853**
Meglumine Amidotrizoate Injection, **1794**
Meglumine Diatrizoate Injection, *see Meglumine Amidotrizoate Injection*
Meglumine Iodipamide Injection, **1795**
Meglumine Iotalamate Injection, **1796**
Meglumine Iothalamate Injection, *see Meglumine Iotalamate Injection*
Melamine, A55
Melphalan, **853**, S76
Melphalan for Injection, **1796**
Melphalan Injection, **1796**
Melphalan Tablets, **1797**
Melting Point, Determination of, A135
Menadiol Phosphate Injection, **1798**
Menadiol Phosphate Tablets, **1798**
Menadiol Sodium Phosphate, **854**, S76
Menadione, **855**, S76, A55
Meningococcal Polysaccharide Vaccine, **2067**
Menotrophin, **855**
Menotrophin for Injection, **1799**
Menotrophin Injection, **1799**
Menthofuran, A55
Menthol, A55
Menthol and Benzoin Inhalation, **1799**
Menthol, Racemic, **1131**
Menthone, A56
Menthyl Acetate, A56
Mepivacaine Hydrochloride, **857**
Meprobamate, **858**
Meptazinol Hydrochloride, **859**, S77
Meptazinol Injection, **1800**
Meptazinol Tablets, **1800**
Mepyramine Maleate, **860**, S77
Mepyramine Tablets, **1801**
Mercaptoacetic Acid, A56
2-Mercaptoethanol, A56
Mercaptopurine, **861**, *see also 6-mercaptopurine*
6-Mercaptopurine, A56
Mercaptopurine Tablets, **1801**
Mercuric Acetate, *see mercury(II) acetate*
Mercuric Acetate Solution, *see mercury(II) acetate solution*
Mercuric Bromide, *see mercury(II) bromide*
Mercuric Bromide Paper, *see mercury(II) bromide paper*
Mercuric Chloride A66, *see also mercury(II) chloride*
Mercuric Chloride, **862**
Mercuric Chloride Solution, *see mercury(II) chloride solution*
Mercuric Iodide, *see mercury(II) iodide*
Mercuric Nitrate, *see mercury(II) nitrate VS; mercury(ii) nitrate*
Mercuric Oxide, *see yellow mercury(II) oxide*
Mercuric Sulphate Solution, *see mercury(II) sulphate solution*
Mercuric Thiocyanate, *see mercury(II) thiocyanate*
Mercuric Thiocyanate Solution, *see mercury(II) thiocyanate solution,*
Mercury, A56
Mercury Compounds, Reactions of, A149
Mercury, Nitric Acid Solution of, A56
Mercury, Reactions of, A149
Mercury Standard Solution (5 ppm Hg), A100
Mercury Standard Solution (100 ppm Hg), A100
Mercury Standard Solution (1000 ppm Hg), A100
Mercury(II) Acetate, A56
Mercury(II) Acetate Solution, A56
Mercury(II) Bromide, A56
Mercury(II) Bromide Paper, A56
Mercury(II) Chloride, A56
Mercury(II) Chloride Solution, A56
Mercury(II) Iodide, A56
Mercury(II) Nitrate, A56
Mercury(II) Nitrate VS, A95
Mercury(II) Oxide, Yellow, A56
Mercury(II) Sulphate Solution, A56
Mercury(II) Thiocyanate, A56
Mercury(II) Thiocyanate Solution, A57
Mesh Aperture for Sieves, A255
Mestranol, **862**
Metalphthalein, *see phthalein purple*
Metanil Yellow, A57
Metanil Yellow Solution, A57
Metaphosphoric Acid, A57
Metaraminol Injection, **1801**
Metaraminol Tartrate, **863**
Metered-dose Preparations for Inhalation, Pressurised, 1436
Metformin Hydrochloride, **864**, S77
Metformin Tablets, **1802**
Methacrylic Acid, A57
Methacrylic Acid–Ethyl Acrylate Copolymer (1:1), **865**
Methacrylic Acid–Ethyl Acrylate Copolymer (1:1) Dispersion 30 per cent, **867**
Methacrylic Acid–Methyl Methacrylate Copolymer **867**
Methacrylic Acid–Ethyl Acrylate Copolymer (1:1) **866**
Methadone, S78
Methadone Hydrochloride, **868**
Methadone Injection, **1802**
Methadone Linctus, **1803**
Methadone Tablets, **1803**
Methanesulphonic Acid, A57
Methanesulphonic Acid, Methanolic, A57

Methanol, A57
Methanol, Acidified, A57
Methanol, Aldehyde-free, A57
Methanol and 2-Propanol Content of Liquid Extracts, 1427
Methanol and 2-Propanol Content of Tinctures, 1456
Methanol, Anhydrous, A57
Methanol, Determination of, A160
Methanol, Deuterated, A33
Methanol, Hydrochloric, A57
Methanol R1, A57
Methanolic Ammonia, A17
Methanolic Hydrochloric Acid, A48
Methanolic Methanesulphonic Acid, A57
Methanolic Potassium Hydrogen Carbonate Solution, A72
Methanolic Potassium Hydroxide, A72
Methanolic Sodium Hydroxide, A80
Methanolic Sodium Hydroxide Solution, A80
Methanolic Sulphuric Acid, A84
Methanolic Tris(hydroxymethyl)-methylamine Solution, A90
Methaqualone, **869**
Methimazole, A57
Methionine, **870**
DL-Methionine, **871**
L-Methionine, A57
Methods of Sterilisation for Parenteral Preparations, 1445
Methohexital Injection, **1804**
Methohexital Sodium for Injection, **1804**
Methohexitone, S78
Methohexitone Injection, *see Methohexital Injection*
Methoserpidine, xxv
Methoserpidine Tablets, xxv
Methotrexate, **872**
Methotrexate Injection, **1804**
Methotrexate Tablets, **1805**
Methotrimeprazine and Salts, *see under Levomepromazine*
Methoxamine Hydrochloride, **873**, S78
Methoxamine Injection, **1805**
2-Methoxyethanol, A57
Methoxyphenylacetic Acid, A57
Methoxyphenylacetic Acid Reagent, A57
Methyl Acetate, A57
Methyl Anthranilate, A57
Methyl Arachidate, A57
Methyl Behenate, *see methyl docosanoate*
Methyl Cinnamate, A58
Methyl Decanoate, A58
Methyl Docosanoate, A58
Methyl Ethyl Ketone, *see butan-2-one*
Methyl Green, A58
Methyl Green-Iodomercurate Paper, A58
Methyl 4-Hydroxybenzoate, A58
Methyl Hydroxybenzoate, **873**, S79
Methyl Isobutyl Ketone, *see 4-methylpentan-2-one*
Methyl Isobutyl Ketone R1, *see 4-methylpentan-2-one R1*
Methyl Laurate, A58
Methyl Methacrylate, A58
Methyl Myristate, A58
Methyl Nicotinate, **874**, S79
Methyl Oleate, A58
Methyl Orange, A58
Methyl Orange Mixed Solution, A58
Methyl Orange Solution, A58
Methyl Orange–Xylene Cyanol FF Solution, A58
Methyl Palmitate, A58
Methyl Parahydroxybenzoate, *see methyl 4-hydroxybenzoate*
Methyl Red, A58
Methyl Red Mixed Solution, A58
Methyl Red Solution, A58
Methyl Salicylate, **874**, A59
Methyl Salicylate Liniment, **1806**
Methyl Salicylate Ointment, **1806**
Methyl Salicylate Ointment, Strong, **1806**
Methyl Stearate, A59
Methyl Thymol Blue, A59
Methyl Thymol Blue Mixture, A59
Methyl *N*-Tosyl-L-argininate Hydrochloride, *see tosyl arginine methyl ester hydrochloride solution*
Methyl Tricosanoate, A59
4-Methylaminophenol Sulphate *A59*
Methylaminophenol–Sulphate Reagent, A59
Methylated Spirit (Ketone-free), Industrial, **875**
Methylated Spirit, Industrial, **875**
Methylated Spirits, Industrial, **875**
Methylatropine Bromide, *see Atropine Methobromide*
Methylatropine Nitrate, *see Atropine Methonitrate*
3-Methylbenzothiazolin-2-one Hydrazone Hydrochloride, A59
Methylbenzothiazolone Hydrazone Hydrochloride, *see methylbenzothiazolin-2-one hydrazone hydrochloride*
2-Methylbutane, A59
3-Methylbutan-1-ol, *see isoamyl alcohol*
2-Methylbut-2-ene, A59
Methylcellulose, **875**
Methylcellulose 450, A59
Methylcellulose Eye Drops, *see Hypromellose Eye Drops*
Methylcellulose Granules, **1806**
Methylcellulose Tablets, **1806**
Methyldopa, **876**, S79
Methyldopa Tablets, **1807**
3-O-Methyldopamine Hydrochloride, A59
4-O-Methyldopamine Hydrochloride, A59
Methyldopate Hydrochloride, **877**, S80
Methyldopate Injection, **1807**
Methylene Blue, A59
Methylene Blue for External Use, *see Methylthioninium Chloride for External Use*
Methylene Chloride, *see Dichloromethane*
Methylene Chloride, Acidified, *see acidified dichloromethane*
N,N′-Methylenebisacrylamide, A59
4,4′-Methylenebis-*N*,*N*-dimethylaniline, A59
4,4′-Methylenebis-*N*,*N*-dimethylaniline Reagent, A59
N-Methylglucamine, A59
Methylhydroxyethylcellulose, *see Hydroxyethylmethylcellulose*
2-Methyl-1,4-naphthoquinone, A59
2-Methyl-5-nitroimidazole, *A60*
Methylparaben, **873**
4-Methylpentan-2-one, A60
4-Methylpentan-2-one R1, A60
Methylpentoses in Polysaccharide Vaccines, Test for, A234
Methylphenobarbital, **878**
Methylphenobarbitone, *see Methylphenobarbital*
Methylpiperazine, *see* N-*methylpiperazine*
N-Methylpiperazine, A60
Methylprednisolone, **879**, S80
Methylprednisolone Acetate, **881**, S80
Methylprednisolone Acetate Injection, **1808**
Methylprednisolone Hydrogen Succinate, **883**
Methylprednisolone Tablets, **1808**
2-Methylpropan-1-ol, A60
2-Methylpropanol, *see 2-methylpropan-1-ol*
2-Methylpropan-2-ol, A60
Methyltestosterone, **885**
Methylthioninium Chloride for External Use, **886**
Methysergide Maleate, **887**, S81
Methysergide Tablets, **1809**
Metoclopramide Hydrochloride, **888**
Metoclopramide Injection, **1810**
Metoclopramide Oral Solution, **1810**
Metoclopramide Tablets, **1811**
Metoprolol, S81
Metoprolol Injection, **1812**
Metoprolol Tartrate, **889**
Metoprolol Tartrate Tablets, **1812**
Metrifonate, **891**
Metronidazole, **893**, S81
Metronidazole Benzoate, **894**
Metronidazole Gel, **1814**
Metronidazole Intravenous Infusion, **1814**
Metronidazole Suppositories, **1815**
Metronidazole Tablets, **1815**
Metyrapone, **895**
Metyrapone (1), S82
Metyrapone (2), S82
Metyrapone Capsules, **1816**
Mexenone, **895**, S82
Mexenone Cream, **1816**
Mexiletine Capsules, **1816**
Mexiletine Hydrochloride, **896**, S83
Mexiletine Injection, **1817**
Mianserin Hydrochloride, **897**, S83
Mianserin Tablets, **1817**
Mice, 14, 1404
Miconazole, **898**
Miconazole Cream, **1818**
Miconazole Nitrate, **900**
Micro-organisms, Collections of, 25, 1415

Micro-organisms, Test for Specified, A243
Microbial Contamination, Tests for, A243
Microbial Quality of Pharmaceutical Preparations, A253
Microcrystalline Cellulose, *see cellulose for chromatography*
Microcrystalline Cellulose, **287**
Microfine Powder, Definition of, A254
Microscopy, Limit Test of Particle Size by, A254
MID, A313
Midazolam, **902**, S83
Midazolam Injection, **1818**
Minocycline Hydrochloride, **903**
Minocycline Tablets, **1819**
Minoxidil, **905**
Mint Oil, Dementholised, **906**
Mitobronitol, **907**, S84
Mitobronitol Tablets, **1820**
Mitoxantrone Hydrochloride,/Mitozantrone Hydrochloride, **908**
Mitozantrone Hydrochloride, *see Mitoxantrone Hydrochloride*
Mixed Botulinum Antitoxin, *see Botulinum Antitoxin*
Mixed Gas-gangrene Antitoxin, **2036**
Mixed Phosphate Buffer pH 4.0, A103
Mixed Phosphate Buffer pH 5.4, A103
Mixed Phosphate Buffer pH 6.8, A103
Mixed Phosphate Buffer pH 6.8, 0.2M, A103
Mixed Phosphate Buffer pH 7.0, A103
Mixed Phosphate Buffer pH 7.0, 0.067M, A103
Mixed Phosphate Buffer pH 7.0, 0.1M, A103
Mixed Phosphate Buffer pH 10, A103
Mixed Phosphate Buffer Solution, 0.067M, *see 0.067M mixed phosphate buffer pH 7.0*
Mixtures, 1441, *see also under name of substance*
Mixtures of the BP, List of, 1441
MLD, A313
MMR/Vac(Live), *see Measles, Mumps and Rubella Vaccine, Live*
Moderately Coarse Powder, Definition of, A254
Moderately Fine Powder, Definition of, A254
Modified-release Capsules, 1422
Modified-release Granules, 1433
Modified-release Tablets, 1453
Moisture, Protected from, Storage Statements, 14, 22, 1404, 1412
Molarity, Definition of, 6, 1396, A92
Molecular Formula, Status of, 4, 1394
Molecular Sieve, A60
Molecular Weight [Mass], by Size-exclusion Chromatography, A127
Molecular Weight [Mass] Distribution in Dextrans, A127
Molecular Weight, Status of, 4, 1394
Molybdenum(VI) Oxide, A60
Molybdovanadic Reagent, A60
Monoethanolamine, **550**
Monofilament Stainless Steel Suture, Sterile, xxvi
Monofilament Sutures, Sterile Synthetic Absorbable, **2161**
Monograph Development, Guidance to Manufacturers, A339
Monograph Development, Mechanism of, A338
Monograph Development, Methods of Analysis, A340
Monographs, Technical Changes to, xxvi
Monostearin, Self-emulsifying, **649**
Monosulfiram, xxv
Monosulfiram Solution, xxv
Mordant Black 11, A60
Mordant Black 11 Mixed Triturate, A60
Mordant Black 11 Solution, A60
Mordant Black 11 Triturate, A60
Mordant Blue 3, A60
Morison's Paste, **1790**
Morphine, S84
Morphine and Atropine Injection, **1820**
Morphine Hydrochloride, **909**, A60
Morphine Mixture, Ammonium Chloride and, xxv
Morphine Mixture, Kaolin and, **1769**
Morphine Oral Suspension, Kaolin and, **1769**
Morphine Sulphate, **910**
Morphine Sulphate Injection, **1820**
Morphine Suppositories, **1821**
Morphine Tablets, **1822**
Morphine Tincture, Chloroform and, **1559**
Moulded Pessaries, 1461
Mouthwashes, 1437
Mouthwashes of the BP, List of, 1437
Moxisylyte Hydrochloride, S84, S119
Moxisylyte Hydrochloride/Thymoxamine Hydrochloride, **912**
Moxisylyte Tablets/Thymoxamine Tablets, **1822**
Multidose Container, A268
Mumps and Rubella Vaccine, Live Measles and, **2066**
Mumps Vaccine, Live, **2069**
Mump/Vac (Live), *see Mumps Vaccine, Live*
Mustine Hydrochloride and Preparations, *see under Chlormethine*
Mycobacteria, Test for A250
Mycoplasmas, Test for Absence of, A248
Myristic Acid, A60
Myristicine, A60

N

Nabumetone, **912**, S85
Nabumetone Oral Suspension, **1823**
Nabumetone Tablets, **1823**
Nadroparin Calcium, **913**
Naftidrofuryl, S85
Naftidrofuryl Capsules, **1824**
Naftidrofuryl Oxalate, **916**
Nalidixic Acid, **917**, S85
Nalidixic Acid Oral Suspension, **1824**
Nalidixic Acid Tablets, **1825**
Nalorphine Hydrochloride, A60
Naloxone Hydrochloride, **918**
Naloxone Injection, **1825**
Naloxone Injection, Neonatal, **1826**
Names of Medicinal Substances and Preparations, A334
Names, Symbols and Atomic Weights of Elements, A311
Nandrolone Decanoate, **919**, S86
Nandrolone Decanoate Injection, **1827**
Nandrolone Phenylpropionate, **919**, S87
Nandrolone Phenylpropionate Injection, **1827**
Naphazoline Hydrochloride, **920**
Naphazoline Nitrate, **921**
Naphthalene, A60
Naphthalene Black 12B, A60
Naphthalene Black Solution, A60
Naphthalene-1,3-diol, A60
Naphthalene-2,7-diol, A60
Naphthalenediol Reagent Solution, A61
Naphthalenediol Solution, A61
α-Naphthol, *see 1-naphthol*
α-Naphthol Solution, *see 1-naphthol solution*
β-Naphthol, *see 2-naphthol*
β-Naphthol Solution, *see 2-naphthol solution*
1-Naphthol, A61
1-Naphthol Solution, A61
1-Naphthol Solution, Strong, A61
2-Naphthol, A61
2-Naphthol Solution, A61
Naphtholbenzein, *see 1-naphtholbenzein*
Naphtholbenzein Solution, *see 1-naphtholbenzein solution*
1-Naphtholbenzein, A61
1-Naphtholbenzein Solution, A61
2-Naphthylacetic Acid, A61
1-Naphthylamine, A61
Naphthylamine, *see 1-naphthylamine*
N-(1-Naphthyl)ethylenediamine Dihydrochloride, A61
Naproxen, **922**, S87
Naproxen Oral Suspension, **1828**
Naproxen Suppositories, **1828**
Naproxen Tablets, **1829**
Napthylethylenediamine Dihydrochloride, *see* N-*(1-naphthyl)ethylenediamine dihydrochloride*
Nasal Drops, 1438, 1439, *see also under name of substance*
Nasal Drops of the BP, List of, 1439
Nasal Powders, 1438
Nasal Preparations, 1437
Nasal Preparations of the BP, Additional Requirements for, 1439
Nasal Preparations, Semi-solid, 1438
Nasal Sprays, 1439, *see also under name of substance*
Nasal Sprays, Liquid, 1438
Nasal Sprays of the BP, List of, 1439
Nasal Sticks, 1439
Nasal Washes, 1439
Natural Light Kaolin, **763**
Natural Vitamin A Ester Concentrate, **1360**
NCIMB, A313

NCPF, A313
NCTC, A313
NCYC, A313
Near Infrared Spectrophotometry, A115
Nebulisation, Liquids for, 1434
Nebulisation of the BP, List of Solutions for, 1436
Nebulisation, Solutions for, 1449
Neiman/Vac, *see Meningococcal Polysaccharide Vaccine*
Neomycin Cream, Hydrocortisone and, **1730**
Neomycin Ear Drops, Hydrocortisone Acetate and, **1731**
Neomycin Ear Drops, Hydrocortisone and, **1731**
Neomycin Eye Drops, **1829**
Neomycin Eye Drops, Hydrocortisone Acetate and, **1732**
Neomycin Eye Drops, Hydrocortisone and, **1732**
Neomycin Eye Ointment, **1830**
Neomycin Eye Ointment, Hydrocortisone Acetate and, **1732**
Neomycin Oral Solution, **1830**
Neomycin Sulphate, **922**
Neomycin Tablets, **1831**
Neonatal Naloxone Injection, **1826**
Neostigmine Bromide, **924**
Neostigmine Injection, **1831**
Neostigmine Methylsulphate, *see Neostigmine Metilsulfate*
Neostigmine Metilsulfate, **924**
Neostigmine Tablets, **1832**
trans-Nerolidol, A61
Neryl Acetate, A61
Nessler Cylinders, A151
Neurovirulence of Live Viral Vaccines, Test for, A231
Neurovirulence of Poliomyelitis Vaccine (Oral), Test for, A232
Neutral Adrenaline Eye Drops/Neutral Epinephrine Eye Drops, **1469**
Neutral Glass, A268
Neutral Insulin, **1754**
Neutral Insulin Injection, **1754**
Neutral Red, A61
Neutral Red Solution, A61
Niacinamide, *see Nicotinamide*
Nickel–Aluminium Alloy A61
Nickel Chloride, *see nickel(II) chloride*
Nickel Chloride Solution, Ammoniacal, A61
Nickel in Polyols, Limit Test for, A154
Nickel Standard Solution (0.1 ppm Ni), A100
Nickel Standard Solution (10 ppm Ni), A100
Nickel Sulphate, *see nickel(II) sulphate*
Nickel(II) Chloride, A61
Nickel(II) Chloride Hexahydrate A61
Nickel(II) Sulphate, A61
Niclosamide **925**, S88
Niclosamide, Anhydrous, **925**
Niclosamide Monohydrate, **926**
Niclosamide Tablets, **1832**
Nicotinamide, **927**, S88
Nicotinamide Tablets, **1833**
Nicotinamide-adenine Dinucleotide, A61
Nicotinamide-adenine Dinucleotide Solution, A62
Nicotinic Acid, **928**, A62
Nicotinic Acid Tablets, **1833**
Nicotinyl Alcohol Tablets, **1834**
Nicotinyl Alcohol Tartrate, **929**
Nicoumalone, S88
Nicoumalone and Preparations, *see under Acenocoumarol*
Nifedipine, **930**, S89
Nifedipine Capsules, **1834**
Nikethamide, **931**, S89
Nikethamide Injection, **1835**
Nile Blue A, A62
Nile Blue A Solution, A62
Nimodipine, **932**
Ninhydrin, A62
Ninhydrin and Stannous Chloride Reagent, A62
Ninhydrin and Stannous Chloride Reagent R1, A62
Ninhydrin Solution, A62
Ninhydrin Solution I, A62
Ninhydrin Solution R1, A62
Ninhydrin Solution R2, A62
Ninhydrin Solution R3, A62
Nitrate Standard Solution (2 ppm NO_3), A100
Nitrate Standard Solution (10 ppm NO_3), A100
Nitrate Standard Solution (100 ppm NO_3), A100
Nitrate-free Water, A91
Nitrates, Reactions of, A149
Nitrazepam, **933**
Nitrazepam Capsules, **1835**
Nitrazepam Oral Suspension, **1836**
Nitrazepam Tablets, **1836**
Nitrendipine, **934**
Nitric Acid, **935**, A62
Nitric Acid, Cadmium- and Lead-free, A62
Nitric Acid, Dilute, A62
Nitric Acid, Fuming, A62
Nitric Acid, Lead-free, A62
Nitric Acid Solution of Mercury, A56
Nitric Acid VS, A95
Nitrile Silica Gel for Chromatography, A77
Nitrile Silica Gel for Chromatography R1, A77
Nitrilotriacetic Acid, A62
Nitrite Standard Solution (20 ppm NO_2), A100
Nitroaniline, *see 4-nitroaniline*
4-Nitroaniline, A62
Nitroaniline Solution, Diazotised, A62
Nitrobenzaldehyde, *see 2-nitrobenzaldehyde*
2-Nitrobenzaldehyde, A62
Nitrobenzaldehyde Paper, A63
Nitrobenzaldehyde Solution, A63
Nitrobenzene, A63
4-Nitrobenzoic Acid, A63
Nitrobenzoyl Chloride, A63
4-Nitrobenzyl Bromide, A63
Nitrobenzyl Chloride, *see 4-nitrobenzyl chloride*
4-Nitrobenzyl Chloride, A63
4-(4-Nitrobenzyl)pyridine, A63
Nitrochromic Reagent, A63
Nitroethane, A63
Nitrofurantoin, **936**, A63
Nitrofurantoin Oral Suspension, **1837**
Nitrofurantoin Tablets, **1837**
Nitrofurazone, **936**
(5-Nitro-2-furyl)methylene Diacetate, A63
Nitrogen, **937**, A63
Nitrogen, Determination of, A161
Nitrogen Dioxide in Medicinal Gases, Determination of, A169
Nitrogen for Chromatography, A63
Nitrogen Monoxide, A63
Nitrogen Monoxide in Medicinal Gases, Determination of, A169
Nitrogen, Oxygen-free, A63
Nitrogen R1, A63
Nitrogen-free Sulphuric Acid, A84
Nitroglycerin Tablets, **1712**
Nitromethane, A63
Nitrosodipropylamine, A63
Nitrosodipropylamine Solution, A63
Nitrotetrazolium Blue, A63
Nitrous Oxide, **938**, A63
Nitro-vanado-molybdic Reagent, A63
Nomenclature of Substances of Natural or Semi-synthetic Origin, A334
Non-absorbable Ligatures, Sterile, *see Non-absorbable Sutures, Sterile*
Non-absorbable Sutures, Sterile, **2163**
Non-aqueous Titration, A155
Non-ionic Emulsifying Wax, **1551**
Non-nitrogen Substituted Barbiturates, Reactions of, A147
Nonadecanoic Acid, A63
Nonan-5-one, A63
Noradrenaline Acid Tartrate, A63
Noradrenaline Acid Tartrate/ Norepinephrine Acid Tartrate, **940**
Noradrenaline Concentrate/ Norepinephrine Concentrate, **1838**
Noradrenaline Hydrochloride/ Norepinephrine Hydrochloride, **941**
Noradrenaline Injection/Norepinephrine Injection, **1838**
Norcholesterol Injection, Iodinated[^{131}I], **2125**
Nordazepam, A63
Norepinephrine, Salts and Preparations, *see under Noradrenaline*
Norethisterone, **942**
Norethisterone Acetate, **943**
Norethisterone Tablets, **1838**
Norfloxacin, **945**
Norgestrel, **946**
DL-Norleucine, A63
Normal Immunoglobulin, **2016**
Normal Immunoglobulin for Intravenous Use, **2018**
Normal Immunoglobulin Injection, **2016**
Normal Saline, *see Sodium Chloride Solution*
Normal Saline Solution for Injection, *see Sodium Chloride Intravenous Infusion*
Normalisation, Definition of, A125, A129

Noroxymorphone, A63
Norpseudoephedrine Hydrochloride, A64
Nortriptyline Capsules, **1839**
Nortriptyline Hydrochloride, **946**
Nortriptyline Tablets, **1839**
Noscapine, 947
Noscapine Hydrochloride, **948**, A64
Notices, vi, xl
Notices, General, 1, 1391
Nov/Ser, *see Gas-gangrene Antitoxin (Novyi)*
Nuclear Magnetic Resonance Spectrometry, A118
Nucleic Acids in Polysaccharide Vaccines, Test for, A233
Nutmeg Oil, **949**
Nystatin, **949**
Nystatin Ointment, **1840**
Nystatin Oral Drops, **1840**
Nystatin Oral Suspension, **1840**
Nystatin Pessaries, **1841**
Nystatin Tablets, **1841**

O

Octadecan-1-ol, A64
Octadecyl 3-(3,5-Di-(1,1-dimethylethyl)-4-hydroxyphenyl)propionate, A64
Octadecylsilyl Silica Gel for Chromatography, A77
Octadecylsilyl Silica Gel for Chromatography, Base-deactivated, A77
Octadecylsilyl Silica Gel for Chromatography R1, A77
Octanoic Acid, **950**, S89, A64
Octanol, *see octan-1-ol*
Octan-1-ol, A64
Octan-2-ol, A64
Octoxinol 10, A64
Octyl Gallate, **950**
Octylamine, A64
n-Octylamine, *see octylamine*
Octylamine Phosphate Buffer pH 3.0, A103
Octyldodecanol, **951**
Octylsilyl Silica Gel for Chromatography, A77
Odour of Volatile Oils, Test for, A175
Odour, Test for, A150
Oestradiol, Salts and Preparations, *see under Estradiol*
Official, Definition of, 3, 1393
Official Standards, 4, 1394
Official Titles, 7, 1397
Oily Cream, **1738**
Oily Phenol Injection, **1867**
Ointment, Emulsifying, **1658**
Ointment, Hydrous, **1738**
Ointment, Simple, **1925**
Ointments, 1458, 1459, *see also under name of substance*
Ointments, Eye, 1430, *see also under name of substance*
Ointments of the BP, List of, 1460
Old Tuberculin, **2096**
Oleamide, A64
Oleic Acid, **952**
Oleoyl Macrogolglycerides, **952**
Olive Oil, **953**, A64
Olive Oil Ear Drops, **1841**
Olive Oil Substrate Emulsion, A64
Omega-3-Acid Ethyl Esters, **954**
Omeprazole, **959**
Omeprazole Sodium, **960**
Omissions from the British Pharmacopoeia, xxv
Opacity, Standard Preparation of, A106
Opalescence of Solution, Degree of, A133
Opalescence, Standard of, A133
Ophthalmic Inserts, 1430
Opiate Linctus for Infants, **1948**
Opiate Squill Linctus, **1947**
Opiate Squill Linctus, Paediatric, **1948**
Opium, **962**
Opium, Raw, *see Opium*
Opium Tincture, **1842**
Opium Tincture, Camphorated, **1843**
Opium Tincture, Concentrated Camphorated, **1843**
Optical Rotation, Definition of, A139
Optical Rotation, Determination of, A139
Optical Rotation, Specific, Determination of, A139
OPV, *see Poliomyelitis Vaccine, Live (Oral)*
Oracet Blue 2R, A64
Oracet Blue B, A64
Oracet Blue B Solution, A64
Oral Drops, 1441, *see also under name of substance*
Oral Emulsions, 1441, *see also under name of substance*
Oral Emulsions of the BP, List of, 1441
Oral Liquids, 1439
Oral Liquids of the BP, Additional Requirements for, 1440
Oral Powders, 1442, *see also under name of substance*
Oral Powders of the BP, Additional Requirements for, 1442
Oral Powders of the BP, List of, 1442
Oral Rehydration Salts, **1843**
Oral Solutions, 1441, *see also under name of substance*
Oral Solutions of the BP, List of, 1441
Oral Suspensions, 1441, *see also under name of substance*
Oral Suspensions of the BP, List of, 1441
Orange Flower Oil, Bitter- **963**
Orange Oil, **964**
Orange Oil, Terpeneless, **965**
Orange Peel, Dried Bitter-, **965**
Orange Peel Infusion, **1844**
Orange Peel Infusion, Concentrated, **1844**
Orange Spirit, Compound, **1844**
Orange Syrup, **1845**
Orange Tincture, **1845**
Orange-flower Oil, Bitter-, **963**
Orcinol, A64
Orciprenaline Injection, xxv
Orciprenaline Oral Solution, **1845**
Orciprenaline Sulphate, **965**
Orciprenaline Tablets, **1845**
Organ Preservation, Solution for, *see Organ Preservation Solutions*
Organ Preservation Solutions, **1846**
Organisation, Pharmacopoeial, A337
Organochlorine Pesticides, Determination of, A185
Organophosphorus Pesticide Residues, Determination A185
Orphenadrine Citrate, **967**, S90
Orphenadrine Hydrochloride, **968**, S90
Orphenadrine Hydrochloride Tablets, **1847**
Orthophosphates, Reactions of, A150
Orthophosphoric Acid, A64
Orthophosphorous Acid, A64
Osmium Tetroxide, A64
Osmium Tetroxide Solution, A64
Osmolality, A145
Ouabain, **968**
Ox Brain, Acetone-dried, A64
Oxalic Acid, A64
Oxalic Acid and Sulphuric Acid Solution, A64
Oxazepam, **969**, S90
Oxazepam Tablets, **1847**
Oxetacaine, **970**, S91
Oxethazaine, *see Oxetacaine*
Oxidised Cellulose, xxvi
Oxidising Substances, Determination of, A174
Oxpentifylline, *see Pentoxifylline*
Oxprenolol, S91
Oxprenolol Hydrochloride, **971**
Oxprenolol Tablets, **1848**
Oxybuprocaine Hydrochloride, **972**
Oxygen, **973**, A64
Oxygen in Medicinal Gases, Determination of, A169
Oxygen-flask Combustion, A156
Oxygen-free Nitrogen, A63
Oxymel, Squill, **1948**
Oxymetazoline Hydrochloride, **974**
Oxymetholone, **975**, S91
Oxymetholone Tablets, **1848**
Oxyphenbutazone, **975**, S92
Oxyphenbutazone Eye Ointment, **1848**
Oxytetracycline, **976**
Oxytetracycline Calcium, **978**
Oxytetracycline Capsules, **1849**
Oxytetracycline Dihydrate, **976**
Oxytetracycline Hydrochloride, **979**
Oxytetracycline Tablets, **1850**
Oxytocin, **981**
Oxytocin Concentrated Solution, **983**
Oxytocin Injection, **1851**
Oxytocin Injection, Ergometrine and, **1661**

P

Paediatric Alimemazine Oral Solution, Strong/Paediatric Trimeprazine Oral Solution, Strong, **1472**
Paediatric Alimemazine Oral Solution/ Paediatric Trimeprazine Oral Solution, **1472**
Paediatric Chloral Elixir, **1552**
Paediatric Chloral Oral Solution, **1552**

Paediatric Codeine Linctus, **1598**
Paediatric Compound Tolu Linctus, **1973**
Paediatric Co-trimoxazole Oral Suspension, **1611**
Paediatric Co-trimoxazole Tablets, **1613**
Paediatric Digoxin Injection, **1639**
Paediatric Digoxin Oral Solution, **1639**
Paediatric Ferrous Sulphate Oral Solution, **1679**
Paediatric Ipecacuanha Emetic, **1760**
Paediatric Ipecacuanha Emetic Mixture, **1760**
Paediatric Ipecacuanha Oral Solution, **1760**
Paediatric Opiate Squill Linctus, **1948**
Paediatric Paracetamol Mixture, *see Paracetamol Oral Suspension*
Paediatric Paracetamol Oral Solution, **1853**
Paediatric Paracetamol Oral Suspension, *see Paracetamol Oral Suspension,*
Paediatric Simple Linctus, **1925**
Paediatric Sulfadimidine Oral Suspension, **1953**
Paediatric Trimethoprim and Sulfamethoxazole, Oral Suspension, **1611**
Paediatric Trimethoprim and Sulfamethoxazole Tablets, **1613**
Paints, 1425, *see also under name of substance*
Paints of the BP, List of, 1425
Palladium Chloride, *see palladium(II) chloride*
Palladium(II) Chloride, A64
Palladium Chloride Solution, A65
Palm Kernel Oil, Fractionated, **986**
Palmitic Acid, A65
Pancreas Powder, A65
Pancreatic Extract, **987**
Pancreatin, **990**
Pancreatin Granules, **1851**
Pancreatin Tablets, **1851**
Pancuronium Bromide, **992**
Pancuronium Injection, **1852**
Papaveretum **993**
Papaveretum Injection **1852**
Papaverine Hydrochloride, **993**, A65
Paper Chromatography, A130
Paracetamol, **994**, S92, A65
Paracetamol, 4-Aminophenol-free, A65
Paracetamol Mixture, Paediatric, *see Paracetamol Oral Suspension*
Paracetamol Oral Solution, Paediatric, **1853**
Paracetamol Oral Suspension, **1854**
Paracetamol Oral Suspension, Paediatric, *see Paracetamol Oral Suspension*
Paracetamol Tablets, **1854**
Paracetamol Tablets, Codeine Phosphate and, **1593**
Paracetamol Tablets, Dextropropoxyphene Hydrochloride and, **1606**
Paracetamol Tablets, Dihydrocodeine and, **1600**
Paracetamol Tablets, Dispersible, **1855**
Paracetamol Tablets, Soluble, **1855**
Paracytic Stomata, A183
Paraffin and Magnesium Hydroxide Oral Emulsion, Liquid, **1857**
Paraffin Emulsion, Liquid, **1856**
Paraffin Gauze Dressing, xxvi
Paraffin, Hard, **995**
Paraffin, Light Liquid, **996**
Paraffin, Liquid, **996**, A65
Paraffin Ointment, **1856**
Paraffin Oral Emulsion, Liquid, **1856**
Paraffin, White Soft, **997**, A65
Paraffin, Yellow Soft, **998**
Paraldehyde, **998**
Paraldehyde Injection, **1857**
Parametric Release, 4, 17, 1394, 1407
Pararosaniline Solution, Decolorised, A65
Paregoric, **1843**
Parenteral Preparations, 1442
Parenteral Preparations, Excipients in, 1443
Parenteral Preparations of the BP, Additional Requirements for, 1444
Parenteral Preparations, Water for Use in Manufacture of, 1445
Parnaparin Sodium, **999**
Particle Size Classification of Powders, A254
Particle Size, Microscopy Limit Test, A254
Particle Size of
Eye Drops, 1429
Semi-solid Eye Preparations, 1429
Particle Size of Powders, A254
Particle-free Water, A91
Particles, Sub-visible, Limit Test for, A205
Particles, Visible, Limit Test for, A205
Particulate Contamination, Limit Tests for, A205
Particulate Contamination, Microscope Method, A206
Particulate Contamination of Parenteral Preparations, 1445
Paste, Morison's, **1790**
Pastes, 1459, *see also under name of substance,*
Pastes of the BP, List of, 1460
Patches, Dissolution Test for Transdermal, A192
Patches, Transdermal, 1460
Patents, vi, xl
PD_{50}, A313
Peanut Oil, **111**
Penetrometry, Measurement of Consistency by, A260
Penicillamine, **999**
Penicillamine Tablets, **1857**
Penicillinase Solution, A65
Pentaerythritol Tablets, **1858**
Pentaerythritol Tetranitrate Tablets, **1858**
Pentaerythrityl Tetrakis[3-(3,5-di-*tert*-butyl-4-hydroxyphenyl)propionate], A65
Pentagastrin, **1001**
Pentagastrin Injection, **1858**
Pentamidine Diisetionate, *see Pentamidine Isetionate*
Pentamidine Injection, **1858**
Pentamidine Isethionate and Preparations, *see under Pentamidine Isetionate*
Pentamidine Isetionate, **1002**, S92
Pentamidine Isetionate for Injection, **1858**
Pentane, *see* n*-pentane*
1-Pentanesulphonic Acid Sodium Salt, *see sodium pentanesulphonate*
Pentan-1-ol, A65
Pentanol, *see pentan-1-ol*
Pentazocine, **1003**
Pentazocine (form A), S93
Pentazocine (form B), S93
Pentazocine Capsules, **1859**
Pentazocine Hydrochloride, **1004**, S93
Pentazocine Injection, **1860**
Pentazocine Lactate, **1004**, S94
Pentazocine Suppositories **1860**
Pentazocine Tablets, **1861**
Pentobarbital, **1005**, S94
Pentobarbital Sodium, **1006**
Pentobarbital Tablets, **1861**
Pentobarbitone, Salts and Preparations, *see under Pentobarbital*
Pentoxifylline/Oxpentifylline, **1007**
tert-Pentyl Alcohol, A65
Peppermint Emulsion, Concentrated, **1862**
Peppermint Essence, **1862**
Peppermint Leaf, **1008**
Peppermint Oil, **1009**
Peppermint Spirit, **1862**
Pepsin, **1010**, A65
Pepsin Powder, A65
Perchloric Acid, A65
Perchloric Acid Solution, A66
Perchloric Acid VS, A95
Percolation, Definition of, A182
Percolation, Production of Extracts by, 1427
Percolation, Production of Tinctures by, 1456
Percut, BCG Vaccine, **2042**
Percutaneous Bacillus Calmette-Guérin Vaccine, **2042**
Perf/Ser, *see Gas-gangrene Antitoxin (Perfringens)*
Perforated Film Absorbent Dressing, xxvi
Periodic–Acetic Acid Solution, A66
Periodic Acid, A66
Periodic Acid Solution, A66
Peritoneal Dialysis Solutions, **1862**
Peritoneal Dialysis, Solutions for, *see Peritoneal Dialysis Solutions*
Permeable Plastic Wound Dressing, xxvi
Peroxide Value, Determination of, A173
Peroxide-free Ether, A42
Peroxyacetic Acid Solution, A66
Peroxymonosulphuric Acid Reagent, A66
Perphenazine, **1011**, S94
Perphenazine Tablets, **1864**
Pertussis Vaccine, **2071**
Pertussis Vaccine, Adsorbed, *see Pertussis Vaccine*
Pertussis Vaccine, Adsorbed Diphtheria, Tetanus and, **2050**
Pertussis Vaccine, Assay of, A230

Peru Balsam, **1012**
Peruvian Rhatany, *see Rhatany Root*
Per/Vac, *see Pertussis Vaccine*
Per/Vac/Ads, *see Pertussis Vaccine*
Pessaries, Disintegration Test for, A187
Pessaries, Moulded, 1461
Pessaries of the BP, List of, 1462
Pesticide Residues, Determination of, A184
Pethidine, S95
Pethidine Hydrochloride, **1013**, S95
Pethidine Injection, **1865**
Pethidine Tablets, **1865**
Petroleum Jelly, White, **997**
Petroleum Jelly, Yellow, **998**
Petroleum, Light, *see petroleum spirit (boiling range, 50° to 70°)*
Petroleum R1, Light, *see petroleum spirit (boiling range, 40° to 60°)*
Petroleum R2, Light, *see petroleum spirit (boiling range, 30° to 40°)*
Petroleum R3, Light, A66
Petroleum Spirit, A66
Petroleum Spirit (boiling range 40° to 60°), Aromatic-free, A66
pH Values, Determination of, A144
Ph.Eur., Definition of, 16, 1406
Pharmacopoeia Commission, Membership of the British, x
Pharmacopoeia, European, A343
Pharmacopoeial Organisation, A337
Pharmacopoeial Requirements, Basis of, xix, A317
Phenacetin, **1014**, A66
Phenanthrene, A66
Phenanthroline Hydrochloride, A66
Phenazone, **1015**, A66
Phenelzine Sulphate, **1015**
Phenelzine Tablets, **1865**
Phenethicillin Capsules, xxv
Phenethicillin Potassium, xxv
Phenethicillin Tablets, xxv
Phenindamine Tablets, **1866**
Phenindamine Tartrate, **1016**
Phenindione, **1016**, S95
Phenindione Tablets, **1866**
Pheniramine Maleate, **1017**, S96
Phenobarbital, **1017**, S96
Phenobarbital Elixir, **1866**
Phenobarbital Injection, **1867**
Phenobarbital Oral Solution, **1866**
Phenobarbital Sodium, **1018**
Phenobarbital Sodium Tablets **1867**
Phenobarbital Tablets, **1867**
Phenobarbitone, Salts and Preparations, *see under Phenobarbital*
Phenol, **1019**, A66
Phenol and Glycerol Injection, **1868**
Phenol in Antisera and Vaccines, A231
Phenol Injection, Oily, **1867**
Phenol, Liquefied, **1020**, A66
Phenol Red, A66
Phenol Red Solution, A66
Phenol Red Solution, Buffered, *see phenol red solution R1*
Phenol Red Solution R1, A66
Phenol Red Solution R2, A66
Phenol Red Solution R3, A66
Phenoldisulphonic Acid Solution, A66
Phenolphthalein, **1020**, A67
Phenolphthalein Solution, A67
Phenolphthalein Solution R1, A67
Phenolphthalein–Thymol Blue Solution, A67
Phenolsulphonphthalein, **1021**
Phenothiazines, Related Substances in, A123
Phenothiazines, Test for Identification of, A123
Phenoxybenzamine Capsules, **1868**
Phenoxybenzamine Hydrochloride, **1022**, S96, A67
2-Phenoxyethanol, A67
Phenoxyethanol, **1022**, *see also 2-phenoxyethanol*
Phenoxymethylpenicillin, **1023**
Phenoxymethylpenicillin Capsules, xxv
Phenoxymethylpenicillin Oral Solution, **1868**
Phenoxymethylpenicillin Potassium, **1025**
Phenoxymethylpenicillin Tablets, **1869**
Phentolamine Injection, **1870**
Phentolamine Mesilate, **1026**
Phentolamine Mesylate, *see Phentolamine Mesilate*
Phenyl Benzoate, A67
Phenyl Silica Gel, A78
Phenyl Silica Gel for Chromatography, A77
Phenylalanine, **1027**, *see L-phenylalanine*
L-Phenylalanine, A67
Phenylbutazone, **1028**
(*E*)-4-Phenylbut-3-en-2-one, A67
N-Phenylcarbazole, A67
p-Phenylenediamine Dihydrochloride, A67
Phenylephrine, **1029**
Phenylephrine Eye Drops, **1870**
Phenylephrine Hydrochloride, **1030**
Phenylephrine Injection, **1870**
α-Phenylglycine, *see DL-phenylglycine*
DL-Phenylglycine, A67
Phenylhydrazine, A67
Phenylhydrazine Hydrochloride, A67
Phenylhydrazine Hydrochloride Solution, A67
Phenylhydrazine–Sulphuric Acid Solution, A67
Phenylmercuric Borate, **1031**
Phenylmercuric Nitrate, **1031**
Phenylpropanolamine Hydrochloride, **1032**
Phenytoin, **1033**, S97
Phenytoin Capsules, **1871**
Phenytoin Injection, **1871**
Phenytoin Oral Suspension, **1872**
Phenytoin Sodium, **1034**
Phenytoin Tablets, **1872**
Phloroglucinol, A67
Phloroglucinol Solution, A67
Pholcodine, **1035**, S97
Pholcodine Linctus, **1873**
Pholcodine Linctus, Strong, **1873**
Phosphate Buffer, 0.025M Standard, A104
Phosphate Buffer pH 2.5, *see buffer solution pH 2.5*
Phosphate Buffer pH 2.5 R1, *see buffer solution pH 2.5 R1*
Phosphate Buffer pH 3.0, A103
Phosphate Buffer pH 3.5, A103
Phosphate Buffer pH 4.0, A103
Phosphate Buffer pH 4.0, Mixed, A103
Phosphate Buffer pH 4.75, A103
Phosphate Buffer pH 4.9, A103
Phosphate Buffer pH 5.4, Mixed, A103
Phosphate Buffer pH 5.8, *see phosphate buffers*
Phosphate Buffer pH 6.0, *see phosphate buffers*
Phosphate Buffer pH 6.2, *see phosphate buffers*
Phosphate Buffer pH 6.4, *see phosphate buffers*
Phosphate Buffer pH 6.6, *see phosphate buffers*
Phosphate Buffer pH 6.8, *see phosphate buffers*
Phosphate Buffer pH 6.8, 0.2M Mixed, A103
Phosphate Buffer pH 6.8, Mixed, A103
Phosphate Buffer pH 7.0, *see phosphate buffers*
Phosphate Buffer pH 7.0, 0.067M Mixed, A103
Phosphate Buffer pH 7.0, 0.1M Mixed, A103
Phosphate Buffer pH 7.0, Mixed, A103
Phosphate Buffer pH 7.2, *see phosphate buffers*
Phosphate Buffer pH 7.4, *see phosphate buffers*
Phosphate Buffer pH 7.5, 0.2M, A103
Phosphate Buffer pH 7.6, *see phosphate buffers*
Phosphate Buffer pH 7.8, *see phosphate buffers*
Phosphate Buffer pH 8.0, *see phosphate buffers*
Phosphate Buffer pH 10, Mixed, A103
Phosphate Buffer Solution pH 2.0, A104
Phosphate Buffer Solution pH 3.0 R1, A104
Phosphate Buffer Solution pH 3.2, A104
Phosphate Buffer Solution pH 3.2 R1, A104
Phosphate Buffer Solution pH 3.5, *see phosphate buffer pH 3.5*
Phosphate Buffer Solution pH 5.5, A104
Phosphate Buffer Solution pH 5.8, A104
Phosphate Buffer Solution pH 6.0, *see citro-phosphate buffer pH 6.0*
Phosphate Buffer Solution pH 6.0 R1, A104
Phosphate Buffer Solution pH 6.0 R2, A104
Phosphate Buffer Solution pH 6.4 R1, *see phosphate-buffered saline pH 6.4*
Phosphate Buffer Solution pH 6.8, *see citro-phosphate buffer pH 6.8*
Phosphate Buffer Solution pH 6.8 R1, *see 0.2M mixed phosphate buffer pH 6.8*

Phosphate Buffer Solution pH 7.0, *see citro-phosphate buffer pH 7.0*
Phosphate Buffer Solution pH 7.0, 0.067M Mixed, *see 0.067M mixed phosphate buffer pH 7.0*
Phosphate Buffer Solution pH 7.0, 0.1M, *see 0.1M mixed phosphate buffer pH 7.0*
Phosphate Buffer Solution pH 7.0 R1, A104
Phosphate Buffer Solution pH 7.0 R2, A104
Phosphate Buffer Solution pH 7.0 R3, A104
Phosphate Buffer Solution pH 7.2, *see citro-phosphate buffer pH 7.2*
Phosphate Buffer Solution pH 7.4, A104
Phosphate Buffer Solution pH 7.5, 0.2M, *see 0.2M phosphate buffer pH 7.5*
Phosphate Buffer Solution pH 7.5, 0.33M, A104
Phosphate Buffer Solution pH 8.0, 0.02M, A104
Phosphate Buffer Solution pH 8.0, 0.1M, A104
Phosphate Buffer Solution pH 8.0, 1M, A104
Phosphate Buffers, A103
Phosphate Standard Solution (5 ppm PO_4), A100
Phosphate Standard Solution (100 ppm PO_4), A100
Phosphate-albumin Buffered Saline pH 7.2, A104
Phosphate-buffered Saline pH 6.4, A104
Phosphate-buffered Saline pH 6.8, A104
Phosphate-buffered Saline pH 7.4, A104
Phosphate-citrate Buffer Solution pH 5.5, A104
Phosphates Enema, **1874**
Phosphates, Limit Test for, A155
Phosphates, Reactions of, A150
Phospholipid, A67
Phosphomolybdic Acid, A68
Phosphomolybdic Acid Solution, A68
Phosphomolybdic Reagent, A68
Phosphomolybdotungstic Reagent, A68
Phosphomolybdotungstic Reagent, Dilute, A68
Phosphoric Acid, *see orthophosphoric acid*
Phosphoric Acid, **1036**
Phosphoric Acid, Concentrated, *see Phosphoric Acid*
Phosphoric Acid, Dilute, **1037**, A68
Phosphoric Vanillin Solution, A90
Phosphorus in Polysaccharide Vaccines, Test for A233
Phosphorus Pentoxide, A68
Phosphotungstic Acid Solution, A68
Phthalaldehyde, A68
Phthalaldehyde Reagent, A68
Phthalate Buffer pH 3.6, A104
Phthalate Buffer Solution pH 4.4, A104
Phthalazine, A68
Phthalein Purple, A68
Phthalic Acid, A68
Phthalic Anhydride, A68
Phthalic Anhydride Solution, A68
Phthalylsulfathiazole, **1037**
Phthalylsulphathiazole, *see Phthalylsulfathiazole*
Physostigmine Eye Drops, xxv
Physostigmine Salicylate, **1038**
Physostigmine Sulphate, **1039**
Phytomenadione, **1040**
Phytomenadione Injection, **1874**
Phytomenadione Tablets, **1875**
Picric Acid, A68
Picric Acid Solution, A68
Picric Acid Solution R1, A68
Picrolonic Acid, A68
Pilocarpine Hydrochloride, **1041**
Pilocarpine Hydrochloride Eye Drops, **1875**
Pilocarpine Nitrate, **1042**, S97
Pilocarpine Nitrate Eye Drops, **1876**
Pimozide, **1043**
Pindolol, **1045**, S98
Pindolol Tablets, **1876**
β-Pinene, A68
Piperazine Adipate, **1046**
Piperazine Citrate, **1047**
Piperazine Citrate Elixir, **1877**
Piperazine Citrate Oral Solution, **1877**
Piperazine Dipicrate Solution, A69
Piperazine Hydrate, **1048**
Piperazine Oestrone Sulphate, *see Estropipate,*
Piperazine Phosphate, **1049**
Piperazine Phosphate Tablets, **1877**
Piperidine, A69
Piperonyl Butoxide CRS, A106
Piroxicam, **1049**
Piroxicam Capsules, **1878**
Piroxicam Gel, **1878**
Pivampicillin, **1050**
Pizotifen, S98
Pizotifen Malate, **1053**, S98
Pizotifen Tablets, **1879**
Plaited Stainless Steel Suture, Sterile, xxvi
Plasma for Fractionation, **2004**
Plasma, Fresh Frozen, xxvi
Plasma, Substrate A69
Plasma Substrate Deficient in Factor V, A69
Plasma Substrate R1, A69
Plasma Substrate R2, A69
Plasminogen, Human, A69
Plaster of Paris, **236**
Plastic Containers and Closures, A272
Plastic Containers for Aqueous Solutions for Intravenous Infusion, A272
Plastic Syringes, Sterile Single-use, A279
Plastic Wound Dressing, Impermeable, xxvi
Plastic Wound Dressing, Permeable, xxvi
Plasticised Poly(vinyl Chloride), Containers of, A281
Platelet Substitute, A69
Platelet-poor Plasma, A69
Plates for Thin-layer Chromatography, A122
Platinum Standard Solution (30 ppm Pt), A100
Pneumococcal Polysaccharide Vaccine, **2073**
Pneumo/Vac, *see Pneumococcal Polysaccharide Vaccine*
Podophyllin, **1053**
Podophyllin Paint, Compound, **1880**
Podophyllum Resin, **1053**
Poldine Methylsulphate, *see Poldine Metilsulfate*
Poldine Metilsulfate, **1054**, S99
Poldine Tablets, **1880**
Poliomyelitis Vaccine, Inactivated, **2075**
Poliomyelitis Vaccine, Live (Oral), **2076**
Poloxamer 124, A70
Poloxamer 188, **1055**, S99
Pol/Vac(Inact), *see Inactivated Poliomyelitis Vaccine*
Pol/Vac(Oral), *see Poliomyelitis Vaccine, Live (Oral)*
Polyacrylamide Gel Electrophoresis, A132
Polyacrylate Dispersion (30 per cent), **1056**
Polyamide 6 Suture, Sterile, *see Non-absorbable Sutures, Sterile*
Polyamide 6/6 Suture, Sterile, *see Non-absorbable Sutures, Sterile*
Poly[(cyanopropyl)methylphenylmethyl-siloxane], A70
Poly(cyanopropyl)(7)(phenyl)(7)-methyl)(86)siloxane, A70
Poly(cyanopropyl)(phenylmethyl)-siloxane, A70
Polycyanopropylsiloxane, A70
Poly(dimethyl)(diphenyl)-(divinyl)siloxane, A70
Poly(dimethyl)(diphenyl)siloxane, A70
Polydimethylsiloxane, A70
Polyether Hydroxylated Gel for Chromatography, A70
Polyethylene, Containers of, A288
Polyethylene Glycol, *see under Macrogol for pharmacopoeial grades*
Polyethylene Glycol 200, A70
Polyethylene Glycol 200 R1, A70
Polyethylene Glycol 300, A70
Polyethylene Glycol 400, A70
Polyethylene Glycol 1000, A70
Polyethylene Glycol 1500, A70
Polyethylene Glycol 20,000, A70
Polyethylene Glycol 20,000 2-Nitroterephthalate, A70
Polyethylene Glycol Adipate, A70
Polyethylene Glycol Succinate, A70
Poly(ethylene Terephthalate) Suture, Sterile, *see Non-absorbable Sutures, Sterile*
Polyethylene with Additives For Containers, A289
Polyethylene without Additives for Containers, A288
Polymethacrylic Resin, see Weak Cationic Resin, A27
Poly[methyl(95)phenyl(5)]siloxane, A70
Polymethylphenylsiloxane, A70
Poly[methyl(94)phenyl(5)vinyl(1)]-siloxane, A70

Polymorphism, A321
Polymyxin and Bacitracin Eye Ointment, **1880**
Polymyxin B Sulphate, **1056**
Polyolefines, Containers of, A285
Polyols, Nickel in, Limit Test for, A154
Polyoxyethylated Castor Oil, A70
Polyoxyethylene 20 Sorbitan Monolaurate, **1058**
Polyoxyethylene 20 Sorbitan Monooleate, **1059**
Polyoxyethylene 20 Sorbitan Monostearate, **1058**
Polyoxyethylene 23 Lauryl Ether, A70
Polyoxyl Castor Oil, **262**
Polyoxyl Castor Oil, Hydrogenated, **263**
Polypropylene, Containers of, A292
Polypropylene Suture, Sterile, *see Non-absorbable Sutures, Sterile*
Polysaccharide Vaccines, Composition of, A233
Polysorbate 20, **1058**, A70
Polysorbate 60, **1058**
Polysorbate 80, **1059**, A70
Polystyrene, S3, S4
Polystyrene 900-1000, A70
Polystyrene Sulphonate, Calcium, **233**
Polystyrene Sulphonate, Sodium, **1194**
Polythiazide, **1060**, S99
Polythiazide Tablets, **1881**
Polyurethane Foam Dressing, xxvi
Polyvidone, *see povidone*
Potable Water, 10, 1400
Potash Alum, **70**
Potash, Caustic, **1068**
Potash Solution, **1885**
Potassium Acetate, **1060**, A70
Potassium Antimonate(v), A70
Potassium Antimonate(v) Solution, A70
Potassium Bicarbonate, *see potassium hydrogen carbonate*
Potassium Bicarbonate, **1061**
Potassium Bicarbonate Solution, Saturated Methanolic, A71
Potassium Borohydride, A71
Potassium Bromate, A71, A92
Potassium Bromate VS, A95
Potassium Bromide, **1062**, A71
Potassium Carbonate, A71
Potassium Carbonate, Anhydrous, *see potassium carbonate*
Potassium Carbonate Sesquihydrate, A71
Potassium Chlorate, A71
Potassium Chloride, **1063**, A71
Potassium Chloride, 0.1M, A71
Potassium Chloride and Dextrose Injection, **1882**
Potassium Chloride and Dextrose Intravenous Infusion, **1882**
Potassium Chloride and Glucose Injection, **1882**
Potassium Chloride and Glucose Intravenous Infusion, **1882**
Potassium Chloride and Sodium Chloride Injection, **1882**
Potassium Chloride and Sodium Chloride Intravenous Infusion, **1882**
Potassium Chloride Concentrate, Sterile, **1881**
Potassium Chloride, Sodium Chloride and Glucose Intravenous Infusion, **1883**
Potassium Chloride, Sodium Chloride and Dextrose Intravenous Infusion, **1883**
Potassium Chloride, Sodium Chloride and Dextrose Injection, **1883**
Potassium Chloride, Sodium Chloride and Glucose Injection, **1883**
Potassium Chloride Tablets, Effervescent, **1883**
Potassium Chloride Tablets, Slow, **1884**
Potassium Chromate, A71
Potassium Chromate Solution, A71
Potassium Citrate, **1064**, A71
Potassium Citrate Mixture, **1884**
Potassium Citrate Oral Solution, **1884**
Potassium Clavulanate, **1064**
Potassium Clavulanate Tablets, Amoxicillin and, **1592**
Potassium Clorazepate, *see Dipotassium Clorazepate*
Potassium Cyanide, A71
Potassium Cyanide Solution, A71
Potassium Cyanide Solution PbT, A71
Potassium Dichromate, A71, A92
Potassium Dichromate Solution, A71
Potassium Dichromate Solution, Dilute, A71
Potassium Dichromate Solution R1 A71
Potassium Dichromate VS, A95
Potassium Dihydrogen Citrate, A71
Potassium Dihydrogen Orthophosphate, A71
Potassium Dihydrogen Phosphate, *see potassium dihydrogen orthophosphate*
Potassium Dihydrogen Phosphate, **1066**
Potassium Dihydrogen Phosphate, 0.2M, A71
Potassium Ferricyanide, *see potassium hexacyanoferrate(III)*
Potassium Ferricyanide Solution, *see potassium hexacyanoferrate(III) solution*
Potassium Ferriperiodate Solution, A71
Potassium Ferrocyanide, *see potassium hexacyanoferrate(II)*
Potassium Ferrocyanide Solution, *see potassium hexacyanoferrate(II) solution*
Potassium Hexacyanoferrate(II), A71
Potassium Hexacyanoferrate(II) Solution, A71
Potassium Hexacyanoferrate(III), A71
Potassium Hexacyanoferrate(III) Solution, A72
Potassium Hexacyanoferrate(III) Solution, Dilute, A72
Potassium Hyaluronate, A72
Potassium Hyaluronate Stock Solution, A72
Potassium Hydrogen Carbonate, *see Potassium Bicarbonate*
Potassium Hydrogen Carbonate, A72
Potassium Hydrogen Carbonate Solution, Saturated, A72
Potassium Hydrogen Phthalate, A72, A92
Potassium Hydrogen Phthalate, 0.2M, A72
Potassium Hydrogen Phthalate VS, A96
Potassium Hydrogen Sulphate, A72
Potassium Hydrogen Tartrate, **1067**, *see also potassium hydrogen (+)-tartrate*
Potassium Hydrogen (+)-Tartrate, A72
Potassium Hydroxide, **1068**, A72
Potassium Hydroxide, 2M Alcoholic, A72
Potassium Hydroxide, Alcoholic, *see ethanolic potassium hydroxide VS*
Potassium Hydroxide, Ethanolic, A72
Potassium Hydroxide in Alcohol (10% v/v), 0.5M, A72
Potassium Hydroxide in Alcohol (60%) VS, *see potassium hydroxide in ethanol (60% v/v) VS*
Potassium Hydroxide in Ethanol (60%) VS, A96
Potassium Hydroxide in Ethanol (90%) VS, A96
Potassium Hydroxide, Methanolic, A72
Potassium Hydroxide Solution, **1885**
Potassium Hydroxide Solution, Alcoholic, A72
Potassium Hydroxide Solution R1, Alcoholic, A72
Potassium Hydroxide VS, A96
Potassium Hydroxide VS, Ethanolic, A96
Potassium Hydroxyquinoline Sulphate, **1068**
Potassium Hydroxyquinoline Sulphate and Benzoyl Peroxide Cream, **1885**
Potassium Iodate, **1069**, A72, A92
Potassium Iodate Tablets, **1886**
Potassium Iodate VS, A96
Potassium Iodide, **1069**, A72
Potassium Iodide and Starch Solution, A72
Potassium Iodide Solution, A72
Potassium Iodide Solution, Dilute, A72
Potassium Iodide Solution, Iodinated, A72
Potassium Iodide Solution, Saturated, A72
Potassium Iodide VS, A96
Potassium Iodobismuthate Solution, A72
Potassium Iodobismuthate Solution, Acid, A72
Potassium Iodobismuthate Solution, Dilute, A72
Potassium Iodobismuthate Solution R1, A72
Potassium Iodobismuthate Solution R2, A73
Potassium Iodoplatinate Solution, A73
Potassium, Limit Test for, A155
Potassium Mercuri-iodide Solution, Alkaline, A73
Potassium Metaperiodate, *see potassium periodate*
Potassium Nitrate, **1070**, A73
Potassium Periodate, A73
Potassium Permanganate, **1071**, A73
Potassium Permanganate and Phosphoric Acid Solution, A73

Potassium Permanganate Solution, Dilute, A73
Potassium Permanganate VS, A96
Potassium Perrhenate, A73
Potassium Persulphate, A73
Potassium Plumbite Solution, A73
Potassium Pyroantimonate, *see potassium antimonate(v)*
Potassium Pyroantimonate Solution, *see potassium antimonate(v) solution*
Potassium, Reactions of, A150
Potassium Salts, Reactions of, A150
Potassium Sodium (+)-Tartrate, A73
Potassium Sorbate, **1071**
Potassium Standard Solution (20 ppm K), A100
Potassium Standard Solution (100 ppm K), A100
Potassium Standard Solution (600 ppm K), A100
Potassium Sulphate, A73
Potassium Tablets, Bumetanide and Slow, **1526**
Potassium Tartrate, *see dipotassium (+)-tartrate*
Potassium Tetrahydroborate, *see potassium borohydride*
Potassium Tetraiodomercurate Solution, A73
Potassium Tetraiodomercurate Solution, Alkaline, A73
Potassium Tetraoxalate, A73
Potassium Thiocyanate, A73
Potassium Thiocyanate Solution, A73
Potato Starch, **1072**
Potency, Estimated, 13, 1403
Potency of Antibiotics, 13, 1403
Potency, Stated, 13, 1403
Potentiometric Determination of Ionic Concentration, A157
Potentiometric Titration, A156
Potentiometry, Ion-selective, A157
Povidone, **1072**, A73
Povidone, Iodinated **1074**
Povidone–Iodine Solution, **1886**
Powdered Cellulose, **288**
Powdered Vegetable Drug, *see name of drug*
Powders, Dusting, 1458, *see also under name of substance*
Powders, Ear, 1426, *see also under name of substance*
Powders, Effervescent, 1442
Powders for Inhalation, 1435, *see also under name of substance*
Powders for Inhalation of the BP, List of, 1436
Powders for Injections, 1444, 1445
Powders for Intravenous Infusions, 1444
Powders for Oral Solutions and Suspensions, 1440
Powders for Rectal Solutions and Suspensions, 1449
Powders, Nasal, 1438, *see also under name of substance*
Powders, Oral, 1442, *see also under name of substance*
Powders, Particle Size of, A254
Powders, Topical, 1457
ppm, Definition of, 6, 19, 1396, 1409, A313
Praziquantel, **1075**
Prazosin, S100
Prazosin Hydrochloride, **1076**
Prazosin Tablets, **1887**
Precipitated Sulphur, A84
Precision of Measurements, 18, 1408
Prednisolone, **1078**, S100, A73
Prednisolone 21-Acetate, A73
Prednisolone Acetate, **1080**
Prednisolone Enema, **1887**
Prednisolone Pivalate, **1081**
Prednisolone Sodium Phosphate, **1083**
Prednisolone Sodium Phosphate Eye Drops, **1888**
Prednisolone Tablets, **1889**
Prednisolone Tablets, Enteric-coated, **1890**
Prednisolone Tablets, Gastro-resistant, **1890**
Prednisone, **1084**, S100
Prednisone Tablets, **1890**
Preface, vii
Pregelatinised Maize Starch, *see Pregelatinised Starch*
Pregelatinised Starch, **1225**
Prekallikrein Activator, Test for, A226
Preparations for Inhalation, 1433
Preparations for Inhalation of the BP, Additional Requirements for, 1435
Preparations for Irrigation, 1436
Preparations for Irrigation of the BP, Additional Requirements for, 1437
Prepared Belladonna, *see Prepared Belladonna Herb*
Prepared Belladonna Herb, **145**
Prepared Calamine **212**
Prepared Chalk **301**
Prepared Hyoscyamus, **711**
Prepared Ipecacuanha, **740**
Prepared Stramonium, **1230**
Preservative Solutions for Blood, Anticoagulant and, **2001**
Pressurised Inhalations, 1436, *see also under name of substance*
Pressurised Inhalations of the BP, List of, 1436
Pressurised Metered-dose Preparations for Inhalation, 1434
Pressurised Pharmaceutical Preparations, 1447
Prilocaine, S101
Prilocaine Hydrochloride, **1086**, S101
Prilocaine Injection, **1891**
Primaquine Diphosphate, *see Primaquine Phosphate*
Primaquine Phosphate, **1087**
Primaquine Tablets, xxv
Primary Aromatic Amines, Reactions of, A147
Primary Aromatic Amino Nitrogen, Determination of, A156
Primary Standards, A92
Primidone, **1088**, S101
Primidone Oral Suspension, **1892**
Primidone Tablets, **1892**
Probenecid, **1089**, S102
Probenecid Tablets, **1893**
Procainamide, S102
Procainamide Hydrochloride, **1089**
Procainamide Injection, **1893**
Procainamide Tablets, **1894**
Procaine Benzylpenicillin for Injection, Fortified/Procaine Penicillin Injection, Fortified, **1895**
Procaine Benzylpenicillin for Injection/ Procaine Penicillin for Injection, **1895**
Procaine Benzylpenicillin Injection, Fortified/Procaine Penicillin Injection, Fortified, **1895**
Procaine Benzylpenicillin Injection/ Procaine Penicillin Injection, **1894**
Procaine Benzylpenicillin/Procaine Penicillin, **1090**
Procaine Hydrochloride, **1092**, A73
Procaine Penicillin and Preparations, *see under Procaine Benzylpenicillin*
Prochlorperazine, S102
Prochlorperazine Injection, **1896**
Prochlorperazine Maleate, **1093**
Prochlorperazine Mesilate, **1094**, S103
Prochlorperazine Mesylate, *see Prochlorperazine Mesilate*
Prochlorperazine Oral Solution, **1897**
Prochlorperazine Tablets, **1897**
Procyclidine, S103
Procyclidine Hydrochloride, **1094**, S103
Procyclidine Injection, **1898**
Procyclidine Tablets, **1898**
Production, Status of, 8, 20, 1398, 1410
Products of Recombinant DNA Technology, **1095**
Progesterone, **1097**, S104
Progesterone Injection, **1899**
Proguanil Hydrochloride, **1098**, S104
Proguanil Tablets, **1899**
Proline, **1099**
Promazine, S104
Promazine Hydrochloride, **1100**, S105
Promazine Injection, **1900**
Promazine Tablets, **1900**
Promethazine, S105
Promethazine Hydrochloride, **1100**
Promethazine Hydrochloride Tablets, **1902**
Promethazine Injection, **1901**
Promethazine Oral Solution, **1901**
Promethazine Teoclate, **1101**
Promethazine Teoclate Tablets, **1903**
Promethazine Theoclate and Preparations, *see under Promethazine Teoclate*
Propan-2-ol, Determination of, A160
Propane-1,2-diol, A73
Propanol, *see propan-1-ol*
Propan-1-ol, A73
Propan-2-ol, A73
Propan-2-ol R1, A74
2-Propanol, *see propan-2-ol*
2-Propanol R1, *see propan-2-ol R1*
Propanolamine, *see 3-Aminopropanol*
Propantheline Bromide, **1102**
Propantheline Tablets, **1903**
Propionaldehyde, A74
Propionic Acid, A74

Propionic Anhydride, A74
Propionic Anhydride Reagent, A74
Propranolol, S105
Propranolol Hydrochloride, **1103**
Propranolol Injection, **1904**
Propranolol Tablets, **1904**
Propyl Acetate, A74
Propyl Gallate, **1104**
Propyl Hydroxybenzoate, **1105**, S106
Propyl 4-Hydroxybenzoate, A74
Propyl Parahydroxybenzoate, *see propyl 4-hydroxybenzoate and Propyl Hydroxybenzoate*
Propylene Glycol, **1106**, *see also propane-1,3-diol*
Propylene Glycol Monostearate, **1107**
Propyliodone, **1108**
Propyliodone Injection, **1905**
Propyliodone Oily Injection, **1906**
Propyliodone Oily Suspension, **1906**
Propyliodone Suspension, **1905**
Propylparaben, **1105**
Propylthiouracil, **1109**, S106
Propylthiouracil Tablets, **1906**
Propyphenazone, **1110**
Protamine Hydrochloride, **1110**
Protamine Sulphate, **1112**, A74
Protamine Sulphate Injection, **1906**
Protected from Light, Definition for Storage Statements, 14, 1404
Protected from Light, Definition of, 12, 22, 1402, 1412
Protected from Moisture, Definition of, 14, 22, 1404, 1412
Protein in Blood Products, Determination of, A161
Protein in Polysaccharide Vaccines, Test for, A233
Prothrombin Complex, Dried, **2012**
Protirelin, **1113**
Protriptyline, S106
Protriptyline Hydrochloride, **1115**
Protriptyline Tablets, **1907**
Proxymetacaine, S107
Proxymetacaine Eye Drops, **1907**
Proxymetacaine Hydrochloride, **1115**, S107
Proxyphylline, **1116**
Pseudoephedrine, S107
Pseudoephedrine Hydrochloride, **1117**, S108
Pseudoephedrine Tablets, **1908**
Pseudomonas aeruginosa, Test for, A244
Psyllium seed, **1117**
Pulegone, A74
Pulsed Spectrometry, A119
Pumice Powder, A74
Purified Hexane, A48
Purified Talc, **1255**
Purified Water, **1367**
Pyrazinamide, **1118**, S108
Pyrazinamide Tablets, **1908**
Pyrethroid Insecticides, Determination of, A185
Pyridine, A74
Pyridine, Anhydrous, A74
Pyridine Bromide Solution, A74
Pyridine-3-carboxaldehyde, A74
Pyridostigmine Bromide, **1119**, S108
Pyridostigmine Injection, **1909**
Pyridostigmine Tablets, **1909**
Pyridoxine Hydrochloride, **1120**, S109
Pyridoxine Tablets, **1910**
2-Pyridylamine, A74
Pyrid-2-ylamine, *see 2-pyridylamine*
Pyridylazonaphthol, A74
Pyridylazonaphthol Solution, A74
(3-Pyridylmethyl)amine, *see 3-(aminomethyl)pyridine*
Pyrimethamine, **1121**, S109
Pyrimethamine Tablets, **1910**
Pyrocatechol, *see catechol*
Pyrogallol, A74
Pyrogallol Solution, Alkaline, A74
Pyrogens in Formulated Preparations, *see appropriate general monograph*
Pyrogens, Test for, A218
Pyroxylin, **1122**
Pyruvic Acid, A74

Q

Qualitative Reactions and Tests, A147
Quillaia, **1122**
Quillaia Bark, **1122**
Quillaia Liquid Extract, **1911**
Quillaia, Powdered, xxv, *see also Quillaia*
Quillaia Tincture, 1911
Quinaldine Red, A74
Quinaldine Red Solution, A74
Quinalizarin, A74
Quinhydrone, A75
Quinidine, A75
Quinidine Bisulphate, **1123**
Quinidine Sulphate, **1124**, A75
Quinidine Sulphate Tablets, **1911**
Quinine, A75
Quinine Bisulphate, **1125**
Quinine Bisulphate Tablets, **1912**
Quinine Dihydrochloride, **1127**
Quinine Hydrochloride, **1128**
Quinine Sulphate, **1129**, A75
Quinine Sulphate Tablets, **1913**
Quinoline, A75
Quinoline Solution, A75
Quinolin-8-ol, S109

R

Rabbit Erythrocyte Suspension, A75
Rabies Antiserum, Fluorescein-conjugated, A75
Rabies Immunoglobulin, **2023**
Rabies Vaccine, **2080**
Rab/Vac, *see Rabies Vaccine*
Racementhol, **1131**
Racemic Camphor, **236**
Racemic Ephedrine Hydrochloride, **1132**
Racemic Menthol, **1131**
Racephedrine Hydrochloride, **1132**
Radioactivity, Definition of Terms, 2103
Radioactivity, Measurement of, 2105
Radiochemical Purity, 2106
Radionuclidic Purity, 2106
Radiopharmaceutical Preparations, General Monograph, 2103
Raney Nickel Catalyst, *see nickel-aluminium alloy*
Ranitidine Hydrochloride, **1133**, S110
Ranitidine Injection, **1914**
Ranitidine Oral Solution, **1915**
Ranitidine Tablets, **1916**
Rapeseed Oil, A75
Raw Opium, *see Opium*
Reaction of Solution and Colour of Certain Indicators, A143
Reactions and Tests, Qualitative, A147
Reagents, Descriptions of, 6, 18, 1396, 1408
Reagents, General, A13
Reagents, Volumetric, A92
Recently Prepared, Definition of, 10, 1400
Recombinant DNA Technology, Products of, **1095**
Recrystallised Imidazole, A50
Recrystallised Iodine Pentoxide, A51
Rectal Capsules, 1449
Rectal Foams, 1449
Rectal Preparations, 1448
Rectal Preparations of the BP, Additional Requirements for, 1449
Rectal Preparations, Semi-solid, 1449
Rectal Solutions, 1449, 1450, *see also under name of substance*
Rectal Solutions of the BP, List of, 1450
Rectal Suspensions, 1449
Rectal Tampons, 1449
Rectified Spirit, **549**
Red Blood Cells, Concentrated, xxvi
Red Cells, xxvi
Red Cinchona Bark, **339**
Red Primary Solution, A133
Reducing Mixture, A75
Reference Buffer Solutions for Determination of pH, A144
Reference Materials and Spectra, 11, 1401
Reference Materials, Chemical and Biological, A106
Reference Preparation, International, 14, 1404
Reference Preparations, European Pharmacopoeia Biological, A106
Reference Solutions for Colour of Solution Test, A134
Reference Spectra of the European Pharmacopoeia, A115
Reference Spectra, Preparation of Infrared, S2
Reference Substances, British Pharmacopoeia Chemical, A106
Reference Substances, European Pharmacopoeia Chemical, A106
Reference Substances, Preparations and Spectra, 23, 1413
Reference Suspensions, A133
Refined Almond Oil, **57**
Refined Sugar, **1235**
Refractive Index, Determination of, A138
Rehydration Salts, Oral, **1843**
Related Substances, Tests for, A319
Relative Density, Determination of, A140
Relative Foam Density of Medicated Foams, 1431

Reserpine, **1134**
Residual Ethylene Oxide and Dioxan, Determination of, A164
Residual solvents, A321
Residual Solvents, Determination of, A163
Residue on Evaporation of Volatile Oils, Test for, A175
Resinified Volatile Oils in Volatile Oils, Test for, A175
Resistance to Crushing of Tablets, A262
Resolution Factor, Definition of, A124, A130
Resolution Power of Ultraviolet and Visible Spectrophotometers, A117
Resorcinol, **1135**, A75
Resorcinol Reagent, A75
Response Factor, Definition of, A320
Retention Volume, Definition of, A126
Retinol, *see under Vitamin A*
Retinol Concentrate (Powder Form), Synthetic, **1362**
Retinol Concentrate (Oily Form), Synthetic, **1361**
Retinol Concentrate (Water-dispersible Form) Synthetic, **1364**
Revision of Monographs, xvi
Rhamnose, *see L-rhamnose*
L-Rhamnose, A75
Rhaponticin, A75
Rhatany Root, **1136**
Rhatany Root, Powdered, xxv, *see also Rhatany Root*
Rhodamine B, A75
Rhubarb, **1137**
Rhubarb, Powdered, xxv, *see also Rhubarb*
Rhubarb Tincture, Compound, **1916**
Ribbon Gauze, X-Ray-Detectable Cotton, xxvi
Ribbon Gauze, X-Ray-Detectable Cotton and Viscose, xxvi
Ribes Nigrum, **187**
Riboflavin, **1138**
Riboflavin Sodium Phosphate, **1139**
Riboflavine, Salts and Preparations, *see under Riboflavin*
Ribose, A75
Ribose in Polysaccharide Vaccines, Test for, A235
Rice Starch, **1140**
Ricinoleic Acid, A75
Rifampicin, **1141**, S110
Rifampicin Capsules, **1916**
Rifampicin Oral Suspension, **1917**
Rifamycin Sodium, **1142**
Ringer–Lactate Solution for Injection, **1936**
Ritodrine Hydrochloride, **1144**, S110
Ritodrine Injection, **1918**
Ritodrine Tablets, **1918**
Rod Gels, A132
Roman Chamomile Flower, *see Chamomile Flowers*
Rotation, Optical, Definition of, A139
Rotation, Optical, Determination of, A139
Rotation, Specific Optical, Determination of, A139
Roxithromycin, **1145**
Rubber Closures for Containers, A276
Rubber Elastic Bandage, Cotton and, xxvi
Rubber Elastic Bandage, Heavy Cotton and, xxvi
Rubella Immunoglobulin, **2024**
Rubella Vaccine, Live, **2082**
Rubella Vaccine, Live Measles, Mumps and, **2066**
Rub/Vac(Live), *see Rubella Vaccine, Live*
Ruthenium Red, A76
Ruthenium Red Solution, A76
Rutin, A76

S

Sabinene, A76
Saccharin, **1147**, A76
Saccharin Sodium, **1148**
Saccharin, Soluble, **1148**
SAL, A264
Sal Volatile Solution, **1484**
Sal Volatile Spirit, **1485**
Salbutamol, **1150**, S111
Salbutamol Injection, **1919**
Salbutamol Pressurised Inhalation, **1920**
Salbutamol Sulphate, **1151**, S111
Salbutamol Tablets, **1921**
Salcatonin and Preparations, *see under Calcitonin (Salmon)*
Salicylaldehyde, A76
Salicylates, Reactions of, A150
Salicylic Acid, **1152**, S111, A76
Salicylic Acid Collodion, **1922**
Salicylic Acid Lotion, xxv
Salicylic Acid Ointment, **1922**
Salicylic Acid Ointment, Coal Tar and, **1957**
Salicylic Acid Paste, Zinc and, **1995**
Saline, Normal, *see Sodium Chloride Solution*
Saline pH 6.4, Phosphate-buffered, A104
Saline pH 6.8, Phosphate-buffered, A104
Saline pH 7.2, Phosphate-albumin Buffered, A104
Saline pH 7.4, Phosphate-buffered, A104
Salmonella, Test for, A244
Salsalate, xxv
Salsalate Capsules, xxvi
Sand, A76
Saponification Value, Determination of, A173
Saturated Methanolic Potassium Bicarbonate Solution, A71
Saturated Methanolic Potassium Hydrogen Carbonate Solution, A72
Saturated Potassium Iodide Solution, A72
Schick Control, **2095**
Schick Test Toxin, **2095**
Scorpion Venom Antiserum, **2036**
Sealed Container, A268
Second-Derivative Spectrophotometry, A118
Secondary Band, Definition of, A122
Secondary Peak, Definition of, A125, A129
Secondary Spot, Definition of, A122
Selegiline Hydrochloride, **1153**
Selenious Acid, A76
Selenium, A76
Selenium Disulphide, *see Selenium Sulphide*
Selenium Standard Solution (1 ppm Se), A100
Selenium Standard Solution (100 ppm Se), A100
Selenium Sulphide, **1154**
Selenium Sulphide Application, **1922**
Selenium Sulphide Scalp Application, **1922**
Selenous Acid, *see selenious acid*
Self-emulsifying Glyceryl Monostearate, 649
Self-emulsifying Mono- and Diglycerides of Food Fatty Acids, **649**
Self-emulsifying Monostearin, **649**
Semi-solid Ear Preparations, 1426
Semi-solid Eye Preparations, 1429
Semi-solid Nasal Preparations, 1438
Semi-solid Preparations, Topical, 1458
Semi-solid Rectal Preparations, 1449
Semicarbazide Acetate Solution, A76
Semicarbazide Hydrochloride, A76
Semipermeable Hydrocolloid Dressing, xxvi
Senega, **1155**
Senega Root, **1155**
Senega Root, Powdered, xxv, *see also Senega Root*
Senna Fruit, Alexandrian, **1156**
Senna Fruit Powdered Alexandrian, xxv, *see also Alexandrian Senna Fruit*
Senna Fruit, Powdered Tinnevelly, xxv, *see also Tinnevelly Senna Fruit*
Senna Fruit, Tinnevelly, **1157**
Senna Granules, Standardised, **1924**
Senna Leaf, **1158**
Senna Leaf Dry Extract, Standardised, 1923
Senna Leaf, Powdered, xxv, *see also Senna Leaf*
Senna Liquid Extract, **1924**
Senna Pods, *see Senna Fruit*
Senna Tablets, **1924**
Sep/Ser, *see Gas-gangrene Antitoxin (Septicum)*
Serine, **1159**, *see also L-serine*
L-Serine, A76
Sertaconazole Nitrate, **1160**
Serum Gonadotrophin, A47
Serum Solution, A76
Serum Stock Solution, A76
Sesame Oil, **1161**
Sets for the Transfusion of Blood and Blood Components, A278, A283
Shampoos, 1424
Shell Pessaries, *see Vaginal Capsules*
Shell Suppositories, *see Rectal Capsules*
Shellac, **1163**
SI Units, A312
SI Units and Equivalents, 25, 1415
SI Units, Use of, 5, 1395

Sialic Acid in Polysaccharide Vaccines, Test for, A235
Sieves, A255
Signal to Noise Ratio, Definition of, A125, A130
Silanised Diatomaceous Earth for Gas Chromatography, *see silanised diatomaceous support*
Silanised Diatomaceous Earth for Gas Chromatography R1, *see silanised diatomaceous support*
Silanised Diatomaceous Support, A34
Silanised Silica Gel H, A78
Silanised Silica Gel HF_{254}, A78
Silica, Colloidal Anhydrous, **1164**
Silica, Colloidal Hydrated, **1164**
Silica Gel, *see silica gel for chromatography*
Silica Gel, Anhydrous, A76
Silica Gel, Butylsilyl, A76
Silica Gel for Chromatography, A77
  Aminopropylmethylsilyl, A77
  Aminopropylsilyl, A77
  Amylose-derivative, A77
  Base-deactivated, End-capped Octadecylsilyl, A77
  Base-deactivated Octadecylsilyl, A77
  Cyanosilyl, A77
  Diol, A77
  Hexylsilyl, A77
  Hydrophilic, A77
  Nitrile, A77
  Octadecylsilyl, A77
  Octylsilyl, A77
  Phenyl, A77
Silica Gel for Chromatography R1, Nitrile, A77
Silica Gel for Chromatography R1, Octadecylsilyl, A77
Silica Gel for Chromatography, Strong-anion-exchange, A77
Silica Gel for Size-exclusion Chromatography, A77
Silica Gel G, A78
Silica Gel GF_{254}, A78
Silica Gel H, A78
Silica Gel H, Silanised, A78
Silica Gel HF_{254}, A78
Silica Gel HF_{254}, Silanised, A78
Silica Gel OD for Chiral Separations, A78
Silica Gel, Phenyl, A78
Silicates, Reactions of, A150
Silicone Elastomer For Closures and Tubing, A298
Silicone Foam Cavity Wound Dressing, xxvi
Silicone Oil Used as a Lubricant, A298
Silicotungstic Acid, A78
Silk Suture, Sterile Braided, *see Non-absorbable Sutures, Sterile*
Silver Compounds, Reactions of, A150
Silver Diethyldithiocarbamate, A78
Silver Manganese Paper, A78
Silver Nitrate, **1165**, A78
Silver Nitrate Solution, A78
Silver Nitrate Solution, Ammoniacal, A79
Silver Nitrate Solution in Pyridine, A79
Silver Nitrate Solution R1, A79
Silver Nitrate Solution R2, A79
Silver Nitrate VS, A96
Silver Oxide, A79
Silver, Reactions of A150
Silver Standard Solution (5 ppm Ag), A100
Simple Eye Ointment, **1925**
Simple Linctus, **1925**
Simple Linctus, Paediatric, **1925**
Simple Ointment, 1925
Sinensetine, A79
Single-dose Container, A268
Size-exclusion Chromatography, A126
Size-exclusion Chromatography, Silica Gel for, A77
Slab Gels, A132
Slow Diclofenac Tablets, **1633**
Slow Lithium Carbonate Tablets, **1782**
Slow Potassium Chloride Tablets, **1884**
Slow Potassium Tablets, Bumetanide and, **1526**
SN_{50}, A313
Snake Venom Antiserum, *see European Viper Venom Antiserum*
Soap, Soft, **1165**
Soap Spirit, **1926**
Soda, Caustic, **1186**
Soda Lime, **1166**
Soda Mint Tablets, **1928**
Soda-lime–Silica Glass, A268
Sodium, A79
Sodium Acetate, **1167**, A79
Sodium Acetate, Anhydrous, A79
Sodium Acetate Solution pH 6.0, Buffered, A104
Sodium Acid Citrate, **1168**
Sodium Acid Phosphate, **1184**
Sodium Alginate, **1168**
Sodium Amidotrizoate, **1169**, S112
Sodium Amidotrizoate Injection, **1926**
Sodium Arsenite VS, A96
Sodium Ascorbate Solution, A79
Sodium Aurothiomalate, **1171**
Sodium Aurothiomalate Injection, **1927**
Sodium Azide, A79
Sodium Benzoate, **1171**
Sodium Bicarbonate, **1172**, *see also sodium hydrogen carbonate*
Sodium Bicarbonate Ear Drops, **1927**
Sodium Bicarbonate Eye Lotion, **1927**
Sodium Bicarbonate Injection, **1927**
Sodium Bicarbonate Intravenous Infusion, **1927**
Sodium Bicarbonate Tablets, Compound, **1928**
Sodium Bismuthate, A79
Sodium Borate, **188**
Sodium Bromide, **1173**
Sodium Butanesulphonate, A79
Sodium Butyl Hydroxybenzoate, **1173**
Sodium Butylparaben, **1173**
Sodium Calcium Edetate, **1174**
Sodium Calcium Edetate Concentrate, Sterile, **1928**
Sodium Calcium Edetate Injection, **1928**
Sodium Calcium Edetate Intravenous Infusion, **1928**
Sodium Calciumedetate and Preparations, *see under Sodium Calcium Edetate*
Sodium Carbonate, A79
Sodium Carbonate, Anhydrous, **1175**, A79, A92
Sodium Carbonate Decahydrate, **1175**
Sodium Carbonate Monohydrate, **1176**
Sodium Carbonate Solution, A79
Sodium Carbonate Solution, Dilute, A79
Sodium Carbonate Solution R1, A79
Sodium Cetostearyl Sulphate, **1177**, A79
Sodium Chloride, **1179**, A92
Sodium Chloride and Dextrose Injection, **1930**
Sodium Chloride and Dextrose Injection, Potassium Chloride and, **1883**
Sodium Chloride and Dextrose Intravenous Infusion, **1930**
Sodium Chloride and Dextrose Intravenous Infusion, Potassium Chloride and, **1883**
Sodium Chloride and Glucose Injection, Potassium Chloride, **1883**
Sodium Chloride and Glucose Injection, **1930**
Sodium Chloride and Glucose Intravenous Infusion, **1930**
Sodium Chloride and Glucose Intravenous Infusion, Potassium Chloride, **1883**
Sodium Chloride Eye Drops, **1929**
Sodium Chloride Eye Lotion, **1929**
Sodium Chloride Injection, **1929**, A79
Sodium Chloride Injection, Potassium Chloride and, **1882**
Sodium Chloride Intravenous Infusion, **1929**
Sodium Chloride Intravenous Infusion, Potassium Chloride and, **1882**
Sodium Chloride Irrigation Solution, **1930**
Sodium Chloride Mouthwash, Compound, **1930**
Sodium Chloride Solution, **1931**, A79
Sodium Chloride Tablets, **1931**
Sodium Cholate, A79
Sodium Chromate[^{51}Cr] Sterile Solution, **2126**
Sodium Citrate, **1180**, A79
Sodium Citrate Eye Drops, **1931**
Sodium Citrate Irrigation Solution, **1931**
Sodium Citrate Solution for Bladder Irrigation, Sterile, **1931**
Sodium Citrate Tablets, **1932**
Sodium Cobaltinitrite, A79
Sodium Cobaltinitrite Solution, A79
Sodium Cromoglicate, **1181**
Sodium Cromoglicate Powder for Inhalation, **1932**
Sodium Cromoglycate and Preparations, *see under Sodium Cromoglicate*
Sodium Cyclamate, **1182**
Sodium Decanesulphonate, A79

Sodium Deoxyribonucleate, A79
Sodium Diatrizoate and Preparations, *see under Sodium Amidotrizoate*
Sodium Diclofenac, *see Diclofenac Sodium*
Sodium Diethyldithiocarbamate, A79
Sodium Diethyldithiocarbamate Solution, A79
Sodium Dihydrogen Orthophosphate, A80
Sodium Dihydrogen Orthophosphate, Anhydrous, A80
Sodium Dihydrogen Orthophosphate Monohydrate, A80
Sodium Dihydrogen Phosphate, *see sodium dihydrogen orthophosphate monohydrate*
Sodium Dihydrogen Phosphate, Anhydrous, **1183**, *see also anhydrous sodium dihydrogen orthophosphate*
Sodium Dihydrogen Phosphate Dihydrate, **1184**
Sodium Dihydrogen Phosphate Monohydrate, **1184**, *see also sodium dihydrogen phosphate monohydrate*
Sodium Dithionite, A80
Sodium Dodecyl Sulphate, A80
Sodium Dodecyl Sulphate VS, A96
Sodium Edetate, *see disodium edetate and disodium edetate VS*
Sodium Etacrynate for Injection, **1933**
Sodium Etacrynate Injection, **1933**
Sodium Ethacrynate Injection, *see Sodium Etacrynate Injection*
Sodium Fluoresceinate, *see fluorescein sodium*
Sodium Fluoride, **1185**, A80
Sodium Formate, A80
Sodium Fusidate, **1185**
Sodium Fusidate Capsules, xxvi
Sodium Fusidate Gauze Dressing, xxvi
Sodium Fusidate Ointment, **1934**
Sodium Glucuronate, A80
Sodium Heptanesulphonate, A80
Sodium Heptanesulphonate Monohydrate, A80
Sodium Hexanesulphonate, A80
Sodium Hexanitritocobaltate(III), *see sodium cobaltinitrite*
Sodium Hydrogen Carbonate, A80, *see also Sodium Bicarbonate*
Sodium Hydrogen Carbonate Solution, A80
Sodium Hydroxide, **1186**, A80
Sodium Hydroxide BET, A215
Sodium Hydroxide, Ethanolic, A80
Sodium Hydroxide LAL, A215
Sodium Hydroxide, Methanolic, A80
Sodium Hydroxide Solution, A80
Sodium Hydroxide Solution, Dilute, A80
Sodium Hydroxide Solution, Methanolic, A80
Sodium Hydroxide Solution, Strong, A80
Sodium Hydroxide VS, A96
Sodium Hydroxide VS, Ethanolic, A97
Sodium Hypobromite Solution, A80
Sodium Hypochlorite Solution, A80
Sodium Hypochlorite Solution (3% Cl), A80
Sodium Hypochlorite Solution, Dilute, **1935**, A80
Sodium Hypochlorite Solution, Strong, **1934**, *see also sodium hypochlorite solution (3% Cl)*
Sodium Hypophosphite, A81
Sodium Iodide, **1187**, A81
Sodium Iodide Injection, **1935**
Sodium Iodide[^{131}I] Capsules for Diagnostic Use, **2127**
Sodium Iodide[^{123}I] Solution, **2128**
Sodium Iodide[^{125}I] Solution, **2129**
Sodium Iodide[^{131}I] Solution, **2129**
Sodium Iodobismuthate Solution, A81
Sodium Iodohippurate[^{123}I] Injection, **2130**
Sodium Iodohippurate[^{131}I] Injection, 2131
Sodium Iotalamate Injection, **1935**
Sodium Iothalamate Injection, *see Sodium Iotalamate Injection*
Sodium Lactate Injection, **1936**
Sodium Lactate Injection, Compound, **1936**
Sodium Lactate Intravenous Infusion, **1936**
Sodium Lactate Intravenous Infusion, Compound, **1936**
Sodium Lactate Solution, **1187**
Sodium Laurilsulfate, *see Sodium Lauryl Sulphate*
Sodium Lauryl Sulphate, **1189**, *see also sodium dodecyl sulphate*
Sodium Mercaptoacetate, *see sodium thioglycollate*
Sodium Metabisulphite, **1189**, A81
Sodium Metaperiodate, *see sodium periodate,*
Sodium Methanesulphonate, A81
Sodium Methoxide VS, A97
Sodium Methyl Hydroxybenzoate, **1190**
Sodium Methyl Parahydroxybenzoate, *see Sodium Methyl Hydroxybenzoate*
Sodium Methylparaben, **1190**
Sodium Molybdate, A81
Sodium Molybdotungstophosphate Solution, A81
Sodium Naphthoquinonesulphonate, *see sodium 1,2-naphthoquinonesulphonate*
Sodium 1,2-Naphthoquinone-4-sulphonate, A81
Sodium Nitrate, A81
Sodium Nitrite, A81
Sodium Nitrite Solution, A81
Sodium Nitrite VS, A97
Sodium Nitroprusside, **1191**, A81
Sodium Nitroprusside–Carbonate Solution, A81
Sodium Nitroprusside for Injection, **1937**
Sodium Nitroprusside Intravenous Infusion, **1937**
Sodium Octanesulphonate, A81
Sodium Octanoate, A81
Sodium Octyl Sulphate, A81
Sodium Oxalate, A81
Sodium Pentanesulphonate, A81
Sodium Perborate, **1192**
Sodium Perchlorate, A81
Sodium Periodate, A81
Sodium Periodate Solution, A81
Sodium Pertechnetate[^{99m}Tc] Injection (Fission), **2132**
Sodium Pertechnetate[^{99m}Tc] Injection (Non-fission), **2134**
Sodium Phosphate Dihydrate, **495**
Sodium Phosphate[^{32}P] Injection, **2135**
Sodium Phosphates Enema, **1874**
Sodium Phosphite, A81
Sodium Picosulfate, **1193**
Sodium Picosulfate Oral Powder, **1938**
Sodium Picosulphate and Preparations, *see under Sodium Picosulfate*
Sodium Picrate Solution, Alkaline, A81
Sodium Polystyrene Sulphonate, **1194**, S112
Sodium Potassium Tartrate, *see potassium sodium (+)-tartrate*
Sodium Propyl Hydroxybenzoate, **1195**
Sodium Propyl Parahydroxybenzoate, *see Sodium Propyl Hydroxybenzoate*
Sodium Propylparaben, **1195**
Sodium Pyrophosphate, A81
Sodium Pyrosulphite, **1189**
Sodium, Reactions of, A150
Sodium Salicylate, **1196**, A81
Sodium Salicylate Mixture, xxvi
Sodium Salicylate Mixture, Strong, xxvi
Sodium Salts, Reactions of, A150
Sodium Standard Solution (50 ppm Na), A100
Sodium Standard Solution (200 ppm Na), A100
Sodium Starch Glycollate, A81
Sodium Starch Glycollate (Type A), **1196**
Sodium Starch Glycollate (Type B), **1198**
Sodium Stibogluconate, **1199**
Sodium Stibogluconate Injection, **1938**
Sodium Sulphate, **1200**, A81
Sodium Sulphate, Anhydrous, **1199**, A81
Sodium Sulphate Decahydrate, *see Sodium Sulphate*
Sodium Sulphide, A81
Sodium Sulphide Solution, A82
Sodium Sulphite, **1201**, A82
Sodium Sulphite, Anhydrous, **1200**, A82
Sodium Sulphite Heptahydrate, **1201**
Sodium (+)-Tartrate, A82
Sodium Tartrate, *see sodium (+)-tartrate*
Sodium Taurocholate CRS, A106
Sodium Tetraborate, **188**, A82
Sodium Tetradecyl Sulphate Concentrate, **1202**
Sodium Tetradecyl Sulphate Injection, **1939**
Sodium Tetradeuteriodimethylsilapentanoate, A82
Sodium Tetraphenylborate, A82
Sodium Tetraphenylborate Solution, A82
Sodium Tetraphenylborate VS, A97
Sodium Thioglycollate, A82

Sodium Thiosulphate, **1203**, A82
Sodium Thiosulphate Injection, **1939**
Sodium Thiosulphate VS, A97
Sodium 3-Trimethylsilylpropane-sulphonate, A82
Sodium Tungstate, A82
Sodium Valproate, **1203**
Sodium Valproate Enteric-coated Tablets, **1941**
Sodium Valproate Oral Solution, **1939**
Sodium Valproate Tablets, **1940**
Soft Capsules, 1421
Soft Extracts, 1427
Soft Paraffin, White, **997**
Soft Paraffin, Yellow, **998**
Soft Soap, **1165**
Softening Time Determination of Lipophilic Suppositories, A263
Solids, Total, Determination of, A180
Solochrome Dark Blue, A82
Solochrome Dark Blue Mixture, A82
Solubility, Definition of Terms Used, 11, 21, 1401, 1411
Solubility in Ethanol of Volatile Oils, Test for, A175
Solubility, Status of, 11, 21, 1401, 1411
Soluble Aspirin Tablets, *see Dispersible Aspirin Tablets*
Soluble Aspirin Tablets, Effervescent, **1493**
Soluble Fluorescein, **601**
Soluble Insulin, **1754**
Soluble Insulin Injection, *see Soluble Insulin*
Soluble Paracetamol Tablets, **1855**
Soluble Saccharin, **1148**
Soluble Starch, A82
Soluble Sulfacetamide, **1238**
Soluble Tablets, 1452
Solutions, *see under name of substance*
Solutions, Buffer, A101
Solutions for Haemodialysis, *see Haemodialysis Solutions*
Solutions for Haemofiltration, *see Haemofiltration Solutions*
Solutions for Nebulisation of the BP, List of, 1436
Solutions for Organ Preservation, *see Organ Preservation Solutions*
Solutions for Peritoneal Dialysis, *see Peritoneal Dialysis Solutions*
Solutions of the BP, List of, 1425
Solutions, Oral, 1441, *see also name of substance*
Solutions, Rectal, 1449
Solutions, Standard, A98
Solutions, Volumetric, A92
Solvent Ether, **552**
Solvents, Determination of Residual, A163
Solvents for Pharmacopoeial Tests, 12, 19, 1402, 1409
Solvents for Use in Ultraviolet and Visible Spectrophotometry, A117
Somatostatin, **1204**
Somatropin, **1206**
Somatropin Bulk Solution, **1209**
Somatropin for Injection, **1941**
Somatropin Injection, **1941**
Sorbic Acid, **1211**, A82
Sorbide Nitrate, Diluted, *see Diluted Isosorbide Dinitrate*
Sorbitan Laurate, **1212**
Sorbitan Monolaurate, *see Sorbitan Laurate*
Sorbitan Mono-oleate, *see Sorbitan Oleate*
Sorbitan Monopalmitate, *see Sorbitan Palmitate*
Sorbitan Monostearate, *see Sorbitan Stearate*
Sorbitan Oleate, **1212**
Sorbitan Palmitate, **1213**
Sorbitan Stearate, **1213**
Sorbitan Trioleate, **1214**
Sorbitol, **1214**, *see also* D*-sorbitol*
D-Sorbitol, A82
Sorbitol 70 per cent (Crystallising), *see Sorbitol Solution (70 per cent) (Crystallising)*
Sorbitol 70 per cent (Non-crystallising), *see Sorbitol Solution (70 per cent) (Non-crystallising)*
Sorbitol Injection, **1944**
Sorbitol Intravenous Infusion, **1944**
Sorbitol Solution (70 per cent) (Crystallising), **1215**
Sorbitol Solution (70 per cent) (Non-crystallising), **1216**
Sotalol Hydrochloride, **1217**, S112
Sotalol Injection, **1944**
Sotalol Tablets, **1945**
Soya Oil, **1218**
Soya Oil, Hydrogenated, **1219**
Soya-bean Oil, *see Soya Oil*
Soya-bean Oil, Hydrogenated, *see Soya Oil, Hydrogenated,*
Soyabean Oil, **1218**
Soyabean Oil, Hydrogenated, **1219**
Spearmint Oil, **1220**
Specific Absorbance, Definition of, A116
Specific Optical Rotation, Determination of, A139
Specific Surface Area, Determination of, A257
Specified Micro-organisms, Tests for, A243
Specified Pathogen-free Flocks, A236
Spectinomycin Hydrochloride, **1221**, S113
Spectinomycin Hydrochloride for Injection, **1945**
Spectinomycin Injection, **1945**
Spectrometry, *see under name of method*
SPF Flocks, A236
Spirit (Ketone-free), Industrial Methylated, **875**
Spirit, Industrial Methylated, **875**
Spirit, Rectified, **549**
Spirit, Surgical, **1955**
Spirits, 1450, *see also under name of substance*
Spirits, Industrial Methylated, **875**
Spirits of the BP, List of, 1450
Spironolactone, **1222**, S113
Spironolactone Tablets, **1946**
Spray-dried Acacia, **32**
Sprays, Ear, 1426
Sprays, Liquid Nasal, 1438
Sprays, Nasal, 1439, *see also under name of substance*
Squalane, A82
Squill, **1223**
Squill, Indian, **1224**
Squill Linctus, Compound, **1947**
Squill Linctus, Opiate, **1947**
Squill Linctus, Paediatric Opiate, **1948**
Squill Liquid Extract, **1947**
Squill Oxymel, **1948**
Squill, Powdered, xxv, *see also Squill*
Squill, Powdered Indian, xxv, *see Squill*
SSI, A313
Stabiliser-free Di-isopropyl Ether, A36
Stabiliser-free Tetrahydrofuran, A85
Stainless Steel Suture, Sterile Monofilament, xxvi
Stainless Steel Suture, Sterile Plaited, xxvi
Stainless Steel Suture, Sterile Twisted, xxvi
Standard 2,6-Dichlorophenolindophenol Solution, Double-strength, A35
Standard Dichlorophenolindophenol Solution, A35
Standard, International, 14, 1404
Standard Phosphate Buffer, 0.025M, A104
Standard Preparation of Opacity, A106
Standard Preparations for Biological Assays, A332
Standard Solutions, A98
Standard Terms, xxi
Standardised Aloes Dry Extract, **1474**
Standardised Frangula Bark Dry Extract, **1699**
Standardised Senna Granules, **1924**
Standardised Senna Leaf Dry Extract, **1923**
Standards, Official, 4, 1394
Standards, Primary, A92
Stannated Hydrochloric Acid, A49
Stannous Chloride, *see tin(II) chloride*
Stannous Chloride Dihydrate, **1224**
Stannous Chloride Solution R1, *see tin(II) chloride solution R1*
Stanozolol, **1225**, S113
Stanozolol Tablets, **1948**
Staphylococcus aureus, Test for, A244
Star Anise, **104**
Starch, A82
Starch, Cassava, **1257**
Starch, Hydrolysed, A82
Starch Iodate Paper, A82
Starch Iodide Paper, A82
Starch Iodide Solution, A82
Starch, Maize **836**
Starch Mucilage, A82
Starch, Potato, **1072**
Starch, Pregelatinised, **1225**
Starch, Rice, **1140**
Starch, Soluble, A82
Starch Solution, A82
Starch Solution, Iodide-free, A83
Starch, Sterilisable Maize, **837**
Starch Substrate, A83

Starch, Tapioca, **1257**
Starch, Wheat, **1369**
Stars, Significance of Chaplet of, 3, 1393
Stated Potency, 13, 1403
Stationary Phase A, A130
Stationary Phase B, A130
Stationary Phase C, A130
Stationary Phases for Liquid Chromatography, A130
Steam Sterilisation, A264
Stearic Acid, **1226**, A83
Stearic Anhydride, A83
Stearoyl Macrogolglycerides, **1226**
Stearyl Alcohol, *see octadecan-1-ol*
Stearyl Alcohol, **1228**
Sterculia, **1228**
Sterculia Granules, **1949**
Sterculia Gum, **1228**
Sterculia, Powdered, xxv, *see also Sterculia*
Stereochemistry, A333
Sterile Absorbent Cotton, **2156**
Sterile Absorbent Viscose Wadding, **2157**
Sterile Amiodarone Concentrate, **1481**
Sterile Catgut, **2158**
Sterile Cetrimide Solution, **1552**
Sterile Clonazepam Concentrate, **1585**
Sterile Co-trimoxazole Concentrate, 1610
Sterile Dopamine Concentrate, **1651**
Sterile Lidocaine Solution, **1779**
Sterile Noradrenaline Concentrate/ Sterile Norepinephrine Concentrate, **1838**
Sterile Potassium Chloride Concentrate, **1881**
Sterile Products, Methods of Preparation of, A264
Sterile Sodium Calcium Edetate Concentrate, **1928**
Sterile Sodium Citrate Solution for Bladder Irrigation, **1931**
Sterile Sutures, *see under name of suture*
Sterile Trisodium Edetate Concentrate, **1983**
Sterilisable Maize Starch, **837**
Sterilisation, Methods of, 10, 1400, A264
Sterility Assurance Level, A264
Sterility, Guidelines on the Test for, A242
Sterility of Formulated Preparations, *see appropriate general monograph*
Sterility of Radiopharmaceutical Preparations 2106
Sterility, Test for, A239
Steroids, Test for Identification of, A123
Steroids, Tetrazolium Assay of, A161
Sterols in Fatty Oils, Determination of, A179
Sticks, 1450
Sticks, Nasal, 1439
Stilboestrol and Preparations, *see under Diethylstilbestrol*
Stomata, Types of, A183
Stomatal Index, Determination of, A183
Storage of Formulated Preparations, *see appropriate general monograph*
Storage of Radiopharmaceutical Preparations, 2107
Storage of Vaccines, 2040
Storage Statements, Status of, 14, 22, 1404, 1412
Stramonium Leaf, **1229**
Stramonium Leaf, Powdered, *see Stramonium Leaf*
Stramonium Leaf, Powdered, xxv
Stramonium, Prepared, **1230**
Strapping, Extension, xxvi
Streptokinase, **1231**
Streptokinase for Injection, **1949**
Streptokinase Injection, **1949**
Streptomycin Injection, **1950**
Streptomycin Sulphate, **1232**, A83
Streptomycin Sulphate for Injection, **1950**
Strip Electrophoresis, A131
Strong Ammonia Solution, **85**
Strong Ammonium Acetate Solution, **1485**
Strong Cation Exchange Resin (Calcium Form), *A27*
Strong Cetrimide Solution, **299**
Strong Coal Tar Solution, **1958**
Strong Ginger Tincture, **1707**
Strong Glutaraldehyde Solution, **645**
Strong Haloperidol Oral Drops, **1723**
Strong Haloperidol Oral Solution, **1723**
Strong Hydrogen Peroxide Solution, *see hydrogen peroxide solution (100 vol)*
Strong Iodine Monochloride Reagent, A51
Strong Methyl Salicylate Ointment, **1806**
Strong 1-Naphthol Solution, A61
Strong Paediatric Alimemazine Oral Solution/Strong Paediatric Trimeprazine Oral Solution, **1472**
Strong Pholcodine Linctus, **1873**
Strong Sodium Hydroxide Solution, A80
Strong Sodium Hypochlorite Solution, **1934**, *see sodium hypochlorite solution (3% Cl)*
Strong Sodium Salicylate Mixture, xxvi
Strong-anion-exchange Silica Gel for Chromatography, A77
Strongly Acidic Ion-exchange Resin, A52
Strongly Basic Anion Exchange Resin, A20
Strontium Chloride, A83
Structures of Substances of Natural or Semi-synthetic Origin, A334
Styrene, A83
Styrene–divinylbenzene Copolymer, A83
Sub-visible Particles, Limit Test for, A205
Subdued Light, Definition of, 12, 1402
Subsidiary Titles, Status of, 7, 1397
Substrate Plasma, *see plasma substrate*
Substrate Plasma R1, *see plasma substrate R1*
Succinate Buffer Solution pH 4.6, A104
Succinic Acid, A83
Succinylsulfathiazole, **1234**
Succinylsulphathiazole, *see Succinylsulfathiazole*
Sucrose, **1235**, A83
Sudan Orange, *see Sudan Yellow*
Sudan Red, A83
Sudan Red G, A83
Sudan Red Solution, A83
Sudan Yellow, A83
Sudan Yellow Solution, A83
Sufentanil Citrate, **1236**
Sugar, Refined, **1235**
Sugars, Lead in, Limit Test for, A154
Suggested Methods, Status of, 13, 1403
Sulfacetamide, S114
Sulfacetamide Eye Drops, **1952**
Sulfacetamide Eye Ointment, **1952**
Sulfacetamide Sodium, **1238**
Sulfacetamide, Soluble, **1238**
Sulfadiazine, **1239**, S114
Sulfadiazine Injection, **1952**
Sulfadimidine, **1240**, S115
Sulfadimidine Injection, **1953**
Sulfadimidine Oral Suspension, Paediatric, **1953**
Sulfadimidine Sodium, **1241**
Sulfadimidine Tablets, **1954**
Sulfadoxine, **1241**
Sulfafurazole, **1241**
Sulfamethizole, **1243**
Sulfamethoxazole, **1244**, S115
Sulfanilamide, *see sulphanilamide*
Sulfasalazine, **1245**
Sulfathiazole, **1246**, *see also sulphathiazole*
Sulfinpyrazone, **1247**
Sulfinpyrazone Tablets, **1954**
Sulfisomidine, **1248**
Sulindac, **1249**, S114
Sulindac Tablets, **1951**
Sulphacetamide, Salts and Preparations, *see under Sulfacetamide*
Sulphadiazine and Preparations, *see under Sulfadiazine*
Sulphadimidine, Salts and Preparations, *see under Sulfadimidine*
Sulphafurazole, *see Sulfafurazole*
Sulphamethizole, *see Sulfamethizole*
Sulphamethoxazole and Preparations, *see under Sulfamethoxazole*
Sulphamethoxazole and Trimethoprim Preparations, *see Co-trimoxazole Preparations*
Sulphamic Acid, A83
Sulphan Blue, A83
Sulphanilamide, A83
Sulphanilic Acid, A83, A92
Sulphanilic Acid Solution, A83
Sulphasalazine, *see Sulfasalazine*
Sulphate Standard Solution (10 ppm SO_4), A100
Sulphate Standard Solution (10 ppm SO_4) R1, A100
Sulphated Ash, Determination of, A166
Sulphates, Limit Test for, A155
Sulphates, Reactions of, A150
Sulphathiazole, *see Sulfathiazole*
Sulphinpyrazone and Preparations, *see under Sulfinpyrazone*

Sulphisomidine, *see Sulfasomidine*
Sulphisoxazole, *see Sulfafurazole*
Sulphite Standard Solution (1.5 ppm SO_2), A100
Sulphomolybdic Reagent R2, A83
Sulphomolybdic Reagent R3, A83
Sulphosalicylic Acid, A83
Sulphur, *see precipitated sulphur*
Sulphur Dioxide, A83
Sulphur Dioxide, Determination of, A166
Sulphur Dioxide R1, A83
Sulphur Dioxide Solution, A84
Sulphur for External Use, **1251**
Sulphur, Precipitated, A84
Sulphur-free Toluene, A88
Sulphuric Acid, **1251**, A84
Sulphuric Acid, 0.25M Alcoholic, A84
Sulphuric Acid, 2.5M Alcoholic, A84
Sulphuric Acid, Dilute, **1252**, A84
Sulphuric Acid, Ethanolic, A84
Sulphuric Acid–Formaldehyde Reagent, A84
Sulphuric Acid, Methanolic, A84
Sulphuric Acid, Nitrogen-free, A84
Sulphuric Acid VS, A97
Sulphurous Acid, *see sulphur dioxide solution*
Sulpiride, **1252**
Sumatra Benzoin, **158**
Sunflower Oil, A84
Superfine Powder, Definition of, A254
Supplementary Chapters, xxiii
Supplementary Chapters, Contents of the, A316
Suppositories, 1448, 1450, *see also under name of substance*
Suppositories, Disintegration Test for, A187
Suppositories of the BP, List of, 1450
Suppositories, Softening Time Determination of Lipophilic, A263
Surface Area, Determination of Specific, A257
Surgical Materials, xxii
Surgical Spirit, **1955**
Suspensions, Oral, 1441, *see also under name of substance*
Suspensions, Rectal, 1449
Suxamethonium Chloride, **1253**
Suxamethonium Chloride Injection, **1955**
Sweet Fennel, **577**
Swelling Index, Determination of, A180
Symbols and Abbreviations, 24, 1414
Symbols, Atomic Weights of Elements, Names and, A311
Symmetry Factor, Definition of, A124, A129
Synonyms, Approved, A289
Synthetic Absorbable Braided Sutures, Sterile, **2159**
Synthetic Absorbable Monofilament Sutures, Sterile, **2161**
Synthetic Retinol Concentrate (Oily Form), **1361**
Synthetic Retinol Concentrate (Powder Form), **1362**
Synthetic Retinol Concentrate (Water-dispersible Form), **1364**
Syringes, Glass, A268
Syringes, Sterile Single-use Plastic, A279
Syringes, Sterile, Single-use Plastic, A279
Syrup, **1956**
Syrup, Invert, **1757**
Syrups, 1450, *see also Oral Liquids and under name of substance*
Syrups of the BP, List of, 1451
Systems Suitability, Chromatographic Tests, A321

T

Tablets, 1451, *see also under name of substance*
  Coated, 1452
  Dispersible, 1452
  Effervescent, 1452
  for Rectal Solutions and Suspensions, 1449
  for Use in the Mouth, 1453
  Gastro-resistant, 1452
  Modified-release, 1453
  Soluble, 1452
  Uncoated, 1451
  Vaginal, 1462
Tablets, Chocolate Basis for, 1453
Tablets, Disintegration Test for, A187
Tablets, Dissolution Test for, A189
Tablets, Friability of Uncoated, A262
Tablets of the BP, Additional Requirements for, 1453
Tablets of the BP, List of, 1453
Tablets, Resistance to Crushing of, A262
Tagatose, *A84*
Talc, *see Purified Talc*
Talc, A84
Talc Dusting Powder, **1956**
Talc, Purified, **1255**
Tamoxifen, S115
Tamoxifen Citrate, **1256**
Tamoxifen Tablets, **1956**
Tamper-evident Container, Definition of, 15, 1405
Tamper-proof Container, A268
Tampons, Medicated, 1456
Tampons, Medicated Ear, 1426
Tampons, Rectal, 1449
Tampons, Vaginal, 1462
Tannic Acid, A84
Tannic Acid Reagent, A84
Tapioca Starch, **1257**
Tar, **1258**
Tar, Coal, **1258**
(+)-Tartaric Acid, A84
Tartaric Acid, **1258**, *see also (+)-tartaric acid*
Tartrates, Reactions of, A150
Taste of Volatile Oils, Test for, A175
Tears, Artificial, **1744**
Technetium[^{99m}Tc] Albumin Injection, **2135**
Technetium[^{99m}Tc] Colloidal Rhenium Sulphide Injection, **2137**
Technetium[^{99m}Tc] Colloidal Sulphur Injection, **2138**
Technetium[^{99m}Tc] Colloidal Tin Injection, **2139**
Technetium[^{99m}Tc] Etifenin Injection, **2140**
Technetium[^{99m}Tc] Gluconate Injection, **2141**
Technetium[^{99m}Tc] Macrosalb Injection, **2142**
Technetium[^{99m}Tc] Medronate Injection, **2144**
Technetium[^{99m}Tc] Microspheres Injection,, **2145**
Technetium[^{99m}Tc] Pentetate Injection, **2146**
Technetium[^{99m}Tc] Succimer Injection, **2147**
Technetium[^{99m}Tc] Tin Pyrophosphate Injection, **2148**
Technical Changes to Monographs, xxvi
Temazepam, **1259**
Temazepam Oral Solution, **1958**
Temperature, Expression of, 5, 19, 1395, 1409
Tenoxicam, **1260**
Terbutaline Sulphate, **1261**
Terbutaline Tablets, **1959**
Terconazole, **1262**
Terfenadine, **1263**
Terminology Used in Vaccines and Certain Other Products, A230
Terpeneless Lemon Oil, **780**
Terpeneless Orange Oil, **965**
α-Terpineol, A84
Terpineol, **1265**
Testosterone, **1265**, S116, A84
Testosterone Decanoate, **1265**, S116
Testosterone Enantate, **1266**
Testosterone Enanthate, *see Testosterone Enantate*
Testosterone Implants, **1960**
Testosterone Isocaproate, **1268**, S116
Testosterone Propionate, **1269**, S117, A84
Testosterone Propionate Injection, **1960**
Tests and Assays, 11, 21, 1401, 1411
Tests, Biological Assays and, 13, 1403, A332
Tests, Qualitative Reactions and, A147
Tetanus and Petussis Vaccine, Adsorbed Diphtheria, **2050**
Tetanus Antitoxin, **2036**
Tetanus Antitoxin for Human Use, *see Tetanus Antitoxin*
Tetanus Immunoglobulin, **2024**
Tetanus Prophylactic, Adsorbed Diphtheria–, **2046**
Tetanus Vaccine, **2083**
Tetanus Vaccine, Adsorbed, **2085**
Tetanus Vaccine, Adsorbed Diphtheria and, **2046**
Tetanus Vaccine, Assay of Adsorbed, A231
Tetanus Vaccine for Adults and Adolescents, Adsorbed **2048**
Tetanus Vaccine, Typhoid and, **2090**
Tetanus–Whooping-cough Prophylactic, Adsorbed Diphtheria–, **2050**

Tetrabutylammonium Bromide, A84
Tetrabutylammonium Dihydrogen Orthophosphate, A84
Tetrabutylammonium Dihydrogen Phosphate, *see tetrabutylammonium dihydrogen orthophosphate*
Tetrabutylammonium Hydrogen Sulphate, A84
Tetrabutylammonium Hydroxide, A85
Tetrabutylammonium Hydroxide in 2-Propanol, A98
Tetrabutylammonium Hydroxide in Propan-2-ol VS, A98
Tetrabutylammonium Hydroxide Solution, A85
Tetrabutylammonium Hydroxide Solution (104 g/l), A85
Tetrabutylammonium Hydroxide VS, A97
Tetrabutylammonium Iodide, A85
Tetrabutylammonium Iodide VS, A98
Tetracaine Eye Drops/Amethocaine Eye Drops, **1961**
Tetracaine Hydrochloride/ Amethocaine Hydrochloride, **1270**
^{12}C-2,3,7,8-Tetrachloro-*p*-dioxin CRS, A106
^{13}C-2,3,7,8- Tetrachloro-*p*-dioxin CRS A106
Tetrachloroethane, A85
Tetracosactide, **1271**
Tetracosactide Injection, **1961**
Tetracosactide Zinc Injection **1962**
Tetracosactrin and Preparations, *see under Tetracosactide*
Tetracycline, **1274**, A85
Tetracycline Capsules, **1963**
Tetracycline Hydrochloride, **1275**
Tetracycline Hydrochloride for Intravenous Infusion, **1964**
Tetracycline Injection, **1964**
Tetracycline Intravenous Infusion, **1964**
Tetracycline Oral Suspension, xxvi
Tetracycline Tablets, **1964**
n-Tetradecane, A85
Tetradecylammonium Bromide, A85
Tetraethylammonium Hydroxide Solution, A85
Tetraethylene Pentamine, A85
Tetraheptylammonium Bromide, A85
Tetrahexylammonium Hydrogen Sulphate, A85
Tetrahydrofuran, A85
Tetrahydrofuran, Stabiliser-free, A85
Tetramethylammonium Chloride, A85
Tetramethylammonium Hydrogen Sulphate, A85
Tetramethylammonium Hydroxide Pentahydrate, A85
Tetramethylammonium Hydroxide Solution, A85
Tetramethylammonium Hydroxide Solution, Dilute, A85
Tetramethyldiaminodiphenylmethane, *see 4,4′-methylenebis-(*N,N-*dimethylaniline)*
Tetramethyldiaminodiphenylmethane Reagent, *see 4,4′-methylenebis-(*N,N-*dimethylaniline) reagent*
Tetramethylethylenediamine, A85
Tetramethylsilane, A86
1,2,3,4-Tetraphenylcyclopenta-1,3-diene, A86
1,2,3,4-Tetraphenylcyclopenta-1,3-dienone, A86
N,N,N′,N′-Tetramethylphenylenediamine Dihydrochloride, A85
Tetraphenylethylene, A86
Tetrazolium Assay of Steroids, A161
Tetrazolium Blue, A86
Tetrazolium Blue Solution, Alkaline, A86
Tet/Ser, *see Tetanus Antitoxin*
Tet/Vac/Ads, *see Adsorbed Tetanus Vaccine*
Tet/Vac/FT, *see Tetanus Vaccine*
Thallium Standard Solution (10 ppm Tl), A100
Thallium(I) Nitrate, A86
Thallium(I) Sulphate, A86
Thallous Sulphate, *see thallium(I) sulphate*
Thallous[^{201}Tl] Chloride Injection, **2150**
Thebaine, A86
Theobroma Oil, **1277**
Theobromine, **1277**
Theophylline, **1278**, S117, A86
Theophylline Hydrate, **1279**
Theophylline Monohydrate, *see Theophylline Hydrate*
Theophylline–Ethylenediamine, *see Aminophylline*
Theophylline–Ethylenediamine Hydrate, *see Aminophylline Hydrate*
Theoretical Plates, Definition of, A124, A126, A129
Thermal Analysis, A145
Thermogravimetry, A145
Thiabendazole and Preparations, *see under Tiabendazole*
Thiamazole, *see methimazole*
Thiamine Hydrochloride, **1279**
Thiamine Injection, **1965**
Thiamine Nitrate, **1280**
Thiamine Tablets, **1965**
Thiamphenicol, **1280**
2-(2-Thienyl)acetic Acid, A86
Thimerosal, **1281**
Thin-layer Chromatography, A122
Thioacetamide, A86
Thioacetamide Reagent, A86
Thioacetamide Solution, A86
Thiobarbituric Acid, A86
Thiobarbituric Acid–Citrate Buffer, A104
Thiodiethanol, see Thiodiglycol, A86
Thiodiglycol, A86
Thioglycollic Acid, *see mercaptoacetic acid*
Thioguanine and Preparations, *see under Tioguanine*
Thiomersal, **1281**, A86
Thiopental, S117
Thiopental Injection, **1966**
Thiopental Sodium, **1282**
Thiopental Sodium for Injection, **1966**
Thiopentone, Salts and Preparations, *see under Thiopental*
Thioridazine, **1283**
Thioridazine (1), S118
Thioridazine (2), S118
Thioridazine Hydrochloride, **1284**
Thioridazine Oral Solution, **1967**
Thioridazine Oral Suspension, **1967**
Thioridazine Tablets, **1968**
Thiotepa, **1285**, S118
Thiotepa for Injection, **1968**
Thiotepa Injection, **1968**
Thiourea, A86
Threonine, **1285**, *see also* L*-threonine*
L-Threonine, A86
Thrombin, A86
Thrombin, Bovine, A86
Thrombin, Human, *see thrombin*
Thrombin Solution, A86
Thrombin Solution, Human, *see thrombin solution*
Thrombokinase Extract, *see thromboplastin reagent*
Thromboplastin Reagent, A87
Thyme, **1286**
Thymine, A87
Thymol, **1288**, A87
Thymol Blue, A87
Thymol Blue Solution, A87
Thymolphthalein, A87
Thymolphthalein Solution, A87
Thymoxamine Hydrochloride, S84, S119
Thymoxamine Hydrochloride and Preparations, *see under Moxisylyte*
Thyroxine Sodium and Preparations, *see under Levothyroxine*
Tiabendazole, **1288**
Tiabendazole Tablets, **1969**
Tiaprofenic Acid, **1289**
Ticarcillin Sodium, **1291**
Ticlopidine Hydrochloride, **1293**
Timolol, S119
Timolol Eye Drops, **1970**
Timolol Maleate, **1295**
Timolol Tablets, **1970**
Tin, A87
Tin(II) Chloride, A87
Tin(II) Chloride Solution, A87
Tin(II) Chloride Solution AsT, A87
Tin(II) Chloride Solution R1, A87
Tin(II) Chloride Solution R2, A87
Tin, Granulated, *see tin*
Tin Standard Solution (0.1 ppm Sn), A100
Tin Standard Solution (5 ppm Sn), A100
Tinctures, 1456, *see also under name of substance*
Tinctures of the BP, List of, 1457
Tinidazole, **1296**
Tinnevelly Senna, *see Senna Leaf*
Tinnevelly Senna Fruit, **1157**
Tinnevelly Senna Fruit, Powdered, xxv, *see also Tinnevelly Senna Fruit*
Tinnevelly Senna Pods, *see Tinnevelly Senna Fruit*
Tinzaparin Sodium, **1297**
Tioguanine, **1297**, S119
Tioguanine Tablets, **1971**
Titan Yellow, A87
Titan Yellow Paper, A87

Titan Yellow Solution, A87
Titanium, A87
Titanium Dioxide, **1298**, A87
Titanium Dioxide Elastic Adhesive Bandage, xxvi
Titanium Standard Solution (100 ppm Ti), A101
Titanium Trichloride, *see titanium(III) chloride*
Titanium Trichloride Solution, *see titanium(III) chloride solution*
Titanium Trichloride–Sulphuric Acid Reagent, *see titanium(III) chloride–sulphuric acid reagent*
Titanium(III) Chloride, A87
Titanium(III) Chloride Solution, A87
Titanium(III) Chloride–Sulphuric Acid Reagent, A87
Titanium(III) Chloride VS, A98
Title, Changes in, Introduction, xxviii
Titles, Abbreviated, A301
Titles of Monographs, 20, 1410
Titles, Official, 7, 20, 1397, 1410
Titration, Non-aqueous, A155
Titrations, Amperometric and Potentiometric, A155
Titrations, Complexometric, A157
Tobramycin, **1299**
Tobramycin Injection, **1971**
α-Tocopherol, *see Alpha Tocopherol*
Alpha Tocopherol, **1300**
RRR-α-Tocopherol, *see RRR-Alpha-Tocopherol,*
RRR-Alpha-Tocopherol, **1302**
α-Tocopherol Acetate, *see Alpha Tocopheryl Acetate*
RRR-α-Tocopherol Acetate, *see RRR-Alpha Tocopheryl Acetate,*
α-Tocopherol Acetate Concentrate (Powder Form), *see Alpha Tocopheryl Acetate Concentrate (Powder Form)*
DL-α-Tocopherol Hydrogen Succinate, *see Alpha Tocopheryl Hydrogen Succinate,*
DL-α-Tocopherol Hydrogen Succinate, *see Tocopheryl Hydrogen Succinate, Alpha*
RRR-α-Tocopherol Hydrogen Succinate, *see RRR-Alpha Tocopheryl Succinate*
Alpha Tocopheryl Acetate, **1303**
RRR-Alpha-Tocopheryl Acetate, **1306**
Alpha Tocopheryl Acetate Concentrate (Powder Form), **1305**
Alpha-Tocopheryl Hydrogen Succinate, **1308**
Alpha Tocopheryl Succinate, S120
Alpha Tocopheryl Succinate Tablets, **1972**
RRR-Alpha-Tocopheryl Succinate, **1310**
Tolazamide, **1312**, S120
Tolazamide Tablets, **1972**
Tolbutamide, **1313**, S120
Tolbutamide Tablets, **1973**
Tolerances on Sieves, A255
Tolnaftate, **1314**
Tolu Linctus, Paediatric Compound, **1973**
Tolu Syrup, **1974**
Tolu-flavour Solution, **1973**
Toluene, A88
Toluene, Sulphur-free, A88
Toluene-3,4-dithiol, *see dithiol*
Toluenedithiol Reagent, *see dithiol reagent*
Toluenesulphonamide, *see toluene-p-sulphonamide*
Toluene-*o*-sulphonamide, A88
Toluene-*p*-sulphonamide, A88
o-Toluenesulphonamide, *see toluene-o-sulphonamide*
p-Toluenesulphonamide, *see toluene-p-sulphonamide*
Toluenesulphonic Acid, *see toluene-p-sulphonic acid*
Toluene-*p*-sulphonic Acid, A88
o-Toluic Acid, A88
o-Toluidine, A88
p-Toluidine, A88
Toluidine Blue, A88
o-Toluidine Hydrochloride, A88
Topical Powders, 1457
Topical Powders of the BP, Additional Requirements for, 1457
Topical Semi-solid Preparations, 1458
Topical Semi-solid Preparations of the BP, Additional Requirements for, 1459
Tosylarginine Methyl Ester Hydrochloride, A88
Tosylarginine Methyl Ester Hydrochloride Solution A88
Tosyl-lysyl-chloromethane Hydrochloride, A88
Tosylphenylalanylchloromethane, A88
Total Ionic Strength Adjustment Buffer R1, A105
Total Permeation Volume, Definition of, A126
Total Solids, Determination of, A180
Total Viable Aerobic Count, Test for, A245
Total-ionic-strength-adjustment Buffer, A105
Tragacanth, **1314**, A88
Tragacanth, Powdered, xxv, *see also Tragacanth*
Tranexamic Acid, **1316**, S121
Tranexamic Acid Injection, **1974**
Tranexamic Acid Tablets, **1974**
Transdermal Patches, 1460
Transdermal Patches, Dissolution Test for, A192
Transparency of Monographs, A321
Tranylcypromine Sulphate, **1317**, S121
Tranylcypromine Tablets, **1975**
Trazodone Hydrochloride, **1318**, S121
Treated Ethyl Acetate, A42
Treated Formamide, A45
Tretinoin, **1319**
Tretinoin Gel, **1975**
Tretinoin Solution, **1976**
Triacetin, **1320**, A88
Triamcinolone, **1321**, S122, A88
Triamcinolone Acetonide, **1322**, S122
Triamcinolone Acetonide Injection, **1977**
Triamcinolone Cream, **1976**
Triamcinolone Dental Paste, **1978**
Triamcinolone Hexacetonide, **1323**
Triamcinolone Ointment, **1977**
Triamcinolone Tablets, **1978**
Triamterene, **1324**
Triamterene and Hydrochlorothiazide Tablets, **1609**
Triamterene Capsules, **1978**
Tribasic Calcium Phosphate, **232**
Tribavirin, **1325**, S122
Tribavirin for Nebulisation **1979**
Tribavirin Solution for Nebulisation, **1979**
Tributyl Orthophosphate, A88
Trichloroacetic Acid, A88
Trichloroacetic Acid Solution, A88
1,1,1-Trichloroethane, A88
Trichloroethylene, A89
Trichlorotrifluoroethane, A89
Triclofos Oral Solution, **1979**
Triclofos Sodium, **1326**, S123
Tricosane, A89
Triethanolamine, **1327**, A89
Triethylamine, A89
Triethylamine Hydrogen Carbonate Solution, A89
Triethylenediamine, A89
Trifluoperazine, S123
Trifluoperazine Hydrochloride, **1328**
Trifluoperazine Tablets, **1980**
Trifluoroacetic Acid, A89
Trifluoroacetic Anhydride, A89
Triglycerides, Medium-chain, **1329**
Trihexyphenidyl Hydrochloride, S13, S123
Trihexyphenidyl Hydrochloride/ Benzhexol Hydrochloride, **1330**
Trihexyphenidyl Tablets/Benzhexol Tablets, **1980**
Trimeprazine, S7, S124
Trimeprazine Tartrate and Preparations, *see under Alimemazine*
Trimethadione, **1331**
Trimethoprim, **1332**, S124
Trimethoprim and Sulphamethoxazole Preparations, *see Co-trimoxazole Preparations*
Trimethoprim Tablets, **1981**
Trimethylchlorosilane, A89
Trimethylpentane, *see 2,2,4-trimethylpentane*
2,2,4-Trimethylpentane, A89
Trimethylpentane R1, A89
N-Trimethylsilylimidazole, A89
Trimipramine Maleate, **1333**, S124
Trimipramine Tablets, **1982**
Trinitrin Tablets, **1712**
2,4,6-Trinitrophenol, *see picric acid*
Triphenylamine, A89
Triphenylethylene, A89
Triphenylmethanol, A89
2,3,5-Triphenyltetrazolium Chloride, A89
Triphenyltetrazolium Chloride Solution, A89
Triprolidine Hydrochloride, **1334**, S125
Triprolidine Tablets, **1982**
Tris Acetate Buffer Solution pH 8.5, A105
Tris–EDTA Buffer pH 8.4, A105

Tris(hydroxymethyl)aminomethane sodium chloride buffer solutions, *see appropriate tris-chloride buffer*
Tris(hydroxymethyl)aminomethane-EDTA buffer, *see tris–EDTA buffer solution pH 8.4*
Tris-chloride Buffer pH 7.4, A105
Tris-chloride Buffer pH 7.5, A105
Tris-chloride Buffer pH 7.5 R1, A105
Tris-chloride Buffer pH 8.1, A105
Tris-chloride Buffer pH 8.6, A105
Tris-EDTA BSA Buffer Solution pH 8.4, A105
Tris-glycine Buffer Solution pH 8.3, A105
Triscyanoethoxypropane, A89
Tris(2,4-di-(1,1-dimethylethyl)phenyl) Phosphite, A89
1,3,5-Tris(3,5-di-(1,1-dimethylethyl)-4-hydroxybenzyl)-1H,3H,5H,-1,3,5-triazine-2,4,6-trione, A89
Tris(hydroxymethyl)aminomethane Solution, *see tris(hydroxymethyl)-methylamine solution*
Tris(hydroxymethyl)aminomethane, *see tris(hydroxymethyl)methylamine*
Tris(hydroxymethyl)methylamine, A89
Tris(hydroxymethyl)methylamine Solution, A89
Tris(hydroxymethyl)methylamine Solution, Methanolic, A90
Trisodium Citrate, **1180**, *see sodium citrate*
Trisodium Edetate Concentrate, Sterile, **1983**
Trisodium Edetate Injection, **1983**
Trisodium Edetate Intravenous Infusion, **1983**
Trisodium Orthophosphate, A90
Trisodium Phosphate Dodecahydrate, *see trisodium orthophosphate*
Tritiated[^{3}H] Water Injection, **2150**
Trometamol, **1334**
Tropicamide, **1335**, S125
Tropicamide Eye Drops, **1983**
Tropine, A90
Trypsin, **1336**, A90
Trypsin for Peptide Mapping, A90
Tryptophan, **1338**, A90
Tuberculin, Old, **2096**
Tuberculin PPD, **2097**
Tuberculin Purified Derivative for Human Use, *see Tuberculin Purified Protein Derivative*
Tuberculin Purified Protein Derivative, **2097**
Tubes Used for Comparative Tests, A151
Tubing Used in Sets for the Transfusion of Blood A283
Tubocurarine Chloride, **1340**
Tubocurarine Injection, xxvi
Tubular Bandage, Elasticated, xxvi
Tub/Vac/BCG(Percut), *see Percutaneous Bacillus Calmette Guérin Vaccine*
Turpentine Liniment, xxvi
Turpentine Oil, **1341**
Twisted Stainless Steel Suture, Sterile, xxvi
Typhoid (Strain Ty 21a) Vaccine, Live (Oral), **2088**
Typhoid and Tetanus Vaccine, **2090**
Typhoid Polysaccharide Vaccine, **2086**
Typhoid/Tet/Vac, *see Typhoid and Tetanus Vaccine*
Typhoid/Vac, *see Typhoid Vaccine*
Typhoid Vaccine, **2088**
Typhoid/Vac(Oral), *see Typhoid (Strain Ty 21a) Vaccine, Live (Oral)*
Typhoid/Vi/Vac, *see Typhoid Polysaccharide Vaccine*
Typhus/Vac, *see Typhus Vaccine*
Typhus Vaccine, **2090**
L-Tyrosine, A90
Tyrosine, *see L-tyrosine*
Tyrosine, **1341**

U

Ultraviolet and Visible Absorption Spectrophotometry, A116
Ultraviolet Lamps for Analytical Purposes, A123
Ultraviolet Light, Definition of, A122
Unbleached Ginger, *see Ginger*
Uncoated Tablets, 1451
Undecanoic Acid, A90
Undecenoic Acid, **1342**
Undecylenic Acid, *see Undecenoic Acid*
Uniformity of Content of Formulated Preparations, *see appropriate general monograph*
Uniformity of Content, Test for, A203
Uniformity of Dose of Formulated Preparations, *see appropriate general monograph*
Uniformity of Mass of Formulated Preparations, *see appropriate general monograph*
Uniformity of Weight [Mass], Test for, A203
Uniformity of Weight of Formulated Preparations, *see appropriate general monograph*
Units, International, xx
Units of Activity of Biological Preparations, A333
Units of Biological Activity, Definition of, 14, 1404
Units, SI, A312
Unsaponifiable Matter, Determination of, A173
Urea, **1343**, A90
Urea Cream, **1984**
Urease-active Meal, A90
Uridine, A90
Urofollitrophin and Preparations, *see under Urofollitropin*
Urofollitropin, **1344**
Urofollitropin for Injection, **1984**
Urofollitropin Injection, **1984**
Urokinase, **1346**
Uronic Acids in Polysaccharide Vaccines, Test for A235
Ursodeoxycholic Acid, **1347**

V

Vaccine Strain, Choice of, 20, 1410
Vaccines, *see under name of vaccine*
Vaccines, General Monograph, **2038**
Vaccines, Terminology of, A230
Vaccines, Tests for, *see under name of test*
Vaginal Capsules, 1462
Vaginal Foams, 1462
Vaginal Preparations, 1461
Vaginal Preparations of the BP, Additional Requirements for 1462
Vaginal Tablets, 1462
Vaginal Tampons, 1462
Valerian, **1348**
Valerian, Powdered, xxv, *see also under Valerian*
Valeric Acid, A90
Validation, Analytical, A341
Validation, Analytical, Glossary of Terms, A342
Valine, **1350**
Valproic acid, S125
Vanadium Standard Solution (0.1% V), A101
Vancomycin Hydrochloride, **1351**
Vancomycin Hydrochloride for Injection, **1985**
Vancomycin Injection, **1985**
Vanillic Acid, A90
Vanillin, **1352**, A90
Vanillin Reagent, A90
Vanillin Solution, Phosphoric, *A90*
Vapour-permeable Adhesive Film Dressing, xxvi
Vapour-permeable Waterproof Plastic Wound Dressing, xxvi
Varicella Immunoglobulin, **2025**
Varicella Vaccine, Live, **2091**
Var/Vac(Live), *see Varicella Vaccine, Live*
Vegetable Drugs, 22, 1412
Vegetable Drugs, Contamination of, 15, 1405
Vegetable Drugs, Form of, 20, 1410
Vegetable Oil, Hydrogenated, **1353**
Ventilated Elastic Adhesive Bandage, xxvi
Verapamil, S126
Verapamil Hydrochloride, **1353**
Verapamil Injection, **1986**
Verapamil Tablets, **1986**
Veratric Acid, A90
Very Fine Powder, Definition of, A254
Vials, Glass, A268
Vigabatrin, **1354**, S126
Vigabatrin Oral Powder, **1987**
Vigabatrin Tablets, **1987**
Vinblastine Injection, **1988**
Vinblastine Sulphate, **1356**
Vinblastine Sulphate for Injection, **1988**
Vincristine Injection, **1988**
Vincristine Sulphate, **1357**
Vincristine Sulphate for Injection, **1989**
Vindesine Sulphate, **1358**
Vinyl Acetate, A90
Vinyl Chloride, A90
2-Vinylpyridine, A90
1-Vinylpyrrolidin-2-one, A90
Viper Venom Antiserum, European, **2032**

Viral Vaccines, Extraneous Agents in, A250
Viscose Gauze, X-Ray-Detectable Cotton and, xxvi
Viscose Primary Dressing, Knitted, xxvi
Viscose Ribbon Gauze, X-Ray-Detectable Cotton and, xxvi
Viscose Wadding, Absorbent, **2156**
Viscose Wadding, Sterile Absorbent, **2157**
Viscosity, Determination of, A140
Visible Absorption Spectrophotometry, Ultraviolet and, A116
Visible Particles, Limit Test for, A205
Vitamin A, **1360**
all-trans-Vitamin A Acetate, A162
Vitamin A, Assay of, A161
Vitamin A Concentrates, *see under Retinol*
Vitamin A Ester Concentrate, Natural, **1360**
Vitamin B_1 Preparations, *see under Thiamine*
Vitamin B_{12} Injection, *see Hydroxocobalamin Injection*
Vitamin B_6, *see Pyridoxine Hydrochloride*
Vitamin B_6 Tablets, *see Pyridoxine Tablets*
Vitamin C and Preparations, *see under Ascorbic Acid*
Vitamin C Injection, *see Ascorbic Acid Injection*
Vitamin C Tablets, *see Ascorbic Acid Tablets*
Vitamin D, *see Ergocalciferol*
Vitamin D_2, *see Ergocalciferol*
Vitamin D_3, *see Colecalciferol*
Vitamin K_1 and Preparations, *see under Phytomenadione*
Vitamins B and C Injection, **1989**
Volatile Oil in Drugs, Determination of, A181
Volatile Oils, Methods for, A175
Volume, Apparent, Determination of, A258
Volume, Extractable, A204
Volumetric Glassware, Requirements for, 18, 1408
Volumetric Reagents, A92
Volumetric Solutions, A92
Preparation and Standardisation, A92
VS, A313, *see also volumetric solutions*

W

Wadding, Absorbent Viscose, **2156**
Wadding, Sterile Absorbent Viscose, **2157**
Warfarin, S126
Warfarin Sodium, **1365**
Warfarin Sodium Clathrate, **1366**
Warfarin Tablets, **1990**
Warnings, 23, 1413, *see also Caution Statements*
Washed Flux-calcined Diatomaceous Filter-aid, A34
Washes, Ear, 1426
Washes, Nasal, 1439
Water, A90
Water, Ammonium-free, *see ammonia-free water*
Water Bath, Definition of 6, 1396
Water-bath, Definition of, 18, 1408
Water BET, A215, A326
Water, Determination of, A167
Water for Buffer Solutions, A101
Water for Chromatography, A91
Water for Diluting Concentrated Haemodialysis Solutions, **1718**
Water for Formulated Preparations, Quality of, 10, 1400
Water for Injections, **1368**, A91
Water for Irrigation, **1991**
Water for Use in Manufacturing Parenteral Preparations, 1445
Water in Medicinal Gases, Determination of, A170
Water in Volatile Oils, Test for, A175
Water LAL, A215, A326
Water, Particle-free, A91
Water, Potable, 10, 1400
Water, Purified, **1367**
Waterproof Plastic Wound Dressing, Vapour-permeable, xxvi
Waters, Aromatic, 1462, *see also under name of substance*
Waters, Aromatic, of the BP, List of, 1462
Wax, Emulsifying, **1658**
Weak Cationic Resin, A27, A91
Weak Copper Sulphate Solution, A32
Weak Ginger Tincture, **1707**
Weight per Millilitre, Determination of, A139
Weight, Test for Uniformity of, A203
Weights and Measures, A312
Weights and Measures, Expression of 5, 1395
Weights, Atomic, 5, 1395
Well Closed Container, A268
Wheat Starch, **1369**
White Beeswax, **142**
White Embrocation, **1992**
White Liniment, **1992**
White Petroleum Jelly, **997**
White Soft Paraffin, **997**
White Squill, *see Squill*
White's Tar Paste, **1994**
Whitfield's Ointment, **1509**
Whooping-cough Prophylactic, Adsorbed Diphtheria– **2050**
Whooping-cough Vaccine, **2071**
Wintergreen and Wintergreen Oil, *see Methyl Salicylate*
Wool Alcohols, **1369**
Wool Alcohols Ointment, **1992**
Wool Fat, **1370**
Wool Fat, Hydrogenated, **1371**
Wool Fat, Hydrous, **1372**
Wool Wax Alcohols, **1369**

X

X-Ray Fluorescence Spectrometry A121
X-Ray-Detectable Abdominal Pad, xxvi
X-Ray-Detectable Cotton and Viscose Gauze, xxvi
X-Ray-Detectable Cotton and Viscose Ribbon Gauze, xxvi
X-Ray-Detectable Cotton Gauze, xxvi
X-Ray-Detectable Cotton Ribbon Gauze, xxvi
X-Ray-Detectable Gauze Pledget, xxvi
X-Ray-Detectable Gauze Swab, xxvi
Xanthan Gum, **1373**
Xanthines, Reactions of, A150
Xanthydrol, A91
Xanthydrol R1, A91
Xanthydrol Reagent, A91
Xanthydrol Solution, A91
Xenon[^{133}Xe] Injection, **2151**
Xylene, A91
o-Xylene, A91
Xylene Cyanol FF, A91
Xylenol Orange, A91
Xylenol Orange Solution, A91
Xylenol Orange Triturate, A91
Xylometazoline, S127
Xylometazoline Hydrochloride, **1375**
Xylometazoline Nasal Drops, **1992**
Xylose, **1376**, *see also D-xylose*
D-Xylose, A91

Y

Yellow Beeswax, **143**
Yellow Fever Vaccine, Live, **2092**
Yellow Mercury(II) Oxide, A56
Yellow Petroleum Jelly, **998**
Yellow Primary Solution, A133
Yellow Soft Paraffin, **998**
Yel/Vac, *see Yellow Fever Vaccine, Live*

Z

Zidovudine, **1377**
Zinc, A91, A92
Zinc Acetate, A91
Zinc Acetate Solution, A91
Zinc Acexamate, **1378**
Zinc, Activated, A91
Zinc and Castor Oil Cream, **1994**
Zinc and Castor Oil Ointment, **1994**
Zinc and Coal Tar Paste, **1994**
Zinc and Hexachlorophene Dusting Powder, **1725**
Zinc and Ichthammol Cream, **1993**
Zinc and Salicylic Acid Paste, **1995**
Zinc Chloride, **1380**, A91
Zinc Chloride–Formic Acid Solution, A91
Zinc Chloride Solution, Iodinated, A91
Zinc Chloride VS, A98
Zinc, Complexometric Titration of, A157
Zinc Cream, **1993**
Zinc Iodide, A91
Zinc Ointment, **1994**
Zinc Ointment, Coal Tar and, **1957**
Zinc Oxide, **1381**, A92
Zinc Paste and Coal Tar Bandage, xxvi
Zinc Paste and Ichthammol Bandage, xxvi
Zinc Paste Bandage, xxvi
Zinc Paste, Calamine and Clioquinol Bandage, xxvi

Zinc Paste, Compound, **1994**
Zinc Powder, A92
Zinc, Reactions of, A150
Zinc Salts, Reactions of, A150
Zinc Shot, A92
Zinc Standard Solution (5 ppm Zn), A101
Zinc Standard Solution (10 ppm Zn), A101
Zinc Standard Solution (25 ppm Zn), A101
Zinc Standard Solution (100 ppm Zn), A101
Zinc Standard Solution (5 mg/ml Zn), A101
Zinc Stearate, **1381**
Zinc Sulphate, **1382**, A92
Zinc Sulphate Eye Drops, **1995**
Zinc Sulphate Lotion, **1995**
Zinc Sulphate VS, A98
Zinc Undecenoate, **1383**
Zinc Undecylenate, *see Zinc Undecenoate*
Zirconium Standard Solution (0.1% Zr), A101
Zirconyl Chloride, A92
Zirconyl Nitrate, A92
Zirconyl Nitrate Solution, A92
Zolpidem Tartrate, **1383**
Zopiclone, **1385**
Zuclopenthixol Acetate, **1386**, S127
Zuclopenthixol Acetate Injection, **1996**
Zuclopenthixol Decanoate, **1387**, S127
Zuclopenthixol Decanoate Injection, **1996**
Zuclopenthixol Hydrochloride, **1388**, S128
Zuclopenthixol Tablets, **1997**